Seizure Tables

EMERGENT MEDICATIONS FOR SEIZURES

Drug	Dose	Comments
Diazepam (Valium)	0.2 mg/kg IV 0.5 mg/kg p.r.	Give q10 min; can repeat up to three IV doses; maximum dose 10 mg
Lidocaine (Xylocaine)	1.5–2.0 mg/kg	Monitor for dysrhythmia while giving slow IV push
Lorazepam (Ativan)	0.05–0.1 mg/kg	IV push over 2 min; can repeat q 20 min; maximum dose 4 mg
Midazolam (Versed)	0.08–0.2 mg/kg	Can give IV, IM, or p.r.; maximum dose 5 mg
Paraldehyde	0.3 ml/kg	1 g/1 ml solution diluted 1:1 with cottonseed, mineral, or olive oil; give p.r. in a glass syringe; maximum dose 5 ml
Phenobarbital (Luminal)	5–10 mg/kg	Give slow IV push over 10 min; repeat dose at 20 and 40 min for total loading dose of 15–20 mg/kg
Phenytoin (Dilantin)	15–20mg/kg	IV piggyback at 0.5–1.0 mg/kg/min while on cardiac monitor; maximum dose 1 g
Thiamylal sodium (Surital)	2 mg/kg	Give slow IV push; if no seizure lysis, repeat in 15 min at 5 mg/kg

ORAL ANTICONVULSANTS

Drug	Maintenance Dose	Comments
Carbamazepine (Tegretol)	15–30 mg/kg/day divided q6–8 hr; maximum dose 1000 mg/day	Desired serum level 4–12 µg/ml; suspension 100 mg/ml; tabs 200 mg; chewable tabs 100mg
Clonazepam (Klonopin)	0.1–0.2 mg/kg/day divided q8 hr; adult maximum dose 20 mg/day	Desired serum level 0.013–0.072 µg/ml; suspension 80 µg/5 ml, 0.1 mg/ml; tabs 0.5, 1.0, 2.0 mg
Ethosuximide (Zarontin)	20–30 mg/kg/day divided q24 hr; maximum dose 1000 mg/day	Desired serum level 40–100 µg/ml; syrup 250 mg/5 ml; caps 250 mg
Mephobarbital (Mebaral)	<5 yr: 16–32 mg q6–8 hr >5 yr: 32–64 mg q6–8 hr	Metabolized to phenobarbital; desired serum level 15–40 µg/ml; tabs 32, 50, 100, 300 mg
Phenobarbital (Luminal)	3–5 mg/kg day divided 12–24 hr; adult dose 200–300 mg/24 hr	Desired serum level 15–40 µg/ml; drops 16 mg/ml; elixir 15 mg/5 ml; 20 mg/5 ml; tabs 8, 15, 30, 60, 100 mg
Phenytoin (Dilantin)	5–10 mg/kg/day divided q12–24 hr; adult dose 200–400 mg/24 hr	Desired serum level 10–20 µg/ml; suspension 30 mg/5 ml, 125 mg/5 ml; chewable tabs 50 mg; caps 30, 100 mg
Primidone (Mysoline)	10–25 mg/kg/day divided q6–8 hr; adult dose 750–1500 mg/day	Metabolized to phenobarbital; desired level 15–40 µg/ml (phenobarbital component); suspension 250 mg/5 ml; tabs 50, 250 mg
Valproic Acid (Depakene)	15–60 mg/kg/day divided q8–24 hr; adult dose 250–750 mg tid	Desired serum level 50–100 µg/ml; syrup 250 mg/5 ml (473 ml); caps 250 mg; do not give syrup with carbonated beverages

PEDIATRIC
EMERGENCY
MEDICINE

PEDIATRIC EMERGENCY MEDICINE

■ ■ ■

Earl J. Reisdorff, MD, FACEP

Associate Professor
College of Human Medicine
Michigan State University
Assistant Residency Director of Education
Michigan State
Emergency Medicine Residency
Lansing, Michigan

Mont R. Roberts, MD, FACEP

Associate Professor
College of Human Medicine
Michigan State University
Assistant Residency Director of Research
Michigan State
Emergency Medicine Residency
Lansing, Michigan

John G. Wiegenstein, MD

Professor and Chief
Section of Emergency Medicine
College of Human Medicine
Michigan State University
Chairman
Department of Emergency Medicine
Ingham Medical Center
Lansing, Michigan

with 165 contributors

W.B. SAUNDERS COMPANY
A Division of Harcourt Brace & Company
Philadelphia ■ London ■ Toronto ■ Montreal ■ Sydney ■ Tokyo

W.B. SAUNDERS COMPANY
A Division of
Harcourt Brace & Company

The Curtis Center
Independence Square West
Philadelphia, Pennsylvania 19106

Library of Congress Cataloging-in-Publication Data

Pediatric emergency medicine / [edited by] Earl J. Reisdorff,
Mont R. Roberts, John G. Wiegenstein.

    p.   cm.

ISBN 0–7216–3281–5

1. Pediatric emergencies.   I. Reisdorff, Earl J.
  II. Roberts, Mont R.   III. Wiegenstein, John G.
  [DNLM: 1. Emergencies—in infancy & childhood.
  WS 200 P37115]

RJ370.P4515 1992   618.92'0025—dc20

DNLM/DLC   91–43069

PEDIATRIC EMERGENCY MEDICINE   ISBN 0–7216–3281–5

Printed in the United States of America

Last digit is the print number: 9   8   7   6   5   4   3

To children—the world's hope,
and to physicians everywhere
who care for ill and injured children.

CONTRIBUTORS

Thomas J. Abramo, MD, FAAP
Assistant Professor of Pediatrics, Eastern Virginia Graduate School of Medicine; Associate Director of Pediatric Emergency Medicine, Children's Hospital of The King's Daughters, Norfolk, Virginia
Cystic Fibrosis

Anthony Albano, MD
Assistant Professor, Department of Surgery, Division of Emergency Medicine, University of Connecticut Health Center, Farmington; Director of Clinical Research, Division of Emergency Medicine, John Dempsey Hospital, University of Connecticut Health Center; Attending Physician, St. Francis Hospital and Medical Center, Hartford, Connecticut
Parathyroid Disorders

Rodney L. Baker, MD
Attending Physician, Emergency Department, Miami Children's Hospital, Miami, Florida
Tricyclic Antidepressants

Theodore M. Barnett, MD
Assistant Professor of Pediatrics, University of Missouri–Kansas City School of Medicine; Attending Physician, Pediatric Emergency Medicine, The Children's Mercy Hospital, Kansas City, Missouri
Seizures and Status Epilepticus

Patricia A. Bayless, MD
Attending Physician, Maricopa Medical Center, Phoenix, Arizona
Jaundice and Hepatitis

John G. Benitez, MD, FACEP
Assistant Professor of Medicine, Division of Emergency Medicine, University of Pittsburgh Medical Center; Fellowship Director, Toxicology Treatment Program, University of Pittsburgh Medical Center; Attending Physician (Toxicology, Emergency Medicine, Hyperbaric Medicine), Presbyterian University Hospital and Montefiore University Hospital, Pittsburgh, Pennsylvania
Acetaminophen

Carol D. Berkowitz, MD
Professor of Clinical Pediatrics, UCLA School of Medicine, Los Angeles; Acting Chair, Department of Pediatrics, Harbor/UCLA Medical Center, Torrance, California
Pediatric Sexual Abuse

Stephen O. Bernardon, MD
Assistant Professor of Emergency Medicine, Emergency Medicine Department at University of Cincinnati, Cincinnati, Ohio
Neonatal Resuscitation

Mananda S. Bhende, MD, FAAP, FACEP
Associate Professor of Pediatrics, University of Pittsburgh; Attending Physician, Emergency Department, Children's Hospital of Pittsburgh, Pittsburgh, Pennsylvania
Diarrhea; Ataxia

Paul Blackburn, DO
Chief Resident, Emergency Medicine Residency; Affiliate Faculty, Michigan State University College of Osteopathic Medicine, East Lansing, Michigan
Dehydration and Fluid Replacement; Electrolyte Disorders

Danny C. Blankenship, MD
Attending Physician, Cardiology, Brookwood Medical Center, Birmingham, Alabama
Congenital Heart Disease

William A. Bonadio, MD
Associate Professor, Medical College of Wisconsin; Attending Physician of Emergency Medicine, Children's Hospital of Wisconsin, Milwaukee, Wisconsin
Diabetes Mellitus

G. Randall Bond, MD
Assistant Professor, Departments of Pediatrics and Internal Medicine, University of Virginia; Medical Director, UVA–Blue Ridge Poison Center, Charlottesville, Virginia
Alcohols; Reptile Bites

Joan Bothner, MD
Assistant Professor of Pediatrics, Section of General and Emergency Pediatrics, University of Colorado School of Medicine; Clinical Director, Emergency Services, The Children's Hospital, Denver, Colorado
Nephrotic Syndrome

Leslie V. Boyer Hassen, MD, FAAP
Assistant Clinical Lecturer, Section of Emergency Medicine (Department of Surgery) and Department of Pediatrics, University of Arizona Health Sciences Center; Staff, University Medical Center and Tucson Medical Center, Tucson, Arizona
Arthropod Envenomation

Margaret Boyer, MD
Chief Resident, Emergency Medicine, Geisinger Medical Center, Danville, Pennsylvania
Heavy Metals

Carolyn R. Burt, BS Educ, DO
Clinical Faculty, Michigan State University College of Medicine, East Lansing; Active Staff, St. Lawrence Hospital, Lansing, Michigan
Dental Emergencies

Lisa Cahill, MD, FAAP, FACEP
Assistant Professor of Emergency Medicine, Medical College of Pennsylvania, Allegheny Campus; Staff, Allegheny General Hospital, Pittsburgh, Pennsylvania
Otitis

Louis A. Cannon, MD, FACC, FACA
Assistant Clinical Professor, Section of Emergency Medicine, Assistant Clinical Professor, Section of Cardiology, Michigan State University College of Human Medicine; Regional Campus, Saginaw, Michigan
Congenital Heart Disease

Stephen V. Cantrill, MD, FACEP
Associate Director, Emergency Medical Services, Denver General Hospital, Denver, Colorado
Aspirated Foreign Bodies

Patrick L. Carolan, MD
Clinical Assistant Professor, Departments of Pediatrics, Family Medicine, and Community Health, University of Minnesota School of Medicine; Staff Physician, Pediatric Emergency Services, Minneapolis Children's Medical Center; Medical Director, Minnesota Sudden Infant Death Center, Minneapolis, Minnesota
Anemia

Ann N. Champoux, MD
Associate Clinical Professor of Pediatrics, University of Washington School of Medicine; Attending Physician, Emergency Department, Children's Hospital and Medical Center, Seattle, Washington
Henoch-Schönlein Purpura; Hemolytic-Uremic Syndrome

Patricia S. Chase, MD
Assistant Director, Ambulatory Services, Children's Hospital of Oakland, Oakland, California
Pneumonia

Michael R. Clark, MD, FACEP
Associate Professor, Michigan State University, Colleges of Human and Osteopathic Medicine; Program Director, Michigan State University Emergency Medicine Residency; Chairman, Department of Emergency Medicine, Sparrow Hospital, Lansing, Michigan
Epistaxis

Richard F. Clark, MD
Assistant Clinical Professor of Medicine, University of California, San Diego; Attending Physician, Emergency Department, University of California, San Diego; Medical Director, San Diego Regional Poison Center, San Diego, California
Organophosphates and Carbamates

Roland B. Clark, MD, FACEP
Chairman, Emergency Department, Brea Community Hospital, Brea, California
Ophthalmologic Emergencies

L. Mason Cobb, MD
Associate Professor of Surgery and Pediatrics, College of Human Medicine, Michigan State University, East Lansing; Associate Staff, Edward W. Sparrow Hospital, Lansing, Michigan
Appendicitis

Bernard A. Cohen, MD
Associate Professor of Pediatrics and Dermatology, Johns Hopkins University School of Medicine; Director of Pediatric Dermatology, Johns Hopkins Hospital, Baltimore, Maryland
Dermatologic Emergencies

Elizabeth Contreras, MD
Director, Pediatric Intensive Care Unit, St. Joseph Mercy Hospital, Pontiac, Michigan
Brain Death and Organ Donation

Arnold G. Coran, MD
Professor of Surgery and Head of the Section of Pediatric Surgery, University

of Michigan Medical School; Surgeon-in-Chief, C. S. Mott Children's Hospital, Ann Arbor, Michigan
Thoracic Trauma; Abdominal Trauma

Richard A. Craven, MD, FACEP

Assistant Professor, Eastern Virginia Graduate School of Medicine, Norfolk, Virginia; Staff Physician with Emergency Physicians of Tidewater at Sentera Norfolk General, Virginia Beach General, Sentera Leigh Memorial, Maryview Medical Center, Portsmouth General, and DePaul General Hospitals, Norfolk, Virginia
Acute Rheumatic Fever

Steven C. Curry, MD

Associate Director, Department of Medical Toxicology, Samaritan Regional Poison Center, Good Samaritan Regional Medical Center, Phoenix, Arizona
Salicylates; Iron; Organophosphates and Carbamates; Anticholinergics

Adrian Dana, MD

Assistant Professor of Pediatrics, Medical College of Pennsylvania, Allegheny Campus; Director, Division of In-patient Pediatrics, and Pediatric Infectious Disease Specialist, Allegheny General Hospital, Pittsburgh, Pennsylvania
Infection-Related Congenital Syndromes

Daniel F. Danzl, MD

Professor and Chair, Department of Emergency Medicine, University of Louisville, Louisville, Kentucky
Hypothermia and Frostbite

Richard C. Dart, MD, PhD

Assistant Professor, University of Arizona Health Sciences Center, Section of Emergency Medicine, Department of Surgery; Director of Clinical Toxicology, University Medical Center, Tucson, Arizona
Arthropod Envenomation

Eric A. Davis, MD, FACEP

Assistant Professor of Medicine, Division of Emergency Medicine, University of Pittsburgh; Medical Director, STAT System, Center for Emergency Medicine; Attending Physician, Emergency Department, Presbyterian University Hospital; Attending Physician, Emergency Department, Montefiore University Hospital, Pittsburgh, Pennsylvania
Cerebral Palsy

Holly W. Davis, MD

Medical Director, Emergency Department, Children's Hospital of Pittsburgh; Associate Professor of Pediatrics, University of Pittsburgh School of Medicine, Pittsburgh, Pennsylvania
Dermatologic Emergencies

Barbara L. Demby, MD

Staff Pediatrician, Tallahassee Memorial Regional Medical Center and Tallahassee Community Hospital, Tallahassee, Florida
Hematuria

Constance J. Doyle, MD, FACEP

Clinical Instructor, Section of Emergency Services, Department of Surgery, University of Michigan, Ann Arbor; Senior Attending Physician, Emergency Department, Foote Hospital, Jackson, Michigan
The Grieving Family

Steven C. Dronen, MD

Associate Professor of Emergency Medicine, University of Cincinnati College of Medicine; Staff Physician, University Hospital, Cincinnati, Ohio
Shock and Fluid Resuscitation

Timothy C. Evans, MD, FACEP

Assistant Professor of Emergency Medicine, Medical College of Pennsylvania, Allegheny Campus; Division of Emergency Medicine, Allegheny General Hospital, Pittsburgh, Pennsylvania
Inflammatory Bowel Disease

David H. Fagin, MD

Assistant Director, Emergency Department, Scottish Rite Children's Medical Center, Atlanta, Georgia
Weakness

Robert A. Felter, MD, FAAP

Associate Professor, Pediatric Chief, Division of Pediatric Emergency Medicine, Northeastern Ohio Universities College of Medicine; Director, Division of Emergency and Trauma Services, Children's Hospital Medical Center of Akron, Akron, Ohio
Hand and Wrist Injuries; Medicolegal Considerations

Paula M. Fontanarosa, MD

Senior Resident, Pediatrics, Children's Hospital Medical Center of Akron, Akron, Ohio
Gynecologic Disorders

Phil B. Fontanarosa, MD, FACEP

Associate Professor, Emergency Medicine, Northeastern Ohio Universities College of Medicine; Attending Physician and Research Director, Department of Emergency Medicine, Akron City Hospital, Akron, Ohio
Gastrointestinal Hemorrhage; Gynecologic Disorders

Bassam M. Gebara, MD

Director, Pediatric Intensive Care Unit, Henry Ford Hospital, Detroit, Michigan
Brain Death and Organ Donation

Marie C. Giarratana, RNP, MS, MPH

Division of Adolescent Medicine, Children's Hospital of Oakland, Oakland; Department of Obstetrics and Gynecology, University of California, San Francisco, San Francisco, California
Adolescent Pregnancy and Obstetric Emergencies

James P. Gillen, MD, FACEP

Clinical Assistant Professor of Surgery (E.M.), Jefferson Medical College, Philadelphia; Residency Director, Associate Physician, Department of Emergency Medicine, Geisinger Medical Center, Danville, Pennsylvania
Immunizations

Susan L. Gin-Shaw, MD, FACEP

Research Coordinator, Emergency Medicine Residency, Maricopa Medical Center, Phoenix, Arizona
Maxillofacial Trauma

Mark G. Goetting, MD

Director, Pediatric Critical Care, William Beaumont Hospital, Royal Oak, Michigan
Brain Death and Organ Donation

Johanna Goldfarb, MD

Assistant Professor of Pediatrics, Case Western Reserve University; Attending, Pediatric Infectious Diseases, Rainbow Babies and Children's Hospital, Cleveland, Ohio
Meningitis

Javier A. Gonzalez del Rey, MD

Fellow, Pediatric Emergency Medicine, University of Cincinnati Medical School, Children's Hospital Medical Center, Cincinnati, Ohio
Phenothiazines

Russell H. Greenfield, MD

Clinical Faculty, Department of Emergency Medicine, Carolinas Medical Center, Charlotte, North Carolina
Bronchiolitis

Stephen R. Guertin, MD

Associate Professor of Pediatrics, Michigan State University College of Human Medicine, East Lansing; Director, Pediatric Intensive Care Unit, E.W. Sparrow Hospital, Lansing, Michigan
Hydrocephalus and Ventricular Shunts

Kelley A. Hails, MD

Clinical Instructor, Section of Emergency Medicine, College of Human Medicine at Michigan State University; Faculty, Michigan State University Emergency Medicine Residency, Lansing, Michigan
Reye's Syndrome; Nutrition

M. Lois Hall, MD

Assistant Clinical Professor of Pediatrics, University of Minnesota; Associate Director of Emergency Services, Children's Hospital of St. Paul, St. Paul, Minnesota
Blood Products and Transfusion; Hereditary Bleeding

William Hardwick, Jr, MD

Assistant Professor, Children's Hospital of Alabama, University of Alabama, Birmingham School of Medicine, Birmingham, Alabama
Theophylline

Martin Harris, MD

Assistant Clinical Professor, Department of Emergency Medicine, Wayne State University School of Medicine; Associate Residency Director, Emergency Medicine Residency, Grace Hospital, Detroit, Michigan
Cocaine

Oliver Hayes, DO

Associate Professor and Chief, Section of Emergency Medicine, Michigan State University, East Lansing; Staff, Ingham Medical Center, Lansing, Michigan
Pelvic and Lower Extremity Injuries

Martin G. Hellman, MD, FAAP, FACEP

Assistant Professor of Pediatrics and Emergency Medicine, Northeastern Ohio University College of Medicine, Rootstown; Attending, Department of Emergency/Trauma Services, and EMS Director for Children's Hospital of Akron, Akron; Flight Physician and Clinical Instructor in Surgery, Metrohealth Hospital Medical Center, Cleveland, Ohio
The Development-Based Examination

Halim M. Hennes, MD, MS

Associate Professor of Pediatrics and Surgery, Medical College of Wisconsin; Pediatric Emergency Medicine Physician, Children's Hospital of Wisconsin, Milwaukee, Wisconsin
Thyroid Disorders

R. N. Hensinger, MD

Professor, Department of Surgery, University of Michigan; Chief, Pediatric Orthopaedics, C. S. Mott Children's Hospital, Ann Arbor, Michigan
Spine and Spinal Cord Trauma

Nancy S. Hilton, MD

Director, Ambulatory Services, Children's Hospital, Oakland, California
Pneumonia

Marion Hoelzer, MD, FACEP

Attending Physician, William Beaumont Hospital, Royal Oak, Michigan
Mushroom and Plant Ingestions

Michele K. Holloway-Nichols, MD

Assistant Professor of Pediatrics, University of Alabama at Birmingham; Attending Physician, Emergency Medicine, Children's Hospital of Alabama, Birmingham, Alabama
Caustic Ingestions

J. Stephen Huff, MD, FACEP

Associate Residency Director, Division of Emergency Medicine, Eastern Virginia Graduate School of Medicine, Norfolk; Staff Physician, Sentera Norfolk General Hospital and DePaul Medical Center, Norfolk, Virginia
Coma; Cerebrovascular Syndrome

Mary Hughes, DO

Assistant Professor, Section of Emergency Medicine, Michigan State University College of Osteopathic Medicine, East Lansing; Attending Physician, Emergency Department, Sparrow Hospital and Ingham Medical Center, Lansing, Michigan
Upper Airway Emergencies; Feeding Problems

Richard C. Hunt, MD, FACEP

Assistant Professor and Chief, Division of Air Medical Services, Department of Emergency Medicine, East Carolina University School of Medicine; Medical Director, EastCare Emergency Air Medical Service, University Medical Center of Eastern Carolina–Pitt County, Greenville, North Carolina
Mammal Bites

Kenneth V. Iserson, MD, MBA, FACEP

Associate Professor of Surgery (Emergency Medicine) and Director, Arizona Bioethics Program, University of Arizona College of Medicine; Chair, Bioethics Committee, and Emergency Physician, University Medical Center, Tucson, Arizona
Pediatric Bioethics

Eugene Izsak, MD, FAAP

Assistant Professor of Pediatrics, Northeastern Ohio Universities College of Medicine, Rootstown; Associate Director, Division of Emergency/Trauma Services, Children's Hospital Medical Center of Akron, Akron, Ohio
Approach to Abdominal Pain

Kenneth Jackimczyk, MD

Program Director, Emergency Medicine Residency, Department of Emergency Medicine, Maricopa Medical Center, Phoenix, Arizona
Genitourinary Trauma

Raymond E. Jackson, MD, FACEP

Residency Director, Emergency Medicine, William Beaumont Hospital, Royal Oak, Michigan
Basic Pediatric Resuscitation

David M. Jaffe, MD

Associate Professor of Pediatrics, Washington University School of Medicine; Director, Division of Emergency Medicine, St. Louis Children's Hospital, St. Louis, Missouri
Pharyngeal Disease; Craniocerebral Trauma

Dietrich Jehle, MD

Director of Emergency Services, Erie County Medical Center, Department of Emergency Medicine, State University of New York at Buffalo, Buffalo, New York
Otitis

Carden Johnston, MD, FAAP

Associate Professor, Pediatrics, University of Alabama at Birmingham; Medical Director, Emergency Medicine, Children's Hospital of Alabama, Birmingham, Alabama
Diphtheria, Pertussis, and Tetanus

Raymond B. Karasic, MD

Associate Professor of Pediatrics, University of Pittsburgh School of Medicine; Fellowship Director, Pediatric Emergency Medicine, Children's Hospital of Pittsburgh, Pittsburgh, Pennsylvania
Measles, Mumps, and Rubella; Chickenpox

Samuel M. Keim, MD

Residency Director, Emergency Medicine, University of Arizona; Staff Attending, University Medical Center, University of Arizona, Tucson, Arizona
Psychiatric Emergencies

Ray E. Keller, MD

Associate, Department of Emergency Medicine, Geisinger Medical Center, Danville, Pennsylvania
Drowning and Near-Drowning

Mark A. Kirk, MD

Clinical Assistant Professor, Department of Medicine, University of North Carolina, Chapel Hill; Assistant Director, Division of Clinical Toxicology, Department of Emergency Medicine, Carolinas Medical Center, Charlotte, North Carolina
Poisoning in Children

Niranjan Kissoon, MD, FRCP(C), FAAP

Associate Professor of Pediatrics, Pediatric Critical Care, University of Florida, Health Science Center; Staff, Pediatric Critical Care, University Medical Center and Wolfson Children's Hospital, Jacksonville, Florida
Airway Management and Ventilatory Support

Jane F. Knapp, MD, FAAP

Associate Professor of Pediatrics, University of Missouri–Kansas City School of Medicine; Director of Emergency Services, Children's Mercy Hospital, Kansas City, Missouri
Pericarditis

Bertha Koomson, MD

Assistant Professor, University of Southern California; Attending Physician, Emergency Department, Children's Hospital of Los Angeles, Los Angeles, California
Pharyngeal Disease

Allan E. Kornberg, MD

Assistant Professor of Pediatrics and Emergency Medicine, State University of New York at Buffalo School of Medicine and Biomedical Sciences; Chief, Division of Emergency Medicine, Children's Hospital of Buffalo, Buffalo, New York
Pancreatitis

Ken J. Kroger, MD

Attending Physician, Sutter General Hospital, Sacramento, California
Upper Extremity Injuries

Jon R. Krohmer, MD, FACEP

Assistant Professor, Section of Emergency Medicine, Michigan State University College of Human Medicine, East Lansing; Assistant Residency Director, Emergency Medicine Residency, Butterworth Hospital; Medical Director, Kent County Emergency Medical Service, Grand Rapids, Michigan
Emergency Medical Systems

Steven E. Krug, MD

Assistant Professor of Pediatrics, Case Western Reserve University School of Medicine; Chief, Division of Pediatric Emergency Medicine, Rainbow Babies and Children's Hospital, Cleveland, Ohio
Back Pain; Syncope

Gloria J. Kuhn, DO, FACEP

Assistant Professor, Department of Emergency Medicine, Wayne State University; Program Director, Emergency Medicine Residency Program, Grace Hospital, Detroit, Michigan
Hallucinogens

Ken Kulig, MD

Clinical Assistant Professor of Surgery, Division of Emergency Medicine and Trauma, University of Colorado Health Sciences Center, Denver; Director, Porter Regional Toxicology Center, Denver, Colorado
Poisoning in Children

Lee L. Labadie, MD, FACEP

Associate Director, Emergency Medicine Residency Program, Maricopa Medical Center, Phoenix, Arizona
Intestinal Obstruction

Ira S. Landsman, MD

Children's Mercy Hospital, University of Missouri School of Medicine, Kansas City, Missouri
Bone Development and Pediatric Considerations

Robert W. Lasek, MD, FACEP

Associate in Emergency Medicine, Geisinger Medical Center; Medical Director, Susquehanna Poison Center, Danville, Pennsylvania
Heavy Metals

Frank W. Lavoie, MD

Associate Professor, Department of Emergency Medicine, University of Louisville, Louisville, Kentucky
Hypothermia and Frostbite

Joseph L. Lelli, MD

Senior Resident in Surgery, St. Joseph Mercy Hospital, Ann Arbor, Michigan
Appendicitis

Mary A. Letourneau, MD

Assistant Professor of Pediatrics, University of Southern California School of Medicine; Attending Physician, Division of Emergency Medicine, Children's Hospital of Los Angeles, Los Angeles, California
Craniocerebral Trauma

Deborah Lubitz, MD

Assistant Professor, Pediatrics, Case Western Reserve School of Medicine; Attending Physician, Pediatric Emergency Medicine, Rainbow Babies and Children's Hospital, Cleveland, Ohio
Management of Orthopedic Injuries

William M. Maguire, MD

Attending Physician, Department of Emergency Medicine, Maricopa Medical Center, Phoenix, Arizona
Mononucleosis; Regional Anesthesia

Ronald F. Maio, DO, MS, FACEP

Instructor, Section of Emergency Medicine, Department of Surgery, University of Michigan; Staff, University of Michigan Medical Center, Ann Arbor, Michigan
Evaluation and Stabilization of the Injured Child

Barbara N. Malone, MD

Assistant Clinical Professor, Department of Otolaryngology, University of Minnesota; Chief of Staff-Elect, Children's Hospital, St. Paul, Minnesota
Foreign Body Ingestion; Neck Masses

Vince Markovchick, MD

Associate Professor of Surgery, Section of Emergency Medicine, University of Colorado; Director of Emergency Medical Services, Denver General Hospital, Program Director, Denver Affiliated Residency in Emergency Medicine, Denver, Colorado
Soft Tissue Injury and Wound Repair

Craig Marsden, MD

Resident, Emergency Medicine, Maricopa Medical Center, Phoenix, Arizona
Genitourinary Trauma

Richard E. Marshall, MD

Professor, Seton Hall University School of Graduate Medical Education; Director of Pediatrics, St. Michael's Medical Center, Newark, New Jersey
Bronchopulmonary Dysplasia

Marcus L. Martin, MD, FACEP

Associate Professor of Emergency Medicine, Medical College of Pennsylvania—Allegheny Campus; Emergency Medicine Residency Director and Senior Attending, Emergency Department, Allegheny General Hospital, Pittsburgh, Pennsylvania
Drug Abuse

Peter T. Mellis, MD

Assistant Professor of Pediatrics, Medical College of Virginia, Virginia Commonwealth University; Director, Section of Pediatric Emergency Medicine, Division of General Pediatrics and Emergency Care, Medical College of Virginia Hospitals, Richmond, Virginia
Congestive Heart Failure

Jorge Montes, MD

Assistant Professor, Department of Pediatrics, Eastern Virginia Graduate School of Medicine; Director, Pediatric Intensive Care Unit, Children's Hospital of The King's Daughters, Norfolk, Virginia
Coma

Gregory P. Moore, MD, FACEP

Associate Director, Emergency Medicine Residency Program, Maricopa Medical Center, Phoenix, Arizona
Intestinal Obstruction

Barbara A. Murphy, MD

Assistant Professor, Emergency Department, Duke University School of Medicine; Staff Physician, Emergency Department, Duke University Medical Center Hospital, Durham, North Carolina
Narcotics and Sedative-Hypnotics

Daniel W. Ochsenschlager, MD

Associate Professor of Pediatrics and Emergency Medicine, George Washington University; Medical Director, Emergency Medical Trauma Center, Children's National Medical Center, Washington, DC
Burns

Timothy J. O'Connor, MD

Assistant Professor of Pediatrics, University of Missouri–Kansas City School of Medicine; Staff Member, Pediatric Emergency Medicine, The Children's Mercy Hospital, Kansas City, Missouri
Myocarditis

Kelly P. O'Keefe, MD

Associate Residency Director, Joint Military Medical Centers Emergency Medicine Residency Program, Wilford Hall USAF Medical Center, San Antonio, Texas
Electrical and Lightning Injuries

Margaret Orcutt Tuddenham, DO, FACOP

Clinical Faculty, Emergency Medicine Residency, Portsmouth Naval Hospital, Portsmouth, Virginia
Cerebrovascular Syndrome

Irene M. O'Shaughnessy, MD

Assistant Professor of Medicine, Medical College of Wisconsin, Division of Endocrinology, Metabolism and Clinical Nutrition; Staff, Froedtert Memorial Lutheran Hospital, Milwaukee, Wisconsin
Thyroid Disorders

Maria Jevitz Patterson, MD, PhD

Professor, Microbiology and Public Health, and Clinical Professor, Pediatrics and Human Development, Michigan State University, East Lansing; Medical Staff, Ingham Medical Center, E.W. Sparrow Hospital, St. Lawrence Hospital, and Lansing General Hospital, Lansing, Michigan
Parasitic Infections

Stephen Penaskovic, MD
Attending Physician, Maricopa Medical Center, Phoenix, Arizona
Leukemia

Elizabeth H. Perry, MD
Assistant Professor, Laboratory Medicine and Pathology, University of Minnesota; Assistant Medical Director, Blood Bank, University of Minnesota Hospital and Clinic, Minneapolis, Minnesota
Blood Products and Transfusion; Hereditary Bleeding

Ann Petru, MD
Assistant Clinical Professor, University of California, San Francisco; Medical Staff, Children's Hospital of Oakland, Oakland, California
Human Immunodeficiency Virus

David A. Poleski, MD
Vice-Chief, Emergency Department, and Chief, Pediatric Emergency Division, William Beaumont Hospital, Royal Oak, Michigan
Adrenal Disorders

N. Heramba Prasad, MD, FACEP
Assistant Professor, Department of Emergency Medicine, East Carolina University School of Medicine; Medical Director, Department of Emergency Medicine, East Carolina University School of Medicine; Attending Physician, Emergency Department, University Medical Center of Eastern North Carolina, Greenville, North Carolina
Marine Animal Envenomation

Maureen C. Prendergast, MD, FACEP
Clinical Instructor, Northwestern University School of Medicine; Staff, Department of Emergency Medicine, Northwestern Memorial Hospital, Chicago, Illinois
Hydrocarbons and Inhalants

Jeffrey Proudfoot, DO
Assistant Clinical Professor, Section of Emergency Medicine, Michigan State University—College of Osteopathic Medicine, East Lansing; Staff, Department of Emergency Medicine, E.W. Sparrow Hospital, Lansing, Michigan
Kawasaki Disease

Wassam M. Rahman, MD
Children's Mercy Hospital, University of Missouri School of Medicine, Kansas City, Missouri
Bone Development and Pediatric Considerations

Marsha D. Rappley, MD
Assistant Professor, Pediatrics and Human Development, College of Human Medicine, Michigan State University, East Lansing, Michigan
Toxic Shock Syndrome

Earl J. Reisdorff, MD, FACEP
Associate Professor, College of Human Medicine, Michigan State University; Assistant Residency Director of Education, Michigan State Emergency Medicine Residency, Lansing, Michigan
Sickle Cell Hemoglobinopathy; Limping, Arthritis, and Orthopedic Infections; Viral Encephalitis

Ronald L. Rhule, DO, FACOEP
Associate Clinical Professor, Michigan State University, College of Human Medicine; Assistant Director, Military Affairs, Michigan State University; Attending Physician, Sparrow Hospital, Lansing, Michigan
Advanced Pediatric Resuscitation

T. J. Rittenberry, MD, FACEP
Assistant Residency Director, University of Illinois Residency in Emergency Medicine, University of Illinois at Chicago; Director of Emergency Medical Education, Illinois Masonic Medical Center, Chicago, Illinois
Ankle and Foot Injuries

Frederick P. Rivara, MD, MPH
Professor of Pediatrics and Adjunct Professor of Epidemiology, University of Washington; Director, Harborview Injury Prevention and Research Center; Attending Physician, Harborview Medical Center and Children's Hospital and Medical Center, Seattle, Washington
Injury Prevention

Mont R. Roberts, MD, FACEP
Associate Professor, College of Human Medicine, Michigan State University; Assistant Residency Director of Research, Michigan State Emergency Medicine Residency, Lansing, Michigan
Limping, Arthritis, and Orthopedic Infections

Michael A. Ross, MD, FACEP
Clinical Instructor, Emergency Medicine Residency, William Beaumont Hospital, Royal Oak, Michigan
Male Genital Disorders

Joseph Salisz, MD
Attending Urologist, Hackley Hospital, Muskegon, Michigan
Male Genital Disorders

Augusta J. Saulys, MD

Formerly Assistant Professor, Department of Pediatrics, University of Chicago Hospitals, Chicago, Illinois; Now Attending Physician, Emergency Department, Children's Hospital of Oakland, Oakland, California
Urinary Tract Infections

Robert W. Schafermeyer, MD, FACEP, FAAP

Clinical Associate Professor of Pediatrics, University of North Carolina School of Medicine, Chapel Hill; Associate Chairman, Department of Emergency Medicine, Carolinas Medical Center, Charlotte, North Carolina
Bronchiolitis

Donna L. Seger, MD, FACEP, ABMT

Assistant Professor of Surgery and Medicine, Division of Emergency Medicine, Vanderbilt University Medical Center; Medical Director, Middle Tennessee Poison Control Center, Vanderbilt University Medical Center, Nashville, Tennessee
Acetaminophen

Brad S. Selden, MD

Staff Physician, Department of Medical Toxicology, Good Samaritan Regional Medical Center, and Department of Emergency Medicine, Maricopa Medical Center, Phoenix, Arizona
Anticholinergics

Sid M. Shah, MD

Clinical Instructor, Michigan State University—Affiliated Emergency Medicine Residency, East Lansing, Michigan
Toxic Shock Syndrome

Richard P. Shugerman, MD

Clinical Assistant Professor, University of Washington School of Medicine; Attending Physician, Emergency Services, Children's Hospital and Medical Center, Seattle, Washington
Dysrhythmias

Jonathan I. Singer, MD

Professor of Emergency Medicine and Pediatrics and Vice Chair and Program Director of Emergency Medicine, Wright State University; Staff Physician, Children's Medical Center, Dayton, Ohio
Fever and Sepsis

Narendra Singh, MD, FRCP(C), FAAP

Assistant Professor of Pediatrics, University of Western Ontario; Staff, Pediatric Emergency, Children's Hospital of Western Ontario, London, Ontario, Canada
Airway Management and Ventilatory Support

John J. Skiendzielewski, MD, FACEP

Director, Department of Emergency Medicine, Geisinger Clinic, Danville, Pennsylvania
Electrical and Lightning Injuries

Edward P. Sloan, MD, FACEP

Assistant Professor, Program in Emergency Medicine, University of Illinois College of Medicine; Attending, Emergency Services, University of Illinois Hospital, and Trauma Emergency Services, Cook County Hospital Trauma Unit, Chicago, Illinois
Ankle and Foot Injuries

Douglas S. Smith, MD, MS

Assistant Professor of Pediatrics, Medical College of Wisconsin; Attending Physician, Emergency Department, Children's Hospital of Wisconsin, Milwaukee, Wisconsin
The Neurologic Examination

Karen K. Smith, MD

Ambulatory Staff Pediatrician, Children's Hospital of Oakland, Oakland, California
Human Immunodeficiency Virus

Kathleen M. Smith, MD

Clinical Assistant Professor, University of Washington, Seattle; Attending Physician, Pediatric Emergency Medicine, Mary Bridge Children's Hospital, Tacoma, Washington
Neck Masses

S. William Snover, MD, FACEP

Associate Clinical Professor of Surgery (Emergency Medicine), Thomas Jefferson University Hospital, Philadelphia; Associate, Department of Emergency Medicine and Department of Hyperbaric Medicine, and Director, Occupational Health Services, Geisinger Medical Center, Danville, Pennsylvania
Smoke Inhalation and Carbon Monoxide Poisoning

Bonnie Sowa, MD

Staff, Emergency Pediatrics: Department of Pediatrics and Division of Emergency Medicine, Henry Ford Hospital, Detroit, Michigan
Vascular Access

Albert W. Sparrow, MD, MPH

Professor of Pediatrics and Human Development, College of Human Medicine, Michigan State University, East Lansing; Active Staff, E. W. Sparrow Hospital, Ingham Medical Center, St. Lawrence Hospital, and MSU Clinical Center, Lansing, Michigan
Murmurs

William H. Spivey, MD
Associate Professor of Emergency Medicine, Medical College of Pennsylvania; Chief, Division of Research; Associate Director, Emergency Department; Director of Fellowships, Medical College of Pennsylvania, Philadelphia, Pennsylvania
Asthma

Barbara Staggers, MD, MPH, FAAP
Director, Division of Adolescent Medicine, Children's Hospital Medical Center of Northern California, Oakland, California
Adolescent Pregnancy and Obstetric Emergencies

R. Daryl Steiner, DO
Associate Clinical Professor, Ohio University College of Osteopathic Medicine; Attending Physician, Department of Emergency Medicine, and Medical Director, Child at Risk Evaluation (C.A.R.E.) Center, Children's Hospital Medical Center of Akron, Akron, Ohio
Apnea

Susan A. Stern, MD
Research Fellow, Department of Emergency Medicine, University of Cincinnati College of Medicine, Cincinnati, Ohio
Shock and Fluid Resuscitation

John E. Stork, MD
Assistant Professor of Pediatrics and Assistant Professor of Medicine, Case Western Reserve University; Chief, Division of Pediatric Nephrology, Rainbow Babies and Children's Hospital, Cleveland, Ohio
Hypertension

Robert M. Street, MD, FRCP(C)
Clinical Assistant Professor and Assistant Residency Director, Emergency Medicine, University of British Columbia; Staff Physician, Vancouver General Hospital, Vancouver, British Columbia, Canada
The Pediatric Patient in the Emergency Department

Robert A. Swor, DO, FACEP
Clinical Instructor, Division of Emergency Services, University of Michigan Medical School, Ann Arbor; EMS Fellowship Director, William Beaumont Hospital, Royal Oak, Michigan
Emergency Medical Systems

Bruce M. Thompson, MD
Clinical Instructor, University of Michigan, Ann Arbor; Vice Chair/Program Director, Emergency Medicine Residency Program, Department of Emergency Medicine, Henry Ford Hospital, Detroit, Michigan
Vascular Access

Christian Tomaszewski, MD
Director of Toxicology Research, Department of Emergency Medicine, Carolinas Medical Center, Charlotte, North Carolina
Poisoning in Children

Karen Villalba, MD
Clinical Instructor, Case Western Reserve University School of Medicine, Cleveland, Ohio
Upper Extremity Injuries

Michele B. Wagner, MA, MD
Assistant Professor, Department of Surgery, Section of Emergency Medicine, Medical College of Georgia and University Hospital, Augusta, Georgia
Sudden Infant Death Syndrome

Laurie Wallace, DO
Teaching Faculty, Botsford General Hospital, Farmington Hills, Michigan
Epistaxis; Post-Tonsillectomy Hemorrhage

Gert-Paul Walter, MD, FACEP
Associate Faculty, New England School of Osteopathic Medicine; Director, Emergency Department, St. Mary's Regional Medical Center, Lewiston, Maine
Pediatric Malignancies

Bradford L. Walters, MD, FACEP
Clinical Faculty, Michigan State University and Wayne State University; Staff, Department of Emergency Medicine, Henry Ford Hospital, Detroit, Michigan
Pain Control in the Emergency Department

Suman Wason, MD, MBA
Adjunct Associate Professor of Pediatrics and Emergency Medicine, University of Cincinnati; Staff, Children's Hospital Medical Center and University Hospital, Cincinnati, Ohio
Caustic Ingestions; Phenothiazines; Theophylline; Tricyclic Antidepressants

Gary S. Wasserman, DO
Professor of Medicine, Department of Pediatrics, University of Missouri–Kansas City School of Medicine; Attending Physician, Pediatric Emergency Medicine; Clinical Toxicologist; and Director of Poison Control Center, The Children's Mercy Hospital, Kansas City, Missouri
Seizures and Status Epilepticus

Kathryn Weise, MD
Assistant Professor, University of Virginia School of Medicine; Staff, Department of Pediatrics, Division of Pediatric Critical Care, University of Virginia Health Sciences Center and Children's Medical Center, Charlottesville, Virginia
Cardiovascular Drug Ingestions

John G. Wiegenstein, MD
Professor and Chief, Section of Emergency Medicine, College of Human Medicine, Michigan State University; Chairman, Department of Emergency Medicine, Ingham Medical Center, Lansing, Michigan

James J. Williams, MD
Staff Physician, Children's Hospital of Oakland; Attending Pediatrician, University of California, San Francisco, San Francisco General Hospital, San Francisco, California
Child Abuse

Alice S. Yih, MD
Attending Physician, Emergency Medicine, Valley Lutheran Hospital, Phoenix, Arizona
Regional Anesthesia

David N. Zull, MD
Associate Professor of Clinical Medicine, Northwestern University Medical School; Associate Chief, Medicine, Northwestern Memorial Hospital, Chicago, Illinois
Anaphylaxis and Allergy-Mediated Disease

PREFACE

Approximately thirty years ago, emergency medicine had its beginning as a discipline. In 1968 the American College of Emergency Physicians was established; in 1980 the American Board of Emergency Medicine (ABEM) certified the first specialists in the specialty. Today nearly 100 residency programs in emergency medicine are approved by the American Board of Medical Specialties. Addressing the need for specialized environments, pediatric emergency medicine fellowships and integrated residency programs in pediatrics and emergency medicine are developing. The subspecialty of pediatric emergency medicine is a reality.

It seems only fitting that a textbook addressed to the practice of this specialized area should emanate from the city where academic emergency medicine had its origin. Michigan State University's Office of Medical Education, Research and Development (OMERAD) served as a catalyst for the development of the content of the emergency medicine specialty and for the certification and recertification process as it exists today. OMERAD continues to collaborate with ABEM in developing the subspecialty of pediatric emergency medicine.

Collectively, the editors have been treating children in the emergency department for 50 years. The authors were chosen primarily from faculty of emergency medicine residencies and pediatric emergency fellowships. It was important to the editors that the information be current and the recommended treatment be consistent with the most accepted expert opinion available at the time of publication. In order to avoid being provincial, attempts were made to obtain respected authors from a wide spectrum of national emergency medicine.

The text is divided into seventeen sections beginning with "Pediatric Emergentology," which includes special considerations in approaching the management of life-threatening conditions. Pediatric resuscitation and airway and shock management are key to this section. Sections 2 to 9, 11, 15, and 16 address anatomic and systemic diseases of children. Section 10 deals with infections in general, with specific diseases highlighted. Emphasis on toxicology and environmental emergencies and trauma is made in sections 12 to 14. The last section covers contemporary topics such as drug abuse, bioethics, and organ donation.

In an attempt to provide easy reference to essential material, frequently used tables are printed inside the front and back covers. The "Therapy at a Glance" feature highlights commonly used medications pertinent to each subject. In addition, signs and symptoms, differential diagnosis, disposition, and documentation considerations are highlighted throughout the text when appropriate. Further explanation of a topic is enhanced in select chapters by the use of in-text references. It is hoped that such efforts make this treatise valuable to every emergency department and hospital library and a useful reference for every teaching program addressing issues in pediatric emergency medicine.

EARL J. REISDORFF, MD, FACEP
MONT R. ROBERTS, MD, FACEP
JOHN G. WIEGENSTEIN, MD

ACKNOWLEDGMENTS

The authors are pleased to acknowledge the tireless efforts of many individuals who contributed to the development of this book. Their "fingerprints," found throughout, have richly enhanced the quality of the text.

At W.B. Saunders, Darlene Pedersen (Editor) believed in and encouraged the project. Kendall Sterling and David Harvey (Manuscript Editors), Bill Preston (Production Manager), Joan Wendt (Designer), Cathy Carroll (Editorial Assistant), and Walt Verbitski (Illustrator) oversaw detailed elements of the work. Les Hoeltzel (Developmental Editor) was instrumental in the completion of the book, acting as consultant, mediator, wise sage, and most of all, friend.

A special thank you is offered to Karen McPherson who served as secretary, typist, and consultant. Her persistence, cheerfulness, and never-waning support were beyond price.

The Chi Medical Library Staff (Barbara Shipman, Ruth Krause, Mary Andrick, Jane Vick, and Director David G. Keddle) were tolerant of numerous requests for obscure information. They were quick to provide support, assistance, and an environment for achievement.

Rianne Anderson wore many hats and was always willing to take on the most menial task with vigor. Dave Courey and Will Waterman provided most of the photographic support for the book, always within a need-it-now deadline. Radiologists Ken Thorp and Bing Tai provided both radiographs and commentary. Dr. Alan Oestreich was gracious in supplying numerous radiographs from Children's Hospital Medical Center in Cincinnati.

We would also like to thank co-workers and residents for their understanding. They never grew restless as energies were being directed away from their interests toward the editing of this book.

Finally, the authors wish to thank the 165 contributors to this project. Their knowledge, compassion, and gift of instruction were freely given.

SPECIAL ACKNOWLEDGMENTS

Thanks to my wife Jane, who led me to an understanding of the creative wonder we call "the child";

To Hannah, who every day of her early life has affirmed her mother's wisdom;

To Rebecca, who I am certain will challenge and instruct with innocence and energy. EJR

To my wife Gina, and to Megan, Monty, and Emma for their inspiration and understanding. MRR

Special thanks to my wife Iris for her understanding and forbearance. JGW

CONTENTS

SECTION ONE

Pediatric Emergentology

CHAPTER 1

The Pediatric Patient in the Emergency Department

Robert M. Street

INTRODUCTION

Illnesses and accidents are a part of growing up. These incidents seldom occur at convenient times. In addition, because working parents are often unable to make office appointments as a result of schedule conflicts, it is no wonder that pediatric visits to emergency departments comprise approximately one third of the total number of ambulatory care visits.

Parents have a variety of reasons for bringing a child to the emergency department.[1–10] In essence, the parents determine what constitutes an "emergency." Fortunately, most of these children are not seriously ill, but even so, the presence of a frightened, crying patient and anxious parents is often stressful for the emergency staff. Adding to this stress is the fact that the history is often nonspecific, and the physical examination may be frustrating and not diagnostic. Physical signs of serious illness may be subtle, and the illness may progress rapidly. Seriously ill children must be differentiated from the much larger group of patients with similar presenting signs but minor illnesses.

Every emergency facility that sees pediatric patients must be equipped and staffed to meet the unique challenges of caring for ill children. The emergency staff must be sensitive to children's dependency on the family and their age-related response to illness. Thus the "patient" is frequently the child *and* the parents. A special relationship evolves from the interaction of the hospital staff, the child, and the parents. This relationship should be encouraged to facilitate the physical assessment and provide a positive experience for all concerned.

THE PEDIATRIC PATIENT

The pediatric patient varies in a number of ways: age, size, development, culture, and disease. The stress that emergency personnel experience when a child presents to an emergency department can be reduced by being prepared to deal with unique relations with both the patient and the physical illness.

Hospitals are frightening places for children and their parents. Children's responses to the emergency department are related to their age and psychological development.[11] Previous surveys[12, 13] have shown that younger patients exhibit more stress than older patients. Gender and previous hospital experience do not affect the level of stress. Preschool- and school-age children tend to verbalize their fears more than older children. Fear of pain is frequently expressed, as is a fear of having to stay in the hospital or a fear of the consequences of their injuries to their bodies in the future. School-age children try stalling tactics more often than those in other age groups and are more curious about the procedure or the facility. The time spent in the emergency department and the person who treats the child do increase the child's stress, but the use of restraints causes much more protest than when restraints are not used. Preteens express fewer fears and more curiosity and are more concerned about their immediate future.

An understanding of some basic principles of child development helps explain a child's reaction to injury or illness and helps the emergency staff deal more effectively with the patient. From infancy to 2 years of age, children learn to act in the world and cannot think about what they are doing. Attachment to parents develops. By 2 months of age, infants can discriminate parents from strangers and mothers from fathers. Children realize their parents exist even when they cannot see them (*object permanence*). Separation from the parent at this stage evokes protest and is strongest between the ages of 12 and 18 months. When an infant is ill, the parents are a primary source of comfort, and separating them will be counterproductive. Maximizing parental contact will minimize the crying and protest responses.

Preschool-age children are beginning to use language and to explore their environment as their senses develop. They are egocentric and do not know that any other viewpoint exists. They focus on the present and have little concept of the future, and they are developing a sense of right and wrong. It follows, then, that these children may want to see and touch the instruments used to examine them. They do not like to be restrained and cannot understand why this might need to be done. Trying to show the child other children who are not crying is not reassuring. Telling the child how long a procedure may take or that it will feel better in a few days has little meaning. Fear of pain is well formed, and a fear of harm to the body is real. Fantasy or "magical thinking" abounds, and having children express any fantasies may help in reducing fear through play.

Children may view an illness or treatment as a form of punishment for something they have done wrong.

School-age children are beginning to establish themselves as members of society and undergo rapid intellectual growth. Preoccupation with fantasy gradually subsides. Thinking remains concrete, with the child dealing only with concrete (not hypothetical) objects and events. It is as important to be a member of a peer group as it is to cooperate and obey. Children in this age group verbalize their fears and are concerned about their bodily integrity. Thus taking time to explain a procedure such as suturing in simple language can make their visit a less frightening experience.

Adolescents have the ability for abstract thinking but are often difficult to communicate with. The adolescent has to deal with the rapid bodily changes that are occurring as well as learn to control emotions of love, hate, and aggression. The previous parental relationship may be replaced by rebellion. Their thinking is egocentric, and physical appearance is important. Late adolescence sees the maturing of bodily drives channeled into constructive activity. They may be uncooperative with the examination and are concerned about their future appearance (for example, their cosmetic appearance after a laceration). Following a treatment plan may be impossible because of poor compliance.

THE PARENTS

The pediatric patient may well be both the child and the parents. Parents play an important role in a child's experience in the emergency department. Sensitivity to this special relationship will result in a better emergency experience for everyone.

Parents bring their children to the emergency department for a variety of reasons. These include a lack of understanding of childhood diseases, proximity to the hospital,[4, 8] convenience,[4, 6] and a belief that the services offered are superior to those at their own doctor's office.[3, 5] Members of all socioeconomic classes[14–16] and families in which both parents work[5] are increasingly using the emergency department as a source of primary care.

The parents may be feeling anxious, frightened, angry, helpless, and even guilty. Cultural and family influences determine how the parents and the child cope. The child and the parents look for support or signals from each other to reassure themselves. Parents with poor coping mechanisms often transfer this to their children, and the behavior can become exaggerated in a time of illness. Adults who are suspicious or distrust the emergency department staff may communicate this to the child. Lying to the child that a procedure will not hurt enhances this mistrust, and the child loses confidence in adults. Some parents see the pain from a procedure such as suturing as a form of punishment. Threatening a child who is misbehaving with a trip to the hospital for "a shot" reinforces the belief that treatment is punishment. Understanding these behaviors and emotions enables staff members to deal effectively with parents, as well as with their own emotions. An opportunity for educating the child and the parents is thus opened.

Children are dependent on their parents for comfort and, whenever possible, they should not be separated during a time of stress. Insisting that parents leave their child may be more harmful than beneficial. Parents who feel uncomfortable staying should not be made to feel guilty when choosing to leave, and they should be kept informed about their child's condition. An exception is when dealing with teenagers, when parents should be excused to allow the teenager needed privacy. Parents also respond to their child's illness.[11, 12] They commonly attempt to quiet the child; this is especially true of parents of boys and preschoolers. Messages of guilt and punishment are more common in parents of school-age and preteen children, whereas feelings of personal guilt are more common in parents of preschoolers.

All parents are concerned regarding their child's injury or illness. Appropriate information[17] to the parents regarding the nature of their child's illness and its treatment, passed on in an understanding manner, serves to reduce anxiety.

THE EMERGENCY STAFF

Understanding the emotional states of parents and their children helps the emergency staff deal with their own reactions. It is common to feel anger toward a parent who is demanding and irate. The parent may be frightened or feeling guilty and may express these emotions as anger. This anger is then misdirected at staff members. In addition, the parent may exhibit a process called *transference*. This is the tendency to act toward staff members as the parent acted toward someone in the past. That is, the parent has transferred feelings that were held toward someone in a previous relationship to the staff members, giving rise to behavior that is inappropriate in the present treatment situation. The identification of these phenomena enables staff members to be more effective in dealing with inappropriate behavior and avoids a senseless confrontation. To effectively deal with the patient, staff members must understand the pathophysiology of pediatric illness and development. Familiarity with childhood diseases and experience in performing necessary procedures provide a more positive experience for patients and their parents. Adequate training and continuing education must be directed toward proficiency in emergency pediatrics.

The Physician

A physician who cares for children in an emergency department must be skilled in the diagnosis and treatment of pediatric disorders. Most children are not seriously ill or injured, but the physician must be alert to subtle signs that may differentiate a child with a potentially serious problem from the majority with milder illnesses. Nonspecialist physicians and many pediatricians working in emergency settings are not trained or equipped to handle serious medical or surgical emergencies. Yet, early intervention by skilled physicians can have a significant effect on outcome.[18]

Physician coverage in emergency departments requires that doctors be trained to deal with both nonurgent and urgent medical and surgical problems.[6, 19–23] Primary care training programs must give adequate time to pediatrics. Emphasis must be given to conditions identified as occurring more commonly, such as central nervous system and respiratory diseases,[24] and to the therapeutic interventions.[25]

All physicians should be trained in pediatric advanced life support. Specialist physicians trained in emergency medicine, pediatrics, or, more recently, pediatric emergency medicine are increasing in number. Physicians must update their knowledge and skills[26] to ensure adequate quality of care. Quality assurance audits should be performed to evaluate care. Physicians must help in education in a wide variety of ways. Informing parents, children, and the public about accident and poisoning prevention, training prehospital care workers who have first contact with the child, and educating administrators, legislators, and fellow colleagues are suggested ways to help. Physicians must also take the time to inform parents of their child's injury or illness and care.[27]

The Nurse

The nurse is often the first member of the emergency staff to see an ill child[28] and must have the clinical skills to identify a serious problem with a nonspecific presentation. This triage process plays an important role in patient care and can be done in a safe and effective way.[29]

As a member of the emergency team, the nurse must be aware of the special problems in dealing with pediatric patients and their families.[30] Being sensitive to the concerns and need of families enables the nurse to be supportive and provide families with information about childhood illness. Promoting high standards of care for children may be aided by the designation of a nursing staff member who coordinates educational activities.[31]

ANATOMY AND PHYSIOLOGY

Accidents are the leading cause of death in children younger than 15 years of age. The basic principles of patient care are similar to those in adults. However, certain aspects of caring for injured children differ from caring for adults and require emphasis.

Infants do not tolerate cold ambient temperatures well, so attention to decreasing heat loss is necessary. The child's airway is anatomically different from, not just smaller than, that of an adult. Airway obstruction is often sudden, and management of a child's airway requires knowledge and skill. Vital signs vary with age and are difficult to memorize; thus an appropriate chart placed in the resuscitation area is helpful. Accuracy in administration of fluids is needed, and the proper amount is based on the child's weight. Recognition of shock can be difficult, and because the child compensates well hemodynamically, "sudden" development of shock is common. Basic procedures such as vascular access are often difficult, and the life-saving technique of intraosseous infusion must be learned.

Traumatic injuries differ in children when compared with those in adults. Head trauma is more common in children, and early intervention can lead to a more favorable outcome.[18] The chest is more compliant, and internal injury may be present with few external signs. Extremity trauma is common, and management of growth plate injuries must be appropriate to avoid potential limb abnormalities. The metabolic demands of children are higher than those in adults, and as for all intravenous therapies, attention to body weight is required for correct calculation of needs.

EMERGENCY MEDICAL SYSTEM CONSIDERATIONS

Between 6% and 10% of all ambulance runs involve pediatric patients.[3, 32, 33] Of these, about half are because of trauma,[2, 33, 34, 35] primarily in adolescent males. Medical emergencies, especially seizures, predominate in younger patients (those younger than 5 years).

The purpose of prehospital care is to provide treatment earlier than would otherwise be possible. This should increase patient survival.[36] Provision of this service requires trained, available personnel who are equipped to deal with such emergencies.

Time spent training prehospital care personnel in pediatric emergencies is less than that devoted to management in adult emergencies.[37] Acquiring and maintaining pediatric skills such as obtaining vital signs and intravenous access is difficult.[38] The use of advanced life support techniques can be associated with prolonged on-scene time.[33] Benefit from advanced prehospital pediatric care has been questioned,[39] but rapid transport to a trauma facility may improve survival.[40]

Future pediatric emergency medical systems should reflect the most common causes of pediatric ambulance runs: trauma (in adolescents) and medical emergencies (in young children). Pediatric-sized equipment must be available. These factors should allow earlier intervention, minimized on-scene time, and improved survival rates.

CLINICAL EVALUATION

A thorough clinical assessment in a child requires a different approach from that in an adult. The basic principles (i.e., a complete history and physical examination) remain the same, but certain aspects pertaining to the pediatric patient require emphasis.

There is a wide variation in what is normal in children. Clinical findings vary with age; thus the examiner must be guided in the approach to history taking and the technique of examination by the child's stage of growth and development. Becoming acquainted with the normal patterns at each stage facilitates an approach that will be more successful at obtaining and interpreting the information gathered.

The history for most children comes from the parents, who may be feeling anxious or guilty. Questions must be asked in such a way as to avoid implicating the parents and reinforcing their guilt. "Where were you when this happened?" or "How did this happen?" may not be the best way to ask about an unwitnessed fall. "Tell me about what happened" allows the parents to give their own account without being implicated as responsible. Obviously, when the history and physical findings are incompatible, a more direct approach is required. When speaking directly to a child, one should maintain eye contact, use a normal tone of voice, and ask simple questions the child can understand. "Does it hurt when you pee?" is better understood than "When was your last bowel movement?" The history should be taken with the parents and child together and their interaction observed. The adolescent's right to privacy must be respected and personal questions saved for a time when the parents are excused.

In many situations, the diagnosis depends on an accurate examination of the child. Every effort must be directed toward obtaining the child's cooperation. When examining the child, use a friendly, positive tone of voice. Commands should be stated simply, and the physician should tell the child what is about to be done (for example, "Please lie down, I'm going to feel your tummy"). Begging and pleading with the child is not productive. If an unpleasant part of the examination is required, it is best left until the end. Explain briefly to the child what is to be done, and complete the examination efficiently, using restraints if needed. For example, when examining the ears, explain to the child that you are going to look in his or her ears with a special light, and it will feel funny, but it will not hurt; this informs the child so that he or she can anticipate your actions. If the parent will need to restrain the child, explain what is required and instruct the parents what to do. Examining the ears in the mother's lap while she holds the child might elicit some protest, but it is usually much less than if the physician examines the child on the bed with a nurse trying to hold the child still.

The physician should allow the parents to remain in the room while examining the child. Much of the examination can be done with the child in a parent's arms. Allowing the child to see and touch instruments such as a stethoscope or a reflex hammer makes these instruments much less frightening, especially when accompanied with a brief explanation or demonstration of their purpose. The child may be reassured and distracted if a few simple toys are available for play.

The order of the examination may have to be individualized. In an infant who is quiet, one should listen to the chest and heart first and examine the ears and throat last. Patience is of paramount importance. A hastily performed assessment may only upset everyone and be counterproductive.

Investigations or procedures should be explained appropriately to the parents and child in understandable terms. One should not lie to a child that "it won't hurt." If restraints are required, they should be used in an efficient, professional manner.

A friendly, unhurried assessment can be accomplished even in a busy emergency department. This will maximize the information gathered while enabling the parents to participate and preventing the child from feeling threatened or fearful.

DIAGNOSTIC EVALUATION

Patients seen in an emergency department often have medical or surgical problems that require laboratory investigation. Judicious selection of laboratory tests and imaging techniques aids in diagnosis while avoiding unnecessary delays and expense. Knowledge of pediatric illnesses is imperative in order to accurately interpret results.

The child younger than 2 years who has a fever and no source of infection is a good example of the limitations of tests.[41–45] Clinically, there may be a paucity of findings. The history and physical examination alone are unreliable as indicators of bacteremia. An elevation in the peripheral white blood cell count and the erythrocyte sedimentation rate suggests the possibility of bacteremia. Although elevations in these indicators may be sensitive, they are not specific and when used in combination may actually lower the positive predictive value. Thus laboratory tests can be used only to assign the patient with positive test values to a high-risk group; treatment cannot be based on these laboratory tests alone.

Children with minor injuries may not require extensive laboratory studies on arrival at the hospital.[46] When radiographs are ordered, they frequently include studies of the skull, chest, pelvis, abdomen, spine, and extremities. Skull films have limited use in children with minor head injuries.[47] Radiographic interpretations by physicians in the emergency department and radiologists agree in 80% to 90% of cases.[48–50] Abnormalities on chest radiographs and missed extremity fractures account for the majority of discrepancies. Simple quality assurance measures can reduce patient morbidity and potential for litigation. The emergency physician's radiographic interpretation should be reviewed within 12 to 24 hours by a radiologist and the clinician notified if a discrepancy exists.

DOCUMENTATION/DISPOSITION

The medical record serves both to document the patient visit and to communicate to others the essential points of the history and physical examination that formed the basis for a diagnosis and treatment plan. The hospital record may be reviewed by those involved in further care of the child or later by those in quality assurance or research activities. Thorough charting is crucial in any medicolegal review, and although there are many arguments for good record keeping, this is the most compelling reason for many health professionals.

It is often difficult to maintain records in a busy department and often almost impossible to make chart entries during a resuscitation. Other members of the emergency staff may make entries on the chart as well. A well-designed chart can help in accuracy and ease of entries. Separating the triage form, nursing notes, and physician charting areas allows each team member access to the record. In cases of resuscitations, a "recorder" should be assigned to document the chain of events. The record should be completed as soon as time permits.

Poor charting continues despite efforts to improve record keeping. Taking a few minutes to complete a record can often save hours of anguish months later when a case must be recalled. Documenting pertinent positives and negatives of the history and physical examination in legible handwriting avoids many problems. Use of diagrams and accepted scoring systems such as the Glasgow Coma Scale decreases the amount of writing while improving communication. Avoiding abbreviations avoids ambiguity. Documentation of laboratory test results and their interpretation lends support to a tentative diagnosis. The therapy initiated and follow-up instructions must be documented. A clear and complete discharge form is necessary.

Written discharge information that has also been explained to parents serves several purposes. Knowing what the child has and what can be expected in the next few days allays many parents' fears of the unknown and may decrease guilt feelings. Written instructions at discharge may help compliance with aspects of treatment that are forgotten after they are explained.

Some patients leave the emergency department before their evaluation is begun or completed.[51, 52] Reasons for this include long waiting times, fear, and anger. Understanding the unique patient-parent dynamics can diffuse the situation and may prevent such instances. If a parent still insists on leaving, documentation of any clinical findings and of the explanation and understanding of the risks of refusing treatment should be made. Nevertheless, parental signature on a "refusal of treatment" or "against medical advice" form is not protection from litigation.

OTHER CONSIDERATIONS
The Emergency Department

An emergency department that provides efficient and comprehensive care requires good design, staffing, and support.[53–61] The layout of the department must ensure easy access for both ambulatory and ambulance patients. The entrance should be clearly marked and adequate space available for parking vehicles and unloading patients. This space should be large enough to allow for oversized vehicles or large numbers of patients, as might occur in a disaster.

Once inside the building, the waiting area, triage desk, and patient areas should be separate. The triage area must allow a private and relatively quiet space for a brief assessment. The waiting area should be designed to avoid overcrowding and noise. Many poor patient-staff encounters result from long, frustrating waits in an overcrowded room. Children should be shielded from the frightening sights and sounds of a busy emergency department, especially if the department takes adult and pediatric patients. A play area with safe toys and equipment may serve as a welcome distraction. A place quiet enough to nurse an infant or to allow a late night nap makes the wait more acceptable. A separate area is ideal for families of the critically ill or injured.

The patient care areas must allow adequate space for examination rooms and nursing stations. The design should enable staff to observe the treatment area with minimal obstructions. The overall design should be functional and pleasant to the eye. Specialized treatment areas, such as a resuscitation room, require extra equipment and may be separated from the general treatment area.

Support services should be located in close proximity to the emergency department. Laboratories, radiology facilities, surgical suites, and intensive care units are often on the same floor level. Importantly, no matter how well staffed, equipped, or designed an emergency department is, team work is the key to making the department function optimally.

References

1. Christoffel KK. Effect of season and weather on pediatric emergency department use. Am J Emerg Med 1985;3:327.
2. Ramenofsky ML, Luterman A, Curreri PW, et al. EMS for pediatrics: Optimum treatment or unnecessary delay? J Pediatr Surg 1983;18:498.
3. Kljakovic M, Allan BC, Reinken J. Why skip the general practitioner and go to the accident and emergency department? NZ Med J 1981;94:49.
4. Christoffel KK, Garside D, Tokich T. Pediatric emergency department utilization in the 1970's. Am J Emerg Med 1985;3:177.
5. Feldman W, Cullum C. The pediatric walk-in clinic: Competition for the private practitioner. Can Med Assoc J 1984;130:1003.
6. Wingert WA. Delivery of emergency care to children: Who is responsible? Pediatrics 1978;62:124.
7. Walschall JM. Why parents use the emergency department for nonemergency care. J Emerg Nurs 1983;9:37.
8. McFarlane JM. Pediatric care in the emergency room. Pediatr Nurs 1976;2:22.
9. Smith RD, McNamara JJ. Why not your pediatrician's office? A study of weekday pediatric emergency department use for minor illness care in a community hospital. Pediatr Emerg Care 1988;4:107.
10. Kushnir T. Parental anxiety and children's attendance at emergency departments in relation to the child's birth order. J Soc Pychol 1984;123:123.
11. Meier EM. The pediatric emergency patient. Emerg Med 1981;13:29.
12. Resnick R, Hergenroeder E. Children and the emergency room. Child Today 1975;4:5.
13. Resnick Gratz R. Children's responses to emergency department care. Ann Emerg Med 1984;13:322.
14. Shaw KN, Selbest SM, Gill FM. Indigent children who are denied care in the emergency department. Ann Emerg Med 1990;19:107.
15. Muller HA. Emergency medicine and the health care needs of the indigent child. Ann Emerg Med 1990;19:156.
16. Alwash R, McCarthy M. Accidents in the home amongst children under 5: Ethnic differences or social disadvantage? Br Med J 1988;296:1450.
17. Baker SP. Prevention of childhood injuries. Med J Aust 1980;1:466.
18. Mayer TA, Walker ML. Pediatric head injury: The critical role of the emergency physician. Ann Emerg Med 1985;14:1178.
19. Baker MD. Physician coverage in the pediatric emergency room. Am J Dis Child 1986;140:755.
20. Jackson RH. Children in accident and emergency departments. Br Med J 1985;291:991.
21. Bushore M. Emergency care of the child. Pediatrics 1987;79:572.
22. American College of Emergency Physicians. The role of the emergency physician in the care of children. Ann Emerg Med 1990;19:435.
23. Eitzen E, Schafermyer PW, Strange GR. The role of the emergency physician in providing pediatric emergency care—a membership survey. Ann Emerg Med 1990;19:532.
24. Kissoon N, Walia MS. The critically ill child in the pediatric emergency department. Ann Emerg Med 1989;18:59.
25. Waschman L, Singleton AF. Assessing the quality of care provided to pediatric patients by emergency room physicians. J Natl Med Assoc 1983;75:31.
26. Duncan B, Banner W, Ruggill J. Emergency drills in a pediatric residency training program. Ann Emerg Med 1983;12:164.
27. Morris RE, Henderson D. Some difficulties encountered in teaching physician-parent communication in a pediatric emergency department. Pediatr Emerg Care 1989;5:86.
28. Bourg PW. The nurse's role. In Barkin RM, Rosen P (eds). Emergency Pediatrics. St Louis, CV Mosby, 1984, pp 6–7.
29. Rivara EP, Wall HP, Wosley P. Pediatric nurse triage: Its efficacy, safety, and implications for care. Am J Dis Child 1986;140:205.
30. Schade J, Passo S. Needs assessment of parents in pediatric ambulatory care. J Amb Care Mgmt 1981;4:23.
31. Fredrichson JM. The pediatric liaison nurse: A new specialist in the emergency department. J Emerg Nurs 1988;14:129.
32. Johnston C, King WD. Pediatric prehospital care in a southern regional emergency medical service system. South Med J 1988;81:1473.
33. Tsai A, Kallsen G. Epidemiology of pediatric prehospital care. Ann Emerg Med 1987;16:284.
34. Fifield GC, Magnuson C, Carr WP, et al. Pediatric emergency care in a metropolitan area. J Emerg Med 1984;1:495.
35. O'Rourke PP. Outcome of children who are apneic and pulseless in the emergency room. Crit Care Med 1986;14:466.
36. Friesen RM, Duncan P, Tweed WA, et al. Appraisal of pediatric cardiopulmonary resuscitation. Can Med Assoc J 1982;126:1055.
37. Seidel JS. Emergency medical services and the pediatric patient: Are the needs being met? Training and equipping emergency medical services providers for pediatric emergencies. Pediatrics 1986;78:808.
38. Gausche M, Henderson DP, Seidel JS. Vital signs as part of the prehospital assessment of the pediatric patient: A survey of paramedics. Ann Emerg Med 1990;19:173.
39. Applebaum D. Advanced prehospital care for pediatric emergencies. Ann Emerg Med 1985;14:656.
40. Haller JA, Shorter N, Miller D, et al. Re-organization and function of a regional pediatric trauma center: Does a system of management improve outcome? J Trauma 1983;23:691.
41. Jaffe DM, Tanz RR, Davis AT, et al. Antibiotic administration to treat possible occult bacteremia in febrile children. N Engl J Med 1987;317:1175.
42. McLellan D, Giebink GS. Perspectives on occult bacteremia in children. J Pediatr 1986;109:1.
43. Carroll WL, Farrell MK, Singer JJ, et al. Treatment of occult bacteremia: A prospective randomized clinical trial. Pediatrics 1983;72:608.
44. Teele DW, Marshall R, Klein JO. Unsuspected bacteremia in young children. Pediatr Clin North Am 1979;26:773.
45. Crocher PJ, Quick G, McCombs W. Occult bacteremia in the emergency department: Diagnostic criteria for the young febrile child. Ann Emerg Med 1985;14:1172.
46. Bryant MS, Tepas JJ, Talbert JL, et al. Impact of emergency room laboratory studies on the ultimate triage and disposition of the injured child. Am Surg 1988;54:209.
47. Masters SJ, McClean PM, Arcarese MS, et al. Skull x-ray examinations after head trauma. N Engl J Med 1987;316:84.
48. Masel JP, Grant PJF. Accuracy of radiological diagnosis in the casualty department of a children's hospital. Aust Paediatr J 1984;20:221.
49. Fleisher G, Ludwig S, McSorley M. Interpretation of pediatric x-ray films by emergency department pediatricians. Ann Emerg Med 1983;12:153.
50. Nolan TM, Oberklaid F, Boldt D. Radiological services in a hospital emergency department—an evaluation of service delivery and radiographic interpretation. Aust Paediatr J 1984;20:109.
51. Dershewitz RA, Paichel W. Patients who leave a pediatric emergency department without treatment. Ann Emerg Med 1986;15:717.
52. Selbst SM. Leaving against medical advice. Pediatr Emerg Care 1986;2:266.
53. Goldman A. Child oriented emergency department design. In Fleisher G, Ludwig S, Henretig FM, et al (eds). Textbook of Pediatric Emergency Medicine. Baltimore, Williams & Wilkins, 1983, pp 1187–1200.
54. Isaacman DJ. Pediatric emergency medicine—current standards of care: Results of a national survey. Ann Emerg Med 1990;19:527.
55. Shah CP. Pediatric emergency services of the future. Can Med Assoc J 1976;21:307.
56. Richmond PW, Evans RC, Sibert JR. Improving facilities for children in an accident department. Arch Dis Child 1987;62:299.
57. Banco L, Powers A. Hospitals: Unsafe environments for children. Pediatrics 1988;82:794.
58. Arensman RM, Falterman KW. Emergency care of the injured child. Postgrad Med 1984;75:257.
59. Ogundipe O. Organization of emergency pediatric units. J Trop Pediatr Environ Child Health 1975;21:64.
60. Liptak GS, Super DM, Baker N, et al. An analysis of waiting times in a pediatric emergency department. Clin Pediatr 1985;24:202.
61. Ramenofsky MD, Morse TS. Standards of care for the critically injured pediatric patient. J Trauma 1982;22:921.

CHAPTER 2

The Development-Based Examination

Martin G. Hellman

INTRODUCTION

The physical examination of infants and children in the emergency department is the most vital aspect of the clinical assessment and diagnostic evaluation. Histories are often incomplete, unclear, or based on a care provider's opinion of the problem. Laboratory studies may be equivocal or misleading. It is crucial that the emergency department physician recognize the severity of the child's condition based on the examination.

Understanding normal growth and developmental milestones aids the emergency department physician in assessment. Unlike adults, children require different examination strategies for various age groups. Knowledge of key points in normal developmental milestones can assist the staff in categorizing the patient's general state of health.

The frequent repetition of the physical examination within various age groups is necessary to understand normal variations in children and to develop a "clinical sense" about the infant's condition. Emergency department physicians who only sporadically see children are at a disadvantage when compared with pediatricians or pediatric emergency physicians who have frequent contact with children of all ages.

The physical examination should be structured to accommodate children at different ages. Each child is different in developing; some may be precocious, whereas others may lag behind. By knowing what to expect of the average child, the emergency department physician can better assess the patient's general status (Table 2–1).

EXAMINATION
The Newborn to 8-Week-Old Infant

The first few months of a child's life are an exciting yet potentially unnerving time for many parents. They may present to the emergency department with a wide range of problems concerning their infants. Family members' beliefs coupled with parental inexperience often lead to emergency department visits for medically "trivial" matters, yet these concerns may seem monumental to the parents. A thorough examination and calm words of reassurance are often the best therapy for parental anxiety.

The evaluation of any infant in the first several months also requires knowledge of the infant's gestational age at delivery. A general guideline is to expect a premature baby to lag behind its expected milestones for chronologic age. The average delay usually corresponds to the number of weeks born prematurely. This lag in developmental milestones gradually narrows over the first 1 to 2 years of life, assuming the child has no compromising medical conditions.[1]

Growth

Growth in the first several months is rapid. Initially, infants lose 6% to 10% of their birth weight in the first week after delivery as a result of fluid losses.[1] By the tenth day, the original birth weight is reattained. Subsequently, an infant's weight increases 15 to 30 gm each day.[2]

Showing an infant's weight gain to parents may help allay fears relating to a variety of topics. Infants will generally not follow normal growth patterns if they have a serious, chronic medical condition. Standard growth charts should be available in the emergency department for this purpose. Visual conformation of acceptable growth should calm worried parents. Conversely, further evaluation can be initiated if growth parameters are declining.

Though the emergency department physician may not be an expert on feeding, a basic understanding of breastfeeding and formula preparation is essential. Problems with either of these procedures may lead to poor weight gain in infancy.

Nursing mothers need to consume increased quantities of fluids above their normal maintenance requirements. The feeding time should be noted, as most infants are satiated after 12 to 15 minutes on each breast.[3] If the child is to be formula fed, one must know that formulas are available in three forms: ready-to-feed, concentrate, and powder. The physician must be able to ascertain whether the parents are preparing the formula correctly.

Developmental Milestones

By 1 to 2 months, infants display the asymmetric tonic neck reflex and will assume the typical "fencer's position" as the head is turned from side to side in the supine position.[1] When the infant is pulled up from the supine position, the head shows a definite lag. Babies begin to turn their heads while prone and start to initiate a "push-up" in the second month.

The key milestone of this age group is the socially responsive smile, which begins at 6 to 8 weeks.[10] Before this, it is difficult to judge an infant's general attitude and interaction with the environment. Subsequently, a young infant can be more easily evaluated for its mental alertness and responsiveness to both objects and human contact.

Physical Examination

The infant should first be watched carefully in the care giver's lap or on the examination table. The infant's activity level, skin color, and position of the extremities at rest should be noted. Full-term infants tend to lie in a flexed attitude, whereas premature babies hold their arms and legs in a more extended posture.

The resting respiratory rate and signs of retraction or flaring should be observed. Any audible sounds denoting respiratory difficulty should be appreciated. Both a central area and a distal extremity can be quickly palpated for capillary refill and skin temperature. The anterior fontanel should be felt lightly for pulsations using the tips of the index and long fingers.

The examination is continued by gently feeling the precordium before auscultating the heart and lung fields. At this age, murmurs not heard at birth first become audible as a result of changes in pulmonary vascular resistance. A stethoscope with a pediatric head should be used, as sounds from several areas may merge together with an adult-sized stethoscope.

After checking for abdominal distention, bowel sounds should be auscultated before the abdomen is palpated for masses. The restless or crying infant may be more cooperative while sucking on a bottle or pacifier.

Checking the genitalia and diaper area for signs of hernias, hydroceles, rashes, or anomalies should always complete the abdominal examination. Feeling for femoral pulses and habitually testing for a dislocatable hip is a good practice.

A thorough funduscopic examination is difficult to perform. Checking for a red reflex is mandatory to exclude tumors. Ear canals are narrow and tortuous, and the tym-

---

TABLE 2–1
PHYSICAL EXAMINATION: GENERAL TIPS
• General status is most important • Reexamine after a short interval • Observe first from afar • Avoid painful procedures until examination finale • Continually interact with the child • Make a walking child walk • Be alert for social smile

panic membranes are difficult to visualize. The neonate's tympanic membrane is positioned more in the horizontal plane, giving it a retracted appearance.[4]

The absence of tears does not always reflect dehydration. Up to 35% of infants do not normally produce tears for the first several months.[5] The oral cavity should be examined for signs of candidiasis or other problems.

Recognition of normal neonatal dermatologic and soft tissue findings is important. Parental questions regarding nevus flammeus, milia, Mongolian spots, and other marks commonly arise. Resolving cephalohematomas may be present for several months.[6]

Neonatal gynecomastia can be seen in both sexes and gradually fades at 2 to 4 months.[7] Emergency department physicians should be acquainted with routine care of the separating umbilicus and be alert for umbilical granulomas.[1]

Female infants may have a whitish, creamy vaginal discharge in the first few weeks. Moreover, a small amount of withdrawal vaginal bleeding can occur in the first week after delivery.[8] Uncircumcised boys need no special treatment except routine cleansing.

A quick but thorough neurologic examination is required. Moro's and stepping reflexes are present at birth, and begin to fade by 3 to 4 months. The knee jerk is the easiest of the deep tendon reflexes to observe.[1]

The 2- to 6-Month-Old Child

During the 2-month to 6-month period, many growth and developmental changes occur (Table 2–2). This stage represents the period just before infants identify "friend or foe." Preference for certain people and objects begins at 6 to 8 months. Therefore, the 2- to 6-month-old should still be nonfearful.

Growth

Rapid weight gain continues throughout this period. Normal healthy infants should double their birth weight by 3 to 4 months. Length also increases rapidly in the first 6 months. Of the average 25- to 30-cm gain in the first year, two thirds comes in the first 6 months. Head circumference also markedly increases from an average 34 to 35 cm at birth to 44 to 45 cm by 6 months.[1, 2]

Developmental Milestones

Gross Motor Skills. Gradually, the infant's head lag when pulled from a supine position diminishes. At 3 months of age, the child's head bobs when placed in a sitting position. By 4 months, the head will be steady in the midline.[10] The stepping reflex fades at 3 to 4 months as infants begin to bear weight on both legs when held under the axilla. Finally, infants begin to roll over from front to back, then later back to front by 5 to 6 months of age.[1]

Sitting without support is just starting at this age. At 4 months, the infant falls over, but by 5 months, he or she can sit in a tripod position for a short length of time. By 6 months of age, most infants are beginning to sit on a firm surface without support.[10]

Fine Motor Skills. Asymmetric movement of the hands and arms gradually fades by 4 months as infants bring their hands to the midline. Grasping keys, rattles, or toys, using the entire palm, becomes possible by 4 to 5 months. At 5 to 6 months, these objects are transferred from hand to hand. By 6 months, these objects are brought to the mouth for exploration.

Language. Laughing, cooing, and babbling all begin after 8 weeks of age. Coupled with the social smile, these traits further enable an infant to interact socially with other people. No discernible words are made until the second half of the first year.[10]

Personal/Social Skills. The social interactive smile is firmly entrenched during this stage. Getting an infant to smile and interact is probably the best way to indicate a normal mental status.

Physical Examination

As with neonates, most of the examination can be done with the infant in the care giver's lap. The child's general activity and respiratory efforts should be observed first. It is best to face the child in a calm, nonthreatening manner. The examiner should try to elicit coos or laughter from the infant while the infant is sitting in the parent's lap. A 12- to 16-week-old infant should easily respond to face-to-face talking or funny sounds ("baby talk"). The infant should react favorably to humorous inflections of the examiner's voice.

Observation of the child's fontanel is best done before any screaming or crying starts. The examiner might have to move to optimize the room's light reflection in order to see pulsations. Obvious pulsations of the anterior fontanel are inconsistent with low hydration status or central nervous system infection. Conversely, noting a sunken or bulging fontanel without pulsations may be ominous.

Using a set of keys or a bright object, the examiner can view the infant's general attitude. The infant should visually follow it in all directions and grasp, transfer, or place the object in the mouth.

Assessment of hydration status can also be accomplished by recognizing moisture on the eyes and lips. Bubbles of saliva, drool on the chin, or tears are also good indicators of adequate hydration.

Listening for audible respiratory noises and watching for retractions or nasal flaring should also be done before the child is agitated. When infants get rhinorrhea from viral upper respiratory infections, it is difficult to distinguish upper from lower airway sounds on auscultation. A helpful technique is to position one's ear near the infant's nose and simultaneously auscultate the lung fields with the stethoscope. Most often, noises heard emanating from the nostrils are the same sounds heard through the stethoscope, thus identifying them as upper airway noises.

A wealth of information about the infant is gathered with minimal physical contact. The examiner may already have a sense regarding the infant's general status. The remaining examination can then be completed, examining the chest and abdomen first, followed by the head and neck.

Auscultation and palpation of the chest and abdomen can be done either in the parent's lap or on the examination table. While on the table, the infant's diaper is removed to allow inspection for diaper rashes or any genital problems. Noting the diaper contents or even a dry diaper yields further information about the baby's hydration status.

Inspecting the tympanic membranes for landmarks and mobility at this age is best accomplished on the examination

TABLE 2–2
DEVELOPMENTAL HIGHLIGHTS: THE 2- TO 6-MONTH-OLD CHILD

Personal skills:	Social smile
Language:	Cooing
Fine motor skills:	Grabs objects
Gross motor skills:	Looks all around

table. The care giver can hold the infant steady by firmly grasping the legs with each hand, holding one thigh above the infant's knee. The pinna is pulled superiorly and laterally to straighten the auditory canal with the examiner's free hand. If motion precludes a good view, another adult can stabilize the arms and head. A quick look at the oropharynx is sufficient to check for moistness or intraoral lesions.

The examination should finish with a succinct neurologic check. Both the Moro and stepping reflexes begin fading by 3 to 4 months of age.[1] The 4- to 6-month-old will bear weight on both legs while being held under the axilla. The sitting posture should be noted, along with a consideration of general muscle tone.

Potential Medical Problems Based on Development

Infants between the ages of 2 and 3 months often present with the acute onset of irritability and crying, although they are afebrile. A self-induced corneal abrasion is always possible at this age because of the infant's random hand movements approaching the midline. A simple fluorescein stain of both eyes will identify the abrasion.

Because some parents are unaware of expected "rolling over" episodes, unattended infants can roll off changing tables, beds, or sofas. These children present with minor head trauma but are usually not seriously hurt.

The 6- to 12-Month-Old Child

The second half of the first year of life marks a time of many growth and developmental milestones (Table 2–3). These changes have an impact on the child's personality and affect the evaluation of potential medical problems. Moreover, emergency department physicians usually find this group of infants the most difficult to examine. These infants cannot vocalize problems yet, but they are old enough to be afraid of strangers and become uncooperative.

Growth

Weight and length gains begin to decelerate during this period and attain a more linear pattern. The parent may become concerned about the child's apparent growth delay. Again, reassurance with growth charts can be useful.

After doubling the birth weight by 3 to 4 months of age, an infant then usually gains the same amount by the age of 1 year, thus approximately tripling birth weight. Therefore 7 kg would be the average weight gain by the first birthday.[1]

Length increase slows after the first 6 months, as only one third of the first year's growth occurs after this time. Head circumference increase tapers off also and averages only a 3- to 4-cm increase during these 6 months.

Primary tooth eruption usually commences at this time. The first tooth commonly appears at between 5 and 9 months of age, and a pattern of one new tooth each month follows.[1, 2] The emergency department physician can refer to the number of teeth for yet another confirmation of normal growth patterns. This can be variable, as some children erupt no teeth until their second year.

Developmental Milestones

Gross Motor Skills. After firmly establishing an erect sitting position, 6- to 8-month-old infants begin to pull themselves up to stand. By 9 to 10 months, most children can stand while holding onto a chair or the wall.[10] Crawling slowly advances to the early stages of walking with help and then finally to independent ambulation.

Fine Motor Skills. Perhaps the most important feat that occurs at this time is the realization of the pincer grasp. Use of the thumb and index finger to grab tiny objects begins at 7 to 8 months. This should be well established by 9 to 10 months.

Language. Nonspecific babbling and cooing gradually evolve into one to two words that are used randomly. Most infants begin with "dada" or "mama" but usually don't associate them with the actual person until they are about 1 year old.

Personal/Social. The onset of memory for objects and persons slowly forms and by 6 to 8 months is well entrenched. After this, children show preference for favorite toys and recognize familiar faces.

Physical Examination

The general examination should begin from outside or across the room. Activity, playfulness, and respiratory rate are noted before approaching the child. Investing 30 to 45 seconds of time determining the child's general status will be crucial later in the examination.

With the child resting in the care giver's lap, the examiner sits facing the child. The general status examination should be continued without getting close too quickly. It is unlikely that a 9- to 12-month-old child will laugh or smile as readily as a 4-month-old infant.

The examiner can shake a key ring or a brightly colored object in all directions. Having the child gaze up, down, and side to side tests both mental status and neck mobility.

Pulsations of the anterior fontanel should be seen if hair does not preclude the view. Though some infants' fontanels are closed by this time, most do not fuse until 9 to 18 months of age.[1]

The child should be able to grab small objects. Watching the mode of grasp and the usual subsequent placement of the object into the mouth gives the examiner additional facts about the infant's general status.

The respiratory rate should be counted and the presence of retractions recognized. Younger infants with respiratory distress usually show substernal and inferior rib retractions. If the infant is too restless while sitting, the care giver can cuddle the child over the shoulder to enable the examiner to get a more accurate view. A true measure of the child's respiratory status may then be ascertained by watching the child's back for rate and retractions.

By this time the examiner should have a good idea about the child's general status, and it is time for a hands-on evaluation. The child should be approached slowly but methodically with the stethoscope. It is best to avoid startling the child by first placing the stethoscope head against the parent's arm or the child's arm or leg. Hopefully, this will reassure the child and delay any crying outbursts for an adequate time.

After listening to the chest, heart, and abdomen, the examiner may be able to deeply palpate the abdomen with the child still in the parent's lap. A good funduscopic

TABLE 2–3
DEVELOPMENTAL HIGHLIGHTS: THE 6- TO 12-MONTH-OLD CHILD

Personal skills:	Begins to fear strangers
Language:	"Dada"/"mama"—nonspecific
Fine motor skills:	Pincer grasp with fingers
Gross motor skills:	Pulls to a stand; walks

examination may be difficult but should be attempted anyway.

The remaining otolaryngologic examination needs the aid of the care giver and some possible restraint. Because this may irritate the child, any further general status observations may be unobtainable.

Before 6 to 8 months of age, infants are difficult to hold motionless in an adult's lap. Parents can usually obtain firm control of older children more successfully. The parent should face the examiner and wrap his or her legs around the child's legs to avoid kicking. Next, the adult should encompass the child's arms securely to prevent movement (Fig. 2–1).

While holding the otoscope with one hand, the examiner can grasp the pinna and gently pull upward and outward to straighten the auditory canal. This is an important step to ensure proper visualization of the entire tympanic membrane. By holding the infant's head against the care taker's chest, the examiner should be afforded the opportunity to carefully inspect the tympanic membranes without undue head movement (Fig. 2–2).

Landmarks and drum mobility are checked after a proper seal is made with the pneumatic otoscope. Erythema or a tympanic membrane blush may be the result of fever, crying, or irritation from cerumen irrigation.

Usually, an adequate peek at the oropharynx is possible without a tongue blade if the child is crying. The gums should be checked for erupting teeth or other oral problems.

The infant can be placed on a table for the examination's conclusion. The abdomen can be observed, then deeply palpated. If the child is crying, waiting a few seconds between screams should allow for deep palpation.

The diaper is then removed to check for rashes or genital problems. When indicated, a digital rectal examination should be done with the small finger until 1 year of age.

The examination should conclude with a test of neurologic

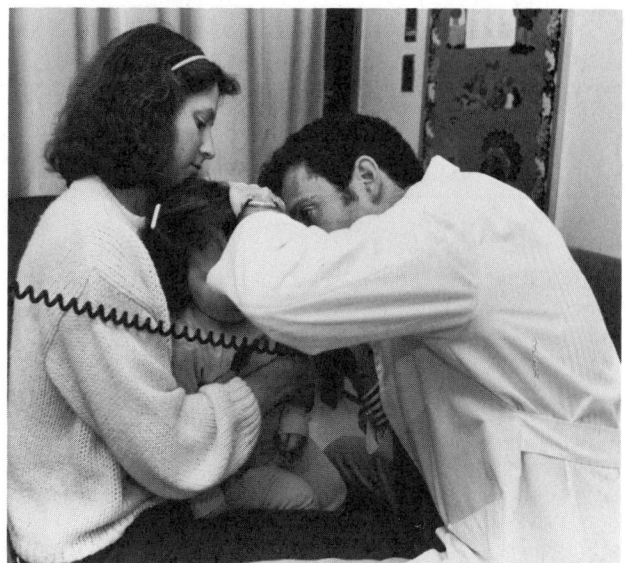

Figure 2–2. Even otoscopy is easier with this gentle holding technique.

function. The parachute reflex starts by 7 to 8 months of age and should be easily elicited by 9 to 10 months. If the child can ambulate, observing him or her walking in the room demonstrates the child's overall status, state of hydration, and level of strength. If doubt exists regarding the child's general condition, one should allow a short interval of time to elapse before reassessing the patient.

Potential Medical Problems Based on Development

The achievement of the pincer grasp midway through this period is a potentially hazardous milestone, as infants have the capability to place small objects into their mouths without the aid of a sibling or parent. Aspiration of food pieces, tiny toys, or other debris becomes possible. Although total airway occlusion is uncommon, it can lead to a disastrous outcome. Ingestion of coins, pins, or other bright things is commonly encountered. Pills or other dangerous toxins are readily eaten by inquisitive infants. Young parents may be unaware of the need to "childproof the home" until after an accident occurs.

Pulling to stand without help can cause a self-induced "nursemaid's elbow" (subluxation of the radial head). Though this entity usually occurs in the 1- to 3-year-old walking child, it can infrequently present with apparent spontaneity in the 7- to 10-month-old infant. These children are generally found after slipping down while holding a crib rail or the side of a sofa or chair.

Naturally, learning to walk implies the risk of falls and bruises. Fractures and serious head trauma are very rare, because the low falling distance precludes a large force. Any fractures occurring in this age group may be the result of child abuse, and emergency department physicians must be wary.

The 1- to 2-Year-Old Child

During this time, physical growth greatly declines as emotional and intellectual achievement take precedence (Table 2–4). Children begin to assert their own independence as they explore the world.[11] Playing with other children at home, at a day care center, or at relatives' homes is common.

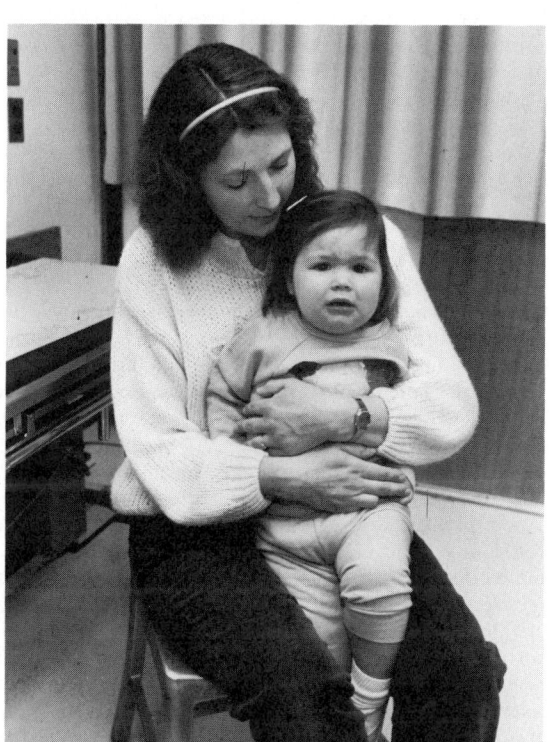

Figure 2–1. By securing the child's legs between the parent's knees, then wrapping the arms around the child, physical examination is easily performed.

TABLE 2–4	
DEVELOPMENTAL HIGHLIGHTS: THE 1- TO 2-YEAR-OLD CHILD	
Personal skills:	Imitation
Language:	Two- to three-word phrases
Fine motor skills:	Scribbles
Gross motor skills:	Walks well

Transmission of viral illnesses is prevalent, and minor traumatic events are routine.

Growth

All growth parameters diminish during the second year. A child gains only 2 to 3 kg in weight and invariably becomes a "picky" eater. This often causes undue worry for nervous parents and may require reassurance by emergency department physicians.

The child's length increases by only one half of the first year's growth. Head circumference enlarges only one sixth as much as the first year's change.

Developmental Milestones

Gross Motor Skills. Walking more steadily and quickly is a daily achievement (see Table 2–4). By the second year's end, children are usually running well, and most can jump in place. Kicking and throwing a ball are other second-year accomplishments.

Fine Motor Skills. Pincer grasp of small objects is well developed. Toddlers begin to scribble with pens or crayons. Building small towers of four to five blocks or cubes is a reasonable goal.[10]

Language. In the second 12 months, most children undergo an almost daily increase in verbal understanding and subsequent usage. The ability to point to one or two body parts is expected by 18 months. Following simple directions becomes the norm for most 2-year-olds. Though great variability exists, toddlers begin to say many different words other than "mama" or "dada."[11]

Personal/Social Skills. Imitation sums up the major advancement of the year. Toddlers watch adults around the house and repeat their actions.[11]

Physical Examination

It is best to observe the child from across or outside the room for a few moments. A child's interactions with parents and surroundings may be the best measure of the general status. Removing the child's shirt allows the examiner to gauge respiratory rate and effort in a nonthreatening manner.

The examination begins with the toddler in the parent's lap. Some children in this age group will be cooperative, but this may not always be the case, especially if the child is ill.

It is best to begin by sitting and facing the child to see if the toddler will follow an object in all directions. Giving a child a crayon and a sheet of paper to gauge activity can be informative. Older toddlers can be asked to point to particular body parts to help judge mental status.

It is important for the examiner to spend a few moments trying to befriend the child. These children may realize they are in a strange situation and may even remember past unpleasant experiences. Allowing a child to hold the stethoscope or otoscope before the examination may be enough to allay the child's fears.

Once a clear general status picture has been obtained, the child should be slowly approached with the stethoscope. Touching the scope's head to the child's arm or leg before touching the chest may decrease the likelihood for instantaneous screaming.

Auscultating both lung fields for air entry and quality of breath sounds is done first. True rales are uncommon findings in young children. It is most important to be cognizant of decreased breath sounds or wheezing. If wheezing is suspected but not audible, the examiner can lightly compress the chest or have the child cough to accentuate any wheezes.

Trying to auscultate for heart rate and cardiac sounds before the toddler cries or screams can be difficult. A normal resting heart rate rules against clinically important dehydration in the sick child. Elevated temperature and pain are other causes of tachycardia in children.

After listening for quality and quantity of bowel sounds, the examiner can use the stethoscope head to palpate the abdomen. Many toddlers become frightened and tense when a hand is placed on their abdomen. By pushing the stethoscope head into all four quadrants, a determination of tenderness, rebound, or guarding can be made.

The examination is continued with a thorough ear, nose, and throat evaluation. The comfortable "wrap-around" technique already described should be used to view the ears. If the oropharynx cannot be seen, gently pinching the nares will force the mouth to open to breathe. Two tongue blades firmly placed on the tongue's anterior tip should overcome any resistance and permit adequate inspection.

The examination can be completed on a table. The diaper should be removed and the skin checked for rashes or unusual markings. The abdomen is palpated if previous examination techniques were not conclusive. When indicated, a digital rectal examination should be performed with the index finger after the parent is informed.

Finally, the toddler is placed on the floor away from the parent. Watching the child ambulate is crucial. It may be necessary to inquire if this is the normal walking pattern. The older toddler may stand and scream. A useful ploy is to stand behind the child, which usually entices the child to walk or run to the care giver.

It is always a matter of concern when a normally walking child will not do this. Conversely, the child's general status is reaffirmed by this behavior.

Potential Medical Problems Based on Development

Ambulation leads to potential problems. Tumbles down stairs or collisions with table corners are commonplace. Again, the younger toddler does not usually fall with enough force to cause fractures. Though uncommon, the older toddler can generate small buckle wrist fractures when falling onto an outstretched hand.

One injury of note is a spiral, or "toddler's," fracture in the leg, usually the tibia. This occurs when the child has one foot firmly planted and suddenly twists. This entity needs consideration with any acute onset of a limping child.

Nursemaid's elbow is at the peak incidence in children at this age. This occurs commonly as care givers hold the toddler's hand while walking. A sudden slip of the child with a subsequent yank on the arm is a common history. The entity can also be self-induced as the toddler grabs hold of furniture while slipping and falling.

Ingestions are prevalent in this age group as toddlers begin to explore parts of the environment. Parents are unaware of the child's physical prowess and may carelessly leave small objects about the house.

The 2- to 5-Year-Old Child

The preschool years encompass the final age grouping in which the emergency department physician can use growth and developmental milestones to aid the examination. By age 6 and beyond, the vast majority of children and adolescents cooperate, and examinations can be done in the usual fashion.

Growth

In both sexes, height and weight increase at a slow linear rate. On average, preschoolers gain 2 kg and grow 6 to 8 cm each year. Head circumference growth is limited during this time, because most of the adult head size is attained in the first 2 years.

Developmental Milestones

Gross Motor Skills. The 2-year-old child should be walking and running well without falling. By age five years, jumping in place or hopping is an expected accomplishment. These attributes can be observed when evaluating a child's general status and strength. They are particularly useful in children with abdominal pain. Performing these tasks helps to exclude peritoneal irritation.

Fine Motor Skills. Preschoolers gradually improve writing and building skills with different toys.[10] Risk of object aspiration or ingestion diminishes through the years but is still a consideration.

Personal/Social Skills. During this phase, preschoolers evolve from being dependent on adults to caring for themselves. Gradually children learn to dress themselves and to manage their own toilet needs. They imitate adult behavior in performing tasks and playing with others.

Language. Substantial progress constantly occurs, thereby enabling children to interact with adults. Two- to three-word phrases are expected at 2 years. The 4- to 5-year-old should be able to carry on a small conversation and can help the examiner focus on any problems. Gradual knowledge of colors and object identification can help determine mental status in the preschooler.

Physical Examination

Depending on the child's nature, the emergency department examiner may have to alter the examination order. If the preschooler appears cooperative and relaxed, the evaluation can proceed from head to toe in a systematic fashion. Conversely, a frightened or crying child should be approached in a manner similar to the toddler. A gown should be provided to keep the child warm and protect an increasing sense of modesty.

The examiner should try to befriend the patient first. The 2- to 3-year-old may respond favorably to holding a small toy or picture. Cheerful, reassuring words can be directed to younger preschoolers while they are sitting in the parent's lap. The ability to communicate with and explain actions to the preschooler is the examiner's most valuable tool.

The older child may choose to sit alone on the examination table. The physician can sit beside the child and begin asking nonthreatening questions. Inquiries about siblings, games, cartoons, or family pets help to put the youngster at ease.

The examiner can measure how interactive the child is and respond accordingly. An ongoing, friendly conversation may clarify the problem and keep the child content. In most cases, the preschooler's communicative skills can help pinpoint the problem areas.

By knowing areas of pain or discomfort, the examiner can initially avoid them. The remainder of the necessary examination can be completed before finally returning to a "trouble" spot. This should help the preschooler tolerate the entire examination better.

The examiner should have a good idea of the child's general condition by this point. This can be continually reevaluated as the evaluation proceeds by monitoring the child's response.

The head and neck examination can initiate the assessment in the cooperative child. Inspection and palpation for rashes, bruises, or enlarged lymph nodes can be done quickly but gently. The funduscopic examination is fairly successful in children at this age. Some children will focus for the necessary interval, but others will not comply. Noting pupillary response or signs of conjunctival irritation is usually simple.

Preschoolers usually like to open their mouths widely for inspection. Some older children enjoy protruding their tongues at parents after being told "this is the only time you're allowed to do this!" This facilitates the examiner's view and retains the child's interest. Children should be encouraged to say "ehh" instead of "ahh." This allows for greater elevation of the soft palate, enabling a better view of the posterior pharynx.

Younger children may need gentle restraint to examine the ears, but this is not usually necessary as they approach school age. Communication of otalgia can aid the examiner to diagnose otitis media or other otic problems. Asymmetric erythema with otalgia may be the first clue to otitis media.

The child's shirt or gown should be removed briefly to inspect for respiratory rate or retractions. As children grow, retractions are usually noted in the suprasternal or neck region. Younger preschoolers usually demonstrate retractions in the inferior rib margins.

Listening for adventitious sounds becomes easier as children become more cooperative. The child can cough or breathe deeply to produce more audible wheezes, if they are present. Comparing both lung fields for diminished breath sounds is more accurate now in children at this age. Percussion for dullness may also be helpful.

New murmurs or abnormal heart sounds not previously heard in infancy are rare in this group. The rate and quality of the pulse are important to note, especially when dehydration is considered.

Abdominal examinations often require much patience. Tightening of the abdominal musculature occurs if the child is crying or afraid. Distracting a child during the evaluation often facilitates a more accurate assessment. This can usually be done by conversing with the child about familiar subjects.

Much of the examination can be performed with the child sitting on the parent's lap, if the child is frightened. It may be helpful to have parents stand next to the child's head to provide reassurance. Until ages 3 to 4 years, most children have a soft, protuberant abdomen because of relatively weak abdominal muscles and a concurrent lordotic lower spine.

After inspection, auscultation should proceed slowly with a warmed stethoscope. Percussion should follow to help delineate masses or excess gas. Palpation often elicits crying or fear, which results in tensing of the muscles. This can hopefully be avoided using several techniques. First, the child should bend the knees to relieve strain on the abdomen. Distracting the child with questions and friendly conversation should put the child at ease. Finally, allowing the child to place one hand over the examiner's hand may diminish the chance of fear or giggling episodes.

Both superficial and deep palpation should be performed in all four quadrants for masses, signs of tenderness, and for rebound. It is best to examine the area of concern last. When necessary, an index finger rectal examination should be explained first to both parents and child. Examination of the genitalia for rashes, discharges, or other abnormalities is usually well tolerated by preschoolers.

The entire surface of the skin should be inspected when any child presents with a rash. Even though the complaint may be referable to an isolated spot, clues about the rash's origin may be found elsewhere.

The preschool child should always be encouraged to walk across the room or around the emergency department. When abdominal pain is being evaluated, the child should jump up and down several times to exclude peritoneal irritation. The ability to ambulate or run eliminates the possibility of serious infection, dehydration, or any serious compromise. Conversely, a child too weak to ambulate normally needs urgent medical attention.

School-age Children (6 Years and Older)

Unless the school-age child has emotional or physical handicaps, examinations are usually well tolerated and less stressful to perform than in younger children. Cooperation is expected, and the capacity to understand and communicate should be anticipated from the child or adolescent.

In this age group, modesty and feelings of privacy should always be considered. Use of gowns, curtains around beds, and closed rooms all enhance the examiner's credibility with the child or teenager.

It is important to obtain all or part of the history from these patients before or during the parents' interview. The child or teenager then feels important, and potential embarrassment is minimized.

Honesty in dealing with this age group is absolutely essential. Explaining the examination and its findings in simple terms may gain the patient's trust. Many children are versed in health terms from school lessons and may understand what is being discussed. They often enjoy looking at their own radiographs.

The emergency department physician must always remember that children and adolescents are still not adults and have needs different from those of adults. Examinations may proceed more quickly and efficiently in these children because of their ability to cooperate and communicate. Attention to the patient's feelings and self-image is important.

THE CHRONICALLY ILL CHILD

A common dilemma for the emergency department physician arises when children with congenital anomalies, mental or physical handicaps, or chronic illnesses are examined. Normal growth and developmental milestones may be absent or delayed. Expected physical examination parameters may be partially or completely altered in all age groups.

Parents or regular care givers often perceive subtle changes in these children that may be unapparent to the examiner. Previous records or laboratory data may be helpful to clarify the situation. Because physical examinations in these children may be inconclusive, additional laboratory tests are often necessary to properly evaluate the child.

Comparing present vital signs, care provider observations, and laboratory data may be the only way to categorize these children. Using developmental milestones to judge the child's general condition may be of little value.

SUMMARY

Examining children of all ages can be a challenge to emergency physicians unfamiliar with the pediatric patient. A fundamental knowledge of growth and developmental milestones can aid the examiner in determining the patient's general status. The examination order may need to be changed based on the child's age and level of cooperation. Each physician should develop a set of routines in order to feel comfortable with and to be consistent in examining infants and children.

References

1. Behrman RE, Vaughn VC, Nelson WE. Nelson Textbook of Pediatrics. 13th ed. Philadelphia, WB Saunders, 1987, pp 6–35.
2. Lowery GH. Growth and Development of Children. 7th ed. Chicago, Year Book, 1978, pp 69–129.
3. Riordan J. A Practical Guide to Breastfeeding. St Louis, CV Mosby, 1983, p 356.
4. Bluestone CD, Stool SE, Scheetz MD. Pediatric Otolaryngology. 2nd ed. Philadelphia, WB Saunders, 1990, pp 119–120.
5. Sjogren H. The lacrimal secretion in newborn, premature and fully developed children. Acta Ophthalmol 1955;33:557.
6. Barness LA. Manual of Pediatric Physical Diagnosis. 5th ed. Chicago, Year Book, 1981, p 221.
7. McKiernan JF, Hull D. Breast development in the newborn. Arch Dis Child 1982;56:525.
8. Green M. Pediatric Diagnosis. 4th ed. Philadelphia, WB Saunders, 1986, p 99.
9. Report of the Task Force on Circumcision. Pediatrics 1989;84:388.
10. Frankenburg WK, Dodds JB. Denver Developmental Screening Test. Denver, University of Colorado Medical Center, 1969.
11. Caplan F, Caplan T. The Second Twelve Months of Life. 5th ed. New York, Putnam Publishing, 1982, pp 238–239.

CHAPTER 3

Emergency Medical Systems

Jon R. Krohmer
Robert A. Swor

INTRODUCTION

The development of emergency medical services (EMS) systems during the past 20 years has made significant improvements in the quality of care afforded patients prior to arrival at a hospital. This improved care has resulted in decreased morbidity and mortality from injuries and illnesses. In the past, pediatric patients were perceived as "little adults" and were treated accordingly. With the growth of pediatric emergency medicine and other pediatric subspecialties, that premise has been proven false. EMS medical directors and administrators, working with pediatric specialists, are realizing the unique issues involved in caring for pediatric patients in the prehospital environment.

EMS SYSTEMS HISTORY

The field stabilization and delivery of a critically ill or injured patient to a hospital is a critical factor in determining that patient's outcome. Physicians in the Napoleonic wars and the Crimean conflict first noted the need to render care on the battlefield during the conflict and that such care could improve the fate of injured soldiers. Sir Hugh Owen-Thomas observed a dramatic improvement in survival from closed femur fractures after splint immobilization. This concept and that of the importance of rapid evacuation evolved dramatically during wartime. A clear relationship was established between the evacuation time and the soldier's survival from traumatic injuries. The utilization of helicopter evacuation in the Korean and Vietnam wars reaffirmed this critical relationship.[1, 2]

The application of these principles of emergency care to the civilian community was a gradual one. Prior to the development of sophisticated EMS systems in the late 1960s and early 1970s, emergency transport of patients to the hospital was performed by funeral directors, because they were the only ones who were able to transport a supine patient. This inherent conflict of interest, the obvious lack of quality medical care, and the concurrent development of emergency medicine as a specialty led to the development of EMS systems.

THE EMS SYSTEM

An EMS system is "an organized system, capable of providing a comprehensive and timely response to an individual's or community's medical emergencies."[3] The original purpose of EMS systems was to treat sudden cardiac death, the leading cause of death in the United States.[4] The development of portable defibrillators and early work by Pantridge in Northern Ireland demonstrated that definitive care for many cardiac patients could be provided at the scene of the emergency. This definitive care, known as *advanced life support (ALS)*, included advanced airway management, defibrillation, and administration of intravenous (IV) fluids and emergency medications. Early projects in the United States demonstrated that a physician surrogate, an emergency medical technician-paramedic (EMT-P, or paramedic), could perform all of these ALS functions. Provision of cardiopulmonary resuscitation (CPR) by basic emergency medical technicians (EMT-As) who had minimal training was also recognized as important. These measures have been proven to save lives, and EMS has become an accepted (and important) component of emergency care.[5–7] Most urban and suburban areas now have ALS service for emergency care. Six phases of care of the pediatric patient have been identified (Table 3–1).[8, 9]

Prevention of injuries is the best method of treatment.[10] Preventive measures include seat belt and child restraint laws, drunk driving laws, flame-retardant clothing, child-resistant containers, and home child-proofing campaigns. Pediatricians, family physicians, and emergency physicians have important roles in educating the public regarding prevention techniques. These physicians are also important in teaching the public about injury and illness recognition. According to Seidel, "early recognition of the pre-arrest state is necessary for the prevention of a catastrophic event."[11] It is estimated that early and appropriate identification of an event could decrease mortality by 42%.[12] Parents and other child care providers are the most immediate bystanders and must be trained in the recognition of an emergency. They must also be trained in how and when to

access appropriate care for the child. That appropriate care may involve going to a pediatrician or family physician or requesting an ambulance.[13] The public must accept the important concept of a universal telephone number (e.g., 911) to access emergency services, including the EMS system. Subsequent education of family members, other care givers, and teachers regarding the appropriate use of EMS must then occur to ensure proper utilization. Critical time may be spent trying to contact a personal physician by telephone for instructions. Likewise, many people request EMS assistance inappropriately, removing valuable resources from availability as a result of unnecessary calls. One study addressing the use of EMS resources for pediatric patients demonstrated a 58% incidence of inappropriate EMS use, with 49% of those judged to need EMS not using it.[14] Finally, pediatricians and family physicians must be prepared to give appropriate urgent aid to their patients if needed and should be aware of the appropriate local emergency care and hospital resources.[13]

Once the initial request for EMS assistance is received, it is the responsibility of the EMS system to ensure that proper resources are dispatched (i.e., individuals who have received proper training and have the necessary equipment to care for the ill or injured child). All prehospital care is considered an extension of emergency department care and as such must operate under the direct supervision of a physician. This is referred to as *medical control*. Most medical control physicians are emergency department–based physicians, as they are most knowledgeable about emergency care in general and prehospital care specifically. As more emphasis is placed on care of the pediatric patient, pediatric emergency physicians (pediatricians with specialized training in emergency medicine or emergency physicians with specialized training in pediatrics) are becoming more common. These physicians, where available, provide an excellent resource for EMS systems. In areas where pediatric emergency physicians are unavailable, other pediatric specialists can be of great assistance to EMS physicians.

Medical control activities can be defined as *off-line* and *on-line* functions. Off-line activities include the development of all protocols, policies, and procedures under which prehospital care providers operate. These include defining, by protocol, the care to be given children in specific situations. It also defines such things as communications issues (the local 911 system, dispatch, and hospital communications), triage decisions, transportation destination decisions (based on available hospital resources), and appropriate equipment use. Off-line considerations also involve prehospital provider education (initial and continuing education) and quality assurance programs. On-line medical control activities involve direct communication (either person-to-person, by radio, or by telephone) between the prehospital care giver and the physician, typically an emergency physician. That physician must have access to specialty consultants such as pediatricians when needed.

PREHOSPITAL PROVIDERS

The major components of any EMS system are the providers of emergency care in the field. Training guidelines have been developed by the United States Department of Transportation (DOT)[15] and have been adopted by most states. There are several levels of prehospital providers who are available to help care for the pediatric patient, with each able to provide increasing levels of care.

Emergency Medical Dispatchers

Emergency medical dispatchers (EMDs) receive approximately 25 hours of training in dispatch techniques to ensure

---

TABLE 3–1

PHASES OF PEDIATRIC EMERGENCY CARE

Prevention and public education
Identification and access to care
Field treatment, triage, and transport
Emergency department care
Inpatient definitive care
Rehabilitation

that the most appropriate prehospital resources are sent to the scene of the emergency. EMDs are also trained to provide care instructions over the telephone such that the caller can begin first aid (e.g., bleeding control, CPR) for the victim before anyone else arrives.

First Responders

First responders, typically police officers and fire fighters, receive approximately 40 to 60 hours of instruction in initial patient assessment and emergency care. The first responder's goal is to immediately recognize life-threatening problems and stabilize the patient, hopefully preventing any further deterioration in the patient's condition until additional care is available.

Basic Emergency Medical Technicians

Basic emergency medical technicians (EMT-As) receive approximately 150 hours of didactic and practical training. They have a better understanding of anatomy, physiology, and pathophysiology than do first responders, allowing for additional assessment and treatment skills. They have the resources and knowledge to provide better airway management, injury stabilization (splinting and bandaging), extrication, immobilization, and transportation. EMT-As do not provide any ALS care.

Intermediate Emergency Medical Technicians

Intermediate EMTs (EMT-Is) have additional training (from 25 to 100 hours) to allow them to provide some level of ALS. That level, however, varies greatly from state to state. Typically, EMT-Is are able to intubate patients and begin intravenous therapy. In some states, they can monitor and defibrillate cardiac patients and deliver limited types of medications.

Paramedics

Paramedics (EMT-Ps) are sometimes referred to as advanced EMTs (Adv EMT-As). These are the most highly trained prehospital providers, undergoing 750 to 2000 hours of training. The didactic training further elaborates medical and traumatic emergencies, cardiac rhythm interpretation, and pharmacology. Paramedics provide advanced airway management (intubation, cricothyrotomy), IV therapy, medication therapy, and cardiac monitoring and defibrillation or cardioversion.

Finally, prehospital care capability has risen in recent years with the development of semi-automatic and automatic defibrillators. These devices automatically analyze the rhythm of a patient in cardiac arrest. If it is a rhythm warranting defibrillation (e.g., ventricular fibrillation or ventricular tachycardia), the machine will charge to a predefined energy level and either automatically deliver the shock (in automatic units) or prompt the operator to push the "shock" button (in semi-automatic units). Because of the shock energy levels defined with these units, these instruments are not indicated in patients younger than 12 years.

PEDIATRIC PREHOSPITAL CARE

For a long time, pediatric patients were regarded as "little adults." This philosophy was applied to emergency care in the prehospital setting. Also, the initial focus of EMS care was to deliver definitive emergency cardiac care at the scene of an emergency. Because pediatric emergency problems are typically not cardiac in origin, pediatric care has traditionally been a neglected portion of an EMS system. Recent emphasis has focused on the special needs of children, their response to stress and medications, and the long-term problems resulting from improper care.[16]

Demographics

The paucity of pediatric cases in EMS systems also diminished interest in pediatric EMS care and made it difficult for EMS providers to maintain what limited knowledge and skills base they had acquired. It is estimated that pediatric patients comprise a small percentage (5% to 10%) of most systems' run volume.[3, 17–19] In contrast to adult emergency care, transport of a critically ill child is easily accomplished by private vehicle, which decreases the system's exposure to the ill child. The number of pediatric patients requiring critical care is similarly low (1.5% to 5%).[20] This lack of significant volume has been an impediment to the development of emergency care strategies in children. However, approximately 30% of the population is younger than 19 years,[21] and up to 30% of visits to large emergency departments are for pediatric patients.[19] This pediatric volume seems to be almost equally divided between medical and traumatic problems,[22] with medical causes occurring primarily in the younger patients and trauma (i.e., motor vehicle accidents) in older children, primarily adolescents.[17–19] With proper public education regarding the appropriate use of EMS resources, the EMS system's pediatric call volume should increase.

Trauma Resuscitation

Preventable injuries and illnesses are the primary cause of morbidity and mortality in children, trauma being the leading cause.[23] Trauma is more commonly fatal than all other causes (e.g., cancer, congenital disease, cardiac disease, and pneumonia) combined.[3, 8, 10, 16] Major causes of accidental death in children include motor vehicle accidents, drowning, fires and burns, poisoning, suffocation, and use of firearms.[24] Accidents requiring medical attention account for more than 21 million injuries to children annually.[10] One fourth of those who die in accidents are children, numbering approximately 25,000 annually.[3, 10] One study indicated that the majority of pediatric trauma deaths (70%) occurred in areas without pediatric tertiary care centers.[11, 19] The importance of proper treatment of pediatric injuries is clear; when properly treated, children recover from traumatic injuries better than do adults.[16]

Cardiopulmonary Resuscitation

Initial studies on pediatric sudden death demonstrated a dismal response to resuscitation in children.[25–27] Events that compromise a child's cardiac status are usually respiratory, commonly resulting in bradycardia and asystole.[11] These respiratory problems include infection, foreign body aspiration, trauma, and toxic ingestion.[11, 28] Approximately 1% of all pediatric EMS calls (0.1% of all EMS calls) in one system were for cardiac arrest.[17, 18] Most pediatric patients in cardiac arrest are found in asystole at the time of EMS arrival. Epidemiologic studies have found that the overall survival rate for pediatric nontraumatic cardiac arrests is 7%; for witnessed arrests, 15%; and for unwitnessed arrests, 3%.[11, 27] In a Milwaukee study, the only cardiac arrests that were successfully resuscitated were those that were witnessed by paramedics.[25]

EMS SYSTEM REVISION

Intense interest in pediatric EMS has been rekindled by federal initiatives. Demonstration projects addressing var-

TABLE 3–2

PREHOSPITAL TRAINING PROGRAMS: PEDIATRIC TOPICS

Topics Covered	Topics Not Covered
Epiglottitis	Dysrhythmias
Croup	Field simulations
Respiratory distress	Envenomation
Asthma	Hypotension
Seizures	Approach to coma
Ingestions/poisonings	Drowning
Child abuse/neglect	Sexual abuse
	ALS procedures
	Diarrhea/dehydration
	Neonatal resuscitation
	Trauma

ALS = Advanced Life Support.

TABLE 3–4

PALS COURSE OUTLINE

Lectures	Skills Stations
Respiratory failure	BLS and BVM ventilation
Shock	Advanced airway management
Cardiopulmonary arrest	Vascular access, fluids, and
Infant and child integration	medications
sessions	Rhythm disturbances
Neonatal resuscitation	Newborn resuscitation
Postresuscitation stabilization	Respiratory failure
and transport	Shock
	Cardiopulmonary arrest

PALS = Pediatric Advanced Life Support.

ious aspects of pediatric prehospital care have been funded by federal grants from the Department of Health and Human Services to many states. These projects have better defined the epidemiology of pediatric emergency care and the types of problems encountered. In particular, pediatric trauma care has evolved as a major priority for EMS systems.[17] For this reason, the initial focus has been on systems of care, similar to the trauma center concept, allowing delivery of a critically injured or ill child to a facility that is able to provide definitive care. These receiving facilities have traditionally been in university-based tertiary care hospitals. Ramenofsky and Morse have demonstrated in one series that a large percentage (53%) of traumatized children would be potentially salvageable if an ideal system using pediatric specialty centers were in place.[16]

TRAINING

The focus of all training programs is the emergency care of the ill and injured adult. Limited information is provided about pediatric care. The U.S. Department of Transportation requires only 6 hours of coursework on pediatric and neonatal care for paramedics.[10, 15] However, in one study of paramedic training programs, 21% had no clinical pediatric training, and 41% had less than 10 hours of total pediatric training (5% had none). Of those paramedic programs surveyed, 22% provided no formal training in pediatric ALS (Table 3–2).[29]

As a result of the work initiated by the federally supported grant programs, much has been done to improve training for prehospital providers in pediatric care. Children's Hos-

pital National Medical Center developed an 18-hour, 3-day series of lectures and skill stations addressing medical emergencies, the care of the injured child, and the special needs of infants (Table 3–3). Special training sessions for course instructors were conducted. This allowed the instructors to take the program back to their areas of the country.[10] Subsequently, 16 states have developed pediatric training courses. All of these courses address pediatric assessment, cardiovascular and respiratory emergencies, trauma, and newborn care. Most are oriented to ALS activities.[30] Additionally, the American Heart Association has developed the 2-day Pediatric Advanced Life Support course (PALS) (Table 3–4),[31] and the American Academy of Pediatrics and the American College of Emergency Physicians have jointly developed the 2-day Advanced Pediatric Life Support course (APLS) (Table 3–5).[32] Training programs currently in existence are also incorporating additional training addressing pediatric care. For example, Basic Trauma Life Support (BTLS) of Michigan has added special components of pediatric airway management and immobilization to both the advanced and basic training programs.[33, 34] The United States Department of Transportation is currently reviewing its training guidelines, hoping to place more emphasis on the pediatric patient. The development of all of these training components is encouraging, but the task of training the large number of prehospital providers currently in practice remains.

PREHOSPITAL CARE PROTOCOLS AND PROCEDURES

Literature that documents a positive effect of any prehospital procedures on patient outcome is limited. Development

TABLE 3–3

CHILDREN'S HOSPITAL NATIONAL MEDICAL CENTER COURSE CONTENT

Emotional needs of the child and family
Pediatric assessment
Medical emergencies
Neurologic emergencies
Respiratory emergencies
Airway management
Cardiopulmonary resuscitation
Trauma assessment and management
Burn management
Child abuse
Sudden infant death syndrome
Newborn assessment

TABLE 3–5

APLS COURSE OUTLINE

Lectures	Skills Stations
Recognition of respiratory failure	Trauma/animal and neonatal laboratory
Cardiopulmonary arrest	Neonatal emergencies
Cardiac dysfunction	Shock and vascular access
Multiple trauma	Respiratory cases
Severe head trauma	Altered level of consciousness
Seizures	Multiple trauma
Medical emergencies	Environmental emergencies
	Megacode
	Radiology laboratory
	Child abuse

APLS = Advanced Pediatric Life Support.

of EMT training in pediatrics has been slow, with little emphasis placed on care at the scene. Harris has stated, however, that 40% of children who die in the prehospital setting require intervention to open the airway and control hemorrhage.[35] In a review of Fresno County, California, Tsai and Kallsen found that 38% of medical patients received ALS interventions.[17] Many systems' protocols call for only basic airway management and rapid transport to an emergency department. Nevertheless, it is becoming clear that paramedics can perform pediatric ALS procedures in a rapid, appropriate fashion.

Basic EMT Skills

Protection of the cervical spine and opening of an airway are two critically important skills in emergency care. As has been shown, a major cause of death in children is upper airway compromise. Simple measures such as the chin-lift and jaw-thrust maneuvers may be lifesaving and can be performed by a rescuer with minimal training.

Despite the rarity of cervical spine injuries in children, the morbidity associated with an unrecognized injury makes appropriate care of an injured child at the scene mandatory. The literature indicates that the proper procedure for immobilization of a child is different from that of an adult. Standard collar and board immobilization may force the child's head and neck into kyphotic flexion, which is precisely the wrong position for a patient with an unstable injury.[36] Proper immobilization of children in vehicle restraint devices must also be emphasized.

Paramedic Skills

Standard ALS procedures include provision of airway support through endotracheal intubation, defibrillation, IV fluid administration, and resuscitative drug administration. The initial rationale for training paramedics to perform these procedures was to resuscitate adults from cardiac arrest. For these reasons, provision of these techniques and procedures for children has not been uniformly applied and has not been shown to be beneficial. The most commonly used procedures in one study were oxygen administration, intravenous line placement, and electrocardiographic (EKG) monitoring. Procedures not performed included needle cricothyroidotomy, needle thoracostomy, cardioversion, defibrillation, and esophageal obturator airway placement.[17]

Intravenous fluid administration is technically more difficult in children, and its value is uncertain in an urban environment. Different studies indicate variable success rates in intravenous line placement in children, with dramatic decreases in success in preschoolers and infants. Tsai and Kallsen documented unsuccessful vascular access in all children younger than 6 years who were in cardiac arrest; intravenous lines were placed successfully in only 30% of non–cardiac arrest patients younger than 1 year.[17] A Milwaukee study demonstrated a low (19%) rate for successful intravenous lines in CPR in children who were younger than 18 months old.[37]

Intraosseous (IO) infusion has recently regained favor in emergency care. It offers a rapid, reliable means of infusing fluids and drugs. The technique is simple, and some authors have demonstrated that it can be easily taught to paramedical personnel.[38] One preliminary study in Utah documented successful placement of an IO line in 10 of 12 patients. All were placed in children younger than 5 years.[39] In a national survey, however, fewer than half of the states indicated current use of IO lines, with an additional third not planning to initiate training in the technique.[40] Serious consideration

needs to be given by ALS systems to the use of this valuable procedure.

Umbilical vein catheterization has also been advocated for use in the prehospital setting, although no data have been published to support its use. Fortunately, the need for resuscitation of neonates appears to occur infrequently in the field.

Alternative methods for medication administration should be emphasized for the pediatric patient. The endotracheal route can be used for several medications (naloxone, atropine, diazepam, epinephrine, and lidocaine). The rectal route of administration of diazepam has been investigated.[41] Also, several anticonvulsants (phenobarbital, lorazepam, midazolam) may be administered intramuscularly.

Many systems allow paramedics to perform endotracheal intubation, but data supporting this approach are limited.[17] Aijian et al. reviewed pediatric intubation in their system, but the number of cases was small (28).[42] Success rates were low in the neonatal and toddler age groups. Other systems have reported their experience, with low rates of intubation documented (4% of all pediatric calls in Milwaukee).[37] The overall success rate for all pediatric patients requiring intubation was 78%, with a 93% rate for those patients in cardiac arrest.[43]

Cricothyroidotomy and percutaneous jet ventilation are taught as part of the paramedic curriculum, although they are rarely performed in the field. Advanced trauma life support guidelines advocate the use of needle cricothyrotomy in patients younger than 12 years old.[44]

EQUIPMENT

Most of the prehospital equipment in use has been developed for adult patients and then used directly or modified for children. There are no studies looking at the effectiveness or usefulness of the equipment, with the exception of the study of spinal immobilization described earlier.[36] Additionally, many EMS systems do not even supply equipment in a size appropriate for pediatric patients. Michigan currently does not mandate that ambulances carry pediatric or infant bag-valve-mask devices, equipment that is imperative to support the resuscitation of an apneic child. Seidel found the most common equipment not carried on ambulances included backboards, correctly sized oxygen masks, appropriate cervical collars, properly sized blood pressure cuffs, pediatric-strength atropine and bicarbonate solutions, and small-gauge IV catheters.[11] A subcommittee of the Prehospital Care Committee of the American Academy of Pediatrics has looked at the indications and use of prehospital equipment, including endotracheal intubation, the pneumatic antishock garment (PASG), IO devices, and immobilization devices. The committee concluded that more information is needed before an educated decision can be made regarding appropriate equipment use in pediatric patients.[45] Equipment should be analyzed for ease of application, success rate, time efficiency, and effectiveness.[45] Until this issue is resolved, a certain amount of appropriate equipment should be available to treat pediatric patients (Table 3–6).[19, 28, 45]

RECEIVING FACILITIES

As emergency medicine, specifically pediatric emergency medicine, has grown, it has been suggested that pediatric emergency care is inadequate nationwide. It has been recommended that systems should be designed to deliver pediatric patients to specialty institutions with the resources to adequately care for them. This mimics the "systems" approach that has been followed for other medical problems (e.g., trauma, burns, high-risk obstetric patients). This would

---

TABLE 3–6

SUGGESTED PEDIATRIC EQUIPMENT LIST

Airway: Suction catheters (No. 6.5, No. 8 French)
      Oral airways
      Laryngoscope blades and endotracheal tubes
Ventilation: Face mask (newborn, infant, child)
      Bag-valve-mask with pop-off valve
      Oxygen mask (infant, child)
Spinal Immobilization: Short backboard
      Cervical collars
      Towel rolls
Circulation: Cardiac monitor (with pediatric paddles)
      Blood pressure cuff (infant, child)
      IV catheter (22- and 24-gauge)
Miscellaneous: Short and long arm boards
      Obstetrics kit
Medications: Special considerations
      Dextrose 25% solution
      Bicarbonate 4.2% solution

---

require that some hospitals be bypassed by ambulances and would further assume that the patient could receive adequate care in an ambulance en route to the specialty institution.

The development of emergency medicine as a specialty and of pediatric emergentology fellowships has improved the quality of care children receive in many emergency departments, as specialty training provides both inpatient and outpatient pediatric training. Many other institutions, however, lack appropriate inpatient support services (personnel and equipment) to care properly for seriously ill or injured children.[8, 16, 46]

The state of California has established guidelines for emergency departments approved for pediatrics (EDAPs) and pediatric critical care centers (PCCCs). Following identification of those resources, prehospital destination protocols identified those patients who should be transferred to certain institutions.[11] The American College of Surgeons has also published guidelines for the "Adult Trauma Center with Pediatric Commitment" and the "Pediatric Trauma Regional Resource Center."[47]

Transport systems have developed because pediatric critical care is not a resource readily available in most hospitals. Both ground and aeromedical systems have become active in the transfer of critically ill and injured patients. These are poorly integrated into most EMS systems but serve to supplement those systems. For the process to work efficiently, transfer agreements must be prospectively established between primary care institutions and the tertiary referral centers.

CONCLUSIONS

The growth and development of EMS in the past 25 years has done much to improve the quality of care and decrease morbidity and mortality of ill and injured persons. Much of the emphasis, however, has been on the adult patient. It is now time in the evolution of EMS to place greater emphasis on the pediatric patient. EMS planners, administrators, and physicians have been addressing patient care and training issues. These activities must continue, along with a closer look at appropriate equipment and its use, as well as the resources available at receiving institutions.

References

1. Stewart RD. Historical perspective. *In* Roush WR (ed). Principles of EMS Systems; A Comprehensive Text for Physicians. Dallas, TX, American College of Emergency Physicians, 1989, pp 5–8.

2. Stewart RD. Historical overview. *In* Kuehl AE (ed). EMS Medical Directors' Handbook, National Association of EMS Physicians. St Louis, CV Mosby, 1989, pp 3–6.

3. Barkin RM. The system and training. Pediatr Emerg Care 1990;6:72.

4. Advanced Cardiac Life Support in Perspective. *In* McIntyre KM, Lewis AJ (eds). Textbook of Advanced Cardiac Life Support. Dallas, TX, American Heart Association, 1987, pp 1–9.

5. Eisenberg MS. Paramedic programs and out-of-hospital cardiac arrest: I. Factors associated with successful resuscitation. Am J Public Health 1979;69:30.

6. Eisenberg MS. Paramedic programs and out-of-hospital cardiac arrest: Impact on community mortality. Am J Public Health 1979;69:39.

7. Eisenberg MS. Out-of-hospital cardiac arrest: Improved survival with paramedic services. Lancet 1980;1:812.

8. Luten RC. The child in the emergency medical services system. ACEP News 1989;9:8.

9. Ramenofsky ML. How can we address the differences in trauma versus illness systems? *In* Emergency Medical Services for Children: Report of the 97th Ross Conference on Pediatric Research. Columbus, OH, Ross Laboratories, 1989, p 51.

10. Eichelberger MR, Stossel-Pratsch G, Mangubat EA. A pediatric emergencies training program for emergency medical services. Pediatr Emerg Care 1985;1:177.

11. Seidel JS. A needs assessment of advanced life support and emergency medical services in the pediatric patient: State of the art. Circulation 1986;74(IV):129.

12. Ramenofsky ML, Luterman A, Quindlen E, et al. Maximum survival in pediatric trauma: The ideal system. J Trauma 1984;24:818.

13. Ludwig S. The parent and the primary care provider in EMS-C. Pediatr Emerg Care 1990;6:77.

14. Santer L, Yamashita T, Krug S. Inappropriate use and unmet need in emergency medical services for children. Pediatr Emerg Care 1990;6:232. Abstract.

15. Department of Transportation Training Guidelines. EMS 1990;19:214.

16. Ramenofsky ML, Morse TS. Standards of care for the critically injured pediatric patient. J Trauma 1982;22:921.

17. Tsai A, Kallsen G. Epidemiology of pediatric prehospital care. Ann Emerg Med 1987;16:284.

18. Applebaum D. Advanced prehospital care for pediatric emergencies. Ann Emerg Med 1985;14:656.

19. Seidel JS, Hornbein M, Yoshiyama K, et al. Emergency medical services and the pediatric patient: Are the needs being met? Pediatrics 1984;73:769.

20. Simon JE. Current problems in the emergency management of severe pediatric illness. *In* Emergency Medical Services for Children: Report of the 97th Ross Conference on Pediatric Research. Columbus, OH, Ross Laboratories, 1989, p 10.

21. Johnston C, King WD. Pediatric prehospital care in a southern regional emergency medical service system. South Med J 1988;81:1473.

22. Luten RC (ed). Access to optimal care for children in the EMS system. *In* Pediatric Resources for Prehospital Care. Pittsburgh, PA, NAEMSP and AAP, 1990, p 2.

23. Holmes JM, Reyes HM: A critical review of urban pediatric trauma. J Trauma 1984;24:253.

24. Matlak ME. Current problems in the management of pediatric trauma. *In* Emergency Medical Services for Children: Report of the 97th Ross Conference on Pediatric Research. Columbus, OH, Ross Laboratories, 1989, p 2.

25. Torphy DE, Minter MG, Thompson BM. Cardiopulmonary arrest and resuscitation in children. Am J Dis Child 1984;138:1099.

26. Ludwig S, Kettrick RG, Parker M. Pediatric cardiopulmonary resuscitation. Clin Pediatr 1984;23:71.

27. Eisenberg M, Bergner L, Hallstrom A. Epidemiology of cardiac arrest and resuscitation in children. Ann Emerg Med 1983;12:672.

28. Foltin G, Salomon M, Tunik M, et al. Developing prehospital advanced life support for children: The New York City experience. Pediatr Emerg Care 1990;6:141.

29. Seidel JS. Emergency medical services and the pediatric patient: Are the needs being met? II. Training and equipping emergency medical services providers for pediatric emergencies. Pediatrics 1986;78:808.

30. Luten RC (ed). Educational courses for prehospital care. *In* Pediatric Resources for Prehospital Care. Pittsburgh, PA, NAEMSP and AAP, 1990, p 25.

31. Chameides L (ed). Textbook of Pediatric Advanced Life Support. Dallas, TX, American Heart Association/American Academy of Pediatrics, 1989.

32. Silverman BK (ed). Advanced Pediatric Life Support Textbook. Dallas, TX, American Academy of Pediatrics/American College of Emergency Physicians, 1989.

33. Instructor's Manual BTLS-A. Grand Rapids, MI, Michigan Chapter BTLS-A, 1990.

34. Instructor's Manual BTLS-B. Grand Rapids, MI, Michigan Chapter BTLS-B, 1990.

35. Harris BH. Creating pediatric trauma systems. J Pediatr Surg 1989;24:149.

36. Herzenberg JE, Hensinger RN, Dedrick DK. Emergency transport and

positioning of young children who have an injury of the cervical spine. J Bone Joint Surg 1989;71A:15.

37. Losek JD, Hennes H, Glaeser P, et al. Prehospital care of the pulseless, nonbreathing pediatric patient. Am J Emerg Med 1987;7:370.
38. Seigler RS, Tecklenburg FW, Shealy R. Prehospital intraosseous infusion by emergency medical services personnel: A prospective study. Pediatrics 1989;84:173.
39. Miner WF, Corneli HM, Bolte RG, et al. Prehospital use of intraosseous infusion by paramedics. Pediatr Emerg Care 1989;5:5.
40. Salassi-Scotter M, Fiser DH. Adoption of intraosseous infusion technique for prehospital pediatric emergency care. Pediatr Emerg Med 1990;6:263.
41. Albano A, Reisdorff EJ, Wiegenstein JG. Rectal diazepam in pediatric status epilepticus. Am J Emerg Med 1989;7:168.
42. Aijian P, Tsai A, Knopp R, et al. Endotracheal intubation of pediatric patients by paramedics. Ann Emerg Med 1988;17:424. Abstract.
43. Losek JD, Bonadio WA, Walsh-Kelly C, et al. Prehospital pediatric endotracheal intubation performance review. Pediatr Emerg Care 1989;5:1.
44. Committee on Trauma. Airway management and ventilation. *In* Advanced Trauma Life Support Instructor Manual. Chicago, IL, American College of Surgeons, 1988, p 37.
45. Luten RC (ed). Equipment. *In* Pediatric Resources for Prehospital Care. Pittsburgh, PA, NAEMSP and AAP, 1990, p 41.
46. Haller JA. Toward a comprehensive emergency medical system for children. Pediatrics 1990;86:120.
47. Committee on Trauma. Planning pediatric trauma care. *In* Resources for Optimal Care of the Injured Patient. Chicago, IL, American College of Surgeons, 1988, p 51.

CHAPTER 4

Neonatal Resuscitation

Stephen O. Bernardon

INTRODUCTION

The emergency physician must be able to manage a variety of problems. Stabilizing a newborn child is one of the most stressful and difficult tasks faced in the emergency department. Birth asphyxia is the most common cause of neonatal morbidity and mortality; consequently, prevention will lead to a successful outcome.

Emergency department exposure to newborns is common. There are 3.8 million infants born every year in the United States.[1] Of these, 35,000 are not born in a hospital setting.[2] Of the 5700 hospitals that have obstetric services, only 5% have neonatal care units capable of handling an intubated newborn.[1] Another 1000 hospitals do not have any obstetric services. Of all infants born in the United States, 4% die at less than 24 hours of age.[3] Of the 1.2% of infants that weigh less than 1500 grams (3 pounds, 5 ounces), 80% require resuscitation.[4] In addition, 3.2% of all births will have Apgar scores less than or equal to 5 (10 being the maximum score), thus requiring resuscitation. Consequently, an emergency physician must have an organized, clear approach to neonatal resuscitation to prevent the most common problem, birth asphyxia.

ANATOMY AND NEWBORN PHYSIOLOGY

Drastic physiologic changes occur in the newborn. Infants must adapt to an environment in which they must rely on themselves for oxygenation and nutrition. The lungs and heart undergo the most significant of changes. The lungs develop in the latter part of pregnancy. In the 24th week of gestation, terminal airways develop; alveoli form between 30 and 32 weeks of gestation.[5] Surfactant, which is a key in reducing the surface tension in the respiratory tree and permitting subsequent airway patency, is initially produced between the 23rd and 24th week of gestation. It is not until the 28th week, and maximally the 34th week, that enough surfactant is present to maintain airway expansion. Thus a reduced quantity of surfactant will impede normal ventilation and oxygenation.

The fetal lungs contain a considerable amount of fluid before delivery. In the birth canal, the infant's chest is compressed with 30 to 250 cm of water pressure, resulting in 7 to 42 ml of fluid exiting the lung.[6] The neonate must exert a negative 40 to 80 cm of water pressure to expand its lungs.[7] This initial breath is stimulated by mild hypoxia and acidosis (asphyxia), cord occlusion, a cold environment, and tactile stimulation. However, severe acidosis, hypoxia, and moderate hypothermia depress this effort. Maternal and fetal factors also play a role in this initiation of ventilation (Table 4–1).

If the stimulus to breathe is blunted for any reason, asphyxia occurs, with a specific physiologic response (Fig. 4–1).[5–11] The respiratory rate increases in depth and frequency for up to 3 minutes of complete asphyxia. This is followed by *primary apnea*, which lasts approximately 1 to 2 minutes. During this time, thrashing movements of the extremities and sinus tachycardia occur. By the end of primary apnea, the pulse decreases to about 100 beats/min. If appropriate sensory stimuli occur, spontaneous respirations can still be induced. If asphyxia progresses, rhythmic gasping begins and is maintained for several minutes. During this time, the infant loses muscle tone; becomes pale, mottled, and cyanotic; and the heart rate falls below 100 beats/min. At the cessation of respirations, *secondary apnea* begins. At this point sensory stimuli cannot induce spontaneous respiration. For every minute that artificial ventilation is delayed after the last gasp, 2 more minutes are required before gasping is reestablished and another 2 to 4 minutes until the onset of spontaneous respiration. A progressively greater degree of brain damage occurs with correspondingly longer periods of asphyxia. Primary and secondary apnea are hard to distinguish at birth. Therefore secondary apnea should always be assumed and the resuscitation approached accordingly.

Once rhythmic respirations are present, residual lung fluid is resorbed. The respiratory rate can range from 60 to 90 breaths/min during the first few hours of life. Then a respiratory rate of 30 to 40 breaths/min with a tidal volume of 15 to 20 ml (6 to 8 ml/kg) is normal.[7]

The circulatory system begins development in the third week of gestation. By the third trimester, blood travels primarily from the fetal body/placenta to the right atrium and into the left atrium through the foramen ovale. Blood from the right ventricle traverses primarily into the aorta through the ductus arteriosus. Because of high resistance in the pulmonary vascular bed, there is a right-to-left shunt (Fig. 4–2).

At birth, changes in vascular resistance are the key to developing a normal adult circulation, as the initial right ventricular and left ventricular pressures are about equal. Two main events initiate this conversion. First, clamping of the umbilical cord increases peripheral vascular resistance and aortic pressure, with a subsequent decrease in the venous return and right atrial pressure. With lung expansion, oxygen tension (Po_2) rises, and carbon dioxide pressure (Pco_2) falls. These two events further stimulate pulmonary vasodi-

TABLE 4–1

FACTORS CONTRIBUTING TO ASPHYXIA

I. Maternal factors
  A. Decreased placental blood flow
    1. Hypertension/toxemia
    2. Renal failure
  B. Intrauterine
    1. Multiple gestation
    2. Malpresentation
    3. Prematurity/postmaturity
    4. Oligohydramnios
    5. Polyhydramnios
  C. CNS depressants
    1. Alcohol
    2. Illegal drugs
    3. Magnesium
  D. Inadeqate gas exchange at placenta
    1. Decreased effective oxygen-carrying capacity
      a. Anemia
      b. Isoimmunization
    2. Maternal hypotension
      a. Hypovolemia
        (1) Dehydration
        (2) Acute hemorrhage
        (3) Placenta previa/abruption
      b. Normovolemia
        (1) Pressure of the uterus on the vena cava
        (2) Maternal hyperventilation
        (3) Spinal/epidural anesthesia
    3. Abnormal uterine contractions
  E. Cord problems
    1. Compression
      a. Compression by presenting part
      b. Prolapsed cord
    2. Thrombosis/hematoma
    3. Rupture/vasa previa
II. Fetal factors
  A. Inadequate fetal circulation
    1. Septic shock
    2. Hypovolemic shock
      a. Fetal-maternal hemorrhage
      b. Twin-twin transfusion
      c. Maldistribution of blood between infant and maternal side of the placenta
    3. Drug-induced (transplacental passage of anesthesia)
    4. Severe congenital heart disease
  B. CNS unresponsiveness to normal respiratory stimuli
    1. Intracranial bleeding
    2. Immaturity
    3. Maternal drugs
    4. Severe CNS anomaly
  C. Normal initiation of respirations with failure of pulmonary expansion
    1. Lung hypoplasia
      a. Diaphragmatic hernia
      b. Congenital
    2. Limitation of respiratory expansion
      a. Severe ascites/hydrops fetalis
      b. Intrapulmonary/abdominal masses
    3. Obstruction of trachea with mucus/meconium
    4. Congenital anomalies of the upper respiratory tract

of body heat, hypoxemia, acidosis, hypercarbia, hypovolemia, or shock can cause the fetal circulation to return.

The normal newborn heart rate can vary between 100 to 200 beats/min during the first 30 minutes of life.[7] It will then stabilize at 120 beats/min, ±50 beats/min. Blood pressure is dependent on weight (Table 4–2). A general rule is if the weight is 1, 2, or 3 kg, the minimum systolic blood pressure will be 40, 50, or 60 mm Hg. The normal intravascular volume is about 80 to 100 ml/kg. However, this will vary depending on when the umbilical cord is clamped and where the infant is in relationship to the mother's perineum. The longer the time to clamping and the lower the infant is in relationship to the perineum, the more blood from the placenta that is autotransfused to the infant.

EMERGENCY MEDICAL SERVICE CONSIDERATIONS

One potential problem that emergency personnel will encounter involves transporting an impending delivery patient in the ambulance or stabilizing a newborn. The airway, breathing, and circulation (ABC) approach used for all patients still applies, but other aspects need to be addressed.

Special instructions can be given from medical control to the ambulance when transporting an imminent delivery. To ensure fetal well-being, the mother's ABCs must be addressed and stabilized. This is accomplished by two simple maneuvers to optimize uterine blood flow and fetal oxygenation. First, because the gravid uterus impedes maternal venous return through inferior vena cava compression, turning the mother into the left lateral decubitus position or gently maneuvering the uterus into the left abdominal quadrant will improve placental profusion. Second, applying oxygen to the mother will maximize fetal oxygenation. If intravenous (IV) access is possible, crystalloids should be started during transport to the emergency department. The medical control physician should receive a report including repeated vital signs and the frequency of contractions. Obtaining a brief maternal history (see Table 4–1) will alert the medical staff to potential problems.

Precipitous birth in the ambulance or in the home does occur. Once the baby is born, a systematic approach must be initiated by the ambulance staff. The ABC approach still applies to the newborn, but with some modifications. Establishing an open airway requires (1) proper positioning in a slight Trendelenburg position; (2) suctioning of the nose and mouth and, when meconium is present, the trachea; and (3) placing an endotracheal tube if necessary. Prevention of heat loss by drying or wrapping the trunk in blankets or a plastic bag (or bubble wrap) should be performed prior to or during infant positioning. Breathing is initiated first by tactile stimulation and, if necessary, by positive-pressure ventilation using either the bag and mask or bag and endotracheal tube. Finally, circulation must be maintained during resuscitation by using chest compressions and medications. Bradycardia results primarily from inadequate ven-

lation with a resulting decrease in pulmonary vascular resistance and pulmonary arterial pressure (Fig. 4–3).

The increasing PO_2 also constricts the ductus arteriosus with the help of sympathomimetic amines and prostaglandin. Consequently, at 24 to 48 hours, the foramen ovale and ductus arteriosus functionally close with discontinuation of the right-to-left shunt. Anatomic closure of these structures occurs at between 1 week and approximately 2 months of life, depending on the neonate's maturity. Stress such as loss

TABLE 4–2

NORMAL NEONATAL BLOOD PRESSURES

Pressure (mm Hg)	Birth Weight (kg)			
	≤1	1–2	2–3	≥3
Systolic	40–60	50–65	50–70	50–80
Diastolic	15–35	20–40	25–45	30–50

From McKluein RE, Ostshmeimer GW. Resuscitation of the newborn. Clin Obstet Gynecol 1987;30:611.

Approximate Times of Physiologic Events in Perinatal Asphyxia

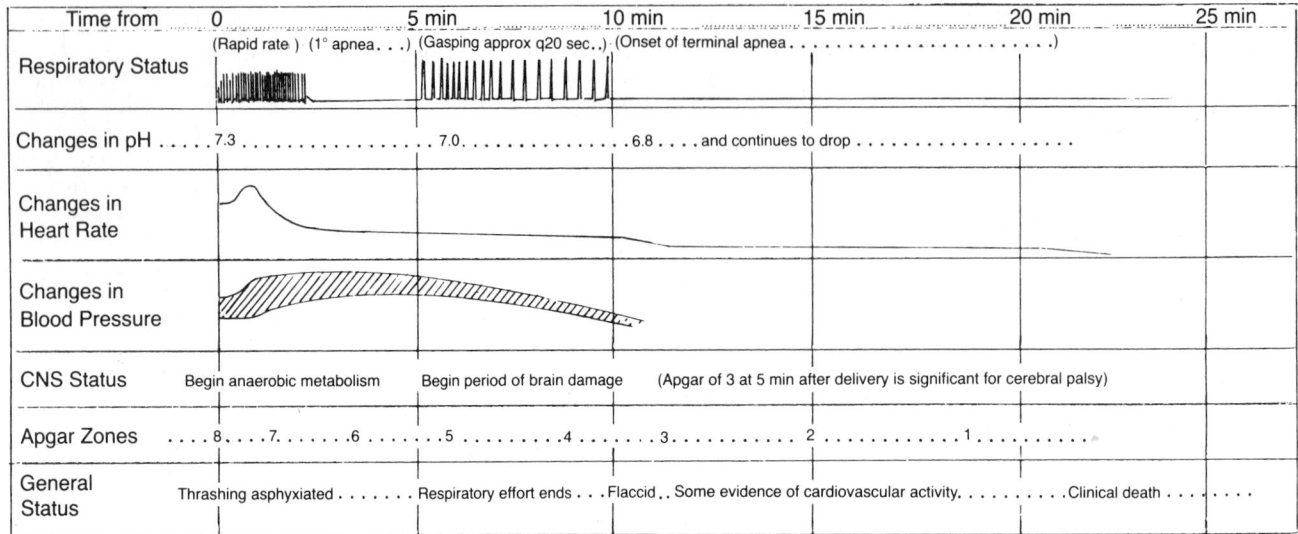

Figure 4–1. The clinical course of every hypoxic or anoxic episode is unique to that setting. This figure represents a compilation of the available data. (From Lamb FS, Rosner MS. Neonatal resuscitation. Emerg Med Clin North Am 1987;5:555.)

tilation and oxygenation. Consequently, complications concerning these areas should be addressed concurrently. Rapid transport to the nearest facility for stabilization is the highest priority.

Emergency Department Preparation

A well-prepared staff can perform a delivery efficiently and effectively. For this to occur, certain personnel, equipment, and medications must be immediately available. Optimally, there should be at least three people designated to aid in newborn resuscitation. The leader should be at the baby's head maintaining airway control and assessing breathing. He or she should evaluate, decide, and act on the newborn's physiologic responses. The second person's sole duty is to monitor the heart rate. This can be performed in two ways: by palpating the umbilical artery pulsations at the cord, or, if this is not successful, performing auscultation at the heart's apex. These data are transmitted to the leader by "tapping out" the heart rate on the side of the resuscitation bed. Then the leader can estimate if the heart rate is above or below 100. To arrive at a more accurate pulse rate, the leader could multiply the number of beats in a 6-second interval by ten. For example, if there are 12 beats in the 6-second period, then the heart rate would be 120 beats/min. The final person is available to assist in establishing IV access or preparation of other materials. A team approach is necessary for successful resuscitation.

A variety of equipment and medications is needed. These should be prepared in anticipation of an impending delivery. Ideally, a "neonatal resuscitation tray" can be opened in the event of a delivery, with most of the needed equipment present on the tray (Table 4–3).[12–16] A circular silicone mask (Laerdal) is absolutely required. This circular mask leaks less and is more efficiently cleaned than other masks. The design is superior, especially when compared with the Rendell-Bater (a triangular molded rubber mask), Ambu-OA, Bennett, and Ohio masks.[17]

Pulse oximetry has been used effectively in newborns.[18] It is accurate in neonates for arterial oxygen saturation (SaO_2) greater than 40% and is unaffected by fetal hemoglobin.[19] By 5 minutes of age, a normal, term, vaginally delivered

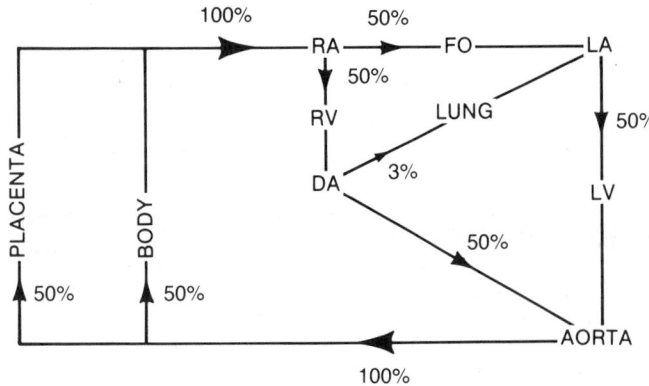

Figure 4–2. Fetal circulation. Flow estimates: >, 100%; >, 50%; >, 3%. DA, Ductus arteriosus; FO, foramen ovale; LA, left atrium; LV, left ventricle; RA, right atrium; RV, right ventricle.

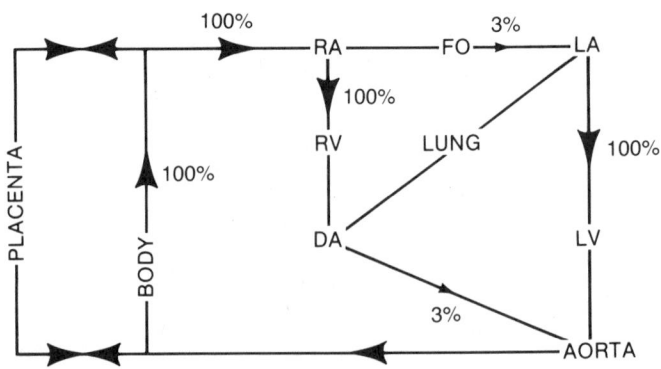

Figure 4–3. Circulation at birth. Flow estimates: >, 100%; >, 3%. DA, Ductus arteriosus; FO, foramen ovale; LA, left atrium; LV, left ventricle; RA, right atrium; RV, right ventricle.

TABLE 4–3

NEONATAL RESUSCITATION SUPPLIES

Suction equipment
  A large and a small bulb syringe
  DeLee mucus trap with No. 10 French catheter for mechanical
    suctioning
  Suction catheters No. 5, 6, 8, and 10 French
  No. 5 and 8 French feeding tube and 20-ml syringe
Bag-mask equipment
  Self-inflating resuscitation bag (500 ml) with oxygen reservoir
    or anesthesia bag with manometer
  Face mask, newborn and premature size (00, 0, 1, 2)
  Oral airways, newborn and premature size (000, 00, 0)
  Oxygen with flow meter and tubing
Equipment
  Laryngoscope with straight blades (0, premature; 1, newborn)
  Extra bulbs and batteries for laryngoscope
  Endotracheal tubes, sizes 2.5, 3.0, 3.5, 4.0 mm
  Small stylet
  Gloves
  Small Magill forceps
Medications
  Epinephrine 1:10,000—3-ml or 10-ml ampules
  Naloxone hydrochloride (Narcan)—0.4 mg/ml or 1.0 mg/ml
  Volume expander—albumin 5% solution, normal saline,
    Ringer's lactate
  Sodium bicarbonate 4.2% (5 mEq/10 ml)—10-ml ampules
  Dextrose 10%—250 ml
  Sterile water—30 ml
  Prepared chart with drug dosages per weight
Miscellaneous
  Prewarmed blankets and towels
  1- to 2-gallon plastic bags (bubble wrap material)
  No. 8 French orogastric tubes
  Radiant warmer
  Stethoscope
  Cardiac monitor with EKG oscilloscope
  Small electrode leads; adhesive tape, ½- to ¾-in width
  Syringes—1, 3, 5, 10, 20, 50 ml
  Needles—25, 21, 18 gauge
  IV catheters—24, 22 gauge
  Butterfly needles—23, 25 gauge
  Umbilical vein catheter
  Umbilical tape
  Umbilical catheters—No. 3.5, 5 French
  Three-way stopcocks
  Chest tubes—No. 8, 10, 12 French with chest tube trays

neonate in room air has a rapid rise in SaO_2 to an average value of 80%.[20] The changes in SaO_2 were more predictive of a newborn response to resuscitation than Apgar scores. This is especially noted in preterm infants, whose immaturity automatically decreases their maximum score.[21] Consequently, if pulse oximetry is available in an emergency

department, it should be modified for newborns and used to monitor resuscitation.

CLINICAL EVALUATION
Initial Evaluation

In 1953 Virginia Apgar devised a scoring system to evaluate infants at 1 minute after birth; a repeat score at 5 minutes has been recommended.[22] This score consists of five objective signs that are easily obtained without interfering with the neonate's care. The signs are heart rate, respiratory effort, muscle tone, reflex irritability, and color. Each sign has a designated value, with 2 being the highest (Table 4–4). By adding the point value for all signs, a total score is derived, with the maximum of 10 indicating a vigorous infant and the minimum of 0 indicating no signs of life. The purpose of this score is to give a general assessment of an infant at birth, monitor the response to resuscitation, compare various hospital approaches to different diseases and subsequent therapy, and predict outcome. However, its value in assessing premature infants and predicting their future outcome has been debated. Time, color, and reflex irritability are partially dependent on the infant's maturity. The greater the degree of prematurity, the lower the score will be, even in a normal premature infant without asphyxia. Moreover, drugs and analgesia given to the mother prior to the delivery will also decrease the point value of these signs. A 5-minute score initially serves as a predictor of future neurologic outcome, especially if the score is between 0 and 3. Nevertheless, the American Academy of Pediatrics (AAP) has issued the following statement: "Substantial cerebral hypoxia leading to cerebral palsy can be presumed only when these criteria are met: Apgar score is 0 to 3 at 10 minutes; infant remains hypotonic for at least several hours; and infant has seizures."[23]

For emergency department purposes, the Apgar score is best used to predict the need for resuscitation and to assess the newborn's response to therapy. This score should be taken every 5 minutes until the newborn is stable. A simple method of remembering the five signs is the following: *A*ctivity or muscle tone, *P*ulse, *G*rimace or reflex irritability, *A*ppearance or color, and *R*espiratory effort (Apgar).

Although many articles have reviewed neonatal resuscitation in detail,[5–16] the American Academy of Pediatrics in 1987 formalized a protocol for neonatal resuscitation (Fig. 4–4). The common theme in this approach is first to *assess*, then *act*, and then *reassess*. This should continue until the infant is stabilized and disposition is made.

As soon as the infant is born, a modified ABC approach is used. Initially, steps are taken to prevent heat loss. Infants lose heat more quickly than adults because of their greater ratio of surface area to body mass. Increased heat loss will increase the metabolic rate, which subsequently increases

TABLE 4–4

APGAR SCORE

Sign	Number of Points		
	0	*1*	*2*
Heart rate	Absent	Slow (below 100 beats/min)	More than 100 beats/min
Respiratory effort	Absent	Slow, irregular	Good, crying
Muscle tone	Flaccid	Some flexion of extremities	Active motion
Reflex irritability	No response	Grimace	Vigorous cry
Color	Pale	Cyanotic	Completely pink

From Apgar V. A proposal for a new method of evaluation of the newborn infant. Anesth Analg 1953; 32:260.

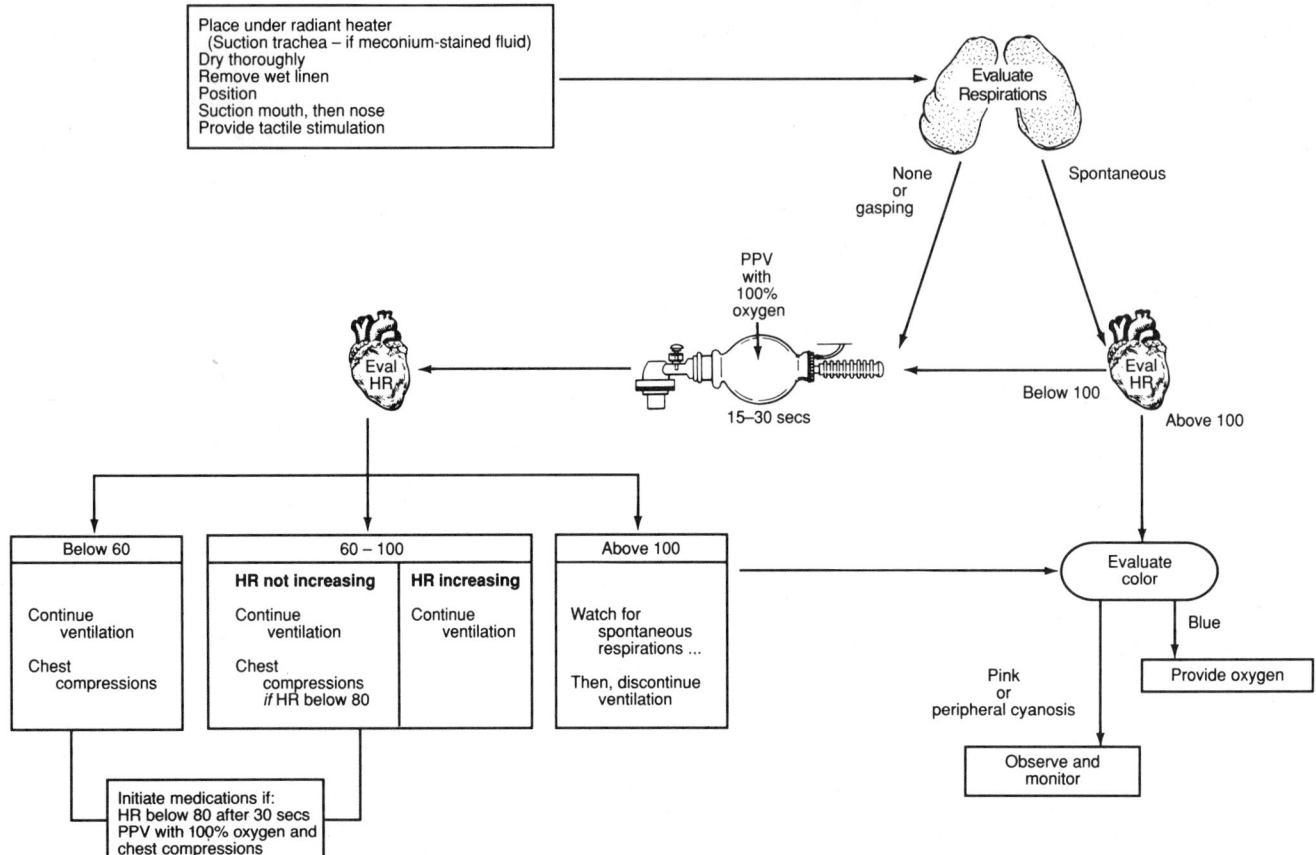

Figure 4–4. Overview of resuscitation in the delivery room. (Reproduced with permission. © From Bloom RS, Cropley C (eds). Textbook of Neonatal Resuscitation, 1987. Chicago, AHA. Copyright American Heart Association.)

oxygen consumption. In asphyxiated infants, this can be disastrous. Consequently, heat loss should be prevented by placing an infant under a radiant warmer or a heat lamp. Drying the child thoroughly and removing wet clothing should follow. Finally, covering the child's torso with some insulating material (e.g., warm blanket, plastic bag, or bubble wrap) and placing a stocking cap on the head will maximize heat retention.

Airway

Next the airway should be opened. This is performed by placing the child in a slight Trendelenburg position with the neck slightly extended. Too much extension or flexion easily occludes the pliable trachea. A rolled towel placed transversely under the shoulders may help in maintaining this position. If there are excessive oral secretions, turning the head to one side will facilitate the use of a bulb syringe to remove the material. The mouth is suctioned first, followed by the nose, because nasal stimulation often causes gasping, which allows oral secretions to be aspirated. A DeLee suction catheter or mechanical suction (maximal wall pressure, 100 mm Hg) can be used. With any kind of suction, stimulating the posterior pharynx is avoided, because early after birth this can cause severe bradycardia or apnea as a result of vagal reflexes.

In 8% to 15% of all pregnancies, and in up to 30% of postterm deliveries, the amniotic fluid is meconium stained.[24] More than 50% of term newborns have meconium in the trachea. Of neonates with meconium in the trachea, 15% have none in the mouth or the pharynx.[25] Prevention of meconium aspiration is important because of potentially lethal complications, including pneumothorax, pneumonitis, and persistent pulmonary hypertension with hypoxia.

Thin, watery meconium without particulate matter requires no special intervention. However, thick, particulate matter requires removal. As soon as the head is delivered at the introitus, a No. 10 French catheter from a DeLee trap or wall suction is used to remove the meconium from the mouth, pharynx, and hypopharynx. Once the infant is on the bed, the trachea should immediately be intubated and suctioned until no meconium remains. Tracheal suctioning can be performed in several ways. First, the physician can use his or her own mouth with a surgical mask as a filter and apply suction. The problem with this method is that the endotracheal tube must be repeatedly taken out to verify the removal of meconium. Second, the end of an endotracheal tube from which the adapter has been removed can be attached to the distal two thirds of a cut No. 10 French DeLee suction trap. This should be secured with tape. Then intubation is performed, and suction is applied orally until no meconium is collected in the trap. A wall suction device can also be modified to fit a DeLee suction trap. Another wall suction method involves using a disposable plastic adapter with a fingertip suction control interdisposed between the endotracheal tube and standard suction tubing.[26]

There are infectious risks to the physician when using oral suction.[27, 28] These include exposure to chlamydia, gonorrhea, group B streptococcus, trichomonas, *Haemophilus influenzae*, cytomegalovirus, herpes simplex, varicella zoster, hepatitis, and human immunodeficiency virus.

Breathing

The next step is to ensure respiration. Usually drying, warming, positioning, and suctioning the newborn are all that is needed to induce respiration. Additional tactile stimulation such as slapping or flicking the soles of the feet and rubbing the infant's back may be needed. This whole process should not take more than 30 seconds.

The next step in the resuscitation process is the physician's evaluation of the infant's respiratory rate, heart rate, and color. These are three key vital signs that should always be reassessed. If there is no response to stimulation, positive-pressure ventilation (PPV) using a bag and mask should be initiated at a rate of 40 breaths/min. If respirations and chest movements are present, the heart rate should be checked. If the heart rate is below 100 beats/min, intervention with PPV should begin. If the heart rate is above 100 beats/min, color is then evaluated. Oxygen should be given if central cyanosis is present in an infant with spontaneous respiration and adequate heart rate. Oxygen is not needed for peripheral cyanosis, which is usually present during the first few minutes of birth. If PPV is required for longer than 2 minutes, an orogastric tube must be inserted. This will decompress the stomach, relieve diaphragmatic pressure, allow full expansion of the lungs, and prevent aspiration of gastric contents.

Circulation

After PPV is initiated for 15 to 30 seconds, the heart rate should be reassessed. If the heart rate is greater than 100 beats/min and spontaneous respirations are present, PPV can be discontinued, with gentle rubbing to provide additional stimulation. If the heart rate is greater than 100 beats/min, but there are no spontaneous respirations, PPV should be continued. If the heart rate is 60 to 100 beats/min and increasing, PPV should be continued. If the heart rate is 60 to 100 beats/min and not increasing, PPV should be continued and airway problems reassessed. If during this time the heart rate is less than 80 beats/min, chest compressions should begin. If the heart rate is less than 60 beats/min after 15 to 30 seconds of PPV, then chest compression should be started and airway problems reassessed. After chest compressions are initiated, a repeat heart rate evaluation should be taken in 30 seconds. If the heart rate is below 80 beats/min, chest compression should be continued and drug therapy and intubation initiated. If the heart rate is more than 80 beats/min, chest compression should be stopped. However, PPV should be continued until the heart rate is greater than 100 beats/min and the infant is breathing spontaneously. Color assessment and administration of oxygen should follow. Assessment of color, heart rate, and ventilation should continue every 15 to 30 seconds until stability is ensured.

When the neonate is either not improving or deteriorating from an improved state, several problems should be considered. The most common problem is inadequate ventilation. This may result from equipment failure (bag-valve-mask leak, lack of oxygen flow, no oxygen reservoir, not enough pressure, mask leak); a blocked airway secondary to improper positioning, accumulation of secretions, choanal atresia, or macroglossia; poor diaphragmatic excursion secondary to gastric distention or diaphragmatic hernia; and pneumothorax. Each problem area should be rechecked and corrected accordingly.

Thus a set procedure should be followed in newborn resuscitation, beginning with warming, drying, positioning, and suctioning; tactile stimulation (a 30-second evaluation); assessment of ventilation, heart rate, and color (a 5- to 10-second evaluation); and appropriate action in regard to physiologic responses. Then, after 15 to 30 seconds of PPV, the heart rate is reassessed. If chest compressions are initiated, the heart rate should be rechecked in 30 seconds, and

if the rate is inadequate, pharmacologic intervention and intubation should follow.

DIAGNOSTIC EVALUATION

Once the neonate is stabilized, there is minimal testing that can be performed and acted on in the emergency department. Laboratory evaluation usually is not necessary unless abnormal symptoms arise; these include grunting, retractions, tachypnea, cyanosis, apnea, and shock. The most common diagnostic procedures are determinations of hemoglobin, hematocrit, and serum glucose. Radiographic evaluation can verify endotracheal tube position and central line placement.

After 34 to 35 weeks of gestation, the umbilical cord hemoglobin is about 16.8 gm/dl.[29] Capillary samples (i.e., heel sticks) can be 2 to 3 gm/dl higher. Anemia is defined as a venous hemoglobin less than or equal to 13 gm/dl or a capillary sample of less than 14.5 gm/dl. Anemia should be treated if symptomatic. However, the criteria for diagnosis and the therapy for polycythemia or hyperviscosity syndrome are controversial. If the venous hemoglobin and hematocrit are greater than 27 gm/dl and 65%, respectively, at 4 to 6 hours of age and the baby is symptomatic, therapy should be started.[30] However, the initiation of this treatment is in the realm of the pediatrician or neonatologist who should be caring for the resuscitated baby by the fourth hour of age.

The initial glucose determination will usually reflect maternal values. However, if stresses such as asphyxia, cold, or hypovolemia are present, glucose stores will be rapidly depleted. By definition, hypoglycemia is a plasma glucose level in a premature infant of less than 25 mg/dl or in a term infant of less than 35 mg/dl within the first 72 hours of age. After 72 hours of age, the plasma glucose concentration should be above 45 mg/dl.[29] The use of a Dextrostick or Accu-Check to diagnose hypoglycemia may be inaccurate. Consequently, a "crash" serum glucose determination should be ordered if symptoms arise. However, if the glucose level as determined by Dextrostick or Accu-Check is less than 40 mg/dl, it is better to treat the infant rather than wait for a serum glucose determination. Emergent treatment of hyperglycemia, defined as a plasma glucose level greater than 150 mg/dl, is unnecessary.[30]

The indications for diagnostic radiographs in the newborn are for evaluation of pulmonary causes of neonatal distress and to verify endotracheal tube and central line placement. If the infant is critically ill and a pneumothorax is considered, treatment should always precede radiographic evaluation.

DIFFERENTIAL DIAGNOSIS

There is a myriad of causes of neonatal distress (Table 4–5), each of which can present with similar signs and symptoms. These include tachypnea, grunting, retractions, apnea, cyanosis, and shock. Most pulmonary causes of neonatal distress can be treated adequately in the emergency department by initially securing the airway with the aid of a bag-valve-mask system, oral airway, or endotracheal intubation. Cardiac, metabolic, and neuromuscular origins need more definitive care by consultants. However, some of these problems, such as hypoglycemia, hypothermia, and complications resulting from maternal narcotic therapy, can be treated acutely. Hypocalcemia usually does not occur until 24 to 48 hours after birth. Blood loss responds to infusion of crystalloid and blood.

TABLE 4–5

DIFFERENTIAL DIAGNOSIS OF NEONATAL DISTRESS

I. Pulmonary causes
  A. RDS (hyaline membrane disease)
  B. Meconium aspiration
  C. Pneumonia
  D. Transient tachypnea of newborn
  E. Persistent fetal circulation
  F. Pneumothorax
  G. Airway obstruction
    1. Upper
      a. Choanal atresia
      b. Macroglossia (i.e., Pierre Robin syndrome)
      c. Other (i.e., tracheal, laryngeal, and esophageal abnormalities)
    2. Lower
      a. Diaphragmatic hernia
      b. Pulmonary hypoplasia
      c. Primary
      d. Associated with renal aplasia (Potter's syndrome), obstructive uropathy, dwarfing syndrome, diaphragmatic hernia
      e. Congenital lung cysts
II. Extrapulmonary causes
  A. Heart
    1. Dysrhythmia
    2. Congenital heart block
    3. Supraventricular tachycardia
    4. Structural defect (i.e., hypoplastic left heart, coarctation of the aorta, transposition of the great vessels)
  B. Metabolic
    1. Any cause of metabolic acidosis
    2. Hypoglycemia
    3. Hypocalcemia
    4. Hypothermia
    5. Sepsis
  C. Blood
    1. Acute loss
      a. Rupture of cord
      b. Incision of placenta during cesarean
      c. Placenta previa/abruption placenta
      d. Internal hemorrhage (i.e., subgaleal, adrenal, pulmonary, intracranial)
      e. Coagulopathy
    2. Chronic loss
      a. Fetal-maternal transfusion
      b. Twin-twin transfusion
      c. Hemolysis
      d. Isoimmunization (erythroblastosis)
      e. Chronic uterine infection
    3. Hyperviscosity syndrome
  D. Neuromuscular disease
    1. Brain
      a. Asphyxia
      b. Maternal drugs
      c. Local and general anesthetics
      d. Analgesias
      e. Addiction (i.e., narcotics)
    2. Spinal cord
      a. Trauma
      b. Werdnig-Hoffmann disease
    3. Phrenic nerve injury
    4. Myasthenia gravis
    5. Myotonic dystrophy

RDS = Respiratory distress syndrome.

THERAPEUTIC INTERVENTION
Ventilation

Ensuring adequate ventilation and oxygenation are the keys to successful stabilization of the neonate. Adjuncts that can improve ventilation and oxygenation include the use of oxygen, PPV, orogastric tube placement, oral airway use, and endotracheal intubation. Chest compressions, intravenous drugs, endotracheal medications, fluid or blood boluses, and pneumothorax decompressions are other interventions used.

Oxygen is used to treat central cyanosis in a neonate who has adequate respirations and a heart rate greater than 100 beats/min. Oxygen should be delivered by tubing or face mask and not by a self-inflating resuscitation bag in which oxygen flow is not continuous. Ideally, oxygen should be heated and humidified, but if it is used only for a few minutes, this is unnecessary. Various oxygen concentrations can be obtained by using tubing at varying distances from the nares or by a simple face mask held loosely or firmly on the face (Table 4–6). When oxygen is used, once the central cyanosis has resolved, the oxygen should be *slowly* withdrawn until the infant remains pink while breathing room air.

Bag-valve-mask ventilation (BVMV) is indicated when the newborn remains apneic after initial procedures are performed and when respirations are insufficient to maintain a heart rate greater than 100 beats/min. The only exception to using BVMV initially is in the infant suspected of having a diaphragmatic hernia. In this case, an endotracheal intubation should be used, as BVMV will increase intragastric air, causing less lung expansion and further asphyxia.

BVMV can be difficult to perform accurately. The mask must adequately cover both nose and mouth without impingement on the eyes. The mask is held firmly at the chin and nose without pressure over the trachea. The neck should be slightly extended. The physician who is controlling the airway should have a clear view of the chest to monitor expansion. If the seal is inadequate, the airway is blocked by secretions or the tongue, or there is not enough pressure from the bag-valve-mask unit, chest expansion will be inadequate. Repositioning the mask and applying more pressure usually corrects the air leak. Repositioning the neonate's neck, suctioning any obstructive secretions in the oropharynx, or using an oral airway will usually correct a blocked airway problem. With a self-inflating bag, pressure can be increased by squeezing the bag maximally until the pressure release valve opens. If this is inadequate (i.e., in severe respiratory distress syndrome), overriding the release valve will give maximum pressure. An anesthesia bag is more difficult to control, because it is not self-inflating and the pressure must be regulated. Initially, the manometer should be set at 30 cm H_2O pressure by adjusting the flow control valve. If this pressure is inadequate, then using the flow control valve to increase the pressure will solve the problem. The manometer should not be watched for specific pressures, but instead the infant should be observed for adequate chest expansion. If the chest still does not rise, a new bag-valve-mask device should be used. The optimal ventilation rate is 40 to 60 times/min. Complications of BVMV are

TABLE 4–6

OXYGEN CONCENTRATION CHART (100% Oxygen at 5 L/Min)

O₂ Concentration	Tubing	Mask
Approx. 80%	½ in from nares	Mask held firmly on face
Approx. 60%	1 in from nares	
Approx. 40%	2 in from nares	Mask held losely on face

Reproduced with permission. © From Bloom RS, Cropley C (eds). Textbook of Neonatal Resuscitation, 1987. Chicago, AHA. Copyright American Heart Association.

hypoxia resulting from inadequate positioning, equipment malfunction, or gastric distention; soft tissue trauma to the face; pneumothorax; and infection. If performed properly, BVMV is usually all that is needed to stabilize the newborn.

An orogastric tube must be placed if BVMV must be used for more than 2 minutes, the patient remains cyanotic, or a congenital diaphragmatic hernia is suspected. A No. 8 French feeding tube and a 20-ml syringe are the only equipment needed. First, the tube length is estimated. The distance from the bridge of the nose to the earlobe, then from the earlobe to the xiphoid process is the length that the feeding tube must transverse. Second, the catheter is inserted through the mouth, rather than the nose, because neonates are obligate nose breathers; the tube is then taped to the cheek. Finally, a syringe is used to decompress the stomach contents, and the end of the catheter is left opened to air. During orogastric tube placement, BVMV is momentarily interrupted but can be resumed with a good face mask seal. Complications of orogastric tube placement include tracheal intubation, esophageal perforation, soft tissue trauma, and infection.

Oral airways are rarely used with BVMV. However, if the tongue blocks the airway, (e.g., in Pierre Robin syndrome [micrognathia, pseudomacroglossia, glossoptosis, high arched or cleft palate]), if bilateral choanal atresia exists, or if chest expansion occurs only with an open mouth, then an oral airway is needed. The proper-size oral airway will fit over the tongue, reaching the posterior pharynx with the flange just outside the lips. The airway is placed by opening the mouth and positioning it directly over the tongue. Reversing the airway when it is in the posterior pharynx is unnecessary in newborns. Complications, which include soft tissue trauma, hypoxia resulting from further obstruction of the airway, or an infection, can be minimized if a gentle technique is used.

Intubation

There are four indications for endotracheal tube placement: ineffective BVMV, BVMV required for more than 2 minutes,[31] suspected diaphragmatic hernia, and meconium aspiration requiring tracheal suctioning. A few important points must be stressed. The endotracheal tube should not be tapered or cuffed (see Table 4–3). The tracheal length of a full-term infant is about 2 to 3 inches, and a preterm newborn's trachea is about half this length. As soon as the endotracheal tube is visualized through the cords, that position should be held and the tube not advanced any further. Some endotracheal tubes have a vocal cord guide at the tip to aid in proper placement. Premature infants usually require a 2.5- to 3-mm tube using a No. 0 straight blade, whereas a term infant usually needs a 3.5- to 4-mm tube using a No. 1 straight blade. If a stylet is used, its tip should not extend beyond the end of the endotracheal tube, and the proximal portion should be secured at the endotracheal tube connector. Hypoxia can be minimized during intubation by providing 5 L of oxygen as close to the mouth as possible through the tubing. Once the endotracheal tube is secured at the mouth, it should be shortened so that only 4 cm remain exiting the mouth. This will decrease the amount of dead space and limit the chance of tube kinking. A maximum of 100 mm Hg of negative pressure should be used when suctioning an endotracheal tube.

Once the decision to intubate has been made, several steps should be taken. The neck should be maintained in a slightly extended position. A towel roll placed transversely at the shoulders may assist in this positioning. While holding the laryngoscope with the left hand, the blade is placed *directly* over the tongue and not in the right corner of the mouth.

While visualizing the oropharynx, the blade is advanced into the vallecula or posterior to the epiglottis. The blade is lifted in the direction the handle is pointing, not rocked or tilted superiorly such that the proximal portion of the blade impinges on the alveolar ridge. This permits visualization of the glottis. Often, mild external tracheal pressure will maximize glottis exposure. Once placed, the appropriately sized endotracheal tube is secured. This entire procedure should be limited to 20 seconds to prevent further hypoxia. Finally, tube placement is verified by observing symmetric chest expansion and noting positive and equal breath sounds in both axillae and the absence of gastric distention or air heard over the stomach. A chest radiograph will assist in verifying placement.

There are complications associated with intubation. These include hypoxia resulting from tube placement in the right main stem bronchus or esophagus or an inordinate amount of time taken to perform the procedure, bradycardia and apnea secondary to hypoxia or to a vagal response from stimulating a posterior pharynx, pneumothorax, injury to the soft tissue, perforation of the esophagus or trachea, and infection. These can be minimized by using a calm, organized approach during the intubation process.

Cardiac Compression

Chest compressions are indicated only if, after 15 to 30 seconds of PPV, the heart rate is less than 60 beats/min or is between 60 and 80 beats/min and not increasing. Chest compressions are stopped when the heart rate is greater than 80 beats/min. There are two techniques for performing chest compressions: the *two-hand technique* and the *two-finger technique*. With the two-hand technique, both hands encircle the chest, and the thumbs, either side by side or one over the other, oppose the sternum (Fig. 4–5). In the two-finger method, the tips of the middle finger and either the index or ring finger on one hand compress the sternum in a perpendicular manner.

The two-hand technique produces a higher cardiac output than the two-finger technique.[32] An explanation for this difference is that cardiac output during closed chest massage is independent of direct cardiac compression but results from increasing the intrathoracic pressure. The two-hand technique may provide a more uniform increase in the intrathoracic pressure and is also less tiring for the person performing the technique than the two-finger method. However, it cannot be used effectively if the infant is larger than the resuscitator's hands or if access to an umbilical cord catheter is needed for medication administration. In these situations, the two-finger method is acceptable.

With either compression technique, the location, depth, and rate of compression are identical. The heart lies beneath the lower one third of the sternum.[33, 34] The lower one third of the sternum lies below a line drawn from nipple to nipple. Compression depth should be one-half to three-fourths inch. During compression, the tips of the fingers or thumbs should remain in contact with the sternum. The rate is 120 beats/min, or 2 compressions per second. Complications of chest compressions include rib fractures, hemorrhage, pneumothorax, and lacerations to the liver from excess pressure over the xiphoid. These complications can be minimized by adhering to strict technique.

PPV should continue at 40 to 60 breaths/min during chest compressions. Either interposed ventilations or simultaneous ventilation with chest compressions can be performed in the intubated baby. However, if BVMV is used and the chest is compressed simultaneously, air flow will enter the stomach rather than the lungs. Three actions can maximize the effectiveness of BVMV and chest compressions: interposing

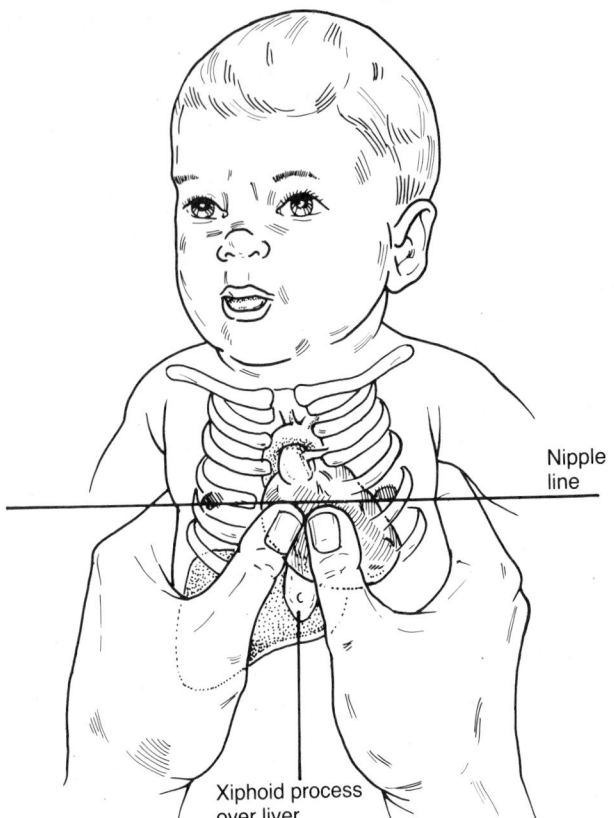

Nipple
line

Xiphoid process
over liver

Figure 4–5. Thaler technique of external cardiac compression for infants. The thumbs are placed on the sternum between the infant's nipples.

a ventilation between every third compression, using an oral gastric tube to decompress the stomach, and intubation of the newborn.

Vascular Access

Intravenous access can be life-saving in the neonate. Failure of the infant to respond to resuscitation is the main indication for its use. A failed IV access attempt at a peripheral site should mandate immediate umbilical vein catheterization. This central site, rather than the umbilical arteries, is the only central access that should be cannulated in the emergency department. The umbilical vein is easy to identify because of its large size, is the easiest to cannulate, and results in the fewest complications when used. If immediate umbilical vein access is desired and the equipment is not available, the umbilical stump is quickly prepped, the umbilical vein identified, and the drug injected directly into the vein through an angiocatheter. The disadvantage to this procedure is that a one-time injection is usually all that is possible and further use of umbilical vein may be lost.

Pneumothorax

Pneumothorax is seen in 10% to 40% of all ventilated newborns. It can also occur after PPV with a bag-valve-mask device, especially when meconium is present. If the infant is in a critical state, needle aspiration should be performed first. To accomplish this, the skin at the second intercostal space in the midclavicular line or at the fourth intercostal space in the anterior axillary line is prepped with a povidone-iodine solution (Betadine) and alcohol. A 22-gauge IV an-

giocatheter attached to a 20-ml syringe is inserted into the pleural space using continuous negative pressure. Once air has been aspirated, the angiocatheter can be connected either to a three-way stopcock to facilitate extraction of pleural air or to IV tubing, with the opposite end of the tube placed under a water-filled container placed below the level of the heart. (If placed above the heart, fluid flows into the pleural space.) Once a pneumothorax has been decompressed with an angiocatheter, a chest tube should be placed. If deterioration continues despite pneumothorax decompression on one side, a needle aspiration of the other side should be performed.

Chest tube placement is performed in the same location and sterile manner as needle aspiration. After a small incision in the skin, a curved hemostat is placed over the rib, using blunt dissection into the intercostal muscles, and then "popped" into the pleural space. If possible, the physician's small finger should verify the entrance into this area. Advancement of the chest tube (No. 10 French for an infant weighing 1500 grams or less, No. 12 French for a larger infant) follows, guided into the pleural space with either a hemostat or a trocar. After it is secured with sutures, dressing, and tape, the tube is connected to an underwater seal with a negative pressure of 10 to 15 cm H_2O. A chest radiograph is made to confirm placement and lung reinflation. Complications of needle or tube thoracostomy include infection, bleeding, laceration or puncture of solid organs, and incorrect tube placement.

Pharmacologic Intervention

Volume expanders and drugs are rarely needed but must be anticipated in the resuscitation of a neonate. IV access is the preferred route, but two medications, epinephrine[35] and naloxone hydrochloride (Narcan), can be given through the endotracheal tube. If using the endotracheal tube route, PPV should be done *after* instilling the drug in order to distribute the drug into the bronchial tree. The endotracheal naloxone dose is the same as the intravenous dose. However, the endotracheal epinephrine dose is double to triple the intravenous dose. Another method to ensure that all the drug enters the respiratory tract and does not remain in the endotracheal tube is to place a No. 5 French suction tube through the endotracheal tube. The drug is administered, and then 0.5 ml of normal saline is flushed through the inner tube.

There are two main indications for drug therapy: (1) a heart rate that is less than 80 beats/min despite adequate ventilation and chest compressions for a minimum of 30 seconds and (2) asytole. Resuscitation medications include epinephrine, volume expanders, sodium bicarbonate, and dopamine. Naloxone and glucose are also used in specific circumstances. Currently, there is no evidence that the use of calcium and atropine in the acute phase of neonatal resuscitation is useful.

Epinephrine

Epinephrine is used when the heart rate remains below 80 beats/min after 30 seconds of adequate ventilation and chest compressions or the heart rate is 0. The dose is 0.1 to 0.3 ml/kg of 1:10,000 solution given rapidly through an IV. The endotracheal dose is two to three times higher. If the heart rate remains below 100 beats/min, the dose can be repeated every 5 minutes.

Volume Expanders

Volume expanders are used if acute blood loss has occurred. Signs of hypovolemia include pallor persisting after adequate oxygenation, weak pulses with a good heart rate, poor response to resuscitation, poor capillary refill, and decreased blood pressure. The initial determination of hemoglobin or hematocrit may be normal. Volume expanders include whole blood (O-negative blood crossmatched with the mother's blood), 5% albumin, other colloids, and crystalloids. The dose is 10 ml/kg given over a 5- to 10-minute period. This can be repeated two to three times if signs of hypovolemia persist. If no improvement occurs, sodium bicarbonate can be used to correct any coexisting metabolic acidosis.

Sodium Bicarbonate

Sodium bicarbonate is indicated whenever there is a documented metabolic acidosis. It may also be beneficial when repeated epinephrine boluses and maximum volume expansion have been given, yet persistent poor perfusion has promoted concurrent metabolic acidosis. Sodium bicarbonate in a 0.5 mEq/ml (4.2%) solution should be given intravenously in 2-mEq/kg doses over a 2-minute period. Rapid administration increases venous irritation with possible extravasation of material and loss of IV access. It also increases the risk of intracranial hemorrhage.

Dopamine

The role of dopamine in initial resuscitation is to increase cardiac contractility, cardiac output, and blood pressure. It is used when the newborn has failed to respond to epinephrine and other drug therapies. The optimal dose is between 5 to 15 µg/kg/min. A simple method for preparing this solution is to place 15 mg/kg of dopamine in 250 ml of D5W or D10W.[36] An infusion of 1 ml/hr equals the dose of 1 µg/kg/min.

Naloxone

Naloxone hydrochloride (Narcan) is indicated when there is severe respiratory depression and a history of maternal narcotic administration within the previous 4 hours. The dose is 0.1 mg/kg of a 0.4-mg/ml or 1.0-mg/ml concentration to be given rapidly intravenously, intramuscularly, subcutaneously, or through an endotracheal tube.[37] This can be repeated if respiratory depression recurs. If naloxone is given to the infant of a drug-addicted mother, it may precipitate seizures.

Glucose

Hypoglycemia can occur during resuscitation but most frequently arises after stabilization. It is common in premature infants and in those who are small for their gestational age, following prolonged and difficult labor, in infants of mothers on ritodrine or terbutaline drips, and in infants of diabetic mothers. Hypoxia, hypothermia, hyperthermia, and sepsis also consume glucose stores. Symptoms may not be present or may vary from simple jitteriness and lethargy to hypotonia, seizures, and cyanosis. The strict definition of hypoglycemia is a plasma glucose level of less than 25 mg/dl in a premature infant and less than 35 mg/dl in a term infant in the first 72 hours of life. However, if the newborn is symptomatic without a known cause and a bedside Dextrostick or Accu-Check glucose determination is less than or equal to 40 mg/dl, therapy should be instituted after a "crash" blood glucose test is made. The dose is 1 to 2 ml/kg of D10W IV push. If symptoms abate, then a continuous infusion of 6 to 8 mg/kg/min should be maintained.[38]

DISPOSITION

All newborns require admission. Consequently, as soon as delivery is anticipated, the pediatrician or neonatologist should be consulted. All resuscitated neonates need not be admitted to an intensive care nursery, especially if the resuscitation required only momentary PPV. However, there are a few situations that require neonatal intensive care monitoring (i.e., ventilator capabilities). These include gestational age less than 30 to 32 weeks; weight less than 1025 grams; use of mechanical ventilation for more than 24 hours; major nonlethal congenital anomalies; neonatal seizures; surgically correctable conditions; asphyxia with multisystem involvement (CNS, pulmonary, renal, gastrointestinal, or hematologic compromise); and persistent cyanosis, hypoxia, or hypoglycemia.[39]

Whenever neonates are transported, even after stabilization, they may deteriorate further because of the environmental stress of transport. Consequently, the situation can be optimized by spending the least amount of time possible in transport either by air or ground.

OTHER CONSIDERATIONS

The legal aspects of neonatal resuscitation are overwhelming. In some states, the physician responsible for the infant's initial care is liable for any damages until the child is 18 years old. In addition to excellent team coordination toward the resuscitation effort, clear and concise documentation must be emphasized. Only through the medical records will the court system be able to judge whether malpractice occurred.

A final topic concerns termination of resuscitation. Currently there are no clear-cut guidelines. However, it is generally considered that problems with inadequate ventilation, shock, and any metabolic disturbance should be corrected and reassessed. Maximal cardiopulmonary resuscitation should continue until a successful outcome is considered impossible. In an apparently normal term infant, this may be after about 1 hour of resuscitation.[12] Current data report a higher mortality rate as the response time from birth becomes longer, although a substantial number of survivors of prolonged resuscitation have had a satisfactory long-term outcome. Ultimately, termination is the responsibility of each emergency physician. It is indeed a serious decision that requires personal forethought regarding what to do when faced with this situation.

References

1. Hospital Statistics, 1989–1990. Chicago, American Hospital Association, 1989.
2. Suille H (ed). Vital Statistics of the U.S. Department of Health and Human Services National Center for Health Statistics. Vol 2. 1987.
3. Infant and Perinatal Mortality Rates, 1976–1980; 1981–1985. Vienna, VA, Maternal and Child Health Studies Project.
4. Bloom RS, Cropley C (eds). Textbook of Neonatal Resuscitation. Chicago, IL, American Heart Association/American Academy of Pediatrics, 1987.
5. Schafermeyer RW. Neonatal resuscitation. In Fleischer G, Ludwig S (eds). Textbook of Pediatric Emergency Medicine. Baltimore, Williams & Wilkins, 1985, pp 31–34.
6. Fanaroff AA, Martin RJ. Diseases of the Fetus and Infant. 4th ed. St. Louis, CV Mosby, 1987, pp 360–368.
7. McKluein RE, Ostshmeimer GW. Resuscitation of the newborn. Clin Obstet Gynecol 1987;30(3):611.
8. Lamb FS, Rosner MS. Neonatal resuscitation. Emerg Med Clin North Am 1987;5:541.
9. Stevenson DK, Frankel PR, Benitz WE. Immediate management of the asphyxiated infant: Facilitating the cardiorespiratory transition from fetus to newborn. J Perinatol 1987; 7:221.
10. Fisher DE, Paton JB. Resuscitation of the newborn infant. In Klaus MN, Fanaroff AA (eds). Care of the High-Risk Neonate. 3rd ed. Philadelphia, WB Saunders, 1986, p 23.
11. Welch KA, Philips JB. Management of the depressed newborn. Clin Obstet Gynecol 1984;27:125.

12. Edwards MC. Delivery room resuscitation of the neonate. Pediatr Ann 1988;17:458.
13. Benitz WE, Sunshine P. Neonatal resuscitation. *In* Nelson MN (ed). Current Therapy, Neonatal Perinatal Medicine. 1985–1986. St. Louis, CV Mosby, 1985, p 360.
14. Stine MJ. Neonatal resuscitation: Review and update. Indiana Med 1985; 78:1001.
15. Boychuk RB. Resuscitation of the newborn. Hawaii Med J 1984;43:79.
16. Britton JR. Resuscitation of the newborn infant. J Emerg Med 1984;2:95.
17. Palme C, Nyström B, Tunell R. An evaluation of the efficiency of face masks in the resuscitation of newborn infants. Lancet 1985;1:207.
18. Brocks TD, Graunstein N. Pulse oximetry for early detection of hypoxemia in anesthetized infants. J Clin Monit 1985;1:135.
19. Deckardt R, Steward DJ. Noninvasive arterial hemoglobin oxygen saturation versus transcutaneous oxygen tension monitoring in the preterm infant. Crit Care Med 1984;12:935.
20. Harris AP, Sendak MJ, Donham RT. Changes in arterial oxygen saturation immediately after birth in the human neonate. J Pediatr 1986;109:117.
21. Maxwell LG, Harris AP, Sendak MJ, Donham RT. Monitoring the resuscitation of preterm infants in the delivery room using pulse oximetry. Clin Pediatr 1987;26:18.
22. Lucky J, Vidyasagar D. The value of Apgar scores. Indian J Pediatr 1987;54:679.
23. Use and abuse of the Apgar score. Committee on Fetus and Newborn. American Academy of Pediatrics. Pediatrics 1986;78:1148.
24. Gregory GA, Gooding CA, Phibbs RH, et al. Meconium aspiration in infants: A prospective study. J Pediatr 1974;85:848.
25. Carson BS, Simmons MA, Bowes WA. Meconium aspiration syndrome following cesarian section. Am J Obstet Gynecol 1978;130:596.
26. Frazer LE. Modified apparatus for aspiration of meconium from the airway. Pediatrics 1982;70:307.
27. Demmler GJ, Brady MT. Cytomegalovirus and neonatal resuscitation. Pediatr Infect Dis 1986; 5:605.
28. Ballard JL, Musial MJ, Myers MG. Hazards of delivery room resuscitation using oral methods of endotracheal suctioning. Pediatr Infect Dis Mar 1989;55:190.
29. Avery GB. Neonatology, Pathophysiology and Management of the Newborn. 2nd ed. Philadelphia, JB Lippincott, 1981.
30. Pernoll ML, Benda GI, Babson SG. Diagnosis and Management of the Fetus and Neonate at Risk. St Louis, CV Mosby, 1986, pp 87–103.
31. Harris V. Face mask resuscitation of the newborn. Indian J Pediatr 1989;54:614.
32. David R. Closed chest cardiac massage in the newborn infant. Pediatrics 1988;81:552.
33. Finholt DA, Kettrick RG, Wagner HR, Swedlow DB. The heart is under the lower third of the sternum. Am J Dis Child 1986;140:546.
34. Phillips GWL, Zideman DA. Relation of infant heart to sternum: Its significance in cardiopulmonary resuscitation. Lancet 1986;1:1024.
35. Lindemann R. Resuscitation of the newborn. Endotracheal administration of epinephrine. Acta Paediatr Scand 1984;73:210.
36. Benitz WE, Frankel LR, Stevenson DK. The pharmacology of neonatal resuscitation and cardiopulmonary intensive care. Part II. Extended intensive care. West J Med 1986;145:47.
37. Naloxone dosages and route of administration for infants and children: Addendum to emergency drug doses for infants and children. Committee on Drugs. Pediatrics 1990;86:484.
38. Benitz WE, Frankel LR, Stevenson DK. The pharmacology of neonatal resuscitation and cardiopulmonary intensive care. Part I. Immediate resuscitation. West J Med 1986;144:704.
39. Bartoletti AL. Defining the indications for neonatal transport in a perinatal referral network. *In* MacDonald MG, Miller MK (eds). Emergency Transport of the Perinatal Patient. Boston, Little, Brown, 1989, pp 332–341.

CHAPTER 5

Basic Pediatric Resuscitation

Raymond E. Jackson

INTRODUCTION

Basic cardiopulmonary resuscitation (CPR) encompasses the concepts and techniques that form the foundation of

---

TABLE 5–1

CAUSES OF CARDIOPULMONARY ARREST IN CHILDREN

Sudden infant death syndrome (SIDS)
Foreign body aspiration
Drownings
Intrinsic upper airway obstruction (supraglottitis)
Status asthmaticus
Intracranial hypertension
Smoke inhalation
Carbon monoxide poisoning
Electric shock
Accidental overdose
Vascular collapse secondary to trauma
Hypovolemia
Sepsis

---

effective emergency care. The purpose of cardiopulmonary resuscitation is to provide artificial circulation of oxygenated blood to the vital organs, especially the heart and brain, in an attempt to halt the degenerative processes associated with ischemia and anoxia until spontaneous circulation can be restored. The goal of resuscitation is to preserve the function of those key organs.[1] Basic life support alone may be lifesaving in some instances. In situations in which more advanced interventions are essential to the resuscitation of a child, basic resuscitation may be of some benefit. The most critical factor in determining the success of resuscitative efforts is the time from arrest to the return of an effective spontaneous circulation.

Cardiac arrest in children is an uncommon event that primarily results from respiratory compromise or as an end-stage manifestation of shock.[2] Less than 2% of all resuscitation patients who present to the emergency department are younger than 10 years, and most pediatric patients with respiratory or cardiac arrest are younger than 1 year (Table 5–1).[3–5] The presenting rhythms are most likely to be asystole, idioventricular rhythm, electromechanical dissociation, or bradycardia.[6–9] In pediatric patients without a history of congenital or acquired cardiac disease or a history of drug ingestion, a primary cardiac event such as ventricular tachycardia or fibrillation is rare.[9–12] This consideration does not alter the initial basic approach to the pediatric patient by the emergency physician. The focus of the pediatric resuscitation is on airway management and, if applicable, rehydration.

OUTCOME

Factors that may determine outcome include the location of the arrest (i.e., in the hospital or in an out-of-hospital setting).[13] Cardiac arrest may be secondary to prolonged anoxic-ischemic times in children who experience an out-of-hospital arrest. Unlike prehospital CPR in adults, prehospital CPR in children seems to have a positive effect on outcome.[7, 13, 14] This may be because of the role of ventilation in improving respiratory acidosis in children, whereas in adults, the time to defibrillation, a relatively more advanced intervention, is the most important factor. An isolated respiratory arrest has a better patient prognosis than a complete cardiac arrest, which has a high mortality rate in all series.[15–18] A patient presenting with bradycardia has a more favorable prognosis than one presenting with asystole.[13, 15] Although the pathophysiologic mechanisms leading to these rhythms are most likely related, asystole probably represents a more severe and prolonged anoxic-ischemic insult. In an experimental asphyxial arrest model in infant piglets, the time elapsed from asphyxiation to asystole was 5 minutes.[19] The pulseless bradycardia patient may retain weak cardiac activity[20] that may respond to ventilation and oxygenation. The resuscitation rate and survival rate of children with these rhythms are similar to those of adults. Successful resuscitation using only ventilation, oxygen, and closed chest compression have the best outcome rate, a reflection of good myocardial viability at the onset of the resuscitation.[13, 16]

The preceding indicators and the rhythm and presence of pulses reflect the duration of the anoxic-ischemic arrest and subsequent resuscitation. Time is the most important variable: resuscitative efforts that last less than 15 minutes have improved short-term survival,[13] and those lasting less than 5 minutes have better long-term outcomes.[9] An initial arterial pH of less than 7.0 is a negative prognostic finding, reflecting the severity of the anoxic-ischemic insult.[7] The final neurologic outcome tends to be poor in prolonged resuscitations, although cases of good neurologic outcome have been documented following up to 30 minutes of closed chest massage.[21]

ANATOMY AND PHYSIOLOGY OF RESUSCITATION

Regardless of the origin of arrest, once the heart has ceased to pump oxygenated blood, a series of biochemical and physiologic events are initiated that can rapidly lead to an irreversible state resulting in obligatory cell death. Therefore rapid application of a technique that supplies an adequate flow of oxygenated blood is crucial.

Hemodynamics

Closed chest compression produces, in the vast majority of cases, a severe low-flow state. In experimental animals, optimal cardiac outputs have ranged from 17% to 27% of the pre-arrest values.[1] The mean cardiac index in a few patients who have had cardiac output determinations during closed chest compression is 0.76 L/min/m^2, which is approximately 25% of the normal resting cardiac index in adults and is even less than that found in severe cardiogenic shock.[22] There are no data on cardiac output in children during closed chest compression.

Successful resuscitation from experimental arrest is strongly dependent on myocardial perfusion.[23–25] Diastolic pressure is the driving force for coronary blood flow during closed chest compression; it may be as high as 20 to 40 mm Hg if closed chest compression is immediately applied at the onset of arrest, but rapidly falls to below 20 mm Hg despite continuous chest compressions.[26, 27] The likelihood of a successful resuscitation attempt is small with a diastolic pressure below 40 mm Hg,[25, 28] because at this pressure coronary blood flow and myocardial perfusion are extremely low, typically around 5% of the pre-arrest values.[29, 30] There is a strong positive linear correlation among diastolic blood pressure, coronary blood flow, and myocardial perfusion.[24, 26, 31] Therefore maneuvers that improve coronary perfusion pressure may improve resuscitation rates. Cerebral blood flow is also low during closed chest compressions.[30, 32] In general, if closed chest compressions can be initiated at the time of collapse, hemodynamic parameters are not as poor as depicted[27, 33] but rapidly deteriorate without adrenergic support.[30]

Mechanism of Flow Generation

How the application of force onto the thoracic cage induces movement of blood is a subject of great interest. A liquid flows in a closed system when a pressure gradient is developed. Flow does occur during closed chest compression, and therefore a pressure gradient is generated by this technique. There are two theories to explain how the pressure gradient develops during chest compressions: the cardiac pump theory and the thoracic pump theory.

The *cardiac pump theory* was first formulated by Kouwenhoven and states that the pressure gradient developed is within the heart, across the valves as with normal spontaneous circulation[34, 35]; this is accomplished by direct compression of the heart between the sternum and spine. A pressure gradient from the aorta to the right atrium would be evident during the actual compression of the chest. Competent cardiac values are an essential component of this theory.[36, 37] Evidence for this theory has been enhanced by high-impulse CPR, which uses a higher force than is normally applied and at a higher rate, with a longer relative time devoted to the compression phase (duty cycle). This results in augmented cardiac output and coronary and cerebral blood flows.[38–40]

The observation that there is no pressure gradient from the aorta to the right atrium during closed chest compression led to the theory that forward flow is generated by a intrathoracic-to-extrathoracic pressure gradient; this is known as the *thoracic pump theory*.[41] During the compression (systolic) phase of standard closed chest compression, all intrathoracic pressures are equal, while at the same time there is a pressure gradient from the intrathoracic arterial vessels to the extrathoracic arterial vessels.[41, 42] Only during the relaxation (diastolic) phase of the cycle does an aorta-to–right atrium pressure gradient develop.[43] This pressure gradient is also the diastolic coronary perfusion pressure, which is the major determinant of coronary blood flow during closed chest compression.

Further evidence supporting the thoracic pump mechanism is obtained from observations with two-dimensional echocardiography in adults during closed chest compression showing that the ventricular volumes do not change with compression and the mitral and aortic valves remain open during compression.[44, 45] Cineangiography in animal models shows that the mitral and aortic valves are incompetent during compression, with no evidence of ventricular compression[24, 45, 46] and a reduction in the cross-sectional diameter of the thoracic aorta during compression.[47] Vascular pressure measurements during adult closed chest compression support the thoracic pump model.[48] Aortic blood flow occurs during compression, whereas pulmonary and coronary blood flow take place during the relaxation phase.[42]

The thoracic pump mechanism generates blood flow by creating an intrathoracic-to-extrathoracic pressure gradient. This is most evident with cerebral blood flow. Valves in the jugular venous system prevent the transmission of intrathoracic pressure to the venous side of the central nervous system (CNS) vasculature during compression.[49] Maneuvers that increase systolic intrathoracic pressures should, in theory, increase the carotid artery–to–jugular vein pressure gradient and, subsequently, cerebral blood flow.[50]

The relative roles of the thoracic pump and direct cardiac compression mechanisms in the generation of blood flow in children probably vary from patient to patient and among different age groups.[48, 51] With the high chest wall compliance found in infants, it is possible that direct cardiac compressions may occur during adequately performed chest compression. Evidence from animal investigations suggests that in the younger patient, direct cardiac compression occurs,[36] and increasing the duration of compression augments flow.[52–54] However, increasing the rate of compressions does not significantly alter flow.[52–54] Maneuvers that increase intrathoracic pressure during compression have limited effect in the experimental model of infant resuscitation.[33]

In older children and adults, who have less chest wall compliance, the thoracic pump mechanism is more likely to be in effect. In this case, increasing the rate of compressions augments cardiac output and increasing intrathoracic pressures may also improve cerebral blood flow. Regardless of the mechanism, increasing the rate and depth of compressions, along with prolonging the relative time of compression, may be beneficial to improving forward flow.

EMERGENCY MEDICAL SERVICE CONSIDERATIONS

It is not known what percentage of pediatric patients who experience an out-of-hospital arrest come to the emergency department by car, rather than by ambulance. In a large urban setting, 1% of all pediatric calls and 0.1% of all ambulance runs involved a pediatric cardiac arrest.[4] The amount of training received by paramedics is minimal, and retention of this training in regard to resuscitation of children is a concern.[4] Ample and precise stocking of the mobile units for emergency pediatric care is often deficient.[4] Pediatric Ambu bags and endotracheal tubes are necessary equipment for every prehospital advanced life support unit. Because early basic cardiopulmonary resuscitation of children may have a beneficial effect, efforts to enhance the quality of prehospital care may positively affect outcome.

THERAPEUTIC INTERVENTION

The initial clinical evaluation of these children is brief and focuses on the presence or abscence of respirations and pulses. Clinical evaluation and patient management are done concurrently.

The application of effective cardiopulmonary resuscitation demands a methodical approach to assess the child's condition rapidly and adequately and ensure effective delivery of care. Table 5–2 lists eight maneuvers that, when performed in a stepwise fashion, enable the care provider to quickly evaluate the need for and intensity of intervention.[55-60]

Establish Unresponsiveness and Obtain Assistance

The first step in assessing a child who has collapsed is to establish the level of responsiveness. This is accomplished by providing some form of noxious stimulus.

Once it has been established that the child is unresponsive, the initial rescuer should call for help and activate the emergency medical service (EMS) system if the arrest has occurred outside the hospital. This step is critical, as it is the time from arrest to the institution of advanced resuscitation procedures (e.g., intubation) that most affects outcome.

TABLE 5–2
APPROACH TO THE UNRESPONSIVE CHILD
1. Establish unresponsiveness.
2. Obtain assistance; activate EMS system.
3. Properly position the patient.
4. Open the airway.
5. Establish breathlessness.
6. Ventilate the patient.
7. Establish presence or absence of pulse.
8. Perform closed chest compressions.

Open the Airway

With loss of muscle tone in the obtunded patient, the tongue may fall back into the oropharynx and cause an upper airway obstruction. The negative pressure generated during inspiratory efforts can force the tongue back into the oropharynx, creating a one-way valve effect and occluding the airway during inspiration. This will manifest as stridor. One of three simple maneuvers is initially used to open the airway and relieve upper airway obstruction.

The *head tilt* is the first maneuver that should be attempted and is accomplished by placing one hand beneath the child's neck and the other hand on the forehead. The neck is then flexed in relation to the thorax and the head extended in relation to the neck (the so-called *sniffing position*). Hyperextension of the neck in relation to the thorax is not helpful and may worsen obstruction. If the head tilt is unsuccessful, the chin lift or jaw thrust should be applied. Both of these maneuvers should be executed along with the head tilt and are very effective in lifting the tongue out of the oropharynx by displacing the mandible, to which the tongue is connected.

The preferred method for opening the airway in young children is the *chin-lift* maneuver, in which the hand that had been supporting the neck is placed under the symphysis of the mandible, which is then lifted forward and up until the teeth barely touch. In a child it is important to be careful not to compress the soft tissues at the base of the tongue, which could increase the obstruction.

The *jaw thrust* also elevates the tongue by means of mandibular displacement. With the rescuer positioned at the head of the patient, the hands are placed at the sides of the victim's face, grasping the angles of the mandible and lifting the mandible forward. The rescuer may rest his or her elbows on the surface on which the patient lies.

Establish Breathlessness and Begin Ventilation

When there is no evidence of air movement or chest expansion, artificial ventilations should be immediately instituted. The rescuer places his or her open mouth around the child's mouth and nose, making an airtight seal, and then forcibly exhales air into the patient's airway. The volume delivered should be 10 to 15 ml/kg. Larger tidal volumes, as well as rapid insufflation, should be avoided because of the danger of creating (1) gastric distention with subsequent regurgitation and aspiration or (2) barotrauma resulting in a pneumothorax. Two breaths are delivered initially, allowing adequate time for exhalation. The rescuer's expired air has an FIO_2 of 16% to 17% and therefore resources that are able to deliver higher oxygen concentrations are needed as soon as possible. With these two initial breaths, the rescuer watches the child's chest to determine whether it rises with each forced inhalation and falls with the end of forced inhalation. Any observed impairment to airflow during rescue breathing indicates either an obstruction of air flow in the upper airway or a serious restriction to lung expansion such as a tension pneumothorax. If lack of chest wall motion is noted or there is a large amount of resistance to flow, the oropharynx must be inspected for an obstruction, and efforts to relieve the obstruction should be executed.

With severe maxillofacial trauma, mouth-to-nose ventilation may be more effective than mouth-to-mouth. This is done by using the jaw-thrust maneuver to lift the tongue from the posterior oropharynx and sealing the mouth shut with the thumb and forefinger during inhalation. The mouth is opened during exhalation to diminish the resistance to airflow. Patients with stomas or tracheostomies are ventilated by placing the mouth over the stoma or tracheostomy tube.

Foreign Body Obstruction

Foreign bodies may cause either partial or complete airway obstruction. With partial airway obstruction, the victim may be capable of air exchange. With good air exchange, the patient may have a cough, although there may be wheezing or stridor between coughs; drooling may be present. As long as adequate air exchange continues, spontaneous coughing and breathing should be encouraged. The rescuer should not interfere with attempts to expel the foreign body. The child with partial airway obstruction and sufficient airway movement should not be turned upside down, as this may drive a tracheal foreign body against the vocal cords.

Poor air exchange is characterized by a weak, ineffective cough, marked respiratory stridor, and respiratory distress. The patient may look ashen, and mental status will be altered. The patient should be managed as for a complete obstruction.

With complete airway obstruction, the child is unable to speak, breathe, or cough. If still conscious, the older child may clutch his or her neck; this is the universal distress signal. In an unconscious victim, a complete obstruction is identified by resistance to artificial ventilation and a lack of rise and fall of the chest with each attempted ventilation.

Maneuvers for Relieving Obstruction. The maneuvers recommended for relieving foreign body obstruction are the finger sweep, back blows, manual thrusts, and direct removal of the object. The sequence in which these maneuvers should be executed is as follows: check the oropharynx and finger sweep; apply back blows; apply manual thrusts; then repeat the cycle until the obstruction is cleared.[58, 61-63] If at any time the object appears in the oropharynx, it is then removed manually. Back blows produce an instantaneous increase in airway pressure, which may result in either partial or complete dislodgement of the foreign body. Manual thrusts develop a lower but more sustained increase in pressure and may further assist in dislodging the object. Combining these techniques appears to be more effective than using any one alone.

The back blow technique is a series of four rapid, sharp blows delivered over the spine and between the scapulae with the heel of the hand. They may be given with the child standing, sitting, or lying and should be applied forcibly and rapidly. Whenever possible, the patient's head should be slightly lower than the chest to enlist the aid of gravity.

The manual thrust method, or Heimlich maneuver, may be used in children older than 1 year. This maneuver consists of four thrusts to the upper abdomen or lower chest. The low chest thrust develops somewhat higher flows and peak pressure. The abdominal thrust can be performed with the child sitting or standing. In a younger child, place a fist between the umbilicus and the xiphoid process and press forcibly upward four times. The rescuer may also be positioned behind the child with the arms wrapped around the waist. After making a fist with one hand, placing the thumb side of the fist into the epigastrium, and grasping the fist with the other hand, the rescuer delivers four quick upward thrusts. A victim who is lying prone must be placed in the supine position before the airway is opened. The rescuer can be either astride or alongside the patient. The heel of one hand is placed in the epigastrium and covered with the heel of the other hand. A quick upward thrust may then be delivered. Complications of abdominal thrusts include rupture or laceration of abdominal viscera.

Chest thrusts are performed in a similar manner when the victim is lying or sitting, with the fist placed directly on the sternum. When the victim is supine, the hands should be placed over the sternum, as in closed chest compression, and compressed four times. The chest thrust is useful, as it may be less likely to cause complications.

If these attempts are unsuccessful, rescue breathing should begin. Direct visualization should be attempted as soon as possible.

Establish Pulselessness and Begin Compressions

After the two initial ventilations, the presence of a pulse is determined by palpating either the carotid or the femoral artery. To palpate the carotid, place the index and middle fingers on the trachea and then slide them between the trachea and the sternocleidomastoid muscle. If no pulse is felt or if the pulse is slow or weak, closed-chest compression should begin immediately.

The closed-chest compression technique varies with the age of the patient.[50, 55, 64, 65] When using two-person CPR in an infant, the chest is grasped with both hands by one rescuer, with the thumbs resting on the lower third of the sternum (Fig. 5-1); the heart lies under the lower third of the sternum in all age groups.[50, 64, 65] The sternum is depressed 2.5 to 4.0 cm at a rate of 100 to 120 compressions/ min. The duty cycle (the percentage of the compression-relaxation cycle spent in compression) should be at least 60%. A ventilation should be delivered after every fifth compression. With only one rescuer, the child should be resting on a hard surface and the sternum compressed with the index and middle fingers. Two ventilations are delivered after every 15 compressions.

In preschool-age children, the same compression rate (100 to 120 compressions/min) and compression depth (2.5 to 4.0 cm) are used. In these children, however, compression is performed with the thenar eminence of one hand.

The school-aged child is placed supine on a firm surface, the xiphoid process is located, and the heel of one hand is placed on the sternum one to two inches cephalad to the xiphoid. The other hand is brought to rest on top of the hand that is on the sternum. The rescuer is positioned over the sternum with the arms straight and the elbows locked and forces the sternum straight downward 3 to 5 cm at a rate of 80 to 120 compressions/min. With two rescuers, a ventilation is delivered after every fifth compression; with one rescuer, two ventilations are delivered after every 15 compressions. Compressions and ventilations are continued until circulation has been restored or efforts are stopped by the physician in charge.

DIAGNOSTIC EVALUATION

Ancillary tests play only a secondary role in the initial management of pediatric resuscitation. A rapid bedside evaluation of the serum glucose level is essential. If there is evidence of a pneumothorax on examination (e.g., decreased breath sounds, subcutaneous emphysema, or difficulty bagging), a chest radiograph can be performed to confirm the clinical suspicion. However, a needle thoracostomy is an appropriate diagnostic and therapeutic maneuver. Continuous observation of the cardiac monitor is essential.

If the resuscitative efforts are successful, the clinician should begin an evaluation to determine the origin of the event. This includes a history and a complete physical examination. A complete blood cell count; determination of electrolyte, calcium, magnesium, blood urea nitrogen (BUN), creatinine, and glucose levels; and measurement of prothrombin partial thromboplastin times should be performed. Blood, urine, and CSF cultures should be obtained if indicated, and a chest radiograph and electrocardiogram should be obtained. Most of these tests will reflect the

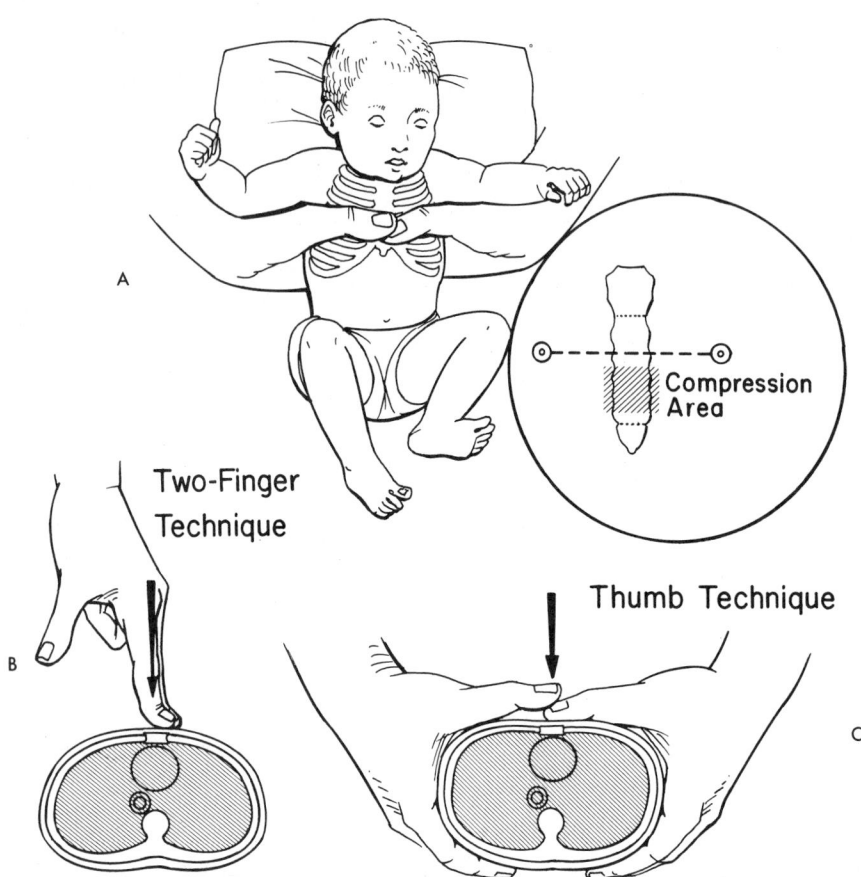

Two-Finger Technique

Thumb Technique

Compression Area

Figure 5–1. CPR hand positions. *A,* Location of compressions in the lower third of the sternum. *B,* Proper finger position. *C,* Proper thumb position. (From Blumer JL. A Practical Guide to Pediatric Intensive Care. 3rd ed. St. Louis, Mosby-Year Book, 1990, p 44.)

underlying condition of the child. Arterial blood gases often indicate a serious respiratory acidosis and possibly concurrent metabolic acidosis.[7]

DOCUMENTATION

The completeness of physician documentation of resuscitative events should differ little from the usual high standard of the typical emergency department visit. Particular attention is paid to the timing of events leading to the discovery of the unresponsive child, the method of transportation, what efforts were made prior to arrival at the hospital, and the times and timing of the resuscitative efforts in the prehospital setting. The emergency department chart should indicate the initial respiratory and cardiac status, airway management, type of cardiac compression, type and timing of interventions, and why each therapeutic decision was made. The timing of invasive procedures should be noted. Flow sheets are helpful in documenting the course of events, with attention paid to the heart rhythm, skin color, presence of pulses, spontaneous respirations, blood pressure, medications, and procedures. A member of the emergency team should be assigned to document these events. The use of audiotaping or bar coding of the events is being explored in both the prehospital and in-hospital resuscitation settings to assess the ease and accuracy of these methods in recording these intensive events.[65a]

An accurate history of the events leading to the arrest are important but often difficult to obtain. If there is more than one physician on duty, a second physician should be with the parents and obtain the history of events leading to the arrest. Any pertinent medical history, such as diabetes, asthma, or cardiac or airway disease, and any medications that the child (or anyone else in the family) may be taking should be elicited. If another physician is unavailable, a nurse should be assigned as the family contact.

The examination should note the general appearance of the child, the presence or absence of cyanosis or pallor, evidence of rigor mortis, and evidence of trauma. Breath sounds should be noted at multiple intervals during the resuscitation. Pupillary reflexes should be noted, although they may not have any predictive value. Any sign of abuse must also be sought.

Results of all interventions, laboratory tests, and radiographs should be documented. Admission to a pediatric intensive care unit after a successful resuscitation is mandatory and often requires transportation to a tertiary care facility accompanied by a transport team. The documentation of the disposition should also be complete and should include the admission or transfer destination and the name of the physician who assumed responsibility for the patient's care. If the patient is transferred, the risk-to-benefit considerations should be documented and patient consent obtained.

OTHER CONSIDERATIONS

Training

Efforts to teach CPR techniques to families of children at risk for cardiac or respiratory events should be encouraged.[66] This may aid in the recognition of a potentially lethal event and may have a positive effect on outcome. All medical personnel should be familiar with and have demonstrated competency in pediatric resuscitation.

Complications of Closed Chest Massage

Complications of closed chest compression include sternal and rib fractures, pulmonary contusion, and pneumothorax. Myocardial contusions, primarily of the right ventricle, have been noted to result in acute right ventricular failure. Hemorrhagic pericardial effusions have also been observed. Gastric distention, erosions, and rupture have occurred.[67] The incidence of liver laceration is approximately 2%. Regurgitation and aspiration pneumonia are frequent complications.[68] Retinal hemorrhages may occur secondary to high jugular venous pressures transmitted to the central retinal vein during closed chest compressions and are not necessarily the result of abuse.[69] Careful performance of basic closed chest technique can diminish, but cannot totally abolish, many of these complications.

Late complications include development of pulmonary edema, electrolyte abnormalities, gastrointestinal hemorrhage, pneumonia, bacteremia from ischemic bowel, and recurrent cardiopulmonary arrest.[70] Anoxic encephalopathy is the major cause of death in resuscitated patients.

Terminating Resuscitative Efforts

Resuscitative efforts should be continued until ventilation and circulation are restored, the patient is transported to a hospital setting, the rescuer becomes exhausted, or a physician resumes responsibility for the patient. The decision by the physician to terminate resuscitation is dependent on the history of events leading to the arrest, the amount of time before onset of resuscitative efforts, the effects of interventions, the heart rhythm at presentation, and the duration of resuscitative efforts. Emotion can also play a role in the decision to halt efforts, potentially prolonging efforts in children. Success in resuscitation is time dependent, with a dismal long-term outcome in efforts that last longer than 30 minutes in patients experiencing normothermic arrest.[13, 21]

Pediatric resuscitation is often an emotionally traumatic event, even for experienced, seasoned emergency personnel. Efforts should be made to provide emotional support not only for the family, but also for the physicians and nurses who aided in the resuscitative efforts.

An autopsy should always be obtained in unsuccessful resuscitation attempts. Child abuse is a haunting consideration in the untimely and unexpected death of a child.

SUMMARY

The pediatric cardiac arrest is an uncommon event that demands exceptional attention to the details of resuscitative technique. Most cases of cardiac arrest follow an episode of respiratory compromise. These are most often a bradycardic-asystolic arrest. Outcomes are generally poor except in patients in whom the resuscitation times were short and the interventions involved were no more than ventilation and compression. Closed chest compression and ventilation offer benefit in children. The mechanism for the generation of blood flow is most likely direct cardiac compression in young infants and either a combination of direct compression and the thoracic pump mechanism or the thoracic pump mechanism only in older children. Improvements in resuscitation in the future will result from efforts that reduce the anoxic-ischemic times. These include training families of children at risk and improvements in prehospital care.

References

1. Jackson R, Freeman S. Hemodynamics of cardiac massage. Emerg Med Clin North Am 1983;1:501.
2. Friesen R, Duncan P, Tweet W, et al. Appraisal of pediatric CPR. Can Med Assoc J 1982;126:1055.
3. DeBard ML. Cardiopulmonary resuscitation: Analysis of six years' experience and review of the literature. Ann Emerg Med 1981;10:408.
4. Foltin G, Salomon M, Tunik M, et al. Developing prehospital advanced life support for children: The New York City experience. Pediatr Emerg Care 1990;6:141.
5. Ludwig S, Fleisher G. Pediatric cardiopulmonary resuscitation: A review and a proposal. Pediatr Emerg Care 1985;1:40.
6. Eisenberg N, Bergner L, Hallstrom A. Epidemiology of cardiac arrest and resuscitation in children. Ann Emerg Med 1983;12:672.
7. Fiser DH, Wrape V. Outcome of cardiopulmonary resuscitation in children. Pediatr Emerg Care 1987;3:235.
8. Torphy DE, Minter MG, Thompson BM. Cardiopulmonary arrest and resuscitation in children. Am J Dis Child 1984;138:1099.
9. Bazilay Z, Somekh E, Boichis H. Pediatric cardiopulmonary resuscitation outcome. J Med 1988;19:229.
10. Vetter VL, Josephson ME, Horowitz LN. Idiopathic recurrent sustained ventricular tachycardia in a young population. Am J Cardiol 1981;47:315.
11. Rocchini AP, Chun PO, Dick M. Ventricular tachycardia in children. Am J Cardiol 1981;47:1091.
12. Pederson DH. Ventricular tachycardia and ventricular fibrillation in children. Circulation 1979;60:977.
13. Nichols DG, Kettrick RG, Swedlow DB, et al. Factors influencing outcome of cardiopulmonary resuscitation in children. Pediatr Emerg Care 1986;2:1.
14. Kowalski R, Thompson BM, Horwitz L, et al. Bystander CPR in prehospital course ventricular fibrillation. Ann Emerg Med 1984;13:1016.
15. Roberts D, Landolfo K, Light RB, et al. Early predictors of mortality for hospitalized patients suffering cardiopulmonary arrest. Chest 1990;97:413–419.
16. Zaritsky A, Nadkarni V, Getson, P, et al. CPR in children. Ann Emerg Med 1987;16:1107.
17. Zaritsky A. Selected concepts and controversies in pediatric cardiopulmonary resuscitation. Crit Care Clin 1980;4:735.
18. Lewis JK, Minter MG, Eshelman SJ, et al. Outcome of pediatric resuscitation. Ann Emerg Med 1983;12:297.
19. Caputo G, Delgado-Paredes C, Swedlow D. Anoxic cardiopulmonary arrest in a pediatric animal model: Clinical and laboratory correlates of duration. Pediatr Emerg Care 1985;1:57.
20. Bocka JJ, Overton DT, Hauser A. Electromechanical dissociation in human beings: An echocardiographic evaluation. Ann Emerg Med 1988;17:450.
21. Davies CR, Carrigan T, Wright JA, et al. Neurologic outcome following pediatric resuscitation. J Neurosci Nurs 1987;19:205.
22. Del Guercio LRM, Coomaraswamy RP, State D. Cardiac output and other hemodynamic variables during external cardiac massage in man. N Engl J Med 1963;269:1398.
23. Sanders AB, Meislin HW, Ewy GA. The physiology of cardiopulmonary resuscitation. JAMA 1985;252:3283.
24. Niemann JT, Haynes KS, Garner D, et al. Postcountershock pulseless rhythms: Response to CPR, artificial cardiac pacing and adrenergic agonists. Ann Emerg Med 1986;15:112–120.
25. Sanders AB, Ewy G, Taft TV. Prognostic and therapeutic importance of the aortic diastolic pressure in resuscitation from cardiac arrest. Crit Care Med 1984;12:871.
26. Ditchey RV, Winkler JV, Rhodes CA. Lack of coronary blood flow during closed-chest resuscitation. Circulation 1982;66:297.
27. Sharff JA, Pantley G, Noel E. Effect of time on regional organ perfusion during two methods of cardiopulmonary resuscitation. Ann Emerg Med 1984;13:649.
28. Redding J. Cardiopulmonary resuscitation: An algorithm and some pitfalls. Am Heart J 1979;98:788.
29. Bellamy RF, DeGuzman LR, Pedersen DC. Coronary blood flow during cardiopulmonary resuscitation in swine. Circulation 1984;69:174.
30. Brown CG, Werman HA. Adrenergic agonists during cardiopulmonary resuscitation. Resuscitation 1990;19:1.
31. Chandra N, Tsitlik J, Weisfeldt M, et al. Augmentation of carotid blood flow during cardiopulmonary resuscitation at high airway pressures simultaneous with chest compressions. Am J Cardiol 1981;98:1053.
32. Jackson RE, Joyce K, Danosi S, et al. Blood flow in the cerebral cortex during cardiac resuscitation in dogs. Ann Emerg Med 1984;13:657.
33. Berkowitz ID, Chantarojanasiri T, Koehler RC, et al. Blood flow during cardiopulmonary resuscitation with simultaneous compression and ventilation in infant pigs. Pediatr Res 1989;26:558.
34. Kouwenhoven WB, Jude JR, Knickerbocker CG. Closed chest cardiac massage. JAMA 1960;173:1064.
35. Jude JR, Kouwenhoven WB, Knickerbocker CG. Cardiac arrest: Report of application of external cardiac massage on 118 patients. JAMA 1961;178:1063.
36. Deshmukh H, Weil M, Gudipati C, et al. Mechanism of blood flow generated by precordial compression during CPR: I. Studies on closed-chest precordial compression. Chest 1989;95:1092.
37. Hackl W, Simon P, Mauritz W, et al. Echocardiographic assessment of mitral valve function during mechanical cardiopulmonary resuscitation in pigs. Anesth Analg 1990;70:350.

38. Newton JR, Glower DD, Wolfe JA, et al. A physiologic comparison of external cardiac massage techniques. J Thorac Cardiovasc Surg 1988; 95:892.

39. Maier GW, Tyson GS Jr, Wolfe JA, et al. The influence of manual chest compression rate on hemodynamic support during cardiac arrest: High-impulse cardiopulmonary resuscitation. Circulation 1986;74(Pt 2):IV51.

40. Maier GW, Tyson GS, Olsen C, et al. The physiology of external cardiac massage: High impulse cardiopulmonary resuscitation. Circulation 1984;70:86.

41. Rudikoff M, Maughan W, Effron M, et al. Mechanism of blood flow during cardiopulmonary resuscitation. Circulation 1980;61:345.

42. Niemann JT, Rosborough J, Hausknecht M, et al. Blood flow without cardiac compression during closed-chest CPR. Crit Care Med 1981;9:380.

43. Niemann JT, Rosborough J, Ung S, et al. Coronary perfusion pressure during experimental cardiopulmonary resuscitation. Ann Emerg Med 1982;11:127.

44. Rich S, Wix H, Shapiro E. Clinical assessment of heart chamber size and valve motion during cardiopulmonary resuscitation by two dimensional echocardiogram. Am Heart J 1981;102:368.

45. Werner J, Greene H, Janko C, et al. Visualization of cardiac valve motion in man during external chest compression using two dimensional echocardiography. Implications regarding the mechanism of blood flow. Circulation 1981;63:1417.

46. Niemann JT, Rosborough JP, Hausknecht M, et al. Pressure synchronized cineangiography during experimental cardiopulmonary resuscitation. Circulation 1981;64:985.

47. Guerci AD, Halperin HR, Beyer R, et al. Aortic diameter and pressure-flow sequence identify mechanism of blood flow during external chest compression in dogs. J Am Coll Cardiol 1989;14:790.

48. Paradis NA, Martin GB, Goetting MG, et al. Simultaneous aortic, jugular bulb, and right atrial pressures during cardiopulmonary resuscitation in humans. Circulation 1989;80:361.

49. Goetting MG, Paradis NA. Right atrial-jugular venous pressure gradients during CPR in children. Ann Emerg Med 1991;20:27.

50. Berkowitz ID, Rogers M. The physiology of cerebral blood flow during cardiopulmonary resuscitation. Can J Anaesth 1988;35:S23.

51. Paradis MA, Martin GB, Rivers EP, et al. Coronary perfusion pressure and return of spontaneous circulation in human cardiopulmonary resuscitation. JAMA 1990;263:1106.

52. Dean JM, Koehler RC, Schleien CL, et al. Age-related effects of compression rate and duration in cardiopulmonary resuscitation. J Appl Physiol 1990;68:554.

53. Fitzgerald K, Babbs C, Frissura H, et al. Cardiac output during cardiopulmonary resuscitation at various compression rates and durations. Am J Physiol 1981;241:H442.

54. Fleisher G, Delgado-Paredes C, Heyman S. Slow versus rapid closed-chest cardiac compression during cardiopulmonary resuscitation in puppies. Crit Care Med 1987;15:939.

55. Standards and guidelines for cardiopulmonary resuscitation (CPR) and emergency cardiac care (ECC). JAMA 1986;255:2905.

56. Melker R. CPR in neonates, infants and children. Crit Care Q 1978;1:49.

57. Rosenberg N. Pediatric cardiac arrest. Emerg Med Clin North Am 1983;1:609.

58. Johnston C, Vacarella JS, McCloskey KA. Pediatric cardiopulmonary resuscitation. Indian J Pediatr 1988;55:715.

59. Tibballs J. Practical aspects of advanced paediatric cardiopulmonary resuscitation. Aust Paediatr J 1980;24:228.

60. Orlowski JP. Pediatric cardiopulmonary resuscitation. Emerg Med Clin North Am 1983;1:3.

61. Steicher FM, Fellini A, Einhorn AH. Acute foreign body laryngeal obstruction: A cause for sudden and unexpected death in children. Pediatrics 1975;48:281.

62. Greensher J. Emergency treatment of the choking child. J Pediatr 1982;70:110.

63. Redding J. The choking controversy. Critique and evidence on the Heimlich maneuver. Crit Care Med 1979;7:475.

64. Finholt DA, Kettrick RG, Wagner HR, et al. The heart is under the lower third of the sternum. Am J Dis Child 1986;140:646.

65. Orlowski JP. Optimum position for external cardiac compression in infants and young children. Ann Emerg Med 1986;15:667.

65a. Burt TW, Bock HC. Computerized MegaCode recording. Ann Emerg Med 1988;17:339.

66. Higgins SS, Hardy CE, Higashino SM. Should parents of children with congenital heart disease and life-threatening dysrhythmias be taught cardiopulmonary resuscitation? Pediatrics 1989;84:1102.

67. Custer JR, Polley TZ, Moler F. Gastric perforation following cardiopulmonary resuscitation in a child: Report of a case and review of the literature. Pediatr Emerg Care 1987;3:24.

68. Bjork R, Snyder B, Campion B, et al. Medical complications of cardiopulmonary arrest. Arch Intern Med 1982;142:500.

69. Goetting MG, Sowa B. Retinal hemorrhage after cardiopulmonary resuscitation in children: An etiologic reevaluation. Pediatrics 1990;85:585.

70. Gaussorgues P, Gueugniaud PY, Vedrinne JM, et al. Bacteremia following cardiac arrest and cardiopulmonary resuscitation. Intensive Care Med 1988;14:575.

CHAPTER 6

Advanced Pediatric Resuscitation

Ronald L. Rhule

INTRODUCTION

A well-trained resuscitation team is mandatory for the greatest chance for patient survival following cardiopulmonary arrest. A core of proficient emergency department nursing staff optimizes performance during the pediatric resuscitation. It is imperative to have specific pediatric "crash" carts with user-friendly information on pediatric drug doses available in the emergency department for the care of the critically ill child.[1, 2]

Emergent cardiopulmonary resuscitation (CPR) in children parallels the adult approach to resuscitation. The ultimate goal of CPR is to reestablish circulatory and ventilatory delivery of necessary metabolic substrates.[2, 3] In children, cardiac arrest is often the end result of a hypoxemic episode and the resulting acidosis (Table 6–1). The terminal cardiac rhythm is usually bradycardia followed by asystole. In the majority of pediatric cardiac arrests, the cascade of factors is respiratory distress, hypoxia, acidosis, bradycardia, and finally asystolic death.[2, 4, 5]

Survival statistics are extremely poor for pediatric cardiac arrests—less than 20% at best.[2, 4] Patients with respiratory arrest have a better survival rate. (Specifically, respiratory arrest has a 32.5% mortality rate, and cardiac arrest has a 90.6% mortality rate.) When resuscitation requires multiple doses of epinephrine or epinephrine coupled with bicarbonate during CPR, there is a low chance of survival (Fig. 6–1).[3, 4, 6–8]

Rapid intervention is mandated when respiratory distress is progressing. If early intervention and aggressive treatment prevent a pulseless state, the outcome of children in cardiac arrest is greatly improved. Therefore a specialized training plan is needed for physicians evaluating and treating children at risk.[3, 4, 9]

In the newborn patient, congenital, infectious, and metabolic catastrophes are the most likely causes of critical illness when the child is brought to the emergency department. In the first year of life, sudden infant death syndrome (SIDS) is the most common cause of death. In addition to SIDS,

TABLE 6–1
CAUSES OF CARDIOPULMONARY ARREST

Childhood arrest
  Usually the result of respiratory decline.
  Progression of hypoxia, acidosis, then arrest.
  The most common dysrhythmia is bradycardia, then asystole.
  Treatment is directed at correcting the respiratory problem.
  Respiratory arrest is treatable; cardiac arrest is usually fatal (>90%).
  Early intervention can improve survival by 70%.
Adult arrest
  Usually caused by cardiac disturbance.
  Most commonly fatal dysrhythmia is ventricular fibrillation.
  Treatment focuses on cardiac disturbances.

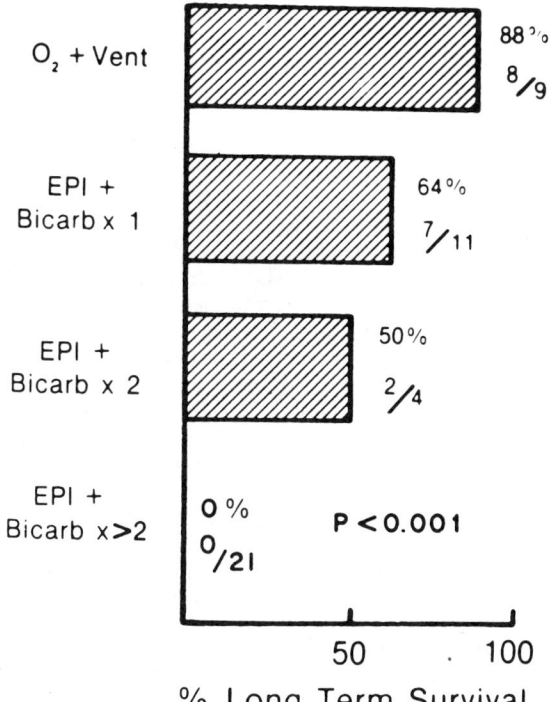

O₂ + Vent — 88% — 8/9

EPI + Bicarb × 1 — 64% — 7/11

EPI + Bicarb × 2 — 50% — 2/4

EPI + Bicarb ×>2 — 0% — 0/21 — P < 0.001

50   100

% Long Term Survival

Figure 6–1. Long-term survival rates based on magnitude of therapy. The increased magnitude of therapy measured by repeated administration of epinephrine and bicarbonate is associated with significantly lower long-term survival rates (P < .001). (From Nichols DG, Kettrick RG, Swedlow DB, et al. Factors influencing outcome of cardiopulmonary resuscitation in children. Pediatr Emerg Care 1986;2:1. © by Williams & Wilkins 1986.)

airway obstruction, infection, and trauma are likely to precipitate life-threatening events. Accidental or intentional trauma is also a cause of cardiac arrest in childhood. Worldwide, an unfortunate result of military conflict is an increased incidence of traumatic pediatric arrests.

The precipitating causes of cardiopulmonary embarrassment in children are manifold (Table 6–2). Most pediatric arrests can be anticipated in the patient with sepsis, respiratory compromise, acidosis, or hypovolemia.

ANTICIPATING THE ARREST

Progressive respiratory insufficiency accounts for 60% of all pediatric cardiopulmonary arrests. This is followed statistically by sepsis, dehydration, hypovolemia, acidosis, hypotension, and then asystole.

Respiratory failure in children is not typically a sudden event; rather, it is the result of a progressive decline. Therefore close monitoring of the respiratory status of critically ill children is warranted. Signs of respiratory obstruction, recruited use of accessory muscles of respiration, and labored breathing all signal respiratory distress. Cyanosis, poor feeding, and weak sucking patterns are also signs of early respiratory decompensation.

Although cardiac arrest is usually secondary to altered respiratory gas exchange, the child's myocardium is unusually resilient to hypoxemia.[5, 10] Correction of the respiratory component may be all that is required to resuscitate the ill child.

Dysrhythmia management is generally simple in pediatric resuscitation. The use of antiarrhythmic medications and defibrillation is unusual. The most frequent dysrhythmias seen are bradycardia and asystole.

Whether the cardiopulmonary arrest results from a pure respiratory decline or originates from hypovolemia, sepsis, or other shock states, the final result is the same: cardiopulmonary arrest (Fig. 6–2).[11] Shock-like syndromes are characterized by inadequate perfusion of tissue with oxygen and other metabolic substrates necessary to meet metabolic demands.[12–14] Ultimately, poor perfusion leads to delayed capillary refill time (>2 seconds), mottling, cyanosis, cool skin, flaccid muscle tone, an altered state of consciousness, and decreased urine output. Urine output is the most sensitive measurement of adequate core perfusion.

EMERGENCY MEDICAL SERVICE CONSIDERATIONS

Emergency medical service (EMS) care of critically ill children can be hampered by inadequately trained personnel and lack of properly sized equipment. The equipment requirements in most locales are aimed at adult care and lack even the basic material for care of children.

TABLE 6–2
PREDISPOSING FACTORS FOR CHILDHOOD CARDIOPULMONARY ARREST

Airway disorders
  Aspiration-obstruction
  Asthma
  Epiglottitis
  Bronchiolitis
  Laryngotracheobronchitis
  Pneumonia
  Suffocation, strangulation, and trauma
  Croup
Cardiovascular disorders
  Hypovolemia-dehydration
  Septic shock
  Congenital heart disease
  Pericarditis-myocarditis
  Congestive heart failure
  Dysrhythmias
Gastrointestinal disorders
  Bowel obstruction or perforation
  Trauma
  Ingestion of penetrating agents or chemicals
  Enterocolitis
  Congenital malformation
Central nervous system disorders
  Meningitis-encephalitis
  Head trauma
  Seizure disorder
  Acute hydrocephalus
  Hemorrhage
  Cerebral anoxia
Metabolic disorders
  Hypoglycemia
  Hypocalcemia-hyperkalemia
  Ingestion of narcotics/depressants
  Ingestion of sedatives/antidysrhythmics
  Diabetic ketoacidosis
Environmental factors
  Hypothermia-hyperthermia
  Child abuse
  Near drowning
  Noxious agent inhalation
  Poisoning
Miscellaneous factors
  Sudden infant death syndrome
  Tumors
  Acquired immunodeficiency syndrome–related disorders
  Major trauma

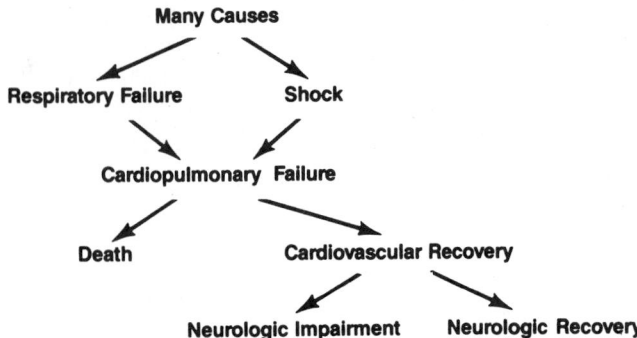

Figure 6–2. Path of various disease states leading to cardiopulmonary failure in children. (From Chameides L (ed). Textbook of Pediatric Advanced Life Support, 1988. Reproduced with permission. Copyright American Heart Association.)

The survival statistics for children requiring prehospital resuscitation reflect a dismal patient prognosis (Table 6–3). The vast majority of pediatric deaths occur in areas that place little emphasis on pediatric prehospital and in-hospital care. The ideal pediatric transport system should be centered around a regionally controlled system and directed by a trained pediatric emergentologist.

The American Academy of Pediatrics Committee on Hospital Care recommends that physician members of a transport team be at least at the senior resident level and that nurses have specific pediatric critical care experience. All levels of transportation must be adequately supplied with appropriately sized equipment. The designation of Emergency Department Approved for Pediatrics (EDAP) or Pediatric Critical Care Center (PCCC) facilitates the efficient care of critically ill children.[15-17]

Communications

Hospital-based communications and the development of protocols necessary for the care of critically ill children are essential. Informational transmissions should contain certain critical elements to facilitate appropriate reception of the critically ill child, including the child's condition, the suspected cause of the condition, most recent vital signs, and the estimated time of arrival (Table 6–4).

CLINICAL EVALUATION

Anticipating respiratory compromise can reduce childhood morbidity and mortality. The physician should interpret tachypnea, bradypnea, apnea, or labored breathing as respiratory embarrassment. Rapid heart rate, decreasing pulse pressure (hypotension), reduced capillary refill rate, and cyanosis are indications of poor cardiopulmonary performance. Increasing cyanosis; mottled skin; flaccid, "rag doll" muscle tone; and an altered level of awareness are grave indicators of impending demise. The CNS manifestations of hypoxia include delirium, confusion, undirected screaming, seizures, and unresponsiveness.

THERAPEUTIC INTERVENTION

The resuscitation team must be commanded by a designated team leader. The leader delegates the performance of tasks to others.[3, 18] In any critically ill child, the first goal of therapeutic intervention is to improve oxygenation. Cerebral and myocardial hypoxia must be corrected if cardiac arrest is to be prevented.

Establishing the Airway

Aggressive establishment of the child's airway and rapidly restoring effective and adequate ventilation are often all that is required to prevent further cardiovascular collapse. Airway management is easily provided by bag and mask ventilation alone. Proper attention must be paid to the potential for stomach distention.[3, 5, 13, 19]

Once ventilation is being provided, the physician should carefully measure the arterial pulses. The brachial, carotid, and femoral pulses are assessed by palpation. The absence of palpable pulses after a 15-second assessment should prompt immediate external cardiac compression (ECC).

TABLE 6–3			
RESULTS OF OUT-OF-HOSPITAL CARDIOPULMONARY RESUSCITATION			
Author	Number of Resuscitations	Number of Survivors (%)	Comments
Torphy et al[19]	92	3 (3.3%)	All survivors responded promptly to in-the-field therapy. Neurologic status of survivors not stated.
Tsai and Kailson*	23	0	
Losek et al†	114	9 (8%)	Only three of the nine survivors were neurologically intact.
Eisenberg et al[6]	119	9 (7%)	Four of eight survivors were drowning victims; two of eight survivors were anaphylactic. Neurologic outcome of survivors not stated.
Ludwig et al‡	34	10 (29%)	Neurologic outcome of survivors not stated.
Rosenberg[10]	18	1 (5.6%)	There were six additional arrest patients who received no prehospital efforts, two of whom survived.
Applebaum§	22	0	Four initially responded, but no long-term survivors
O'Rourke‖	—	34 (Admitted to ICU after prehospital resuscitation)	Seven discharged from ICU; one of seven expired out of hospital; one of seven had moderate neurologic impairment; all others had profound neurologic impairment.

*Tsai A, Kailson G. Epidemiology of pediatric prehospital care. Ann Emerg Med 1987;16:284.
†Losek JD, Hennes H, Glaeser P, et al. Prehospital care of the pulseless, nonbreathing pediatric patient. Am J Emerg Med 1987;5:370.
‡Ludwig S, Kettrick RG, Parker M. Pediatric cardiopulmonary resuscitation: A review of 130 cases. Clin Pediatr 1984;23:71.
§Applebaum D. Advanced prehospital care for pediatric emergencies. Ann Emerg Med 1985;14:656.
‖O'Rourke PP. Outcome of children who are apneic and pulseless in the emergency room. Crit Care Med 1986;14:466.

TABLE 6–4

ELEMENTS OF HOSPITAL-BASED COMMUNICATION

Essential information
  Name, age, and weight (or Broselow estimate)
  Current illness or reason for transportation
  Significant past medical history
  All medications being given:
    All IVs: drip rates, number, and type of IV lines
    Fluid type, infusion rates, type of infusers being used
  Current vital signs:
    Heart rate, blood pressure, respiratory rate, temperature
    Capillary refill, distal pulses, etc
    Mental status: level of awareness, wakefulness, and activity
      level (responsiveness)
    Vital sign flow sheets
    Ventilation settings (if intubated)
    Estimated time of arrival
Additional information
  Laboratory data
  All radiographs
  Provide telephone numbers of physicians and family
    members significant to the child
  Permission to treat, if available
  Detailed transfer data (COBRA transfer sheets)
  Organ donation information

Before any attempt at securing endotracheal manipulation of the airway, the tissues of the oropharynx are lifted away from the posterior structures, using the chin-lift or jaw-thrust maneuvers. If the child is breathing spontaneously, the respiratory effort is supported.

Endotracheal Intubation

Initial management of the pediatric airway requires proper positioning of the head and neck. The pediatric airway is positioned more anteriorly than that in an adult and is surrounded by soft cartilage and a relatively large tongue.[20, 21] The child's head should be placed in the "sniffing position" with slight flexion of the neck and extension of the head. Using this alignment, the airway is positioned for intubation, for facilitating spontaneous respirations, and for bag-mask ventilation.

Bag-mask ventilation performed without a nasogastric tube causes gastric distention. This can be minimized by applying finger pressure over the cricoid cartilage (known as the *Sellick maneuver*). This procedure occludes the esophagus, thereby limiting the amount of air passing to the stomach.[22]

The most secure and stable control of the airway is provided by the endotracheal (ET) tube. This provides an uninterrupted and efficient passage of air and maximizes ventilation, prevents passage of air into the stomach, and provides a route for the administration of essential resuscitative drugs. The size of the ET tube depends on the patient's age and, most importantly, the size of the patient's airway diameter. The ET tube size can be estimated by adding 16 to the child's age (up to 16) and dividing the total by four.[21] Neuromuscular blocking agents can facilitate the ease of intubation.

Drug Therapy

The primary agents used for advanced resuscitation include fluids, oxygen, epinephrine, atropine, sodium bicarbonate, and glucose (Table 6–5). Ancillary medications include lidocaine, naloxone, bretylium, procainamide, tromethamine, and 5% albumin. These agents comprise the first line of resuscitation drugs.[3, 4, 7, 23, 24]

Drug doses are calculated according to the weight of the child in kilograms. However, when the child enters the emergency department in extremis, an accurate measurement is not always possible. In the absence of a known, accurate recent weight and in the pressure and urgency of the moment, the child's precise weight may be unavailable. However, some methods can assist in determining the weight for drug dosing.

TABLE 6–5

PRIMARY DRUGS USED IN ADVANCED RESUSCITATION

Drug	Patient Age (Estimated Weight)				
	Newborn (3 kg)	6 Mo (7 kg)	1 Yr (10 kg)	6 Yr (20 kg)	10 Yr (30 kg)
Epinephrine (1:10,000) (0.1 mg/ml) IV,IO*					
Standard dose	0.3 ml (0.03 mg)	0.7 ml (0.07 mg)	1.0 ml (0.1 mg)	2.0 ml (0.2 mg)	3.0 ml (0.3 mg)
High dose	6 ml (0.6 mg)	14 ml (1.4 mg)	20 ml (2.0 mg)	40 ml (4.0 mg)	60 ml (6.0 mg)
Atropine (0.1 mg/ml)† IV,IO	1.0 ml (0.1 mg)	1.0 ml (0.1 mg)	2.0 ml (0.2 mg)	4.0 ml (0.4 mg)	6.0 ml (0.6 mg)
Lidocaine (10 mg/ml) IV,IO,ET	0.3 ml (3.0 mg)	0.7 ml (7.0 mg)	1.0 ml (10 mg)	2.0 ml (20 mg)	3.0 ml (30 mg)
Bicarbonate‡ 4.2% solution (0.5 mEq/ml) 8.4% solution (1.0 mEq/ml)	6 ml (3 mEq) 4.2% solution	7 ml (7 mEq) 8.4% solution	10 ml (10 mEq)	20 ml (20 mEq)	30 ml (30 mEq)
Glucose D25W§ D50W	6 ml (D25W)	14 ml (D25W)	20 ml (D25W)	20 ml (D50W)	30 ml (D50W)

*Epinephrine (1:10,000): standard dose, 0.01 mg/kg IV push (IVP) (0.1 ml/kg); high dose: 0.20 mg/kg IVP (2.0 ml/kg). High-dose epinephrine protocols are not standard; they can be used when the physician feels that such a protocol is potentially lifesaving.
†Atropine: 0.02 mg/kg IVP (0.2 ml/mg); minimum dose is 0.1 mg (1.0 ml).
‡Sodium bicarbonate use in cardiac arrest is controversial. The 4.2% solution (0.5 mEq/ml) is used in children younger than 3 mo.
§Use D25W in children <1 year. To make D25W, put 9 ml D50W in 11 ml D5W to make 20 ml D25W.

A standardized growth curve should be posted in the major resuscitation area; the fiftieth percentile curve will yield an approximate drug dose based on the child's estimated age (Table 6–6). Another useful method is to measure the child from head to extended foot using the Broselow tape. This tape provides estimated weight and drug dosages for pediatric patients based on their length and is reliable in the child with normal body habitus. A comparison of actual body weights with Broselow tape estimates confirms acceptable approximation of body weight for drug dosing. Metered levels of drugs and endotracheal tubes can be determined using this device. Lubitz et al. studied the Broselow tape and concluded that a highly accurate estimation of weight is rapidly obtained in both the prehospital and emergency department setting.[24]

Another useful device is a preprinted drug dosage chart based on weight. These charts are attached to the front of the patient's chart, providing ready information on defibrillation dose, endotracheal tube size, and drug doses. Emergidose, a pocket-sized pediatric medication reference card, provides similar information and can be displayed for use at the bedside.[25]

Fluids

An aggressive fluid challenge is unlikely to be detrimental to the arrested patient in any circumstance. A bolus of 20 ml/kg of lactated Ringer's solution is indicated. If the challenge exceeds 30 to 40 ml/kg, colloid solutions must be considered. Colloid solutions should be given at a similar dose rate in doses of 10 to 20 ml/kg. The total circulating blood volume in the pediatric patient is 80 ml/kg, and large fluid boluses may be calculated using this figure.

The simplest method of administering the fluid is to place the solute in a 50- to 60-ml syringe and push the calculated volume into the patient. This is easy and safe as long as 5% dextrose solution is avoided. The 5% dextrose solution is not a fluid volume expander and can cause cell lysis in the pediatric patient.[26, 27]

Epinephrine

Epinephrine is the single most effective drug used in cardiac arrest. The primary benefits are derived from its alpha-adrenergic effects, and the result is increased coronary artery and cerebral blood flow during CPR.

The standard dose for epinephrine is 0.01 mg/kg (0.1 ml/kg of a 1:10,000 solution). High-dose epinephrine therapy is considered to be 0.2 mg/kg (2.0 ml/kg of a 1:10,000 solution). Epinephrine may also be given in single bolus doses of 0.01 mg/kg intravenously every 5 minutes during resuscitation. Sodium bicarbonate should not be given in the same line as it may inactivate the epinephrine. Though epinephrine is absorbed through the tracheobronchial tree, larger doses may be required endotracheally to achieve the same hemodynamic effect achieved with an intravenous dose.[28]

High-dose epinephrine has been studied by Goetting and Paradis, who state that the preceding recommendations may be underestimated.[29] Some authors suggest that substantially elevated doses are not only tolerated, but may also enhance the resuscitation outcome.[29–33] In their study, Goetting and Paradis demonstrated that high-dose epinephrine increased survivability. After two standard epinephrine doses failed, a dose of 0.2 mg/kg (2.0 ml/kg of a 1:10,000 solution) was given. All 14 survivors in this study developed sinus tachycardia in response to the epinephrine that lasted at least 15 minutes; none developed life-threatening tachyarrhythmias.[29]

Given the apparent success high-dose epinephrine and the lack of significant side effects in survivors, it is likely that the high-dose schedule may become integrated into pediatric arrest algorithms.

When epinephrine is intravenously infused, it has a dose-related action. The lower doses (0.3 µg/kg/min) have mainly beta-adrenergic effects—that is, increases in heart rate, contractility, pulse pressure, and systolic blood pressure. Doses of more than 0.3 µg/kg/min result in greater degrees of alpha-adrenergic action as noted by a rise in both the systolic and diastolic blood pressure.

Atropine

Atropine sulfate is a parasympatholytic agent that accelerates pacemakers at both the atrioventricular and sinoatrial level. Atropine is recommended for the treatment of third-degree atrioventricular block, hypotensive bradycardia, and asystole. The dose for atropine is 0.02 mg/kg, with a minimum dose of 0.10 mg and a maximum total dose of 1.0 mg. Regular doses may be repeated at 5-minute intervals until the maximum total dose is achieved.

Although endotracheal administration is advocated, the efficacy is in doubt. Endotracheal atropine produces peak serum levels that are only approximately one ninth of that produced by the same dose of intravenous atropine.[34]

Atropine can be given during resuscitation without concern about abolishment of the pupillary response. After atropine is given, the pupillary response remains intact, causing only slight to moderate dilation of the pupil.[35]

Sodium Bicarbonate

The role of sodium bicarbonate in advanced pediatric resuscitation is controversial. A cardiopulmonary arrest produces a metabolic acidosis resulting from anaerobic metabolism. An excess of hydrogen ions and accumulation of lactate occurs. The poor systemic blood flow and inadequate ventilation lead to a mixed respiratory and metabolic acidosis. Once CPR occurs, the improvement in ventilation and systemic circulation is insufficient to correct this metabolic catastrophe. Only when spontaneous circulation returns does the mounting pH gradient between central venous and arterial blood disappear.

During an arrest, the venous CO_2 content is dependent

			TABLE 6–6													
			AVERAGE WEIGHT AND ENDOTRACHEAL TUBE SIZE FOR PEDIATRIC PATIENTS													
	Premature Infant	Term Newborn	1 Mo	3 Mo	6 Mo	1 Yr	2 Yr	3 Yr	4 Yr	5 Yr	6 Yr	7 Yr	8 Yr	9 Yr	10 Yr
Weight (kg)	1.5	3.0	4.0	5.5	7.0	10	12	14	16	18	20	22	25	28	30
Endotracheal tube size	2.5–3.0	3.5	3.5	4.0	4.0	4.0	4.5	5.0	5.5	5.5	5.5	5.5	6.0	6.0	6.0

on metabolic production, whereas the arterial content is reduced by increasing the cardiac output. Arterial blood gases measure ventilatory function but do not reflect the adequacy of tissue perfusion. By measuring the venous blood gas in this situation, a more accurate reflection of the metabolic status is ascertained.

Sodium bicarbonate buffers excess hydrogen ions by ultimately producing water and carbon dioxide. If respiration is inadequate, carbon dioxide cannot be removed, and no effective buffering occurs. When sodium bicarbonate is used, it is given intravenously (1 mEq/kg) as a bolus. Efforts during advanced resuscitation are better directed at reestablishing both adequate circulation and ventilation than at administering bicarbonate sodium.

Lidocaine

Lidocaine is the agent of choice for supression of ventricular ectopic activity. The use of lidocaine is somewhat limited, as ventricular fibrillation is seen in less than 10% of pediatric arrests. Lidocaine not only supresses discharge from ectopic foci, it also elevates the fibrillation threshold without influencing myocardial contractility.

Lidocaine is used in children with ventricular tachyarrythmia and ventricular fibrillation. The initial bolus of 1 mg/kg is usually followed by continuous infusion. However, a continuous infusion should never be started unless there is restoration of spontaneous circulation. In the absence of spontaneous circulation, lidocaine metabolism is slowed, and lidocaine toxicity rapidly develops.

The recommended dose is 1 mg/kg, repeated in 10 to 15 minutes if needed. A continuous infusion of lidocaine is easily made by placing 300 mg (15 ml of 2% solution) of lidocaine in 250 ml of D5W given at a rate of 20 to 50 µg/kg/min (1.0 to 2.5 ml/kg/hr). Children are particularly sensitive to lidocaine toxicity. Lidocaine-induced seizures should be treated with diazepam or phenobarbital.

Tromethamine

Tromethamine (THAM) is an organic amine that readily crosses lipid membranes. It buffers both the intracellular and extracellular spaces. Unlike bicarbonate, when ventilation is fixed, tromethamine is able to lower the PCO_2. A substantial limitation to tromethamine is that it is renally excreted, and renal blood flow is markedly reduced during pediatric cardiac arrest.

The dose range for acidosis associated with cardiac arrest in children is 3.5 to 6.0 ml/kg as an intravenous infusion. This dose can be given through a peripheral intravenous (IV) line and should be infused over a 3- to 5-minute interval.

Defibrillation

Defibrillation is the untimed, electrically induced depolarization of cardiac muscle that allows an organized beat to be initiated. Synchronous depolarization follows the same principal, with the energy being discharged in time with the RS complex.

Paddle Size

Three paddle sizes are available for children: a 4.5-cm paddle for infants and 8-cm and 13-cm paddles for larger children. The larger adult electrode paddles minimize transthoracic impedance. Increased paddle size should be used when the child's thorax is large enough to permit adequate electrode-to-chest contact with the entire paddle surface. This limits sparking and burning of the skin and permits maximum effective electrical delivery to the myocardium.

The transition from the smaller paddle size to the larger size occurs at a patient weight of about 10 kg, or 1 year of age. An adult-sized paddle has decreased transthoracic impedance when compared with a pediatric paddle. Therefore it is recommended that the largest paddle size possible be used for the pediatric defibrillation effort.

The transthoracic impedance for the pediatric paddles is 108 ohms (range, 61 to 212 ohms). Using adult paddles in the same children decreased transthoracic impedance to 59 ohms (range, 29 to 101 ohms). Large paddles and use of an adequate conductive medium facilitate defibrillation and cardioversion in children, with minimal burning and maximum transcardiac depolarization.

Paddle Location

Defibrillation is most effective when the heart is situated between the paddles, thereby minimizing transthoracic impedance through the heart muscle. Although anterior and posterior placement is acceptable, this is difficult to achieve and limits safety during a resuscitation attempt.

The recommended placement is to position one paddle on the upper right chest at the midclavicular line and the other paddle lateral to the left nipple, below the nipple line, at the anterior axillary line. This placement, coupled with the largest paddle size acceptable, provides for the least resistance and maximum effective energy delivery.

Energy Dose

All energy doses are weight related. The synchronized cardioversion dose of 0.5 to 1.0 joules (watt-seconds) per kilogram is recommended for supraventricular tachycardia. If supraventricular tachycardia continues, the dose can be increased to 2.0 J/kg. A lidocaine bolus (1.0 mg/kg) administered before cardioversion is safe and easy to deliver and improves effective conversion.

Electrode Contact

The least resistance to electrical delivery provides the most advantage in defibrillation procedures. Skin has a high resistance, so in order to provide a low-impedance interface, highly conductive electrode gels or creams are used. Using an electrode paste results in a lowered transthoracic impedance when compared with electrode creams. Sonographic gels and other lubricating lotions are not recommended, as they are poor conductors and may explode.

Saline-soaked pads are avoided, as their conductivity is variable and may cause sparking across the chest wall. Prepared, individually packed, presoaked lubricated gel sponges are available and are excellent. However, if the chest wall becomes slippery, CPR may be hampered.[3, 29, 30]

TREATMENT ALGORITHMS
Supraventricular Tachycardia

Supraventricular tachycardia (SVT) is an accelerated rhythm that is usually paroxysmal and originates at the level of the bundle of His or through an accessory pathway. This rhythm can result from a reentry mechanism and can produce profound hypotension.

Diagnosis

The typical heart rate is 260 beats/min, with a range from 240 beats/min to more than 300 beats/min (Fig. 6–3). The rhythm is regular with a normal QRS duration. In the infant

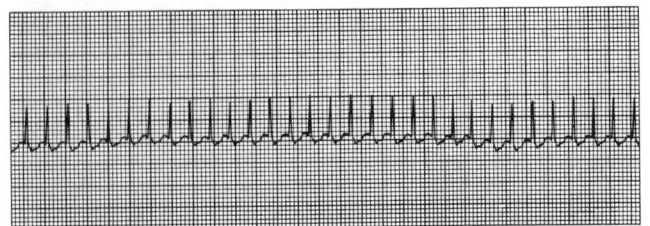

Figure 6–3. Supraventricular tachycardia in an infant. The heart rate is 320 beats/min. (From Chameides L (ed). Textbook of Pediatric Advanced Life Support, 1988. Reproduced with permission. Copyright American Heart Association.)

and newborn, this can be difficult to distinguish from sinus tachycardia, especially in the presence of a high fever or dehydration. Radiographs may show pneumonia consistent with sepsis or cardiomegaly. The heart rate in sinus tachycardia is usually less than 200 beats/min and may have R wave–to–R wave variation; in SVT the R wave–to–R wave interval is regular. Sinus tachycardia rates are usually less than 200 beats/min, whereas the supraventricular tachycardia rate is usually greater than 230 beats/min.

Therapy

Synchronized cardioversion (0.5 to 1.0 J/kg) is recommended for patients with cardiovascular instability from supraventricular tachycardia (Fig. 6–4). Subsequent levels should be 2.0 J/kg. The cardioversion should be preceded by a sedative dose of diazepam (0.2 mg/kg) or midazolam (0.07 mg/kg IV) given every 5 minutes as needed. The largest paddle size that will accommodate the child's chest without sparking should be used.

The treatment of supraventricular tachycardia in the infant without hemodynamic compromise begins with a vagal maneuver. This is most safely attempted by applying an ice water–soaked washcloth to the face for 20 seconds. If this is unsuccessful, drug therapy can begin. Either digoxin or procainamide can be used intravenously (Fig. 6–4). With increased use in children, adenosine (37.5 μg/kg given as a rapid IV push) may become the agent of choice. Adenosine can be used as a first-line agent in adolescents (Fig. 6–5). Verapamil, beta blockers, or synchronous cardioversion can also be used, but these interventions are usually not necessary in the stable patient.

Verapamil is given at a dose of 0.1 to 0.2 mg/kg administered slowly over 1 to 2 minutes. Concomitant use with intravenous propranolol should be done with extreme caution. There is an elevated instance of tachyarrythmias in patients with Wolff-Parkinson-White (WPW) syndrome. Up to 20% of the patients with WPW syndrome will present with atrial fibrillation. Whether the QRS complex is wide or narrow depends on which tract the impulse is conducted through. In more than 80% of cases, reentrant SVT occurs with the impulse passed along the normal atrioventricular conducting system.

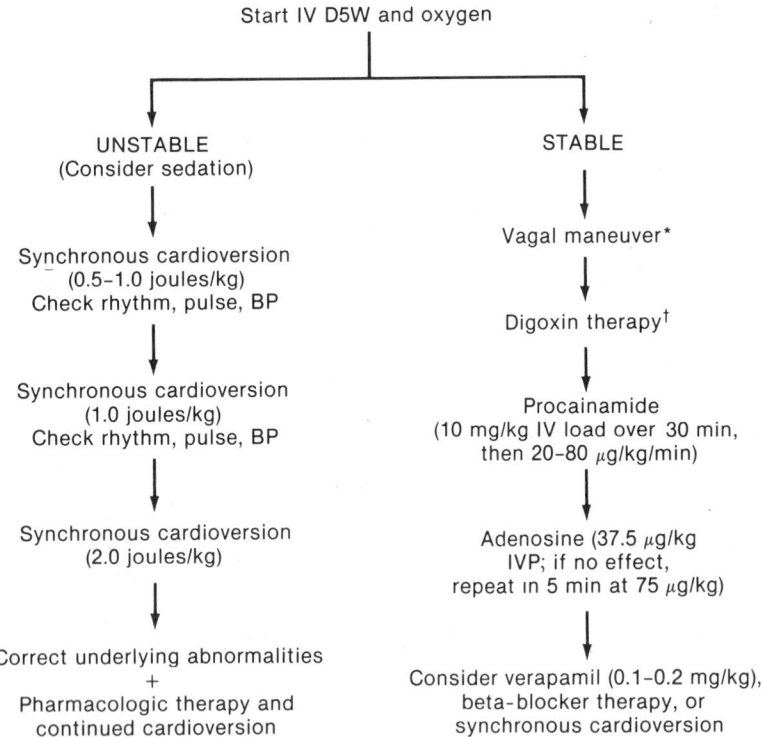

* Apply ice water–soaked washcloth to the face for 20 seconds.

† Digoxin loading: half of the total dose is given immediately; the other half is given over the next 24 hours.

Total digoxin dose:

Full term	20–30	μg/kg
1–24 mo	30–50	μg/kg
2–5 yr	25–35	μg/kg
5–10 yr	15–30	μg/kg
< 10 yr	8–12	μg/kg

Figure 6–4. Algorithm for treatment of **paroxysmal supraventricular tachycardia (PSVT) in an infant.**

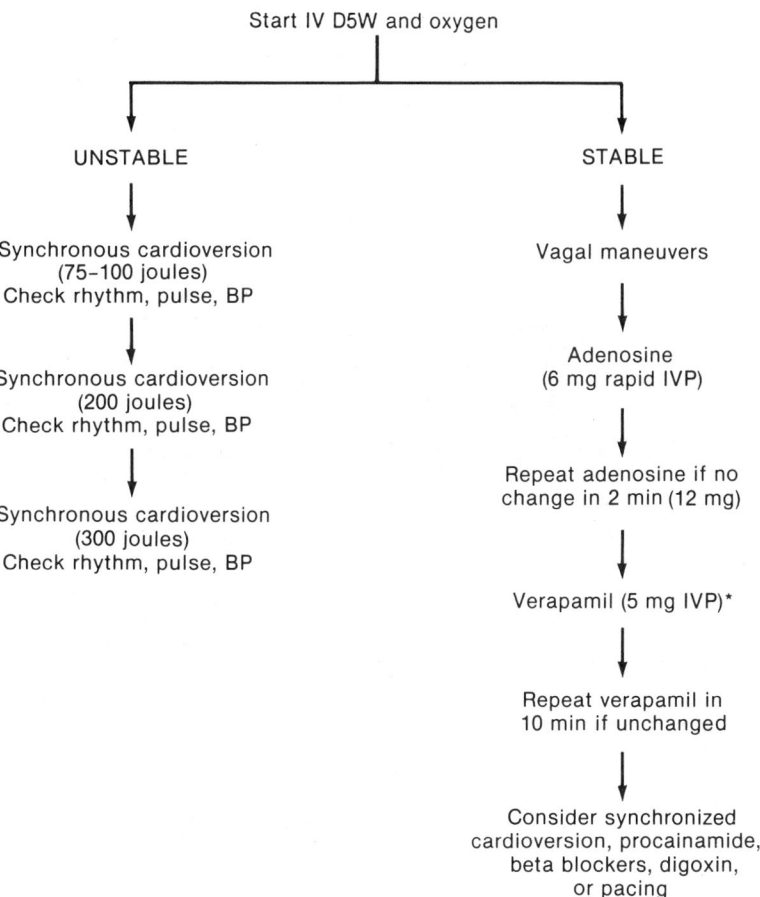

Start IV D5W and oxygen

UNSTABLE

Synchronous cardioversion
(75–100 joules)
Check rhythm, pulse, BP

Synchronous cardioversion
(200 joules)
Check rhythm, pulse, BP

Synchronous cardioversion
(300 joules)
Check rhythm, pulse, BP

STABLE

Vagal maneuvers

Adenosine
(6 mg rapid IVP)

Repeat adenosine if no
change in 2 min (12 mg)

Verapamil (5 mg IVP)*

Repeat verapamil in
10 min if unchanged

Consider synchronized
cardioversion, procainamide,
beta blockers, digoxin,
or pacing

Figure 6–5. Algorithm for treatment of **PSVT in an adolescent**.

* Verapamil should not be used if the patient is in atrial fibrillation and has Wolff–Parkinson–White syndrome. Maximum total dose is 20 mg.

Atrial fibrillation with a rapid ventricular response is best treated with cardioversion. Intravenous procainamide or digoxin therapy is an excellent alternative. Procainamide can be given intravenously at a rate of 20 to 80 μg/kg/min. Cardiovascular collapse can occur in the hydrated child when administering verapamil.

Ventricular Tachycardia

Hypoxia, acidosis, dehydration, and a variety of toxins (i.e., caffeine, theophylline, phencyclidine, and other stimulants) can induce ventricular tachycardia in children. This rhythm originates in the ventricles and is poorly tolerated. Ventricular rates can range from 120 beats/min to more than 360 beats/min. The slower rates are better tolerated, but the accelerated rates can lead to low-output failure and possibly to ventricular fibrillation.

Diagnosis

The QRS complex is typically greater than 0.08 seconds, and the rate is at least 120 beats/min and regular (Figs. 6–6 and 6–7). Wide QRS tachyarrhythmias in children must be considered ventricular tachycardia until proven otherwise. P waves are often not apparent. When P waves are present, they may be dissociated from the QRS pattern. The T waves are usually opposite in polarity to the QRS.

Therapy

If the child's circulation is compromised, synchronized cardioversion (0.5 to 1.0 J/kg) is used (Fig. 6–8). Lidocaine

(1.0 mg/kg) given as a bolus before cardioversion improves the success rate. Infusion therapy with lidocaine 20 to 40 μg/kg/min may help to maintain sinus rhythm. If cardioversion needs to be repeated, 2.0 J/kg is used. Consideration must be given to the hydration status. Hypovolemia and circulatory collapse are important considerations in the pathogenesis of terminal rhythm changes in the critically ill child.

Bradycardia

One of the most common causes of bradycardia in children is hypoxemia. In addition to intrinsic conduction from

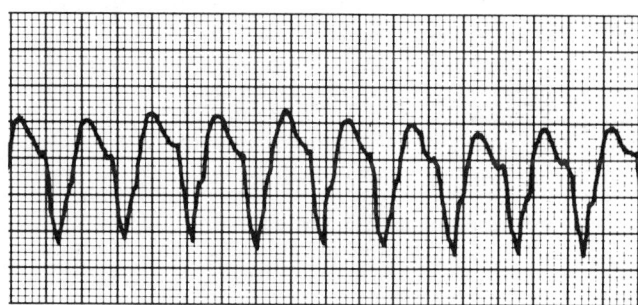

Figure 6–6. Ventricular tachycardia. The rhythm is regular at a rate of 158 beats/min. The QRS complex is wide. No evidence of atrial depolarization is seen. (From Chameides L (ed). Textbook of Pediatric Advanced Life Support, 1988. Reproduced with permission. Copyright American Heart Association.)

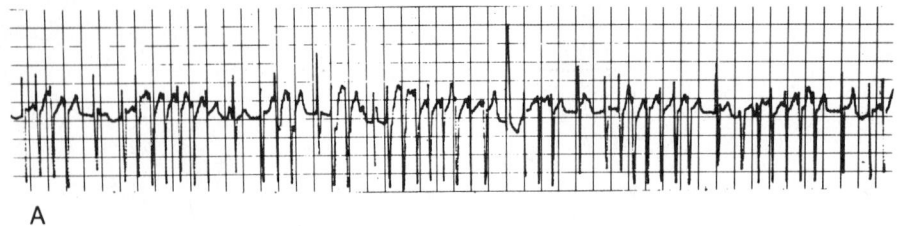

A

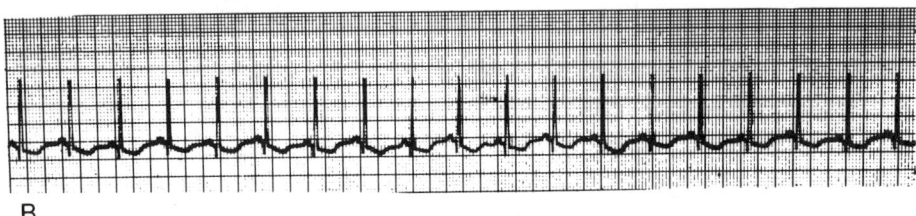

B

Figure 6–7. This figure demonstrates rapid ventricular tachyarrhythmia with a rate of 440 beats/min at times. There is a sinus capture beat (upright QRS in the middle of the tracing), several fusion beats, atrioventricular dissociation, and a QRS complex during tachycardia that is completely different from that found in sinus rhythm. Electrophysiology studies showed that this rhythm originated in the left ventricular apex. (From Long WA. Fetal and Neonatal Cardiology. Philadelphia, WB Saunders, 1990, p 517.)

congenital heart disease, acidosis and hypotension interfere with the normal function of the sinus and atrioventricular nodes. Sinus bradycardia and sinus nodal arrest with a slow junctional rhythm are common rhythm patterns seen in the severely ill child. The various atrioventricular blocks are common terminal rhythms in children with cardiopulmonary arrest.

Diagnosis

On monitor, the P wave and QRS relationship may be lost, and the associated slow rate may not demonstrate any P wave. The QRS duration may be normal or wide.

Therapy

The first steps in treating bradycardia are to maintain the airway, oxygenate the patient, ensure adequate glucose delivery, support the heart rate with chest compressions, and provide pharmacologic support with atropine (Fig. 6–9). Isoproterenol may also be used; a simple infusion can be prepared by adding 0.6 mg/kg of isoproterenol to 100 ml of D5W. Infusing the solution at a rate of 1 ml/hr will deliver 0.1 μg/kg/min.

Atropine is instrumental in the early treatment of bradycardia. The cardiac output in children is rate dependent, and in the young child (less than 6 months of age), rates below 80 beats/min must be treated. The recommended dose is 0.02 mg/kg, with a minimum dose of 0.1 mg and a maximum dose of 2.0 mg/kg. Atropine is safe for endotracheal administration, but endotracheal atropine may be ineffective during advanced resuscitation.[34]

Atropine is also used in the treatment of organophosphate ingestion in children. Organophosphates are powerful inhibitors of acetylcholinesterase. A salivation, lacrimation, urination, and defecation (SLUD) reaction can be seen. Atropine blocks the action of acetylcholine on parasympathetic receptors; this situation may require extremely high doses of atropine. In cases of moderate to severe poisoning, a test dose of 0.05 mg/kg is given. This dose should be given slowly intravenously and repeated every 15 minutes until the muscarinic symptoms are relieved and signs of mild atropinization (mydriasis, dry mouth, tachycardia) appear.[1, 3, 35]

Ventricular Fibrillation

Ventricular fibrillation is a quivering of the heart muscle with no circulatory contribution, producing a massive oxygen drain on the heart muscle. It is a coarse or fine disturbance reflecting chaotic myocardial electrical activity. The lead placement and cord attachment to the monitor must be secure, and the lead selector on the monitor must be set to the leads applied to the patient. For example, if the monitor is set on "paddle," the paddles must be applied to the patient for an accurate reading.

The treatment of this disruptive, chaotic depolarization of the heart is multiple unsynchronized defibrillations. Defibrillation can be lethal to a child who is not in ventricular fibrillation. If electrode leads are loosely applied, the physician may wrongly suspect ventricular fibrillation and defibrillate the child.

Diagnosis

With ventricular fibrillation, there are no identifiable complexes. There is an irregular, wandering isoelectric line with no established rhythm and no P wave or QRS wave. Determining whether a rhythm is fine ventricular fibrillation or coarse ventricular fibrillation is dependent on the height of the isoelectric waves (Figs. 6–10 and 6–11). Coarse ventricular fibrillation appears as choppy, irregular waves of variable height, whereas fine ventricular fibrillation reveals a smoother, generally lower, close-to-isoelectric-line pattern.

Therapy

Rapid and repeated defibrillations are indicated once ventricular fibrillation has been established. If the episode is witnessed, the child should be defibrillated immediately. If this is not effective, defibrillation should be repeated, followed by continuous CPR (Fig. 6–12).

Asystole

Asystole is found in the pulseless, apneic child in extremis. This devastating rhythm is associated with the highest morbidity rate.

Diagnosis

Asystole is essentially a straight line on the monitor; occasionally, isolated P waves can be seen (Fig. 6–13). Leads should be frequently checked when asystole occurs, as lead displacement mimics asystole.

Text continued on page 48

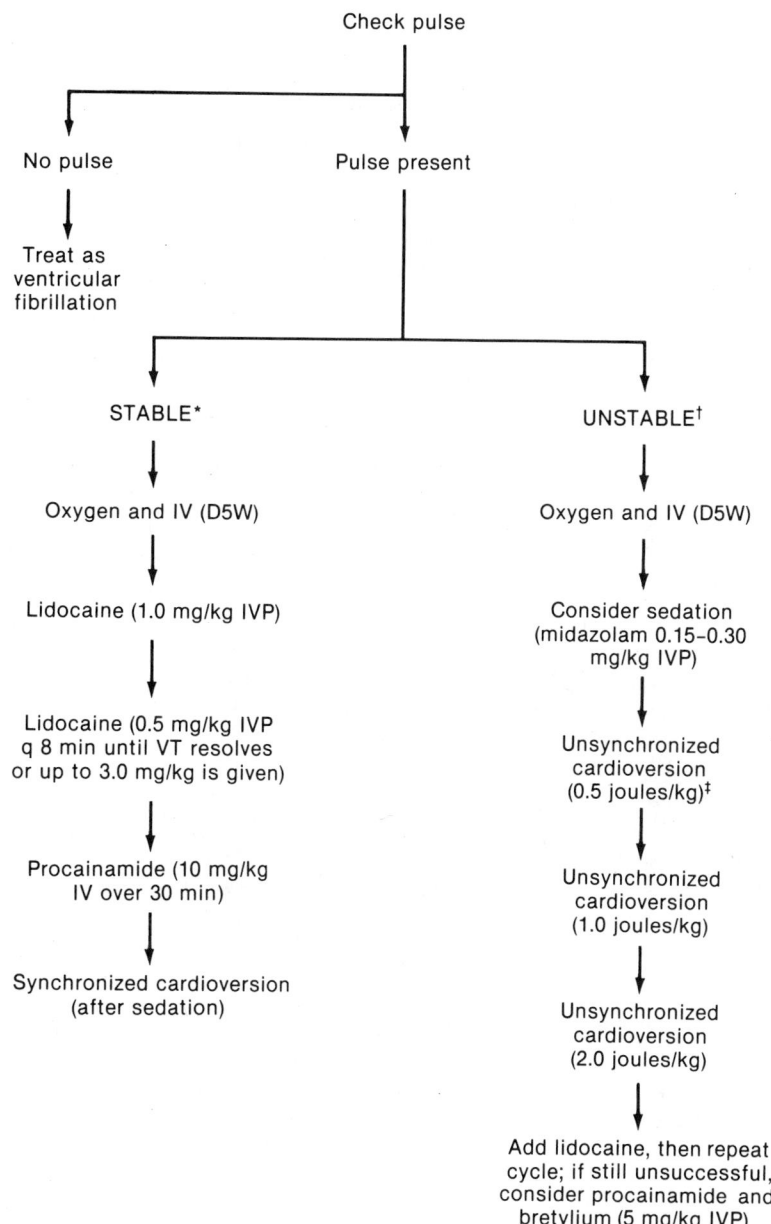

Check pulse

No pulse   Pulse present

Treat as
ventricular
fibrillation

STABLE*   UNSTABLE†

Oxygen and IV (D5W)   Oxygen and IV (D5W)

Lidocaine (1.0 mg/kg IVP)   Consider sedation
                                     (midazolam 0.15–0.30
                                     mg/kg IVP)

Lidocaine (0.5 mg/kg IVP   Unsynchronized
q 8 min until VT resolves   cardioversion
or up to 3.0 mg/kg is given)   (0.5 joules/kg)‡

Procainamide (10 mg/kg   Unsynchronized
IV over 30 min)   cardioversion
                                     (1.0 joules/kg)

Synchronized cardioversion   Unsynchronized
(after sedation)   cardioversion
                                     (2.0 joules/kg)

                                     Add lidocaine, then repeat
                                     cycle; if still unsuccessful,
                                     consider procainamide and
                                     bretylium (5 mg/kg IVP)

*If at any time the patient becomes unstable, move to the "unstable" algorithm.

†Instability is indicated by chest pain, dyspnea, hypotension, pulmonary edema, or ischemia.

‡Once ventricular tachycardia has resolved, begin an IV infusion of the antiarrhythmic agent that aided the resolution of ventricular tachycardia. If the patient is hypotensive, lidocaine is used first, then bretylium, and then procainamide. Phenytoin should be used in place of procainamide if the QT interval is prolonged. (Lidocaine infusion: 20–50 μg/kg/min; procainamide infusion: 20–80 μg/kg/min.)

Figure 6–8. Algorithm for treatment of **ventricular tachycardia**.

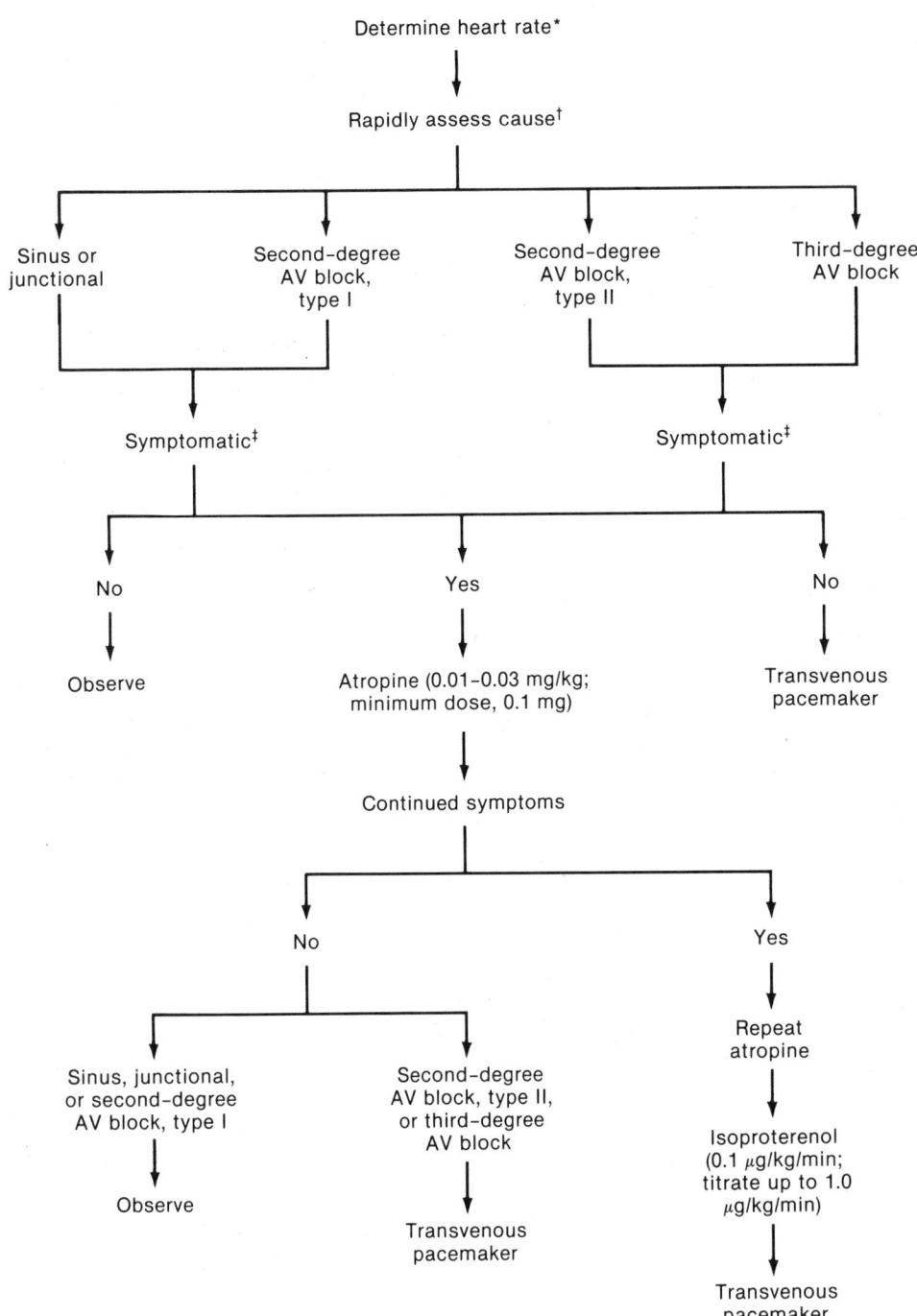

*Bradycardia is age dependent and generally well tolerated.

†Address potential causes of bradycardia, including respiratory distress, acidosis, and vagal stimulation.

‡Symptoms include hypotension, PVCs, altered mental status, chest pain, dyspnea, or ischemia.

Figure 6–9. Algorithm for treatment of **bradycardia**.

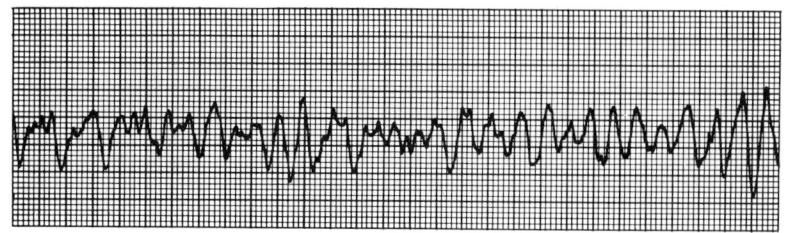

Figure 6–10. Ventricular fibrillation. With coarse ventricular fibrillation, there are high-amplitude waveforms that vary in size, shape, and rhythm, representing chaotic ventricular electrical activity. (From Chameides L (ed). Textbook of Pediatric Advanced Life Support, 1988. Reproduced with permission. Copyright American Heart Association.)

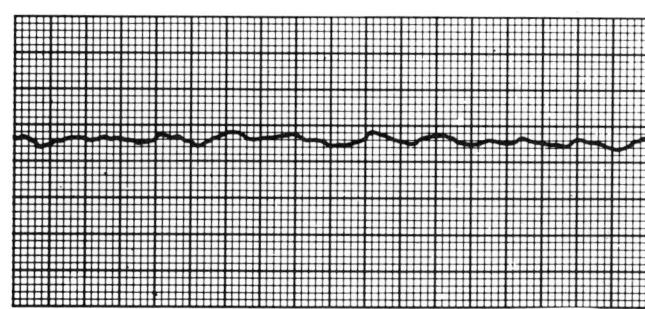

Figure 6–11. Ventricular fibrillation. With fine ventricular fibrillation, there is reduced electrical activity. (From Chameides L (ed). Textbook of Pediatric Advanced Life Support, 1988. Reproduced with permission. Copyright American Heart Association.)

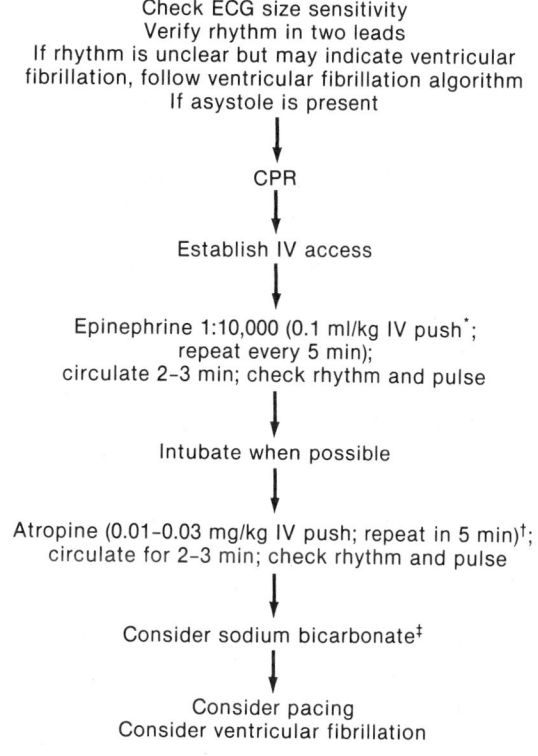

Check ECG size sensitivity
Verify rhythm in two leads
If rhythm is unclear but may indicate ventricular
fibrillation, follow ventricular fibrillation algorithm
If asystole is present

CPR

Establish IV access

Epinephrine 1:10,000 (0.1 ml/kg IV push*;
repeat every 5 min);
circulate 2–3 min; check rhythm and pulse

Intubate when possible

Atropine (0.01–0.03 mg/kg IV push; repeat in 5 min)†;
circulate for 2–3 min; check rhythm and pulse

Consider sodium bicarbonate‡

Consider pacing
Consider ventricular fibrillation

* High-dose epinephrine: 2 ml/kg (0.2 mg/kg) IV push after two standard doses have failed.

† Atropine: minimum dose, 0.1 mg IVP.

Figure 6–12. Algorithm for treatment of **ventricular fibrillation** and pulseless ventricular tachycardia.

‡ The dose for sodium bicarbonate, if used, is 1 mEq/kg IV push initially, then 0.5 mEq/kg q 10 min.

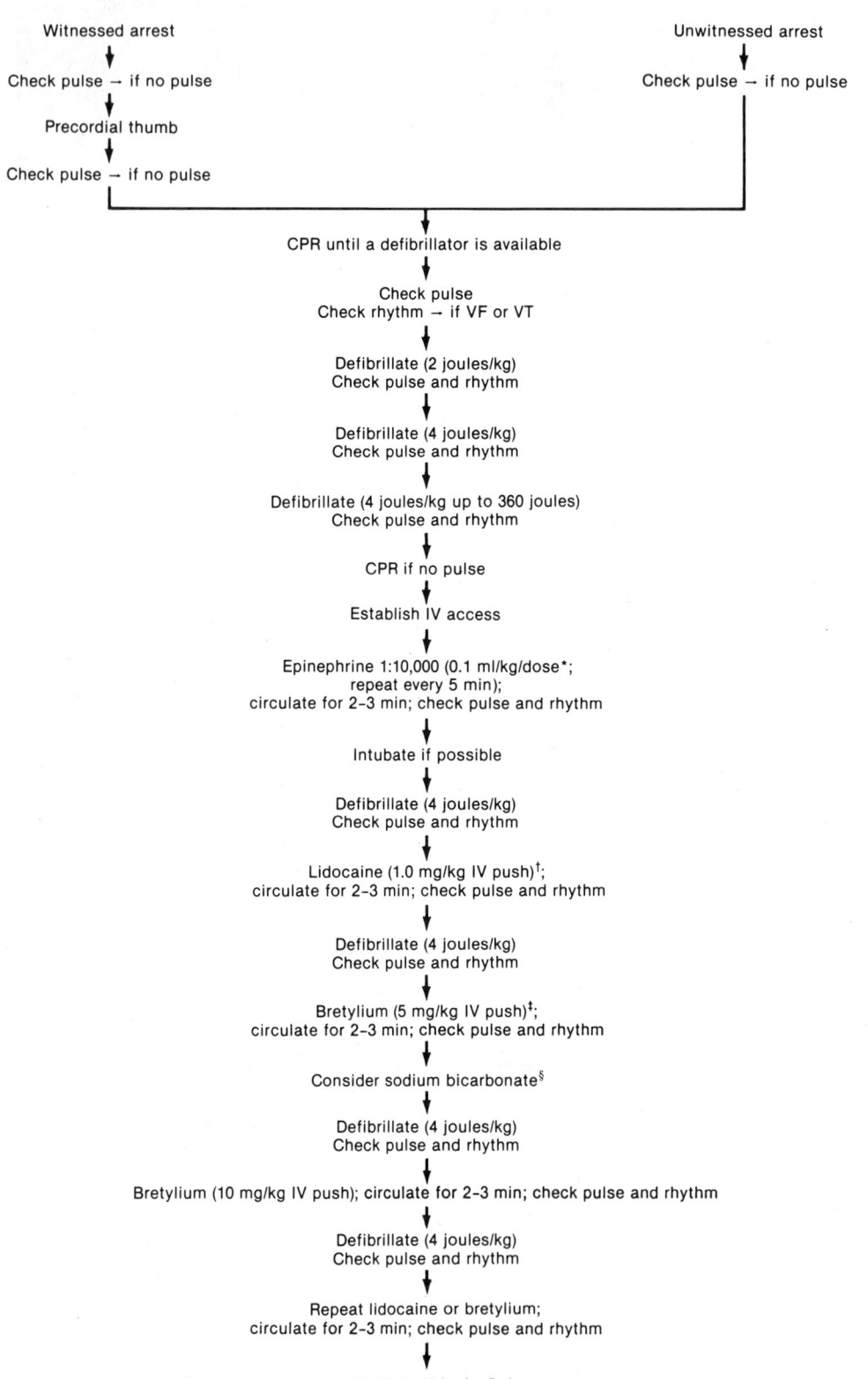

Witnessed arrest
↓
Check pulse → if no pulse
↓
Precordial thumb
↓
Check pulse → if no pulse

Unwitnessed arrest
↓
Check pulse → if no pulse

CPR until a defibrillator is available
↓
Check pulse
Check rhythm → if VF or VT
↓
Defibrillate (2 joules/kg)
Check pulse and rhythm
↓
Defibrillate (4 joules/kg)
Check pulse and rhythm
↓
Defibrillate (4 joules/kg up to 360 joules)
Check pulse and rhythm
↓
CPR if no pulse
↓
Establish IV access
↓
Epinephrine 1:10,000 (0.1 ml/kg/dose*;
repeat every 5 min);
circulate for 2–3 min; check pulse and rhythm
↓
Intubate if possible
↓
Defibrillate (4 joules/kg)
Check pulse and rhythm
↓
Lidocaine (1.0 mg/kg IV push)[†];
circulate for 2–3 min; check pulse and rhythm
↓
Defibrillate (4 joules/kg)
Check pulse and rhythm
↓
Bretylium (5 mg/kg IV push)[‡];
circulate for 2–3 min; check pulse and rhythm
↓
Consider sodium bicarbonate[§]
↓
Defibrillate (4 joules/kg)
Check pulse and rhythm
↓
Bretylium (10 mg/kg IV push); circulate for 2–3 min; check pulse and rhythm
↓
Defibrillate (4 joules/kg)
Check pulse and rhythm
↓
Repeat lidocaine or bretylium;
circulate for 2–3 min; check pulse and rhythm
↓
Defibrillate (4 joules/kg)
Check pulse and rhythm

*If high-dose epinephrine is used, give 2 ml/kg of 1:10,000 solution after two standard doses have failed.

[†]Lidocaine: maximum dose, 3 mg/kg.

[‡]Bretylium: maximum dose, 30 mg/kg.

[§]If used, the dose for sodium bicarbonate is 1.0 mEq/kg IV push initially, then 0.5 mEq/kg q 10 min.

Figure 6–13. Algorithm for treatment of **asystole**.

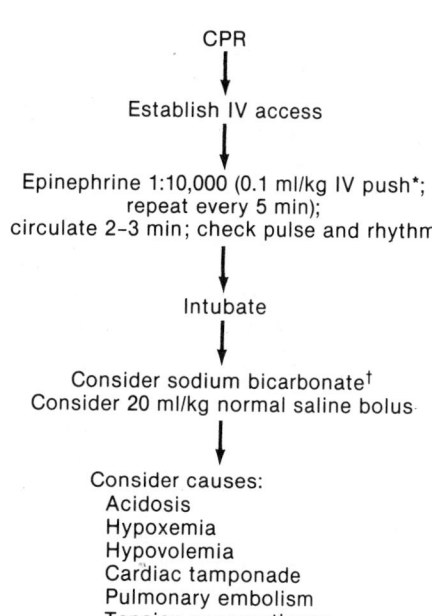

CPR

↓

Establish IV access

↓

Epinephrine 1:10,000 (0.1 ml/kg IV push*;
repeat every 5 min);
circulate 2–3 min; check pulse and rhythm

↓

Intubate

↓

Consider sodium bicarbonate†
Consider 20 ml/kg normal saline bolus

↓

Consider causes:
  Acidosis
  Hypoxemia
  Hypovolemia
  Cardiac tamponade
  Pulmonary embolism
  Tension pneumothorax

* High-dose epinephrine: 2 ml/kg (0.2 mg/kg) IV push after two standard doses
have failed. The effectiveness of high-dose epinephrine therapy is
uncertain. It should be used only when the physician feels that it is
potentially lifesaving.

Figure 6–14. Algorithm for treatment of **electromechanical dissociation**.

† The dose for sodium bicarbonate, if used, is 1.0 mEq/kg IV push initially,
then 0.5 mEq/kg q 10 min.

Therapy

The patient receives continuous cardiac monitoring. Glucose, epinephrine, atropine, and bicarbonate are given. If a fine ventricular fibrillation is suspected, the ventricular fibrillation algorithm is followed.

Electromechanical Dissociation

Electromechanical dissociation (EMD) is observed, organized electrical activity on a cardiac monitor without a palpable pulse or blood pressure. The diagnosis of EMD has a poor patient prognosis. Several conditions may mimic this fatal rhythm: severe hypovolemia, tension pneumothorax, massive pulmonary embolus, cardiac tamponade, and myocardial rupture (Fig. 6–14).[3, 36]

OTHER CONSIDERATIONS

Tort Law

In the context of the resuscitative effort, the physician is acting to save a life with limited background information and often no ability to obtain a medical history. The Good Samaritan Act protects the lifesaving efforts of individuals providing care in areas other than the emergency department. The exposure to potential liability is present in probably the worst case in which a physician could be placed.

The standard of care has been implied in the performance of Pediatric Advance Life Support guidelines. It is the duty of the physician to approach these standards. Though debatable, it is implied that a person certified as a provider by the American Heart Association to deliver advanced pediatric life support is held to the guidelines as a standard of care.[37–39]

The current prevailing laws in most states requires the first responder to initiate CPR to the best of his or her training and continue this effort until the patient is seen by a physician who can then determine whether the effort should be terminated. In most cases, the information concerning a living will or wishes of the patient is unknown, and in such cases the responder should provide the maximum care possible until the effort exceeds the rescuer's ability to continue.

Determining when to terminate resuscitation efforts is a complex ethical, physical, and psychological issue. Most CPR teams provide CPR far beyond any reasonable hope for recovery of the victim.[38–41]

TABLE 6–7

COBRA GUIDELINES

Actions	Comments
Adopt antidumping policies	Hospitals must adopt and enforce policies that comply with the law
Provide immediate screening	Method of payment cannot act as impediment to treatment
Maintain records	Transfer records must be maintained for 5 years
Physicians on call	Staff physicians are required to "back up" the emergency department
Post signs	Patient rights sign must be conspicuously placed
Provide ancillary services	All normal services must be available
Make special units available	If the hospital has a special unit, it must be made available to the patient
"Whistleblower" protection	No hospital may penalize a physician for reporting a transfer of an unstable patient

TABLE 6–8

BRAIN DEATH DOCUMENTATION*

	No. 1	No. 2
A. Date of examination		
B. Time of examination		
C. Coma of established cause and absence of hypothermia (below 32°C) and central nervous system depressant drugs		
1. Body temperature		
2. Toxicology studies (when indicated)		
3. Unresponsiveness to intensely painful stimuli (e.g., supraorbital pressure)		
4. No spontaneous muscular movements and no evidence of decerebrate or decorticate posturing or shivering (in the absence of muscle relaxants) NOTE: Spinal reflex activity may persist after death		
D. Cranial nerve reflexes and responses		
1. Pupils light-fixed		
2. Absent corneal reflexes		
3. Absent response to airway stimulation (e.g., pharyngeal and endotracheal suctioning)		
4. Absent ocular response to head turning (no eye movement)		
5. Absent ocular response to irrigation of the ears with ice water (25–50 ml), head upright at 30 degrees (no eye movement)		
E. Absence of spontaneous breathing movements for at least 5 minutes after stopping ventilatory support. Ventilate with pure oxygen for 5 minutes at arterial PCO_2 of 35 mm Hg before withdrawal of the ventilator, followed by passive flow of oxygen		
1. $PaCO_2$ at end of apnea test		
2. PaO_2 at end of apnea test		
II. Ancillary tests—if a confirmatory test is desired, only one study (EEG or isotope flow study) is needed		
A. Evidence of brain death by radioisotope scan or cerebral angiogram may supercede items I-C-1, I-C-2, I-E		
B. An isoelectric electroencephalograph		

*The patient must be observed in the hospital during treatment of potentially correctable abnormalities (e.g., hypovolemic shock). Two clinical examinations must be performed:
1. The observation period should be at least 6 hours if the cause of coma is clearly defined.
2. If the cause of coma is unknown or if hypoxic ischemic injury is suspected, at least 24 hours of clinical observation is recommended. A shorter observation time is sufficient if an ancillary test (EEG or flow study) is done.

Note: If a significant depressant drug or hypothermia is present, an isotope flow study is preferable to the EEG if a confirmatory test is desired.

TABLE 6–9

THERAPY AT A GLANCE

Drug	Solution	Dose		Comments
Epinephrine	1:10,000			If 1:1000 is used, it must be diluted.
Standard dose	(0.1 mg/ml)	0.01 mg/kg	0.1 ml/kg	Give q 5 min IV/IO; ET administration has limited effect.
High dose		0.2 mg/kg	2.0 ml/kg	Only use after two standard doses have failed.
Atropine	0.1 mg/ml	0.02 mg/kg	0.2 ml/kg	Minimum dose: 0.1 mg (1.0 ml). Maximum dose for infants and children: 1 mg; for adolescents: 2 mg. More may be required for toxin-induced bradycardia. Give IV or IO. ET has limited effect.
Sodium bicarbonate	4.2% (0.5 mEq/ml) 8.4% (1.0 mEq/ml)	1 mEq/kg	2.0 ml/kg 4.2% 1.0 ml/kg 8.4%	Children younger than 3 mo should receive 4.2% solution. Give IV or IO. Use in cardiac arrest is controversial.
Lidocaine	10% (10 mg/ml) 20% (20 mg/ml)	1 mg/kg	0.10 ml/kg 10% 0.05 ml/kg 20%	Use for ventricular dysrhythmias. Use only IV bolus therapy during cardiac arrest.
Procainamide	100 mg/ml (10%) 500 mg/ml	10–15 mg/kg over 30 min	0.10–0.15 ml/kg	Discontinue drug if hypotension develops or the QRS complex widens.
Phenytoin	50 mg/ml	5 mg/kg	0.1 ml/kg	Maximum infusion rate: 1 mg/kg/min. Tissue necrosis can occur with extravasation.
Bretylium	50 mg/ml	5 mg/kg	0.1 ml/kg	IV only. Second dose is 10 mg/kg. Can cause vomiting.
Adenosine	3 mg/ml	37.5 µg/kg	0.013 ml/kg	Give rapid IV push; repeat dose in 5 minutes is 0.025 ml/kg (75.0 µg/kg).
Verapamil	2.5 mg/ml	0.2 mg/kg	0.08 ml/kg	Maximum 3 doses. Avoid use in WPW-associated atrial fibrillation.
Digoxin	0.25 mg/ml (adults) 0.10 mg/ml (children)	Total IV loading dose (µg/kg): Term 20–30 1–24 mo 30–50 2–5 yr 25–35 5–10 yr 15–30 >10 yr 8–12		Give half of the total loading dose as a slow IV push. The remainder is given over 24 hours.
Propranolol	1 mg/ml	0.01–0.15 mg/kg	0.01–0.15 ml/kg	Slow IV push; maximum total single dose is 10 mg.
Normal saline	0.9 solution		10–20 ml/kg	Use 10 ml/kg in newborns. Use up to 40 ml/kg total in EMD.
Glucose	D50W (0.50 gm/ml) D25W (0.25 gm/ml)	0.5–1.0 g/kg	1–2 ml/kg 2–4 ml/kg	Use D25W solution in children younger than 1 yr. To make 20 ml of D25W, combine 9 ml of D50W with 11 ml of D5W.
Diazepam	5 mg/ml	0.2 mg/kg	0.04 ml/kg	Use for seizure lysis or sedation. Do not use ET. Can use IV, IO, or rectal.
Midazolam	5 mg/ml	0.15 mg/kg	0.03 ml/kg	Use for seizure lysis or sedation. Can give IV, IO, or rectal.

ET = Endotracheal tube; IO = intraosseous; IV = intravenous; WPW = Wolff-Parkinson-White syndrome; EMD = electromechanical dissociation.

TABLE 6–10

THERAPY AT A GLANCE: CONTINUOUS INFUSIONS

Drug	Solution	Drip Preparation	Infusion Rate
Epinephrine	1:1000 (1 mg/ml)	0.6 mg per body weight in kg is added to D5W to make a total solution volume of 100 ml	1 ml/hr = 0.1 µg/kg/min Dose range: 0.1–1.0 µg/kg/min
Isoproterenol	1:5000 (1 mg/5 ml)	0.6 mg per body weight in kg is added to D5W to make a total solution volume of 100 ml	1 ml/hr = 0.1 µg/kg/min Dose range: 0.1–1.0 µg/kg/min
Dopamine	40 mg/ml	6 mg per body weight in kg is added to D5W to make a total solution volume of 100 ml	1 ml/hr = 1.0 µg/kg/min Dose range: 2.0–20 µg/kg/min
Dobutamine	250-mg vial	6 mg per body weight in kg is added to D5W to make a total solution volume of 100 ml	1 ml/hr = 1.0 µg/kg/min Dose range: 5–20 µg/kg/min
Lidocaine	20 mg/ml (2%)	Add 300 mg to D5W to make a total of 250 ml solution	1 ml/hr = 20 µg/kg/min Dose range: 20–50 µg/kg/min
Procainamide	100 mg/ml	Add 300 mg to D5W to make a total of 250 ml of solution	1 ml/hr = 20 µg/kg/min Dose range: 20–80 µg/kg/min

Cobra

The Consolidated Omnibus Reconcilation Act (COBRA) legislation of 1985 (updated in 1988) has broad implications involving the care of the critically ill child. This also affects transfers from one institution to another and mandates a screening examination with stabilization of the patient (Table 6–7). The current COBRA law requires that a patient who registers to be seen in the emergency department must be seen, evaluated, and stabilized prior to discharge, referral, or transfer. Anything less than total compliance with this statute constitutes a breach of duty. Although the original intent of the law was to monitor patients participating in Medicare and Medicaid, it has been interpreted as a standard of care for all patients visiting any emergency department in the United States.

Under COBRA, transfers are considered appropriate when the target facility has the personnel and space required for the subject patient. The hospital of origin must send a copy of the patient's medical records, and qualified personnel must accompany the patient.

Brain Death

Most institutions have provisions and guidelines for determining brain death in children. Brain death occurs when cerebral functions are irreversibly absent, and the patient lacks both receptive and responsive ability. Brain stem dysfunction is evidenced by absent pupillary, corneal, oculocephalic, oculovestibular, orophayngeal, and respiratory reflexes. After extensive resuscitative attempts, irreversibility is recognized when the reason for the coma is established, and the observation period is sufficient to confirm nonresponsiveness. The period of observation varies depending on the circumstances involved. Forms should be used to document the basic elements used to determine brain death (Table 6–8).[42–45]

Living Wills

The state in which the emergency department is located establishes directives as to the status of living wills and advanced directives as they apply to the concept of pediatric resuscitation.[40, 41]

Although not likely to apply to the pediatric patient, laws in many states affect the ability of the EMS system and emergency departments to provide unrestrained resuscitation. The Do Not Resuscitate (DNR) bills limit the code efforts.

References

1. Sullivan JJ, Guyatt GH. Simulated cardiac arrests for monitoring quality of in-hospital resuscitation. Lancet 1986;Sept 13:201.
2. Ludwig S, Kettrick R. Resuscitation—pediatric basic and advanced life support. Life support emergencies, section 1. In Fleisher G, Ludwig S (eds). Textbook of Pediatric Emergency Medicine. 2nd ed. Baltimore, Williams & Wilkins, 1988.
3. Chameides L (ed). Textbook of Pediatric Advanced Life Support. American Heart Association, 1990.
4. Zaritsky A, Nadkami V, Getsen P, et al. CPR in children. Ann Emerg Med 1987;16:1107.
5. Lamb R, Rosner MS. Neonatal resuscitation. Emerg Med Clin North Am 1987;5:541.
6. Eisenberg M, Bergner L, Hallstrom A. Epidemiology of cardiac arrest and resuscitation in children. Ann Emerg Med 1983;12:672.
7. Tibballs J. Practical aspects of advanced paediatric cardiopulmonary resuscitation. Aust Paediatr J 1988;24:228.
8. Friesen RT, Duncan P, Tweed WA, et al. Appraisal of pediatric cardiopulmonary resuscitation. Can Med Assoc J 1987;126:1055.
9. Chameides L, Zaritsky A. Advanced pediatric life support: ABC with a difference. Emerg Med Rep 1988;79:446.
10. Rosenberg NM. Pediatric cardiopulmonary arrest in the emergency department. Am J Emerg Med 1984;2:497.
11. Holbrook PR, Mickell J, Pollack KNM, et al. Cardiovascular resuscitation drugs for children. Crit Care Med 1980;8:588.
12. Ludwig S, Fleisher G. Pediatric cardiopulmonary resuscitation: A review and a proposal. Pediatr Emerg Care 1985;1:40.
13. Sanders AB, Meislin MW, Ewy GA. The physiology of cardiopulmonary resuscitation. An update. JAMA 1984;252:3283.
14. Pearson JW, Redding JS. Peripheral vascular tone on cardiac resuscitation. Anesth Analg 1965;44:746.
15. Haller JA Jr, Shorter N, Miller D, et al. Organization and function of a regional pediatric trauma center: Does a system of management improve outcome? J Trauma 1983;23:691.
16. Ludwig S, Selbst S. A child-oriented emergency medical services system. Curr Probl Pediatr 1990;20:109.
17. Henderson DP. The Los Angeles pediatric emergency care system. J Emerg Nurs 1988;14:96.
18. Otto CW, Yakaitis RW, Blitt CD. Mechanism of action of epinephrine in resuscitation from asphyxial arrest. Crit Care Med 1981;9:321.
19. Torphy DE, Minter MG, Thompson BM. Cardiorespiratory arrest and resuscitation of children. Am J Dis Child 1984;138:1099.
20. Echenhoff JE. Some anatomic considerations of the infant larynx influencing endotracheal anesthesia. Anesthesiology 1951;12:401.
21. Smith RM. Endotracheal Intubation: Anesthesia for Infants and Children. St. Louis, CV Mosby, 1984, p 164.
22. Sellick BA. Cricoid pressure to control regurgitation of stomach contents during induction of anesthesia. Lancet 1961;2:404.
23. Zaritsky A. Selected concepts and controversies in pediatric cardiopulmonary resuscitation. Crit Care Clin North Am 1988;4:735.
24. Lubitz DS, Seidel JS, Chameides L, et al. A rapid method for estimating weight and resuscitation drug dosages from length in the pediatric age group. Ann Emerg Med 1988;17:576.
25. Okstein CJ, Odal M, Kelly RW. Emergency drug dosage guides. Pediatrics 1988;82:119.
26. Standards and guidelines for cardiopulmonary resuscitation (CPR) and emergency cardiac care (ECC). JAMA 1980;244:453.
27. Standards and guidelines for cardiopulmonary resuscitation (CPR) and emergency cardiac care (ECC). JAMA 1986;255:2933.
28. Ralston SH, Tacker WA, Showen L, et al. Endotracheal versus intravenous epinephrine during electromechanical dissociation with CPR in dogs. Am Emerg Med 1985;14:1044.
29. Goetting MG, Paradis NA. High-dose epinephrine improves outcome from pediatric cardiac arrest. Am Emerg Med 1991;20:22.
30. Koscove EM, Paradis NA. Successful resuscitation from cardiac arrest using high-dose epinephrine therapy. JAMA 1988;259:3031.
31. Goetting MG, Paradis NA. High dose epinephrine in refractory pediatric cardiac arrest. Crit Care Med 1989;17:1258.
32. Callaham M, Barton C, Hayser S. Potential adverse effects of high-dose epinephrine in human survivors of cardiac arrest. Abstract. Am Emerg Med 1990;19:479.
33. Barton CW, Callaham M. High-dose epinephrine significantly improves resuscitation rates in human victims of cardiac arrest. Abstract. Am Emerg Med 1990;19:490.
34. Prete MR, Hannan CJ, Burkle FM. Plasma atropine concentrations via intravenous, endotracheal, and intraosseous administration. Am J Emerg Med 1987;5:101.
35. Goetting MG, Contreras E. Systemic atropine administration during cardiac arrest does not cause fixed and dilated pupils. Ann Emerg Med 1991;20:55.
36. Walsh CK, Krongrad E. Terminal cardiac electrical activity in pediatric patients. Am J Cardiol 1983;51:557.
37. Mample FE, Weigel CJ: Good Samaritan Laws—who needs them: The current state of Good Samaritan Protection in the United States. South Tex Law J 1981;8:327, 351.
38. Lipkin RJ. Beyond good samaritans and moral monsters: An individualistic justification of the general legal duty to rescue. UCLA Law Rev 1983;14:252, 253, 262.
39. Feuerhelm KW. Taking notice of Good Samaritan and Duty to Rescue Laws. J Contemp Law 1984;11:219.
40. Beauchamp TL, Childres TF. Principles of Biomedical Ethics. 2nd ed. New York, Oxford University Press, 1983.
41. Schowalter JE, Ferholt JB, Mann NM. The adolescent patient's decision to die. Pediatrics 1973;51:97.
42. Schwartz JA, Baxter J, Brill DR. Diagnosis of brain death in children by radionuclide cerebral imaging. Pediatrics 1984;73:14.
43. Oro JJ. Determination of death by neurological criteria. Mo Med 1989;86:628.
44. Alvarez LA, Moshé SL, Belman AL, et al. EEG and brain death determination in children. Neurology 1988;38:227.
45. Fackler JC, Troncoso JC, Gioia FR. Age-specific characteristics of brain death in children. Am J Dis Child 1988;142:999.

CHAPTER 7

Airway Management and Ventilatory Support

Niranjan Kissoon
Narendra Singh

INTRODUCTION

Children with life-threatening illnesses comprise a small number of visits to the emergency department.[1] However, in these patients, primary respiratory failure or respiratory failure secondary to other organ involvement is usually the final common pathway leading to morbidity and mortality. Maintenance of airway patency and the provision of adequate ventilation are therefore the most important lifesaving measures in pediatric emergency medicine. It is imperative that all physicians involved in the delivery of emergency care to children be adept at emergency airway management.

Maneuvers to maintain airway patency should be undertaken in a stepwise fashion, with initial simple measures such as positioning and oropharyngeal toilet. More invasive procedures such as intubation and cricothyroidotomy require additional skills and should be attempted by those who are most experienced. Airway maintenance should be conducted in a calm, efficient manner by adequately trained staff. Training should include both lectures and skill stations for the greatest benefit.

ANATOMY AND PHYSIOLOGY

The need to provide airway support in the child poses a tremendous challenge under emergency conditions. A thorough working knowledge of the anatomy and physiology of the child's airway is the first step in the successful management of the pediatric airway. Failure to appreciate airway differences between the adult and child may result not only in unsuccessful attempts at airway support but also in significant morbidity and possibly mortality.

The anatomy of the airway of the child differs from that of the adult in certain aspects unrelated to size (Table 7–1). These differences are likely to lead to airway compromise, especially in the young child, and render airway support more difficult. Because the infant's head is proportionally larger than that of the adult or older child, the size of the occiput and the lack of neck muscle tone are much more likely to force the cervical spine into a flexed position and therefore increase the chance of airway obstruction.[2] The nostrils are also small in proportion to the trachea, and because infants younger than 3 months are obligate nose breathers, obstruction of the nostrils is more likely to cause respiratory difficulty. The tongue is proportionally larger in the child, making the oral cavity and oropharynx smaller. Less muscle tone in both the mandible and tongue allows for greater posterior displacement of the tongue and, therefore, airway obstruction. In fact, the nasal and oral cavity accounts for 50% of the total respiratory resistance.[4] Vascular gums and poorly anchored teeth are also a problem since bleeding is more likely to occur during vigorous attempts at intubation.

The epiglottis is relatively longer and stiffer and is U or V shaped when compared with that in the adult.[4] It also

TABLE 7–1

DIFFERENCES IN THE PEDIATRIC AIRWAY WHEN COMPARED WITH THAT IN THE ADULT

Anatomic Differences	Clinical Significance
1. Proportionally larger head	Increases neck flexion and obstruction
2. Smaller nostrils	Increases airway resistance
3. Larger tongue	Increases airway resistance
4. Decreased muscle tone	Airway obstruction by tongue
5. Epiglottitis—longer, stiffer, more horizontal	Increases airway obstruction
6. Larynx more anterior	Difficult to perform blind intubation
7. Cricoid ring is narrowest portion	Cuffed tubes not recommended
8. Shorter trachea	Increases right main stem intubation
9. Airway more narrow	Increases airway resistance

Physiologic Differences	Adult	Infant
RR (breaths/min)	15	40
Tidal volume (ml/kg)	6	6
Vital capacity (ml/kg)	70	35
Total lung capacity (ml/kg)	86	63
O_2 consumption	3.5	6.4

projects more posteriorly at an angle of 45°, compared with that in the adult, which is more vertical and closer to the base of the tongue. All these features make epiglottic enlargement more hazardous in the pediatric patient. The larynx is located higher in the child, with the vocal cords more concave and at a more anteroinferior incline.[2] This makes the vocal cord much more difficult to visualize and blind nasotracheal intubation almost impossible.

The airway lumen also differs in that the cricoid ring is the narrowest part of the airway in the infant and child. It is completely enclosed in cartilage and is therefore not a yielding structure like other parts of the airway. Because of this unique feature, children younger than 8 years of age usually do not require a cuffed endotracheal tube, as the narrow cricoid area provides a physiologic seal.[2] The trachea is also short in the child, making intubation of the right main stem bronchus a frequent complication.[5] In addition, the softer and more compliant nature of the trachea makes airway obstruction more likely with overextension or overflexion of the cervical spine. The tracheal lumen of the child is lined by ciliated columnar epithelium,[2] which is much more likely to accumulate edema. Because airway resistance is inversely related to the fourth power of the radius (Poiseuille's law), small changes in the airway diameter can have a profound effect on airway resistance in the child.

Apart from anatomic disadvantages such as a barrel-shaped chest and more flattened diaphragm, a number of physiologic differences between the adult and child place children at a tremendous respiratory disadvantage. Despite similar tidal volumes in both groups, the respiratory rate of the infant is higher, and minute ventilation is almost twice that of the adult. This increase in minute ventilation is associated with an oxygen consumption of 6.4 ml/kg/min in the infant, compared with 3.5 ml/kg/min in the adult.[6] The infant also has a limited respiratory reserve as a result of the higher ratio of alveolar ventilation to functional residual capacity, higher closing volumes, and higher oxygen consumption. Because of the higher metabolic rate and limited respiratory reserve in children, respiratory decompensation in pediatric patients requires aggressive intervention and hence leaves little time for deliberation.

INDICATIONS FOR AIRWAY SUPPORT

The major indication for airway support in the emergency department is for the provision of ventilation to alleviate respiratory failure (Table 7–2). In fact, respiratory failure accounts for 50% of admissions to the critical care unit[7] and is the third leading cause of death in infants.[8] In many cases, respiratory insufficiency and respiratory failure may be caused by primary disorders of the respiratory system. Other major causes are diseases of the respiratory pump or derangement of other organ systems. For example, the patient with head trauma may hypoventilate as a result of the primary injury or as a result of seizures. In addition, head trauma may lead to an inability to protect the airway because of poor cough and diminished gag reflexes, pulmonary aspiration, and airway compromise as a result of tracheal compression or posterior displacement of the tongue. Patients in shock may also require airway support for ventilation in order to decrease the work of the respiratory muscles.[9]

APPROACH TO THE PEDIATRIC AIRWAY
Basic Airway Management

Although airway management often necessitates endotracheal intubation, simple maneuvers may aid in creating a patent airway and alleviate the need for immediate endotracheal intubation. The most important initial maneuvers are the clearing of foreign material from the oropharynx and proper positioning of the patient. Clearance of the oropharynx is best done by suctioning under direct visualization of the oral cavity, rather than by blind sweeping techniques, which may result in further obstruction. Proper positioning of the patient is critical, because in children with an altered sensorium, the tongue commonly causes airway obstruction (Fig. 7–1A). It may fall into the posterior pharynx because of the lack of tone in the supporting muscles, or it may be pulled toward the airway with each respiratory effort. In addition, the cervical spine adopts a semiflexed position, narrowing the distance between the tongue and the posterior pharynx, with the epiglottis gravitating toward the glottis. An overflexed or overextended cervical spine also results in airway compromise either because of anterior displacement of the posterior pharynx or because of posterior displacement of the tongue (Fig. 7–1B).

TABLE 7–2	

INDICATIONS FOR ENDOTRACHEAL INTUBATION

1. Cardiopulmonary resuscitation
2. Need to maintain a patent airway
   a. Airway obstruction (croup, epiglottitis)
   b. Ineffective cough and gag reflex (altered sensorium)
3. Need to improve respiratory effort
   a. Poor effort
      (1) central (drugs, infection, trauma)
      (2) spinal cord (trauma)
      (3) chest wall deformity (kyphosis)
   b. Normal effort but overwhelming demand
      (1) Upper airway disease (croup, epiglottitis)
      (2) Lower airway disease (bronchiolitis, asthma, pneumonia)
4. Need to control other systems
   a. Elevated intracranial pressure—hyperventilation
   b. Shock—remove respiratory effort
   c. Drug overdose—airway protection during gastric lavage

Positioning the Child

Simple maneuvers (see Fig. 7–1) may elevate the tongue and open the airway. The head-tilt/chin-lift maneuver is performed by placing one hand on the victim's forehead and tilting the head backward, with the other hand lifting the bony portion of the patient's chin (Fig. 7–1C). This is most effective in the unconscious patient.[10] An alternative is the jaw-thrust maneuver, which is performed by gripping the angle of the mandible with both hands and pulling forward, while at the same time tilting the head backward. The triple airway maneuver is similar to the head-tilt/jaw-thrust maneuver, with the third component being retraction of the lower lip with the thumb, thereby opening the mouth (Fig. 7–1D). Overextension should be avoided, as it can further increase airway obstruction and is contraindicated in the patient with a possible cervical spine injury.

ESTABLISHMENT OF A PHARYNGEAL AIRWAY
Oropharyngeal Airway

The oropharyngeal airway is also useful in maintenance of airway patency in the unconscious patient since it brings

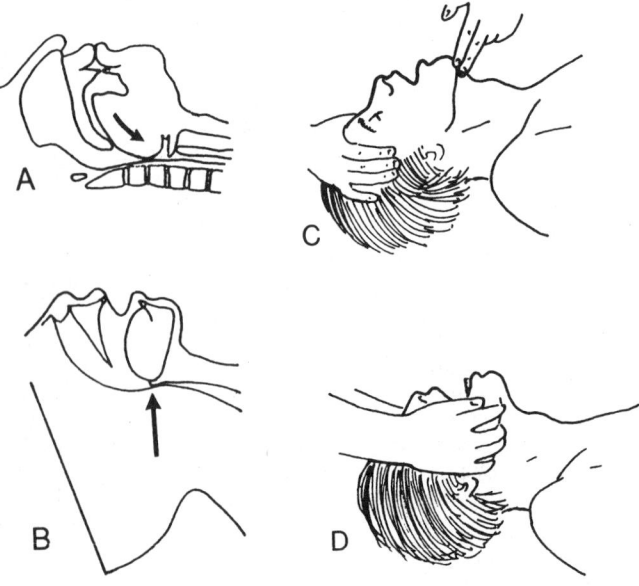
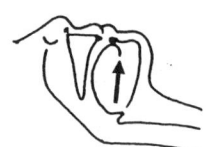
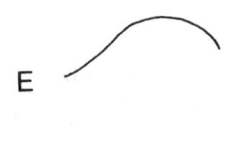

Figure 7–1. Establishing patency of the airway. *A,* Unconscious patient with posterior displacement of the tongue obscuring vision. *B,* Overextension of the cervical spine, causing airway obstruction. *C,* Head-tilt/chin-lift maneuver. *D,* Triple airway maneuver. *E,* The patent airway.

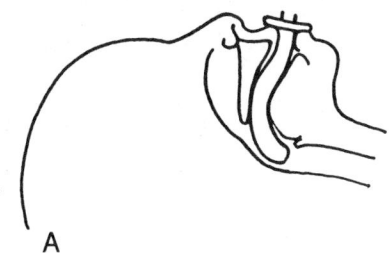

Figure 7–2. Correct positioning of the oral (A) and nasopharyngeal (B) airway.

the tongue forward (Fig. 7–2A). The length required for the oropharyngeal airway is determined by the distance from the angle of the mouth to the angle of the mandible. An appropriately sized airway is inserted by placing it in the mouth with the curve concave superiorly. The tip is then curved toward the larynx by rotating it through 180° in order to avoid pushing the tongue posteriorly. It can also be inserted by depressing the tongue with a wooden tongue blade and then inserting the airway to follow the natural curve of the tongue. Meticulous care must be taken, as trauma to the lips and teeth may occur, and in conscious patients, laryngospasm or vomiting may be induced. The conscious patient with cough and gag reflexes is unlikely to tolerate an oropharyngeal airway, and hence such an airway should not be placed.

Nasopharyngeal Airway

Another option in the semiconscious patient or in the conscious patient with mild or moderately enlarged adenoids is the soft nasopharyngeal airway (Fig. 7–2B). The length of airway required is the distance from the ala nasi to the angle of the mandible. The size of the nostril determines the airway diameter; however, if after adequate lubrication there is resistance to insertion of the airway, a smaller size should be used. These should not be inserted in patients with a cerebrospinal fluid leak, nasal bleeding, or hemorrhagic diathesis or those who are undergoing anticoagulant therapy. Complications resulting from placement of nasopharyngeal airway include epistaxis and initiation of vomiting and laryngospasm.

Placement of a nasopharyngeal or oropharyngeal airway may be adequate for airway support in the spontaneously breathing patient. Under these circumstances, oxygen may be delivered to the patient by nasal cannula or plastic mask. Masks commonly used include simple, partial rebreathing, and non-rebreathing masks and Venturimasks.[2] The partial rebreathing mask can be used to deliver oxygen in concentrations greater than 50%, with concentrations as high as 100% possible with the total non-rebreathing mask. The Venturimask is designed to deliver varying concentrations of oxygen and is useful in situations where hyperoxia must be avoided.[2] Infants may not tolerate these masks, however, and therefore placement of a plastic hood that fits over the head and neck is often more useful. Patients with respiratory insufficiency who require assistance using a bag-valve-mask apparatus will usually need to undergo endotracheal intubation.

ENDOTRACHEAL INTUBATION

A correctly placed endotracheal tube is the most effective way of providing adequate gas exchange. Endotracheal intubation is fraught with complications and is likely to fail if medical personnel are not skilled and appropriate equipment and medications are not readily available.

Equipment
Suction Catheters

Suctioning of the upper airway is often necessary to adequately clear the airway, both for improved ventilation and to facilitate endotracheal intubation. Three types of suction catheters are commonly used (Fig. 7–3). The soft suction catheter is used for nasal and oropharyngeal secretions, decompression of the stomach, and endotracheal suctioning. The dental and tonsillar tip catheters are rigid, which limits their usefulness. The dental tip is appropriate for large particulate debris in the airway, and the tonsillar tip is effective for secretions and blood. Familiarity with the suctioning technique and attention to detail are necessary in order to limit complications. Suction pressures of 70 to 100 mm Hg[11] are effective in clearing secretions but are not high enough to damage the mucous membranes. Vigorous suctioning of the nasal and oropharyngeal cavities should be avoided, as this may induce hypoxia and epistaxis.[12, 13] Hypoxia during endotracheal suctioning can be avoided by

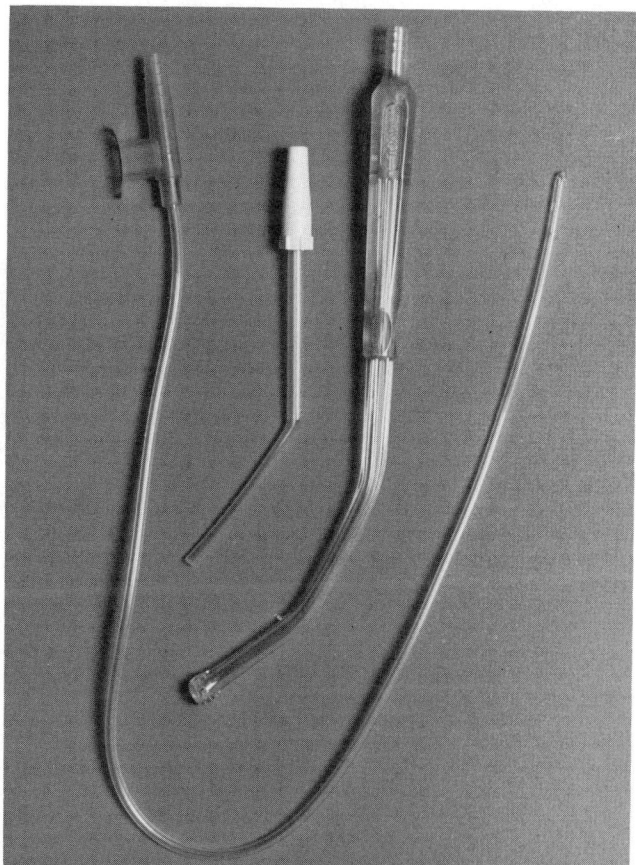

Figure 7–3. Suction catheters. Left to right: soft, dental tip, and tonsillar tip.

adequate pre-oxygenation and by limiting suctioning time to 10 seconds.[14, 15] Suctioning of the nasal cavity should also be avoided in patients with basilar skull fractures because of the risk of introducing the catheter into the intracranial vault.[16]

Endotracheal Tubes

Choosing the appropriate-size endotracheal tube is critical, as a tube that is too small may be inadequate for ventilation, and a tube that is too large may be difficult to insert and may traumatize the airway, leading to long-term complications such as subglottic stenosis.[17, 18] The correct diameter of the tube can be estimated from the age of the patient (Table 7–3). In addition, a rough estimate of the tube diameter required can be gained from the diameter of the nares or of the little finger of the patient. Because these are only guidelines, it is important when proceeding with intubation that tubes one size smaller and one size larger be immediately available (Fig. 7–4). In children older than 8 years of age, the epiglottis is the narrowest part of the airway; if required, a cuffed endotracheal tube can be used (see Fig. 7–4). However, as a general rule, cuffed tubes should not be used in children except when high ventilatory pressures are anticipated, as in children with asthma, pneumonia, adult respiratory distress syndrome (ARDS), or major chest trauma. For cuffed tubes, a half size smaller than recommended by the formula should be used.

Because the infant's trachea is short, it is important to attempt to predict the length of endotracheal tube required for intubation (see Table 7–3). The formula provides an estimate of the distance from the midtrachea to the teeth or nares. However, the position of the head can significantly influence the tube position in the trachea. Flexion of the head causes the endotracheal tube to be pushed downward, increasing the chances of endobronchial intubation; extension causes the endotracheal tube to be pulled up, increasing the risk of dislodgement.[19]

Laryngoscope Blades

There are two main types of laryngoscope blades: straight and curved (Fig. 7–5). The straight blade is preferred in

TABLE 7–3
ESTIMATING ENDOTRACHEAL TUBE AND LARYNGOSCOPE SIZE

Age (Years)	Tube Size (mm)	Blade Size
Premature	2.5–3.0	Miller 0
Newborn	3.0–3.5	Miller 1
1–2	4.0–4.5	Miller 1.5
3–4	4.5–5.0	Miller 2
5–6	5.0–5.5	Miller 2
6–7	5.5–6.0	Miller 2
7–8	6.0–7.5	Miller 2

$$\text{Tube size: Internal diameter (mm)} = \frac{16 + \text{age (years)}}{4}$$

For proper position: Oral: Tube length (cm) = 12 + age/2
Nasal: Tube length (cm) = 15 + age/2

infants and children, because the larynx is more anteriorly placed. Airway visualization is accomplished by using the straight blade to elevate the epiglottis, whereas the curved blade rests behind the epiglottis and permits visualization of the vocal cords by upward pull along the axis of the handle.

Stylet

Most intubations can be done without the use of a stylet, but it may be needed to guide the endotracheal tube into the anteriorly placed larynx. Precautions should be taken to prevent trauma from both the stylet and the stiffened tube. The stylet should be introduced into the tube 0.5 to 1.0 cm proximal to the end of the tube. Because the tube is stiff, intubation should be as gentle as possible, as the risks of bleeding or perforation of the trachea or esophagus is increased.

Forceps

A Magill forceps is used to position the endotracheal tube in the larynx during nasotracheal intubation. It is often needed because the larynx is anteriorly placed and the tube

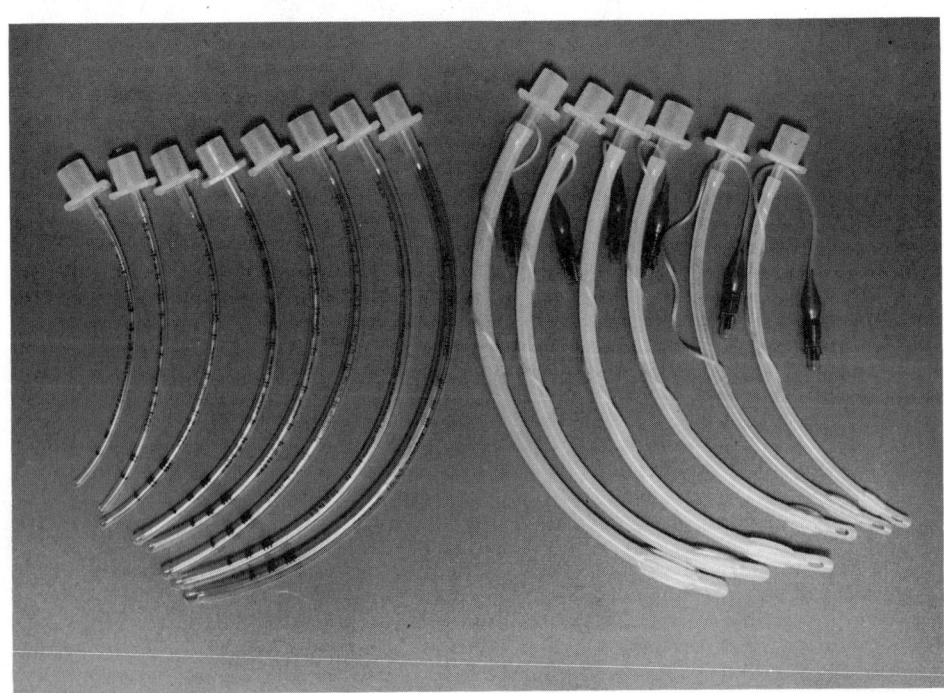

Figure 7–4. Various sizes of endotracheal tubes. *Left,* Uncuffed tubes. *Right,* Cuffed tubes.

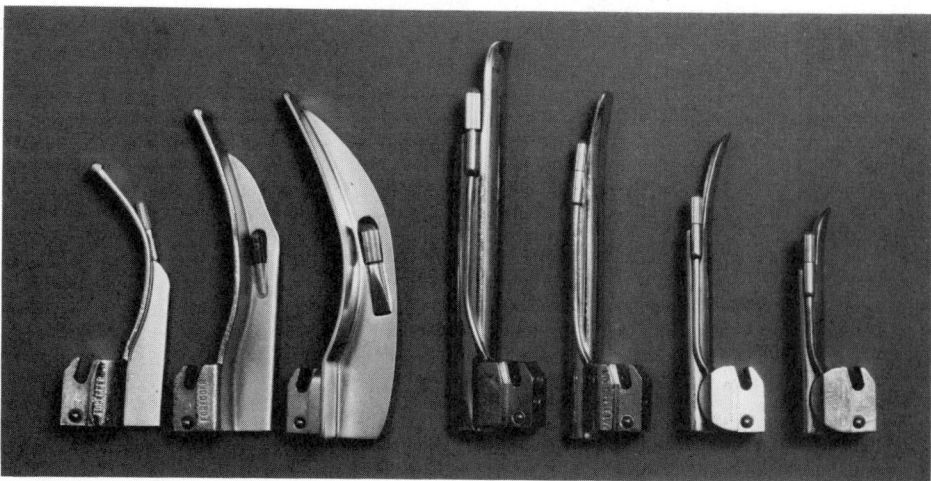

Figure 7–5. Various sizes of laryngoscope blades. *Left,* Curved blades. *Right,* Straight blades.

must be picked up in the posterior pharynx and guided through the vocal cords. In all cases, trauma can be avoided by visualization of the forceps when opening and closing them and during forceps removal from the oral cavity.

Bag-Valve-Mask Apparatus

Successful application of bag and mask ventilation relies on proper positioning of the child and attaining a good seal over the nose and mouth while avoiding pressure on the eyes. The mask should preferably be made of clear material so that any foreign material in the airway, such as vomitus, can be visualized. There are several bag-mask apparatuses available. Although most of these meet the minimum standards set by the Canadian Standards Association[20] and the American Standards for Testing of Material,[21] many are less than ideal.[22, 23] The anesthesia bag is able to deliver 100% oxygen and provides visual clues that the seal is proper; however, it requires additional skill for correct use.[24] Failure to deliver 100% oxygen, as well as improper functioning of pop-off valves are the common deficiencies of the currently available devices.[22–25] However, such devices are adequate for use in the emergency department, as long as staff members are cognizant of their limitations and are trained in their use.

DRUGS TO FACILITATE INTUBATION

In patients with impending or frank cardiac arrest, intubation is urgently required and may be conducted without the use of medications. In most instances, however, time is available to properly prepare the patient for intubation. Intubation in an awake patient has many disadvantages and is fraught with failure. On the other hand, intubation performed with patients in a fully relaxed state facilitates the procedure,[26–30] decreases pain and discomfort, and lowers elevated intracranial pressure.[31–34] Sedation or neuromuscular blockade is helpful in assisting intubation (Table 7–4).

Sedating Agents
Benzodiazepines

Most conscious patients requiring intubation should be sedated to alleviate anxiety. The benzodiazepine most frequently used is diazepam, but midazolam is being used with increasing frequency. Diazepam results in sedation of slow onset; however, it produces anesthetic induction at higher doses. Midazolam has anxiolytic, hypnotic, and antegrade amnesic properties.[35, 36] It has a faster onset of action and

shorter duration of effect when compared with diazepam. However, it has not been as widely used in the emergency department. Although cardiovascular and respiratory depression may occur with these medications, it is usually less severe than that occurring with the alternatives (e.g., barbiturates) (see Table 7–4).

Opiates

The two most frequently used narcotics are fentanyl and morphine. Fentanyl is more potent and has a more rapid onset and shorter duration of effect than morphine.[37] Both narcotics have the potential to cause respiratory depression that can be reversed with naloxone. In patients with an airway that is difficult to establish, narcotics are preferred for sedation, because the resultant respiratory depression can be reversed. Fentanyl also produces less hypotension than morphine and may be useful in patients with borderline intravascular volume.[37–39] Chest wall rigidity may occur with fentanyl administration but can be prevented by slow administration and is reversed with naloxone or a muscle relaxant.[37, 38, 40, 41] Although there is extensive experience with morphine use in the emergency department, there is limited experience with fentanyl use in facilitating endotracheal intubation.

Barbiturates

Thiopental is a short-acting barbiturate with a rapid onset of action resulting in unconsciousness within 10 to 20 seconds.[42] It is advantageous in patients with elevated intracranial pressure, as it reduces intracranial pressure by decreasing the cerebral metabolic rate for oxygen consumption.[42–45] The major disadvantage is hypotension, which occurs as a result of both vasodilation and myocardial depression.[42, 43] To avoid hypotension, the drug is administered slowly at a lower dose and is not used in hemodynamically unstable patients.

Ketamine

Ketamine produces rapid sedation, amnesia, and analgesia[36, 37, 40] as a result of central dissociation of the cerebral cortex. Its sympathomimetic effect results in increased heart rate, blood pressure, and cardiac index.[46, 47] It also increases pulmonary compliance and decreases airway resistance and bronchospasm in patients with reactive airway disease.[47] Ketamine does not produce significant respiratory depression except in those situations when it is given as a

TABLE 7-4						
COMMONLY USED SEDATING AGENTS						
Sedation	**Dose**	**Onset**	**Duration**	**Advantages**	**Disadvantages**	**Clinical Uses**
Benzodiazepines						
Diazepam	0.2–0.5 mg/kg	1–3 min	10–20 min	Good amnesia Little hemodynamic effect Anti-epileptic	No analgesic effect Respiratory depression Venous thrombosis	Elective intubation Seizure condition
Midazolam	0.05–0.15 mg/kg	1–3 min	30–80 min	Good amnesia Short duration Anti-epileptic	Respiratory depression	Elective intubation Seizure condition
Opiates						
Fentanyl	30–150 μgm/kg	1–2 min	30 min–4 hr	Rapid onset Short duration Little hemodynamic effect Reversible with naloxone Analgesic effect	Risk of chest wall rigidity Respiratory depression	Airway obstruction Elective intubation
Morphine	0.1–0.2 mg/kg	2–5 min	4–6 hr	Analgesic effect Reversible with naloxone	Hypotension Respiratory depression Histamine release	Airway obstruction Elective intubation
Barbiturates						
Thiopental	2–5 mg/kg	Rapid	10–30 min	Rapid onset Short duration Decreases ICP	Hypotension Contraindicated in porphyria Increases bronchospasm No analgesic effect	Raised ICP (head injuries or meningitis) Rapid-sequence induction
Ketamine	1–2 mg/kg	Rapid	10–20 min	Rapid onset Beneficial in hypotension Bronchodilation Analgesia and amnesia	Increases ICP Increases secretions Dreams and hallucinations	Hypotension Reactive airway disease

ICP = Intracranial pressure.

rapid intravenous bolus. However, it increases intracranial[48] and intraocular pressure and may cause numerous psychic sensations, including hallucinations, vivid dreams, and occasionally frank delirium. Lorazepam has been most effective in preventing the unpleasant dreams and the psychic sensation following ketamine use.[47] Ketamine also increases salivary and tracheobronchial secretions, which may be decreased by the prophylactic administration of atropine.

Muscle Relaxants
Depolarizing Agents

Succinylcholine is one of the most commonly used muscle relaxants (Table 7–5). However, it has a number of disadvantages, including clinically significant bradycardia, which may be followed by tachycardia and hypotension.[49] Other cardiovascular side effects include nodal rhythm and ventricular ectopic beats.[49] However, these effects can be diminished by the prior administration of atropine. Pulmonary edema and hemorrhage has developed in infants following both intramuscular and intravascular succinylcholine.[50] Succinylcholine increases intragastric pressure ten times more commonly in adults than in children; children with an incompetent cardioesophageal sphincter may have regurgitation and aspiration.[51, 52] It also elevates intraocular and intracranial pressure and should be avoided in patients with penetrating eye injuries, as it may result in extrusion of the vitreous.[53] Myoglobinemia occurs more frequently in children than in adults but is of minimal clinical significance. Malignant hyperthermia and masseter spasm[54] are uncommon complications.

There have been numerous reports of hyperkalemia after administration of succinylcholine.[55–66] These reports involved patients with upper motor neuron lesions such as spinal cord transection, and tetanus and burns[55]; massive trauma[57]; neuromuscular disease[56]; and severe intra-abdominal sepsis.[60] The potassium-releasing action of succinylcholine begins by 5 to 15 days after injury and persists for 2 to 3 months in patients who have sustained burns or trauma and perhaps for 3 to 6 months in patients with upper motor neuron lesions.[61] Therefore in the acutely injured child, there is no evidence to suggest succinylcholine is contraindicated. Pretreatment with diazepam has been shown to decrease the degree of muscular fasciculation as well as the elevation in potassium.[62]

Nondepolarizing Agents

Pancuronium is one of the more commonly administered long-acting neuromuscular blocking agents.[67] It causes less histamine release and less bronchospasm than other paralyzing agents[67] and therefore is the drug of choice in asthmatics. After administration there is often an increase in heart rate and blood pressure.[67] Because of its long half-life, pancuronium should be used only in situations in which prolonged artificial ventilation of the child is possible. Tubocurarine chloride causes more histamine release than pancuronium and therefore should be avoided in asthmatics. Tubocurarine chloride frequently may result in hypotension as a result of histamine release, direct vasodilation, or myocardial depression.

Both atracurium and vecuronium are intermediate-acting, nondepolarizing neuromuscular blocking agents.[68–70] The

TABLE 7–5						
COMMONLY USED MUSCLE RELAXANTS						
Drug	**Dose**	**Onset**	**Duration**	**Advantages**	**Disadvantages**	**Clinical Uses**

Depolarizing agent
  Succinylcholine
	Infants: 2 mg/kg
	Children: 1 mg/kg
		30–60 sec	3–12 min	Rapid onset
				Short duration
				May be administered
				  IM
					CV: Bradycardia,
					  hypotension,
					  dysrhythmias
					R: Pulmonary edema,
					  pulmonary
					  hemorrhage
					GI: Increased
					  intragastric
					  pressure
					Eye: Increased
					  intraocular
					  pressure
					Other: Hyperkalemia,
					  myoglobinuria,
					  malignant
					  hyperthermia,
					  masseter spasm
						Rapid-sequence
						  induction
						Elective intubation

Nondepolarizing
LONG-ACTING
  Pancuronium
	Neonate
	  0–1 wk: 30 µgm/kg
	  1–2 wk: 60 µgm/kg
		1–5 min	50–90 min	Reversible
				Little hemodynamic
				  effect
					Histamine release
					Long acting
						Status asthmaticus

Defasciculating dose	0.01 mg/kg					

Paralyzing dose	Neonate
	  0–1 wk: 0.03 mg/kg
	  1–2 wk: 0.06 mg/kg
	  2–4 wk: 0.09 mg/kg
	Infants and older
	  children
	  0.1–0.15 mg/kg					

Tubocurarine chloride	0.25–0.5 mg/kg	1–5 min	50–90 min	Reversible	Myocardial depression Histamine release Hypotension	Elective intubation
Defasciculating dose	0.025 mg/kg					
Paralyzing dose INTERMEDIATE-ACTING	0.25–0.5 mg/kg					

Atracurium	0.4 mg/kg	2.5–4 min	20–45 min	Reversible
				Little hemodynamic
				  effect
					Histamine release
					Hypotension with large
					  dose or rapid
					  administration
						Hemodynamic
						  instability

Vecuronium	0.1 mg/kg	1–4 min	30–60 min	Reversible
				Short acting
				Minimal histamine
				  release
				Minimal hemodynamic
				  effect
						Hemodynamic
						  instability

CV = Cardiovascular; GI = gastrointestinal; IM = intramuscular; R = respiratory.

distinct advantage of these agents lies in the lack of cardiovascular adverse effects. A large dose of atracurium given rapidly may cause a moderate amount of histamine release and transient hypertension.[43] Vecuronium, however, does not produce any histamine-related adverse effects. Both of these drugs are also useful in patients with hemodynamic instability.

Additional Drugs

Lidocaine in an intravenous dose of 1.0 to 1.5 mg/kg before intubation suppresses the cough reflex, lowers increased intracranial pressure, and prevents increases in blood pressure, making the drug ideal for control of intracranial pressure during intubation and suctioning.[71] To be effective, however, it should be given 3 minutes prior to intubation. Atropine may be used in an attempt to block vagal stimulation during intubation, prevent bradycardia

commonly associated with succinylcholine, and minimize airway secretions.

TECHNIQUE OF INTUBATION
Orotracheal Intubation

Successful intubation can only be achieved when the medical personnel and patient are properly prepared and the appropriate equipment is in place (Table 7–6). Intubation should be conducted by the most experienced person available in a calm and orderly fashion. All patients should receive cardiorespiratory monitoring along with blood pressure and oximetry monitoring.

Proper positioning of the head and neck is important to place the mouth, pharynx, and larynx in optimal alignment for intubation. The sniffing position, with the head extended on the neck and the neck slightly flexed in relation to the trunk, is ideal. A common pitfall during this procedure is

TABLE 7–6
SEQUENCE OF INTUBATION
1. Have drugs and equipment available.
2. Use sniffing position to align the airway.
3. Preoxygenation: Awake: 100% by mask.
Apneic: 100% bag and mask.
4. Sedation.
5. Preoxygenation—establish ability to ventilate.
6. Administer muscle relaxant.
7. Open mouth—scissors maneuver.
8. Insert laryngoscope and sweep tongue to left.
9. Suctioning may be required.
10. Visualize cords.
11. Insert endotracheal tube from right side.
12. Ascertain correct position.

either failure to flex the cervical spine or hyperextending the cervical spine by allowing the head to hang over the edge of the bed. In the traumatized patient with the potential for cervical spine injury, mobilization of the head should be done without in-line traction.[72]

Preoxygenation is essential in all patients in an attempt to provide adequate oxygen reserve for the procedure. This is especially true in young infants, in whom a high oxygen consumption may deplete stores and result in bradycardia. In the awake patient, administration of 100% oxygen by mask for 5 minutes is adequate. In the apneic patient, bag and mask ventilation with 100% oxygen is required for a minimum of 3 minutes. Adequate sedation with a rapid-acting agent is preferred in the awake child. A muscle relaxant should only be administered after confirmation that adequate ventilation can be achieved using a bag-valve-mask apparatus.

A common reason for failure to intubate is an improperly performed laryngoscopy. With the right thumb on the lower teeth and the index finger on the upper teeth, the mouth is opened with the scissors maneuver. The laryngoscope handle should be grasped with the left hand and the blade introduced into the right side of the child's mouth. The tongue is displaced toward the left side by moving the laryngoscope toward the center of the mouth.

There are two techniques for advancing the laryngoscope blade to visualize the vocal cords. A straight laryngoscope blade may be introduced all the way and then gradually withdrawn until the vocal cords become visible. With this technique, the epiglottis often falls back and occludes the view of the vocal cords and should be elevated with the blade (Fig. 7–6A). The second method involves gradually introducing a curved blade until the epiglottis is visualized. The curved blade is inserted into the vallecula; traction along the body of the laryngoscope (forward and upward without rotating the wrist) will elevate the epiglottis and allow visualization of the cords (Fig. 7–6B). Regardless of the method used, after visualization of the cords, the orotracheal tube is inserted at the right corner of the mouth below and to the right of the laryngoscope blade, with the concavity toward the ceiling, and advanced gently through the vocal cords.

Trauma to the teeth and gums can be avoided by proper traction along the body of the laryngoscope without rotating the wrist over the upper jaw (Fig. 7–6C). Because the larynx is anteriorly placed, gentle cricoid pressure (Sellick's maneuver) may be required to bring the cords into view. Another common error is to insert the tube within the concavity of the blade, thereby obstructing the field of vision. Insertion

of the tube to the right of the blade may be facilitated by having an assistant retract the right corner of the mouth.

Failure to intubate the patient within a reasonable time period should be followed by withdrawal of the laryngoscope and tube and administration of oxygen by bag-valve-mask ventilation. As a guideline, the physician should take a deep breath prior to introduction of the laryngoscope into the oropharynx. If the intubation is not completed when the physician can no longer hold his or her breath, the tube should be withdrawn and bag-valve-mask ventilation reinstituted.

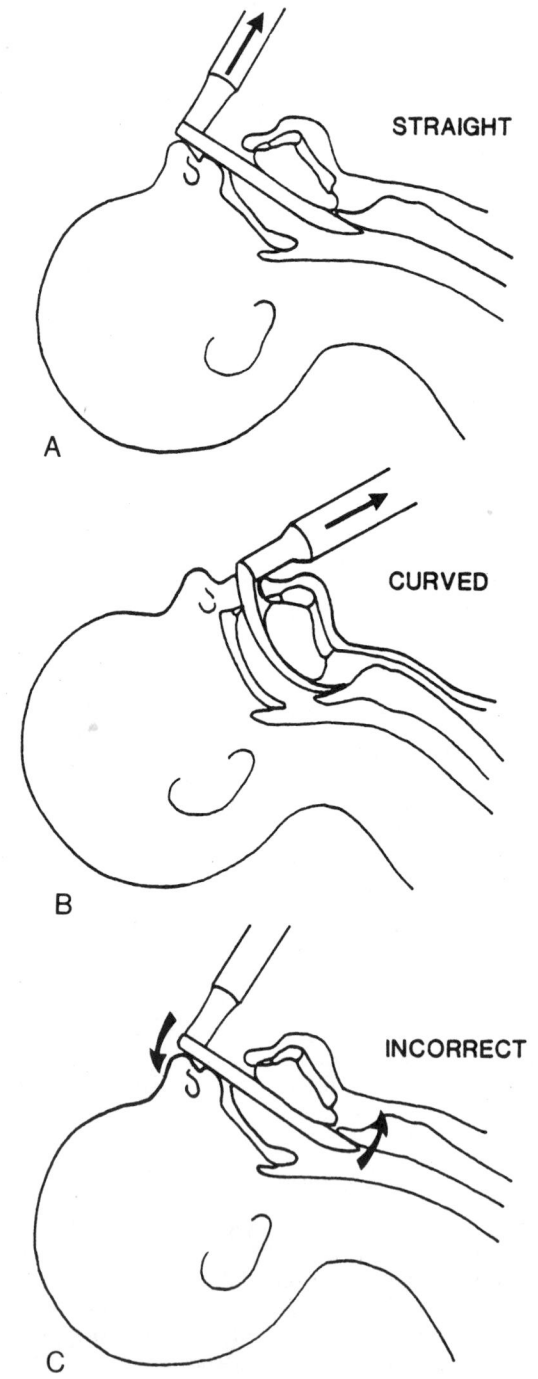

Figure 7–6. Technique of laryngoscopy. A, The straight blade elevates the epiglottis. B, The curved blade rests in the vallecula. C, Improper technique resulting in trauma.

Nasotracheal Intubation

Nasotracheal intubation requires more expertise than orotracheal intubation and should not be attempted in emergency situations by unskilled physicians. It is a useful procedure if intubation is required for a prolonged period in the conscious patient, as the nasotracheal position protects the tube from being bitten. This placement also provides better immobilization of the tube and easier suctioning and applies less pressure on the posterior larynx. It is contraindicated in patients with a fracture of the cribriform plate, a nasal deformity, or bleeding disorders or in patients on anticoagulant therapy.

Nasotracheal intubation can be performed by one of two techniques. The first method involves lubricating the tube and passing it through the nares into the posterior pharynx. With the laryngoscope in place, the tube is visualized in the pharynx and picked up by Magill forceps. Its insertion through the vocal cords is then facilitated by having an assistant advance the tube through the nares.

The second method involves placing an orotracheal tube as the first step. A second tube is then lubricated and inserted through the other naris. The orotracheal tube is then positioned to the left side of the oral cavity and artificial ventilation continued. The nasal tube is then visualized by direct laryngoscopy and held by Magill forceps. The nasal tube is placed alongside the oral tube as it enters the vocal cords. The assistant then removes the oral tube, and the nasal tube is inserted between the cords by the physician and advanced by the assistant as described in the first method.

Once the tube is in place, it is important to quickly ascertain its position, as right main stem intubation is a common complication. There are a number of methods available to confirm tube position (Table 7–7). The "gold standard" is visualization of the tube as it enters the cords. End-tidal CO_2 monitoring is now being used and is quite reliable.[73] A noninvasive method has also been introduced (Trach-Mate intubation system; McCormack Laboratories, Inc.) that utilizes an endotracheal tube with a magnetic strip. This strip is detected by an instrument placed in the suprasternal notch that provides an audible sound. In the emergency situation, however, visualization of the tube as it passes through the cords, proper aeration of both sides of the chest, and confirmation of position by chest radiography are the most common methods used.

If the endotracheal tube position in the trachea cannot be confirmed by these methods and the patient's condition is deteriorating, the tube should be removed and bag-valve-mask ventilation commenced. Intubation can then be reattempted after adequate preoxygenation.

INTUBATION IN SPECIAL CLINICAL SITUATIONS

Gastric Distention

The acutely injured child who presents to the emergency department should be assumed to have a full stomach and is at risk for aspiration (Table 7–8). Precautions are necessary to prevent pulmonary aspiration of stomach contents. A rapid-sequence intubation is indicated and consists of preoxygenation, sedation, muscle paralysis, and cricoid pressure to prevent aspiration (Table 7–9). Appropriate medical personnel, drugs, and equipment should be available before the initiation of intubation.

Preoxygenation with 100% oxygen (by mask in the spontaneously breathing patient and by bag-mask ventilation in the apneic patient) is necessary to establish an oxygen reserve during the period of apnea. Premedication with atropine blunts vagal stimulation, and administration of lidocaine suppresses the cough reflex and prevents elevation of blood pressure and intracranial pressure. If succinylcholine is being used, fasciculations must be prevented by pretreatment with a small dose of a nondepolarizing blocking agent. In children younger than 4 years, this may not be required, as fasciculation is not a problem. After premedication, a proper seal with the mask should be ascertained. Gentle cricoid pressure is then applied by an assistant, followed by administration of the sedating and paralyzing agents. Bag-mask ventilation is continued until full relaxation is attained; then the patient is intubated. After this, cricoid pressure is released, ventilation is initiated, and the stomach is decompressed with the use of a nasogastric tube. The sedating and paralyzing agent used for rapid-sequence induction may vary depending on the diagnosis and the hemodynamic state of the patient.

Hypovolemia

Airway support for the provision of adequate ventilation is useful in patients with shock, as a large fraction of the cardiac output is shunted toward the respiratory muscles.[9] Provision of assisted ventilation will result in relaxation of respiratory muscles and, hence, diversion of blood to vital organs. In the hypovolemic patient, drugs that decrease peripheral vascular resistance may potentiate hypotension and should be avoided. Ketamine is a useful drug in this situation, as it often increases the heart rate, blood pressure, and cardiac output.[47]

Elevated Intracranial Pressure

In patients with increased intracranial pressure, intubation and hyperventilation are necessary both for airway protection and to decrease intracranial pressure. Rapid-sequence induction (see Table 7–9) is recommended to decrease intracranial pressure and prevent pulmonary aspiration. Lidocaine is used to suppress the cough reflex and prevent elevations in blood pressure and intracranial pressure. Thiopental is the sedating agent of choice, as it diminishes the cerebral metabolic rate for oxygen and lowers intracranial pressure.[42–45] If the patient is hypovolemic, half the recommended dose of thiopental may be given slowly, or diazepam may be used. Ketamine should be avoided, as it may exacerbate the rising intracranial pressure.[48] If succinylcholine is being used, a defasciculating dose of pancuronium is required in children older than 4 years. After paralysis and before intubation, hyperventilation is recommended to decrease the $Paco_2$ and intracranial pressure.[74]

Status Asthmaticus

Most asthmatic patients require intubation as a result of impending respiratory failure caused by muscle fatigue. Adequate preoxygenation with 100% oxygen administered by mask should be provided. Excessive tracheal stimulation may further increase bronchospasm, and thus the use of local lidocaine is recommended. Because of its bronchodi-

---

TABLE 7–7

METHODS TO ASCERTAIN CORRECT POSITION OF ENDOTRACHEAL TUBE

Direct vision of tube between cords
Auscultation of chest and epigastrium
Symmetric chest movements
Stable vital signs
Endotracheal CO_2 monitoring
Trach-Mate magnetic detector
Chest radiograph

TABLE 7–8

SUGGESTED DRUGS FOR INTUBATION IN SPECIAL SITUATIONS

Patient Condition	Drugs	Dose (mg/kg IV)	Precautions
Full stomach	Atropine	0.01–0.02 (min 0.1 mg–max 1 mg)	
	Pancuronium (defasciculating dosage)	0.01	
	Thiopental	2–4	
	Succinylcholine	1–2	
	or Pancuronium	0.1–0.15	
	or Vecuronium	0.1	
Hypovolemic	Atropine	0.01–0.02	Avoid thiopental
	Ketamine	1–2	Avoid narcotics
	Succinylcholine	1–2	
	or Pancuronium	0.1–0.15	
	or Vecuronium	0.1	
Increased ICP	Atropine	0.01–0.02	Avoid ketamine
	Pancuronium (defasciculating dosage)	0.01	
	Lidocaine	1–1.5	
	Thiopental	2–4	
	Succinylcholine	1–2	
	or Pancuronium	0.1–0.15	
	or Vecuronium	0.1	
Status asthmaticus	Atropine	0.01–0.02	Avoid narcotics*
	Ketamine	1–2	Avoid succinylcholine*
	Pancuronium	0.1–0.15	
Airway obstruction	No muscular paralysis		
Awake	Inhalation anesthetic (nitrous oxide/oxygen)		
Obtunded	No drugs; bag and mask ventilation and intubation		
Anxious and hypoxic	Inhalation anesthetic (nitrous oxide/oxygen)		
	If no inhalation anesthesia, then morphine or fentanyl		

*Relatively contraindicated.

lator action, the sedating agent of choice is ketamine.[47] Narcotics are relatively contraindicated, as they may cause histamine release and can theoretically increase bronchospasm.[40] Thiopental should be avoided, as it may further increase bronchospasm. Pancuronium is the muscle relaxant of choice because of minimal histamine release and reduced incidence of bronchospasm.

Airway Obstruction

Failure to manage the airway properly in acute airway obstruction can lead to significant morbidity and mortality. For the awake patient who has some respiratory reserve,

TABLE 7–9

RAPID-SEQUENCE INDUCTION

Equipment and drugs available
Preoxygenation with 100% O$_2$
Premedication
  Atropine, 0.01–0.2 mg/kg (min 0.1 mg)
  Lidocaine, 1–1.5 mg/kg IV
  Defasciculating agent—pancuronium, 0.01 mg/kg
Achieve mask seal
  Bag-mask ventilation of apneic patient
Cricoid pressure (by assistant)
Sedating agent
Muscle relaxant
Intubate; then release cricoid pressure
Begin bag ventilation
Decompress the stomach

procedures that increase patient anxiety should be avoided. Therefore blood sampling, separating the child from the parents, and repeated examinations should be avoided. The patient should be allowed to remain with the parents and should be given oxygen in as comfortable a position as possible. Individuals such as anesthesiologists, otolaryngologists, and critical care specialists should be consulted as soon as possible. Ideally the patient should have the airway secured with the use of an inhalational anesthetic.

For the patient who is obtunded as a result of hypoxia, hypercarbia, or respiratory fatigue, bag-valve-mask ventilation is often adequate as an interim measure. Intubation should be attempted by the most experienced person, keeping in mind that if this fails, bag-valve ventilation should be reinstituted and additional help summoned. Patients who are hypoxic may be anxious and uncooperative. Under these circumstances, bag-valve-mask ventilation may be difficult. Muscle relaxants are absolutely contraindicated if personnel or facilities are unavailable to secure a surgical airway. Abolishing the patient's own respiratory drive by paralysis, followed by inability to secure the airway, is a potentially fatal situation. If appropriate personnel are not immediately available, fentanyl or morphine may be helpful to facilitate ventilation, as reversal with naloxone is possible if ventilation is not secured.

THE DIFFICULT AIRWAY

Arbitrarily, an airway may be considered difficult when a competent clinician who has had 12 months of anesthesia or critical care training is unable to intubate a patient following three attempts.[2] Difficulty securing the airway may be a result of simple errors in technique (Table 7–10). Malalignment of the mouth, pharynx, and larynx is a common problem and is usually caused by inadequate extension of the head on the neck or inadequate flexion of the neck on the trunk. If the mouth is inadequately opened and the laryngoscope blade is not used to sweep the tongue to the left, visualization of the cords becomes difficult. Another pitfall is use of leverage instead of traction along the body of the laryngoscope. This provides less exposure of the cords and usually results in trauma to the teeth and gums. Introduction of the tube in the visual field is another common error. Inadequate or improper sedation or muscle relaxation may render intubation challenging; however, if the airway is difficult to secure, sedation should be used judiciously and neuromuscular relaxation avoided.

A truly difficult airway may result from a number of anatomic problems, including limited access to the oropharynx or nasopharynx, poor visualization of the larynx, and diminished cross-sectional area of the larynx or trachea.[75] Access to the mouth may be limited because of facial trauma, burns, edema of the lips, a small mandible, and temporomandibular joint disease. Small nares, nasal trauma, fracture of the cribriform plate, deviated septum, large adenoids, and polyps may limit access to the nasal cavity. Poor visualization of the larynx may be a result of a small oral cavity, a large tongue, edema of the oropharynx, an unstable cervical spine, or a short, rigid neck. Narrowing of the airway as a result of intrinsic causes (e.g., subglottic stenosis or croup) or external compression may make advancement of the tube into the trachea difficult. This may often necessitate the use of a smaller tube or, more infrequently, the use of a surgical airway.

Approach to a Difficult Airway

Because the anatomy of each airway is different, an individualized approach is necessary (Table 7–11). On the basis of the history of the presenting illness, previous intubations, and a quick examination, one can determine where the difficulty may lie. The approach used to secure the airway will be dictated by the urgency of the clinical situation. In all cases, the approach to be used should be planned and all necessary equipment be available. An alternative plan should always be considered in advance if the first one fails. The numerous procedures used to facilitate intubation of the difficult airway can be conveniently classified into simple and special procedures.

Simple Procedures

External pressure on the cricoid ring often brings an anteriorly placed larynx into view. When it is difficult to

---

TABLE 7–11

METHODS USED TO SECURE THE DIFFICULT AIRWAY

Simple procedures
  Cricoid pressure
  Identify landmarks
  Stylet
  Blind intubation
Special procedures
  Fiberoptic bronchoscopy
  Retrograde catheter technique
  Needle cricothyroidotomy
  Emergency cricothyroidotomy

---

visualize the cords, identification of landmarks such as the epiglottis and the arytenoid cartilages can often be helpful. The esophageal surface of the larynx is characterized by being convex in both sagittal and transverse sections. Because the mucosa is loosely attached to the underlying surface, it appears as transverse folds[67] and hence if this surface is exposed, the laryngoscope blade has been introduced too far.

A stylet may be used to shape the endotracheal tube to the natural curvature of the oropharynx. The stylet should not protrude beyond the end of the tube, which should be introduced gently because of the high risk of complications such as submucosal dissection, hemorrhage, hematoma, tracheal and esophageal perforation, pneumothorax, and pneumomediastinum. The stylet should not be used if the larynx or other landmarks cannot be visualized.

Blind Nasal Intubation. Blind nasal intubation can be used in the cooperative, spontaneously breathing older patient in whom direct laryngoscopy is difficult. After explanation of the procedure to the patient, both nostrils should be sprayed with cocaine 4% or a mixture of lidocaine and phenylephrine. A lubricated tube is then inserted through the nares into the oropharynx. The cervical spine is flexed and the head extended, with the mandible pulled upward using the left hand. When entry into the airway occurs, the patient usually coughs, and a clear tubular breath sound is audible. Several attempts may be necessary, during which manipulation of the cervical spine and mandible may be required in order to secure the tube beyond the cords. This procedure is difficult in the active, uncooperative child. Blind nasal intubation is contraindicated with bleeding, tumors, or abscesses above the glottis because of the risk of trauma and rupture.[33] In addition, manipulation of the cervical spine should be avoided in patients with potential cervical spine injuries.

Special Procedures

Fiberoptic Bronchoscopy. Fiberoptic bronchoscopy is rapidly replacing other conventional methods for difficult intubations. This method is useful not only for securing a difficult airway but also for diagnostic purposes. This technique can provide immediate, safe, and accurate diagnosis of croup, epiglottitis, paralysis of the vocal cords, subglottic stenosis, and hemangioma, with the immediate option of intubation.[76, 77] Tube position can also be confirmed during bronchoscopy, thus decreasing the chance of right main stem intubation.

Pediatric flexible bronchoscopes are available with a 3.5-mm outer diameter and a suction channel to clear blood and secretions to enhance visualization. The fiberoptic scope is lubricated and passed through the endotracheal tube. After instillation of xylocaine into the oropharynx, the scope

---

TABLE 7–10

COMMON PITFALLS OF OROTRACHEAL INTUBATION

Errors in technique
  Inappropriate equipment
  Improper positioning
  Inadequate opening of mouth
  Failure to sweep the tongue to the left
  Improper traction to visualize cords
  Inadequate suctioning
  Endotracheal tube obliterates visual field
Anatomic problems
  Limited access to oropharynx or nasopharynx (e.g., facial trauma)
  Poor visualization of larynx (e.g., large tongue)
  Small cross-sectional area of larynx (e.g., croup)

is passed through the nose and the vocal cords. The tube is then advanced over the scope through the cords and positioned above the carina.

Failure to intubate may be a result of secretions, blood, edema, fogging of the scope, or improper technique. Transient bradycardia, hypoxia, and epistaxis may occur during the procedure. This procedure is contraindicated in patients with severe nasal obstruction or posterior pharyngeal bleeding and in apneic patients in the emergency setting. The oral route is an alternative in situations in which the nasal route is difficult or contraindicated. This technique requires considerable skill and is rarely used in the emergency department.

Retrograde Catheter Technique. The retrograde catheter technique was first described in 1960[78] and has since undergone some modification.[79, 80] This method is used in patients whose glottis is not completely obstructed, when direct laryngoscopy and blind nasal intubation have failed, and when fiberoptic bronchoscopy is unavailable. After local anesthetic infiltration over the cricoid membrane, a puncture is made with a needle (Fig. 7–7). The size of the needle is determined by whether a guide wire or an epidural catheter is used. In the pediatric patient, the guide wire is preferable. The wire is then visualized in the posterior pharynx with a laryngoscope and can be retrieved with a Magill forceps. The wire is then passed through the side hole of the endotracheal tube into the lumen. The endotracheal tube is then introduced through the vocal cords over the guide wire, which is then removed. For a nasotracheal tube, a suction catheter is passed through the nose and retrieved through the mouth. The guide wire is then tied to the suction catheter and is pulled through the nose. The endo-

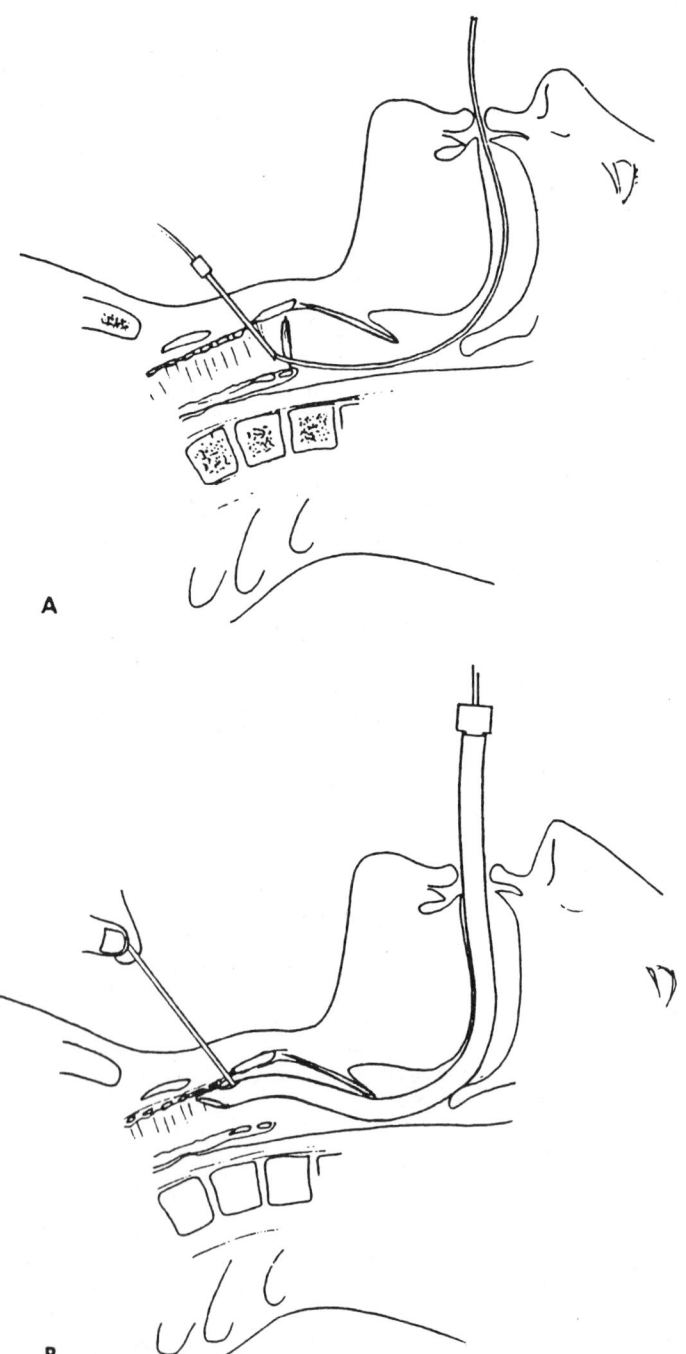

A

B

Figure 7–7. Retrograde intubation using a catheter threaded from the larynx by cricothyroid membrane puncture. (From Clinton JE, Ruiz E. Trauma Life Support Manual 1982, unpublished.)

tracheal tube can then be introduced through the nose over the guide wire. This technique has been successfully used in a 30-month-old child.[79]

Needle Cricothyroidotomy. In situations in which intubation is not possible (e.g., trauma, infection, presence of a foreign body, allergies, edema, or burns in the upper airway) a needle cricothyroidotomy[81] offers an easy, rapid, but temporary, method for securing the airway (Fig. 7–8).

After administration of 100% oxygen by mouth and subcutaneous infiltration of 1% lidocaine over the cricoid membrane, a 14- or 16-gauge angiocatheter attached to a 3-ml syringe is inserted through the membrane. The angiocatheter is inserted in a slightly caudal angle while applying negative pressure to the syringe until there is a free flow of air. The catheter is then introduced into the trachea and the needle removed. A 3.0 endotracheal tube adaptor (15

mm) will fit on the angiocatheter, and bag ventilation and oxygenation can be instituted.

With transtracheal ventilation, expiration occurs passively through the vocal cords unless there is a complete obstruction. In this case a stopcock may be used and occluded intermittently to allow for expiration and to provide better ventilation. Alternatively, another catheter may be inserted to allow for expiration. Transtracheal jet ventilation has also been used and limits the CO_2 accumulation.[82] However, a number of complications may result during this procedure. In the infant and young child, difficulty in locating the surface landmarks may result in procedure failure and the following complications[83]: bleeding, perforation of the esophagus or submucosa, mediastinal emphysema, infection, fistula formation, edema, and damage to the vascular and neural structures. Pneumothorax, pneumomediastinum, and pneumopericardium may also occur infrequently.

Emergency Cricothyroidotomy. This procedure is rarely indicated and ideally should be performed by an experienced surgeon[84] if attempts using conventional methods to secure an airway in patients with critical airway obstruction have been futile. After installation of a local anesthetic, a transverse incision is made over the skin and subcutaneous tissue of the cricothyroid membrane. Blunt dissection is carried out until the cricothyroid membrane is exposed. A transverse incision 0.5 to 1.0 cm long is made through the membrane. The endotracheal tube or tracheostomy tube can then be inserted through this hole and ventilation initiated.

Complications inherent in this technique include bleeding, pneumothorax, emphysema, injury to the laryngeal structures, laceration to the esophagus, and later subglottic stenosis, especially in children.[85]

MECHANICAL VENTILATION

Mechanical ventilation remains an important modality for the support of the critically ill pediatric patient, as more than 50% of pediatric intensive care unit admissions are a result of respiratory failure.[7] Mechanical ventilation is also important during the emergency treatment of conditions such as elevated intracranial pressure, cardiac failure, lower respiratory tract disease, and shock. In many cases, the initiation of ventilation takes place in the emergency department after endotracheal intubation and before admission to critical care units. Therefore those involved in emergency care should have the basic knowledge and skill to provide ventilatory support.

Indications

There are numerous indications for initiation of mechanical ventilation (Table 7–12); however, its primary use is in patients with respiratory failure, which results from the inability to meet the demand for O_2 delivery and CO_2 removal. Respiratory failure or insufficiency may be primary (resulting from lung failure) or secondary (resulting from pump failure).

Lung failure is due to parenchymal lung disease causing either inadequate alveolar gas delivery or inadequate gas exchange between alveoli and blood. The resultant effect is inadequate oxygenation, although adequate CO_2 removal may be achieved by increasing respiratory rate or tidal volume.

Pump failure is due to diseases of the central nervous system, respiratory muscles, and thoracic cage and is characterized by hypoventilation and hypercarbia. Hypoxia is also present and is primarily due to dilution of the alveolar O_2 by a high P_{CO_2}.

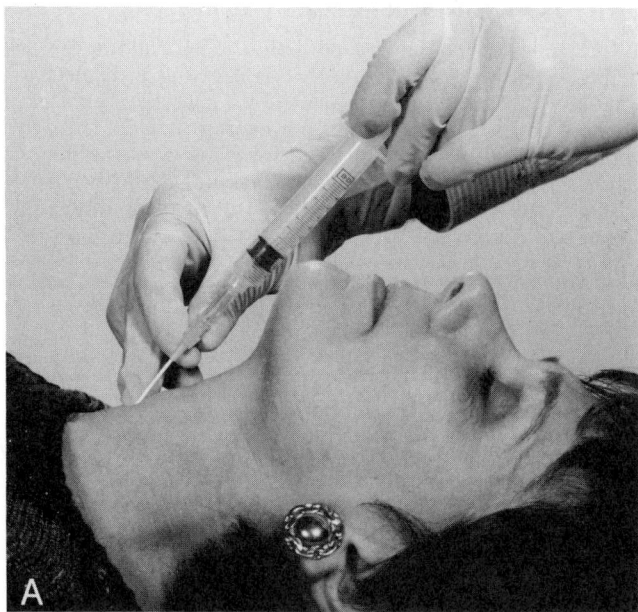

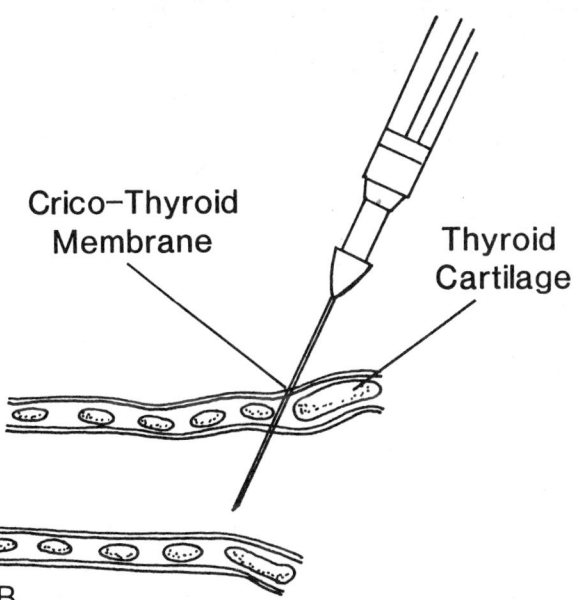

Crico–Thyroid Membrane

Thyroid Cartilage

B

Figure 7–8. The needle cricothyroidotomy. The technique for this procedure is demonstrated with an adult (A). The needle should enter between the thyroid and the cricothyroid cartilages, puncturing the cricothyroid membrane (B).

TABLE 7–12

GUIDELINES FOR INITIATING MECHANICAL VENTILATION

Neonates and infants (pressure-limited ventilator)
  Respiratory rate: 30–40 breaths/min (higher if required)
  Inspiratory time (I:E ratio): 1:2
    May change with higher respiratory rate
    May change with different disease states
  Peak inflating pressure (PIP)—two methods of determining:
    Start low (16 mm Hg), then increase quickly in small
      increments (2 mm Hg) until excursion is good
    Use a bag and manometer and determine optimal PIP for
      good chest excursion
  PEEP: Start at 3–4 cm H_2O (increase if needed)
  FIO_2: 5% to 10% above preintubation FIO_2 (adjust using
    oximetry and PaO_2)
Older children (volume-limited ventilator)
  Respiratory rate: Normal for age (higher if required)
  Inspiratory time (1:E ratio): 1:2
  Tidal volume (V_T): 10–12 ml/kg*
  PEEP: 3–4 cm H_2O (increase if needed)
  FIO_2: 5% to 10% above preintubation FIO_2 (adjust using
    oximetry and PaO_2)

*Set pressure limits on ventilator.

Classification of Positive-Pressure Mechanical Ventilators

An understanding of the simple classification of ventilators is useful for rational use in different clinical situations. The two most important criteria for classifying ventilators are based on initiation of inspiration and expiration (Fig. 7–9). Ventilators can initiate the inspiratory phase in a preset time (controller) or in response to the patient's spontaneous inspiratory effort (assistor) or a combination of both (assistor/controller). In the last case, the ventilator assists the patient's inspiratory effort, but in the absence of an effort, it delivers a breath in a predetermined time period.

The second mode of classification is based on parameters used to limit inspiration and allow expiration. These parameters include time (time-limited), volume (volume-limited), pressure (pressure-limited), and flow (flow-limited). Time-limited and volume-limited ventilators are the most commonly used in pediatrics; however, both have the ability to limit the peak inspiratory pressure (i.e., pressure-limited). Pressure-limited ventilators are generally used in infants and neonates weighing less than 10 kg, and volume-limited

ventilators are used in the older pediatric patient. There are advantages and disadvantages to the use of either device. With the volume-limited mode, an inspiratory pressure alarm may be used to limit excessive inflating pressures, possibly limiting barotrauma.

Common Modes of Mechanical Ventilation
Controlled Mechanical Ventilation

During controlled mechanical ventilation (CMV), the patient is unable to partake in any phase of respiration (Fig. 7–10). Hyperventilation, sedation, or paralysis is often required in order to be able to fully control the patient's respiratory effort. This method is used in situations when respiratory efforts are not desirable (e.g., in patients with shock or increased intracranial pressure).

Intermittent Mandatory Ventilation

Intermittent mandatory ventilation (IMV) allows the patient to breathe spontaneously while assisting with mechanical breaths. This decreases the need for excessive ventilatory support and is a good mode for weaning patients from the ventilator. It also avoids the need for excessive sedation and paralysis. The mechanical breaths may not be in synchrony with the spontaneous breaths, however, thereby increasing the risk of high airway pressures.

Synchronized (Assistor) Intermittent Mandatory Ventilation

During synchronized intermittent mandatory ventilation (SIMV), spontaneous inspiratory effort triggers the mechanical ventilator and provides assistance for this phase of inspiration. The inspiratory effort provided by the ventilator at a preset frequency is in synchrony with the patient's effort, thereby avoiding the higher peak pressures that may occur with IMV.

Pressure Support Ventilation

Pressure support ventilation (PSV) is used with spontaneously breathing patients; each inspiratory effort triggers the ventilator to provide positive pressure to a preset level. The major advantage of this mode is the synchrony of the breath-to-breath assistance which results in patient comfort and may be advantageous for weaning from mechanical

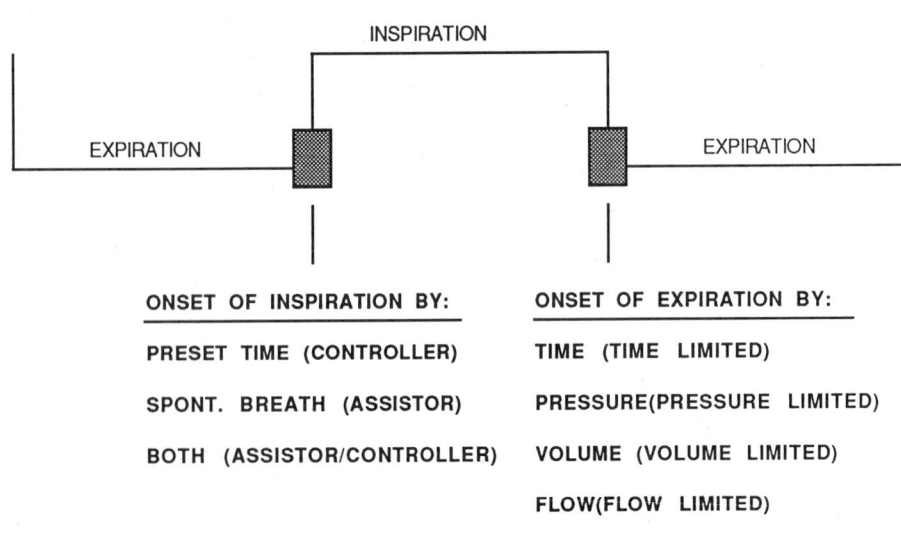

ONSET OF INSPIRATION BY:

PRESET TIME (CONTROLLER)

SPONT. BREATH (ASSISTOR)

BOTH (ASSISTOR/CONTROLLER)

ONSET OF EXPIRATION BY:

TIME (TIME LIMITED)

PRESSURE(PRESSURE LIMITED)

VOLUME (VOLUME LIMITED)

FLOW(FLOW LIMITED)

Figure 7–9. Classification of mechanical ventilation on the basis of initiation of inspiration and expiration.

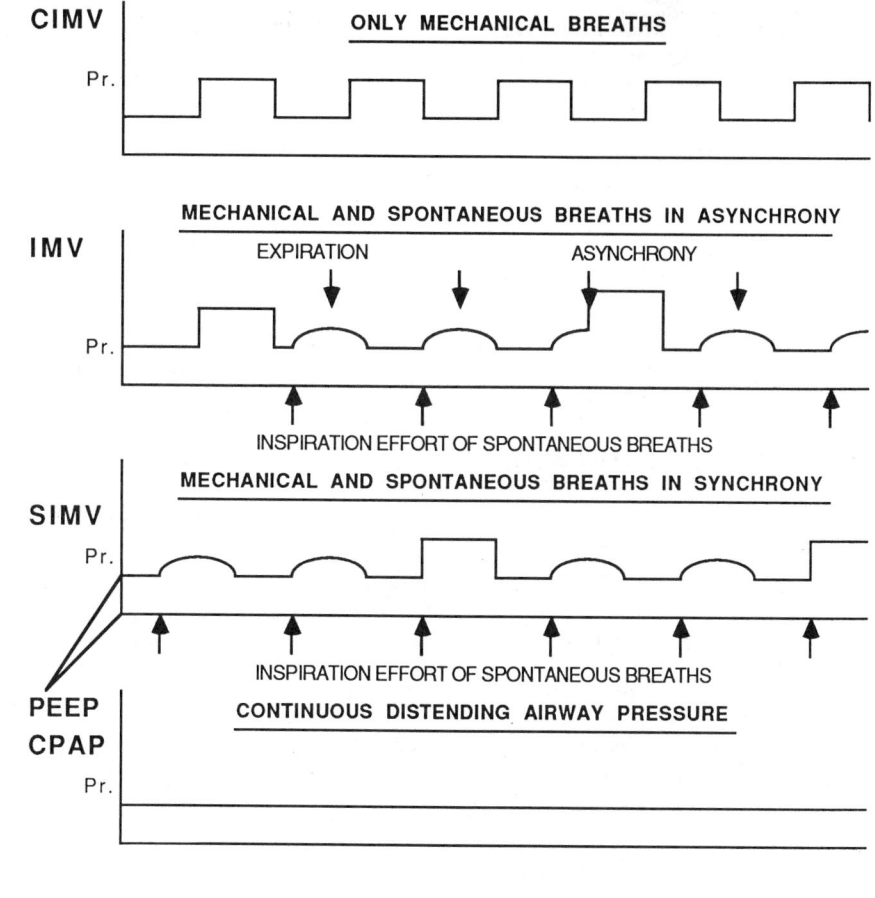

Figure 7–10. Various modes of mechanical ventilation.

VENTILATOR SENSES INSPIRATORY EFFORT THEN TRIGGERS AT A PRESET PRESSURE

ventilation. When compared with SIMV and continuous positive airway pressure (CPAP), PSV has been shown to decrease oxygen consumption, which is probably due to decreased ventilatory work.[86]

Continuous Positive Airway Pressure

CPAP is the application of a continuous distending airway pressure in the absence of mechanical breaths. Positive end-expiratory pressure (PEEP) refers to the same continuous pressure occurring in the presence of mechanical breaths. This mode is useful in disease states characterized by decreasing lung compliance and functional residual capacity (FRC). Application of PEEP recruits poorly ventilated and atelectatic alveoli, improving the FRC and lung compliance. The end effect is improved ventilation to areas of adequate perfusion, resulting in improved oxygenation and decreased oxygen requirement.

Initiating Mechanical Ventilation

Emergency physicians should be familiar with the ventilators used in their departments. Once the decision to provide assisted ventilation has been made, the appropriate choice of mode of ventilation will depend on several factors. Patients weighing less than 10 kg are generally ventilated using a pressure-limited mode; patients weighing more than 10 kg are ventilated using a volume-limited mode.

In the pressure-limited mode, assessment of the required inflating pressure can often be difficult. This can be done in two ways: (1) starting at a low inflating pressure and increasing quickly in small increments until the desired chest excursion is achieved or (2) use of a bag-valve apparatus connected to a manometer to determine the peak pressure required to achieve good chest excursion before placing the child on a ventilator. Adequate inflating pressure is ensured by chest excursion and appropriate patient monitoring. Though the normal tidal volume of spontaneous breathing is 7 to 8 ml/kg, the tidal volume delivered during volume ventilation is 10 to 12 ml/kg. This higher tidal volume requirement is a result of increased dead space due to the disease process and increased CO_2 production due to respiratory failure.

Patient Monitoring During Mechanical Ventilation

All patients should be monitored closely during mechanical ventilation in order to optimize therapy and avoid

TABLE 7–13

MONITORING DURING MECHANICAL VENTILATION

Clinical
  Cyanosis
  Tachycardia
  Tachypnea
  Accessory muscles
  Decreased air entry
Chest Radiograph
  Endothracheal tube position
  Lung disease
  Barotrauma/pneumothorax
Invasive
  Arterial blood gas
Noninvasive
  Pulse oximetry
  Transcutaneous P_{CO_2} and P_{O_2} (Ptc_{CO_2} and Ptc_{O_2})
  Capnometry (end-tidal CO_2)

complications (Table 7–13). Clinical parameters, although useful, are often subjective, and therefore other modes of monitoring are utilized. Chest radiography is useful to determine endotracheal tube position and lung pathology but is of limited value in assessment of ventilation. Arterial blood gas analysis is the most commonly used method of monitoring the adequacy of oxygenation and ventilation. This, however, is invasive and intermittent and has therefore prompted development of more sophisticated continuous, noninvasive monitoring.

Pulse oximetry is the most widely used noninvasive technique that combines plethysmography with oximetry. The resultant beat-to-beat display is extremely accurate.[87] Oximetry is less effective in peripheral hypoperfusion and is inaccurate in the presence of carboxyhemoglobin, sulfhemoglobin, methemoglobin, and high ambient light.[88]

Transcutaneous measurement of P_{O_2} (Ptc_{O_2}) and P_{CO_2} (Ptc_{CO_2}) provides an estimate of the arterial Pa_{O_2} and Pa_{CO_2}. In hemodynamically stable patients, the Ptc_{O_2} is slightly lower than the Pa_{CO_2} and the Ptc_{CO_2} is higher than the Pa_{CO_2}. In shock states, however, transcutaneous gas tensions are more dependent on the cardiac index than on arterial gas tension.[89] Therefore Ptc_{O_2} and Ptc_{CO_2} serve as a sensitive but nonspecific indicator of both tissue perfusion and oxygenation.

Measurement of the expired CO_2 (end-tidal CO_2 or $etCO_2$) by capnometry provides a measure of the efficiency of CO_2 transport to the lungs and excretion through the lungs.[90] The $etCO_2$ is normally 2 to 5 mm Hg less than the Pa_{CO_2}.

TABLE 7–14

GUIDELINES FOR WEANING AND DISCONTINUING MECHANICAL VENTILATION

Reversal or adequate recovery from primary disease
Clinically acceptable conditions
  Minimal pulmonary secretion
  Good cough and gag reflex
  Good cardiac, renal, hepatic, and metabolic function
  Good nutritional status
Cardiopulmonary reserve
  Normal pH, P_{O_2}, P_{CO_2}
  PEEP ≤ 4 cm H_2O
  FIO_2 ≤ 40%
  Vital capacity > 15 ml/kg
  Acceptable lung compliance/dead space
  Maximal inspiratory force > 30 cm H_2O

In the presence of pulmonary hypoperfusion (cardiac arrest, low cardiac output), there is less CO_2 delivery to the lungs, and therefore there is a decrease in $etCO_2$.[89] Complications such as endotracheal tube extubation, obstruction, or disconnection from the ventilator are quickly reflected in a lower $etCO_2$.

The noninvasive techniques provide the following advantages: early warning of cardiopulmonary deterioration, rapid assessment of efficacy of ventilator change, decreased need for blood gases during monitoring and weaning, and early detection of mechanical complications.

Weaning from Mechanical Ventilation

Weaning from mechanical ventilation is rarely done in the emergency department. However, if weaning is to be successfully undertaken, several conditions should be met (Table 7–14). In most cases, sufficient resolution of the primary disease does not occur in the emergency department, and weaning is undertaken in the critical care setting.

References

1. Kissoon N, Walia M. The critically ill child in the pediatric emergency department. Ann Emerg Med 1989;18:30.
2. Finucane BT, Santora AH. Principles of Airway Management. Philadelphia, FA Davis, 1988, pp 220–257.
3. Eckenhoff JE. Some anatomic considerations of the infant larynx influencing endotracheal anesthesia. Anesthesiology 1951;12:401.
4. Kubota Y, Toyoda Y, Nagat M, et al. Tracheobronchial angles in infants and children. Anesthesiology 1986;64:374.
5. Fearon B, Whalen JS. Tracheal dimensions in the living infant. Proceedings of the 47th annual meeting of the American Broncho-esophagological Association, Montreal Canada 1967;LXXX:964.
6. Rothstein P. Respiratory physiology in the pediatric patient. ASA refresher courses in anesthesiology 1980;8:155.
7. Gregory GA. Respiratory failure in the child. Clin Crit Care Med 1981;3:VII.
8. Wegman ME. Annual summary of vital statistics. Pediatrics 1983;72:755.
9. Aubier M, Viires N, Suyllia G, et al. Respiratory muscle contribution to lactic acidosis in low cardiac output. Am Rev Respir Dis 1982;126:648.
10. American Heart Association Standards and Guidelines for cardiopulmonary resuscitation (CPR) and emergency cardiac care (ECC). JAMA 1986;255:2905.
11. Kuzenski BM. Effect of negative pressure on tracheobronchial trauma. Nurs Res 1978;27:260.
12. Petersen GM, Pierson DJ, Hunter PM. Arterial oxygen saturation during nasotracheal suctioning. Chest 1979;76:283.
13. Naigow D, Powaser MM. The effect of different endotracheal suction procedures on arterial blood gases in a controlled experimental model. Heart Lung 1977;6:808.
14. Barnes CA, Kirchhoff KT. Minimizing hypoxemia due to endotracheal suctioning: A review of the literature. Heart Lung 1986;15:164.
15. Fell T, Cheney FW. Prevention of hypoxia during endotracheal suction. Ann Surg 1971;174:24.
16. Bouzarth WF. Intracranial nasogastric tube insertion. Editorial. J Trauma 1978;18:810.
17. Supance JS, Reilly JS, Doyle W, et al. Acquired subglottic stenosis following prolonged endotracheal intubation. Arch Otolaryngol 1982;108:727.
18. Parkin J, Stevens M, Jung A. Acquired and congenital subglottic stenosis in the infant. Ann Otolaryngol 1976;85:573.
19. Comardy PA, Goodman LR, Lavinge F, et al. Alteration of endotracheal tube position: flexion and extension of the neck. Crit Care Med 1976;4:8.
20. Resuscitators can -2168.7-M83. Rexdale, Ontario, Canada, Canadian Standards Association, 1983, p 11.
21. Standard specification for minimum performance and safety requirements of resuscitators intended for use with humans: F920–985. Philadelphia, American Society for Testing and Materials Committee in Standards, 1985, p 292.
22. Connors R, Kissoon N, Tiffin N, et al. Evaluation of physical and functional characteristics of pediatric resuscitators. Clin Invest Med 1990;13:B105.
23. Connors R, Kissoon N, Tiffin N, et al. Evaluation of physical and functional characteristics of infant resuscitators. Clin Invest Med 1990;13:B105.
24. Kanter RK. Evaluation of bag-mask-ventilation in resuscitation of infants. Am J Dis Child 1957;141:761.
25. Finer NN, Burrington KJ, Fadel A, et al. Limitations of self-inflating resuscitators. Pediatrics 1986;77:47.

26. Yamamoto LG, Yim G, Britten A. Rapid sequence anesthesia induction for emergency intubation. Pediatr Emerg Care 1990;6:200.

27. Thompson JD, Fish S, Ruiz E. Succinylcholine for endotracheal intubation. Ann Emerg Med 1982;11:526.

28. Roberts DJ, Clinton JE, Ruiz E. Neuromuscular blockade for critical patients in the emergency department. Ann Emerg Med 1986;15:152.

29. Stoelting RK. Endotracheal intubation. *In* Miller RD (ed). Anesthesia. 2nd ed. New York, Churchill Livingstone, 1986, pp 523–552.

30. DeGarmo BH, Dronen S. Pharmacology and clinical use of neuromuscular blocking agents. Ann Emerg Med 1983;12:48.

31. Cohen DE, Broennle AM. Emergency department anesthetic management. *In* Fleischer GR, Ludwig SL (eds). Textbook of Pediatric Emergency Medicine. 2nd ed. Baltimore, Williams & Wilkins, 1988, pp 53–65.

32. Pavlin EG. Anesthesia for the traumatized patient. Can Anaesth Soc J 1983;30:527.

33. Backofen JE, Rogers MC. Emergency management of the airway. *In* Rogers MC (ed). Textbook of Pediatric Intensive Care. Baltimore, Williams & Wilkins, 1987, pp 57–79.

34. Weiskopf RB, Fairley HB. Anesthesia for major trauma. Surg Clin North Am 1982;62:31.

35. Reves JG, Fragen RJ, Vinik HR, et al. Midazolam: Pharmacology and uses. Anesthesiology 1984;63:310.

36. Gerecke M. Chemical structure and properties of midazolam compared with other benzodiazipines. Br J Clin Pharmacol 1983;156:115.

37. Marshall BE, Wollman H. General anesthetics. *In* Gilman AG, Goodman LS, Rall TW, Murad F (eds). Goodman and Gilman's The Pharmacologic Basis of Therapeutics. 7th ed. New York, MacMillan, 1985, pp 276–301.

38. Chudnofsky CR, Wright SW, Dronen SC, et al. The safety of fentanyl in the emergency department. Ann Emerg Med 1989;18:635.

39. Bailey PL, Wilbrink J, Zwanikken P, et al. Anesthetic induction with fentanyl. Anesth Analg 1985;64:48.

40. Bailey PL, Stanley TH. Pharmacology of intravenous narcotic anesthetics. *In* Miller RD (ed). Anesthesia. 2nd ed. New York, Churchill Livingstone, 1986, pp 745–797.

41. Klausen JM, Caspi J, Lelcuk S, et al. Delayed muscular rigidity and respiratory depression following fentanyl anesthesia. Arch Surg 1988;123:66.

42. Way WL, Tevor AJ. Pharmacology of intravenous non-narcotics anesthetics. *In* Miller RD (ed). Anesthesia. 2nd ed. New York, Churchill Livingstone, 1986, pp 799–833.

43. Intravenous anesthetics. *In* Dripps RD, Eckenhoff JE, Vandam LD (eds). Introduction to Anesthesia, The Principle of Safe Practice. Philadelphia, WB Saunders, 1988, pp 141–155.

44. Rockoff MA. Brain resuscitation—barbiturates and other anesthetic agents. Arch Neurol 1984;4:408.

45. Michersfelder JD, Milde JH, Stundt TM. Cerebral protection by barbiturate anesthesia. Arch Neurol 1976;33:345.

46. Clements JA, Nimmo WS. Pharmacokinetics and analgesic effect of ketamine in man. Br J Anaesth 1981;53:27.

47. White PF, Way W, Trevor A. Ketamine-Its pharmacology and therapeutic uses. Anesthesiology 1982;56:119.

48. Takeshita H, Okuda Y, Sari A. The effects of ketamine on cerebral circulation and metabolism in man. Anesthesiology 1972;36:69.

49. Brandom B, Cook D. Muscle relaxants in children. Semin Anesth 1985; IV:41.

50. Cook DR, Westman H, Rosenfeld L, et al. Pulmonary edema in infants: Possible association with intramuscular succinylcholine. Anesth Analg 1981;60:220.

51. Andersen N. Changes in intragastric pressure following the administration of suxamethonium. Br J Anaesth 1961;34:363.

52. Salem MR, Wong AY, Lin YH. The effect of suxamethonium on the intragastric pressure in infants and children. Br J Anaesth 1972;44:166.

53. Cook D. Muscle relaxants in infants and children. Anesth Analg 1981;60:335.

54. Barnes PK. Masseter spasm following intravenous suxamethonium. Br J Anaesth 1973;45:759.

55. Schaner PJ, Brown RL, Kirksey TD, et al. Succinylcholine-induced hyperkalemia in burned patients. Anesth Analg 1969;48:764.

56. Brooke MM, Donovon WH, Stolov WC. Paraplegia: Succinylcholine-induced hyperkalemia and cardiac arrest. Arch Phys Med Rehab 1978;59:306.

57. Mazze RI, Escue HM, Houston JB. Hyperkalemia and cardiovascular collapse following administration of succinylcholine to the traumatized patient. Anesthesiology 1969;31:540.

58. Tobey RE, Jacobsen DM, Kahle CT, et al. Serum potassium response to muscular relaxants in neural injury. Anesthesiology 1972;37:332.

59. Genever EE. Suxamethonium-induced cardiac arrest in unsuspected pseudo-hypertrophic muscular dystrophy: A case report. Br J Anaesth 1971;43:984.

60. Kolschutter B, Baur H, Rolts F. Suxamethonium-induced hyperkalemia in patients with severe intra-abdominal infections. Br J Anaesth 1976;48:557.

61. Gronert GA, Theye RA. Pathophysiology of hyperkalemia induced by succinylcholine. Anesthesiology 1975;43:89.

62. Fahmy NR, Malek NS, Lappas DG. Diazepam prevents some adverse effects of succinylcholine. Clin Pharmacol Ther 1979;26:395.

63. Royston D, Wilkes RG. True anaphylaxis to suxamethonium chloride. Br J Anaesth 1978;59:611.

64. List WFM. Succinylcholine-induced cardiac arrhythmias. Anesth Analg 1971;50:361.

65. Wong AL, Brodsky JB. Asystole in an adult after a single dose of succinylcholine. Anesth Analg 1978;57:135.

66. Whittaker M. Genetic aspects of succinylcholine sensitivity. Anesthesiology 1970;32:143.

67. Bennet EJ, Daughety MJ, Bowyer DE, Stephen CR. Pancuronium bromide: Experiences in 100 pediatric patients. Anesth Analg 1971;50:798.

68. Fisher DM, Miller RD. Neuromuscular effects of vecuronium (ORG NC45) in infants and children during N_2O, halothane anaesthesia. Anesthesiology 1983;58:519.

69. Brandom BW, Rudd GD, Cook DR. Clinical pharmacology of atracurium in pediatric patients. Br J Anaesth 1983;55:117S.

70. Brandom BW, Woelfel SK, Cook DR, et al. Clinical pharmacology of atracurium in infants. Anesth Analg 1984;63:309.

71. Hamill JF, Bedford RF, Weaver DC, et al. Lidocaine before endotracheal intubation: Intravenous or laryngotracheal? Anesthesiology 1981;55:578.

72. Bivins HG, Ford S, Bezmalonovicz, et al. The effects of axial traction during orotracheal intubation of the trauma victim with an unstable cervical spine. Ann Emerg Med 1988;17:25.

73. Sayah AJ, Peacock WF, Overton DT. Value of end-tidal CO_2 measurement in the detection of esophageal intubation during cardiac arrest. Abstract. Ann Emerg Med 1989;18:459.

74. Bruge DA. Effects of hyperventilation on cerebral blood flow and metabolism. Clin Perinatol 1984;11:673.

75. Salem MR, Mathrubhutham MD, Bennet EJ. Difficult intubation. N Engl J Med 1976;29:879.

76. Rucker RW, Silva WJ, Worcester CC. Fiberoptic bronchoscopic nasotracheal intubation in children. Chest 1979;76:56.

77. Fan LL, Flynn JW. Laryngoscopy in neonates and infants: experience with the flexible fiberoptic bronchoscope. Laryngoscope 1981;91:451.

78. Butler FS, Cirillo AA. Retrograde tracheal intubation. Anesth Analg 1960;39:333.

79. Borland LM, Swan DM, Leff S. Difficult pediatric endotracheal intubation: A new approach to the retrograde technique. Anesthesiology 1981;55:577.

80. Bourque D, Levesque P. Modification of retrograde guide for endotracheal intubation. Anesth Analg 1974;53:1013.

81. Jacobs BH. Emergency percutaneous transtracheal catheter and ventilator. J Trauma 1972;12:50.

82. Attia RR, Battit GE, Murphy JD. Transtracheal ventilation. JAMA 1975;234:1152.

83. Kress TD, Balasubramaniam S. Crycothyroidotomy. Ann Emerg Med 1982;11:197.

84. Johnson DG, Jones R. Surgical aspects of airway management in infants and children. Surg Clin North Am 1976;56:263.

85. Aberdeen E, Downes JJ. Artificial airways in children. Surg Clin North Am 1974;54:1155.

86. Kanak R, Fahey PJ, Vanderwort C. Oxygen cost of breathing: Changes dependent upon mode of mechanical ventilation. Chest 1985;87:126.

87. Yelderman M, New W Jr. Evaluation of pulse oximetry. Anesthesiology 1983;59:349.

88. Lysak SZ, Prough DS. Anesth Clin North Am 1987;5:821.

89. Tremper KK, Shoemaker WC. Transcutaneous oxygen monitoring of critically ill adults with and without low flow shock. Crit Care Med 1981;9:706.

90. Swedlow DB. Capnometry and capnography: The anesthesia disaster early warning system. Semin Anesth 1986;5:194.

CHAPTER 8

Vascular Access

Bruce M. Thompson
Bonnie Sowa

INTRODUCTION

Vascular access is the most frequently used invasive procedure in pediatric emergency practice[1, 2] and is important for diagnostic sampling. In the critically ill or injured child, vascular access is imperative after airway control. Some patients may require more invasive or extensive monitoring, including arterial or central venous pressure lines to determine the degree of respiratory failure or shock. All emergency department providers must be skilled in the techniques of pediatric vascular access.

Obtaining vascular access in children can be difficult, time consuming, and frustrating.[2–4] Physicians who are unfamiliar with evolving techniques and who rarely start intravenous (IV) lines in children can expect to have less success and to require more time than those who do the procedures frequently. The urgency and anxiety inherent with the resuscitation of a sick child build markedly as time passes. As a result, establishing vascular access on the sickest children is often technically the most difficult. The difficulty may be heightened in premature or multiple handicapped children who have undergone prior hospitalizations and extensive procedures.

The timing of vascular access and the invasiveness of the techniques employed should be determined by the condition and acuity of the presenting child.[2, 3, 5] In a stable child who needs simple vascular access and sampling, the physician can start venipuncture peripherally and work proximally along the extremities until success occurs. For the critically ill or injured child, highly reliable, albeit more invasive, techniques for stabilization should be used.[5] The use of time-directed algorithms reduces the time to vascular access,[6] and once vascular access is established, efforts can be redirected to diagnosing and treating the critically ill child.

The child presenting in shock needs aggressive fluid resuscitation, which requires the use of short, larger bore catheters.[7] In general, the largest diameter catheter possible should be used. In shock, when vessel size is constricted, the dilatation of vessels using the guide wire technique will permit a much larger catheter size to be used.[8]

Anything as valuable and as difficult to obtain as pediatric vascular access should be tightly secured. In the sickest children, the catheters should be sewn in place and then taped securely. Appropriate arm or leg boards and sufficient restraint of other extremities are especially important in children capable of vigorous movement.

ANATOMY AND PHYSIOLOGY

Anatomically, body proportions and depth of subcutaneous fat play an important role in choosing peripheral access sites. Body proportions constantly change from the time of birth until approximately 12 years of age, at which time the body attains adult proportion (Fig. 8–1). The most marked change occurs in the relative proportions of the head to the total body stature. In the infant, the head accounts for one fourth of the total body stature. The large surface area of the infant head, along with typically scant hair and the superficial nature of the scalp veins, make these vessels readily accessible for peripheral venous access.

Body proportion influences the choice of site for central venous access as well. In both infants and young children, the neck is a short, stubby structure located between a large head and a barrel-shaped thorax. Thus central access through the jugular and subclavian veins may be more difficult to obtain. In the older child, the head, neck, and thorax achieve adult proportions, making these veins more available.

Unique to the anatomy of the newborn are the umbilical vessels that provide rapid access to the central circulation. After approximately 2 weeks of age, as the umbilical cord shrivels, dries, and eventually falls off, these vessels can no longer be cannulated.

The veins of the extremities lie within subcutaneous fat layers, the depth of which is age dependent. The infant has proportionately more fat than muscle, making it more difficult to locate peripheral veins within the thick subcutaneous tissue of the extremities. From 1 year to 7 years of age, there is a decrease in the thickness of the subcutaneous layer, making the peripheral extremity veins more accessible.[9]

With respect to physiologic differences, as a patient loses intravascular volume, the body compensates by constricting peripheral vessels in an attempt to increase vascular resistance. This maintains cardiac output and the essential volume of the central circulation. Although this phenomenon occurs in all age groups, it is more dramatic in young children. As a result they are relatively tolerant to fluid loss. Infants sustaining severe fluid loss develop marked peripheral vascular constriction, making access to peripheral vessels nearly impossible.

The local complications of peripheral venous access generally correlate with the related watershed area of a particular vein. A small-caliber vein in an infant may drain a relatively larger area of an extremity when compared with a vein of similar size in an adult. Hence thrombosed vessels

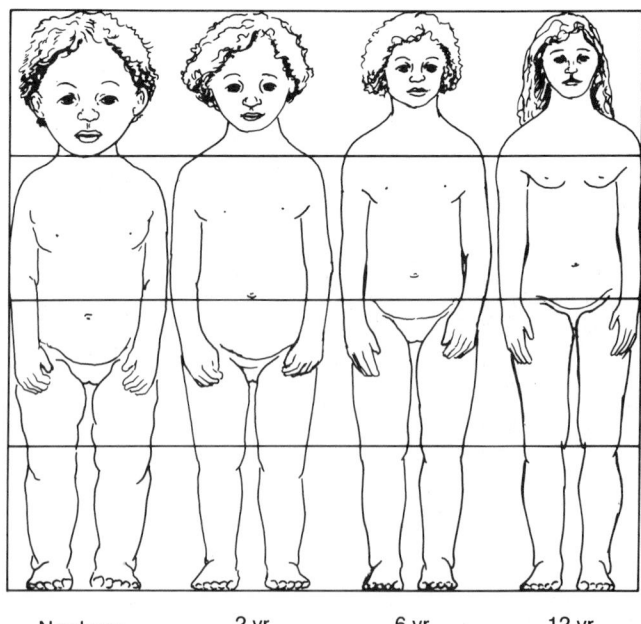

Figure 8–1. Changes in body proportions from birth to 12 years of age. (Redrawn from Robbins WJ, Brody S, Hogan AG, et al. Growth. New Haven, CT, Yale University Press, 1928.)

Newborn   2 yr   6 yr   12 yr

and veins "sacrificed" through the classic cutdown technique may create more serious complications for young children than for older children and adults.

Although complications associated with central venous access may be more frequent in young children, the types of complication are identical to those seen in adults and older children.[10] For any age group, complications of central venous access are generally more serious and more rapidly recognized than those of peripheral venous access (Table 8–1).

PRIORITIES IN VASCULAR ACCESS
Routine Vascular Access

Vascular access in the stable child should be approached in a stepwise manner. Techniques that are the least invasive and have the lowest morbidity should be attempted first.[2] Thus percutaneous venipuncture is attempted before a cutdown, and distal peripheral veins of the extremities are used before more proximal veins.

The initial approach to vascular access in the stable child is percutaneous cannulation of the distal peripheral veins of the extremities, including scalp veins in the infant. If establishment of access fails at these sites, the percutaneous technique is attempted more proximally on the extremities until successful. Ultimately it may be necessary to proceed to more invasive techniques, including percutaneous cannulation of central veins using the Seldinger technique or cutdown (Fig. 8–2).

In the ambulatory child it is undesirable to place a catheter in the lower extremity, thus preventing the child from walking. In the infant, the lower extremity or scalp is preferable to the upper extremity, which the baby uses for self-comforting.

Emergency Vascular Access

In the child who has impending cardiorespiratory failure or is in actual arrest, immediate vascular access is mandatory, preferably at a central site. Guidelines for priorities in venous access in the unstable child have been established.[11] Percutaneous peripheral venous catheterization is often futile because of poor perfusion and vascular collapse. A maximum of less than 90 seconds or no more than three attempts should be allotted for peripheral placement alone. Prefera-

TABLE 8–1
GENERAL COMPLICATIONS OF INTRAVASCULAR PUNCTURE OR CANNULATION
Damage to surrounding nonvascular structures
Laceration or direct injury to vessels
Cannulation of wrong vessel
Hematoma or extravasation of fluid
Thrombosis and clot embolization
Air embolization
Embolization of catheter tip
Phlebitis, catheter infection, or sepsis

bly, peripheral access should be attempted simultaneously with central approaches (Fig. 8–3).

If an endotracheal tube is in place before vascular access is obtained, this route can be used for the administration of the *ALIEN* drugs (*a*tropine, *l*idocaine, *i*soproterenol, *e*pinephrine, and *n*aloxone). However, absorption of drugs from the respiratory tract is erratic, with peak drug levels that are much lower than those obtained from vascular routes.[12–14] Therefore, after vascular access is obtained, drugs given initially through the endotracheal tube should be readministered intravenously, if clinically indicated, and all subsequent doses should be given intravenously.

For the child younger than 6 years, the intraosseous route is the vascular access site of choice. The venous plexus within the bone marrow provides direct access to the central circulation.[15] All resuscitation fluids and medications given intravenously can be administered through an intraosseous line.[16]

In unstable children older than 6 years, the femoral vein is the access site of choice. If cannulation of the femoral vein is unsuccessful (after attempting both legs), the next possible sites for vascular access are influenced by the presence or absence of cardiopulmonary resuscitation (CPR). If CPR is in progress, cannulation of the saphenous veins is attempted next. Both the femoral and saphenous sites remove activity from the thoracic area, minimizing interference with the operators performing chest compression. If CPR is not in progress, cannulation of the external jugular vein, followed by the internal jugular and the subclavian veins, is attempted. The order of attempts should be modified according to the experience of the operator.

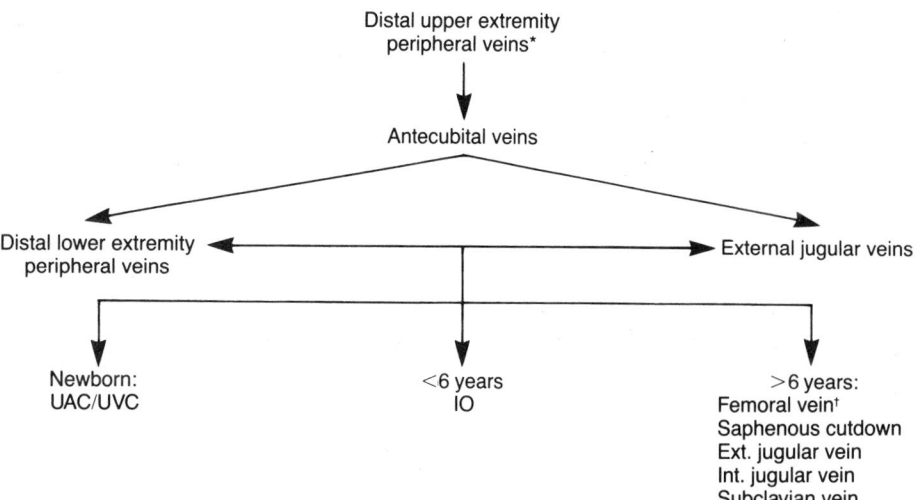

Figure 8–2. Priorities for vascular access in the stable child.

*All attempts are percutaneous unless otherwise indicated.
†The priority of access sites may vary with the operator's experience.

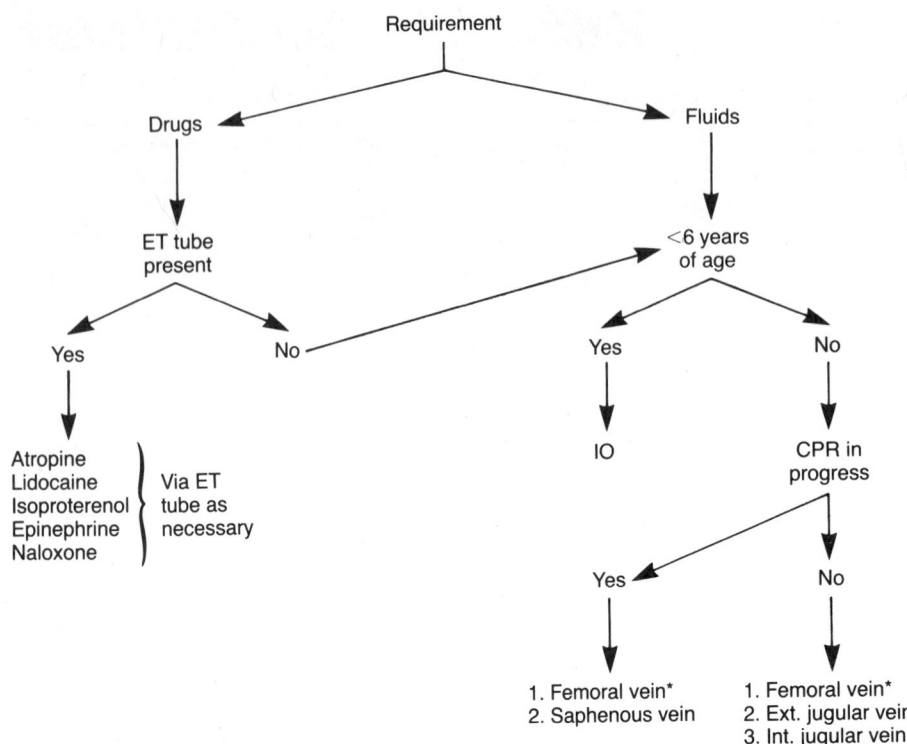

Figure 8–3. Priorities for vascular access in the unstable child. (Reproduced with permission. © From Chameides L (ed). Textbook of Pediatric Advanced Life Support, 1988. Copyright American Heart Association.)

*The priority of access sites may vary with the operator's experience.

Long-Term Vascular Access

For children needing long-term IV access, the child's disease state, previous IV access history, and type of infusate must be taken into consideration. The pediatric use of Broviac and similar catheter devices is limited to chronic conditions such as cancer, infection, and long-term alimentation.[17, 18]

VASCULAR ACCESS PRINCIPLES

Fluid Flow in Tubing and Catheters

The Ohm's Law for Fluid Flow states that the flow of an ideal fluid is

$$\mathscr{F} = \frac{P_1 - P_2}{R},$$

where $\mathscr{F}$ = volume flow rate (volume/time), P_1 = pressure at upstream and tube end, P_2 = pressure at downstream tube end, $P_1 - P_2$ = pressure difference, and R = effective resistance to flow.

When using a standard IV delivery system, P_1 can be increased by raising the IV container higher above the patient or by squeezing or pressurizing a plastic IV bag. Under ideal flow conditions, the resistance depends on the diameter and length of the tube, as well as the viscosity of the fluid.

The flow pattern of a liquid within a tube affects the pressure gradient and rate of flow. In a straight tube with uniform walls, a fluid tends to flow in smooth layers. The layer nearest the wall is essentially at rest. The velocity of flow increases progressively to a maximum at the central axis of the vessel. The average flow rate is approximately one half the maximum speed found at the center. This flow pattern is known as *laminar flow* and represents a minimal energy loss or resistance. If there is a partial obstruction or the velocity exceeds a certain critical level, the laminar pattern develops eddies, which increase resistance and significantly lower the flow velocity. Such turbulent flow patterns exist following any abrupt change in tubing size or in bends or kinks in the IV tubing or vessel. Turbulence may also cause hemolysis of red blood cells (RBCs) when sampling is done using a vacuum container or with excessive syringe suction. Gentle syringe withdrawal of a sample using larger caliber catheters or needles minimizes turbulence and hemolysis.

Other frictional forces exist within the fluid itself. The molecular adhesive force that opposes movement or flow is known as *viscosity*. Physiologic saline solutions have a lower viscosity and thus flow much faster than complex colloid solutions such as blood or plasma. Within a given pressure gradient, volume flow is inversely proportional to the viscosity. In small laminar flow tubes where wall friction is not significant, Poiseuille found that pure liquids like water approximate ideal flow.[19]

Two key relationships are immediately apparent: First, increasing the standard length of tubing from the IV bag to the catheter with extension tubing will reduce flow velocity by a proportional amount (i.e., doubling the IV tubing length will cut flow in half). Most importantly, the volume flow rate is dependent on the *fourth power* of the tubing radius. Therefore to increase the rate of flow, it is most efficient to increase the size of the catheter or IV tubing; doubling the diameter of a catheter will increase flow by a factor of 16. In practice, the shortest, largest diameter catheter possible should be used for fluid resuscitation. Actual flow measurements for a variety of catheters, pressures, and fluids have been established (Table 8–2).[20]

Viscosity becomes important with the rapid transfusion of blood products in resuscitation. The viscosity of water at room temperature is 0.01 poise (dyne-sec/cm²). Whole blood at body temperature has a viscosity of 0.03 to 0.05 poise—three to five times the viscosity of water (Fig. 8–4).[21] Most

TABLE 8–2
COMPARATIVE AVERAGE FLOW RATES (ML/MIN)

Catheter	Tap Water at 200 mm Hg	Diluted PRBCs at 200 mm Hg	Tap Water Gravity	Diluted PRBCs, Blood Warmer at 200 mm Hg	PRBCs at 200 mm Hg
Central Venous Catheters					
USCI No. 9 French introducer					
Internal diameter, 0.117 in; length 5½ in	566 (±16)	343 (±21)	247 (±2)	218 (±26)	124 (±2)
USCI No. 8 French introducer					
Internal diameter, 0.104 in; length 5½ in	540*	324 (±23)	243 (±5)	—	—
Deseret angiocatheter					
Gauge, 14; length, 5¼ in	341 (±6)	210 (±7)	157 (±6)	171 (±9)	63 (±6)
Peripheral Venous Catheters					
IV extension tubing					
Internal diameter, 0.12 in; length, 12 in	500 (±21)	312 (±1)	222 (±4)	—	—
Argyle Medicut					
Gauge, 14; length, 2 in	484 (±8)	287 (±21)	194 (±5)	192 (±15)	96 (±6)
Argyle Medicut					
Gauge, 16; length, 2 in	353 (±4)	220 (±5)	151 (±3)	—	—

*95% confidence interval not calculated because all three trials resulted in 11.1 sec for 100-ml flow.
From Mateer JR, Thompson BM, Aprahamian C, Darin JC. Rapid fluid resuscitation with central venous catheters. Ann Emerg Med 1983;12:151.

blood banks only have cooled packed RBC units available for resuscitation. The viscosity of such cold packed RBCs is markedly higher. The viscosity of the packed cells can be reduced by warming and dilution. To quickly and easily warm the RBCs and reduce the blood viscosity, the packed cells are reconstituted to their original volume by infusing warmed crystalloid solution into the blood bag (Fig. 8–5). Significant hemolysis is not seen.[20] Such warmed, diluted packed cells approximate the viscosity of whole blood at body temperature. If multiple units of blood are to be transfused, additional blood warming techniques should be used. Most blood warmers reduce the rate of fluid flow significantly by increasing the length to heat exchange and decreasing the diameter of tubing in the warmer.[20]

Blood is a complex fluid that does not precisely follow Poiseuille's Law. In high-pressure, high-flow states, the viscosity of blood is found to decrease with increased fluid pressure; doubling the pressure will more than double the rate of flow.[22] This is thought to be because of the tendency of RBCs to accumulate near the central axis of the catheter, where the flow is the fastest.

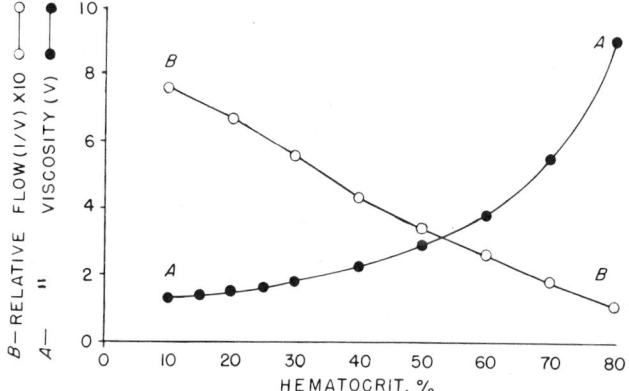

Figure 8–4. Curve A: Relative viscosity (V) for bloods with various hematocrits. Curve B: Relative flow rates for bloods with various hematocrits. The curve was constructed by taking the reciprocals (1/V) of points on curve A. In order to use the same vertical scale, these were then multiplied by 10. (From Castle WB, Jandl JH. Blood viscosity and blood volume: Opposing influence upon oxygen transport in polycythemia. Semin Hematol 1966;3:193.)

It is important to emphasize that when large-bore IV tubing is used to supply fluid to a smaller catheter, the resistance caused by the length of IV tubing is usually negligible when compared with the resistance created by the catheter. The internal diameters of larger bore IV tubing are essentially equal to the internal diameters of the largest catheters now available for specialized applications requiring massive fluid resuscitation. Pressure infuser units have had limited application in children and should be used only with great care.

NEEDLE DEVICES
Scalp Vein or "Butterfly" Needles

The simplest devices, known as the *scalp vein* or *butterfly needles*, are an adaptation of common disposable needles. These "butterflies" require absolute immobilization of the metallic needle within the cannulated vein to prevent extravasation, subcutaneous infusion, or vascular injury.

Catheter-Over-the-Needle Devices

The catheter-over-the-needle device was developed in the late 1950s by the Rochester Products Company and was known as the *Rochester needle*.[23] Improvements in cannulating needles and catheter plastics and the development of extremely small-gauge catheter devices continue. The catheter-over-the-needle device is currently the most common device used for intermediate-duration vascular access.

Catheter-Through-the-Needle Devices

George Doherty,[24] an anesthesiologist, developed the catheter-through-the-needle device, in which a larger, thin-walled needle is introduced into the vessel, and a smaller catheter is placed through the needle into the vessel. The needle is then either pulled back and guarded or removed entirely. Because the catheter is advanced through and past the sharp bevel of the needle, such catheters are always at risk of being sheared off and embolized.

Guide Wire–Dilator-Catheter Devices

In 1953, Seldinger reported a method of catheter placement using a "pilot needle" through which a sterile guide

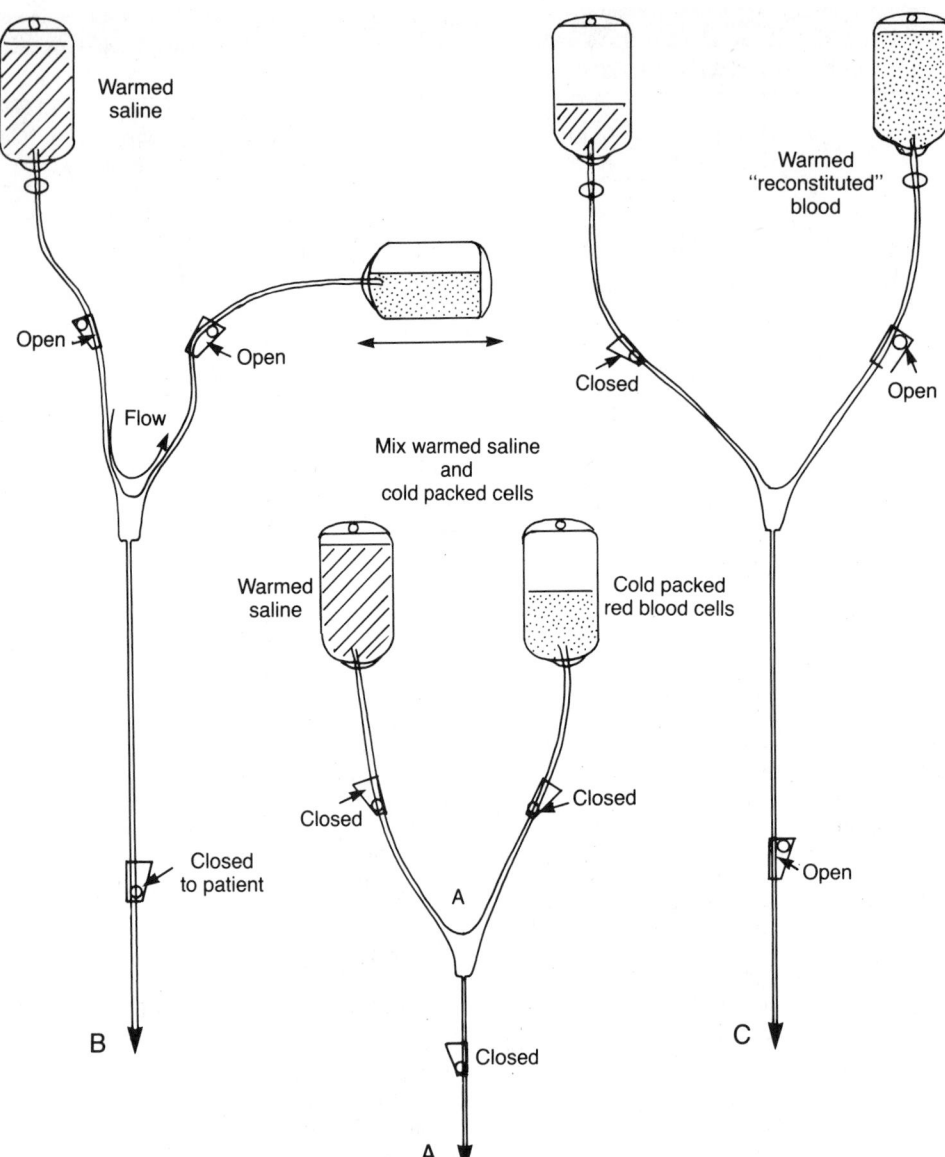

Figure 8–5. Procedure for warming and lowering the viscosity of cold packed red blood cell units for rapid administration. Warmed saline is mixed with cold packed red blood cells.

wire was introduced into the vessel.[25] The pilot needle was removed, and a long catheter was threaded over the guide wire and into the vessel. The guide wire was then removed and the infusion begun. This technique was an important advancement and is the basis of all modern central venous access devices. The technique is safer, more versatile, and more reliable than direct catheter access techniques.[8]

Minor Bone Marrow Needles

The technique of bone marrow, or intraosseous, infusion was commonly used in children in the 1940s and 1950s. Initial studies were done using spinal needles and bone marrow biopsy needles,[26] but an array of specialized bone-penetrating needles have since been developed, particularly for intraosseous infusion in emergency situations.[27]

MODIFIED SELDINGER TECHNIQUE

The modern modified Seldinger device uses a thin-walled needle through which a matched flexible guide wire is threaded into the vein (Fig. 8–6). The needle is replaced by the dilator and catheter sheath with the guide wire and

dilator removed. An extensive array of specialized catheters are available that can be advanced through the catheter sheath for specialized monitoring. These include Swan-Ganz catheters, thermistor catheters, mixed venous sampling catheters, and pacing catheters.

Indications

In situations requiring large catheter insertion, the modified Seldinger technique is the safest and most efficient method (Table 8–3).[8] A significant advantage of the Seldinger technique is the use of a smaller introducer needle, which reduces the amount of damage caused by the needle entering the vessel or adjacent structures. In general, the Seldinger technique is faster and has a lower morbidity than cutdown approaches[8] and is especially valuable when attempting central venous access.

In cases in which the patient is not in profound shock but requires central venous pressure monitoring, a small-diameter catheter can be introduced. If the patient's clinical condition deteriorates, a sterile guide wire may be reintroduced through the monitoring catheter and a larger bore dilator and sheath placed to allow fluid resuscitation.

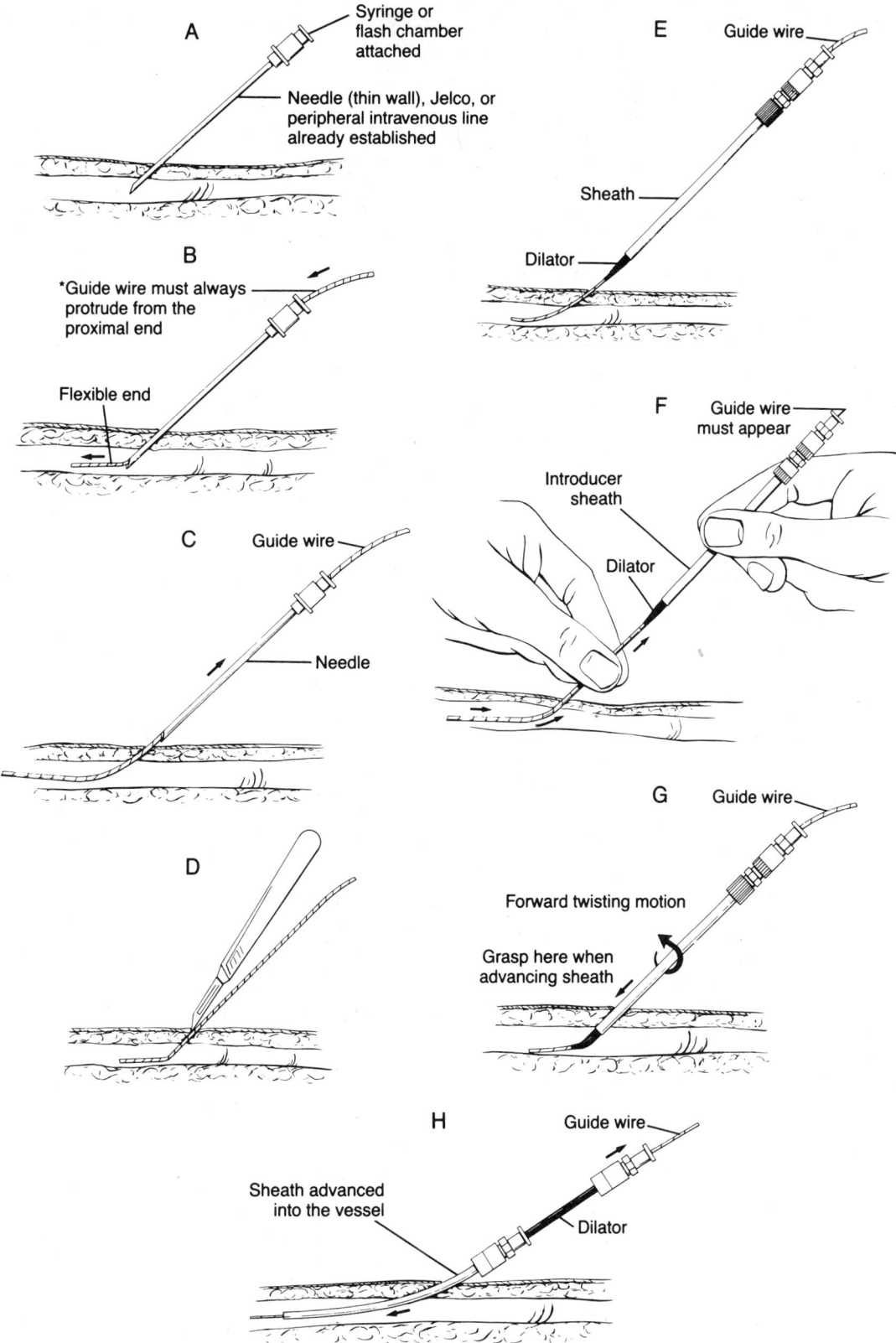

A   Syringe or
flash chamber
attached

Needle (thin wall), Jelco, or
peripheral intravenous line
already established

B

*Guide wire must always
protrude from the
proximal end

Flexible end

C   Guide wire

Needle

D

E   Guide wire

Sheath

Dilator

F   Guide wire
must appear

Introducer
sheath

Dilator

G   Guide wire

Forward twisting motion

Grasp here when
advancing sheath

H   Guide wire

Sheath advanced
into the vessel

Dilator

Figure 8–6. Procedure for placement of a Seldinger guide wire catheter. *A,* The selected vessel is cannulated. *B,* The guide wire is threaded through the vessel, flexible end first, into the lumen of the vessel. *C,* The needle is removed so that only the wire enters the vessel. *D,* The skin entry site is enlarged with a No. 11 scalpel. *E,* The catheter sheath and the dilator are threaded over the wire and advanced to the skin. The wire must be visible through the back of the device. *F,* If the proximal wire is not visible, it is pulled from the skin through the catheter until it appears at the back of the catheter. *G,* The sheath and the dilator are advanced as a unit into the skin with a twisting motion. It is best to grasp the unit at the junction of the sheath and the dilator to prevent bunching up of the sheath. *H,* Once the sheath and the dilator are well within the vessel, the wire guide and the dilator are removed. (From Roberts J, Hedges J (eds). Clinical Procedures in Emergency Medicine. Philadelphia, WB Saunders, 1985.)

				Intracatheters		**Venous Catheters**				**Catheter Introducers**			
Age (yr)	**Weight (kg)**	**Butterfly Needles (gauge)**	**Over-the-Needle Cathe- ters (gauge)**	**Catheter (gauge)**	**Needle (gauge)**	**French Size**	**Length (cm)**	**Wire Diameter [mm (in)]**	**Needle (gauge)**	**French size**	**Length (cm)**	**Wire Diameter [mm (in)]**	**Needle (gauge)**
<1	<10	21, 23, 25	20, 22, 24	22	19	3.0	8	0.46 (0.018)	21	4.0	6	0.53 (0.021)	20
										4.5	6	0.53 (0.021)	20
1–12	10–40	16, 18, 20	16, 18, 20	18	16	4.0	12	0.53 (0.021)	20	5.0	13	0.64 (0.025)	19
										5.5	13	0.64 (0.025)	19
										6.5	13	0.64 (0.025)	19
>12	>40	16, 18, 20	14, 16, 18	16	14	5.0	20	0.89 (0.035)	18	7.0	13	0.89 (0.035)	18
						6.3	20		18	8.0	13	0.89 (0.035)	18

TABLE 8–3

EQUIPMENT FOR VENOUS CANNULATION

Reproduced with permission. © From Chameides L (ed). Textbook of Pediatric Advanced Life Support, 1988. Copyright American Heart Association.

Occasionally, central venous catheters will be malpositioned. Reinsertion of a guide wire through the catheter and the withdrawal of the catheter and the guide wire to a point beyond the malposition will often allow the guide wire to be properly advanced and the catheter reintroduced over it.

Equipment
Needles and Guide Wires

Introducer needles have a tapered hub to allow the guide wire to pass smoothly into the lumen (Fig. 8–7). Attempts to pass a guide wire through a standard needle can be more difficult, but if a standard peripheral IV catheter is in place, a guide wire may be introduced through it.

Guide wires are made of stainless steel alloy wire coiled tightly about a central core mandrel wire, which terminates approximately 2 to 3 cm from each end.[28] The tip ends are either straight or J shaped and, without the mandrel wire, are soft and compliant. They are usually packed in a plastic ring with the J tip and wire introducer loaded for use. The opposite end is commonly in a straight, soft-tip configuration. The use of a J wire or straight wire is largely dependent on operator preference. When a large-caliber straight vein is to be entered, the straight-tipped guide wire works extremely well. If there will be difficulty in turning, twisting, or manipulating the guide wire around corners or through valves, the J wire is used. The straight wire is introduced by passing the straight tip through the tapered introducer needle and advancing the wire centrally. The J wire can be advanced in two ways. Each J wire comes with a plastic sheath that straightens the wire for passage into the introducer needle. Alternately the J wire may be bent distally with opposing fingers of the introducing hand, which straightens the J wire at its curved end for presentation to the catheter hub. In either case, the wire should pass easily through the introducer needle and into the vein. When resistance is felt, it usually indicates malposition. The guide wire is removed at that time and blood flow reestablished with the introducer needle before reinserting the wire. With the guide wire in place, the introducer needle is removed and the appropriate catheter-introducer device advanced.

Catheter Sheaths

For hemodynamic monitoring, a simple small catheter can be advanced. This is acceptable for low-flow infusions, drug administration, and monitoring. For large-bore infusions, a catheter sheath with an introducer-dilator is used to dilate the vein to the appropriate size. Originally this device was used in angiography procedures requiring catheter changes.[29] Many modifications of this basic device have been made, including the addition of side ports, which allows central as well as sheath administration of fluid or medications.[20] For rapid fluid resuscitation, such side ports create considerable turbulence and actually slow the total flow that can be administered through the sheath. Multiple-lumen catheters are available for critical care and alimentation applications.

Cautions

Catheters should be advanced only when the end of the guide wire is in full view. Failure to follow proper technique may result in the guide wire being lost inside the patient, with considerable consequent morbidity. Complications specific to the Seldinger technique are few and include wire migration and trauma, and defective or damaged guide wire tips.

PERIPHERAL PERCUTANEOUS ACCESS

Many sites are available for peripheral venous access in the infant and child. Sites include the veins on the dorsal surface of the hands and feet and those in the antecubital fossa (Fig. 8–8). In addition, in children younger than 1 year, the scalp provides a plexus of readily visible and accessible veins. In general, distal veins should be used first. Veins above the eyes and those overlying joints should be avoided.

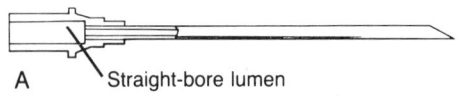

A Straight-bore lumen

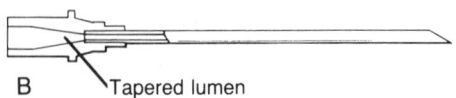

B Tapered lumen

Figure 8–7. Introducing needles. *A,* An ordinary needle with a straight-bore lumen. *B,* A Seldinger needle with a tapered lumen. (From Roberts J, Hedges J (eds). Clinical Procedures in Emergency Medicine. Philadelphia, WB Saunders, 1985.)

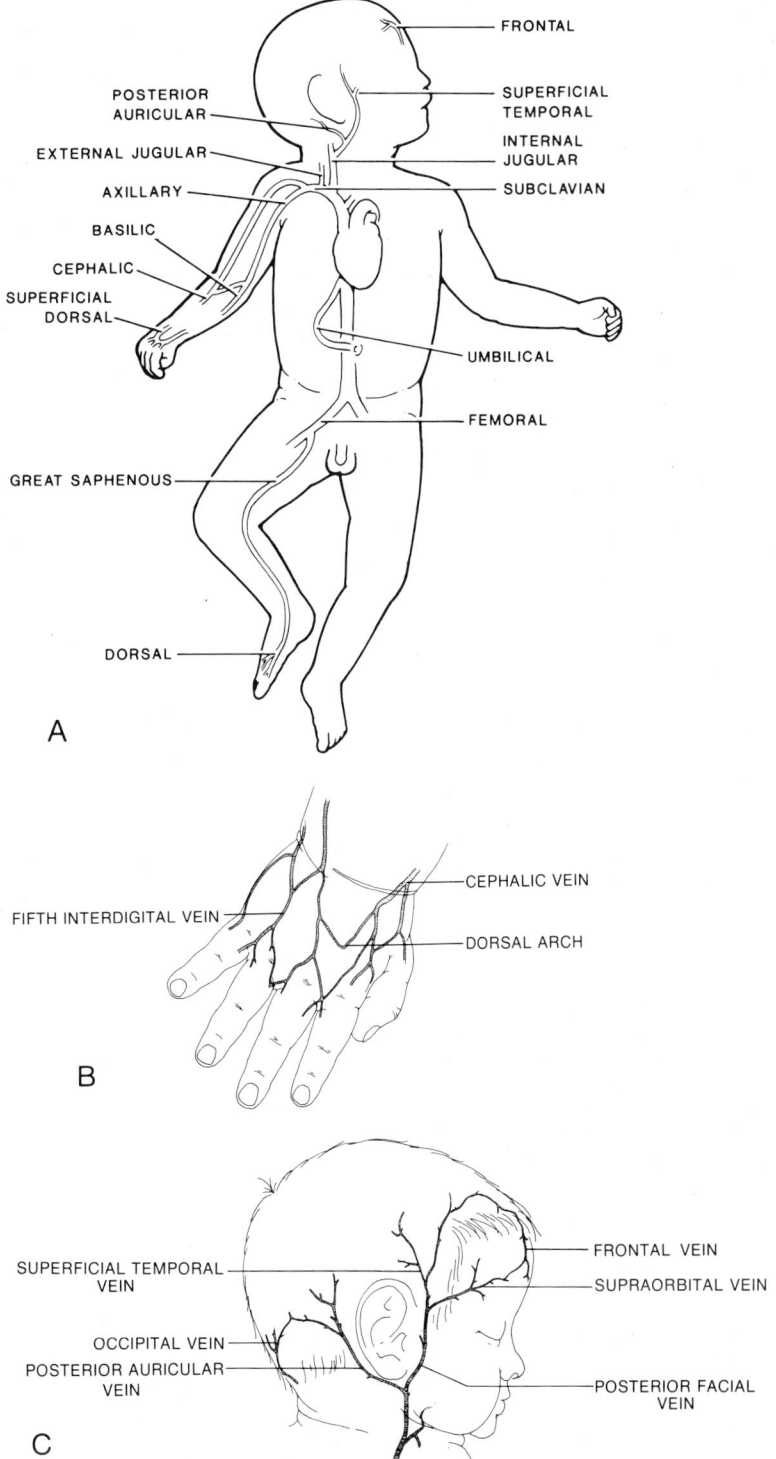

Figure 8–8. *A*, Venous access sites in the neonate and young infant. (From Roberts JR, Hedges JR (eds). Clinical Procedures in Emergency Medicine. 2nd ed. Philadelphia, WB Saunders, 1991, p 273.) *B*, Venous distributions on the dorsum of the hand. (From Hughes W, Buescher E (eds). Pediatric Procedures. 2nd ed. Philadelphia, WB Saunders, 1985, p 98.) *C*, Venous distribution on the scalp. (From Hughes W, Buescher E (eds). Pediatric Procedures. 2nd ed. Philadelphia, WB Saunders, 1980, p 95.)

Although the peripheral venous network of the child is similar to that of the adult, the veins tend to be less visible, especially in the young child. Often the choice of a particular vein for cannulation is based more on touch than on actual visualization. Veins within subcutaneous tissue can be identified by a "spongy" quality when compared with the more firm texture of the surrounding tissue.

A venous tourniquet placed proximally on the extremity aids in the identification of more distally located veins. A rubber band around the scalp or extremity provides adequate venous stasis without occluding arterial flow. A pediatric blood pressure cuff and a thin surgical drain can also serve as tourniquets. In infants, tourniqueting sometimes blanches the distal extremity, making the identification and cannulation of peripheral veins difficult. A fiber-optic transilluminator placed on the palmar or plantar aspect of the hands and feet may be useful for finding veins on the dorsal surfaces.[30]

Locally applied 2% nitroglycerin ointment induces local venodilation when applied to the superficial veins of the dorsum of the hand.[31] It is a safe and effective method for facilitating IV access.[32]

After the site for percutaneous cannulation of a peripheral vein is chosen and before venipuncture is attempted, the site must be fully immobilized. Proper immobilization is the key to a successful pediatric procedure. Some operators prefer to immobilize an extremity with their nondominant hand while performing the procedure with the other. This method affords the feeling of complete control. The main disadvantage is in having only one hand available for the procedure. An alternative method secures the extremity to a board or sandbag. The arm or leg should be firmly but gently taped both distal and proximal to the desired cannulation site. A gauze pad placed under the tape overlying the skin prevents adhesive attachment and subsequent painful removal of the tape. The most distal part of the extremity must always be visible for monitoring perfusion (Fig. 8–9).

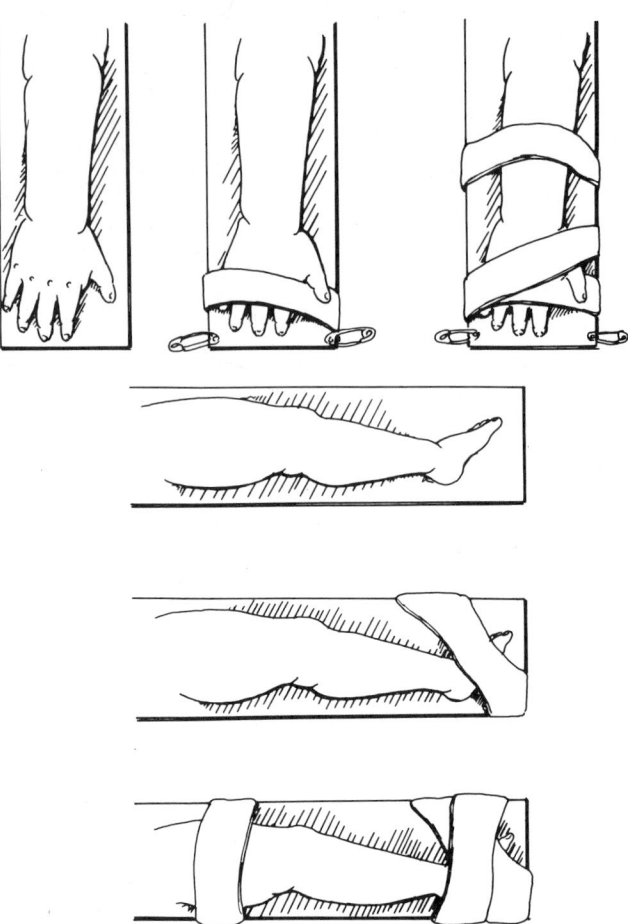

Figure 8–9. Method for securing an extremity to a board or sandbag. The toes and fingers must be visible for monitoring perfusion. (From Hughes W, Buescher E (eds). Pediatric Procedures. 2nd ed. Philadelphia, WB Saunders, 1980.)

Equipment

The equipment required for peripheral percutaneous access consists of the following:

Butterfly needle, 21 to 27 gauge
Angiocatheter, 18 to 24 gauge
Tourniquet
IV tubing and fluid
Arm/leg board
Tape
Aseptic solution
Plastic medicine cup
Transilluminator (optional)
Sand bag (optional)

Technique

1. The site is properly immobilized and the patient adequately restrained.

2. The site is cleaned with an aseptic solution. (If the scalp is to be used, a small area of surrounding hair must be shaved to allow for secure taping of the cannula or butterfly needle).

3. A syringe containing saline is used to flush the cannula or butterfly needle and tubing.

4. With the needle at a 10- to 20-degree angle to the skin surface, a puncture is made 3 to 5 mm distal to the point of entry into the vessel securing the needle in the subcutaneous tissue before it enters the vein. The vein can be entered from the side, from a bifurcation, or from directly above the vessel.[33]

5. Once the vein is entered, a small amount of blood flashes into the catheter hub or butterfly tubing. If a catheter is used, it is advanced 0.5 to 1.0 mm further to ensure its position within the lumen; then the stylet needle is removed and advanced into the vessel through its entire length. If a butterfly needle is used, once the vein is entered and blood flashes back into the tubing, the needle is not advanced further. If both sides of the vein are punctured, it is unlikely that the vessel will be successfully cannulated.

6. The butterfly needle or catheter is firmly secured with tape. To further protect the site, the catheter or butterfly is covered with a plastic medicine cup, which allows direct visualization of the puncture and surrounding area.

Intravenous fluid should flush easily. If there is resistance or fluid infiltration within the surrounding subcutaneous tissue, the device should be removed and the procedure attempted at another site. Often a single vein will have several potential cannulation sites, and starting at the most distal part allows the physician to move proximally to other sites if necessary.

Complications

Infiltration of intravenous fluid into the subcutaneous tissue is a common complication of peripheral percutaneous venous lines. Associated problems range from local edema to severe tissue necrosis. Tissue damage is related to the type of fluid being infused, the extent and location of the infiltration, and the promptness of intervention.[34] As soon as an extravasation of fluid is recognized, the infusion should be discontinued and the catheter removed. For mild infiltrations, warm packs can be applied to the involved area; elevation of the extremity aids in resolution. Severe infiltrations with toxic infusates require surgical evaluation. Other potential complications include hematoma formation, infection, and air embolism.[34–36]

Teaching Model

The peripheral percutaneous technique can be taught using the following equipment:

Butterfly needle, 21 to 27 gauge
Angiocatheter, 18 to 24 gauge
IV fluid and tubing
Syringe
Placenta
Latex gloves
Metal pan
Absorbent pads

Universal precautions for the handling of blood products and human tissue should be strictly followed. As much blood as possible is drained from the placenta. The prepared placenta is positioned with the amniotic surface visible on absorbent pads in the metal pan. The amniotic surface of the placenta has numerous arteries and veins that are superficially located and easily visible.

The procedure for venous cannulation as outlined earlier should be attempted with both butterfly needles and angiocatheters on the vessels on the amniotic surface of the placenta. However, there will be no flashback of blood. Placement can be confirmed by using the syringe to flush IV fluid through the catheter or butterfly needle. If correctly placed, the fluid will flow without resistance, and the vessel will dilate.

CENTRAL CIRCULATORY ACCESS

Access to the central circulation of a child may be necessary because of difficulty in cannulating peripheral veins or the need to perform specialized pressure monitoring, pacing, or hyperalimentation (Table 8–4). There are a number of approaches to cannulating the central circulation (Table 8–5). Each physician should use the approach that is the safest and technically the most successful in their experience (Table 8–6).

Hemodynamic Monitoring

Central vascular access using the subclavian or internal jugular veins is employed to measure the central venous

TABLE 8–4

INDICATIONS FOR CENTRAL VENOUS CANNULATION

Inability to cannulate peripheral veins
Volume loading for hypovolemic shock
Cardiorespiratory arrest—central drug administration
Central venous or Swan-Ganz pressure monitoring
Transvenous pacemaker access
Severe burns
Need for prolonged indwelling catheter placement
   (hyperalimentation, antibiotic administration, chemotherapy)
Central hemodialysis access
Infusion of concentrated or irritative solutions
Other unstable cardiac or circulatory conditions

TABLE 8–5

APPROACHES TO THE CENTRAL VENOUS CIRCULATION

Umbilical vein	Internal jugular vein
External jugular vein	Posterior approach
Femoral vein	Anterior approach
Subclavian vein	Middle approach
Infraclavicular approach	Basilic, cephalic, and axillary
Supraclavicular approach	veins

pressure (CVP) of critically ill patients.[37] The key to accurate measurements of CVP is the proper placement of the catheter tip. Ideally, the tip should lie within the superior vena cava at the entrance to the right atrium. Discordant values may indicate a malposition of the catheter tip within the internal jugular vein[37, 38] or advancement of the tip into the right ventricle.[39] Catheter tip placement should be confirmed radiographically before interpreting CVP measurements.

A number of additional factors affect the accuracy of CVP measurements.[40–43] First, readings must be obtained in a consistent manner, using the same patient position and at an identical reference level on the patient. A reference point should be marked on the patient's skin for this purpose. Second, measurements must be taken at rest and during exhalation, as coughing, straining, and positive-pressure ventilation can significantly raise intrathoracic pressure and factitiously raise the CVP. Third, low pressure readings can result from valve-like obstruction of the catheter by clots or by contact with the vessel wall. Fourth, measurements may also be affected by air bubbles in the CVP line and by concurrent central fluid infusion. Several authors have de-

TABLE 8–6

RECOMMENDATIONS OF THE CENTRAL VENOUS CATHETER TASK FORCE, JULY, 1989

1. Central venous catheters (CVCs) should be placed only when potential benefits outweigh the inherent risks.
2. Catheter tips should not be placed or allowed to migrate into the heart (exception: pulmonary artery catheters).
3. Catheter tip position should be confirmed by radiograph and rechecked periodically.
4. CVCs should be placed *only by trained personnel* well-versed in anatomic landmarks, proper techniques, and potential complications and their treatment.
5. Until authorized (certified) to place CVCs independently, trainees must be closely supervised by qualified personnel and monitored thereafter to ensure continued competence.
6. Operators performing CV catheterizations should be familiar with equipment, insertion sites, and catheter type, size, and length.
7. Family and nursing personnel caring for patients with CVCs should understand and be alert to signs of CVC complications.
8. Manufacturers should include specific labeling and instructions to address the use of the device and potential complications. Operators should read the specific technique required by each device and review warnings and other information needed for safe and efficient utilization.
9. Except in emergencies, catheterization should be performed with full aseptic technique including universal precautions (hand washing, sterile gloves, masks, gowns, goggles, and a suitable antiseptic prep solution). Catheters placed in a less than sterile fashion should be replaced as soon as medically feasible.

From FDA CV Catheter Task Force. Precautions necessary with central venous catheters. FDA Drug Bull 1989; July:15.

scribed varying "normal" ranges of CVP readings,[44, 45] as follows:

Low	Less than 5 cm H_2O
Normal	5 to 12 cm H_2O
High	Greater than 12 cm H_2O

Although the interpretation of CVP measurement is affected by cardiac decompensation, pulmonary embolus, restrictive pericarditis, pulmonary stenosis, and pericardial tamponade, these conditions occur infrequently in children. In general, measurements and changes in the CVP are reflective of the child's fluid status.

A low CVP reading is reflective of low right atrial pressure and usually indicates decreased blood return to the right heart. Various forms of distributive shock (septic, anaphylactic, and neurogenic) can also be indicated by low CVP measurements.

A high CVP reading may reflect cardiac decompensation in a normovolemic patient or overhydration in a patient with normal cardiac status. Past medical history regarding childhood pulmonary or cardiac conditions is helpful in interpreting these values.

Patient care is influenced by initial CVP readings and CVP changes in response to fluid challenges.[46] This permits precise adjustment of the rate of fluid administration in hypovolemia. The changes in CVP resulting from a fluid infusion are a more important indication than any single CVP reading.

Swan-Ganz catheter measurements of pulmonary artery wedge pressure are most reflective of the actual volume status of a patient.[47] Such measurements permit the optimization of fluid status for patients with cardiac or renal decompensation and any form of distributive shock. These catheters are placed using a dilator and a centrally placed catheter sheath. The catheters are inserted fluoroscopically or with hemodynamic monitoring using aseptic technique.

UMBILICAL VESSEL CATHETERIZATION

Umbilical vessel (arterial and venous) catheterization is a common procedure used to stabilize and monitor critical newborns. The umbilical vein (UV) offers rapid access to the central venous circulation for fluid and drug administration and blood sampling. Cannulation of the umbilical artery (UA) provides the same vascular access and, in addition, allows continuous monitoring of blood pressure and arterial blood gases. In the emergency situation, either vessel is an acceptable source of vascular access, although the UV is easier to cannulate.[48]

Umbilical vessels are most easily cannulated in newborns, although UV catheters have been successfully placed in infants up to 2 weeks of age. As the infant ages, the umbilical vein thromboses with the drying of the cord. Successful advance of the catheter into the inferior vena cava from an older umbilical vessel may also be hindered by closure of the ductus venosus, an embryologic vessel connecting the umbilical vein, portal vein, and inferior vena cava that involutes after birth to become the ligamentum venosum.[49] Applying saline-soaked gauze to the dried cord and transecting the cord close to the abdominal wall are often helpful when cannulating an umbilical vein in an older infant. To prevent embolization, care must be taken to remove clot formed within the vessel lumen before inserting the catheter.

Insertion of an umbilical vessel catheter for routine parenteral fluid or blood sampling is inappropriate. Umbilical catheters should not be inserted in the presence of omphalitis or abdominal wall skin lesions. Placement of a UA or UV catheter is generally contraindicated in the presence of abdominal distention that is suggestive of necrotizing enterocolitis or impaired intestinal circulation.[50]

Equipment

Umbilical vein catheterization requires the following equipment:

No. 3.5 or 5.0 French umbilical catheter
Three-way stopcock
Syringe
Umbilical tape
Adhesive tape
Cutdown tray

The equipment is assembled and flushed with saline before beginning the procedure.

Complications

Although umbilical vessel catheterization has become a standard procedure in the resuscitation and monitoring of the critically ill neonate,[48, 49, 51] complications have been associated with placement and maintenance. Complications occur both during or immediately after placement and with long-term use.

Immediate complications of line placement include hemorrhage; air embolism; ischemia to bowel, kidney, or extremities; and perforations. Hemorrhage most commonly occurs from a dislodged line; secure suturing of the catheter and frequent checking of the line are mandatory. The risk of air embolism can be minimized by careful flushing of the catheter and tubing with IV fluid and use of a three-way stopcock. Ischemia may respond to catheter repositioning or replacement or may require removal. Perforations of the umbilical vein, bladder, liver, colon, and pericardium have been described.[51–54] Once suspected, perforation requires immediate surgical evaluation.

Additional complications associated with long-term umbilical catheter use include portal vein thromboses, portal hypertension, hepatic abscess, sepsis, thrombotic embolism, hepatic calcification, necrotizing enterocolitis, systemic hypertension, hematuria, and aneurysm formation.[52, 55–57]

Technique

1. The umbilical stump and periumbilical area are cleaned with an antiseptic solution and draped with sterile towels.

2. Umbilical tape is looped around the base of the cord, and a surgical half-knot is tied; this knot can later be tightened to control bleeding. The umbilical stump is cut to a length of 1 to 2 cm. The three umbilical vessels—two small, constricted, thick-walled umbilical arteries and a single, larger, thin-walled umbilical vein—should be identified. In the newborn, the UV is the freely bleeding vessel. Because the UV is the more easily cannulated lumen, catheterization should be attempted in this vessel first (Fig. 8–10).

3. The umbilical stump is grasped between the thumb and forefinger with gauze; alternately, the cut edge may be held with a forceps or hemostat from the cutdown tray. The catheter is held with either a forceps or the fingers while the catheter is inserted into the UV.

The catheter should insert easily and should never require force to advance. In the emergency situation, catheter insertion should be limited to approximately 5 cm below the skin surface or only the length needed to achieve a free backflow of blood, thereby minimizing the risk of mechanical or pharmacologic injury to the liver.[48, 52] A reference graph can be used to determine either position (Fig. 8–11).

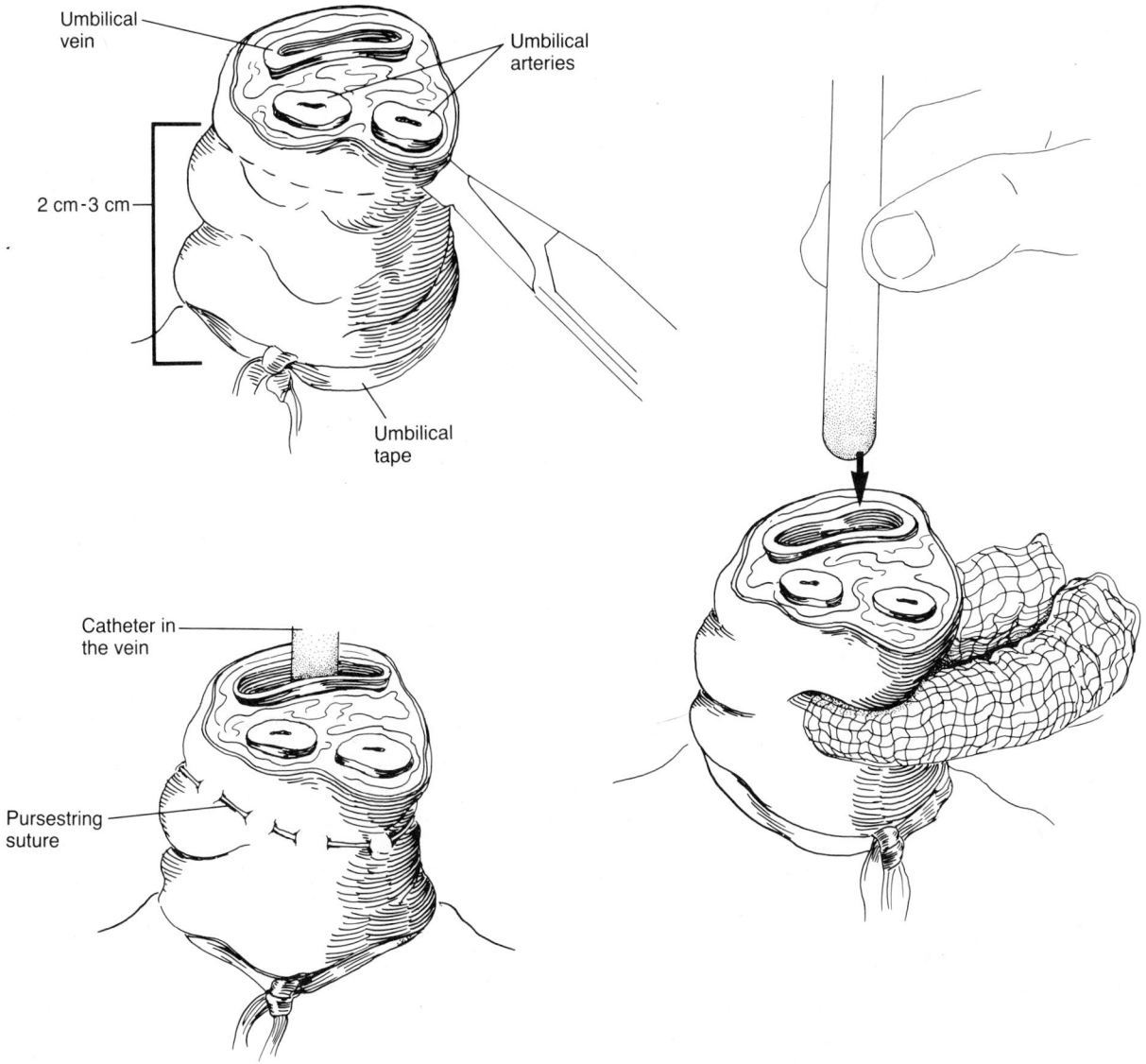

Figure 8–10. Technique for insertion of an umbilical vein catheter.

4. After catheter position is determined, the umbilical tape is tightened. A pursestring suture is then placed around the edge of the umbilical stump while avoiding disruption of the other cord vessels. Once tightened, a knot is made, leaving both ends of the suture long.

5. The suture ends are used to tie square knots on alternating sides up the catheter for 3 to 5 cm, further anchoring it in place. A piece of tape is placed perpendicularly across the catheter and suture.

6. Catheter position should be confirmed radiographically, if possible, before infusion.

Teaching Model

Human umbilical cords can be used as a model to teach the umbilical vessel catheterization technique. Required equipment includes the following:

5-cm length of umbilical cord
Styrofoam cup
Metal pan
Dyed saline
Latex gloves

The umbilical cord is inserted through a small slit in the bottom of an inverted styrofoam cup, which holds the cord tightly and acts as the abdominal wall. The cord and cup setup is placed in a metal pan to prevent spillage of blood products still within the cord. Vessel identification and catheterization technique can be demonstrated as discussed. Once the catheter is inserted into the vein, intraluminal position can be verified by infusing dyed saline through the catheter and observing the fluid coming out the vein of the cut end of the cord within the cup. The catheter is secured and sutured to the cup for additional practice. Universal precautions for the handling of human tissue and blood products should be followed.

EXTERNAL JUGULAR VEIN ACCESS

The external jugular vein is formed by the posterior facial and auricular branch veins, which join together just below the ear and behind the angle of the mandible (Fig. 8–12). It crosses down obliquely across the surface of the sternocleidomastoid (SCM) muscle and then penetrates through the deep fascia just above the clavicle. This vein is often overlooked during the initial minutes of resuscitation. Once

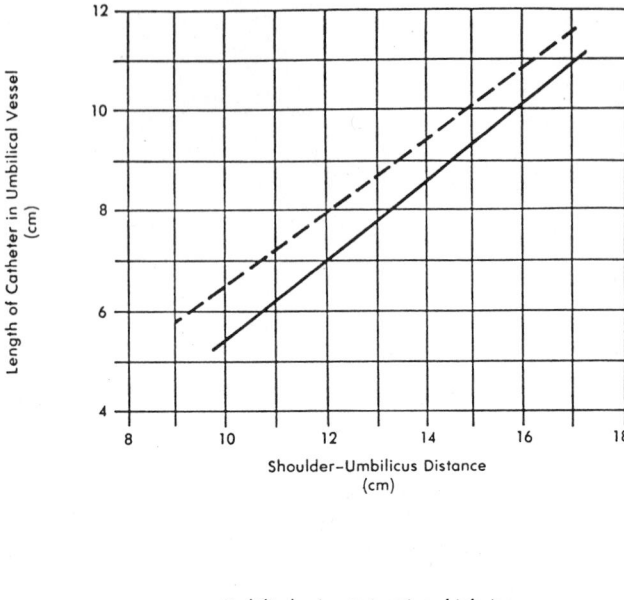

— — — — Umbilical vein—to junction of inferior
vena cava and right atrium

———— Umbilical artery—to bifurcation of aorta

Figure 8–11. Determination of catheter length for UAC/UVC placement. The shoulder-umbilicus distance is the perpendicular distance
between parallel lines at the level of the umbilicus and through the
distal ends of the clavicles. The length of the umbilical stump must
be added. (From Klaus MH, Fanaroff AA. Care of the High-Risk
Neonate. Philadelphia, WB Saunders, 1986, p 36.)

the airway is secured, if no IV access has been obtained, the
external jugular vein should be used. It is often an inviting
target, especially in the young infant, as it is the largest
peripheral vein available.[58] The child should be placed in
the Trendelenburg position with the neck extended slightly,
if not contraindicated, to reveal the vein. One finger placed
proximally on the vein to fill it and another placed more
cephalad on the vein to straighten it will fix the vein in place
to assist penetration. If *any* peripheral access is all that is
needed, the vein is usually cannulated with a catheter-over-
the-needle device. An external jugular line may be considered a central venous cannulation in patients in cardiac
arrest because of the proximity of this site to the superior
vena cava and heart.[58, 59]

When other methods of central venous access have been
unsuccessful or are contraindicated, it is often possible to
cannulate the central circulation through the external jugular vein.[58–61] The success rate is improved by the use of a J
tipped guide wire, which can be rotated, gently advanced,
and withdrawn until the guide wire passes into the central
circulation.[62, 63] Nonetheless, such cannulations are often time
consuming and difficult.[58–62] Cannulation rates from 76% to
100% have been reported in adults but may be reduced in
children.[58–62]

The most frequent complication of this technique is the
formation of hematomas, as the vessel is extremely superficial and a needle may easily pass through both walls.[58, 59]
Because the entry site is visible, direct pressure over the area
of the hematoma will stop further bleeding. These catheters
should be sewn in place to prevent dislodgement.

Technique

1. The child is placed supine in the 20- to 30-degree
Trendelenburg position with the head turned away from

the puncture site. The right side may be preferred if an
attempt to pass a guide wire and cannulate the subclavian
vein is to be made.

2. The patient should be adequately restrained.

3. The area is scrubbed thoroughly with antiseptic solution.

4. The external jugular vein is identified. Placing a finger
on it proximally may cause increased filling and allow easier
entry.

5. The skin is punctured about 1 cm distal to the point
where the vein is to be entered.

6. The needle is advanced superficially. The clinician
should attempt to "pick up" the superior wall of the vein
with the tip of the needle and obtain flashback of blood or
blood flow.

7. The catheter is advanced, or the guide wire is inserted
centrally. A long catheter and dilator may be advanced
centrally and the dilator and guide wire removed. After
establishing flow, the catheter should be hooked up to a
manometer for CVP monitoring.

8. The catheter is sutured in place, and ointment and a
sterile dressing are applied.

9. A chest radiograph is obtained to check for complications and proper line placement.

FEMORAL VEIN ACCESS

Femoral vein access is the technique of choice in children
older than 3 years who cannot be promptly cannulated
peripherally.[2, 5, 6] The obvious advantage of this technique is
that the procedure area is located away from any resuscitative efforts involving the airway or chest compressions.
Because the femoral vein is a large-caliber, high-flow vessel,
the chance of vascular thrombosis is remote (Fig. 8–13).[64]

The femoral vein lies just medial to the artery in the
femoral canal below the inguinal ligament. This can be

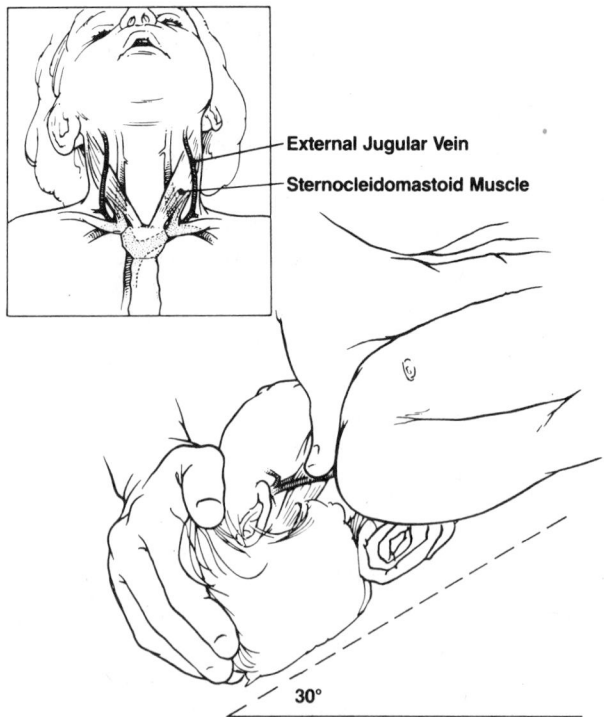

Figure 8–12. Technique for finding the external jugular vein. (Repro-
duced with permission. © From Chameides L (ed). Textbook of
Pediatric Advanced Life Support, 1988. Copyright American Heart
Association.)

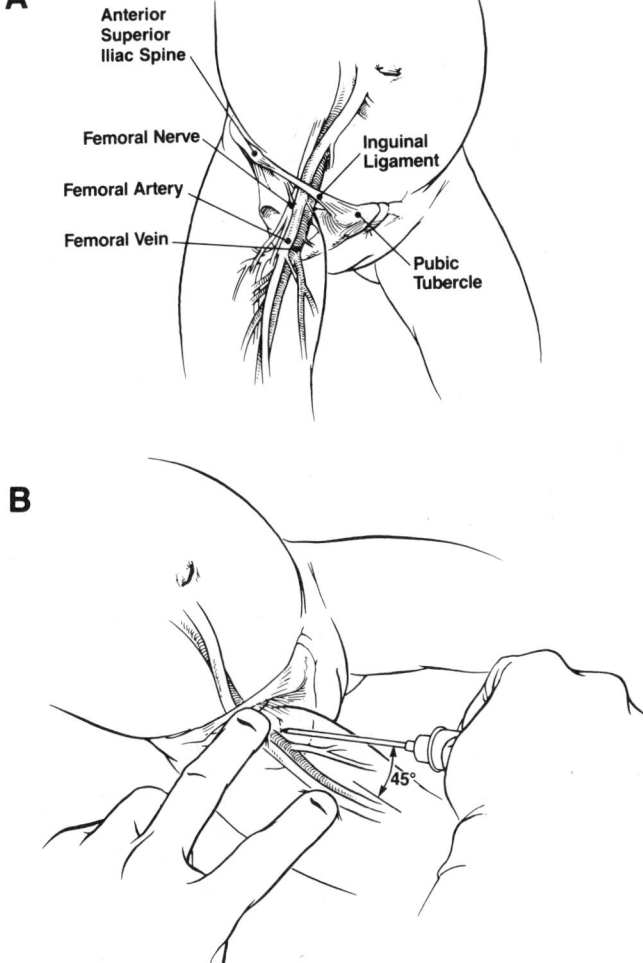

A

Anterior
Superior
Iliac Spine

Femoral Nerve

Femoral Artery

Femoral Vein

Inguinal
Ligament

Pubic
Tubercle

B

45°

Figure 8–13. *A,* Femoral vein anatomy. *B,* Technique for cannulating the femoral vein. (Reproduced with permission. © From Chameides L (ed). Textbook of Pediatric Advanced Life Support, 1988. Copyright American Heart Association.)

remembered by using the mnemonic *NAVEL* (*n*erve, *a*rtery, *v*ein, *e*mpty space, and *l*ymphatics), which lists structures from lateral to medial on the leg. Alternatively, in the pulseless child who is undergoing chest compressions, papable pulsations are usually felt over the femoral vein rather than the artery.[65] The insertion of the needle should be made at that point.

Complications

The operator must take care not to advance the needle above the inguinal ligament, which can lead to peritoneal puncture and peritonitis. Other complications of this approach include hip joint injury and sepsis, as well as cannulation or injury to the femoral artery. Delayed complications of sepsis from femoral lines occur.[64–67] Improved success rates and fewer complications are associated with the Seldinger technique.

Technique

1. The child is restrained, placing the leg in slight external rotation.
2. The femoral artery is identified by palpation; the vein

is just medial to the pulse. During CPR, pulsations may be most prominent over the vein, and needle puncture should be attempted at the pulse point. Alternately, the midpoint between the anterosuperior iliac spine and pubic symphysis may be used as the insertion point.

3. The area is scrubbed thoroughly with antiseptic solution.

4. Universal precautions are followed; hands are washed and sterile gloves worn.

5. The skin insertion point may be anesthetized with 0.5 to 1.0 ml of local anesthetic (1% lidocaine).

6. The needle, attached to a syringe, should puncture the skin 1 fingerbreadth below the inguinal ligament and medial to the femoral artery. The needle is slowly advanced at a 45-degree angle until free blood flow is obtained.

7. The catheter is advanced, or the guide wire is inserted centrally. A long catheter sheath and dilator are advanced centrally, the dilator and guide wire are removed, and IV therapy is established.

8. The catheter is sutured in place. A sterile dressing is applied.

SUBCLAVIAN AND INTERNAL JUGULAR ACCESS

The use of the subclavian and internal jugular veins in pediatric practice is not as frequent as in adults. In low-flow states (cardiac arrest and shock), central venous access provides a significant advantage over peripheral access for drug delivery.[68] The subclavian and internal jugular veins can be accessed with high success and low complication rates.[69–71] When hemodynamic monitoring or cardiac pacing is a consideration, the internal jugular or supraclavicular techniques offer the most direct access to the superior vena cava.[72]

The clinical situation influences the technique chosen (Table 8–7). Vascular access should be obtained on the same side as penetrating or blunt thoracic trauma, thus avoiding the complications of a second and iatrogenic pneumothorax. The exception to this is a penetrating injury above the clavicle. In this instance, if there is a significant risk of great vessel injury, cannulation of potentially disrupted vessels may be harmful.[7] If no significant thoracic trauma is suspected, most practitioners use a right-sided approach, which affords the most direct entry to the central circulation and eliminates injury to the thoracic duct.[72, 73] Furthermore, the

TABLE 8–7
CONTRAINDICATIONS TO SUBCLAVIAN VENIPUNCTURE
Distorted local anatomy*
Chest wall deformities
Extremes of weight
Vasculitis
Prior long-term subclavian cannulation
Prior injection of sclerosing agents
Suspected superior vena cava injury
Suspected subclavian vessel injury*
Previous radiation or surgery*
Pneumothorax†
Bleeding disorders
Anticoagulant therapy
Combative patient
Inexperienced, unsupervised physician

*Clinician may cannulate contralateral side.
†Clinician may cannulate ipsilateral side.
From Dronen SC. Subclavian venipuncture. *In* Roberts J, Hedges JR (eds). Clinical Procedures in Emergency Medicine. Philadelphia, WB Saunders, 1985.

dome of the right lung is slightly lower anatomically and perhaps less liable to injury.[73]

The sites for all approaches to the internal jugular and subclavian veins should be widely prepped on the side of the procedure. If one site is unsuccessful, the next one will be already prepared and ready for placement. Subsequent approaches should be attempted on the original side until successful. The possibility of an iatrogenic pneumothorax should be eliminated before attempting access on the opposite side.

The patient should be placed in the 15- to 30-degree Trendelenburg position to increase venous return and lessen the risk of air embolism. The Trendelenburg position, the Valsalva maneuver, and the use of the pneumatic antishock garment may be used to distend the internal jugular but probably not the subclavian veins.[74]

Although turning the head to the opposite side does not change the anatomic position of the subclavian vein, it is still recommended, because it lessens patient contamination of the venipuncture site and prevents the child from observing a potentially frightening procedure.[73] Abducting the arm and placing the patient on a towel roll to force the shoulders backward are seldom necessary, and may actually make the procedure more difficult.[75, 76]

Subclavian Vein Technique
Infraclavicular Approach

The subclavian vein has as its origin the axillary vein at the edge of the first rib. It joins the internal jugular vein to form the innominate vein, which continues into the superior vena cava and into the right atrium (Fig. 8–14). This confluence is the anatomic target area for the supraclavicular approach to subclavian vein cannulation. The subclavian vein lies below the medial third of the clavicle, and this anatomic relationship is used in performing the infraclavicular approach.

The infraclavicular approach was first described in 1952.[77] Early reports in children indicated that the complication rate was higher with this technique, and it should not be used in children younger than 2 years.[78, 79] However, more recent studies in children using a refined technique and equipment with experienced personnel have shown complication rates comparable to those in adults.[80, 81] The Seldinger technique should be used for all infraclavicular subclavian cannulations.

The infraclavicular approach is indicated in patients requiring central venous access or after unsuccessful attempts at peripheral or femoral access. With the infraclavicular approach, the clinician must adapt the landmarks and penetration depth to the size of the child. The infraclavicular approach is more difficult during the performance of CPR. Chest wall movements caused by closed chest compression and positive-pressure ventilation lower the success rate and increase the complication rate.[82] Ambulatory or awake patients find the technique more comfortable than IV techniques requiring precise neck placement.

Complications. Numerous complications of the infraclavicular approach have been described in children. Pneumothorax is the most common major complication of this approach. Although pneumothorax is seen more frequently in the infraclavicular approach when compared with the supraclavicular and internal jugular approaches, the incidence of pneumothorax remains low with experienced operators. Operator experience is considered the most important factor in the development of complications.[83, 84]

The complication of unrecognized bleeding is common to all approaches but may have greater significance when it

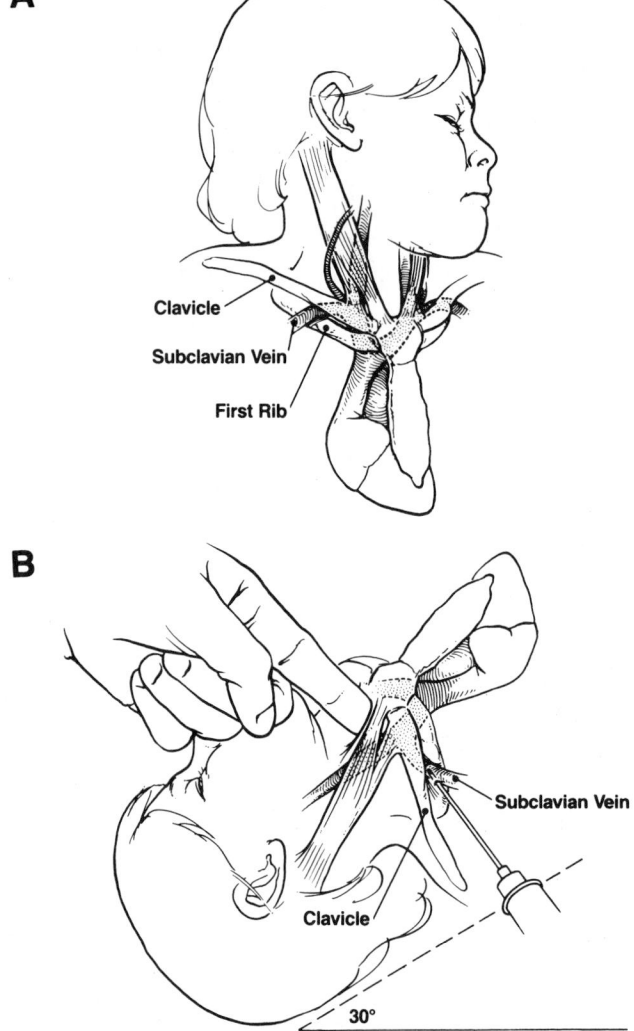

Figure 8–14. *A*, Subclavian vein anatomy. *B*, The infraclavicular approach to subclavian vein cannulation. (Reproduced with permission. © From Chameides L (ed). Textbook of Pediatric Advanced Life Support, 1988. Copyright American Heart Association.)

occurs within the chest. Such bleeding is usually self-limited but in anticoagulated patients can be significant. Routine radiograph surveillance after central venous catheter placement should detect this condition.

Supraclavicular Approach

The supraclavicular approach was first described by Yoffa in 1965.[85] Using this technique, the needle enters the innominate vein at the confluence of the internal jugular and subclavian veins. The needle is advanced above the clavicle from an insertion 0.5 to 1.0 cm lateral to the lateral border of the SCM muscle and 1 cm cephalad to the clavicle. The anatomy is better seen when the awake patient raises the head slightly to define the SCM muscle. The needle is aimed at the contralateral nipple, which enables the angle of insertion to conform to the chest wall habitus and keeps the needle tip away from the subclavian artery and pleural dome. As with the internal jugular approach, the supraclavicular approach is aided by placing the patient in the Trendelenburg position, which distends the vessel superiorly and lowers the risk of air embolism. The right side is preferred because of its direct route to the SVC, the lower pleural dome, and no risk of injury to the left-sided thoracic duct.[82, 85]

Direct comparisons of the supraclavicular with the infraclavicular subclavian approach show the risks and benefits to be similar (Table 8–8).[82, 86, 87] Successful puncture occurs within 1 to 3 cm of needle insertion. For children in shock, frequently a needle thrust will not yield a flashback of blood. From its deepest point, the syringe should be withdrawn very slowly with slight negative pressure while observing for intermittent blood return. Once the needle is withdrawn to the skin entrance, it may be redirected, after rechecking the landmarks, until cannulation is obtained. When free blood flow is obtained, the Seldinger technique is employed to advance first a guide wire and then the catheter-dilator centrally. As with all central thoracic techniques, a chest radiograph must be obtained to note the position of the catheter and to check for complications.

A major advantage of this technique during CPR is that the operator can stand between the person managing the airway and the individual doing chest compression. The insertion is through a relatively motionless area, with the needle tracking away from the dome of the pleura. Because of its superficial location, there is less risk of laceration and injury to other structures during CPR.[82]

Complications. The reported complication rates for the supraclavicular approach have been low (0% to 6%), with an overall rate of 1.3%.[72] Pneumothorax and subclavian artery puncture are the two most important complications, but careful definition of surface landmarks and strict adherence to proper technique decrease these risks.

The supraclavicular technique used in children has a comparable success rate and a reduced complication rate when compared with the infraclavicular technique.[72] The number of directly comparable studies in children is limited because of the relative novelty of the approach.

The supraclavicular subclavian vein approach has the lowest catheter malposition rate when compared with the infraclavicular and internal jugular techniques. In studies where malposition has been reported, the overall rate is 1.1%. The highest rate of malposition was reported as 7%.[82] This study compared the success rate of supraclavicular and infraclavicular catheter placement during CPR using randomly assigned approaches. The infraclavicular approach yielded a 26% malposition rate.

Internal Jugular Cannulation

The internal jugular vein drains the head, beginning at the superior jugular bulb, courses caudally, and runs parallel to the internal carotid artery and the spinal accessory, vagus, and hypoglossal nerves. More distally, it is enclosed in the carotid sheath but maintains its anterior and lateral relationship to the other structures. The internal jugular vein lies beneath the SCM muscle at the level of the thyroid cartilage. The internal jugular lies directly under the apex of the triangle formed by the two heads of the SCM muscle and joins the subclavian vein under the clavicle.

The use of the internal jugular vein for venous access in children has paralleled the development and invasiveness of pediatric intensive care over the past 15 years. In general, this technique carries less risk of pneumothorax and undetected hemorrhage than does the infraclavicular subclavian approach. It may be technically more difficult to perform, and the success rate may be less than with the subclavian approaches.

The internal jugular approach is contraindicated when neck trauma causes bleeding and loss of landmarks. Gaining access to the insertion site is difficult if the patient is in a cervical collar for spinal immobilization. Afterward, a conscious child may have difficulty keeping the neck immobilized and the catheter in proper position. In children with known coagulopathies, the posterior internal jugular approach is preferred, because hemorrhage can be controlled by direct compression over the area. In cardiac arrest, the internal jugular approaches are preferred by some because

---

TABLE 8–8

SUBCLAVIAN VERSUS INTERNAL JUGULAR TECHNIQUES

Technique	Advantages	Disadvantages
Basilic (peripheral) puncture with long central catheter placement	Low incidence of major complications Performed under direct visualization of vein	Greater incidence of minor complications of infection, phlebitis, and thrombosis Hinders free movement of arms More difficult to place catheter in correct position for central venous pressure monitoring
Internal jugular puncture	Good external landmarks Lesser risk of pneumothorax than with subclavian puncture Bleeding can be recognized and controlled Malposition of catheter is uncommon Almost a straight course to the superior vena cava on the right side Carotid artery easily identified	"Blind" procedure Has a slightly higher incidence of failures than subclavian More difficult and inconvenient to secure
Infraclavicular subclavian puncture	Good external landmarks	Higher incidence of complications, especially in hypovolemic shock "Blind" procedure Increased complication risk in children younger than 2 yr
Supraclavicular subclavian puncture	Good landmarks Less risk of pneumothorax than with infraclavicular puncture Most practical method of inserting a central line in cardiorespiratory arrest Malposition of catheter is uncommon	"Blind" procedure

Modified from Knopp R, Dailey RH. Central venous cannulation and pressure monitoring. J Am Coll Emerg Phys 1977;6:358.

they are away from the movement and activity of chest compressions. The approaches to the internal jugular vein have been organized into three groups defined by their relationship to the SCM muscle (Fig. 8–15).[88]

Technique

1. The child should be restrained in a 20- to 45-degree Trendelenburg position with the head turned away from the puncture site. A small towel may be placed under the shoulders to hyperextend the head.

2. The area is scrubbed widely and thoroughly with antiseptic solution.

3. Universal precautions should be followed; hands are washed and gloves worn.

4. The skin insertion site may be anesthetized with 1% lidocaine.

5. The anatomic landmarks are identified, including both heads of the SCM muscle and clavicle. Using the specific approaches listed later, the needle, attached to a syringe, is inserted through the skin in the proper orientation while gentle suction is maintained with the syringe. A flashback or free flow of blood is evidence of vessel cannulation. If no blood is obtained, the needle is withdrawn to the skin entrance, the angles of insertion are redirected, and the technique is repeated until successful. In children with hypovolemic shock, blood flow may be intermittent, and blood may be seen only on slow withdrawal.

6. When the free flow of blood is attained, the syringe is disconnected and the hub of the needle immediately occluded with the thumb to prevent air embolization.

7. With the patient in exhalation, the sterile guide wire is inserted into the vessel to the proper insertion distance in the central circulation.

8. The needle is removed, and a small 2- to 4-mm skin incision is made at the insertion point. The dilator or catheter sheath is placed over the guide wire and advanced, and the guide wire and dilator are removed. Appropriate sampling is obtained and the IV tubing attached. The IV is opened momentarily to clear blood from the catheter. The IV bag should be dropped below the level of the patient and observed for backflow of blood. If this does not occur, the catheter may no longer be in the vessel, warranting catheter removal.

9. The catheter is sutured in place. Antiseptic ointment and sterile dressing are applied.

10. An anteroposterior chest radiograph is made to check for complications and line placement.

BASILIC AND CEPHALIC VEIN CENTRAL ACCESS

The basilic and cephalic veins are routinely used for peripheral vascular access in children and adults. However, as a means of obtaining central vein cannulation without fluoroscopic guidance in an emergency, these approaches have limited application. The Seldinger technique and numerous other methods have been used to improve access to the central venous system.[89–91] Failure rates ranging from 2% to 40% have been reported.[89, 90] In general, the rate of successful advancement to the central circulation is lower in children than in adults. An alternate central venous route should be used.

COMPLICATIONS OF CENTRAL CATHETERS
Early Complications

Numerous complications can result from subclavian and internal jugular venipuncture (Table 8–9). The early com-

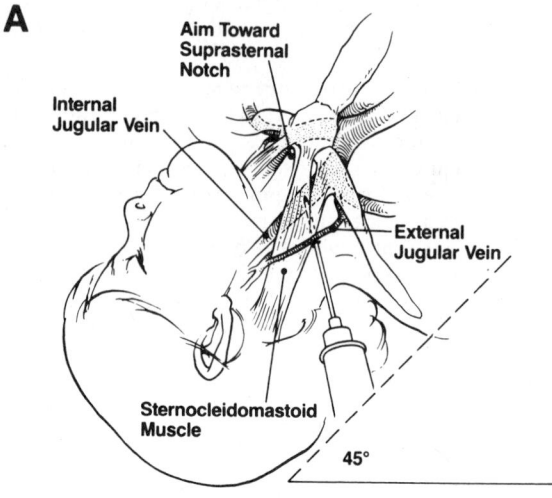

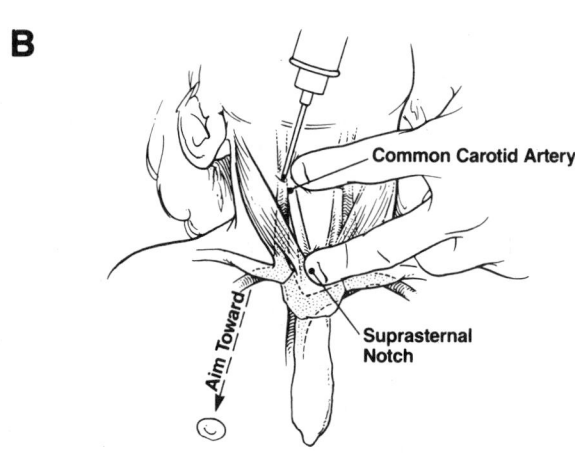

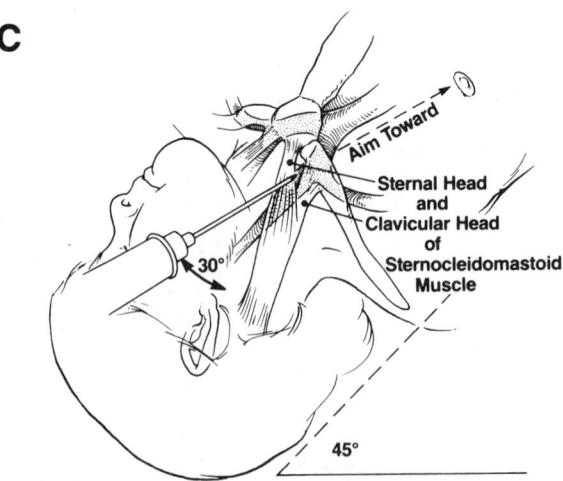

Figure 8–15. The posterior *(A)*, central *(B)*, and anterior *(C)* approaches to cannulating the internal jugular vein. (Reproduced with permission. © From Chameides L (ed). Textbook of Pediatric Advanced Life Support, 1988. Copyright American Heart Association.)

TABLE 8–9
COMPLICATIONS OF SUBCLAVIAN AND INTERNAL JUGULAR VENIPUNCTURE

Pulmonary
  Pneumothorax
  Hemothorax
  Hydrothorax
  Hemomediastinum
  Hydromediastinum
  Tracheal perforation
  Endotracheal cuff perforation
  Intrathoracic catheter fragmentation
Vascular
  Air embolus
  Subclavian artery puncture
  Pericardial tamponade
  Thrombophlebitis
  Catheter embolus
  Volume depletion
  Arteriovenous fistula
  Superior vena cava obstruction
  Thoracic duct laceration
Infectious
  Generalized sepsis
  Local cellulitis
  Osteomyelitis
  Septic arthritis
Neurologic
  Phrenic nerve injury
  Brachial plexus injury
Miscellaneous
  Dysrhythmias
  Ascites
  Catheter knotting
  Catheter malposition

From Dronen SC. Subclavian venipuncture. *In* Roberts J, Hedges JR (eds). Clinical Procedures in Emergency Medicine. Philadelphia, WB Saunders, 1985.

plications of subclavian or internal jugular catheters are often related to operator skill and to difficulties in finding and cannulating the vein. These include dysrhythmias; pneumothorax; hydrothorax; chylothorax; hemothorax; hydromediastinum; air embolus; catheter fragment embolization; cardiac perforation; and lacerations to the trachea, vessel, or esophagus.[92–96] The most serious technical error is the failure to occlude the end of the catheter or sheath when disconnecting the syringe and attaching the IV tubing.[97] This can result in a fatal air embolism. A characteristic, ominous "sucking sound" may be an important diagnostic sign of venous air embolism during the insertion of a central venous catheter.[95, 97] When followed by symptoms of air hunger, tachypnea, wheezing, hypotension, or a classic "mill wheel" murmur, the diagnosis is confirmed. If air embolism does occur, the patient should be immediately placed in the left lateral decubitus position. A syringe attached to the catheter or sheath should be used to aspirate the air.[95] All central venous catheters should be connected to the IV line with a screw-on fitting to prevent air embolism and exsanguination by accidental dislodgement.

Iatrogenic pneumothorax is an uncommon complication. It is rarely life threatening unless the child has a pneumothorax on the contralateral side. A pneumothorax must be excluded or confirmed after every central venous canulation attempt involving the subclavian or internal jugular vein. A pneumothorax is easily treated by catheter aspiration of the pneumothorax (CASP)[98] or placement of an appropriate-size thoracostomy tube. A pneumothorax must be treated immediately with needle decompression. A catheter-over-the-needle device such as an angiocatheter is ideal for this procedure, as it can be safely left in place as a vent until a chest tube can be inserted.[7]

Early complications that are detectable on immediate and serial upright chest radiographs include hydrothorax, hemothorax, chylothorax, hydromediastinum, tracheal and esophageal penetration or laceration, catheter knot formation, fragment embolization, and cardiac perforation.[95, 96]

Dysrhythmias caused by catheter irritation are easily treated by withdrawing the catheter into the superior vena cava. Additional dysrhythmias may be caused by cardiac disease, hypoxia, or toxic ingestions.[99]

Late Complications

Late complications include venous thrombosis, thrombophlebitis, and catheter-related bacteremia and sepsis. The frequency of delayed complications is inversely related to the patient's age.[96, 100] The risk of catheter colonization and sepsis is reduced by meticulous inspection and cleaning of the IV site.[101–103] Elective rotation of IV sites every 48 to 72 hours reduces complications and may permit the reuse of the same vein after 4 to 7 days.[104]

A number of studies have examined the significance of positive catheter tip cultures and central venous catheter–related bacteremia in the diagnosis of sepsis.[103–105] The simultaneous quantitative blood culture technique has been shown to correlate with catheter-related bacteremia.[106] A fivefold or greater increase in bacterial concentration in catheter blood compared with peripheral blood is a useful criterion for diagnosing catheter-related bacteremia in patients with long-term catheters.[107]

Catheter removal is recommended in children with catheter-related bacteremia and hypotension, shock, or septic emboli. However, more recent studies have demonstrated successful treatment of central venous catheter sepsis while leaving the catheters in situ.[108–110] Streptococcal and fungal infections are more resistant; removal of long-term catheters may ultimately be required to clear these infections.[107, 111]

Thrombus formation associated with central venous catheters in infants and children has been carefully studied.[112] Real-time echocardiography was used to show catheter tip thrombi in 16 of 350 patients with long-term catheter access. Thrombus formation was most often related to prematurity and the use of total parenteral nutrition by continuous infusion; it did not correlate with the duration of catheterization. Although there appears to be some benefit to thrombolytic and surgical clot removal, few randomized studies with statistical power have been published.[113–115] Nevertheless, the incidence of catheter thrombus formation is significant, and if cardiopulmonary decompensation, sepsis, or catheter malfunction occurs, an echocardiographic examination is indicated.[116]

VENOUS CUTDOWNS

When the peripheral or central venous circulation cannot be accessed by percutaneous techniques or intraosseous placement, access can be obtained by venous cutdown. Cutdown may also be necessary in children who are obese, chronically ill, multiply impaired, or "veinless" as a result of multiple previous attempts with resultant scarring over peripheral access sites.

The venous cutdown technique is an essential skill for all emergency physicians.[117] It is time consuming even in the most experienced hands,[118] and as a result, venous cutdown is inappropriate as a first-line maneuver when rapid access is essential.[118] In addition to being time consuming, traditional cutdown technique involves venesection with resultant loss of the vein for future cannulation.

Two variations of the traditional cutdown are the modified guide wire and mini-cutdown techniques.[119, 120] The modified guide wire technique decreases time to access and also allows for placement of larger bore catheters.[120] A 10-gauge catheter can successfully be placed using the mini-cutdown technique.[121] Both techniques avoid ligation of the proximal vein, thereby preserving the vein for future cannulation.[120, 122]

Access Sites

The most commonly used vessel for cutdown in children is the greater saphenous vein (Fig. 8–16).[118] From its origin on the medial border of the foot, the greater saphenous vein travels along the periosteum of the tibia anterior to the medial malleolus and then superiorly along the medial aspect to the thigh, where it joins the femoral vein just distal to the inguinal ligament.[123] There are several sites along the greater saphenous vein available for cutdown. The most distal site requires an incision 1 to 2 cm anterior and superior to the medial malleolus. Several characteristics of the distal greater saphenous vein make the ankle a preferred cutdown site; these include a consistent location, a relatively large diameter, no adjacent important structures, and elasticity.[124]

Similarly, predictable anatomic location, accessibility, and large caliber make the proximal vein at the groin an ideal site for cutdown.[125] In the adult, an incision is made 5 to 6 cm distal to a line drawn between the anterosuperior iliac spine and the pubic tubercle along the middle and medial one third of the thigh. For children, the location must be adjusted for size.

A less commonly used site for proximal saphenous vein cutdown is at the level of the knee. The incision site is made 1 to 4 cm (5 to 10 cm in the adult) below the joint line along the medial ridge of the tibia. This area contains no other significant structures, and the caliber allows adequate access.[126]

Additional sites for cutdown in children include the external jugular vein and the veins of the antecubital fossa of the upper extremity. Although these veins are superficially located, they are technically more difficult to cannulate by cutdown.[117] In addition, these sites have important structures located in the immediate area of incision that dissection could easily damage.

Traditional Cutdown

The technique for a traditional venous cutdown will be described for the distal saphenous vein. The same technique applies for other sites.

Equipment

Necessary equipment for the traditional cutdown technique includes the following:

Local anesthetic, if necessary
Aseptic solution
Sterile drapes
4 × 4 gauze sponges
Small hemostat
Curved Kelly hemostat
Scalpel with No. 10 blade
Scalpel with No. 11 blade or iris scissors
Vein dilator/introducer (optional)
Plastic catheter device
Suture
IV fluid and tubing

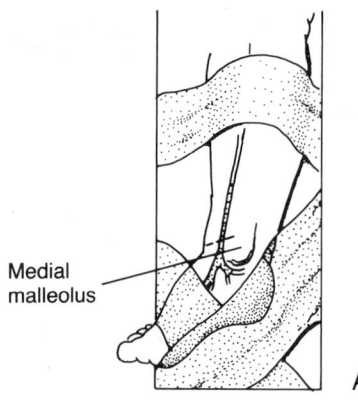

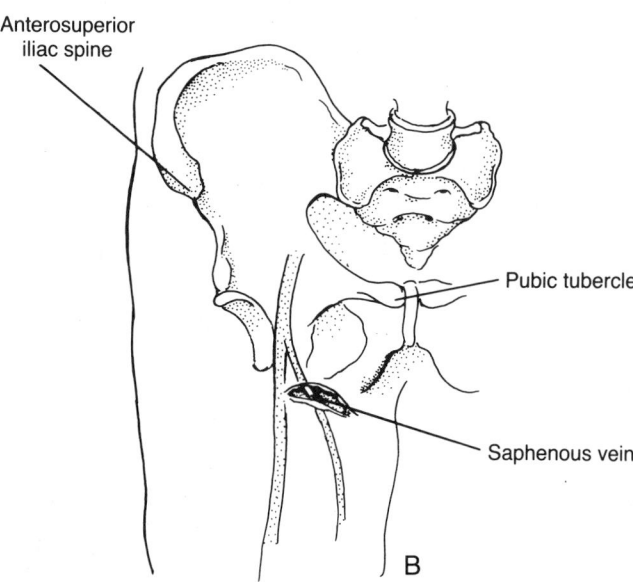

Figure 8–16. Sites for venous cutdown along the great saphenous vein. *A,* Distal, at the ankle. (From Chameides L (ed). Textbook of Pediatric Advanced Life Support, 1988, p 43. Dallas, American Heart Association. Copyright American Heart Association.) *B,* Proximal, at the groin. (From Dronen SC, Yee AS, Tomlanovich MC: Proximal saphenous vein cutdown. Ann Emerg Med 1981;10:328.)

Technique

1. The child is restrained with the site exposed and easily accessible.

2. The site is cleaned with aseptic solution, and sterile drapes are applied. Local anesthesia can be used.

3. The skin is incised to the subcutaneous tissue.

4. Blunt dissection parallel to the vessel is used to identify the vein. For the distal saphenous vein, one should "scoop" along the periosteum with the curved hemostat to lift the vein off the bone (Fig. 8–17).

5. Two ligatures are placed beneath the vein. A small longitudinal incision is made in the vein between the ligatures. Gentle traction of the ligatures will prevent bleeding into the site, as well as stabilize the vein.

6. The catheter is inserted into the vein. A vein introducer or mosquito hemostat placed in the venotomy may be helpful to lift the vein wall and aid catheter insertion. A makeshift vein introducer can be made by bending the bevel tip of an 18-gauge needle 90 degrees using a needle holder.

7. The proximal ligature is relaxed to allow passage of the catheter within the vessel.

8. The clinician should aspirate with a syringe to check position.

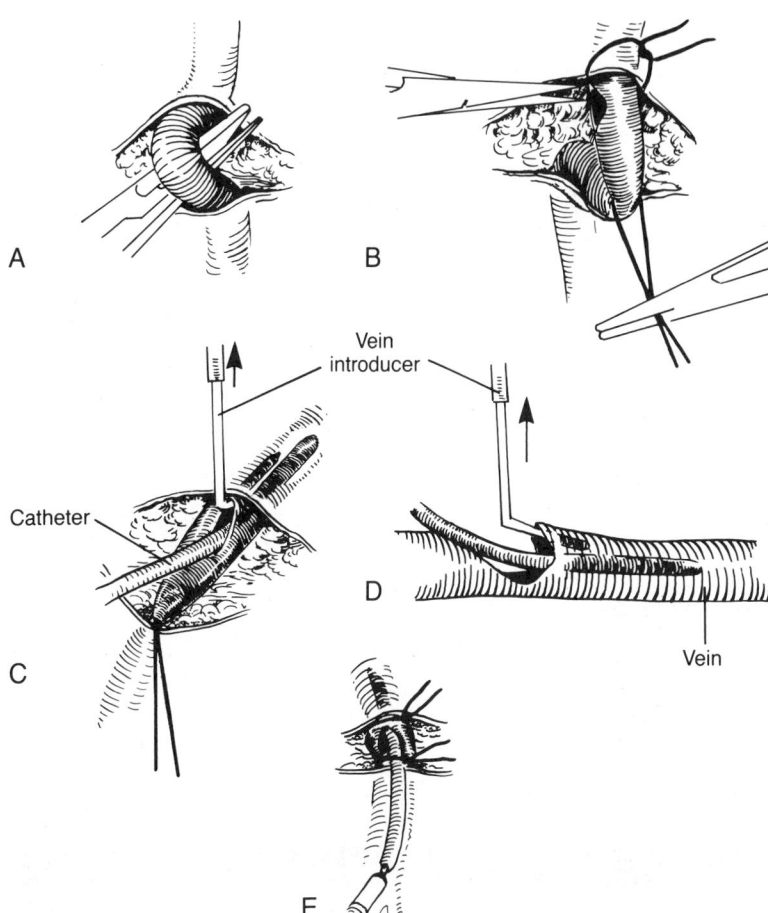

Figure 8–17. Method for traditional greater saphenous vein cutdown.

9. With attachment of the IV tubing, fluids should flow freely.

10. The distal vein is ligated, and the proximal vein is secured to the catheter with the other ligature.

11. The skin is sutured and a sterile dressing applied.

Modified Guide Wire Cutdown

The modified guide wire cutdown method uses the Seldinger (wire-dilator-catheter) technique. It allows passage of a larger catheter through a small venotomy under direct visualization of the vein.[120]

Equipment

The modified guide wire cutdown uses the same equipment listed for the traditional cutdown, with the addition of a catheter with an introducer guide wire.

Technique

1. The vein is located and prepared as in the traditional technique (see steps 1 through 4 of the traditional cutdown technique).

2. The vein is elevated on the hemostat.

3. The No. 11 blade or iris scissors is used to make a small 1- to 2-mm venotomy in the vein site.

4. The wire-dilator-catheter unit is passed through the venotomy and into the vessel lumen using the Seldinger technique.

5. The wire and dilator are removed.

6. If necessary, ligatures can be passed to control bleeding around the venotomy.

7. The catheter is secured.

8. The skin is sutured; a sterile dressing is applied.

Mini-cutdown

In the mini-cutdown technique the vein is punctured under direct visualization using a standard percutaneous venous catheter.

Equipment

The mini-cutdown uses the same equipment as the traditional cutdown, with the addition of a catheter-over-the-needle device or a catheter-through-the-needle device.

Technique

1. The vein is located and prepared as in the traditional technique (see steps 1 through 4 of the traditional cutdown technique).

2. At a distance away from the cutdown incision, a separate skin puncture is made with the catheter-needle-device, which is then advanced into the cutdown field (Fig. 8–18). The vein can also be cannulated through the skin incision.

3. Under direct vision the vein is punctured, and the catheter is threaded into the vessel lumen.

4. The needle is removed.

5. IV fluids and infusion are begun.

6. The catheter is secured by sutures and tape.

7. The skin is sutured and a sterile dressing applied.

Complications

Complications of venous cutdown include local bleeding, infection, sepsis, phlebitis, embolization, wound dehiscence, and injury to associated structures.[119] The incidence of complications is reduced when the catheter enters through a

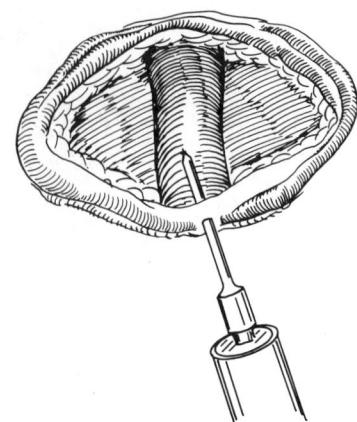

Figure 8–18. "Mini"-cutdown technique showing a separate entry site. (Redrawn from Roberts JR, Hedges JR (eds). Clinical Procedures in Emergency Medicine. Philadelphia, WB Saunders, 1985, p 302.)

separate puncture rather than through the cutdown incision itself.[127] The use of locally applied antibiotic ointment decreases the infectious complications from venous cutdowns.[128] Complications can be further minimized by removing cutdown lines that were started in the emergency department within the previous 24 hours.[129]

During the traditional cutdown technique, the vein can be

inadvertently transected. When using the modified guide wire technique, the wire can be errantly inserted into the vein wall, dissecting the adventitia rather than entering the lumen.[120] In addition, perforation of the posterior wall by a wire or needle can occur.

INTRAOSSEOUS INFUSIONS

In 1922, the bone marrow route was proposed for injecting fluids and drugs into the circulation.[15] In 1940, the first clinical studies of intraosseous (IO) infusion were published.[130, 131] Tocantins' research and publications strongly advocated the technique,[130–136] and in the 1940s and 1950s it gained wide acceptance. It was used frequently during the Korean War,[137] but as intravenous technology improved in the 1950s and 60s, the IO technique fell into obscurity; it was largely forgotten.

In the 1980s, physicians began to carefully examine the timeliness of the resuscitation process in children. In 1984, Rosetti and coworkers reported a 3-year retrospective study regarding IV access in children presenting in cardiac arrest.[3] Despite at least two experienced operators attempting vascular access simultaneously, the results showed that in more than 6% of cases, IV access was never attained, even when the resuscitation effort was stopped after more than 45 minutes. The mean time to IV access in patients in whom a line was eventually established was 7.8 minutes, but almost one fourth of the cases required 10 minutes or more to establish access.

		Failed Infusions			
TABLE 8–10					
MAJOR STUDIES OF INTRAOSSEOUS INFUSION*					
Author (Date)	**Number of Successful Infusions**	**Number**	**%**	**Complications Noted**	
Arbeiter (1944)	35	8	18.66	0	
Bailey (1944)	60	?		1	Posterior sternal perforation
Behr (1944)	60	?		1	Osteomyelitis
Bielstein (1944)	58	?		0	
Clement (1947)	65	?		3	Osteomyelitis
Couder (1948)	100+	?		0	
Dardinski (1945)	?	?		1	Mediastinitis
Ellison (1944)	40	?		0	
Elston (1947)	97	15	13.4	1	Subcutaneous abscess
Giraud (1945)	20	?		0	
Gunz (1945)	35	1	2.9	3	Osteomyelitis
Heinild (1947)	982	18	1.8	5	Osteomyelitis
Heyrouti (1947)	310	?		0	
Higgins (1947)	120	?		0	
Massey (1950)	72	12	14.3	1	Osteomyelitis
Meola (1944)	326	0	0	1	Arterial thrombosis
O'Neill (1942)	116	?		1	Posterior sternal perforation
Pillar (1954)	35	?		1	Subcutaneous sloughing, 2° level
Quilligan (1946)	45	?		1	
Ravitch (1943)	?	?		1	Anterior mediastinitis
Reich (1945)	35	?		0	
Reisman (1944)	?	?		1	Subcutaneous abscess
Romero (1945)	77	?		0	
Rooney (1944)	100	2	2.0	2	Osteomyelitis
Sondergaard (1946)	750	?		5	Osteomyelitis
Sutton (1947)	200	?		0	
Texter (1948)	300	25	7.7	2	Osteomyelitis, 1 subcutaneous abscess
Tocantins (1943)	79	9	10.2	2	Osteomyelitis, 1 subcutaneous abscess
Valdes (1977)	15	2	11.8	0	
Williams (1948)	138	?		1	Osteomyelitis
Total	4270	89	2.1	27	Osteomyelitis
				10	Other

*Complete reference information for the studies cited in the table can be found in the source given below.
From Rosetti VA, Thompson BM, Miller J, et al. Intraosseous infusion: An alternative route of pediatric intravascular access. Ann Emerg Med 1985;14:886.

In 1985, Rosetti et al. presented a review of 30 IO studies in the world literature involving 4359 attempts (Table 8–10).[26] There was a 2.1% failure rate, and osteomyelitis was reported in only 27 cases (0.6%). This low rate of infection is remarkable, because most cases involved prolonged IO infusion. Multiple studies involving IO access have confirmed its safety and effectiveness,[138–144] studied the rates of absorption,[145–153] investigated the effect on bone marrow,[153, 154] and eliminated most of the concern regarding fat and bone embolization (Table 8–11).[155–157]

Several studies of IO infusions have mapped the return of fluids from the long-bone medullary sinusoids through the nutrient and emissary veins to the vena cava.[15, 158, 159] The intramedullary marrow provides rapid and complete delivery of fluids and drugs comparable to that provided by a similar size IV cannula in a similar position.[26] The marrow can be considered a rigid vein that is not collapsible in shock but is also not distensible during pressure infusion. As the patient matures to adulthood, the vascular red marrow changes to a less vascular yellow marrow that is infiltrated with fat cells. As a result, many sites that are available in young children (Table 8–12) are not available in the adult, leaving the iliac crests, the sternum, and the distal tibias as the only viable sites.[144] In infants, the proximal tibia or distal tibia and femur are routinely used; but the os calcis and the femoral greater trocanter have also been used. The proximal tibia is the first choice for IO access in the child.[11]

The risks associated with sternal puncture preclude its routine use in the small child. IO cannulation should not be done through a grossly infected site, thereby decreasing the possibility of seeding the infection to the marrow. IO infusion is contraindicated in extremities with known or suspected fractures and relatively contraindicated in children with osteopetrosis or osteogenesis imperfecta.[144]

IO access is an excellent source for obtaining samples for most blood chemistry tests, blood cell counts, and blood cultures.[160–162] Bone marrow blood does not correlate with arterial blood gases, having a pH intermediate to that found in arterial and venous samples.[160]

The IO technique is easily mastered and can be quickly and reliably performed using a variety of specially designed bone marrow needles. If necessary, the technique can be

---

TABLE 8–11

MEDICATIONS REPORTED TO HAVE BEEN ADMINISTERED VIA THE INTRAOSSEOUS ROUTE

Agent	Site	Rate/Dose	Response	Subject
Ampicillin	Tibia	*	An initial dose was administered during the treatment of meningitis.	6-month-old infant
Atropine	Tibia	0.03 mg/kg of a 0.01% solution	The mean plasma concentration of atropine administered IO was significantly higher than that of ET administration at 5 min and was greater than that of IV and ET administrations for the samples collected from 5–30 min. The IO route can provide an alternative to the IV administration of atropine.	Pigtail macaque
Dextran	Iliac crest	*	Treatment of shock associated with mesenteric thrombosis.	Human male
Diazepam	Tibia	0.1 mg/kg	Diazepam blood concentrations were identical from both IO and IV administration over a 20-min time interval. Both routes were efficacious in suppressing seizures induced by pentylenetetrazol.	Domestic swine
Diazepam	Tibia	1.0 mg	Cessation of seizure activity within 1 min of administration.	6-month-old infant
Digoxin	Iliac crest	*	In a patient with rheumatic mitral stenosis with rapid atrial fibrillation, it was noted that the patient was adequately digitalized in the expected length of time.	*
Dopamine and dobutamine	Tibia	10 μg/kg/min	Blood pressure elevation within seconds from infusion.	6-month-old infant
Epinephrine Ephedrine	Tibia	0.5 mg in 3 ml NS; 50 mg in 10 ml NS	The mean time to initial effect (increased blood pressure) of IO injections of either epinephrine or ephedrine was 17.3 sec; mean time to 90% maximum effect was 45 sec.	Female calves
Insulin and glucose	Manubrium	120 units insulin followed by D5W at 11 ml/min	15 min following completion of infusion the patient came out of coma. Circulatory status temporarily improved, but the patient eventually expired.	25-year-old
Levarterenol	*	*	It was noted that the physiologic vasopressor effects of levarterenol became manifest as quickly as one would expect in a direct IV infusion. The magnitude of vasopressor effect was directly proportional to the rate of infusion.	Human
Phenytoin	Tibia	17 mg/kg	Resolution of seizure activity reported after a bolus was administered IO. A plasma phenytoin concentration drawn 60 min postinjection was 28 μg/ml.	2-year-old child
Sodium bicarbonate	Tibia	1.0 mg/kg	IO route was a rapid and effective alternative for venous access	Domestic swine
Sodium pentothal	Iliac crest	0.5 gm	When sodium pentothal was administered, it was observed that the second stage of anesthesia was reached as quickly as if the same dose had been given IV.	Human male
Sodium pentothal	*	*	During World War II, sodium pentothal was used extensively on the battlefield as intramarrow-induced anesthesia.	*

Abbreviations: ET = Endotracheal, IO = intraosseous, IV = intravenous, NS = normal saline.
*No information provided.
†On histologic examination of the marrow, only minimal damage was evident in the cells surrounding the injection site.
Reprinted with permission from Mofenson H, Tascone A, Caraccio T. Guidelines for Intraosseous Infusion. J Emerg Med 1988;6:145. Copyright 1988, Pergamon Press Ltd.

TABLE 8–12

INTRAOSSEOUS INFUSION

I. Indications
   A. After 90 seconds or three attempts at peripheral access in a child younger than 3 years in shock or impending arrest.
   B. When other methods fail.
   C. Laboratory sampling when venous and arterial sampling is unsuccessful.
II. Contraindications
   A. Active infection at the insertion site.
   B. Known or suspected fracture of the same bone or extremity.
   C. Known or suspected osteogenesis imperfecta.
   D. Known or suspected osteopetrosis.
III. Sites (children)

Sites (children)	Advantages
Proximal tibia	Rapidity of access
Distal femur	Reliability of access
Distal tibia	Safety
Sternum (adolescents and adults)	Not affected by hypovolemia or shock
Iliac crest	Effective for all drugs and fluids
Greater trocanter	

IV. Complications
   Extravasation of fluid/drugs
   Local cellulitis
   Osteomyelitis
   Sepsis
   Fracture at infusion site
   Compartment syndrome
   Injury to growth plate
   Toxic injury to marrow
   Fat or bone marrow embolization
   Specific complications
   With sternal approach only
      Mediastinitis
      Pneumothorax
      Death
   With iliac approach
      Peritonitis
   With greater trochanter approach
      Septic arthritis

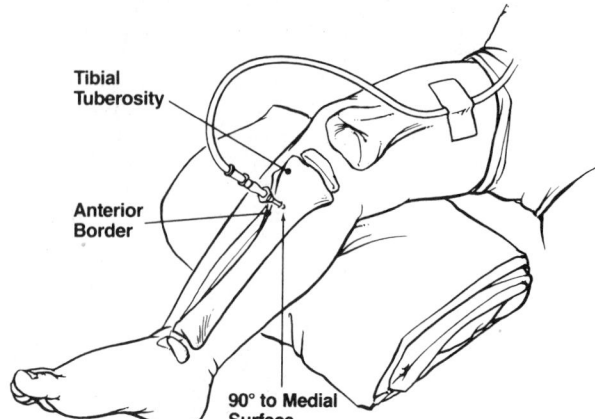

Figure 8–19. Intraosseous cannulation technique. (Reproduced with permission. © From Chameides L (ed). Textbook of Pediatric Advanced Life Support, 1988. Copyright, American Heart Association.)

2. Following universal precautions, hands are washed and sterile gloves worn.

3. The insertion point is identified (0.5 to 2 cm below the tibial tuberosity on the medial side of the anterior tibia). Some believe the needle should be inserted at or just below the tibial tuberosity to increase success and lessen the chance of fracture.[164]

4. The tip of the needle is directed away from the growth plate by aiming slightly caudad from the perpendicular.

5. The skin is initially penetrated and the needle tip seated on the periosteal bone site while firm control is maintained with the other hand.

6. The needle is advanced using a firm boring or screwing motion until a decrease in resistance is felt, indicating marrow penetration.

7. Placement is confirmed by aspirating the bone marrow using a 1- to 3-ml syringe.

8. Standard IV tubing is attached. Drugs and fluids can be administered by gravity or pressure infusion.

9. The infusion of 2 to 3 ml of heparinized saline or other flush solution will clear the needle of rapidly clotting marrow blood and bone spicules.

10. A curved clamp (hemostat) is placed tip down against the skin to support the needle and limit movement.

11. A radiograph can be obtained to check marrow placement.

The distal femur is another commonly used IO site in children. Insertion is made in the midline 2 to 3 cm above the external condyles, and the needle is directed slightly cephalad from the perpendicular to avoid injury to the growth plate. The cortex of the femur at this point is only slightly thicker than that at the tibial insertions. The distal tibia can also be used in older children and adults.[144] The needle is inserted approximately 1 cm proximal to the medial malleolus and posterior to the saphenous vein. The needle is directed perpendicular and slightly cephalad to the skin edge. Though both malleoli have been used, the medial site is technically easier.

The sternum should be avoided in small children, but in adolescents and adults not requiring CPR, it is the easiest of the remaining sites to access. The sternal marrow matures at approximately age 3 and remains an active and reliable bone marrow site throughout adulthood. Complications after use of this site are dramatic and have yielded the only fatalities attributed solely to IO infusion.[165] With care, however, the sternum can be used safely.

successful using the short Rosenthal, Osgood, or Illinois bone marrow biopsy needles or a common spinal needle. Newly developed needles have made the procedure easier to perform and have improved success rates.[163] Parents may find the technique more invasive than an IV line and should not usually be present during the procedure.

Equipment

IO infusion requires the following equipment:

Povidone-iodine prep solution
IO infusion needles (various types)
1- to 3-ml syringe for sampling (optional)
3- to 5-ml syringe with isotonic flush solution (optional)
Curved mosquito or Kelly clamp
Antiseptic ointment
Tape

Technique

The technique is most commonly performed at the proximal tibia (Fig. 8–19), but the principles of the technique apply to any site.

1. The procedure site is prepped with povidone-iodine and then properly supported, immobilized, and draped to allow anatomic orientation.

The remaining available sites are technically more difficult and fraught with complications. Although the iliac crests are excellent marrow sites throughout life, these are difficult to access on a supine patient. Attempts at obtaining access have the potential risk of peritoneal perforation. The greater trocanter is also technically difficult to access and carries significant risk of penetration and contamination of the hip joint.

Multiple cortical punctures reduce the effectiveness of IO infusion.[166] If a puncture fails to function, the original needle may be left in place with the stylet and another attempted placement made. Preferably, a second puncture should be made in a different extremity or in a bone more proximal to the original site of puncture.

Despite the successful use of prolonged IO infusion in the past, normal IV access should be substituted for IO access as soon as possible.[26] This eliminates those complications associated with prolonged placement. A radiograph should be obtained to check placement of the IO device for proper patient care, quality assurance, and medicolegal considerations.[164]

Complications

Considering the invasive nature of the technique, IO infusion has a remarkably low rate of complications.[26] The most frequent complication is undoubtedly the extravasation of medication and fluids as a result of malplacement or loose IO needles.[26] Once detected, the infusion should be stopped and the needle removed. Localized cellulitis or subcutaneous abscesses occur in less than 1% of cases and are seen most frequently with prolonged placements. Sepsis and osteomyelitis can occur at the infusion site and are associated with prolonged placement, ongoing bacteremia or sepsis, and the use of hypertonic infusion.[26]

As part of the standard technique the needle is placed away from the growth plate to avoid injury. No serious bone deformity has been associated with IO placement. Concern has been raised regarding the effect of medication, fluids, and blood products being rapidly infused through the marrow.[153, 154] Although a transient reduction of cellularity occurs, once the infusion is stopped, the marrow reconstitutes itself, and within weeks it appears virtually normal.[154] Bone embolization has not been documented. Fat embolization occurs microscopically but is clinically insignificant.[155–157] Alert patients have reported a sensation of dull, deep pain when fluids are infused under great pressure. Pain decreases with a corresponding reduction in the rate and pressure of infusion.

Compartment syndrome and fractures at the puncture sites have been reported.[167, 168] Fracture risks may be reduced by careful adherence to accepted techniques, routine radiography of all placements, and protection of weakened bones.[164] Death has occurred in rare instances and is associated with sternal puncture leading to mediastinitis, hydrothorax, or injury to the great vessels.[165] Avoidance of the sternal approach eliminates these serious complications.

ARTERIAL CATHETERIZATION

Percutaneous peripheral arterial catheterization serves several functions. It is a means for continuously monitoring blood pressure, and the arterial line provides ready access to arterial blood for arterial blood gas analysis and other frequently needed laboratory studies, eliminating the need for multiple arterial punctures.[169] Arterial catheterization can be successfully performed on pediatric patients in the emergency department with few complications, thereby aiding initial resuscitation and stabilization.[170]

The preferred site for arterial catheterization is the radial artery. Other potential peripheral arterial sites include the dorsalis pedis, posterior tibial, and temporal arteries.

Complications

The most commonly reported complication of arterial cannulation is ischemic damage to the extremities.[171] Varying degrees of ischemia have occurred, ranging from necrosis of small areas of skin to necrosis of the fingertips. Below-the-elbow amputation secondary to necrosis from a radial line has been reported in a premature infant.[172] Cannulation of the temporal artery minimizes the risk of skin necrosis because of the rich vascularity and collateral circulation of the scalp.[173]

Thrombosis occurs in approximately 50% of the arterial vessels cannulized. In a series of 53 peripheral arterial lines, 27 (51%) became obstructed. All vessels recannulized spontaneously, the majority at between 7 and 14 days. Young age and increased duration of cannulation were identified as factors predisposing to thrombotic obstruction.[174] Additional complications include emboli, pseudoaneurysm formation,[175] sepsis, and hemorrhage.

Arterial catheters require continuous infusion of a heparinized isotonic solution, avoidance of forceful flushing and air bubbles, a firmly secured cannula, and frequent direct visualization of the catheter and attached lines.[176] Catheters should be removed if any of the following conditions occur: persistent skin blanching, erythema over the catheter tip, clot formation (inability to withdraw blood or loss of blood pressure tracing), or leakage around the insertion site.[173]

Equipment

Arterial catheterization requires the following equipment:

Arterial catheter
18-gauge needle
T connector
Three-way stopcock
Syringe
Isotonic heparinized flush
Tape
Arm/leg board
Suture material (optional)
Arterial pressure monitor (optional)

Technique

1. The clinician should assemble the T connector, three-way stopcock, and syringe and flush them with heparinized saline.

2. The radial arteries on both sides should be palpated for site selection. A modified Allen's test will assess the adequacy of collateral flow from the ulnar artery.[177] In infants the use of a transilluminator may aid in visualizing the artery.[178, 179] The wrist is supinated and extended to 45 to 60 degrees over a small roll of gauze and taped or held securely in place. The skin is prepped with an antiseptic solution.

3. The skin is punctured with an 18-gauge needle a few millimeters distal to the point where the catheter will enter the artery. The optimal site for penetration of the catheter into the artery is at the level of the radial styloid. The catheter and stylet are introduced at a 15- to 30-degree angle through the skin puncture toward the artery. The younger the child, the less acute the angle of entry must be.[173]

4. The catheter and stylet are advanced until the vessel is punctured. The stylet is removed, and if good pulsatile flow

occurs, the catheter is advanced through its entire length into the artery (Fig. 8–20).

5. If the vessel has been transfixed, the catheter is slowly withdrawn until free pulsatile flow occurs, and then the catheter is carefully advanced into the artery.

6. The line is firmly secured with tape or suture.

7. The extremity should be restrained with tape with the fingertips and puncture site exposed.

Alternative techniques for radial artery cannulation include arterial cutdown[180] and percutaneous guide wire methods.[8]

EMERGENCY MEDICAL SERVICE CONSIDERATIONS

Attempts to resuscitate pediatric cardiac arrest victims are usually unsuccessful.[181–183] Abysmal results were seen in a 2-year retrospective study of pediatric cardiac arrest patients in the excellent Milwaukee County Paramedic System.[181] Few pediatric arrest victims had IV access in the field, which was partly the result of a desire to not delay transport to the hospital. It may also have been a response to the reality of

the difficulty of pediatric vascular access in this setting. These findings led to the trend for specialized training in pediatric emergencies for EMS personnel.

In 1987, a preliminary study of prehospital IO infusion was reported.[184] Soon other EMS studies of IO infusion confirmed the low complication and relatively high success rates obtained without significant delays for vascular access.[185, 186]

A method of paramedic training in the IO technique using chicken legs has been described.[187] This model has been recommended by the American Heart Association and the American Academy of Pediatrics and has been adapted for use in Pediatric Advanced Life Support courses.

MEDICOLEGAL IMPLICATIONS OF VASCULAR ACCESS

The techniques for obtaining vascular access in children are associated with risks and complications. In general, the more invasive the technique, the more likely the chance of a complication and, usually, the more serious that complication will be. For this reason it is important for both the parent or legal guardian of a minor and the patient to be well informed about procedures that need to be done, including possible complications. Consent should be obtained to perform such procedures. Provided that obtaining informed consent does not delay the delivery of care, consent should be obtained when risky procedures are to be performed or when choices between alternative methods of treatment exist.[188] There is no obligation to obtain informed consent when immediate vascular access procedures are necessary for the treatment of life- and limb-threatening conditions or when obtaining informed consent will delay delivery of care.

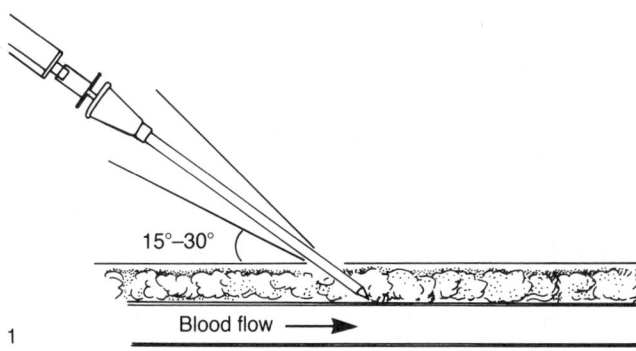

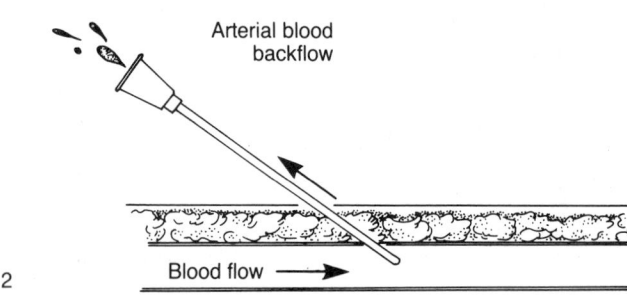

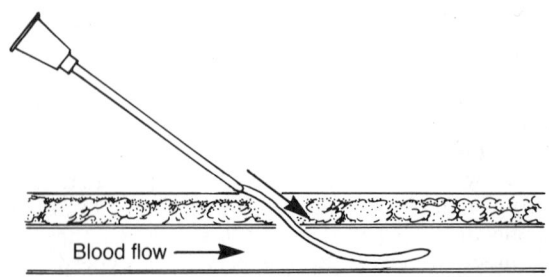

Figure 8–20. Radial artery cannulation technique—single wall puncture. (Redrawn from Hughes WT, Buescher ES. Pediatric Procedures. 2nd ed. Philadelphia, WB Saunders, 1980, p 83.)

References

1. Larkin M. IV therapy yesterday and today with a look to the future. Natl Intraven Ther Assoc 1979;2:40.
2. Zimmerman JJ, Strauss RH. History and current application of intravenous therapy in children. Pediatr Emerg Care 1989;2:120.
3. Rosetti V, Thompson BM, Aprahamian C, et al. Difficulty and delay in intravascular access in pediatric arrests. Abstract. Ann Emerg Med 1984;13:406.
4. Orlowski JP. My kingdom for an intravenous line. Am J Dis Child 1984;138:803.
5. Chameides L (ed). Textbook of Pediatric Advanced Life Support. Dallas, TX, American Heart Association, 1988, p 37.
6. Kanter RK, Zimmerman JJ, Strauss RH, et al. Pediatric emergency intravenous access: Evaluation of a proposal. Am J Dis Child 1986;140:132.
7. Committee on Trauma, American College of Surgeons. Advanced Trauma Life Support Course Manual. Chicago, American College of Surgeons, 1988.
8. Dailey RH. Use of wire-guided (Seldinger-type) catheters in the emergency department. Ann Emerg Med 1983;12:489.
9. Rudolph AM, Hoffman JI (eds). Pediatrics. Norwalk, CT, Appleton & Lange, 1987, p 79.
10. Feliciano DV, Mattax KL, Grahim JM, et al. Major complications of percutaneous subclavian vein catheters. Am J Surg 1979;138:869.
11. Chameides L (ed): Textbook of Pediatric Advanced Life Support. Dallas, American Heart Association, 1988, p. 44.
12. Quinton DN, O'Bryne G, Aitkenhead AR. Comparison of endotracheal and peripheral intravenous adrenaline in cardiac arrest. Lancet 1987;1:828.
13. Orlowski JP, Gallagher JM, Porembka DT. Intratracheal epinephrine is unreliable. Abstract. Crit Care Med 1988;16:389.
14. Brickman K, Rega P, Guinness M. Comparison of intraosseous, intratracheal, and central venous administration of lidocaine in pigs. Abstract. Ann Emerg Med 1988;17:435.
15. Drinker CK, Drinker KR, Lund CC. The circulation in the mammalian bone marrow. Am J Physiol 1922;62:1.
16. Orlowski JP, Porembka DT, Gallagher JM, et al. Study of intravenous and peripheral intraosseous infusions of emergency drugs. Am J Dis Child 1990;144:112.
17. Gauderer MWL, Stellato TA, Izant RJ. Broviac Silastic catheter insertion

in children: A simplified direct subclavian approach. J Pediatr Surg 1982;17:580.

18. Davis SJ, Thompson JS, Edney JA. Insertion of Hickman catheters: A comparison of cutdown and percutaneous techniques. Am J Surg 1984;50:673.

19. Poiseuille JLM. Recherches expérimentales sur le mouvement des liquides dans les tubes de très-petits diamètres, Mem Present Divers Savants l'Acad Sci l'Institut France 1846;9:433.

20. Mateer JR, Thompson BM, Aprahamian C, Darin C. Rapid fluid resuscitation with central venous catheters. Ann Emerg Med 1983;12:149.

21. Pirofsky B. The determination of blood viscosity in man by a method based on Poiseuille's Law. J Clin Invest 1953;32:292.

22. Milnor WR. Principles of hemodynamics. *In* Mountcastle VB (ed). Medical Physiology. 14th ed. St Louis, CV Mosby, 1988, pp 1017–1022.

23. Lundy JS. Plastic stylet for plastic needles. Mayo Clinic Proc 1958;33:458.

24. Gritsch JH, Ballinger CM. The value of indwelling catheters in intravenous therapy—description of a new needle and catheter set. JAMA 1959;171:281.

25. Seldinger SI. Catheter replacement of the needle in percutaneous arteriography. Acta Radiol Diagn (Stockh) 1953;39:368.

26. Rosetti VA, Thompson BM, Miller J, et al. Intraosseous infusion: An alternative route of pediatric intravascular access. Ann Emerg Med 1985;14:885.

27. Glaeser PW, Losek JD. Intraosseous needles: New and improved. Pediatr Emerg Care 1988;4:135.

28. Schwartz AJ, Horrow JC, Jones DR, et al. Guidewires—a caution. Crit Care Med 1981;4:347.

29. Desilets DT, Hoffman R. A new method of percutaneous catheterization. Radiology 1965;85:145.

30. Gerbitz S. Transillumination helps nurses find veins. Nursing 1974;74:12.

31. Hecker JF, Lewis GHB, Stanley H. Nitroglycerine ointment as an aid to venepuncture. Lancet 1983;1:332.

32. Roberge R, Kelly M, Evans TC, et al. Facilitated intravenous access through local application of nitroglycerine ointment. Ann Emerg Med 1987;16:546.

33. Clarke TA, Reddy PG. Intravenous infusion technique in the newborn. Clin Pediatr 1979;18:550.

34. MacDonald MG, Chou MM. Preventing complications from lines and tubes. Semin Perinatol 1986;10:224.

35. Hildebrand WL, Schreiner RL, Yacko MS, et al. Placing a needle in an infant's scalp vein. Am Fam Phys 1980;21:139.

36. Willis J, Duncan C, Gottschalk S. Paraplegia due to peripheral venous air embolus in a neonate. Pediatrics 1981;67:472.

37. Wilson JN, Grow JB, Demong CV, et al. Central venous pressure in optimal blood volume maintenance. Arch Surg 1962;85:563.

38. Hemosura B. Management of pressure during intravenous therapy. JAMA 1966;195:181.

39. Dunbar RD, Mitchell R, Lavine M. Aberrant locations of central venous catheters. Lancet 1981;1:711.

40. Knopp R, Dailey RH. Central venous cannulation and pressure monitoring. J Am Coll Emerg Phys 1977;6:358.

41. James PM, Meyers RT. Central venous pressure monitoring. Misinterpretations, abuses, indications, and a new technique. Ann Surg 1972;175:693.

42. Wilson J, Owens J. Pitfalls in monitoring central venous pressure. Hosp Med 1970;6:86.

43. Notterman DA. Invasive hemodynamic monitoring. *In* Zimmerman SS, Gidea JH (eds). Critical Care Pediatrics. Philadelphia, WB Saunders, 1985, pp 43–54.

44. Debrunner F, Buhler F. Normal central venous pressure: Significance of reference point and normal range. Br Med J 1969;3:148.

45. Guyton A, Jones C. Central venous pressure: Physiological significance and clinical implications. Am Heart J 1973;86:431.

46. Weil MH, Shubin H, Rosoff L. Fluid repletion in circulatory shock. Central venous pressure and other practical guides. JAMA 1965;192:668.

47. DeLaurentis D, Hayes M, Matsumoto T. Does central venous pressure accurately reflect hemodynamic and fluid volume patterns in the critical surgical patient. Am J Surg 1973;126:415.

48. Klaus MH, Fanaroff AA. Care of the High-Risk Neonate. Philadelphia, WB Saunders, 1986, p 36.

49. Moore KL. The Developing Human: Clinically Oriented Embryology. 4th ed. Philadelphia, WB Saunders, 1988, pp 325–329.

50. Prinz SC, Cunningham MD. Umbilical vessel catheterization. J Fam Pract 1980;10:885.

51. Kitterman JA, Phibbs RH, Tooley WH. Catheterization of umbilical vessels in newborn infants. Pediatr Clin North Am 1970;17:895.

52. Chameides L. Textbook of Pediatric Advanced Life Support. Dallas, TX, American Heart Association, 1988, p 74.

53. Dmochowski RR, Crandell SS, Corrieve JN: Bladder injury and uroascites from umbilical artery catheterization. Pediatrics 1986;77:421.

54. Walker D, Pellett JR: Pericardial tamponade secondary to umbilical vein catheters. J Pediatr Surg 1972;7:79.

55. Omene JA, Odita JC, Diakparomre MA: The risks of umbilical vessel catheterization in a neonatal intensive care unit. Afr J Med Med Sci 1979;8:115.

56. Drucker DE, Greenfield LJ, Ehrlich F, et al: Aorto-Iliac aneurysms following umbilical artery catheterization. J Ped Surg 1986;21:725.

57. MacDonald MG, Chou MM: Preventing complications from lines and tubes. Sem Perinatol 1986;10:224.

58. Humphrey MJ, Blitt CD: Central venous access in children via the external jugular vein. Anesthesiology 1982;57:50.

59. Craig RG, Jones RA, Sproul GJ et al: The alternate methods of central venous system catheterization. Am Surg 1968;34:131.

60. Belani KG, Buckley JJ, Goron JR et al: Percutaneous cervical central venous line placement: A comparison of the internal and external jugular vein routes. Anesth Analg 1980;59:40.

61. Schwartz AJ, Jobes R, Levy WJ, et al. Intrathoracic vascular catheterization via the external jugular vein. Anesthesiology 1982;56:400.

62. Blitt DC, Wright WA, Pretty WC. Central venous catheterization via the external jugular vein: A technique employing the J-wire. JAMA 1974;229:817.

63. Blitt CD, Carlson GL, Wright WA, et al. J-wire versus straight wire for central venous system cannulation via the external jugular vein. Anesth Analg 1982;61:536.

64. Bosch DT, Kengeter JP, Beling CA. Femoral venipuncture. Am Surg 1950;79:722.

65. Coletti RH, Hartjen B, Gozdziewskia SL, et al. Origin of canine femoral pulses during standard CPR. Abstract. Crit Care Med 1983;11:218.

66. Agnes RS, Arendar GM. Septic arthritis of the hip: A complication of femoral venipuncture. Pediatrics 1966;38:837.

67. Fuchs HJ, Genett G, Klehr U, et al. Percutaneous puncture of the femoral vein for hemodialysis: Report of 5,000 punctures. Dtsch Med Wochenschr 1977;102:1280.

68. Barsan WG, Hedges JR, Nishiyama H, et al. Differences in drug delivery with peripheral and central venous injections. Am J Emerg 1986;4:1.

69. Linos DA, Muchta P Jr, Van Heerden JA. Subclavian vein: A golden route. Mayo Clin Proc 1980;55:315.

70. Abraham E, Shapiro M, Podalsky S. Central venous catheterization in the emergency setting. Crit Care Med 1983;11:515.

71. Dronen SC. Central venous catheterization in the emergency setting. Crit Care Med 1984;12:540.

72. Dronen SC. Subclavian venipuncture. *In* Roberts J, Hedges JR (eds). Clinical Procedures in Emergency Medicine. Philadelphia, WB Saunders, 1985, pp 304–321.

73. Land RE. Anatomic relationship of the right subclavian vein. Arch Surg 1971;102:178.

74. Bazaral M, Harlan S. Ultrasonographic anatomy of the internal jugular vein relevant to percutaneous cannulation. Crit Care Med 1981;9:30.

75. Borja AR. Current status of infraclavicular subclavian vein catheterization. Ann Thorac Surg 1972;13:615.

76. Moosman DA. The anatomy of the infraclavicular subclavian vein catheterization and its complications. Surg Gynecol Obstet 1973;136:17.

77. Aubaniac R. L'injection intraveineuse sous-claviculiare. Avantages et techniques. Press Med 1952;60:1456.

78. Mogil R, Delaurentis D, Rosemond G. Infraclavicular venipuncture. Arch Surg 1967;95:320.

79. Groff DB, Ahmed N. Subclavian vein catheterization in the infant. J Pediatr Surg 1974;9:171.

80. Venkataraman ST, Ott RA, Thompson AE. Percutaneous infraclavicular subclavian vein catheterization in critically ill infants and children. J Pediatr 1988;113:480.

81. Irwin G, Fifield G, Clinton J. Emergency catheterization of the superior vena cava in pediatric patients. Am J Emerg Med 1984;2:494.

82. Dronen S, Thompson B, Nowak R, et al. Subclavian vein catheterization during cardiopulmonary resuscitation. A prospective comparison of the supraclavicular and infraclavicular approaches. JAMA 1982;247:3227.

83. Westreich M. Preventing complications of subclavian vein catheterization. J Am Coll Emerg Phys 1978;17:368.

84. Herbst C. Indications, management and complications of percutaneous subclavian catheters. Arch Surg 1978;113:1421.

85. Yoffa D. Supraclavicular subclavian venipuncture and catheterization. Lancet 1965;2:614.

86. Brahos GJ, Cohen MJ. Supraclavicular central venous catheterization: Technique and experience in 250 cases. Wis Med J 1981;80:36.

87. Sterner S, Plummer DW, Clinton J, et al. A comparison of the supraclavicular approach and the infraclavicular approach for subclavian vein catheterization. Ann Emerg Med 1986;15:421.

88. DeFalque RJ. Percutaneous catheterization of the internal jugular vein. Anesth Analg 1974;53:116.

89. Lumley J, Russell WJ. Insertion of central venous catheters through arm veins. Anaesth Intensive Care 1975;3:101.

90. Webre DR, Arens JF. Use of the cephalic and basilic veins for introduction of central venous catheters. Anesthesiology 1973;38:389.

91. Bridges BB, Carden E, Takacs FA. Introduction of central venous pressure catheters through arm veins with a high success rate. Can Anaesth Soc J 1979;26:128.

92. Matz R. Complications of determining the central venous pressure. N Engl J Med 1965;273:703.

93. Smith-Wright DL, Green TP, Lock JE, et al. Complications of vascular catheterization in critically ill children. Crit Care Med 1984;12:1015.

94. Scott WL. Complications associated with central venous catheters. Chest 1988;91:1221.

95. Feliciano D, Mattox K, Graham J, et al. Major complications of percutaneous subclavian vein catheters. Am J Surg 1979;138:869.

96. FDA CV Catheter Task Force. Precautions necessary with central venous catheters. FDA Drug Bulletin 1989; July:15.

97. Peters JL, Armstrong R. Air embolism occurring as a complication of central venous catheterization. Ann Surg 1978;197:375.

98. Vallee P, Sullivan M, Richardson H, et al. Sequential treatment of simple pneumothorax. Ann Emerg Med 1988;9:936.

99. Daniels SR, Hannon DW, Meyer RA, et al. Paroxysmal supraventricular tachycardia: A complication of jugular central venous catheters in neonates. Am J Dis Child 1984;138:474.

100. Eichelberger MR, MacDonald MG, Ward J. General principles of central venous catheterization. In Fletcher MA, MacDonald MB, Avery GB (eds). Atlas of Procedures in Neonatology. Philadelphia, JB Lippincott, 1983, pp 173–178.

101. Corso JA, Agostinella R, Brandiss MW. Maintenance of venous polyethylene catheters to reduce risk of infection. JAMA 1969;210:2075.

102. Stillman RM, Soliman F, Garcia L, et al. Etiology of catheter association sepsis. Arch Surg 1977;112:1497.

103. Maki DG, Weise EC, Saraffin HW. A semiquantitative culture method for identifying intravenous catheter related infection. N Engl J Med 1977;296:1305.

104. MacDonald MG. Aseptic preparation. In Fletcher KA, MacDonald MG, Avery GB (eds). Atlas of Procedures in Neonatology. Philadelphia, JB Lippincott, 1983, pp 11–17.

105. Wing EJ, Norden CW, Shadduck RK, et al. Use of quantitative bacteriologic techniques to diagnose catheter-related sepsis. Arch Intern Med 1979;139:482.

106. Raucher HS, Hyatt AC, Barzilai A, et al. Quantitative blood cultures in the evaluation of septicemia in children with Broviac catheters. J Pediatr 1984;104:29.

107. Flynn P, Shenep J, Stokes D, et al. In situ management of confirmed central venous catheter-related bacteremia. Pediatr Infect Dis 1987;729.

108. Wang EEL, Prober CG, Ford-Jones L, et al. The management of central venous catheter infections. Pediatr Infect Dis 1984;3:110.

109. Hiemanz J, Skelto J, Pizzo PA. Perspective on the management of catheter related infections in cancer patients. Pediatr Infect Dis 1986;5:6.

110. Nahata M, King D, Powell D, et al. Management of catheter-related infections in pediatric patients. J Parenter Enter Nutr 1988;12:58.

111. Fleer A, Verhoef J, Hernandez AP. Coagulase-negative staphylococci as nosocomial pathogens in neonates: The role of host defense, artificial devices, and bacterial hydrophobicity. Am J Med 1986;80:161.

112. Ross P, Ehrenkranz R, Kleinman C, et al. Thrombus associated with central venous catheters in infants and children. J Pediatr Surg 1989;24(3):253.

113. Lawson M, Bottino JC, Hurtubise MR, et al. Use of urokinase to restore the patency of occluded central venous catheters. Am J IV Ther Clin Nutr 1982;10:29.

114. Winthrop AI, Wesson DE. Urokinase in the treatment of occluded central venous catheters in children. J Pediatr Surg 1984;19:536.

115. Olsen MM, Blumer JL, Gauderer MWL, et al. Streptokinase dissolution of a right atrial thrombus. J Pediatr Surg 1985;20:19.

116. Mendoza GJB, Soto A, Brown EG, et al. Intracardiac thrombi complicating central total parenteral nutrition: Resolution without surgery or thrombolysis. J Pediatr 1986;108:610.

117. Knopp R. Venous cutdowns in the emergency department. J Am Coll Emerg Phys 1978;7:439.

118. Iserson KV, Criss EA. Pediatric venous cutdowns: Utility in emergency situations. Pediatr Emerg Care 1986;2:231.

119. Roberts JR, Hedges JR. Clinical Procedures in Emergency Medicine. Philadelphia, WB Saunders, 1985, p 301.

120. Shockley LW, Butzier DJ. A modified wire-guided technique for venous cutdown access. Ann Emerg Med 1990;19:393.

121. Hansbrough JF, Cain TL, Millikan JS. Placement of 10 gauge catheter by cutdown for rapid fluid replacement. J Trauma 1983;23:231.

122. Shiu MH. A method for conservation of veins in the surgical cutdown. Surg Gynecol Obstet 1972;134:315.

123. Hollinshead W. Textbook of Anatomy. 34th ed. New York, Harper & Row, 1974, p 363.

124. Randolph J. Technique for insertion of plastic catheter into saphenous vein. Pediatrics 1959;24:631.

125. Dronen SC, Yee AS, Tomlanovich MC. Proximal saphenous vein cutdown. Ann Emerg Med 1981;10:328.

126. Preston G, Rosenberg N. Emergency venous access and cannulation. Ann Emerg Med 1982;11:642.

127. Simon RR, Brenner BE (eds). Emergency Procedures and Techniques. 2nd ed. Baltimore, Williams & Wilkins, 1987, p 380.

128. Moran JM, Atwood RP, Rowe MI. A clinical and bacteriologic study of infections associated with venous cutdowns. N Engl J Med 1965;272:554.

129. Bogen JE. Local complications in 167 patients with indwelling venous catheters. Surg Gynecol Obstet 1960;110:112.

130. Tocantins LM. Rapid absorption of substances injected into the bone marrow. Proc Soc Exp Biol Med 1940;45:292.

131. Tocantins LM, O'Neil JF. Infusion of blood and other fluid into the circulation via the bone marrow. Proc Soc Exp Biol Med 1940;45:782.

132. Tocantins LM, O'Neil JF. Infusion of blood and other fluid into the circulation via the bone marrow. Surg Gynecol Obstet 1941;73:281.

133. Tocantins LM, O'Neil JF, Price AH. Infusions of blood and other fluids via the bone marrow in traumatic shock and other forms of peripheral circulatory failure. Ann Surg 1941;114:1085.

134. Tocantins LM, O'Neil JF, Jones HW. Infusions of blood and other fluids via the bone marrow. Application in pediatrics. JAMA 1941;117:1229.

135. Tocantins LM, Price AH, O'Neil JF. Infusions via the bone marrow in children. Pa Med J 1943;46:1267.

136. Tocantins LM, O'Neil JF. Complications of intraosseous therapy. Ann Surg 1945;122:266.

137. Turkel H. Intraosseous infusion. Letter. JAMA 1953;151:1108.

138. Glaeser PW, Losek JD. Emergency intraosseous infusions in children. Am J Emerg Med 1986;4:34.

139. McNamara RM, Spivey W, Sussman C. Pediatric resuscitation without an intravenous line. Am J Emerg Med 1986;4:31.

140. Parrish GA, Turkewitz D, Skiendzielewski JJ. Intraosseous infusions in the emergency department. Am J Emerg Med 1986;4:59.

141. McNamara RM, Spivey WH, Unger HD, et al. Emergency applications of intraosseous infusion. J Emerg Med 1987;5:97.

142. Spivey WH. Intraosseous infusions. J Pediatr 1987;111:639.

143. Wagner MB, McCabe JB. A comparison of four techniques to establish intraosseous infusion. Pediatr Emerg Care 1988;4:87.

144. Fisher D. Intraosseous infusion. N Engl J Med 1990;322:1579.

145. Shoor PM, Berryhill RE, Benumof JK. Intraosseous infusion: Pressure-flow relationship and pharmacokinetics. J Trauma 1979;19:772.

146. Berg RA. Emergency infusion of catecholamines into bone marrow. Am J Dis Child 1984;138:810.

147. Thompson BM, Rossetti V, Miller J, et al. Intraosseous administration of sodium bicarbonate: An effective means of pH normalization in the canine model. Abstract. Ann Emerg Med 1984;13:405.

148. Spivey WH, Lathers CM, Malone DR, et al. Comparison of intraosseous central and peripheral routes of sodium bicarbonate administration during CPR in pigs. Ann Emerg Med 1985;14:1135.

149. Spivey WH, Unger HD, McNamara RM, et al. The effect of intraosseous sodium bicarbonate on bone in swine. Ann Emerg Med 1987;16:773.

150. Walsh-Kelly CM, Bereus RJ, Glaeser PW, et al. Intraosseous infusion of phenytoin. Am J Emerg Med 1986;4:523.

151. Prete MR, Hannan CJ, Burkle FM. Plasma atropine concentration via intraosseous, endotracheal, and intravenous administration. Am J Emerg Med 1987;5:101.

152. Orlowski JP, Porembka DT, Gallagher JM, Van Lente F. Comparison study of intraosseous, central-intravenous, and peripheral intraosseous infusions of emergency drugs. Am J Dis Child 1990;144:112.

153. Wallden L. On injuries of bone and bone-marrow after intraosseous injections: A experimental investigation. Acta Chir Scand 1947;96:152.

154. Brickman KR, Rega P, Koltz M, et al. Analysis of growth plate abnormalities following intraosseous infusion through the proximal tibial epiphysis in pigs. Ann Emerg Med 1988;17:121.

155. Wile UJ, Schamberg IL. Pulmonary fat embolism following infusions via the bone marrow. J Invest Dermatol 1942;5:173.

156. Bisgard JD, Baker C. Experimental fat embolism. Am J Surg 1970;47:466.

157. Orlowski JP, Julius CJ, Petras RE, et al. Safety of intraosseous infusions: Risks of fat and bone marrow emboli to the lungs. Crit Care Med 1988;16:388.

158. Doan CA. The circulation of the bone marrow. Contrib Embryol 1922;1427.

159. Root WS. The flow of blood through bones and joints. In Hamilton WF (ed). Handbook of Physiology. Vol 2. Baltimore, Williams & Wilkins, 1966, p 1651.

160. Brickman K, Rega P, Guinness M. A comparative study of intraosseous, intravenous and intraarterial pH changes during hypoventilation in dogs. Abstract. Ann Emerg Med 1987;16:510.

161. Orlowski JP, Porembka DT, Gallagher JM, et al. The bone marrow as a source of laboratory studies. Ann Emerg Med 1989;18:1348.

162. Fainstein V, Hopfer RL, Trier P, et al. Bone marrow cultures: Their value in diagnosing fungal and mycobacterial infection in patients with cancer. J Infect Dis 1981;144:79.

163. Glaeser PW, Losetc JD. Intraosseous needles: New and improved. Pediatr Emerg Care 1988;4:135.

164. Melker R, Miller G, Geaven P, et al. Complications of intraosseous infusions. Letter to the editor. Ann Emerg Med 1990;19:731.

165. Turkel H. Deaths following sternal puncture. JAMA 1954;156:992.

166. Brickman K, Rega P, Chou M. Comparison of serum phenobarbital levels after single verse multiple attempts at intraosseous infusion. Ann Emerg Med 1990;19:31.

167. Rimar S, Westry J, Rodriquez R. Compartment syndrome in an infant following emergency intraosseous infusion. Clin Pediatr 1988;27:259.

168. LaFleche F, Milzman D. Iatrogenic bilateral tibial fractures after interosseous infusion attempts in a 3 month infant. Ann Emerg Med 1989;18:1099.

169. Bucci G, Scalamandre A, Savignon P, et al. Crib-side sampling of blood from the radial artery. Pediatrics 1966;37:497.

170. Saladino R, Bachman D, Fleisher G. Arterial access in the pediatric emergency department. Ann Emerg Med 1990;19:382.

171. Samaan HA. The hazards of radial artery pressure monitoring. J Cardiovasc Surg 1971;12:342.

172. Johnson FE, Sumner DS, Strandness DE. Extremity necrosis caused by indwelling arterial catheters. Am J Surg 1976;131:375.

173. Randel SN, Tsang BH, Wung J. Experience with percutaneous indwelling peripheral arterial catheterization in neonates. Am J Dis Child 1987;141:848.

174. Miyasaka K, Edmonds JF, Conn AW. Complications of radial artery lines in the paediatric patient. Can Anaesth Soc J 1976;23:9.

175. Cohen A, Reyes R, Kirk M, et al. Osler's nodes, pseudoaneurysm formation, and sepsis complicating percutaneous radial artery cannulation. Crit Care Med 1984;12:1078.

176. Galvis AG, Donahoo JS, White JJ. An improved technique for prolonged arterial catheterization in infants and children. Crit Care Med 1976;4:166.

177. Chameides L (ed). Textbook of Pediatric Advanced Life Support. Dallas, TX, American Heart Association, 1988, p 45.

178. Cole FS, Todres ID, Shannon DC. Technique for percutaneous cannulation of the radial artery in the newborn infant. J Pediatr 1978;92:105.

179. Pearse RG. Percutaneous catheterization of the radial artery in newborn babies using transillumination. Arch Dis Child 1978;53:549.

180. Pfenninger J, Bernasconi G, Sutter M. Radial artery catheterization by surgical exposure in infants. Intensive Care Med 1982;8:139.

181. Torphy DE, Minter MG, Thompson BM. Cardiorespiratory arrest and resuscitation in children. Am J Dis Child 1984;138:1099.

182. Rosenberg NM. Pediatric cardiopulmonary arrest in the emergency department. Am J Emerg Med 1984;2:497.

183. Eisenberg M, Bergner L, Hallstrom A. Epidemiology of cardiac arrest and resuscitation in children. Ann Emerg Med 1983;12:672.

184. Stroup C. Intraosseous infusion: Pre-hospital use in the critically ill pediatric patient. J Emerg Med Serv 1987;5:38.

185. Seigler R, Tecklenberg F, Shealey R. Prehospital intraosseous infusion by emergency medical service personnel. A prospective study. Pediatrics 1989;84:173.

186. Zimmerman J, Coyne M, Logsdon M. Implementation of intraosseous infusion technique by aeromedical transport programs. J Trauma 1989;29:1.

187. Walter G, Clark M. A practical method of teaching emergency intraosseous infusion. Am J Emerg Med 1990;8:272.

188. Fish RM, Ehrhardt ME. Preventing Emergency Malpractice. Medical Economics Books, Oradell, NJ, 1989, p 24.

CHAPTER 9

Shock and Fluid Resuscitation

Susan A. Stern
Steven C. Dronen

INTRODUCTION

Shock is a clinical syndrome that has been recognized for more than 200 years. In spite of this long history, a clear definition and understanding of this complex pathophysiologic state has only recently emerged. Early descriptions and definitions emphasized macroscopic parameters such as blood pressure and the general appearance of the patient. The term *shock* was used initially by Henri Francois Le Dran in 1743 to describe the progressive collapse of vital organ functions after injury or surgery. As early as 1917, clinicians recognized that although hypotension was one of the most constant findings in shock, it was not the cause.[1] In 1930, Blalock demonstrated that traumatic shock was due to hypovolemia.[2] Later, he redefined shock as "a peripheral circulatory failure, resulting from a discrepancy in the size of the vascular bed and the volume of the intravascular fluid." Over the next two decades, the development and refinement of techniques to measure cardiac output in seriously ill and injured patients provided a better understanding of the hemodynamic changes that occur during shock. More recently the focus of shock research has shifted from these gross hemodynamic parameters to the cellular and subcellular changes that occur. Based on the most recent research, shock may be more accurately defined as a clinical syndrome characterized by inadequate tissue perfusion resulting in widespread cellular dysfunction.[1-4]

EPIDEMIOLOGY

Shock is not a primary pathophysiologic entity. Hence it always occurs as the result of some other illness or injury. Trauma and infection are the most common causes of morbidity and mortality in the pediatric population. Correspondingly, the most common forms of shock in pediatric patients are hypovolemic (hemorrhagic) and distributive (septic). Cardiogenic and obstructive shock are seen less often in the pediatric population than in adults. Children rarely suffer from the conditions that predispose to the development of these types of shock (e.g., myocardial infarction, pulmonary embolism, systemic hypertension, and arrhythmia).

Acute hypovolemia is the most common cause of shock in the pediatric age group. The two principal causes of hypovolemic shock in children are (1) fluid and electrolyte depletion as a result of diarrhea and vomiting and (2) blood loss consequent to trauma. Infectious gastroenteritis with subsequent hypovolemic shock is a leading cause of worldwide infant mortality. Five to eight million children die annually throughout the world as a result of hypovolemic shock from infectious gastroenteritis. Although acute gastroenteritis and subsequent hypovolemia are common in the United States, they are generally successfully treated with volume infusion. In the United States, the most common cause of morbidity and mortality in the pediatric age group is trauma. Accidents account for close to 50% of all deaths in children from ages 1 to 14 years, and hemorrhagic shock is most often the cause.[5-9]

Hypovolemic shock can also occur as a result of massive fluid extravasation, such as occurs with large burns and peritonitis. Other less common causes of hypovolemic shock in children include excessive renal fluid losses resulting from diabetes insipidus or tubular damage, metabolic abnormalities such as diabetic ketoacidosis, adrenogenital syndrome, and other salt-depleting disorders.[7] Unique causes of hemorrhagic shock in the newborn include occult hemorrhage secondary to coagulation deficiencies and birth trauma, transplacental hemorrhage from fetus to mother, and twin-to-twin transfusion syndrome.[10-12]

Septic shock is the most common form of distributive shock in children. The overall incidence of septic shock has been steadily increasing during the past 50 years. In the United States, there is currently an estimated incidence of 200,000 cases of septic shock per year and 100,000 deaths annually from this disorder. Septic shock is the most common cause of death in intensive care units in the United States. Ironically, this upsurge is a reflection of recent medical progress in the treatment of life-threatening injuries and illnesses, which has resulted in a growing number of immunocompromised patients at risk for developing sepsis and subsequent shock.[13-16] In spite of these recent medical advances, the mortality from septic shock remains high in both children and adults. Pediatric studies have demonstrated case fatality rates for septic shock ranging from 45% to 98%.[17]

In the neonate, septic shock is the most common of all shock states. This is a reflection of the fact that the neonate is a relatively immunocompromised host. Neonatal sepsis occurs in approximately 1 in 1000 full-term live births and 1 in 250 premature births. The risk is increased by a number of factors, including prematurity, prolonged rupture of membranes, and maternal chorioamnionitis.[18, 19] The mortality rate associated with neonatal sepsis varies from 15% to greater than 50%, with increasing mortality when septic shock develops.[20–22]

Septic shock occurs most commonly in immunocompromised children and is often a hospital-acquired entity. It does occur in previously healthy unhospitalized children, but much less often. Host factors predisposing to sepsis and septic shock include the presence of indwelling arterial, venous, or urinary catheters; invasive medical and surgical procedures; malnutrition; immunosuppressive chemotherapy; and malignancies.

Cardiogenic shock is relatively uncommon in children. It occurs most frequently in children with known congenital heart disease, often following surgical repair of the cardiac defect. Other causes of cardiogenic shock in the pediatric age group include impaired cardiac function from dysrhythmias; drug intoxication; late sepsis; inflammatory processes (myocarditis); ischemic infarction (Kawasaki's disease); infiltrative cardiomyopathies; and metabolic derangements, including acidosis, hyperthermia, and hypoglycemia. Cardiogenic shock may also develop in previously healthy children following asphyxial episodes such as near-drowning and near–sudden infant death syndrome.[7, 8, 23, 24]

Obstructive shock is also uncommon in the pediatric age group. The most probable causes of obstructive shock in children include pericardial tamponade and tension pneumothorax secondary to trauma. Massive pulmonary embolism, atrial thrombus or myxoma, and dissecting thoracic aortic aneurysm are other possible origins, although these are extremely rare in the pediatric population (Table 9–1).

TABLE 9–1

DIFFERENTIAL DIAGNOSIS OF SHOCK

Classification	Common Causes
Hypovolemic	Hemorrhage
	Gastrointestinal losses
	Renal losses
	Plasma losses
	Burns
	Peritonitis
	Sepsis
	Adrenal insufficiency
Distributive	Sepsis
	CNS/spinal cord injury
	Drug intoxication
	Anaphylaxis
Cardiogenic	Arrhythmias
	Drug intoxication
	Congenital defect
	Hypoxic or ischemic injury
	Metabolic derangements
	Cardiomyopathy
	Kawasaki's disease
Obstructive	Cardiac tamponade
	Tension pneumothorax
	Pulmonary embolus

PATHOPHYSIOLOGY

In simplest terms, shock represents a breakdown in the physiologic processes governing cellular perfusion. Under normal circumstances the cardiovascular system delivers metabolic substrate to the cell and removes waste products under finely balanced neuroendocrine control. Cardiac contractility, circulating blood volume, and vasomotor tone, along with many other variables, are continually regulated to ensure the adequacy of cellular perfusion. When one or more of these variables is altered significantly, others compensate. When compensation is inadequate, shock ensues.

Shock is commonly described as occurring in three stages according to the degree of physiologic responsiveness. These three stages are compensated, uncompensated, and irreversible shock. Although it is convenient to discuss shock as though it occurs in stepwise fashion, it is more likely an uninterrupted process of progressive deterioration in cellular perfusion culminating in death.

In compensated shock, the body's intrinsic compensatory mechanisms are able to maintain cardiac output, systemic arterial blood pressure, and vital organ perfusion at normal or near-normal levels. In uncompensated shock, the compensatory responses are no longer able to maintain adequate tissue perfusion, and cardiovascular dysfunction and impaired cellular respiration result. Irreversible shock occurs when there has been such widespread cellular damage that the organism dies in spite of the institution of appropriate therapy.

Regardless of the origin of shock, the final common pathway is tissue ischemia and injury resulting from widespread cellular dysfunction. The primary pathophysiologic events and compensatory responses may vary somewhat, however, depending on the cause. The discussion that follows applies primarily to hypovolemic shock. Those features unique to distributive, cardiogenic, and obstructive shock will be discussed separately.

Hypovolemic Shock

The primary pathophysiologic event in hypovolemic shock is a reduction in circulating blood volume. This may occur secondary to acute hemorrhage or as the result of extracellular fluid losses occurring with dehydration. The reduction in circulating blood volume causes a fall in preload and a diminished stroke volume and cardiac output. Preservation of a normal blood pressure under these circumstances is dependent on enhancement of the pumping function of the myocardium and resistance of the systemic vasculature. These functions are dependent on an increase in endogenous catecholamines. The initial fall in blood pressure inhibits the afferent discharge of baroreceptors in the aortic arch and carotid sinus, and the decrease in blood volume inhibits the discharge of stretch receptors of the right atrium. This decrease in baroreceptor discharge results in stimulation of the sympathetic nervous system by the midbrain. At the same time, the initial reduction in tissue perfusion associated with a decrease in effective blood volume stimulates the afferent discharge of chemoreceptors in the aortic arch and carotid bodies, which further activates the sympathetic nervous system. This increase in sympathetic tone results in release of epinephrine and norepinephrine from the heart, blood vessels, and adrenal medulla. The child's cardiovascular system is particularly sensitive to catecholamine release and responds with a profound increase in venomotor tone. Heart rate and myocardial contractility are subsequently increased and yield an increase in cardiac output.[25, 26]

The regulation of cardiac output in the infant differs from that in the older child. Although the determinants of stroke volume and cardiac output are the same, their relative contributions differ. The myocardium of the young infant has relatively less contractile tissue per unit mass and exhibits a disorganized pattern of muscle fiber arrangement. This results in a myocardium that is less responsive to inotropic autonomic stimulation than that of older children and adults. Also, children can tolerate much greater heart rates than adults because of excellent coronary vasculature and relatively smaller stroke volumes. These physiologic differences result in a greater dependence on preload to increase stroke volume and on heart rate to increase cardiac output in the younger child.[7, 27]

The increase in sympathetic outflow also results in an increase in venous tone, as well as constriction of the arteriolar resistance vessels. Because 60% or more of the total circulating blood volume may reside in the venous capacitance system, an autotransfusion-like effect is created. Venous return to the heart is augmented, resulting in an increase in the end-diastolic volume and, consequently, an increase in stroke volume and cardiac output. This autotransfusion-like response is rapid but can only compensate for a volume loss of approximately 15%.[28]

The arteriolar constriction caused by catecholamine release is organ selective. Blood flow is preferentially shunted to the heart and brain and away from the skin, muscles, and gastrointestinal tract. The blood flow to the liver is also reduced, but this reduction is less than that to the peripheral tissues. Renal blood flow is preserved with small to moderate volume loss; however, with larger volume loss, renal vessels also constrict. This increase in arteriolar constriction results in an increase in the total peripheral resistance and in diastolic pressure.[25, 28–30]

This initial vasoconstrictive response results in extracellular fluid mobilization. The direction of fluid movement between the intravascular space and the interstitium is dependent on Starling's forces, which include the capillary and interstitial hydrostatic pressures and the capillary and interstitial oncotic pressures. The capillary hydrostatic and interstitial oncotic pressures tend to drive fluid into the interstitium, whereas the capillary oncotic and interstitial hydrostatic pressures tend to keep fluid in the vascular compartment. Normally these forces are balanced so that there is little or no net movement of fluid between the vascular compartment and the interstitium. During the early or compensated phase of shock, however, there is a decrease in capillary hydrostatic pressure secondary to both a decrease in effective circulating volume and precapillary arteriolar vasoconstriction. As a result, there is a net movement of protein-free fluid from the interstitium to the vascular space. This phenomenon of transcapillary refill results in an increase in intravascular volume and a decrease in the interstitial fluid compartment. Extracellular fluid mobilization occurs over a 6- to 12-hour period and therefore does not account for large volume changes in the earliest phase of shock.[25, 28, 31–33]

In addition to the immediate and effective increase in sympathetic tone, there are also delayed but important endocrine responses to the shock state. These hormonal responses are mediated through the sympathoadrenal and pituitary endocrine systems.

The renin-angiotensin system is a complex endocrine unit that is activated by a decrease in the effective blood volume and consequent diminished renal blood flow. Renin, a product of the renal juxtaglomerular cells, causes an increase in the production of angiotensin I, which is subsequently converted to angiotensin II. Angiotensin II is a potent vasoconstrictor and a major stimulus for aldosterone release from the adrenal cortex. Angiotensin II also potentiates the action of corticotropin (adrenocorticotropic hormone, or ACTH)

on the adrenal cortex and epinephrine release from the adrenal medulla.[25, 28, 34]

Aldosterone concentration is increased during stress and shock. Aldosterone is released from the adrenal cortex, specifically by the cells of the adrenal zona glomerulosa. The synthesis and release of aldosterone during shock are stimulated primarily by angiotensin II and corticotropin and, to a lesser extent, by an increase in the serum potassium concentration. Aldosterone is the most potent mineralocorticoid released from the adrenal cortex. It causes an increase in sodium and water retention and potassium excretion by the kidneys and therefore acts to increase the intravascular volume.[25, 28, 35, 36]

Corticotropin is released by chromophobe cells of the anterior pituitary, and elevated levels are found with any sort of stress, including shock; it then acts on cells of the adrenal zona fasciculata to stimulate cortisol production (in addition to stimulating aldosterone secretion). Cortisol in turn has a variety of metabolic effects, including increasing glucose production and potentiating the actions of epinephrine and glucagon.[25, 28, 35, 36]

Antidiuretic hormone (ADH), or vasopressin, is also elevated during the shock state; it is released from the posterior pituitary in response to the decrease in effective circulating blood volume. The main action of ADH is to increase the reabsorption of solute-free water in the distal tubules and collecting ducts of the kidneys. Vasopressin also stimulates peripheral vasoconstriction and hepatic glycogenolysis and gluconeogenesis.[25, 28, 35, 36]

The plasma concentration of glucagon rises in response to any type of shock. Glucagon is secreted by the alpha cells of the pancreas. The primary mechanism for the increase in glucagon in shock is sympathetic stimulation of the alpha cells of the pancreas. Glucagon, like the catecholamines, causes an increase in liver gluconeogenesis, glycogenolysis, and lipolysis. The net effect is an increase in hepatic glucose production and ketogenesis.[25, 28, 35, 36]

Insulin is an anabolic hormone synthesized by the beta cells of the pancreas. During the acute stages of shock, when hepatic gluconeogenesis and glycogenolysis are maximally stimulated, the secretion and concentration of insulin are generally low. In the recovery phase, however, insulin levels rise and are important in rebuilding and repairing injured tissues.[25, 35, 36]

These complex neuroendocrine reflexes allow the child to tolerate relatively large volume losses before exhibiting overt signs of shock. At approximately 25% to 30% of blood volume loss, however, these compensatory mechanisms begin to fail. The intense local vasoconstriction that initially acted to maintain vital organ perfusion begins to cause local ischemia. As tissue perfusion fails and ischemia worsens, cellular respiration is compromised, and cells shift from aerobic to anaerobic metabolism. With anaerobic metabolism predominating, there is a significant decrease in cellular adenosine triphosphate (ATP) levels, and energy-dependent cell functions deteriorate. One of the most important energy-dependent functions to be affected is the sodium-potassium pump. This pump is responsible for maintaining low intracellular sodium and high-intracellular potassium concentrations. The pump extrudes three sodium ions from the cell for every two potassium ions it takes into the cell. Cellular ATP provides the energy needed for this ion transport. As shock progresses and ATP levels fall, this pump fails, and sodium leaks into and potassium leaks out of cells. Water enters the cell passively with sodium, further aggravating the extracellular fluid deficit of the shock state. The result is cellular swelling and ultrastructural changes in cellular organelles such as mitochondria and lysosomes.[23, 25, 28, 37, 38]

Calcium homeostasis is dependent on an ATP-driven

membrane pump. The intracellular concentration of calcium is normally 0.1 μmol/L, as opposed to an extracellular concentration of 1 mmol/L. This large concentration gradient enables calcium to function effectively as a second messenger for stimulus-response coupling in many biologic processes. As with the sodium-potassium pump, tissue ischemia and the resultant decline in cellular ATP levels impair the function of the calcium adenosine triphosphatase (ATPase) pump. Intracellular and intramitochondrial calcium concentrations increase while extracellular concentration decreases. The increased intracellular calcium concentration causes disturbances in cellular physiology and morphology, including separation of cell junctions, alterations in the cytoskeleton leading to changes in cell shape and in organelle orientation, and uncoupling of oxidative phosphorylation in the mitochondria, further depleting the cell's energy stores. The elevation of intracellular calcium concentration also leads to activation of membrane phospholipases that produce additional cell and organelle membrane damage; lysosomal damage and mitochondrial membrane damage result in the release of acid hydrolases and additional decreases in energy production, respectively. The plasma hypocalcemia that results impairs the function of contractile tissue, including that of cardiac and smooth muscle.[23, 25, 28, 39–43]

As shock progresses and cellular respiration is further compromised, acid-base disturbances develop. The most frequently encountered acid-base abnormality after mild to moderate trauma with compensated shock is a respiratory alkalosis. Hypoxic and hypotensive stimulation of the aortic and carotid chemoreceptors, metabolic acidosis, and pain produce respiratory center stimulation leading to hyperventilation. As shock progresses, however, and anaerobic metabolism predominates, there is a large increase in lactic acid production, and a metabolic acidosis develops. Initially this metabolic acidosis is partially compensated by the respiratory alkalosis. A mild acidosis may actually have a beneficial effect on peripheral perfusion in that it shifts the oxyhemoglobin dissociation curve to the right and therefore enhances oxygen delivery to the tissues. With continued tissue ischemia, however, lactate levels rise, and acidosis worsens. Excess lactate concentrations have been shown to have a strongly positive correlation with mortality in shock. Serial lactate levels are an even better prognostic indicator of survival after shock and can provide an early objective evaluation of the patient's response to therapy. The adverse effects of acidosis include a decrease in myocardial contractility, a decrease in sensitivity to catecholamines, an increase in catecholamine release, and a predisposition to cardiac arrhythmias.[25, 43–46]

As shock progresses, ischemia worsens and cellular damage becomes more widespread. The inadequate tissue perfusion characteristic of the shock state leads to failure of cellular respiration; this results in decreased energy production and ultimately in the failure of energy-dependent cellular functions. The normal ion concentration gradients are disrupted, which leads to further abnormalities in cellular morphology and physiology, including extensive membrane disruption and activation of membrane phospholipases. The activated membrane phospholipases release fatty acids and promote prostaglandin formation, which stimulates tissue inflammation and additional injury. Damaged lysosomes release large quantities of acid hydrolases into the cell cytoplasm, which causes further cell injury, and injured cells themselves release large quantities of waste products into the circulation. In addition to lysosomal enzymes, lactate, and other waste products, ischemic cells release potent secondary vasoactive mediators, including arachadonic acid metabolites, kinins, histamine, serotonin, and vasoactive peptides. These mediators, which likely evolved as an adaptive response to injury, perpetuate the shock state through a variety of mechanisms. They alter vascular tone, induce platelet aggregation and thrombus formation, increase capillary permeability, decrease myocardial contractility, and lead to redistribution of blood away from the vital organs.[23, 25, 28]

Distributive Shock

Distributive shock occurs when vascular resistance abnormalities result in a maldistribution of blood flow. The intravascular volume is normal, but the capacity of the vascular system is greatly expanded. This maldistribution of flow results in inadequate tissue perfusion in the presence of normal or even high cardiac output. The most common causes of distributive shock in children include sepsis, central nervous system injury, anaphylaxis, and drug ingestions (tranquilizers, barbiturates, antihypertensive medications, and smooth muscle relaxants).[47]

Septic shock is most commonly associated with bacterial infections, although the syndrome may also develop from fungal, viral, protozoal, or other infections. In adults, septic shock is most commonly observed with gram-negative sepsis. Although gram-negative sepsis and septic shock are also seen in the pediatric population, infants and children are susceptible to and more often affected by organisms that rarely cause sepsis in the adult population, specifically *Haemophilus influenzae, Neisseria meningitidis*, and gram-positive organisms such as *Staphylococcus aureus*, group B streptococcus, and pneumococcus. The incidence of infection with these organisms varies with age. In a review of bacterial sepsis in children, *H. influenzae* type b was the most commonly isolated pathogen and was responsible for 22% of sepsis episodes; 13% of these patients developed septic shock. Gram-negative bacilli accounted for 16% of sepsis and occurred primarily in immunocompromised patients.[13, 14, 23, 48, 49]

Septic shock develops when a host organism undergoes an unregulated immunologic response to invading microorganisms or the microbial toxins they produce. This results in the host's production of a large array of vascular mediators and activation of certain protein systems that themselves cause cell damage. Some of these mediators and protein systems include arachidonic acid metabolites; bradykinin; histamine; interleukin-1; and the complement, coagulation, and fibrinolytic pathways. In septic shock, these mediators appear to play a primary role in the pathogenesis of the shock state. The overall effect is unregulated vasodilation and microscopic clotting that produces a mismatch of blood flow and oxygen requirements at the cellular level. Ultimately the organism experiences a decrease in systemic vascular resistance that is not fully compensated for by an increase in the cardiac output. Although septic shock is considered a classic form of distributive shock, during the course of the syndrome, one often also observes evidence of hypovolemia resulting from poor fluid intake or increased water losses secondary to fever, hyperventilation, vomiting, or diarrhea.[15, 16, 25, 50]

Cardiogenic Shock

Cardiogenic shock is characterized by a primary abnormality in cardiac function. Acute circulatory failure results from a marked decline in myocardial contractility. Unlike other forms of shock, intrinsic compensatory responses may be either nonexistent, such as an increase in stroke volume, or harmful, such as arteriolar constriction. The increase in arteriolar and venous resistance intended to normalize blood pressure causes an increase in afterload and therefore an increase in the left ventricular work load. The compensatory increase in heart rate increases the myocardial oxygen requirement and at the same time impairs myocardial oxygen supply. The "compensatory" increase in sodium and water retention results in an increase in the central blood volume, which subsequently elevates left ventricular pressure and volume and impairs subendocardial blood flow. Thus the body's intrinsic response to a decreased cardiac output further diminishes ventricular function. Because of this self-perpetuating cycle, compensated states of cardiogenic shock are rarely encountered.[7, 8, 23]

Obstructive Shock

Obstructive shock results when a normally functioning heart is unable to produce an adequate cardiac output in the presence of a normal intravascular volume because of mechanical obstruction. The mechanical obstruction may block flow through the heart, lungs, or aorta. These patients manifest the same compensatory mechanisms associated with hypovolemic shock but fail to improve with aggressive fluid resuscitation.

EMERGENCY MEDICAL SERVICE CONSIDERATIONS

In recent years the concept of field stabilization of trauma and shock victims has been popularized despite the fact that the primary pathophysiologic events generally cannot be controlled or corrected in the field. Universally accepted goals of prehospital treatment are control of obvious hemorrhage, maintenance of a patent airway, adequate ventilation, and rapid delivery to the site of definitive therapy. Some would argue that attempts should also be made in the field to restore the circulating blood volume and to improve blood pressure. Two somewhat controversial prehospital interventions that have been widely adopted in an attempt to achieve these goals are the application of the pneumatic antishock garment (PASG) and the infusion of intravenous fluid.

Originally developed by Crile in 1903 to prevent postural hypotension in neurosurgical patients, the PASG became widely used during the Vietnam War for the treatment of shock victims during air evacuation. After the war, the device was enthusiastically adopted by civilian ambulances and emergency departments because of its reported ability to raise blood pressure in shock victims. PASGs are widely used in the prehospital management of shock, and many municipalities mandate that they be carried on their ambulances.[51–57]

Previously, PASG was assumed to raise blood pressure through the translocation of blood from the lower extremities to the central circulation. More recent studies suggest that the observed increase in blood pressure is instead the result of an increase in peripheral resistance. Although considerable effort has been expended elucidating the PASG's mechanism of action, little data have been accumulated documenting their efficacy. There is to date no evidence to suggest that small and transient increases in blood pressure improve outcome in victims of shock. A large clinical trial has been conducted in an urban setting comparing outcomes in adult hemorrhagic shock victims with and without use of the PASG. Although the PASG-treated patients in this study did manifest an improvement in blood pressure, they failed to demonstrate any improvement in morbidity, mortality, or length of hospital stay.[55, 58–62]

Accepted uses for the PASG include hypovolemic, neurogenic, anaphylactic, and septic shock with hypotension,

pelvic fractures, multiple lower extremity fractures, lower extremity soft tissue bleeding, and abdominal or retroperitoneal bleeding. The PASG also functions as a pressure dressing for external bleeding sites of the lower extremities and help to tamponade internal hemorrhage. Acting as a pneumatic splint, it immobilizes fractures and prevents further bleeding secondary to excessive motion of the fractured bones. This is especially important with long-bone fractures and retroperitoneal bleeding from pelvic fractures. Several case reports demonstrate the value of the PASG in the stabilization of retroperitoneal hemorrhage secondary to pelvic fracture in pediatric patients.[28, 63, 64]

The only absolute contraindications to the use of the PASG are pulmonary edema and known or suspected ruptured diaphragm. Relative contraindications include pregnancy, penetrating abdominal and thoracic trauma, and evisceration of abdominal contents. In pregnancy, the PASG may be used as long as only the legs are inflated.[28, 63, 65]

The PASG should only be deflated when adequate fluid resuscitation has resulted in stabilization of vital signs. Deflation should be gradual, in a stepwise manner. The abdominal compartment is deflated first, and vital signs are rechecked. If the blood pressure decreases by more than 5 mm Hg, the deflation should be discontinued and further fluid replacement begun until the blood pressure is restored. Once the abdominal compartment is deflated, each leg is deflated separately in the same manner.[28, 63, 65]

Prehospital intravenous fluid therapy is also a controversial topic. Proponents of prehospital fluid therapy argue that skilled paramedics can place intravenous lines with minimal or no delay in transport and can infuse large volumes of saline prior to arrival in the emergency department. Opponents claim that delays in transport occur commonly and that fluid infusion cannot keep pace with the bleeding rate in severe hemorrhage. At the present time there is insufficient evidence for either position. The ability to rapidly start intravenous lines, however, is particularly suspect in the pediatric population. It is likely that prehospital fluid therapy does not affect outcome in the vast majority of cases, but it may be valuable given a specific combination of hemorrhage severity and distance from the hospital. Until conclusive data for a particular position can be obtained, it is reasonable to place intravenous lines while enroute to the hospital whenever possible. This avoids potentially lethal delays in the field and grants the patient the potential benefits of prehospital fluid therapy.

CLINICAL EVALUATION

History

Early recognition of the child in shock, along with prompt institution of appropriate therapy, is essential for a good outcome. The exquisite ability of a previously healthy child to compensate for the hypoperfusion state, however, often makes the diagnosis of early shock difficult. The history of the illness or injury that precipitated the shock state is important for both diagnosis and treatment. A recent history of trauma, vomiting, or diarrhea may be helpful in establishing the diagnosis of hypovolemic shock. A history of recent fever, chills, jaundice, or exposure to others with similar symptoms may assist in the diagnosis of septic shock. The possibility of a toxic ingestion or exposure should always be considered. The physician should elicit the parents' assessment of the child's recent oral intake and urinary output. An assessment of the child's level of activity is equally important; a newborn in early shock may present only with decreased oral intake and irritability. Details of the duration of illness and the rapidity of onset are essential. The patient's past medical history should be established, including any previous occurrence of a similar illness, the presence of an underlying immunosuppressive disorder, or congenital heart disease. In neonates, the perinatal history is essential; a history of premature rupture of membranes, maternal chorioamnionitis, or significant intrapartum blood loss may be suggestive of sepsis or hypovolemia. In the trauma victim, the precise mechanism of injury must be established. Certain mechanisms of injury are associated with specific injury patterns. Deceleration injuries, for example, may be associated with transection of the thoracic aorta. Pelvic and lower extremity fractures commonly occur in pedestrians struck by automobiles. The clinical course after the injury is also important. The child who becomes hypotensive shortly after trauma has likely sustained a drastic injury with a large amount of hemorrhage that will necessitate aggressive resuscitation and early surgical intervention. Because successful therapy of the shock state often requires immediate intervention, the clinician must elicit this history simultaneously with the physical examination and initiation of therapy.

Physical Examination

The physical signs seen during the early or compensated phase of shock are a manifestation of increased sympathetic tone. With a relatively small amount of volume loss (less than 15% of total blood volume), the only sign of shock may be a slight increase in heart rate. As volume loss and sympathetic outflow increase, other signs develop. These include pallor; cool, moist skin; anxiety; hyperventilation; and additional increases in heart rate. With a 15% to 25% volume loss, adrenergic stimulation is nearly maximal. Total peripheral resistance and diastolic blood pressure increase, resulting in a decrease in the pulse pressure, although mean arterial pressure remains normal. Mottling, pallor, and delayed capillary refill, all evidence of poor skin perfusion, are observed. Because the child's skin is thinner and lacks the more stratified epithelium characteristic of adult skin, the effects of increased vasomotor tone are more obvious in children. This accounts for the extreme mottling classically seen in early shock in children.

With 25% to 30% volume loss, the clinical picture becomes more dramatic and easily recognizable. Blood pressure is decreased even in the supine position, and the pulse pressure is markedly narrowed. The patient becomes agitated, which is evidence of poor central nervous systen perfusion. If the shock state persists or worsens, increasing hypotension develops along with confusion and lethargy (Table 9–2).

TABLE 9–2

CLINICAL MANIFESTATIONS OF HEMORRHAGIC SHOCK

Blood Loss (%)	Clinical Manifestations
<15	Increase in heart rate; no change in blood pressure
15–25	Pallor (or mottling of skin with increasing blood loss); diaphoresis; delayed capillary refill; further increases in heart rate; decrease in pulse pressure; increase in diastolic pressure; no change in mean arterial pressure; increasing anxiety; hyperventilation
25–30	Above manifestations, plus: pulse pressure markedly narrowed; mean arterial pressure decreased; increasing agitation and confusion
>30	Marked hypotension; acidosis; decreasing level of consciousness

The initial assessment of the child in shock should be rapid and systematic. The purpose is twofold: to evaluate end-organ perfusion and to detect any acutely life-threatening but treatable lesion. This initial evaluation for circulatory failure should be performed within the first moments of the child's arrival in the emergency department. The examination includes evaluation of respiratory rate and mechanics, heart rate, peripheral pulses, blood pressure, skin, and CNS perfusion.[25, 28, 66]

Normal heart rates and blood pressures in children vary widely according to age. Although a number of charts are available that summarize the normal ranges of heart rate and blood pressure for children of varying ages, there are some general rules for normal estimates that are easily memorized. The upper limits of normal for heart rates are as follows: less than 140/min for infants, less than 120/min for preschool children, and less than 100/min for school-age children. An estimate of the normal systolic blood pressure can be obtained by adding 80 to twice the child's age in years. The normal diastolic blood pressure is two thirds of the normal systolic pressure.[25, 28, 66]

Peripheral pulses should be evaluated for rate, volume, and symmetry. Pulse volume is related to pulse pressure. As shock progresses, the pulse pressure decreases and so does the pulse volume—hence the description of a weak and thready pulse in hypovolemic shock. A widened pulse pressure, and therefore a bounding pulse, is characteristic of early septic shock. Asymmetric pulses (for example, femoral pulses that are noticeably weaker than brachial pulses) may indicate the presence of a congenital defect such as coarctation of the aorta.[25, 28, 66]

Evaluation of the child's respiratory status is also an important part of the initial examination of the child in shock. Tachypnea without respiratory distress, or "quiet tachypnea," is common in shock. This is a compensatory mechanism that results from stimulation of the respiratory center by the metabolic acidosis and hypoperfusion characteristic of shock. A slow respiratory rate in an acutely ill child is an ominous sign that may be seen in late decompensated shock, hypothermia, respiratory muscle fatigue, and CNS depression or injury. Labored respirations may indicate underlying pulmonary parenchymal disease, airway obstruction, or chest wall injury in the trauma patient.[7, 25, 28, 47]

Temperature is another important parameter to measure when evaluating a child in shock. Protection from thermal stress is often overlooked during the emergent evaluation and resuscitation of the child with circulatory failure. Thermoregulation in pediatric patients, especially infants, is not as effective as that in adults. Infants lose body heat rapidly because of their relatively large body surface area-to-mass ratio. The development of hypothermia greatly increases oxygen consumption and energy expenditure and thus impairs the child's homeostatic mechanisms. In one study of pediatric septic shock, a temperature of less than 37°C was associated with 100% mortality. In another study, trauma patients who were hypothermic had significantly higher mortality rates than trauma patients with similar injuries who were normothermic. On the other hand, young children with sepsis and hypoperfusion may develop temperatures approaching 41°C; in febrile patients prompt antipyretic therapy is necessary to decrease the metabolic requirements on an already stressed cardiovascular system. Thus continuous temperature monitoring and maintenance of euthermia is essential for the care of critically ill children, especially infants and neonates.[7, 28, 67, 68]

While rapid cardiopulmonary assessment is being performed, the physician should observe the child's general appearance. The child's level of activity and response to the environment, particularly to parents and medical personnel, are important. For example, a young child who seems to tolerate frightening or painful procedures is usually more ill than one who fights an examination. Other signs of hypovolemia that may be helpful are a sunken anterior fontanelle, delayed capillary refill, dry mucous membranes, and sunken eyes. Hemorrhage or petechiae may indicate intravascular coagulation or septic emboli.

After initial evaluation, resuscitation, and stabilization of the patient, a more complete head-to-toe physical examination should be performed, including examination of the heart for evidence of congenital heart disease or an acute myocardial process, a complete neurologic examination, and close inspection for any focus of infection.

The trauma patient should be closely evaluated for any injuries that are not immediately obvious. As many as 25% of patients admitted to major trauma centers with serious injuries have at least one injury that is missed at the time of initial evaluation. The patient should be completely undressed and a systematic assessment of the entire body surface area performed to ensure that no wounds are overlooked. Recognition of occult bleeding requires a thorough physical examination with close attention to the sometimes subtle signs of major hemorrhage. Occult but significant internal hemorrhage occurs in five main areas: the chest, abdomen, retroperitoneum, pelvis, and femurs. Pain, swelling, or ecchymosis in any of these areas should alert the physician to the possibility of internal hemorrhage. It is important to recognize that cumulative blood loss from multiple sites of injury can quickly add up to a significant proportion of the total blood volume. For example, 10% of the total blood volume may be lost for each pelvic ring fracture, and a femur fracture may cause a loss of 20% of the blood volume.[69–71]

Infants with inadequate perfusion may exhibit a unique syndrome known as *sclerema neonatorum*. These infants develop a diffuse, rapidly spreading, nonedematous hardening of their subcutaneous tissues. Their skin is cool, smooth, often mottled, and adherent to the subcutaneous tissues. Although the infant's subcutaneous tissues undergo unique pathologic changes, the basic pathophysiology appears to be similar to shock states in older patients. This syndrome carries a poor prognosis, and only a few survivors have been described.[7, 28, 72]

Diagnostic Evaluation and Monitoring

Although blood pressure measurement is generally regarded as an important part of the evaluation of the patient in shock, standard blood pressure measurement techniques can be unreliable in small children. Because of the wide range of extremity size in the pediatric age group, blood pressure cuffs are often too large or too small relative to the extremity circumference, and measured pressures will therefore be falsely low or falsely elevated, respectively. This error is easily avoided by using the proper size cuff—one that covers two thirds of the distance between the child's shoulder and the olecranon process.[28]

In vasoconstricted children, intravascular arterial pressures measured directly by strain-gauge transducers may be significantly higher than when measured by auscultated or palpated cuff pressures. This phenomenon is a result of the elevated vascular resistance in shock patients, which may dampen or eliminate the Korotkoff sounds and distal pulses. The wide variability of normal blood pressure ranges, along with the inexactitudes of cuff pressure measurements, underscores the importance of following serial blood pressure measurements and not basing therapeutic decisions on individual determinations. A peripheral arterial line is indicated for the unstable child who requires continuous blood

pressure monitoring and will remain in the emergency department or intensive care unit for an extended period of time.[7, 28]

Continuous cardiac monitoring for heart rate and rhythm should be instituted as soon as possible in all shock patients. The change in heart rate is a useful guide in shock resuscitation. In hypovolemia with the absence of other abnormality, the heart rate should decrease with adequate volume replacement. Patients should be observed for the presence of any arrhythmias. Arrhythmias may contribute to or even be the cause of shock, although more commonly arrhythmias result from hypoxia or electrolyte abnormalities that occur during shock. Dysrhythmias are most frequently seen in children with shock related to cardiac surgery and drug intoxication.

Frequent measurement of urine output is a useful index of renal perfusion and therefore of overall central perfusion. In all children with hypoperfusion that does not immediately resolve with volume replacement therapy, a catheter should be placed into the bladder for the accurate measurement of urine output. A normal urine output is 1 to 2 ml/kg/hr; a urine output of less than 1 ml/kg/hr, in the absence of renal disease, is a sign of poor perfusion.[25, 28, 73]

In addition to core temperature, surface temperature monitoring is an important but seldom measured parameter. It has been demonstrated that in the presence of a constant ambient temperature, a fall in effective circulating blood volume that results in peripheral vasoconstriction causes an increase in the central-to-peripheral temperature gradient. Thus the central-to-peripheral temperature gradient provides the clinician with another simple, noninvasive method for the ongoing evaluation of perfusion in the hypovolemic patient.[7, 28, 73–75]

Although central venous pressure (CVP) and pulmonary artery catheter measurements are not usually necessary in the initial stages of shock resuscitation, they may be of great benefit during prolonged resuscitation. In the absence of significant cardiac or pulmonary disease, CVP can be used as a reasonable estimate of left ventricular filling pressure. Changes in CVP can be used as an indicator of the heart's ability to pump the volume of blood presented to it and of the adequacy of fluid resuscitation. The absolute CVP measurement is not as useful as the changes or trends in CVP during resuscitation. The initial CVP is usually low in hypovolemic patients but rises as intravascular volume is replaced. If the CVP remains the same in spite of volume replacement, regardless of the initial measurement, it is likely the patient is still hypovolemic. Central venous pressure measurement may also be useful in diagnosing pump dysfunction. The presence of an elevated CVP or a CVP that rises with the rapid administration of fluids without an increase in blood pressure is indicative of poor pump function, whether from primary myocardial deficiency or mechanical obstruction (e.g., pericardial tamponade or pulmonary embolus).[25, 28, 43, 73]

Pulmonary artery catheterization was first described for the use in children in 1971. It is not generally indicated in the management of early shock. It is of greatest use in shock states that do not respond as expected to volume replacement, or when volume replacement must be more carefully guided, as in cardiogenic shock, head trauma, and (often) sepsis. It is also indicated when volume resuscitation requirements exceed 50 to 70 ml/kg. All patients in shock have some element of myocardial dysfunction, and hypotension in the presence of large volume fluid resuscitation mandates intravascular monitoring.[28, 73]

The appropriate use of laboratory tests can provide valuable diagnostic information and guidance for ongoing shock resuscitation. The most important initial blood test in the patient suspected of hemorrhagic shock is the type and crossmatch. Hemoglobin and hematocrit determinations may not be helpful in early hemorrhagic shock, because the extracellular fluid mobilization phase and subsequent equilibration requires approximately 6 hours. An hematocrit of less than 35%, even in the early stage of shock, is nonetheless significant and indicates either severe hemorrhage or a preexisting anemia. In the neonate, the normal hematocrit is 50% to 60%, and hematocrits less than 40% indicate significant blood loss or anemia. Serial hematocrits performed over several hours are useful in detecting ongoing hemorrhage and guiding blood transfusion.[25, 28]

Arterial pH and gas partial pressure measurements are important parameters to follow in the shock state. Arterial Po_2 is often low with shock, even without obvious clinical evidence of hypoxia. Arterial pH should be determined to evaluate the presence and severity of acidosis or alkalosis. Arterial Pco_2 is used to evaluate the patient's ventilation status. These parameters can help assess the need for endotracheal intubation, ventilatory assistance, and subsequent adjustment of the respiratory settings.

Electrolytes should also be monitored in children with shock. Serial blood glucose measurements are especially important in newborn infants in shock because of the increased frequency of hypoglycemia and its complications. Serum sodium, potassium, and chloride levels should be followed closely during resuscitation, as imbalances may develop quickly, particularly when large amounts of fluid are administered. Blood urea nitrogen and creatinine levels are followed as part of the ongoing renal function evaluation.

The serum lactate level is an excellent index of the severity of shock and tissue anoxia. Serial lactate determinations can provide objective evaluation of the patient's response to therapy. An increasing level indicates a worsening of the shock state in spite of therapy and is a poor prognostic sign. Unfortunately, rapid serum lactate determinations are unavailable in the emergency department setting and therefore have limited clinical usefulness.[44, 45]

An elevated white blood cell count may indicate the presence of infection, but also occurs in the face of trauma and other major stress. It is not uncommon to see an abnormally low white blood cell count in septic infants. Evaluation of the coagulation system—including prothrombin time (PT), partial thromboplastin time (PTT), platelet count, fibrinogen, and fibrin degradation products—is essential in shock, as coagulopathies may develop with all types of shock. Cultures of blood, urine, sputum, cerebrospinal fluid, and abscess fluid should be obtained to identify any focus of infection and guide antimicrobial therapy. A chest radiograph and any other imaging study that may be relevant should be obtained.

THERAPEUTIC INTERVENTION

Hypovolemic Shock

The major goals in the initial management of hemorrhagic shock are control of the hemorrhage, restoration of the circulating blood volume, maintenance of adequate oxygen delivery, and correction of the underlying cause of shock. Hemorrhage control may be easily accomplished when the site of bleeding is accessible to simple manual compression. Usually, however, this is not the case, and surgical intervention is required.

The initial emergency department intervention must be simultaneously focused toward correction of the underlying volume deficit and restoration of adequate tissue oxygenation. Often, undue attention is given to reversal of hypotension, which is in fact a secondary rather than a primary pathophysiologic event. If the volume deficit is corrected and the tissues are adequately oxygenated, the blood pressure will return to normal.

Optimizing tissue oxygenation is in many respects the central goal of shock therapy, as the underlying pathophysiologic derangement of shock is inadequate tissue perfusion. Cellular survival will not improve with volume expansion unless the blood oxygen content is adequate. Improving tissue oxygenation begins with an assessment of the patency of the airway and the adequacy of ventilation. Supplemental oxygen administration and frequent oximetry monitoring are standard during shock. Respiratory failure is uncommon in the early phase of shock, but as shock progresses, respiratory muscle dysfunction may develop and lead to hypoventilation and hypoxemia. The cause of this respiratory muscle dysfunction is multifactorial. It may result from poor perfusion of the respiratory muscles themselves or from acidosis, fatigue, or electrolyte abnormalities. The physician must be aware that children fatigue rapidly. Respiratory compensation is usually maximal until complete and sometimes alarmingly rapid deterioration occurs. It is therefore essential to repeatedly assess the patient's oxygenation and ventilation status. The physician must be prepared to intubate the child in acute circulatory failure. Indications for intubation are the following: a Pao_2 less than 50 mm Hg with an Fio_2 of 50%, a $Paco_2$ greater than 50 mm Hg, a severe metabolic acidosis (which is indicative of inadequate respiratory effort and compensation), severe pulmonary edema, marked respiratory distress with an increasing respiratory rate, inability of the patient to protect the airway, and the need for hyperventilation, as in the presence of a head injury with increased intracranial pressure.[7, 28, 65, 76]

The other critical and interrelated aspect of shock therapy is restoration of an effective circulating blood volume. Rapid expansion of the blood volume clearly improves outcome in hemorrhagic shock. To a certain extent, this is true whether the fluid administered is crystalloid, colloid, whole blood, or blood components. This is a reflection of the Fick equation, which quantitatively describes oxygen consumption (Vo_2) as the product of three variables: blood flow (Q), hemoglobin concentration, and the fractional unloading of oxygen ($Sao_2 - Svo_2$).

$$Vo_2 = Q \times 1.39 \, Hgb \times (Sao_2 - Svo_2)$$

Thus even if the hemoglobin and the fractional unloading of oxygen remain constant, an increase in the effective circulating volume will increase critical organ blood flow and oxygen transport. Therefore a primary goal of shock therapy is to restore volume.[77, 78]

The amount and type of volume expander used depends primarily on the clinical status of the patient and, to a lesser extent, on individual or institutional preference. Until the 1960s, transfusion with whole blood was the gold standard of therapy for hemorrhagic shock. It was assumed that whole blood infusion resulted in precise replacement of the fluid that had been lost. This practice came into question, however, when investigators demonstrated the presence of an interstitial fluid deficit and the phenomenon of transcapillary refill during hemorrhagic shock. Multiple investigations of various resuscitation regimens followed. One such study used a modified Wiggers model to evaluate the effects of various fluids on survival rates of animals in hemorrhagic shock. The resuscitation regimens that yielded maximal survival rates used a combination of shed blood and crystalloid. The investigators hypothesized that the sodium-containing electrolyte solutions expanded the extracellular space, whereas the blood did not, and that this expansion was essential for optimal resuscitation.[37, 77, 79, 89]

It should be pointed out that the animal models used by

the majority of shock investigators did not replicate the pathophysiologic or clinical chain of events commonly occuring in human hemorrhagic shock. The conclusions of these studies are therefore suspect. Since the 1970s, however, the demand for blood products and the associated costs have escalated dramatically. In addition there has been a growing awareness of the potential for the transmission of serious and even life-threatening diseases through blood transfusions. Therefore it has generally become accepted, although not proven, that asanguinous fluids are the agents of choice for initial resuscitation of shock.

Considerable controversy exists, however, concerning which asanguinous fluid is most appropriate: colloid or crystalloid. Studies have not produced convincing evidence that either agent is superior to the other. Much of the colloid-crystalloid debate revolves around the effect of these various fluid types on the lung. Colloid supporters argue that preservation of the plasma colloid oncotic pressure (PCOP) is essential to prevent the collection of fluid in the pulmonary interstitium. They argue that large-volume crystalloid infusion causes hemodilution of serum proteins and decreases PCOP by one half to one third of normal values. Theoretically a fall in the intravascular oncotic pressure creates a gradient that favors movement of fluid out of the intravascular space into the pulmonary interstitium. Analysis of the Starling microvascular forces, however, indicates that this assumption is incorrect. Decreases in PCOP as a result of crystalloid administration are only one fourth as important as increases in hydrostatic pressure in increasing fluid exchange. This is because the pulmonary capillary endothelia are normally more "leaky" than the systemic capillary endothelia and permit considerable flow of fluid, including plasma proteins, between the capillaries and the interstitium. As a result the interstitial oncotic pressure of the lung is relatively high, typically about 70% of intravascular values. As PCOP decreases, interstitial oncotic pressure decreases proportionally, so the difference between the two, which is what governs fluid exchange, changes little.[37, 77, 81–83]

Colloid supporters also argue that because colloids remain primarily in the intravascular compartment, they are more effective in elevating blood volume and result in shorter resuscitation times and the development of less peripheral edema than crystalloids. Systemic capillaries behave differently from pulmonary capillaries. Systemic capillary endothelia are less "leaky" and more restrictive of protein filtration. The systemic interstitial oncotic pressure is therefore only 20% to 30% of the intravascular values. This results in a much larger transcapillary oncotic gradient and makes the peripheral tissues much more sensitive to protein hemodilution. This is manifested clinically in patients who receive large volumes of crystalloid by the development of marked peripheral edema 2 to 3 days following resuscitation.[37, 77, 81–83]

Crystalloid supporters point out that although the use of crystalloids results in greater peripheral edema formation, this does not appear to have any harmful consequences, and there is no correlation between peripheral edema and pulmonary edema. They also argue that balanced salt solutions are needed to effectively treat the interstitial fluid deficit associated with hypovolemic shock.[81–86]

A critical review of the experimental and clinical studies comparing crystalloid and colloid resuscitation fails to reveal a superior efficacy of one asanguinous solution over the other. Because there is no proven advantage to either therapy, and because crystalloids are readily available and much less expensive than colloids, crystalloids are recommended as the agent of choice for the initial shock resuscitation. Additional studies continue on alternative infusion solutions, including dextran, hypertonic saline, hetastarch, and stroma-free hemoglobin. At present, however, there is

no justification for the routine use of these solutions in children.

At the present time crystalloids, specifically 0.9 normal saline (NS) and lactated Ringer's solution (LR), are the solutions most commonly used in shock resuscitation. Sodium and chloride ions are present in 0.9 NS in a concentration of 154 mEq/L, a concentration significantly higher than found in plasma. The concentrations of sodium (130 mEq/L) and chloride (109 mEq/L) in LR more closely reflect the normal physiologic state. LR also contains 4 mEq/L of potassium, 3 mEq/L of calcium, and 28 mEq/L of lactate. The theoretic advantage of LR is that the lactate is rapidly converted to bicarbonate by the liver and may tend to buffer any metabolic acidosis accompanying the shock state. Also, patients are less likely to develop hyperchloremic acidosis with LR infusion than with 0.9 NS infusion. Studies in animals and in humans, however, have shown that in resuscitation from hemorrhagic shock with either 0.9 NS or LR, there is essentially no difference in the volumes required, in the serum pH, or in serum electrolyte levels. Both 0.9 NS and LR are appropriate solutions for initial infusion in shock resuscitation.[81, 87–89]

The initial crystalloid bolus administered to the patient in hypovolemic shock should be equal to approximately one fourth of the patient's total blood volume or 20 ml/kg. If severe shock with hypotension or acidosis is present, the child should receive a bolus equal to approximately one half of the total blood volume or 40 ml/kg. Additional fluid replacement is then guided by the patient's response to the initial infusion. If the child's pulse, systolic blood pressure, and diastolic blood pressure do not improve within 5 to 10 minutes after receiving the initial fluid bolus, a second bolus of equal volume is indicated. In patients whose losses have been controlled and in whom the bolus infusion has improved their clinical status, the infusion rate may be slowed to 5 ml/kg/hr for several hours of close observation, until the child has received the calculated amount of fluid required to replace the loss. A child with hypovolemic shock often requires at least 40 to 60 ml/kg of intravenous fluid in the first hour of resuscitation.[7, 23, 28, 90]

The principle of fluid resuscitation is to administer a volume bolus, reassess the patient, and then give additional boluses with frequent reassessment. It is important to monitor resuscitation as it proceeds to prevent overinfusion of fluid or inadequate fluid replacement. A frequent error in fluid resuscitation from hypovolemic shock in children is inadequate volume replacement. The resuscitation phase of shock is similar to the initial development of shock in that pulse and blood pressure normalize before the volume deficit has been completely corrected. Therefore a normal blood pressure and pulse do not guarantee adequate volume resuscitation. Adequate resuscitation is reflected by an improvement in the patient's skin color and temperature, a decrease in the capillary refill time, and an improvement in mental status, along with a decrease in heart rate and an increase in the mean arterial pressure and pulse pressure.

When treating hemorrhagic shock, blood loss of up to 20% of the total blood volume may be replaced solely with crystalloids at a volume of 3 ml of crystalloid per milliliter of blood loss. The 3:1 rule is based on the empiric observation that three times as much crystalloid is required to achieve an effect comparable to isovolemic blood replacement. Patients who have experienced blood loss of 20% to 40% of their blood volume, or those with continuing signs of shock in spite of aggressive resuscitation with 40 ml/kg or more of crystalloid, will probably require blood transfusion. In this situation it is often possible to wait for fully typed and crossmatched blood, but this decision must be individualized based on the assessment of ongoing blood loss and the efficiency of the local blood bank in performing cross-matches. When in doubt, it is advisable to use type-specific blood. Concerns are frequently raised about the safety of this practice, but several large studies have provided clear evidence that transfusion of type-specific blood is safe. In all likelihood, failure to provide timely replacement of red cells poses a much greater risk to the patient than does the transfusion of type-specific blood.[7, 28, 65, 71, 90–93]

More aggressive therapy is mandated in the uncompensated shock patient, who probably has at least a 40% to 50% volume deficit. Infusion of large volumes of asanguinous fluids without blood transfusion will result in profound hemodilution, a dramatic decrease in oxygen carrying capacity, and considerable dilution of plasma clotting factors. In uncompensated and moribund shock patients, it is appropriate to begin transfusion immediately with type O blood. A type and crossmatch should always be drawn before the administration of type O blood.[7, 28, 65, 71, 90–93]

To determine the volume of blood to be transfused, one must first estimate the patient's total blood volume. A child's blood volume is equal to 80 ml/kg.

$$\text{Blood volume (ml)} = 80 \text{ ml/kg} \times \text{body weight (kg)}$$

For example, a 30-kg child has an estimated total blood volume of 2400 ml. In patients who require blood transfusion, both blood products and crystalloid should be administered. When using whole blood for volume replacement, the volume administered should equal one half the blood loss. The remaining 50% volume loss should be replenished with crystalloid in the amount of 3 ml per milliliter of blood to be replaced. For example, a 30-kg child with an estimated 50% blood loss (1200 ml) would receive 600 ml of whole blood and 1800 ml of crystalloid. Currently, transfusion of packed red blood cells (PRBCs) is the standard means by which red cell mass is increased in the hemorrhagic shock patient, because whole blood is not as readily available as PRBCs. Whole blood is generally substituted with one half the volume of PRBCs; the child in this example would receive 300 ml of PRBCs. The whole blood and crystalloid should be infused in boluses of 20 ml/kg and the PRBCs in boluses of 10 ml/kg. Although these are helpful guidelines, the amount of blood and crystalloid replacement is best governed by frequent reassessment of the patient's clinical status with the end point being stabilization of vital signs and evidence of improved peripheral perfusion.[23, 28, 65, 71]

Adequate replacement of the circulating red cell mass in the patient with hemorrhagic shock may require transfusion of large volumes of stored blood. This has a number of potential physiologic consequences. Platelet number and function are rapidly diminished during red blood cell storage, and dilutional thrombocytopenia is usually associated with massive transfusion. Coagulation factors are also depleted, and the development of a hemorrhagic diathesis is a potentially life-threatening complication of massive fluid and blood resuscitation. Timely administration of platelets and fresh frozen plasma may prevent this complication. Routine protocols for the infusion of platelets and plasma based on the number of units of red cells transfused were once routine but are no longer recommended. Transfusion of these agents should be based on clinical evidence of impaired hemostasis and abnormalities of the PT, PTT, and platelet count.[25, 28, 43, 65, 94, 95]

Hypocalcemia is another potential complication of massive transfusion. Each unit of PRBCs contains approximately 20 ml of citrate solution, which in vivo binds to ionized calcium. Fortunately, citrate is rapidly metabolized by the tricarboxylic acid cycle, and therefore only large doses are toxic. Nevertheless, serum calcium levels should be monitored closely during blood transfusions, as hypocalcemia may further aggravate the shock state.[25, 28, 43, 65, 94, 95]

Potassium levels are significantly elevated in banked blood because of leakage from intact cells with impaired sodium-potassium pumps and the small amount of cell lysis and death that invariably occurs during collection and storage of blood. Although it is logical to assume that hyperkalemia might occur secondary to massive transfusion, it is generally not seen. On transfusion, the sodium-potassium pump deficiency is rapidly corrected, and potassium is absorbed. In addition, the metabolic alkalosis often associated with massive blood transfusion results in the movement of potassium into the cells.[94, 95]

Acid-base abnormalities are common in shock and may be aggravated with massive blood transfusion. Banked blood is acidic because of the lactate accumulation during storage. Most of the lactate, however, is converted to bicarbonate in a single pass through the liver, resulting in a posttransfusion alkalosis rather than an acidosis.[94, 95]

If a metabolic acidosis does exist, however, treatment should be directed primarily at correcting the underlying cause of the acidosis. In the shock state, this generally involves improving tissue perfusion and oxygenation with aggressive fluid resuscitation. Controlled studies have failed to demonstrate a beneficial effect with bicarbonate therapy, and there are several potential adverse effects, including the development of hypernatremia, hypokalemia, hyperosmolarity, and volume overload, as well as a leftward shift of the oxyhemoglobin dissociation curve and a subsequent decrease in tissue oxygen delivery. Sodium bicarbonate therapy should be reserved for those patients who exhibit a persistent metabolic acidosis (pH less than 7.15 or base deficit greater than or equal to 10 mEq/L) in spite of having received appropriate fluid therapy. In those cases, sodium bicarbonate should be administered as a slow intravenous bolus of 1 to 2 mEq/kg and a repeat arterial blood gas obtained. If severe acidosis persists, subsequent boluses of 0.5 mEq/kg may be given. The sodium bicarbonate may be given full strength (1 mEq/ml) in children older than 6 months. A dilute solution of 0.5 mEq/ml, however, should be used in children younger than 6 months to decrease the osmotic load.[96–99]

Hypothermia is a frequent and serious complication of massive blood transfusion. Hypothermia results in an increase in oxygen consumption and shifts the oxyhemoglobin dissociation curve to the left, thereby making less oxygen available to the already underperfused tissues. This complication is prevented by infusing both blood and crystalloids through a fluid warmer whenever massive fluid resuscitation is indicated.[28, 94, 95]

Septic Shock

Septic shock is a complex, rapidly evolving process that may progress to death within hours. A successful outcome is dependent on early recognition with prompt institution of aggressive treatment. The resuscitation strategy for septic shock differs slightly from that of hemorrhagic shock and is a reflection of the difference in the underlying pathophysiology of these two shock states.

As in hypovolemic shock, the initial goal of resuscitation is to restore an effective circulatory volume. An initial fluid bolus of 20 ml/kg of crystalloid should be rapidly infused and the patient's response closely monitored. If the patient's vital signs do not improve within 5 to 10 minutes, another fluid bolus should be administered. If the patient's hemodynamic parameters have not normalized after having received approximately 50 ml/kg of crystalloid, invasive monitoring is indicated. Unlike hemorrhagic shock, pulmonary artery catheter monitoring is frequently required early in septic shock to help guide therapy. This is because of the significant impairment of left ventricular function characteristic of septic shock; the myocardium typically does not respond as well to fluid administration. Volume is infused until the pulmonary capillary wedge pressure reaches 15 to 18 mm Hg. This ensures adequate ventricular filling without leading to pulmonary edema.[7, 14, 100–102]

Patients who remain hypotensive despite volume restoration require inotropic therapy. Dopamine is the inotropic agent of choice in septic shock because of its beta-agonist effects on the myocardium, its alpha vasoconstrictive effects on the peripheral vasculature, and its augmentation of splanchnic renal blood flow. If the systemic vascular resistance is elevated, dobutamine is preferred, because it lacks the peripheral vasoconstrictive effects of dopamine. Both dopamine and dobutamine infusions should be titrated to maintain a near-normal blood pressure. In patients with profound hypotension and myocardial depression unresponsive to high doses of dopamine or dobutamine, norepinephrine is indicated. Again, the infusion should be titrated to normalize the blood pressure (Table 9–3).[14, 100, 102–107]

In addition to restoration of organ perfusion, the other primary goal in the treatment of septic shock is identification and eradication of the infectious source. Hemodynamic stabilization may not actually be possible until the bacterial population is significantly reduced. The emergency physician must perform a thorough search for the source of infection. Appropriate cultures including blood, urine, sputum, and cerebrospinal fluid should be obtained. Any apparent wounds should be cultured. Antibiotics should be administered as soon as cultures are taken. The selection of the antibiotic regimen is based on the spectrum of organisms likely to cause sepsis in that particular patient. This will vary with the patient's age and baseline state of health.

During the first 2 months of life, group B streptococcus, coliforms, and *Listeria monocytogenes* are the most common causes of sepsis. *N. meningitidis, H. influenzae,* and *Streptococcus pneumoniae* emerge as the most frequent causes of sepsis by age 3 months. Immunocompromised or neutropenic patients are commonly infected with *Pseudomonas aeruginosa*. If an abdominal or pelvic source of infection is suspected, the antibiotic regimen must be effective against anaerobes (Table 9–4).

The most common cause of death in septic shock is acute respiratory distress syndrome leading to the development of noncompliant and atelectatic lungs. As the work of breathing is increased, the oxygen demand increases from 3% to 5% to up to 25%, further compromising oxygen supply to the tissues and mandating early institution of mechanical ventilation. This decreases the work of respiration and the associated oxygen consumption and improves tissue oxygenation and pH.[108, 109]

One of the most widely debated issues in the treatment of septic shock has been the use of corticosteroids. The potential benefits of corticosteroid therapy include cell membrane and lysosomal stabilization, inhibition of complement-induced granulocyte aggregation, inhibition of the cellular release of arachidonic acid metabolites, and feedback inhibition of corticotropin secretion and, therefore, prevention of endorphin release. High-dose corticosteroid therapy has been found to be beneficial in some animal models of septic shock. The first human, double-blind, randomized, placebo-controlled trial of corticosteroid therapy in patients with septic shock was published in 1976. In this study the mortality rate was 10% in the corticosteroid-treated patients versus 38% in the control group. Methodologic and statistical objections were raised, however, and the steroid controversy continued. More recently, three large clinical trials demonstrated no differences in mortality between corticosteroid- and placebo-treated patients. The largest of these was a placebo-controlled, double-blind, randomized trial in which 382 patients with severe sepsis or septic shock received methylprednisolone or placebo. There was no difference in the prevention or reversal of shock or in overall mortality between the two groups. Another multicenter trial enrolled 223 patients with clinical signs of sepsis and a normal sensorium. Again, mortality rates were not statistically different between the control and steroid-treated groups. A smaller, partially blinded study of 59 patients with severe septic shock also failed to demonstrate a difference in mortality between groups. In this study, however, the patients treated with steroids within 4 hours after the onset of shock had a significantly higher incidence of shock reversal at 24 hours after diagnosis. Significantly, these studies did demonstrate a higher morbidity from secondary infection in the steroid-treated groups. On the basis of these most recent trials, corticosteroids should not be used in the treatment of septic shock except when there is documented or suspected adrenal insufficiency.[110–114]

The most recent potential therapy being investigated for septic shock is anti-endotoxin immunotherapy. Endotoxin, a lipopolysaccharide in the membrane of gram-negative bacteria, is the proposed initial mediator of many of the systemic responses and sequelae in patients with septic shock secondary to gram-negative bacteremia. It is therefore theorized that the binding and subsequent inhibition of endotoxin by an antisera may prevent the adverse manifestations of septic shock. The results of a randomized double-blind study comparing placebo with polyclonal immune serum in

---

TABLE 9–3

PEDIATRIC RESUSCITATION MEDICATIONS

Drug	Dose	Action
Dopamine	2–5 μg/kg/min	Dopaminergic effects predominate
	5–10 μg/kg/min	Inotropic dose; beta₁ receptor stimulation increases in a dose-related fashion
	>10 μg/kg/min	Pressor dose; alpha receptor stimulation increases in a dose-related fashion
Dobutamine	2–20 μg/kg/min	Inotropic effects predominate
Epinephrine	0.05–0.50 μg/kg/min	Inotropic and pressure effects: Low dose: greater beta₁ and beta₂ effects High dose: greater alpha effects
Norepinephrine	0.05–1.0 μg/kg/min	Potent alpha and beta₁ agonist; little beta₂ effect compared with epinephrine; produces marked increases in systemic vascular resistance

TABLE 9–4

COMMON PATHOGENS OF PEDIATRIC SEPTIC SHOCK AND RECOMMENDED ANTIMICROBIAL REGIMENS

Patient Population	Common Pathogens	Antibiotic
Age		
<2 weeks	Group B streptococcus	Ampicillin
	Coliforms	+
	Listeria monocytogenes	cefotaxime
2 to 8 weeks	Group B streptococcus	Ampicillin
	Coliforms	+
	Listeria monocytogenes	cefotaxime or ceftriaxone
	Streptococcus pneumoniae	
2 months to 9 years	*S. pneumoniae*	Cefotaxime or ceftriaxone
	Haemophilus influenzae	
	Neisseriae meningitidis	
	Staphylococcus aureus	
>9 years	*S. pneumoniae*	Cefotaxime or ceftriaxone
	Neisseriae meningitidis	
	S. aureus	
Immunocompromised host	*S. aureus*	Vancomycin
	Pseudomonas spp.	+
	Coliforms	antipseudomonal third-generation cephalosporin (ceftazidime)
		+
		aminoglycoside
Urinary tract source	*Escherichia coli*	Ampicillin
		+
		aminoglycoside

the treatment of gram-negative bacteremia were published in 1982. The mortality in the control group was significantly higher than in the immune serum-treated group (39% vs. 22%). In patients with septic shock, mortality was sigificantly decreased from 77% in the control group to 44% in the treatment group. Unfortunately, the production and use of polyclonal antiserum has some difficulties. First, vaccinating serum donors with the heat-inactivated cells of *Escherichia coli* is associated with mild toxicity. Second, the antibody content of the antisera preparations vary. Third, there is a finite risk of transmitting infection with pooled human blood. The development and use of monoclonal antibodies, however, would avoid all of these difficulties.[100, 101, 115]

Most recently, a double-blind, placebo-controlled, randomized, multicenter trial was conducted to evaluate the efficacy of HA-1A, a monoclonal IgM antibody that binds endotoxin, in the treatment of patients with gram-negative sepsis. In this trial, the anti-endotoxin also significantly reduced mortality in patients with sepsis and gram-negative bacteremia.[116] Unfortunately not all studies demonstrate such positive results, and additional trials to confirm these results are needed.[100, 101, 117, 118]

Other potential therapies for septic shock include opiate antagonists, arachidonic acid inhibitors, toxic oxygen scavengers, and endotoxin antiserum. Endogenous endorphins are released in response to stress in all types of shock and can cause profound hypotension. Animal studies using naloxone, an opiate antagonist, have shown improvement in cardiac function and reversal of hypotension. The results of human studies have been inconsistent, however, and have not confirmed the animal study data. Although several human studies have demonstrated improvement in mean arterial pressure with naloxone therapy, these same studies have failed to show increases in survival. Although naloxone is a relatively safe drug, serious side effects have been documented, including episodes of hypotension, hypertension, ventricular arrhythmia, and acute pulmonary edema. On the basis of these clinical trials, the use of naloxone in

septic shock should be considered investigational and is not recommended as routine therapy.[7, 25, 100, 101, 119–121]

Metabolites of arachidonic acid, prostaglandins, thromboxane, and leukotrienes are clearly involved in the pathophysiology of septic shock. The use of indomethacin and ibuprofen, nonsteroidal anti-inflammatory agents, have been studied in animal models of septic shock. In all species studied, including primates, a significant improvement in survival has been demonstrated with the administration of these drugs following induction of septic shock.[25, 100, 101]

Oxygen free radicals and related species are important mediators of tissue injury. Superoxide dismutase, catalase, and vitamin E, as well as other oxygen free radical scavengers are currently under investigation for therapeutic use in septic shock.[25, 100, 101]

The basic principles of the treatment of septic shock include adequate fluid resuscitation, inotropic support as needed, early antibiotic therapy, and the eradication of septic foci. However, despite the use of potent antibiotics and aggressive supportive care, the mortality of septic shock remains unacceptably high.

References

1. Archibald EW, McLean WS: Observations upon shock with particular reference to the condition as seen in war surgery. Ann Surg 1917; 66:280.
2. Blalock A. Experimental shock, the cause of the low blood pressure produced by muscle injury. Arch Surg 1930; 20:959.
3. Shires TG, Canizaro PC, Carrico CJ. Shock. *In* Schwartz SI, Shires GT, Spencer FC, Storer EH (eds). Principles of Surgery. New York, McGraw-Hill, 1979, pp 135–179.
4. Holcroft JW, Blaisdell FW. Shock: Causes and management of circulatory collapse. *In* Sabiston DC (ed). Textbook of Surgery. Philadelphia, WB Saunders, 1986, pp 38–63.
5. Carpenter CCJ. Oral rehydration: Is it as good as parenteral therapy. N Engl J Med 1982; 306:1103.
6. Accident Facts. Chicago, National Safety Council, 1981.
7. Wetzel RC. Shock in neonates and children. *In* Hardaway RM (ed). Shock: The Reversible Stage of Dying. Littleton, CO, PSG Publishing Co, 1988, pp 261–280.

8. Perkin RM, Levin DL. Shock in the pediatric patient. Part 1. J Pediatr 1982; 101:163.

9. King DR. Trauma in infancy and childhood: Initial evaluation and management. Pediatr Clin North Am 1985; 325:1299.

10. Shiller JG. Shock in the newborn caused by transplacental hemorrhage from fetus to mother. Pediatrics 1957; 20:7.

11. Becker AH, Glass H. Twin-to-twin transfusion syndrome. Am J Dis Child 1963; 106:134.

12. Kirkman HN, Riley HD. Posthemorrhagic anemia and shock in the newborn: A review. Pediatrics 1957; 24:97.

13. Ellner JJ. Septic shock. Pediatr Clin North Am 1983; 30:365.

14. Zimmerman JJ, Dietrich KA. Current perspectives on septic shock. Pediatr Clin North Am 1987; 34:131.

15. Parker MM, Parillo JE. Septic shock: Hemodynamics and pathogenesis. JAMA 1983; 250:3324.

16. Parillo JE, Parker MM, Natanson C, et al. Septic shock in humans. Advances in the understanding of pathogenesis, cardiovascular dysfunction, and therapy. Ann Intern Med 1990; 113:227.

17. Jacobs RF, Sowell MK, Moss MM, Fiser DH. Septic shock in children: Bacterial etiologies and temporal relationships. Pediatr Infect Dis J 1990; 9:196.

18. Pryor RW, Kline MW, Matson JR. Septic shock: Principles of management in the emergency department. Pediatr Emerg Care 1989; 5:193.

19. Kanter RK, Weiner LB. Pediatric life-threatening infections. In Shoemaker WC, Ayres S, Grenvik A, et al (ed). Textbook of Critical Care. Philadelphia, WB Saunders, 1989, pp 825–829.

20. Weintzen RL, McCracken GH. Pathogenesis and management of neonatal sepsis and meningitis. Curr Probl Pediatr 1977; 8:1.

21. Freedman RM, Ingram DL, Gross I, et al. A half century of neonatal sepsis at Yale. Am J Dis Child 1981; 135:140.

22. Miller MK, Pan JSC. Life-threatening infections in the newborn. In Shoemaker WC, Ayres S, Grenvik A, et al (ed). Textbook of Critical Care. Philadelphia, WB Saunders, 1989, pp 817–825.

23. Witte MK, Hill JH, Blumer JL. Shock in the pediatric patient. Adv Pediatr 1987; 34:139.

24. Lucking SE, Pollack MM, Fields AI. Shock following generalized hypoxic-ischemic injury in previously healthy infants and children. J Pediatr 1986; 108:359.

25. Gann DS, Amaral JF. Pathophysiology of trauma and shock. In Zuidema GD, et al (ed). The Management of Trauma. Philadelphia, WB Saunders, 1985, pp 37–105.

26. Guyton AC. Arterial pressure regulation: Rapid pressure control by nervous reflexes and other mechanisms. In Guyton AC (ed). Textbook of Medical Physiology. Philadelphia, WB Saunders, 1986, pp 244–256.

27. Friedman WF. The intrinsic physiologic properties of the developing heart. Prog Cardiovasc Dis 1972; 15:87.

28. Mayer T. Management of hypovolemic shock. In Mayer TA (ed). Emergency Management of Pediatric Trauma. Philadelphia, WB Saunders, 1985, pp 39–52.

29. Slater GI. Sequential changes in distribution of cardiac output in hemorrhagic shock. Surgery 1973; 73:714.

30. Zeifach BW, Bronek A. The interplay of central and peripheral factors in irreversible hemorrhagic shock. Prog Cardiovasc Dis 1975; 18:147.

31. Pruitt BA Jr, Moncrief JA, Mason AD Jr. Efficacy of buffered saline as the sole replacement fluid following acute measured hemorrhage in man. J Trauma 1967; 7:767.

32. Moss GS, Saletta JD. Traumatic shock in man. N Engl J Med 1974; 290:724.

33. Drucker WB, Chadwick CDJ, Gann DS. Transcapillary refill in hemorrhagic shock. Arch Surg 1981; 116:1344.

34. Lefer AM, Hock CE. Vascular mediators in circulatory shock. In Hardaway RM (ed). Shock: The Reversible Stage of Dying. Littleton, CO, PSG Publishing Co, 1988, pp 102–123.

35. Campbell ITG, Newbegin HE. Endocrine aspects of shock. In Hardaway RM (ed). Shock: The Reversible Stage of Dying. Littleton, CO, PSG Publishing Co, 1988, pp 91–102.

36. Trachte GJ. Endocrinology of shock. In Altura BM, Lefer AM, Schumer W. Handbook of Shock and Trauma. Vol 1: Basic Science. New York, Raven Press, 1983, pp 337–354.

37. Carico CG, et al. Fluid resuscitation following injury: Rationale for the use of balanced salt solutions. Crit Care Med 1976; 4:46.

38. Illner H, Shires GT. The effect of hemorrhagic shock on potassium transport in skeletal muscles. Surg Gynecol Obstet 1980; 150:17.

39. Carpenter MS, et al. Ionized calcium and magnesium in the baboon: Hemorrhagic shock and resuscitation. Circ Shock 1976; 5:163.

40. Trunkey DD, Carpenter MA, Holcroft TJ. Ionized calcium and magnesium: The effect of septic shock in the baboon. J Trauma 1976; 16:633.

41. Carafoli E. Membrane transport and the regulation of the cell calcium levels. In Trump BF, Cowley RA (eds). Pathophysiology of Shock, Anoxia, and Ischemia. Baltimore, Williams & Wilkins, 1982, pp 95–112.

42. White BC. Mitochondrial oxygen use and ATP synthesis: Kinetic effects of Ca^{++} and $HPO_4{-2}$ modulated by glucocorticoids. Ann Emerg Med 1980; 9:396.

43. Mannix FL. Hemorrhagic Shock. In Rosen P, et al (ed). Emergency Medicine: Concepts and Clinical Practice. St Louis, CV Mosby, 1988, pp 179–202.

44. Peretz DI, Scott HM, Duff J, et al. The significance of lactic acidemia in the shock syndrome. Ann NY Acad Sci 1965; 119:1133.

45. Vincent JL, Philippe D, et al. Serial lactate determinations during circulatory shock. Crit Care Med 1983; 11:449.

46. Broder G, Weil MH. Excess lactate: Index of reversibility of shock in human subjects. Science 1964; 143:1457.

47. Crone RK. Acute circulatory failure in children. Pediatr Clin North Am 1980; 27:525.

48. Naqvi AH, Chundu KR, Friedman AD. Shock in children with gram-negative bacillary sepsis and Hemophilus influenzae type b sepsis. Pediatr Infect Dis 1986; 5:512.

49. DuPont HL, Spink WW. Infections due to gram-negative organisms: An analysis of 860 patients with bacteremia at the University of Minnesota Medical Center 1958–1966. Medicine 1969; 48:307.

50. Parillo JE. The cardiovascular pathophysiology of sepsis. Ann Rev Med 1989; 40:469.

51. Crile GW. Blood Pressure in Surgery: Experimental and Clinical Research. Philadelphia, JB Lippincott, 1903, pp 288–291.

52. Gardner WJ, Storer J. The use of the G-suit in control of intraabdominal bleeding. Surg Gynecol Obstet 1966; 123:797.

53. Cutler BS, Daggett W. Application of the G-suit to the control of hemorrhage in massive trauma. Ann Surg 1971; 173:511.

54. Kaplan BC, Civetta JM, Nagel EL, et al. The military anti-shock trouser in civilian pre-hospital emergency care. J Trauma 1973; 13:843.

55. Bickell WH, Pepe PE, Bailey ML, et al. Randomized trial of pneumatic antishock garments in the prehospital management of penetrating abdominal injuries. Ann Emerg Med 1987; 16:653.

56. Davis SM. Antishock trousers: A collective review. J Emerg Med 1986; 4:145.

57. McSwain NE. Pneumatic anti-shock garment: State of the art. Ann Emerg Med 1988; 17:506.

58. Mattox KL, Bickell WH, Pepe PE, Mangelsdorff AD. Prospective randomized evaluation of anti-shock MAST in post traumatic hypotension. J Trauma 1986; 26:779.

59. Mackerzie RC, Christensen JM, Lewis FR. The prehospital use of external counterpressure: Does MAST make a difference? J Trauma 1984; 10:882.

60. Mattox KL, Bickell W, Pepe PE, et al. Prospective MAST study in 911 patients. J Trauma 1989; 29:1104.

61. Kaback KR, Sanders AB, Meislin H. MAST suit update. JAMA 1984; 252:2598.

62. Henneman PL. MAST controversy. Letter. J Trauma 1987; 27:1095.

63. Frumkin K. The pneumatic anti-shock garment. In Roberts JR, Hedges JR (ed). Clinical Procedures in Emergency Medicine. Philadelphia, WB Saunders, 1985, pp 403–414.

64. Brunette DD, Fifield G, Ruiz E. Use of pneumatic antishock trousers in the management of pediatric pelvic hemorrhage. Pediatr Emerg Care 1987; 3:86.

65. Trunkey DD, Sheldon GF, Collins JA. The treatment of shock. In Zuidema GD, et al (ed). The Management of Trauma. Philadelphia, WB Saunders, 1985, pp 105–127.

66. Recognition of respiratory failure and shock: Anticipating cardiopulmonary arrest. In Chameides L (ed). Textbook of Pediatric Advanced Life Support. American Heart Association and American Academy of Pediatrics, 1988, pp 3–9.

67. Pollack MM, Fields AI, Ruttimann UE. Distributions of cardiopulmonary variables in pediatric survivors and nonsurvivors of septic shock. Crit Care Med 1985; 13:454.

68. Jurkovich GJ, Greiser WB, Luterman A, Curreri PW. Hypothermia in trauma victims: An ominous predictor of survival. J Trauma 1987; 27:1019.

69. Chan RN, Ainscow D, Sikorski JM. Diagnostic failures in the multiply injured. J Trauma 1980; 20:674.

70. Dove DB, Stahl WM, Del Guercio LRM. A five year review of deaths following urban trauma. J Trauma 1980; 20:760.

71. Kallen RJ, Lonergan JM. Fluid resuscitation of acute hypovolemic hypoperfusion states in pediatrics. Pediatr Clin North Am 1990; 37:287.

72. Warwick WJ, Ruttenberg HD, Quie PG. Sclerema neonatorum—a sign, not a disease. JAMA 1963; 184:680.

73. Edmonds JF, Barker GA, Conn AWL. Concepts in cardiovascular monitoring in children. Crit Care Med 1980; 8:548.

74. Ibsen B. Treatment of shock with vasodilators measuring skin temperature on the big toe. Dis Chest 1967; 52:425.

75. Aynsley-Green A, Pickering D. Use of central and peripheral temperature measurements in care of the critically ill child. Arch Dis Child 1974; 49:477.

76. Shock. In Barkin RM, Rosen P (ed). Emergency Pediatrics. St Louis, CV Mosby, 1990, pp 26–39.

77. Shires GT. Pathophysiology and fluid replacement in hypovolemic shock. Ann Clin Res 1977; 9:144.

78. Carey LC, Lowery ND, Cloutier CT. Hemorrhagic shock. Curr Probl Surg 1971; 3:48.

79. Dillon JL, et al. A bio-assay of treatment of hemorrhagic shock. Arch Surg 1966; 93:537.

80. Virgilio RN, Smith DE, Zurins CK. Balanced electrolyte solutions: Experimental and clinical studies. Crit Care Med 1979; 7:98.
81. Tranbaugh RF, Lewis FR. Crystalloid vs. colloid for fluid resuscitation of hypovolemic patients. Adv Shock Res 1983; 9:203.
82. Peters RM, Hargens AR. Protein vs. electrolytes and all of the Starling forces. Arch Surg 1981; 116:1293.
83. Guyton AC, Lindsey AW. Effect of elevated left atrial pressure and decreased plasma protein concentration on the development of pulmonary edema. Circ Res 1959; 1:649.
84. Tranbaugh RF, Elings VB, Christensen JM, Lewis FR. Determinants of pulmonary interstitial fluid accumulation after trauma. J Trauma 1982; 22:820.
85. Moss GS, Lowe RJ, Jilek J, Levine HD. Colloid or crystalloid in the resuscitation of hemorrhagic shock: A controlled clinical trial. Surgery 1981; 89:434.
86. Moss GS, Siegel DC, Cochin A, et al. Effects of saline and colloid solutions on pulmonary function in hemorrhagic shock. Surg Gynecol Obstet 1971; 130:53.
87. Cervera AL, Moss G. Dilutional re-expansion with crystalloid after massive hemorrhage: Saline versus balanced electrolyte solutions for maintenance of normal blood volume and arterial pH. J Trauma 1975; 15:498
88. Coran AG, Ballantine TV, Horwitz DL, et al: The effect of crystalloid resuscitation in hemorrhagic shock on acid-base balance: A comparison between normal saline and Ringer's lactate solutions. Surgery 1971; 69:874.
89. Lowery BD, Loutier CT, Carey LC. Electrolyte solutions in resuscitation in human hemorrhagic shock. Surg Gynecol Obstet 1971; 133:273.
90. Fluid Therapy and Medications. *In* Chameides L (ed). Textbook of Pediatric Advanced Life Support. American Heart Association and American Academy of Pediatrics, 1988, pp 47–48.
91. Dronen SC. Plasma and volume expanders. *In* Barsan WG, Jastremski MS, Syverud SA (eds). Emergency Drug Therapy. Philadelphia, WB Saunders, 1991, pp 50–55.
92. Blumberg N, Bove JR. Uncross-matched blood for emergency transfusion: One year's experience in a civilian setting. JAMA 1978; 240:2057.
93. Barnes A. Transfusion of universal donor and uncrossmatched blood. Bib Haematol 1980; 46:132.
94. Sohmer PR, Dawson RB. Transfusion therapy in trauma: A review of the principles and techniques used in the MIEMS program. Am Surg 1979; 79:109.
95. Schiffer CA. Transfusion therapy in the critical care setting. *In* Shoemaker WC, Ayres S, Grenvik A, et al (eds). Textbook of Critical Care. Philadelphia, WB Saunders, 1989, pp 903–910.
96. Wilson RF. Acid-base abnormalities in clinical shock. *In* Hardaway RM (ed). Shock: The Reversible Stage of Dying. Littleton, CO, PSG Publishing Co, 1988, pp 78–90.
97. Stapcoole PW. Lactic acidosis: The case against bicarbonate therapy. Ann Intern Med 1986; 105:276.
98. Kearns T, Wolfson AB. Metabolic acidosis. Emerg Med Clin North Am 1989; 7:823.
99. Narins RG, Cohen JJ. Bicarbonate therapy for organic acidosis: The rare case for its continued use. Ann Intern Med 1987; 106:615.
100. Putterman C. Modern approaches to the therapy of septic shock. Am J Emerg Med 1990; 8:152.
101. Parrillo JE, Parker MM, Natanson C, et al. Septic shock in humans (NIH conference). Ann Intern Med 1990; 113:227.
102. Shine KI, Kuhn M, Young LS, Tillisch JH. Aspects of the management of shock. Ann Intern Med 1980; 93:723.
103. Desjars P, Pinaud M, Potel G, et al. A reappraisal of norepinephrine therapy in human septic shock. Crit Care Med 1987; 15:134.
104. Schaer GL, Fink MP, Parrillo JE. Norepinephrine alone versus norepinephrine plus low-dose dopamine: Enhanced renal blood flow with combination pressor therapy. Crit Care Med 1985; 13:492.
105. Vincent JL, Roman A, Kahn RJ. Dobutamine administration in septic shock: Addition to a standard protocol. Crit Care Med 1990; 18:689.
106. Meadow D, Edwards D, Wilkins RG, et al. Reversal of intractable septic shock with norepinephrine therapy. Crit Care Med 1988; 16:663.
107. Jardin F, Sportiche M, Bazin M, et al. Dobutamine: A hemodynamic evaluation in human septic shock. Crit Care Med 1981; 9:329.
108. Parrillo JE. Cardiovascular pathophysiology of sepsis. Ann Rev Med 1989; 40:469.
109. Karakusis PH. Considerations in the therapy of septic shock. Med Clin North Am 1986; 70:933.
110. Schumer W. Steroids in the treatment of clinical septic shock. Ann Surg 1976; 184:333.
111. Bone RC, Fisher CJ, Clemmer TP, et al. A controlled clinical trial of high-dose methylprednisolone in the treatment of severe sepsis and septic shock. N Engl J Med 1987; 317:653.
112. Hinshaw L, Peduzzi P, Young E, et al. Effect of high-dose glucocorticoid therapy on mortality in patients with clinical signs of systemic sepsis. N Engl J Med 1987; 317:659.
113. Sprung CL, Caralis PV, Marcial EH, et al. The effects of high-dose corticosteroids in patients with septic shock. N Engl J Med 1984; 311:1137.

114. Sheagren JN. Septic shock and corticosteroids. Letter. N Engl J Med 1981; 305:456.
115. Ziegler EJ, McCutchan JA, Fierer J, et al. Treatment of gram-negative bacteremia and shock with human antiserum to a mutant Escherichia coli. N Engl J Med 1982; 307:1125.
116. Ziegler EJ, Fisher CJ, Sprung CL, et al. Treatment of gram-negative bacteremia and septic shock with HA-1A human monoclonal antibody against endotoxin. N Engl J Med 1991; 324:431.
117. Aitchison JM, Arbuckle DD: Anti-endotoxin in the treatment of severe surgical septic shock: Results of a randomized double blind trial. S Afr Med J 1985; 68:787.
118. Adhikari M, Coovadia HM, Gaffin SL, et al. Septicaemic low birthweight neonates treated with human antibodies to endotoxin. Arch Dis Child 1985; 60:382.
119. Groeger JJ, Carlon GC, Howland HS. Naloxone in septic shock. Crit Care Med 1983; 11:650.
120. DeMaria A, Carven DE, Heffernan JJ, et al. Naloxone versus placebo in the treatment of septic shock. Lancet 1985; 1:1363.
121. Roberts DE, Dobson KE, Hall KW, et al. Effects of prolonged naloxone infusion in septic shock. Lancet 1988; 2:699.

CHAPTER 10

Dehydration and Fluid Replacement

Paul Blackburn

INTRODUCTION

The concept of fluid and electrolyte replacement for dehydration began during a cholera epidemic in England in the early 1830s. Debate centered around the pathogenesis and treatment of cholera. Because a constant finding in most patients was "black, thick, cold blood," most treatments involved attempts at removal of the unknown toxins through bloodletting and purgatives.[1] A physician and chemist named O'Shaughnessy recorded a classic description of dehydration and shock[1] and studied the blood of cholera victims in his laboratory. He found that the blood had lost "a large portion of its water" and further described losses of alkali and salts.[2] Another physician, Latta, is credited with the first attempts at intravenous rehydration. While attending a moribund patient, in whom all attempts at oral and rectal rehydration had failed, Latta intravenously administered a solution of 51 mEq/L sodium, 33 mEq/L chloride, and 14 mEq/L bicarbonate, with dramatic favorable results.[3] However, intravenous rehydration did not gain acceptance because of the limited comprehension of fluid balance, electrolyte pathophysiology, and infectious disease. The solutions used were impure, unsterile, and hypotonic. Once rehydrated, patients resumed their gastrointestinal fluid losses. The fluid quantities needed to treat patients were unknown.[1] It is not surprising, then, that despite Latta's success, it was not until a greater understanding of fluid and electrolyte physiology, acid-base balance, and the clinical application of rehydration[4] that replacement therapy became commonplace.

Despite advances in fluid management, significant morbidity and mortality remain. In the United States there are approximately 500 deaths annually in children 1 month to 4 years old as a result of imbalances caused by diarrhea.[5] Worldwide, at least 5 million children younger than 5 years die annually because of fluid losses caused by diarrhea.[6, 7]

The emergency department physician routinely sees children with fluid and electrolyte disturbances. Children with gastroenteritis, pyloric stenosis with protracted vomiting, cystic fibrosis, postoperative ileostomy, and cardiac or renal disease can all develop disturbances that may require emergent intervention.[8, 9]

RENAL DEVELOPMENT AND NEONATAL PHYSIOLOGY

Embryology

Some of the unique physiologic features of the neonate are the regulation of energy metabolism, thermogenesis,[9] and the initial factors of the "dormant fetal organs"—the lungs, gut, and kidneys.[10] The human kidney that persists into adulthood is the metanephros. Development begins the fifth week of gestation from the ureteric bud and evolves through two intermediates, pronephros and mesonephros. Glomeruli are produced by the ninth to twelfth gestational weeks, and urine is produced.[11]

Nephrogenesis continues through 36 weeks' gestation and is then complete for life. Each kidney will contain about 1 million nephron units. If the infant is born prematurely, nephrogenesis continues until 36 weeks' gestational age.[12] The fetal kidney is essentially "dormant," as it is not required for fluid and electrolyte balance; the placenta provides this function. As a result, fetal metabolic balance reflects maternal homeostasis.[13]

As the fetus produces urine, it voids into the amniotic sac, providing amniotic fluid volume. The amount of urine contributed to the amniotic fluid is important. Anuric fetuses (i.e., as a result of bilateral renal agenesis or high-grade obstruction) can be born in proper homeostatic balance. However, the resulting oligohydramnios produces a characteristic constellation of abnormalities, including pulmonary hypoplasia, known as *Potter's syndrome*.[14]

Renal Function

Fetal renal blood flow is about 5% of cardiac output, compared with 20% to 25% in adults. The glomerular filtration rate is also low at birth. Both renal blood flow and the glomerular filtration rate double by 2 weeks of age in the term infant and reach adult values by age 2 years.[15–17]

Renal concentrating abilities are poor at birth. Serum antidiuretic hormone (ADH) levels are low, and the kidneys are hyporesponsive to the ADH that is present. The renal medullary architecture is immature, with short nephrons and marked variation in nephron size. Because of the neonate's high anabolic rate, little urea is excreted, resulting in decreased medullary solute accumulation. The short nephron tubules and decreased medullary urea concentration limit the countercurrent multiplier and exchange mechanisms responsible for urine concentration.[18] Because of this, the newborn infant can concentrate urine to a maximum of less than 700 mOsm/kg, in contrast to adult values of 1200 mOsm/kg.[19] This means that greater fluid loads are required to excrete any given solute load, and that the child may be more prone to water deficit (dehydration). Adult renal concentrating abilities are achieved by 1 to 2 years of age.[20]

In contrast to the limited renal concentrating ability, the dilutional capability of the neonate is excellent. Despite this, both premature and term infants have difficulty excreting hypotonic fluid loads.[21, 22] This is especially evident the first 3 days of life in low-birth-weight and premature infants[21, 22] and persists through 5 weeks of postnatal life. There exists, then, the possibility of fluid overload and hyponatremia.

The renin-angiotensin system is hyperfunctioning in the newborn. This is a result of low blood pressure and renal blood flow, with tubular sodium wasting, especially in premature infants of less than 34 weeks' gestation.[23–25] The hyperfunctioning renin-angiotensin system contributes to increased blood flow and maintenance of systemic blood pressure. Plasma aldosterone is elevated, increasing sodium retention[26] and helping prevent hypokalemia during early life when the glomerular filtration rate is low.[27] However, maximized from the outset, there may be limited reserve for episodes of hypotension or hypoperfusion.[28]

Acid-Base Balance

Infants demonstrate incomplete renal acid-base homeostasis, being influenced by such factors as stress of delivery, ambient temperature, and diet.[29] The infant normally exists in a state of slight metabolic acidosis, which may become significant in 10% of premature infants between the first and second week of life.[18] This delayed metabolic acidosis is noted especially in low-birth-weight infants and is characterized by a blood pH less than 7.25, total serum CO_2 less than 21 mEq/L, or a base deficit greater than 8 mEq/L.[30] This acidosis has several etiologies. Bicarbonate reabsorption is diminished in the renal proximal tubule,[31] and the distal tubular excretion of some acids is reduced because of a lack of urinary buffers. In addition, ammonia production is decreased in the immature kidney. Premature infants are unable to maximally acidify urine, with urine pH after birth maintained above 6.0.[18] Regardless of prematurity, by 1 month of age the urine becomes maximally acidified.[24] Acid-base homeostatic mechanisms reach adult capabilities by 2 years of age.[18]

Fluid Balance

Maintenance fluid requirements in the newborn are based on insensible losses, volume of urine required to excrete solute load, and fluid retained for growth. These requirements are based on caloric expenditure per kilogram body weight. Neonates have higher requirements. The ambient temperature and humidity, motor activity, congenital defects, skin trauma, and crying can profoundly affect insensible losses.[13, 32] For example, a 1°C body temperature elevation results in a 10% increase in caloric expenditure.[33]

Total body water (TBW) changes greatly during maturation, both in gross amount and in the ratio between extracellular water (ECW) and intracellular water (ICW). Total body water is about 94% of fetal body weight in the third gestational month and declines to 78% at term.[34]

The extracellular water volume greatly exceeds intracellular water volume in early gestation but declines as intracellular water increases, especially after birth. This is probably a reflection of postnatal improvement in renal function.[34] Overhydration of the neonate or failure to allow extracellular water contraction increases the risk of a significant patent ductus and necrotizing enterocolitis.[35, 36] Intracellular water increases parallel to body weight in the first weeks of prenatal life. After this time, the ratio changes more quickly, and by 3 months of age intracellular exceeds extracellular water.[37, 38]

Electrolytes

The primary extracellular electrolytes are the cation sodium and the anion chloride. Proteins and bicarbonate contribute to anions to a lesser extent. The primary intracellular electrolytes are the cations potassium and magnesium and the anion phosphate (organic and inorganic) (Fig. 10–1).[34]

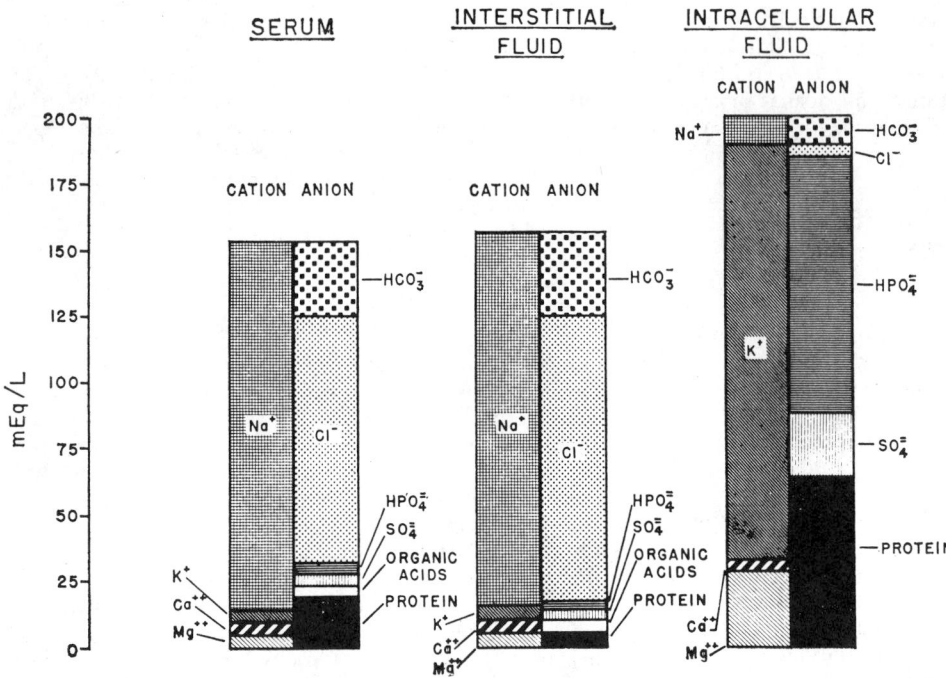

Figure 10–1. Differences in the composition of intracellular and extracellular fluids. (From Nelson WE, Behrman RE, Vaughan VC (eds). Nelson Textbook of Pediatrics. Philadelphia, WB Saunders, 1987, p 176.)

FLUID HOMEOSTASIS

Water is essential for existence, and its loss results in death within days.[39] Pediatric maintenance water requirements are related to insensible losses, volume of urine required to excrete solute load, and fluid retained for growth. These maintenance requirements are based on caloric expenditure per body surface area or kilogram weight and are the result of loss of water from heat production. Heat and water loss are proportional to body surface area.

Fluid Requirements

Estimates of fluid requirements based on surface area are accurate regardless of body size.[40] However, body weight is a more familiar measure to use for the physician, is easily measured, does not require a nomogram at hand (Fig. 10–2), and can be used to estimate the surface area in children with normal height-for-weight relationships (Table 10–1). If using body weight, there is a need for a reduction in dose with increasing age and size.[40]

The infant's surface-to-mass ratio is five times greater than that of an adult. This means more heat per unit of mass must be produced to remain in thermal balance.[41] Because of the increased heat loss there is a proportionately increased water loss. The human infant must ingest larger amounts of water per unit body weight (equivalent to 10% to 15% of body weight) than the adult (2% to 4%), but the two are approximately equal in caloric expenditure.[39]

Water Sources

Most water absorption occurs in the duodenum and jejunum, although water is also absorbed throughout the gastrointestinal tract to some degree.[42] Absorption occurs primarily by passive diffusion following active transport of sodium.[43] A small amount of water is endogenously created by carbohydrate and fat metabolism, yielding approximately 12 ml water per 100 calories metabolized. Smaller amounts of water can be obtained from sources such as nebulized inspired gas during mechanical ventilation (10 to 15 ml/kcal/day) and "preformed" water from tissue catabolism during disease states or times of catabolic stress.[42] Water rapidly equilibrates throughout the intracellular and vascular compartments to maintain a homeostatic balance.[40]

Water Losses

Water loss occurs from urinary excretion of solute loads, from water loss in the gastrointestinal tract, and from insensible losses through the lungs and skin. Urinary water excretion is proportional to the metabolic rate. Because infant kidneys receive a high solute load and have a low concentrating ability, more water is required to excrete waste.[19] This makes infants more prone to develop a water deficit, or dehydration.

The gastrointestinal system accounts for 5% of normal daily losses. The gastrointestinal tract provides the most frequent challenges to water homeostasis because of the frequency of vomiting and diarrhea in children. Fluid and electrolyte losses occur in diarrhea; in vomiting not only is there fluid loss, but also oral intake of further fluids is precluded.

Controlling Mechanisms

Despite much variability of intake, plasma osmolality (the concentration of solute particles) remains an almost constant 285 to 295 mOsm/kg water.[43] Thirst is the volitional control of fluid intake and is one of the primary mechanisms used to regulate the plasma osmolarity. Thirst is stimulated by osmoreceptor and volume receptors, along with possible interactions with angiotensin II and antidiuretic hormone (ADH).[42, 43] The other primary control mechanism complementing thirst is the secretion of ADH. ADH increases the permeability of the renal collecting ducts, promoting resorption of water.[42, 43]

DEHYDRATION

Dehydration is a state of negative water balance. This negative balance can result from either inadequate fluid

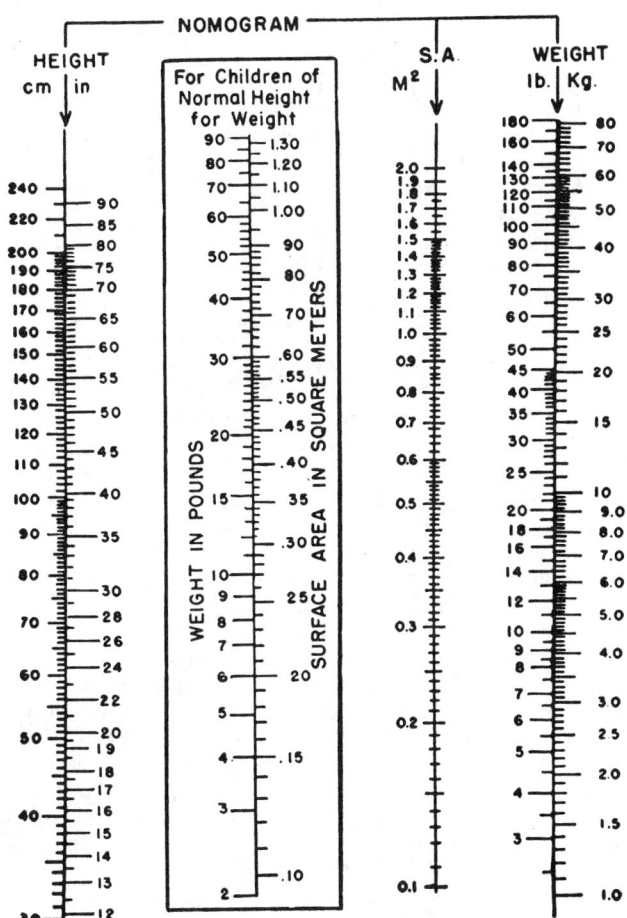

Figure 10–2. Nomogram for the estimation of surface area. The surface area is indicated at the point at which a straight line that connects the height and weight levels intersects the surface area column. If the patient is roughly of average size, the surface area can also be determined from weight alone (enclosed area). (From Nelson WE, Behrman RE, Vaughan VC (eds). Nelson Textbook of Pediatrics. Philadelphia, WB Saunders, 1987, p 1521. Nomogram modified by CD West from the data of E Boyd.)

intake or excessive losses (Table 10–2). Dehydration resulting from purely decreased intake is rare. Children with impaired thirst, anorexia, physical restraints, or in a comatose state can have a decreased intake, but the regulatory mechanisms (especially ADH release) are activated and fluid is conserved. Increased losses are from insensible, renal, and gastrointestinal sources.

TABLE 10–1
WATER REQUIREMENTS*

Body Weight (kg)	Water Requirement/Day
≤10	100 ml/kg
11–20	1000 ml + 50 ml/kg for each kilogram above 10 kg
>20	1500 ml + 20 ml/kg for each kilogram above 20 kg
Adults	2000–2400 ml/day

*For water maintainance based on total body surface area, 2000 ml/M² is recommended

TABLE 10–2
ETIOLOGY OF DEHYDRATION

Reduced intake
  Anorexia
  Coma
  Fluid restriction
Increased loss
  Gastrointestinal
    Vomiting
    Diarrhea
    Enterocutaneous fistula or drains
  Renal
    Osmotic diuresis
    Diuretic administration
    Adrenal insufficiency
    Chronic renal failure
    Salt-losing nephropathy
    Postobstructive diuresis
    Central or nephrogenic diabetes inspidus
  Skin and respiratory
    Heat exposure
    Cystic fibrosis
    Inflammatory skin disease
    Burns

From Awazu M, Kon V, Barakat AY. Volume disorders. *In* Ichikawa I (ed). Pediatric Textbook of Fluids and Electrolytes. Baltimore, Williams & Wilkins, 1990, p 121.

Insensible Losses

Increased insensible losses are seen with inflammatory skin conditions such as burns, pemphigus, and exfoliative dermatitis. Dehydration is more common in the child with cystic fibrosis because of high perspiration sodium concentrations and resulting passive fluid loss. Tachypnea and fever are other sources of insensible fluid loss.

Renal Losses

Renal water loss can occur despite normal renal function. Osmotic diuretics (glucose, mannitol, radiocontrast media) in large amounts can cause significant water loss. Diuretics (furosemide, thiazides, ethacrynic acid) inhibit sodium and water resorption, resulting in both diuresis and natriuresis. Adrenal insufficiency can cause hypovolemia with associated hyponatremia, hyperkalemia, and acidosis as a result of the inability to reabsorb sodium or excrete potassium and hydrogen ion.

Hypotonic fluid loss occurs in central or nephrogenic diabetes insipidus. Excessive loss of water caused by renal tubular dysfunction can be secondary to chronic pyelonephritis, medullary cystic disease, postobstructive diuresis, sickle cell disease, hypokalemia, and hypercalcemia.

Gastrointestinal Losses

Water loss from the gastrointestinal tract is the most common cause of dehydration in the child. Vomiting or nasogastric suction results in loss of acidic fluid, usually resulting in a metabolic alkalosis. Because potassium is in all gastrointestinal fluids, gastrointestinal losses are usually accompanied by potassium depletion.

CLINICAL EVALUATION

The magnitude of dehydration is accurately assessed by weight loss, but this information is rarely available to the clinician. Instead, clinical estimates must be made based on symptoms and physical examination. This can be inaccurate, as patients with identical fluid deficits but differing osmolar loads will present differently. For example, the child with hypernatremic dehydration will appear to have a less severe deficit than the child with hyponatremic dehydration. In young infants a weight loss of up to 5% is considered mild dehydration, 5% to 10% is moderate, and greater than 15% is severe. Severe dehydration is usually associated with circulatory failure.

Degree of dehydration =

$$\frac{[\text{Pre-illness weight (kg)}-\text{admission weight}]}{\text{Pre-illness weight}} \times 100$$

History

The clinical history should optimally document a pre-illness weight and the type and frequency of fluid losses (Table 10–3). Urine output is usually low in dehydrated patients, except in some low-birth-weight infants who have poor renal concentrating abilities. Continued urinary output despite dehydration should suggest intrinsic renal disease, diabetes mellitus, or diabetes insipidus.

Dehydration is a balance between intake and output, and it is important to investigate the type and quantity of oral intake. Tap water has virtually no sodium and can contribute to hyponatremia. Homemade electrolyte solutions are generally inconsistently prepared and can be dangerous to the child.[44, 45]

Physical Examination

The child with mild dehydration may have thirst only (Table 10–4). Most children with moderate to severe dehydration appear ill. This appearance ranges from restlessness and lethargy to coma with circulatory collapse. Children with severe dehydration can present with nuchal rigidity resembling meningeal infection.

The skin is evaluated for the turgor by pinching the skin and subcutaneous tissues with the index finger and thumb. Turgor is related to capillary filling after pinching and can be decreased with significant dehydration; however, it may be normal in the well-nourished but dehydrated child. Evaluation for turgor should not be performed over the anterior chest and the abdomen to avoid being misled by taut skin secondary to abdominal distention. Normal skin retracts immediately. Children with hypernatremic dehydration may present with velvet-like or doughy skin (Table 10–5).

TABLE 10–3

HISTORICAL DATA REQUIRED IN ESTIMATING MAGNITUDE AND TYPES OF DEFICIT AND IN PLANNING DEFICIT THERAPY

Intake–during period of illness
  Quantity and how given
  Kind: water, electrolyte, protein, drugs
Output—during period of illness
  Quantity
  Kind: urine, vomiting, diarrhea, sweat, drainage
Balance
  Weight change
General medical
  Age
  Cardiovascular, respiratory, renal, or central nervous
    system

From Nelson WE, Behrman RE, Vaughan VC (eds). Nelson Textbook of Pediatrics. Philadelphia, WB Saunders, 1987, p 195.

The anterior fontanelle should be examined, if present. If it is depressed, dehydration is strongly suggested. The eyes appear sunken, with darkened periorbital areas. Tears may be decreased or absent. Intraocular pressure by palpation is decreased. Clinical assessment of mucous membranes can be misleading. Mucous membranes will be dry in dehydration, but prolonged mouth breathing or tachypnea may mimic dehydration.

With severe dehydration, shock may be present as manifested by hypotension, tachycardia, and cyanosis. Skin color and capillary refill should be assessed but interpreted with consideration to the ambient temperatures.

DIAGNOSTIC EVALUATION

Laboratory evaluation will help assess the type of deficit and therapy required, but serial evaluations are of greater importance. No laboratory test is specific for dehydration. Therapy should be initiated while laboratory studies are pending.

The serum sodium reflects the ratio between body water and sodium and is not an evaluation of the total body sodium content. In fact, the total body sodium is usually decreased in all dehydrated patients, including those with hypernatremia. Serum potassium is not a reflection of body stores, as it is primarily an intracellular cation. Serum levels can be elevated despite intracellular deficits in renal failure, acidosis, and cellular damage. The serum chloride will permit calculation of the anion gap and will reflect unmeasured anions. The bicarbonate level gives an indication as to presence of acidemia or alkalemia. The blood urea nitrogen (BUN) and creatinine levels may be elevated because of a decreased glomerular filtration rate. This is a result of decreased renal perfusion and is described as *prerenal azotemia*.

The urinalysis may show a variety of abnormal findings secondary to dehydration and should be repeated once rehydration and recovery have occurred. These findings may include proteinuria, red and white blood cells, and casts (both hyaline and granular). The specific gravity should be high proportionate to the degree of dehydration to exclude intrinsic renal disease. The specific gravity is used to follow the effectiveness of fluid replacement therapy.

DIFFERENTIAL DIAGNOSIS

Dehydration is typically divided into three types based on the serum sodium concentration. *Hyponatremic* dehydration implies a serum sodium less than 130 mEq/L; *isonatremic* dehydration is a sodium between 130 to 150 mEq/L. *Hypernatremic* dehydration is present when sodium exceeds 150 mEq/L. Serum osmolality is largely a reflection of serum sodium, and for this reason the three types of dehydration are often referred to as *hypotonic, isotonic,* and *hypertonic* dehydration. Neverthelesss, the terms *osmolality* and *tonicity* are not exactly interchangeable, as the tonicity does not always reflect sodium changes. With uremia or diabetic ketoacidosis, the serum is hypertonic owing to levels of urea and glucose, respectively, and the serum sodium may be low.

Concepts to aid in the understanding of fluid and electrolyte disturbances are (1) the total body amounts of water and solute and their relative relationship and (2) the distribution of water and solute between body compartments (i.e., intracellular versus extracellular).

Hyponatremic Dehydration

Hyponatremic dehydration results from a proportionately greater loss of sodium and potassium when compared with

TABLE 10–4

CLINICAL ASSESSMENT OF SEVERITY OF DEHYDRATION

Signs and Symptoms	Mild Dehydration	Moderate Dehydration	Severe Dehydration
General appearance and condition:			
Infants and young children	Thirsty; alert; restless	Thirsty; restless or lethargic but irritable to touch or drowsy	Drowsy; limp, cold, sweaty, cyanotic extremities; may be comatose
Older children and adults	Thirsty; alert; restless	Thirsty; alert; postural hypotension	Usually conscious; apprehensive; cold, sweaty, cyanotic extremities; wrinkled skin of fingers and toes; muscle cramps
Radial pulse	Normal rate and strength	Rapid and weak	Rapid, feeble, sometimes impalpable
Respiration	Normal	Deep, maybe rapid	Deep and rapid
Anterior fontanel	Normal	Sunken	Very sunken
Systolic blood pressure	Normal	Normal or low	Less than 90 mm; may be unrecordable
Skin elasticity	Pinch retracts immediately	Pinch retracts slowly	Pinch retracts very slowly (>2 sec)
Eyes	Normal	Sunken (detectable)	Grossly sunken
Tears	Present	Absent	Absent
Mucous membranes	Moist	Dry	Very dry
Urine flow	Normal	Reduced amount and dark	None passed for several hours; empty bladder
% Body weight loss	4%–5%	6%–9%	10% or more
Estimated fluid deficit	40–50 mL/kg	60–90 mL/kg	100–110 mL/kg

From Nelson WE, Behrman RE, Vaughan VC (eds). Nelson Textbook of Pediatrics. Philadelphia, WB Saunders, 1987, p 196.
Modified from World Health Organization guide.

water. This type of dehydration most commonly results from the intake of hypotonic solutions in an attempt to replace gastrointestinal losses. The initial effect is for the intracellular fluid to become hyperosmolar in relation to the extracellular fluid as sodium is lost. Water then moves intracellularly. As water equilibrates across the cell membrane, both extracellular and intracellular spaces become hypotonic, and extracellular (intravascular) volume is reduced. The result is decreased organ perfusion and more severe symptoms of dehydration.

Isonatremic Dehydration

Isonatremic dehydration is the most common type of dehydration and occurs as a result of equal losses of solute

and water. The most common cause of isonatremic dehydration is gastrointestinal fluid loss, although urinary losses and decreased fluid intake may also contribute. Because the net loss is isotonic, there is no osmolar gradient between the extracellular and intracellular fluid. There is no redistribution between fluid compartments, and the resultant fluid loss is entirely from the extracellular fluid. This means a reduction in plasma volume and circulating blood volume.[46]

Hypernatremic Dehydration

Hypernatremic dehydration is caused by a greater loss of water than solute. The extracellular fluid becomes contracted and hypertonic. Fluid shifts from the intracellular to the

TABLE 10–5

EFFECTS OF TYPE OF DEHYDRATION ON PHYSICAL SIGNS

	Isonatremic Dehydration (Proportionate Loss of Water and Sodium)	Hyponatremic Dehydration (Loss of Sodium in Excess of Water)	Hypernatremic Dehydration (Loss of Water in Excess of Sodium)
ECF Volume	Markedly decreased	Severely decreased	Decreased
ICF Volume	Maintained	Increased	Decreased
Physical Signs			
Skin			
Color*	Gray	Gray	Gray
Temperature	Cold	Cold	Cold or hot
Turgor†	Poor	Very poor	Fair
Feel	Dry	Clammy	Thickened, doughy
Mucous membrane	Dry	Slightly moist	Parched‡
Eyeball	Sunken and soft	Sunken and soft	Sunken
Fontanel	Sunken	Sunken	Sunken
Psyche	Lethargic	Coma	Hyperirritable
Pulse*	Rapid	Rapid	Moderately rapid
Blood pressure*	Low	Very low	Moderately low

ECF = Extracellular fluid; ICF = intracellular fluid.
*Signs of shock rather than of dehydration itself.
†Reflects magnitude of fluid loss from ECF.
‡Tongue often has shriveled appearance owing to loss of cellular fluid.

extracellular compartment, resulting in extracellular fluid expansion at the cost of intracellular volume. Both the intracellular and extracellular fluids ultimately become hyperosmolar. Circulation is well maintained, and the degree of dehydration is underestimated. The intracellular dehydration can be so severe that brain cells can contract in volume, tearing bridging vessels and resulting in a subdural or subarachnoid hemorrhage. The child may appear to have meningeal signs and symptoms of a central nervous system infection such as nuchal rigidity, irritability, a high-pitched cry, and seizures.

Hyperglycemia and hypocalcemia frequently accompany hypernatremic dehydration. Hyperglycemia is thought to be due to either stress or decreased glucose uptake by the dehydrated cells[47]; the origin of the hypocalcemia is unknown.[48]

THERAPEUTIC INTERVENTION

Fluid and electrolyte therapy is broadly divided into two categories: deficit replacement and maintenance. Maintenance needs assume normal water requirements are directly proportional to caloric expenditure. One milliliter per kilogram of water is required for every kilocalorie of energy expended. Therefore maintenance fluid can be calculated from the body weight in kilograms (see Table 10–3).

Deficit Replacement

The treatment plan for the dehydrated patient is developed at the time of the examination. Ideally, the physician would know the exact percentage dehydration, the magnitude of sodium and potassium loss, and the acid-base status. However, these values are often unknown when therapy is initiated. No laboratory test is so important that therapy for the dehydrated child should be withheld.

Children with mild to moderate dehydration can be appropriately managed with oral replacement therapy. Parenteral therapy is indicated for rapid intravascular volume replacement in a child with shock or for ongoing losses from continued vomiting or diarrhea. Although the intravenous route is preferred, replacement fluids have been given intraperitoneally, subcutaneously, and intraosseously. Parenteral deficit therapy is divided into three phases: initial therapy, repletion or restoration therapy, and final (early recovery) phase.

Initial Therapy

The goal of initial treatment is to restore circulating volume and increase tissue perfusion, especially renal perfusion (Table 10–6). The crystalloid of choice should have a sodium concentration approximating that of serum and should contain dextrose to provide a metabolic substrate. Ill children have high metabolic demands and store little glycogen, making them especially prone to hypoglycemia. The most appropriate choices for immediate infusion are isotonic saline with 5 gm/dl glucose (D5/0.9 NS) and LR with 5 gm/dl glucose (D5 LR). These solutions are usually readily available in emergency departments. Other choices may include plasma expanders (albumin, hetastarch) or whole blood.

The crystalloid solution should be infused in a 20- to 30-ml/kg volume as rapidly as possible to the hypoperfused patient or over a 1-hour period in the less critically ill child. If adequate circulation and clinical response does not occur, an additional 20- to 30-ml/kg bolus can be given. Only rarely will a third bolus be needed.

If severe acidosis is present, it can be addressed in either

TABLE 10–6	
THERAPY AT A GLANCE: REHYDRATION STRATEGIES	
Phase	**Strategy**
Initial	20–30 ml/kg bolus D5/0.9 NS or D5 LR May repeat twice if necessary 5% albumin, 0.9% NS, LR, and whole blood are alternatives
Restorative	Maintenance fluids + deficit fluids + ongoing losses − initial phase fluids administered = total fluid replacement 50% total fluids administered over first 8 hours (D5/0.45 NS or D5/0.9 NS) 50% total fluids administered over subsequent 16 hours Correct acidosis if severe (initial or restorative phase)
Final	Oral therapy if possible (exception: hypernatremic dehydration)—restoration of body potassium

LR = Lactated Ringer's solution; NS = normal saline.

the initial or repletion phases. In the initial treatment phase, administration of bicarbonate may help correct pH while renal acid excretion is subnormal as a result of decreased perfusion. The lactate or acetate in intravenous solutions may not be readily convertible to bicarbonate in the child with decreased perfusion and may, in fact, worsen the acidosis. Adding 26 ml of 7.5% sodium bicarbonate solution to 750 ml 0.9% chloride, then increasing the final volume to one liter with D5W will result in a solution containing 140 mEq/L sodium, 115 mEq/L chloride, and 25 mEq/L bicarbonate per liter.[49]

Once circulation and perfusion have been reestablished, serum electrolytes will guide fluid and electrolyte therapy in both the restoration and final phases of therapy. The initial therapy will tend to normalize serum sodium except in hypertonic dehydration, in which the sodium may paradoxically rise by an unknown mechanism.

Potassium replacement need not be initiated in the initial treatment phase and should be withheld until renal function is established (Table 10–7). The only exception is the severely hypokalemic patient or if there are conditions known to cause extreme potassium depletion (e.g., diabetic ketoacidosis).

Repletion or Restoration Therapy

The restorative phase encompasses the first 24 hours of the patient's stay in the hospital and in most cases begins when the patient reaches the inpatient floor. Sodium and water alterations are gradually corrected. During the initial treatment, potassium replacement need not begin unless the patient is severely hypokalemic or is known to have a condition leading to extreme potassium depletion.

Fluid replacement is determined by maintenance requirements plus deficit replacement, in addition to ongoing losses. Serial electrolyte determinations guide sodium correction.

TABLE 10–7		
ELECTROLYTE REQUIREMENTS		
Sodium	=	2–3 mEq/100 kcal
Potassium	=	2–3 mEq/100 kcal
Chloride	=	2–5 mEq/100 kcal

Patient monitoring should include body weight and urine output. To manage severe acidosis in the restorative phase, the guidelines for sodium bicarbonate administration in Table 10–8 may be followed.

Hyponatremic Dehydration. Hyponatremic dehydration results from a proportionately greater loss of sodium than water. The initial treatment is identical to that of isonatremic and hypernatremic dehydration. The restorative phase is identical to that of isonatremic dehydration except for replacing sodium deficit. The additional sodium is administered over several days as volume is expanded, and as the sodium returns to normal, the body fluids become isonatremic. Thus the patient continues to be treated similarly to the patient with isonatremic dehydration, requiring isotonic fluids. Sodium deficit is calculated by the following formula:

$$\text{Sodium deficit in (mEq)} = (135 \text{ mEq/L} - \text{measured serum Na}^+) \times \text{Total body water}$$

The value 135 mEq/L represents the desired goal of sodium repletion, the low-normal value. Sodium is primarily an extracellular cation but exerts osmotic effects on both extracellular and intracellular compartments. Using total body water in calculating the deficit allows for this osmotic effect and for repletion of intracellular sources. Because of dehydration, total body water should be estimated at 50% to 55% measured body weight, rather than the usual 60%.

The serum sodium need not be rapidly raised unless the patient has symptoms of water intoxication (e.g., seizures). Symptoms are unusual unless the serum sodium falls below 120 mEq/L. If rapid correction is necessary, a 3% hypertonic sodium chloride solution (513 mEq/L of Na$^+$) can be administered intravenously at a rate of 1 ml/min to a maximum of 12 ml per kilogram of body weight.[50] The rise in sodium of 2 mEq/L/hr or less to a level of 120 mEq/L is considered safe. The desired serum sodium in this case is lower than the "low-normal" serum sodium of 135 mEq/L. An association between rapid, complete correction of hyponatremia and central pontine myelinolysis has been reported, though the relationship is unclear.

The addition of hypertonic saline expands extracellular volume to a lesser extent than an equal amount of isotonic solution. The extracellular expansion occurs as a result of intracellular volume loss; thus total body volume changes little. The rate of fluid administration is reduced after hypertonic saline infusion to allow equilibration of water and sodium levels.

Isonatremic Dehydration. Losses of fluid and solute are proportionate in isonatremic dehydration. Because the goal of the restorative phase is to continue replenishment of sodium and water deficits, a solution similar to that used in the initial treatment is continued. A 0.9% sodium chloride solution with 5 gm/dl dextrose (D5/0.9% NS) is a satisfactory choice, although 0.45% isotonic saline with added dextrose (D5/0.45 NS) can also be used.

Total fluids needed in the restorative phase will equal maintenance and deficit requirements, in addition to ongoing losses. One half of the total fluid amount should be given during the first 8 hours (subtracting the "initial phase" fluid amount) and the remaining one half of the fluid total over the next 16 hours.

Some feel that only two thirds of the needed fluids should be administered over the first 24 hours. This would theoretically prevent volume overload later as sodium shifts extracellular. This extracellular sodium shift is in response to potassium intracellular movement as potassium is replenished and acidosis is corrected.

Potassium is lost in amounts equivalent to those of sodium in isonatremic dehydration, but it cannot be replaced at a similar rate, or dangerous hyperkalemia can result. When renal function is assured, potassium may be added to the intravenous solution in a concentration of 20 to 40 mEq/L.

Hypernatremic Dehydration. Hypernatremic dehydration is a result of a proportionately greater loss of water than sodium. The total body sodium deficit is usually small, and extracellular volume is well maintained, so that the amounts of water and sodium to be administered are less than in hyponatremic or isonatremic dehydration.

Hypernatremic dehydration can result in permanent neurologic injury from cerebral hemorrhage, vascular thrombosis, or subdural hemorrhage induced by a dehydrated, contracting brain that shrinks and tears bridging vessels. Seizures are common with hypernatremic dehydration, even without pathologic cerebral findings.

In hypernatremic dehydration, water leaves brain cells, which respond by attempting to raise intracellular osmolarity by increasing concentrations of glucose, sodium and potassium. Proteins break down to form idiogenic osmoles.[51] During rehydration, water crosses the cell membrane rapidly, whereas solute equilibration can take hours to days. This inequity between water and solute movement may lead to cerebral edema and seizure activity. The mechanism of rehydration seizures in hypernatremic dehydration is unclear, but the predilection can be reduced by correcting the sodium and water abnormalities over a 48-hour period. If seizures occur during rehydration, the rehydration fluid should be discontinued, and 3 to 5 ml/kg of 3% sodium chloride solution (or hypertonic mannitol) infused. This should control the seizures.

Suitable solutions for restorative therapy in hypernatremic dehydration are 5% dextrose solution with 0.33% isotonic saline and 25 mEq/L potassium chloride (D5/0.33% NS with 25 mEq/L KCl) or a 5% dextrose solution with 0.45% isotonic saline and 25 mEq/L potassium chloride (D5/0.45% NS with 25 mEq/L KCl).[40] Some investigators theorize that a relative insulin deficiency is present in some cases of hypernatremia and therefore a 2% or 3% dextrose solution, rather than a 5% dextrose solution, should be used instead.[52]

Whatever solution is chosen, the crucial factor is gradual, continuous replacement over 48 hours of calculated maintenance plus deficits and ongoing losses. Treatment should not decrease the sodium by more than 2 mEq/hr or more than 10 mEq/L per 24-hour period.[53, 54] Ultimately, the clinical response should dictate the reduction in sodium.

Administration of large amounts of fluid in hypernatremic dehydration may result in extracellular fluid expansion before any correction of acidosis or chloride loss. This could lead to edema and congestive heart failure, requiring digitalization. In addition, hypernatremic dehydration may result in renal tubular injury with resultant azotemia and loss of urine-concentrating ability.[54]

Hypocalcemia is often seen with hypernatremic dehydra-

TABLE 10–8

SODIUM BICARBONATE DOSING

Arterial pH	Sodium Bicarbonate
7.2	0.3–0.7 mEq/kg
7.1	0.5–1.0 mEq/kg
7.0	1.0–1.5 mEq/kg

Bicarbonate should be administered over 2 hours, and then the pH should be reassessed.

Modified with permission from Awazu M, Davarajan P, Stewart C, et al. Maintenance therapy and treatment of dehydration and overhydration. *In* Ichikawa I (ed). Pediatric Textbook of Fluids and Electrolytes. Baltimore, Williams & Wilkins, 1990, p 418

TABLE 10–9				
ORAL ELECTROLYTE SOLUTION COMPOSITION				
	Sodium (mEq/L)	Potassium (mEq/L)	Chloride (mEq/L)	Carbohydrate (g/dl)
Rehydration solutions				
World Health Organization formulation	90	20	80	2.0 (glucose)
Rehydralyte	75	20	65	2.5 (glucose)
Maintenance solutions				
Pedialyte	45	20	35	2.5 (glucose)
Lytren	50	25	45	2.0 (glucose)
Resol	50	20	50	2.0 (glucose)
Infalyte	50	20	40	2.0 (glucose)
Ricelyte	50	25	45	30 (glucose polymers)

tion and may be prevented by administering appropriate amounts of potassium. If hypocalcemia is already present, it will require calcium replacement.

Final (Early Recovery) Phase

The final phase of rehydration occurs from 24 hours to 4 days after hospitalization. Body stores of potassium, fat, carbohydrate, and protein are restored. Oral intake is usually begun but may not be possible in the child with ongoing vomiting or diarrhea or in one requiring the remaining slow correction of hypernatremic dehydration.

ORAL REHYDRATION THERAPY

Oral rehydration therapy (ORT) is used extensively in the Third World but is not commonly employed in the United States. The majority of dehydrated children can be rehydrated orally. Contraindications are severe dehydration, shock, intractable vomiting, and profuse diarrhea. There are no age restrictions, and no special monitoring is required.

Water absorption is a passive, unidirectional flow from bowel lumen to blood, driven by osmotic forces and solute movement.[55] Sodium flux is central to many intestinal processes.[56] It determines which oral rehydration solution should be used as well as the subsequent success of therapy. Gut epithelial cells expel two sodium ions for each potassium absorbed. This maintains a low intracellular sodium concentration and, thus, a favorable gradient for absorption. Co-transportation with sodium is a common mechanism, en-

hancing the absorption of monosaccharides and amino acids as well as water. Conversely, glucose and the hexoses augment sodium absorption. Chloride absorption passively follows sodium.

Diarrhea is fecal loss beyond normal amounts and may result from decreased absorption (osmotic agents), increased water secretion (secretory diarrhea), or a combination of both. In secretory diarrhea, crypt epithelial cells of the gut actively secrete chloride, and water follows. Water is primarily absorbed by the epithelial cells on the villous tips in the gut, which are usually unaffected in secretory diarrhea. This, coupled with an increased chloride permeability at the villous tip, allows even children with enterotoxin-induced secretory diarrhea to be successfully rehydrated with oral glucose-electrolyte solutions.[57]

Two types of oral electrolyte solutions exist, varying primarily with regard to sodium concentration. Rehydration solutions contain 60 to 90 mEq/L sodium, and maintenance solutions contain 40 to 60 mEq/L sodium (Table 10–9).

The World Health Organization (WHO) rehydration solution was developed in the 1970s to treat cholera-associated dehydration and contains 90 mEq/L sodium. This oral rehydrating solution can also be safely used in children with nonsecretory diarrhea if sufficient free water is also provided. The majority of diarrhea in developed nations is nonsecretory, and hypernatremia has been reported in young children given WHO rehydrating solution for nonsecretory diarrhea.[58] Therefore maintenance solutions with 40 to 60 mEq/L sodium are often used to maintain fluid and electrolyte balance after rehydration and to prevent further dehydration.

TABLE 10–10				
COMPOSITION OF CLEAR LIQUID BEVERAGES				
Fluid	Sodium (mmol/L)	Potassium (mmol/L)	Carbohydrate (gm/100 mL)	Osmolarity (mmol/L)
Beef broths	110–248	2.5–17	—	300–390
Chicken broths	140–251	1.5–8.2	—	380–500
Apple juice	0.1–3.5	24–32	12	650–734
Grape juice	0.8–2.8	31–44	15	1170–1190
Colas	1.3–1.7	0.1	10.4–11.3	390–750
Gingerale	0.8–5.5	0.1–1.5	5.3	520–560
7-Up	5–5.5	1.0–2.0	7.4	520–550
Kool-Aid	0.5–1.2	0.1–1.8	10.6	250–590
Popsicles	4.7–5.6	0.5–2.0	NA	670–720
Jell-O	22–27	1.3–2.0	15.8	570–640
Tea (unsweetened)	0	5	0	—
Gatorade	20	3	4.6	330

NA = Not available.
From Casteel HB, Fiedorek SC: Oral rehydration therapy. Pediatr Clin North Am 1990; 37(2):304.

Most liquid rehydration solutions contain citrate as their base. The WHO formulation is a powder requiring reconstitution and uses bicarbonate as a base. Both citrate and bicarbonate are equally effective in treating the acidosis infants develop from fecal bicarbonate loss and decreased renal excretion of hydrogen ion. On reconstitution, the bicarbonate in the WHO solution produces a brownish discoloration.

Although sucrose can be used,[59, 60] 2.0% to 2.5% solutions of glucose remain the standard. Higher concentrations of glucose result in osmotic diarrhea from carbohydrate malabsorption. Higher concentrations of carbohydrate do not result in higher absorption of sodium.

Hydrolyzed wheat- and rice-based oral electrolyte solutions appear to be superior to glucose oral solutions in rehydrating patients. In addition, rice-based rehydrating solutions may decrease the frequency and volume of stools.[61]

The concentrations of sodium in juices, soda, flavored gelatin, and sports drinks are either excessive or insufficient, making them inappropriate for treatment of dehydration (Table 10–10). Likewise, homemade solutions prepared with household measuring devices can result in inconsistently prepared solutions that can be dangerous to the child.[44, 45]

Oral rehydration therapy is similar to parenteral rehydration with an initial treatment and subsequent restorative phase. Many empiric regimens exist, differing mostly in the amount of fluid administered. They do not differ greatly regarding solutions or schedule of administration.

The WHO regimen recommends administration of its rehydration solution at a rate of 100 ml/kg for 4 hours, followed by 50 ml/kg of water or breast milk for the next 2 hours. If the child is still dehydrated, the WHO formula is given at 50 ml/kg over the next 6 hours. If the child is then hydrated, the WHO rehydration solution is administered at a rate of 100 ml/kg for 24 hours. It is an absolute requirement that liquids with free water be concomitantly administered.[62, 63]

After rehydration therapy, maintenance solution is given at a rate of 150 ml/kg/day. This amount can be increased if stools persist, supplemented freely with breast milk, or alternated in volume amounts with soy formula.[62, 63] Exclusive administration of oral electrolyte solution should not persist beyond 24 hours, and if a rehydration solution is to be used as maintenance therapy, free water must be supplied.

References

1. Consnett JE. The origins of intravenous fluid therapy. Lancet 1989;1:768.
2. O'Shaughnessy WB. Experiments on the blood in cholera. Lancet 1831;1:490.
3. Latta T. Relative to the treatment of cholera by the copious injections of aqueous and saline fluids into the veins. Lancet 1831;2:274.
4. Sellands AW, Shaklee AD. Indications of acid intoxication in adriatic cholera. Philippine J Surg 1911;6(Sec B):53.
5. Ho MS, Glass RI, Pinsky PF, et al. Diarrheal deaths in American children, are they preventable? JAMA 1988;260:3281.
6. Carpenter CCJ, Greenough WB, Pierce NF. Oral rehydration therapy— the role of polymeric substrates. N Engl J Med 1988;319:1346.
7. Snyder JD, Merson MH. The magnitude of the global problem of acute diarrhoeal disease: A review of active surveillance data. Bull WHO 1982;60:605.
8. Filler RM. The newborn and young infant. In Dudrick SJ, Daue AE, Eiseman B, et al (eds). Manual of Preoperative and Postoperative Care. Philadelphia, WB Saunders, 1983, p 307.
9. Chesney RW, Zelikovic I. Pre- and postoperative fluid management in infancy. Pediatr Rev 1989;3:343.
10. Jaykka S. The problem of dormant fetal organs: The kidneys, lungs, and the gut. Biol Neonate. 1961;3:343.
11. Avner ED, Ellis D, Ichikawa I, et al. Normal neonates and the maturational development of homeostatic mechanisms. In Ichikawa I (ed). Pediatric Textbook of Fluids and Electrolytes. Baltimore, William & Wilkins, 1990, p 107.
12. Yared A. Regulation of renal blood flow and glomerular filtration rate.
In Ichikawa I (ed). Pediatric Textbook of Fluids and Electrolytes. Baltimore, William & Wilkins, 1990, p 46.
13. Bell EF, Oh W. Fluid and electrolyte management. In Avery GB (ed). Neonatology Pathophysiology and Management of the Newborn. Philadelphia, JB Lippincott, 1987, p 777.
14. Behrman RE, Vaughan VC (eds). The urinary system, nephrologic diseases. In Nelson Textbook of Pediatrics. Philadelphia, WB Saunders, 1987, p 1126.
15. Robillard JE, Kulvinskas C, Sessions C, et al. Maturational changes in the fetal glomerular filtration rate. Am J Obstet Gynecol 1975;122:601.
16. Guignard JP, Torrado A, Da Cunho O, et al. Glomerular filtration rate in the first three weeks of life. J Pediatr 1975;87:268.
17. Fawer CL, Torrado A, Guignard JP. Maturation of renal function in full-term and premature neonates. Helv Paediatr Acta 1979;34:11.
18. Avner ED, Ellis D, Ichikawa I, et al. Normal neonates and the maturational development of homeostatic mechanisms. In Ichikawa I (ed). Pediatric Textbook of Fluids and Electrolytes. Baltimore, Williams & Wilkins, 1990, pp 114, 115.
19. Hansen JDL, Smith CA. Effects of withholding fluid in the immediate postnatal period. Pediatrics 1953;12:99.
20. Polacek E, Vocel J, Neugebauerova L, et al. The osmotic concentrating ability in healthy infants and children. Arch Dis Child 1965;40:291.
21. Calcagno PL, Rubin MI, Weintraub DH, et al. Studies on the renal concentrating and diluting mechanisms in the premature infant. J Clin Invest 1954;33:91.
22. Leake RD, Zakauddin S, Trygstad CW. The effects of large volume intravenous fluid infusion on neonatal renal function. J Pediatr 1976;89:968.
23. Sulyok E, Nemeth M, Tenyi I, et al. The possible role of prostaglandins in the hyperfunction of the renin-angiotensin-aldosterone system in the newborn. Br J Obstet Gynecol 1979;86:205.
24. Sulyok E, Nemeth M, Tenyi I, et al. Postnatal development of renin-angiotensin-aldosterone system, RAAS, in relation to electrolyte imbalance in premature infants. Pediatr Res 1979;13:817.
25. Godard C, Geering J, Geering K, et al. Plasma renin activity related to sodium balance, renal function and urinary vasopressin in the newborn infant. Pediatr Res 1979;13:742.
26. Spitzer A. The role of the kidney in sodium homeostasis during maturation. Kidney Int 1982;21:539.
27. Honour JW, Valman HB, Shackleton CHL. Aldosterone and sodium homeostasis in preterm infants. Acta Paediatr Scand 1977;66:103.
28. Avner ED, Ellis D, Ichikawa I, et al. Normal neonates and the maturational development of homeostatic mechanisms. In Ichikawa I (ed). Pediatric Textbook of Fluids and Electrolytes. Baltimore, Williams & Wilkins, 1990, p 109.
29. Sulyok E, Heim T, Soltesz G, et al. The influence of maturity on renal control of acidosis in newborn infants. Biol Neonate 1972;21:418.
30. Schwartz GJ, Haycock GB, Edelmann CM, et al. Late metabolic acidosis: A reassessment of the definition. J Pediatr 1979;95:102.
31. Svenningsen NW, Aronson AS. Postnatal development of renal concentration capacity as estimate by DDAVP-test in normal and asphyxiated neonates. Biol Neonate 1984;25:230.
32. Avner ED, Ellis D, Ichikawa I, et al. Normal neonates and the maturational development of homeostatic mechanisms. In Ichikawa I (ed). Pediatric Textbook of Fluids and Electrolytes. Baltimore, Williams & Wilkins, 1990, p 116.
33. Dubois EF. The basal metabolism in fever. JAMA 1921;77:352.
34. Bell EF, Oh W. Fluid and electrolyte management. In Avery GB (ed). Neonatology: Pathophysiology and Management of the Newborn. Philadelphia, JB Lippincott, 1987, p 775.
35. Bell EF, Warburton D, Stonestreet BS, et al. Effect of fluid administration on the development of symptomatic patent ductus arteriosus and congestive heart failure in premature infants. N Engl J Med 1980;302:598.
36. Bell EF, Warburton D, Stonestreet BS, et al. High-volume fluid intake predisposes premature infants to necrotizing enterocolitis. Lancet 1979;2:90.
37. Friis-Hansen B. Changes in body water compartments during growth. Acta Paediatr Scand (Suppl) 1957;110:1.
38. Friis-Hansen B. Body water compartments in children: Changes during growth and related changes in body composition. Pediatrics 1961;28:169.
39. Behrman RE, Vaughan VC (eds). Nutrition and nutritional disorders. In Nelson Textbook of Pediatrics. Philadelphia, WB Saunders, 1987, p 113.
40. Feld LG, Kaskel FJ, Schoeneman MJ. The approach to fluid and electrolyte therapy in pediatrics. Adv Pediatr 1988;35:497.
41. Darrow DC. The significance of body size. Am J Dis Child 1959;98:416.
42. Simmons CF, Ichikawa I. External balance of water and electrolytes. In Ichikawa I (ed). Pediatric Textbook of Fluids and Electrolytes. Baltimore, Williams & Wilkins, 1990, pp 23, 24.
43. Behrman RE, Vaughan VC (eds). General considerations in the care of sick children. In Nelson Textbook of Pediatrics. Philadelphia, WB Saunders, 1987, p 174.
44. Hendrata L. Spoons for making glucose-salt solutions. Lancet 1976;1:612.
45. Levine MM, Hughes TP, Black RE, et al. Variability of sodium and sucrose levels of simple sugar/salt oral rehydration solutions prepared under optimal and field conditions. J Pediatr 1980;97:324.
46. Awazu M, Kon V, Barakat AY. Volume Disorders. In Ichikawa I (ed).

Pediatric Textbook of Fluids and Electrolytes. Baltimore, Williams & Wilkins, 1990, p 122.

47. Hogan GR. Hypernatremia—problems in management. Pediatr Clin North Am 1976;23:569.

48. Awazu M, Kon V, Barakat AY. Volume disorders. *In* Ichikawa I (ed). Pediatric Textbook of Fluids and Electrolytes. Baltimore, Williams & Wilkins, 1990, p 124.

49. Behrman RE, Vaughan VC (eds). General considerations in the care of sick children. *In* Nelson Textbook of Pediatrics. Philadelphia, WB Saunders, 1987, p 197.

50. Behrman RE, Vaughan VC (eds). General considerations in the care of sick children. *In* Nelson Textbook of Pediatrics. Philadelphia, WB Saunders, 1987, p 198.

51. Thurston JH, Hauhart RE, Dirges JA. Taurine: A role in osmotic regulation of mammalian brain and possible clinical significance. Life Sci 1980;26:1561.

52. Finberg L. Treatment of dehydration in infancy. Pediatr Rev 1981;3:113.

53. Awazu M, Devarajan P, Stewart CL, et al. "Maintenance" therapy and treatment of dehydration and overhydration. *In* Ichikawa I (ed). Pediatric Textbook of Fluids and Electrolytes. Baltimore, Williams & Wilkins, 1990, p 420.

54. Behrman RE, Vaughan VC (eds). General considerations in the care of sick children. *In* Nelson Textbook of Pediatrics. Philadelphia, WB Saunders, 1987, p 199.

55. Soergell KH, Whalen GE, Harris JA. Passive movement of water and sodium across the human small intestinal mucosa. J Appl Physiol 1968;24:40.

56. Schultz S, Frizzell RA, Nellans NH. Ion transport of mammalian small intestine. Ann Rev Physiol 1974;36:51.

57. Casteel HB, Fiedorek SC. Oral rehydration therapy. Pediatr Clin North Am 1990;37:295.

58. Bhargava S, Sachdev HPS, Das Gupta B, et al. Oral rehydration of neonates and young infants with dehydrating diarrhea: Comparison of low and standard sodium content in oral rehydration solutions. J Pediatr Gastroenterol Nutr 1984;3:500.

59. Sack DA, Chowdhury AMAK, Eusof A, et al. Oral rehydration in rotavirus diarrhea: A double-blind comparison of sucrose with glucose electrolyte solution. Lancet 1978;2:280.

60. Sack DA, Islam S, Brown KH, et al. Oral therapy in children with cholera: A comparison of sucrose and glucose electrolyte solutions. J Pediatr 1980;96:20.

61. Pizarro D, Posada G, Sandi L, et al. Rice-based oral electrolyte solutions for the management of infantile diarrhea. N Engl J Med 1991;324:517.

62. Booth IW, Levine MM, Harris JT. Oral rehydration therapy in acute diarrhea in childhood. J Pediatr Gastroenterol Nutr 1984;3:491.

63. World Health Organization. A Manual for the Treatment of Acute Diarrhea. WHO/CDD/SER/80.2 Geneva, World Health Organization, 1980.

CHAPTER 11

Electrolyte Disorders

Paul Blackburn

INTRODUCTION

Electrolyte abnormalities are seen daily by the emergency physician. Electrolytes define a child's metabolic homeostasis and direct the physician's emergency department treatment. In children, electrolyte disturbances are often found in conjunction with fluid disorders, and the two are therefore interrelated.

SODIUM

Sodium is the primary extracellular cation and represents almost half the osmotically active particles maintaining intra-vascular and interstitial volumes. About two thirds of sodium is freely exchangeable; the remainder is sequestered in bone. The fetus contains a larger total body and exchangeable sodium pool as a result of the proportionately greater amounts of cartilage, connective tissue, and extracellular fluid and the smaller amount of low-sodium-containing muscle tissue.[1]

The extracellular sodium level is approximately 145 mEq/L; the intracellular level is 12 mEq/L. This transmembrane gradient is maintained by the magnesium-dependent, energy-requiring, sodium-potassium adenosine triphosphatase (ATPase) pump. Inhibitors of the pump include calcium and cardiac glycosides.

The amount of total body sodium is a result of a dynamic balance between intake and excretion. There is no specific regulatory mechanism for sodium ingestion such as the thirst mechanism for water intake. However, large changes in sodium values, such as occur in salt-wasting syndromes, may result in salt craving, and aldosterone may help regulate intestinal sodium absorption to a small extent.

Sodium requirements are 1 to 2 mEq/kg/day in full-term infants, whereas premature infants require approximately 4 mEq/kg/day.[2] This results from the premature infant's high renal fractional excretion of sodium, which resolves within about 2 weeks postnatally. A positive sodium balance is required for active growth, and term infants are able to do this even on relatively low sodium breast milk. Cow's milk has a relatively high sodium content.

Excretion

Sodium excretion occurs in feces, sweat, and urine, but the kidney is the major regulatory organ. Fecal losses are usually minimal unless profuse diarrhea is present, when sodium losses may reach 10 mEq/kg/day in absolute losses.[3] Sweat is not a primary sodium regulator, but does involve active transport and loss of water and electrolytes through specialized skin glands. The normally low sodium losses in sweat can be increased in patients with cystic fibrosis or Addison's disease.

Regulation

Renal sodium regulation is referred to in terms of the glomerulotubular balance, or balance between the glomerular filtration rate (GFR) and tubular reabsorption. Normally, alternations in GFR are compensated for by tubular absorption, and sodium homeostasis is unaffected. A useful test, both conceptually and in the evaluation of certain disorders, is the fractional excretion of sodium, or FE_{Na}. The FE_{Na} is that fraction of sodium in the final urine that was filtered by the glomerulus and not reabsorbed. It is easily calculated by urine and plasma evaluations.

$$\frac{(U_{Na}/P_{Na})}{(U_{Cr}/P_{Cr})} \times 100 = FE_{Na}\ (\%),$$

where U_{Na} = urine sodium concentration, P_{Na} = plasma sodium concentration, U_{Cr} = urine creatinine concentration, and P_{Cr} = plasma creatinine concentration.

The FE_{Na} is normally 1% to 2%. Large dietary alterations may change this value slightly, but new steady states are achieved within about 3 days. Newborns, especially premature infants less than 34 weeks, have a high fractional excretion of sodium (up to 5%), which usually approaches 1% within 2 months of postnatal life. Critically ill premature infants may have an FE_{Na} of up to 15%,[2] which may result in a negative sodium balance and hyponatremia.

Approximately two thirds of filtered sodium is reabsorbed

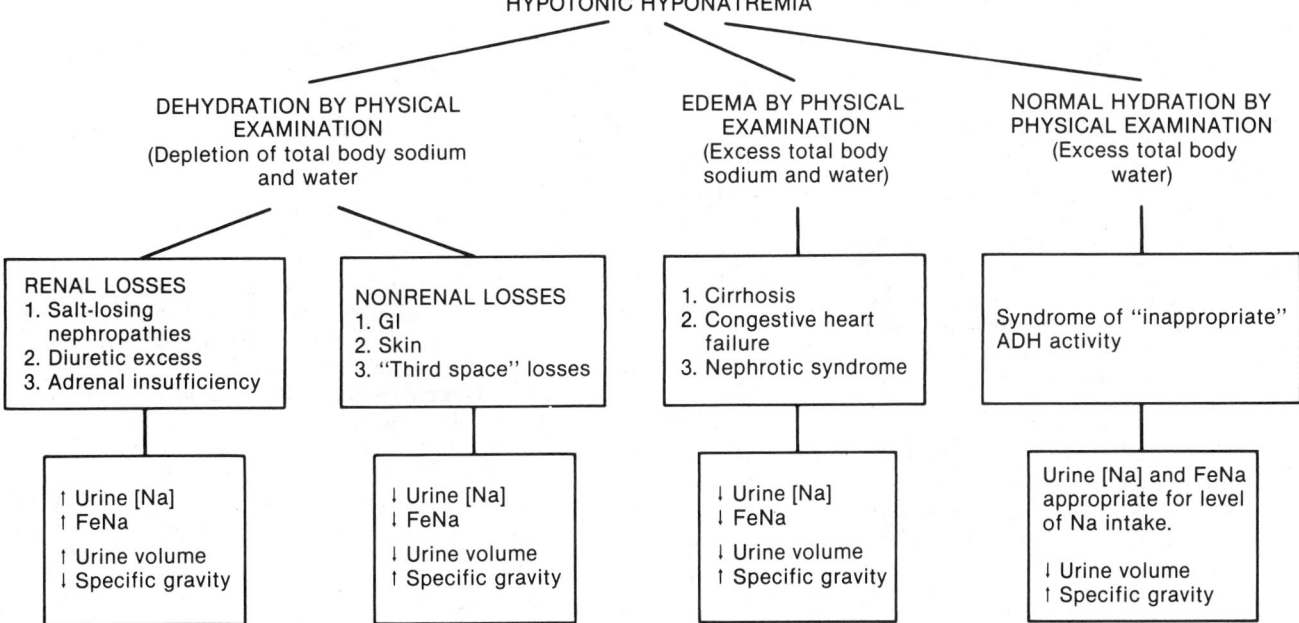

Figure 11–1. Algorithm for the differential diagnosis of hyponatremia. FE_{Na} = Fractional excretion of sodium. (Redrawn from Feld LG, Kaskel FJ, Schoeneman MJ. The approach to fluid and electrolyte therapy in pediatrics. Adv Pediatr 1988;35:497.)

in the proximal tubule, probably by active transport. Sodium reabsorption in the loop of Henle occurs in the ascending limb as sodium follows chloride. Reabsorption at this site is essential for the maintenance of the countercurrent multiplier system and subsequent urine-concentrating ability and water balance. The so-called *loop diuretics* block chloride reuptake and thus promote a natriuresis. The *distal tubule* and *collecting ducts* provide fine regulation of sodium balance under the regulatory influences of aldosterone and antidiuretic hormone.

Hyponatremia

Alterations in serum sodium concentrations usually reflect abnormalities in the control of water balance. The serum sodium level is always determined by the ratio of sodium to water and does not indicate the absolute amount of either substance (Fig. 11–1).

Hyponatremia (serum sodium level less than 130 mEq/L) is a common clinical problem indicating a relatively decreased amount of sodium in relation to water in the extracellular space. Slowly progressing, chronic hyponatremia may be asymptomatic with values less than 120 mEq/L. Conversely, higher mortality is seen with rapidly developing hyponatremia. In general, sodium levels below 120 mEq/L should be treated promptly.

The pathophysiologic mechanism involves the intracellular movement of water into brain cells, producing swelling. This leads to CNS symptoms that include lethargy and hypothermia, depressed deep tendon reflexes, pathologic reflexes, pseudobulbar palsies, and seizures (Table 11–1).

Pseudohyponatremia refers to a low serum sodium level by laboratory measurement, when in fact the sodium content

of the water phase is normal. Normal serum is 93% water and 7% solids, mostly lipids and protein. If the 7% fraction becomes larger, the amount of water used to measure sodium is smaller, resulting in a falsely low measurement. Increased amounts of triglycerides and protein falsely indicate decreased sodium and may be seen in the child with nephrotic syndrome or hypothyroidism. An elevated glucose level will also lower the serum sodium measurement (1.6 mEq/L for each 100 mg/dl increase in glucose beyond 100 mg/dl).[4]

Isotonic Hyponatremia

Isotonic hyponatremia refers either to pseudohyponatremia or to the hyponatremia resulting from the rapid administration of isotonic sodium-free fluids, such as dextrose-

TABLE 11–1	
SYMPTOMS AND SIGNS OF HYPONATREMIA	
Symptoms	**Signs**
Lethargy, apathy	Abnormal sensorium
Disorientation	Depressed deep tendon reflexes
Muscle cramps	Cheyne-Stokes respiration
Anorexia, nausea	Hypothermia
Agitation	Pathological reflexes
	Pseudobulbar palsy
	Seizures

From Ichikawa I. Pediatric Textbook of Fluids and Electrolytes. Williams & Wilkins, Baltimore, 1990.

containing solutions, in large amounts. This cause of hyponatremia is usually evident.

Hypertonic Hyponatremia

Hypertonic hyponatremia usually results from infusions of hypertonic solutions such as 10% dextrose or mannitol. The resultant extracellular shift of water causes hyponatremia, although the osmolarity is elevated because of the concentrations of the osmotically active glucose or mannitol.

Hypotonic Hyponatremia

Hypotonic hyponatremia is a below-normal sodium concentration with decreased osmolarity of body fluids. Hypotonic hyponatremia only results with adequate fluid intake or fluid retention in the presence of sodium losses exceeding intake. The physical examination reveals a normally hydrated, a dehydrated, or an edematous child. These categories assist in evaluating the hypotonic hyponatremic child and determining the necessary therapy.

Hypotonic Hyponatremia With Normal Hydration. This is a dilutional hyponatremia, often not appreciated on physical examination because of the apparent lack of volume changes. Causes include excessive fluid administration in normal infants receiving dilute formulas[5] and late hyponatremia in premature infants.[6] However, the primary cause of this dilutional hyponatremia in children is the syndrome of inappropriate secretion of antidiuretic hormones (SIADH). SIADH must be suspected in any child whose urine osmolarity exceeds the serum osmolarity. Treatment in nonemergent cases consists of fluid restriction to insensible losses or less. If emergent therapy is required (in patients with seizures, neurologic complications, or a serum sodium level less than 120 mEq/L), hypertonic saline is administered. The goal of hypertonic saline therapy is not to replace deficits but to provide solute for obligatory renal excretion and concomitant loss of free water. The following formula is used to correct hyponatremia with hypertonic saline:

$$(\text{sodium desired} - \text{sodium observed}) \times 0.6 \times \text{wt (kg)} = \text{Na}^+ \text{ mEq}$$

Hypertonic saline (3%) contains 513 mEq/L of sodium or 0.5 mEq/ml. Therefore the volume to be administered is twice the milliequivalent of sodium desired. Half the calculated dosage of sodium needed is given over 1 to 2 hours, the sodium and clinical status are reassessed, and the remainder is administered if necessary.

Example: Sodium desired = 120 mEq/L
Sodium observed = 110 mEq/L
Body weight = 10 kg

$(120 \text{ mEq/L} - 110 \text{ mEq/L}) \times 0.6 \times 10 \text{ kg} = 60 \text{ mEq Na}^+$

$60 \text{ mEq Na}^+/513 \text{ mEq Na}^+/\text{L} = 0.12 \text{ L} = 120 \text{ ml } 3\% \text{ saline}$

Administer 60 ml over 1 to hours
Reassess
Administer remaining 60 ml if necessary
Reassess

In addition to hypertonic saline administration, judicious use of diuretics to increase loss of free water may be beneficial. Additional hypertonic saline may be needed to offset ongoing sodium losses.[7] Administration of glucocorticoid may be considered in patients with SIADH, if sodium retention is due to aldosterone suppression.

Hypotonic Hyponatremia With Dehydration. Hypotonic hyponatremia with dehydration is a depletional hyponatremia, inferring loss of sodium that is out of proportion to the net loss of water. Patients with this form of hyponatremia are more prone to hypovolemia and shock with less provocation than are patients with other forms of hyponatremia because of extracellular hypoosmolarity and depletion.

Physical examination and urinalysis will assist in determining whether the cause of hypotonic hyponatremia with dehydration is renal or nonrenal. Children with renal causes (salt-losing nephropathies, diuretic overuse, adrenal insufficiency) have urine with a high sodium content and a high FE_{Na}. Children with nonrenal causes (gastrointestinal losses and "third spacing"; skin losses, as in cystic fibrosis patients; or spinal fluid loss from myelomeningocele) have a low urine sodium, a low FE_{Na}, low urine output, and a high specific gravity. The administration of fluid and electrolytes in hypotonic hyponatremia with dehydration is discussed in Chapter 10; in the adrenal insufficiency patient who presents similarly to a patient with acute oliguric renal failure (azotemic, acidotic, hyponatremic, and hyperkalemic), restricting the fluid and sodium intake would be devastating.[8] Instead, vigorous fluid resuscitation with 5% dextrose with 0.9% normal saline (NS) (20 ml/kg) administered intravenously over 30 to 60 minutes should be carried out.

Hypotonic Hyponatremia With Edema. Hypotonic hyponatremia results from the retention of sodium and disproportionately greater amounts of water. A decreased effective circulating blood volume, with the body perceiving intravascular volume contraction, impairs the nephron's ability to concentrate urine and results in antidiuretic hormone (ADH) release and activation of the renin-angiotensin system. Renal water excretion is impaired, sodium retention is stimulated, and salt and water retention is perpetuated. The causes include cirrhosis of the liver, congestive heart failure, and the nephrotic syndrome and usually result in peripheral edema. Examination of the urine shows decreased urine volume, high specific gravity, decreased urine sodium, and a decreased FE_{Na}.

Therapy consists of salt and fluid restriction and judicious use of diuretics. In addition, children with nephrotic syndrome may benefit from hypertonic albumin (1 gm/kg) given over 1 hour, up to three times per day.[9]

Hypernatremia

Hypernatremia, which is a serum sodium level greater than 150 mEq/L, occurs when serum sodium is increased in proportion to water in the extracellular fluid. As with hyponatremia, derangements result from salt or water imbalance, alone or in combination. Physical examination will assess hydration status, dividing hypernatremia into categories of either dehydration or edema (Fig. 11–2).

Hypernatremia with dehydration occurs with water losses proportionately greater than sodium; evidence of volume contraction is present if total body depletion of sodium has occurred. Chronic renal disease, postobstructive uropathy, and diabetes insipidus consist of concentrating defects with continuing inappropriate loss of water and sodium despite dehydration. Urine output is large, with a low specific gravity. Nonrenal water losses may occur from gastrointestinal sources, the respiratory tract, skin surface, and decreased intake. The urine output is low with a high specific gravity, except in the premature infant, who may not be able to produce a concentrated urine.

If diuretics are the etiologic agent, they should be discontinued. Hormonal replacement is mandatory in patients with adrenal insufficiency. However, caution must be exercised when correcting hypernatremia. Vigorous rehydration does not allow time for intracellular reequilibration, and cerebral edema with increased intracranial pressure, seizures, stupor, and death may occur. In general, the type of rehydration

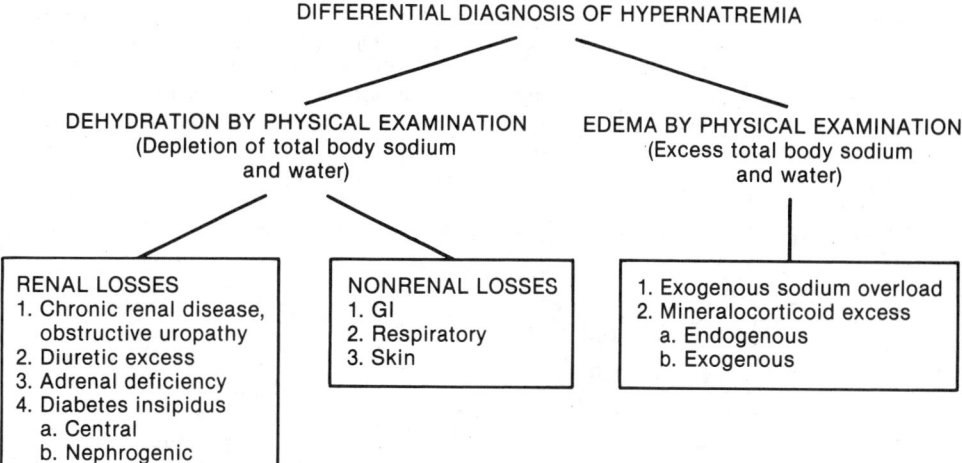

DIFFERENTIAL DIAGNOSIS OF HYPERNATREMIA

DEHYDRATION BY PHYSICAL EXAMINATION
(Depletion of total body sodium
and water)

EDEMA BY PHYSICAL EXAMINATION
(Excess total body sodium
and water)

RENAL LOSSES
1. Chronic renal disease,
   obstructive uropathy
2. Diuretic excess
3. Adrenal deficiency
4. Diabetes insipidus
   a. Central
   b. Nephrogenic

NONRENAL LOSSES
1. GI
2. Respiratory
3. Skin

1. Exogenous sodium overload
2. Mineralocorticoid excess
   a. Endogenous
   b. Exogenous

Figure 11–2. Algorithm for the differential diagnosis of hypernatremia. (Redrawn from Feld LG, Kaskel FJ, Schoeneman MJ. The approach to fluid and electrolyte therapy in pediatrics. Adv Pediatr 1988;35:497.)

solution is not as important as the proper volume and rate of administration.[10]

If the physical examination reveals an edematous child with hypernatremia, the physician should consider either sodium overload or mineralocorticoid excess. Sodium overload is uncommon and is usually iatrogenic, and a careful history easily reveals the cause in most cases. Administration of hypertonic saline (3% or 5%), hypertonic sodium bicarbonate, or improperly mixed powdered oral rehydration supplements can lead to sodium overload. Rapid treatment is necessary with 5% dextrose in water, in conjunction with a loop diuretic to induce natriuresis.[11] The infusion rate depends on the rate and amount of diuresis, the rate of serum sodium decline, and the neurologic status. The serum sodium level should not decline by more than 2 mEq/L/hr, in order to avoid central pontine myelinolysis. Cerebral edema secondary to vigorous fluid administration must be avoided. Dialysis may be required for patients with congestive heart failure and oliguria unresponsive to initial therapy.

Mineralocorticoid excess (endogenous or as a result of excessive intake) usually increases the sodium to high-normal levels only. With endogenous excess, treatment entails salt restriction and correction of the primary underlying disorder. Therapy of excess exogenous mineralocorticoid requires salt restriction and modification of replacement therapy.

CHLORIDE

Chloride is the predominant extracellular anion. Comprising approximately 45 mEq/kg at birth, the total body chloride decreases to 35 mEq/kg at 1 year of age and maintains a value of 33 mEq/kg throughout adulthood.[12] Only small amounts are intracellular.

Regulation

Chloride closely parallels the sodium ion in both intake and excretion. In fact, chloride absorption is probably linked to sodium absorption. Renal chloride transport may also be active. Inhibiting this active chloride transport mechanism is the mechanism of action of the diuretics furosemide, bumetanide, and ethacrynic acid.[13]

Because chloride metabolism closely parallels sodium metabolism in most clinical situations, the serum chloride will most often reflect the serum sodium. Thus hyperchloremia is most often present with hypernatremia, and hypochloremia is often present with hyponatremia.[14]

Hypochloremia can result from either prolonged diminished chloride intake or altered chloride excretion, usually in relation to metabolic alkalosis. Feeding a child chloride-deficient milk for a protracted period (several months) will result in a child with weakness, lethargy, decreased appetite, and failure to thrive. Laboratory analysis may show a hypokalemic metabolic alkalosis and depletion of chloride. The electrolyte abnormalities are rapidly reversed with chloride supplementation, but long-term sequelae, such as behavioral abnormalities, may occur.[15]

Hypochloremia may also result from altered renal excretion of chloride in acid-base disturbances. Although chloride levels are not directly related to renal hydrogen ion excretion, chloride will increase or decrease inversely to bicarbonate, which does change as a result of hydrogen ion disturbances. Therefore hypochloremia is typically seen in metabolic alkalosis.

To correct metabolic alkalosis, chloride must usually be administered. Chloride administration will result in urinary excretion of bicarbonate and correction of the alkalosis. In a similar fashion, metabolic acidosis with potassium deficiency must have the chloride deficit corrected before the potassium can be restored.

Excessive losses of chloride in relation to sodium can also occur with protracted vomiting or gastric suctioning, secretory diarrhea, and the rare entity of congenital chloride diarrhea. A pathologic defect in the chloride-bicarbonate exchange mechanism of the ileum and colon leads to secretory diarrhea presenting at birth and is invariably associated with hydramnios and numerous electrolyte imbalances.[16]

Hyperchloremia results primarily from renal conservation of chloride ions in excess of sodium and potassium. It may occur with increased chloride absorption in renal tubular acidosis or with formation of alkaline urine during correction of metabolic alkalosis.

The most beneficial way to use the serum chloride is to measure the patient's anion gap. This is calculated as follows[17]:

$$\text{Anion gap} = (Na^+ + K^+) - (Cl^- + HCO_3^-)$$

A normal anion gap is 8 to 16 mEq/L and reflects unmeasured endogenous or exogenous anions such as phosphates, sulfates, proteins, and organic acids, which exceed unmeasured cations such as magnesium and calcium.

An increased anion gap, a major tool in the evaluation of acid-base disorders, may be the only chemical evidence of acidosis in patients suffering from a mixed acid-base disorder.[18] An increased anion gap, therefore, strongly suggests metabolic acidosis. A helpful mnemonic for causes of increased anion gap metabolic acidosis is MUDPILES: *Methanol, Uremia, Diabetes mellitus (ketoacidosis), Paraldehyde overdosage, Iron and Isoniazide, Lactic acidosis, Ethanol or Ethylene glycol,* and *Salicylate toxicity or Starvation.*

A decreased anion gap is seen less frequently. Lithium ingestion (unmeasured cation), multiple myeloma (cationic proteins), and loss of albumin (anionic at pH 7.4) in patients with nephrotic syndrome will all result in a decreased anion gap.[15]

POTASSIUM
Physiology

Potassium derangements (normal serum values are 3.5 to 5.0 mEq/L) can result in widespread physiologic dysfunction, including death. Though potassium is the primary intracellular cation, clinical estimation of potassium balance is dependent on extracellular values. Although serum values are easily obtained, they do not reflect total body potassium stores. Serum values may reflect transcellular shifts of the ion without any net gain or loss of total body stores.

The total body potassium content is approximately 50 mEq/L in the adult male.[19] Approximately 50% to 70% of potassium is found in muscle tissue, less than 0.5% in plasma, and 7% to 8% in bone and connective tissue.[20] The total body potassium varies with age, sex, lean body mass, and rate of growth.[19, 21] There is an inverse relationship between plasma potassium and gestational age.[22] Newborns require potassium for growth.

High intracellular potassium concentrations are required for growth, protein and nucleic acid synthesis,[23] acid-base balance,[24, 25] and intracellular-extracellular gradients for membrane potential generation and impulse formation.

The steep transmembrane potential of cells is generated and maintained by the sodium-potassium ATPase pump, actively extruding three sodium ions for every two potassium ions inwardly transported. This unequal exchange results in an overall intracellular negative charge and creates an environment favoring outflow of potassium down the concentration gradient. The activity of the sodium-potassium ATPase pump is highest in excitable and transporting tissues (nervous tissue and kidney).[26, 27]

Acid-base balance and potassium transcellular shifts are integrally related. Acidemia (i.e., an increase in extracellular hydrogen ion concentration) produces potassium release from intracellular tissues and an increase in plasma potassium. Alkalemia (a decrease in extracellular hydrogen ion concentration) results in intracellular shifts of potassium and a subsequent decrease in serum potassium concentration. For every 0.1 unit change in blood pH, the plasma potassium concentration inversely changes 0.3 to 1.3 mEq/L.[28] Acute onset and metabolic acid-base disorders result in larger potassium shifts than respiratory and chronic changes.

Plasma bicarbonate concentration changes reciprocally alter serum potassium levels independent of blood pH.[29, 30] For example, in patients with asthma (acidic serum pH and elevated serum bicarbonate levels), the serum potassium level is lower than in those with a metabolic acidosis (acidic serum pH and low serum bicarbonate level). This implies a net inward movement in asthma and a linked outward movement in metabolic acidosis, with lower and higher serum potassium levels, respectively.[31]

Insulin promotes potassium uptake, particularly by cardiac and skeletal muscle, adipose tissue, nervous tissue, and hepatocytes, thus lowering serum concentrations.[32] This effect is thought to be unrelated to insulin's intracellular transport of glucose.[33]

Catecholamines produce a biphasic response in serum potassium levels, independent of other hormonal or renal influences.[34–36] An initial rise in potassium levels is followed by a fall below baseline levels.[37] Conversely, beta blockers are associated with increases in serum potassium levels following exercise,[38] possibly as a result of impaired cellular uptake.[36] Aldosterone stimulates secretion of potassium at the distal renal tubule, colon, and salivary glands and induces potassium uptake at nontransport tissue sites.[39]

The kidney is the primary site of chronic potassium regulation and balance. The kidney cannot achieve extreme adjustments in potassium conservation as rapidly as sodium; however, the speed of adaption may depend on the baseline potassium level and the amount of deviation.[40]

Potassium is freely filtered at the glomerulus, with approximately half of the potassium being passively reabsorbed in the proximal tubule.[41, 42] Because only 10% to 25% of the filtered load is ultimately excreted, it is evident that the potassium in the urine results from secretion rather than glomerular filtration. This occurs in the distal tubule[42] and collecting ducts.[43]

Control of net secretion of potassium is poorly understood. Transcellular movement across the luminal membrane is passive and depends on membrane permeability and chemical and electrical gradients. The electrical gradient is established by coordinated potassium secretion and sodium reabsorption. In addition, hypokalemia and kaliuresis are often seen with systemic alkalosis.[44]

The gastrointestinal tract is a major regulator of potassium. An intake of 1 to 2 mEq/kg/day is recommended, but intake varies widely.[44] Potassium is well absorbed in the upper gut,[45] whereas secretion, paralleling nephron secretion, occurs in the colon.[46, 47] Aldosterone increases absorption of sodium while increasing secretion of potassium.[46, 48] The colon also increases potassium secretion in response to potassium loading.[46] The colonic mucus is rich in potassium, and diarrhea or increased mucus in the stool can lead to potassium losses.[47, 49]

Sweat contains approximately 5 to 25 mEq/L potassium, a level that may be elevated in the presence of cystic fibrosis or hyperaldosteronism.[44]

Hypokalemia

Hypokalemia is usually defined as a serum potassium level less than 3.5 mEq/L. Hypokalemia can be caused by decreased total body stores resulting from decreased intake or increased loss (renal, gastrointestinal, integumentary). However, a decreased serum potassium level can be evident, despite adequate total body stores, as a result of transcellular shifting; this is seen in alkalemia, insulin-induced intracellular movement, pseudohypokalemia of leukemia, and familial hypokalemic periodic paralysis. Potassium is practically impossible to delete from the diet. However, administering parenteral fluids without potassium for prolonged periods can produce hypokalemia.

Increased renal losses can result from many factors. Diuretic use constitutes the most common cause of renal potassium wasting, and all classes of diuretics contribute to renal losses. Potassium wasting from diuretics is a result of an increased volume of filtrate in the distal tubule, stimulating potassium secretion. Additionally, loop and thiazide diuretics create an alkalotic environment, thereby stimulating the intracellular shift of potassium. Diuretics are often administered in edema-forming conditions (congestive heart failure, nephrotic syndrome) where decreased circulating volume stimulates hyperaldosteronism. This results in increased potassium secretion.[50] Therefore the child with chronic disease may have multiple factors contributing to potassium imbalance: use of diuretics, elevated aldosterone levels, inadequate potassium intake, or enhanced gastrointestinal losses.

The kidney is also a mediator of potassium loss in a variety of other conditions, including tubular disorders (renal tubular acidosis), endocrinopathies, excessive renin-angiotensin production, renal vascular disease, renin-producing tumors such as hemangiopericytoma[51] and Wilms' tumor,[52] and hypomagnesemia.

Antibiotics can contribute to renal kaliuresis and subsequent hypokalemia. The penicillins (including carbenicillin and nafcillin)[53-55] are administered as sodium salts and are nonreabsorbable ions; both stimulate potassium secretion in the distal tubule. Polymyxin B,[56] the aminoglycosides,[57, 58] and amphotericin B also cause hypokalemia.

Leukemia is frequently associated with hypokalemia. The etiology of hypokalemia is multifactorial and may include decreased intake, antibiotic-induced wasting, increased uptake by rapidly multiplying cells, mineralocorticoid effect of steroid therapy, and osmotic diuresis employed with some chemotherapeutic agents (e.g., cisplatin).[59]

Diabetic ketoacidosis is associated with profound losses of total body potassium that may not become evident until intracellular shifting occurs with resolving acidosis.[60] This depletion is a result of many factors: osmotic diuresis of hyperglycemia, vomiting, extracellular fluid depletion with secondary hyperaldosteronism, and urinary ketones presenting to the distal renal tubule as nonreabsorbable anions.[61]

Hypokalemic periodic paralysis is a form of transcellular shift of potassium characterized by intermittent attacks of muscle weakness and paralysis lasting for hours. Hypokalemic periodic paralysis usually presents in the first two decades of life. During an attack, the serum potassium will abruptly shift intracellularly, and propagation of the muscle action potential does not occur. An intracellular potassium shift can be triggered by glucose, insulin, a high carbohydrate–low potassium diet, certain mineralocorticoids, stress, trauma, or alcohol. Typically, the attack is the morning after a day of vigorous activity followed by a large evening meal. Treatment with a carbonic anhydrase inhibitor may be more effective than that with potassium supplements or potassium-sparing diuretics in eliminating severe attacks.[62]

The gastrointestinal tract is the primary site of extrarenal loss of potassium. Hypokalemia can result from protracted vomiting or nasogastric suctioning, but not from direct gut loss of potassium; gastric secretions contain only 10 to 20 mEq/L potassium.[21, 63] Rather, the volume contraction and metabolic alkalosis caused by hydrogen ion loss increase renal potassium excretion. Secondary hyperaldosteronism increases distal tubular potassium secretion. The metabolic alkalosis increases distal tubular intracellular potassium and causes increased delivery of tubular bicarbonate; both factors favor potassium secretion. This is demonstrated in the infant with pyloric stenosis who is classically dehydrated, alkalotic, and hypokalemic.[59]

Colonic potassium losses can be substantial. Colonic mucus is rich in potassium (100 to 140 mEq/L). With diarrhea and volume contraction, secondary hyperaldosteronism stimulates renal and colonic potassium secretion.[59] Marked potassium loss can occur with villous adenomas of the colon and rectum[64, 65]; non–insulin-secreting islet cell adenomas of the pancreas[66]; ureterosigmoidostomies, biliary drainage, and enterocutaneous fistulae[28]; laxative abuse; and toluene abuse.

Clinical Manifestations

Symptoms and signs of hypokalemia generally do not appear until serum concentrations fall below 3.0 mEq/L.[8]

Both the acuteness of change and the serum level affect the severity of symptoms. Chronic losses can be well tolerated.

The history of the child with suspected hypokalemia should include information regarding the pattern of childhood growth, the presence or absence of chronic illness, the use of medications (diuretics, steroids, antibiotics, insulin, laxatives), a surgical history (e.g., ureterosigmoidostomy), and the symptoms of the current disturbance (e.g., skeletal muscle weakness, polyuria).[67] Physical examination should include growth indices; blood pressure measurement; observation of edema, if present; assessment of neural and muscular function; and a cardiac evaluation. Laboratory studies should, at a minimum, include measurement of serum electrolyte levels and arterial blood gases and an electrocardiogram.

Hypokalemia leads to an elevated intracellular-to-extracellular potassium ratio, thereby creating a state of relative hyperpolarization of cells. Nerve conduction is slowed, as is muscle contraction, which is manifested as muscle weakness. This is first noted in limb muscles, but trunk and respiratory muscles may be profoundly involved, resulting in respiratory arrest and death. Smooth muscle paralysis may manifest as a paralytic ileus. Lethargy, confusion, areflexia, hypotension, and autonomic instability may also be present.

Cardiac abnormalities of conduction and rhythm, particularly premature atrial contractions and premature ventricular contractions are common. Children taking digoxin who are hypokalemic are more likely to develop arrhythmias.[68] Characteristic electrocardiographic manifestations include ST depression, diminished T wave amplitude, and the appearance of a U wave. Sodium retention and edema regularly occur with hypokalemia. Metabolic disturbances with hypokalemia are common and include suppression of insulin release (with subsequent glucose intolerance)[69] and growth failure.

Treatment

Mild hypokalemia should be treated in patients with hypercalcemia,[70] hypomagnesemia,[71] or cardiac disease, especially those taking digoxin.[61, 72] Therapy is instituted empirically, because intracellular potassium cannot be easily measured, and no relationship necessarily exists between intracellular and extracellular potassium. Urine output should be ensured before potassium replenishment, and deficits should be replaced over several days, avoiding large doses. Electrocardiographic monitoring must be available when rapid administration is attempted.[8] Mild hypokalemia may respond simply to dietary supplementation.

With moderate hypokalemia, oral replacement of deficits is adequate and safe.[8] A dose of 3 mEq/kg/day in addition to maintenance is sufficient.

Parenteral potassium supplementation should be reserved for those patients with severe hypokalemia (e.g., resulting from neuromuscular or cardiac disturbances, diabetic ketoacidosis, administration of amphotericin B) or those unable to take oral preparations.[67] Intravenous potassium concentration should be limited to 40 mEq/L and administered no faster than 0.5 to 1.0 mEq/kg/hour.[8] In patients with severe ongoing loss, diabetic ketoacidosis, or life-threatening symptoms, higher concentrations (40 to 100 mEq/L) can be administered at up to 2 mEq/kg/hour.[73] Constant electrocardiographic monitoring and frequent measurements of serum potassium levels are mandatory.

Hyperkalemia

Hyperkalemia is a serum potassium concentration greater than 6.0 mEq/L in the newborn and greater than 5.5 mEq/L in the older child and adult.

Unlike hypokalemia, in which factitious values are uncommon, pseudohyperkalemia is quite common and must be excluded before the diagnosis of hyperkalemia is established and treatment initiated. Clotting in the test tube results in potassium release from leukocytes and platelets[4, 74]; this can be avoided by using a heparinized test tube. Intracellular leakage also occurs from hemolysis or abnormal membrane permeability of red blood cells.

Venipuncture can factitiously elevate potassium levels. Excessive forearm squeezing to delineate veins can significantly elevate serum potassium, probably as a result of muscular release during exercise. Excessive squeezing of an infant's heel or a too-rapid transfer of blood through a small-gauge needle will hemolyze the specimen and result in higher potassium values. Transfer of the specimen in a cold environment promotes potassium leakage by inhibiting the sodium-potassium ATPase pump.[75]

Increased potassium loads (exogenous or endogenous) do not normally contribute to dangerously elevated levels of potassium in persons with normal excretory mechanisms; however, patients with impaired renal function are at significant risk.[75]

Exogenous sources of potassium may include transfusion of old stored blood,[76] use of salt substitutes,[77, 78] and administration of potassium penicillin (1.7 mEq potassium per million units) or other potassium-containing drugs.[75]

Endogenous potassium loads may come from any source of acute tissue breakdown: trauma, burns, major surgery, rhabdomyolysis, intravascular coagulation, sickle cell hemolytic crisis, massive gastrointestinal bleeding, or chemotherapeutic destruction of large tumor masses.[74]

Medications may contribute to hyperkalemia. Potassium-sparing diuretics are primarily used in conjunction with other diuretics to diminish loss, but may also be used in cirrhosis. Spironolactone is a competitive inhibitor of aldosterone, whereas triamterene and amiloride block sodium uptake in the distal renal tubule. Succinylcholine, a depolarizing agent, causes release of potassium and inhibits membrane repolarization (cellular potassium uptake).[79] This is especially noticeable in patients with acute tissue necrosis, rhabdomyolysis, neuromuscular disease, tetanus, or renal failure.[80]

Digitalis overdose may cause severe hyperkalemia by inhibiting sodium-potassium exchange by sodium-potassium ATPase and leakage of potassium extracellularly.[81] Infusions of hyperosmotic solutions such as mannitol or hypertonic saline[82] and diabetic hyperglycemia may increase serum potassium.[83, 84] Transcellular redistribution in acid-base disorders is one of the major causes of hyperkalemia. In children, the most common cause is metabolic acidosis.[74]

Mineralocorticoid deficiency of any cause may elevate potassium levels. Addison's disease (primary adrenal insufficiency) is notable for salt wasting, but potassium retention can be pronounced.[85] This is more likely to be seen in patients receiving inadequate dosages of mineralocorticoid replacement therapy.[85] Congenital defects in enzymatic synthesis of aldosterone, such as 21-hydroxylase deficiency, may lead to diminished mineralocorticoid production and subsequent hyperkalemia with salt wasting, virilization, and failure to thrive.[86] A pseudohypoaldosteronism (in the presence of elevated aldosterone levels) that does not respond to mineralocorticoid therapy has been reported. Children usually outgrow this by the age of 4 years.[87]

The kidney is the primary regulator of potassium balance, and hyperkalemia may result from any acute or chronic excretory disorder. Potassium equilibrates to normal limits in chronic disorders by renal and extrarenal mechanisms. Surviving nephrons markedly increase their ability to secrete potassium; however, transient potassium loads may be poorly tolerated in this impaired condition.[75] Total body stores are normal to reduced in patients with chronic renal insufficiency.

The adverse consequences of hyperkalemia are a result of the altered transmembrane potential of resting cell membranes. The increased extracellular potassium reduces the resting membrane potential toward threshold levels. Although initially enhancing depolarization, conduction velocity is then slowed, and tissue excitability is reduced.

Clinical Manifestations

Hyperkalemia is often asymptomatic, and a thorough history and physical examination are required. Mandatory information in the history includes growth patterns, a history of chronic illnesses (adrenal disease, renal failure, diabetes mellitus), and medication usage (beta blockers, potassium-sparing diuretics, digoxin).[88] Similarly, the physical examination may be unremarkable or may only reveal muscle weakness. A review of growth indices, vital signs (particularly blood pressure), and any signs of chronic illness should be sought.

Progressive hyperkalemia results in paresthesia, followed by muscle weakness and, potentially, an ascending flaccid paralysis. The muscles of the head, trunk, and respiratory system are usually spared.

Laboratory tests should include a complete blood cell count (to exclude sickle cell anemia, leukemia, anemia, or chronic renal failure) and determination of glucose, bicarbonate, creatinine, and electrolyte levels. If the potassium level is elevated, repeat testing may be required to exclude factitious hyperkalemia. Urinalysis may show an abnormal pH or specific gravity, casts, red blood cells, or large amounts of protein, indicating intrinsic renal disease.

An electrocardiogram is required immediately. The heart is especially vulnerable to hyperkalemia, and sudden death may occur. Cardiac toxicity generally develops at serum potassium levels of 7 mEq/L. This is generally the critical value at which specific therapy to treat the hyperkalemia must be initiated.[8, 89] The electrocardiogram will show predictable changes: tall, peaked T waves are followed by a prolonged PR interval and widening of the QRS complex. At potassium concentrations greater than 8 mEq/L, the P wave amplitude decreases and may disappear as the atria stand still.[87] Ventricular conduction time continues to prolong, and the broadened QRS begins to merge with the peaked T wave, creating the classic sine wave of hyperkalemia.[68] This may herald the initiation of ventricular fibrillation or asystole.

Treatment

Acute hyperkalemia is a medical emergency. Therapy must be initiated immediately when the patient has skeletal muscle symptoms or cardiac abnormalities. Potassium concentrations between 6 to 7 mEq/L may not require immediate temporizing therapeutic measures in some cases; limiting potassium intake and increasing potassium excretion may be sufficient.[8] Treatment of hyperkalemia falls into three broad, sequential categories: reversing the membrane effects of hyperkalemia; enhancing the transcellular shift of potassium intracellularly; and removing potassium from the body.[8, 88]

A 10% calcium gluconate solution administered intravenously, 0.5 to 1.0 mg/kg over 2 to 5 minutes, will reverse the membrane effects of hyperkalemia (Table 11–2). Constant electrocardiographic monitoring is essential. A second dose may be given after 5 to 10 minutes if no result is seen.[89] The effect of calcium is transient, lasting from 30 to 60 minutes.

TABLE 11–2

TREATMENT OF HYPERKALEMIA

1. Membrane—reversing effects
   a. 10% calcium gluconate, 0.5–1.0 mg/kg IV over 2–5 min
      1. May repeat in 5–10 min
      2. Duration of action 30–60 min
      3. EKG monitoring
2. Transcellular shifting of potassium
   a. Sodium bicarbonate, 1–2 mEq/kg IV over 5–10 min
      1. May repeat in 15 min
      2. Duration of action up to 2 hr
      3. EKG monitoring
   b. Glucose, 0.5 to 1.0 gm/kg IV over 30 min
      1. May repeat as needed
      2. Duration of action 4–6 hr
      3. May administer regular insulin IV (1 unit/3 gm glucose or 1 unit/kg)
      4. Glucose monitoring
3. Potassium elimination
   a. Diuretics
   b. Ion exchange resin (sodium polystyrene sulfonate) 1 gm/kg
      1. Retention enema, 0.5 to 1.0 gm/kg over 30–45 min
         (a) Sorbitol 20%–25% solution, 3 mL/gm resin
      2. Orally: 0.5 to 1.9 gm/kg
         (a) Water, 3–4 ml/gm resin
         (b) Sorbitol 70% solution or dextrose 10% solution
   c. Dialysis
      1. Preferably hemodialysis
      2. Peritoneal dialysis

Intracellular shifting of potassium can be accomplished through the use of both bicarbonate and glucose (with or without insulin). Alkalinization of blood with bicarbonate can result in a rapid (5 to 10 minutes) shift of potassium intracellularly that persists for up to 2 hours. Administration of 1 to 2 mEq/kg of sodium bicarbonate intravenously over 5 to 10 minutes is recommended. This may be repeated if no effect is noted in 15 minutes. Transient electrocardiographic improvement is usually seen almost immediately.[8]

Glucose (0.5 to 1.0 mg/kg) is given intravenously over 30 minutes. The onset of action is within 30 minutes and may last several hours. In the absence of diabetes, this may stimulate endogenous insulin and avoid the need for exogenous insulin administration; nevertheless, many physicians administer regular insulin (1 unit IV for every 3 gm of glucose). Alternatively, 1 unit/kg may be given intravenously.[89] Glucose may be administered as often as necessary, monitoring possible complications such as hyperglycemia (without insulin) or hypoglycemia (with insulin).[8, 88]

If renal function is adequate, loop diuretics may be administered. The mainstay of therapy, however, is the ion exchange resin, sodium polystyrene sulfonate (Kayexalate), administered orally or as a retention enema. The resin exchanges potassium for sodium in a ratio of 1:1; administration of 1 gm/kg of resin should lower serum concentration by 1 mEq/L. The effect on potassium removal is variable[90] and is not specific for potassium; therefore potassium, magnesium, and calcium levels must be monitored, and frequent electrocardiographic monitoring is recommended. The preferential route of resin administration is by retention enema, 0.5 to 1.0 gm/kg with sorbitol (20% to 25% solution, 3 ml solution per gram of resin), optimally retained over 30 to 45 minutes. If given orally, the dose is 0.5 to 1.0 gm/kg, given in 3 to 4 ml of water per gram of resin. A 70% sorbitol solution or 10% dextrose solution should also be given, when the oral route is used, to avoid constipation.[91]

The resin should cause a decrease in serum potassium within 4 to 6 hours and may be repeated every 4 to 6 hours as needed.[8] Caution is necessary when administering ion exchange resins. Potassium exchange for sodium and osmotic catharsis from sorbitol or dextrose has resulted in severe hypernatremic dehydration. If the above measures are not successful in lowering the serum potassium, dialysis may be necessary.[8, 89, 91]

MAGNESIUM

Magnesium is the fourth most abundant cation in the body[92] and plays a vital role in neuromuscular function, growth, and enzymatic processes, particularly glycolysis and ATPase stimulation. Sixty percent of magnesium is stored in bone, and approximately one third of the magnesium in bone is freely exchangeable.

Only 1% of magnesium is extracellular. The remaining portion is found intracellularly, primarily in muscle (approximately 30%) and the liver. Only a fraction of the intracellular magnesium is exchangeable (20% to 30%), with the majority bound to proteins, RNA, and adenosine triphosphate (ATP).[92]

Extracellular levels are maintained at a low level within a narrow range. The average serum level is identical for both children and adults: 2.0 mg/dl (1.7 mEq/L), with a range of 1.7 to 2.8 mg/dl (1.4 to 2.3 mEq/L).[93]

Absorption

Magnesium intake is variable, with most diets resulting in excess intake of the minimum requirement of 3.6 mg/kg/day (12 mg magnesium = 1.0 mEq = 0.5 mmol).[92] Absorption occurs in the jejunum and ileum, with enhanced absorption in the presence of vitamin D, parathyroid hormone, calcitrol, and increased calcium absorption. Decreased absorption occurs in the presence of calcium, phosphorus, and increased intestinal motility.

Regulation

Magnesium is regulated primarily by the kidney, but excretion is affected by nonrenal factors. For example, a diet low in magnesium results in decreased excretion. Elevated parathyroid hormone levels in hyperparathyroidism can lead to magnesium wastage. Magnesium is 90% to 99% reabsorbed in the kidney tubules,[93] paralleling sodium and calcium reabsorption. There is competition for transport between the divalent cations calcium and magnesium. Approximately one third of total magnesium intake is renally excreted. Increased excretion can occur through the use of diuretics (loop, thiazide, osmotic, or mercurial), extracellular volume expansion, calcium loading, and glucagon.[92]

Hypomagnesemia

Hypomagnesemia is a common occurrence in hospitalized patients.[94] Probably the most common cause of hypomagnesemia is diuretic administration or use of medications leading to increased magnesium excretion (aminoglycosides, cisplatin, cyclosporins).[95] Prolonged administration of magnesium-free intravenous fluids, as in infants undergoing surgery, may lead to hypomagnesemia, as may malabsorption syndromes, hypoparathyroidism, hypercalciuria, renal tubular acidosis, primary aldosteronism, and alcoholism.[92] Early neonatal tetany may be mild and transient, whereas the hypocalcemia of late neonatal tetany will fail to respond to calcium therapy until magnesium levels are corrected.[93]

Hypomagnesemia presents clinically as neuromuscular irritability: tremors, tetany, seizures, tachycardia, and arrhythmias. Weakness or personality changes may also be evident. Because magnesium is primarily an intracellular ion, symptoms may not correlate with serum levels. Hypomagnesemia causes hypocalcemia through inhibition of parathyroid hormone (PTH) synthesis or release and also inhibits PTH action on skeletal sites; thus hypomagnesemia and hypocalcemia often coexist.

Treatment

Magnesium should be administered only after adequate renal function has been established. Cardiac monitoring should be performed during intravenous administration, and serum levels should be reassessed to avoid toxicity. Magnesium should never be given undiluted and should be infused intravenously slowly, and calcium gluconate should be nearby for administration if toxicity occurs.

For infants with hypomagnesemic tetanus, intravenous or intramuscular magnesium is given in a dose of 5 to 10 mg/kg (0.4 to 0.8 mEq/kg). This can be given as 0.01 to 0.02 ml/kg of a 50% solution that contains 500 mg/ml. A 10% solution can also be used (0.05 to 0.10 ml/kg). For the child with severe hypomagnesemia and tetany, some authors recommend an initial dose of 25 mg/kg. Cutaneous flushing, nausea, vomiting, and hypocalcemia can occur from magnesium administration.

Under less severe circumstances, oral supplementation of magnesium can be administered at a rate of 1 to 3 mEq/kg/day (12 to 36 mg/kg/day). All magnesium salts (chloride, citrate, gluconate) can be diluted with water.[96]

Hypermagnesemia

Hypermagnesemia is defined as a serum level greater than 5 mg/dl and most commonly occurs as a result of renal failure. Hypermagnesemia can also occur in the absence of decreased renal function, in children born to preecclampsic mothers on magnesium therapy,[97] and with overuse of magnesium-containing antacids,[98] enemas, or laxatives. Iatrogenic hypermagnesemia can occur from intravenous fluids.

Symptoms do not generally occur until serum magnesium levels exceed 5 mg/dl. Hyporeflexia and weakness precede neuromuscular blockade and paralysis. Respiratory depression with hypoxia, hypotension, bradycardia or tachycardia, drowsiness, or coma may occur. The electrocardiogram may reveal atrioventricular block or QT prolongation. Coma or death usually occurs with serum levels of 15 mg/dl or greater.[92]

The effects of hypermagnesemia are rapidly reversed with intravenous calcium. When administering calcium, cardiac monitoring is necessary. Calcium must be administered with extreme caution in the digitalized patient. It is incompatible with sodium bicarbonate in solution, causing precipitation.

A 10% solution calcium chloride (100 mg/ml = 1.36 mEq/ml) is given in an intravenous dose of 20 to 30 mg/kg slowly; the maximum single dose is 500 mg. This may be repeated every 10 minutes as needed.[99] A 10% solution calcium gluconate (100 mg/ml = 0.45 mEq/ml) is given as a 100-mg/kg intravenous dose slowly; the maximum single dose is 1 gm. This may be repeated every 10 minutes as needed. For less emergent circumstances, calcium gluconate may be given orally 500 mg/kg/day every 6 hours.[99]

The effect of intravenous calcium is transient, and definitive therapy includes elimination of the source of magnesium and possibly the use of dialysis.

PHOSPHORUS

In evaluating phosphorus levels, the clinician must be aware of terminology, methods of measurement, and what fraction of phosphorus is actually being measured. The quantitation of phosphate in biologic samples is usually performed as and expressed in terms of the total elemental phosphorus concentration.[15] The serum phosphorus represents a much smaller fraction. Phosphorus is primarily an intracellular ion, playing essential roles in energy production (ATP, creatine phosphorate), structural elements (sphingolipids, nucleotides, phosphoproteins), and in enhancing intracellular enzyme activity. The hydroxyapatite crystals of bone are the largest reservoir of phosphorus. Phosphate derangements may manifest as metabolic bone disease.

Organic phosphates comprise about two thirds of extracellular phosphates, are insoluble in acid, and therefore are not measured in routine serum phosphorus determinations. The remaining extracellular phosphorus is inorganic, acid-soluble, and usually measured by a calorimetric method. This acid-soluble fraction is commonly referred to as the *serum phosphorus*.

The serum phosphorus is often expressed in relation to adult values. This can be misleading, as values vary greatly with age. In children, the serum phosphorus levels of the newborn (1.4 to 2.8 mmol/L) increase during the first week of life (2.0 to 3.3 mmol/L), and then gradually decline through childhood to adult levels (1.0 to 1.3 mmol/L).

Phosphate Metabolism

Phosphate is well absorbed in the proximal small intestine. The major sources of dietary phosphorus are milk, milk products, and animal products. Absorption is stimulated by phosphate depletion, vitamin D and its metabolites, and PTH. Absorption is decreased by any binders in the gut such as aluminum, magnesium, calcium, and the hormone thyrocalcitonin.

Breast-fed infants (breast milk phosphate concentration, 150 to 220 mg/dl) and those children on prolonged hyperalimentation without phosphate supplementation may develop hypophosphatemia of dietary origin. Overt rickets may be seen in breast-fed neonates as a result of hypophosphatemia of dietary origin and having less well mineralized bones at birth.

As with other electrolytes, the most important control of phosphate metabolism occurs in the kidney. Phosphate is freely filtered at the glomerulus and is almost entirely reabsorbed in the proximal tubule. This normally results in nearly phosphate-free urine. The amount of phosphorus normally excreted is minimal.

Parathyroid hormone is the primary hormone affecting tubular resorption of phosphate; it reduces reabsorption of phosphate, leading to phosphaturia. Calcitriol (1,25-$(OH)_2D_3$) is the most active vitamin D metabolite and responds to decreased phosphorus by increasing tubular resorption of phosphate.

The renal transport of phosphate will appear to follow sodium in certain instances; extracellular fluid expansion and diuretic administration will result in phosphaturia.

Administration of glucose and insulin results in decreased plasma phosphorus, probably as a result of glucose phosphorylation and intracellular transport. Hyperglycemia results in phosphaturia. Inorganic phosphorus (HPO_4^{-2}, $H_2PO_4^-$) is the principal urinary buffer and thus plays a key role in acid-base balance. An alkaline urine results in increased phosphate reabsorption. Systemic acidosis results in an intracellular shift of phosphorus, and diabetic ketoacidosis can result in profound hypophosphatemia. Paradoxically, alkalosis also causes intracellular phosphate shift.

Hypophosphatemia

Hypophosphatemia indicates decreased circulating levels of inorganic phosphorus below an age-related range. It is usually mild to moderate and is asymptomatic, and its causes are many.

Decreased intake can occur with starvation, malabsorption, sustained vomiting, and antacid administration. Dietary phosphorus deficiency is rare. Sustained intravenous alimentation without phosphate supplementation can lead to hypophosphatemia. The premature, low-birth-weight infant being breast-fed needs phosphate; a reduction in serum phosphorus of only 1 mg/dL below normal may result in rickets.[100]

Increased renal excretion can occur with hyperparathyroidism, renal tubular defects, diminished reabsorption (potassium deficiency, oncogenic osteomalacia), extracellular volume expansion, or diuretic administration.[101, 102] Hypophosphatemia also occurs in recipients of renal transplants.[102]

Leukemia has been associated with hypophosphatemia, presumably as a result of increased needs in rapid cellular proliferation. A "hungry bone" syndrome has been described in rickets, in which therapy can result in acute hypophosphatemia.[102]

Clinical Manifestations

Symptoms of mild hypophosphatemia include proximal muscle weakness, with or without tenderness.[103] Hypotonia may exist, but deep tendon reflexes are normal. Neurologically, severe hypophosphatemia may result in a metabolic encephalopathy with irritability, paresthesia, memory loss, confusion, seizures, coma, and death. Acute respiratory failure may occur, and cardiomyopathy or myocardial dysfunction may be present. Muscle weakness and rhabdomyolysis have occurred. Renal tubular defects may occur, and hydrogen ion excretion is impaired. Chronic hypophosphatemia may lead to bone pain and fractures. Hemolytic anemia may occur at phosphorous levels below 0.5 mg/dl as a result of decreased red blood cell ATP and reduced conformability, with splenic destruction.[104]

Treatment

Oral phosphate supplementation is indicated in moderate or severe hypophosphatemia or with symptomatic hypophosphatemia that is not life threatening. The goal is to administer 1 to 3 gm elemental phosphate daily in divided doses to maintain the serum phosphorus level above 3.5 mg/dl.[105]

Parenteral administration of phosphate varies depending on the clinical situation. When administering phosphate parenterally, calcium, potassium, and phosphate levels must be monitored. Normal renal function must be ensured to prevent a hypocalcemic crisis or hypokalemia, and blood pressure must be monitored to avert hypotension. These solutions are usually hypertonic and require dilution.

Parenteral phosphate is always indicated when serum phosphorus is less than 1 mg/dl. In symptomatic children, 3 to 4 mg/kg is administered over the first 6 hours, unless there is concomitant hypercalcemia. In the presence of hypercalcemia, only 1 mg per kilogram phosphate should be given.[105]

In asymptomatic children with recent-onset hypophosphatemia, 2.5 mg per kilogram elemental phosphorus (potassium salt) diluted in half-normal saline is given over 6 hours.[105] For asymptomatic children with long-standing hypophosphatemia, 5 mg per kilogram elemental phosphorus (potassium salt) is recommended over the same time period.[105]

Hyperphosphatemia

Hyperphosphatemia may result from increased exogenous or endogenous sources, decreased glomerular filtration rate, or artifactually. Large dietary phosphate loads may result in infants being fed cow's milk. Intravenous phosphate loads may be received in old blood transfusions or in phosphate therapy for hypercalcemia. Phosphate-containing enemas have caused hyperphosphatemia and hypocalcemic cardiac arrest.[106]

Endogenously, cell lysis with release of intracellular phosphate may lead to hyperphosphatemia in a variety of conditions: cytotoxic cell lysis (especially lymphomas and leukemia), burns, and rhabdomyolysis (infection, trauma, toxins). Hypothyroidism and pseudohypoparathyroidism increase phosphate reabsorption.

A decrease in the glomerular filtration rate of 25% or more will result in phosphate retention, a reciprocal decline in calcium, and secondary hyperparathyroidism.[101] In the young infant, any reduction of the glomerular filtration rate, especially in the presence of phosphorus loading, will result in hyperphosphatemia. More importantly, the reciprocal hypocalcemia may result in latent or manifest tetany. Tetany may also occur after an acute phosphate load. Spurious serum phosphorus elevations can occur with hemolysis of the collected specimen.

Clinical Manifestations

The primary clinical consideration in hyperphosphatemia is that of systemic symptoms secondary to the reciprocal hypocalcemia and extraskeletal calcification.

The product of calcium and phosphorus needs evaluation to anticipate the possibility of soft tissue calcification. In children, a calcium × phosphorus value exceeding 60 to 70 mg/dl[2] may result in soft tissue calcification, including precipitation of calcium phosphate crystals in the kidney, leading to renal failure.[106]

Treatment

If the symptoms of hyperphosphatemia are a result of the reciprocal hypocalcemia, therapeutic measures for hypocalcemia should be instituted (see Chapter 55).

If renal function is diminished, several approaches to hyperphosphatemia can be used. Prevention of phosphorus ingestion or dietary restriction is the first step. Second, intestinal binding compounds can be administered. Aluminum and magnesium preparations can be alternated in order to diminish the possible side effect of diarrhea. Calcium salts are also effective. Finally, dialysis may be used in severe or refractory cases.

References

1. Nelson WE, Behrman RE, Vaughan VC (eds). General considerations in the care of sick children. *In* Nelson Textbook of Pediatrics. Philadelphia, WB Saunders, 1987, p 176.
2. Arner ED, Ellis D, Ichikawa I, et al. Normal neonates and the maturational development of homeostatis mechanisms. *In* Ichikawa I (ed). Pediatric Textbook of Fluids and Electrolytes. Baltimore, Williams & Wilkins, 1990, p 111.
3. Simmons CF, Ichikawa I. External balance of water and electrolytes. *In* Ichikawa I (ed). Pediatric Textbook of Fluids and Electrolytes. Baltimore, Williams & Wilkins, 1990, p 24.
4. Naris RG, Jones ER, Storm MC, et al. Diagnostic strategies in disorders of fluid, electrolyte, and acid-base homeostasis. Am J Med 1982;72:496.
5. David R, Ellis D, Gartner JL. Water intoxication in normal infants: Role of antidiuretic hormone in pathogenesis. Pediatrics 1981;68:349.
6. Sulyok E, Kovacs L, Lichardus B, et al. Late hyponatremia in premature infants: Role of aldosterone and arginine vasopressin. J Pediatr 1985;106:990.

7. Hantman D, Rossier B, Zohlman R. Rapid correction of hyponatremia in the syndrome of inappropriate secretion of antidiuretic hormone. Ann Intern Med 1973;78:870.
8. Feld LG, Kaskel FJ, Schoeneman MJ. The approach to fluid and electrolyte therapy in pediatrics. Adv Pediatr 1988;35:497.
9. Weiss RA, Schoeneman MJ, Griefer I. Treatment of severe nephrotic edema with albumin and furosemide. NY J Med 1984;84:384.
10. Finberg L. Pathogenesis of lesions in the central nervous system in hypernatremic states. I. Clinical observations of infants. Pediatrics 1959;25:40.
11. Feig PU, McCurdy DK. The hypertonic state. N Engl J Med 1977;297:1444.
12. Yoshioka T, Iitaka K, Ichikawa I. Body fluid compartments. In Ichikawa I (ed). Pediatric Textbook of Fluids and Electrolytes. Baltimore, Williams & Wilkins, 1990, p 19.
13. Burg MB. Tubular chloride transport and the mode of action of some diuretics. Kidney Int 1976;9:189.
14. Nelson WE, Behrman RE, Vaughan VC (eds). General considerations in the care of sick children. In Nelson Textbook of Pediatrics. Philadelphia, WB Saunders, 1987, p 188.
15. Nelson WE, Behrman RE, Vaughan VC (eds). General considerations in the care of sick children. In Nelson Textbook of Pediatrics. Philadelphia, WB Saunders, 1987, p 188.
16. Holmberg L, Perheentupa J, Launiala K, et al. Congenital chloride diarrhea. Arch Dis Child 1977;52:255.
17. Emmett M, Narins RE. Clinical use of the anion gap. Medicine 1977;56(1):38.
18. Shaffer MA. Acid-base homeostasis. In Rosen P, Baker FJ, Barkin RM, et al (eds). Emergency Medicine Concepts and Clinical Practice. Vol II. St. Louis, CV Mosby, 1988, p 1954.
19. Pierson RN, Lin DH, Phillips RA. Total body potassium in health: Effects of age, sex, height, and fat. Am J Physiol 1974;226(1):206.
20. Edelman IS, Liebman J. Anatomy of body water and electrolytes. Am J Med 1959;27:256.
21. Flynn MA, Woodruff L, Clark J, et al. Total body potassium in normal children. Pediatr Res 1972;6:239.
22. Sulyok E, Nemeth M, Tenyi I, et al. Relationship between maturity, electrolyte balance and the function of the renin-angiotensin-aldosterone system in newborn infants. Biol Neonate 1979;35:60.
23. Lubin M. Intercellular potassium and macromolecular synthesis in mammalian cells. Nature 1967;213:451.
24. Adler S, Fraley DS. Potassium and intracellular pH. Kidney Int 1977;11:433.
25. Tannen RL. Relationship of renal ammonia production and potassium homeostasis. Kidney Int 1977;11:453.
26. Katz AI. Renal Na-K-ATPase: Its role in tubular sodium and potassium transport. Am J Physiol 1982;242:F207.
27. Thomas RL. Electrogenic sodium pump in nerve and muscle cells. Physiol Rev 1972;52(3):563.
28. Nelson WE, Behrman RE, Vaughn VC (eds). General considerations in the care of sick children. In Nelson Textbook of Pediatrics. Philadelphia, WB Saunders, 1987, p 180.
29. Fraley DS, Adler S. Isohydric regulation of plasma potassium by bicarbonate in the rat. Kidney Int 1976;9:333.
30. Fraley DS, Adler S. Correction of hyperkalemia by bicarbonate despite constant blood pH. Kidney Int 1977;12:354.
31. Adrogne HJ, Modias NE. Changes in plasma potassium concentration during acute acid-base disturbances. Am J Med 1981;71:456.
32. Kunan RT, Stein JH. Disorders of potassium metabolism. In Early LE, Gottschalk CW (eds). Strauss and Welt's Diseases of the Kidney Third Edition. Boston, Little, Brown, 1979, p 1581.
33. Zierler KL. Effect of insulin on potassium efflux from rat muscle in the presence and absence of glucose. Am J Physiol 1960:198:1066.
34. Bia MJ, Defronzo RA. Extrarenal potassium homeostasis. Am J Physiol 1981;240(4):F257.
35. Defronzo RA, Bia MJ, Birkhead G. Epinephrine and potassium homeostasis. Kidney Int 1981;20:83.
36. Rosa RM, Silva P, Young JB, et al. Adrenergic modulation of extrarenal potassium disposal. N Engl J Med 1980;300(8):431.
37. D'Silva JH. The action of adrenaline on serum potassium. J Physiol 1935;86:219.
38. Carlsson E, Fellenius E, Lundborg P. Beta adrenoreceptor blockers, plasma potassium, and exercise. Lancet 1978;2:424.
39. Bia MJ, Tyler KA, Defronzo RA. Regulation of extrarenal potassium homeostasis by adrenal hormones in rats. Am J Physiol 1982; 242(6):F641.
40. Rabinowitz L, Sarason RL, Yamauchi J, et al. Time course of adaptation to altered K intake in rats and sheep. Am J Physiol 1984;247:F607.
41. Jamison RL, Work J, Schafer JA. New pathways for potassium transport in the kidney. Am J Physiol 1982;242(4):F297.
42. Malnic G, Klose RM, Giebisch G. Micropuncture study of renal potassium exertion in the rat. Am J Physiol 1964;206:674.
43. Grantham JJ, Burg MB, Orloff J. The nature of transtubular Na and K transport in isolated rabbit renal collecting tubules. J Clin Invest 1970;49:1815.
44. Nelson WE, Behrman RE, Vaughan VC (eds). General considerations

45. Turnberg LA. Electrolyte absorption from the colon. Gut 1970;11:1049.
46. Bastl LP, Binder HJ, Hayslett JP. Role of glucocorticoid and aldosterone in maintenance of colonic cation transport. Am J Physiol 1980;238:F181.
47. Phillips SF. Absorption and secretion by the colon. Gastroenterology 1969;56:966.
48. Fisher KA, Binder HJ, Hayslett JP. Potassium secretion by colonic mucosal cells after potassium adaptation. Am J Physiol 1976;231(4):987.
49. Bastl C, Hayslett JP, Binder HJ. Increased large intestinal secretion of potassium in renal insufficiency. Kidney Int 1977;12:9.
50. Satlin LM, Schwartz GJ. Disorders of potassium metabolism. In Ichikawa I (ed). Pediatric Textbook of Fluids and Electrolytes. Baltimore, Williams & Wilkins, 1990, p 220.
51. Eddy RL, Sanchez SA. Renin-secreting renal neoplasm and hypertension with hypokalemia. Ann Int Med 1971;75:725.
52. Voute PA, van der Meer J, Staugaard-Kloosterziel W. Plasma renin activity in Wilms tumor. Acta Endocrinol (Copenh) 1971;67:197.
53. Brunner FP, Frick PG. Hypokalemia, metabolic aklaosis, and hypernatremia due to "massive" sodium penicillin therapy. Br Med J 1968;4:550.
54. Klastersky J, VanderKelen B, Daneau D, et al. Carbenicillin and hypokalemia. Ann Int Med 1973;78:774.
55. Stapleton FB, Nelson B, Vats TS, et al. Hypokalemia associated with antibiotic treatment. Am J Dis Child 1976;130:1104.
56. Rodriguez V, Green S, Bodey GP. Serum electrolyte abnormalities associated with the administration of polymyxin B in febrile leukemic patients. Clin Pharmacol Ther 1969;11:106.
57. Cronin RE, Bulger RE, Southern P, et al. Natural history of aminoglycoside nephrotoxicity in the dog. J Lab Clin Med 1980;95(3):463.
58. Holmes AM, Hesling CM, Wilson TM. Drug induced secondary hyperaldosteronism in patients with pulmonary tuberculosis. Q J Med 1970;39(154):299.
59. Satlin LM, Schwartz GJ. Disorders of potassium metabolism. In Ichikawa I (ed). Pediatric Textbook of Fluids and Electrolytes. Baltimore, Williams & Wilkins, 1990, p 223.
60. Beigelman PM. Potassium in severe diabetic ketoacidosis. Am J Med 1973;54(4):419.
61. Satlin LM, Schwartz GJ. Disorders of potassium metabolism. In Ichikawa I (ed). Pediatric Textbook of Fluids and Electrolytes. Baltimore, Williams & Wilkins, 1990, p 221.
62. Ewanixk JS, Engel WK, Griggs RL, et al. Acetazolamide prophylaxis in hypokalemic periodic paralysis. N Engl J Med 1968;278(11):582.
63. Witten TA, Bickel JG. Potassium in gastric juice. Gastroenterology 1970;59(2):330.
64. Babior BM. Villous adenoma of the colon. Am J Med 1966;41:615.
65. Schrock LG, Polk HC. Rectal villous adenoma producing hypokalemia. Am Surg 1974;40(1):54.
66. Verner JV, Morrison AB. Islet cell tumor and syndrome of refractory watery diarrhea and hypokalemia. Am J Med 1958;25:374.
67. Satlin LM, Schwartz GJ. Disorders of potassium metabolism. In Ichikawa I (ed). Pediatric Textbook of Fluids and Electrolytes. Baltimore, Williams & Wilkins, 1990, pg. 227.
68. Fisch C. Relation of electrolyte disturbances to cardiac arrhythmias. Circulation 1973;47:408.
69. Satlin LM, Schwartz GJ. Disorders of potassium metabolism. In Ichikawa I (ed). Pediatric Textbook of Fluids and Electrolytes. Baltimore, Williams & Wilkins, 1990, p 224.
70. Aldinger JA, Samaan NA. Hypokalemia with hypercalcemia. Ann Intern Med 1977;87:571.
71. Dyckner T. Ventricular extrasystoles and intracellular electrolytes before and after potassium and magnesium infusions in patients on diuretic treatment. Am Heart J 1979;97:12.
72. Kassirer JP, Harrington JI. Diuretics and potassium metabolism: A reassessment of the need, effectiveness and safety of potassium therapy. Kidney Int 1977;11:505.
73. Satlin LM, Schwartz GJ. Disorders of potassium metabolism. In Ichikawa I (ed). Pediatric Textbook of Fluids and Electrolytes. Baltimore, Williams & Wilkins, 1990, p 228.
74. Defronza RA, Bia MJ, Smith D. Clinical disorders of hyperkalemia. Ann Rev Med 1982;33:521.
75. Satlin LM, Schwartz GJ. Disorders of potassium metabolism. In Ichikawa I (ed). Pediatric Textbook of Fluids and Electrolytes. Baltimore, Williams & Wilkins, 1990, p 229.
76. Bostic O, Duvernay WFC. Hyperkalemic cardiac arrest during transfusion of stored blood. J Electrocardiol 1972;5(4):407.
77. Haddad A, Strong E. Potassium in salt substitutes. N Engl J Med 1975;292:1082.
78. Sopko JA, Freeman RM. Salt substitutes as a source of potassium. JAMA 1977;238(7):608.
79. Gronert GA, Theye RA. Pathophysiology of hyperkalemia induced by succinylcholine. Anesthesiology 1975;43(1):89.
80. Cooperman LH. Succinylcholine-induced hyperkalemia in neuromuscular disease. JAMA 1970;213(11):1867.
81. Smith TW, Wilkerson JT. Suicidal and accidental digoxin ingestion. Circulation 1971;44:29.
82. Satlin LM, Schwartz GJ. Disorders of potassium metabolism. In Ichikawa

I (ed). Pediatric Textbook of Fluids and Electrolytes. Baltimore, Williams & Wilkins, 1990, p 230.

83. Ammon RA, May WS, Nightingale SD. Glucose-induced hyperkalemia with normal aldosterone levels. Ann Intern Med 1978;89:349.

84. Goldfarb S, Cox M, Singer I, et al. Acute hyperkalemia induced by hyperglycemia: Hormonal mechanisms. Ann Intern Med 1976;84:426.

85. Daughaday WH, Rendleman D. Severe symptomatic hyperkalemia in an adrenalectomized woman due to enhanced mineralocorticoid requirement. Ann Intern Med 1967;66:1197.

86. Satlin LM, Schwartz GJ. Disorders of potassium metabolism. *In* Ichikawa I (ed). Pediatric Textbook of Fluids and Electrolytes. Baltimore, Williams & Wilkins, 1990, p 231.

87. Satlin LM, Schwartz GJ. Disorders of potassium metabolism. *In* Ichikawa I (ed). Pediatric Textbook of Fluids and Electrolytes. Baltimore, Williams & Wilkins, 1990, p 232.

88. Satlin LM, Schwartz GJ. Disorders of potassium metabolism. *In* Ichikawa I (ed). Pediatric Textbook of Fluids and Electrolytes. Baltimore, Williams & Wilkins, 1990, p 233.

89. Dobrin RS, Larsen CD, Holliday MA. The critically ill child: Acute renal failure. Pediatrics 1971;48(2):286.

90. Scherr L, Ogden DA, Mead AW, et al. Management of hyperkalemia with a cation exchange resin. N Engl J Med 1961;264(3):115.

91. Satlin LM, Schwartz GJ. Disorders of potassium metabolism. *In* Ichikawa I (ed). Pediatric Textbook of Fluids and Electrolytes. Baltimore, Williams & Wilkins, 1990, p 234.

92. Nelson WE, Behrman RE, Vaughan VC (eds). General consideration in the care of sick children. *In* Nelson Textbook of Pediatrics. Philadelphia, WB Saunders, 1987, pp 181, 182.

93. Key LL, Carpenter TO. Metabolism of calcium, phosphorus, and other divalent ions. *In* Ichikawa I (ed). Pediatric Textbook of Fluids and Electrolytes. Baltimore, Williams & Wilkins, 1990, p 106.

94. Wong ET, Rude RK, Singer FR, et al. A high prevalence of hypomagnesium and hypermagnesemia in hospitalized patients. Am J Clin Pathol 1983;79(3):348.

95. Carpenter TO, Key LL. Disorders of the metabolism of calcium, phosphorus, and other divalent ions. *In* Ichikawa I (ed). Pediatric Textbook of Fluids and Electrolytes. Baltimore, Williams & Wilkins, 1990, p 260.

96. Carpenter TO, Key LL. Disorders of the metabolism of calcium, phosphorus, and other divalent ions. *In* Ichikawa I (ed). Pediatric Textbook of Fluids and Electrolytes. Baltimore, Williams & Wilkins, 1990, p 261.

97. Rasch DK, Huber PA, Richardson CJ, et al. Neurobehavioral effects of neonatal hypermagnesemia. J Pediatr 1982;100(2):272.

98. Humphrey M, Kennon S, Pramanik A. Hypermagnesemia from antacid administration in a newborn infant. J Pediatr 1981;98:313.

99. Barkin RM, Rosen P (eds). Appendix D: Formulary. *In* Emergency Pediatrics: A Guide to Ambulatory Care. St Louis, CV Mosby, 1990, p 720.

100. Key LL, Carpenter TO. Metabolism of calcium, phosphorus, and other divalent cations. *In* Ichikawa I (ed). Pediatric Textbook of Fluids and Electrolytes. Baltimore, Williams & Wilkins, 1990, p 105.

101. Nelson WE, Behrman RE, Vaughan RC (eds). General considerations in the care of sick children. *In* Nelson Textbook of Pediatrics. Philadelphia, WB Saunders, 1987, p 190.

102. Carpenter TO, Key LL. Disorders of the metabolism of calcium, phosphorus, and other divalent ions. *In* Ichikawa I (ed). Pediatric Textbook of Fluids and Electrolytes. Baltimore, Williams & Wilkins, 1990, p 257.

103. Carpenter TO, Key LL. Disorders of the metabolism of calcium, phosphorus, and other divalent ions. *In* Ichikawa I (ed). Pediatric Textbook of Fluids and Electrolytes. Baltimore, Williams & Wilkins, 1990, p 255.

104. Carpenter TO, Key LL. Disorders of the metabolism of calcium, phosphorus, and other divalent ions. *In* Ichikawa I (ed). Pediatric Textbook of Fluids and Electrolytes. Baltimore, Williams & Wilkins, 1990, p 256.

105. Carpenter TO, Key LL. Disorders of the metabolism of calcium, phosphorus, and other divalent ions. *In* Ichikawa I (ed). Pediatric Textbook of Fluids and Electrolytes. Baltimore, Williams & Wilkins, 1990, p 258.

106. Carpenter TO, Key LL. Disorders of the metabolism of calcium, phosphorus, and other divalent ions. *In* Ichikawa I (ed). Pediatric Textbook of Fluids and Electrolytes. Baltimore, Williams & Wilkins, 1990, p 259.

CHAPTER 12

Sudden Infant Death Syndrome

Michele B. Wagner

DEFINITIONS

Sudden unexpected death in infants: A disease of theories.[1]

The sudden infant death syndrome: A bustling ignorance?[2]

Sudden infant death syndrome: Is the confusion ending?[3]

'Near-miss' or 'near-myth' for sudden infant death syndrome?[4]

Infantile apnea, home monitoring, and SIDS: Go back to go.[5]

In few other areas of medicine are such titles found, reflecting so much uncertainty after so prolonged a period of research into a type of death affecting up to 2 in every 1000 children born in industrialized countries. The decision whether to call SIDS a *disease* or a *syndrome* and whether to use the terms *near-miss episode*, *infantile apnea*, or *apparent life-threatening event*, even before beginning a discussion of the topic, reflect the uncertainties dominant in this field.

For those who are not involved in the care of these children and their families, the profusion of terms seems bewildering. In reality, each term has a clear meaning; the very real confusion in this field derives from the degree of overlapping of the syndromes described and the frequent misuse of the terms.

Sudden Infant Death Syndrome

Sudden infant death syndrome (SIDS) is the sudden death of any infant or young child that is unexpected according to the history and in which a thorough postmortem examination fails to demonstrate an adequate cause of death.[6] To call this a *syndrome* implies a common cause, rather than simply a commonality of physical and historical findings. However, this term was incorporated into the ninth edition of the International Classification of Diseases (1975)[7] and is so widely used that it is probably futile to attempt any change.

In 1989, the National Institutes of Health (NIH) assembled a group of experts to revise the definition; the most recent version adds that a death can be attributed to SIDS only after "an investigation of the death scene and a review of the case history."[8] The major remaining difficulties are the retrospective nature of the definition and the imprecision of the term *unexpected*. As Thach has pointed out, "in SIDS we are unable to distinguish between absence of symptoms and failure to detect symptoms."[9]

Sudden Unexpected Infant Death

The term *sudden unexpected infant death* (SUID) may be used when no autopsy has been performed. Any epidemiologic study of such cases purporting to illuminate the causes of SIDS is misleading. However, this term may be used in investigations of "preventable unexpected infant deaths."[10]

SIDS Sibling

SIDS sibling merely refers to the surviving twin or subsequent sibling of a child who has died from SIDS. When these children are followed with any purpose other than psychological evaluation or support of the family, this term implies that part of the cause of SIDS deaths is hereditary. At this time, there is insufficient evidence to support this view.

Near-Miss or Near-SIDS Episode

The terms *near-miss* and *near-SIDS episodes* were widely (and interchangeably) used for episodes in which a previously healthy and normal infant was found, generally during sleep, with depressed or absent respirations, cyanosis, or hypotonia, and in which vigorous stimulation or cardiopulmonary respiration (CPR) was necessary to end the episode. Especially in the early years of SIDS research, it seemed logical that infants with apparent severe apneic episodes of unknown cause were "survivors" of SIDS[11]; in fact, the term *SIDS survivors* was used in early reviews.[12] The shortcomings of these terms are that they imply that the episode would have resulted in death had intervention not occurred, and that the same mechanism is involved as in SIDS cases. In addition, the terms are often used to imply that surviving or subsequent infants in these families are at increased risk of SIDS.

Infantile Apnea

The American Academy of Pediatrics defines prolonged infantile apnea as "cessation of breathing for at least 20 seconds or a briefer episode of apnea associated with bradycardia, cyanosis, or pallor."[13] In 1981, the National SIDS Foundation proposed this term as an alternative for near-SIDS.[14] However, the terms are clearly not synonymous; the term *infantile apnea* should be used only when apnea has been documented as a cause of the episode.

Apparent Life-Threatening Episode

An apparent life-threatening episode (ALTE) is "an episode that is frightening to the observer and is characterized by some combination of apnea (central or occasionally obstructive), color change (usually cyanotic or pallid but occasionally erythematous or plethoric), marked change in muscle tone (usually marked limpness), choking, or gagging."[15] This term, first defined by an NIH Consensus Conference in 1986, has several advantages. First, it merely describes the nature of the episode; because the infant has often fully recovered by the time medical care is sought, an ALTE is defined by the conclusion reached by the bystander. In addition, this term makes no assumptions regarding the origin of the event. Because of this neutrality, the term has met with some resistance in the SIDS community.

Much of the research into the causes of SIDS has been hampered by the low incidence of the syndrome. Even in a prospective study involving several thousand infants, no more than a handful can be expected to die from SIDS. This number is so small that the chance of finding statistically significant results is almost negligible. Because prospective studies of hundreds of thousands of infants are impractical, researchers have turned to the evaluation of ALTE infants or SIDS siblings. Interpretation of findings obtained in this way depends on acceptance of the hypotheses that an ALTE is indeed a "missed SIDS" and that SIDS siblings share certain risk factors or pathologic processes with their dead brothers and sisters.

HISTORICAL CONSIDERATIONS

Descriptions of sudden unexpected infant deaths date back to biblical times, when they were called "overlaying" and assumed to be caused by suffocation by an adult sharing the bed. This term was in common use until the beginning of the twentieth century. By 1950, infant mortality in the United States had decreased to one fourth of the rate in 1900,[16] and these apparently inexplicable deaths began to make up a significant proportion of postneonatal infant mortality. At the same time, decreased bed sharing by adults and infants made accidental suffocation seem an unlikely cause of death in many cases. As an overreaction to earlier beliefs and to some obviously unfounded accusations of infanticide or neglect in specific instances, the paradigm most widely accepted in the SIDS community in the 1970s and 1980s essentially excluded accidental suffocation as a cause of SIDS. These conclusions were largely based on a 1954 report by Woolley[17] of some uncontrolled studies purporting to show that even small infants are capable of movement to clear their airway. This paradigm has, in turn, been recently challenged.

The years since the 1960s have seen the development of a "SIDS establishment" made up of SIDS researchers and families who have experienced the shock and grief of sudden infant deaths or of frightening, apparently life-threatening episodes. The existence of such an establishment has provided a support system for thousands of families. However, it has also created resistance to findings that appear to contradict long-held beliefs. Some of these beliefs include the following:

1. The cause of all or most SIDS deaths is an apneic episode during sleep.
2. The cause of (most) SIDS deaths is the same as that of (most) apparent life-threatening episodes.
3. Home apnea monitoring prevents subsequent deaths in infants who have experienced an apparent life-threatening event.
4. SIDS siblings have a higher rate of SIDS deaths than "normal" infants.
5. It is possible to predict whether a SIDS sibling has a higher risk of SIDS than "normal" infants.
6. Home apnea monitoring prevents subsequent deaths in SIDS siblings.

Most of these statements are at best unproven; some have been proven false.

SUDDEN INFANT DEATH SYNDROME
Epidemiology
Rate

In industrialized countries, SIDS is one of the leading causes of death in infants between the ages of 1 month and 1 year, with a reported rate of autopsy-confirmed SIDS deaths of 0.3[18] (Hong Kong) to 6.3[19, 20] (New Zealand) per 1000 live births. In the United States, the rate of SIDS is currently reported to be about 1.7 per 1000.[21] SIDS is responsible for approximately 40% of postneonatal deaths[21] and is the leading cause of postneonatal death in normal-birth-weight infants.[22] In the United States the relative risk for black infants has been reported to be two to three times that for white infants[23, 24]; however, in the U.S. Collaborative Perinatal Project, this excess risk disappeared after adjusting for maternal education and family income.[25] In contrast to many other industrialized nations, not all SIDS cases in the United States undergo autopsy. However, the median autopsy rate increased from 82% in 1980 to 93% in 1985, although in some states less than half of all SIDS cases were undergoing autopsy.[26] The overall infant mortality has continued to decline in most industrialized countries, but the SIDS rate has remained virtually unchanged and in some countries has increased. In the United States, the rate decreased from 1.43 per 1000 in 1979 to 1.17 per 1000 in 1988.[27] Although sudden unexpected deaths certainly occur in older children and adolescents, these rarely remain unexplained after autopsy; one study gives a rate of completely unexplained deaths of only 0.13 per 1000.[28] Deaths unexplained after autopsy are equally rare in adults; the exception is a syndrome of unexpected nocturnal death that seems to occur primarily in young adults of Laotian extraction.[29]

Age

Most SIDS deaths occur in children less than 1 year of age. By convention, a sudden unexpected death in a child younger than 1 month or older than 1 year is not classified as SIDS. (One of the few studies of sudden deaths in healthy term neonates gave a rate of 0.12 unexplained deaths per 1000 live births,[30] a rate similar to that found after infancy.) SIDS deaths peak around 3 months of age, and 80% of these deaths occur before 5 months of age.[31] It is this peak that distinguishes SIDS deaths from the other common causes of death in the first year of life; in deaths from congenital anomalies and infections, the peak occurs in the first month of life.[32] However, the single peak in SIDS may be the result of the summation of several causes of death, with peaks at different ages.[33]

Seasonal and Daily Variation

In most countries, SIDS deaths occur more frequently during the winter months.[34, 35] Some, but not all, of this effect can be attributed to seasonal variations in the month of birth.[36] This seasonal variation has prompted many researchers to look for an infectious cause of death. Many studies also demonstrate an increased proportion of SIDS deaths on weekends, in contrast to all other causes of death[37–40]; this finding is difficult to explain under any theory of causation.

Circumstances of Death

Infants are usually found dead during periods of presumed sleep (i.e., during naps or at night), and death appears to be silent. Except for the fact that younger infants are generally fed just before being put to bed, there seems to be no association with feeding times. The presumption that SIDS deaths occur during sleep rather than during waking is supported by the fact that SIDS deaths in infants less than 2 months old appear to occur evenly throughout the day and night, whereas there is a heavy predominance of nocturnal deaths after 2 months of age.[41]

Risk Factors

Epidemiologic studies have found an increased risk in males and in low-birth-weight and premature infants[25]; presumably these factors are responsible for the increased rate in twin births.[38] Data show a rate of autopsy-confirmed SIDS of almost 11 per 1000 in infants who had previously been in the neonatal intensive care unit[42] and a rate of 11% in infants with bronchopulmonary dysplasia.[43] There is also an increased risk of SIDS in infants of young mothers.[25, 38] All these factors are also found in deaths from infections, accidents, and other causes, but not in deaths attributed to congenital malformations.[44] An association has been found

in many studies between an increased risk for SIDS and the following factors: neonatal pathologic abnormality, need for resuscitation at birth, poor medical follow-up after birth, decreased interval between pregnancies, and maternal smoking and drug habits. Again, these risk factors are also found in infants dying from known causes. The concern in the 1980s relating to the association between SIDS and the diphtheria-tetanus-pertussis (DTP) vaccine appears to have been unfounded.[45, 46]

Risk of Recurrence in a SIDS Sibling

The recurrence risk of SIDS in a family was previously considered to be four to ten times that of the general population, whereas the risk for a surviving twin was considered to be increased by a factor of 20. More recent studies have given relative risks of 1.85,[47] 3.7,[48] and 6.0[49] for all subsequent siblings after a SIDS death. This issue is important in the management of these siblings, as they have been investigated in depth as a high-risk group for SIDS. Using a baseline risk of 2 per 1000 and a relative risk of 6 gives a risk of 1.2% in subsequent siblings; this is a clear indication for close attention to these families but makes it difficult to justify monitoring these infants en masse. Consequently much effort has gone into attempting to identify subgroups at higher risk. Little data are available concerning twins; however, it appears that the risk in a surviving twin is within the same range as that for subsequent siblings.[50] Two series of twin infants dying suddenly and simultaneously have been described in the literature, but in many of these cases, the scene investigation was inadequate to exclude nonaccidental or infectious causes of death.[51, 52]

Previous ALTE

Only a minority of SIDS victims have been reported to have a previous history of a "near-miss" episode or ALTE. In the National Institute of Child Health and Human Development SIDS study, 7.7% of mothers of SIDS infants and 3.0% of control mothers reported such an episode.[21]

Scoring Systems

A number of attempts have been made to develop scoring systems to identify infants in the general population who are at higher risk of SIDS. These have used the criteria already identified in epidemiologic studies and have been successful in identifying a small group of infants in which the risk of SIDS is markedly increased (in one study, up to 10%[53]). However, only a minority of subsequent SIDS victims could be identified by these criteria. Scoring systems with higher sensitivity also have an unacceptably high false-positive rate.[54] Some intervention studies have been conducted that appear to decrease subsequent morbidity and mortality (from all causes) in these high-risk groups through improved preventive care, including home health visits.[55]

Etiology

Since 1970, the consensus has gradually shifted from the belief that SIDS deaths occur in perfectly healthy babies to the belief that the infants involved suffered from chronic illness that may have made them less able to resist the ultimate insult. No truly new theory of SIDS has been developed since 1980, probably because of the large number of theories proposed earlier. Theories generally fall into one of six categories: respiratory/ventilatory, cardiovascular, autonomic/temperature, infectious, metabolic, or miscellaneous.

Respiratory/Ventilatory Causes

Theoretic central apnea causes include congenital apnea and apnea acquired as a result of an infection such as respiratory syncytial virus. Theoretic obstructive apnea causes involve multiple factors, such as the anatomy of the infant airway, pathologic narrowing secondary to an upper respiratory infection, and laryngeal spasm secondary to reflux of gastric contents.

Cardiovascular Causes

Theoretic cardiovascular causes include fatal dysrhythmias, conduction abnormalities (e.g., long QT syndrome), and anaphylactic reactions (e.g., to cow's milk proteins or other substances).

Autonomic/Temperature Causes

The "autonomic instability" of infants has been cited by some authors, but no convincing mechanism of death has been proposed. Hypothermic deaths probably occur, but the widespread distribution of SIDS makes this unlikely as a major cause. Hyperthermic deaths, secondary either to overheating or to loss of cooling mechanisms in some infants, probably also occur. Malignant hyperthermia has been proposed as a mechanism for SIDS deaths,[56] but no prospective study has been carried out, and the low rate of familial recurrence makes this an unlikely cause.

Infectious Causes

Multiple infectious causes have been considered, including infantile botulism, respiratory syncytial virus, and cytomegalovirus.

Metabolic Causes

Metabolic causes include thiamine, vitamin C, vitamin D, vitamin E, and selenium deficiency states; hypo- or hypernatremia, hypo- or hyperkalemia, hypo- or hypermagnesemia, and hypo- or hypercalcemia; and hypoglycemia. Much research into these factors has shed little light on the subject. A relatively recent addition to this category is the group of diseases collectively known as *inborn errors of metabolism*. However, these are more plausibly considered as a differential diagnosis to SIDS than as a cause.

Miscellaneous Causes

Miscellaneous theoretic causes are legion. Most involve a precipitating factor that results in a cause of death under one of the previous categories; an example is the use of nonprescription phenothiazines, which is hypothesized to result in a variant of malignant hyperthermia.[57] None of these causal theories are supported to any major degree by existing evidence. There is also a "nihilistic" view that SIDS does not exist as a syndrome; according to this perspective, all deaths presently classified as SIDS are attributable to a specific cause.

None of the diseases discussed earlier has been established as a "cause" for SIDS. However, almost all of them must be considered in the differential diagnosis, a fact that explains the difficulty of the diagnosis, even after autopsy, and probably also the wide variations in reported SIDS rates in different countries.

Anatomy and Physiology
Neonatal and Infant Airway

Several aspects of the anatomy of neonates and infants make the theory of obstructive apnea plausible, including the need for active upper airway muscle control to maintain an open airway.[58] Airway obstruction resulting from the laryngeal chemoreflex[33] or other mechanisms resulting in laryngospasm have been discussed; support for these theories comes from the known increased susceptibility of young infants to develop laryngospasm during general anesthesia (2.5% of infants 1 to 3 months of age in the study by Olsson and Hallen).[59] However, laryngospasm is generally believed to resolve as asphyxia increases, and therefore an additional mechanism must be invoked to explain the fatal outcome in SIDS. A malignant variant of the infant breath-holding response[9] ("cyanotic or pallid breath-holding spell") has also been suggested as a possible cause of death, although in its usual form this behavior is seen in infants older than 9 months. Nevertheless, one center reported on a series of 30 infants younger than 6 months with a severe form of this disorder.[60] Simplistic earlier theories, (e.g., neonates are "obligatory nasal breathers"[61]) have largely been disproved.[62, 63]

Two arguments can be made against these theories as a group. The first is that in older children with obstructive apnea, the diagnosis is generally made after a prolonged period of failure to thrive and sleep disturbances, with marked physical findings including cor pulmonale[64]; this is not true of SIDS babies. The second argument is that in normal infants, these anatomic peculiarities are most marked in newborns and diminish progressively thereafter; it is therefore difficult for these theories to account for the peak age of death in SIDS. There has been one report of a small series of infants with ALTE episodes who subsequently developed obstructive sleep apnea, but this is clearly not the norm.[65]

Ventilatory Control in Infants

For many years the theory of central apnea during sleep as the predominant cause of SIDS held center stage both in research and in the public mind. Because of its popularity, and because it is testable, it has also reached a point that many rival theories have not: it has been found *not* to be helpful in identifying infants at risk of SIDS or ALTE episodes. The hypothesis that there is a pathologic continuum ranging from the extreme of Ondine's syndrome (lifelong central hypoventilation during sleep)[66, 67] to the brief apneic episodes and periodic breathing observed during sleep in normal infant and adults is plausible. It has been tested with both pneumographic or polysomnographic recordings in normal newborn and older infants, in ALTE infants, and in SIDS siblings. No differences have *consistently* been found among these groups. Periodic breathing has been found to be common in normal infants.[68, 69] Some studies have found that pneumograms of infants with reported ALTE can predict a recurrent episode[70]; most have not achieved even that much.[71–74] However, no study has been able to predict which infants in a tested group will subsequently die of SIDS. In all groups, there have been infants who have died despite being on a home apnea monitor.[71, 72, 74] The cumulative effect of this research has been to produce a new consensus in the SIDS research community regarding the use of home apnea monitors in at-risk infants.

Study design has been a major problem in SIDS research. Because of the low incidence of SIDS in the general population, most prospective apnea studies comparing infants who subsequently died of SIDS with matched controls have suffered from small sample sizes (10 to 20). The risk of type II error (falsely concluding that there is no difference between the two groups) is therefore extremely high. Those studies that compare SIDS infants to a larger "normal" population are more satisfactory in their design, but have also failed to find significant differences between SIDS infants and controls. Many studies have used the material at hand in a monitoring program and have compared a mixed group of SIDS siblings and ALTE infants to "normal controls"; conclusions from such studies must be viewed with skepticism.

Cardiac Manifestations

Two types of cardiac dysfunction may cause sudden and silent death: ventricular dysrhythmias and conduction disturbances. In addition, the two may be related, as in the long QT syndrome.

A large prospective nonintervention study, involving more than 9000 term infants, is being conducted by Southall and colleagues. Electrocardiograms (EKGs) and pneumographic monitoring have shown no evidence of any obvious dysrhythmias or respiratory abnormalities in the infants in this group who subsequently died of SIDS.[75, 76]

The search for conduction abnormalities in SIDS infants has also been fruitless. Studies have been based on small numbers of infants[77, 78] or have been done in the immediate neonatal period only.[79] The QT interval appears to be extremely variable immediately after birth,[80] and therefore neonatal studies would not necessarily detect a long QT syndrome. A prospective study is under way in Italy to address this question.[81] This theory is appealing in that at least some deaths could be preventable by routine EKG screening in children at vulnerable ages. However, in the congenital forms of long QT syndrome, manifestations in infancy are extremely uncommon and death extremely rare.[82] Additionally, Guntheroth has argued that most dysrhythmias in childhood, including supraventricular and ventricular tachycardias, are well tolerated.[83]

Autopsy Findings

An autopsy performed on an infant with suspected SIDS should have three aims: to exclude another cause of death, to document the "typical" SIDS findings, and to add to the established body of knowledge about SIDS deaths. Because of the extensive differential diagnosis in sudden unexpected infant deaths, the recommended autopsy protocols are complex, expensive, and time consuming and may be beyond the capability of coroners in many areas. One review of autopsies performed over a 2-year period documented the virtual absence of certain important procedures, such as measurement of carboxyhemoglobin levels. Overall in this study, less than half of the autopsies met the published state requirements, and only 11% included any report of a scene investigation.[84]

"Typical" findings in SIDS have generally been described as the absence of any other abnormality susceptible of causing death and the combination of pulmonary "congestion," pulmonary edema, and thymic and other intrathoracic petechiae. Beginning in 1980, a group of pathologists began a double-blind study that showed that there was no difference between SIDS and non-SIDS infants in the prevalence of pulmonary congestion or pulmonary edema; however, thymic petechiae were found only in SIDS infants (approximately half) and not in the control infants.[85] Intrathoracic petechiae, in the absence of petechiae elsewhere, have long been considered a marker for SIDS. Evidence from animal

studies and autopsy results suggests that these findings are also found (although to a lesser degree) in infants dying after documented airway obstruction.[86-88]

In addition to these gross findings, seven abnormalities have been proposed as typical of SIDS.[89] These were described by Naeye as markers of chronic hypoxia in SIDS babies and have served as the justification for much research into possible mechanisms of recurrent apnea in these infants. However, many of these findings have not been confirmed by independent investigators. Only the abnormal retention of periadrenal brown fat, increased hepatic erythropoiesis, and abnormalities of glomic tissue in the carotid body have been reproducible,[90] and there is still disagreement about their significance.

A study in 1987 suggested that fetal hemoglobin was elevated in infants dying of SIDS.[91] However, a subsequent study was unable to confirm these findings.[92] A number of articles have reported various abnormalities of pulmonary surfactant in SIDS infants[93-95]; the significance of these findings is unknown.

Autopsy research into the etiology of SIDS has been hampered by limited knowledge about the normal state of the infant heart, lung, and brain stem at different postconceptional and postnatal ages. For example, there are still inadequate data on the maturation of the cardiac conduction system in normal infants to interpret apparently anomalous findings at autopsy.[96] The most recent evidence indicates that the range of variation in the conduction system in infants dying from known causes is so wide that none of the conduction theories can be supported by autopsy data at this time.[97, 98]

Differential Diagnosis (A "Diagnostic Dustbin")[99]

The autopsy criteria for SIDS are complex. It is essential that the conditions under which the death occurred be fully investigated. However, this is probably the requirement least often met, even in countries such as Britain and Norway, where a 90% to 100% autopsy rate of suspected SIDS deaths has been the rule for many years. Retrospective reviews evaluating autopsy findings and investigation of the household and circumstances of death, showed that only about 17%[10] of the deaths previously classified as SIDS could be described as "completely unexplained." It is important to exclude both abuse and familial disorders in families in which two or more apparent SIDS deaths have occurred[100]; Wigglesworth has recommended that all such deaths be investigated by a pediatric pathologist.[101]

Infection

Apart from the obvious infectious causes of death, which should be excluded by a standard autopsy protocol, several organisms have been suggested as a possible cause of sudden infant death. These include cytomegalovirus, *Clostridium botulinum* (infant botulism), and *Clostridium difficile*. However, epidemiologic and autopsy studies have been unable to establish a link in the majority of cases.[102, 103] No large-scale study has been carried out concerning *Clostridium botulinum* infection.

Respiratory syncytial virus (RSV) is a more plausible etiologic agent, as it is known to cause apnea and produces upper respiratory symptoms (commonly described in SIDS cases) that may not initially appear severe.[104, 105] However, two reviews of infants with RSV infection showed that two thirds to three fourths of infants developing apnea were premature, and the preponderance of infants hospitalized for RSV-associated apnea were younger than 2 months old.[106, 107] RSV must be excluded in suspected SIDS and

ALTE cases, but it is unlikely that unrecognized RSV infection accounts for more than a small proportion of SIDS deaths. One of these studies also indicated that infants suffering from RSV with apnea did not appear to be at risk for subsequent apneic episodes.[106]

A study of normal infants has shown no increase in the number of apneic episodes during upper respiratory tract infections.[108] However, supporting evidence that respiratory infection is at least a concurrent event in SIDS was provided by a study showing grossly raised concentrations of lung immunoglobulins in SIDS cases.[109]

Inborn Errors of Metabolism

In the last half of the 1980s, inborn errors of metabolism became a major concern in the differential diagnosis of SIDS.[110, 111] In principle these diseases should be easily differentiated from the classic SIDS scenario by the preterminal phase (failure to thrive, period of vomiting, and altered mental status prior to death). They have therefore been emphasized as an important differential diagnosis in both SIDS and ALTE, rather than as a possible cause of "true" SIDS deaths. The significance of these deficiencies is that they are hereditary, making it essential to screen even asymptomatic siblings.

Accidental and Nonaccidental Death

Controversy and often frank hostility are prompted by the suggestion that a significant number of SIDS deaths are the result of child abuse, homicide, or neglect. At this time, even the suggestion that a scene investigation should be part of the routine evaluation of SIDS deaths results in criticism from SIDS investigators and the parents of SIDS infants.[112]

Several unrelated studies have suggested that a variable proportion of deaths initially classified as SIDS (after autopsy) may be accidental or homicidal deaths; these studies took place in Sheffield, Britain (12/115)[10, 113]; and Arkansas, (8/170)[114]; and Brooklyn, N.Y. (24/26).[115] In Sweden, a country with a homogeneous society and a low rate of autopsy-confirmed SIDS deaths (0.44 per 1000), 12% of the infants studied were sharing a bed with one or two adults, often following heavy alcohol consumption by the adults.[38] Even after excluding the Brooklyn series on the basis of socioeconomic conditions and high rates of infant mortality and child abuse, the remaining studies strongly suggest that nonaccidental causes have been neglected in recent years, often to the detriment of children born subsequently in the family.

The combination of unsatisfactory autopsies and inadequate scene investigation has caused concern in the SIDS research community. One researcher concluded that "all postperinatal deaths should be examined in very great depth in a few centers that have the time and skill to do so; epidemiologic studies should be based only on data from these centers; and journals should be encouraged to accept only those studies on the sudden infant death syndrome in which every child has been examined by a paediatric pathologist and been subject to a neutral confidential inquiry."[99]

Emergency Medical Service Considerations

The essential contributions of Emergency Medical Service (EMS) personnel in a situation of suspected SIDS death are effective resuscitation, rapid transport, and the collection of on-scene evidence. These requirements are unfortunately largely incompatible.

Resuscitation. The truism in pediatric arrests—that if on-scene resuscitation is ineffective, there is little chance that later efforts will succeed—also applies to SIDS cases. As in any pediatric resuscitation, rapid vascular access can be obtained by intraosseous infusion.

On-Scene Evidence. There can be no suggestion that resuscitation and transport should be delayed even by 1 minute in order to gather information. However, the emergency medical technicians (EMTs) and paramedics will automatically observed details that may be crucial in interpretation of autopsy results, and they should share this information with emergency department staff. These details include the position in which the child was found, and the child's exact location, particularly whether he or she had been asleep in an adult bed, with an adult or older child, or in an inappropriate piece of furniture. Details of this kind, if withheld from a coroner, can make accurate diagnosis of the cause of death almost impossible. Prehospital care personnel find SIDS cases emotionally upsetting and discussing the episode may be helpful to them.

Emergency Department Management

The unexpected death of a child is one of the most traumatic events that can occur in a family. EMS personnel and emergency department staff members also react with shock and grief to such an event. Guntheroth points out that "these two considerations—expectations of the possibilities of death and the opportunity to place the infant in the care of a physician—are denied to the parents of SIDS victims."[116] In addition, the diagnostic uncertainty inherent in a suspected SIDS death makes the situation almost intolerable to the surviving family members. Most parents of SIDS infants will eagerly adopt the conventional wisdom regarding SIDS and infant apnea, and it is probably inappropriate to burden them with the multiple diagnoses that may be under consideration.

The emergency department physician must be prepared to answer at least a few questions about SIDS (the term *sudden unexpected death* would probably be preferable, but many parents will spontaneously use the expression *SIDS death*). Discussion must be kept simple; almost no information given immediately after such an event will be retained in a coherent form. Basic information may include the approximate number of SIDS deaths in the United States, the average age of death, and some simple theories about the cause of death. In this situation, it is important to stress that these deaths are generally silent; to the parents this will imply that the child felt no pain. Psychological or pastoral help must be offered, and information about hospital or community support groups is valuable.

Parents should not be told that any subsequent siblings will need home monitoring. If the parents ask, the clinician should briefly say that all subsequent siblings should be carefully followed.

A history must be obtained from the parents while they are in the emergency department; this is probably the last chance for an accurate history, unless there is a SIDS research program in the community or the local public health department has the resources for a home visit. The parents are generally willing to talk, often over and over again, about what happened; gentle questioning can elicit a number of important details (Table 12–1).

Medicolegal Considerations

Autopsy. The 1974 SIDS Act made available funds for the development of regional centers for autopsies for SIDS deaths, but in practice it has not had much impact. Many

TABLE 12-1
HISTORY OF THE EPISODE (SIDS OR ALTE)

I. Description of the event
  Hour of discovery
    Location (home or elsewhere, cot or bed, other piece of furniture)
    Time since child was last seen or heard
    Appearance of the child when last seen
    Any sounds since last seen
    Time of last feeding; normal appetite?
    Circumstances of discovery (Routine check? "Felt something was wrong"?)
    Position of the child when found (prone, supine; covered or uncovered)
    Appearance: respiration, heart beat; color, tone, temperature, skin (moist or dry); blood, secretions, or vomitus in nose or mouth
    Intervention (vigorous stimulation, mouth-to-mouth ventilation, CPR)
    Time before intervention begun? By whom?
    Duration of intervention
    Condition of child after intervention
II. Immediate history (last 24–48 hr)
  Illness or unusual symptoms, medications, vaccinations
  Last meal, any changes in eating patterns or appetite
  Any changes in sleeping habits or usual routine
  Changes in behavior
III. Personal history
  Usual details on pregnancy, delivery, neonatal problems
  Feeding habits, feeding problems, reflux, choking spells
  Sleep routines, unusual respiration during sleep
  Psychomotor development
  Past illnesses, hospitalizations, medications, immunizations
  History of similar events
  History of seizures, breath-holding spells, syncope, apnea
IV. Family history
  History of previous SIDs or sudden unexpected infant death
  Seizures, breath-holding spells, syncope, apnea, snoring, heart disease

states have legislation mandating autopsies in such cases, but often funds are not provided to support this requirement. Even when specific legislation does not exist, in most states an apparent SIDS death is by definition a matter for the coroner. Therefore it is important to obtain an autopsy on each case of suspected SIDS. Both from a legal standpoint and for the protection of surviving or subsequent children, it is essential to exclude cases of fatal child abuse and accidental deaths. A number of well-defined disease entities can present as sudden unexpected death in infants, and a significant proportion of these involve the possibility of risk to existing family members or subsequent siblings. These include meningitis, RSV pneumonia, inborn errors of metabolism, and cardiac anomalies.

Most family members will understand and accept the need for an autopsy. They should be told that an autopsy may identify some other cause of death, which might be helpful in evaluating children born subsequently or, as in cases of meningitis, may mandate prophylactic antibiotic treatment for other family members. The value of autopsy data in research efforts to save other children can also be mentioned.

The emergency department physician should not sign a death certificate in these circumstances unless the coroner has agreed to perform the autopsy. If the family has a pediatrician or other family physician who does not believe that an autopsy is necessary and is willing to sign the certificate, then the situation is more difficult. However, citing the differential diagnoses in cases of sudden infant death may convince the other physician of the importance of this requirement.

Several detailed protocols for autopsy of a suspected SIDS death have been published.[101] Local protocols should be established in cooperation with the coroner. However, sam-

ples of blood and cerebrospinal fluid should be obtained for culture as quickly as possible; nasal swabs or aspirates are important for viral cultures; and if there is a history of diarrhea, stool samples should also be obtained.

Social Services. Investigation into the circumstances of a sudden unexpected death in a child must be governed by two contradictory principles: the need to determine whether the circumstances are suggestive of homicidal or accidental death and the equally important need to support grieving family members who may feel guilty for not having "done something" to prevent the death. At the same time, the emergency department physician and other staff members are usually themselves stricken by the child's death and may feel guilt because resuscitation attempts failed. Under these circumstances, it is easy to go to one of two extremes: to overtly or covertly accuse the family of being negligent or abusive, or to feel such sympathy toward the parents that even basic historical information is not gathered.

Support Groups. Unless the circumstances of the death or physical findings are so suggestive of homicide that immediate police and social services notification is required, the family of a child dying suddenly and unexpectedly must receive the benefit of every doubt. Narratives by parents demonstrate repeatedly that even though the term *SIDS* is widely known and understood, the casual comments of hospital staff members, neighbors, and friends can appear to accuse the family of neglect. The essence of the definition of SIDS is that it is "unexpected" even to a physician, and in a significant number of SIDS cases, the infant had been seen that day or the previous day by a physician, with no untoward finding. Parents need this reassurance, as they will hear contrary remarks from neighbors, acquaintances, and possibly even family members or other medical personnel. Immediate support from a family that has been through the same situation is one of the most helpful things that can be offered to the parents and siblings of a SIDS victim.

Most areas in the United States have SIDS support groups readily available. If one cannot be found through hospital social services or in the telephone directory listings, information can be obtained through the National Foundation for Sudden Infant Death Syndrome, 8240 Professional Place, Landover, Maryland, 20785–2246. The toll-free telephone number is 1–800–221–SIDS.

APPARENT LIFE-THREATENING EPISODES

Most emergency department physicians dealing with children will sooner or later become involved in one or more cases of SIDS deaths in their emergency department. However, personal observation of an ALTE is considerably less likely. An emergency physician is more often presented with a distraught (or embarrassed) family saying, "My child stopped breathing." In most of these cases, the baby will look perfectly well. It is essential to accept the parents' evaluation of the episode and to respond to their anxieties.

Acceptable epidemiologic studies of ALTE distinguish between explained and unexplained episodes and also between apparently major and probably minor episodes, the latter probably corresponding to a benign incident causing undue parental anxiety. The NIH Consensus Statement,[15] after a review of the available evidence, claims that approximately half of all ALTE episodes have no cause found, despite extensive workup. However, one review of 2779 infants in Belgium demonstrated a treatable cause for the event in 61% of cases, with only 14% being termed "unexplained and apparently severe."[117] None of the infants placed on home monitors in this series subsequently died of SIDS.

Clinical Evaluation
Documented Life-Threatening Episode

A life-threatening episode is defined by required continued stimulation or CPR or by the child being acidotic, hypothermic, or hypotonic on arrival in the emergency department. Resuscitative measures are as indicated by the infant's presentation, and there is no debate about the need for admission. As a rule, the more aggressive the treatment needed on admission to the emergency department, the greater the probability of finding a serious underlying disorder (i.e., infection, seizure, trauma, metabolic derangement).

The next responsibility of the emergency department physician is to obtain an accurate history from the parents (see Table 12–1). The parents must be reassured, and it must be made clear that little information about the cause of the event is immediately available. Discussion about the need for later treatment, such as home monitoring, is best deferred.

The Well-Appearing Child

The well-appearing child is by far the most common presentation to the emergency department. The caregivers usually state that the child was not breathing when found but now looks healthy and happy; a careful physical examination discloses no abnormalities. The parents are not sure what happened, because the room was dark, and they were too alarmed to get a proper look at the child. They think the child was not breathing, was limp when picked up, or could not be easily aroused.

The emergency department physician should attempt to determine whether a true ALTE has occurred. This should not be confused with the workup to find the cause of the episode; when the infant looks well on arrival, it is extremely unlikely that the cause will be determined in the emergency department. The history of the episode is all-important, and a minute-by-minute description of the event must be obtained from those caregivers who observed the episode. The parents should be asked about specific reasons for alarm that might have led to overreaction, such as a family history of SIDS or having recently heard about a SIDS death. It should be determined why the parents went to see the child at that particular moment, whether they heard an unusual sound or "just stopped by."

Pseudo-ALTEs are frequent and include deep sleeping, shallow breathing with or without sighs, and periodic breathing. A pneumogram performed during hospitalization may be able to demonstrate this behavior and reassure the parents.

Differential Diagnosis

Several conditions may present as an ALTE (Table 12–2). Probably the most common cause of an apparent apneic or hypotonic episode is gastroesophageal reflux (GER). Again, a careful history is the most useful diagnostic tool. GER with aspiration, and sometimes with larygospasm,[118] is a common cause of explained ALTE (40% to 50% in some series).[117, 119] Congenital malformations or functional abnormalities may be found in some cases. GER may be a more common cause of ALTE in awake than in sleeping children, but the difference does not seem to be significant.[119] Asymptomatic GER is extremely common in normal infants and should not be assumed to be the cause of an ALTE without full investigation. Ideally, documentation of laryngospasm or significant desaturation[120] during an episode of GER is required for diagnosis.

TABLE 12–2
DIFFERENTIAL DIAGNOSIS OF AN ALTE
Cardiovascular causes
Cardiomyopathy
Congenital anomalies
Dysrhythmias
Vasovagal episode
Child abuse
Attempted homicide (suffocation)
Munchausen syndrome by proxy
Subdural hematoma
Gastroesophageal reflux (GER)*
With apnea (laryngospasm or central)
With aspiration
Infection
Meningitis
Respiratory infection (including RSV)*
Sepsis
Metabolic/endocrine causes
Hypocalcemia
Hypoglycemia
Hypothyroidism
Inborn errors of metabolism
Reye's syndrome
Neurologic causes
Brain tumor (causing apnea)
Breath-holding spell
Seizure*
Respiratory causes
Congenital alveolar hypoventilation
Obstructive apnea

*Most common diagnoses.

Far less common, but of great importance because of the implications for further care of the infant, is child abuse. Only a small number of investigated ALTEs have a simple demonstrated cause, such as a subdural hematoma resulting from direct abuse. Much more difficult to diagnose are those cases resulting from attempted suffocation or drug administration, either as attempted homicide or as a particularly dangerous form of Munchausen's syndrome by proxy. There is no evidence that a significant number of ALTE episodes are the result of abuse; however, a number of case reports[121, 122] have delineated the type of episode that requires close investigation, sometimes including closed-circuit camera observation during hospitalization.[123, 124] Criteria for such investigation include multiple episodes in one child or in one family, particularly when the same family member reports witnessing all episodes. Administration of drugs has been reported in a variable number of cases; reasons for such action may be an intention to harm, but may also be the result of accident or ignorance of the possible effects (e.g., promethazine).[125, 126] Both careful history taking and toxicologic analysis are important.

Cyanotic or pallid breath-holding spells occasionally occur in young infants. An extensive study found that 25% of patients presented before the age of 6 months.[127] In children in this age group, it is more difficult to elicit the history of surprise or frustration that seems to trigger the episodes, and consequently these cases may be misdiagnosed as seizure or idiopathic apnea until the child grows older.

It is impossible to give precise information regarding the prevalence of these causes, as they vary greatly from one area to another and depend in particular on the referral patterns of infants with ALTE episodes within a medical community.

Diagnostic Evaluation
Emergency Department Tests

No test that can be performed in an emergency department can determine whether a child with a reported ALTE can safely be discharged home. Consequently only those tests that can be done more expeditiously in the emergency department while the child is awaiting admission should be performed. These generally do not include anything more extensive than an EKG and basic blood tests (complete blood cell count, serum glucose, electrolytes), although these are rarely diagnostic.[128]

In the infant with a severe episode of prolonged cyanosis, acidosis, or hypotonia, the most important differential diagnosis is infection, and the appropriate tests, including a chest radiograph and cultures of the blood, urine, and CSF, should be performed. If there is evidence of altered mental status, a search for metabolic abnormalities, toxins, and intracerebral injury must also be undertaken.

Parental support must not be neglected; a survey of infants with an episode severe enough to require emergency department evaluation indicates unsurprisingly that a majority of such parents rank such an event as "one of the most difficult in their lives."[129] All parental reports of this type of event must be taken seriously, even when the infant appears well on arrival in the emergency department. Often a careful discussion of the event will help to allay parents' fears and at the same time will provide essential information for evaluation of the child. If it is difficult to gauge the degree of parental anxiety, the simple question, "What do you think would have happened if you had not found the child at that moment?" will often encourage them to express their fears.

Clinical Investigation

A number of protocols for investigation of an ALTE have been published (Table 12–3).[4, 130, 131] There is debate concerning the routine use of barium swallow as a diagnostic tool. Many researchers consider this test to be insufficiently sensitive and specific; the sensitivity of a barium swallow alone for detecting symptomatic aspiration appears to be as low as 20%.[132] Some authorities recommend routine esophageal pH monitoring[119] in all infants with an ALTE during sleep.

A normal result on an electroencephalogram (EEG) of course does not exclude a seizure disorder. There is increasing evidence suggesting that subclinical seizures are an important cause of apneic episodes in newborns[133, 134]; these may also, although more rarely, occur in older children.[135] One follow-up study of infants monitored for a severe ALTE during sleep showed that 11 of the 76 infants developed a seizure disorder despite initial normal EEG results.[73]

Holter monitoring is unlikely to result in definite diagnosis unless symptoms or results of previous tests suggest a cardiac abnormality.[136]

Pneumography/Polysomnography. A pneumogram is a low-speed recording, similar to that obtained by a Holter monitor, of the EKG and respiration measured by thoracic impedance. It will generally not demonstrate pure obstructive apnea. Although there is universal agreement that prolonged central apnea (more than 20 seconds) is abnormal, it is unclear whether such an episode always justifies home monitoring. At this time, there is no evidence that shorter apneic episodes or even large amounts of periodic breathing are a cause for concern.

Polysomnography was the initial method used to evaluate "near-miss" infants and SIDS siblings but has been largely replaced by pneumography. It involves recording an EEG (six to eight leads), respiration (using one or two nasal thermistors and thoracic and abdominal impedance), an EKG, eye movement monitor, and an electromyogram (EMG). It is now primarily a research tool used to study different types of apnea in various sleep stages. As part of the evaluation of an ALTE infant, polysomnography is

TABLE 12–3	
INVESTIGATION OF AN ALTE	
Routine	**When Indicated**
Accident/injury	
Toxicologic studies (serum, urine)	Cerebral CT scan
	Rib and long-bone radiographs
	Bone scintigram
Cardiac causes	
EKG	Holter monitoring
Infectious causes	
Sepsis evaluation (CBC, chest radiograph, urinalysis, and urine culture)	Lumbar puncture
	Virology studies (nasopharyngeal swabs)
	Liver enzymes, ammonia
Gastrointestinal causes	
	Barium swallow
	Esophageal pH monitoring
Metabolic/endocrine causes	
Serum glucose and electrolytes	Thyroid studies
	Amino acid chromatogram
	Organic acids
Neurologic causes	
	Cerebral CT scan
	EEG
Respiratory causes	
Pneumogram	Polysomnogram
	Lateral neck radiograph
	Laryngoscopy

indicated if obstructive apnea is strongly suspected, when the pneumogram is inconclusive, or to exclude neurologic abnormalities.

Long-Term Management
Apnea Monitors

Apnea monitors are typically reserved for the relatively small number of ALTE infants with no demonstrable treatable cause for an episode that required resuscitation or vigorous stimulation.[15] Similar guidelines have been developed in Britain.[137] In the group of infants with ALTE requiring resuscitation, the subsequent mortality as reported by one SIDS research center is extremely high. However, all deaths occurred while the infants were in the monitoring program,[71, 73] although noncompliance with the monitor may have been a factor in some instances. It is clear that parents of these children must be skilled in cardiopulmonary resuscitation and aware of the significant risk of death despite apnea monitoring. The NIH Consensus Statement says merely that in this group, lives can be saved with home monitoring.[15]

Those involved in SIDS and ALTE management have known families who were so anxious about a subsequent sibling that they stayed up all night watching the infant for months. Severe parental anxiety of this type is recognized by many centers as an acceptable indication for monitoring. However, there is no evidence that home monitoring in infants with less severe ALTE episodes or in SIDS siblings will prevent subsequent sudden unexpected death (Tables 12–4 and 12–5).[138–148] Impedance monitors, the type most commonly used, do not detect obstructive apnea or shallow breathing unless bradycardia occurs. In addition, parents must be made aware of the possible risk of home monitors; one fatal electrocution has been associated with their use.[149] The FDA has recently published a safety alert for caregivers regarding risks of apnea monitors.[150] Emery, among many

	TABLE 12–4		
	DEATHS IN INFANTS ON HOME APNEA MONITORS (DETAILED REPORTS)		
Study	**Patient Description**	**Number Monitored**	**Deaths**
Duffty and Bryan[138] (Toronto, 1982)	72 "idiopathic apnea"	All	0
Hodgman et al[139] (California, 1982)	17 "prolonged apnea"	None	0
Rosen et al[72] (Houston, 1983)	26 "life-threatening apnea"	All	2 (1 while briefly off monitor; 1 "pad" monitor)
Ariagno et al[140] (California, 1983)	156 "near miss"	137 monitored 19 not monitored	0 1
Rahilly and Symonds[74] (Australia, 1984)	92 "near miss"	All	1 (at 16 months after monitor discontinued)
MacKay[141] (England, 1984)	24 "near miss"	All	0
Oren et al[73] (Boston, 1986)	76 ALTE with resuscitation	All	10 (4 "delay in response"; 4/11 with seizure disorder)
Oren et al[142] (Boston, 1987)	73 recurrent ALTE	All	5 (no information on status of monitor)
Dunne and Matthews[143] (Ireland, 1987)	73 "near miss"	52 monitored 21 not monitored	1 (briefly off monitor while in hospital) 1
Rowland et al[144] (Massachusetts, 1987)	110 "primary apnea"	All	0
Oren et al[71] (Boston, 1989)	51 "apnea of infancy"	All	7 (4/7 "delay in resuscitation"; only 3 cases autopsied)

others, has pointed out that "cardiorespiratory monitoring should not be an isolated measure, although a monitoring device may be used as a means of facilitating consultations with some parents."[100]

Some investigators have used xanthines to treat excessive infantile apnea. Although their effectiveness in treating apnea in premature infants is clear, it is less clear whether they improve long-term outcome in older infants.[151]

Treatment of GER

In infants with documented apneic or bradycardic episodes caused by GER, a monitor may be recommended in conjunction with the usual methods of treatment (upright position, thickening of foods). If xanthines are used for treatment of apnea, they may worsen the GER.[152] One author has reported two subsequent SIDS deaths in a group of 51 infants with severe GER-associated apnea who underwent fundoplication.[153]

Other Considerations

Additional treatment may be indicated by the evaluation of the infant. The rare child with apnea resulting from a seizure disorder may need an apnea monitor as well as antiseizure medications. One center has documented an extraordinarily high mortality rate in a small group of infants with seizure-related apnea,[73] despite monitoring.

EVALUATION OF AN INFANT ON AN APNEA MONITOR

Management of Apnea Alarms

Home apnea monitoring of infants uses a system of three electrodes (or, more rarely, a belt) in order to monitor both cardiac activity and respiration. Isolated cardiac monitoring in these cases is insufficient, as bradycardia is a late and preterminal manifestation of apnea in infants. Monitors should allow for at least two different types of alarm signals (loose electrode and cardiac/apnea alarm) and for a method of indicating what alarm has sounded (cardiac or respiratory) through alarm lights that remain on until reset. Other kinds of monitoring systems include mattress systems, easily purchased by parents but not widely used in research or monitoring centers, and microphone systems to detect breathing; the latter are in experimental use in the United Kingdom. Parents must be able to change the sensitivity of the monitor and be able to set the apnea alarm (generally at 20 seconds, as normal infants may have apneas of that duration). The

	TABLE 12–5	
	DEATHS IN INFANTS ON HOME APNEA MONITORS (LARGE-SCALE REPORTS)	
Study	**Description**	**Deaths/Number Monitored**
Ward et al[145] (California, 1986)	31 apnea programs	7/1841 monitored 4/1565 not monitored
Kahn et al[117] (Belgium, 1988)	2779 ALTE patients	0/200 monitored 0/2579 not monitored
Kelly[146] (Boston, 1988)	13,401 "near miss" patients, SIDS sibs	21/1445 monitored 19/11,943 not monitored
Meny et al[147] (Baltimore, 1988)	765 infants on home monitors	10/765 monitored
Light and Sheridan[148] (Hawaii, 1989)	1000 infants with apnea of prematurity or ALTE	17/1000 monitored

ideal home monitor should have either a power alarm failure or a backup battery system in case of power failure.

Criteria for physician-controlled home monitoring include a severe ALTE episode documented to be either of apneic origin or of unknown cause. Monitoring in general is discontinued after a 2-month period has passed without alarms and after documentation of no unusual apneas on pneumogram or polygraphy. An asymptomatic sibling monitored because of parental anxiety is often removed from the monitor at between 6 and 9 months of age, if that is beyond the age of the previous child's death. Occasionally, infants remain on the monitor after 1 year of age because of persistent apnea. However, as infants grow and develop psychomotor control, keeping them on the monitor becomes a test of the parents' ingenuity and patience.

Parents must be taught how to respond to monitor alarms and must be able to perform CPR, although gentle stimulation of the infant or mouth-to-mouth ventilation is generally all that is required to terminate an apneic episode. Careful recording of all alarms is indispensable, and continued parent education is therefore required in a responsible monitoring program. In many areas, however, monitors may be purchased over the counter. Parents who have purchased such monitors may present to the emergency department with little knowledge of how to respond to alarms. Only one limited review of reported alarms has been conducted; the authors were skeptical of the "true alarms" reported by the family, as no bradycardia was recorded in these cases.[154]

Parental attitudes toward apnea monitors are generally positive, in spite of the severe constraints on family life created by the monitor. These constraints include the difficulty of finding baby sitters who are willing to accept the responsibility of the monitor. In deprived home situations, the caregivers may be incapable of proper use of the monitor. In some investigations of deaths in infants for whom home monitors had been prescribed, the equipment had been "just turned off" or was gathering dust in a corner.

History of the Episode

An infant on a home apnea monitor may be brought to the emergency department when an alarm sounds either because the parents are inexperienced, or because they believe that it was a true alarm requiring significant resuscitative measures. Infants with an episode of severe idiopathic apnea have a relatively high recurrence rate of such apneic episodes[139, 140]; such recurrences are associated with a high mortality rate, as previously discussed. It is therefore extremely important to obtain an accurate history of the episode, both to reassure the parents and for the sake of the child.

The episode or family history justifying the use of a home apnea monitor may be helpful in determining the importance of the present episode. If this is a relatively minor event similar to previous ones, no treatment other than gentle stimulation was required, and the child is normal on careful physical examination, then hospitalization may not be indicated. Obtaining this historical information will also help identify those children who are on a monitor either without a physician's care or whose families have recently moved with the monitor but with no physician follow-up—a fairly frequent event in this highly mobile country.

Similar historical information, although in an abbreviated form, must be obtained as in a SIDS or ALTE (see Table 12–1). If the infant appears well, the emergency department visit may be an educational experience for the parents, who must be taught to look at the infant and not just at the monitor when the alarm sounds. Parents often concentrate on the monitor alarm and may shake the infant or even

start CPR without further investigation. If adequate information about the episode is unavailable, it must be treated as a genuine apneic event. It is important to find out whether the monitor was recently checked and, if so, by whom. The evaluation will depend on the infant's condition, the parents' description of the event, and the opinion of the physician who prescribed the monitor and is following the child.

Disposition

As a general principle, any episode that so alarmed the parents that they brought their child to the emergency department probably justifies hospitalization. This is obviously true in the case of an episode with documented cyanosis or hypotonia or when vigorous stimulation or CPR was needed. If the child is febrile or has an upper respiratory infection, these are also generally considered reasons for hospital observation.

Some children may be brought to the emergency department after a relatively minor episode, or the parents may even volunteer that they thought this was a "false alarm." In these cases it is important to try to discover the underlying reasons for the visit. The parents may be seeking information that they cannot obtain from other sources. They may be overwhelmed with false alarms and need technical assistance. They may be asking whether the monitor can be removed. Such information and assistance should be available relatively easily in most areas of the country; if there is no hospital department or pediatrician familiar with the problems of home monitoring, a local SIDS support group can often provide effective help.

Although rare, well-documented cases of Münchausen's syndrome by proxy have occurred in families with a monitored infant. This must be suspected in situations when multiple alarms are reported, particularly when one person is always or often present, and when claims that resuscitation was necessary cannot be corroborated.

References

1. Collins JD, Piper PJ. Sudden unexpected death in infants: A disease of theories. Wisc Med 1961;60:571.
2. Matthews T. The sudden infant death syndrome—a bustling ignorance? Editorial. Ir Med J 1986;79:206.
3. Naeye RL. Sudden infant death syndrome: Is the confusion ending? Mod Pathol 1988;1:169.
4. Simpson H, MacFadyen UM, Paton JY. 'Near-miss' or 'near-myth' for sudden infant death syndrome? Clinical observations on 57 infants. Aust Paediatr J 1986;22(suppl):47.
5. Little GA. Infantile apnea, home monitoring, and SIDS: Go back to go. Editorial. J Perinatol 1987;7:83.
6. Beckwith JB. Discussion of terminology and definition of sudden infant death syndrome. *In* Bergman AB, Beckwith JB, Ray CG, (eds). Sudden Infant Death Syndrome. Proceedings of the Second International Conference on Causes of Sudden Death in Infants. Seattle, University of Washington Press, 1970.
7. Hunter JC. The federal SIDS support network in perspective. Ann NY Acad Sci 1988;533:155.
8. Zylke JW. Sudden infant death syndrome: Resurgent research offers hope. News. JAMA 1989;262:1565.
9. Thach BT. The potential role of airway obstruction in sudden infant death syndrome. *In* Culberton JL, Krous HF, Bendell RD (eds). Sudden Infant Death Syndrome: Medical Aspects and Psychological Management. Baltimore, Johns Hopkins University Press, 1988, pp 62–93.
10. Taylor EM, Emery JL. Categories of preventable unexpected infant deaths. Arch Dis Child 1990;65:535.
11. Guntheroth WG. Crib Death. The Sudden Infant Death Syndrome. 2nd ed. New York, Futura Publishing Company, 1989, p 110.
12. Mandell F, Belk B. Sudden infant death syndrome. The disease and its survivors. Postgrad Med 1977;62:193.
13. American Academy of Pediatrics, Task Force on Prolonged Infantile Apnea. Prolonged infantile apnea: 1985. Pediatrics 1985;76:129.
14. Friedman SF, Bergman AB, Mandell F, et al. Statement on terminology from the National SIDS Foundation. Pediatrics 1981;68:543.
15. National Institutes of Health Consensus Development Conference on

Infantile Apnea and Home Monitoring, Sept 29 to Oct 1, 1986. Pediatrics 1987;79:292.

16. Behrman RE, Vaughan VC, eds. Nelson Textbook of Pediatrics, 13th ed. Philadelphia, WB Saunders, 1987, p 155.

17. Woolley PV. Mechanical suffocation during infancy: Relation to total problem of sudden death. J Pediatr 1945;26:572.

18. Lee NN, Chan YF, Davies DP, et al. Sudden infant death syndrome in Hong Kong: Confirmation of low incidence. Br Med J 1989;298:721.

19. Borman B, Fraser J, de Boer G. A national study of sudden infant death syndrome in New Zealand. NZ Med J 1988;101:413.

20. Nelson EA, Williams SM, Taylor BJ, et al. Postneonatal mortality in south New Zealand: Necropsy data review. Paediatr Perinat Epidemiol 1989;3:375.

21. Hoffman HJ, Damus K, Hillman L. Risk factors for SIDS. Results of the National Institute of Child Health and Human Development SIDS Cooperative Epidemiological Study. Ann NY Acad Sci 1988;533:13.

22. Dollfus C, Patetta M, Siegel E, Cross AW. Infant mortality: A practical approach to the analysis of the leading causes of death and risk factors. Pediatrics 1990;86:176.

23. Bergman AB, Ray CG, Pomery MA, et al. Studies of the sudden infant death syndrome in King County, Washington. III. Epidemiology. Pediatrics 1972;49:860.

24. Naeye RL, Ladis B, Drage JS. Sudden infant death syndrome: A prospective study. Am J Dis Child 1976;130:1207.

25. Kraus JF, Greenland S, Bulterys M. Risk factors for sudden infant death syndrome in the US Collaborative Perinatal Project. Int J Epidemiol 1989;18:113.

26. Sudden infant death syndrome as a cause of premature mortality—United States, 1984 and 1985. JAMA 1988;260:3255.

27. Wegman ME. Annual summary of vital statistics—1988. Pediatrics 1989;84:943.

28. Driscoll DJ, Edwards WD. Sudden unexpected death in children and adolescents. J Am Coll Cardiol 1985;5:118B.

29. Furst G. Sudden, unexpected, nocturnal deaths among Southeast Asian refugees. Am J Forensic Med Pathol 1982;3:277.

30. Polberger S, Svenningsen NW. Early neonatal sudden infant death and near death of full-term infants in maternity wards. Acta Paediatr Scand 1985;74:861.

31. Goyco PG, Beckerman RC. Sudden infant death syndrome. Curr Probl Pediatr 1990;20:297.

32. Peterson DR, Van Belle G, Chinn NM. Epidemiological comparisons of the Sudden Infant Death Syndrome with other major components of infant mortality. Am J Epidemiol 1979;110:699.

33. Thach BT, Davies AM, Koenig JS. Pathophysiology of sudden upper airway obstruction in sleeping infants and its relevance for SIDS. Ann NY Acad Sci 1988;533:314.

34. Peterson DR, Sabotta EE, Strickland D. Sudden infant death syndrome in epidemiological perspective: Etiologic implications of variation with season of the year. Ann NY Acad Sci 1988;533:6.

35. Helweg-Larsen K, Bay H, Mac F. A statistical analysis of the seasonality in sudden infant death syndrome. Int J Epidemiol 1985;14:566.

36. Osmond C, Murphy M. Seasonality in the sudden infant death syndrome. Paediatr Perinat Epidemiol 1988;2:337.

37. Murphy MFG, Campbell MJ, Jones DR. Increased risk of sudden infant death syndrome in older infants at weekends. Br Med J 1986;293:364.

38. Norvenius SG. Sudden infant death syndrome in Sweden in 1973–1977 and 1979. Acta Paediatr Scand [Suppl] 1987;333:1.

39. Mitchell EA, Stewart AW. Deaths from sudden infant death syndrome on public holidays and weekends. Aust NZ J Med 1988;18:861.

40. Kaada B, Sivertsen E. Sudden infant death syndrome during weekends and holidays in Norway in 1967–1985. Scand J Soc Med 1990;18:17.

41. Wagner M. Enquete epidemiologique sur la mort subite inopinee du nourrison en Seine-Maritime. 1978–1981. Thesis, Faculty de Medecine de Rouen, 1983, p 95.

42. Sells CJ, Neff TE, Bennett FC, Robinson NM. Mortality in infants discharged from a neonatal intensive care unit. Am J Dis Child 1983;137:44.

43. Werthammer J, Brown ER, Neff RK, Taeusch HW. Sudden infant death syndrome in infants with bronchopulmonary dysplasia. Pediatrics 1982;69:301.

44. Babson SG, Clarke NG. Relationship between infant death and maternal age. J Pediatr 1983;103:391.

45. Hoffman HJ, Hunter JC, Damus K, et al. Diphtheria-tetanus-pertussis immunization and sudden infant death: Results of the National Institute of Child Health and Human Development Cooperative Epidemiological Study of Sudden Infant Death Syndrome risk factors. Pediatrics 1987;79:598.

46. Griffin MR, Ray WA, Livengood JR, Schaffner W. Risk of sudden infant death syndrome after immunization with the diphtheria-tetanus-pertussis vaccine. N Engl J Med 1988;319:618.

47. Peterson DR, Sabotta EE, Daling JR. Infant mortality among subsequent siblings of infants who died of sudden infant death syndrome. J Pediatr 1986;108:911.

48. Irgens LM, Skjaerven R, Peterson DR. Prospective assessment of recurrence risk in sudden infant death syndrome siblings. J Pediatr 1984;104:349.

49. Guntheroth WG, Lohmann R, Spiers PS. Risk of sudden infant death syndrome in subsequent siblings. J Pediatr 1990;116:520.

50. Beal S. Sudden infant death syndrome in twins. Pediatrics 1989;84:1038.

51. Smialek JE. Simultaneous sudden infant death syndrome in twins. Pediatrics 1986;77:816.

52. Bass M. The fallacy of the simultaneous sudden infant death syndrome in twins. Am J Forensic Med Pathol 1989;10:200.

53. Lewak N. Sudden infant death syndrome risk factors. Clin Pediatr 1979;18:404.

54. Peters TJ, Golding J. Prediction of sudden infant death syndrome: An independent evaluation of four scoring methods. Stat Med 1986;5:113.

55. Carpenter RG, Gardner A, Harris J, et al. Prevention of unexpected infant death. A review of risk-related intervention in six centers. Ann NY Acad Sci 1983;533:96.

56. Ellis FR, Halsall PJ, Harriman DG. Malignant hyperpyrexia and sudden infant death syndrome. Br J Anaesth 1988;60:28.

57. Stanton AN: Sudden infant death syndrome and phenothiazines. Letter. Pediatrics 1983;71:986.

58. Mathew O. Maintenance of upper airway patency. J Pediatr 1985;106:863.

59. Olsson GL, Hallen B. Laryngospasm during anesthesia. A computer-aided incidence study in 136,929 patients. Acta Anaesth Scand 1984;28:567.

60. Southall DP, Talbert DG. Mechanisms for abnormal apnea of possible relevance to the sudden infant death syndrome. Ann NY Acad Sci 1988;533:329.

61. Tonkin S. Sudden infant death syndrome: Hypothesis of causation. Pediatrics 1975;55:650.

62. Rodenstein DOL, Perlmutter N, Stanescu DC. Infants are not obligatory nasal breathers. Am Rev Respir Dis 1985;131:343.

63. Miller MJ, Martin RJ, Carlo WA, et al. Oral breathing in newborn infants. J Pediatr 1985;107:465.

64. Brouillette RT, Fernback SK, Hunt CE. Obstructive sleep apnea in infants and children. J Pediatr 1982;100:31.

65. Guilleminault C, Souquet M, Ariagno RL, et al. Five cases of near-miss sudden infant death syndrome and development of obstructive sleep apnea syndrome. Pediatrics 1984;73:71.

66. Guilleminault C, McQuitty J, Ariagno RL, et al. Congenital central alveolar hypoventilation syndrome in six infants. Pediatrics 1982;70:684.

67. Armstrong D, Sachis P, Bryan C, Becker L. Pathological features of persistent infantile sleep apnea with reference to the pathology of sudden infant death syndrome. Ann Neurol 1982;12:169.

68. Waite SP, Thoman EB. Periodic apnea in the full-term infant: Individual consistency, sex differences and state specificity. Pediatrics 1982;70:79.

69. Richards JM, Alexander JR, Shinebourne EA, et al. Sequential 22-hour profiles of breathing patterns and heart rate in 110 full-term infants during their first 6 months of life. Pediatrics 1984;74:763.

70. Rahilly PM. Pneumographic studies: Predictors of future apnoeas but not sudden infant death in asymptomatic infants. Aust Paediatr J 1989;25:211.

71. Oren J, Kelly DH, Shannon DC. Pneumogram recordings in infants resuscitated for apnea of infancy. Pediatrics 1989;83:364.

72. Rosen CL, Frost JD, Harrison GC. Infant apnea: Polygraphic studies and follow-up monitoring. Pediatrics 1983;71:731.

73. Oren J, Kelly D, Shannon DC. Identification of a high-risk group for sudden infant death syndrome among infants who were resuscitated for sleep apnea. Pediatrics 1986;77:495.

74. Rahilly PM, Symonds PF. Simplified pneumographic monitoring of infants at risk from sudden infant death syndrome. Arch Dis Child 1984;59:351.

75. Stevens V, Wilson AJ, Southall DP, et al. Analysis of the heart rate and breathing patterns of infants destined to suffer sudden infant death syndrome: Probability density function analysis. Pediatr Res 1985;19:1327.

76. Waggener TB, Southall DP, Scott LA. Analysis of breathing patterns in a prospective population of term infants does not predict susceptibility to sudden infant death syndrome. Pediatr Res 1990;27:113.

77. Weinstein SL, Steinschneider A. QT and R-R intervals in victims of the sudden infant death syndrome. Am J Dis Child 1985;139:987.

78. Sadeh D, Shannon DC, Abboud S, et al. Altered cardiac repolarization in some victims of sudden infant death syndrome. N Engl J Med 1987;317:1501.

79. Southall DP, Arrowsmith WA, Stebbens V, Alexander JR. QT interval measurements before sudden infant death syndrome. Arch Dis Child 1986;61:327.

80. Schwartz PJ. The quest for the mechanisms of the sudden infant death syndrome: Doubts and progress. Circulation 1987;75:677.

81. Schwartz PJ, Segantini A. Cardiac innervation, neonatal electrocardiography and SIDS. Ann NY Acad Sci 1988;533:210.

82. Schwartz PJ, Periti M, Malliani A. The long Q-T syndrome. Am Heart J 1975;89:378.

83. Guntheroth WG. Crib Death. The Sudden Infant Death Syndrome. 2nd ed. New York, Futura Publishing Company, 1989, pp 168, 169.

84. Samuels BN, Rubio-Freidberg S. A review of Georgia SIDS autopsy reports for a 2-year period. J Med Assoc Ga 1989;78:615.

85. Valdes-Dapena M. Sudden infant death syndrome: Overview of recent

research developments from a pediatric pathologist's perspective. Pediatrician 1988;15:222.

86. Krous HF, Jordan J. A necropsy study of distribution of petechiae in non-sudden infant death syndrome. Arch Pathol Lab Med 1984;108:75.

87. Krous HF. The microscopic distribution of intrathoracic petechiae in sudden infant death syndrome. Arch Pathol Lab Med 1984;108:77.

88. Beckwith B. Intrathoracic petechial hemorrhages: A clue to the mechanism of death in sudden infant death syndrome? Ann NY Acad Sci 1988;533:37.

89. Naeye RL. Sudden infant death. Sci Am 1980;242:52.

90. Valdes-Dapena M. A pathologist's perspective on possible mechanisms in SIDS. Ann NY Acad Sci 1988;533:31.

91. Giulian GG, Gilbert EF, Moss RL. Elevated fetal hemoglobin levels in sudden infant death syndrome. N Engl J Med 1987;316:1122.

92. Zielke HR, Meny RG, O'Brien MJ, et al. Normal fetal hemoglobin levels in the sudden infant death syndrome. N Engl J Med 1989;321:1359.

93. Gibson RA, McMurchie EJ. Decreased lung surfactant disaturated phosphatidylcholine in sudden infant death syndrome. Early Hum Dev 1988;17:145.

94. Hill CM, Brown BD, Morley CJ, et al. Pulmonary surfactant. II. In sudden infant death syndrome. Early Hum Dev 1988;16:153.

95. James D, Berry PJ, Fleming P, Hathaway M. Surfactant abnormality and the sudden infant death syndrome—a primary or secondary phenomenon? Arch Dis Child 1990;65:774.

96. James TN. Sudden death in babies. New observations in the heart. Am J Cardiol 1968;22:477.

97. Ho SY, Anderson RH. Conduction tissue and SIDS. Ann NY Acad Sci 1988;533:176.

98. Thiene G. Problems in the interpretation of cardiac pathology in reference to SIDS. Ann NY Acad Sci 1988;533:191.

99. Emery JL. Is sudden infant death syndrome a diagnosis? Or is it just a diagnostic dustbin? Editorial. Br Med J 1989;299:1240.

100. Emery JL. Families in which two or more cot deaths have occurred. Lancet 1986;1:313.

101. Wigglesworth JS, Keeling JW, Rushton DI, et al. Pathological investigations in cases of sudden death. J Clin Pathol 1987;40:1481.

102. Coumbe A, Fox JD, Briggs M, et al. Cytomegalovirus and human herpesvirus-6 in sudden infant death syndrome: An in situ hybridization study. Pediatr Pathol 1990;10:483.

103. Cooperstock MC, Steffen E, Yolken R, Onderdonk A. Clostridium difficile in normal infants and sudden infant death syndrome: An association with infant formula feeding. Pediatrics 1982;70:91.

104. Anas NG, Boettrich C, Hall CB, Brooks JG. The association of apnea and respiratory syncytial virus infection in infants. J Pediatr 1982;101:65.

105. Pickens DL, Schefft GL, Storch GA, Thach BT. Characterization of prolonged apneic episodes associated with respiratory syncytial virus infection. Pediatr Pulmonol 1989;6:195.

106. Church NR, Anas NG, Hall CB, Brooks JG. Respiratory syncytial virus-related apnea in infants. Am J Dis Child 1984;138:247.

107. Bruhn FW, Mokrohisky ST, McIntosh K. Apnea associated with respiratory syncytial virus infection in young infants. J Pediatr 1977;90:382.

108. Southall DP, Stebeens VA, Alexander JR, et al. Cardiorespiratory patterns occurring in infants during and after recovery from respiratory tract infection. Pediatrics 1986;78:37.

109. Forsyth KD, Weeks SC, Koh L, et al. Lung immunoglobulins in the sudden infant death syndrome. Br Med J 1989;298:23.

110. Howat AJ, Bennett MJ, Variend S. Defects of metabolism of fatty acids in the sudden infant death syndrome. Br Med J [Clin Res] 1985;290:1771.

111. Harpey JP, Charpentier C, Coude M, et al. Sudden infant death syndrome and multiple acyl-coenzyme A dehydrogenase deficiency, ethylmalonic-adipic aciduria, or systemic carnitine deficiency. J Pediatr 1987;110:881.

112. Suffocation and sudden infant death syndrome. Letters. Br Med J 1989;299:178.

113. Emery JL. Infanticide, filicide and cot death. Arch Dis Child 1985;60:505.

114. Perrot LJ, Nawojczyk S. Nonnatural death masquerading as SIDS (sudden infant death syndrome). Am J Forensic Med Pathol 1988;9:105.

115. Bass M, Kravath RE, Glass L. Death-scene investigation in sudden infant death. N Engl J Med 1986;315:100.

116. Guntheroth WG. Crib Death. The Sudden Infant Death Syndrome. 2nd ed. New York, Futura Publishing Company, 1989, p 257.

117. Kahn A, Rebuffat E, Sottiaux M, Blum D. Management of an infant with an apparent life-threatening event. Pediatrician 1988;15:204.

118. Leape LL, Holder TM, Franklin JD, et al. Respiratory arrest in infants secondary to gastroesophageal reflux. Pediatrics 1977;60:924.

119. Sacre L, Vandenplas Y. Gastroesophageal reflux associated with respiratory abnormalities during sleep. J Pediatr Gastroenterol Nutr 1989;9:28.

120. See CC, Newman LJ, Berezin S, et al. Gastroesophageal reflux-induced hypoxemia in infants with apparent life-threatening event(s). Am J Dis Child 1989;143:951.

121. Rosen CL, Frost JD, Glaze DG. Child abuse and recurrent infant apnea. J Pediatr 1986;109:1065.

122. Meadow R. Suffocation, recurrent apnea, and sudden infant death. J Pediatr 1990;117:351.

123. Rosen CL, Frost JD, Bricker T, et al. Two siblings with recurrent cardiorespiratory arrest: Munchausen syndrome by proxy or child abuse? Pediatrics 1983;71:715.

124. Southall DP, Stebens VA, Rees SV, et al. Apnoeic episodes induced by smothering: two cases identified by covert surveillance. Br Med J 1987;294:1637.

125. Hickson GB, Altemeier WA, Martin ED, Campbell PW. Parental administration of chemical agents: a cause of apparent life-threatening events. Pediatrics 1989;83:772.

126. Shnaps Y, Frand M, Rotem Y, Tirosh M. The chemically abused child. Pediatrics 1981;68:119.

127. Lombroso CT, Lerman P. Breathholding spells (cyanotic and pallid infantile syncope). Pediatrics 1967;39:563.

128. Lewis JM, Ganick DJ. Initial laboratory evaluation of infants with 'presumed near-miss' sudden infant death syndrome. Am J Dis Child 1986;140:484.

129. Light MJ, Sheridan MS. Psychosocial impact of emergency apnea. Am J Dis Child 1987;141:668.

130. Gould JB, James O. Management of the near-miss infant: A personal perspective. Ped Clin North Am 1979;26:857.

131. Jeffery HE, Rahilly P, Read DJC. Multiple causes of asphyxia in infants at high risk of sudden infant death. Arch Dis Child 1983;58:92.

132. MacFadyen UM, Hendry GM, Simpson H. Gastro-oesophageal reflux in near-miss sudden infant death syndrome or suspected recurrent aspiration. Arch Dis Child 1983;58:87.

133. Watanabe K. Apneic seizures in the newborn. Am J Dis Child 1982;136:980.

134. Monod N, Peirano P, Plouin P, et al. Seizure-induced apnea. Ann NY Acad Sci 1988;533:411.

135. Watanabe K, Hara K, Hakamada S, et al. Seizures with apnea in children. Pediatrics 1982;79:87.

136. Woolf PK, Gewitz MH, Preminger T, et al. Infants with apparent life threatening events. Cardiac rhythm and conduction. Clin Pediatr (Phila) 1989;28:517.

137. Monitoring and sudden infant death syndrome: An update. Report from the Foundation for the Study of Infant Deaths and the British Paediatric Respiratory Group. Arch Dis Child 1990;65:238.

138. Duffty P, Bryan MH. Home apnea monitoring in 'near-miss' sudden infant death syndrome (SIDS) and in siblings of SIDS victims. Pediatrics 1982;70:69.

139. Hodgman JE, Hoppenbrouwers T, Geidel S, et al. Respiratory behavior in near-miss sudden infant death syndrome. Pediatrics 1982;69:785.

140. Ariagno RL, Guilleminault C, Korobkin R, et al. 'Near-miss' for sudden infant death syndrome infants: a clinical problem. Pediatrics 1983;71:726.

141. MacKay M, Abreu E, Silva FA, et al. Home monitoring for central apnoea. Arch Dis Child 1984;59:136.

142. Oren J, Kelly DH, Shannon DC. Familial occurrence of sudden infant death syndrome and apnea of infancy. Pediatrics 1987;80:355.

143. Dunne K, Matthews T. Near-miss sudden infant death syndrome: Clinical findings and management. Pediatrics 1987;79:889.

144. Rowland TW, Donnelly JH, Landis JN. Infant home apnea monitoring. A five-year assessment. Clin Pediatr (Phila) 1987;26:383.

145. Ward SL, Keens TG, Chan LS, et al. Sudden infant death syndrome in infants evaluated by apnea programs in California. Pediatrics 1986;77:451.

146. Kelly DH. Home monitoring for the sudden infant death syndrome: The case for. Ann NY Acad Sci 1988;533:158.

147. Meny RG, Blackmon L, Fleischmann D. Sudden infant death and home monitors. Am J Dis Child 1988;142:1037.

148. Light MJ, Sheridan MS. Home monitoring in Hawaii: The first 1,000 patients. Hawaii Med J 1989;48:304.

149. Katcher ML, Shapiro MM, Guist C. Severe injury and death associated with home infant cardiorespirator monitors. Pediatrics 1986;78:775.

150. Food and Drug Administration. FDA safety alert: Important tips for apnea monitor users. February 16, 1990. HFZ-240.

151. Hunt CE, Brouillette RT. Methylxanthine treatment in infants at risk for sudden infant death syndrome. Ann NY Acad Sci 1988;533:119.

152. Vandenplas Y, De Wolf D, Sacre L. Influence of xanthines on gastroesophageal reflux in infants at risk for sudden infant death syndrome. Pediatrics 1986;77:807.

153. St Cyr JA, Ferrara TB, Thompson T, et al. Treatment of pulmonary manifestations of gastroesophageal reflux in children two years of age or less. Am J Surg 1989;157:400.

154. Krongrad E, ONeill L. Near miss sudden infant death syndrome episodes? A clinical and electrocardiographic correlation. Pediatrics 1986;77:811.

CHAPTER 13

The Grieving Family

Constance J. Doyle

INTRODUCTION

Historically, in preindustrial societies (and now in developing countries), multiple child deaths within a single family were not unusual. There were multiple incidences of children dying from malnutrition, infectious disease, and trauma. Only a few children in any family could be expected to survive to adulthood. Childhood death and mourning occurred in the home with the comfort and support of the extended family. Children saw death as part of the life process. However, with the current use of funeral parlors and with the dying process taking place in the hospital, children are isolated from the process of death.

In today's industrialized society, childhood death is rare, and survivors often feel isolated and unusual if a child in the family dies. Death often occurs in the hospital or in the hospital emergency department after an accident or sudden catastrophe. Emergency physicians not only must deal with the resuscitation, notification, and support of the next of kin, they must also notify certain authorities if a violent death has occurred. The physician may need to interview the family members to ascertain whether child abuse or neglect has occurred. At some facilities, the emergency physician is also the deputy medical examiner and may order a postmortem examination with or without the family's consent. The physician may also have the additional burden of requesting organ donation.

Medicine has become adept at prolonging the time of death, which may not prolong meaningful or comfortable life. There is much attention paid in residency training programs to the subject of resuscitation, but little attention given to dying and bereavement, particularly pertaining to sudden death.

There is little in modern life that prepares us for the complicated process of grieving. Children and the weak are isolated from the process of dying and bereavement.[1] There are additional societal barriers to and isolation of survivors if the death is caused by suicide, homicide, or AIDS. There is little continuity of support from the hospital or emergency department with families after the death.

CIRCUMSTANCES OF DEATH IN THE EMERGENCY DEPARTMENT

Emergency physicians confront death more often than family physicians and cardiologists.[2] Death in the emergency department is not an unusual occurrence, and sudden deaths occur more commonly in the emergency department than elsewhere. Sixty-five percent of the deaths in the emergency department are unexpected.[3] Emergency physicians must perform the resuscitation, then meet with a family they do not know.[2] The physician and the lay public may define death differently. The physician may surmise that death occurred out of the hospital; the patient may not be "dead" to the family until pronounced dead by the physician.

The emergency physician's ability to interact with grieving families is dependent on many variables. These include the number and acuteness of other patients in the emergency department that need attention, the circumstances sur-

rounding the death, the difficulty of the resuscitation, and the level of the physician's fatigue, sensitivity, skill, and experience. The physician's personal experience with loss and grief will affect his or her interaction with the grieving family. Cultural and ethnic biases of both the physician and the family also influence the interaction.[4]

Children are the family's and society's future. In older patients who have lived a "full life," death is easier to understand as part of the life process. The age of the patient and whether prevention was possible will have an impact on the physician and nursing staff. If staff members have children who are of similar ages to that of the deceased, a parallel may be drawn. The unfairness of young and violent deaths increases the difficulty of grieving. If death is in the context of illegal activity, such as drug dealing, or if there was an intentional overdose or suicide, feelings of anger may surface.[4]

Support of the family by hospital chaplains, social workers, nursing personnel who are not involved in the resuscitation effort, and community clergy can take an additional burden off the medical resuscitation team. A liaison can also facilitate communication between the resuscitation team and the family during the period of resuscitation.

Physicians are trained to save lives, and having a patient die may represent a personal failure. Many physicians have entered the medical profession for altruistic reasons and wish to help others. They may be influenced by an unconscious need for power over illness and death.[5]

The circumstances of the child's death, the manner of support for the family, and perhaps the need to support the dying child will have an impact on those in the emergency department. When resuscitation begins in the field, and when the child is brought to the emergency department, immediate access to old records and to the family's physician may be unavailable. Resuscitation efforts in cases of expected deaths may continue unnecessarily while a terminal illness is confirmed. Paramedical personnel have limited protocols in which they may either not initiate or stop resuscitation. In addition, the on-line medical control physician may have insufficient data to allow paramedics to confirm death and console the family. Private physician instruction regarding what must be done at the death of a terminally ill child in the home may not be conveyed to local on-line medical control authority. Families may have no resource other than the emergency number 911 when death occurs. There is no universal recognition of a "do not resuscitate" or a living will in adults, and even less so in children, who do not have the legal ability to convey their wishes to the medical profession. In addition, there may be problems identifying the individual who has died as the same person who signed the living will. Other concerns, when the death appears to be other than natural and a living will is presented, have yet to be addressed.

A chronically ill child may present to the emergency department during an exacerbation of an illness. The staff members should become familiar with the course of treatment of that child. When the child seems the most ill, both the attending physician and the family can be asked about the desirability of resuscitation measures. The child's desires should also be heard. Chronically ill children have some awareness that they are dying, but this may not be expressed to their family. Facilitating that communication can help the child say good-bye to the family. When a child is terminally ill, communication between the private physician and the emergency department staff and guidelines as to the degree of resuscitation that is to be undertaken will aid the emergency staff in treating terminal illness humanely. It should not be assumed, when a child has the diagnosis of an ultimately fatal illness, that aggressive treatment is unwarranted under some circumstances. For instance, during chemotherapy, the patient may become extremely ill but, with aggressive therapy, recover from that particular episode. The emergency team can be guided by medical records, private physician recommendations, and input from the family. Depending solely on a discouraged family's requests, without additional information, may not be in the best interest of the patient.

Though a chronic illness exists, death may still be unexpected. The family will need additional reassurance that unexpected events occur and that those events are not predictable.

Sudden Infant Death Syndrome

Sudden infant death syndrome (SIDS) is often encountered in the emergency department. Because of the emotional nature of an infant's sudden death and the unknown downtime, resuscitation may begin even when efforts will be futile. It is difficult for paramedical personnel to declare death at the scene and support the family in the home. The police and the medical examiner must also be involved in these cases to ensure that no abuse or neglect has occurred.

Support of the family should begin in the emergency department. Efforts to allay guilt, arrange for an autopsy that can confirm SIDS, and provide contact with support groups for the parents can be coordinated in the emergency department. The family may have tremendous anger, some of which may be directed toward the medical personnel, especially if the infant is not resuscitated. The infant's physician may also be the target of anger, particularly if the child has recently been examined. Additional information for the medical examiner can also be gathered at this time.

Miscarriage

The emergency department is a common place to treat early and sometimes late miscarriages. The diagnosis of pregnancy may be concurrent with the spontaneous abortion. The pregnancy may also be known, and several trips to the emergency department with vaginal bleeding or pain may occur before the abortion becomes inevitable. In a busy emergency department, physicians may not be sensitive to the loss of a child or a potential child as represented by a miscarriage. Support of the parents and connection with support resources may not be offered.

Occasionally the late miscarriage represents a deliberate attempt to abort the pregnancy, and an investigation may be warranted by the medical examiner or the police. There are times when a birth has occurred, and the mother will present as having a bleeding problem. The physician must determine whether the birth of a live infant in need of support has been hidden and whether the medical examiner should investigate. Stillbirth may occur in the emergency department if the mother is unaware of her pregnancy. If the stillbirth occurs outside the hospital, the mother and infant may be brought to the emergency department. The mother may need medical treatment for any complications related to the birth, and both parents should be supported and made aware of resources to help them through the grieving process. This situation is both the loss of an expected birth and the death of an child not yet known. The parents may want to hold the infant or take a picture of the child.

Unexpected Death

Acute sudden deaths in apparently healthy people; traumatic deaths caused by motor vehicle accidents, falls, or other trauma; and death caused by violence, including child abuse, present unique challenges to the emergency department. These include the difficulty of resuscitation, the investigation when abuse or neglect has occurred, and the notification and support of family members. Grieving is more difficult in sudden deaths, suicides, and violent deaths, yet many emergency departments have few resources dedicated to handling this problem.

Suicides and deaths during illegal drinking or drug-related activities evoke strong reactions in families and caregivers. The emergency team may have difficulty remaining objective under such circumstances.

THE EMERGENCY DEPARTMENT ENVIRONMENT

The emergency team must have an organized, consistent response to resuscitation and sudden death and a plan to address the needs of grieving families. In the chaos of the emergency department, it is difficult to find a quiet place for families to wait during resuscitative efforts and to grieve afterward. It may be difficult for the physician to spend much time with a family if there are other patients who require urgent attention; one source suggests that the physician plan to spend 15 to 20 minutes with the family.[6] When the department is busy, it may be difficult to provide a support person who can serve as a liaison between the medical team and the family. The department should plan to have an organized group of resource individuals (e.g., chaplain staff members, social workers, nurses, or other sensitive, compassionate individuals familiar with emergency processes) who can communicate with the family; offer support; keep the family updated regarding resuscitation efforts; facilitate contacts with resources for grieving help; and, finally, support the family in viewing, holding the body, and making final arrangements, including organ donation. The physician, as team leader, should inform the family of resuscitative efforts that have been made and tell them about the death. The physician can support the family in other phases of the emergency department grieving process as time and patient load allow.

If the preterminal child is to receive supportive efforts only and is not to be admitted, or if there will be some delay in admission, it is helpful to have a quiet, private area for the family to be with the child during the dying process. Even if the child is unconscious, the near-death literature suggests that hearing and some form of a knowing or "seeing" process exists.[7-9]

As more families observe field resuscitation and feel that they can choose the manner of care delivered to the child, there will be increasing pressure for individuals to be with and support their loved one during the dying process. Hospice and inpatient wards for the terminally ill support this, allowing the family to be present. Some families may wish to be present during resuscitation from a sudden death. When the family wishes to be with or support their child during the resuscitation, the medical efforts should not be disrupted; the family should have full support from a compassionate individual who is not part of the resuscitation team.

If the family wishes to be present during resuscitation, the attempt will be easier for emergency team members if intubation and intravenous lines are placed before the family comes into the room.[10] The family should be briefed as to what the resuscitation process entails and what is occuring at the time they enter the room. It is not merely an "observation," but provides support for the dying family member. In one survey, some 64% of family members present during resuscitation felt that their presence was helpful to the dying person. Many felt that their grieving was easier and that they had said "good-bye" before the person was pronounced dead.[10] However, the resuscitation may be more difficult for staff members because of emotions expressed by the family. Educational seminars for staff members may alleviate anxiety about the practice of admitting the family into the resuscitation room.

Stress-relieving sessions help staff members cope with and vent their feelings. Pediatric codes are difficult for staff members, and it may be helpful to have a stress debriefing after a pediatric death or other difficult, stressful events.[11]

ANATOMY OF GRIEVING AND SUPPORT

Emergency physicians care for children who die and mothers who experience miscarriage and support grieving families. Emergency physicians also see children who mourn significant losses, who have physical and psychological manifestations to those losses, and anniversary reactions to those losses.

The initial contact with survivors has a significant impact on their grief.[12] Altered mourning and blocked grief reactions can have significant pathologic and psychological morbidity for the individual and the family. This may happen when expressions of grief are blocked by platitudes (i.e., trite remarks that do not invite further expression of grief). The survivors' emotional needs cannot be adequately expressed or met when grief is masked by their use of alcohol or other drugs and when the death is unusually stressful to the bereaved (e.g., sudden, violent, or pediatric deaths).[13] In addition, any psychopathology already present in the family will tend to be magnified. Marital and familial discord is common following a pediatric death. Unresolved guilt may lead to lasting emotional difficulty, including substance abuse and refusal to have subsequent children.[14] Blame by spouses and relatives is not unusual; this is particularly magnified in divorced spouses. Mourning the death of a child lasts much longer than the commonly recognized 1 year.

Children and siblings are often left out of the acute phase of grieving at the hospital; they are usually protected from the full expression of the trauma by both medical staff and families. Parents and other family members may be so distraught that little comfort is offered to surviving children. Children may need to be included in the acute grieving and support process with other family members. Children may also have a mystical and distorted picture of death that warrants additional counseling. Children who have disordered mourning may have a pervasion of unexplainable sadness the rest of their lives.

There is a delicate balance between the rights of a family to grieve and a legal investigation. In violent deaths, or where abuse or neglect has occurred, staff members' feelings must not interfere with the family's need to grieve, regardless of who may be at fault. The legal system will ultimately determine guilt or innocence.

Acute grief reactions from a sudden death include shock, denial, anger, guilt, intense sadness, and disbelief. The family may exibit all or only a few of these in the emergency department. Cultural and ethnic background will modify the expression of grief. The grieving process is also affected by the notion of the completeness of life: had the patient experienced a "full" life? In pediatric deaths, the perception is that life has been terminated prematurely. The patient may not have been at peace with himself or herself or with the world. Teens and young adults undergo the natural turmoil of forming a personal identity; death of a teen may leave a family with feelings of guilt if peace and harmony were not achieved with the teen prior to death. The family's perception of the patient's pain or disfigurement will also affect the grief reaction. The emergency team can do much

to allay this discomfort by positive statements that the patient felt "little pain" or that the patient was "probably unconscious and did not suffer." Fantasies of what happened may be much worse than the reality. Relating to the family all that is known about the accident and the resuscitative efforts help to give an accurate picture of events.

Emergency staff members have many duties in addition to resuscitation and care for the dying patient. The family is another "patient" that must have additional attention. Emergency personnel have constraints imposed on them by living patients who need urgent medical attention. Preferably, staff members who are not part of the resuscitation team can serve as a liaison between the emergency team and the family. Those individuals should be compassionate, work well with those who have different ethnic and religious beliefs, and understand emergency procedures as well as the grief process. Facilitators can transmit valuable medical information to the resuscitation team and keep the family informed of the resuscitation effort. They can assist in contacting additional family members, people from local churches, and support groups. The liaison can also assist with paperwork for organ donation and in locating a funeral home. At times when there are large numbers of family or friends, the liaison can help with crowd control and in locating a quiet area where friends and family may wait together. In some situations (i.e., divorced families), there may be hostilities between family members such that two separate waiting areas are needed. In general, however, divorced parents can wait in the same room and be informed of the death together.

The facilitator can accompany the family to support the dying patient or to view or hold the body. The expression of grief, even if loud, should not be blunted as long as there is no physical destruction or danger to staff members or patients. It may be necessary for the family to mourn in another place outside the hearing of other patients in the emergency department. Platitudes and grief-limiting phrases such as, "Pull yourself together," "It's God's will," and "You have other children," reflect bias or discomfort on the part of the liaison and may be inconsistent with the beliefs and needs of the family. Emergency personnel should be aware of their own biases, level of fatigue, and the family's reaction to anticipated loss.

Ideally the family will know of the emergency and begin to anticipate a loss when the EMS system is activated. In cases in which the deceased is at a different location, such as school, the family will be notified by phone to come to the hospital. They should not be informed about the death over the phone except in unusual circumstances (e.g., great geographic distance or when the informed family member has a handicap that makes it difficult to leave the home). In those instances, one should ensure that family support is available at the time of notification. In some communities, the police will assist with personal notification.

When the family arrives, they should be met by the facilitator and taken to a quiet area out of the emergency department waiting area. They should be informed of treatment or resuscitation if it is ongoing. If the treating physician is able to speak to the family and leave the patient, he or she should do so. If the physician cannot leave the patient, the liaison can serve as a communication link between the emergency team and the family. The task of announcing the death belongs to the physician as head of the emergency team. If the family's private physician is present, he or she may wish to accompany the emergency physician to tell the family. The words died or dead should be used to avoid the confusion that the patient has "gone" or "been taken" somewhere else. The family should be given details of the circumstances surrounding the death and what treatment was initiated. The family should be informed if any investigation by the medical examiner, a child abuse evaluation, or other legal investigation will be necessary. They should be asked if they would like to see the body, to say good-bye, or to hold or touch the deceased. Touching or holding surviving family members by medical personnel depends on the comfort of both staff members and the family. Physical touch at times of need can be greatly comforting and calming.

Viewing the body reinforces the realization that the child has died. When children request to see the body, they should be included in the viewing.[12] Even if the body is mutilated or bloody, emergency staff can facilitate viewing by appropriate placement of towels and sheets and by wiping away vomitus and blood. Family should be informed of what they will see before being escorted to the room. When there are many family members, or when the space is needed in the emergency department, another site will need to be located for family viewing and good-byes. Some families will wish to stay with the deceased for a long time; they should not be hurried.[12] Staff members' bias and feelings about "what is right" for each individual family may need to be expressed privately in a debriefing session. Staff attitudes about illegal activities, drug overdose or suicide, drinking, and child abuse should not burden the family at the time of grieving.

Dealing with significant others may present some difficulty for staff members. Attempts to assist grieving in an unbiased manner may be difficult. In most states, significant others have no legal right to see the deceased or to even obtain information at or from the hospital. If the legal family is willing (and they should be encouraged to do so), these individuals can be included as family members in the grieving process at the hospital. The grieving process is greatly facilitated for these individuals if they are included. Teenagers have significant close ties to peers, and these peers may come to the hospital when a catastrophe occurs. With family permission and guidance, they can be included to some extent in the acute processes. Lovers, both of the opposite and the same sex, will face a genuine loss and a need to grieve, regardless of staff or family acceptance of their life-style. The family may not be aware of the teen's relationships until the time of death.

A significant amount of staff time can be spent in completing paperwork; assisting in funeral home contact; discussing choices regarding autopsy and organ donation; notifying other family and the personal physician; and having the family say good-bye to the deceased. The liaison can take a tremendous part of this burden from emergency department staff.

Survivors need community resource information and information on symptoms of the grief response. The family should be assured that symptoms of sleep disturbances, depression, anorexia, mood swings, difficulties in concentration and interest, anger and guilt, overwhelming sorrow, and numbness are normal reactions. Families should be encouraged to call with any questions concerning the death, and support group information should be offered. Some emergency departments have developed bereavement packages or booklets with grief and support information that can be given to the family. Sympathy cards and a follow-up call can let the family know of support.

Anniversary reaction to significant losses may occur in subsequent years and present to the emergency department as vague symptoms related to stress, anxiety, or depressive episodes. Children may have grief reactions to losses of family, significant animals, and friends and to moving.

An organized plan for handling acute grief in the emergency department can greatly facilitate normal mourning, allow families to begin to face the realities of their loss, and serve as a conduit to community resources for grieving support.

References

1. Cutter F. Coming to Terms with Death. Chicago, Nelson-Hall, 1974.
2. Schmidt TA, Tolle SW. Emergency physicians' responses to families following patient death. Ann Emerg Med 1990;19:125.
3. Tolle SW, Bascom PB, Hickam DH, Bensen JA Jr. Communication between physicians and surviving spouses following patient deaths. J Gen Intern Med 1986;1:309.
4. Sciabbarrasi J. Death and dying in the emergency department. Presented at ACEP Scientific Assembly, San Francisco, CA, 1990.
5. Wiener JM. Response of medical personnel to the fatal illness of a child. *In* Schoenberg B, Carr A, Peretz D, Kutscher A (eds). Loss and Grief. New York, Columbia University Press, 1970.
6. Breaking the worst news: When a child dies suddenly. Emerg Med 1989; 21:74. March 30.
7. Moody RA. Life After Life. Covington, GA, Mockingbird Books, 1975.
8. Moody RA. Reflections on Life After Life. New York, Bantam Books, 1977.
9. Atwater PMH. Coming Back to Life. New York, Ballentine, 1988.
10. Doyle CJ, Post H, Burney R. Family participation during resuscitation: An option. Ann Emerg Med 1987;16:673.
11. Mitchell JT, Bray GP. Emergency Services Stress. Englewood Cliffs, NJ, Prentice-Hall, 1990.
12. Dubin WR, Sarnoff JR. Sudden unexpected death: Intervention with the survivors. Ann Emerg Med 1986;15:54.
13. Bowlby J. Loss. *In* Bowlby J (ed). Attachment and Loss. Vol III. New York, Basic Books, 1980.
14. Singer JI. Emergency department response to the death of a child. Presented at ACEP Scientific Assembly, San Francisco, CA, 1990.

Reading Resources

About Grief. S Deerfield, MA, Channing Bete, 1986.
Cassell EJ. On being and becoming dead. Soc Res 1972;39:528.
Davies P. Grief. New York, Carol Communications, 1988.
Evans A. If a Child Must Die . . . N Engl J Med 1968;278:138.
Friedman R, Gradstein B. Surviving Pregnancy Loss. Boston, Little, Brown, 1982.
Grollman E. Explaining Death to Children. Boston, Beacon Press, 1967.
Harrison SI, Davenport CW, McDermott JF. Children's reactions to bereavement. Arch Gen Psych 1967;17:593.
Howell D. A child dies. J Ped Surg 1976;1:2.
James J, Cherry F. The Grief Recovery Handbook. New York, Harper & Row, 1988.
Johnson EA. As Someone Dies. Santa Monica, CA, Hay House, 1987.
Kapleau P. The Wheel of Life and Death. New York, Doubleday, 1989.
Karofsky PS. Death of a high school hockey player. Physician Sports Med 1990;18:2.
Koenig R. Handling grief in the emergency department. Emerg Med Serv 1975 August.
Krementz J. How It Feels When a Parent Dies. New York, Alfred A Knopf, 1988.
Kubler-Ross E. On Children and Death. New York, Collier Books, 1983.
Kubler-Ross E. On Death and Dying. New York, Collier Books, 1969.
Kubler-Ross E. Living with Death and Dying. New York, Collier Books, 1981.
Kubler-Ross E. Working it Through. New York, Collier Books, 1982.
Levine S. Who Dies? New York, Anchor Books, 1982.
Lukas C, Seiden H. Silent Grief: Living in the Wake of Suicide. New York, Bantam Books, 1987.
Lund D. Death and Consciousness. New York, Ballantine, 1985.
Orbach I. Children Who Don't Want to Live. San Francisco, Jossey-Bass, 1988.
Pincus L. Death and the Family. New York, Schocken Books, 1974.
Powers G. Humanizing hospital experiences. Am J Dis Child 1948;76:365.
Sarnoff-Schiff H. The Bereaved Parent. New York, Penguin Books, 1977.
Scholl S. Death and the Humanities. Associated University Press, Cranbury, NJ, 1984.
Stearns AK. Coming Back. New York, Ballantine, 1988.
Stearns AK. Living Through Personal Crisis. New York, Ballantine, 1984.
Vore DA. A child's view of death. South Med J 1974;67:383.

Support Resources

American Association of Suicidology, 2459 S Ash St, Denver, CO, 80222. (303) 692–0985.
Compassionate Friends. PO Box 3696, Oak Brook, IL, 60522–9803. (708) 990–0010. A source for literature for grieving parents; has chapters and support groups in many locations. Some of its literature would also be useful in adult grieving.

Concern for Dying, 250 W. 57th St, New York, NY, 10107. Conducts conferences on death and dying. Distributes the living will. Newsletter.

The Guild for Infant Survival, PO Box 3841 Davenport, IA, 52808. (319) 326–4653. Provides information and consolation to families who have lost a child to SIDS. Support groups in many areas.

Mothers Against Drunk Drivers (MADD), 5330 Primrose, Suite 146, Fair Oaks, CA, 95628. Provides support for families who have lost a member in an accident involving a drunk driver. Literature is available. There are regional and state groups.

National Hospice Organization, 1901 N Fort Meyer Dr, Arlington, VA, 22209.

National SIDS Clearinghouse, 1555 Wilson Blvd, Suite 600, Rosslyn, VA, 22209. (730) 538–0480. Provides information and literature on sudden infant death syndrome.

National Sudden Infant Death Syndrome Foundation, Metro Plaza, Suite 103, 8200 Professional Place, Landover, MD, 20785. (301) 459–3388 or (800) 221–SIDS. Support chapters in many locations. Publications are available.

Our Newsletter, Jean Kollantai, PO Box 1064, Palmer, AK, 99645. Newsletter for parents who have lost one or more children from a multiple birth.

Parents of Murdered Children. 1739 Bella Vista, Cincinnati, OH, 45237. (513) 242–8025 or 721–LOVE. Newsletter and support through local chapters.

CHAPTER 14

Child Abuse

James J. Williams

INTRODUCTION

The recognition of child abuse is dependent on the examining physician's suspicion that it may exist.[1] The physician must be aware of the range of injuries with which abused children present to the emergency department. A high index of suspicion and proficient interview and examination skills are therefore required. The emergency department has become one of the most utilized community resources for social and medical problems.[2] Missing the diagnosis of child abuse, particularly in children under 12 months of age, risks repeated injuries to the child or possible fatality; on the other hand, an inappropriate diagnosis may result in unnecessary and potentially traumatic intervention. To protect children and prevent repeated injury, the physician must be able to identify the child who may have been abused, report clinical suspicions to protective services, and work with the family and authorities to prevent further injury.

BACKGROUND

Child abuse is poorly understood. Its antecedents lie in societies that have historically tolerated violence and denied agency to women and children.[3, 4] Child abuse emerged as a public concern despite denial of its existence and its assignment to the realm of family privacy.[5] By the nineteenth century, there was a growing recognition that children deserve special protections. Post–Civil War America saw the establishment of foundling homes and the Society for the Prevention of Cruelty to Children.[6, 7] Child labor laws were passed, and courts began to develop juvenile divisions. Women's movements advocated children's rights in tandem with their own. Such movements were responsible for many

of the child welfare reforms during this period, including the development of the social service profession.[8, 9] Child welfare workers had struggled with child abuse long before medicine rediscovered it in the mid twentieth century. In 1946, the radiologist John Caffey argued that a subdural hematoma and a long-bone fracture, found in association in the same infant, resulted from trauma, even when no history of injury could be obtained.[10] In 1962, C. Henry Kempe coined the phrase *battered child syndrome*, and the attention of medicine was finally drawn to the problem.[11]

For children younger than 12 months of age, physical abuse is still among the leading causes of death. Homicide of children between the ages of 1 and 4 years accounts for 10% of all deaths.[12–15] The latest concern, the rising number of infants born to drug-addicted mothers, has overwhelmed the medical and protective services systems. In 1986, more than 2.4 million abuse reports were made to protective service agencies in the United States, a rate of more than 3 reports per 100 children.[16] A national survey reported an even higher rate.[17] Nevertheless, child abuse remains underreported. Homicide and child neglect fatalities have been misdiagnosed and incorrectly reported as sudden infant death syndrome, and deaths due to natural causes or accidental injury.[18–21] Some physicians do not report child abuse, even when it is suspected. Individuals may be reluctant to become involved with the criminal justice system or may doubt the ability of protective service agencies to protect children.[22–25] Physicians themselves disagree on what acts of discipline constitute abuse and when these acts should be reported.[26] Most U.S. pediatric residency programs provide inadequate training for house staff in child abuse recognition and reporting.[27] Finally, varying definitions of child abuse have led to imprecise statistics.[28]

DEFINITIONS

Child abuse is a broad category of conditions in which an injury occurs to a child as the result of family dysfunction or a breakdown in the parent-child interaction. Physical abuse is any inflicted injury that significantly jeopardizes the child's safety, impairs physical functioning, and is accompanied by physical evidence of injuries. It accounts for about 25% of child abuse reports. Unrelated male care providers are responsible for a large number of fatal child abuse cases.

Child neglect is the failure to provide for the child's basic needs (i.e., an adequate level of care with respect to food, clothing, shelter, hygiene, medical attention, or supervision). Neglect is responsible for more than 60% of the case reports and for more child deaths than physical abuse.

Sexual abuse is the use of the child for sexual activities or economic gain, such as pornography and prostitution. It accounts for 15% of all child abuse reports. Children and adolescents are developmentally immature and neither fully comprehend the nature of sexual activity nor possess the autonomy for consent. Most sexually abusive activity occurs in the home.

Emotional abuse is the destruction or impairment of the child's self-development and social competence. Though reported as the sole form of abuse in 5% of cases, emotional abuse and exploitation is the context in which all forms of child maltreatment occur.[29] Child abuse implies not only physical injury, but also an attack on the child's self-image as good and lovable. The long-term consequences of emotional abuse have the greatest destructive effects on the child's development.

RISK FACTORS

Although there are no reliable profiles with which to predict abusive families, awareness of factors associated with child abuse may alert the physician to its possibility.[30] Abusive families are socially isolated and display violent behavior patterns.[31–33] A man in such a family who abuses the woman is more likely to abuse the child.[34] Abusive families are found in all socioeconomic and ethnic groups, but the predominance of reports originate from situations where poverty adds to an already reduced sense of community responsibility for children.[35, 36] Families experiencing unemployment and economic deprivation are more likely to be involved with social welfare, police, and health agencies and, therefore, are more likely to be reported.[37] However, most socially and economically stressed families do not abuse their children. Although research on the causes of abusive behaviors is limited, abusive parents and care providers are more likely to be inadequately nurtured adults. They may be young with an unwanted pregnancy, mentally ill, or chemically addicted.[17, 38–45] Stressed parents who poorly understand child development are more likely to choose corporal punishment and harsh alternatives to manage the child's behavior.[46] Abusive parents have been found to have had negative and harmful childhood experiences several times more often than nonabusive parents.[47] Nonabusive parents who were raised in abusive homes differ from abusive parents in significant ways. The nonabusive parents report having more extensive social supports and, as children, were more apt to find a supportive relationship with a nonabusive adult. They have fewer ambivalent feelings about childbearing and are better able to express their feelings about their childhood.[48]

Child-related factors are also involved in abuse. Most abused children are young, with two thirds under 3 years of age. Adolescents are another age group likely to experience violent abuse resulting in serious physical injury.[49, 50] Children who are perceived as different or difficult are at greater risk for abuse. Twins and children with handicapping conditions (birth defects, mental retardation, chronic illness) may impose additional stresses on the family.[51–53]

There is an association between parental drug or alcohol addiction and child abuse.[54–56] Addiction is found in a high number of families reported for abuse and neglect.[57] Increased levels of violence are shared in both substance-abusing and child-abusing families.[58–60] The poverty and social isolation, the personality traits (e.g., depression, poor self-image), and erratic behavior attributed to alcoholics and drug abusers are similar to descriptions of child-abusing or neglectful parents. Addicted parents may suffer from the effects of the drugs (e.g., hallucinations, seizures, and criminal behaviors). These effects prevent them from meeting the physical and emotional needs of their children. The child is also at risk for injury and abuse from other persons in the household. Children born after being exposed to maternal drug abuse add to the addicted parent's stress by being more difficult to interact with and feed. The parent may leave the responsibility to others or may abandon the child.

CLINICAL EVALUATION

Suspicion of nonaccidental trauma arises when there is a disclosure of abuse, abnormal parental attitudes or behavior, a discrepant history, or characteristic physical findings of injury.

History

The account of the injury is often the first and best indication that the child may have been abused. Only a *reasonable suspicion* of abuse, not certitude, is needed to begin the reporting process. Raising the question of abuse when faced with an injured child is awkward,[61] and conducting

the interview requires diplomacy. The parents may be uncooperative or untruthful and uncomfortable with their abusive behaviors, yet angry and fearful. However, the parents may also be innocent of having inflicted the injury, and the inference of abuse may have a devastating impact. Therefore it is important at the outset to inform them of the reason for the interview. Negative and punitive feelings of medical personnel are counterproductive if expressed to the parents. It is better to redirect energies toward caring for the injured child. The parents should be allowed to express their feelings and maintain self-esteem. The physician should support their desire to do what is best for the child. However, they should be informed of the physician's obligation to ensure the child's protection from harm and to report cases of suspected abuse.

A detailed description of the conditions surrounding the injury should be obtained from each care provider involved at the scene (i.e., who, what, when, where, how, height of fall, surface of impact, and who was present). The physician should interview the child, if the child is able to talk. Separating those who were present may result in different stories. Changing or contradictory stories, not consistent with the injury, may suggest abuse. The main statements should be quoted verbatim. The goal of the interview is to obtain a spontaneous account with few prompting questions.[62]

An unexplained delay between the time of the injury and the attempt to obtain medical care is often associated with abusive injury. Most parents promptly seek medical care when their child is injured.

Direct disclosures of abuse are uncommon, but occur when the injured child reveals the identity of the perpetrator during the interview or to a trusted adult. Disclosures also occur when one parent accuses another adult, usually absent, of injuring the child. When a parent admits to causing some injuries but not others, the statement should be regarded as an admission. Indirect disclosures occur, for example, when the parent admits feeling "out of control" around the child but denies acting on the impulse.

Discrepant histories are recognized when the mechanisms of trauma are understood. A history of a single injury from an accidental fall is not supported by the finding of multiple injuries at different stages of healing. Likewise, a history of a minor injury is contradicted by finding injuries to several areas, particularly bilateral lesions, or finding injuries that are more severe than the history would suggest. Injured children sometimes present for care without an explanation from their care providers, or an injury is discovered in the course of an evaluation for an unrelated problem. Most nonabusing parents freely discuss the details of their child's injury with the physician, but the lack of an explanation, by itself, is not a firm indication of abuse. The person who caused the injury may not be the one who brought the child for care.

The parents' behavior and emotional reaction to the child's injury should be observed. Most parents feel distressed when their child has been injured, but abusive parents may be focused on something else. Whether they appear to be intoxicated or drugged should also be noted.[63] The parent's inability to attend to the child's affective signals may suggest dysfunctional patterns.[64–68] Abusive parents have unrealistic expectations of the child's abilities that often conflict with the child's actual abilities during certain developmental periods, such as toilet training.[69] Many expect the child to fulfill their adult emotional needs and harbor strong beliefs on the use of corporal punishment as a disciplinary technique. The force used on the child may reflect the parents' over-reliance on physically controlling behaviors.[70]

The injury and its history are best evaluated within a

context that considers the capabilities of the child. Familiarity with age-appropriate accidental injuries and their possible mechanisms is required (Table 14–1).[71, 72] For example, the history of a 4-month-old child who sustains rib fractures by crawling off a tabletop is unlikely, since a 4-month-old is incapable of crawling. The injured child should be directly observed to see if the action attributed to self-injury is possible. Blaming the injured child (self-inflicted trauma) or another child for the injury is common. Children themselves can be "battering" and self-destructive, and some are victims of punitive childrearing.[73–75] An evaluation of the "abusing" child's capabilities is needed.

An experienced social worker should take a detailed psychosocial history. Information regarding the family dynamics and home environment is vital both in determining the safety of returning the child to the home and in formulating a treatment plan for the family. The possibility that some mothers of child victims are themselves experiencing physical abuse from their male partners needs to be explored.[76] Risk assessment is an individualized process, made in collaboration with the social worker, police, and other professionals involved in the case.[77]

Physical Findings

Bruises

The cutaneous tissues are the most commonly injured site in physical abuse.[78] The child's age and the location of the injuries may indicate the cause (Table 14–2). Bruises are not expected on any part of an infant's body who is not yet walking. Falls from beds and changing tables produce bruises that are not serious. Toddlers and children usually have some bruises over bony prominences, such as the shins, knees, and foreheads, from falls and collisions. Bruises over central and soft parts of the body, such as the buttocks, upper thighs, back, inner arms, cheeks of the face, and

TABLE 14–2

LOCATION OF CUTANEOUS INJURIES IN THE YOUNG CHILD

Possibly Accidental Cause	Probably Nonaccidental Cause
Shins and knees	Buttocks
Hips (iliac crests)	Inner aspects of thighs
	Genitalia, perineum, rectum
Prominences of the spine	Abdomen
	Chest
Forehead and chin	Cheeks, neck, ears
Facial scratches in infant	
Lower arms	Inner aspects of upper arms
Elbows	

abdomen, are less likely to be accidental (Fig. 14–1). Bruises over the ears may result from pinches or blows. Bilaterally located bruises are unlikely to be accidental. Bruises located near the pubic area, genitalia, and rectum raise the possibility of sexual abuse.

The pattern or shape of the bruises may suggest the origin. When the force of the blow is sufficient to rupture capillaries, an impression of the hitting object may be seen. Slapping with the open hand may leave a characteristic outline of parallel linear marks (Fig. 14–2). Oval bruises on the upper arm and chest may be fingertip marks indicating forcible grabbing or violent shaking. The possibility of associated rib and long bone fractures should be excluded. Bruises around the neck suggest strangulation. Whip and loop marks with wire, cord, or rope leave linear bruises of uniform depth that follow curved body surfaces (Fig. 14–3).

TABLE 14–1

COMMON ACCIDENTAL INJURIES BY AGE

Age Group	Type of Accidental Injury Expected
Infants (birth to 12 mo)	Birth trauma: Skull fracture Cephalohematoma Clavicle, humerus, femur fracture Falls/being dropped: Soft tissue injury Simple skull fracture
Toddler (10 mo to 3 yr)	Collision and fall injuries: Soft tissue injuries to bony prominences Superficial cuts Clavicle, distal radius/ulna, skull fracture Toddler's fracture of tibia Splash burns to anterior body surface Hand injury: Distal phalangeal soft tissue injury/fracture
Young child (3 to 5 yr)	Collision and fall injuries: Distal radius/ulna, clavicle fracture Simple or depressed skull fracture Soft tissue injuries to bony prominences

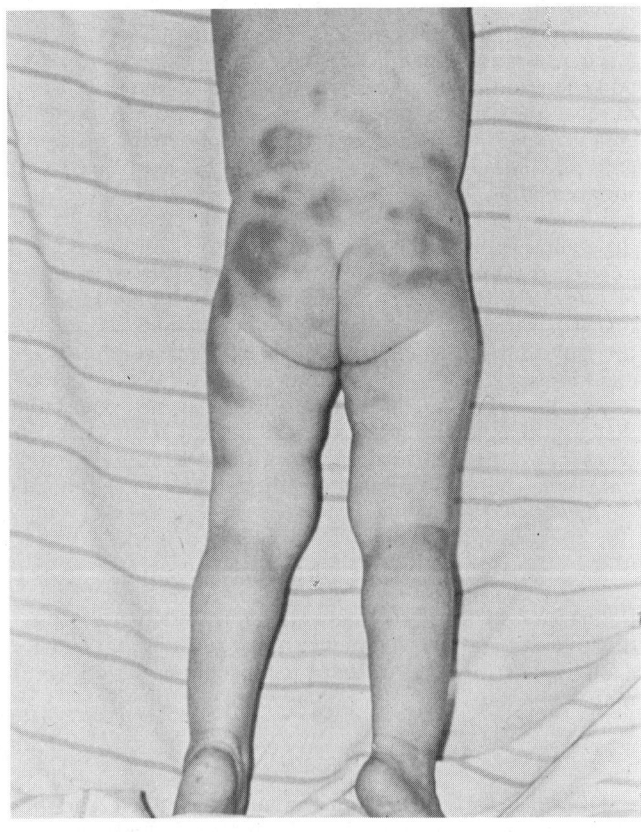

Figure 14–1. Bruises inflicted on the lower back and buttocks. (From Schmitt B. The Visual Diagnosis of Non-Accidental Trauma and Failure to Thrive. Prepared in cooperation with the American Academy of Pediatrics, 1979.)

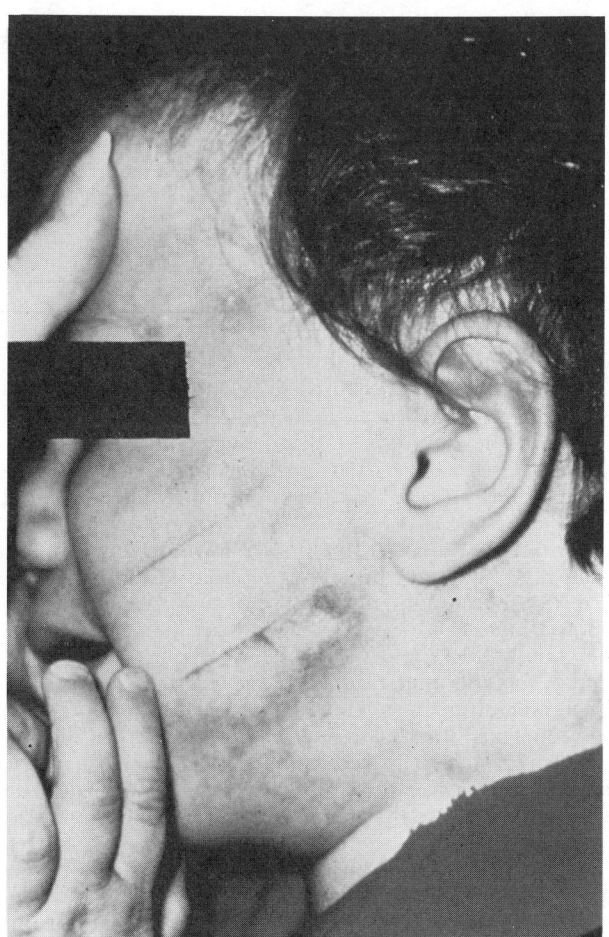

Figure 14–2. Slap mark with fingers outlined on the face. (From Schmitt B. The Visual Diagnosis of Non-Accidental Trauma and Failure to Thrive. Prepared in cooperation with the American Academy of Pediatrics, 1979.)

The injury caused by a looped wire is elliptical in shape; a belt mark is broad and linear, and the impression of the eyelets and buckle may be seen. Scarring may result if the skin was broken. Restraint marks appear as deep cuts or burns at the ends of extremities and on the torso. Injuries around the mouth, such as bruised lips and a torn frenulum, occur from forcing a bottle, pacifier, or finger into the child's mouth to stop crying. Sharp instruments used inside the mouth have resulted in perforation of the pharynx.[79] Gag marks, sometimes mistaken for impetigo, appear at the corners of the mouth (Fig. 14–4).

Bites are an uncommonly inflicted injury. They leave a distinctive oval mark in which tooth impressions appear as bruises facing each other (Fig. 14–5). Abuse-related bites have been attributed to an animal or to another child. The "rule of three" (i.e., a distance >3.0 mm between the maxillary canines in the wound indicates an adult attacker) can be applied but may be misleading if applied in an unqualified way.[80] An experienced forensic odontologist should be consulted. Bites inflicted during sexual assault may leave a visible central suction mark. High-quality photography with a rigid ruler visible in the frame should document the wound.

Estimating the age of bruises is possible, as they undergo recognizable color changes with hemoglobin degradation and healing (Table 14–3).[81] An estimate of age is often necessary to check the consistency of the history, but inter-

pretation should be cautious, as only a general estimate of age is possible. Bruises in infants change color more rapidly than those in older age groups. Infant bruises may be red or red-blue during the first 24 hours and change to a yellow color as early as the third to fifth day. An older child may take 7 to 10 days for these changes to occur. Injuries with greater amounts of bleeding, deep bleeding with loculation of blood, or repetitive trauma at the same site may show delayed appearance or healing of the bruise; such bruises will change color at the periphery first. In child death cases, the "bruise" may be due to postmortem pooling of blood. A skin biopsy can establish the lesion age in doubtful cases.

Burns

Abusive burn injuries occur by splashing, immersion, and branding with hot liquids or objects (Table 14–4). They account for 8% to 16% of all abusive injuries.[82, 83] Burns may be the result of extreme neglect in a significant number of cases. The peak age range for such injuries is 13 to 24 months.

Splash burns are caused when hot liquids are pulled down from tables or stoves or are thrown on the child. Accidental and inflicted splash burns are usually indistinguishable from one another. They appear as several noncontiguous areas of full- or partial-thickness burns that have irregular borders and surrounding satellite lesions caused by splattering. As the hot liquid runs off the body, a cascade, or arrowhead, pattern may develop, permitting an analysis of the child's body relative to the direction of flow of the hot liquid. If the child's clothes were covering the area at the time of the

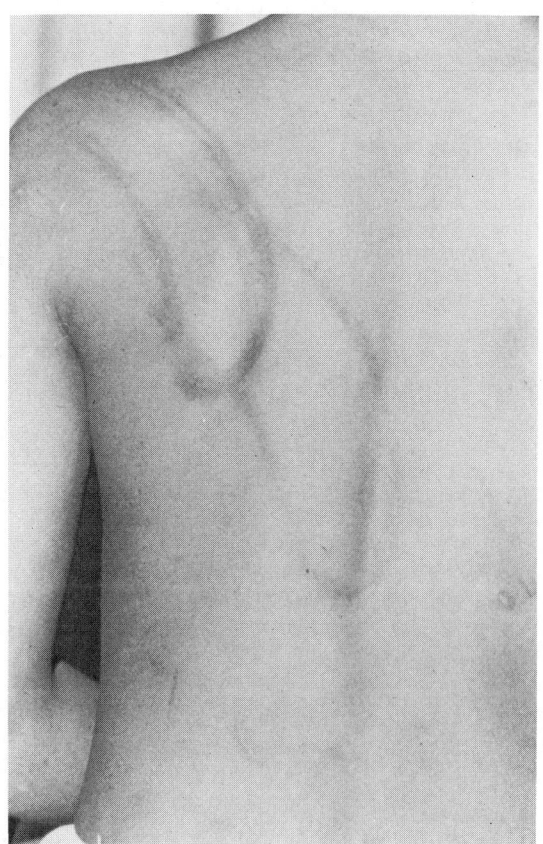

Figure 14–3. Whip marks produced by a wire loop. (From Schmitt B. The Visual Diagnosis of Non-Accidental Trauma and Failure to Thrive. Prepared in cooperation with the American Academy of Pediatrics, 1979.)

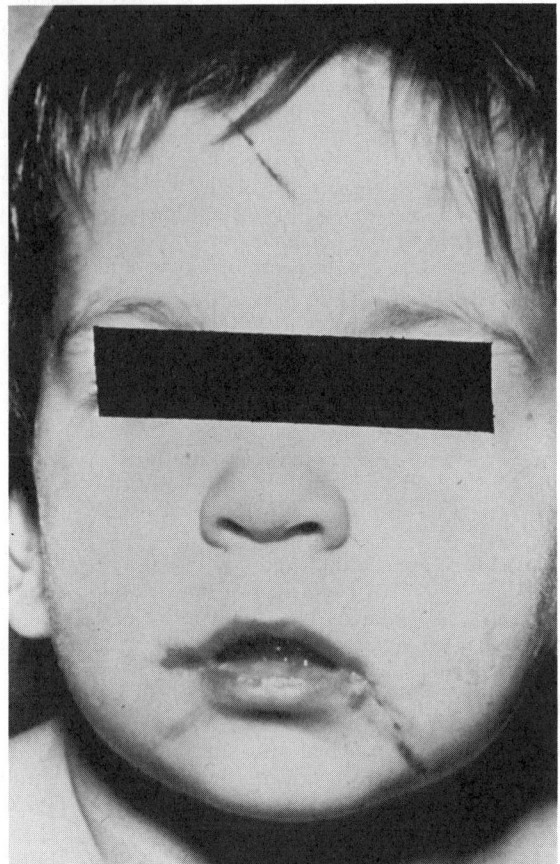

Figure 14–4. Gag marks. (From Schmitt B. The Visual Diagnosis of Non-Accidental Trauma and Failure to Thrive. Prepared in cooperation with the American Academy of Pediatrics, 1979.)

burn, the injury may be more extensive because of prolonged contact with the hot liquid. The burns may present initially as several large, bullous lesions. Differentiation from a staphylococcal (bullous) impetigo and the scalded skin syndrome is made by history, culture, and Gram stain.

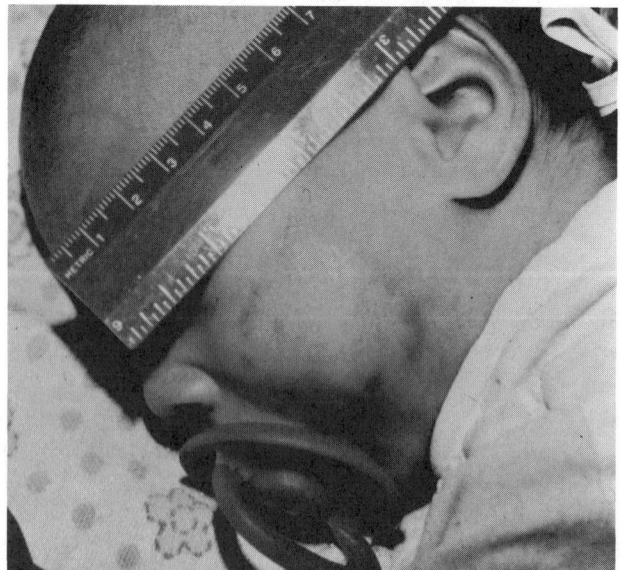

Figure 14–5. Human bite marks. (From Braham R, Morris M. Textbook of Pediatric Dentistry. Philadelphia, BC Decker, Inc, 1985.)

TABLE 14–3	
ESTIMATION OF THE AGE OF CUTANEOUS BRUISES	
Estimated Age (Days)	**Appearance**
0–1	Swollen, tender
0–2	Red, blue, purple
3–6	Blue, green
6–10	Green, brown
10–14	Tan, yellow
14–30	Faded to clear

Immersion burns are caused by scalding liquids (Fig. 14–6). The depth of the burn is related to the liquid's temperature and the duration of the contact. Most home water heaters are set between 60°C and 65°C (140°–150°F). Water at 65°C will cause a full-thickness burn to adult skin in only 2 seconds, whereas 30 seconds are required to produce a similar burn at 55°C.[84, 85] Immersion burns occur to children under 3 years of age and are often inflicted for noncompliance with toilet training. They are of uniform depth in the exposed areas, with sharp skin demarcation at the water line. The buttocks and perineum may be involved, or if a hand or foot was immersed, there may be a glove or stocking distribution of the burn. If the palms, soles, or buttocks were pressed against the cooler sides or bottom of a bathtub, the central areas may be spared from injury while the surrounding skin is burned. A child who thrashed about while immersed will have a combination of splash and immersion burns.

Branding burns are caused by contact with a hot object and are common inflicted burns.[86] They may be shapeless or take the form of the object, such as a heater grate, curling iron, or the smoldering end of a cigarette (Figs. 14–7 and 14–8). An inflicted cigarette burn creates a deep circular ulcer on the skin, 5 to 10 mm in diameter, but the burn of an accidental contact is single, superficial, and linear in shape.

The history of the burn must be evaluated with the child's developmental level in mind. Branding and immersion burns of the hands can result from childhood exploratory behavior. Children more than 15 to 18 months of age have been able to climb into tubs, pull open a water control valve, and tumble into the hot water, usually burning themselves around the face and torso. Older children can climb into the tub and turn a circular knob, but if the child was standing, the expected burns will be of the splash type to the anterior parts of the feet.

Other Skin Injuries

Injuries around the scalp and face are common in child abuse, accounting for one third of the injuries in one large study.[82] Scalp injuries may be caused by violent, sudden hair pulling. Traumatic alopecia, unlike alopecia areata, appears as a diffuse, nondiscrete area that is incompletely bald and contains broken hairs of various lengths within it and no loose hairs at the periphery (Fig. 14–9). If the force was severe enough, the scalp may have been lifted off the calvarium, resulting in a subgaleal hematoma. An underlying skull fracture with spinal fluid leakage may resemble a subgaleal hematoma. Computed tomography (CT) should be used to assess these injuries.[87]

Facial and external eye injuries frequently result from accidents and are seldom diagnostic of abuse. Facial fractures are uncommon in abuse but, when they occur, often involve the mandible.[88] Eye injuries often occur in physical abuse and include orbital and lid ecchymosis and hematoma,

TABLE 14–4		
CHARACTERISTICS OF ACCIDENTAL AND INTENTIONAL BURNS		
	Accidental	**Intentional**
History	Burn compatible with physical findings	Burn not compatible with history
		Burns blamed on sibling
		Unrelated adult seeks medical care
		Differing accounts
		Treatment delay >24 hr
		Prior "accidents" or absence of parental concern
Location	Usually front of body	Trunk of body
		Buttocks, perineum, genitalia
	Random; injury specific	Ankles, wrists
		Palms, soles
Pattern	Associated irregular splash burns	Sharply demarcated borders with normal skin
		Stocking/glove distribution
	Partial thickness	Full thickness
	Asymmetric	Symmetric
		Burn older than history indicates
		Burn neglected/infected
	One traumatic event	Numerous lesions of varying age
		Pattern of burning instrument discernible
		Large area with uniform burn (forced contact)

From: Reece RM, Grodin MA. Recognition of nonaccidental injury. *In* Alpert JJ, Guyer B (eds). Symposium on injuries and injury prevention. Pediatr Clin North Am 1985;32(1):48.

hyphema, anisocoria, subconjunctival hemorrhage, retinal hemorrhage, papilledema, and sixth nerve palsy (Fig. 14–10).[89] Bilateral periorbital hematomas do not occur without prior injury. Leakage of blood from a basilar skull fracture or subgaleal hematoma should be excluded in cases of "racoon eyes." Assessment of visual fields and acuity is required as part of the evaluation.

Differential Diagnosis

Certain uncommon conditions must be considered in children with skin injuries (Table 14–5). An underlying bleeding disorder should be excluded with bruising, although a bleeding disorder and child abuse can certainly coexist.[90] In addition to coagulation studies, factor VIII and IX assays should be considered to exclude mild degrees of hemophilia.[91] The partial thromboplastin time alone is not a sensitive screening test. It can be prolonged after minor viral infections in children, extensive tissue injury to the brain, and when there is difficulty obtaining blood as a result of clotting in the syringe.[92–94] Other systemic conditions, such as osteogenesis imperfecta, vitamin K deficiency, hypersensitivity vasculitis, erythema multiforme, and bleeding secondary to salicylate ingestion, also cause easy bruising.[92, 95–101] Impetigo, insect bites, and puncture wounds should be excluded when a cigarette burn is suspected. Self-inflicted injuries are seen in children with depression, severe mental retardation, certain congenital syndromes, and factitious illness.[73, 102] Ethnic medical customs, used as home remedies for minor ailments, have also been mistaken for child abuse. The Southeast Asian folk practice of dermabrasion, Cạo Gío or Qí Sa ("to scratch the wind"), produces bruises over the thorax and back.[102, 103] Cupping and moxibustion produce superficial burns.[104] Mongolian spots are deep brown to blue-black dermal melanin deposits that are mistaken occasionally for bruises.[105] Such spots are distributed over the lumbosacral areas of infants and toddlers in dark-skinned peoples and in 10% of white infants. They usually fade completely by the first year but may persist into adolescence.[106] Differentiating traumatic alopecia from tinea capitis, seborrhea, and atopic dermatitis is made by finding no evidence of scalp inflammation or scaling and by a negative result on microscopic examination for hyphae and negative fungal culture. Trichotillomania, or self-induced traumatic hair loss, is a disorder seen in older children and young adults.[107] Rarely, a neuroblastoma will present with periorbital ecchymoses.

HEAD INJURIES

Head injuries are the main cause of death and morbidity in child abuse.[108–110] Child victims often present in a delayed fashion with a history of a minor injury or with no explanation. Infants under 2 years of age are particularly vulnerable to severe injury, with the peak incidence at 6 months of age. Survivors are at risk for mental retardation, cerebral palsy, blindness, and seizures.[111, 112] Nonambulatory infants rarely sustain accidental intracranial injuries.[113, 114] Head injury should be excluded in all children who are suspected of being abused.

Certain anatomic features of infants increase their vulnerability to inflicted head injury.[115–117] Shaking and impact, or a combination of the two, are the mechanisms of abuse-related head injuries.[118, 119] The direct impact of forces on the infant's thin and pliable skull tends to be transferred to the underlying brain rather than absorbed by fracture formation, as in adults.[120, 121] Severe shaking produces rotational forces that tear the intracranial veins bridging the comparatively large subarachnoid space in which the brain sits (Fig. 14–11). The whiplash effect of shaking on the brain is accentuated by the inability of the infant's weak neck muscles to dampen the motions. When the skull's limit of pliability is exceeded in impact injury, the resulting fracture is often extensive and frequently of the bursting type, extending for considerable distances, with wide separation and comminution of the fragments (Fig. 14–12). Features suggestive of great force include multiple fractures, complex (branching) fracture, nonparietal skull fracture, depressed skull fracture, fracture length greater than 3 mm, growing fractures, involvement of more than one cranial bone, and associated intracranial injury. Depressed skull fractures are caused by contact with projecting objects, not flat surfaces. Plain ra-

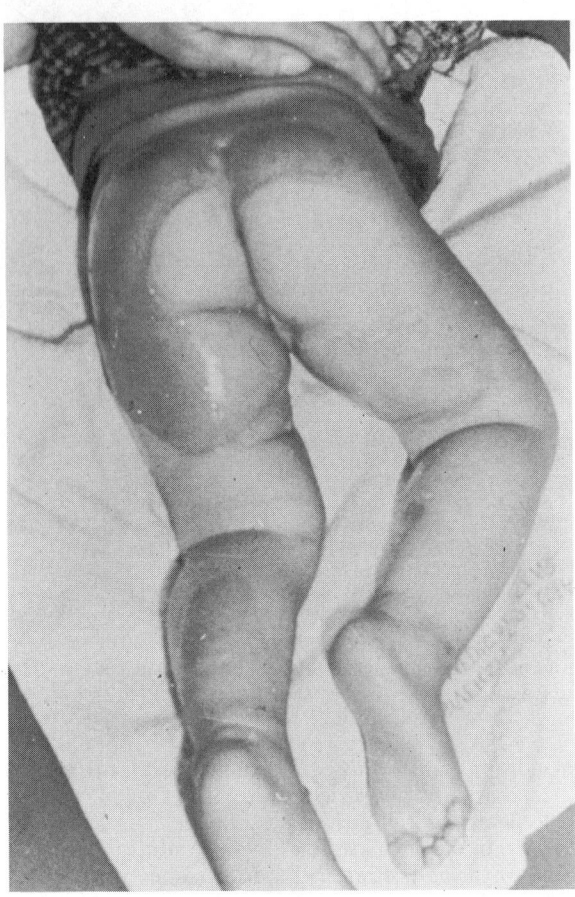

Figure 14–6. Immersion burns sparing the buttocks. (From Schmitt B. The Visual Diagnosis of Non-Accidental Trauma and Failure to Thrive. Prepared in cooperation with the American Academy of Pediatrics, 1979.)

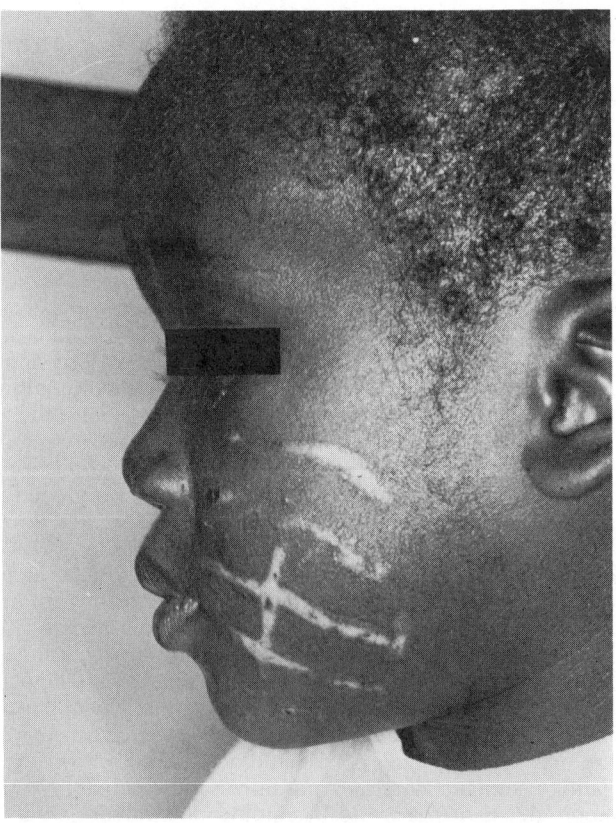

Figure 14–7. This 2-year-old had inflicted burns from a heating grate on the face, back, and buttocks.

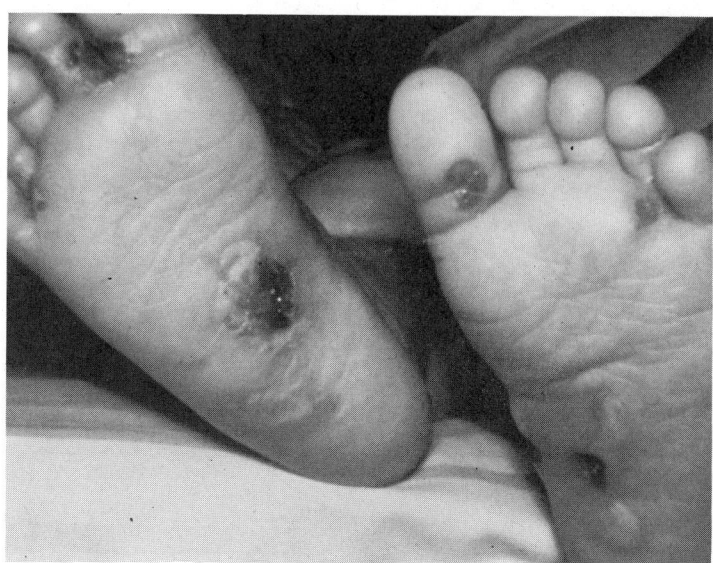

Figure 14–8. Cigarette burns. (From Schmitt B. The Visual Diagnosis of Non-Accidental Trauma and Failure to Thrive. Prepared in cooperation with the American Academy of Pediatrics, 1979.)

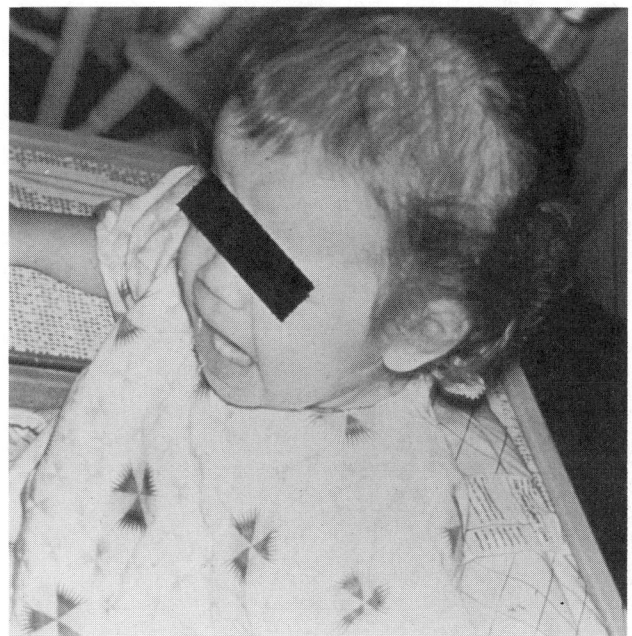

Figure 14–9. Inflicted hair loss (traumatic alopecia). (From Schmitt B. The Visual Diagnosis of Non-Accidental Trauma and Failure to Thrive. Prepared in cooperation with the American Academy of Pediatrics, 1979.)

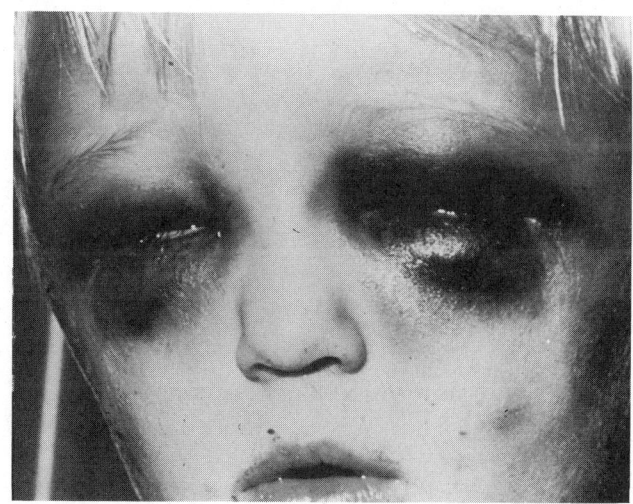

Figure 14–10. Periorbital ecchymoses from direct blows to the eyes. (From Schmitt B. The Visual Diagnosis of Non-Accidental Trauma and Failure to Thrive. Prepared in cooperation with the American Academy of Pediatrics, 1979.)

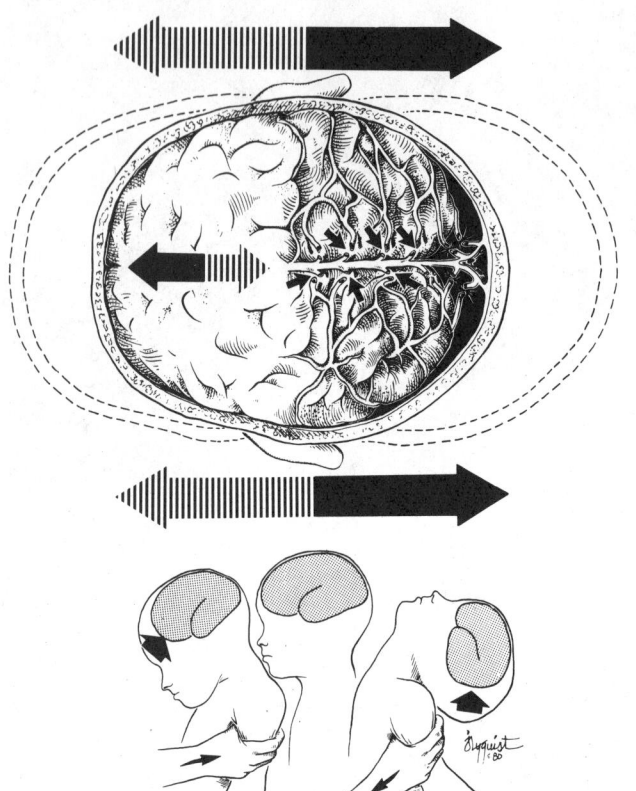

Figure 14–11. Rapid shaking of the head produces shearing forces that tear the veins bridging the cortex from the dura to the venous sinuses. (From Spivack BS. Biomechanics of non-accidental trauma. *In* Ludwig S, Kornberg AE (eds). Child abuse: A Medical Reference. 2nd ed. New York, Churchill Livingstone, 1992, p 71.)

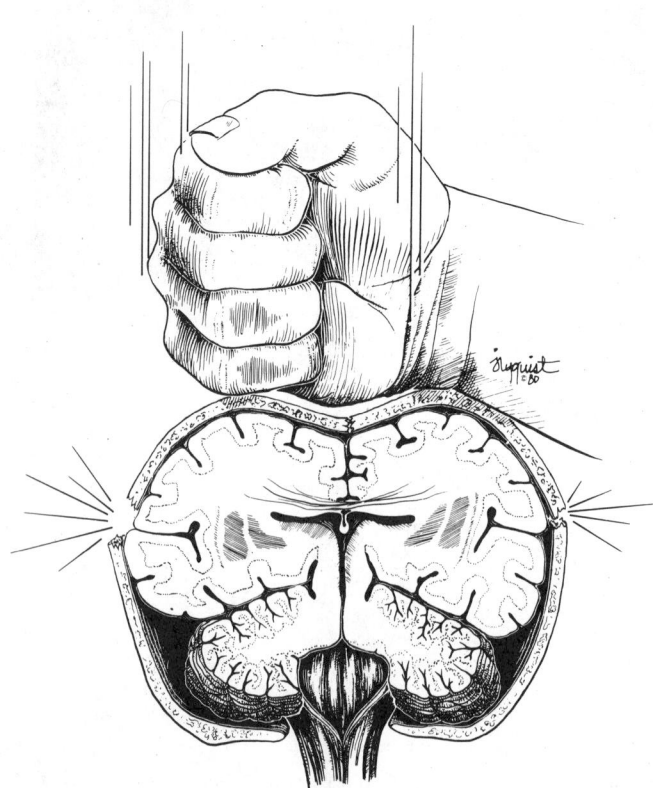

Figure 14–12. Direct cranial impact can result in "bursting" fractures with underlying brain injury. (From Ellerstein NS (ed). Child Abuse and Neglect: A Medical Reference. New York, Churchill Livingstone, 1981, p 75.)

TABLE 14–5

DIFFERENTIAL DIAGNOSIS OF SKIN LESIONS IN CHILD ABUSE

Finding and Differential Diagnosis	Differential Studies
Bruising	
Trauma	
Hemophilia	Prothrombin time, partial thromboplastin time, factor VIII and IX assays
von Willebrand disease	Bleeding time, von Willebrand factor antigen and ristocetin cofactor
Idiopathic thrombocytopenic purpura	CBC, platelet count
Neuroblastoma with periorbital ecchymoses	CT scan
Mongolian spots	History (ethnicity)
Coin rubbing	History (ethnic custom)
Osteogenesis imperfecta	Plasma osteocalcin, radiographic bone density
Local erythema, bullae	
Burn	
Staphylococcus impetigo	Culture, Gram stain
Photosensitivity reaction	History of sensitizing agent
Herpes simplex/zoster	Culture, scrape, and stain lesion
Hair loss	
Traumatic alopecia	Clinical appearance
Tinea capitis	Potassium hydroxide examination Fungal culture
Alopecia areata	Clinical appearance
Seborrhea, eczema	Clinical appearance

diography is preferred in identifying skull fractures, except for basilar fractures.[122]

Subdural hematoma, cerebral edema, and brain contusions are among the lesions produced by abusive trauma. (Figs. 14–13 through 14–15). Clinical signs of cerebral compression may evolve rapidly, with immediate loss of consciousness, or more slowly, within days after injury. Increased intracranial pressure may present as changes in behavior, consciousness, and respiratory pattern. Altered consciousness, a sensitive early sign of intracranial injury, should be tested in infants through visual alertness and following, purposeful movements (grasping and head control), and pain response (ability to cry). Acute subdural hematomas do not occur spontaneously but indicate prior trauma by impact force with or without violent shaking. Nonacute subdural collections may present in children as developmental delays or cerebral palsy.

A complete and rapid examination of the ocular fundi is an essential part of the emergency department evaluation in suspected head injury. Retinal hemorrhages may be the only physical sign of abuse in a comatose child[123] and occur in infants who have sustained shaking-impact trauma.[118] The severity of the hemorrhage correlates generally with the degree of the acute neurologic injury.[124, 125] Associated metaphyseal fractures of the long bones, rib fractures, and grab marks on the skin may be seen if the infant was gripped around the arms or thorax during shaking. Cervical spine injuries occur in association with shaking-impact injury cases.

The "tin ear syndrome," a particular type of impact head trauma, consists of the clinical triad of unilateral ear bruising, ipsilateral cerebral edema, and retinal hemorrhages. Blunt trauma to the ear, resulting in rotational acceleration forces

to the brain and tearing of the cortical veins, is the mechanism.[126]

CT without contrast is the preferred means for assessing brain injury on an emergent basis. A normal CT scan does not exclude thin layers of blood located high over the convexities of the cerebral hemispheres or petechial hemorrhages in the brain parenchyma, both of which may be seen readily on a magnetic resonance imaging (MRI) scan. CT is superior to MRI in delineating subarachnoid hemorrhage; CT findings reflect a combination of severe shaking and impact forces.[110, 127, 128] Subdural hematomas are most frequently found between the hemispheres and may also extend over the cerebral convexities in the posterior parietal and occipital regions.[129–131] There is often a mass effect from the hematoma and loss of gray-white matter differentiation. MRI is superior to CT in subacute and chronic situations and may diagnose injuries that are beyond the capabilities of CT.[132, 133]

Differential Diagnosis

Retinal hemorrhages occur frequently in the newborn period but usually resolve within the first month of life.[134–136] Retinal hemorrhages are caused by a sudden rise in intracranial pressure from intracranial bleeding, an intracranial mass, suddenly raised intrathoracic or intraabdominal pressures (resuscitation), infection (subacute bacterial endocarditis), and coagulopathy (leukemia, thrombocytopenia).[137] They are also seen in infants with meningitis complicated by subdural empyema, brain abscess, or venous sinus thrombosis.[131] The Latin-American folk practice of caida de mollera, or the "fallen fontanelle," may cause subdural hematoma and retinal hemorrhages.[138] (In this folk remedy, the child is held up by the ankles and shaken vigorously in an attempt to raise a sunken fontanelle.) Subdural hematoma, hydrocephalus, and subsequent developmental delay have developed in infancy as the result of precipitous vaginal delivery of large babies and breech deliveries.[139] Bloody cerebrospinal fluid (CSF) may be ascribed to a traumatic lumbar puncture. CSF should be centrifuged and examined for xanthochromia, which indicates that the bleeding came from the central nervous system. Intracranial injury must be distinguished from other nervous system diseases such as meningitis, toxic ingestions, seizure disorders, and acute metabolic disease.

SKELETAL INJURIES

Fractures in child abuse are related to the age of the child and the forces applied to an immature skeletal system. Radiography is the most accurate and direct method to support the diagnosis in skeletal injury. Guidelines for radiographic surveys vary with the age of the child (Table 14–6).

Skeletal trauma occurs in one fifth to one third of all abuse cases, with more than half of the fractures occurring in children under 12 months of age.[140] Fractures are rarely present without other signs of abuse or neglect. Fractures are unexpected in infants who are not yet walking, as infants cannot exert sufficient force to fracture a bone. The long bones of the extremities are the most common site injured in abuse, followed by the skull and the ribs.

In long-bone injuries, fractures to the midshaft (diaphyseal) are several times more frequent than to the ends (metaphyseal-epiphyseal) of the bone.[141] Diaphyseal fractures are often the result of abuse when they occur in children under 3 years of age.[142] They are also more frequently spiral than transverse in configuration. A nondisplaced spiral fracture may occur in the toddler whose leg is trapped under his or her body during a fall, but this also occurs when the child has been pushed or the leg has been violently twisted by an adult (Fig. 14–16). The amount of force required to

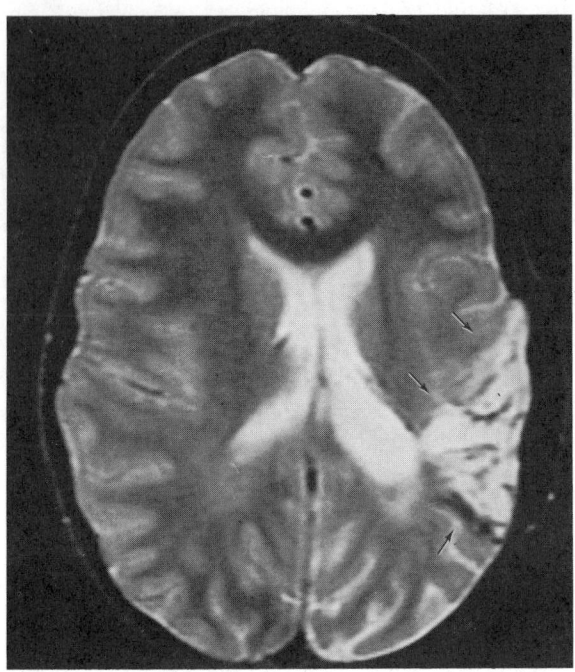

Figure 14–13. Magnetic resonance imaging (MRI) scan of a 2-year-old child reveals a large area of encephalomalacia of the left posterior temporal and parietal regions *(arrows)* resulting from direct impact to the head.

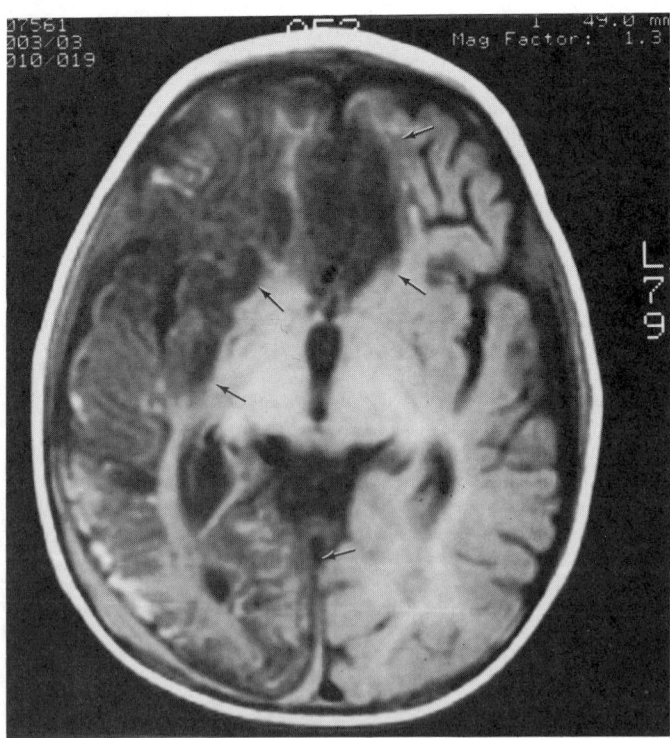

Figure 14–14. MRI scan of a 6-month-old child who presented 3 weeks earlier with a history of a fall from a couch at home and a chief complaint of respiratory irregularity that rapidly progressed to respiratory arrest. There is massive infarction of the entire right cerebral hemisphere and the medial frontal pole of the left hemisphere *(arrows)*. The thalamus and basal ganglia on both sides have been preserved. There is also a subdural hematoma over the right convexity.

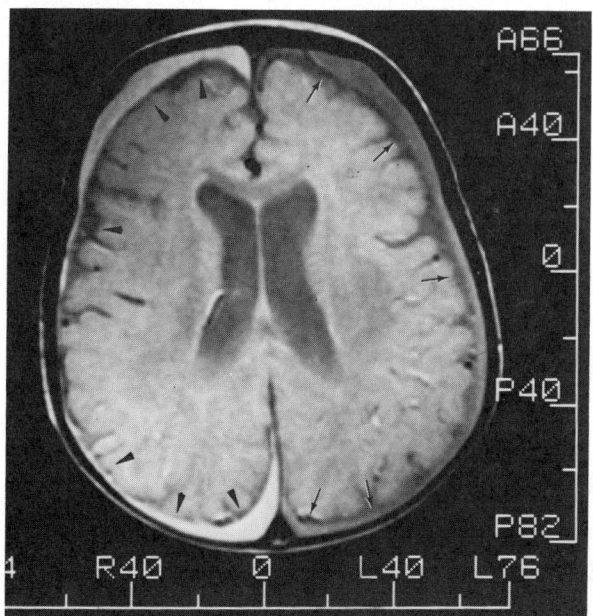

Figure 14–15. MRI scan of an 11-month-old child whose history was an unwitnessed fall from a changing table to a carpeted floor. The scan shows bilateral subdural hematomas, with the high signal intensity on the right *(arrowheads)* indicating a subacute injury and the lower-signal-intensity fluid on the left *(arrows)* indicating an older injury that likely occurred at a different point in time.

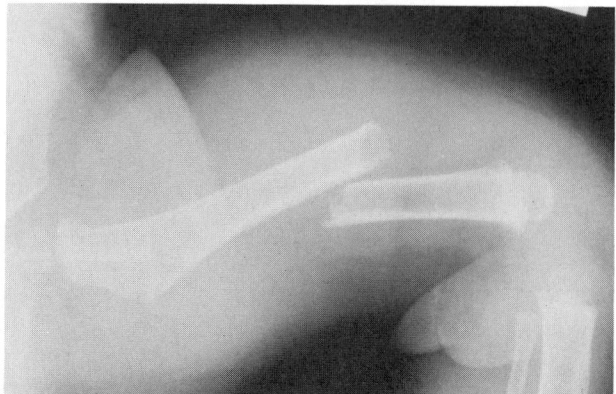

Figure 14–16. Radiograph of a 15-month-old child with a transverse midshaft fracture to the left femur.

fracture the midshaft of an infant's femur requires a major acceleration-deceleration injury, such as a motor vehicle accident or a heavy weight falling on the limb.[143, 144] Falls from heights of less than 90 cm (36 inches) are unlikely to produce these injuries.[114]

Epiphyseal-metaphyseal fractures occurring beyond the newborn period are virtually diagnostic of abuse, because they cannot occur from accidental falls. Commonly injured sites are the distal humerus and femur and proximal tibia (Fig. 14–17). These fractures occur more often to infants but may be seen in any abused child up to 5 years of age. Metaphyseal fractures are produced by acceleration-deceleration forces acting at the ends of the limb, by way of severe twisting, pulling, and shaking.[10, 87, 115] Rough play and accidental falls may produce minor injury but not a meta-

physeal fracture. Histologically, the injury is a fracture through the bony, not cartilaginous, side of the whole metaphyseal-epiphyseal plate.[145] The terms *corner fracture* and *bucket handle fracture* refer to the projected radiographic image of portions of a continuous ring of bone that has been fractured, although they may actually be avulsed fragments. Cartilaginous fractures with epiphyseal separation also occur, though less commonly, when massive forces are applied. Periosteal new bone formation, the result of traumatic separation of the periosteum around the bone shaft, is frequently associated with such fractures.

Rib fractures that occur in the absence of documented major trauma or underlying bone disease should be considered the result of abuse. Minor falls rarely cause fractures to the pliant rib cage of the infant. Posterior rib fractures near the costovertebral articulations are the most common inflicted rib fractures in infants. They occur during shaking episodes when the care provider violently grabs and compresses the chest.[87] Anterior and midaxillary rib fractures occur more often from direct blows to the older child's anterior chest and sternum (Fig. 14–18). Acute rib fractures are difficult to identify. Callus formation is often the first radiographic indication of an injury. In the acute situation, oblique and coned views of clinically suspicious areas may be helpful. An anteroposterior projection with reduced kilovoltage to visualize bone structures should be used for screening of infants for posterior rib fractures.[146] A second radiograph 2 weeks later is advised if a rib fracture is suspected clinically but not seen initially.[147] Radionuclide bone scanning is not considered a means of primary screening for rib fractures.[148]

Most abuse-related clavicular fractures are midshaft and indistinguishable from accidental fractures. However, lateral clavicular fractures, particularly those involving the acromion or scapula, are a result of violent traction forces on the arms.[149] Vertebral injuries in child abuse are usually caused by violent flexion-extension of the spine during shaking.[150] Fractures of the metacarpals or metatarsals result from deliberate stepping on the child's hands or feet (Fig. 14–19).

An estimate of the age of a given fracture is possible and may be critical to the diagnosis of child abuse (Table 14–7).[87, 151] A fracture with early periosteal new bone is, at a minimum, 7 to 10 days old. A fracture with loss of sharpness in the fracture line is 2 to 3 weeks old. A fracture with obliteration of the fracture line by a firmly calcified callus is 3 to 6 weeks old. Remodeling of the fracture, seen in the smoothing of the callus, can begin as early as 3 to 4 months after the initial injury and may continue for more than 1

TABLE 14–6

THE SKELETAL SURVEY IN CHILD ABUSE

1. Conventional radiography of the skull and thoracolumbar spine, extremities (including shoulders, hands, and feet), and ribs.
2. The radionuclide bone scan is not an appropriate *screen* for the physically abused child, but may be used when radiographic findings are equivocal.
3. The indication *varies* with the age and nature of the abuse:
   a. All children 24 months or younger with suspected physical abuse or neglect
   b. Children younger than 5 years with other evidence of physical abuse or neglect
   c. Consider extending the age for children with physical and mental handicaps with suspected physical abuse
   d. Site-specific examination in children older than 5 years
   e. Repeat radiographic examination in 2 weeks if initial examination is negative but the physical findings point to a bony injury
   f. Not indicated in isolated sexual abuse

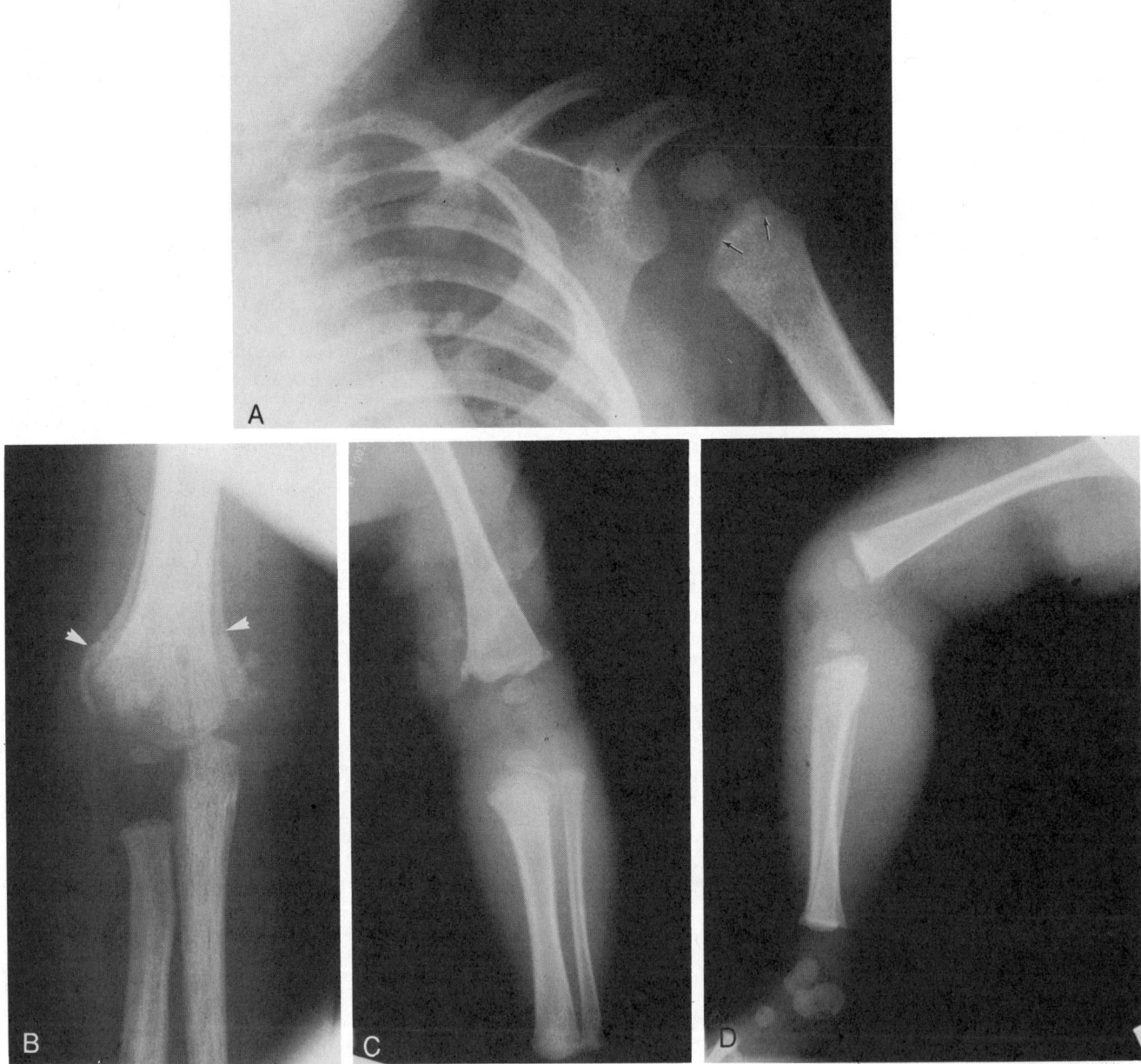

Figure 14–17. Radiographs of multiple corner fractures in a 6-month-old child. *A,* Left proximal humeral metaphysis. *B,* Right distal humerus, also with considerable periosteal new bone formation *(white arrows). C* and *D,* Right distal femur and proximal tibia, respectively.

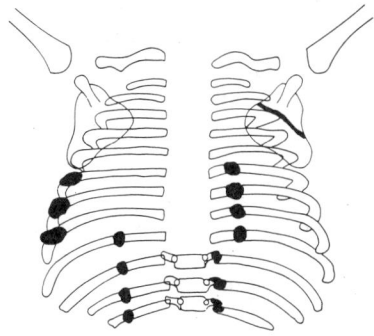

Figure 14–18. Common sites of rib injuries from blows to the chest: the costochondral junctions; near the midaxillary line; the costovertebral articulations; the sternum; and the scapula. (From Hilton SvW, Edwards DK, Hilton JW. Practical Pediatric Radiology. Philadelphia, WB Saunders, 1984, p 461.)

year. In all these stages, fractures in an infant will heal more rapidly than in an older child or adult. Injuries to large long bones take longer to heal than to small bones.

Differential Diagnosis

Fractures resulting from birth trauma usually carry a history of traumatic delivery and appear to be unifocal and without additional injuries that are typical of abuse; periosteal new bone develops at the site within 2 weeks of delivery.[152, 153] Rib fractures, in the absence of underlying bone disease, are uncommon after properly performed cardiopulmonary resuscitation.[154] Subperiosteal new bone is not specific to trauma and may be seen in osteomyelitis and metabolic disorders. Bone or metabolic diseases, such as syphilis,[155, 156] vitamin C or D deficiencies,[156, 157] Menkes' syndrome,[158] vitamin A toxicity, and infantile cortical hyperostosis[159] mimic typical findings of physical abuse. Fortunately, these conditions are rare (Table 14–8).

VISCERAL INJURIES

The frequency of visceral injury in child abuse is thought to be underreported because only severe injuries are recognized. These injuries carry a high mortality rate because of delayed recognition.[160] The initial presenting abdominal symptoms may be vague and thus may mislead the physician into diagnosing a benign condition. The spectrum of injury in abused children is similar to that in accident victims. The abused child with visceral trauma is typically between 18 months and 5 years of age.[161, 162] The injuries occur as the result of blunt trauma to the child's weak abdominal wall from rapidly decelerating or crushing blows. Fixed structures in the midabdomen, such as the small bowel, liver, and pancreas, are especially vulnerable to injury when forced against the spinal column.[163, 164] Punches or violent kicks may cause shearing of organs from their vascular pedicles and mesenteric attachments. The lower thorax and lungs have also been involved. Bruising of the abdominal wall may not be visible, even with extensive internal injuries. Accidental injuries occur to older children who fall while bicycling and during rough play in contact sports. Crush injuries from automobile and pedestrian collisions are another source. Visceral injury should be suspected in children who present with tenderness, bruises, distention, hematuria, and low or falling hematocrit levels, or when neurologic impairment makes the abdominal examination unreliable.[165] Pneumo-

peritoneum, hemoperitoneum, and peritonitis must be quickly excluded.

Perforations of hollow organs present soon after injury with signs of peritonitis. Pneumoperitoneum should be suspected on clinical grounds, as free air is not always seen on plain radiographs.[166] Intramural hematomas of the small bowel are a common lesion in child abuse and suggest prior injury.[167] Often, with intestinal hematoma the child takes several days to present with symptoms of intestinal obstruction. Oral contrast radiography is preferred for intramural small bowel hematomas and often demarcates the obstructing mass defect. In acute cases, the coiled-spring appearance of barium may be seen as the opposing mucosal folds of small bowel are draped and compressed over the expanding mass.[168]

Pancreatitis and resulting pancreatic pseudocysts in children are caused by prior injury and usually present in a delayed manner.[169] The child may have an acute abdomen or few symptoms on initial presentation. Other injured children present subacutely over the next several days to weeks, with gradual development of symptoms of fever, vomiting, and abdominal or back pain. By this time, an upper abdominal mass may be found on examination.[170] Serum amylase and lipase levels are usually elevated. Radiography typically shows the mass effect of the pseudocyst displacing the stomach or duodenum, but ultrasonography is the preferred mode for the evaluation. In a few cases, pancreatitis has been associated with the late complication of fat necrosis in tubular bones, sometimes mistaken for osteomyelitis.[171]

CT is considered the examination of choice in suspected injury to solid organs.[172] Significant, though not life-threatening, injuries to solid organs, especially the liver, appear to be as frequent as small bowel injuries.[173] These injuries may remain unrecognized unless studied by CT or accompanied by significant bleeding (Fig. 14–20).

POISONING

Accidental ingestion of poison is not usually considered to be the result of abuse; nevertheless, severe family disorganization may be related to repeated episodes. These children may live in homes where the parents do not provide a safe environment.

There is a growing incidence of children exposed to

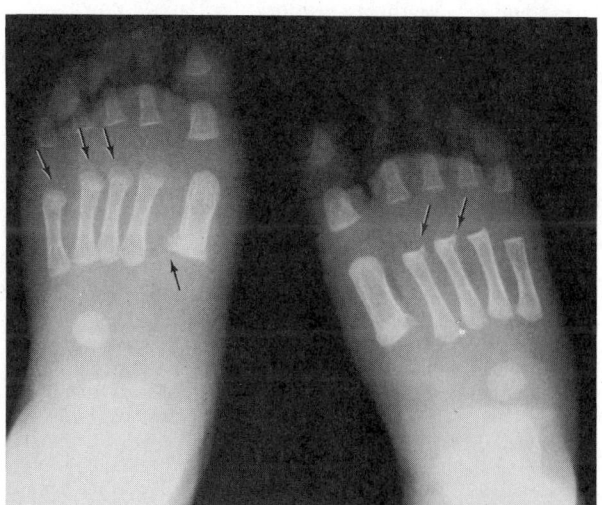

Figure 14–19. Radiograph of a 2-month-old child with fractures of the metaphyses of the distal right second and third metatarsals, proximal left first, and distal third through fifth metatarsals.

TABLE 14–7

ESTIMATING THE AGE OF FRACTURES IN INFANTS

Estimated Age	Findings
0–10 days	Soft tissue swelling
7–14 days	Calcification of callus at fracture site* Periosteal new bone formation†
2–3 weeks	Loss of fracture line definition
3–6 weeks	Hard callus formation, obliteration of fracture line
>3 months	Remodeling

*Rib fractures will take longer (15 to 20 days).

†The rate of metaphyseal-epiphyseal fracture healing may be much faster than indicated above for cancellous or cortical bone.

Note: Repetitive injury will prolong these stages. Skull fractures cannot be dated in the manner given above.

alcohol and drugs by accidental ingestion, passive inhalation of the smoked substance, deliberate poisoning, and accepting drugs from another child.[174–177] Drugs and alcohol have been used by substance-abusing care providers to quiet an annoying or crying child,[178, 179] and toxic ingestions occurring under these conditions are underreported. In the "morning-after syndrome," children develop ethanol intoxication, hypoglycemia, and convulsions after consuming drinks left unattended after a party in the home.[180] Cocaine, which can cause severe convulsions, has also been ingested in a similar manner.[181] Abuse of drugs or alcohol should be considered in any child who presents with a new onset of seizures or in any child whose death is unexplained.

MUNCHAUSEN SYNDROME BY PROXY

Munchausen syndrome by proxy (MBP) refers to clinical situations in which parents repeatedly fabricate or induce illnesses in their children and present the children for invasive and often painful procedures to attract attention to the parents themselves.[182] Children have died or been seriously injured in this way. The presenting parent is usually the mother, who appears to be a model of self-sacrificing care and is familiar with medical tests and terminology. The parent and child have a history of using a series of health facilities.

MBP primarily involves children under 6 years of age; after that, the child is less likely to cooperate in the deception. Poisonings are involved in many cases of MBP.[183] In fact, the first report of MBP involved a child who died after receiving toxic doses of salt during the first 14 months of life.[184] There are no limits to the variety of poisons and methods parents will use to injure their children. Reported substances include laxatives, propranolol, chloral hydrate, ipecac, petroleum distillate, phenothiazines, barbiturates, salicylates, acetaminophen, warfarin, pine oil, insulin, imipramine, and furosemide.[185–196] The diagnosis of MBP should be considered in any child who has repeated or persistent illnesses that do not follow the usual course or cause of disease and whose illness does not recur when the child is separated from the parent. Other warning signs include a parent's indifference to the child's illness or a parent who seems to want to have procedures performed on the child.

CHILD NEGLECT

Neglect covers a broad array of child maltreatment and is the most potentially lethal form of child abuse.[197] It is more indolent and less obvious and its negative outcomes seem less immediately severe to the public and to protective services agencies. No consensus on the definition of neglect exists, nor is there agreement on criteria describing neglectful childrearing. The vast numbers of child neglect cases are related to poverty; nevertheless, neglect and poverty are not equivalent.[198]

Failure to thrive (FTT) has historically been classified as a form of child neglect when organic causes have been excluded. This is neither accurate nor helpful. Collectively, the various forms of FTT occur in 3% to 5% of infants. FTT is defined as weight below two standard deviations for age and an inappropriate weight for height or a falling weight curve (crossing percentile lines) occurring in a child under 2 years of age. Weight is the first growth measurement to slow, but height and head circumference also lag if the problem is severe.

FTT is a pediatric disease in which there are two extreme forms on a continuum of growth failure. Organic origins are at one end of the continuum, and disturbed parent-child interactions at the other.[199–202] The latter includes multiple etiologic factors: physical or mental illness of the mother; early childhood developmental dysfunctions resulting from prior abuse, neglect, or sexual exploitation; poverty; retardation; educational limitations of the parents; and lack of social support within the family. Other factors, such as maternal drug addiction, marital violence, and multiple siblings, are also known to be involved. Responsibility for child neglect in many cases must be expanded beyond the individual and family level to include the "neglect of neglect" found in social and educational agencies and public policy-making institutions.[203–205] Most children with FTT are neither physically abused nor intentionally neglected.

Children with FTT need a thorough dietary assessment to document the malnutrition.[206, 207] Laboratory investigations are rarely helpful without specific indicators from the clinical evaluation.[208] A complete blood cell count, serum albumin determination, urinalysis, assessment of thyroid function, and radiographs for bone age should be performed initially to confirm the absence of underlying conditions. Further

TABLE 14–8

DIFFERENTIAL DIAGNOSIS OF SKELETAL LESIONS

Diagnosis	Differential Studies
Trauma	History
Birth trauma	History
Scurvy	Nutrition history, long-bone radiographs; rare in infants <6 mo old
Vitamin A toxicity	Nutrition history, vitamin A levels
Rickets	Nutrition history, wrist radiograph, alkaline phosphatase
Congenital syphilis	Serology, physical stigmata
Prostaglandin E therapy	History
Infantile cortical hyperostosis	Mandibular involvement, metaphyseal sparing, alkaline phosphatase
Leukemia	CBC, platelet count, bone marrow analysis
Metastatic neuroblastoma	Bone marrow analysis
Osteogenesis imperfecta	Family history, blue sclerae, bone biopsy, skeletal radiographs
Osteomyelitis	History
Menkes' syndrome	Hair analysis, serum copper and ceruloplasmin levels, long-bone radiographs
Mucolipidosis II	Facial appearance, fibroblast studies

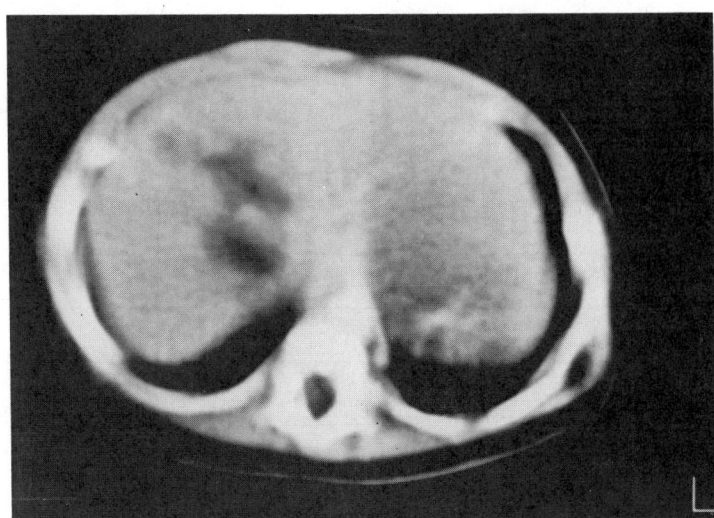

Figure 14-20. Computed tomographic (CT) scan of the abdomen in a 10-week-old infant with multiple areas of low attenuation within the liver and spleen consistent with extensive contusions.

laboratory tests should be deferred pending a trial of diet therapy and environmental change. Infants younger than 6 months with growth failure should be hospitalized, as severe malnutrition in infancy can result in decreased brain growth and lower intelligence.[209] The diagnosis of interactional FTT is supported by a negative clinical examination and negative laboratory findings, by evidence of rapid weight gain during a change in environment, and by close observations of the mother-infant interaction.[210, 211] The child may avoid eye contact, avoid smiling or vocalization, show a lack of interest in the environment, and respond negatively to attempts to be comforted. Observations of parent-child interactions during meals and at other times provide critical information and form the basis of long-term treatment. Patience and skill are needed in working with parents, because they are characteristically inattentive to the child's needs and deny that the child is ill.

Neglect has also presented as developmental delay and behavioral problems in a child who is otherwise without identifiable physical problems. Just as there are underfed infants, there are also understimulated and emotionally neglected infants. Just as growth failure leads to consideration of disturbed parent-child interaction, so the presence of developmental delay, without other physical conditions, should lead to consideration of emotional neglect and understimulation. The child's care providers, home environment, birth, and early history should be evaluated.

THE MEDICAL RECORD

The medical chart serves as the physician's record to be used by protective services and the legal system in their efforts to ensure protection for the child. The main points of the child and parent histories should be recorded verbatim, when possible. Discrepancies and contradictions should be carefully noted. Positive physical findings should be drawn and located on a diagram of the body, and color photographs of the injury are valuable for documentation. Multiple photographs should be taken with a rigid metric ruler in the frame for reference and properly identified with the patient's name and medical record number, date, and name of the photographer.

CHILD ABUSE REPORTING

Every state has a statute for discovering and stopping child abuse, and every statute has a reporting requirement.[212–214] The laws for each state are similar in many ways,

and in all jurisdictions, the reporting requirement is a key part. Most child abuse reporting laws require physicians to report *reasonable suspicions* of abuse, thereby requiring them to exercise professional judgment in determining whether a report is required in a given case. Physicians who report in good faith are generally immune from civil and criminal liability. In fact, penalties are allocated for *not* reporting suspected abuse.[215] In some states, new reporting laws in cases of prenatal drug exposure remove the element of professional judgment by making drug exposure alone, and sometimes a positive drug test alone, the basis of a mandatory report. Physicians must be familiar with local child protection and abuse reporting laws and procedures. Suspected child abuse or neglect reports should be made immediately to the legally designated agency by telephone and by written report (Fig. 14–21). In cases of serious injury or when there is concern that the parents will flee with an injured child, the report should be made to the police for immediate action.

PREVENTION AND TREATMENT

Efforts to prevent and treat child abuse have been hampered by the inability to accurately predict the risk of abuse; similar difficulties exist for child neglect. Health care professionals are often unable to provide clear and specific outcomes of neglect to the courts and public agencies.

In practice, treatment and prevention of abuse or neglect begin in tandem with the first professional encounter in the emergency department. Determining whether the child is in danger of permanent damage is of immediate concern. When hospitalization is not indicated, appropriate medical and protective service follow-up should be in place before the child leaves the emergency department. Long-term treatment and supervision of abusive and neglectful families should be carried out under the guidance of a multidisciplinary team, involving medicine, law, social welfare, psychology, and nursing professionals.

The home health visitors approach advocated by Kempe has been the most effective measure in reducing the incidence of abuse in high-risk families.[216, 217] This program, though underutilized, can be easily implemented using local community organizations. Treatment approaches limited to counseling do not reduce the subsequent incidence of abuse. Direct support services, including decent housing, job training, employment, and financial help, have rarely been offered by protective services but could make a major difference in the stability of many families and in the protection of the children at risk.[218, 219]

SUSPECTED CHILD ABUSE REPORT

To Be Completed by Reporting Party
Pursuant to Penal Code Section 11166

A. CASE IDENTI-FICATION

TO BE COMPLETED BY INVESTIGATING CPA

VICTIM NAME: _____

REPORT NO./CASE NAME: _____

DATE OF REPORT: _____

B. REPORTING PARTY

NAME/TITLE

ADDRESS

PHONE ( )   DATE OF REPORT   SIGNATURE OF REPORTING PARTY

C. REPORT SENT TO

☐ POLICE DEPARTMENT   ☐ SHERIFF'S OFFICE   ☐ COUNTY WELFARE   ☐ COUNTY PROBATION

AGENCY   ADDRESS

OFFICIAL CONTACTED   PHONE ( )   DATE/TIME

D. INVOLVED PARTIES

VICTIM

NAME (LAST, FIRST, MIDDLE)   ADDRESS   BIRTHDATE   SEX   RACE

PRESENT LOCATION OF CHILD   PHONE ( )

SIBLINGS

	NAME	BIRTHDATE	SEX	RACE		NAME	BIRTHDATE	SEX	RACE
1.					4.				
2.					5.				
3.					6.				

PARENTS

NAME (LAST, FIRST, MIDDLE)   BIRTHDATE   SEX   RACE   NAME (LAST, FIRST, MIDDLE)   BIRTHDATE   SEX   RACE

ADDRESS   ADDRESS

HOME PHONE   BUSINESS PHONE ( )   HOME PHONE   BUSINESS PHONE ( )

E. INCIDENT INFORMATION

IF NECESSARY, ATTACH EXTRA SHEET OR OTHER FORM AND CHECK THIS BOX. ☐

1. DATE/TIME OF INCIDENT   PLACE OF INCIDENT   *(CHECK ONE)*   ☐ OCCURRED   ☐ OBSERVED

IF CHILD WAS IN OUT-OF-HOME CARE AT TIME OF INCIDENT, CHECK TYPE OF CARE:

☐ FAMILY DAY CARE   ☐ CHILD CARE CENTER   ☐ FOSTER FAMILY HOME   ☐ SMALL FAMILY HOME   ☐ GROUP HOME OR INSTITUTION

2. TYPE OF ABUSE: *(CHECK ONE OR MORE)*   ☐ PHYSICAL   ☐ MENTAL   ☐ SEXUAL ASSAULT   ☐ NEGLECT   ☐ OTHER

3. NARRATIVE DESCRIPTION:

4. SUMMARIZE WHAT THE ABUSED CHILD OR PERSON ACCOMPANYING THE CHILD SAID HAPPENED:

5. EXPLAIN KNOWN HISTORY OF SIMILAR INCIDENT(S) FOR THIS CHILD:

SS 8572 (REV. 7/87)

INSTRUCTIONS AND DISTRIBUTION ON REVERSE

DO NOT submit a copy of this form to the Department of Justice (DOJ). A CPA is required under Penal Code Section 11169 to submit to DOJ a Child Abuse Investigation Report Form SS-8583 if (1) an active investigation has been conducted and (2) the incident is **not** unfounded.

Police or Sheriff-WHITE Copy; County Welfare or Probation-BLUE Copy; District Attorney-GREEN Copy; Reporting Party-YELLOW Copy

Figure 14-21. *A,* Sample suspected child abuse report to be filled out by the reporting party.

DOJ 900   84 89220

MEDICAL REPORT—SUSPECTED CHILD ABUSE	HOSPITAL

INSTRUCTIONS: ALL PROFESSIONAL MEDICAL PERSONNEL ARE REQUIRED BY SECTION 11166 OF THE PENAL CODE TO COMPLETE THIS FORM IN CONJUNCTION WITH THE SS 8572 SUSPECTED CHILD ABUSE REPORT WHERE CHILD ABUSE, AS DEFINED BY SECTION 11165 OF THE PENAL CODE, IS SUSPECTED. THE REPORTS, DOJ 900 AND SS 8572, MUST BE SUBMITTED TO A POLICE OR SHERIFF'S DEPARTMENT, OR A COUNTY PROBATION OR WELFARE DEPARTMENT WITHIN 36 HOURS. PROFESSIONAL MEDICAL PERSONNEL MEANS ANY PHYSICIAN AND SURGEON, PSYCHIATRIST, PSYCHOLOGIST, DENTIST, RESIDENT, INTERN, PODIATRIST, CHIROPRACTOR, LICENSED NURSE, DENTAL HYGIENIST OR ANY OTHER PERSON WHO IS CURRENTLY LICENSED UNDER DIVISION 2 (COMMENCING WITH SECTION 500) OF THE BUSINESS AND PROFESSIONS CODE. EACH PART OF THE FORM MUST BE COMPLETED UNLESS INAPPLICABLE. IN FILLING OUT THIS FORM, NO CIVIL LIABILITY ATTACHES AND NO CONFIDENTIALITY IS BREACHED.

I. GENERAL INFORMATION   Print or type

PATIENT'S NAME   HOSPITAL ID NO.

ADDRESS	CITY	COUNTY	STATE	PHONE

AGE	BIRTHDATE	RACE	SEX	DATE AND TIME OF ARRIVAL	MODE OF TRANSPORTATION	DATE AND TIME OF DISCHARGE

ACCOMPANIED TO HOSPITAL BY: NAME   ADDRESS   CITY   STATE   RELATIONSHIP

PHONE REPORT MADE TO	ID NO.	DEPARTMENT	PHONE	RESPONDING OFFICER/AGENCY

NAME OF: ☐ FATHER ☐ STEPFATHER	ADDRESS	CITY	COUNTY	HOME PHONE	BUS. PHONE	AGE/DOB

NAME OF: ☐ MOTHER ☐ STEPMOTHER	ADDRESS	CITY	COUNTY	HOME PHONE	BUS. PHONE	AGE/DOB

SIBLINGS: LAST NAME, FIRST	DOB	LAST NAME, FIRST	DOB	LAST NAME, FIRST	DOB

II. MEDICAL EXAMINATION

A. History   1. EXPLANATION OF INJURIES BY PARENT OR PERSON ACCOMPANYING CHILD (LOCATION, DATE, TIME AND CIRCUMSTANCES)

2. PATIENT'S STATEMENT EXPLAINING INJURY (PARAPHRASE)

3. PATIENT'S EMOTIONAL REACTION TO EXAMINATION (SUBMISSIVE, COMPLIANT, ETC.)

4. PREVIOUS HISTORY OF CHILD ABUSE (IF KNOWN)

B. Sexual Assault   Perform exam only if necessary.
(use California OCJP 923/925 Report Form for Sexual Assault)

1. ACTS COMMITTED: NOTE—COITUS, FELLATIO, CUNNILINGUS, SODOMY

2. DURING ASSAULT
☐ VAGINAL PENETRATION (HOW)   EJACULATION: ☐ VAGINAL ☐ ORAL ☐ ANAL   ☐ OTHER:

☐ ANAL PENETRATION (HOW)   ☐ CONDOM USED ☐ VOMITED ☐ LOSS OF CONSCIOUSNESS ☐ OTHER:

3. AFTER ASSAULT:
☐ WIPED/WASHED ☐ BATHED ☐ DOUCHED ☐ VOMITED ☐ CHANGED CLOTHES ☐ BRUSHED TEETH ☐ DEFECATED ☐ OTHER:

C. Physical Examination	DATE AND TIME OF EXAM	DATE AND TIME OF ASSAULT	BP	PULSE	RESP.	TEMP

HEIGHT	WEIGHT	HEAD CIRCUM	LAST TETANUS	KNOWN ALLERGIES	CURRENT MEDICATION

DIAGNOSTIC DATA

Check if indicated and incorporate results in written examination at left

☐ X-rays (skull, chest, longbone, full skeletal)

☐ Bleeding, coagulation, tourniquet, tests

☐ Funduscopic

☐ Other

INVESTIGATING AGENCY

Figure 14–21 *Continued B,* Sample medical report for suspected child abuse.

DOJ 900

DATE	HOSPITAL ID NO.	HOSPITAL

PHYSICAL EXAMINATION (CONTINUED) LOCATE AND DESCRIBE IN DETAIL ANY INJURIES OR FINDINGS: TRAUMA, BRUISES, ERYTHEMA, EXCORIATIONS, LACERATIONS, WOUNDS. TRACE OUTLINE USED AND INDICATE LOCATION OF WOUNDS/LACERATIONS USING 'X' FOR SUPERFICIAL, 'O' FOR DEEP; SHADE FOR BRUISES OR BURNS. BESIDE EACH INJURY INDICATED NOTE COLOR, SIZE, PATTERN, TEXTURE, AND SENSATION. WRITE OVER UNUSED OUTLINES. DESCRIBE IN DETAIL SHAPE OF ARM OR OTHER BRUISES WHICH MAY INDICATE FORCE.

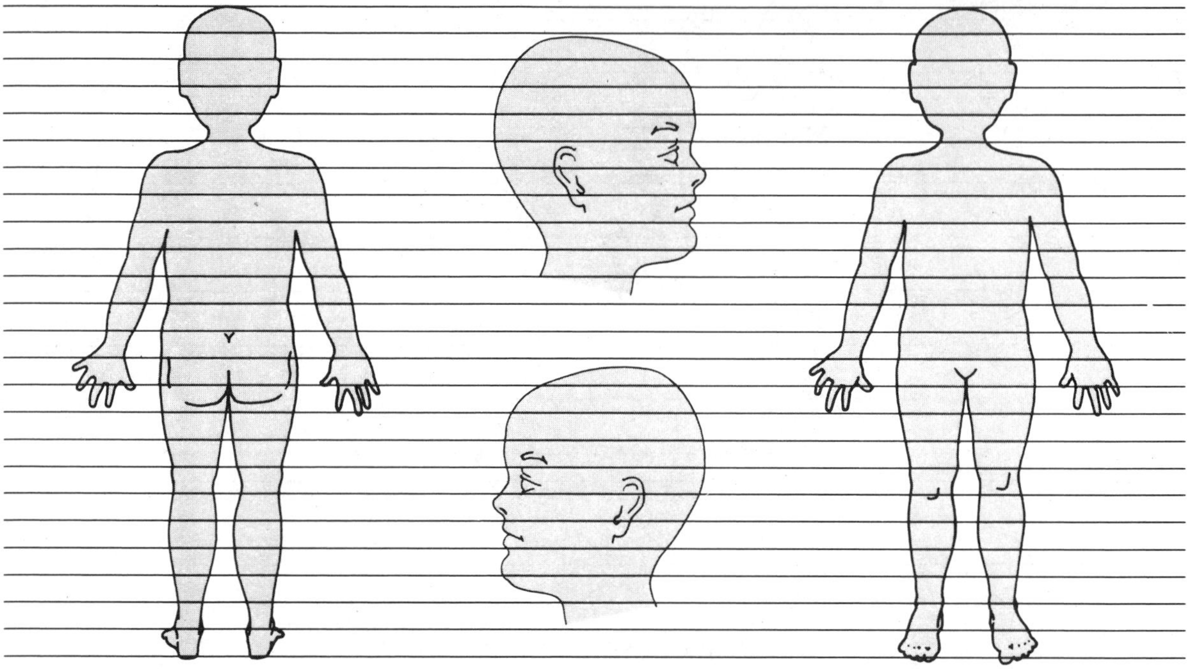

D. PELVIC   A PELVIC EXAMINATION SHOULD NOT BE PERFORMED UNLESS THE PARENT, GUARDIAN OR MINOR CONSENT OR UNLESS NECESSARY AS PART OF TREATMENT. SEE DEPARTMENT OF HEALTH REGULATIONS TITLE 22, DIVISION 2, VICTIMS OF SEXUAL ASSAULT. SAME INSTRUCTIONS AS GENERAL PHYSICAL; IN ADDITION, NOTE PUBIC HAIR COMBINGS WHERE INDICATED, DRIED SECRETIONS AND RECENT INJURIES TO HYMEN, TRACE AND OUTLINE AS ABOVE.

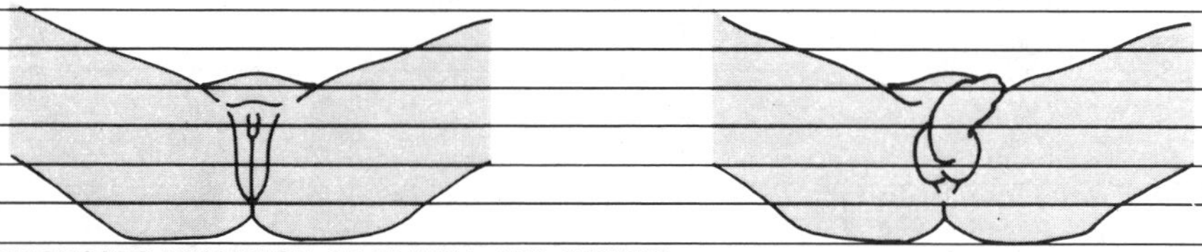

V. SPECIMENS

STAINS/FOREIGN MATERIALS (WHEN INDICATED)

LOOSE HAIR ____	FINGERNAIL SCRAPINGS ____
BLOOD ____	DIRT OR GRAVEL ____
THREADS ____	VEGETATION ____
GRASS ____	CLOTHING ____
DRIED SECRETIONS ____	

	SLIDES	SWABS
VAGINAL	____	____
RECTAL	____	____
ORAL	____	____
ASPIRATES/ WASHINGS	____	____
BITE MARKS	____	____
OTHER:	____	____

PATIENT'S SAMPLES. TIME OF COLLECTION AT MD DISCRETION

BLOOD	____
HAIR FROM HEAD	____
SALIVA	____
HAIR FROM PUBIC AREA	____

III. DIAGNOSTIC IMPRESSION OF TRAUMA AND INJURIES

IV. TREATMENT/DISPOSITION OF PATIENT

A. ☐ GC CULTURE   ☐ VDRL   ☐ PREGNANCY TEST   ☐ POST COITAL ESTROGEN   ☐ VD PROPHYLAXIS   ☐ OTHER:

☐ MOTILE SPERM: ☐ PRESENCE   ☐ ABSENCE   ☐ NOT TAKEN   ☐ FAMILY ASSESSMENT BY: ☐ NOT ORDERED

B. ORDERS:

C. DISPOSITION: ☐ ADMIT   TRANSFERRED TO:

☐ RELEASED   ACCOMPANIED BY: NAME   ADDRESS   RELATIONSHIP

D. FOLLOW-UP WITHIN:

☐ MEDICAL

____ HRS   ____ DAYS

☐ SOCIAL SERVICES

____ HRS   ____ DAYS

☐ PRIVATE MD

____ HRS   ____ DAYS

☐ OTHER

____ HRS   ____ DAYS

I HAVE RECEIVED THE INDICATED ITEMS AS EVIDENCE AND A COPY OF THIS REPORT.

OFFICER: ID NO.:   DATE:

NURSE   SIGNATURE OF EXAMINATION PHYSICIAN

INVESTIGATING AGENCY

Figure 14–21 *Continued C,* Sample report to be filled out by the investigating agency.

THE PHYSICIAN WITNESS

Immediate legal intervention to stop child abuse can include removing the child from the abusive home with temporary or permanent placement in foster care or returning the child to the home with court-ordered supervision by the child protective service system. On occasion, the physician must participate in legal hearings as part of this intervention.[220] The knowledge the physician brings to the courtroom can clarify whether abuse is the probable diagnosis and may be of critical importance for the child's protection. The physician should always insist on a conference with the attorney before the hearing date to clarify the attorney's expectations of the medical evidence and of the physician's role in court. The usual medical opinions in child abuse cases concern the diagnosis, the possible causes of injury, and the mechanisms of injury. The physician should review the medical record and inform the attorney of the level of certitude of the diagnosis. It is also important to determine whether the physician will function as an expert witness or simply recount the facts. An expert medical witness is expected to give an opinion based on the facts and the scientific literature. The physician should know the details of the case and should review them before testifying. It is not the physician's role to testify for one side or the other, despite the adversarial qualities of court proceedings, but to relate the facts and conclusions in a neutral manner.

References

1. Sgroi SM. Sexual molestation of children: The last frontier in child abuse. Children Today 1975;4:18.
2. Holter JC, Friedman SB. Child abuse: Early case finding in the emergency department. Pediatrics 1968;42:128.
3. Schleper-Hughes N, Stein HF. Child abuse and the unconscious in American popular culture. In Schleper-Hughes N (ed). Child Survival: Anthropological Perspectives on the Treatment and Maltreatment of Children. Boston, MA, D Reidel, 1987, pp 339–358.
4. Rush F. The Best Kept Secret: Sexual Abuse of Children. New York, McGraw-Hill, 1980, pp 16–73.
5. Bloch H. Abandonment, infanticide, and filicide: An overview of inhumanity to children. Am J Dis Child 1988;142:1058.
6. English PC. Pediatrics and the unwanted child in history: Foundling homes, disease, and the origins of foster care in New York City, 1860–1920. Pediatrics 1984;73:699.
7. Antler J, Antler S. From child rescue to family protection: The evolution of the child protective movement in the United States. Children Youth Service Rev 1979;1:177.
8. Gordon L. Heroes of Their Own Lives: The Politics and History of Family Violence. New York, Viking, 1988, pp vii, 250–299.
9. Bordin R. Woman and Temperance: The Quest for Power and Liberty, 1873–1900. Philadelphia, Temple University Press, 1981, 162.
10. Caffey J. Multiple fractures in the long bones of infants suffering from chronic subdural hematoma. AJR 1946;56:163.
11. Kempe CH, Silverman FN, Steele BF, et al. The battered child syndrome. JAMA 1962;181.
12. Christoffel KK. Violent death and injury in US children and adolescents. Am J Dis Child 1990;144:697.
13. Waller AE, Baker SP, Szocka A. Childhood injury deaths: National analysis and geographic variations. Am J Public Health 1989;79:310.
14. Mayer T, Walker ML, Johnson DG. Causes of morbidity and mortality in severe pediatric trauma. JAMA 1981;245:719.
15. Christoffel KK, Zieseri EJ, Chiaramonte J. Should child abuse and neglect be considered when a child dies unexpectedly? Am J Dis Child 1985;139:876.
16. American Humane Association. Highlights of Official Child Neglect and Abuse Reporting 1986. Denver, CO, The American Humane Association, 1988, p 6.
17. Straus MA, Gelles RJ, Steinmetz SK. Behind Closed Doors: Violence in the American Family. Garden City, NY, Doubleday, 1980, pp 3–28.
18. Griest KJ, Zumwalt RE. Child abuse by drowning. Pediatrics 1989;83:41.
19. Roberts J, Golding J, Keeling J. Is there a link between cot death and child abuse? Br Med J 1984;289:798.
20. Minford AMB. Child abuse presenting as apparent "near miss" sudden infant death syndrome. Br Med J 1981;282:521.
21. Jason J, Carpenter MM, Tyler CW. Underrecording of infant homicide in the United States. Am J Public Health 1983;73:195.
22. Saulsbury FT, Campbell RE. Evaluation of child abuse reporting by physicians. Am J Dis Child 1985;139:393.
23. James J, Womack WM, Strauss F. Physician reporting of sexual abuse of children. JAMA 1978;240:1145.
24. McDonald AE, Reece RM. Child abuse: Problems of reporting. Pediatr Clin North Am 1979;26:785.
25. Sanders RW. Resistance to dealing with parents of battered children. Pediatrics 1972;50:653.
26. Morris JL, Johnson CF, Clasen M. To report or not to report: Physician's attitudes toward discipline and abuse. Am J Dis Child 1985;139:194.
27. Dubowitz H. Child abuse programs and pediatric residency training. Pediatrics 1988;82(suppl):477.
28. Smith JE, Rachman SJ, Yule B. Non-accidental injury to children: II. Methodological problems of evaluative treatment research. Behav Res Ther 1984;22:367.
29. Navarre EL. Psychological maltreatment: The core component of child abuse. In Brassard MR, Germain R, Hart SN (eds). Psychological Maltreatment of Children and Youth. Elmsford, NY, Pergamon Press, 1987, pp 45–56.
30. Levanthal JM, Garber RB, Brady CA. Identification during the postpartum period of infants who are at risk of child maltreatment. J Pediatr 1989;114:481.
31. Straus MA, Gelles RJ, Steinmetz SK. Behind Closed Doors: Violence in the American Family. Garden City, NY, Anchor/Doubleday, 1980, pp 123–152.
32. Finkelhor D. Psychological, cultural and family factors in incest and sexual abuse. J Marriage Family Counseling 1978;4:41.
33. Wright K. Sociocultural factors in child abuse. In Bass BA, Wyatt GE, Powell GJ (eds). The Afro-American Family Assessment: Treatment and Research Issues. New York, NY, Grune & Stratton, 1982, pp 237–261.
34. Besharov DJ, Dempsey PL, Dudley RG, et al. 1988 Report of the Child Fatality Review Panel. New York, The City of New York Human Resources Administration, 1989.
35. Gabarino J. What kind of society permits child abuse? Infant Mental Health J 1980;1:270.
36. Gabarino J. An ecological approach to child maltreatment. In Pelton LH (ed). The Social Context of Child Abuse and Neglect. New York, NY, Human Sciences Press, 1981, pp 228–267.
37. Daniel JH, Hampton RL, Newberger EH. Child abuse and accidents in black families: A controlled comparative study. Am J Orthopsychiatry 1983;53:645.
38. Showers J, Johnson CF. Child development, child health and child rearing knowledge among urban adolescents: Are they adequately prepared for the challenges of parenthood? Health Educ 1985;16:37.
39. Straus MA. Ordinary violence, child abuse, and wife beating: What do they have in common? In Finkelhor D, Gelles RJ, Hotaling GT, Straus MA (eds). The Dark Side of Families: Current Family Violence Research. Beverly Hills, CA, Sage, 1983, pp 213–234.
40. Altemeier WA, O'Connor S, Vietze PM, et al. Behavioral pediatrics: Antecedents of child abuse. Pediatrics 1982;100:823.
41. Dubowitz H. Prevention of child maltreatment: What is known. Pediatrics 1989;83:570.
42. Gabarino J. Preventing childhood injury: Developmental and mental health issues. Am J Orthopsychiatry 1988;58:25.
43. Jones DPH. The untreatable family. Child Abuse Negl 1987;11:409.
44. Famularo R, Stone K, Barnum R, Wharton R. Alcoholism and severe child maltreatment. Am J Orthopsychiatry 1986;56:481.
45. Listernick R, Christoffel K, Pace J, Chiramonte J. Severe primary malnutrition in US children. Am J Dis Child 1985;139:1157.
46. Johnson CF, Showers J. Injury variables in child abuse. Child Abuse Negl 1985;9:205.
47. Kaufman J, Zigler E. Do abused children become abusive parents? Am J Orthopsychiatry 1987;57:186.
48. Friedrich WN, Wheeler KK. The abusing parent revisited: A decade of psychological research. J Nerv Ment Dis 1982;170:577.
49. Rosenthal JA. Patterns of reported child abuse and neglect. Child Abuse Negl 1988;12:263.
50. O'Carroll PW. Homicides among black males 15–24 years of age, 1970–1984. MMWR 1988;37(SS-1):53.
51. Groothuis JR, Altemeier WA, Robarge J, et al. Increased child abuse in families with twins. Pediatrics 1982;70:769.
52. White R, Benedict MI, Wulff L, Kelley M. Physical disabilities as risk factors for child maltreatment: A selected review. Am J Orthopsychiatry 1987;57:93.
53. Jaudes P, Diamond L. Neglect of chronically ill children. Am J Dis Child 1986;140:655.
54. Mayer J, Black R. The relationship between alcoholism and child abuse and neglect. In Seixas FA (ed). Currents in Alcoholism. Vol II. New York, Grune & Stratton, 1977, pp 429–444.
55. Mayer J, Black R, Zakian A. The relationship between opiate abuse and child abuse and neglect. In Lowinson JH (ed). Critical Concerns in the Field of Drug Abuse. Proceedings of the National Drug Abuse Conference. New York, Marcel Dekker, 1976, pp 755–758.
56. Bays J. Substance abuse and child abuse: Impact of addiction on the child. Pediatr Clin North Am 1990;37:881.
57. Black R, Mayer J. Parents with special problems: Alcoholism and opiate addiction. Child Abuse Negl 1980;4:45.

58. Leonard KE, Jacob T. Alcohol, alcoholism and family violence. *In* Van Hasselt VB, Morrison RL, Bellack AS, et al (eds). Handbook of Family Violence. New York, Plenum Press, 1988, pp 383–406.

59. Pernhanen K. Alcohol and crimes of violence. *In* Kissin B, Begleiter H (eds). The Biology of Alcoholism. Vol 4: Social Aspects of Alcoholism. New York, Plenum Press, 1976, pp 351–444.

60. Amaro H, Zukerman B, Cabral H. Drug use among adolescent mothers: Profile of risk. Pediatrics 1989;84:144.

61. Sanders RW. Resistance to dealing with parents of battered children. Pediatrics 1972;50:853.

62. Council on Scientific Affairs. AMA diagnostic and treatment guidelines concerning child abuse and neglect. JAMA 1985;254:796.

63. Kaplan S. Psychopathology of parents of abused and neglected children and adolescents. J Am Acad Child Adolesc Psychiatry 1983;22:238.

64. Rossen DW, Leob LS, Jura MB. Differentiation of organic from non-organic failure to thrive syndrome in infancy. Pediatrics 1980;66:698.

65. Massie HN, Campbell K. The Massie-Campbell Scale of Mother-Infant Attachment Indicators During Stress. Detroit, MI, Wayne State University Press, 1980.

66. Bavolek SJ, Henderson HL. Teaching nurturing parenting skills. Missing/Abused 1989;5:3.

67. Burgess R, Conger R. Family interaction patterns related to child abuse and neglect. Child Abuse Negl 1977;1:269.

68. Dietrich KN, Starr RH, Weisfield GE. Infant maltreatment: Caretaker-infant interaction and developmental consequences at different levels of parenting failure. Pediatrics 1983;72:532.

69. Schmitt BD. Seven deadly sins of childhood: Advising parents about difficult developmental phases. Child Abuse Negl 1987;11:412.

70. Fontana VJ, Robison E. Observing child abuse. J Pediatr 1984;105:655.

71. McCormick MC, Shapiro S, Starfield BH. Injury and its correlates among one year old children. Am J Dis Child 1981;135:159.

72. Rivara FP, Kamitsuka MD, Quan L. Injuries to children younger than one year of age. Pediatrics 1988;81:93.

73. Putnam N, Stein M. Self-inflicted injuries in childhood: A review and diagnostic approach. Clin Pediatr 1985;24:514.

74. Adelson L. The battering child. JAMA 1972;222:159.

75. Crittenden PM, Craig SE. Developmental trends in the nature of child homicide. J Interpersonal Violence 1990;5:202.

76. McKibben L, De Vos E, Newberger EH. Victimization of mothers of abused children: A controlled study. Pediatrics 1989;84:531.

77. Craft JL, Clarkson CD. Case disposition recommendations of attorneys and social workers in child abuse investigations. Child Abuse Negl 1985;9:165.

78. Ellerstein NS. The cutaneous manifestations of child abuse and neglect. Am J Dis Child 1979;133:906.

79. McDowell HP, Fielding DW. Traumatic perforation of the hypopharynx—an unusual form of abuse. Arch Dis Child 1984;59:888.

80. Levine LJ. Bite marks in child abuse. *In* Sanger RG, Bross DC (eds). Clinical Management of Child Abuse and Neglect: A Guide for the Dental Professional. Chicago, IL, Quintessence, 1984, pp 53–59.

81. Wilson EF. Estimation of the age of cutaneous contusions in child abuse. Pediatrics 1977;60:751.

82. Johnson CF, Showers J. Injury variables in child abuse. Child Abuse Negl 1985;9:207.

83. Hight DW, Bakalar HR, Lloyd JR. Inflicted burns in children. JAMA 1979;242:517.

84. Moritz AR, Henriques FC. Studies of thermal injury: The relative importance of time and temperature in the causation of cutaneous burns. Am J Pathol 1947;23:695.

85. Feldman KW, Schaller RT, Feldman JA, McMillon M. Tap water scalds in children. Pediatrics 1978;62:1.

86. Showers J, Garrison KM. Burn abuse: A four-year study. J Trauma 1988;28:1581.

87. Kleinman PK. Diagnostic Imaging of Child Abuse. Baltimore, Williams & Wilkins, 1987, pp 159–199.

88. Becker DB, Needlemann HL, Kotelchuck M. Child abuse and dentistry: Orofacial trauma and its recognition by dentists. Am J Dent Assoc 1978;97:24.

89. Harley RD. Ocular manifestations of child abuse. Pediatr Ophthalmol Strabismus 1980;17:5.

90. Johnson CF, Coury DL. Bruising and hemophilia: Accident or child abuse? Child Abuse Negl 1988;12:409.

91. Hathaway WE, Assmus SL, Montgomery RR, Dubansky AS. Activated partial thromboplastin time and minor coagulopathies. Am J Clin Pathol 1979;71:22.

92. O'Hare AE, Eden OB. Bleeding disorders and non-accidental injury. Arch Dis Child 1984;59:860.

93. Sarnaik AP, Stringer KD, Jewell PF, et al. Disseminated intravascular coagulation with trauma: Treatment with exchange transfusion. Pediatrics 1979;63:337.

94. Taylor GP. Severe bleeding disorders in children with normal coagulation tests. Br Med J 1982;284:1851.

95. Paterson CR. Osteogenesis imperfecta in the differential diagnosis of child abuse. Child Abuse Negl 1981;1:449.

96. Carpentieri U, Gustavson LP, Haggard ME. Misdiagnosis of neglect in a child with bleeding disorder and cystic fibrosis. South Med J 1978;71:854.

97. Waskerwitz S, Christoffel KK, Hauger S. Hypersensitivity vasculitis presenting as suspected child abuse: case report and literature review. Pediatrics 1981;67:283.

98. Owen SM, Durst RD. Ehlers-Danlos syndrome simulating child abuse. Arch Dermatol 1984;120:97.

99. Roberts DLL, Pope FM, Nicholls AC, Narcisi P. Ehlers-Danlos syndrome type IV mimicking nonaccidental injury in a child. Br J Dermatol 1984;111:341.

100. Adler R, Kane-Nussen B. Erythema multiforme. Confusion with child battering syndrome. Pediatrics 1983;72:718.

101. Hurwitz A, Castells S. Misdiagnosed child abuse and metabolic disorders. Pediatr Nurs 1987;13:33.

102. Gellis SS, Feingold M. Cạo Gío (pseudo-battering in Vietnamese children). Am J Dis Child 1976;130:857.

103. Golden SM, Duster MC. Hazards of misdiagnosis due to Vietnamese folk medicine. Clin Pediatr 1977;16:949.

104. Asnes RS, Wisotsky DH. Cupping lesions simulating child abuse. J Pediatr 1981;99:267.

105. Kirschner RH, Stein RJ. The mistaken diagnosis of child abuse: A form of medical abuse? Am J Dis Child 1985;139:873.

106. Cole HN, Hubler WR, Lund HZ. Persistent, aberrant mongolian spots. Arch Dermatol Syph 1950;61:244.

107. Muller SA, Winkelmann RK. Trichotillomania: A clinicopathologic study of 24 cases. Arch Dermatol 1978;105:535.

108. Hobbs CJ. Skull fracture and the diagnosis of child abuse. Arch Dis Child 1984;59:246.

109. Billmire ME, Myers PA. Serious head injury in infants: Accident or abuse? Pediatrics 1985;75:340.

110. Merten DF, Osborne DRS. Craniocerebral trauma in the child abuse syndrome. Pediatr Ann 1982;12:882.

111. Martin HP, Breezley P, Conway EF. The development of abused children. Adv Pediatr 1974;21:25.

112. Frank Y, Zimmerman R, Leeds NMD. Neurological manifestations in abused children who have been shaken. Dev Med Child Neurol 1985;27:312.

113. Kravitz H, Driessen G, Gomberg R, et al. Accidental falls from elevated surfaces in infants from birth to one year of age. Pediatrics 1969;44:869.

114. Helfer RE, Slovis TL, Black M. Injuries resulting when small children fall out of bed. Pediatrics 1977;60:533.

115. Caffey J. On the theory and practice of shaking infants: Its potential residual effects of permanent brain damage and mental retardation. Am J Dis Child 1972;124:161.

116. Caffey J. The whiplash shaken infant syndrome: Manual shaking by the extremities with whiplash-induced intracranial and intraocular bleedings, linked with residual permanent brain damage and mental retardation. Pediatrics 1974;54:396.

117. Harwood-Nash DC. Craniocerebral trauma in children. Curr Probl Radiol 1973;3:3.

118. Alexander R, Sato Y, Smith W, Bennett T. Incidence of impact trauma with cranial injuries ascribed to shaking. Am J Dis Child 1990;144:724.

119. Bruce DA, Zimmerman RA. Shaken impact syndrome. Pediatr Ann 1989;18:482.

120. Zumwalt RE, Hirsch CS. Pathology of fatal child abuse and neglect. *In* Helfer RE, Kempe RS (eds). The Battered Child. Chicago, University of Chicago Press, 1987, pp 247–285.

121. Hardman JM. The pathology of traumatic brain injuries. *In* Thompson RA, Green JR (eds). Advances in Neurology 1979;22:15.

122. Saulsbury FT, Alford BA. Intracranial bleeding from child abuse: The value of skull radiographs. Pediatr Radiol 1982;112:175.

123. Harley RD. Ocular manifestations of child abuse. J Pediatr Ophthalmol Strabismus 1980;17:5.

124. Wilkinson WS, Han DP, Rappley MD, Owings CL. Retinal hemorrhage predicts neurologic injury in the shaken baby syndrome. Arch Ophthalmol 1989;107:1472.

125. Lambert SR, Johnson TE, Hoyt CS. Optic nerve sheath and retinal hemorrhages associated with the shaken baby syndrome. Arch Ophthalmol 1986;104:1509.

126. Hanigan WC, Peterson RA, Njus G. Tin ear syndrome: Rotational acceleration in pediatric head injuries. Pediatrics 1987;80:618.

127. Alexander R, Crabbe L, Sato Y, et al. Serial abuse in children who are shaken. Am J Dis Child 1990;144:58.

128. Duhaime AC, Gennarelli TA, Thibault LE, et al. The shaken baby syndrome: A clinical, pathological, and biomechanical study. J Neurosurg 1987;66:409.

129. Zimmerman RA, Bilaniuk LT, Bruce D, et al. Computed tomography of craniocerebral injury in the abused child. Radiology 1979;130:687.

130. Cohen RA, Kaufman RA, Myers PA. Cranial computed tomography in the abused child with head injury. AJR 1986;146:97.

131. Ludwig S, Warman M. Shaken baby syndrome: A review of 20 cases. Ann Emerg Med 1984;13:104.

132. Levin AV, Magnusson MR, Rafto SE, Zimmerman RA. Shaken baby syndrome diagnosed by magnetic resonance imaging. Pediatr Emerg Care 1989;5:181.

133. Alexander R, Schor DP, Smith WL Jr. Magnetic resonance imaging of intracranial injuries from child abuse. J Pediatr 1986;109:975.

134. Baum JD, Bulpitt CJ. Retinal and conjunctival hemorrhage in the newborn. Arch Dis Child 1970;45:344.

135. Sezen F. Retinal hemorrhages in newborn infants. Br J Ophthalmol 1970;55:248.

136. Levin S, Janive J, Mintz M, et al. Diagnostic and prognostic value of retinal hemorrhages in the neonate. Obstet Gynecol 1980;55:309.

137. Tomasi LG, Rosman P. Purtscher retinopathy in the battered child syndrome. Am J Dis Child 1975;129:1335.

138. Guarnaschelli J, Lee J, Pitts FW. Fallen fontanelle (caida de mollera): A variant of the battered child syndrome. JAMA 1972;222:1545.

139. Abroms IF, McLennan JE, Mandell F. Acute neonatal subdural hematoma following breech delivery. Am J Dis Child 1977;131:192.

140. McClelland CQ, Kingsbury GH. Fractures in the first year of life: A diagnostic dilemma. Am J Dis Child 1982;136:26.

141. Merten DF, Radkowski MA, Leonidas JC. The abused child: A radiologic reappraisal. Radiology 1983;146:377.

142. Anderson WA. The significance of femoral fracture in children. Ann Emerg Med 1982;11:174.

143. Dalton HJ, Slovis T, Helfer RE, et al. Undiagnosed abuse in children younger than three years with femoral fracture. Arch Dis Child 1990;144:875.

144. Rivara F, Kamitsuka M, Quan L. Injuries to children younger than one year of age. Pediatrics 1988;81:93.

145. Kleinman PK. The metaphyseal lesion in abused infants: A radiologic-histopathologic study. AJR 1986;146:895.

146. Kleinman PK, Marks SC, Adams VI, Blackbourne BD. Factors affecting visualization of posterior rib fractures in abused infants. AJR 1988;150:635.

147. Thompson BM, Finger W, Tonsfeldt D. Rib radiographs for trauma: Useful or wasteful? Ann Emerg Med 1986;15:261.

148. Pickett WJ, Faleski EJ, Chacko A, Jarrett RV. Comparison of radiographic and radionuclide skeletal surveys in battered children. South Med J 1983;76:207.

149. Kogutt MS, Swischuk LE, Fagan CJ. Patterns of injury and significance of uncommon fractures in the battered child syndrome. AJR 1974;121:143.

150. Swischuk LE. Spine and spinal cord trauma in the battered child syndrome. Radiology 1969;92:733.

151. Swischuk LE. Radiology of the skeletal system in child abuse and neglect. In Ellerstein NS (ed). Child Abuse and Neglect: A Medical Reference. New York, John Wiley & Sons, 1981, pp 263–269.

152. Ekengren F, Bergdahl S, Ekström G. Birth injuries to the epiphyseal cartilage. Acta Radiol [Diagn] 1978;19:197.

153. Cumming WA. Neonatal skeletal fractures: Birth trauma or child abuse? J Can Assoc Radiol 1979;30:30.

154. Feldman KW, Brewer DK. Child abuse, cardiopulmonary resuscitation fractures. Pediatrics 1984;73:339.

155. Fiser RH, Kaplan J, Holder JC. Congenital syphilis mimicking the battered child syndrome: How does one tell them apart. Clin Pediatr 1972;11:305.

156. Hirsch M, Mogle P, Markli Y. Neonatal scurvy. Pediatr Radiol 1976;4:251.

157. Berant M, Jacobs T. A pseudo-battered child. Clin Pediatr 1966;5:230.

158. Adams PC, Strand RD, Bresnan MJ, et al. Kinky hair syndrome: Serial study of radiological findings with emphasis on the similarity to the battered child syndrome. Radiology 1974;112:401.

159. Caffey J. Infantile cortical hyperostosis: A review of the clinical and radiographic features. Proc R Soc Med 1957;50:347.

160. Caniano DA, Beaver BL, Boles ET. Child abuse: An update on surgical management in 256 cases. Ann Surg 1986;203:219.

161. Radkowski MA, Merten DF, Leonidas JC. The abused child: Criteria for the radiologic diagnosis. RadioGraphics 1983;3:262.

162. Cooper A, Floyd T, Barlow B, et al. Major blunt abdominal trauma due to child abuse. J Trauma 1988;28:1483.

163. Philipart AI. Blunt abdominal trauma in childhood. Surg Clin North Am 1977;57:151.

164. Wolley MW, Mahour GH, Sloan T. Duodenal hematoma in infancy and childhood: Changing etiology and changing treatment. Am J Surg 1978;136:8.

165. Taylor GA, Eichelberger MR, Potter BM. Hematuria: A marker of abdominal injury in children after blunt abdominal trauma. Ann Surg 1988;208:688.

166. Cobb LM, Vinocur CD, Wagner MD, Weintraub WH. Intestinal perforation due to blunt trauma in children in an era of increased nonoperative treatment. J Trauma 1986;26:461.

167. Kirks DR. Radiological evaluation of visceral injuries in the battered child syndrome. Pediatr Ann 1983;12:888.

168. Felson B, Levine J. Intramural hematoma of the duodenum: A diagnostic roentgen sign. Radiology 1954;63:823.

169. Kleinman PK, Raptopoulos VD, Brill PW. Occult nonskeletal trauma in the battered-child syndrome. Radiology 1981;141:393.

170. Bongiovi JJ, Logosso RD. Pancreatic pseudocyst occurring in the battered child syndrome. J Pediatr Surg 1969;4:220.

171. Neuer FS, Roberts FF, McCarthy V. Osteolytic lesions following traumatic pancreatitis. Am J Dis Child 1977;131:738.

172. Taylor GA, Fallat ME, Potter BM, Eichelberger MR. The role of computed tomography in blunt abdominal trauma in children. J Trauma 1988;28:1660.

173. Sivit CJ, Taylor GA, Eichelberger MR. Visceral injury in battered children: A changing perspective. Radiology 1989;173:659.

174. Shnaps Y, Frand M, Tirosh M. The chemically abused child. Pediatrics 1981;68:119.

175. Bateman DA, Heagarty MC. Passive freebase cocaine ("crack") inhalation by infants and toddlers. Am J Dis Child 1989;143:25.

176. Schwartz RH, Einhorn A. PCP intoxication in seven young children. Pediatr Emerg Care 1986;2:238.

177. Weinberg D, Lande A, Hilton N, Kerns D. Intoxication from accidental marijuana ingestion. Pediatrics 1983;71:848.

178. Schwartz RH, Peary P, Mistretta D. Intoxication of young children with marijuana: A form of amusement for "pot"-smoking teenage girls. Am J Dis Child 1986;140:326.

179. Ernst AA, Sanders WM. Unexpected cocaine intoxication presenting as seizures in children. Ann Emerg Med 1989;18:774.

180. Schwartz R. Hypoglycemia. In Behrman R, Vaughan V (eds). Nelson Textbook of Pediatrics. Philadelphia, WB Saunders 1987, p 1269.

181. Rivkin M, Gilmore HE. Generalized seizures in an infant due to environmentally acquired cocaine. Pediatrics 1989;84:1100.

182. Rosenberg D. Web of deceit: A literature review of Munchausen syndrome by proxy. Child Abuse Negl 1987;11:547.

183. Dine MS, McGovern ME. Intentional poisoning of children—an overlooked category of child abuse: Report of seven cases and review of the literature. Pediatrics 1982;70:32.

184. Meadow R. Munchausen syndrome by proxy: The hinterland of child abuse. Lancet 1977;2:343.

185. Fenton AC, Wailoo MP, Tanner MS. Severe failure to thrive and diarrhea caused by laxative abuse. Arch Dis Child 1988;63:978.

186. Warwick GL, Boulton-Jones JM. Recurrent cardiovascular collapse due to surreptitious ingestion of propranolol. Br Med J 1989;298:294.

187. Lansky LL. An unusual case of childhood chloral hydrate poisoning. Am J Dis Child 1974;127:275.

188. Feldman KW, Christopher DM, Opheim KB. Munchausen syndrome—bulimia by proxy: Ipecac as a toxin in child abuse. Child Abuse Negl 1989;13:257.

189. Saulsbury FT, Chobanian MC, Wilson WG. Child abuse: Parenteral hydrocarbon administration. Pediatrics 1984;73:719.

190. Dine MS. Tranquilizer poisoning: An example of child abuse. Pediatrics 1965;36:782.

191. Rendle-Short J. Nonaccidental barbiturate poisoning of children. Lancet 1978;2:1212.

192. Pickering D. Salicylate poisoning: The diagnosis when its possibility is denied by the parents. Acta Paediatr 1964;53:501.

193. Hickson GB, Greene JW, Craft LT. Apparent intentional poisoning of an infant with acetaminophen. Am J Dis Child 1983;137:917.

194. White ST. Surreptitious warfarin ingestion. Child Abuse Negl 1985;9:349.

195. Hill RM, Barer J, Hill LL, Butler CM. An investigation of recurrent pine oil poisoning in an infant by the use of gas chromatographic–mass spectrometric methods. J Pediatr 1975;87:115.

196. Bauman WA, Yalow RS. Child abuse: Parenteral insulin administration. J Pediatr 1981;99:588.

197. Cantwell HB. Child neglect. In Kempe CH, Helfer RE (eds). The Battered Child. Chicago, University of Chicago Press, 1980, pp 183–197.

198. Pelton LH. Child abuse and neglect: The myth of classlessness. Am J Orthopsychiatry 1978;48:608.

199. Helfer RE. The neglect of our children. Pediatr Clin North Am 1990;37:923.

200. Ayoub CC, Milner JS. Failure to thrive: Parental indicators, types, and outcomes. Child Abuse Negl 1985;9:491.

201. Homer C, Ludwig S. Categorization of failure to thrive. Am J Dis Child 1981;135:848.

202. Berwick DM. Nonorganic failure to thrive. Pediatr Rev 1980;1:265.

203. US House of Representatives, Committee on Children, Youth, and Families. Abused Children in America: Victims of Official Neglect. Report 100-260, 100th Congress, 1st Session, 1987: pp XV and 15–16.

204. Wolock I, Horowitz B. Child maltreatment as a social problem: The neglect of neglect. Am J Orthopsychiatry 1984;54:530.

205. Helfer RE. The litany of smoldering neglect of children. In Helfer RE, Kempe RS (eds). The Battered Child. Chicago, University of Chicago Press, 1987, pp 301–311.

206. Suskind RM, Varma RJ. Assessment of nutritional status of children. Pediatr Rev 1984;5:195.

207. Baker JP, Detsky AS, Wesson DE. Nutritional assessment: A comparison of clinical judgment and objective measurements. N Engl J Med 1982;306:969.

208. Sills RH. Failure to thrive: The role of clinical and laboratory evaluation. Am J Dis Child 1979;132:967.

209. Winick M, Rosso P. The effect of severe early malnutrition on cellular growth of human brain. Pediatr Res 1980;3:181.

210. Dietrich KN, Starr RH, Weisfield GE. Infant maltreatment: Caretaker-infant interaction and developmental consequences at different levels of parenting failure. Pediatrics 1983;72:532.
211. Casey PH, Bradley R, Wortham B. Social and non-social home environments of infants with non-organic failure to thrive. Pediatrics 1984;73:348.
212. Myers JEB, Peters WD. Child Abuse Reporting Legislation in the 1980s. Denver, CO, American Humane Association, 1987, p 1.
213. Myers JEB. A survey of child abuse and neglect reporting statutes. J Juvenile Law I 1986:4.
214. Besharov DJ. What physicians should know about child abuse reporting laws. *In* Ellerstein NS (ed): Child Abuse and Neglect: A Medical Reference. New York, John Wiley & Sons, 1981, pp 21–49.
215. Landeros v. Flood: 17 California 3d 399, 551 P.2d 389, 131 Cal Rptr 1976:69.
216. Kempe CH. Approaches to preventing child abuse: The health visitor's concept. Am J Dis Child 1976;130:941.
217. Olds DL, Henderson CR, Chamberlin R, Tatelbaum R. Preventing child abuse and neglect: A randomized trial of nurse home visitation. Pediatrics 1986;78:65.
218. Caldwell RA, Bogat GA, Davidson WS. The assessment of child abuse potential and the prevention of child abuse and neglect. Am J Comm Psych 1988;16:609.
219. Meddin BJ. The services provided during a child abuse and/or neglect case investigation and the barriers that exist to service provision. Child Abuse Negl 1985;9:175.
220. Leake HC, Smith DJ. Preparing for and testifying in a child abuse hearing. Clin Pediatr 1977;16:1057.

CHAPTER 15

Pediatric Sexual Abuse

Carol D. Berkowitz

INTRODUCTION

Child sexual abuse is a problem that has been recognized with increasing frequency since the early 1980s.[1, 2] It is now believed to account for about 20% of the over 1 million cases of child abuse reported each year in the United States.[3] Although the task of medical assessment of the acutely assaulted patient has often fallen on the emergency physician, the increasing demand for medical evaluations of chronically abused children has necessitated involvement of the emergency physician in the assessment of these more problematic children. The emergency department physician may specifically be asked by law enforcement or child protective services to perform an examination, or the abuse may be suspected or detected during an evaluation for some other medical complaint. Functional complaints, such as recurrent abdominal pain or headache; behavioral problems, such as enuresis; and psychosocial problems, such as suicide gestures may all be manifestations of child sexual abuse.[4, 5] In order to perform an appropriate and adequate assessment, the physician should obtain and record a medical history, including a history of the abuse; perform a complete physical examination; obtain the necessary laboratory studies; exchange pertinent information with appropriate agencies; and be available for court testimony if the need arises.

CLINICAL EVALUATION
Medical History

The medical history should include details specific to the allegations of the abuse, as well as questions related to the general health and well-being of the child. Although the physician is an ideal interviewer, time constraints and lack of expertise may preclude the physician from conducting the interview.[6] Because of the forensic nature of the interview, care must be taken not to contaminate the information by using leading questions.[7, 8] It is totally acceptable, and sometimes preferable, for the "disclosure" interview to be carried out by a social worker.[6] Alternatively, it is completely appropriate for the physician to ask the child, "Do you know why you are here?" or "Can you tell me what happened?" The child's statements should be recorded verbatim. The medical record may be entered into evidence, and the child's statements are then admitted, not for "the truth of the matter," but because they assisted the physician in rendering an opinion.[9]

The disclosure statements should include who did what, how often, and the last time any abuse occurred. It is critical to realize that these disclosures often are only partial, and children frequently are imprecise regarding time.

Included in the history of the abuse should be an assessment of the symptoms, both physical and behavioral, that may be related to the abuse. One should inquire about episodes of vaginal bleeding or discharge. A history of enuresis and urologic symptoms such as dysuria and urinary tract infections should be noted. Age of menarche, date of last menstrual period, and type of sanitary protection should be recorded. Stooling problems such as encopresis, hematochezia, constipation, and the use of enemas or suppositories should also be noted. One should also inquire about genitourinary or anorectal trauma or surgery.[10]

Other behavioral areas about which to make specific inquiries include masturbation (quantify if possible), sexually provocative or pseudomature behavior, sleep disturbances, and nightmares. These issues are obviously less relevant in an adolescent patient who has undergone an isolated episode of acute assault.[5, 11, 12, 13]

The general medical history should also be obtained, noting relevant birth history; previous medical problems, including hospitalizations, fractures, and operations; immunizations; developmental history; family history; and social history, including an assessment of with whom the child lives.

The medical history is important for two reasons. First, it de-emphasizes the genitalia as the focus of attention, a therapeutically important phenomenon for the chronically molested child. Second, it ensures the absence of any medical condition that might offer an alternative explanation for the physical findings, if any.

The medical history should be recorded in the routine manner, including pertinent negatives. Additional information is frequently obtained after an acute assault, and these inquiries are often noted on standard rape protocols. Such inquiries serve to determine the likelihood of recovering forensic material, and include showering, douching, and toothbrushing after the assault.

Medical Examination

The patient should undergo a thorough physical examination.[7, 10] Again, the purpose of this is twofold: to de-emphasize a genital focus and to make certain there is no other medical explanation for the genital findings. Traumatic injuries such as bruises and slap or grip marks should be recorded, although these are uncommon in a child who has been chronically abused. It is also important to make a careful neurologic assessment, particularly of the lower extremities, since spinal cord lesions may affect anal sphincter tone.

The anogenital area should be carefully assessed. One

should be familiar with a number of techniques that facilitate the examination.[14-17] First, the examination is generally confined to visualization of the external genitalia. Internal ("pelvic") examinations are usually reserved for postmenarchal females or abused children with suspected penetrating or internal trauma. Adequate visualization may be facilitated by appropriate positioning of the child and by the use of magnification. Stirrups are usually reserved for older or obese children. Young infants and toddlers are often most comfortable seated on the mother's lap, with the mother abducting the infant's legs (Fig. 15–1). Older children may be examined in the supine frog-leg position (Fig. 15–2). Visualization of the hymen is accomplished by separation of (spreading) or traction on (grasping the labia majora with thumb and index finger and pulling forward) the labia (Fig. 15–3). The prone knee-chest position is advocated by some as further facilitating visualization (Fig. 15–4); it is the only position in which the cervix can be visualized. Magnification tools, such as a hand-held magnifying glass or the colposcope, also help define anatomy.[18, 19] In addition, the colposcope is useful if equipped with a camera for recording the genital findings. Toluidine blue applied to the genital area is selectively absorbed by areas of microtrauma that might otherwise be undetectable.[20]

It is useful for the physician to examine the genital area of all children, so as to appreciate the range of normal anatomy. The genitalia of abused young boys virtually never show any telltale evidence of abuse. Prepubescent girls who have been abused may likewise heal with no residua, or may show evidence of scarring or disruption of the hymen. There are also many forms of abuse that in no way injure the hymen.

It is important for the physician to appreciate that the contour and configuration of the hymen change with age.[14] In infants the effect of placentally transferred maternal hormones is readily apparent and the hymen is thick, red, and scalloped (Fig. 15–5). These changes gradually resolve over 2 to 3 years and the hymen takes on a thinner, more fragile appearance (Fig. 15–6). The hymen itself is most often crescentic or annular in appearance, although there may be other variations such as septate or imperforate hymen (Fig. 15–7). Puberty brings a surge of estrogen, and as a result the hymen once more becomes thickened and scalloped (Fig. 15–8). A white physiologic discharge usually appears. Scars and changes in the postpubertal hymen may be difficult to detect or may not be present even in the face of penetration, because of the resistance of the thickened, estrogenized hymen to trauma.

The size of the hymenal orifice may provide the first clue to penetration. In *nonabused* children the opening has a linear relationship to their age: a rough approximation is 1 mm per year of age.[21] Other investigators feel that the orifice should not be greater than 5 mm in a prepubertal child.[22, 23] The measurement should be horizontal, with the child supine in a frog-leg position. Values for vertical diameters and size in a knee-chest position are available, but their significance and applicability to a population of abused children is unclear.[24]

The shape of the hymen should be noted and any irregularities recorded. Irregularities may appear as indentations; these may represent healed lacerations and are distinctly unusual in nonabused children when in the lower portion of the hymen.[25, 26] Localized areas of thickening may also represent healed injury. It is important to be certain that the thickening is real and not merely hymen flipped over on itself. Tethering of the hymen to the perihymenal tissue may also occur after trauma. Elasticity of tissues is lost. Attenuation or reduction in the amount of hymenal tissue is particularly significant and suggests previous repeated penetration (Fig. 15–9).[26] Frequently the remaining hymen is not only reduced in amount but also thickened (Fig. 15–10).[27] Bands of scar tissue may span from the hymen to the perihymenal tissue, but these should not be confused with the very common periurethral support bands, which are generally symmetric and at the 11:00 and 1:00 positions of the hymen (Fig. 15–11). Some physical findings such as erythema are nonspecific; they may occur with abuse, but are also seen with other conditions such as irritation or inflammation.

Changes seen with acute trauma are less problematic than those found with previous or chronic abuse. Acute changes include hematomas, bruises, and lacerations.[14] Microtrauma (small areas of abrasion) are noted in the region of the posterior fourchette, even in women who consent to intercourse.[28] This microtrauma may be detected only with the aid of magnification or toluidine blue.[20]

Changes in the anal area may occur with acute or previous repeated penetration in about 50% of victims.[29-31] Acutely, one may see fissures that are characteristically external to the dentate line, or hematomas (Fig. 15–12). Changes in anal tone consisting of anal spasm or marked anal dilatation may be noted after acute penetration. These acute changes may resolve with no residual scarring.[29] Changes reported with repeated or traumatic anal penetration include distortion in the contour of the normally circular or elliptic anal orifice (Fig. 15–13). Rugae may be reduced in number but thickened in appearance. Conversely, the scarred skin in the perianal area may appear thin and atrophic, like scar tissue in other areas.[32] Sometimes this atrophy leads to easy visibility of purple veins below the surface.[33, 34] However, such venous pooling may be noted in nonabused children who have been kept in a prone knee-chest position for 5 minutes.[35] Hemorrhoids are a very unusual finding in children, but their relationship to sexual abuse is undefined. Anal dilatation also is frequently noted in nonabused children if they are maintained for 5 minutes in a prone knee-chest position, especially if there is stool in the rectal ampulla.[35] Immediate anal dilatation, especially if the patient is in a prone or lateral decubitus position, no stool is present, or the dilatation exceeds 2 cm, is highly indicative of previous repeated anal penetration.[33, 34] The anal wink may be suppressed after repeated anal penetration.[29]

COLLECTION OF FORENSIC MATERIAL

Patients who have been acutely assaulted should be evaluated for forensic material.[7, 10] The methods to use in collecting these specimens are usually specifically defined in rape protocols.[36] In general, specimens are collected from the throat, rectum, and vagina. A Wood light assists the examiner in finding semen that may be on body surfaces. Swabs should be thoroughly air-dried to prevent the overgrowth of normal flora and subsequent destruction of evidence. Fluid in the vaginal pool should be examined directly for motile sperm. Specimens are evaluated for a number of markers that verify the presence of semen and that may help identify or eliminate a suspect. "Rape kits" generally outline in detail the proper way to collect specimens, and the physician should gather the evidence in the prescribed manner. This evidence should be initialed and passed directly to the law enforcement officer handling the case.

Documentation of the physical findings is imperative. This can best be accomplished with meticulous descriptive recording and the use of drawings and photography. Most colposcopes are equipped with photographic potential; if not, pictures can be obtained using cameras fitted with a macrolens.

Text continued on page 175

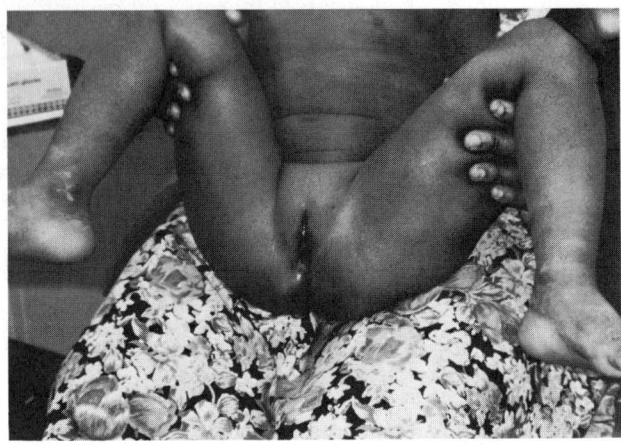

Figure 15–1. Infant with legs abducted seated on the mother's lap.

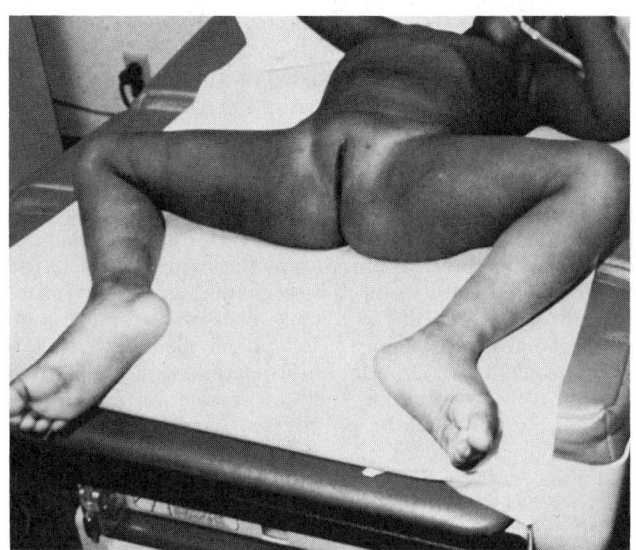

Figure 15–2. Child lying supine in the frog-leg position.

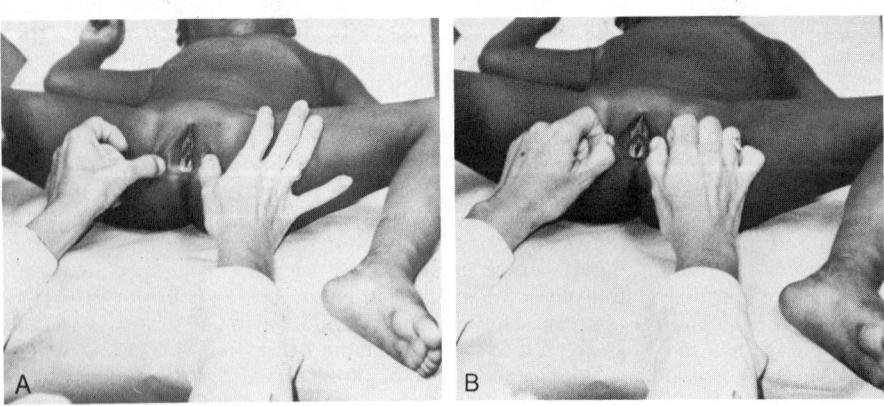

Figure 15–3. Visualization of the hymen using *(A)* separation of the labia and *(B)* traction of the labia.

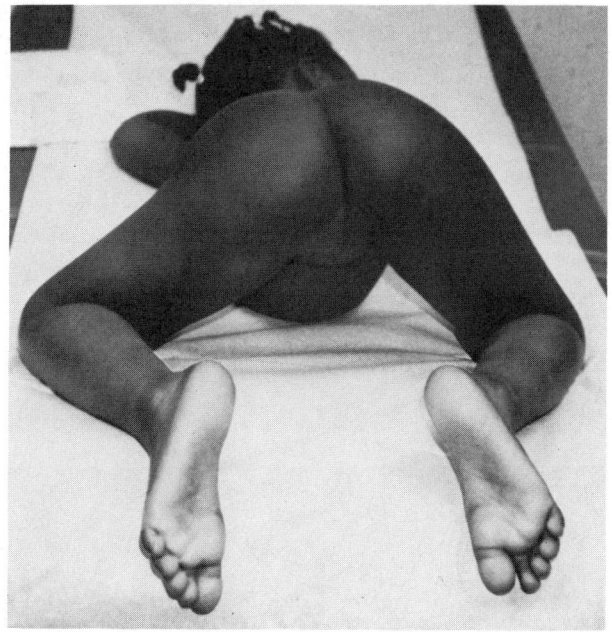

Figure 15–4. Child lying in the prone knee-chest position.

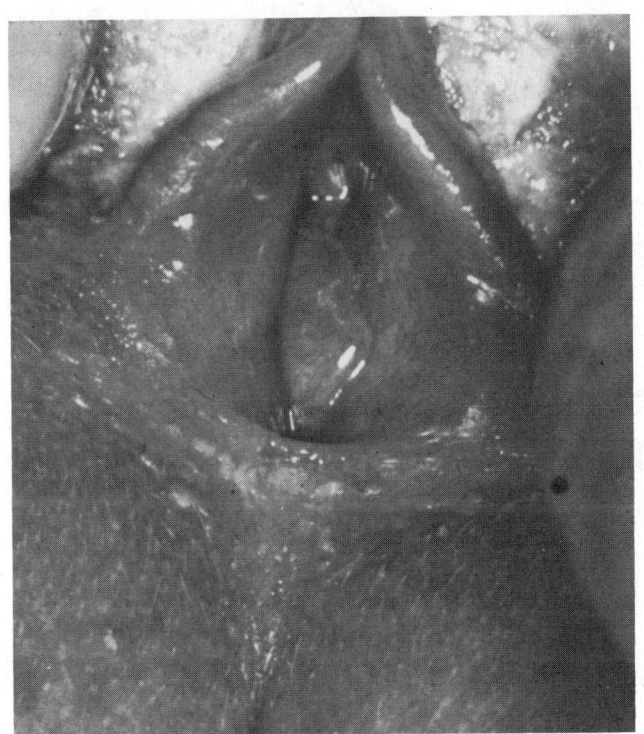

Figure 15–5. Newborn infant. The hymen is full and covers the orifice.

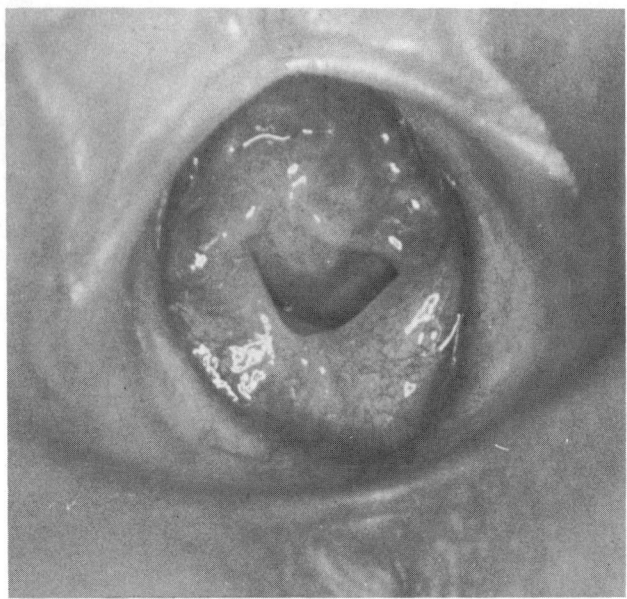

Figure 15–6. Hymen in a 5-year-old child. It is thin, fine, elastic, and annular.

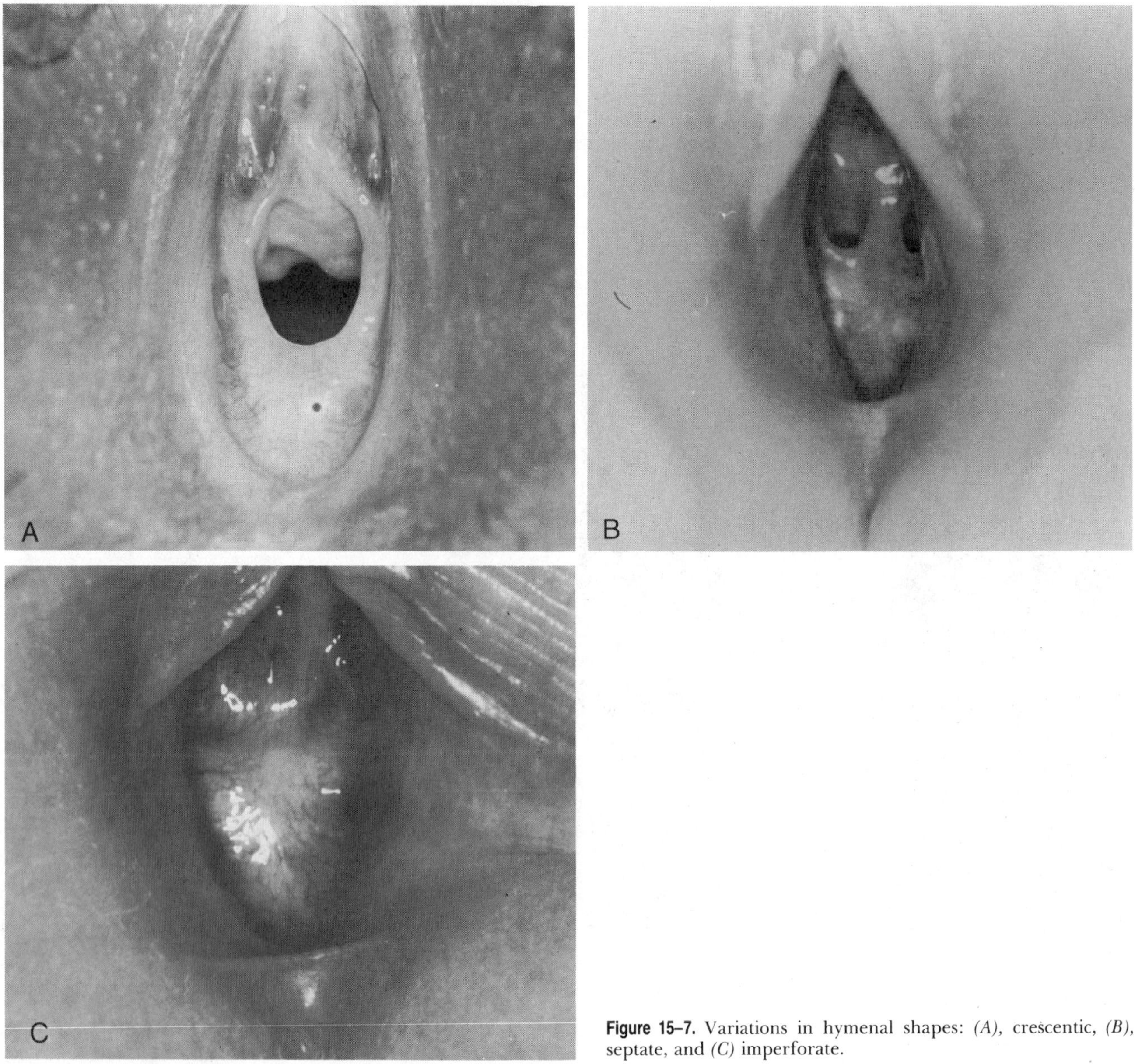

Figure 15–7. Variations in hymenal shapes: *(A)*, crescentic, *(B)*, septate, and *(C)* imperforate.

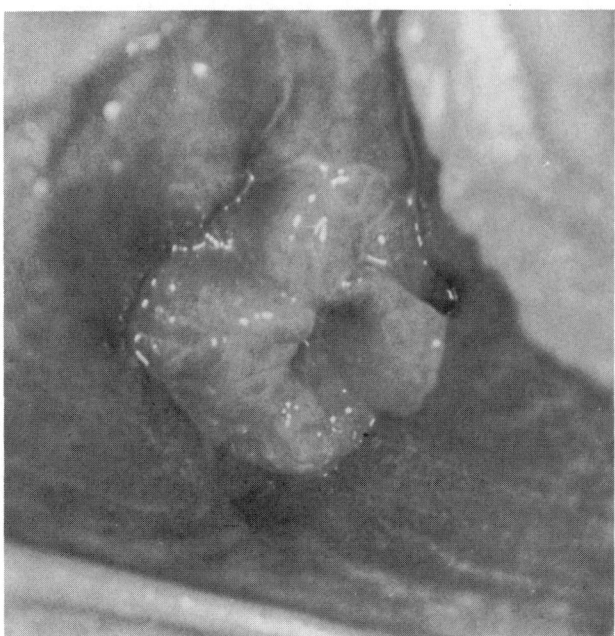

Figure 15–8. Hymen of an adolescent female. It is thickened and scalloped, covering the hymenal orifice.

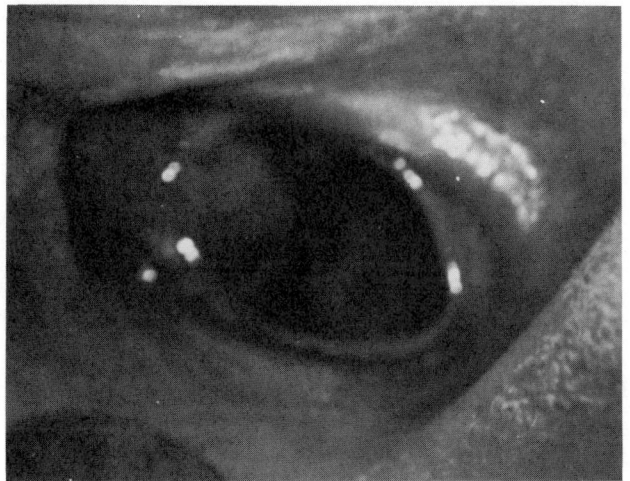

Figure 15–9. Attenuated hymenal remnant in a 10-year-old child who had been repeatedly sexually abused.

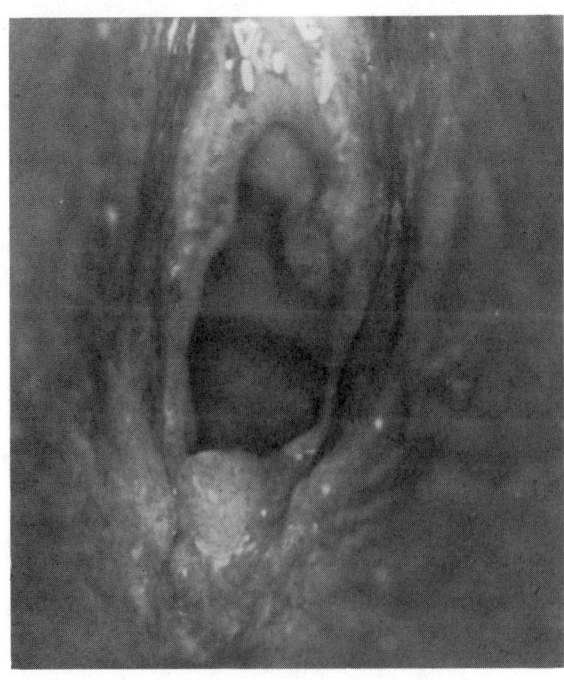

Figure 15–10. Attenuated irregular hymen with thickened scar tissue at the 6:00 position.

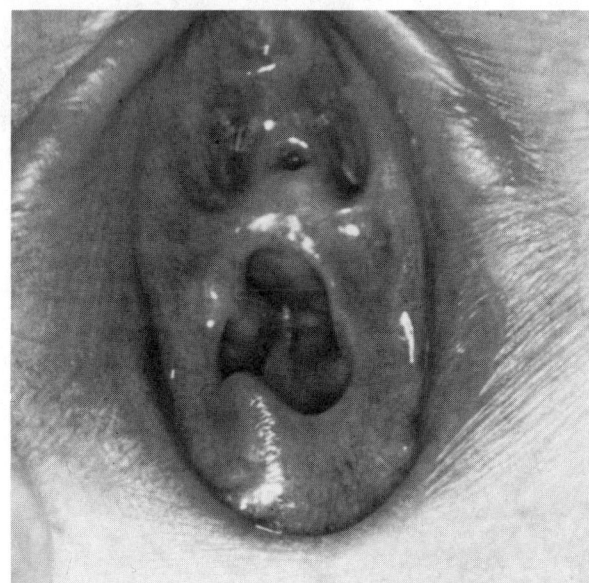

Figure 15–11. Periurethral bands are a normal finding, not a sign of scarring.

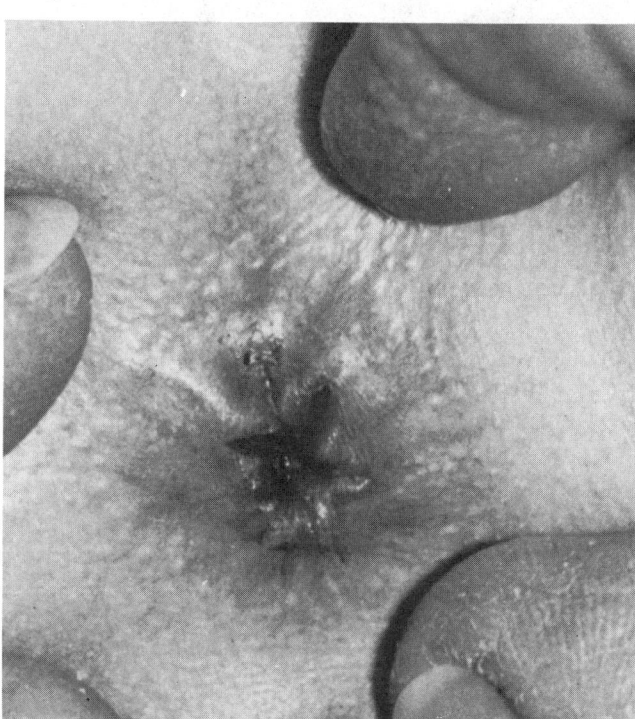

Figure 15–12. Multiple perianal fissures in a 3-month-old infant after anal penetration.

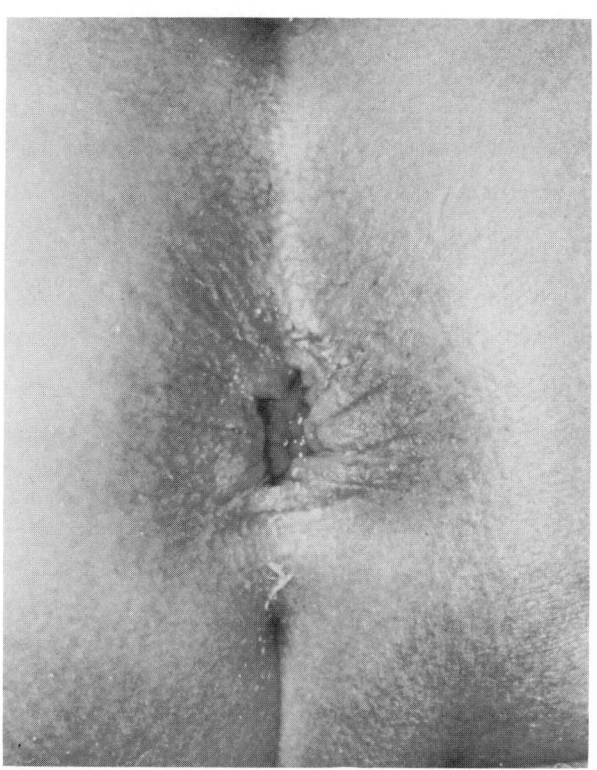

Figure 15–13. Distorted appearance of the anus in a chronically molested 8-month-old infant.

SEXUALLY TRANSMITTED DISEASES

Children who have been sexually abused should be evaluated for sexually transmitted diseases, particularly *Neisseria gonorrhoeae* and *Chlamydia trachomatis*. The decision to evaluate for other diseases, such as syphilis, HIV infection and *Trichomonas* infection must be based on clinical considerations.[7, 10]

REPORTING CHILD SEXUAL ABUSE

All U.S. states require that cases in which child sexual abuse is suspected be reported.[7, 10] It is not incumbent on the physician to conduct a comprehensive evaluation to determine whether the abuse occurred or the identity of the perpetrator. A disclosure about abuse, physical findings consistent with abuse, pregnancy, or a sexually transmitted disease all warrant reporting. Less specific evidence, such as behavioral changes noted, nonspecific genital findings (e.g., erythema), or vaginal discharges, may warrant further assessment before notification of law enforcement or child protective agencies. The primary responsibility of the physician is to initiate the chain of events that will ensure the safety of the child. However, it is important to keep in mind that even the investigation of child sexual abuse may be a trying and traumatic event for the family.

THERAPEUTIC INTERVENTION

Medical intervention is rarely needed unless the patient has been acutely assaulted. After acute assaults, prophylaxis for sexually transmitted diseases should be offered. The currently recommended regimen includes ceftriaxone as a single injection (125 mg up to 45 kg and 250 mg above 45 kg). Prophylaxis for infection with *Chlamydia* is given with erythromycin, 40 to 50 mg/kg/day in four divided doses for 7 days. Individuals over the age of 8 years may receive doxycycline, 100 mg twice a day for 7 days. In postmenarchal girls, pregnancy counseling should be offered, with all options discussed. Pregnancy prophylaxis can be given with Ovral (0.05 mg ethinyl estradiol and 0.5 mg norgestrel), 2 tablets with a repeat dose 12 hours later.

Rarely the assault results in significant genital injuries for which surgical repair is needed. Consultation with the gynecology service should be considered in these cases.

Children who have been chronically abused rarely need medical treatment unless they have contracted a sexually transmitted disease. They, like victims of acute assaults, benefit from psychologic counseling.[37] It is appropriate for the emergency department staff to maintain a roster of local agencies that provide these services to sexual abuse victims.

TESTIFYING IN COURT

Even after evaluating the patient, securing the appropriate consultative services, initiating needed management and referrals, and reporting the case to protective services and law enforcement agencies, the physician may find that his or her involvement does not end. The testimony of the examining physician is often key to the courtroom case.[7, 10, 38] There are a number of different courts in which child abuse cases are heard: family court (for divorce and custody issues), dependency court (investigating the ability of parents to care for and protect the child), and criminal court (determining the guilt or innocence of the perpetrator). In any of these cases, the physician should review the records and discuss the findings with the attorney who issued the subpoena before going to court. Child abuse cases frequently arouse conflicting and intense emotions, and it is helpful for the physician who is testifying to remember that the purpose is to share with the court the truth as determined by the medical findings related to the abuse.

CONCLUSION

The emergency physician is in a unique position as the first person to evaluate the child. He or she may not only be responsible for gathering the evidence to corroborate the child's story, but may also be able to begin the process of emotional recovery for the child.

References

1. National Center on Child Abuse and Neglect. Study Findings—Study of National Incidence and Prevalence of Child Abuse and Neglect 1988. Washington, DC, US Dept of Health and Human Services, 1988.
2. Durfee M. Los Angeles, Los Angeles County Department of Health Services, Child Abuse Prevention Program, 1990.
3. Krugman R. Recognition of sexual abuse in children. Pediatr Rev 1986;8:25.
4. Seidel JS, Elvik SL, Berkowitz CD, et al. Presentation and evaluation of sexual misuse in the emergency department. Pediatr Emerg Care 1986;2:157.
5. Gomes-Schwartz B, Horowitz JM, Sauzier M. Severity of emotional distress among sexually abused preschool, school-age, and adolescent children. Hosp Community Psychiatry 1985;36:503.
6. Newberger E. Pediatric interview assessment of child abuse. Challenges and opportunities. Pediatr Clin North Am 1990;37:943.
7. De Jong AR, Finkel MA. Sexual abuse of children. Curr Probl Pediatr 1990;20:489.
8. Meyers JEB. Role of physician in preserving verbal evidence of child abuse. J Pediatr 1986;109:409.
9. Capraro VJ. Sexual assault of female children. Ann NY Acad Sci 1967;142:817.
10. Berkowitz CD: Sexual abuse of children and adolescents. Adv Pediatr 1987;34:275.
11. MacFarlane K. Please No, Not my child . . . Coping with Sexual Abuse of Your Preschool Child. Los Angeles, Children's Institute International, 1985.
12. Yates A. Children eroticized by incest. Am J Psychiatry 1982;139:482.

13. Hunter RS, Kilstrom N, Loda F. Sexually abused children: Identifying masked presentations in a medical setting. Child Abuse Negl 1985;9:17.

14. Chadwick DL, Berkowitz CD, Kerns DL, et al. Color Atlas of Child Sexual Abuse. Chicago, Year Book, 1989.

15. Herman-Giddens ME, Frothingham TE. Prepubertal female genitalia: Examination for evidence of sexual abuse. Pediatrics 1987;80:203.

16. Emans SJ, Goldstein DP. The gynecologic examination of the prepubertal child with vulvovaginitis: Use of the knee-chest position. Pediatrics 1980;65:758.

17. McCann J, Voris J, Simon M, Wells R. Comparison of genital examination techniques in prepubertal girls. Pediatrics 1990;85:182.

18. Woodling BA, Heger A. The use of the colposcope in the diagnosis of sexual abuse in the pediatric age group. Child Abuse Negl 1986;10:111.

19. McCann J. Use of the colposcope in childhood sexual abuse examinations. Pediatr Clin North Am 1990;37:863.

20. McCauley J, Gorman RL, Guzinski G. Toluidine blue in the detection of perianal lacerations in pediatric and adolescent sexual abuse victims. Pediatrics 1986;78:1039.

21. Goff CW, Burke KR, Rickenback C, Buebendorf DP. Vaginal opening measurement in prepubertal girls. Am J Dis Child 1989;143:1366.

22. Cantwell HB. Vaginal inspection as it relates to child sexual abuse in girls under thirteen. Child Abuse Negl 1983;7:171.

23. Tipton AC: Child sexual abuse: Physical examination techniques and interpretation of findings. Adolesc Pediatr Gynecol 1989;2:10.

24. Heger A, Emans SJ. Introital diameter as the criterion for sexual abuse. Pediatrics 1990;85:22.

25. Adams JA, Ahmad M, Phillips P. Anogenital findings and hymenal diameter in children referred for sexual abuse examination. Adolesc Pediatr Gynecol 1988;1:123.

26. Emans SJ, Woods ER, Flagg NT, et al. Genital findings in sexually abused, symptomatic and asymptomatic girls. Pediatrics 1987;79:778.

27. Woodling BA, Kossoris PD. Sexual misuse: Rape, molestation and incest. Pediatr Clin North Am 1981;28:481.

28. Norvell MK, Benrubi GI, Thompson RJ. Investigation of microtrauma after sexual intercourse. J Reprod Med 1984;29:269.

29. Paul DM. The medical examination in sexual offenses against children. Med Sci Law 1977;17:251.

30. Spencer MJ, Dunklee P. Sexual abuse of boys. Pediatrics 1986;78:133.

31. Ellerstein NS, Canavan JW. Sexual abuse of boys. Am J Dis Child 1980;134:255.

32. Woodling BA. Sexual abuse and the child. Emerg Med Serv April 1986;17.

33. Hobbs CJ, Wynne JM. Buggery in childhood: A common syndrome of child abuse. Lancet 1986;2:792.

34. Hobbs CJ, Wynne JM. Sexual abuse of English boys and girls: The importance of anal examination. Child Abuse Negl 1989;13:195.

35. McCann J, Voris J, Simon M, et al. Perianal findings in prepubertal children selected for non-abuse: A descriptive study. Child Abuse Negl 1989;13:211.

36. Sproles ET. The Evaluation and Management of Rape and Sexual Abuse: A Physician's Guide. Rockville, MD, National Center for Prevention and Control of Rape, US Dept of Health and Human Services, Public Health Services, NIMH, 1985.

37. Sgroi SM. Handbook of Clinical Intervention in Child Sexual Abuse. Lexington, MA, Lexington Books, DC Health, 1982.

38. Chadwick DL. Preparation for court testimony in child abuse cases. Pediatr Clin North Am 1990;37:955.

SECTION TWO

Cardiovascular Disease

CHAPTER 16

Congenital Heart Disease

Louis A. Cannon
Danny C. Blankenship

INTRODUCTION

Abnormalities in cardiovascular structure or function that are present at birth or develop during normal maturation comprise a group of conditions known as *congenital heart disease* (CHD). These malformations are often genetic or multifactorial in origin and may represent an arrest in embryogenesis, exposure to toxins, or exposure to infectious agents. CHD is predominantly a male disorder, with the exception of patent ductus arteriosus (PDA) and atrial septal defect (ASD), which are predominant in females. CHD affects approximately 0.8% of live births, a figure that probably underrepresents the true prevalence of the disorder, as patients who often present later in life with mitral valve prolapse, ASD, or bicuspid aortic valve are not usually included in these statistics.[1]

Congenital cardiovascular anomalies may be associated with other cardiovascular or somatic anomalies.[2] The fetal alcohol syndrome is often associated with ventricular septal defect (VSD), microcephaly, micrognathia, microphthalmia, growth retardation, and developmental delays.[3] Maternal exposure to rubella during pregnancy is associated with multiple cardiovascular anomalies including PDA, pulmonic or aortic stenosis, and ASD, as well as cataracts, deafness, and microcephaly.[4]

The emergency physician should know the noncardiac anomalies associated with CHD so that associated conditions (e.g., hypercalcemia associated with supravalvular aortic stenosis or syncope secondary to complete heart block in corrected tetralogy of Fallot) may be recognized and treated correctly (Table 16–1).

ANATOMY AND PHYSIOLOGY
Fetal Circulation

In utero, most of the fetal cardiac output is delivered to the placenta as a result of the placenta's lower vascular resistance; here oxygen, carbon dioxide, and nutrient ex-change occurs. Blood, about 80% saturated with oxygen, is returned to the fetus by the umbilical vein. Most of this flow bypasses the liver through the ductus venous (Fig. 16–1) and flows into the inferior vena cava, where it mixes with a smaller amount of deoxygenated blood returning from the lower extremities. Blood then enters the right atrium and is directed by the eustachian valve to the foramen ovale, where approximately one third of the flow enters the left atrium, mixing with a small amount of blood returning from the lungs. This preferential shunting of inferior vena caval blood to the left heart results in selective flow of oxygenated blood to the coronary and cerebral circulations through the ascending aorta. The remaining desaturated inferior vena caval flow mixes with superior vena caval and coronary sinus return and enters the right ventricle and main pulmonary artery. Because the pulmonary vascular resistance (PVR) is high, most of the flow passes through the ductus arteriosus into the descending aorta, where it returns to the placenta by two umbilical arteries.

Circulatory Changes at Birth

The major hemodynamic change at birth is the shift of flow from the placenta to the lungs. Expansion of the lungs with the first few breaths causes a sudden reduction in the PVR, a drop in the pulmonary artery pressure, and an increase in pulmonary blood flow. The increased left atrial pressure caused by the increased pulmonary venous return, plus the decreased right atrial pressure resulting from interruption of placental flow through the ductus venosus, results in a left-greater-than-right interatrial pressure difference. This leads to functional closure of the foramen ovale as the septum primum is pressed against the septum secundum, usually resulting in eventual fusion of the two septa by 1 year of age. Interruption of the umbilical cord results in an increase in the systemic vascular resistance (SVR) with removal of the low-resistance placental circulation. Interruption of placental flow also results in closure of the umbilical arteries, which form the remnant ligamentum teres hepatis, ligamentum venosum, and umbilical ligaments. Increased arterial oxygen saturation and the release of bradykinins from the expanded lungs result in functional closure of the ductus arteriosus, which forms the remnant ligamentum arteriosum.

Embryology

Cardiac development and the environmental and genetic influences on maldevelopment are complex. Formation of the various cardiac structures depends on a rather intricate,

TABLE 16–1

CONGENITAL CARDIOVASCULAR DISEASE AND ASSOCIATED ABNORMALITIES

Cardiac Abnormality	Associated Noncardiac Abnormality	Syndrome
Supravalvular aortic stenosis	Hypercalcemia Elfin facies Inguinal hernias Dental anomalies	Williams'
Atrial septal defect with prolonged atrioventricular conduction	Thumb deformities Abnormal carpal bones, scapula, radius, ulna	Holt-Oram
Pulmonary/aortic stenosis Hypertrophic cardiomyopathy Complete heart block	Lentigines EKG changes Ocular hypertelorism Pulmonary stenosis Abnormal genitals Retarded growth Deafness—sensorineural	Leopard
Aortic insufficiency	Multiple fractures Blue sclerae	Osteogenesis imperfecta
Atrioventricular canal defects Ventricular septal defects	Mental retardation Simian crease Short neck Phalangeal hypoplasia	Down
Coarctation of aorta Aortic stenosis	Shield chest Webbed neck Pectus excavatum Phenotypic females	Turner's
Pulmonary valve stenosis Atrial septal defect	Short stature Webbed neck Mental retardation Pectus excavatum	Noonan's

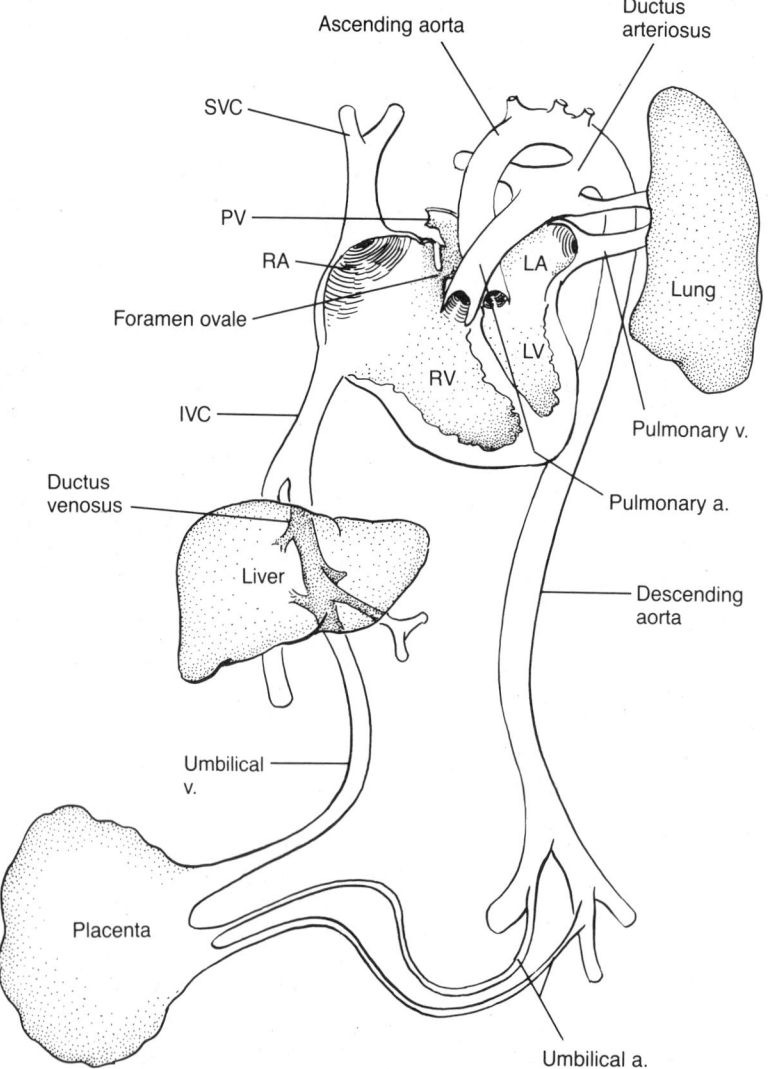

Figure 16–1. Diagram of the fetal circulation showing the four sites of shunt: placenta, ductus venosus, foramen ovale, and ductus arteriosus. Intravascular shading is in proportion to oxygen saturation, with the lightest shading representing the highest Po_2. The numerical value inside the chamber or vessel is the Po_2 for that site in mm Hg. The percentages outside the vascular structures represent the relative flows in major tributaries and outlets for the two ventricles. The combined output of the two ventricles represents 100%. IVC = Inferior vena cava; LA = left atrium; LV, left ventricle; PV = pulmonary vein; RA = right atrium; RV = right ventricle; SVC = superior vena cava. (Modified from Guntheroth WG, et al. Physiology of the circulation: Fetus, neonate and child. *In* Kelley VC (ed). Practice of Pediatrics. Vol. 8. Philadelphia, Harper & Row, 1982–83, p. 70.)

interdependent, and progressive sequence of differential growth. Most cardiac defects form between the third and seventh gestational week as the primitive heart tube divides into the typical four-chambered structure. Most abnormalities occur during this period and include cardiac position abnormalities (dextrocardia), chamber partition abnormalities (atrioventricular canal defects; atrial or ventricular septal defects), valve malformation (Ebstein's anomaly; stenotic or regurgitant tricuspid, pulmonic, mitral, or aortic lesions), truncal partitioning and rotation abnormalities (tetralogy of Fallot; transposition of the great arteries; truncus arteriosus), and pulmonary venous drainage abnormalities (partial or total anomalous pulmonary venous return).

EMERGENCY MEDICAL SERVICE CONSIDERATIONS

Paramedics called to the scene to aid a child in distress should follow routine protocols. Distress in a pediatric patient should not be assumed to have a cardiac origin, even if a diagnosis of CHD is known. Respiratory embarrassment is still the primary concern during decompensation. Resuscitation attempts should be directed at establishing an airway and supporting breathing before administration of cardiac drugs is considered. The child with CHD will usually assume a position that reduces the work of breathing (e.g., squatting or a knee-to-chest position). Attempts should be made to transport the patient in this position. The presence of a family member may be helpful during transport to alleviate the child's anxiety, which can further contribute to decompensation.

SPECIFIC ABNORMALITIES OF STRUCTURE AND FUNCTION

Coarctation of the Aorta

Coarctation of the aorta (COA) accounts for about 8% of all congenital heart defects and may be minimally or overtly symptomatic from birth.[5] Coarctation is frequently associated with a bicuspid aortic valve and is the most common cardiovascular abnormality associated with Turner's syndrome.

Pathophysiology

Variation in the extent and location of the aortic coarctation will influence the presence and severity of symptoms and its association with other cardiac defects (Fig. 16–2). *Postductal COA* is most common and is usually a focal, hourglass-shaped stenotic lesion distal to the ductus arteriosus and the left subclavian artery. It is less frequently associated with other cardiac defects, is microscopically characterized by thickening of the aortic media, and usually does not produce symptoms in infancy. *Preductal COA* exists as either a focal or long stenotic segment of the aorta proximal to the ductus arteriosus. This is frequently associated with other cardiac defects (PDA, VSD, and transposition of the great arteries) and usually produces heart failure symptoms during infancy.

Many patients with COA have an abnormal bicuspid aortic valve that may become stenotic or regurgitant. Significant hypertension proximal to the stenotic lesion may cause ventricular dysfunction from pressure overload, formation of cerebral aneurysms, and development of intercostal collaterals, which cause rib notching.

Persistent flow across the ductus arteriosus in patients with severe preductal COA may cause a *differential cyanosis pattern*, in which deoxygenated blood from the right ventricular pulmonary circuit perfuses the lower half of the body. Variation in the blood flow to the upper extremities depends

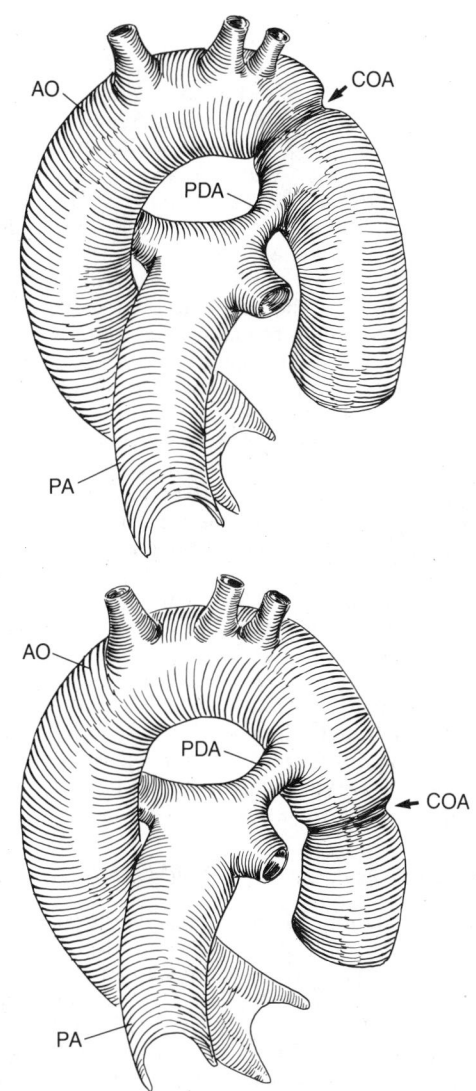

Figure 16–2. Two types of coarctation of the aorta (COA) in relation to the patent ductus arteriosus (PDA). Type A is preductal; type B is postductal. PA = Pulmonary artery; AO = aorta.

on the origin of the subclavian arteries relative to the coarctation. Diminished pulses and blood pressure gradients may not always be prominent or even appreciated in the lower extremities, especially in the presence of severe heart failure and decreased cardiac output.

The Symptomatic Infant With COA

Clinical Evaluation. The symptomatic infant with COA usually presents with congestive heart failure (CHF) and failure to thrive. These infants are usually pale, irritable, weak, and tachypneic and feed poorly. Lower extremity (differential) cyanosis may exist if right-to-left ductal flow is present. A prominent left ventricular heave, S_3 gallop, pulmonary rales, and hepatomegaly are usually present. A nonspecific systolic murmur over the precordium and back may be generated by the coarctation itself. A variety of systolic and diastolic murmurs may be produced by an accompanying VSD, PDA, or stenotic or regurgitant bicuspid aortic valve. A blood pressure differential and diminished pulses may be noted in the lower extremities and between the left and right arm, depending on the location and severity of the coarctation. These blood pressure and pulse differences may be seen only after a low-flow CHF state is ameliorated with digitalization and diuretic therapy.

Diagnostic Evaluation. The electrocardiogram usually reveals a rightward QRS axis with right ventricular hypertrophy (RVH). This pattern reflects the increased right ventricular afterload prenatally as it contributes blood flow through the PDA to the aorta. With an accompanying VSD or persistent PDA, the RVH pattern may persist. The chest radiograph reveals marked cardiomegaly with pulmonary venous congestion and edema.

Therapeutic Intervention. Medical care includes oxygen, diuretic, and digitalis therapy. Antibiotics are needed to prevent the development of endarteritis and aortitis.

CHF poorly responsive to medical therapy usually requires surgical repair. Resection of the coarcted segment with end-to-end anastomosis or various patch aortoplastic procedures may be used. A persistent PDA, if present, is also ligated. The type and timing of repair of other defects, such as a VSD, depends on multiple hemodynamic and technical factors. Periprocedural antibiotics should be administered when appropriate to prevent the development of endarteritis and aortitis.

Prognosis. The onset of CHF symptoms during infancy, seen most frequently in patients with preductal COA, often results in early death if not corrected. Postsurgical residual obstruction or restenosis may occur, especially in those who had surgery during infancy. Postsurgical follow-up should also include attention to the development of upper extremity hypertension, stenotic or regurgitant bicuspid aortic valve disease, and CHF symptoms. The periprocedural use of antibiotics will minimize endocarditis and aortitis.

The Asymptomatic Child With COA

Clinical Evaluation. Depending on the degree of stenosis or the presence of associated cardiac defects, COA may have few symptoms. Other than the infrequent complaints of headache and lower extremity fatigue or claudication, COA may be silent and may be discovered only after evaluation of an asymptomatic hypertensive patient. The most distinctive feature on physical examination is the blood pressure differential between the upper and lower extremities. Systolic hypertension above the 95th percentile for age is usually noted, along with a diminished, absent, or delayed femoral pulse. Although COA is commonly an associated finding in Turner's syndrome, most children experience normal growth and development into adulthood. A prominent apical left ventricular heave, a suprasternal systolic thrill, and a precordial or intrascapular murmur from the coarctation itself may be present. A systolic ejection murmur, ejection click, or the decrescendo diastolic murmur of aortic insufficiency may be heard in patients with associated bicuspid aortic valve disease.

Diagnostic Evaluation. The chest radiograph may reveal a minimally enlarged heart, dilatation of the ascending aorta, rib notching between the fourth and eighth ribs (in children over 5 years of age), and the aortic arch figure-of-three sign on overpenetrated films (Fig. 16–3), produced by the prominent aorta reflecting prestenotic and poststenotic dilatation. The electrocardiogram may be normal or demonstrate a change from right to left ventricular hypertrophy with a leftward QRS axis.

Therapeutic Intervention. Definitive surgical therapy is the treatment of choice for asymptomatic COA occurring during the first decade of life. Hypertensive crises can be managed by intravenous nitroprusside or other afterload-reducing agents. Prophylactic antibiotics and good dental hygiene are important in preventing endocarditis and aortitis, both before and after corrective surgery.

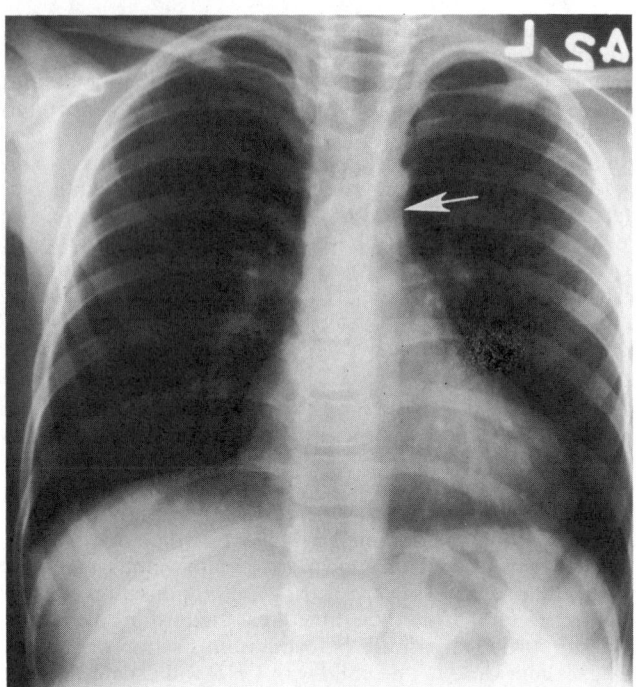

Figure 16–3. Coarctation of the aorta in a 6-year-old boy with upper extremity high blood pressure. On plain films, an indentation of the aortic density at the narrowing gives a figure-of-three sign *(arrow)*. The most definitive imaging is by magnetic resonance (MR). Already at this age, the patient also shows rib-notching of the undersurfaces of several posterior upper ribs. (Courtesy of A. Oestreich, M.D., Cincinnati, OH.)

Elective resection or various aortoplastic procedures are usually performed during the first decade of life, often just before the child begins school. Balloon angioplasty has also been successfully used, both in native and recurrent COA after surgical repair.

Paraplegia secondary to spinal cord ischemia during cross-clamping of the aorta occurs infrequently. A transient rebound hypertension may be seen during the first week after surgical repair and is probably the result of sympathetic nervous system hyperactivity and a transient rise in plasma renin activity; it may be prevented by early beta blocker use.[6]

Angiotensin converting enzyme inhibitors or other intravenous antihypertensive agents may also be used, but long-term antihypertensive therapy is seldom required. The post-coarctectomy syndrome (also known as necrotizing mesenteric arteritis) occasionally occurs and is characterized by abdominal pain, distention, fever, and leukocytosis during the first postoperative week. This syndrome is thought to be caused by an arteritis resulting from hemodynamic flow and pressure changes to the mesentery and in severe cases may lead to melena and the need for resection of gangrenous infarcted bowel. Delayed enteral feedings, nasogastric tube decompression, and control of rebound hypertension usually minimize this potential problem.

Prognosis. Autopsy studies in patients with uncorrected COA indicate a marked increased risk for hypertensive cardiovascular disease, hypertensive encephalopathy, intracranial bleeding, aortic dissection and rupture, and premature death. Studies have shown better survival rates, decreased rates of complications, and less persistent hypertension when surgical repair is performed at an early age. The average age of death in patients with coarctation of the aorta who do not elect to undergo surgery is 34 years.[7]

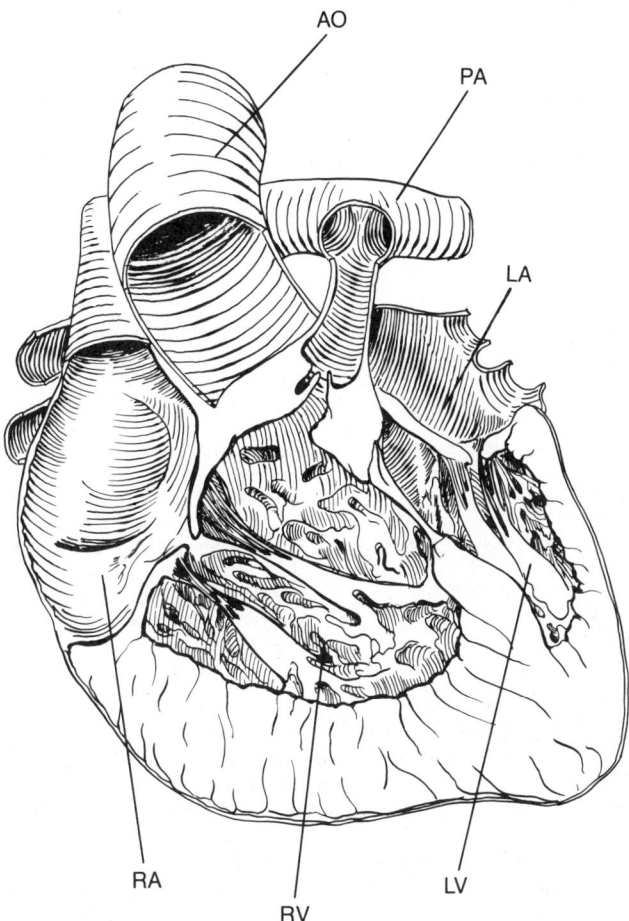

Figure 16–4. Tetralogy of Fallot. Note the right ventricular outflow obstruction, right ventricular hypertrophy, ventricular septal defect, and overriding aorta. AO = Aorta; PA = pulmonary artery; RA = right atrium; RV = right ventricle; LV = left ventricle; LA = left atrium.

Tetralogy of Fallot
Pathophysiology

Tetralogy of Fallot is the most common cardiac malformation responsible for cyanosis in children over 1 year of age and accounts for approximately 10% of all forms of congenital heart disease.[8]

There are four anatomic anomalies responsible for this condition: right ventricular outflow obstruction, right ventricular hypertrophy, ventricular septal defect, and overriding aorta (Fig. 16–4). The degree of obstruction to right ventricular outflow is the principal determinant of the degree of symptoms; severe right ventricular outflow obstruction will cause blood to flow through the path of least resistance (i.e., the ventricular septal defect), which causes right-to-left shunting, hypoxia, and increasing right ventricular pressures. This additional increase in right heart pressure causes worsening of the right-to-left shunt and may exacerbate cyanosis. This cycle of right-to-left shunting must be broken to allow blood to pass through the pulmonary circuit to alleviate hypoxia and symptoms.

Occasionally the degree of right ventricular obstruction is not severe, and cyanosis is not a prominent component of the patient's symptoms. These so-called *pink* or *acyanotic tets* exhibit the physiology of simple ventricular septal defects early in life; however, the degree of right ventricular obstruction often increases and may be progressive.

Clinical Evaluation

Dyspnea and cyanosis associated with exertion or feedings are common, and children will naturally assume a squatting position during periods of dyspnea, thereby increasing systemic vascular resistance, decreasing shunting, and increasing flow through the pulmonary tree. However, spells of intense cyanosis may develop that are resistant to squatting or rest and are responsible for significant morbidity and mortality. Progressive hypoxia may progress to syncope, seizures, cerebrovascular accidents, and death.[9] This is a common reason for presentation to the emergency department, and attention should immediately be focused on reducing hypoxia and the right-to-left shunt.

Children may also present with failure to thrive. Cardiac examination often reveals a right ventricular lift, a single second heart sound, and a systolic ejection murmur originating from the pulmonary artery that may be either soft during periods of cyanosis or so loud that it is palpable. A continuous murmur may indicate a PDA, an anomaly that may accompany the tetralogy of Fallot.

Diagnostic Evaluation

The chest radiograph shows a characteristic wooden shoe– or boot-shaped appearance *(coeur en sabot)* caused by right ventricular prominence and a poorly developed pulmonary vasculature (Fig. 16–5). A right-sided aortic arch may be present.

The electrocardiogram shows a right axis deviation and right ventricular hypertrophy. Postsurgical electrocardio-

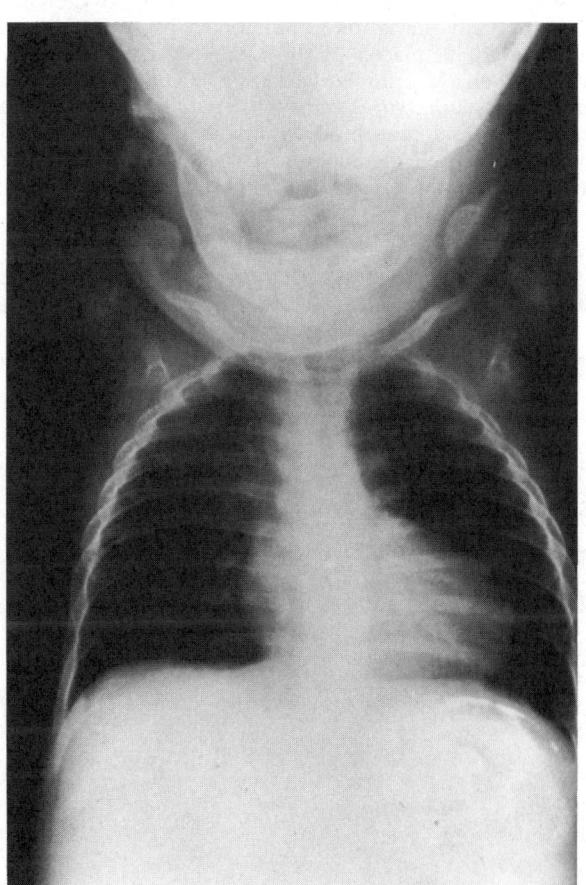

Figure 16–5. Chest radiograph of a child with tetralogy of Fallot, demonstrating the typical boot-shaped deformity (coeur en sabot).

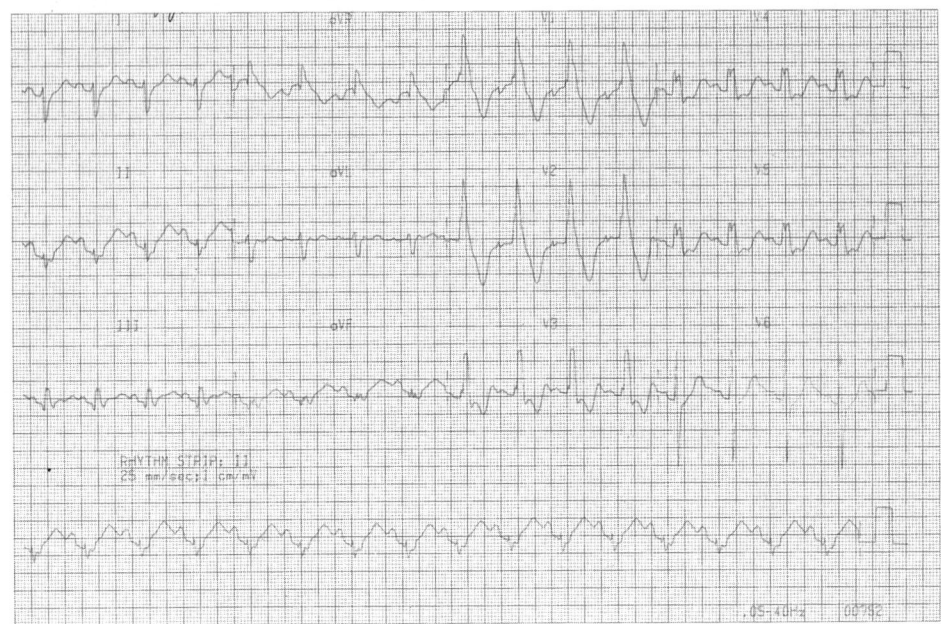

Figure 16–6. Electrocardiogram of a 10-year-old boy who underwent corrective surgery at an early age for single ventricle syndrome with transposition of the great arteries. It shows characteristics common to many patients with congenital heart disease, such as a wide right bundle branch block, first-degree atrioventricular (AV) block, atrial abnormality, right axis deviation, and probable right ventricular hypertrophy.

grams often reveal a bifascicular block involving a wide and often bizarre right bundle branch block (RBBB) configuration (Fig. 16–6).

Therapeutic Intervention

Treatment of a cyanotic spell centers on oxygenation, relaxation, and alleviation of pulmonary hypertension. The child should be placed in the knee-to-chest position and given oxygen. Morphine alleviates anxiety, decreases pulmonary artery pressure, and can be readily reversed. Occasionally, general anesthesia, intubation, and vasopressors may be needed. If metabolic acidosis develops, bicarbonate should be administered. Beta blockers may be helpful in

small doses to slow the ventricular rate. The hematocrit should be kept at 55% to 65% by phlebotomy.

A thorough search for the origin of decompensation should be made. Infections, dehydration, hyperviscosity from thrombocytosis, change in medications, and unusual exertion are often responsible for decompensation. Complications associated with tetralogy of Fallot include cerebral thrombosus (in patients less than 2 years of age), infectious endocarditis, brain abscesses (in patients over 2 years of age), and congestive heart failure.

The Blalock-Taussig shunt is the most common procedure used to alleviate the symptoms of tetralogy (Table 16–2). The procedure involves anastomosis of the right subclavian artery to the ipsilateral branch of the pulmonary artery to

TABLE 16–2			
SURGICAL TREATMENTS FOR COMMON CONGENITAL HEART DISEASES			
Procedure	**Disease**	**Correction**	**Complications**
Blalock-Taussig anastomosis	Tetralogy of Fallot	Subclavian to pulmonary artery	Endocarditis Heart failure
Potts or Waterson	Tetralogy of Fallot	Descending or ascending aorta to pulmonary artery	Endocarditis Heart failure
Glenn	Ebstein's anomaly	Superior vena cava to pulmonary artery	Heart failure
Fontan	Triscuspid atresia	Right atrium to pulmonary artery	Heart failure SVC syndrome
Rashkind	Tricuspid atresia Transposition of the great arteries	Interatrial septostomy	Endocarditis Heart failure
Mustard	Transposition of the great arteries	Atrial baffle	Endocarditis Heart failure
Jantene	Transposition of the great arteries	Arterial switch	Endocarditis Heart failure Right or left ventricular outflow obstruction
Rastelli	Persistent truncus arteriosus	Homograft from right ventricle to pulmonary artery Ventricular septal defect closure	Endocarditis Valvular insufficiency Right ventricular outflow obstruction Outgrowth of conduit
Norwood	Hypoplastic left ventricle	Staged correction	Endocarditis Heart failure

improve flow to the pulmonary circuit. Other less commonly used procedures involve anastomosis of the ascending aorta (Waterson) or descending aorta (Potts) to the pulmonary artery. Successful shunts will produce a continuous machinery type murmur and predispose to development of infective arteritis.

Definitive correction alleviates right ventricular outflow tract obstruction and corrects the ventricular septal defect. Hypoplasia of the pulmonary arteries often limits repair, and shunt procedures may help to increase pulmonary arterial flow and thereby enlarge the pulmonary vessels.

Prognosis

After successful operations, patients are generally in good health and able to lead relatively unrestricted lives. Younger patients should undergo a palliative anastomosis until definitive repair can be made. Older patients should undergo early definitive repair.

Ebstein's Anomaly
Pathophysiology

Ebstein's anomaly is created by downward displacement of the tricuspid valve into the lower portion of the right ventricular cavity (Fig. 16–7). The extent of displacement corresponds to the degree of impairment as the upper portion of the ventricle becomes dilated and atrialized, leaving only the small lower cavity to function as a normal ventricle.[10] In more than 50% of patients, an atrial septal defect coexists, or right atrial dilatation causes the foramen ovale to stay patent or widen, creating variable degrees of right-to-left shunting and cyanosis.[11]

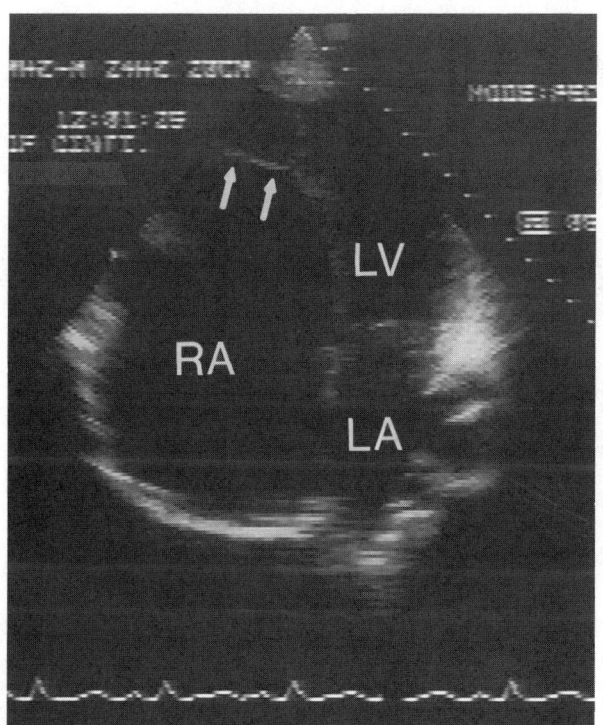

Figure 16–7. Two-dimensional echocardiogram of a patient with Ebstein's anomaly. Note the displacement of the tricuspid valve toward the ventricular apex *(arrows)* with right atrial enlargement. RA = Right atrium; LA = left atrium; LV = left ventricle.

Clinical Evaluation

The symptoms associated with Ebstein's anomaly may vary widely, from fatigue and palpitations to severe debilitation with dyspnea, cyanosis, and congestive heart failure. In the neonate, tricuspid regurgitation may be severe. However, as pulmonary pressures decline, the degree of tricuspid regurgitation diminishes, heart size decreases, and symptoms of heart failure abate.

Supraventricular tachycardias are common as a result of the association of accessory pathways with the Wolff-Parkinson-White (WPW) syndrome type B.[12] Coexistent anatomic anomalies often include atrial septal defects, pulmonary stenosis, ventricular septal defects, congenitally corrected transposition, and PDA.

Diagnostic Evaluation

Radiographic evaluation shows varying degrees of right atrial enlargement and cardiomegaly. Electrocardiography reveals a right bundle branch configuration either alone or in association with WPW type B. Wide P waves and PR prolongation are common (Fig. 16–8).

Therapeutic Intervention

Arrhythmia control and treatment of hypoxia and cyanosis are important. Surgical treatment is rarely necessary, and patients tend to do poorly postoperatively. Occasionally a Glenn procedure is used to anastomose the right pulmonary artery to the superior vena cava to alleviate the volume overload of the right atrium and ventricle. Most patients survive into the third decade without serious impairment.[10]

Tricuspid Atresia
Pathophysiology

Tricuspid atresia is characterized by agenesis of the tricuspid orifice with no communication between the right atrium and ventricle. The right ventricle becomes hypoplastic, and circulation to the pulmonary arteries is dependent on interatrial communication through an atrial septal defect, with pulmonary artery flow by way of a VSD or PDA. This syndrome is often accompanied by other anomalies, including transposition of the great arteries (TGA), pulmonary stenosis, or persistent left superior vena cava.[13]

Clinical Evaluation

Many infants with tricuspid atresia fail to survive even the first weeks of life because of persistent hypoxemia. Cyanosis, clubbing, and failure to thrive dominate the clinical picture. Usually a pansystolic or systolic ejection murmur is heard at the left sternal border. The second heart sound is classically single because of lack of development of the pulmonary elements.

Diagnostic Evaluation

Deficient pulmonary arterial shadows are noted, along with a straight right heart border, similar to that seen in tetralogy of Fallot. The electrocardiogram reveals the classic combination of right atrial enlargement, left axis deviation, and left ventricular hypertrophy. These findings in a cyanosed infant are strongly suggestive of tricuspid atresia.

Therapeutic Intervention

Cardiac catheterization is diagnostic as well as temporarily therapeutic, as balloon atrial septostomy (Rashkind proce-

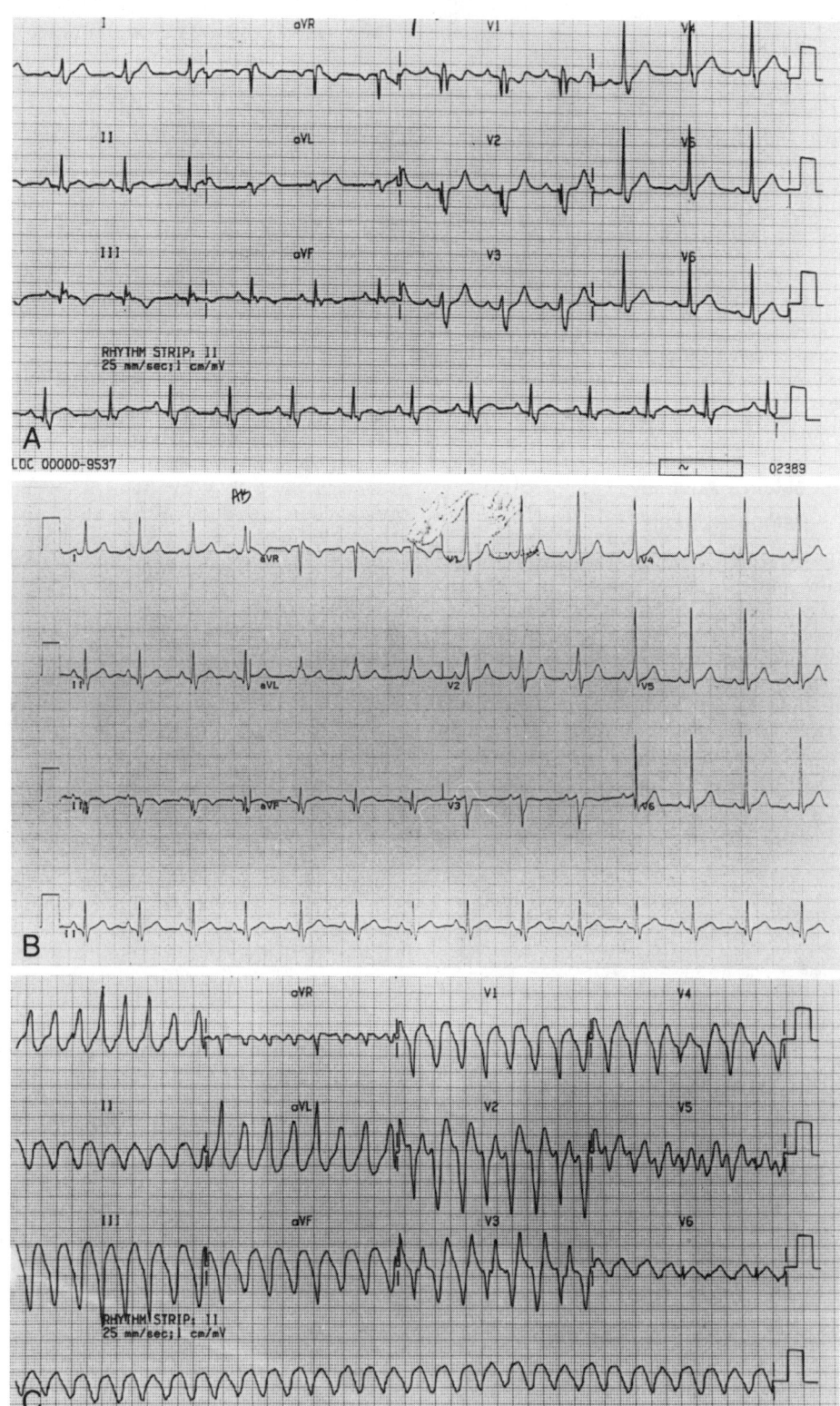

Figure 16–8. Electrocardiograms of a patient with Ebstein's anomaly. *A*, A wide, bizarre, atypical right bundle branch pattern. There is evidence of right atrial enlargement. *B* (same patient) shows a short P-R interval and delta waves that are seen best in V₁ and V₂. (Actually, leads V₁ and V₃ are transposed in this tracing.) This suggests ventricular pre-excitation through an accessory pathway. *C* shows a wide complex rhythm with precordial concordance of a wide QRS pattern from V₁ to V₆. Closer inspection in leads aVR and aVL and in V₆ shows an occasional narrow complex beat (first and fourth from the end of V₆). Although these beats would typically indicate fusion beats in ventricular tachycardia, in this instance they may indicate both orthodromic (narrow complex) and antidromic (wide complex) conduction through both the AV node and accessory pathway, respectively. Note the bizarre right bundle branch and delta wave in the right precordial leads, consistent with accessory pathway and Wolff-Parkinson-White syndrome.

dure) may widen or create an interatrial communication. This is performed by inflating a balloon in the interatrial septum, often through a patent foramen ovale. This increases flow to the left atrium, alleviates right heart symptoms, and improves pulmonary blood flow by taking advantage of other associated lesions such as a VSD or PDA.[14]

Infusion of prostaglandins in the neonate may be lifesaving by avoiding closure of a PDA. Alprostadil (formerly called prostaglandin E[1], or PGE[1]) should be administered immediately in doses ranging from 0.01 to 0.05 µg/kg/min; overdose may cause respiratory suppression or complete apnea. After infancy, however, medical management is supportive until definitive surgery can be performed.

A prosthetic conduit (Fontan procedure) can be placed between the right atrium and pulmonary artery to improve pulmonary blood flow and minimize right-to-left shunting of blood. This procedure can only be performed if the pulmonary arteries are of adequate size and pulmonary vascular resistance is relatively normal.[15]

Prognosis

Surgical improvement is not as successful as with tetralogy of Fallot.[16] Patients often have postoperative superior vena caval syndrome, as well as right and left heart failure.[17] Only 50% of patients survive to the second decade after successful operations.[16]

Patent Ductus Arteriosus
Pathophysiology

A PDA is necessary for survival in utero. It can be harmful in infants who fail to thrive because of left-to-right shunt and pulmonary hypertension, or it may be life-sustaining in infants with certain congenital anomalies with decreased pulmonary flow (e.g., complete transposition of the greater arteries or tricuspid atresia). The ductus arteriosus connects the aorta to the left pulmonary artery just distal to the left subclavian artery. Although the exact stimulus for closure is unknown, prostaglandins are intimately involved. Alprostadil can be given to infants to keep the ductus open, and prostaglandin inhibitors such as indomethacin can be used to promote its closure.[18] Appreciable left-to-right shunting often complicates the care of premature infants who weigh less than 1500 gm and may contribute to congestive heart failure and respiratory distress unresponsive to routine medical therapy.[19]

Clinical Evaluation

Parents often seek medical attention because of the child's failure to thrive or because of dyspnea that occurs during feedings. Physical examination reveals a characteristic thrill and "continuous" murmur at the left upper sternal border and interscapular area posteriorly. Although said to be continuous, the murmur is usually heard prominently during systole, peaks during the second heart sound, and decrescendoes through all or a part of diastole until the gradient for flow between the aorta and pulmonary artery diminishes in mid to late diastole. If severe pulmonary hypertension or systemic hypotension is present, the diastolic component of the murmur may be absent, as the higher pulmonary pressures do not permit a gradient for significant amounts of flow to take place between the aorta and the pulmonary tree.

Radiographic findings include a prominent pulmonary artery and aortic shadows with pulmonary vascular enlargement. Left atrial and left ventricular hypertrophy predominate as delayed electrocardiographic findings.

Therapeutic Intervention

In conditions such as pulmonary stenosis, tricuspid atresia, and hypoplastic left ventricle, the patent ductus may be the only mechanism for flow to the pulmonic or systemic circuits. Closure in these instances can be catastrophic; alprostadil should be administered immediately in doses ranging from 0.01 to 0.05 µg/kg/min. Overdose may cause respiratory suppression or complete apnea. Because patency of the ductus arteriosus reverts circulation to the prenatal state, administration of alprostadil is often lifesaving and rarely, if ever, absolutely contraindicated, especially when the exact anatomy is unknown, as is often the case when a decompensating patient presents to the emergency department.

Persistent pathologic patency of the ductus arteriosus is not in itself life-threatening until the excess of left-to-right flow eventually creates either right heart failure or an excessive right-to-left shunt. Bacterial endarteritis may involve a patent ductus; fever and signs of embolization may be present. Prostaglandin inhibitors such as indomethacin may permit pharmacologic closure, but surgery may be necessary. Surgical ligation of a patent ductus is a low-risk operation if heart failure has not yet developed.

Many patients survive without physical limitations until later in life, when heart failure or endarteritis supervenes. However, these complications may also take place at a younger age.

Atrial Septal Defects
Pathophysiology

ASDs are the most common congenital heart defect noted in adults but rarely cause serious disability in infants or children. There are three main types of ASD: *ostium primum*, which is a type of endocardial cushion defect, often involving the atrioventricular valves; *ostium secundum* (Fig. 16–9), which

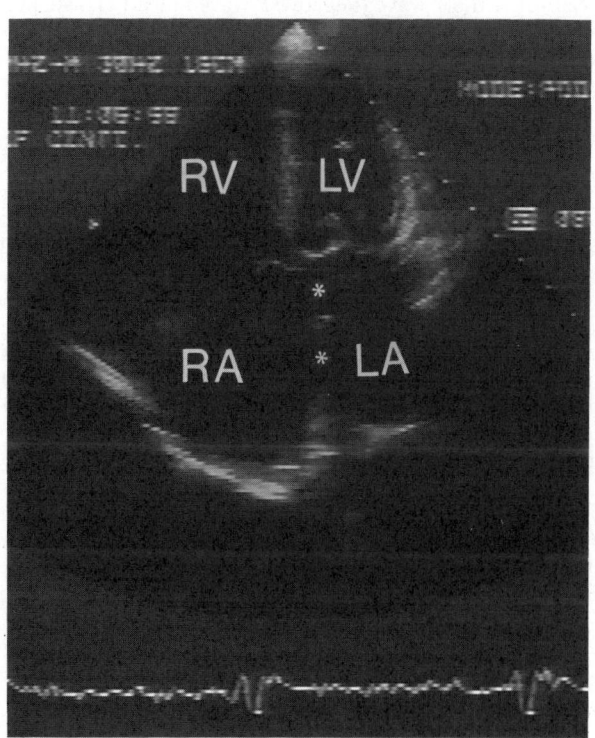

Figure 16–9. Note the lack of echogenic structure in the areas of the interatrial septum (*), indicating an atrial septal defect. RA = Right atrium; LA = left atrium; RV = right ventricle; LV = left ventricle.

exists along the area of the foramen ovale; and *sinus venosus*, which occurs in the upper part of the atrium near the superior venae cavae and is often associated with partial anomalous pulmonary venous return. The left atrium usually has a higher pressure than the right side, and therefore blood shunts from left to right at the time of peak atrial pressures near the end of ventricular and atrial systole.

Clinical Evaluation

There are occasional reports of heart failure, pneumonia, and failure to thrive in infancy, but serious disability early in life is rare unless a significant anomaly (e.g., anomalous pulmonary venous return or an atrioventricular valve anomaly) coexists. In adults or older children, atrial arrhythmias, pulmonary artery hypertension, and heart failure may develop. Somatic anomalies are commonly associated with ASDs. Any suspicion of an ASD should prompt a thorough physical examination, as ASD is often associated with somatic anomalies (see Table 16–1). Endocarditis is a consideration when fever exists, especially if mitral valve prolapse or a cleft mitral valve *(ostium primum)* is present.

Physical examination often reveals an increase in the tricuspid closure sound, a midsystolic pulmonary ejection murmur from increased flow or a mid-diastolic rumble. There may be a prominent right ventricular impulse with accentuation of pulmonary closure. The classic fixed or widely split second heart sound may be absent early in life until pulmonary vascular resistance falls.

Diagnostic Evaluation

Radiographs may show enlargement of the right atrium and ventricle, as well as prominent pulmonary vasculature. The electrocardiogram shows a classic left axis deviation with rSR′ or rsR′ in ostium primum ASD and lack of left axis deviation with or without the incomplete right bundle branch block pattern in ostium secundum defects. Left axis deviation of the P wave (negative P wave in lead III) strongly supports the diagnosis of sinus venosus ASD. In these patients, anomalous pulmonary venous return with a left-to-right shunt must also be a consideration.

Therapeutic Intervention

Management of patients presenting with heart failure should be supportive until an accurate diagnosis can be made by echocardiography or cardiac catheterization. Early operative repair is ideal.

Operation is usually performed by insertion of a patch or by direct suturing. Operative mortality in uncomplicated ASDs is less than 1%. Surgery should be performed with caution in patients with trivial shunts (ratio of pulmonary to systemic flow, <1.5:1.0) or in patients with severe pulmonary artery hypertension (ratio of pulmonary to systemic resistance, >0.7:1.0).[20]

The prognosis for children with uncomplicated ASDs is excellent. Surgery should be performed early if a large shunt exists. Infections should be treated promptly, and infectious endocarditis should be suspected for all children with fever or unexplained decompensation.

Aortic Valve Stenosis
Pathophysiology

Obstruction to left ventricular outflow may take place at the level of the aortic valve or at the supravalvular or subvalvular levels. The common factor, obstruction to ventricular outflow, may precipitate myocardial infarction from the increased oxygen demands of a failing hypertrophied ventricle, pulmonary edema, or left-to-right shunt through a patent foramen ovale or PDA. Cardiovascular anomalies that coexist in up to 20% of cases of aortic stenosis include a PDA, coarctation of the aorta, and branch pulmonic stenosis.

Clinical Evaluation

Aortic stenosis at any level may be a medical emergency, and delay in diagnosis may be catastrophic. Although some patients tolerate this lesion remarkably well, others quickly decompensate. A history of dyspnea with feedings and general failure to thrive may be appreciated in infants with severe obstruction. Aortic stenosis may even present as a medical emergency in the first few hours of life.

A characteristic elfin appearance with mental retardation and hypercalcemia is commonly noted in patients with supravalvular obstruction (Williams syndrome); however, no characteristic appearance is noted for valvular or subvalvular stenosis. The precordium is hyperactive, with a palpable precordial systolic thrill and left ventricular lift. An aortic valve opening snap along with a diminished closing sound suggests a valvular origin for stenosis. A distinct aortic valve closure sound and a lack of an opening snap is characteristic of subvalvular or supravalvular aortic stenosis rather than a valvular anomaly. A loud, harsh, ejection systolic murmur is best heard at the base of the heart, and an early diastolic murmur may indicate the presence of concomitant aortic insufficiency. Aortic closure may be delayed or may not be heard until after the pulmonic sound.

Left ventricular hypertrophy or poststenotic dilatation of the ascending aortic root may be seen radiographically. The electrocardiogram is highly variable and often shows left ventricular predominance with hypertrophy and strain pattern.

Therapeutic Intervention

There is no definitive medical therapy for decompensated aortic stenosis. Any decompensation should prompt urgent cardiologic consultation for intervention (balloon valvuloplasty) or surgical therapy. Patients with mild to moderate degree of obstruction (0.5 to 1.2 cm²/M²) may be observed closely and treated symptomatically. Prophylactic antibiotic treatment should be advised, and strenuous activity, afterload reduction, and inotropes should be avoided.

Balloon aortic valvuloplasty is a nonsurgical option performed in the cardiac catheterization laboratory by inflating a balloon across the stenotic aortic valve to stretch and crack the deformed leaflets. Though aortic insufficiency may occasionally be created, the procedure is generally safe and effective, at least temporarily.

Operation should be considered for any symptomatic child with critical stenosis (valve area < 0.5 cm²/M²). The decision to operate in cases of mild to moderate obstruction with or without symptoms is controversial. The mortality rate is less than 2% in centers with experienced surgeons when the aortic valve ring is not hypoplastic.[21]

Prognosis

Patients who become symptomatic with moderate or critical stenosis should have surgery or valvuloplasty before life-threatening decompensation takes place. After surgical valve replacement, most patients can lead normal, active lives. They should be maintained on chronic anticoagulation therapy if a mechanical prosthesis is used, and appropriate antibiotics should be administered for endocarditis prophylaxis.

Hypertrophic Cardiomyopathy
Pathophysiology

Hypertrophic cardiomyopathy (HCM) has multiple synonyms, including idiopathic hypertrophic subaortic stenosis (IHSS), and may be obstructive or nonobstructive depending on the varying degrees of hypertrophy and the anatomic relationship in the left ventricle. When confined to the septum (Fig. 16–10), the hypertrophy limits left ventricular outflow similar to a subvalvular obstruction, whereas in other circumstances, the hypertrophy is confined to the apical region. The disorder occurs at all ages and is associated with an increased risk of sudden death. It is transmitted by an autosomal dominant pattern with a variable degree of penetrance and expressivity.[22]

Clinical Evaluation

Many children are asymptomatic but receive evaluation because of a striking murmur. Others experience dyspnea and shortness of breath on exertion with angina and weakness. Patients with Noonan's syndrome and leopard syndrome may develop hypertrophic cardiomyopathy, and physical findings supportive of these syndromes should be noted (see Table 16–1). The pulse is brisk and may be bifid because of the obstruction to outflow in midsystole. The murmur is systolic, has a crescendo-decrescendo pattern, enhances markedly with the Valsalva maneuver or on standing, and diminishes with squatting or maneuvers that increase afterload. The aortic sound is preserved without evidence of an opening snap, thereby helping to differentiate this murmur from valvular aortic stenosis.

The radiographic examination is usually normal, and electrocardiographic findings are variable. Signs of left ventricular hypertrophy may be present, as may a pseudoinfarct pattern with prominent Q waves noted in the inferior leads.

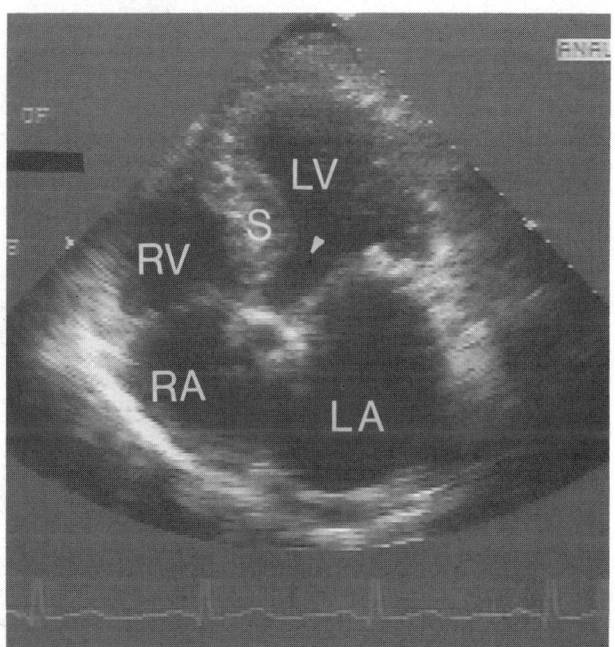

Figure 16–10. Two-dimensional echocardiogram of a patient with a localized septal form of hypertrophic cardiomyopathy. The hypertrophied ventricular septum partially obstructs the left ventricular outflow tract *(arrowhead)* during ventricular systole. RA = Right atrium; LA = left atrium; RV = right ventricle; LV = left ventricle; S = interventricular septum.

Therapeutic Evaluation

Medical therapy centers on increasing preload, decreasing contractility, and lowering heart rates. Because tachycardia shortens diastole, further decreasing the time available for filling of the hypertrophied noncompliant ventricle, pharmacologic agents that slow heart rate (e.g., beta blockers or verapamil) have been found to be quite effective. If arrhythmias are problematic, diisopyramide and amiodarone may be used, taking advantage of diisopyramide's negative inotropic as well as antiarrhythmic effects.[23] Digitalis and isoproterenol are contraindicated, because they increase contractility and worsen obstruction. Diuretics are also contraindicated unless heart failure occurs, as lower ventricular volumes often increase the intraventricular gradient.

Atrial fibrillation may be life-threatening if an atrial systolic "kick" is needed to fill the noncompliant, stiff left ventricle. Immediate cardioversion in the emergency department is often lifesaving. Digitalis may be used cautiously if there is no response to beta blockers or verapamil. Surgical myectomy is reserved for the minority of patients with incapacitating symptoms, recurrent syncope, and disabling angina. The prognosis of patients with hypertrophic cardiomyopathy is highly variable and dependent on response to medications, the presence of heart failure, and life-threatening arrhythmias.

Pulmonary Valve Stenosis
Pathophysiology

Patients with pulmonary valve stenosis may lead normal lives or may be incapacitated by the symptoms produced from right ventricular obstruction. In cases of severe obstruction, right-to-left shunting through a patent foramen ovale occurs, and cyanosis is common. Valvular stenosis is the most common form of right ventricular obstruction and is especially common in patients with Noonan's syndrome. The leaflets may be compliant and pliable with commissural fusion, or the valve itself may be dysplastic, thickened, and immobile. The degree of obstruction and the resultant gradient are the important physiologic determinants.

Diagnostic Evaluation

The chest radiograph often shows a normal-sized heart, normal vascularity, occasional poststenotic dilatation, or prominence of the left pulmonary artery. In patients with severe stenosis, there may be right atrial or right ventricular enlargement and decreased pulmonary vasculature. The electrocardiogram shows right atrial and right ventricular hypertrophy in severe cases, but is usually normal.

Therapeutic Intervention

Medical management alone is all that is needed in the majority of cases, and treatment is supportive. The course is generally favorable and does not require limitation of activities.[24] In patients with severe stenosis with compliant, pliable leaflets and commissural fusion, a valvuloplasty may be performed. In patients with a dysplastic, thickened valve, surgery is required. Prophylactic treatment for infective endocarditis is required in all cases of pulmonary stenosis.

Surgery for pulmonary stenosis is a low-risk, high-yield procedure. In patients with a dysplastic valve and malformed right ventricular outflow tract, a patch may also be needed to widen the right ventricular outflow tract.

Prognosis

The prognosis for patients with mild to moderate pulmonary stenosis is favorable. Close observation should be maintained during the child's first decade, as a small number of patients may worsen. The prognosis for critical pulmonary stenosis is dependent on the adequacy of pulmonary valvuloplasty or surgery; both are low-risk procedures.

Dextrocardia

Dextrocardia is a malposition of the heart such that the apex is pointed to the right side of the chest. This definition does not refer to the position of the great vessels or the ventricles. *Kartagener's syndrome* is associated with dextrocardia, immotile cilia, sinusitis, and reversal of the abdominal viscera. The reversal of abdominal and chest organs is termed *situs inversus. Dextroversion* refers to rightward displacement of the left chest contents as a result of right chest collapse or from compressive left-sided forces, such as tension pneumothorax. Isolated dextrocardia without reversal of abdominal viscera is seen in association with other severe congenital anomalies.

The chest radiograph shows the heart apex oriented toward the right chest. This may be surprisingly difficult to diagnose as a result of the usual tendency for physicians to place the radiograph on the viewing board with the heart on the left side. If the left and right markers are not checked, the radiographic diagnosis may be elusive.

The electrocardiogram shows inversion of the usually upright complexes in limb lead I. Precordial leads V_1 to V_6 reveal decreasing R-wave progression. Recording the limb leads in the wrong position will create the same limb lead changes as dextrocardia; however, the precordial leads will show normal R-wave progression, thus differentiating dextrocardia from lead misplacement.

Transposition of the Great Arteries
Pathophysiology

TGA accounts for 5% to 7% of all congenital cardiac malformations.[25] It is more common in male infants and often presents with progressive cyanosis from birth. It is inevitably lethal without medical and surgical therapy.

TGA is a malformation in which the aorta arises from the right ventricle and the pulmonary artery arises from the left ventricle as a result of abnormal development of the truncoconal septum. Because of this malformation, hypoxemic blood is recirculated back to the systemic circulation while hyperoxemic blood is recirculated within the pulmonary circuit. Survival after birth depends on a communication between the two parallel circuits, with intercirculatory mixing through a defect such as a patent foramen ovale (PFO), VSD, or PDA. Other associated defects, such as tricuspid artresia, pulmonary left ventricular outflow tract obstruction, and coarctation of the aorta, may also occur. The degree of cyanosis, pulmonary hypertension, and congestive heart failure are influenced by the amount of intercirculatory mixing through the intra- or extracardiac communications. Infants with poor mixing (i.e., those with an intact ventricular septum, a closed VSD, or a small PFO) may have marked cyanosis from birth; infants with better mixing (i.e., those with a large VSD or PDA) may have less cyanosis, but marked heart failure. The presence of associated obstruction to pulmonary flow may exacerbate the degree of cyanosis but impede the development of pulmonary hypertension. Regardless, unless intercirculatory mixing is improved by medical or surgical intervention, progressive hypoxia, heart failure, acidemia, hypoglycemia, hypothermia, and death will occur.

Clinical Evaluation

The majority of infants with TGA are born large for gestational age and become dyspneic and progressively cy-

anotic during the first week of life. Tachypnea, congestive heart failure, and growth retardation develop, with the timing and severity dependent on the associated defects. An array of physical findings may be present, including cyanosis, clubbing, rales, hepatomegaly, bounding pulses (caused by a PDA), and a systolic or continuous murmur (caused by an associated VSD, pulmonary stenosis, or PDA). Pulmonary hypertension may be diagnosed by the presence of a right ventricular heave, a loud second heart sound, or early diastolic murmur of pulmonary insufficiency. Cyanosis is usually progressive and may precipitously worsen if the PDA closes or during stress and crying-induced hypoxic spells. Differential cyanosis, in which the legs are more cyanotic than the upper extremities, may be observed if reversed pulmonary-to-systemic shunting occurs across a PDA. However, the degree of cyanosis may be less marked or may even be subtle if there is sufficient mixing of the pulmonary and systemic circulations through a large foramen ovale, a large VSD, or persistent opening of the PDA. Oxygenation is usually improved at the expense of increased pulmonary hypertension or congestive heart failure.

Polycythemia and arterial oxygen desaturation are usually present. Small increases in arterial oxygen tension with supplemental 100% oxygen are suggestive of poor intracirculatory mixing. Simultaneous blood gas readings from the upper and lower extremities (or the umbilical artery) may confirm the differential cyanosis pattern suspected on physical examination.

Diagnostic Evaluation

The chest radiograph typically reveals a characteristic oval or egg-shaped heart (Fig. 16–11) with a narrow cardiac base in the frontal projection (as a result of superimposition of

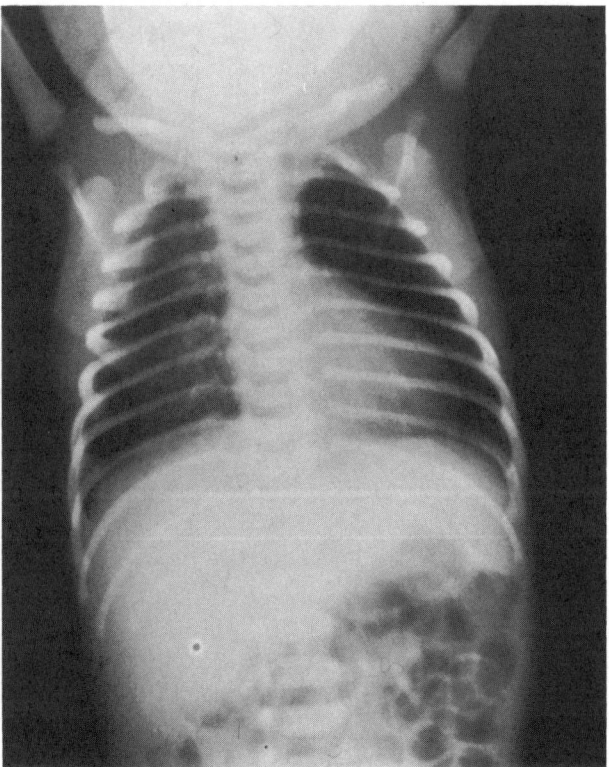

Figure 16–11. Chest radiograph of a child with transposition of the great arteries. Note the broad-based, egg-shaped heart with narrow mediastinum caused by superimposition of the aorta and pulmonary artery.

the aortic and pulmonary trunk shadows) and hypoplasia of the thymus because of the associated stress and cyanosis. Progressive cardiomegaly and increased vascular markings are common.

The electrocardiogram may be normal in the newborn, but right axis deviation, right or biventricular hypertrophy and P-pulmonale soon develop. Arrhythmias are infrequent before surgery but are common after palliative or corrective procedures.

Therapeutic Intervention

A tachypneic and cyanotic neonate with suspected TGA is a medical emergency. Supplemental oxygen, maintenance of a normal body temperature, and correction of hypoglycemia or metabolic acidemia are beneficial. Digoxin and diuretic therapy may help in infants with evidence of congestive heart failure. Intravenous alprostadil administered in the early neonatal period may keep the PDA open and improve intracirculatory mixing and tissue oxygenation. These efforts should be followed by transfer to a cardiac center where a confirmatory emergency catheterization can be performed.

Initial palliative treatment in the neonate usually involves balloon atrial septostomy, or the *Rashkind procedure,* which improves intracardiac mixing of the pulmonic and systemic circulations. This is followed 3 to 12 months later by either a definitive atrial baffle *Mustard procedure* or a *Senning procedure* creating a serial pulmonary-to-systemic circulation pattern, with the left and right ventricles remaining as the pulmonary and systemic ventricles, respectively.[26] The *Jantene procedure* involves switching the transposed aorta and pulmonary artery to the normal left and right ventricular outflow, respectively, with reimplantation of the coronary arteries from the right to the reconstructed left ventricular systemic outflow channel.

Prognosis

Most surgical survivors lead active lives during childhood, and the 15-year survival rate is 70%.[27] The growing number of survivors with surgically corrected TGA presents a unique set of problems during childhood and adolescence. Brady- and tachyarrhythmias are commonly seen in patients who have undergone atrial baffling procedures. Palpitations, light-headedness, or syncope may result from these arrhythmias, and there is a presumed arrhythmogenic basis for the sudden unexplained deaths in 2% to 9% of this population. Furthermore, long-term concerns exist for the development of infective endocarditis, right (systemic) ventricular failure, tricuspid regurgitation, suture line anastomotic stenosis, and obstruction to the surgically altered venous return to the heart.

Anomalous Pulmonary Venous Connections
Pathophysiology

Anomalous pulmonary venous connections, in a variety of patterns, account for 1% to 2% of all congenital heart defects.[28] Partial anomalous pulmonary venous connection (PAPVC) occurs when one or more, but not all, of the pulmonary veins drain into the right atrium or its venous contributories. PAPVC usually involves the right pulmonary veins, with pulmonary venous return to the superior vena cava, the right atrium, or the inferior vena cava. Anomalous connections of the left pulmonary veins may drain into a persistent left superior vena cava or coronary sinus.

Total anomalous pulmonary venous connections (TAPVC)

occurs when all the pulmonary veins drain into the right atrium. To sustain life there must be an interatrial communication through an ASD, PFO, or VSD. The magnitude of the increased recirculation through the lungs is dependent on the number of anomalous pulmonary veins, the size of the septal defect or PFO, and the pulmonary vascular resistance. The systemic cardiac output in TAPVC is dependent on the size of the interatrial right-to-left communication. Increased pulmonary blood flow plus the occasional added obstruction of the pulmonary venous return to the right heart may result in pulmonary hypertension, right-to-left shunting with cyanosis, and CHF.

TAPVC can be divided into supracardiac, cardiac, and infracardiac types with or without accompanying obstruction of the anomalous pulmonary venous return. An intrinsic obstruction may develop secondary to progressive pulmonary arteriole hypertrophy, intimal proliferation, or pulmonary hypertension. Extrinsic obstruction may be seen with infracardiac types.

Partial Anomalous Pulmonary Venous Connection

Clinical Evaluation. Depending on the nature of the anomalous connections and the resulting hemodynamics, patients with PAPVC may remain asymptomatic until adulthood or may present during infancy with cyanosis, CHF, frequent pneumonia, or death.

Children with PAPVC are usually asymptomatic but may subsequently develop cyanosis and exertional dyspnea during their third and fourth decades as a result of chronic pulmonary hypertension and increasing right-to-left shunting. Straining, crying, or swallowing transiently increases intra-abdominal pressure and may cause impingement of an anomalous intracardiac vein by the esophagus, resulting in transient cyanosis in some patients.

Baseline cyanosis, however, is usually absent. A split S_2, a systolic pulmonary outflow murmur at the left upper sternal border, and a diastolic tricuspid flow murmur at the left lower sternal border may be present.

Diagnostic Evaluation. The chest radiograph usually reveals increased pulmonary vascularity and cardiomegaly, reflecting increased pulmonary flow and enlargement of the main pulmonary artery, right atrium, and right ventricle. Other radiographic features may also suggest the actual site of anomalous connection. A crescent-shaped vertical shadow in the right lower lung field may be seen with the *scimitar syndrome* (Fig. 16–12), which is associated with anomalous connection of the right pulmonary veins to the inferior vena cava. (The anomaly is named after the characteristic shape of the scimitar sword.) This may be accompanied by hypoplasia of the right lung and dextroposition of the heart. Pulmonary infections are commonly seen in patients with the scimitar syndrome.

A prominent supracardiac shadow may be seen at 3 to 4 months of age with anomalous drainage of the left pulmonary veins into a persistent left superior vena cava (vertical vein). This malformation, together with the *innominate* vein and right superior vena cava, produces a *figure-of-eight* or *"snowman"* appearance of the heart. Anomalous connections to the superior vena cava are suggested by dilatation above the right atrial shadow.

The electrocardiogram may be normal or show evidence of right ventricular hypertrophy or right bundle branch block. A sinus venosus ASD is associated with anomalous pulmonary venous return. The electrocardiogram characteristically shows a low atrial or junctional rhythm.

Therapeutic Intervention. The usual medical management of CHF and pulmonary infection is indicated. Childhood exercise should not be restricted, and prophylaxis for bacterial endocarditis is not routinely needed.

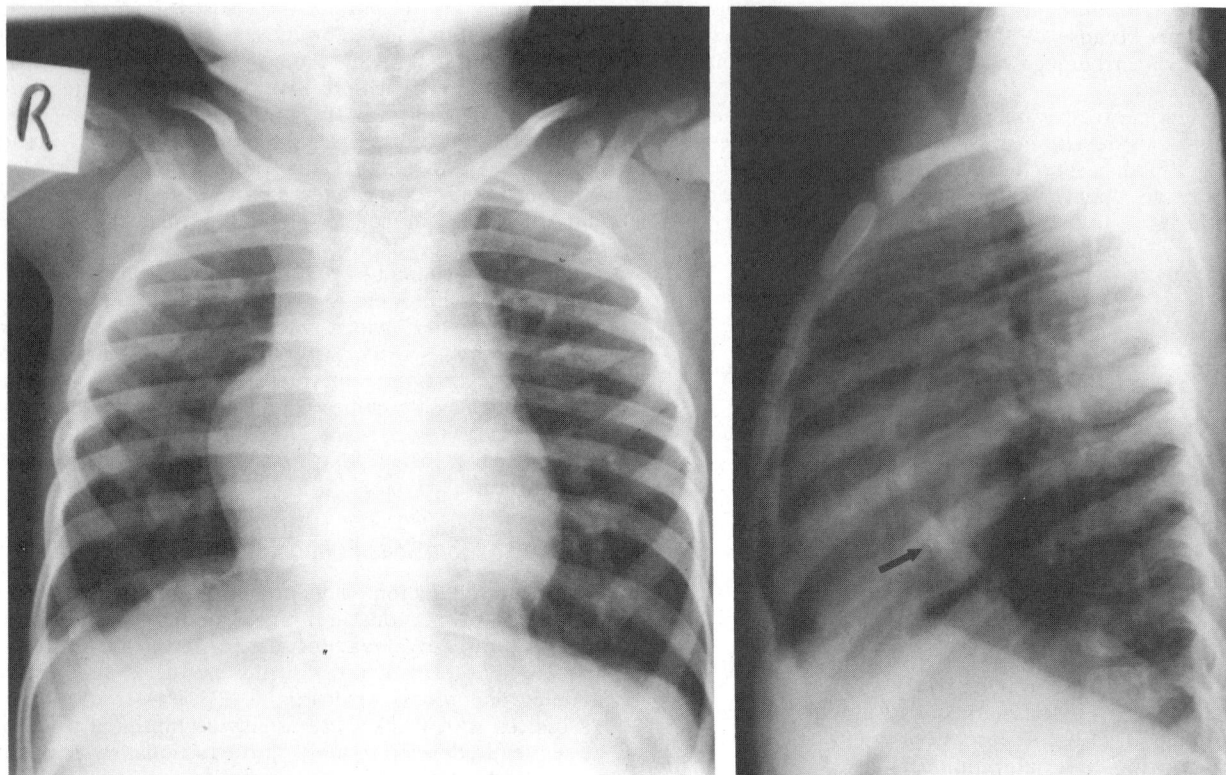

Figure 16–12. The scimitar-shaped vessel *(arrow)* on the lateral film of this 2½-year-old girl is typical of an anomalous pulmonary vein partially draining the lungs into the inferior vena cava below the diaphragm in the scimitar syndrome. The dextroposition of the heart and smaller right lung are also a part of this venolobar syndrome. (Courtesy of L. Young, M.D., Loma Linda, CA, and A. Oestreich, M.D., Cincinnati, OH.)

A significant left-to-right shunt with a ratio greater than 1.5:1 or 2:1 is an indication for surgical correction, usually at 4 to 5 years of age. The corrective procedure depends on the site of the anomalous connection but usually requires cardiopulmonary bypass with diversion of the anomalous pulmonary flow into the left atrium. Anomalous right pulmonary connections to the inferior vena cava in *scimitar syndrome* cases may be eliminated by resection of the involved lobes of the right lung without connecting the anomalous vein to the heart. Postoperative superior vena caval obstruction may rarely occur, but overall mortality is usually less than 1%. Postoperative supraventricular arrhythmias typical of the sick sinus syndrome may be seen, especially with correction of an associated sinus venosus ASD.

Prognosis. Patients with only one anomalous pulmonary vein with an intact septum usually have only a small left-to-right shunt and, therefore, an excellent prognosis. The natural history of symptomatic, uncorrected patients is unknown, but is probably similar to the largely uncomplicated early course of patients with an ASD. Dramatic improvement and a near-normal life span are expected postoperatively in symptomatic patients who have not already developed significant pulmonary hypertension.

Total Anomalous Pulmonary Venous Connection

Clinical Evaluation. Clinical findings in TAPVC are variable, depending on the adequacy of life-sustaining, interatrial shunting and the pulmonary vasculature hemodynamics. The clinical course is often divided according to whether pulmonary venous obstruction is present or absent.

Without pulmonary venous obstruction, mild cyanosis, CHF, tachypnea, feeding difficulties, and growth retardation develop as the neonate matures. A right ventricular heave, hepatomegaly, and multiple cardiac sounds (a quadruple or quintuple rhythm) may be heard, including a loud S_1, a widely fixed-split S_2, a systolic pulmonic ejection murmur at the left upper sternal border, an S_3, and a diastolic tricuspid flow murmur.

With pulmonary venous obstruction, marked cyanosis, respiratory distress, and growth failure are seen in the early neonatal period but usually not during the first 12 hours of life. A split S_2, hepatomegaly, rales, and an S_3 may be present, but a cardiac murmur and right ventricular heave are often absent.

Regardless of the presence or absence of obstruction, all the venous blood returns to the right atrium, so both anomalous systems require interatrial, interventricular, or ductal communication to sustain life.

Diagnostic Evaluation. Chest radiographs of children without pulmonary venous obstruction are similar to those of patients with PAPVC. However, in those with pulmonary venous obstruction, the heart size may appear normal, despite radiographic evidence of pulmonary edema.

The electrocardiogram may reveal a rightward QRS axis, right atrial hypertrophy, ventricular hypertrophy, and an incomplete right bundle branch block pattern.

Therapeutic Intervention. Supplemental oxygen, diuretics, digitalis, and mechanical ventilation with positive end-expiratory pressure (PEEP) may be needed during initial management. Balloon or blade atrial septostomy are palliative procedures that improve interatrial mixing. However, these should not significantly delay the more definitive surgical correction.

Corrective surgery is generally indicated. Surgical mortality is high, between 10% and 50%, but is still better than with medical management alone. Obstruction of anastomotic sites may occur, requiring future surgeries.[29] Postoperative supraventricular arrhythmias, including the sick sinus syndrome, may occur.

Prognosis. Most untreated patients with TAPVC die by 1 year of age. The degree of interatrial shunting and pulmonary vascular hemodynamic properties influence the course of individual cases. The long-term postoperative prognosis depends on the degree of pulmonary hypertension present at the time of surgery, thus favoring early surgical correction before pulmonary vascular occlusive disease develops.

Persistent Truncus Arteriosus
Pathophysiology

Persistent truncus arteriosus (PTA) accounts for less than 1% of all congenital heart malformations and without early surgical correction is usually fatal during childhood. PTA is characterized by a single arterial trunk that emanates from the base of the heart and supplies the pulmonary, systemic, and coronary circulations. This defect is caused by maldevelopment of the truncal ridges, which normally fuse and separate the truncal lumen into the ascending aorta and main pulmonary artery channels. Normal development of the truncal ridges also contributes to formation of the upper ventricular septum; maldevelopment accounts for the supracristal or infundibular VSD that is always present with a PTA. As a result, the undivided truncus receives blood from and often overrides both ventricles. A single truncal valve with a variable number of deformed cusps develops and may be functionally insufficient or, rarely, stenotic. Several anatomic variants of PTA may exist and are classified according to the origin of the main, left, and right pulmonary arteries.

The resulting increased pulmonary blood flow and the potential for truncal valvular insufficiency provides the pathophysiologic basis for biventricular hypertrophy, cardiac enlargement, hypertensive pulmonary obstructive vascular disease, CHF, and cyanosis. A functional stenosis of the pulmonic vasculature may develop; this protects the lungs from pulmonary edema and hypertensive obstructive changes but results in increased right-to-left shunting and progressive cyanosis. Although PTA usually occurs as an isolated cardiovascular malformation, associated extracardiac anomalies may include a right or interrupted aortic arch, an absent ductus arteriosus, an aberrant subclavian artery, a secundum ASD, PAPVC, coronary abnormalities, tricuspid valve malformations, skeletal deformities, hydroureter, and bowel malrotation.

Clinical Evaluation

The development, severity, and timing of PTA symptoms depends on the volume of pulmonary blood flow and the amount of truncal valve insufficiency. Dyspnea, poor feeding, CHF, and variable degrees of cyanosis are seen within the first weeks of life. The cyanosis may actually decrease or disappear during the first weeks after birth as the pulmonary vascular resistance decreases, permitting increased left-to-right shunting. A loud single S_2, rales, hepatomegaly, jugular venous distention, and an S_3 may be present. A harsh systolic regurgitant murmur and thrill from the VSD is usually present along the left sternal border. Bounding pulses; a wide pulse pressure; an active precordium; and a high-pitched, early diastolic, decrescendo murmur may be present if truncal valve insufficiency exists. An apical low-pitched diastolic mitral murmur may be present because of the increased pulmonary flow.

The chest radiograph usually reveals moderate cardiomegaly and increased pulmonary vascular markings. When present, a right aortic arch and increased pulmonary vascular markings may be seen. The electrocardiogram may reveal biventricular hypertrophy, a slightly rightward axis, and, occasionally, left atrial enlargement.

Therapeutic Intervention

Medical supportive therapy is limited to diuretics, digitalis, and endocarditis prophylaxis. Most patients with uncorrected PTA die of CHF within the first year of life, particularly if truncal valvular insufficiency coexists. Palliative pulmonary artery banding may help protect the pulmonary vascular bed from hypertensive obstructive changes. However, the *Rastelli procedure* represents a more definitive corrective approach. The VSD is closed in a fashion that enables the left ventricle to eject into the truncus, and a valved homograft or synthetic conduit is placed from the right ventricle to the pulmonary artery, which has been excised from the truncus.

Coexisting truncal valvular insufficiency may require reconstructive valvuloplasty. Corrective surgery is usually done at 1 or 2 years of age, before significant pulmonary vascular obstructive disease develops. Successful surgical correction during infancy will eventually require insertion of a larger conduit as somatic growth continues. Postoperative progression of truncal valvular insufficiency, CHF, and pulmonary vascular disease may be seen. Uncorrected PTA results in death during early childhood, usually from CHF, pulmonary vascular obstructive disease, or endocarditis.

Complete Atrioventricular Canal Defect
Pathophysiology

Complete atrioventricular (AV) canal or endocardial cushion defect accounts for 2% of all congenital heart malformations and may be associated with *Down syndrome*.[30]

A complete AV canal defect consists of a primum type ASD (i.e., defect in the lower portion of the atrial septum), a membranous VSD, and a common AV valve with a cleft in the septal and anterior leaflet of the tricuspid and mitral portions, respectively. A partial or incomplete AV canal defect is similar, but with an intact ventricular septum. Both types are characterized by increased pulmonary blood flow because of left-to-right shunting and by variable degrees of tricuspid and mitral regurgitation because of the abnormally cleft AV valves.

Clinical Evaluation

Symptoms usually develop during infancy and are characterized by bouts of pulmonary edema, respiratory infections, tachycardia, tachypnea, and failure to thrive. Examination may reveal a hyperdynamic precordium; a loud S_1 and split S_2 with P_2 accentuation; a harsh III/VI to IV/VI holosystolic, left-to-right regurgitant murmur with a palpable thrill at the left lower sternal border; and a separate crescendo-descrescendo systolic murmur at the left upper sternal border from increased pulmonary flow. Pulmonary rales, an S_3 gallop, and hepatomegaly suggest congestive heart failure. A diastolic rumbling murmur at the left upper sternal border and the apex may be heard because of flow through the abnormal tricuspid and mitral valves, respectively. Cyanosis or clubbing is usually not seen except in children and young adults who develop occlusive pulmonary vascular disease from chronic pulmonary hypertension.

Diagnostic Evaluation

The chest radiograph is characterized by cardiomegaly and increased pulmonary vascular markings with a prominent main pulmonary artery. The electrocardiogram usually reveals a normal sinus rhythm with first-degree AV block, right atrial enlargement, left atrial enlargement, a leftward QRS axis between −60 and −135 degrees, some degree of right bundle branch block and right ventricular hypertrophy, and left ventricular hypertrophy.

Therapeutic Intervention

Routine diuretic and digitalis therapy is indicated for CHF. Antibiotic and supportive therapy for recurrent pulmonary infections and prophylactic antibiotic treatment for bacterial endocarditis are indicated.

Pulmonary artery banding offers adequate palliation to many patients who have large left-to-right shunts and are unresponsive to medical therapy. Early corrective surgery between a few months and several years of age involves patch closure of the ASD and VSD and reconstruction of the cleft mitral valve.[31] Postsurgical complications may include development of subaortic stenosis and arrhythmias, which may require pacemaker or medical anti-arrhythmic therapy.

Prognosis

When left untreated, the majority of patients will die within the first several years of life. Those who survive to childhood, adolescence, or young adulthood usually develop symptomatic pulmonary hypertension with a right-to-left shunt.

Ventricular Septal Defect
Pathophysiology

VSD is the most common congenital heart defect, accounting for approximately 20% of all cases of congenital heart disease.[25] Defects in the ventricular septum may occur in various sizes and anatomic locations. They may occur in the muscular or membranous septum, above the crista supraventricularis (supracristal or subpulmonic), or just below the common AV canal in patients with complete AV canal defects and an associated primum type ASD. The resulting hemodynamics largely depend on the size, not the location, of the defect. A small VSD offers a high resistance to left-to-right shunting, resulting in a small increase in pulmonary flow and pressure, and often closes spontaneously during the first year of life. The resistance to left-to-right shunting in larger VSDs is dependent on the level of pulmonary vascular resistance. The high pulmonary pressures in infants with larger VSDs delays the normal fall in pulmonary vascular resistance after birth, delaying the onset of pulmonary edema until 6 to 8 weeks of age. Gradually progressive and irreversible increases in pulmonary vascular resistance may occur with the development of pulmonary vascular obstructive disease in patients with large, uncorrected VSDs.

Clinical Evaluation

A small VSD may have minimal hemodynamic or clinical consequences. However, delayed growth and development, recurrent pneumonias, CHF, and decreased exercise tolerance are usually seen in infancy with larger VSDs. A hyperdynamic precordium and a regurgitant holosystolic murmur with or without a thrill may be present at the lower left sternal border. Larger shunts across a VSD may be suggested by an accentuated pulmonic sound at the left upper sternal border or by an apical mitral diastolic murmur created by the combined systemic and shunt flow through the normal mitral valve. Pulmonary rales, hepatomegaly, and an S$_3$ heart sound may be present in patients with accompanying CHF. Development of the *Eisenmenger complex* with reversed right-to-left shunting, cyanosis, and decreased exercise tolerance is an ominous sign and usually does not occur until the second decade of life.

Diagnostic Evaluation

Increased pulmonary vascularity and cardiomegaly involving the left atrium, left ventricle, and even the right ventricle may be seen depending on the size of the VSD and the amount of left-to-right shunting. The radiographic or electrocardiographic presence of left atrial enlargement helps distinguish a VSD from an ASD. End-stage pulmonary hypertension with Eisenmenger's physiology is characterized by prominent main and perihilar pulmonary arteries and oligemia of peripheral lung fields. A serial decrease in the patient's baseline cardiomegaly may be noted as the volume of left-to-right shunting decreases or reverses.

Patients with small VSDs may have a normal electrocardiogram. Moderate to large VSDs usually create left atrial and left or biventricular hypertrophy.

Therapeutic Intervention

Small VSDs with a pulmonary-to-systemic flow ratio of less than 1.5:1 usually do not require surgery. Normal physical activity without exercise restriction is allowed in the absence of pulmonary hypertension. Close monitoring for CHF symptoms, particularly during infancy, and symptomatic treatment with digitalis and diuretic therapy is indicated. Early recognition and appropriate antibiotic therapy for pulmonary infections is essential. Good dental hygiene and antibiotic prophylaxis for infective endocarditis are indicated both before and after corrective surgery.

Large VSDs with pulmonary-to-systemic flow ratios greater than 2:1, CHF unresponsive to medical management, recurrent pneumonias, and progressive increases in the pulmonary vascular resistance are all indications for surgical repair. Direct patch or suture closure of the defect under cardiopulmonary bypass is preferably done on symptomatic infants or electively before 2 to 4 years of age in more stable patients.[32] Some infants with large VSDs may develop significant infundibular pulmonary stenosis also requiring surgery. Aortic regurgitation may also develop as a result of prolapse of one or more of the aortic cusps into a supracristal VSD. Corrective surgery is contraindicated and is of no benefit in older patients with severe pulmonary hypertension or in those with the *Eisenmenger* complex.

Prognosis

Patients with small VSDs of minimal hemodynamic consequence do well, with no change in life expectancy. For those requiring surgical correction, the low operative mortality rate and occasional conduction system abnormalities usually permit normal growth, development, and activity into adulthood. Appropriate medical or surgical therapy can usually prevent the complications of endocarditis, cerebral abscesses or thrombosis, and the development of the Eisenmenger complex.

Hypoplastic Left Ventricle Syndrome

Anomalies comprising this group of disorders are characterized by underdevelopment of the left cardiac chambers, particularly the left ventricle. Infants often present with heart failure during the first week of life. The anomaly is seen more often in males. Symptoms include heart failure, systemic hypoperfusion, and a cardiac murmur.

The electrocardiogram often shows right axis deviation because of lack of development of the left heart. Though findings on chest radiographs are often nonspecific, echocardiography is diagnostic.

Medical therapy is supportive only, and the anatomic defects are unfortunately only poorly amenable to surgical interventions.

References

1. Mitchell SC, Korones SB, Berendes HW. Congenital heart disease in 56,109 births. Incidence and natural history. Circulation 1971;43:323.
2. Greenwood RD, Rosenthal R, Parisi L, et al. Extracardiac abnormalities in infants with congenital heart disease. Pediatrics 1975;55:485.
3. Ouelette EM, Rosett HL, Rossman MP, Wiener L. Adverse effects on offspring of maternal alcohol abuse during pregnancy. N Engl J Med 1977;297:528.
4. de la Cruz MV, Munoz-Castellanos L, Nadal-Ginard S. Extrinsic factors in the genesis of congenital heart disease. Br Heart J 1971;33:203.
5. Nadus AS, Fyler DC. Pediatric Cardiology. 3rd ed. Philadelphia, WB Saunders, 1972.
6. Gidding SS, Rocchini AP, Beekman R, et al. Therapeutic effect of propranolol on paradoxical hypertension after repair of coarctation of the aorta. N Engl J Med 1985;312:1224–1229.
7. Maron BJ. Aortic Isthmus Coarctation. In Roberts WC (ed). Adult Congenital Heart Disease. Philadelphia, FA Davis, 1987.
8. Engle MA. Cyanotic congenital heart disease. Am J Cardiol 1976;37:283.
9. Morgan BC, Gunteroth WG, Blume RS, et al. A clinical profile of paroxysmal hyperpnea in cyanotic congenital heart disease. Circulation 1965;31:66.
10. Watson H. Natural history of Ebstein's anomaly of the tricuspid valve in childhood and adolescence. An international cooperative study of 505 cases. Br Heart J 1974;36:417.
11. Genton E, Blount SG. The spectrum of Ebstein's anomaly. Am Heart J 1967;73:395.
12. Kastor JA, Goldrier BN, Josephson ME, et al. Electrophysiologic characteristics of Ebstein's anomaly of the tricuspid valve. Circulation 1975;52:987.
13. Dick M, Fyler DC, Nadas AS. Tricuspid atresia: Clinical course in 101 patients. Am J Cardiol 1975;36:327.
14. Kyger ER, Reul GJ, Sandiford FM, et al. Surgical palliation of tricuspid atresia. Circulation 1975;52:685.
15. Tatooles CJ, Ardekani R, Miller RA, Serratto M. Operative repair of tricuspid atresia. Thorac Surg 1976;6:499.
16. Williams WG, Rubis L, Fowler RS, et al. Tricuspid atresia: Results of treatment in 160 children. Am J Cardiol 1976;38:235.
17. William DB, Kiernan PD, Schaff HV, Danielson GK. The hemodynamic response to dopamine and nitroprusside following right atrium–pulmonary artery bypass (Fontan procedure). Ann Thorac Surg 1982;34:51.
18. Friedman WF, Hirschklau MJ, Printz MP, et al. Pharmacologic closure of patent ductus arteriosus in the premature infant. N Engl J Med 1976;295:596.
19. Jones RWA, Pickering D. Persistent ductus arteriosus complicating the respiratory distress syndrome. Arch Dis Child 1977;52:274.
20. Cohn LH, Morrow AG, Braunwald E. Operative treatment of atrial septal defect: Clinical and haemodynamic assessments in 1975 patients. Br Heart J 1967;29:725.
21. Fisher RD, Mason DT, Morrow AG. Results of operative treatment in congenital aortic stenosis. J Thorac Cardiovasc Surg 1970;59:218.
22. Maron BJ, Mulvihill JJ. The genetics of hypertrophic cardiomyopathy. Ann Intern Med 1986;105:610–613.
23. Maron BJ, Bonon RO, Cannon RO, et al: Medical progress. Hypertrophic cardiomyopathy: Interrelation of clinical manifestation, pathophysiology and therapy. Part 2. N Engl J Med 1987;316:844.
24. Nadas AS (ed). Pulmonary stenosis, aortic stenosis, ventricular septal defect: Clinical course and indirect assessment. Circulation 1977;56:1.
25. Keith JD, Rowe RD, Vlad P. Heart disease in infancy and childhood. New York, Macmillan, 1978.
26. Williams WG, Trusler GA, Kirklin JW, et al. Early and late results of a protocol for simple transposition leading to an atrial switch (Mustard) repair. J Thorac Cardiovasc Surg 1988;95:717.
27. Castaneda AR, Trusler GA, Paul MH, et al. The early results of treatment of simple transposition in the current era. J Thorac Cardiovasc Surg 1988;95:14.
28. Clarke DR, Stark J, De Leval M, et al. Total anomalous pulmonary venous drainage in infancy. Br Heart J 1977;39:436.
29. Yee ES, Turley K, Hsieh WR, et al. Infant total anomalous pulmonary venous connection: Factors influencing timing of presentation and operative outcome. Circulation 1987;76(suppl 3):83.
30. Fyler DC. Report of the New England Regional Infant Cardiac Program. Pediatrics 1980;65(suppl 12):375.
31. Williams WM, Guyton RA, Michalik RE, et al. Individualized surgical management of complete atrioventricular canal defect. J Thorac Cardiovasc Surg 1983;86:838.
32. Weidman WH, Blount SG, DuShane JW, et al. Clinical course in ventricular septal defect. Circulation 1977;56(suppl 1):56.
33. Norwood WI, Lang P, Castenada AR, et al. Experience with operations for hypoplastic left heart syndrome. J Thorac Cardiovasc Surg 1981;82:511.

CHAPTER 17

Murmurs

Albert W. Sparrow

INTRODUCTION

Heart murmurs are often heard in infants, children, and adolescents, both during routine office examinations and during assessment in the emergency department. The frequency with which the presence of a murmur is recognized is dependent on the examiner's experience, the care in performing the auscultatory examination, the patient's physical state, and the lack of ambient noise. Murmur discovery and the subsequent educated analysis of its origin are critical skills for the emergency physician; it is necessary to differentiate pathologic from physiologic murmurs and organic from functional murmurs.

DEFINITIONS

The American College of Cardiology and the American Heart Association recognized that cardiovascular physical assessment is ever changing. To improve communication, The Bethesda Conference Committee on Standardized Terminology has published a glossary of terms,[1] some of which are given here.

Murmur. A murmur is a relatively prolonged series of auditory vibrations of varying intensity (loudness), frequency (pitch), quality, configuration, and duration. The murmur is produced by structural changes and hemodynamic events occurring in the heart or blood vessels. Thus a murmur can be physiologically defined as audible turbulence in flow as contrasted with, but physiologically identical to, palpable turbulence characteristic of a thrill over the precordium or great blood vessels. The terms *systolic, diastolic,* and *continuous* further define murmurs and are related to the cardiac cycle during which the murmur is heard.

Intensity (Loudness). Murmurs are graded from 1 to 6 according to their loudness. A grade 1 murmur is very faint and is often described as being audible only by the cardiologist. A grade 2 murmur is also faint but can be readily heard. A grade 3 murmur is moderately loud but is not associated with a thrill. A grade 4 murmur is loud and is associated with a thrill in the same area. Grade 5 and 6 murmurs are loud and are both associated with a thrill. A grade 5 murmur can be heard with the stethoscope just off the chest; a grade 6 murmur can be heard with the stethoscope 1 to 2 cm off the chest.

Frequency (Pitch). The predominant frequency band (pitch) of the murmur may vary from very high to very low and is determined by auscultation with the diaphragm and the bell of the stethoscope.

Quality. The particular tonal effect of a murmur is characterized by a descriptive term such as *blowing, harsh, rumbling,* or *musical.*

Configuration (Shape). *Crescendo* means that the loudness of the murmur increases progressively, and *decrescendo* means that the loudness decreases progressively. *Crescendo-decrescendo (diamond-shaped)* describes a murmur in which the loudness increases then decreases in progressive fashion. The word *plateau* suggests that the loudness remains relatively constant throughout.

PHYSIOLOGIC MURMURS

Physiologic murmurs by definition are murmurs that are not associated with any anatomic or pathologic abnormality. They are common in the pediatric age group, occurring in approximately 50% of children. Thus the emergency physician who treats children should be able to differentiate physiologic from pathologic murmurs.

The physiologic murmur is often referred to as *functional, normal, innocent, benign, inorganic,* or *innocuous.* When conversing with other physicians, the term *physiologic* is most apt, but when communicating with parents, the terms *innocent, normal,* and *functional* are better understood. The common thread in these terms and concepts is the absence of underlying heart disease or congenital abnormality. These murmurs are thought to result from the turbulence generated at the origin of the great arteries.[2] The great arteries originate from the ventricles at an angle and are considerably more narrow than the ventricles beneath. The resulting turbulence is more likely to be heard in the child because of the thin chest wall and the relative proximity of the heart beneath the chest wall.

The clinical features of the physiologic outflow murmur include early systolic presentation (except venous hum), short duration, low intensity (grade 1 or 2), low or occasionally medium pitch, a crescendo-decrescendo pattern, poor transmission (isolated), and lack of association with other cardiovascular abnormalities. Physiologic murmurs originate from both the right and the left heart structures. The clinical classification of the physiologic murmur is dependent on its origin (Table 17–1).

Still's Murmur

Still's murmur is the most common physiologic murmur and is characterized by a vibratory quality often likened to a groan, a frog's croak, or a low-pitched buzz or hum.[3] It is quite distinctive and is usually heard at the lower left sternal border with the patient in the supine position. This murmur is thought to originate from turbulent flow in the left ventricular outflow tract. Doppler echocardiography studies have shown that the origin of Still's murmur is related to the relative smallness of the ascending aorta combined with the concomitant increase in aortic flow velocity.[4] It is most often heard at 3 to 6 years of age but can be present from infancy to adolescence; it can be heard in 50% of children.

Pulmonary Ejection Murmur

The next most common physiologic murmur is the pulmonary ejection murmur, characteristically heard at the second left intercostal space with the patient in the supine position. It is harsh in quality, medium- to high-pitched, and quite different from the Still's murmur both in quality and location. This murmur is caused by turbulent flow from the right ventricular outflow tract and is heard most often between the ages of 8 and 14 years but can also be heard in infants and young children. In a study of vibratory functional murmurs, a lower prevalence of such murmurs was noted in children at 4500-m elevations.[5] The presumed higher hematocrit at higher elevations may alter blood flow patterns, making functional murmurs less frequent. Vibratory murmurs are uncommon in patients with polycythemia or cyanosis.

Supraclavicular Arterial Murmur

The supraclavicular arterial physiologic murmur is heard about the clavicle, most often on the right, and is caused by turbulence at the branching sites of the brachiocephalic vessels. The murmur is of low intensity, short, low-pitched, and harsh in quality. It can be heard in one third of children ages 4 to 14 years and is heard frequently in adolescents.

Venous Hum

The venous hum is the only physiologic murmur not confined to systole. This is a continuous murmur heard throughout the cardiac cycle. It may be loud (grade 3) and characteristically varies with position, being heard best with the patient in the sitting position. It progressively diminishes as the child returns to the supine position, where it disappears. The murmur sounds like a hum and is heard at the base of the heart, in the supraclavicular area, and in the neck, most often on the right. It is heard most often in children 3 to 5 years of age (50%) but can also be heard at 2 years of age and well into early adolescence. This murmur is caused by turbulence of flow created in the great venous system at the junction of the right subclavian-innominate vein and the superior vena cava. In addition to positional variation, this murmur is accentuated by head rotation and respirations.

Other Causes

Less common conditions may cause physiologic murmurs (Table 17–2). Some of these murmurs are not associated with pathologic abnormalities (cardiorespiratory murmurs, exertion murmurs, "athlete's heart"); some are associated

TABLE 17–1			
PHYSIOLOGIC MURMUR CLASSIFICATION			
Murmur Type	**Phase**	**Location**	**Patient Age at Occurrence (%)**
Classical vibratory (Still's)	Systolic	Mid left lower sternal border	3–6 yr (50%)
Pulmonary ejection	Systolic	Mid left upper sternal border	8–14 yr
Supraclavicular carotid bruit	Systolic	Right supraclavicular area	4–14 yr (33%)
Venous hum	Continuous	Bilateral bases and supraclavicular area	3–6 yr (60%)

TABLE 17–2

LESS COMMON TYPES OF PHYSIOLOGIC MURMURS

Murmurs caused by straight back
  syndrome
Murmurs caused by pectus excavatum
Cardiorespiratory murmurs
Hemic murmurs
Exertion murmurs
Athlete's heart
Abdominal bruit
Femoral-carotid bruit

with only insignificant deviations from the norm (straight back syndrome, pectus excavatum). Only the hemic murmur, when associated with severe anemia, requires intervention. Abdominal, femoral, and carotid bruits in children and adolescents are most often benign and are related only to vascular anatomic variations.

The straight back syndrome and pectus excavatum can occur alone or together and cause turbulent flow in the right ventricular outflow tract as a result of compromise of the chest's anteroposterior diameter. The cardiorespiratory murmur is a bruit heard only during inspiration in systole and heard best at the apex; it is caused by increased right ventricular filling. The hemic murmur and exertion murmur result from rapid ejection, whereas athlete's heart murmur results from slow, increased stroke volume; these causes of physiologic murmurs result in left ventricular outflow turbulence. The murmur of neonatal (insignificant) pulmonary stenosis is a low-intensity, often long ejection systolic murmur heard best at the base and in the back bilaterally. It is heard in the neonatal period and may persist in infants up to 6 months of age. It is caused by turbulence produced by the relative underdevelopment of the branch pulmonary arteries in the neonate and premature infant. Abdominal and femoral bruits may be heard in the older child and adolescent and are similar to those heard in adults, although they are much less frequent. In children, these bruits are caused by arterial constriction or angulation, rather than by aneurysms or atherosclerotic plaque, as in adults.

All physiologic murmurs are made louder and more obvious by alterations in the physiologic state that are associated with increased cardiac output (e.g., fever, agitation, anxiety, and exercise) (Table 17–3). Thus the clinical presentation in the emergency department is likely to exaggerate the easily heard physiologic murmur or make obvious the subtle or previously missed physiologic murmur. Fever in the ill child is probably the most common cause of concern or referral for evaluation of a physiologic murmur, as the murmur is accentuated by one to two grades because of the associated increase in cardiac output. With careful reevaluation, the emergency physician can reduce the need for these referrals.

CLINICAL EVALUATION

Children are rarely brought to the emergency department because of a heart murmur, particularly not a physiologic murmur. Thus a murmur must be evaluated in relationship to the history of the current illness or immediate emergency. The murmur is noted during the physical examination, which is focused on the system involved in the presenting problem. The examiner may need to elicit additional information to evaluate the significance of this unexpected finding. Important historical points include a previous history of heart disease or heart murmur; a history of prematurity, if the patient is an infant, as patent ductus arteriosus is much more common in the premature infant; a history of small size for gestational age, as infants with congenital heart disease are more likely to be small; the presence of a genetic abnormality or an identifiable syndrome such as Down syndrome, which is complicated by congenital heart disease in 50% of cases; the presence of other congenital abnormalities, as malformations tend to involve multiple systems, and 25% of children with congenital heart disease have associated extracardiac anomalies;[6] a history of failure to thrive, poor weight gain, frequent and recurrent lower respiratory infection, or asthma, all of which may have a congenital heart lesion as an underlying cause, especially when significant left-to-right shunts are present; and finally, the presence of intermittent or previously unrecognized central cyanosis, which is likely to be caused by congenital heart disease with an associated right-to-left shunt.

The examiner uses the patient history and a focused physical examination to determine whether the diagnosis of congenital heart disease is correct. It may be unclear initially whether the newly discovered murmur is physiologic or pathologic. Distinguishing physiologic from pathologic murmurs may be difficult for the inexperienced examiner and, at times, confusing for the more experienced clinician. Therefore a grading scale has been developed to aid in differentiating the two. The diagnosis of congenital heart disease is suggested when one major criterion or two minor criteria are present (Table 17–4).

In general, most grade 1 and 2 systolic murmurs are functional and their characteristics can be easily learned. However, any grade 1 or 2 pansystolic or late systolic murmur is of more concern and can be recognized with experience and careful auscultation. Also important to the examiner is the usual diagnostic unimportance of subtle abnormalities in the chest radiograph, electrocardiogram (EKG), blood pressure, or second heart sound. These findings are diagnostically significant when seen together.

DIAGNOSTIC EVALUATION

After a careful history and cardiac examination, further diagnostic laboratory assessment should be considered. The clinician must evaluate the cost versus the benefit of per-

TABLE 17–3

PATHOPHYSIOLOGIC ALTERATIONS CAUSING INCREASED CARDIAC OUTPUT

Hyperthyroidism	Fever
Pregnancy	Hypertension
Anemia	Arteriovenous fistula
Emotion	Heart block

TABLE 17–4

CRITERIA FOR THE DIAGNOSIS OF CONGENITAL HEART DISEASE

Major	Minor
Systolic murmur of grade 3 or louder	Systolic murmur < grade 3
Any pansystolic murmur	Abnormal chest radiograph
Late systolic murmur	Abnormal EKG
Any diastolic murmur	Abnormal blood pressure
Congestive heart failure	Abnormal second sound
Cyanosis	

forming an EKG, a chest radiograph, and an echocardiogram. In the majority of children with murmurs, the history and physical examination should be sufficient to identify the physiologic murmur. When the diagnosis is in doubt, particularly if the child is at high risk for either congenital heart disease or acquired heart disease (i.e., as a result of acute rheumatic fever or bacterial endocarditis), an EKG and a chest radiograph will provide additional information. An emergency echocardiogram to distinguish between the physiologic and pathologic murmur is almost never warranted. Furthermore, the quality of these studies—often obtained at night or on weekends by technicians unfamiliar with the equipment and interpreted by inexperienced personnel— may be poor, thereby adding confusion instead of clarity.

In assessing the value of the echocardiogram in the initial evaluation of heart murmurs in children, several investigators[7, 8] have shown that clinical diagnosis by a pediatric cardiologist is an accurate means of distinguishing between physiologic and pathologic murmurs. Echocardiography is not indicated when a clinical diagnosis of physiologic murmur has been made by a pediatric cardiologist. The echocardiogram and the EKG are valuable primarily in making specific diagnoses when heart disease is suspected clinically.

DISPOSITION

When a pathologic murmur is suspected, admission of the child for further diagnostic evaluation and for consultation with a pediatric cardiologist is indicated. Outpatient management with reevaluation of the child by the primary care provider is another alternative when reliable follow-up is available. The latter option recognizes that the child is best examined on numerous occasions, concentrating on the bruit in question under varied physiologic circumstances (fever, normothermia, and high or normal cardiac output). If uncertainty as to the significance of the murmur persists, outpatient evaluation by a pediatric cardiologist is the next step. In general, the younger the child, the greater the need for early definitive diagnosis. This is particularly true in the neonate and in the infant younger than 6 months of age. The signs and symptoms in and status of these infants can change drastically over short periods of time, and thus management should be conservative, with admission or immediate consultation for the young infant.

In summary, as Rosenthal[9] aptly expressed, "the heart is a pump, not a music box." Any malfunction may aberrate the expected sounds, but the clinician cannot rely on murmurs alone for a diagnosis. Careful history taking, a focused physical examination, appropriate diagnostic studies, and thoughtful synthesis of all pertinent data will usually distinguish between the physiologic and the pathologic murmur.

References

1. Report of the Bethesda Conference on Standardized Terminology. JAMA 1967;200:1041.
2. Stein PD, Sbach HN. The aortic origin of innocent murmurs. Am J Cardiol 1977;39:665.
3. Still GH. Common Disorders and Diseases of Childhood. 3rd ed. London, Oxford University Press, 1918, p 495.
4. Schwartz ML, Goldberg SJ, Wilson N, et al. Relation of Still's murmur, small aortic diameter and high aortic velocity. Am J Cardiol 1986;57:1344.
5. Miao C, Zuberbuhler JS, Zuberbuhler JR. Genesis of vibratory functional murmurs. Am J Cardiol 1987;60:1198.
6. Greenwood RD, Rosenthal A, Ponsi L, et al. Extracardiac anomalies in infants with congenital heart disease. Pediatrics 1975;55:485.
7. Newberger JM, Rosenthal A, Williams RG, et al. Non-invasive tests in the initial evaluation of heard murmurs in children. N Engl J Med 1983;308:61.
8. Smythe JF, Teixerira OHP, Vlad P, et al. Initial evaluation of heart murmurs: Are laboratory tests necessary? Pediatrics 1990;86:497.
9. Rosenthal A. How to distinguish between innocent and pathologic murmurs in childhood. Pediatr Clin North Am 1984;31:6.

CHAPTER 18

Dysrhythmias

Richard P. Shugerman

INTRODUCTION

The diagnosis and emergent management of pediatric dysrhythmias is generally perceived as an uncommon event. In recent years, however, improved cardiovascular surgical techniques have led to a much larger surviving population of children with congenital heart disease who are at risk for a variety of dysrhythmias. Although there are no firm incidence figures on the number of emergency department visits for such children each year, many pediatric cardiologists believe the numbers are rising and will continue to rise as the population of surviving children increases.[1]

In addition to this growing population, there remains a significant group of children who present with dysrhythmias and have structurally normal hearts. For both groups of children, those with and without structural heart disease, a framework for management has evolved that recognizes the unique features of pediatric cardiac and respiratory physiology. An awareness of these features can provide a rational basis for the increasingly more common management of pediatric dysrhythmias in the emergency department.

CONCEPTUAL FRAMEWORK

Prior to the 1970s, much of the emergency management of pediatric dysrhythmias was based on extrapolation of adult information. Pediatric dysrhythmias were generally conceptualized as disorders of cardiac physiology alone. Aside from the administration of drugs on a per-kilogram basis, pediatric dysrhythmias were generally treated using Adult Cardiac Life Support guidelines developed for adult populations. Although considerable overlap still exists for a number of dysrhythmias, there has developed an increased awareness of the differing origins and manifestations of many adult and pediatric dysrhythmias.

This difference is most striking in the case of cardiopulmonary arrest. Primary cardiac disorders are the cause of arrest for 80% of out-of-hospital cases involving pulseless, nonbreathing adults.[2, 3] In contrast, several reviews have found primary cardiac disorders to be the cause of arrest in less than 10% of out-of-hospital cases of pulseless, nonbreathing children.[2–4] The origin of arrest in the majority of these children is a primary respiratory event.[5] Cardiac arrest in a pediatric patient most commonly results from prolonged hypoxia and acidosis secondary to respiratory failure.[6] A primary cardiac cause for pediatric cardiopulmonary arrest is rare.

The electrocardiographic correlates of cardiac arrest are also strikingly dissimilar for pediatric and adult populations. For example, ventricular fibrillation is commonly found in a significant number of out-of-hospital incidents involving pulseless, nonbreathing adults but has been found in only 6% of similar incidents involving out-of-hospital pulseless, non-breathing children.[2, 3]

A study of terminal cardiac electrical activity in 100 dying hospitalized children demonstrated the scarcity of ventricular fibrillation and other tachyarrhythmias as a precursor to death in pediatric patients.[7] In this study, 78% of children progressed to asystole through a terminal sequence composed entirely of bradycardic phenomena. Sixteen percent of these children had episodes of ventricular tachycardia or fibrillation with bradycardic arrest as the final electrical sequence. Only 6% died in unremitting ventricular fibrillation, and none of these had structurally normal hearts. Older and larger children were significantly more likely to develop tachyarrhythmias than were newborns and smaller children in this study.

The authors of the study suggest that this paucity of tachyarrhythmias in dying children may relate to cardiac mass and developmental aspects of the autonomic nervous system. Animal studies from the early 1900s support the theory that a critical cardiac mass is required to initiate and maintain ventricular fibrillation, and the relatively small hearts of infants and children may be less prone to fibrillation on this basis.[8]

The profound parasympathetic predominance found in the developing autonomic nervous system of newborns and infants has also been postulated as a factor for the frequency of bradycardic events in these children. Subsequent development of sympathetic input has been suggested as a factor not only in the increase in ventricular fibrillation with age,[9] but also in the decrease in incidence of SIDS with age.[1]

Studies such as these have led to unique guidelines for the management of certain pediatric dysrhythmias. These guidelines stress the importance of proper airway management and recognition of the parasympathetic predominance in pediatric patients. Many other dysrhythmias have not been studied exclusively in children, and their management remains based on extrapolation of data derived from adult populations. For all pediatric dysrhythmias detailed in this chapter, however, the prerequisites of management are a stable airway, good oxygenation, and adequate ventilation.

SINUS NODE DYSFUNCTION

The sinus node is a small structure located at the junction of the superior vena cava and the right atrium. It is composed primarily of pacemaking cells; these cells have the highest rate of spontaneous depolarization of all pacemaking cells in the heart. Under normal conditions, the sinus node functions as the origin of the cardiac impulse. It is extensively innervated with both sympathetic and parasympathetic fibers. Sympathetic stimulation increases the rate of spontaneous depolarization and increases the speed of conduction through the sinus node out to the atrial tissue. Parasympathetic stimulation decreases the rate of spontaneous depolarization and decreases the speed of sinus node conduction. Congenital, surgical, and nonsurgically acquired damage to the sinus node, drug-induced changes in sinus node conduction times, and alterations in autonomic input are all recognized causes of sinus node dysfunction. Many of the derangements they cause are clinically inapparent, but some alterations in sinus node function cause a patient to become symptomatic (e.g., syncope, seizures, dizziness, or exercise intolerance) or result in abnormalities on the standard electrocardiogram.

Diagnosis

There are no universally accepted criteria for making the diagnosis of sinus node dysfunction in children. The most commonly accepted criteria that are apparent on the surface electrocardiogram are sinus bradycardia, severe sinus arrhythmia, sinus arrest, and brady-tachyarrhythmias.

Sinus bradycardia is defined as a heart rate lower than the lower limits of normal for age (Table 18–1). There is considerable disagreement over how much variability during

sleep is acceptable and which method is preferred for obtaining normal values.

The most widely accepted guidelines for the diagnosis of sinus bradycardia in children, obtained on a standard electrocardiogram (EKG), are as follows: heart rate < 100 beats/min in children < 3 years of age; heart rate < 60 beats/min in children 3 to 9 years of age; heart rate < 50 beats/min in children 9 to 16 years of age; heart rate < 40 beats/min in children > 16 years of age.[10]

Sinus arrhythmia is a phasic irregularity of the heart beat that increases with inspiration and decreases with expiration.[11] The P wave axis is normal, and the RR interval may vary by as much as 10% to 100% of the preceding RR interval. The term *sinus arrhythmia* is misleading, as the variation in rhythm is considered a variant of normal. *Severe sinus arrhythmia*, however, is not a normal variant and is characterized by variation in the RR interval of greater than 100%.[12]

Sinus arrest results from failure of the sinus node to generate an impulse. With extended sinus arrest, subsidiary pacemakers located in the atria, atrioventricular node, or ventricles may depolarize, resulting in an escape rhythm.

The amount of time between beats that is required to make the diagnosis of sinus arrest is unclear and appears to vary with age. In one report of healthy 7- to 11-year-old children studied with 24-hour monitoring, the mean length of the longest sinus pause was 1.36 ± 0.23 seconds.[13] The authors suggest that pauses in excess of two standard deviations from this mean (i.e., > 1.82 seconds) may be taken as evidence of sinus arrest in this age group.

Brady-tachyarrhythmias are defined as episodes of alternating bradycardia and supraventricular tachycardia. The bradycardia may be sinal, atrial, or junctional in origin. The supraventricular tachycardia is usually the result of a reentry phenomenon.[14]

Pathophysiology and Clinical Features

Among the disorders of cardiac conduction in children, sinus node dysfunction is perhaps the most difficult to conceptualize, as it is a constellation of findings rather than a single dysrhythmia. Sinus node dysfunction may result from abnormalities in automaticity, innervation, or conduction within the sinus node. The electrophysiologic basis for the rhythm disturbance varies with the underlying disorder.

In children, the vast majority of cases of sinus node dysfunction are a direct result of cardiac surgery. The location, blood supply, and innervation of the sinus node make it especially vulnerable to injury. The surgical procedures most commonly resulting in sinus node dysfunction are those involving the atria (e.g., Mustard or Fontan procedures).[14] Less commonly, sinus node dysfunction may be seen in children with congenital heart defects that have not been surgically repaired;[15, 16] it is rarely seen in children with structurally normal hearts.[16]

Alterations in autonomic tone may cause transient sinus node dysfunction in otherwise healthy children. Such alterations may result from endotracheal intubation, pharyngeal suctioning, nasogastric tube placement, and the Valsalva maneuver.

Drugs may also alter sinus node function either directly or through changes in autonomic tone. Common culprits include digoxin, quinidine, beta blockers, and verapamil.

Therapeutic Intervention

Sinus node dysfunction rarely requires treatment in the pediatric emergency department, as the majority of children with sinus node dysfunction are asymptomatic. If a patient

		TABLE 18–1	
		NORMAL CARDIAC VALUES FOR AGE	
Age	Heart Rate, Beats/min	PR Interval, sec	QRS Duration, sec
Newborn	93–154 (123)	0.08–0.16 (0.11)	0.03–0.07 (0.05)
1–2 days	91–159 (123)	0.08–0.14 (0.11)	0.03–0.07 (0.05)
3–7 days	91–166 (129)	0.07–0.14 (0.10)	0.03–0.07 (0.05)
1–4 wk	107–182 (148)	0.07–0.14 (0.10)	0.03–0.08 (0.05)
1–3 mo	121–179 (149)	0.07–0.13 (0.10)	0.03–0.08 (0.05)
3–6 mo	106–186 (141)	0.07–0.15 (0.11)	0.03–0.08 (0.05)
6–12 mo	109–169 (134)	0.07–0.16 (0.11)	0.03–0.08 (0.05)
1–3 yr	89–151 (119)	0.08–0.15 (0.11)	0.04–0.08 (0.06)
3–5 yr	73–137 (108)	0.09–0.16 (0.12)	0.04–0.08 (0.06)
5–8 yr	65–133 (100)	0.09–0.16 (0.12)	0.04–0.08 (0.06)
8–12 yr	62–130 (91)	0.09–0.17 (0.13)	0.04–0.09 (0.06)
12–16 yr	60–119 (85)	0.09–0.18 (0.14)	0.04–0.09 (0.07)

*Values shown are the 2nd to 98th percentile; mean values are given in parentheses. From Garson A, Bricker JT, McNamara DG. The Science and Practice of Pediatric Cardiology. Vol II. Philadelphia, Lea & Febiger, 1990, p 714.

is symptomatic, however, the initial treatment involves diagnosis and treatment of any of the correctable causes for sinus node dysfunction. Particular attention should be paid to oxygenation and ventilation in the pediatric patient with symptomatic bradycardia. Failure of these measures requires acute medical management with intravenous atropine (0.04 mg/kg). Second-line treatments include intravenous isoproterenol drip (0.05 to 0.5 µg/kg/min) or temporary transvenous pacing for rhythms unresponsive to either medication.

Sinus node dysfunction diagnosed in the emergency department, whether symptomatic or asymptomatic, warrants referral to a pediatric cardiologist for further evaluation. Permanent pacemaker implantation is indicated for children with sinus node dysfunction and symptomatic bradycardia.[17]

DISORDERS OF ATRIOVENTRICULAR CONDUCTION

Many of the disorders of atrioventricular conduction are directly related to disorders of the atrioventricular (AV) node. The AV node is a small, flattened structure located interatrially at the base of the atrial septum.[18, 19] It is composed of pacemaker cells, myocardial cells, and Purkinje cells and is innervated extensively by sympathetic and parasympathetic fibers. Parasympathetic stimulation prolongs conduction through the AV node, whereas sympathetic stimulation shortens it. Like all pacemaker cells, the pacemaker cells of the AV node are capable of spontaneous depolarization. This pacemaking function, however, is rarely required, as the rate of spontaneous depolarization of pacemaker cells in the AV node is much slower than that of pacemaker cells in the sinus node.

The PR interval on a standard EKG is generally assumed to reflect conduction time through the AV node. Using His bundle electrocardiography, however, the PR interval can be divided into three distinct entities reflecting (1) conduction time from the sinus node to the AV node, (2) conduction time through the AV node, and (3) conduction time from the His bundle to the ventricles. Using His bundle electrocardiography, conduction through the AV node is the largest component of the PR interval and the site at which the majority of disorders of AV conduction are found.[20] AV conduction abnormalities may also involve disorders of interatrial conduction or His-Purkinje conduction or may include a combination of disorders of all three.

First Degree AV Block
Diagnosis

First degree AV block is present when the PR interval is prolonged beyond the upper limit of normal for age (see Table 18–1). This interval is measured from the beginning of the P wave to the beginning of the R inflection and is most easily visualized in standard lead II or precordial lead V_1.

Pathophysiology and Clinical Features

The PR interval represents three distinct conduction intervals. Most commonly, a prolongation of the AV nodal conduction interval is responsible for prolonging the PR interval. This may occur transiently secondary to variations in autonomic tone, in which case it is a normal finding.[20]

A consistently prolonged PR interval, however, suggests an underlying pathologic abnormality. Congenital cardiac defects such as atrial septal defect,[21] a single ventricle, and Ebstein's anomaly are associated with first degree AV block, likely as a result of structural damage to the AV node. Infectious diseases such as endocarditis, rheumatic fever, scarlet fever, and rubella may be the cause of acquired first degree AV block.[20] Drugs such as digitalis and verapamil may also cause acquired first degree AV block.

Therapeutic Intervention

First degree AV block does not require emergent treatment, as it does not cause clinical instability.

Second Degree AV Block
Diagnosis

Second degree AV block may present in two forms. Type I second degree AV block is characterized by a progressive prolongation of the PR interval until eventually a P wave is not conducted to the ventricles. Type II second degree AV block is characterized by generally normally conducted P waves and, intermittently, an abrupt loss of conduction to the ventricles.

Pathophysiology and Clinical Features

Type I second degree AV block, also known as *Wenckebach block*, is by far the most common form of second degree AV block in pediatric patients. The conduction delay most often occurs within the AV node. Type I second degree AV block occurs in 6% of young adults during sleep[22] and occasionally in trained athletes at rest.[23, 24] It may also be indicative of an underlying pathologic abnormality such as drug toxicity (digitalis, calcium channel blockers, beta blockers, and quinidine are most common) or an infectious disease (e.g., rheumatic fever, scarlet fever, or myocarditis). Cardiac surgery involving the AV nodal area may also results in type I second degree AV block. As a rule, type I second degree AV block is not thought to be a risk factor for progression to complete third degree AV block.

Type II second degree AV block is a less common dysrhythmia in the pediatric patient, and its prognosis is less benign. The conduction defect is usually distal to the AV node and involves the His bundle or bundle branches. It is most frequently seen in children who have undergone cardiac surgery and has a significant potential to progress to complete AV block.[25, 26]

Therapeutic Intervention

There is no specific treatment for type I or type II second degree AV block other than correction of the underlying disorder. In a patient taking cardiac medications, serum drug levels should be determined and medications withheld until drug toxicity is excluded. In the rare event that either rhythm is accompanied by symptoms, intravenous atropine (0.04 mg/kg) or isoproterenol drip (0.05 to 0.5 µg/kg/min) may be useful in the acute setting, along with consideration of temporary pacing.

For the otherwise healthy, asymptomatic patient with type I second degree AV block and no obvious underlying cause, elective referral to a pediatric cardiologist for further evaluation is a reasonable measure. Because of the potential for progression to complete AV block, a patient with previously undiagnosed type II second degree AV block, even if asymptomatic, warrants hospitalization and cardiology consultation.

Third Degree AV Block
Diagnosis

The diagnosis of complete or third degree AV block is made when the EKG reveals P waves and QRS complexes that occur independent of one another. Typically the P wave rate is faster than that of the QRS complex.

Pathophysiology and Clinical Features

Complete heart block may be congenital or acquired. Congenital complete heart block occurs in 1 of every 20,000 live births.[27] Most infants (50% to 70%) with congenital complete heart block have structurally normal hearts;[27] however, there is a strong association with maternal connective tissue disease and transplacental passage of maternal antibodies to tissue ribonucleoproteins.[28–30] Infants with congenital complete heart block and associated cardiac defects may have undergone surgery to correct transposition of the great arteries, an AV canal, or tricuspid atresia.

Acquired complete heart block is most commonly a result of cardiac surgery. Other causes include rheumatic heart disease, myocarditis, and diphtheria.

The location of the block and the resting heart rate appear to have some prognostic significance in terms of development of symptoms. Children with a block located above the His bundle recording site, whether the block is congenital or acquired, appear less likely to develop symptoms than

children with a block below the His bundle recording site;[31, 32] however, some studies have challenged the wisdom of management decisions based solely on this finding.[33]

Children with congenital complete heart block and resting heart rates greater than 50 beats/min appear less likely to develop symptoms than children with congenital complete heart block and resting heart rates less than 50 beats/min.[33, 34] Nevertheless, it appears that the heart rate alone (independent of the location of the AV block) is the most important determinant for the placement of a pacemaker.[35]

Therapeutic Intervention

It is rare to make acute management decisions for complete heart block in the emergency department. Typically, congenital heart block is discovered in utero or at delivery, and decisions regarding the need for cardiac pacing are made during the newborn stage. As discussed earlier, infants with congenital heart block and a heart rate less than 50 beats/min are candidates for cardiac pacing,[17, 33–35] as are infants with congenital heart block and a wide QRS complex.[17, 36]

Acquired heart block is most commonly seen after cardiac surgery, and decisions regarding the need for pacing are generally made during the immediate postoperative period. Permanent pacing is recommended in children whose heart block persists for 14 days after surgery despite temporary pacing.[17, 32, 37]

If decisions regarding the acute management of children with complete AV block are made in the emergency department, they are most likely to be in the setting of an unpaced, previously asymptomatic child who acutely develops symptoms. The association of symptoms with complete AV block is a definite indication for pacing.[17] Prior to the placement of a temporary pacer, acute therapy may be attempted with intravenous atropine (0.04 mg/kg) or isoproterenol drip (0.05 to 0.5 µg/kg/min).

DISORDERS OF INTRAVENTRICULAR CONDUCTION

Intraventricular conduction defects may occur because of disorders of the distal His bundle, disorders of the right or left bundle branches, or disorders of ventricular muscle repolarization. Disorders of the distal His bundle generally present clinically as complete AV block, and their management has been discussed earlier. Disorders of the bundle branches usually present clinically as prolongation of the QRS complex with morphologic changes in the QRS complex that are dependent on the bundle branch involved. Disorders of ventricular muscle repolarization present clinically as prolongation of the QT interval.

Right Bundle Branch Block
Diagnosis

The diagnosis of complete right bundle branch block (RBBB) is made when the QRS complex is prolonged for age (see Table 18–1), an RSR′ pattern is seen in the right chest leads (V_1 and V_{4R}), and a slurred S wave is seen in standard lead I and the left chest leads (V_5 and V_6).

The diagnosis of incomplete RBBB is made when the QRS morphology is the same as that for complete RBBB, but the QRS duration is normal.

Pathophysiology and Clinical Features

RBBB is the most common of the intraventricular conduction disorders and in children usually results from open heart surgery, typically repair of a ventricular septal defect, tetralogy of Fallot, or a complete AV canal.[38-40]

A number of nonsurgical conditions are associated with RBBB in children, including myotonic dystrophy,[41] Duchenne's muscular dystrophy,[42] cardiomyopathy, nonoperated congenital heart disease, and myocarditis. Rarely, RBBB is found in an otherwise healthy child as an isolated, inherited defect.[43, 44]

Incomplete RBBB is commonly seen in patients with an atrial septal defect. The characteristic EKG pattern is likely a result of ventricular hypertrophy rather than a true conduction defect.[45] In a small percentage of children, incomplete RBBB may be found in an otherwise normal heart and may represent a variant of normal.[46, 47]

Therapeutic Intervention

In the emergency department, RBBB is generally an incidental finding. RBBB does not produce symptoms and does not require treatment. If the history, physical examination, chest radiograph, and EKG fail to identify one of the causes listed earlier, referral to a pediatric cardiologist for further evaluation on an outpatient basis is warranted.

Left Bundle Branch Block
Diagnosis

The diagnosis of left bundle branch block (LBBB) is made when the QRS is prolonged for age, a dominant S wave is seen in lead V_1, and a dominant R wave is seen in lead V_6.

Pathophysiology and Clinical Features

In children, the vast majority of LBBB is a result of cardiac surgery, typically of the aortic valve. Nonsurgical causes are the same as those for RBBB. Unlike in RBBB, there appears to be a small but significant risk for progression to complete AV block.

Therapeutic Intervention

In the emergency department, LBBB is generally an incidental finding. It does not produce symptoms and does not require treatment. However, if the diagnosis of LBBB is made in the emergency department, referral to a cardiologist for a complete evaluation and consideration of pacing is warranted because of the potential for progression to complete AV block.

Fascicular Block

Shortly after separation of the His bundle into the left and right bundle branches, the left bundle branch separates into the anterior and posterior fascicles. Disorders of conduction in either of these fascicles may occur, resulting in asymmetric depolarization of the ventricles and an abnormal QRS complex. This condition is known as *hemifascicular block*.[48]

The diagnosis of anterior or posterior left hemifascicular block is difficult to make on a standard EKG and is rarely an issue in the pediatric emergency department.

Disorders of conduction in the right bundle branch, combined with disorders of conduction in one or both fascicles, may also occur, resulting in disorders known as *bifascicular* or *trifascicular block*, respectively. As in the case of hemifascicular block, these disorders are difficult to diagnose on standard EKG and are rarely seen in the pediatric emergency department.

Prolonged QT Interval
Diagnosis

The diagnosis of prolonged QT interval is made when the corrected QT interval (QT_c) is greater than 0.44 seconds. The corrected QT interval can be determined by the following formula:

$$QT_c = \frac{QT \text{ interval}}{\sqrt{RR \text{ interval}}}$$

The QT interval is measured from the initial Q inflection to the end of the T wave.

Pathophysiology and Clinical Features

Prolongation of the QT interval is caused by abnormal repolarization of ventricular muscle. The electrophysiologic basis for this abnormal repolarization is unknown at the cellular level. Features of the syndrome have been duplicated in dogs who have undergone ablation of the right stellate ganglion.[49] This has led some authors to postulate that the primary abnormality is one of disordered sympathetic input to the heart.[50]

Clinically, children with the long QT syndrome are a diverse group. Most commonly, the disorder is inherited, and it may or may not be associated with deafness. Children with hereditary long QT syndrome and deafness generally demonstrate a pattern of autosomal recessive inheritance (Jervell and Lange-Neilsen syndrome).[51] Children with hereditary long QT syndrome without deafness generally demonstrate autosomal dominant inheritance (Romano-Ward syndrome).[52, 53] The disorder may also be congenital without a clearly established pattern of inheritance.[54]

Less commonly, the long QT syndrome may be an acquired phenomenon in children. The most common cause of acquired long QT syndrome in children is antiarrhythmic medication such as quinidine,[55] procainamide, and amiodarone. Other medications that prolong the QT interval include phenothiazines, lithium, and tricyclic antidepressants. A prolonged QT interval may also be caused by electrolyte disorders, myocarditis, and severe liver disease. It is also a recognized complication of patients who have experienced extreme weight loss (e.g., those on very low calorie diets[56] and possibly those with anorexia nervosa).[57]

Therapeutic Intervention

Children with the long QT syndrome typically present to the pediatric emergency department with unexplained syncope[50, 58] or new onset of seizures.[59] Occasionally they present with sudden death in a previously healthy individual following exercise or emotional trauma.[50, 58]

Any child with the long QT syndrome, whether the syndrome is congenital or acquired, is at risk for sudden death as a result of malignant ventricular arrhythmias such as ventricular tachycardia or torsades de pointes. Because of the potential morbidity and mortality from a missed diagnosis of long QT syndrome, a standard EKG with measurement of the QT_c is warranted in the emergency department evaluation of any child with unexplained syncope or new-onset, afebrile seizures.

If the diagnosis of long QT syndrome is made, the child should be referred to a pediatric cardiologist for further evaluation and long-term monitoring. Although there is some controversy regarding the need for treatment in asymptomatic patients,[54, 60] symptomatic patients are treated with long-term beta-blocking agents either alone or in combination with other antiarrhythmic medications. Intractable symptoms may require pacemaker implantation, left stellate ganglionectomy, or implantation of an automatic defibrillator.

Extrasystole
Atrial Extrasystole

Diagnosis. Atrial extrasystoles, or premature atrial contractions (PACs), are characterized by premature P waves that usually are of different morphology than those occurring during sinus conduction. The premature P wave may be conducted to the ventricles with a resultant normal QRS complex or an aberrant QRS complex, or the P wave may not be conducted to the ventricles at all. Depending on the effect that the PAC has on the sinus node pacemaker cells, there may or may not be a compensatory pause between the premature P wave and the next sinus P wave.

Pathophysiology and Clinical Features. PACs may arise from premature depolarization anywhere within the atria. They are usually benign in children, and their cause is unknown. Rarely, PACs may be indicative of an underlying pathologic abnormality such as hypoxia, electrolyte disturbances, drug toxicity, or chronic atrial enlargement.

The incidence of benign PACs in healthy children varies with the study cited and ranges from 0.68%[61] to 14%[62] in newborns and from 13%[63] to 21%[13] in older children. Infrequent benign PACs have been reported in as many as 56% of healthy young adults.[22]

Therapeutic Intervention. In an otherwise healthy child in whom pathologic causes have been excluded, PACs are most likely benign, do not produce symptoms, and do not require treatment. In a child with PACs and a history of syncope, referral to a pediatric cardiologist for 24-hour monitoring is warranted, as PACs are known to initiate tachyarrhythmias in susceptible patients.[64]

Ventricular Extrasystole

Diagnosis. Ventricular extrasystoles, or premature ventricular contractions (PVCs), are characterized by premature QRS complexes that are different in morphology from the regular QRS complex and are usually prolonged in duration. Usually, but not always, there is a fully compensatory pause before the next regularly conducted sinus beat.

It is important to differentiate PVCs from PACs. Because a significant percentage of PACs are conducted aberrantly in children, one cannot rely on a prolonged QRS duration to always distinguish the two. PACs should, however, always be preceded by a P wave. The P wave may be buried in the preceding T wave and thus be difficult to find. If, however, after careful review of the preceding T wave, no P wave is identified and the QRS complex has a different morphology from the regular QRS complex, the complex is a PVC.[60]

PVCs may regularly alternate with normal QRS complexes so that every other QRS complex is a PVC (bigeminy) or every third QRS complex is a PVC (trigeminy). Two consecutive PVCs without an intervening normal QRS complex is called a *ventricular couplet*. Three or more consecutive PVCs without an intervening normal QRS complex is known as *ventricular tachycardia*.

PVCs may all have the same morphology, in which case they are known as *uniform*. PVCs with different morphology are known as *multiform*. When a normal beat is conducted from one ventricle and a PVC is conducted from the other ventricle at the same time, the sum of their vectors will likely produce a QRS complex that is different morphologically from the normal beat and from the PVC. Such a QRS complex is called a *fusion beat* and is not indicative of multiform PVCs. If the QRS complex in question is preceded by a P wave, fusion between a normal beat and a PVC is possible, and the PVCs may still be uniform. If the QRS complex in question is not preceded by a P wave, fusion could not have occurred with a normal beat, and the PVCs are then identified as multiform.[60]

Pathophysiology and Clinical Features. PVCs may arise from premature depolarization anywhere within the ventricles. The actual electrophysiologic basis for these rhythms is unknown.

Pathologic causes of PVCs in children are numerous but can be divided into four categories: metabolic derangements, drugs, infections, and congenital heart disease. Metabolic derangements include electrolyte abnormalities, hypoxia, acidosis, and hypoglycemia. Drugs that cause PVCs include digitalis, tricyclic antidepressants, quinidine, anesthetic agents, and phenothiazines. Nicotine, caffeine, and stimulants have also been implicated. Infectious causes include myocarditis, rheumatic fever, and endocarditis.

The reported incidence of PVCs varies with the age of those studied and the type of study performed. When 24-hour electrocardiograms were used, PVCs were recorded in none of 134 healthy newborn infants,[62] in only 1 of 104 healthy 7- to 11-year-old children,[13] but in 25 of 50 healthy young adults.[22] The reasons for this variability are unclear. As a rule, however, PVCs appear to be less common in healthy children than PACs.[60]

Like PACs, most PVCs in healthy children appear to be benign. No significant sequelae have been demonstrated in long-term follow-up of healthy, asymptomatic children with normal hearts and isolated uniform PVCs, bigeminy, or trigeminy that were suppressed with exercise.[65]

There is limited information on the significance of multiform PVCs or couplets in children. Some evidence suggests that these rhythms are more common in children with structural heart disease and that even in children with normal hearts, they have the potential for malignant degeneration.[60]

Therapeutic Intervention. A careful search for any of the pathologic causes listed earlier should be undertaken for any child who presents to the emergency department with PVCs. An otherwise healthy child with a normal heart and no pathologic source who presents with asymptomatic uniform PVCs, bigeminy, or trigeminy may be referred on an elective basis to a pediatric cardiologist for exercise testing and further evaluation. A child with multiform PVCs or couplets or a child with hemodynamically significant uniform PVCs, bigeminy, or trigeminy should be treated with an antiarrhythmic.

Tachycardias
Sinus Tachycardia

Diagnosis. Sinus tachycardia is present when the heart rate is faster than the upper limit of normal for age (see Table 18–1) and a P wave precedes every QRS complex. At very high rates, sinus tachycardia may be difficult to distinguish from supraventricular tachycardia. Some features of sinus tachycardia that may aid in the differential diagnosis include the following:

1. Sinus tachycardia is rarely seen with heart rates greater than 220 beats/min.
2. In sinus tachycardia, there is usually some variation in the heart rate from beat to beat; in supraventricular tachycardia, the heart rate is frequently fixed.
3. In sinus tachycardia, treatment of the underlying causes listed in the next section will usually lower the rate.

Pathophysiology and Clinical Features. Sinus tachycardia is a compensatory rhythm that is generally provoked by one of three major categories of problems: increased metabolic needs (fever, infection, exercise); low cardiac output (hypovolemia, poor pump function); or direct stimulation of the heart (medications, anxiety, pain).

Therapeutic Intervention. Sinus tachycardia is corrected by treating the underlying cause.

Supraventricular Tachycardia

Diagnosis. The diagnosis of supraventricular tachycardia (SVT) can be difficult to make. In general, SVT is present when the heart rate is regular but faster than the upper limit of normal for age (see Table 18–1), the QRS complex duration is normal, and sinus tachycardia has been excluded.

With the exception of exclusion of sinus tachycardia, none of these criteria are absolute, as the surface EKG findings of SVT can be quite variable. As a rule, the rhythm is regular. SVT with associated second or third degree AV block is rare, but does occur. P waves may or may not be present. They have been identified in as many as 56%[66] and in as few as 10%[67] of children with SVT. The QRS complex should be narrow but has been reported to be prolonged in up to 8% of patients studied.[66]

Pathophysiology and Clinical Features. SVT is a relatively common problem in children and is seen frequently in the pediatric emergency department. Estimates of its prevalence range from as low as 1 in every 25,000 children[68] to as high as 1 in every 250 children.[69] By most accounts, it appears to be increasing in frequency as better methods of detection are developed and more children survive cardiac surgery.

The demographic features of children with SVT are somewhat variable depending on the patient population studied. In the largest reported series of children with SVT, Garson et al.[66] studied the first episode of SVT in 217 children and described demographic and prognostic features; approximately half of the 217 children were male and half female. The children ranged in age from 1 day to 17.5 years, with a median age of 24 months. SVT appeared by 3 months of age in 34% of the children and by 1 year of age in 43%. Children with onset of SVT at less than 4 months of age were more likely to present in congestive heart failure but were also more likely to have structurally normal hearts than were children whose SVT began after the age of 4 months.

For the group as a whole, 60% of the children had structurally normal hearts and no predisposing factors to which the SVT could be attributed. Seventeen percent had normal hearts but some predisposing factor to which the SVT was attributed; these factors included stimulant medications, cardiomyopathy, myocarditis, and other infections. Twenty-three percent of the children had structural heart disease to which the SVT was attributed. Children with Ebstein's anomaly and transposition of the great vessels appeared to be overrepresented (i.e., the percentages of such children in this study group were greater than corresponding percentages in the general population).

With the advent of electrophysiologic studies, there has been an explosion of information regarding the mechanisms of initiation and maintenance of SVT in children.[69–74] In general, children with SVT fall into two major mechanistic categories: those with tachycardia secondary to a reentry phenomenon and those with tachycardia secondary to an ectopic focus with increased automaticity. Children with SVT secondary to a reentry phenomenon may be further subdivided into two other mechanistic categories: those whose reentry occurs over a bypass tract between the atria and ventricles (e.g., Wolff-Parkinson-White syndrome or Lown-Ganong-Levine syndrome) and those whose reentry occurs

without a bypass tract (e.g., sinus node or AV node reentry). Children with SVT secondary to an ectopic focus may also be further subdivided into two mechanistic categories: those whose ectopic focus is located in the atria (e.g., atrial ectopic tachycardia) and those whose ectopic focus is located in the region of the AV node and His bundle (e.g., junctional ectopic tachycardia).

The most common form of SVT in children appears to be tachycardia secondary to reentry with a bypass tract. This form occurs in approximately one half of all children with SVT. The remaining half are equally divided between those with tachycardia secondary to reentry without a bypass tract and those with tachycardia secondary to an ectopic focus with abnormal automaticity.[69]

Therapeutic Intervention. Determination of the exact mechanism for SVT in an individual child is a complicated procedure that frequently requires electrophysiologic studies. Although many pediatric cardiologists consider this information crucial for long-term management, it has little practical significance in the acute treatment of these children in the pediatric emergency department. Decisions in the emergency department should be based on the hemodynamic status of the patient.

Any child who presents to the emergency department with SVT and signs of significant hemodynamic compromise should be treated with synchronized direct current (DC) cardioversion. Hypotension is a common side effect of almost all of the intravenous antiarrhythmics available for the treatment of SVT and may not be tolerated by a child already showing signs of significant hemodynamic compromise. In addition, the time required for placement of an intravenous line in these children may be prohibitively long.

The energy delivered during cardioversion should be 0.5 joules/kg, and the clinician must ensure that the synchronized mode has been selected. For a child with SVT who is already taking digoxin, pretreatment with lidocaine (1 mg/kg) is recommended by some authors to protect against ventricular fibrillation.[75]

Clinicians have a much broader array of therapeutic options for children who present with SVT but without evidence of cardiac compromise. The fact that these children are tolerating the rhythm dictates that the therapy chosen should have the smallest potential for complications.

Maneuvers to increase vagal tone are simple, noninvasive, and inexpensive and are both safe and effective in the treatment of SVT. In an older child, vagal maneuvers such as carotid sinus massage, the Valsalva maneuver, or gagging should be the initial line of therapy. Ocular pressure should not be used because of the potential for retinal damage. Infants and younger children who cannot cooperate with vagal maneuvers should have vagal tone elicited by use of the diving reflex.

The diving reflex, an oxygen-conserving reflex consisting of peripheral vasoconstriction and vagally mediated bradycardia, has demonstrated efficacy in the treatment of SVT in children.[76–81] Numerous techniques have been used to elicit the reflex, including placement of a cold washcloth or bag of ice on the infant's face for 10 to 15 seconds, as well as actual submersion of the infant's face in a basin of ice and water for 6 to 7 seconds. Successful cardioversion has been reported with each method. There is no available information to indicate whether one technique is superior to another. Although there are reports that the diving reflex may initiate ventricular tachycardia in adults,[82, 83] there are no reported complications of its use in children.

Failure of these maneuvers requires progression to more invasive therapy with a higher risk of complications. Adenosine is an excellent therapeutic option that is only slightly more invasive than vagal maneuvers and relatively low in significant complications. It is an extremely rapidly acting agent with strong but very brief depressant effects on the SA and AV nodes and an estimated half-life of 10 to 15 seconds. It has been used for the treatment of SVT in both children and adults[84–89] and has been effective in terminating SVT in up to 87% of children studied.[84] Side effects, both cardiac (sinus bradycardia, AV block, sinus arrest) and noncardiac (flushing, wheezing, and vomiting) have been reported relatively commonly. Only one study has reported symptoms that required treatment: a child with Down syndrome, pulmonary hypertension, and sinus node dysfunction required temporary pacing for symptomatic bradycardia following adenosine administration.[86] Otherwise, the extremely short half-life of the agent has rendered essentially all complications benign.[86, 87]

In the uncompromised infant or child with SVT, adenosine is an excellent second line of treatment. Adenosine should be given as a rapid intravenous bolus in a dose of 0.05 mg/kg. For refractory SVT, subsequent doses should be increased by 0.05 mg/kg with each dose to a maximum dose of 0.25 mg/kg.

Failure of vagal maneuvers, the diving reflex, and adenosine may be an indication for the use of digoxin in the treatment of SVT in children. For many years, digoxin has been the mainstay of treatment in the uncompromised child because of its high degree of efficacy and low incidence of complications. However, some cardiologists have questioned its use in children because of complications known to occur in adults.

In adults with SVT, primarily those with SVT resulting from Wolff-Parkinson-White (WPW) syndrome, digoxin can increase the risk of ventricular fibrillation by facilitating conduction across the bypass tract during periods of atrial fibrillation or flutter.[90, 91] For this reason, digoxin is contraindicated in the long-term management of adults whose SVT is caused by the WPW syndrome.

Because the diagnosis of WPW syndrome can only be made when a patient is in a normal sinus rhythm, some investigators have recommended that digoxin should not be used in the acute management of any patient in SVT if there is no previous EKG tracing in sinus rhythm to exclude WPW syndrome.[92, 93] The increased risk of ventricular fibrillation if the patient eventually requires electrical cardioversion is an additional contraindication to the use of digoxin in the acute setting.

Despite this controversy, many pediatric cardiologists continue to recommend digoxin as a second-line agent for children in whom vagal maneuvers have failed; this is based on its safe track record in children over many years.[75] The risk of ventricular fibrillation, even in children with WPW syndrome, appears to be exceedingly low, because the precursor rhythm, atrial fibrillation, is very uncommon in the pediatric population.

With the introduction of adenosine, digoxin may best be viewed as a third-line agent for the treatment of SVT in the uncompromised child. The patient should appear well enough to tolerate the SVT for the additional 2 to 6 hours that digoxin frequently requires for effect. Digoxin may be given orally in a dose of 0.025 mg/kg initially, followed by 0.0125 mg/kg 8 hours later and an additional 0.0125 mg/kg given 8 hours after the second dose for a total digitalizing dose of 0.05 mg/kg. If, after conversion to sinus rhythm, WPW syndrome is identified on the EKG, digoxin should be discontinued and some other medication for chronic management begun.

A number of other medications have also been used for the acute treatment of SVT in children. All have merit in particular settings but have significant side effects that limit their usefulness in other situations.

Verapamil (0.1 mg/kg IV) is an extremely effective agent for the treatment of SVT in children and works primarily by slowing conduction through the AV node.[94] There are numerous reports, however, of severe hemodynamic side effects with the use of verapamil in infants; these include hypotension, profound sinus bradycardia, varying degrees of AV block, and asystole.[95, 96] For this reason, verapamil is not recommended in the treatment of SVT in children younger than 1 year. It is also contraindicated in any patient who is already taking a beta blocker, who has significant sinus node dysfunction, or who is in severe congestive heart failure. For any other uncompromised child who has SVT and is older than 1 year, verapamil is a safe and effective medication.

Phenylephrine (0.01 to 0.1 mg/kg IV) has been used to elicit vagally mediated bradycardia through an increase in systemic blood pressure. However, its efficacy in very young children has been questioned, and there are concerns regarding its potential for decreasing cardiac output.[69]

Propranolol (0.02 to 0.1 mg/kg IV) has also been used in the acute management of SVT in children because of its depressant effects on the AV node. However, it may be less efficacious than other medications described.[97, 98] The potential for hypoglycemia in very young children and for a sustained decrease in cardiac output as a result of sinus bradycardia in any child has limited its use in the pediatric emergency department.[75]

Ventricular Tachycardia

Diagnosis. Ventricular tachycardia is present when three or more premature ventricular contractions are seen together without an intervening normal QRS complex. The ventricular rate is fast, generally greater than 120 beats/min. The atrial rate is frequently difficult to determine, as P waves may be buried in the QRS complexes. If P waves are discernible, dissociation from the ventricular rate is common.

As previously described in the section on premature ventricular contractions, the QRS complex during a PVC, and thus during ventricular tachycardia, should always have a different morphology than that of the normal QRS complex. The duration of the QRS complex should also be prolonged; however, this finding is not absolute. Ventricular tachycardia has been described in infants with very rapid conduction through the ventricles that allowed a QRS duration as low as 0.045 seconds.[60]

If the QRS complex is prolonged, SVT with aberrant conduction may be present. However, SVT in children is rarely conducted aberrantly.[66] Until proven otherwise, a wide complex tachycardia in children should always be treated as ventricular tachycardia.

Therapeutic Intervention. For all patients with ventricular tachycardia, a rapid search for the cause should be undertaken. Particular attention should be paid to the possibility of metabolic derangements, drug ingestions, or infection. Adequate oxygenation and ventilation must be assured and determination of serum electrolytes performed quickly. The acute presentation of seizures and ventricular tachycardia in a previously healthy child should immediately suggest the possibility of tricyclic antidepressant ingestion. A previous history of fever and respiratory symptoms is suggestive of myocarditis.

The acute management of the child with ventricular tachycardia is dictated by the patient's hemodynamic status. If the patient shows signs of hemodynamic compromise, the treatment is immediate synchronized DC cardioversion. The energy dose is 0.5 joules/kg and may be doubled with each shock to a maximum of 2 joules/kg. If cardioversion is unsuccessful, lidocaine (1 mg/kg IV bolus) should be given and cardioversion attempted again.

In the child without hemodynamic compromise and in whom correctable causes for the ventricular tachycardia have been excluded, treatment should begin with lidocaine (1 mg/kg IV bolus followed by a drip at 20 to 40 µg/kg/min). If lidocaine fails to convert the rhythm and the child's hemodynamic status remains stable, immediate consultation with a pediatric cardiologist is warranted. Medical management at this point can be quite varied depending on the cause of the rhythm disturbance.

Procainamide (10 mg/kg IV drip over 30 minutes) can be used for ventricular tachycardia refractory to lidocaine. It should not be used, however, in patients in whom the ventricular tachycardia is a result of quinidine toxicity or long QT syndrome.[60]

Phenytoin (10 to 15 mg/kg IV, at a rate no faster than 50 mg/minute) has been recommended for ventricular tachycardia caused by digoxin toxicity if digoxin antibodies are not readily available. Phenytoin has also been recommended as treatment for both the seizures and the dysrhythmias associated with tricyclic antidepressant ingestion.

Lastly, propranolol (0.025 to 0.1 mg/kg IV) may be used; however, propranolol is not recommended unless facilities for temporary pacing are available in the event of symptomatic bradycardia.[60]

Atrial Flutter

Diagnosis

Atrial flutter is present when P waves are seen in a characteristic sawtooth or undulating pattern on the surface EKG at rates higher than the upper limits of normal for age (see Table 18–1). Flutter waves are seen best in standard leads II, III, and VF. The rate of flutter waves is typically 300 beats/min in infants and children, although rates as high as 500 beats/min have been reported. Flutter waves may be conducted to the ventricles in ratios of 1:1, 2:1, 3:1, or 4:1.

In infants, atrial flutter has been reported without the typical sawtooth pattern of flutter waves on the standard EKG. Dunnigan et al.[99] reported on six infants evaluated for tachycardia, in whom the standard EKG and rhythm strip showed no evidence of flutter waves. In each case, the transesophageal atrial EKG revealed atrial flutter with 2:1 conduction.

Pathophysiology and Clinical Features

Atrial flutter is a form of supraventricular tachycardia in which the rhythm disturbance is confined solely to the atrial tissue. Although the exact electrophysiologic mechanism is unknown, abnormal automaticity of ectopic tissue is not thought to be the basis for this rhythm, and thus it is not classified as an atrial ectopic tachycardia. The electrophysiologic basis of the characteristic EKG pattern is unclear.

Atrial flutter is primarily a disorder of children with congenital heart disease. In a large collaborative study of 380 patients with atrial flutter, Garson et al.[100] found that 81% of the patients had congenital heart disease, and the vast majority had already undergone corrective surgery. Six percent of the patients had a cardiomyopathy as the basis for the rhythm disturbance, and only 7% had structurally normal hearts. The mean age at onset was 10.3 years.

Therapeutic Intervention

Atrial flutter is generally treated with synchronized DC cardioversion. The energy dose is 0.5 joules/kg and may be doubled with each subsequent shock to a maximum of 2 joules/kg. Acute medical management of atrial flutter with digoxin is frequently unsuccessful.

Atrial Fibrillation

Diagnosis

Atrial fibrillation is identified by an irregular atrial rate with an undulating baseline and an irregular ventricular response. Atrial rates are in the range of 350 to 600 beats/min, and ventricular response is generally greater than 150 beats/min.

Pathophysiology and Clinical Features

Atrial fibrillation is a primary atrial disorder in which multiple different waves of electrical activity are generated within the atria at the same time. The electrophysiologic basis of the rhythm is unknown. Enlargement of the atrial tissue is thought to contribute to the disorder but is not present in all cases.

Atrial fibrillation in children is even less common than atrial flutter. It is seen most often in children who have undergone surgical repair of congenital heart disease, but it is also seen in children with cardiomyopathy, endocarditis, and rheumatic heart disease.[101]

Therapeutic Intervention

Atrial fibrillation may be difficult to control. For the patient with signs of hemodynamic compromise, synchronized DC cardioversion is the preferred treatment. As with atrial flutter and SVT, the energy dose is 0.5 joules/kg, which may be doubled with each dose to a maximum of 2 joules/kg. Medical management with digoxin may be attempted in the stable patient; however, it should be avoided if the patient has WPW syndrome. Verapamil (0.1 mg/kg IV) may slow the ventricular rate in patients with rapid conduction and improve ventricular filling; however, it, too, should be avoided in patients with WPW syndrome and in children less than 1 year of age, on beta-blocker medication, or with severe congestive heart failure.

Ventricular Fibrillation

Diagnosis

The EKG in patients with ventricular fibrillation shows low- or high-amplitude wave forms of varying size, shape, and rhythm with no discernible P, QRS, or T waves. High-amplitude wave forms are called *coarse ventricular fibrillation*. Low-amplitude wave forms are called *fine ventricular fibrillation*. Fine ventricular fibrillation may be of such low amplitude that it can be mistaken for asystole if multiple leads are not checked.

Pathophysiology and Clinical Features

Ventricular fibrillation is characterized by chaotic, uncoordinated ventricular depolarizations that generate no cardiac output. The electrophysiologic basis of ventricular fibrillation is unknown. It has been postulated that there is a critical mass of myocardium required to initiate and maintain ventricular fibrillation.[8] The relatively small hearts of infants and children may be less prone to fibrillation on this basis. This may help to explain the scarcity of ventricular fibrillation in the pediatric population.

Ventricular fibrillation is seen most commonly in children with structurally abnormal hearts.[7] In a previously healthy child, spontaneous ventricular fibrillation may be caused by the long QT syndrome,[54, 58] acute myocarditis, or a toxic ingestion.

Therapeutic Intervention

Ventricular fibrillation is a lethal rhythm that must be treated acutely. Cardiopulmonary resuscitation should be initiated and continued until electrical defibrillation can be administered. Although the optimal emergency dose for children in ventricular fibrillation is unknown, the current recommendation is to begin with 2 joules/kg, increasing to 4 joules/kg if the first shock is unsuccessful.[6] Although it should not be allowed to delay defibrillation, establishment of an adequate airway to optimize oxygenation and ventilation is essential.

References

1. Perry JC, Garson A. Diagnosis and treatment of arrhythmias. Adv Pediatr 1989;36:177.
2. Losek JD, Hennes H. Prehospital countershock treatment of pediatric asystole. Am J Emerg Med 1989;7:571.
3. Eisenberg M, Bergner L, Hallstrom A. Epidemiology of cardiac arrest and resuscitation in children. Ann Emerg Med 1983;12:672.
4. Ludwig S, Fleisher G. Pediatric cardiopulmonary resuscitation: A review and a proposal. Pediatr Emerg Care 1985;1:40.
5. Orlowski JP. Pediatric cardiopulmonary resuscitation. Emerg Med Clin North Am 1983;1:3.
6. Chameides L (ed). Textbook of Pediatric Advanced Life Support. Dallas, TX, American Heart Association, 1988, p 61.
7. Walsh CK, Krongrad E. Terminal cardiac electrical activity in pediatric patients. Am J Cardiol 1983;51:557.
8. Garrey WE. The nature of fibrillary contraction of the heart—its relation to tissue mass and form. Am J Physiol 1914;33:397.
9. Reder RF, Rosen MR. The role of the sympathetic nervous system in sudden cardiac death. Drug Ther 1978;8:41.
10. Kugler JD. Sinus node dysfunction. In Gillette PC, Garson A (eds). Pediatric Arrhythmias: Electrophysiology and Pacing. Philadelphia, WB Saunders, 1990, pp 250–300.
11. Nadas AD, Flyer DC. Pediatric Cardiology. Philadelphia, WB Saunders, 1982, p 63.
12. Garson A, Gillette PC, McNamara DG. A Guide to Cardiac Dysrhythmias in Children. New York, Grune & Stratton, 1980, p 117.
13. Southall DP, Johnston F, Shinebourne EA, et al. 24-hour electrocardiographic study of heart rate and rhythm patterns in a population of healthy children. Br Heart J 1981;45:281.
14. Gillette PC, Kugler JD, Garson A, et al. Mechanisms of cardiac arrhythmias after the Mustard operation for transposition of the great arteries. Am J Cardiol 1980;45:1225.
15. Radford DJ, Izukawa T. Sick sinus syndrome: Symptomatic cases in children. Arch Dis Child 1975;50:879.
16. Beder SD, Gillette PC, Garson A, et al. Symptomatic sick sinus syndrome in children and adolescents as the only manifestation of cardiac abnormality or associated with unoperated congenital heart disease. Am J Cardiol 1983;51:1133.
17. Frye RL, Collins JJ, DeSanctis RW, et al. Special report: Guidelines for permanent pacemaker implantation, May 1984. J Am Coll Cardiol 1984;4:434.
18. Anderson RH, Ho SY. The conduction system of the human heart. In Harrison RJ, Holmes RL (eds). Progress in Anatomy. Vol 1. New York, Cambridge University Press, 1981, pp 163–181.
19. Roberts NK, Castleman KR. Morphology of the atrioventricular node, bundle and proximal bundle branches: A study employing computerized reconstruction. Anat Rec 1979;195:699.
20. Roberts NK. Atrioventricular conduction and intraventricular conduction. In Roberts NK, Gelland H (eds). Cardiac Arrhythmias in the Neonate, Infant, and Child. Norwalk, CT, Appleton-Century-Crofts, 1983, pp 233–252.
21. Anderson PAW, Rogers MC, Canent RV, et al. Atrioventricular conduction in secundum atrial septal defects. Circulation 1973;48:27.
22. Brodsky M, Wu D, Denes P, et al. Arrhythmias documented by 24 hour continuous electrocardiographic monitoring in 50 male medical students without apparent heart disease. Am J Cardiol 1977;39:390.
23. Meytes I, Kaplinsky E, Yahini JH, et al. Wenckebach A-V block: A frequent feature following heavy physical training. Am Heart J 1975;90:426.
24. Lightfoot PR, Sasse L, Mandel WJ, et al. His bundle electrograms in healthy adolescents with persistent second degree A-V block. Chest 1973;63:358.
25. Kelly DT, Brodsky SJ, Krovetz LJ. Mobitz type II atrioventricular block in children. J Pediatr 1971;79:972.
26. Ross BA. First and second degree atrioventricular block. In Gillette PC, Garson A (eds). Pediatric Arrhythmias: Electrophysiology and Pacing. Philadelphia, WB Saunders, 1990, pp 301–305.
27. Michaelsson M, Engle MA. Congenital complete heart block: An international study of the natural history. Cardiovasc Clin 1972;4:85.
28. Reed BR, Lee LA, Harmon C, et al. Autoantibodies to SS-A/Ro in infants with congenital heart block. J Pediatr 1983;103:889.
29. Scott JS, Maddison PJ, Taylor PV, et al. Connective-tissue disease, antibodies to ribonucleoprotein, and congenital heart block. N Engl J Med 1983;309:209.
30. Taylor PV, Scott JS, Gerlis LM, et al. Maternal antibodies against fetal cardiac antigens in congenital complete heart block. N Engl J Med 1986;315:667.
31. Kelly DT, Brodsky SJ, Mirowski M, et al. Bundle of His recordings in congenital complete heart block. Circulation 1972;45:277.
32. Driscoll DJ, Gillette PC, Hallman GL, et al. Management of surgical complete atrioventricular block in children. Am J Cardiol 1979;43:1175.
33. Karpawich PP, Gillette PC. Congenital complete atrioventricular block: Clinical and electrophysiologic predictors of need for pacemaker insertion. Am J Cardiol 1981;48:1098.
34. Dewey RC, Capeless MA, Levy AM. Use of ambulatory electrocardiographic monitoring to identify high-risk patients with congenital complete heart block. N Engl J Med 1987;316:835.
35. Kugler JD, Danford DA. Pacemakers in children: An update. Am Heart J 1989;117:665.
36. Pinsky WW, Gillette PC, Garson A, et al. Diagnosis, management, and long-term results of patients with congenital complete atrioventricular block. Pediatrics 1982;69:728.
37. Ross BA, Pinsky WW, Driscoll DJ. Complete atrioventricular block. In Gillette PC, Garson A (eds). Pediatric Arrhythmias: Electrophysiology and Pacing. Philadelphia, WB Saunders, 1990, pp 306–316.
38. Krongrad E. Postoperative arrhythmias in patients with congenital heart disease. Chest 1984;85:107.
39. Kay EB, Nogukira C, Mendelsohn D, et al. Corrective surgery for tetralogy of Fallot. Circulation 1961;24:1342.
40. Vetter VL, Horowitz LN. Electrophysiologic residua and sequelae of surgery for congenital heart defects. Am J Cardiol 1982;50:588.
41. Komajda M, Frank R, Vedel J, et al. Intracardiac conduction defects in dystrophia myotonica. Br Heart J 1980;43:315.
42. Sanyal SK, Johnson WW. Cardiac conduction abnormalities in children with Duchenne's progressive muscular dystrophy: Electrocardiographic features and morphologic correlates. Circulation 1982;66:853.
43. Husson GS, Blackman MS, Rogers MC, et al. Familial congenital bundle branch system disease. Am J Cardiol 1973;32:365.
44. Esscher E, Hardell LI, Michaelsson M. Familial, isolated, complete right bundle-branch block. Br Heart J 1975;37:745.
45. Sung RJ, Tamer DM, Agha AS. Etiology of the electrocardiographic pattern of "incomplete right bundle branch block" in atrial septal defect: An electrophysiologic study. J Pediatr 1975;87:1182.
46. Moore EN, Boineau JP, Patterson DF. Incomplete right bundle-branch block: An electrocardiographic enigma and possible misnomer. Circulation 1971;44:678.
47. Burch GE, Depasquale NP. Electrocardiography in the diagnosis of congenital heart disease. Philadelphia, Lea & Febiger, 1967.
48. Ewing L. Bundle-branch and fascicular blocks. In Gillette PC, Garson A (eds). Pediatric Arrhythmias: Electrophysiology and Pacing. Philadelphia, WB Saunders, 1990, pp 317–327.
49. Yanowitz F, Preston JB, Abildskov JA. Functional distribution of right and left stellate innervation to the ventricles: Production of neurogenic electrocardiographic changes by unilateral alteration of sympathetic tone. Circ Res 1966;18:416.
50. Schwartz PJ, Periti M, Malliani A. Fundamentals of clinical cardiology: The long Q-T syndrome. Am Heart J 1975;89:378.
51. Jervell A, Lange-Nielsen F. Congenital deaf-mutism, functional heart disease with prolongation of the Q-T interval and sudden death. Am Heart J 1957;54:59.
52. Romano C, Gemme G, Pongiglione R. Aritmie cardiache rare delléta pediatrica. Clin Pediatr 1963;45:656.
53. Ward OC. A new familial cardiac syndrome in children. J Irish Med Assoc 1964;54:103.
54. Moss AJ. Prolonged QT-interval syndromes. JAMA 1986;256:2985.
55. Reynolds EW, Vander Ark CR. Quinidine syncope and the delayed repolarization syndromes. Mod Concepts Cardiovasc Dis 1976;55:117.
56. Moss AJ. Caution: Very-low-calorie diets can be deadly. Ann Intern Med 1985;102;121.
57. Isner JM, Roberts WC, Heymsfield SB, et al. Anorexia nervosa and sudden death. Ann Intern Med 1985;102:49.
58. Weintraub RG, Gow RM, Wilkinson JL. The congenital long QT syndromes in childhood. J Am Coll Cardiol 1990;16:674.
59. Grospe SM, Choy M. Hereditary long Q-T syndrome presenting as epilepsy: Electroencephalography laboratory diagnosis. Ann Neurol 1989;25:514.
60. Garson A. Ventricular arrhythmias. In Gillette PC, Garson A (eds).

Pediatric Arrhythmias: Electrophysiology and Pacing. Philadelphia, WB Saunders, 1990, pp 427–500.

61. Salice P, Segantini A, Locati E, et al. The prognosis of premature atrial beats in infancy. Circulation 1983;68(III):395.
62. Southall DP, Richards J, Mitchell P, et al. Study of cardiac rhythm in healthy newborn infants. Br Heart J 1980;43:14.
63. Scott O, Williams GJ, Fiddler GI. Results of 24 hour ambulatory monitoring of electrocardiogram in 131 healthy boys aged 10 to 13 years. Br Heart J 1980;44:304.
64. Dunnigan A, Benditt DG, Benson DW. Modes of onset ("initiating events") for paroxysmal atrial tachycardia in infants and children. Am J Cardiol 1986;57:1280.
65. Jacobsen JR, Garson A, Gillette PC, et al. Premature ventricular contractions in normal children. J Pediatr 1978;92:36.
66. Garson A, Gillette PC, McNamara DG. Supraventricular tachycardia in children: Clinical features, response to treatment, and long-term follow-up in 217 patients. J Pediatr 1981;98:875.
67. Nadas AS, Daeschner CW, Roth A, et al. Paroxysmal tachycardia in infants and children: Study of 41 cases. Pediatrics 1952;9:167.
68. Keith JD, Rowe RD, Vlad P. Heart disease in infancy and childhood. New York, Macmillan, 1967, p 1056.
69. Ludomirsky A, Garson A. Supraventricular tachycardia. In Gillette PC, Garson A (eds). Pediatric Arrhythmias: Electrophysiology and Pacing. Philadelphia, WB Saunders, 1990, pp 380–426.
70. Gillette PC. The mechanisms of supraventricular tachycardia in children. Circulation 1976;54:133.
71. Garson A, Gillette PC. Electrophysiologic studies of supraventricular tachycardia in children. I. Clinical electrophysiologic correlations. Am Heart J 1981;102:233.
72. Garson A, Gillette PC. Electrophysiologic studies of supraventricular tachycardia in children. II. Prediction of specific mechanism by noninvasive features. Am Heart J 1981;102:383.
73. Wu D, Denes P, Amat-Y-Leon F, et al. Clinical, electrocardiographic and electrophysiologic observations in patients with paroxysmal supraventricular tachycardia. Am J Cardiol 1978;41:1045.
74. Mehta AS, Casta A, Wolff GS. Supraventricular tachycardia. In Roberts NK, Gelband H (eds). Cardiac Arrhythmias in the Neonate, Infant and Child. Norwalk, CT, Appleton-Century-Crofts, 1983, pp 105–146.
75. Garson A. Medicolegal problems in the management of cardiac arrhythmias in children. Pediatrics 1987;79:84.
76. Whitman V, Friedman Z, Berman W, et al. Supraventricular tachycardia in newborn infants: An approach to therapy. J Pediatr 1977;91:304.
77. Bisset GS, Gaum W, Kaplan S. The ice bag: A new technique for interruption of supraventricular tachycardia. J Pediatr 1980;97:593.
78. Hamilton J, Moodie D, Levy J. The use of the diving reflex to terminate supraventricular tachycardia in a 2-week-old infant. Am Heart J 1979;97:371.
79. Grahame IFM, Hann IM. Use of the diving reflex to treat supraventricular tachycardia in an infant. Arch Dis Child 1978;53:515.
80. Sperandeo V, Pieri D, Palazzolo P, et al. Supraventricular tachycardia in infants: Use of the "diving reflex." Am J Cardiol 1983;51:286.
81. Wildenthal K, Atkins JM. Use of the "diving reflex" for the treatment of paroxysmal supraventricular tachycardia. Am Heart J 1979;98:536.
82. Pickering T, Bolton-Maggs P. Treatment of paroxysmal supraventricular tachycardia. Lancet 1975;1:340.
83. Condry P, Jain A, Marshall R, et al. Ventricular tachycardia caused by the diving reflex. Lancet 1975;2:1263.
84. Greco R, Musto B, Arienzo V, et al. Treatment of paroxysmal supraventricular tachycardia in infancy with digitalis, adenosine-5'-triphosphate, and verapamil: A comparative study. Circulation 1982;66:504.
85. Belhassen B, Pelleg A. Adenosine triphosphate and adenosine: Perspectives in the acute management of paroxysmal supraventricular tachycardia. Clin Cardiol 1985;8:460.
86. Overholt ED, Rheuban KS, Gutgesell HP, et al. Usefulness of adenosine for arrhythmias in infants and children. Am J Cardiol 1988;61:336.
87. Till J, Shinebourne EA, Rigby ML, et al. Efficacy and safety of adenosine in the treatment of supraventricular tachycardia in infants and children. Br Heart J 1989;62:204.
88. Rossi AF, Burton DA. Adenosine in altering short- and long-term treatments of supraventricular tachycardia in infants. Am J Cardiol 1989;64:685.
89. Clarke B, Rowland E, Barnes PJ, et al. Rapid and safe termination of supraventricular tachycardia in children by adenosine. Lancet (I) 1987;1:299.
90. Sellers T, Bashore TM, Gallagher JJ. Digitalis in the pre-excitation syndrome: Analysis during atrial fibrillation. Circulation 1977;56:260.
91. Wellens HJ, Durrer D. Effect of digitalis on atrioventricular conduction and circus-movement tachycardias in patients with Wolff-Parkinson-White syndrome. Circulation 1973;47:1229.
92. Benson DW, Dunnigan A. Disturbances of cardiac rhythm. In Moller JH, Neel WA (eds). Fetal, Neonatal and Infant Cardiac Disease. Norwalk, CT, Appleton & Lange, 1990, pp 835–868.
93. Jedeikin R, Gillette PC, Garson A, et al. Effect of ouabain on the anterograde effective refractory period of accessory atrioventricular connections in children. J Am Coll Cardiol 1983;1:869.
94. Porter CJ, Garson A, Gillette PC. Verapamil: An effective calcium blocking agent for pediatric patients. Pediatrics 1983;71:748.
95. Epstein ML, Kiel EA, Victorica BE. Cardiac decompensation following verapamil therapy in infants with supraventricular tachycardia. Pediatrics 1985;75:737.
96. Abinader E, Borochowitz A, Berger A. A hemodynamic complication of verapamil theraphy in a neonate. Helv Paediatr Acta 1981;36:451.
97. Denes P, Cummings JM, Simpson R, et al. Effects of propranolol on anomalous pathway refractoriness and circus movement tachycardias in patients with preexcitation. Am J Cardiol 1978;41:1061.
98. Barrett PA, Jordan JL, Mandel WJ, et al. The electrophysiologic effects of intravenous propranolol in the Wolff-Parkinson-White syndrome. Am Heart J 1979;98:213.
99. Dunnigan A, Benson W, Benditt DG. Atrial flutter in infancy: Diagnosis, clinical features, and treatment. Pediatrics 1985;75:725.
100. Garson AJ, Bink-Boelkens M, Hesslein PS, et al. Atrial flutter in the young: A collaborative study of 380 cases. J Am Coll Cardiol 1985;6:871.
101. Radford DJ, Izukawa T. Atrial fibrillation in children. Pediatrics 1977;59:250.

CHAPTER 19

Congestive Heart Failure

Peter T. Mellis

INTRODUCTION

Congestive heart failure (CHF) in infants and young children challenges the physician's ability to recognize and stabilize the patient with significantly altered physiologic status. The frequency of the initial presentation of heart disease in children in the emergency department is low. More than 80% of children who develop CHF do so in the first year of life, predominantly as a result of congenital heart disease.[1] The physical manifestations of CHF are characteristically age related and overlap those of a number of more common diseases of noncardiac origin. Therefore a basic understanding of the physiology of the major types of congenital and acquired heart disease and their expected age-related presentation is essential in guiding emergency management.

ANATOMY AND PHYSIOLOGY
Definitions

The function of the heart is to pump blood to tissue beds to provide for substrate delivery and uptake. The vascular tree serves to distribute blood to, and drain blood from, tissue beds in a balanced fashion. Dysfunction of either or both components of the circulatory system may result in its failure. Circulatory failure is therefore a state in which the circulatory system is (1) unable to maintain the level of tissue perfusion required by metabolic demands (*heart failure*), (2) unable to provide adequate venous tissue drainage (*circulatory congestion*), or (3) a combination of the two (*congestive heart failure*).

Physiologic Mechanisms

The adequacy of circulatory function results from a complex interaction of physiologic factors affecting *cardiac output*

TABLE 19–1

PHYSIOLOGIC FACTORS AFFECTING CARDIAC OUTPUT

Physiologic Factor	Definition	Pathophysiologic State
Preload	Venous diastolic filling pressure	Volume overload
Contractility	Intrinsic mechanical myocardial performance	Decreased inotropic state
Afterload	Pressure load against myocardial work	Pressure overload
Autonomic control	Neurohumoral stimulation of myocardium and vascular tree	Dysrhythmias

(i.e., the product of heart rate and stroke volume) and *vascular resistance*, which reflects the distribution and drainage of blood within the pulmonary and systemic circuits (Fig. 19–1). Four such physiologic factors are described: preload, contractility, afterload, and automaticity (Table 19–1). *Preload* refers to end-diastolic ventricular filling pressure or volume to be ejected by the heart. *Contractility*, or inotropic state, refers to the biochemical and ultrastructural limits to myocardial performance. The interrelationship of cardiac output, preload, and contractility is classically expressed by the Frank-Starling relationship (Fig. 19–2). *Afterload* refers to the impedance the myocardium must work against secondary to both structural and dynamic vascular resistance. *Automaticity* refers to both extrinsic and intrinsic neurohumoral regulation of heart rate.

Hemodynamic States

Two major hemodynamic states may result in the clinical manifestations of CHF in infants and children; each is the consequence of disease processes resulting in compromise of the physiologic mechanisms by which cardiac function is maintained. High-output states typically result from volume overloading conditions such as the left-to-right shunt of a patent ductus arteriosus or a ventricular septal defect. Low-output states may result from pressure overloading conditions such as the left-sided heart obstruction of coarctation of the aorta, the depressed inotropic state of the cardiomyopathies, or dysrhythmias such as supraventricular tachycardia (Table 19–2).

Left-sided heart failure results in increased left-sided end-diastolic pressure, giving rise to pulmonary venous congestion, lung edema, and ultimately arterial hypertension with secondary right-sided heart failure. Right-sided heart failure results in increased right-sided end-diastolic pressure, giving rise to systemic venous congestion and decreased forward flow with secondary left-sided heart failure. In each case, biventricular failure ultimately occurs.

Acute heart failure is manifested by signs of cardiogenic shock with limited compensatory response, as may occur with the sudden onset of mitral or aortic papillary muscle dysfunction following myocardial infarction resulting from Kawasaki disease. Chronic heart failure is characterized by prominent findings of compensatory responses with no or minimal evidence of inadequate cardiac output, as may occur with the gradual onset of mitral or aortic valvular insufficiency following rheumatic fever. Thus the time course over which the primary disease process has altered myocardial volume or pressure-loading conditions will determine the degree of efficacy of compensatory responses.

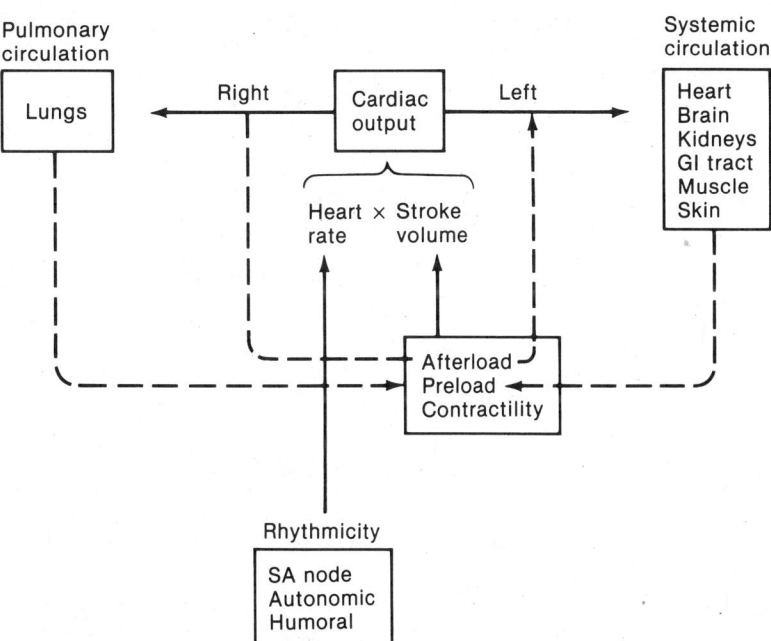

Figure 19–1. Schematic representation of the systemic and pulmonary circulation with major physiologic determinants of cardiac output.

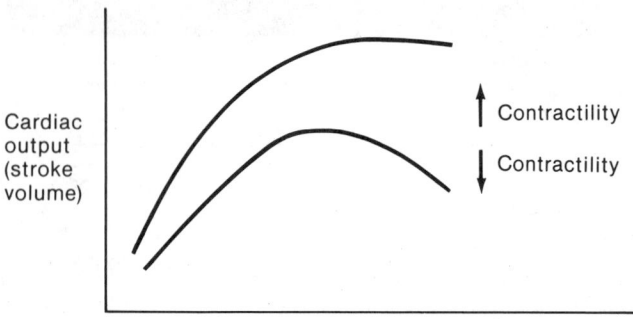

Figure 19–2. Schematic representation of the Frank-Starling relationship between cardiac output and preload with fixed heart rate and afterload. The effect of varying contractile states is illustrated.

Developmental Effects and Etiology

Predictable changes in circulatory physiology occur after birth and have a profound impact on the time of presentation and course of the child with CHF caused by congenital heart disease (Table 19–3). The onset of respiration after birth results in a rise in arterial blood oxygen saturation with concomitant structural and physiologic changes. The first response is closure of the ductus arteriosus shortly after birth, removing the connection between the ascending aorta and the left main pulmonary artery. This has major implications in patients with congenital abnormalities such as coarctation of the aorta, in which a distal patent ductus arteriosus is the major route of lower body perfusion. The second response is a fall in pulmonary vascular resistance during the first 6 weeks of life. This may result in the development of a significant systemic-to-pulmonary left-to-right shunt at any level of the circuit where an interconnection occurs. Beyond the first year of life, acquired causes of heart failure predominate. Acquired heart disease, as well as renal, pulmonary, and metabolic diseases, also has a predictable time of presentation with CHF, though to a lesser degree than congenital heart disease (Table 19–4). These diseases must be considered for their noncardiac complications. In particular, rheumatic fever has reemerged as the major preventable cause of heart failure in children over 2 years of age.[2] Therefore the age of the child at the time of presentation with CHF offers a useful diagnostic clue to the cause of heart failure.

Compensatory Responses

The mechanisms by which the performance of the failing heart is modulated are responsible for many of the physical manifestations of CHF in infants and children. The efficacy of these compensatory responses is greater when CHF has occurred gradually. Adrenergic effects are the major compensatory mechanisms by which cardiac output is maintained in infants. These are primarily the result of an increased

---

TABLE 19–2
CORRELATION OF PHYSIOLOGY WITH ORIGIN OF CHF

Pathophysiologic State	Mechanism of Disease	Origin of CHF
High output Volume overload	Left-to-right shunt	Ventricular septal defect Patent ductus arteriosus Truncus arteriosus Arteriovenous malformation
	Valvular regurgitation	Aortic insufficiency Pulmonary insufficiency
	Pulmonary venous obstruction	Anomalous pulmonary venous return
	Hematologic	Severe anemia (sickle cell disease)
Low output Pressure overload	Left ventricular outflow tract obstruction	Hypoplastic left heart syndrome (aortic atresia) Coarctation of the aorta Aortic stenosis
	Systemic hypertension	Renal failure Pheochromocytoma
	Pulmonary hypertension	Bronchopulmonary dysplasia Cystic fibrosis
Decreased inotropic state	Infection	Myocarditis Endocarditis Sepsis (meningococcemia)
	Inflammation	Cardiomyopathies (muscular dystrophy) Acute rheumatic fever Collagen-vascular disease Kawasaki disease
	Infarction	Anomalous left main coronary artery
	Ingestion	Beta blockers Calcium channel blockers
	Metabolic	Glycogen storage diseases Endocardial fibroelastosis Thyroid disease
Altered autonomic regulation	Dysrhythmias	Supraventricular tachycardia Complete heart block
Mechanical restriction	Tamponade	Pericarditis Cardiac neoplasm (tuberous sclerosis)

Note: One or more pathophysiologic mechanisms may apply to a given disease causing CHF. For purposes of clarity, the major mechanism is indicated.

TABLE 19-3

RELATIONSHIP OF AGE TO PRESENTATION OF CHF FROM CONGENITAL HEART DISEASE

Age	Origin of CHF
1–7 days	Hypoplastic left heart syndrome
	Transposition of the great vessels
	Coarctation of the aorta with distal patent ductus arteriosus
	Less common:
	Anomalous pulmonary venous return
	Aortic stenosis (critical)
	Pulmonary stenosis (critical)
	Arteriovenous fistula
	Supraventricular tachycardia
1–6 wk	Coarctation of the aorta with distal patent ductus arteriosus
	Transposition of the great vessels
	Endocardial cushion defect
	Patent ductus arteriosus (premature infant)
6 wk to 6 mo	Ventricular septal defect
	Patent ductus arteriosus
	Supraventricular tachycardia
	Anomalous left main coronary artery

level of circulating catecholamines of adrenal origin.[3] Beta-adrenergic stimulation results in increased heart rate and contractile state. Cardiac output in young infants is particularly dependent on heart rate; bradycardia is an ominous finding indicative of inadequate tissue oxygenation. Alpha-adrenergic stimulation results in systemic vasoconstriction and decreased perfusion of less vital organ systems such as skin, skeletal muscle, gastrointestinal tract, and kidneys. Regional circulation effects include the autoregulation of blood flow to preserve perfusion of the heart and brain at the expense of less vital organ systems. Pulmonary effects include preservation of oxygenation and ventilation by increased minute ventilation, primarily by tachypnea, in response to the increased lung fluid resulting from left-sided failure. Renal effects are primarily caused by decreased renal blood flow. Augmentation of preload by fluid and sodium retention occurs through both intrinsic proximal tubular and renin-angiotensin–mediated distal tubular reabsorptive

TABLE 19-4

TYPICAL AGE OF PRESENTATION WITH CHF CAUSED BY ACQUIRED AND PRIMARY MYOCARDIAL DISEASE

Age	Origin of CHF
Infancy (0–12 mo)	Bronchopulmonary dysplasia
	Endocardial fibroelastosis
	Glycogen storage disease
	Congenital hypothyroidism
	Sickle cell (acute sequestration)
Early childhood (1–4 yr)	Viral myocarditis
	Kawasaki disease
School age (5–12 yr)	Rheumatic carditis
	Chronic renal failure (hypertension)
Adolescence (13–18 yr)	Rheumatic valvular disease
	Muscular dystrophy
	Cystic fibrosis
	Sickle cell (chronic anemia)

Note: Broad variation exists for age of onset of most listed disease entities. For purposes of illustration of age-related distribution, each has been listed only at its peak age of presentation with CHF.

mechanisms. Oxygen transport effects include improved tissue oxygenation, as indicated by a shift to the right in the oxygen-hemoglobin dissociation curve, and, in disease states associated with chronic hypoxemia, a higher hemoglobin concentration. Mechanical effects include ventricular dilatation and hypertrophy, which preserve cardiac output at the expense of increased myocardial oxygen consumption. Because these changes occur only after a significant period of myocardial insufficiency, dilatation and hypertrophy are evidence of compromised cardiac performance with limited ability to respond to further circulatory demands.

Finally, the ability of the infant to augment or maintain cardiac output by these compensatory mechanisms is limited relative to the older child and adult. This limitation stems from the compromise of diastolic filling time with increasing tachycardia,[4] an increased myocardial wall stiffness,[5] and a decreased ability to augment stroke volume with a given degree of preload[6] relative to the adult myocardium. Consequently, most children who present with CHF do so during infancy, when developmentally least able to tolerate increased volume or pressure loads, and thus are at greatest risk for cardiac decompensation.

EMERGENCY MEDICAL SERVICE CONSIDERATIONS

The objective of prehospital care is to stabilize the acutely ill patient for expeditious transport to a capable facility. Therefore the emphasis for the emergency medical service (EMS) provider caring for children at risk for heart failure must be placed on recognizing cardiopulmonary decompensation and stabilizing vital functions. It is unlikely that CHF will be recognized in the young child before arrival in the emergency department, unless the child has been previously diagnosed as having heart disease.

Identifying the early signs of respiratory failure is the first priority. These findings should prompt the prehospital provider to administer high-flow oxygen and place the child on a cardiac monitor. If conscious, the child should be transported in an upright position of comfort. Assisted ventilation with 100% oxygen is indicated for the unresponsive child with evidence of respiratory failure.

Signs of poor peripheral perfusion indicate shock. As long as transport is not delayed, vascular access may be obtained. However, the prehospital provider must be cautioned against giving large amounts of intravenous fluid if there has been no history of volume loss. Attention should always be paid to avoiding hypothermia and hyperthermia when transporting infants.

Reassessment should be performed while en route, and medical control should be contacted with a report of vital signs, respiratory and perfusion parameters, and response to therapy. Whenever possible, medical control by a designated pediatric emergency center is indicated for the critically ill infant.

CLINICAL EVALUATION
Symptoms

Recognition presents the principal challenge for the emergency practitioner in the management of CHF in infants and children. Characteristically, the history is the key to timely identification of the child with CHF. The principal work of infancy is feeding, with the essential consequence of growth. Feeding problems are frequently noted by parents for days or weeks before symptoms of CHF are present in infants at rest. The normal duration of feeding is less than 15 minutes, but the infant with CHF will feed slowly and fitfully, often over 30 to 60 minutes, and appear fatigued and short of breath during and afterward. Weight gain is slow as a result of inadequate total caloric intake and increased metabolic demands. The normal growth rate in early infancy is 30 gm per day, but infants with CHF often have a growth rate of less than 10 gm per day. Chronic cough and wheezing are common respiratory complaints in older infants and children with CHF secondary to increased interstitial lung fluid. Exertional dyspnea and orthopnea may be easily recognized in older children, but may be manifested in infants only as decreased motor activity and irritability when the infant is recumbent. Excessive sweating, particularly about the forehead and scalp, is a frequent parental complaint and results from increased adrenergic tone.

The history must also include identification of associated complaints such as fever, mental status changes, and rash. Information regarding prior heart disease and surgery, acute or chronic respiratory disease, and renal, hematologic, and neuromuscular disorders is also essential. Current and recent medications and their doses should be identified. A careful history regarding the neonatal period and the risk for bronchopulmonary dysplasia is essential for infants. The presence of congenital limb or facial abnormalities may be a clue to associated heart disease. The potential for ingestion of cardiotoxic drugs should be assessed when acute CHF occurs in age groups at risk. A history of prior streptococcal pharyngitis may be elicited for older children with evidence of CHF. If the child is acutely ill, the history should be obtained by another physician, rather than deferred while the patient is stabilized.

Signs

The physical signs of CHF primarily reflect the adequacy of cardiac output and the type and degree of compensatory responses. These signs are classically categorized into three groups: compensatory responses, venous congestion, and, in the decompensated state, cardiogenic shock (Table 19–5). From a practical standpoint, the physical assessment of the child at risk for circulatory failure should be accomplished in two stages. Initially, a directed cardiorespiratory assessment should be performed in the acutely ill child to determine the child's physiologic status and establish intervention priorities (Fig. 19–3). If the child is stable, the physical examination is completed, and further evaluation may follow on an elective basis. If the child is at risk for decompensation (e.g., in poorly compensated cardiogenic shock), immediate intervention is performed to stabilize physiologic parame-

TABLE 19–5
PRINCIPAL PHYSICAL FINDINGS OF CHF IN CHILDREN
Compensatory responses
Tachycardia
Diminished peripheral pulses
Delayed capillary refill time
Pulmonary venous congestion
Tachypnea
Increased work of breathing
Wheezes
Rales (late)
Systemic venous congestion
Hepatomegaly
Periorbital edema (late)
Cardiac dysfunction
Gallop rhythm
Hypotension (late)

ters; this is followed by frequent reassessments. The complete physical examination and workup are subsequently performed as patient resuscitation progresses.

Tachycardia is the principal compensatory response to impaired cardiac function. Resting heart rates of 160 beats/min or more in children younger than 2 years and of 100 beats/min or more in older children are typically present in CHF. Heart rates greater than 220 beats/min virtually always represent supraventricular tachycardia in children. Bradycardia is an unequivocal sign of cardiac decompensation in infants and young children and demands immediate intervention. The heart rate should be continuously monitored in children with symptomatic CHF both as a guide to the adequacy of therapy and to detect dysrhythmias.

Palpation of pulses should be performed early in the evaluation of patients at risk for circulatory dysfunction. Special attention should be paid to simultaneous palpation of proximal and distal pulses in both the upper and lower extremities to detect a pulse gradient. In infants the carotid pulse may be difficult to palpate as a result of a short neck, and thus the brachial and femoral sites are preferred for comparison with distal pulses. Diminished peripheral pulses are suggestive of systemic vasoconstriction as a compensatory response to inadequate cardiac output. Bounding peripheral pulses may indicate a high-output failure state; this may occur in a large left-to-right shunt, as in a patent ductus arteriosus. Diminished lower extremity pulses with normal upper extremity pulses suggest obstruction to aortic flow (e.g., coarctation of the aorta). Diminished central pulses are consistent with a decompensated shock state and are usually accompanied by hypotension. *Pulsus alternans* refers to a regular, alternating, beat-to-beat variability in pulse amplitude and is a late finding of decompensated myocardial function.

The skin should be inspected and palpated. Pallor and mottling may indicate peripheral systemic vasoconstriction as a result of anemia or impaired cardiac function. Cyanosis indicates skin perfusion with deoxygenated blood resulting from intracardiac right-to-left shunting or severe pulmonary edema. Central cyanosis is best detected in the mucous membranes and is not usually clinically evident until the oxygen saturation of hemoglobin has fallen below 75%. A delayed capillary refill time suggests decreased skin perfusion. Normal capillary refill time is less than 2 seconds and is most reliably assessed at the thenar or hypothenar eminence of the palm or the heel with the extremity held at the level of the heart. Cool distal extremities also suggest peripheral vasoconstriction. Changes in capillary refill time may be followed as a guide to therapy. Notably, skin findings may also reflect peripheral vasoconstriction resulting from exposure to cold temperature and thus must be interpreted in the context of environmental conditions.

Tachypnea and increased work of breathing are the principal signs of pulmonary venous congestion seen in left-sided heart failure. In early CHF, minute ventilation can be maintained in the presence of decreased effective tidal volume by increasing the respiratory rate alone. With progression, retractions and nasal flaring occur, reflecting the increased muscular effort required for air entry into poorly compliant lungs with interstitial edema. Grunting respirations are evidence of increased patient-generated positive end-expiratory pressure against a closed glottis in order to maintain alveolar distention. Wheezing may be a prominent physical finding in the infant with CHF; it results from compression of small airways by distended pulmonary vasculature and bronchial edema.[7] Rales are less commonly appreciated in infants than in older children and adults with CHF, perhaps because of a relatively smaller tidal volume. The absence of rales should not be interpreted as an indi-

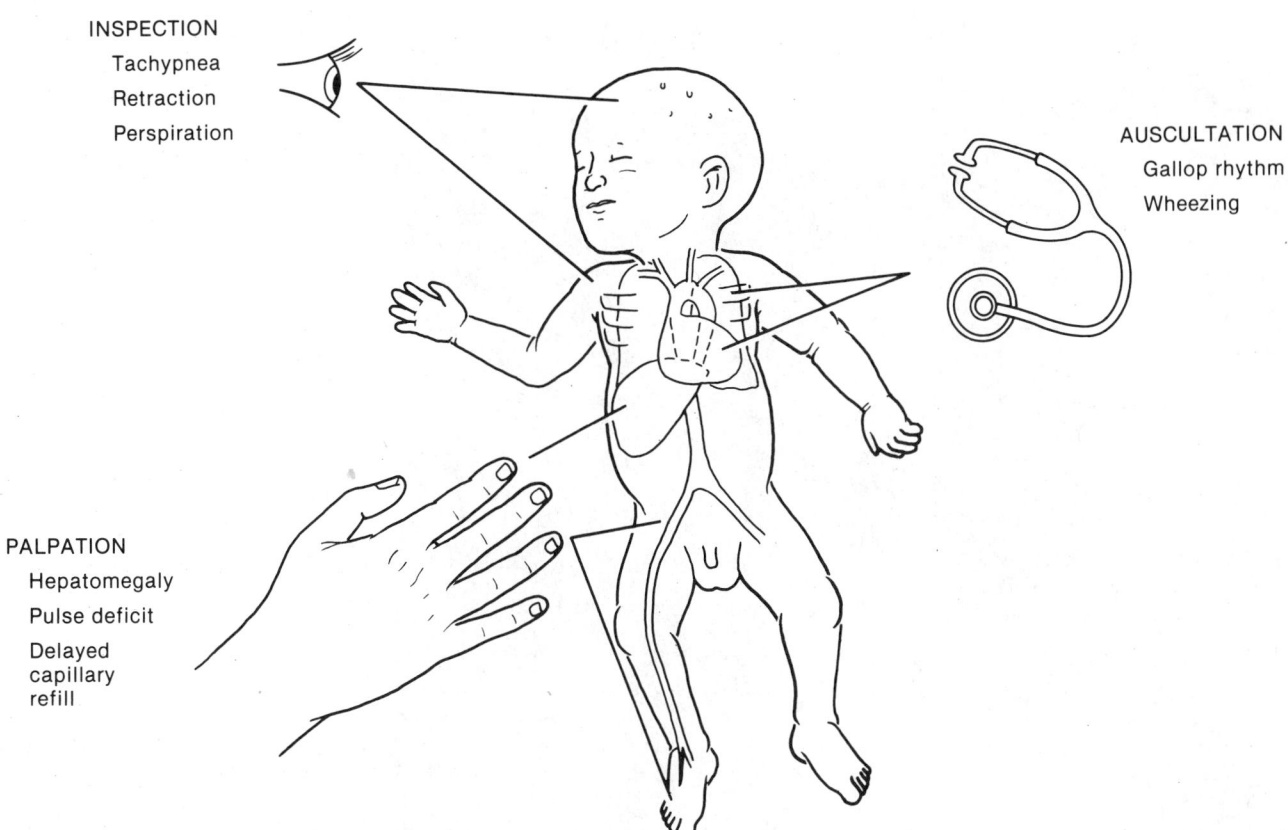

INSPECTION
Tachypnea
Retraction
Perspiration

AUSCULTATION
Gallop rhythm
Wheezing

PALPATION
Hepatomegaly
Pulse deficit
Delayed capillary refill

Figure 19–3. Principal physical findings of congestive heart failure in infancy.

cation that pulmonary edema is not present; the presence of rales suggests an advanced degree of pulmonary edema with fluid-filled alveoli.

Hepatomegaly is the principal sign of systemic venous congestion seen in infants and children with CHF. It is seen in disease states resulting in either left- or right-sided heart failure, which in turn results in increased ventricular end-diastolic volume and fluid retention. The liver edge is normally palpable at, or 1 cm below, the right costal margin in early infancy. Care must be taken to approach the liver from below the level of the umbilicus in order to palpate the rounded edge. Tenderness from distention of the capsule may be appreciated in older children. Distended peripheral veins may be noted in the hands or scalp, but prominent jugular veins are difficult to appreciate because of the typically short neck in small children. Peripheral edema is an unusual and late manifestation of CHF in children, possibly as a result of the lower resting central venous pressure and greater resistance of tissues to stretch in infancy. Periorbital edema is more likely to be present in young children than pedal edema, which is usually seen in older children and adults with CHF.

Blood pressure measurement is an important ongoing guide to the degree of compensation in the setting of inadequate cardiac function. Animal studies utilizing a hypovolemic shock model have shown that blood pressure is well maintained in the infant mammal compared with the adult, despite a marked fall in cardiac output.[8] Hypotension is a late finding in pediatric shock, regardless of the cause, and is evidence of a decompensated state, following which deterioration to cardiac arrest may occur precipitously. Blood pressure measurements in all extremities are useful when there is clinical suspicion of coarctation of the aorta, suggested by lower extremity hypotension with upper extremity hypertension.

The cardiac examination must be interpreted in the context of other physical findings suggestive of inadequate cardiac function. A *precordial thrill* may be appreciated with significant intracardiac shunt lesions but is typically absent in the presence of decreased cardiac function. The presence or absence of a heart murmur is not central to the identification of CHF but may be a clue to its origin. A systolic murmur of grade III or more or any diastolic murmur is suggestive of significant cardiac disease (e.g., intracardiac shunting or valvular dysfunction). However, a murmur occurring in the presence of significant underlying heart disease may soften as cardiac output declines.

A gallop rhythm is frequently noted with CHF in infancy, but its presence does not necessarily indicate a decompensated state. An S_3 gallop occurs as a result of decreased ventricular compliance and is often associated with well-compensated volume overload states such as left-to-right shunts. Similarly, an S_4 gallop results from decreased atrial compliance. However, because extra heart sounds may be heard in normal children, care must be taken to interpret their significance within the framework of the complete physical assessment.

DIAGNOSTIC EVALUATION
Radiographs

Although the diagnosis of CHF is made on clinical grounds, the chest radiograph frequently provides essential information necessary to confirm the clinical impression. The finding of an enlarged cardiac silhouette on an inspiratory, upright chest radiograph provides objective evidence of impaired myocardial function. This may represent ventricular dilatation, pericardial effusion, or both. The *cardiothoracic index* is defined as the ratio of the sum of maximal

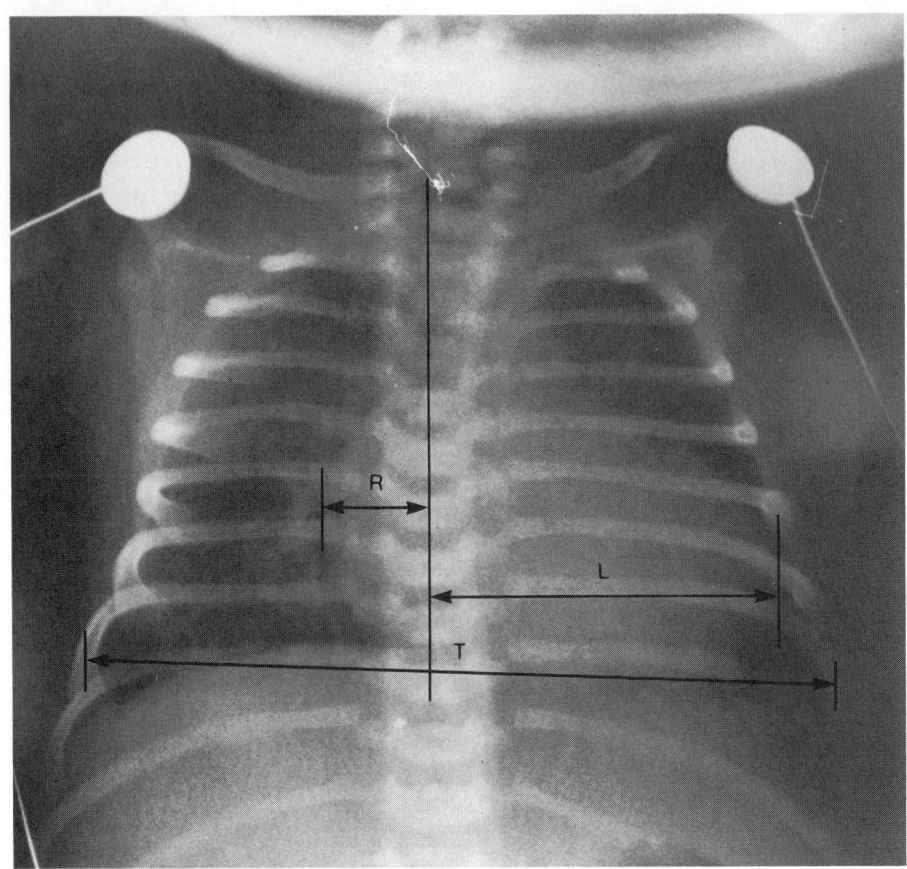

Figure 19–4. The cardiothoracic index (CT) is determined by dividing the cardiac width (R + L) by the thoracic width (T). This supine chest radiograph of a 4-week-old infant with coarctation of the aorta had a CT of 0.64.

distances between right and left heart borders and the midline to that of the intrathoracic diameter measured at the level of the dome of the right hemidiaphragm (Fig. 19–4). A cardiothoracic index greater than 0.55 in infants or 0.50 in children 2 years or older, with good inspiratory effort, is suggestive of cardiomegaly.[9] The normal thymic shadow of infancy is identified by its sail-like appearance in the right chest and its anterior location on a lateral radiograph. The heart size may remain normal in the presence of early, well-compensated CHF of many causes, obstruction of pulmonary venous return, and cardiac tamponade.

Other typical radiographic findings in patients with CHF reflect pulmonary congestion. These include enlarged central vascular markings, fine peripheral interstitial markings reflecting engorged lymphatic vessels, and the hazy granular pattern of pulmonary edema. Pleural effusions may also be seen with CHF, particularly in association with volume overload states such as renal failure. Atelectasis and hyperinflation are findings common to both cardiac and respiratory disease. Because the markings of vascular congestion often resemble pulmonary infiltrates, and because the two processes may coexist, the chest radiograph may not differentiate between CHF and pneumonia. Comparison with prior and subsequent radiographs is routinely indicated.

Arterial Blood Gases

Arterial blood gases provide important information regarding the respiratory and perfusion status of the child with CHF. The development of respiratory alkalosis is characteristic of well-compensated CHF with volume overloading conditions caused by intrapulmonary right-to-left shunting and ventilation-perfusion mismatch. Respiratory acidosis accompanies the development of overt pulmonary edema. Metabolic acidosis indicates severe compromise of systemic perfusion resulting from anaerobic metabolism and the accumulation of lactic acid.

Serum Studies

Electrolyte abnormalities are common in patients with CHF. Hyponatremia frequently develops as a result of increased water retention relative to sodium, a renal compensatory effect. Hyperkalemia may occur in the presence of poor tissue perfusion and metabolic acidosis. The use of loop diuretics frequently results in hypochloremia, hypercarbia, and hypokalemia.

Severe hypoglycemia may complicate CHF in infants as a result of depletion of hepatic glycogen stores.[10] Early identification with laboratory confirmation and aggressive correction may significantly improve myocardial function. Calcium may be administered to correct hypocalcemia in patients with CHF and antagonize toxic calcium channel blocker ingestion; this may also be followed by rapid improvement in cardiac function.

Acute or chronic severe anemia results in a high-output failure state that may be corrected with improvement of the oxygen-carrying capacity. Superimposed anemia may aggravate an already inadequate tissue perfusion state resulting from underlying heart disease.

Noninvasive Cardiac Studies

The 12-lead electrocardiogram (EKG) is rarely useful in the identification of CHF but may provide valuable information regarding underlying heart disease. Most importantly, bradydysrhythmias and tachydysrhythmias may be specifically diagnosed, permitting early directed treatment. Ventricular chamber hypertrophy and atrial enlargement are suggested by abnormalities in the P and QRS complex axes, anterior forces, and P waves. Abnormal Q waves indicating myocardial infarction and ST-T changes consistent with ischemia may be seen with congenital aberrant left main coronary artery and Kawasaki disease. Acute pericarditis is often accompanied initially by ST elevation without abnormal Q waves, followed by T-wave inversion, low-voltage QRS complexes, and normalization of ST segments. Low voltages with T-wave abnormalities are also seen with myocarditis.

The echocardiogram provides invaluable diagnostic information regarding cardiac structure and function in a non-invasive fashion. The identification of abnormal cardiac anatomy, measurement of ventricular function and cardiac output, detection of intracardiac shunting, and estimation of chamber pressure relationships are readily performed by an experienced pediatric cardiologist. Of additional importance to the emergency practitioner, however, is the rapid detection of pericardial fluid for which emergent intervention may be required.

DIFFERENTIAL DIAGNOSIS

The principal challenge in the recognition of heart failure in the infant and young child is the differentiation of pulmonary from cardiac disease as a result of their overlapping clinical features. Respiratory illnesses such as pneumonia, bronchiolitis, and asthma are prevalent in this age group, whereas the incidence of cardiac disease is low. The findings of tachycardia, tachypnea, increased work of breathing, rales, and wheezing are common to diseases of the heart and lungs. Hyperinflation of the lungs resulting from obstructive pulmonary disease may produce a palpable liver edge below the right costal margin. Diagnostic heart sounds may not be clearly audible in young infants because of rapid, noisy respirations and lack of cooperation. Obvious cyanosis usually suggests cardiac disease with right-to-left shunting, although this finding may be present in late respiratory failure. A markedly positive response to supplemental oxygen supports the diagnosis of underlying pulmonary disease. Similarly, significant improvement in oxygenation with positive-pressure ventilation suggests a primary respiratory disorder. Not uncommonly, cardiac and respiratory disease may coexist. A child with well-compensated CHF is often rendered symptomatic by a middle or lower tract respiratory infection, making identification of underlying heart disease more difficult.

The second problem for the physician caring for the acutely ill child is the differentiation of cardiogenic shock from shock resulting from other causes. Inappropriate fluid resuscitation may result in cardiovascular collapse. In the absence of a hypovolemic or distributive mechanism for shock, careful consideration must be given to decompensated heart failure as the cause. The rapid initial cardiorespiratory assessment must include perfusion parameters and an estimation of liver size. Serial reassessment is mandatory with fluid resuscitation. A chest radiograph obtained early in the management of the child in shock may reveal cardiomegaly.

Determination of the primary disease process, of which inadequate cardiac output is but one manifestation, is the third challenge posed by the child with CHF. Renal, hematologic, endocrine, infectious, and immune-mediated causes of CHF must be considered because of their noncardiac complications (Fig. 19–5).

THERAPEUTIC INTERVENTION
Initial Resuscitation

The priorities for the initial management of the child with symptomatic heart failure are directed toward optimization of (1) oxygenation and ventilation, (2) cardiac function, and (3) monitoring for complications and associated problems (Table 19–6).

Warmed and humidified oxygen in the highest possible concentration is always indicated initially. Young infants should be placed in a 100% oxygen hood and older children in an appropriately sized non-rebreather mask until actual oxygen requirements are defined. However, the response to oxygen therapy should be carefully monitored and the dose adjusted. Two special situations merit specific concern in the setting of congenital heart disease. First, infants with large left-to-right shunts can acutely deteriorate because of a decrease in pulmonary vascular resistance produced by an increase in Pao_2. Second, the ductal-dependent systemic perfusion of coarctation of the aorta may be severely compromised by closure of the ductus in response to hyperoxemia.

Upright positioning with the head and chest elevated 45 to 90 degrees will improve the intrapulmonary match of ventilation and perfusion. Maintenance of the lower extremities in a dependent position will decrease excessive preload and thus reduce pulmonary venous congestion. The use of an infant seat with appropriate restraints will achieve this purpose. However, in patients with cardiogenic shock and hypotension, the head should not be elevated above the level of the heart. Rotating tourniquets, three extremities at a

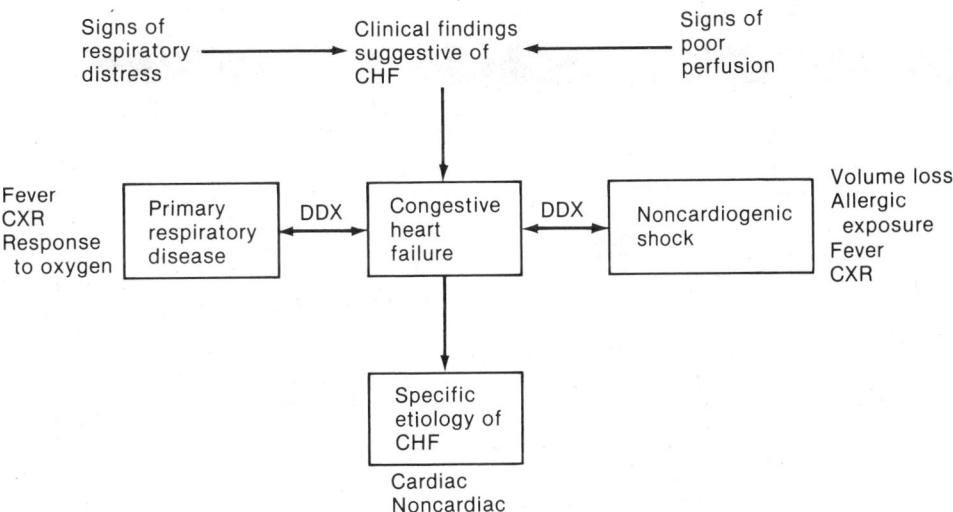

Figure 19–5. Differential diagnostic approach to the child with suspected CHF.

TABLE 19–6

OVERVIEW OF TREATMENT OF CHF IN CHILDREN

Prehospital phase	Emergency department phase II
Recognition of shock and respiratory failure	Complete examination
High-flow oxygen	Consider furosemide, 2 mg/kg IV, if diuresis <3 ml/kg/hr
Assist ventilation, if indicated	
Appropriate positioning	Consider Foley catheter
Monitor, keep warm	Mechanical ventilation with paralysis, if indicated
IV access if trained personnel available	Consult pediatric cardiologist
Contact medical control	Consider digoxin if stable
Reassess en route	Contact appropriate pediatric inpatient unit
Emergency department phase I	Reassess frequently
Obtain history	**Emergency department phase III**
Initial cardiopulmonary assessment	Consider furosemide, 5 mg/kg IV, if diuresis <3 ml/kg/hr
100% oxygen	
Assist ventilation if indicated	Correct anemia slowly
Appropriate positioning	Consider central venous access
Monitor, keep warm	
IV access, restrict fluids	Consider catecholamine infusion if indicated
Correct hypoglycemia	
Furosemide, 1 mg/kg	Consider prostaglandin infusion if indicated
Chest radiograph	
Arterial blood gas	Admit/transport to appropriate pediatric inpatient unit
Blood count, electrolytes	
Reassess frequently	

time and changed every 15 minutes, may also be useful in reducing venous return.

Aggressive monitoring is essential to aggressive management. Continuous monitoring of the heart rate with the ability to produce a paper tracing allows for titration of therapy to response and early detection of dysrhythmias. Preset monitoring of the blood pressure by oscilloscopic means every 5 to 15 minutes with appropriate cuff size is also necessary. The pulse oximeter, which senses peripheral oxygen saturation rather than central oxygen delivery, may be misleading. Absent or low readings may reflect peripheral vasoconstriction. Oxygen saturation in the normal range may give false reassurance regarding actual oxygen delivery and provides no information regarding oxygen requirements.

Serial monitoring of temperature should be performed. Hypothermia and hyperthermia are treated specifically.

Vascular access for drug delivery must be obtained early in anticipation of decompensation. Fluids must be restricted to two thirds maintenance needs and weight, intake, and output recorded. A blood glucose level should be obtained early and treatment of hypoglycemia initiated with 0.5 gm/kg of glucose. An arterial blood gas determination made while the patient is receiving supplemental oxygen, measurement of serum electrolytes, a complete blood cell count, and a chest radiograph are routinely indicated. Type and cross-match for correction of severe anemia may be necessary acutely. To avoid exacerbating fluid overload, packed red blood cells are typically given in 5-ml/kg aliquots over 2 to 4 hours to achieve a target hematocrit of 45%. If volume overload and agitation secondary to the hypoxia of pulmonary edema are present, judicious use of morphine sulfate (0.05 mg/kg IV) may be useful to increase venous capacitance.

Mechanical ventilation is indicated in decompensated cardiogenic shock to treat severe pulmonary edema and decrease the work of breathing imposed on the failing myocardium. The adverse myocardial effects of severe acidosis (pH < 7.20) are best treated initially by endotracheal intubation and hyperventilation to achieve a pH of 7.35 and a Pco_2 of 30 mm Hg. Although atelectasis and ventilation-perfusion mismatch are improved with positive-pressure ventilation, care must be taken to avoid excessive positive end-expiratory pressure (>10 mm Hg) as this may decrease venous return and right ventricular volume and thus lower the cardiac output. After documentation of adequate ventilation, severe and persistent metabolic acidosis may be treated with sodium bicarbonate in 1-mEq/kg aliquots given slowly. Care must be taken to avoid an excessive sodium load and cerebral edema from osmotic shifts caused by rapid infusion of hypertonic sodium bicarbonate. Aminophylline may be used to treat severe bronchospasm associated with pulmonary edema, but care must be taken to monitor carefully for dysrhythmias.

Early treatment of the precipitating cause of CHF will result in a more rapid response to therapy. Hypertension should be treated aggressively in patients with CHF, and careful serial monitoring of blood pressure should be performed. Infectious processes, particularly of the respiratory tract, are common triggers for exacerbation of CHF. In the febrile child with heart failure, cultures and radiographs should be obtained as indicated by the history and physical examination and antibiotic therapy begun if there is evidence of infection. Toxic ingestion presenting as heart failure should be treated with gastrointestinal decontamination and supportive care. Inflammatory causes of heart failure may also require specific treatment (e.g., IV immune globulin for Kawasaki disease).[11] Dysrhythmias also require treatment.

TABLE 19–7

DIURETIC THERAPY FOR CHF IN CHILDREN

Class	Drug	How Supplied	Dose	Adverse Effects
Loop diuretic	Furosemide (Lasix)	10-mg/ml vials	1 mg/kg IV; may repeat at 2 mg/kg, then 4 mg/kg at hourly intervals ×2 to achieve diuresis	Rapidly acting Potassium, sodium depletion Volume depletion
	Bumetanide (Bumex)	0.25-mg/ml vials	0.1–0.2 mg/kg IV	As above More potent
Thiazide diuretic	Hydrochlorothiazide (Hydrodiuril)	25-, 50-mg tablets	2–4 mg/kg/day po div tid	Slow onset of effect Potassium depletion
Aldosterone antagonist	Spironolactone (Aldactone)	25-mg tablets	2 mg/kg/day po div tid	Very slow onset Potassium sparing

Note: As described above, potassium loss occurs with loop and thiazide diuretics. Chloride loss resulting in metabolic alkalosis is also seen. Both hypokalemia and alkalosis predispose the patient to digitalis toxicity.

Diuretic Therapy

Rapidly acting diuretics will prompt an abrupt decrease in excessive preload and pulmonary congestion. The agents of choice for initial therapy are the loop diuretics (Table 19–7). These drugs rapidly inhibit sodium and chloride reabsorption in the ascending limb of the loop of Henle, interfering with renal concentrating ability. Because they are highly protein bound, these agents work best by IV push. The most commonly used loop diuretic is furosemide (Lasix) at an initial dose of 1 mg/kg. A urinary flow in excess of 3 ml/kg/hour within 1 hour is the desired end point; a Foley catheter is indicated in infants to monitor output. If the urinary response is inadequate, the dose is doubled at hourly intervals to a maximum of 4 mg/kg/dose until diuresis is initiated. Marked hypokalemia may be seen with diuresis, and thus serum potassium must be carefully monitored.

An alternative loop diuretic for use in refractory pulmonary edema is bumetanide (Bumex). This drug has a mechanism of action similar to that of furosemide but has 40 times the potency with proportionally less ototoxicity.[12] Nevertheless, there is limited experience with parenteral bumetanide in children.

Other classes of diuretics have a more gradual onset of action and thus are less suited to the acute management of CHF. These are generally used in oral form for chronic heart failure. The thiazides inhibit tubular reabsorption of sodium and chloride and may induce potassium depletion and metabolic alkalosis. The aldosterone antagonists have an onset of action over several days but possess a potassium-sparing effect and are thus useful in combination with other diuretics administered chronically. All patients on diuretic therapy with evidence of volume loss or heart failure should have serum electrolyte levels determined.

Digitalis Therapy

The cardiac glycosides (e.g., digitalis) are the positive inotropic agents of first choice for most children with CHF not complicated by cardiogenic shock. The effect of digitalis is to increase intracellular calcium, resulting in an improved contractile state. The specific mechanism involves inhibition of the sodium-potassium adenosine triphosphatase (ATPase) pump at the myocardial cell membrane. This results in an intracellular accumulation of sodium, which competes with calcium for efflux through a similar pump mechanism.

Digoxin is the preferred form for use in children because of its excellent oral absorption and rapid renal elimination. The intravenous and oral routes of administration are preferred in acute and chronic CHF, respectively, for their more predictable pharmacokinetics. The intramuscular route is to be avoided because of unpredictable absorption and severe pain on injection. The parenteral preparation of digoxin contains 100 μg/ml. The oral preparation contains 50 μg/ml and is administered by dropper.

The loading dose of digoxin is expressed as a *total digitalizing dose* (TDD), calculated on a microgram-per-kilogram basis. In the acutely ill child with CHF, it is preferable to reliably deliver the TDD by the intravenous route. Half of the TDD is given initially, followed by 25% of the TDD at 8 and 16 hours later. As a result of pharmacodynamic differences between young infants and older children, the recommended TDD varies with age (Table 19–8). The TDD should be reduced in the presence of renal failure, inflammatory myocardial disease, and electrolyte or acid-base imbalances. If the oral route is used in the more chronic setting, the calculated TDD is increased by 20% to account for decreased bioavailability.

Because of a narrow therapeutic index, great care must

		TABLE 19–8	
AGE-RELATED DIGOXIN DOSAGES IN CHILDREN			
Age	TDD (IV)	Maintenance (IV)	
Neonate (preterm)	20 μg/kg	4 μg/kg q 24 hr	
Newborn (term)	30 μg/kg	4–5 μg/kg q 12 hr	
1–24 mo	40 μg/kg	5–10 μg/kg q 12 hr	
2–10 yr	35 μg/kg (max 2.0 mg)	5–10 μg/kg q 12 hr (max 0.125 mg)	

Notes: TDD = Total digitalizing dose of digoxin, given over 16–24 hr in a total of 3 divided doses. The IV route is preferred in acute CHF; po dosages are 20% greater. IV preparation = 100 μg/ml; po preparation = 50 μg/ml. Dosage should be reduced in patients with renal impairment, hypokalemia, or myocarditis.

be taken to avoid errors of dosage. Specifically, the TDD should be calculated in terms of total micrograms per kilogram and total micrograms, and each dose should be calculated at the appropriate time in both micrograms and milliliters. This dose should be confirmed by another physician and reviewed in person with the nurse administering the drug. Continuous cardiac monitoring during intravenous digoxin therapy is an essential component of care.

The child receiving acute digoxin therapy must be assessed for a therapeutic digitalis effect. Most importantly, clinical signs of improvement in terms of compensatory responses to CHF indicate a positive effect; these signs include resolution of tachycardia, tachypnea, and hepatomegaly, with improvement of peripheral perfusion and urinary output. EKG evidence of a digitalis effect includes prolongation of the PR interval, shortening of the QT_c interval, and ST segment depression.

The maintenance dose of digoxin is 12.5% of the TDD given at 12-hour intervals, the first dose given 12 hours after the TDD is completed. If CHF is early or mild, the child may be placed on the maintenance regimen, and full digitalization will be achieved within 5 days.

Digitalis toxicity may present variably with anorexia, nausea, vomiting, lethargy, worsening of CHF, and dysrhythmias. Toxicity is more likely in the presence of deteriorating renal function, hypokalemia, and inflammatory cardiac disease. Dysrhythmias may occur in the absence of other symptoms of toxicity. The emergence of any new conduction disturbance in a patient on digoxin must be interpreted as a sign of toxicity. Although bradydysrhythmias are more common than tachydysrhythmias in children, the full spectrum of conduction disorders may be seen. In acute pediatric ingestions, lack of symptoms or EKG findings and a serum digoxin level less than 2.0 ng/ml are predictive of a benign outcome.[13]

Treatment of digitalis toxicity starts with supportive care and discontinuation of the drug. A serum potassium level less than 2.5 mEq/L should prompt replacement therapy by a route appropriate for the degree of symptomatology, particularly in the setting of diuretic therapy. However, care must be taken to monitor for hyperkalemia, which is an ominous sign. Atropine, phenytoin (Dilantin), and lidocaine may be used to treat the rhythm disturbances that accompany digitalis toxicity (Table 19–9).

A temporary transvenous pacemaker may be required for severe bradycardia. Refractory ventricular fibrillation has been reported following synchronized cardioversion, and therefore cardioversion should be reserved for the unstable patient with a digitalis-induced supraventricular dysrhythmia, using the lowest possible energy settings. Parenteral magnesium sulfate has also been described as an effective temporizing treatment for severe digitalis toxicity.[14]

TABLE 19–9

TREATMENT OF DIGITALIS TOXICITY

Discontinue digitalis
Correct hypokalemia (K$^+$ <2.5 mEq/L) slowly; beware of hyperkalemia*
Gastrointestinal decontamination
   Gastric lavage if recent, large ingestion
   Activated charcoal, repeated pulses
Management of dysrhythmias

Modality	Indication
Atropine 0.02 mg/kg	Sinus bradycardia
Phenytoin 10–15 mg/kg	Supraventricular and ventricular dysrhythmias
Lidocaine, 1 mg/kg, infusion 25–50 µg/kg/min	Ventricular ectopy
Magnesium sulfate 20 mg/kg	
Transvenous pacemaker	Temporizing second and third degree heart block
Cardioversion, 0.25 J/kg	Supraventricular tachycardia; beware of ventricular tachycardia
Fab fragments	Refractory dysrhythmias
Number of vials = $\dfrac{\text{body load (mg digoxin)}}{0.6 \text{ mg/vial}}$	Rising serum potassium > 5.0 mEq/L

*Hyperkalemia can occur with acute digoxin toxicity. Potassium should be administered extremely cautiously. If hyperkalemia exists, calcium should never be used, as it potentiates the toxic effects of digoxin.

The treatment of choice for life-threatening digitalis toxicity is intravenous anti-digoxin antibody fragment (Fab) therapy.[15] Indications include ingestion of more than 4 mg of digoxin by a young child, ventricular or bradydysrhythmias unresponsive to drug therapy, or a serum potassium level greater than 5 mEq/L in the presence of toxicity.

Catecholamine Therapy

The critically ill infant with a low cardiac output may, in the absence of an obstructive lesion, require inotropic support by continuous infusion. With their rapid onset of action and short half-life, these agents are easy to titrate for the desired effect. All improve myocardial contractility through a beta-agonist effect, with a variable alteration in systemic vascular resistance. However, all may cause life-threatening dysrhythmias, and therefore these agents are best given by secure, preferably central, intravenous access through an infusion pump with continuous monitoring of heart rate, blood pressure, and urinary output. Great care must be taken in calculating infusion concentrations and rates in the emergency department to avoid major complications (Table 19–10). Arterial and central venous access for hemodynamic monitoring are required as soon as the child can be transported to the intensive care environment. These agents have significant drug interaction with tricyclic antidepressants and the monoamine oxidase inhibitors.

Isoproterenol is the drug of choice for the initial treatment of atropine-resistant bradycardia. Tachydysrhythmias are a frequent complication because of its potent beta$_1$-agonist effect. Hypotension may occur as a result of systemic vasodilation, and myocardial oxygen requirements are increased.

Dopamine has differing, dose-related effects that have proved valuable in a variety of situations. At low doses (2 to 5 µg/kg/min), selective improvement in renal perfusion is the dominant effect. At intermediate doses (5 to 10 µg/kg/min), a positive inotropic effect is seen without compromise of renal perfusion. At higher doses (10 to 20 µg/kg/min), vasoconstriction caused by the increasing alpha-agonist effect is seen. In the presence of systemic hypotension caused by cardiogenic shock, the starting dose of dopamine is 10 µg/kg/min with rapid titration upward to effect.

Dobutamine is a relatively selective beta$_1$ agonist with a greater inotropic than chronotropic effect. Thus cardiac output is improved with less risk of tachydysrhythmias and a smaller rise in myocardial oxygen consumption than seen with older agents. There is no direct effect on systemic vascular tone. Renal perfusion, therefore, is not selectively enhanced. Dobutamine has emerged as the drug of choice for inotropic augmentation when there is no need to augment vascular tone.

Epinephrine is a potent, nonselective alpha and beta agonist and is most useful when there is a need to augment both myocardial contractility and vascular tone. Dysrhythmias are common and severe systemic vasoconstriction universal.

Prostaglandin Therapy

Alprostadil (prostaglandin E$_1$) is effective in preserving patency of the ductus arteriosus in selected infants with congenital heart disease.[16] Alprostadil improves oxygenation in the presence of pulmonary outflow tract obstructive

TABLE 19–10

CATECHOLAMINE DOSES IN PEDIATRIC CARDIOGENIC SHOCK

Drug	Dose	Effects
Dopamine	2–50 µg/kg/min	Dose-dependent effects
	2–5 µg/kg/min	Renal vasodilation
	5–10 µg/kg/min	Inotropic effect
	10–20 µg/kg/min	Vasoconstriction

Dobutamine	2–40 µg/kg/min	Inotropic effect
		  Less tachycardia
		  No effect on peripheral vascular tone
		  No effect on renal perfusion

Epinephrine	0.05–1.00 µg/kg/min	Tachydysrhythmias Vasoconstriction
Isoproterenol	0.05–0.50 µg/kg/min	Chronotropic effect Tachydysrhythmias Systemic vasodilation Myocardial ischemia

Rules for rapid calculation of infusion concentration and rate:
  Dopamine/dobutamine: Add 6 mg/kg to 100 ml D5W; 1 ml/kg/hr will give 1 µg/kg/min.
  Epinephrine/isoproterenol: Add 0.6 mg/kg to 100 ml D5W; 1 ml/kg/hr will give 0.1 µg/kg/min.

lesions (e.g., critical pulmonary stenosis) by increasing pulmonary blood flow through the ductus. In transposition of the great vessels, ductal flow results in greater mixing of pulmonary and systemic blood and, thus, improved oxygenation. Finally, in left-sided obstructive lesions such as coarctation of the aorta, ductal flow may be essential to preserve perfusion of the lower body.

Significant adverse effects may result from inappropriate use of alprostadil. These include apnea, fever, hypotension, and seizures. Hypotension is potentiated with sepsis. Pulmonary perfusion is markedly reduced by a patent ductus with total anomalous pulmonary venous return, resulting in cyanosis. Consequently, alprostadil should be given only in consultation with a pediatric cardiologist. The recommended initial dose is 0.05 µg/kg/min and is gradually reduced as the patient is stabilized.

Vasodilator Therapy

Recognition of the positive effects of a reduction in vascular tone on cardiac output and vascular congestion has added an important tool to the management of heart failure. Decreasing systemic vascular resistance (afterload) for a given contractile state, heart rate, and preload will result in an increase in cardiac output. Increasing systemic venous capacitance results in decreased filling pressures (preload), giving rise to decreased pulmonary and systemic venous congestion. Because the compensatory responses to heart failure typically lead to augmentation of both preload and afterload, vasodilator therapy would seem to offer a great advantage. Most pediatric experience has been with sodium nitroprusside and phentolamine, although the nitrates and calcium channel blockers are being used increasingly.

The manipulation of these factors in the absence of precise knowledge regarding their contribution to heart failure in a given child may lead to severe hypotension. This may result from collapse of arteriolar tone or from excessive reduction in preload, resulting in inadequate cardiac output. Emergency department use of vasodilators in children, therefore, is not recommended. These drugs should initially be used in the pediatric intensive care unit setting after failure of conventional therapy and accompanied by invasive hemodynamic monitoring. When used in combination with positive inotropic agents, the vasodilators offer the ability to fully manipulate the major physiologic factors contributing to cardiac output.

DISPOSITION

Children presenting to the emergency department with newly diagnosed CHF or significant exacerbation of preexisting chronic failure should be admitted to the hospital (Fig. 19–6). Inpatient care is necessary both for diagnostic evaluation and for monitoring cardiac function. A pediatric cardiologist should always be consulted to assist in assessment, resuscitation, and disposition.

The decision in this situation is whether to admit the patient to a pediatric intensive care unit or to a monitored floor. In the presence of impending respiratory failure, cyanosis, cardiogenic shock, or dysrhythmia, the child should be transferred, after stabilization, to a regional pediatric intensive care unit with pediatric cardiology and cardiothoracic surgical capability. On the other hand, if the child presented with mild compensatory CHF responses and responded well to initial management with oxygen, positioning, and diuresis, then admission to a monitored inpatient floor unit is most appropriate.

The nature of the underlying disease will also affect this

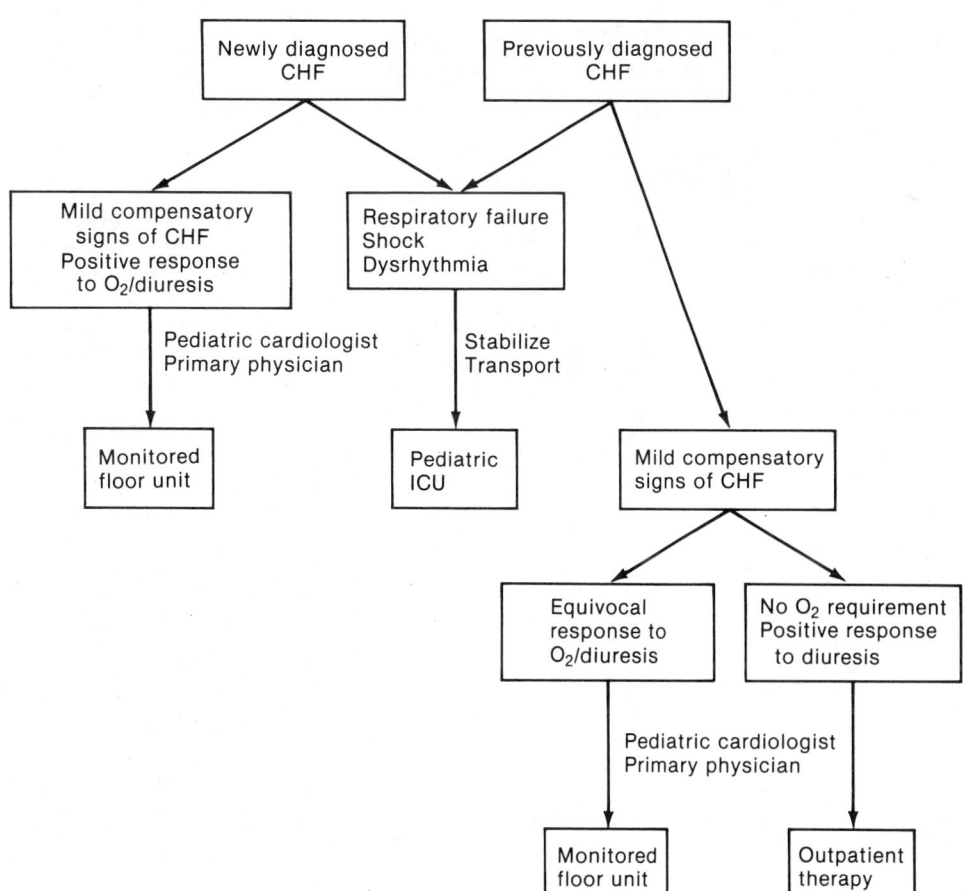

Figure 19–6. Disposition tree for the child with CHF.

decision. In all cases, the disposition decision should be made in conjunction with the primary physician. The child with an acute exacerbation of previously recognized CHF presents a more difficult disposition decision; criteria for admission to the pediatric intensive care unit are the same as for the newly diagnosed child. The underlying disease process, triggering factors, and likelihood of deterioration must be known before a discharge plan from the emergency department can be contemplated. In this case, the input from the primary care physician and cardiologist are essential at the time of the emergency department visit. A previous lack of follow-up, inadequate transportation, return visits for similar complaints, prior history of acute deterioration, and lack of parental understanding of the disease process all make outpatient management unfeasible. Conversely, adequate oxygenation on room air, an excellent response to diuresis without electrolyte abnormalities, reversible underlying triggering factors, a good relationship with a primary care physician, and appropriate parental assessment skills make outpatient therapy possible.

References

1. Fyler DC, Buckley LP, Hellenbrand WE, et al. Report of the New England Regional Infant Cardiac Program. Pediatrics 1980;65(suppl, part 2):375.
2. Veasy LG, Wiedmeier SE, Orsmond GS, et al. Resurgence of acute rheumatic fever in the intermountain area of the United States. N Engl J Med 1987;316:421.
3. Lebowitz EA, Novick JS, Rudolph AM. Development of myocardial sympathetic innervation in the fetal lamb. Pediatr Res 1972;6:887.
4. Kirkpatrick SE, Nabiloff J, Pitlick PT, et al. The influence of poststimulation potentiation and heart rate on the fetal lamb heart. Am J Physiol 1977;233:H269.
5. McPherson RA, Kramer MF, Covell JW, et al. A comparison of the active stiffness of fetal and adult cardiac muscle. Pediatr Res 1976;10:660.
6. Romero TE, Friedman WF. Limited left ventricular response to volume overload in the neonatal period: A comparative study with the adult animal. Pediatr Res 1979;13:910.
7. Rudolph AM. Diagnosis and treatment: Respiratory distress and cardiac disease in infancy. Pediatrics 1965;35:999.
8. Schwaitzberg SD, Bergman KS, Harris BH. A pediatric trauma model of continuous hemorrhage. J Pediatr Surg 1988;23:605.
9. Maresh MM, Washburn AH. Size of the hearts of normal children: II. Roentgen ray studies. Am J Dis Child 1938;56:33.
10. Benzing G III, Schubert W, Hug G, et al. Simultaneous hypoglycemia and acute congestive heart failure. Circulation 1969;49:209.
11. Newburger JW, Takahashi M, Burns JC, et al. The treatment of Kawasaki syndrome with intravenous gamma globulin. N Engl J Med 1986;315:341.
12. Chemtob S, Kaplan BS, Sherbotie JR, et al. Pharmacology of diuretics in the newborn. Pediatr Clin North Am 1989;36:1231.
13. Lewander WJ, Gaudreault P, Einhorn A, et al. Acute pediatric digoxin ingestion. Am J Dis Child 1986;140:770.
14. French JH, Thomas RG, Siskind AP, et al. Magnesium therapy in massive digoxin intoxication. Ann Emerg Med 1984;13:562.
15. Wenger TL, Butler VP, Haber E, et al. Treatment of severely digitalis-toxic patients with digoxin-specific antibody fragments. J Am Coll Cardiol 1985;5:118A.
16. Freed MD, Heymann MA, Lewis AB, et al. Prostaglandin E₁ in infants with ductus arteriosus–dependent congenital heart disease. Circulation 1981;64:899.

CHAPTER 20

Pericarditis

Jane F. Knapp

INTRODUCTION

The pericardium may be affected by a variety of conditions in isolation, as a component of myocarditis, or as a manifestation of systemic disease. The true incidence of pericardial inflammation is unknown, because it is often subclinical or is an unrecognized feature of systemic illness or infection noted on postmortem examination.[1] At one children's hospital, pericardial disease of all origins accounted for 67 admissions over a 12-year period.[2] The incidence of pericardial constriction in children ranges from 0.7% to 13.0% of all cases of pericarditis.[3, 4] Early aggressive pericardial drainage has reduced the mortality rate from purulent pericarditis to 0% to 28%.[5, 6]

ANATOMY AND PHYSIOLOGY

The visceral and parietal pericardial membranes combine to form the tough fibrous sac that surrounds the heart and forms the pericardium. The space between the two layers is the pericardial cavity, which in children normally contains 10 to 15 ml of fluid.[7] The pericardium, along with its fluid, lubricates the moving surfaces of the heart, holds the heart in a fixed position, and isolates the heart from other structures in the thorax, thus preventing adhesions or spread of infection.[8] Physiologically the pericardium helps to prevent cardiac hypertrophy and regulates interaction between the stroke volumes of the ventricles. Sensory innervation to the parietal pericardium is supplied by the vagus and phrenic nerves.

Inflammation of the pericardium can result in either accumulation of fluid in the pericardial space or thickening and constriction of the fibrous sac. When effusion occurs, the nature of the fluid depends on the origin of the illness and may be serous, fibrinous, purulent, or hemorrhagic. The effect of the fluid on myocardial function and the ultimate production of cardiac tamponade is dependent on the state of the myocardium, the nature of the fluid, the rate of the fluid accumulation, and the pressure-volume relationships of the pericardial space (Fig. 20–1). There is normally a slight decrease in systolic arterial pressure during inspiration. With cardiac tamponade, this normal phenomenon is accentuated, and pulsus paradoxus is observed.[9]

Pericardial pressure-volume curves show that the pericardial pressure rises steadily as fluid accumulates and lowers when fluid is removed.[10] The rate of pressure rise is a function of both the speed of accumulation and the compliance of the pericardium. When fluid accumulates slowly, large volumes can be accommodated because of the gradual rate of expansion of the pericardium. When fluid accumulates rapidly, a marked elevation in intrapericardial pressure may occur with smaller amounts. In either situation, once the steep portion of the pericardial pressure-volume curve is reached, an additional small accumulation of fluid can produce a fatal cardiac tamponade.[11] The primary hemodynamic problem is restriction of right ventricular filling. As the restriction increases, ventricular stroke volume and cardiac output fall. To maintain cardiac output, reflex tachycardia and peripheral vasoconstriction occur. With further

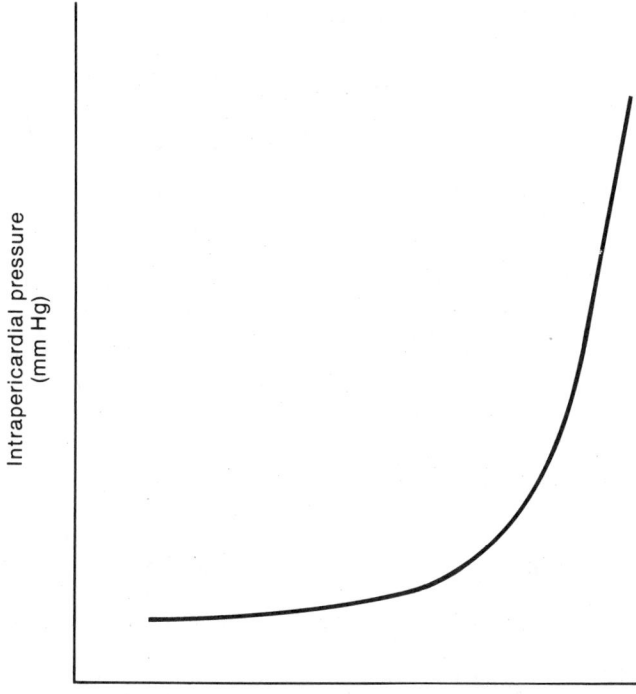

Figure 20–1. Example of an intrapericardial pressure-volume relationship. The steep portion of the curve represents the point where small increments in volume can produce marked increases in intrapericardial pressure.

decompensation, systemic arterial blood pressure and pulse pressure fall. Therapy is aimed at restoring cardiac output and relieving the tamponade with pericardiocentesis. Systemic hypovolemia appears to lower the slope of the pressure-volume curve measured during tamponade but does not change the resting pericardial pressure. By lowering the slope of the pericardial pressure curve, hypovolemia may mask a tamponade that will become clinically apparent with fluid resuscitation. Hypervolemia increases the resting pericardial pressure and raises the slope of the pericardial pressure-volume curve.

Constrictive pericarditis refers to dense thickening and adhesion of the pericardium as sequelae of previous inflammation. The course of constrictive pericarditis depends on the extent, intensity, rate of development, and primary sites of constriction.[12] It has been described in both acute and chronic forms, with multiple origins. Hemodynamically, constrictive pericarditis prevents proper diastolic filling of the ventricles, with a resultant decrease in cardiac output. Sufficient compression of the heart will produce a cardiac tamponade. Pericardial effusion can occur with constrictive pericarditis, and nonrestrictive pericardial fibrosis can occur with effusion.

EMERGENCY MEDICAL SERVICE CONSIDERATIONS

The early diagnosis of pericardial effusion is important in preventing cardiac tamponade. Cardiac tamponade, when present, requires immediate diagnosis and treatment. These are important considerations in the prehospital care setting. Pericardial effusion with possible tamponade should be considered in patients with penetrating trauma to the left side of the chest and when the cardiovascular examination

reveals muffled or distant heart sounds, a friction rub, or neck vein distention. Medical control should recommend establishing vascular access and maintaining circulation with fluid resuscitation and vasopressors until the tamponade can be relieved.

CLINICAL EVALUATION
History

The presentation of pericardial disease varies depending on the cause. Frequently it is seen in conjunction with myocardial or endocardial disease, and the two may be difficult to differentiate. It is also important to realize that when other symptoms of systemic illness dominate the clinical picture, concomitant pericarditis may be easily obscured or unrecognized (Table 20–1).

Overall, chest pain is the most common presenting complaint. Its reported frequency with purulent pericarditis varies from 15% to 80%.[13] The pain is a sharp, stabbing sensation that radiates over the left neck, shoulder, and back. It is usually pleuritic, worsening with cough or deep inspiration. Characteristically the pain is exaggerated by lying down and relieved by sitting up, especially leaning forward. Infants or young children may present with fever, lethargy and cough or other evidence of concurrent infection. Pericarditis may also present with such nonspecific symptoms as weight loss, malaise, fatigue, weakness, or anorexia.

The duration of illness may be short, as with a fulminant purulent pericarditis, or chronic. A history of prolonged high fever, rash, red eyes, and sore mouth is characteristic of Kawasaki disease.

A history of previous or chronic illness should be obtained. Patients with rheumatologic or inflammatory bowel disease may present with complaints of exacerbation of their illness (e.g., pain in the joints or abdomen). Children who have had mediastinal radiation for intrathoracic malignancy are at risk for constrictive pericarditis.[14] Renal dialysis patients can develop uremic pericarditis. Nephrotic patients may also present with pericardial effusion as a complication of their illness.

Penetrating chest trauma should alert the clinician to the possible presence of a hemorrhagic effusion, and a history of previous trauma or surgery may indicate the possibility of infection or adhesions with constriction of the pericardium. Blunt chest trauma has also been implicated in pericardial effusion and infection.[15]

The family history should include the presence of peri-

TABLE 20–1
SIGNS AND SYMPTOMS OF PERICARDIAL DISEASE

Respiratory	Nonspecific
Chest pain	Malaise
Cough	Lethargy
Dyspnea	Fatigue
Circulatory	Weakness
Quiet precordium	Anorexia
Muffled or distant heart sounds	Weight loss
Friction rub	Fever
Narrow pulses	
Jugular venous distention	
Pulsus paradoxus	
Cardiomegaly	
EKG changes	
Hepatomegaly	
Peripheral edema	

carditis or other chronic infections or debilitating disease. A familial syndrome of camptodactyly, arthritis, and pericarditis (CAP syndrome) has been described.[16–18]

Physical Examination

The patient's vital signs are frequently altered. These changes can include fever, tachycardia, tachypnea, or alterations in blood pressure. Tachypnea has been noted to be the earliest and most common physical finding of effusion in adults.[1] Pulsus paradoxus suggests significant fluid accumulation. A paradoxical pulse greater than 20 mm Hg in a child with pericarditis is a reliable indicator of the presence of cardiac tamponade; a pulse of 10 to 20 mm Hg is equivocal.[19] To determine the degree of pulsus paradoxus, the systolic pressure is measured during expiration. As the manometer is allowed to fall, the point when the systolic pressure is heard equally well during inspiration and expiration is then recorded. The difference between the two readings is the degree of paradox. With the current use of blood pressure monitors for measurement, the presence of pulsus paradoxus can be easily missed.

Children with pericarditis frequently have physical findings indicative of concurrent infection. These may include a skin infection, abscess, or rash such as found with varicella, Rocky Mountain spotted fever, or meningococcemia. Findings associated with upper respiratory infection or pneumonia frequently accompany *Haemophilus influenzae* purulent pericarditis.

During the cardiorespiratory examination, physical evidence of pericardial effusion and cardiac compromise should be sought. During respiratory examination, the child may exhibit dyspnea and cough, and during cardiac examination, there is a quiet precordium, and heart sounds are distant or muffled. The pericardial friction rub is pathognomonic of pericarditis but is not always present or may be audible only intermittently or after the effusion has been relieved. The typical sound of a rub is that of a to-and-fro, high-frequency murmur.[20] It does not necessarily have any correlation with the cardiac cycle. Frequently the rub is heard better with the patient leaning forward or kneeling.[21] The rub may be amplified by placing the diaphragm of the stethoscope firmly on the chest. Other findings on physical examination include narrow pulses and jugular venous distention.

With a chronic condition, ascites and hepatomegaly can be observed during the abdominal examination. There may also be peripheral edema. Evidence of other systemic illness may include an assessment of the patient's nutritional state, joint involvement, or lymphadenopathy. Flexion contractures of the fingers and coxa vara along with arthritis and pericarditis are features of the familial CAP syndrome.

DIAGNOSTIC EVALUATION

Echocardiography

Echocardiography is the primary diagnostic modality for pericardial disease, because it is sensitive, portable, and noninvasive.[1] It is especially useful in children in differentiating between pericarditis with effusion and myocarditis with cardiac dilatation, as this distinction cannot always be made on clinical grounds alone. Effusions as small as 15 ml can be identified.[22] Echocardiography is indicated in any patient in whom the diagnosis of pericarditis is being considered based on clinical signs, physical findings, the presence of cardiomegaly on chest radiograph, or electrocardiographic changes consistent with pericardial disease. Two-dimensional echocardiography is also of value in directing pericardiocentesis when needed for diagnostic or therapeutic

purposes and for assessing the evolution or reaccumulation of fluid. Computed tomographic (CT) scanning is a sensitive technique for the evaluation of pericardial thickening and effusion but offers no advantages over echocardiography.[23]

Electrocardiography

The electrocardiographic changes produced by pericardial disease can be attributed to three different factors: (1) the presence of an effusion, (2) the "injury" to the superficial myocardium caused by the presence of fluid or fibrin, and (3) superficial myocarditis.[24]

The electrocardiographic abnormalities of pericarditis evolve through several distinct stages that reflect different clinical and pathologic phases of the disease (Table 20–2).[24–26] Subepicardial myocardial damage produces time-dependent changes in the ST segment and T wave. As a rule, T wave changes follow those of the ST segment. Initially, elevation of the ST segment occurs in many limb and precordial leads, particularly those representing the left ventricle (I, II, aVL, V_5, and V_6). Within 2 to 3 days, the ST segment approaches normal. At this stage, the T wave is small but still upright. During this transitional phase, abnormalities may be undetectable on the electrocardiogram (EKG). Two to four weeks after the onset, T waves become sharply inverted as a result of myocardial inflammation (Fig. 20–2). At this stage, the ST segment is usually isoelectric. These changes may persist for 1 to 2 months. Dysrhythmias are relatively rare with acute disease. Permanent EKG abnormalities occur most frequently after purulent, tuberculous, and constrictive pericarditis. Sinus tachycardia is the most common dysrhythmia, but atrial fibrillation and flutter and supraventricular tachycardia have also occurred. P wave abnormalities indicative of intra-atrial conduction disturbances have been noted, and first degree heart block has been reported in a child with constrictive pericarditis.[2] Children with constrictive pericarditis show flattening to depression of the ST and T waves and low voltage.[2]

Pericardial effusion may also produce low QRS voltages. Low voltages occur when QRS amplitude in every one of the limb leads is 5 mm or less.[26] Low voltage is usually a result of a short-circuiting in the electrical impulse caused by the increased amount of pericardial fluid. If the voltage remains low after the removal of the fluid, it is probably a result of the insulating effect of fibrin.[27] Cyclic variations (electrical alternans) in amplitude of the QRS complex may also be noted. Subtle variations in the amplitude of the QRS complexes are associated with a large effusion, whereas marked variations are associated with cardiac tamponade.

The incidence and severity of the EKG changes in pericarditis depend on the origin of the disease. Patients with chronic effusion may have no signs of pericarditis except for low voltage and low T wave amplitude.[28] The typical pattern with ST segment and T wave changes occurs in almost all pediatric patients.[29]

Although acute myocardial infarction is rare in childhood, it is important to note that it produces EKG findings similar to those of pericarditis. However, in acute myocardial infarction the changes are more localized, ST segment and T wave changes occur simultaneously, and Q waves are present.[19, 26]

Radiography

Cardiomegaly is not always seen on the chest radiograph. With large effusions, an enlarged water bottle–shaped cardiac silhouette is present (Fig. 20–3). In contrast, with constrictive pericarditis, the heart may appear small and exhibit calcification. The lung fields are usually normal.

⊙ TABLE 20–2		
EKG CHANGES RELATED TO CLINICAL STAGE OF ILLNESS		
EKG Change	**Pathologic Phase**	**Clinical Phase**
ST elevation in leads I, II, aVL, V_5, V_6	Subepicardial damage	Initial
ST normal	Transitional phase	2–3 days
T wave small but upright		
T wave sharply inverted (see Fig. 20–2)	Myocardial inflammation	2–4 wk
ST isoelectric		May persist for 1–2 mo
ST flattening or depression	Constrictive	Variable
T wave depression		
Low voltage		

Ancillary Studies

Other laboratory tests should be chosen to establish or confirm the cause of pericardial disease. Frequently, the erythrocyte sedimentation rate is elevated, and the C-reactive protein is positive. Immunoglobulin E (IgE) levels may be elevated in Kawasaki disease. In purulent pericarditis, the peripheral white blood cell count is usually elevated. Cultures should be obtained prior to starting antibiotic therapy when possible. The diagnosis of purulent pericarditis should be established by culture analysis and examination of pericardial fluid obtained by pericardiocentesis.[30] Blood culture results are positive in 40% to 80% of cases of purulent pericarditis depending on the organism.[31, 32]

DIFFERENTIAL DIAGNOSIS

Most episodes of acute benign pericarditis appear to be associated with viral illness.[7] Viruses that cause pericarditis include coxsackievirus, influenza, echovirus, adenovirus, varicella, Epstein-Barr, mumps, and hepatitis B.[32–36]

Purulent pericarditis most frequently occurs in children less than 4 years of age.[37] Most cases result from hematogenous spread from another site of infection such as cellulitis, abscess, pneumonia, epiglottitis, meningitis, septic arthritis, or osteomyelitis.[5, 32, 38, 39] *Staphylococcus aureus* is the most frequent causative organism of purulent pericarditis in children.[37, 40, 41] It is usually associated with pneumonia accompanied by empyema, acute osteomyelitis, or soft tissue infection or occurs in the initial postoperative period following open heart surgery.[42] *Haemophilus influenza* type B is the second most common cause of purulent pericarditis in children. Most children are found to have had symptoms of an upper respiratory infection in the preceding 5 to 12 days.[43] *H. influenza* pericarditis has also been observed in conjunction with meningitis, epiglottitis, and pneumonia.[39] *Neisseria meningitidis* is a third important cause of purulent pericarditis in children[37] and has been found in conjunction with meningococcal meningitis. Cardiac abnormalities occur in approximately 8% of patients with Lyme disease, usually during the second stage of the illness. Myopericardial involvement may result in conduction disturbances, ventricular dysfunction, or arrhythmias. Fifty percent of the patients are febrile at the time of onset of cardiac manifestations. In most cases the abnormalities resolve within 3 to 6 weeks.

Many other bacterial causes have been reported (Table 20–3).[5, 44–46] *Mycobacterium tuberculosis*, once a common cause of acute pericarditis in the United States, is now more often responsible for chronic pericardial disease.[42]

Fungal disease such as histoplasmosis, coccidiomycosis, and blastomycosis may also cause pericardial disease. Other fungal organisms such as *Aspergillus* and *Candida* are more serious considerations in patients who are immunosuppressed or are in the postoperative period after cardiac surgery.

Other infectious causes of pericarditis are rare in the United States (see Table 20–3).[47, 48]

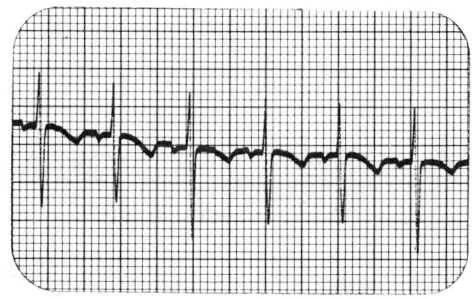

Figure 20–2. Precordial lead demonstrating a sharply inverted T wave characteristic of myocardial inflammation with pericarditis and effusion.

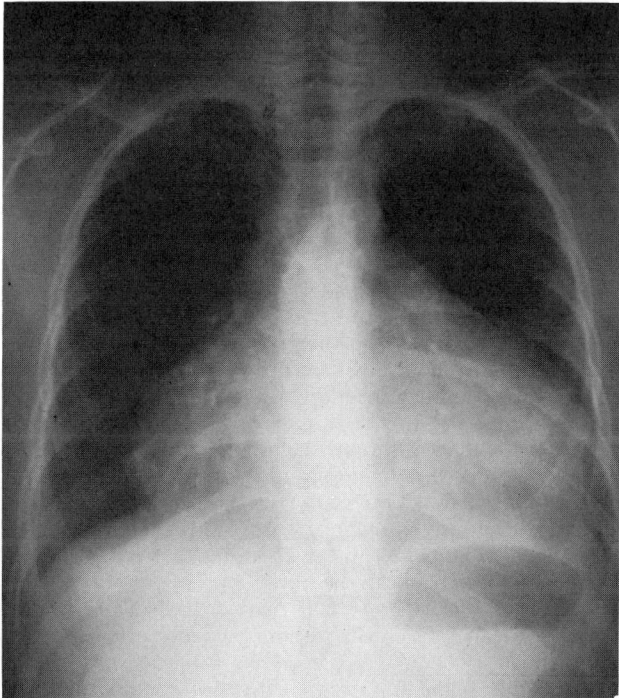

Figure 20–3. A 7-year-old girl with acute pericardial effusion, showing a typical "water bottle" configuration to the central silhouette. The diagnosis is rapidly confirmed by ultrasonography. (Courtesy of A. Oestreich, M. D., Cincinnati, OH.)

TABLE 20–3	
CAUSES OF PERICARDITIS	
Infectious Causes	**Noninfectious Causes**
Viral	Kawasaki disease
Coxsackievirus B	Trauma—blunt or
Influenza types A and B	penetrating
Mumps	Metabolic—uremia,
Echoviruses	myxedema
Adenoviruses	Neoplasm
Epstein-Barr	Postirradiation
Hepatitis viruses	Connective tissue disorders:
Varicella	JRA, systemic lupus
Cytomegalovirus	erythematosus,
Rubeola	dermatomyositis,
HIV	periarteritis nodosa
Bacterial	Inflammatory bowel disease
Staphylococcus aureus	Rheumatic fever
Haemophilus influenzae b	Postpericardiotomy
Neisseria meningitidis	syndrome
Neisseria gonorrhea	Hypersensitivity to drugs
Streptococcus pneumoniae	Familial syndrome
Streptococcus sp.	
Salmonella	
Francisella tularensis	
Pseudomonas	
Listeria	
Anaerobes	
Enteric bacilli	
Nocardia	
Rickettsia	
Borrelia burgdorferi (Lyme	
disease)	
Mycobacteria	
Fungal	
Histoplasmosis	
Coccidioidomycosis	
Candida	
Blastomycosis	
Other	
Parasites	
Protozoa	

Uremic pericarditis may be seen in chronic renal dialysis patients. It may also be a feature of end-stage chronic renal disease.[49]

Neoplasms such as leukemia, lymphosarcoma, and Hodgkins disease can directly invade the pericardium and produce inflammation and effusion.[50, 51] Pericarditis can also occur from therapeutic mediastinal radiation for neoplastic disease.[14] Myocardial involvement has been described in children with human immunodeficiency virus (HIV) infection, and pericardial disease has been observed in adults.[52–55] In these cases the pericarditis was nonspecific, associated with Kaposi's sarcoma, or caused by *Mycobacterium tuberculosis* or *Cryptococcus* organisms.[56, 57]

Cardiovascular symptoms, including pericarditis, usually appear in the second stage or subacute phase of Kawasaki disease about 7 to 10 days after the onset of illness. Many times the diagnosis is not made until this time, when desquamation of the palms and soles begins to occur.[58] Clinical signs of pericarditis can be rare, and hence the use of echocardiography is important diagnostically.[59] Most effusions resolve spontaneously without evidence of constrictive pericarditis.[60]

Pericarditis is an important feature of rheumatic fever, systemic-onset juvenile rheumatoid arthritis, and systemic lupus erythematosis.[61–63] It also occurs in conjunction with inflammatory bowel disease, though this is rare.[64–67]

Hemorrhagic effusion with the potential complication of

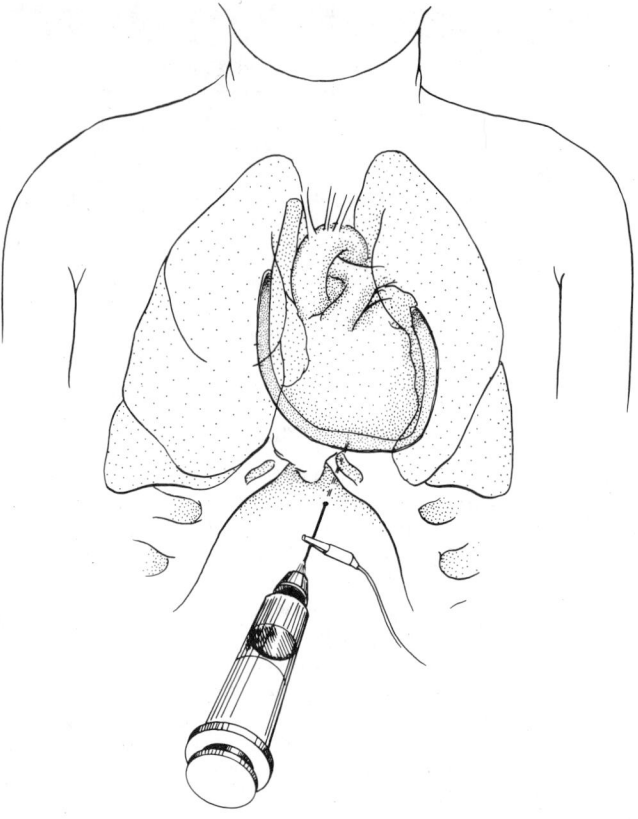

Figure 20–4. Pericardiocentesis technique showing the position of the needle.

tamponade must be considered in all cases of penetrating or severe blunt trauma to the chest.

THERAPEUTIC INTERVENTION

Management of pericarditis is determined by the origin of the illness. All patients must be immediately assessed for the presence of cardiac tamponade. In patients with penetrating chest trauma, especially on the left, this is of critical importance. If tamponade is present, pericardiocentesis (Figure 20–4) is immediately undertaken to relieve the tamponade and restore cardiac output (Table 20–4). Pericardiocentesis is most likely to be effective in patients with effusions greater than 200 ml.[68] When cardiac function is compromised by the presence of effusion that cannot be immediately removed, it is important to consider fluid resuscitation and the use of vasopressors to restore cardiac output.

The treatment of viral pericarditis is symptomatic and supportive. Bed rest is important until evidence of inflammation disappears, and the patient should be observed for evidence of cardiac decompensation or tamponade. Salicylates may be used for fever, inflammation, and analgesia, although patients can become resistant to their effect, even

TABLE 20–4
INDICATIONS FOR PERICARDIOCENTESIS
Emergent
Cardiac tamponade from any cause
Urgent
Culture and diagnosis of infectious origin of effusion

TABLE 20-5

THERAPY AT A GLANCE

Organism	Antibiotic Therapy
Staphylococcus aureus	Nafcillin—150 mg/kg/day IV divided q 6 hr for 3 wk *or* For methicillin-resistant organisms: Vancomycin—40 mg/kg/day IV divided q 6 hr for 3 wk
Haemophilus influenzae type B	Ampicillin—150 mg/kg/day IV divided q 6 hr *and* Chloramphenicol–50–75 mg/kg/day IV divided q 6 hr for 10–14 days *or* Cefuroxime—150 mg/kg/day IV divided q 6 hr for 10–14 days *or* Ceftriaxone—100 mg/kg/day IV divided q 12 hr for 10–14 days *or* Cefotaxime—200 mg/kg/day IV divided q 6 hr for 10–14 days
Pneumococcus, Meningococcus, Group A *Streptococcus*	Penicillin G—150,000 U/kg/day IV divided q 4–6 hr for 10–14 days *or* For penicillin G–resistant organisms: Vancomycin (see above)
Coliform bacilli	Gentamicin—6 mg/kg/day IV divided q 8 hr for 21 days *or* Cephalosporins
Anti-inflammatory Agents	
Aspirin: 80–90 mg/kg/day in three to four divided doses Prednisone: 1–2 mg/kg/day in divided doses Indomethacin: 0.5–2.5 mg/kg/day in two to four divided doses, tapered after the patient has been asymptomatic for 5–7 days	

at doses causing symptoms of salicylate toxicity. Aspirin is given in a dosage of 80 to 90 mg/kg/day in three or four divided doses. Steroids have also been effective in controlling symptoms but are difficult to withdraw without causing remission and may cause undesirable side effects in the dosages required. Prednisone is started at 1 to 2 mg/kg/day. Indomethacin has also been used with success, especially in patients refractory to aspirin. The suggested dose is 0.5 to 2.5 mg/kg/day in two to four divided doses, with a maximum daily dose of 100 mg.[69] The dose is tapered after the patient has been asymptomatic for 5 to 7 days (Table 20–5). Recurrence of disease is not uncommon.

A combination medical and surgical approach is indicated in the management of purulent pericarditis. Therapy begins with a careful search for the causative organism to aid in the choice of antibiotic (see Table 20–3). The duration of antibiotic therapy is 4 to 6 weeks, depending on the patient's clinical response. Early surgical drainage is preferred over pericardiocentesis to break loculations and remove thick fluid, but there is debate concerning the preferred method of pericardial drainage. Proponents of pericardiectomy believe it lessens the risk of constrictive pericarditis as a sequela, whereas those who favor pericardiostomy believe it is just as effective and uses a simpler technique.[70–73]

Constrictive pericarditis occurs as a sequela of pericarditis, developing weeks to months following the acute illness. Although many causes have been determined, including infections, trauma, uremia, radiation, and rheumatic fever, in more than 50% of cases the origin cannot be determined.[74] It is estimated that constrictive pericarditis will develop in 4% to 16% of patients who have had purulent pericarditis.[32, 40]

Postpericardiotomy syndrome is characterized by fever, chest pain, and pleural and pericardial effusion seen 1 to 2 weeks following open heart surgery in approximately 15%

of patients.[41, 75] It must be distinguished from other causes of postoperative fever or cardiomegaly. Patients will generally respond well to anti-inflammatory therapy (see Table 20–5).

DISPOSITION

Patients with pericardial disease should be admitted to the hospital for observation and treatment (Table 20–6). Admission to the intensive care unit is indicated for the treatment of sepsis or septic shock, when congestive heart failure or cardiac arrhythmias are present, or if the development

TABLE 20-6

DISPOSITION FOR PATIENTS WITH PERICARDITIS

Admit
All patients with acute pericarditis
All patients with exacerbation of chronic pericarditis

Admit to ICU
Patients with sepsis
Patients with septic shock
Patients with conduction disturbances
Patients with congestive heart failure or respiratory distress
Patients with impending tamponade

Consider Consultation With:
Surgeon for patients with bacterial pericarditis, traumatic effusions
Cardiologist for all patients
Rheumatologist for patients with pericarditis of inflammatory origin
Infectious disease specialist for patients with pericarditis of infectious origin

of cardiac tamponade is a concern. Early cardiology consultation is recommended in all cases, and immediate surgical consultation is important in the treatment of purulent pericarditis. Other specialists may need to be consulted depending on the origin of the illness.

References

1. Sternbach GL. Pericarditis. Ann Emerg Med 1988;17:214.
2. Strauss AW, Santa-Maria M, Goldring D. Constrictive pericarditis in children. Am J Dis Child 1975;129:822.
3. Simcha A, Taylor JFN. Constrictive pericarditis in childhood. Arch Dis Child 1972;46:515.
4. Keith JD, Rowe RD, Vlad P. Pericarditis Heart Disease in Infancy and Childhood. 2nd ed. New York, Macmillan, 1967, pp 970–975.
5. Sinzobahamvya N, Ikeogu MO. Purulent pericarditis. Arch Dis Child 1987;62:696.
6. Fyfe DA, Hagler DJ, Puga FJ, Driscoll DJ. Clinical and therapeutic aspects of Haemophilus influenzae pericarditis in pediatric patients. Mayo Clin Proc 1984;59:415.
7. Gersony WM, Hordof AJ. Infective endocarditis and diseases of pericardium. Pediatr Clin North Am 1978;25:831.
8. Holt JP. The normal pericardium. Am J Cardiol 1970;26:455.
9. Golinko RJ, Kaplan N, Rudolph AM. The mechanism of pulsus paradoxus during acute pericardial tamponade. J Clin Invest 1963;42:249.
10. Morgan BC, Guntheroth WG, Dillard DH. Relationship of pericardial to pleural pressure during quiet respiration and cardiac tamponade. Circ Res 1965;16:493.
11. Shabetai R, Fowler NO, Guntheroth WG. The hemodynamics of cardiac tamponade and constrictive pericarditis. Am J Cardiol 1970;26:480.
12. Somerville W. Constrictive pericarditis with special reference to the change in natural history brought about by surgical intervention. Circulation 1968;37 and 38(suppl):V-102–V-111.
13. Feigin RD, Cherry JD. Pediatric Infectious Disease. 2nd ed. Philadelphia, WB Saunders, 1987, p 418.
14. Greenwood RD, Rosenthal A, Cassady R, et al. Constrictive pericarditis in childhood due to mediastinal irradiation. Circulation 1974;50:1033.
15. Callanan DL, Morriss MJ, Kaplan SL, et al. Constrictive pericarditis due to Streptococcus sanguis. South Med J 1981;74:377.
16. Martinez-Lavin M, Buendia A, Delgado E, et al. A familial syndrome of pericarditis, arthritis, and camptodactyly. N Engl J Med 1983;309:224.
17. Laxer RM, Cameron BJ, Chaisson D, et al. The camptodactyly-arthropathy-pericarditis syndrome: Case report and literature review. Arthritis Rheum 1986;29:439.
18. Bulutlar G, Yaziz H, Ozdogan H, Schreuder I. A familial syndrome of pericarditis, arthritis, camptodactyly, and coxa vara. Arthritis Rheum 1986;29:436.
19. Nelson D. Pocketbook of Pediatric Antimicrobial Therapy 1989–1990. 8th ed. Baltimore, Williams & Wilkins, 1989, pp 32–33.
20. Phillips JH, Burch GE. Selected clues in cardiac auscultation. Am Heart J 1962;63:1.
21. Fowler NO, Manitasas GT. Infectious pericarditis. Prog Cardiovasc Dis 1973;16:323.
22. Horowitz MS, Schultz CS, Stinson EB, et al. Sensitivity and specificity of echocardiographic diagnosis of pericardial effusion. Circulation 1974;50:239.
23. Isner JM, Carter BL, Bankoff MS, et al. Computed tomography in the diagnosis of pericardial heart disease. Ann Intern Med 1982;97:473.
24. Surawicz B, Lasseter KC. Electrocardiogram in pericarditis. Am J Cardiol 1970;26:471.
25. Spodick DH. Electrocardiogram in acute pericarditis. Am J Cardiol 1974;33:470.
26. Park MK, Guntheroth WG. How to Read Pediatric ECGs. Chicago, Year Book, 1981, pp 77–78.
27. Lepeschkin E: Modern Electrocardiography. Vol 1. Baltimore, Williams & Wilkins, 1955, pp 453–458.
28. Bedford ED. Chronic effusive pericarditis. Br Heart J 1964;26:499.
29. Nadas AS, Levy JM. Pericarditis in children. Am J Cardiol 1961;7:109.
30. Moss AJ, Adams FH. Heart disease in infants, children, and adolescents. Baltimore, Williams & Wilkins, 1984, pp 584–594.
31. Naraqui S, Kabins S. Acute meningococcal pericarditis without meningitis. Arch Intern Med 1975;135:314.
32. Van Reken D, Strauss A, Hernandez A, Feigin RD. Infectious pericarditis in children. J Pediatr 1974;85:165.
33. Seddon DJ. Pericarditis with pericardial effusion complicating chickenpox. Postgrad Med J 1986;62:1133.
34. Williams AJ, Freemont AJ, Barnett DB. Pericarditis and arthritis complicating chickenpox. Br J Clin Pract 1983;37:226.
35. Hudgins JM. Infectious mononucleosis complicated by myocarditis and pericarditis. JAMA 1976;234:2626.
36. Hirschman SZ, Hammer GS. Coxsackie virus myopericarditis: A microbiological and clinical review. Am J Cardiol 1974;34:224.
37. Feldman WE. Bacterial etiology and mortality of purulent pericarditis in pediatric patients. Am J Dis Child 1979;133:641.
38. Rane HS, Lahari KR, Desai AG. Pyo-pericarditis in children. Indian J Pediatr 1984;51:305.
39. Kresch MJ. Pericarditis complicating Haemophilus epiglottitis. Pediatr Infect Dis 1985;4:559.
40. Boyle JD, Pearce ML, Guze LB. Purulent pericarditis: Review of literature and report of eleven cases. Medicine 1961;40:119.
41. Gersony WM, McCracken GH. Purulent pericarditis in infancy. Pediatrics 1967;40:224.
42. Pinsky WW, Friedman RA, Jubelirer DP, Nihill MR. Infectious pericarditis. In Feigin RD, Cherry JD (eds). Textbook of Pediatric Infectious Diseases. 2nd ed. Philadelphia, WB Saunders, 1987, pp 415–426.
43. Echeverria P, Smith EWP, Ingram D, et al. Haemophilus influenzae B pericarditis in children. Pediatrics 1975;56:808.
44. Haggman DL, Rehm SJ, Moodie DS, Mackenzie AH. Nontyphoidal salmonella pericarditis: A case report and review of the literature. Pediatr Infect Dis 1986;5:259.
45. Marin-Garcia J, Gooch WM, Coury DL. Cardiac manifestations of Rocky Mountain spotted fever. Pediatrics 1981;67:358.
46. Pinsky WW, Friedman RA, Jubelirer DP, Nihill MR. Infectious pericarditis. In Feigin RD, Cherry JD (eds). Textbook of Pediatric Infectious Diseases. 2nd ed. Philadelphia, WB Saunders, 1987, pp 415–426.
47. Ibarra-Pérez C, Green L, Calvillo-Juárez M, Vargas de la Cruz J. Diagnosis and treatment of rupture of amebic abscess of the liver into the pericardium. J Thorac Cardiovasc Surg 1972;64:11.
48. Baldwa VS, Gupta K, Sanghvi S, Gupta BS. Amoebic pericarditis—an unusual complication of liver abscess. J Assoc Physicians India 1986;34:449.
49. Bailey GL, Hampers CL, Hager EB, Merrill JP. Uremic pericarditis: Clinical features and management. Circulation 1968;38:582–591.
50. Battle CU, Bonfiglio TA, Miller DR. Pericarditis as the initial manifestation of acute leukemia: Report of a case. J Pediatr 1969;75:692.
51. Berg M, Wilander E, Eriksson A. Case report: Mediastinal lymphosarcoma simulating pericarditis. Acta Paediatr Scand 1975;64:873.
52. Acierno LJ. Cardiac complications in acquired immunodeficiency syndrome (AIDS): A review. J Am Coll Cardiol 1989;13:1144.
53. Steinherz LJ, Brochstein JA, Robins J. Cardiac involvement in congenital acquired immunodeficiency syndrome. Am J Dis Child 1986;140:1241.
54. Joshi VV, Gadol C, Connor E, et al. Dilated cardiomyopathy in children with acquired immunodeficiency syndrome: A pathologic study of five cases. Hum Pathol 1988;19:69.
55. Joshi VV, Pawel B, Connor E, et al. Arteriopathy in children with acquired immune deficiency syndrome. Pediatr Pathol 1987;7:261.
56. Roldan EO, Moskowitz L, Hensley GT. Pathology of the heart in acquired immunodeficiency syndrome. Arch Pathol Lab Med 1987;111:943.
57. D'Cruz IA, Sengupta EE, Abrahams C, et al. Cardiac involvement, including tuberculous pericardial effusion, complicating acquired immune deficiency syndrome. Pediatr Pathol 1987;7:261.
58. Crowley DC. Cardiovascular complications of mucocutaneous lymph node syndrome. Symp Pediatr Cardiol 1984;31:1321.
59. Rowe RD, Rose V. Kawasaki disease: Canadian update. Can Med Assoc J 1985;132:25.
60. Hicks RV, Melish ME. Kawasaki syndrome. Pediatr Clin North Am 1986;33:1151.
61. Majeed HA, Shaltout A, Yousof AM. Recurrences of acute rheumatic fever. Am J Dis Child 1984;138:341.
62. Brewer E Jr. Juvenile rheumatoid arthritis—cardiac involvement. Arthritis Rheum 1977;20:231.
63. Chang RW. Cardiac manifestations of SLE. Clin Rheum Dis 1982;8:197.
64. Granot E, Rottem M, Rein AJ. Carditis complicating inflammatory bowel disease in children. Eur J Pediatr 1988;148:203.
65. Thompson DG, Lennard-Jones JE, Swarbrick ET, Bown R. Pericarditis and inflammatory bowel disease. Q J Med 1979;8:93.
66. Mowat NAG, Bennet PN, Finlayson JK, et al. Myopericarditis complicating ulcerative colitis. Br Heart J 1974;36:724.
67. Frid C, Bjarke B, Eriksson M. Myocarditis in children with inflammatory bowel disease. J Pediatr Gastroenterol Nutrition 1986;5:964.
68. Krikorian JG, Hancock EW. Pericardiocentesis. Circulation 1978;65:808.
69. Sherry DD, Patterson MWH, Petty RE. The use of indomethacin in the treatment of pericarditis in childhood. J Pediatr 1982;100:995.
70. Morgan RJ, Stephenson LW, Woolf PK, et al. Surgical treatment of purulent pericarditis in children. J Thorac Cardiovasc Surg 1983;85:527.
71. Driscoll DJ, Rhodes KH. Treatment of purulent pericarditis—a comment. J Thorac Cardiovasc Surg 1983;85:531.
72. Cheatham JE Jr, Grantham RN, Peyton MD, et al. Hemophilus influenzae purulent pericarditis in children. J Thorac Cardiovasc Surg 1980;79:933.
73. Adebo OA, Adebonojo SA. Purluent pericarditis in children. J Thorac Cardiovasc Surg 1984;88:312.
74. Spodick DH. Acute Pericarditis. New York, Grune & Stratton, 1959.
75. Engle MA, Zabriskie JB, Senterfit LB, Ebert PA. Postpericardiotomy syndrome: A new look at an old condition. Mod Concepts Cardiovasc Dis 1975;XLIV(11):59.

CHAPTER 21

Acute Rheumatic Fever

Richard A. Craven

INTRODUCTION

Acute rheumatic fever (ARF) is a nonsuppurative inflammatory disease with lesions involving primarily the heart, joints, subcutaneous tissues, and central nervous system.[1, 2] It is a sequela of the infection of the upper respiratory tract by Lancefield group A beta-hemolytic streptococcus.[3]

The disease was first described in the seventeenth century, when it was known as *acute articular rheumatism*. That same century, Thomas Sydenham used the term *chorea* to describe the peculiar spasmodic movements of children with central nervous system involvement. In 1812, William Charles Wells noted the association of rheumatism and carditis and characterized the subcutaneous nodules often associated with the disease. Jean-Baptiste Bouillard, in 1836, gave the first clinical description of heart disease in patients with rheumatoid arthritis. It was not until 1880 that the association between the antecedent pharyngitis and rheumatic fever development was noted by J. K. Fowler.[2] However, the bacterial origin of the pharyngitis was not discovered until 50 years later.

At the beginning of the twentieth century, ARF was established as an entity occurring after infection with scarlet fever. In 1904, Ludwig Aschoff gave his classic description of the myocardial rheumatic lesion, now known as the *Aschoff body*. In 1939, 8 years after the streptococcal origin of ARF was revealed, continuous antibiotic prophylaxis against the streptococcal bacteria was found to prevent ARF recurrences. A few years later, Denny and Wannamaker noted that primary prevention of ARF could be accomplished by treatment of the streptococcal pharyngitis.[2] They called the streptococcus the "chain that links the heart to the throat."

INCIDENCE AND PREVALENCE

The incidence of rheumatic fever in the United States has declined dramatically since the advent of antibiotics. From 1943 to 1945, there were 388 cases per 100,000 population; in the 1980s, this decreased to 0.5 to 1.9 cases per 100,000.[4–8] Similarly, ARF was the leading cause of death in individuals 5 to 20 years old in the 1920s, with an average of 10 deaths per 100,000 people[9]; this rate has decreased to 0.01 deaths per 100,000 population in the 1980s.[6, 10] Nevertheless, in India, the Middle East, and urbanized South Africa, ARF is the leading cause of cardiovascular morbidity and mortality for the young and middle-aged.[4]

ARF typically affects those 6 to 15 years of age.[5, 11–13] Although there is no clear gender predilection, there is a female preponderance in cases of pure chorea occurring after puberty.[14] Socioeconomic factors are important in the development of ARF.[2, 6, 15–18] There is an increased incidence in areas of crowded living conditions, as demonstrated in military camps. Populations with lower standards of living or with less access to medical care are at increased risk for developing ARF. In addition, the incidence of ARF is higher during the cooler months of the year. Although a family history of ARF may occur in affected individuals, there is actually a limited genetic predisposition for developing the disease.[19]

Several theories have been proposed to explain the decline in the incidence of ARF since the 1940s.[4, 6, 8, 10, 20] Antibiotics have been used both in the treatment of streptococcal pharyngitis (primary prevention) and in the continued prophylaxis against recurrences (secondary prevention). Although the use of antibiotics accelerated the decreased incidence of ARF, as well as the incidence of pathologic murmurs, there was actually a decline in the number of cases of ARF before widespread antibiotic use. Other theories cite less crowded and better living conditions as reasons for the decreased incidence of ARF. Access to medical care has also improved with rural health plans and the establishment of federally subsidized health care programs. Arguments against these theories are supported by the recent outbreaks of ARF in six states.[5, 12, 13, 21–23] These were simultaneous yet multifocal outbreaks in areas that were not poverty stricken or inaccessible to medical care. Finally, similar diseases, incorrectly diagnosed as ARF in the past, are now easily differentiated by more accurate diagnostic regimens.

Factors involving the streptococcal bacteria have also been studied.[4, 8] The frequency of group A beta-hemolytic streptococcal infections has actually not changed since the 1940s.[3] Although never proven, the possibility of decreased "rheumatogenicity" of the organism has been proposed.[23, 24] The likelihood of a less virulent strain has also been raised, causing less person-to-person transmission.[25] Susceptible patients with streptococcal pharyngitis infections remain untreated in this country, while the incidence of ARF continues to decline.[22]

The attack rates for ARF range from 0.4% in the endemically occurring, open population to 3.0% during epidemics or in crowded situations.[1, 26] The discontinuance of the rheumatic fever registry by health departments, however, makes attack rates difficult to monitor.[21] It is believed that ARF is more likely to occur after more severe forms of streptococcal throat infection, although 50% of the patients with ARF in the Utah outbreak did not have a sore throat during the 2-month period before the onset of their illness.[1, 5]

The recurrence, or secondary attack rate, of ARF has increased from 5 to up to 50 per 100 infections and is thought to be related to the virulence of the reactivating infection.[18] The higher frequency of recurrence is found in those with a history of rheumatic carditis.[18, 27] ARF still causes significant morbidity and mortality in developing countries. In any patient, heart valve damage may be chronic and progressive, producing disability, cardiac failure, and even death.[28, 29]

ANATOMY AND PHYSIOLOGY
Pathophysiology

Four factors are required in order to develop ARF: the presence of group A beta-hemolytic streptococcus, a susceptible host, persistence of the organism, and infection of the upper respiratory tract.[30] Historically, ARF sufferers were children who appeared ill and suffered a succession of upper respiratory tract infections. They presented with pallor and failure to thrive, a poor appetite, mild fever, joint and muscle pains, and often nosebleeds. The diagnosis of ARF was not suspected until the telltale murmur of mitral regurgitation appeared.[9]

The exact pathogenesis of rheumatic fever remains unclear. Typically, there is a sequence of tonsillitis caused by group A beta-hemolytic streptococcus, followed by a latent period of 1 to 2 weeks, and then the appearance of clinical symptoms caused by the nonsuppurative sequelae. Although the disease is not caused by the spread of the streptococcus throughout the body, the exact mechanism of inducing ARF is poorly understood.[6]

The bacteria, *Streptococcus pyogenes*, is a gram-positive coccus with a cell wall composed of M proteins and exhibiting fimbriae, which allows it to adhere to epithelial cells. It is a member of the Lancefield group A, as determined by the antigenic properties of the carbohydrate in its cell wall. There are more than 60 types of M protein, and certain ones confer resistance to phagocytosis, thus increasing the virulence of the organism.[25] Although some serotypes predominate in patients with ARF, none are found to be truly *rheumatogenic*.[31–34]

The streptococcus produces several biologically active substances.[25] Hemolysins are toxic to red blood cells, platelets, granulocytes, and lysosomes; examples are types O and S. Hemolysin O is antigenic, and the presence of antistreptolysin O (ASO) antibodies denote a recent infection with streptococcus. The erythrogenic toxin produces the characteristic rash of scarlatina. The streptococcus produces enzymes that help the spread of the infection; examples are the anti-DNA enzymes (deoxyribonuclease, or DNase) A, B, C, and D and streptokinase. Antibodies against DNase B are also used as markers of recent infection and are especially useful in confirming the diagnosis of ARF in a patient who may not have ASO antibodies. The streptokinase causes clot lysis and is used to dissolve coronary artery thrombosis.

Several theories of the pathogenesis of acute rheumatic fever have been proposed.[35–38] The immunopathogenic theory is based on an exaggerated immune response by the infected patient. The streptococcal antigens produce B-cell sensitization, T-cell sensitization, or both, which stimulate the production of antistreptococcal antibodies. Immune complexes are then formed that cross-react with cardiac sarcolemmal antigens, which resemble streptococcal antigens. This results in a valvular and perivalvular myocardial inflammatory response.

High titers of antibodies and increased frequency of antibodies to soluble cardiac antigens in patients with ARF and rheumatic heart disease (RHD) have been demonstrated.[39] These *heart-reactive antibodies* (HRA) persist in these patients and are thought to contribute to an exaggerated immune response to certain antigens. It is speculated that the HRA are important in the formation of immune complexes that activate complement, either from damaged tissue or in the circulation, to produce immunoregulation changes or direct tissue damage.

The role of lymphoid elements in the pathogenesis of ARF has also been studied. The predominant constituents of Aschoff bodies, valvular lesions, and subcutaneous nodules are lymphoid elements. A decrease in total T lymphocytes, helper-inducer cells, and helper-suppressor ratios in ARF patients has been noted; these decreases persisted for years.[40] During periods of disease activity these alterations are accentuated, with an associated hyporesponsiveness of blast transformation. Although the role these lymphoid elements play in producing the clinical sequelae of ARF is still unclear, monitoring T-cell function may be important in following disease activity.

Another host factor may be important in the development of ARF.[41] A vitamin D–binding protein, known as a *group-specific component* (Gc), is present in B lymphocytes and has an affinity for the actin that is released by damaged tissue. In one population, there was a strong association between patients possessing a specific allele for Gc production and the development of ARF. If B-cell function is directed by the Gc allele, then the exaggerated B-cell activity seen in patients with ARF may be directly related to the particular Gc allele they possess.

Other support for an immunologic origin for rheumatic fever comes from studies suggesting that patients with HLA type DR4 are predisposed to develop both ARF and chronic rheumatic valvular heart disease.[42a] In addition, there is less risk of developing ARF in patients classified as streptococcal carriers. Their lack of an immunologic response to the presence of streptococcus may eliminate the formation of immune complexes necessary to develop the sequelae of ARF.

Other unproven theories include mechanisms that involve direct tissue invasion by the organism, toxic effects from the products of the streptococcus, or even a serum sickness–like reaction. Nevertheless, the exact mechanism by which group A streptococcus induces ARF is still unclear.

PATHOLOGY

Acute rheumatic fever results in nonsuppurative, exudative, and proliferative inflammatory lesions of connective tissue, especially in the heart, joints, blood vessels, and subcutaneous tissue. In the heart, all layers (endocardium, myocardium, and pericardium) may be involved; hence the term *rheumatic pancarditis*.[19] Early changes include edema of the ground substance, collagen fiber fragmentation, lymphocytic infiltration, and fibrinoid deposition. The pathognomonic feature of cardiac involvement is a perivascular focus of inflammation termed the *Aschoff body*, which is characterized microscopically by an area of central necrosis surrounded by mononuclear and giant multinuclear cells, sometimes called *Anichkov's myocytes*.[1] Endocardial involvement can result in a verrucous valvulitis, which leads to serious permanent damage to the affected valves. The mitral valve is most commonly involved, followed by the aortic and tricuspid valves and, much less commonly, the pulmonic valve.[19] When other valves are affected, there will be evidence of mitral involvement.[29] The acute phase is characterized by edema and deformity of the valve leaflets, whereas fibrous thickening and adhesions typify the chronic phase of valvulitis.[42b] Rheumatic pericarditis, although distinguished by a serofibrinous effusion and fibrin deposition, produces no pericardial constriction.[19, 43, 44]

Joint involvement in ARF is characterized by a fibrinous infiltration of the synovial membrane, accompanied by a serous effusion. Unlike rheumatoid arthritis, there is no joint destruction or pannus formation, and complete recovery is expected.[16, 19, 45, 46] Subcutaneous tissue involvement is characterized by nodule formation. These resemble the Aschoff body microscopically, with a central area of fibrinoid necrosis surrounded by an area of fibroblasts and histiocytes. There may be inconsistent areas of cellular degeneration and hyalinization of blood vessels in the central nervous system. These lesions are not uncharacteristic of rheumatic fever, however, and there is no clinical correlation with their presence and the patient's symptoms.[1]

EMERGENCY MEDICAL SERVICE CONSIDERATIONS

In the prehospital setting, the care of a patient with ARF is mainly supportive. The patient should be placed on a cardiac monitor and given supplemental oxygen, and intravenous access should be established. Decompensation of the cardiovascular system may occur, requiring more aggressive treatment. Patients with pulmonary edema may require intravenous furosemide (1 mg/kg, up to a maximum of 6 mg/kg) and morphine sulfate (0.1 to 0.2 mg/kg, up to a maximum of 15 mg). Dysrhythmias should be treated according to Advanced Cardiac Life Support protocols.[47] In the patient with severe airway compromise, an endotracheal tube should be placed and ventilations controlled. Communication with the medical command base is essential when dealing with an unstable patient.

CLINICAL EVALUATION

The history and physical findings in the patient with ARF will vary depending on the site of involvement, the stage of the disease, and the severity of illness. Acute rheumatic fever follows an upper respiratory infection with group A beta-hemolytic streptococcus; however, in up to 75% of patients with these infections, symptoms are mild or nonexistent. The onset of ARF is variable, occurring an average of 19 days following infection; those patients with *pure* chorea often present several weeks later.[1, 2, 48–50]

Vital Signs

Approximately 90% of patients with ARF will have an elevated temperature of 38.3°C to 40.0°C (101°F to 104°F).[12] Although fever is one of the minor criteria, it follows no characteristic pattern and is usually absent in patients presenting with only chorea.[16, 50] Tachycardia is expected, and carditis should be suspected in the sleeping patient with a pulse greater than 100 beats/min.[16] Patients can also present with bradycardia, at times severe enough to cause Stokes-Adams attacks.[51, 52] Patients with aortic stenosis from rheumatic heart disease may have pulsus alternans (a regular rhythm with alternating strong and weak beats) or parvis et tardus (a dampening of the arterial pulse).[29] The *irregularly irregular* pulse of atrial fibrillation may be seen in patients with chronic rheumatic fever.[53] The respiratory rate is often normal but may be increased because of fever, anxiety, the presence of congestive heart failure, or the use of salicylates.[16] The blood pressure is usually normal but may be low with severe congestive heart failure. With aortic regurgitation, widened pulse pressure is seen.

Skin

One of the major criteria for the diagnosis of ARF is the finding of subcutaneous nodules.[30, 54–56] These are pea sized, firm, painless, and freely movable and are found over bony prominences, especially the olecranon. They occur in only 2% of ARF patients but are often present in patients with severe carditis. The nodules typically appear several weeks after the onset of the attack of ARF and persist for 1 or 2 weeks.[16, 50]

Another major criterion is the presence of erythema marginatum.[55, 56] The rash consists of nonpruritic, painless, pink papules on the trunk or inner aspects of the extremities. It spreads outward with distinct margins and central clearing, described as a *smoke rings* or *chicken wire* pattern.[16] The rash occurs in less than 15% of ARF patients and usually begins a few days after the onset of arthritis.[5, 12] It is often evanescent but may appear off and on for months.[1] The rash is believed to be caused by a vasomotor phenomenon and has no correlation with the activity of the disease or its response to treatment.[19]

Other skin findings include pallor (which may be striking), cyanosis, or jaundice.[57] Jaundice is secondary to increased systemic venous pressure from tricuspid regurgitation. Erythema papulatum is a rare finding, occurring in less than 0.2% of patients with ARF. It consists of keratotic, erythematous papules found on the extensor surfaces of the elbows and knees and lasting from 6 to 8 days.[16]

Head, Eye, Ear, Nose, and Throat

Though ARF is preceded by a streptococcal pharyngitis, it is unusual for a patient to present with a sore throat as part of the symptom complex. Although once thought to be common, the incidence of epistaxis is decreasing, being present in less than 4% of patients with their first attack of ARF and in only 9% of those with recurrent attacks.[11, 48] Other findings include soft palate petechiae, Roth's spots, and conjunctival hemorrhages. Cervical adenopathy may persist from the antecedent pharyngitis. The presence of congestive heart failure can cause jugular venous distention and generalized facial edema.[16] Prominent arterial pulses may be noted with aortic regurgitation, whereas tricuspid regurgitation may produce jugular venous pulsation.[29]

Respiratory Symptoms

Dyspnea will be present in patients with congestive heart failure and is a cardinal feature of symptomatic mitral stenosis. With mitral regurgitation or aortic stenosis, dyspnea will be a late finding. The patient may complain of pleuritic chest pain, and a cough may be present as a result of rheumatic pneumonitis or lobar pneumonia.[57] Mitral stenosis produces pulmonary venous hypertension, which can present as hemoptysis. On auscultation, the lungs can be clear or have localized or generalized rales.[16]

Cardiovascular Symptoms

The patient may complain of chest pain. With the presence of pericarditis, this pain may be severe, sudden, and related to inspiration and change in position. Chest pain may also be ischemic in origin.[58] Valvular lesions such as aortic regurgitation, mitral stenosis, or aortic stenosis may also produce chest pain. Dysrhythmias can produce palpitations.

Carditis is one of the major manifestations of ARF.[55] It usually occurs within 3 weeks of the onset of the attack and is present in 40% to 50% of initial attacks, being more frequent in younger patients.[59] Although carditis may be asymptomatic, it is associated with a more serious prognosis in patients with ARF.[19, 60] The duration of carditis varies from 6 weeks to 6 months, with longer durations in patients with *chronic* rheumatic fever. The hallmarks of carditis include cardiac murmurs, cardiomegaly, pericardial friction rubs, and congestive heart failure.[28, 29, 61]

The murmur in ARF carditis is produced by structural changes in the valve. It may be a new murmur or represent a distinct change in a preexisting murmur. Three types are recognized: apical systolic, apical mid-diastolic, and basal diastolic.[19, 28] Acute mitral regurgitation produces the apical systolic murmur, a loud, blowing, high-pitched sound that is increased when the patient lies on the left side. The apical mid-diastolic, or Carey-Coombs, murmur is low pitched and is caused by rapid flow across the mitral valve with an associated valvulitis. If present, it confirms the significance of the aforementioned apical systolic murmur. The stethoscope's bell is needed to hear this murmur, which may be transient. The basal diastolic murmur is high pitched and blowing and is heard along the left sternal border after expiration and with the patient leaning forward; it is caused by aortic regurgitation.[62]

Cardiomegaly will be present in 50% to 55% of patients with carditis and should be clinically suspected with a diffuse or displaced apical impulse.[14] As mentioned, the patient with carditis may present with frank congestive heart failure, having rales, jugular venous distention, peripheral edema, and an S_3 gallop.[63]

Six percent to 13% of patients with ARF develop a

pericardial friction rub.[10, 14] This is a superficial scratching sound at the base and left sternal border and is usually heard in both systole and diastole. When present, the rub is associated with acute valvulitis and signifies a severe form of rheumatic carditis.

Gastrointestinal Symptoms

The signs and symptoms of ARF may include abdominal pain or hepatomegaly.[16] Hepatomegaly can result from congestive heart failure or valvular disease; occasionally it is a result of prolonged treatment with corticosteroids.[64] The patient may also complain of diffuse abdominal pain with generalized tenderness. Frequently the pain will be accompanied by rigidity and abdominal distention, mimicking an acute abdominal condition.

Musculoskeletal Symptoms

Involvement of the musculoskeletal system includes the major manifestation of arthritis, the minor manifestation of arthralgia, and uncommon sign of tenosynovitis.[55, 65] From 50% to 75% of patients with ARF have migratory polyarthritis.[1, 6, 16] The joints are swollen, warm, and red and have a limited range of motion, and the patient complains of pain that is disproportionate to the physical findings. The large joints are affected, with the elbows, knees, ankles, and wrists most commonly involved. The arthritis improves dramatically with administration of salicylates, but even if untreated will spontaneously resolve in 3 to 4 weeks.[2, 19] The severity of the arthritis and the severity of any associated carditis are inversely related.[1]

When arthritis is absent, the presence of arthralgia is used as a minor criteria for ARF.[55] This is joint pain without any objective findings and must not be confused with localized myalgias. Tenosynovitis has also been reported in adults with ARF.[66, 67] It typically affects the dorsal aspects of the wrists, hands, or ankles and may be associated with arthritis.

Neuropsychiatric Symptoms

Another major manifestation of ARF is Sydenham's chorea, also known as *St. Vitus' dance*. It is present in up to 30% of patients and may be the sole major manifestation in 5% to 15%.[5, 7, 11–13] It is rare in patients younger than 3 years old but may be found in adolescent females. It is exaggerated during pregnancy.[19] Chorea may appear after a long latent period, from 1 to 3 months after the antecedent streptococcal infection, thus making the diagnosis of ARF more difficult. In patients with *pure* chorea there are no previous or concurrent rheumatic manifestations; however, these patients have a higher incidence of subsequent rheumatic heart disease.[1] The chorea presents initially as subtle personality changes and progresses to ataxia, weakness, jerky speech patterns, and difficulty with fine motor tasks. This is followed by the appearance of sudden, aimless, spasmodic movements, which then dominate the clinical picture.[16] The chorea mainly affects the face and upper extremities, with up to 10% of patients exhibiting unilateral symptoms only (hemichorea). Other features may include a darting tongue, pronator sign, or the choreic hand (hyperextension of the fingers and metacarpophalangeal joints with thumb abduction and wrist flexion). The chorea may last from a few weeks to years, but the usual duration is 2 to 4 months. Despite a dramatic clinical presentation, the chorea leaves no permanent neurologic sequelae.[14, 19, 68]

Psychiatric symptoms may be seen in ARF and are most often associated with the chorea. These include emotional lability, personality and behavioral changes, and occasionally psychosis.

DIAGNOSTIC EVALUATION

Because the incidence of ARF has decreased since the 1940s, the diagnosis may not be readily apparent to the physician. In addition, ARF has varied clinical presentations, and there is no specific diagnostic test for it. The criteria set forth by T. Duckett Jones, and modified by the American Heart Association, serve as the basis for diagnosing acute rheumatic fever (Table 21–1).[55] Although these criteria are not infallible, they do minimize both over and underdiagnosing of the disease.

Laboratory findings in ARF can be as varied as the clinical symptoms. Throat cultures should be analyzed prior to any antibiotic therapy. Eight percent to 15% of ARF patients will have group A *Streptococcus* organisms present in their pharynx. This low culture rate is thought to be a result of the latent period between the pharyngeal infection and the onset of ARF symptoms.[5, 11, 15] Because there are few organisms present in the throat, multiple cultures should be obtained.

Although the presence of leukocytosis is helpful as a minor manifestation of ARF, the absolute white blood cell count varies.[16] Rheumatic fever patients often have a mild normochromic, normocytic anemia. The blood urea nitrogen level may also be elevated. In addition, patients often have an elevated level of aspartate aminotransferase (AST; previously called serum glutamic-oxaloacetic transaminase, or

---

TABLE 21–1

MODIFIED JONES CRITERIA FOR GUIDANCE IN THE DIAGNOSIS OF RHEUMATIC FEVER

Major Manifestations
Carditis
Polyarthritis
Chorea
Erythema marginatum
Subcutaneous nodules

Minor Manifestations
Clinical
   Previous rheumatic fever or rheumatic heart disease
   Arthralgia
   Fever
Laboratory
   Elevated acute phase reactants:
      Erythrocyte sedimentation rate
      C-reactive protein
      Leukocytosis
   Prolonged PR interval
Plus:
Supporting evidence of preceding streptococcal infection:
   Increase in antistreptolysin O (ASO) antibody titers
   Increase in other streptococcal antibodies
      (antideoxyribonuclease B, [anti DNase B] heart-reactive
      antibodies, or others using the streptozyme test, including
      ASO, antihyaluronidase, antistreptokinase, anti-DNase B,
      and antinicotinamide adenine dinucleotidase).
Positive throat culture for group A *Streptococcus*
Recent scarlet fever

The presence of two major criteria or of one major and two minor criteria indicates a high probability of the presence of rheumatic fever if supported by evidence of a preceding streptococcal infection. The absence of the latter should make the diagnosis doubtful, except in situations in which rheumatic fever is first discovered after a long latent period from the antecedent infection (i.e., Sydenham's chorea or low-grade carditis).

SGOT), but the levels are inconsistent in rheumatic carditis and do not correlate with disease activity.[61, 69, 70]

During the acute phase of ARF, although nonspecific, an elevated erythrocyte sedimentation rate (>20 mm/hr) is found in more than 85% of children and in virtually all adults with ARF.[5, 11, 12, 50, 61] The C-reactive protein level is a sensitive, though nonspecific, indicator of inflammation.[16] Unlike the sedimentation rate, the C-reactive protein level is less often influenced by exogenous factors such as anemia, but may be elevated in a patient with only rheumatoid congestive heart failure.[71]

According to the revised Jones Criteria, evidence of an antecedent streptococcal infection is important when making the diagnosis of ARF.[54, 55, 72] Several tests are specific for streptococcus by detecting antibodies to the bacteria. Anti-streptococcal antibody levels are usually elevated in patients with ARF, except after prolonged latency periods as in *pure chorea* or insidious rheumatic carditis. Once a test demonstrates antistreptococcal antibodies, there is no need to repeat it, as there is no correlation between the elevation and duration of the antibody titer and the severity or persistence of the illness.[2] Additionally, the rate of decline of the antibody titer is independent of the course of the illness. However, the diagnostic yield can be increased by testing for several antibody types.[1] For example, more than 95% of patients with ARF will have an elevation in at least one antibody titer when a battery of three different antibody tests are used.[73]

The most widely used test is for detection of ASO. In the child, a titer of more than 333 units is considered elevated; adult titers exceeding 200 units are elevated.[55, 74] Of patients with ARF, 65% to 90% have elevated ASO titers.[5, 11, 12] Patients may have normal titers during the early stages of ARF or if they present with pure chorea or "chronic" carditis, as these typically have prolonged latent periods.[55] The anti-deoxyribonuclease B (anti-DNase B) test detects antibodies to DNase B. Although a specific test, it can be falsely negative and vary seasonally or geographically. High titers of anti-DNase B are also found in patients with glomerulonephritis or streptococcal skin infections, while ASO titers in these same patients remain normal.[5, 12, 74]

ASO and anti-DNase B are also part of the antistreptozyme battery (ASTZ), a sensitive agglutination test that detects extracellular streptococcal antigens adsorbed to red blood cells. In addition, the ASTZ includes antistreptokinase (ASK), antihyaluronidase (ASH), and antinicotinamide adenine dinucleotidase (anti-NADase). The ASTZ is considered positive if the titer is greater than 200 units/ml (or greater than 1:200 dilutions). Unfortunately the ASTZ is not as well standardized as the ASO test.[74, 75] Finally, one can test for antibodies that cross-react with myocardial sarcolemmal and group A streptococcal membranes. This is the heart reactive antibody (HRA) test and is considered positive at greater than 1:10 dilutions. The HRA levels decline rapidly in the first 2 months to reach zero by 5 years, making it a more useful test in early stages of ARF.[31]

In addition to the antibody tests, other laboratory and radiographic tests may be helpful in establishing the diagnosis of ARF. A chest radiograph will assess the pulmonary vasculature and may show left atrial enlargement as a result of valvular damage. In addition, cardiomegaly may be present with congestive heart failure or pericardial effusions or from other diseases in young people. Patients with rheumatic carditis may also have normal cardiac silhouettes. Nonsegmental, diffuse, bilateral pulmonary infiltrates produced by rheumatic pneumonitis or other pneumonias or even congestive heart failure can also be seen.[76] Radiographs of the extremities may be useful, if only one joint is affected, to exclude trauma, foreign bodies, or underlying infection.[16]

As mentioned, there is no joint destruction in ARF. Echocardiography is used to detect inaudible valvular regurgitation, as well as the presence of pericarditis, myocarditis, valvulitis, and pericardial effusions.[5, 77, 78] Serial echocardiograms are useful in following the course of cardiac involvement.[79]

An electrocardiogram (EKG) should be performed in all patients with ARF. Prolongation of the PR interval (greater than 0.20 sec) is a minor manifestation found in 15% to 25% of patients with ARF[5, 11, 12] and is thought to be caused by heightened vagal tone.[51] It is not an indicator of carditis, nor does it have any prognostic significance. Other conduction abnormalities found on EKG include second and third degree blocks.[80–84] Dysrhythmias, including atrial fibrillation, junctional rhythms, and ventricular tachycardias, may occur.

Arthrocentesis of an involved joint may exclude other causes of arthritis such as gout or infection. The synovial fluid in ARF-affected joints contains an average of 16,000 white blood cells (WBCs) per cubic millimeter, about 90% of which are polymorphonuclear neutrophils (PMNs). Electroencephalograms done on patients with chorea have had conflicting results.[85]

DIFFERENTIAL DIAGNOSIS

Distinguishing ARF from other entities can be difficult at times because of the diverse manifestations of the illness (Table 21–2).[86–106] The differential diagnosis will vary with the presenting complaint, especially if the physician is dealing with only a single clinical feature. Diagnostic errors arise both from failure to use the revised Jones Criteria (see Table 21–1), and from noncritical reliance on the criteria, resulting in a misdiagnosis of a major disease.

The organic murmurs found in ARF should be differentiated from functional murmurs.[29] In general, functional murmurs are short in duration, with no overlap with normal cardiac sounds. Functional murmurs are vibratory in quality,

---

TABLE 21–2

DIFFERENTIAL DIAGNOSIS OF ARF

Arthralgias	**Carditis**
Nonspecific limb pain	Functional murmur
Patellar chondromalacia	Congenital valvular disorders
Osteochondroses (Legg-Calvé-Perthes disease)	Infectious endocarditis
	Atrial myxomas
Ankylosing spondylitis	
Toxic synovitis	**Chorea**
	Tics
Arthritis	Tremors
Juvenile rheumatoid arthritis	Athetosis
Serum sickness	Dystonia from drugs
Subacute bacterial endocarditis	Huntington's chorea
	Wilson's disease
Systemic lupus erythematosus	
Leukemia	**Erythema marginatum**
Osteomyelitis	Erythema annulare centrifugum
Trauma	
Postrubella arthritis	Tinea corporis
Lyme arthritis	Erythema chronicum migrans
Tuberculosis	
Meningococcemia	**Prolonged PR interval**
Penicillin hypersensitivity	Idiopathic
Gonococcal arthritis	Myocarditis
Hepatitis	Hyperkalemia
Yersinia enterocolitis	Digoxin toxicity
Kawasaki syndrome	Quinidine toxicity
Sickle cell disease	Profound hypoxemia
Other infections (i.e., *Mycoplasma*)	

will change with position changes, and be louder with increased heart rates, fever, or in patients with a thin chest wall. Functional murmurs are found along the upper or lower left sternal borders and often radiate to the neck.

Erythema marginatum, if present, can be confused with other rashes. In particular, erythema annulare centrifugum will persist for months, with new crops appearing. Tinea corpus will have scaling and a raised edge with central clearing, and fungi will be present on a wet preparation. The rash of Lyme disease, erythema chronicum migrans, shows rapid expansion and is accompanied by pruritus or a burning sensation.

THERAPEUTIC INTERVENTION

The treatment of ARF is primarily supportive, with the use of salicylates, antibiotics, and possibly steroids. Specific treatment is required for the complications of ARF (e.g., diuretics for congestive heart failure).[107, 108] The disease is considered active in the presence of joint symptoms, a new organic murmur, an enlarging heart, subcutaneous nodules, a sleeping pulse of more than 100 beats/min, or an elevated erythrocyte sedimentation rate.[2, 16] About 75% of the cases will abate within 6 weeks, and by 12 weeks about 90% of the cases will have resolved. Less than 5% of patients will have active disease for more than 6 months.[19, 53]

The patient with ARF should be placed on bed rest for 2 weeks if no carditis is present, followed by 2 weeks of gradual ambulation. Patients who have carditis but no cardiomegaly should remain on bed rest for 4 weeks, followed by 4 weeks of gradual ambulation. These time periods should be extended to 6 weeks if carditis is accompanied by cardiomegaly. Patients with congestive heart failure should remain on bed rest until the failure has resolved, and gradual ambulation should take place slowly over the next 3 months.[1, 2, 16]

Antibiotics are recommended for all patients in the initial treatment of ARF.[10, 19, 109] The goal is to eliminate any group A streptococcus from the pharynx. Penicillin is the drug of choice; for those allergic to penicillin, erythromycin should be used (Table 21–3).

Anti-inflammatory agents are useful in controlling the joint and cardiac manifestations of ARF. However, they should not be used if the diagnosis of ARF is uncertain, as they may interfere with the natural progression of the patient's disease, making a definitive diagnosis impossible.

Instead, other analgesics should be used until the physician is certain the patient has ARF.[2]

Salicylates are the anti-inflammatory drugs of choice, and aspirin is the most commonly used (see Table 21–3).[1, 2, 16, 19, 30, 109] Aspirin should be given to those patients with arthritis or carditis uncomplicated by cardiomegaly or CHF. It may cause bleeding episodes, hypersensitivity reactions, or potential hepatotoxicity with high doses. Chronic salicylate use may also cause tinnitus and mental status changes. Aspirin should not be used in patients in the third trimester of pregnancy. The possible association with Reye's syndrome in patients with viral illnesses must also be remembered.

Adrenal corticosteroids are also used in the treatment of ARF and are indicated for patients with carditis, cardiomegaly, congestive heart failure, or an inability to tolerate salicylates or in whom salicylate treatment has failed to control inflammation.[1, 2, 16, 19, 109] Steroids may be useful in controlling chorea in patients showing signs of an inflammatory process.[110] Prednisone is the steroid of choice. Gastric ulceration, hypokalemia (when steroids are used concurrently with diuretics), and adrenal insufficiency are the risks of steroid use.

Haloperidol is used to control chorea.[111] The abnormal movements are thought to be controlled by haloperidol's inhibition of the functional overactivity of dopamine on the striatal neurons.[112] The dose in children is 0.01 to 0.03 mg/kg/day in four divided doses; adults may receive 2 to 5 mg/day divided in three doses. Young patients are prone to extrapyramidal reactions, however, and occasional blood dyscrasias have occurred with the use of haloperidol. Chorea has been treated with barbiturates or reserpine in the past, but these drugs are not currently recommended.

The patient with mild congestive heart failure may only need bed rest, fluid restriction, and supplemental oxygen. Patients with more severe disease may require a diuretic such as furosemide. Digoxin may be helpful but must be used with caution because of the increased digitalis sensitivity in patients with carditis. Finally, the use of morphine sulfate as a preload reducer may be indicated.

Atropine is useful for patients with severe bradycardia or heart block with a slow ventricular response. Bradycardia may temporarily require external cardiac pacing or isoproterenol. Extreme cases may require transvenous pacing. Lidocaine is indicated for stable ventricular tachycardia; procainamide is the drug of second choice. Unstable ven-

TABLE 21–3
THERAPY AT A GLANCE

Penicillin—Drug of choice	
Penicillin G benzathine	Patient Weight
1.2 million units IM	>90 lb
900,000 units IM	61–90 lb
600,000 units IM	30–60 lb
300,000 units IM	<30 lb
Penicillin V: 25–50 mg/kg/day po in four divided doses for 10 days	
Erythromycin—for penicillin-allergic patients	
Erythromycin estolate: 20–40 mg/kg/day po divided in two to four doses for 10 days (maximum 1 gm/day)	
Erythromycin ethylsuccinate: 40 mg/kg/day po divided in two to four doses for 10 days (maximum 1 gm/day)	
Aspirin	
First 1–2 wk: 100 mg/kg/day po divided in four to six doses (maximum 5 gm/day); may increase to 150 mg/kg/day to control arthritis	
Following 4–6 wk: 50–75 mg/kg/day in four divided doses	
Prednisone	
First 1–2 wk: 2 mg/kg/day po in one to two doses	
After 1–2 wk: 1 mg/kg/day, then begin gradual tapering over 2 weeks	
Salicylates should be given during the tapering phase to prevent post-therapeutic rebounds and continued for 2 to 4 weeks after the steroid is stopped.	

tricular tachycardia requires synchronized cardioversion, whereas pulseless ventricular tachycardia or ventricular fibrillation requires defibrillation followed by epinephrine and lidocaine.[47]

PROGNOSIS

The mortality rate for ARF has markedly decreased since the 1950s. The current 10-year mortality rate is 4%, compared with a 10-year mortality rate of 20% to 30% prior to 1950. The only long-term sequela of ARF is rheumatic heart disease.[1] Patients can be expected to recover fully if they do not have carditis or if PR interval prolongation is the sole cardiac manifestation. In other patients, the incidence of residual disease is proportional to the severity of the carditis. Hence only 30% of patients with mild carditis (apical systolic murmur of mild mitral regurgitation without pericarditis or congestive heart failure) still have an organic murmur at 10-year follow-up. Patients with basal or apical diastolic murmurs (moderate carditis) have a 40% incidence of organic murmurs at 10 years. Patients with severe carditis (murmurs accompanied by congestive heart failure or pericarditis) have a 68% to 70% incidence of residual heart disease after 10 years.[1, 19] The occurrence of mitral stenosis within 5 years is associated with a high morbidity and mortality rate. Insidious development of mitral stenosis has less morbidity and mortality and is primarily seen in women or in those with initially mild mitral valvulitis.[19] Patients presenting with pure chorea have a high incidence of late-developing rheumatic heart disease, possibly because an acute carditis initially present had resolved prior to their being diagnosed with ARF. Because each recurrence of ARF puts the patient at risk for developing carditis, prognosis has been greatly improved by preventing recurrent attacks. Nevertheless, rheumatic heart disease is neither modified nor prevented by the use of salicylates or steroids.[1]

PREVENTION

In 1950, Floyd W. Denny presented convincing evidence that ARF was prevented by penicillin therapy for the antecedent pharyngitis.[8] In 1984, the American Heart Association reaffirmed these findings and added erythromycin as an alternative therapy for the penicillin-allergic patient.[113] Thus primary prevention—that is, the diagnosis and treatment of streptococcal pharyngitis—is of paramount importance in the prevention of ARF. Unfortunately, up to one third of cases of ARF follow subclinical streptococcal infections. In the Utah outbreak of ARF in 1985, 50% of patients had no recall of an antecedent sore throat.[5]

The diagnosis of streptococcal pharyngitis is impossible using only the clinical examination. Classic symptoms include a sudden sore throat, painful swallowing, headache, nausea, vomiting, and cough. These are accompanied by tonsillopharyngeal erythema and exudate, palatal petechiae, fever, cervical adenitis, and occasionally a scarlatiniform rash.[3] It is unlikely for an older adult or a child younger than 3 years to have either streptococcal pharyngitis or ARF.[1]

The gold standard for diagnosing streptococcal pharyngitis is the throat culture. Its advantage is that it has up to a 95% negative predictive value; treatment is safely withheld if the culture is negative. Conversely, there can be up to a 10% false-negative rate, depending on the technique of sampling and plating, and the culture is relatively expensive. In addition, the culture does not differentiate between an acute infection and the carrier state.[8, 73, 114] Carriers, up to 20% of whom are children, usually show no symptoms of infection or subsequent evidence of an immunologic response to the bacteria. They are also less likely to transmit

the disease and have a low risk of developing ARF.[25] Because adequate prophylaxis against ARF mandates early treatment of the pharyngitis, increasing streptococcal antibody titers cannot be used to differentiate carriers from patients with acute infections, because titer levels must be measured at least 2 weeks apart.

Rapid streptococcal antigen tests have become popular.[8] In these tests, chemical (i.e., nitrous acid) or enzymatic (i.e., pronase) technique is used to extract the group-specific carbohydrate from the cell wall of the group A *Streptococcus* organism. Latex agglutination, coagglutination, or precipitant techniques are then used to detect the carbohydrate. These tests are rapid and highly specific, with sensitivities ranging from 80% to 90%.[73, 114] Like pharyngeal cultures, antigen tests do not differentiate the acute infection from the carrier state. In addition, the false-negative rate can be as high as 20%.

A rapid streptococcal test is recommended first in suspected cases. If the result is positive, then treatment is warranted. If the result of the rapid test is negative, the throat should be cultured and the patient treated only if the culture is positive.[3, 25] Penicillin is the drug of choice, and the key to eliminating streptococcus is by prolonged, rather than short-term, treatment with high-dose penicillin.[25] For the penicillin-allergic patient, erythromycin is recommended (see Table 21–3). Acceptable, but not recommended, alternatives include amoxicillin, dicloxacillin, oral cephalosporins, and clindamycin. Antibiotics not acceptable in the treatment of streptococcal pharyngitis include sulfonamides, tetracyclines, trimethoprim, and chloramphenicol.[3] Follow-up care is imperative in the patient with a previous history or family history of ARF, as such patients are at greatest risk for recurrence. In addition, patients with continued or recurrent symptoms should receive follow-up care.

Once the patient has had ARF, it is important to prevent recurrent episodes. This secondary prevention is aimed at stopping upper respiratory tract infections caused by group A *Streptococcus* organisms. Unfortunately, no single regimen is entirely effective in eradicating the streptococcus from the oropharynx or in preventing recurrent attacks of rheumatic fever.[3] Furthermore, additional therapy is needed for prophylaxis against bacterial endocarditis.

Risk factors for recurrent ARF include the time since the previous attack, the number of previous attacks, and the likelihood of exposure to group A streptococcus.[3] The risk for recurrent ARF is decreased with increased time since the previous attack, and a patient's risk increases with multiple attacks of ARF. The likelihood of exposure to streptococcus is increased among school teachers, health care workers, parents of young children, military recruits, and those in crowded living conditions. Furthermore, patients who have had carditis are at an increased risk for recurrent episodes during the ARF attack. These recurrences can also cause further cardiac and valvular damage. Interestingly, patients who did not develop carditis in the first episode of ARF also did not develop it during recurrent attacks.[27]

The preferred treatment for secondary prevention of ARF is parenteral penicillin.[113, 115] It should be given every 3 weeks to patients with a history of carditis and every 3 to 4 weeks in all others. Oral antibiotics may be given, but there is a higher rate of recurrence with their use, and therefore they should only be used in patients at lower risk for recurrent attacks (i.e., those in late adolescence or when 5 years have elapsed since the previous episode). Penicillin V is the drug of choice, but it may cause the emergence of resistant alpha streptococci in the pharynx, potentially increasing the risk of acquiring bacterial endocarditis. Sulfadiazine is recommended for the penicillin-allergic patient, and erythromycin

---

TABLE 21-4

ANTIBIOTIC DOSING IN SECONDARY PREVENTION OF ARF

Penicillin G benzathine	Patient Weight
1.2 million units IM	>90 lb
900,000 units IM	61–90 lb
600,000 units IM	30–60 lb
300,000 units IM	<30 lb

Oral agents (less effective)
Penicillin V: 125 to 250 mg po bid
Sulfadiazine: 1 gm po qd
(for patients less than 60 lb, 0.5 gm po qd)
Erythromycin: 250 mg po bid

---

is reserved for patients allergic to both penicillin and sulfa (Table 21-4).

Prophylaxis should continue for at least 5 years beyond the last attack of ARF and until patients are at least in their early 20s. Continuance of prophylaxis beyond this is considered on an individual basis. Most clinicians recommend continuing prophylaxis in persons with rheumatic heart disease, even after valve replacement. Lifelong prophylaxis is effective.[3]

Patients with rheumatic valvular disease are predisposed to develop bacterial endocarditis from dental procedures, surgical procedures, and instrumentation involving mucosal surfaces.[116] Because rheumatic fever prophylaxis regimens are inadequate in protecting against the development of bacterial endocarditis, additional antibiotics are recommended (Table 21-5). Indications for prophylaxis include oral surgery or dental procedures causing gingival bleeding, surgical procedures of the upper respiratory tract or ear or involving respiratory mucosa, and genitourinary or gastrointestinal tract procedures. Although oral regimens are safer and more convenient, parenteral regimens are more effective. Parenteral dosing is especially recommended for patients currently on oral prophylactic rheumatic fever therapy, with prosthetic heart valves, or with a past history of endocarditis. Because most diagnostic and dental procedures are accompanied by bacteremia of short duration, a single dose of parenteral antibiotic is probably adequate; patients judged to be at higher risk may be given one or two follow-up doses at 8- to 12-hour intervals.

DISPOSITION

All patients with ARF should be placed on bed rest, and serial examinations must be performed to detect complications. Certainly the presence of CHF, dysrhythmias, or organic murmurs warrants hospitalization. Patients with a monarticular arthritis may also be admitted in order to rule out an infectious process and closely follow the clinical course. All patients with known rheumatic valvular disease should be admitted as well. Finally, patients with severe chorea may require admission until the chorea is under better control.

Many patients can be adequately treated by their primary care physician while hospitalized. Cardiology consultation should be obtained for patients with carditis, dysrhythmias, congestive heart failure, or an organic murmur. A rheumatologist or orthopedist may be needed to perform joint aspirations or for help in differentiating ARF from other inflammatory joint conditions. Dermatology consultation may be helpful in distinguishing erythema marginatum from other similar skin lesions.

OTHER CONSIDERATIONS

Although prevention of ARF relies on the diagnosis and treatment of the antecedent pharyngitis, there is an interest

---

TABLE 21-5

PREVENTION OF BACTERIAL ENDOCARDITIS

	Adult Dosage	Child Dosage
Dental and Upper Respiratory Procedures		
Oral		
Penicillin V	2 gm 1 hr before and 1 gm 6 hr after procedure	>60 lb: adult dose <60 lb: ½ adult dose
For penicillin allergy		
Erythromycin	1 gm 1 hr before and 500 mg 6 hr after procedure	20 mg/kg 1 hr before and 10 mg/kg 6 hr after procedure
Parenteral		
Ampicillin	2 gm IM or IV 30 min before procedure	50 mg/kg IM or IV 30 min before procedure
plus		
Gentamicin	1.5 mg/kg IM or IV 30 min before procedure	2.0 mg/kg IM or IV 30 min before procedure
For penicillin allergy		
Vancomycin	1 gm IV infused *slowly over 1 hr* beginning 1 hr before procedure	20 mg/kg IV infused *slowly over 1 hr* beginning 1 hr before procedure
Gastrointestinal and Genitourinary Procedures		
Oral		
Amoxicillin	3 gm 1 hr before and 1.5 gm 6 hr after procedure	50 mg/kg 1 hr before and 25 mg/kg 6 hr after procedure
Parenteral		
Ampicillin plus gentamicin in doses as above		
For penicillin allergy		
Vancomycin in doses as above		
plus		
Gentamicin in doses as above		

From Abramowicz M. Handbook of Antimicrobial Therapy. New Rochelle, NY, The Medical Letter, 1990, pp 84–85.

in developing a polyvalent vaccine against the illness.[1] The vaccine is based on the M-protein serotypes of the bacteria; however, there is still difficulty in separating type-specific M determinants from non–type-specific M-protein moieties. The use of an effective vaccine could further reduce the already low incidence of ARF.

References

1. Bisno AL. Nonsuppurative poststreptococcal sequelae: Rheumatic fever and glomerulonephritis. *In* Mandell GL, Douglas RG, Bennett SE (eds). Principles and Practice of Infectious Disease. New York, John Wiley & Sons, 1985, pp 1133–1138.
2. Markowitz M. Rheumatic fever. In Behrman RE, Vaughan VC III (eds). Nelson Textbook of Pediatrics. Philadelphia, WB Saunders, 1987, pp 539–543.
3. Dajani AS. Rheumatic fever prevention revisited. Pediatr Infect Dis J 1989;8:266.
4. Bisno AL, Shulman ST, Dajani AS. The rise and fall (and rise?) of rheumatic fever. Editorial. JAMA 1988;259:728.
5. Veasy LG, Wiedmeier SE, Orsmond GS, et al. Resurgence of acute rheumatic fever in the intermountain area of the United States. N Engl J Med 1987;316:421.
6. Markowitz M. Rheumatic fever in the eighties. Pediatr Clin North Am 1986;33:1141.
7. Land MA, Bisno AL. Acute rheumatic fever: A vanishing disease in suburbia. JAMA 1983;249:895.
8. Bisno AL. The rise and fall of rheumatic fever. JAMA 1985;254:538.
9. Bland EF. Rheumatic fever: The way it was. Editorial. Circulation 1987;76:1190.
10. Massell BF, Chute CG, Walker AM, et al. Penicillin and the marked decrease in morbidity and mortality from rheumatic fever in the United States. N Engl J Med 1988;318:280.
11. Bitton Y, Joseph A, Weinhouse E, et al. Review of 222 cases of acute rheumatic fever in southern Israel (1974–1983). Pediatr Cardiol 1986;7:199.
12. Hosier DM, Craenen JM, Teske DW, et al. Resurgence of acute rheumatic fever. Am J Dis Child 1987;141:730.
13. Wald ER, Dashefsky B, Feidt C, et al. Acute rheumatic fever in western Pennsylvania and the tristate area. Pediatrics 1987;80:371.
14. Bland EF, Jones TD. Rheumatic fever and rheumatic heart disease: A twenty year report on 1000 patients followed since childhood. Circulation 1951;4:836.
15. Berrios X, Quesney F, Morales A, et al. Acute rheumatic fever and poststreptococcal glomerulonephritis in an open population: Comparative studies of epidemiology and bacteriology. J Lab Clin Med 1986;108:535.
16. Markowtiz M, Gordis L. Rheumatic Fever. 2nd ed. Philadelphia, WB Saunders, 1972, pp 19–22, 61–79, 90–114.
17. Perry CB. Incidence of rheumatic fever. Letter. Br Med J 1990;300:122.
18. Neutze JM. Rheumatic fever and rheumatic heart disease in the Western Pacific region. NZ Med J 1988;101:404.
19. Stollerman GH. Acute rheumatic fever and its managment. *In* Hurst JW (ed). The Heart, New York, McGraw-Hill, 1986, pp 1306–1313.
20. Rodnan GP (ed). Primer on rheumatic diseases. JAMA 1973;224(suppl):74.
21. Acute rheumatic fever—Utah. Morbidity and Mortality Weekly Report 1987;36:108.
22. Kaplan EL, Hill HR. Return of rheumatic fever: Consequences, implications and needs. Editorial. J Pediatr 1987;111:244.
23. Kaplan EL, Markowitz M. Rheumatic fever in the United States: No longer a disease of the past. NZ Med J 1988;101:402.
24. Martin DR. Rheumatogenic streptococci revisited. NZ Med J 1988;101:394.
25. Dobson SR. Group A streptococci revisited. Arch Dis Child 1989;64:977.
26. Hutten-Czapski P. Acute rheumatic fever—no epidemic in Ontario. Can J Public Health 1989;80:71.
27. Majeed HA, Shaltout A, Yousof AM. Recurrences of acute rheumatic fever: A prospective study of 79 episodes, Am J Dis Child 1984;138:341.
28. Schlant RC. Altered cardiovascular function of rheumatic heart disease. *In* Hurst JW, Logue RB (ed). The Heart. 4th ed. New York, McGraw-Hill, 1978, p 1965.
29. Vandenbelt RJ, Ronan JA, Bedynek JL (eds). Cardiology: A Clinical Approach. Chicago, Year Book, Inc. 1979, p 216.
30. Kashani IA. Acute rheumatic fever: A review of the pathogenesis, diagnosis and modified approach to Jones Criteria and management. Paediatrician 1981;10:158.
31. Zabriskie JB, Hus KC, Seigal BC. Heart reactive antibody associated with rheumatic fever: Characterization and diagnostic significance. Clin Exp Immunol 1970;7:147.
32. Lennon D, Martin D, Wong E, et al. Longitudinal study of poststreptococcal disease in Auckland; rheumatic fever, glomerulonephritis, epidemiology and M-typing 1981–86. NZ Med J 1988;101:396.
33. Majeed HA, Khuffash FA, Mohsen A, et al. The rheumatogenic and nephritogenic strains of group A streptococcus: The Kuwait experience. NZ Med J 1988;101:398.
34. Neutze JM. Third international conference on rheumatic fever and rheumatic heart disease. NZ Med J 1988;101:387.
35. Cairns LM. The immunology of rheumatic fever. NZ Med J 1988;101:388.
36. Schoenfeld AE, Rubenstein A, Raviv U. Immunoglobulins in rheumatic fever. Isr J Med Sci 1968;4:815.
37. Stollerman GH, Lewis AJ, Shultz I, et al. Relationships of immune response to group A streptococci to the course of acute, chronic, and recurrent rheumatic fever. Am J Med 1956;20:163.
38. Williams RC Jr. Host factors in rheumatic fever and heart disease. Hosp Pract 1982;17:125.
39. Shastry P, Naik S, Joshi M, et al. Persistence of heart-reactive antibodies (HRA) in acute rheumatic fever (ARF) and rheumatic heart disease (RHD) patients. J Clin Lab Immunol 1988;27:87.
40. Hafez M, El-Shannawy F, El-Salab SH, et al. Studies of peripheral blood T lymphocytes in assessment of disease activity in rheumatic fever. Br J Rheumatol 1988;27:181.
41. Bahr GM, Eales LJ, Nye KE, et al. An association between Gc (vitamin D–binding protein) alleles and susceptibility to rheumatic fever. Immunology 1989;67:126.
42a. Rajapakse CNA, Halim K, Al-Orainey I, et al. A genetic marker for rheumatic heart disease. Br Heart J 1987;58:659.
42b. Levy MJ, Edwards JE. Anatomy of mitral insufficiency. Prog Cardiovasc Dis 1962;5:119.
43. Bernstein B. Pericarditis in juvenile chronic arthritis. Arthritis Rheum 1977;20(suppl):241.
44. Van Reken D, Strauss A, Hernandez A, et al. Infectious pericarditis in children. J Pediatr 1974;85:165.
45. Goldenberg DL, Cohen AS. Acute infectious arthritis: A review of patients with non-gonococcal joint infections (with emphasis on therapy and prognosis). Am J Med 1976;60:369.
46. Kantor TB, Tanner M. Rubella arthritis and rheumatoid arthritis. Arthritis Rheum 1962;5:378.
47. American Heart Association. Textbook of Advanced Cardiac Life Support. Dallas, TX, 1987, pp 99–109.
48. Feinstein AR, Spagnvolo M. The clinical patterns of acute rheumatic fever: A reappraisal. Medicine 1962;41:279.
49. Herman J. A family physician's experience with rheumatic fever and acquired valvular heart disease. J Clin Epidemiol 1988;41:417.
50. Massell BF, Fyler DC, Roy SB. The clinical picture of rheumatic fever: Diagnosis, immediate prognosis, course, and therapeutic implications. Am J Cardiol 1958;1:436.
51. Keith JD. Overstimulation of the vagus nerve in rheumatic fever. Q J Med 1938;7:29.
52. Stern VS. Stokes-Adams attacks in a child. Fr Heart J 1944;6:66.
53. Stollerman GK. Rheumatic fever. *In* Braunwald E (ed). Heart Disease—A Textbook of Cardiovascular Medicine. Philadelphia, WB Saunders, 1980, pp 1724–1746.
54. Markowitz M. Evolution and critique of changes in Jones Criteria for the diagnosis of rheumatic fever. NZ Med J 1988;101:392.
55. Stollerman GH, Markowitz M, Taranta A, et al. Jones Criteria (revised) for guidance in the diagnosis of rheumatic fever. Circulation 1965;32:664.
56. Tadzinski LA, Ryan ME. Diagnosis of rheumatic fever: A guide to the criteria and manifestations. Postgrad Med 1986;79:295.
57. Nemir RL. Rheumatic pneumonia. *In* Kendig EL, Chernick V (ed). Disorders of the Respiratory Tract in Children. 3rd ed. Philadelphia, WB Saunders, 1977, p 1006.
58. Kalaeva VA. Myocardial ischemia in rheumatic coronaritis in children. Pediatriia 1974;74:85.
59. Wee AST, Goodwin SF. Acute rheumatic fever and carditis in older adults. Lancet 1966;2:239.
60. Feinstein AR, Di Massa R. Prognostic significance of valvular involvement in acute rheumatic fever. N Engl J Med 1959;260:1001.
61. Barnert AL, Terry EE, Persellen RH. Acute rheumatic fever in adults. JAMA 1975;232:925.
62. Frahm CJ, Braunwald E, Morrow AG. Congenital aortic regurgitation: Clinical and hemodynamic findings in four patients. Am J Med 1961;31:63.
63. Feinstein AR, Arevalo AC. Manifestations and treatment of congestive heart failure in young patients with rheumatic heart disease. Pediatrics 1964;33:661.
64. Schadler JG. Chronic salicylate administration in juvenile rheumatoid arthritis: Aspirin "hepatitis" and its clinical significance. Pediatrics 1978;62(suppl):916.
65. Nelson AM. Joint pain in children. When is it serious? Postgrad Med 1969;85:141.
66. Cherian S, Tabatabai MF, Cummings NA. Rheumatic fever and gonococcal pharyngitis in the adult. South Med J 1979;72:319.
67. McDonald EC, Weisman MH. Articular manifestations of rheumatic fever in adults. Ann Intern Med 1978;89:417.
68. Lavy S, Lavy R, Brand A. Neurological and electroencephalographic abnormalities in rheumatic fever. Acta Neurol Scand 1964;40:76.

69. Massie RW, Stahlman M. Serum oxaloacetic transaminase activity in acute rheumatic fever. J Dis Child 1958;95:469.

70. Nydick I, Tang J, Stollerman GH, et al. The influence of rheumatic fever on serum concentration of the enzyme glutamic oxaloacetic transaminase. Circulation 1955;12:795.

71. Elster SK, Braunwald E, Wood HF. A study of C-reactive protein in the serum of patients with congestive heart failure. Am Heart J 1956;51:533.

72. Padmavati S, Gupta V. Reappraisal of the Jones Criteria: The Indian experience. NZ Med J 1988;101:391.

73. Bisno AL, Ofek I. Serologic diagnosis of streptococcal infection; comparison of a rapid hemagglutination technique with conventional antibody tests. Am J Dis Child 1974;127:676.

74. Burdash NM, Teti G, Hund P. Streptococcal antibody tests in rheumatic fever. Ann Clin Lab Sci 1986;16:163.

75. Kaplan EL, Huwe BB. The sensitivity and specificity of an agglutination test for antibodies to streptococcal extracellular antigens: A quantitative analysis and comparison of the streptozyme test with the anti-streptolysin O and anti-deoxyribonuclease B tests. J Pediatr 1980;96:367.

76. Curry GC. Plain chest radiography of rheumatic heart disease. Cardiol Clin 1983;1:597.

77. Burgess J, Clark R, Kamigaki M, et al. Echocardiographic findings in different types of mitral regurgitation. Circulation 1973;48:97.

78. Schienken RM, Kerber RE. Echocardiographic abnormalities in acute rheumatic fever. Am J Cardiol 1976;38:458.

79. Kay HH, Tynan M, Hunter S. Validity of echocardiographic estimates of left ventricular size and performance in infants and small children. Br Heart J 1971;37:371.

80. Clarke M, Keith JD. Atrioventricular conduction in acute rheumatic fever. Br Heart J 1972;43:472.

81. Mirowski M, Rosinstein BJ, Markowitz M. A comparison of atrioventricular conduction in normal children and in patients with acute rheumatic fever, glomerulonephritis, and acute febrile illness. Pediatrics 1965;33:334.

82. Reddy DV, Chun LT, Yamamoto LG. Acute rheumatic fever with advanced heart block. Clin Pediatrics 1989;28:326.

83. Salversen HA. Complete heart block in the course of rheumatic infection. Acta Med Scand 1932;78:189.

84. Weller SDV. Complete A-V dissociation in acute rheumatism. Br Heart J 1951;13:102.

85. Ertugal A, Renda Y, Saraciar M, et al. Electroencephalographic study in acute rheumatic arthritis. Am Heart J 1976;91:163.

86. Alpert E, Isselbacher KJ, Schur PH. The pathogeneses of arthritis associated with viral hepatitis: Complement component studies. N Engl J Med 1971;285:184.

87. Cooper LZ, Ziring PR, Weiss HJ, et al. Transient arthritis after rubella vaccination. Am J Dis Child 1979;118:218.

88. Holmes KK, Counts GW, Beaty HN. Disseminated gonococcal infection. Ann J Med 1971;74:979.

89. Jones MC. Arthritis and arthralgia in infection with Mycoplasma pneumonia. Thorax 1970;25:748.

90. Laitinen O, Leirisalo M, Allander E. Rheumatic fever and Yersinia arthritis: Criteria and diagnostic problems in a changing disease pattern. Scand J Rheumatol 1975;4:145.

91. Lambert HP. Syndrome with joint manifestation in association with Mycoplasma pneumonia infection. Br Med J 1968;3:156.

92. Leino R, Kalliomaki JL. Yersiniosis as an internal disease. Ann Intern Med 1974;81:458.

93. Litt IF, Edberg SC, Finberg L. Gonorrhea in children and adolescents: A current review. J Pediatr 1974;85:595.

94. Meislin AG, Rothfield N. Systemic lupus erythematosus in childhood. Analysis of 42 cases, with comparative data on 200 adult cases followed concomitantly. Pediatrics 1968;42:37.

95. Meisner HC, Gellis SE, Milliken JF. Lyme disease first observed to be aseptic meningitis. Am J Dis Child 1982;136:465.

96. Molteni RA. The differential diagnosis of benign and septic joint disease in children. Clin Pediatr 1978;17:19.

97. Nelson JD. The bacterial etiology and antibiotic management of septic arthritis in infants and children. Pediatrics 1972;50:437.

98. Norris DG, Colon AR, Stickler GB. Systemic lupus erythematosis in children. Clin Pediatr 1977;16:774.

99. Silva J Jr, Wilson K. Disseminated gonococcal infections (DGI). Cutis 1979;24:601.

100. Thayer WS. On the cardiac complications of gonorrhea. Bull Johns Hopkins Hosp 1922;33:361.

101. Waldvogel FA, Medoff G, Swartz MN. Osteomyelitis: A review of clinical features, therapeutic considerations and unusual aspects. Part 1. N Engl J Med 1970;282:98.

102. Weinstein MP, Hall CB. Mycoplasma pneumonia infection associated with migratory polyarthritis. Am J Dis Child 1974;127:125.

103. Woodward TE, McCrumb FR Jr, Carey TN, et al. Viral and rickettsial causes of cardiac disease, including the coxsackie virus etiology of pericarditis and myocarditis. Ann Intern Med 1960;53:1130.

104. Keith JC. Congenital mitral insufficiency. Prog Cardiovasc Dis 1962;5:264.

105. Lortscher RH, Towes WH, Nora JJ, et al. Atrial myxoma presenting as rheumatic fever. Chest 1974;66:303.

106. Steere AC, Batsford WP, Weinberg M, et al. Lyme carditis: Cardiac abnormalities of lyme disease. Ann Intern Med 1989;93:8.

107. Alsop RF. The intracardiac pacemeker in acute rheumatic carditis. Letter. N Engl J Med 1969;281:1075.

108. Falk RH, Zoll PM, Zoll RH. Safety and efficacy of non-invasive cardiac pacing: a preliminary report. N Engl J Med 1983;309:1166.

109. Done AK, Ely RS, Ainger LE, et al. Therapy of acute rheumatic fever. Pediatrics 1955;15:522.

110. Green LN. Corticosteroids in the treatment of Sydenham's chorea. Arch Neurol 1978;35:53.

111. Shenker DM, Grossman HJ, Klawans HL. Treatment of Sydenham's chorea with haloperidol. Dev Med Child Neurol 1973;15:19.

112. Naidu S, Narasimhachari N. Sydenham's chorea: A possible presynaptic dopaminergic dysfunction initially. Ann Neurol 1989;8:445.

113. Shulman ST, Amren DP, Bisno AL, et al. Prevention of rheumatic fever: A statement of health professionals by the Committee on Rheumatic Fever and Infective Endocarditis of the Council on Cardiovascular Disease in the Young. Circulation 1984;70:1118A.

114. Kaplan EL. Rapid detection of group A streptococcal antigen for the clinician and the epidemiologist: Accurate? Cost-effective? Useful? NZ Med J 1988;101:401.

115. Lue HC, Wu MH, Hsieh KH, et al. Rheumatic fever recurrences: Controlled study of 3-week versus 4-week benzathene penicillin prevention programs. J Pediatr 1986;108:299.

116. Shulman ST, Amren DP, Bisno AL, et al. Prevention of bacterial endocarditis: A statement for health professionals by the Committee on Rheumatic Fever and Bacterial Endocarditis of the Council of Cardiovascular Diseases in the Young of the American Heart Association. Am J Dis Child 1985;139:232.

CHAPTER 22

Myocarditis

Timothy J. O'Connor

INTRODUCTION

The diagnosis of myocarditis, an inflammation of the muscular walls of the heart, is difficult to make.[1] The patient with myocarditis may have no cardiac signs or symptoms or may present in profound shock or as sudden death.[2-8] Because of the variety of symptoms that can occur and the existence of other illnesses that may mimic myocarditis, the diagnosis is often missed. Even when the alert clinician considers myocarditis, definitive diagnosis may be elusive. Though myocarditis is a relatively uncommon diagnosis made in the emergency department, there is histologic evidence of myocarditis in 4% to 10% of routine autopsies.[2, 9] It is thought that in the majority of patients, myocarditis is asymptomatic and, in fact, of little consequence.

INFECTIOUS CAUSES

There are multiple infectious and noninfectious causes of myocarditis.[10-14] The most common causes in North America are viruses, and of these, the coxsackieviruses are responsible for the majority of cases. Males are more commonly affected than females, though pregnancy is also a risk factor.[15, 16] Although viral myocarditis may present at any age, it has a bimodal age distribution. Infants less than 6 months of age and older children and adolescents are the two groups most commonly affected.[9]

Chagas' disease is caused by the protozoan *Trypanosoma cruzi* and is transmitted in the excreta of reduviid or triatomine bugs. The disease occurs commonly in Central and South America and has an acute, latent, and chronic phase. The acute phase typically affects infants and young children. It may be suggested by a nodular skin lesion at the initial site of infection (chagoma) or by painless unilateral palpebral edema (Romana sign). The disease affects multiple organs, but myocarditis is the usual cause of death in 5% to 10% of those affected. The latent phase lasts 10 to 40 years. The chronic phase mainly affects the heart and gastrointestinal tract; cardiac conduction disturbances are common.[17]

Diphtheria toxin causes myocarditis in the second week of the disease.[18] The conduction system is commonly affected.[19, 20] Carditis may occur with or without coronary artery aneurysm in patients with Kawasaki disease[21] and is a major manifestation of rheumatic fever.

Myocarditis may also occur in Lyme disease. The diagnosis is suggested by history of tick bite, erythema chronicum migrans, arthritis, and facial palsy or other neurologic manifestations. As in diphtheritic myocarditis, the conduction system is commonly involved. In the absence of a known tick bite or erythema chronicum migrans, Lyme disease may be confused with acute rheumatic fever. Third degree heart block, temporomandibular joint arthritis, or meningoencephalitis are all suggestive of Lyme disease. Valvular disease, aspirin-responsive arthritis, chorea without other neurologic manifestations, or erythema marginatum with evidence of preceding streptococcal infection suggests acute rheumatic fever.[13]

ANATOMY AND PHYSIOLOGY

The heart lies within a serous cavity defined by the fibrous pericardium. The myocardium is lined internally by a layer of endothelium and connective tissue known as the endocardium. The heart is innervated by the cardiac plexus located near the inferior end of the trachea. Fibers from the cardiac plexus innervate, among other things, the sinoatrial (SA) and atrioventricular (AV) nodes. Electrical impulses travel from the SA node to the AV node to the ventricles through the His-Purkinje system.[22]

Myocarditis may affect the myocardium, the His-Purkinje system, or both. Also, because myocarditis may be focal or diffuse, the pathophysiology may differ significantly among patients. Diffuse involvement of the myocardium may cause heart failure because of poor contractility, or the overfilling and distention of an involved ventricle may prevent adequate filling of the other ventricle. Alternatively, small focal lesions may be of little consequence unless they are arrhythmogenic. The arrhythmias seen with myocarditis are protean and include all degrees of heart block, ventricular tachycardia, and ventricular fibrillation.[23]

In addition, myocarditis is often not an isolated entity. Other associated conditions include pericarditis, pericardial effusion, and cardiac tamponade. Other organ systems may also be affected either primarily (by the causative agent) or secondarily as a consequence of heart failure.

EMERGENCY MEDICAL SERVICE CONSIDERATIONS

Definitive diagnosis of myocarditis in the field is unnecessary. Basic principles of emergency supportive care should be followed, and specific attention should be given to assessment of the respiratory and cardiac systems.

The history obtained depends on the presenting symptom. The older child or adolescent may present with chest pain, palpitations, syncope, dyspnea, or sudden collapse. The infant may present with fever or poor feeding or may just not "look right" to the mother. Certain questions should be

asked if circumstances allow. Where is the symptom located? What is the quality and intensity of the symptom? Under what circumstances did it occur? Is there anything that aggravates or alleviates it? When did the symptom begin, and how long does it last? What other symptoms occur with it?[24] Has the patient ever been hospitalized or had any surgery? Does the patient have any history of heart disease or other medical illness? Has the patient had a fever recently? Is the patient taking any medications or using any illegal drugs? What medications are kept in the home? Has the patient recently sustained any physical or emotional trauma? Has urine output been normal? Has there been any travel outside North America?

After performing a physical examination and instituting appropriate life support measures, the emergency medical services team should confer with medical control. It is important that the patient's general appearance, mental status, vital signs, color, and capillary refill be accurately assessed and reported. In addition, pupillary findings may be a clue to drug ingestion or an unsuspected neurologic problem. Results of the heart, lung, and abdominal examination should be reported, as should any evidence of heart disease (rales, muffled or loud heart sounds, murmurs, rubs, gallops, jugular venous distension, hepatomegaly, or evidence of abnormality on the cardiac monitor).

Intervention in the field should be concentrated on airway support, oxygenation, and ventilation. Early assisted ventilation is indicated for the infant or child who shows signs of respiratory fatigue (grunting, retractions, poor air exchange, lethargy) and does not respond to 100% oxygen inhalation. All patients should be placed on a cardiac monitor. Intravenous (or intraosseous) access should be established rapidly in patients with life-threatening arrhythmias or shock. Rapid blood glucose assessment should be considered in infants in significant distress. The patient should be continuously monitored during expedient transport to an appropriate facility.

CLINICAL EVALUATION
History

A patient who presents with a history of fever, lethargy, pallor, shortness of breath, and palpitations should alert the physician to the possibility of myocarditis.[25] If, on examination, the patient has tachycardia out of proportion to the fever, tachypnea, rales, softened heart sounds, a gallop, hepatomegaly, delayed capillary refill, and abnormalities on the electrocardiogram (EKG), the diagnosis of myocarditis should be strongly suspected.[26, 27] Unfortunately, this "classic" presentation for myocarditis is the exception, and the signs and symptoms may be more subtle.[28] A high index of suspicion is the clinician's best asset in making the diagnosis of myocarditis.

In the infant, myocarditis will often present with signs of congestive heart failure. These infants usually have difficulty feeding. Often there is a preceding upper respiratory infection or gastroenteritis. Alternatively, myocarditis may present with signs of cardiogenic shock with or without fever. This can easily be confused with the more common diagnoses of hypovolemic or septic shock. Sometimes the diagnosis is considered only after evidence of congestive heart failure occurs after bolus intravenous fluid administration. Often, cardiomegaly or EKG findings will provide the important clue. Epidemics of myocarditis have been reported, usually occurring in newborn infants and usually secondary to coxsackievirus group B.[19, 28]

Older children or adolescents are less likely to present in shock unless they are having a significant arrhythmia. They may report a recent upper respiratory, gastrointestinal, or flu-like illness. Typical complaints include fatigue, dyspnea, palpitations, myalgias, or chest pain, which may be pericardial or anginal in character.[29] The patient may or may not appear ill.[23] Older children are more likely than infants to have a nonviral cause of their myocarditis, although a viral origin is most common in both groups. Both infants and older children may present with sudden death as the only manifestation of their disease.

Because myocarditis is not one of the common causes of syncope, fatigue, chest pain, fever, or dyspnea, much of the history obtained is directed at finding other, more common causes of these symptoms. Other conditions such as pneumonia may coexist with myocarditis and make the diagnosis even more difficult.

Physical Examination

Although physical findings may be absent or minimal, a thorough physical examination should be completed to search for evidence to either support the diagnosis of myocarditis or make another diagnosis more likely. Myocarditis may present as right or left ventricular failure, or both. Any evidence of arrhythmia or muffled heart sounds supports the diagnosis. A pericardial friction rub is more typical of pericarditis, but myocarditis and pericarditis often coexist. Hypertension, evidence of drug abuse, thyromegaly, evidence of chest trauma, discrepancies between upper and lower extremity blood pressures, or evidence of carbon monoxide poisoning are just a few examples of findings that would make another diagnosis more likely.

DIAGNOSTIC EVALUATION

There is no test with a high sensitivity and specificity for myocarditis (Table 22–1). To diagnose myocarditis in the emergency department, the most useful tests are the chest radiograph, the EKG, and, if available, the echocardiogram. Unfortunately, all may be normal, despite the presence of myocarditis; however, in symptomatic patients with myocarditis, at least one of the three would be expected to be abnormal.[15] Although chest pain in the child or adolescent is rarely of cardiac origin, unexplained chest pain should prompt a chest radiograph and an EKG.[29]

Radiography

On the chest radiograph, an enlarged cardiac silhouette strongly suggests cardiac disease. The cause of the enlargement may be pericardial effusion, cardiomegaly, or a combination of the two. Pulmonary edema, hepatomegaly, or pneumonia may also be present.

Cardiac Monitoring

The patient with suspected myocarditis should be placed on a cardiac monitor. Every effort should be made to document transient arrhythmias. In addition, the clinician must be alerted to potentially dangerous arrhythmias. A 12-lead EKG should also be performed. Findings suggestive of myocarditis include heart block, atrial or ventricular arrhythmia, small or absent Q waves in the lateral precordial leads, diffusely low voltages of the QRS complexes, ST segment changes, or T-wave flattening or inversion.

Echocardiography

Echocardiography is extremely helpful in determining the cause of an enlarged cardiac silhouette. It can detect chamber enlargement or pericardial effusion and can be helpful in excluding congenital heart disease. Chamber enlargement and a decreased ejection fraction in the absence of other structural abnormalities is suggestive of myocarditis. Although echocardiography may lend strong support to the diagnosis if results are positive, a negative study does not exclude myocarditis. However, a normal echocardiogram does reassure the clinician that the pumping ability of the heart is intact.

Cardiac Enzymes

Cardiac enzymes may be elevated depending on the amount of myocardial necrosis.[30] Serial evaluation of enzymes and of the erythrocyte sedimentation rate may be helpful in following the course of the patient with myocarditis.

Pericardiocentesis

Pericardiocentesis may be lifesaving in the presence of cardiac tamponade. The diagnosis of cardiac tamponade

TABLE 22–1	
DIAGNOSTIC CONSIDERATIONS IN MYOCARDITIS	
Test	**Suggestive Findings**
Chest radiograph	Enlarged cardiac silhouette
	Pulmonary edema
Cardiac monitoring	
Single lead	Dysrhythmias, including first, second, and third degree atrioventricular blocks, ventricular tachycardia, and ventricular fibrillation
12-Lead	Small or absent Q waves in the lateral precordial leads
	Low-voltage QRS complexes
	T-wave flattening or inversion
Echocardiography	
Real-time study	Chamber enlargement
	Pericardial effusion
	Decreased ejection fraction
Laboratory evaluation	
Creatine kinase	Elevated or high MB fraction
Erythrocyte sedimentation rate	Elevated
Viral and bacterial cultures	Detection of causative organism
Viral titers	Acute and convalescent titers required
Myocardial biopsy	Requires cardiology consultation

should be based on the physical examination, and pericardiocentesis should not be delayed in the critically ill or acutely worsening patient with possible cardiac tamponade. Cardiac tamponade is suggested by softening heart sounds, decreased pulse pressure, jugular venous distention, worsening capillary refill, and a worsening mental status. The pericardial fluid should be evaluated for viral and bacterial infection.

Laboratory Evaluation

Laboratory evaluation should include a complete blood cell count, erythrocyte sedimentation rate, and cardiac isoenzymes. Although the MB fraction of creatine kinase (formerly called creatine phosphokinase) is commonly elevated in patients with myocarditis, a normal value does not exclude the diagnosis. In fact, values are usually within normal limits in patients with rheumatic carditis.[31] Aerobic and anaerobic blood cultures; viral cultures of the throat, feces, and urine; and any pericardial or pleural fluid cultures should be followed. Viral origin is not excluded by failure to isolate the virus, and isolation of the virus from noncardiac tissue may suggest, but does not prove, causation.[15] Acute and convalescent viral titers may also be helpful; a fourfold rise in titers is considered significant.[19] Neonates with coxsackievirus type B myocarditis will often have multiorgan involvement. In these patients, laboratory evidence of encephalomyelitis, pancreatitis, nephritis, or hepatitis may be found.[25]

Biopsy

Radionuclide imaging is not indicated in the emergency setting, but this study may localize the sites of myocardial involvement and allows for a guided myocardial biopsy.[32, 33] Also, it has the advantage of being much less invasive and posing less radiation risk to the patient than angiocardiography.[34] Cardiac catheterization with myocardial biopsy is an inpatient procedure that should be performed by a pediatric cardiologist.

Although biopsy would seem to be both sensitive and specific for making the diagnosis of myocarditis, it is far from being a perfect test.[35, 36] Because myocarditis may be localized, even multiple biopsy specimens may contain only normal myocardium, giving a false-negative result.[9] The specificity of the test also suffers, because there is no precise pathologic definition of myocarditis.[2]

Finally, cardiac catheterization and biopsy are potentially dangerous, especially when the heart is already prone to arrhythmia. The decision to perform cardiac catheterization should be made by a cardiologist. The procedure is often reserved for the patient with atypical findings in whom another diagnosis, such as anomalous origin of the left coronary artery, is being considered.

DIFFERENTIAL DIAGNOSIS

It is difficult for the emergency physician to make the diagnosis of myocarditis without evidence of cardiomegaly on chest radiograph or abnormalities on the EKG (Table 22–2). Patients with hypoplastic left heart syndrome present in the first week of life with cardiomegaly, weak peripheral pulses, and signs of congestive failure. The EKG is usually normal. The prognosis is extremely poor.[37]

Coarctation of the aorta also presents with congestive failure in infancy. Although differences in upper and lower extremity pulses and blood pressures are expected, these differences may be difficult to appreciate during heart failure. However, EKG findings of right ventricular hypertrophy in younger infants and left ventricular hypertrophy

TABLE 22–2
DIFFERENTIAL DIAGNOSIS OF MYOCARDITIS*
Younger child (<3 yr)
Hypoplastic left ventricle syndrome
Coarctation of the aorta
Anomalous origin of the left coronary artery
Pompe's disease (Glycogen storage disease type II)
Sepsis
Older child (>10 yr)
Cocaine abuse
Hyperthyroidism

*Pericarditis can coexist with myocarditis in several conditions.

in older infants suggest the diagnosis. Inverted T waves in the left precordial leads are also common. Older children with this diagnosis seldom develop congestive heart failure.

Patients with anomalous origin of the left coronary artery also present in infancy with heart failure. These patients are usually asymptomatic in the first few weeks of life. Because the left coronary artery arises from the pulmonary trunk instead of the aorta, the myocardium is poorly perfused and poorly oxygenated. The EKG suggests anterolateral myocardial infarction with deep Q waves and inverted T waves in leads I, AVL, V_5, and V_6. In some cases it may show left ventricular hypertrophy and strain or complete left bundle branch block. Patients with myocarditis may also have infarct patterns on EKG; an anterolateral infarct pattern mandates further studies to exclude anomalous left coronary artery.[38]

In Pompe's disease (glycogen storage disease, type II), the infant presents with heart failure at between 2 and 6 months of age. Skeletal muscle weakness, hypotonia, a large tongue, and hyporeflexia are often present. Because this is an autosomal recessive disorder, a sibling may also be affected. EKG findings of extraordinarily enlarged QRS voltages and a shortened PR interval are diagnostic.

Supraventricular tachycardia is usually characterized by heart rates greater than 220 beats/min (often 250 to 350 beats/min) that are very regular. There is often no history of fever or significant dehydration. Tachypnea, poor feeding, diaphoresis, and irritability are common. It is usually easily differentiated from myocarditis because of the extremely high heart rates. Patients with myocarditis may have sinus tachycardia, with heart rates up to 220 beats/min. However, in atypical cases, the diagnosis may not be obvious.[39]

Although sepsis in the infant is usually not accompanied by cardiomegaly or EKG findings other than sinus tachycardia, it often presents with fever, tachypnea, and poor capillary refill of greater than 2 seconds. In the absence of hepatomegaly, an infant with these findings is much more likely to have sepsis than isolated myocarditis. However, the latter diagnosis is still a possibility. Poor myocardial function or myocarditis may also result from sepsis.

The differential diagnosis changes for the older child and adolescent. Cocaine may produce fever, tachycardia, ischemic changes on EKG, arrhythmias, and even sudden death. Tricyclic antidepressants may also cause fatal arrhythmias, and amphetamines and other drugs may mimic myocarditis. Therefore a drug screening test and a thorough history of possible drug exposure are essential.

Hyperthyroidism may present with fever, tachycardia, and palpitations. The chest radiograph and EKG are usually normal. The patient will often have other findings suggesting hyperthyroidism.

THERAPEUTIC INTERVENTION

In some instances, treatment directed toward the causative agent has been beneficial. Examples include antitoxin and antibiotic therapy for diphtheria, amphotericin B therapy for *Candida* infections, and nifurtimox for acute Chagas' disease.[17, 18] However, the majority of cases are of viral origin, and the treatment of these patients is supportive (Table 22–3).

Adequate oxygenation and ventilation should be maintained. The patient should not exercise and should, as a general rule, stay in bed during the acute phase of the illness.[38, 40] Cardiac tamponade, if present, should be treated by pericardiocentesis.[41]

Fluid administration should be judicious. In the emergency setting, fluid boluses of 10 to 20 ml/kg are often given to the infant in shock. If myocarditis is suspected and the history suggests dehydration, a 10 ml/kg fluid bolus should be given. It is essential that the patient be reassessed immediately after the fluid bolus. If the patient's heart failure worsens, then inotropic and diuretic support are indicated. However, if the patient improves (i.e., heart rate, capillary refill, mental status, and color begin to normalize), additional boluses may be given if indicated. The patient should be reassessed after every therapeutic maneuver. The clinician must attempt to achieve adequate filling pressures (to maximize cardiac output) without greatly increasing pulmonary edema or cardiac work. Invasive monitoring with a central venous catheter or even a pulmonary artery catheter can be helpful.

The most useful inotropic agents for the acute treatment of myocarditis without significant heart block in the emergency department setting are dopamine and dobutamine. Dopamine has the added advantage of augmenting renal blood flow and urine output. The dose of dopamine is 2 to 15 µg/kg/min by a constant infusion. Lower doses are preferred if good cardiac output can be maintained, as the beneficial effect of dopamine on the renal vessels is gradually lost as doses increase between 10 and 20 µg/kg/min.

Dobutamine does not increase heart rate or ventricular irritability as dopamine can. It may be used in combination with low-dose dopamine infusions in order to take advantage of the inotropic effect of both drugs and the renal effect of dopamine. Patients who are unresponsive to dopamine may be treated with a continuous infusion of epinephrine.[42, 43]

If high-grade AV block has occurred, a continuous infusion of isoproterenol may be used. However, it should be used with caution in patients with myocarditis, as it may precipitate more serious arrhythmias. Transvenous pacing is a reasonable alternative for the patient with symptomatic heart block.[44]

Digitalis may be used for both inotropic support and control of atrial arrhythmia. The inflamed myocardium may be more sensitive to digitalis, and cardiology consultation is recommended prior to its use.

Furosemide is the most appropriate diuretic in the emergency setting. Fluid overload may occur as the renin-angiotensin-aldosterone system responds to decreased cardiac output or as a result of iatrogenic fluid administration or both. Furosemide, 1 to 2 mg/kg, will usually result in a prompt diuresis.

Urine output should be maintained at a minimum of 1 ml/kg/hr. Daily determinations of weight, electrolyte levels, and urine specific gravity are also helpful in assessing fluid status. In general, intravenous fluids should be infused at two thirds to three fourths of the calculated "maintenance" rate as long as adequate urine output can be maintained. Ongoing fluid losses (e.g., from diarrhea or fever) should be replaced.

Arrhythmias should be managed by standard therapy, but lidocaine infusion dosage should be adjusted downward in a patient with heart failure.

Any aggravating factors such as anemia, electrolyte abnormalities, hypoglycemia, or malnutrition should also be corrected.[15] Antibiotics are generally not indicated for viral myocarditis, but in the infant in whom sepsis is a consideration, antibiotic coverage is appropriate. In the critically ill patient with heart failure, stressful procedures such as lumbar puncture should be postponed until the patient's condition has stabilized.

If all of these measures have been carried out and cardiac output is still unacceptable, afterload reduction with nitroprusside or captopril may be helpful. This, too, should be done by a physician specializing in care of critically ill children. Patients on a nitroprusside infusion should have

---

TABLE 22–3

MYOCARDITIS THERAPY AT A GLANCE

Agent	Dose	Administration
Fluid Bolus		
0.9% Normal saline	10–20 ml/kg	IV bolus over 15 minutes
Inotropy		
Dopamine	2–15 µg/kg/min	Continuous infusion
Dobutamine	5–20 µg/kg/min	Continuous infusion
Digoxin (use with caution)*	Term infant: 20–30 µg/kg 1–24 mo: 30–50 µg/kg 2–5 yr: 25–35 µg/kg 5–10 yr: 15–30 µg/kg >10 yr: 8–12 µg/kg	This amount represents the digitalizing dose. Half the dose is initially given in an IV push over 5 minutes. The rest is given over 24 hours as clinically indicated
Blood pressure support		
Dopamine	5–20 µg/kg/min	Continuous infusion
Epinephrine	0.1–1.0 µg/kg/min	Continuous infusion
Atrioventricular block		
Isoproterenol	0.1–1.0 µg/kg/min	Continuous infusion
Pacemaker		
Diuresis		
Furosemide	1 mg/kg	IV push

*Do not exceed the maximum recommended adult dose. Caution is advised in patients with metabolic abnormalities, decreased cardiac output, or impaired renal function.

their blood pressure continuously monitored by an indwelling arterial catheter.

The role of immunosuppressive therapy in viral myocarditis is undetermined. There is evidence that much of the damage done by viruses to the myocardium is the result of an autoimmune phenomenon. However, human studies evaluating the efficacy of immunosuppressive agents in viral myocarditis have had mixed results. Animal studies suggest that steroids given early in the course of myocarditis worsen the disease.[9, 45a]

If myocarditis has a nonviral cause, certain other medications may be of benefit, depending on the origin.[45] Steroids are helpful in acute rheumatic carditis, but their role is unclear in other forms of myocarditis.[46] Antibiotics are helpful in Lyme carditis. In diphtheritic myocarditis, antitoxin therapy and antibiotics are essential.

DISPOSITION

Virtually all patients with the diagnosis of acute myocarditis require admission to the hospital for stabilization and observation. Ideally, the hospital should be equipped with a pediatric intensive care unit. Adequate monitoring equipment and equipment necessary for defibrillation and pericardiocentesis should be readily available. All patients should be followed by a pediatric cardiologist during the hospitalization and indefinitely thereafter. When the patient is discharged, restriction of activity for several weeks is usually recommended.[47]

Patient prognosis is generally worse for the infant than for the older child[15] and varies depending on the causative agent. Myocarditis may be recurrent or chronic, and there is evidence that a subset of patients develop cardiomyopathy later in life.[9, 25, 48–52] Some cases of endocardial fibroelastosis are thought to result from previous myocarditis,[19] but most patients who survive the acute illness have few or no long-term sequelae.[15]

OTHER CONSIDERATIONS

Because of the great variety of organisms that may cause myocarditis, consultation with an infectious disease expert may be indicated for both diagnostic and therapeutic assistance. Isolation of the patient may be necessary, and public health considerations may need to be addressed. There may be a role for extracorporeal membrane oxygenation in selected cases,[53] but experience is limited.

SUMMARY

Myocarditis is a frequently unrecognized and asymptomatic condition. However, in its more severe forms myocarditis may be damaging to the heart of the infant, child, or adolescent and result in significant morbidity and mortality. A high index of suspicion is of paramount importance in making the diagnosis.

References

1. Stedman's Medical Dictionary. 23rd ed. Baltimore, Williams & Wilkins, 1976, p 915.
2. Noren GR, Staley NA, Bandt CM, Kaplan EL. Occurrence of myocarditis in sudden death in children. J Forensic Sci 1977;22:188.
3. Neuspiel DR. Sudden death from myocarditis in young athletes. Mayo Clin Proc 1986;61:226.
4. Neuspiel DR, Kuller LH. Sudden and unexpected natural death in childhood and adolescence. JAMA 1985;254:1321.
5. Wentworth P, Jentz LA, Croal AE. Analysis of sudden unexpected death in southern Ontario, with emphasis on myocarditis. Can Med Assoc J 1979;120:676.
6. Molander N. Sudden natural death in later childhood and adolescence. Arch Dis Child 1982;57:572.
7. Topaz O, Edwards JE. Pathologic features of sudden death in children, adolescents, and young adults. Chest 1985;87:476.
8. de Sa DJ. Isolated myocarditis as a cause of sudden death in the first year of life. Forensic Sci Int 1986;30:113.
9. Kerelakes DJ, Parmley WW. Myocarditis and cardiomyopathy. Curriculum Cardiol 1984;108:1318.
10. Grayston JT, Mordhorst CH, Wang S. Childhood myocarditis associated with *Chlamydia trachomatis* infection. JAMA 1981;246:2823.
11. Fujiwara H, Chen C, Fujiwara T, et al. Clinicopathologic study of abnormal Q waves in Kawasaki disease (mucocutaneous lymph node syndrome). Am J Cardiol 1980;45:797.
12. Frid C, Bjarke B, Eriksson M. Myocarditis in children with inflammatory bowel disease. J Ped 1986;5:964.
13. Steere AC, Batsford WP, Weinberg M, et al. Lyme carditis: Cardiac abnormalities of Lyme disease. Ann Intern Med 1980;93:8.
14. Walsh TJ, Hutchins GM. Postoperative *Candida* infections of the heart in children: Clinicopathologic study of a continuing problem of diagnosis and therapy. J Pediatr Surg 1980;15:325.
15. Woodruff JF. Viral myocarditis—a review. Am J Pathol 1980;101:427.
16. Hohn AR, Stanton RE. Myocarditis in children. Pediatr Rev 1987;9:83.
17. Wittner M. Trypanosomiasis. *In* Feigin RD, Cherry JD (eds). Textbook of Pediatric Infectious Diseases. 2nd ed. Philadelphia, WB Saunders, 1987, p 2079.
18. Feigen RD, Stechenberg BW. Diphtheria. *In* Feigin RD, Cherry JD (eds). Textbook of Pediatric Infectious Diseases. 2nd ed. Philadelphia, WB Saunders, 1987, p 1138.
19. Harris LC, Powell G, Brown OW III. Primary myocardial disease. Pediatr Clin North Am 1978;25:847.
20. Favara BE, Franciosi RA. Diphtherial myocardiopathy. Am J Cardiol 1972;30:423.
21. Hiraishi S, Yashiro K, Oguchi K, et al. Clinical course of cardiovascular involvement in the mucocutaneous lymph node syndrome. Am J Cardiol 1981;47:323.
22. Hollinshead WH. Textbook of Anatomy. 3rd ed. Hagerstown, Harper & Row, 1974, p 491.
23. Wenger NK, Abelmann WH, Roberts WC. Myocarditis. *In* Hurst JW, Logue RB, Rackley CE, et al (eds). The Heart. 6th ed. New York, McGraw-Hill, 1986, p 1158.
24. Morgan WL Jr, Engel GL. The approach to the medical interview. *In* Morgan WL Jr, Engel GL (eds). The Clinical Approach to the Patient. Philadelphia, WB Saunders, 1969, p 35.
25. Hirshman SZ, Hammer GS. Coxsackie virus myopericarditis. Am J Cardiol 1974;34:224.
26. Wagner H. Cardiac disease in congenital infections. Clin Perinatol 1981;8:481.
27. Bonadio WA, Losek JD. Infants with myocarditis presenting with severe respiratory distress and shock. Pediatr Emerg Care 1987;3:110.
28. Friedman RA, Duff DF. Myocarditis. *In* Feigin RD, Cherry JD (eds). Textbook of Pediatric Infectious Diseases. 2nd ed. Philadelphia, WB Saunders, 1987, p 393.
29. Hoyer MH, Fischer DR. Acute myocarditis simulating myocardial infarction in a child. Pediatrics 1991;87:250.
30. Rizzotti P, Cocco C, Burlina A Jr, et al. Macro creatine kinase type 2: A marker of myocardial damage in infants? Clin Biochem 1985;18:239.
31. Haffejee IE, Coutts P, Moosa A. Serum MB-creatine kinase is not elevated in active rheumatic carditis. J Trop Med Hyg 1984;87:215.
32. Matsuura H, Ishikita T, Yamamoto S, et al. Gallium-67 myocardial imaging for the detection of myocarditis in the acute phase of Kawasaki disease (mucocutaneous lymph node syndrome): The usefulness of single photon emission computed tomography. Br Heart J 1987;58:385.
33. Saji T, Matsuo N, Hashiguchi R, et al. Radionuclide imaging for assessment of myocarditis and postmyocarditic state in infants and children. Jpn Heart J 1985;26:413.
34. Bjorkhem G, Evander E, White T, Lundstrom N. Myocardial scintigraphy with 201-thallium in pediatric cardiology: A review of 52 cases. Pediatr Cardiol 1990;11:1.
35. Schmaltz AA, Apitz J, Hort W, Maisch B. Endomyocardial biopsy in infants and children: Experience in 60 patients. Pediatr Cardiol 1990;11:15.
36. Takahashi O, Kamiya T, Echigo S, et al. Myocarditis in children—clinical findings and myocardial biopsy findings. Jpn Circ J 1983;47:1298.
37. Moller JH. Essentials of Pediatric Cardiology. 2nd ed. Philadelphia, FA Davis, 1978.
38. Greenwood RD, Nadas AS, Fyler DC. The clinical course of primary myocardial disease in infants and children. Am Heart J 1976;92:549.
39. Gillette PC, Smith RT, Garson A Jr, et al. Chronic supraventricular tachycardia: A curable cause of congestive cardiomyopathy. JAMA 1985;253:391.
40. Tilles JG, Elson SH, Shaka JA, et al. Effects of exercise on coxsackie A9 myocarditis in adult mice. Proc Soc Exp Biol Med 1964;117:777.
41. Tan AH, Mah PK, Chia RL. Cardiac tamponade in acute rheumatic carditis. Ann Rheum Dis 1983;42:699.
42. Zaritsky A, Chernow B. Use of catecholamines in pediatrics. J Pediatr 1984;105:341.
43. Bollaert PE, Bauer P, Audibert G, et al. Effects of epinephrine on

hemodynamics and oxygen metabolism in dopamine-resistant septic shock. Chest 1990;98:949.

44. Onouchi Z, Shigemoto H, Kiyosasa N, et al. Stokes-Adams attacks due to acute nonspecific myocarditis in childhood. Jpn Heart J 1980;21:307.

45. Newburger JW, Takahashi M, Burns JC, et al. The treatment of Kawasaki syndrome with intravenous gamma globulin. N Engl J Med 1986;315:341.

45a. Tomioka N, Kishimoto C, Matsumori A, et al. Effect of prednisolone on acute viral myocarditis in mice. J Am Coll Cardiol 1986;7:868.

46. French WJ, Criley JM. Caution in the diagnosis and treatment of myocarditis. Am J Cardiol 1984;54:445.

47. Oda T, Hamamoto K, Morinaga H. Sequelae of nonrheumatic myocarditis in children: A follow-up study. Jpn Circ J 1980;44:817.

48. Nishikawa T, Sekiguchi M, Kunimine Y, et al. An infant with dilated cardiomyopathy confirmed as myocarditis by endomyocardial biopsy. Heart Vessels 1987;3:108.

49. Dec GW, Palacios IF, Fallon JT, et al. Active myocarditis in the spectrum of acute dilated cardiomyopathies. N Engl J Med 1985;312:885.

50. Kawai C, Matsumori A, Hisayoshi F. Myocarditis and dilated cardiomyopathy. Ann Rev Med 1987;38:221.

51. Okuni M, Usami H. Cardiomyopathy and myocarditis in children. Heart Vessels 1985;1(Suppl):30.

52. Menahem S. Viral myocarditis and dilated cardiomyopathy in early childhood. Br Heart J 1987;58:420.

53. Splaingard ML, Frazier OH, Jefferson LS, et al. Extracorporeal membrane oxygenation: Its role in the survival of a child with adenoviral pneumonia and myocarditis. South Med J 1983;76:1172.

CHAPTER 23

Hypertension

John E. Stork

INTRODUCTION

Hypertension may be encountered in the emergency department either as an acute, symptomatic, and potentially life-threatening problem or as a serendipitous finding during routine monitoring of vital signs in an asymptomatic patient. In both instances, there is a need for evaluation and therapy.

Hypertension is the largest single risk factor for premature death and disability among the adult population. Prevalence rates have been estimated to be from 15.7 per 100 population for white females to 28.6 per 100 population for black males.[1] Although the incidence in children is much lower, longitudinal studies have shown that childhood hypertension is a highly significant predictor of adult hypertension.[2] A single blood pressure reading in the emergency department is no substitute for repeated measurements by the primary care pediatrician over time; nonetheless, an elevated reading in an asymptomatic child requires referral and follow-up. Measurement of blood pressure in all children in emergency departments is a current recommendation of the Task Force on Blood Pressure Control of the National Heart Lung and Blood Institute (NHLBI).[3] If hypertension is confirmed, long-term management may have significant preventive benefits.

Severe hypertension with complications requires emergent therapy. This is not always straightforward in the acutely ill child. The effects of hypertension and antihypertensive therapy on cerebral perfusion are unclear, particularly in the injured brain, and management remains problematic. Careful consideration of the hemodynamic consequences of antihypertensive therapy, as well as the side effects associated with therapy, is vital.

BLOOD PRESSURE EVALUATION

Normal Values

Blood pressure varies with age and size, and evaluation of blood pressure requires age-specific norms (Table 23–1). Values are available for healthy children from several epidemiologic studies and provide a starting point for evaluation of blood pressure in critically ill children. Norms have been compiled and published in a cooperative study by the NHLBI (Figs. 23–1 through 23–6).[3]

Blood Pressure Measurement

Auscultation of Korotkoff sounds has long been the standard indirect method for determination of blood pressure. For valid measurements, cuff size must be carefully matched to arm size, and a wide range of cuffs should be available in the emergency department. In infants, auscultation of the Korotkoff sounds may be difficult. Other methods, such as Doppler detection of the pulse as occlusion is released or the primitive flush technique, provide only a systolic determination and are marginal at best. Oscillometric devices such as the Dinamap monitor work well in infants and provide consistent readings, which is particularly useful in following trends over time.[4] Comparisons with direct intra-arterial monitoring show good correlation, but in one neonatal intensive care unit (Rainbow Babies and Children's Hospital, Cleveland), the Dinamap tended to overestimate the blood pressure in sick infants, with the greatest difference seen in systolic readings and only minimal difference in diastolic. Other studies have had varying results, although in general the Dinamap has been shown to be adequate for clinical use.

The emotional state of the child is also important in the determination of blood pressure, but this is difficult to control in the emergency setting. Repeated determinations over time can be very helpful in evaluating dubious readings.

CLINICAL PRESENTATION

Hypertension can present in one of several patterns. The child may be asymptomatic, particularly if the hypertension is chronic and elevations have been gradual. With the grad-

TABLE 23–1

CLASSIFICATION OF HYPERTENSION BY AGE GROUP

Age Group	Significant Hypertension (mm Hg)	Severe Hypertension (mm Hg)
Newborn (7 days)	Systolic BP ≥ 96	Systolic BP ≥ 106
Newborn (8 to 30 days)	Systolic BP ≥ 104	Systolic BP ≥ 110
Infant (<2 yr)	Systolic BP ≥ 112 Diastolic BP ≥ 74	Systolic BP ≥ 118 Diastolic BP ≥ 82
Children 3–5 yr	Systolic BP ≥ 116 Diastolic BP ≥ 76	Systolic BP ≥ 124 Diastolic BP ≥ 84
6–9 yr	Systolic BP ≥ 122 Diastolic BP ≥ 78	Systolic BP ≥ 130 Diastolic BP ≥ 86
10–12 yr	Systolic BP ≥ 126 Diastolic BP ≥ 82	Systolic BP ≥ 134 Diastolic BP ≥ 90
Adolescents 13–15 yr	Systolic BP ≥ 136 Diastolic BP ≥ 86	Systolic BP ≥ 144 Diastolic BP ≥ 92
16–18 yr	Systolic BP ≥ 142 Diastolic BP ≥ 92	Systolic BP ≥ 150 Diastolic BP ≥ 98

From Report of the Second Task Force on Blood Pressure Control in Children. Pediatrics 1987;79:1. Reproduced by permission of Pediatrics.
BP = Blood pressure.

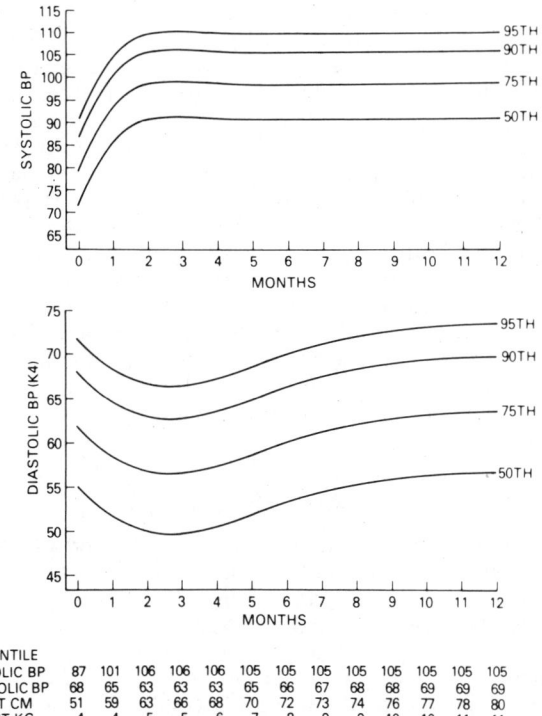

90TH PERCENTILE													
SYSTOLIC BP	87	101	106	106	106	105	105	105	105	105	105	105	105
DIASTOLIC BP	68	65	63	63	63	65	66	67	68	68	69	69	69
HEIGHT CM	51	59	63	66	68	70	72	73	74	76	77	78	80
WEIGHT KG	4	4	5	5	6	7	8	9	9	10	10	11	11

Figure 23–1. Age-specific percentiles of blood pressure (BP) measurements in boys from birth to 12 months of age. Korotkoff phase IV (K4) used for diastolic BP. (From Report of the Second Task Force on Blood Pressure Control in Children. Pediatrics 1987; 79:1. Reproduced by permission of Pediatrics.)

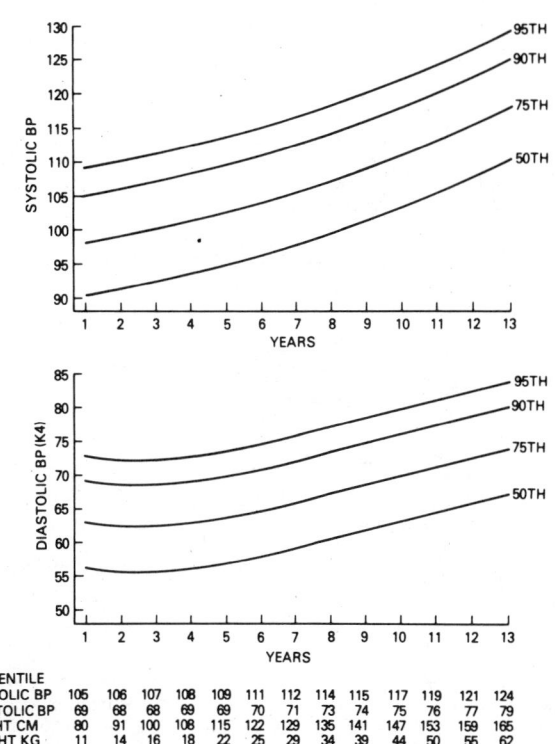

90TH PERCENTILE													
SYSTOLIC BP	105	106	107	108	109	111	112	114	115	117	119	121	124
DIASTOLIC BP	69	68	68	69	69	70	71	73	74	75	76	77	79
HEIGHT CM	80	91	100	108	115	122	129	135	141	147	153	159	165
WEIGHT KG	11	14	16	18	22	25	29	34	39	44	50	55	62

Figure 23–3. Age-specific percentiles of BP measurements in boys from 1 to 13 years of age. Korotkoff phase IV (K4) used for diastolic BP. (From Report of the Second Task Force on Blood Pressure Control in Children. Pediatrics 1987; 79:1. Reproduced by permission of Pediatrics.)

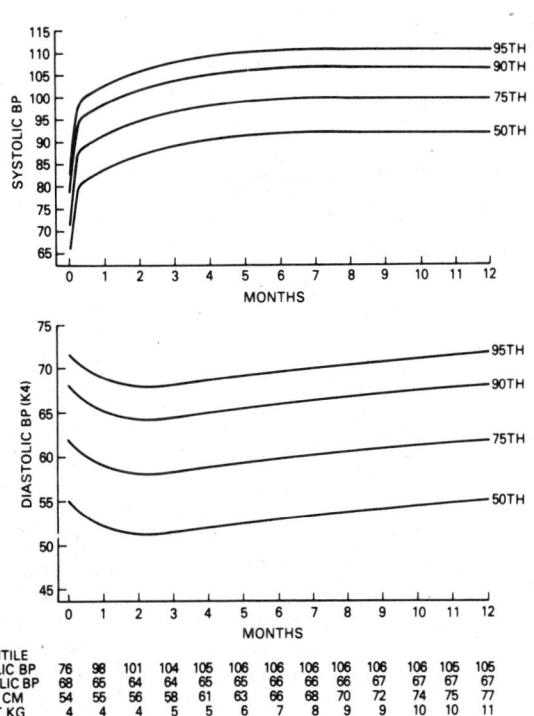

90TH PERCENTILE													
SYSTOLIC BP	76	98	101	104	105	106	106	106	106	106	106	105	105
DIASTOLIC BP	68	65	64	64	65	65	66	66	66	67	67	67	67
HEIGHT CM	54	55	56	58	61	63	66	68	70	72	74	75	77
WEIGHT KG	4	4	4	5	5	6	7	8	9	9	10	10	11

Figure 23–2. Age-specific percentiles of BP measurements in girls from birth to 12 months of age. Korotkoff phase IV (K4) used for diastolic BP. (From Report of the Second Task Force on Blood Pressure Control in Children. Pediatrics 1987; 79:1. Reproduced by permission of Pediatrics.)

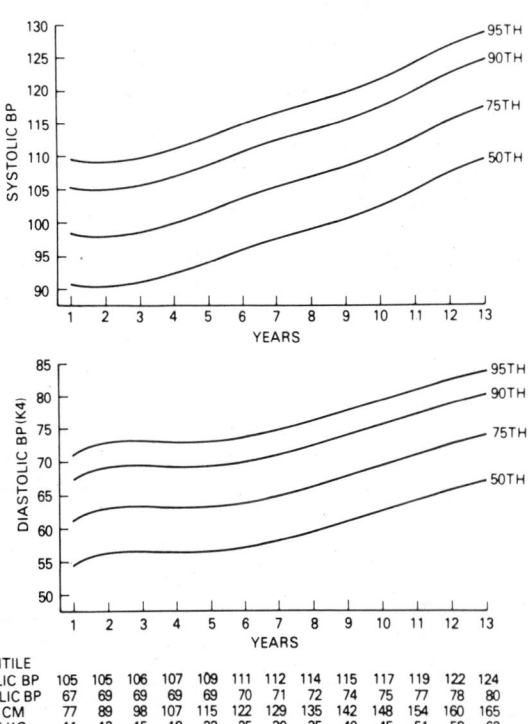

90TH PERCENTILE													
SYSTOLIC BP	105	105	106	107	109	111	112	114	115	117	119	122	124
DIASTOLIC BP	67	69	69	69	69	70	71	72	74	75	77	78	80
HEIGHT CM	77	89	98	107	115	122	129	135	142	148	154	160	165
WEIGHT KG	11	13	15	18	22	25	30	35	40	45	51	58	63

Figure 23–4. Age-specific percentiles of BP measurements in girls from 1 to 13 years of age. Korotkoff phase IV (K4) used for diastolic BP. (From Report of the Second Task Force on Blood Pressure Control in Children. Pediatrics 1987; 79:1. Reproduced by permission of Pediatrics.)

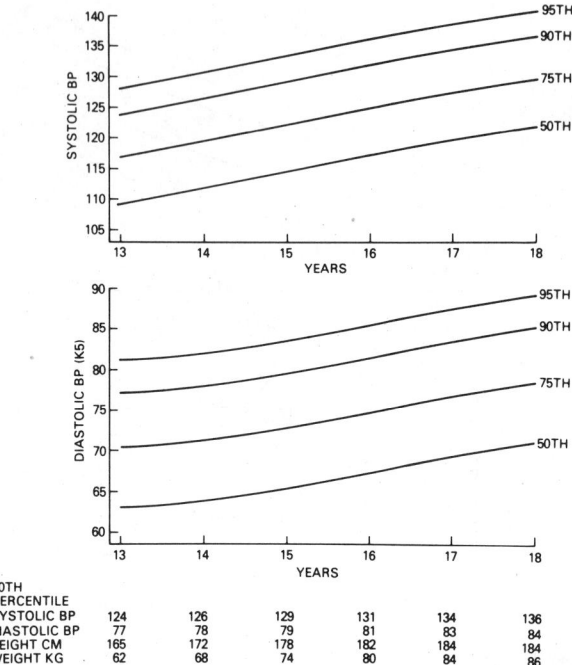

90TH PERCENTILE						
SYSTOLIC BP	124	126	129	131	134	136
DIASTOLIC BP	77	78	79	81	83	84
HEIGHT CM	165	172	178	182	184	184
WEIGHT KG	62	68	74	80	84	86

Figure 23–5. Age-specific percentiles of BP measurements in boys from 13 to 18 years of age. Korotkoff phase IV (K5) used for diastolic BP. (From Report of the Second Task Force on Blood Pressure Control in Children. Pediatrics 1987; 79:1. Reproduced by permission of Pediatrics.)

ual onset of hypertension, vital organs, including the brain, develop a tolerance for increased blood pressures because of a shift in the autoregulatory mechanism toward higher pressures.[5] *Hypertensive encephalopathy*, or diffuse cerebral dysfunction caused by acute hypertension, is the most com-

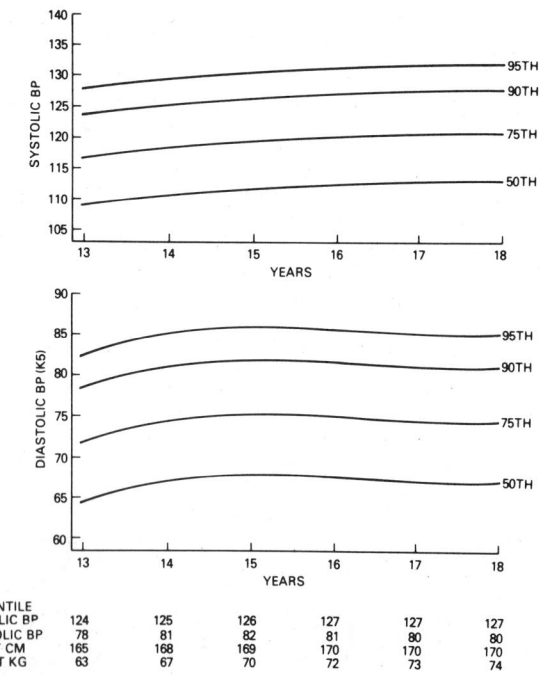

90TH PERCENTILE						
SYSTOLIC BP	124	125	126	127	127	127
DIASTOLIC BP	78	81	82	81	80	80
HEIGHT CM	165	168	169	170	170	170
WEIGHT KG	63	67	70	72	73	74

Figure 23–6. Age-specific percentiles of BP measurements in girls from 13 to 18 years of age. Korotkoff phase IV (K5) used for diastolic BP. (From Report of the Second Task Force on Blood Pressure Control in Children. Pediatrics 1987; 79:1. Reproduced by permission of Pediatrics.)

mon presentation of acute hypertension in children. Early signs include a vague headache for several days, followed by nausea, visual abnormalities, confusion, changes in consciousness, and focal neurologic signs. Seizures occur in as many as 92% of children and may occur without warning.[6, 7] *Malignant hypertension* refers to severe hypertension with retinal changes and papilledema and is associated with widespread fibrinoid necrosis of arterioles. Hypertensive encephalopathy, congestive heart failure, pulmonary edema, and renal insufficiency are usually present and can progress rapidly if untreated. In *accelerated hypertension*, blood pressure elevations and retinopathy are similar, but there is no papilledema. The presentation of hypertension in infants is usually nonspecific. Neurologic symptoms ranging from irritability to seizures are common. Congestive heart failure with pulmonary edema and respiratory distress is also a common presentation.

PATHOPHYSIOLOGY

The primary determinants of arterial blood pressure are the cardiac output and systemic vascular resistance. The cardiac output is determined by cardiac contractility, heart rate, and vascular volume. Hypertension can result from alterations in any of these factors or in a combination of factors. For example, hypertension in patients with chronic renal failure is predominantly a result of volume overload and responds well to diuretics or even dialysis, if needed. With pheochromocytoma, excessive catecholamine production results in increased peripheral resistance; vascular volume is diminished as a result of pressure diuresis.

Severe hypertension may be acute or may complicate underlying chronic hypertension. The factors responsible for conversion of stable hypertension to malignant hypertension are unclear. One theory is that sodium depletion stimulates renin release, initiating a further pressure diuresis and a circular cascade leading to the vascular damage of malignant hypertension.[8] Interestingly, volume depletion, rather than volume overload, is characteristic of malignant hypertension. Thus additional diuresis or fluid restriction may not be appropriate unless there are clear signs of volume overload–mediated hypertension.

Hypertension and the Brain

Cerebral blood flow remains constant over a wide range of systemic blood pressures as a result of autoregulation. Unfortunately, understanding of this complicated system, particularly in patients with central nervous system abnormality, is incomplete. The effects of various antihypertensive agents on the cerebral circulation have also been incompletely studied, and data are particularly scant for the pediatric population.

Cerebral blood flow is autoregulated in both normotensive and chronically hypertensive adults.[9] A lower limit to autoregulation, below which cerebral blood flow decreases, clearly exists. However, the upper limit appears to be less well defined. Because chronic hypertension induces structural changes in the cerebral vessels, the autoregulatory curve is shifted to the right. Thus patients with chronic hypertension are able to tolerate higher levels of systemic arterial pressure, at least acutely. These vascular changes ultimately lead to an increased risk of cerebrovascular disease (e.g., stroke). Chronic antihypertensive therapy partially reverses these structural changes.[10] However, vigorous acute therapy can lead to cerebral ischemia and catastrophe if systemic blood pressure is rapidly lowered below the autoregulatory threshold, which may be at normotensive pressures for that particular patient as a result of the shift in autoregulation.[11] This problem is greatest in the elderly, but also potentially exists in pediatric patients with long-term chronic hypertension.

The effects of intracranial pathology on cerebral autoregulation are unclear. Cerebral perfusion depends on the cerebral perfusion pressure (CPP), which is the difference between systemic blood pressure and intracranial pressure (ICP). Cushing's reflex attempts to maintain CPP in the presence of increased ICP by raising the systemic blood pressure. In the presence, and within the limits, of intact autoregulation, Cushing's reflex may be beneficial, as increased systemic pressure leads to autoregulatory vasoconstriction, thereby limiting further rises in ICP and maintaining normal perfusion.[12] Antihypertensive therapy in this situation is detrimental, particularly if vasodilators are used. Drugs such as sodium nitroprusside also dilate the cerebral circulation, which further increases ICP as systemic pressure is lowered, thus leading to decreases in CPP. To support this, induced hypertension has been used with some limited success in patients with head trauma and increased ICP.[13] Nevertheless, there is clear evidence that arterial hypertension in children with head trauma is a poor prognostic sign.[14] If autoregulation is abnormal in the area of a cerebral lesion, an increased systemic pressure will lead to increased perfusion and ICP, thereby initiating a cycle of rising ICP and systemic pressure.

Hypertension can also occur with CNS disease as a result of generalized sympathetic discharge; such increases in pressure may not carry the same "protective" implications as Cushing's reflex. Patients with subarachnoid and intracerebral bleeding are at increased risk of rebleeding in the presence of hypertension. In these situations it has been recommended that antihypertensive therapy should be instituted gradually and in concert with measures to decrease ICP in an attempt to maintain CPP.

Early studies of hypertensive encephalopathy theorized that with rising systemic blood pressure, autoregulatory vasoconstriction ultimately leads to inadequate cerebral perfusion. Direct observation of pial arteries was thought to support this theory, as there appeared to be segmental regions of intense vasoconstriction,[15] known as *sausage strings*. Further evaluation, however, has led to an opposite view: that as systemic blood pressure rises above the limits of autoregulation, "breakthrough" vasodilation occurs, with resultant local cerebral edema.[16-18] The "sausage strings" are now thought to represent areas of reasonably normal caliber vessel interspersed with areas of vasodilation. This view is supported by several factors. If the vasoconstriction theory is true, patients with chronic hypertension and a shifted autoregulatory curve might be expected to be more prone to develop encephalopathy; in fact, the reverse is true, and children with relatively mild, acute elevations in blood pressure are most likely to become encephalopathic. Second, intracranial pressure is increased in hypertensive encephalopathy,[19] and because this is easily reversible with therapy, it would seem likely to be a result of breakthrough and increased intracranial flow, rather than ischemic damage. The presence of increased ICP raises additional concerns with respect to therapy. Vasodilators are commonly used as first-line drugs in hypertensive encephalopathy, but as already mentioned, these agents also dilate the cerebral circulation and could further increase ICP, possibly leading to decreases in CPP.

Differentiation of hypertensive encephalopathy from intracranial pathology with secondary elevation of blood pressure can be difficult but is of extreme importance, as therapies may differ. A careful history, with attention to the possibility of trauma, is important. A computed tomographic (CT) scan may be necessary, as well as a lumbar puncture if there is any indication of CNS infection. Ultimately, a rapid clearing of defects in response to careful lowering of the blood pressure will confirm hypertensive encephalopathy.

CLINICAL EVALUATION

Although severe hypertension in adults is most commonly a complication of essential hypertension, in children, particularly before adolescence, hypertension is usually secondary to another condition (Table 23–2). Consideration of the diagnostic possibilities is helpful in orienting history taking and evaluation (Table 23–3). The chronicity of hypertension should also be estimated during the initial evaluation. Patients with underlying chronic hypertension are less likely to develop acute symptoms but are also less tolerant of acute drops in blood pressure. Previously normal children are more likely to develop serious symptoms, such as hypertensive encephalopathy, with moderate elevations in blood pressure. Evidence of end-organ damage, such as retinal changes, or left ventricular hypertrophy are indicative of chronic hypertension. This can often be determined on physical examination, although funduscopic examination and echocardiography may be required (Table 23–4).

A full evaluation of hypertension is beyond the purview of the emergency department. Emergency therapy and sta-

TABLE 23–2
COMMON CAUSES OF SEVERE HYPERTENSION IN CHILDREN

Renal
  Acute glomerulonephritis
    Poststreptococcal
    Henoch-Schönlein purpura
  Hemolytic-uremic syndrome
  Systemic lupus erythematosus
  Chronic glomerulonephritis
    Focal and segmental glomerulosclerosis
    Membranoproliferative glomerulonephritis
  Renovascular
  Vesicoureteral reflux with scarring
  Renal dysplasia
  Obstructive uropathy
  Polycystic kidney disease
  Wilms' tumor
  End-stage renal disease
  Renal transplantation
CNS disease
  Increased intracranial pressure
  Head trauma (even without elevated intracranial pressure)
  Spinal cord lesions
Tumors
  Neurofibromatosis
  Neuroblastoma
  Pheochromocytoma
  Adrenal adenoma
Drugs and ingestions
  Steroids
  Cyclosporine A
  Oral contraceptives
  Sympathomimetics
  Amphetamines
  Cocaine
  Phencyclidine
  Lead poisoning
  Licorice
Coarctation of the aorta
Miscellaneous
  Burns
  Immobilization
Essential hypertension

TABLE 23-3

HISTORICAL INFORMATION TO ELICIT

Information	Relevance
Family history of hypertension, preeclampsia, toxemia, renal disease, tumors	Important in essential hypertension, inherited renal disease, and some endocrine diseases (e.g., familial pheochromocytoma with multiple endocrine adenopathy II)
Family history of early complications of hypertension and/or atherosclerosis	Suggests likely course of hypertension and/or presence of other coronary artery disease risk factors
Neonatal history	Use of umbilical artery catheter suggests need to evaluate renal vasculature and kidneys
Headaches, dizziness, epistaxis, visual problems	Nonspecific symptomatology, usually not etiologically helpful
Abdominal pain, dysuria, frequency, nocturia, enuresis	May suggest underlying renal disease
Joint pains/swelling, facial or peripheral edema	Suggests connective tissue disease and/or other forms of nephritis
Weight loss, failure to gain weight with good appetite, sweating, flushing, fevers, palpitations	In combination, symptoms suggest pheochromocytoma
Muscle cramps, weakness, constipation	May suggest hypokalemia and hyperaldosteronism
Age of onset of menarche, sexual development	May be helpful in suggesting hydroxylase deficiencies
Ingestion of prescription and over-the-counter drugs, contraceptives, illicit drugs	Drug-induced hypertension

From Report of the Second Task Force on Blood Pressure Control in Children. Pediatrics 1987; 79:11. Reproduced by permission of Pediatrics.

bilization of the hypertensive child is not dependent on many of the sophisticated studies required for a comprehensive evaluation of hypertension and therefore, should not be delayed.

Renal Disease

Renal disease is the most common cause of hypertension, both acute and chronic, in children. Hypertension is common in acute nephritis such as poststreptococcal glomerulonephritis, and hypertensive encephalopathy with seizure may be the initial presentation. Sodium retention and volume expansion secondary to a diminished glomerular filtration rate are probably responsible for the acute rise in blood pressure.[20, 21] Findings consistent with acute nephritis include periorbital edema, hematuria and red blood cell (RBC) casts, and mild to moderate proteinuria. Levels of complement components C3 and C4 are low in the majority of patients, and serologic tests for streptococcal exposure are usually positive, even though there may not be a clear history of an antecedent streptococcal infection. Other primary glomerular diseases, particularly focal and segmental glomerulosclerosis and membranoproliferative glomerulonephritis, may cause hypertension. Systemic diseases with renal involvement, such as hemolytic-uremic syndrome (HUS),[22] systemic lupus erythematosus (SLE), and Henoch-Schönlein purpura

TABLE 23-4

FINDINGS TO LOOK FOR ON PHYSICAL EXAMINATION

Physical Findings	Relevance
General	
Pale mucous membranes, facial or pretibial edema	Renal disease
Pallor, evanescent flushing, increased sweating at rest	Pheochromocytoma vs. hyperdynamic essential hypertension
Café au lait spots, neurofibromas	Neurofibromatosis
Moon face, hirsutism, buffalo hump, truncal obesity, striae	Cushing's syndrome
Webbing of neck, low hairline, wide-spaced nipples, wide carrying angle	Turner's syndrome
Elfin facies, poor growth, retardation	Williams' syndrome
Thyroid enlargement	Hyper- or hypothyroidism
Cardiovascular	
Absent or delayed femoral pulses, low leg pressure relative to arm BP	Aortic coarctation
Heart size, rate, rhythm, murmurs; respiratory difficulty; hepatomegaly	Murmur—coarctation; tachycardia and/or arrhythmia—pheochromocytoma; large heart or heart failure—prolonged or severe hypertension
Bruits over great vessels	Arteritis or arteriopathy
Abdomen	
Epigastric bruit	Renovascular diseases isolated or associated with Williams' syndrome or neurofibromatosis, or arteritis
Unilateral or bilateral masses	Wilms' tumor, neuroblastoma, pheochromocytoma, polycystic kidneys, other tumors
Neurologic	
Hypertensive funduscopic changes	Chronic hypertension
Bell palsy	Chronic hypertension
Neurologic deficits (e.g., hemiparesis)	Chronic or severe acute hypertension with stroke

From Report of the Second Task Force on Blood Pressure Control in Children. Pediatrics 1987; 79:11. Reproduced by permission of Pediatrics.

(HSP), are also commonly associated with hypertension. With both SLE and HUS, it may be difficult to distinguish hypertensive encephalopathy from neurologic involvement of the disease.

Renovascular disease results in hypertension as a result of baroreceptor-mediated stimulation of renin production and, ultimately, increased production of angiotensin II. Angiotensin II produces hypertension both by direct vasoconstriction and through stimulation of aldosterone secretion. Increases in aldosterone promote sodium retention transiently, after which sodium balance is reestablished, although at an increased plasma volume, possibly accompanied by hypertension.

It may be difficult to diagnose renovascular disease. Fibromuscular dysplasia is the most common cause of renovascular disease in children.[23] In children with neurofibromatosis, paraspinal tumors can cause renal artery stenosis.

Presence of an abdominal bruit is an inconstant finding. A marked difference in renal size on ultrasound may be helpful if disease is unilateral. Peripheral levels of renin are not helpful. A nuclear flow scan of the kidneys is also of limited benefit, as autoregulatory vasodilation of the involved kidney minimizes abnormalities of flow. The accuracy of the renal scan may be improved by pretreatment with an angiotensin converting enzyme inhibitor,[24] which disrupts renal autoregulation and magnifies flow discrepancies in an involved kidney. Ultimately, renal angiography, with sampling of renal venous plasma for renin, may be necessary for diagnosis.

Thromboembolic involvement of the kidney secondary to placement of umbilical artery catheters has been implicated in neonatal hypertension.[25, 26] Demonstrating a clot by ultrasound may be of diagnostic benefit; however, emboli often involve the small vessels of the kidney and may not be seen with ultrasound. Renal vein thrombosis, although rare, tends to occur in infants of diabetic mothers, particularly after difficult labor with fetal distress, and may cause hypertension.[27] In contrast to adults, renal vein thrombosis in infants usually causes renal infarction. Physical signs include marked enlargement of the kidney and gross hematuria.

Other forms of chronic renal disease are associated with hypertension; these include renal scarring from infection, most commonly in children with vesicoureteral reflux,[28] renal dysplasia, obstructive uropathy,[29] and polycystic kidney disease. Ultrasound is valuable in diagnosing these conditions. Reflux is best detected with voiding cystourethrography, whereas intravenous pyelography is most useful for detection of renal scarring. Increased renin production by an involved kidney probably accounts for hypertension in these patients.[30]

Renal involvement with Wilms' tumor[31, 32] or with nephroblastomatosis can also be associated with hypertension. Children with end-stage renal disease may be hypertensive; this can be caused by their underlying renal disease or may be associated with volume changes. Hypertension is also common after renal transplantation.[33] Acute elevations can be a sign of acute rejection,[34] whereas more chronic elevations can be secondary to anastomotic narrowing, chronic rejection, or the effects of drugs, primarily steroids and cyclosporine.

Central Nervous System Disease

Hypertension is commonly seen with central nervous system disease. *Cushing's triad* refers to hypertension, bradycardia, and bradypnea and is a sign of increased intracranial pressure.[35] This reflex is protective to some extent, as the body attempts to maintain CPP against the increased ICP. Common lesions responsible for increased ICP include tumor, hydrocephalus, subarachnoid hemorrhage, intraparenchymal hemorrhage, head trauma, and CNS infections. Hypertension may also occur in head trauma without increased ICP because of a generalized hyperadrenergic state.[36] The presence of tachycardia instead of bradycardia helps to distinguish this form of hypertension from that occurring in Cushing's triad. The distinction is important, as there are significant therapeutic implications. Quadriplegia has also been associated with severe hypertension caused by spinal reflexes resulting in increased autonomic discharge.[37]

Tumors and Endocrine Causes

Several childhood tumors are associated with hypertension. Neuroblastoma can cause hypertension secondary to increased catecholamine release. A similar mechanism can cause hypertension in neurofibromatosis, and involvement of the renal nerves may result in renal artery stenosis. Pheochromocytoma, a tumor of the adrenal medulla, also causes hypertension through catecholamine release.[38] Hypertension may be episodic or sustained; there may be additional signs of catecholamine release such as tachycardia, flushing, palpitations, anxiety, sweating, and chest pain. Measurement of urinary catecholamine metabolites and plasma catecholamines is helpful in diagnosis, although critical illness and stress can also cause elevations. A nuclear scan using metaiodobenzylguanidine, an iodinated catecholamine, can be helpful in finding a pheochromocytoma, which can occur in sites other than the adrenal medulla.[39] Adrenal cortical tumors can cause hypertension because of increased cortisol production[40]; the same is true of other adrenal disorders such as congenital adrenal hyperplasia.[41] Primary hyperaldosteronism is a rare cause of hypertension, as are renin-secreting tumors. Other endocrine causes include hyperparathyroidism, other causes of hypercalcemia, and hyperthyroidism.

Drug Toxicity

Many drugs and toxins have been associated with severe hypertension. Steroids, when given as a large intravenous bolus, can result in acute hypertension because of volume expansion. Nonsteroidal anti-inflammatory agents and oral contraceptives can have similar effects on sodium balance and volume. In children with underlying chronic hypertension, over-the-counter medications containing phenylephrine and pseudoephedrine can cause serious elevation of blood pressure.[42] Other sympathomimetics, such as albuterol aerosols used in respiratory distress, may also cause hypertension. Cyclosporine A can cause hypertension not only in renal transplant patients, but also in patients with other organ transplants, such as liver or pancreas. The mechanism seems to involve aldosterone-like activity by cyclosporine. Ingestion of drugs, including antidepressants, ergot alkaloids, phencyclidine,[43] cocaine, and amphetamines can result in acute hypertension, whereas poisoning with heavy metals, most commonly lead, can lead to chronic elevations of blood pressure. Finally, although rare, ingestion of large amounts of licorice containing glycorrhizic acid can cause hypertension through mineralocorticoid-like effects.[44]

Other Causes

Coarctation of the aorta is the most common cause of hypertension in the first year of life and is the cause for as much as 2% of secondary hypertension occurring in children and adolescents.[45] Diagnosis can be made on physical examination by noting a gradient between upper and lower extremity blood pressure; this can be confirmed by echocardiography. The origin of the hypertension is similar to that in renal artery stenosis (i.e., decreased renal perfusion pressure resulting in increased renin production).

Hypertension is frequently seen in children with burn injury and may be caused by generalized sympathetic discharge.[46] Stress and anxiety of any kind can result in hypertension, which is usually transient and controlled by reassurance or sedation. Immobilization following orthopedic surgery in children has also resulted in hypertension,[47] which may be related to changes in calcium balance, as calcium is an important determinant of smooth muscle tone. Hypertension has also been noted in up to 43% of formerly premature neonates who survived with bronchopulmonary dysplasia.[48] The pathophysiology is, at present, undetermined.

Although most severe hypertension in childhood is secondary, primary hypertension does occur, particularly in later adolescence. In the absence of other causes, and particularly with a strong family history, primary hypertension should be considered in patients in this age group.

THERAPEUTIC INTERVENTION

Several keys to management must be stressed. The cause of the hypertension is not the first concern, although some estimate of origin can be useful in selecting appropriate pharmacologic therapy. In patients with neurologic signs and symptoms, however, every attempt should be made to distinguish hypertensive encephalopathy from hypertension secondary to intracranial pathology (Table 23–5). Additionally, evidence of renal disease, (e.g., hematuria and proteinuria) suggests hypertension as a cause rather than a consequence of neurologic dysfunction. If the situation is unclear, antihypertensive therapy should not be delayed until CT scans are obtained. However, such therapy should be gradual and controlled, with an initial aim to decrease pressures to within the autoregulatory envelope. Decreasing the blood pressure is clearly an urgent concern in the setting of hypertensive encephalopathy or malignant hypertension, but overly vigorous therapy can adversely affect perfusion of vital organs, even in the absence of overt hypotension, especially if blood pressure elevations have been chronic.

Drug therapy should be limited to the minimum necessary, with the aim of a modest, *controlled* decrement in blood pressure. More potent agents such as sodium nitroprusside should be reserved until continuous direct monitoring of arterial pressure is available. Neurologic status must also be carefully and serially evaluated. Anticonvulsants should be used when hypertensive encephalopathy presents with sei-

CHARACTERISTICS OF THE IDEAL ANTIHYPERTENSIVE AGENT

Rapid onset of action
Rapid reversibility of action
Potent
No effect on cardiac output or renal or cerebral blood flow
Decreases systemic vascular resistance
Minimal side effects

zures; however, control of the blood pressure is the definitive therapy.

Unfortunately, no drug possesses all of the characteristics of the ideal antihypertensive agent for hypertensive emergencies (Table 23–6), but with care, rational therapeutic choices can be made. The route of administration also deserves some discussion. In general, the parenteral route is preferred for emergent therapy (i.e., in the presence of life-threatening complications such as neurologic involvement and congestive heart failure). Sublingual therapy has recently gained some favor and is useful as a temporary route while intravenous access is obtained. The oral route should be reserved for patients with accelerated but asymptomatic hypertension. Once the acute elevation in blood pressure is controlled, consideration should be given to ongoing therapy. Plans should be made for substitution of an oral agent with continued improvement in blood pressure control. In some situations the need for therapy may be self-limited, whereas in others, chronic treatment may be needed.

Antihypertensive Agents

Almost every antihypertensive agent has at some time been advocated for use in hypertensive emergencies in adults (Table 23–7). Less information exists for children, and most of the agents have never been specifically approved for pediatric use.

Direct Vasodilators

Sodium nitroprusside is the drug of first choice in emergent hypertension. Its mode of action is by direct vasodilation. Onset is rapid, and the duration of action is short, thus requiring administration by continuous infusion pump. Continuous intra-arterial monitoring of blood pressure is mandatory, and use of sodium nitroprusside should be reserved for the intensive care unit. It is extremely potent, and there is essentially no "floor" to its action—that is, extreme hypotension can easily be induced. The solution is light sensitive and must be mixed daily. The rapidity of onset and decay allows precise titration for control of blood pressure.[49] The drug should be started at a low dose (0.5 μg/kg/min), with dosage gradually increased. Metabolism produces cyanide, with detoxification by the liver resulting in thiocyanate, which is then cleared by the kidneys. Thiocyanate accumulation, particularly in patients with renal failure, constitutes a major side effect of the drug. The major symptoms of thiocyanate toxicity are neurologic, and thiocyanate levels should be monitored in patients receiving prolonged therapy with sodium nitroprusside. Cyanide can also accumulate, especially in the presence of hepatic disease. An unexplained metabolic acidosis in a patient receiving large doses of sodium nitroprusside may indicate cyanide toxicity. Sodium nitroprusside also causes cerebral vasodilation, which could increase ICP in some patients.[50]

Diazoxide is a potent direct vasodilator that is structurally similar to the thiazide diuretics.[51] It is highly protein bound

DIFFERENTIATION OF HYPERTENSIVE ENCEPHALOPATHY AND NEUROLOGIC DISEASE

	Hypertensive Encephalopathy	Subarachnoid Bleed	Intracerebral Hemorrhage
Onset	Days	Sudden	Sudden
Symptoms and signs	Nausea, vomiting, seizures; headache for hours to days	Stiff neck; sudden "worst headache of life"	Dense fixed loss
Level of consciousness	Progressive obtundation	Alert to coma	Coma
Fundi	Hemorrhages, exudates, and papilledema sometimes seen	May have subhyaloid hemorrhage	May have subhyaloid hemorrhage

TABLE 23–7

AGENTS FOR TREATMENT OF ACUTE HYPERTENSION

Drug	Route	Dosage	Onset of Action	Duration of Action	Side Effects	Contraindications
Sodium nitroprusside	Continuous IV infusion	0.5 μg/kg/min titrated to a maximum of 10 μg/kg/min	<30 sec	During infusion	Thiocyanate toxicity, cyanide toxicity; hypotension	Hepatic failure; caution in renal failure
Diazoxide	IV bolus or minibolus	1–3 mg/kg q5 to 15 min	1–5 min	Varies; <12 hr	Hyperglycemia, reflex tachycardia, salt retention	
Hydralazine	IV or IM	0.15–0.2 mg/kg, repeated q 6 hr	10–20 min	3–6 hr	Headache, nausea, vomiting, reflex tachycardia	
Labetalol	IV	0.5–2 mg/min as continuous infusion; stop when goal BP reached; repeat q 6 hr	1–5 min	Varies; about 6 hr	Hypotension, bronchospasm	Asthma, first-degree heart block
Nifedipine	Sublingual or PO	1–10 mg q 2–4 hr	10–15 min	2–3 hr	Headache; dose difficult to measure in young children	
Propranolol	IV or PO (PO preferred)	0.5–1 mg/kg q 6 hr	20–30 min IV	8 hr	Arrythmogenic when used IV; CNS depression, decreased cardiac output, renal blood flow; bronchospasm	Asthma, CHF, diabetes
Minoxidil	PO	0.1–0.2 mg/kg q 8–24 hr	1 hr	8 hr	Reflex tachycardia, salt and water retention, hirsutism (chronic)	Diuretic often needed
Captopril	PO	0.5–1 mg/kg tid	1 hr	8 hr	Rash, proteinuria (rare): Renal insufficiency in renovascular disease	Bilateral renal artery disease

and has been traditionally been given as a rapid intravenous (IV) bolus to limit removal by binding during the first pass. Duration of action is significantly longer than that of sodium nitroprusside. Given as a bolus, diazoxide is less controllable than sodium nitroprusside, although there is a "floor" to its action. Its use has largely been supplanted by sodium nitroprusside, although administration by mini-bolus has recently been advocated as allowing improved control.[52] Hyperglycemia resulting from inhibition of insulin action is another side effect.

Hydralazine has long been used in pediatrics, and many clinicians are familiar with the drug. Its potency is significantly less than that of sodium nitroprusside, although onset of action is reasonably rapid (10 to 20 minutes) when given parenterally. Intramuscular injection has been a widely used route in the past. The drug does cause significant reflex tachycardia and when used chronically has often been combined with a beta blocker. Hydralazine increases cardiac work, which can be serious following myocardial infarction, but this is rarely a problem in children. Use of hydralazine should probably be limited to less emergent hypertension because of the variability of response. Hydralazine can be useful in the emergency department setting and is less likely to result in overly vigorous decreases in blood pressure.

Minoxidil is a potent orally active agent that can be used in accelerated hypertension. The onset of action is within 1 hour, with a peak effect at 4 to 8 hours. There is some reflex tachycardia. Major adverse effects include marked salt and water retention, and concomitant therapy with a diuretic is necessary. Significant hirsutism is a long-term problem.

Calcium Channel Blockers

Nifedipine has been used with increasing frequency in acute hypertension and is particularly valuable in the emergency department or in the field, as it can be conveniently given sublingually. Decrements in blood pressure are modest, and overtreatment is unusual. Action is by vasodilation secondary to blockade of calcium channels in vascular smooth muscle. The onset of action is within 10 to 15 minutes when given sublingually; duration of action is short, and repeat dosing may be required in 1 to 2 hours. Variable absorption and action have sometimes been reported. Side effects are minimal, although cerebral vasodilation can cause headache. Unfortunately, pediatric experience is limited, and dosing can be problematic. The drug is a viscous liquid contained in 10-mg capsules, and administration of a smaller dose, as required in young children, necessitates cutting the capsule and attempting to measure the viscous liquid in a syringe. A sustained-release form is now available for more chronic oral use. Other calcium channel blockers such as verapamil are rarely used in hypertension because of their cardiac depressant effects. Additional agents are currently being developed and marketed, but again, pediatric experience is limited.

Alpha- and Beta-Adrenergic Blockers

Beta blockers, of which propranolol is the prototype, have been used intravenously for treatment of acute hypertension, but propranolol, when used intravenously, may cause arrythmias. Other disadvantages include decreased cardiac contractility, central nervous system depression, and diminished renal blood flow. Asthma is a strong contraindication because of the risk of bronchospasm. Oral dosing is generally preferred. Beta blockade may be of benefit in diminishing the reflex tachycardia associated with vasodilators.

Alpha-adrenergic blockers are of limited use. Phentolamine, a direct alpha-adrenergic blocker with both alpha$_1$- and alpha$_2$-blocking activity is occasionally useful in disorders associated with excessive catecholamine production (e.g., pheochromocytoma). The onset of action is rapid, and the duration is brief. Surgical removal of pheochromocytomas is particularly difficult, as blood pressure may increase drastically with manipulation of the tumor and then plummet with removal. Careful attention must be paid to preoperative fluid balance to minimize postoperative hypotension. Prazosin is a postsynaptic alpha$_1$ blocker that has no role in hypertensive emergencies. Labetalol is an interesting agent with both alpha- and beta-blocking activity. Used intravenously, labetalol has an onset of action within 5 minutes and a duration of action of 3 to 6 hours, and can be used in the treatment of acute hypertension.[53] There is limited published pediatric experience. Labetalol has no effect on cardiac output, although, as with beta blockers, it may cause bronchospasm and should be avoided in patients with pulmonary disease. Several dosing regimens can be used, but continuous intravenous infusion is convenient and associated with few side effects. A continuous drip is begun at a dose of 0.5 to 2.0 mg/min. Blood pressure is monitored carefully, and the drip is interrupted when the desired reduction in blood pressure is achieved. The same dosage can then be repeated in 3 to 6 hours as the drug is cleared. Labetalol can be given without direct arterial pressure measurements by using a Dinamap set to cycle frequently.

Centrally Acting Agents

Methyldopa is rarely used for acute hypertension because of its unpredictable onset. In addition, it causes significant sedation, which can cause difficulties in evaluating neurologic function. Oral clonidine has been used for accelerated hypertension in adults but again, sedation is a problem, unless this effect is specifically desired.

Angiotensin Converting Enzyme Inhibitors

Captopril and enalapril inhibit angiotensin converting enzyme, thereby lowering blood pressure by inhibiting conversion of angiotensin I to angiotensin II and by inhibiting metabolism of bradykinin. This duality of action explains the usefulness of these agents in low-renin hypertension, as well as in high-renin states. Although not specifically approved, captopril has been used with increasing frequency in neonatal hypertension and has been effective and well tolerated.[54] A potential risk is acute renal failure, which can occur if bilateral renovascular disease is present. In this situation renal function is dependent on renal vasodilation through autoregulation. This system requires an intact renin angiotensin system and is disrupted by angiotensin converting enzyme inhibition.

Onset of action of angiotensin converting enzyme inhibitors is too slow to allow their use in emergent hypertension. There are intriguing data, however, showing that angiotensin converting enzyme inhibitors shift the cerebral autoregulatory curve to the left, thereby improving tolerance to low blood pressure.[55] These agents are of great value in chronic treatment of hypertension.

Diuretics

Concomitant diuretic therapy is often necessary to prevent reflex salt and water retention when vasodilators are used. In general, a loop diuretic such as furosemide or bumetanide is needed. In steroid-induced hypertension, diuretic treatment may be sufficient, as the primary defect is salt and water retention. However, diuretics are more useful for chronic antihypertensive therapy and have a limited role in the emergency setting.

DISPOSITION AND PROGNOSIS

Specific admission criteria are difficult to determine. Obviously acute hypertension with symptoms or complications (e.g., hypertensive encephalopathy or malignant hypertension) requires admission to an intensive care unit, where direct arterial pressure monitoring and controlled therapy with potent intravenous agents are available. The child with severe but asymptomatic hypertension also warrants admission, as response to antihypertensive agents can be variable, and careful titration may be needed. Severe hypertension has been defined by the NHLBI as pressures greater then the 99th percentile for age.[3] Modest elevations of blood pressure in an asymptomatic child do not necessitate admission and may in fact not represent hypertension. Blood pressure is often labile, and the emergency department generally has an upsetting influence on a child. These children should be referred for further evaluation. Diagnosis of mild to moderate hypertension is best done by the primary pediatrician and should be based on repeated measurements. Current recommendations are that blood pressure readings above the 95th percentile for the age on three separate occasions warrants further evaluation. Pressure readings between the 90th and 95th percentile are termed *high normal* and are often explained by increased height, with weight proportional to height.[3]

The outcome of hypertension depends primarily on the underlying disease. Prior to the advent of adequate antihypertensive therapy, malignant hypertension and hypertensive encephalopathy were associated with major morbidity and mortality. With appropriate and urgent therapy, patient outcome is significantly improved. Hypertensive encephalopathy secondary to acute poststreptococcal glomerulonephritis tends to resolve without serious sequelae, given prompt control of blood pressure. Prolonged antihypertensive therapy is occasionally needed, but this is unusual. Patients with hemolytic-uremic syndrome and Henoch-Schönlein purpura similarly tend to do well; neonatal hypertension likewise has a good prognosis. In a cohort of infants with significant hypertension during their initial neonatal intensive care unit stay, all were normotensive and off medications at 2 years of age.

Longitudinal studies of long-term therapy in children with chronic hypertension are presently ongoing. There is potential for significant improvements in cardiovascular risk factors by early and appropriate preventive therapy.

References

1. Roberts J. Blood pressure levels of persons 6–74 years. DHEW publ. no. (HRA) 78-1648 203, 1977.

2. Shear CL, Burke GL, Freedman DS, et al. Value of childhood blood pressure measurements and family history in predicting future blood pressure status: Results from 8 years of follow-up in the Bogalusa Heart Study. Pediatrics 1986;77:862.
3. Report of the Second Task Force on Blood Pressure Control in Children—1987. Pediatrics 1987;79:1.
4. Park MK, Menard SM. Accuracy of blood pressure measurement by the Dinamap monitor in infants and children. Pediatrics 1987;79:907.
5. Strandgaard S, Olesen J, Skinhoj E, et al. Autoregulation of brain circulation in severe arterial hypertension. Br Med J 1973;1:507.
6. Trompeter RS, Smith RL, Hoare RD, et al. Neurologic complications of arterial hypertension. Arch Dis Child 1982;57:913.
7. Still JL, Cotton D. Severe hypertension in childhood. Arch Dis Child 1967;42:34.
8. Houston MC. Pathophysiology, clinical aspects and treatment of hypertensive crises. Prog Card Dis 1989;32:99.
9. Paulson OB, Waldemar G, Schmidt JF, et al. Cerebral circulation under normal and pathologic conditions. Am J Card 1989;63:2C.
10. Strandgaard S. Autoregulation of cerebral blood flow in hypertensive patients. The modifying influence of prolonged antihypertensive treatment on the tolerance to acute drug-induced hypotension. Circulation 1976;53:720.
11. Barry DI. Cerebrovascular aspects of antihypertensive treatment. Am J Cardiol 1989;63:14C.
12. Plets C. Arterial hypertension in neurosurgical emergencies. Am J Cardiol 1989;63:40C.
13. Muizelaar JP. Induced arterial hypertension in the treatment of high ICP. Presented at the 7th international symposium on intracranial pressure and brain injury. Ann Arbor, MI, 1988.
14. Kanter RK, Carroll JB, Post EM. Association of arterial hypertension with poor outcome in children with acute brain injury. Clin Pediatr 1985;24:320.
15. Byrom FB. Pathogenesis of hypertensive encephalopathy and its relation to the malignant phase of hypertension. Lancet 1954;2:201.
16. MacKenzie ET, Strandgaard S, Graham DI. Effects of acutely induced hypertension in cats on pial arteriolar caliber, local cerebral blood flow, and the blood brain barrier. Circ Res 1976;34:435.
17. Auer L. The sausage-string phenomenon in acutely induced hypertension—arguments against the vasospasm theory in the pathogenesis of acute hypertensive encephalopathy. Eur Neurol 1978;17:166.
18. Johansson B, Strandgaard S, Lassen NA. On the pathogenesis of hypertensive encephalopathy: The hypertensive "breakthrough" of autoregulation of cerebral blood flow with forced vasodilation, flow increase, and blood brain barrier damage. Circ Res 1974;35:167.
19. Griswold WR, Viney J, Mendoza SA, et al. Intracranial pressure monitoring in severe hypertensive encephalopathy. Crit Care Med 1981;9:573.
20. Eisenberg S. Blood volume in patients with acute glomerulonephritis as determined by radioactive chromium tagged red cells. Am J Med 1959;27:241.
21. Powell HR, Rotenberg E, Williams AL, et al. Plasma renin activity in acute post-streptococcal glomerulonephritis and the hemolytic uremic syndrome. Arch Dis Child 1974;49:802.
22. Loirat C, Sonsino E, Varga Moreno A, et al. Hemolytic-uremic syndrome: An analysis of the natural history and prognostic features. Acta Paediatr Scand 1984;73:505.
23. Stanley P, Gyepes MT, Olson DL. Renovascular hypertension in children and adolescents. Radiology 1978;129:123.
24. Fommei E, Ghione S, Palla L, et al. Renal scintigraphic captopril test in the diagnosis of renovascular hypertension. Hypertension 1987;10:212.
25. Vailis GN, Brouillette RT, Scott JP, et al. Neonatal aortic thrombosis: Recent experience. J Pediatr 1986;109:101.
26. Adelman RD. Neonatal hypertension. Pediatr Clin North Am 1978;25:99.
27. Duncan RE, Evans AT, Martin LW. Natural history and treatment of renal vein thrombosis in children. J Pediatr Surg 1977;12:639.
28. Holland NH, Kotchen T, Bhathena D. Hypertension in children with chronic pyelonephritis. Kidney Int 1975;8S:243.
29. Munoz A, Pascual JF. Arterial hypertension in infants with hydronephrosis. Am J Dis Child 1977;131:38.
30. Savage JM, Dillon MJ, Shah V, et al. Renin and blood pressure in children with renal scarring and vesicoureteric reflux. Lancet 1978;2:441.
31. Baum ES, Morgan EM. Wilms' tumor. Pediatr Ann 1983;12:357.
32. Ganguly A, Gribble J, Tyne B, et al. Renin secreting Wilms' tumor with severe hypertension: Report of a case and brief review of renin secreting tumors. Ann Intern Med 1973;79:835.
33. Ingelfinger JR. Hypertension in children with ESRD. In Fine RN, Gruskin AB, (eds). End Stage Renal Disease in Children. Philadelphia, WB Saunders, 1984.
34. Bennett WM, McDonald WJ, Lawson RK. Post-transplant hypertension: Studies of cortical blood flow and the renal pressor system. Kidney Int 1974;6:99.
35. Cushing H. Some experimental and clinical observations concerning states of increased intracranial tension. The Mütter Lecture for 1901. Am J Med Sci 1902;124:375.
36. Simard JM, Bellefleur M. Systemic arterial hypertension in head trauma. Am J Cardiol 1989;63:32C.
37. Naftchi NE, Tuckman J. Hypertensive crises in spinal man. Am Heart J 1979;97:536.
38. Stackpole RH, Melicow MM, Uson AC. Pheochromocytoma in children: Report of 9 cases and review of the first 100 published cases with follow-up studies. J Pediatr 1963;63:315.
39. Sisson JC, Frager MS, Valk TW, et al. Scintigraphic localization of pheochromocytoma. N Engl J Med 1981;305:12.
40. Loridan L, Senior E. Cushing's syndrome in infancy. J Pediatr 1969;75:349.
41. New MI, Levine IS. Adrenocortical hypertension. Pediatr Clin North Am 1978;25:67.
42. Horowitz JD, Howes JD, Cristophidis N, et al. Hypertensive responses induced by phenylpropanolamine in anorectic and decongestant preparations. Lancet 1980;1:60.
43. Eastman JW, Cohen SN. Hypertensive crisis and death associated with phencyclidine poisoning. JAMA 1975;231:1270.
44. McNicholl B, Kilroy MK. Transient hypertensive encephalopathy: Possible relation to licorice. J Pediatr 1969;74:963.
45. Ingelfinger JR. Hypertension and hypotension. In Ichikawa I (ed). Pediatric Textbook of Fluids and Electrolytes. Baltimore, Williams & Wilkins, 1990.
46. Popp MG, Silberstein EB, Srivastava LS. A pathophysiologic study of the hypertension associated with burn injury in children. Ann Surg 1981;193:817.
47. Turner MC, Ruley EJ, Buckley KM, et al. Blood pressure elevation in children with orthopedic immobilization. J Pediatr 1979;95:989.
48. Abman SH, Warady BA, Lum GM, et al. Systemic hypertension in infants with bronchopulmonary dysplasia. J Pediatr 1984;104:928.
49. Gordillo-Paniagua G, Velasquez-Jones L, Martini R, et al. Sodium nitroprusside treatment of severe arterial hypertension in children. J Pediatr 1975;87:799.
50. Davis RF, Douglas ME, Heenan TJ. Brain tissue pressure measurement during nitroprusside infusion. Crit Care Med 1981;9:17.
51. McCrory WW, Kohut EC, Lewy JE, et al. Safety of intravenous diazoxide in children with severe hypertension. Clin Pediatr 1979;18:661.
52. Ram CVS, Kaplan NM. Individual titration of diazoxide dosage in the treatment of severe hypertension. Am J Cardiol 1979;43:627.
53. Vlachakis ND, Maronde RF, Maloy JW, et al. Pharmacodynamics of intravenous labetalol and follow-up therapy with oral labetalol. Clin Pharmacol Ther 1985;38:503.
54. Bifano E, Post EM, Springer J, et al. Treatment of neonatal hypertension with captopril. J Pediatr 1982;100:143.
55. Barry DI, Jarden JO, Paulson OB, et al. Cerebrovascular aspects of converting enzyme inhibition. I. Effects of intravenous captopril on spontaneously hypertensive and normotensive rats. J Hypertens 1984;2:589.

SECTION THREE

Pulmonary Disease

CHAPTER 24

Apnea

R. Daryl Steiner

INTRODUCTION

Sudden infant death syndrome (SIDS) is "the sudden death of any infant or young child which is unexpected by history and in which a thorough postmortem examination fails to demonstrate an adequate cause for death."[1] This poorly understood, mysterious, and tragic entity affects approximately 8000 infants yearly in the United States and is responsible for 45% of all postperinatal infant deaths and 20% of all deaths in infants age 8 days to 14 years. SIDS ranks second in incidence only to accidents as a cause of death in childhood.[2] To reduce the incidence of SIDS, focus has been placed on the antecedent event of SIDS, apnea, hoping that intervention at this point will prevent the tragic outcome of SIDS.

Any discussion involving the significance of apnea and its relationship to SIDS is controversial because of the confusion often surrounding the identification of the patients to be studied. These infants often present to the physician after being first observed by an anxious, untrained observer. The resulting heterogeneous group of infants makes review of this subject difficult.

Despite the similarities between the infant who has suffered an apneic episode and the infant who has died from SIDS, several investigators have failed to find that healthy infants who were prospectively monitored and who subsequently died of SIDS had any monitored evidence of apnea or bradycardia.[3,4]

The incidence of apneic episodes is difficult to determine, largely because the reports are made by untrained, nonmedical observers. There is no evidence that the number of children with prolonged apneic episodes is growing.

The American Academy of Pediatrics' Task Force on Prolonged Apnea has defined apnea as "the cessation of breathing for at least 20 seconds or a briefer episode of apnea associated with bradycardia, cyanosis, or pallor."[4] This definition eliminates short pauses in the respiratory cycle that occur normally. Even with this clarification, apnea's association with SIDS remains as the terms *near-miss SIDS* and *aborted SIDS* continue to be used. To eliminate this unwarranted connection between apnea and SIDS, the National Institutes of Health (NIH) in 1986 published a consensus statement that the reported episodes of apnea be known as *apparent life-threatening events* (ALTEs).[5] Implied in

an ALTE is a breakdown in the normal control mechanisms maintaining ventilation and preventing or terminating apnea.

PHYSIOLOGY

The respiratory control system guards against hypoxemia and hypercapnia, changing the frequency of respiration and the tidal volume by varying the timing of inspiratory or expiratory flow in response to metabolic demands or variations in impedance to air flow. The regulation of breathing involves the interaction of respiratory muscles in the upper airway and thorax and their action on the passive elements in the thorax. Adequate minute ventilation is modulated by the carotid body, chemoreceptors in the central medulla, and the afferent limb of the vagus nerve.

Several factors unique to the newborn increase the newborn's vulnerability to the effects of hypoventilation. Anatomically, the hypopharynx is shallower, the tongue and epiglottis located more cephalad, and the mandible more mobile than in adults. In addition, the newborn's rib cage is more compliant, which results in a relatively lower functional residual capacity. The functional residual capacity serves as a reservoir for oxygen in the body; this falls rapidly during periods of apnea.

The young infant is continuously developing, and so are the systems that control the function of respiration. Infants normally have a respiratory pattern that consists of alternating periods of regular breathing and respiratory pauses of up to 10 seconds in length, which are associated with no color change. This respiratory pattern is termed *periodic breathing* and is most often noted during sleep. It is considered to be normal if it comprises no more than 3% of the sleep time. However, the significance of periodic breathing that comprises more than 10% of sleep time is unclear.

Infants also demonstrate simple respiratory pauses. These pauses are only 5 to 15 seconds in duration, are not accompanied by a change in color or muscle tone, and are often associated with a sigh or a Valsalva maneuver.

Sucking and swallowing require that the infant has established a prompt airway defense mechanism. This defense mechanism results in a maneuver that begins with secretion or swallowed food coming into contact with the glottis and results in choking with repeated swallowing and a brief period of stridor. When the airway defense maneuver is associated with flushing or cyanosis, it is often mistaken for an ALTE.

When a prolonged period of apnea is the presenting symptom, it need not be the primary symptom (Table 24–1). Acute illnesses such as meningitis, sepsis, respiratory syncytial virus (RSV) pneumonia, and pertussis often have apnea as the presenting complaint.

The infant may also have a chronic condition that is associated with varying periods of apnea. The most common

TABLE 24–1

DIFFERENTIAL DIAGNOSIS OF INFANTILE APNEA

Normal respiratory variation
  Periodic breathing
  Respiratory pauses
  Airway defense maneuver

Acute illness
  Sepsis
  Meningitis
  Respiratory syncytial virus
  Pertussis
  Traumatic intracranial hemorrhage

Chronic illness
  Gastroesophageal reflux
  Seizures

Defective respiratory control
  CNS anomalies
  CNS immaturity
  Drugs
  Chronic hypoxia

chronic illness that is associated with apneic episodes is a seizure disorder. Along with prolonged apnea, the infant often will present with a history of color change and an alteration in muscle tone. These seizures can occur during sleep as well as during waking hours.

Gastroesophageal reflux is another chronic condition that may have associated apnea. The apnea results when the gastric contents contact and stimulate the receptors in the esophagus and larynx. Infants are likely to demonstrate a period of apnea, and the increased vagal activity in some infants produces bradycardia and cyanosis.

Occasionally a chronic condition involving a primary defect in the respiratory control centers causes apnea. These defects may result in failure to initiate contraction of the muscles of respiration, coordinate the contraction-relaxation cycle of the upper airway musculature, or maintain an appropriate rate and depth of respiration (Ondine's curse) or in the failure of sleep arousal when prolonged apnea induces hypoxia. Such dysfunction may be caused by anatomic aberrations, such as Arnold-Chiari malformation, or may be a result of chronic central nervous system hypoxia from chronic lung disease (bronchopulmonary dysplasia) or anemia.

Apnea of prematurity is attributed to a primary defect in the respiratory control center. This typically involves an infant born prematurely who demonstrates an increased frequency of periodic breathing. Both the apnea and periodic breathing resolve by the chronologic age of 1 to 2 months.

Airway anatomy may also account for apnea caused by chronic illness. The anatomic defects of Pierre-Robin syndrome, micrognathia, and hyperglossia and the structural deficiency of the airway in tracheal malacia, combined with the infant's normally shallow hypopharynx and mobile mandible, result in periods of apnea that may be considered ALTEs.

CLINICAL EVALUATION

A detailed history will determine subsequent management. It is essential to determine the state of consciousness prior to the event. Events that occur when the infant is awake are likely to be benign. The duration of the episode is also of key importance, as an episode lasting less than 20 seconds is not pathologic. The presence of pallor or cyanosis indicates

that the period of apnea was significantly severe, placing the infant at increased risk for recurrence. Additionally, any change in the infant's muscle tone, either flaccidity or hypertonicity, indicates the need for further evaluation in order to differentiate an episode of primary apnea from a seizure disorder. If the episode was related to feeding, management might be directed toward the treatment of gastroesophageal reflux rather than primary apnea. Finally, what was needed to resuscitate the infant to the current state of arousal? Vigorous or prolonged resuscitative efforts indicate a concerning event.

Though the parents' observations of the episode must be regarded seriously, they must also be interpreted accurately. Parental response and interpretation of the events are influenced by the parents' knowledge and apprehension. Krongrad and O'Neill[6] reported parents' responses to home electrocardiographic (EKG) monitoring of 20 infants considered to be at high risk for apnea. The parents reported 93 true alarms that they believed to be life threatening. On review of these monitor recordings, none of the reported events were associated with an abnormal EKG.[6]

Physical findings may provide clues to underlying conditions that are the primary cause of the apneic episode. A compromised respiratory status with evidence of dyspnea and air hunger suggests an acute respiratory process. Poor peripheral perfusion with prolonged capillary refill and mottling may signify an overwhelming infection. A child who is active, bright-eyed, alert, and vigorously moving about may have suffered a benign feeding-associated choking episode, not an ALTE. Abrasion and contusions may indicate a trauma-related apneic episode. A congenital anomaly, especially one involving the face, should alert the examiner to the distinct probability of an anatomic cause for the apneic episode.

DIAGNOSTIC EVALUATION

The laboratory evaluation is used to differentiate apnea secondary to an underlying condition from primary apnea. A complete blood cell count may exclude an underlying anemia or suggest an infective process. A normal blood glucose level eliminates hypoglycemia as a cause. In blood gas evaluation particular attention is paid to the bicarbonate value. A chronic hypoventilation condition exists if the bicarbonate level is high; the event is considered acute if the bicarbonate level is low. Though toxic ingestions are rare causes of apnea in this age group, a blood and urine screening test may uncover a toxic agent.

Apnea that is related to a primary cardiac process is better defined by a chest radiograph. A barium swallow should only be done to evaluate the possibility of gastroesophageal reflux. If trauma is suspected, a skeletal survey will identify occult fractures.

Ancillary studies helpful in the evaluation of a child who has suffered an ALTE include an EKG to evaluate the existence of a rhythm disturbance and an electroencephalogram (EEG) to document a seizure disorder.

The final decision that must be made is whether the infant can safely be sent home or should be admitted (Table 24–2). Clearly, not all of these infants require hospitalization. Hospitalization "just to be safe" may only serve to unnecessarily increase parental anxiety for those infants in whom the episodes are not pathologic. However, hospitalization for a 48-hour period does allow continuous cardiorespiratory monitoring to document any recurrence and also allows time to obtain the results of all studies and confirm the absence of serious acute illness. Hospitalization also gives the staff the time to address the parental anxiety that often accompanies this frightening event.

TABLE 24–2

ADMISSION CRITERIA FOR PATIENTS WITH APNEA

Indicators of a serious event
  Cardiopulmonary resuscitation needed to resuscitate infant
  Failure of infant to respond to initial stimulation
  Delayed onset of crying
  Gasping respiration once respiration is initiated
Indicators of a benign event
  Resumption of normal, quiet respirations
  Vigorous response to initial stimulation
  Alert mental status following resuscitation
  Event associated with feeding

Once the infant is hospitalized, continuous 12- to 24-hour monitoring is performed. This can be accomplished by either pneumography or polysomnography. The pneumogram is a simultaneous recording of the EKG and the respiration pattern using the chest impedance measurements. The polysomnograph, however, simultaneously records the EEG, EKG, electrooculogram, electromyogram, and two-channel respiratory functions. Initially, the pneumogram and polysomnogram were designed as research tools, not as clinical screening tools, and the value of such monitoring in infants is unclear. In the group of 1157 infants studied by the Southhall group, none of the six infants who suffered a sudden death had an abnormal monitor record.[3] The value of physiologic monitoring seems to be in detecting periodic breathing, picking up short periods of apnea, and recording the frequency of each; thereby better defining the need for pharmacotherapy.

Therapy for the child with infantile apnea is directed at the underlying disease process. Therefore antibiotics are prescribed for the infant suffering from an infectious process, and anticonvulsants are used to treat seizures. General supportive therapy is maintained when there are signs of shock. Antireflux measures are implemented for the infant with gastroesophageal reflux.

Specific therapy for apnea is most useful when directed toward stimulation of a defective central nervous system control center. If this defect is documented, methylxanthine therapy is started in the form of theophylline. The methylxanthines are general central nervous system stimulants and thereby stimulate the respiratory control centers. Theophylline is effective at blood levels of between 8 to 10 μg/ml. This blood level can be safely achieved with a dose of 10 mg/kg initially, followed by a dose of 2 to 4 mg/kg every 6 hours. Paradoxically, theophylline for the treatment of one cause of apnea may exacerbate other causes of apnea. The methylxanthines tend to lower the esophageal muscle tone and thereby contribute to gastroesophageal reflux. In addition, methylxanthines lower the seizure threshold, making a seizure disorder more difficult to manage.

HOME MONITORING

Home monitoring may be a useful alternative to prolonged hospital stays for the infant with occasional brief episodes of apnea. Its use, however, may produce undesirable consequences. No study has confirmed that home monitor use prevents SIDS. Nevertheless, anecdotal experiences show that apnea may be terminated by the apnea alarm sounding and the parents responding to revive their infant. However, some infants have died, despite the prompt use of cardiopulmonary resuscitation when the alarm sounded. Failure of the infant to respond to cardiopulmonary resuscitation may be in part a result of the fact that home monitors measure respiratory activity by using electrical impedance to detect chest wall movement. Thus, a child with obstructive apnea would go undetected until hypoxia and fatigue cause cessation of chest wall movement; this may be too late to effect resuscitation.

Once initiated, monitoring should be continued until the infant is at least 6 months of age, a febrile upper respiratory illness passes without apnea, or the infant has been apnea free for 2 months.

References

1. Beckwith JB. Discussion of terminology and definition of sudden infant death syndrome. *In* Bergman AB, Beckwith JB, Ray CG (eds). Proceedings of the Second International Conference on Causes of Sudden Death in Infants. Seattle, University of Washington Press, 1970, pp 14–22.
2. Bergman AB, Ray CG, Pomeroy MA, et al. Studies of the sudden infant death syndrome in King County, Washington. III. Epidemiology. Pediatrics 1971;49:860.
3. Southall DP, Richards JM, Rhoden KJ, et al. Prolonged apnea and cardiac arrhythmias in infants discharged from neonatal intensive care units: Failure to predict an increased risk for sudden infant death syndrome. Pediatrics 1982;70:844.
4. American Academy of Pediatrics. Task force on prolonged apnea. Pediatrics 1985;76:129.
5. National Institutes of Health Consensus Development Conference Statement. Infantile apnea and home monitoring. Vol 6, No 6. Bethesda, MD, US Dept of Health and Human Services, 1986.
6. Kongrad E, O'Neill L. Near miss sudden infant death syndrome episodes? A clinical and electrocardiographic correlation. Pediatrics 1986;77:811.

CHAPTER 25

Asthma

William H. Spivey

INTRODUCTION

Asthma is one of the most common problems seen in the emergency department. It accounts for more than 27 million physician visits annually and is the most common chronic illness in the pediatric population.[1, 2] The incidence ranges from a high of 12% in males, blacks, and Hispanics under the age of 12 years to approximately 8% for all groups during adolescence.[3, 4]

In addition to the morbidity, there has been an increase in the mortality rate from acute asthma documented in the United States and other countries.[5–10] The cause for this increase is unclear, but retrospective studies have indicated that many of these deaths were preventable.[11, 12] Underestimation of the severity of the attack, delay in treatment, and underutilization of beta agonists and corticosteroids have all been implicated as contributing factors.[11]

PATHOPHYSIOLOGY

Asthma is characterized by a hyperreactive airway with reversible obstruction. Airway obstruction in asthma is a multifactorial process consisting of bronchial smooth muscle changes, inflammation, and mucus plugging. Bronchial smooth muscle may become hypertrophied over time and develop both central and peripheral spasm during acute attacks. Acute bronchoconstriction may be induced by agents such as histamine, slow-reacting substance of anaphylaxis, and prostaglandin D_2.[13] Infection, stress, and allergies stimulate the release of these agents, which may lead to inflammation and edema of the lining of the airway (Fig. 25–1).[14] As part of this response, there is an increase in mucus production, and inflammatory cells are secreted into the lumen of the airway.[15] This produces mucus plugging, with further obstruction of the airway. The obstructed airways close prematurely and increase the airway resistance. This leads to a decrease in flow and volume of air exchanged, hyperaeration of the lungs, and increased work of breathing. As the obstruction worsens, a ventilation-perfusion mismatch develops. The patient then hyperventilates, and the CO_2 decreases. As the asthma worsens, CO_2 increases, oxygen decreases, a metabolic and respiratory acidosis develops, and the child begins to fatigue.[16] This is compounded by a loss of fluid from the lungs as a result of the tachypnea, leading to dehydration and thickened respiratory mucus. Right ventricular strain, pulmonary hypertension, and decreased left ventricular filling may also occur.

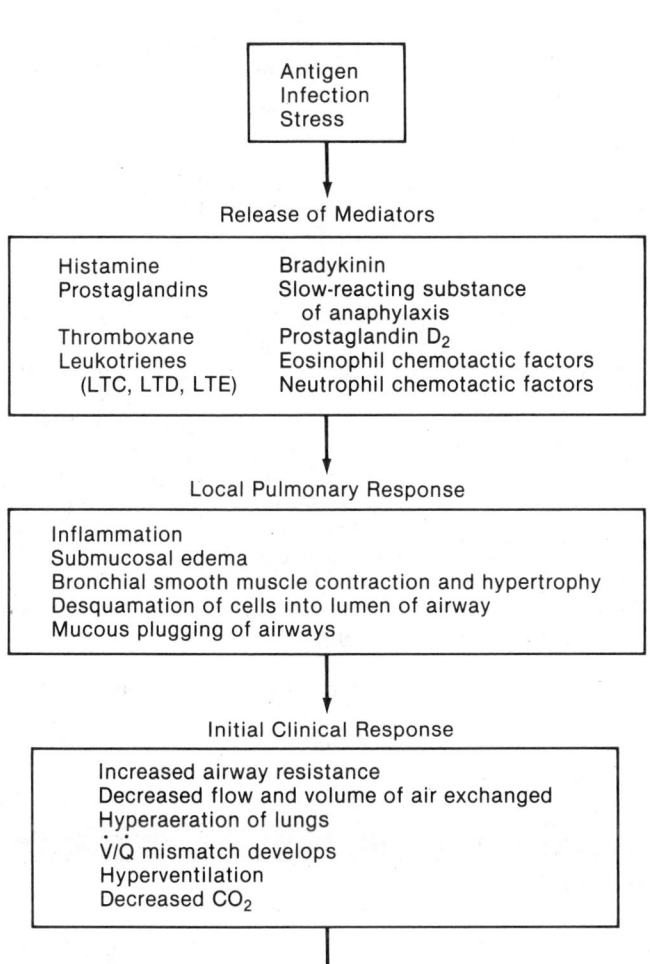

Figure 25–1. Pathophysiology of asthma.

Bronchospasm may be induced by a wide variety of causes such as viral infections, allergens, exercise, drugs, weather, and emotion.[17–19] Viral infections of the upper airway are believed to precipitate asthma by increasing inflammation, mucus production, and airway reactivity.[17, 20] The relationship between acute exacerbations of asthma and viral illness in children has long been recognized. In one study of 6165 children with lower respiratory illness, approximately 30% had wheezing.[21] Wheezing was most commonly seen in children less than 2 years of age, but also occurred in 19% of children over 9 years of age. A prospective study of 32 children ages 1 to 5 years evaluated episodes of acute wheezing and viral respiratory infections. Of the 139 acute asthma attacks, 58 (42%) occurred during a viral respiratory infection.[22] The development of constitutional symptoms is closely related to acute episodes of asthma. Symptoms such as malaise, mucus production, or cough are likely to be associated with wheezing when the patient is infected with a virus.[23]

Several factors determine the effect of a viral illness on lung function. They include the patient's age, sex, underlying airway hyperresponsiveness, severity of the respiratory tract infection, and the respiratory virus itself. Young children, especially males, are more prone to episodes of bronchospasm with a viral illness. The most common infectious agents are respiratory syncytial virus, parainfluenza, adenovirus, and *Mycoplasma pneumoniae*.[24–26]

Bacterial infections do not play a significant role in producing acute asthma attacks. Although a lobar pneumonia may produce wheezing and bronchospasm, for the most part there is little correlation between asthma and bacterial organisms cultured from tracheal aspirations.[27]

Inhalation of an allergen is a common source of acute bronchospasm.[28–31] The allergen may precipitate an immediate reaction, thought to be caused by an immunoglobulin E (IgE) reaction with the allergen, leading to mast cell degranulation and release of mediators of anaphylaxis, which produce bronchospasm. A delayed reaction may occur as an immunoglobulin G (IgG)-mediated response, which involves activation of the complement system and an inflammatory response.[13]

The airway reaction induced by exercise is not a direct result of the exercise, but is thought to be secondary to the inhalation of cold air and the airway's response to a loss of heat.[32, 33] Although most children wheeze to some degree after exercise, some may wheeze both during and after exercise. The airway response to changes in weather is poorly understood but may be caused by changes in barometric pressure or humidity.[34] The response caused by emotion is also incompletely understood. It may be a result of central nervous system input from the vagus nerve directly to peripheral airways.

Drugs such as aspirin and nonsteroidal anti-inflammatory agents may exacerbate asthma.[35, 36] The mechanism for this is thought to be the blockage of prostaglandin production by these agents, which in turn leads to a buildup of leukotrienes.[37] Leukotrienes act like slow-reacting substance of anaphylaxis and lead to an inflammatory response.

EMERGENCY MEDICAL SERVICE CONSIDERATIONS

Emergency medical care in the field should focus on providing oxygen, treating life-threatening disease, and, if possible, initiating bronchodilator therapy. The patient should be placed on 4 L of oxygen and a brief history obtained. This is necessary to confirm that the shortness of breath is indeed a result of bronchospasm and not caused by aspiration of a foreign body, epiglottitis, or tension pneumothorax.

If possible, bronchodilators should be given in the field. Subcutaneous epinephrine, subcutaneous terbutaline, or a nebulized beta agonist may be used. If these are not available, the patient's own nebulizer may be used.

CLINICAL EVALUATION

When first presenting to the emergency department with an acute asthma attack, the patient should be placed on 4 L of oxygen and a brief series of specific questions asked. These questions should focus on the duration of the current attack, use of medications, history of steroid dependence, previous hospitalizations, and preceding symptoms, as follows:

When did the wheezing start?
What medications are used, when were they last used, and has the patient been complaining?
Has the patient ever been on steroids?
When was the last emergency department visit for asthma?
Has the patient ever been hospitalized for asthma? If so, how long ago?
Has the patient ever been intubated and required a ventilator?
Have there been preceding symptoms such as fever, productive cough, rhinitis, or contact with known allergies?

Once the patient has improved, a detailed history may be obtained. More information regarding the severity of this attack in comparison with previous attacks should be obtained, along with information about the patient's usual time course for improvement. History regarding environmental exposure and the family history of asthma or atopic disease are also important.

The physical examination is also brief initially, focusing on the overall degree of distress and respiratory symptoms, and includes the following:

Observation of general appearance—position of the child (sitting vs. leaning forward), nasal flaring, use of accessory muscles, cyanosis or diaphoresis
Auscultation of the lungs for movement of air, inspiratory and expiratory wheezing, prolonged expiratory phase, equal breath sounds, and evidence of rales
Examination for evidence of pulsus paradoxus (greater than 10–mm Hg drop in systolic pressure with inspiration in moderate to severe asthmatics)

Once the patient has improved, a more detailed physical examination should include evaluation of the eyes, ears, nose, pharynx, and neck. The heart should be auscultated for evidence of a murmur and the lungs reevaluated for rales or evidence of pneumonia.

Wheezing may not always be present with obstructive airway disease. Patients with severe asthma and reduced airflow often have few sounds on auscultation of the lungs. Wheezes may not be heard until after initial therapy and clinical improvement. Wheezing may also not occur if the obstruction is mild. In mild cases, the only symptom may be coughing as a result of increased mucus production.

Several systems for scoring the severity of asthma and following clinical improvement have been devised. They commonly use skin color, breath sounds, use of accessory muscles, expiratory wheezing, and cerebral function (Table 25–1). Scoring systems do not replace experienced clinical judgment but do provide a standardized method for following improvement in asthmatics by different observers.[38]

DIAGNOSTIC EVALUATION

Few diagnostic studies are of any real value in the pediatric asthmatic patient. A peak expiratory flow rate (PEFR) or forced expiratory volume (FEV) is useful in determining the severity of the attack and gauging improvement. However, most children under the age of 7 years are unable to cooperate sufficiently to use these tests. The predicted PEFR may be calculated using the following formula:

Males: PEFR × height (cm) − 500 = L/min
Females: PEFR × height (cm) − 400 = L/min

If the PEFR does not improve to at least 65% of normal, the patient should be considered for admission.[39]

A chest radiograph is not indicated for most cases of acute asthma. Exceptions include patients with rales or focal findings on auscultation, those with failure to improve with therapy, or those experiencing the first attack. Unless there are complications, the chest radiograph will only show a mild hyperaeration of the lungs with an increase in anteroposterior diameter and flattening of the diaphragm.

Arterial blood gas measurements are also not indicated in uncomplicated asthma. If the patient is either severely short of breath or does not improve, however, they may prove useful. In mild asthma, there is little or no change in partial oxygen pressure (PO_2), while CO_2 decreases and pH increases. As the obstruction worsens, PO_2 decreases, partial carbon dioxide pressure (PCO_2) increases, and pH decreases (Table 25–2). A child who is acidotic and has a PCO_2 of 40 mm Hg or greater is in danger of respiratory failure and should be intubated.

Other than determination of theophylline level, few blood tests provide any useful information. Determination of the theophylline level is useful not only to confirm compliance

TABLE 25–1			
CLINICAL ASTHMA SCORE			
	Score		
	0	**1**	**2**
PaO_2	70–100 in room air	<70 in room air	<70 in 40% oxygen
Cyanosis	None	In air	In 40% oxygen
Respiratory breath sounds	Normal	Unequal	Decreased to absent
Accessory muscle use	None	Moderate	Maximal
Expiratory wheezing	None	Moderate	Marked
Cerebral function	Normal	Depressed or agitated	Coma

Adapted from Wood BW, Downes JJ, Lecks HI. A clinical scoring system for the diagnosis of respiratory failure. Am J Dis Child 1972; 123:227. Copyright 1972, American Medical Association.

TABLE 25–2			
ARTERIAL BLOOD GAS CHANGES IN ASTHMA			
Airway Obstruction	Po$_2$	Pco$_2$	pH
Mild	Normal	Decreased	Increased
Moderate	Decreased	Normal or decreased	Normal or increased
Severe	Decreased	Increased	Decreased

with medications, but also to adjust dosing regimens to keep up with the growth and development of the child.

The white blood cell count is neither sensitive nor specific for pneumonia and is normally elevated slightly in asthma because of stress and demargination. Eosinophilia greater than 250 to 400 cells/mm^3 is common in asthma but rarely used as a diagnostic test. Electrolyte and glucose levels do not change appreciably during asthma and are of no value.

Sputum cultures and Gram stain tests are rarely useful, as bacterial superinfection is rare. Eosinophilia of the sputum is commonly seen in asthma but is not often used to make a diagnosis.

DIFFERENTIAL DIAGNOSIS

The differential diagnosis for asthma changes with the age of the child (Table 25–3).[40] Causes of wheezing in infants can be divided into three categories: infection, aspiration, or congenital abnormality. The most common cause of wheezing in infants is infection. This is usually a result of viral bronchitis, which produces an inflammatory response and narrowing of the airway. It is difficult to differentiate between bronchiolitis and asthma at the first presentation of a child under 1 year of age. Symptoms such as fever, cough, and coryza suggest a viral infection, whereas a family history of asthma and no viral symptoms suggest an initial asthma attack. Several episodes of wheezing during the first 2 years of life is highly suggestive of asthma.

In addition to viral infections, a bacterial pneumonia may also produce wheezing. As in a viral infection, an inflammatory response is produced by the bacteria, which leads to airway narrowing and wheezing.

Although more common in older children, aspiration should be considered in infants. Aspiration of formula or food will produce either a bilateral or a unilateral inflammatory response. The infant may have a low-grade fever but usually does not present with the increased secretions seen with a viral illness. If the wheezing is unilateral, aspiration of a foreign body should be suspected.

During the early months of life, an infant may also present with wheezing caused by a congenital defect. Congenital

TABLE 25–3	
DIFFERENTIAL DIAGNOSIS OF ASTHMA	
Infants	Children
Bronchiolitis	Bronchiolitis
Pneumonia	Pneumonia
Aspiration	Foreign body aspiration
Congestive heart failure	Pneumothorax
Tracheoesophageal fistula	Pulmonary edema or embolism
	Congestive heart failure
	Cystic fibrosis
	Hyperventilation
	Neoplasm (pulmonary or mediastinal)

heart defects may lead to congestive heart failure that presents as wheezing. The presence of a heart murmur or a history of failure to thrive should alert the physician to consider a heart defect as the source of the problem. A tracheoesophageal fistula produces a clinical picture similar to that of aspiration, but with tracheoesophageal fistula, the child may have coughing during feeding or difficulty with feeding.

Children can present with many of the same diseases that mimic asthma in infants. Infection, foreign body aspiration, and congestive heart failure produce wheezing in both infants and older children. As the child ages, other diagnoses should be considered. Cystic fibrosis may begin to present as wheezing and coughing. A pulmonary embolus, although rare, may present as chest pain, tachypnea, tachycardia, and wheezing. A child with increasing fatigue, night sweats, weight loss, or failure to thrive should be examined for the possibility of pulmonary or mediastinal neoplasm.

A pneumothorax may present with chest pain, tachypnea, and wheezing. A spontaneous pneumothorax may be seen in older children who smoke marijuana or other drugs and then perform a Valsalva maneuver. This increases the thoracic pressure, leading to the rupture of a bronchus and subsequent pneumothorax. Hyperventilation may produce wheezing and usually occurs in school age children or adolescents. The wheezing is usually caused by voluntary upper airway narrowing and is associated with numbness of the hands and perioral area. It usually follows a stressful event.

A physician should suspect the possibility of a nonasthma origin in the adolescent who presents with the first episode of wheezing. The diagnosis of asthma is usually made during the first 12 years of life, and adolescents who appear in the emergency department with a sudden onset of wheezing should be closely questioned for systemic complaints, and a social history should be obtained.

THERAPEUTIC INTERVENTION

General Measures

Increased hospitalization and mortality results from failure to both recognize the severity of the attack and provide aggressive treatment. It is important for the emergency physician to carefully evaluate the patient with asthma, especially while therapy is administered and during the periods between aerosol treatments.

Oxygen (4 L/min) should be administered by nasal cannula to patients with mild or moderate asthma. More severe asthma requires high-flow, humidified oxygen delivered by face mask and cardiac monitoring. Continuous pulse oximetry is not necessary in mild to moderate cases of asthma, but in severe cases it will help to ensure that the patient is adequately oxygenated and is not deteriorating.

Hydration helps to mobilize secretions that may otherwise become sticky and plug the bronchioles. Oral hydration is adequate for most asthmatic patients, but those requiring intravenous medications or those who are likely to require admission should have an intravenous line started to provide hydration and vascular access.

Beta Agonists

The first line of pharmacologic therapy is a rapid-acting beta agonist (Table 25–4). Beta agonists may be divided into beta$_1$- and beta$_2$-receptor stimulators. Beta$_1$-receptor stimulation produces an increase in chronotropic and inotropic effects on the heart.[41] Beta$_2$-receptor stimulation results in bronchodilation, inhibition of mast cell degranulation, decreased bronchial secretions, increased clearance of mucus by cilia, vasodilation, and skeletal muscle tremor.[42] When the beta$_2$-adrenergic receptor on a cell surface is stimulated, it activates adenyl cyclase, which in turn converts intracellular adenosine triphosphate (ATP) to cyclic adenosine monophosphate (AMP). Cyclic AMP acts to regulate intracellular calcium movement and thus smooth muscle relaxation.[42] Increased cyclic AMP also inhibits mast cell degranulation.

Parenteral and nebulized drugs may be either combination beta$_1$ and beta$_2$ agonists or beta$_2$-selective agents. The beta$_2$-selective agents produce fewer cardiac effects and have increased in popularity in recent years.[43–46]

The choice of parenteral or nebulized therapy depends on the age and cooperation of the patient. Young children and infants in many cases can be treated with nebulized beta agonists using a face mask, rather than subcutaneous injections. Older children are usually able to cooperate with a nebulizer and do not require subcutaneous injections. This eliminates the fear of coming to the hospital for treatment and the exacerbation of bronchospasm that occurs with crying after an injection.

Nebulized agents should be administered using 6 L/min of oxygen. This helps correct hypoxemia resulting from a ventilation-perfusion mismatch.[47] Nebulized therapy may be used for all asthmatic patients, even severely obstructed children, as long as there is adequate air movement. They work as well as parenteral agents, regardless of the severity of the disease.[48]

The optimal dose of nebulized agents and the frequency with which they should be administered continue to be controversial. Most investigators recommend that these drugs be given every 20 to 30 minutes and not more frequently than every 20 minutes, a recommendation that is also supported by the drugs' manufacturers. However, some studies have shown beneficial effects in severely ill children using either continuous nebulization or high doses of nebulized drugs.[49]

Several studies have reported a beneficial effect of continuously nebulized terbutaline in severely ill children.[49–51] In one study terbutaline (2 mg/hr) was administered by continuous nebulized treatment. The PCO_2 decreased in all the patients, but the greatest decrease (15 mm Hg in 8.7 hr) was seen in that group with a PCO_2 of 45 mm Hg or greater.[49] Another study reported 12 children who received between 1.0 and 12.0 mg/hr of continuous nebulized terbutaline.[51] All children improved, and none experienced significant side effects. The mean duration of therapy was 8.3 hr (range, 1 to 24 hr). Although other beta agonists could be given as continuous therapy, terbutaline has been most widely studied. Continuous therapy has not been studied in the emergency department for shorter periods of time.

In addition to continuous nebulized therapy, higher than currently recommended doses of beta agonists may offer an advantage in severely obstructed children. One study comparing low-dose albuterol (0.05 mg/kg) and high-dose albu-

---

TABLE 25–4

THERAPY AT A GLANCE

Parenteral agents

Epinephrine (Adrenalin)—Dose: 0.01 ml/kg of 1:1000, given subcutaneously; maximum dose, 0.35 ml. May be repeated every 20 min up to three times. Side effects include tachycardia, hypertension, and tremor. (Use diminishing.)

Sus-Phrine—1:200; Dose: 0.005 ml/kg. Long-acting form of epinephrine administered subcutaneously after the patient has cleared. It helps to prevent a recurrence of wheezing. Side effects include tachycardia and tremor.

Terbutaline (Brethine)—Dose: 0.01 ml/kg of 1 mg/ml given subcutaneously; maximum dose, 0.25 ml. May be repeated every 20 min. Side effects include tachycardia and tremor. (More selective than epinephrine.)

Theophylline—Dose: 6–7 mg/kg loading dose; 1.2 mg/kg/hr maintenance for those under 10 yr old; 0.8 mg/kg/hr maintenance for those over 10 yr old. Side effects include tachycardia, tremor, vomiting, and seizures.

Isoproterenol—Dose: 0.1 µg/kg/min, increased by 0.1 µg/kg/min every 15 min until patient is improved or tachycardic. Side effects include tachycardia.

Ketamine—Dose: 0.5–2.0 mg/kg. May be given every 30 min. Side effects include tachycardia, postanesthetic hallucinations.

Steroids—Methylprednisolsone (Solumedrol): 1–2 mg/kg q 6 hr. Hydrocortisone (Solu-Cortef): 4–5 mg/kg q 6 hr. Side effects: none for acute or short-term use.

Nebulized agents

Metaproterenol 5% (Alupent)—Dose: 0.1 ml for those under 2 yr old; 0.2 ml for those 2–9 yr; 0.3 ml for those over 9 yr old. Mixed with 2.5 ml saline in nebulizer. May be repeated every 20 min. Side effects include tachycardia (mild).

Isoetharine 1% (Bronkosol)—Dose: 0.25–0.5 ml. Mixed with 2.5 ml saline in nebulizer. Not to be given less than 20 min apart. Side effects include tachycardia (mild).

Albuterol (Salbutamol) 0.5% (5 mg/ml)—Dose: 0.2 ml for those less than 2 yr old; 0.4 ml for those 2–9 yr; 0.6 ml for those over 9 yr old. Side effects include tachycardia (mild).

Terbutaline (Brethine)—Dose: 0.03–0.05 ml/kg (1 mg/ml) mixed in 2.5 ml saline in nebulizer. Given every 4 hr. Has also been reported as a continuous therapy using 2 mg/hr. Side effects include tachycardia.

Atropine—Dose: 0.01–0.03 ml/kg (0.01 mg/kg) mixed in 2.5 saline in nebulizer. Used every 3–4 hr. Side effects include tachycardia.

Drugs for intubation

Pancuronium—Defasciculating dose: 0.01 mg/kg IV. Give 5 min before succinylcholine. Side effects include respiratory depression. Don't use pancuronium in children under 5 yr old.

Succinylcholine—Dose: 1–2 mg/kg IV. Produces total paralysis for 5 min. Side effects include respiratory arrest and bradycardia. Pretreat with atropine (0.02 mg/kg IV) to prevent bradycardia, unless patient is tachycardic.

Diazepam—Dose: 0.1–0.2 mg/kg IV. Administered prior to intubation for sedation and amnesia. Side effects include respiratory depression and hypotension.

terol (0.15 mg/kg) given as a nebulized treatment every 15 minutes demonstrated significantly greater improvement in forced vital capacity and asthma symptoms, with decreased hospitalization time in children receiving the high dose of albuterol.[52] There was no difference in adverse effects, blood pressure, white blood cell count, or serum potassium level. Thus for patients with severe asthma who respond poorly to standard doses of conventional therapy, higher doses of beta agonists may be beneficial.[53, 54] If high doses are used, however, they should be used under constant observation and monitoring for adverse effects.

In general, nebulized beta agonists have a wide margin of safety, especially when compared with parenteral agents.[55–58] The adverse side effects seen with nebulized beta agonists are further minimized when a beta$_2$-selective agent is used. However, all of the beta agonists have side effects that should be monitored for and prevented if possible. The most common side effects included anxiety, tremor, nausea, vomiting, and tachycardia. These effects are seen less commonly in young children and may be minimized by using the recommended doses of beta agonist. The nebulized route allows a smaller dose of the drug to be given, as it acts directly on the lung and thus has fewer systemic effects. In one study comparing different routes of metaproterenol administration, the nebulized route had the fewest side effects; there was actually a decrease in heart rate, rather than an increased tachycardia.

The hypokalemic effect of catecholamines has been well documented.[59, 60] This is especially true for epinephrine and norepinephrine.[61] The nebulized beta agonists have been shown to produce a small decrease in serum potassium. Metaproterenol, albuterol, isoethrane, and atropine all produce a small decrease in serum potassium, with metaproterenol producing the greatest (0.56 mg/L)[62, 63] The clinical effects of this, especially in otherwise healthy children, are minimal in the emergency department but may require potassium replacement if the child is admitted for prolonged therapy.

Hypophosphatemia occurs in patients who are treated with bronchodilator therapy.[64] This is not an acute drop in the early hours of therapy, but instead occurs over the first 24 to 48 hours. Hypophosphatemia is important because it has been reported as a cause of respiratory muscle fatigue.[65, 66] Most of these measurements have been done in adults; there are currently few data available in children to guide phosphorus monitoring and replacement.

Ketamine

Ketamine has been described in several studies for use in severe asthma.[67–69] It is a dissociative anesthetic that increases catecholamine levels and produces bronchial smooth muscle relaxation in patients with pulmonary dysfunction.[70, 71] The intravenous (IV) dose of ketamine used ranges between 0.5 and 2.0 mg/kg.[72] Additional doses may be given as needed. Clinical improvement is usually seen within 1 to 2 minutes and lasts approximately 20 to 30 minutes. Ketamine may be used in conjunction with other therapies such as aminophylline and isoproterenol, but infusions of beta-adrenergic drugs may need to be decreased to prevent a potentiation of cardiac effects by ketamine.

Ketamine should be reserved for use in severely ill children who are likely to be intubated. Ketamine with succinylcholine effectively combines an anesthetic and a paralyzing agent and may be used for the intubation of a patient with severe asthma.[69] Ketamine does have several side effects that limit its use. It produces increased bronchial secretions, which may be aspirated if the patient is not intubated or not frequently suctioned; this may be minimized by predosing

with atropine. It has mild direct myocardial depressant effects but increases circulatory catecholamines, which stimulates the cardiovascular system. Ketamine produces an increase in heart rate, cardiac index, mean arterial pressure, and central venous pressure. A major disadvantage of ketamine is the postanesthetic emergence reaction it produces. This is characterized by alterations in mood, an extracorporeal state in which the patient feels dissociated from his or her body, and vivid dreams or hallucinations. This reaction is seen in approximately 10% of children and adolescents and may be minimized by sedation with a benzodiazepine.[72]

Theophylline

Theophylline is a mainstay of management for outpatient asthma, but its role in the acute management of asthma is not as well defined.[73] Its onset of action is slow (thought to be at least several hours), and consequently its benefits are often not seen until after the patient has left the emergency department or has been admitted. This raises the question of whether it should even be administered in the emergency department, as it has little acute effect and is given in combination with other beta agonists, which may increase toxicity. Even though its benefit may not be seen in the emergency department, the earlier theophylline is started, the earlier the beneficial effects will be seen after discharge or in the hospital. If the patient does not respond well to beta agonists, theophylline therapy should be started in the emergency department and given in conjunction with nebulized beta agonists. When using theophylline and beta agonists, close attention should be given to potential toxic effects such as nausea, vomiting, irritability, agitation, and seizures.

When a patient who is taking theophylline presents to the emergency department with an asthma attack, a determination of the amount of medication should be made and the patient given theophylline according to the following regimen:

1. No theophylline—a loading dose of 6 to 7 mg/kg IV of aminophylline or 5 to 6 mg/kg po of theophylline, followed by a maintenance infusion.
2. Subtherapeutic or questionable compliance—half loading dose, followed by a maintenance infusion; wait for determination of theophylline level.
3. Therapeutic dose—start maintenance infusion, but wait for determination of theophylline level before bolus.

A loading dose of aminophylline (85% theophylline) is given over 20 minutes. This is followed by a maintenance infusion of 1.2 mg/kg/hr in children under 10 years of age and 0.8 mg/kg/hr in children older than 10 years. This dose is higher than adults, because the serum half-life of theophylline in children is 2.5 hours, compared with 4.6 hours in adults.[74]

If the serum theophylline level has been determined, the dose of aminophylline necessary to increase the serum theophylline to therapeutic levels (10 to 20 µg/ml) can be determined by the following formula:

$$\text{Change in level (µg/ml)} = (\text{bolus dose in mg/V}_d) \times 0.85,$$

where V_d is the volume of distribution that equals 0.5 L/kg and 0.85 is the percentage of theophylline in aminophylline. This formula may be also used to calculate the initial loading dose.

Another quick formula often used is: 1 mg/kg of theophylline raises the serum concentration by approximately 2 µg/ml. An alternative to intravenous loading is oral loading in the emergency department. The oral loading dose is 6 to

7 mg/kg as a single dose, followed by 4 to 5 mg/kg every 6 hours. Within 3 hours after an oral dose of theophylline, the same blood levels are achieved as with an intravenous dose.[75] Children who receive an intravenous loading dose of aminophylline and a maintenance infusion should be closely monitored for tachycardia and changes in blood pressure.

Isoproterenol

If the patient has been aggressively treated with beta$_2$ agonists, oxygen, and fluid but is not improving, intravenous isoproterenol should be started. The starting dose is 0.1 µg/kg/min and may be increased every 15 minutes by 0.1 µg/kg/min until the patient improves or side effects such as tachycardia become unacceptable. If possible, an arterial line should placed in the emergency department in children receiving isoproterenol, or arrangements should be made for immediate transfer to an intensive care unit for placement of an arterial line.

Steroids

Intravenous steroids administered in the emergency department improve asthma over the next 24 to 36 hours. Several studies have demonstrated an improvement in forced vital capacity, hypoxemia, and clinical scoring in children receiving intravenous steroids when compared with placebo.[76] It is unclear, however, whether steroids have a significant effect on patients while in the emergency department. In general, reversal of an inflammatory process does not occur for 1 to 2 hours, so it is unlikely that clinically significant improvement will be seen immediately with steroids. Like theophylline, the earlier steroids are administered, the earlier the beneficial effects will be seen.

The recommended dose of methylprednisolone (Solu-Medrol) is 1 to 2 mg/kg every 6 hours. Hydrocortisone (Solu-Cortef) (4 to 5 mg/kg every 6 hours) may also be used. If the patient improves in the emergency department and is discharged, a tapering dose of steroids should be added to the therapeutic regimen. A 7- to 10-day taper is adequate for most children. In steroid-dependent children, the tapering period will be longer and is best directed by the patient's pediatrician. Adverse side effects with intravenous steroids or with a short tapering course of steroids are uncommon.

Mechanical Ventilation

If pharmacologic intervention fails and respiratory failure occurs, the patient should be intubated and placed on a respirator. Respiratory failure may be defined as a Pco_2 of 55 to 60 mm Hg or over 40 mm Hg with exhaustion. Hypercapnea, lethargy, agitation, cyanosis, tachycardia, and bradycardia are manifestations of respiratory failure and indications for intubation. Intubation necessitated by respiratory failure in an acute asthmatic patient is difficult and requires careful attention to heart rate and tissue oxygenation. If time permits, the stomach should be emptied using a nasogastric tube. The child may be paralyzed by administering pancuronium (0.01 mg/kg) IV plus atropine (0.02 mg/kg) to prevent bradycardia. The atropine may be omitted if the patient is tachycardic. Children under 5 years should not receive pancuronium, but do need atropine. Because these patients are frequently agitated, they often require paralysis and sedation. Five minutes after the patient receives pancuronium, succinylcholine (1 to 2 mg/kg) is administered for paralysis. Diazepam (0.1 to 0.2 mg/kg) may be administered for sedation and to induce amnesia even prior to succinylcholine administration. The patient should be hyperventilated with 100% oxygen, and cricoid pressure should be administered during intubation to prevent regurgitation and aspiration. As with any intubation, proper equipment, including suction, proper endotracheal tube, stylet, laryngoscope, and bag mask, is essential.

Once the patient is intubated, he or she should be placed on a volume-controlled ventilator and given neuromuscular paralyzing agents and sedation as necessary. The mortality rate for children on a ventilator is less than 2%, with morbidity rates ranging from 15% to 82%.[77] This includes pneumomediastinum, pneumothorax, atelectasis, and dysrhythmias.

DISPOSITION

Children who continue to wheeze after three beta-agonist treatments are admitted. Fluids, steroids, aminophylline, and observation for several hours in the emergency department generally do not provide significant improvement in children who have not improved after three beta-agonist treatments.

The following parameters indicate the need for admission:

Symptoms for more than 24 hours
Marked retractions
Failure to clear after three treatments with a beta agonist
Any respiratory distress after three treatments
PEFR less than 65% of predicted after treatment and
   less than 40% of predicted after first treatment
Evidence of fatigue
Abnormal arterial blood gases
Severe shortness of breath
Return visit for wheezing within 24 hours.
Poor history of compliance.

If improved, the child may be discharged with bronchodilator therapy. Bronchodilators may be prescribed in an oral form such as tablets or syrup or as a metered-dose inhaler for direct pulmonary delivery of the drug. The metered-dose inhalers may be used by children over 6 years of age and are especially good for episodic asthma attacks. Inhalers require good coordination to inhale the drug to maximize effects. Patients prescribed a metered-dose inhaler should be carefully instructed to keep the inhaler several inches from the mouth when using it. If the inhaler is held too closely to the mouth, most of the drug will be deposited in the pharynx, where it has no effect. Short tubes or spacers between the patient and inhaler may be used to ensure that proper distance is maintained and to help direct the flow of nebulized particles. In order to maximize the effectiveness of a metered-dose inhaler, a collapsible reservoir (Inspir-Ease) may be used. A dose of the inhaler is released into the cylindrical reservoir, which is then compressed as the patient inhales. This eliminates the coordination and proper spacing that are required to use metered-dose inhalers and maximizes drug delivery to the lungs. If the asthma attack is an isolated episode, a 7- to 10-day course of the bronchodilator may be prescribed. In children, asthma is frequently precipitated by a viral upper respiratory illness, which produces inflammation and narrowing of the airways. Consequently, it is necessary to dilate the airways until the patient has recovered from the viral illness. The decision to start a patient on long-term therapy for asthma is better made by the family physician or pediatrician.

If theophylline is used, an oral or intravenous loading dose of aminophylline should be given in the emergency department and maintenance therapy continued at home. Theo-Dur sprinkles are easy to administer to small children, whereas sustained-release preparations are acceptable for older children. Beta agonists such as metaproterenol (Alupent) or albuterol (Ventolin) may be given in syrup form or in an inhaler in place of theophylline. The inhalers are particularly useful in older children, as they are used as needed for wheezing. If the child is on steroids or has been difficult to clear in the emergency department, a short course of steroids (prednisone, 1 to 2 mg/kg/day) may be needed for 5 to 7 days. If a child develops an exacerbation of asthma and is already on theophylline or a beta agonist, the dose may be increased to 1½ times the normal dose for the first day, with the normal dose regimen followed afterward.

In addition to ensuring that the patient is given adequate bronchodilator therapy prior to discharge, the emergency physician should make an attempt to find out what started the asthma attack. New pets, exposure to known allergins or drugs, and emotional stress should be considered. Failure to identify and remove a bronchogenic stimulus may lead to future outpatient therapy and readmission.

Finally, careful follow-up instructions should be given as follows:

1. All medications should be taken as directed. (Instructions should be given as to when and how to take medications.)
2. Keep the child quiet and avoid exercise.
3. Encourage drinking plenty of clear liquids.
4. Avoid things that precipitate an asthma attack (e.g., pets, dust, foods or medications, and exposure to cold).
5. Return immediately if breathing becomes difficult, wheezing returns, or there are restlessness, color changes, or an inability to take medication.
6. Call your doctor tomorrow for follow-up.

Good follow-up should be arranged for patients discharged from the emergency department. The family physician or pediatrician should be informed of the visit so that he or she can keep a record of the frequency of emergency department visits and the changes in therapy initiated in the emergency department.

OTHER CONSIDERATIONS
Potential Pitfalls

Unlike adults, children rarely have baseline wheezing. When a child is treated in the emergency department, the lungs should be completely clear prior to discharge. Only in rare cases will baseline wheezing be the norm. Discharging a child who is wheezing but improving will likely result in a return visit to the emergency department and a child who is clinically much worse. If in doubt, it is better to admit a child than take a chance that the wheezing will clear at home.

Once a child has cleared and is being discharged, make sure he or she is able to get the prescribed medications immediately, not the next day. A delay of 10 to 12 hours is almost certain to produce rebound bronchospasm and result in admission. If necessary, dispense several doses of the medication to ensure that the patient has enough medication until the parents can get a prescription filled.

Anticipated Advances

The use of continuous nebulized beta agonists has a beneficial effect in patients who have been admitted to the hospital or intensive care unit. The role of this therapy in the emergency department, however, has not been defined. Another potentially beneficial treatment is the use of helium with nebulized beta agonists. Helium has a lower density and viscosity than air and penetrates the lungs better than air or oxygen. It may be more effective in delivering nebulized drugs to the small airways than conventional methods. Several recent studies have demonstrated a beneficial

effect on PEFR when magnesium sulfate is administered intravenously to patients with moderate to severe asthma.[78, 79] In one study, PEFR was shown to improve by 25% after a 20-minute infusion of magnesium sulfate (1.2 gm). The number of admissions to the hospital was also significantly less for those patients receiving magnesium.[78] The response was thought to be caused by relaxation of bronchial smooth muscle induced by magnesium.[80] There are no studies of the use of magnesium sulfate to treat acute asthma in children. Consequently, the potential benefit and drug dosage are unknown. In adult studies, 1.2 to 2.0 gm of intravenous magnesium sulfate have been administered over 20 minutes. This therapy is indicated for those patients who do not have moderate to severe asthma and respond well to beta agonists.

An allergy to magnesium sulfate and hypotension are specific contraindications. Adverse side effects include burning at the site of infusion, a feeling of warmth, and a decrease in blood pressure. A potential adverse effect is rebound bronchospasm as serum magnesium levels decrease after an infusion. Levels return to baseline within 24 hours, and therefore a rebound may be possible. Magnesium should be viewed as a temporizing measure for short-term PEFR improvement until beta agonists, steroids, and theophylline have a chance to work.

References

1. Skoner DP, Fischer TJ, Gormley C, et al. Pediatric predictive index for hospitalization in acute asthma. Ann Emerg Med 1987;16:25.
2. Parcel GS, Gilman SC, Nader PR, Bunce H. A comparison of absentee rates of elementary school children with asthma and nonasthmatic schoolmates. Pediatrics 1988;64:878.
3. Hen J. An overview of pediatric asthma. Pediatr Ann 1986;15:92.
4. Cropp GJA. Special features of asthma in children. Chest 1985;87(suppl):55.
5. Sears MR, Rea HH, Fenwick J, et al. Deaths from asthma in New Zealand. Arch Dis Child 1986;61:6.
6. Bonner JR. The epidemiology and natural history of asthma. Clin Chest Med 1984;5:557.
7. Hodgkin JE. United States audit of asthma therapy. Chest 1986;90(suppl):62.
8. Stolley PD. Asthma mortality: Why the United States was spared an epidemic of deaths due to asthma. Am Rev Respir Dis 1973;107:306.
9. Mitchell EA. Is current treatment increasing asthma mortality and morbidity? Thorax 1989;44:81.
10. Robin ED. Death from bronchial asthma. Chest 1988;93:614.
11. British Thoracic Association. Death from asthma in two regions of England. Br Med J 1982;285:1251.
12. Sears MR, Rea HH, Rothwell RPG, et al. Asthma mortality: Comparison between New Zealand and England. Br Med J 1986;293:1342.
13. Kolski GB. Allergic emergencies. In Fleisher G (ed). Textbook of Pediatric Emergency Medicine. Baltimore, Williams & Wilkins, 1988, p 649.
14. McFadden. Pathophysiology of asthma. In Fishman AP (ed). Pulmonary Disease and Disorders. New York, McGraw-Hill, 1980, p 568.
15. Saunders NA, McFadden ER. Asthma–an update. Disease-A-Month 1978;24:1.
16. Stempel DA, Mellon M. Management of acute severe asthma. Pediatr Clin North Am 1984;31:879.
17. Gurwitz D, Mindorff C, Levison H. Increased incidence of bronchial reactivity in children with a history of bronchiolitis. J Pediatr 1981;98:551.
18. McFadden ER. Pathogenesis of asthma. J Allergy Clin Immunol 1984;73:413.
19. Nadel JA. Inflammation and asthma. J Allergy Clin Immunol 1984;73:651.
20. Halperin SA, Eggleston AA, Beasley P, et al. Exacerbations of asthma in adults during experimental rhinovirus infection. Am Rev Respir Dis 1985;132:976.
21. Minor TE, Dick EC, Baker JW, et al. Rhinovirus and influenza A infections as precipitants of asthma. Am Rev Respir Dis 1976;113:149.
22. McIntosh K, Ellis EF, Hoffman LS, et al. The association of viral and bacterial respiratory infections with exacerbations of wheezing in young asthmatic children. J Pediatr 1973;82:578.
23. Horn MEC, Gregg I. Role of viral infection and host factors in acute episodes of asthma and chronic bronchitis. Chest 1973;63:44S.
24. Bronchiolitis in infancy and childhood. Editorial. Br Med J 1980;16:428.
25. Tabachnik E, Levison H. Infantile bronchial asthma. J Allergy Clin Immunol 1981;67:339.
26. Pullan CR, Hey EN. Wheezing, asthma, and pulmonary dysfunction 10

years after infection with respiratory syncytial virus in infancy. Br Med J 1982;284:1665.

27. Berman SZ, Mathison DA, Stevenson DD, et al. Transtracheal aspiration studies in asthmatic patients in relapse with "infective" asthma and in subjects without respiratory disease. J Allergy Clin Immunol 1975;56:206.

28. Zweiman B, Schoenwetter WF, Pappano JE, et al. Patterns of allergic respiratory disease in children with a past history of bronchiolitis. J Allergy Clin Immunol 1971;48:283.

29. Sly RM. Evolving views of asthma: Past and present. In Tinkelman DG, Falliers CJ, Naspitz CK (eds). Childhood Asthma: Pathophysiology and Treatment. New York, Marcel Dekker, 1987, p 85.

30. Falliers CJ. Asthma or variable obstructive intrabronchial disease (VOID). Ann Allergy 1984;53:113.

31. McNichol KN, Williams HE. Spectrum of asthma in children. I. Clinical and physiological components. II. Allergic components. III. Psychological and social components. Br Med J 1973;4:7.

32. Scoggin C. Exercise-induced asthma. Chest 1985;87:S48.

33. Deal EC, McFadden ER, Ingram HR, et al. Effects of atropine on the potentiation of exercise-induced bronchospasm by cold air. J Appl Physiol 1978;45:238.

34. Deal EC, McFadden ER, Ingram RH, et al. Hyperpnea and heat flux: Initial reaction sequence in exercise-induced asthma. J Appl Physiol 1979;46:476.

35. McDonald JR, Mathison DA, Stevenson DD. Aspirin intolerance in asthma. J Allergy Clin Immunol 1972;50:198.

36. Tan Y, Collins-Williams C. Aspirin-induced asthma in children. Ann Allergy 1982;48:1.

37. Szczekli A, Gryglewski RJ, Czerniawska-Mysik G. Clinical patterns of hypersensitivity to nonsteroidal anti-inflammatory drugs and their pathogenesis. J Allergy Clin Immunol 1977;60:276.

38. Rose CC, Murphy JG, Schwartz JS. Performance of an index predicting the response of patients with acute bronchial asthma to intensive emergency department treatment. N Engl J Med 1984;310:573.

39. Beer S, Laver J, Karpuch J, et al. Prodromal features of asthma. Arch Dis Child 1987;62:345.

40. Simons FE, Chernick V. Principles of diagnosis and treatment of lower respiratory tract disease. In Bierman CW, Pearlman DS (eds). Allergic Diseases of Infancy, Childhood, and Adolescence. Philadelphia, WB Saunders, 1980, p 504.

41. Robertson C, Levison H. Bronchodilators in asthma. Chest 1985;87:S64.

42. Schneid CR, Honeyman TW, Fay FS. Mechanisms of β-adrenergic relaxation of smooth muscle. Nature 1979;277:32.

43. Becker AB, Nelson NA, Simons FE. Inhaled salbutamol (albuterol) vs injected epinephrine in the treamtent of acute asthma in children. J Pediatr 1983;102:465.

44. Adverse reactions of drugs. Med Lett Drugs Ther 1979;2:5.

45. Speer F, Tapay NJ. Syncope in children following epinephrine. Ann Allergy 1970;28:50.

46. Nelson HS. Beta adrenergic agonists. Chest 1982;82:S33.

47. McFadden ER, Lyons HA. Arterial-blood gas tension in asthma. N Engl J Med 1968;278:1027.

48. Bolte RG. Nebulized β-adrenergic agents in the treatment of acute pediatric asthma. Pediatr Emerg Care 1986;2:250.

49. Moler FW, Hurwitz ME, Custer JR. Improvement in clinical asthma score and PaCO$_2$ in children with severe asthma treated with continuously nebulized terbutaline. J Allergy Clin Immunol 1988;81:1101.

50. Portnoy J, Aggarwal J. Continuous terbutaline nebulization for the treatment of severe exacerbations of asthma in children. Ann of Allergy 1988;60:368.

51. Aggarwal J, Portnoy J. Continuous terbutaline inhalation for the treatment of severe asthma. Abstract. J Allergy Clin Immunol 1986;77:185.

52. Schuh S, Parkin P, Rajan A, et al. High- versus low-dose, frequently administered, nebulized albuterol in children with severe, acute asthma. Pediatrics 1989;83:513.

53. Robertson CF, Smith F, Beck R, et al. Response to frequent low doses of nebulized salbutamol in acute asthma. Pediatrics 1985;106:672.

54. Lee H, Evans HE. Lack of cardiac effect from repeated doses of albuterol aerosol: A margin of safety. Clin Pediatr 1986;25:349.

55. Larsson S, Svedmyr N. Bronchodilating effect and side efects to β$_2$-adrenoreceptor stimulants by different modes of administration (tablets, metered aerosol, and combinations thereof). A study with salbutamol in asthmatics. Am Rev Respir Dis 1977;116:861.

56. Van Reterghem D, Lamont H, Elinck W, et al. Intravenous versus nebulized terbutaline in patients with acute severe asthma: A double-blind randomized study. Ann Allergy 1987;59:313.

57. Bloomfield P, Carmichael J, Petrie GR, et al. Comparison of salbutamol given intravenously and by intermittent positive pressure breathing in life-threatening asthma. Br Med J 1979;1:848.

58. Maguire GP, Emirgil C. Bronchodilator and side effects of different modes of administration of metaproterenol: inhaled, oral and in combination. Am J Med Sci 1986;291:168.

59. Silva P, Spokes K, Epstein FH. Catecholamines and potassium homeostasis. Kidney Int 1977;12:544.

60. Rosa RM, Silva P, Young JB, et al. Adrenergic modulation of extrarenal potassium disposal. N Engl J Med 1980;302:431.

61. Todd EP, Vick RL. Kalemotropic effect of epinephrine: Analysis with adrenergic agonists and antagonists. Am J Physiol 1971;220:1964.

62. Gelmont DM, Balmes JR, Yee A. Hypokalemia induced by inhaled bronchodilators. Chest 1988;94:763.

63. Swenson ER, Aitken ML. Hypokalemia occurs with inhaled albuterol. Am Rev Respir Dis 1985;131(4, pt 2):A99.

64. Brady HR, Ryan F, Cunningham J. Hypophosphatemia complicating bronchodilator therapy for acute severe asthma. Arch Intern Med 1989;149:2367.

65. Aubier M, Murciano D, Lecocguic Y, et al. Effect of hypophosphatemia on diaphragmatic contractility in patients with acute respiratory failure. N Engl J Med 1985;313:420.

66. Fiaccadori E, Del Canale S, Vitali P, et al. Skeletal muscle energetics, acid-base equilibrium and lactate metabolism in patients with severe hypercapnia and hypoxemia. Chest 1987;92:883.

67. Rock MJ, De La Rocha SR, L'Hommedieu S. Use of ketamine in asthmatic children to treat respiratory failure refractory to conventional therapy. 1986;14:514.

68. Fisher MM. Ketamine hydrochloride in severe bronchospasm. Anaesthesia 1977;32:771.

69. L'Hommedieu CS, Arens JJ. The use of ketamine for the emergency intubation of patients with status asthmaticus. Ann Emerg Med 1987;16:568.

70. Cabanas A, Souhrada FJ, Aldrete JA. Effects of ketamine and halothan on normal and asthmatic smooth muscle of the airway in guinea pigs. Can Anaesth Soc J 1980;27:47.

71. Huber FC, Reves JG, Gutierrez J, et al. Ketamine: Its effect on airway resistance in man. South Med J 1972;65:1176.

72. Elliot E, Hanid TK, Arthur JH, et al. Ketamine anesthesia for medical procedures in children. Arch Dis Child 1976;51:56.

73. Tinkelman DG. Theophylline—use and misuse in pediatric asthma. Hosp Pract 1988;23:179.

74. Zaske DE, Miller KW, Strem EL, et al. Oral aminophylline therapy. Increased dosage requirements in children. JAMA 1977;237:1453.

75. Carrier JA, Shaw RA, Porter RS, et al. Comparison of intravenous and oral routes of theophylline loading in acute asthma. Ann Emerg Med 1985;14:1145.

76. Younger RE, Gerber PS, Herrod GH, et al. Intravenous methylprednisolone efficacy in status asthmaticus of childhood. Pediatrics 1987;80:225.

77. Dworkin G, Kattan M. Mechanical ventilation for status asthmaticus in children. J Pediatr 1989;114(4):545.

78. Skobellof EM, Spivey WH, McNamara RM, Greenspon L. Intravenous magnesium sulfate for the treatment of acute asthma in the emergency department. JAMA 1989;262:1210.

79. Okayama H, Takashi A, Okayama M, et al. Bronchodilating effect of intravenous magnesium sulfate in bronchial asthma. JAMA 1987;257:1076.

80. Spivey WH, Skobeloff EM, Levin RM. Effect of magnesium chloride on rabbit bronchial smooth muscle. Ann Emerg Med 1990;19:1107.

CHAPTER 26

Upper Airway Emergencies

Mary Hughes

INTRODUCTION

The child who presents to the emergency department with upper airway disease demands prompt and aggressive management to prevent unnecessary morbidity and mortality. Epiglottitis, spasmodic croup, laryngotracheobronchitis, and bacterial tracheitis involve different therapeutic approaches and present different levels of risk for airway obstruction (Tables 26–1 and 26–2).

ANATOMY OF THE UPPER AIRWAY

The supraglottic space is that area of the pharynx above the vocal cords and includes the epiglottis (Fig. 26–1). The

TABLE 26–1

RAPID DIFFERENTIAL DIAGNOSIS OF UPPER AIRWAY EMERGENCIES

	Spasmodic Croup	Viral Laryngotracheobronchitis	Bacterial Tracheitis	Epiglottitis
Age	1–3 yr	3 mo–3 yr	>3 yr (often 5–10 yr)	2–5 yr
Season	Fall/winter	Fall/winter	Fall/winter	Fall/winter/spring
Duration of prodrome	Short Sudden onset Usual at night	Hours to days	Hours to days	Minutes or hours
Temperature	Usually normal	Usually normal	Usually elevated to 102° F or greater	Usually elevated
Radiographic findings	Subglottic narrowing often normal	Subglottic narrowing— steeple sign	Subglottic narrowing may show foreign body material in trachea on radiograph	Swollen epiglottis Normal subglottic area
White blood cell count	Normal	Normal	Elevated; high percentage of bands	Elevated; left shift
Endoscopic findings	Pale, watery swelling	Subglottic edema No secretions	Purulent secretions in tracheobronchial tree Pseudomembranes	Red, swollen epiglottis No exudate
Causative agent(s)	Possibly allergic	Parainfluenza type 1; less often types 2, 3	*Staphylococcus aureus* Streptococcal sp. Miscellaneous	*Haemophilus influenzae* type b
Presence of:				
Stridor	Yes	Yes	Yes	Yes
Barking cough	Yes	Yes	Yes	No
Drooling	No	No	No	Yes
Tripod posture	No	No	No	Yes
Retractions	No	Occasionally	Yes	Yes
Patient appears toxic	No	Occasionally	Yes	Yes
Patient requires intubation and ICU care	No	Rarely yes	Routinely yes	Routinely yes
Patient responds to:				
Cool mist	Yes	Maybe	No	No
Racemic epinephrine	No	Yes	No	No

epiglottis is a thin cartilaginous structure covered on the entire anterior surface and the superior one third of the posterior surface by loosely adherent stratified squamous epithelium. This creates a large potential space for the accumulation of fluid during inflammatory processes. With epiglottitis this fluid accumulation, coupled with the inherently smaller supraglottic space in infants and children, leads to rapid airway obstruction. The infant epiglottis is elongated and omega shaped (Ω), with some redundancy of the aryepiglottic folds. In addition, it is made of elastic cartilage that is less rigid than the hyaline cartilage that composes the adult epiglottis. The infant epiglottis lies at the level of the second or third cervical vertebra, which potentially allows for easy direct visualization of the swollen epiglottitis if the child merely opens the mouth. The adult epiglottis, in contrast, is opposite the body of the fifth cervical vertebra.[1–3]

The subglottic space is that area of the larynx beginning at the vocal cords and extending to the inferior margin of the cricoid cartilage. The cricoid cartilage rigidly encircles this portion of the airway, which makes it susceptible to narrowing by relatively small amounts of inflammatory reaction.[2]

EMERGENCY MEDICAL SERVICE CONSIDERATIONS

The child who presents to emergency medical service (EMS) personnel awake but with obvious respiratory distress

TABLE 26–2

MANAGEMENT OF UPPER AIRWAY EMERGENCIES

	Spasmodic Croup	Viral LTB	Bacterial Tracheitis	Epiglottitis
Intubation	No	About 6% of patients	Yes	Yes
Humidified oxygen	Rarely	Sometimes	Yes	Yes
Mist	Yes	Yes	No	No
Helium-oxygen mixture	No	Maybe	No	No
Racemic epinephrine	No	Yes*	No	No
Steroids	No	Yes	No	No
ICU care	No	Sometimes	Yes	Yes

*If needed, admit patient to hospital.

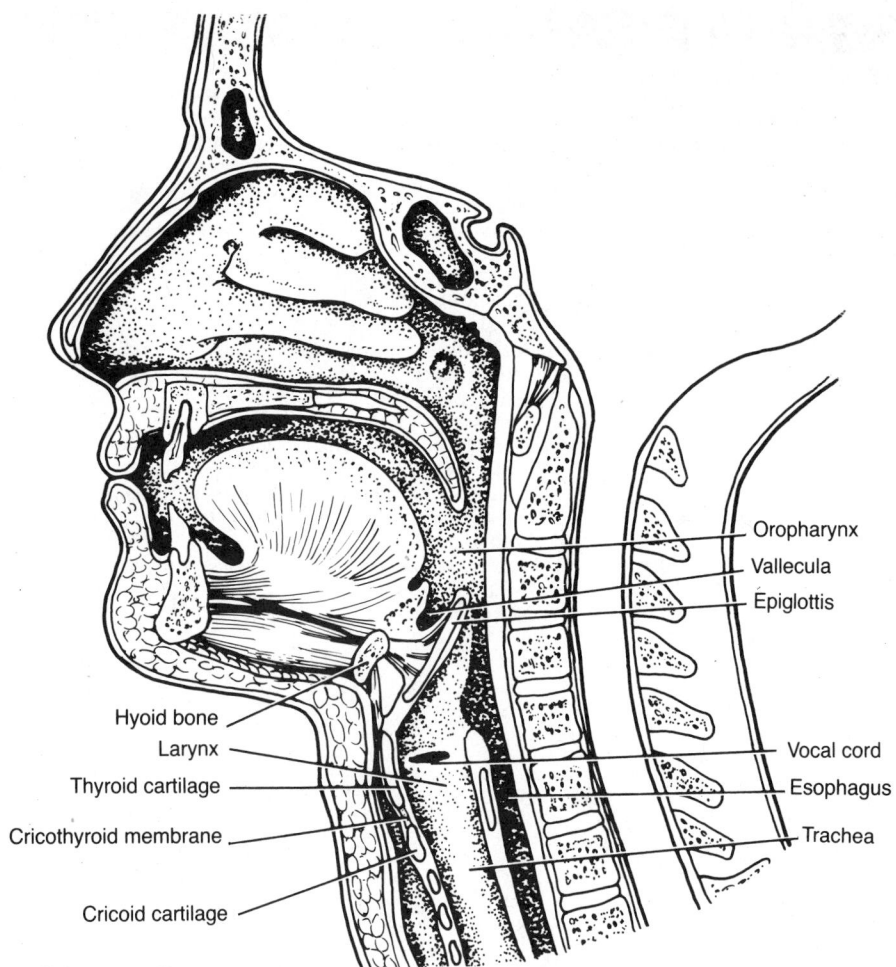

Figure 26–1. Sagittal view of the airway. (Redrawn from Rosen PR, Baker FJ, Barkin RM, et al. (eds). Emergency Medicine: Concepts and Clinical Practice. St. Louis, CV Mosby, 1983, p 29.)

warrants quick and skillful assessment, appropriate treatment, and prompt, nonfrightening transport to the nearest medical care facility equipped to handle airway difficulties. Often assessment, treatment, and history gathering occur simultaneously.

EMS personnel must obtain the essential facts, including (1) onset of distress, including whether abrupt or gradual, time of day, and activity occurring with the child at the time of onset; (2) the possibility of foreign body aspiration (e.g., small toys in the crib or play area or whether the child was playing unattended); (3) recent state of health, including history of signs and symptoms of an upper respiratory infection (runny nose, cough, sore throat, or possible earache); (4) determination of the presence of a fever or a history of a fever in the last several days; (5) any prior history of the same type of complaint; and (6) any treatment provided to the child prior to notifying EMS personnel.

Essential Physical Assessment

Essential physical assessment should include the position assumed by the patient in attempting to maintain oxygenation (e.g., an upright, tripod, or supine position), the presence or absence of drooling, the voice character, and whether there is any audible stridor or visible cyanosis. Respiratory rates in children vary widely with age (Table 26–3). Generally, children who are in distress initially respond with tachypnea. Terminal respiratory distress is often marked by a slow respiratory rate. Mental obtundation, confusion, combativeness, or agitation are often a hallmark of severe cerebral hypoxia.[4]

Treatment

Treatment of all children who are awake with respiratory distress should be nonthreatening to prevent further respiratory demand on an already compromised system. Every effort should be made to keep the child calm and in the position that provides maximum comfort and respiratory function. Allowing the child to be held by a parent often limits agitation. Administration of oxygen is essential to hypoxic children, but the parent may be allowed to hold the mask within inches of the child's face, rather than strapping it to the child's head and thus threatening an already compromised child. Intravenous lines are frequently not

TABLE 26–3
AVERAGE RESPIRATORY RATES OF PEDIATRIC PATIENTS

Age (yr)	Mean Rate (While Awake)
0.5–1	64
1–2	35
2–4	31
4–6	26
6–8	23
8–10	21
10–12	21
12–14	22

From Kendig EL Jr, Chernick V (eds). Disorders of the Respiratory Tract in Children. 4th ed. Philadelphia, WB Saunders, 1983.

essential. Prehospital attempts to establish vascular access in environments with poor lighting and inadequate personnel may do additional harm. Cardiac monitoring should be considered and attempted if it can be done without increased agitation of the child.

Communicating With Medical Control

The EMS provider should present the following information to medical control in an organized fashion: the estimated time of arrival; the age of the child; the chief complaint, with a brief description of the essential historical facts and the initial assessment; current medications taken by and allergies of the child; and treatment provided in the field, either by parents or EMS personnel, and the response. EMS personnel should also query medical control for any other orders or treatment that should be instituted prior to arrival of the patient in the emergency department.

DIFFERENTIAL DIAGNOSIS FOR STRIDOR

The differential diagnosis for stridor in children includes several disease entities. Infectious processes of the supraglottic airway that may lead to stridor are those diseases that cause swelling of these spaces; these include epiglottitis, diphtheria, infectious mononucleosis, and retropharyngeal abscess. Noninfectious causes include inflammatory edema secondary to allergic reactions or other causes, foreign body aspiration, and tumors.

Stridor secondary to involvement of the subglottic airway may have one of several causes, and differential diagnosis should include the following:

Spasmodic croup
Laryngotracheobronchitis
Laryngotracheitis
Bacterial tracheitis
Foreign body aspiration
Angioneurotic edema
Congenital or acquired tracheal stenosis
Tumors

EPIGLOTTITIS

Incidence

Epiglottitis is a disease of young children, primarily those between the ages of 2 and 5 years.[5-13] It is characterized by a male preponderance (male-to-female ratio approximately 3:2)[3, 5-7, 13] and carries a 0% to 10% mortality rate depending on the reported series.[5-13] The incidence of epiglottitis varies with the geographic location but in large series studies accounts for approximately 1 of every 1000 to 2000 pediatric hospital admissions.[7, 13-15] Seasonal incidence seems to vary with geographic location, but in most studies reporting a seasonal incidence, epiglottitis occurred most often during the spring months, in combination either with late fall and winter or with summer.[5-10, 12, 13]

Etiology

Epiglottitis in children is caused almost exclusively by *Haemophilus influenzae* type b (Hib).[5, 6, 11, 12, 16] It is rare to have supraglottitis with bacteremia secondary to other organisms in children. Isolated cases occur involving *Streptococcus pneumoniae*,[8, 9] group A beta-hemolytic streptococcus,[17] *Staphylococcus aureus*,[14] other *Haemophilus* species,[6, 17, 18] and group C beta-hemolytic *streptococci*.[19]

Clinical Evaluation

In the child over the age of 2 years, epiglottitis is a dramatic, life-threatening disease that has a fulminant, fatal course if not recognized and treated aggressively. The classic presentation involves the 2- to 5-year-old child, more often male, who presents with a rapid onset of respiratory distress and who has been ill less than 24 hours and often less than 12 hours. Typically the disease is characterized by a high fever of 39°C to 40°C, a toxic appearance, and obvious respiratory distress with inspiratory stridor, if not overt respiratory embarrassment or failure. The child usually prefers to sit with the head extended, rather than lie supine, and will drool rather than swallow saliva because of severe pain with swallowing. The child, if verbal, may demonstrate a muffled or guttural voice, and the older child will complain of a severe sore throat. Cough is rarely part of the initial presentation. Mental status changes compatible with hypoxia include irritability, lethargy, or combativeness. Tachycardia out of proportion to the fever is a reflection of the hypoxic status of the patient.[5, 7, 8, 10, 12, 20, 21] Occasionally the child with acute epiglottitis will present with pulmonary edema or will develop pulmonary edema immediately after intubation.[22-24]

Nearly 25% of cases of epiglottitis occur in children less than 2 years of age.[5, 7, 8, 12, 25] Epiglottitis often presents a different clinical picture in the child under 2 years old when compared with the classic presentation of the 2- to 5-year-old child just described. Often there is a prodrome in excess of 12 hours; this may include anorexia and vomiting or rhinitis and a croupy cough. Nearly 50% of patients in one study presented with a croupy cough.[5] The majority of children less than 2 years old with epiglottitis had inspiratory stridor and appeared in respiratory distress, but nearly 50% were not clinically thought to be "toxic" on initial presentation.[5, 25] Nearly 25% were afebrile on presentation,[5] although other authors reported a high fever (40°C).[25] Few children younger than 2 years prefer the sitting position; most have a normal voice, and drooling is present only in 50% of patients.[5, 25]

Physical Examination

The direct examination of the oropharynx in the awake child suspected of having acute epiglottitis is controversial. Bottenfeld reported that three of 19 patients admitted for epiglottitis suffered respiratory arrests during direct visualization of the oropharynx.[11] All were successfully resuscitated. Another report described an 18-month-old child who suffered a respiratory arrest secondary to crying during an attempt at establishing an intravenous line; this report inferred that any maneuver that causes crying may precipitate a respiratory arrest.[26] Other investigators reported several patients who suffered respiratory arrests, thought to be precipitated by the use of a tongue depressor to examine the oropharynx.[6, 14]

Protocols range from absolute prohibition of direct examinations to recommendations that such examinations be performed on all patients with the suspected diagnosis of epiglottitis.[8, 11, 12, 21, 26-28] Direct visualization under general anesthesia by an anesthesiologist or otolaryngologist prior to intubation is routinely performed to confirm the diagnosis.[11, 27]

A prospective study of children who presented with stridor evaluated the role of direct inspection of the epiglottis in children suspected of having laryngotracheitis.[28] If the child was suspected of having epiglottitis, direct examination was deferred until a pediatric anesthesiologist was in attendance. Of the 155 patients studied, six had a final diagnosis of epiglottitis.

A sequential method was used in the study, beginning with a light and asking the child to open his or her mouth; then progressing to a light and tongue blade, including depressing the posterior third of the tongue, taking care to avoid the epiglottis; and then on to direct laryngoscopy, first with the child upright and then supine if unsuccessful. The sequence was terminated when the epiglottitis was visualized. Use of restraint was permitted. No cases of respiratory arrest occurred, and two clinically unsuspected cases of epiglottitis were diagnosed by this method.[28]

Diagnostic Evaluation
Laboratory Tests

The diagnosis of epiglottitis is based on clinical suspicion, and confirmation is made in the operating room under general anesthesia by an experienced anesthesiologist or otolaryngologist. Typically, the complete blood cell (CBC) count reveals an elevated white blood cell (WBC) count, often with a shift to the left.[5, 8, 10, 12] WBC counts can range from 10,000 to 44,000 with a significant percentage of band cells.[8, 14]

Laboratory tests usually performed in children with epiglottitis include a CBC count with differential, blood cultures with sensitivity, urine counterimmunoelectrophoresis (CIE), and often a culture of the epiglottic surface. Occasionally arterial blood gas measurements are obtained.

Blood cultures are routinely obtained and are positive for *H. influenzae* type b in children not on prior antibiotic therapy in 80% to 100% of cases.[5, 29] In contrast to blood cultures, the microorganisms obtained from cultures of the epiglottis vary widely and often consist of normal respiratory flora. Often cultures obtained from the blood and epiglottis do not produce the same organisms.[6, 13, 14, 21] Serum and urine CIE results, when obtained, add little to information obtained from blood cultures.[30]

Capillary or arterial blood gases are occasionally obtained at the time of intubation.[30] The arterial-alveolar (a-A) oxygen tension gradient was measured in several children with epiglottitis both before and after intubation. It was found to be nearly always below the lower limit of normal.[31] The hypoxemia was alleviated by providing the patient with a minimum of 30% humidified oxygen.[31]

Radiologic Studies

Soft tissue radiographs of the neck are often diagnostic of epiglottitis but should never delay definitive airway management in the child who needs airway control emergently. Although the characteristic clinical pictures of epiglottitis, bacterial tracheitis, and laryngotracheitis are so different that radiographs are unnecessary to aid in the differentiation, in actuality, the clinical overlap of these diseases is considerable, and occasionally radiographic studies provide further definition.[11, 30, 32, 33]

The appearance of acute epiglottitis on radiographic examination of the soft tissues of the neck is characteristically described as the *thumbprint* or *smudge sign* when looking at the epiglottitis on the lateral projection (Fig. 26–2). The vallecula is narrowed, and the swollen epiglottis and aryepiglottic folds seem to fill the entire hypopharynx. There is evidence of inspiratory obstruction on an inspiratory radiograph.[7, 11, 33]

In studies in which lateral neck radiographs were performed, a 100% correlation with the clinical diagnosis was reported.[11, 32, 34, 35] However, in patients with endoscopically documented epiglottitis, Sendi and Crysdale reported only 79% of patients with positive radiographs;[12] Murrage et al. reported 92% with positive radiographs.[16]

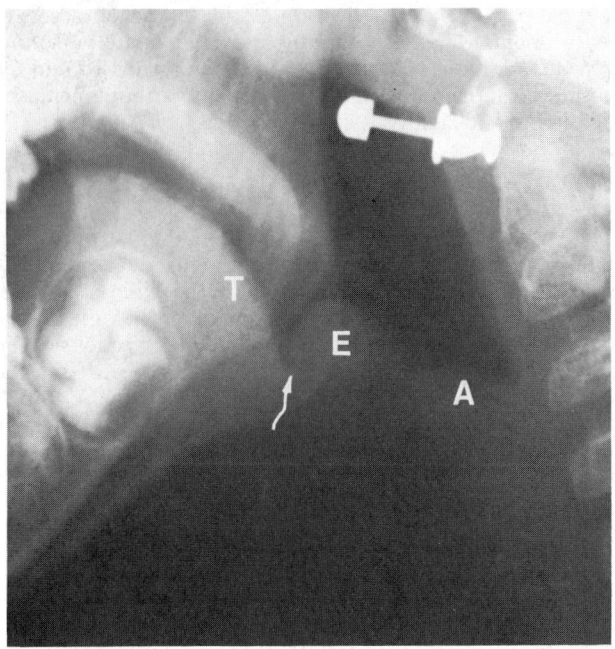

Figure 26–2. Epiglottitis in a 2-year-old child with drooling and high fever; a highly characteristic radiograph of this dangerous condition. The epiglottis (E) is found immediately posterior to the tongue (T), their junction marked by the arrow. This epiglottis is short and squat (thumbprint sign) rather than the normal tall and thin. Behind the epiglottis, the aryepiglottic folds (A) are swollen into the piriform sinus, being convex upward rather than the normal concave upper margin. (Courtesy of A. Oestreich, M.D., Cincinnati, OH.)

If radiographs are to be performed, several factors must be considered:

1. Radiographs should not delay definitive airway control in patients who need it emergently.[9, 33]
2. Once the diagnosis of epiglottitis is suspected, the child should always be attended by a physician skilled at airway management until the diagnosis is excluded.[9, 12, 21]
3. Radiographic studies should be performed with the child sitting up; forcing the child to lie supine may precipitate complete obstruction.[9, 12, 21]
4. Oxygen should be provided to those that need it clinically.
5. If agitation should occur secondary to attempts to obtain the radiographic studies, the attempt should be discontinued. Parents should be allowed to be present if their presence contributes to a more calm child.

General Approach

From the prehospital encounter to the securing of an artificial airway, the child with epiglottitis should be managed gently, with minimal amounts of distress and agitation. Epiglottitis remains a cause of sudden death in children, and written protocols that involve EMS personnel, emergency department personnel, radiologists, otolaryngologists, anesthesiologists, and pediatricians are essential. When death occurs, it is usually in the first several hours of the disease presentation.

Prehospital Management

EMS personnel should be taught the "four Ds" for the clinical diagnosis of epiglottitis, namely: dysphagia, dysphonia, drooling, and distress.[36] Suspicion should be heightened if the history is one of a sudden onset of illness in the febrile child with inspiratory stridor and minimal to no cough. EMS personnel should assess for the possibility of foreign body aspiration.

Considerations of EMS transport include the following:

1. Awareness that respiratory arrest may occur at any time.

2. If respiratory arrest occurs, management of the airway by bag-valve-mask will usually provide adequate oxygenation for transport to the hospital. Attempts at intubation may be extremely difficult. If endotracheal intubation is attempted, a tube one size smaller than normally used is recommended.[20, 33, 37]

3. Transport of the child should be in the position that maximizes air exchange for the child, often on the lap of a parent. Parents should be informed of the need for a calm demeanor.

4. Oxygen should be provided and is often tolerated if the parent holds the device close to, but not over, the child's face.

5. No attempts should be made to start an intravenous line or otherwise antagonize the child who is still breathing independently.

6. Physical examination of the oral pharynx in the child suspected of having epiglottitis is strictly prohibited.

7. Constant attention should be paid to recognize complete obstruction.

8. Transport should be without lights and siren if these agitate the child; otherwise they may be used.

Airway Management and Oxygen Therapy

Sudden death from epiglottitis is more often caused by hypoxia than by complete airway obstruction.[10, 38] Airway protection is the single most important aspect of management of the child with epiglottitis.[6] Once epiglottitis is confirmed, the child must be provided with an artificial airway. This is best performed in the operating room under induction anesthesia with halothane and oxygen by an anesthesiologist with an otolaryngologist in attendance.[11, 35, 39, 40] Neuromuscular paralytic agents are generally not used, because often the only landmark seen are the bubbles emanating from the narrow region of the trachea, which helps guide tube position.[41, 42] Occasionally pressure on the chest is necessary to produce bubbles.[43] A curved blade for intubation should be used with Magill forceps to guide the tube.[41] Once deep anesthesia is obtained, the child should be examined directly, nasotracheally intubated with a tube one size smaller than normally used for the size of the child, and oxygenated.[11, 20] Occasionally it is necessary to intubate the child orotracheally, oxygenate, and then change the tube to a nasotracheal tube. If intubation cannot be accomplished, tracheostomy should be performed by the otolaryngologist. Prior to this, a percutaneous translaryngeal ventilation may be required as a temporizing measure.[43]

Once the tube is secured, an intravenous line should be established, blood and epiglottis cultures obtained, routine laboratory tests performed, and intravenous antibiotics commenced. Prior to arousal, the child should be restrained to prevent accidental extubation. If intubation is to be required for more than 72 hours, standard tracheostomy may be considered.[6, 11, 20, 39, 44] A chest radiograph should be taken to verify tube placement.

Humidified oxygen with a minimum FIO_2 of 30% should be provided to all children with epiglottitis.[8, 13, 31, 33, 44] Once the airway is secured, aggressive hourly pulmonary toilet with normal saline and tracheal suction should be employed.[39] Pulse oximetry may be used to monitor oxygen saturation.[45]

The most serious error in the treatment of the child with epiglottitis is assuming that the airway will remain patent. Successful management of the child with epiglottitis without definitive airway control or otherwise known "observation" and including oxygen, humidity, intensive care monitoring, and intravenous antibiotics is reported in a small percentage of the cases in the literature. Of these patients, a high percentage went on to require airway management, and several developed abrupt respiratory arrest necessitating an emergent intubation or tracheostomy in the intensive care unit under less than ideal circumstances and with less than ideal outcomes. As there is no way to predict which children are likely to suffer a respiratory arrest, this course seems inherently risky.[10–12, 21, 34, 46, 47]

Drug Therapy

Antibiotics

Intravenous antibiotic therapy is essential in the treatment of children with epiglottitis and should be started as soon as intravenous access is obtained. The majority of children are infected and are often bacteremic with *H. influenzae* type b. Antibiotic coverage must be appropriate to treat this invasive organism until the culture and sensitivity results can direct the most appropriate therapeutic regimen. In general, antibiotic therapy should be guided by known sensitivities of *H. influenzae* type b in the region in which one practices.

Cefuroxime in doses ranging from 75 to 200 mg/kg/day[12, 21, 48] divided every 8 hours are recommended in the initial management of epiglottitis. An alternative regimen is a combination of ampicillin (200 mg/kg/day) with chloramphenicol (100 mg/kg/day), both divided and given every 6 hours.[30, 49] When the child is discharged from the hospital, appropriate antibiotics should be continued to complete a 10-day course.[12, 21]

Steroids

Steroids are controversial in the treatment of epiglottitis. A study regarding the duration of hospital stay and prevention of tracheostomy found no differences between the patients who received steroids and those who did not.[10]

Sedation

Sedation of the child with acute respiratory distress prior to transport to the operating room for general anesthesia is contraindicated. Once the child's airway has been secured, sedation is nearly always essential to maintain the tube position and function.

Complications

The most feared and serious complication of epiglottitis is respiratory arrest with subsequent death or permanent neurologic impairment. It may be precipitated by agitation[26] or direct inspection of the oral pharynx.[11] Of 1193 patients reviewed, 3.5% suffered death or permanent neurologic sequelae.[5–15, 21, 34, 50] Accidental extubation or tube obstruction is fairly common and occurs in 10% to 23% of patients, despite constant monitoring in a critical care setting.[6, 9, 11, 12, 16, 21, 23, 37, 39]

Abnormal chest radiographs occur in 10% to 50% of patients. The most common abnormality is an infiltrate, followed distantly by pulmonary edema, atelectasis, pleural effusion, and extrapulmonary air.[35, 37, 39, 48, 50, 51]

Although not as common, secondary foci of infection caused by *H. influenzae* type b have been reported in patients with epiglottitis. These include meningitis, septic arthritis, pericarditis, cervical adenitis, septic shock, and paraglottic laryngitis.[15, 51, 52–55]

Prevention and Prophylaxis

The advent of the Hib vaccine, recommended for all children as a series starting at 2 months of age, should prevent a substantial number of cases of epiglottitis. Encapsulated *H. influenzae* type b bacteria cause nearly all cases of epiglottitis, and the Hib vaccine has a demonstrated 90% protective efficacy in prevention of all forms of invasive *H. influenzae* type b infection in a 4-year follow-up period.[56–58]

The American Academy of Pediatrics Committee on Infectious Diseases recommends the following prophylactic treatment for contacts of patients with invasive *H. influenzae* type b infection: rifampin (20 mg/kg/day, maximum 600 mg) in a single dose given daily for 4 consecutive days to all household contacts, including adults, in those households that have at least one contact under the age of 49 months.[59] The index patient should also be given prophylaxis. Rifampin prophylaxis therapy should be started within 7 days of exposure to the index patient, but prophylaxis is not recommended for pregnant women or in households in which all contacts are older than 48 months.

CROUP SYNDROMES

Croup syndromes are those diseases involving the subglottic tissues of the upper airway and are divided into three distinct groups: spasmodic croup, viral laryngotracheobronchitis, and bacterial tracheitis. These diseases have different origins, clinical courses, and responses to treatment but usually present with some combination of inspiratory stridor, barky cough, fever, hoarseness, and varying degrees of respiratory distress (Table 26–1).

Spasmodic Croup

Spasmodic croup is a disease of uncertain origin that often presents with a sudden onset of inspiratory stridor and barky cough in the middle of the night. Spasmodic croup is more prevalent in the fall and winter in the 1- to 3-year-old child. There is a strong male preponderance and a predisposition to recurrence in allergic families.[49, 60–62]

Although the origin of spasmodic croup is unknown, the symptoms are related to noninflammatory edema within the submucosa of the subglottic trachea.[49] Pale, watery swelling without inflammatory edema is seen.[41, 61] In children with recurrent croup (defined as three or more episodes of croup), there is a familial predisposition, an association with airway hyperactivity affecting both the inspiratory and expiratory limbs of the flow volume loop, and significantly lower serum immunoglobulin A (IgA) levels when compared with asthmatic and normal children.[63]

Clinical Evaluation

Spasmodic croup is characterized by a barky cough and inspiratory stridor. It generally has a sudden onset in the middle of the night and prompts frantic visits to the emergency department, with the symptoms nearly resolved by the time of arrival.

The physical examination of the child with spasmodic croup generally reveals an afebrile child with a completely normal examination, with the exception of inspiratory stridor and a barky cough. Signs and symptoms of ear, nose, throat, or pulmonary infections are notably absent.[49, 60, 61]

Diagnostic Evaluation

Rarely are any diagnostic studies performed on the child with spasmodic croup. Soft tissue neck radiographs might be expected to show steepling of the subglottic airway (Fig. 26–3), but in fact radiographic studies are usually normal.[61]

Therapeutic Intervention

Spasmodic croup responds readily to humidification, cool air, and reassurance. Often, after a car ride in the cool night air to the hospital, the child is nearly normal. Despite this, a thorough history and physical examination should be performed to exclude other, more serious problems.[41, 64]

Hospitalization is rarely needed, but the clinician must be ready at all times to provide airway support for these children if indicated. Racemic epinephrine is of little value in the treatment of this disease. These children are likely to have a recurrence later the same night, as well as on the following three or four nights. Humidification with a cool-mist vaporizer and antihistamines may be of some value in preventing the recurrence.[41, 64]

Disposition

As hospitalization for spasmodic croup is rare, the child's parent or attendant should be given the following instructions (assuming the child has no other infections and is well at the time of discharge):

1. Observe the child for development of signs or symptoms of respiratory distress (e.g., noisy breathing, rapid breathing, retractions, or color changes). If these develop, recheck with the emergency department.
2. Place a cool-mist vaporizer at the child's bedside for the next four to five nights.
3. If the child develops noisy breathing despite the vaporizer, take the child to a cool air environment (i.e., outside) or steam up the bathroom and allow the child to breathe

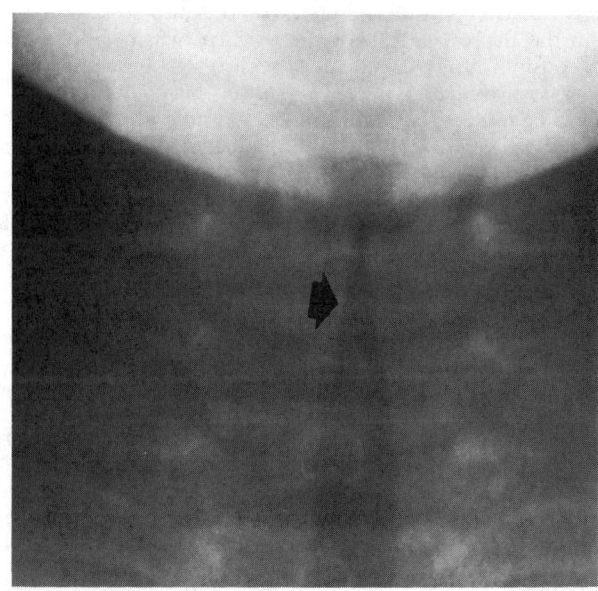

Figure 26–3. The symmetric subglottic narrowing *(arrow)* evident in the anteroposterior film of this child's airway is typically for croup and has been described as the steeple sign. In patients without subglottic narrowing, the trachea interface with the undersurface of the true vocal cords is nearly horizontal. (Courtesy of A. Oestreich, M.D., Cincinnati, OH.)

this mist. If there is no improvement after 20 to 30 minutes or the child's condition worsens, recheck with the emergency department.

4. Report any fever to the family doctor or the emergency department.

Viral Laryngotracheobronchitis

Laryngotracheobronchitis (LTB) is the most common croup syndrome[49] and is a relatively common disease entity.[65] Though some clinicians feel that LTB is a separate entity from laryngotracheitis, most use the terms interchangeably.[66]

LTB affects children of all ages but is more common in the 3-month to 3-year-old population, with the highest incidence in the second year of life.[67, 68] There is a 1.4 to 2.3:1 male-to-female ratio.[67, 68] LTB has a biannual occurrence peak, with the largest peak beginning in September and ending in December and the second peak beginning in January and ending in March.[67]

Origin

Almost all cases of LTB are viral, and the most frequent virus involved is parainfluenza type 1. Parainfluenza virus types 2 and 3 have also been implicated, as have influenza virus, respiratory syncytial virus, adenovirus, rhinovirus, coxsackievirus, and echovirus.[60, 69, 70] *Mycoplasma pneumoniae* has also been recovered.[67]

Clinical Evaluation

The patient with LTB generally presents with a history of a mild upper respiratory infection for 1 to 2 days preceding the development of a hoarse, barky, cough and inspiratory stridor. The symptoms are often worse at night and generally disappear in 5 to 7 days. The child often has a mild fever of 38.3°C to 39.4°C.[49, 71] Physical examination usually reveals mild respiratory distress with a normal-appearing pharynx. Retractions may be present, and the child has clear breath sounds.[49] The intensity of the stridor is a poor indicator of the severity of the obstruction.[71] Restlessness and agitation may indicate serious hypoxemia, rather than anxiety.[71] Patients with stridor and without sternal or chest wall retractions on admission are routinely discharged within 48 hours and recover rapidly and spontaneously without artificial airway placement or administration of racemic epinephrine.[68] Children demonstrating sternal and chest wall retractions at rest on admission experience longer hospitalizations, frequently receive medical intervention such as mist therapy or racemic epinephrine, and have a 6% risk of requiring artificial respiratory support.

The subglottic tissues are generally intensely red and swollen, and the patient may have small patches of secretions that are easily wiped away without leaving eroding or bleeding mucosal surfaces, necrosis, ulcerations, or membranes. Because the subglottic trachea is surrounded by a ring of cartilage, swelling caused by inflammation can only occur by encroaching on the airway.[64] The child is rapidly compromised by any process that causes inflammatory swelling or spasm of the subglottic space.[1]

Diagnostic Evaluation

A child with LTB on soft tissue neck radiographs often has the classic "steeple" sign of subglottic narrowing.[32, 36, 72, 73] However, in a significant percentage of patients, the soft tissue radiographs are normal.[74-76] Dynamic inspiratory and expiratory films may show overdistention of the hypopharynx and narrowing of the trachea on inspiration and ballooning of the cervical trachea on exhalation.[72] The epiglottis and surrounding tissues should appear normal. A complete blood cell count may show the white blood cell count to be normal or slightly elevated.[36, 76]

Therapeutic Management

Patients with LTB have been variously classified in the literature to standardize their severity when comparing various treatment modalities (Tables 26–4 and 26–5). The croup score was initially devised by Taussig and coworkers to categorize patients with croup and gives arbitrary point scores to color, air entry, retractions, level of consciousness, and stridor.[77]

Approximately 5% to 10% of children who present to the emergency department with LTB will require admission,[49] and 1% to 6% will require intubation.[49, 68] The need for intubation is established when the clinical examination reveals severe respiratory distress manifested by increasing tachycardia, tachypnea, chest retractions, cyanosis, exhaustion, agitation, or confusion.

Therapy for viral LTB, once the clinician is assured that the patient is not in need of an artificial airway, may take one of several different forms. Therapy should be based on the child's clinical picture and may require any of the following: oxygen therapy, mist treatment with humidification, racemic epinephrine, helium-oxygen mixtures, and steroids (Table 26–6).

Oxygen Therapy. Oxygen should be offered to all children being initially treated for croup or LTB if their pulse oximetry suggests hypoxia. Oxygen will not correct the obstruction but will alleviate some of the symptoms associated with hypoxemia.[71] Oxygen should be provided in a manner that does not agitate the child.

Mist Treatment. Mist treatment is a mainstay in LTB therapy. Bourchier et al.[78] studied the use of high humidity versus normal humidity in patients with croup and found

TABLE 26–4				
CROUP SCORE				
	0	**1**	**2**	**3**
Color	Normal	Dusky	Cyanotic in room air	Cyanotic in 30% to 40% O_2
Air entry	Normal	Mildly decreased	Moderately decreased	Substantially decreased
Retractions	None	Mild	Moderate	Severe
Level of consciousness	Normal	Restless	Lethargy (depressed)	Obtunded
Stridor	None	Mild	Moderate	Severe or absent in the presence of severe obstruction

Modified from Taussig LM, Castro O, Beaudry PH, et al. Treatment of laryngotracheobronchitis (croup). Am J Dis Child 1975;129:790–793. Copyright 1975, American Medical Association.

TABLE 26–5

STAGES OF CROUP AND THEIR USUAL MANAGEMENT

Total Croup Score	Classification	Usual Treatment
0–4	Mild	Mist. Home care to include vaporizer and careful observation.
5–6	Mild to moderate	Mist. If good response, as above. If poor response or mitigating circumstances such as long transport, young age, unreliable caregivers, then hospitalize.
7–8	Moderate	Hospital admission unless patient responds well to mist, has reliable caregivers, and resides close to hospital. Give oxygen and racemic epinephrine if admitted.
9–14	Severe	Oxygen, racemic epinephrine aerosol while team is mobilized to provide artificial airway. Occasionally, if good patient response to treatment, patient may be observed only. Steroids may be indicated.
15	Terminal	Oxygen, racemic epinephrine, establishment of artificial airway, steroids.

Any child with a score of 3 in one category is automatically classified as having severe disease.

Modified from Battaglia JD. Severe croup: The child with fever and upper airway obstruction. Pediatr Rev 1986;7:231 (reproduced by permission of Pediatrics, copyright 1986); and Davis HW, Gartner JC, Galvis AG, et al. Acute upper airway obstruction: Croup and epiglottitis. Pediatr Clin North Am 1981;28:859.

no difference between the two in improvement of physical signs over the first 12 hours in the treatment of children with mild croup.[78] Nevertheless, if used in moderate amounts, increased humidity should be harmless. Cold, dry air should be avoided during the treatment of patients with croup.[79]

Racemic Epinephrine. Racemic epinephrine is advocated for children with moderate to severe LTB. The usual dose is 0.25 to 0.50 ml of a 2.25% racemic epinephrine solution

TABLE 26–6

UPPER AIRWAY EMERGENCY: THERAPY AT A GLANCE

Epiglottitis
Airway management by intubation
Oxygen
Intravenous antibiotics
  Cefuroxime, 75–200 mg/kg/day divided every 8 hours
    or
  Ampicillin, 200 mg/kg/day divided every 6 hours
    and
  Chloramphenicol, 100 mg/kg/day divided every 6 hours

Spasmodic croup
Humidification by cool mist

Laryngotracheobronchitis (LTB)
Airway management by intubation if clinically indicated
Oxygen
Humidification by cool mist
Racemic epinephrine, 0.25–0.5 ml of 2.25% solution
  diluted 1:8 and administered by aerosol; used in
  patients with moderate to severe croup; and, if used,
  necessitates hospital admission
Helium-oxygen mixture: 20% to 30% oxygen combined
  with 80% to 70% helium
Dexamethasone, 0.3 mg/kg administered intramuscularly.
Acetaminophen, 15 mg/kg given rectally every 4 hours for
  fever control

Bacterial Tracheitis
Airway management with suction and intubation if
  indicated
Oxygen therapy
Intravenous antibiotics
  Cefuroxime, 75 to 200 mg/kg/day divided every 8 hours
    or
  Nafcillin, 50 to 100 mg/kg/day divided every 6 hours
    and
  Chloramphenicol 100 mg/kg/day divided every 6 hours

diluted 1:8 and administered either by aerosol alone or through patient-triggered intermittent positive pressure breathing (IPPB). In children with croup scores greater than 4, racemic epinephrine solution given by IPPB was more effective initially than normal saline given by IPPB, but relapses were routine 2 hours after treatment. In addition, many treatments were often necessary over the course of the disease to prevent the need for intubation or tracheostomy.[77] Racemic epinephrine did not alter the course of the disease process or the duration of hospital stay, but did provide clinical improvement. Westley et al. also noted that there was no significant difference in the respiratory rate or heart rate at any time in a study between groups receiving normal saline or racemic epinephrine.[80] A randomized prospective study comparing the efficacy of racemic epinephrine given by nebulization alone versus nebulization with IPPB found a highly significant reduction in croup scores over time with administration of racemic epinephrine by either route.[81] There was no significant difference demonstrated in the croup score reduction between the two methods of delivery or in the order of the delivery. Acute improvement was obtained with racemic epinephrine, but there was no difference at 90 and 120 minutes, with either method of delivery, between the mean croup scores and the pretreatment scores. It was also noted that nebulization alone was better tolerated than nebulization with IPPB in younger patients. Nebulization is simpler to use and less expensive and eliminates the potential risk of a pneumothorax associated with IPPB therapy. Epinephrine 1:1000 (5 ml) provides an equivalent dose of active epinephrine and has been successfully substituted for racemic epinephrine.[82] If racemic epinephrine is used in the emergency department to treat a patient with LTB, it necessitates admission of the child and observation.[76]

Helium-oxygen Mixtures. Helium is a low-density inert gas that can be substituted for nitrogen to decrease the force necessary to move the gas through the airways. When provided a mixture of 20% to 30% oxygen and 80% to 70% helium in an intensive care unit setting, patients with croup refractory to racemic epinephrine had immediate improvement, with near-immediate recurrence of symptoms if the mixture was removed. No patients in these studies using helium-oxygen inhalation required intubation or tracheostomy, and a minimal number of racemic epinephrine treatments were used.[83, 84]

The limitations of helium-oxygen mixtures include the high expense of helium, the high concentrations required (minimum 60%), and the temporizing, not curative property of treatment. A helium mixture only "buys time" to allow the underlying condition to resolve spontaneously. Though not curative for upper airway obstructions, it does seem to alter the dynamics of respiration significantly and allows obstructed children to breath much easier in a near-immediate fashion. Helium-oxygen mixtures are useful in patients in whom racemic epinephrine is contraindicated (e.g., those with tetralogy of Fallot).[84]

Steroids. The use of steroids in LTB is controversial, and many studies have had variable results. Kairys and coworkers performed meta-analysis on nine randomized studies[85] and noted that a positive difference in clinical improvement and a lower incidence of endotracheal intubation occurred in those patients who received steroids.

A prospective double-blind study evaluating the use of dexamethasone in the management of LTB was conducted.[86] Patients were evaluated and randomly received 0.3 mg/kg of dexamethasone or normal saline intramuscularly on admission and 2 hours later. Modified croup scores were performed initially and every 2 hours. The patients who received dexamethasone had significantly improved croup scores, required fewer racemic epinephrine treatments, and had shorter hospital stays.

Studies in which dexamethasone in doses of 0.3 mg/kg or greater was used demonstrated beneficial effects, whereas those in which less than 0.3 mg/kg of dexamethasone or its equivalent was used failed to demonstrate any significant improvement.[76, 86–92]

Disposition

The treatment of patients with LTB is multifaceted. The clinical decision as to which children require hospital admission and which can be safely managed at home is as much art as science and lies with the physician-provider.[3, 76, 93] The following considerations are used to determine the need for admission:

Stridor at rest
Evidence of exhaustion
Toxicity
Respiratory distress
Need to use racemic epinephrine
Dehydration
Significant respiratory compromise
Unreliable care providers

If admission criteria are absent and the physician feels that the patient may be safely discharged from the emergency department, the following information should be provided to the child's parent:

1. Laryngotracheobronchitis is generally caused by viruses, which antibiotics will not help. It usually lasts 5 to 7 days.

2. If the child develops difficulty in breathing, retractions, color changes, or altered behavior, return to the emergency department immediately. Do not hesitate to call an ambulance.

3. Temperature may be controlled with acetaminophen (15 mg/kg).

Bacterial Tracheitis

Bacterial tracheitis, also termed *pseudomembranous croup*[94] and *membranous laryngotracheobronchitis*,[95] is characterized by bacterial infection of the subglottic airway causing obstruction as a result of subglottic edema and copious mucopurulent secretions.[94–99] These secretions often become inspis-

sated, forming casts of the bronchopulmonary tree and occasionally the gastrointestinal tract, and may mimic a foreign body aspiration on soft tissue radiographs of the neck.[95, 100, 101]

Bacterial tracheitis is actually more common than epiglottitis but less frequent than viral LTB. There is an approximately 2:1 male-to-female ratio,[94–100, 102, 103] with a preponderance in the fall and winter reported.[96, 98]

Origin

Bacterial tracheitis is caused most often by *S. aureus*. There are reports of cases of bacterial tracheitis secondary to infection by *S. pneumoniae*, alpha-hemolytic streptococci, group A streptococci, *Klebsiella* organisms, *Pseudomonas* organisms, *Escherichia coli*, *H. influenzae*, *Branhamella (Moraxella) catarrhalis* and the viruses parainfluenza and influenza.[94–98, 100–103]

Clinical Evaluation

Bacterial tracheitis is characterized by an insidious onset with an upper respiratory infection picture prior to the onset of stridor. The child usually presents with a history of an upper respiratory infection prodrome for hours to days, followed by a high fever (over 38.9°C [102.0°F]) and evidence of respiratory distress. Often the child has a barky or brassy cough but, unlike patients with viral LTB, generally has a high fever and looks toxic. Children with bacterial tracheitis generally do not demonstrate drooling. The child with bacterial tracheitis is usually older than the child with LTB or epiglottitis, with the average age generally somewhat more than 3 years.[94, 96–98, 101] Sudden onset of respiratory distress and obstruction is common and may be repetitive secondary to the generation of large volumes of tenacious secretions, which often become inspissated.

Bacterial tracheitis has a significant morbidity and mortality. Of 65 patients reviewed with bacterial tracheitis, nine (14%) suffered cardiopulmonary arrest, and four of these died.[95–103]

The physical examination of the child with bacterial tracheitis often reveals a toxic-appearing febrile child with marked respiratory distress, including stridor, retractions, and cyanosis. This condition can progress to respiratory arrest. At the time of intubation, copious mucopurulent secretions exuding from the trachea are often noted and must be cleared prior to establishing an airway. Cultures of the secretions should be obtained as they are cleared, but this should not delay airway management. Patients with bacterial tracheitis should have aggressive airway management first, followed by a complete physical examination and laboratory and diagnostic studies. Direct endoscopy or bronchoscopy of the airway reveals subglottic narrowing, purulent secretions, and mucus casts.[94–98, 100–103]

Diagnostic Evaluation

The diagnosis of bacterial tracheitis is often based on clinical suspicion; confirmation is made at the time of intubation. Laboratory data, usually obtained after the airway is secured, aid in the ongoing management of the child in the intensive care unit. Typically, a complete blood cell count, when performed, demonstrates an elevated white cell count with 10% to 64% band cells. Cultures of the purulent secretions obtained from the airway often reveal *S. aureus* but may also show numerous streptococcal species, *Klebsiella*, *Pseudomonas*, or *H. influenzae*. If viral cultures are done, parainfluenza and influenza will occasionally be documented.[96–98, 100]

Soft tissue radiographs of the neck are often performed

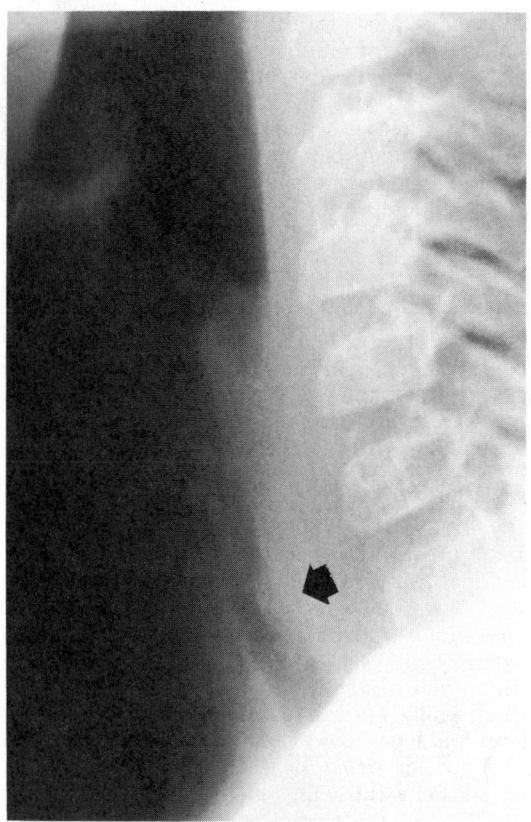

Figure 26–4. Note the characteristic abnormal soft tissue density *(arrow)* within the posterior lumen of the cervical trachea of this 6-year-old boy with membranous (bacterial) croup. Such a membrane is potentially dangerous if it becomes lodged in the glottis after a cough. (Courtesy of A. Oestreich, M.D., Cincinnati, OH.)

in the child with bacterial tracheitis to determine the cause of the stridor in patients not requiring immediate artificial airway support. As with epiglottitis, radiographs should never delay airway management in the child who needs it emergently. The appearance of bacterial tracheitis on soft tissue radiographs of the neck almost uniformly shows subglottic narrowing and often demonstrates foreign body material in the trachea (Fig. 26–4). This foreign body material is often a cast of the airway secondary to inspissated secretions.[94–103] Concommitant pneumonia as demonstrated on a chest radiograph is found in approximately 50% of patients with a diagnosis of bacterial tracheitis.[96–99, 101]

Therapeutic Intervention

Patients who demonstrate severe respiratory distress should undergo immediate airway management with removal of secretions and intubation. Such patients often demonstrate rapid clinical improvement when secretions are removed, only to relapse within several hours because of reaccumulation of these secretions. For this reason, children with bacterial tracheitis should be managed in an intensive care unit setting with intubation, oxygen, and aggressive pulmonary toilet. Despite this, endotracheal tube obstruction may occur, prompting some authors to recommend tracheostomy because of the greater ease of cleaning and suctioning.[94] Repeated therapeutic bronchoscopies are often necessary to maintain a patent airway.

Antibiotic coverage for *S. aureus* is essential, and often a second antibiotic is added to broaden the coverage to include *Streptococcus* species, *H. influenzae*, *Klebsiella* and *Pseudomonas*

organisms, and *B. (M.) catarrhalis*. The average duration of hospitalization ranges from 3 to 48 days in reported studies.[95–97, 103]

Disposition

All patients with bacterial tracheitis should be managed with intubation and intravenous antibiotics. The child should be admitted to an intensive care unit.

References

1. Cramblett HG. Croup (epiglottitis; laryngitis; laryngotracheobronchitis). *In* Kendig EL, Chernick V (eds). Disorders of the Respiratory Tract in Children. Philadelphia, WB Saunders, 1971, pp 140–141, 353–360.
2. Fried MP. Controversies in the management of supraglottitis and croup. Pediatr Clin North Am 1979;26:931.
3. Daum RS, Smith AL. Epiglottitis (supraglottitis) *In* Feigin RD, Cherry JD (eds). Textbook of Pediatric Infectious Diseases. 2nd ed. Philadelphia, WB Saunders, 1987, pp 224–237.
4. Kendig EL Jr, Chernick V (eds). Disorders of the Respiratory Tract in Children. 4th ed. Philadelphia, WB Saunders, 1983, pp 62–63.
5. Brilli RJ, Benzing G, Cotcamp DH. Epiglottitis in infants less than two years of age. Pediatr Emerg Care 1989;5:16.
6. Briggs RJ, Atenau MM. Acute epiglottitis in children. Otolaryngol Head Neck Surg 1980;88:665.
7. Baxter JD. Acute epiglottitis in children. Laryngoscope 1967;77:1358.
8. Berenberg W, Kevy S. Acute epiglottitis in childhood. A serious emergency, readily recognized at the bedside. N Engl J Med 1958;258:870.
9. Baines DB, Wark H, Overton JH. Acute epiglottis in children. Anaesth Intens Care 1984;13:25.
10. Johnson GK, Sullivan JL, Bishop LA. Acute epiglottitis. Review of 55 cases and suggested protocol. Arch Otolaryngol 1974;100:333.
11. Bottenfield GW, Arcinue EL, Sarnaik A, Jewell MR. Diagnosis and management of acute epiglottitis—report of 90 consecutive cases. Laryngoscope 1980;90:822.
12. Sendi K, Crysdale WS. Acute epiglottitis: Decade of change—a 10-year experience with 242 children. J Otolaryngol 1987;16:196.
13. Vetto RR. Epiglottitis. Report of thirty-seven cases. JAMA 1960;173:88.
14. Bass JW, Steele RW, Wieke RA. Acute epiglottitis. A surgical emergency. JAMA 1974;229:671.
15. Faden HS. Treatment of *Haemophilus influenzae* type B epiglottitis. Pediatrics 1979;63:402.
16. Murrage KJ, Janzen VD, Ruby RR. Epiglottitis: Adult and pediatric comparisons. J Otolaryngol 1988;17:194.
17. Lacroix J, Ahronheim G, Arcand, P, et al. Group A streptococcal supraglottitis. J Pediatr 1986;109:20.
18. Trollfors B, Brorson JE, Claesson B, Sandberg T. Invasive infections caused by *Haemophilus* species other than *Haemophilus influenzae*. Infection 1985;13:12.
19. Schwartz RH, Knerr RJ, Hermansen K, Wientzen RL. Acute epiglottitis caused by β-hemolytic group C streptococci. Am J Dis Child 1982;136:558.
20. Lewis JK, Gartner JC, Galvis AG. A protocol for management of acute epiglottitis. Clin Pediatr 1978;17:494.
21. Crysdale WS, Sendi K. Evolution in the management of acute epiglottitis: A 10-year experience with 242 children. Int Anesthesiol Clin 1988;26:32.
22. Lee SC, Meislin H, Iserson KV. Epiglottitis presenting as acute pulmonary edema. Ann Emerg Med 1985;14:60.
23. Travis KW, Todres ID, Shannon DC. Pulmonary edema associated with croup and epiglottitis. Pediatrics 1977;59:695.
24. Kanter RK, Watchko JF. Pulmonary edema associated with upper airway obstruction. Am J Dis Child 1984;138:356.
25. Singer, JI, McCabe JB. Epiglottitis at the extremes of age. Am J Emerg Med 1988;6:228.
26. Tarnow-Mordi WO, Berrill AM, Darby CW, et al. Precipitation of laryngeal obstruction in acute epiglottitis. Br Med J 1985;290:629.
27. Williams PAD, Armitage EN, Fisher NGS, Hatcher CW. Precipitation of laryngeal obstruction in acute epiglottitis. Br Med J 1985;290:1007.
28. Mauro RD, Poole SR, Lockhart CH. Differentiation of epiglottitis from laryngotracheitis in the child with stridor. Am J Dis Child 1988;142:679.
29. Butt W, Shann F, Walker C, et al. Acute epiglottitis: A different approach to management. Crit Care Med 1988;16:43.
30. Hodge KM, Ganzel TM. Diagnostic and therapeutic efficiency in croup and epiglottitis. Laryngoscope 1987;97:621.
31. Costigan DC, Newth CJL. Respiratory status of children with epiglottitis with and without an artificial airway. Am J Dis Child 1983;137:139.
32. Rapkin RH. The diagnosis of epiglottitis: Simplicity and reliability of radiographs of the neck in the differential diagnosis of the croup syndrome. J Pediatr 1972;80:96.
33. Grodin MA. Epiglottitis. J Emerg Med 1983;1:13.

34. Vernon DD, Sarnaik AP. Acute epiglottitis in children: A conservative approach to diagnosis and management. Crit Care Med 1986;14:23.
35. Kimmons HC, Peterson BM. Management of acute epiglottitis in pediatric patients. Crit Care Med 1986;14:278.
36. Diaz JH. Croup and epiglottitis in children: The anesthesiologist as diagnostician. Anesth Analg 1985;64:621.
37. Zulliger JJ, Garvin JP, Schuller DE, et al. Assessment of intubation in croup and epiglottitis. Ann Otol Rhinol Laryngol 1982;91:403.
38. Adair JC, Ring WH. Management of epiglottitis in children. Anesth Analg 1975;54:622.
39. Breivik H, Klaastad O. Acute epiglottitis in children. Br J Anaesth 1978;50:505.
40. Arndal H, Andreassen UK. Acute epiglottitis in children and adults. Nasotracheal intubation, tracheostomy or careful observation? Current status in Scandinavia. J Laryngol Otol 1988;102:1012.
41. Battaglia JD. Severe croup: The child with fever and upper airway obstruction. Pediatr Rev 1986;7:PIR 227–PIR 233.
42. Fearon BW, Bell RD. Acute epiglottitis: A potential killer. Can Med Assoc J 1975;112:760.
43. Rosen P, Barkin RM: Respiratory distress in the child. J Emerg Med 1985;3:157.
44. Schenck NL. Airway intervention in croup and epiglottitis: The changing role of the otolaryngologist. ORL 1978;86:513.
45. Gussack GS, Tacchi EJ. Pulse oximetry in the management of pediatric airway disorders. South Med J 1987;80:1381.
46. Bass JW. Routine tracheotomy for epiglottitis: what are the odds? J Pediatr 1973;83:510.
47. Rothstein P, Lister G. Epiglottitis—duration of intubation and fever. Anesth Analg 1983;62:785.
48. Barson WJ, Miller MA, Marcon MJ, et al. Cefuroxime therapy for bacteremic soft-tissue infections in children. Am J Dis Child 1985;139:1141.
49. McLain LG. Croup syndrome. Am Fam Physician 1987;36:207.
50. Wald E, Reilly JS, Bluestone CD, Chiponis D. Sulbactam/ampicillin in the treatment of acute epiglottitis in children. Rev Infect Dis 1986; suppl 5:S617–S619.
51. Molteni RA. Epiglottitis: Incidence of extraglottic infections; report of 72 cases and review of the literature. Pediatrics 1976;58:526.
52. Friedman EM, Healy GB, Damion J, McGill TJI. Supraglottitis and concurrent *Haemophilus* meningitis. Ann Otol Rhinol Laryngol 1985;94:470.
53. Gonzalez C, Gartner JC, Casselbrant ML, Kenna MA. Complication of acute epiglottitis. Int J Pediatr Otorhinolaryngol 1986;11:67.
54. LaScolea LJ Jr, Rosales SV, Welliver RC, Ogra PL. Mechanisms underlying the development of meningitis or epiglottitis in children after *Haemophilus influenzae* type b bacteremia. J Infect Dis 1985;151:1162.
55. Healy GB, Hyams VJ, Tucker GF Jr. Paraglottic laryngitis in association with epiglottitis. Ann Otol Rhinol Laryngol 1985;94:618.
56. Centers for Disease Control. Polysaccharide vaccine for prevention of *Haemophilus influenzae* type b disease. MMWR 1985;34:201.
57. Committee on Infectious Diseases. *Haemophilus* type b polysaccharide vaccine. Pediatrics 1985;76:322.
58. Daum RS, Granoff DM. A vaccine against *Haemophilus influenzae* type b. Pediatr Infect Dis 1985;4:355.
59. Committee on Infectious Diseases. Revision of recommendation for use of Rifampin prophylaxis of contacts of patients with *Haemophilus influenzae* infection. Pediatrics 1984;74:301.
60. Baugh R, Gilmore BB Jr. Infectious croup: A critical review. Otolaryngol Head Neck Surg 1986;95:40.
61. Davison FW. Acute laryngeal obstruction in children. JAMA 1959;171:1301.
62. Hide DW, Guyer BM. Recurrent croup. Arch Dis Child 1985;60:585.
63. Zach MS. Airway reactivity in recurrent croup. Eur J Respir Dis 1983;64(suppl 128):81.
64. Cherry JD. Croup (laryngitis, laryngotracheitis, spasmodic croup, and laryngotracheobronchitis). *In* Feigin RD, Cherry JD (eds). Textbook of Pediatric Infectious Diseases. Philadelphia, WB Saunders, 1987, pp 237–250.
65. Broniatowski M. Croup. Ear Nose Throat 1985;64:12.
66. Cherry JD. The treatment of croup: Continued controversy due to failure of recognition of historic, ecologic, etiologic and clinical perspectives. J Pediatr 1979;94:352.
67. Denny FW, Murphy TH, Clyde WA Jr, et al. Croup: An 11-year study in a pediatric practice. Pediatrics 1983;71:871.
68. Wagener JS, Landau LI, Olinsky A, Phelan PD. Management of children hospitalized for laryngotracheobronchitis. Pediatr Pulmonol 1986;2:159.
69. Stool SE. Croup syndrome: historical perspective. Pediatr Infect Dis J 1988;7:S157.
70. Levison H, Tabachnik E, Newth CJL. Wheezing in infancy, croup, and epiglottitis. Curr Prob Pediatr 1982;12:1.
71. Couriel JM. Management of croup. Arch Dis Child 1988;63:1305.
72. Currarino G, Williams B. Lateral inspiration and expiration radiographs of the neck in children with laryngotracheitis (croup). Radiology 1982;145:365.
73. Corkey CWB, Barker GA, Edmonds JF, et al. Radiographic tracheal diameter measurements in acute infectious croup: An objective scoring system. Crit Care Med 1981;9:587.
74. Goel KM. Are neck radiographs necessary in the management of croup syndrome? Arch Dis Child 1984;59:908.
75. Stankiewicz JA, Bowes AK. Croup and epiglottitis: A radiologic study. Laryngoscope 1985;95:1159.
76. Postma DS, Jones RO, Pillsbury HC III. Severe hospitalized croup: Treatment trends and prognosis. Laryngoscope 1984;94:1170.
77. Taussig LM, Castro O, Beaudry PH, et al. Treatment of laryngotracheobronchitis (croup). Am J Dis Child 1975;129:790.
78. Bourchier D, Dawson KP, Fergusson DM. Humidification in viral croup: A controlled trial. Aust Paediar J 1984;20:289.
79. Henry R. Moist air in the treatment of laryngotracheitis. Arch Dis Child 1983;58:577.
80. Westley CR, Cotton EK, Brooks JG. Nebulized racemic epinephrine by IPPB for the treatment of croup. Am J Dis Child 1978;132:484.
81. Foget JM, Berg IJ, Gerber MA, Cherter CB. Racemic epinephrine in the treatment of croup: Nebulization alone versus nebulization with intermittent positive pressure breathing. J Pediatr 1982;101:1028.
82. Remington S, Meakin G. Nebulised adrenaline 1:1000 in the treatment of croup. Anesthesia 1986;41:923.
83. Nelson DS, McClellan L. Helium-oxygen mixtures as adjunctive support for refractory viral croup. Ohio State Med J 1982;78:729.
84. Duncan PG. Efficacy of helium-oxygen mixtures in the management of severe viral and post-intubation croup. Can Anaesth Soc J 1979;26:206.
85. Kairys SW, Olmstead EM, O'Connor GT. Steroid treatment of laryngotracheitis: A meta-analysis of the evidence from randomized trials. Pediatrics 1989;83:683.
86. Leipzig B, Oski FA, Cummings CW, et al. A prospective randomized study to determine the efficacy of steroids in treatment of croup. J Pediatr 1979;94:194.
87. James JA. Dexamethasone in croup. Am J Dis Child 1969;117:511.
88. Eden AN, Larkin VD. Experience and reason. Briefly recorded. Pediatrics 1964;33:768.
89. Eden AN, Kaufman A, Yu R. Corticosteroids and croup. Controlled double-blind study. JAMA 1967;200:133.
90. Bass JW, Bruhn FW, Merritt WT. Corticosteroids and racemic epinephrine with IPPB in the treatment of croup. J Pediatr 1980;96:173.
91. Kuusela AL, Vesikari T. A randomized double-blind, placebo-controlled trial of dexamethasone and racemic epinephrine in the treatment of croup. Acta Paediatr Scand 1988;77:99.
92. Hawkins DB, Crockett DM, Shum TK. Corticosteroids in airway management. Otolaryngol Head Neck Surg 1983;91:593.
93. Goldhagen JL. Croup: Pathogenesis and management. J Emerg Med 1983;1:3.
94. Henry RL, Mellis CM, Benjamin B. Pseudomembranous croup. Arch Dis Child 1983;58:180.
95. Denneny JC III, Handler SD. Membranous laryngotracheobronchitis. Pediatrics 1982;70:705.
96. Jones R, Santos JI, Overall JC Jr. Bacterial tracheitis. JAMA 1979;242:721.
97. Sofer S, Duncan P, Chernick V. Bacterial tracheitis—an old disease rediscovered. Clin Pediatr 1983;22:407.
98. Liston SL, Gehrz RC, Siegel LG, Tilelli J. Bacterial tracheitis. Am J Dis Child 1983;137:764.
99. Liston SL, Gehrz RC, Jarvis CW. Bacterial tracheitis. Arch Otolaryngol 1981;107:561.
100. McKenzie M, Norman MG, Anderson JD, Thiessen PN. Upper respiratory tract infeciton in a 3-year-old girl. J Pediatr 1984;105:129.
101. Han BK, Dunbar JS, Striker TW. Membranous laryngotracheobronchitis (membranous croup). AJR 1979;133:53.
102. Hefelfinger DC. Croup vs epiglottitis vs tracheitis. JAMA 1981;246:1087.
103. Edwards KM, Dundon C, Altemeier WA. Bacterial tracheitis as a complication of viral croup. Pediatr Infect Dis 1983;2:390.

Bronchiolitis

Russell H. Greenfield
Robert W. Schafermeyer

INTRODUCTION

Bronchiolitis is an acute lower respiratory tract infection common in young children, particularly those less than 6 months of age. The disease generally occurs during the winter or early spring[1-7] and has an incidence of approximately 11.6 per 100 children per year[1]; respiratory syncytial virus is the most common causative organism.[8-10] An increase in the incidence of bronchiolitis has been associated with passive smoke and crowded living conditions.[8, 10-13] A significant number of patients with a history of bronchiolitis will develop bronchospastic disease later in life.[14-28] The infection produces inflammatory obstruction of the small airways and reactive airways disease.[14-19] Clinically, patients present with cough, tachypnea, dyspnea, and wheezing, often associated with retractions and nasal flaring. Although the clinical course is usually mild, with resolution in 1 to 2 weeks, patients may develop hypoxia, dehydration, pneumothorax, or congestive heart failure. A small number of infants will develop respiratory failure requiring ventilatory support. Death occurs in 1% to 7%[9, 29] of all patients, primarily in infants less than 6 months of age and in children with preexisting pulmonary and cardiac diseases.[14, 30] The primary focus of treatment is provision of supportive care, rapid identification and treatment of the child in early respiratory failure, and careful observation.

ANATOMY AND PATHOPHYSIOLOGY

The differences between the anatomy of the respiratory tract of a child and that of an adult help explain pathologic conditions that are relatively specific to the pediatric population. Cartilage, ciliated cells, and mucous glands are all present at birth, and there is tracheobronchial mucous secretion in the infant. The conducting airways of the infant are small and more easily obstructed at the level of the larynx and tracheobronchial tree than are those in the adult. Smooth muscle is present even in the peripheral lung zones from birth, allowing bronchospasm to occur at a very young age. As obstruction increases, the expiratory phase of respiration increases, and wheezing is heard. As obstruction becomes more severe, wheezing may disappear, and cyanosis may occur. Chest wall retractions are much greater in infants than in adults because of the greater pliability of the supporting structures. As the turbulence of inspiratory and expiratory air flow increases, the work of breathing likewise increases, and the accessory muscles of respiration—the intercostals, sternocleidomastoids, and abdominal muscles—are recruited to assist with breathing.

The normal resting respiratory rate of an infant is approximately 40 breaths/min. The rate decreases as body size increases, finally reaching the adult rate of about 12 breaths/min. Patients with respiratory distress will have increased respiratory rates and can lose significant amounts of fluid from the lungs. A slow respiratory rate in a patient with respiratory distress is an ominous finding and portends impending respiratory arrest.

EMERGENCY MEDICAL SERVICE CONSIDERATIONS

Management of the child with respiratory distress in the field begins with recognition. Respiratory failure is easily identified in a patient who is cyanotic, bradypneic or severely tachypneic, or stridorous or exhibits altered mental status. More subtle findings include head bobbing, grunting, nasal flaring, intercostal retractions, prolonged expiration, and poor muscle tone. Paramedics and field personnel must suspect possible foreign body aspiration with obstruction, infectious airway compromise (croup and epiglottitis), reactive airway disease (asthma and bronchiolitis), and toxin-induced respiratory distress (smoke inhalation, carbon monoxide).

Supplemental oxygen should be administered to the patient after it has been determined that the airway is patent. Oxygen should be delivered using an oxygen hood; high-flow oxygen using tubing or a mask should be used for children less than 2 years of age. Patients older than 2 years can have oxygen administered with a mask at a rate of 6 L/min, whereas children older than 6 years may tolerate administration by nasal cannula at a rate of 2 to 6 L/min. If a nonrebreather mask is used, the flow rate should be 12 to 15 L/min. The child should be allowed to maintain a position of comfort to prevent possible acute airway obstruction. Should respiratory failure ensue, ventilations should be assisted with a bag-mask apparatus and endotracheal intubation considered. The base station should be contacted early in the care of any child with respiratory distress.

DIAGNOSTIC EVALUATION

Laboratory Tests

The white blood cell count may be elevated to more than 12,000/mm³, usually because of lymphocytosis.[31] Urine specific gravity may be increased, and electrolyte abnormalities may be present, reflecting dehydration secondary to fever, tachypnea, and decreased intake of fluids.

Pulse oximetry should be performed on all ill-appearing children, and oxygen saturation should be maintained above 90%. Once patients have been placed in the position of comfort and airway patency and adequate ventilation have been ensured, arterial blood gases should be measured if marked respiratory distress is exhibited. Hypoxia occurs in a large percentage of patients as a result of inflammation and accumulation of exudative debris in the tracheobronchial tree. Several studies have shown arterial oxygen saturation (SaO_2) values ranging from 74% to 95%, with a mean level of 87% on room air.[9] The initial reading did not represent the lowest level occurring during the course of the illness. The range at hospital discharge was 83% to 98%; the partial arterial pressure of oxygen (PaO_2) level was in the low 50– to 60–mm Hg range.[9] The partial carbon dioxide pressure (PCO_2) is lowered initially as patients hyperventilate. As the obstructive process worsens, CO_2 retention occurs in the infant and the severely ill patient, especially when the respiratory rate exceeds 60 breaths/min.[9] A PCO_2 greater than 65 mm Hg carries a grave prognosis.[32]

Blood cultures should be obtained from all patients who appear toxic, have temperatures over 38.9°C, and have lobar or segmental infiltrates on chest radiograph. Several studies have stressed the findings of bacterial and viral coinfections in children hospitalized with respiratory syncytial virus (RSV) infections, most commonly with *Streptococcus pneumoniae*.[33, 34] Viral cultures of nasal washings and the throat may be obtained for isolation of RSV. Documentation of the infection should precede therapy with ribavirin if possible, as quantification of RSV will help monitor the response of the patient to ribavirin therapy.[35, 36]

Fluorescent monoclonal antibody stains of nasopharyngeal specimens appear to be more sensitive and more specific than cell cultures for RSV.[37–39] Two commercial agents are available: an indirect fluorescent antibody test and an enzyme-linked immunoassay. Both are as sensitive and specific as cultures.

Studies utilizing immunoelectrophoresis have shown markedly elevated levels of immunoglobulins E (IgE) and G (IgG) in children with RSV infections and wheezing, suggesting that a hypersensitivity reaction is responsible for bronchospasm. One study of infants with bronchiolitis noted that 60% of the patients had elevated levels of immunoglobulin A (IgA).[28, 40]

Pulmonary function tests may be difficult to perform in young children. However, in older children and adults, increased total lung volume and residual volume, decreased compliance, hypoxemia, and an increase in the work of breathing can be determined.[32, 41, 42] Bronchiolitis causes residual parenchyma and airway damage in the majority of infants, and many of these patients will develop abnormalities in peak expiratory flow rates, forced expiratory volume in 1 second (FEV_1),[42] and gas exchange.[43] Some patients will demonstrate increased airway reactivity as a result of their illness.[21, 22, 25–28]

Radiographic Studies

Hyperinflation with flattened diaphragms is the most common finding on chest radiograph, although areas of atelectasis and patchy infiltrates are occasionally seen. The infiltrates resemble interstitial pneumonia or peribronchial thickening[14, 44] and may be indistinguishable from those seen in asthma. Inspiratory and expiratory radiographs or a lateral decubitus radiograph may be useful in the evaluation of foreign body aspiration that may mimic bronchiolitis.[19]

A barium swallow may be helpful in selected patients to rule out the presence of a vascular ring, foreign body, or tracheoesophageal fistula, especially in the wheezing patient who does not appear ill, has no sign of infection, and does not improve by the third or fourth day. It may be necessary to perform this procedure earlier in the course of the illness if the index of suspicion for one of these entities is high.[45] A barium swallow is also indicated in the evaluation of the patient with recurrent bronchiolitis.

DIFFERENTIAL DIAGNOSIS

Differentiating between bronchiolitis and asthma can be difficult. Asthma is a disease of the lower airways characterized by bronchospasm, mucus plugging, mucosal edema, and inflammation (Table 27–1). There is usually a history of recurrent episodes of wheezing and therapeutic response to bronchodilator therapy, and there may be a family history of asthma or allergic conditions. There is often a history of recent upper respiratory tract infection. On physical examination the physician may see wheezing, nasal flaring, intercostal retractions, and a prolonged expiratory phase. In the majority of patients, bronchospasm responds rapidly to the administration of sympathomimetics. It may be extremely difficult, if not impossible, to differentiate between bronchiolitis and asthma during the first presentation of a child less than 2 years of age.

Upper respiratory tract illnesses may mimic bronchiolitis in the child under two years of age. *Mycoplasma, chlamydia,* and viral infections can also present as bronchiolitis.[4, 44] Wheezing may also be present in the early stages of pertussis.[44] Patients with pertussis commonly have increased res-

---

TABLE 27–1
DIFFERENTIAL DIAGNOSIS OF BRONCHIOLITIS
Asthma
Mycoplasma, Chlamydia, viral infections
Tracheobronchial foreign body aspiration
Tracheobronchial polyps
Tumors
Laryngomalacia
Cysts
Vascular rings
Anomalous pulmonary vascular return
Congestive heart failure
Irritant gas exposure (smoke inhalation)

piratory tract secretions associated with an uncontrollable cough and inspiratory whoop, although the whoop is usually absent in children less than 6 months of age.

Foreign bodies in the tracheobronchial tree or esophagus can cause airway obstruction and wheezing. There is usually a more sudden onset of wheezing with no history of preceding upper respiratory tract illness and no therapeutic response to bronchodilators. Patients with foreign bodies in the esophagus may present with dysphagia and drooling. Inspiratory and expiratory chest radiographs or a lateral decubitus radiograph may show air trapping consistent with a foreign body in the tracheobronchial tree.

Polyps in the tracheobronchial tree and tumors or cysts of the mediastinum or respiratory tract may present in a fashion similar to bronchiolitis.[45] Children with laryngomalacia may also present with respiratory distress.

A vascular ring compressing the trachea can present with wheezing, hyperinflation, and areas of atelectasis on chest radiograph. This condition should be suspected if there are repeated attacks of bronchiolitis. Patients with anomalous pulmonary venous return may exhibit wheezing and have areas of hyperinflation as well. Wheezing may also be a component of congestive heart failure.[46] A murmur may be heard, and heart size is usually increased.

Any irritant gas exposure, including smoke inhalation injury, may produce a pathophysiologic picture similar to that of bronchiolitis.[32] Patient history, evidence of burns, and carbonaceous sputum should help determine this as a cause of respiratory distress.

THERAPEUTIC INTERVENTION

The child with bronchiolitis who is discharged home should require only symptomatic and supportive care. Caregivers should give the child small, frequent feedings and keep the child well hydrated. The child should be placed in a position of comfort and secretions cleared as needed by bulb syringe suction. Depending on the child's response to treatment in the emergency department, therapy with bronchodilators may be continued on an outpatient basis in selected cases.

If the providers are having difficulties following discharge instructions or the child is not taking fluids well or develops respiratory distress, the patient should be taken to a medical facility immediately. Although therapy for patients with bronchiolitis is primarily supportive, frequent reevaluation of the patient is important, as a small but significant number of patients become dehydrated and hypoxemic and even require ventilatory assistance.

Humidified oxygen at a fraction of inspired oxygen (FIO_2) of 30% to 40% delivered by hood, mask, or incubator is the most useful of the supportive therapies available for bronchiolitis, as up to 80% of infants with this disease have some degree of hypoxia.[31, 47] Humidity should be added to the oxygen to decrease the drying effect on the respiratory tract and secretions. However, a mist tent should not be used, because the large water particles may act as an irritant. The tent may also make it more difficult for nursing personnel to observe the patient for apnea or increasing respiratory distress.[48]

The need for intubation is a clinical judgment based mainly on the patient's course.[15, 49–53] Guidelines for intubation include a partial oxygen pressure (PO_2) less than 50 mm Hg on supplemental oxygen, a PCO_2 greater than 50 mm Hg, an inability to protect the airway, severe metabolic acidosis with insufficient respiratory compensation, or significant change in mental status.

Premature infants who develop respiratory failure secondary to RSV infection may require mechanical ventilation with high minute ventilation, high tidal volumes of 10 to 15 ml/kg, and slow intermittent mandatory ventilation (IMV) rates of 16 to 22 breaths/min.[54, 55] Some patients may require sedation. Expiratory time constants are often prolonged in these patients to allow full emptying of the lungs.[56]

Assessing the state of hydration is important in the young child, as dehydration can occur rapidly, leading to shock and death. Abnormal fluid losses occur from tachypnea, fever, and diarrhea. In addition, there is decreased fluid intake and increased risk of aspiration in the severely tachypneic patient.[19] Dehydration associated with bronchiolitis is usually isotonic with a normal serum sodium level.

Intravenous fluids should be administered only if oral intake is inadequate or respiratory distress precludes safe oral rehydration. Total maintenance fluid requirements may be decreased if humidified oxygen is used.[57, 58]

Replacement of fluid deficit is based on the magnitude of dehydration determined by physical examination and laboratory data. Assuming normal renal function, initial rehydration should take place over 30 minutes as a fluid bolus in the moderately to severely dehydrated child, using 20 ml/kg of 0.9% normal saline (NS) or lactated Ringer's solution (LR). If the response is poor, a repeat bolus of 20 ml/kg may be administered over 20 to 30 minutes. In the presence of rapidly continuing losses or suspected cardiac or renal problems, or if the patient cannot be stabilized, central venous pressure or pulmonary artery wedge pressure may need to be monitored.

Maintenance and deficit fluids can be replaced by a combination of 0.45% NS and 0.25% NS at a rate sufficient to maintain normal vital signs and urine output, assuming that the patient has isotonic dehydration. Some patients will have increased secretion of antidiuretic hormone and can be overhydrated; input and output, daily weight, urine specific gravity, and serum sodium should be accurately monitored.

A trial of bronchodilator therapy is indicated in infants and children with bronchiolitis, as many of these patients will have reactive airways.[44, 46] If the patient does not improve, bronchodilator therapy should cease, as repeated administration may be harmful to the patient.[57]

Multiple studies have been performed comparing inhaled beta agonists with subcutaneous epinephrine injection. These studies show that inhaled beta-agonist therapy is at least as effective as epinephrine and may actually be safer because of the adverse effects associated with epinephrine use (including palpitations, transient hypertension, dysrhythmias, and lactic acidosis). Although a number of inhaled sympathomimetic agents are available, inhaled albuterol in a dose of 0.05 mg/kg every 20 minutes can be used.[59] Bronchodilation may last as long as 4 to 6 hours with this agent. Hypokalemia is a reported adverse effect associated with the use of inhaled albuterol. Young children usually

can be given this therapy using a mouthpiece, but administration of aerosolized beta agonists to an infant should be done with a mask.

Many physicians still prefer to use a trial dose of 0.01 ml/kg of 1:1000 epinephrine administered subcutaneously in children older than 6 months of age (maximum of 0.35 ml/dose) (Table 27–2). Doses may be repeated every 20 minutes to a total of three if there is partial response to the initial administration and the heart rate remains below 180 beats/min. Vital signs and serum glucose levels should be monitored. If there is no response, epinephrine therapy is discontinued. Terbutaline (0.005 to 0.010 ml/kg) can also be given subcutaneously and is more beta$_2$ specific than epinephrine.

Aminophylline is also useful in selected cases. Aminophylline may be administered orally in a dose of 4 to 5 mg/kg every 6 hours after an initial load of 6 to 7 mg/kg as a single dose, or it may be loaded intravenously in a dose of 5 to 6 mg/kg over 30 minutes. A loading dose raises the blood level of aminophylline 2 µg/ml for every milligram per kilogram administered.[60] If theophylline is already present in the blood stream, particularly at levels greater than 8 µg/ml, the pharmacokinetics change such that a loading dose of 5 mg/kg will raise levels more than an increment of 10 µg/ml. Intravenous maintenance aminophylline doses range from 0.8 to 1.2 mg/kg/hr (0.6 to 0.9 mg/kg/hr for theophylline). In the emergency setting, when levels are not immediately available, adjustments are made

---

TABLE 27–2
BRONCHIOLITIS THERAPY AT A GLANCE

Place patient in position of comfort
Humidified 30%–40% oxygen
Intubation and mechanical ventilation based on:
  Clinical judgment
  PO_2 <50 mm Hg on supplemental oxygen
  PCO_2 >50 mm Hg
  Inability to protect airway
  Severe metabolic acidosis with insufficient respiratory compensation
  Altered mental status

Maintain adequate hydration
  Oral fluid administration if deemed safe (respiratory rate <60 breaths/min)
  Intravenous fluid administration with inadequate oral intake or moderate to severe dehydration
    20 ml/kg normal saline or Ringer's lactate over 20–30 min
    Repeat 20 ml/kg bolus if inadequate response
    After vital signs and other parameters of dehydration have stabilized, initiate maintenance fluid administration

Drug therapy
  Aerosolized beta agonists (Example: albuterol 0.05 mg/kg/20 min; may repeat in 20 min if there is improvement)
    or
  Epinephrine 0.01 ml/kg 1:1000 given subcutaneously; may repeat in 20 min if there is improvement; do not repeat if there is no therapeutic response
  Aminophylline (if good response to sympathomimetics)
    Oral: initial load, 6–7 mg/kg, followed by 5 mg/kg every 6 hr
    IV: 5 mg/kg load, followed by maintenance drip of 0.8–1.2 mg/kg/hr (0.6–0.9 mg/kg/hr for theophylline)
  Ribavirin, 0.8 mg/kg/hr by continuous aerosol administration for 12–18 hours per day for 3–7 days

TABLE 27–3

ADMINISTRATION OF AMINOPHYLLINE BASED ON TIME OF LAST AMINOPHYLLINE DOSE

Time Since Last Dose	Dose
>24 hr	Full loading dose
8–24 hr	Half loading dose
<8 hr (12 hr for sustained-release capsules)	Maintenance only

based on the timing of the last aminophylline dose (Table 27–3).

The preferred times for having theophylline levels measured are before treatment, 1 hour after the loading dose, and 6 hours after initiating maintenance therapy.[61–64] The optimal serum level has been shown to be between 10 and 20 μg/ml in most patients. Nausea and vomiting have been reported with levels less than 20 μg/ml,[65, 66] and cardiac dysrhythmias may occur with levels less than 20 to 40 μg/ml. With levels greater than 40 μg/ml, focal or generalized seizures, often without antecedent symptoms, have been reported.[66–68]

Rapid intravenous (IV) injections of aminophylline may produce dizziness, precordial pain, or dysrhythmias. Other adverse reactions associated with aminophylline use include irritability, restlessness, nervousness, tachycardia, and convulsions (acute toxicity). Aminophylline should be used with caution in patients with diabetes, peptic ulcer disease, and hyperthyroidism (Table 27–4).[69, 70] Aminophylline enhances elimination of phenytoin (Dilantin) and decreases the effects of lithium. Intravenous use of aminophylline is contraindicated in patients allergic to ethylenediamine.

Ribavirin, a synthetic nucleoside (guanosine) analogue, possesses inhibitory activity against many DNA/RNA viruses. When given as an aerosol over extended periods of time, ribavirin has resulted in decreased viral shedding, improved arterial oxygenation, and a more rapid clinical recovery for infants with lower respiratory tract disease secondary to RSV.[35, 36, 71–73] Symptoms of upper respiratory tract infection are unchanged.[73, 74]

Ribavirin administration is indicated for the treatment of moderately to severely ill children with documented RSV infection who require at least 3 days of hospitalization. It is also indicated for children at risk for severe and possibly fatal RSV infections (e.g., those with congenital heart disease, bronchopulmonary dysplasia, or immunodeficiency).

Ribavirin is given at a dose of 0.8 mg/kg/hr by continuous aerosol administration for 12 to 18 hours per day for 3 to 6 days. Aerosolization of a 20-mg/ml concentration of ribavirin should be delivered through an SPAG-2 small-particle gen-

erator at flow rates of 4 L/min[54] for 12 to 18 hours per day for 3 to 7 days. Ribavirin is available as a powder for reconstitution; each vial contains 6 gm of sterile lyophilized ribavirin. Use of ribavirin for infants and children on ventilators requires special setups, as the ribavirin may precipitate in ventilator lines.[14, 54, 74] The special setup includes a blender, SPAG-2 collision generator ventilator, and special in-line filters.[54, 55] When delivered as an aerosol, ribavirin appears to have minimal toxicity. Rash and conjunctivitis are the most commonly noted adverse effects.[74, 75] Oral administration has been associated with decreased red blood cell counts and transient elevations in bilirubin, but these complications have not been noted with aerosol use.[75]

Antibiotics are of no proven benefit in uncomplicated cases of bronchiolitis.[14, 31] However, they are recommended for severely ill patients with infiltrates on chest radiograph when the diagnosis is unclear.[48] Antibiotic use in patients with documented RSV infection may become more common because of the significant incidence of bacterial coinfection.[33, 34]

Steroids are of no proven benefit in bronchiolitis,[19] but given the pathophysiology of bronchiolitis, they may play a role in the treatment of severely ill patients and patients with bronchiolitis obliterans. Ipratropium bromide was found to be beneficial in one study, but these results have not been confirmed by subsequent investigations.[76]

DISPOSITION

Children less than 6 months of age may be discharged home if there are no signs of hypoxia, respiratory distress, or dehydration. Similarly, children older than 6 months may be discharged home if there is only a mild elevation in the respiratory rate and no signs of distress or hypoxia. If a patient is to be discharged, the parents or care provider must be reliable, live within reasonable distance of a medical facility, and be able to contact medical personnel if the patient's condition worsens.

Patients with respiratory distress and a respiratory rate

TABLE 27–4

FACTORS INFLUENCING THEOPHYLLINE LEVELS[69, 70]

Increased Metabolism	Decreased Metabolism
Childhood	Liver disease
Phenobarbital	Congestive heart failure
Methylxanthine pretreatment	Upper respiratory infection
	Obesity
Valproic acid	Erythromycin
Rifampin	Age <6 mo
Carbamazepine	Cimetidine
	Propranolol
	Flu vaccination

TABLE 27–5

CONSIDERATIONS FOR ADMISSION

All patients meeting the following criteria or circumstances require admission:
  Respiratory rate >60 breaths/min with respiratory distress
  Apneic episode
  Signs of hypoxia (cyanosis, lethargy, restlessness, depressed level of consciousness, PCO_2 >50 mm Hg, PO_2 <50 mm Hg, severe retractions, head bobbing)
  Poor feeding
  Dehydration
  Second emergency department visit within 24 hours, or third visit within 48 hours
  Premature infant <6 mo of age with history of apnea
  Moderate respiratory distress within first 2 days of illness
  Unreliable parent or caretaker
  Long travel distance to medical care

All patients meeting the following criteria should be admitted to an intensive care unit:
  Shock
  Severe dehydration
  Respiratory rate >65 breaths/min and signs of respiratory distress or altered mental status
  PCO_2 >50 mm Hg
  PO_2 <50 mm Hg
  Mechanical ventilation required

greater than 60 breaths/min, signs of hypoxia, or evidence of dehydration should be admitted to the hospital (Table 27–5). If there is any question about the reliability of the parent or provider or if the family must travel a long distance to get to medical assistance, admission should be considered.

All patients with severe dehydration, shock, signs of severe respiratory distress (respiratory rate >65 breaths/min), altered mental status, Pco_2 greater than 50 mm Hg, or Po_2 less than 50 mm Hg or those in need of mechanical ventilation should be admitted to an intensive care unit. Consultation with a pediatrician, neonatologist, or appropriate subspecialist should be undertaken.

Transfer criteria vary according to the age of the patient, severity of illness, and ability of the hospital to provide personnel and equipment to adequately care for the patient. If the medical personnel are unskilled in the management of these patients or the appropriate size and type of ventilators are not available, patients requiring intensive care should be transferred to better equipped centers.

References

1. Denny FW, Clyde WA Jr. Acute lower respiratory tract infections in nonhospitalized children. J Pediatr 1986;108:535.
2. MacDonald NE. RSV update: Time to alter your clinical approach? Respir Dis 1985;6:11.
3. MacDonald NE, Hall CB, Suffin SC, et al. Respiratory syncytial viral infections in infants with congenital heart disease. N Engl J Med 1982;307:397.
4. Barkin RM, Rosen P (eds). Emergency Pediatrics. St Louis, CV Mosby, 1987, p 588.
5. Denny FW, Collier AM, Henderson FW, et al. The epidemiology of bronchiolitis. Pediatr Res 1977;11:234.
6. Eller JJ. Comments on epidemiologic patterns of bronchiolitis. Pediatr Res 1977;11:247.
7. Henderson FW, Clyde WA, Collier AM, et al. The etiologic and epidemiologic spectrum of bronchiolitis in pediatric practice. Pediatrics 1979;95:183.
8. Carlsen KH, Larsen S, Bjerve O, et al. Acute bronchiolitis: Predisposing factors and characteristics of infants at risk. Pediatr Pulmonol 1987;3:153.
9. Wohl MEB, Chernick V. State of the art—bronchiolitis. Am Rev Respir Dis 1978;118:759.
10. Knight V. Common viral respiratory illnesses. *In* Isselbacher KJ, Adam RD, Braunwald E (eds). Harrison's Principles of Internal Medicine. 9th ed. New York, McGraw-Hill, 1980, p 782.
11. McConnochie KM, Roghmann KJ. Parental smoking, presence of older siblings, and family history of asthma increase risk of bronchiolitis. Am J Dis Child 1986;140:806.
12. McConnochie KM, Roghmann KJ. Wheezing at 8 and 13 years: Changing importance of bronchiolitis and passive smoking. Pediatr Pulmonol 1989;6:138.
13. Douglas J. Air pollution and respiratory infections in children. Br J Prev Soc Med 1966;20:1.
14. Wohl ME. Bronchiolitis. Pediatr Ann 1986;15:307.
15. Costrini NV, Thomson WM. Manual of Medial Therapeutics. 22nd ed. Boston, Little, Brown, 1977, p 135.
16. Green M, Turton CW. Bronchiolitis and its manifestations. Eur J Resp Dis 1982;63(suppl 121):36.
17. Hall CB, Hall WJ, Speers DM. Clinical and physiologic manifestations of bronchiolitis and pneumonia. Am J Dis Child 1979;133:798.
18. Illingsworth RS. Common Symptoms of Disease in Children. 3rd ed. Oxford, England, Blackwell Scientific, 1971, p 146.
19. Reece RM. Bronchiolitis. *In* Reece RM, Chamberlain JW (eds). Manual of Emergency Pediatrics. 2nd ed. Philadelphia, WB Saunders, 1978, p 416.
20. Carlsen KH, Larsen S, Orstavik I. Acute bronchiolitis in infancy: The relationship of later recurrent obstructive airway disease. Eur J Respir Dis 1987;70:86.
21. Duiverman EJ, Neijens HJ, Van Strik R, et al. Lung function and bronchial responsiveness in children who had infantile bronchiolitis. Pediatr Pulmonol 1987;3:38.
22. Gurwitz D, Mindorff C, Levison H. Increased incidence of bronchial reactivity in children with a history of bronchiolitis. J Pediatr 1981;98:551.
23. McConnochie KM, Roghmann KJ. Bronchiolitis as a possible cause of wheezing in childhood: New evidence. Pediatrics 1984;74:110.
24. McConnochie KM, Roghmann KJ: Predicting clinically significant lower respiratory tract illness in childhood following mild bronchiolitis. Am J Dis Child 1985;139:625.
25. Nagayama Y, Sakurai N, Nakahara T, et al. Allergic predisposition among infants with bronchiolitis. J Asthma 1987;24:9.
26. Sims DG, Downham M, Gardner PS, et al. Study of 8 year old children with a history of respiratory syncytial virus bronchiolitis in infancy. Br Med J 1978;1:11.
27. Weiss ST, Tager IB, Munoz A, et al. The relationship of respiratory infections in early childhood to the occurrence of increased levels of bronchial responsiveness and atopy. Am Rev Respir Dis 1985;131:573.
28. Welliver RC, Sun M, Rinaldo D, et al. Predictive value of respiratory syncytial virus–specific IgE responses for recurrent wheezing following bronchiolitis. J Pediatr 1986;109:776.
29. Downes JJ, Wood DW, Striker TW, et al. Acute respiratory failure in infants with bronchiolitis. Anesthesiology 1968;29:426.
30. Bruhn RW, Mokrohisky ST, McIntosh K. Apnea associated with respiratory syncytial virus infection in young infants. J Pediatr 1977;90:382.
31. Vaughan VC, McKay RJ, Behrman RE (eds). Textbook of Pediatrics. 10th ed. Philadelphia, WB Saunders, 1979, p 1201.
32. Bates DV, Maclem PT, Christie RV. Respiratory Function in Disease. 2nd ed. Philadelphia, WB Saunders, 1971, p 417.
33. Korrppi M, Leinonen M, Koskela M, et al. Bacterial coinfection in children hospitalized with respiratory syncytial virus infections. Pediatr Infect Dis 1989;8:687.
34. Tristam DA, Miller RW, McMillan JA, et al. Simultaneous infection with respiratory syncytial virus and other respiratory pathogens. Am J Dis Child 1988;142:834.
35. Hall CB, McBride JT, Gala CL, et al. Ribavirin treatment of respiratory syncytial viral infections in infants with underlying cardiopulmonary disease. JAMA 1985;254:3047.
36. Taber LH, Knight V, Gilbert BE, et al. Ribavirin aerosol treatment of bronchiolitis associated with respiratory syncytial virus infection in infants. Pediatrics 1983;72:613.
37. Kadi Z, Dali S, Bakouri S, et al. Rapid diagnosis of respiratory syncytial virus infection by antigen immunofluorescence detection with monoclonal antibodies and immunoglobulin M immunofluorescence test. J Clin Microbiol 1986;24:1038.
38. Freymuth F, Quibriac M, Petitjean J, et al. Comparisons of two new tests for rapid diagnosis of respiratory syncytial virus infections by enzyme-linked immunosorbent assay and immunofluorescence techniques. J Clin Microbiol 1986;24:1013.
39. Bui RHD, Molinaro GA, Kettering JD, et al. Virus-specific IgE and IgG antibodies in serum of children infected with respiratory syncytial virus. J Pediatr 1987;110:87.
40. McIntosh K, Master HB, Orr I, et al. The immunologic response to infection with respiratory syncytial virus in infants. J Infect Dis 1978;138:24.
41. McConnochie KM, Mark JD, McBride JT, et al. Normal pulmonary function measurements and airway reactivity in childhood after mild bronchiolitis. J Pediatr 1985;107:54.
42. Taussig LM. Clinical and physiologic evidence for the persistence of pulmonary abnormalities after respiratory illnesses in infancy and childhood. Pediatr Resus 1977;11:216.
43. Kattan M, Keens TG, Lapierre JG, et al. Pulmonary function abnormalities in symptom-free children after bronchiolitis. Pediatrics 1977;59:638.
44. Welliver RC. Bronchiolitis: Update for managing patients this winter. J Respir Dis 1982;3:19.
45. Rudolph AM, Barnett HL, Einhorn AH (eds): Pediatrics. 16th ed. New York, Appleton-Century-Crofts, 1977, p 346.
46. Tercier JA. Bronchiolitis: A clinical review. J Emerg Med 1983;1:119.
47. Turner R, Hendley JO. Dealing with bronchiolitis in your office practice. J Resp Dis 1980;1:68.
48. Ellis EF. Therapy of acute bronchiolitis. Pediatr Res 1977;11:263.
49. Petty TL, Ashbaugh DG. The adult respiratory distress syndrome. Chest 1971;60:233.
50. Zschoche DA. Comprehensive Review of Critical Care. St Louis, CV Mosby, 1976, p 96.
51. Newth CJ. Recognition and management of respiratory failure. Pediatr Clin North Am 1979;26:617.
52. Outwater KM, Crone RK. Management of respiratory failure in infants with acute viral bronchiolitis. Am J Dis Child 1984;138:1071.
53. Chameides L (ed). Textbook of Pediatric Advanced Life Support. Dallas, TX, American Heart Association, 1988, p 16.
54. Demers RR, Parker J, Frankel LR, et al. Administration of ribavirin to neonatal and pediatric patients during mechanical ventilation. Respir Care 1986;31:1188.
55. Frankel LR, Lewiston NJ, Smith DW, et al. Clinical observations on mechanical ventilation for respiratory failure in bronchiolitis. Pediatr Pulmonol 1986;2:307.
56. Martinez F, Morgan WJ. Time constant analysis of partial expiratory flow volume (PEFV) curves in normals and infants with bronchopulmonary dysplasia or bronchiolitis. Am Rev Respir Dis 1985;131:262.
57. Mellins RB. Bronchiolitis—comments on pathogenesis and treatment. Pediatr Resus 1977;11:268.
58. Graef JW. Manual of Pediatric Therapeutics. 2nd ed. Boston, Little, Brown, 1980, pp 371–372.
59. Schuh S, Parkin P, Rajan A, et al. High versus low dose frequently administered, nebulized albuterol in children with severe, acute asthma. Pediatrics 1989;83:6, 513.

60. Rothstein RJ. Intravenous theophylline therapy in asthma: A clinical update. Ann Emerg Med 1980;9:327.
61. Weinberger M, Hendeles L, Ahrens R. Pharmacologic management of reversible obstructive airways disease. Med Clin North Am 1981;65:579.
62. Weinberger M, Matthay RA, Ginshansky EJ, et al. Intravenous aminophylline dosage: Use of serum theophylline measurement for guidance. JAMA 1976;235:2110.
63. Emerman CL, Nowak RM, Tomlanovich MO, et al. Theophylline concentrations in the emergency treatment of acute bronchial asthma. Am J Emerg Med 1983;1:12.
64. Fox J, Hicks P, Feldman BR, et al. Theophylline blood levels as a guide to intravenous therapy in children. Am J Dis Child 1982;136:928.
65. Jacobs MH, Senior RM, Kessler G. Clinical experience with theophylline: Relationship between dosage, serum concentration, and toxicity. JAMA 1976;18:1983.
66. Zwillich CW, Sutton FD, Heff TA, et al. Theophylline-induced seizures in adults: Correlation with serum concentrations. Ann Intern Med 1975;82:784.
67. Yarnell PR, Chu NNS. Focal seizures and aminophylline. Neurology 1975;25:819.
68. Hendeles L, Bighley L, Richardson RH, et al. Frequent toxicity for IV aminophylline infusion in critically ill patients. Drug Intell Clin Pharm 1977;11:12.
69. Ogilvie RI. Clinical pharmacokinetics of theophylline. Clin Pharmacokinet 1978;3:267.
70. Southall DP, Stebbens VA, Alexander JR, et al. Cardiorespiratory patterns occurring in infants during and after recovery from respiratory tract infection. Pediatrics 1986;78:37.
71. Caramia G, Palazzini E. Efficacy of Ribavirin aerosol treatment for respiratory syncytial virus bronchiolitis in infants. J Intern Med Res 1987;15:227.
72. Conrad DA, Christenson JC, Waner JL, et al. Aerosolized ribavirin treatment of respiratory syncytial virus infection in infants hospitalized during an epidemic. Pediatr Infect Dis J 1987;6:151.
73. Hall CB, McBride JT. Vapors, viruses, and views: Ribavirin and respiratory syncytial virus. Am J Dis Child 1986;140:331.
74. Barry W, Cockburn F, Cornall R, et al. Ribavirin aerosol for acute bronchiolitis. Arch Dis Child 1986;61:593.
75. Janai HK, Marks MI, Zaleska M, et al. Ribavirin: Adverse drug reactions, 1986 to 1988. Pediatr Infect Dis J 1990;9:209.
76. Seidenberg J, Masters IB, Hudson I, et al. Effect of ipratropium bromide on respiratory mechanics in infants with acute bronchiolitis. Aust Paediatr J 1987;23:169.

CHAPTER 28

Bronchopulmonary Dysplasia

Richard E. Marshall

INTRODUCTION

The original report of bronchopulmonary dysplasia (BPD) in 1967 described four radiographic stages in patients who required respirator treatment for hyaline membrane disease (HMD). Stage 1 occurred at 2 to 3 days of life and was identical to severe HMD. Stage 2 was found between 4 and 10 days of life and was characterized by complete opacification of both lung fields. In stage 3, occurring between 10 and 20 days, radiolucent cystic areas were surrounded by areas of irregular density. During stage 4, after 1 month, the cystic radiolucent areas became enlarged.

The author would like to thank Jane Carl for expert secretarial assistance in preparation of the manuscript.

Since this initial description, it has become clear that many patients with BPD do not go through these discrete radiologic states. Stages 1 and 2 of BPD are often indistinguishable from recuperation from HMD. Even though it is still difficult to formulate a definition of BPD that has universal acceptance, the definition proposed by Bancalari and coworkers, with modifications, highlights the most important features of this disorder (Table 28–1). First, it is seen in patients who have required ventilatory assistance within the first week of life for at least 24 hours. Usually these patients have required the ventilator for more than a day. Not all of these patients are preterm infants with HMD; they may be term infants with persistent pulmonary hypertension or meconium aspiration. Perhaps the most important difference between the original description of BPD and the current definition is the time of onset. The current definition of BPD does not include patients who are younger than 28 days; it is too difficult to distinguish between recuperation from HMD and early BPD. Unless there is a persistent oxygen requirement with clinical and radiographic evidence of pulmonary disease, there is no BPD.

There has been an attempt to grade the severity of BPD. This index reflects the clinical and radiologic characteristics of patients who had required mechanical ventilation and were evaluated at 21 days of age. The clinical parameters include respiratory rate, dyspnea as reflected in retractions, fraction of inspired oxygen (FIO_2) requirement for a partial arterial oxygen pressure (PaO_2) of 50 to 70 mm Hg, degree of hypercapnea, and growth rate in grams per day. Radiographic criteria are cardiovascular abnormalities, hyperexpansion, emphysema, fibrosis or interstitial abnormalities, and a subjective impression of the severity of disease.

INCIDENCE

Because there is still variation in defining what constitutes BPD, it is difficult to obtain completely accurate data about the true incidence of BPD. One survey examined seven reports of infants with BPD who had respiratory distress syndrome (RDS). All of the 620 patients had radiographic evidence of BPD, and about half had clinical evidence of BPD as well. Of those recovering from RDS, 18% developed BPD. A survey of 16 neonatal centers for oxygen dependence at 3 to 4 weeks of age found a 20% rate of occurrence of BPD in those patients recovering from RDS. Patients studied with birth weights between 750 and 1500 gm had a 12.2% incidence of BPD.

PATHOGENESIS

Oxygen toxicity and barotrauma from positive-pressure ventilation are generally thought to be the most important causes of BPD. From a clinical perspective, infants who are not exposed to oxygen do not develop BPD. Correlative data show that BPD is associated with longer exposure to high concentrations of oxygen. There is compelling evidence

TABLE 28–1
DEFINITION OF BRONCHOPULMONARY DYSPLASIA
Ventilator required for at least 24 hours during first week of life
Clinical respiratory distress for at least 28 days with tachypnea and/or retractions
Supplemental oxygen required for at least 28 days
Abnormal chest radiographs showing increased density and/or cystic changes

implicating barotrauma as an important cause of BPD. Infants who are on negative-pressure ventilators or constant positive airway pressure (CPAP) rarely develop BPD. There is a higher incidence of BPD in those patients who develop air leaks, a known complication of high positive-pressure ventilation. A correlation has also been shown between high peak-inspiratory pressures (>35 cm H_2O) and an increased incidence of BPD.

Although many other potentially important risk factors may be associated with the development of BPD, there are two additional determinants that deserve particular attention: the duration of oxygen therapy and lung immaturity. If infants do not initially develop RDS, they will not be susceptible to the risks of trauma from oxygen and barotrauma. The immature lung may have properties that make it particularly vulnerable to the injuries that characterize BPD. Another important variable is the length of oxygen exposure. The longer the exposure to oxygen and barotrauma, the higher the risk for BPD.

PATHOPHYSIOLOGY

The early pathologic changes in BPD during the first week of life are similar to those found in HMD. There is an exudative reaction with edema and hyaline membranes, and as BPD evolves, there are major changes in both the bronchial tree and the interstitial space. Microscopic changes in the bronchial tree include loss of cilia. Gross changes include bronchial stenosis, tracheomalacia, and bronchomalacia. In addition, there is cystic dilatation of distal air spaces. Further changes may include thickening of the walls of pulmonary arterioles and changes in ventricular size.

There are multiple changes in pulmonary function associated with these pathologic changes, including the following:

Interstitial fibrosis and obliterative bronchiolitis
Increased airway resistance; decreased lung compliance; ventilation-perfusion mismatch
Increased work of breathing; increased basal metabolic rate; decreased Pao_2; increased Pco_2
Bronchospasm

CLINICAL COURSE

There are three paths that the BPD patient can follow. First, patients can slowly recover from their chronic lung disease. Gradual weight gain will become apparent as their oxygen requirements slowly decline. Second, some patients will have a fulminant rapid course leading to an early death. These patients may have major problems with air leaks that seem to hasten their demise. The third category of patients are those who have BPD that persists for months and about whom it is too early to determine what their outcome will be. Clearly, the major determinant in their survival is the severity of their BPD and how much oxygen and ventilatory assistance they require, but there are additional clinical parameters that seem to affect survival. Those patients who are likely to survive manage to gain weight on a suitable diet. Patients with hypochloremic metabolic alkalosis die more frequently than those without such problems. Progressive neurologic deterioration is associated with fatal BPD and right-sided heart failure. Intractable seizures in BPD patients have been associated with rapidly progressive neurologic deterioration and death. Viral or bacterial infections can lead to rapid deterioration and death in marginally compensated BPD patients.

DIAGNOSTIC EVALUATION

The cardiopulmonary status of BPD patients must be monitored closely (Table 28–2). In the early phases of monitoring a patient, arterial blood gas measurements may be required to optimize supplemental oxygen concentration and ventilator settings. Chest radiographs are obtained as required by the clinical condition of the patient. Early radiographs will show persistence of hazy infiltrates (Fig. 28–1A). As BPD progresses, there will be more cystic changes (Fig. 28–1B).

Monitoring of blood pressure and cardiac status is necessary. BPD patients with systolic blood pressures above 113 mm Hg are at greater risk of dying. In addition there are at least two reasons for following the cardiac status with echocardiograms. First, there may be unexpected cardiac disease, and second, echocardiograms can give information about the presence of pulmonary hypertension, which is known to be associated with BPD.

Monitoring weight is a vital part of following the BPD patient, as such patients are usually in delicate fluid balance, and unexpected weight gain may suggest the need for more diuretics or less fluid intake. If a BPD patient is not slowly gaining weight, nutritional therapy may need reevaluation. Without adequate nutrition, the likelihood of a good outcome is poor.

THERAPEUTIC INTERVENTION

The cardiopulmonary management of the BPD patient is based on supplying adequate oxygen (Table 28–3). Hypoxemia can be common during sleep and feedings in the BPD infant. If there is hypoxemia, then airway constriction is present, and therefore it is recommended that the arterial oxygen saturation be maintained above 90% as measured by the oximeter and that the hemoglobin be kept above 13 gm/dl.

Although oxygen remains the mainstay of therapy for BPD, four classes of drugs have also been shown to be beneficial: methylxanthines, beta$_2$ agonists, diuretics, and steroids (Table 28–4). The mexthylxanthines, theophylline and caffeine, have been shown to increase pulmonary compliance and decrease airway resistance in BPD patients. A number of studies have examined the short-term effects of beta$_2$ agonists administered by aerosols. These studies have shown an increase in lung compliance and a decrease in airway resistance after administration of aerosolized beta agonists. These effects peaked within 30 to 60 minutes after administration and were gone by 3 to 4 hours. Furosemide, a diuretic, has been shown to improve airway resistance and compliance in the BPD patient.

Corticosteroids have also been used to treat BPD, but their use remains controversial. There is little doubt that steroids

---

TABLE 28–2

DIAGNOSTIC STUDIES FOR BRONCHOPULMONARY DYSPLASIA

Cardiopulmonary
  Arterial blood gas measurements; oxygen saturation measurement
  Chest radiographs
  Echocardiogram

Nutrition
  Weight
  Blood chemistry studies

Neurologic imaging and cultures for infections performed as clinically indicated

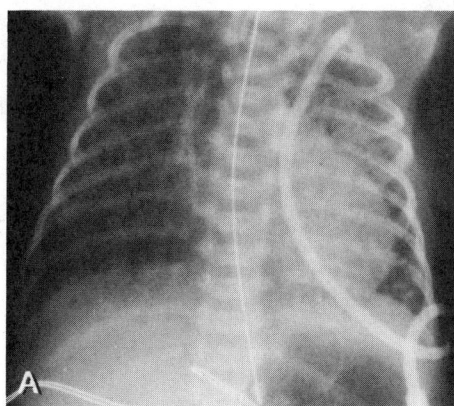
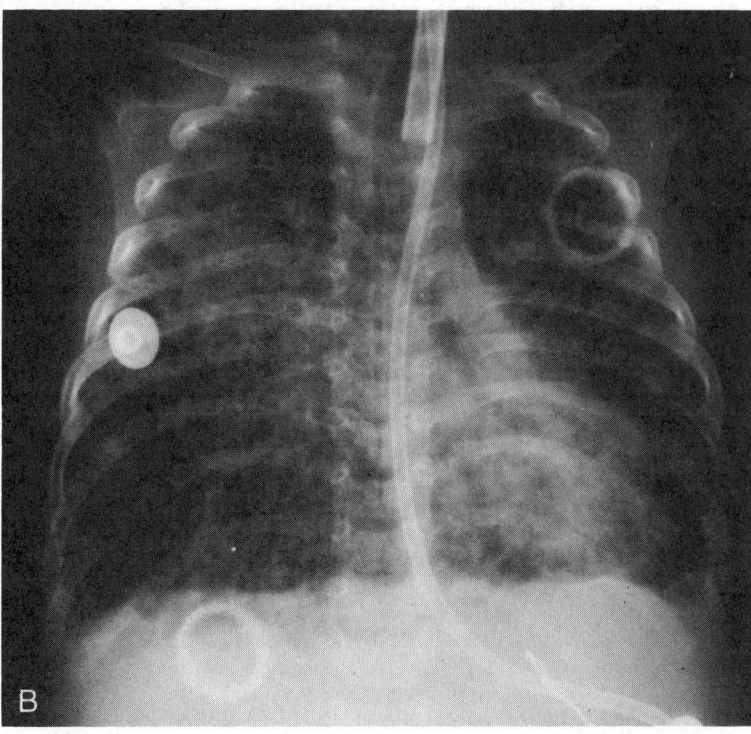

Figure 28–1. Development of bronchopulmonary dysplasia as demonstrated on chest radiographs at 18 days (smaller view) and 5 months (larger view) of a male infant requiring supplemental oxygenation. The smaller view *(A)* shows the "hazy" early stage; the later view *(B)* shows the streaky, bubbly pattern of the established stage, as well as the wide trachea that often accompanies long-term infantile respiratory disease. (Courtesy of A. Oestreich, Cincinnati, OH.)

can improve pulmonary function acutely in BPD patients, as they cause a rapid increase in compliance and a decrease in total pulmonary resistance. Some studies have also shown that some patients can be weaned from the ventilator more rapidly with steroids. However, it is still unclear whether mortality and hospitalization time are decreased. There is some concern about complications of steroid use, which include hyperglycemia, infection, and suppression of the adrenal-pituitary axis.

Nutrition is a difficult problem for BPD patients. It is known that BPD patients have a higher oxygen consumption than controls, perhaps because of an increase in the work of breathing associated with BPD. Moreover, growth failure is not uncommon in BPD patients. The goal is to overcome the need for more calories in patients who have an unusual sensitivity to changes in fluid intake. If too much fluid is given to a BPD patient, there can be a rapid deterioration in cardiopulmonary status with weight gain and edema. Clearly, the nutritional plan must be individualized, but certain guidelines can be recommended. Initially, if the patient cannot tolerate enteral feedings, hyperalimentation

should be maintained. Once enteral feedings are begun, more concentrated formulas (24 kcal/oz) supplemented with medium-chain triglyceride (MCT) oil or glucose polymers can be tried. All of these problems can be complicated by the presence of gastroesophageal reflux (GER). There is controversy as to whether patients with BPD have a greater incidence of GER and whether fundoplication and gastrostomy should be performed.

Infections can cause rapid deterioration in BPD patients. It is important to consider otitis media and urinary tract infection as potential causes of cardiopulmonary decompensation in the BPD patient. The BPD patient should be immunized against common childhood infections while still in the neonatal unit.

DISCHARGE CRITERIA FOR THE BPD PATIENT REQUIRING HOME OXYGEN THERAPY

It is difficult to determine precisely when to discharge a BPD patient who needs home oxygen therapy. There are

---

TABLE 28–3

MANAGEMENT OF BRONCHOPULMONARY DYSPLASIA

Cardiopulmonary management
    Ventilatory support
    Oxygen supplementation
    Chest physiotherapy
    Medications: bronchodilators, diuretics, and steroids

Nutritional management
    Parenteral feedings
    Enteral feedings
    Special needs: gastroesophageal reflux

Neurodevelopmental management: appropriate stimulation; environmental and motor sedation

Infection: immunizations and treatment

TABLE 28–4

THERAPY FOR BRONCHOPULMONARY DYSPLASIA

Bronchodilator
    Theophylline, 8–10 mg/kg/24 hr, to achieve a serum level between 10 and 20 µg/ml

Aerosols: beta-adrenergic agonists
    Metaproterenol (Alupent) as 5% solution, 0.25–0.5 mg/kg q 4–6 hr
    Isoetharine (Bronksol) as 0.25% solution, 0.1–0.2 mg/kg q 4–6 hr

Diuretic
    Furosemide, 1 mg/kg/24 hr

Steroids
    Dexamethasone, 0.5 mg/kg/day initially for 3–7 days; weaning from this level is highly variable

TABLE 28–5

OUTCOME FOR PATIENTS WITH BRONCHOPULMONARY DYSPLASIA

Mortality: 26% die within the first several years of life

Morbidity
  Pulmonary
    50% need hospitalization for lower tract disease in first few years
    25% to 50% have persistent abnormalities in pulmonary function tests
  Neurodevelopmental: highly variable outcomes for patients with cerebral palsy, mental retardation, and visual and auditory deficits

three distinct components that must be in place to plan for an effective discharge. First, the patient must be stable and able to feed. The flow rate of the oxygen delivered should not exceed 1 L/min. The gestational age should be at least 40 weeks.

Next, the family should be prepared for the complex care that they must provide. There should be space for the needed equipment. A telephone and transportation for the many necessary outpatient appointments are required. One important way to help the parents make the transition to home care is to have them stay at the hospital for several days prior to discharge and provide total care to the child.

Finally, the family must have identified a coordinator of their outpatient care who can answer any questions. This person can be either a physician or a nurse, but must be available at all times.

HOME MANAGEMENT OF THE BPD PATIENT REQUIRING OXYGEN THERAPY

The requirements for effective home care pose a major responsibility for the family. Over time, most families become more comfortable with the many burdens imposed by such care. Perhaps the most important need is to find one identifiable resource person whom the family can turn to for guidance and support. This person must make sure that oxygen supplies are adequate and that the necessary monitoring devices are available. In addition, the family must understand how to give the medicines required and how to recognize serious side effects. The family must be sensitive to changes in pulmonary status that can be caused by viral infections or fluid overload. Once there is an acute change in respiratory status, the family must contact the resource person immediately.

PATIENT OUTCOME

The outcome for the BPD patient is somewhat variable (Table 28–5). The mortality rate is close to 25%. Pulmonary morbidity includes hospitalization for lower respiratory infections in the first 2 years in about 50% of cases. Abnormal pulmonary function tests have been noted during the first few years of life, and one report describes abnormal results in pulmonary function tests—including airway obstruction, airway hyperreactivity, and hyperinflation—in surviving teenagers and young adults. The clinical significance of these abnormalities is unclear. Neurodevelopmental outcomes are highly variable.

Selected References

Abman SH, Accurso FJ, Bowman CM. Unsuspected cardiopulmonary abnormalities complicating bronchopulmonary dysplasia. Arch Dis Child 1984;59:966.

Bancalari E, Abdenour GE, Feller R, Gannon J. Bronchopulmonary dysplasia: Clinical presentation. J Pediatr 1979;95:819.

Blanchard PW, Brown TM, Coates AL. Pharmacotherapy in bronchopulmonary dysplasia. Clin Perinatol 1987;14:881.

Brudno DS, Parker DH, Slaton G. Response of pulmonary mechanics to terbutaline in patients with bronchopulmonary dysplasia. Am J Med Sci 1989;297:166.

Campbell LR, McCallister W, Volpe JJ. Neurologic aspects of bronchopulmonary dysplasia. Clin Pediatr 1988;27:7.

Davis J, Sinkin RA, Aranda JV. Drug therapy for bronchopulmonary dysplasia. Pediatr Pulmonol 1990;8:117.

Edwards DK, Dyer WM, Northway WH. Twelve years experience with bronchopulmonary dysplasia. Pediatrics 1977;59:839.

Garg M, Kukrzner SI, Bautista DB, Keens TG. Clinically unsuspected hypoxia during sleep and feeding in infants with bronchopulmonary dysplasia. Pediatrics 1988;81:635.

Goetzman BW. Understanding bronchopulmonary dysplasia. Am J Dis Child 1986;140:332.

Goodman G, Perkin RM, Anas N, et al. Pulmonary hypertension in infants with bronchopulmonary dysplasia. J Pediatr 1988;112:67.

Groothuis JR, Rosenberg AA. Home oxygen promotes weight gain in infants with bronchopulmonary dysplasia. Am J Dis Child 1987;141:992.

Kao L, Durand DJ, Phillips BL, Nickerson BG. Oral theophylline and diuretics improve pulmonary mechanics in infants with bronchopulmonary dysplasia. J Pediatr 1987;111:439.

Kao LC, Warburton D, Sargent CW, et al. Furosemide acutely decreases airway resistance in chronic bronchopulmonary dysplasia. J Pediatr 1983;103:624.

Knapp MA. Bronchopulmonary dysplasia: A review for the pediatrician. Curr Prob Pediatr 1989;19:177.

Koops BL, Abman SH, Accurso FJ. Outpatient management and follow-up of bronchopulmonary dysplasia. Clin Perinatol 1984;11:101.

Markstead T, Fitzhardinge PM. Growth and development in children recovering from bronchopulmonary dysplasia. J Pediatr 1981;98:597.

Mayes L, Perkett E, Stahlman MT. Severe bronchopulmonary dysplasia: A retrospective review. Acta Paediatr Scand 1983;72:225.

McCann EM, Lewis K, Deming DD, et al. Controlled trial of furosemide therapy in infants with chronic lung disease. J Pediatr 1985;106:957.

Northway WH, Moss RB, Carlisle KB, et al. Late pulmonary sequelae of bronchopulmonary dysplasia. N Engl J Med 1990;323:1793.

Northway WH, Rosan RC, Porter DY. Pulmonary disease following respirator therapy of hyaline membrane disease. N Engl J Med 1967;276:357.

Philip AGS. Oxygen plus pressure plus time: The etiology of bronchopulmonary dysplasia. Pediatrics 1975;55:44.

Sauve RS, McMillan DD, Mitchell L, et al. Home oxygen therapy: Outcome of infants discharged from NICU on continuous treatment. Clin Pediatr 1989;28:113.

Sauve RS, Singhai N. Long-term morbidity of infants with bronchopulmonary dysplasia. Pediatrics 1985;76:725.

Stern L. The role of respirators in the etiology and pathogenesis of bronchopulmonary dysplasia. J Pediatr 1979;95:867.

Taghizadeh A, Reynolds EOR. Pathogenesis of bronchopulmonary dysplasia following hyaline membrane disease. Am J Pathol 1976;82:241.

Toce SS, Farrell PM, Leavitt LP, Edwards DK. Clinical and roentgenographic scoring system for assessing bronchopulmonary dysplasia. Am J Dis Child 1984;138:581.

Yu VYH, Orgill AA, Lim SB, et al. Growth and development of very low birth weight infants recovering from bronchopulmonary dysplasia. Arch Dis Child 1983;58:791.

CHAPTER 29

Pneumonia

Patricia S. Chase
Nancy S. Hilton

Respiratory infections account for the majority of visits to any pediatric emergency department. Children may experience as many as ten or more respiratory infections each year in early childhood. Certain environmental factors—including day-care attendance,[1] inhaled pollutants from cigarette smoke[2] or wood-burning stoves,[3] poverty,[4] malnutrition, and crowded living conditions[5]—may increase the incidence and severity of respiratory infections in some children.

Most upper respiratory infections are clinically insignificant and require only symptomatic and supportive care. Their frequency is so great, however, that a relatively infrequent complication like pneumonia is a common diagnosis.[6] The incidence of pneumonia is estimated to be 20 per 1000 in infants younger than 1 year and 40 per 1000 in preschool children, dropping gradually to 9 per 1000 in 9- to 15-year-olds.[7] In one study evaluating febrile infants younger than 3 months of age, pneumonia was diagnosed in 7.5% of cases[8]; in another study evaluating children 2 years and younger, pneumonia accounted for 13% of the final diagnoses.[9] In less developed countries, although the incidence of childhood pneumonia may be comparable to that in more industrialized nations, its significance is much greater, as the mortality rates are 10 to 50 times higher. Complications of acute respiratory infections, in certain parts of the world, account for more than one third of all deaths among children younger than 5 years.[10]

The definitive etiologic diagnosis of pneumonia is difficult. Although diagnostic and therapeutic capabilities have improved in recent years, many patients still receive empiric antimicrobial therapy without the responsible organism being identified.[11] Invasive procedures such as bronchoscopy, transtracheal aspiration, or lung biopsy are reserved for severely ill or immunocompromised patients.[12] Therefore radiographic results, the clinical history, the physical examination, and the age of the patient become the most important factors in the decision-making process in the evaluation and treatment of the infant or child with pneumonia.

Basic treatment goals should be (1) to adequately treat the most likely etiologic agents to avoid morbidity and mortality from untreated disease, and (2) to use a selective approach to antibiotic therapy to avoid the dangers of drug toxicity, superinfection, and excessive cost.[13]

PATHOPHYSIOLOGY

Pneumonia is an acute inflammation of the lungs resulting from the invasion and replication of one or more of a variety of infectious agents or from direct injury to lung tissue by a noxious agent.[14] Organisms colonizing the upper respiratory tract replicate and directly invade or are aspirated into the lower respiratory tree. A less common mode is the hematogenous seeding of the lung parenchyma by organisms such as Haemophilus influenzae type b. Viral agents are capable of damaging normal cells lining the respiratory tract, thereby decreasing their defense mechanisms and increasing the risk of secondary infection. This may explain the mode of infection in patients who develop bacterial pneumonia following varicella, influenza, or rubeola.[15] Studies have verified that upper respiratory viral infections often precede or coincide with bacterial lower respiratory infections.[16, 17] This should be suspected in any child who appears to worsen while recovering from a viral respiratory infection.

ORIGIN

Common causes of acute pneumonia in infants and children are diverse and include the common respiratory viruses, Mycoplasma pneumoniae, Streptococcus pneumoniae, H. influenzae type b, and Chlamydia trachomatis. The likely organism responsible in any given patient depends on the age of

the patient, host factors, season of the year, epidemiology of viruses in the community, and clinical presentation.

In the newborn period, pneumonia is usually caused by organisms acquired from the mother's genital tract during or before delivery. Group B streptococci and enteric gram-negative bacteria especially, Escherichia coli and Klebsiella pneumoniae, are the most important pathogens; Listeria monocytogenes, other gram-positive cocci, and viruses (especially cytomegalovirus and herpes simplex virus) are less common causes.[18]

In infants 1 to 4 months of age, pneumonia is caused by community-acquired viruses and bacteria or by one of the agents implicated in the afebrile infant pneumonitis. Afebrile infant pneumonitis was first described by Beem and Saxon in 1977 as a consequence of perinatal acquisition and infection with C. trachomatis.[19] Other organisms, including Ureaplasma urealyticum, Mycoplasma hominis, Pneumocystis carinii, and cytomegalovirus, have since been shown to cause a similar clinical picture.[20]

After the first few months of life and up to about 4 or 5 years of age, most pneumonias are caused by viruses. Respiratory syncytial virus (RSV) accounts for most infections and is the most common viral agent recovered in a number of studies of lower respiratory infections in childhood.[16, 17] Parainfluenza, influenza types A and B, adenovirus, and rhinovirus have also been associated with childhood viral pneumonia.[21]

Bacterial pneumonia occurring after the neonatal period is caused primarily by S. pneumoniae and H. influenzae type b; the latter is more commonly seen in infants and children younger than 5 years but rarely may occur at any age. Staphylococcus aureus, although a rather rare cause, is extremely important, as it can produce a fulminant pneumonia with rapid deterioration. The majority of cases of primary staphylococcal pneumonia occur in the first year of life.[22] Other agents less commonly seen include Streptococcus pyogenes, Branhamella (Moraxella) catarrhalis, and Legionella pneumophilia.

The incidence of bacterial pneumonia reported in studies of pediatric pneumonia ranges from 3% to 19% depending on the diagnostic criteria and laboratory tests used.[16, 23] Studies using bacterial antigen detection from the urine generally find a higher incidence of bacterial pneumonia than do studies based on positive blood cultures. Overall, between 10% and 30% of cases of childhood pneumonia occurring in industrialized nations are caused by bacterial pathogens.[24] However, among malnourished children in less developed countries, more than 60% of all cases of pneumonia are caused by bacteria, primarily S. pneumoniae and H. influenzae type b.[25] Thus there remains a need for a highly sensitive, noninvasive diagnostic test to detect bacterial pneumonia in children.

M. pneumoniae is an important and common cause of treatable pneumonia in children older than 5 years. Between 9% and 21% of pneumonias occurring in school aged children are caused by this agent.[26] This disease has little seasonal variation, as do the viral entities, but may occur in epidemic proportion in communities or groups.[27] Although clinically recognized pneumonia occurs in only 3% to 10% of infected persons, it accounts for up to 20% of all cases of pneumonia in the general population and should always be considered in an older child or adolescent with a lower respiratory infection.[28–30]

The aforementioned organisms account for the majority of lower respiratory infections in otherwise normal children. However, other less common bacteria or viral or fungal agents may cause pneumonia in the immunocompromised or chronically ill child.

Patients with chronic respiratory disease, congenital heart

disease, sickle cell anemia, or immunodeficiency states, including the acquired immunodeficiency syndrome (AIDS), deserve special consideration when presenting with fever or lower respiratory symptoms. Pneumonia in these high-risk patients may be life threatening and for the most part should be managed in the hospital.

Tuberculosis must be considered in every child with pneumonia. Those at particularly high risk for this infection include immunodeficient hosts; children who have recently immigrated from less developed countries where tuberculosis is endemic; and children from poor urban areas where tuberculosis is still prevalent. Nevertheless, this infection can occur in a child from any socioeconomic class, and a skin test is an easy but essential way to exclude it. In some children, especially those who are immunodeficient or gravely ill, hypersensitivity may be impaired, and skin tests can be falsely negative.

CLINICAL EVALUATION

The presentation of pneumonia depends primarily on the age of the child and the causative agent. Neonates have limited responses to infection and may present with very nonspecific signs of illness. Lethargy, poor feeding, or decreased muscle tone, with or without fever, may be the only clues to the diagnosis of pneumonia in an extremely ill infant. In the neonate, a chest radiograph should be part of the workup for sepsis, even when pulmonary findings such as rales and tachypnea are absent.

Chlamydial pneumonitis, seen between 3 and 12 to 16 weeks of life, usually begins with nasal congestion followed by a stacatto cough and tachypnea. Of the affected infants, 95% are afebrile and 50% will have concurrent or previous conjunctivitis.[31] Physical examination usually reveals diffuse rales with or without wheezing, which may persist for several weeks regardless of treatment.

The older infant or young child with viral or bacterial pneumonia usually presents with fever, tachypnea, cough, wheezing, stridor, nasal flaring, grunting, or cyanosis. Classically, the child with bacterial pneumonia presents with the abrupt onset of high fever and lower respiratory symptoms; the physical examination reveals signs of localized pulmonary consolidation. The child with viral pneumonia characteristically presents with the gradual onset of respiratory symptoms, which may include wheezing and stridor, and a low-grade fever.[24] However, the clinical presentation of most young children with pneumonia, whether bacterial or viral, is varied and is difficult to categorize based on symptoms and signs alone, generally necessitating further diagnostic evaluation.

The typical picture of mycoplasmal pneumonia in the older child begins with the gradual onset of fever (range 38.4°C to 39.0°C), malaise, and headache, followed by a nonproductive cough, rales, and wheezing.[26, 32] Symptoms may last several weeks, despite therapy, and may produce abnormalities in pulmonary function for as long as 3 years after the initial infection.[28]

Children with tuberculosis classically present with the gradual onset of cough, loss of appetite, weight loss, and fever with or without night sweats. However, they may also present with a history of nonresolving respiratory infections or with a clinical picture indistinguishable from that of acute bacterial or viral pneumonia.

When a child presents with pneumonia, one of the primary tasks for the clinician is to attempt to make a distinction between viral and bacterial pathogens. Some characteristic findings in the major categories of etiologic agents (Table 29–1) can be used as guidelines. However, when signs and symptoms overlap, as they do frequently, the clinician must still decide whether to treat the child with antibiotics, based on his or her "best guess" as to the source of the pneumonia. Even after extensive investigation, no pathogen is identified in 40% to 50% of cases of childhood pneumonia, and in 14% to 53% of patients more than one pathogen is found.[18]

Infections caused by *Bordetella pertussis* may mimic chlamydial pneumonitis; the two conditions commonly occur in the same age group and may initially present with similiar clinical pictures, with signs of upper respiratory infection, cough, and tachypnea. However, in the child with pertussis, the cough becomes progressively more severe, with a paroxysmal pattern; an inspiratory whoop sometimes develops and, when present, is almost diagnostic. However it may be absent in very young infants. Prolonged coughing attacks may lead to cyanosis, emesis, and, in severe cases, anoxia. Pneumonia, when present, is discovered during the paroxysmal stage and the chest radiograph shows a bronchopneumonic pattern.[33] The white blood cell count is characteristically elevated, with a marked lymphocytosis. Infants are at risk for aspiration secondary to feeding problems and usually require hospitalization for supportive care, which includes oxygen, intravenous hydration, and cardiorespiratory monitoring. Erythromycin therapy shortens the period of communicability and may reduce the length of symptoms.

Foreign body aspiration is a well-recognized event in pediatric patients between the ages of 6 months and 5 years.[34] The child who has inhaled a foreign body, usually food, may arrive in the emergency department with acute coughing and wheezing. The chest radiograph demonstrates asymmetric obstructive emphysema[35] often best demonstrated by bilateral decubitus views. If the event goes unnoticed and the object is not removed, pneumonia will result distal to the obstruction, and the clinical picture will closely resemble that of bacterial pneumonia. Thus in young children, foreign bodies should be considered, especially in cases of delayed or incomplete resolution after treatment.

Chronic aspiration with secondary pneumonia occurs in children with neuromuscular dysfunction, gastroesophageal reflux, congenital tracheoesopagheal fistulas, and central nervous system disorders. The organisms involved are typically aerobic and anaerobic bacteria that inhabit the mouth and upper gastrointestinal tract. These bacteria are usually sensitive to penicillin, though penicillin-resistant organisms are occasionally involved.[36]

Chemical pneumonitis can result from the ingestion of petroleum distillates and other hydrocarbons. Aspiration may occur during the ingestion or may be secondary to emesis. Except in situations where large volumes have been ingested, it is best not to induce emesis or use lavage. If respiratory symptoms are present after an ingestion, the child should be admitted for observation. Appearance on chest radiograph may lag behind the clinical picture.

History

A careful history and thorough physical examination are critical in the diagnosis of pneumonia in children. Often the clinical evaluation is more important in deciding on management plans than are chest radiographs and laboratory tests. One must ascertain whether the patient has an underlying or chronic illness (e.g., asthma, cystic fibrosis, sickle cell disease); defects in the immune function, including those associated with infection with the human immunodeficiency virus (HIV); congenital heart disease, bronchopulmonary dysplasia, or gastroesophageal reflux; or has had recent infection with measles. All of these conditions can predispose a child to more severe or more frequent pneumonias.

Recent exposure to tuberculosis is important to determine. Day-care or intrafamilial exposures to *H. influenzae* or viral

				Afebrile	
	Viral	**Bacterial**	**Mycoplasma**	**Pneumonitis**	**Tuberculosis**
Age	Any, but usually 2 wk–5 yr	Any, but especially under 2 mo	5–15 yr	3–16 wk	Older than 4 mo
Onset	Gradual	Abrupt	Gradual	Gradual	Gradual to acute
Symptoms	Cough, tachypnea	Cough, tachypnea	Cough	Cough, tachypnea	Weight loss, cough
Fever	Low-grade	High	Low-grade	Usually none	Variable
Physical findings	Diffuse rales, wheezing, or stridor	Rales, decreased breath sounds	Rales, decreased breath sounds	Diffuse rales, wheezing	Variable
Laboratory findings	Normal or slightly elevated WBC count	Elevated WBC count	Normal WBC count, positive cold agglutinins	Eosinophilia, IgM positive for Chlamydia, positive	Nonspecific WBC count, positive purified protein derivative tuberculin test
Chest radiogrpah findings	Hyperaeration, interstitial infiltrates	Lobar or segmented infiltrates, pleural effusion	Lobar or patchy interstitial infiltrates	Interstitial infiltrates, hyperaeration (bilateral)	Hilar adenopathy, infiltrates, pleural effusions
Causative agents	Respiratory synctial virus, parainfluenza, influenza types A and B	*S. pneumoniae, Haemophilus influenzae* (rarely, group B *Streptococcus, Staphylococcus aureus*) Under age 2 mo: group B *Streptococcus,* enterics	*Mycoplasma pneumoniae*	*Chlamydia, Ureaplasma urealyticum, Pneumocystis carinii* cytomegalovirus.	*Mycobacterium tuberculosis*
Treatment	Symptomatic	*Oral:* Amoxicillin, cefaclor, trimethoprim-sulfamethoxazole, erythromycin-sulfasoxazole *Parenteral:* Cefuroxime, ceftriaxone, ampicillin	Erythromycin Tetracycline (if older than 8 years)	Erythromycin (for *Chlamydia*)	Isoniazid ± rifampin ± third drug

infections should also be ascertained. Preceding or concurrent upper respiratory symptoms are common with viral pneumonias. However, bacterial pneumonia often follows a viral process, so that the presence of these symptoms are not particularly indicative of a purely viral infection. A gradual onset of illness usually typifies a viral or mycoplasmal process (or chlamydial in an infant), whereas the sudden onset or worsening of symptoms may be a harbinger of a more serious bacterial process.

Cough is usually, but not always, present. In the infant and younger child, the cough is almost always nonproductive, though the older child or adolescent may produce sputum. Chest pain, usually pleuritic, may be a major complaint; it occurs most commonly with bacterial pneumonias but may occur with any pneumonia associated with severe coughing.

Gastrointestinal symptoms are not unusual and may occasionally predominate. Anorexia is common, as is vomiting, which often follows coughing episodes. Abdominal pain, which may mimic an acute abdomen or appendicitis, classically occurs with lower lobe infiltrates, presumably by irritation of pleura adjacent to the diaphragm. Meningismus may also occur occassionally in children with upper lobe infiltrates.

Physical Examination

The most crucial part of the physical examination is the overall general appearance and behavior of the child. Signs of toxicity and anxiety may signify bacteremia or sepsis associated with bacterial pneumonia or may be caused by hypoxemia, which can occur with moderate to severe viral or bacterial pneumonia, especially in infants. Some degree of dehydration commonly occurs in all forms of pneumonia as a result of anorexia, vomiting, and increased fluid needs with fever and tachypnea.

Fever is usually present in children with pneumonia (except in the infant with afebrile pneumonitis syndrome or in a child recently given antipyretics). If the temperature is normal, patients rarely have an abnormal chest radiograph, regardless of other chest findings.[37] Although a fever over 40°C may suggest a bacterial process, the association is not absolute, as viruses cause the majority of all high fevers and bacterial pneumonia may also occur with temperatures below 39°C.

Tachypnea is the best single predictor of pneumonia in children.[38] Some infants may demonstrate few abnormal results in their physical examination other than an elevated respiratory rate. Tachycardia generally accompanies the increase in rate of breathing. Because fever itself can elevate the respiratory rate, it is important to observe the respiratory rate after the fever is lowered or to look for an elevated respiratory rate that is out of proportion to fever.

Signs of respiratory distress that are often present, to variable degrees, include nasal flaring, grunting, retractions, or cyanosis. The chest examination may be completely normal. Rales, either localized or diffuse, are a sign of alveolar involvement, but may be absent. Decreased breath sounds and dullness to percussion may occasionally be elicted in children and are suggestive of localized consolidation.

A thorough general physical examination, in addition to the chest examination, is vital. A search for generalized lymphadenopathy and hepatosplenomegaly is important. If gastrointestinal symptoms are prominent, the abdomen should be carefully examined for masses and tenderness. Certain bacteria, especially *H. influenzae* type b and *S. aureus*, tend to seed several sites of infection simultaneously, and pneumonia caused by these agents may occur with concomitant foci of infection elsewhere, most importantly the meninges, joints, and bones. In the ill-appearing infant with a pneumonia likely caused by one of these agents, a careful search for other foci is warranted; often a lumbar puncture is necessary to exclude meningitis if a clinical suspicion exists.

DIAGNOSTIC EVALUATION
Radiology

In an emergency department setting, radiographic examination of the chest is essential to the diagnosis and management of pneumonia. Infiltrates signify inflammation of the lung, the very definition of pneumonia.

Practitioners who work in office or clinic settings, know their patients, and can ensure close follow-up often diagnose pneumonia "clinically" based on a constellation of findings gathered from the history and physical examination. Studies compared pre-radiograph diagnosis and management plans based on clinical findings with final diagnoses made after radiographic results were known. These studies revealed that in 10% to 20% of cases, changes in diagnoses or in treatment plans were made based on the radiographic diagnosis—mostly in "ruling in" a diagnosis and instituting therapy that was not planned based on the clinical evaluation. In patients with a consistent pattern of signs and symptoms, there was a greater than 90% chance that the clinical diagnoses agreed with the radiographic findings.[39, 40]

Tachypnea has the highest positive predictive value for an abnormal radiograph. Rales, as a solitary finding, predicts an abnormal radiograph in 33% of patients.[38]

Similarly, another study showed that if a child had one or more of several findings—cyanosis, decreased breath sounds, dullness to percussion, grunting, flaring, retractions, rales, stridor, or tubular breath sounds—there was a greater than 1-in-3 chance that there would be a significant finding on the chest radiograph. Conversely, if a patient had a constellation of findings limited to wheezing, prolonged expiration, and rhonchi associated with cough, there was little likelihood of an infiltrate on the radiograph.[37]

In summary, an infant or child should undergo chest radiography for suspected pneumonia if he or she is acutely ill with respiratory distress or is febrile with associated tachypnea, rales, or decreased breath sounds.

Finding an infiltrate on the chest radiograph is the "gold standard" for the diagnosis of pneumonia (Fig. 29–1). Subsegmental, segmental, or lobar consolidation is generally indicative of a bacterial process, whereas hyperaeration with perihilar or diffuse interstitial infiltrates suggests a viral process (Fig. 29–2).[41] Chlamydial pneumonia in the infant

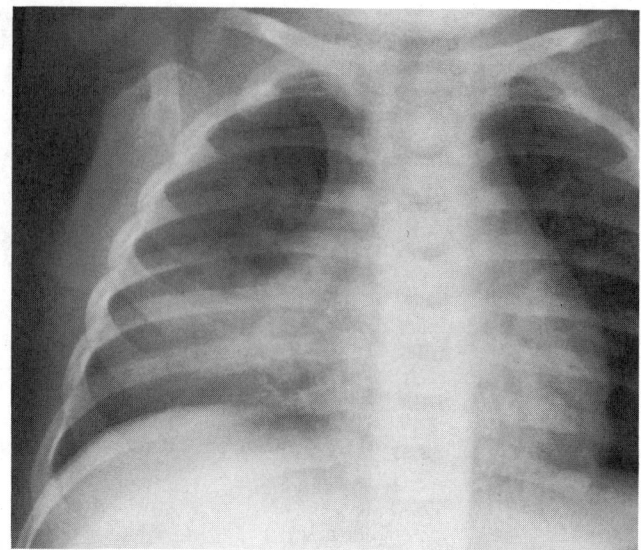

Figure 29–1. The round soft tissue density adjoining the heart in this 10-month-old girl obliterates the heart contour (silhouette sign) and contains some branching air bronchograms medially. The pattern is typical for a lobar pneumonia. (Courtesy of A. Oestreich, M.D., Cincinnati, OH.)

usually appears with diffuse bilateral interstitial infiltrates associated with hyperaeration.[42] Mycoplasmal pneumonia does not have such a "classic" radiographic appearance. It tends to cause a unilateral lower lobe infiltrate that may be patchy, segmental, or lobar in extent; however, early in the course, the pattern may be interstitial.[26, 43]

However, the diagnosis of pneumonia based on radiographic results is quite subjective, and significant interobserver variability exists when trying to determine the origin using chest radiographic findings.[44, 45] McCarthy et al. showed poor interobserver agreement between and among pediatricians and radiologists in trying to decide the origin (viral or bacterial) of pneumonia based on the radiographic findings.[44] In only 6 of 21 cases of etiologically proven pneumonia did all observers agree on the probable origin.

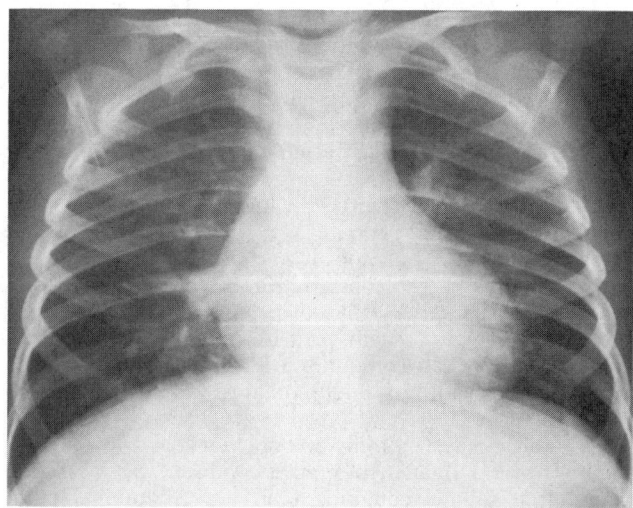

Figure 29–2. The patchy, streaky, and peribronchial nonuniform lung densities in the chest of this 2-year-old girl with cough, congestion, and low-grade fever is typical of interstitial viral pneumonia. A virus was identified: it was measles pneumonia. (Courtesy of A. Oestreich, M.D., Cincinnati, OH.)

Another study of the origin of pediatric pneumonia based on extensive bacterial and viral tests, including bacterial antigen detection in the urine, found much overlap between the type of infiltrates and the origin of pneumonia.[16] Alveolar infiltrates were found in 67% of viral cases and in 42% of bacterial cases. The remaining patients with proven bacterial pneumonia had interstitial infiltrates. One third to one half of bacterial pneumonias would have been missed if the diagnosis had been based on the chest radiograph alone (Fig. 29–3).[16, 46]

Studies of seriously ill infants with proven *H. influenzae* pneumonia have revealed that in up to 25% of cases, the radiographic findings were deceptive and demonstrated patchy or bronchopneumonic infiltrates that were often bilateral or multilobar. These findings are characteristic of a viral process.[47–49]

Findings highly specific for bacterial processes are moderate to large pleural effusions, pneumatoceles, and lung abscesses. Small to moderate parapneumonic pleural effusions (often seen only in decubitus views) occur in up to 20% of children with viral or mycoplasmal pneumonia; rarely do large ones develop.[50] Patients with sickle cell disease are an exception in that they may develop severe mycoplasmal pneumonia associated with large effusions.[51] Pleural effusions are particularly common when pneumonia is caused by *H. influenzae* type b (seen in 25% to 75% of cases[47–49]) or by *S. aureus* (seen in more than 75% of cases[52]). Other important causes of parapneumonic pleural effusions include *S. pneumoniae*, in which large, often sterile effusions may develop during treatment,[53] and *Mycobacteria tuberculosis*.

An empyema, or frank pus in the pleural space, can occur with any bacterial agent, especially *S. aureus* and *H. influenzae*, and appears to be a progression of untreated pleural infection.[54] Radiographs taken in the decubitus position may show failure of the pleural fluid to "layer out" as a result of the loculation of thick pus in the pleural space.

Pneumatoceles are thin-walled, air-filled cysts that may appear initially but are more likely to occur during the course of a bacterial pneumonia. Once thought to primarily occur in pneumonias caused by *S. aureus* and *K. pneumoniae*, pneumatoceles can appear following infection with a variety of bacterial agents, including *S. pneumoniae* and *H. influenzae*.[55] They usually resolve over months. Rarely they rupture, causing a sudden pneumothorax. Lung abscesses are partially fluid-filled, thick-walled cavities more than 2 cm in diameter that usually are caused by the aspiration of a mixture of aerobic and anaerobic bacteria.[36, 56]

Laboratory Tests

Laboratory tests may guide the ordering of a chest radiograph or serve as an adjunct to the radiograph and clinical picture in determining the probable origin of pneumonia in a child.

Acute-Phase Reactants

The complete blood cell count is the most common test ordered. It is important to check the hemoglobin to assess possible undiagnosed sickle cell disease or another serious underlying disorder. However, the white blood cell (WBC) count is the most useful parameter found in the blood count. In general, a WBC count greater than 15,000 to 20,000 cells/mm³ increases the probability of a bacterial origin of pneumonia. The higher the WBC count, the more likelihood there is of a rapid response to antibiotic therapy, indicative of a probable bacterial cause.[57, 58]

The WBC count is usually not elevated in children with chlamydial or mycoplasmal pneumonia, though those with disease caused by *C. trachomatis* may have a moderate eosinophilia.[31] The WBC count in children with tuberculosis may be normal, may show an increase in the percentage of

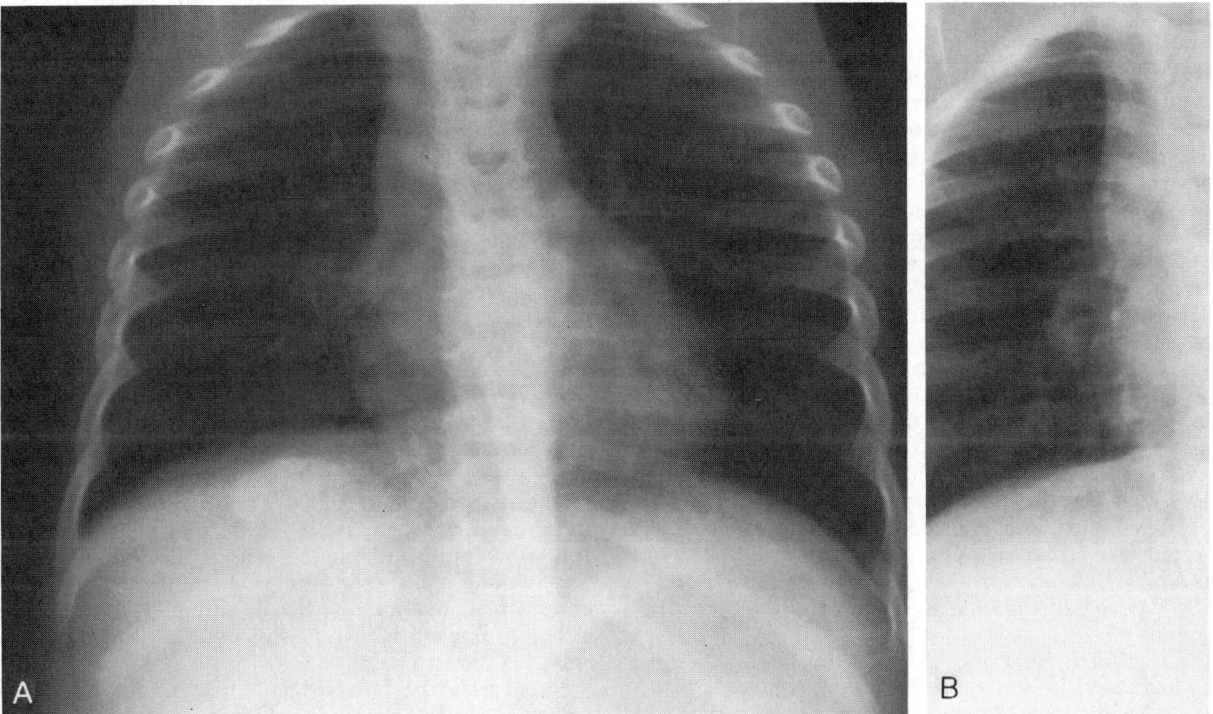

Figure 29–3. One of the hiding places of lobar pneumonia is the right lower lobe behind the diaphragm. *A*, The solid pneumonia of this 14-month-old girl is seen overlying the medial right ribs 9 to 11 where there should be only branching blood vessels, as on the earlier film *(B)*. (Courtesy of A. Oestreich, M.D., Cincinnati, OH.)

lymphoctyes, or, less commonly, may be quite elevated and mimic that seen in bacterial pneumonia.

Other acute-phase reactants, though less clinically utilized, have also been studied as to their usefulness in deciphering the origin of pneumonia. McCarthy et al. found that an elevated erythrocyte sedimentation rate (over 30 mm/hr) was the most sensitive indicator of bacterial pneumonia, bacteremia, or other serious bacterial infection.[59] In another study, a positive C-reactive protein test was found to be better than an elevated WBC count, erythrocyte sedimentation rate, or temperature as a predictor of a probable bacterial origin.[23]

Cultures

Sputum and nasopharyngeal cultures are of limited usefulness in searching for the origin of pneumonia in most children.[60] Infants and young children do not, in general, produce sputum. If they do, it generally becomes contaminated by upper respiratory bacterial flora. Adolescents may, on occasion, produce adequate sputum specimens. Gram stains of these specimens can be helpful if considering a bacterial etiology, as a plethora of gram-positive diplococci, sometimes easily seen, indicate pneumococcal infection. The absence of a predominant bacteria on the Gram stain suggests the possibility of mycoplasmal infection. Cultures of such specimens may be useful, but may be also be contaminated.[24]

S. pneumoniae, H. influenzae type b, and S. aureus may be part of the "normal flora" of the oro- and nasopharynx in healthy children. Studies have shown that the colonization rates for these organisms depend on the time of year and the incidence of infections in household or day-care contacts; such infections can involve greater than 50% of children.[60, 61] In a study of Nigerian children with bacterial pneumonia verified by lung taps (needle aspiration of the lung), pharyngeal cultures were found to be misleading in determining the etiologic diagnosis. In about one third of cases, similiar organisms were identified by needle aspiration of the lung and culture of the pharnyx; in another third, different pathogenic organisms were identified from the two sources; and in yet another third, the pharyngeal cultures were falsely negative.[62] Thus there is little correlation between upper respiratory bacteria and lower respiratory pathogens. Viruses, unlike bacteria, are rare colonizers of the nasopharnyx, with the exception of herpes virus and adenovirus.[24] Thus positive viral cultures of the nasopharynx are usually significant and occasionally may be warranted.

Culturing a bacterial pathogen from the blood of a patient with pneumonia is considered proof of the origin. However, this occurs in a small percentage of patients with pneumonia (3% to about 20% in various studies).[63] Even in patients with pathogens cultured from lung tap specimens, concurrent positive blood cultures are unusual. Only 13% of the Nigerian children with severe pneumonia and positive lung taps in the previously mentioned study had positive blood cultures.[62] Bacteremia does not seem to be a common or constant occurrence in children with bacterial pneumonia. H. influenzae type b pneumonia may be an exception, as some studies show positive blood culture rates of up to 75% in hospitalized children with pneumonia caused by this organism. This is not surprising, as the likely pathogenesis of this type of pneumonia is seeding of infection from bacteremia.[48]

In severely ill or immunocompromised patients presenting with pneumonia, other, more invasive techniques may be warranted when ascertaining the etiologic agent is of vital importance. Transtracheal aspiration is safe in adults but has not been widely used in children.[64] Needle aspiration of the lung is also a safe technique in experienced hands, and

is quite useful when studying pneumonia in less developed countries, where the incidence of bacterial infection is much higher than in more developed countries.[62, 65] These techniques are not generally performed by the pediatrician or emergency physician and should be reserved for critically ill children and performed only after consultation with a pulmonologist or infectious disease expert.

Parapneumonic pleural fluid, when present in sufficient amounts to be obtained by thoracentesis (greater than 10 mm on a lateral decubitus chest radiograph[6]), is an excellent source of information. Sixty to eighty percent of pleural fluid cultures will reveal the offending organism.[52, 66] Thoracentesis should be considered in any child with a moderate to large pleural effusion, both as a key to diagnosis and as a therapeutic manuver to relieve mechanical impairment of respiration. Fluid should be sent for microbiologic, hematologic, and chemical evaluation, including bacterial, fungal, and AFB culture; gram staining; bacterial antigen tests; WBC count; and determination of pH, glucose, lactate dehydrogenase (LDH), and protein content.[52] Exudates associated with bacterial pneumonia usually produce an elevated WBC count (more than 50,000 cells/mm^3) with a preponderance of polymorphonuclear leukocytes, a decreased glucose level (less than 40 mg/dl), and elevated levels of LDH (greater than 200 IU) and protein.[67] Decreased pH (less than 7.4) is also seen with bacterial infections; a pH less than 7.0 to 7.2 usually signifies significant inflammation and the need for a tube thoracostomy.[68] If pus is aspirated, the diagnosis is empyema, and further analysis, except for Gram stain and cultures, are unnecessary. Common noninfectious causes of pleural effusion that must be considered in the differential diagnosis include transudates associated with congestive heart failure, nephrotic syndrome, and overhydration. Less common causes include neoplasms and autoimmune disorders.

Diagnostic Adjuncts

Other, less invasive tests have been studied in trying to decipher the puzzle of what causes a specific pneumonia in children. Bacterial antigen tests of the urine of patients with pneumonia are promising. Ramsey et al. found a 24% incidence of pneumococcal or H. influenzae type b antigenuria using latex agglutination in children with lower respiratory infections, only 2% of whom had positive blood cultures. A comparison group of healthy children had an antigenuria rate of 4%, but 16% of children with otitis showed antigen in their urine.[69] Using counterimmunoelectrophoresis (CIE) assays, Turner and coworkers found that 26% of outpatients with pneumonia had antigen in their urine.[70] In another study also using CIE techniques, 17 of 98 patients with pneumonia were found to have pneumococcal or H. influenzae type b antigen found in their urine, whereas only 3% had positive blood cultures. More important, none of 32 control patients or 19 patients with otitis had detectable antigen.[16] Bacterial antigen tests on nasopharyngeal secretions appear to be much less reliable because of the high frequency of false-positive results.[71] Neither of these bacterial antigen tests can be routinely recommended for outpatients with pneumonia. Urine antigen tests may have a role in the diagnostic evaluation of the seriously ill child with pneumonia who is admitted to the hospital, although one study has questioned the specificity and sensitivity of these tests.[72]

Rapid tests based on antigen detection in nasopharyngeal secretions in the diagnosis of RSV and chlamydial pneumonia are now available and widely used. There are two types of tests for RSV: the immunofluorescent test and the enzyme-linked immunosorbent assay (ELISA). The immunofluorescent test is slightly more sensitive and specific than the ELISA, but both will detect RSV in greater than 80% to 90% of the cases verified by culture.[73]

Chlamydial pneumonia can be diagnosed by culture of the nasopharynx or by specific antibody titers; an elevated anti-*Chlamydia* immunoglobulin M (IgM) titer is diagnostic. Recently, direct fluorescent antibody tests, commonly used in the diagnosis of urethral or conjunctival infections, have been studied on nasopharyngeal secretions. This may prove a useful test; it is both sensitive and specific, identifying *C. trachomatis* in more than 90% of infected infants with proven chlamydial pneumonitis.[74, 75]

Mycoplasmal pneumonia is difficult to diagnose rapidly. Because *M. pneumoniae* cultures are not widely available, the only certain way to make the diagnosis is by awaiting a fourfold rise in serologic titers; a single titer greater than 1:64 is suggestive.[27] Some success with a DNA probe test on nasopharyngeal specimens has been reported.[76] However, the only generally available test that can help with the rapid diagnosis is the cold agglutinins test. A serum titer of 1:32 or greater is considered positive and is present in one third to three fourths of patients infected with *M. pneumoniae*. However, it is nonspecific and may be positive in viral infections as well.[77] A rapid "bedside" version of this test can be done by adding 0.3 to 0.4 ml of blood to a lavender hematology tube that contains a small amount of ethylene-diaminetetraacetic acid (EDTA) or to a prothrombin tube that contains sodium citrate. The tube is then placed in ice water for 15 to 30 seconds and examined for the presence of coarse floccular agglutination, which disappears when the tube is rewarmed.[26, 78]

THERAPEUTIC INTERVENTION

General principles of therapy for any infant or child with pneumonia include the following:

1. If any sign of respiratory distress or anxiety exists, check for hypoxemia by using pulse oximetry or measuring arterial blood gases. The latter is useful in infants with impending respiratory failure with an elevated Pco_2. If the oxygen saturation or Po_2 is low, humidified oxygen is provided by mask or hood to maintain adequate blood oxygen content.

2. Dehydration should be considered, and if signs are present, the child is rehydrated orally or parenterally.

3. Antipyretics (acetaminophen) are used to lower elevated temperatures.

4. If there is associated wheezing and bronchospasm, aerosolized or oral beta-adrenergic agents are given.

5. Cough suppressants are avoided unless coughing is so severe that the patient has severe musculoskeletal pain or cannot rest. They are then used sparingly and intermittently.

Any infant or child seen in the emergency department in whom the diagnosis of pneumonia is entertained should have a chest radiograph (Fig. 29–4). A CBC count and blood culture should be obtained in most younger children with infiltrates on the chest radiograph and in any child or adolescent who appears seriously ill. A skin test for tuberculosis should be considered.

Based on the clinical presentation and general appearance of the patient, the radiographic findings, and the WBC count, the clinician must make a best guess as to the clinical syndrome and proceed accordingly. The nontoxic child with a low-grade fever, streaky or perihilar infiltrate, and normal WBC count probably has viral pneumonia and can usually be managed symptomatically with close follow-up. Bacterial pneumonia typically presents with a greater degree of fever and toxicity, a higher WBC count, and, more commonly, a lobar or segmental consolidation. It should be treated with antibiotics and close follow-up or hospitalization depending on the degree of respiratory distress and toxicity. Unfortunately, many children do not fit into one of these two groups and will have some of the features of both bacterial and viral infections. In these cases, it is best to treat the child with antibiotics, as the possibility of a bacterial origin cannot be ignored. This is particularly true in the emergency setting, when close follow-up cannot be ensured.

Any toxic-appearing child, with or without respiratory distress, or any very young infant should be admitted. Other indications for admission include the following:

Age (less than 3 to 6 months)
Respiratory distress
Hypoxemia and the need for supplemental oxygen
Inability to tolerate oral fluids or medications
Underlying disease (sickle cell anemia, carcinoma, immunodeficiency, etc.)
Moderate to large pleural effusion
Empyema
Lung abscess
Lack of response to ambulatory management
Psychosocial factors (i.e., concern about compliance or follow-up)

Cefuroxime is a good choice for the initial antibiotic management of the hospitalized child or infant out of the newborn period. It is effective against *S. pneumoniae*, *H. influenzae*, and *S. aureus*, and increasing experience confirms it to be safe and efficacious in children.[79] Ampicillin is an alternative if beta-lactamase–resistant *H. influenzae* is not prevalent in the community and the likelihood of a staphylococcal origin is low. Neonates should be started on broad-spectrum antibiotics that are effective against both the gram-negative enterics and the group B streptococci and other gram-positive organisms; the combination of ampicillin and an aminoglycoside (commonly gentamicin) provides this coverage. If staphylococcal pneumonia is strongly considered in any infant or child, nafcillin (or a similar antibiotic), an effective cephalosporin, or vancomycin should be considered. Immunodeficient or neutropenic children with pneumonia need to be started on extremely broad antibiotic coverage in consultation with their subspeciality physicians. In any hospitalized child with pneumonia, if the origin of the pneumonia becomes evident by culture results or other means, then antibiotic therapy can be changed to the most appropriate and specific drug (e.g., penicillin for pneumococcal pneumonia).

Most older infants and children with pneumonia can be managed as outpatients with close follow-up. Patients with presumed bacterial pneumonia or patients in whom the clinical picture and radiograph are not characteristic of a viral process should be treated with oral antibiotics. Because the most important bacterial pathogens causing outpatient pneumonia in the young child are *S. pneumoniae* and *H. influenzae*, amoxicillin is a good choice for the initial management.[80] In areas where *H. influenzae* resistance rates to ampicillin are high (30% in some parts of the United States) or in ill-appearing children, an alternative antibiotic with action against beta-lactamase–producing bacteria should be considered; these include cefaclor, trimethoprim-sulfamethoxazole, erythromycin-sulfisoxazole (Pediazole), amoxicillin-clavulanate (Augmentin) or cefixime (Table 29–2). Older children may be treated with penicillin if bacterial pneumonia is strongly suspected or with erythromycin if the clinical picture is either consistent with mycoplasmal infection or unclear.[81] Erythromycin is the treatment of choice for mycoplasmal pneumonia[82] and is effective against most, but not all, pneumococci. Unfortunately, however, its pro-

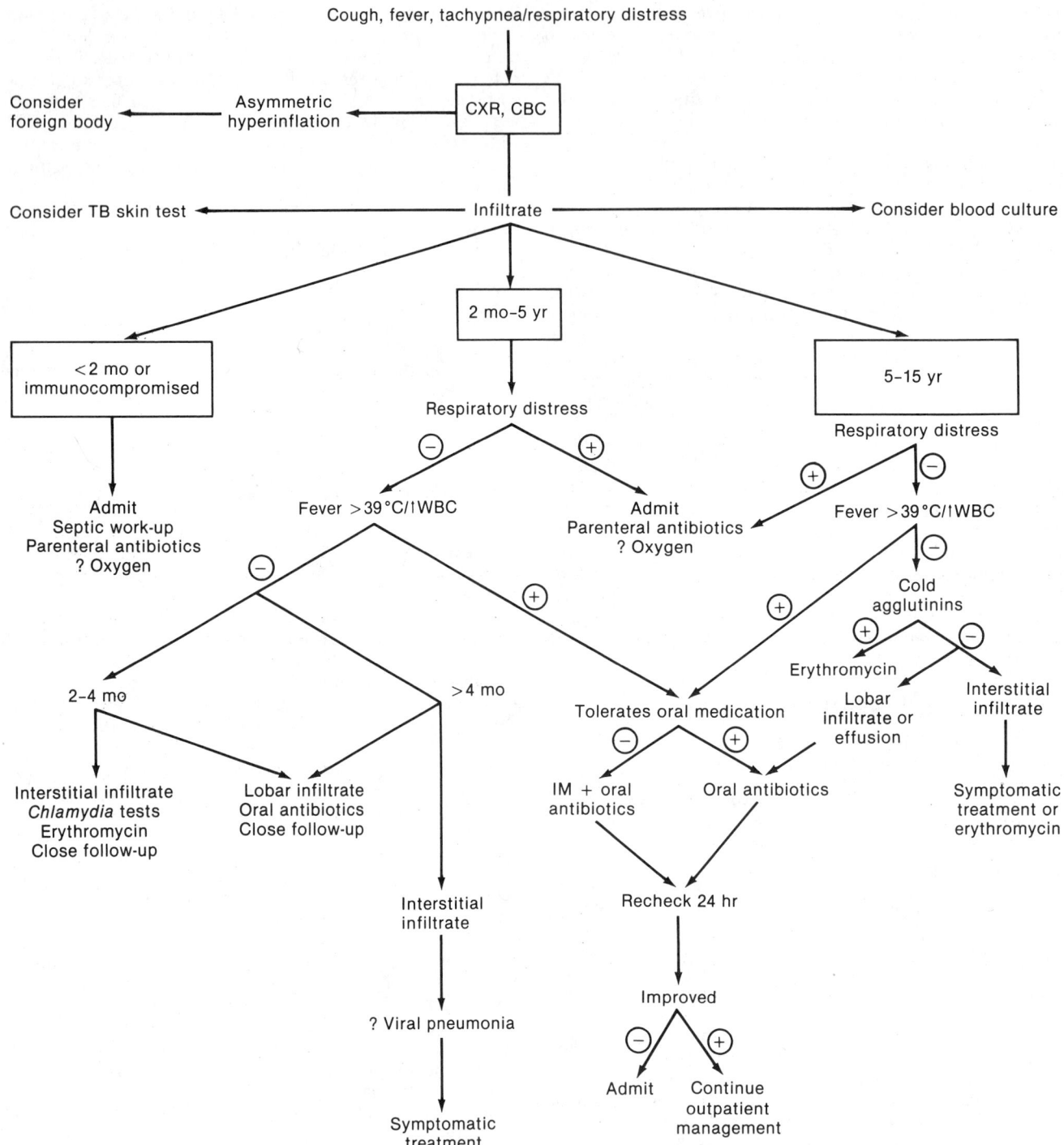

Figure 29–4. Algorithm for the management of pneumonia. (From Hilton NS. Pneumonia. *In* Rosen P, Baker FJ, Barkin RM, et al (eds). Emergency Medicine: Concepts and Clinical Practice. Vol. 2. 2nd ed. St Louis, CV Mosby, 1988, p 2255.)

pensity to cause nausea and vomiting limits its usefulness in some children. Tetracyline is an alternative for pneumonia likely caused by *M. pneumoniae,* but it should not be given to children younger than 8 years.[83]

A practical option in the emergency or office setting when there is a concern about a sick child's initial ability to tolerate oral medication (a common concern with severe coughing) is to administer an initial dose of an intramuscular long-acting antibiotic. Ceftriaxone is a good choice, because it has a long half-life and is effective against *S. pneumoniae, H. influenzae* (including ampicillin-resistant strains), and *S. au-*

reus.[84] Procaine-penicillin, though its spectrum is less broad, is an alternative with a long record of clinical efficacy. After 12 to 24 hours, the child may begin oral antibiotic therapy.

Any ill-appearing child with pneumonia should be seen again in 24 hours, especially if receiving an initial intramuscular dose of antibiotic, to ensure improvement. In the clinic or office setting, where practitioners know their patients, phone follow-up may be sufficient. Often the child with "classic" pneumococcal pneumonia will be surprisingly improved after 1 day. If a child is worse at 24- to 48-hour follow-up, the physician must consider the following possi-

TABLE 29–2

ANTIBIOTIC REGIMEN FOR PATIENTS WITH PNEUMONIA

	Infants/Young Children	Older Children
Oral Agents		
Amoxicillin	40 mg/kg/day divided in three doses	250–500 mg tid
Ampicillin	75–100 mg/kg/day divided in four doses	250–500 mg qid
Erythromycin	40–50 mg/kg/day divided in four doses	250–500 mg qid
Cefaclor	40 mg/kg/day divided in three doses	250–500 mg tid
Amoxicillin-clavulanate potassium (Augmentin)	40 mg/kg/day divided in three doses	250 mg tid
Penicillin V potassium	25–50 mg/kg/day divided in four doses	250–500 mg qid
Tetracycline	20–40 mg/kg/day divided in four doses	250–500 mg qid
Erythromycin ethylsuccinate-sulfisoxazole acetyl (Pediazole)	40–50 mg/kg/day (divided in four doses)	
Trimethoprim-sulfamethoxazole (TMP-SMX)	8 mg/kg TMP per 40 mg/kg SMX (divided in two doses)	One double-strength tablet bid
Parenteral Agents		
Cefuroxime	75–150 mg/kg/day divided q 8 hr IV	
Ampicillin	100–200 mg/kg/day divided q 6 hr IV	
Ceftriaxone	50–75 mg/kg/day divided q 12–24 hr IV or IM	
	50–75 mg/kg, single dose, IM (maximum 1.5 gm)	
Penicillin G procaine	25–50,000 U/kg, single dose, IM (maximum 1 million U)	
Penicillin G	25–100,000 U/kg/day divided 4–6 hr IV	
Gentamicin	5–7.5 mg/kg/day divided q 8 hr IV or IM	
Nafcillin	100 mg/kg/day divided q 6 hr IV	

bilities: (1) the organism is resistant to the chosen antibiotic, (2) the child was noncompliant or could not tolerate the drug, or (3) the child has a viral pneumonia that is progressing.[85] The diagnoses of tuberculosis, staphylococcal pneumonia, foreign body aspiration, recurrent aspiration, or occult asthma should also be entertained. Depending on the degree of toxicity of the child, the physician may elect to repeat the chest radiograph, change the medication, admit the child, or continue the same treatment regimen with close follow-up.

Infants presenting with symptoms and signs of the afebrile pneumonitis syndrome should be treated with erythromycin for at least 14 days and be managed according to their clinical status. Those who present with respiratory distress, hypoxemia, poor feeding, or severe coughing should be admitted for close observation. The nontoxic, mildly ill infant with presumed chlamydial pneumonia can be initially managed as an outpatient if close follow-up can be ensured.

Otherwise healthy children with uncomplicated pneumonia should be seen at the end of their treatment course; 10 days is usually sufficient. These children do not need a follow-up chest radiograph, which often continues to show infiltrates for 4 to 6 weeks, despite clinical cure.[86] However, children with recurrent pneumonia, those with underlying illnesses, or those with prolonged symptoms (except cough, which can last long after other symptoms have resolved) should be followed closely by their primary care doctor and should have repeat radiographs 4 to 6 weeks after their infection.

Subspeciality consultation should also be requested in the child with underlying immunodeficiency, sickle cell disease, or cancer or in the severely ill child who does not respond to normal management. Severely ill infants or infants with underlying medical problems admitted with RSV pneumonia may be candidates for ribavirin therapy after consultation with infectious disease or pulmonary experts.[87, 88]

Instructions to Parents

Parents or guardians of infants and children being discharged from the emergency department with the diagnosis of pneumonia should be carefully taught to administer any prescribed medication according to the physician's discharge plans. Signs of increasing respiratory distress, including increasing respiratory rate, retractions, grunting, cyanosis, poor feeding, or decreased activity, should likewise be reviewed; if any of these occur, the child should be reexamined by his or her own physician or returned to the emergency department as soon as possible. A definite follow-up plan should be arranged and agreed to by the family.

References

1. Denny FW, Collier AM, Henderson FW. Acute respiratory infections in day care. Rev Infect Dis 1986;8:527.
2. Committee on Environmental Hazards. Involuntary smoking—a hazard to children. Pediatrics 1986;77:755.
3. Morris K, Morganlander M, Coulehan JL, et al. Wood-burning stoves and lower respiratory tract infection in American Indian children. Am J Dis Child 1990;144:105.
4. Gardner G, Frank AL, Tabor LH. Effect of social and family factors on viral respiratory infection and illness in the first year of life. J Epidemiol Community Health 1984;38:42.
5. Denny FW. Acute respiratory infections in children: Etiology and epidemiology. Pediatr Rev 1987;9:135.
6. Long S. Treatment of acute pneumonia in infants and children. Pediatr Clin North Am 1983;30:297.
7. Murphy TF, Henderson FW, Clyde WA, et al. Pneumonia: An eleven-year study in a pediatric practice. Am J Epidemiol 1981;113:12.
8. Klein JO, Schlesinger PC, Karasic RB. Management of the febrile infant three months of age or younger. Pediatr Infect Dis 1984;3:75.
9. Fosarelli PD, DeAngelis C, Winkelstein J. Infectious illnesses in the first two years of life. Pediatr Infect Dis 1985;4:153.
10. Stansfield S. Acute respiratory infections in the developing world: Strategies for prevention, treatment and control. Pediatr Infect Dis 1987;6:622.
11. Steele R. Update on managing this winter's pediatric pneumonias. J Respir Dis 1987;8:63.
12. Georges P. The child with pneumonia: Diagnostic and therapeutic considerations. Pediatr Infect Dis 1988;7:453.
13. Dorowitz G, Mandell G. Empiric therapy for pneumonia. Rev Infect Dis 1983;5:540.
14. Hilton NS. Pneumonia. In Rosen P, Baker FJ, Barkin RM, et al (eds). Emergency Medicine: Concepts and Clinical Practice. Vol 2. 2nd ed. St Louis, CV Mosby, 1988, pp 2251–2257.
15. Connor E, Powell K. Fulminant pneumonia caused by concomitant

infection with influenza B virus and *Staphylococcus aureus*. J Pediatr 1985;106:447.

16. Turner RB, Lande AE, Chase P, et al. Pneumonia in pediatric outpatients: Cause and clinical manifestations. J Pediatr 1987;111:194.

17. Paisley JW, Lauer BA, McIntosh K, et al. Pathogens associated with acute lower respiratory tract infection in young children. Pediatr Infect Dis 1984;3:14.

18. Pneumonia in childhood. Editorial. Lancet 1988; 1:741.

19. Beem MO, Saxon EM. Respiratory-tract colonization and a distinctive pneumonia syndrome in infants infected with *Chlamydia trachomatis*. N Engl J Med 1977;296:306.

20. Stagno S, Brasfield D, Brown M, et al. Infant pneumonitis associated with cytomegalovirus, *Chlamydia, Pneumocystis* and *Ureaplasma*. Pediatrics 1981;68:322.

21. Denny FW, Clyde WA. Acute lower respiratory infections in non-hospitalized children. J Pediatr 1986;108:635.

22. Chartrand SA, McCracken GH. Staphylococcal pneumonia in infants and children. Pediatr Infect Dis 1982;1:19.

23. McCarthy DL, Frank AL, Ablow RC, et al. Value of C-reactive protein in differentiation of bacterial and viral pneumonias. J Pediatr 1978;92:454.

24. Wald ER. Management of pneumonia in outpatients. Pediatr Infect Dis 1984; S3:521.

25. Shann F. Etiology of severe pneumonia in children in developing countries. Pediatr Infect Dis 1986;5:247.

26. Broughton RA. Infections due to *Mycoplasma pneumoniae* in childhood. Pediatr Infect Dis 1986;5:71.

27. Azimi PH, Chase PA, Petru A. Mycoplasmas: Their role in pediatric disease. Curr Probl Pediatr 1984;14:1.

28. Cassell GH, Cole BC. Mycoplasmas as agents of human disease. N Engl J Med 1981;304:80.

29. Denny FW, Clyde WA, Glezen WP. *Mycoplasma pneumoniae* disease: Clinical spectrum, pathophysiology, epidemiology, and control. J Infect Dis 1971;123:74.

30. Foy HM, Kenny GE, McMahan R, et al. *Mycoplasma pneumoniae* in the community. Am J Epidemiol 1970;93:55.

31. Rettig PJ. Infections due to *Chlamydia trachomatis* from infancy to adolescence. Pediatr Infect Dis 1986;5:449.

32. Saboto AR, Martin AJ, Marmion BP, et al. *Mycoplasma pneumoniae*: Acute illness, antibiotics and subsequent pulmonary function. Arch Dis Child 1984;59:1034.

33. Ryan ME, Spahr R, Wolf S. Common bacterial pneumonitis in infants. Postgrad Med 1986;79:132.

34. Blazer S, Naveh Y, Friedman A. Foreign body in the airway. Am J Dis Child 1980;134:68.

35. Blumhagen J, Wesenberg R, Brooks J, Cotton E. Endotracheal foreign bodies. Clin Pediatr 1980;19:480.

36. Brook I, Finegold SM. Bacteriology of aspiration pneumonia in children. Pediatrics 1980;65:1115.

37. Zukin DD, Hoffman JR, Cleveland RH, et al. Correlation of pulmonary signs and symptoms with chest radiographs in the pediatric age group. Ann Emerg Med 1986;15:792.

38. Leventhal JM. Clinical predictors of pneumonia as a guide to ordering chest roentgenograms. Clin Pediatr 1982;21:730.

39. Alario AJ, McCarthy PL, Markowitz R, et al. Usefulness of chest radiographs in children with acute lower respiratory tract disease. J Pediatr 1987;III:187.

40. Grossman LK, Caplan SE. Clinical, laboratory and radiological information in the diagnosis of pneumonia in children. Ann Emerg Med 1988;17:43.

41. Griscom NT. Pneumonia in children and some of its variants. Radiology 1988;167:297.

42. Tipple MA, Beem MO, Saxon EM. Clinical characteristics of the afebrile pneumonia associated with *Chlamydia trachomatis* infection in infants less than 6 months of age. Pediatrics 1979;63:192.

43. Mansel JK, Rosenow EC, Smith TF, Martin JW. *Mycoplasma pneumoniae* pneumonia. Chest 1989;95:639.

44. McCarthy PL, Spiesel SZ, Stashwick CA, et al. Radiographic findings and etiologic diagnosis in ambulatory childhood pneumonias. Clin Pediatr 1981;20:686.

45. Bettenay FAL, deCampo JF, McCross DB. Differentiating bacterial from viral pneumonias in children. Pediatr Radiol 1988;18:453.

46. Courtoy I, Lande AE, Turner RB. Accuracy of radiographic differentiation of bacterial from nonbacterial pneumonia. Clin Pediatr 1989;28:261.

47. Jacobs NM, Harris VJ. Acute *Haemophilus* pneumonia in childhood. Am J Dis Child 1979;133:603.

48. Ginsburg CM, Howard JB, Nelson JD. Report of 65 cases of *Haemophilus influenzae* b by pneumonia. Pediatrics 1979;64:283.

49. Asmar BI, Slovis TL, Reed JO, Dajani AS. *Haemophilus influenzae* type b pneumonia in 43 children. J Pediatr 1978;93:389.

50. Fine NI, Smith LR, Sheedy PF. Frequency of pleural effusions in mycoplasma and viral pneumonias. N Engl J Med 1970;283:790.

51. Shulman ST, Bartlett J, Clyde WA, Ayoub EM. The unusual severity of mycoplasmal pneumonia in children with sickle-cell disease. N Engl J Med 1972;287:164.

52. Freij BJ, Kusmiesz H, Nelson JD, McCracken GH. Parapneumonic effusions and empyema in hospitalized children: A retrospective review of 227 cases. Pediatr Infect Dis 1984;3:578.

53. Ledbetter EO. The many faces of pneumococcal pneumonia. Contemp Pediatr 1988; 5:50.

54. McLaughlin FJ, Goldmann DA, Rosenbaum DM, et al. Empyema in children: clinical course and long-term follow-up. Pediatrics 1984;73:587.

55. Amitai I, Mogle P, Godfrey S, Aviad I. Pneumatocele in infants and children. Clin Pediatr 1983;22:420.

56. Brook I, Finegold SM. Bacteriology and therapy of lung abscess in children. J Pediatr 1979;94:10.

57. McCarthy PL, Tomasso L, Dolan TF. Predicting fever response of children with pneumonia treated with antibiotics. Clin Pediatr 1980;19:753.

58. Shuttleworth DB, Charney E. Leukocyte count in childhood pneumonia. Am J Dis Child 1971;122:393.

59. McCarthy PL, Jekel JF, Dolan TF. Comparison of acute-phase reactants in pediatric patients with fever. Pediatrics 1978;62:716.

60. Todd JK. Bacteriology and clinical relevance of nasopharyngeal and oropharyngeal cultures. Pediatr Infect Dis 1984;3:159.

61. Loda FA, Collier AM, Glezen WP, et al. Occurrence of *Diplococcus pneumoniae* in the upper respiratory tract of children. J Pediatr 1975;87:1087.

62. Silverman M, Stratton D, Diallo A, Egler LJ. Diagnosis of acute bacterial pneumonia in Nigerian children. Arch Dis Child 1977;52:925.

63. Marks MI. Pediatric pneumonia: Viral or bacterial? J Resp Dis 1982;3:108.

64. Davidson M, Tempest B, Palmer DL. Bacteriologic diagnosis of acute pneumonia. JAMA 1976;235:158.

65. Mimica I, Donoso E, Howard JE, Ledermann GW. Lung puncture in the etiological diagnosis of pneumonia. Am J Dis Child 1971;122:278.

66. Chonmaitree T, Powell KR. Parapneumonic pleural effusion and empyema in children. Clin Pediatr 1983;22:414.

67. Light RW, MacGregor I, Luchsinger PC, Ball WC. Pleural effusions: The diagnostic separation of transudates and exudates. Ann Intern Med 1972;77:507.

68. Light RW, Girard WM, Jenkinson SG, George RB. Parapneumonic effusions. Am J Med 1980;69:507.

69. Ramsey BW, Marcuse EK, Foy HM, et al. Use of bacterial antigen detection in the diagnosis of pediatric lower respiratory tract infections. Pediatrics 1986;78:1.

70. Turner RB, Hayden FG, Hendley JO. Counterimmunoelectrophoresis of urine for diagnosis of bacterial pneumonia in pediatric outpatients. Pediatrics 1983;71:780.

71. Rusconi F, Rancilio L, Assael BM, et al. Counterimmunoelectrophoresis and latex particle agglutination in the etiologic diagnosis of presumed bacterial pneumonia in pediatric patients. Pediatr Infect Dis J 1988;7:781.

72. Isaacs D. Problems in determining the etiology of community-acquired childhood pneumonia. Pediatr Infect Dis 1989;8:143.

73. McIntosh K. Respiratory syncytial virus infections in infants and children: Diagnosis and treatment. Pediatr Rev 1987;9:191.

74. Paisley JW, Lauer BA, Melinkovich P, et al. Rapid diagnosis of *Chlamydia trachomatis* pneumonia in infants by direct immunofluorescence microscopy of nasopharyngeal secretions. J Pediatr 1986;109:653.

75. Hammerschlag MR. Chlamydial infections. J Pediatr 1989;114:727.

76. Hata D, Kuze F, Mochizuki Y, et al. Evaluation of DNA probe test for rapid diagnosis of *Mycoplasma pneumoniae* infections. J Pediatr 1990;116:273.

77. Cherry JD, Welliver RC. *Mycoplasma pneumoniae* infections of adults and children. West J Med 1976;125:47.

78. Griffin JP. Rapid screening for cold agglutinins in pneumonia. Ann Intern Med 1969;70:701.

79. Nelson JD. Cefuroxime: A cephalosporin with unique applicability to pediatric practice. Pediatr Infect Dis 1983;2:394.

80. Grossman M, Klein JO, McCarthy PL, et al. Consensus: Management of presumed bacterial pneumonia in ambulatory children. Pediatr Infect Dis 1984;3:497.

81. Teele D. Pneumonia: Antimicrobial therapy for infants and children. Pediatr Infect Dis 1985;4:330.

82. McCracken GH. Current status of antibiotic treatment for *Mycoplasma pneumoniae* infections. Pediatr Infect Dis 1986;5:167.

83. The choice of antimicrobial drugs. Med Lett Drug Ther 1990;32:41.

84. Dagan R, Phillip M, Watemberg N, Kassis I. Outpatient treatment of serious community-acquired pediatric infections using once daily intramuscular ceftriaxone. Pediatr Infect Dis J 1987;6:1080.

85. Gooch WM. Bronchitis and pneumonia in ambulatory patients. Pediatr Infect Dis J 1987;6:137.

86. Grossman LK, Wald ER, Nair P, Papiez J. Roentgenographic follow-up of acute pneumonia in children. Pediatrics 1979;63:30.

87. Committee on Infectious Diseases. Ribavirin therapy of respiratory syncytial virus. Pediatrics 1987;79:475.

88. Hall CB. Ribavirin: Beginning the blitz on respiratory viruses? Pediatr Infect Dis 1985;4:668.

CHAPTER 30

Cystic Fibrosis

Thomas J. Abramo

INCIDENCE

The overall incidence of cystic fibrosis is difficult to ascertain because of failure to detect cases with subtle presentations and because of neonatal deaths, miscarriages, and late-diagnosed cases. The disease frequency in whites is estimated to be 1 in 2000 live births, with the gene frequency approximately 1 in 20. In about 1 in 500 marriages there is a 25% risk of cystic fibrosis with each pregnancy. In blacks, cystic fibrosis occurs in 1 in 18,000 live births. Cystic fibrosis is an autosomal recessive trait; the cystic fibrosis factor is located on the long arm of chromosome 7. In the near future, specific allele defects in the cystic fibrosis gene will be determined, as will the resulting defective protein in each patient. When the specific defect is known for each patient, gene surgery may be possible to correct the deficiency, perhaps in the prenatal period.

PATHOPHYSIOLOGY
Mechanism

Until recently, the fundamental defect for cystic fibrosis was presumed to be a dysfunction of the sodium chloride ion transport channel. The theory presumed that there was a defect in sodium transport and an aberration of chloride transport followed. Defective ion transport across epithelial surfaces has been demonstrated. Studies using mucous membrane cells exposed to hypertonic saline show that in cystic fibrosis patients, sodium enters the cells readily, but the chloride ion lags behind, suggesting a blocked chloride channel.

Normally salt is conserved by the reabsorption of sodium from the sweat glands. In cystic fibrosis patients, the chloride cannot follow the sodium, and thus some sodium must remain. This results in a salty taste of the skin in these patients. The cystic fibrosis patient therefore is susceptible to hyponatremic dehydration.

In most cystic fibrosis patients, the initial exocrine system affected is the pulmonary tract. In the healthy respiratory tract, sodium is reabsorbed across the epithelial membrane, and water follows it into the circulation in response to stress, trauma, exercise, or illness. To prevent the inspissation of normal secretions, the respiratory epithelial cells secrete chloride into the lumen and water follows. In cystic fibrosis patients, the ability to reabsorb the sodium and water is functionally intact, but chloride secretion is defective. This inability to secrete chloride into the respiratory tract causes the dehydration of these secretions, hampering normal pulmonary clearance. The inspissated secretions predispose the respiratory tract to infection.

Pulmonary Involvement

The earliest pulmonary involvement is uncertain. Hypertrophy and hyperplasia of the mucous glands may develop first, followed by chronic bacterial colonization. Conversely, hypertrophy of the mucous-secreting system may result from an initial viral infection. Inflammation of the small airways is the earliest finding after the onset of the infectious process. Bronchial lesions occur more commonly than parenchymal lesions in cystic fibrosis patients more than 4 months of age at necropsy.

Infection promotes the inflammatory response, with resultant recruitment of phagocytes to the inflammation site. The release of lytic enzymes contributes to hypertrophy and hyperplasia of the mucous system. Goblet cells replace the respiratory ciliated cells and squamous metaplasia occurs. This process leads to exposure to bacterial antigens that may trigger an allergic response. Inflammatory mediators cause bronchoconstriction and stimulate mucus production. There is also evidence that the exoproduct of *Pseudomonas* plays an important role. The pigments and certain cell components of *Pseudomonas aeruginosa* interfere with cell-mediated immunity. In addition, with pseudomonal infection, mucin secretion is promoted and ineffective opsonins are produced. This process leads to bronchiectasis and mucopurulent plugging.

The progression of tissue damage and altered structural components results in destroyed airway structure and bronchiectasis. In the cystic fibrosis patient, the proportion of bronchial lung volumes are increased 10% to 20%. The bronchiectatic lung may occupy 50% of the entire lung volume. There is an increase in bronchial volume with a reduction of lung parenchyma in the upper lobes, which also contain increased cystic lesions.

Bronchiolitis, mucopurulent airway plugging, and chronic bronchitis are obstructive changes found in all age groups. Bronchiectatic dilation of the airways at the expense of lung parenchyma is a dominating component of lung pathology and increases with progression of the disease process. Bronchiolar stenosis, scarring, and pneumonias are nonobligatory changes occurring more in advanced disease.

Bronchial wall stability is determined by structural factors (which are affected in cystic fibrosis) and the smooth muscle tone of the bronchioles. In cystic fibrosis there is an increase in smooth muscle tone, resulting in obstruction of the airway. Though bronchodilators may relieve the bronchospastic airway obstruction, they may also increase airway wall instability. Increased bronchial smooth muscle tone has been shown to vary with the individual and appears to be more dependent on mucosal inflammation; allergy has a coexistent effect. Airway hyperreactivity appears to be beneficial at times, increasing bronchial smooth muscle tone to compensate for bronchiectatic airway wall instability.

In the first year of life, there is a high degree of structural airway instability. Patients present with obstructive type respiratory symptoms that are aggravated by the airway wall instability. In cystic fibrosis patients, lung disease presents in early infancy with bronchiolitis-like symptoms; in older patients, a suppurative airway pattern is seen. These stages are separated by a benign interval during the toddler stage, when the airway wall instability of early infancy is no longer present and bronchiectasis is not significant.

Gastrointestinal Involvement

Although the most damaging complications in cystic fibrosis are pulmonary, gastrointestinal involvement is often the first to be recognized. The pancreas is the most commonly affected gastrointestinal organ in patients with cystic fibrosis. Pancreatic lesions are the result of the obstruction of the ducts and ductules in the pancreas by secretions that form concretions. This occurs in the earliest stage of life for the cystic fibrosis patient.

Cardiac Involvement

Advanced pulmonary disease leads to hypoxemia, causing marked pulmonary vascular changes. Pulmonary vessels dilate and new vessels are formed around these bronchiectatic airways. As a result, bronchopulmonary shunting occurs which results in increasing hypoxemia. This causes pulmonary vasoconstriction, which results in increased smooth muscle development in the vascular bed. This muscularization progresses as the shunting continues, with the muscularization involving the normally nonmuscular smaller arteries. Ultimately this results in profound pulmonary hypertension leading to right ventricular hypertrophy.

Reproductive System Involvement

In male cystic fibrosis patients, puberty is delayed. The head of the epididymis is normal, but the body is absent. The vas deferens is usually absent, and the sperm are unable to pass from the testes.

Females have a delay in menarche of about 2 years. The reproductive tract is anatomically normal, and the infertility that occurs is a result of anovulatory cycles caused by chronic illness. The cervical mucus is thick, forming a barrier to sperm penetration.

Growth and Nutrition

The typical cystic fibrosis patient has a voracious appetite, but poor weight gain and height development. Nutrient and calorie absorption are below the average requirement. In the emergency setting, it is important to inquire about the last known weight of the patient, the appetite status of the patient, and the use of pancreatic enzymes, nighttime nasogastric tube feeding, and total parenteral hyperalimentation.

The growth pattern in the cystic fibrosis patient is substantially diminished. The infant appears scrawny, with little subcutaneous fat. As the patient grows, there is a catch-up period, followed again by a decrease in weight and height as the disease progresses.

INFECTIOUS AGENTS
Viruses

Viral infections in the normal infant can cause airway reactivity and poor pulmonary function later in childhood in the predisposed patient. Cystic fibrosis patients do not appear to have an increased susceptibility to viral infections. However, they do develop more serious symptoms than other children. Significant complications can result from illness caused by influenza type A and respiratory syncytial virus.

Bacteria

During the first 2 years of life, viral infections affect the respiratory epithelial cell matrixes. This viral-induced mucosal damage is an important prerequisite for bacterial infection. The organism recovered most consistently in the first bacterial bronchopulmonary infections is *Staphylococcus aureus*. *S. aureus* binds to the respiratory epithelial fibronectin (an epithelial cell surface glycoprotein). The resulting loss of surface fibronectin enhances the adherence of *Pseudomonas* organisms to the epithelial cells. Thus the pattern of colonization of the respiratory system is (1) *S. aureus* binds to and damages the cell surface; (2) the denuded cell surface is exposed, allowing *P. aeruginosa* to adhere; and (3) once the colonization of *P. aeruginosa* has occurred, the mucoid type of *P. aeruginosa* is elaborated. The mucoid *P. aeruginosa* is noninvasive but localizes the bacterial toxins and immune complexes on discrete regions. Pseudomonads release cilioinhibitory factors that destroy the respiratory cilia. *P.*

aeruginosa also releases a protease that stimulates the respiratory epithelial cells to release mucin.

The initial pseudomonal colonization of cystic fibrosis patients is with *P. aeruginosa*. This colonization occurs within the first decade of life. Once this has occurred, clearance of this bacteria from the pulmonary system is impossible, despite potent antibiotic regimens. Though this bacteria is initially the non–mucoid producer, it converts to the mucoid-producing strain. When taken from sputum and grown in vitro, the strain reverts to a non–mucoid-producing strain. Eventually there is colonization with *Pseudomonas cepacia*, which correlates with advanced disease.

Mycobacteria

Infection by mycobacteria is rare in cystic fibrosis patients. Because hypoxemia is prevalent in the cystic fibrosis patient, colonization and growth of *Mycobacterium tuberculosis* is suppressed. In one survey of 700 cystic fibrosis patients, only two cases of active tuberculosis were noted during an 18-year span.

Fungi

The two major fungal agents associated with infection in cystic fibrosis patients are *Candida* and *Aspergillus*. The candidal infection is more a colonization phenomenon than a true infectious process.

Aspergillus can cause either true invasion or a hypersensitivity pneumonitis. About 10% of cystic fibrosis patients have sputum containing *Aspergillus*. Invasive presentation in cystic fibrosis patients is rare, but occurs in the terminal phases. Allergic bronchopulmonary aspergillosis (ABPA) tends to occur more in patients with reactive airway disease who are older than 2 years. The criteria for diagnosis of ABPA include pulmonary infiltrates with prominent central bronchiectasis on radiograph, wheezing, a positive *Aspergillus* culture, a positive *Aspergillus* skin test, and the presence of *Aspergillus* precipitating antibodies and *Aspergillus*-specific immunoglobulin E (IgE), usually occurring with increasing total IgE. Fever, an increased erythrocyte sedimentation rate, and eosinophilia further support the diagnosis of ABPA.

DIAGNOSIS

Currently, 58% of cystic fibrosis patients are diagnosed in the first year of life (Table 30–1). The mean delay between the initial symptom and the final diagnosis is 15 to 25 months. Cystic fibrosis usually presents during infancy but may also present in older age groups. The classic case is a child who tastes salty to the parents; has a history of frequent pneumonia; has frequent large, greasy, loose stools; has a voracious appetite; coughs up green sputum; and has a barrel chest.

Pulmonary Presentation
Infancy

The normal infant will experience two to four upper respiratory infections during infancy. The normal infant will also have an episode of either bronchiolitis or pneumonia once during this time. However, frequent bouts of pneumonia are suggestive of cystic fibrosis. The appearance on chest radiograph of hyperinflation with upper right lobe disease strongly suggests cystic fibrosis, as the typical radiographic appearance in infants is a hyperinflated lung pattern with a right upper lobe pneumonia. Pneumonia with a serious course and a prolonged recovery, staphylococcal

TABLE 30–1

CYSTIC FIBROSIS DIAGNOSTIC SYSTEM

Major Criteria
Sweat chloride level greater than 60 mEq/L in patients younger than 20 years or greater than 80 mEq/L in adults
Chronic obstructive pulmonary disease with *Pseudomonas* airway infection
Unexplained obstructive azoospermia

Minor Criteria
Sweat chloride level greater than 40 mEq/L in patients younger than 20 years or greater than 60 mEq/L in adults
Family history of classic cystic fibrosis
Exocrine pancreatic insufficiency in patients younger than 20 years
Unexplained obstructive pulmonary disease in patients younger than 20 years
Unexplained azoospermia

The diagnosis is established by the presence of two major criteria or one major and one minor criterion. The two criteria must involve different organ systems.
From Stern RC, Boat TF, Doershuk CF. Obstructive azoospermia as a diagnostic criterion for the cystic fibrosis syndrome. Lancet 1982; 1:1401. © by The Lancet Ltd.

pneumonia, or *Pseudomonas* infection also suggests the presence of cystic fibrosis.

Childhood

The typical presentation in childhood is one of recurrent pneumonias, thoracic hyperinflation (barrel chest), and asthma that is difficult to control. The appearance of pansinusitis is a consistent finding in cystic fibrosis and appears later in childhood. Nasal polyps may suggest cystic fibrosis, as does the recovery of mucoid *P. aeruginosa*. Clubbing may be present in this age group.

Gastrointestinal Presentation

Infancy

The most common presenting sign of cystic fibrosis in infancy is a meconium ileus (Table 30–2), estimated to occur in 10% to 30% of patients. This is followed in frequency by rectal prolapse, which occurs in 20% of patients. The meconium ileus occurred in the neonatal period in the vast majority of older children who present with this sign. The area of involvement is usually at the ileocecal valve. A variation of this, called the *meconium plug syndrome*, occurs distal to the ileocecal valve. This tends to be a transient obstruction and can also occur in infants who do not have cystic fibrosis. About 15% of infants with cystic fibrosis develop the meconium plug syndrome.

Prolonged neonatal jaundice may be related to cystic fibrosis. The more typical presentation of cystic fibrosis in the early months of life is failure to thrive, maldigestion, and steatorrhea. At this stage, an infant may present with anorexia, lethargy, and vomiting associated with decreasing oral intake. Measurement of serum electrolyte levels demonstrates hyponatremia, hypokalemia (variable), and hypochloremia with subsequent metabolic alkalosis. Less commonly a child may develop a fat-soluble vitamin deficiency.

Childhood

The presence of malabsorption and maldigestion in children is highly suggestive of cystic fibrosis. The approximate incidence of cystic fibrosis is 85% in children presenting with

such symptoms. A protein or fat deficiency is also highly suggestive of cystic fibrosis. Rectal prolapse can occur as the initial presenting complaint, even after infancy. Intussusception is uncommon after infancy but is more frequent among cystic fibrosis patients. Portal hypertension and unexplained cirrhosis, though uncommon, are occasionally the first clinical manifestations of cystic fibrosis.

Initial Diagnosis

A laboratory test to confirm cystic fibrosis in the emergency setting is not currently available. A long sequence of tests must be performed on an outpatient or inpatient basis.

Prenatal Diagnosis

The mutation gene for cystic fibrosis has been located, which allows detection of the carrier state even in those families without prior gene expression. Prenatal detection will soon be available for families with identified carriers. Until these genetic probes are further refined, the current detection technique in the prenatal state uses the assay of a number of microvillar enzymes. These enzymes are depressed in patients with cystic fibrosis, possibly because of impaired pancreatic maturation.

Sweat Test

The sweat test is the primary test to confirm the diagnosis of cystic fibrosis. The sweat chloride levels in most patients will confirm the diagnosis, but there are limitations with this assay. The physiology of sweat production is aberrant in patients with cystic fibrosis. Sweat begins as an isotonic

TABLE 30–2

CLINICAL FEATURES OF CYSTIC FIBROSIS AT DIAGNOSIS

Age and Clinical Feature	Approximate Incidence (%)
0–2 years	
Meconium ileus	10–15
Obstructive jaundice	
Hypoproteinemia/anemia	
Bleeding diathesis	
Heat prostration/hyponatremia	
Failure to thrive	
Steatorrhea	85
Rectal prolapse	20
Bronchitis/bronchiolitis	
Staphylococcal pneumonia	
2–12 years	
Malabsorption	85
Recurrent pneumonia/bronchitis	60
Nasal polyps	6–36
Intussusception	1–5
13 years +	
Chronic pulmonary disease	70
Clubbing	
Abnormal glucose tolerance	20–30
Diabetes mellitus	7
Chronic intestinal obstruction	10–20
Recurrent pancreatitis	
Focal biliary cirrhosis	15–25
Portal hypertension	2–5
Gallstones	4–14
Aspermia	98

From MacLusky I, Levison H. Cystic fibrosis. *In* Chernick V (ed). Kendig's Disorders of the Respiratory Tract in Children. 5th ed. Philadelphia, WB Saunders, 1990, p 701.

TABLE 30-3
INDICATIONS FOR SWEAT TESTING

Pulmonary
  Chronic or productive cough
  Recurrent or chronic pneumonia or infiltrates
  Recurrent bronchiolitis
  Atelectasis
  Hemoptysis
  Infection with *Pseudomonas* (mucoid)
  Staphylococcal pneumonia
Gastrointestinal
  Meconium ileus, meconium plug syndrome
  Steatorrhea, malabsorption
  Rectal prolapse
  Childhood cirrhosis, portal hypertension, bleeding
    esophageal varices
  Hypoprothrombinemia beyond newborn period
Other
  Family history of cystic fibrosis
  Failure to thrive
  Salty taste when kissed
  Nasal polyps
  Heat prostration with unexplained hypochloremic alkalosis
  Pansinusitis
  Aspermia in mature males

Individuals with cystic fibrosis may initially present with any of these signs or symptoms.
From Behrman RE, Vaughan VC. Nelson Textbook of Pediatrics. 13th ed. Philadelphia, WB Saunders, 1987, p 929.

solution in the secretory coil of the sweat gland. As this isotonic solution moves through the duct, sodium is pumped into the tissue by a sodium pump. In patients with cystic fibrosis, the cells appear to be impermeable to the normal passive flow of the chloride in the sweat fluid, resulting in a high concentration of chloride in the sweat. The retention of the chloride causes a resulting reflux of sodium into the sweat fluid.

Sweat testing can be done at almost any age, but the earliest that adequate sweat production can be obtained is at 1 month of age (Table 30–3). Diagnostic sweat chloride values are > 50 mEq/L in children and 60 mEq/L in adults. However, an abnormal sweat chloride level can also result from other conditions, which must be considered before the diagnosis of cystic fibrosis is confirmed.

Assessment of Pancreatic Function

Pancreatic function can be assessed directly or indirectly. The direct method uses duodenal intubation and analysis of secretions. Indirect assessment is done by measuring fecal fat and by pancreatic substrate assay screening tests.

CLINICAL EVALUATION

The evaluation of the cystic fibrosis patient in the emergency department must address the presenting problem and review other affected organ systems. The physician must take a detailed respiratory history. The type of cough and its duration are important to ascertain. The normal color of the patient's sputum, any change in sputum color, and any change in sputum quality and quantity should be noted.

The evaluation should involve detailed questioning about recent antibiotic use and recent hospitalization. The usual colonization of the sputum should be determined; most parents and patients will know the result of the last sputum culture. The clinician should also ask about current medications for pulmonary and gastrointestinal disease processes,

including bronchodilators, steroids, and insulin. Any changes in the dosing of these drugs should be noted.

DIAGNOSTIC EVALUATION
Pulmonary Function

Initially cystic fibrosis affects the peripheral airways and results in airway obstruction, gas trapping, atelectasis, and ventilation-perfusion mismatching. As the disease progresses, the pulmonary disease becomes more restrictive, with gas trapping as the predominant feature.

Pulmonary function testing is usually performed in children who are at least 5 years of age. Air trapping, with increased residual volume and an increase in the residual volume–to–total lung capacity ratio, is present when there is small airways disease.

There is a decline in forced expiratory volume in 1 second (FEV_1) followed by a decreased forced vital capacity. In numerous studies, the average rate of decline of the maximal midexpiratory flow was 8% to 10% each year.

Arterial Blood Gases

As cystic fibrosis progresses, a ventilation-perfusion mismatch occurs. The resulting hypoxemia is one of the earliest signs of increasing pulmonary disease and occurs even prior to pulmonary function abnormalities. The child with cystic fibrosis will be able to maintain normal Po_2 levels by increasing minute ventilation to the less affected lung areas. Eventually, as the disease progresses, this compensatory mechanism is overwhelmed, leading to progressive hypoxemia. Hypercapnia usually signifies advanced disease and has an extremely poor prognosis.

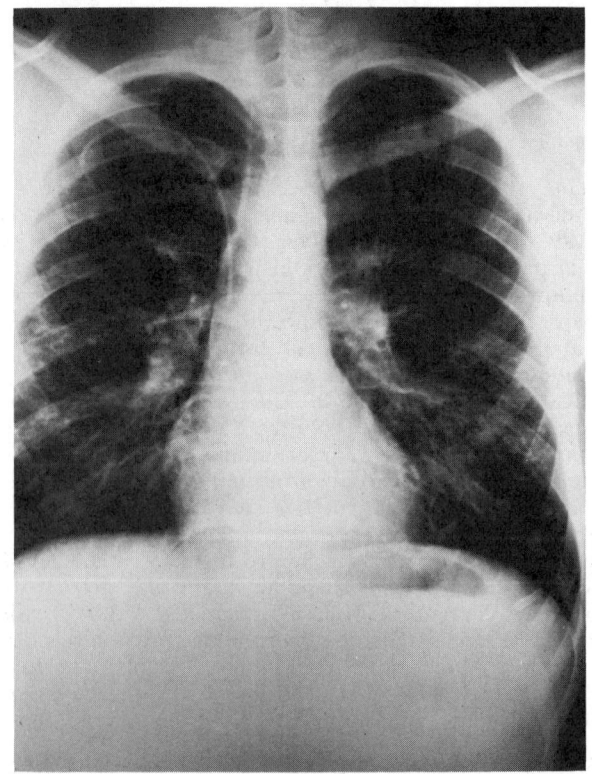

Figure 30–1. Poor clearance of thickened secretions with associated pulmonary infections leads to bronchiectasis and alteration of the lung parenchyma. Radiographically, diffuse coarse reticular changes are seen. (Courtesy of Bing Tai, M.D.)

TABLE 30–4

DRUGS USED IN THE TREATMENT OF CYSTIC FIBROSIS

Drugs	Route	Dose	Schedule
Antibiotics			
Penicillins			
Amoxicillin	po	50–100 mg/kg/day	q 6 hr
Cloxacillin	po/IV	50–200 mg/kg/day	q 6 hr
Ticarcillin	IV	200–300 mg/kg/day	q 4–6 hr
Piperacillin	IV	200 mg/kg/day (max 24 gm/day)	q 6 hr
Cephalosporins			
Cephalexin	po	50–100 mg/kg/day	q 6 hr
Ceftazidime	IV	200 mg/kg/day (max 12 gm/day)	q 6 hr
Aminoglycosides			
Gentamicin*	IV	10 mg/kg/day	q 8 hr
Tobramycin*	IV	10 mg/kg/day	q 8 hr
Others			
Cotrimoxazole			
Trimethoprim }	po	8 mg/kg/day	q 6–12 hr
Sulfamethoxazole }		40 mg/kg/day	

Trimethoprim }	IV	5–10 mg/kg/day
		25–50 mg/kg/day (max adult
		  dose 640 mg trimethoprim/
		  day)
			q 6–12 hr

Sulfamethoxazole }			
Chloramphenicol	po/IV	50–100 mg/kg/day	q 6 hr
Ciprofloxacin	po	1500 mg/day (adults)	q 12 hr
Bronchodilators			
Salbutamol (2-mg or 4-mg tabs)	po	0.1–0.15 mg/kg/dose	q 6 hr
Metered aerosol (100 μg/puff)	Inhalation	1–2 puffs	q 4–6 hr
0.5% solution	Inhalation	0.01–0.03 ml/kg/dose	q 4–6 hr
Terbutaline			
Metered aerosol (250 μg/puff)	Inhalation	1–2 puffs	q 4–6 hr
1% solution	Inhalation	0.03 ml/kg/dose (max 1 ml)	q 4–6 hr
Metaproterenol			
Metered aerosol (750 μg/puff)	Inhalation	1–2 puffs	q 4–6 hr
5% solution	Inhalation	0.01–0.02 ml/kg/dose (max 1 ml)	q 4–6 hr
Fenoterol			
Metered aerosol (200 μg/puff)	Inhalation	1–2 puffs	q 4–6 hr
0.1% solution	Inhalation	0.01–0.03 ml/kg/day (max 1 ml)	q 4–6 hr
Ipratropium bromide			
Metered aerosol (20 μg/puff)	Inhalation	2 puffs	q 6–8 hr
Theophylline* (anhydrous)	po or IV	18–24 mg/kg/day	
Short-acting po preps			q 6 hr
Long-acting po preps			q 8–12 hr
Mucolytics			
N-acetylcysteine (20% solution)		1–2 ml	q 8 hr
Cromolyn Sodium			
1% solution	Inhalation	2 ml	q 6 hr
Sclerosing Agents			
Quinacrine	Intrapleural	100 mg in 50 ml normal saline	1/day × 3 days

*Increased drug clearance in patients with cystic fibrosis requires close monitoring of drug levels.

From MacLusky I, Levison H. Cystic fibrosis. *In* Chernick V (ed). Kendig's Disorders of the Respiratory Tract in Children. 5th ed. Philadelphia, WB Saunders, 1990, p 709.

Chest Radiographs

The initial radiographs are usually normal, but as the disease progresses, hyperinflation and peribronchial thickening are seen. Increased air trapping and bronchiectasis occur in the upper lobes first (Fig. 30–1). Next, pulmonary infiltrates appear as nodular shadows with segmental or lobar atelectasis. With hyperexpansion, there is flattening of the diaphragm, thoracic kyphosis, and bowing of the sternum. In advanced disease, cystic lesions may form, usually in the apical areas. These apical cysts can lead to development of a spontaneous pneumothorax.

Sputum Bacteriology

Bacteria cultured from expectorated sputum reflect the colonizing flora in the lower respiratory system. Therefore a quantitative sputum culture should be obtained during any emergency visit. Sputum cultures will guide antibiotic therapy for the acute exacerbation of cystic fibrosis.

THERAPEUTIC INTERVENTION
Pulmonary Therapy

The emergency care of the patient with cystic fibrosis is often directed toward improving the compromised respiratory status. In the child with respiratory distress, beta-agonist aerosols may provide initial relief (Table 30–4). The regimen for aerosolized beta agonists is dependent on the state of the patient and the pulmonary response to the agent.

Many cystic fibrosis patients who require treatment will need antibiotics for control of pulmonary bacterial colonization and infection. The antibiotic choice should be made in concert with the physician who will be involved in the care of the child outside the emergency department.

Anti-inflammatory Agents

Elevated immune complexes and complement activation occur in those patients with chronic *Pseudomonas* infection. Patients who have persistently low immunoglobulin levels have better lung function, fewer hospitalizations for pulmonary exacerbations, less colonization by *P. aeruginosa*, improved weight for age, and a slower decline in pulmonary function than do age-matched patients with normal or increased immunoglobulin levels. This may be because of an altered antigen access at the mucosal level, resulting in no immune complex formation.

Decreased levels of immunoglobulin G (IgG) result from decreased pulmonary inflammation. Nonsteroidal anti-inflammatory drugs (NSAIDs) decrease this response and provide benefit. Steroids are used in patients with cystic fibrosis to treat reactive airway responses and allergic aspergillosis.

Postural Drainage

Postural drainage is used to remove mucus. Goblet cells and mucous glands produce voluminous amounts of thick, purulent secretions that lead to hyperinflation and increase the risk of infection. Infection causes more secretion, thus establishing a self-perpetuating cycle. Postural drainage, breathing exercises, and exercise therapy facilitate secretion removal and halt disease progression. Methods of postural drainage include gravity drainage, gravity drainage with percussion, or gravity drainage with percussion and vibration.

COMPLICATIONS
Pulmonary Complications
Upper Respiratory Tract

Nasal polyps are present in 7% to 36% of cystic fibrosis patients and occur more often in late childhood and early adolescence. The development of facial sinus opacification occurs in all cystic fibrosis patients. Organisms that colonize the sinuses are the same as those that colonize the lower respiratory tract (i.e., *Haemophilus influenzae*, *S. aureus*, *P. aeruginosa*, and anaerobes). Antibiotics have a minimal role in therapy because of poor penetration and the development of microbial resistance. The risk of development of otitis media and middle ear diseases is not increased in the cystic fibrosis patient.

Lower Respiratory Tract

The thick, tenacious mucus that is produced in the cystic fibrosis patient always produces some small amount of peripheral airway obstruction. Any viral or bacterial infection or ineffective clearing of secretions will lead to marked airway trapping. This will show on chest radiograph as hyperexpansion, and bronchospasm occurs clinically. Infants tolerate atelectasis poorly because of the minimal development of collateral airway transmission. Therapy involves broad-spectrum antibiotics and intensified chest physiotherapy with postural drainage.

Bronchiectasis

The pulmonary progression of cystic fibrosis may eventually lead to bronchiectasis, which usually presents with diffuse findings. A small percentage of patients may develop localized areas of involvement. The patient may present with symptoms of malaise and persistent fever. Occasionally, surgical resection of the affected lobe may be warranted.

Pneumothorax

As pulmonary disease progresses, there is increased air trapping and microabscesses form. This results in apical bullae that may rupture, causing a pneumothorax. The incidence of pneumothorax is between 1% and 23% in patients older than 13 years. The average recurrence rate is about 43%. The mortality rate for patients who develop a pneumothorax is high, about 30% to 60% over a 6-month to 3-year span. The pneumothorax may reflect a progression of the disease; treatment is only a temporary measure.

A small pneumothorax of less than 10% by volume may be managed conservatively and often is asymptomatic. The typical presentation of a significant pneumothorax involves sudden arm, chest, or neck pain with dyspnea. Hemoptysis may precede the pneumothorax because of a pleural tear allowing bleeding into a subpleural bleb, which communicates with the airways.

The acute onset of severe dyspnea and cyanosis suggests a tension pneumothorax. The incidence of tension pneumothorax in cystic fibrosis patients is rare, possibly because of stiff, noncompliant lungs that are incapable of collapse. A pneumothorax in the severely compromised cystic fibrosis patient can precipitously cause death.

The diagnosis of pneumothorax is established by radiograph. The physical examination may reveal hyperresonance to percussion and decreased breath sounds on the affected side. The patient may have tachypnea, retractions (out of proportion to the usual clinical state), and cyanosis. Mediastinal shift is not consistently found in cystic fibrosis patients.

Hemoptysis

The presence of blood-streaked sputum is not unusual in the cystic fibrosis patient with moderate pulmonary involvement. The triggering mechanism is often a paroxysmal cough caused by bronchial infections leading to increased secretions. Treatment requires aggressive antibiotic therapy to suppress the infection. This occurs more often with increasing age, and about 60% of cystic fibrosis patients will develop hemoptysis at some time.

Massive hemoptysis can be life-threatening. The precise definition of severe hemoptysis varies but is usually defined as expectoration of 300 ml or more of blood in 24 hours. Bleeding episodes may be voluminous, involving volumes of 300 to 2500 ml during one episode. The incidence of severe hemoptysis is about 5%, with a mean age of occurrence of 18 to 21 years. There is a 45% recurrence rate in patients who survive the first episode. The immediate mortality rate is 11%.

Treatment for hemoptysis is supportive. The patient must be stabilized with appropriate intravenous fluids and blood products. Chest physiotherapy should be stopped. If the prothrombin time is prolonged, vitamin K is administered. The use of aspirin or other NSAIDs should be stopped. Patients are evaluated by bronchoscopy, followed by bronchial angiography to locate the bleeding site. Selective bronchial artery embolization has been used for patients with massive hemoptysis. Surgical resection of an affected lobe is reserved for life-threatening cases.

Pulmonary Infection

There is no set method for determining antibiotic therapy in cystic fibrosis patients. The choice of agents will depend on several factors. It must be remembered that these patients are constantly colonized with certain flora in the respiratory system, and antibiotics are usually reserved for moderate to severe exacerbations.

The signs of a pulmonary exacerbation include weight loss, increased cough, increased sputum production, increased fatigue, decreased appetite, and a decreased exercise tolerance. These all suggest a bacterial origin. Oral antibiotics are given over a 2-week period. If there is no improvement, an intravenous, multiple-antibiotic regimen and chest physiotherapy are required for 10 days to 21 days. Indicators of improvement are improved pulmonary function, increased appetite, increased weight, decreased respiratory rate, and decreased sputum production.

Antibiotics can also be administered in aerosolized form. Numerous centers have used antibiotics in an aerosol delivery system with good results. Cystic fibrosis patients should also receive a flu vaccine before the start of the flu season. When patients are in an influenza type A epidemic environment, regardless of whether they have been vaccinated, they should receive amantadine (maximum 200 mg per day).

The principal cause of death in cystic fibrosis patients is the progressive pulmonary disease secondary to colonization with *P. aeruginosa* or *P. cepacia. Pseudomonas* species have the capability to develop antibiotic resistance.

Respiratory Failure

Progression of cystic fibrosis will result in increasing hypoxemia. The compensatory mechanism is to increase the minute ventilation. This will increase the Po_2 and maintain the Pco_2 at a normal level. Eventually, the patient will be unable to increase his or her minute ventilation. This results in an increased Pco_2. The only therapy that will overcome this is assisted ventilation, which will not be of long-term benefit to the patient.

Cardiac Complications
Cor Pulmonale

Cor pulmonale is hypertrophy of the right ventricle resulting from pulmonary disease. In cystic fibrosis, progressive pulmonary inflammation and resulting hypoxemia lead to pulmonary revascularization and subsequent pulmonary hypertension. This eventually leads to right ventricular hypertrophy.

When the pulmonary disease is severe enough to cause cor pulmonale, the signs and symptoms of pulmonary disease (cyanosis, tachypnea, and tachycardia) may make clinical assessment of the severity of the cardiac changes difficult. The auscultation of heart sounds for an increased pulmonary component and right ventricular impulse may be masked because of the increased chest diameter from hyperinflation. The hyperinflation causes a flattening of the diaphragm, which makes the assessment of hepatomegaly difficult. The diagnosis of cor pulmonale is assisted by echocardiography.

The treatment of cor pulmonale is difficult. Supplemental oxygen is used. By maintaining the oxygen tension above 60 mm Hg, the pulmonary vasoconstriction induced by hypoxia is partially relieved, thereby improving myocardial contractility. In children and adolescents, supplemental oxygen does not suppress the hypoxic drive as in adult chronic obstructive pulmonary disease (COPD) patients.

Hypervolemia and pulmonary edema can occur in cystic fibrosis patients, and therefore diuretics (furosemide, 1 mg/kg IV) are beneficial in right-sided heart failure. With long-term diuretic use, sodium and potassium depletion can occur, which will result in increased viscosity of the pulmonary secretions.

The prognosis for patients with overt heart failure is poor. The survival time for patients who develop the signs of cor pulmonale is usually 30 months after the initial symptoms.

Hypertrophic Osteoarthropathy

Hypertrophic osteoarthropathy has four characteristic features: clubbing of the digits; periostitis of the ends of the long bones with new bone formation; arthritis; and autonomic dysfunction such as flushing, blanching, and sweating. Hypertrophic osteoarthropathy may occur as a primary problem or as a complication of a suppurative pulmonary process. The age of presentation is usually in the late teens to early adulthood.

Clinical manifestations involve swelling of the knee, ankle, and wrist joints. The patient may describe an aching pain, tenderness, and swelling along the long-bone shafts. The commonly affected bones are the tibia, fibula, radius, ulna, femur, humerus, metacarpals, and metatarsals. The tarsals, carpals, vertebrae, ribs, and scapula are rarely involved. The pain may worsen with cold exposure, after activity, and with exacerbations of pulmonary infections. The pain is alleviated with rest and oxygen. The diagnosis is usually made by radiographs; findings are periosteal elevation and layering along the shafts of the long bones.

There has been a new arthritis characterized in children with cystic fibrosis who are 2 to 10 years of age. There are recurrent attacks of painful swelling of large joints, sometimes associated with an erythematous rash lasting up to 10 days and unrelated to pulmonary infection. Laboratory tests for rheumatologic disease are negative. The erythrocyte sedimentation rate is normal, and no radiologic abnormalities are present. The arthritis appears to be related to immune complex formation. The condition improves dramatically with salicylates and rest.

The treatment for hypertrophic osteoarthritis begins with treatment of the underlying pulmonary infection. The pain may be relieved with aspirin or NSAIDs. Steroids have not been shown to be of benefit.

Gastrointestinal Complications
Pancreas

Pancreatic insufficiency occurs in the first three decades of life. The pancreatic secretions in cystic fibrosis patients are low in volume and in enzyme and bicarbonate levels. This even occurs in patients without steatorrhea. Maldigestion of fats and protein occur when lipase levels are below 2% of normal, resulting in steatorrhea.

The usual presenting syndrome is protein-calorie malnutrition. The infant is usually sickly, with a protuberant abdomen, poor muscle development, and progressive failure to thrive, accompanied by an unsatisfied appetite. The parent describes the stool as frequent, foul, greasy, and bulky. Approximately 5% of cystic fibrosis patients present with hypoproteinemia, edema, and anemia as a result of severe malnutrition.

Cystic fibrosis patients can develop pancreatitis. The patient with residual pancreatic function may experience recurrent pancreatitis. The diagnosis is difficult to establish because of other causes of abdominal pain in the cystic fibrosis patient. The treatment requires parenteral fluids, nasogastric suction, and pain relief. Pancreatitis may be recurrent, but once the residual function is lost, these attacks will cease.

Another complication is diabetes mellitus. The incidence

of diabetes mellitus is about 7% to 12% in adult cystic fibrosis patients. This occurs from continuing pancreatic fibrosis and is expressed as a decreased glucose tolerance and elevated glycosylated hemoglobin; ketoacidosis is rare.

Hepatobiliary System

In 2% to 6% of cystic fibrosis patients, there is clinical evidence of hepatobiliary involvement. The liver involvement associated with obstructive jaundice in the neonatal period takes 2 to 6 months to resolve. Fatty infiltration occurs in 30% to 60% of older children. The incidence of focal biliary cirrhosis is 10%, with 2% of these patients developing multilobar cirrhosis with progressive portal hypertension (with hypersplenism and esophageal varices). Some patients may progress to liver failure.

Gallbladder

Abnormal gallbladder function as determined by ultrasound or cholangiography occurs in about 30% of patients. About 5% to 10% of patients have gallstones, with 4% having clinical symptoms. The symptoms include biliary colic, cholecystitis, and cholangitis.

Bile Duct

Percutaneous transhepatic cholangiography performed in patients with clinical and biochemical evidence of hepatic disease often shows stricture of the distal bile duct. Patients with symptoms of recurrent or persistent right upper quadrant or epigastric pain require surgical correction.

Intestine

Two major intestinal complications are meconium ileus and recurrent distal intestinal obstruction syndrome. Meconium ileus occurs within the first 48 hours of life, with an incidence of 15% in all cystic fibrosis patients. Treatment is dependent on the severity of the initial presentation and the patient's response to conservative management.

Recurrent distal intestinal obstruction occurs in 10% to 20% of patients. Intestinal obstruction appears related to the combination of abnormal intestinal contents resulting from pancreatic insufficiency, abnormal intestinal secretion with increased intestinal mucous adherence, and decreased intestinal motility resulting in fecal stasis. This tends to occur more in the patient with pancreatic insufficiency. The usual presentation is intermittent, crampy, lower abdominal pain. Fecal loading of the colon and terminal ileum is seen on abdominal radiographs, despite the history of regular defecation. This distal intestinal obstruction syndrome may become complicated by a volvulus and intussusception.

The treatment of an intestinal obstruction is primarily nonsurgical. The moderate use of acetylcysteine by enema may disimpact the fecal material, and the use of an oral stool softener (mineral oil or docusate sodium [Colace]) may prevent recurrence. Mineral oil and Colace should not be used together. Severe cases have been treated with enteral GoLytely, a nonabsorbable polyethylene glycol agent that causes little electrolyte or fluid shift transluminally.

Rectal Prolapse

Rectal prolapse occurs in 20% of cystic fibrosis patients. The most common age involved is between 6 months and 24 months. Rectal prolapse has a high tendency for recurrence. It is caused by poor muscle tone secondary to malnutrition, abnormal intestinal motility, bulky stools resulting from steatorrhea, and increased intra-abdominal pressure caused by coughing. Rectal prolapse will resolve with adequate pancreatic supplements. There is little need for surgical correction.

Gastroesophageal Reflux

There have been increasing reports of gastroesophageal reflux in cystic fibrosis patients. This appears to increase as pulmonary disease worsens, possibly because of increasing intra-abdominal pressure and decreasing muscle tone associated with coughing. Treatment is supportive and includes propping the head up during sleep, and using antacids and H_2-receptor blockers.

Suggested Readings

Andersen DH. Cystic fibrosis of the pancreas and its relation to celiac disease. A clinical and pathological study. Am J Dis Child 1938;56:344.

Corey M, Levinson H, Crozien D. 5–10 year course of pulmonary function in cystic fibrosis. Am Rev Respir Dis 1976;114:1085.

di Sant'Agnese PA, Darling RC, Perera GA, et al. Abnormal electrolyte composition of sweat in cystic fibrosis of the pancreas. Pediatrics 1953;12:549.

di Sant'Agnese PA, Hubbard VS. The gastrointestinal tract. In Taussig LM (ed). Cystic Fibrosis. New York, Thieme-Stratton, 1984, pp 212–229.

Lester L. Complication of cystic fibrosis pulmonary disease. Semin Respir Med 1985;4:285.

Marks MI. The pathogenesis and treatment of pulmonary infections in patients with cystic fibrosis. J Pediatr 1981;98:173.

Mischler E. Treatment of pulmonary disease in cystic fibrosis. Semin Respir Med 1985;6:271.

Moss A. The cardiovascular system in cystic fibrosis. Pediatrics 1982;70:728.

Orenstein DM. Diagnosis of cystic fibrosis. Semin Respir Med 1985;6:252.

Tablan OC, Chorba TL, Schidlow DV, et al. Pseudomonas cepacia colonization in patients with cystic fibrosis: Risk factors and clinical outcome. J Pediatr 1985;107:382.

Wood RE, Boat TF, Doershuk CF. State of the art—cystic fibrosis. Am Rev Respir Dis 1976;113:833.

CHAPTER 31

Aspirated Foreign Bodies

Stephen V. Cantrill

INTRODUCTION

Foreign body aspiration is a problem seen mainly in the pediatric age group, with approximately 90% of cases occurring in patients 15 years of age or younger.[1] Eighty percent of foreign body aspirations occur in children 3 years of age or younger.[2] Patients presenting with a foreign body aspiration may range from a child presenting with a chronic cough to a child who is cyanotic, apneic, and pulseless. There are approximately 2000 deaths per year as a result of foreign body aspiration, thus making it the leading cause of home-related deaths in children younger than 6 years.[3] The incidence of death resulting from foreign body aspiration in children is 0.8 per 100,000 in the age group of birth to 9 years, with 95% of cases occurring in children age 4 years or younger. Fortunately, the incidence has been decreasing over the years,[3] which may be because of increased awareness of potential foreign body hazards by caregivers, consumer groups, and toy manufacturers, as well as the passage of federal legislation such as the Consumer Products Safety Act of 1979 governing toys and other articles intended for children under the age of 3 years.

In children, the peak incidence of foreign body aspiration occurs between the ages of 1 and 2 years. Several considerations contribute to vulnerability in this age group: lack of dentition for adequate food grinding; unflagging curiosity; proximity to the ground, where small objects may be found; and a desire to experience the world through placing as much of it as possible into the mouth, with an inability to discriminate between potentially dangerous objects and food, which may be safely eaten.[4] Children in this age group also have a lack of coordination of swallowing mechanisms and often perform additional activities while eating and swallowing (playing, walking, running, laughing), leading to a lack of concentration on the material in the mouth.

In most studies of foreign body aspiration in children, males outnumber females by approximately 2:1. In the younger age groups, there has been a higher risk of death from foreign body aspiration for nonwhites than for whites: for infants younger than 12 months, nonwhites have twice the incidence of whites, whereas in the 1- to 4-year-old age group, the rate for nonwhites is 1.7 times that of whites.[5]

In younger children, edible objects are most commonly aspirated, with nonedible materials (most commonly metal or plastic objects) being more frequently aspirated by those older.[6, 7] In fatal aspirations, the most common foods involved are hot dogs, hard candy, nuts, and grapes, accounting for more than 40% of food-related deaths.[8] Apples, seeds, and raw carrots are also frequently seen in children presenting with foreign body aspiration. The vast majority of aspirated foreign bodies are composed of radiolucent materials, with numbers in the 90% range commonly reported.[9, 10]

Foreign body aspiration represents a challenging clinical problem; up to 24% of children initially seen by a physician for foreign body aspiration are incorrectly diagnosed and managed.[11] The evaluation of foreign body aspiration is made difficult by the fact that the aspiration itself is often not witnessed by an adult.[9, 12] This, combined with the intermittent nature and frequent delay in the development of symptomatology (hours to days) following an aspiration, results in patient evaluation by a physician within 24 hours of the aspiration event in only 20% to 46% of cases.[10, 13, 14] In fact, up to 17% of children with foreign body aspiration may not present until 30 days after the incident.[15] Even in cases where foreign body aspiration has been suspected, fatal outcomes have been reported after prolonged evaluation and observation.[16]

ANATOMY AND PHYSIOLOGY

In foreign body aspiration, any of the larger passages of the airway may be involved, but most aspirated foreign bodies, because of their small size, pass down the trachea, coming to rest in a main stem bronchus, where they are not an immediate life threat.[17] Approximately 80% to 90% of aspirated foreign bodies lodge in the bronchial tree, with 70% of these lodging in the right main stem bronchus.[18] This higher incidence of involvement on the right is partially because the right main stem branches off from the trachea at a more gentle angle on the right than on the left (in the older child and adult, at a 25-degree angle on the right, as opposed to a 45-degree angle on the left). However, in the infant, both sides branch off from the trachea at a 55-degree angle, so this cannot be the sole explanation. Other contributing factors have been sought, but a fully adequate explanation has not yet been found.

From 2% to 12% of nonlethal foreign body aspirations result in laryngeal obstruction. Although a rarer form of foreign body aspiration, laryngeal foreign body aspiration is far more life threatening because of the high incidence of respiratory compromise. Tracheal foreign body aspiration is also seen, but it is infrequent, comprising 3% of foreign body aspirations in one study.[11] Laryngeal and tracheal foreign bodies tend to produce an acute obstruction, whereas those in a bronchus tend to result in a subacute presentation.

Bronchial foreign bodies may cause obstruction through one of four different mechanisms:[20]

1. *Check valve*: Air is allowed to pass to lung areas distal to the obstruction but is not exhaled. This results in hyperinflation of areas distal to the obstruction.
2. *Stop valve*: No air can pass in either direction. This results in atelectasis in areas distal to the obstruction.
3. *Ball valve*: Air is allowed to be expelled from areas distal to the obstruction, but no air can pass into those areas. This also results in distal atelectasis.
4. *Bypass valve*: Airflow is allowed in both directions, but it is decreased, resulting in limited aeration.

Obviously, the younger the child, the smaller the components of the airway. This implies that for any given foreign body, a younger child is at increased risk for a more significant obstruction. Also, in the child the mucous membranes are more fragile and are softer and looser, resulting in increased risk of obstruction from postaspiration edema or inflammation.[21]

Unrelieved complete airway obstruction will result in death by asphyxiation. Initially there is an increase in blood pressure, pulse, and attempts at respiration. This is followed by a rising $PaCO_2$, and a falling PaO_2 and pH. Following 3 to 4 minutes of obstruction, the blood pressure, pulse, and respiratory efforts diminish. These cease after 8 to 10 minutes, with the cardiac rhythm passing from a sinus rhythm to a nodal bradycardia, then to an idioventricular rhythm, culminating in asystole or ventricular fibrillation. If the obstruction is removed within the first few minutes, there is usually complete recovery with no long-term effects.

The anatomy of the upper airway of the child has a direct impact on the acute management of complete upper airway obstruction. In the adult, a cricothyrotomy may be the technically easiest way to provide an airway when obstruction is present at the level of the larynx or above. This area in the young child (age 5 or less) represents the narrowest segment of the upper airway, essentially precluding the performance of this procedure. In these situations, a tracheostomy, which is technically a more difficult and time-consuming procedure, may be the preferred approach.

EMERGENCY MEDICAL SERVICE CONSIDERATIONS

First aid for the child with an aspirated foreign body requires no special tools and may be performed by bystanders, as well as by those with training in prehospital care. If the child is not in respiratory distress but is symptomatic (e.g., coughing) from a partial obstruction, he or she should be allowed to continue to cough in an attempt to clear the foreign body.[22, 23] The upper airway may be inspected by opening the airway with the tongue-jaw lift, and removing the foreign body digitally if visualized. Blind probing is discouraged, as it risks converting a partial obstruction to a complete obstruction.

If the obstruction continues or if the child is in obvious

respiratory distress, immediate attempts to expel the foreign body are necessary. Infants should be placed in a 60-degree head-down position (e.g., supported by the rescuer's thigh or forearm), and four back blows should be quickly delivered between the scapulae with the heel of the hand. If this technique does not result in expulsion of the foreign body, the child should be placed in a supine position, and four chest compressions delivered using a technique similar to that used in external cardiac massage for this age group. Following these efforts, the mouth should be inspected for the presence of the offending foreign body, which should be carefully removed if it is visible. If the child is apneic, attempts should be made at ventilation (mouth-to-mouth, mouth-to-mouth-and-nose, or bag-valve-mask). If ventilation is unsuccessful, the back blows and chest compressions should again be attempted.

In smaller children older than 1 year of age, six to ten manual abdominal thrusts delivered with the heel of the hand to the supine child in the midline area between the navel and the lower ribs should be the initial maneuver.[23] Some caution should be exercised in performing the abdominal thrusts, as traumatic liver damage has been reported with overly aggressive performance of this procedure. If the obstruction is not relieved, the airway should be opened as noted earlier, visually seeking the offending foreign body. No blind finger sweeps should be used, as this may further impact the obstructing foreign body.

In older children, the standard adult Heimlich maneuver may be attempted with the patient in the standing, sitting, or supine position. Again, if the Heimlich maneuver is unsuccessful, the airway should be opened and attempts made to remove the foreign body if it is visible.

In either age group, the initial efforts, if unsuccessful, should be repeated. If they remain unsuccessful, mouth-to-mouth or mouth-to-mouth-and-nose ventilation efforts by the rescuer should commence while attempts are made to activate the emergency medical services system.[22] If ventilation cannot be successfully accomplished, this series of intervention steps should be repeated.

CLINICAL EVALUATION

The clinical evaluation of the pediatric patient with an aspirated foreign body may be simple and straightforward when the history and physical examination are indicative of this problem and diagnostic studies are confirmatory. Unfortunately, the data often are not suggestive of foreign body aspiration. In as many as 25% of cases, no history of foreign body aspiration can be elicited, even in retrospect.[14] Some have reported this to be true in as many as 50% of cases.[12] The actual foreign body aspiration may also have taken place at an historically remote time. The patient may initially cough, gag, choke, wheeze and develop stridor and even cyanosis, and then become asymptomatic for a period ranging from minutes to months.[14] These patients may also be asymptomatic at the time of presentation (57% in one series).[9] Many also have a normal physical examination at the time of presentation. Thus it may often be a difficult task for the physician to arrive at the correct diagnosis of aspirated foreign body. Because of the wide diversity of presentations and the frequent lack of hard clinical data indicating the presence of a foreign body aspiration, the possibility of an aspirated foreign body must be considered in the differential diagnosis any time an emergency physician cares for a child with acute or chronic airway complaints. To do less may result in a significant number of missed foreign bodies, which historically have been misdiagnosed 24% of the time.[11]

History

Clinical evaluation of the patient with a potential foreign body aspiration begins with eliciting a history of the possible aspiration. This may be simple if the aspiration is of recent occurrence, the patient is old enough to participate in the history, or the aspiration was witnessed by those caring for the child. The history surrounding the aspiration may be more difficult if the event is historically remote, the child cannot give a history because of his or her young age, or the aspiration was not witnessed. The course of the aspiration should be established and the patient examined for the presence of any cyanosis, stridor, drooling, coughing, wheezing, vomiting, dysphonia, muffled voice, or respiratory distress. The nature of the possible aspirate should be pursued; vegetable matter mandates more aggressive attempts at removal because of severe inflammatory response it may provoke. For the subacute presentation, a complete respiratory history should be taken, including episodes of spasmodic coughing, fever, and dyspnea. Cough is the most common symptom, being present in 40% to 80% of children with foreign body aspiration.[2, 10, 14, 24]

Physical Examination

The physical examination of the patient with an aspirated foreign body may be markedly abnormal or completely normal. Observation of the patient may reveal the use of accessory muscles of respiration along with nasal flaring and intercostal retractions, all of which indicate a significant degree of obstruction. The presence of cyanosis is worrisome and mandates immediate intervention. The respiratory rate is commonly increased in patients with foreign body aspiration. These patients may also present with a fever, especially if the aspiration occurred more than 24 hours prior to presentation.[24]

Careful evaluation of the respiratory tree may be helpful in supporting the diagnosis of foreign body aspiration (Table 31–1). Marked dysphonia may be present and may indicate a laryngotracheal foreign body.[25] A muffled voice may be present with a bronchial foreign body as a result of diminution of tidal volume. Stridor should be sought. It may be seen in about 60% of patients with a laryngotracheal foreign body,[2] but is also present in 10% to 15% of those presenting with a bronchial foreign body.[14] Stridor only on inspiration may indicate partial obstruction above the larynx. Wheezing is commonly present, being seen in 75% of patients with a

TABLE 31–1
Signs and Symptoms of Foreign Body Aspiration

Signs/Symptoms	Location of Foreign Body		
	Larynx	Trachea	Bronchi
Hoarseness	✓		
Aphonia	✓		
Odynophagia	✓		
Drooling	✓		
Cough	✓	✓	✓
Hemoptysis	✓	✓	✓
Stridor	✓	✓	✓
Wheezing	✓	✓	✓
Dyspnea	✓	✓	✓
Unilateral decreased breath sounds			✓
Airway obstruction	✓	✓	✓
Sudden death	✓	✓	✓

From Kenna MA, Bluestone CD. Foreign bodies in the air and food passages. Pediatr Rev 1988;10:25. Reproduced by permission of Pediatrics. Copyright 1988.

bronchial foreign body and in up to 50% of those with a laryngotracheal foreign body.[24] It may be unilateral, especially in bronchial foreign bodies. Careful auscultation may reveal decreased breath sounds, either generalized or unilateral, the latter being indicative of a bronchial foreign body.

The most commonly seen manifestations of foreign body aspiration include cough, wheezing and decreased breath sounds. This triad may be seen in as many as 40% of patients, with each component being present in up to 75% of children with foreign body aspiration.[24] It is important, however, to note the inverse of this conclusion: this triad will *not* be present in up to 60% of patients with an aspirated foreign body.

Children who present with a chronic aspirated foreign body may be found to have productive cough, hemoptysis, fever, pneumonia, atelectasis, bronchiectasis, pulmonary abscess, pneumothorax, or pneumomediastinum, all of which

also represent complications of a missed diagnosis of foreign body aspiration. If any of these entities are encountered and their origin is unclear, the diagnosis of aspirated foreign body must be considered and further diagnostic efforts undertaken.

The majority of children who have aspirated a foreign body will not present in marked respiratory distress; however, if there is any question of respiratory compromise, supplemental oxygen therapy should be considered during the evaluation. These patients should also be closely monitored, as the foreign body may become dislodged at any time, resulting in complete airway obstruction.[16]

DIAGNOSTIC EVALUATION

If there is any suspicion of foreign body aspiration based on the history or physical examination, chest radiographs should be obtained. These should include anteroposterior views in both inspiration and expiration and a lateral view. If the patient cannot cooperate to allow an expiratory view, a forced-expiratory view may be obtained by using gentle force with a lead-gloved hand over the upper abdomen of the child while the radiograph is taken (Fig. 31–1).[17] These films may demonstrate the presence of a radiopaque foreign body, but this will be the exception, as several studies have demonstrated only a 10% incidence of foreign bodies seen on the plain radiographs.[9, 10] Aluminum and plastic foreign bodies may sometimes be seen in overpenetrated views.[14] The two anteroposterior views should be carefully compared for indirect evidence of aspirated foreign body. Obstructive emphysema (air trapping) with a mediastinal shift away from the obstructed side is evidence of a probable foreign body at the bronchial level. Atelectasis caused by air resorption distal to a complete bronchial occlusion, with subsequent mediastinal shift toward the side of involvement, may also indicate the presence of a foreign body. If a good expiratory view cannot be obtained, left-side and right-side-down lateral decubitus films may be obtained instead of the single expiratory view.[12] On these views, if the down-side decubitus lung remains inflated, it is indicative of air trapping on that side, and a foreign body may be present.

Chest radiography, though helpful, has its definite limitations. In one series, 24% of children with foreign body aspiration had normal inspiratory and expiratory chest studies.[9] Another series also demonstrated 24% false-negative inspiratory, expiratory, and lateral studies.[26] This study also showed that 24% of children with suspected foreign body aspiration who had no evidence of a foreign body on rigid bronchoscopy showed evidence of air trapping on their chest radiographs. This study concludes that inspiratory, expiratory, and lateral chest radiographs have a sensitivity of 68%, a specificity of 67%, and an accuracy (compared with bronchoscopy) of 67% in the diagnosis of foreign body aspiration.

In certain situations, other forms of chest radiography may prove of benefit. Chest fluoroscopy may be helpful, especially if other plain films prove difficult to obtain. Fluoroscopy may show transient unilateral overinflation or mediastinal shift.[17] This procedure, however, rarely contributes any additional information if the standard chest radiographs are available. Xeroradiography has been used to identify airway architecture and the shape of the foreign body but involves increased amounts of radiation.[17] It has little to add in the initial diagnostic evaluation. When an area of lung consolidation is encountered, ultrasound or overpenetrated radiographs may demonstrate bronchiectasis within the area in question, which is consistent with foreign body aspiration.[27]

Lateral soft tissue radiographs of the neck may reveal the foreign body in the airway or in the cervical esophagus in

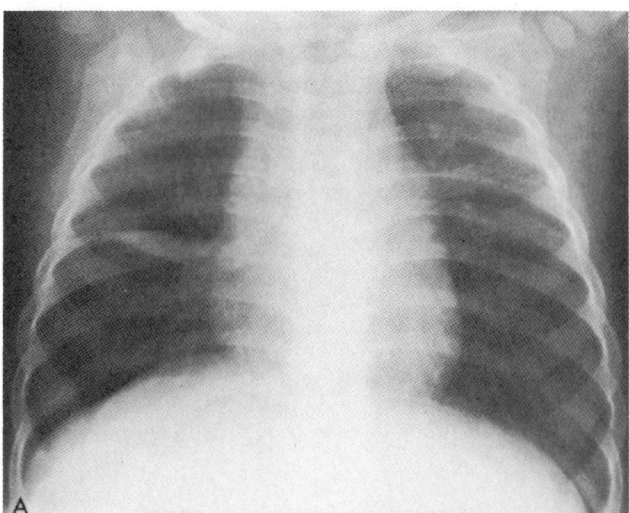

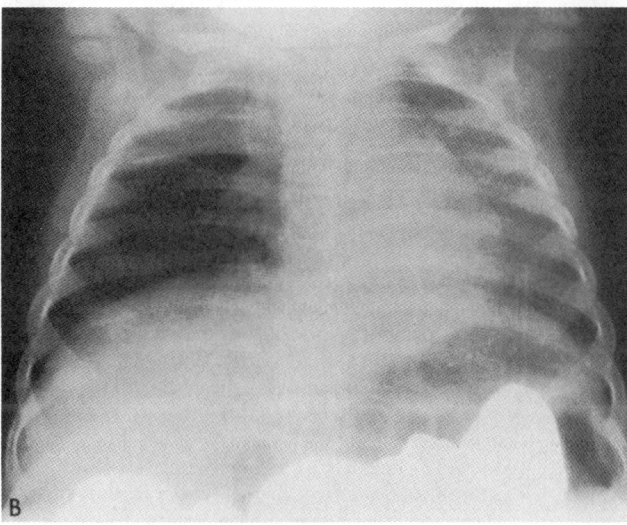

Figure 31–1. This 18-month-old boy presented with wheezing. *A,* Admission chest radiograph, revealing a patch of plate-like atelectasis on the right. *B, Assisted* expiratory radiograph taken 6 days later shows mediastinal shift to the left and virtually complete collapse of the lung except for the right middle and lower lobes. The metallic density across the abdomen is a leaded, gloved fist assisting expiration. A piece of bean was removed from the bronchus intermedius. (From Edwards DK. The child who wheezes. *In* Hilton S von W, Edwards DK, Hilton JW (eds). Practical Pediatric Radiology. Philadelphia, WB Saunders, 1984, p 59.)

the neck.[19, 25] Subglottic obstruction may be evidenced by ballooning of the hypopharynx.[14] Air in, or widening of, the retropharyngeal soft tissues may indicate perforation.

The ventilation-perfusion lung scan may be helpful in evaluating potential chronic foreign body aspiration.[17] This study may demonstrate matching ventilation and perfusion defects in the area of the lung obstructed by the foreign body. In cases of recurrent pneumonia where a chronic foreign body is suspected, a bronchogram may reveal its presence.

All children with a suspected aspirated foreign body should be accompanied whenever they are sent out of the emergency department for any reason. If the patient shows any evidence of airway compromise, portable radiographic studies in the emergency department should be considered, or at minimum, the patient should be accompanied and supervised by an individual experienced in dealing with pediatric airway problems who has the necessary resuscitation equipment close at hand.[19]

Pulse oximetry may assist in determining the adequacy of the child's ventilation. Arterial blood gas measurements may also demonstrate hypoxia from inadequate ventilation. Hypercapnia may indicate a significant ventilatory obstruction and may also indicate tiring of the patient, an ominous sign mandating rapid intervention. Abnormalities in the white blood cell count (elevated in 58% of patients) and the erythrocyte sedimentation rate (elevated in 63% of patients) have been reported,[11] but are so nonspecific that they are of little help.

Although many modalities are available to assist in making the diagnosis of foreign body aspiration, the physician is most likely to make the correct diagnosis by having a high index of suspicion for aspirated foreign body, taking a complete history, performing a careful physical examination, and utilizing inspiratory and expiratory chest radiographs. Additional studies should be ordered only when needed. If the presence of an aspirated foreign body cannot be absolutely excluded on the basis of the history, physical examination, and radiographic studies, and when any one of these three areas is strongly indicative or any two are suggestive of foreign body aspiration, diagnostic and therapeutic rigid bronchoscopy should be strongly considered.[16]

DIFFERENTIAL DIAGNOSIS

An esophageal foreign body may cause a presentation similar to that of an aspirated foreign body because of posterior tracheal compression by the foreign body in the esophagus. These patients may present with a major complaint of dysphagia and difficulty handling secretions, although these symptoms may also be seen with laryngeal foreign bodies. Plain radiographs of the neck, a barium swallow, or esophagoscopy will be most helpful in diagnosing this entity.[28]

Asthma may be difficult to differentiate from foreign body aspiration. If the history of reactive airway disease is in question, inspiratory and expiratory chest radiographs may be indicated. Early bronchoscopy may be required to exclude the possibility of aspirated foreign body in the child with asthma who does not respond appropriately to treatment or who deteriorates despite aggressive therapy.[2, 25]

Many infectious diseases may be confused with foreign body aspiration. Epiglottitis may present with similar respiratory distress, but the rapid course, drooling, high fever, and toxic appearance may help with differentiation. If there is doubt, direct visualization of the epiglottis should be performed under carefully controlled conditions. Croup may also be confused with foreign body aspiration to the degree that children initially diagnosed as croup are later

discovered to actually have aspirated a foreign body, especially if the aspiration was not witnessed. As with asthma, early bronchoscopy should be considered for those children diagnosed as having croup who do not improve or who deteriorate in spite of appropriate therapy.

Both peritonsillar and retropharyngeal abscesses may also present with a degree of airway obstruction, but careful examination of the oropharynx will confirm the diagnosis. Diphtheria may present with inspiratory stridor, causing the physician to consider foreign body aspiration; however, the presence of the gray, membrane-like exudative tonsillitis and posterior pharyngeal membrane make clear its diagnosis. Although rare, infectious mononucleosis has been reported as presenting as upper airway obstruction because of tonsillar swelling.[29] The history and physical examination will assist in differentiating it from foreign body aspiration. Bronchitis, laryngotracheitis, and pneumonia may also present with airway symptomatology. Foreign body aspiration should be considered when contemplating any of these entities as a possible explanation for any airway compromise.

Allergic reactions, with swelling of the pharynx, glottis, and larynx, may be difficult to differentiate from foreign body aspiration. Other manifestations such as rash and swelling of the face and lips may help differentiate these two entities, but direct visualization of the airway may be necessary to exclude the presence of a foreign body.

Tracheal stenosis caused by past endotracheal intubation may present with airway compromise years after the insult to the airway. The history of previous intubation may be of some help in excluding foreign body aspiration, but direct visualization may be required.

Hemangiomata may present with relative airway obstruction. This entity may be suspected based on patient or family history and the presence of other mucocutaneous lesions.

Functional airway obstruction has been reported but is a rare entity.[30] This diagnosis should be made only by careful exclusion of all other disease processes that may produce airway distress.

THERAPEUTIC INTERVENTION

Children with aspirated foreign bodies may present with a spectrum of symptoms ranging from no symptoms at all to full cardiopulmonary arrest. For those in the latter category, initial treatment should be as outlined in the section, "Emergency Medical Services Considerations," followed by standard pediatric resuscitative efforts. If the patient has respiratory compromise, but is still breathing spontaneously, 100% oxygen should be administered and immediate efforts initiated to mobilize an anesthesia and rigid bronchoscopy team. Concurrently, appropriate resuscitative equipment should be made immediately available.

For the stable patient who has been diagnosed or is suspected of having aspirated a foreign body, arrangements should be initiated for diagnostic and therapeutic rigid bronchoscopy. This procedure remains the gold standard of therapy, with extraction rates of nearly 100% having been reported.[31] When bronchoscopy is performed it should be a complete examination, as two or more aspirated foreign bodies are present in 5% of foreign body aspirations.[11, 32]

Conservative management consisting of bronchodilator treatment and postural drainage has been used for the treatment of peripheral, nonorganic foreign body aspirations that are less than 24 hours old.[33] This remains somewhat controversial and is considered by some as being no longer an appropriate mode of therapy.[14, 34]

Complications following bronchoscopic removal are rare. Postinstrumentation edema may be present and may be treated with intravenous steroids and inhaled racemic epinephrine,[12] although there are no studies demonstrating the efficacy of this treatment regimen in this setting. After foreign body removal there may also be granulation tissue formation, bleeding, and postobstruction infection. These entities usually resolve with little difficulty. There are usually no permanent negative effects of foreign body aspiration unless bronchiectasis had developed and progressed to the saccular stage prior to foreign body removal.[17]

DOCUMENTATION

Documentation for the patient with a demonstrated foreign body in the airway is straightforward and consists of the appropriate history, physical examination, radiographic results, laboratory results, and transfer of care to the accepting admitting physician. Vital signs should be recorded periodically during the child's stay in the emergency department, with a final set determined and recorded immediately prior to transport to the inpatient unit or operating room.

The patient who is to be discharged from the emergency department and in whom the possibility of an aspirated foreign body was entertained represents a more difficult problem. Basically, the chart should clearly reflect why the emergency physician does not feel that there is a foreign body present at the time of discharge. The history should be complete and should include significant negative indicators. The documented physical examination should include a detailed description of the examination of the entire airway. All radiographic interpretations, as well as any other ancillary data, should be represented on the chart. Vital signs should have been taken and recorded periodically during the patient's stay. Any abnormal values should be directly addressed by the physician and should cause reconsideration of the appropriateness of the decision to discharge, especially if the abnormal value is the respiratory rate. There should be a clear discussion in the assessment section of why it is safe for the patient to go home. Discharge instructions for the caregiver should be clearly noted, including instructions for follow-up and criteria for returning to the emergency department. Finally, the physician should review the record and consider the possibility that the assessment may be incorrect. Will the record support the assessment that has been made concerning the child's illness? If it will not, the disposition should be carefully reevaluated.

DISPOSITION

The child who has experienced a short episode of choking or obstruction but who at the time of evaluation is free of any respiratory symptoms or physical findings related to the incident, and in whom the examining physician has no suspicion of any retained foreign body in the airway, may be discharged and followed closely as an outpatient. The supervising caregiver should be given careful instructions about follow-up—when to return and under what conditions to activate the emergency medical services system. It may be appropriate at this time to also instruct the caregiver on the techniques of the back blow and manual chest thrust for infants and the abdominal thrust for older children.[35]

Children who have sustained significant airway obstruction with evidence of hypoxia or other complications should be admitted for observation. Children in whom there is either a demonstrated foreign body in the airway or any suspicion that a foreign body may exist in the airway should be admitted for definitive therapy and management.

PREVENTION

Many cases of foreign body aspiration are preventable. Parents should be instructed as to those foods that are inappropriate for young children and should withhold peanuts, raw carrots, chunks of apples, and similar foods until after the child's molars have erupted. Cutting these foods into smaller pieces is not adequate. Parents must understand that enabling their young child to have access to these inappropriate foods may represent a form of child neglect and in some cases intentional child abuse.[36]

References

1. Adeyemo AO, Bankole MA. Foreign bodies in the tracheobronchial tree: Management and complications. J Natl Med Assoc 1986;78:511.
2. Esclamado RM, Richardson MA. Laryngotracheal foreign bodies in children: A comparison with bronchial foreign bodies. Am J Dis Child 1987;141:259.
3. National Safety Council. Accident facts. Chicago, 1984, p 81.
4. Reilly JS. Prevention of aspiration in infants and young children: Federal regulations. Ann Otol Rhinol Laryngol 1990;99:273.
5. US Department of Health, Education, and Welfare. Vital and health statistics. HRA publication no 74–1853. Washington, DC, Government Printing Office, 1974; March.
6. Schloss MD, Pham-Dang H, Rosales JK. Foreign bodies in the tracheobronchial tree: A retrospective study of 217 cases. J Otolaryngol 1983;12:212.
7. Svensson G. Foreign bodies in the tracheobronchial tree: Special references to experience in 97 children. Int J Pediatr Otorhinolaryngol 1985;8:243.
8. Harris CS, Baker SP, Smith GA, et al. Childhood asphyxiation by food: A national analysis and overview. JAMA 1984;251:2231.
9. Losek JD. Diagnostic difficulties of foreign body aspiration in children. Am J Emerg Med 1990;8:348.
10. Blazer S, Naveh Y, Friedman A. Foreign body in the airway: A review of 200 cases. Am J Dis Child 1980;134:68.
11. Steen KH, Zimmermann T. Tracheobronchial aspiration of foreign bodies in children: A study of 94 cases. Laryngoscope 1990;100:525.
12. Friedman EM. Caustic ingestions and foreign bodies in the aerodigestive tract of children. Pediatr Clin North Am 1989;36:1403.
13. Pyman C. Inhaled foreign bodies in childhood. Med J Aust 1971;1:62.
14. Kim IG, Brummitt WM, Humphry A, et al. Foreign body in the airway: A review of 202 cases. Laryngoscope 1973;83:347.
15. Kenna MA, Bluestone CD. Foreign bodies in the air and food passages. Pediatr Rev 1988;10:25.
16. Humphries CT, Wagener JS, Morgan WJ. Fatal prolonged foreign body aspiration following an asymptomatic interval. Am J Emerg Med 1988;6:611.
17. Cotton E, Yasuda K. Foreign body aspiration. Pediatr Clin North Am 1984;31:937.
18. Lima JA. Laryngeal foreign bodies in children: A persistent, life-threatening problem. Laryngoscope 1989;99:415.
19. Kent SE, Watson MG. Laryngeal foreign bodies. J Laryngol Otol 1990;104:131.
20. Chatterji S, Chatterji P. The management of foreign bodies in air passages. Anesthesia 1972;27:390.
21. Barkin RM. Pediatric airway management. Emerg Med Clin North Am 1988;6:687.
22. Wolf AD. Current first aid recommendations for the choking child. Pediatr Rev 1990;12:54.
23. American Academy of Pediatrics, Committee on Accident and Poison Prevention. First aid for the choking child, 1988. Pediatrics 1988;81:740.
24. Wiseman NE. The diagnosis of foreign body aspiration in childhood. J Pediatr Surg 1984;19:531.
25. Gay BB Jr, Atkinson GO, Vanderzalm T, et al. Subglottic foreign bodies in pediatric patients. Am J Dis Child 1986;140:165.
26. Svedstrom E, Puhakka H, Kero P. How accurate is chest radiography in the diagnosis of tracheobronchial foreign bodies in children? Pediatr Radiol 1989;19:520.
27. Seibert RW, Seibert JJ, Williamson SL. The opaque chest: When to suspect a bronchial foreign body. Pediatr Radiol 1986;16:193.
28. Handler SD, Beaugard ME, Canalis RF, et al. Unsuspected esophageal foreign bodies in adults with upper airway obstruction. Chest 1981;80:234.
29. Dailey RH. Acute upper airway obstruction. Emerg Med Clin North Am 1983;1:261.
30. Cormier YF, Camus P, Desmueles MJ. Nonorganic acute upper airway obstruction. Am Rev Respir Dis 1980;121:147.
31. Kosloske AM. Bronchoscopic extraction of aspirated foreign bodies in children. Am J Dis Child 1982;126:924.
32. McGuirt WF, Holmes KD, Feehs R, et al. Tracheobronchial foreign bodies. Laryngoscope 1988;98:615.
33. Campbell DN, Cotton EK, Lilly JR. A dual approach to tracheal foreign bodies in children. Surgery 1982;91:178.
34. Kosloske AM. Tracheobronchial foreign bodies in children: Back to the bronchoscope and a balloon. Pediatrics 1980;66:321.

35. Barkin RM, Rosen P. Emergency Pediatrics—A Guide to Ambulatory Care. 3rd ed. St Louis, CV Mosby, 1990, p 646.
36. Friedman EM. Caustic ingestions and foreign body aspirations: An overlooked form of child abuse. Ann Otol Rhinol Laryngol 1987;96:709.

CHAPTER 32

Anaphylaxis and Allergy-Mediated Disease

David N. Zull

INTRODUCTION

Anaphylaxis is an acute multisystem allergic reaction that follows an exposure to a foreign substance. Manifestations of anaphylaxis may occur singly or in various combinations and include urticaria, angioedema, hypotension, laryngeal edema, bronchospasm, and gastroenteritis. If immediate treatment is not initiated, such reactions may be fatal, particularly if laryngeal edema or shock are present. Even such nuisance symptoms as lip swelling or urticaria may be harbingers of a severe reaction in progress and should be treated aggressively.[1–7]

The overall incidence of anaphylaxis is unknown, although it is estimated that 20% of the population will have urticaria sometime in life. More specifically, following exposure to penicillin, Hymenoptera stings, or iodinated contrast media, up to 1% of the population experience a systemic reaction, and approximately 0.002% die from anaphylaxis.[8–10]

The incidence of anaphylaxis increases with age because of repeated exposures and subsequent sensitization to various antigens over a lifetime. This incidence tends to peak in young to middle-aged adults, although fatalities are more likely in older adults. In the pediatric population, adolescents are the principal group at risk for anaphylaxis; while reactions are uncommon in young children and rare in infants, anaphylactic fatalities are reported annually in these groups.[11, 12] Hymenoptera sting reactions provide an example of the effects of age. By virtue of exposure, patients younger than 19 years comprise 90% of sting victims, yet more than 90% of fatalities occur in patients older than 19 years.[9]

ANATOMY AND PHYSIOLOGY

The massive release of chemical mediators (i.e., histamine, leukotrienes, platelet activating factor) from mast cells and basophils throughout the body results in the clinical manifestations of anaphylaxis. If antigen–immunoglobulin E (IgE) interaction on the mast cell surface results in this reaction, the reaction is called *anaphylactic*; if IgE does not play a role in mediator release, the reaction is referred to as *anaphylactoid* (Fig. 32–1).

For an IgE-mediated reaction to occur, there must be prior exposure to an antigen, at which time B lymphocytes are stimulated to transform into plasma cells and produce IgE and other immunoglobulins. Genetic predisposition and frequency of exposure play a role in the amount and specificity of IgE produced. In order to stimulate the immune system, either the antigen must be a complete protein (e.g., bee venom, foods), or hapten formation, in which an immunologically inactive molecule binds to a host protein, thereby becoming immunogenic, must occur (e.g., penicillin and other antibiotics). Sensitization occurs when IgE binds by its Fc fragment to the surface of tissue mast cells and circulating basophils. On reexposure to the antigen, cellular mediators will be released if the antigen cross-links two adjacent IgE molecules by their Fab arms. This cell membrane interaction results in release of preformed cytoplasmic granules containing histamine, kallikreins, and chemotactic factors and stimulates the production and release of leukotrienes, prostaglandins, and platelet activating factor.[1–6, 13, 14]

Anaphylactoid reactions are clinically identical to anaphylaxis, but the sudden release of chemical mediators is not dependent on an antigen-IgE interaction. Opiates, iodinated contrast media, and muscle relaxants can have a direct effect on mast cells and basophils, resulting in degranulation. Complement activation by immune complex formation or by direct stimulation results in release of C3a and C5a, which also causes mast cell degranulation (i.e., plasma, immunoglobulins, and other blood products). Reactions to aspirin and nonsteroidal anti-inflammatory drugs are also classified as anaphylactoid and probably result from inhibition of prostaglandin synthesis and promotion of leukotriene production. Lastly, physical factors such as exercise and cold exposure may result in mast cell degranulation by a direct effect that is not immunologic.[13, 15]

The chemical mediators released from mast cells and basophils cause vasodilation and increased capillary permeability, resulting in tissue swelling and edema (Fig. 32–2). If tissues in the oropharynx are affected, laryngeal edema, tongue swelling, and uvular swelling may occur (Fig. 32–3). Mediator release in the skin will result in urticaria if the upper dermis is affected or in angioedema if the lower dermis is involved. Edema of the intestinal mucosa may also occur, leading to cramping, vomiting, and diarrhea (Fig. 32–4). The hypotension of anaphylaxis results from vasodilation and fluid third spacing. Bronchospasm is mediated by the bronchoconstrictor effects of leukotrienes, although mucosal edema may also play a role.[14]

Antihistamines competitively inhibit histamine at its vascular and smooth muscle receptors but have no effect on mediator release. The mechanism of action of steroids in anaphylaxis appears to be multifactorial and includes reduction of capillary permeability, anti-inflammatory effects, enhancement of tissue responsiveness to catecholamines, reduction in leukotriene production, and inhibition of mediator release.[16]

EMERGENCY MEDICAL SERVICE CONSIDERATIONS

The base station physician should inquire about possible precipitants such as medications (including over-the-counter preparations), foods, or bee stings. The patient may complain of dyspnea, hoarseness, a sensation of a foreign body in the throat, or dysphagia, suggesting laryngeal edema. A complaint of dizziness or confusion may be related to hypotension.

Using telemetry, the physician should try to ascertain whether the patient's reaction is allergy mediated and if it is life threatening. The rescue team should look for flushing, urticaria, and swelling of the lips, tongue, and uvula. The patient may be hypotensive, wheezing, stridorous, retracting, or drooling. If there is any suggestion of airway involvement or hypotension, the patient should receive epinephrine

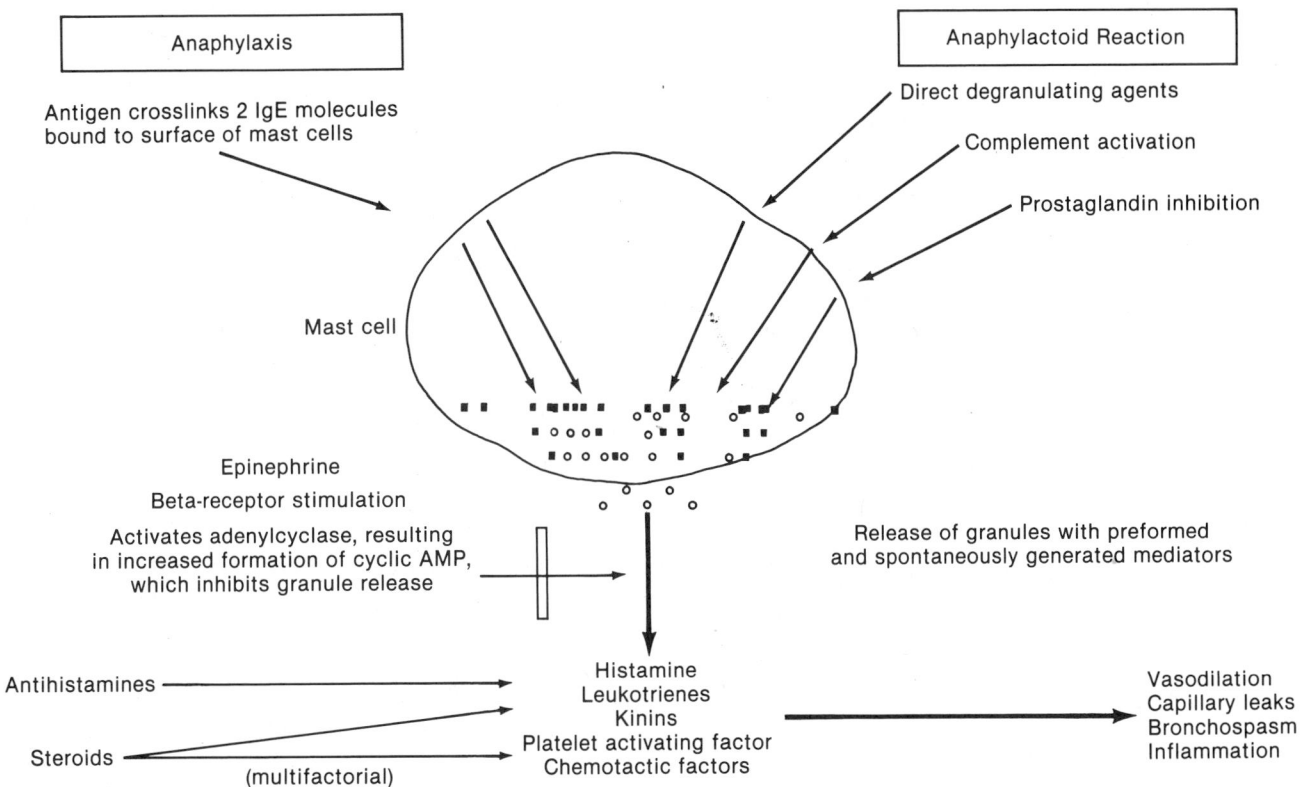

Figure 32–1. The pathophysiology of allergic reactions. Anaphylactic reactions are IgE mediated; anaphylactoid are not.

(1:1000 dilution, 0.01 ml/kg up to 0.4 ml), subcutaneously or intramuscularly (IM).

Concomitant to the expedient administration of epinephrine, the rescuer should start an intravenous (IV) line of 0.9 normal saline (NS) or lactated Ringer's (LR) solution and give a 20-ml/kg bolus of fluid if the patient is hypotensive. If shock is refractory to a repeated fluid bolus or if airway obstruction progresses, the epinephrine dose should be

repeated. The rescuer should intubate if airway obstruction is imminent; otherwise the child is kept upright, like a patient with epiglottitis (if the blood pressure allows), and promptly transported. Administration of diphenhydramine (1 mg/kg IM or IV) may be a useful adjunct if sedation is not

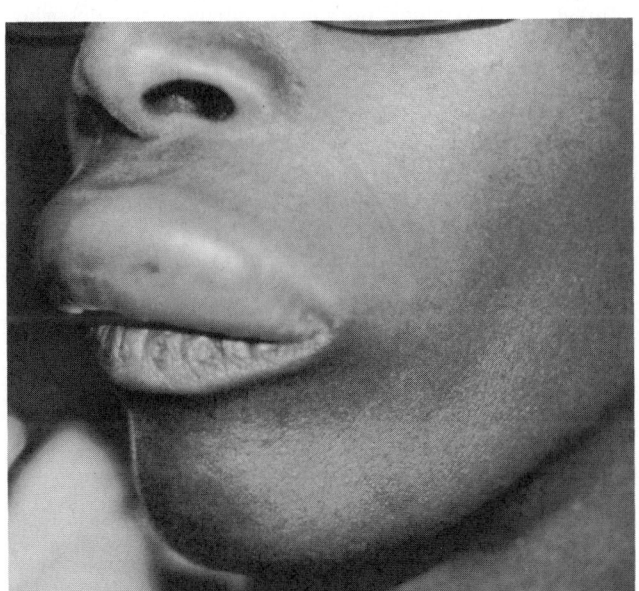

Figure 32–2. Marked angioedema of the upper lip developing suddenly after oral penicillin. Concomitant uvular edema occurred without laryngeal involvement.

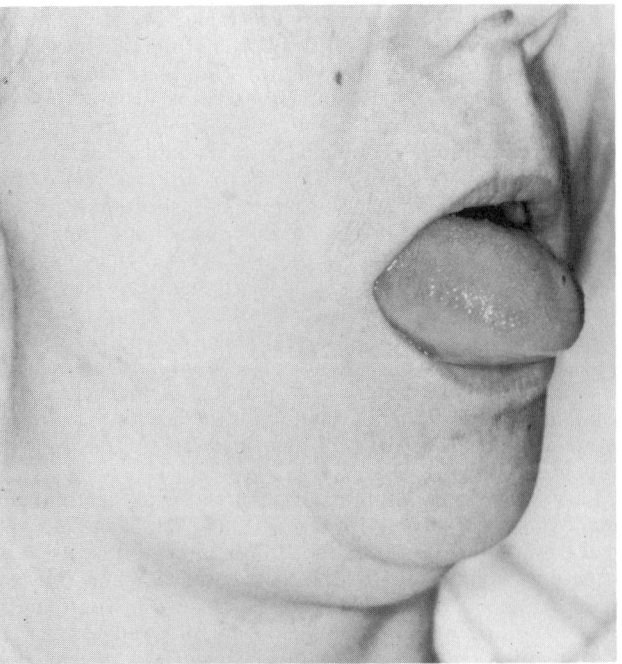

Figure 32–3. Acute angioedema of the tongue after ingestion of peanuts. Concomitant uvular and laryngeal edema also developed.

Reaction	Symptom	Sign
Laryngeal edema	Throat tightness Hoarseness, dysphagia Foreign body sensation	Inspiratory stridor Retractions, cyanosis Drooling Sudden death Edema of uvula, tongue, lips
Vascular collapse	Syncope, coma, dizziness Sudden death	Tachycardia, hypotension
Bronchospasm	Dyspnea, cough Chest tightness	Wheezing, retractions
Urticaria	Pruritus, flushing, warmth	Raised migratory wheels
Angioedema	Nonpruritic tingling Swollen sensation	Swelling of lips, face, hands Nonpitting, tingling No warmth or erythema
Gastroenteritis	Cramping, vomiting Diarrhea, tenesmus, blood	Mild tenderness, distention
Conjunctivitis	Itching, tearing	Edema, erythema
Rhinitis	Sneezing, congestion, tearing	Mucosal edema, rhinorrhea

Figure 32–4. Clinical manifestations of anaphylaxis.

contraindicated. Removal of a stinger or any topical allergen should also be done.

CLINICAL EVALUATION

The onset of anaphylaxis is often dramatic, beginning immediately or within minutes of antigen exposure. Most reactions begin within 30 minutes, although delays of 2 to 3 hours are not unusual if the antigen is administered orally. Rarely, allergic reactions have been described days after a bee sting.[17] The shorter the interval from exposure to reaction onset, the more severe the reaction; in fact, instantaneous anaphylaxis may mimic sudden cardiac death.

Symptoms and signs of anaphylaxis usually peak within several minutes of onset, but often persist for hours afterward. Resolution of symptoms may be as brief as a few minutes even without therapy or persist beyond 24 hours despite intensive treatment. Fewer than 5% of patients demonstrate a biphasic course in which there is recrudescence of symptoms within 24 hours of initial resolution.[18]

The parenteral route of antigen exposure usually leads to the most immediate and life-threatening reactions, but antigen exposure by any route may lead to anaphylaxis. Routes of exposure, in descending order of reaction severity, are intravenous, intra-arterial, intramuscular, subcutaneous, intradermal, oral, conjunctival, vaginal, rectal, and cutaneous. Intermittent administration of a drug or other antigen increases the risk of sensitization, although in many cases there is no history of previous exposure.[3, 6]

Immediately before the development of any manifestations of anaphylaxis, patients often complain of certain premonitory symptoms, such as pruritus of the palms and soles, generalized warmth, tingling of the lips and tongue, a lump in the throat, tightness in the chest, or a feeling of impending doom.

Laryngeal edema is the principal cause of death from anaphylaxis, accounting for up to 70% of fatalities.[19] Laryngeal edema may be the only manifestation of anaphylaxis, sometimes mimicking foreign body aspiration or sudden death. Angioedema of adjacent tissues such as the tongue, uvula, and lips often develops concomitantly and serves as a warning of potential laryngeal involvement. The patient may tolerate significant oropharyngeal edema without risk of obstruction; however, even small amounts of laryngeal or epiglottal swelling may be lethal. The child suspected of having an allergic reaction and who complains of hoarseness, dysphagia, or a lump in the throat should be promptly treated with epinephrine, even if the oropharyngeal examination is normal. Although lateral neck films or indirect laryngoscopy may be useful, treatment should not be delayed while awaiting the results of these studies.

Hypotension is a common component of the anaphylactic syndrome, accounting for up to 25% of reported fatalities.[19] Patients may present with syncope or sudden death secondary to shock, without other manifestations of anaphylaxis, leading to delays in diagnosis and treatment. Often the hypotension is mild and rapidly corrected by epinephrine and intravenous fluids.[20–22]

Patients with anaphylaxis may present with cough, wheezing, shortness of breath, bronchospasm, and lower airway edema. Although the wheezing is generally mild, severe status asthmaticus may occur in patients with preexisting asthma. Noncardiogenic pulmonary edema is also described in anaphylaxis, but it is a rare phenomenon usually associated with drugs used in anesthesia or developing as a terminal event.[7, 23]

Urticaria and angioedema occur in more than 90% of patients with anaphylaxis. Urticaria are raised, erythematous wheals covering most of the body in wandering, pruritic patches. By distinction, angioedema is characterized by non-pitting edematous areas of skin and mucous membranes that lack erythema and remain fixed in location, especially on the face, mucous membranes, and hands. Patients with angioedema complain of tingling and a swollen sensation without itching or pain. Diffuse flushing of the skin may be seen as the first manifestation of anaphylaxis prior to or in place of urticaria and angioedema.[24, 25] Nonrespiratory mucous membrane involvement may sometimes be prominent and include intense rhinitis, nasal obstruction, sneezing, conjunctivitis, and chemosis.

Cardiac involvement in anaphylaxis has been described as featuring ventricular arrhythmias, nonspecific ST-T wave changes, and even myocardial infarction. Although stimulation of H_2 receptors in the heart has been hypothesized as a mechanism of cardiac toxicity, it is more likely that hypotension, hypoxia, and overzealous epinephrine therapy result in myocardial ischemia.[26–28]

Genitourinary involvement, although rare, has been described in anaphylaxis and is manifested by urinary urgency and uterine contractions. Neurologic symptoms such as disorientation, coma, and seizures result from hypotension, although there may be an increased incidence of stroke related to anaphylactic bee sting reactions in adults.[15, 19] Fever and adenopathy are not features of anaphylaxis and usually suggest an infectious process or a delayed allergic phenomenon such as serum sickness.[17]

Gastrointestinal manifestations include nausea, vomiting, diarrhea, and rarely, hematochezia.

ETIOLOGIC FACTORS

Penicillin, Hymenoptera stings, and iodinated contrast media constitute the most common causes of fatalities from anaphylaxis, with foods and nonsteroidal anti-inflammatory drugs increasingly recognized in the outpatient setting (Table 32–1).

Antibiotics

Penicillin and its derivatives (i.e., ampicillin, dicloxacillin) account for more than 100 anaphylactic deaths annually in the United States. Most penicillin-related deaths are by the parenteral route. Although 1% of the population is estimated to be sensitive to penicillin, most manifestations involve rash or urticaria alone. Of 100,000 administrations of penicillin, 14 to 40 will cause life-threatening anaphylaxis, and one or two will cause death.[8, 29]

Ampicillin or amoxicillin cause more skin rashes than other penicillins, especially in patients with infectious mononucleosis. Although the mechanism of the ampicillin rash does not appear to be immunologic, other penicillin derivatives should not be administered unless they have been used safely subsequent to the ampicillin reaction or the patient has undergone a skin test.[5]

Cephalosporins are often used as an alternative antibiotic

TABLE 32–1

SUGGESTED DOCUMENTATION

History
    What: All ingestions, exposures and activities in the previous 6 hr.
    Allergic history: Asthma, hives, rhinitis, drugs, foods.
    Time: Onset of symptoms and interval to time of arrival.
    Symptoms: Hoarseness, dysphagia, foreign body sensation in the throat, drooling, or respiratory distress; dizziness or loss of consciousness.

Examination
    Blood pressure and vital signs at 3- to 5-min intervals until stabilized.
    Lip, uvular, soft palate, or tongue edema.
    Listen for stridor or wheezing.
    Note changes in physical findings at 15-min intervals.

Treatment
    Time, dosage, and response of treatment in the field.
    Time, dosage, and response of treatment in the emergency department.

Disposition
    If patient is going home:
        Note resolution of clinical signs and symptoms.
        Note adequate observation period.
        Document discussion with the patient and family about avoidance of potentially offending agents.
        Outpatient treatment plan should be documented in detail and follow-up physician contacted.

---

in penicillin-allergic patients; however, 5% to 16% of patients will experience a cross-reaction. First-, second-, and third-generation cephalosporins all cross-react with penicillin in a similar manner, and the severity and likelihood of reactions are greater in patients who have had fulminant anaphylaxis to penicillin. As a result, cephalosporins should be used cautiously in penicillin-allergic patients.[30] Of the newer agents, imipenem cross-reacts with penicillin, whereas aztreonam does not.[30]

Anaphylaxis resulting from other classes of antibiotics is unusual. For example, ciprofloxacin has a 1% incidence of skin rash, but anaphylaxis is estimated to occur in 1.2 per 100,000 prescriptions.[31] Sulfonamides and trimethoprim are common causes of rash, urticaria, and serum sickness, but not of anaphylaxis. Vancomycin produces diffuse flushing from histamine release, called *red-man syndrome*, but rarely causes anaphylaxis.[32] There are reports of anaphylactic reactions to chloramphenicol, tetracycline, gentamicin, and clindamycin (parenteral route). Even topical antibiotics like bacitracin and neomycin have been reported to cause anaphylaxis.[33, 34]

Envenomation

Hymenoptera stings constitute the second most common cause of life-threatening anaphylaxis in the United States, resulting in more than 50 deaths annually. The order Hymenoptera includes the families Apoidae (honeybees, bumblebees), Vespidae (yellow jackets, hornets, and wasps) and Formicoidae (fire ants, harvester ants). The yellow jacket is the most commonly incriminated stinging insect, followed by honeybees, hornets, wasps, and bumblebees. The honeybee is the only stinging insect that leaves its stinger, leading to evisceration and death.[20, 35] Although honeybees do not sting unless the hive is threatened, the species known as the African ("killer") bee is very aggressive, stinging indiscriminantly en masse. In mid 1990, the species crossed the Mexican border and is expected to migrate north at a rate of 200 miles per year; however, their migration is limited to areas with mean winter temperatures of at least 60°F.[36, 37]

In some parts of the southeastern and south central United States, another imported insect has become the most common cause of insect sting anaphylaxis: the fire ant. Like the African bee, the fire ant is aggressive, stinging en masse, but it is unique in that it leaves numerous sterile pustules at sting sites. As with other Hymenoptera, 1% of people stung develop anaphylaxis.

The majority of stings occur in the late summer, especially in children. Bright clothing, food, and fragrance attract the insects. Anaphylaxis is most likely to occur from stings to the head and neck region. Surprisingly, large local reactions are not predictive of subsequent anaphylactic risk in children. However, systemic reactions usually predict anaphylaxis on subsequent exposure; such reactions often are worse in adults and milder in children.[20, 35] Other uncommon causes of anaphylaxis include bites or stings from kissing bugs, bedbugs, jellyfish, snakes, and gila monsters.[38]

Contrast Media

Iodinated contrast media constitute the third most common cause of fatal anaphylaxis in the United States, with 40 to 50 deaths reported annually. Anaphylactoid reactions occur in 1% to 2% of patients studied, with fatalities in 1 to 10 per 100,000. Prior contrast media reactions, atopy, dehydration and any systemic illness increase the risk of such reactions. Pretreatment with prednisone and diphenhydramine reduces the incidence and severity of radiocontrast media reactions, whereas nonionic contrast media provides only partial protection.[10]

Food

In the outpatient setting, foods probably constitute the most common cause of mild anaphylaxis, yet fatalities are not unusual.[39] In older children and adults, shellfish, fish, nuts, legumes, and seeds are commonly implicated in food-induced anaphylaxis. In infants and younger children, cow's milk, eggs, and soy products are common causes. Although food allergy is more common in young children (0.3%), it tends to be mild, and most children outgrow it by age 2 or 3 years.[40, 41] Other foods, as well as food additives such as sulfites and tartrazine, may result in anaphylaxis. Exercise appears to be a requisite factor in some food reactions.[42]

Pharmacologic Agents

Aspirin and the nonsteroidal anti-inflammatory drugs (NSAIDs) are an increasingly recognized cause of anaphylaxis. Although their use is most prevalent in young adults, pediatric use is expected to increase with Food and Drug Administration (FDA) approval of ibuprofen and naproxen use in children. Aspirin, NSAIDs, and tartrazine all cross-react, but acetaminophen and the nonacetylated salicylates do not. Patients with an atopic history are at greater risk of anaphylaxis or an exacerbation of preexisting asthma.[43, 44]

Many complete protein antigens may precipitate anaphylaxis, including insulin (animal and human), toxoids, vaccines (egg products), allergy extracts, blood products, L-asparaginase, chymopapaine, streptokinase, and seminal fluid.[5, 13] Numerous therapeutic agents given intravenously may result in anaphylaxis, including morphine, anesthetic induction and paralyzing agents, thiamine, vitamin K, protamine, and hydrocortisone.[5-7]

Only about 1% of adverse reactions to local anesthetics are thought to be true allergy; the majority of these are related to the preservative methyparaben or the ester group anesthetics (procaine, tetracaine, benzocaine). Reactions to the amide group of agents (lidocaine, bupivacaine, mepivacaine) are rare, and therefore the use of lidocaine without preservatives (cardiac lidocaine) is safe in most patients with a history of an adverse reaction. If true anaphylaxis occurred and the agent is unknown, skin testing with cardiac lidocaine may be necessary.[45] Allergy to topical tetracaine-adrenaline-cocaine (TAC) has never been reported, but excessive use may result in seizures.[46]

Physical Factors

Physical factors may also provoke anaphylaxis. Exercise, alone or in conjunction with food or NSAID ingestion, is an underrecognized cause of anaphylaxis. Although it is more common in atopic patients during hot, humid weather, it is not predictable or reproducible in most patients. Preventive measures include stopping exercise at the first hint of pruritus and avoiding food or medications for at least 4 hours before exercise. Exercising with a partner and carrying an epinephrine autoinjector is prudent.[42, 47] Cold exposure is another physical factor that can precipitate urticaria and mild anaphylaxis.

In 25% of patients, no identifiable cause of anaphylaxis is found, despite evaluation by an allergist. Steroid and antihistamine prophylaxis is effective, but epinephrine kits are a mainstay in therapy.[48]

DIAGNOSTIC EVALUATION

There is little role for laboratory tests in the initial assessment and treatment of a patient with anaphylaxis. Eosino-philia is usually absent. Peak expiratory flow and blood gas measurements may be useful in patients with bronchospasm and respiratory distress. If hereditary angioedema is suspected, low serum complement levels may be diagnostic.[49]

DIFFERENTIAL DIAGNOSIS

Upper airway obstruction in the young child is a difficult diagnostic situation. Foreign body aspiration is a primary consideration if symptoms are acute and skin manifestations are absent. The history of events just prior to onset (e.g., playing or eating alone), unilateral wheezing, and the lack of oropharyngeal edema should increase the suspicion of foreign body aspiration.[50] Acute epiglottitis, retropharyngeal abscess, or croup may be confused with angioedema of the larynx and supraglottic region, but the presence of fever and pain with erythema and exudate on examination should distinguish these entities. Occasionally, older children feign stridor and dyspnea, but treatment should not be withheld unless indirect laryngoscopy can be performed safely.[51] Anaphylaxis should be a primary consideration in any child with unexplained hypotension, even if other manifestations of an allergic reaction are absent. Such patients may present with syncope or coma.[5, 6]

Hereditary angioedema (HAE) may mimic anaphylaxis, presenting with acute upper airway obstruction, angioedema of the skin, and gastrointestinal symptoms. HAE is an autosomal dominant disorder, caused by a C1 esterase inhibitor deficiency that results in episodes of spontaneous complement activation and subsequent chemical mediator release. Attacks usually begin in adolescence and may recur throughout life, precipitated by stress and trauma. A family history of death in a young person from laryngeal obstruction may be elicited. Severe abdominal pain mimicking an acute abdomen is a classic feature of this disease, whereas urticaria is absent. An attack of hereditary angioedema does not respond to epinephrine and antihistamines. Fresh frozen plasma, however, may abort an acute episode, and danazol has been successful as prophylaxis.[49]

Scombroid fish poisoning presents with acute urticaria, nausea, vomiting, headache, and dysphagia. This reaction occurs subsequent to ingestion of fish with a high histidine content (e.g., mahi-mahi, tuna), which liberates histamine on spoiling.[52] The Chinese restaurant syndrome, occurring secondary to ingestion of monosodium glutamate, may cause flushing, but the prominent headache is distinguishing.[53]

Serum sickness is an allergic reaction that may resemble anaphylaxis manifesting with acute urticaria. However, serum sickness is a delayed reaction to prolonged antigen exposure in which antigen-IgG complexes are formed, and complement fixation occurs. The presence of joint pains, lymphadenopathy, nephritis, and especially fever differentiate serum sickness from anaphylaxis. Urticaria pigmentosa and systemic mastocytosis are rare causes of anaphylactoid symptoms and present with flushing and hypotension.[54]

Acute urticaria and status asthmaticus are in a sense local forms of anaphylaxis and should be treated with similar urgency.

THERAPEUTIC INTERVENTION

Epinephrine is the cornerstone of therapy of anaphylaxis, taking advantage of both alpha-adrenergic and beta-adrenergic effects. Stimulation of beta receptors on mast cells increases the production of cyclic adenosine monophosphate (AMP), thereby inhibiting further release of chemical mediators. Beta-adrenergic effects also produce bronchodilation, as well as positive inotropic and chronotropic effects on the heart. Stimulation of alpha receptors causes vasoconstriction, which results in a rise in systemic blood pressure and a decrease in angioedema of the skin and mucous membranes.[5, 6, 20, 28]

Epinephrine (1:1000 dilution) is administered in a dose of 0.01 ml/kg, to a maximum of 0.3 ml, subcutaneously or intramuscularly; the intramuscular route is preferred if hypotension or airway compromise exists (Table 32–2). This dose should be repeated at 10- to 20-minute intervals depending on the patient's response. Standard supportive measures should be initiated concomitantly; these include establishment of an intravenous line (infusing 0.9 NS or LR), supplemental oxygen, and cardiac monitoring.[5, 6, 20]

Epinephrine by the intravenous route is rarely necessary but should be considered in a patient with imminent airway obstruction or hypotension unresponsive to fluid resuscitation and intramuscular epinephrine. The intravenous route of epinephrine should be used with great caution, as overzealous use may lead to ventricular arrhythmias, myocardial ischemia, and extremity gangrene. An epinephrine drip is prepared by diluting 1.0 mg of epinephrine in 250 ml of D5W, infused at 0.05 to 0.20 µg/kg/min. In an adolescent or adult in extremis, 1.0 ml of 1:10,000 epinephrine is diluted in 10 ml of normal saline and given in a slow IV push over 5 to 10 minutes. Once a clinical response is demonstrated, intermittent subcutaneous or IM doses are given.[28, 55]

The patency of the upper airway and the patient's hemodynamic status require constant monitoring, as death from anaphylaxis usually results from laryngeal edema or shock (Table 32–3). A complaint of hoarseness, dysphagia, or a lump in the throat, even without the presence of stridor, drooling, or neck retractions, should be approached aggressively. Any degree of angioedema of the uvula, soft palate, tongue, or lips should alert the physician to anticipate laryngeal edema.

If complete airway obstruction occurs or if respiratory distress worsens despite parenteral epinephrine, the patient should be intubated orally to directly visualize the anatomy. If supraglottic edema obscures the airway, cricothyrotomy (in older children and adults) or needle cricothyrostomy (in children younger than 6 years) with percutaneous transtracheal ventilation should be performed. In the uncooperative, awake, older child, nasotracheal intubation may be attempted before or concomitant to surgical airway interven-

tion. Nebulized racemic epinephrine may also be attempted while preparing for intubation, but the physician should realize that its benefits are transient.[6, 55]

Anaphylactic shock should be treated with concomitant epinephrine and fluid resuscitation. Normal saline or LR should be administered in a bolus of 20 ml/kg (up to 1 L), wide open, followed by a second bolus over 15 to 60 minutes, depending on the initial response.[21, 22] Insertion of a urinary catheter and a central venous pressure (CVP) line is recommended to follow the volume status if the patient remains unstable. Placing the patient in the Trendelenburg position or applying the pneumatic antishock garment (PASG) are other adjuncts to raise the blood pressure.[56] If hypotension is refractory to these measures, epinephrine (0.05 to 0.20 µg/kg/min) or dopamine (5 to 20 µg/kg/min) by infusion may be lifesaving.[28, 57] Naloxone in large doses may also ameliorate anaphylactic shock.[58, 59]

Antihistamines should be administered to all patients with anaphylaxis. Diphenhydramine can be given intramuscularly, intravenously, or orally depending on the severity of the reaction. The standard dose is 1 mg/kg repeated at 4-hour intervals. If sedation is undesirable, the dose should be reduced to 0.5 mg/kg. Patients in extremis may require up to 2 mg/kg per dose, given slowly over 3 minutes to avoid paradoxic hypotension.[1, 2, 6]

H_2 receptor antagonists have not been routinely used in anaphylaxis because of concerns that H_2-receptor blockade on mast cells may aggravate mediator release. However, clinical experience suggests that combined use of H_1 and H_2 antihistamines or use of H_2 antagonists alone may play a role in the therapy of anaphylaxis. Cimetidine has been shown to be as effective or more effective than diphenhydramine (as well as less sedative) in the treatment of acute urticaria.[60] In addition, refractory anaphylactic shock has responded to cimetidine. The recommended dose is 5 mg/kg, up to 300 mg, at 6-hour intervals.[6, 15, 60-62]

Corticosteroids should be administered in all patients with moderate to severe anaphylaxis. Immediate steroid treatment in the emergency department has been demonstrated to be beneficial in patients with status asthmaticus, and similar benefits might be inferred for patients with anaphylaxis.[63] Rationales for steroid therapy include reduction of angioedema and bronchial inflammation, prevention of delayed reexacerbation of anaphylaxis, and improved respon-

---

TABLE 32–2

TREATMENT OF ANAPHYLAXIS: THERAPY AT A GLANCE

Epinephrine
1. Mild episode: 0.01 ml/kg up to 0.3 ml (1:1000 dilution) subcutaneously; repeat at 20-minute intervals.
2. Moderate to severe episode: 0.01 ml/kg up to 0.3 ml SC; repeat at 10- to 20-minute intervals.
3. Resistant shock or imminent airway obstruction:
   a. Infant or small child: prepare a drip of 1 mg in 250 ml D5W and infuse at a rate of 0.05–0.20 µg/kg/min.
   b. Older child or adult: dilute 1 ml of cardiac epinephrine (1:10,000) in 10 ml normal saline and push over a 5- to 10-minute interval. May repeat dependent on response.

Volume expansion: Normal saline or lactated Ringer's, initial bolus of 20 ml/kg (up to 1 L), wide open; repeat dependent on response. When stabilized, subsequent fluid bolus slowed to 1- to 2-hour intervals.

Antihistamines
1. Diphenhydramine: 1 mg/kg (0.5–1.5 mg/kg range) given IV, IM, or by mouth depending on the severity of the reaction. The dose may be repeated at 4-hour intervals dependent on response and sedative side effects.
2. Cimetidine: 5 mg/kg (up to 300 mg) by intravenous infusion, repeated at 6-hour intervals. Reserved for refractory cases. May be used alone or in combination with diphenhydramine.

Corticosteroids: Methylprednisolone, 2–3 mg/kg (up to 125 mg), or hydrocortisone, 8–9 mg/kg (up to 500 mg), IV, repeated at 4- to 6-hour intervals.

Local measures: Flick off bee stinger; place a loose tourniquet proximal to an injection or sting site; wash off any topical exposure; apply ice or inject epinephrine 0.005 ml/kg (1:1000) about the inoculation site.

TABLE 32–3

TREATMENT OF ANAPHYLAXIS: SPECIAL SITUATIONS

I. Laryngeal edema and imminent airway obstruction
    A. Upright posture; humidified air; avoid sedative agents; indirect laryngoscopy contraindicated in the small child.
    B. If progressing despite initiating epinephrine IM or subcutaneously, begin intravenous infusion as noted above; methylprednisolone should also be given in bolus.
    C. If immediately available, consider racemic epinephrine to buy time while preparing to open an airway surgically.
    D. If complete or imminent airway obstruction:
        1. Smaller child or infant: Oral intubation preferred so as to directly visualize the anatomy; if the airway is obscured by edema, needle cricothyrostomy with percutaneous transtracheal ventilation may be expedient.
        2. Older child and adult: Oral intubation is preferred, but nasotracheal intubation may be attempted in an awake, uncooperative patient; if the airway is obscured by edema, proceed with cricothyrotomy.
II. Refractory hypotension
    A. Administration of epinephrine and volume expansion (see Table 32–2).
    B. Place a second IV line or consider a central venous pressure line; oxygen, cardiac monitoring, and a urinary catheter are other important adjuncts.
    C. Trendelenburg positioning.
    D. Pneumatic antishock garment inflation.
    E. Vasopressors: Epinephrine, 0.05–0.20 μg/kg/min; dopamine, 5–20 μg/kg/min.
    F. Cimetidine, 5 mg/kg (up to 300 mg) IV every 6 hr.
    G. Naloxone, 0.05–0.10 mg/kg bolus, repeated as needed if there is a clinical response.
    H. Glucagon, 1–2 mg IV over 4 min if patient is on beta blockers.
III. Resistant bronchospasm
    A. Administration of epinephrine and volume expansion (see Table 32–2).
    B. Albuterol by nebulization at 30- to 180-min intervals or constantly.
    C. Aminophylline: Loading dose, 5.6 mg/kg in 100 ml saline or D5W intravenous infusion over 30 min.
    D. Ipratropium by nebulization.
    E. Glucagon, 1–2 mg IV over 4 min if patient is on beta blockers.
    F. Intubation and ventilation if fatigued.

---

siveness of the beta-adrenergic receptors. Recommended dosages include, for methylprednisolone, 2 to 3 mg/kg (up to 125 mg) or, for hydrocortisone, 7 to 8 mg/kg (up to 500 mg) at 6-hour intervals.[5, 6, 15, 16]

Bronchospasm in anaphylaxis usually responds to epinephrine alone; however, aerosolized albuterol, intravenous aminophylline, and steroids may be necessary in more refractory cases.

Patients with cardiac disease and those on beta blockers present special treatment situations, although these are rarely encountered in the pediatric population. Intravenous epinephrine and overzealous fluid resuscitation should be avoided in the child with cardiomyopathy or congenital heart disease.[28] Patients on beta blockers may be resistant to epinephrine, showing a net alpha-adrenergic effect. In this situation, glucagon given in a dose of 1 to 2 mg intravenously over 5 minutes may have great benefit, presumably by stimulating adenylcyclase activity by receptors separate from the beta receptors. Pure beta agonists such as subcutaneous terbutaline or intravenous isoproterenol may have benefit, as may intravenous atropine or aerosolized ipratropium, for bronchospasm and bradyarrhythmia resulting after epinephrine therapy in the beta-blocked patient.[57, 64]

Lastly, measures to prevent further absorption of an antigen should not be overlooked. A loose tourniquet should be placed above the injection site, the honeybee stinger

---

TABLE 32–4

PITFALLS IN DIAGNOSIS AND TREATMENT

1. Failure to recognize common etiologic factors such as foods and medications (especially over-the-counter-drugs like aspirin and NSAIDs).
2. Failure to carefully review all events 4 to 6 hr prior to onset.
3. Failure to recognize that patients may lack the full anaphylactic syndrome, sometimes presenting with shock or airway obstruction as the only symptom or sign.
4. Ignoring symptoms of hoarseness, dysphagia, or lump in the throat. Even if the physical examination is normal, early airway obstruction can be missed.
5. Failure to carefully examine the pharynx or failure to recognize uvular or other pharyngeal edema as a harbinger of laryngeal involvement.
6. Overzealous use of intravenous epinephrine in moderate anaphylaxis, exceeding dosage recommendations with subsequent cardiovascular toxicity.
7. Failure to use intravenous epinephrine in patients with refractory shock or imminent airway obstruction.
8. Exceeding dosage recommendations for diphenhydramine, leading to oversedation.
9. Inadequate emergency department observation time in patients going home, failing to recognize that a small percentage of patients will have delayed recrudescence of the anaphylactic syndrome.
10. Failure to use corticosteroids early in patients with moderate to severe anaphylaxis.
11. Failure to warn patient and family about possible cross-reacting agents (aspirin, NSAIDs and tartrazine; penicillin and cephalosporins).
12. Prescribing new medications (i.e., antibiotics) to a patient who has just recovered from anaphylaxis. If recurrence of symptoms occurs, the inciting cause will be difficult to determine.

flicked off (not squeezed), and 0.005 ml/kg epinephrine 1:1000 injected at the inoculation site. The physician should consider charcoal administration and gastric emptying for ingested antigens.

DISPOSITION

All patients with life-threatening presentations such as severe hypotension or upper airway obstruction (even if there is complete resolution in the emergency department) should be admitted to the hospital (Table 32–4). Patients with a slow or incomplete response to therapy, as well as those who have an exacerbation of symptoms in the emergency department, should also be admitted. Patients with residual upper airway angioedema or hypotension should be observed in an intensive care unit.

Patients who have a complete and rapid clinical response to treatment and who have not had life-threatening manifestations of anaphylaxis may be discharged home after an additional observation period of 2 to 3 hours in the emergency department. Patients who are sent home must have follow-up by their pediatrician within 48 hours and should be discharged on a 2-day course of prednisone 1 to 2 mg/kg (up to 40 mg) daily. The patient and family should be carefully instructed to avoid all possible inciting agents. If avoidance is impossible (i.e., in cases of idiopathic or bee sting anaphylaxis), a prescription for and instruction in the use of an epinephrine autoinjector pen may be appropriate.

References

1. Corren J, Schocket AL. Anaphylaxis: A preventable emergency. Postgrad Med 1990;87:167.
2. Lucke WC, Thomas TH. Anaphylaxis: Pathophysiology, clinical presentations, and treatment. J Emerg Med 1983;1:83.
3. Kelly JF, Patterson R. Anaphylaxis: Course, mechanisms, and treatment. JAMA 1974;227:1431.
4. Terr AI. Anaphylaxis. Clin Rev Allergy 1985;3:3.
5. Weiszer I. Allergic emergencies. In Patterson R (ed). Allergic Diseases: Diagnosis and Management. 3rd ed. Philadelphia, JB Lippincott, 1985, pp 418–439.
6. Lindzon RD, Silvers WS. Anaphylaxis. In Rosen P, Baker FJ, Barkin RM, et al (eds). Emergency Medicine: Concepts and Clinical Practice. 2nd ed. St Louis, CV Mosby, 1988, pp 203–231.
7. Fisher M. Anaphylaxis. Dis Mon 1987;33(8):433.
8. Idsoe O, Gruthe T, Wilcox RR, et al. Nature and extent penicillin side reactions with particular references to fatalities from anaphylactic shock. Bull WHO 1968;38:159.
9. Parrish HM. Analysis of 460 fatalities from venomous animals in the United States. Am J Med Sci 1969;245:129.
10. Greenberger PA. Contrast media reactions. J Allergy Clin Immunol 1984;74:600.
11. Leung AK. Anaphylaxis to DPT vaccine. J R Soc Med 1985;78:175.
12. Jarmoc LM, Primack WA. Anaphylaxis to cutaneous exposure to milk protein in a diaper rash ointment. Clin Pediatr 1987;26(3):154.
13. Sheffer AL. Anaphylaxis. J Allergy Clin Immunol 1985;75:227.
14. Wasserman SI. Mediators of immediate hypersensitivity. J Allergy Clin Immunol 1983;72:101.
15. Wasserman SI, Marquardt DI. Anaphylaxis. In Middleton E, Reed CE, Ellis EF, et al (eds). Allergy: Principles and Practice. 3rd ed. St Louis, CV Mosby, 1988, pp 1365–1376.
16. Lieberman P, Erffmeyer JE. Corticosteroids in the treatment of allergic diseases. In Patterson R (ed). Allergic Diseases Diagnosis and Management. 3rd ed. Philadelphia, JB Lippincott, 1985, pp 759–792.
17. Reisman RE, Livingston A. Late-onset allergic reactions, including serum sickness after insect stings. J Allergy Clin Immunol 1989;84:331.
18. Stark BJ, Sullivan TJ. Biphasic and protracted anaphylaxis. J Allergy Clin Immunol 1986;78:76.
19. Barnard JH. Studies of 400 Hymenoptera sting deaths in the United States. J Allergy Clin Immunol 1973;52:259.
20. Patterson R, Valentine M. Anaphylaxis and related allergic emergencies including reactions due to insect stings. JAMA 1982;248:2632.
21. Smith PL, Kagey-Sobotka A, Bleecker ER, et al. Physiologic manifestations of human anaphylaxis. J Clin Invest 1980;66:1072.
22. Silverman HJ, Van Hook C, Haponik EF. Hemodynamic changes in human anaphylaxis. Am J Med 1984;77:341.
23. Carlson RW, Schaeffer RC, Puri VK, et al. Hypovolemia and permeability pulmonary edema associated with anaphylaxis. Crit Care Med 1981;9:883.
24. Ligresti DJ. Anaphylaxis. Clin Dermatol 1986;4(1):40.
25. Monroe EW, Jones HE. Urticaria: An updated review. Arch Dermatol 1977;113:80.
26. Booth BH, Patterson R. Electrocardiographic changes during human anaphylaxis. JAMA 1970;211:627.
27. Levine HD. Acute myocardial infarction following wasp sting. Am Heart J 1976;91:365.
28. Barach EM, Nowack RM. Epinephrine for treatment of anaphylactic shock. JAMA 1984;25:2118.
29. O'Leary MR, Smith MS. Penicillin anaphylaxis. Am J Emerg Med 1986;4:241.
30. Saxon A, Beall-Gelden N, Rohr AS, et al. UCLA conference: Immediate hypersensitivity reactions to beta-lactam antibiotics. Ann Intern Med 1987;107:204.
31. Davis H, McGoodwin E, Greene-Reed T. Anaphylactoid reactions reported after treatment with ciprofloxacin. Ann Intern Med 1989;111:1041.
32. Polk RE, Healy DP, Schwartz LB, et al. Vancomycin and the red-man syndrome: Pharmacodynamics of histamine release. J Infect Dis 1988;157:502.
33. Palchick BA, Funk EA, McEntire JE, et al. Anaphylaxis due to chloramphenicol. Am J Med Sci 1984;288:43.
34. Goh CL. Anaphylaxis from topical neomycin and bacitracin. Austr J Dermatol 1986;27:125.
35. Settipane GA, Boyd GK. Anaphylaxis from insect stings: Myth, controversy, and reality. Postgrad Med 1989;86(2):273.
36. Taylor OR. Health problems associated with African bees. Ann Intern Med 1986;104:267.
37. Crawford MH. Research news: Briefing: Africanized bees near Texas border. Science 1990;247:284.
38. Piacentine J, Curry SC, Ryan PJ. Life-threatening anaphylaxis following a gila monster bite. Ann Emerg Med 1986;15:959.
39. Yunginger JW, Sweeney KG, Sturner WQ, et al. Fatal food-induced anaphylaxis. JAMA 1988;260:1450.
40. Amlot PL, Kemeny DM, Zachary C, et al. Oral allergy syndrome (OAS): Symptoms of IgE-mediated hypersensitivity to foods. Clin Allergy 1987;17(1):33.
41. Anderson JA. Adverse reaction to foods. In Bierman CW, Pearlman DS (eds). Allergic Diseases from Infancy to Adulthood. 2nd ed. Philadelphia, WB Saunders, 1988, pp 130–140.
42. Novey HS, Fairshter RD, Salness K, et al. Postprandial exercise-induced anaphylaxis. J Allergy Clin Immunol 1983;71:498.
43. Stevenson DD. Diagnosis, prevention, and treatment of adverse reactions to aspirin and nonsteroidal anti-inflammatory drugs. J Allergy Clin Immunol 1984;74:617.
44. Sandler RH. Anaphylactic reactions to zomepirac. Ann Emerg Med 1985;14:171.
45. Swanson JG. Assessment of allergy to local anesthetics. Ann Emerg Med 1983;12:316.
46. Bonadio WA. TAC: A review. Pediatr Emerg Care 1989;5(2):128.
47. Sheffer AL, Austen KF. Exercise-induced anaphylaxis. J Allergy Clin Immunol 1984;73:699.
48. Wiggins CA, Dykewicz MS, Patterson R. Idiopathic anaphylaxis: A review. Ann Allergy 1989;62:1.
49. Moore GP, Hurley WT, Pace SA. Hereditary angioedema. Ann Emerg Med 1988;17:1082.
50. Blazer S, Naveh Y, Friedman A. Foreign body in the airway: A review of 200 cases. Am Rev Dis Child 1980;134:68.
51. Snyder HS, Weiss E. Hysterical stridor: A benign cause of upper airway obstruction. Ann Emerg Med 1989;18:991.
52. Russell FE, Maretic Z. Scombroid poisoning: mini-review with case histories. Toxicon 1986;24(10):967.
53. Zautcke JL, Schwartz JA, Mueller EJ. Chinese restaurant syndrome: a review. Ann Emerg Med 1986;15(10):1210.
54. Travis WD, Li CY, Bergstralh EJ, et al. Systemic mast cell disease. Medicine 1988;67:345.
55. American Heart Association. Standards for CPR and ECC: Pediatric advanced life support. JAMA 1986;255:2961.
56. Oertel T, Loehr MM. Bee-sting anaphylaxis: The use of the military antishock trousers. Ann Emerg Med 1984;13:459.
57. Perkin RM, Anas NG. Mechanisms and management of anaphylactic shock, not responding to traditional therapy. Ann Allergy 1985;54:202.
58. Gullo A, Romano E. Naloxone and anaphylactic shock. Lancet 1983;1(8328):819.
59. Barsan WG, Hedges JR, Syverud SA. Hemodynamic effects of naloxone in anaphylactic shock. Resuscitation 1986;13:223.
60. Moscati RM, Moore GP. Comparison of cimetidine and diphenhydramine in the treatment of acute urticaria. Ann Emerg Med 1990;19:12.
61. Raper RF, Fisher MM. Profound reversible myocardial depression after anaphylaxis. Lancet 1988;1:386.
62. Mayumi H, Kimura S, Asana M, et al. Intravenous cimetidine as an effective treatment for systemic anaphylaxis and acute allergic skin reactions. Ann Allergy 1987;58:447.
63. Littenberg B, Gluck EH. A controlled trial of methylprednisolone in the emergency treatment of acute asthma. N Engl J Med 1986;314:150.
64. Zaloga GP, DeLacey W, Homboe E, et al. Glucagon reversal of hypotension in a case of anaphylactoid shock. Ann Intern Med 1986;105:65.

SECTION FOUR

Digestive System

CHAPTER 33

Approach to Abdominal Pain

Eugene Izsak

INTRODUCTION

Children presenting to the emergency department with abdomen-related complaints make up 9% to 10% of all pediatric emergency visits. This does not include extra-abdominal conditions, which may also present as abdominal pain. When pain is the major complaint, a parent's frequent concern is the potential for surgery. The emergency physician treating the child has many decisions to make and interventions to consider before the question of surgery is answered with certainty.

Abdominal pain may arise from one of three sources: intra-abdominal, extra-abdominal, or a systemic disease. The four intra-abdominal sources are distention of a hollow viscus, stretching of the capsule of a solid organ, peritoneal inflammation, or organ ischemia. Extra-abdominal sources of pain arise outside the abdominal wall musculature (i.e., in the genitourinary system). Finally, systemic diseases such as diabetic ketoacidosis, sickle cell vasoocclusive crisis, arthropod envenomations, poisonings, and porphyria may also cause abdominal pain.

Traumatic conditions tend to damage the solid organs more frequently than hollow organs because of the relatively weak and thin abdominal wall protecting the solid organs and the more cartilaginous ribs protecting the hollow organs. The solid organs of a child are more abdominal in position and thereby are even more likely to absorb the energy of an impact. Chronic conditions (e.g., Crohn's disease) tend not to be surgical problems, unlike acute conditions such as appendicitis. Sudden problems are usually infectious in origin or are problems requiring surgical correction. Gastroenteritis, pelvic inflammatory disease, viral syndromes, pneumonias, or urinary tract infections comprise the majority of cases with an infectious cause. Problems requiring surgery can be broken down into the four broad categories of obstruction, perforation, peritonitis, or masses.

INITIAL EVALUATION

The first step in evaluating the patient is to assess cardiovascular stability, especially in regard to tissue perfusion. In children, this is best accomplished by assessing perfusion to the largest organ, the skin, by measuring capillary refill and skin temperature. In addition, perfusion to the brain is crudely monitored by the level of consciousness, along with the level of activity and interaction with the environment. Finally, perfusion to the kidneys is measured by quantifying urine output. The pulse rate and blood pressure may be helpful if hypotension or tachycardia exists; however, these parameters may be misleading. Tachycardia may be secondary to hypovolemia, temperature elevation, anxiety, or pain. The blood pressure may be near normal despite marked hypovolemia because of the excellent compensatory mechanisms in the young patient.

Once stability is ensured, a brief history and physical examination directed to the presenting complaint is in order (Table 33–1). Questions that elicit the location and character of pain, acuity of onset, and progression of symptoms are essential. A medical history of past problems, surgeries, and the presence of systemic disease is warranted.

A brief abdominal examination is then performed, centering on inspection, auscultation, and then palpation, with the potentially painful procedures last. A rectal examination should be included in all evaluations of abdominal pain and a pelvic examination performed when appropriate. Signs of peritoneal irritation can be elicited by having the child jump, by striking the heels, or by rocking the pelvis.

DIAGNOSTIC EVALUATION
Radiology

Plain radiographs may be diagnostic in certain conditions, such as a fecalith in a child with right lower quadrant pain (appendicitis), a ruptured viscus, a bowel obstruction, or

---

TABLE 33–1

CLINICAL EVALUATION OF ABDOMINAL PAIN

Onset
  Explosive: catastrophic, such as rupture
  Gradual: appendicitis
  Intermittent: intussusception
Location
  Diffuse: visceral, early appendicitis, peritonitis, obstruction, diabetic ketoacidosis, sickle cell vasoocclusive crisis
  Right upper quadrant: liver, gallbladder
  Left lower quadrant: spleen, stomach, left lower lobe pneumonia
  Right lower quadrant: appendix, cecum
  Left lower quadrant: sigmoid, descending colon
Radiation: Limited value
  Left shoulder: left diaphragm, spleen
  Genitals: ureteral colic
Associated symptoms: nausea, vomiting, diarrhea, loss of appetite, fluid losses, constipation, obstipation, urinary symptoms, pulmonary symptoms, gynecologic symptoms

pneumonia. Plain radiographs may suggest other conditions such as a mass, intussusception, or medial displacement of the stomach bubble from a splenic hematoma. In addition to plain radiographs, other imaging procedures such as barium enema, computed tomographic (CT) scans, and ultrasound are considered as directed by the history and physical examination.

Laboratory Tests

A complete blood cell count can be helpful in the child with anemia and can reveal hemoconcentration in the dehydrated child. An elevated white blood cell count may only help to confirm a disease that is suggested by the history and physical examination, but a normal white blood cell count does not exclude significant disease. A urinalysis can be helpful in assessing dehydration or providing evidence of infection or genitourinary disease.

A pregnancy test, preferably one sensitive to 25 mIU human chorionic gonadotropin, is mandatory in all adolescent females of child-bearing ages with abdominal pain in order to determine pregnancy, both intrauterine or ectopic, as the cause of pain.

DIFFERENTIAL DIAGNOSIS

The differential diagnosis of abdominal pain is extensive and changes with age (Table 33–2). Appendicitis is seen more in preadolescents and adolescents, whereas intussusception is commonly seen in children under 2 years of age. In addition to age, the frequency of certain conditions should be considered when arriving at a specific diagnosis in a child.

THERAPEUTIC INTERVENTION

Management of the child often precedes the establishment of the diagnosis. If the child is hemodynamically unstable

TABLE 33–2
DIFFERENTIAL DIAGNOSIS OF ABDOMINAL PAIN BY PREDOMINANT AGE

0–2 years
Aerophagia
Colic
Epiplocele (epigastric hernia)
Gastric duplication
Hemolytic-uremic syndrome
Hereditary angioneurotic edema
Hernia, incarcerated inguinal
Hernia, incarcerated umbilical
Hirschsprung's disease
Intussusception
Kawasaki disease
Lactose intolerance
Lead poisoning
Malrotation
Necrotizing enterocolitis
Pseudoobstruction
Sepsis
Urachal cyst, infected

2–12 years
Abdominal epilepsy
Abdominal migraine
Acute rheumatic fever
Aerophagia
Allergic-tension fatigue syndrome
Appendiceal intussusception
Chronic recurrent abdominal pain of childhood
Constipation
Cystic fibrosis (meconium ileus equivalent)
Diabetes mellitus
Familial mediterranean fever
Functional pain
Gall bladder disease
Hemolytic-uremic syndrome
Hereditary angioneurotic edema
Hypoglycemia
Infectious mononucleosis
Inflammatory bowel disease
Ingestion
Kawasaki disease
Lead poisoning
Lymphoma
Mesenteric adenitis
Nephrotic syndrome
Pancreatitis
Parasitosis

Peritonitis, primary
Pharyngitis
Renolith
Reye syndrome
Rocky Mountain spotted fever
Sickle cell anemia

Teens
Abdominal epilepsy
Abdominal migraine
Acute rheumatic fever
Allergic-tension fatigue syndrome
Appendiceal intussusception
Cystic fibrosis (meconium ileus equivalent)
Dysmenorrhea
Ectopic pregnancy
Endometriosis
Epididymitis
Erythromycin-induced cholestasis
Familial mediterranean fever
Fitz-Hugh-Curtis syndrome
Functional pain
Gallbladder disease
Hematocolpos
Hematometra
Henoch-Schönlein purpura
Hypoglycemia
Infectious mononucleosis
Inflammatory bowel disease
Irritable bowel syndrome
Lymphyoma
Mesenteric adenitis
Mittelschmerz
Ovarian torsion
Pancreatitis
Pelvic inflammatory disease/tuboovarian abscess
Porphyria
Pregnancy
Renolith
Rocky Mountain spotted fever
Sickle cell anemia
Superior mesenteric artery syndrome
Systemic lupus erythematosis
Wegener granulomatosis

All Ages
Abscess

Addison's disease
Adhesions with secondary obstruction
Appendicitis
Ascites
Biliary disease
Black widow spider bite
Brain tumor
Child abuse
Coarctation of the aorta
Dysrhythmias
Electrolyte disturbances
Food poisoning
Fracture (hip, rib)
Gastroenteritis
Geophagia
Glomerulonephritis
Heavy metal poisoning
Hepatitis
Herpes zoster
Hyperlipoproteinemia
Hyperthyroidism
Leukemia
Masses/neoplasms
Meckel's diverticulum
Medications/illicit drugs
Omentum torsion
Ovarian cysts
Ovarian neoplasm
Pericarditis
Pneumonia
Pneumomediastinum
Pneumothorax
Postoperative adhesions
Pyelonephritis
Small bowel obstruction
Spherocytosis
Testicular torsion
Testicular appendage torsion
Trauma
Tuberculosis of the spine
Typhoid
Ulcers
Urinary tract infection
Varicella
Ventriculoperitoneal shunt infection

From Buchert GS. Abdominal pain in children: An emergency practitioner's guide. Emerg Med Clin North Am 1989;7(3):506.

because of fluid losses, immediate intravenous access and fluid resuscitation take precedence. Further stabilization may require gastric decompression with nasogastric tube insertion and Foley catheter insertion for monitoring fluid resuscitation and collecting specimens. Appropriate antibiotic coverage or initial treatment of ingested toxins should also be considered. Early medical or surgical consultation is mandatory for coordinated evaluation and management.

CHAPTER 34

Appendicitis

L. Mason Cobb
Joseph L. Lelli

INTRODUCTION

Appendicitis is the most common cause of emergency laparotomy in children. Ironically, it is also the most commonly missed surgical diagnosis. The longer the time from the onset of symptoms to appendectomy, the greater the risk of perforation.[1, 2] The incidence of perforated appendicitis ranges from 30% to 80% in children; negative explorations for appendicitis (laparotomy with a normal appendix) range from 5% to 25%.[3–5] More than one third of patients with perforation have been previously seen by a physician prior to presenting with perforation.[1, 3, 6] Approximately 80,000 children (from a total population of 62 million children) are diagnosed with appendicitis in the United States each year. If 40% are perforated, then 32,000 children per year will suffer increased morbidity, although mortality is rare. Early diagnosis in the emergency department is essential to decrease the incidence of appendiceal perforation.

Sporadic reports of appendiceal inflammation occurred after a postmortem description in 1554 of a 7-year-old girl.[7] Several reports gave accurate descriptions of appendicitis and appendectomy in the 1880s.[8, 9] These included McBurney, whose 1889 description stated that "the seat of greatest pain, determined by the pressure of one finger has been very exactly between an inch and a half and two inches from the anterior spinous process of the ilium, on a straight line down from that process to the umbilicus."[10]

Since the 1960s, death from appendicitis has become rare with the use of more sophisticated antibiotics, improved fluid management, and advances in critical care medicine. Nevertheless, the late 1980s saw an increased rate of perforated appendicitis because of delays in diagnosis.[11, 12] Prompt recognition of this condition remains the most critical factor in outcome.[3, 11]

ANATOMY AND PHYSIOLOGY

In most medical illustrations, the appendix lies inferomedial to the cecum. This actually occurs only 20% of the time. The child's appendix is retrocecal or retrocolic in 75% of cases.[13] In a small number of cases, the colon is nonrotated,

and the appendix can be anywhere in the peritoneal cavity.[14] The appendiceal artery is an end artery, and thrombosis caused by surrounding inflammation can lead to rapid gangrene and perforation.

The appendix is a secretory organ lined with mucosa. Typically, the precipitating event of appendicitis is lumenal obstruction, with subsequent swelling secondary to secretions. As the swelling progresses, venous return is compromised, the mucosa becomes ulcerated, and bacterial translocation leads to inflammation.

The appendix is relatively short and the lumen relatively wide in the infant; only 0.5% to 2.0% of cases of childhood appendicitis occur in children younger than 2 years.[15, 16] In children younger than 3 years, perforation occurs prior to diagnosis 71% to 94% of the time.[12, 15] This may be because of the inability of the toddler to give a history[17] or because the relatively short appendix in this age group tends to perforate sooner.

Younger children frequently present with generalized peritonitis.[14, 15] Children younger than 5 years have a poorly developed omentum that cannot "wall off" a perforated appendix into a localized abscess as easily as can the omentum in older children.[17] In addition, the normally protuberant abdomen and thin musculature in this age group do not easily produce "board-like" rigidity.[15]

The T9 and T10 dorsal nerve roots innervate the appendix,[18] and therefore the initial aching pain of appendicitis is in the middle region of the abdomen. As inflammation progresses, the parietal peritoneum is secondarily inflamed. This produces a sharp, well-localized pain.[18] Flank pain, costovertebral angle tenderness, right upper quadrant tenderness, back pain, and well-localized abdominal pain are all possible, depending on the location of the inflamed appendix and adjacent peritoneum. Peritoneal pain is more exquisite, and with peritoneal inflammation small amounts of movement can be excruciating. Reflex muscle spasm in the abdominal muscles or in the psoas muscle can produce an altered gait known as the *appendicitis shuffle*.

PREHOSPITAL CARE

It is unusual for emergency medical personnel to transport children with appendicitis. Ambulance transport is more likely in cases of septic shock resulting from late recognition of this serious condition.

The emergency medical technician should recognize septic shock in a child with lethargy, impaired sensorium, and a poor response to stimuli. Whether to use a "scoop-and-run" approach with minimal treatment at the scene and rapid delivery to the emergency department or to stabilize the child at the scene is a choice that must be individualized. If stabilization at the scene is elected, an intravenous (IV) line should be started. However, IV access will likely be problematic, even under ideal circumstances, in a child in the field with septic shock caused by a perforated appendix. Transport to the emergency department should not be delayed significantly by attempts to establish IV access. Ideal solutions to use in this situation include D5 lactated Ringer's solution (D5LR) or D5/.9 normal saline (D5NS). If the child is hypotensive, a bolus of 20 ml/kg of crystalloid solution should be given immediately, with the infusion continued at 6 to 10 ml/kg/hr.[19]

CLINICAL EVALUATION

The "classic" history occurs in only 25% of cases of pediatric appendicitis[20, 21] and starts as dull, poorly localized epigastric or periumbilical pain that changes into localized right lower quadrant pain. The initial pain may be described as intermittent cramps. The character of the localized pain is unrelenting, increasing, and exacerbated by movement or pressure. Physiologically, this represents the shift from visceral to somatic or parietal pain. The patient prefers to lie still, and the pain is increased when the car strikes bumps during the ride to the hospital. Walking is almost always uncomfortable and may be impossible.

Vomiting usually occurs after the onset of pain and is typically isolated to one or two episodes. Anorexia, though common, is not universal. A fever is preceded by the pain localizing to the right lower quadrant.

Localized pain is present in 75% to 92%,[1, 22] vomiting in 70% to 75%,[1, 3, 22] dysuria in 7%,[22] and anorexia in 33% to 74% of cases.[4] Upper respiratory tract infections are seen in 20% of children with appendicitis,[3] and diarrhea is seen in 10% to 25% of cases.[1, 3, 17] Fever may occur in as few as 60% of cases.[1]

Unfortunately, no particular point in the history is pathognomonic.[3, 20-22] The best indicator from the history is steady but increasing localized pain with difficulty walking.[1, 3, 17, 23] Nevertheless, the mnemonic, Plan Now To Fly, representing Pain, Nausea (and vomiting), Tenderness, and Fever, may be useful (Table 34–1).

Examining the abdomen of a child requires a technique different from that used in the adult examination. A child must develop trust for the examiner. Thirty seconds of age-appropriate conversation and a generally nonthreatening approach can assist in obtaining a useful examination. When an adequate examination is not possible because of an inability to gain the child's cooperation, sedation may be used.[17] A short-acting barbiturate alone or a narcotic with or without a benzodiazapine may be useful. A combination of midazolam and nalbuphine or morphine, 0.1 mg/kg each, in a single syringe given intramuscularly (IM) or per rectum, is effective.[24] Most surgeons prefer to be consulted prior to the administration of any sedative or narcotic.

A systematic examination, with the abdominal component last, facilitates the physical assessment. The most tender part of the abdomen should be examined last, following a light scouting examination for rigidity. Palpating the abdomen carefully and slowly with the diaphragm of the stethoscope is less threatening to the child. This is an excellent method to assess intra-abdominal tension and distention once the examiner is familiar with the technique. Usually distention associated with appendicitis occurs with perforation or obstruction hours to days after rupture. Distention accompanying appendicitis is usually seen 2 or more days after the onset of symptoms.

The patient should be observed walking. It is rare to have a completely normal gait with appendicitis. A child bent at the waist and limping on the right foot is said to have the "appendicitis shuffle." If asked to jump, the child frequently cannot comply. The child with appendicitis typically lies still, often with the right leg flexed at the hip because of peritoneal inflammation. Writhing suggests a diagnosis other than appendicitis.

The patient with appendicitis appears toxic, which is difficult to describe objectively. Eye contact may be poor and the emotional reaction blunted, and there is a "glassy" appearance to the eyes. Consistent with this quiet affect, children with appendicitis do not tend to cry.

Bowel sounds are usually decreased, especially if perforation has occurred.[1, 15] With gastroenteritis and often with constipation, bowel tones are normal or increased.[15] With perforation and obstruction, the examiner may hear rushes, succussion splashes, and tinkling.

Tenderness is the most common finding but is not specific to appendicitis.[3, 4, 21] A ruptured appendix may even be nontender in 11% of children.[4] Classic appendiceal tenderness is well localized and associated with the rebound phenomenon in most children.[17, 22] The rebound phenomenon is observer-biased and is best elicited by a single finger or stethoscope pressure applied slowly and steadily and then stopped momentarily. The rapid release of pressure should not startle the child and thereby elicit a false-positive interpretation by the examiner. Referred tenderness phenomenon (Rovsing's sign) is seen in 25% of cases.[1] It should be elicited in the same way as primary tenderness, but with palpation in the left lower quadrant, tenderness is experienced in the right lower quadrant.

The incidence of psoas and obturator signs is variable (30% and 15%, respectively[1]) and may be difficult to interpret in the child. Pain elicited by "punching" the patient's heel while they are supine is difficult to differentiate from the discomfort produced by the maneuver itself.

A right lower quadrant mass that is minimally tender and slightly movable suggests constipation with stool in the cecum. A similar mass in the sigmoid colon palpated in the left iliac fossa helps to confirm this. A periappendiceal abscess is usually ill-defined, fixed, and extremely tender. In most cases, this finding means perforation has occurred. The mass may be obscured by guarding.

A rectal examination is essential, and coordination with the surgeon and other physicians should minimize the number of examinations. The rectal examination may contribute to the diagnosis in up to 79% of cases[25] and may also confirm other causes of abdominal pain such as constipation, ovarian cyst, or salpingitis.

Examination of the rectum is best done with the child in a lithotomy position, with the examiner slowly inserting the finger while talking to the child. A bimanual examination, similar to a pelvic examination in the female, allows the examiner to feel masses or "stagnant" bowel loops efficiently as a result of the shallow pelvis of a child. Differentiation between true peritoneal tenderness and rectal discomfort from the examination may be difficult.

Abnormal vital signs may include fever. A temperature of more than 38°C is likely, and it may reach 40°C. Tachycardia (25% over the normal rate for age) is usually seen but is nonspecific.

The hydration status, degree of sepsis, and vital organ function, particularly renal function, is important. A careful chest examination may prevent a patient with a lower lobe pneumonia from undergoing appendectomy.

TABLE 34–1			
SIGNS AND SYMPTOMS OF APPENDICITIS (PLAN NOW TO FLY)			
Pain	**Nausea**	**Tenderness**	**Fever**
Localized	Vomiting	Localized: early phase	>38.5°C usual
Crescendo	(usually one to two	Generalized: late phase	40°C if rupture has
Increases with movement	times)		occurred
	Anorexia		

In children with worrisome but nonspecific findings, the number of unnecessary explorations can be decreased by intensive, in-hospital observation.[5] One study showed that with close observation and frequent serial examinations, the diagnosis can be made with 95% accuracy.[5] No in-hospital perforations were seen with this approach, and the overall perforation rate was 27%. When observation facilities are not available in the emergency department, intensive inpatient observation may be required.

The child younger than 2 years with appendicitis presents a diagnostic problem. Physicians have misdiagnosed this condition in as many as 66% of cases at the time of hospitalization, contributing to delays in treatment in patients in this young age range.[6, 12, 14, 15, 17]

Intussusception, systemic sepsis, and gastroenteritis in the toddler have similar presentations. Fever and vomiting were present in 81% of infants and toddlers with appendicitis, but only 62% had pain. In almost half of the patients with pain (45%), the pain was colicky.[15] The only reliable physical finding was abdominal distention; localized tenderness was inconsistent. Sedation to facilitate examination is particularly useful in this age group.[17]

In most cases the very young have a left shift in the white blood cell (WBC) count differential, although the actual WBC count may be only 3000 to 10,000/mm^3 in 40% of patients.[15] Because of the difficulty in diagnosing this condition, 71% to 94% of children younger than 2 years have perforation by the time of operation.[13–15, 17] Unfortunately, the morbidity and mortality from perforation is also higher in this age group.[4, 12, 15]

DIFFERENTIAL DIAGNOSIS

Appendicitis is frequently confused with other conditions (Table 34–2). Misdiagnosis, defined as a normal appendix at laparotomy, may occur in 20% to 30% of cases.[12, 22, 26, 27] Delays in diagnosing appendicitis lead to a high rate of perforation. In a review of 344 cases from Hong Kong, 97 (28%) were perforated or gangrenous (late appendicitis) by the time of operation.[12] A preadmission delay of more than 37 hours occurred in 72% of patients with late appendicitis.

Of these, 53% were delays caused by parents, and 47% represented failure to diagnose the condition at initial presentation by medical practitioners. Other series report a 53% incidence of late appendicitis in Texas,[4] 32% in Chicago,[1] 37% in Los Angeles,[7] and 40% in St. Louis.[22] Parental delays in seeking medical attention for the child contribute to a higher rate of perforation, the risk of which greatly increases 12 hours after the onset of symptoms.[6]

A child with Meckel's diverticulitis tends to have a more toxic appearance than a child with appendicitis. The tenderness from Meckel's diverticulitis may be poorly localized. Intussusception is unusual in the child older than 15 months, and the typical finding is an empty right lower quadrant with a palpable psoas muscle. A sausage-shaped mass is felt less commonly. Later, obstruction and distention without point tenderness is more common.

Of all cases of child abuse, 15% present with an acute abdomen. Abused children are usually infants or toddlers. Typically, the history is vague, and the tenderness is poorly localized. The child may be passive and withdrawn. Rectal examination may demonstrate poor sphincter tone, fissures, or a small degree of prolapse, reflecting sexual abuse.

Primary peritonitis (i.e., from extra-abdominal sources) can mimic appendicitis. The tenderness is usually more diffuse, and distention may be more prominent. Primary peritonitis causes 13% to 17% of childhood peritonitis.[28] It occurs secondary to infection, often of an unidentified extraperitoneal organ, with bacterial invasion of the abdominal cavity.[29] The most common causes are pneumococcal pneumonia and systemic streptococcal infection.[28] It is more common in children who are immunosuppressed, nephrotic, or cirrhotic. A subset of cases of primary peritonitis occur in children with ventriculoperitoneal shunts with infection in the abdominal portion of the shunt catheter.[28]

Leukemic children can develop necrosis of the cecum, called *leukemic ileocecitis*. This condition has a high mortality.

Systemic disease with abdominal pain or paralytic ileus may mimic appendicitis. Children with pneumonia will frequently have rales, decreased breath sounds, and depressed diaphragmatic motion. Petechiae can be seen with Henoch-Schönlein purpura. Bloody stools and lethargy may be seen with either intussusception or hemolytic-uremic syndrome.

It is possible for an appendix to become inflamed in an inguinal hernia sac. Conversely, an incarcerated hernia or torsed cryptorchid testicle can closely mimic appendiceal pain. Therefore a careful inguinal examination is important.

Adnexal conditions, particularly in the postpubertal female, notoriously mimic appendicitis.[30, 31] With pelvic inflammation, symptoms take 2 to 3 days to develop; fever and chills are more common and vomiting is less common.[17] The rectal examination (and pelvic examination, if appropriate) may be diagnostic. Appendicitis is misdiagnosed more often in women because of the difficulty in differentiating it from pelvic disease,[20] even in prepubertal girls. In a study from the United Kingdom, the accuracy rate (suspected appendicitis versus true appendicitis) was 86% in boys younger than 11 years, but only 67% in girls of the same age.

Sickle cell anemia with pain crisis usually has a similar, recurrent pattern of pain[32] and may be triggered by various stressors. On examination, the only discriminating finding in sickle cell crisis may be normal bowel tones.

Solid tumors (e.g., lymphomas of the intestine, rhabdomyosarcomas and teratomas of the retroperitoneum, Wilms' tumors, and neuroblastomas) can be confused with a periappendiceal mass.[33] Typically, a tumor is better circumscribed and less tender than an abscess.

Gastroenteritis and constipation are common causes of abdominal pain requiring differentiation from appendicitis. Gastroenteritis may have profuse diarrhea and fecal leuko-

---

TABLE 34–2

DIFFERENTIAL DIAGNOSIS

Primary considerations
  Gastroenteritis
  Constipation
  Intussusception
  Primary peritonitis
  Ileus
  Lower lobe pneumonia
  Ectopic pregnancy
  Mesenteric adenitis
Secondary considerations
  Henoch-Schönlein purpura
  Hemolytic-uremic syndrome
  Inguinal hernia
  Torsed cryptorchid testicle
  Tubo-ovarian abscess
  Salpingo-oophoritis
  Sickle cell crisis
  Abdominal tumors (lymphomas, neuroblastomas, etc.)
  Intra-abdominal abscess
  Omental torsion
  Acute intermittent porphyria
  Sepsis
  Meckel's diverticulitis
  Leukemic ileocecitis

cytes on a stool smear. The abdominal pain is usually cramp-like, with intervals of relief. Tenderness may be located throughout the lower abdomen, and bowel tones are usually hyperactive. There may be minor, diffuse peritoneal signs, probably because of bacterial translocation or generalized serositis.

Constipation is the most common condition mistaken for appendicitis. The stool pattern may be normal, which erroneously leads to early exclusion of constipation as the diagnosis. Constipation can sometimes cause a slightly impaired gait. It may also be associated with McBurney's point tenderness and, infrequently, the rebound phenomenon, probably because of an inflamed, distended cecum or anterior peritoneal irritation. With constipation, the white blood cell count and, rarely, the band cell count may be elevated. Typically, there is less incidence of tachycardia and fever when compared with appendicitis, and more importantly, the pain from constipation is colicky in character. The patient can usually move comfortably, and there is no toxic appearance. Palpable, doughy masses in the iliac fossae that are minimally tender aid in the diagnosis of constipation.

The signs and symptoms of mesenteric adenitis closely approximate those of acute appendicitis.[31, 34] This condition frequently has a viral prodrome. The tenderness associated with mesenteric adenitis may be more diffuse and tends not to progress or localize. Mesenteric adenitis, proven by positive mesenteric node cultures, is probably both rare and over-diagnosed.[5, 29, 34]

Of children with a normal appendix at laparotomy, 7% to 21% have another condition requiring surgery.[10, 29, 35] This confirms the difficulty in making an accurate preoperative diagnosis but reinforces the need for an aggressive approach to abdominal pain. When 12 to 48 hours have lapsed from the onset of symptoms, there is an increased risk of perforation and its complications.[2, 6, 17] In the final analysis, a negative laparotomy is safer than a perforated appendix.

DIAGNOSTIC EVALUATION
Laboratory Studies

Experience proves that the diagnosis of appendicitis is fraught with clinical inaccuracy.[3, 6, 7, 12, 20, 21, 26, 36] Although no specific laboratory test is diagnostic, such information may be useful. Of children with appendicitis at the time of laparotomy, only 4% had a normal WBC count and a normal band cell count.[37] Leukocytosis or a left shift (increased immature polymorphonuclear neutrophils) is not specific for appendicitis. WBC counts above 14,000 to 16,000/mm³ may be associated with gangrene and perforation,[1, 37] warranting aggressive pursuit of a correct diagnosis. The erythrocyte sedimentation rate may not be elevated until 24 hours after symptoms begin, when perforation may have already occurred.[6] The C-reactive protein (CRP) level is elevated earlier in the course of the illness. One series showed that the CRP level was elevated in all patients with acute appendicitis who had symptoms present for 12 or more hours.[38] However, 50% of patients with no identifiable cause of abdominal pain also had an elevated CRP level.[38] A negative CRP result determined less than 12 hours after the onset of symptoms does not exclude the diagnosis of appendicitis.

The urine frequently contains white blood cells or bacteria, as the inflamed appendix may be near the bladder.[39] A urine Gram stain test showing gram-negative rods is a strong indicator of a urinary tract infection, rather than appendicitis.

Aggressive preoperative resuscitation is essential for an optimal outcome.[16, 40] If the patient has been repeatedly vomiting or has been symptomatic for more than 18 hours,

serum electrolytes, creatinine, and urine specific gravity should be measured. In the child with suspected perforation, a serum bicarbonate level of less than 22 mEq/L suggests metabolic acidosis and the need for aggressive fluid resuscitation. Evaluation of the creatinine and blood urea nitrogen (BUN) is also useful in the septic, dehydrated child at risk for renal failure.

Radiologic Studies

Most radiologic studies do not by themselves diagnose appendicitis, though they can enhance the clinical assessment. Plain radiographs are helpful less than 50% of the time[41]; contrast studies and ultrasound are more useful. Radiographic findings associated with appendicitis include a fecalith (7% to 12%), gas in the appendix (2%), a sentinel loop (20%), right lower quadrant mass effect (12% to 33%), loss of properitoneal flank stripe (5%), and cecal deformity (5%).[41] Other than the fecalith, none of these findings are specific for appendicitis (Fig. 34–1). A fecalith in a patient with abdominal pain is an indication for appendectomy because of the high rate of perforation.[42] The sentinel loop in appendicitis is localized and slightly distended.

Constipation typically has a stippled appearance in the cecum without other signs of appendicitis. Nevertheless, these findings may also be seen in some cases of appendicitis. Multiple air-fluid levels throughout the abdomen and without accompanying distended bowel loops suggest gastroenteritis. A chest radiograph may show a lower lobe pneumonia (Fig. 34–2).

The barium enema can be used to diagnose appendicitis.[43–46] Perforation from this procedure is rare.[44] One report involving 48 subjects had no false-positive or false-negative

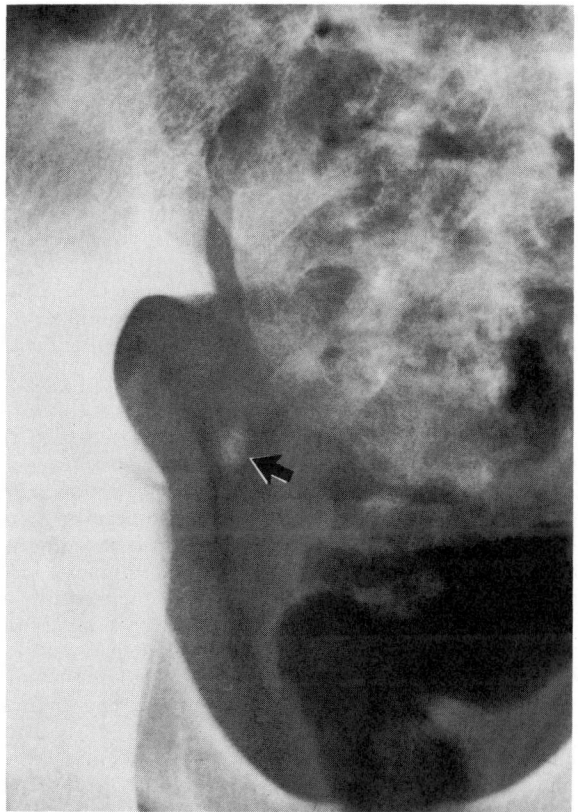

Figure 34–1. Arrow demonstrates an appendicolith in the right lower quadrant. Appendicitis was confirmed at laparotomy. (Courtesy of Dr. Kenneth Thorp.)

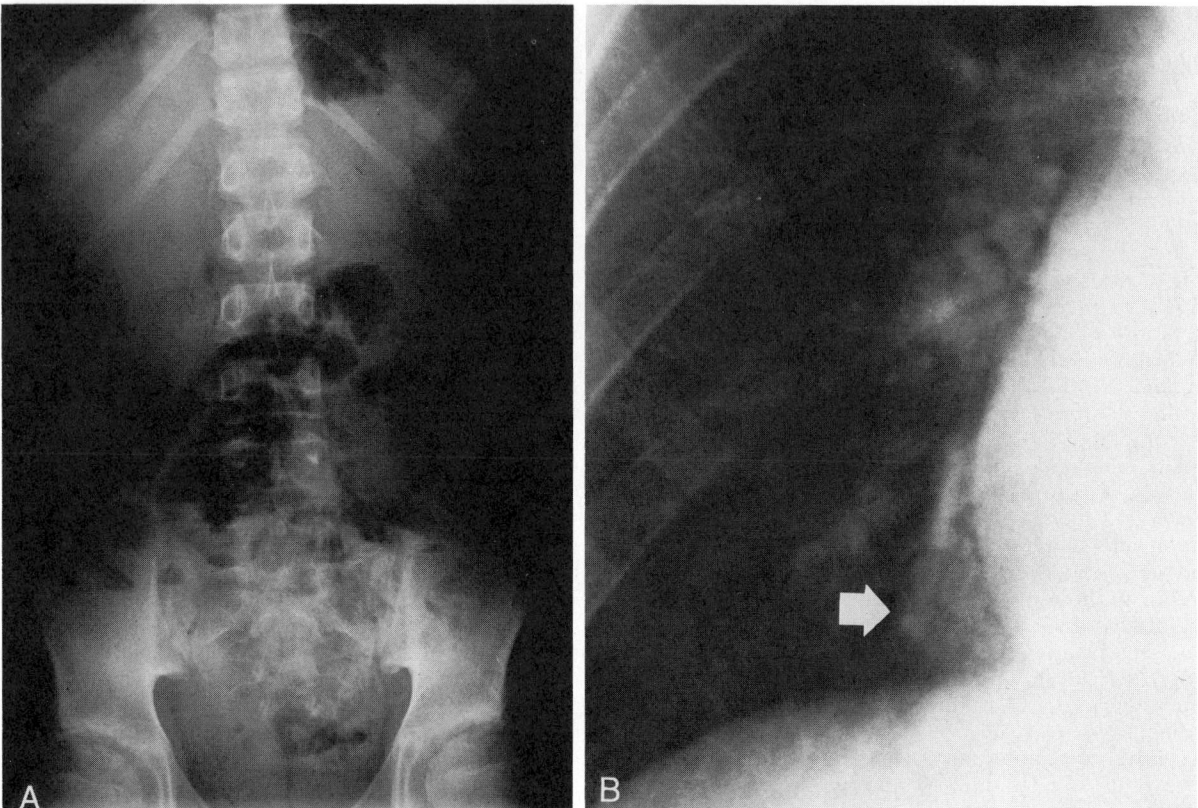

Figure 34–2. This 10-year-old boy was thought to have appendicitis. The flat plate of the abdomen *(A)* shows a mild adynamic ileus. The chest radiograph *(B)* shows a small, localized infiltrate in the right lower lobe *(arrow)*, which proved to be the cause of the pain.

results. This procedure is recommended in problem cases, particularly in young children and those with chronic illnesses, in whom accurate diagnosis is both important and difficult.[46]

Ultrasound also enhances the ability to diagnose appendicitis in difficult cases. One investigator reported that the sensitivity of ultrasound was greater in equivocal cases than in those with definite clinical findings.[47] In equivocal cases, ultrasonic evaluation correlated with surgically proven appendicitis in 96% of patients and was 94% correct in patients without appendicitis.[47] Ultrasound was accurate in women, and reliably differentiated pelvic disease from appendicitis.[48]

THERAPEUTIC INTERVENTION

Acute appendicitis is a surgical emergency. Intravenous fluid resuscitation and urgent operative intervention are the mainstays of therapy.[1, 7, 16] Fluid resuscitation can be accomplished with D5/.45 NS saline in patients who have not been vomiting excessively. In patients with large fluid losses from vomiting, D5/.9 normal saline (D5NS) or D5 lactated Ringer's (D5LR) solution should be administered. Potassium chloride (usually 20 to 30 mEq/L) should be added to replace any potassium losses. The potassium can be added immediately; the risk of hyperkalemia from unrecognized renal failure is extremely low.

A child who has been vomiting for 24 hours may require significant fluid replacement. Hypochloremic alkalosis, particularly in the younger child, may require increased potassium and fluid administration. Emesis-induced hypochloremic, hypokalemic metabolic alkalosis may need correction with sodium chloride and potassium chloride to achieve a chloride concentration of 100 to 110 mEq/L prior to surgery.

With peritonitis, third space fluid losses must also be considered. An additional one fourth of the maintenance requirement of D5NS or D5LR should be infused for each abdominal quadrant with signs of peritonitis.[48]

A thorough examination of the abdomen is performed under anesthesia prior to laparotomy. If no abdominal mass is felt, a transverse skin incision is made over McBurney's point. The wound may be closed, but delayed primary closure results in a decreased rate of infection in the ruptured appendix.[1, 7, 22] Criteria for delayed primary closure may include perforation and obesity. Unless there is a well-localized abscess cavity, the abdomen is not drained.[1, 49, 50]

Laparoscopy is increasingly being used both diagnostically and therapeutically in cases of abdominal pain and appendicitis. The surgeon individualizes those cases in which laparoscopy is preferable to open appendectomy.

A perforated appendix can be removed in most patients. In rare cases where removal is hazardous, the appendiceal abscess is drained with suction drains through the lateral edge of the open wound or through a separate stab incision.[51] An interval appendectomy should be performed after 4 to 6 weeks.

The wound infection rate in nonperforated appendicitis is about 5%.[16, 22] Use of perioperative antibiotics is controversial; however, they have been shown to decrease the wound infection rate to approximately 2%.[5, 7, 52–54] Perioperative antibiotics in nonperforated appendicitis should be administered preoperatively and continued postoperatively for 24 hours. One review of prophylactic antibiotics recom-

---

TABLE 34–3

APPENDICITIS: THERAPY AT A GLANCE

Fluid replacement
  Initial bolus: 20 ml/kg D5NS or D5LR
  Maintenance infusion: 6–10 ml/kg/hr D5/.2 NS
Sedation and analgesia
  Midazolam: 0.1 mg/kg per rectum or IM
  Nalbuphine: 0.1 mg/kg per rectum or IM
  Morphine: 0.1 mg/kg IM
Antibiotics
  Cefoxitin
    Children over 3 months of age: 80–160 mg/kg/day
      divided q 4–6 hr
    Adult: 1–2 g q 6–8 hr
  Ampicillin: 100 mg/kg/24 hr divided q 6 hr
  Gentamicin: 5 mg/kg/24 hr
  Clindamycin: 40 mg/kg/24 hr

---

mends one dose of cefoxitin (Table 34–3) preoperatively, with three doses after surgery.[55] However, cefoxitin may be less effective than combinations of aminoglycosides, synthetic penicillins, and metronidazole in treating perforated appendicitis.[56]

Most postoperative complications occurring with appendicitis are infections related to perforation.[1, 3, 57] Early appendicitis is usually associated with *Escherichia coli* infection. As necrosis and gangrene progress, anaerobes are more likely to be recovered, especially *Bacteroides fragilis*.[54, 56, 58] In the child with a suspected perforated appendix, antibiotics for treating anaerobic organisms are required.[22] Preoperative administration of triple antibiotics such as ampicillin (100 mg/kg/24 hr), gentamicin (5 mg/kg/24 hr), and clindamycin (40 mg/kg/24 hr) has been used since the mid 1970s.[54] Combinations of synthetic penicillins, expanded-spectrum cephalosporins, and metronidazole are frequently used with good results.[59–62] For children with a perforated appendix, antibiotic administration should be continued for at least 1 week postoperatively.[1, 12, 55] Perioperative use of antibiotics in children with a perforated appendix should result in a wound infection rate of 7% and an incidence of intra-abdominal abscesses of 7%.[54, 57, 63]

Some cases of perforation will wall off by themselves. If the child is otherwise healthy, oral antibiotics (metronidazole or a cephalosporin) can be given at home and an interval appendectomy performed later.[51, 64] The risk of recurrent appendicitis is 5% to 20% if the appendectomy is not performed.[51] Any evidence of recrudescence or evolving peritonitis is an indication for earlier surgery.

OUTCOME

Patients with nonperforated appendicitis are usually able to eat within 24 hours of laparotomy and have an average hospital stay of less than 3 days. Children can usually return to school in 1 week and back to athletic activities in 2 to 3 weeks.

Late or perforated appendicitis significantly increases morbidity. Wound infections usually occur from mixed aerobic and anaerobic organisms and are treated with open drainage.[57] Intestinal obstruction or ileus within the first week usually resolves with nasogastric suction. Surgical drainage of abscesses in children is not as necessary as in adults.[1] However, antibiotic coverage for anaerobic organisms may be needed for an additional 1 to 2 weeks. Ultrasound or CT-guided needle drainage can also be used.[27] An increased incidence of female sterility with a perforated

appendix has been postulated; however, scientific and epidemiologic work refutes this contention.[65]

Pylephlebitis is a rare but sometimes fatal complication of appendicitis.[66] It results from the spread of appendiceal inflammation along the mesenteric veins through the portal system. This may cause diffuse liver abscesses, leading to subsequent portal vein thrombosis and portal hypertension. Death from this condition is less common since the advent of antibiotics.[66]

As in-hospital stays become shorter, more patients with postoperative complications will appear in the emergency department. These complications are usually related to an infectious process. Wound infections are diagnosed by fever, tenderness, and swelling of the incision. Deep infections may not show redness or fluctuance. Intra-abdominal abscesses may present with fever, sepsis, ileus, and diffuse tenderness. The WBC count, band cell count, and CRP level are usually elevated. Ultrasound or CT scan can be diagnostic.[27]

Some wound abscesses may be treated with drainage but without antibiotics. Because some postoperative complications may be life threatening, early involvement of the surgeon is requisite.

DOCUMENTATION

Documentation in the medical record should include the time course of each major symptom (Table 34–4). All symptoms should be listed, with attention to the anatomic and chronologic description of pain. The systems review should be elicited and, where relevant, documented. Concomitant diseases and medical conditions should be noted.

The physical examination should be described in enough detail to support the final diagnosis. In particular, details concerning tenderness and the presence of peritoneal signs should be noted. The overall condition of the child, especially regarding hydration and possible sepsis, should be recorded. An interpretation of the radiographic and laboratory findings should also be included. The times of the emergency physician's discussion with the surgeon and the surgeon's first contact with the child should be documented.

Following discussion with the surgeon, the management plan should be documented, including antibiotic treatment, fluid therapy, and timing of surgery and admission.

DISPOSITION

If appendicitis is strongly suspected, laparotomy is indicated. In cases in which appendicitis is a consideration but the clinical presentation is not clear enough to warrant appendectomy, the child should be hospitalized. Serial phys-

---

TABLE 34–4

DOCUMENTATION AND DISCHARGE INSTRUCTIONS

Documentation
  Time course of major symptoms
  Anatomic and chronologic description of pain
  Peritoneal signs
  Hydration status
  Presence of sepsis
  Physician-physician and physician-patient interaction times
  Laboratory and radiographic findings
  Managment plan
Discharge instructions
  Scheduled recheck with family or emergency department
    physician in 8–12 hr
  Return immediately if condition worsens
  Eat or drink nothing before re-examination

ical examinations and repeat WBC counts should be performed. Increased tenderness, pain localizing to the right lower quadrant, or evidence of peritonitis support the diagnosis of appendicitis requiring laparotomy.

Not all children with abdominal pain require admission. If the history, physical examination, and laboratory evaluation support a less serious diagnosis, the child can be sent home and scheduled for a reexamination. A recheck by the same examiner 8 to 12 hours later is ideal. If the patient is to be reevaluated, he or she should not eat or drink between examinations, so that if surgery is required, the stomach will be empty. The signs and symptoms of appendicitis should be explained to the parents and child. If any new signs or symptoms suggesting appendicitis appear, or if the condition worsens in any way, the child must be seen immediately.

SUMMARY

Appendicitis is a source of significant morbidity in childhood. Most of this morbidity is associated with the ruptured appendix. A significant number of children are sent home from the emergency department with an acutely inflamed appendix; this is especially true in younger children, in whom the morbidity is greater and the diagnosis more difficult to determine. In all children with abdominal pain, clinical suspicion of appendicitis, a complete history, and serial physical examinations are essential for the early diagnosis of this condition.

Appropriate use of available diagnostic modalities may facilitate the early recognition of this surgical emergency. Ideally, stronger clinical suspicion on the part of the primary care physician will lead to earlier referral to the emergency department or to a surgeon.

References

1. Samelson SL, Reyes HM. Management of perforated appendicitis in children—revisited. Arch Surg 1987;122:691.
2. Deck KB, Pettitt BJ, Harrison MR. The length-time correlate in appendicitis. JAMA 1980;244:806.
3. Rappaport WD, Peterson M, Stanton C. Factors responsible for the high perforation rate seen in early childhood appendicitis. Am Surg 1989;55:602.
4. McFee AS, Rogers W. Diagnosing appendicitis in the pediatric patient. Infect Surg 1982;42.
5. White JJ, Santillana M, Haller JA. Intensive in-hospital observation: A safe way to decrease unnecessary appendectomy. Am Surg 1975;41:793.
6. Brender JD, Marcuse EK, Koepsell TD, et al. Childhood appendicitis: Factors associated with perforation. Pediatrics 1985;76:301.
7. Meade RH. The evolution of surgery for appendicitis. Surgical history. Surgery 1964;55:741.
8. Hall RJ. Suppurative peritonitis due to ulceration and perforation of the vermiform appendix: Laparotomy; resection of the vermiform appendix, toilette of the peritoneum: drainage, recovery. NY Med J 1886;43:662.
9. Fitz RH. Perforating inflammation of the vermiform appendix, with references to its early diagnosis and treatment. Am J Med Sci 1886;2:321.
10. McBurney C. Experience with early operative interference in cases of disease of the vermiform appendix. NY Med J 1889;50:676.
11. Cacioppo JC, Diettrich NA, Kaplan G, et al. The consequences of current constraints on surgical treatment of appendicitis. Am J Surg 1989;157:276.
12. Lau WY, Fan ST, Yip WC, et al. Acute appendicitis in children. Aust NZ J Surg 1987;57:927.
13. Ellis H. Clinical Anatomy: A Revision and Applied Anatomy for Clinical Students. 7th ed. Oxford, Blackwell Scientific, 1983, p 76.
14. Bartlett RH, Eraklis AJ, Wilkinson RH. Appendicitis in infancy. Surg Gynecol Obstet 1970;130:99.
15. Grosfeld JL, Weinberger M, Clatworthy HW Jr. Acute appendicitis in the first two years of life. J Pediatr Surg 1973;8:285.
16. Janik JS, Firor HV. Pediatric Appendicitis: A 20-year study of 1,640 children at Cook County (Illinois) Hospital. Arch Surg 1979;114:717.
17. Graham JM, Pokorny WJ, Harberg FJ. Acute appendicitis in preschool age children. Am J Surg 1980;139:247.
18. Aach RD. Abdominal pain. *In* MacBryde CM, Blacklow R (eds). Signs and Symptoms. Fifth ed. Philadelphia, JB Lippincott, 1979, pp 165–179.
19. Rowe MI, Pettitt BJ. Management of the critically ill patient. *In* Welch KJ, Randolph JG, Ravitch MM, et al (eds). Pediatric Surgery. 4th ed. Chicago, Year Book, 1986.
20. Lewis FR, Holcroft JW, Boey J, et al. Appendicitis: A critical review of diagnosis and treatment in 1,000 cases. Arch Surg 1975;110:677.
21. Teicher I, Landa B, Cohen M, et al. Scoring system to aid in diagnosis of appendicitis. Ann Surg 1983;198:753.
22. Bower RJ, Bell MJ, Ternberg JL. Controversial aspects of appendicitis management in children. Arch Surg 1981;116:885.
23. Anand KJS, Carr DB. The neuroanatomy, neurophysiology, and neurochemistry of pain, stress and analgesia in newborns and children. Pediatr Clin North Am 1989;36:795.
24. Snodgrass WR, Dodge WF. Lytic/"DPT" cocktail: Time for rational and safe alternatives. Pediatr Clin North Am 1989;36:1285.
25. Bonello JC, Abrams JS. The significance of a "positive" rectal examination in acute appendicitis. Dis Colon Rectum 1979;22:97.
26. Ochsner A. The conservative treatment of appendiceal peritonitis. New Orleans Med Surg J 1934;87:32.
27. Gilmore OJ, Browett JP, Griffin PH, et al. Appendicitis and mimicking conditions. A prospective study. Lancet 1975,2;421.
28. Ein SH. Primary peritonitis in pediatric surgery. *In* Welch KJ, Randolph JG, Ravitch MM, et al (eds). Pediatric Surgery. 4th ed. Chicago, Year Book, 1986, pp 976, 977.
29. Bell MJ, Bower RJ, Ternberg JL. Appendectomy in childhood. Analysis of 105 negative explorations. Am J Surg 1982;144:335.
30. Thal ER, Guzzetta PC, Krupski WC, et al. Morbidity of appendectomy in patients with acute salpingitis. Am Surg 1977;43:403.
31. Herrington JL Jr. Acute suppurative mesenteric lymphadenitis. Am Surg 1969;35:405.
32. Kevy SV. Surgical implications of hematologic disorders. *In* Welch KJ, Randolph JG, Ravitch MM, et al (eds). Pediatric Surgery, 4th ed. Chicago, Year Book, 1986, p 110.
33. Stevenson RJ. Abdominal masses. Surg Clin North Am 1985;65:1481.
34. Asch MJ, Amoury RA, Touloukian RJ, et al. Suppurative mesenteric lymphadenitis: A report of two cases and review of the literature. Am J Surg 1968;115:570.
35. Knight PJ, Vassy LE. Specific diseases mimicking appendicitis in childhood. Arch Surg 1981;116:744.
36. Douville EC, Birinyi LK, Stevenson FJ. Complicated appendicitis in children. Surgery 1986;33.
37. Bower RJ, Bell MJ, Ternberg JL. Diagnostic value of the white blood count and neutrophil percentage in the evaluation of abdominal pain in children. Surg Gynecol Obstet 1981;152:424.
38. Thimsen DA, Tong GK, Gruenberg JC. Prospective evaluation of C-reactive protein in patients suspected to have acute appendicitis. Am Surg 1989;55:466.
39. Arnbjornsson E. Bacteriuria in appendicitis. Am J Surg 1988;155:356.
40. Schwartz MZ, Tapper D, Solenberger RI. Management of perforated appendicitis in children. The controversy continues. Ann Surg 1983;197:407.
41. Shimkin PM. Radiology of acute appendicitis. AJR 1978;130:1001.
42. Copeland EM, Long JM. Elective appendectomy for appendiceal calculus. Surg Gynecol Obstet 1970;130:439.
43. Soter CS. The use of barium in the diagnosis of acute appendiceal disease; a new radiological sign. Clin Radiol 1968;19:410.
44. Garcia C, Rosenfield NS, Markowitz RI, et al. Appendicitis in children. Accuracy of the barium enema. Am J Dis Child 1987;141:1309.
45. Smith DE, Kirchmer NA, Stewart DR. Use of the barium enema in the diagnosis of acute appendicitis and its complications. Am J Surg 1979;138:829.
46. Lewin GA, Mikity V, Wingert WA. Barium enema: An outpatient procedure in the early diagnosis of acute appendicitis. J Pediatr 1978;92:451.
47. Larson JM, Peirce JC, Ellinger DM, et al. The validity and utility of sonograph in the diagnosis of appendicitis in the community setting. Am J Radiol 1989;153:687.
48. Filston HC, Izant RJ. The Surgical Neonate. Norwalk, CT, Appleton-Century-Crofts, 1985, p 15.
49. Haller JA, Shaker IJ, Donahoo JS, et al. Peritoneal drainage versus non-drainage for generalized peritonitis from ruptured appendicitis in children. A prospective study. Ann Surg 1973;177:595.
50. MacKellar A, Mackay AJ. Wound and intraperitoneal infection following appendicectomy for perforated or gangrenous appendicitis. Aust NZ J Surg 1986;56:489.
51. Buntain WL, Custer D. Management of the ruptured pediatric appendix: A place for the interval appendectomy. Contemp Surg 1984;24:23.
52. Winslow RE, Dean RE, Harley JW. Acute nonperforating appendicitis. Efficacy of brief antibiotic prophylaxis. Arch Surg 1983;118:651.
53. Wright JE. Appendicitis in childhood: Reduction in wound infection with preoperative antibiotics. Aust NZ J Surg 1982;52:127.
54. Gilbert SR, Emmens RW, Putnam TC. Appendicitis in children. Surg Gynecol Obstet 1985;161:261.
55. Kaiser AB. Antimicrobial prophylaxis in surgery. N Engl J Med 1986;315:1129.
56. Leigh DA, Simmons K, Norman E. Bacterial flora of the appendix fossa in appendicitis and postoperative wound infection. J Clin Pathol 1974;27:997.

57. Marchildon MB, Dudgeon DL. Perforated appendicitis: Current experience in Childrens Hospital. Ann Surg 1977;185:84.
58. Brook I. Bacterial studies of peritoneal cavity and postoperative surgical wound drainage following perforated appendix in children. Ann Surg 1980;192:208.
59. Stone HH, Strom PR, Fabian TC, et al. Third-generation cephalosporins for polymicrobial surgical sepsis. Arch Surg 1983;118:193.
60. Drusano GL, Warren JW, Saah AJ, et al. A prospective randomized controlled trial of cefoxitin versus clindamycin-aminoglycoside in mixed anaerobic-aerobic infections. Surg Gynecol Obstet 1982;154:715.
61. Kortelainen P, Huttunen R, Kairaluoma MI, et al. Single-dose intrarectal metronidazole prophylaxis against wound infection after appendectomy. Am J Surg 1982;143:244.
62. Saario I, Arvilommi H, Silvola H. Comparison of cefuroxime and gentamicin in combination with metronidazole in the treatment of peritonitis due to perforation of the appendix. Acta Chir Scand 1983;149:423.
63. Fine M, Busuttil RW. Acute appendicitis: Efficacy of prophylactic preoperative antibiotics in the reduction of septic morbidity. Am J Surg 1976;135:210.
64. Foran B, Berne TV, Rosoff L. Management of the appendiceal mass. Arch Surg 1978;113:1144.
65. Puri P, McGuinness EPJ, Guiney EJ. Fertility following perforated appendicitis in girls. J Pediatr Surg 1989;24:547.
66. Slovis TL, Haller JO, Cohen HL, et al. Complicated appendiceal inflammatory disease in children: Pylephlebitis and liver abscess. Radiology 1989;171:823.

CHAPTER 35

Gastrointestinal Hemorrhage

Phil B. Fontanarosa

INTRODUCTION

Few other pediatric medical emergencies are more frightening for the child, more alarming for the parents, or require more skillful clinical judgment by the physician than acute gastrointestinal (GI) hemorrhage. Although the episode may vary in severity from minor anorectal bleeding to exsanguinating variceal hemorrhage, the majority of cases of GI bleeding in infants and children are mild.[1] Consequently, the potential severity of the problem can be easily underestimated, thereby placing some children at risk for unrecognized serious hemorrhage.[2]

PATHOPHYSIOLOGY

The majority of cases of pediatric GI hemorrhage occur secondary to direct damage to the GI tract mucosa and usually involve inflammation or erosion extending to the mucosal vasculature.[3] Potential causes of the underlying mucosal lesion are myriad and include chemical (e.g., peptic ulcer disease), infectious (e.g., bacterial colitis), or drug-induced (e.g., aspirin) processes; stress-related processes; vascular malformations; elevated portal pressures (e.g., esophageal varices); allergic disorders (e.g., milk allergy); ischemic processes (e.g., intussusception); structural abnormalities (e.g., Meckel's diverticulum, polyps); local trauma (e.g., anal fissure, Mallory-Weiss syndrome); and hemorrhagic disorders.[1, 3, 4]

Upper GI hemorrhage is usually associated with hematemesis, melena, or both. Hematemesis, or vomited blood, localizes the bleeding site proximal to the ligament of Treitz (esophagus, stomach, or proximal duodenum). It occurs in one half to two thirds of cases of upper GI hemorrhage, but its absence does not exclude an upper GI bleeding source.[5, 6] Hematemesis may be bright red or have a "coffee grounds" appearance, with the character of emesis dependent on the mixture of blood with stomach contents and the time of vomiting relative to the time of bleeding. Bright red, bloody emesis signifies ongoing or recent hemorrhage, whereas darker or "coffee grounds" emesis suggests that the bleeding has slowed or stopped. "Coffee grounds" emesis indicates that blood has been residing in the stomach for a period of time and that gastric acid has degraded heme to hematin.[7]

Melena is black, pasty, tarry, foul-smelling stool that results from alteration of blood by bacteria and digestive enzymes. The character and color of digested blood depends on the amount, rapidity, and site of bleeding, as well as on the speed of transport through the GI tract. Approximately 60 to 100 ml of blood are necessary to produce a melanotic stool,[8] and at least 4 hours are required for the appearance of melena after an acute bleeding episode.[7, 9] In 90% of cases, melanotic stool is a result of an upper GI bleeding source, although distal small intestinal or right-sided colonic bleeding may produce melena, provided the GI transit time is sufficiently prolonged.[8, 10]

Hematochezia, or the passage of bright red or maroon stool through the rectum, generally originates in the colon or anorectal region. Less commonly, hematochezia is associated with a serious episode of brisk, upper GI bleeding and rapid bowel transit time. Dark red blood with mucus in the stool resembling currant jelly suggests vascular compromise of the intestine and is classically associated with intussusception.[11, 12] The passage of small amounts of bright red blood through the rectum, usually described as *streaking the stool*, is the most common reason pediatric patients present with GI bleeding and usually represents an anorectal disorder.

Hemodynamic Response

The hemodynamic response to hemorrhage includes an increase in cardiac output, improved cardiac contractility, an elevated heart rate, and peripheral vasoconstriction. Mechanisms that help restore lost circulatory volume include intense arteriolar and venular vasoconstriction, interstitial fluid shift into the intravascular space, contraction of the venous capacitance system, and salt and water retention on the renal level.[13]

The observable hemodynamic response to blood loss depends on the amount of hemorrhage, the underlying health of the patient, and, most importantly, the rapidity of blood loss. If acute blood loss is not overwhelming, early signs of hemorrhagic shock may be subtle or even undetectable. Because of the resiliency of the pediatric cardiovascular system, children can maintain nearly normal blood pressure even in the presence of serious hemorrhage.[13] Except for cool skin temperature and an elevated heart rate for age, signs of hemodynamic compromise may be subtle, even with as much as a 15% reduction in blood volume. By the time frank signs of shock appear (e.g., hypotension, significant tachycardia, and evidence of decreased cardiac output), 25% to 30% of blood volume has been lost.[14, 15]

EMERGENCY MEDICAL SERVICE CONSIDERATIONS

As with all prehospital emergencies, initial priorities for the pediatric patient with acute GI hemorrhage include airway, breathing, and circulation. Cool skin temperature and mild tachycardia may be the only observable signs, if any, in the early stages of hemorrhagic shock. Even though hypotension is a late sign, blood pressure must be accurately determined. A blood pressure cuff of appropriate size (i.e., width 20% larger than arm diameter) must be used to avoid an error in blood pressure measurement.[14, 16]

Gaining intravenous (IV) access is perhaps the most challenging aspect of prehospital management of pediatric GI hemorrhage. Inserting IV lines is difficult enough under ideal conditions in the emergency department, and doing so in the field may be impossible when confronted with a frightened, uncooperative, volume-depleted child. Intravenous access should be established en route to the hospital and should not delay transport. For life-threatening hemorrhage requiring immediate resuscitation, insertion of an intraosseous line may be used as a temporizing measure if IV access is unobtainable.[17–20]

Although somewhat controversial, the pediatric pneumatic antishock garment (PASG) is included in many prehospital protocols for the bleeding, hypotensive child. The PASG does not autotransfuse significant amounts of blood from the legs to the central circulation; instead, it augments preload, increases systemic vascular resistance, and mobilizes small amounts of blood to the upper body above the device.[21–24] Hemodynamic responses include improved blood pressure, improved carotid artery perfusion, and increased upper body blood flow. The PASG has been shown to be effective in helping to control GI hemorrhage,[25–27] and it may enhance the ability of prehospital providers to start IV lines.[28]

Patients with hematemesis should have their heads elevated 30 degrees to lessen the chance of aspiration.[29] Although the Trendelenburg position is often used for patients in shock, it provides little benefit in the management of hemorrhage and should be avoided. The Trendelenburg position has minimal effect on blood pressure and central venous pressure, causes a decrease in cardiac stroke volume, and increases the potential for aspiration and respiratory difficulty.[30, 31]

Substantial heat loss and significant hypothermia can occur rapidly in exposed children, compounding the acidosis and poor perfusion caused by the GI hemorrhage. Measures to ensure heat conservation (e.g., limiting exposure and covering the patient with blankets) should be routinely employed.

Early communication with the medical control physician and advanced notification of the destination hospital are essential for prehospital decision making, for preparation of the emergency department for patient arrival, for ensuring availability of necessary consultants (e.g., gastroenterologists and surgeons), and for alerting key support services, such as the blood bank and intensive care unit, of the impending need for their services.

CLINICAL EVALUATION

History

Fortunately, most children presenting to the emergency department with GI bleeding have lost only small amounts of blood and are usually hemodynamically stable. In many cases, historical features provide important diagnostic information. Several key areas should be explored.

The physician should determine whether the patient truly has GI tract bleeding. Not all patients with red emesis or black stools have GI hemorrhage. A number of common substances may color the GI contents and simulate bleeding. Beets, red dye, rifampin, or food coloring (such as occurs in Jello, Kool-Aid, candy, soft drinks, and some antibiotic syrups) may give the appearance of bloody emesis or stool. Intake of iron, bismuth (Pepto-Bismol), blueberries, black licorice, grapes, spinach, charcoal, or black food coloring may simulate melena.[32]

The possibility of a nongastrointestinal bleeding source should also be considered. Epistaxis, dental procedures, maxillofacial or oral trauma, pharyngitis, or hemoptysis may cause small amounts of blood to be swallowed, with subsequent apparent hematemesis. Blood in the diaper of a female infant may also pose diagnostic difficulties, as the bladder, vagina, and anorectum are all possible bleeding sources.[12]

The volume and character of bleeding must be assessed, but the history may be an unreliable estimate of the magnitude of bleeding. For example, as little as 10 ml of blood is enough to color toilet water red[10]; conversely, exsanguinating GI hemorrhage can occur without obvious bleeding from the stomach or rectum, although this is rare.[5, 8] Furthermore, because parents may overestimate or exaggerate the volume of blood loss, asking them to relate the amount of observed bleeding to familiar measurements (such as a teaspoonful, cupful, or quart) can be helpful to approximate the amount of blood lost.[1] The character of GI bleeding (e.g., whether emesis or stool was bright red or dark) may suggest the nature and rapidity of bleeding.

Associated gastrointestinal symptoms should be evaluated. The presence of abdominal pain, especially that which increases just prior or corresponds to acute bleeding, suggests a mucosal lesion such as an erosion or ulceration or a more complex problem such as intestinal ischemia.[40] On the other hand, major GI hemorrhage, such as from esophageal varices, often occurs without significant abdominal pain. Although antecedent vomiting is a nonspecific symptom, an episode of protracted vomiting or severe wretching preceding hematemesis suggests a Mallory-Weiss tear; precedent emesis is only noted in 60% of such cases.[41, 42] Symptoms such as fever, chills, and bloody diarrhea suggest an invasive bacterial infection.

The medical history, underlying medical conditions, bleeding disorders, medications, and family history should be determined. Preexisting GI disorders (e.g., peptic ulcer disease, inflammatory bowel syndrome, or liver disorders), as well as prior episodes of GI hemorrhage, may provide important clues to the origin of the current episode and frequently suggest a possible bleeding source. Recent significant stressful events, including surgery, birth trauma, burns, and accidental trauma, are associated with stress ulcerations.[40] Unexplained bruising or frequent minor episodes of gum bleeding or epistaxis may indicate an undiagnosed bleeding disorder.

A history of medications and any other ingested substances is essential. Aspirin, nonsteroidal anti-inflammatory drugs (NSAIDs), anticoagulants (warfarin), iron preparations, steroids, chemotherapeutic agents, and alcohol are possible contributing factors in bleeding in older children. Introduction of new milk formula can cause bleeding in infants. A family history of ulcer disease, polyposis syndromes, or inflammatory bowel disease should stimulate consideration of these possibilities.

Finally, although the majority of patients with GI hemorrhage have a history of hematemesis, "coffee grounds" emesis, hematochezia, or melena, GI bleeding should also be considered whenever a patient presents with symptoms of volume depletion (e.g., syncope, dizziness, confusion, weakness, or diaphoresis), unexplained hypotension, tachycardia, or anemia.

Physical Examination

Assessment of cardiovascular stability is the most important aspect of the physical examination. Vital signs revealing hypotension or significant resting tachycardia in a previously healthy child usually indicate significant hemorrhage, generally involving a 25% to 30% loss of blood volume.[4, 14] In older children, a systolic blood pressure of less than 100 mm Hg and a resting pulse rate of more than 100 beats/min suggest at least a 20% reduction in blood volume.[43] An orthostatic pulse rate increase of more than 20 beats/min or a systolic blood pressure decrease of more than 10 mm Hg is a sensitive indicator of volume depletion.[43] The respiratory rate is usually increased in response to hypoperfusion and tissue acidosis. Mild temperature elevations of 37.8°C to 39.0°C (100°F to 102.2°F) are common. Newborns in shock appear lethargic, usually have pale, mottled, or slightly gray skin, and often have a decreased temperature.[44]

The physical examination may provide clues to the underlying process. A careful evaluation of the oral cavity and nasopharynx may reveal an unsuspected source of bleeding in the nose or throat. Dermatologic examination may disclose jaundice, palmar erythema, and spider angiomas associated with liver disease or petechiae and purpura suggestive of coagulation disorders. Significant lymph node enlargement may reflect underlying malignancy. The abdominal examination is usually nonspecific, but may reveal tenderness, ascites, organomegaly, masses, or signs of obstruction. Rectal examination is mandatory to evaluate local lower tract abnormality, to palpate for masses, to observe the color and appearance of stool, and to test nonbloody stool for occult blood.

DIAGNOSTIC EVALUATION
Laboratory Studies

A complete blood cell (CBC) count should be obtained in all patients with acute GI bleeding. Although isolated hemoglobin and hematocrit readings are unreliable in evaluating the actual amount of acute blood loss, serial measurements provide an objective means of following the rate of bleeding. The hematocrit level depends on the severity of hemorrhage, the rate of dilution of remaining blood by physiologic equilibration, the amount of exogenous fluid administration, and underlying hematologic status. An initial normal hematocrit reading in the presence of significant bleeding usually indicates that blood loss has occurred too rapidly for equilibration, which does not take place until at least 4 to 8 hours after an acute bleeding episode.[12] A low initial hematocrit reading implies either that blood loss has occurred more slowly or that an acute bleeding episode is superimposed on chronic blood loss or underlying anemia. A platelet count should be obtained to evaluate for the presence of thrombocytopenia. An elevation in the white blood cell (WBC) count (10,000 to 20,000 cells/mm³) is common but may also be present with infectious causes of acute bleeding.

The presence of heme protein can be verified by the Hemoccult (guaiac) or Hematest (toluidine blue O) assay. False-positive results are associated with ingestion of iron preparations, red fruits and meats, iodide, and chlorophyll-containing tablets,[33–35] whereas false-negative results may occur with ingestion of vitamin C or certain antacids and with dehydrated stool specimens.[33, 36, 37] In addition, because the acidic pH diminishes the sensitivity of guaiac slides,[38] test cards specifically marketed for use with gastric aspirates (e.g., Gastroccult) are more reliable and should be used.[33, 39]

Coagulation studies are indicated in all patients with acute GI bleeding. The prothrombin time and partial thromboplastin time provide a baseline determination of coagulation, may disclose unsuspected clotting abnormalities, measure the degree of coagulation dysfunction in hepatic disease, and provide an indicator for the need for administration of clotting factors. If GI hemorrhage is secondary to coagulopathy or disseminated intravascular coagulation, tests to determine bleeding time, thrombin time, and levels of fibrinogen and fibrinolytic split products should also be ordered.

Renal function and electrolyte studies provide information regarding the patient's underlying metabolic status. Elevation of the blood urea nitrogen (BUN) is common in acute upper GI bleeding and may reach 40 to 50 mg/dl in patients with previously normal renal function. This elevation in BUN level results from the digestion of blood with absorption of a high protein load from hemoglobin breakdown and increased urea synthesis. In cases of severe hemorrhage, hypovolemia and reduced renal perfusion contribute to the elevation. Liver function tests and serum ammonia levels should be obtained in patients with bleeding associated with underlying or suspected liver disease.

Arterial blood gas measurements may demonstrate metabolic acidosis and increased base deficit in patients with hypovolemia and inadequate tissue perfusion and are also helpful in monitoring oxygenation and ventilation in cases complicated by respiratory insufficiency.

Blood type determination and crossmatch are the two most important laboratory procedures in patients with acute GI hemorrhage. The blood bank should be notified of the impending need for blood as soon as possible so that two to four units of type-specific or crossmatched whole blood can be available during the acute resuscitation phase.

Nasogastric Tube Insertion

Insertion of a nasogastric (NG) tube is essential to detect an upper GI source of bleeding. A bloody aspirate is diagnostic of upper GI bleeding, whereas a clear initial aspirate followed by aspiration of nonbloody bilious material effectively excludes active bleeding from the esophagus or stomach.[45] A negative gastric aspirate generally suggests a lower GI bleeding source but can also occur with an upper GI lesion that has stopped bleeding or with actively bleeding postpyloric lesions associated with significant pylorospasm.[42]

Endoscopy

Esophagogastroduodenoscopy is the optimal diagnostic procedure to determine the cause, location, and severity of upper GI bleeding and will identify the bleeding site in 75% to 90% of children and infants.[46–49] Endoscopy accurately determines the site, size, and number of lesions; assesses the rate of bleeding; predicts the likelihood of rebleeding; provides information to guide management; and can provide diagnosis and therapy with a single procedure.[50–52] Endoscopy is most useful in the actively bleeding but hemodynamically stable patient and is relatively contraindicated in unstable patients and those with unrelenting, massive hemorrhage.

Proctoscopy, flexible fiberoptic sigmoidocolonoscopy, or both should be among the first diagnostic procedures performed in children with significant lower GI hemorrhage.[11, 47] These procedures can accurately and reliably identify or exclude anorectal or colonic bleeding in the majority of cases if performed within 24 hours of the bleeding episode and can also provide coagulation for small bleeding sites, removal of foreign bodies or polyps, and diagnostic biopsy.[53, 54] Colonoscopy is relatively contraindicated in patients with rapid lower GI bleeding because of poor visualization and the associated risk of colon perforation.

Radiographic Studies

Supine and upright or lateral decubitus abdominal plain films are necessary in all children with GI bleeding in order to exclude obstruction, perforation, and masses. Chest radiographs are useful to detect free air, exclude aspiration, provide a baseline study in patients with underlying pulmonary or cardiac disease, or verify central venous catheter position.

Contrast radiographic studies, including an upper GI series, small bowel series, and barium enema, are not indicated in the acute evaluation of GI bleeding. Contrast studies are diagnostic in less than 30% of cases, typically fail to detect mucosal lesions (such as gastritis or a Mallory-Weiss tear), do not provide an estimate of bleeding severity, and interfere with subsequent endoscopic, colonoscopic, and angiographic examinations.[55] The notable exception is the use of single-contrast enema in cases of suspected intussusception. If performed within 24 hours of onset, the procedure is usually diagnostic, demonstrating 90% to 95% of cases with typical ileo-colic intussusception, and is frequently curative, achieving successful hydrostatic reduction in 60% to 80% of patients.[40, 56–58]

Radionuclide imaging is effective for documenting GI bleeding, although it seldom provides a definitive diagnosis. Radionuclide scanning is useful to detect active, low-grade, or intermittant lower GI bleeding; is more sensitive but less specific than angiography; and is valuable both in selecting candidates for angiography and in providing a target area of bleeding for the angiographer. Technetium Tc 99m–labeled autologous red blood cells (^{99m}Tc–RBC) is the preferred agent for radionuclide imaging in most cases of lower GI hemorrhage, having a 95% sensitivity and 91% specificity.[46]

Radionuclide imaging is the diagnostic procedure of choice for the detection of Meckel's diverticulum.[59–63] The "Meckel scan" consists of intravenous injection of technetium Tc 99m pertechnetate, a radionuclide that has an affinity for parietal cells and that concentrates in gastric mucosa. Because nearly 90% of bleeding Meckel's diverticulae are lined with heterotopic gastric mucosa,[64] a persistent focus of tracer within the lower abdomen, especially the right lower quadrant, strongly suggests the diagnosis. Meckel's scan is indicated for any child younger than 3 years who presents with bright red, painless rectal bleeding. The surgically proven accuracy is 88%, with 85% sensitivity and 92% specificity.[61, 63, 65, 66]

Even though the use of angiography has declined with the increasing sophistication and availability of endoscopy and noninvasive studies, selective celiac angiography may be valuable for establishing the diagnosis, localizing the bleeding site, and providing treatment in selected cases. Angiography should be considered for massive bleeding, when medical control of bleeding is unsuccessful, or when endoscopy fails to reveal the source of significant hemorrhage. Active blood loss exceeding 0.5 to 2.0 ml/min is required for optimal visualization and accurate diagnosis.[46] Angiography also affords the capability for intra-arterial infusion of vasoconstrictive agents such as vasopressin and for transcatheter embolization therapy, if needed.[46, 47]

DIFFERENTIAL DIAGNOSIS

Gastrointestinal hemorrhage may originate from any site along the digestive tract. More than half of all episodes of pediatric GI bleeding occur from the colorectal area, one third are located in the small intestine, and approximately 10% are from an upper GI source (i.e., above the ligament of Treitz).[46, 67] However, upper GI bleeding accounts for 90% of all episodes of *major* GI hemorrhage in children.[29] The differential diagnosis of GI hemorrhage is generally considered from the standpoint of upper and lower causes and is strongly age dependent (Tables 35–1 and 35–2).

Newborn (Birth to 30 Days)

Gastrointestinal bleeding in neonates (birth to 1 month) most commonly occurs within the first 48 hours of birth, usually stops spontaneously and permanently within the next 24 hours, and often has no readily identifiable origin.[2, 46] Commonly there is unanticipated rectal bleeding, or blood is suctioned from the infant's stomach during routine postnatal care.[2] Although the sudden onset of bloody emesis or rectal bleeding in the newborn produces major anxiety among parents, pediatricians, and hospital personnel, the origins and outcome tend to be benign.[40] In most cases, severe congenital or intrinsic gastrointestinal disease is not present, and surgery is seldom required.[40, 62]

In the first few days of life, hematemesis or dark rectal bleeding may result from maternal blood ingested during delivery; this is termed the *swallowed blood syndrome*. The Apt test is useful to differentiate fetal from maternal hemoglobin. Blood from the newborn's stomach is diluted (one part specimen to five parts water) and centrifuged, and the supernatant is mixed with 1 ml of 0.2 normal sodium hydroxide (NaOH). Fetal hemoglobin is resistant to reduction and retains a pink color, whereas adult hemoglobin is rapidly reduced and turns brown.[2, 40, 46, 68]

Hemorrhagic disease of the newborn is rare among term infants in the United States and is an infrequent cause of neonatal GI bleeding. A transient deficiency of vitamin K–dependent factors is accentuated between the second and fifth day of life and results in generalized bleeding involving the skin, respiratory tract, genitourinary tract, and central nervous system, as well as the GI system. Peripartum maternal use of aspirin, phenytoin, phenobarbital, promethazine, or cephalothin has been associated with altered platelet function, decreased vitamin K–dependent clotting factors, and coagulopathy.[2, 11]

There is increased risk for the development of gastric

TABLE 35–1

CAUSES OF UPPER GASTROINTESTINAL BLEEDING IN CHILDREN BY AGE[1, 2, 4, 12]

Newborn (0–30 days)	Toddler (< 2 Yr)	Preschool (2–6 Yr)	6 Yr to Adolescence
Ingested maternal blood	Stress ulceration	Stress ulcerations	Peptic ulcer disease
Bleeding diathesis	Gastritis	Gastritis/duodenitis	Gastritis
Stress ulceration	Esophagitis	Esophagitis	Esophagitis
Hemorrhagic gastritis	Pyloric stenosis	Esophageal varices	Esophageal varices
Esophagitis	Mallory-Weiss syndrome	Mallory-Weiss syndrome	Mallory-Weiss syndrome
Intestinal duplication	Vascular malformation	Foreign body	Inflammatory bowel disease
Vascular malformation		Vascular malformation	Hemophilia
		Hemophilia	Vascular malformation
			Medications

TABLE 35–2

CAUSES OF LOWER GASTROINTESTINAL BLEEDING IN CHILDREN BY AGE[1, 2, 4, 11, 12]

Newborn (0–30 days)	Toddler (< 2 Yr)	Preschool (2–6 Yr)	6 Yr to Adolescence
Ingested maternal blood	Anal fissure	Infectious colitis	Inflammatory bowel disease
Bleeding diathesis	Infectious colitis	Juvenile polyp	Infectious colitis
Infectious colitis	Intussusception	Anal fissure	Juvenile polyp
Colitis caused by milk/soy protein allergy	Meckel's diverticulum	Intussusception	Hemolytic-uremic syndrome
	Milk allergy	Meckel's diverticulum	Henoch-Schönlein purpura
Necrotizing enterocolitis	Juvenile polyp	Inflammatory bowel disease	Anal fissure
Intussusception	Intestinal duplication	Henoch-Schönlein purpura	Hemorrhoids
Meckel's diverticulum	Hemolytic-uremic syndrome	Hemolytic-uremic syndrome	Polyposis syndrome
Midgut volvulus		Pseudomembranous enterocolitis	Pseudomembranous enterocolitis
Vascular malformation	Vascular malformation		
Lymphonodular hyperplasia	Inflammatory bowel disease		
Hirschsprung's disease			

ulceration in premature and newborn infants with low Apgar scores, birth trauma, sepsis, hypotension, and respiratory failure. With the application of diagnostic endoscopy in neonates with GI bleeding, these stress-related ulcers, as well as gastritis, gastric erosions, and peptic ulcers, are being documented with increasing frequency.[69]

Lower GI bleeding in neonates most commonly results from anal fissures or iatrogenic anorectal trauma but may also be caused by infectious diarrhea, intestinal duplication, or vascular malformation.[40] In newborns with significant lower GI bleeding, necrotizing enterocolitis (NEC) and midgut volvulus must also be considered.

NEC is a relatively frequent cause of lower GI bleeding in newborns. The syndrome usually occurs within the first 2 weeks and is associated with high morbidity and mortality rates. Characteristic findings include abdominal distention, fever, and moderate rectal bleeding, although signs of sepsis may predominate.[70, 71] Plain abdominal films showing pneumatosis cystoides intestinalis or portal air are diagnostic.[46]

Malrotation as a cause of lower GI bleeding in newborns and infants carries the most urgent need for surgical correction because of the potential for midgut volvulus and consequent development of total midgut gangrene.[58] Clinical findings include abrupt onset of vomiting and abdominal distention, usually occurring in a previously healthy baby. Early, the stool is streaked with blood; later, as intestinal ischemia progresses, the stool may become frankly bloody. Plain abdominal radiographs may be normal, and contrast studies are often required for diagnosis.[72]

Infants (30 Days to 2 Years)

During the first 2 years of life, significant upper GI bleeding is uncommon; when present, it is usually the result of peptic ulcer disease, esophagitis, or gastric erosions.[48] Nearly 80% of peptic ulcers occurring in infants are secondary to other primary diseases, such as intracranial abnormality, steroid use, sepsis, or congenital heart disease.[40, 51]

Three disorders—anal fissure, intussusception (Fig. 35–1), and Meckel's diverticulum—are responsible for nearly 75% of instances of GI hemorrhage in infants.[62] Anal fissure is the most common cause of passage of bright red blood through the rectum. The stool is typically coated with blood, and the majority of patients have a history of recent alteration of bowel habits. Inspection of the anal canal reveals the fissure.

Intussusception, or the telescoping of a segement of bowel into the adjacent segment, is the second most common cause of GI hemorrhage in this age group and occurs with greatest frequency in patients between the ages of 8 and 18

months.[57, 58] The typical history is sudden onset of intermittent episodes of crying, obvious distress, and abdominal pain in a previously healthy infant. The majority of patients have guaiac-positive or "currant jelly" stool containing mucus, which results from mucosal ischemia and is rarely massive. Abdominal distention is usually present, and an abdominal mass is palpable in the right abdomen in two thirds of patients.[40]

Meckel's diverticulum is the most common cause of massive lower GI bleeding in a previously healthy infant.[46] The anomaly occurs in approximately 2% of the population, most commonly presents at about 2 years of age, and is usually located within two feet of the ileocecal junction.[46] Hemorrhage from Meckel's diverticulum, which results from peptic ulceration associated with the presence of ectopic gastric mucosa in the small bowel, is often painless and classically appears brick red.[73]

Other common considerations for lower GI bleeding in this age group include infectious diarrhea (e.g., from *Salmonella*, *Shigella*, or *Campylobacter*), food sensitivities (most frequently cow's milk or soy protein intolerance), and foreign body ingestion.

Younger Children (2 to 6 Years)

In patients aged 2 to 6 years, gastric ulcers, gastritis, and inflammation of the duodenum account for most instances of upper GI hemorrhage.[48] Less common causes include Mallory-Weiss tear, esophageal varices, foreign body ingestion, and vascular malformation.

Polyps are the single most common cause of substantial lower GI hemorrhage during early childhood.[11, 40, 67] Referred to as *juvenile* or *retention polyps*, these hamartomas most frequently occur in the colon, are often multiple, and lack malignant potential.[74] The prevalence of juvenile polyps peaks between 5 and 6 years of age and becomes uncommon after adolescence (Fig. 35–2). The characteristic bleeding is painless and bright red, is often associated with bowel movements, and is usually not massive. Nearly 20% of polyps are palpable on digital rectal examination.[40]

Along with Meckel's diverticulum, intussusception, infectious diarrhea, and anal fissure, another important cause of GI bleeding in this age group is Henoch-Schönlein purpura (HSP). HSP is a systemic vasculitis associated with edema and hemorrhage into the abdominal wall. GI symptoms, which often precede the cutaneous findings, include gross GI bleeding (30%), massive GI hemorrhage (5% to 10%), and abdominal pain (60%).[29] Other possible causes of GI bleeding include the hemolytic-uremic syndrome, intestinal hemangiomas, and lymphonodular hyperplasia.

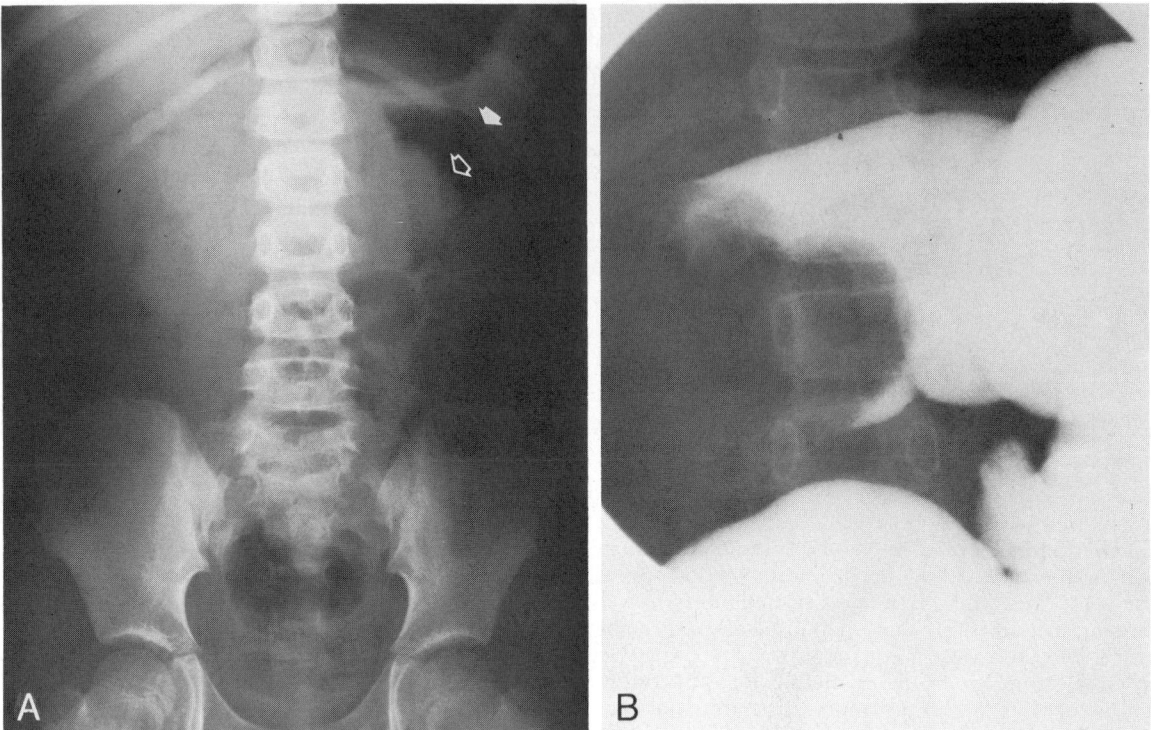

Figure 35–1. A 6-year-old girl with acute crampy abdominal pain (and with known cystic fibrosis). On plain film *(A)*, there is a lack of normal cecal gas in the right lower quadrant, as well as a strong suggestion of a round soft tissue mass of intussusceptum *(open arrow)* within transverse colon gas *(closed arrow)*. Contrast enema revealed intussusception, which was reduced hydrostatically by barium enema. *B* shows the intussusceptum reduced to the midtransverse colon, clasped by barium. (Courtesy of A. Oestreich, M.D., Cincinnati, OH.)

Older Children and Adolescents (6 to 18 Years)

Duodenal ulcer is the most common cause of upper GI bleeding in patients aged 6 to 18 years, followed by gastric erosions, esophagitis, and esophageal varices.[48] Unlike infants, children of this age are likely to have primary peptic ulcer disease.[75, 76] Although abdominal pain is the most common complaint, 30% of older children with ulcers have GI bleeding as the initial manifestation of the disease.[49]

Esophagitis most commonly results from gastrointestinal reflux but may also be caused by infections or chemical agents. Infectious esophagitis is associated with *Candida albicans*, herpes zoster and herpes simplex, and group A beta-hemolytic streptococci.[48] Ingestion of aspirin, alcohol, and NSAIDs, as well as accidental corrosive ingestion, have all been implicated in producing severe erosive gastritis.

Hemorrhage from esophageal varices is usually abrupt, massive, and painless, unless the patient has concomitant gastritis, pancreatitis, or hepatitis. Although most patients with variceal hemorrhage have previously documented liver disease, some experience massive hematemesis as the initial manifestation of unsuspected portal hypertension.[77] Extrahepatic obstruction with portal vein thrombosis is the cause of portal hypertension in nearly two thirds of patients.[78–81] The remaining one third have parenchymal liver disorders such as alpha₁-antitrypsin deficiency, cystic fibrosis, hepatitis, hepatic fibrosis, or biliary atresia with cirrhosis.[40]

With the increased use of endoscopy for diagnosis of upper GI bleeding, there have been several reports of the Mallory-Weiss syndrome in children.[82–84] Antecedent vomiting, retching, or paroxysmal coughing or hiccoughing may produce the characteristic linear tear of the gastroesophageal junction, although nearly half of these lesions are not associated with an identifiable history of forceful straining.

In addition to the previously discussed causes of lower GI hemorrhage, the differential diagnosis of acute lower GI bleeding in adolescents includes inflammatory bowel disease. Though the onset of Crohn's disease in children may be subtle, in nearly 70% of patients, the illness is manifested with abdominal pain, diarrhea, and fever, whereas approximately 30% of patients present with hematochezia.[85] The majority of patients with ulcerative colitis experience the passage of small amounts of blood and mucus through the rectum.[85] Approximately 10% of children present with fulminant colitis characterized by fever, abdominal cramps, and severe bloody diarrhea. Less commonly, ulcerative colitis causes massive, refractory GI hemorrhage.[29, 40]

MANAGEMENT AND THERAPEUTIC INTERVENTION

All patients with significant GI hemorrhage should have their blood pressure, pulse, and cardiac rhythm monitored continuously from the time they enter the emergency department; they should also receive supplemental oxygen and have a urinary catheter inserted to accurately measure urine output. In some patients, central venous or pulmonary artery catheterization may be required for hemodynamic monitoring. Flow sheets are recommended to document the type and volume of fluid administered, the hemodynamic parameters, and the laboratory data.

If signs of volume depletion or shock are present, resuscitation measures should be undertaken rapidly and aggressively. Two large-gauge intravenous catheters should be inserted and 20 ml/kg of 0.9 normal saline (NS) or lactated Ringer's (LR) solution infused rapidly (Table 35–3). If blood pressure rises and peripheral circulation improves, the IV rate should be slowed to avoid serious fluid overload. If signs of shock persist after the initial bolus, an additional 20 ml/kg of 0.9 NS or LR should be rapidly administered.

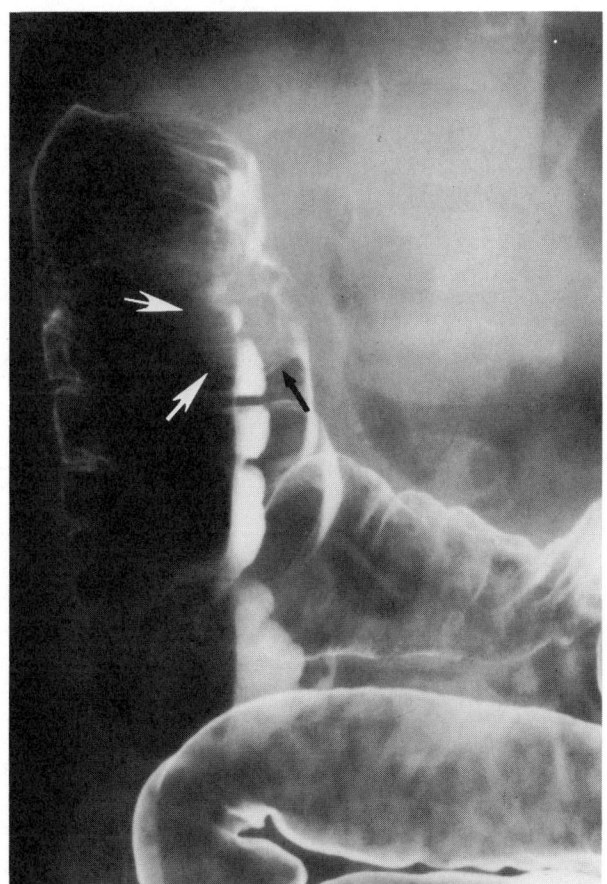

Figure 35–2. Arrows point to a typical juvenile polyp just beyond the hepatic flexure in a 2-year-old girl with 4 weeks of rectal bleeding, as shown on air-barium double-contrast enema. (Courtesy of A. Oestreich, M.D., Cincinnati, OH.)

Blood should be given to patients who remain in shock after the second bolus, to those with massive bleeding, and to any patient with a 35% to 40% loss of blood volume. Whole (preferably fresh) blood should be employed acutely to expand volume and replace red cells. Further replacement with packed cells is indicated after initial stabilization has been accomplished. Platelets, fresh frozen plasma, or vitamin K (1 mg per year of age up to 10 mg) should be given as needed to correct underlying coagulation disorders.

Upper GI Hemorrhage

Although gastric lavage is considered a standard therapeutic measure for upper GI hemorrhage, its efficacy in controlling bleeding remains unproven.[47, 86] Although cause

---

TABLE 35–3

GASTROINTESTINAL HEMORRHAGE: THERAPY AT A GLANCE

For hypovolemia or clinical shock:
  20 ml/kg 0.9 normal saline or lactated Ringer's solution.
For coagulopathy:
  Vitamin K: 1 mg per year of age (up to 10 mg) intramuscularly
For vasoconstriction:
  Vasopressin: 0.3 U/kg in 2 ml/kg (D5W) given IV over 20 minutes; continuous infusion is 0.2 to 0.4 U/1.73 m²/min

---

and effect have not been clearly established, gastric lavage is associated with cessation of bleeding in approximately 85% of patients with upper GI lesions.[87]

The choice of lavage fluid is also controversial. Because of the potential for water intoxication, some authors recommend that only isotonic saline be employed. However, because only small amounts of water are absorbed from the stomach, the risk of this complication appears minimal, and either tap water or saline may be used.[7, 29] Also, even though iced saline experimentally decreases gastric blood flow and enhances vasoconstriction, it appears to be no more effective than room-temperature lavage fluid in promoting hemostasis and carries the risk of producing hypothermia in young children.[88, 89] Finally, adding norepinephrine, vasopressin, or bicarbonate to the lavage fluid has not been proven to be effective.[7, 40, 47]

Most patients can be lavaged effectively with a vented, sump-type NG tube of appropriate size (No. 12 French in small children, No. 16 French in older children). If the gastric aspirate returns significant amounts of bright red blood or clots or if there is difficulty with return of lavage fluid, the NG tube should be removed and replaced with a larger gauge orogastric tube for lavage. If the gastric return does not begin clearing within 20 to 30 minutes, there is little benefit in continuing lavage, and other therapeutic interventions should be planned.

Urgent surgical intervention is occasionally required and should be considered for upper GI hemorrhage associated with unrelenting hemorrhage, when more than 85 ml/kg of blood are transfused within 1.5 hours,[90] in the presence of intestinal perforation or vascular compromise, or with recurrence of hemorrhage after initial cessation.

If bleeding slows or ceases, endoscopy should be performed to determine the type of lesion present. Upper GI bleeding sources are generally categorized as either mucosal (erosion, ulceration, or inflammation) or variceal. Because nearly 25% of patients with peptic ulcers will have recurrent hemorrhage, those identified as being at high risk for rebleeding should be considered for endoscopic therapy, which usually consists of ablation of the ulcer base and coagulation of visible vessels at the ulcer base or margin.[47]

Peptic ulcers endoscopically determined to be low risk for rebleeding, as well as the majority of superficial mucosal lesions (e.g., those caused by esophagitis, gastritis, or duodenitis), are managed medically. Useful pharmacologic agents include those that neutralize gastric acid, suppress acid production, or enhance mucosal protection. A high-potency liquid antacid is considered first-line therapy and should be given every 1 to 2 hours to maintain a gastric pH level ≥ 5.[47, 91] H_2-receptor antagonists (cimetidine, ranitidine) appear useful for inhibition of gastric acid secretion in children, but controlled studies examining their effectiveness in acute GI bleeding in children have not been performed.[92–94] Likewise, whether combined treatment with H_2 blockers and antacids is superior to treatment with antacids alone remains unproven.

Newer agents (e.g., sucralfate, which adheres to the gastric mucosa and forms a protective barrier at the ulcer site[95, 96]; misoprostol, a cytoprotective prostaglandin analogue[97, 98]; and omeprazole, which blocks acid secretion by inhibiting the parietal cell proton pump[99–101]) appear promising in adults, but their safety and clinical effectiveness in children have not been established.

Therapy for upper GI hemorrhage secondary to gastroesophageal varices includes vasopressin infusion, balloon tamponade, and possibly endoscopic sclerotherapy. Intravenous vasopressin decreases portal pressures and blood flow but must be used cautiously, with the patient monitored carefully.[102] Potential side effects are significant and include hypertension, dysrhythmias, reduced cardiac output, and limb ischemia.[47] The initial dose is 0.3 U/kg diluted in 2 ml/kg of D5W given over 20 minutes, followed by a continuous infusion of 0.2 to 0.4 U/1.73 m^2/min, if needed.[2, 47]

Balloon tamponade with the Sengstaken-Blakemore tube should be considered for massive variceal hemorrhage or for significant bleeding that continues despite resuscitation and vasopressin infusion. The procedure is a high-risk one and should only be considered as a temporizing measure until more definitive therapy can be performed. Major complications include mucosal ulceration, esophageal rupture, aspiration pneumonia, and asphyxiation.

Lower GI Hemorrhage

The management of lower GI hemorrhage differs in several respects from that of upper GI hemorrhage. In the majority of cases, rectal bleeding is self-limited, and only rarely does lower GI hemorrhage produce hemodynamic instability or necessitate emergency transfusion.[1] However, when compared with upper GI bleeding, there is a greater likelihood that significant lower GI hemorrhage will represent a lesion that requires surgery. Consequently, after achieving stabilization by appropriate resuscitation measures and excluding an upper GI bleeding source, the main management priorities are to identify those cases of lower tract hemorrhage associated with intestinal obstruction or vascular compromise and to obtain prompt surgical consultation. The most common indications for urgent laparotomy include Meckel's diverticulum; failed hydrostatic reduction of intussusception; midgut volvulus, intestinal obstruction, perforation, or vascular compromise; and unremitting, massive hemorrhage.

The management of nonsurgical causes of lower GI bleeding is dependent on the specific diagnosis. For example, significant bleeding from juvenile polyps may require semiurgent endoscopic hemostasis or removal. If bacterial colitis is suspected by clinical examination and supported by Wright's stain of a stool smear or stool culture, antibiotic therapy may be indicated. For rectal fissures, healing is usually uneventful if stool softeners are employed to alleviate constipation, and local measures to improve perineal hygiene are maintained.

DISPOSITION

Admission to the intensive care unit is indicated for any patient with hemodynamic compromise, orthostasis, active bleeding, suspected massive bleeding (≥85 ml/kg blood loss), low initial hematocrit level (<25%), coexistence of another medical disorder, involvement of another body system, or evidence of coagulopathy.[3] Hemodynamically stable patients with relatively minor hemorrhage that has ceased may be considered for admission to a closely monitored hospital unit. Prior to admission to a hospital floor, the patient should be observed in the emergency department for a reasonable period (at least 1 hour) to ensure that bleeding does not recur.[7]

Patients may be considered for outpatient management if the bleeding episode is minor and resolved, if the specific cause of the bleeding can be clearly identified and is deemed to be insignificant (e.g., anal fissure), if the parents are reliable, and if timely follow-up is arranged.

References

1. Boyle JT. Gastrointestinal bleeding. *In* Fleisher GR, Ludwig S (eds). Textbook of Pediatric Emergency Medicine. 2nd ed. Baltimore, Williams & Wilkins, 1988, pp 171–179.

2. Steinhorn DM, Berman WF. Gastrointestinal hemorrhage. *In* Hoekelman RA (ed). Primary Pediatric Care. St Louis, CV Mosby, 1987, pp 974–978.

3. Shandling B. The digestive system. *In* Nelson WE, Behrman RE, Vaughan VC (eds). Textbook of Pediatrics. 13th ed. Philadelphia, WB Saunders, 1987, pp 767–770.

4. Barkin RM, Rosen P. Gastrointestinal hemorrhage: Hematemesis and rectal bleeding. *In* Barkin RM, Rosen P (eds). Emergency Pediatrics. 3rd ed. St Louis, CV Mosby, 1990, pp 199–206.

5. Janz TJ. Acute gastrointestinal bleeding. Emerg Care 1989;5:28.

6. Pingleton SK. Gastrointestinal hemorrhage. Med Clin North Am 1983;67:1215.

7. Barson WG, Baker PB. Upper gastrointestinal disorders. *In* Rosen P, Baker FJ, Barkin RB, et al (eds). Emergency Medicine—Concepts and Clinical Practice. 2nd ed. St Louis, CV Mosby, 1988, pp 1403–1431.

8. Isselbacher KJ, Richter JM. Hematemesis, melena, and hematochezia. *In* Braunwald E, Isselbacher KJ, Petersdorf RG, et al (eds). Harrison's Principles of Internal Medicine. 11th ed. New York, McGraw-Hill, 1987, pp 180–183.

9. Shaffner JA. Acute gastrointestinal bleeding. Med Clin North Am 1986;70:1055.

10. Schneiderman DJ, Cello JP. Upper gastrointestinal bleeding. *In* Callaham ML (ed). Current Therapy in Emergency Medicine. Toronto, BC Decker, 1987, pp 576–582.

11. Steffan RM, Wylie R, Sivak MV, et al. Colonoscopy in the pediatric patient. J Pediatr 1989;115:507.

12. Nakayama DK, Bishop HC. Pediatric gastrointestinal problems. *In* Callaham ML (ed). Current Therapy in Emergency Medicine. Toronto, BC Decker, 1987, pp 990–996.

13. Simon J. Shock syndromes. *In* Nelson WE, Behrman RE, Vaughan VC (eds). Textbook of Pediatrics. 13th ed. Philadelphia, WB Saunders, 1987, pp 217–220.

14. Jorden RC, Barkin RM. Multiple trauma. *In* Rosen P, Baker FJ, Barkin RB, et al (eds). Emergency Medicine—Concepts and Clinical Practice. 2nd ed. St Louis, CV Mosby, 1988, pp 159–177.

15. Moylan JA. Fluid and nutritional support for the injured child. *In* Randolph JG (ed). The Injured Child: Surgical Management. Chicago, Year Book, 1979, pp 58–65.

16. Kirkendall WM. Recommendations for human blood pressure determination by sphygmomanometers. Circulation 1967;36:980.

17. McNamara RM, Spivey WH, Unger HD, et al. Emergency applications of intraosseous infusion. J Emerg Med 1987;5:97.

18. Hoezler MF. Recent advances in intravenous therapy. Emerg Med Clin North Am 1986;4:487.

19. Rosetti VA, Thompson BM, Miller J, et al. Intraosseous infusion: An alternative route of pediatric intravenous access. Ann Emerg Med 1985;14:885.

20. Cameron JL, Fontanarosa PB, Passalaqua AM. A comparative study of peripheral to central circulation delivery times between intraosseous and intravenous injection using a radionuclide technique in normovolemic and hypovolemic canines. J Emerg Med 1989;7:123.

21. Ransom KJ, McSwain NE. Physiologic changes of antishock trousers in relationship to external pressure. Surg Gynecol Obstet 1984;158:488.

22. Niemann JT, Stapczynski JS, Rosborough JP, et al. Hemodynamic effects of pneumatic external counterpressure in canine hemorrhagic shock. Ann Emerg Med 1983;12:661.

23. Hanke BK, Bivins HG, Knopp R, et al. Antishock trousers: A comparison of inflation techniques and inflation pressures. Ann Emerg Med 1985;14:636.

24. Bivins HG, Knopp R, Tiernan C, et al. Blood volume displacement with inflation of antishock trousers. Ann Emerg Med 1982;11:409.

25. Gardner WJ, Storer J. The use of the G-suit in control of intraabdominal bleeding. Surg Gynecol Obstet 1966;123:792.

26. Milles G, Carlson S, Carlson EE. Use of the G-suit in treatment of acute massive upper gastrointestinal hemorrhage. Ill Med J 1975;147:533.

27. Pelligra R, Sandberg EC. Control of intractable abdominal bleeding by external counterpressure. JAMA 1979;241:780.

28. McSwain NE. Pneumatic anti-shock garment: State of the art 1988. Ann Emerg Med 1988;17:506.

29. Boyle JT, Watkins JB. Gastrointestinal emergencies. *In* Fleisher GR, Ludwig S (eds). Textbook of Pediatric Emergency Medicine. 2nd ed. Baltimore, Williams & Wilkins, 1988, pp 688–707.

30. Bivins HG, Knopp R, dos Santos PA. Blood volume distribution in the Trendelenberg position. Ann Emerg Med 1985;14:641.

31. Sibbald WJ, Nigel AM, Paterson AM, et al. The Trendelenberg position: Hemodynamic effects in hypotensive and normotensive patients. Crit Care Med 1979;7:218.

32. Stillman AE. Black heme-positive stools without gastrointestinal hemorrhage J Pediatr 1982;100:414.

33. Gogel HK, Tandberg D, Strickland RG. Substances that interfere with guaiac card tests. Am J Emerg Med 1989;7:474.

34. Lifton LJ, Kreiser J. False positive stool occult blood tests caused by iron preparations. A controlled study and a review of the literature. Gastroenterology 1982;83:860.

35. Wiener SL. Red fruits causing false-positive occult blood tests in stool. N Engl J Med 1975;293:408.

36. Jaffe RM, Kasten B, Young DS, et al. False-negative stool occult blood test caused by ingestion of ascorbic acid (vitamin C). Ann Intern Med 1975;83:824.

37. Wells HJ, Pagano JF. "Hemoccult" test: Reversal of false-negative results due to storage. Gastroenterology 1977;72:1148.

38. Layne EA, Mellow MH, Lipman TO. Insensitivity of guaiac cards for detection of blood in gastric juice. Ann Intern Med 1981;94:774.

39. Rosenthal P, Thompson J, Singh M. Detection of occult blood in gastric juice. J Clin Gastroenterol 1984;6:119.

40. Oldham KT, Lobe TE. Gastrointestinal bleeding in children: A pragmatic update. Pediatr Clin North Am 1985;32:1247.

41. Saylor JL, Tedesco FJ. Mallory-Weiss syndrome in perspective. Am J Dig Dis 1975;20:1131.

42. Grove K, Klofas ES. Acute gastrointestinal hemorrhage. Top Emerg Med 1990;12:9.

43. Silverman A, Roy CC. Gastrointestinal tract. In Kempe CH, Silver HK, O'Brien D, et al (eds). Current Pediatric Diagnosis and Treatment 1987. 9th ed. Norwalk, CT, Appleton & Lange, 1987, pp 522–551.

44. Burrington JD. Pediatric emergencies. In Kempe CH, Silver HK, O'Brien D, et al (eds). Current Pediatric Diagnosis and Treatment 1987. 9th ed. Norwalk, CT, Appleton & Lange, 1987, pp 666–671.

45. Luk GD, Bynum TE, Hendrix TR. Gastric aspiration localization of gastrointestinal hemorrhage. JAMA 1979;241:576.

46. Stevenson RJ. Gastrointestinal bleeding in children. Surg Clin North Am 1985;65:1455.

47. Hyams JS, Leichter AM, Schwartz AN. Recent advances in diagnosis and treatment of gastrointestinal hemorrhage in infants and children. J Pediatr 1985;106:1.

48. Caulfield M, Wylie R, Sivak MV, et al. Upper gastrointestinal tract endoscopy in the pediatric patient. J Pediatr 1989;115:339.

49. Ament ME, Berquist WE, Vargas J, et al. Fiberoptic upper intestinal endoscopy in infants and children. Ped Clin North Am 1988;35:141.

50. Storey DW, Bown SG, Swain CP, et al. Endoscopic prediction of recurrent bleeding in peptic ulcers. N Engl J Med 1981;305:915.

51. Peterson WL, Barnett CC, Smith HJ, et al. Routine early endoscopy in upper gastrointestinal tract bleeding. A randomized, controlled trial. N Engl J Med 1981;304:925.

52. NIH Consensus Conference: Therapeutic endoscopy and bleeding ulcers. JAMA 1989;262:1369.

53. Williams CB, Laage NJ, Campbell CA, et al. Total colonoscopy in children. Arch Dis Child 1982;57:49.

54. Hassall E, Barclay GN, Ament ME. Colonoscopy in childhood. Pediatrics 1984;73:594.

55. Morris DW, Levine GM, Soloway RD, et al. Prospective, randomized study of diagnosis and outcome in acute upper gastrointestinal bleeding: Endoscopy versus standard radiology. Am J Dig Dis 1975;20:1103.

56. Ravitch MM, McCune RM. Intussusception. In Ravith MM (ed). Pediatric Surgery. 3rd ed. Chicago, Year Book, 1978, pp 989–993.

57. Ein SH, Stephens CA. Intussusception: 354 cases in 10 years. J Pediatr Surg 1971;6:16.

58. Arcari FA. Abdominal emergencies. In Tintinalli JE, Krome RL, Ruiz E (eds). Emergency Medicine—A Comprehensive Study Guide. 2nd ed. New York, McGraw-Hill, 1988, pp 467–471.

59. Duszynski DO, Jewett TC, Allen JE. Tc-99m Na pertechnetate scanning of the abdomen with particular reference to small bowel pathology. AJR 1971;113:258.

60. Sfakianakis GN, Conway JJ. Detection of ectopic gastric mucosa in Meckel's diverticulum and in other aberrations by scintigraphy. J Nucl Med 1982;22:732.

61. Sfakianakis GN, Haase GM. Abdominal scintigraphy for ectopic gastric mucosa: A retrospective analysis of 143 studies. AJR 1982;138:7.

62. Berman WF, Holtzapple PG. Gastrointestinal hemorrhage. Pediatr Clin North Am 1975;23:885.

63. Conway JJ. Radionuclide diagnosis of Meckel's diverticulum. Gastrointest Radiol 1980;5:209.

64. Jewett TC, Duszynski DO, Allen JE. The visualization of Meckel's diverticulum with Tc-99m pertechnetate. Surgery 1970;68:567.

65. Riddlesberger MM. Evaluation of the gastrointestinal tract in the child: CT, MRI, and isotope studies. Pediatr Clin North Am 1988;35:281.

66. Cooney DR, Duszynski DO, Camboa E, et al. The abdominal technetium scan—A decade of experience. J Pediatr Surg 1982;17:611.

67. Spencer R. Gastrointestinal hemorrhage in infancy and childhood: 476 cases. Surgery 1964;55:718.

68. Apt L, Downey WS. "Melena" neonatorum: The swallowed blood syndrome. A simple test for the differentiation of adult and fetal hemoglobin in bloody stools. J Pediatr 1955;47:6.

69. Chang MH, Wang TH, Hsu JY, et al. Endoscopic examination of the upper gastrointestinal tract in infancy. Gastrointest Endosc 1983;143:569.

70. Kosloske A. Pathogenesis and prevention of necrotizing enterocolitis: A hypothesis based on personal observation and a review of the literature. Pediatrics 1984;74:1086.

71. Kliegman R, Faranoff A. Necrotizing enterocolitis. N Engl J Med 1984;310:1093.

72. Andrassey RJ, Mahour GH. Malrotation of the midgut in infants and children. Arch Surg 1981;116:158.

73. Seagram CG, Louch RE, Stephens CA, et al. Meckel's diverticulum: A 10 year review of 218 cases. Can J Surg 1968;34:566.

74. Ward JA, Otherson HB. The juvenile polyp of the colon. Am J Surg 1968;34:566.

75. Nord KS, Rossi TM, Lebenthal E. Peptic ulcer in children. Am J Gastroenterol 1981;75:153.

76. Nord KS, Lebenthal E. Peptic ulcer in children. Am J Gastroenterol 1980;73:75.

77. Shandling B. Portal hypertension and varices. In Nelson WE, Behrman RE, Vaughan VC (eds). Textbook of Pediatrics. 13th ed. Philadelphia, WB Saunders, 1987, p 849.

78. Martin L. Changing concepts of management of portal hypertension in children. J Pediatr Surg 1972;7:559.

79. Fonkalsrud EW. Surgical management of portal hypertension in childhood. Arch Surg 1980;115:1042.

80. Altman RP, Krug J. Portal hypertension—American Academy of Pediatrics Surgical Section Survey—1981. J Pediatr Surg 1982;17:567.

81. Fonkalsrud EW, Myers NA, Robinson MJ. Management of extrahepatic portal hypertension in childhood. Ann Surg 1974;180:487.

82. Cannon RA, Lee G, Cox KL. Gastrointestinal hemorrhage due to Mallory-Weiss syndrome in an infant. Pediatr Gastroenterol Nutr 1985;4:323.

83. Ross LA. Mallory-Weiss syndrome in a 10-month-old infant. Am J Dis Child 1979;133:1069.

84. Lamiell JM, Weyandt TB. Mallory-Weiss syndrome in two children. J Pediatr 1978;92:583.

85. Billar JA. Ulcerative colitis and Crohn's disease. In Gellis SS, Kagan BM (eds). Current Pediatric Therapy. Philadelphia, WB Saunders, 1988, pp 207–209.

86. Moss G. Technique of iced saline lavage in upper gastrointestinal hemorrhage. Am J Surg 1971;122:565.

87. Peterson WL. Gastrointestinal hemorrhage. In Wyngaarder JB, Smith LH (eds). Cecil's Textbook of Medicine. 18th ed. Philadelphia, WB Saunders, 1988, pp 796–800.

88. Himal HS, Watson WW, Jones CW, et al. The management of bleeding gastric erosions: The role of gastric hypothermia. Br J Surg 1975;62:221.

89. Ponsky JL, Hoffman M, Swayngum DS. Saline irrigation in gastric hemorrhage: The effect of temperature. J Surg Res 1980;28:204.

90. Cox K, Ament ME. Upper gastrointestinal bleeding in children and adolescents. Pediatrics 1979;63:408.

91. Peterson WL, Sturdevant RA, Frankl HD, et al. Healing of duodenal ulcer with an antacid regimen. N Engl J Med 1977;297:341.

92. Goudsouzian N, Cote CJ, Liu LM, et al. The dose-response effects of oral cimetidine on gastric pH and volume in children. Anesthesiology 1981;55:533.

93. Zeldis JB, Friedman LS, Isselbacher KJ. Ranitidine: A new H_2 receptor antagonist. N Engl J Med 1983;309:1368.

94. Fedeli G, Anti M, Rapaccini GL, et al. A controlled study comparing cimetidine treatment to intensive antacid regimen in the therapy of duodenal ulcer. Dig Dis Sci 1979;24:758.

95. Nagashima R. Mechanisms of action of sucralfate. J Clin Gastroenterol 1981;3:117.

96. Nagashima R. Development and characteristics of sucralfate. J Clin Gastroenterol 1981;3:103.

97. Dipalma JR. Misoprostol: A prostaglandin for peptic ulcer disease. Am Fam Physician 1989;40:217.

98. Brand DL, Roufail WM, Thompson AB, et al. Misoprostol, a synthetic PGE analog in the treatment of duodenal ulcers—a multicentre double-blind study. Dig Dis Sci 1985;30(suppl):147.

99. Abramowicz M (ed). Omeprazole. Med Lett Drugs Ther 1990;32:19.

100. Decktor DL, Robinson MG. Omeprazole. Drug Ther 1990;20:54.

101. Goustavsson S, Adami HO, Loof L, et al. Rapid healing of duodenal ulcers with omeprazole: Double blind dose-comparative trial. Lancet 1983;2:214.

102. Chojkier M, Groszman BJ, Atterbury CE, et al. A controlled comparison of continuous intra-arterial and intravenous infusions of vasopressin in hemorrhage from esophageal varices. Gastroenterology 1979;77:540.

CHAPTER 36

Inflammatory Bowel Disease

Timothy C. Evans

INTRODUCTION

Ulcerative colitis (UC) and Crohn's disease (CD) are often wrongly considered to be diseases of adults. This fallacy persists even though more than 20% of all patients with inflammatory bowel disease (IBD) are younger than 21 years. The youngest reported patient with UC was 14 months old; the youngest patient with CD was 2 years old. Between 1% and 5% of cases of IBD are diagnosed in patients younger than 10 years old. Though these two chronic diseases adversely affect the pediatric population, definitive diagnosis may not be made until long after the onset of initial symptoms. Occasionally physicians are not aware that IBD may present in childhood and adolescence, and therefore they do not order the necessary test (i.e., barium enema or colonoscopy) to make the diagnosis. Children may be reluctant to discuss their bowel habits, and parents are frequently unaware of these habits. Neither children nor their physicians easily connect the occasionally subtle extraintestinal manifestations of IBD with a bowel disorder. These extraintestinal manifestations may be the presenting complaint in IBD and may precede bowel symptoms by months to years.

The origin of IBD is unknown. The annual incidence ranges from 2 to 20 new cases per 100,000 population per year. The incidence of UC varies from 3 to 15 cases per 100,000 annually, whereas its prevalence ranges from 40 to 225 per 100,000. These figures have remained stable (or may have decreased slightly) during the past several decades. Conversely, the incidence and prevalence for CD appears to have increased dramatically since the 1960s. The annual incidence is 0.5 to 6.3 new cases per 100,000 population per year, with a prevalence of 10 to 100 per 100,000 persons annually.

The risk of acquiring either disease is similar in males and females. The most common age of onset is between 15 and 30 years. Both diseases are more common in whites than in nonwhites. Black Americans and Native Americans are at low risk. People of Jewish origin have a higher than expected frequency of either disease, particularly if they were born in Europe or the United States. In fact, the diseases are more likely to be found in individuals who are of American or Northern European descent. In addition, newly diagnosed patients are frequently found to have a family member with IBD.

ANATOMY AND PHYSIOLOGY

Ulcerative colitis is an inflammatory condition confined to the mucosa of the colon. Rarely does this inflammation extend into the submucosa or the deeper layers of the muscularis propria and serosa. The disease involves the rectum in 95% of patients. Proximal extension is variable but is more frequent in children. The severity of the inflammatory process is also greater in children.

Histologically, both acute and chronic inflammation of the colonic mucosa is present. Microabscesses in the base of the crypts of the villi ("crypt abscesses") and mucosal ulcerations appear. With extension of these ulcerations, pseudopolyps are produced. These pseudopolyps are islands of intact mucosa surrounded by the denuded mucosa; they indicate severe disease.

Toxic megacolon is the most severe manifestation of UC. In this condition the inflammatory process extends through the mucosa to enter the submucosa and the deeper muscular layers of the colon. This produces a loss of colonic motor tone and colonic dilatation. Further progression into the serosa may lead to perforation.

The prominent clinical features of UC can be predicted from the pathologic changes within the colon. Extensive colonic mucosal damage interferes with the colon's ability to reabsorb water and sodium, which leads to profuse watery diarrhea. Ulcerations and vascular engorgement produce colonic bleeding. These ulcerations also account for the numerous leukocytes present in the rectal mucus. Because the pathologic process is usually confined to the intestinal mucosa, the patient will rarely localize pain or develop the complications of perforation or fistula formation. This is more common in patients with CD.

CD involves transmural inflammation of any segment of the intestinal tract from the oropharynx to the anus. More than half of all cases demonstrate involvement of the terminal ileum, and therefore the term *terminal ileitis* has been used synonomously with CD. The rectum is also involved in more than 50% of cases. The upper gastrointestinal tract is involved in up to 30% of children. Diseased areas may be separated from normal-appearing bowel; these areas are called *skip lesions* or *skip areas*. Whether these locations are actually disease free is uncertain.

Histologically, the diagnosis of CD is determined by the presence of inflammation in all layers of the affected organ. This inflammation is most marked in the submucosa. Granulomas are seen throughout the bowel wall and may also be present in lymph nodes, mesentery, peritoneum, liver, lung, bone, and skeletal muscle. Crypt abscesses may be seen but are more characteristic of UC.

As with UC, the mucosal inflammation in CD leads to bloody diarrhea. The transmural inflammation may lead to stricture formation and bowel obstructions. Bowel obstruction is promoted by serosal and mesenteric inflammation, which produces fibrotic peritoneal and mesenteric adhesions. Fistulas are produced as ulcerations burrow through the serosa. These fistulas most often end blindly as abscess cavities; they may develop into fistulous tracts to other portions of the gastrointestinal system or to the genitourinary or skin structures.

A pathognomonic feature distinguishing UC from CD has not been found. Although certain pathologic features tend to distinguish the two, in about 20% of cases it is impossible to make a definite diagnosis based simply on histology.

CLINICAL EVALUATION

UC may present in infancy but more commonly occurs after the age of 11 years and peaks in the late teen years. Most children have a chronic course characterized by intermittent episodes, whereas 10% to 20% experience continuous symptoms, and 10% suffer only one, occasionally fulminant, episode. Overall the course is more severe in children because of a higher incidence of pancolitis and greater disease extension following onset.

Information gathered during history taking should include the frequency and appearance of diarrhea, the presence of abdominal pain or tenesmus, and the presence of anorexia, vomiting, fever, weight loss, and delayed puberty or growth retardation. Information concerning family members with IBD should be sought. A recent travel history should be obtained, and exposure to contaminated food or water should be documented.

In childhood, UC presents in one of three ways. Sixty percent of children present with mild diarrhea and rectal bleeding of insidious onset. Occasionally these children complain of abdominal cramping prior to, and relieved by, defecation. These children experience fewer than four bowel movements daily, are not anemic or hypoalbuminemic, and show no evidence of hypovolemia. The physical examination is typically unremarkable.

The second type of presentation includes bloody diarrhea, tenesmus, low-grade fever, weight loss, mild anemia, and hypoalbuminemia. The abdomen may be diffusely tender without evidence of peritoneal irritation.

In the most severe presentation, the patient has more than six bloody bowel movements daily, is febrile, and exhibits evidence of hypovolemia. The abdominal examination reveals diminished bowel sounds, tympany, and generalized tenderness without peritoneal signs. These patients are anemic because of blood loss, iron deficiency, and bone marrow suppression. They are also hypoalbuminemic as a result of decreased protein intake, a protein-losing enteropathy, and diminished albumin synthesis.

The most important intestinal complications of UC are massive colonic hemorrhage, toxic megacolon, and carcinoma. Massive colonic hemorrhage requiring repeated rapid blood transfusions occurs in less than 5% of UC patients and in most instances spontaneously abates. Emergent colectomy for hemorrhage control is occasionally necessary.

Toxic megacolon develops in only 2% to 5% of children with UC but has a mortality rate of up to 25%. Hypokalemia, barium enemas, and antidiarrheal agents may precipitate the development of toxic megacolon. These children are severely ill, and their abdomens become increasingly distended, tympanitic, and tender. Radiographs usually reveal a transverse colon more than 6 or 7 cm in diameter, although toxic megacolon has occurred in colons measuring as little as 4 cm.

Perforation is the most serious and common complication of toxic megacolon and is indicated by a sudden increase in abdominal pain and girth, the presence of fever, and rebound tenderness. These signs and symptoms may be masked if the patient is taking corticosteroids. Perforations in UC rarely occur in the absence of toxic megacolon and account for nearly one third of the deaths related to UC.

Patients with UC are at higher risk than the general population for the development of colorectal carcinoma. Malignancy accounts for one third of all deaths attributed to UC. However, the risk of developing carcinoma is minimal in patients who have had the disease for less than 8 to 10 years. The incidence of cancer rises rapidly in patients who have had UC for more than 10 years, regardless of the age of the patient. Patients with isolated rectal or left-sided UC are at less risk for developing cancer than those patients with pancolitis, although they are still at greater risk than the general population.

Unlike the initial presentation of UC, which may be dramatic, the onset of CD is usually insidious and its initial signs and symptoms quite subtle, delaying the diagnosis for months to years in most cases. Therefore a thorough history and physical examination are essential. Historical information needed is similar to that required for the patient with presumed UC. However, emphasis should be placed on information concerning weight loss, growth retardation, and delayed sexual maturation. The presence of any of these indicates malabsorption and malnutrition, which are more frequently seen in CD than in UC. Subtle extraintestinal manifestations of CD may be the presenting complaint in some of these children. A careful physical examination may reveal the presence of perirectal or perianal lesions, which are clues to the presence of CD.

The typical patient with CD is a young adult with right lower quadrant pain, diarrhea, and a low-grade fever. The child with CD usually presents between the ages of 8 and 13 years and in some cases has this typical presentation; the diagnosis is relatively easily made in this circumstance. Unfortunately, however, this classic presentation is usually not seen.

Regardless of the symptoms at presentation, the triad of abdominal pain, fever, and diarrhea is seen in most children at some time during the course of the disease. Abdominal pain is seen in nearly 90% of children, tends to be located in the periumbilical region, and occurs after meals. Direct abdominal tenderness is not as frequent but may be present in the right lower quadrant.

Diarrhea is noted in more than 80% of children with CD. It is a particularly pronounced feature of children with diffuse small bowel involvement and produces lactose intolerance and anorexia. This combination promotes weight loss, a prominent finding in CD.

Low-grade fever is present in 40% to 80% of patients and in some instances may be unrecognized. Fever above 38.7°C is unusual in the absence of complications.

Intestinal complications of CD occur with a frequency equal to that of UC. Perianal skin tags and anal fistulas, fissures, and abscesses are uncommon in UC but are seen in between 25% and 50% of patients with CD. Strictures can occur in any segment of the intestinal tract and may lead to obstruction, stasis, bacterial overgrowth, and malabsorption.

Intestinal carcinoma appears in CD, although less frequently than in UC. Several reviews indicate that patients with CD have a 43- to 114-fold increased risk of small intestine cancer when compared with the general population. The risk of colon cancer is increased from 6.4 to 20 times. However, no standard recommendations concerning routine surveillance screening exist.

The extraintestinal manifestations of UC and CD are similar in type but differ in frequency (Table 36–1). Fever is seen in both but may go unrecognized; high fever may indicate a complication. Weight loss, growth retardation, growth arrest, and delayed sexual maturation are probably the result of malnutrition and may be the earliest manifestations of the disease. Chronic caloric insufficiency is the most frequent explanation for these symptoms. Many children with IBD do not exhibit malabsorption, hormonal imbalances, or excessive gastrointestinal losses. The amelioration of these signs of IBD may often be accomplished through vigorous nutritional support, particularly in patients with CD.

Arthralgias and arthritis typically affect the large joints of

TABLE 36–1

EXTRAINTESTINAL MANIFESTATIONS IN PEDIATRIC INFLAMMATORY BOWEL DISEASE

Manifestation	Ulcerative Colitis (%)	Crohn's Disease (%)
Fever	40	22–83
Impaired growth/delayed maturation	5–25	15–75
Arthritis/arthralgias	9–25	9–35
Oral ulcers	2	6–20
Dermatologic lesions		
Pyoderma gangrenosum	1–5	1–2
Erythema nodosum	4	6–15
Renal calculi	5–6	6
Hepatobiliary disease	4–8	4–8
Ocular involvement	4	4–13

the lower limbs. Though this may parallel and reflect bowel disease in adults, such a parallel has not been clearly demonstrated in children. Ankylosing spondylitis and sacroiliitis occur rarely in children.

Aphthous stomatitis, or multiple or recurrent ulcers in the oropharynx, may accompany early IBD or exacerbations of the disease process. Dermatologic manifestations may also reflect disease activity. Pyoderma gangrenosum is more prevalent in UC, whereas erythema nodosum is more common in CD.

Renal calculi affect 5% to 6% of pediatric patients with inflammatory bowel disorders. In CD, fat malabsorption in the distal small bowel promotes oxalate absorption and the formation of oxalate stones. Uric acid stones tend to be seen in UC.

Hepatic dysfunction is present in a large percentage of patients with IBD. This is usually manifested as clinically insignificant mild liver function abnormalities. The diagnosis of IBD is an important consideration in children with chronic liver disease of unclear origin. Although cholelithiasis is more frequent in adults with CD than in the general population, symptomatic gallstones are rare in children.

Significant eye involvement in children with IBD is rare, although transient, asymptomatic uveitis may be seen in up to 30%.

LABORATORY EVALUATION

In most instances, the role of the emergency physician is not to make the diagnosis of IBD, but to rule out the potentially life-threatening complications of these disorders. The emergency physician should also begin the laboratory evaluation necessary to differentiate IBD from other, more easily treated, disease states.

Blood tests should include a complete blood cell (CBC) count to evaluate for anemia, leukocytosis, and thrombocytosis or thrombocytopenia. The erythrocyte sedimentation rate may be useful as a marker of active disease. Gastrointestinal losses of potassium should be evaluated by determining serum electrolyte levels. The presence of azotemia and liver function abnormalities should be assessed, and a measure of nutritional status as reflected by the serum albumin should be obtained.

Infectious agents must be excluded. Therefore a stool specimen should be obtained and enteric pathogen culture, toxin assay for *Clostridium difficile*, and parasitic culture (*Giardia lamblia, Entamoeba histolytica*) tests performed.

The primary role of radiographic evaluation in the emergency department is in the use of flat and upright abdominal radiographs to diagnose the complications of IBD. These complications include partial or complete bowel obstruction, toxic megacolon, and perforation. Plain films may also show bowel wall thickening or loss of the normal haustral fold pattern in UC or intraabdominal masses with small intestine displacement in CD. Further radiologic evaluation is obtained with an air-contrast barium enema. Double-contrast studies are well tolerated in children and are more sensitive than single-contrast studies. However, they should be reserved for patients with mild or moderate disease, because they may precipitate toxic megacolon or perforation in patients with severe disease. Because of the frequency with which CD affects the small intestine, an upper gastrointestinal series with small bowel follow-up is advocated to help differentiate CD from UC. This should be performed when the diagnosis of CD is considered or when a patient presents with upper gastrointestinal symptoms.

Endoscopy provides direct examination of the colon and permits biopsies of involved tissues; thereby allowing for a full evaluation of the extent of the disease and surveillance for dysplasia. It may be diagnostic when radiographic studies are negative or equivocal and allows for evaluation of specific radiographic abnormalities such as a stricture or mass. Colonoscopy is more sensitive than barium enema in detecting the early mucosal changes of IBD and in determining the extent of disease. However, it should not be performed in patients with severe disease because of the risk of inducing a complication.

By using clinical, radiologic, endoscopic, and histologic findings, UC and CD can be distinguished from one another in 85% to 90% of cases. The remaining cases are designated as *indeterminate colitis*.

DIFFERENTIAL DIAGNOSIS

A large number of children will experience abdominal pain, diarrhea, and fever at some time during childhood. The vast majority of these episodes are benign and self-limited and do not require aggressive diagnostic studies or therapy. Those children who present with severe or recurrent symptoms, however, do require investigation. In most instances, the role of the emergency physician is to exclude infections as the cause of symptoms and to decide whether the child requires operative intervention (Table 36–2).

The clinician must be vigilant in excluding colonic infections that mimic UC. In most instances, viral gastroenteritis is a self-limited process that is not associated with hematochezia or fecal leukocytes. Stool cultures for enteric pathogens (e.g., *Escherichia, Salmonella, Shigella, Campylobacter*), ova, and parasites usually exclude most common bacterial and parasitic pathogens. A history of recent antibiotic use suggests the *Clostridium difficile* toxin. In immunocompromised patients or homosexual males, a more aggressive search for causative agents (i.e., viruses and protozoans) should be instituted.

Patients with *Yersinia enterocolitica* infection may present with symptoms identical to those of CD confined to the

---

TABLE 36–2

DIFFERENTIAL DIAGNOSIS OF INFLAMMATORY BOWEL DISEASES

Infectious organisms
  Bacterial
    Salmonella
    Shigella
    Campylobacter jejuni
    Clostridium difficile
    Yersinia enterolitica
    Escherichia coli—invasive and toxigenic
    Aeromonas hydrophilia
  Parasitic
    Entamoeba histolytica
    Giardia lamblia
  Organisms causing "gay bowel"
    Herpes simplex virus
    Neisseria gonorrhea
    Chlamydia trachomatis
    Cryptosporidium
    Cytomegalovirus

Protein sensitivity
  Casein
  Soy

Miscellaneous
  Appendicitis
  Meckel's diverticulum
  Hemolytic-uremic syndrome
  Henoch-Schönlein purpura
  Irritable bowel syndrome

terminal ileum; a stool culture can differentiate between the two diseases. However, such patients are sometimes mistakenly diagnosed as having appendicitis. Patients with appendicitis tend to have less diarrhea, a more rapid course and more pain, and more right lower quadrant tenderness than those with CD.

Allergic colitis generally presents in infancy. Prompt resolution of the symptoms after removal of the allergen from the diet is the hallmark of the disease.

The hemolytic-uremic syndrome is characterized by renal failure, hemolytic anemia, and thrombocytopenia. In nearly one half of cases, abdominal pain and bloody diarrhea may be present, dominating the clinical picture.

The irritable bowel syndrome is distinguished by irregular bowel habits, abdominal pain, diarrhea, and the absence of demonstrable abnormality. Fever and hematochezia are uncharacteristic.

Diverticular disease is rarely present in children but in adults is manifest by abdominal cramping, diarrhea, fever, and occasionally, massive hemorrhage.

THERAPEUTIC INTERVENTION

The aim of therapy in both UC and CD is to induce and maintain a remission. This is more easily achieved in UC than in CD. The immediate goal for the emergency physician is to correct fluid and electrolyte abnormalities and to detect the potentially life-threatening medical and surgical complications of these diseases. Nasogastric suctioning should be instituted in those patients with intractable vomiting and in patients with bowel obstruction or toxic megacolon.

Medical Management

Medical management of IBD attempts to alleviate symptoms and control inflammation. Therapy is largely empirical. The medications used for both UC and CD are similar, but their efficacies vary depending on the cause and location of the inflammation (Table 36–3).

Sulfasalazine combines the anti-inflammatory properties of an aspirin derivative (5-aminosalicylic acid, or 5-ASA) with a sulfonamide antibiotic (sulfapyridine) to treat UC. Clinical trials have subsequently demonstrated the efficacy of this agent in the treatment of mild to moderately severe UC and in maintaining remissions in UC. Sulfasalazine is also effective in treating mild to moderately severe CD, particularly if the CD is confined to the colon. It is not

TABLE 36–3

INFLAMMATORY BOWEL DISEASE: THERAPY AT A GLANCE

Agent	Dosage
Sulfasalazine	50–100 mg/kg/day PO divided qid to maximum 3 gm/day
5-ASA	
Enema	1–4 gm
Suppository	200 mg to 1 gm bid–tid
Prednisone	1–2 mg/kg/day to maximum 40–60 mg/day
Hydrocortisone hemisuccinate enema	50–100 mg q day or bid
Prednisone phosphate enema	20–40 mg q day or bid
Azathioprine	1–2 mg/kg/day
6-Mercaptopurine	1–5 mg/kg/day
Cyclosporine	5.0–7.5 mg/kg/day
Metronidazole	10–20 mg/kg/day divided tid to maximum 1500 mg/day

effective in preventing relapses in CD. Sulfasalazine dosage for children is 50 to 100 mg/kg/day delivered in four divided doses to a maximum dosage of 2 to 3 gm/day. The usual starting dosage of 25 mg/kg/day should be gradually increased over several weeks to this therapeutic range. The usual adult dosage is 4 to 6 gm/day. All patients receiving sulfasalazine require folic acid supplementation, because this drug interferes with the intestinal absorption of folate.

The 5-ASA component is the active ingredient in sulfasalazine. Both 5-ASA and sulfapyridine, when given orally, are rapidly absorbed in the proximal small intestine and do not reach the distal small bowel or colon in an active state. However, sulfasalazine administered orally is delivered intact to the colon, where the two component parts are liberated. The sulfapyridine is completely absorbed and metabolized, but the 5-ASA is poorly absorbed and lingers in prolonged contact with the inflamed colonic mucosa.

Between 15% and 45% of patients suffer an adverse reaction to sulfasalazine. These adverse reactions include anorexia, nausea, vomiting, headache, and reversible oligospermia. Other patients suffer hypersensivity reactions such as a rash, anaphylaxis, or hemolytic anemia. Most of these reactions are caused by the sulfapyridine moiety.

Attempts have been made to deliver the active ingredient (5-ASA) to the site of inflammation without incurring the undesirable side effects of sulfapyridine. 5-ASA enemas have been found to be as effective as sulfasalazine enemas and more effective than hydrocortisone enemas in the treatment of UC located distal to the splenic flexure. They are also effective in maintaining disease remission. In ulcerative proctitis, 5-ASA suppositories have proven effective. These salicylic acid derivatives should not be used in patients with aspirin hypersensitivity but are otherwise well tolerated. These topical forms of 5-ASA have received FDA approval for use in the United States in the treatment of mild to moderate distal ulcerative colitis and proctitis. However, the use of topical salicylic acid derivatives in the treatment of Crohn's proctitis or perianal CD has not yet been approved, and these preparations have not been studied in enough patients to determine their efficacy.

Corticosteroids are a mainstay of therapy for both UC and CD. They are effective when given orally, parenterally, and rectally. In UC, oral dosing is useful for attacks of mild to moderate severity. More severe exacerbations should be treated with intravenous steroids. Ulcerative proctitis and proctosigmoiditis have been successfully managed with topical steroids. Steroid enemas are administered once or twice daily and should be retained for at least 2 hours.

Corticosteroids are the preferred treatment for CD. They are effective in disease affecting both the large and small intestine. Remission rates range from 70% to 92%. Interestingly, clinical remission may not be associated with endoscopic resolution of the disease.

Although immunosuppressive therapy has been used in the treatment of IBD since the early 1960s, its efficacy has not been clearly demonstrated. The use of azathiaprine and 6-mercaptopurine in the management of UC is limited because of their toxicity and because surgery can be curative. Those patients who are poor surgical risks, refuse surgical intervention, have failed optimal medical management, or have suffered the complications of medical therapy may benefit from immunosuppressants. Once instituted, immunosuppressant therapy must be continued for at least 3 to 6 months to observe benefits.

The use of immunosuppressants in CD is controversial. Azathioprine and 6-mercaptopurine may be helpful in treating patients with fistulas, patients who are steroid dependent, or patients who relapse quickly after a course of medical therapy or surgical resection. They also may be effective

---

TABLE 36-4

ADMISSION CRITERIA FOR PATIENTS WITH IBD

Severe episode
Intractable symptoms:
    Pain
    Nausea
    Vomiting
    Rectal bleeding
Complications:
    Perforation
    Toxic megacolon
    Obstruction
Initial diagnosis of
    IBD

---

prophylactic agents. Potential side effects include pancytopenia, pancreatitis, and hypersensitivity reactions. Therapy should be maintained for at least 3 to 6 months before efficacy can be assessed.

Several studies have demonstrated a beneficial effect of cyclosporin A in the treatment of CD. Unfortunately, a high incidence of side effects was noted. As a result, cyclosporine should be used only in controlled trials or in critical situations when other treatment modalities have failed.

Metronidazole has been successfully used in the treatment of perianal involvement in CD. Anecdotal evidence suggests that it may also be beneficial in children with colonic involvement. Side effects include nausea, anorexia, fatigue, paresthesias, and a disulfiram-like reaction when alcohol is ingested concomitantly.

Nutritional Management

Because of the frequency with which growth retardation and delayed maturation affect children with IBD, nutritional counselling is mandatory. General dietary restrictions are not recommended. Rather, a diet that appeals to the patient, contains adequate protein and calories to compensate for enteric protein losses and increased catabolic rates, and avoids substances that worsen symptoms should be encouraged.

Both intravenous and enteral nutritional support have been demonstrated to decrease symptoms, resolve inflammatory masses, close fistulae, accelerate weight gain and linear growth, and reduce postoperative morbidity in patients with CD. Parenteral nutrition is usually used for 2 to 6 weeks and produces remission in 70% to 80% of children. Enteral supplementation may be used for months.

Elemental diets containing monosaccharides, amino acids, and minerals may be used to manage acute episodes of active inflammation in CD. These diets may also be effective in producing remission.

Surgical Management

Surgical resection of the entire colon is curative in UC and will eliminate most of the extraintestinal manifestations of the disease. The indications for colectomy include (1) life-threatening complications such as colonic perforation or documented colon cancer; (2) potentially life-threatening complications not corrected by aggressive medical management, such as toxic megacolon or uncontrolled colonic hemorrhage; and (3) conditions in which there is no immediate risk of death but the cumulative morbidity is high (e.g., severe UC, refractory extraintestinal involvement including uveitis and pyoderma gangrenosum, and conditions related to the adverse effects of long-term steroid therapy).

Surgical resection is not curative in CD. In fact, CD has a tendency to recur shortly after surgery, and therefore surgical intervention is reserved for patients with complicated or refractory disease. Surgery should be considered in patients with bowel obstruction resulting from strictures or adhesions, those with fistula formation or excessive rectal bleeding unresponsive to medical management, those with abscesses, those with extraintestinal complications (including growth failure) unresponsive to conventional therapy, and those suffering from adverse reactions related to medical management.

DISPOSITION

In most instances patients with IBD who present to the emergency department require admission. The decision to admit is easily made when symptoms are severe or there is evidence of shock. Admission is also mandated in nutritionally depleted patients and in those with a complication requiring aggressive medical or surgical intervention. Patients not known to have IBD but in whom the disease is suspected to be likely should probably be admitted for further diagnostic studies. Noncompliant patients should also be admitted (Table 36–4).

Outpatient management of patients known to have IBD may be attempted in attacks of mild to moderate severity. All of these patients should be instructed to return if symptoms worsen or become intractable or if abdominal pain or girth increases. Follow-up arrangements should be made prior to discharge from the emergency department.

The emergency department record should reflect a thorough history, a physical examination directed at those organ systems likely to be affected by these diseases, appropriate laboratory evaluations, and the patient's medical response to

---

TABLE 36-5

DOCUMENTATION FOR PATIENTS WITH IBD

History
    Abdominal pain—location, precipitants
    Diarrhea—frequency, appearance, nocturnal
    Tenesmus
    Associated symptoms—fever, vomiting, anorexia, weight loss, growth or sexual retardation
    Family history
    Travel history
Physical examination
    Vital signs, including orthostatic changes
    Weight, including weight change, if known
    Complete physical examination with emphasis on eyes, oral mucosa, abdominal and rectal examination, skin lesions
Laboratory evaluation
    Complete blood cell count with differential
    Platelet count
    Type and crossmatch
    Electrolytes, blood urea nitrogen, creatinine
    Albumin
    Liver function tests
    Enteric pathogen culture of stool specimen
    Abdominal radiographs
Interventions and response to interventions
    Intravenous fluids
    Nasogastric suction
    Broad-spectrum antibiotics in patients with suspected perforation
Discharge instructions
    Return with continued or increased pain, vomiting, rectal bleeding, abdominal distention
    Medications as prescribed
    Follow-up arrangements

all interventions (Table 36–5). In those instances in which admission is unnecessary, discharge instructions should be clearly recorded and follow-up arrangements explicitly conveyed.

Selected References

Boeckman CR, Stone R, Schueller K. Crohn's disease in children. Am J Surg 1981;142:567.
Booth IW, Harries JT. Inflammatory bowel disease in childhood. Gut 1984;25:188.
Brinberg DE, Berkeley BE. Crohn's disease. A comprehensive approach to management. Postgrad Med 1989;86(5):257.
Danzi JT. Extraintestinal manifestations of idiopathic inflammatory bowel disease. Arch Intern Med 1988;148:297.
Farraye FA, Peppercorn MA. Advances in the management of ulcerative colitis and Crohn's disease. Consultant 1988;28(10):39.
Fonkalsrud EW. Inflammatory bowel disease in children. Surg Clin North Am 1981;61(5):1125.
Gazzard B. Long term prognosis of Crohn's disease with onset in childhood and adolescence. Gut 1984;25:325.
Lenaerts C, Roy CC, Vaillancourt M, et al. High incidence of upper gastrointestinal tract involvement in children with Crohn's disease. Pediatrics 1989;83:777.
Mayberry JF, Rhodes J. Epidemiological aspects of Crohn's disease: A review of the literature. Gut 1984;25:886.
Mock DM. Growth retardation in chronic inflammatory bowel disease. Gastroenterology 1986;91:1019.
Murphy MS, Eastham EJ, Nelson R, et al. Intestinal permeability in Crohn's disease. Arch Dis Child 1989;64:321.
Nord HJ. Complications of inflammatory bowel disease. Hosp Pract 1987;22:65.
Passo MH, Fitzgerald JF, Brandt KD. Arthritis associated with inflammatory bowel disease in children. Relationship of joint disease to activity and severity of bowel lesions. Dig Dis Sci 1986;31(5):492.
Peppercorn MA. Advances in drug therapy for inflammatory bowel disease. Ann Intern Med 1990;112:50.
Puntis J, McNeish AS, Allan RN. Long term prognosis of Crohn's disease with onset in childhood and adolescence. Gut 1984;25:329.
Ruderman WB, Farmer RG. Current management of inflammatory bowel disease. Radiol Clin North Am 1987;25(1):221.
Sack DM, Peppercorn MA. Drug therapy of inflammatory bowel disease. Pharmacotherapy 1983;3:158.
Sanderson IR, Walker-Smith JA. Crohn's disease in childhood. Br J Surg 1985;587.
Seidman EG, Roy CC, Weber AM, et al. Nutritional therapy of Crohn's disease in childhood. Dig Dis Sci 1987;32(12 Dec suppl):82S.
Stringer DA. Imaging inflammatory bowel disease in the pediatric patient. Radiol Clin North Am 1987;25(1):93.
Whelan G. Epidemiology of inflammatory bowel disease. Med Clin North Am 1990;74(1):1.

CHAPTER 37

Intestinal Obstruction

Lee L. Labadie
Gregory P. Moore

INFANTILE HYPERTROPHIC PYLORIC STENOSIS

Pyloric stenosis occurs at a rate of three cases per 1000 live births and is seen more often in males. Hypertrophic pyloric stenosis has some familial tendency. There is a high concordance rate (67%) in monozygotic twins.

Environmental factors also play a role, as hypertrophic pyloric stenosis usually does not present at birth; the char-

acteristic lesion is rarely found in premature infants and fetuses. Some interesting associations occur. For instance, this disease strikes first-born male infants most often. Likewise, elevated maternal age is a factor only for primigravidas. Mothers who formerly used doxylamine succinate–pyridoxine hydrochloride (Bendectin) had an increased risk of having a child with hypertrophic pyloric stenosis.

Elevated serum gastrin levels have been found in infants with hypertrophic pyloric stenosis. Because gastrin increases pyloric smooth muscle contractility, a causal link may exist. Hypergastrinemia has also been implicated as a common factor in the development of associated anomalies of the genitourinary tract. In one series, the incidence of anomalies of the upper urinary tract in infants with hypertrophic pyloric stenosis was 20.6%.

Pathologically, there is diffuse hypertrophy and hyperplasia of the pyloric smooth muscle. The lumen is narrowed to a fine channel that obstructs easily. The antral region is elongated, thickened to as much as twice its normal size, and has a cartilaginous consistency. The muscular thickening extends proximally, well into the antrum, and ends distally at the point where the duodenum begins. The stomach is hypertrophic as a result of outflow tract obstruction.

Clinical Evaluation

Clinically, the diagnosis of hypertrophic pyloric stenosis should be suspected in all 2- to 3-week-old infants who present to the emergency department vomiting. Three days to 5 months are the extremes for the age of onset. The vomiting is initially nonprojectile and occurs during or shortly after feeding time. The vomitus consists solely of gastric contents, is occasionally brownish or blood-tinged, and is almost always free of bile. Projectile vomiting ensues about 1 week after the onset of symptoms. The infant is usually quite hungry, often taking another feeding immediately after vomiting. Bowel movements are diminished as a result of the limited amount of food actually reaching the small intestine. A history of poor weight gain or even weight loss is common.

The physical examination often reveals gastric peristaltic waves coursing from the left upper quadrant to the right. The degree of dehydration varies among patients. The diagnosis of hypertrophic pyloric stenosis can be made confidently by palpating an "olive" in the upper abdomen. Palpation is performed with only the tips of the index and middle fingers in a gentle up-and-down fashion under the edge of the liver. The hypertrophic pyloric tumor or olive is firm, nontender, and freely mobile, tending to squirt away under the examining fingers. This mass is pathognomonic and can be felt by an experienced examiner in 70% to 90% of infants with hypertrophic pyloric stenosis.

Palpation can be facilitated by first evacuating the stomach with a No. 10 French nasogastric tube or a large-bore (No. 12 to 14 French) orogastric tube. The amount of fluid aspirated should be recorded; an amount of 90 to 150 ml is highly suggestive of a gastric outlet obstruction. The nasogastric tube may be attached to continuous gentle suction, but the orogastric tube should be removed after aspiration. Feeding the child a warm sugar-water solution or Pedialyte relaxes the abdominal musculature, as does flexing the thighs to 90 degrees. Alternatively, the child's head can be elevated slightly.

Once the olive is palpated, no further diagnostic workup is necessary, and attention can be given to preoperative stabilization. Prolonged vomiting with loss of hydrogen and chloride ions can lead to profound hypochloremic metabolic alkalosis. In severe cases, the bicarbonate level can rise to more than 35 mEq/L, and the chloride level can fall to 65 to 75 mEq/L. A drop in serum potassium can be expected as a result of intracellular shifts caused by the alkalemia and increased aldosterone production from dehydration. Potassium and sodium are also lost in emesis.

The rehydration fluid of choice is D5/.9 normal saline (NS), usually administered at 1.5 times the maintenance dose. This will prevent the occurrence of seizures resulting from hyponatremia and hypoglycemia. Normal saline (0.9) is used for fluid boluses as needed. For the infant who presents early in the course of the disease without significant dehydration, D5/.45 NS administered at the maintenance rate is adequate. Potassium chloride (3 to 5 mEq/kg/day or 20 to 40 mEq/L IV fluid) is added after adequate urine output has been established.

Diagnostic Evaluation

Diagnostic imaging is indicated when pyloric stenosis is highly suspected, but no mass is palpable. Abdominal plain films may reveal a dilated, air-filled stomach and minimal intestinal gas. However, ultrasound is the ideal modality, as it is painless, noninvasive, and relatively quick and easy to perform. Ultrasound measurements of the thickened pylorus correlate well with those made intraoperatively. Transverse scanning with a high-resolution machine produces a target or "bull's-eye" appearance, signifying a hypoechoic ring of hypertrophied pyloric muscle around the echogenic central mucosa. Longitudinal scanning produces an image that resembles the uterine cervix.

An upper gastrointestinal (GI) series remains the "gold standard" and is the mandatory follow-up study when the ultrasound is negative. A thin mixture of barium is used to outline the pyloric canal. The classic "string sign," a single line of barium exiting a narrowed, elongated, pyloric canal, is diagnostic. Gastric retention of barium with vigorous peristalsis, the shoulders of the muscular olive, and eccentric indentation (pyloric tilt) are also seen. *Railroad tracking* refers to parallel lines of barium seen within the pyloric canal (as opposed to a single one). Rapid gastric emptying essentially excludes the diagnosis of hypertrophic pyloric stenosis. The major advantage of an upper GI series is that other conditions that mimic pyloric stenosis, such as gastroesophageal reflux, malrotation with duodenal bands, antral web, and hiatal hernia, can be diagnosed. Prior to the induction of general anesthesia, any residual barium should be aspirated from the stomach.

Differential Diagnosis

The differential diagnosis of hypertrophic pyloric stenosis includes gastroenteritis, hiatal hernia, antral web, pyloric duplication, gastroesophageal reflux, and malrotation with duodenal bands. Gastroenteritis can often be distinguished by the presence of diarrhea, and the remainder are differentiated by radiographic studies. At times, adrenal insufficiency simulates pyloric stenosis, in both age of onset and symptoms. However, the absence of a palpable tumor, coupled with atypical laboratory findings (metabolic acidosis, hyperkalemia, and elevated urinary sodium), aid in the differentiation.

Therapeutic Intervention

The treatment of hypertrophic pyloric stenosis is surgical, but the procedure is not emergent; fluid and electrolyte resuscitation should take place first. The Fredet-Ramstedt pyloromyotomy is usually performed. Because the intestinal lumen is not entered in this procedure, feedings can begin in small amounts 6 to 8 hours postoperatively. Medical

management has higher mortality and complication rates and has thus been abandoned.

INTUSSUSCEPTION

Intussusception is the telescoping or invagination of one segment of the intestine into the lumen of another immediately adjacent segment. The receiving, or intussuscepting, segment is called the *intussuscipiens*, and the received, or intussuscepted, portion is known as the *intussusceptum*. Intussusception is the leading cause of intestinal obstruction in children 3 months to 6 years of age.

Intussusception can occur at any time in life, but the idiopathic form is primarily a disease of childhood, especially infancy. Sixty percent to 65% of patients are younger than 1 year, and 80% are younger than 2 years. In newborns and in patients older than 3 years, intussusception is rare. Peak occurrence is in infants 3 to 12 months of age, with the average age being about 7 to 8 months. Intussusception has also occurred in the fetus.

The origin of intussusception is unknown in 90% to 95% of children. However, in patients younger than 1 month and older than 3 years, pathologic lesions such as polyps, tumors, duplications, hemangiomas, and Meckel's diverticulum serve as the lead point with some regularity. In adults, a mechanical cause, such as a tumor, is found in 90% of cases.

Ninety-five percent of intussusceptions are located in the ileocecal area and are called *ileocolic intussusceptions*. The ileocecal area contains the terminal ileum and the cecum, which have disproportionate diameters and differential autonomic innervation, which may precipitate cecal antiperistalsis.

Ileoileal and colocolic intussusceptions are uncommon. Occasionally, an ileoileal intussusception of the terminal ileum may itself prolapse through the ileocecal valve, a condition known as *ileoileocolic intussusception*. The use of such compound designations can be confusing and is not particularly helpful. The main point is that more proximal intussusceptions do occur. They are more difficult to diagnose and frequently resist hydrostatic reduction.

Two conditions that predispose the patient to idiopathic intussusception deserve special mention. The first of these is Henoch-Schönlein purpura (HSP). In one series, intussusception was found in 3% of 183 hospitalized HSP patients and was the most common surgical complication. Fifty percent of the intussusceptions involved the small bowel alone, and none were reducible by barium enema. The second predisposing condition is cystic fibrosis. In these patients, barium enema reduction is unlikely, but easy manual reduction at surgery can be anticipated. In both HSP and cystic fibrosis, intussusception occurs almost exclusively in patients older than 3 years.

Peutz-Jehger syndrome is a rare cause of intussusception in older children; in this case, the hamartomatous polyps act as the lead point. Similarly, familial polyposis coli and juvenile polyposis can also cause intussusceptions, and the vermiform appendix may occasionally initiate an intussusception. Intestinal lymphosarcoma can give rise to a rare form of chronic nonstrangulating intussusception and should be suspected in all children older than 6 years with intussusception. Blunt abdominal trauma has also been known to cause intussusception.

Postoperative intussusception in children most commonly follows procedures involving retroperitoneal dissection (e.g., resection of Wilms' tumor) or extensive handling of intra-abdominal viscera (e.g., abdominoperineal pull-through for imperforate anus). The vast majority of postoperative intussusceptions involve the small bowel alone, and thus barium enema is usually nondiagnostic. The characteristic symptom complex includes abdominal distention, bilious vomiting, and increasing nasogastric aspirate. Abdominal pain is variable and is often attributed to the recent operation. On occasion, transient small bowel intussusception is observed during surgery.

Intussusception is believed to begin with intestinal spasm. Just distal to this spasm there is relaxation, allowing the longitudinal muscle fibers to draw the contracted portion of bowel into the relaxed portion. This continues on until the tethering mesentery of the intussusceptum halts the process, usually somewhere in the transverse colon. Compression of the mesentery at the point of invagination (where the bowel wall undergoes a sharp U-turn) occurs from the start, leading to immediate venous compression, venous stasis, and edema. The goblet cells pour copious amounts of mucus into the intestinal lumen. The engorged, hyperemic intestinal mucosa seeps blood, which mixes with the mucus to form the "currant-jelly stool" seen in 60% of patients. Venous obstruction and edema increase, while arterial inflow remains constant. Eventually, tissue pressure finally exceeds arterial pressure, and necrosis ensues. Bacterial proliferation at the site occurs well before actual ischemia and is undoubtedly the cause of the frequently observed high fever. Spontaneous sloughing of the intussusceptum with approximation of viable bowel, though rare, does occur.

Clinical Evaluation

The typical history of intussusception involves a previously healthy, 7-month-old male infant who cries out in a paroxysm of pain, draws up both legs, and vomits (nonbilious). Passage of a formed or perhaps thin liquid stool provides relief, only to have the pain recur in about 20 minutes. The pattern continues, with the child often appearing perfectly normal between attacks of pain and vomiting. Within several hours, however, apathy or even lethargy ensues in the intervals between the colicky abdominal pain. Blood or mucus is passed rectally within 12 to 24 hours. Vomiting may become bilious or even feculent. Eventually the child becomes pale, diaphoretic, and febrile (up to 41°C). If the condition is left untreated, death will occur in 2 to 5 days from overwhelming sepsis and dehydration.

Intussusception has also presented in an atypical, painless manner, with the clinical picture dominated by altered mental status. In such children, the diagnosis may be significantly delayed. The exact reason for the "painless" intussusception is unknown. In one report, a 10-month-old infant with intussusception presented in a coma. Naloxone therapy resulted in drastic improvement in the child's level of arousal. No evidence of opioid ingestion existed, and the child subsequently was found to have an intussusception, which was successfully reduced surgically. The comatose state may have been induced by increased secretion of an endogenous opioid, which would also account for the diminished abdominal pain.

On physical examination, the abdomen is initially soft and nontender but later becomes distended. Intussusception, in the classic form of a sausage-shaped mass, is palpable in 85% to 95% of patients. It is usually located in the upper right quadrant, but may be felt in any quadrant. A digital rectal examination is performed to check for the presence of blood, a mass (which is sometimes more readily palpable on rectal or bimanual rectal abdominal examination), or rectal prolapse, which may actually represent the leading edge of the intussusceptum.

Diagnostic Evaluation

Plain abdominal radiographs may show the head of the intussusceptum projecting into the air-filled colon, a finding seen in approximately 60% of patients. When intussusception is strongly suspected, a barium or water-soluble contrast enema should be performed without delay. Contraindications include shock, peritoneal signs, radiographic evidence of perforation, and, possibly, radiographic evidence of a high-grade bowel obstruction. Contrast enema is successful in reducing 67% to 75% of all intussusceptions and has an even higher rate of success in intussusceptions of short duration.

Controversy still exists as to whether hydrostatic reduction should be attempted in the presence of obstruction. The view of many radiologists is that although contrast enema reduction is often unsuccessful in reducing the intussusception, a significant number of patients who undergo the procedure can be spared an operation, and the use of a water-soluble contrast medium makes the procedure essentially risk free. From the surgeon's standpoint, the appearance of intestinal obstruction provides an early warning about the complicated, incarcerated, or gangrenous nature of the intussusception. Hydrostatic reduction in such situations carries a risk of perforation, which will necessitate a laparotomy, and therefore any attempts at hydrostatic reduction of an intussusception should always be done in consultation with a surgeon (Table 37–1).

Ultrasound has also been used to diagnose intussusception. The characteristic findings include (1) a target, or "bull's-eye," configuration consisting of two rings of low echogenicity separated by an intermediate hyperechoic ring seen on the cross-sectional image of the intussuscepted bowel; and (2) a doughnut configuration consisting of a hypoechoic rim and a dense central echogenic core seen on the cross section near the apex of the intussusception.

Another nonoperative diagnostic method is air reduction. In a large Japanese series, this technique had a success rate of 81%. In this study, the diagnosis of intussusception was initially made on clinical grounds, and the adequacy of reduction was determined by abdominal auscultation.

Indications for surgery include shock, peritonitis, perforation, and irreducibility by nonoperative means.

TABLE 37–1
PROTOCOL FOR CONTRAST ENEMA REDUCTION OF INTUSSUSCEPTION

1. Consult a surgeon, who places the operating room on standby.
2. Perform nasogastric suction and administer IV fluids; consider sedation and antibiotics.
3. Insert a nonlubricated No. 20–24 French Foley catheter in the rectum, inflate balloon 5–10 ml, and pull down against levators.
4. Compress buttocks tightly and tape them together; wrap legs.
5. Allow the contrast agent to flow by gravity into the colon from a height of not more than 1 m.
6. Do not palpate abdomen during procedure
7. Use fluoroscope intermittently
8. Abandon the attempt if the contrast column is stationary and its outline unchanging for 10 min.
9. Reduction is complete when there is:
   —Free flow of barium well into the small bowel
   —Expulsion of feces and flatus with contrast material
   —Disappearance of the mass
   —Improvement in the child's condition

Differential Diagnosis

The differential diagnosis of intussusception includes any condition that causes intestinal obstruction or lower gastrointestinal bleeding. The intestinal hemorrhage of Henoch-Schönlein purpura may be associated with a similar type of colicky abdominal pain or even vomiting. In the presence of preexisting gastroenteritis, the diagnosis of intussusception may be obscured. The bloody stools and abdominal cramps of invasive enterocolitis can usually be differentiated from intussusception, because the pain is less severe and regular, there is diarrhea, and the infant appears ill between bouts of pain.

HIRSCHSPRUNG'S DISEASE

Hirschsprung's disease, also known as *congenital megacolon, congenital aganglionosis,* or *aganglionic megacolon,* is characterized by the absence of parasympathetic ganglion cells in Auerbach's (myenteric) plexus and Meissner's (submucosal) plexus in the intestinal tract. In the classic form of the disease, involvement is limited to the rectosigmoid colon and rectum, including the internal anal sphincter. This so-called *short-segment* version constitutes about 80% to 90% of cases of Hirschsprung's disease. On occasion, ganglia may be absent in more proximal segments of the colon, the entire colon, the small intestine, or even the entire gastrointestinal tract. In such instances, the disease is known as *long-segment aganglionosis.* Regardless of the exact location of aganglionosis, however, the basic problem is a lack of coordinated orderly intestinal motility, which produces varying degrees of functional obstruction.

Hirschsprung's disease occurs in approximately 1 per 5000 live births and is a fairly common cause of intestinal obstruction, especially among newborns. Males are more frequently affected, and incidence is increased in children with Down syndrome. Imperforate anus is occasionally noted, and in this instance, diagnosing Hirschsprung's disease can be difficult. Some infrequently associated anomalies include Klinefelter's syndrome, urologic malformations, hypertrophic pyloric stenosis, achalasia, congenital deafness, and congenital rubella syndrome.

The pathophysiology of Hirschsprung's disease is related to a lack of normal propulsive peristalsis. The aganglionic rectosigmoid is usually narrow and nonhypertrophied, with normal tonus. Just proximal to this is a funnel-shaped "transitional zone" best characterized as oligoganglionic and having some degree of orderly motility. Preceding this is normal colon, which appears quite abnormal as a result of massive dilation with retained feces. Muscular hypertrophy (as a result of the normal colon's attempts to evacuate itself) and edema add to the enlargement. The proximal intestine is increased in diameter and length. The internal anal sphincter contracts instead of relaxing to the stimulus of rectal distention, further impairing defecation.

Clinical Evaluation

The presentation of Hirschsprung's disease varies. In newborns, the spectrum may range from complete obstruction with bilious vomiting and abdominal distention to delayed passage of meconium with mild constipation. Digital rectal examination may result in explosive evacuation of meconium. Most affected infants are full term, of normal birth weight, and otherwise healthy. In time, failure to thrive may occur. When left untreated for a number of years, Hirschsprung's disease produces a classic clinical picture: a child who is ill-appearing, with thin limbs and other evidence of malnutrition, despite a markedly protuberant abdomen with a flared-out lower rib cage. Physical examination reveals palpable abdominal fecalomas and an empty rectum. There is a history of chronic constipation and infrequent bowel movements.

The most serious complication of Hirschsprung's disease in the neonate is the development of ulcerative enterocolitis. This was formerly uniformly fatal and is still the usual cause of death in an infant with unrelieved intestinal obstruction. The markedly elevated intraluminal pressure in the proximal normal colon results in decreased total colonic blood flow, as well as shunting of blood away from the mucosa. Venous congestion and engorgement of the veins and lymphatics, with subsequent bowel wall edema, eventually lead to mucosal necrosis. This is manifested clinically by the sudden onset of gross abdominal distention and explosive, foul-smelling diarrhea. Enteric organisms invade the blood stream. Ulcerative enterocolitis often pursues a rapidly progressive course, and death from combined hypovolemic and septic shock is the ultimate outcome unless prompt intravenous fluids and antibiotic therapy are given. Amazingly, this condition responds promptly to simple decompression by rectocolic irrigation.

Chronic diarrhea may be the dominant symptom and represents liquid stool flowing around a fecal impaction or a subacute form of enterocolitis. Bouts of constipation usually intervene between episodes of diarrhea. A protein-losing enteropathy may develop. Cecal or appendiceal perforation presenting as peritonitis with pneumoperitoneum is a rare complication. Acute appendicitis in the newborn, normally an uncommon occurrence, is often associated with Hirschsprung's disease.

Diagnostic Evaluation

The diagnosis of Hirschsprung's disease is suspected in any infant who fails to pass meconium within the first 48 hours of life. A barium enema, performed on an unprepped bowel, is used as a screening test. The appearance of the typical cone-shaped transition zone is diagnostic; once this is seen, the examination is stopped. Unfortunately, the transition zone is more readily demonstrable in older children than in neonates. Other findings include normal to slightly diminished caliber of the aganglionic segment and a saw-toothed or spiculated appearance to the rectum, representing abnormal peristaltic contractions. In the absence of these findings, the only diagnostic clue may be colonic barium retention for 2 to 3 days.

If the contrast study is nondiagnostic, a rectal biopsy of the mucosa and submucosa is performed. This can be done at the bedside and does not require anesthesia. The use of acetylcholinesterase histochemistry on mucosa and submucosa biopsy specimens increases diagnostic accuracy.

Differential Diagnosis

The differential diagnosis of Hirschsprung's disease depends on the age of the patient at presentation. In the newborn, meconium ileus, meconium plug syndrome, and neonatal small left colon syndrome are the most important considerations. Barium enema usually distinguishes these conditions from Hirschsprung's disease and in the latter two, can be curative. Meconium ileus occurs only in the presence of cystic fibrosis. A rectal biopsy is indicated in meconium plug syndrome, as Hirschsprung's disease occasionally presents with a meconium plug. In neonatal small left colon syndrome, weeks to months may be required before the left colon attains a normal caliber.

For older children, the major disease entity to consider is

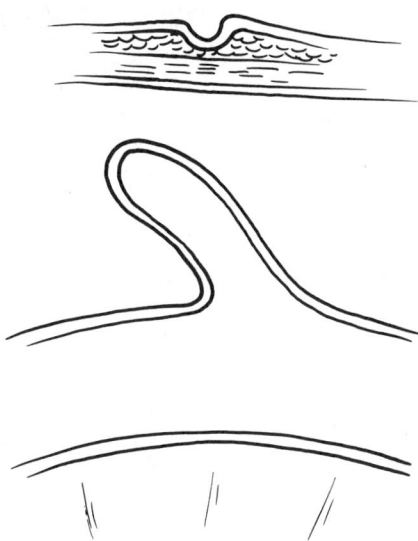

Figure 37–1. Simple Meckel's diverticulum. (Modified from Amoury RA. Meckel's diverticulum. *In* Welch KJ, et al (eds). Pediatric Surgery. 4th ed. Vol 2. Chicago, Year Book, 1986.)

chronic functional constipation. These children are usually distinguishable from those with Hirschsprung's disease, because they are well nourished and healthy appearing. The onset of bowel troubles is usually around age 2 years or the time of toilet training. These children have a history of fecal soilage or encopresis. Rectal examination reveals a dilated rectum packed with hard feces; barium enema shows a dilated rectum and normal motility. At times personality disorders may be evident in the parent or child. Rectal biopsy confirms the presence of ganglion cells.

Therapeutic Intervention

The treatment of classic Hirschsprung's disease is primarily surgical. Colostomy in early infancy can prevent the sequela of ulcerative enterocolitis. Definitive surgical repair with a rectal pull-through procedure is delayed until 12 to 18 months of age in the infant or until the return of good nutritional status in the older child. The goal of surgery is to relieve functional obstruction by bringing normal ganglionated bowel as far down into the aganglionic rectum as possible.

MECKEL'S DIVERTICULUM

Meckel's diverticulum is the most common congenital anomaly of the gastrointestinal tract, occurring in 1% to 2% of the general population. Meckel's diverticulum arises from failure of the omphalomesenteric duct to close, an event that usually occurs at 5 to 7 weeks gestational age. If the duct fails to totally close, an umbilical-fecal fistula occurs. Proximal closure of the duct results in an umbilical sinus, and distal closure of the duct results in Meckel's diverticulum. In 74% of cases, the diverticulum has a free end (Fig. 37–1), but often there is a fibrous cord connecting the structure to the umbilicus (Fig. 37–2).

Meckel's diverticulum is a true diverticulum, containing all layers of the bowel wall and a distinct blood supply. It is found within 100 cm proximal to the ileocecal valve in 90% of cases and is usually about 4 to 6 cm long.

Clinical Evaluation

The majority of Meckel's diverticula remain asymptomatic throughout patients' lives. The complication rate of the diverticulum is 25% to 40%, although some studies show complication rates of 4% to 8%.

Symptomatic manifestation occurs before age 30 years in 70% of patients and in 40% to 80% of patients occurs before age 10 years. Complications primarily involve obstruction, hematochezia, and diverticulitis.

Obstruction is the most common presentation of Meckel's diverticulum in children if intussusception is also present. The clinical appearance is indistinguishable from obstruction resulting from other causes. Intussusception occurring with the diverticulum as the leading edge is the most common cause of obstruction. Another common cause of obstruction resulting from Meckel's diverticulum is herniation through or volvulus around a persistent fibrous cord (Fig. 37–3). Obstruction caused by Meckel's diverticulum increases the risk for bowel infarction.

Gastrointestinal bleeding is a common presentation of Meckel's diverticulum in children, especially in those younger than 2 years. When all causes of lower GI bleeding in children are evaluated, Meckel's diverticulum is the responsible factor in up to 50% of cases. Hemorrhage is usually painless and sudden, although it may be periodic. Thus Meckel's diverticulum should be suspected in any anemic child. Hemorrhage may cause hypovolemic shock, but exsanguination is rare. Rectal bleeding is usually red. Melena may be present if the gut transit time is slow. Bleeding is caused by ulceration at the base of the diverticulum or on the contralateral ileal wall, where tissues eventually erode.

Inflammation (diverticulitis) accounts for 20% of symptomatic patients. It is found most often in children younger than 10 years (mean, 8 years old) and in adults older than 20 years. Its presentation is similar to that of acute appendicitis. Unfortunately, 7% to 50% of patients suffer a perforated diverticulum before surgery, with resultant peritonitis. Meckel's diverticulum should be expected if the course of "appendicitis" is chronic, recurrent, protracted, or associated with gastrointestinal bleeding. Because of confusion

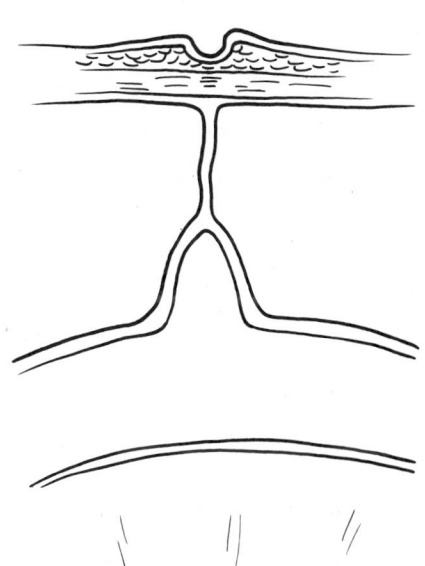

Figure 37–2. Meckel's diverticulum attached to the abdomen by a fibrous remnant. (Modified from Amoury RA. Meckel's diverticulum. *In* Welch KJ, et al (eds). Pediatric Surgery. 4th ed. Vol 2. Chicago, Year Book, 1986.)

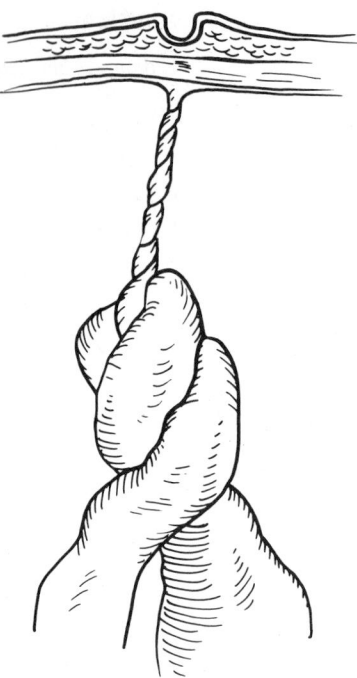

Figure 37–3. Volvulus of Meckel's diverticulum. (Modified from Amoury RA. Meckel's diverticulum. *In* Welch KJ, et al (eds). Pediatric Surgery. 4th ed. Vol 2. Chicago, Year Book, 1986.)

with other entities, Meckel's diverticulum is only infrequently diagnosed preoperatively.

Diagnostic Evaluation

Routine ancillary studies are generally unhelpful, although plain radiographs may demonstrate an obstruction (Fig. 37–4). The diagnostic aid of choice is the technetium Tc 99m pertechnetate nuclear isotope scan, also known as *Meckel's scan.* Technetium Tc 99m has an affinity for parietal cells found in gastric mucosa. The sensitivity of the scan varies from 75% to 100%; its specificity is 80%. A higher incidence of true positive results is elicited if cimetidine is administered 24 hours prior to the study. By blocking histamine, cimetidine prevents secretion (and increases concentration) of Tc 99m from gastric mucosa. False-positive results are elicited in patients with hemangiomas, abdominal aneurysms, hydronephrosis, lymphoma, Peutz-Jeghers syndrome, small bowel ulcers, and intussusception. False-negative results may also be caused by absent gastric mucosa, necrosis of the diverticulum, rapid hemorrhage with dilution of isotope activity, confusion with normal structures, and absorption of barium. Barium studies should be avoided until after a Meckel's scan has been performed. Though barium enema identifies Meckel's diverticulum in only 4% to 22% of patients, it may be helpful in diagnosing other problems. Arteriograms and computed tomography (CT) scans are used when suspicion remains high for Meckel's diverticulum and the result of the Meckel's scan is negative.

Therapeutic Intervention

The treatment of symptomatic Meckel's diverticulum is surgery (i.e., either bowel resection or diverticulotomy). Prior to operation, the physician should stabilize existing hypovolemia, consider antibiotic prophylaxis, and administer an H_2-receptor blocker.

MALROTATION AND MIDGUT VOLVULUS

Anomalies of rotation and fixation represent a form of bowel obstruction that is difficult to conceptualize. The primitive gut forms during the fourth week of embryonal life and consists of three divisions: the foregut, the midgut, and the hindgut. The largest of these, the midgut, is the only portion that undergoes rotation. At between 4 and 10 weeks of gestation, it takes on the shape of a loop that herniates extraembryonically into the umbilical cord. At 10 to 12 weeks, the midgut loop reenters the peritoneal cavity and during the process rotates 270 degrees in a counterclockwise direction around the superior mesenteric artery. This gives rise to the normal C-shaped configuration of the duodenum and results in the cecum coming to rest in the right lower quadrant of the abdomen (Fig. 37–5).

Midgut rotation can arrest at any point, thus giving rise to a spectrum of rotational anomalies. The term *malrotation* is a misnomer, as rotation has actually commenced in the normal fashion but has simply not been completed. Two main clinical varieties are recognized. In *nonrotation,* the duodenojejunal junction lies to the right of the spine, and the ascending colon and cecum remain to the left (Fig. 37–6). This arrangement, if not associated with an abdominal wall defect or diaphragmatic hernia, actually tends to be asymptomatic because of a fairly broad-based mesenteric attachment. In *incomplete* or *mixed rotation,* the cecocolic loop rotates 180 degrees to the epigastrium (or right upper

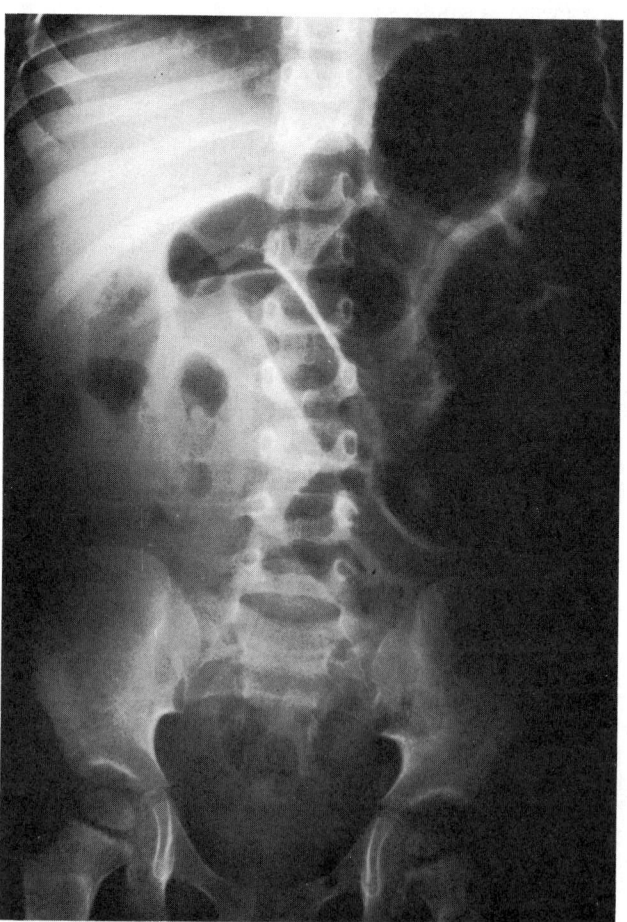

Figure 37–4. Supine radiograph demonstrating obstruction due to a volvulus of Meckel's diverticulum. (Modified from Amoury RA. Meckel's diverticulum. *In* Welch KJ, et al (eds). Pediatric Surgery. 4th ed. Vol 2. Chicago, Year Book, 1986.)

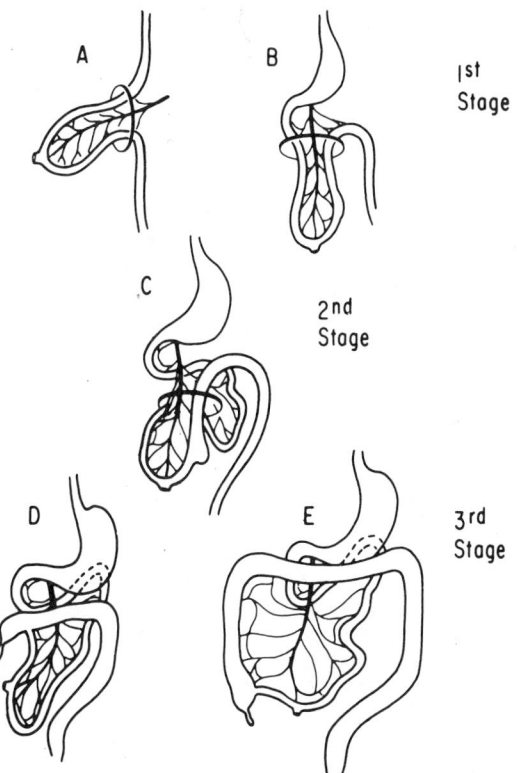

Figure 37–5. Normal intestinal rotation. Gestational age of 6 weeks *(A)*, 8 weeks *(B)*, 9 weeks *(C)*, 11 weeks *(D)*, and 12 weeks *(E)*. (Modified from Snyder WH Jr, Chaffin L. Embryology and pathology of the intestinal tract: Presentation of 40 cases of malrotation. Ann Surg 1954; 140:368.)

quadrant) but fails to descend into the right lower quadrant (see Fig. 37–6). Dense peritoneal bands (Ladd's bands) cross from the malpositioned right colon, across the duodenum, to the right lateral abdominal wall. An extremely narrow mesenteric attachment of the midgut to the posterior abdominal wall is located in the vicinity of these bands. This configuration predisposes to clockwise volvulus of the midgut. Furthermore, Ladd's bands can obstruct the duodenum by themselves.

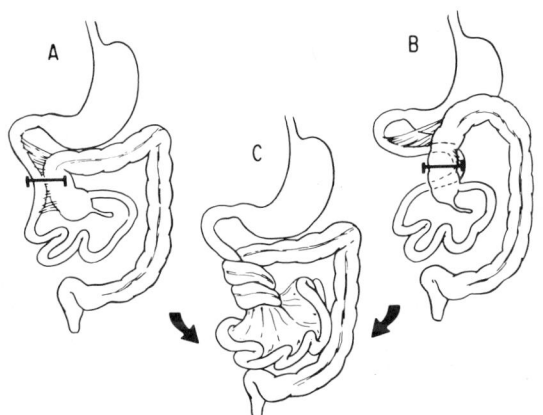

Figure 37–6. Pathophysiology of midgut volvulus with malrotation. If there is a narrow mesenteric attachment of the midgut, either nonrotation *(A)* or incomplete rotation *(B)* may develop midgut volvulus *(C)*. (Modified from Snyder WH Jr, Chaffin L. Embryology and pathology of the intestinal tract: Presentation of 40 cases of malrotation. Ann Surg 1954; 140:368.)

The cause of malrotation is unknown. There is an association with congenital diaphragmatic hernia and abdominal wall abnormalities (omphalocele and gastroschisis). An association with Hirschsprung's disease and intestinal atresias has also been found.

Most patients with symptomatic malrotation present in infancy. The age of presentation is frequently under 1 month, and many of these present in the first week of life; midgut volvulus has even been known to occur in utero. Six percent to 20% present after 1 year of age. Older children tend to have a longer course of vague, antecedent symptoms such as intermittent nonbilious vomiting and chronic abdominal pain.

Clinical Evaluation

The clinical hallmark of acute midgut volvulus is the sudden onset of bilious vomiting. The vomiting may be projectile and on occasion may have a "coffee grounds" appearance or contain frank blood. The presence of abdominal distention or a palpable mass is variable. Older children will typically complain of colicky abdominal pain. Stools are usually absent, but, if present, will be positive on guaiac tests. The presence of bright red blood passed through the rectum implies intestinal ischemia. Hypovolemia, shock, and sepsis can occur.

Diagnostic Evaluation

The best diagnostic aid in the case of acute midgut volvulus is a high index of suspicion. Leukocytosis with a left shift may be present, but generally routine laboratory studies are not helpful. Abdominal plain films sometimes help by demonstrating a double-bubble sign, which consists of air-fluid levels in both the stomach and in the distended duodenum. Often the abdomen is gasless. In an infant with bilious vomiting and a gasless abdomen, midgut volvulus should always be considered. Distended loops of small bowel are only occasionally seen, because the point of obstruction is the third portion of the duodenum. When present, distended bowel may imply intestinal gangrene, as the resorption of intestinal gas from a closed-loop obstruction ceases when the volvulus is tight enough to block venous outflow.

Definitive diagnosis of midgut volvulus requires contrast studies. A barium enema may provide indirect evidence by showing an ectopically placed right colon and cecum. Unfortunately, delineating the end of the colon from the beginning of the small bowel can be difficult in young infants. Moreover, a normal cecal position does not always exclude the possibility of malrotation and of volvulus, and a "high" or mobile cecum is a common finding in many asymptomatic infants. An upper GI series is a quicker, more direct approach. The risk of aspiration is small when barium is injected directly into the stomach through a nasogastric tube. Duodenal obstruction is readily viewed, and a classic "corkscrew" pattern is sometimes seen.

Therapeutic Intervention

The treatment of malrotation with midgut volvulus is surgical. Rapid diagnosis is critical to preserve intestinal viability. Obstruction of venous outflow initially leads to intestinal edema, which in turn produces compromise of arterial inflow as swollen loops of bowel twist about the superior mesenteric artery and the dense peritoneal bands. Ischemia and gangrene may develop in 1 to 2 hours if the volvulus is not reduced, leading to loss of the entire length of the jejunum and ileum, as well as the ascending colon. This is generally incompatible with survival or at best necessitates life-long total parenteral nutrition. Hence, malrotation with midgut volvulus is one of the most emergent obstructive conditions in children.

Nasogastric suction and intravenous hydration should be initiated when entertaining the possibility of midgut volvulus. The initial nasogastric aspirate should be quantitated. If abdominal plain films are diagnostic, contrast studies are deferred, and the child is taken directly to the operating room. On opening the abdominal cavity, volvulus is readily apparent and is reduced by twisting the entire midgut in a counterclockwise direction. Ischemic-appearing bowel often "pinks up" rapidly on reduction. Ladd's bands are lysed, and the cecum is relocated to the left upper quadrant (the so-called *Ladd procedure*). An incidental appendectomy is performed to avoid the later confusion of appendicitis presenting on the left side of the abdomen.

Ladd's Bands

Duodenal obstruction by Ladd's bands can occur acutely or chronically as a result of malrotation. The acute form behaves much like midgut volvulus, except that there is less propensity for vascular compromise. The chronic form may be associated with a partially obstructing volvulus and is characterized by malnutrition. Bilious vomiting is the presenting symptom in both forms, and a double-bubble sign may be seen on abdominal radiographs. An upper GI contrast study is diagnostic.

Mesocolic Hernia

Another malrotational abnormality associated with obstruction is a mesocolic hernia. Nonfixation of the colonic and duodenal mesenteries leads to the formation of potential hernia pouches that transiently and recurrently entrap the bowel, causing partial obstruction. Such internal hernias are either right- or left-sided and can at times incarcerate and strangulate. Patients typically have repeated episodes of colicky abdominal pain and vomiting that spontaneously subside. An upper GI study with small-bowel follow-through during an episode can be diagnostic, showing the intestines bunched together as if enveloped by a sac.

Cecal Volvulus

Cecal volvulus requires a mobile cecum and is a disorder of nonfixation rather than of pure malrotation. It most commonly occurs as an axial twisting of the cecum, ascending colon, and terminal ileum, and therefore the term *cecal volvulus* is actually a misnomer. Occasionally the cecum may fold acutely in an anterior and cephalic direction onto the ascending colon, a condition known as *cecal bascule*.

Cecal volvulus is extremely rare in children. It is less common than sigmoid volvulus, which is also very rare in children. Presenting symptoms include pain, distention, constipation or obstipation, and vomiting. Frequently there is a preexistent underlying illness, and many patients have undergone prior laparotomy.

Abdominal plain films may show a large air-filled loop of colon occupying the left upper quadrant, along with a picture of typical small-bowel obstruction. A "bird's beak" deformity, coupled with nonvisualization of the cecum, is the characteristic finding on barium enema. In contrast to sigmoid volvulus, nonoperative decompression of cecal volvulus is potentially dangerous, and surgical reduction is usually necessary.

INCARCERATED HERNIA

Incarcerated abdominal wall hernias can be inguinal, femoral, or umbilical, but inguinal hernias are the most common.

Most patients with inguinal hernias present in the first year of life, and approximately one third of children are younger than 6 months of age at operation. More males are affected than females. In males the hernia occurs on the right in approximately 60%, on the left in 25%, and bilaterally in 15%. Females have bilateral inguinal hernias more often than do males. Children who present with a left inguinal hernia stand a 41% chance of developing a right inguinal hernia, whereas children presenting with a right inguinal hernia stand only a 14% chance of having left-sided involvement. The vast majority of inguinal hernias are indirect hernias, as direct hernias usually occur after repair of a previous indirect hernia.

The anatomic basis of an indirect inguinal hernia is a patent processus vaginalis peritonea. During the third month of gestation in the male, this process develops as an outpouching of the peritoneum in the region of the internal inguinal ring. It descends the inguinal canal into the scrotum and is later followed by the testis. This process remains patent until the time of birth and frequently until 1 year of age. In children with a unilateral indirect inguinal hernia, the process is patent in the contralateral side 50% to 60% of the time. A patent processus becomes a true hernia only when it contains some part of the abdominal viscera.

Incarceration of an inguinal hernia is common in children. Apparently the relative narrowness of the internal ring prevents trapped viscera from returning to the peritoneal cavity. In a study of 2764 patients with hernias, 12.7% of hernias were incarcerated, strangulated, or both at the time of admission. Of the patients with incarceration, 69% were infants less than 1 year old.

It is desirable to reduce an incarcerated inguinal hernia nonoperatively if possible. Sedating the child and using the Trendelenburg position while gently manipulating the hernia from below is an effective technique. The use of an ice pack on the groin to reduce edema may be counterproductive. The total time that a hernia has been incarcerated is not an important factor in determining whether to attempt nonoperative reduction. Likewise, the presence of obstruction is not an absolute contraindication. However, nonoperative reduction should be avoided (especially by the nonsurgeon) in any patient with unstable vital signs, evidence of peritoneal irritation, significant erythema of the groin, or any other signs of strangulation. Although not absolutely necessary, most surgeons prefer to admit a child whose hernia has been successfully reduced nonoperatively. It is a good practice to seek immediate surgical consultation on all children with incarcerated inguinal hernias, regardless of whether they can be nonoperatively reduced.

In children, strangulation and infarction of the hernia contents can progress fairly rapidly. Impaired venous and lymphatic drainage through the tightly compressing inguinal canal leads to edema of the herniated organ, which further compromises its arterial supply. In the case of a hollow viscus, perforation and peritonitis occur once gangrene is present. Hypovolemic shock from vomiting caused by obstruction can occur concomitantly with septic shock. In girls, in whom sliding hernias are common, the ovary and fallopian tube may become strangulated. Infant boys are at minimal risk for testicular infarction.

Clinical Evaluation

The diagnosis of incarcerated inguinal hernia is generally easy in the unclothed child. A somewhat tense, fluctuant, nonmobile mass is present in the inguinal region and may extend down into the scrotum. The mass may or may not be tender. The child is often irritable or may be lethargic if bowel ischemia is present.

A bimanual digital rectal-abdominal examination, with the rectal finger advanced to the area of the internal ring and the abdominal finger overlying it, allows the examiner to palpate the contents of the hernia sac. This is felt as a markedly increased thickness between the opposing fingers, a finding not encountered with acute hydrocele of the spermatic cord.

In addition to hydrocele, the differential diagnosis of a firm groin mass includes suppurative inguinal or femoral lymphadenitis and torsion of an undescended testis. Transillumination is generally not helpful in distinguishing a hydrocele (because thin-walled infant intestine illuminates well), and aspiration of a suspected one is not recommended. Inflamed inguinal or femoral lymph nodes are frequently located below the inguinal ligament, and there is evidence of recent infection in their watershed area. Careful palpation of the scrotum, revealing absence of a testicle on the ipsilateral side of a groin mass, should provide a clue to torsion of an undescended testis.

The diagnosis of a nonincarcerated inguinal hernia in the child is more challenging. Often there is no visible bulge, only a history of one seen transiently by the parents or perhaps by the pediatrician. Lifting the infant upright may cause the abdominal contents to descend into the hernia sac. Alternatively, stretching the infant out in a supine position (legs extended, arms held straight overhead) can result in the infant struggling to get free, forcing contraction of the abdominal wall musculature and thereby increasing intraperitoneal pressure. Older children can be asked to blow up a balloon, preferably while standing. Palpation of the inguinal region may reveal a dilated external ring or the so-called *silk glove sign*. The latter is the name given to the sensation of smoothness the examiner feels—as if two pieces of silk are being rubbed together—when rolling the spermatic cord in a direction perpendicular to the course of the inguinal canal. This sensation is thought to be created by the thickness of the hernia sac rubbing against the pubic tubercle. If a nonincarcerated inguinal hernia is found or the possibility of an occult one exists, the parents should be educated about the signs and symptoms of incarceration, and a prompt referral to a pediatric or general surgeon should be made.

Femoral and Umbilical Hernias

Femoral hernias are extremely rare in children and are the only hernias that occur in girls more often than boys. Nevertheless, inguinal hernias are still more common in girls than are femoral hernias. Femoral hernias are difficult to diagnose preoperatively and tend to incarcerate. Umbilical hernias, on the other hand, are very common in children and rarely incarcerate. Most umbilical defects less than 1.5 cm in diameter close spontaneously by age 9 or 10 years. Repair before that time is done chiefly for cosmetic reasons but usually is not performed prior to age 4 or 5 years. Unlike in children, umbilical hernias frequently incarcerate in adults.

NECROTIZING ENTEROCOLITIS

Necrotizing enterocolitis (NEC) is primarily seen in premature infants in the setting of a newborn intensive care unit. There are between 2200 and 40,000 cases annually. NEC accounts for 15% of the deaths after 1 week of age in infants with birth weight below 1500 gm and can produce strictures that later on lead to intestinal obstruction.

The basis of the disease seems to be ischemic or hypoxemic insult to the intestinal mucosa. Bacterial invasion of the denuded mucosa follows, with subsequent gram-negative septicemia and intestinal necrosis. The most commonly involved sites are the terminal ileum and the colon. Infants who have not been fed develop NEC less frequently; the addition of substrate formula to the intestinal lumen is a critical step in promoting bacterial proliferation and mucosal invasion.

Clinical Evaluation

The clinical features of NEC are nonspecific. Lethargy, temperature instability, and abdominal distention frequently occur. Gastric retention or vomiting is common, with emesis or nasogastric aspirates eventually becoming bilious. Gross or occult rectal bleeding is often seen, but diarrhea is surprisingly infrequent. Stool specimens often test positive for reducing substances. The white blood cell count may be elevated or decreased, and thrombocytopenia is common.

Diagnostic Evaluation

Radiographic examination of the abdomen initially reveals multiple gas-filled loops of intestine and air-fluid levels. Later, pneumatosis intestinalis can develop. This is the name given to intramural intestinal gas and is a clinical hallmark of NEC. It is thought to represent gas resulting from bacterial fermentation. Pneumatosis intestinalis may be associated with portal vein gas, which is seen as an arborizing pattern in the right upper quadrant. This finding indicates severe disease. Occasionally a gasless abdomen may be encountered.

Therapeutic Intervention

Management of NEC consists of nasogastric suction, careful fluid management, parenteral nutrition, close observation, and antibiotic therapy. Antimicrobial therapy is directed at *Escherichia coli, Klebsiella,* and *Clostridia.* Gentamicin or kanamycin plus ampicillin and clindamycin are reasonable choices. Aggressive fluid resuscitation may be necessary. Medical management should continue for 7 to 14 days, depending on the severity of the disease. Other than pneumoperitoneum, indications for surgery are somewhat sketchy. Some clinicians advocate surgery for any child who is either not improving or deteriorating on conservative therapy.

Long-term sequelae of NEC include the development of intestinal strictures in 11% to 36% of patients. Strictures usually occur within 1 to 6 months after the acute episode of NEC. Presentation may be fulminant, with vomiting and abdominal distention, or subtle, with diarrhea, malabsorption, and failure to thrive.

POSTOPERATIVE ADHESIVE SMALL-BOWEL OBSTRUCTION

Postoperative adhesive small-bowel obstruction is responsible for about 7% of the intestinal obstructions seen in infants and children. The overall risk of developing adhesive small-bowel obstruction (SBO) after laparotomy in infants and children approaches 2%. Regardless of the nature of the previous illness or type of prior abdominal surgery, in most cases the obstruction is caused by a single adhesion.

The interval between previous operation and the onset of obstructive symptoms ranges from 2 days to 10 years. Most adhesive SBOs occur within the first 3 to 6 postoperative months, and the vast majority occur within 2 years. In the early postoperative period obstruction may be caused by intussusception and not just by a paralytic ileus, whereas after 2 weeks, adhesions are the most likely cause.

The clinical features of adhesive SBO include sudden onset of crampy abdominal pain followed by anorexia, nausea, and vomiting. Bowel movements usually cease shortly after the onset of symptoms, but diarrhea may be present, implying partial obstruction. The child often has a decreased level of activity or even lethargy. Physical examination may reveal abdominal distention and hyperactive, high-pitched bowel sounds with borborygmi. Distended small intestine generally produces diffuse, poorly localized tenderness that improves with proximal decompression by suction tube. Loops are occasionally palpable or even visible.

Supine and upright abdominal radiographs reveal dilated gas-filled loops of small intestine. Air in the colon usually indicates a partial obstruction. In infants, it is notoriously difficult to distinguish whether a gas-filled loop is colon or small bowel, and only by demonstrating gas in the rectum is it possible to be certain that there is gas in the colon. A prone cross-table lateral film is sometimes helpful in this respect. An upper GI contrast study is also helpful, especially in questionable cases. Barium is generally safe when there is no clinical evidence of perforation; an upright chest radiograph should be done prior to the study.

Prompt surgical consultation is mandatory whenever the diagnosis of adhesive SBO is considered. Delays can result in intestinal necrosis. Emergency department management consists of fluid resuscitation, nasogastric suction, and general preoperative care. Surgical management consists of enterolysis and occasionally, resection of gangrenous bowel may be necessary.

DUPLICATIONS

Duplications may occur virtually anywhere in the gastrointestinal tract. They are relatively rare lesions, and when encountered, they are most commonly found in the ileum, especially near the ileocecal valve, and the esophagus.

Mediastinal duplications (esophagus and stomach, also known as *neurenteric cysts*) are often associated with cervical and upper thoracic vertebral malformations such as hemivertebrae and anterior spina bifida. Complete duplication of the colon and rectum is frequently associated with doubling of the genitalia and of the bladder and urethra, exstrophy of the bladder, spina bifida, omphalocele, and other lesions. Small-bowel duplications may occasionally be associated with intestinal atresias.

The clinical presentation of duplications depends largely on their type of mucosal lining. Communicating intestinal duplications that contain ectopic gastric mucosa may present with peptic ulceration and gastrointestinal hemorrhage. Spherical cystic duplications may become large enough to cause obstruction and should always be considered in the differential diagnosis of a vomiting infant or child with a palpable, solid abdominal mass; may also act as the lead point for an intussusception or form the apex of a volvulus. Thoracic duplications characteristically produce respiratory symptoms and dysphagia early in life. Abdominal gastric and duodenal duplications usually present with vomiting and an upper abdominal mass and may be confused with pyloric stenosis.

Most patients with duplications present in early childhood or infancy, but some may not become symptomatic until much later in life. Chronic intermittent vomiting caused by recurring partial obstruction is the usual course in older patients. A large mass resembling the feces-filled megacolon of Hirschsprung's disease is occasionally palpable.

The diagnosis of enteric duplication is difficult to make preoperatively. Thoracic duplications are the type easiest to diagnose, frequently appearing as a posterior mediastinal mass on chest radiograph. Technetium scanning images those duplications that contain ectopic gastric mucosa. An upper GI contrast series may show stenosis or compression by an extrinsic mass. For most abdominal duplications, ultrasonography is more expedient and provides greater detail than conventional contrast radiography. The surgical management of duplications is quite variable and depends largely on the location.

GASTRIC VOLVULUS

Gastric volvulus is an abnormal rotation of one part of the stomach around another part. It is an extremely rare condition but is nonetheless an important one to consider, as it represents an acute pediatric surgical emergency and presents in an atypical fashion in the very young.

The clinical features of acute gastric volvulus depend on the degree of rotation and obstruction. In general, torsion of the stomach of up to 180 degrees results in partial obstruction with vomiting that may or may not be bilious and does not lead to vascular compromise. Torsion beyond 180 degrees causes complete obstruction and strangulation of the gastric vasculature. The resulting clinical picture in adults is known as the *triad of Borchardt* and consists of nonproductive retching, acute localized epigastric pain and distention, and the inability to pass a nasogastric tube. However, these components are difficult to assess in children. On occasion, infants and children will present with sudden respiratory distress or gastrointestinal bleeding (both upper and lower). In the newborn, persistent regurgitation and vomiting are common. At times the distended stomach is palpable, giving the impression of an epigastric mass.

Roentgenographic evaluation is crucial in diagnosing acute gastric volvulus. In mesenterioaxial volvulus, abdominal plain films show a spherical, markedly distended stomach on the supine projection and double fluid levels on the upright view. The superiorly located fluid level is in the antrum, and the inferiorly located one is in the fundus. Also seen on the upright film, and occasionally on the supine film, is a characteristic "bird's beak" at the esophagogastric junction. This finding is also readily seen on contrast examination. Barium may not get beyond the esophagogastric junction, which is located in the normal position, but if it does, the upside-down orientation of the stomach is confirmed, and the degree of obstruction can be documented.

Radiographic diagnosis of organoaxial gastric volvulus is more difficult. Often there is no spherically dilated stomach on supine abdominal plain films, and the upright view typically shows just one air-fluid level. On barium study, the stomach is positioned horizontally, with the esophagogastric junction situated lower than normal. The bird's beak sign is usually absent, but the esophagogram may show a spiral twist or distal esophageal obstruction. Occasionally the stomach may lie above the diaphragm.

Acute gastric volvulus is a true surgical emergency. Nasogastric suction should be initiated, if possible, and intravenous fluids begun. After a brief period of resuscitation, the patient is taken directly to the operating room, where the volvulus is reduced and gastropexy is performed.

ANNULAR PANCREAS

Annular pancreas is a rare lesion but is perhaps the most common form of external compression on the second portion of the duodenum. Annular pancreas consists of a thin, flat ring of histologically normal pancreatic tissue surrounding the descending duodenum. In annular pancreas, the ventral bud of the developing pancreas winds around the duodenum prior to fusing with the dorsal bud. Despite this bizarre anatomic arrangement, an annular pancreas usually functions normally, barring the development of pancreatitis or obstruction of the duct of Wirsung.

The finding of annular pancreas is frequently associated with malrotation and Down syndrome. Also seen with high frequency is intrinsic duodenal stenosis or atresia at the same level as the annular pancreas. Associations with congenital heart disease (primarily tetralogy of Fallot), esophageal atresia, and imperforate anus have also been noted. Infrequently associated conditions include partial situs inversus and congenital absence of the gallbladder.

The annular pancreas can be asymptomatic. The age of onset of obstructive symptoms varies and is sometimes delayed until adulthood. Many pediatric cases present in the newborn period with complete duodenal obstruction, often after the first feeding. Because the duodenum is most often compressed at a point distal to the ampulla of Vater, bilious vomiting is the hallmark symptom. Abdominal distention is typically minimal. There may be failure to pass meconium or an abrupt cessation of stooling. The degree of dehydration varies, but dehydration is frequently accompanied by metabolic alkalosis. A more insidious form of chronic partial duodenal obstruction may also occur, in which older children may be accused of having psychogenic abdominal pain or vomiting.

The diagnosis of annular pancreas is often not made until surgery. Abdominal plain films may show the double-bubble sign characteristic of duodenal obstruction. An upper GI series reveals the point of obstruction but not necessarily the exact cause. Ultrasound can reliably diagnose duodenal obstruction, even prenatally in pregnancies complicated by polyhydramnios in the third trimester.

The surgical management of annular pancreas consists of a bypass procedure. The standard operation is a retrocolic duodenojejunostomy.

GASTROINTESTINAL OBSTRUCTIONS IN THE IMMEDIATE POSTNATAL PERIOD

Conditions causing obstruction in the immediate postnatal period are rarely seen by emergency medicine practitioners (Table 37–2). Nonetheless, it is important to have an awareness of these causes of obstruction, particularly for emergency physicians at hospitals with heavily used obstetrics services. It is common for a mother and her newborn baby to be discharged within 24 to 36 hours after normal spontaneous vaginal delivery. Such infants may arrive at the

---

TABLE 37–2

CAUSES OF INTESTINAL OBSTRUCTION IN THE IMMEDIATE POSTNATAL PERIOD

Esophageal atresia, with or without tracheoesophageal fistula
Congenital gastric outlet syndrome
  Pyloric membrane and atresia
  Antral membrane and atresia
Congenital microgastria
Duodenal atresia
Duodenal stenosis
Duodenal diaphragm or web
Preduodenal portal vein
Jejunoileal atresia
Jejunoileal stenosis
Meconium ileus
Megacystis-microcolon-intestinal hypoperistalsis syndrome
Colonic atresia
Neonatal small left colon syndrome
Meconium plug syndrome
Imperforate anus

---

emergency department in the first week of life for problems not apparent at the time of the initial postnatal screening examination.

Many of the disorders previously discussed can present in the early postnatal period, especially Hirschsprung's disease, malrotation with midgut volvulus, necrotizing enterocolitis, and annular pancreas. Pyloric stenosis is uncommon in the first week of life, and intussusception in a neonate is extremely rare. However, inguinal hernia is often discernible in newborns and may even incarcerate. Duplications and gastric volvulus are rare but may present early in life.

Jejunoileal Atresia

Of the conditions listed in Table 37–2, the most common is probably jejunoileal atresia, with a reported incidence of 1 in 330 to 1 in 1500 live births. Atresia of the jejunum and ileum is much more common than stenosis and is characterized by maternal polyhydramnios, bilious vomiting, jaundice, and failure to pass meconium in the first day of life. Bilious vomiting is slightly more common in jejunal atresia, whereas abdominal distention occurs with greater frequency in patients with ileal atresia.

Radiographic findings of jejunoileal atresia include thumb-sized intestinal loops ("rule of thumb") and air-fluid levels. A barium enema will demonstrate a microcolon. An upper GI series is not indicated in atresia (complete obstruction) but can be helpful in jejunoileal stenosis (incomplete obstruction). Operative management includes resection or modification of the blind proximal atretic segment of intestine and anastomosis to the distal segment.

Anorectal Malformation

Anorectal malformations occur in multiple varieties and have an overall incidence of 1 per 5000 live births. Fistulas between the rectum and genitourinary tract are common. Other congenital anomalies may be associated with anorectal malformation, including *v*ertebral defects, *a*nal atresia, *tr*acheo*e*sophageal fistula, and *r*adial and *r*enal anomalies (known as the VATER complex). Diagnosis is usually apparent on examination of the perineum.

Meconium Ileus

Meconium ileus is seen almost exclusively in patients with cystic fibrosis. Meconium ileus results from the production of hyperviscous secretions by the small intestinal mucous glands, which renders the meconium formed in utero thick, tenacious, and tar-like, with a low water content. This abnormally sticky meconium adheres firmly to the small intestinal mucosa, producing intraluminal obstruction.

Meconium ileus may be simple or complicated. In the simple form, pellets of meconium obstruct the terminal ileum, and dark green, tarry meconium packs the proximally dilated ileum. Meconium ileus is said to be complicated when it is associated with intestinal volvulus, atresia, perforation, necrosis, calculus, pseudocyst, or meconium peritonitis. The simple form can be diagnosed and often treated by enema with a hyperosmolar contrast medium, but the complicated form usually requires surgery.

Meconium ileus must be distinguished from the meconium plug syndrome, which, along with the neonatal small left colon syndrome, probably represents a continuum of transient neonatal colonic motility dysfunction. Meconium plug syndrome is not associated with cystic fibrosis but is frequent among infants of diabetic mothers; it is a fairly common cause of neonatal colonic obstruction. Its name results from the characteristic plug of inspissated meconium, usually located in the splenic flexure. Radiographic findings may also be similar to those in Hirschsprung's disease, with a small lumen and a "pseudo" transition zone distal to the plug and a dilated, meconium-filled colon proximal to the plug. Contrast enema is usually curative, as well as diagnostic, in meconium plug syndrome.

Duodenal Obstruction

Congenital duodenal obstruction of all types is relatively rare (1 in 10,000 to 40,000 live births). Approximately 25% of small-bowel atresias are found in the duodenum. Duodenal atresia is at least four times more common than duodenal stenosis, but stenosis occurs more often in the duodenum than in other portions of the gastrointestinal tract and may go undetected until adulthood. Membranous or diaphragmatic duodenal obstruction may elongate and take the form of a "wind sock" as a result of peristalsis and high proximal intraluminal pressure. The double-bubble sign on the abdominal radiograph is the key radiographic finding.

Colonic Atresia

Colonic atresia is another rare form of neonatal intestinal obstruction. Infants may take several feedings normally before developing marked abdominal distention and bilious vomiting. Stools are unsustained or absent. Barium enema is diagnostic, and surgical management involves colostomy initially, with subsequent anastomosis in 3 to 6 months.

Megacystis-Microcolon-Intestinal Hypoperistalsis

Megacystis-microcolon–intestinal hypoperistalsis syndrome (MMIHS) is a rare disorder of intestinal motility that is frequently fatal. It is also known as *Sieber syndrome* or *chronic idiopathic intestinal pseudo-obstruction syndrome*. The clinical features of MMIHS include a massively distended, nonobstructed urinary bladder, a malrotated microcolon, and absent or ineffective peristalsis. The bowel is shortened and dilated proximally, but ganglion cells are present throughout. No mechanical cause for the obstruction is found, and decompressive surgical procedures do not restore intestinal motility. The origin of this condition is unknown. Pharmacologic stimulators of peristalsis have not been effective, and long-term total parenteral nutrition is required.

Selected References

Andrassy RJ, Isaacs H, Weitzman JJ. Rectal suction biopsy for the diagnosis of Hirschsprung's disease. Ann Surg 1981;193(4):419.

Andrassy RJ, Mahour GH. Malrotation of the midgut in infants and children: A 25-year review. Arch Surg 1981;116:158.

Atwell JD, Levick P. Congenital hypertrophic pyloric stenosis and associated anomalies in the genitourinary tract. J Pediatr Surg 1981;16(6):1029.

Barr LL, Stansberry SD, Swischuk LE. Significance of age, duration, obstruction and the dissection sign in intussusception. Pediatr Radiol 1990;20:454.

Blumhagen JD, Maclin L, Krauter D, et al. Sonographic diagnosis of hypertrophic pyloric stenosis. AJR 1988;150:1367.

Boley SJ, Brandt LJ, Frank MS. Severe lower intestinal bleeding: Diagnosis and treatment. Clin Gastroenterol 1981;10:65.

Boley SJ, Dinari G, Cohen MI. Hirschsprung's disease in the newborn. Clin Perinat 1978;5(1):45.

Bowerman RA, Silver TM, Jaffe MH. Real-time ultrasound diagnosis of intussusception in children. Radiology 1982;143:527.

Breaux CW, Georgeson KE, Royal SA, et al. Changing patterns in the diagnosis of hypertrophic pyloric stenosis. Pediatrics 1988;81(2):213.

Brown CK, Olshaker JS. Meckel's diverticulum. Am J Emerg Med 1988;6(2):157.

Burke J. Femoral hernia in childhood. Ann Surg 1967;166(2):287.

Cameron AEP, Howard ER. Gastric volvulus in childhood. J Pediatr Surg 1987;22(10):944.

Carter R, Brewer LA, Hinshaw DB. Acute gastric volvulus: A study of 25 cases. Am J Surg 1980;140:99.

Cole BC, Dickinson SJ. Acute volvulus of the stomach in infants and children. Surgery 1971;70(5):707.

Dalinka MK, Wunder JF. Meckel's diverticulum and its complications, with emphasis on roentgenologic demonstrations. Radiology 1973;106(2):295.

Debartolo HM, Small-van Heerde JA. Meckel's diverticulum. Ann Surg 1976;183:30.

DeLorimier AA, Fonkalsrud EW, Hays DM. Congenital atresia and stenosis of the jejunum and ileum. Surgery 1969;65(5):819.

DeVries PA, Cox KL. Surgery of anorectal anomalies. Surg Clin North Am 1985;65(5):1139.

Ein SH, Shandling B, Reilly BJ, et al. Hydrostatic reduction of intussusception caused by lead points. J Pediatr Surg 1986;21(10):883.

Ein SH, Stephens CA, Minor A. The painless intussusception. J Pediatr Surg 1976;11(4):563.

Ein SH, Stephens CA, Shandling B, et al. Intussusception due to lymphoma. J Pediatr Surg 1986;21(9):786.

Ellis DG, Clatworthy HW. The meconium plug syndrome revisited. J Pediatr Surg 1986;1(1):54.

Feller RA. Nontraumatic surgical emergencies in children. Emerg Med Clin North Am 1991;9(3):589.

Festen C. Postoperative small bowel obstruction in infants and children. Ann Surg 1982;16(5):580.

Filston HC, Kirks DR. Malrotation—the ubiquitous anomaly. J Pediatr Surg 1981;6(4, suppl 1):614.

Firor HV. The many faces of Meckel's diverticulum. South Med J 1980;73:1507.

Fonkalsrud EW, deLorimier AA, Clatworthy HW. Femoral and direct inguinal hernias in infants and children. JAMA 1967;192(7):597.

Forman HP, Leonidas JC, Kronfeld GD. A rational approach to the diagnosis of hypertrophic pyloric stenosis: Do the results match the claims? Pediatr Surg 1990;25(2):262.

Franken EA, Kac SCS, Smith WL, et al. Imaging of the acute abdomen in infants and children. AJR 1989;153:921.

Fuchs S, Jaffe D. Vomiting. Pediatr Emerg Care 1990;6(2):164.

Ghory MJ, Sheldon CA. Newborn surgical emergencies of the gastrointestinal tract. Surg Clin North Am 1985;65(5):1083.

Grosfeld JL, O'Neill JA. Enteric duplications in infancy and childhood: An 18-year review. Ann Surg 1970;172(1):83.

Heij HA, Niessen GJCM. Annular pancreas associated with congenital absence of the gallbladder. J Pediatr Surg 1987;22(11):1033.

Hickey WF, Corson JM. Squamous cell carcinoma arising in a duplication of the colon: Case report and literature review. Cancer 1981;47(3):602.

Howell CG, Vozza F, Shaw S, et al. Malrotation, malnutrition, and ischemic bowel disease. J Pediatr Surg 1982;17(5):469.

Idowu J, Aitken DR, Georgeson KE. Gastric volvulus in the newborn. Arch Surg 1980;115:1046.

Janik JS, Ein SH, Filler RM, et al. An assessment of the surgical treatment of adhesive small bowel obstruction in infants and children. J Pediatr Surg 1981;16(3):225.

Janik JS, Ein SH, Mancer K. Intestinal stricture after necrotizing enterocolitis. J Pediatr Surg 1981;16(4):438.

Jedd MB, Melton LJ, Griffin MR, et al. Factors associated with infantile hypertrophic pyloreic stenosis. Am J Dis Child 1988;142:334.

Jona JZ, Werlin SL. The megacystis microcolon intestinal hypoperistalsis syndrome: Report of a case. J Pediatr Surg 1981;16(5):749.

Kalayoglu M, Sieber WK, Rodnan JB, et al. Meconium ileus: A critical review of treatment and eventual prognosis. J Pediatr Surg 1971;6(3):290.

Khamapirad T, Athey PA. Ultrasound diagnosis of hypertrophic pyloric stenosis. J Pediatr 1983;102(1):23.

Kirks DR, Swischuk LE, Merten DF, et al. Cecal volvulus in children. AJR 1981;136:419.

Klein MD, Coran AG, Wesley JR, et al. Hirschsprung's disease in the newborn. J Pediatr Surg 1984;19(4):370.

Kliegman RM, Fanaroff AA. Neonatal necrotizing enterocolitis: A nine-year experience. Am J Dis Child 1981;135:603.

Leonidas JC. Treatment of intussusception with small bowel obstruction: Application of decision analysis. AJR 1985;145:665.

Mackey WC, Dineen P. A fifty year experience with Meckel's diverticulum. Surg Gynecol Obstet 1983;156:56.

Martin LW, Torres AM. Hirschsprung's disease. Surg Clin North Am 1985;65(5):1171.

Merrill JR, Raffensperger JG. Pediatric annular pancreas: Twenty years' experience. J Pediatr Surg 1976;11(6):921.

Mollitt DL, Ballantine EVN, Grosfeld JL. Postoperative intussusception in infancy and childhood: Analysis of 119 cases. Surgery 1979;86(3):402.

Moore GP, Burkle FM. Isolated axial volvulus of Meckel's diverticulum. Am J Emerg Med 1988;6(2):137.

Morgan WW, White JJ, Stumbaugh S, et al. Prophylactic umbilical hernia repair in childhood to prevent adult incarceration. Surg Clin North Am 1970;50(4):839.

Neblett WW, Pietsch JB, Holcomb GW. Acute abdominal conditions in children and adolescents. Surg Clin North Am 1985;65(5):1331.

O'Neill JA. Neonatal necrotizing enterocolitis. Surg Clin North Am 1981;61(5):1013.

Ong NT, Beasley SW. The leadpoint in intussusception. J Pediatr Surg 1990;25(6):640.

Ong NT, Beasley SW. Progression of intussusception. J Pediatr Surg 1990;25(6):644.

O'Mara CS, Wilson TH, Stonesifer GL, et al. Cecal volvulus: Analysis of 50 patients with long-term follow up. Ann Surg 1979;189(6):724.

Pang LC. Intussusception revisited: Clinicopathologic analysis of 261 cases, with emphasis on pathogenesis. South Med J 1989;82(2):215.

Philippart AI, Reed JO, Georgeson KE. Neonatal small left colon syndrome: Intramural not intraluminal obstruction. J Pediatr Surg 1975;10(5):733.

Powell DM, Biemann O, Smith CD. Malrotation of the intestines in children: The effect of age on presentation and therapy. J Pediatr Surg 1989;24(8):777.

Puri P, Guiney EJ, O'Donell B. Inguinal hernia in infants: The fate of the testis following incarceration. J Pediatr Surg 1976;11(3):451.

Rachmel A, Rosenback Y, Amir J, et al. Apathy as an early manifestation of intussusception. Am J Dis Child 1983;137:701.

Ricketts RR, Pettitt BJ. Management of Hirschsprung's disease in adolescents. Am Surgery 1989;55(4):219–225.

Rowe MI, Clatworthy HW. Incarcerated and strangulated hernias in children: A statistical study of high-risk factors. Arch Surg 1970;101:135.

Schwartz MZ, Richardson CJ, Hayden CK, et al. Intestinal stenosis following successful medical management of necrotizing enterocolitis. J Pediatr Surg 1980;15(6):890.

Shandling B, Auldist AW. Punch biopsy of the rectum for the diagnosis of Hirschsprung's disease. J Pediatr Surg 1972;7(5):546.

Sieber WK, Girdany BR. Functional intestinal obstruction in newborn infants with morphologically normal gastrointestinal tracts. Surgery 1963;53(3):357.

Simpson AJ, Leonidas JC, Krasna IH, et al. Roentgen diagnosis of midgut malrotation: Value of upper gastrointestinal radiographic study. J Pediatr Surg 1972;7(2):243.

Singer J. Altered consciousness as an early manifestation of intussusception. Pediatrics 1979;64(1):93.

Stevenson RJ. Gastrointestinal bleeding in children. Surg Clin North Am 1985;65(6):1455.

Stevenson RJ. Non-neonatal intestinal obstruction in children. Surg Clin North Am 1985;65(5):1217.

Swenson O, Sherman JO, Fisher JH, et al. Diagnosis of congenital megacolon: An analysis of 501 patients. J Pediatr Surg 1973;8(5):587.

Takada Y, Aoyama K, Goto T, et al. The association of imperforate anus and Hirschsprung's disease in siblings. J Pediatr Surg 1985;20(3):271.

Tamanaha K, Wimbish K, Talwalkar YB, et al. Air reduction of intussusception in infants and children. J Pediatr Surg 1987;111(5):733.

Tenebein M, Wiseman NE. Early coma in intussusception: Endogenous opioid induced? Pediatr Emerg Care 1987;3(1):22.

Wang GD, Liu SJ. Enema reduction of intussusception by hydrostatic pressure under ultrasound guidance: A report of 377 cases. J Pediatr Surg 1988;23(9):814.

Wayne ER, Campbell JB, Kosloske AM, et al. Intussusception in the older child—suspect lymphosarcoma. J Pediatr Surg 1976;11(5):789.

Ziprkowski MN, Teele RL. Gastric volvulus in childhood. AJR 1979;132:921.

CHAPTER 38

Foreign Body Ingestion

Barbara N. Malone

INTRODUCTION

Young children are naturally curious, and the mouth is a common place to evaluate objects. Factors that contribute to the high incidence of foreign body ingestion in young children include the lack of molars for fine chewing prior to 3 years of age, a child's lack of fear, and the encouragement of older siblings in the "discovery" process.

Incidence and Prevalence

Eighty percent of foreign body ingestions occur in children. Coins are reported to comprise 15% to 52% of ingested foreign bodies. Meat impactions are rare in children unless a congenital anomaly, such as a tracheoesophageal fistula predisposing to narrowing, is present or there is mental or neurologic impairment. Sharp objects and batteries are the most dangerous ingested foreign bodies, as they can cause perforation of the soft esophageal wall. The majority of ingestions are unwitnessed; and therefore a high index of suspicion is required regarding the possibility of foreign body ingestion (Table 38–1).

ANATOMY

There are five areas of narrowing within the esophagus; these are the most likely regions in which a foreign body may lodge. Two areas, the cricopharyngeus muscle at the level of the sixth cervical vertebra and the gastroesophageal junction, account for 95% of foreign body impactions. These two regions are characterized by a thickened muscular band that contributes to less pliability of the esophageal lumen, leading to easier impaction. Other regions include the thoracic inlet correlating to the first thoracic vertebra, the area juxtaposed to the aortic knob, and the level of the esophagus corresponding to the tracheal bifurcation where the left main stem bronchus crosses the esophagus, causing a relative narrowing.

The esophageal introitus or opening is posterior and slightly superior to the laryngeal inlet. Therefore objects lodged in the introitus (the level of the cricopharyngeus muscle) may become dislodged and be aspirated into the trachea. Second, the wall between the esophagus and trachea is soft, and therefore a large object in the esophagus may cause tracheal compression and result in significant respiratory symptoms. As a result of these factors, even esophageal foreign bodies that appear stable require expeditious removal.

EMERGENCY MEDICAL SERVICE CONSIDERATIONS

The level of foreign body obstruction, the degree of obstruction, and the amount of distress determine the timing and course of intervention of foreign body ingestion. The American Academy of Pediatrics has made specific recommendations in the treatment of the choking child. Methods of foreign body removal in which there is no control of the airway are discouraged unless there is no choice and the airway is markedly compromised. The following methods should be avoided:

Back pounding
Postural drainage
Finger probing of the mouth
Heimlich maneuver
Bronchodilators

A child's natural protective airway reflexes are better than any maneuver provided by someone else. Therefore, if a child's airway is uncompromised, the physician should not perform any manipulation, but instead should maintain close observation. If a child is cyanotic or in obvious distress, a series of steps are undertaken to regain control of the airway. These especially apply to foreign bodies obstructing the glottis or introitus or those impacted in the esophagus and compressing the airway. More advanced maneuvers include the following:

1. Placing the child in a head-down, prone position and administering back blows
2. Delivering chest thrusts
3. Removing the foreign body with forceps if it can be directly visualized in the mouth or pharynx
4. Administering cardiopulmonary resuscitation if manipulating the foreign body fails
5. Repeating the process if unsuccessful

The child should be expeditiously transported to the hospital, where the foreign body can be extracted. The child should be transported in an upright position, with close attention paid to the airway, and if there are any signs of respiratory distress, the child should receive oxygen. Needle cricothyroidotomy can be used as a temporizing measure in the apneic child.

CLINICAL EVALUATION

Foreign body ingestion should be considered in the differential diagnosis of any child with a history of gagging, choking, coughing, or vomiting. The specific presenting symptoms depend on the type of foreign body, site of obstruction, degree of obstruction, and duration of the foreign body's presence. Because the majority of esophageal foreign bodies lodge at the level of the cricopharyngeus muscle, airway symptoms often accompany the symptoms of drooling and dysphagia because of the proximity of the glottis and trachea.

Patients with foreign bodies at the midesophageal level may present with dysphagia and throat or chest pain. If the foreign body is retained for a prolonged period, symptoms of perforation with mediastinitis may develop. Similarly, retained foreign bodies at the gastroesophageal junction may perforate into either the chest or peritoneal cavity.

Many patients with foreign body obstruction are asymptomatic, especially if they tend to eat a liquid or soft diet. Early symptoms of foreign body obstruction may include dysphagia, poor feeding, the inability to handle secretions, and vomiting. Late symptoms appear after weeks to months of foreign body retention and include weight loss, failure to thrive, and infectious symptoms.

The physical examination may be normal, or the child may demonstrate drooling and the inability to swallow or handle secretions. Stridor or wheezing may be present if glottic compromise or tracheal compression result from esophageal foreign body obstruction.

DIAGNOSTIC EVALUATION

All children suspected of ingesting a foreign body require radiologic evaluation, including a lateral neck radiograph as well as anteroposterior and lateral chest radiographs (Fig. 38–1). A lateral neck radiograph (Fig. 38–2) will distinguish a tracheal foreign body from one in the esophagus. Chest radiographs will illustrate the level of lower foreign bodies and evaluate for pneumothorax, mediastinitis, or aspiration pneumonia. Cricopharyngeal foreign body obstruction has been missed because the neck was excluded from the radiologic examination. If there is a delay in endoscopic removal of the object, radiographs should be repeated to evaluate for possible distal migration.

Radiopaque foreign bodies are easily visible. Those that are semiopaque or lucent may be suggested by periesophageal inflammation and proximal ballooning of the hypopharynx and esophagus secondary to obstruction. Radiographic studies of the chest in the lateral and anteroposterior positions may help if there is a second foreign body, making treatment by endoscopic removal more efficacious (Fig. 38–3).

Contrast studies (e.g., barium swallow) are often not recommended unless a child is not a surgical candidate. Such studies risk aspiration with complete esophageal impaction. Contrast also impairs visualization of the foreign body during endoscopic removal.

DIFFERENTIAL DIAGNOSIS

Children with foreign body obstruction may exhibit drooling, dysphagia, and an inability to handle secretions. How-

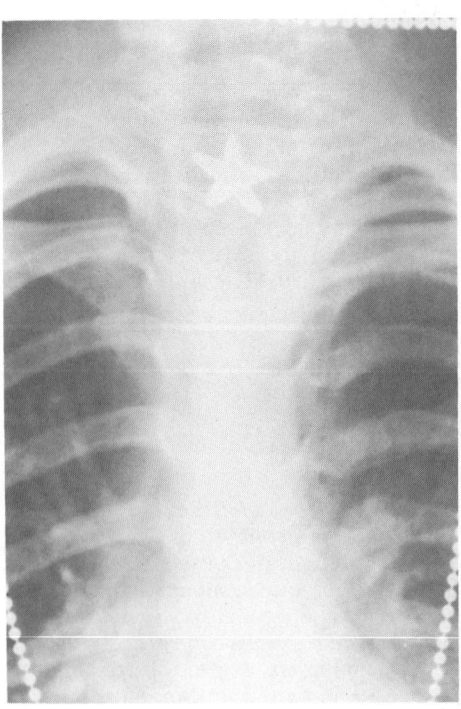
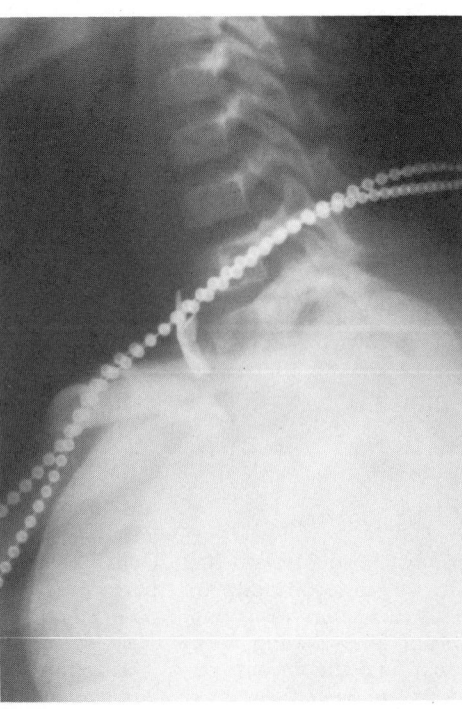

Figure 38–1. The swallowed metallic star in this 6-year-old girl illustrates the typical orientation of a flat swallowed coin or other object in the esophagus, namely, in the coronal plane (so that it is in profile on lateral view and en face on frontal view).(Courtesy of A. Oestreich, M.D., Cincinnati, OH.)

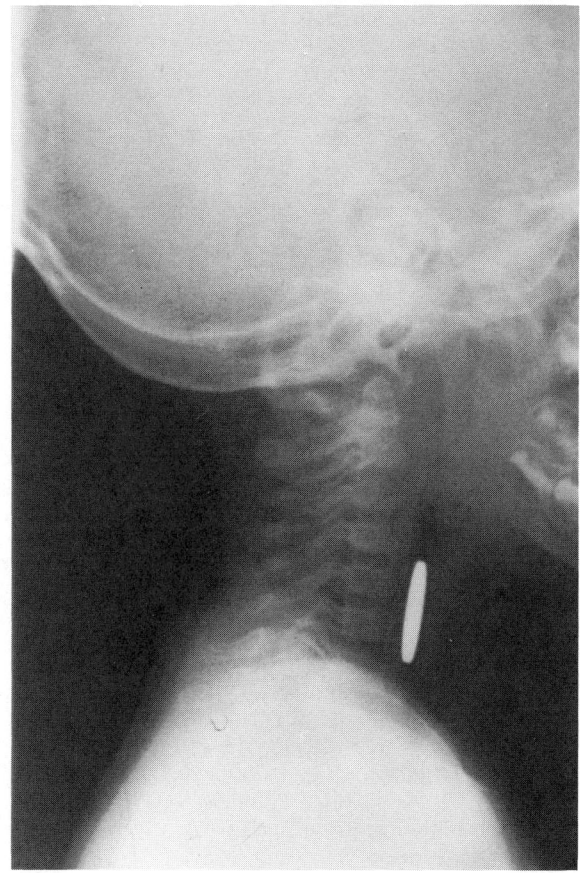

Figure 38–2. Occasionally a lateral neck radiograph alone is sufficient to distinguish a tracheal foreign body from an esophageal foreign body.

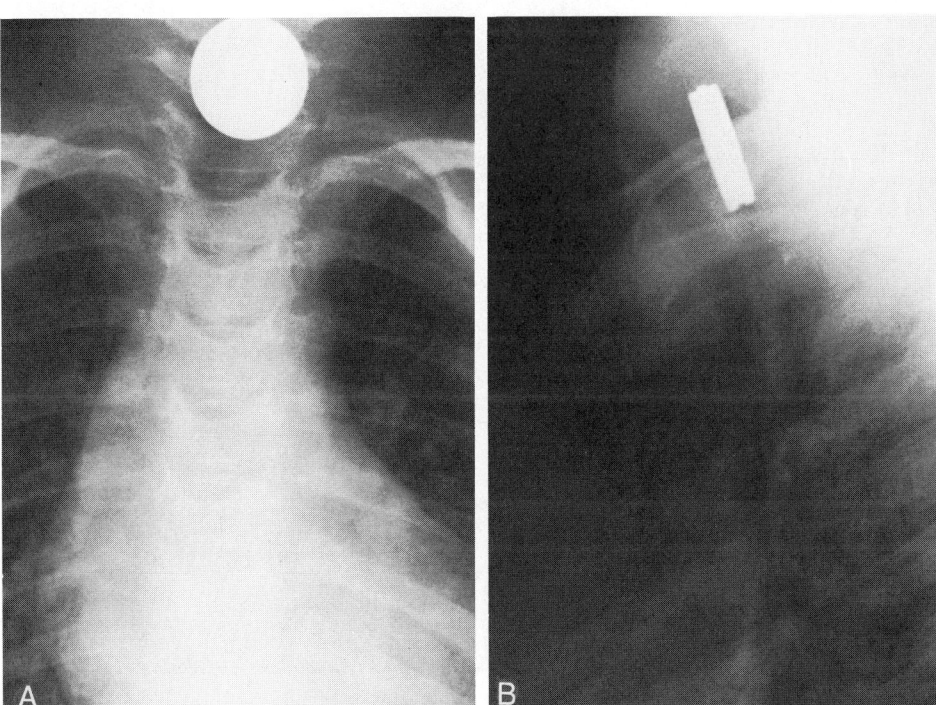

Figure 38–3. *A*, Posteroanterior radiograph suggests the presence of a single coin. However, on the lateral radiograph *(B)*, three coins are found to be at the level of the cricopharyngeal narrowing.

TABLE 38–1

COMMON ERRORS IN MANAGEMENT OF ESOPHAGEAL FOREIGN BODIES

1. Absence of positive history
2. Absence of confirmatory radiographs
3. Inadequate radiographs
4. Omission of foreign body ingestion from primary differential diagnosis
5. Errors created by inexperienced consultants
6. Inappropriate use of instruments for removal of foreign bodies
7. Inappropriate or delayed methods of removal
8. Inexperienced endoscopist
9. Inadequate communication between the endoscopist and anesthesiologist
10. Expecting only one foreign body
11. Expecting the foreign body to lodge in the "usual" place
12. Parental ignorance or negligence

ever, acutely ill children with tonsillitis and epiglottitis may present with similar symptoms. Children with glottic compromise or tracheal compression secondary to foreign body ingestion must be differentiated from those with bronchitis, acute reactive airway disease, or other causes of airway obstruction.

THERAPEUTIC INTERVENTION

Medical management of esophageal foreign body obstruction is limited mainly to meat impactions. Glucagon is given intravenously in a dose of 0.03 to 0.10 mg/kg and may contribute to increased pliability of the esophageal wall and passage of the impaction. The dose may be repeated once. If glucagon therapy is unsuccessful, surgical intervention should be instituted.

Impacted foreign bodies in the esophagus are usually removed by endoscopy. Rigid and flexible esophagoscopy have both been advocated, and general anesthesia is required in children for proper muscular tone relaxation, cooperation, and airway control. An open rigid system is often preferable for objects lodged proximally at the esophageal introitus. In these cases the airway must be protected, as an object may be easily dislodged and fall anteriorly. Flexible endoscopy is more advantageous for distally impacted foreign bodies and for those lodged in the stomach.

Fogarty catheters have been used to remove esophageal foreign bodies in the radiology suite. Such removal may be applied successfully in selected cases. General anesthesia is not required if the child is cooperative and the airway protected at the level of sedation required to ensure cooperation. Catheter removal should only be used for single blunt objects that have been lodged for a brief period of time, thereby minimizing the risk of perforation. With the catheter technique there is a risk of foreign body aspiration, because the object is not firmly grasped with forceps.

Coins, the most common object ingested by children, and other blunt plastic objects that are impacted should be removed expeditiously to avoid perforation or fistula formation. If a coin has passed into the stomach, observation for 3 to 4 weeks may be indicated in the asymptomatic patient. Once past the duodenum, most objects are passed easily.

When button type batteries are lodged in the esophagus, urgent removal is warranted. Battery obstruction usually occurs in children younger than 5 years, as such batteries average 21 mm in diameter, and the esophogi of older children are generally too large to allow obstruction. A moist

environment causes the electrolyte solutions in these batteries to be released, and these alkaline solutions may create liquefaction necrosis and lead to perforation. If lodged in the esophagus, the battery should be urgently removed under direct vision. The child should then be observed and evaluated with a contrast study in 24 to 36 hours and again in 10 to 14 days. If eschar or inflammation is noted, the child should be observed for at least another 24 to 48 hours. If perforation is suspected, a similar period of observation is warranted. The child may be treated prophylactically with broad-spectrum antibiotics during the observation period. Steroids are not recommended, as they may mask the symptoms and signs of perforation and impending infection. If the battery is passed into the stomach either naturally or endoscopically, watchful waiting is advocated for 3 to 4 weeks to allow passage. Once the battery is in the intestine, fecal material surrounding the battery will protect the bowel wall from perforation (Fig. 38–4). If the object persistently traverses the gut, as evidenced on radiographs, no intervention is necessary.

Sharp objects that are ingested require special consideration. The most common of these is the open safety pin. Sharp objects often require urgent endoscopic removal, with the major goal being to avoid perforation. It must be remembered that *advancing* points perforate, and *trailing* points do not. After removal of the foreign body, the child should be monitored for signs of perforation, including chest and back pain, fever, tachycardia (higher than the rate expected for the level of fever), subcutaneous air, and mediastinal widening or air on chest radiograph (Fig. 38–5).

Those children without predisposing factors for obstruction should be evaluated with a barium swallow 1 to 2 weeks after foreign body removal. This is to evaluate for stricture

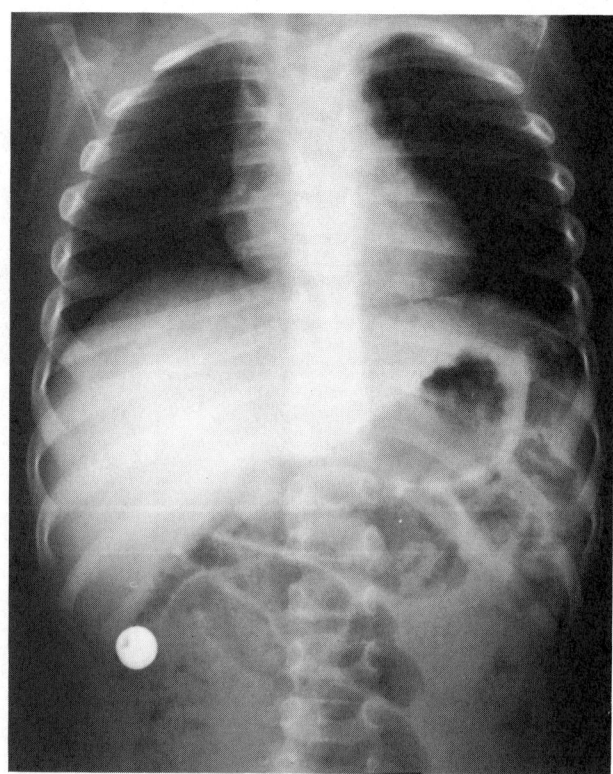

Figure 38–4. Radiographic evaluation of the chest and abdomen may be required to locate a foreign body. This button battery is in the intestine, eliminating the need for endoscopic removal. (Courtesy of A. Oestreich, M.D., Cincinnati, OH.)

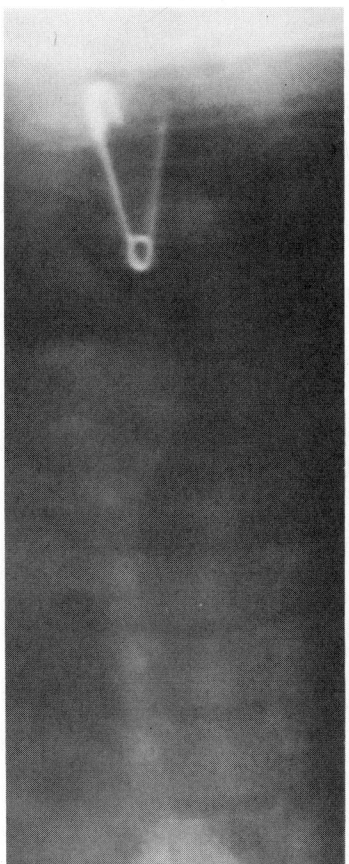
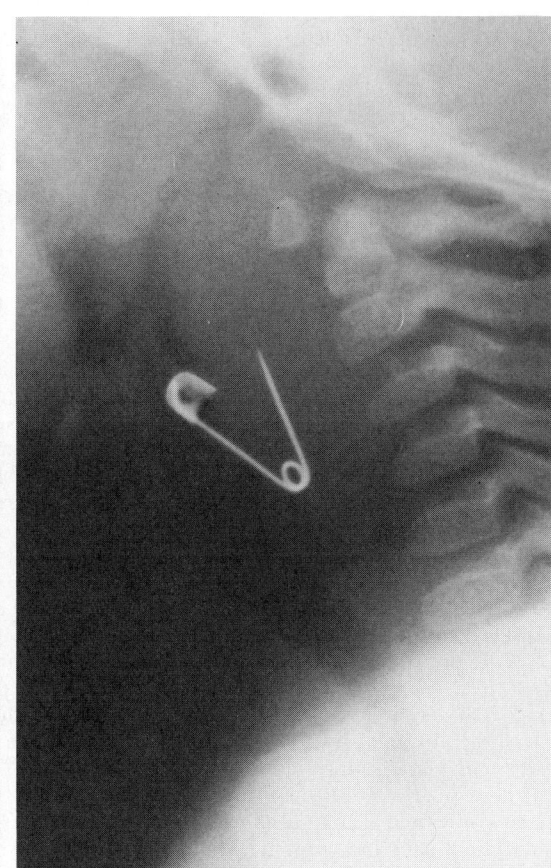

Figure 38–5. This 10-month-old boy with choking and gagging is revealed to have swallowed an open safety pin. It is in the right piriform sinus, with its tip pentrating now-swollen retro-pharyngeal tissues. (Courtesy of A. Oestreich, M.D., Cincinnati, OH.)

that may require further therapeutic intervention. The use of meat tenderizers to dissolve meat impactions should be avoided. This practice has resulted in the fatal complication of dissolution of the esophageal wall and mediastinitis.

DISCHARGE CRITERIA

The time of discharge after endoscopic removal of a foreign body depends on the ease of removal, the amount of damage to the esophageal wall, the presence or absence of airway edema, and the ability to handle secretions and tolerate oral intake. Discharge may be considered 6 to 12 hours following the uncomplicated removal of a blunt esoph-ageal foreign body present for only a short duration, or when the child can tolerate oral intake.

Selected References

Cohen SR. Unusual presentations and problems created by mismanagement of foreign bodies in the aerodigestive tract of the pediatric patient. Ann Otol Rhinol Laryngol 1981;90:315.

Friedman EM. Foreign bodies in the pediatric aerodigestive tract. Pediatr Ann 1988;17:640.

Mofenson HG, Greensher J. Management of the choking child. Pediatr Clin North Am 1985;32:183.

Phillips JJ, Patel P. Swallowed foreign bodies. J Laryngol Otol 1988;102:235.

Savitt DL, Wason S. Delayed diagnosis of coin ingestion in children. Am J Emerg Med 1988;6:378.

Webb WA. Management of foreign bodies of the upper gastrointestinal tract. Gastroenterology 1988;94:204.

CHAPTER 39

Diarrhea

Mananda S. Bhende

INTRODUCTION

Acute diarrhea is a global problem and is recognized as a leading cause of mortality and morbidity, especially in de-veloping countries.[1-3] In developing countries there are approximately 1.5 billion episodes (or 3.3 episodes per child) and 4 million deaths annually in children younger than 5 years.[2, 3]

In North America the annual rate is about 0.9 episodes per child, unless the child attends a day-care center, a risk factor that increases the diarrhea attack rate to 4.5 episodes annually in some centers.[4] One 10-year survey demonstrated that about 500 American children die of diarrheal disease each year.[5, 6] Nevertheless, there has been a dramatic reduc-tion in mortality rates from greater than 75% in 1832 to 0% to 2% during the period from 1966 to 1979.[1]

PATHOPHYSIOLOGY
Pathogenesis

Intestinal absorption is a two-stage process; ions and water enter the enterocyte through the luminal surface and exit through the basolateral membrane. Sodium (Na^+) enters the enterocyte by the following active and passive processes:

1. Na^+ diffuses down its electrochemical and concentration gradient.

2. Na^+ and chloride (Cl^-) are transported by a carrier mechanism accounting for the bulk of NaCl absorption in the small intestine and are blocked by cyclic adenosine monophosphate (cAMP).

3. Na^+ coupled to organic solutes such as glucose and amino acids is absorbed. This property continues to function in diarrheal illness and forms the basis of oral rehydration therapy.

4. The bulk flow of water between and through the cell straps additional Na^+ and Cl^- molecules in the flowing stream, referred to as *solvent drag action.*[4, 7, 8]

During the second stage of absorption, Na^+ is pumped out of the enterocyte by a Na^+-K^+ adenosine triphosphatase (ATPase) pump that is situated in the basolateral membrane. This keeps the intracellular Na^+ level low and establishes a steep electrochemical gradient for entry of Na^+ from the intestinal lumen.[4, 7, 8]

The gastrointestinal mucosa is more permeable to water in young infants than in adults. This can cause greater fluid and electrolyte losses when there is an increased osmotic load, which occurs during diarrhea.[9] Four principal pathophysiologic processes—secretory, cytotoxic, osmotic, and dysenteric—contribute individually or collectively to diarrhea. These tend to produce different types of diarrhea with varying fluid and electrolyte losses, which can have significant management implications.[9]

These processes can also alter intestinal motility, leading to a functional ileus. Luminal dilation leads to visceral abdominal pain and vomiting. Delayed gastric emptying also contributes to vomiting,[9] so much so that in rotaviral diarrhea, vomiting can often be the presenting symptom.

Stool composition can vary among different diarrheal states. The cholera stool contains about 88 mmol/L of Na^+, whereas the rotaviral stool contains only 37 mmol/L. Also the rotaviral stool is acidic, containing only 6 mmol/L of HCO_3.[10] These differences are important factors in formulating replacement therapy in diarrhea.

Secretory Diarrhea

Acute secretory diarrhea[4, 7–9] is caused by enterotoxins produced by infectious agents such as *Escherichia coli, Vibrio cholerae,* clostridia, some staphylococci, *Shigella,* and *Salmonella* and by metabolic or exogenous toxic agents. The endotoxins cause secretion of fluids and electrolytes from the crypt cells and also block the absorption of Na^+ and Cl^- by the carrier mechanism. They do not block glucose-coupled Na^+ absorption.

Cytotoxic Diarrhea

Cytotoxic diarrhea[4, 7–9] is usually caused by viral agents such as rotavirus and is characterized by destruction of mucosal cells of the villi. The virus blocks the Na^+-K^+ ATPase pump at the basolateral membrane, resulting in an intracellular buildup of Na^+, causing cell lysis. The villi shorten, decreasing the surface area of the small intestine and thereby decreasing absorption capacity. The rapid enterocyte turnover produces an immature mucosa with reduced brush border enzymes, and consequently absorption is impaired. In addition, the secretory crypt cells remain intact, resulting in a proportional increase in secretory ability and a marked decrease in the absorptive function of the small intestinal mucosa.

Osmotic Diarrhea

Osmotic diarrhea[4, 7–9] occurs most often in malabsorption syndromes, the most common of which is lactose intolerance. If the concentration of a malabsorbed substance is high enough, the substance will be osmotically active, and enough water will be drawn into the lumen to maintain isotonicity, resulting in loose diarrheal stools. This also occurs in cytotoxic and secretory diarrheas because of the impaired ability of the intestine to absorb nutrients and electrolytes. Substances such as magnesium sulphate and sorbitol also cause loose stools, because they are not absorbed and exert osmotic forces that draw fluid into the intestine.

Dysenteric Diarrhea

In dysenteric diarrhea[4, 7–9] there is invasion of the mucosa and submucosa of the colon and terminal ileum by infectious agents such as *Salmonella, Shigella, Yersinia,* and *Campylobacter* and by enteroviruses. The invasion and inflammation cause edema, mucosal bleeding, and leukocyte infiltration, resulting in exudation of blood and leukocytes into the lumen. This causes loose, runny stools, often containing blood and mucus.

Pathophysiologic Effects
Dehydration

Dehydration results from net loss of fluid when total output exceeds total intake.[11–15] This is likely to occur with severe vomiting or diarrhea. Moderate (5% to 10% weight loss) or severe (>10% weight loss) dehydration can result in decreased blood volume, with significant secondary effects. It can also result in prerenal azotemia, which, when severe or prolonged, can be accompanied by decreased renal conservation of water, or the decreased ability to excrete an acid load. Severe dehydration can cause tissue hypoperfusion, resulting in lactic acidosis.

Electrolyte Imbalance

Electrolyte imbalance results from net losses or gains of electrolytes relative to water losses.[11–15] *Hyponatremia* occurs when losses contain Na^+ and intake contains little or no Na^+, resulting in *hypotonic dehydration* (Na^+ <130 mEq/L). When serum Na^+ decreases, water moves into the cells at the expense of the vascular compartment. These patients have a greater compromise of vascular volume and therefore are clinically "drier" than their weight would suggest. They may present in shock.

Hypernatremia occurs when losses contain water in excess of Na^+ or when intake consists of fluids high in Na^+ (e.g., boiled skim milk, bouillon, or homemade salt-water solution). This results in *hypertonic dehydration* (Na^+ > 150 mEq/L). In this case water moves from the cells into the vascular compartment, thus sparing the vascular compartment at the expense of the intracellular compartment. Therefore the clinical signs of dehydration may be deceptively mild.

Isotonic dehydration (Na^+ 130 to 150 mEq/L) results when the net losses are isotonic but still exceed intake. With prolonged (>48 to 72 hours) isotonic losses, serum proteins exert some osmotic effect and draw water out of the cells and into the vascular compartment.

Gastrointestinal losses contain potassium (K^+), and most fluids offered are low in K^+. In order to maintain serum levels, K^+ is drawn out of cells in exchange for Na^+. Acidosis causes K^+ to leave the cell in exchange for H^+, and the K^+

is lost in the urine. Thus the serum K^+ level does not reflect total body K^+. *Acidosis*[11-15] results from increased bicarbonate losses from the gastrointestinal (GI) tract, starvation ketosis, lactic acidosis caused by hypoperfusion of tissues, and phosphate and sulphate retention with prerenal azotemia.

Additional Fluid Losses

Increased insensible water losses from the skin occur with fever. Hourly losses amount to 12% of hourly maintenance for each centigrade degree of fever above 38°C. Dehydrated patients usually try to compensate for metabolic acidosis by increasing their respiratory rates. Hourly losses caused by hyperventilation amount to about 25% of hourly fluid requirement with P_{CO_2} in the range of 30 mm Hg. Losses are increased only for the duration of the fever and tachypnea.

CLINICAL EVALUATION
History

The initial evaluation of all children with acute diarrhea should begin with a thorough history and physical examination.[16] The history should reconstruct the child's total intake, type of intake, and output during the course of the illness. The character, frequency, and volume of stools and emesis should be noted. Blood in the stool indicates a bacterial origin in about 50% of cases.[9] The history should also include general activity level, urine output, weight loss, use of antibiotics or any other medications, day-care attendance, travel history, household pets, dietary changes, and any similar illness in other family members. Also, it is important to know whether anyone else known to the patient became acutely ill after consumption of a particular food item. A history of intake of raw milk, poorly prepared or stored poultry and salads, and certain fish and of exposure to other potential sources of enterotoxin (e.g., untreated water) should be obtained.[9] Associated symptoms such as rash, abdominal pain, tenesmus, or urinary problems and underlying conditions such as previous GI surgery, ulcerative colitis, neoplasms, and immunodeficiency syndromes should be noted.[16]

Physical Examination

The physical examination should begin with the global assessment of the child, paying particular attention to the state of hydration. Heart rate, respiratory rate, temperature, and blood pressure all give an idea not only of hydration status, but also of the general level of illness. These should be measured and recorded. Tachycardia, hypotension, hyperpnea, and tachypnea all indicate dehydration. Orthostatic changes, especially a pulse increase of more than 25 beats/min, may indicate hypovolemia.[17] A fever normally indicates an infectious origin. An accurate weight should be obtained. This can be used to calculate the amount of weight loss and the percentage of dehydration if a recent weight is available. It also serves as a baseline for monitoring weight loss or gain during the course of the illness.

Hydration status is also reflected in moistness of mucous membranes, appearance of the anterior fontanelle (in young infants), tearing, sunken eyes, skin turgor, capillary refill, presence or absence and quality of peripheral pulses, and skin temperature.[9, 11, 13, 14] In one study[18] the main indicators of mild to moderate dehydration were decreased perfusion, deep breathing, decreased skin turgor, elevated urea levels, and acidosis. Lethargy, sunken eyes and fontanelle, dry

mouth, and absence of tears corresponded poorly to the degree of dehydration.

A thorough abdominal examination should be performed to note if there is abdominal distention, which can occur with ileus or peritonitis. A scaphoid abdomen indicates severe dehydration. Auscultation may reveal high-pitched sounds of peristaltic rushes found in dysenteric and secretory diarrheas. A rectal examination should also be performed.

Usually the child is designated as being mildly, moderately, or severely dehydrated. Traditional criteria[11, 13-19] have no statistical basis and at best give an approximate degree of dehydration.

Mild dehydration (5% weight loss in infants, 3% in the older child) is characterized by increased pulse rate, decreased tearing, dry mucous membranes, and slight oliguria. *Moderate dehydration* (10% weight loss in infants, 6% in the older child) is manifested by increased severity of previously listed signs, decreased skin turgor, and a sunken fontanelle and eyes. *Severe dehydration* (15% weight loss in infants, 9% in the older child) presents with a marked increase in the severity of previously listed signs, decreased blood pressure, mottled skin color, and signs of shock.

The degree of dehydration reflects the state of the vascular and interstitial compartments only.[11, 13, 14] The clinical signs tend to underreflect water losses in hypernatremic dehydration and overreflect water losses in hyponatremic dehydration, because in the former the water moves from the cells into the vascular space, with the reverse being true in the latter. Clinical signs will also underreflect actual water losses in prolonged diarrhea and are unreliable in the presence of precipitous losses.[11]

DIAGNOSTIC EVALUATION

Several laboratory studies can assist in the assessment of the dehydrated child.[20-27] No laboratory data are necessary before treatment of a dehydrated child can begin.

Serum Electrolytes. The serum Na^+ indicates the type of dehydration, whether hypotonic ($Na^+ < 130$ mEq/L), isotonic (Na^+ 130 to 150 mEq/L), or hypertonic ($Na^+ > 150$ mEq/L). Serum K^+ does not necessarily reflect total body K^+; an electrocardiogram (EKG) can give a better estimate. Flattened T waves suggest significant depletion.

Serum Glucose. Determination of serum glucose level is useful in excluding diabetes as an underlying condition and also in excluding hypoglycemia especially in small infants, as hypoglycemia can be a cause of significant mortality and morbidity.[21]

Blood Urea Nitrogen and Creatinine. The blood urea nitrogen (BUN) level is elevated in patients with prerenal azotemia but will be falsely low if the child has not ingested protein in the preceding 24 hours. It is not an accurate method for assessing hydration status in children with dehydration caused by gastroenteritis.

Hemoglobin/Hematocrit. Hemoglobin and hematocrit levels will be increased as a result of hemoconcentration during dehydration.[24] Because these can be assessed only if prehydration numbers are available, the use of these measures is generally limited. The complete blood cell (CBC) differential in a child with shigellosis often displays a left shift.

Venous Blood Gases. Determination of the bicarbonate level is useful, as acidosis is usually present with dehydration, especially in infants. The P_{CO_2} level will indicate the degree of compensation and secondary pulmonary insensible water losses if the patient is hyperventilating.

Urine. The urine specific gravity gives a good indication of hydration, unless there is underlying renal disease and the kidneys cannot concentrate the urine.[24] Urine ketones indicate starvation. Pyuria may indicate underlying pyelonephritis in infants.

Stool. Examination of the stool can be helpful in determining the diagnosis.[25–28] The presence of blood and neutrophils (demonstrated by methylene blue stain) indicates a probable bacterial infection. Seventy percent of patients with neutrophils in their stool have a bacterial infection, and 90% of patients with bacillary dysentery have neutrophils in their stool. The presence of reducing substances (demonstrated on Clinitest) and a low pH are indicative of lactose malabsorption.

A stool culture can identify *E. coli, Salmonella, Shigella, Campylobacter, Yersinia,* and *Clostridium difficile* organisms. However, the vast majority of acute diarrheal illnesses are viral, and stool cultures are not routinely indicated. Stool cultures are indicated if there is high fever, bloody diarrhea, tenesmus, severe or persisting symptoms, a history of recent travel or known exposure to bacterial agents, and if fecal leukocytes are present. Stools for ova and parasites should be obtained if parasites are a consideration. An enzyme-linked immunosorbent assay (ELISA) for rotavirus is available.

General Approach

Urinalysis is useful in determining the degree of dehydration. Other laboratory tests are typically unnecessary if the patient is not clinically dehydrated and can be treated symptomatically. When a patient is clinically dehydrated and rehydration is required in the emergency department, there is a high prevalence of laboratory abnormalities.[29]

DIFFERENTIAL DIAGNOSIS

The most common causes of diarrhea are (1) gastrointestinal infections caused by bacterial or viral agents; (2) parenteral infections, such as otitis and urinary tract infections, with associated gastrointestinal symptoms; (3) antibiotic treatment; and (4) dietary disturbances with a secondary lactase deficiency (Table 39–1). Bacterial diarrheas have a summer predominance and can be caused by a variety of agents such as *Salmonella, Shigella, Yersinia, Campylobacter, Aeromonas, E. coli,* and *V. cholerae*[25–28, 30–38] Usually the patients are febrile and have tenesmus and frequent small stools containing blood and mucus. Viral diarrhea is by far the most common.[35, 39, 40] It is normally more watery, and patients present with vomiting, which can occur even prior to the onset of diarrhea.[9] Rotavirus is the most common pathogen, though Norwalk virus and adenovirus can also cause diarrhea.[41–43] Children attending day-care centers have an increased incidence of diarrhea, especially from highly contagious organisms such as *Shigella, Giardia,* and rotavirus.[4, 25] Parasitic infections with *Giardia* and *Entamoeba histolytica* also cause diarrhea.[44]

Food poisoning is defined as an incident in which two or more persons experience a similar illness involving the gastrointestinal tract after ingestion of common food or water.[45–49] It can be produced by food or water contaminated with bacteria such as *Shigella, Salmonella,*[50] *E. coli,*[51] *Yersinia,*[51] and *Campylobacter*[52]; by bacterial enterotoxins produced by, for example, *Staphylococcus aureus,*[53] *Bacillus cereus,* and *Clostridium perfringens*[54]; by viruses such as rotavirus and Norwalk virus[25, 45, 55]; and by parasites such as *Giardia* and *E. histolytica.*[56] Food poisoning can also be caused by chemical toxins produced by heavy metals such as cadmium[25]; by ciguatera, tetrodotoxin, and scombroid toxin, which are all caused by consumption of contaminated fish[25, 45, 57, 58, 59]; by monosodium

TABLE 39–1
DIFFERENTIAL DIAGNOSIS

Infections—most common of all causes
  Viral: Rotavirus
  Bacterial: *Salmonella, Shigella, Yersinia, Campylobacter*
  Parasitic: *Giardia lamblia, Entamoeba histolytica*
Malabsorption
  Secondary to lactase deficiency—most common
  Cystic fibrosis
Dietary disturbances
  Starvation
  Overfeeding
Anatomic abnormalities
  Intussusception
  Hirschsprung's disease
Inflammatory bowel disease
  Regional enteritis
  Ulcerative colitis
Systemic illness
  Hyperthyroidism
  Congenital adrenal hyperplasia
  Immune deficiency syndromes
Food poisoning—food- or water-borne
  Bacterial, viral, parasitic
  Bacterial enterotoxins: *Staphylococcus aureus, B. cereus, Clostridium*
  Chemical:
    Heavy metals
    Fish: ciguatera, tetrodotoxin, scombroid
    Poisonous mushrooms
Miscellaneous
  Antibiotic-related disease
  Hemolytic-uremic syndrome
  Drug withdrawal
  Psychogenic disease

glutamate, an additive found in many foods, particularly Chinese[25] food; and by various poisonous mushrooms.[25, 45, 49] Chemically food-poisoned patients can also present with neurologic symptoms such as paresthesias, numbness, reversal of hot-cold sensations, and reactions caused by histamine release.[25, 45]

Antibiotic-associated diarrhea is common in children[9, 17] and is caused by a change in bowel flora. Usually, discontinuation of the medication is sufficient to eliminate the symptoms. In a small number of patients with antibiotic-induced diarrhea, a severe, potentially fatal form of colitis, known as *pseudomembranous enterocolitis,* may develop. Pseudomembranous enterocolitis is caused by the toxin produced by *Clostridium difficile.*[9, 16, 25] These patients appear toxic and have bloody diarrhea. This is uncommon in early childhood.[16]

Intussusception classically presents in a child younger than 2 years as colicky abdominal pain, "currant jelly" stools, and, in fewer than half of cases, an abdominal mass. This diagnosis should be ruled out in any infant presenting with bloody diarrhea and intermittent severe colic. The patient with intussusception may be more lethargic than would be indicated by the degree of dehydration and usually is not febrile. If intussusception is suspected, a barium enema, which can also be therapeutic,[16] is indicated.

Hemolytic-uremic syndrome is uncommon but is life threatening and should be recognized. Patients are usually younger than 3 years and have a history of presumed viral gastroenteritis followed by bloody stools, severe anemia, thrombocytopenic purpura, and hematuria caused by nephritis. These patients can present with hypertension and renal failure.[16]

Patients with Hirschsprung's disease, short-bowel syndrome, inflammatory bowel diseases (e.g., ulcerative colitis or regional enteritis) can all present with diarrhea. Patients with malabsorptive syndromes such as cystic fibrosis present with large fatty stools. Patients with hyperthyroidism, congenital adrenal hyperplasia, neoplasms, or immune deficiency can have diarrhea as a complication of their underlying disease process.[16]

Bloody diarrhea in febrile children usually has an infectious origin[9, 16, 25]; febrile children with nonbloody diarrhea usually suffer from viral enteritis or parenteral infection. Afebrile children with bloody diarrhea can have life-threatening conditions such as hemolytic-uremic syndrome, intussusception, and pseudomembranous enterocolitis, whereas afebrile children with nonbloody diarrhea may have viral infections, antibiotic-induced diarrhea, or malabsorption.[16]

THERAPEUTIC INTERVENTION

The most important clinical consideration in a patient with diarrhea is whether the patient is dehydrated.[60-69] Though dehydration literally means loss of water, in the clinical setting it means loss of water and electrolytes. The actual weight loss is the best indication of the actual fluid deficit. If a patient is deemed "5% dry," the deficit is about 50 ml/kg. Daily maintenance fluid requirements are as follows:

Children weighing <10 kg: 100 ml/kg/day
Children weighing 11 to 20 kg: 1000 ml + 50 ml/kg for each kilogram over 10 kg
Children weighing >20 kg: 1500 ml + 20 ml/kg/day for each kilogram over 20 kg

For electrolyte maintenance, requirements are 3 mEq/kg/day for Na^+ and 2 mEq/kg/day for K^+.

There are three stages in the treatment of diarrheal dehydration: (1) rehydration, which is divided into an emergency phase, for the patient in shock, and a repletion phase; (2) maintenance after hydration is achieved; and (3) early refeeding. These stages may merge into each other quickly.

Staging Therapy
Mild Dehydration

Patients with mild dehydration (i.e., who are well hydrated or minimally dry) should be given maintenance hydration solutions (Pedialyte, Ricelyte) with Na^+ (about 40 to 50 mEq/L) and small, frequent feeds (for the vomiting patient) or "ad lib" feeds every 2 to 4 hours (for the patient with diarrhea) (Table 39–2). Usually the child is soon advanced to regular formula and feeds.

Mild to Moderate Dehydration

Patients with mild to moderate isotonic dehydration (5% to 10%)[60-69] should be rehydrated in the emergency department or in the hospital; smaller infants should be considered for admission because of the risk of sudden decompensation. Fluid deficits can be replaced orally or intravenously. If they improve markedly, have normal laboratory values, and have no ongoing losses, older infants and children may be considered for close follow-up and sent home.

Moderate to Severe Dehydration

Patients with moderate to severe dehydration (10% to 15%)[11, 14, 60-69] should receive rapidly administered, intravenous fluids. An isotonic solution such as Ringer's lactate or normal saline should be used as an intravenous bolus (20 to 30 ml/kg). A decrease in tachycardia, an ability to feel peripheral pulses, an increase in blood pressure, and brisk

TABLE 39–2
DEHYDRATION: THERAPY AT A GLANCE
Recognize dehydration: Mild (5%), moderate (10%), severe (15%), shock (>15%)
No dehydration or minimally dry
Make sure patient can take po glucose electrolyte solutions (Pedialyte, Ricelyte)
Very close follow-up with discharge instructions
Mild to moderate dehydration
Monitor; laboratory tests: electrolytes, BUN, blood gases, blood glucose, urinalysis
Rapid rehydration in emergency department if no contraindications (renal, heart, lung disease)
Rehydration IV or po
Start with 20 ml/kg/hr of D5NS or oral rehydration solution (Na^+ 75–90 mEq/L)
Continue 10–15 ml/kg/hr for another 2–3 hr
Type of IV fluid depends on serum Na^+
Admit or discharge (see Table 39–4)
Moderate to severe dehydration
Monitor; laboratory tests as above
Rehydration—usually IV or po
Calculate deficit (10% = 100 ml/kg, etc.)
Start with 20 ml/kg/hr D5NS or oral rehydration solution (Na^+ 75–90 mEq/L)
Admit and continue replacement in hospital
Shock
Immediate IV access; monitor; administer O_2 IV fluid boluses 20 ml/kg RL or NS
Continue boluses until improvement of shock
Laboratory tests as above
Continue replacement in hospital
Careful clinical monitoring
Accurate recording of intake and output
Add potassium
Monitor glucose to guide IV fluids
Drugs
Antidiarrheal/antiemetic drugs *not* indicated
Antimicrobials
Shigella: TMP-SMX—8 mg/kg TMP, 40 mg/kg SMX in bid doses
Campylobacter: Erythromycin 40 mg/kg/day
Salmonella: Ampicillin or amoxicillin, only if indicated

BUN = Blood urea nitrogen; NS = normal saline; RL = Ringer's lactate; TMP-SMX = trimethoprim-sulfamethoxazole.

capillary refill all indicate that the patient is no longer in shock, and repletion of deficit can then be continued by the intravenous or oral route. These patients should be admitted to the hospital.

Intravenous Rehydration Therapy

Intravenous rehydration therapy is indicated for the patient in shock or with impending shock (moderate to severe dehydration), for the lethargic patient, for severe ongoing stool losses about 5 to 10 ml/kg/hour, for intractable vomiting, and for the very small infant.

Outpatient parenteral therapy is not commonly practiced. However, it is feasible if the emergency department has an observation or holding area. For many years, fluid deficits were corrected slowly, but now the aim is to accomplish full repletion in 8 to 24 hours, except in patients with hypertonic dehydration. Rapid rehydration is contraindicated for children with renal, heart, or pulmonary disease, as they may be unable to handle large fluid loads[11, 64]; it is more useful in acute than in chronic diarrhea. The patient can be started with D5 normal saline (NS) at a rate of 20 ml/kg/hour. In most cases, the solution is changed to D5/.45NS at a rate of

10 to 15 ml/kg/hour for an additional 2 to 3 hours. This provides a fluid total of approximately 40 to 60 ml/kg, which is adequate to rehydrate a mildly to moderately dehydrated child.[11, 64] The dextrose is omitted if the serum glucose level is high or the child has glucose in the urine. Potassium is added to the fluids if there are flat T waves on the EKG and definitely after urine output is established. Hypokalemia can occur after rapid rehydration when K^+ has not been added to the fluids.[67]

Hypertonic and hypotonic dehydrated patients should be admitted to the hospital.[9, 11] Patients with severe hypotonic dehydration ($Na^+ < 120$ mEq/L) who present with seizures may need a rapid increase of serum Na^+ to a level of 120 to 125 mEq/L to stop the risk of seizures; this is accomplished by using 3% saline ($Na^+ = 513$ mEq/L). The Na^+ needed is equal to

$$(125 - [\text{observed } Na^+]) \times 0.6 \times (\text{weight in kilograms})$$

replaced over 1/2 to 1 hour,[11] or about 4 ml/kg of 3% saline can be given. In cases of hypertonic dehydration, the initial treatment of shock is the same, but later fluids must be given such that the level of Na^+ does not drop quickly, as this can precipitate seizures. Bicarbonate usually does not need to be replaced, because in most cases acidosis corrects with rehydration.

Oral Rehydration Therapy

Oral rehydration therapy (ORT) is based on the phenomenon that during all types of diarrhea, cotransport of sodium with an organic anion such as glucose remains intact. Absorption of glucose and the anion leads to water absorption secondarily.[70] The World Health Organization (WHO) solution contains Na^+ (90 mmol/L), K^+ (20 mmol/L), Cl^- (80 mmol/L), base (30 mmol/L), and glucose (111 mmol/L). It can be used in all age groups, including neonates,[71] and in patients with hypotonic, isotonic, and hypertonic dehydration. In hypernatremia, oral therapy may be superior to intravenous therapy, because the latter causes seizures during correction. The American Academy of Pediatrics recommends that rehydration solutions contain Na^+ in a concentration of 75 to 90 mEq/L and that maintenance solutions contain Na^+ in a concentration of 40 to 60 mEq/L.

Regular glucose electolyte solutions supply the electrolytes and water to correct dehydration but do not decrease stool output and have essentially no nutritive value. Rice-based and wheat-based[72] ORT solutions are more efficacious than standard ORT solutions in correcting rehydration and decreasing stool output.

Clear liquids that are often used at home, such as juices, sodas, and jello, are inappropriate for the treatment of acute diarrhea, as they contain little Na^+ and have a high carbohydrate content.[73, 74] This increases the osmotic load and actually aggravates the diarrhea. In particular, apple juice contains sorbitol, in addition to sugar, and increases stool output.

Contraindications to oral therapy include shock, impending shock, intractable vomiting, severe lethargy, or high purging rates of about 5 to 10 ml/kg/hour.[14] ORT can be conducted in an emergency department observation area.

Refeeding

The prevalent method of delayed refeeding of diarrheal patients to provide "gut rest" is probably unnecessary and may have deleterious effects on the nutritional status of children with diarrhea.[75, 76] The classic approach has been to provide gut rest, followed by administration of clear fluids and gradual reintroduction of a lactose-free diet.[75, 76]

Several studies have shown that early feeding (i.e., immediately after hydration) hastens mucosal recovery, causes weight gain, and shortens the duration of illness, even though it can increase stool output.[77–83] Breast milk is well tolerated throughout episodes of diarrhea and decreases the volume and number of stools, and therefore breast feeding should be continued throughout the illness.[84]

Another question is whether feeds should be introduced gradually, at half strength and then full strength, or if they should be started immediately at full strength. Some studies show that reintroduction of full-strength feeds is beneficial, keeps the patient in a positive nutritional balance, and does not worsen the course of the disease.[85]

Controversy exists over the use of lactose-free foods, such as soy, versus cow's milk–based formula. Some patients with severe and prolonged diarrhea develop lactose intolerance,[86–90] but the majority of children tolerate lactose well.[91, 92] Currently available information does not suggest that lactose should be routinely eliminated from the diet of all infants recovering from diarrhea.

For children who eat solids, the BRAT (*B*ananas, *R*ice, *A*pplesauce, *T*oast) diet, along with wheat noodles and potatoes, can be started as soon as the infant will eat it. Foods high in starches and low in fat should be used, and early refeeding should be tempered with common sense. The patient should be watched for lactose intolerance (i.e., large stools that show the presence of reducing sugars). Such patients should be fed lactose-free formulas for 2 weeks.

Drug Therapy
Antidiarrheal Agents

Many compounds are available for the symptomatic treatment of patients with diarrhea. Kaolin-pectin (Kaopectate) is an adsorbent and increases the form of the stool.[25, 93]; it is safe but minimally effective. Other agents such as diphenoxylate (Lomotil) and loperamide[94] (Imodium) alter intestinal motility. They may worsen symptoms caused by *Shigella* or *Salmonella* infection by allowing the enteropathogens to be in contact with the intestinal mucosa for a longer period of time; they may also accelerate the development of pseudomembranous enterocolitis. There is also a potential for overdosage with opiate-like effects; fatalities in children have occurred. Bismuth subsalicylate (Pepto-Bismol) inhibits intestinal secretions and is effective in traveler's diarrhea; one study showed it to be effective in children with acute diarrhea.[95] Potential problems relate to the absorption of salicylates and the fact that bismuth causes the stools to be black. Antiemetics are rarely effective, can cause serious side effects, and should be avoided. Antidiarrheal compounds are not recommended for routine use in children.[9, 16, 25, 96]

Antimicrobial Agents

Antimicrobial agents are administered to selected patients with gastroenteritis to shorten the clinical course and decrease the excretion of the causative organism.[25, 97, 98] Stool specimens should be cultured and tested for antibiotic sensitivity of the suspected pathogen. Antibiotics should not be used as empiric therapy for gastroenteritis of unknown origin. Antibiotic therapy is always indicated for diarrhea caused by *Shigella*, *V. cholerae* and enteroinvasive *E. coli* (traveler's diarrhea), because it can effect a bacterial and clinical cure. Trimethoprim-sulfamethoxazole is the drug of choice for all these children. In adults with cholera, tetracycline is the drug of choice.[25, 97, 98]

Treatment of gastroenteritis caused by *Salmonella* infection is indicated in young, immunocompromised hosts (e.g., those with cancer or sickle cell disease).[99] Mild gastroenteritis caused by *Salmonella* should not be treated, as treatment prolongs the carrier state. Young patients with *Salmonella* infection should also have blood specimens cultured.

Diarrhea caused by *Campylobacter* infection should be treated, especially if there is a high fever or bloody or severe diarrhea. Treatment reduces fecal excretion and shortens the clinical course. Erythromycin is the drug of choice.

Protozoa-induced diarrhea should be treated with appropriate agents, but this form of diarrhea is usually chronic.[25]

No antiviral agents are available to treat viral diarrheas.

CHRONIC DIARRHEAS

Chronic diarrheas[16, 100] are a less frequent cause of visits to the emergency department. However, worsening symptoms or frustration, especially during weekends when the primary care provider may not be available, may cause the parents to bring the child into the emergency department. It is important to differentiate children with urgent conditions from those who can be referred back to their physician. A stool culture should be obtained in urgent cases.

Bacterial infection, secondary lactose deficiency, and starvation may cause persistence of what seems to be a viral diarrhea in the child who has been kept on a clear liquid diet for several days. This persistence may cause the patient to return to the emergency department. A stool specimen should be cultured and the stool tested for a low pH and the presence of reducing substances. These two factors, if present, indicate lactose intolerance. All milk and milk products should be withheld in such patients for 2 weeks. The patient who has been starving should be gradually started back on a regular diet.

PREVENTION

Vaccines for rotavirus and for *Shigella*, enterotoxic *E. coli*, and *Campylobacter* infection are all in the experimental

---

TABLE 39–3
DISCHARGE INSTRUCTIONS

1. Begin with clear liquids
   Pedialyte, Lytren, Ricelyte are preferred, especially in smaller children
   Older children may be given Gatorade, Jell-O water, or diluted cola
   DO NOT give plain water or juices
   Give large amounts of fluid every 3–4 hr if patient has only diarrhea. If vomiting is present, give small sips (1–2 tsp) q 10 min and then slowly increase amount and decrease frequency
2. Start refeeding within 8–12 hr and never later than 24 hours, even if diarrhea is present
   Full-strength regular formula; some start with diluted formula and then go to full strength
   If diarrhea is prolonged, start with soy formula; switch to soy if stooling is markedly increased after administration of regular formula
   If soy formula is started, keep on it for 1–2 wk.
3. If the child can tolerate solids, give bananas, rice, applesauce, toast, noodles, potatoes; temper refeeding with common sense; no fried foods
4. Return or call physician if:
   Diarrhea and vomiting are increasing in amount or frequency
   Diarrhea lasts >3 days, vomiting >1 day
   Stool is bloody or vomitus is green
   Signs of dehydration develop (i.e., dry mucous membranes, fatigue and lethargy, weight loss, decreased urination, decreased tearing, sunken eyes)

TABLE 39–4
ADMISSION CRITERIA

1. Shock
2. Moderate or severe dehydration
3. Mild to moderate dehydration
   If there is no emergency department facility to rehydrate, admit the child
   If, after rehydration in the emergency department, admit the child if any of the following are present:
   No clinical improvement
   Abnormal laboratory data (Na^+ <130, >150; acidosis; blood urea nitrogen >20)
   Ongoing losses during hydration
   Toxic appearance
   Child is less than 6 mo old
   Follow-up is not reassured
   Care and supervision at home are doubtful
4. Hypertonic, hypotonic dehydration
5. Underlying conditions—immunodeficiency, hemoglobinopathies, neoplasms, etc.

---

stages.[101] If these can be shown to be safe, effective, and inexpensive, they can probably be incorporated into the primary health care immunization program.[101]

Careful food and water selection can decrease the risk of acquiring traveler's diarrhea. Carbonated water and boiled water are the safest for consumption, and uncooked vegetables and undercooked meat or fish should be avoided.[101]

The Centers for Disease Control do not recommend chemoprophylaxis for children.[102, 103] Breast feeding during the first 13 weeks of life has been found to protect against gastrointestinal illness beyond the period of breast feeding.[104]

DISPOSITION

Patients with acute diarrhea who are well hydrated or minimally dry may be orally hydrated and sent home with explicit discharge instructions (Table 39–3). All children with mild to moderate dehydration should be rehydrated in the emergency department, if possible, or in the hospital. If the child is hydrated in the emergency department and has marked clinical improvement, no laboratory abnormality (e.g., Na^+ < 130 mEq/L, Na^+ > 150 mEq/L, blood urea nitrogen > 25, HCO_3^- < 15, or serum pH < 7.3), and no ongoing losses, and if close follow-up and a good social situation can be assured, the patient may be discharged. Follow-up with the private physician or the emergency department physician should be arranged. Parents should be educated about signs of dehydration and instructed about when to return. All patients with moderate to severe dehydration or shock; small infants younger than 6 months; toxic, immunocompromised children; and children with hypotonic or hypertonic dehydration should be admitted to the hospital (Table 39–4).

References

1. Hirschhorn N. The treatment of acute diarrhea in children: A historical and physiological perspective. Am J Clin Nutr 1980;33:637.
2. Claeson M, Merson MH. Global progress in the control of diarrheal diseases. Pediatr Infect Dis J 1990;9:345.
3. Snyder JD, Merson MH. The magnitude of the global problem of acute diarrhoeal disease: A review of active surveillance data. Bull WHO 1982;60(4):605.
4. Rhoads JM, Powell DW. Diarrhea. *In* Walker WA, Durie PR, Hamilton JR, et al (eds). Pediatric Gastrointestinal Diseases. Philadelphia, BC Decker, 1991, pp 62–78.
5. Ho MS, Glass RI, Pinsky PF, et al. Diarrheal deaths in American children: are they preventable? JAMA 1988;260(22):3281.
6. Too many deaths from diarrhea. Editorial. JAMA 1988;7(2):3329.

7. Banwell J. Pathophysiology of diarrheal disorders. Rev Infect Dis 1990;12(suppl):30.
8. Ghishan FK. The transport of electrolytes in the gut and the use of oral rehydration solutions. Pediatr Clin North Am 1988;35(1):35.
9. DeWitt TG. Acute diarrhea in children. Pediatr Rev 1989;11(1):6.
10. Molla AM, Sarker SA, Molla A. Stool electrolyte content and purging rates in diarrhea caused by rotavirus, enterotoxigenic E. coli, and V. cholerae in children. J Pediatr 1981;98(5):835.
11. Davis HW. Acute gastroenteritis and dehydration. Children's Hospital of Pittsburgh Emergency Department Orientation Manual 1991, pp 1–15.
12. Kooh SW, Metcoff J. Physiologic considerations in fluid and electrolyte therapy with particular reference to diarrheal dehydration in children. J Pediatr 1963;62:107.
13. Dell RB. Pathophysiology of dehydration. In Winters RW (ed). The Body Fluids in Pediatrics. Boston, Little, Brown, 1973, pp 134–154.
14. Kallen RJ. The management of diarrheal dehydration in infants using parenteral fluids. Pediatr Clin North Am 1990;37(2):265.
15. Boineau FG, Lewy JE. Maintenance fluids and the management of diarrheal dehydration. Pediatr Ann 1981;10:280.
16. Fleisher GR. Diarrhea. In Fleisher G, Ludwig S (ed). Textbook of Pediatric Emergency Medicine. 2nd ed. Baltimore, Williams & Wilkins, 1988, pp 133–137.
17. Fuchs SM, Jaffe DM. Evaluation of the "tilt test" in children. Ann Emerg Med 1987;16:386.
18. Mackenzie A, Barnes G, Shann F. Clinical signs of dehydration in children. Lancet 1989;2:605.
19. Chameides L (ed). Textbook of Pediatric Advanced Life Support. Dallas, TX, American Heart Association, 1988.
20. Poole SR. Criteria for measurement of dehydration. Letter to editor. Ann Emerg Med 1990;19:730.
21. Bennish ML, Azad AK, Rahman O, Phillips RE. Hypoglycemia during diarrhea in childhood. N Engl J Med 1990;322(19):1357.
22. Amin SS, Jusniar B, Suharjono. Blood urea nitrogen (BUN) in gastroenteritis with dehydration. Paediatr Indones 1980;20:77.
23. Bonadio WA, Hennes HH, Machi J, Madagame E. Efficacy of measuring BUN in assessing children with dehydration due to gastroenteritis. Ann Emerg Med 1989;18:755.
24. Francesconi RP, Hubbard RW, Szlyk PC, et al. Urinary and hematologic indexes of hypohydration. J Appl Physiol 1987;62(3):1271.
25. Pickering LK, Cleary TG. Approach to patients with gastrointestinal infections and food poisoning. In Feigin RD, Cherry JD (eds). Textbook of Pediatric Infectious Diseases. 2nd ed. Philadelphia, WB Saunders, 1987, pp 622–651.
26. Guerrant RL, Shields DS, Thorson SM, et al. Evaluation and diagnosis of acute infectious diarrhea. Am J Med 1985;78(suppl 6B):91.
27. Bishop WP, Ulshen MH. Bacterial gastroenteritis. Pediatr Clin North Am 1988;35(1):69.
28. Radetsky M. Laboratory evaluation of acute diarrhea. Pediatr Infect Dis J 1986;5(2):230.
29. Bhende MS, Davis HW, Karasic RB, Fuchs SM. High prevalence of laboratory abnormalities in children with clinical dehydration. Abstract. Ann Emerg Med 1991; 20:448.
30. Snyder JD. Bacterial infections. In Walker WA, Durie PR, Hamilton JR, et al. Pediatric Gastrointestinal Diseases. Philadelphia, BC Decker, 1991, pp 527–537.
31. Rennels MB, Levine MM. Classical bacterial diarrhea: Perspectives and update—Salmonella, Shigella, Escherichia coli, Aeromonas and Plesiomonas. Pediatr Infect Dis J 1986;5(1):S91.
32. Marks MI, Pai CH, Lafleur L, et al. Yersinia enterocolitica gastroenteritis: A prospective study of clinical, bacteriologic and epidemiologic features. J Pediatr 1980;96(1):26.
33. Drumm B, O'Brien A, Cutz E, Sherman P. Campylobacter pyloridis-associated primary gastritis in children. Pediatrics 1987;80(2):192.
34. Challapalli M, Tess BR, Cunningham, DG et al. Aeromonas-associated diarrhea in children. Pediatr Infect Dis J 1988;7(10):693.
35. Kotloff KL, Wasserman SS, Steciak JY, et al. Acute diarrhea in Baltimore children attending an outpatient clinic. Pediatr Infect Dis J 1988;7(2):753.
36. Guerrant RL, Lohr JA, Williams EK. Acute infectious diarrhea I: Epidemiology, etiology and pathogenesis. Pediatr Infect Dis J 1986;5(2):353.
37. Nelson JD. Etiology and epidemiology of diarrheal diseases in the United States. Am J Med 1985;78(suppl 6B):76.
38. Silverman A. Common bacterial causes of bloody diarrhea. Pediatr Ann 1985;14(1):39.
39. Barnes GL. Intestinal viral infections. In Walker WA, Durie PR, Hamilton JR, et al. (eds). Pediatric Gastrointestinal Diseases. Philadelphia, BC Decker, 1991, pp 538–545.
40. Hamilton JR. Viral enteritis. Pediatr Clin North Am 1988;35(1):89.
41. Steinhoff MC. Rotavirus: The first five years. J Pediatr 1980;96(4):611.
42. Krajden M, Brown M, Petrasek A, Middleton P. Clinical features of adenovirus enteritis: A review of 127 cases. Pediatr Infect Dis J 1990;9(9):636.
43. Lew JF, Glass RI, Petric M, et al. Six-year retrospective surveillance of gastroenteritis viruses identified at ten electron microscopy centers in the United States and Canada. Pediatr Infect Dis J 1990;9(10):709.
44. Farthing MJG. Parasitic and fungal infections of the digestive tract. In Walker WA, Durie PR, Hamilton JR, et al (eds). Pediatric Gastrointestinal Diseases. Philadelphia, BC Decker, 1991, pp 546–556.
45. Ellenthorn MJ, Barceloux DG. Foodborne toxins. In Medical Toxicology: Diagnosis and Treatment of Human Poisoning. New York, Elsevier, 1988, pp 1172–1188.
46. Bean NH, Griffin PM, Goulding JS, Ivey CB. Foodborne disease outbreaks: A 5-year summary. 1983–1987. MMWR 1990;39:15.
47. Waites WM, Arbuthnott JP. Foodborne illness: An overview. Lancet 1990;336:722.
48. Todd E. Epidemiology of foodborne illness: North America. Lancet 1990;336:788.
49. Roberts D. Sources of infection: Food. Lancet 1990;336:859.
50. Baird-Parker AC. Foodborne salmonellosis. Lancet 1990;336:1231.
51. Doyle MP. Pathogenic Escherichia coli, Yersinia enterocolitica, and Vibrio parahaemolyticus. Lancet 1990;336:1111.
52. Skirrow MB. Campylobacter. Lancet 1990;336:921.
53. Tranter HS. Foodborne staphylococcal illness. Lancet 1990;336:1044.
54. Lund BM. Foodborne disease due to bacillus and Clostridium species. Lancet 1990;336:982.
55. Appleton H. Foodborne viruses. Lancet 1990;336:1362.
56. Casemore DP. Foodborne protozoal infection. Lancet 1990;336:1427.
57. Ho AM, Fraser IM, Todd ECD. Ciguatera poisoning: A report of three cases. Ann Emerg Med 1986;15:1225.
58. McGuigan MA, Wason S. Ciguatera. Clin Toxicol Rev 1980;3:1.
59. Morgan MRA, Fenwick GR. Natural foodborne toxicants. Lancet 1990;336:1492.
60. Finberg L. Treatment of dehydration in infancy. Pediatr Rev 1981;3(4):113.
61. Barkin RM. Treatment of the dehydrated child. Pediatr Ann 1990;19(10):597.
62. Gottlieb RP. Dehydration and fluid therapy. Emerg Med Clin North Am 1983;1(1):113.
63. Kallen RJ, Lonergan, JM. Fluid resuscitation of acute hypovolemic hypoperfusion states in pediatrics. Pediatr Clin North Am 1990;37(2):287.
64. Rosenstein BJ, Baker MD. Pediatric outpatient intravenous rehydration. Am J Emerg Med 1987;5(3):183.
65. Moineau G, Newman J. Rapid intravenous rehydration in the pediatric emergency department. Pediatr Emerg Care 1990;6(3):186.
66. Rahman O, Bennish ML, Alam AN, Salam MA. Rapid intravenous rehydration by means of a single polyelectrolyte solution with or without dextrose. J Pediatr 1988;113(4):654.
67. Malone DR, McNamara RM, Malone RS, et al. Hypokalemia complicating emergency fluid resuscitation in children. Pediatr Emerg Care 1990;6(1):13.
68. Harrison HE. Dehydration in infancy: Hospital treatment. Pediatr Rev 1989;11(5):139.
69. Goepp JG, Hirschhorn B. Fluid therapy of diarrhea: Industrialized countries. In Walker WA, Durie PR, Hamilton JR, et al (eds). Pediatric Gastrointestinal Diseases. Philadelphia, BC Decker, 1991, pp 1567–1576.
70. Mahalanabis D. Oral rehydration therapy: Physiological basis. In Gracey M (ed). Diarrhoeal Disease and Malnutrition: A Clinical Update. New York, Churchill Livingstone, 1985, pp 145–157.
71. Pizarro D, Posada G, Mata L. Treatment of 242 neonates with dehydrating diarrhea with an oral glucose-electrolyte solution. J Pediatr 1983;102(1):153.
72. Alam AN, Sarker SA, Molla AM, et al. Hydrolysed wheat-based oral rehydration solution for acute diarrhoea. Arch Dis Child 1987;62:440.
73. Finberg L. Oral rehydration: Finding the right solution. Contemp Pediatr 1987:61.
74. Snyder JD. Use and misuse of oral therapy for diarrhea: Comparison of US practices with American Academy of Pediatrics recommendations. Pediatrics 1991;87(1):28.
75. Brown KH, MacLean WC Jr. Nutritional management of acute diarrhea: An appraisal of the alternatives. Pediatrics 1984;73(2):119.
76. Committee on Nutrition. Oral fluid therapy and posttreatment feeding following enteritis. In Forbes GB, Woodruff CW (eds.). Pediatric Nutrition Handbook. 2nd ed. Elk Grove Village, IL, American Academy of Pediatrics, 1985, pp 274–279.
77. Santosham M, Foster S, Reid R, et al. Role of soy-based, lactose-free formula during treatment of acute diarrhea. Pediatrics 1985;76:292.
78. Isolauri E, Vesikari T, Saha P, Viander M. Milk versus no milk in rapid refeeding after acute gastroenteritis. J Pediatr Gastroenterol Nutr 1986;5:254.
79. Brown KH, Gastanaduy AS, Saavedra JM, et al. Effect of continued oral feeding on clinical and nutritional outcomes of acute diarrhea in children. J Pediatr 1988;112:191.
80. Armitstead J, Kelly D, Walker-Smith J. Evaluation of infant feeding in acute gastroenteritis. J Pediatr Gastroenterol Nutr 1989;8:240.
81. Margolis PA, Litteer T, Hare N, Pichichero M. Effects of unrestricted diet on mild infantile diarrhea: A practice-based study. Am J Dis Child 1990;144:162.
82. Dugdale A, Lovell S, Gibbs V, Ball D. Refeeding after acute gastroenteritis: A controlled study. Arch Dis Child 1982;57:76.
83. Hjelt U, Paerregaard A, Peterson W, et al. Rapid versus gradual feeding

in acute gastroenteritis in childhood; energy intake and weight gain. J Pediatr Gastroenterol Nutr 1989;8(1):75.

84. Khin-Maung-U, Nyunt-Nyunt-Wai, Myo-Khin, et al. Effect on clinical outcome of breast feeding during acute diarrhoea. Br Med J 1985;290:587.

85. Placzek M, Walker-Smith JA. Comparison of two feeding regimes following acute gastroenteritis in infancy. J Pediatr Gastroenterol Nutr 1984;3(2):245.

86. Penny ME, Paredes P, Brown KH. Clinical and nutritional consequences of lactose feeding during persistent postenteritis diarrhea. Pediatrics 1989;84(5):835.

87. Ransome-Kuti O. Lactose intolerance. In Gracey M (ed). Diarrhoeal Disease and Malnutrition: A Clinical Update. New York, Churchill Livingstone, 1985, pp 102–117.

88. Sack DA, Rhoads M, Molla A, et al. Carbohydrate malabsorption in infants with rotavirus diarrhea. Am J Clin Nutr 1982; 36:1112.

89. Torres-Pinedo R, Lavastida M, Rivera CL, et al. Studies on infant diarrhea I: A comparison of the effects of milk feeding and intravenous therapy upon the composition and volume of the stool and urine. J Clin Invest 1966;45(4):469.

90. Rajah R, Pettifor JM, Noormohamed M, et al. The effect of feeding four different formulae on stool weights in prolonged dehydrating infantile gastroenteritis. J Pediatr Gastroenterol Nutr 1988;7:203.

91. Groothuis JR, Berman S, Chapman J. Effect of carbohydrate ingested on outcome in infants with mild gastroenteritis. J Pediatr 1986;108:903.

92. Haffejee IE. Cow's milk-based formula, human milk, and soya feeds in acute infantile diarrhea: A therapeutic trial. J Pediatr Gastroenterol Nutr 1990;10(2):193.

93. Berschneider HM, Powell DW. Prospect for antidiarrhoeal therapy in acute diarrhoeas. In Gracey M (ed). Diarrhoeal Disease and Malnutrition: A Clinical Update. New York, Churchill Livingstone, 1985, pp 128–143.

94. Motala C, Hill ID, Mann MD, Bowie MD. Effect of loperamide on stool output and duration of acute infectious diarrhea in infants. J Pediatr 1990;117(3):467.

95. Soriano-Brucher H, Avendano P, O'Ryan M, et al. Bismuth subsalicylate in the treatment of acute diarrhea in children: A clinical study. Pediatrics 1991;87(1):18.

96. Antidiarrhoeal drugs (not) for children. Noticeboard. Lancet 1991;337:169.

97. Williams EK, Lohr JA, Guerrant RL. Acute infectious diarrhea II: Diagnosis, treatment and prevention. Pediatr Infect Dis J 1986;5(4):458.

98. Ashkenazi S, Cleary TG. Antibiotic treatment of bacterial gastroenteritis. Pediatr Infect Dis J 1991;10(2):140.

99. St Geme III JW, Hodes HL, Marcy SM, et al. Consensus: Management of Salmonella infection in the first year of life. Pediatr Infect Dis J 1988;7(9):615.

100. Fitzgerald JF. Management of the infant with persistent diarrhea. Pediatr Infect Dis 1985;4(1):6.

101. Levine MM. Immunization against infectious diarrhoeas. In Gracey M (ed). Diarrhoeal Disease and Malnutrition: A Clinical Update. New York, Churchill Livingstone, 1985, pp 183–200.

102. Nahlen BL, Parsonnet J, Preblud SR, et al. International travel and the child younger than two years II: Recommendations for prevention of travelers' diarrhea and malaria chemoprophylaxis. Pediatr Infect Dis J 1989;8(11):735.

103. Du Pont HL. Nonfluid therapy and selected chemoprophylaxis of acute diarrhea. Am J Med 1985;78(suppl 6B):81.

104. Howie PW, Forsyth JS, Ogston SA, et al. Protective effect of breast feeding against infection. Br Med J 1990;300:11.

CHAPTER 40

Pancreatitis

Allan E. Kornberg

INCIDENCE AND MORTALITY

The incidence of pancreatitis in the United States and England has been reported as being between 1.5 and 10 cases per 100,000 population.[1–3] Many patients have pancreatitis secondary to other disorders, and thus the incidence is dependent on how hard the diagnosis is sought. In a prospective study of acute pancreatitis, the described incidence was much higher: 28.1 per 100,000.[4] In adults, the incidence is related to the incidence of alcoholism in the population under study.[5]

Pancreatitis is much less common in children than in adults.[6, 7] Even in major pediatric referral centers, acute pancreatitis as a primary diagnosis is seen only a few times per year. Reasons for the reduced incidence in childhood are multifactorial. One obvious factor is that the two most common origins of acute pancreatitis in adults—cholelithiasis and alcoholism—are uncommon in children.

Mortality rates for pancreatitis are variable and highly dependent on the population studied and the relative frequencies of underlying origins. In a population with an incidence of pancreatitis of 10 per 100,000, the mortality rate was 1 per 100,000.[2] Another reference quotes the mortality rate from an individual attack of pancreatitis to be less than 5%.[8] In adults, the mortality rate is 1.6 times higher for initial attacks than for recurrences.[3]

ANATOMY AND PHYSIOLOGY

The pancreas is a long, narrow, thin gland that in the healthy adult is approximately 12 to 15 cm long and weighs between 70 and 110 gm.[9] The head is enveloped by the curvature of the duodenum[10]; the tail reaches as far as the spleen, and the body is anterior to the aorta and vertebral column. The stomach covers the pancreas. The main pancreatic duct and the common bile duct enter the duodenum at the sphincter of Oddi. A normal variant has an accessory pancreatic duct entering the duodenum as a smaller opening just proximal to the sphincter of Oddi. The pancreas is a fixed and retroperitoneal organ and does not have a capsule.

Enterokinase, an enzyme formed in the duodenum, converts trypsinogen to trypsin.[11] Trypsin in turn converts the proenzyme form of other pancreatic proteases to the active form. The pancreatic acinar cells secrete lipase and amylase in their active forms. Pancreatic exocrine function has great reserve; regardless of the cause of pancreatic insufficiency, malabsorption does not occur unless enzyme secretion is less than 10% of normal. Pancreatic islets, which contain the endocrine tissue of this gland, make up less than 1% of the weight of the pancreas. These cells release insulin and glucagon directly into the circulation, thereby regulating carbohydrate metabolism.

The vagus nerve plays a role in inducing pancreatic enzyme secretion. Cholecystokinin, secretin, gastrin, and vasoactive intestinal polypeptide, all hormones of the upper gastrointestinal tract, provoke pancreatic exocrine secretion. Insulin exerts a positive effect on pancreatic exocrine secretion, whereas glucagon exerts a negative effect.

PATHOLOGY AND PATHOGENESIS

Acute hemorrhagic pancreatitis refers to extensive destruction of pancreatic tissue caused by release of enzymes into the gland parenchyma. Microscopically there is a proteolytic destruction of parenchyma, necrosis with hemorrhage of blood vessels, fat necrosis, and an inflammatory infiltration that is initially neutrophil predominant. Grossly, gray-white areas of parenchymal necrosis, hemorrhage, and white areas of fat necrosis are seen.

Direct extension of activated pancreatic enzymes and inflammatory cells can cause aseptic peritonitis, pleural effusion, or pneumonia.[12, 13] Pseudocysts, which are sterile fluid collections within or adjacent to the pancreas or to other abdominal organs, frequently complicate acute pancreatitis. Abscesses within and about the pancreas may develop.

Distant lesions occasionally complicate pancreatitis; injury by circulating lipase is incriminated.[14] Subcutaneous fat necrosis has been described.[15, 16] Lytic lesions of bone and arthritis from fat necrosis have been reported.[17-19] Distant lesions frequently occur secondary to circulating lipase in the weeks after initial abdominal symptoms. Distant fat necrosis is diagnosed clinically in less than 1% of cases; however, in one postmortem series it was noted in 10% of patients dying from pancreatitis.[20]

Several different events may initiate the process leading to acute pancreatitis. In cases of blunt abdominal trauma, the fixed retroperitoneal location of the pancreas predisposes it to injury. Infections of the pancreas may cause direct inflammation. Obstruction of the pancreatic duct with secretion of pancreatic juices has been offered as a cause in some cases.[21] Other theories include reflux of duodenal contents or reflux of bile retrograde into the pancreas. Regardless of the inciting event, the final common pathway for acute pancreatitis is the activation of pancreatic proenzymes. Trypsin plays a major role as an activator of other proteases. Typically, trypsinogen converted to trypsin is quickly inactivated by a trypsin inhibitor present in the pancreas.[22] If more proteases are being activated than inhibited, then pancreatitis can proceed.

CAUSES OF ACUTE PANCREATITIS IN CHILDREN

There are many causes of pediatric acute pancreatitis (Table 40–1). Trauma is one of the most frequent origins, causing as many as one third of all cases.[6, 7, 23, 24] Blunt trauma is a more common cause than penetrating trauma. One of the more common mechanisms of trauma-induced pancreatitis, especially in young children, is child abuse.[23, 24]

Infections are another frequent cause of pancreatitis in children. Mumps can cause mild pancreatitis, but elevation of serum amylase levels can also occur from isolated parotitis. When abdominal pain is present with mumps, pancreatitis should be suspected. Only rarely has severe hemorrhagic pancreatitis been reported with mumps.[25] Enteroviral disease[26, 27] and Epstein-Barr virus[28, 29] have been implicated as causes for pancreatitis. *Mycoplasma pneumoniae* infection has been reported to cause pancreatitis in children.[30] Leptospirosis, although rare in the United States, has been described as an infectious cause of pancreatitis.[31] Ascaris, also a rare infection in the United States, is the leading cause of pancreatitis in children in endemic parts of the third world.[32, 33] The worms traverse from the duodenum into the pancreatic duct, causing obstruction. Malaria has been reported to be associated with pancreatitis,[34] and congenital rubella has been described as causing pancreatitis.[35]

Biliary tract disease is one of the two most common causes of pancreatitis in the United States; it is less common in children but still occurs often enough to warrant consideration in every case.[7, 36] Although not all cases of gallstones in children are related to hematologic disease, an evaluation for hemolysis is appropriate.

As a group, drugs are one of the most frequent etiologic categories for acute childhood pancreatitis.[37] Valproic acid (Depakene), an anticonvulsive agent, causes pancreatitis in addition to its known hepatotoxicity, that is sometimes fatal.[38, 39] Among the chemotherapeutic agents, asparaginase has been most frequently associated with pancreatitis, which can be severe.[40]

Many other medications have been suggested as causes of pancreatitis.[41-43] Nevertheless, if the pancreatitis is suspected of being drug induced, one should still consider an underlying illness capable of causing pancreatitis.

Malnutrition has also been associated with pancreatitis.[44] When a starved child is refed, pancreatitis sometimes super-

TABLE 40–1

CAUSES OF ACUTE PANCREATITIS IN CHILDREN

Trauma	Metabolic-endocrine
Blunt	Malnutrition, with refeeding
Penetrating	after
Child abuse	Hypercalcemia
Infectious	Reye's syndrome
Mumps	Hyperlipidemia
Enterovirus	Hyperparathyroidism
Hemolytic streptococcus	Cystic fibrosis
Salmonella	Miscellaneous
Hepatitis A and B	Henoch-Schönlein purpura
Mycoplasma pneumoniae	Systemic lupus erythematosus
Infectious mononucleosis	Perforated duodenal ulcer
Leptospirosis	Kawasaki disease
Influenza A virus	Juvenile tropical pancreatitis
Measles	Uremia
Typhoid fever	Scorpion venom
Ascaris	Hereditary
Malaria	Idiopathic
Rubella	
Biliary tract obstruction	
Cholelithiasis	
Congenital duodenal stenosis	
Choledochal cyst	
Tumor	
Drugs	
Steroids	
Thiazides	
Sulfonamides	
Azathioprine	
Alcohol	
Valproate	
Tetracycline	
Borate	
Estrogen	
Asparaginase	
Furosemide	
Cimetidine	
Diazoxide	
Enalapril	
Nitrofurantoin	
Sulindac	

venes.[45] Pancreatitis can be associated with Reye's syndrome, although Reye's syndrome has decreased in frequency since 1980.[46, 47]

The association of hyperlipidemia and pancreatitis is well known in adults, and it is generally thought that the increase in serum lipids precedes pancreatitis.[48] Hyperlipidemia is less common in children, but may still cause pancreatitis when present. Recognizing hyperlipidemia is also important, as it affects the patient's long-range risk for cardiovascular disease.

Hyperparathyroidism in children has been described as being complicated by pancreatitis.[49] The pancreas is also typically involved in cystic fibrosis. Acute pancreatitis sometimes occurs in patients with this disorder, usually before complete pancreatic exocrine failure develops.[50]

Pancreatitis rarely complicates Henoch-Schönlein purpura,[51] but it should be considered in the child complaining of abdominal pain associated with Henoch-Schönlein purpura. Other, more common origins such as intussusception should also be considered in such children. Pancreatitis has also been described in Kawasaki disease.[52]

The only naturally occurring substance known to cause pancreatitis is the venom of the scorpion genus *Tityus*, which has caused death in children.[53]

Pancreatitis can also be inherited in an autosomal dominant fashion with incomplete penetrance. It presents in childhood with a course typical of acute pancreatitis, except that it is recurrent.[54, 55]

CLINICAL EVALUATION

Abdominal pain is the most consistent symptom of pancreatitis and is present in nearly all cases. Its absence may be an ominous sign if related to shock and obtundation.[56] The pain is usually localized to the epigastrium but can radiate to either upper quadrant or to the back, including the left scapula. The pain is steady, knife-like, or boring and is exacerbated in the supine position. Children have difficulty describing the quality of pain. The pain may have developed over less than 1 hour or over several days. It varies in severity but is usually quite intense.

Nausea and vomiting are frequently associated with the abdominal pain. In severe cases, the patient may appear pale and diaphoretic, complaining of dizziness. Fever is frequently present and is usually of low or moderate grade. Persistent high fever is suggestive of bacterial superinfection.

Patients with pancreatic pain prefer not to move. They either sit or, more commonly, lie on their side with the knees flexed. Localized epigastric tenderness, typically severe, is present. Early in the course of acute pancreatitis, rebound tenderness and a rigid, board-like abdomen are absent because of the retroperitoneal location of the pancreas. Bowel sounds may be decreased. A complete paralytic ileus or signs of peritoneal irritation suggest more extensive disease and are accompanied by leakage of destructive pancreatic juices to the peritoneum. A pleural effusion suggests spread of disease across the diaphragm.

Mild jaundice is sometimes present, and it is appropriate to check for an associated parotitis. An epigastric mass is unusual in acute pediatric pancreatitis and suggests a pseudocyst. Hepatosplenomegaly is sometimes present.

Rarely, evidence of spreading pancreatic hemorrhage can be seen as a bluish-brown discoloration in the flanks (Grey Turner's sign) or the periumbilical area (Cullen's sign). These are only seen several days after initial symptoms.

Signs of intravascular volume depletion may be present. Among the factors causing this are fluid losses from vomiting and diarrhea, third-space loss of plasma into the retroperitoneal and peritoneal spaces, collection of fluid in the intestines from ileus, and hemorrhage. "Distributive" shock may also play a role as a result of the release of circulating vasoactive substances. Signs of tetany from hypocalcemia are rarely present.

DIAGNOSTIC EVALUATION
Laboratory Studies

Total serum amylase measurement remains the laboratory test most frequently used to make the diagnosis of pancreatitis.[57–60] Amylase determination is readily available and relatively easy to perform in most clinical laboratories. Only about 40% of total serum amylase originates from the pancreas; most of the rest is of salivary gland origin.[61] In approximately 10% of cases of acute pancreatitis, the total serum amylase remains normal.[59, 62] Serum amylase tends to rise in the first several hours to half day of clinical symptoms in acute pancreatitis and remains elevated for 1 to 4 days.[57, 58]

Amylase is also sometimes elevated in disorders other than pancreatitis, thereby leading to diagnostic confusion, particularly in conditions associated with abdominal pain (Table 40–2).[1, 21, 60, 63, 64] One study primarily using adult patients

TABLE 40–2
NONPANCREATIC CONDITIONS ASSOCIATED WITH ELEVATED SERUM AMYLASE
Side effect of endoscopic retrograde cholangiopancreatography (ERCP)
Anorexia nervosa
Appendicitis
Biliary tract disease
Bowel infarction
Burns
Carbon monoxide poisoning
Diabetic ketoacidosis
Head trauma
Hepatitis
Intestinal obstruction
Macroamylasemia
Perforated peptic ulcer
Peritonitis
Pneumonia
Pregnancy
Renal failure
Ruptured ectopic pregnancy
Salivary gland disorders
Salpingitis
Shock

demonstrated a sensivity of 95% for total serum amylase and a specificity of 86% to 89%.[39] In general, serum amylase appears to be slightly more sensitive than specific for acute pancreatitis.

When first described, measurement of the renal clearance of serum amylase, when compared with that of creatinine clearance, was thought to be a more accurate test for acute pancreatitis than spot serum amylase measurement.[65] This ratio is calculated as:

$$\frac{amylase_u}{amylase_s} \times \frac{creatinine_s}{creatinine_u} \times 100$$

and is expressed as a percentage. In adults, the ratio averages 3%, with ranges of 1% to 4% reported as normal.[21, 66] No normative values have been reported in childhood. It has been suggested that the elevated ratios seen in acute pancreatitis are caused by decreased renal absorption of the relatively small amylase protein (molecular weight, 55,000) during acute pancreatitis.[67] Unfortunately, the sensitivity and specificity of this test are no better than those of more conventional tests, and the ratio has not found a role as a standard diagnostic test.[68, 69]

Lipase is found naturally only in the pancreas. Hence, an elevated lipase level is more specific for pancreatitis than total serum amylase, although it is usually found to be less sensitive.[57–60, 62] In acute pancreatitis, the lipase level rises less rapidly than the total serum amylase, although it tends to stay elevated for longer periods (i.e., up to 7 to 10 days). Lipase determination is not done routinely in all patients with suspected pancreatitis, in part because its assay is more difficult and less available. A lipase determination may be useful in selected cases, however, particularly when amylase results do not conform to clinical expectations.

Other laboratory tests that are appropriate in managing pancreatitis include determinations of serum electrolye, glucose, and calcium levels. Tests to determine liver transaminase, alkaline phosphatase, and direct and indirect bilirubin levels also are relevant. A complete blood cell count, blood urea nitrogen and creatinine tests, and determination of serum lipid levels may also be indicated.

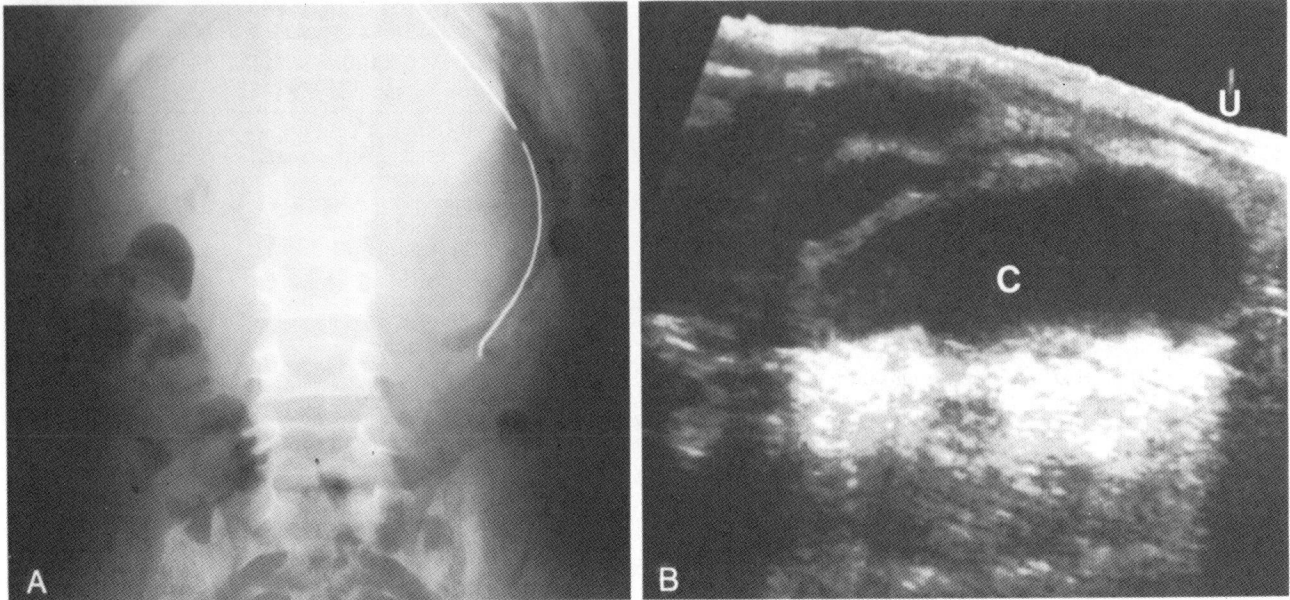

Figure 40–1. This 6-year-old girl fell from a bicycle 1 month before these images were taken. At the time of radiographic evaluation, she was diagnosed as having traumatic pancreatitis with vomiting and had abdominal distention. The abdominal radiograph *(A)* shows a soft tissue density in the midabdomen, displacing the stomach to the left. At the midline, longitudinal ultrasonography *(B)* revealed an anechoic, fluid-filled cyst *(C),* which was a pancreatic pseudocyst. U, Umbilicus. (Courtesy of A. Oestreich, M.D., Cincinnati, OH.)

Radiologic Tests

A plain abdominal radiograph series is routinely ordered when a diagnosis of pancreatitis is considered. This study frequently has a normal result but may demonstrate "sentinel" loops of distended intestine overlying the pancreas.[70] A paralytic ileus involving a larger portion of the intestine may be seen. A diffuse haziness representing ascites may be noted. Calcifications, which may be present in chronic pancreatitis, can be visualized. If a pancreatic abscess has developed, an air-fluid level or multiple bubbles may be present.[13, 71] The absence of free intraperitoneal air should be documented, as other intra-abdominal catastrophes, including intestinal perforation, are part of the differential diagnosis.

Nonspecific abnormalities should be searched for on the chest radiograph. These include pulmonary edema, pneumonitis, and pleural effusion.

Ultrasonography and abdominal computed tomography (CT) are the mainstays of diagnostic imaging for pancreatitis (Figs. 40–1, 40–2). They are of value in making the diagnosis, assessing severity, and examining for associated abdominal disorders.[72–77] Ultrasound does not use ionizing radiation and thus is without known side effects. It is less expensive than CT and can be done at the patient's bedside. Ultrasound is the imaging modality of choice for evaluating the biliary tract for gallstones or other abnormalities, which are a major cause of pancreatitis (Fig. 40–1).[78]

When available, CT is the technique of choice for imaging the pancreas (Fig. 40–2), as it provides greater anatomic detail than ultrasound. Additionally, ultrasound has a significant rate of unsatisfactory examination results; this is because of patient obesity, excessive bowel gas (especially with coexisting ileus), and overlying dressings and stomas. In a series of 908 patients, 14% had technically unsatisfactory results on ultrasound.[76] By comparison, in a series of 300 patients thought to have pancreatitis, only 1% had technically unsatisfactory CT studies.[79] Ultrasound has been reported to have positive and negative predictive values for pancrea-

titis of 83% and 86%, respectively, compared with 88% and 93% for CT.[76] Nevertheless, CT is not 100% diagnostic for acute pancreatitis. Ultrasound and CT are complementary methods in the evaluation of possible acute pancreatitis. Ultrasound has some advantages, as already described, but in the setting of possible pancreatitis associated with blunt abdominal trauma, an urgent CT scan is most appropriate as a result of the greater anatomic detail that can be obtained.

DIFFERENTIAL DIAGNOSIS

Disorders that clinically mimic acute pancreatitis are typically those that present with acute upper abdominal pain, especially epigastric pain, and include the following:

Abdominal abscess
Appendicitis
Biliary tract disease
Ectopic pregnancy
Hepatitis
Intestinal obstruction/perforation
Mesenteric ischemia
Peptic ulcer disease
Pneumonia
Pyelonephritis
Renal colic

Some of these disorders cause an elevated serum amylase level (see Table 40–2), but pancreatitis can be present with a normal level of serum amylase. Although biliary tract disease is less common in children than in adults, it may still occur and should be considered in any child with acute upper abdominal pain. Cholelithiasis can coexist with pancreatitis. Pneumonia can also present with substantial abdominal pain and without peritoneal signs, especially in young children. Any condition presenting with acute abdominal findings can be clinically confused with pancreatitis.

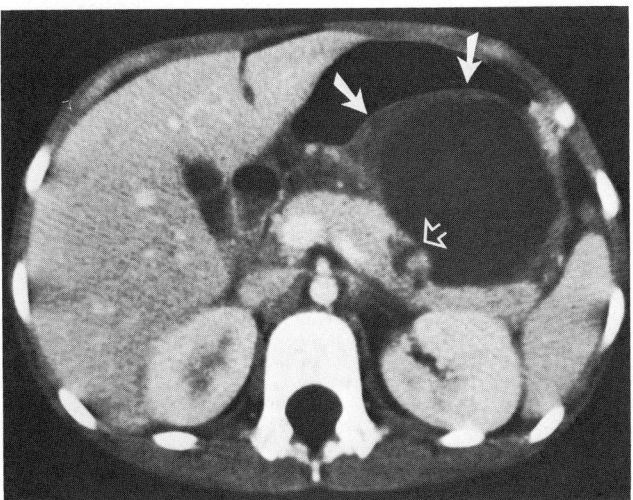

Figure 40–2. CT scan demonstrates a large pancreatic pseudocyst (*solid arrows*). A presumed communication with the pancreatic duct is demonstrated (*open arrow*).

Most of the disorders that make up the differential diagnosis for acute pancreatitis require abdominal surgery.

PROGNOSTIC CONSIDERATIONS

In their classic work, Ranson and colleagues attempted to assess which patients with pancreatitis were at increased risk for death or a complicated course; data were derived from 100 adult patients. The study was later prospectively applied to 200 adults with pancreatitis, 207 with alcoholism, and 51 with biliary tract disease.[80] Five risk factors were assessed at admission: age over 55 years; white blood cell count more than 16,000/mm³; blood glucose level of more than 200 mg/dl; lactate dehydrogenase (LDH) greater than 350 IU/L; and aspartate aminotransferase (AST; previously called serum glutamic-oxaloacetic transaminase, or SGOT) greater than 250 IU/L. Six additional risk factors were assessed during the first 48 hours of hospitalization: hematocrit decline of more than 10%; blood urea nitrogen (BUN) rise of more than 5 mg/dl; serum calcium less than 8 mg/dl; arterial oxygen pressure less than 60 mm Hg; base deficit greater than 4 mEq/L; and estimated fluid sequestration of more than 6 L. Only 1 of 162 patients (0.6%) with two or fewer criteria was seriously ill or eventually died, whereas 24 of 38 patients (63%) with three or more criteria were seriously ill or eventually died.

This same group of investigators also found that poor prognosis was related to a severe first attack or to a small number of preceding attacks and to a lower serum amylase level on admission.[81] Other investigators have found no correlation between serum amylase and severity of pancreatitis, although this was based on seeing no increase in morbidity or mortality with higher values.[1, 62] One study found no rise in serum amylase levels in 10% of patients dying from pancreatitis.[82]

Another group of investigators studied adults primarily with biliary tract disease–associated pancreatitis; eight prognostic criteria, similar to the eleven described earlier, were developed, but these were not age dependent.[83] Again, three or more positive criteria suggested a more difficult course.

No formal criteria have been developed for prognostic indicators in children with pancreatitis. One group of investigators applied eight of the original 11 Ranson criteria (excluding age, base deficit, and fluid sequestration criteria) retrospectively to 49 children with pancreatitis.[24] Most of the patients with a complicated course, as well as the only patient who died, had three or more risk factors. There was some overlap among patients, and statistical significance was not determined. Ranson's criteria, with modification, may have some prognostic value in pediatric pancreatitis patients, but there is no adequate clinical evidence to demonstrate this.

THERAPEUTIC INTERVENTION

Generally, all pediatric patients with the suspected diagnosis of pancreatitis are admitted to the hospital. Rarely, children with mild recurrent pancreatitis can be discharged from the emergency department. This is especially true if pain is mild and the child can tolerate food.

If evidence of intravascular volume depletion is noted, 20 ml/kg of an isotonic solution (Ringer's lactate or normal saline) should be rapidly given intravenously. Patients are placed on a nothing-by-mouth regimen. This is important in the emergency department as well, as the differential diagnosis includes disorders requiring emergent operative therapy.

Nasogastric suction is routinely employed, although data regarding its efficacy are lacking.[84] Certainly in patients with nausea, vomiting, gastric distention, or paralytic ileus, gastric suctioning seems rational. When acute surgical abdominal disorders have been excluded and symptomatic relief of abdominal pain has been deemed appropriate, narcotic analgesia is indicated. Meperidine is likely to cause less spasm of the sphincter of Oddi than morphine or codeine and is the analgesic drug of choice.

Hypocalcemia and hyperglycemia, if present, should be treated, although patients with mild cases may be treated initially with observation. Routine administration of H₂ blockers has not been shown to be valuable.[85] Nonetheless, if blood is noted in gastric contents, it would seem reasonable to administer H₂ blockers along with antacids. It has been hypothesized that administration of anticholinergic drugs reduces pancreatic secretions and hence ameliorates pancreatitis. However, this has not been proven in clinical trials.[7, 86]

Prophylactic antibiotics are not routinely indicated in the management of acute pancreatitis.[7, 87] However, if bacterial infection is suspected (based on persistent high fever, elevated white blood cell count, systemic toxicity, radiographic evidence, and, especially, culture results from percutaneous aspirate or laparotomy), antibiotic coverage should be instituted. Gram-negative enteric, staphylococcal, and anaerobic organisms should be covered.[77] One regimen includes ampicillin, clindamycin, and an aminoglycoside (Table 40–3).

Refeeding of children hospitalized with acute pancreatitis can be considered when pain has subsided in the absence of narcotic analgesia. Meals should be small, high in carbohydrates, and low in fat and protein. If pain recurs on refeeding, food should be withdrawn and reinstituted when the pain has subsided again. For children expected to be without enteral intake for more than approximately 1 week, total parenteral nutrition should be considered.

OTHER CONSIDERATIONS
Complications

Systemic complications sometimes supervene in the course of pancreatitis. If shock is present, central venous monitoring, volume repletion, and administration of pressors are appropriate. If adult respiratory distress syndrome (ARDS) develops, monitoring of oxygenation and chest radiographs are mandatory. Intubation, ventilation, and positive end-expiratory pressure may be needed. For renal failure, fluid

---

TABLE 40–3

ACUTE PEDIATRIC PANCREATITIS: THERAPY AT A GLANCE

Fluid replacement
  Initial bolus: 20 ml/kg of Ringer's lactate or normal saline
  Maintenance fluid: Start with 1.5 to 2 times usual
    maintenance, 2250 to 3000 ml/m²/day of D5/.3NS with 20
    to 30 mEq/L KCl
Analgesia
  Meperidine, 1 mg/kg IM
Antibiotics (not usually indicated)
  Ampicillin, 100 mg/kg/day, divided every 6 hours, IV
  Clindamycin, 30 to 40 mg/kg/day, divided every 8 hours, IV
  Gentamycin, 5 to 7.5 mg/kg/day, divided every 8 hours, IV

---

restriction is necessary, and dialysis should be considered. Gastrointestinal bleeding may require the administration of blood, endoscopy, or (rarely) surgery.

In general, therapy for acute pancreatitis is expectant and supportive. Surgery should be considered when the diagnosis is uncertain, infection is present, or deterioration occurs during intensive care unit (ICU) care (to look for treatable causes), and for surgically correctable biliary tract disease.

Pseudocysts of the pancreas occur not infrequently during the course of acute pediatric pancreatitis.[74, 88, 89] Many are associated with blunt abdominal trauma. An abdominal mass is palpable in some cases. The serum amylase level may remain elevated well beyond the typical first few days usually seen in acute pancreatitis. Sonography and CT are extremely valuable in making the diagnosis. Some pseudocysts resolve spontaneously. If pancreatic abscess is suspected, laparotomy with drainage is the standard approach.

Consultation

Pediatric general surgical consultation is frequently obtained for children with pancreatitis because of the many diseases requiring surgery that are a major part of the differential diagnosis. Gastroenterologists are also sometimes consulted in the care of children with pancreatitis. If gastrointestinal bleeding occurs, endoscopy is required.

Child Abuse

Blunt abdominal trauma is one of the leading causes of pancreatitis in children. Most pancreatitis related to accidental trauma in children occurs in association with automobile accidents or contact sports.[7] However, in preschool-age children with pancreatitis who do not have a diagnosable underlying medical condition and who have not experienced obvious severe accidental trauma, the possibility of child abuse should be considered.

The association of pediatric pancreatitis and child abuse has been well described.[23, 24, 90–92] One series of 49 children with pancreatitis described trauma as the cause in 33% of all cases.[24] Of all the children in the series, 10% (five) were victims of child abuse.

Risk Management

Because pancreatitis is an uncommon pediatric disorder, malpractice cases involving this disease are uncommon. One area of potential concern is failure to correct a surgically treatable abdominal disorder when pancreatitis is the presumed diagnosis. Early in the course of managing presumed

pancreatitis, and also if a patient deteriorates in spite of standard therapy, experienced pediatric surgical consultation should be obtained.

References

1. Young M. Acute diseases of the pancreas and biliary tract. Management in the emergency department. Emerg Med Clin North Am 1989;7:555.
2. O'Sullivan JN, Nobrega FT, Morlock CG, et al. Acute and chronic pancreatitis in Rochester, Minnesota, 1940–1969. Gastroenterology 1972;62:373.
3. Corfield AP, Cooper MJ, Williamson RCN. Acute pancreatitis: A lethal disease of increasing incidence. Gut 1985;26:724.
4. The Copenhagen pancreatitis study group. An interim report from a prospective epidemiological multicenter study. Scand J Gastroenterol 1981;16:305.
5. McEntree GP, Gillen P, Peel AL. Alcohol-induced pancreatitis. Social and surgical aspects. Br J Surg 1987;74:402.
6. Buntain WL, Wood JB, Woolley MM. Pancreatitis in childhood. J Pediatr Surg 1978;13:143.
7. Jordan SC, Ament ME. Pancreatitis in childhood and adolescents. J Pediatr 1977;91:211.
8. Regan PT, Go VLW. Pancreatic diseases. In Stein JH (ed). Internal Medicine. 2nd ed. Boston, Little, Brown, 1987, p 261.
9. Ermak TH, Grendell JH. Anatomy, histology, embryology, and developmental anomalies. In Sleisenger MH, Fordtran JS (eds). Gastrointestinal Disease. Philadelphia, WB Saunders, 1989, p 1765.
10. Anderson JE (ed). Grant's Atlas of Anatomy. 8th ed. Baltimore, Williams & Wilkins, 1983.
11. Go VLW. Pancreatic secretion. In Stein JH (ed). Internal Medicine. 2nd ed. Boston, Little, Brown, 1987, p 36.
12. Siegelman SS, Copeland BE, Saba GP, et al. CT of fluid collections associated with pancreatitis. AJR 1980;134:1121.
13. Poppel MH. The roentgen manifestations of pancreatitis. Semin Roentgenol 1968;3:227.
14. Lee PC, Howard JM. Fat necrosis. Surg Gynecol Obstet 1979;148:785.
15. Schrier RW, Melmon KL, Fenster LF. Subcutaneous nodular fat necrosis in pancreatitis. Arch Intern Med 1965;116:832.
16. Swerdlow AB, Berman ME, Gibbel MI, et al. Subcutaneous fat necrosis associated with acute pancreatitis. JAMA 1960;173:765.
17. Goluboff N, Cram R, Ramgotra B, et al. Polyarthritis and bone lesions complicating traumatic pancreatitis in two children. Can Med Assoc J 1978;118:924.
18. Keating JP, Shackelford GD, Ternberg JL. Pancreatitis and osteolytic lesions. J Pediatr 1972;81:350.
19. Neuer FS, Roberts FF, McCarthy V. Osteolytic lesions following traumatic pancreatitis. Am J Dis Child 1977;131:738.
20. Scarpelli DG. Fat necrosis of bone marrow in acute pancreatitis. Am J Pathol 1956;32:1077.
21. Soergel KH. Acute pancreatitis. In Sleisenger MH, Fordtran JS (eds). Gastrointestinal Disease. Philadelphia, WB Saunders, 1989, p 1816.
22. Pubols MH, Bartelt DC, Greene LJ. Trypsin inhibitor from human pancreas and pancreatic juice. J Biol Chem 1974;249:2235.
23. Pena SDJ, Medovy H. Child abuse traumatic pseudocyst of the pancreas. J Pediatr 1973;83:1026.
24. Ziegler DW, Long JA, Philippart AI, et al. Pancreatitis in childhood. Experience with 49 patients. Ann Surg 1988;207:257.
25. Feldstein JD, Johnson FR, Kallick CA, et al. Acute hemorrhagic pancreatitis and pseudocyst due to mumps. Ann Surg 1974;180:85.
26. Ursing B. Acute pancreatitis in coxsackie B infections. Br Med J 1973;3:524.
27. Capner P, Lendrum R, Jeffries DJ, et al. Viral antibody studies in pancreatic disease. Gut 1975;16:866.
28. Lifschitz C, LaSala S. Pancreatitis, cholecystitis, and choledocholithiasis associated with infectious mononucleosis. Clin Pediatr 1981;20:131.
29. Werbitt W, Mohsenifar Z. Mononucleosis pancreatitis. South Med J 1980;71:1094.
30. Mardh P, Ursing B. The occurrence of acute pancreatitis in Mycoplasmae pneumoniae infection. Scand J Infect Dis 1974;6:167.
31. Bell MJ, Ternberg JL, Feigen RD. Surgical complications of leptospirosis. J Pediatr Surg 1978;13:325.
32. Louw JH. Abdominal complications of Ascaris lumbricoides infestation in children. Br J Surg 1966;53:510.
33. Gilbert MG, Carbonell ML. Pancreatitis in childhood associated with ascariasis. Pediatrics 1964;33:589.
34. Johnson RC, DeFord JW, Carlton PK. Case report: Pancreatitis complicating falciparum malaria. Postgrad Med 1977;6:181.
35. Bunnell CE, Monif GRG. Interstitial pancreatitis in the congenital rubella syndrome. J Pediatr 1972;80:465.
36. Auldist AW. Pancreatitis and choledocholithiasis in childhood. J Pediatr Surg 1972;7:78.
37. Mallory A, Kern F. Drug induced pancreatitis: A critical review. Gastroenterology 1980;78:813.

38. Allen RJ, Coulter DL. Valproic acid induced pancreatitis in children. Pediatrics 1980;65:1194.
39. Batalden PB, VanDyne BJ, Cloyd J. Pancreatitis associated with valproic acid therapy. Pediatrics 1979;64:520.
40. Land VJ, Sutow WW, Fernback DJ, et al. Toxicity of L-asparaginase in children with advanced leukemia. Cancer 1972;30:339.
41. Isenberg JN. Pancreatitis, amylase clearance and azathioprine. J Pediatr 1978;93:1043.
42. Steinberg WM, Lewis JH. Steroid induced pancreatitis: Does it really exist? Gastroenterology 1981;81:799.
43. Elmore MF, Rogge JS. Tetracycline induced pancreatitis. Gastroenterology 1981;81:1134.
44. Danus O, Urbena AM, Valenzuela I, et al. The effect on pancreatic exocrine function in the marasmic infant. J Pediatr 1970;77:334.
45. Gryboski J, Hillemeir C, Kocoshis S, et al. Refeeding pancreatitis in malnourished children. J Pediatr 1980;97:441.
46. DeVivo DC, Keating JP. Reye's syndrome. Adv Pediatr 1975;22:175.
47. Ellis GH, Mirkin LD, Mills MC. Pancreatitis and Reye's syndrome. Am J Dis Child 1979;133:1014.
48. Cameron JL, Capuzzi DM, Zuidema GD, et al. Acute pancreatitis with hyperlipemia. Evidence for a persistent defect in lipid metabolism. Am J Med 1974;56:482.
49. Daum F, Rosen JF, Boldy SJ. Parathyroid adenoma, parathyroid crisis, and acute pancreatitis in an adolescent. J Pediatr 1973;83:275.
50. Schwachman J, Lebenthal E, Khaw KT. Recurrent acute pancreatitis in patients with cystic fibrosis with normal pancreatic enzymes. Pediatrics 1975;55:86.
51. Garner JA. Acute pancreatitis as a complication of anaphylactoid purpura. Arch Dis Child 1977;52:971.
52. Stoler J, Biller J, Grand R. Pancreatitis in Kawasaki disease. Am J Dis Child 1987;141:306.
53. Bartholomew C. Acute scorpion pancreatitis in Trinidad. Br Med J 1970;1:666.
54. Appel MF. Hereditary pancreatitis. Arch Surg 1974;108:63.
55. Kattwinkel J, Lapey A, diSant'Agnese PA, et al. Hereditary pancreatitis: Three new kindreds and a critical review of the literature. Pediatrics 1973;51:55.
56. Toffler AH, Spiro HM. Shock or coma as the predominant manifestation of painless acute pancreatitis. Ann Intern Med 1962;57:655.
57. Eckfeldt JH, Kolars JC, Elson MK, et al. Serum tests for pancreatitis in patients with abdominal pain. Arch Pathol Lab Med 1985;109:316.
58. Kolars JC, Ellis CJ, Levitt MD. Comparison of serum amylase pancreatic isoamylase and lipase in patients with hyperamylasemia. Dig Dis Sci 1984;29:289.
59. Steinberg WM, Goldstein SS, Davis ND, et al. Diagnostic assays in acute pancreatitis. A study of sensitivity and specificity. Ann Intern Med 1985;102:576.
60. Tietz NW, Huang WY, Rauh DF, et al. Laboratory tests in the differential diagnosis of hyperamylasemia. Clin Chem 1986;32:301.
61. Heffernon JJ, Fridhandler L, Berk JE, et al. Assay of amylase and isoamylase activities in serum and urine. Modification in methods and range of normal values. Am J Gastroenterol 1977;67:473.
62. Clavien PA, Robert J, Meyer P, et al. Acute pancreatitis and normoamylasemia. Not an uncommon combination. Ann Surg 1989;210:614.
63. Crist DW, Cameron JL. The current management of acute pancreatitis. Adv Surg 1987;20:69.
64. Rosenblum JL. Pancreatitis. In Feigin RD, Cherry JD (eds). Textbook of Pediatric Infectious Disease. Philadelphia, WB Saunders, 1987, p 750.
65. Levitt MD, Rapoport M, Cooperband SR. The renal clearance of amylase in renal insufficiency, acute pancreatitis and macroamylasemia. Ann Intern Med 1969;71:919.
66. Warshaw AL, Fuller AF. Specificity of increased renal clearance of amylase on diagnosis of acute pancreatitis. N Engl J Med 1975;292:325.
67. Levitt MD, Cooperband SR. Increased renal clearance of amylase in acute pancreatitis. N Engl J Med 1975;292:364.
68. Levine RI, Glauser FL, Berk JE. Enhancement of the amylase-creatinine clearance ratio in disorders other than acute pancreatitis. N Engl J Med 1975;292:329.
69. Levitt MD, Johnson SG. Is the C_{am}/C_{cr} ratio of value for the diagnosis of pancreatitis? Gastroenterology 1978;75:118.
70. Davis S, Parbhoo SP, Gibson MJ. The plain abdominal radiograph in acute pancreatitis. Clin Radiol 1980;31:87.
71. Woodward S, Kelvin FM, Rice RP, et al. Pancreatic abscess: importance of conventional radiology. AJR 1981;136:871.
72. Attar B, Levendoglu H, Causay N. Prognostic value of CT scanning in acute pancreatitis. Gastroenterology 1988;94:A15.
73. Block S, Maier W, Bittner R, et al. Identification of pancreas necrosis in severe acute pancreatitis: Imaging procedures versus clinical staging. Gut 1986;27:1035.
74. Cox KL, Ament ME, Sample WF, et al. The ultrasonic and biochemical diagnosis of pancreatitis in children. J Pediatr 1980;96:407.
75. Fleischer AC, Parker P, Kirchner SG, et al. Sonographic findings of pancreatitis in children. Radiology 1983;146:151.
76. Van Dyke JA, Stanley RJ, Berland LL. Diagnosis and treatment. Pancreatic imaging. Ann Intern Med 1985;102:212.
77. Warshaw AL, Gongliang J. Improved survival in 45 patients with pancreatic abscess. Ann Surg 1985;202:408.
78. Cooperberg PL, Burhenne HJ. Real time ultrasonography. Diagnostic technique of choice in calculus gallbladder disease. N Engl J Med 1980;302:1277.
79. Freeny PC, Marks WM, Ball TJ. Impact of high resolution computed tomography of the pancreas on utilization of endoscopic retrogade cholangiopancreatography and angiography. Radiology 1982;142:35.
80. Ranson JHC, Rifkind KM, Turner JW. Prognostic signs and nonoperative peritoneal lavage in acute pancreatitis. Surg Gynecol Obstet 1976;143:209.
81. Ranson JHC, Pasternak BS. Statistical methods for quantifying the severity of clinical acute pancreatitis. J Surg Res 1977;22:79.
82. Peterson LM, Brooks JR. Lethal pancreatitis: A diagnostic dilemma. Am J Surg 1979;137:491.
83. Osborne DH, Imrie CW, Carter DC. Biliary surgery in the same admission for gallstone-associated pancreatitis. Br J Surg 1981;68:758.
84. Sarr MG, Sanfey H, Cameron JL. Prospective randomized trial of nasogastric suction in patients with acute pancreatitis. Surgery 1986;100:500.
85. Regan PT, Malagelada JR, Go VLW. A prospective study of the antisecretory and therapeutic effects of cimetidine and glucagon in human pancreatitis. Mayo Clin Proc 1981;56:449.
86. Soergel KH. Medical treatment of acute pancreatitis. What is the evidence? Gastroenterology 1978;74:620.
87. Howes R, Zuidema GD, Cameron JL. Evaluation of prophylactic antibiotics in acute pancreatitis. J Surg Res 1975;18:197.
88. Pokorny WJ, Raffensperger JG, Harberg FJ. Pancreatic pseudocysts in children. Surg Gynecol Obstet 1980;151:182.
89. Cooney DR, Grosfeld JL. Operative management of pancreatic pseudocysts in infants and children. A review of 75 cases. Ann Surg 1975;182:590.
90. Cooper A, Floyd T, Barlow B, et al. Major blunt abdominal trauma due to child abuse. J Trauma 1988;28:1483.
91. Sivit CJ, Taylor GA, Eichelberger MR. Visceral injury in battered children. Radiology 1989;173:659.
92. Slovis TL. Pancreatitis and the battered child syndrome. Report of two cases with skeletal involvement. Am J Radiol 1975;125:456.

CHAPTER 41

Jaundice and Hepatitis

Patricia A. Bayless

JAUNDICE

Jaundice is the condition of hyperbilirubinemia manifested by bile pigment deposited in the skin and mucous membranes. There are many causes of this condition in the pediatric population. Differentiation is simplified by a review of historical detail, a careful physical examination, and selective use of biochemical and radiologic studies. Differential diagnoses are grouped according to the type of hyperbilirubinemia (unconjugated versus conjugated) and the age of the patient. Knowledge of the anatomy and physiology of the liver and an understanding of hepatocyte ultrastructure and function are critical.

Anatomy and Physiology

The liver performs multiple homeostatic functions: carbohydrate metabolism, lipid and steroid metabolism, protein and amino acid metabolism, and hematopoiesis. In addition, the liver is responsible for the metabolism and elimination of other endogenous and exogenous substances such as heme, toxins, and drugs. The catabolism of heme-containing compounds provides the substrate for production of bilirubin, the principal pigment of bile (Fig. 41–1). Jaundice may

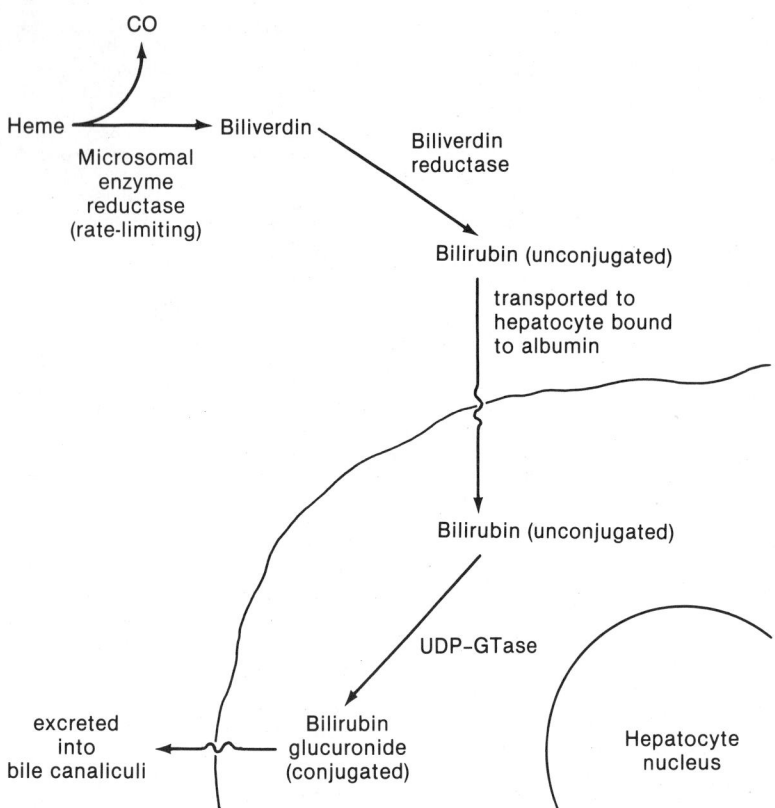

Figure 41–1. Schematic representation of bilirubin metabolism.

be caused by overproduction of bilirubin, abnormal bilirubin metabolism, hepatocellular disease, or cholestasis.

Differential Diagnosis

The list of diseases that may cause or be associated with hyperbilirubinemia and jaundice is extensive. Working through the differential diagnosis is a less formidable task when the age of the patient is considered. Two age groups are considered: neonates (up to 8 to 12 weeks) and older infants and children.

Neonatal Jaundice

Newborns exhibit relative hepatic insufficiency that resolves within the first 4 to 6 weeks of life. Up to 97% of healthy term infants have biochemical hyperbilirubinemia, and approximately 65% are clinically jaundiced. A review of several large studies of normal neonates showed the 50th percentile of bilirubin values to be 6 mg/dl; 6% of infants had levels greater than 12 mg/dl. In the older child and adult, a level of greater than 2 mg/dl results in jaundice, whereas in infants jaundice is produced by a level greater than 5 mg/dl.

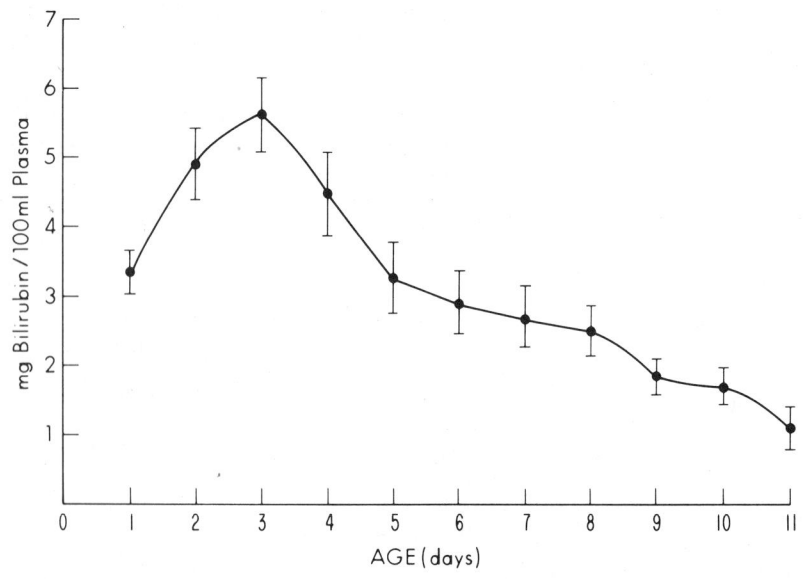

Figure 41–2. Mean total daily bilirubin concentrations in sera from 29 normal term human newborn infants. Vertical bars represent one SE of the mean. (From Gartner LM, Lee K, Vaisman S, et al. Development of bilirubin transport and metabolism in the newborn rhesus monkey. J Pediatr 1977; 90:513.)

Newborns have a biphasic pattern of "physiologic" jaundice (Fig. 41–2). One study in healthy newborns found that unconjugated hyperbilirubinemia (>12.9 mg/dl) was significantly associated with breast-feeding, the percentage of weight lost after birth, maternal diabetes, Oriental race, induction of labor with oxytocin, decreasing gestational age, and male sex. The cause of jaundice associated with breast-feeding has eluded investigators. It is suspected that a factor in the breast milk of certain women enhances the entero-hepatic circulation of bilirubin in the infant.

Prolonged unconjugated hyperbilirubinemia can lead to the development of kernicterus. The serum concentration of unconjugated bilirubin exceeds the capacity of serum proteins to bind it. As a result, the unconjugated bilirubin diffuses across the blood-brain barrier. The precise blood level at which the unbound bilirubin will be toxic for an individual infant is unpredictable, and the necessary duration of exposure is unknown. The unconjugated bilirubin tends to be concentrated in midbrain structures and in cerebellar and cranial nerve nuclei.

Clinical signs and symptoms of kernicterus appear at 2 to 5 days in the term infant and at up to the seventh day in a premature neonate. The manifestations may resemble other systemic illnesses, such as sepsis. The infant appears lethargic, with poor feeding and loss of the Moro reflex, but may also appear gravely ill. By the age of 2 to 3 months, the child may actually improve, with resolution of neurologic signs. However, by 1 year of age, opisthotonos, convulsions, and other movement disorders reappear and may progress until the child is 3 years old.

The bilirubin level at which to treat newborns for unconjugated hyperbilirubinemia is controversial. The level at which most neonatologists recommend an evaluation and treatment is 12 mg/dl. About 50% of these infants will not have an apparent cause of or condition responsible for the jaundice. The definition of physiologic jaundice cannot be based simply on serum bilirubin levels but must also take into account the various other factors associated with hyperbilirubinemia in the neonate. Therefore the decision to treat is not necessarily dependent on the origin of the jaundice (Table 41–1).

Jaundice in the newborn may also be a sign of systemic disease or of anatomic anomalies that require immediate recognition and treatment. These conditions may be revealed by unconjugated or conjugated hyperbilirubinemia. When present within the first week of life, the prognosis for infants with elevated bilirubin levels is ominous if the condition remains untreated (Table 41–2). Conjugated hyperbilirubinemia is more likely to occur within the first 4 weeks of life; a smaller number of cases present at 5 to 8 weeks and a few as late as 4 months (Table 41–3). Along with jaundice, the infant also develops dark urine, clay-colored stools, hepatomegaly, and splenomegaly.

Biliary atresia in the neonate is usually divided into extrahepatic atresia, or hypoplasia, and intrahepatic biliary hypoplasia, or biliary dysgenesis. Biliary atresia is the most common hepatic cause of morbidity in infancy and early childhood. It is suspected that biliary atresia is a continuum of a single disease that has been poorly characterized. In fact, most investigators believe that a viral infection or other toxic insult results in progressive obliteration of the extrahepatic bile ducts, with variable intrahepatic bile duct injury. Hepatocytes appear to develop relatively normally. Biliary atresia is surgically correctable if the common hepatic duct is patent up to the level of the porta hepatis, contains bile, and is in continuity with the main intrahepatic bile ducts. Otherwise, the child who survives beyond the first 4 to 6 months of life will suffer the progressive effects of cirrhosis and fat malabsorption. These children require liver transplantation.

Infant and Childhood Jaundice

In later infancy and childhood, unconjugated jaundice is likely the result of hemolytic disorders, Gilbert's disease, or Crigler-Najjar syndrome. Conjugated hyperbilirubinemia can be caused by hepatocellular injury or obstruction. The

---

TABLE 41–1

GUIDELINES FOR SUSPECTING PATHOLOGIC (NONPHYSIOLOGIC) JAUNDICE IN THE NEONATE

Jaundice appearing within 24 hours and rapidly increasing (>5 mg/dl/day)
Persistence of jaundice >7–10 days in a term, otherwise healthy infant
Onset of jaundice after the first week of life
Elevated levels in an infant with few of the significant associated factors mentioned in text

---

TABLE 41–2

CAUSES OF NEONATAL UNCONJUGATED HYPERBILIRUBINEMIA THAT REQUIRE URGENT IDENTIFICATION AND TREATMENT

Hemolytic disorders, such as ABO/Rh incompatibility, defects of red cell membranes; red blood cell enzyme deficiencies, and ingestion of hemolytic agents
Increased red blood cell mass (polycythemia), as in placental transfusion, twin-to-twin transfusion, infants of diabetic mothers, late clamping of cord
Hypoxia
Hypoglycemia
Hypothyroidism
Dehydration
Galactosemia
Fructosemia
Administration of drugs competing with bilirubin for hepatic excretion
Meconium retention
High intestinal obstruction
Sepsis
TORCH
Congenital syphilis

TORCH = Toxoplasmosis, rubella, cytomegalovirus, herpes simplex.
From Mowat A. Liver Disease in Childhood. London, Butterworth, 1979.

TABLE 41–3

CAUSES OF CONJUGATED HYPERBILIRUBINEMIA IN INFANCY

Structural defects
    Bile duct anomalies
    Polycystic disease
    Vascular lesions
    Chromosomal abnormalities
Metabolic defects
    Infections
    Posthemolytic disorders
    Toxic or deficiency disorders
        Parenteral nutrition
        Drugs/toxins
    Familial syndromes (e.g., Dubin-Johnson)
    Neonatal hepatic necrosis
    Idiopathic

From Mowat A. Liver Disease in Childhood. London, Butterworth, 1979.

most frequent cause of hepatocellular injury is viral hepatitis A, but chronic active hepatitis, Wilson's disease, and other metabolic or nutritional disorders must also be considered. Cholelithiasis is more common in older children than in neonates.

Biliary tract disease may present with conjugated hyperbilirubinemia in children. A 20-year review of pediatric cholelithiasis showed that it is a disease of young infants and adolescents but is infrequent in children ages 1 to 11 years. Overall, the most common symptom was vomiting (60% of cases), followed by abdominal pain (50%), but not necessarily localized to the right upper quadrant. In infants, jaundice was the most common symptom (90%), whereas in the total population of patients, jaundice was present about 25% of the time. The most common condition associated with pediatric cholelithiasis in the infant-to-adolescent age group was hemolytic disease.

Infants with cystic fibrosis may develop conjugated hyperbilirubinemia because of obstruction of both the extrahepatic bile duct and the intrahepatic bile ductule. This is thought to be a result of the abnormally viscous mucus that is secreted into their lumens. There are also associated, but less clearly defined, toxic and dietary problems that may cause hepatocellular damage. Obstructive jaundice is rare in newborns and is frequently associated with meconium ileus. Up to 20% of children and adolescents with cystic fibrosis develop cirrhosis. They may also exhibit hepatosplenomegaly, esophageal varices, and occasionally hepatic encephalopathy.

Children with sickle cell disease frequently have associated liver disease. Hepatomegaly is present in nearly all patients, along with elevated serum bilirubin and hepatic transaminase levels. Jaundice is frequently detectable. The serum bilirubin may be mostly unconjugated or conjugated. If 90% is unconjugated, this may be attributed to rapid hemolysis. If more than 10% is conjugated, there is usually hepatocellular damage or an abnormality of the biliary tract. Children with sickle cell disease who present with conjugated hyperbilirubinemia may be experiencing sickle cell crisis or have hepatitis. A limited study reviewed 11 children with sickle cell disease and acute onset of jaundice. None had cholelithiasis proven by ultrasound, and none had received transfusions. This group was matched to a control group of children without sickle cell disease but with the same clinical presentation and positive serologic markers for hepatitis A. Half of the children in the study group were found to have positive serologic markers for hepatitis A, and none had markers for hepatitis B.

Clinical and Diagnostic Evaluation

When jaundice is recognized in the child, the emergency department physician should screen for any treatable diseases. It is also important to screen for viral agents (e.g., hepatitis viruses) that may cause jaundice in order to prevent transmission to other children and family members.

For the infant with jaundice, the physician must review several historical details with the parent. Included among these are maternal infections or diseases, breast-feeding, premature birth, and external ecchymoses or hematoma from birth trauma. The presence of hepatosplenomegaly should be sought during the physical examination. The color of the infant's stool should be determined and any recent change in stool color noted by the parent.

Initial laboratory studies should include determinations of total and fractionated serum bilirubin and serum transaminase levels. Hyperbilirubinemia can be divided into unconjugated (indirect) and conjugated (direct) forms. Normal bilirubin values, except in the newborn, can be defined as a total bilirubin level of <1.5 mg/dl in direct form. Unconju-

TABLE 41–4
ADDITIONAL DIAGNOSTIC LABORATORY TESTS FOR EVALUATION OF THE INFANT WITH HYPERBILIRUBINEMIA

Hemoglobin and reticulocyte count
Red blood cell morphology tests
Test to determine blood group of mother and child
Direct Coombs' test on infant's red blood cells
Test to determine maternal antibodies and hemolysins
Viral and bacterial cultures (blood/urine/cerebrospinal fluid)
Viral serology tests (hepatitis screen, TORCH, VDRL)
Metabolic and hormonal screens (thyroxine, thyrotropin, sweat chloride, urine or serum amino acids)
Genetic screen (alpha$_1$-antitrypsin)

gated hyperbilirubinemia is defined as an elevated total bilirubin level with less than 15% in the direct form. Conjugated hyperbilirubinemia is defined as an elevated total bilirubin level with a more than 15% to 30% direct fraction; this is always considered abnormal. Prothrombin time and albumin values are useful indicators of hepatic protein synthesis function. The degree and type of jaundice and the pattern of liver function test results are guides to identifying the origin of liver dysfunction. If disease other than primary hepatic disease is suspected, other diagnostic tests can be included (Table 41–4).

For older infants and children, the history and physical examination are also important. The same initial screening studies are required. In those patients in an active bone growth stage, the alkaline phosphatase value is less useful, as it is elaborated by bone growth.

Noninvasive radiologic studies that may be useful include computed tomography, ultrasound, and nuclear imaging studies. These are generally well tolerated by the pediatric patient. Computed tomography and ultrasound may elucidate a choledochal cyst or other mass lesion in the right upper quadrant of the abdomen. Ultrasound is effective for determining the presence of gallstones and is also sensitive in demonstrating ascites. Radionuclide scanning suggests biliary atresia if no isotope reaches the duodenum.

Therapeutic Intervention

Management of unconjugated hyperbilirubinemia in the neonate depends on the origin (Fig. 41–3). In a healthy-appearing neonate with some of the aforementioned risk factors for physiologic jaundice, the physician may elect to follow serial bilirubin values in consultation with a pediatrician. Some pediatricians' offices and neonatal units may use a hand-held ictometer, which correlates well with serum bilirubin levels. Exchange transfusion may be recommended for conditions with a high rate of red cell lysis. The transfusion removes any sensitized red blood cells, can correct anemia caused by loss of red blood cells, and removes circulating unconjugated bilirubin that is bound to albumin in the serum. Phototherapy stimulates alternate pathways for bilirubin conjugation that ordinarily do not contribute. Pharmacologic acceleration of normal metabolic pathways for bilirubin excretion can be accomplished pharmacologically (i.e., enzyme induction); phenobarbital is the most widely accepted agent. Results from additional studies determine whether the infant will require antibiotics or other therapy for underlying systemic disease. For otherwise healthy newborns who are being breast-fed, a regimen that eliminates breast milk for 24 to 48 hours may be tried. Formula is substituted and increased fluids such as Pedialyte are recommended. The mother may continue to use a breast

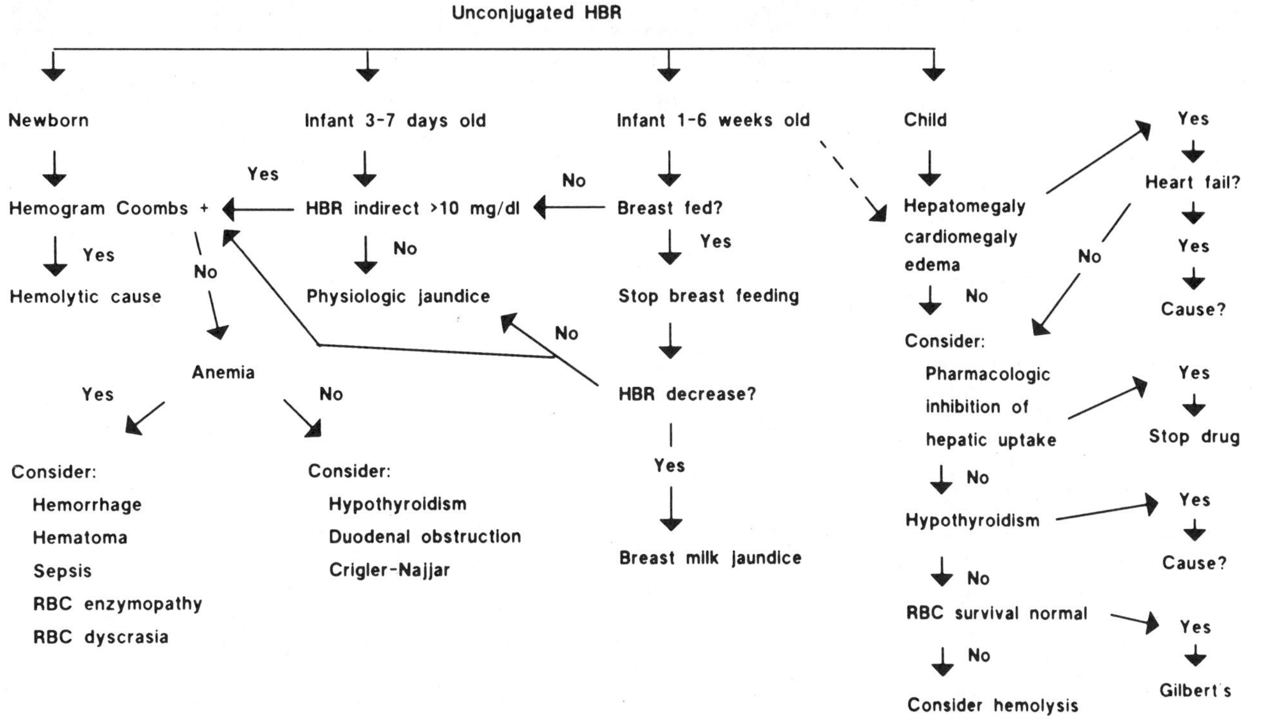

Unconjugated HBR

Newborn

Infant 3-7 days old

Infant 1-6 weeks old

Child

Yes

Hemogram Coombs +

Yes ← HBR indirect >10 mg/dl ← No ← Breast fed?

Heart fail?

Yes

Hepatomegaly
cardiomegaly
edema

No

Yes

Hemolytic cause

No

Yes

Physiologic jaundice

Yes

Stop breast feeding

No

Cause?

No

Anemia

No

HBR decrease?

Consider:

Yes

Pharmacologic
inhibition of
hepatic uptake

Yes

Yes

No

Stop drug

Consider:

Hemorrhage

Hematoma

Sepsis

RBC enzymopathy

RBC dyscrasia

Consider:

Hypothyroidism

Duodenal obstruction

Crigler-Najjar

Yes

Breast milk jaundice

Hypothyroidism

No

Yes

Cause?

No

RBC survival normal

Yes

No

Consider hemolysis

Gilbert's

Figure 41-3. The approach to determining the cause of unconjugated hyperbilirubinemia is age dependent. (From Colón AR. Textbook of Pediatric Hepatology. 2nd ed. Chicago, Year Book, 1990, p 17.)

pump in the interim and may resume breast-feeding if bilirubin levels are decreasing.

Treatment of conjugated hyperbilirubinemia is unnecessary, as this compound does not cross the blood-brain barrier. Investigation should be directed at determining the origin of the jaundice (Fig. 41–4). It is important to emphasize follow-up for the infant with persistently elevated bilirubin levels.

HEPATITIS

Hepatitis is simply inflammation of the liver. Multiple infectious agents, in addition to numerous chemical agents,

can cause hepatitis. The major role of the physician is to identify the causative agent and interrupt its transmission. Although hepatitis A virus (HAV) does not have any long-term sequelae, hepatitis B virus (HBV) infection in childhood is considered the major predisposing factor to primary hepatocellular carcinoma.

The hepatitis viruses have been divided into five distinctive viral entities. Type A virus (HAV) is implicated in most childhood epidemics in the United States. A major concern has been the spread of HAV in day-care centers. The risk is greater if there are large numbers of children who are not toilet trained. Typically, the disease is traced back to the day-care center when a worker, parent, or other family

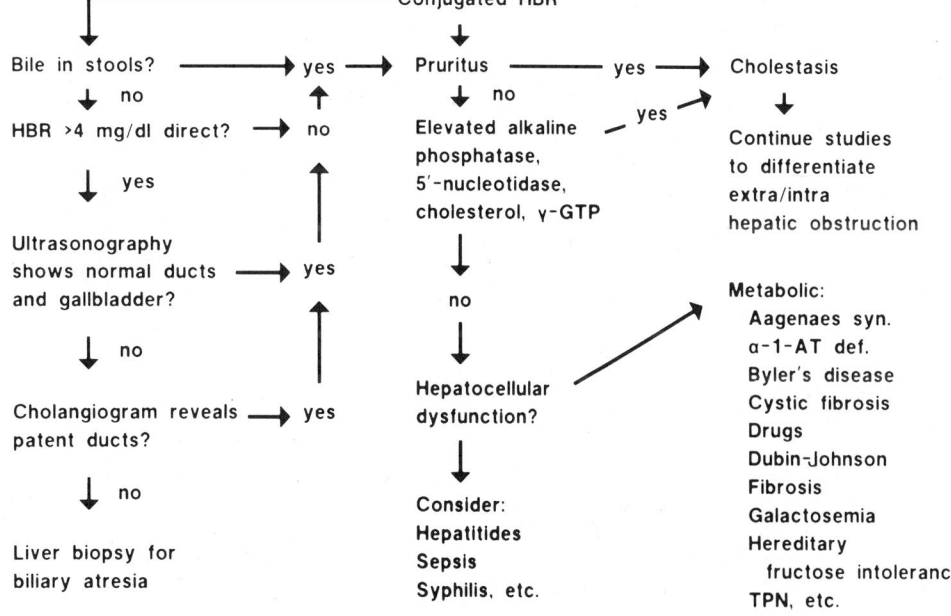

Figure 41-4. The approach to determining the cause of conjugated hyperbilirubinemia more greatly considers anatomic etiologies and hepatocellular dysfunction. (From Colón AR. Textbook of Pediatric Hepatology. 2nd ed. Chicago, Year Book, 1990, p 18.)

TABLE 41–5		
RECOMMENDATION FOR PRE- AND POSTEXPOSURE IMMUNIZATION FOR HEPATITIS A AND B		
Group	Preexposure/Timing	Postexposure/Timing
Hepatitis A		
Contact with active case of hepatitis A (household, sexual, care provider, day care or epidemic exposure)	None	0.2 ml/kg/, <2 weeks after exposure, one dose 0.5 ml weight <25 kg 1.0 ml weight 25–50 kg 2.0 ml for adults
Before travel to endemic areas	0.5 ml/kg q 4–6 mo	Same as above
Hepatitis B		
Health care workers with blood or needle-stick exposure; hemodialysis staff and patients; homosexual sexually active men; clients and staff at developmentally disabled institutions; IV drug abusers; recipients of certain blood products; household and sexual contacts of HBV carriers; travelers to endemic areas	No HBIG Vaccine: 1 ml IM >10 yr old × 3 doses 0.5 ml IM <10 yr old × 3 doses Complete series within 6 months	If completed vaccination series, test for anti-HBs If low, give HBIG (0.6 ml/kg) once and booster dose of vaccine
Perinatal exposure (mother is HBV+)		HBIG, 0.5 ml IM, within 12 hr of birth Vaccine: 0.5 ml IM, within 7 days of birth and at 1 and 6 mo (at different site than HBIG administered)
Percutaneous or mucosa exposure If source is positive or suspected to be positive		HBIG, 0.06 ml/kg IM or 5 ml for adult, as single dose within 24 hours Vaccine: 1 ml IM >10 yr old, 0.5 ml IM <10 yr old—within 7 days of exposure and at 1 and 6 mo
If source is unknown or suspicion is low that source is positive		No HBIG Initiate vaccination series

member of a child becomes jaundiced. Hepatitis A infection is anicteric in 80% of children younger than 4 years old, but 75% of adults develop jaundice. Care for the child or adult is generally supportive, with the main focus on prevention of further spread of the disease. In day-care centers, maximal hygienic practices, such as hand washing and cleansing of diaper-changing surfaces, should be enforced. Prompt immunization with immunoglobulin for the children and their adult caregivers must be initiated (Table 41–5). This strategy has proven successful in curbing outbreaks of hepatitis A. Once a child is exposed, the parent should not move them to another day-care facility until the epidemic is controlled.

Hepatitis type B virus is not a risk in day-care centers, even if one is exposed to a child who is a chronic carrier. However, it has been well established that children in institutionalized settings are at greater risk for exposure. Hepatitis B immunization is recommended for both the clients and providers at such institutions. Another group at significant risk for contracting HBV are infants born to HBV-infected or carrier mothers. Women who are intravenous drug abusers should be screened prenatally.

Hepatitis B is not considered endemic in the United States when compared with other countries. Early infection with HBV predisposes the patient to the carrier state, to cirrhosis, and to primary hepatocellular carcinoma. Hepatitis B immunization is recommended for neonates at risk and for other children who are in endemic areas (see Table 41–5).

Non-A/non-B hepatitis has now been characterized into three different viral particles. These are referred to as types C (transfusion related), D (delta agent), and E (water-borne epidemic). A screening assay for hepatitis type C (HCV) is available. Most blood banks in the United States have also

initiated screening. Albumin and immune serum globulin are risk free, but pooled plasma and prothrombin factor concentrate may contain the type C virus. Many hemophiliac children have been infected.

Hepatitis type D (HDV) only seems to be present when HBV is present. Theories have been proposed that HDV requires HBV to enter and leave the hepatocyte but can replicate independently once inside the cell. There is no direct screening test for HDV, because the circulating virus is encapsulated in an HBV envelope. The presence of HDV tends to make the hepatitis more severe in both children and adults.

Type E hepatitis is rare in the United States and is poorly understood. It does not seem to be associated with chronicity, but does seem to cause considerable fetal wastage and disease in pregnant women.

Clinical and Diagnostic Evaluation

The pediatric patient with hepatitis usually presents with gastroenteritis or a flu-like syndrome. This may progress to jaundice and acholic stools. Frequently infants and young children may develop only hyperbilirubinemia and not clinical jaundice.

The diagnosis of hepatitis is accomplished by appropriate serum assays; many facilities have a standard panel for the detection of HAV and HBV infections. Liver function tests should also be performed to determine the degree of hepatic injury, which may necessitate hospitalization.

It is important to have a mechanism to follow up the hepatitis assay in patients discharged from the emergency department. This is usually done by a hospital infection control nurse or public health officer. Discharge instructions should include strict hygiene guidelines to prevent further exposure in the home or community.

Once the type of hepatitis virus is identified, passive or active immunization is recommended (see Table 41–5). Generally, the emergency department is not the place to administer prophylaxis. Contacts can be referred to public and community health clinics or offices for administration of the immunoglobulin and vaccines. When hepatitis is identified as type B, C, or D, the patient should have regularly scheduled follow-up for at least 6 to 12 months to be sure that the episode resolves and does not evolve into carrier status or chronic hepatitis.

Selected References

Balistreri WF. Viral hepatitis. Pediatr Clin North Am 1988;35(3):637.
Child Day Care Infectious Disease Study Group. Public health considerations of infectious disease in child day care centers. Pediatrics 1984;105(5):683.
Chow CB, Lau TTY, Chang WK. Acute viral hepatitis: Aetiology and evolution. Arch Dis Child 1989;64:211.
Friesen CA, Roberts CC. Cholelithiasis—clinical characteristics in children. Clin Pediatr 1989;28(7):294.
Hadler SC, McFarland L. Hepatitis in day care centers: Epidemiology and prevention. Rev Infect Dis 1986;8(4):548.
Maisels J. Neonatal jaundice. Semin Liver Dis 1988;8(4):148.
Maisels MD, Gifford K, Antle CE, et al. Jaundice in the healthy newborn infant: A new approach to an old problem. Pediatrics 1988;81(4):505.
Mallouh AA, Asha MI. Acute cholestatic jaundice in children with sickle cell disease: Hepatic crises or hepatitis? Pediatr Infect Dis J 1988;7:689.
Shapiro CN, McCaig LF, Gensheimer KF, et al. Hepatitis B virus transmission between children in day care. Pediatr Infect Dis J 1989;8:870.
Smego RA, Halsey NA. The case for routine hepatitis B immunization in infancy for populations at increased risk. Pediatr Infect Dis J 1987;6:11.
Tabor E. Etiology, diagnosis and treatment of viral hepatitis in children. Adv Pediatr Infect Dis 1988;3:19.

CHAPTER 42

Reye's Syndrome

Kelley A. Hails

EPIDEMIOLOGY

Reye's syndrome is a rapidly progressive postviral syndrome characterized by vomiting and deteriorating mental status. The overall incidence in the United States is 0.58 to 2.8 cases per 100,000 population younger than 18 years.[1,2] The highest incidence, reaching 3.5 cases per 100,000 population younger than 18 years, has been reported in Colorado, Georgia, Iowa, Michigan, Nebraska, Ohio, South Dakota, and Utah.[1–5] Reye's syndrome remains a deadly disease, although mortality rates have dropped from 80% in 1963[6] to 30% in the 1980s.[7–10]

Reye's syndrome follows a mild viral prodrome in more than 90% of children. The antecedent illness is primarily a respiratory illness in about 70% of patients,[1,7–9,11] varicella in 15% to 30%,[1,7,8] and a diarrheal illness in 2% to 15%.[1,7–9,11] Other less specific viral prodromes, including a fever or a nonvaricella rash, may occur in up to 10% of patients.[7–9] There is no difference between the antecedent illness in children who develop Reye's syndrome and that in those who do not.[12]

Both sexes are affected equally. In 90% of cases, patients are 15 years old or younger, and most cases occur in children 4 to 12 years old. The average age in children who have primarily respiratory prodromal illness is 8 to 11 years. Children who present with rash, fever, or diarrheal prodrome have a mean age of 6 years.[1] Diarrheal prodromes are especially common in infants who develop Reye's syndrome.[13]

More than 90% of cases occur in white children[1,7,8,10,11]; suburban and rural children are most frequently affected.[3,14] Black children who are affected fall disproportionately into the age group of 1 year old or younger.[1,7,13] Infants with Reye's syndrome tend to come from mostly urban, lower socioeconomic groups.[13]

A voluntary surveillance system to assess the U.S. incidence of Reye's syndrome was established by the Centers for Disease Control (CDC) in 1968. From 1967 to 1973, between 11 and 83 cases were reported annually.[15] From 1974 to 1983 the number of reported cases increased to a peak of 548 cases in 1980.[1] Since that time, the number of cases has been steady at about 200 cases per year[7–9] until 1987, when it dropped precipitously to less than 40 cases annually through 1989.[10,11]

ETIOLOGY

Despite three decades of research, the origin of Reye's syndrome remains unclear. The most plausible hypothesis suggests that a combination of viral, host, and exogenous toxic factors are responsible.[2]

Viral Factors

The existence of an antecedent viral illness in almost all cases is well documented.[1,7–9] Most data suggest that viruses, especially influenza types A and B and varicella, are related to the onset of Reye's syndrome.[2] The highest reported incidence in the United States occurred during years of primary influenza types A (H_1N_1) and B activity.[1,2] In addition, the majority of cases occur in the months of peak influenza activity—January, February, and March.[1,2,9,10]

Influenza type B virus has been recovered from the nasopharynx, serum, and visceral organs of numerous children with Reye's syndrome.[2,16] Reye's syndrome occurs in 1 of every 2000 influenza type B infections in children.[3,17] Children who have influenza type B–associated Reye's syndrome have a median age of 11 years, paralleling the median age at attack of influenza type B.[2,18]

Influenza A, particularly H_1N_1 viruses ("Russian flu"),[4,14,19] has also been associated with endemic Reye's syndrome. Reye's syndrome occurs in 1 of 33,000 influenza A infections in children.[17]

Varicella virus is associated with 15% to 30% of cases,[1,7,8] and antibodies to varicella have been isolated from the serum of Reye's syndrome patients.[20] These cases occur primarily in late winter and spring, the period of peak varicella activity.[1,2] Reye's syndrome occurs in 0.3 to 0.9 cases per 100,000 varicella infections.[2,17,21] Varicella-related Reye's syndrome affects younger children (mean age, 6 years), paralleling the mean age at attack of varicella.[2,18,21,22] These patients present in stage 0 more often than in stages I through V (Table 42–1).[12]

Seventeen other viruses have been implicated in the prodromal illness.[2,17,23,24] These include adenovirus, coxsackievirus types A and B, cytomegalovirus, echovirus, Epstein-Barr virus, herpes simplex virus, mumps, parainfluenza, respiratory syncytial virus, rotavirus, rubella, and rubeola (measles). In addition, in two cases systemic bacterial infection with *Haemophilus influenzae* has been associated with Reye's syndrome, although concurrent viral infections could not be ruled out.[25,26]

Stage	Sign and Symptoms
	TABLE 42-1
	CLINICAL STAGING OF REYE'S SYNDROME
0	Alert, wakeful, vomiting (must develop encephalopathy greater than or equal to stage I during the illness), liver dysfunction
I	Difficult to arouse, lethargic, sleepy, vomiting, liver dysfunction
II	Delirious, combative, confused, liver dysfunction
III	Obtunded, decorticate posturing, pupillary light reflexes intact, ± seizures, liver dysfunction
IV	Obtunded, decerebrate posturing, fixed pupils, seizures
V	Comatose; flaccid; areflexic; apneic; fixed, dilated pupils; liver function often normalized

From Hurwitz ES, Nelson DB, Davis C, et al. National surveillance for Reye syndrome: A five-year review. Pediatrics 1982;70:895. Reproduced by permission of Pediatrics.

Host Factors

A genetic predisposition to Reye's syndrome has been sought. Although it is not associated with an HLA antigen type, Reye's syndrome has been reported in twins, in siblings, and in the offspring of first-cousin marriages.[17, 18, 20, 27, 28] Episodes mimicking Reye's syndrome occur in children with defects in ureagenesis and fatty acid metabolism.[2, 18, 29]

Exogenous Toxic Factors

Many exogenous toxins have been linked with Reye's syndrome. Exposure to isopropyl alcohol, lead, methyl bromide, paint, insecticides and their emulsifiers, insect repellents, and even acetaminophen has been reported in patients with Reye's syndrome.[2, 15, 17, 30, 31] The clinical similarities of Reye's syndrome to Jamaican vomiting sickness, which is caused by eating the unripe fruit of the akee tree, have implicated hypoglycin A.[6, 18, 32] Aflatoxin, a mycotoxin produced by many species of fungi, has also been implicated in the development of Reye's syndrome.[18, 33, 34] Aflatoxin toxicity, which is indistinguishable from Reye's syndrome, is endemic in northeastern Thailand.

Aspirin is the drug most often implicated in the development of Reye's syndrome. Salicylate toxicity is clinically similar to Reye's syndrome in that both produce hepatic dysfunction with encephalopathy.[35] An association between Reye's syndrome and aspirin use in the antecedent illness has been well documented.[15, 36] Case-control studies in the United States indicate that from 59% to 95% of patients had been given aspirin during the antecedent illness.[8, 12, 37–39] Less than half of the controls had been given salicylates; acetaminophen was more frequently used in this group.

A dose-response relationship between Reye's syndrome and aspirin has also been demonstrated.[40] Children on chronic salicylate therapy for connective tissue disease or juvenile rheumatoid arthritis are at increased risk.[41–43] This strong association between aspirin use and Reye's syndrome development prompted warnings concerning the use of aspirin in the treatment of influenza and varicella in children.[44–46] In 1986, the Food and Drug Administration mandated a package label warning.[47] Because of these efforts, fewer children are receiving aspirin during illnesses that may precede Reye's syndrome.[48–50] The decreased incidence of Reye's syndrome parallels the decreased use of aspirin in young children, lending further support to the connection between the two.[51–53]

PATHOLOGY AND PATHOGENESIS

The pathologic abnormalities indicative of Reye's syndrome are found primarily in the liver and brain. Grossly, the liver is swollen, tense, and pale yellow. Microscopically, fatty infiltration of hepatocytes is diffuse and particularly marked at portal areas. There is a characteristic absence of inflammation or necrosis. Diffuse cerebral edema may be visualized grossly by flattening of the cerebral gyri, reduction of ventricular size, or internal herniations. The brain demonstrates cytotoxic cerebral edema microscopically with astrocyte swelling, decreased extracellular space, and, again, a characteristic absence of inflammatory cells.[54]

Biochemical assays show a severe reduction in activity of all mitochondrial enzymes.[17, 55–57] These include the urea cycle enzymes ornithine carbamoyltransferase (OCTase), carbamoyl phosphate synthetase (CPSase), and pyruvate dehydrogenase. Decreased OCTase and CPSase may result in hyperammonemia, the hallmark of Reye's syndrome[15, 58, 59] (Fig. 42–1). In addition, exaggerated lipolysis, evidenced by elevated serum free fatty acids and abnormalities in carnitine metabolism, suggests defective mitochondrial beta oxidation of fatty acids.[15, 51, 57] This triggers intracellular fat accumulation and may, with hyperammonemia, contribute to cerebral edema.[15, 57] Mitochondrial injury also impairs glyconeogenesis. This, along with increased anaerobic glycolysis and glucagon-mediated glycogenolysis, accounts for the hepatocellular glycogen depletion seen.[57]

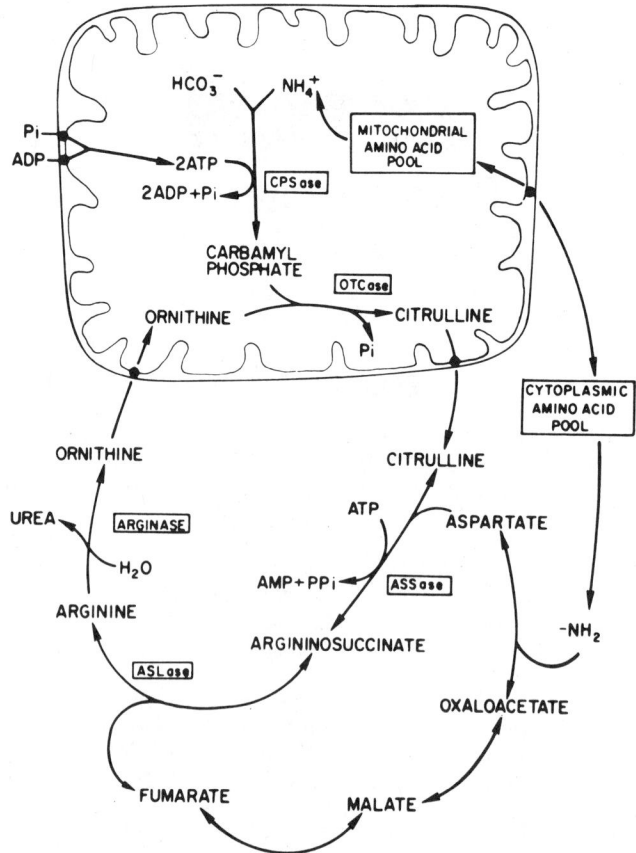

Figure 42–1. The urea cycle. Interruption of pathways that lead to release of urea results in accumulation of excess ammonia. (From Rockoff MA, Pascucci RC. Reye's syndrome. Emerg Med Clin North Am 1983;1:88.)

EMERGENCY MEDICAL SERVICE CONSIDERATIONS

Prehospital assessment should focus on the child's level of consciousness. Intervention in the field should be aimed at those children who have a decreased level of consciousness. A combative child may need physical restraint to prevent injury to self or others. The airway is a primary concern in any child with altered consciousness and should be fully assessed. The child should be placed on oxygen, intravenous access established, and a blood sample obtained for glucose determination. An intravenous D5W or D10W solution should then be instituted. Dextrose, 0.5 to 1.0 gm/kg/dose administered as a 25% solution, and naloxone (Narcan), 0.01 mg/kg (up to 2 mg), should be given intravenously in any child with a decreased level of consciousness unrelated to trauma. Persistent seizures should be controlled with diazepam, 0.5 to 1.0 mg intravenously, repeated at 2- to 5-minute intervals.

CLINICAL EVALUATION

Reye's syndrome develops following typical childhood viral illnesses. A history of respiratory or gastrointestinal illness, varicella, or other rash in the preceding 3 to 7 days is usual.[1, 7–9, 15] The mean onset is 4 days following varicella, and 5½ days following other illnesses.[12] A history of salicylate use during the viral prodrome should be sought. Profuse and persistent vomiting begins as the infectious symptoms are resolving. The child may complain of headache. Vomiting usually persists for less than 24 hours and is associated with, or closely followed by, a change in the child's mental status. As intracranial pressure rises, quiet, withdrawn, or lethargic behavior may progress to delirium, obtundation, seizures, and coma with catastrophic speed.

Fever is not usually part of the syndrome but may be present. Kussmaul respirations are common. Papilledema is usually not found because of the rapid rate of rise in intracranial pressure. Meningeal signs such as nuchal rigidity are absent. Hepatomegaly occurs in up to 50% of children at some time during their clinical course, but the absence of jaundice differentiates Reye's syndrome from hepatitis. Focal neurologic abnormalities are unusual, but generalized neurologic changes are progressive as cerebral edema worsens (see Table 42–1). Seizures occur in 30% of patients.[17] Progression to brain death may occur; maximum progression usually occurs within 48 to 60 hours of onset (Fig. 42–2). Reversal of progression may occur at any stage.

Infants with Reye's syndrome typically present with tachypnea, respiratory distress, seizures, and apnea.[13, 17] Vomiting is rare, and prodromal viral illness is much less common than in older children, thereby confounding the diagnosis. Hepatomegaly and hypoglycemia are more prominent than in older children. The death rate is higher in infants, and Reye's syndrome may present as "near-miss" sudden infant death syndrome (SIDS).[13, 17, 60, 61]

Staging

Clinical staging of Reye's syndrome helps direct management and predict outcome. Several staging systems have been suggested, including the Glasgow Coma Scale.[30, 62] The staging system recommended by the National Institutes of Health (NIH)[30, 63] consists of five progressive levels of neurologic compromise, stages I through V. The CDC recommends a sixth stage, stage 0, in which patients with mild Reye's syndrome present in an alert and wakeful state[1, 12] and later progress to a higher stage (see Table 42–1). Up to 75% of children present in stages I and II.[8–10] Since the

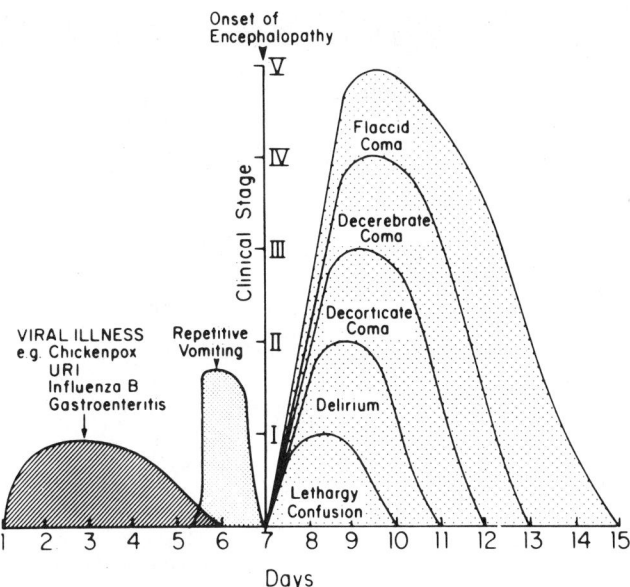

Figure 42–2. Clinical course of Reye's syndrome and rostrocaudal progression of encephalopathy. (From Sarnaik AP. Diagnosis and management of Reye's syndrome. Compr Ther 1982;8:48.)

1970s, the percentage of children who progress to stage V has decreased dramatically, from 74% in 1974 to 30% in 1988.[1, 8, 10]

LABORATORY EVALUATION

Results of liver function tests are abnormal in all cases. Transaminase levels are elevated, with aspartate aminotransferase (AST; previously called serum glutamic-oxaloacetic transaminase, or SGOT) and alanine aminotransferase (ALT; previously called serum glutamate pyruvate transaminase, or SGPT) levels between 2 and 100 times normal.[6, 17, 18, 57] The AST measurement is probably the most sensitive screening tool.[57] Lactic dehydrogenase (LDH) levels are elevated, but serum alkaline phosphatase and bilirubin levels are usually normal.[17, 57] Creatine kinase (CK) may be elevated, particularly in later stages[12, 57, 64]; the MB band may also be elevated.[30, 57] Prothrombin time is usually prolonged by 3 to 10 seconds, and there may be a severe coagulopathy.[17]

Serum ammonia is frequently elevated to a level two to ten times normal (Table 42–2).[17, 65] Blood ammonia levels usually peak within 4 hours of admission and are predictive of disease severity and patient survival.[12, 13, 64–67] Ammonia levels less than five times normal are associated with 100% survival.[65] Hyperammonemia is very transient, however, and can be missed.[17, 54]

Although hypoglycemia was once considered to be a hallmark of Reye's syndrome,[6] it is well established that blood glucose levels may be normal or even elevated.[57] Hypoglycemia secondary to depleted glycogen stores occurs in severe cases, most frequently in infants and young children.[6, 13, 17]

The complete blood cell (CBC) count is usually normal, although the white blood cell (WBC) count may be over 20,000 as a result of stress and acidosis.

The acid-base findings are characteristically those of a mixed disturbance.[27, 57] Typically there is a primary respiratory alkalosis as a result of Kussmaul respirations, with arterial $P_{CO_2} \leq 25$ mm Hg. A primary metabolic (lactic) acidosis related to disturbances in oxidative metabolism is also present, with serum bicarbonate usually ≤ 15 mEq/L; pH is often in or near the normal range.

TABLE 42–2

LABORATORY STUDIES USEFUL IN THE DIAGNOSIS AND MANAGEMENT OF REYE'S SYNDROME

Primary studies
  Liver function tests: aspartate aminotransferase (SGOT),
    alanine aminotransferase (SGPT), lactate dehydrogenase,
    creatine kinase, prothrombin time, ammonia
  Glucose test
  Electrolyte tests: sodium, potassium, chloride, CO_2, calcium,
    phosphorus
  Renal function tests: blood urea nitrogen, creatine, urinalysis
  Arterial blood gas measurements
  Complete blood cell count; type and crossmatch blood for
    red blood cells and plasma
  Amylase and bilirubin measurements
  Toxicology screen (serum and urine)
Adjunctive studies
  Chest radiograph
  Electrocardiogram
  Cranial computed tomography scan
  Lumbar puncture

Many other laboratory abnormalities have been noted in Reye's syndrome. Azotemia may occur as a result of dehydration from vomiting. Hyperamylasemia may also occur.[27, 57, 68] Pancreatitis occurs in approximately 9% of patients[27, 68] and probably explains the hyperamylasemia.[57] Uric acid levels may be elevated. Hypophosphatemia may occur, and serum free fatty acids are elevated.

Adjunctive Tests

If lumbar puncture is performed, the cerebral spinal fluid (CSF) is usually normal; the glucose level may be low if severe hypoglycemia is present.[1, 17] There is an absence of inflammatory cells (Table 42–3). Lumbar puncture is indicated only when it is necessary to rule out meningitis or encephalitis. The intracranial hypertension that occurs in later stages of Reye's syndrome greatly increases the risk of herniation and brain stem compression.[69–71] Thus, if the emergency physician elects to perform lumbar puncture, the use of mannitol prior to performing the lumbar puncture must be considered.[69] Cranial computed tomography (CT) scans may demonstrate diffuse cerebral edema and may be particularly helpful in patients presenting in stage III or higher, in those with atypical presentations, or in those with focal findings.[30]

TABLE 42–3

CENTERS FOR DISEASE CONTROL CASE DEFINITION OF REYE'S SYNDROME

1. Acute noninflammatory encephalopathy with either
    —Fatty metamorphosis of the liver, diagnosed by biopsy
     or autopsy, or
    —A three-fold or greater rise in serum aspartate
     aminotransferase, alanine aminotransferase, or ammonia
2. CSF, if obtained, with 8 or fewer leukocytes per cubic
   millimeter
3. No other more reasonable explanation for the cerebral or
   hepatic abnormalities

From Hurwitz ES, Nelson DB, Davis C, et al. National surveillance for Reye syndrome: A five-year review. Pediatrics 1982;70:895. Reproduced by permission of Pediatrics.

DIFFERENTIAL DIAGNOSIS

A wide differential diagnosis must be considered in children or infants with vomiting, progressive coma, and elevated serum transaminase levels (Table 42–4).[32] Children who present early, in stages 0 or I, may appear to have gastroenteritis. Generalized viral syndromes, such as varicella and adenovirus infections, may cause liver damage and encephalopathy.[17, 30, 72–74] CNS infection (e.g., encephalitis or meningitis) should be considered. Shock from bacterial sepsis or dehydration may also cause diagnostic difficulties.[17, 72, 74] In addition, many toxins or ingestions may mimic Reye's syndrome.[74–76]

Metabolic abnormalities producing encephalopathy include hepatitis (before the onset of jaundice), pancreatitis, diabetic ketoacidosis, and hypoglycemia.[74] In infants, inborn errors of metabolism are important possibilities. These include defects of the urea cycle and fatty acid oxidation, organic acidurias, amino acidurias, carnitine deficiency, and fructosemia.[72, 74, 77–79] Reye's syndrome must also be considered in what appears to be "near-miss" SIDS.[13, 17, 60, 61, 72] Unwitnessed head trauma, particularly that associated with the battered child syndrome, may produce a constellation of signs and symptoms that may be confused with Reye's syndrome in children of any age.[80]

THERAPEUTIC INTERVENTION
General Measures

All patients in whom Reye's syndrome is suspected should receive an intravenous infusion of 10% glucose solution and 0.2% to 0.45% sodium chloride.[17, 69, 72, 81–83] This corrects hypoglycemia and minimizes proteolysis and lipolysis, decreasing ammonia and fatty acid accumulation.[17] Hypertonic

TABLE 42–4

DIFFERENTIAL DIAGNOSIS OF REYE'S SYNDROME

Infection
  Gastroenteritis with dehydration
  Severe generalized viral infection (varicella or adenovirus)
  Meningitis
  Septicemia with shock
  Fulminant hepatitis
Drugs or toxins
  Acetaminophen
  Aflatoxin
  Emulsifiers
  Hypoglycins
  Insecticides
  Intramuscular injections
  Isopropyl alcohol
  Phenothiazine antiemetics
  Salicylates
Metabolic disorders
  Fulminant hepatic failure
  Pancreatitis
  Diabetic ketoacidosis
  Hypoglycemia
Genetic disorders
  Urea defects
  Fatty acid oxidation defects
  Carnitine deficiency
  Organic acidurias
  Amino acidurias
  Fructose intolerance
Other
  "Near miss" sudden infant death syndrome
  Battered child syndrome

glucose administration to patients in the early stages of disease may prevent disease progression.[5] Maintaining blood glucose levels at 150 to 200 mg/dl is recommended.[17, 72, 81] Potassium, 30 mEq/L as chloride or phosphate, may be added to the intravenous fluids.[30, 69] After correction of dehydration, fluid therapy should be restricted to two-thirds maintenance requirements,[17, 72, 81] maintaining serum osmolarity at 300 to 320 mOsm/kg.[30, 72, 83, 84] Vitamin K, 0.1 mg/kg given by intramuscular or slow intravenous injection, should be given if prothrombin time is prolonged. Fresh frozen plasma is given for clinical bleeding or severe coagulopathy.[30, 69, 84, 85] Seizures should be controlled with intravenous diazepam followed by phenytoin. Body temperature should be kept at normal.[30, 69, 84] Patients in stage 0 or I can often be managed by these conservative measures alone.

Infants or children who present in stage II or higher require more extensive monitoring and intensive care. Endotracheal intubation and control of mechanical hyperventilation is routine for all patients in stage III or higher.[30, 69, 72, 82] Elective intubation may be indicated in patients in stage II as well.[17] If sedation is necessary for intubation, morphine sulfate (0.1 mg/kg IV) or diazepam (0.15 mg/kg IV) should be used.[81] Increases in intracranial pressure associated with endotracheal intubation or suctioning may be abated by administering intravenous lidocaine (1.0 to 1.5 mg/kg) 3 minutes prior to the procedure.

Direct monitoring of intracranial pressure (ICP) is indicated for the management of severe encephalopathy.[17, 30, 72, 81, 82, 85–87] A subarachnoid or subdural bolt or an intraventricular cannula may be used. The insertion of a subarachnoid bolt may be quickly accomplished at the bedside by an experienced neurosurgeon. Cerebral perfusion pressure (CPP) should also be monitored. Cerebral perfusion pressure (CPP = mean arterial pressure (MAP) − ICP) is a better guide to prognosis and management than ICP.[88] The objective is to maintain ICP at less than 20 mm Hg and CPP in the range of 50 to 90 mm Hg.[17, 30, 69, 72, 81, 83]

Reduction of Cerebral Edema

Cerebral edema, leading to intracranial hypertension and brain stem compression, is the key cause of morbidity and mortality in patients with Reye's syndrome.[69] Clinically, patients in stage II and higher require therapeutic intervention directed at reducing ICP. One measure used to reduce ICP is elevation of the head of the bed to 30 to 45 degrees.[17, 30, 69, 72, 81] Stimulation or unnecessary handling should be kept to a minimum, as these increase ICP.

Mechanical Hyperventilation

Endotracheal intubation and controlled mechanical hyperventilation are mainstays in the manipulation of ICP and cerebral blood flow (CBF). Maintaining Pco_2 between 25 and 30 mm Hg is recommended to reduce both ICP and CBF to acceptable levels.[17, 30, 69, 72, 81, 82, 84] Pao_2 should be kept at above 100 mm Hg to maintain tissue oxygenation and limit hypoxemic rises in CBF[17, 69, 81] without causing severe cerebral vasoconstriction.

Osmolar Therapy

Osmolar therapy is indicated in comatose patients in stage II and higher.[69] The cytotoxic cerebral edema of Reye's syndrome is very sensitive to hyperosmolar agents, making such agents extremely effective in inducing cerebral dehydration.[69, 81] Mannitol (0.25 to 1.0 gm/kg) is administered as a 20% solution over 5 to 15 minutes through a centrally placed venous catheter. Therapy should be begun at an intravenous dose of 0.25 gm/kg.[30, 81, 82, 84, 85] This dose may doubled in 20 minutes if the first dose is unsuccessful.[81] The lowest effective dose should be utilized, as fluid and electrolyte wasting increases with higher doses. Mannitol dosing may be repeated at 4- to 6-hour intervals.[30, 69, 83] Acute elevations in ICP, as evidenced by neurologic deterioration or indicated on an ICP monitor, should be treated by hyperventilation with 100% oxygen, additional doses of mannitol, and, if necessary, furosemide (1 mg/kg).[30, 69, 82, 85] The central venous pressure (CVP) should be maintained at 2 to 4 mm Hg with volume expanders, and plasma osmolarity should be kept at 300 to 320 mOsm/L to avoid secondary renal failure.[30, 69, 81, 83]

Other Modalities

The use of high-dose infusion of barbiturates or "barbiturate coma" to decrease ICP is still being debated. Barbiturates may reduce cerebral edema, promote collateral blood flow, and lower cerebral metabolism, thereby resulting in lowered ICP.[89] Cerebral edema in Reye's syndrome may be refractory to the conventional methods used to reduce ICP; the use of high-dose pentobarbital has been recommended by some.[30, 69, 72, 81, 83, 85] Pentobarbital may be administered as a loading dose of 3 to 5 mg/kg IV bolus, followed by a 1 to 2 mg/kg hourly dose or continuous infusion until levels of 25 to 40 μg/ml are achieved.[69, 81, 85] Barbiturates should be used only in conjunction with mannitol osmotherapy and mechanical hyperventilation, and only if more conventional therapies fail to reduce ICP effectively.[69] Barbiturate use in Reye's syndrome remains very controversial.[82, 84, 90]

Induction of hypothermia, to a core temperature of 32°C, is another modality that has been used to lower the cerebral metabolic rate and blood flow. Hypothermia is used only when all other forms of therapy, including high-dose pentobarbital infusions, fail.[81] Hypothermia is of doubtful value at best and increases the risk of infection.[30, 69, 81] Therefore it is not a modality to be instituted in the emergency department.

The use of steroids to decrease the cytotoxic cerebral edema of Reye's syndrome is controversial.[72, 81, 85, 91] A loading dose of 0.5 mg/kg of dexamethasone, followed by maintenance doses of 0.25 mg/kg every 6 hours, has been used.[17, 85] However, steroids are not routinely recommended.

Decompressive craniotomy is a drastic measure indicated if all other measures fail.[72, 83, 85] Children who survive are often severely neurologically handicapped.[85] Neomycin sulfate enemas or lactulose may help clear ammonia[30, 84, 91] but are of questionable value in improving the encephalopathy. Therapies that have been tried without success include peritoneal dialysis, exchange transfusions, hemodialysis, insulin-glucose infusions, and amino acid supplementation.[30, 91] Charcoal hyperperfusion, intravenous levodopa, and total body washout have also been suggested.

CLINICAL COURSE

Children with Reye's syndrome may improve or recover completely at any stage short of brain death. Recovery may occur spontaneously or with therapy; this characteristic makes the evaluation of therapeutic efficacy extremely difficult. With recovery, histologic and biochemical abnormalities resolve completely, with no evidence of residual liver damage. The illness may vary from 6 hours to 10 days in length, but usually is less than 5 days (see Fig. 42–2).[17]

Recognized prognostic indicators help identify which patients may progress to coma, and which will recover. In patients presenting in stage I encephalopathy, those who have clearly elevated transaminase levels, a blood ammonia level of more than 100 µg/dl, and a prothrombin time prolonged more than 3 seconds are at risk for progression to coma.[17, 82] In children presenting in stage II to IV encephalopathy, factors indicating poor prognosis include age less than 1 year, rapid progression of symptoms, ammonia level more than six times normal, and CK level more than 10 times normal.[17] In addition, the onset of seizures in patients in stage III may indicate a poor prognosis. A 100% survival rate can be expected in patients in whom the peak ammonia level is less than five times normal.[65]

Death is caused by intractable brain swelling and intracranial hypertension. Mortality rates have dropped from 80% initially to 30% in the 1980s.[7–10] This probably is a result of improved recognition and treatment of the syndrome in early stages, as well as advances in pediatric critical care medicine. Mortality rates in children younger than 2 years are probably higher.[17, 92, 93]

Complications include infection, renal failure, and pancreatitis, which occurs in up to 1 of 11 patients.[27, 68] However, most Reye's syndrome victims recover without sequelae. Ten percent develop mild neurologic sequelae,[7] including emotional instability, visuomotor imperception, fine motor incoordination, difficulties with sequencing and concept formation, and short attention span.[69, 94] Short- and long-term memory may be affected.[95] Children who have experienced severe or repeated episodes of intracranial hypertension may have profound neurologic sequelae,[20] but such sequelae occur in only 2% of Reye's syndrome survivors.[7] The frequency and severity of neurologic sequelae are increased in infants and young children.[13, 20]

One should document the relevant history, physical examination, and results of diagnostic studies. Any changes in the child's status, especially the neurologic condition, must be recorded. Therapeutic intervention and the patient's response should be noted (Table 42–5).

DISPOSITION

Reye's syndrome is an explosive disease in which rapid deterioration occurs without warning. All patients suspected of having Reye's syndrome should be expeditiously admitted to a fully equipped pediatric intensive care unit capable of ongoing ICP monitoring.[17, 30, 69]

PITFALLS

A history of salicylate ingestion should be sought in every child with a recent viral illness and a primary complaint of vomiting and lethargy. The emergency or primary care physician should not be led astray by a negative history of aspirin ingestion. Many over-the-counter preparations contain aspirin and are a source of "hidden salicylates," which parents may not be aware of.[96] Some products such as Pepto-Bismol, which is commonly used for upset stomach, nausea, or diarrhea, contain salicylates in a combined form and may not list aspirin as an ingredient. Pepto-Bismol contains a significant amount of salicylate in the recommended children's dose. Older children may be at particular risk through self-medication.[97] Children traveling abroad may be prescribed medications containing salicylates and may develop Reye's syndrome.[98] Reye's syndrome can also occur in the absence of salicylate use.

A second pitfall to avoid is the use of phenothiazine antiemetics in children in whom the diagnosis of Reye's syndrome has not been excluded. Phenothiazines were used in a significant number of children who were later diagnosed as having Reye's syndrome. These agents may delay diagnosis and are probably ineffective in treating the pernicious vomiting of Reye's syndrome.[30, 99] In addition, prochlorperazine may predispose the child to autonomic collapse.[100]

References

1. Hurwitz ES, Nelson DB, Davis C, et al. National surveillance for Reye syndrome: A five-year review. Pediatrics 1982;70(6):895.
2. Sullivan-Bolyai JZ, Corey L. Epidemiology of Reye syndrome. Epidemiol Rev 1981;3:1.
3. Corey L, Rubin RJ, Thompson TR, et al. Influenza B-associated Reye's syndrome: Incidence in Michigan and potential for prevention. J Infect Dis 1977;135:398.
4. Luscomb FA, Monto A, Baublis J. Mortality due to Reye's syndrome in Michigan: Distribution and longitudinal trends. J Infect Dis 1980;142:363.
5. Lichtenstein PK, Heubi JE, Daugherty CC, et al. Grade I Reye's syndrome. A frequent cause of vomiting and liver dysfunction after varicella and upper-respiratory-tract infection. N Engl J Med 1983;309(3):133.
6. Reye RDK, Morgan G, Baral J. Encephalopathy and fatty degeneration of the viscera. A disease entity in childhood. Lancet 1963;2:749.
7. Barrett MJ, Hurwitz ES, Rogers MF, et al. The National Reye Syndrome Surveillance System, 1983. MMWR CDC Surveill Summ 1984;33(3):9SS.
8. Reye syndrome—United States, 1984. MMWR 1985;34(1):13.
9. Reye's syndrome surveillance—United States, 1986. MMWR 1987;36(41):689.
10. Reye's syndrome surveillance—United States, 1987 and 1988. MMWR 1989;38(18):325.
11. Reye's syndrome surveillance—United States, 1989. MMWR 1991;40:88.
12. Holtzhauer FJ, Campbell RJ, Hall LJ, et al. Reye's syndrome. An epidemiologic analysis of mild disease. Am J Dis Child 1986;140(12):1231.
13. Huttenlocher PR, Trauner DA. Reye's syndrome in infancy. Pediatrics 1978;62:84.
14. Sullivan-Bolyai JZ, Marks JS, Johnson D, et al. Reye syndrome in Ohio, 1973–1977. Am J Epidemiol 1980;112:629.
15. Heubi JE, Partin JS, Schubert WK. Reye's syndrome: Current Concepts. Hepatology 1987;7(1):155.
16. Rao BL, Phadke MA, Joshi AS. Reye's syndrome associated with influenza A and B virus. Indian Pediatr 1982;19(8):719.
17. Mowat AP. Reye's syndrome—a continuing enigma. Adverse Drug React Acute Poisoning Rev 1987;4:211.
18. Keating JP. Reye syndrome. In Feigin RD, Cherry JD (eds). Textbook of Pediatric Infectious Diseases. 2nd ed. Philadelphia, WB Saunders, 1987, p 1845.
19. Reye syndrome—United States. MMWR 1979;28:97.
20. Chu AB, Nerurkar LS, Witzel N, et al. Reye's syndrome. Salicylate metabolism, viral antibody levels, and other factors in surviving patients and unaffected family members. Am J Dis Child 1986;140(10):1009.
21. Guess HA, Broughton DD, Melton LJ, et al. Population-based studies of varicella complications. Pediatrics 1986;78:723.
22. Preblud SR, Orenstein WA, Bart KJ. Varicella: Clinical manifestations, epidemiology and health impact in children. Pediatr Infect Dis 1984;3(6):505.
23. Orlowski JP, Campbell P, Goldstein S. Reye's syndrome: A case control study of medication use and associated viruses in Australia. Cleve Clin J Med 1990;57(4):323.
24. Edwards KM, Bennett SR, Garaner WL, et al. Reye's syndrome associated with adenovirus infections in infants. Am J Dis Child 1985;139(4):343.

TABLE 42–5

DOCUMENTATION FOR PATIENTS WITH REYE'S SYNDROME

History	Clinical course
Presenting complaint	Clinical stage of llness
Vomiting	Neurologic
Behavioral changes	deterioration
Seizures	Seizures
Apnea	Therapy
Recent viral illness	Intubation
Salicylate use	Medication
Physical examination	Elevation of head of
Level of consciousness	bed
Jaundice	
Nuchal rigidity	
Hepatomegaly	
Diagnostic studies	
Aspartate aminotransferase level	
Ammonia level	
Blood glucose level	

25. Sundwall DA, Bergeson ME, Ortiz A. Reye syndrome associated with Haemophilus influenzae infection. Clin Pediatr 1980;19(5):357.
26. Dajani AAS, Asmar BL, Thiumoorthi MC. Systemic Haemophilus influenzae disease: An overview. J Pediatr 1979;94:355.
27. DeVivo DC, Keating JP. Reye's syndrome. Adv Pediatr 1976;22:175.
28. Linneman CC, Shea L, Partin JC, et al. Reye's syndrome: Epidemiologic and viral studies, 1963–1974. Am J Epidemiol 1975;101:517.
29. Glasgow AM. Reye's syndrome mimickers. J Natl Reye Syndrome Found 1980;1:105.
30. Rockoff MA, Pascucci RC. Reye's syndrome. Emerg Med Clin North Am 1983;1(1):87.
31. Rozee KR, Lee SHS, Crocker JFS, et al. Is a compromised interferon response an etiological factor in Reye's syndrome? Can Med Assoc J 1982;126:789.
32. Crocker JF. Reye's syndrome. Semin Liver Dis 1982;2(4):340.
33. Stora C, Dvorackova I, Ayraud N. Aflatoxin and Reye's syndrome. J Med 1983;14(1):47.
34. Ryan NJ, Hogan GR, Hayes AW, et al. Aflatoxin B: Its role in the etiology of Reye's syndrome. Pediatrics 1979;64:71.
35. Snodgrass WR. Salicylate toxicity. Pediatr Clin North Am 1986;33:381.
36. Hurwitz ES. Reye's syndrome. Epidemiol Rev 1989;11:249.
37. Hall SM, Plaster PA, Glasgow JFT, et al. Preadmission antipyretics in Reye's syndrome. Arch Dis Child 1988;63(7):857.
38. Forsyth BW, Horwitz RI, Acompora D, et al. New epidemiological evidence confirming that bias does not explain the aspirin/Reye's syndrome association. JAMA 1989;261:2517.
39. Hurwitz ES, Barrett MJ, Bregman D, et al. Public Health Service study of Reye's syndrome and medications. Report of the main study. JAMA 1987;257(14):1905.
40. Pinsky PF, Hurwitz ES, Schonberger LB, et al. Reye's syndrome and aspirin. Evidence for a dose-response effect. JAMA 1988;260(5):657.
41. Young RSK, Torenti D, Williams RH, et al. Reye's syndrome associated with long-term aspirin therapy. JAMA 1984;251:754.
42. Rennebohm RM, Heubi JE, Daugherty CC, et al. Reye's syndrome in children on salicylate therapy for connective tissue disease. J Pediatr 1985;107:877.
43. Remington PL, Shabino CL, McGee H, et al. Reye syndrome and juvenile rheumatoid arthritis in Michigan. Am J Dis Child 1985;139:870.
44. National surveillance for Reye's syndrome, 1981: Update. Reye's syndrome and salicylate usage. MMWR 1982;31:53.
45. Surgeon General's advisory on the use of salicylates and Reye syndrome. MMWR 1982;31:289.
46. Committee on Infectious Diseases. Aspirin and Reye syndrome. Pediatrics 1982;69:810.
47. Mortimer EA. Reye's syndrome, salicylates, epidemiology, and public health policy. JAMA 1987;257(14):1941.
48. Remington PL, Rowley D, McGee H, et al. Decreasing trends in Reye syndrome and aspirin use in Michigan, 1979 to 1984. Pediatrics 1986;77(1):93.
49. Taylor JP, Gustafson TL, Johnson CC, et al. Antipyretic use among children during the 1983 influenza season. Am J Dis Child 1985;139(5):486.
50. Banco L. Use of aspirin and Reye's syndrome. Am J Dis Child 1987;141(3):240.
51. Kilpatrick-Smith L, Hale DE, Douglas SD. Progress in Reye syndrome: Epidemiology, biochemical mechanisms, and animal models. Dig Dis 1989;7:135.
52. Barrett MJ, Hurwitz ES, Schonberger LB, et al. Changing epidemiology of Reye syndrome in the United States. Pediatrics 1986;77(4):590.
53. Arrowsmith JB, Kennedy DL, Kuritsky JN, et al. National patterns of aspirin use and Reye syndrome reporting, United States, 1980 to 1985. Pediatrics 1987;79(6):858.
54. Pranzatelli MR, DeVivo DC. Pharmacology of Reye syndrome. Clin Neuropharmacol 1987;10(2):96.
55. DeVivo DC. How common is Reye's syndrome? N Engl J Med 1983;309(3):179.
56. Mitchell RA, Arcinue EL, Partin JC, et al. Quantitative evaluation of the extent of hepatic enzyme changes in Reye syndrome compared with normal liver or with non-Reye liver disorders: Objective criteria for animal models. Pediatr Res 1985;19(1):19.
57. Brown RE, Forman DT. The biochemistry of Reye's syndrome. CRC Crit Rev Clin Lab Sci 1982;17(3):247.
58. Brown T, Hug G, Lansky L, et al. Transiently reduced activity of carbamyl phosphate synthetase and ornithine transcarbamylase in livers of children with Reye's syndrome. N Engl J Med 1976;294:861.
59. Snodgrass PJ, DeLong GR. Urea-cycle enzyme deficiencies and an increased nitrogen load producing hyperammonemia in Reye's syndrome. N Engl J Med 1976;294:855.
60. Richmond DA, Stair T. Reye's syndrome. Ann Emerg Med 1982;11a:379.
61. Glasgow JFT. Clinical features and prognosis of Reye's syndrome. Arch Dis Child 1984;59(3):230.
62. Duncan CC, Ment LR, Shaywitz BA. Evaluation of level of consciousness by the Glasgow Coma Scale in children with Reye's syndrome. Neurosurgery 1983;13(6):650.
63. Lovejoy FH, Smith AL, Bresnan MJ, et al. Clinical staging in Reye syndrome. Am J Dis Child 1974;128:36.
64. Morens DM, Sullivan-Bolyai JZ, Slater JE, et al. Surveillance of Reye syndrome in the United States, 1977. Am J Epidemiol 1981;114:406.
65. Fitzgerald JF, Clark JH, Angelides AG, et al. The prognostic significance of peak ammonia levels in Reye syndrome. Pediatrics 1982;70(6):997.
66. Huttenlocher PR. Reye's syndrome: Relationship of outcome to therapy. J Pediatr 1972;80:845.
67. Newman SL, Caplan DB, Camp VM, et al. Prolactin and the encephalopathy of Reye's syndrome. Lancet 1979;2:1097.
68. Glick TH, Likosky WH, Levitt LP, et al. Reye's syndrome: An epidemiologic approach. Pediatrics 1970;46:371.
69. Sarnaik AP. Diagnosis and management of Reye's syndrome. Compr Ther 1982;8(10):47.
70. Trauner DA. Treatment of Reye's syndrome. Ann Neurol 1980;7:2.
71. Frewen TC, Kissoon N. Cerebral blood flow and brain oxygen extraction in Reye syndrome. J Pediatr 1987;110(6):903.
72. Mowat AP. Reye's syndrome: 20 years on. Br Med J 1983;286:1999.
73. Myers MG. Hepatic cellular injury during varicella. Arch Dis Child 1982;57:317.
74. Gauthier M, Guay J, Lacroix J, et al. Reye's syndrome. A reappraisal of diagnosis in 49 presumptive cases. Am J Dis Child 1989;149(10):181.
75. Partin JS, Daugherty CC, McAdams AJ, et al. A comparison of liver ultrastructure in salicylate intoxication and Reye's syndrome. Hepatology 1984;4(4):687.
76. Makela AL, Lang H, Koppela P. Toxic encephalopathy with hyperammonemia during high-dose salicylate therapy. Acta Neurol Scand 1980;61:146.
77. Greene CL, Blitzer MG, Shapira E. Inborn errors of metabolism and Reye syndrome: Differential diagnosis. J Pediatr 1988;113:156.
78. Taubman B, Hale DE, Kelley RI. Familial Reye-like syndrome: A presentation of medium-chain acyl-coenzyme A dehydrogenase deficiency. Pediatrics 1987;19(3):382.
79. Hsia YE. Changing trends of inborn errors in Reye's syndrome: Rarity is relative. Hepatology 1990;11(2):327.
80. Conradi S, Brissie R. Battered child syndrome in a four year old with previous diagnosis of Reye's syndrome. Forensic Sci Int 1986;30(2–3):195.
81. Swedlow DB, Schreiner MS. Management of Reye's syndrome. Crit Care Clin 1985;1(2):285.
82. Partin JC. Management of Reye's syndrome. Pediatr Ann 1985;14(7):511, 514.
83. Balistreri WF. Reye Syndrome. In Behrman RE, Vaughn VC (eds). Nelson's Textbook of Pediatrics. 13th ed. Philadelphia, WB Saunders, 1987.
84. Trauner DA. What is the best treatment for Reye's syndrome? Arch Neurol 1986;43(7):729.
85. Shaywitz BA, Lister G, Duncan CC. What is the best treatment for Reye's syndrome? Arch Neurol 1986;43(7):730.
86. Shaywitz BA, Rothstein P, Venes JL. Monitoring and management of increased intracranial pressure in Reye syndrome: Results in 29 children. Pediatrics 1980;66:198.
87. Trauner DA, Brown F, Ganz E, et al. Treatment of elevated intracranial pressure in Reye syndrome. Ann Neurol 1978;4:275.
88. Jenkins JG, Glasgow JFT, Black GW, et al. Reye's syndrome: Assessment of intracranial monitoring. Br Med J 1987;294:337.
89. Marshall LF, Shapiro HM, Rauscher A, et al. Pentobarbital therapy for intracranial hypertension in metabolic coma. Crit Care Med 1978;6:1.
90. Frewen TC, Swedlow DB, Watcha M, et al. Outcome in severe Reye syndrome with early pentobarbital coma and hypothermia. J Pediatr 1982;100(4):663.
91. Riela AR, Roach ES. Reye's syndrome: Twenty years in perspective. NC Med J 1983;44(6):351.
92. Orlowski JP, Gillis J, Kilham HA. A catch in the Reye. Pediatrics 1987;80(5):638.
93. Reye syndrome. Wkly Epidemiol Rec 1990;29:225.
94. Brunner RL, O'Grady DJ, Partin JC, et al. Neuropsychologic consequences of Reye syndrome. J Pediatr 1979;95:706.
95. Quart EJ, Buchtel HA, Sarnaik AP. Long-lasting memory deficits in children recovered from Reye's syndrome. J Clin Exp Neuropsychol 1988;10(4):409.
96. Szap MD. Hidden salicylates. Am J Dis Child 1989;143(2):142.
97. Hurwitz ES. The changing epidemiology of Reye's syndrome: Further evidence for a public health success. JAMA 1988;260:3178.
98. Donaldson M, Fleming P. Reye's syndrome in children travelling abroad. Lancet 1988;2(8619):1073.
99. Barnhart ER (ed). Physician's Desk Reference. 45th ed. Oradell, NJ, Medical Economics Data 1991, p 2098.
100. Jones R, Thompson JA. Intravenous calcium treatment of refractory hypotension in Reye's syndrome. Arch Neurol 1984;41(7):786.

CHAPTER 43

Nutrition

Kelley A. Hails

INTRODUCTION

Pediatric malnutrition is a leading cause of childhood morbidity and mortality worldwide. Not only is pediatric malnutrition the most prevalent illness of children in the developing world, it has been discovered in up to half of hospitalized children in the United States.

The emergency department is frequently used as a gateway to health care, particularly by families of lower socioeconomic status. Thus the emergency physician may be the first, or perhaps the only, physician to evaluate such children. In addition, children with chronic diseases often are frequent emergency department visitors.

NUTRITIONAL REQUIREMENTS

Nutritional requirements vary greatly with the changing energy needs of growing children. Some essential nutrients must be provided in the diet on a daily basis, whereas others are stored in the body and need to be replaced only periodically. Essential nutrients include water, calories, vitamins, and minerals. Calories are supplied in the form of carbohydrates, proteins, and fats. The Recommended Dietary Allowance (RDA) of an essential nutrient is the level of intake of that nutrient considered to be adequate to meet the known nutritional needs of a healthy individual.

Water

Water is the major component of body tissues, comprising from up to 75% of body weight in infancy to 60% of body weight in adulthood. Water has the highest daily turnover of any body component. Balance depends on fluid intake, the protein and mineral content of the diet, the solute load, the metabolic rate, the respiratory rate, and the body temperature. Infants daily consume 10% to 15% of their body weight in fluids, compared with about 3% consumed by adults. Most of the solid foods consumed by infants and children are also high in water content.

Calories

Energy is supplied to the body in the form of calories derived from carbohydrates, proteins, and fats. The distribution of energy use varies with age. Daily energy intake per kilogram body weight is high at birth, decreases during the first 6 months of life, and increases thereafter to a peak at 15 months. After 15 months, energy intake gradually decreases. Energy needs in the first year of life are 105 to 115 kcal per kilogram body weight.

Carbohydrates

Carbohydrates are the chief source of dietary calories. In infancy, 35% to 65% of calories are supplied by carbohydrates, principally lactose, the predominant carbohydrate in breast milk. In older children, 58% of calories are supplied by carbohydrates. Metabolism of carbohydrates yields 4 kcal of energy for each gram of carbohydrate ingested. Carbo-

hydrates are stored chiefly as glycogen in the liver and muscles and make up no more than 1% of total body weight. An inadequate intake of carbohydrates leads to hypoglycemia, ketosis, and excessive protein catabolism.

Protein

Essential amino acids, which include threonine, valine, leucine, isoleucine, lysine, tryptophan, phenylalanine, methionine, and histidine, must be supplied in the diet. Protein provides these amino acids along with nitrogen, both of which are necessary for growth. Proteins are responsible for body tissue synthesis and maintenance of muscle mass and constitute 20% of adult body weight. Proteins are also necessary for enzymatic, hormonal, and immunologic regulation. In infancy and childhood, protein should make up 7% to 16% of caloric intake. Proteins, like carbohydrates, supply 4 kcal per gram ingested.

Fats

Fats are the most concentrated source of energy in the diet, supplying 9 kcal per gram of fat ingested. Fat should supply about 35% of a child's dietary calories. It is stored in the body as adipose tissue and is essential for cell membrane integrity and storage of fat-soluble vitamins.

Essential fatty acids (EFAs) are precursors of prostaglandins and must be supplied in the diet. The primary EFAs are linolenic acid, linoleic acid, and arachidonic acid. Neonates, especially those born prematurely, are prone to EFA deficiency as a result of low amounts of adipose tissue and high energy needs.

The body fat content of a term infant is 11% and increases to 23% by 1 year of age. Body fat then decreases and protein stores increase by 2 years of age.

Vitamins

Vitamins are organic compounds that function in the body as cofactors and catalysts for cell function and replication. Fat-soluble vitamins include vitamins A, D, E, and K; water-soluble vitamins include vitamins C and B complex. A well-rounded diet will usually prevent vitamin deficiencies in individuals who have no metabolic abnormalities.

Minerals

Minerals are inorganic nutrients that make up two distinct groups: macronutrients and micronutrients. *Macronutrients* comprise a matrix of water and solvents in which all biochemical and physiologic functions take place. Macronutrients include water; the cations sodium, potassium, calcium, and magnesium; and the anions chloride, phosphorus, and sulfur. *Micronutrients* are those inorganic ions that activate or moderate enzyme functions; these are termed *trace minerals*. Iron, iodine, and cobalt appear in important organic complexes. Other trace elements found in the body include copper, zinc, selenium, fluoride, silicon, boron, aluminum, nickel, arsenic, lead, manganese, molybdenum, and lithium. Several national dietary and health surveys have shown that vitamin or mineral deficiencies are rare, with the exception of iron deficiency.

FEEDING AND DIET
First Year of Life

The first year of life is a period of rapid growth and development that creates unique nutritional requirements. Breast milk or commercially prepared infant formulas are usually the sole source of energy and nutrients in the first few months of life. Semisolid foods such as cereals are usually introduced into the diet at 4 to 6 months of age, and soft table foods are introduced at approximately 1 year of age. These dietary changes closely follow developmental changes in the infant's ability to suck, swallow, and chew.

Breast Milk

Breast milk is recommended by the American Academy of Pediatrics as the sole source of nutrients during the first 4 to 6 months of life. Breast milk imparts both passive and active immunity, protecting the infant from atopic conditions and infectious disease. Secretory immunoglobulin A (IgA) is present in large amounts in colostrum (the milk produced during the latter part of pregnancy and the first 2 to 4 days after birth) and breast milk. Immunoglobulins G and M (IgG and IgM) are also found in breast milk and help confer passive immunity. Lactoferrin and lysozyme in breast milk inhibit the growth of enteric pathogens. Other antimicrobial agents in breast milk are granulocytes, T lymphocytes, B lymphocytes, complement, and several antibacterial and antiviral factors. Mortality and morbidity rates for breast-fed infants are lower than those for formula-fed infants. Breast-fed infants have fewer episodes of upper respiratory tract infections, otitis media, and diarrhea when compared with infants who are fed formula.

Breast-fed infants may be more energy efficient and require relatively fewer calories than formula-fed infants. Colostrum is thicker and more yellow than later breast milk. It is high in cellular antimicrobials and secretory IgA and provides important early passive immunity. Colostrum and transitional milk make up breast milk during the first 2 weeks of life and are high in proteins and fat-soluble vitamins. Mature breast milk is higher in calories, lactose, fat, and water-soluble vitamins than either colostrum or transitional milk.

Lactose is the predominant carbohydrate in breast milk, although glucose and galactose are also found. Proteins are found in human milk in lower concentrations than in bovine milk (0.9% versus 3.4%, respectively). Human milk proteins are made of casein and whey fractions in a ratio of 4:6, compared with a ratio of 8:2 in bovine milk. This 4:6 ratio allows for a lower "curd tension" and better digestibility.

Vitamins, with the possible exception of vitamin D, are present in breast milk in adequate concentrations to prevent deficiencies. The levels of water-soluble vitamins are directly influenced by maternal diet, whereas the levels of fat-soluble vitamins are less easily altered.

Mineral levels in human milk are significantly lower than those in bovine milk, resulting in a lower renal solute load. Sodium, potassium, and magnesium levels are one third those in bovine milk; calcium and phosphorus levels vary. The iron content of human milk is equal to that of bovine milk but is lower than that of commercial formulas. However, because of the high concentrations of vitamin C and lactose in human milk, the efficiency of iron absorption is nearly 50% in human milk, compared with 10% in bovine milk and 4% in commercial formulas. Fluoride levels are low and are not affected by maternal intake. Dental caries, however, are rare in breast-fed infants.

Disadvantages. The disadvantages of breast-feeding are limited to physiologic jaundice and the ingestion of toxins in breast milk. Physiologic breast milk jaundice is thought to be a result of the inhibitory effects of a progesterone metabolite on bilirubin conjugation. The jaundice appears after the third day of life and peaks in the first week and is usually associated with bilirubin levels of 10 to 27 mg/dl. It is treated by temporarily withholding breast milk or by short-term phototherapy and does not represent a threat to the healthy infant.

Infant Formulas

Breast-feeding may not be practical or even safe for some infants. There are several contraindications to breast-feeding, including maternal eclampsia, severe infection, tuberculosis, severe heart disease, thyrotoxicosis, diabetes mellitus, chronic renal disease, and severe puerperal depression; mastitis is not a contraindication.

Commercially prepared infant formulas are an alternative to breast milk. Infants fed standard infant formulas demonstrate no significant differences in long-term growth or development when compared with infants fed breast milk. Commercially prepared infant formulas account for 65% to 70% of U.S. infants' intake in the first 4 months of life.

Standard infant formulas are stable mixtures of emulsified fats, proteins, carbohydrates, vitamins, and minerals (Table 43–1). The Infant Formula Act of 1980 regulates the composition of infant formulas sold in the United States. Most formulas supply 20 calories per ounce. The American Academy of Pediatrics recommends formulas with a caloric distribution of 30% to 54% fat, 7% to 18% protein, and the remainder from carbohydrates.

Fluoride supplementation is recommended for infants fed formula or breast milk. However, when fluoridated tap water is used to dilute concentrated formulas, fluoride supplementation is unnecessary. In addition, iron supplementation is recommended by the American Academy of Pediatrics after 4 months of age because of depleted neonatal iron stores. Most formulas contain 1 mg/L of iron, and iron-fortified formulas contain 10 to 12 mg/L of iron.

Low-Birth-Weight Infants

Preterm and low-birth-weight infants have special nutritional needs that differ from those of full-term infants. Higher energy intake is necessary for adequate growth. These infants require 119 to 181 kcal/kg/day and approximately 3 gm/kg/day of protein to maintain growth and adequate nutritional status.

Preterm human milk is uniquely suited to the preterm or low-birth-weight infant and differs substantially in content from term human milk. Term human milk supplies insufficient protein, electrolytes, calcium, and phosphate for low-birth-weight infants.

Vitamin requirements of low-birth-weight infants are greater than those of full-term infants because of lower body stores, higher growth rates, decreased gastrointestinal vitamin absorption, and lower daily milk intake. Preterm human milk and formulas for premature infants have higher vitamin contents than term milk and standard formulas.

Weaning and Mixed Feeding

Weaning breast-fed infants is a gradual process accomplished by replacing one breast-feeding at a time with a formula feed offered by bottle or cup (Table 43–2). Weaning usually begins at age 5 to 6 months and is more easily accepted by an infant who has already been spoon-fed some solid foods. By age 5 to 6 months, an infant can sit with support and has developed the neuromuscular control of the head and neck necessary for spoon-feeding.

New foods should be introduced singly and in small amounts; they are best accepted if diluted or of thin consistency. Spoon-feeding should start with low-protein foods such as cereal, as weaning infants are still taking in adequate protein in breast milk or formula.

TABLE 43-1

INFANT FORMULA COMPARISON

	Infant Formula Act 1980[a]		Breast milk	Similac	Enfamil	SMA	PM 60/40	Isomil	Nursoy	Proso-bee	Isomil SF	Pregest-imil	Nutrami-gen	Porta-gen
	Mini-mum	Maxi-mum												
Calorie per ounce			~22	20	20	20	20	20	20	20	20	20	20	20
Carbohydrate % of calories*			38 (35–44)	43	41	43	41	40	40	40	40	54	54	46
Lactose			100	100	100	100	100							2
Corn syrup solids										100	100	85		72
Sucrose								50					100	
Modified tapioca starch								50				15		26
Protein (gm/100 kcal)*	1.8	4.5	1.5	2.2	2.2	2.2	2.2	3.0	3.0	3.0	3.0	2.8	2.8	3.5
% of calories			7 (6–8)	9	9	9	9	12	12	12	12	11	11	14
Bovine milk 60:40 whey:casein				100										
Soy protein isolate					100	100	100							
Casein hydrolysate								100	100	100	100			
Sodium caseinate												100	100	100
Fat (gm/100 kcal)	3.3	6.0	6	3.6	3.8	3.6	3.8	3.6	3.6	3.6	3.6	2.7	2.6	3.2
% of calories*	30	54	56 (35–58)	48	50	48	50	48	48	48	48	35	35	40
Soybean oil				60	45	15		60	15	45	60			
Coconut oil				40	55	27	60	40	27	55	40			
Corn oil							40					60	100	12
Oleo oil						33			33					
Medium chain triglyceride oil												40		88
% Linoleic acid as total calories	2.7		6–15	16	13	13	13	16	13	12	16	13	21	3.5
E:PUFA ratio (IU vitamin E/gm polyunsaturated fatty acid)	0.7:1		1:1	1:1	2:1	2:1	1:1	1:1	2:1	2:1	1:1	1.6:1	0.7:1	8.1:1
Calcium: Phosphorus ratio	1.1:1	2.0:1	1.4–2.4:1	1.3:1	1.5:1	1.3:1	2:1	1.4:1	1.5:1	1.3:1	1.4:1	1.5:1	1.3:1	1.3:1
Na⁺/K⁺ mEq/100 kcal	0.87/2.0	2.6/5.1	1.1/2.04	1.0/2.1			0.98/2.1	0.7/1.5	1.4/2.0	1.3/2.8	1.9/3.0	1.4/2.0	2.0/2.8	2.0/2.8	2.0/3.2
Iron (mg/100 kcal)	0.15	2.5	0.13–0.2	0.2 (1.8)†	0.16 (1.9)†	1.9	0.38	1.8	1.9	1.9	1.8	1.9	1.9	1.9
Osmolality (mOsm/kg H₂O)		400	300	290	300	300	260	250	224	200	150	350	320	220
Renal solute load (mOsm/L)				108	100	92	92	126	120	130	126	120	120	150

*Sources are listed below including their percentage contribution to the specific nutrients.
†Formula with iron added.
Reproduced, with permission, from Queen PM, Wilson SE. Growth and nutrient requirements of infants. *In* Grand RJ, Sutphen JL, Dietz WH (eds.). Pediatric Nutrition: Theory and Practice. Stoneham, MA, Butterworth, 1987, pp 331, 332.

Minor First-Year Feeding Problems

Overfeeding. Overfeeding should be avoided, as an overfed infant can become an obese child and adult, leading to a lifetime of health problems. In the first and second week of life, excessive caloric intake leads to loose, diarrheal stools.

TABLE 43-2

NUMBER AND AMOUNT OF FEEDS, BIRTH TO 12 MO OF AGE

Age	No. of feeds per 24 hours	Amount consumed per feed
Birth–2 wk	6–10	2–3 oz (60–90 ml)
2–6 wk	6–8	4–5 oz (120–150 ml)
6 wk–3 mo	5–6	5–6 oz (150–180 ml)
3–4 mo	4–5	6–7 oz (180–210 ml)
4–8 mo	3–4	7–8 oz (210–240 ml)
8–12 mo	3	7–8 oz (210–240 ml)

Based on Barness LA. Nutrition and nutritional disorders. *In* Behrman RE, Vaughan VC III (eds). Nelson Textbook of Pediatrics. 13th ed. Philadelphia, WB Saunders, 1987, pp 133, 134.

Abdominal distention, vomiting, and excessive weight gain can result from diets too high in fat or carbohydrates.

Vomiting. A distinction must be made between "spitting up," or regurgitation of small mouthfuls of food shortly after eating, and vomiting, or the complete emptying of the stomach usually some time after eating. Regurgitation is a natural occurrence during the first 6 months of life. It can be minimized by adequately "burping" infants and by placing them on their right side or abdomen with the head elevated for a nap after eating. Vomiting is common in infancy and is often caused by aerophagia. Aerophagia is rare in breast-fed infants.

Rumination, an infantile psychoneurosis, also should be distinguished from vomiting. This habit affords the infant oral gratification by voluntarily bringing part of the feed back into the mouth by way of curling the tongue into a funnel and rhythmically thrusting the mandible forward and backward. Thickening the feeds, propping the infant up after feeding, and diverting the infant's attention will help to reduce the symptoms.

Constipation. Constipation is identified by the nature of the stool (i.e., small and hard), not by stool frequency. Constipation can be caused by anal fissures, which are usually alleviated by relief of irritation, or by Hirschsprung's disease, also known as aganglionic megacolon, which is suggested by infantile constipation with an absence of stool in the rectum.

Constipation is rare in breast-fed infants. Formula-fed infants whose diets are high in fat and protein but deficient in bulk may become constipated. For these infants, increasing the amount of fluid or sugar by adding one to two teaspoons of Karo syrup to eight ounces of water may be helpful. However, in infants older than 4 months, adding bulk to the diet in the form of cereal, vegetables, or fruit is preferable.

Diarrhea. Diarrhea is the passage of frequent loose or watery stools. Breast-fed infants have loose, greenish-yellow stools for the first 4 to 6 days of life; these stools then change to soft "milk stools." Breast-fed infants have less frequent stools than do formula-fed infants.

Diarrhea in a breast-fed infant should be considered to have an infectious origin until proved otherwise. Enteral infections that frequently cause diarrhea in infants include rotavirus, *E. coli* infection, and infections caused by other pathogens. Parenteral infections such as pyelonephritis and otitis media cause diarrhea through mechanisms that are poorly understood.

Colic. Some infants younger than 3 months are particularly susceptible to a symptom complex known as *colic.* The attack begins suddenly with inconsolable screaming, facial flushing, and occasional circumoral pallor. The abdomen is distended or tense, the legs are drawn up with the thighs flexed against the abdomen, the feet are cold, and the hands are clenched. The attack may last from 2 minutes to several hours. Attacks usually occur in the evening and are recurrent. The infant is usually not consoled by feeding or fondling.

The actual cause of colic is unknown, but it is doubtful that colic has a pathologic condition underlying it. When severe abdominal pain occurs, as in intussusception, the child demonstrates blanching and faintness, neither of which are part of the colic symptom complex.

Sometimes relief may be obtained by holding the infant upright or prone across the lap or on a warmed blanket. The physical examination should rule out intussusception, strangulated hernia, infections, or other sources of discomfort. Usually there is spontaneous recovery; colic rarely persists after the age of 3 months.

Second Year of Life

By 1 year of age, most infants have settled into a schedule of three to four meals per day and can manage to spoon-feed themselves. In the second year of life, a slowing growth rate causes a reduced caloric requirement, which manifests as a toddler's lack of interest in food. The diet tends to be balanced over several days, and self-selection of foods should be encouraged. Bovine milk can be introduced into the diet after the age of 1 year.

Minor Second-Year Feeding Problems

Baby Bottle Tooth Decay. Baby bottle tooth decay (BBTD) is a rampant form of dental caries affecting the maxillary incisors and molars that occurs before the age of 2 years. It is the most frequent caries problem described in children younger than 3 years. The period at which children are most susceptible to this problem is the second year of life. Caries are caused by infection with *Streptococcus mutans.* The precipitating factor is night-time or nap-time bottle-feeding with a sweetened liquid. Commonly reported bottle contents include juice, soft drinks, and milk. BBTD occurs exclusively

from bottle-feeding, and children who sleep with a bottle beyond the age of 1 year are at risk.

VEGETARIAN DIETS

Vegetarian diets can supply all needed nutrients when the diet is carefully selected from all the vegetable classes. Vegetables are high in fiber, vitamins, and minerals. The benefits of a vegetarian diet may include lowered serum cholesterol and a lowered risk of appendicitis, diverticulosis, and degenerative diseases. Vegetarians who consume milk are known as *lactovegetarians;* those who consume eggs are *ovovegetarians;* those who consume neither are *vegans.* Vegans may develop vitamin B_{12} deficiency and deficiencies of trace minerals. Vegan-like diets for infants and children pose special nutritional problems, but lactovegetarian, lacto-ovo-vegetarian, and semivegetarian diets are satisfactory. Despite an adequate nutritional intake, vegetarian infants may not grow as rapidly as omnivores during the first 2 years of life.

NUTRITIONAL DISORDERS AND DEFICIENCIES

The diagnosis of malnutrition is based on an adequate assessment of nutritional status. The child's growth must be evaluated for any present or past deviations from normal by comparison with standard growth charts.

Disorders of Inadequate Intake
Failure to Thrive

Failure to thrive (FTT) is a clinical syndrome characterized by inadequate growth, indicated by weight that is at or below the third to fifth percentile on standard growth charts or is less than 80% to 85% of the median weight for age. It occurs primarily in infants and toddlers and is a consequence of physical problems, psychosocial problems, or a combination of the two.

In children with FTT, deviation from normal weight is usually more marked than deviation from normal height, particularly when FTT is caused primarily by psychosocial factors. Motor and language development are usually delayed, and the child may appear withdrawn or apathetic.

Factors that increase the risk of FTT can be psychosocial or organic. Psychosocial risk factors include early separation of the mother from the infant, interference with mother-infant bonding, parental social isolation, marital problems, and depression. Children who were unwanted, who are being raised by a single parent, or whose mothers were 17 or younger at the time of the birth of their first child are also at risk. Altered social interactions between the care provider and child are common. The child is often perceived by the parent to be behaviorally difficult or sickly. Mealtimes are often disruptive, and feeding problems are common. Poverty is a prominent additional risk factor because of food shortage and generalized family strain. Organic problems that may contribute to FTT include congenital anomalies, prematurity, and medical illness.

When a child is suspected of having FTT, a thorough physical examination is necessary to search for signs of neglect or abuse. Emergency department laboratory evaluation for FTT should include a complete blood cell count, urinalysis, urine culture, evaluation of blood urea nitrogen (BUN) or creatinine, and chest radiograph. In addition, a tuberculin test, a free erythrocyte protoporphyrin/lead (FEP/Pb) test, stool studies, a sweat chloride test, and tests to determine the levels of serum albumin and urine reducing substances should be considered. However, laboratory tests are rarely helpful in making the diagnosis.

Hospitalization may be necessary to provide the child with adequate nutrition, stimulation, and affection. Indications for hospitalization include concomitant illness or dehydration, signs of abuse or neglect, or failed outpatient management.

Marasmus

Marasmus is the severely malnourished state resulting from inadequate caloric intake. Marasmus can occur as a result of child neglect, metabolic abnormalities, or congenital malformations that make feeding difficult.

In patients with marasmus, the skin loses turgor and subcutaneous fat and becomes wrinkled and loose. The face may continue to appear relatively normal, as fat is lost last from the cheeks. The abdomen may be flat or distended. Initial constipation may be followed by "starvation diarrhea" with small, frequent, mucus-containing stools. The muscles become atrophied and hypotonic. The child exhibits apathy and indifference to the environment. Extremity edema may occur, particularly if protein malnutrition predominates. Cyanosis may be present, along with low blood pressure and muffled heart sounds. Because the basal metabolic rate is slowed, bradycardia and subnormal temperatures occur. Deficiencies of vitamins A, B, C, and D and mineral deficiencies are often associated with marasmus.

Most commonly marasmus occurs in combination with protein deficiency, a state known as *protein-calorie malnutrition* (PCM). PCM is common in chronically ill hospitalized children.

In both marasmus and PCM, the hemoglobin level is characteristically reduced, often to the 9- to 10-gm/dl range. The white blood cell count may be low, normal, or increased. Serum electrolyte studies characteristically show hyponatremia, hypokalemia, and mildly decreased bicarbonate. Serum total protein and albumin levels should be measured to assess protein status. Assessment of immune status by total lymphocyte count and skin tests for delayed hypersensitivity should also be performed.

Children with marasmus and PCM deceptively appear dehydrated, although they are not. Overzealous rehydration may aggravate water and salt overload, and congestive heart failure and sudden death may result. Lowering daily sodium intake significantly reduces the incidence of heart failure.

Treatment is aimed at a gradual increase in calories in a form tolerated by the child. Oral alimentation can be used in most children. Lactose intolerance is assumed and lactose-free, mixed carbohydrates used. Initial energy intake should be low: 25 kcal/kg/day in infants and 50 kcal/kg/day in older children. These may be increased by 25-kcal/kg/day increments every day as tolerated by the child. Response is rapid in children who recover.

Anorexia Nervosa

Anorexia nervosa is a chronic disease of self-induced inadequate nutritional intake and subsequent starvation. It occurs primarily in teenage women and occurs in 1 per 100 to 200 female adolescents.

The characteristic clinical picture in anorexia nervosa is a loss of more than 20% of body weight, aversion to food, preoccupation with thoughts of food, and severe body image distortions. Amenorrhea is always present in female patients, and in 40%, menses ceased before the decision to diet was made. Hypothermia, bradycardia, lanugo, and constipation are common; sleep disturbances and motor restlessness also occur. Most frequently, patients are middle class, female, hard-working overachievers between the ages of 15 and 20 years.

Effective management is contingent on prompt nutritional rehabilitation, pharmacologic therapy with tricyclic antidepressants, and supportive psychotherapy.

Disorders of Excessive Intake
Obesity

Obesity, or the excessive intake of calories in relation to energy expenditure, also constitutes a form of malnutrition. Obesity is one of the most common childhood nutritional disorders and occurs in 5% to 20% of children. It appears to be influenced by genetic, physiologic, environmental, and psychological factors. The best predictor of adult obesity is obesity at 6 to 16 years of age.

Bulimia

Bulimia is a disorder in which binge eating is alternated with periods of attempted weight loss. It occurs primarily in adolescent women but is not strongly associated with amenorrhea. The binge-eating periods are characterized by rapid consumption of high-calorie food in a short time, usually less than 2 hours. Binges are recurrent and are terminated by abdominal pain, sleep, social interruption, or self-induced vomiting. They are often followed by depression and self-deprecating thoughts. Binges are interspersed with periods during which the patient attempts to lose weight using restrictive diets, amphetamines, cathartics, diuretics, and self-induced vomiting.

Esophagitis and Mallory-Weiss tears occur after prolonged vomiting. Elevated amylase levels and pancreatitis may develop. During the weight loss attempts, hypokalemia and hypochloremic alkalosis may be severe as a result of vomiting or the use of cathartics and diuretics. Patients with electrolyte imbalances should be monitored for arrhythmias, which can be fatal. Calcium, magnesium, and phosphorus levels may be altered by laxative abuse.

Bovine Milk Allergy

Mothers of young infants with recurrent diarrhea are frequently concerned about whether their infant may have a milk allergy. The prevalence of allergy to bovine milk has been reported to be 0.3% to 7.5%. Bovine milk allergy is caused by a sensitivity to the primary protein in bovine milk, beta-lactoglobulin. Infants at high risk for developing allergy may be identified at birth by the presence of elevated immunoglobulin E (IgE) levels in the cord blood.

Symptoms of milk allergy may develop rapidly within 48 hours or slowly over a period of 2 to 30 days after ingesting bovine milk or milk-based formulas. The infant usually presents during the first 6 weeks of life with diarrhea or mucous or bloody stools and occasionally with vomiting or FTT. Respiratory symptoms such as rhinorrhea or wheezing are common, and the skin may be affected with eczema or urticaria.

Definitive diagnosis is made with a skin test. Bovine milk allergy must be differentiated from lactase deficiency and lactose intolerance by a lactose tolerance test. Enteral infection should be excluded by stool cultures.

Treatment is aimed at eliminating bovine milk protein from the diet and substituting soy-based or hydrolyzed casein formulas, such as Pregestimil or Nutramigen. Most children outgrow bovine milk allergy by 2 years of age.

Imbalances of Specific Dietary Nutrients
Protein Deficiency

Caloric imbalances most often involve a combination of nutrients rather than a single nutrient. However, protein is the most likely caloric nutrient to be involved in an isolated deficiency state. Protein deficiency is usually superimposed on total energy malnutrition in PCM.

Kwashiorkor is a state of protein deficiency occurring in the presence of adequate caloric intake, or a lowered dietary protein–to-energy ratio. The diet of children who develop kwashiorkor is often similar to that of those who develop marasmus; the critical difference is often infection, which decreases the body's protein utilization and precipitates kwashiorkor.

Kwashiorkor can progress rapidly over 2 to 3 weeks to an advanced state, as the metabolic rate (and thus the amino acid requirement) is maintained by the adequate energy intake. During periods of protein insufficiency, amino acids preferentially maintain serum immunoglobulins, whereas transport proteins such as albumin are catabolized.

The child with kwashiorkor develops peripheral edema and sometimes ascites. There may be a feeble pulse, low blood pressure, or muffled heart sounds. Hepatomegaly, considered a hallmark of kwashiorkor, develops as fat, normally used in the production of lipoproteins, is sequestered in the liver. The child's hair becomes downy, light-colored, soft, and sparse. It may develop patchy or striped areas of discoloration, known as the *flag sign*. The skin develops a "flaky paint" appearance, easily peeling away to leave raw areas.

As in PCM, the hemoglobin level is reduced, and the white blood cell count is variable. Serum electrolyte levels demonstrate hyponatremia and hypokalemia, and serum total protein and albumin levels are markedly depressed. Liver function tests may be abnormal, particularly serum bilirubin (elevated) and prothrombin time (increased). A total lymphocyte count should be performed to evaluate the immune status.

The treatment of kwashiorkor is similar to the treatment of marasmus, with the addition of potassium supplements of up to 5 mEq/kg/day for the first week in children.

Avitaminosis A

Vitamin A, or retinol, is a fat-soluble vitamin that acts as a retinal photosensitivity pigment and maintains tissue integrity by stabilizing cell membranes and controlling epithelial differentiation (Table 43–3). It is supplied in milk, butter, egg yolks, fish, and meat livers. Pro-vitamin A carotenoids, such as carotene, are supplied in dark green leafy vegetables and carrots.

Avitaminosis A remains the most widespread and serious nutritional disorder leading to blindness in India, Africa, Southeast Asia, Central America, and South America. In developed countries, children with chronic malabsorptive diseases or chronic mineral oil ingestion may not absorb adequate amounts of vitamin A, despite an adequate diet. Premature infants are at risk because of low serum levels and low liver stores of vitamin A.

Hypervitaminosis A

Hypervitaminosis A may be caused by acute or chronic ingestion of vitamin A. Acute vitamin A toxicity is manifested by vomiting, drowsiness, a bulging fontanelle, and papilledema suggestive of pseudotumor cerebri. Chronic hypervitaminosis A occurs over weeks to months of excess ingestion. Children develop anorexia, pruritus, hair loss, and desquamation of the palms and soles. Increased intracranial pressure and hepatomegaly may occur.

Thiamine (B₁) Deficiency

Vitamin B_1 (thiamine) is required for the synthesis of acetylcholine, and deficiency results in impaired nerve conduction. Thiamine is supplied in milk, cereals, fruits, vegetables, and eggs.

Thiamine deficiency is known as *beriberi*. Early manifestations are apathy, anorexia, and abdominal discomfort. Peripheral neuritis with paresthesias of the feet, decreased tendon reflexes, and loss of vibration sense indicate a more advanced deficiency state. Hoarseness caused by laryngeal nerve impingement by an enlarged left atrium is characteristic.

The presence of cardiac involvement distinguishes *wet beriberi* from *dry beriberi*. Early cardiac signs are cyanosis and dyspnea. Cardiac enlargement occurs in more than 50% of patients, and the electrocardiogram (EKG) shows sinus tachycardia, inverted T waves, and low voltage, all of which rapidly reverse with treatment. In the 1970s there was a recurrence of beriberi heart disease in young Japanese teenagers whose diets consisted of soft drinks, noodles, and polished rice.

Infantile beriberi may be treated with thiamine, 25 mg intramuscularly and 25 mg intravenously. Adolescent beriberi should be treated according to the severity of the disease. Fulminant cardiovascular collapse caused by wet beriberi, termed *shoshin*, should be treated aggressively with immediate high-dose thiamine (50 to 100 mg IV push) (Table 43–3). Beriberi usually reverses rapidly and completely with treatment.

Pyridoxine (Vitamin B₆) Deficiency

Vitamin B_6 includes pyridoxine, pyridoxal, and pyridoxamine. Vitamin B_6 is a precursor to a coenzyme necessary for glycogen and fatty acid metabolism. It is necessary for brain and nerve cell functioning, and deficiency leads to seizures and peripheral neuropathy. Pyridoxine is found in nearly all plant and animal food sources, and therefore nutritional deficiency is rare.

Four clinical disturbances related to vitamin B_6 deficiency are recognized: microcytic anemia; dermatitis, including

---

TABLE 43–3

VITAMIN DEFICIENCY STATES: THERAPY AT A GLANCE

Vitamin Deficiency	Clinical State	Treatment
Vitamin A	Keratomalacia Xerophthalmia	Vitamin A, 50,000–100,000 IU IM or po *or* Vitamin A, 5000 IU po daily
Vitamin B₁ (thiamine)	Beriberi	Thiamine, 25 mg IM and 25 mg IVP *or* Thiamine, 10 mg IM or po daily
	Shoshin	Thiamine, 50–100 mg IVP
Vitamin B₆ (pyridoxine)	Seizures	Pyridoxine, 100 mg IM
Vitamin C	Scurvy	Ascorbic acid, 100–200 mg IM or po daily
Vitamin D	Rickets	Vitamin D, 15,000 μg po *or* Vitamin D₃, 50–100 μg po daily
Vitamin K	Coagulopathy Hemorrhage	Vitamin K, 1 mg IM Fresh frozen plasma, 10–20 ml/kg

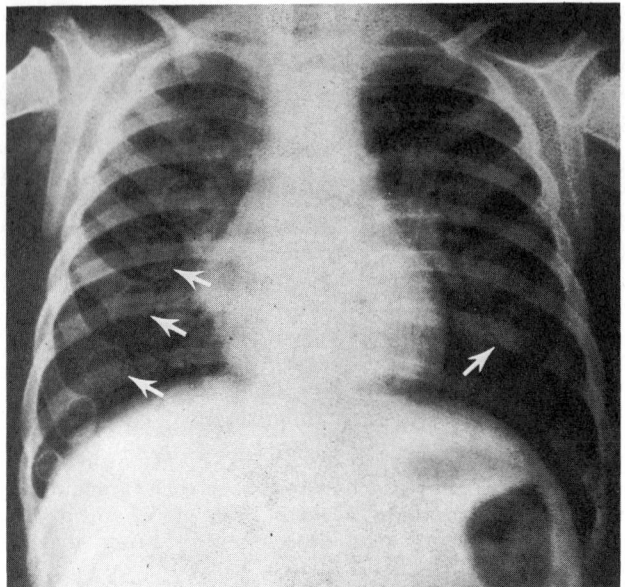

Figure 43–1. Scorbutic rosary *(arrows)* in a 7-month-old baby. (From Wimberger H. Klinisch-radiologische Diagnostik von Rachitis, Skorbut und Lues congenita in Kindesalter. Ergebnisse der innere Medizin u. Kinderheilkunde 1925;88.)

weight loss, and irritability. A low-grade fever is usually present, and a mild anemia is common. The classic features of scurvy are the result of defective collagen formation, especially in bone, cartilage, and teeth. In addition, the intercellular tissue of capillaries is also defective. Together these defects result in spontaneous hemorrhages and defective bone ossification. Subperiosteal hemorrhages, seen as edematous swelling and tenderness at the ends of the tibia and femur, are a classic sign and are caused by periosteal loosening. There is generalized tenderness of the long bones, especially the legs, and the infant assumes a frog-leg position to avoid pain. The infant appears apprehensive when picked up or when the diaper is changed. Knobby swelling of the costochondral junction and the anterior ends of the ribs produces a scorbutic rosary (Fig. 43–1). The sternal plate subluxates, causing depression of the sternum and a sharp angle at the costochondral junction. This angulation helps differentiate the *scorbutic beads* from the *rachitic rosary* seen in patients with vitamin D deficiency. The gums are characterized by purplish spongy swelling, and the teeth are loose. Bleeding from the gums, periorbital ecchymosis, and proptosis from retro-orbital hematomas are common, but hemorrhages into the skin, epistaxis, and gastrointestinal bleeding are rare in infantile scurvy.

The diagnosis is most reliably made by the radiographic appearance of the long bones (Fig. 43–2). The cortex is seen as a thin white line, but the trabeculae are lost, giving the

cheilosis, glossitis, and facial seborrhea; peripheral neuritis; and infantile seizures. Peripheral neuropathy occurs predominantly in patients who are receiving the pyridoxine antagonist isoniazid (INH) for tuberculosis or in patients who are receiving other hydrazides (such as the antihypertensive agent hydralazine). Milk has a low vitamin B$_6$ content, and in addition, vitamin B$_6$ is destroyed by heat. For this reason, infant formulas are commonly fortified with heat-stable pyridoxine hydrochloride. Infants whose mothers received large doses of pyridoxine during pregnancy are also at risk for seizures because of pyridoxine dependency. These may occur at any time from several hours to 6 months after birth. Pyridoxine dependency can also result from ingestion of daily supplements of 200 mg of pyridoxine for more than a month (see Table 43–3).

Infants with seizures should be suspected of having vitamin B$_6$ deficiency or dependency if more common causes of infantile seizures can be excluded. If deficiency is suspected, 100 mg of pyridoxine may be injected intramuscularly.

Vitamin C Deficiency

Vitamin C is water soluble and is a reducing agent. It functions as a cofactor in the hydroxylation of proline, which is required for collagen synthesis. Vitamin C is also required for normal functioning of osteoblasts and fibroblasts. Vitamin C is supplied by many fresh fruits and vegetables (see Table 43–3).

Vitamin C deficiency, or scurvy, is observed in infants receiving either unsupplemented bovine milk or breast milk from vitamin C–deficient mothers. Alternatively, deficiency may be precipitated in infants whose mothers ingested large amounts of vitamin C during pregnancy. Children who have a high carbohydrate diet also seem to be susceptible. The need for vitamin C is increased by febrile illnesses, particularly infectious and diarrheal illnesses, by cold exposure, and by iron deficiency.

Scurvy occurs in infants 6 to 24 months of age and is rare in newborns. It is first manifested by symptoms of anorexia,

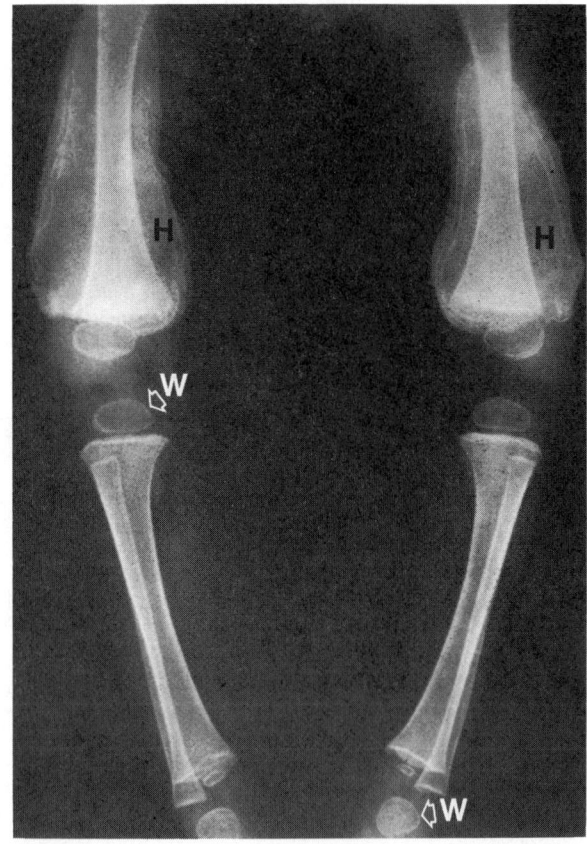

Figure 43–2. Scurvy in an 8-month-old boy, with classic findings, including the Wimberger sign (W, *arrow*), which is the thin white line of the zone of provisional calcification around otherwise osteoporotic epiphyses; bilateral epiphyseal slips laterally at the distal femurs; and the markedly vigorous periosteal hemorrhage (H) now beginning to calcify at its margins. (From Wimberger H. Klinisch-radiologische Diagnostik von Rachitis, Skorbut und Lues congenita in Kindesalter. Ergebnisse der innere Medizin u. Kinderheilkunde 1925; 88.)

bones a ground-glass appearance. A dense white line (Fraenkel's line) forms proximal to the epiphyseal plate. The epiphysis has the appearance of being ringed with white ink.

Scurvy is easily prevented with a diet that includes citrus fruits and juices. Treatment with a daily dose of 100 to 200 mg or more of ascorbic acid, orally or parenterally, produces rapid healing.

Vitamin D Deficiency

Vitamin D is a fat-soluble vitamin that regulates calcium and phosphorus metabolism. Two forms are of chief importance. Vitamin D_2, or ergocalciferol, is the primary dietary and therapeutic source of vitamin D. In the diet, vitamin D is supplied primarily in fish liver oils, eggs, butter, and margarine. Because of the low natural vitamin D content of milk, bovine milk and infant formulas are commonly fortified with vitamin D. Vitamin D_3, or cholecalciferol, is naturally present in human skin and is activated photochemically by sunlight.

Clinical vitamin D deficiency is termed *rickets*. A resurgence of rickets has been noted in recent years. An insufficient diet, inadequate exposure to sunlight, premature birth, and dark skin color are all risk factors. Prolonged breast-feeding also places infants at risk because of the low vitamin D content of breast milk. In addition, children with malabsorption disorders and children receiving phenytoin or phenobarbital therapy are also predisposed.

Rickets results from the body's attempt to maintain a normal serum calcium level. Normal bone reabsorption is followed by replacement with uncalcified osteoid in both the epiphysis and the subperiosteal shaft areas. At the bone ends, this creates a wide, irregular zone between the metaphysis and epiphysis. This zone then becomes compressed, leading to flaring at the bone ends. The softened shaft may become distorted or easily fractured.

Clinical signs of rickets include craniotabes, or a *"Ping-Pong ball"* sensation caused when pressing firmly over the occiput in infants; sweating about the head; palpably enlarged costochondral junctions (rachitic rosary) (Fig. 43–3); pigeon breast deformity; and thickening of the wrists and ankles as a result of epiphyseal flaring. Greenstick fractures are common and can occur with minimal trauma. Muscle hypotonia may also occur and may cause a protuberant abdomen. Rickets may often be complicated by respiratory tract infections, including bronchitis, bronchopneumonia, and atelectasis. Concomitant iron deficiency may also occur. Hypocalcemia may lead to tetany if the serum calcium levels fall below 7.0 to 7.5 mg/dl.

Radiographs demonstrate a widened epiphyseal junction and cupping and fraying of the metaphyseal ends (Fig. 43–4). Greenstick fractures may be seen. Laboratory studies typically demonstrate a normal or low serum calcium level, a markedly reduced serum phosphate level, and a high level of serum alkaline phosphatase.

Treatment with oral cholecalciferol will produce rapid healing within several weeks. Recommended dosage is 50 to 150 μg of cholecalciferol daily (see Table 43–3). Alternatively, the administration of 15,000 μg of cholecalciferol in a single dose without further therapy may achieve more rapid healing.

Vitamin K Deficiency

Vitamin K is fat soluble and facilitates clotting factor synthesis in the coagulation cascade. Vitamin K is supplied in soybeans, alfalfa, spinach, tomatoes, and kale and is endogenously synthesized by the intestinal flora in the form of vitamin K_2. Breast milk has a low vitamin K content.

Vitamin K deficiency should be considered in all patients with hemorrhagic disturbances, as deficiency results in hypoprothrombinemia and bleeding. Deficiency may be caused by factors that limit vitamin K synthesis in the intestine (e.g., diarrhea or prolonged antibiotic use). Drugs such as dicumarol or salicylic acid may prevent the liver from using vitamin K to synthesize prothrombin. Dietary deficiency, especially in breast-fed infants, and low prenatal stores may contribute to hemorrhagic disease of the newborn.

Three forms of infantile vitamin K deficiency have been described. The classic form, *hemorrhagic disease of the newborn*, presents in infants 2 to 5 days old. Generalized bleeding into the skin, gastrointestinal tract, umbilical cord, and

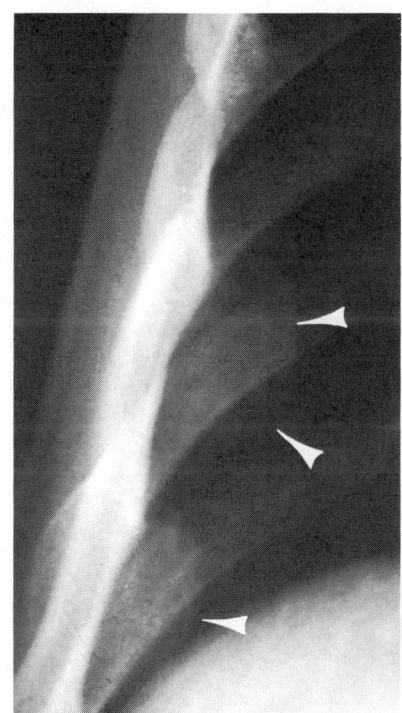
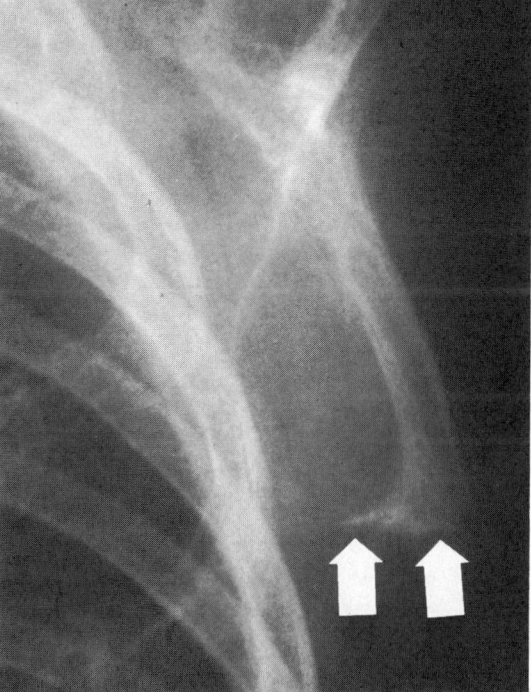

Figure 43–3. Findings of rickets on the chest radiograph in this 3-year-old child include the bulbous expansion of anterior rib ends *(arrowheads)*, known as rachitic rosary, and the irregular, frayed inferior margin of the scapula *(arrows)*. (Courtesy of A. Oestreich, M.D., Cincinnati, OH.)

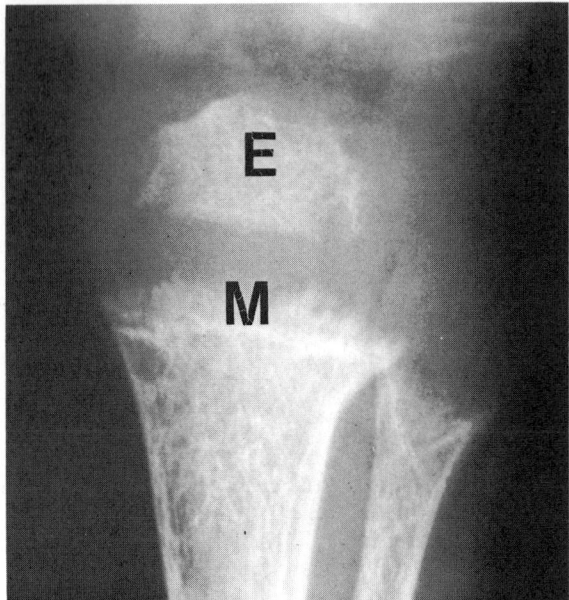

Figure 43–4. In this young child with nutritional rickets, note the frayed, unsharp physeal margin of the metaphysis (M); the wide space between metaphysis and epiphysis (E), with the soft tissue composed of physis plus uncalcified osteoid; and the unsharp margins of the epiphysis, also covered with unossified osteoid on its hemispheric surface. The proximal fibular metaphysis is also cupped. These are all characteristic of established rickets. (Courtesy of A. Oestreich, M.D., Cincinnati, OH.)

central nervous system occurs. An early form may present in infants born to mothers exposed to drugs that alter vitamin K metabolism (e.g., warfarin, phenytoin, and barbiturates). A late form may present after 1 month of age in infants with underlying diseases such as cystic fibrosis, biliary atresia, alpha₁-antitrypsin deficiency, and hepatitis.

Prophylactic parenteral administration of 1 mg of vitamin K at birth is recommended for all infants, especially those who will be breast-fed. This practice has sharply decreased the incidence of hemorrhagic disease of the newborn. Coagulopathy caused by vitamin K deficiency is treated with 1 mg vitamin K intravenously; this improves the coagulopathy within a few hours and completely corrects it within 24 hours. Intramuscular administration of vitamin K should be avoided in patients with hemorrhagic coagulopathy because of the risk of hematoma formation at the injection site. In patients with life-threatening hemorrhage, giving 10 to 20 ml/kg fresh frozen plasma will rapidly boost all vitamin K–dependent coagulation factors (see Table 43–3).

Iron Deficiency

Iron deficiency is the most common nutritional disturbance found among American children of all ages. Data from United States Department of Agriculture food consumption surveys indicate that 82% of 1- to 2-year-old children and 38% of 3- to 5-year-old children consume less than 70% of the recommended dietary allowance of iron.

Although breast milk contains less iron than bovine milk, iron from breast milk is better absorbed. Breast-fed infants rarely develop iron deficiency in the first 6 months of life. However, after 6 months of age, breast-feeding does not protect against iron deficiency.

Iron deficiency anemia manifests as general weakness, headaches, fatigue, anorexia, and pica. The child appears pale, and the spleen is palpably enlarged in 10% to 15% of

patients. Because this form of anemia is hypochromic, a reduction in the hemoglobin level precedes a decrease in the packed cell volume (hematocrit). All red cell indices (mean corpuscular volume, mean corpuscular hemoglobin, and mean corpuscular hemoglobin concentration) are reduced. The serum iron level is reduced, and total iron-binding capacity is increased. The free erythrocyte protoporphyrin (FEP) is an accurate estimate of iron deficiency; the higher the FEP, the more severe the iron deficiency.

A child with iron deficiency anemia should receive 5 to 9 mg/kg/day of oral ferrous sulfate divided into three doses between meals. Blood transfusion is rarely indicated except in patients with severe cardiovascular compromise and congestive heart failure resulting from severe anemia (hemoglobin < 4 gm/dl).

Selected References

American Academy of Pediatrics Committee on Nutrition. Commentary on breast-feeding and infant formulas, including standards for formulas. Pediatrics 1976;57:278.

American Academy of Pediatrics Committee on Nutrition. Fluoride supplementation: Revised dosage schedule. Pediatrics 1979;63:150.

American Academy of Pediatrics Committee on Nutrition. The promotion of breast-feeding. Pediatrics 1982;69:654.

American Academy of Pediatrics Committee on Nutrition. Soy protein formulas: Recommendations for use in infant feeding. Pediatrics 1983;72:359.

American Academy of Pediatrics Committee on Nutrition. Vitamin and mineral supplement needs in normal children in the United States. Pediatrics 1980;66:1015.

Anderson SA, Chinn HI, Fischer KD, et al. History of current status of infant formulas. Am J Clin Nutr 1982;35:381.

Armistead J, Kelly D, et al. Evaluation of infant feeding in acute gastroenteritis. J Pediatr Gastroent Nutr 1989;8:240.

Beaton GH, Chery A. Protein requirements of infants: A reexamination of concepts and approaches. Am J Clin Nutr 1988;48:1403.

Bleyer WA, Skinner AL. Fatal neonatal hemorrhage after maternal anticonvulsant therapy. JAMA 1976;235:626.

Chandra RK. Immunologic aspects of human milk. Nutr Rev 1978;36:265.

Coursin DB. Convulsive seizures in infants with pyridoxine deficient diets. JAMA 1954;154:406.

Cunningham AS. Morbidity in breast-fed and artificially fed infants. J Pediatr 1977;90:726.

Driggers DA, Reeves JD, Lo EY, Dallman PR. Iron deficiency in one-year-old infants: Comparison of results of a therapeutic trial in infants with anemia or low-normal hemoglobin values. J Pediatr 1981;98:753.

English P. Failure to thrive without organic reason. Pediatr Ann 1978;7:774.

Garza C, Schanler RJ, Butte NF, Motil KJ. Special properties of human milk. Clin Perinatol 1987;14:11.

Goose D, Gittus E. Infant feeding methods and dental caries. Public Health 1968;82:72.

Hambraeus L. Proprietary milk versus human breast milk in infant feeding. Pediatr Clin North Am 1977;24:17.

Hope PL, Hall MA, Millward-Sadler GH, Normand IC. Alpha-1-antitrypsin deficiency presenting as a bleeding diathesis in the newborn. Arch Dis Child 1982;57:68.

Jacobs K, Dwyer JT. Vegetarian children: Appropriate and inappropriate diets. Am J Clin Nutr 1988;48:811.

Jeliffe DB, Jeliffe EFT. The uniqueness of human milk. Am J Clin Nutr 1971;24:968.

Jung AL, Carr SL. A soy protein formula and a milk-based formula: A comparative evaluation in milk-tolerant infants showed no significant differences. Clin Pediatr 1977;16:982.

Kawai C, Wakabayashi A, Matsumura T, Yui Y. Reappearance of beriberi heart disease in Japan. A study of 23 cases. Am J Med 1980;69:383.

Kotelchock M, Newberger EH. Failure to thrive: A controlled study of familial characteristics. J Am Acad Child Psychiatr 1983;22:322.

Kruger DM, Lyne ED, Kleerekoper M. Vitamin D deficiency rickets. A report on three cases. Clin Orthop 1987;224:277.

Lane PA, Hathaway WE. Vitamin K in infancy. J Pediatr 1985;106:351.

Leung SSF, Lui S, Davies DP. Energy intake from birth to 2 years. Lancet 1988;8595:1161.

Martinez GA, Dodd DA, Samartgedes JA. Milk feeding patterns in the United States during the first 12 months of age. Pediatrics 1981;68:863.

McLaren DS. Energy needs of infants. Lancet 1988;8626–7:1494.

McMillan JA, Landaw SA, Oski FA. Iron sufficiency in breast-fed infants and the availability of iron from human milk. Pediatrics 1976;58:686.

Newberger EH, Reed RB, Daniel JH, et al. Pediatric social illness: Toward an etiologic classification. Pediatrics 1977;60:175.

Nutrition Committee of the Canadian Paediatric Society and Committee on Nutrition of the American Academy of Pediatrics. Breast-feeding. Pediatrics 1978;62:591.

Periera GR, Barbora NM. Controversies in neonatal nutrition. Pediatr Clin North Am 1986;33:65.

Pereira GR, Zucker AH. Nutritional deficiencies in the neonate. Clin Perinatol 1986;13:175.

Rossouw JE. Kwashiorkor in North America. Am J Clin Nutr 1989;49:588.

Rudolf M, Arulanantham K, Greenstein RM, et al. Unsuspected nutritional rickets. Pediatrics 1980;66:72.

Shapiro LR, Crawford PB, Clark MJ, et al. Obesity prognosis: A longitudinal study of children from the age of 6 months to 9 years. Am J Public Health 1984;74:968.

Sills RH. Failure to thrive: The role of the clinical and laboratory evaluation. Am J Dis Child 1978;132:967.

Smith NT, Rios E. Iron metabolism and iron deficiency in infancy and childhood. Adv Pediatr 1974;21:239.

Stahlberf MR, Savilahti E. Infantile colic and feeding. Arch Dis Child 1986;61:1232.

Stark O, Atkins E, Wolff OH, Douglas JW. Longitudinal study of obesity in the National Survey of Health and Development. Br Med J 1981;283:13.

Sutherland JM, Glueck HI, Gleser G. Hemorrhagic disease of the newborn. Breast feeding as a necessary factor in the pathogenesis. Am J Dis Child 1967;113:524.

Walker-Smith J, Harrison M, Kilby A, et al. Cows' milk–sensitive enteropathy. Arch Dis Child 1978;53:375.

Welsh JK, May JT. Anti-infective properties of breast milk. J Pediatr 1979;94:1.

World Health Organization. Energy and protein requirements. WHO Tech Rep Ser 1985;724.

Zachman RD. Retinol (vitamin A) and the neonate: Special problems of the human premature infant. Am J Clin Nutr 1989;50:413.

CHAPTER 44

Feeding Problems

Mary Hughes

INTRODUCTION

Feeding problems are rarely an emergency, but difficulties with feeding caused by different disease processes will have implications for the emergency physician. Feeding difficulties produced by transfer dysphagia, coughing or choking with feeding, and gastrointestinal motility disorders may all be seen by the emergency physician. More serious disorders may even cause vomiting.

DISORDERS CAUSING TRANSFER DYSPHAGIA

Transfer dysphagia is difficulty moving food from the lips to the upper esophagus. Multiple conditions may affect the ability of a child to adequately take in nutrients, including diseases that cause oral pain and congenital facial malformations.

Diseases Causing Oral Pain
Aphthous Ulcers

Aphthous ulcers (canker sores) are lesions that may recur in a given child, have no known origin, and may present as a solitary sore or as diffuse oral lesions. Aphthous ulcers are commonly found on the mucosal surfaces adjacent to the gingiva and on the ventral tongue surface. Treatment is generally symptomatic, with the application of cold. Topical anesthetics applied prior to eating help to control pain. The sores are self-limited and generally last less than 14 days.

Candidiasis

Oral candidiasis may present in neonates who contract the disease on passage through an infected birth canal and affects up to 5% of newborns. The causative agent is *Candida albicans*. Oral candidiasis can also be acquired from the mother during breast-feeding and from bottles and nipples that are improperly cleaned and sterilized.

The typical lesion is a white or cream-colored plaque that leaves an underlying inflamed mucosal surface on its removal. Lesions may occur as small patches or cover the entire oral pharynx in coalescing patches. Other sites of infection with *C. albicans*, such as the diaper area or other intertriginous areas, should be sought.

Oral nystatin in doses of 100,000 U (1 ml) applied to each buccal surface four times daily for 1 week is the recommended treatment (Table 44–1). Reinfection may be prevented by searching for the source and treating it concomitantly. Parents should dispose of all nipples and pacifiers used prior to infection.

Herpangina

Herpangina is a viral illness caused primarily by coxsackievirus type A and occasionally by other enteroviruses. Patients with herpangina present with sudden onset of fever, headache, sore throat, myalgias, and malaise. The typical oral lesions begin as a small papule, progress to a vesicle, and then ulcerate. Transmission is generally mouth-to-mouth or feces-to-mouth. It is rapidly contagious, has an

TABLE 44–1	
FEEDING DISORDERS: THERAPY AT A GLANCE	
Condition	**Treatment**
Oral candiadiasis	Nystatin suspension, 1 ml (100,000 U) to each buccal surface qid for 7 days
	Gentian violet, 1% solution painted on involved surfaces (stains purple)
Herpes gingivostomatitis (postnatal)	Acyclovir suspension, 2.5 ml five times daily (only used if patient is immunocompromised)
Trench mouth	Penicillin V potassium suspension, 30–50 mg/kg/day divided every 6 hr
Esophagitis (of any origin)	Antacids, 5–12 ml, 1 and 3 hours pc and hs
	or
	Cimetidine, 20–40 mg/kg/day
	or
	Bethanechol, 8.7 mg/m²/24 hr given ac and hs
	or
	Metoclopramide; 1- to 6-yr-olds: 0.1 mg/kg/dose given ac and hs 6- to 12-yr-olds: 2.5–9 mg/dose
Esophageal candidiasis	Antacids, 5–12 ml, 1 and 3 hr pc and hs
	or
	Cimetidine, 20–40 mg/kg/day
	and
	Nystatin, 2–6 ml four times daily
	or
	Ketoconazole (in children >2 yr old), 3.3–6.6 mg/kg/day
Esophageal herpes	Antacids, 5–12 ml, 1 and 3 hours pc and hs
	or
	Cimetidine, 20–40 mg/kg/day
	and
	Acyclovir, 5 mg/kg every 8 hours IV

incubation period of approximately 2 to 7 days, and lasts 3 to 6 days.

Treatment is generally symptomatic and includes analgesics, antipyretics, and topical anesthetics used judiciously prior to feeding. Resolution usually occurs within 3 to 5 days. During the acute phase, oral secretions and feces are infectious, and the feces may remain contagious for weeks after the clinical illness has disappeared.

Herpes Simplex

The initial attack of herpes simplex virus type 1 is generally associated with fever, malaise, lymphadenopathy, and severe oral pain and occasionally requires hospital admission as a result of the inability to maintain hydration and nutritional needs.

The lesions in primary or initial infections are often widespread in the intraoral and perioral regions. Recurrent lesions are unilateral at or near the vermilion border in most cases and tend to recur at or near the same site. Exposure to sun, fever, stress (including premenstrual stress), respiratory tract infection, and trauma may all precipitate recurrent lesions. Diagnosis is made by a Tzanck test or herpes simplex culture.

Treatment of postnatal herpes gingivostomatitis is most often symptomatic and includes antipyretics, analgesics, cold fluids, and foods. Occasionally intravenous acyclovir has been used in the treatment of severe herpes gingivostomatitis. Oral acyclovir is generally not recommended unless the patient is immunocompromised, but if oral acyclovir therapy is necessary, the usual dose is 2.5 ml acyclovir suspension five times daily.

Cheilosis

Cheilosis is a painful fissure at the corner of the mouth. It can be caused by dehydration, fever, wind chapping, repeated wetting and drying of the lips, contact sensitivity to chemicals or foods, chronic *Candidiasis* infection, or iron deficiency anemia. Treatment is based on identifying and correcting the underlying cause, and symptomatic relief is generally provided with a bland ointment that may or may not contain antibiotics.

Behçet's Disease

Behçet's disease is a vascular inflammatory disease that presents with ulcerative stomatitis, genital ulcerations, and ocular inflammation, most often manifested as uveitis. It is a rare cause of ulcerative stomatitis in children. Its history is that of exacerbation and remission, and treatment is nonspecific.

Trauma

Perioral or intraoral trauma may make adequate oral fluid and nutrient intake difficult. Oral or rectal analgesics and diet modification may be necessary. If these are insufficient to maintain hydration status, hospital admission is required until the child can demonstrate the ability to maintain sufficient nutritional intake.

Trench Mouth

Vincent's infection, or acute necrotizing ulcerative gingivitis, is a severe intraoral infection occurring secondary to spirochetes. This disease is seen more commonly in patients with poor oral hygiene and may occur in epidemics in institutions for children.

Patients generally present with complaints of severe oral pain, foul breath, and blood-streaked sputum and may develop a fever. Cervical lymphadenopathy generally occurs. The typical lesion is a punched-out ulcer covered by a gray pseudomembrane. Treatment consists of dental cleaning by a professional and administration of antibiotics; penicillin is the antibiotic of choice. Occasionally dental or gingival surgery may be necessary to repair damage caused by this disease.

Hand-Foot-and-Mouth Disease

Coxsackievirus A is the usual cause of hand-foot-and-mouth disease. The classic lesions are vesicles located in the mouth and on the hands and feet. The oral lesions rapidly erode to ulcers and generally clear in 4 to 5 days. This is a disease of the summer months and may present with a low-grade fever. Treatment is symptomatic.

Facial Malformations
Cleft Palate

The incidence of cleft palate in the United States is approximately 1 in every 1500 births. Cleft palate can range in severity from a bifed uvula to lateral or median clefting of the entire hard and soft palate. Generally the most severe defects cause significant feeding difficulties early in life because of the inability to generate the normal amount of negative pressure intraorally, leading to inefficient sucking and excessive air swallowing.

Breast-feeding should be attempted if possible. If not, a palatal prosthesis, placed to encourage growth of the maxilla, and an ordinary nipple are often sufficient to allow feeding. A variety of cleft palate nipples exist; these are designed to occlude the palatal gap and decrease the amount of negative pressure needed to suck and swallow effectively. Frequent burping is essential during feeding. If the child is not able to maintain nutrition with a modified nipple, then feeding with a rolled-edged spoon (to deliver the milk to the back of the tongue) or tube feeding should be undertaken. Cleft lip repairs are often accomplished at 3 to 4 months of age and cleft palate repairs at approximately 18 months of age, depending on other needs of the patient.

Thyroglossal Cyst

Thyroglossal duct cysts are developmental anomalies that may occur at several sites along the thyroglossal duct. They are one of the more common causes of cystic swellings in the neck, but also can occur as high as the base of the tongue. Thyroglossal duct cysts may become enlarged, causing feeding difficulties primarily due to esophageal compression or actual obstruction in the posterior pharynx. Surgical excision is recommended if feeding difficulties exist.

Micrognathia (Pierre Robin Syndrome)

Pierre Robin syndrome, characterized by micrognathia secondary to mandibular hypoplasia, causes posterior tongue displacement, which can in turn cause occlusion of the posterior oral pharynx. Associated anomalies can include a cleft palate or eye and ear defects.

Nursing or feeding the child with Pierre Robin syndrome in the prone position will help the tongue to fall forward, thus preventing respiratory difficulties during feeding. If this is unsuccessful, feedings may be given slowly with a Breck feeder spoon or, in severe cases, with a feeding tube.

Sucking helps develop the mandible and should be encouraged in all children with Pierre Robin syndrome.

DISORDERS CAUSING COUGHING OR CHOKING
Tracheoesophageal Fistula With Esophageal Atresia

Children with tracheoesophageal anomalies generally present with difficulties at birth. Maternal hydramnios is common. Children with tracheoesophageal fistulas (TEF) and esophageal atresia (EA) present clinically with copious secretions in the oral pharynx and require frequent suctioning. Any child with profuse oral secretions should be examined prior to oral feeding. This examination should include the attempted passage of a fairly large catheter into the stomach with aspiration of contents to ensure that the catheter has actually entered the stomach. In children with TEF and EA, the catheter will not pass into the stomach (Fig. 44–1). Coughing, choking, and cyanosis often occur with the first attempt at feeding. TEF without EA is fairly rare and may not cause problems until the patient is several months of age. Often there is a history of intermittent coughing and choking related to feeding, difficulty breathing during or after feeding, or perceived difficulty sucking. The diagnosis of this type of TEF is made by an esophagogram, but more than one esophagram may be necessary to confirm the suspected diagnosis.

Children who have TEF with EA generally undergo surgical repair and reconstruction as soon as medically feasible while being nourished parenterally. All children with EA have some abnormality of esophageal motility or associated dysphagia. Reflux esophagitis may also occur and may require an antireflux procedure. Other postoperative complications may include strictures (which may be recurrent and require bougienage), nocturnal regurgitation, and aspiration pneumonia.

Feeding difficulties are common among children who have undergone repair of EA, and a significant percentage of these children are growth retarded. One study examined 124 children who had undergone repair of both TEF and EA using either primary anastomosis or esophagostomy. In the group that underwent primary anastomosis, 61% were considered by parents to be slow to feed, 33% had episodes of coughing and choking associated with feeding, 20% refused feeding episodically, and 17% had episodes of vomiting. Numbers were similar in the esophagostomy group. Both groups had significant growth retardation, and a high number of children had to undergo esophageal dilation at some point, with many treated emergently for foreign body obstruction of the esophagus. Choking often occurred if feeding was hurried and could often be prevented with increased fluid intake and use of a slower pace at mealtime. Although symptoms disappeared in two thirds of the patients in both groups by the age of 7 years, one third still reported symptoms associated with particular foods.

Respiratory complications following TEF-EA repair are frequent and often present as recurrent bronchitis or pneumonia, most often in children younger than 8 years. Almost uniformly, these complications occur in children with an esophageal stricture. Various factors cause aspiration pneumonia, including disordered motility of the esophagus, strictures of the esophagus, and gastroesophageal reflux caused by an incompetent gastroesophageal sphincter.

Gastroesophageal reflux is also a complication of TEF-EA repair, and recurrent acute respiratory disease or frequent episodes of esophagitis, refusal to eat, or choking and vomiting with feeding may necessitate a surgical antireflux procedure.

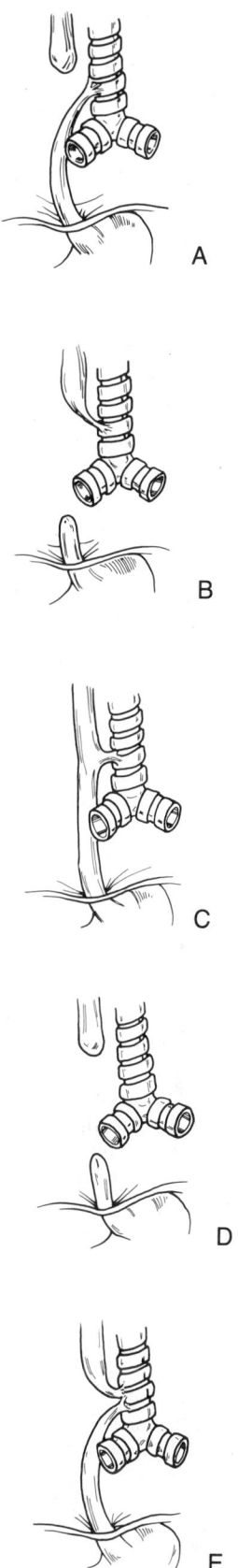

Figure 44–1. Tracheoesophageal anomalies. *A,* Esophageal atresia with distal tracheoesophageal fistula is the most common type. *B,* Esophageal atresia with proximal tracheoesophageal fistula is the most rare. *C,* Tracheoesophageal fistula without esophageal atresia. *D,* Esophageal atresia without tracheoesophageal fistula. *E,* Esophageal atresia with proximal and distal tracheoesophageal fistulas.

Extrinsic Masses

Extrinsic masses compressing the esophagus along its route may cause difficulty with swallowing in the newborn. Respiratory distress is often the primary symptom. Teratomas and cystic hygromas are the most common types of masses in the cervical region. Esophageal duplications, although rare, are the second most common type of posterior mediastinal masses occurring in children. Congenital anomalies associated with esophageal duplications include vertebral abnormalities and secondary alimentary tract malformations. Carinal node enlargement, as might be seen with lymphoma, tuberculosis, or histoplasmosis, may also compress the esophagus and cause dysphagia or choking. Esophageal webs are a rare cause of dysphagia when solid foods are added to the diet.

Gastroesophageal Reflux

Gastroesophageal reflux (GER) is defined as a retrograde flow of gastric material into the esophagus. GER may be the result of one or more of the following factors: abnormally low gastroesophageal sphincter (GES) pressure (in which GER is often spontaneous, transient, and not associated with swallowing), delayed gastric emptying, abnormal lower esophageal motility, or a transient increase in intra-abdominal pressure.

Most newborns have occasional symptoms related to GER, but rarely is the vomiting significant enough to cause difficulties. Occasionally GER will lead to reflux esophagitis as a result of the frequency and duration of episodes. The child with GER generally presents with effortless regurgitation, often of large portions, of the previous feeding but does not look clinically ill.

The evaluation of symptomatic GER may include a study to document the presence of reflux and grade its severity. Monitoring pH in the distal esophagus on an ambulatory basis over a 24-hour period can determine those children with significant disease who might be expected to benefit from medical therapy or a surgical procedure.

GES pressure may be measured using esophageal manometry. In children older than 3 years with reflux documented by pH or scintigraphic evaluation, a low GES pressure correlates with delayed gastric emptying. Children 6 years of age and older with GER and delayed gastric emptying are more likely to have significant reflux esophagitis than are similarly afflicted children younger than 3 years.

Esophagoscopy may be needed to evaluate the child for esophagitis. Children older than 6 years with overt esophagitis have significantly delayed gastric emptying when compared with children without esophagitis.

Therapy for GER must be individualized. In patients with uncomplicated GER, all that is required is reassurance of the parents and observation of the child. After feeding, the child should be placed in an upright prone position. Formal immobilization (on a Herbst board) at a 30-degree posture, along with frequent small feedings, often resolves the symptoms. Documented esophagitis requires the use of antacids, H$_2$ antagonists, or agents to enhance gastrointestinal motility.

In most infants GER resolves by 6 to 7 weeks of age, and 90% of infants are symptom free by age 18 months. Surgical intervention is only rarely necessary and is reserved for those patients with significant disease (e.g., bleeding esophagitis, recurrent pneumonias, esophageal strictures unrelieved by dilation, intractability of symptoms, and Barrett's epithelium) who respond poorly to medical treatment.

Reflux Esosphagitis

Infants with esophagitis often present with frequent regurgitations that include blood-tinged secretions. Such infants may be generally irritable, colicky, or demonstrate failure to thrive. Older children may complain of heartburn, halitosis, or a foul taste that is more prominent when the child is supine. Esophagitis may indicate that the child has pathologic GER. Patients who develop bleeding esophagitis secondary to GER should be considered early for definitive operative therapy. Anemia may occur secondary to chronic blood loss.

Treatment is based on the underlying cause and may include positional therapy, antacids, H$_2$ antagonists, or agents to stimulate gastrointestinal motility.

Esophageal Foreign Bodies

Swallowed foreign bodies are common in children between the ages of 1 and 4 years. The most common objects swallowed by children in the United States are toy parts and discs such as coins, buttons, and batteries. Patients with true esophageal foreign bodies often present with increased salivation, vomiting, odynophagia, or refusal to eat.

Esophageal foreign bodies should be removed as soon as possible. Swelling secondary to edema at the site makes it unlikely that a lodged object will pass spontaneously. Fiberoptic endoscopy is the method of choice for removal of esophageal foreign bodies that cannot be advanced or withdrawn by other means.

Retroesophageal Abscess

Retroesophageal abscess generally results from the extension of a retropharyngeal abscess inferiorly; more rarely it may be secondary to esophageal perforations, foreign body ingestion, diphtheria, pleuritis, pericarditis, or ulceration with erosion secondary to intubation. These usually present with dyspnea, cough, dysphagia, and neck swelling. Palpation of the neck may elicit pain, swelling, or subcutaneous air. Soft tissue radiographs are often diagnostic. Treatment includes surgical drainage and antibiotics.

Esophageal Candidiasis and Herpes Simplex

Patients with esophagitis caused by *C. albicans* infection or herpes simplex virus usually present with dysphagia, odynophagia, retrosternal chest pain, weight loss, and often nausea and vomiting. Fever is common with herpes simplex esophagitis. Although these forms of esophagitis are most commonly seen in children with underlying immunocompromising conditions, occasional cases are reported in patients without such underlying factors. In one review, approximately 50% of patients with esophageal candidiasis did not have concomitant oral thrush. Oral herpes simplex is occasionally associated with esophageal herpes in the immunocompetent host. Concomitant infection with herpes simplex virus and *C. albicans* is not uncommon in those with severe immunocompromise.

Esophagoscopy can provide a definitive diagnosis by allowing direct visualization and by obtaining material for stains and culture. Esophageal candidiasis often appears as multiple raised white plaques covering a friable red mucosa. Herpes simplex esophagitis often causes vesicles or discrete ulcers with raised yellow rims of exudate.

Treatment of herpes simplex esophagitis may include antacids, H$_2$ blockers, and acyclovir (5 mg/kg every 8 hours). Treatment of esophageal candidiasis may include antacids, H$_2$ blockers, and oral nystatin or ketoconazole. Amphotericin B should be reserved for deep-seated or systemic candidal infections.

Hiatal Hernia

Hiatal hernias are congenital anomalies that often present in infancy. There are two types: *sliding* (most common), in which a portion of the stomach and the abdominal portion of the esophagus herniate into the thoracic cavity, and *paraesophageal*, in which the lower esophagus remains in the abdomen and the cardiac portion of the stomach herniates into the thoracic cavity (Fig. 44–2). The primary symptoms of a sliding hiatal hernia occur secondary to GER and subsequent esophagitis. These may include "coffee-ground" emesis secondary to bleeding esophagitis; constipation, if vomiting is severe; and iron deficiency anemia secondary to repeated bouts of hematemesis. A significant percentage of children with GER have a hiatal hernia, but many patients with a hiatal hernia are asymptomatic and severe GER often occurs without an associated hiatal hernia.

Patients with paraesophageal hernias may present with abdominal pain, distention, vomiting, and early satiety. The risk of strangulation and infarction of the herniated portion of the stomach is high, and therefore surgery is advocated. Diagnosis of a hiatal hernia is made by barium swallow with fluoroscopy. Esophagoscopy may be used to confirm esophagitis or the presence of strictures. Gastric scintigraphy, when performed by skilled clinicians, may also be useful.

Treatment of the sliding hiatal hernia is directed at the GER and associated esophagitis, rather than at the hernia itself. Treatment includes thickened feedings and maintenance of the 30-degree upright prone position, especially after feedings and often 24 hours a day. Frequent use of antacids, cimetidine (20 to 40 mg/kg/day), bethanechol (8.7 mg/m²/day, ac and hs), or metoclopramide (0.1 mg/kg/dose ac and hs) may be necessary. Surgical repair is reserved for those patients with severe esophagitis unresponsive to medical therapy, esophageal strictures, recurrent aspiration pneumonia, cardiorespiratory arrest, and unremitting asthma secondary to frequent aspiration and for patients

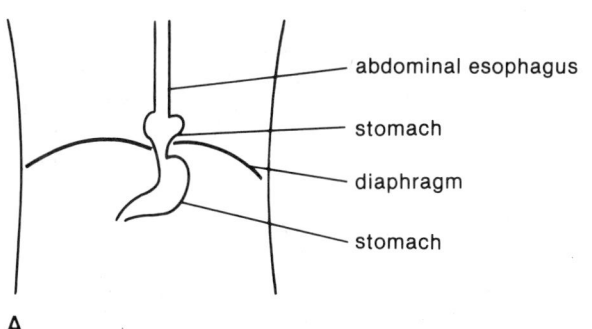

who fail to maintain nutritional status while receiving medical therapy.

GASTROINTESTINAL MOTILITY DISORDERS

Motility disorders cause disordered propulsion of food and may be regional or diffuse. Smooth muscle disorders can lead to decreased intraluminal pressure in the bowel and delayed transit of its contents, bacterial overgrowth, and malabsorption syndromes.

Nerve damage or abnormalities such as occur with achalasia, Hirschsprung's disease, or Riley-Day syndrome may alter gastrointestinal transit time, leading to nausea, vomiting, diarrhea or constipation, malabsorption, and bacterial overgrowth. Symptoms may vary.

Achalasia

Also known as *megaesophagus*, achalasia is a lack of gastroesophageal sphincter relaxation with deglutition, causing functional obstruction at the level of the gastroesophageal junction. The primary deficiency is in the number of ganglion cells at the level of the gastroesophageal sphincter. Achalasia is seen more commonly in adults and adolescents; only 10% of achalasia patients are children.

Signs and symptoms of achalasia include dysphagia, regurgitation of undigested food, cough from food overflow into the trachea, failure to thrive, retrosternal chest pain, recurrent aspiration pneumonia, and a history of mucus and saliva found on the pillow in the morning.

The diagnosis is made on barium swallow, which demonstrates a dilated esophagus with a distinct narrowing at the distal end, disordered peristalsis, and poor esophageal emptying. Standard chest radiographs may reveal air-fluid levels in the esophagus if obtained with the patient in the upright position. Treatment may include esophageal dilation or a Heller procedure, in which the muscles at the cardioesophageal junction are divided.

Cricopharyngeal Dysfunction

Cricopharyngeal dysfunction results from spasm of the superior esophageal sphincter or cricopharyngeal muscle during swallowing and may cause intermittent dysphagia. Pressure may be so elevated that a posterior diverticulum occurs in the pharynx. Treatment is myotomy of the cricopharyngeal muscle.

Bulbar Palsy

Bulbar palsy often presents with dysphagia secondary to poor sucking ability and difficulty in chewing. It is often associated with spastic cerebral palsy. Pseudobulbar palsy often causes incoordination of swallowing as a result of striated muscle dysfunction secondary to abnormalities of central control in the brain stem.

Transient Pharyngeal Muscle Dysfunction

Transient pharyngeal muscle dysfunction is often associated with cerebral palsy but may also be caused by delayed normal development. Choking with feeding, cough, and dribbling of formula are present, and aspiration can be prevented by gavage until the muscle dysfunction resolves.

Riley-Day Syndrome

Riley-Day syndrome, also known as *familial dysautonomia*, is an autosomal recessive disease, found primarily in Ash-

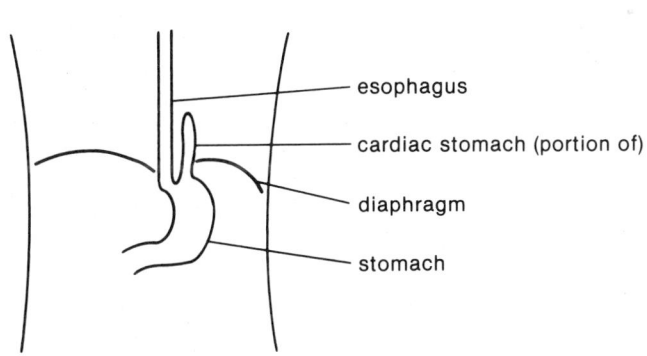

A

- abdominal esophagus
- stomach
- diaphragm
- stomach

B

- esophagus
- cardiac stomach (portion of)
- diaphragm
- stomach

Figure 44–2. A sliding hiatal hernia *(A)*, the most common type, is characterized by a portion of both the stomach and abdominal esophagus moving into the thoracic cavity. A paraesophageal hiatal hernia *(B)* is characterized by the abdominal esophagus remaining in the peritoneal cavity, and the cardia of the stomach entering the thoracic cavity.

kenazic Jews, in which there is a disturbance in autonomic and peripheral sensory function.

Swallowing is poorly coordinated, and thus choking, vomiting, and aspiration are frequent. Pneumonia is recurrent and often leads to respiratory failure, which subsequently may cause premature death.

Other clinical symptoms resulting from autonomic dysfunction include increased salivation and sweating; decreased tears and absence of corneal sensation, leading to corneal ulcers; decreased deep tendon reflexes; abnormalities in thermal and blood pressure regulation; decreased taste; and urinary incontinence. Treatment is aimed at the frequent respiratory tract infections and prevention of corneal ulcers.

Prader-Willi Syndrome

Prader-Willi syndrome includes hypotonia, mental retardation, hypogonadism, and obesity. Feeding difficulties are secondary to congenital hypotonia, which lessens with age. Children with Prader-Willi syndrome develop increased appetites by 2 or 3 years of age, leading to marked obesity. These children generally demonstrate a narrow bifrontal diameter with almond-shaped eyes and a triangular mouth. The diagnosis should be suspected in boys with hypotonia and undescended testicles.

DISORDERS CAUSING VOMITING
Pyloric Stenosis

Pyloric stenosis is the most common cause of intestinal obstruction in infancy and is a result of diffuse hypertrophy and hyperplasia of the smooth muscle of the antrum of the stomach and the circular pyloric muscles. Pyloric stenosis is more likely in full-term infants, and the male-to-female ratio is approximately 4:1 to 5:1. It occurs in approximately 1 in 500 births, and 15% of children have a positive family history.

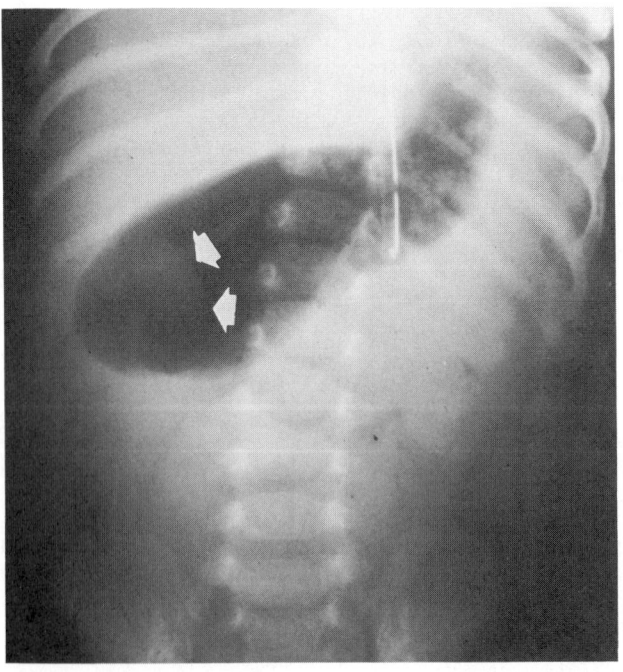

Figure 44–3. The thick muscle *(arrows)* of hypertrophic pyloric stenosis may be recognized on plain film on occasion, as in this infant in a left-side-down decubitus view. (Courtesy of A. Oestreich, M.D., Cincinnati, OH.)

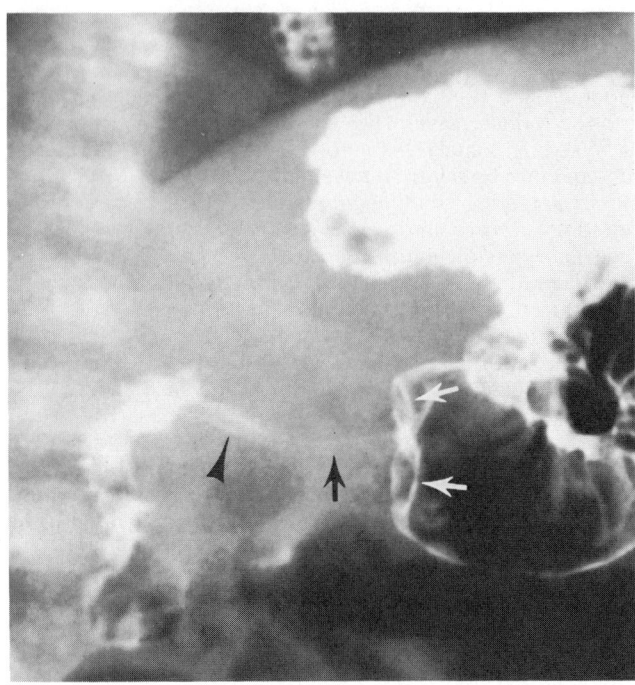

Figure 44–4. Classic appearance on barium study of hypertrophic pyloric stenosis in a vomiting 1-month-old boy. The white arrows indicate the impressions (shoulder sign) of hypertrophic muscle on the antrum (which suffices for diagnosis). The long, thin pylorus *(black arrow, arrowhead)* demonstrates the string sign, of which the more distal pylorus shows the twin lines of a railroad track sign *(arrowhead)*. (Courtesy of A. Oestreich, M.D., Cincinnati, OH.)

Children with pyloric stenosis generally present with nonbilious vomiting at between 2 and 4 weeks of life. The vomiting gradually increases in frequency and becomes projectile as complete obstruction of the gastric outlet channel ensues, generally by the age of 4 to 6 weeks (Fig. 44–3). The vomit may be bloody, and constipation generally follows. Failure to thrive is a common finding. These children are continuously ravenously hungry, eating voraciously even after vomiting. Clinically, upper abdominal distention and left-to-right peristaltic waves are seen, and a 1.5- to 2.0-cm olive-sized mass may be palpated in the epigastrium or to the right of the midline, especially immediately following vomiting. Dehydration, metabolic alkalosis, and hypokalemia are frequent results of pyloric stenosis.

Diagnosis of pyloric stenosis is made in nearly 90% of patients by palpating the olive-sized mass. If a palpable mass is not felt, a barium swallow will demonstrate the "string sign" (i.e., the unchanging elongation and narrowing of the antrum and pylorus) (Fig. 44–4). Abdominal ultrasound may also demonstrate the pyloric mass (Fig. 44–5). Treatment of pyloric stenosis is correction of the fluid and electrolyte abnormalities and then surgical pyloromyotomy.

Congenital Intestinal Obstruction

Congenital intestinal obstruction may be caused by a variety of disorders, the most common being intestinal atresia or stenosis, malrotation, meconium ileus, and Hirschsprung's disease.

Clinically patients with intestinal obstruction present with the classic triad of bilious vomiting, abdominal distention, and constipation. Depending on the level of the obstruction, vomiting will be an early or late finding and may or may not be forceful. Distention will be progressively more marked

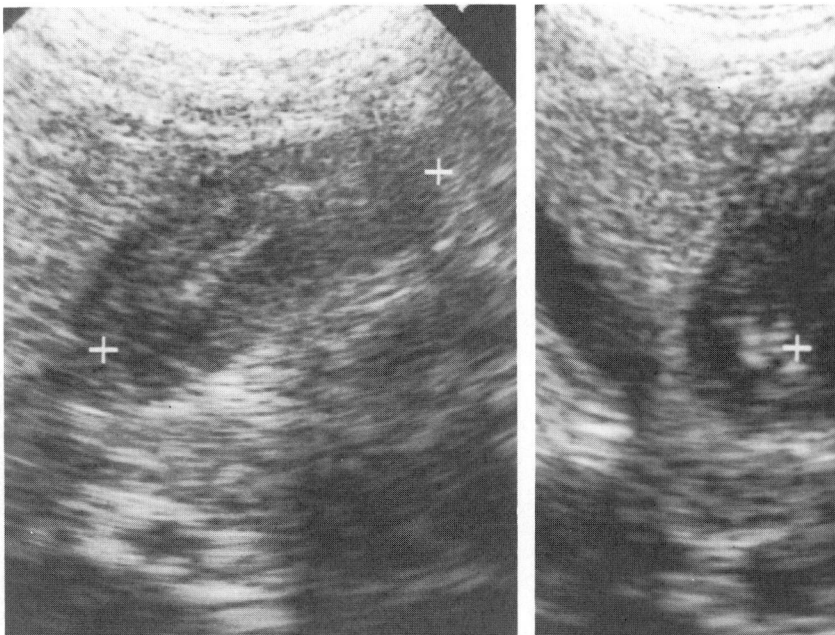

Figure 44–5. Classic appearance on ultasound study of hypertrophic pyloric stenosis in a vomiting 6-week-old boy. The longitudinal sausage of pyloric muscle measures well over the "required" 1.9 cm in length; the muscle width of the en face "doughnut" of thick pyloric muscle is well over 3.5 mm in width. (Courtesy of A. Oestreich, M.D., Cincinnati, OH.)

with more distal obstruction. Diseases such as duodenal atresia are often associated with Down syndrome, but others have no associated disorders. Children with intestinal obstruction secondary to meconium ileus should be examined for cystic fibrosis.

Infants with complete atresia may pass meconium, often of a lighter color because of the absence of bilirubin, prior to the onset of inability to pass stool. Children with intestinal obstruction often look well until late in the course of their disease, so a high index of suspicion must be maintained in any child presenting with the classic triad. Diagnosis is often made by an erect anteroposterior abdominal film, which will demonstrate dilation, air-fluid levels, or abnormal gas patterns, depending on the level of obstruction.

Intussusception

Intussusception is the telescoping of a proximal piece of bowel into a more distal piece. It is most often ileocolic but may be ileoileal or colocolic. The most common age of occurrence is 3 to 12 months, but intussusception can occur in children up to the age of 6 years. It is more common in males than females.

Intussusception generally presents in the previously healthy child with a sudden onset of severe, crampy abdominal pain associated with screaming and drawing up of the legs. These episodes may last for 5 to 10 minutes and resolve spontaneously. Between spasms the child appears normal. The pain increases in frequency and often is associated with emesis. Initially, the child may have a normal bowel movement, but this progresses to "cranberry" or "currant-jelly" stools. Frequently there is a palpable sausage-shaped mass in the abdomen in the right upper quadrant or epigastrium and an empty right lower quadrant. A rectal examination generally obtains bloody mucus.

Once a clinical diagnosis of intussusception is suspected, the child should undergo rapid fluid resuscitation. Treatment is reduction of the intussuscepting segments (Fig. 44–6). Early in the course of the disease, if the child has no evidence of peritoneal irritation, the diagnosis can be made with a barium enema by using hydrostatic pressure fluoroscopy without abdominal pressure. With this technique, 75%

of early intussusceptions can be reduced. If not treated, the child with intussusception will develop fever and shock and will ultimately die.

Volvulus

Malrotation of the gut about the superior mesenteric artery causes severe problems in the first year of life. It is twice as common in males as in females and frequently produces symptoms in the first 2 months of life. It often leads to midgut volvulus, which progresses to intestinal obstruction and dead bowel if not treated emergently. Approximately 80% of patients develop symptoms in the first month of life, with sudden onset of bilious vomiting and rapid clinical deterioration. Abdominal distention is often localized to the upper abdomen, and peristaltic waves are visible to the examiner. Currant-jelly stools may occur secondary to vascular compromise of the gut. If not treated urgently, volvulus will lead to sepsis, perforation, and peritonitis. If the child is acutely obstructed, a history and physical examination and an upright plain radiograph of the abdomen are all that are needed to take the patient to surgery. Diagnosis may be aided by an upper gastrointestinal series, which will demonstrate obstruction and an abnormal contour in the area near the duodenal jejunal juncture, with very little barium passing beyond this point.

The mortality rate for midgut volvulus is approximately 35%, and therefore treatment with IV fluids, electrolyte replacement, and laparotomy are urgent. In midgut volvulus it is possible to lose almost all of the absorptive surface of the small bowel, thus creating a short-gut syndrome in which the patient cannot be maintained on enteral nutrition.

Hirschsprung's Disease

Hirschsprung's disease, also called *congenital megacolon* or *aganglionic megacolon*, occurs in approximately 1 in 5000 live births and is a result of a developmental dysplasia of the hindgut that produces an absence or deficiency of ganglion cells of the myenteric plexuses of the rectum and distal colon. The loss of inhibitory innervation results in contracted and obstructed aganglionic gut. The condition occurs pre-

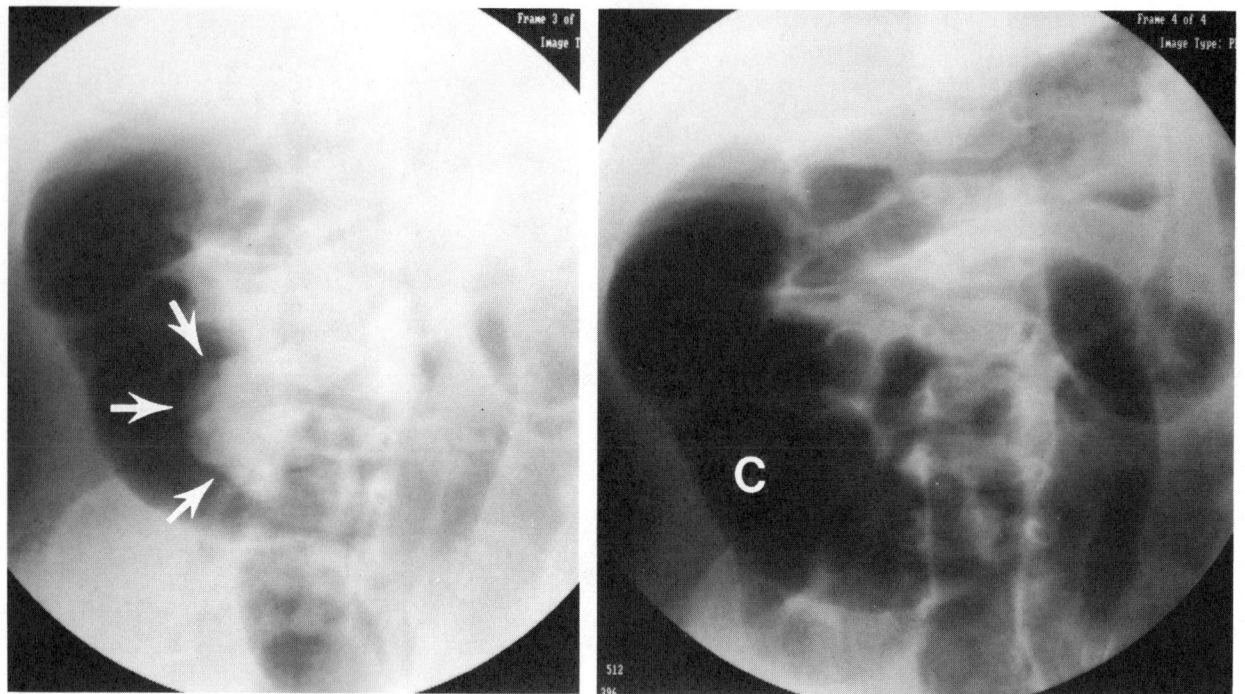

Figure 44–6. The last two views from a successful air enema reduction of intussusception in a 1-year-old who had presented with vomiting. In the left view, air surrounds the intussusceptum *(arrows)* in the left side of the cecum; in the right view, the intussusceptum has been reduced, the cecum (C) is air filled, and the distal ileal loops are also air filled. (Courtesy of A. Oestreich, M.D., Cincinnati, OH.)

dominantly in males, and most have only a short segment of bowel that is so affected. The clinical symptoms often relate to the length of bowel that is aganglionic. Down syndrome may be associated with this disease.

Clinically the patient's disease process may range from acute neonatal obstruction to chronic constipation. Most infants with Hirschsprung's disease will have a delay of more than 24 hours before passage of the first meconium stool.

Pain is generally not a feature of Hirschsprung's disease unless perforation occurs or enterocolitis develops. Unless the affected segment is very short, fecal incontinence does not occur. Children with long narrow segments of aganglionic bowel usually present with intestinal obstruction at birth, whereas those with short narrow segments generally present with intermittent constipation, thus delaying diagnosis. Diagnosis is made by barium enema, which will demonstrate a distal narrow segment running for a variable length, beginning at the rectum, and above this narrowed segment the colon will be markedly dilated.

The management of Hirschsprung's disease is designed to relieve intestinal obstruction, restore normal peristalsis, and preserve the integrity of the external anal sphincter. A colostomy may be required as a temporary measure; then the aganglionic section is removed, and a reanastomosis is undertaken.

Selected References

Friedland GW, Sunshine P, Zboralske FF. Hiatal hernia in infants and young children: A 2- to 3-year follow-up study. J Pediatr 1975;87:71.

Hacker JF, Cattau EL. Management of gastrointestinal foreign bodies. AFP 1986;34:101.

Ildstad ST, Tollerud DJ, Weiss RG, et al. Duplications of the alimentary tract. Ann Surg 1988;208:184.

Illingworth RS. Sucking and swallowing difficulties in infancy: Diagnostic problem of dysphagia. Arch Dis Child 1969;44:655.

Milla PJ. Gastrointestinal motility disorders in children. Pediatr Clin North Am 1988;35:311.

Puntis JWL, Ritson DG, Holden CE, et al. Growth and feeding problems after repair of oesophageal atresia. Arch Dis Child 1990;65:84.

Sondheimer JM. Gastroesophageal reflux: Update on pathogenesis and diagnosis. Pediatr Clin North Am 1988;35:103.

Tack ED, Perlman JM, Bower RJ, McAlister WH. Pyloric stenosis in the sick premature infant. Clinical and radiologic findings. Am J Dis Child 1988;142:68.

Utian HL, Lond DCH, Thomas RG. Cricopharyngeal incoordination in infancy. Pediatrics 1969;43:402.

Wheeler RR, Peacock JE, Cruz JM, Richter JE. Esophagitis in the immunocompromised host: Role of esophagoscopy in diagnosis. Rev Infect Dis 1987;9:88.

SECTION FIVE

Renal and Genitourinary System

CHAPTER 45

Hematuria

Barbara L. Demby

INTRODUCTION

Hematuria is common to many disorders but is pathognomonic of virtually none. It may be gross (urine is discolored) or microscopic (urine is of normal color), painless or uncomfortable; it may occur throughout the void or only during part of the void, be accompanied by other signs and symptoms or be entirely asymptomatic, or be intermittent or persistent.

In the pediatric population (younger than 20 years old) glomerulonephritis is the most common cause of hematuria, accounting for up to 50% of all cases, and urinary tract infection (UTI) is the second most common cause. In children, no cause for the hematuria is found in 9% to 22% of cases.

It is estimated that in between 4% and 6% of healthy school-age children asymptomatic hematuria is found on testing a single urine specimen. However, repeated testing performed over 6 to 12 months decreases this prevalence to 0.5% to 1.0%. The presence of asymptomatic microhematuria in the school-age population is not influenced by age or gender.

Gross hematuria is uncommon in children, with a frequency of 0.13% and a female-to-male predilection of 4:1. The presence of hematuria in an otherwise asymptomatic and healthy child is rarely indicative of serious illness. It is estimated that 50% to 75% of patients with asymptomatic microscopic hematuria have benign hematuria.

The physician will encounter the occasional patient and parent who are alarmed after seeing dark or bloody urine, as well as patients who are unaware that increased numbers of red blood cells (RBCs) are present in their urine. In most cases there is no direct correlation between the degree of hematuria and the seriousness of its origin. Microhematuria may signify a serious disease, whereas gross bleeding may be relatively benign.

DEFINITION

The continued presence of blood in sequential urine samples tested over several weeks is considered significant.

A consistent approach is needed to compare separate specimens. One method is to take a 15-ml urine sample, centrifuge it at 1500 rpm for 5 to 10 minutes, discard the supernatant, resuspend the sediment in 1 to 2 ml of residual urine, and place a uniform drop of this onto the microscope slide. More than 5 RBCs per high power field is considered significant microhematuria. Gross hematuria occurs when the number of RBCs present in the urine is sufficient to produce urine discoloration visible without magnification.

ANATOMY

Once the presence of blood in the urine has been confirmed, the anatomic site of the bleeding must be defined. RBCs can be added to the urine at any point along the urinary tract, from the glomeruli through the urethra.

Symptom Clues. Glomerular origin is suggested by oliguria, anuria, edema, hypertension, proteinuria, and RBC casts. Bleeding from the ureters, bladder, or urethra is suggested by dysuria, urgency, frequency, and flank pain. Polyuria is suggestive of obstructive uropathy, hypoplastic or dysplastic kidneys, chronic pyelonephritis, or polycystic kidney disease. Abdominal or flank pain may indicate an obstructive uropathy, nephrolithiasis, hydronephrosis, Henoch-Schönlein purpura, a renal tumor (e.g., Wilms'), acute pyelonephritis, or, if bilateral, polycystic kidney disease.

Historical Clues. A history of a skin or respiratory tract infection 1 to 3 weeks prior to the onset of hematuria may suggest poststreptococcal glomerulonephritis. Gross hematuria with, or 1 to 2 days after, a respiratory tract infection is suggestive of immunoglobulin A (IgA) nephropathy.

Color Clues. Red urine indicates bleeding from the lower urinary tract or the renal pelvis. Brown, rust-colored, or tea-colored urine is indicative of glomerular bleeding.

Pattern Clues. Urine that is uniformly bloody indicates glomerular bleeding, whereas blood that is seen only at the initiation or termination of voiding indicates bleeding from the lower urinary tract.

Shape Clues. Distorted RBCs tend to be glomerular in origin. RBCs that appear undistorted when viewed through the microscope originated distal to the glomerulus.

Miscellaneous Clues. Upper urinary tract bleeding is suspected if RBC or white blood cell (WBC) casts are present or proteinuria is greater than 2+ (approximately 150 mg/dl). The presence of blood clots suggests lower urinary tract bleeding. Rarely, structures outside the urinary tract, such as tumors, cysts, or diverticuli, may cause bleeding into the urinary tract.

PHYSIOLOGY

RBCs are normally excreted in the urine at a rate of up to 600,000 cells each day, or as many as 25,000 cells per hour. Hematuria is considered significant with an excretion rate of 30,000 RBCs per hour, which would be equivalent to approximately 2 to 8 RBCs per high power field.

The following five patterns of hematuria are recognized:

Type 1: Persistent microscopic hematuria
Type 2: Intermittent microscopic hematuria
Type 3: Persistent macroscopic (gross) hematuria
Type 4: Intermittent macroscopic hematuria
Type 5: Persistent microscopic hematuria with intermittent macroscopic hematuria

Types 1 and 2 comprise the majority of cases of hematuria seen in the pediatric population. Type 3 is seen in patients with acute glomerulonephritis, Alport's syndrome, hydronephrosis, polycystic kidney disease, UTI, trauma, and hemoglobinopathy. Types 4 and 5 are found in patients with IgA nephropathy, idiopathic benign hematuria, and hypercalciuria.

CLINICAL EVALUATION

Because of the many possible causes of hematuria in the child presenting to the emergency department, it is imperative that a brief, thorough history and physical examination be performed prior to ordering any laboratory tests or invasive procedures.

History

Important points to be covered during history taking include the onset of the hematuria, presence or absence of associated symptoms (e.g., dysuria, urgency, frequency, abdominal or flank pain, or edema), the pattern of bleeding, and the color of the urine. Any history of trauma, whether accidental or intentional, must be ascertained. The possibility of physical or sexual abuse must be considered. Recent or concurrent respiratory tract infections should also be noted. The presence of any urethral or vaginal discharge should be ascertained and a menstrual history obtained. It is also important to note any drug ingestions and whether such ingestion was acute or chronic, accidental or intentional, or consisted of a prescription drug, an illicit drug, or over-the-counter medication. A history of recent athletic activity or strenuous exertion should also be obtained.

A past medical history should include any hemoglobinopathy (e.g., sickle cell disease), coagulopathy (e.g., thrombocytopenia or hemophilia), chronic or systemic disease (e.g., systemic lupus erythematosus, diabetes mellitus), recent or chronic respiratory tract or skin disorders, congenital anomalies, past episodes of hematuria, UTI, pyelonephritis, hypercalciuria, or urinary tract stones. A family history of hematuria, nephritis, renal failure, deafness or hearing loss, renal stones, sickle cell disease or other hemoglobinopathy, hemophilia or other coagulopathy, renal anomalies, oxalosis, hypercalciuria, cystinuria, or renal tumors is significant. A travel history, especially of travel to tropical zones, is important to obtain.

Physical Examination

Vital signs are crucial to the physical examination. It is especially important to ascertain whether the patient is febrile or hypertensive. Any evidence of trauma, whether accidental or intentional, must be sought. The possibility of physical or sexual abuse must be considered. Foreign bodies and areas of tenderness should be sought. The abdomen and flanks must be examined carefully for masses, as well as for hepatomegaly and splenomegaly. The extremities should be examined to detect edema or joint involvement. Skin findings, such as rashes, petechiae, purpura, and pallor, and involvement of the mucous membranes can give important clues to the diagnosis. The examiner should also palpate for enlarged lymph nodes and an enlarged bladder (especially in males after voiding). A thorough examination of the genitalia and anus must be performed.

DIAGNOSTIC EVALUATION

In the emergency department the goal is to identify those causes of hematuria that are acutely dangerous to the patient and thus require immediate diagnosis and treatment (Table 45–1). These include trauma, acute glomerulonephritis, tumors, pyelonephritis, hemolytic-uremic syndrome, toxins, obstruction of the urinary tract, sickle cell nephritis, hemophilia, and thrombocytopenia.

Urinalysis

The first study to perform is the urinalysis, which typically consists of determination of urine pH and specific gravity; a dipstick test for blood (sometimes separated into determinations for RBCs and WBCs); determination of protein, glucose, and ketone levels; and microscopic examination of the urine to confirm the presence of any RBCs or WBCs and to search for cellular elements and casts. The presence of RBC casts in the urine specimen suggests a glomerular source for the bleeding; however, the absence of casts does not exclude glomerular origin.

The most sensitive method for detecting blood in the urine uses a reagent strip (dipstick) impregnated with orthotolidine-peroxide and enhanced with 6-methoxyquinolone. The presence of hemoglobin (or any oxidizing agent) causes the strip to turn blue. The dipsticks most commonly used (Chemstrip, Multistix, or Labstix) are quite sensitive and will detect between 0.02 and 0.03 mg/dl of hemoglobin or myoglobin. This correlates to approximately 2 to 8 RBCs per high power field in a fresh, uncentrifuged sample; more than 2 to 5 RBCs per high power field in a fresh, centrifuged sample; and an RBC excretion rate of approximately 10,000 RBCs per hour.

The false-negative rate of these dipsticks is 0.9%. One cause of false-negative dipstick tests for blood is urine that contains a high concentration of ascorbic acid. False-negative dipstick results have also been associated with high urinary pH and low specific gravity. A false-positive result (which is unusual) may occur when another oxidizing agent is present in the urine and is seen in heavily infected urine in which large amounts of bacterial peroxidase are being produced. A true-positive result on a dipstick test may indicate hematuria, myoglobinuria, or hemoglobinuria. Thus a positive urine dipstick test must be confirmed by microscopic examination of the urine. If no RBCs are seen microscopically in a fresh urine sample, then the possibility of hemoglobinuria or myoglobinuria must be considered.

If the urine appears discolored but the dipstick test is negative, the absence of blood must be confirmed by microscopic examination of the urine before it can be concluded that no blood is present. If the absence of blood in a discolored urine sample is confirmed by microscopic evaluation, then other causes of discolored urine, such as dyes, berries, and drugs (Fig. 45–1), should be considered.

TABLE 45–1

DIFFERENTIAL DIAGNOSIS

Renal diseases
  Glomerular diseases
    Glomerulonephritis (proliferative lesions)
      Postinfectious (poststreptococcal, postviral, including
        infectious mononucleosis)
      Henoch-Schönlein purpura (HSP)
      Systemic lupus erythematosus (SLE)
      IgA nephropathy (Berger's disease)
      Syphilis
      Mesangioproliferative disease
      Mesangiocapillary disease
      Focal proliferative disease
      Rapidly progressive disease
      Membranoproliferative disease
    Glomerulopathy (nonproliferative lesions)
      Familial nephritis (Alport syndrome and variants such as
        Drash syndrome)
      Vasculitis (hemolytic-uremic syndrome)
      Membranous nephropathy
      Nephrosclerosis
      Hypercalciuria
      Focal and segmental glomerulosclerosis
      Familial hematuria
      Idiopathic benign hematuria
      Lipoid nephrosis (minimal change disease)
  Nonglomerular diseases
    Interstitial nephropathy
      Infectious (tuberculosis, pyelonephritis)
      Acute tubular necrosis (ATN)
      Metabolic (nephrocalcinosis)
      Drug-induced (aspirin and other nonsteroidal anti-
        inflammatory drugs, phenacetin, phenytoin and other
        anticonvulsants, anticoagulants, penicillins,
        cephalosporins)
    Vascular and hematologic diseases
      Malformations
      Thrombosis (venous or arterial)
      Sickle cell nephropathy
      Coagulation disorder (hemophilia, thrombocytopenia,
        anticoagulant medications)
    Neoplastic diseases
      Wilms' tumor
      Others (leukemias)
    Developmental diseases
      Simple cysts
      Polycystic kidney disease
      Multicystic disease
  Medullary sponge kidney

Postrenal diseases
  Renal pelvis
    Vascular abnormalities
      Malformations
      Papillary necrosis
    Hydronephrosis
    Nephrolithiasis
    Trauma
    Ureteral pelvic junction (UPJ) obstruction
  Ureteral diseases
    Nephrolithiasis
    Inflammation (chemical or infectious [usually an infection of
      the urinary tract, but may also be seen in acute
      appendicitis])
  Bladder diseases
    Inflammation (bacterial, viral, radiation, schistosomal)
    Obstruction
    Stones
    Drugs (Cyclophosphamide)
    Tumors
    Inflammatory pseudotumor (pseudosarcoma)
    Trauma
    Foreign body
  Urethral diseases
    Inflammation
    Trauma
    Diverticula
    Friable condylomata
    Foreign body
  Prostatic disease
    Inflammation
  Other diseases
    Exercise-induced hematuria
    Pseudohematuria
      Red-diaper syndrome
      Genital or anal bleeding
      Bleeding from circumcision
      Factitious
    Pigmenturia
      Porphyria hemoglobinuria
      Myoglobinuria
      Foods (beets, blackberries, rhubarb)
      Drugs (chloroquine, quinine, daunorubicin, doxorubicin,
        rifampin, sulfamethoxazole, phenazopyridine)

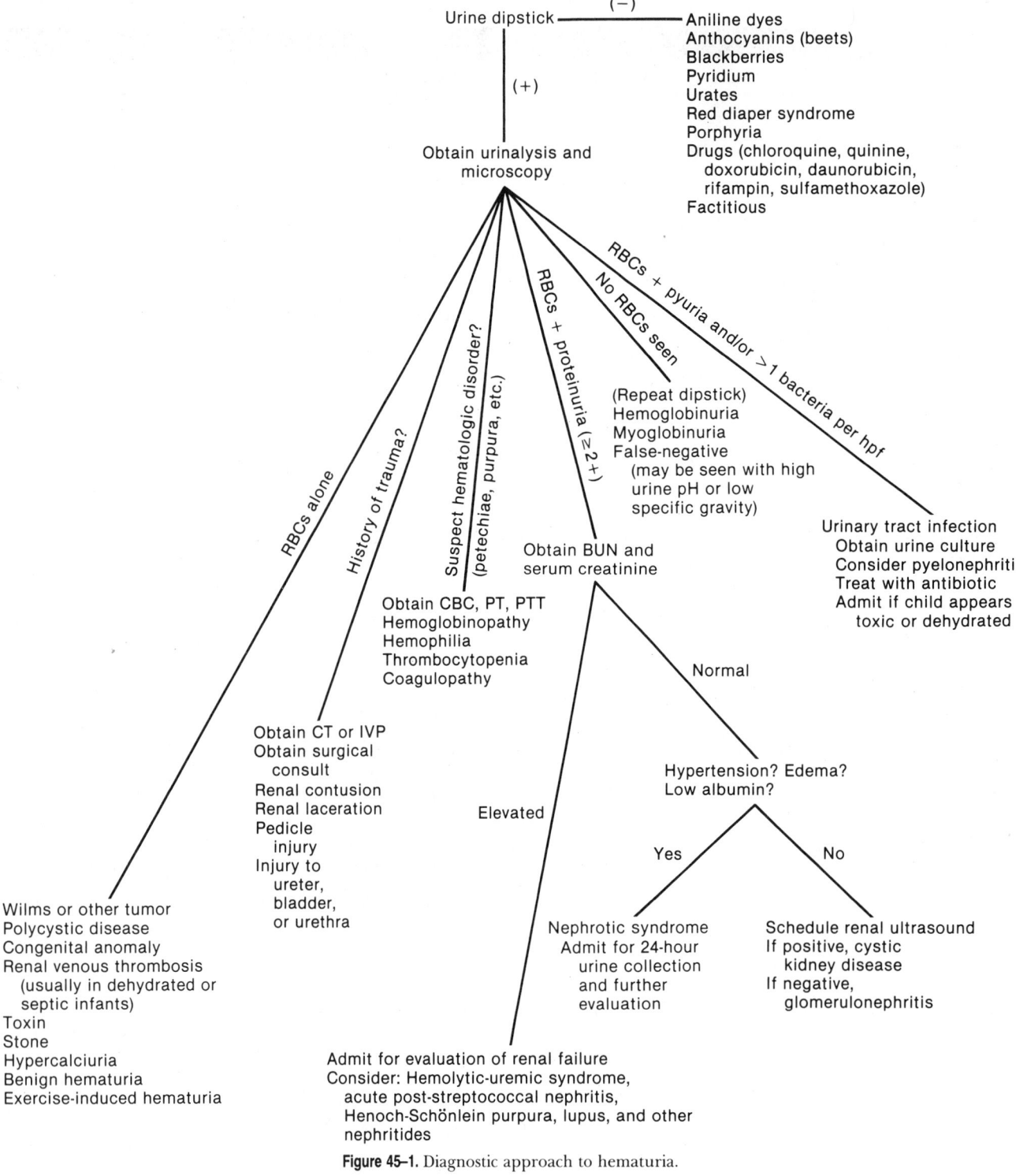

Patient presents with red or dark urine, trauma, or complaints
related to the urinary tract

Urine dipstick ———— (−) ———— Aniline dyes
Anthocyanins (beets)
Blackberries
Pyridium
Urates
Red diaper syndrome
Porphyria
Drugs (chloroquine, quinine,
doxorubicin, daunorubicin,
rifampin, sulfamethoxazole)
Factitious

(+)

Obtain urinalysis and
microscopy

RBCs + pyuria and/or > 1 bacteria per hpf
No RBCs seen
RBCs + proteinuria (≥ 2+)
Suspect hematologic disorder? (petechiae, purpura, etc.)
History of trauma?
RBCs alone

(Repeat dipstick)
Hemoglobinuria
Myoglobinuria
False-negative
(may be seen with high
urine pH or low
specific gravity)

Obtain BUN and
serum creatinine

Obtain CBC, PT, PTT
Hemoglobinopathy
Hemophilia
Thrombocytopenia
Coagulopathy

Urinary tract infection
Obtain urine culture
Consider pyelonephritis
Treat with antibiotic
Admit if child appears
toxic or dehydrated

Normal

Obtain CT or IVP
Obtain surgical
consult
Renal contusion
Renal laceration
Pedicle
injury
Injury to
ureter,
bladder,
or urethra

Hypertension? Edema?
Low albumin?

Elevated

Yes   No

Wilms or other tumor
Polycystic disease
Congenital anomaly
Renal venous thrombosis
(usually in dehydrated or
septic infants)
Toxin
Stone
Hypercalciuria
Benign hematuria
Exercise-induced hematuria

Nephrotic syndrome
Admit for 24-hour
urine collection
and further
evaluation

Schedule renal ultrasound
If positive, cystic
kidney disease
If negative,
glomerulonephritis

Admit for evaluation of renal failure
Consider: Hemolytic-uremic syndrome,
acute post-streptococcal nephritis,
Henoch-Schönlein purpura, lupus, and other
nephritides

Figure 45–1. Diagnostic approach to hematuria.

If proteinuria (greater than 2+ on the dipstick test) is found along with hematuria, the prognosis is worse than if either occurs separately. The amount of protein must be quantitated, preferably using a urine sample collected over 24 hours. However, a protein-to-creatinine ratio can be calculated on a "spot" urine sample.

If proteinuria is seen in addition to hematuria, measurements of the blood urea nitrogen (BUN), serum creatinine, and serum albumin should be obtained. If the BUN and creatinine levels are elevated, the patient should be admitted for evaluation of renal failure. The differential diagnosis includes hemolytic-uremic syndrome, acute poststreptococcal glomerulonephritis, Henoch-Schönlein purpura, systemic lupus erythematosus, and other nephritides. Depending on the circumstances of the particular patient's case, a throat culture, C3 complement titers, antistreptococcal enzyme (ASO) titers, antinuclear antibody titers, or anti-DNA antibody titers may be ordered.

If the BUN and serum creatinine levels are within normal limits but the albumin level is low and the patient exhibits symptoms of nephrotic syndrome (e.g., hypertension, edema) the child should be admitted for 24-hour urine collection and further diagnostic evaluation. If these symptoms are absent, imaging studies such as an intravenous pyelogram (IVP), computed tomography, or renal ultrasound should be scheduled to exclude cystic kidney disease and other structural anomalies. If the results of these studies are normal, the diagnosis of glomerulonephritis must be considered.

If the child has pyuria or bacteriuria in addition to hematuria, a urine culture is indicated. Gross hematuria occurs in 5% to 10% of children with urinary tract infection. The frequency of microscopic hematuria in UTI is unknown. However, it is rare to see microscopic hematuria as the only sign of a UTI, and thus a urine culture is unlikely to be useful in the child with no other signs or symptoms of a urinary tract infection. If the child has a high fever, a toxic appearance, or flank pain, the diagnosis of pyelonephritis must be considered, and the child should probably be admitted for intravenous antibiotic therapy. However, if these findings are absent, the child can usually be sent home with a prescription for an oral antibiotic (e.g., sulfamethoxazole) and a follow-up examination scheduled in 24 to 72 hours for a repeat urine culture and possibly further diagnostic tests (e.g., renal ultrasound or a voiding cystourethrogram).

If a hematologic disorder is suspected by past or family history or other signs of bleeding (e.g., petechiae or purpura) are present, a complete blood cell (CBC) count should be ordered to determine if the patient is anemic or thrombocytopenic. The prothrombin time (PT) and partial thromboplastin time (PTT) should also be determined.

If the patient with hematuria has a history of trauma, especially penetrating trauma, an urgent surgical consultation is indicated. There may be a disruption of the urinary tract anywhere from the kidney to the urethra, which will show as an extravasation of dye on an IVP and usually mandates immediate surgical exploration and repair. A computed tomography (CT) scan may be ordered in conjunction with or instead of the IVP, depending on its availability and the discretion of the surgical consultant. Obtaining an IVP in all patients with hematuria who have sustained blunt trauma is controversial. Some authors mandate its use in all patients with significant blunt abdominal trauma, whereas others feel that it is indicated only in the presence of gross hematuria or microscopic hematuria associated with hypotension, abdominal signs, severe head injury, or fracture of the pelvis or spine.

If hematuria is seen without proteinuria, pyuria, bacteriuria, signs of bleeding, or evidence of trauma, other causative factors must be considered. These include Wilms' tumor or other tumors, polycystic disease, congenital anomalies, renal venous thrombosis (usually seen in dehydrated or septic infants), toxins, urinary stones (Fig. 45–2), and hypercalciuria. These conditions may require a renal ultrasound, IVP, or quantitation of urinary calcium. Only after these causes have been excluded can the clinician diagnose benign (familial) hematuria or exercise-induced hematuria.

DISPOSITION

The need for urgent admission usually depends on the underlying cause. Several causes generally require admission (Table 45–2).

DISCHARGE INSTRUCTIONS

The discharge instructions given to the patient and the parents will vary widely depending on the cause of the hematuria. If a urinary tract infection is found, the patient will generally be given an oral antibiotic with instructions to schedule a follow-up examination with a private physician within 48 hours for a repeat urinalysis and urine culture. If a familial syndrome is suspected, not only will the patient be asked to follow up with a physician for repeat urine screening, but the parents and siblings will also need to be tested. Hearing tests may also be advisable for the patient and family members. If a developmental or anatomic abnormality is suspected, the patient should be referred to a private physician for the scheduling of an appropriate imaging study, usually a renal ultrasound. If exercise-induced hematuria is the cause, the patient should be asked to "take it easy" for the next several days. In all instances, the patient should be sent to his or her physician within 48 hours for a repeat urinalysis and should be told to return to the emergency department if there is any worsening of signs or symptoms.

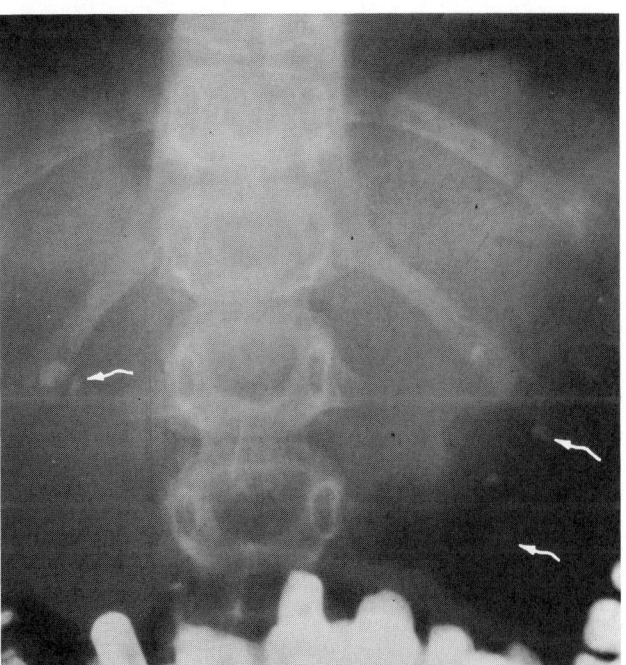

Figure 45–2. Radiograph illustrates multiple opaque renal stones (*arrows*) seen incidentally during barium enema in a 12-year-old boy with renal tubular acidosis and hyperparathyroidism. (Courtesy of A. Oestreich, M.D., Cincinnati, OH.)

TABLE 45–2
INDICATIONS FOR HOSPITAL ADMISSION IN PATIENTS WITH HEMATURIA
Trauma
Acute glomerulonephritis
Toxins
Pyelonephritis
Tumors
Hemolytic-uremic syndrome
Urinary obstruction
Urinary lithiasis
Sickle cell nephritis
Severe pain
Severe dysuria
Coagulopathy
Evidence of renal failure
Hypertension
Evidence of nephropathy
Evidence of systemic disease (i.e., systemic lupus erythematosus)
Dehydration
Anuria or oliguria
Electrolyte abnormalities
Profound blood loss
Toxic appearance
Suspicion of physical or sexual abuse

Selected References

Bloom KJ. An algorithm for hematuria. Clin Lab Med 1988;8:577.

Clarkson AR, Woodroffe AJ, Bannister KM, et al. The syndrome of IgA nephropathy. Clin Nephrol 1984;21:7.

Kraus SE, Siroky MB, Babayan RK, Krane RJ. Hematuria and the use of nonsteroidal anti-inflammatory drugs. J Urol 1984;132:288.

Mariani AJ, Luangphinith S, Loo S, et al. Dipstick chemical urinalysis: An accurate cost-effective screening test. J Urol 1984;132:64.

Stapleton FB. Nephrolithiasis in children. Pediatr Rev 1989;11:21.

Wyker AW. Standard diagnostic considerations. *In* Gillenwater JY, Grayhack JT, Howards SS, Duckett JW (eds). Adult and Pediatric Urology. 2nd ed. St Louis, Mosby-Year Book, 1991, p 68.

CHAPTER 46

Nephrotic Syndrome

Joan Bothner

INTRODUCTION

Nephrotic syndrome is a clinical syndrome resulting from massive urinary losses of protein, the origin of which may be one of a variety of underlying glomerular disorders. The current criteria for the diagnosis of nephrotic syndrome are proteinuria greater than 40 mg/m^2/day (or urine dipstick test >2+) and hypoalbuminemia (usually less than 2.5 gm/dl), often associated with edema and hypercholesterolemia. Hypertension and renal insufficiency are unusual in pediatric nephrotic syndrome. Causes of nephrotic syndrome in the pediatric age group are numerous (Table 46–1) and can be divided into primary and secondary forms. Ninety percent of cases of childhood nephrotic syndrome are primary (not related to an underlying disorder), and of these, 80% to 85% are the result of minimal-change disease.

The incidence of nephrotic syndrome is estimated to be 2 per 100,000 per year in the United States, with a similar incidence seen in the United Kingdom. The incidence is slightly higher in black, Asian, and Arab children for reasons that are unclear. A history of atopy or allergy is often present, and increased immunoglobulin E (IgE) levels are seen. Recent viral infections and immunization have also been implicated in the development of nephrotic syndrome.

PATHOPHYSIOLOGY

The primary abnormality seen in nephrotic syndrome is increased permeability of the glomerular capillary basement membrane, which leads to proteinuria. The acellular glomerular basement membrane is the major impediment to the flow of proteins and macromolecules and possesses anionic surface charges as a result of the presence of glycosaminoglycans. Cationic molecules are preferentially allowed to pass, whereas albumin and other anionic molecules are hindered. The true pathogenesis of the defect seen in minimal-change disease is unknown but is hypothesized to be related to a decrease in anionic surface charges in the basement membrane. The negative charge on the erythrocytes and platelets is reduced in minimal-change disease, and mononuclear cells from patients with minimal-change disease may produce circulating factors that induce a reduction in glomerular polyanion. A second pathogenetic mechanism may be an increase in pore size in the basement membrane, which allows passage of larger molecules. The primary result of these proposed alterations is albuminuria, but other proteins are also excreted.

Effects of Proteinuria

The major effect of the proteinuria described is hypoalbuminemia. The selectivity of the proteinuria correlates with the extent of the alteration of the glomerular permeability characteristics and can help to identify minimal-change disease without biopsy and predict initial response to steroid therapy. The quantity of proteinuria is nonspecific. The hypoalbuminemia is a result of massive renal losses, but hepatic synthesis of albumin is actually increased, possibly because of the stimulus of decreased oncotic pressure. Renal

TABLE 46–1
CAUSES OF PEDIATRIC NEPHROTIC SYNDROME
A. Primary nephrotic syndrome
1. Minimal-change disease
2. Focal glomerulosclerosis
3. Membranoproliferative glomerulonephritis
4. Membranous glomerulonephritis
5. Mesangial proliferative glomerulonephritis
6. Congenital nephrotic syndrome
B. Nephrotic syndrome as a manifestation of underlying disease (secondary nephrotic syndrome)
1. Infections—TORCH agents, poststreptococcal glomerulonephritis, hepatitis B, malaria, acquired immunodeficiency syndrome
2. Systemic disease—systemic lupus erythematosus, diabetes mellitus, Henoch-Schönlein purpura, sickle cell anemia
3. Neoplasia—Wilms' tumor, lymphoma
4. Renal disease—hemolytic-uremic syndrome, rapidly progressive glomerulonephritis
5. Allergic reactions—envenomations, serum sickness, poison plants
6. Drug exposure—heroin, heavy metals

TORCH = *T*oxoplasmosis, *r*ubella, *c*ytomegalovirus, and *h*erpes simplex.

catabolism of albumin, usually an extrarenal event, is increased by five times and, along with the inability of hepatic synthesis to keep up with losses, leads to edema.

Other proteins lost include vitamin D–binding globulin and bound hydroxyvitamin D, which leads to osteomalacia and altered vitamin D metabolism. The loss of thyroxin-binding globulin can lead to hypothyroidism. Transferrin loss may lead to iron deficiency anemia. Loss of immunoglobulin G (IgG) and factor B play a role in increased susceptibility to infection and defective opsonization. Decreased levels of antithrombin III and plasminogen increase the risk of thrombosis and lead to abnormal fibrinolysis. Several proteins are increased in nephrotic syndrome, possibly secondary to the overall increased hepatic protein production induced by hypoalbuminemia and decreased colloid oncotic pressure. These include antifibrinolysins, coagulation factors V and VIII, and lipoproteins, which contribute to altered clotting mechanisms and increased thrombotic tendencies.

The classic hypothesis for the edema seen in nephrotic syndrome is altered Starling forces resulting from decreased colloid oncotic pressure, which activate the renin-angiotensin-aldosterone system and ultimately lead to sodium and water retention and resultant edema. Evidence that some nephrotic patients have normal or low renin and aldosterone levels and normal or increased blood and plasma volumes has led to the hypothesis that the edema is caused by increased blood volume and decreased colloid oncotic pressure in the presence of impaired renal function.

Hyperlipidemia is a well-described feature of nephrotic syndrome. Serum cholesterol levels are consistently elevated and are inversely related to serum albumin levels. Hyperlipidemia may be affected by age, diet, steroid use, or diuretic therapy, and its significance in later atherosclerotic coronary vascular disease and progression of glomerulosclerosis is unknown.

CLASSIFICATION OF NEPHROTIC SYNDROME

Many glomerular diseases may present as nephrosis. The majority (more than 90%) of cases in children are primary or idiopathic. The primary forms have distinguishing clinical as well as characterized morphologic differences that permit precise classification from biopsy specimens when evaluated under light, immunofluorescent, or electron microscopy. The primary glomerular diseases that evoke the nephrotic syndrome in children are minimal-change disease, focal glomerulosclerosis, membranoproliferative glomerulonephritis, membranous glomerulonephritis, and mesangial proliferative glomerulonephritis.

Minimal-Change Disease

Minimal change disease (MCD), also known as *minimal-change nephrotic syndrome*, *lipoid nephrosis*, and *nil disease*, accounts for 75% to 80% of prepubertal disease. The age of onset is usually less than 10 years, with a median age of 3 years. There is a male-to-female ratio of 2:1. The typical presentation is one of dependent edema, which is initially periorbital, later becoming generalized. Proteinuria is selective, and microscopic hematuria occurs in 10% to 20% of patients. Hypertension is unusual, occurring in only 10% to 15% of patients. Renal function is normal, as is the serum C3 level. Progression to end-stage renal disease is rare. About 95% of patients are initially steroid responsive. The presence of gross hematuria is rare and should prompt investigation for another underlying lesion. Urine output may be decreased or normal, and the urine is concentrated.

Focal Glomerulosclerosis

Focal glomerulosclerosis (FGS) accounts for 6% to 12% of cases of nephrotic syndrome in children. The age at onset is usually 1 to 10 years, with a median of 6 years, and there is a slight male preponderance. Proteinuria is poorly selective. The reported incidence of hematuria varies, but hematuria occurs in most patients and is usually microscopic. Hypertension is present in 25% to 50% of patients, and 20% of patients present with asymptomatic proteinuria. Renal insufficiency is present in 25% to 40% of patients, response to steroids is variable (20% to 60% reported), and progression to end-stage renal disease occurs within 5 years in 20% to 30% of patients and within 10 years in 50%. Recurrence after renal transplantation is the rule. The histologic finding of FGS is seen in pediatric patients in association with nephrotic syndrome and vesicoureteral reflux, drug abuse (heroin), acquired immunodeficiency syndrome (AIDS), sickle cell disease, type I glycogen storage disease, malignancies, Henoch-Schönlein purpura, and Alport's syndrome.

Membranoproliferative Glomerulonephritis

Membranoproliferative glomerulonephritis (MPGN) accounts for 5% to 7% of cases of pediatric nephrotic syndrome, and only 50% of patients with MPGN present in a nephrotic state. The incidence increases after 6 years of age and is most prevalent between the ages of 10 years and 20 years; females slightly outnumber males. Distinctive features include hematuria (50% to 80%), which may be macroscopic; hypertension (35% to 50%); and decreased serum C3 level (75% to 80%). Evidence of renal insufficiency is present in almost half of patients, anemia is common (possibly a reflection of chronic disease), and proteinuria is moderately to poorly selective. Microscopy reveals enlarged and lobular glomeruli with proliferation of mesangial cells and resultant "tram track" appearance. Crescent formation is seen in severe cases because of a proliferation of epithelial cells. The response to steroids is poor, and end-stage renal disease develops in 50% to 70% of patients within 10 years. MPGN is associated with multiple secondary diseases leading to nephrotic syndrome, including systemic lupus erythematosus, sickle cell disease, hepatitis B, hemolytic-uremic syndrome, endocarditis, ventriculoatrial shunt infection, and malaria.

Membranous Glomerulonephritis

Membranous glomerulonephritis (MGN) is unusual in children, accounting for only 1% to 2% of cases of pediatric nephrotic syndrome. Onset usually occurs in adolescence. Hypertension is unusual, occurring in less than 10% of patients. Hematuria occurs in 80% of patients and is macroscopic in 20%. Renal function at presentation is normal, as is serum C3 level. Patients have a poor response to steroids, and 20% develop end-stage renal disease. MGN is most often associated with infections, including syphilis, malaria, and poststreptococcal disease. It is prevalent in young black males and is associated with hepatitis B infection. It also occurs with systemic lupus erythematosus, sickle cell disease, Fanconi's anemia, drugs (heavy metals, captopril) and has occurred de novo following renal transplantation. Pathologic findings include thickened basement membranes without cellular proliferation and thickened glomerular capillary walls as a result of deposition of immune complexes in the glomerular basement membrane.

Mesangial Proliferative Glomerulonephritis

Mesangial proliferative glomerulonephritis is characterized by a mild proliferation of the mesangial matrix with mesangial immunoglobulin M (IgM) deposition and is thought by some to be a progression in the spectrum of minimal-change disease. It accounts for 2% of cases of idiopathic nephrotic syndrome. Renal function and serum C3 levels are normal. Hematuria occurs in 80% of patients, and hypertension is unusual. Steroid sensitivity is usual, and a frequently relapsing course is common.

Nephrotic Syndrome in Infancy

Nephrotic syndrome that presents in the first year of life deserves special mention. True idiopathic congenital nephrotic syndrome is rare, occurs during the first 3 months of life, and accounts for 1.5% of all cases of pediatric nephrotic syndrome. Affected infants are usually premature and small for gestational age.

Nephrotic syndrome is commonly associated with umbilical hernias. The placenta is often large and edematous, and elevated levels of alpha-fetoprotein are usually found in the amniotic fluid. Infants may present with poor feeding, vomiting, failure to thrive, and malnutrition, as well as with frank edema, which may take weeks to develop. Some affected infants are found as a result of neonatal screening for hypothyroidism. Proteinuria is present at birth, and hematuria is common. Severe infections, including pneumonia, meningitis, sepsis, and urinary tract infections, affect 80% of infants in the first year of life, and decreased renal function becomes apparent by the second birthday, along with hypertension and uremia. The incidence of thromboembolic phenomena approaches 10%, with involvement of the peripheral arteries, renal and pulmonary veins, and the sagittal sinus. Profound developmental delay may be seen, along with seizures caused by metabolic abnormalities. Infants are often hypothyroid, iron deficient, vitamin D deficient, and severely immunocompromised.

Other causes of nephrotic syndrome in the first 3 months of life include congenital infections (toxoplasmosis, cytomegalovirus, rubella, herpes, and syphilis), toxins, systemic lupus erythematosus, Wilms' tumor, renal vein thrombosis, hemolytic-uremic syndrome, nail-patella syndrome, and XY gonadal dysgenesis. Nephrotic syndrome presenting after the age of 6 months is usually idiopathic; histologic studies have revealed MCD, FGS, and diffuse mesangial sclerosis. There is usually a response to steroids and to cytotoxic agents, although no studies have been done on infants younger than 1 year. All patients who present under 1 year of age need referral to a pediatric nephrologist, along with renal biopsy for optimal diagnosis and management.

CLINICAL EVALUATION

The most common clinical presentation of nephrotic syndrome in pediatric patients is that of minimal-change disease. The typical patient is a young male who presents with asymptomatic edema that had first been periorbital and perhaps attributed to an allergy or sinus problem. Flu-like symptoms may have preceded the presentation, as nausea, vomiting, and anorexia are often symptoms of bowel edema. An allergy history may be evident, and the child may have recently been immunized. Urine output may be decreased, and the urine may seem concentrated. Hypertension is rarely seen but, when present, may be a result of increased intravascular fluid volume with a chronic glomerulonephritis or may reflect an excessive vasoconstrictive response to decreased circulating plasma volume. Children with ascites may present with nausea and vomiting, and respiratory distress, although rare, may accompany ascites or pleural effusions. Pericardial effusions are rare. Overall, edema with minimal symptomatology is the most common presentation.

DIAGNOSTIC EVALUATION

Laboratory evaluation (Table 46–2) in nephrotic syndrome can be divided into several categories: studies needed for diagnosis, studies that help gauge severity, studies that may delineate origin, and studies necessary to evaluate for the presence of the many complications associated with nephrotic syndrome. Studies necessary for diagnosis include a urinalysis for quantitative protein (usually 3-4+ on a dipstick test) and serum protein and albumin determinations. Baseline laboratory determinations should also include serum electrolytes, blood urea nitrogen, creatinine, cholesterol, and a complete blood cell count to assess hemoconcentration and possible thrombocytosis. Complement levels should be determined in patients who are hypertensive, have macroscopic hematuria, or exhibit evidence of impaired renal function. Cholesterol and triglyceride levels help determine severity, and the serum C3 level will be decreased in patients with MPGN, systemic lupus erythematosus, and poststreptococcal glomerulonephritis. Urine should be evaluated for the presence of hematuria, and the presence of macroscopic hematuria should prompt investigation for underlying causes other than minimal-change disease. Sickle cell anemia should be ruled out. Also of note is the presentation of acute poststreptococcal glomerulonephritis as nephrotic syndrome in patients with sickle cell disease. In patients with atypical presentations (i.e., with severe hypertension or evidence of renal insufficiency), laboratory evaluation to delineate the origin of the underlying disorder should include serum tests for hepatitis and syphilis and quantification of serum antistreptolysin O (ASO), antinuclear antibodies (ANA), and immunoglobulins.

Common laboratory abnormalities include hyponatremia (secondary to hyperlipidemia and dilution) and hypocalcemia. Mild elevation of the erythrocyte sedimentation rate can be seen. Anemia is rare, and an elevated white blood cell count may be indicative of infection. Serum IgM and IgE levels may be increased, although the serum IgG level is uniformly low. Serum blood urea nitrogen and creatinine levels are normal or only mildly elevated secondary to hypovolemia. Twenty-four–hour urine collections for quantification of proteinuria reveal protein excretion in excess of 40 mg/m²/hour or 50 mg/kg/24 hr.

DIFFERENTIAL DIAGNOSIS

The accurate diagnosis of a patient who presents with "classic" nephrotic syndrome with proteinuria, hypoalbu-

---

TABLE 46–2
NEPHROTIC SYNDROME: THERAPY AT A GLANCE

A. Newly diagnosed, stable patient
  1. Mild sodium restriction
  2. Tuberculin skin test
  3. Prednisone, 60 mg/m²/day divided after consultation with follow-up physician tid until remission, then 40 mg/m² every other day
B. Patient with refractory edema
  1. Mildly decreased serum albumin and hemodynamically stable: furosemide, 1 mg/kg/day, or hydrochlorothiazide, 1 mg/kg/day
  2. Significantly depressed serum albumin: 1 gm/kg 25% albumin IV over several hours; may be followed by judicious use of diuretic to establish urine flow
C. Hypovolemic patient
  1. Fluid resuscitation with 20 ml/kg isotonic fluid if intravascular volume depletion is evident
  2. Intravenous infusion of 1 gm/kg 25% albumin, repeated as needed

minemia, and generalized edema is no problem. Differentiating between minimal-change disease and the other causes of idiopathic nephrotic syndrome is possible by carefully evaluating the child for hypertension, gross hematuria, and renal insufficiency. The secondary causes of nephrotic syndrome are often evident by their primary mode of presentation (i.e., Henoch-Schönlein purpura, hemolytic-uremic syndrome). The presence of significant proteinuria (3+ to 4+ on a dipstick test) confirms a renal origin of edema.

The evaluation of the child who presents with generalized edema without proteinuria includes a careful history and physical examination, with attention to possible ingestion or toxic exposure and relation to menstrual cycle in adolescent females. Thorough cardiovascular evaluation for the presence of congestive heart failure or pericarditis is essential and should include evaluation for tachycardia, tachypnea, rales, hepatomegaly, muffled heart tones, jugular venous distention, and pulsus paradoxus. Edema may also be seen with certain gastrointestinal disorders, including liver failure, severe hepatitis, biliary atresia, cirrhosis, chronic protein malnutrition, protein-losing enteropathy, and cystic fibrosis. Edema formation with these conditions is usually more insidious in onset. Localized edema, as seen with trauma, cellulitis, urticaria, thrombophlebitis, and lymphedema, is not seen in nephrotic syndrome. Edema associated with severe allergic reactions is evident by history and presentation.

THERAPEUTIC INTERVENTION

The management of patients with nephrotic syndrome is contingent on their mode of presentation, as the problems and complications seen in new-onset patients differ from those seen in patients who are on chronic therapy for their disease. The major problems seen in newly diagnosed patients include edema, hypovolemia, infection, and thrombotic phenomena. The edema in nephrotic syndrome is often bothersome but not debilitating and can often be controlled with salt restriction. Severe edema that is associated with gastrointestinal or respiratory symptoms, decreased activity, or skin irritation is an indication for management with diuretics. Furosemide, 1 to 2 mg/kg/day in divided doses, is effective and is often combined with a potassium-sparing diuretic in order to prevent severe kaliuresis. Hydrochlorothiazide, 1 mg/kg/day, can also be used. Diuretics are ineffective when the serum albumin level is below 1.5 gm/dl, and in patients with severe hypoalbuminemia and edema, therapy with salt-poor albumin (1 gm/kg of 25% albumin IV given over 4 hours), followed by furosemide, is indicated (see Table 46–3). The effect of intravenous albumin is transient, lasting only 24 to 48 hours. Careful evaluation of intravascular fluid volume is essential before the institution of any diuretic therapy to avoid further contraction and resultant hypovolemic shock. Long-term sequelae of diuretic use include metabolic alkalosis, hyperglycemia, hyperuricemia, hyperlipidemia, and interstitial nephritis, which may ultimately worsen the patient's renal disease. Thrombosis and acute renal failure have been linked to overly aggressive diuresis. Metolazone, a diuretic with its site of action at the distal tubule, is given in a dose of 0.1 to 0.4 mg/kg/day combined with furosemide; this combination has been shown to increase natriuresis and decrease edema more effectively than furosemide alone and may be used in cases of severe edema resistant to furosemide therapy.

Hypovolemia is often associated with vomiting and diarrhea, decreased intake secondary to illness, sepsis, and overzealous diuretic administration. The evaluation of a nephrotic patient for evidence of hypovolemia can be difficult in the presence of significant peripheral edema and must include documentation of heart rate, perfusion, blood pressure, mental status, and urine output. Blood pressure may be increased because of reflex vasoconstriction. Early signs of hypovolemia include abdominal pain, and laboratory evaluation reveals increases in hemoglobin and hematocrit. Initial treatment of symptomatic hypovolemia is intravenous administration of 20 ml/kg of isotonic fluid to restore circulating intravascular volume. Additional therapy includes intravenous infusion of 25% albumin (1 gm/kg) with addition of diuretics as necessary to establish urine output.

Infection must be suspected and excluded in any febrile child with nephrotic syndrome and, if present, should be treated promptly and aggressively. Common infections include cellulitis of edematous skin, peritonitis, sepsis, meningitis, pneumonia, and urinary tract infections. Infection is the leading cause of death in nephrotic children, despite advances in antibiotic therapy. The most common pathogen is *Streptococcus pneumoniae*; other pathogens include *Haemophilus influenzae*, *Klebsiella*, alpha streptococcus, and *Escherichia coli*. Some studies have implicated an increased incidence of peritonitis caused by gram-negative organisms. In one study, the clinical symptoms of patients with peritonitis included abdominal pain (98%), fever (95%), rebound tenderness (85%), and nausea and vomiting (71%). A complete blood cell count, urine culture, and blood culture should be obtained in all patients suspected of having an infection, and empiric antibiotic treatment should be started. Current recommendations for choice of antibiotics based on known common pathogens include ampicillin and gentamicin or a broad-spectrum cephalosporin. A diagnostic peritoneal tap should be performed in any child suspected of having peritonitis.

Children with nephrotic syndrome are also at risk for thrombotic complications because of hyperviscosity associated with hypovolemia and a generalized hypercoagulable state. Hypercoagulability is believed to be caused by increased plasma fibrinogen, decreased antithrombin III, increased platelet count, and platelet hyperfunction. Thrombosis has occurred at both arterial and venous sites, including the deep leg and renal veins, as well as in the subclavian, axillary, brachial, pulmonary, femoral, carotid, and cerebral arteries. Renal vein thrombosis is more common in adults than in children and presents with flank pain, hematuria, and evidence of decreased renal function. Evaluation includes renal ultrasound and contrast-enhanced computed tomography (CT) scan. Magnetic resonance imaging (MRI) may also be utilized. Cerebral artery thrombosis appears to be more common than cerebral venous thrombosis. Initial treatment includes heparinization followed by oral anticoagulation. Urokinase has been successfully used in patients with severe pulmonary thrombosis. Symptoms of pulmonary thrombosis include tachycardia, tachypnea, cyanosis, hemoptysis, elevated blood pressure, and right bundle branch block shown on electrocardiogram (EKG). Diagnosis is made by arteriography or ventilation-perfusion scanning.

Acute renal failure has been described in patients with nephrotic syndrome, usually in association with hypovolemia and circulatory collapse, but it may also occur with bilateral renal vein thrombosis or a nephrotoxic injury. Renal failure resulting from intravascular volume depletion is treated with intravenous albumin and plasma volume expanders, with cautious administration of diuretics to establish urine flow. Renal failure has also occurred without evidence of volume depletion and is postulated to be secondary to increased intrarenal edema and resultant decreased glomerular filtration. Treatment demands prompt recognition and institution of diuretic therapy; steroids have also been beneficial. Recovery usually occurs.

The mainstay of chronic therapy in nephrotic syndrome,

specifically in minimal-change disease, is glucocorticoids. The aim of therapy is to induce remission of proteinuria. More than 90% of nephrotic pediatric patients respond to an initial course of prednisone, although 60% relapse. The initial dosage of prednisone in uncomplicated nephrotic syndrome that fits the clinical spectrum of minimal-change disease is 60 mg/m²/day or 2 mg/kg/day (maximum 80 mg) in divided doses until remission occurs. Remission is defined as absence of proteinuria on a urine dipstick test for 2 to 3 consecutive days. Most patients achieve remission by 1 to 2 weeks after institution of therapy, and after remission occurs, the dose is reduced to 40 mg/m² on alternate days for an additional 4 weeks. Evidence suggests that a continued gradually tapered dose rather than cessation of prednisone at this point leads to a lower rate of relapse. A relapsing course is typical, with 50% to 80% of patients relapsing two or more times within the first 6 months of diagnosis; these are known as *frequent relapsers*.

Cytotoxic agents have been used in nephrotic syndrome for more than 30 years, and indications for their use include steroid resistance, a frequently relapsing course, steroid dependence, and significant steroid toxicity. Because of their inherent significant toxicity, these agents should be used only under the direct supervision of a pediatric nephrologist. Cyclophosphamide, 2.0 to 2.5 mg/kg/day over a 6- to 12-week period and usually used in conjunction with alternate-day steroid therapy, has been shown to increase the length of time between relapses in patients with a frequently relapsing course. Results in patients with steroid resistance are not as clear. A course of cyclophosphamide may also increase responsiveness to steroids in later relapses. Chlorambucil, 0.1 to 0.2 mg/kg/day with a maximum cumulative dose of 10 mg/kg, has also been used but has not been shown to be any more effective than cyclophosphamide.

Cyclosporin has been introduced as a promising therapeutic agent, with its mechanism of action being suppression of T-cell function by interfering with interleukin-2 production. Current recommended doses are 4 to 7 mg/kg/day given with alternate-day, low-dose steroid therapy. Preliminary results have demonstrated the induction of remission in steroid-resistant and frequently relapsing patients. The stability of long-term remission remains to be determined. A significant side effect is impairment of renal function, and abnormalities of facial growth and unconjugated hyperbilirubinemia have occurred in children.

Nonsteroidal anti-inflammatory agents are not recommended in pediatric patients, for although they have been demonstrated to decrease proteinuria, their mechanism of action is by decreasing glomerular filtration. A tuberculin skin test should be placed before the institution of steroid therapy, and children should not be immunized with attenuated viral vaccines during therapy with steroids or cytotoxic agents. Any exposure to varicella should be treated with varicella-zoster immune globulin.

DISPOSITION

Children who present to the emergency department with new-onset nephrotic syndrome and who fit the clinical description of minimal-change disease may usually be discharged home with follow-up arranged with their private physician. A tuberculin skin test placed in the emergency department may hasten definitive therapy with steroids. Children older than 6 years who present with hypertension, hematuria, or evidence of impaired renal function should be admitted for further evaluation to elucidate the underlying cause of their disease (Table 46–3). Mildly symptomatic edema may be managed conservatively, and patients with mild dehydration and hypoalbuminemia may be treated with

TABLE 46–3
ADMISSION CRITERIA IN PEDIATRIC NEPHROTIC SYNDROME
Newly diagnosed patients with unusual clinical presentation
Suspicion of systemic infection
Evidence of thrombotic event
Significant hypovolemia and dehydration
Acceleration of hypertension
Evidence of increasing renal insufficiency
Refractory edema
Respiratory distress
Severe hypoalbuminemia

oral fluid replacement. Subspecialty consultation should be sought in patients with evidence of dehydration with significant hypoalbuminemia or refractory edema. Absolute indications for admission include evidence or suspicion of infection, respiratory distress, evidence of thromboembolism, severe dehydration, and renal insufficiency.

Discharge instructions to parents should include warnings regarding fever, cough, tachypnea, anorexia, abdominal pain, chest pain, vomiting, increasing edema, and decreasing urine output (Table 46-4). They should be advised to inform their physician of any suspected exposures to measles or varicella, or any unexplained behavioral changes. The side effects of all discharge medications should be carefully explained. The parents should be advised about any planned immunizations and instructed to allow the child full activity as tolerated. Dietary advice should include mild salt restriction and adequate protein intake.

OTHER CONSIDERATIONS

Renal biopsy is indicated in children younger than 1 year, children over 6 yrs, or adolescents; in nephrotic syndrome with unusual characteristics (e.g., evidence of impaired renal function); in patients unresponsive to 6 weeks of steroid therapy; and in frequently relapsing or steroid-dependent patients. Complications of renal biopsy that may be seen in the emergency department include macroscopic hematuria (5%), which usually resolves spontaneously within 2 days, perirenal hematomas (1%), and hematuria requiring transfusion (0.5% to 2.0%). Other complications include arteriovenous (AV) fistulas, puncture of viscera or major renal vessels, infection, and sepsis. Pneumothorax, pancreatitis, and renal pelvis perforation with resultant urinoma have also occurred. AV fistulas are characterized by a bruit heard over the biopsy site, hypertension, persistent hematuria, and an increase in pulse pressure. The mortality rate is less than 0.1%. Pain and mild bleeding at the biopsy site are also common.

A peritoneal tap is indicated for diagnosis of suspected peritonitis or, rarely, for relief of respiratory distress secondary to a large amount of ascitic fluid. The procedure may be performed with the child sitting or in a lateral decubitus position. The best site for entry into the peritoneal cavity is the midline, just above or below the umbilicus. After sterile preparation of the intended site, the skin is anesthetized with 1% lidocaine. The skin is then punctured perpendicular to the abdominal wall, moved laterally a short distance (a "Z track"), and then advanced until a pop is felt. An 18-, 20-, or 22-gauge over-the-needle catheter attached to a syringe should be used. As soon as decreased resistance is appreciated, fluid should be withdrawn into the syringe to verify placement in the peritoneal cavity. The needle and catheter are then slowly advanced with continued aspiration, the needle is then removed from the catheter, and the

TABLE 46–4

DISCHARGE INSTRUCTIONS IN PEDIATRIC NEPHROTIC SYNDROME

Maintain low-salt diet
Immediately contact health care provider in case of fever, abdominal pain, chest pain, difficulty breathing, nausea and vomiting, or increased headache
Avoid active chickenpox and notify health care provider of exposure
Maintain normal activity as tolerated
Avoid live virus vaccines (MMR)
Perform daily urine dipstick tests for protein after therapy is begun
Review side effects of discharge medication

MMR = measles, mumps, rubella.

catheter is attached to a stopcock, tubing, and large syringe apparatus. Fluid can then be freely aspirated and the patient safely positioned to allow maximum withdrawal. Potential complications include bleeding, infection, and perforation of abdominal contents. Pulmonary effusions rarely require thoracentesis for symptomatic relief.

Selected Readings

Assar R, Pitel P, Lammer N, et al. Acute poststreptococcal glomerulonephritis and sickle-cell disease. Child Nephrol Urol 1989;9:176.

Churg J, Habib R, White RHR. Pathology of the nephrotic syndrome in children. A report for the International Study of Kidney Diseases in Children. Lancet 1970;1:1299.

Diaz-Buxo J, Donadio J Jr. Complications of percutaneous renal biopsy: An analysis of 1,000 consecutive biopsies. Clin Nephrol 1975;4:223.

Habib R, Kleinknecht C, Gubler MC, et al. Idiopathic membranoproliferative glomerulonephritis in children: report of 105 cases. Clin Nephrol 1973;1:194.

Hoyer JR, Anderson CE. Congenital nephrotic syndrome. Clin Perinatol 1981;8:333.

International Study of Kidney Disease in Children. Nephrotic syndrome in children: Prediction of histopathology from clinical and laboratory characteristics at the time of diagnosis. Kidney Int 1978;13:159.

International Study of Kidney Disease in Children. The primary nephrotic syndrome in children: Identification of patients with minimal change nephrotic syndrome from initial response to prednisone. J Pediatr 1981;98:561.

Kaysen GA, Gambestoglio J, Felts J, et al. Albumin synthesis, albuminuria, and hyperlipidemia in nephrotic patients. Kidney Int 1987;31:1368.

Kher K, Sweet M, Makker S. Nephrotic syndrome in children. Curr Probl Pediatr 1988;18:197.

Koskimies O, Vilski J, Rapola J, et al. Long-term outcome of primary nephrotic syndrome. Arch Dis Child 1982;57:544.

Mahan JD Jr, Hoyer JR, Vernier RL. Nephrotic syndrome in the first year of life. In Cameron J, Glassock R (eds). The Nephrotic Syndrome. New York, Dekker, 1988, pp 401–422.

Makker SP, Heymann W. The idiopathic nephrotic syndrome: a clinical re-evaluation of 148 cases. Am J Dis Child 1981;56:517.

Schnaper H. The immune system in minimal change nephrotic syndrome. Pediatr Nephrol 1989;3:101.

Trompeter R. Immunosuppressive therapy in the nephrotic syndrome in children. Pediatr Nephrol 1989;3:194.

CHAPTER 47

Henoch-Schönlein Purpura

Ann N. Champoux

INTRODUCTION

Henoch-Schönlein purpura (HSP) is a systemic vasculitis in which the principal clinical manifestations involve the skin, joints, gastrointestinal (GI) tract, and kidneys. It may be the most common vasculitic syndrome affecting children. Some authors believe that the characteristic visceral manifestations may occur without the skin lesions; hence the term *Henoch-Schönlein syndrome*. Other names include anaphylactoid purpura, allergic purpura, and allergic vasculitis.

This disease has a predilection for children and young adults. Its peak incidence is between the ages of 4 to 5 years, but it has been reported in infants as young as 6 months. The incidence of HSP among children younger than 15 years is approximately 0.2 to 1.0 per 10,000 per year. Boys are affected more frequently than girls by a ratio of approximately 1.5:1; most patients are white. There appears to be a seasonal incidence, with more reported cases in the winter and early spring. It is unusual for more than one family member to develop the syndrome.

Although HSP has been recognized as a distinct clinical entity for more than a century, its origin remains uncertain. Although a history of preceding infection or fever is frequently obtained, a specific pathogen has not been consistently demonstrated. Some causal or precipitating factors implicated have included infections (*Streptococcus*, *Mycoplasma pneumoniae*, hepatitis B), numerous drugs (aspirin, antibiotics), food allergens (chocolate, milk, eggs, wheat, beans), insect bites, vaccinations, and exposure to cold.

PATHOPHYSIOLOGY

HSP represents a small-vessel vasculitis involving the capillaries as well as the postcapillary arterioles and venules. There is leukocytic and lymphocytic infiltration, necrosis of vessel walls, and extravasation of red cells into surrounding tissue. These abnormalities account for the clinical findings in the affected areas of skin, GI tract, and other organs. Deposits containing immunoglobulin A (IgA), C3, fibrin, and fibrinogen have been detected in the purpuric skin, GI tract, and the kidney.

Kidney pathology in patients with HSP has received much attention, and many similarities have been found with the kidney abnormalities seen in IgA nephropathy (Berger's disease). As in IgA nephropathy, there is great variability in the morphologic changes observed in the kidney.

CLINICAL EVALUATION

The clinical manifestations in HSP are a consequence of the underlying vasculitis, and therefore, virtually any organ may be affected. The common target organs are the skin, joints, kidneys, and GI tract, with less likely targets being the scrotal sac, nervous system, heart, and lungs (Table 47–1). The syndrome usually presents in an otherwise healthy child and is associated with a preceding upper respiratory tract infection in as many as two thirds of patients. The

---

TABLE 47–1

SIGNS AND SYMPTOMS OF HSP

Skin
  Palpable purpuric rash primarily over buttocks and legs
  Maculopapular or urticarial rash initially in some patients
  Subcutaneous edema over hands and feet
GI tract
  Episodic abdominal pain and vomiting
  GI bleeding
  Intussusception
  Perforation
Joints
  Large-joint swelling and pain
Kidneys
  Microscopic hematuria or gross hematuria
  Nephritis or nephrotic syndrome
  Renal failure

---

onset may be acute, with the simultaneous appearance of several symptoms, or gradual, with manifestations appearing over several weeks. The skin, joint, and GI manifestations of HSP may occur in any order. Rash is the first sign in more than half of the patients. Two thirds may develop simultaneous involvement of the skin, GI tract, and joints within the first few days. In the remaining one third, the abdominal and joint symptoms may precede the purpura by several weeks. In a given patient, the involved target organs usually manifest during the initial 3 months; however, a new target organ may rarely become involved up to a year later.

Skin

The skin is a major target organ in many vasculitis syndromes and is involved in nearly 100% of patients with HSP. The rash most frequently consists of small, palpable, purpuric spots that appear in crops that may coalesce to form large ecchymotic areas. Pinpoint petechiae may also be present. In one third of the patients this rash may be preceded by a maculopapular or urticarial rash that evolves to the characteristic purpuric eruption within 48 hours in most patients. Sometimes vesicles or bullae are seen. The purpuric lesions progress in the usual manner of ecchymosis, changing from red to purple to brown. The rash in HSP is usually characteristic in its distribution, with involvement confined to the area below the waist, mainly the buttocks and lower legs. The trunk is usually spared, but limited involvement may be seen on the hands, elbows, and face. The purpura, which appears to be gravity dependent, resolves more quickly with bed rest; it then reappears in fresh crops when the patient resumes ambulation. The rash has a median duration of 14 days but may be transient and recurrent for several months or even years.

Subcutaneous edema is seen in 25% to 35% of children and consists of localized, painless, nonpitting swelling, usually over the dorsal aspects of the hands or feet. This edema may also affect the scalp, forehead, periorbital area, or perineum, where it is generally quite painful. Children under 2 years of age are more likely to develop this edema and are also more likely to exhibit an urticarial rather than purpuric rash. Infants with HSP may have edema as their only cutaneous manifestation.

GI Tract

Gastrointestinal manifestations are seen in 50% to 90% of children. The most common complaint (found in 50% to 80% of patients) is episodic abdominal pain that at times is severe. Occasionally the pain is continuous. Vomiting accompanies the abdominal pain in the majority of patients, but

hematemesis is present in less than 10%. Approximately one half of the patients have evidence of GI bleeding ranging from occult blood loss to gross GI hemorrhage. Bleeding does not generally occur in the absence of abdominal pain. Massive GI bleeding (found in 5% to 10% of patients) is self-limited and is generally not associated with a drop in hemoglobin concentration.

GI symptoms result from edema of the bowel wall and hemorrhage secondary to vasculitis; this has been verified by endoscopic correlation and pathologic specimens. Uncommonly, jejunal or ileal infarction and perforation may ensue. Intussusception occurs in 3% to 6% of children with HSP, with the lead point located in a hemorrhagic section of bowel. Other abdominal organs, such as the pancreas and gallbladder, can be affected by the vasculitis, resulting in abdominal pain and vomiting. In 20% of patients, the abdominal pain and GI bleeding may precede the appearance of cutaneous purpura and joint manifestations by days to weeks, thus resulting in an incorrect diagnoses. The GI complications of intussusception and massive hemorrhage appear to be more common in older children.

Joints

Joint complaints occur in 50% to 75% of children. Large joints such as the knees and ankles are the most frequently affected, although the hands, feet, and elbows are occasionally involved. Swelling is usually periarticular, rather than an actual joint effusion. Joint pain varies from mild to incapacitating.

Joint symptoms are not the result of intraarticular bleeding, and accordingly these joints are usually without significant erythema or warmth. Joint manifestations are nonmigratory and transient, resolving within several days. There may be recurrences of joint involvement, but there is no residual joint damage. Like the purpura, the arthalgia abates with bed rest, only to reappear with ambulation. Joint swelling is the first sign of HSP in 25% of patients.

Kidneys

Occurring in 50% of patients, the renal manifestations of HSP are potentially the most serious aspect of the syndrome and the only one likely to become chronic. The spectrum of renal manifestation is broad, ranging from transient microscopic hematuria (the most common finding) to acute nephritis, nephrotic syndrome, or renal failure. Episodic gross hematuria occurs in 30% to 40% of those with renal involvement, mild to moderate proteinuria or a nephrotic syndrome occurs in 25%, a transient reduction in glomerular filtration rate occurs in 20%, and progressive renal failure occurs in 5%. Hypertension occurs in 10% to 25% of patients and is rarely observed in the absence of nephritis. Renal manifestations tend to be more common and more severe in older children. There appears to be an increased incidence of renal involvement in those with severe GI involvement. Some have found a positive correlation between frequent episodes of purpura during the initial months of the disease and the subsequent severity of the nephritis, whereas others have not. Most of the renal manifestations present during the first month, and more than 90% of patients who eventually develop serious renal disease show signs within the first 3 months. However, the first sign of renal disease leading to chronic nephritis or nephrotic syndrome may occasionally occur months or years after the initial episode, frequently coincident with a new episode of purpura. The renal involvement rarely precedes the rash or other features of HSP.

The patient with isolated microscopic hematuria has a uniformly good prognosis, whereas 10% to 20% of patients with hematuria and proteinuria have persistent long-term urinary abnormalities. In about half of the children with hematuria and heavy proteinuria, or with nephrotic syndrome with or without nephritis, the disease may progress to chronic renal insufficiency. However, a patient is unlikely to progress to end-stage renal disease when at 3 months the urinalysis results are normal or demonstrate only hematuria and mild proteinuria or at 15 months the patient is no longer nephrotic or nephritic.

Miscellaneous

Acute scrotal swelling with severe pain, tenderness, and purpura occurs in up to 10% of males. This is a result of the vasculitis, which may affect the scrotal sac, spermatic cord, epididymis, and testes. This involvement has not been reported to occur before the onset of the rash and is therefore not easily confused with testicular torsion.

Neurologic symptoms occur in about 5% of patients as a result of cerebral vasculitis, subarachnoid and intracranial hemorrhage, and CNS disturbances secondary to hypertension. The patient may have, in order of decreasing frequency, seizures, headache (with or without hypertension), altered mental status, hemiparesis, facial nerve palsy, and optic neuritis.

Other uncommon manifestations of HSP include pulmonary hemorrage, carditis, and parotitis.

CLINICAL COURSE

With the exception of nephritis, HSP is an acute illness lasting from several days to several weeks. Most children have an illness lasting 2 to 4 weeks. In younger patients the illness tends to follow a shorter course, with fewer recurrences and fewer renal and GI manifestations.

One or more recurrences are seen in 30% to 50% of the patients; these usually consist of a recurrence of the rash and abdominal pain. Recurrences of joint symptoms and hematuria are seen in a smaller number of children. On rare occasions, hematuria may appear for the first time during a recurrence. Patients with nephritis are more likely to develop recurrences. The majority of recurrences occur within 3 months after the initial episode and are a milder version of the original episode.

DIAGNOSTIC EVALUATION

The diagnosis of HSP is based on clinical findings. Laboratory tests are generally aimed at excluding other disorders associated with purpura, such as thrombocytopenia, coagulation disorders, or malignancies.

The complete blood cell (CBC) count usually shows a normal hemoglobin concentration unless there has been significant GI blood loss. There may be moderate leukocytosis with a left shift in the differential cell count. Thrombocytosis is seen in two thirds of the patients and is frequently associated with abdominal pain and GI bleeding. An increased erythrocyte sedimentation rate is seen in three fourths of the patients and is not associated with any of the clinical features.

Bleeding and clotting studies are normal. Results of antinuclear antibody (ANA) tests and rheumatoid factor tests are negative, and complement levels are normal. In half of the patients, the serum IgA level is elevated early in the course, but this does not appear to correlate with any of the clinical features. IgG levels are normal.

In difficult cases, a skin biopsy of a purpuric lesion may help establish the diagnosis by revealing the characteristic deposits of IgA, C3, and fibrin.

The urinalysis may show gross or microscopic hematuria, red blood cell or granular casts, or the presence of protein.

Usually the blood urea nitrogen (BUN) and creatinine levels are normal, but on occasion they may be elevated. In patients with renal failure or nephrotic syndrome, electrolyte disturbances may be seen.

Abdominal radiographs may show dilated loops with air-fluid levels and a thickened small bowel wall. An abnormal bowel gas pattern and a soft tissue mass may indicate the presence of an intussusception; this can then be confirmed by a barium enema. The stool contains occult blood in 80% of the patients with GI complaints.

DIFFERENTIAL DIAGNOSIS

When a patient has the characteristic rash in conjunction with GI, joint, and possibly renal involvement, the diagnosis of HSP is straightforward. However, the diagnosis is somewhat more difficult in the 50% of patients in whom the rash is the only initial finding, or in the one third of patients in whom the abdominal pain and joint manifestations precede the characteristic rash. A similar purpuric rash may be seen in the patient with thrombocytopenia, coagulation disturbances, septicemia, malignancy, and hemolytic-uremic syndrome (Table 47–2). The clinical presentation and specific laboratory abnormalities help in differentiating these conditions from HSP. Patients with acute poststreptococcal glomerulonephritis may also have a similar purpuric rash and renal abnormalities, but C3 levels are low.

A positive ANA test and decreased C3 and C4 levels help in the diagnosis of systemic lupus erythematosus (SLE), which may also have similar skin, joint, and renal manifestations. A wide variety of infections, as well as allergic or drug-related eruptions, may mimic the early urticarial or maculopapular rash of HSP. When joint symptoms present prior to the skin or abdominal manifestations, juvenile rheumatoid arthritis, polyarteritis nodosa, rheumatic fever, and serum sickness must be considered. The causes of an acute abdomen must be addressed when abdominal pain and GI bleeding occur early in the course of HSP. Intussusception should be considered at all stages of the disease when abdominal pain and GI bleeding are present. In patients with nephropathy, the differential diagnosis includes SLE, IgA nephropathy, subacute bacterial endocarditis, acute and membranoproliferative glomerulonephritis, and Goodpasture's disease.

THERAPEUTIC INTERVENTION

Therapy for HSP is directed at treating the sequelae of the vasculitis, as specific intervention in the pathogenesis of the disease is not yet available. Most patients require nothing more than maintenance of hydration, adequate nutrition, and symptomatic relief. Analgesics such as acetaminophen or nonsteroidal anti-inflammatory drugs may be helpful for joint pain and soft tissue complaints. In a patient with

TABLE 47–2	
DIFFERENTIAL DIAGNOSIS OF HSP	
Idiopathic thrombocytopenic purpura	Polyarteritis nodosa
	Rheumatic fever
Coagulation disturbances	Serum sickness
Septicemia	Intussusception
Malignancy	IgA nephropathy
Hemolytic-uremic syndrome	Goodpasture's disease
Acute poststreptococcal glomerulonephritis	Subacute bacterial endocarditis
Systemic lupus erythematosus	
Juvenile rheumatoid arthritis	

bleeding, salicylates or other drugs that interfere with platelet function should be avoided.

Repeated abdominal examinations, monitoring of vital signs and stools for occult blood, and serial hemoglobin determinations should be used to detect evidence of obstruction, perforation, or GI hemorrhage. Intussusception should be considered and a barium enema performed in the patient with abdominal pain, bloody stools, and an abdominal mass. Surgical intervention is required if there is severe hemorrhage, perforation, or an intussusception that does not reduce with barium.

The nephropathy should be managed by close supervision of fluid status and serum electrolytes, and hypertension should be controlled in the patient with renal failure or nephrotic syndrome. The indications for renal biopsy vary but may include profuse proteinuria (>1.0 gm/24 hr), nephrotic syndrome, proteinuria and hematuria accompanied by hypertension or impaired renal function, and persistent urinary abnormalities.

Corticosteroid therapy has been used in HSP, but its indications and efficacy are controversial. Uncontrolled studies of steroid therapy suggest that soft tissue swelling and joint and GI manifestations are favorably affected. When GI manifestations have been severe, steroids have provided impressive relief of abdominal colic and GI hemorrhage. However, the benefit of steroid use in patients with only mild abdominal pain is questioned because of the self-limited nature of the pain and the possibility that steroid use may mask the development of more ominous abdominal signs. Some investigators feel the reduction in abdominal pain after steroid therapy indicates reduced bowel edema and thus a theoretically lessened risk for intussusception.

If steroid therapy is desired, prednisone is used in a dosage of 1 to 2 mg/kg/day for 1 week, followed by a gradually tapered dosage over the next week. Recurrence of abdominal pain and mild GI bleeding is not uncommon as steroids are tapered. Corticosteroids should be used to treat important manifestations caused by localized vasculitis and bleeding involving other organs such as the central nervous system, lungs, and testes. Steroids do not appear to alter the duration of the illness or the frequency of relapse and do not influence the purpura or the outcome of nephritis.

It has yet to be demonstrated that any form of therapy, including cytotoxic drugs, alters the outcome of HSP nephritis. However, in those patients with severe renal involvement early in the course of their disease, a trial of cytotoxic drugs (cyclophosphamide, azathioprine) in varying combinations with steroids, dipyridamole, anticoagulants, and plasma exchange may reduce the likelihood of the development of chronic renal disease or progressive renal failure.

DISPOSITION

Most patients with HSP may be discharged. Hospitalization should be considered for those with significant abdominal pain, frank GI bleeding, significant renal manifestations, or central nervous system symptoms (Table 47–3).

If the patient is sent home, close follow-up is required. The patient should be told of the possibility of recurrence and that new target organs may become involved in the ensuing few weeks. The patient must be warned about the possibility of worsening GI manifestations with increased bleeding or obstruction. Follow-up physical examinations should include a stool test for occult blood and, if indicated, measurement of the hemoglobin concentration. If a child has more than just microscopic hematuria and mild proteinuria, a consultation with a nephrologist should be obtained. Even in those with normal results on the initial urinalysis,

TABLE 47–3
DOCUMENTATION AND DISPOSITION

Documentation
  History of GI bleeding or abdominal pain
  History of hematuria
  History of joint swelling and pain
  Vital signs and perfusion status
  Rash and distribution
  Abdominal examination findings
  Joint findings
  Stool test for occult blood
  Urinalysis results
Disposition
  Admit
    Significant dehydration
    Severe abdominal pain
    Frank GI bleeding
    Possible abdominal obstruction or perforation
    Severe nephritis or nephrotic syndrome; renal failure
    CNS symptoms
  Discharge
    Most patients can be discharged with follow-up within the next few days
    Inform patient that all symptoms are likely to worsen
    Inform patient that new target organs may become involved
    Warn patient of possibility of recurrence
    Recommend serial urinalysis for several months
    Advise patient to return if he or she appears sicker (i.e., dehydrated, worsening GI bleeding, increased abdominal pain, decreased urine output)

serial urinalyses for at least a 3-month period are necessary and extremely important. All patients with nephrotic syndrome or nephritis deserve prolonged observation, as clinical deterioration can occur even after several years.

The short-term prognosis is excellent for the majority of patients with HSP. The acute morbidity and mortality are the results of renal involvement and GI manifestations of massive hemorrhage and intussusception. In patients with neurologic manifestations, the mortality rate is as high as 10%. The long-term outlook is based primarily on the outcome of the renal involvement; 5% of those with HSP nephritis develop end-stage renal disease.

Selected References

Austin HA, Barlow JE. Henoch-Schönlein nephritis: Prognostic features and the challenge of therapy. Am J Kidney Dis 1983;2:512–520.

Belman AL, Leicher CR, Moske SL, et al. Neurologic manifestations of Schönlein-Henoch purpura: Report of three cases and review of the literature. Pediatrics 1985;75:687.

Byrn JR, Fitzgerald JF, Northway JD, et al. Unusual manifestations of Henoch-Schönlein syndrome. Am J Dis Child 1976;130:1335.

Counahan R, Winterborn MH, White RHR, et al. Prognosis of Henoch-Schönlein nephritis in children. Br Med J 1977;20:11.

Farine M, Poucell S, Geary DL, et al. Prognostic significance of urinary findings and renal biopsies in children with Henoch-Schönlein nephritis. Clin Pediatr 1986;25:257.

Levinsky RJ, Barratt TM. IgA immune complexes in Henoch-Schönlein purpura. Lancet 1979;2:1100.

Meadow SR. The prognosis of Henoch-Schönlein nephritis. Clin Nephrol 1978;9:87.

Meadow SR, Glasgow EF, White RH, et al. Schönlein-Henoch nephritis. Q J Med 1972;163:241.

Rosenblum ND, Winter HS. Steroid effects on the course of abdominal pain in children with Henoch-Schönlein purpura. Pediatrics 1987;79:1018.

Saulsbury FT. Henoch-Schönlein purpura. Pediatr Dermatol 1984;1:195.

Silber DL. Henoch-Schönlein syndrome. Pediatr Clin North Am 1972;19:1061.

Zurowska AM, Wryolkowa T, Uszycka-Karcz M. Henoch-Schönlein nephritis in children—a clinicopathological study. Int J Pediatr Nephrol 1985;6:183.

CHAPTER 48

Hemolytic-Uremic Syndrome

Ann N. Champoux

INTRODUCTION

Hemolytic-uremic syndrome (HUS) is characterized by the triad of microangiopathic hemolytic anemia, thrombocytopenia, and acute renal failure (Table 48–1). It is a multisystem disorder occurring primarily in infants and young children and frequently follows a prodrome of bloody diarrhea. HUS is the most common cause of acute renal failure in children.

In a summary of 21 series, the mean age of patients with HUS in the United States was 4 years, compared with a mean age of 1.9 years for patients outside the United States. The incidence is equal in the two sexes. HUS occurs in blacks, but only infrequently. It occurs more commonly in the summer and fall, and the incidence appears to be increasing.

During the past decade, it has become clear that HUS is a heterogeneous entity with several discrete clinical variants. The HUS triad represents the final pathway for a number of pathogenic processes with diverse origins. The classic form of HUS seen in infants and young children is preceded by a diarrheal illness and has a good prognosis; relapses are rare. Another clinical variant is HUS associated with shigellosis in which the patient is toxic, often with evidence of disseminated intravascular coagulation, and has a poor prognosis. *Pneumococcus*-associated HUS is another important variant characterized by a positive Coombs' test and high morbidity and mortality rates. Familial patterns of HUS may occur through an autosomal recessive mode and are associated with a 68% mortality rate. Non–diarrhea-associated HUS frequently follows a relapsing or progressive course and has a poor outcome.

Etiologic or predisposing factors implicated in HUS have included bacterial causes (*Shigella dysenteriae, Escherichia coli, Salmonella typhi, Campylobacter jejuni, Streptococcus pneumoniae, Yersinia,* and others); viral causes (coxsackievirus, echovirus, adenovirus, influenza, and others); medications (oral contraceptives, chemotherapy medications, penicillin); and other precipitants such as pregnancy, malignant hypertension, and

renal transplantation. The majority of cases, however, were unexplained until 1983, when the association of classic HUS with infection by verotoxin-producing *E. coli* was recognized in 60% of cases. In Argentina, the largest endemic area for HUS, the majority of cases are associated with infection by a variety of different serotypes of verotoxin-producing *E. coli*. In the Pacific Northwest of the United States, 60% of HUS cases are associated with a single serotype (*E. coli* 0157:H7). The *E. coli* organism appears to be spread by both person-to-person contact and contaminated food. The incubation period is usually a few days, although it may be as long as 2 weeks.

PATHOPHYSIOLOGY

It is believed that injury to the endothelial cells of the renal microvasculature is the initial pathogenic event. In classic HUS where there is a gastroenteritis prodrome, it is thought that this primary insult may be caused by bacterial toxins, most commonly the verotoxin-producing *E. coli* organism. This verotoxin has similarities to the Shiga toxin that has been implicated in outbreaks of HUS associated with *Shigella* infection. This verotoxin is thought to gain access to the circulation and damage the renal vascular endothelium by inhibiting protein synthesis in these cells, thereby causing cell death. This is probably then followed by fibrin deposition and the development of a microangiopathic hemolytic anemia whereby red blood cells and platelets are mechanically damaged by the fibrin strands as the cells attempt to pass through the narrowed vessels. Microthrombi then form, and there is additional anoxic damage caused by adherence of the platelets to the altered capillary walls and simultaneous activation of the coagulation system. In addition to the mechanical destruction of the red blood cells and platelets by the fibrin strands, there is probably also direct toxic damage to the red cell and platelet membranes. This is supported by the lack of correlation between the severity of the vascular injury and the degree of hemolysis or the degree of thrombocytopenia. In addition, platelet counts may return to normal levels before the resolution of the glomerular fibrin deposits.

In most cases of classic HUS, the microangiopathy mainly involves the kidneys, but similar changes may be seen in the capillaries of the brain, gastrointestinal (GI) tract, and other organs.

CLINICAL EVALUATION
The Prodrome

Several days or weeks before the onset of HUS, a diarrheal illness with bloody, watery stools occurs in 94% of the patients. This is often associated with vomiting and crampy abdominal pain, and a low-grade fever may be present. Less frequently, the prodrome is an upper respiratory tract infection. Often, a "silent" period of 1 to 14 days follows, during which time the diarrhea improves. The acute phase of the HUS then begins abruptly with the sudden onset of hemolysis and renal failure.

Clinical Manifestations

The typical child with HUS appears ill and pale, with episodes of irritability alternating with drowsiness. The patient is often edematous and may be dehydrated. Oliguria is usually present but is masked by watery diarrhea. Vital signs may demonstrate a low-grade fever. Hypertension may be present in as many as 80% of patients and is usually related to fluid overload; however, it may persist in up to one half

TABLE 48–1	
SIGNS AND SYMPTOMS OF HUS	
Triad of HUS:	Microangiopathic hemolytic anemia
	Thrombocytopenia
	Acute renal failure
Prodome:	Bloody diarrhea, vomiting, abdominal pain
Syndrome:	Symptoms
	Oliguria
	Abdominal pain
	Signs
	Ill-appearing, pale, edematous
	Hypertension
	Irritability, drowsiness, seizures, coma
	Abdominal distention/rectal bleeding

of patients after the blood volume is normalized. The hypertension may contribute to the development of encephalopathy and cardiac failure. The skin may show petechiae or bruising in 30% to 40% of patients, although these findings are generally not marked. Frank bleeding is rare, with the exception of bleeding from the GI tract. The remainder of the examination may show multisystem involvement, with the renal, GI, and nervous systems being the most frequently involved.

HUS frequently is not diagnosed in the emergency department. Ten to thirty percent of patients are initially admitted with a neurologic diagnosis (encephalitis, meningitis), 30% with a cardiac presentation and diagnosis (congestive heart failure, edema, hypertension), 10% to 25% with a renal diagnosis (oliguria, hematuria), 10% with anemia, and 5% to 15% with an acute abdomen.

Renal Findings

Urine output may occasionally be normal, but oliguria or anuria is usually present. The urine may be red or brown in color. Acute renal failure usually develops simultaneously with the onset of hemolysis, although there is no correlation between the degree of azotemia and that of anemia. The patient may then develop complications of acute renal failure, which can include fluid overload, hypertension, pulmonary edema, acidosis, and electrolyte abnormalities. There is great variability in the degree of renal impairment. Mildly affected patients have decreased or increased urine output but are not anuric.

GI Findings

The GI signs and symptoms in HUS may be striking and may occur before the appearance of the characteristic triad. Severe abdominal pain is present in 17% to 46% of patients. HUS can mimic an acute abdomen in 20% of cases, and appendectomies and emergency barium enemas have been unnecessarily performed before a correct diagnosis was made. HUS has also mimicked ulcerative colitis.

In the patient with HUS, the physical examination may reveal abdominal distention, peritoneal signs, rectal bleeding, or rectal prolapse. There have been reported cases of fulminant colitis, bowel perforation, gangrene of the bowel, toxic megacolon, and intussusception. Involvement of the mesenteric blood vessels by the microangiopathic process may be responsible for these severe complications. Hepatosplenomegaly is present in as many as 50% of the patients. There may be clinical and biochemical hepatitis with mild jaundice. Cholelithiasis and pancreatic involvement have been reported.

Neurologic Findings

In 20% to 50% of patients, there are serious neurologic manifestations, with seizures and coma accounting for the majority. The seizures are usually generalized, brief, and occur within the first 48 hours of admission. Occasionally, the seizures will precede the admission and will be the main presenting complaint. Although the risk of CNS involvement is reduced by early control of hypertension and correction of uremia, hyponatremia, and hypocalcemia, severe CNS dysfunction may still occur. This may be explained by the neuropathologic finding in some patients showing involvement of the cerebral vessels in the microangiopathic process, with resultant vascular compromise, cerebral infarctions, thrombosis, or hemorrhage. In addition to seizures and coma, other neurologic manifestations seen in HUS include hemiparesis, cortical blindness, decerebrate posturing, behavioral changes, eye involvement (nerve palsy, vitreous and retinal hemorrhages), and ataxia.

The presence of neurologic symptoms is a major factor in determining prognosis. Only one third of those with neurologic manifestations fully recover, with the remainder experiencing significant morbidity (hemiparesis, seizures, cortical blindness, optic atrophy) and mortality. In addition, there is an increased incidence of residual hypertension and chronic renal failure in children with neurologic involvement, suggesting that their HUS is more severe.

Cardiopulmonary Findings

Cardiac involvement has included cardiomyopathy, cardiac aneurysm, and myocarditis. Tachycardia, electrocardiographic (EKG) disturbances, and cardiac enlargement are seen in as many as one half of patients. Myocardial dysfunction with congestive heart failure and pulmonary edema is usually the result of volume overload, hypertension, and metabolic derangement but may also be related to microvascular disease.

DIAGNOSTIC EVALUATION
Complete Blood Cell Count

Microangiopathic hemolytic anemia is one of the important diagnostic features of HUS. The hemoglobin level generally varies from 3 to 10 gm/dl and is accompanied by microscopic evidence (i.e., fragmented red blood cells, helmet cells, burr cells, and schistocytes) of intravascular erythrocyte destruction on a peripheral smear. Hemolysis occurs rapidly. The hemoglobin may fall 4 to 5 gm/dl within a few hours. Repeat hemolytic episodes may occur over a period of days to weeks. A platelet count of less than 100,000/mm³ is present on admission in most patients, but the duration of the thrombocytopenia may be brief. Thrombocytopenia rarely persists for more than 2 weeks, and the degree of thrombocytopenia has no prognostic significance and does not seem to bear any temporal relationship to the course of the renal disease. Except for GI bleeding, there are usually no hemorrhagic complications, despite low platelet counts. A reticulocytosis and a leukocytosis with a left shift are usually present. The serum haptoglobin concentrations are low.

Renal Studies

Renal failure is evidenced by increased blood urea nitrogen (BUN) and creatinine levels. In most, but not all patients, renal failure is proportionally related to hemolysis. Urinalysis results are abnormal; protein, blood, and, on occasion, casts and pyuria are present. Other abnormalities indicative of renal dysfunction include metabolic acidosis, hypo- or hyperkalemia, hyponatremia, hypocalcemia, hyperphosphatemia, and hyperuricemia.

Other Studies

Except in rare cases, results of direct and indirect Coombs' tests are negative. The prothrombin time, partial thromboplastin time, and fibrinogen levels are usually normal. In examining the complement system, the C3, C4, and total hemolytic complement (CH$_{50}$) levels may be low or normal. Liver enzyme levels may be elevated, and serum bilirubin levels may be increased.

The stool frequently contains fecal leukocytes. A stool specimen should be sent for bacterial culture, looking especially for verotoxin-producing E. coli. This should be pursued early in the course of the illness, as this pathogen may be rapidly cleared from the stool.

A cranial computed tomographic (CT) or magnetic resonance imaging (MRI) scan should be considered in those patients with significant neurologic symptoms; it may show diffuse cerebral edema, infarctions, and hemorrhages.

A barium enema may be necessary to better define lower GI tract abnormality. The study may reveal "thumbprinting," spasm, ulceration, and narrowing of the lumen.

DIFFERENTIAL DIAGNOSIS

The triad of microangiopathic hemolytic anemia, nephropathy, and thrombocytopenia following an acute diarrheal illness is sufficient to permit the diagnosis of HUS. The clinical triad seen in HUS may also be seen in many other disease states, including overwhelming sepsis, disseminated intravascular coagulation, malignant hypertension, collagen vascular diseases, and thrombotic thrombocytopenic purpura (Table 48–2). Coagulation studies that generally have normal results in HUS will have abnormal results in patients with sepsis and disseminated intravascular coagulation. Patients with collagen vascular disease can be differentiated by hemolytic anemia that is positive on the Coombs' test and is not microangiopathic.

If renal abnormalities are the main initial findings, then other causes of acute renal failure must be considered, including glomerulonephritis, interstitial nephritis, obstructive nephropathy, renal vein thrombosis, and severe dehydration. Other forms of hemolytic anemia, such as those caused by an intrinsic red cell enzyme defect, may initially resemble HUS, causing dark red urine and abnormal urinalysis results. When petechiae are present, the diagnosis of idiopathic thrombocytopenia should be considered. Because the abdominal symptoms and signs may precede the characteristic triad of HUS, the clinician must also consider in such cases the differential diagnosis of an acute abdomen. In a patient with seizures, the differential diagnosis includes CNS abnormalities caused by infection, metabolic abnormalities, head trauma, drug ingestion, tumors, and vascular accidents.

THERAPEUTIC INTERVENTION
Administration of Fluids and Electrolytes

Inappropriate administration of fluids when oliguria is wrongly suspected to be prerenal may result in severe complications. Unless dehydration is present, fluids should be restricted to insensible losses (500 ml/m²/24 hours) plus urinary and GI losses (Table 48–3). Dialysis is generally needed to manage the significantly edematous and hyponatremic patient. Hyperkalemia, the result of renal failure and red blood cell hemolysis, should be carefully monitored. An EKG should be obtained, looking for peaked T waves or

---

TABLE 48–2

DIFFERENTIAL DIAGNOSIS OF HUS

Overwhelming sepsis	Severe dehydration
Disseminated intravascular coagulation	Idiopathic thrombocytopenia
	Intussusception
Malignant hypertension	Peritonitis
Collagen vascular disease	Colitis
Thrombotic thrombocytopenia	CNS infection
Glomerulonephritis	Drug ingestion
Renal vein thrombosis	

TABLE 48–3

HEMOLYTIC-UREMIC SYNDROME: THERAPY AT A GLANCE

Fluid replacement:	Insensible losses, 500 ml/m²/24 hr, plus urinary and GI losses.
Hyperkalemia therapy:	Sodium polystyrene sulfonate, 1 gm/kg po or pr
	Sodium bicarbonate, 1 mEq/kg IV
	1 U insulin/3 gm glucose (½ U insulin/kg IV)
Red cell replacement:	5–10 ml/kg prbc slowly
Hypertension control:	Oral or sublingual nifedipine, 0.25–0.50 mg/kg/dose
	Hydralazine, 0.2 mg/kg/dose IV
	Diazoxide, 5 mg/kg/dose IV
Seizure control:	Diazepam, 0.1–0.2 mg/kg/dose IV
	Phenytoin, 10 mg/kg load IV

---

other signs of cardiotoxicity. If there are no EKG changes, the hyperkalemia can be treated by a cation-exchange resin (sodium polystyrene sulfonate [Kayexalate], 1 gm/kg po or pr). If the hyperkalemia is severe, the patient may need intravenous treatment with sodium bicarbonate (1 mEq/kg), glucose with insulin (1 U regular insulin per 3 gm glucose to ½ U insulin per kilogram), or 10% calcium gluconate (1 ml/kg). The patient should then be prepared for dialysis. Hypocalcemia may need treatment with intravenous calcium or dialysis.

Red Cell Replacement

A slow transfusion of 5 to 10 ml/kg of packed red blood cells should be given if the hemoglobin concentration is less than 5 gm/dl, if the hemoglobin concentration is less than 8 gm/dl and falling rapidly, or if there are signs of cardiac failure. Extreme caution should be exercised during the transfusion so that the added fluid load does not result in worsening of the hypertension and circulatory congestion.

Platelet Transfusion

Thrombocytopenia rarely requires specific therapy. Platelet transfusion should be considered in a child who is actively bleeding, when the platelet count is less than 50,000/mm³, or when there is a need for an invasive central vascular procedure.

Control of Azotemia

Approximately half of the patients will require dialysis. Peritoneal dialysis is preferable to hemodialysis in infants and young children, as peritoneal access is easier and safer. Some researchers advocate early dialysis in those with anuria or oliguria for more than 24 hours. Others use dialysis in those with BUN levels greater than 100 mg/dl or when there is congestive heart failure, encephalopathy, hyperkalemia, or refractory hypertension.

Control of Hypertension

Hypertension that persists after the correction of volume overload should be treated with antihypertensive drugs. The hypertension may respond to oral or sublingual nifedipine (0.25 to 0.50 mg/kg/dose), captopril (0.2 to 2.0 mg/kg/dose po), or propranolol (0.2 to 0.3 mg/kg/dose po). If the hypertension is persistent, parenteral hydralazine (0.2 mg/kg/dose), diazoxide (5 mg/kg/dose IV), or sodium nitroprusside (1 to 3 mg/kg/day IV) should be considered.

Neurologic Symptoms

Seizures will usually respond to diazepam (0.1 to 0.2 mg/kg/dose IV) followed by an intravenous loading dose of phenytoin (10 mg/kg). The patient with worsening CNS status may require intubation and treatment for increased intracranial pressure (i.e., hyperventilation, mannitol, and fluid restriction).

Cardiopulmonary Symptoms

Although most of the cardiopulmonary symptoms will resolve with treatment and control of volume overload, some patients may require therapy with digoxin or pressors. In addition, a central venous pressure line may be necessary to assess fluid status.

Specific Treatments

A variety of specific agents have been used alone or in combination. Although antibiotic treatment would seem to be logical when the disorder is caused by bacteria, it is thought that this may lead to a worse outcome by increasing the release of verotoxin from the dying bacteria. Corticosteroids, prostacycline infusion, vitamin E, and antiplatelet agents do not seem to be of any value. Anticoagulants have not been shown to be beneficial in controlled studies. Fibrinolytic agents have been used in an attempt to lyse microthrombi, but there is no evidence that these agents are effective. Controlled studies show no benefit from the use of fresh frozen plasma or plasmapheresis, although there are encouraging anecdotal reports, and many advocate the use of these agents in "nonclassic" HUS or in patients with a progressive course. There have been no controlled clinical trials involving the use of intravenous immunoglobulin G (IVIG) infusion. However, in a preliminary study, IVIG was associated with improved thrombocytopenia, a shortened period of oliguria, and improved long-term morbidity and mortality rates.

DISPOSITION

All patients with the probable diagnosis of HUS require hospitalization for evaluation and treatment (Table 48–4). There have been many attempts to predict outcome based on symptoms and laboratory data at presentation. The type of HUS appears to be a major determinant of prognosis. Those with classic HUS who have a short diarrheal prodrome have much lower morbidity and mortality rates than those with HUS and a genetic predisposition, *Shigella* infection, or pneumococcal sepsis. Mildly affected patients have an excellent prognosis. CNS and cardiovascular disturbances appear to contribute to a poor prognosis. Some have suggested that an initial oliguria period of more than 2 weeks is associated with a high likelihood of residual renal insufficiency. However, others have not agreed. Laboratory data, including the degree of anemia and thrombocytopenia and the degree of elevation of BUN and creatinine levels, have

TABLE 48–4
DOCUMENTATION AND DISPOSITION

Documentation:	History of bloody diarrhea
	Time of last void
	Blood pressure
	Level of alertness
	Signs of cardiac failure
	Peritoneal signs
	Laboratory findings
	Fluid management
Disposition:	All patients with HUS should be admitted
	Consult nephrologist
	Monitor household members

not correlated with outcome. A serum calcium level of less than or equal to 7.6 mg/dl associated with a urine output of less than 0.4 ml/kg/hr over a 24-hour period was shown to have a 90% positive predictive value of a poor outcome.

The mortality rate for patients with this disease has decreased from 40% during the first decade of its description to 4% to 7% by the mid 1980s. Significant morbidity still exists, however, in 10% to 20% of patients in the form of neurologic sequelae, chronic renal failure, or hypertension. Close follow-up is indicated in patients with residual renal abnormalities or persistent hypertension. Recurrence of the disease in its classic form is rare.

Selected References

Cleary TG. Cytoxin-producing *Escherichia coli* and the hemolytic-uremic syndrome. Pediatr Clin North Am 1988;35:485.

Dolislager D, Tune B. The hemolytic-uremic syndrome. Am J Dis Child 1978;132:55.

Fong JSC, De Chadarevian JP, Kaplan BS. Hemolytic-uremic syndrome: Current concepts and management. Pediatr Clin North Am 1982;4:835.

Hahn JS, Havens PL, Higgins JJ. The neurological complications of hemolytic uremic syndrome. J Child Neurol 1989;4:108.

Havins PL, O'Rourke P, Hahn J, et al. Laboratory and clinical variables to predict outcome in hemolytic-uremic syndrome. Am J Dis Child 1988;142:961.

Kaplan BS, Cleary TG, Obrig TG. Recent advances in understanding the pathogenesis of the hemolytic uremic syndromes. Pediatr Nephrol 1990;4:276.

Kaplan BS, Drummond KN. The hemolytic-uremic syndrome is a syndrome. N Engl J Med 1978;298:964.

Kaplan BS, Katz J, Krawitz S, et al. An analysis of the results of therapy in 67 cases of the hemolytic uremic syndrome. J Pediatr 1971;78:420.

Kaplan BS, Proesmans W. The hemolytic-uremic syndrome of childhood and its variants. Semin Hematol 1987;24:148.

Kaplan BS, Thomson PD, DeChadarevian JP. The hemolytic-uremic syndrome. Pediatr Clin North Am 1976;23:761.

Karmali MA, Petric M, Lim C, et al. The association between idiopathic hemolytic uremic syndrome and infection by verotoxin-producing *Escherichia coli*. J Infect Dis 1985;151:775.

Levin M, Barratt TM. Haemolytic uraemic syndrome. Arch Dis Child 1984;59:397.

Levin M, Walters MDS, Barratt TM. Hemolytic uremic syndrome. Adv Pediatr Infect Dis 1989;4:51.

Neill MA, Tarr PI, Clausen CR, et al. *Escherichia coli* 0157:H7 as the predominant pathogen associated with the hemolytic uremic syndrome: A prospective study in the Pacific Northwest. Pediatrics 1987;80:37.

Siegler RL. Management of hemolytic-uremic syndrome. J Pediatr 1988;112:1014.

Spika JS, Parsons JE, Nordenberg D, et al. Hemolytic uremic syndrome and diarrhea associated with *E. coli* 0157:H7 in a day care center. J Pediatr 1986;109:287.

CHAPTER 49

Urinary Tract Infections

Augusta J. Saulys

INTRODUCTION

According to some estimates, by the age of 11 years, 3% of girls and 1% of boys will have had a urinary tract infection (UTI). At any one time, 2% of preadolescent girls and 0.03% of boys have a UTI. Outside of the neonatal period (during which time 75% of UTI's are diagnosed in male infants), the ratio of girls to boys with UTI is roughly 10:1. The occurrence of asymptomatic infection and its significance is a topic of interest, as a sizeable population of children (2% of school-age girls by some estimates) have such infection. Within the past 15 years, recognition of two important concepts has allowed for the better identification of children likely to suffer significant morbidity from UTI. The first of these concepts is that most renal abnormalities secondary to UTI occur in patients whose genitourinary systems have a preexisting functional or anatomic obstruction. Second, most cases of reflux (which is thought to be responsible for a subset of UTI-associated renal disorders) result from a primary defect of the ureterovesical junction and not from bladder neck obstruction or meatal stenosis, as was once thought.

PATHOPHYSIOLOGY

The urinary tract begins with the kidneys and ends with the external urethral meatus and includes all elements of the collecting system and bladder in between. Normally urine within the urinary tract is sterile; the exception is in the lower urethra (in females and, to a much lesser extent, in males), where some bacterial organisms are often detectable. The route by which infections get established in the urinary tract is largely dependent on the age and immunocompetence of the child.

Routes of Establishment

UTI is thought to occur most commonly by the *hematogenous route* in at least three subsets of patients: neonates, children with a bacterial focus elsewhere, and immunocompromised patients. In neonates it is thought that bacteremia-sepsis results in secondary renal contamination and subsequent infection. This is supported by data showing that 31% of neonates with UTI also had a positive blood culture for the same organism.

In children with a bacterial focus elsewhere (e.g., prosthetic heart valves, osteomyelitis, or infected burns), hematogenous seeding may also result in a UTI. In immunocompromised patients, both of the previously listed mechanisms above may result in a UTI.

UTI is thought to occur by the *ascending route* from the perineal area in most other situations. In addition, any functional or anatomic obstruction to the urinary tract not only predisposes to infections, but also makes them that much more difficult to eradicate.

Causative Agents

Because the usual source of bacteria causing ascending UTI is the perineum, the most common organisms responsible are the Enterobacteriaceae, gram-negative enterics such as *Escherichia coli* that cause up to 90% of acute pediatric UTIs and account for up to 80% of recurrent infections. The specific breakdown of causative agents tends to vary with age and predisposing factors, just as the route of establishment tends to do. For example, in neonates the organisms isolated tend to be *E. coli* in 74% of cases, *Klebsiella* in 7%, *Pseudomonas* in 7%, and *Proteus* in 4%. In preschool and school-age children, *E. coli* organisms cause almost all acute infections. In hospitalized children, those with frequent UTI recurrence, and in boys, infection with *Proteus* and *Pseudomonas* tends to be relatively more frequent. Aerobic gram-positive cocci, previously discounted as contaminants, have recently been recognized as true urinary tract pathogens. In addition to group D streptococci (enterococci), *Staphylococcus aureus*, *Streptococcus viridans*, and *Staphylococcus saprophyticus* have been shown to be responsible for UTI in up to 40% of adolescent girls.

Viral origins of UTI have not been commonly documented, possibly because of the technical difficulties associated with isolation. Adenovirus types 11 and 21 have been associated with hemorrhagic cystitis. Fungal UTI is a consideration in immunocompromised children, especially those who have been treated with repeated courses of antibiotics and/or urinary tract manipulation.

CLINICAL EVALUATION

Infants present with vague nonspecific complaints, as up to about age 2 months the localization of any infection is difficult. Signs and symptoms may include fever, irritability, jaundice, vomiting, abdominal distention, or mass. Occasionally even the more chronic complaint of failure to thrive can be associated with UTI.

As children get older, symptoms get more specific and are generally referrable to the urinary tract. In addition to those already mentioned, symptoms may include frequency, dribbling, dysuria, enuresis, and flank pain. The differential diagnosis for symptoms referrable to the urinary tract should also include urethritis from bubblebath as an irritant, retained vaginal foreign bodies, vaginitis from sexual abuse, poor perineal hygiene, and occlusive underwear.

The distinction between lower versus upper UTI (i.e., cystitis vs. pyelonephritis) is sometimes attempted on the basis of signs and symptoms. This is difficult and also of questionable utility. However, an accurate diagnosis is crucial, because upper and lower UTI, as undistinguishable as they are initially, must be treated and followed up with equal degrees of aggressiveness.

Some minor congenital anomalies on clinical examination (preauricular pits, other ear deformities, supernumerary nipples) are thought by some to be associated with a greater incidence of urinary tract abnormalities, and thus a careful search for these and their attendant complications (UTI) is required.

DIAGNOSTIC EVALUATION
Urinalysis and Culture

The definition of what actually constitutes a UTI varies depending on various attendant conditions: how the sample is collected, the time of day during which it is obtained, and whether symptoms are associated.

The quantitative urine culture is the gold standard for diagnosis. The precise colony count that constitutes a positive culture is a matter of some continuing debate but depends to a large extent on how the sample is collected. Because of attendant morbidity, accurate diagnosis of UTI is crucial in children.

Traditionally it was thought that the presence of $>10^5$ colonies of a single bacterial species per milliliter of clean voided specimen were diagnostic of UTI. This was true in 80% of patients after one such sample collection and in 96% of patients after two such samples. Particularly in younger children who are not yet toilet trained and in whom the adequate cleansing of the perineum is problematic, the clean-catch method of obtaining a sample is inadequate for most situations. Clean-catch bag samples, although the easiest and least invasive method of obtaining urine samples from infants, are not very accurate; one study cites that of 53 positive bagged urine cultures, only 7.5% were confirmed to have bacteriuria by suprapubic aspiration. Thus this method of collecting urine for culture has no place in the emergency department.

In infants and children who are not yet toilet trained, the best method for obtaining urine is to get it directly from the bladder, either by suprapubic tap (Fig. 49–1) or catheterization. The suprapubic aspiration method is a simple procedure involving povidone-iodine (Betadine) preparation of the suprapubic area, introduction of a 22-gauge needle attached to a syringe at a 30-degree cephalic angle, and slow aspiration after penetration of the abdominal skin. In infants the procedure is particularly safe, because the bladder is an intra-abdominal organ during the first several months of life. The most common complication is hematuria (3.2%). The general success rate is greater than 90%. A suprapubic urine culture is considered to contain significant bacteria if bacterial organisms are present.

Catheterization of the urethra in order to obtain a urine specimen is also a reliable, if not a more "palatable," method of obtaining urine when compared with suprapubic aspiration. The periurethral area is prepped with povidone-iodine and sterile water, and a sterilely lubricated feeding tube or urethral catheter is introduced until urine is obtained. Uncircumcised infants can theoretically present some difficulties, as can infants weighing less than 2500 grams, in whom the smallest generally available catheter (No. 5 French) may cause some urethral trauma. Otherwise the urine obtained in this manner is considered positive if >1000 colonies of a particular organism are present per milliliter of urine. Complications include urethral trauma and iatrogenic introduction of bacteria, which occur in up to 3% of patients.

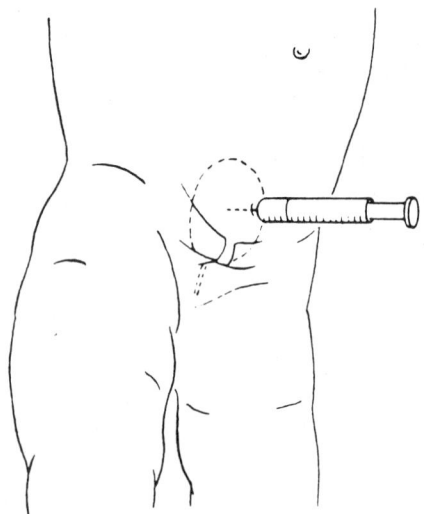

Figure 49–1. Suprapubic aspiration in the neonate. (From Roberts JR, Hedges JR. Clinical Procedures in Emergency Medicine. 1st ed. Philadelphia, WB Saunders, 1985, p 815.)

Other variables that may influence the final colony count obtained in a urine culture include the timing of the urine sample. Normal diurnal variation in urine concentration usually results in the highest colony counts from the first morning void specimen. In the emergency department this is not really of practical significance. In a child who has high fluid intake and frequency caused by a UTI, the colony count may also be below strict criteria for infection, even though the patient has a true UTI.

Another frequent source of error is the inappropriate handling of a urine sample once it is obtained. A urinalysis should be done within several minutes of collection, before cellular elements have had the opportunity to degenerate. Although a specimen can be refrigerated at 4°C to 5°C for up to 1 week without altering the quantitative results of the culture, keeping the specimen at room temperature for even 20 minutes can falsely elevate colony counts.

Bacteriostatic or bactericidal agents used in cleaning of the perineum before obtaining clean-catch or catheterized samples may have falsely low colony counts if these agents contaminate the sample. A child on antimicrobial agents, for whatever reason, may have antimicrobial bladder concentrations that are high enough to cause falsely low bacterial colony counts on culture.

Urinalysis, if kept in the proper perspective, can also be an important adjunct in evaluating the child with a possible UTI. It should never be used independently of the urine culture during the evaluation of a child who may have an infection of the urinary tract. The urinalysis should be done as soon as possible after obtaining the sample, as many cellular elements quickly degenerate. The search for pyuria and its significance also depend on a variety of attendant conditions. First, white blood cells (WBCs) may originate outside of the urinary tract, especially from the perineum. Usually samples so contaminated will also include many epithelial cells and fibers. Misidentification of cells may also occur; for example, renal tubular cells may easily be mistaken for WBCs during a less experienced microscopist's examination. The number of WBCs per high power field also depends on how a particular urine sample was prepared. In some cases, as in girls with recurrent UTI, a white cell inflammatory response is often not developed, and pyuria may be absent, even in the presence of a true UTI. There are also a variety of conditions in which pyuria is present in the absence of a true UTI. These include inflammation of adjacent structures (e.g., appendix or fallopian tube); severe dehydration, usually to the extent that granular casts are also present; nephritis; and chemical inflammation of the urinary tract (as commonly occurs from certain cancer chemotherapeutic agents). Loss of concentrating ability during acute UTI, especially in infants, will decrease the relative number of WBCs in a urine sample.

Chemical tests performed on urine dipsticks can be useful provided the limitations are appreciated. The nitrite test is based on the fact that most urinary pathogens (*E. coli, Proteus, Klebsiella, Enterobacter, Salmonella*) convert dietary nitrate to nitrite when they are present in the urine. Although a positive nitrite test will almost always signify a UTI, a negative test may be falsely so; this can result from inadequate intake of dietary nitrate, from a urine that is too dilute (i.e., not the first morning specimen), and most importantly, from infections caused by organisms that do not cause the nitrate conversion (*S. saprophyticus, Pseudomonas,* and enterococci). The leukocyte esterase test is a sensitive indicator of the presence of the equivalent of at least 6 WBCs per high power field; because WBCs are fairly unstable and lyse under a variety of conditions, this test is a useful indicator of their presence. It is important to note the previously discussed conditions in which UTI may not result in pyuria, however.

Together, the nitrite test and leukocyte esterase test have a sensitivity of 86.2% if either or both tests are positive. When used as a screening tool to predict those urines that will be negative by culture method, this combination provides 97.2% predictive value when both tests are negative. The clinician can then decide which samples to culture and which do not require it.

THERAPEUTIC INTERVENTION FOR SUSPECTED UTI

Neonates (≤2 Months)

History. Nonspecific complaints are typical and include fever, irritability, and poor feeding. It is important to specifically question the parents about the character of the urinary stream and the quality of the urine.

Evaluation. The physical examination should carefully assess the infant's vital signs (including blood pressure and position on the growth curve compared with birth weight), color (to exclude jaundice), the appearance of the genitourinary area (to exclude anomalies), and should document whether the male child has been circumcised and whether bladder distention or other abdominal mass is present. A urine sample (obtained by suprapubic tap or catheter) should be collected for urinalysis; it should be sent for culture even if the urinalysis results are unremarkable. Usually the patient will also be febrile. Since the source of infection may be presumed to be hematogenous, a blood culture; lumbar puncture for culture, chemistries, cell count, and Gram stain; measurement of electrolytes, blood urea nitrogen (BUN), creatinine, and glucose; and a complete blood cell count are done. It is useful to collect the urine sample before the other invasive procedures are begun, as even the act of drawing blood will frequently induce the infant to void.

Radiology. In the acute emergency department situation, radiologic procedures are indicated if acute obstruction is suspected (i.e., from abdominal mass or poor urinary stream); ultrasonography of the abdomen and pelvis are usually all that are required in this setting. Otherwise an intravenous pyelogram (IVP) and a voiding cystourethrogram (VCUG) can be scheduled during inpatient stay (if response to antibiotic therapy is poor) or at follow-up. Many investigators recommend waiting 6 weeks after clearing of the infection to prevent the confounding effect of infection-associated inflammatory changes in the collecting system.

Drug Therapy. Generally intravenous ampicillin and gentamicin or ampicillin and cefoxitin, the same agents used for treatment of presumptive neonatal sepsis, are appropriate (Table 49–1). Thus infants of this age should be initially treated as inpatients. As soon as all other culture results are negative, consideration can be given to appropriate oral antibiotic therapy on an outpatient basis with close follow-up. Repeat urine cultures should be sterile after 2 days of antibiotic therapy, and the child should no longer appear septic.

Toxic Children Younger Than 5 Years

History. The history gets more specific as a child gets older and may include fever, irritability, and emesis, as well as frequency, dribbling, dysuria, enuresis, and flank pain. The state of hydration, ability to drink, and presence or absence of vomiting are often key factors deciding admission.

Evaluation. A careful, complete physical examination should include assessment of vital signs, especially blood pressure, as well as signs of urinary tract obstruction. A urine sample (obtained by suprapubic tap, catheter, or supervised clean catch in the continent child) should be sent for urinalysis and culture (even if the urinalysis seems

TABLE 49–1

URINARY TRACT INFECTION: THERAPY AT A GLANCE	
Age Group	**Regimen**
Neonates	Ampicillin, 100 mg/kg/day, q 12 hr if patient is younger than 7 days; q 8 hr if patient is 7 days or older *plus* Gentamicin, 5 mg/kg/day, q 12 hr if patient is younger than 7 days; 7.5 mg/kg/day q 8 hr if patient is 7 days or older *or* Cefotaxime, 100 mg/kg/day q 8 hr Drug therapy for UTI in the neonatal period (<2 mo of age) is given parenterally because of the presumptive hematogenous acquisition of the infection.
Older infants, children, and adolescents	Sulfisoxazole, 100–150 mg/kg/day q 6–8 hr Trimethoprim (TMP)-Sulfamethoxazole (SMX), 10 mg/kg/day TMP and 40 mg/kg/day SMX q 12 hr Amoxicillin, 40 mg/kg/day q 8 hr Ampicillin, 50–100 mg/kg/day q 6 hr Amoxicillin–clavulanic acid, 50 mg/kg/day q 8 hr Cefaclor, 30 mg/kg/day q 6–8 hr Cefadroxil, 30 mg/kg/day q 6–8 hr Cephalexin, 50 mg/kg/day q 6 hr The above antibiotics are administered orally to children with uncomplicated UTI. The drug of choice because of ease of administration and relative lack of resistance is TMP-SMX.
Adolescents with uncomplicated UTI	TMP-SMX, 240 mg TMP and 1200 mg SMX (three double-strength tablets) po × 1 Amoxicillin, 1.5–3.0 gm po × 1 Gentamicin or other aminoglycoside, usual dose × 1 IM Single-dose therapy, when studied in adults was effective in uncomplicated cases of UTI in which symptoms of infection were of short duration. Most studies in pediatrics are not directly applicable to UTI in adolescents, but because of high noncompliance in this age group, single-dose therapy might be appropriate in some situations.

unremarkable); electrolytes, BUN, and creatinine are measured to assess renal function. Abnormalities involving the complete blood cell count, erythrocyte sedimentation rate, and C-reactive protein are supportive of the diagnosis, although they do not provide definitive evidence of upper urinary tract involvement; blood culture is generally not useful except in the immunocompromised patient. Most infections in this age group are not hematogenously spread.

Treatment. Therapy should include intravenous hydration and parenteral antibiotics as long as the oral intake is poor and until there is a therapeutic response (usually after several days). In the toxic patient, initial broad-spectrum therapy with a penicillin and aminoglycoside should be considered, because the infection may be caused by a less common organism (Table 49–1). After therapeutic response is achieved, dehydration is corrected, and culture and sensitivity results are available, then the appropriate oral therapy can be initiated. The total usual duration of intravenous and oral antibiotics necessary for eradication of even a renal parenchymal infection in the absence of obstruction is 7 to 10 days.

Follow-up. Follow-up should include a repeat culture 2 days after the initiation of therapy, again after the therapeutic course is complete, and just prior to the necessary radiologic evaluation. Some authorities recommend culturing urine every 3 months for 1 year following first-time UTI; thereafter yearly intervals are considered adequate. Radiologic evaluation after resolution of acute infection is mandatory in first well-documented UTIs of both boys and girls in this age group because of the frequency of subsequent renal damage inflicted on growing genitourinary systems.

Nontoxic Children Younger Than 5 Years

History. The history is more likely to include elements consistent with urethritis, such as use of bubblebaths, wearing of occlusive clothing, and poor perineal hygiene in children who go to the bathroom on their own; the possibilities of sexual abuse or masturbation must also be explored. A new onset of incontinence is a frequent complaint.

Evaluation. Evaluation should include an appropriately collected urine sample for culture and urinalysis.

Treatment. Therapy may be begun with oral antibiotic agents (amoxicillin or trimethoprim-sulfamethoxazole) if the urinalysis is suggestive of infection; a culture should be obtained even if the urinalysis is unremarkable. Phenazopyridine may also be prescribed for relief of symptoms at a dose of 1.5 mg/kg po after meals and at bedtime. Duration of therapy should be 7 to 10 days (Table 49–1).

Follow-up. Follow-up is similar to that in the toxic child. Repeat cultures of urine should be obtained after 2 days of antibiotic therapy and then again after the full course is completed. Again, because of frequent recurrence, culturing at the time of radiologic evaluation (after 6 weeks), then every 3 months for 1 year, and then yearly thereafter is used by many pediatricians for follow-up. Radiologic evaluation should be the same as for the toxic child younger than 5 years.

Children Older Than 5 Years

The same elements of the history, physical examination, and treatment for children younger than 5 years also apply to those older than 5 years. The primary difference lies in the controversy surrounding whether these children need aggressive radiologic evaluation. Current belief is that girls of this age with a first-time uncomplicated UTI do not need aggressive radiologic evaluation. A documented UTI in a boy of any age, however, warrants radiologic evaluation. Because of frequent recurrences, the same schedule for follow-up culturing applies as for the younger child.

Adolescents

History. The history should include questions regarding sexual activity (and thus sexually transmitted disease) and, in females, the possibility of pregnancy must always be considered when symptoms referrable to the urinary tract are described.

Evaluation. The evaluation should include a urinalysis and clean-catch or straight catheter urine culture (used particularly in females who may be menstruating or whose genitourinary hygiene may preclude obtaining a noncontaminated sample).

Treatment. Therapy can include amoxicillin or trimethoprim-sulfamethoxazole as the preferred agents; if the symptoms have been of short duration (less than 3 days), then single-dose therapy in this often noncompliant population can be used (Table 49–1).

Follow-up. Radiologic evaluation is usually unnecessary, but periodic culturing may be useful and the child is usually best followed by the pediatrician or gynecologist.

Selected References

Abbott GD. Neonatal bacteriuria: A prospective study in 1,460 infants. Br Med J 1972;1:267.

Alon U, Berant M, Pery M. Intravenous pyelography in children with urinary tract infection and vesicoureteral reflux. Pediatrics 1989;83(3):332.

Aronson AS, Gustafson B, Svenningsen NW. Combined suprapubic and clean voided urine examination in infants and children. Acta Paediatr Scand 1973;62:396.

Burns MW, Burns JL, Krieger JN. Pediatric urinary tract infection: Diagnosis, classification and significance. Pediatr Clin North Am 1987;34(5):1111.

Crain EF, Gershel JC. Urinary tract infections in febrile infants younger than 8 weeks of age. Pediatrics 1990;86(3):363.

Durbin WA, Peter G. Management of urinary tract infections in infants and children. Pediatr Infect Dis 1984;3(6):564.

Feld LG, Greenfield SP, Ogra PL, et al. Urinary tract infections in infants and children. Pediatr Rev. 1989;11(3):71.

Ginsburg CM, McCracken GH. Urinary tract infections in young infants Pediatrics 1982;69:409.

Klevan JL, DeJong AR. Urinary tract symptoms and urinary tract infection following sexual abuse. Am J Dis Child 1990;144:242.

Kunin CM. Urinary tract infections in children. Hosp Practice 1986;11:91.

Lindberg U, et al. Asymptomatic bacteriuria in schoolgirls: Clinical and laboratory findings. Acta Paediatr Scand 1975;64:425.

Marshall FF. Urinary incontinence in children. Pediatr Rev 1984;5(7):209.

Nelson JD, Peters PC. Suprapubic aspiration of urine in premature and term infants. Pediatrics 1965;36:132.

Pryles CV, Lustik B. Laboratory diagnosis of urinary tract infection. Pediatr Clin North Am 1974;18:233.

Siegel SR, et al. Urinary tract infection in infants and preschool children. Am J Dis Child 1980;134:369.

CHAPTER 50

Male Genital Disorders

Michael A. Ross
Joseph A. Salisz

MALE GENITAL ANATOMY

In the uncircumcised male the foreskin of the penis extends over the glans penis, forming the preputial orifice, which lies over the urinary meatus (Fig. 50–1). The foreskin forms a sulcus where it meets the corona of the glans.

The glans is a continuation of the single anterior erectile body, the corpus spongiosum, which surrounds the anterior urethra. The larger paired bodies of the corpus cavernosum lie posteriorly. The erectile bodies are covered by the thick tunica albuginia. The deep dorsal vein, dorsal artery, and nerve lie deep to the foreskin and superficial to the corpus cavernosum, whereas the profunda artery runs through the body of the cavernosum and is connected to the deep dorsal vein by penetrating arteriovenous shunts.

The superficial fascia of the penis contains no subcutaneous fat. It is continuous with the perineal, or Colles', fascia, the scrotal fascia, or dartos layer, and the subcutaneous fascia of the abdominal wall, or Camper's fascia. Any process occurring under this continuum, such as cellulitis, may spread to the extent of its boundaries, from the anus to the clavicles. The dartos layer of the scrotum contains many muscle fibers, which contract with exposure to the cold and anxiety.

The scrotum contains the paired testes, which in a standing resting state lie with their inferior pole angled slightly in a posterior and outward position (Fig. 50–2). The cremasteric muscle of the spermatic cord is a continuation of the internal oblique muscle. The testes and epididymis are suspended in the scrotum by the spermatic cord. The C-shaped epididymis is applied to the posterior portion of the testis. The appendix testis and the appendix epididymis arise from the superior portion of the testis and the head of the epididymis.

Surrounding the testis is the thick tunica albuginia. Encasing this is the two-layered tunica vaginalis. Normally, the investing layers of the tunica vaginalis hold the testis in a relatively fixed position. The bell-clapper deformity is caused by a congenitally high investment of this tunica vaginalis, which allows greater mobility (Fig. 50–3).[1] This anatomic variant is usually bilateral and increases the tendency for the testes to torse. A persistent, patent processus vaginalis allows a direct inguinal hernia to form, especially in premature infants and those with familial predispositions. Fluid collection in the tunica vaginalis leads to a hydrocele.

PHIMOSIS AND PARAPHIMOSIS

At birth 95% of males have physiologic adhesions that prevent complete retraction of the prepuce. In uncircumcised males this percentage decreases to 80% at 6 months, 50% at 1 year, and 10% at 3 years. The separation becomes complete by early adolescence, at which time the production of smegma increases.[2] Retraction of the foreskin in the infant or young child for cleaning or examination may cause undue pain or bleeding and may lead to secondary scarring and true adhesions. This unnecessary practice is to be discouraged.[2,3] When the child is 4 years old, he can be safely shown how to gently retract the foreskin and wash while bathing. Smegma, or desquamated epithelial cells that collect between

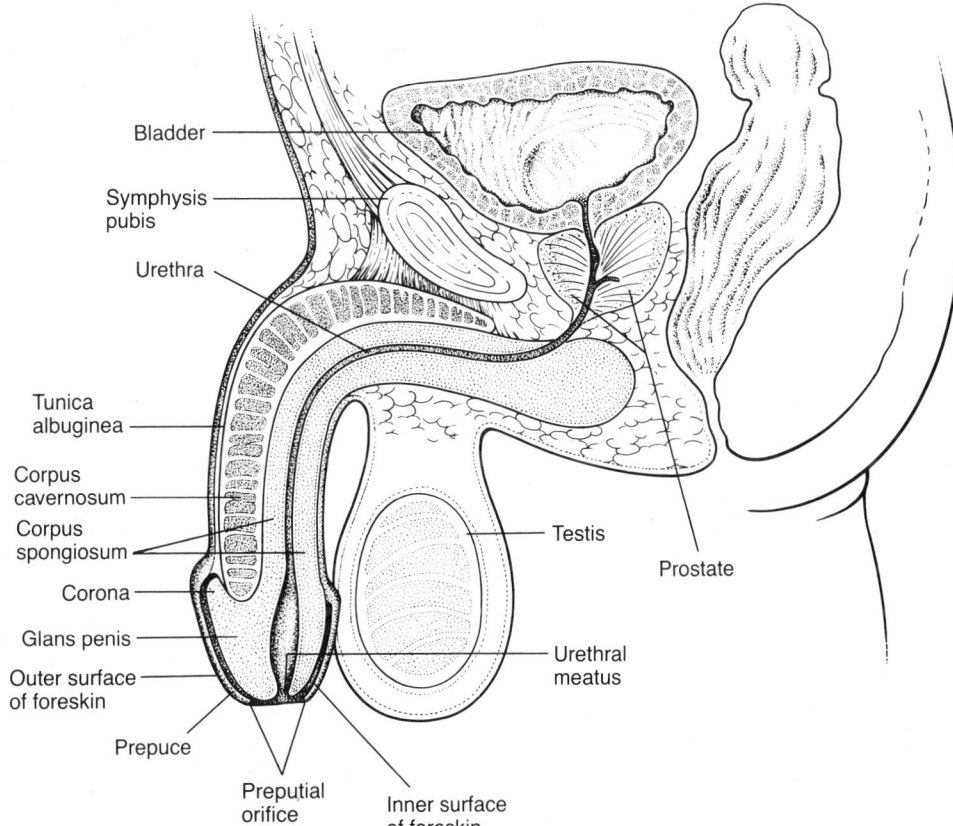

Figure 50–1. Male genital anatomy.

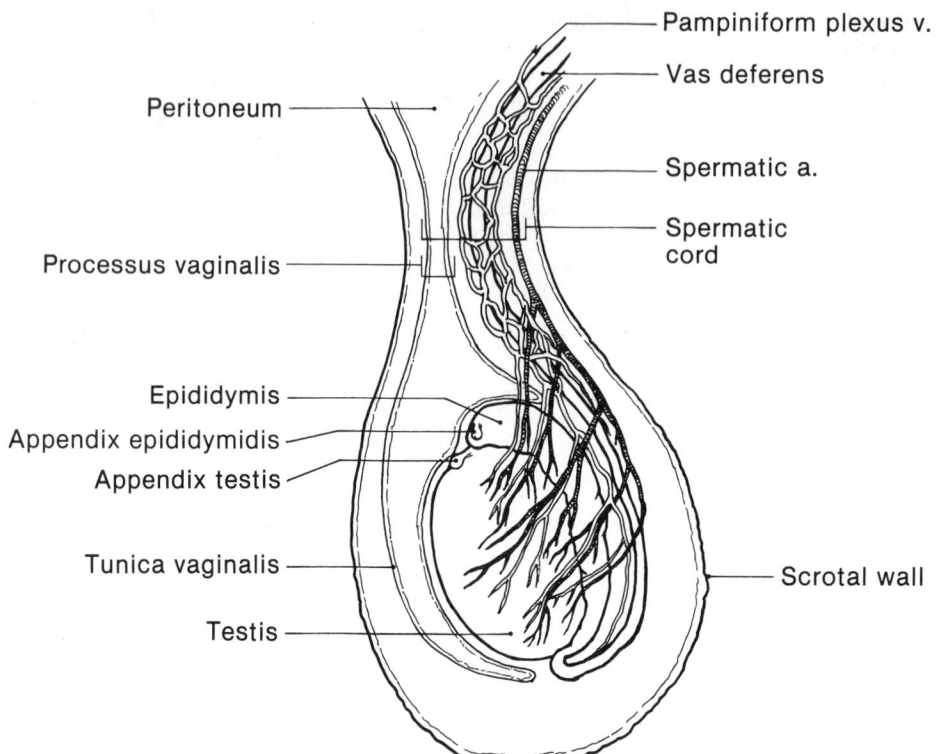

Figure 50–2. The scrotal contents.

the glans and prepuce, may be mistaken for pus and be a source of anxiety.

True phimosis is a constriction of the preputial orifice preventing the foreskin from being retracted over the glans. This is not to be confused with what has been called *physiologic phimosis*, the normal adhesion described earlier. Phimosis is uncommon in children. When it does occur it may be the result of chronic inflammation from trauma, infection, allergy, or chemical irritation.[3] If acute urinary retention has occurred as a consequence of phimosis, having the child try to urinate while sitting in a tub of warm water may facilitate bladder emptying. Referral to a urologist or gently opening the preputial orifice with the tip of a hemo-

stat, being careful not to enter the urethral orifice, may be required. This may also be of help when inserting or removing a catheter in a patient with a tight preputial orifice. Uncomplicated phimosis may be managed by outpatient referral.

Paraphimosis occurs when the uncircumcised foreskin is retracted behind the glans and is not returned. The narrower preputial foreskin acts like a tourniquet, causing venous congestion and edema of the distal penis. If left untreated, this may lead to necrosis of the distal penis.

Treatment consists of application of cold compresses and steady manual compression to decrease the distal swelling. This may be done using a latex glove half filled with crushed

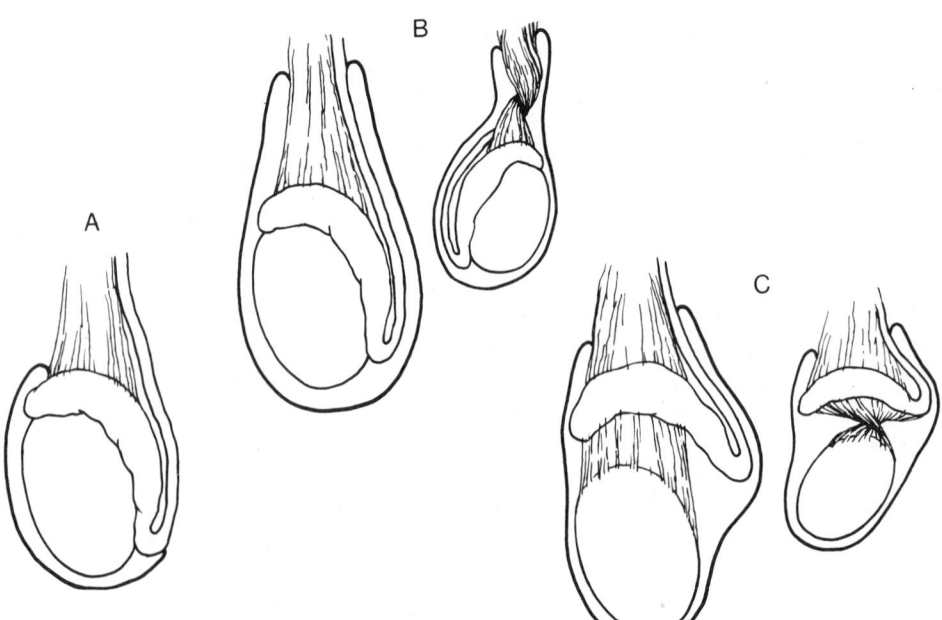

Figure 50–3. *A,* The normal position of the testis and tunica vaginalis. *B,* Testicular torsion. *C,* Torsion between the testicle and epididymis.

ice and water and tied at its end. The thumb is invaginated, and the lubricated phimotic penis is steadily held in this opening for 5 to 10 minutes. Reduction of the phimosis may be attempted by placing both thumbs over the tip of the glans and the index and middle fingers over the edematous distal foreskin and applying steady pressure over the glans to force it back in, much like turning a sock inside out (Fig. 50–4). A dorsal penile nerve block may help. The nerve block is performed with 1% lidocaine without epinephrine, infiltrated subcutaneously along the base of the dorsum of the penis.[4]

If manual reduction fails, the constricting band of foreskin is vertically incised with a scalpel, using local anesthesia and

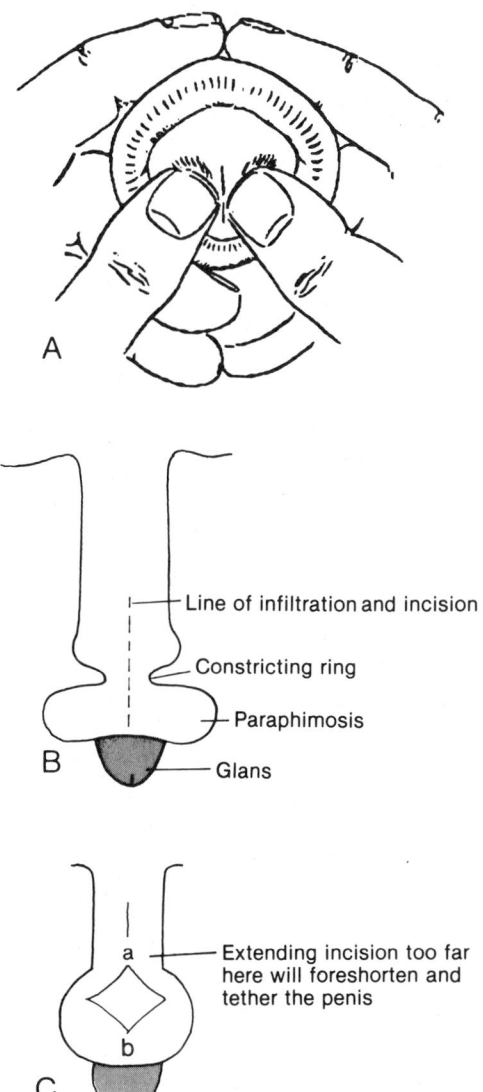

Figure 50–4. *A*, Manual reduction of paraphimosis is accomplished by combined traction and compression of the foreskin with simultaneous counter-pressure against the glans penis. *B*, The surgical treatment of this condition involves infiltration with local anesthetic (without epinephrine) and a dorsal slit that does not injure the penile shaft or glans. *C*, When the constricting paraphimosis is incised completely, the foreskin edges will relax laterally, producing a diamond-shaped defect. The apices of the dorsal slit (a and b) are approximated. (*A*, From Kelalis PP, King LR, Belman AB. Clinical Pediatric Urology. 2nd ed. Philadelphia, WB Saunders, 1985, p. 827. *B* and *C*, From Roberts JR, Hedges JR. Clinical Procedures in Emergency Medicine. 2nd ed. Philadelphia, WB Saunders, 1991, pp. 884, 885.)

Labels in figure:
- Line of infiltration and incision
- Constricting ring
- Paraphimosis
- Glans
- Extending incision too far here will foreshorten and tether the penis

sedation. The incision is opened laterally and closed on itself horizontally with absorbable suture (Fig. 50–4).[4] This should be followed by elective outpatient circumcision in a few weeks.

BALANITIS

Balanitis, or inflammation of the glans penis, and balanoposthitis, or inflammation of the glans and preputial foreskin, occur more commonly in older boys. Both conditions are local forms of cellulitis caused by trauma or poor hygiene. The infected area is red, swollen, and tender and may be treated with an oral antibiotic such as cefaclor or cephalexin. Local hygiene and warm compresses are beneficial, and a topical antibiotic ointment such as neomycin should be applied three times per day.

PRIAPISM

Priapism is an abnormally prolonged, painful erection of the penis not accompanied by sexual desire. It usually involves engorgement of the corpora cavernosa, often without involvement of the corpus spongiosum or glans penis. It may lead to prolonged pain, acute urinary retention, and, if untreated, impotence. However, impotence is not as common following priapism in children as following that in adults.[5,6]

The origin of primary, or idiopathic, priapism is unclear. Secondary priapism may be caused by sickle cell anemia or leukemia but may also be seen after local trauma, congenital syphilis, or retroperitoneal fibrosarcomas.[7] Therapy should be directed to the underlying cause.

Priapism occurs in 2.4% to 5.0% of patients with sickle cell anemia, the pediatric group accounting for about 60% of cases.[8] Factors that precipitate priapism in these patients include mild acidosis associated with hypoventilation during sleep, normal erections during rapid eye movement (REM) sleep, masturbation, sexual intercourse, local trauma, and infection.[7]

Many earlier therapies are no longer practiced because they are physiologically unsound. These include hot and cold compresses, spinal anesthesia, aspiration, local or systemic anticoagulants or fibrinolytics, and hormonal therapy.[5,7] On presentation, any cause of sickling should be identified and treated. A blood sample should be obtained for hemoglobin electrophoresis if sickle cell anemia is suspected but undiagnosed. Intravenous hydration, alkalinization, and analgesic therapy should be initiated. If there is no improvement in 12 hours, "hypertransfusion" should be carried out over the next 2 to 4 hours in an effort to double the patient's hematocrit concentration or increase the hemoglobin level to more than 10 gm/dl.[9] The amount of blood needed for this can be calculated by the following equation:[10]

$$\text{Volume of blood needed to double the hematocrit} = \frac{\text{Patient's hematocrit} \times \text{Patient's blood volume}}{\text{Hematocrit of transfused blood}}$$

This hypertransfusion is followed by 24 hours of observation for improvement. If there is none, a shunting procedure is performed.[5] Usually a fistula or shunt is placed between the cavernous bodies and the glans penis, corpus spongiosum, or saphenous vein.[7,11,12] Exchange transfusion performed preoperatively to lower the hemoglobin S level to 30% or less decreases the postoperative morbidity.[8]

Leukemia is a rare cause of priapism in children. Chronic granulocytic leukemia, which comprises roughly 5% of childhood leukemias, accounts for about 50% of reported cases. Sludging is caused by the increased white cell mass. Treatment is directed at the leukemia and consists of chemotherapy, hydration, and analgesics. If this fails or pain control becomes difficult, shunting procedures are used.[13, 14]

PENILE STRANGULATION

Any time a young male presents with pain, swelling, or redness of the distal penis, the "penile tourniquet syndrome" should be considered. The "tourniquet" is usually a human hair, string, or any of a number of other materials, and is often invisible. It may be placed accidentally, during play, incidental to circumcision, for punishment, or for more dubious reasons. Ninety-seven percent of all patients are younger than 12 years, the average age being 2.5 years.[15] Human hair constricts each time it gets wet and dries out and eventually becomes encysted and hidden in epithelium. Initially this may lead to urinary retention and foreskin injury. Later, gangrene, a "wasp waist" deformity of the penis, or a urethral stricture or fistula may occur. Unfortunately, the band is easily missed at examination, and the risk of morbidity increases with time. Treatment consists of removing the band using a hemostat and scissors. If there is any question of a remaining band a perpendicular incision should be made over the depressed area.[15–18] In two thirds of reported cases, hair was removed before complications developed. All patients should have urologic follow-up.

PENILE FOREIGN BODIES

The insertion of penile foreign bodies takes place most commonly in adolescent males. Assorted objects may be placed for reasons of self-stimulation or exploration. Full evaluation requires urethrography,[19, 20] and urologic consultation is often required for removal and treatment. The possibilities of psychiatric abnormality and sexual abuse should also be considered.[21, 22]

PENILE TRAUMA

When a hurried, careless boy zips his penile foreskin or scrotum into his zipper, the emergency physician is faced with a delicate crisis. The sliding piece of the zipper consists of an anterior and posterior plate connected by a median bar, which looks like the "nose" of the piece. Using the tip of a bone cutter, the physician cuts this median bar, separating the two plates and thus freeing the entrapped skin (Fig. 50–5).[23, 24]

Dog bites to the genitalia are an uncommon but well-documented phenomenon. Typically an unsupervised male infant is left with a dog. The dog may tear off the diaper and lick or chew the genitalia, thinking the child is prey.

Proper wound management with irrigation and appropriate debridement is the cornerstone of therapy. Deep lacerations, amputations, or urethral injuries should be managed by a urologist. Antibiotic prophylaxis covering *Pasteurella multocida* should be considered.[25]

As a rule, penile lacerations should be explored. If there is any question as to the depth of injury, a urologic consultation should be obtained. If a urethral injury is considered, a urethrogram should be performed.

Toilet seat injuries are unique to the 2- to 4-year-old age group. Typically the toddler is voiding alone when the seat falls on his penis. This painful blunt injury may be associated with bleeding, swelling, and urinary retention. Emergency management consists of control of bleeding using direct pressure and control of pain. Urethrography and urologic consultation are often needed. The child may regress in his toilet training and develop a fear of toilets. Injury prevention through proper supervision, pediatric toilet seat inserts, step stools, or the use of "potty chairs" may be recommended.

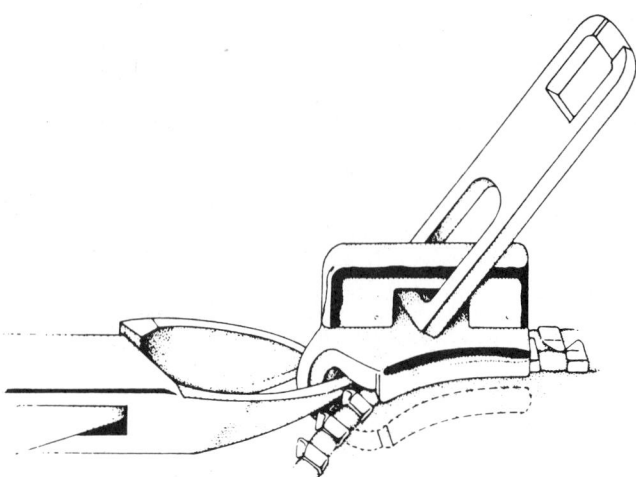

Figure 50–5. When loose skin is caught in the teeth of a zipper, one can release it quickly and without risk to the patient by cutting the diamond that holds the slider together with a bone cutter or a pair of wire clippers. (From Emergency Medicine, October 15, 1982, p 215.)

THE PAINFUL SCROTUM
Testicular Torsion

During testicular torsion the spermatic cord twists and venous drainage is obstructed, resulting in testicular engorgement, arterial shutdown, tissue ischemia, and (later) infarction. A delay in diagnosis may result in loss of a testis. Semen production can be adversely affected by as little as 4 hours of ischemia. The critical time period from onset of torsion to ischemic damage resulting in measurable testicular atrophy is approximately 6 hours.[26–28] However, a longer duration of symptoms does not always clearly correlate with testicular loss.[28] Partial torsion and intermittent torsion-detorsion may allow for longer periods of symptoms prior to testicular infarction.

A painful swollen scrotum must be considered a surgical emergency unless torsion can rapidly be excluded. It is the responsibility of the emergency physician to swiftly evaluate and refer the child to a urologist.

Technologic advancements, including scrotal ultrasound and nuclear scanning, have resulted in fewer unnecessary surgical explorations.[29] No single test, however, yields a definite diagnosis in the evaluation of the acutely painful scrotum. Final judgment should rarely be the sole responsibility of the emergency physician (Table 50–1).

Clinical Evaluation

Prepubertal children rarely present with epididymitis. Acute torsion of a testis or one of its appendages is more common. Excluding neonates, the peak age range of presentation of testicular torsion is 14 to 17 years.[26–30]

A complete history should be obtained from the patient and the parents regarding the patient's age, suddenness of onset of pain, duration of symptoms, previous history of similar episodes, presence of urinary symptoms, and any history of trauma. The boy usually recalls a sudden onset of unilateral scrotal pain followed by swelling, usually blamed on some mild traumatic event. In fact, the incidence of preceding trauma is 5% to 6% and should not dissuade the physician from a diagnosis of torsion.[31] Occasionally, the pain may awaken the patient from sleep. Many experience abdominal pain, nausea, and emesis, and more than 50%

TABLE 50-1

THE PAINFUL SCROTUM

	Testis Torsion	Epididymo-orchitis	Appendiceal Torsion
Signs and symptoms			
Pain	Severe, acute onset	Gradual (84% present later than 12 hours)	Usually gradual
Location	Testis, with radiation to groin and abdomen	Localized to testis and epididymis, sometimes groin	Appendix or general scrotum
Similar previous pain	Frequent	Uncommon, unless previous epididymitis	Occasional
Fever (>99.5°F)	"Rare" in up to 66% of patients	38% to 40%	"Rare" in up to 58%
Emesis	Frequent	Rare	Rare
Dysuria	Rare	Common	Rare
Physical examination	Testis may be horizontal, high riding, swollen, exquisitely tender	Testis and epididymis are firm, tender, swollen; scrotum is red and warm (>70%)	Testis is usually normal; distinct firm mass separate from epididymis at upper pole; blue dot sign; swollen scrotum
Laboratory findings			
Leukocytosis (>10,000)	34%	44% to 54%	33%
Pyuria/UTI	10%	24% to 61%	8%
Blood flow			
Doppler/nuclear scan	Decreased	Increased	Normal or increased

may recall a previous history of similar testicular pain.[1] Unfortunately, the history is nonspecific (Table 50–1).

The physical findings in testicular torsion vary with their duration. Testicular tenderness is always present, except in very late instances and in cases of neonatal torsion that have a prenatal origin.[1, 32] Scrotal edema is usually present, though not invariably, but is not specific for torsion. Because of shortening of the cord, the testis may be "high riding" and in a transverse position.[33]

If one of the twists is less than 360 degrees, the epididymis may be displaced anteriorly. Occasionally, the knot of the twisted cord can be palpated posterior to the elevated testis. The cremasteric reflex is often absent in testicular torsion.[1, 29]

In testicular torsion the entire testis and epididymis are tender. In contrast, the tenderness of epididymitis is restricted to the epididymis in its early stages, but may progress to involve the entire scrotal contents, as in epididymo-orchitis or abscess. Signs of infection such as fever, pyuria, and urethral discharge may point toward epididymo-orchitis but will not entirely eliminate the diagnosis of torsion.

The *blue dot sign* is a firm pea-sized nodule with point tenderness, seen to be bluish in light-skinned patients, that is located on the upper pole of the testis or epididymis. It suggests a torsion of the appendix rather than the testis. However, edema soon masks the finding, and reliance on the blue dot sign to exclude the diagnosis of torsion should be the responsibility of the urologic consultant.

Torsion can recur in a previously surgically fixed testis.

Diagnostic Evaluation

The Doppler ultrasonic stethoscope works on the principle that blood flow in an artery reflects sound waves in a pulsatile fashion. The sound waves are emitted from a probe placed over the lower pole of the testis, and the echoes from the spermatic artery are monitored either with an amplifying stethoscope or with a graph-paper flowmeter.[29, 34–36] Some investigators have criticized this technique, saying that the inflamed scrotum of patients with underlying torsion often yielded very strong pulsatile echo patterns that reflected the increased blood supply in the scrotal wall.[37, 38] Some claim that this mistake can be avoided by using funicular compression, or compressing the testicular vessels at the level of

the scrotal inlet while monitoring the presumed spermatic arterial pulse.[30, 34] Proponents have admitted that Doppler ultrasonography is a beneficial adjunct but is not the precise diagnostic tool it was thought to be.[39]

Nuclear medicine imaging of the acute scrotum is used most commonly to further confirm that the intrascrotal abnormality is not testicular torsion. Static and dynamic imaging techniques are used to track the intravascular flow of technetium pertechnetate (Tc 99m), which is intravenously injected. In torsion, the flow is diminished in comparison with the opposite nontorsed testis. Increased flow to the affected side indicates an inflammatory condition such as epididymitis. Torsed appendages may also give an increased flow picture, because the response is inflammatory without decreasing spermatic artery inflow. The study yields an occasional false-positive result, but false-negative results are rare. A false diagnosis of torsion may occur if there is an overlying hydrocele or an avascular area, such as an abscess, because these intrascrotal masses will appear relatively "cold" on the images. In addition, scan interpretation is difficult in a child with a small scrotum. Nevertheless, the accuracy of these scans at detecting the absence of torsion has been reported to be near 100% in many series.[27–30, 39–43]

Ultrasonic imaging has been accepted as an excellent method to assess the traumatized testis. However, it cannot accurately evaluate the painful, swollen scrotum. Newer equipment combining ultrasonic probes and Doppler analysis with computer enhancement may yield visualization of intratesticular vessels, and reveal patency.

The clinical diagnostic abilities of the emergency physician should be used as screening tools. The physician's responsibility to a patient with acute scrotal pain is to rapidly obtain helpful information by recording the patient history, performing the physical examination, and obtaining a white blood cell count, urinalysis and urine culture, and, if appropriate, analysis of urethral discharge. A urologic consultation should then be obtained.

The morbidity associated with false-positive surgical explorations is minimal, and the cost of missing a torsion is high. Deciding not to surgically explore the scrotum places the patient at very great risk. Indications for surgery in the acutely painful scrotum, therefore, are liberal enough to permit a certain percentage of false-positive explorations while allowing correction of all torsed testes. All of those patients whose initial examination suggests torsion, as well as those whose elapsed time since onset of symptoms is close to 6 hours, should be operated on and excluded from any investigation that will take additional time.

When the diagnosis of torsion appears less likely and when time permits, the radionuclide testicular scan may provide additional objective evidence excluding the diagnosis of torsion.[27-30, 39-45] The emergency physician must be mindful of the importance of time. If testicular torsion is a possibility, these tests should be ordered in conjunction with urologic consultation.

Epididymitis

Epididymitis, or inflammation of the epididymis, has been reported in children from 1 to 18 years old. Two thirds of pediatric cases occur in children 12 to 18 years of age. It is extremely uncommon in those younger than 6 years.[40] Older boys may admit to sexual activity, and in these the pathogens involved may have been sexually transmitted and associated with urethritis. Epididymitis may occur in patients with anatomically or functionally abnormal urinary tracts that predispose them to infections.

Clinical Evaluation

The onset of pain and swelling resulting from an inflammatory process is usually more insidious than that resulting from a vascular event such as occurs in torsion. Patients presenting with epididymitis may complain of a progressive discomfort gradually worsening over a period of a few days. Less than half have constitutional symptoms of fever or chills, and even fewer complain of dysuria or urethral discharge.[40]

The tenderness of epididymitis is restricted to the epididymis in its early stages. If the physician is fortunate to examine the patient early, point tenderness is often located over the lower pole of the epididymis, distinctly separate from the testis. Localized edema may also be present, and comparison with the opposite epididymis is extremely helpful. These findings later progress to involve the entire scrotal contents, as in epididymo-orchitis or abscess, and make differentiation from torsion much more difficult. Prehn's sign, or decreased pain with elevation of the testis, has been touted as an indication of epididymitis but is unreliable in children.[27-29] Signs of infection such as fever, pyuria, and urethral discharge may suggest epididymitis, but their reliability is also poor.[1, 27, 29, 40]

Diagnostic Evaluation

The white blood cell count may be elevated and show an increase in band cells. The urinalysis may reveal pyuria and bacteriuria. A urine sample for culture should be obtained in the emergency department, but results will not play a role in the initial diagnosis.

If the clinical picture is not that of torsion, a nuclear testicular scan can be used to document normal or increased blood flow to the involved testis as a result of inflammation. This can be both diagnostically and medicolegally beneficial.

Because of the infrequency of epididymitis in children and its confusion with torsion of the testis, diagnosis should be based on the history and physical examination in only the most obvious cases and should also be confirmed by the urologist. In those cases in which diagnosis is not obvious, nuclear scanning may be used if time permits.

Therapeutic Intervention

Treatment is aimed at decreasing the inflammatory process and fighting the infection. The dependent position of the testis causes pain, impedes lymphatic drainage, and may retard improvement. Bed rest and scrotal elevation will assist recovery. Analgesics, especially those with anti-inflammatory properties, should be prescribed. Symptomatic relief (i.e., by application of ice packs and sitz baths) may be helpful. Cultures should be obtained prior to beginning antibiotics. Antibiotics should be started empirically and should be based on the patient's history. If the patient is sexually active, a tetracycline (e.g., doxycycline) is appropriate. If there is coincident urinary infection, trimethoprim-sulfamethoxazole combination therapy treats most pathogens.[28]

The timing in caring for epididymitis is not as critical as that for torsion. However, the infection is still a threat to the child's testis. Many of these infections will progress, requiring hospitalization and parenteral antibiotics.

Torsed Appendages

The incidence of torsion of the appendix testis or epididymis peaks during prepuberty. Because it causes vascular compromise to the appendage, pain is usually sudden, and patients present early. The child may present later, however, with a more gradual onset of symptoms.[46]

The blue dot sign may be the only pathognomonic finding excluding torsion.[47] There is point tenderness at the upper pole of the testis or epididymis, and the physician may be able to identify the blue, pea-sized, tender nodule that represents the ischemic appendage.[48]

If the diagnosis is a torsed appendage, treatment is symptomatic, with bed rest and anti-inflammatory drugs. If the diagnosis is in doubt, nuclear scanning may be appropriate if time permits; otherwise surgical exploration is required.[47, 49]

Incarcerated Hernia

If a loop of bowel, mesenteric fat, appendix, or other intra-abdominal organ becomes entrapped within the inguinal canal, a patient may present with an acutely painful scrotum. If the organ becomes fixed in this position, the hernia becomes incarcerated; if ischemic conditions result, the hernia is said to be *strangulated.*

The age at presentation is usually less than 3 years, and many of these patients present with a history of known hernia or communicating hydrocele that is being observed.[50] The onset of symptoms may be sudden or gradual, and nausea and vomiting usually overshadow the scrotal complaints.[46]

Swelling and pain may be present in the scrotum but will most likely be greater in the inguinal region. Abdominal distention, vomiting, and peritoneal signs may accompany the local signs. Placing the patient in Trendelenburg's position and gently attempting reduction of the groin mass may reduce the hernia, but an incarcerated hernia must never be reduced forcibly.[51] Immediate surgical consultation should be obtained.

Other Causes

Henoch-Schönlein purpura is a pediatric vasculitis involving many systems. Dermal purpuric lesions, abdominal pain, renal abnormalities, and arthralgias characterize the syndrome. Scrotal involvement has been reported in as many as 38% of patients and may be the initial manifestation.[44, 52, 53] The testis is usually palpably normal in the thickened, tender, erythematous scrotum.

Fat necrosis in the scrotum of obese prepubertal boys after exposure to severe cold and mild perineal trauma has been described.[54] A palpable, firm, tender mass adjacent to a normal testis identifies this condition.

Intraperitoneal abnormalities may cause acute scrotal swelling.[55] Peritoneal inflammation, such as that associated with appendicitis or an infected ventriculoperitoneal shunt, has been described as a cause of scrotal swelling in infants with a patent processus vaginalis. One patient with a ruptured spleen reportedly presented with an enlarging scrotal hematoma.[56]

Mumps orchitis may occur preceding or following the onset of parotitis.[57] It is the most common complication of mumps infection and may result in testicular atrophy. Treatment is symptomatic.[58]

PAINLESS SCROTAL CONDITIONS
Undescended Testis

If the testis is not palpable or if positioning it in the dependent portion of the scrotum without tension is difficult, the parents should be instructed to consult a urologist. The diagnosis of an absent or undescended testis implies a higher than normal risk of future infertility[59] and malignant degeneration.[60] The risk of both may be reduced by early correction of testicular position.

Hernia and Hydrocele

The testis descends through the inguinal canal into the scrotum during the third trimester of pregnancy. An outpouching of peritoneum called the *tunica vaginalis* extends into the scrotum alongside the spermatic vessels and vas deferens within the cord (Fig. 50–2). This tongue of peritoneum usually closes at birth or shortly after, but it may remain patent.[61]

Most commonly, the inguinal canal allows peritoneal fluid to fill the tunica vaginalis alongside the testis, creating a painless translucent mass, called a *hydrocele*, that may obscure the testicular examination. Continued patency may yield a scrotal mass with variable size, becoming larger when the baby cries or strains for defecation. At times, when the child is quiet, it may be invisible. This communicating hydrocele is essentially a potential inguinal hernia—that is, a defect in the anterior abdominal wall through which intra-abdominal contents may course.[62] Mesenteric fat, bowel, bladder, and other organs may herniate through the patent channel.[62]

Varicocele

Varicoceles are abnormally dilated veins of the pampiniform plexus draining the testis. They present in pubertal boys as nontender masses within the scrotum situated above the gonad and feel like a "bag of worms" on physical examination. A smaller ipsilateral testis may be found. The mass usually "deflates" with the patient in a supine or Trendelenburg position.[63]

Idiopathic varicoceles are known to be associated with adult male subfertility, the pathophysiology of which is unknown. Because not all men with varicoceles are subfertile, the management of adolescent varicoceles is controversial.[63]

Testicular Tumors

The incidence of testicular neoplasms in children is approximately 1 per 100,000 males.[64] Tumors of the testis usually present as painless, firm, non-transilluminating, nodular masses obscuring the normal palpable architecture. Germ cell tumors, the most common of which is the yolk sac tumor, account for 75%; most affected children present before 2 years of age. The most common nongerminal tumor is the Leydig cell tumor, with an incidence that peaks at 4 years of age. These tumors are usually benign. Hydroceles

may be a concurrent finding and may obscure the diagnosis. Ultrasound is a useful diagnostic tool to differentiate scrotal masses and to examine the testis with an overlying hydrocele.[65] Definitive diagnosis rests on surgical exploration.

Idiopathic Scrotal Edema

In a rare instance, when all acute causes of scrotal swelling are excluded, a child may be left with an edematous scrotum; a normal testis, epididymis, and cord; and minimal or no tenderness. If the urologist has evaluated this patient, and if all indicated tests including ultrasonography and technetium scan are normal, the child may have idiopathic scrotal edema.

BLUNT SCROTAL TRAUMA

Children younger than 10 years rarely suffer injury to the testes during blunt scrotal trauma, probably because of the testes' small size and mobility. In addition, prior to puberty, a strong cremasteric reflex pulls the testes out of the scrotum at the least threat. However, during puberty, the testes rapidly approach adult size, and the cremasteric reflex lessens. Testicular injury occurs when the gonad is caught between the imposing object and the pubic or ischial bone. Males aged 10 to 30 years sustain the highest incidence of all kinds of traumatic injuries, including those involving the scrotum and its contents.[66] These usually occur during either sports activities or motor vehicle accidents. Falls, straddle injuries, and kicks to the groin are additional causes.

Several types of injury to the testis and epididymis may occur, ranging from contusion to rupture. Because of the mobility and suspension of the organ, a traumatic event can twist the testis on its cord or displace it out of the scrotum.

In its pendulous portion, the anterior urethra dips toward the perineum and resides close to the base of the scrotum. It is subject to injury from the same forces that play a role in testicular trauma. A blow directed to the base of the scrotum, as in a straddle injury, can entrap the urethra against the pubic arch, resulting in contusion or disruption, either complete or incomplete (Fig. 50–6).

Testicular rupture and torsion of the spermatic cord are the potentially most serious injuries sustained during blunt scrotal trauma. Unfortunately, the various injuries are not always discernible by physical examination. Scrotal ecchymosis, edema, and tenderness often preclude palpable definition of the injured part. In addition, even if anatomy is identifiable, torsion and contusion may appear identical. If properly diagnosed in a timely fashion, both torsion and testicular rupture[67] may be successfully corrected.

Clinical Evaluation

Children may not be reliable historians, particularly regarding accidents involving the genitalia. They are often embarrassed and consequently may minimize the event surrounding the injury, not only when talking to the physician, but also when talking to the parents. Many of these patients present late in the course of the problem and make differentiation even more difficult. In general, however, major injuries yield major symptoms. The boy may be in extreme pain, with nausea and lightheadedness. He may find walking difficult and may have urinary retention related to the pain.

Testicular rupture usually presents with edema of the scrotum that obliterates the skin folds. Ecchymosis is usually present and is often confined to the involved side. The testis is tender and swollen, and normal landmarks are not usually palpable.

Often a mass within the scrotum that does not transilluminate and may appear ecchymotic indicates an associated

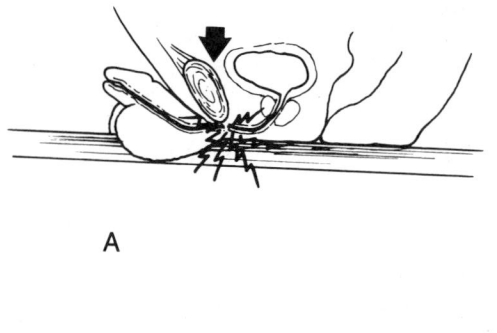

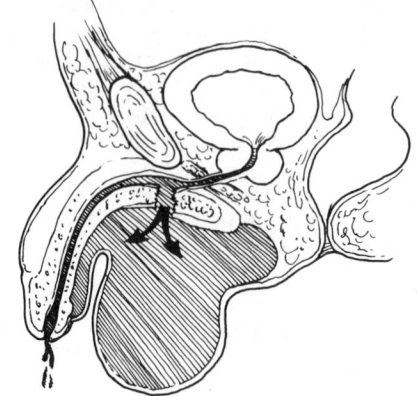

Figure 50–6. A straddle injury can result in a urethral tear. *A,* Downward forces *(arrow)* cause the urethra to become trapped against the pubic arch. *B,* With a urethral disruption, blood and urine *(arrows)* can diffuse into the scrotum and perineum.

hematocele, or blood contained within the tunica vaginalis. Testicular rupture should be excluded by means other than physical examination. Although it is true that greater force is required to rupture the testis than to cause contusion, an underlying abnormality such as a tumor can allow minimal trauma to fracture the tunica albuginea. This must be considered when the injury appears to be out of proportion to the inciting event.[66–70]

Trauma is reported to be a significant cause of torsion by many authors.[31, 71, 72] Presumably, a force applied in a specific direction can cause the testis to twist on its suspensory cord. The findings can be similar to those seen in nontraumatic torsion, and in addition, abrasions and ecchymosis may be present.

Testicular dislocation should be considered in any patient with an empty, normally developed hemiscrotum. This injury occurs most commonly as a result of a motorcycle accident. If no reliable history is available, absence of a testis in the scrotum, until disproved, must be perceived as displacement either into the inguinal canal or, more commonly, superficial to the external oblique fascia.

The urethra may be injured by a compressive force to the base of the scrotum against the underside of the ischial rami (Fig. 50–6). This most commonly occurs as a result of a straddle injury[73] and causes contusion or some degree of disruption. It should be suspected in any patient with blunt trauma to the scrotum or perineum, with blood in the urine or at the urethral meatus, or with difficulty in voiding. It should also be considered when a bruise involves the base of the scrotum or penis (Fig. 50–7).[74]

Therapeutic Intervention

The severity of scrotal injury can be difficult to determine based on the history and physical examination. Because severe injuries are likely to have the best possible outcome with early surgical correction, nearly all of these patients should have immediate urologic consultation.

The examiner should categorize patients into one of three groups: those with obvious intrascrotal injury, those with no identifiable abnormality, and those with indeterminate injury. A scrotal mass may obscure the testicular examination. The mass may be a hematocele, which does not transilluminate, or a reactive hydrocele, which does transilluminate. Scrotal ultrasonography can help evaluate the integrity of the testis.[75] If there is any question of torsion, however, a nuclear medicine scan is even more helpful in evaluating the blood flow to the testis. Again, the 6-hour time constraint applies.

If a urethral injury is suspected because of difficulty in voiding, blood at the urethral meatus, hematuria, or the proximity of the injury, a catheter should not be inserted, and a retrograde urethrogram should be performed to exclude disruption. If the urethrogram is normal, the patient probably has a urethral contusion, and the family should be counseled on urologic follow-up and the possibility of future stricture formation. Disrupted urethras should be treated with suprapubic tube urinary diversion to allow healing of the injury.[73]

If a major injury has been disproved, ice packs, bed rest, and pain management are appropriate.

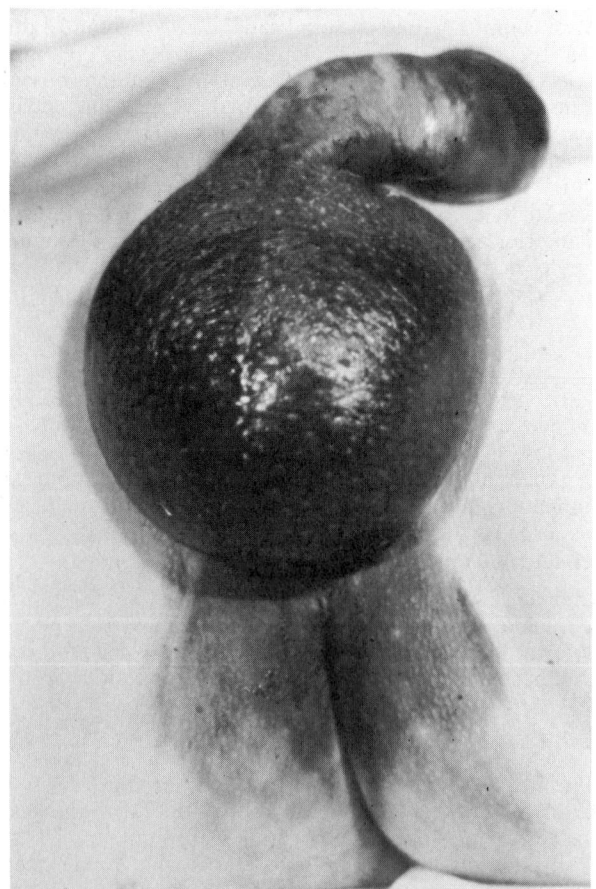

Figure 50–7. This child sustained a urethral injury. Ecchymosis of the scrotum and perineum is highly suggestive of a urethral disruption. (Courtesy of Dr. Evan J. Kass.)

PENETRATING TRAUMA
Bullet and Knife Wounds

All gunshot and knife wounds to the scrotum should be explored surgically,[76] and therefore immediate urologic consultation is required. In the emergency department, hemostasis should be obtained with pressure, if possible, and appropriate broad-spectrum antibiotics should be started. Tetanus prophylaxis should also accompany any penetrating trauma.[76–78]

Minor Lacerations

Small lacerations deserve careful inspection for deeper injuries. If the child is uncooperative, an anesthetic may be required for in-depth examination of the wound. However, if the child is cooperative and the dartos muscle layer of the scrotum is intact, the wound should be cleansed and debrided, if necessary, and closed in one layer with absorbable suture under local anesthesia. Injuries through the dartos layer should be repaired surgically.

Major Penetrating Injuries

Severe puncture wounds can result from straddling sharp objects (i.e., as when climbing over picket or hurricane fencing). Consideration of deeper injury should direct operative investigation.

Major demasculinating or degloving injuries of the genitalia are unusual in childhood.[79] If they occur, however, emergency treatment includes hemostasis, resuscitation, antibiotics, and stabilization of the wound with immediate urologic referral. Occasionally, amputated parts are reimplantable and should accompany the patient to the operating room.[80] The amputated part should be placed on saline-soaked gauze inside a clean bag. This bag should be placed on ice within a second bag. Shortage of skin for closure of defects can be a problem,[81] and therefore no debridement should be performed in the emergency department.

BURNS

Perineal burns are not unusual in the pediatric population but most commonly occur in association with burns involving other areas. Therapy is essentially the same as for those involving other body regions and is dependent on the origin.[82]

Isolated burns to the genitalia may occur, such as when a toddler pulls a cup of scalding liquid from the table, dumping it into his lap. In addition, scald burns to the scrotum, perineum, penis, and buttocks are occasionally inflicted by intentional or accidental immersion in hot water.

Heat-induced burns, if they are limited first- or second-degree burns, should be initially cooled with water. Application of topical burn ointment is then appropriate, along with symptomatic care. If the injury is more extensive, initial management includes urethral catheterization, fluid resuscitation, parenteral antibiotics, tetanus prophylaxis, and pain management. Urologic consultation should be obtained.[78] Debridement, skin grafting, and future reconstruction may be required. Genital burns are usually an indication for hospitalization.

INFECTIONS
Folliculitis

Folliculitis of the scrotum is common in postpubertal males. The small, suppurative, infected hair roots are usually self-limiting and will drain spontaneously. However, if accompanied by cellulitis or fluctuance, they may require surgical drainage. Staphylococcal and streptococcal organisms are the usual pathogens, and appropriate antibiotic therapy should be administered.

Fournier's Gangrene

Fournier's gangrene, an idiopathic necrotizing fasciitis that spreads rapidly and is associated with a high rate of morbidity and mortality, has been described in children.[83–85] Many of these patients have a predisposing immunologic defect, a minor disruption of the skin, or a perirectal process. They may present with minimal symptoms or in profound sepsis. Fever, chills, and rigor may accompany a state of delirium and confusion. On physical examination, various degrees of fluctuance, erythema, and edema are present involving the scrotum, penis, and perineum. The line of demarcation may advance posteriorly to the perirectal spaces, anteriorly to the abdominal wall, and laterally to the thighs. Crepitus caused by subcutaneous gas indicates infection by anaerobic organisms. Often, multiple gram-positive and gram-negative organisms are responsible, and an adequate multiple-drug regimen should be started immediately. Coverage for anaerobes, including *Bacteroides fragilis*, must be included. Surgical drainage and debridement should be instituted as soon as possible.

References

1. Parker RM, Robison JR. Anatomy and diagnosis of torsion of the testicle. J Urol 1971;106:243.
2. Oster J. Further fate of the foreskin: Incidence of preputial adhesions, phimosis, and smegma among Danish schoolboys. Arch Dis Child 1968;43:200.
3. Osborn LM, Metcalf TJ, Mariani EM. Hygienic care in uncircumcised infants. Pediatrics 1981;67:365.
4. Roberts JR, Hedges JR. Clinical Procedures in Emergency Medicine. Philadelphia, WB Saunders, 1985, pp 809–813.
5. Seeler RA. Intensive transfusion therapy for priapism in boys with sickle cell anemia. J Urol 1973;110:360.
6. Rifkind S, Waisman J, Thompson R, Goldfinger D. RBC exchange pheresis for priapism in sickle cell disease. JAMA 1979;242:2317.
7. Resnick MI, Holland JM, King LR, Grayhack JT. Priapism in boys: Management with cavernosaphenous shunt. Urology 1975;5:492.
8. Kinney TR, Harris MB, Russell MO, et al. Priapism in association with sickle hemoglobinopathies in children. J Pediatrics 1975;86:241.
9. Broderick GA, Lue TF. Priapism and the physiology of erection. AUA Update Series 1988;29(VII):226.
10. Baron M, Leiter E. The management of priapism in sickle cell anemia. J Urol 1978;119:610.
11. Winter CC. Priapism treated by modification of creation of fistulas between glans penis and corpora cavernosa. J Urol 1979;121:743.
12. Noe HN, Wilimas J, Jerkins GR. Surgical management of priapism in children with sickle cell anemia. J Urol 1981;126:770.
13. Steinhardt GF, Steinhardt E. Priapism in children with leukemia. Urology 1981;18:604.
14. Altebarmakian VK, Rabinowitz R, Rana SR, Ettinger LJ. Transglandular cavernosum-spongiosum shunt for leukemic priapism in childhood. J Urol 1980;123:287.
15. Haddad FS. Penile strangulation by human hair: Report of three cases and review of the literature. Urology 1982;37:375.
16. Bashir AY, El-Barbary M. Hair coil strangulation of the penis. J R Coll Surg Edinb 1980;25:47.
17. McClure WJ, Gradinger GP. Hair strangulation of the glans penis. Plast Reconstr Surg 1985;76:120.
18. Sheinfeld J, Cos LR, Erturk E, Cockett ATK. Penile tourniquet injury due to a coil of hair. J Urol 1985;133:1042.
19. Sandler CM, Corriere JN. Urethrography in the diagnosis of acute urethral injuries. Urol Clin North Am 1989;16:283.
20. Pierce JM. Disruptions of the anterior urethra. Urol Clin North Am 1989;16:329.
21. Geist RF. Sexually related trauma. Emerg Med Clin North Am 1988;6:439.
22. Kenney RD. Adolescent males who insert genitourinary foreign bodies: Is psychiatric referral required? Urology 1988;32:127.
23. Saraf P, Rabinowitz R. Zipper injury of the foreskin. Am J Dis Child 1982;136:557.

24. Oosterlinck W. Unbloody management of penile zipper injury. Eur Urol 1981;7:365.
25. Donovan JF, Kaplan WE. The therapy of genital trauma by dog bite. J Urol 1989;141:1163.
26. Ransler CW III, Allen TD. Torsion of the spermatic cord. Urol Clin North Am 1989;9:245.
27. Bartsch G, Frank S, Marberger H, Mikuz G. Testicular torsion: Late results with special regard to fertility and endocrine function. J Urol 1980;124:375.
28. Snyder HM III, Caldamone AA, Duckett JW Jr. Scrotal pain/swelling. In Fleisher GR, Ludwig S (eds). Textbook of Pediatric Emergency Medicine. Baltimore, Williams & Wilkins, 1988, pp 279–285.
29. Haynes BE, Bessen HA, Haynes VE. The diagnosis of testicular torsion. JAMA 1983;149:2522.
30. Kogan SJ. Acute and chronic scrotal swellings. In Gillenwater JY, Grayhack JT, Howards SS, Duckett JD (eds). Adult and Pediatric Urology. Chicago, Year Book, 1987, pp 1947–1974.
31. Elsharty S, Pranikoff K, Magoss IV, Sufrin G. Traumatic torsion of the testis. J Urol 1984;132:1155.
32. Jerkins GR, Noe NH, Hollenbach RS, Allen RG. Spermatic cord torsion in the neonate. J Urol 1983;129:121.
33. Angell JC. Torsion of the testicle: A plea for diagnosis. Lancet 1963;1:19.
34. Pedersen JF, Holm HH, Hald T. Torsion of the testis diagnosed by ultrasound. J Urol 1975;113:66.
35. Levy BJ. The diagnosis of torsion of the testicle using the Doppler ultrasonic stethoscope. J Urol 1975;113:63.
36. Milleret R, Liaras H. L'auscultation a l'aide des ultra-sons dans les torsions du testicule. J Chir 1974;107:35.
37. Nasrallah PF, Manzone D, King LR. False negative Doppler examinations in testicular torsion. J Urol 1977;118:194.
38. Perri AJ, Morales JO, Feldman AE. Necrotic testicle with increased blood flow on Doppler ultrasonic examination. Urology 1976;8:265.
39. Rodriguez DD, Rodriguez WC, Rivera JJ, et al. Doppler ultrasound versus testicular scanning in the evaluation of the acute scrotum. J Urol 1981;125:343.
40. Gislason T, Noronha RFX, Gregory JG. Acute epididymitis in boys: A 5-year retrospective study. J Urol 1980;124:533.
41. Golimbu M, Florio FE, Al-Askari S, et al. Value of scrotal scanning. Urology 1985;25:89.
42. Stage KH, Schoenvogel R, Lewis S. Testicular scanning: Clinical experience with 72 patients. J Urol 1981;125:334.
43. Kogan SJ, Lutzker LG, Perez LA, et al. The value of the negative radionuclide scrotal scan in the management of the acutely inflamed scrotum in children. J Urol 1979;122:223.
44. Stein BS, Kendall AR, Harke HT, et al. Scrotal imaging in the Henoch-Schönlein syndrome. J Urol 1980;124:568.
45. Kogan SJ, Levitt SB. Re: Imaging techniques and testicular abnormalities. Letter. J Urol 1984;131:559.
46. Klauber GT, Sant GR. Disorders of the male external genitalia. In Kelalis PP, King LR, Belman AB (eds). Clinical Pediatric Urology. Philadelphia, WB Saunders, 1985, pp 825–863.
47. Koff SA, DeRidder P. Conservative management of intrascrotal appendiceal torsion. Urology 1976;8:482.
48. Dresner ML. Torsed appendage. Diagnosis and management: Blue dot sign. Urology 1973;1:63.
49. Holland JM, Graham JB, Ignatoff JM. Conservative management of twisted testicular appendages. J Urol 1981;125:213.
50. Genitourinary diseases. In Barkin RM, Rosen P (eds). Emergency Pediatrics: A Guide to Ambulatory Care. St Louis, CV Mosby, 1987, pp 504–507.
51. Raffensperger JG. Inguinal hernia. In Raffensperger JG (ed). Swenson's Pediatric Surgery. Norwalk, CT, Appleton & Lange, 1990, pp 121–134.
52. Loh HS, Jalan OM. Testicular torsion in Henoch-Schönlein syndrome. Br Med J 1974;2:96.
53. O'Regan S, Robitaille P. Orchitis mimicking testicular torsion in Henoch-Schölein's purpura. J Urol 1981;126:834.
54. Koster LH, Antoon SJ. Fat necrosis in the scrotum. J Urol 1980;123:599.
55. Udall DA, Drake DJ Jr, Rosenburg RS. Acute scrotal swelling: A physical sign of primary peritonitis. J Urol 1981;125:750.
56. Sujka SK, Evans EJ, Nigam A. Delayed rupture of the spleen presenting as a scrotal hematoma. J Trauma 1986;26:85.
57. Johnson JH. Acquired lesions of the penis, the scrotum and the testis. In Williams DI, Johnson JH (eds). Paediatric Urology. London, Butterworth Scientific, 1982, pp 467–475.
58. Preblud SR. Infectious diseases: Mumps. In Gellis SS, Kagan BM (eds). Current Pediatric Therapy. Philadelphia, WB Saunders, 1986, pp 577–578.
59. Fonkalsrud EW. Undescended testes. In Welch KJ, Randolph JG, Ravitch MM, (eds). Pediatric Surgery. Chicago, Year Book, 1986, pp 793–807.
60. Kogan SJ. Cryptorchidism. In Kelalis PP, King LR, Belman AB (eds). Clinical Pediatric Urology. Philadelphia, WB Saunders, 1985, pp 864–887.
61. Shrock P. The processus vaginalis and gubernaculum: Their raison d'être redefined. Surg Clin North Am 1971;51:1263.
62. Rowe MI, Lloyd DA. Inguinal hernia. In Welch KJ, Randolph JG, Ravitch MM (eds). Pediatric Surgery. Chicago, Year Book, 1986, pp 779–793.
63. Kass EJ. Evaluation and management of the adolescent with a varicocele. AUA Update Series 1990;9(lesson 12):89–96.
64. Brosman SA. Tumors: Male genital tract. In Kelalis PP, King LR, Belman AB (eds). Clinical Pediatric Urology. Philadelphia, WB Saunders, 1985, pp 1202–1219.
65. Friedman SG, Rose JG, Winston MA. Ultrasound and nuclear medicine evaluation in acute testicular trauma. J Urol 1981;125:748.
66. Munter DW, Faleski EJ. Blunt scrotal trauma: Emergency department evaluation and management. Am J Emerg Med 1989;7:227.
67. Cass AS. Testicular trauma. J Urol 1983;129:299.
68. Rao KG. Traumatic rupture of testis. Urology 1982;20:624.
69. Schuster G. Traumatic rupture of the testicle and a review of the literature. J Urol 1982;127:1194.
70. Zivkovic SM, Janjic G. Traumatic rupture of the testis and epididymis. J Pediatr Surg 1980;15:287.
71. Cos LR, Rabinowitz R. Trauma-induced testicular torsion in children. J Trauma 1982;22:244.
72. Kursh ED. Traumatic torsion of testicle. Urology 1981;17:441.
73. Pierce JM. Disruptions of the anterior urethra. Urol Clin North Am 1989;16:329.
74. McDougal WS, Persky L. Urethral injuries. In Libertino JA (ed). International Perspectives in Urology: Traumatic Injuries of the Genitourinary System. Baltimore, Williams & Wilkins, 1981, pp 59–83.
75. Fournier GR, Laing FC, McAninch JW. Scrotal ultrasonography and the management of testicular trauma. Urol Clin North Am 1989;16:377.
76. McAninch JW, Kahn RI, Jeffrey RB, et al. Major traumatic and septic genital injuries. J Trauma 1984;24:291.
77. Donovan JF, Kaplan WE. The therapy of genital trauma by dog bite. J Urol 1989;141:1163.
78. Firlit CF. Injury to the genitalia in children. In Cass AS (ed). Genitourinary Trauma. Boston, Blackwell Scientific, 1988, pp 269–283.
79. Grewal SS, Dalal SS, Singh S. Traumatic degloving of penis. Br J Urol 1982;54:296.
80. Jordan GH, Gilbert DA. Management of amputation injuries of the male genitalia. Urol Clin North Am 1989;16:359.
81. McAninch JW. Management of genital skin loss. Urol Clin North Am 1989;16:387.
82. McDougal WS, Persky L. Traumatic injuries of the external genitalia. In Libertino JA (ed). International Perspectives in Urology: Traumatic Injuries of the Genitourinary System. Baltimore, Williams & Wilkins, 1981, pp 39–57.
83. Jones RB, Hirschmann JV, Brown GS, Tremann JA. Fournier's syndrome: Necrotizing subcutaneous infection of the male genitalia. J Urol 1979;122:279.
84. Redman JF, Yamauchi T, Higginbothom WE. Fournier's gangrene of the scrotum in a child. J Urol 1979;121:827.
85. Gibson TE. Idiopathic gangrene of the scrotum with report of a case and review of the literature. J Urol 1930;23:125.

SECTION SIX

Obstetrics and Gynecology

CHAPTER 51

Adolescent Pregnancy and Obstetric Emergencies

Marie C. Giarratana
Barbara Staggers

INTRODUCTION

Adolescent pregnancy has become a major public health problem since the 1970s. The National Center for Health Statistics reports that from 1970 to 1985, the pregnancy rate in the 10- to 14-year-old group remained stable at 1.2 to 1.3 births per 1000, while there was an increase of 41% (from 22.4 to 31.6 births per 1000) for adolescents aged 15 to 19 years during this same 15-year period. For black adolescents, the birth rate of unmarried mothers decreased by 8% between 1970 and 1985 (from 96.9 per 1000 to 88.8 per 1000); for the white adolescent population, the birth rate increased by 88% (from 10.9 per 1000 in 1970 to 20.5 per 1000 in 1985).

There are approximately 1.6 million teenage pregnancies per year in the United States. One fifth of these pregnancies occur within 1 month of initiation of sexual activity, and 50% occur within the first 6 months following initiation of sexual activity. An adolescent woman under 15 years of age in the United States is five times more likely to have given birth than an adolescent woman of similar age in any other developed country.

Emergency departments and outpatient clinics are often where the teen first presents with obstetric and gynecologic problems, and thus primary care providers should be knowledgeable about the health care of young women. The physician must be able to assess, triage, and manage the pregnant adolescent, who often falls into the high-risk category for prenatal obstetric care.

Competent diagnosis and management require familiarity and experience with procedures used in the evaluation and management of adolescent women. Obstetric and gynecologic issues are an integral aspect of the medical care for adolescent females and involve the legal issue of minors and their right to confidentiality in health care delivery. The type of care a pregnant adolescent chooses to access may have much to do with the laws in her state of residence. A minor's rights include the right to seek an abortion without parental permission, often an option many teens wish to explore when they learn they are pregnant.

PSYCHOSOCIAL ASPECTS

In United States society adolescents must cope with developmental stages that are often in conflict with societal norms. The role of an adolescent is often not clearly defined, and adolescents may resort to sexual activity (with resultant pregnancy) as a means of establishing their identity. Annually, more than 1 million young women under 20 years of age in the United States become pregnant, with a large proportion of these births being to young unmarried adolescents between the ages of 14 and 16 years.

Adolescence is a dynamic period of life characterized by rapid growth and change. The transition from childhood to adulthood involves the completion of developmental tasks. The timing of the sequence of events involved in physiologic and psychosocial maturation varies with each individual.

Adolescents display a varied range of physiologic and psychosocial maturation within a given age group. Similarly, a group of 14-year-olds will be quite different from a group of 18-year-olds. The differences involve decision-making skills, the ability to abstract, contraceptive utilization, and risk assessment. Assessment of developmental or maturational level (physiologic or psychosocial) is critical when attempting to understand the pregnant adolescent.

Physiologic Development

The physiologic aspects of adolescence and puberty include the development of secondary sex characteristics, the development of reproductive capacity, and the establishment of sexual dimorphism. These pubertal changes develop in a defined course and occur within a range of time for onset, growth spurt, and peak height velocity, with some variation in the age of onset and completion of growth.

The average age of menarche in the United States is 12.5 years for white adolescent females and 11.8 years for black adolescent females. This is approximately 2 years younger than the average age of menarche in the year 1900. Thus young adolescent females are entering and completing pubertal development at an earlier age, and this earlier physiologic development can place young females at risk for engaging in behaviors that could potentially result in pregnancy.

The adolescent female who attains adult physiologic status earlier than her male or female counterparts experiences psychosocial developmental needs at an earlier time. The young adolescent female with a physiologically mature body may have limited cognitive experience and skills, increased needs pertaining to autonomy and independence (including heterosexual initiative), an older peer social network, and a social environment that encourages adult behavior.

Factors Contributing to Adolescent Pregnancy

Although many factors contribute to adolescent pregnancy, there are three main components to the developmental framework: inability to experience normal developmental stages of growth; low self-esteem and depression; and sexual messages from the media. The number of single-parent, female-headed families more than doubled between the years 1959 and 1983. Often, adolescents from single-parent families have to assume more responsibility. Because the single parent must work long hours, adolescents may have the responsibility of caring for siblings or performing household chores. This may lead to a lack of opportunities to experience the normal developmental stages of youth. In an attempt to seek attention from adults and to foster independence and adulthood, the adolescent may become pregnant.

Furthermore, during the early-adolescence stage, when concrete thinking is typical, adolescents possess limited cognitive ability to think in terms of the future and the consequences of their actions. Most adolescents who have not completed the early-adolescence stage know little about the implications of having a baby. Adolescent parents must struggle with being both an adolescent and an adult. Raising a child results in less time for personal development and networking with peers. Adolescent parents cannot maintain the expected independence, because they are in need of emotional and financial support from family and friends.

The inability to experience normal adolescent developmental stages may lead to low self-esteem and depression. Chronic depression is directly linked to adolescent pregnancy. Adolescents seek the acceptance and affection of others to affirm self-worth and develop self-esteem. Often, adolescents look to newborn infants to provide affection and acceptance. Members of the opposite sex are often sought to fill voids and heal the wounds caused by depression and low self-esteem.

Adolescents spend more time watching television than they do in school. Sexually explicit behaviors are demonstrated through the media, and television shows are replete with profanity and violence. Adolescents may assimilate the behaviors exhibited on television. Television shows may suggest that promiscuity is acceptable, thereby resulting in increased rates of adolescent pregnancy as well as sexually transmitted diseases.

Pregnancy is associated with significant physical and emotional changes and complicates the ongoing developmental process of adolescence. The pregnant adolescent must cope with the physiologic changes of pregnancy, as well as the later changes brought on with lactation. Important features of obstetric health care include the nutritional health of the adolescent, mental health care assessment, and health care support and educational needs. The health care provider must have an understanding of the unique features of puberty and pregnancy and the stress each places on adolescent development.

EMERGENCY MEDICAL SERVICE CONSIDERATIONS

Addressing maternal survival is absolutely necessary for fetal survival. The stabilization of maternal vital signs through the early recognition of hypoxia or hypotension is crucial. In the field, the prehospital care provider must perform a rapid initial survey of airway, breathing, and circulation. A more complete physical examination follows to determine additional injury and establish baseline neurologic function. A brief history, including a history of any recent vaginal bleeding or discharge, should be obtained. A secondary survey should note the fundal height and any evidence of uterine contractions or irritability. Vaginal bleeding or other discharge should be noted. Nitrazine strip testing should be reserved for management in the emergency department with a sterile speculum. The detection of fetal movement should be documented and fetal heart rate assessed, including quality, rate, and location. Fetal bradycardia of less than 100 to 110 beats/min is evidence of uterine irritability. The obstetric patient should be positioned on her left side to enhance venous return. When spinal injury is a possibility, the patient should be securely immobilized against a backboard prior to this positioning.

Initiation of intravenous access with a large-bore peripheral catheter should be performed and an isotonic solution of 0.9% normal saline or Ringer's lactate (LR) should be infused. Supplemental oxygen should be administered, and the patient should be rapidly transported to the nearest facility capable of managing obstetric complications.

CLINICAL EVALUATION

The pregnant adolescent patient presenting to the emergency department for care should have a focused history based on the chief complaint. Data relevant to the obstetric patient should also be gathered. Such information includes the patient's parity as well as the quality and timing of the last menstrual period. A history of lower abdominal pain, vaginal bleeding, or fever is particularly important.

A more routine screening examination and a more comprehensive history can then be obtained. The nutritional status and eating habits of the pregnant adolescent as well as a drug history (including tobacco use) are also important (Table 51–1). A psychosocial assessment should be performed, with special consideration given to the maturity level of the teen. The patient's coping and problem-solving abilities should be assessed, as well as sources of support from family, friends, and the father of the infant. The teen's educational plans and current level of education are important. The sources of financial support for the patient and for the infant should be ascertained.

The physical examination should include an assessment of vital signs, giving particular attention to any orthostatic changes in pulse and blood pressure. Hypertension in pregnancy is particularly serious and may suggest preeclampsia. The examination may also detect abnormally low or increased weight gain during a pregnancy, anemia, or other evidence of chronic illness.

DIAGNOSTIC EVALUATION
Diagnosis of Pregnancy

The main function of human chorionic gonadotropin (HCG) is to support the corpus luteum. HCG takes an active role approximately 8 days after ovulation, when it can first be detected in maternal blood. The survival of the corpus luteum is totally dependent on HCG, and the survival of the fetus is dependent on the steroids from the corpus luteum until the seventh week of pregnancy. At the seventh to tenth week of pregnancy, the fetus is supported less by the corpus luteum and more by the placenta.

HCG is secreted by the syncytiotrophoblast and reaches a

TABLE 51–1

APPROACH TO THE PREGNANT ADOLESCENT

A. Histories should include all information pertinent to any pregnant woman, along with specific information pertaining to adolescents
   1. Nutritional status and eating habits
   2. Drug history, including tobacco use
   3. Psychosocial assessment, with special consideration given to:
      a. Maturity level
      b. Coping and problem-solving abilities
      c. Family support, significant other, and friend support systems
      d. Educational plans, present level of education
      e. Childbirth education plans
      f. Financial support of teen and infant
      g. Help with infant's care
      h. Involvement of the father
      i. Teen's perception of her and the infant's needs
B. The physical examination should include the usual components for any pregnant woman. It is important to rigorously screen for the following:
   1. Low or increased weight gain
   2. Anemia
   3. Poor eating habits
   4. Development of adolescent high-risk, pregnancy-induced hypertension
   5. Signs and symptoms of adolescent preterm labor
C. Antepartum Laboratory Tests
   1. Blood type and Rh factor
   2. Antibody screening and identification
   3. Complete blood cell count
   4. Gonorrhea and *Chlamydia* screen
   5. Pap smear
   6. Rubella titer
   7. Urinalysis or urine culture and stain as indicated
   8. Syphilis testing
   9. Alpha-fetoprotein test for selected women: obtain at 15 to 18 weeks' gestation when there is a history of neural tube defect or when the woman is in a high-risk geographic area
   10. Glucose-6-phosphatase dehydrogenase (G6PD) deficiency assessment: done on women of black or Middle Eastern descent, especially if there is a history of severe anemia
   11. Glucose screen—obtain initially and repeat at 24 to 28 weeks
   12. Hepatitis B antigen
   13. Routine cervical cultures: gonorrhea, *Chlamydia,* herpes simplex
   14. HIV titer for high-risk groups
   15. Renal function tests; determination of blood urea nitrogen, creatinine, and uric acid levels; screening of all patients with hypertension, renal disease, or hypertensive disorders of pregnancy
   16. Thyroid studies as indicated

maximal level of 50,000 to 100,000 mIU/ml at 10 weeks of gestation. Maternal levels of circulating HCG at the time of the first missed period are approximately 100 mIU/ml. By 10 to 20 weeks, HCG levels drop to 10,000 to 20,000 mIU/ml.

Highly sensitive monoclonal antibody immunologic tests that detect the presence of HCG in maternal urine and blood have replaced the old bioassay tests. Blood HCG levels are helpful in two clinical situations: trophoblastic disease and ectopic pregnancy. In early pregnancy there is the characteristic sequential appearance of HCG, followed by beta-HCG and then alpha-HCG. The ratio of beta-HCG to total HCG remains constant in a normal early pregnancy. Trophoblastic disease is distinguishable by high levels of circulating HCG that are up to 3 to 100 times those found in a normal pregnancy. In an ectopic pregnancy, the circu-

lating levels of HCG do not rise as they do with a normal gestational pregnancy. Measuring the rate of rise of HCG is a useful diagnostic indicator for ectopic pregnancy. When measuring two beta-HCG levels 48 hours apart, the percentage of HCG rise should be at least 66% over a period of 48 hours.

Antepartum Laboratory Screening

The pregnant adolescent patient will need routine antepartum laboratory screening. The blood type and Rh factor must be determined to evaluate the need for immunization with Rh immune globulin if the patient is Rh negative. A complete blood cell count, urinalysis, fasting glucose test, rubella titer, and Pap smear should also be obtained. Certain patients may also need other specific tests performed. The alpha-fetoprotein level should be measured at 15 to 18 weeks' gestation in women who have a history of a neural tube defect or in those patients in a high-risk geographic population for such defects. Glucose-6-phosphatase dehydrogenase (G6PD) deficiency assessment should be done in women of black, Mediterranean, or Middle Eastern descent, especially if there is a history of severe anemia. Cervical cultures for gonorrhea, chlamydia, and herpes simplex virus should be done if cervicitis is present. High-risk groups should be tested for hepatitis B antigen and should be counseled regarding the need for assessment of infection with the human immunodeficiency virus (HIV). Other tests to be considered include VDRL, renal function, uric acid, and thyroid function tests.

OBSTETRIC COMPLICATIONS
Ectopic Pregnancy

In an ectopic pregnancy, the fertilized ovum implants in tissue other than the endometrium. Approximately 95% of these implantations occur in the fallopian tube. The rate of occurrence can vary from 1 in 64 pregnancies to 1 in 241 pregnancies, depending on the population studied. Currently there are 70,000 cases per year in the United States. In the decade from 1970 to 1980, the rate of ectopic pregnancy increased threefold, with 36% of these pregnancies occurring in 15- to 24-year-old women.

The medical history may include the classic triad (seen in 70% of patients) of amenorrhea (for a period of 7 to 10 weeks), abdominal pain (can be localized, diffuse, or referred to the shoulder), and abnormal vaginal bleeding (irregular bleeding, spotting, or heavy bleeding).

The physical examination should include an assessment of vital signs, including orthostatic blood pressure and pulse reading; careful abdominal and gynecologic evaluation; and costovertebral angle assessment.

A pregnancy test should be performed in the stable adolescent patient when ectopic pregnancy is suspected from the clinical evaluation. The initial test is usually a qualitative serum HCG test; a complete blood cell count and urinalysis are also indicated. If the results of the qualitative pregnancy test are positive, a quantitative beta-HCG test should immediately be obtained. The quantitative HCG is used as a baseline for serial evaluation in the patient with no or minimal symptoms. It is also useful in determining the indications for and the interpretation of pelvic ultrasonography.

Pelvic ultrasonography can be diagnostic in the evaluation of the pregnant patient with abdominal pain or other clinical findings suggestive of ectopic pregnancy. If the estimated gestation time is 6 weeks or more or the patient is found to have a beta-HCG level greater than or equal to 6500 mIU/ml, the pelvic ultrasound should reveal an intrauterine gestational sac if the pregnancy is normal. When no intrauterine gestational sac is seen with this HCG level, the pelvic ultrasound has an 85% positive predictive value in the diagnosis of ectopic pregnancy. Detection of an intrauterine gestational sac has also become possible using transvaginal probe-guided ultrasonography, and reliable results have been obtained with HCG levels greater than 1300 mIU/ml.

Additional diagnostic tests can include culdocentesis. Culdocentesis should be performed only after consultation with an obstetrician and preferably by an experienced specialist. Many investigators suggest that a culdocentesis should be performed before the symptomatic patient is considered for outpatient management, and the patient should then be followed with serial beta-HCG tests. If the culdocentesis yields blood, then a laparoscopy is performed (Table 51–2). A negative culdocentesis does not exclude ectopic pregnancy, but it does exclude a ruptured ectopic pregnancy or a ruptured and bleeding ovarian cyst as a cause for the patient's symptoms.

Serial measurement of quantitative beta-HCG levels has become popular as a means of following the asymptomatic or minimally symptomatic patient suspected of having a possible ectopic pregnancy. An HCG level that does not increase by 66% every 48 hours during early pregnancy is suggestive of an abnormal pregnancy. Management of such patients should be carried out with the consultation of an obstetrician.

TABLE 51–2

INTERPRETATION OF CULDOCENTESIS FLUID

Aspirated Fluid	Condition and Suggested Differential Diagnosis
Clear, serous, straw-colored (usually only a few milliliters)	Normal peritoneal fluid
Large amount of clear fluid	Ruptured or large ovarian cyst (fluid may be serosanguineous); pregnancy may be coexistent Ascites Carcinoma
Exudate with polymorphonuclear leukocytes	Pelvic inflammatory disease Gonococcal salpingitis Chronic salpingitis
Purulent fluid	Bacterial infection Tubo-ovarian abscess with rupture Appendicitis with rupture Diverticulitis with perforation
Bright red blood	Ruptured viscus or vascular injury Recently bleeding ectopic pregnancy (ruptured or unruptured) Bleeding corpus luteum Intra-abdominal injury Liver Spleen Other organs Ruptured aortic aneurysm
Old, brown, nonclotting blood	Ruptured viscus Ectopic pregnancy with intraperitoneal bleeding over a few days or weeks Old (days) intra-abdominal injury (e.g., delayed splenic rupture)

From Roberts JR, Hedges JR. Clinical Procedures in Emergency Medicine. 2nd ed. Philadelphia, WB Saunders, 1991.

Initial management of the patient with a suspected ectopic pregnancy depends on the patient's stability. Patients with evidence of acute blood loss or hypovolemia require two large-bore peripheral intravenous catheters, supplemental oxygen, and cardiac monitoring. The unstable patient in shock should have a nasogastric tube and Foley catheter inserted, and immediate consultation with an obstetrician should be obtained for emergency laparotomy. In the unstable patient, surgery should not be delayed for diagnostic testing. Transfusion of packed red blood cells and other blood products may be necessary. Stable patients may have a laparoscopy performed followed by laparotomy, whereas unstable patients usually require immediate surgery with salpingectomy. Smaller ectopic pregnancies may be removed by salpingotomy, with preservation of the tube and possible preservation of fertility in that tube.

An adnexal mass is palpated in 30% to 50% of patients with ectopic pregnancy, and adnexal tenderness is present in 72% to 98%. Uterine enlargement is found on physical examination in 30% of patients with ectopic pregnancy.

Differential Diagnosis

Ectopic pregnancy should be included in the differential diagnosis of all abnormal vaginal bleeding, even in the absence of abdominal pain. The patient with a positive pregnancy test result may have had a spontaneous abortion or an incomplete abortion. Both ectopic pregnancy and spontaneous abortion may have a nondiagnostic ultrasound associated with a positive pregnancy test, vaginal bleeding, and lower abdominal pain. The pregnant patient may also have a ruptured corpus luteal cyst with or without bleeding, appendicitis, ovarian torsion, pelvic inflammatory disease, or gastroenteritis mimicking ectopic pregnancy.

Given the potentially fatal outcome of ectopic pregnancy, it is imperative for clinicians to remember that early diagnosis and management are essential. If the ectopic pregnancy can be diagnosed prior to rupture, there is decreased morbidity and improved reproductive potential if the ovarian duct can be preserved.

Hemorrhage Early in Pregnancy

The causes of bleeding early in pregnancy include ectopic pregnancy, hydatidiform mole (choriocarcinoma), spontaneous abortion (miscarriage), implantation bleeding, carcinoma of the cervix, cervical polyp, fibroid polyp, and vaginal ulceration. Of these, the most life-threatening is an ectopic pregnancy. Nevertheless, bleeding from other causes can be significant. Approximately 20% of women have abnormal bleeding early in pregnancy. Of these, half have an early spontaneous abortion. In the other half, bleeding early in the pregnancy does not necessarily imply an unsuccessful pregnancy. The term *abortion* refers to delivery of a fetus prior to a time when it can survive. Typically this is a fetus of less than 20 weeks' gestation and weighing less than 500 gm. Often a fetus has been dead for more than 2 weeks before vaginal bleeding occurs.

Threatened Abortion

Any bleeding early in pregnancy should be considered a threatened abortion unless another cause can be specifically identified. When a threatened abortion is suspected, a pelvic examination should be performed, specifically assessing the amount of bleeding and integrity of the cervical loss. With a threatened abortion, bleeding is usually slight, no tissue is seen in the vagina, and the cervical loss is closed (Table 51–3). The hemoglobin level should be checked. If it is uncertain

TABLE 51–3

CLINICAL DIAGNOSIS OF ABORTION

Type Abortion	Fever	Complaint of Abdominal Cramps	Bleeding (amt)	Tissue Passed Vaginally	On Examination		
					Tissue in Vagina	Status of Internal Cervical Os	Uterine Size
Threatened	None	Slight	Slight	None	None	Closed	Commensurate with "dates"
Inevitable	None	Moderate	Moderate	None	None	Open with membranes or tissue bulging	Commensurate with "dates"
Incomplete	None	Severe	Severe	Placental or fetal tissue	Possibly	Open with tissue in cervical canal	Smaller than "dates"
Complete	None	None	Minimal	Complete placenta and fetus	Possibly	Closed with no tissue in cervical canal	Smaller than "dates"
Missed	None	No cramps; no life felt; no fetal heart tones (Doptone)	Brownish discharge; heavy if disseminated intravascular coagulation present	None	None	Closed	Smaller than expected and not enlarging

Modified from Cavanagh D, Woods RE, O'Connor TCF, Knuppel RA. Obstetric Emergencies. 3rd ed. Philadelphia, JB Lippincott, 1982.

whether the patient is pregnant, an HCG determination should be made. If an ectopic pregnancy is a diagnostic consideration, a pelvic ultrasound should be considered; transvaginal monitoring should be used if bleeding occurs very early in the pregnancy. In addition, culdocentesis should be considered.

Treatment for a threatened abortion includes 48 hours of bed rest with no heavy lifting and increased oral intake of fluids. All patients with a threatened abortion should be reexamined in 24 to 48 hours.

Inevitable Abortion

An *inevitable abortion* is characterized by dilatation of the internal os of the cervix. This can occur any time during early pregnancy. With opening of the internal os, there is often increased uterine cramping, heavier vaginal bleeding, and occasionally a sudden discharge of fluid resulting from rupture of the amniotic sac. Hospitalization is necessary, especially if the pregnancy is beyond the 12th week. The patient's hemoglobin level should be assessed and the blood type determined in anticipation of the potential need for blood transfusion. Narcotics can be given for pain control, and obstetric consultation should be urgently obtained.

Incomplete and Complete Abortions

Incomplete or *complete abortion* implies that some or all, respectively, of the fetal tissue has been delivered. In an incomplete abortion there is still some tissue in the cervical canal. In a complete abortion all placenta and fetal tissue has been passed, and the cervical os is closed.

Missed Abortion

A *missed abortion* is the retention of the products of conception for 4 weeks or more after the death of an embryo or fetus. Missed abortions usually terminate spontaneously within 4 weeks after fetal death. Disseminated intravascular coagulation can occur.

Third-Trimester Bleeding

There are three significant causes of third-trimester bleeding: abruptio placentae, placenta previa, and spontaneous abortion. Lower genital tract bleeding or systemic coagulopathy also cause third-trimester bleeding. It is essential that the pediatric emergency physician view third-trimester bleeding as a serious emergency threatening the life of both the mother and the baby. A vaginal speculum examination for third-trimester bleeding should be avoided in the emergency department because of the possibility of inducing severe uncontrolled hemorrhage. These procedures are best performed by an obstetrician with a double setup who is capable of performing an immediate cesarean section if necessary.

Abruptio Placentae

In abruptio placentae, the placenta prematurely separates from the endometrium. It is characterized by severe abdominal and pelvic pain and tenderness on palpation. The placental separation is associated with hemorrhage into the subplacental space (the area between the uterus and the placenta). In some cases the presentation is vaginal bleeding; in others, the subplacental hemorrhage may be concealed. Disseminated intravascular coagulation may accompany abruptio placentae.

Placenta Previa

In placenta previa, the placenta is implanted in the lower uterine wall. Painless bleeding in small amounts occurring over a short period most often accompanies this emergency. The small amount of bleeding does not diminish the need for rapid evaluation, as massive hemorrhage can commence at any time.

Therapeutic Intervention

Treatment of third-trimester bleeding requires emergency obstetric consultation. The patient should be evaluated for signs of hypoglycemia as evidenced by supine or postural hypotension. If hypoglycemia is present, an infusion of crystalloid or whole blood is indicated through a large-bore intravenous catheter. Laboratory studies to be performed include a complete blood cell count, coagulation studies (including a prothrombin time, partial thromboplastin time, and fibrinogen level), and a platelet count. Blood urea nitrogen and serum creatinine levels should also be determined. The patient should be crossmatched for administration of at least four units of red blood cells. Fetal heart tones should be monitored continuously. A bladder catheter should be inserted and a urinalysis performed.

The patient with third-trimester bleeding requires immediate hospitalization. The need for an emergency cesarean section is determined by an obstetrician; fetal bradycardia increases the urgency of this situation.

DISPOSITION

The pregnant adolescent is often characterized as being at high risk. This is based on maternal-child health data demonstrating that pregnant adolescents are predisposed to the following: higher maternal-infant mortality rates, lower birth rates, anemia, preeclampsia, problems with uterine sizing and determining gestational age, and multiple socioeconomic problems.

Often the emergency department is the first medical contact for the pregnant adolescent. This contact often occurs as late as at the time of active labor. When an adolescent accesses care late in the third trimester, providers of adolescent obstetric care should enroll the pregnant teen immediately in a perinatal care program. Such a program offers high-risk adolescent obstetric and gynecologic care, case management of the teen, psychosocial support, and immediate nutritional assessment and support.

Selected References

Anderson M, Irwin C, Synder D. Abnormal vaginal bleeding in adolescents. Pediatr Ann 1986;10:697–707.

Bearinger LK. Study group report on the impact of television on adolescent views of sexuality. J Adolesc Health Care 1990;1:71–75.

Bidwell RJ, Deisher RW. Adolescent sexuality: Current issues. Pediatr Ann 1991;20:293.

Braverman PK, Strasburger VC. Why adolescent gynecology? Pediatr Clin North Am 1989;36(3):471–487.

Brooks-Gunn J. Antecedents to and consequences of variations in girls' maturational timing. J Adolesc Health Care 1988;9:1–11.

Brooks-Gunn J, Furstenberg FF: Adolescent sexual behavior. Am Psychol 1989;44:249.

Brown JD, Childers KW, Waszak CS. Television and adolescent sexuality. J Adolesc Health Care 1990;11:62–70.

Claessens EA, Cowell CA. Dysfunctional uterine bleeding in the adolescent. Pediatr Clin North Am 1984;24:30.

Coupey SM, Ahlstrom P. Common menstrual disorders. Pediatr Clin North Am. 1989;36(3):551.

Easley HA, Olive DL, Holman JF. Contemporary evaluation of suspected ectopic pregnancy. J Reprod Med 1987;32(12):901–906.

Emans SJ, Goldstein DP. Contraception in Pediatric and Adolescent Gynecology. Boston, Little, Brown, 1990.

Fayez JA. Dysfunctional uterine bleeding in the emergency room. Hosp Phys 1987; April:27–33.

Fisher M. Adolescent sexuality: Overview and implications for the pediatrician. Pediatr Ann 1991;20:6.

Greydanus DE. Adolescent sexuality: An overview and perspective for the 1980s. Pediatr Ann 1982;11:714–726.

Hockberger RS. Ectopic pregnancy. In Hochbaum SR (eds). Obstetric and gynecologic emergencies. Emerg Med Clin North Am 1987;5(3):481–493.

Kegeles S, Millstein SG, Adler MR, et al. The transition to sexual activity and its relationship to other risk behaviors. J Adolesc Health Care 1987;8:308.

Levine M. The pediatrician as the primary adolescent gynecologist. Pediatr Ann 1986;7:495–498.

Lewis CL, Lewis MA. Peer pressure and risk-taking behaviors in children. Am J Public Health 1984;74:580.

McAnarney ER. Adolescent pregnancy and childbearing—new challenges. Pediatrics 1985;75:973–975.

McAnarney ER. Young maternal age and adverse neonatal outcome. Am J Dis Child 1987;141:1053.

McAnarney ER, Hendee WR. Adolescent pregnancy and its consequences. JAMA 1989;262:74–77.

Miller KA, Field CS. Adolescent pregnancy: Critical review for the clinician. Semin Adolesc Med 1985;1:195–212.

Olds DL, Henderson CR, Tatelbaum R, et al. Improving the delivery of prenatal care and outcomes of pregnancy: A randomized trial of nurse home visitation. Pediatrics 1986;77:16–28.

Orr DP, Wilbrandt ML, Brack CJ, et al. Reported sexual behaviors and self-esteem among young adolescents. Am J Dis Child 1989;143:86.

Sanfilippo J. Overview: Adolescent gynecology. Pediatr Ann 1986;15:499.

Silber TJ. Ethical and legal issues in adolescent pregnancy. Clin Perinatal 1987;14:265.

Spivak H, Weitzman M. Social barriers faced by adolescent parents and their children. JAMA 1987;258:1500–1504.

Stevens-Simon C, White MM. Adolescent pregnancy. Pediatr Ann 1991;20:322–331.

Strasburger VC. Adolescent sexuality and the media. Pediatr Clin North Am 1989;36:747–773.

Talbot CW. The gynecologic examination of the pediatric patient. Pediatr Ann 1986;7:501–508.

CHAPTER 52

Gynecologic Disorders

Phil B. Fontanarosa
Paula M. Fontanarosa

GYNECOLOGIC EXAMINATION

Clinical evaluation of the pediatric patient with a gynecologic complaint requires patience, sensitivity, and a gentle but appropriately complete examination. The gynecologic examination of children tends to be deferred for reasons of shyness, modesty, and embarrassment by the patient. There is often a certain degree of anxiety and reluctance on the part of the parents and perhaps uneasiness on the part of the physician. However, a careful genital examination is essential and often provides key diagnostic clues that may be easily overlooked if an inadequate examination is performed.

General Physical Examination

Regardless of the specific presenting complaint, a general physical examination should be performed to search for findings that may be related to the gynecologic problem. Moreover, a gentle and thorough physical examination allows the child to become familiar with the physician. It also enables the physician to establish a rapport with and instill confidence in both the child and her parent.

Approach

When examining the child's genitalia, the comfort, developmental stage, and preparation of the patient must be considered. Toddlers or preschool children in the preoperational stage of cognitive development may view the procedure as punishment, and simple explanations should be offered. The concrete operational thought exhibited by school-age children enables them to understand a cause-and-effect relationship. Older patients with formal operational development are able to infer empathy and intent and are usually the most cooperative. Providing explanations, drawing diagrams, answering questions, and allowing the child to view and touch the instruments greatly increases cooperation.[1] The older child should be invited to hold the examination instruments until they are needed, thereby enlisting her active participation in the examination.

Most children prefer to have a parent present during the genital examination. Mothers are generally helpful during the examination of younger girls and provide a sense of familiarity and security. In fact, most young children will readily cooperate for genital inspection if they can be held on their mother's lap. However, for adolescent girls, the parent's presence detracts from privacy, and the physician should request that the parent leave the room during the examination, especially when the presenting complaint relates to sexual activity, sexually transmitted diseases, or the possibility of pregnancy. Teenage girls are most comfortable being examined by a female physician but usually cooperate with a male physician with a female nurse present.

Genital Inspection

Genital inspection is performed with the prone child in the knee-chest position or the supine child in the frog-legged position.[2-4] Separation of the labia and simultaneous depression of the perineum provides adequate visualization of the mons pubis, labia, clitoris, urethra, hymen, and anus. Careful inspection of the perineum and vaginal introitus constitutes a sufficient examination in the majority of prepubertal girls. Vaginal discharge, bleeding, trauma, irritation, and ulceration, as well as labial adhesions, imperforate hymen, and urethral prolapse are easily recognized with a genital inspection.

The majority of gynecologic disorders in premenarchial children do not require visualization of the entire vagina or cervix or a bimanual examination. Speculum and manual vaginal examinations are uncomfortable and unnecessary for most premenarchial girls. In prepubertal girls, the posterior vaginal fornix is short, the cul-de-sac is virtually nonexistent, and it is difficult to advance the examining finger high enough to vaginally palpate pelvic structures.

If vaginal inspection is inadequate, especially when foreign body, trauma, or pelvic or abdominal mass is suspected, rectovaginal palpation should be performed. The rectal examination is often the best method for evaluation of the pelvic cavity, because the thin rectovaginal septum allows examination of the vaginal tract. In the prepubertal child, the cervix is normally palpable as a small firm mass of tissue anterior to the rectum, but the ovaries and uterus are usually not palpable.[5] Rectoabdominal palpation is also useful to delineate localized areas of tenderness and lower abdominal and adnexal masses.

When complete examination of the vaginal vault is necessary, a well-lubricated pediatric vaginoscope is the optimal method for visualization. Makeshift instruments, such as narrow, standard-length nasal speculums or pediatric laryngoscopes or otoscopes, have been employed but are generally inadequate to expose the upper vagina and cervix.

Sexually active teenagers presenting with abdominal pain or gynecologic complaints require a careful, complete pelvic examination that includes a speculum examination along with bimanual pelvic and rectovaginal palpation. Providing detailed explanations and maintaining an empathetic, supportive approach are essential.[5, 6]

VAGINAL DISCHARGE AND VULVOVAGINITIS

Vulvovaginitis accounts for nearly 70% of gynecologic disorders in the pediatric age group.[7] Familiarity with the age-dependent causes and the clinical features of this disorder facilitates accurate diagnosis and proper therapy. In the majority of cases, the diagnosis can be established reliably from the history and from careful inspection of the vulva and vagina along with microscopic examination and cultures of the vaginal discharge (Table 52–1).

Vaginal Specimen Collection and Evaluation

In prepubertal or peripubertal girls, sterile cotton-tipped swabs premoistened with nonbacteriostatic normal saline are gently inserted into the vagina to obtain material for microscopic smears and cultures. Alternatively, 2 to 3 ml of nonbacteriostatic saline may be introduced and then aspirated through the hymenal opening using a soft plastic medicine dropper, small pipette, or tapered eye dropper. For postpubertal patients, the use of standard culture techniques is appropriate.

The following microscopic procedures should be performed routinely on vaginal secretions: pH determination using nitrazine or similar paper, 10% potassium hydroxide (KOH) preparation, normal saline wet mount, and Gram stain.

Indications for specific cultures are determined by the age of the patient, the specific presenting complaint, and findings from the history and physical examination.

Prepubertal Vulvovaginitis

Preadolescent females have an increased susceptibility to genital infection when compared with older girls. Vulvovaginitis occurs primarily because of poor perineal hygiene combined with a vulnerable anatomic and hormonal status.[7] Factors predisposing young girls to genital infection include small labial folds that fail to protect the vulvar mucosa from contamination; a relatively short distance between the rectum and vagina; low levels of circulating estrogen, rendering the mucosa susceptible to irritation or infection; alkaline pH of vaginal secretions that create a hospitable environment for bacteria; less than fastidious genital hygiene; and the proclivity of young girls to touch the perineum with unclean hands.[8-10]

Complaints suggestive of vulvovaginitis vary with the child's age. Infants may cry with voiding or simply be irritable; toddlers may scratch or rub the perineum or pull at their diapers; older children may complain of vaginal burning, itching, or odor. The appearance of discharge or spotting on the child's underwear or a complaint of dysuria is frequently the initial sign of the problem.

Nonspecific Vulvovaginitis

Nonspecific vulvovaginitis is the most frequently encountered premenarchal genital disorder. Contributing factors include inadequate perineal cleansing after urination, improper perineal wiping following bowel movement (i.e., back to front rather than front to back), and failure to change soiled underclothing.

On examination, the vaginal introitus typically appears edematous and erythematous and is tender. Vaginal discharge is usually mucoid and thin. Cultures yield mixed, nongonorrheal, pyogenic bacteria unrelated to a specific disease and are unnecessary unless abuse is suspected or the problem is chronic or recurrent.

TABLE 52–1

DIAGNOSTIC FEATURES OF VAGINAL INFECTION

Agent	Discharge	Odor; pH	Other Symptoms/Signs	Diagnosis
Normal vaginal examination	Variable, usually scant Clear or white, nonhomogeneous, floccular	None; <4.5	None	Normal epithelial cells; lactobacilli predominant
Candida albicans	White, scant to moderate, curd-like, "cheesy," adherent plaques	None usually; pH usually <4.5	Vulvar itching and/or irritation, dysuria frequent, pruritus (4+), erythema of vaginal epithelium, introitus	Hyphae on potassium hydroxide examination. Leukocytes, epithelial cells; yeast, mycelia, or pseudomycelia in up to 80%
Trichomonas vaginalis	Profuse, frothy, yellow-green or gray, homogeneous	Foul-smelling; pH >5.0 (5.2–5.5)	Profuse purulent discharge, vulvar itching, dysuria frequent, pruritus, low abdominal pain, "strawberry cervix," punctate vaginal hemorrhages, erythema of vaginal and vulvar epithelium, colpitis macularis	Leukocytes, motile trichomonads seen in 80% to 90% of symptomatic patients, less often in the absence of symptoms
Bacterial vaginosis (*Gardnerella vaginalis*)	Moderate; gray, white, or clear; homogeneous; low viscosity; uniformly coating vaginal walls	Fish-like and foul, increased when mixed with potassium hydroxide; pH >4.7 (5.0–5.5)	No dysuria, slight pruritus	Few leukocytes, lactobacilli outnumbered by profuse mixed flora, nearly always including *G. vaginalis* plus anaerobic species on Gram stain, bacteria-coated epithelial cells on wet prep
Neisseria gonorrheae	Purulent, but usually not prominent	None usually; pH <6.0	Occasional dysuria, not usually pruritic; partner has discharge or dysuria	Gram-negative intracellular diplococci suggestive; confirm with culture
Chlamydia trachomatis	Purulent	None usually; pH >4.5	Dysuria often; no pruritus; partner has discharge or dysuria	Purulent material in endocervix, >10 WBCs per field (oil immersion)

Management involves education to improve perineal hygiene, warm sitz baths, washing with mild soap and water, and frequent changes of white cotton undergarments. Secondary infection may improve with local use of intravaginal nitrofurazone or triple sulfa creams nightly for 2 weeks. Severe cases with weeping dermatitis may benefit from collodial oatmeal soaks or Burrow's solution compresses.

Allergic or Contact Vaginitis

Contact vaginitis may cause a clinical presentation similar to that of vulvovaginitis but typically is associated with perineal itching and irritation. Common offending agents include soaps, bubblebaths, powders, perfumes, laundry detergents, and rubberized or nylon underwear. For patients with a history of nocturnal itching accompanied by persistent vaginal discharge, rectal infestation with pinworms (*Enterobius vermicularis*) must be excluded. Therapy for allergic vaginitis involves removal of the causative factor, avoidance of nylon undergarments, warm sitz baths, and topical corticosteroid cream (fluocinolone 0.01%) to relieve pruritic symptoms (Table 52–2).

Foreign Body Vaginitis

The presence of purulent, blood-tinged vaginal discharge, especially if accompanied by vaginal pain and odor, suggests a vaginal foreign body. Toilet paper fragments are the most common foreign material present in young children, but coins, marbles, beads, toys, safety pins, pen caps, paper clips, and small household objects have also been inserted vaginally during self-stimulation or curious self-exploration.[7, 11]

Rectovaginal palpation and endoscopic inspection of the vaginal canal are the best means of localization. In selected cases, ultrasonography may prove useful when a vaginal foreign body has migrated into adjacent tissues. Although plain abdominal or pelvic radiographs have been used for identification of radiopaque objects, several factors argue against their routine use. First, only a minority of vaginal foreign bodies are radiographically detectable. Second, routine studies often fail to adequately image the entire vagina. Third, abdominal radiographs deliver needless radiation exposure to the ovaries. Finally, even when diagnosed by plain radiographs, foreign body removal and complete vaginal inspection are required and often necessitate direct vaginal visualization under anesthesia.

TABLE 52–2

GYNECOLOGIC DISORDERS: THERAPY AT A GLANCE

Condition	Treatment
Sexually transmitted diseases	See Table 52–4
Allergic vaginitis	Fluocinolone 0.01%, tid
Dysfunctional uterine bleeding	
Moderate	Estrogen-progestin combination (e.g., Ortho-Novum 1/50 or Noslestrin 1/50, one tablet po four times daily for 5 days)
Severe	Conjugated estrogen, 25–40 mg IV every 4 hours for up to six doses
Dysmenorrhea	Aspirin, 650 mg po four times daily, or ibuprofen, 400 mg po every 6 hours, or naproxen, 375–500 mg every 6–8 hours
Labial adhesions	Estrogen cream applied twice daily for 2 weeks

All vaginal foreign bodies must be removed. If the child is cooperative, the majority of objects can be retrieved relatively easily. For blunt or rounded objects, the physician should perform rectal palpation and gently guide the foreign body toward the introitus. Other objects may be grasped with thin nasal forceps guided by vaginoscopy. Gentle vaginal irrigation through a soft rubber catheter is helpful for removal of paper products. In uncooperative patients or in those with inaccessible, breakable, sharp, or embedded foreign bodies, sedation or general anesthesia is required for safe removal under direct vision and for complete vaginal inspection to exclude associated trauma.

Systemic Illness

Nongenital infectious diseases in remote body sites may be transmitted to the perineal area and produce discomfort, discharge, and itching. Contaminated hands of the patient or parent can facilitate spread. Upper respiratory tract, throat, ear, or skin infections with streptococcal or staphylococcal organisms can produce a secondary vaginitis. Vaginal lesions may also result from other systemic infections that have dermatologic manifestations, including measles, chickenpox, scarlet fever, or blood dyscrasias. Recent antibiotic therapy (particularly with penicillins or tetracyclines), diabetes mellitus, obesity, and occlusive tight nylon undergarments increase the susceptibility to vaginal yeast infections.[12, 13]

Sexually Transmitted Diseases

Sexually transmitted diseases (STDs) such as gonorrhea, chlamydia, trichomoniasis, and herpes infections are decidedly uncommon in prepubertal children beyond the neonatal period. The presence of an STD in this age group virtually always indicates sexual contact and should strongly suggest sexual abuse.[14] However, rare exceptions do exist. The hygienic habits of young girls, close nonsexual contact, fomites, and newborn exposure to an infected maternal vagina could potentially result in infection with organisms traditionally considered sexually transmitted. For instance, trichomoniasis may theoretically be acquired from wet toilet seats and swimming pools; on occasion, Chlamydia trachomatis in young children may represent a persistent perineally acquired infection that may last until age 3 years.[7, 14]

Prepubertal girls with gonorrheal or chlamydial infection usually demonstrate a thick, greenish-yellow, pruritic vaginal discharge. Infection is limited to the vagina, because lack of endocervical gland development prevents harboring of the organism.[15] Vulvar discomfort, dysuria, and urinary frequency are common symptoms.

Other Causes of Prepubertal Vaginitis

Premenarchal vulvovaginitis may result from a variety of other causes, including bacterial, protozoan, and viral infections; chemical, allergic, and physical agents; and enteric illnesses (Table 52–3). Other conditions producing vulvar lesions and secondary vaginitis include molluscum contagiosum, poison ivy, and tinea versicolor. Bacterial vaginosis and candidiasis may occur but are far more common in older females.

Postpubertal Vulvovaginitis

Estrogen secretion during puberty produces substantial alterations in the female genital tract. The vagina and cervix lengthen and thicken. The vaginal flora acquires increased numbers of lactobacilli. The resulting bacterial metabolism contributes to the development and maintenance of an acidic pH, which normally suppresses local vaginal infections. Whereas the majority of vulvovaginitis in prepubertal children is generally nonspecific, vaginitis in adolescents is usually caused by a specific organism. Except for physiologic leukorrhea, bacterial vaginosis, and Candida albicans vaginitis, the majority of episodes of vulvovaginitis in postpubertal females are, unfortunately, sexually transmitted.[10]

Physiologic Leukorrhea

With the advent of menarche and associated estrogen stimulation of vulvovaginal and cervical glands, vaginal secretions increase considerably, producing physiologic leukorrhea. The discharge is usually clear or white, has no odor, and occurs in the absence of any vaginal irritation. The quantity of leukorrhea varies during the menstrual cycle and increases with sexual excitement. At times, the condition is first noticed as stains in laundered underwear, because washing heats the proteinacious discharge and leaves a yellow discoloration.[16]

Microscopic examination of vaginal secretions reveals numerous epithelial cells, mucus, and few leukocytes, but no

TABLE 52–3

ETIOLOGIC FACTORS IN PREMENARCHAL VULVOVAGINITIS

Specific infections	Nonspecific mixed infections
Neisseria gonorrheae*	Poor perineal hygiene
Trichomonas vaginalis*	Skin infections
Chlamydia trachomatis*	Respiratory infections
Herpes simplex*	Urinary tract infection
Bacterial vaginosis	Intestinal parasites
(Gardnerella)	Physical, chemical, and allergic
Candida albicans	agents
Hemolytic streptococci	Vaginal foreign bodies
Corynebacterium diphtheriae	Sandbox sand
Streptococcus pneumoniae	Medications
Shigella flexneri	Vulvar deodorant sprays
Amebiasis	Nylon, rayon underclothing
Chickenpox	Soaps, laundry detergents
Molluscum contagiosum*	Bubblebath preparations
Condylomata acuminata*	

*Sexual abuse should be suspected.

pathogens. If the patient is not sexually active, cultures are unnecessary.

Physicians should reassure patients that leukorrhea is normal during puberty and does not represent any abnormality or infection. Recommendations for those with heavy discharge include good perineal hygiene, loose cotton underwear, avoidance of underwear at night to allow air drying, and use of a panty liner during the day. Tampons should be avoided because of the theoretical risk of toxic shock syndrome.[17]

Bacterial Vaginosis

Formerly called *nonspecific vaginitis*, *Haemophilus-associated vaginitis*, *Corynebacterium vaginitis*, and *Gardnerella-associated vaginitis*, bacterial vaginosis is one of the most common causes of abnormal vaginal discharge, occurring in 30% to 50% of young women.[18, 19] It is unclear whether bacterial vaginosis represents a sexually transmitted infection. The syndrome is associated with risk factors common to sexually transmitted diseases, such as increased incidence with multiple sexual partners and occurrence soon after intercourse with a new partner. However, a single sexually transmitted pathogen has not been identified, and male sexual partners are usually asymptomatic.[20]

The causative factor in bacterial vaginosis consists of an overgrowth of anaerobic bacteria resulting from alterations in the vaginal microflora. The predominant organism, *Gardnerella vaginalis*, is a common vaginal inhabitant, but with disease, the number of organisms increases dramatically.[16] *Gardnerella*, a pleomorphic, facultative, anaerobic coccobacillus, is involved synergistically with anaerobic organisms to produce the "fishy amine" vaginal discharge characteristic of the disorder. Increased concentrations of *Mycoplasma hominis*, *Ureaplasma urealyticum*, and anaerobic bacteria also have been documented in patients with bacterial vaginosis.

Typical presenting symptoms include a foamy or pasty, grayish-white, malodorous vaginal discharge, occasionally accompanied by pruritis, dysuria, and dyspareunia. Clinical findings include a homogeneous white vaginal discharge without significant vulvovaginal inflammation.

The diagnosis of bacterial vaginosis can be made with reasonable certainty in a patient with vaginal discharge who has the following signs:[21] characteristic white homogeneous discharge; pH of vaginal secretions greater than 4.5; saline preparation or Gram-stained smear revealing "clue cells"—vaginal epithelial cells coated with many gram-negative organisms, causing the cells to have a granular appearance and indistinct borders; alteration of normal vaginal flora (i.e., normally predominant lactobacilli are replaced by bacteria with morphology consistent with *G. vaginalis*); and detection of a distinct "fishy" odor when one to two drops of 10% KOH is mixed with vaginal secretions. Cultures are unnecessary for the diagnosis but should be obtained in sexually active patients to exclude chlamydial and gonorrheal infections.

Metronidazole is the treatment of choice, as it effectively reduces the number of anaerobic bacteria and allows reestablishment of normal flora, with a 70% to 90% cure rate.[14, 22] Patients must avoid alcohol while taking metronidazole because of the disulfiram-like effect of the drug. Ampicillin is the primary alternative agent for pregnant or metronidizole-allergic patients but is effective in only 40% to 50% of cases.[20] Oral tetracyclines and sulfonamide-containing vaginal creams are ineffective. Routine treatment of asymptomatic sexual partners is not recommended, but evaluation for trichomoniasis and other STDs is reasonable.

Candida albicans *Vaginitis*

Candida albicans is a normal inhabitant of the vagina in the majority of postpubertal females. Vulvovaginal candidiasis generally is not acquired sexually and usually is not found in the presence of healthy vaginal mucosa. Rather, candidal vaginitis results from endogenous overgrowth and proliferation of this yeast-like fungus and most commonly occurs when drugs, environmental changes, or disease alters normal vaginal defenses.

Specific factors predisposing to candidal infection include eradication of normal oral flora (e.g., from antibiotic therapy); increased epithelial cell glycogen content (e.g., from diabetes, pregnancy, oral contraceptives); excess vulvar moisture (e.g., from obesity; tight, occlusive, nylon undergarments; poor perineal hygiene); lowered host mechanisms (e.g., from corticosteroid therapy, anemia, chronic illness, malignancy); local factors (e.g., abrasions of the vaginal mucosa); and exposure to infected sources (e.g., contaminated soaps and douche bags, sexual transmission from a colonized male).[16,19]

The predominant symptoms are intense vulvar pruritus, burning with urination, and a thick, white vaginal discharge. Examination reveals vulvovaginal erythema and white cottage cheese–like curds or thrush-like plaques ("thrush patches") adherent to the vaginal mucosa.[16] At times, the inner thighs, labia, and perianal area are contiguously involved, and pruritic lesions ("id reactions") may occasionally be noted on the fingers.[23]

Microscopic examination of vaginal secretions in 10% KOH preparation, saline, or Gram stain reveals fungal forms with yeast buds, hyphae, or pseudohyphae along with white blood cells (WBCs). Fungal culture on Nickerson's or Sabouraud's media is confirmatory, but routine cultures are unnecessary for diagnosis and may detect asymptomatic carriers who do not require treatment.

Treatment should be instituted on clinical grounds for patients with symptomatic, characteristic-appearing vulvovaginitis or pseudohyphae with inflammatory cells on microscopic examination. Intravaginal miconazole, clotrimazole, or butoconazole are the recommended first-line agents.

SEXUALLY TRANSMITTED DISEASES

Sexually transmitted diseases (STDs) are a major health problem among sexually active adolescents, with more than 1 million cases reported annually in teenagers.[23] By age 18, 58% of all teenage girls are sexually experienced.[24] The combination of early sexual activity and multiple sex partners leads to a high frequency of STDs in adolescents.[24–27]

In diagnosing and managing sexually active teenagers with gynecologic complaints, the physician should follow certain principles:

- Obtaining an accurate sexual history is often difficult. With their uncertain, new sexual consciousness, teenagers may be fearful, embarrassed, and reluctant to disclose information fully.
- Direct, specific questions about sexual activity should be asked.
- Patients should be assured of confidentiality regarding information related to sexual problems.
- Cultures should be used liberally. Many patients harboring STDs (notably those with chlamydial infections) may have relatively minor symptoms.
- The physician should be alert for STD complications. Teenagers with STDs have a high rate of complications because of delays in seeking treatment.

- Searching for concomitant infections is important. Coinfection with other STDs is common in sexually active teenagers.
- High-risk sexual behaviors (i.e., multiple partners, unprotected intercourse) are associated with an increased risk of contracting other serious infections, such as HIV infection, chronic hepatitis B, and syphilis.
- The physician should provide referral for timely gynecologic follow-up and to appropriate agencies for education, counseling, and prevention of STDs.
- Sexual partners must be identified and evaluated. Partners should not be treated empirically without examination, cultures, and counseling.

Trichomonas vaginalis

Trichomonas vaginalis infection is one of the most common sexually transmitted diseases in adolescents and has a 10% to 33% prevalence in STD clinic populations.[16, 19] Sexual transmission of the organism is well established, with the risk of infection increasing with both the frequency of sexual activity and number of sexual partners. Trichomoniasis is thought to be sexually acquired in almost all cases and commonly occurs along with other STDs. However, because trichomonads can survive in sponges, washcloths, and urine, nonsexual fomite spread (e.g., through wet toilet seats, hot tubs, towel sharing) have been postulated but are unproven.[7, 16]

Infection with *T. vaginalis* typically causes a profuse, yellow-green, malodorous, mucopurulent or seropurulent vaginal discharge, vulvar pruritus, dysuria, and dyspareunia. The vaginal mucosa is inflamed, and the cervix may have petechial or friable lesions ("strawberry cervix") that bleed easily when touched.[28]

The diagnosis is confirmed by finding motile trichomonads and WBCs on microscopic examination of vaginal secretions in normal saline. The overall sensitivity of the saline wet-mount examination is approximately 60%,[29] with false-negative results common in patients who are chronic carriers or have recently used a chemical douche. A vaginal culture is the most reliable method of diagnosis but is not routinely performed by most laboratories.

Metronidazole is the treatment of choice for trichomoniasis and is usually curative. A single 2.0-gm dose is as effective as week-long regimens and has fewer side effects.[14, 22] Because metronidazole is potentially teratogenic, it should not be used during early pregnancy. Pregnant women with trichomoniasis may be treated with intravaginal clotrimazole, which may improve symptoms but has low cure rates.

Chlamydia trachomatis

Chlamydial infection is the most common sexually transmitted disease in the United States today, affecting 20% of sexually active adolescent and adult women each year and frequently occurring concomitantly with other STDs.[30] The causative agent, *Chlamydia trachomatis*, is responsible for a variety of disorders in females, including cervicitis, salpingitis, pelvic inflammatory disease, perihepatitis, and urethritis. In addition, the effects of chlamydial infections on childbearing potential are devastating. For example, each year more than 50,000 women sustain involuntary sterility following chlamydial salpingitis.[31,32] Moreover, the risk of ectopic pregnancy more than doubles following chlamydial salpingitis.[33]

The majority of patients infected with *C. trachomatis* present with vaginal discharge and dysuria, but many females are asymptomatic. Typical clinical findings consist of malodorous, mucopurulent discharge and an erythematous,

friable cervix. A positive "swab test"—yellow discharge on a white swab inserted into the endocervix, indicating purulent endocervical mucus—is commonly noted with chlamydial cervicitis but can also represent gonococcal or herpes infection.[34]

Gram stain of endocervical secretions reveals more than 10 WBCs per high power field. A McCoy cell culture is the most reliable method of establishing the diagnosis but is expensive, labor intensive, and time consuming, with results unavailable for 2 to 3 days.[35] Newly developed antigen detection assays using monoclonal antibodies or enzyme-linked immunofluorescence are rapid, convenient, and inexpensive.

Because the results of diagnostic studies for STDs are usually unavailable for at least 24 to 48 hours, the treatment regimen for sexually active teenagers with mucopurulent cervicitis should include effective coverage for both *Chlamydia* and *Neisseria gonorrheae* (Table 52–4). Doxycycline is the treatment of choice for chlamydial infections. Pregnant patients and those allergic to tetracyclines should receive erythromycin.

Neisseria gonorrheae

With more than 500,000 cases reported annually in North American teenagers and an estimated equal number of unreported cases, *Neisseria gonorrheae* infections pose a major health risk to sexually active teenagers.[23] One in every five sexually active adolescent girls has or has had gonorrhea, and 5000 teenage girls are absent from high school each day because of gonorrheal infection.[23, 30, 36]

The clinical presentation of *N. gonorrheae* infection varies widely. Patients may be asymptomatic or have severe vaginal and cervical inflammation with purulent discharge. Common presenting complaints include profuse, purulent, yellow vaginal discharge that appears 3 to 5 days after exposure; dysuria, frequency, and urgency; vulvar pruritus; lower abdominal pain; and abnormal vaginal bleeding. Physical examination findings include low-grade fever, lower abdominal tenderness, central cervical erythema, and mucopurulent cervicitis. A Gram stain of cervical discharge that reveals intracellular gram-negative diplococci and WBCs is highly suggestive of gonorrheal infection, but culture is required to definitively establish the diagnosis. Enzyme immunoassays have also become available to aid in diagnosis.

Parenteral ceftriaxone is the currently recommended treatment for uncomplicated gonorrheal infection and is effective even against strains resistant to penicillin and tetracycline.[14, 37–39] For patients with penicillin or cephalosporin allergy, parenteral spectinomycin or oral ciprofloxacin are reasonable choices. In addition, all patients require doxycycline for *Chlamydia* coverage. For pregnant adolescents with suspected concurrent gonorrheal-chlamydial infection, erythromycin is an acceptable alternative.

Pelvic inflammatory disease (PID), local infections (e.g., the Bartholin gland or periurethral duct abscess), and the disseminated arthritis-dermatitis syndrome affect 10% to 20%, 1% to 2%, and 2% to 3%, respectively, of untreated adolescents.[23]

Herpes Simplex Virus

Herpes simplex virus (HSV) is a common cause of genital ulcers in sexually active pubertal females. The highest incidence of herpes genital infections occurs in 15- to 19-year-olds. Approximately 10% of sexually active teenagers have positive results on herpes cultures.[23] Herpes simplex virus type 2 (HSV-2) is responsible for the majority of herpetic genital infections, is readily transmitted sexually, and is

TABLE 52–4

TREATMENT OF VULVOVAGINITIS AND SEXUALLY TRANSMITTED DISEASES

Bacterial vaginosis
Premenarchal: Metronidazole, 15 mg/kg/day in three divided doses for 10 days
Postmenarchal: Metronidazole,* 500 mg twice daily for 7 days
or
Ampicillin, 500 mg orally four times daily for 10 days
or
Clindamycin, 300 mg orally twice daily for 7 days

Candida albicans infection
Premenarchal: Gentian violet (0.5%), 1 ml vaginally at bedtime for 10 days
Postmenarchal: Miconazole suppository, 200 mg vaginally at bedtime for 3 days
or
Clotrimazole vaginal tablets, 200 mg at bedtime for 3 days
or
Butaconazole (2% cream), 5 gm intravaginally at bedtime for 3 days
or
Nystatin vaginal cream or tablets, twice daily for 10–14 days

Trichomonas vaginalis infection
Premenarchal: Metronidazole, 15 mg/kg/day orally in three divided doses for 10 days
Postmenarchal: Metronidazole, 2.0 gm orally in a single dose or 500 mg orally twice daily for 10 days

Chlamydia trachomatis infection
Patients < 8 years old: Erythromycin, 40 mg/kg/day orally in three divided doses for 7 days
Patients > 8 years old: Doxycycline, 100 mg orally twice daily for 7 days

Neisseria gonorrheae infection
Patients weighing < 45 kg: Ceftriaxone,* 125 mg IM in a single dose
or
Spectinomycin, 40 mg IM in a single dose
or
Amoxicillin, 50 mg/kg orally in a single dose *plus*
Probenecid, 25 mg/kg (maximum 1 gm) orally in a single dose
Patients weighing > 45 kg: Ceftriaxone,* 250 mg IM in a single dose
or
Spectinomycin, 2 gm IM in a single dose
or
Ciprofloxacin, 500 mg orally in a single dose
and
Doxycycline, 100 mg orally twice daily for 7 days
or
Tetracycline, 500 mg orally four times daily for 10 days

Herpes simplex virus infection
Postmenarchal
Initial episode: Acyclovir, 200 mg orally five times daily for 10–14 days
Severe cases: Acyclovir, 5 mg/kg IV every 8 hours for 5–7 days

*Drug of choice.

---

extremely contagious. Herpes simplex virus type 1 (HSV-1) primarily causes oral and ocular infections and accounts for only a small proportion (10%) of all genital herpes infections.

Initial symptoms begin 2 to 8 days after exposure and consist of perineal pain, swelling, and paresthesias. Patients with primary infection often have systemic symptoms of viremia, including fever, malaise, myalgia, and headache. Within 48 hours, the characteristic lesions appear; these consist of multiple groups of painful vesicles located on the mucocutaneous genital surfaces and occasionally on the vagina or cervix. The lesions, which are associated with intense pain, burning, itching, and lymphadenopathy, ultimately rupture, ulcerate, and heal spontaneously within 2 to 3 weeks.

Recurrence of genital herpes occurs in 60% to 90% of patients and usually is less severe than the primary episode.[34, 40] Symptoms include groin pain, paresthesias, and itching, followed by the appearance of the characteristic vesicles. Systemic symptoms are usually absent, and the lesions heal within 10 to 14 days.

The diagnosis of HSV infection is confirmed by viral isolation in tissue culture. Tzanck smear, Wright's stain, and a Pap smear may demonstrate giant cells or intranuclear inclusion bodies characteristic of HSV infection but lack adequate sensitivity for routine use. Serologic studies are unreliable for diagnosing acute genital infection but are useful to identify previous infection.

Management of genital HSV infection includes good perineal hygiene; sitz baths; analgesics, if necessary; antibiotics, if secondary skin infection occurs; and acyclovir. Oral acyclovir shortens the symptomatic period, reduces the number and healing time of lesions, and decreases pain and constitutional symptoms.[22, 42] Topical acyclovir is less effective than the oral form and offers no additional benefit.[42] Patients who are severely ill, have extensive lesions, are immunocompromised, or have complications from HSV infection (e.g., urinary retention) should be admitted for intravenous acyclovir.

VAGINAL BLEEDING

Vaginal bleeding is an alarming symptom for children and their parents. A thorough history usually provides definite clues to the origin. Physicians should obtain a detailed description of the bleeding in terms of onset, duration, previous episodes, and cyclic patterns. In general, the estimates of bleeding provided by anxious patients and parents are unreliable. The physician should inquire about events associated with bleeding, such as accidental trauma, the possibility of a vaginal foreign body, and topical or systemic medications. Associated symptoms should be sought, including abdominal or pelvic pain; vaginal itching, discharge, or odor; dysuria, frequency, or hematuria; diarrhea or hematochezia; easy bruising or bleeding from other sources (nose, gums); and associated dizziness, weakness, or syncope.

In postmenarchal females, a detailed menstrual history should be obtained. The physician should also determine the age at menarche, menstrual cycle characteristics (i.e., regularity, duration, flow pattern), date and normalcy of last menstrual period, and associated symptoms, such as pain. A history of sexual experience, contraceptive use, previous pregnancies, and abortions is also important.

Neonatal Vaginal Bleeding

Bloody or blood-tinged vaginal discharge during the first 2 weeks after birth usually signifies withdrawal from circulating maternal estrogen. The bleeding is usually of short duration, requires no specific treatment, and typically disappears within 10 days after birth.[7, 43]

Minor Prepubertal Vaginal Bleeding

In premenarchal girls, vaginal bleeding usually represents a localized vaginal or uterine problem. The most common cause of vaginal bleeding prior to menarche is a vaginal foreign body. Other causes include vulvovaginal infections, pruritus-induced excoriations, trauma, sexual abuse, tumors, coagulation disorders, and hormonal imbalances.[44] Childhood vaginal bleeding may also result as a consequence of precocious puberty but should be readily recognized by the appearance of associated sex characteristics. Occasionally, bleeding may result from exogenous hormones, such as when the curious toddler inadvertently ingests the mother's oral contraceptives. Vaginal and ovarian tumors are extremely rare in childhood but should be considered if an abdominal mass is present. Finally, the possibility of a nongynecologic bleeding source should be considered. Blood in the diaper or on the perineum may be the result of a urinary or gastrointestinal disorder.

Postpubertal Vaginal Bleeding

In pubertal females, most episodes of vaginal bleeding are due to menstruation. Abnormal bleeding most commonly results from menstrual irregularities, but pregnancy and its related complications should always be considered as a possibility.

Menstruation

In the United States, menarche usually occurs between the ages of 11 and 16 years, with a mean age of 12.7 years.[44] Various genetic, social, economic, and general health factors influence the age of menarche. However, by age 14, nearly 95% of all females have experienced the onset of menstruation.[45] Onset of menses before age 10 years (precocious puberty) and absence of menses beyond age 16 years (primary amenorrhea) should be considered abnormal and require thorough investigation by the primary care physician and gynecologic endocrinologist.[46]

"Normal" menstrual cycles are 21 to 35 days in length with a 2- to 8-day flow, but wide variations in this pattern frequently occur during the first 2 to 4 years after menarche. Although abnormal vaginal bleeding in postpubertal females can have a wide variety of causes, the most commonly encountered origins include dysfunctional bleeding and pregnancy and its related complications (Table 52–5).

Dysfunctional Uterine Bleeding

Anovulatory dysfunctional uterine bleeding is exceedingly common during adolescence and is the most likely cause of menstrual irregularities. Dysfunctional bleeding is a product of anovulatory cycles with continuous estrogen stimulation and resulting endometrial hyperplasia. Because more than half of menstrual cycles during the first postmenarchal year are anovulatory, menstrual irregularities are almost expected among pubertal girls.[23, 44] In general, an average of 20 months is required for the establishment of normal menstrual cycles after menarche.[47, 48]

Teenage menstrual irregularities may include the following: normal bleeding at irregular intervals (metrorrhagia); excessive bleeding at irregular intervals (menometrorrhagia); frequent menses, such as cycles less than 21 days apart (polymenorrhea); infrequent menses, such as cycles

TABLE 52–5
CAUSES OF ABNORMAL VAGINAL BLEEDING IN PUBERTAL FEMALES

Dysfunctional uterine bleeding	Intrauterine devices
Complicated intrauterine pregnancy (e.g., threatened abortion)	Vaginal adenosis
	Cervical carcinoma
Ectopic pregnancy	Endometrial polyps
Vulvovaginitis	Anticoagulant medications
Pelvic inflammatory disease	Blood dyscrasias
Vaginal foreign bodies	Adrenal insufficiency
Mittelschmerz	Thyroid disorders
Local genital trauma	Obesity
Coitus	Severe weight loss
Sexual abuse	Psychological stress
Oral contraceptives	

greater than 40 days apart (oligomenorrhea); and excessive bleeding, such as saturating more than six pads or ten tampons within 24 hours (menorrhagia or hypermenorrhea).

The typical clinical presentation is a teenager with irregular, heavy, painless bleeding, an unremarkable pelvic examination, and mild anemia. Acute bleeding may be substantial, and patients may display orthostatic hypotension. Physicians should obtain hemoglobin and hematocrit values to evaluate for underlying anemia, a platelet count to exclude thrombocytopenia, and, in sexually active adolescents, a pregnancy test to detect unsuspected pregnancy.

Dysfunctional bleeding is a diagnosis of exclusion and requires that more serious causes of abnormal menses be evaluated. In addition, even though a reasonable amount of time must be allowed for establishment of a full ovulatory cycle, adolescent menstrual disorders are not always self-limited and must be carefully followed by a gynecologist. If dysfunctional bleeding persists for more than 4 years, patients will likely experience future menstrual irregularities, have decreased reproductive potential, and be at increased risk for uterine neoplasm.[46]

Patients with minimal or mild bleeding and a normal hemoglobin concentration should be reassured and referred to a gynecologist. Patients with moderate bleeding and mild anemia but without evidence of hypovolemia (i.e., normal orthostatic vital signs) need pharmacologic intervention. Hormonal therapy with an estrogen-progestin combination (Ortho-Novum 1/50; Norlestrin 1/50) at a dose of one tablet orally four times daily for 5 days is usually effective. Bleeding decreases within 1 day and usually stops within 3 to 5 days.[5, 6] Patients with rapid or severe bleeding and evidence of hemodynamic compromise require circulatory resuscitation, gynecologic consultation, hospitalization, and administration of high-dose conjugated estrogens (25 to 40 mg IV every 4 hours, to a maximum of six doses) until bleeding stops.[5, 6] For rare cases refractory to these measures, dilatation and curettage may be necessary.

Ectopic Pregnancy

All menstruating females of childbearing age with abnormal vaginal bleeding or abdominal pain must be considered to have an ectopic pregnancy until proven otherwise. Although the typical age of patients with ectopic pregnancy is between age 20 and 30 years, the disorder is well known in teenagers.[49] With the ever-increasing prevalence of pelvic inflammatory disease and salpingitis among teenagers (both well-known risk factors for ectopic pregnancy), there may be a corresponding increase in the incidence of ectopic pregnancy among teens.

Other Causes

Other causes of postpubertal vaginal bleeding are generally identical to those encountered in vaginal bleeding in adults and include local trauma, vaginal foreign body, infection, disorders of the hypothalamic-pituitary-ovarian axis, and, rarely, polyps or tumors.

PELVIC PAIN

Acute lower abdominal and pelvic pain is a common complaint in pediatric patients and presents a difficult diagnostic problem. In postpubertal teenage girls, the differential diagnosis of pelvic pain is extensive and includes medical, surgical, urologic, and gynecologic disorders (Table 52–6).

Differentiating between a gynecologic and a nongynecologic cause of lower abdominal pain is often difficult. Several concepts regarding acute pelvic pain may prove helpful in the clinical evaluation. Sudden or abrupt pelvic pain suggests a serious abnormality, such as ruptured ectopic pregnancy, ovarian torsion, or ruptured ovarian cyst. Gradual onset of pain is more suggestive of an inflammatory process, such as pelvic inflammatory disease, a leaking nonhemorrhagic ovarian cyst, or an unruptured ectopic pregnancy. Gradually increasing pain associated with vaginal bleeding may be related to threatened or inevitable abortion or dysmenorrhea.

In all females of childbearing age, it is essential to obtain a reliable pregnancy test to identify or exclude pregnancy or its related complications. The gynecologic emergencies of greatest concern to the physician in the evaluation of patients with acute pelvic pain are ectopic pregnancy and pelvic inflammatory disease. Other commonly encountered causes for acute pelvic pain include ruptured ovarian cyst and dysmenorrhea.

Pelvic Inflammatory Disease

Pelvic inflammatory disease (PID) is an ascending infection involving the uterus and fallopian tubes and is more accurately described as endometritis-salpingitis-parametritis–pelvic peritonitis, or ESP. When adjusted for age and sexual experience, the incidence of PID is highest among teenage females.[27] For example, the risk of contracting salpingitis in sexually active 15-year-old girls is 1 in 8, compared with 1 in 80 in women aged 24 years.[27, 50]

Pelvic inflammatory disease carries the potential for serious complications and is a well-known cause of sterility. Approximately 13% of patients become infertile after a severe episode of PID; 35% do so after the second episode; more than 50% are infertile after three or more episodes.[51, 52] It is estimated that PID has caused sterilization of nearly 300,000 teenage girls during the past 15 years.[23]

TABLE 52–6

DIFFERENTIAL DIAGNOSIS OF ACUTE PELVIC PAIN IN ADOLESCENTS

Pelvic inflammatory disease	Pelvic adhesions
Ectopic pregnancy	Mesenteric lymphadenitis
Intrauterine pregnancy	Acute appendicitis
Threatened abortion	Acute peritonitis
Septic abortion	Inflammatory bowel disease
Hemorrhagic ovarian cyst	Acute cystitis
Mittelschmerz	Acute pyelonephritis
Ovarian tumor	Pelvic thrombophlebitis
Ovarian torsion	

TABLE 52–7

PELVIC INFLAMMATORY DISEASE: INDICATIONS FOR HOSPITALIZATION

All adolescents
First episode of PID
Nulligravida patient
Temperature greater than 38°C
Pregnancy
Pelvic or tubo-ovarian abscess suspected or confirmed
Evidence of peritonitis
Intrauterine device in place
Failed outpatient therapy
Noncompliance or inability to tolerate oral medications (e.g., vomiting)
Possibility of surgical lesion—appendicitis, ectopic pregnancy
Any suspicion of sexual abuse
Underlying immunocompromised state
Uncertain diagnosis of pelvic pain requiring further evaluation

---

Pelvic pain is the most common presenting symptom. The pain is usually dull, continuous, gradually progressive, located bilaterally in the lower abdomen, and often has been present for 1 to 2 days by the time of presentation. Associated presenting symptoms include fever, chills, vaginal discharge, menstrual irregularities, and dyspareunia. Characteristic examination findings include tachycardia, fever, abdominal tenderness and guarding, tenderness with motion of the cervix and uterus, and adnexal tenderness with palpation. Leukocytosis and elevation of the erythrocyte sedimentation rate (ESR) occur but are not required for diagnosis. In one study of patients with laparoscopically proven salpingitis, nearly half had a normal WBC count, and 25% had a normal ESR.[53]

Neisseria gonorrheae infection accounts for 40% to 60% of cases of PID, with infection with *Chlamydia trachomatis*, gram-negative bacilli, and anaerobes accounting for most of the remaining cases.[14, 36, 54] Approximately 30% to 50% of patients with gonoccocal PID have concomitant chlamydial infection.[14, 33] Adolescents with features indicating an acute, clinically significant episode of PID require hospital admission for aggressive therapy to reduce complications and maximize long-term fertility (Table 52–7).

Dysmenorrhea

Although not life-threatening, dysmenorrhea, or pain associated with menses, is a common gynecologic problem. Ten percent to 30% of females are unable to carry out their usual activities during their menstrual cycle because of menstrual pain.[5] Dysmenorrhea results from prostaglandin-mediated increases in uterine contractility. Progesterone withdrawal during ovulatory cycles appears to enhance prostaglandin synthesis. These factors help to explain the strong association of dysmenorrhea with ovulatory menstrual cycles and the relatively low prevalence of the disorder during the first 6 to 18 months after menarche (when menstrual cycles are typically anovulatory).

Patients with dysmenorrhea experience dull, cramping, lower abdominal pain that radiates to the back and thighs and is associated with menstruation. The pain usually commences within 1 to 4 hours of the onset of menstruation and continues for 24 to 48 hours. Associated symptoms may include nausea, vomiting, diarrhea, thigh pain, and headache. Fatigue, emotional lability, bloating, weight gain, and edema frequently occur. Results of physical and pelvic examinations are normal, but these examinations must be performed to exclude other causes of pelvic pain. Laboratory studies are indicated to exclude unsuspected pregnancy and evaluate for possible pelvic infection.

Management consists of reassurance and symptomatic treatment with hot baths, heating pads, relaxation, and medications to inhibit prostaglandin synthesis.[5, 6] Aspirin (650 mg four times daily), the first-line agent, is inexpensive and effective in many patients but may cause increased bleeding. Nonsteroidal anti-inflammatory drugs (e.g., ibuprofen, 400 mg every 6 hours, or naproxen, 375 to 500 mg initially, followed by 250 mg every 6 to 8 hours) are indicated for dysmenorrhea unrelieved by aspirin and may be even more effective if initiated a day before the onset of menses.

Ovarian Cyst

Ovarian cysts are a relatively uncommon yet important cause of abdominal pain in postpubertal females. Two types of ovarian cysts occur with each menstrual cycle: follicular cysts, during the first 2 weeks, and corpus luteum cysts, during the last 2 weeks.[55] Other types of ovarian cysts include those caused by corpus luteum of pregnancy, endometriosis, or neoplasm and dermoids.

The patient with acute ovarian cyst rupture presents with abrupt onset of well-defined, unilateral pelvic pain. Rupture of a graafian follicle with ovulation occurs at midcycle, releases follicular fluid into the peritoneal cavity, and produces dull, aching, unilateral pain that lasts from several minutes to a few hours (mittelschmerz).

Hemorrhagic ovarian cysts generally cause sudden, sharp abdominal pain accompanied by significant local tenderness, guarding, and evidence of peritoneal irritation. In stable patients, differentiation from ruptured ectopic pregnancy requires serum pregnancy testing and possibly pelvic ultrasonography or laparoscopy. For hemodynamically unstable patients, vigorous cardiovascular resuscitation and arrangements for immediate laparotomy are necessary.

CONGENITAL PROBLEMS
Mucocolpos and Hematocolpos

On occasion, the vagina of infants with complete vaginal obstruction caused by an imperforate hymen or a transverse vaginal septum may become grossly distended with mucus from the cervical glands, producing mucocolpos. The disorder causes dilatation of the vagina and may simulate a lower abdominal mass.[56]

In other cases, congenital vaginal obstruction may remain asymptomatic until puberty, when retained menstrual blood produces vaginal and uterine distention, termed *hematocolpos*, that causes lower abdominal pain and a pelvic mass.[3, 56] Mucocolpos and hematocolpos both require surgical correction with excision of a portion of the imperforate hymen, but such correction is not an emergency department procedure.

Labial Adhesions

Labial adhesions are among the most common gynecologic problems in childhood and are usually diagnosed in patients 1 to 5 years old. Labial adhesions, or *synechiae vulvae*, represent an acquired attachment of the medial labial surfaces. Maternal estrogen cornifies the labial epithelium and allows separation, but in the absence of hormone, the labia are free to fuse. Withdrawal of maternal estrogen and the normally low level of estrogen in children combined with minor trauma or irritation stimulate the labia minora to fuse in a posterior-to-anterior direction.[57]

Adhesions may be discovered incidentally during routine examination, or the parent may complain that the child's vagina is "closing up."[5] Examination reveals a flat plane of tissue covering the urethral meatus and introitus, a small pinpoint opening below the clitoris, and a central, vertical translucent line of fusion.[57] Estrogen cream applied directly to the labia twice daily for 2 weeks allows spontaneous separation without precocious sexual development. Surgical separation is rarely required. Parental support and reassurance are important.

Urethral Prolapse

Urethral prolapse involves protrusion of distal urethral mucosa through the urethral meatus. Most cases occur in girls between the ages of 2 and 10 years, with blacks affected more often than whites. Patients usually present with painless vaginal bleeding (which may be erroneously interpreted as menstruation or hematuria), often accompanied by dysuria. Examination reveals a nontender, soft, red or purplish, circular periurethral mass that measures 1 to 2 cm in diameter. The urethral lumen is located in the center of the mass and appears as a small central dimple. For patients with prolapse and healthy mucosal tissue, warm sitz baths should be instituted and timely urologic follow-up arranged. The presence of dark red or black mucosa indicates thrombosed, necrotic tissue and signals the need for prompt urologic evaluation and surgical intervention.

References

1. Brewster AB: Chronically ill hospitalized children's concepts of their illness. Pediatrics 1982;69:355.
2. McCann J, Voris J, Simon M, et al. Comparison of genital exam techniques in prepubertal girls. Pediatrics 1990;85:182.
3. Cowell CA. The gynecologic examination of infants, children, and young adolescents. Ped Clin North Am 1981;28:247.
4. Emans SJ, Goldstein DP. The gynecologic examination of the prepubertal child with vulvovaginitis: Use of the knee-chest position. Pediatrics 1980;65:758.
5. Paradise J. Pediatric and adolescent gynecology. *In* Fleisher GR, Ludwig S (eds). Textbook of Pediatric Emergency Medicine. 2nd ed. Baltimore, Williams & Wilkins, 1988, pp 709–735.
6. Barkin RM, Rosen P (eds). Gynecologic disorders. *In* Emergency Pediatrics—A Guide to Ambulatory Care. 3rd ed. St. Louis, CV Mosby, 1990, pp 543–559.
7. Bacon JL. Pediatric vulvovaginitis. Adolesc Pediatr Gynecol 1989;2:86.
8. Hammerschlag MR, Alpert S, Rosner I, et al. Microbiology of the vagina in children: Normal and potentially pathogenic organisms. Pediatrics 1978;62:57.
9. Caprano VJ, Gallego MB. Vulvovaginitis in children. Pediatr Ann 1974;3:74.
10. Joffe A. Vaginal discharge. *In* Hockelman CJ (ed). Primary Pediatric Care. St Louis, CV Mosby, 1987, pp 1111–1114.
11. Paradise JE, Willis ED. Probability of vaginal foreign body in girls with genital complaints. Am J Dis Child 1985;139:472.
12. Huffman JW. Gynecologic problems in childhood. Pediatr Ann 1981;10:165.
13. Altchek A. Vulvovaginitis, vulvar skin disease, and pelvic inflammatory disease. Pediatr Clin North Am 1981;28:397.
14. Centers for Disease Control. 1989 Sexually transmitted diseases treatment guidelines. MMWR 1989;38:1.
15. Huffman J. Vulvovaginitis. *In* Feigin RD, Cherry JD (eds). Textbook of Pediatric Infectious Disease. 2nd ed. Philadelphia, WB Saunders, 1987, pp 555–573.
16. Rosenfeld WD, Clark J. Vulvovaginitis and cervicitis. Pediatr Clin North Am 1989;36:489.
17. Greydanus DE. Vaginitis in the adolescent. Pediatr Emerg Casebook 1986;4:1.
18. Connell EB, Tatum HJ. Sexually Transmitted Diseases: Diagnosis and Treatment. Durant, OK, Creative Infomatics, 1985, pp 6–102.
19. Paavonen J, Stamm WE. Lower genital tract infections in women. Infect Dis Clin North Am 1987;1:179.
20. Holmes KK, Handsfield HH. Sexually transmitted diseases. *In* Wilson JD, Braunwald E, Isselbacher KJ, et al (eds). Harrison's Principles of Internal Medicine. 12th ed. New York, McGraw-Hill, 1991, pp 524–532.
21. Amsel R, Totten PA, Spiegel CA, et al. Nonspecific vaginitis: Diagnostic criteria and microbial and epidemiologic associations. Am J Med 1983;74:14.

22. Abramowitz M. Treatment of sexually transmitted diseases. Med Lett Drugs Ther 1990;32:5.
23. McAnarney ER, Greydanus DE. Adolescence. *In* Kempe CH, Silver HK, O'Brien D, et al (eds). Current Pediatric Diagnosis and Treatment. 9th ed. Norwalk, CT, Appleton & Lange, 1987, pp 213–252.
24. Werner MJ, Biro FM. Contraception and sexually transmitted diseases in adolescent females. Adolesc Pediatr Gynecol 1990;3:127.
25. Orr DP, Wibrandt ML, Brack CJ, et al. Reported sexual behaviors and self esteem among young adolescents. Am J Dis Child 1989;143:89.
26. Bell T, Hein K. Adolescents and sexually transmitted diseases. *In* Holmes K, Mardh PA, Sparling P, et al (eds). Sexually Transmitted Diseases. New York, McGraw-Hill, 1984, pp 73–84.
27. Labadie LL, Rhule RL. Management of genital infections. Emerg Med Clin North Am 1987;5:443.
28. Fouts AC, Kraus SJ. Trichomonas vaginalis: Reevaluation of its clinical presentation and laboratory diagnosis. J Infect Dis 1980;141:137.
29. Krieger JN, Tam MR, Stevens CE, et al. Diagnosis of trichomoniasis. JAMA 1988;259:1223.
30. Huffman J. Gynecologic infections in childhood and adolescence. *In* Feigin RD, Cherry JD (eds). Textbook of Pediatric Infectious Diseases. 2nd ed. Philadelphia, WB Saunders, 1987, pp 555–563.
31. Graham JM, Blanco JD. Chlamydia infections. Primary Care 1990;17:85.
32. Lindner LE, Geerling S, Nettum JA, et al. Clinical characteristics of women with chlamydial cervicitis. J Reprod Med 1988;33:684.
33. Chow JM, Yokenura ML, Richwald GA, et al. The association between chlamydia trachomatis and ectopic pregnancy. JAMA 1990;263:3164.
34. Wasserheit JN, Holmes KK. Sexually transmitted diseases in women. Emerg Med Clin North Am 1985;3:47.
35. Custodio DE, Henschen RR. Sexually transmitted diseases. Top Emerg Med 1990;13(1):66.
36. Wilfert C, Gutman L. Sexually Transmitted Diseases. *In* Feigin RD, Cherry JD (eds). Textbook of Pediatric Infectious Diseases. 2nd ed. Philadelphia, WB Saunders, 1987, pp 595–607.
37. LeSaux N, Ronald AR. Role of ceftriaxone in sexually transmitted diseases. Revi Infect Dis 1989;11:299.
38. Judson FN. Management of antibiotic-resistant Neisseria gonorrhoeae. Editorial. Ann Intern Med 1989;110:5.
39. Crump JRC, Engleberg NC. Sexually transmitted diseases: 1990 treatment update. Drug Therapy 1990;20:25.
40. Kalter D, Rosen T. Sexually transmitted diseases. Emerg Med Clin North Am 1985;3:693.
41. Arvin A. Oral therapy with acyclovir in infants and children. Pediatr Infect Dis J 1987;6:56.
42. Corey L, Benedetti J, Critchlow C, et al. Treatment of primary first episode genital herpes with acyclovir: Results of topical, intravenous, and oral therapy. J Antimicrob Ther 1983;12:79.
43. Singleton AF. Vaginal discharge in children and adolescents. Clin Pediatr 1980;19:799.
44. Hochbaum SR. Vaginal bleeding. Emerg Med Clin North Am 1987;5:429.
45. Sizonenko PC. Endocrinology in preadolescents and adolescents. Am J Dis Child 1978;132:704.
46. Carrington ER. Pediatric gynecology. *In* Willson JR, Carrington ER (eds). Obstetrics and Gynecology. 8th ed. St Louis, CV Mosby, 1987, pp 36–51.
47. Greydanus DE, McAnarney ER. Menstruation and its disorder in adolescence. Curr Probl Pediatr 1982;12:1.
48. McDonough PG, Gambrell RD. The adolescent gynecologic patient and her problems. Clin Obstet Gynecol 1979;22:491.
49. Honigman B. Ectopic pregnancy. *In* Rosen P, Baker RM, Barkin RM, et al (eds). Emergency Medicine—Concepts and Clinical Practice. St Louis, CV Mosby, 1988, pp 1591–1603.
50. Westrom L. Incidence, prevalence, and trends in acute pelvic inflammatory disease and its consequences in industrialized countries. Am J Obstet Gynecol 1980;138:880.
51. Washington AE, Sweet RL, Shafer MB. Pelvic inflammatory disease and its sequelae in adolescents. J Adolesc Health Care 1985;6:293.
52. St John RK, Brown ST. International symposium on pelvic inflammatory disease. Am J Obstet Gynecol 1980;135:845.
53. Jacobson L, Westrom L. Objectivized diagnosis of acute pelvic inflammatory disease. Am J Obstet Gynecol 1969;105:1088.
54. Moy JG, Clasen ME. The patient with gonococcal infection. Primary Care 1990;17:59.
55. Young G. Pelvic pain. *In* Rosen P, Baker RM, Barkin RM, et al (eds). Emergency Medicine—Concepts and Clinical Practice. St Louis, CV Mosby, 1988, pp 1573–1580.
56. Dewhurst J. Genital tract obstruction. Pediatr Clin North Am 1981;28:331.
57. Capraro VJ, Greenberg F, Greenberg H. Adhesions of the labia minora. Obstet Gynecol 1972;39:65.

SECTION SEVEN

Endocrine Emergencies

CHAPTER 53

Diabetes Mellitus

William A. Bonadio

INTRODUCTION

Diabetes mellitus is the most common endocrine disorder of childhood. Type I, or insulin-dependent diabetes mellitus (IDDM), is a syndrome of abnormal intermediary metabolism with altered utilization of carbohydrate, fat, and protein caused by a deficiency of insulin secretion (insulinopenia).

The prevalence rate of this disorder is estimated to be approximately 2 per 1000 school-age children, with new cases appearing most commonly during the autumn and winter seasons. Symptoms of newly recognized diabetes usually manifest when insulin-secreting reserve is below 20% of normal and consist of polyuria, polydipsia, polyphagia, and weight loss. The duration of symptoms varies but is generally 1 to 2 months.

HYPOGLYCEMIC REACTION

A hypoglycemic reaction is the most common acute complication of insulin therapy in childhood diabetes and results from an inappropriate balance among insulin effect, energy intake, and energy expenditure. This imbalance results in a relative excess of insulin, which causes an acute decline in the serum glucose level. Common causes include errors in insulin dosage, inadequate caloric intake for a given dose of insulin, and exercise without compensatory increased caloric intake or decreased insulin supplementation.

Symptoms

The symptoms of hypoglycemic reaction usually develop suddenly when compared with those of diabetic ketoacidosis (DKA), which develop over hours to days. These symptoms are caused by activation of the sympathetic nervous system, which may result in trembling, sweating, apprehension, and tachycardia; and by neuroglycopenia, which results in lethargy, confusion, seizures, and coma.

Differential Diagnosis

In the setting of documented hypoglycemia in a diabetic child with resolution of symptoms after administration of glucose, the diagnosis of hypoglycemic reaction is usually straightforward. If hypoglycemia is not present, the differential diagnosis includes seizure disorder, cardiac arrhythmia, toxic ingestion, meningitis or some other intracranial process, and anxiety attack.

The differential diagnosis of hypoglycemia in the child who is not diabetic is extensive; some of the more common causes of hypoglycemia include hyperinsulinism caused by beta-cell tumors of the pancreas; hepatic enzyme deficiencies; deficiencies in pituitary and adrenal hormones, which regulate glucose homeostasis; ketotic hypoglycemia; ingestion of drugs and toxins (ethyl alcohol, salicylates); Reye's syndrome; and severe malnutrition. Ketotic hypoglycemia is the most common cause of hypoglycemia in children, accounting for more than half of all cases; onset is usually between 18 months and 5 years of age. The origin of this specific disorder is unclear, but it has been noted to accompany periods of illness, vomiting, or deprivation of food.

Therapeutic Intervention

When hypoglycemic reaction is suspected in a child known to be diabetic, a blood sample should be tested to determine the serum glucose concentration. In addition, rapid measurement of the serum glucose concentration using a glucose oxidase strip (Dextrostix) should be performed at the bedside prior to administering therapy. Acute management of this condition in the conscious patient includes oral administration of a food source containing 10 to 20 gm of carbohydrate (e.g., orange juice or a candy bar); symptomatic improvement is usually noted within minutes. If the patient is vomiting or has altered consciousness, intravenous access should be obtained and a bolus infusion of D50W (1 to 2 ml/kg, up to a maximum dose of 20 ml) administered; when intravenous access cannot be readily obtained, glucagon (0.5 mg) should be administered intramuscularly. Most patients with a hypoglycemic reaction who experience resolution of symptoms after administration of therapy can be discharged from the outpatient setting. It is essential to perform a thorough history and physical examination to identify factors that may have induced the hypoglycemic episode and to make appropriate adjustments in insulin dose or diet to prevent additional hypoglycemic episodes.

DIABETIC KETOACIDOSIS

DKA is the most common acute complication requiring hospitalization of children with diabetes mellitus. It is a serious condition, with an overall mortality rate of 5% to 15% and accounting for 70% of diabetes-related deaths in children younger than 10 years. Approximately 15% to 30% of children with newly diagnosed IDDM present with ketoacidosis.

Pathophysiology

DKA is an abnormal metabolic condition initiated by a deficiency (either relative or absolute) of insulin, with resultant aberrations in glucose production and disposition. In children, DKA is most commonly precipitated by a usually ill-defined physiologic stress, such as infection or vomiting, which renders the normal dose of insulin inadequate. As a result of insulin insufficiency, there is an increase in the plasma concentration of the counterregulatory hormones glucagon, epinephrine, norepinephrine, cortisol, and growth hormone. A catabolic state is produced in the peripheral tissues, with mobilization of long-chain fatty acids from adipose stores. Glycogenolysis occurs in the liver, with oxidation of fatty acids and the production of acetoacetic and beta-hydroxybutyric acids. The end result is hyperglycemia and ketoacidosis.

These metabolic derangements have a significant impact on intermediary metabolism. Hyperglycemia and ketonemia induce an osmotic diuresis, resulting in total-body fluid depletion approximating 10% body weight. Ketoacid formation and dehydration combine to produce metabolic acidosis, often of profound magnitude. In addition to fluid depletion, significant deficits of electrolytes (sodium, 8 to 10 mEq/kg; potassium, 5 mEq/kg; chloride, 5 to 7 mEq/kg), and the minerals phosphorus (4 mEq/kg) and calcium occur. Therapy is directed toward correction of these derangements and any underlying precipitating factor that is identified.

Differential Diagnosis

DKA is characterized by hyperglycemia, metabolic acidosis, ketonemia, glycosuria, and ketonuria; fewer than 10% of children with DKA are comatose at the time of presentation. This condition must be differentiated from other causes of metabolic acidosis with an increased anion gap, including hypoglycemia, uremia, lactic acidosis, salicylate intoxication, and meningitis or other intracranial processes, all of which may present with similar symptoms.

Clinical Evaluation

The diagnosis of DKA is usually straightforward when a patient with known diabetes presents with hyperglycemia and metabolic acidosis. In addition, examination can reveal the following symptoms:

Hyperglycemia
Metabolic acidosis
Ketonemia
Glycosuria
Ketonuria
Dehydration
Kussmaul's respiration
Abdominal pain
Fever
Vomiting

It is important that clinical evaluation be directed toward identifying and treating any underlying condition, such as infection, that may have precipitated the episode of diabetic ketoacidosis.

Therapeutic Intervention

Replenishing the fluid deficit is the single most important measure in treating DKA. Parenterally administered fluid

therapy corrects dehydration caused by the osmotic diuresis; improved peripheral perfusion ameliorates metabolic acidosis, enhances glucose excretion by restoring glomerular filtration, and decreases the plasma concentration of the various counterregulatory hormones. Rehydration should be initiated as soon as the diagnosis of DKA has been established. During the first hour of therapy, the patient should receive an intravenous bolus infusion of 500 ml/m² of either 0.9% normal saline (NS) or lactated Ringer's solution (LR); during the next 12 hours, approximately 50% of the remaining volume deficit is replaced with 0.45% NS to replenish total-body sodium stores depleted by the osmotic diuresis (Table 53–1). A 5% dextrose solution should be added to the crystalloid solution when the blood glucose level decreases to the range of 250 to 300 mg/dl, both to avoid hypoglycemia and to prevent a too-rapid decline in serum osmolality.

Total-body potassium stores are depleted secondary to both the osmotic diuresis and hyperaldosteronism induced by dehydration. The administration of insulin and glucose

TABLE 53–1
DKA MANAGEMENT PROTOCOL

	Outpatient
Admission:	Analysis of complete blood cell count; serum glucose, electrolytes, blood urea nitrogen, pH, osmolarity; urinalysis.
Hour 1:	Parenteral fluids: 500 ml/m² lactated Ringer's solution.
	Regular insulin: 0.1 U/kg intravenous bolus infusion, and 0.1 U/kg/hr.*
Hour 2:	Repeat analysis of serum glucose, electrolytes, pH.
	Parenteral fluids: 200 ml/m² 0.45% normal saline solution† with potassium phosphate (20 mEq/L) and potassium chloride (20 mEq/L).‡
	Regular insulin: 0.1 U/kg/hr.*
Hour 3:	Repeat analysis of serum glucose, electrolytes, pH.
	If serum pH <7.35 and bicarbonate <20 mEq/L, repeat fluid and insulin therapy as per hour 2.
	If serum pH ≥7.35 or bicarbonate ≥20 mEq/L, give oral fluids ad lib; if tolerated, and abnormal clinical findings resolve, discharge.
Hour 4:	Repeat analysis of serum glucose, electrolytes, pH.
	If serum pH <7.35 and bicarbonate <20 mEq/L, hospitalize.
	If serum pH ≥7.35 or bicarbonate ≥20 mEq/L, give oral fluids ad lib; if tolerated, and abnormal clinical findings resolve, discharge; if patient is unable to tolerate oral fluids or abnormal physical findings persist, hospitalize.
	Inpatient
Hours 4–24:	Analysis of serum glucose, electrolytes, pH q 1–2 hr.
	Parenteral fluids: 3000 ml/m² 0.45% normal saline solution† with potassium phosphate (20 mEq/L) and potassium chloride (20 mEq/L).
	Regular insulin: 0.1 U/kg/hr continuous intravenous infusion.
	When serum pH ≥7.35 and patient is able to tolerate oral feeding, begin diet and subcutaneous insulin administration.

*Can be administered either by intramuscular injection or continuous intravenous infusion.

†5% Dextrose solution in 0.45% normal saline when serum glucose concentration is 250–300 mg/dl.

‡Potassium supplementation should be undertaken only after urine output is established.

will exacerbate hypokalemia because of the resulting intracellular influx of potassium. Therefore potassium should be added after the initial hour of fluid therapy if urine output has been established. Phosphorus depletion is also common secondary to renal losses and can exacerbate resistance to the action of insulin. Phosphate supplementation is important to promote the formation of 2,3-diphosphoglycerate, which will shift the oxygen-dissociation curve to the right, releasing oxygen to the tissues and correcting acidosis. Administration of half of the potassium supplement in the form of potassium phosphate can reduce the potential for chloride overload, which can occur with treatment of DKA and can aggravate acidosis.

Use of sodium bicarbonate to correct metabolic acidosis is controversial. Paradoxical cerebral acidosis can occur when sodium bicarbonate is administered because of the formation and diffusion of CO_2 from the systemic circulation into the central nervous system. Rapid administration of sodium bicarbonate can also cause an acute intracellular influx of potassium and exacerbate hypokalemia. In general, the metabolic acidosis of DKA will gradually correct with replenishment of fluid deficit and insulin supplementation; administration of sodium bicarbonate should not be used except in instances of severe acidosis (serum pH less than or equal to 7.0), in which myocardial depression can occur.

Insulin is the major anabolic hormone of the body and affects target cells in the liver, adipocytes, and muscle. Insulin must be administered for the resolution of ketoacidosis to occur; it lowers the plasma concentration of the counterregulatory hormones, inhibits the effects of glucagon on the liver, inhibits the peripheral catabolism of fatty acids and amino acids, and enhances utilization of glucose as a fuel source for target tissues. Only regular insulin should be used for the treatment of DKA.

Insulin supplementation should commence following the initial hour of fluid therapy. At that point, fluid replenishment will have improved peripheral perfusion and acid-base status, both of which will augment the action of insulin. During the first hour of therapy, regular insulin is administered as a single parenteral bolus infusion (0.1 U/kg) and then by continuous parenteral infusion at a rate of 0.1 U/kg/hr. If necessary, insulin can be administered hourly by intramuscular injection. Both intramuscular injection and continuous parenteral infusion are safe and effective means of providing insulin during the treatment of DKA. If the serum glucose concentration continues to fall below the range of 150 to 200 mg/dl despite the addition of 5% dextrose to parenteral fluids, administration of additional glucose in the form of 10% dextrose solution should be used instead of decreasing the rate of insulin infusion. This is essential to inhibit ketoacid production and continue the correction of metabolic acidosis.

Monitoring Progress

The effectiveness of therapy for DKA is best monitored by closely following trends in vital signs, fluid intake and output, neurologic status, plasma glucose levels, and acid-base status, initially on an hourly basis. Inhibition of ketogenesis, which is essential to the resolution of DKA, is reflected by both decreasing serum glucose levels and increasing serum bicarbonate levels with an associated lowering of the anion gap. Resolving hyperglycemia alone does not denote the resolution of DKA; there must be concomitant resolution of metabolic acidosis to signify the cessation of ketoacid production.

Complications

Potential complications of treatment of DKA include hypoglycemia, hypokalemia, and cerebral edema. Hypoglycemia can result from insulin supplementation without adequate glucose administration. The serum glucose concentration should be monitored closely; when the serum glucose level declines to the range of 250 to 300 mg/dl, a 5% dextrose solution should be added to parenteral fluids.

Hypokalemia can result from both the correction of metabolic acidosis and the administration of insulin and glucose. The serum potassium concentration should also be monitored closely and potassium added early in the course of therapy after urine output has been established.

Hyperosmolarity should be corrected slowly, as a too-rapid decline may predispose the patient to cerebral edema, the major complication of therapy for DKA in children. Clinically apparent cerebral edema is an uncommon complication of DKA that usually manifests after several hours of seemingly uncomplicated treatment with improvement in hydration, acid-base status, and serum glucose concentration. Drowsiness, headache, papilledema, and neurologic abnormalities may develop; these can progress to coma and cerebral herniation syndrome. The development of cerebral herniation has been associated with higher rates of parenteral fluid administration and development of the syndrome of inappropriate antidiuretic hormone secretion. Treatment involves prompt administration of the osmotic diuretic mannitol.

Outpatient Management of DKA

The outpatient management of DKA employs all of the previously mentioned therapeutic measures for restoring glucose homeostasis and intermediary metabolism to a normal state. When this method of "abbreviated" treatment for DKA is used for selected patients, there is a greater than 90% rate of resolution of metabolic acidosis after 3 hours of therapy. The metabolic parameters on admission accurately predict the outcome of patients with DKA during the initial 3 hours of therapy: almost all patients with admission serum pH greater than or equal to 7.20 or a bicarbonate concentration greater than or equal to 10 mEq/L experience resolution of metabolic acidosis within 3 hours of initiating therapy, can tolerate oral feeding, and can be discharged from the outpatient setting with little risk of relapse or other complication. By contrast, nearly all patients with admission serum pH less than 7.20 and a bicarbonate concentration less than 10 mEq/L will have persistence of acidosis after 3 hours of therapy, necessitating hospitalization for further treatment. The admission serum glucose concentration is predictive of the duration of therapy necessary to resolve metabolic acidosis in patients with an initial serum pH greater than or equal to 7.20 or a bicarbonate concentration greater than or equal to 10 mEq/L. Those with a serum glucose concentration less than 500 mg/dl usually require 2 hours of therapy to resolve metabolic acidosis, whereas those with a serum glucose concentration greater than 500 mg/dl usually require 3 hours of therapy to resolve metabolic acidosis. The longer duration of therapy required in patients with more marked hyperglycemia may reflect a greater degree of dehydration, thus necessitating prolonged fluid replenishment to restore glomerular filtration.

Based on the average deficits accrued by patients with DKA, approximately one third of the fluid deficit and one half of the sodium deficit are replenished after 3 hours of outpatient therapy.

HYPEROSMOLAR COMA

Nonketotic hyperosmolar coma is a rare complication of unknown origin in childhood diabetes. It consists of nonketotic acidosis, marked hyperglycemia, severe dehydration with marked hyperosmolarity, and altered mental status and other neurologic abnormalities. There is an increased association between this condition and preexisting neurologic damage in children. Management consists of fluid and electrolyte therapy similar to that used in the treatment of DKA. It is recommended that one half the usual dose of insulin supplementation used to treat DKA (0.05 U/kg/hr) be administered to prevent a too-rapid decline in serum glucose concentration and serum osmolarity.

Selected References

Barrett EJ, DeFonzo RA. Diabetic ketoacidosis: Diagnosis and treatment. Hosp Pract 1984;19:89.

Bonadio WA, Gutzeit MF, Losek JD, Smith DS. Outpatient management of diabetic ketoacidosis. Am J Dis Child 1988;142:448.

Connell FA, Louden JH. Diabetes mortality in persons under 45 years of age. Am J Public Health 1983;73:1174.

Foster DW, McGarry JD. The metabolic derangements and treatment of diabetic ketoacidosis. N Engl J Med 1983;309:159.

Krane EJ. Diabetic ketoacidosis: Biochemistry, physiology, treatment, and prevention. Pediatr Clin North Am 1987;34:935.

CHAPTER 54

Thyroid Disorders

Halim M. Hennes
Irene M. O'Shaughnessy

ANATOMY AND PHYSIOLOGY

Disorders of the thyroid gland are seen in childhood. Congenital hypothyroidism (cretinism) is estimated to affect 1 in 4000 live births with a male to female ratio of 1:4. Hyperthyroidism is also seen in children, usually as a manifestation of Graves' disease.

The thyroid gland consists of two symmetric, pear-shaped lobes connected in front of the second, third, and fourth tracheal rings by the isthmus; it is enclosed in a thin capsule that is well adhered to the gland. At birth, the gland weighs approximately 2 gm. The weight increases by 1.0 to 1.5 gm each year during childhood and adolescence. Because of its small size, the gland is often difficult to palpate in infants; but it is almost always palpable in school-age children. In adults, it weighs almost 20 gm and is considered the largest endocrine gland in the body.

Two important hormones are secreted by the gland: thyroxine (T_4) and triiodothyronine (T_3). Biologically, T_3 is three to four times more potent than T_4. Only 20% of T_3 is secreted by the thyroid, with the remaining portion being produced through deiodination of T_4 in the liver, kidney, and peripheral tissue. These hormones have a significant effect on almost all body tissues, organs, and other endocrine glands. Both hormones are largely protein-bound, however; only 0.4% of T_3 and 0.04% of T_4 circulate in the metabolically active "free" or unbound form.

The thyroid function is regulated through the hypothalamic-pituitary axis and intrathyroidal autoregulation. Thyroid-stimulating hormone (TSH) is secreted by the anterior pituitary and controls the release of thyroid hormone. Release of thyroid hormone is further regulated through hypothalamic neural control, which includes one stimulating factor, thyrotropin releasing hormone (TRH), and two inhibitory factors, somatostatin and dopamine. TRH decreases the sensitivity of the anterior pituitary to the negative feedback effect of T_3. Intrathyroidal autoregulation is dependent on iodide supply to the gland.

In the tissue, thyroid hormone function is accomplished through various mechanisms that result in significant enhancement of intracellular events and alteration in cell function (Table 54-1).

HYPERTHYROIDISM

Hyperthyroidism results from an increased concentration of circulating thyroid hormone. In children, Graves' disease (diffuse toxic goiter) is the most common cause.

Graves' disease is an autoimmune disease caused by autoantibodies to the TSH receptor on thyroid tissue. These antibodies appear as a result of an antigen-specific cell defect. An association between HLA-DR3 and HLA-B8 has also been observed. Graves' disease is often associated with other autoimmune disorders such as pernicious anemia, idiopathic adrenal insufficiency, myasthenia gravis, and insulin-dependent diabetes mellitus.

Neonatal or congenital Graves' disease is a rare transient disorder occurring in infants whose mothers had hyperthyroidism during pregnancy or a history of hyperthyroidism. Neonatal hyperthyroidism is caused by transplacental passage of thyroid-stimulating antibodies (TSAbs), and remission usually parallels the disappearance of TSAbs from the circulation. In contrast to Graves' disease in other age groups, neonatal Graves' disease affects male and female infants equally. The clinical course is variable, and spontaneous resolution occurs in most cases by 3 months of age

TABLE 54-1

FUNCTION OF THE THYROID HORMONES IN THE TISSUE

System	Effect
Metabolic	Carbohydrate and fat metabolism are enhanced. The rate of protein synthesis and catabolism is increased. The basal metabolic rate increases 60% to 100% in all body tissues except the brain, retina, testes, and lungs.
Growth	Development and maturation of the brain are promoted during fetal and early postnatal life, as well as skeletal development.
Cardiovascular	Blood flow increases secondary to increased metabolism; subsequently, cardiac output and heart rate increase. Thyroid hormone also causes an increase in blood volume, strength of heart beat, and a wide pulse pressure.
Neurologic	Levels of several neurotransmitters, including tyrosine, dopamine, and tryptophan, are affected. Adrenergic and cholinergic receptors are also modulated.
Gastrointestinal	Appetite, secretion of digestive juices, and intestinal motility are increased.
Musculoskeletal	Muscle weakness, fine tremor, and sluggish deep tendon reflexes are associated with hormone excess. Delayed tendon relaxation is seen in hypothyroidism.
Endocrine	Insulin secretion, parathyroid hormone release, ACTH production, and glucocorticoid secretion are all increased.

but may rarely persist beyond 6 months. Clinical features are usually present at birth, but if TSH-inhibiting antibodies are also present, the onset of clinical features may be delayed by several weeks (Table 54–2).

Clinical Evaluation

Systemic manifestations of excessive circulating thyroid hormone involves multiple organ systems, as described (in Table 54–3). The extent and severity of these manifestations are related in part to the underlying cause of hyperthyroidism and, to a far greater extent, to the duration of hyperthyroidism.

Diagnostic Evaluation

In children with classic signs and symptoms, hyperthyroidism is easily confirmed with an elevated free T_4 level or total T_3 level by radioimmunoassay (RIA). TSH concentration is invariably suppressed. With the introduction of third-generation TSH assay, the measurement of TSH has become an extremely useful tool in the diagnosis of hyperthyroidism and has made TSH stimulation testing unnecessary.

Elevated levels of TSAb are present in most patients with Graves' disease and appear to correlate with disease activity. Other proteins, including thyroglobulin and antithyroid antibodies, are usually elevated, but it is rarely necessary to measure them.

Thyroid radioiodine uptake studies are considered diagnostic tools in Graves' disease and are useful to differentiate hyperthyroidism caused by Graves' disease (high 4-hour and 24-hour uptake) from that caused by thyroiditis (high 4-hour, low 24-hour uptake).

Differential Diagnosis

In children, hyperthyroidism is almost always caused by diffuse toxic goiter (Graves' disease). Less common causes of hyperthyroidism include neonatal hyperthyroidism, functioning solitary thyroid nodule (Plummer's disease), and thyrotoxicosis factitia; transient hyperthyroidism can also occur as an early manifestation of chronic lymphocytic thyroiditis (Hashimoto's thyroiditis). Rarely, childhood hyperthyroidism can be caused by hyperfunctioning thyroid carcinoma or acute suppurative thyroiditis or may occur as one manifestation of polyostotic fibrous dysplasia (McCune-Albright syndrome) (Fig. 54–1).

Therapeutic Intervention

There is no consensus regarding the preferred method of treatment of Graves' disease in children. Some clinicians prefer antithyroid drugs, others consider surgery to be most appropriate, and a third group uses radioiodine. However,

TABLE 54–2

CLINICAL FEATURES OF NEONATAL HYPERTHYROIDISM

System	Clinical Manifestation
General	Prematurity, hyperthermia, tachypnea (greater than 40)
Ocular	Exophthalmos
Cardiovascular	Tachycardia (greater than 160), cardiac decompensation
Neurologic	Irritability, tremulousness
Gastrointestinal	Diarrhea, vomiting, hepatosplenomegaly
Growth	Failure to thrive
Endocrine	Goiter (may not be present)

TABLE 54–3

CLINICAL MANIFESTATIONS OF GRAVES' DISEASE

System	Clinical Manifestation
Skin	Moist, warm skin; fine hair
Ocular	Exophthalmos, eyelid retraction and eyelid lag
Muscular	Diminished muscle strength; poor endurance and motor hyperactivity (tremulousness)
Cardiovascular	Tachycardia, palpitations and systolic hypertension, cardiac failure
Neurologic	Emotional disturbances (emotional lability) or deteriorating school performance
Gastrointestinal	Excessive appetite (with no change in weight or weight loss)
Growth	Accelerated growth; advanced bone age
Endocrine	Thyromegaly

most thyroidologists prefer antithyroid drugs as their initial choice of therapy.

Antithyroid Drugs

The recommended antithyroid drugs are propylthiouracil (PTU) and methimazole (Tapazole). These drugs have both intrathyroidal and extrathyroidal effects, which include an inhibition of a number of processes including thyroglobulin iodination, a coupling reaction between iodotyrosines to form iodothyronines (T_3 and T_4), and the conversion of T_4 to the more potent T_3 (PTU only). They also exert a direct effect on the immune system. The starting dose for PTU is 5 to 7 mg/kg/day divided into three doses and for methimazole, 0.5 to 0.7 mg/kg/day divided into three doses. Clinical improvement usually occurs within 7 to 8 days. The dosage may be gradually decreased to the lowest effective dose, or L-thyroxine supplementation may be provided. Careful monitoring of T_3, T_4, and TSH levels is important. Both T_3 and T_4 should be maintained in the euthyroid range. An elevated TSH level suggests an overdose of medication. With drug therapy, the actual remission rate is higher in children than in adults (approximately 50%), and there is evidence suggesting that the remission rate is 25% every 2 years. Drug therapy may then be continued indefinitely.

Adverse reactions occur with antithyroid drug therapy in 1% to 5% of patients and include fever, rash, urticaria, arthralgias or frank arthritis, nephritis, and carditis. Adverse reactions occur more frequently with higher drug doses. Agranulocytosis is a more serious yet reversible toxic reaction that occurs in approximately 0.5% of patients and usually develops within the first 3 months of therapy. Routine monitoring of the white blood cell count in all patients on antithyroid drug therapy is not useful, because agranulocytosis occurs quite abruptly. When antithyroid drugs are discontinued, the clinical course is one of gradual improvement over days to weeks. All patients taking antithyroid drugs should be advised that if fever, pharyngitis, mouth sores, or other symptoms of infection develop, they should stop taking the drug immediately and call their physician.

A beta-adrenergic blocking agent such as propranolol is a useful adjunct in the management of children with severe hyperthyroidism. Symptoms caused by potentiated catecholamine action, including tachycardia, tremor, excessive sweating, lid lag, and stare, are usually well controlled with propranolol (Table 54–4).

Surgical Management

The preferred surgical treatment for Graves' disease is subtotal thyroidectomy. It offers the advantage of rapid

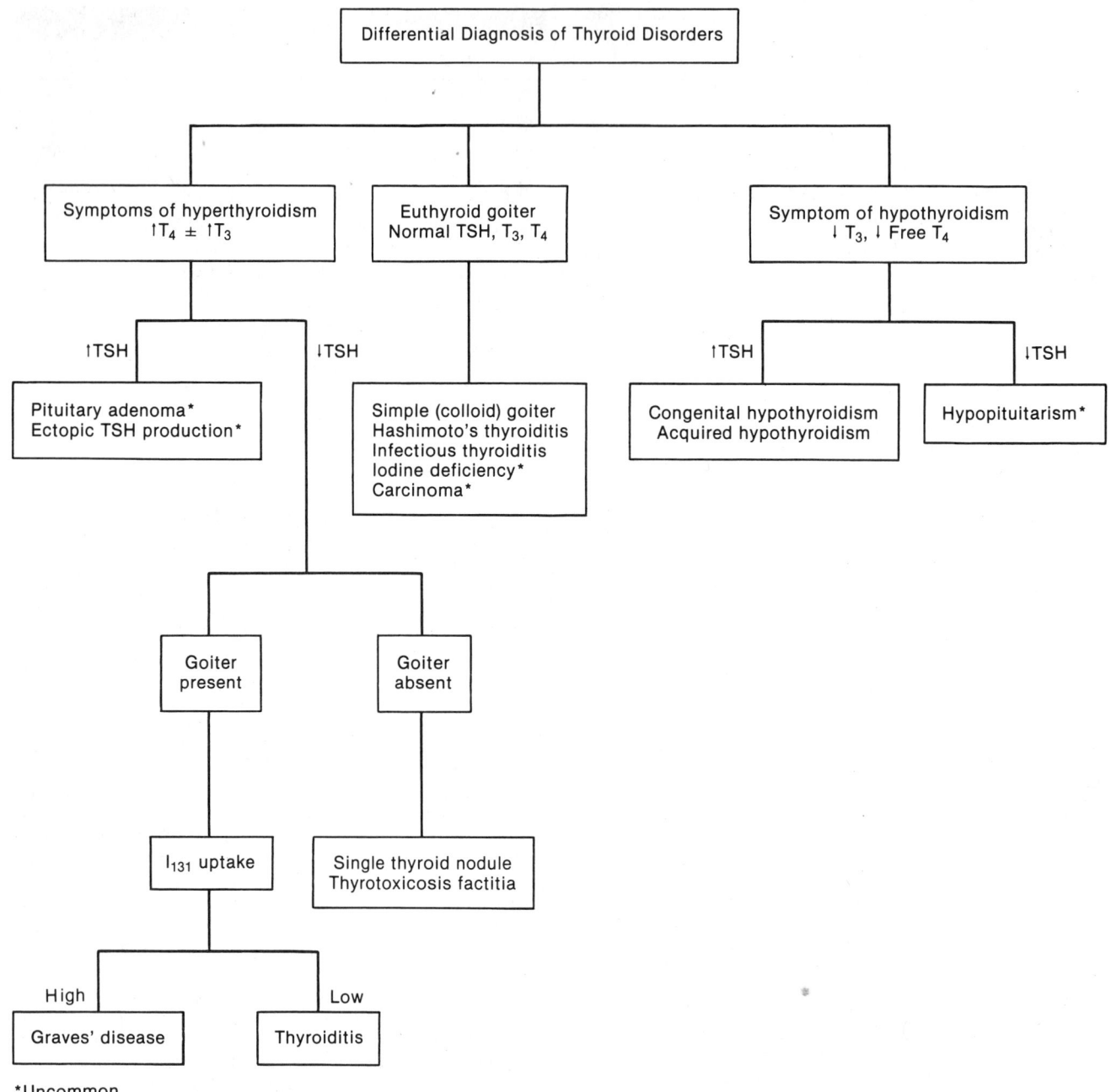

Figure 54–1.

TABLE 54–4				
MEDICATIONS FOR THE TREATMENT OF HYPERTHYROIDISM				
Drug	**Dose**	**Route**	**Side Effects**	**Contraindications**
Propylthiouracil	5–7 mg/kg/day	Orally q 8 hr	Agranulocytosis, rash, arthralgia, fever, neuritis, hepatitis, lupus-like syndrome	Dose should be reduced to minimum during pregnancy
Methimazole	0.5–0.7 mg/kg/day	Orally q 8 hr	Similar to propylthiouracil	Not recommended during pregnancy
Propranolol	4 mg/kg/day	Orally q 6 hr	Hypoglycemia, bradycardia, hypertension	Asthma, heart block
Iodine	2–3 drops of saturated KI solution	Orally q 8 hr	Fever, rash, vasalitis, conjunctivitis, eosinophilia granulocytosis	Past history of sensitivity

improvement but has the disadvantages of a surgical procedure. Iodine solution (Lugol's solution) or potassium iodide (SSKI) should be administered 10 to 14 days prior to surgery to reduce thyroid vascularity. Complications of subtotal thyroidectomy include transient hypocalcemia, hypoparathyroidism, recurrent laryngeal nerve injury, and temporary tracheostomy.

Radioiodine Therapy

Because of the complications of both surgery and antithyroid drug therapy, some physicians prefer high-dose radioiodine as the initial treatment for Graves' disease in children and adolescents. In one study, one radioiodine treatment effectively eliminated hyperthyroidism in 85% of patients; two treatments were required in 9%, and three treatments were required in less than 1%. Adjunctive therapy to alleviate severe symptoms of thyrotoxicosis is indicated while awaiting the definitive effects of radioiodine therapy; this may include administration of SSKI or Lugol's solution and beta-adrenergic blockade. Treatment with antithyroid drugs is not indicated prior to radioiodine therapy. Although specific data in children are unavailable, in adults control of hyperthyroidism is generally observed beginning approximately 2 months after radioactive iodine administration. Hypothyroidism is a common complication of radioiodine, occurring in up to 50% of patients.

Neonatal Graves' disease requires vigorous therapy because it is associated with high morbidity and mortality. Therapy includes sedatives, digitalization, and administration of propylthiouracil or methimazole and iodide. Propylthiouracil is preferable to methimazole, as it inhibits the peripheral conversion of T_4 to T_3, and also inhibits thyroid hormone synthesis. Iodides potentiate the propylthiouracil inhibition of hormone synthesis and block thyroid hormone release. Propylthiouracil should be administered in dosages of 5 to 10 mg/kg/day in divided doses at 8-hour intervals. Lugol's solution is given in doses of one drop (about 8 mg iodine) every 8 hours. If a therapeutic response is not observed within 24 to 48 hours, the dose of both drugs can be increased 50% to 100%. In the absence of congestive heart failure, propranolol hydrochloride is useful in controlling sympathetic overactivity; the recommended dosage is 3 mg/kg/day at 8- to 12-hour intervals.

Disposition

Most patients with hyperthyroidism can be treated for minor nonthyroidal illness (e.g., otitis media, upper respiratory tract infection) as outpatients. Admission may be warranted for certain illnesses or complications, and the decision to admit the child should always be made after a consultation with an endocrinologist is obtained.

THYROID STORM

Thyroid storm (thyrotoxic crisis) is a life-threatening syndrome characterized by acute multisystem failure. In children, thyroid storm is extremely uncommon with only two cases reported in the pediatric literature.

Pathophysiology

The exact mechanism that results in sudden release of T_3 and T_4 from the thyroid follicles is unclear. Several precipitating factors, such as sepsis, radioactive I^{131} therapy, surgery, emotional trauma, and sudden withdrawal of thyroid-blocking agents, are implicated in the pathogenesis of thyroid storm. Secondary to any of these factors, there is a sudden surge of T_3 and T_4, resulting in significant exacerbation of hyperthyroidism and the development of signs and symptoms of a hypermetabolic state. Infection appears to be the most common precipitating factor of thyroid storm.

Clinical Evaluation

The diagnosis of thyroid storm is often unclear at the time of presentation, as several other disease entities (e.g., sepsis, malignant hyperthermia, pheochromocytoma, cocaine toxicity, anticholinergic poisoning, and adrenal crisis) may mimic thyrotoxic crisis.

History of thyroid disease and the presence of goiter are usually the necessary clues for considering the diagnosis. Hyperpyrexia ($\geq 41°C$), dyspnea, tachycardia, and systolic hypertension with wide pulse pressure are frequent findings (Table 54–5).

Diagnostic Evaluation

Serum levels of free T_4 or T_3 RIA, TSH, and electrolytes should be determined. A complete blood cell count, blood culture, urinalysis, and urine culture should also be obtained. Values of T_3, T_4, and T_3 resin uptake will be elevated above the normal range but are usually indistinguishable from those seen in uncomplicated thyrotoxicosis.

An electrolyte imbalance may result from vomiting and diarrhea. A chest radiograph and electrocardiogram should be obtained to evaluate heart size and determine the presence of tachyarrhythmias or congestive heart failure.

Therapeutic Intervention

The management of patients in thyrotoxic crisis should be carried out in the intensive care unit after stabilization in the emergency department.

Initial Stabilization

During the initial stabilization, emergency department management should be directed toward maintaining the advanced life support procedures. Intravenous access should be secured with a large-bore catheter and hypovolemia corrected with LR or NS given as a rapid fluid bolus of 20 ml/kg; this may be repeated as necessary until adequate blood pressure is maintained. Fever is reduced with acetaminophen and if the temperature is greater than 40°C, a cooling blanket may be needed.

TABLE 54–5
CLINICAL MANIFESTATIONS OF THYROTOXIC CRISIS
Fever
Hyperthermia greater than 38.5°C and accompanied by excessive diaphoresis
Cardiovascular manifestations
Tachycardia (out of proportion to fever)
Signs and symptoms of congestive heart failure
Systolic hypertension with wide pulse pressure
Hypotension secondary to dehydration
Gastrointestinal manifestations
Nausea, vomiting, diarrhea, hepatomegaly, and jaundice (secondary to congestive heart failure)
Central nervous system manifestations
Confusion, apathy, coma, or seizure
Endocrine manifestations
Goiter, ophthalmopathy

Treatment of Hyperthyroidism

PTU, 10 to 20 mg/kg/day in four divided doses given by a nasogastric tube, will stop iodide organification and reduce intrathyroidal conversion of T_4 to T_3. Methimazole (0.6 to 0.7 mg/kg/day every 8 hours) is an alternative to PTU; it also blocks new hormone synthesis but lacks the ability to inhibit T_4 conversion to T_3. Lugol's solution, 2 to 3 drops orally every 8 hours, or sodium iodide, 125 to 250 mg/day by intravenous drip over 24 hours, will inhibit the proteolysis of colloid and the subsequent release of T_4 and T_3 into the circulation but must be given after PTU has already been administered. Glucocorticoids have been observed to inhibit T_4 conversion to T_3; also there is some theoretical evidence that a state of relative adrenal insufficiency may coexist secondary to increased catabolism during thyrotoxic crisis. Dexamethasone (0.2 mg/kg bolus) may be administered intravenously in the acute phase, followed by 0.1 mg/kg every 6 hours (Table 54–6).

Treatment of Hyperdynamic Circulation

The hyperdynamic cardiovascular state can be controlled with a beta-adrenergic blocking agent such as propranolol (0.01 to 0.03 mg/kg) administered by a slow intravenous push every 10 to 15 minutes until the tachycardia has resolved (total maximum dose should not exceed 5 mg). The maintenance dosage is 4 mg/kg/day orally in four divided doses. If the patient is in congestive heart failure, propranolol is contraindicated; instead, digitalization and maintenance digoxin are indicated.

HYPOTHYROIDISM

Congenital hypothyroidism is the major thyroid disease in the newborn and may be caused by agenesis or aberrant descent of the thyroid or by an enzymatic deficiency in the synthesis of thyroid hormone. Secondary and tertiary hypothyroidism are rare. Congenital hypothyroidism is an important preventable cause of mental retardation. Its prevalence of 1 per 4500 newborn infants is fairly consistent worldwide. It is most common in infants of Asian and Hispanic background (1 per 3000), less common in whites (1 per 5000), and least frequent in black infants (1 per 32,000). Female infants are affected twice as frequently as males. Most cases are sporadic, but thyroid dysgenesis is the cause of decreased thyroid function in the majority of infants with permanent congenital hypothyroidism.

Acquired hypothyroidism, or hypothyroidism that develops in a child who was previously euthyroid, may be caused

TABLE 54–6

SUMMARY OF MANAGEMENT

Target	Intervention
Hormone synthesis inhibitors	Propylthiouracil, 6 to 10 mg/kg/day by nasogastric tube every 8 hr *or* Methimazole, 0.6 to 0.7 mg/kg/day by nasogastric tube every 8 hr Dexamethasone, 0.2 mg/kg IV bolus
Hormone secretion inhibitors	Lugol's iodine, two to three drops every 8 hr orally *or* Sodium iodide, 250 mg/kg by continuous IV infusion
Beta-adrenergic blockers	Propranolol, 0.01 to 0.03/kg IV over 10 to 15 min

TABLE 54–7

CLINICAL FEATURES OF HYPOTHYROIDISM

System	Clinical Manifestation
Skin	Pale, dry, scaly skin; sparse, brittle hair; increased mucopolysaccharide accumulation in the subcutaneous tissue
Muscular	Pseudohypertrophy
Central nervous	Apathy; delayed tendon relaxation
Gastrointestinal	Constipation
Growth	Slow growth; mild obesity; delayed dentition
Endocrine	Delayed puberty; menorrhagia or metrorrhagia; precocious puberty in females (rare)

by a wide variety of defects. Classification is based on the presence or absence of a goiter. Hashimoto's disease, or lymphocytic thyroiditis, is the most common acquired thyroid disorder in children and adolescents.

Clinical Evaluation

Signs and symptoms of congenital hypothyroidism usually manifest themselves prior to or during the period in the newborn nursery. These may include a prolonged gestation period, an infant who is large for gestational age, a large posterior fontanel, respiratory distress, hypothermia, peripheral cyanosis, hypoactivity, poor feeding, delay in onset of stooling, abdominal distention with vomiting, prolonged physiologic icterus, and edema. Other features that may be recognizable at 2 to 3 weeks of age include unusual facies, umbilical hernia, an enlarged tongue, and dry skin. These manifestations progress if hypothyroidism remains untreated. Retardation of physical and mental development becomes greater during the following months, and by 3 to 6 months of age the clinical picture is fully developed.

The clinical presentation of acquired hypothyroidism will depend on the child's age at onset and the extent of gland dysfunction (Table 54–7).

Diagnostic Evaluation

The initial screening of any patient with suspected hypothyroidism should include measurement of serum total T_4 and TSH concentrations. Because occasional alterations in serum binding proteins may result in high or low total T_4 concentrations, free T_4 concentrations should be measured if laboratory findings do not correlate with the clinical impression. In juvenile hypothyroidism caused by a defect primarily in the thyroid gland, as in Hashimoto's thyroiditis, serum levels of T_4 and T_3 are low and TSH in serum is greater than 25 μU/ml. Both antimicrosomal and antithyroglobulin antibody titers are commonly elevated in Hashimoto's thyroiditis.

Ultrasound imaging is a valuable diagnostic tool for the differential diagnosis of diffuse thyroid disorders in children. Radioactive iodine uptake studies may be helpful in distinguishing transient toxic thyroiditis or chronic lymphocytic thyroiditis from Graves' disease.

During acute nonthyroidal illness, serum T_3, T_4, free T_3, and free T_4 levels are usually decreased without a subsequent increase in TSH (euthyroid sick syndrome). This state of secondary hypothyroxinemia was noted to be more prominent in patients receiving glucocorticoids or dopamine, both of which are known to inhibit the release of TSH from the pituitary gland. In adults, this syndrome is associated with increased mortality. However, no increase in mortality rates has been observed among critically ill children with euthyroid sick syndrome.

Therapeutic Intervention

Whatever the cause of hypothyroidism, full replacement therapy with thyroid hormone is indicated. The treatment of choice is levothyroxine sodium given orally.

Replacement therapy should be started immediately after biochemical confirmation of the diagnosis of hypothyroidism is obtained. The daily dose of levothyroxine is determined by age and body weight: during the first 6 months of age, the dose is 8 to 10 μg/kg (25 to 50 μg); from 6 months to 12 months of age, the dose is 5 to 8 μg/kg (50 to 75 μg), with gradual reduction to 3 to 4 μg/kg/day (or 100 μg/m^2/day). Infants can be safely given the full replacement dose of T_4 at the time of diagnosis unless they have congenital heart disease and are at risk for cardiac decompensation. Because of rapid weight gain during infancy, the serum T_4 should be measured and the dose of levothyroxine adjusted at 1 month, 3 months, and 6 months of age and yearly thereafter. The goal of therapy is to provide the correct amount of T_4 for optimal physical and intellectual development. In infants with primary hypothyroidism, the TSH concentration should be decreased to less than 5.8 μU/ml after 1 month of age and to less than 4.0 μU/ml by 1 year of age. To achieve this, T_4 concentrations will be high by adult standards and should be interpreted in light of age-matched standards. For patients with central hypothyroidism, one must rely on T_4 concentrations and the clinical impression when assessing the dose.

In children with congenital hypothyroidism, the prognosis for physical growth is excellent. Maintenance of serum thyroxine levels in the upper half of the normal range results in normal growth patterns. Early treatment also improves the prognosis for mental development in neonates with hypothyroidism. Ninety percent of children treated within 45 days of birth were found to have normal IQ values when measured at 4 to 7 years of age.

THYROIDITIS

Thyroiditis is one of the most common endocrine disorders of childhood. Chronic lymphocytic thyroiditis, also known as Hashimoto's thyroiditis, is by far the most frequent cause of goiter in childhood; less common causes include colloid or simple goiter, infectious thyroiditis (acute suppurative and subacute viral), dyshormonogenesis, goitrogen, neoplasia, anatomic abnormalities, and iodine deficiency. Most commonly, thyroiditis is associated with euthyroid function but may occasionally result in transient or permanent thyroid dysfunction. Chronic lymphocytic thyroiditis is an autoimmune, inflammatory process resulting from altered humoral and cell-mediated immunity. Commonly assayed immunoglobulins include antithyroglobulin and antimicrosomal antibodies, which are present in virtually all patients with chronic lymphocytic thyroiditis. However, these are not specific for this disease and may be found with other autoimmune diseases such as Graves' disease. Other autoimmune disorders seen with increased frequency in children with chronic lymphocytic thyroiditis include diabetes mellitus, hypoadrenocorticism, hypoparathyroidism, myasthenia gravis, and pernicious anemia. More than 50% of patients with juvenile diabetes mellitus also have thyroid dysfunction.

Clinical Evaluation

The clinical presentation of children with chronic lymphocytic thyroiditis is that of an asymptomatic goiter. Most children are euthyroid initially. A smaller number of children will have laboratory evidence of hypothyroidism, subclinical hypothyroidism, or, rarely, transient thyrotoxicosis. Transient or permanent hypothyroidism may follow an initial euthyroid period, but spontaneous resolution of thyroiditis may occur in up to 50% of affected children.

Diagnostic Evaluation

The initial screening of thyroid function should include measurement of serum total T_4 and TSH concentrations and of serum T_3 concentration if the patient appears to have hyperthyroidism. Both antimicrosomal and antithyroglobulin antibody titers should be measured.

Therapeutic Intervention

Replacement therapy with levothyroxine is indicated for all patients with hypothyroidism. Thyroxine therapy is also indicated in euthyroid children with large goiters, obstructive symptoms, or cosmetic disfigurement or an increased TSH level. Careful clinical follow-up may be chosen for those children with normal or slightly enlarged thyroid glands, positive antibody titers, and normal thyroid function studies.

Selected References

Aiello DP, DuPlessis AJ, Pattishall EG III, Kulin HE. Thyroid storm. Presenting with coma and seizures in a 3-year-old girl. Clin Pediatr 1989;28:571.

Bachrach LK, Foley TP Jr. Thyroiditis in children. Pediatr Rev 1989;11:184.

Buckingham BA, Costin G, Roe TF, et al. Hyperthyroidism in children. A reevaluation of treatment. Am J Dis Child 1981;135:112.

Collen RJ, Landaw EM, Kaplan SA. Remission rates of children and adolescents with thyrotoxicosis treated with antithyroid drugs. Pediatrics 1980;65:550.

Croom RD, Thomas CG, Reddick RL, et al. Autonomously functioning thyroid nodules in childhood and adolescence. Surgery 1987;102:1101.

Dunn JT. Choice of therapy in young adults with hyperthyroidism of Graves' disease. A brief, case-directed poll of fifty-four thyroidologists. Ann Intern Med 1984;100:891.

Fisher DA, Klein AH. Thyroid development and disorders of thyroid function in the newborn. N Engl J Med 1981;304:702.

Galaburda M, Rosman NP, Haddow JE. Thyroid storm in an 11-year-old boy managed by propranolol. Pediatrics 1975;53:920.

Hayles AB. Problems of childhood Graves' disease. Mayo Clin Proc 1972;47:850.

Levy WJ, Schumacher OP, Gupta M. Treatment of childhood Graves' disease. A review with emphasis on radioiodine treatment. Cleve Clin J Med 1988;55:373.

Lippe BM, Landaw EM, Kaplan SA. Hyperthyroidism in children treated with long term medical therapy: Twenty-five percent remission every two years. J Clin Endocrinol Metab 1987;64:1241.

Reiter EO, Root AW, Rettig K, Vargas A. Childhood thyromegaly: Recent developments. J Pediatr 1981;99:507.

Safa AM, Schumacher OP, Rodriguez-Antunez A. Long-term follow-up results in children and adolescents treated with radioactive iodine (131 I) for hyperthyroidism. N Engl J Med 1975;292:167.

Smith CS, Howard NJ. Propranolol in treatment of neonatal thyrotoxicosis. J Pediatr 1973;83:1046.

Sobel EH, Saenger P. Hypothyroidism in the newborn. Pediatr Rev 1989;11:15.

Szabo SM, Allen DB. Thyroiditis. Differentiation of acute suppurative and subacute. Clin Pediatr 1989;28:171.

Zakarija M, McKenzie JM, Banovac K. Clinical significance of assay of thyroid-stimulating antibody in Graves' disease. Ann Intern Med 1980;93:28.

Zuker AR, Chernow B, Fields AI, et al. Thyroid function in critically ill children. J Pediatr 1985;107:552.

CHAPTER 55

Parathyroid Disorders

Anthony Albano

INTRODUCTION

Fewer than 200 cases of primary hyperparathyroidism in children under 16 years of age have been reported in the literature, and only 28 cases of neonatal hyperparathyroidism have been reported. Primary hyperparathyroidism with childhood onset occurs more frequently in males than in females, but the female-to-male ratio is greater if onset is in adulthood. In addition, primary hyperparathyroidism in children under 1 year of age appears to be almost exclusively caused by parathyroid hyperplasia. This is in contrast to parathyroid adenomas, which are responsible for more than 90% of cases of primary hyperparathyroidism in patients older than 1 year.

Hypoparathyroidism can arise from multiple causes, including congenital forms consisting of isolated aplasia or hypoplasia of the parathyroids, and can also be associated with dysmorphic syndromes. Isolated aplasia or hypoplasia of the parathyroid gland may be familial. Hypoparathyroidism may also result from extrinsic causes, such as surgical removal or irradiation of the parathyroid glands. Heavy metals may also adversely affect parathyroid functions, as has been documented in Wilson's disease.

ANATOMY AND PHYSIOLOGY
Parathyroid Hormone

The parathyroid glands are small, oval endocrine glands usually consisting of two pairs, one pair situated on the posterior surface of the thyroid gland on each side. The chief, or principal, cells of the parathyroid gland secrete parathyroid hormone (PTH).

The major factor affecting the release of PTH is the extracellular fluid calcium concentration. Low calcium levels enhance release of PTH, and elevated serum calcium suppresses release. Vitamin D or its metabolites also likely play a role in feedback control of PTH. Parathyroid hormone synthesis can be reduced by the presence of 1,24-dihydroxyvitamin D. Control of calcium homeostasis involves the interaction of PTH and vitamin D on target tissues. PTH acts on renal tissues to increase active reabsorption of calcium by the distal nephron, to decrease phosphate absorption in the proximal nephron, and to induce synthesis of 1,25-dihydroxyvitamin D_3 by the activation of 1-alpha-hydroxylase. Urinary excretion of sodium, potassium, and bicarbonate is increased, with a subsequent decrease in excretion of ammonium ion and hydrogen ion. Unopposed PTH effects produce hypercalcemia, hypophosphatemia, and hypocalciuria.

Vitamin D

Vitamin D has two active forms: vitamin D_2 (ergocalciferol) and vitamin D_3 (cholecalciferol). Vitamin D_2 is the plant equivalent of vitamin D_3. Vitamin D_3 may be synthesized in the skin and can also be obtained by ingestion of fish liver oils, butter, and eggs.

The mechanism of action of the active vitamin D metabolites is similar to that of the other sterol hormones. The major role of 1,25-dihydroxyvitamin D_3 $(1,25(OH)_2D_3)$ is to mediate intestinal calcium absorption in the duodenum and phosphate absorption in the jejunum. PTH release may be affected by a feedback loop involving $1,25(OH)_2D_3$.

Other Factors Influencing Calcium Metabolism

The calcium flux in the kidney parallels that of sodium. Factors that increase sodium loss, such as administration of loop diuretics, usually cause calcium loss. Factors that cause an increase in tubular sodium resorption, such as hypovolemia, usually increase calcium absorption. Calcium deposition into bone and soft tissues is promoted by an exogenously administered phosphate load or occurs secondary to a metabolic hyperphosphatemia.

Calcitonin is a hormone produced in the C cells of the thyroid gland. Calcitonin's primary action appears to be an inhibition of skeletal osteoclast function.

Neoplastic diseases are associated with hypercalcemic states. The hypercalcemia associated with malignancy has been reported both with solid tumors, such as medulloblastoma, and with hematopoietic neoplasms, such as lymphoblastic leukemia. The mechanism of hypercalcemia in many of these cases is related to increased bone resorption by metastatic tumor cells.

Normal Calcium Metabolism

Fetal calcium requirements increase significantly following the onset of skeletal mineralization, usually in about the eighth week of gestation. The parathyroid gland is active in the fetus and responds to ambient calcium levels; this is evidenced by the occurrence of hypoparathyroidism in infants of hyperparathyroid mothers and of neonatal hyperparathyroidism in cases of maternal hypoparathyroidism. Following delivery, serum calcium begins to drop within the first few hours of life. If the infant is fed cow's milk, which has a lower calcium-to-phosphorus ratio than breast milk, the greatest change in serum calcium usually is seen at 3 to 5 days of life. Neonatal hypocalcemia may be defined as occurring within 48 to 72 hours of delivery and is usually seen in preterm infants. Other risk factors include birth asphyxia, phototherapy for hyperbilirubinemia, maternal diabetes, a maternal history of anticonvulsant medication, and maternal hyperparathyroidism.

Current milk-based formulas usually contain sufficient calcium and vitamin D for the normal term infant; however, human milk may not be completely adequate, especially as a sole supply of vitamin D. Children with nutritional rickets secondary to vitamin D deficiency present more commonly with a history of exclusive breast-feeding without vitamin D supplementation. Thus current recommendations for breast-fed infants call for supplementation of 400 International Units (IU) of vitamin D every day.

HYPOPARATHYROIDISM
Clinical Evaluation

The signs and symptoms of hypoparathyroidism are the signs and symptoms of hypocalcemia. Increased neuromuscular irritability is commonly seen, giving rise to the classic Chvostek's sign, which is a facial twitch caused by a tap over the facial nerve approximately 2 cm anterior to the ear, and Trousseau's sign, which is carpopedal spasm produced by approximately 3 minutes of limb ischemia induced by tourniquet. The usefulness of these physical signs is limited by their low sensitivity and specificity and by the patient's age.

The central nervous system presentations of hypocalcemia include seizures, psychiatric illness, movement disturbances, dementia, and even mental retardation. Optic neuritis and papilledema have been reported as complications of hypocalcemia resulting from hypoparathyroidism. The cardiovascular effects of hypocalcemia may produce bradycardia and left ventricular failure.

The ocular manifestations of hypocalcemia include keratitis, conjunctivitis, and cataracts. Hypoparathyroid patients have a higher incidence of candidal infections of the skin and gastrointestinal tract, which may be related to a T-cell immunodeficiency. The physical examination should note signs of autoimmune dysfunction (such as candidiasis) or signs of pseudohypoparathyroidism. Hypocalcemia occurring during enamel formation leads to an increased incidence of dental caries as a result of defective enamel.

Diagnostic Evaluation

Following the correction of symptomatic hypocalcemia, the underlying cause of the disorder must be sought. Blood should be collected for analysis of serum albumin, calcium, magnesium, phosphate, alkaline phosphatase, sodium, potassium, chloride, and venous carbon dioxide. Renal function should be assessed by the serum blood urea nitrogen and creatinine values.

Radiologic evaluation of the extremities may reveal signs of abnormal mineralization. Serum parathyroid hormone levels are sometimes useful and should be evaluated with careful clinical correlation. The N-terminal portion of the hormone is the active form, and assays that reflect evaluation of this portion are the most useful.

Hypocalcemia causes prolongation of the QT interval as a result of prolongation of the ST segment. The duration of the T wave is unchanged. With the exception of hypothermia, there are no other extrinsic causes of QT prolongation that do not change the duration of the T wave. The initial minor electrocardiographic changes may progress to complete heart block or ventricular fibrillation.

Hepatic disease, malabsorption syndromes, chronic renal failure, pernicious anemia, achlorhydria, and multiple endocrine deficiencies may all be associated with hypoparathyroidism. An appropriate laboratory evaluation to exclude these conditions must be made on an individual basis.

If causes of hypocalcemia such as hypoalbuminemia or hypomagnesemia are eliminated, then abnormalities involving the PTH–vitamin D axis should be considered (Fig. 55–1).

Differential Diagnosis
Hypocalcemia

There are many causes of hypocalcemia (Table 55–1). Approximately 35% of serum calcium is bound to protein, with about 55% remaining free. It is this 55% of ionized serum calcium that is referred to in hypocalcemia, as the total serum calcium may be low with a normal ionized calcium. This is most often seen in hypoalbuminemia where a decrease in the serum albumin of 1 gm/dl will produce a reduction in the serum calcium level of 0.8 mg/dl.

An exogenous phosphate load (e.g., as occurs with administration of an adult or pediatric phosphate enema or with medicinal phosphate used as a treatment for diabetic ketoacidosis) has been reported to cause hypocalcemia. The endogenous phosphate load from severe rhabdomyolysis may cause a fall in the serum calcium level and precipitation of calcium phosphate in the tissues.

Oncologic treatments are associated with calcium defects.

TABLE 55–1
DIFFERENTIAL DIAGNOSIS FOR HYPOCALCEMIA

I. Hypoparathyroidism
II. Renal insufficiency
III. Acute pancreatitis
IV. Malignancy
  A. Osteoblastic metastases
  B. Tumor lysis syndrome
  C. Medications
    1. Mithramycin
    2. Cisplatin
    3. Methotrexate
V. Medications
  A. Anticonvulsants
  B. Phosphates
  C. Blood products (citrates)
  D. Albumin
  E. Ethylenediaminetetra-acetate (EDTA)
VI. Anion chelation
  A. Fluoride
  B. Citrate
  C. Oxalate
  D. Bicarbonate
  E. Phosphate
VII. Vitamin D deficiency
  A. Dietary deficiency
  B. Malabsorption
  C. Anticonvulsant therapy
  D. Hepatic insufficiency
VIII. Hypoalbuminemia

Renal damage from cisplatin has been associated with hypomagnesemia and hypocalcemia. Methotrexate has been reported to cause a malabsorption syndrome resulting in hypocalcemia. The acute tumor lysis syndrome usually results from the lysis of a large tumor load. Metabolic abnormalities occur as a result of the release of intracellular metabolites, which include uric acid, potassium, and phosphorus, and hyperphosphatemia produces a resultant hypocalcemia.

The administration of blood products may be associated with hypocalcemia. This is because of the citrate ion present in many blood products (e.g., fresh frozen plasma or packed red blood cells), as well as the albumin present in blood products, both of which bind the ionized serum calcium.

Burns from hydrofluoric acid can result in the fluoride ion binding with calcium and producing a severe acute hypocalcemia. Several deaths have been reported from the hypocalcemia of hydrofluoric acid burns.

A growing body of evidence indicates that critically ill children may have an associated ionized hypocalcemia. The origin of this hypocalcemia remains unclear, but in critically ill children it should be treated.

Magnesium metabolism and calcium metabolism are intimately related. Hyperparathyroidism, which often causes magnesium wasting and magnesium deficiency, impairs PTH release. Thus any cause of hypomagnesemia places a patient at risk for hypoparathyroidism. Hypocalcemia that is unresponsive to other modes of therapy may respond once the patient's magnesium levels have been restored to normal.

Hypoparathyroidism

Hypocalcemia may also occur as a failure of the homeostatic mechanisms involving parathyroid hormones or vitamin D. This hypoparathyroidism can be clarified by origin (Table 55–2). *Transient hypofunction* of the parathyroid glands is seen in both early and late neonatal hypocalcemia. Isolated

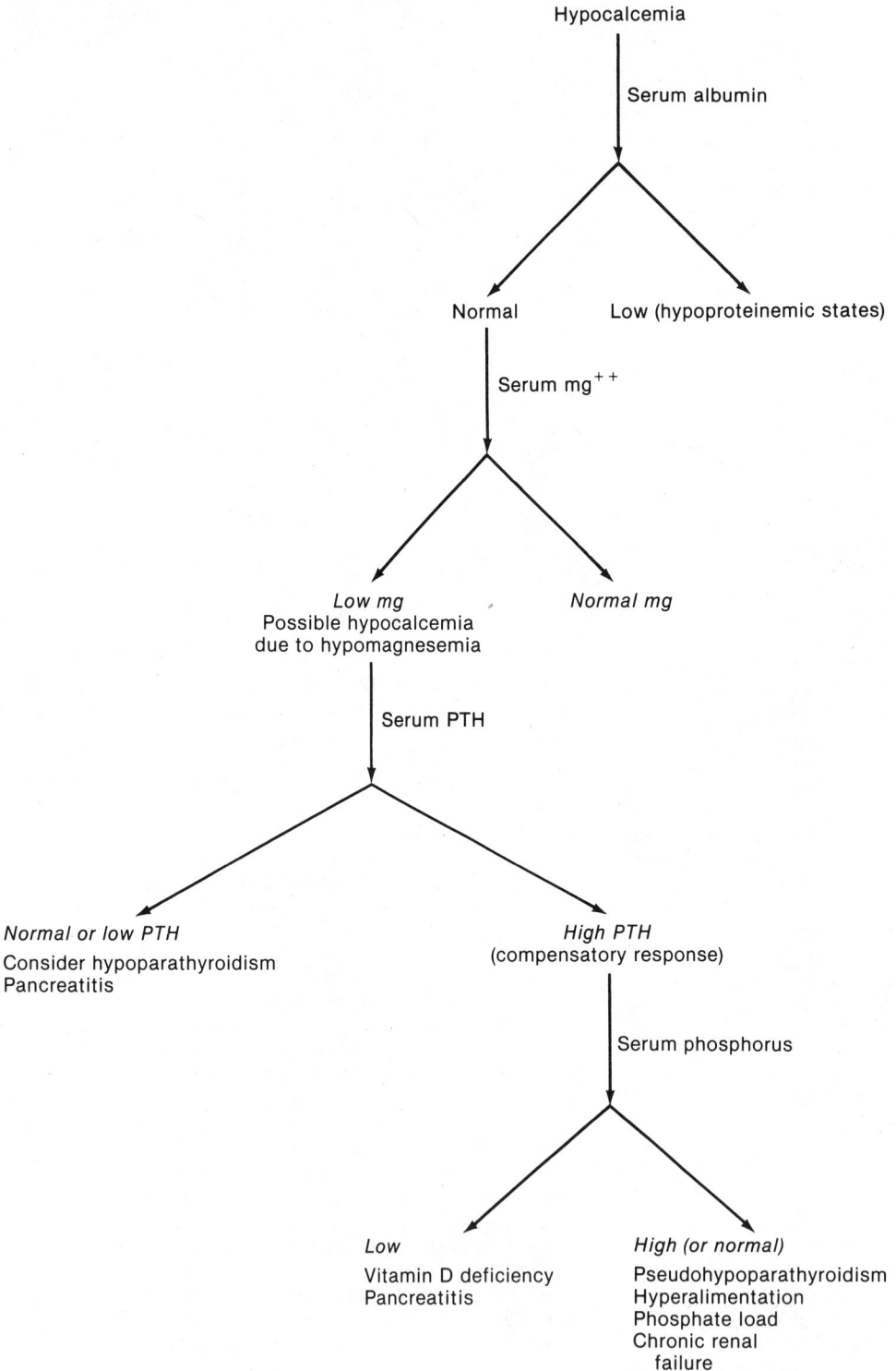

Figure 55–1. Algorithm for the initial evaluation of hypocalcemia.

TABLE 55–2

CLASSIFICATION OF HYPOPARATHYROIDISM

I. Pseudohypoparathyroidism (end-organ resistance)
II. Parathyroid gland injury
  A. Postoperative removal or manipulation
  B. Postirradiation
  C. Infiltrative/depositive
    1. Amyloidosis
    2. Wilson's disease
    3. Hemochromatosis
III. Acquired hypofunction (other categories)
  A. Hypomagnesemia
  B. Pancreatitis
IV. Neonatal hypocalcemic conditions
  A. Secondary hypoparathyroidism
  B. Early neonatal hypocalcemia
  C. Late neonatal hypocalcemia
V. Idiopathic hypoparathyroidism
  A. Isolated (multiple forms)
  B. Associated with polyendocrine failure
  C. Associated with dysmorphic syndromes

---

aplasia of the parathyroid glands is termed *idiopathic hypoparathyroidism*. Idiopathic hypoparathyroidism may occur in many congenital forms. *Congenital aplasia* or *hypoplasia* of the parathyroid glands may be associated with malformation complexes such as the DiGeorge syndrome, which is a triad of thymic hypoplasia, hypoparathyroidism, and congenital cardiac anomalies. *Congenital hypoparathyroidism* may be associated with teratogens, most notably maternal alcohol or retinoic acid use. Maternal exposure to iodine 131 has also been reported to cause hypoparathyroidism.

The parathyroid glands may also be damaged from exogenous physical causes such as surgical manipulation or removal. Metal deposition, as in hemochromatosis secondary to blood transfusion in patients with thalassemia or copper deposition in Wilson's disease, or infiltrative processes such as amyloidosis may all cause parathyroid insufficiency.

Target organ resistance to parathyroid hormone is termed *pseudohypoparathyroidism*. The associated laboratory findings include hypocalcemia and an increased concentration of immunoreactive parathyroid hormone. Albright's hereditary osteodystrophy is a hypoparathyroid state associated with end-organ resistance to PTH; its characteristics include short stature, round facies, mental retardation, brachydactyly, short fourth metacarpals and metatarsals, subcutaneous and basal ganglia calcifications, and hypoplasia of the dental enamel leading to dental abscesses. The term *pseudopseudohypoparathyroidism* refers to the presence of the phenotypical characteristics of Albright's dystrophy without the hypoparathyroidism.

Therapeutic Intervention

Acute hypocalcemia is a medical emergency often manifested by seizure activity, tetany, or electrocardiographic (EKG) changes. Restoration of serum calcium is necessary and is performed by intravenous (IV) infusion of calcium.

Elemental calcium is commonly available as two solutions. Calcium chloride solution contains more calcium on a molar basis than calcium gluconate. However, it also causes more tissue injury if extravasation occurs. Calcium chloride is supplied in 10-ml ampules of a 10% solution, which contains 1.36 mEq/ml; this is the equivalent of 27.3 mg of elemental calcium per milliliter. Calcium gluconate is also supplied in 10-ml ampules of a 10% solution. It contains 0.45 mEq/ml of calcium, which is the equivalent of 9 mg of elemental calcium. Both calcium solutions require a 1:5 dilution in 5% dextrose water (D5W). These solutions should not be mixed with bicarbonate, as precipitation of calcium carbonate will occur. The administration of IV calcium should be accompanied by cardiac monitoring. Treatment of hypocalcemic emergencies may be performed by the administration of 10% calcium chloride, 20 mg (0.2 ml) per kilogram IV over the course of 2 to 10 minutes. The maximum individual dose is 5 ml (500 mg). Further supplementation is guided by serum calcium concentration. Caution must be used when administering calcium to patients receiving digitalis preparations, because hypercalcemia may exacerbate digitalis cardiotoxicity. If there is minimal response to the IV calcium infusion, then magnesium supplementation should be considered.

Magnesium supplementation may be performed either intravenously or intramuscularly. A 50% magnesium sulfate solution is available for intramuscular injection, with the dose being 20 to 50 mg/kg every 4 hours up to four doses. An intravenous infusion at the same dose, but using a 20% magnesium sulfate solution containing 0.8 mEq/ml, may accomplish the same goal and should be infused over 3 to 5 minutes (Table 55–3).

The goal of therapy in chronic hypocalcemia is to increase gastrointestinal absorption of calcium while avoiding hypercalciuria. This may be accomplished by oral calcium supplementation and possibly by vitamin D therapy. In addition, the use of a thiazide diuretic or sodium restriction may be helpful. These efforts should be coordinated by a pediatric endocrinologist (Table 55–4).

HYPERPARATHYROIDISM
Clinical Evaluation

The manifestations of hyperparathyroidism are those of hypercalcemia. The signs and symptoms of hypercalcemia may be somewhat dependent on the underlying cause of the elevated serum calcium. However, these symptoms usually

---

TABLE 55–3

MEDICATIONS USEFUL FOR TREATMENT OF ACUTE HYPOCALCEMIA

Drug	Dose	Route	Limiting Dose
Calcium chloride (10%)	0.2 ml/kg q 10 min	IV over 2–10 min in a 1:5 dilution in D5W	500 mg = 5 ml/dose q 10 min
Calcium gluconate (10%)	1.0 ml/kg/dose q 10 min	IV over 10 min in a 1:5 dilution in D5W	10–20 ml/dose q 10 min
Magnesium sulfate (20%)	0.1–0.25 ml/kg/dose for one to two doses	IV over 3–5 min	1 gm/day

---

TABLE 55–4

ADMISSION CRITERIA FOR HYPOCALCEMIA

1. Symptomatic hypocalcemia
   Increased neuromuscular irritability
   Grand mal seizures
   Psychiatric disturbances
   Movement disturbances
   Dementia
2. Significant systemic manifestations
   Congestive heart failure
   Bradycardia
   Keratitis or conjunctivitis
3. Newly diagnosed or suspected metabolic bone disease or hypoparathyroidism
4. Asymptomatic hypocalcemia with unreliable home situation

---

are the result of disturbances in the CNS, neuromuscular, renal, or gastrointestinal (GI) systems.

The CNS alterations of hypercalcemia include psychiatric disturbances, which may range from subtle personality changes or depression to blatant psychosis. Disturbances in memory and orientation may be noted. Neuromuscular symptoms may include muscle weakness and depressed deep tendon reflexes. Twitching of isolated muscles may progress to grand mal seizures.

Renal colic may be a presenting symptom of hyperparathyroidism, as may painless hematuria. Bone and joint pain may indicate osteitis fibrosa, in which cavities form in the interior of bones.

The classic GI disturbances of hyperparathyroidism include constipation, nausea, and abdominal pain. Constipation may be ablated by rehydration but is usually a result of a decrease in GI motility secondary to hypercalcemia. Pancreatitis or ulceration of the GI tract may also cause abdominal pain and obscure the clinical picture.

Precipitation of calcium in soft tissues may be associated with pruritus, whereas precipitation in the soft tissues of the eye may cause a keratopathy that can be a threat to vision.

The cardiovascular effects of hypercalcemia include a positive inotropic effect on nonischemic cardiac muscle that produces a shortened systolic duration. Hypertension is associated with hyperparathyroidism.

The serum calcium concentrations in patients with primary hyperparathyroidism usually correlate with the severity of symptoms. Patients may be asymptomatic or may present with the consequences of chronic hypercalcemia and hypercalciuria, such as nephrocalcinosis, renal calculi, or renal failure. A minority of persons will present in hypercalcemic crisis with seizures and an extreme elevation of serum calcium.

Diagnostic Evaluation

The laboratory evaluation of hypercalcemia includes measurement of the serum concentrations of calcium, ionized calcium (if possible), albumin, electrolytes, phosphorus, and PTH (preferably the N-terminal). The initial evaluation of hypercalcemia may begin in the emergency department, but definitive evaluation is usually delayed because of the unavailability of serum PTH assays and other diagnostic tests (Fig. 55–2).

Hypercalcemia may produce chronic renal failure secondary to interstitial calcium deposition with chronic interstitial nephritis and tubular dysfunction. Microscopic or gross hematuria with or without renal colic and polyuria may be seen. In children the most common cause of renal calculus

formation is urinary stasis and infection, although 6% of renal calculi in children may be caused by hyperparathyroidism. Other urologic complications of hyperparathyroidism and hypercalciuria include nephrolithiasis, nephrocalcinosis, and defective urine-concentrating ability or acidification. Serum cortisol and thyroid function tests are adjuncts to diagnosis. Although the bone and joint pain of hypercalcemia may be caused by osteitis fibrosa, tumor metastases must be excluded. Radiographs of painful musculoskeletal anatomy are indicated (Fig. 55–3). Increasing hypercalcemia is associated with a shortening of the QT interval, a shortening of the ST segment, and an increased incidence of dysrhythmias. This is aggravated in patients receiving digitalis preparations. More long-standing hypercalcemia may produce deposition of calcium in cardiac tissues.

Differential Diagnosis
Hypercalcemia

Physiologic states that involve increased resorption of bone, such as hyperparathyroidism, prolonged immobilization, hypervitaminosis, and neoplasm, may all be causes of hypercalcemia (Table 55–5). The hypercalcemia of malignancy may be caused either by metastases that directly stimulate bone resorption or by tumor secretion of a PTH-like factor. The increased metabolism of hyperthyroidism may result in a bone resorptive state that may cause hypercalcemia. Both hyperthyroidism and hypothyroidism have been associated with hypercalcemia. The resorptive hypercalcemia of immobilization is often seen in children placed in long-leg casts. Vitamin A intoxication may occur in ado-

---

TABLE 55–5

CAUSES OF HYPERCALCEMIA

I. Primary hyperparathyroidism
   A. Inheritable
      1. Multiple endocrine neoplastic syndromes
      2. Neonatal
      3. Various familial syndromes (hypocalciuric-hypercalcemia)
   B. Sporadic
      1. Adenomas
      2. Hyperplasia
      3. Carcinomas
II. Neoplasia
   A. Osteolysis from metastases to bone
   B. Humoral mediators
III. Granulomatous diseases
   A. Sarcoidosis
   B. Tuberculosis
   C. Berylliosis
   D. Coccidioidomycosis
   E. Other
IV. Chemical
   A. Thiazide
   B. Lithium
   C. Vitamins A and D
   D. Milk-alkali syndrome
V. Endocrinopathies
   A. Hyperthyroidism
   B. Hypothyroidism
   C. Addison's disease
   D. Pheochromocytoma
VI. Miscellaneous
   A. Infants of hypoparathyroid mothers
   B. Acute renal failure
   C. Idiopathic hypercalcemia of infancy
   D. Immobilization hypercalcemia

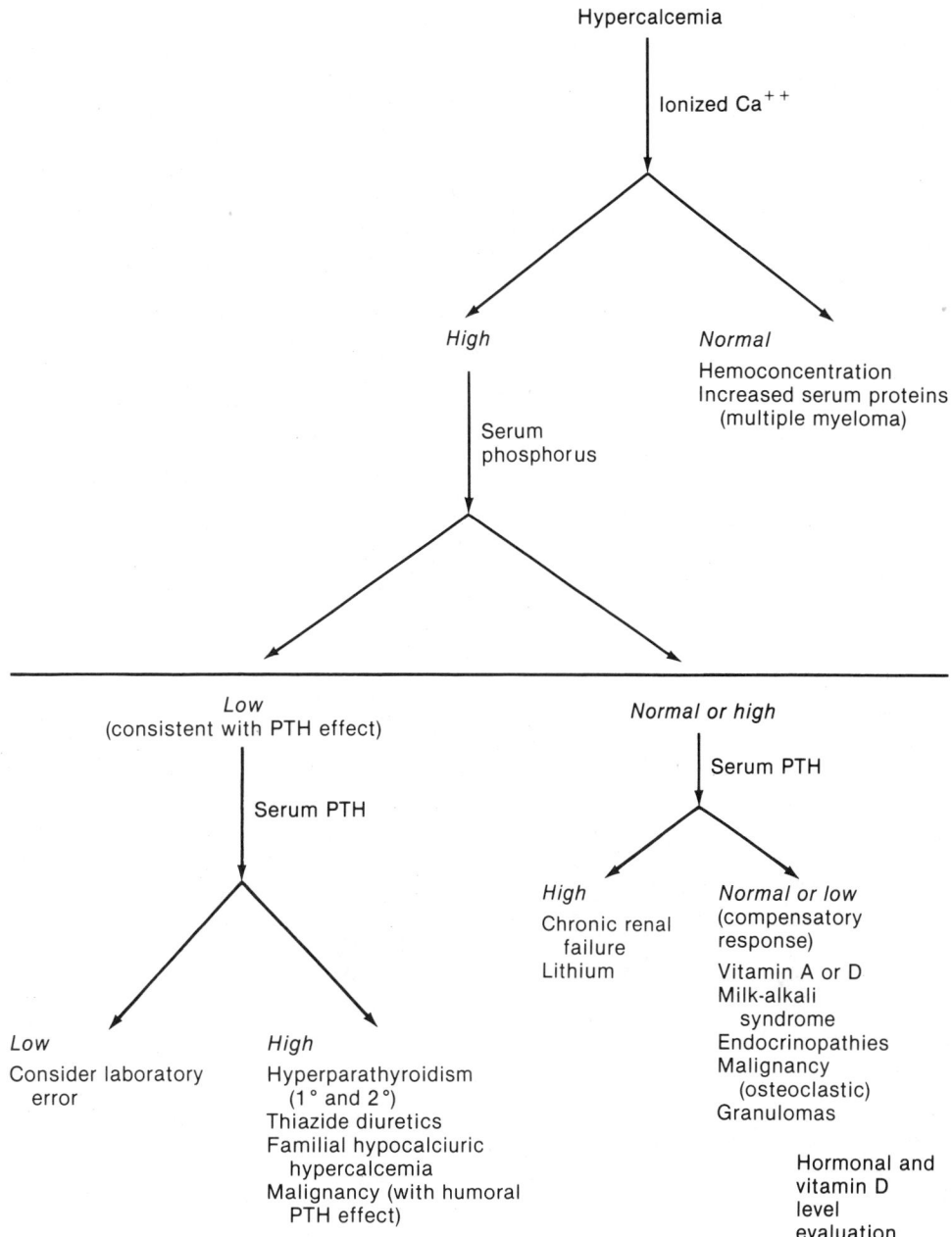

Figure 55–2. Algorithm for the initial evaluation of hypercalcemia.

lescents or adults taking doses greater than 50,000 IU daily, and pharmacologic doses of vitamin A cause osteoclastic bone resorption. These patients may be under treatment for a skin disorder or may simply be taking large doses of vitamins. Treatment consists of cessation of vitamin A intake and possibly hydration and diuresis.

GI hyperabsorption of calcium may cause elevations in the serum calcium level. The milk-alkali syndrome results from ingestion of large amounts of absorbable antacids, usually calcium carbonate or calcium bicarbonate, used in the treatment of peptic ulcer disease or gastritis. In addition to hypercalcemia, renal insufficiency, hypocalciuria, metabolic alkalosis, and hypophosphatemia may be seen.

The familial hypocalciuric-hypercalcemic syndrome is distinct from primary hyperparathyroidism, especially in its mode of treatment. These patients have few symptoms and signs, and urologic and GI manifestations are rare. The outcome of surgical intervention has been unsatisfactory, in contrast to the benefits of surgery seen in patients with

primary hyperparathyroidism. Following subtotal parathyroidectomy, normocalcemia is rare.

Adrenal insufficiency may occasionally be associated with hypercalcemia, although the exact cause of hypercalcemia in Addison's disease is poorly understood. Sarcoidosis, tuberculosis, berylliosis, and other granulomatous disorders are also associated with hypercalcemia, which may be related to increased vitamin D metabolism in the granulomas. Lithium may induce a state of hypercalcemia, although the mechanism is poorly understood. The thiazide diuretics may also cause hypercalcemia by decreasing renal excretion of calcium. Hypercalcemia can be associated with chronic renal failure, although hypocalcemia is more commonly seen. Hypercalcemia may also be induced by overenthusiastic calcium supplementation during hyperalimentation. The "blue diaper syndrome" is a complex of familial hypercalcemia, with nephrocalcinosis and indicanuria. Subcutaneous fat necrosis of the newborn is associated with hypercalcemia, although the underlying mechanism is not understood. In

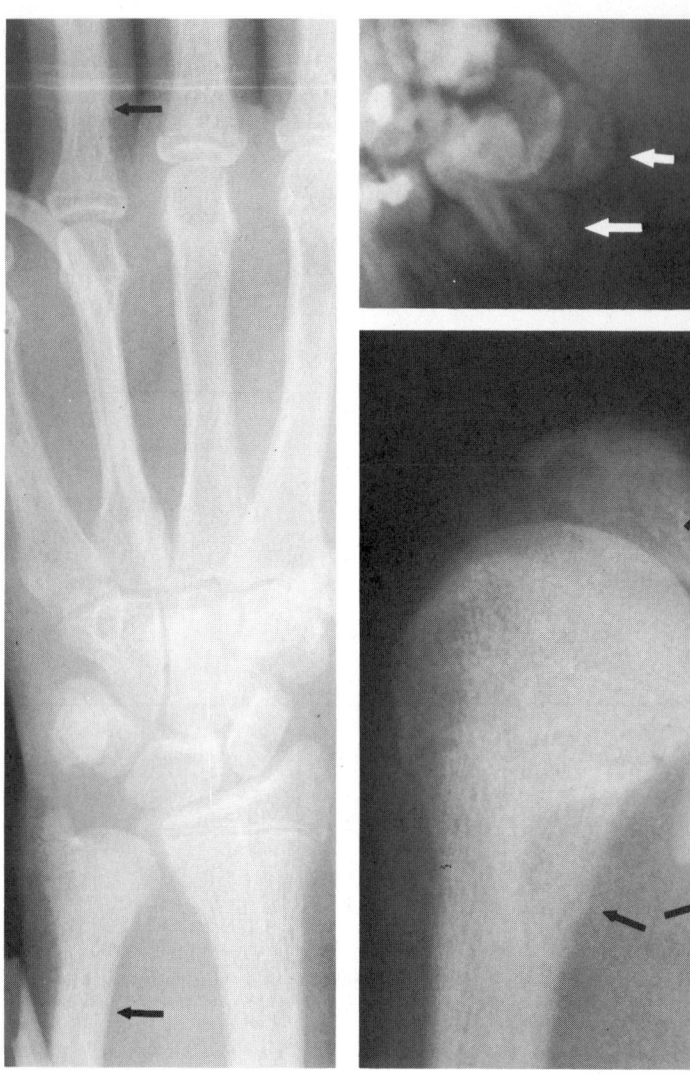

Figure 55–3. The skeleton of this teen-age girl with primary hyperparathyroidism demonstrates many sites of washed-out cortex *(black arrows),* coarse trabeculae, and lack of lamina dura *(white arrows)* around crypts of unerupted teeth and around roots of erupted teeth, all basic radiologic signs of this metabolic disease. (Courtesy of A. Oestreich, M.D., Cincinnati, OH.)

the general population, at least 75% of the cases of hypercalcemia are caused either by primary hyperparathyroidism or by malignancy.

Hyperparathyroidism

Primary hyperparathyroidism can be divided into several different types. The first of these is neonatal hyperparathyroidism, which usually presents within the first 3 months of life. These infants may present with severe hypercalcemia that manifests itself as muscular hypertonia, respiratory distress, and skeletal demineralization seen radiographically as osteopenia and severe subperiosteal resorption. Long-bone fractures secondary to osteopenia may be present and may be the presenting complaint. Rib fractures and marked dehydration may contribute to respiratory distress in these infants. This variant of primary hyperparathyroidism is associated with inheritance.

In the neonate, hyperparathyroidism appears to be exclusively caused by parathyroid hyperplasia. Approximately 80% of cases of childhood and adult primary hyperparathyroidism have a solitary parathyroid adenoma as the cause of the hypercalcemia. Parathyroid hyperplasia appears to be responsible for aproximately 10% to 15% of cases of primary hyperparathyroidism. Parathyroid carcinomas account for less than 1% of primary hyperparathyroidism and are extremely rare in children.

TABLE 55–6			
MEDICATIONS AND TREATMENTS USED IN THE ACUTE TREATMENT OF HYPERCALCEMIA			
Drug	**Dose**	**Route**	**Comments**
Normal saline (0.9% NaCl)	20 ml/kg 1 L/1.73 m²	IV over 1 hr	Usual adult dose is 1–2 L; may re-bolus at ½ initial trial if poor therapeutic response; this does not include maintenance fluids
Furosemide	1–2 mg/kg	IV every 2–4 hr	Volume repletion is mandatory before the use of loop diuretics; serum K⁺ and Mg²⁺ values must be closely followed
Dialysis		Peritoneal or hemodialysis	Especially useful if renal function is compromised

TABLE 55–7

SUBACUTE TREATMENT OF HYPERCALCEMIA

Drug	Dose	Route	Comments
Calcitonin	4 U/kg	IV	Acts in 6–12 hr; may repeat dose in 12 hr
Mithramycin	20–30 mg/kg	IV over 8 hr	Acts in 12–36 hr; may repeat in 2 days; hepatic, renal, and bone marrow toxicity
Prednisolone	1 mg/kg/day	IV over 3 days	Following a 3-day course, a tapering dose is recommended
Ethane hydroxydiphosphate	5–10 mg/kg/day	IV	

Hyperparathyroidism may also be inheritable. Inheritable causes include the multiple endocrine neoplasia (MEN) syndromes, which occur in up to 50% of adults who present with primary parathyroid hyperplasia. The inheritance of the MEN syndromes is autosomal dominant, but the inheritance of other familial hyperparathyroid disorders is unclear. MEN type I consists of primary parathyroid hyperplasia or adenoma associated with thyroid, pituitary, pancreatic, and adrenal neoplasms. In MEN type II, medullary carcinoma of the thyroid gland and pheochromocytoma are associated with primary hyperparathyroidism. Although the MEN syndromes are more common in adolescents and adults, all patients presenting with hyperparathyroidism must be evaluated to exclude the inheritable MEN disorders. Thus evaluation of the patient's relatives becomes a consideration in cases of hyperparathyroidism.

Therapeutic Information

The first step in management of the acute hypercalcemic crisis is rehydration, assuming at least 5% dehydration. Normal saline (0.9 NS) is the fluid of choice, and infusion restores the extracellular volume, promotes a natriuresis, and causes a calciuresis. Following volume loading, 0.45% NS may be used to promote diuresis. Replenishment of the extracellular volume is necessary for the effectiveness and safety of loop diuretic therapy. Administration of a loop diuretic such as furosemide promotes calciuria if the patient's fluid volume has been replenished. The thiazide diuretics have an anticalciuric affect and should be avoided. Monitoring the serum potassium and magnesium levels is necessary, as hypokalemia and hypomagnesemia are complications of loop diuretic therapy. Glucocorticoids decrease intestinal calcium absorption, bone remodeling, and renal tubular resorption of calcium. These effects are minimal in the short term. Therefore glucocorticoids are not useful in primary hyperparathyroidism but may be useful in lymphoma, multiple myeloma, or tumors metastatic to bone. Glucocorticoids are also helpful in countering hypercalcemia caused by vitamin D intoxication or exogenous vitamin D production, as in cases of sarcoidosis. Dialysis is useful in severe cases of hypercalcemia or when renal function is compromised. Unfortunately, there are no established guidelines as to when dialysis should be performed. Intravenous infusion of phosphate may be used for extreme cases but is fraught with the dangers of hyperphosphatemia and calcium precipitation in the soft tissues. Chelating agents such as ethylenediamine-tetra-acetate (EDTA) may also be used for extreme situations, but the therapeutic-toxic margin is small, and the calcium complexes formed must be excreted renally or removed by dialysis. The chelating agent itself may be toxic to the kidney, and its use should be avoided if there is a concurrent deterioration in renal function (Table 55–6).

Therapy for subacute or chronic hypercalcemia includes chemotherapy aimed at some of the metabolic pathways that produce hypercalcemia. Calcitonin is now available for such therapy (Table 55–7). Mithramycin lowers serum calcium by blocking osteoclast function, thereby decreasing the amount of calcium released from the bone reservoir. However, with prolonged treatment this drug is toxic to bone marrow, kidney, and liver. Mithramycin acts within 12 hours, and its effects last several days. Ethane hydroxydiphosphate (EHDP) is another osteoclast suppressor that is available in both oral and intravenous forms.

Definitive treatment of primary hyperparathyroidism is usually surgical. Medical management of this disorder is usually reserved for those patients who are poor surgical risks.

Referral of the asymptomatic child to a pediatric endocrinologist is mandatory. Investigation of other family members for some of the familial syndromes, including the MEN syndromes, is prudent. Symptomatic children with hypercalcemia should be admitted for treatment and evaluation (Table 55–8). Hypercalcemic children with no definite symptomatology but with significant radiographic findings should also be hospitalized.

RENAL OSTEODYSTROPHY

Chronic renal failure in children is associated with metabolic bone disease. This syndrome involves elements of osteomalacia and osteitis fibrosa in association with chronic

TABLE 55–8

ADMISSION CRITERIA FOR HYPERCALCEMIA

1. Any symptomatic patient:
    Psychiatric disturbances
    Disorientation
    Disturbances of memory
    Muscle weakness
    Depressed tendon reflexes
    Muscular irritability
    Grand mal seizures
    Renal colic
    Arthralgias
    Constipation
    Abdominal pain
    Nausea and vomiting
    Pruritus
    Vision loss
2. Any patient with physical signs:
    Hypertension
    Keratopathy
3. Suspected hyperparathyroidism or malignancy
4. Significant laboratory abnormalities:
    Renal failure
    Electrocardiographic abnormalities
    Abnormal radiographic findings
5. Asymptomatic patient with a poor social situation or poor follow-up

renal failure. Although hemodialysis and chronic ambulatory peritoneal dialysis are both effective in managing renal failure, neither has any substantial advantage in controlling the metabolic bone disease of renal failure. Treatment of the bone disease may include dietary phosphate restriction and calcium carbonate supplements. Calcium carbonate supplements are useful to reduce excess phosphate intake and supply extra calcium. Replacement therapy with vitamin D or vitamin D metabolites also helps promote growth.

Renal osteodystrophy, like osteogenesis imperfecta, presents with multiple fractures caused by poor bone mineralization.

Selected References

Allen DB, Friedman AL, Hendricks SA. Asymptomatic primary hyperparathyroidism in children. Am J Dis Child 1986;140:819.

Allo M, Thompson NW, Harness JK, et al. Primary hyperparathyroidism in children, adolescents, and young adults. World J Surg 1982;6:771.

Alon U, Chan JCM. Hypocalcemia from deficiency of and resistance to parathyroid hormone. Adv Pediatr 1985;32:439.

Anast CS, Winnacker JL, Forte LR, et al. Impaired release of parathyroid hormone in magnesium deficiency. J Clin Endocrinol Metab 1976;42:707.

Avioli LV. The therapeutic approach to hypoparathyroidism. Am J Med 1974;57:34.

Cardenas-Rivero N, Chernow B, Stoiko MA, et al. Hypocalcemia in critically ill children. J Pediatr 1989;114:946.

Cervera A, Corral MJ, Gomez-Campdera FJ, et al. Idiopathic hypercalcuria in children. Acta Paediatr Scand 1987;76:271.

Cogan MG, Covey CM, Arieff AI, et al. Central nervous system manifestations of hyperparathyroidism. Am J Med 1978;65:963.

Dent DM, Miller JL, Klaff L, et al. The incidence and cause of hypercalcemia. Postgrad Med J 1987;63:745.

Fuhrman BP. Hypocalcemia in critical illness in children. J Pediatr 1989;114:990.

Grantmyre EB. Roentgenographic features of primary hyperparathyroidism in infancy. J Can Assoc Radiol 1973;24:257.

Harris SS, D'Ercole AJ. Neonatal hyperparathyroidism: The natural course in the absence of surgical intervention. Pediatrics 1989;83:53.

Hauser GJ, Gale AD, Fields AI. Immobilization hypercalcemia: Unusual presentation with seizures. Pediatr Emerg Care 1989;5:105.

Haussler MR, McCain TA. Basic and clinical concepts related to vitamin D metabolism and action. N Engl J Med 1977;297:974.

Kainer G, Chan JCM. Hypocalcemic and hypercalcemic disorders in children. Curr Probl Pediatr 1989;19:493.

Malek RS, Kelalis PP. Urologic manifestations of hyperparathyroidism in childhood. J Urol 1976;115:717.

Mannix H Jr. Primary hyperparathyroidism in children. Am J Surg 1975;129:528.

Mohanlal D, Pettifor JM, Moodley GP. Serum calcium and phosphate disturbances during rehydration in acute dehydrating gastoenteritis. J Pediatr Gastroenterol Nutr 1987;6:252.

Murtaza A, Khan SR, Butt KS, et al. Hypocalcemia and hyperphosphatemia in severely dehydrated children with and without convulsions. Acta Paediatr Scand 1988;77:251.

Norman ME, Mazur AT, Borden S, et al. Early diagnosis of juvenile renal osteodystrophy. J Pediatr 1980;97:226.

Olinger ML. Disorders of calcium and magnesium metabolism. Emerg Med Clin North Am 1989;764:795.

Patterson KL, Klopovich P. Metabolic emergencies in pediatric oncology: The acute tumor lysis syndrome. JAPON 1986;4:19.

Rapaport D, Ziv Y, Rubin M, et al. Primary hyperparathyroidism in children. J Pediatr Surg 1986;21:395.

Ross AJ, Cooper A, Attie MF, et al. Primary hyperparathyroidism in infancy. J Pediatr Surg 1986;21:493.

Rude RK, Oldham SB, Singer FR. Functional hypoparathyroidism and parathyroid hormone end-organ resistance in human magnesium deficiency. Clin Endocrinol 1976;5:209.

Sanchez GJ, Venkataraman PS, Pryor RW, et al. Hypercalcitoninemia and hypocalcemia in acutely ill children: Studies in serum calcium, blood ionized calcium, and calcium-regulating hormones. J Pediatr 1989;114:952.

Scholz DA, Purnell DC. Asymptomatic primary hyperparathyroidism: 10 year prospective study. Mayo Clin Proc 1981;56:473.

Sivula A, Ronni-Sivula H. Natural history of treated primary hyperparathyroidism. Surg Clin North Am 1987;67:329.

Specker BL, Tsang RC. Vitamin D in infancy and childhood: Factors determining vitamin D status. Adv Pediatr 1986;33:1.

Thomsen RJ. Subcutaneous fat necrosis of the newborn and idiopathic hypercalcemia. Arch Dermatol 1980;116:1155.

Troughton O, Singh SP. Heart failure and neonatal hypocalcemia. Br Med J 1972;4:76.

Wolfson BJ, Capitanio MA. The wide spectrum of renal osteodystrophy in children. CRC Crit Rev Diagn Imag 1987;27:297.

CHAPTER 56

Adrenal Disorders

David A. Poleski

INTRODUCTION

Adrenal crisis occurs when there is a failure of cortisol and aldosterone production by the adrenal cortex. Adrenal insufficiency is a relative lack of cortisol or aldosterone and is the more common condition encountered in pediatric emergentology.

ANATOMY AND PHYSIOLOGY

The management of adrenal disorders in the emergency department requires a basic understanding of adrenal steroidogenesis. The adrenal cortex secretes mineralocorticoids, glucocorticoids, and androgens (Fig. 56–1). Disease of the adrenal cortex results in varying degrees of reduced production of mineralocorticoids, glucocorticoids, and androgens. With certain enzyme deficiencies, such as 21-OH deficiency, there is an overproduction of androgens because of the shunting of precursors into the androgen pathway, which can result in a virilizing syndrome.

Few disorders of the adrenal medulla are likely to be diagnosed in the emergency department. Most are tumors such as neuroblastomas, ganglioneuromas, ganglioneuroblastomas, and pheochromocytomas (Fig. 56–2). These disorders are rare.

CLINICAL EVALUATION

The signs and symptoms of adrenal disease in children are related to the relative lack or overproduction of adrenal hormones. Cortical over- or underproduction of androgens, mineralocorticoids, or glucocorticoids and medullary overproduction of catecholamines result in recognizable symptoms suggestive of adrenal disease.

There are many causes of adrenal insufficiency. In children the important causes include genetic enzyme defects, particularly 21-OH deficiency, discontinuation of long-term adrenal suppressive doses of steroids, and adrenal hemorrhage and destruction resulting from overwhelming sepsis as occurs with the Waterhouse-Friderichsen syndrome. Other causes of adrenal disease are rare and are unlikely to be seen in the emergency department.

Signs of adrenal insufficiency are fever, nausea, vomiting, altered mental status, hypotension, shock, hyponatremia, hyperkalemia, and hypoglycemia (Table 56–1). Other entities, particularly sepsis, can mimic adrenal crisis. When the diagnosis is in doubt, the patient should be treated for adrenal crisis and the exact diagnosis determined later.

Certain factors are important in determining whether the previously mentioned signs and symptoms are caused by an adrenal abnormality. A history of chronic steroid use or of identified adrenal disease (e.g., Addison's disease or a congenital enzyme defect) should be sought. The clinical findings of ambiguous genitalia (Fig. 56–3), increased pigmentation, and emaciation are suggestive of underlying adrenal disease, as are the physical findings of Cushing's syndrome (truncal obesity, buffalo hump, plethora, purplish atrophic striae, short stature, hypertension). In Cushing's syndrome,

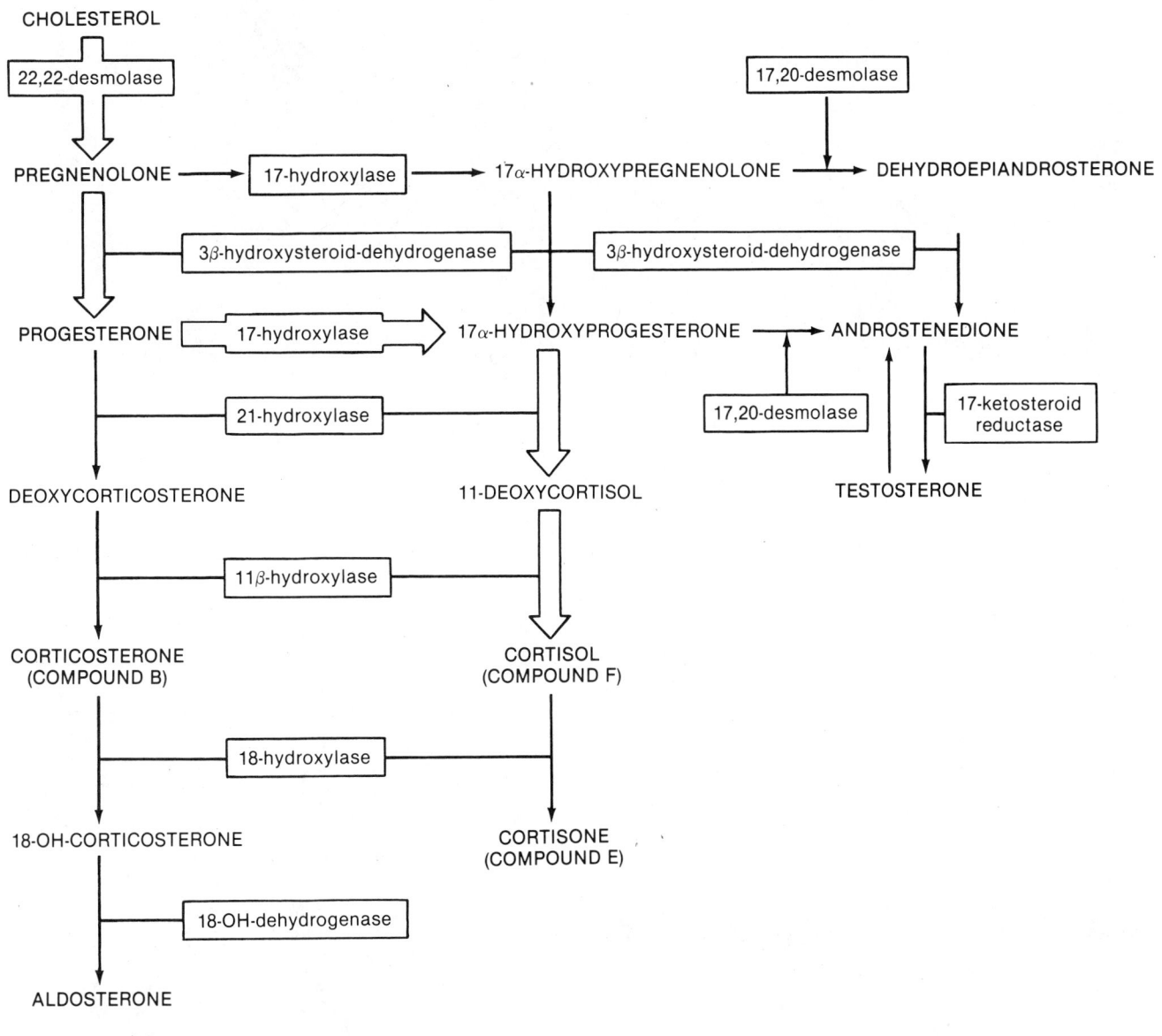

SYNTHESIS OF ADRENAL STEROIDS

Figure 56–1. Schematic representation of adrenal steroid production.

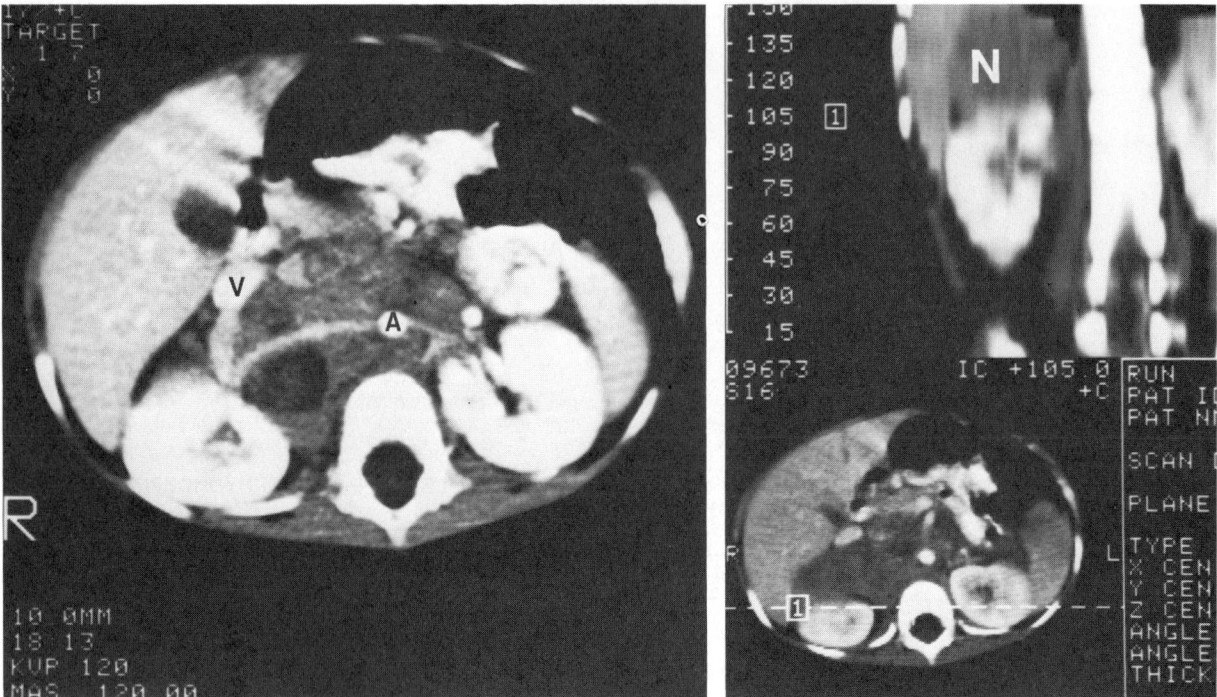

Figure 56–2. A large abdominal mass (neuroblastoma) in this 4-year-old girl is depicted on axial CT and coronal reconstruction (where the tumor, N, is shown above the contrast-enhanced right kidney). The engulfment and displacement of vessels such as the inferior vena cava (V), aorta (A), and renal arteries stretching to either side of the aorta are clearly shown. (Courtesy of A. Oestreich, M.D., Cincinnati, OH.)

adrenal hormones are produced in excess, usually because a pituitary adenoma is present. Adrenal insufficiency is seldom a problem in Cushing's syndrome unless the exogenous administration of steroids is abruptly halted.

Medullary overproduction of catecholamines can occur as a result of adrenal tumors. Excessive diaphoresis, hypertension, flushing, thirst, and polyuria should alert the clinician to the possibility of an adrenal neuroblastoma, ganglioneuroma, ganglioneuroblastoma, or pheochromocytoma, particularly if an abdominal mass is palpable. Nonspecific findings such as fever, weight loss, anorexia, and anemia may be present in advanced disease. Some adrenal tumors that secrete vasoactive intestinal peptides may cause chronic watery diarrhea and hypokalemia. Although adrenal tumors are rare, the hypertension caused by excessive catecholamine production requires blood pressure determination in all children seen in the emergency department.

TABLE 56–1
CLINICAL EVALUATION FOR ADRENAL DISEASE

History	Physical Findings
Fever	Hypotension
Nausea/vomiting	Cachexia
Lethargy	Hyperpigmentation
Diarrhea	Altered mental status
Polydipsia	Ambiguous genitalia
Polyuria	
Weakness	
Anorexia	
Adrenal surgery	
Radiation therapy	
History of cancer	
Family history of congenital adrenal disease	
Chronic steroid use	
Diaphoresis	
Flushing	

DIAGNOSTIC EVALUATION

Important studies in managing suspected adrenal insufficiency include determination of electrolyte and glucose levels. Other studies that assist in management are a complete

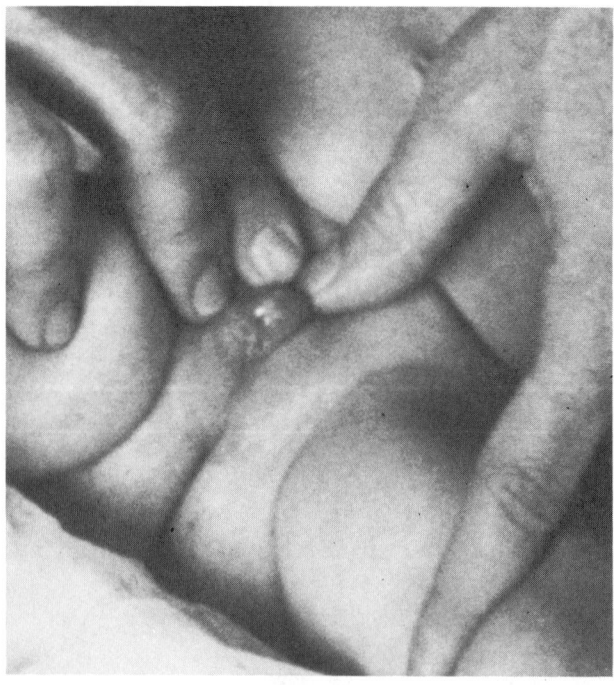

Figure 56–3. Virilized infant with 21-OH deficiency. Note the hypertrophied clitoris and fused labia. On further evaluation this child was noted to have a uterus (rectal examination) and ovaries and was a genetic female.

blood cell (CBC) count and blood urea nitrogen (BUN), creatinine, and arterial blood gas determinations. The white blood cell (WBC) count may help determine whether the cause of adrenal insufficiency is overwhelming sepsis; if this is suspected, blood cultures should be obtained and antibiotic therapy started. BUN, creatinine, and arterial pH determinations can help ascertain the degree of volume loss and serve as guidelines during fluid replacement and acidosis management. Radiographs are of little help in the emergency department setting.

THERAPEUTIC INTERVENTION

The treatment of acute adrenal insufficiency addresses the problems of volume depletion, acidosis, hyponatremia, hyperkalemia, hypoglycemia, and deficiency of glucocorticoids and mineralocorticoids (Table 56–2). Initial fluid replacement should be with 0.9% normal saline (NS) or lactated Ringer's (LR) solution in 20-ml/kg boluses until the shock is corrected. To correct hypoglycemia, 25% glucose can be given in an initial dose of 1.0 ml/kg. Once hypoglycemia is corrected, maintenance infusions of D5W with 0.9% NS should be started, with adjustments in the amount of sodium and glucose based on frequent glucose and electrolyte determinations. Potassium should not be given initially. As volume is replaced and the acidosis corrected, the potassium level should decrease. Volume alone should correct acidosis; sodium bicarbonate is generally not needed. Maintenance potassium should be added to the intravenous fluid when the potassium level has fallen to normal limits. Hyperkalemia rarely needs to be treated as a primary problem in adrenal crisis unless cardiac arrhythmias are noted.

Replacement of glucocorticoids and mineralocorticoids is a mainstay of treatment in adrenal crisis, although correction of shock is the first priority. Ideally, glucocorticoids should be administered simultaneously with volume replacement. Mineralocorticoid administration can be delayed and is not an immediate need. Initial glucocorticoid replacement with hydrocortisone (50 mg IV) should be administered as soon as adrenal crisis in a child is suspected, followed by a 50–mg/m²/24-hour continuous infusion. Deoxycorticosterone acetate (DOCA), 1 to 2 mg IM, is used to provide mineralocorticoid replacement. Extra blood should be obtained and stored prior to administering this therapy in order to do the cortisol and adrenal enzyme assays necessary to accurately diagnose the etiology of the adrenal insufficiency.

TABLE 56–2

ADRENAL CRISIS: THERAPY AT A GLANCE

Fluid replacement
  Initial bolus, 20 ml/kg of 0.9% NS or Ringer's lactate; repeat 20-ml/kg boluses until shock state is corrected. D5 NS should be started for maintenance once shock is corrected.
Hypoglycemia
  25% glucose, 1 ml/kg initially and repeat as necessary depending on blood glucose levels.
Mineralocorticoid replacement
  Deoxycorticosterone acetate (DOCA), 1–2 mg IM.
Glucocorticoid replacement
  Hydrocortisone, 50 mg IV followed by a maintenance infusion of 50 mg/m²/24 hr.
Antibiotics (if sepsis suspected)
  Ceftriaxone, 100 mg/kg/day divided into two doses if child is older than 2 mo.
  Ampicillin, 200 mg/kg divided into six doses, and gentamicin, 5 mg/kg divided into two doses, if child is younger than 2 mo.

TABLE 56–3

DISCHARGE INSTRUCTIONS FOR PATIENTS WITH ADRENAL DISORDERS

1. Any child with known adrenal disease who has been seen for another problem such as otitis, pharyngitis, or upper respiratory tract infection should be instructed to double all maintenance steroids.
2. Patient should follow up with regular doctor as soon as possible.
3. Patient should return immediately if symptoms worsen prior to follow-up.

Finally, whenever sepsis or any infection is suspected as the stress precipitating acute adrenal insufficiency, antibiotics should be administered and the appropriate cultures obtained. Ceftriaxone, 100 mg/kg/day divided into two doses with an initial dose of 50 mg/kg, provides adequate coverage for *Haemophilus influenzae*, *Streptococcus pneumoniae* and *Neisseria meningitidis* for children over 2 months of age. Ampicillin, 200 mg/kg/day divided into 4-hour doses, and gentamicin, 5 mg/kg/day divided into 12-hour doses, can be used for children under 2 months of age. Empiric treatment of septic shock with glucocorticoids is not recommended unless adrenal insufficiency is suspected or the patient is known to be on chronic or tapering doses of steroids.

DISPOSITION

Any child who presents to the emergency department with acute adrenal insufficiency should be admitted to the hospital. Children with suspected adrenal tumors (i.e., with symptoms of abdominal mass, weight loss, anorexia, hypertension, etc.) should also be admitted for further diagnostic studies. Attempting to make a definitive diagnosis in the emergency department is not appropriate. If a child with known adrenal disease is seen for another problem (e.g., otitis media, pharyngitis, or upper respiratory tract infection), instructions on discharge should include doubling of all maintenance steroids that the patient may be taking in order to prevent stress-precipitated adrenal insufficiency.

If discharged from the emergency department, patients with known adrenal disease should always be instructed to follow up with the physician who monitors them for their adrenal-related problems as soon as possible (Table 56–3). Emergency department physicians should not manipulate doses of maintenance steroids without close consultation with a pediatric endocrinologist.

OTHER CONSIDERATIONS

Although this is unlikely, emergency physicians may be the first to diagnose ambiguous genitalia in a neonate with a virilizing form of congenital adrenal hyperplasia (most commonly caused by a 21-hydroxylase deficiency (Fig. 56–3). An important facet of treatment for this disorder is sex assignment. Immediate problems such as a salt-losing crisis should be treated in the emergency department, but sex assignment should never be done in the emergency setting.

If a patient has adrenal disease or is at risk for adrenal insufficiency (e.g., a chronic steroid user) but does not have a medical information bracelet, one should be recommended.

Extra tubes of blood must always be obtained when adrenal disease is suspected, so that various tests (i.e., cortisol levels, 17-OH progesterone levels, and other enzyme assays) can be obtained after the immediate crisis has been treated.

Selected References

Addison T. Disease of the Supra-Renal Capsules. London, Samuel Highley, 1855.

Bravo E, Gifford R. Pheochromocytoma: Diagnosis, localization and management. N Engl J Med 1984;311:1298.

Cacciari E, Balsamo A, Cassio A, et al. Neonatal screening for congenital adrenal hyperplasia. Arch Dis Child 1983;58:803.

Drucker S, New M. Disorders of adrenal steroidogenesis. Pediatr Clin North Am 1987;34:1053.

Hochberg Z, Benderly A, Zadik Z. Salt loss in congenital adrenal hyperplasia due to 11-β-hydroxylase deficiency. Arch Dis Child 1984;59:1092.

Leshin M. Acute adrenal insufficiency: Recognition, management and prevention. Urol Clin North Am 1982;9:229.

Migeon C. Diagnosis and management of congenital adrenal hyperplasia. Hosp Pract 1977;12:75.

Winter J. Current approaches to the treatment of congenital adrenal hyperplasia. J Pediatr 1980;97:81.

Winterer J, Chrousos G, Loriaux D, et al. Effect of hydrocortisone dose schedule on adrenal steroid secretion in congenital adrenal hyperplasia. J Pediatr 1985;106:137.

SECTION EIGHT

Hematology and Oncology

CHAPTER 57

Blood Products and Transfusion

M. Lois Hall
Elizabeth H. Perry

CROSSMATCHING AND ORDERING BLOOD PRODUCTS

Pediatric emergency physicians may require the use of blood products in three settings: to reestablish circulating cardiovascular volume, to increase oxygen delivery to the tissues during resuscitation of patients in shock, and to improve hemostasis in patients with coagulopathies.

ABO red blood cell antigens and antibodies are the most important antigens and antibodies in blood transfusion; immediate intravascular hemolysis occurs when incompatible red blood cells are transfused. *Blood type* refers to the presence or absence of antigens A and B on an individual's red blood cells. Naturally occurring immunoglobulin M (IgM) antibodies are found in the serum of normal individuals whose red cells lack one or both of these antigens. Crossmatch procedures assess the agglutination reaction between antibodies and antigens when the red cells and serum of donors and recipients are mixed. If a patient is transfused with ABO-incompatible red blood cells, then a hemolytic reaction occurs as a result of activation of the complement system by IgM antibodies.

An individual's red cells may have A and B antigens (type AB), A antigen only (type A), B antigen only (type B), or no A or B antigens (type O) (Table 57–1). Donor reagent sera may give weaker reactions with red cells from neonates, because antigens are not fully developed at birth. Red cell antigens are fully developed by 2 to 4 years of age.

There are some subgroups of the A and B antigens that only rarely cause clinically significant crossmatch incompatibilities (e.g., the A_2 antigen). The "Bombay," or O_h, phenotype is a rare blood group without A and B antigens.[1, 2] Bombay serum agglutinates A and B red cells and also reacts strongly with group O red cells. A person known to have the Bombay phenotype should be completely crossmatched and transfused only with O_h blood.

After determining the ABO blood type, the next most important transfusion issue is the Rh (or D antigen) status. The terms *Rh-positive* (D+) and *Rh-negative* (D−) refer to the presence or absence of D antigen on red cells. Individuals without D antigen do not have anti-D antibodies in their serum unless previously exposed to red cells with D antigen. Formation of anti-D antibodies occurs 50% to 100% of the time after transfusion of a single unit of Rh-positive cells to an Rh-negative recipient.[3, 4] Rh-incompatible transfusions occurring after this initial transfusion may result in a delayed hemolytic transfusion reaction as a result of anti-D immunoglobulin G (IgG) antibodies (see "Transfusion Reactions"). Rh-negative females of childbearing age are at risk for pregnancies complicated by erythroblastosis fetalis if they have developed anti-D antibodies from prior transfusions or have had a prior pregnancy with an Rh+ fetus, which results in formation of anti-D antibodies 8% of the time.[5] Because D antigens are immunogenic, all donors and recipients are tested for the presence or absence of D antigen, and Rh+ cells should not be transfused into Rh− individuals. If a transfusion is urgently required in an Rh-negative patient and ABO-compatible, Rh-negative blood is unavailable, the use of Rh-positive blood products may be the only alternative. Rh immune globulin (RhIG) may be given to these patients to prevent the formation of anti-D antibodies after transfusions of blood components containing small amounts of red blood cells (RBCs) such as platelets or granulocytes. In massive transfusions of packed RBCs, RhIG is not practical, because so much is required (20 µg/ml of RBCs) that hemolysis of the transfused cells results in symptoms such as hemoglobinuria. Hemolytic disease of the newborn (erythroblastosis fetalis) remains the most clinically significant complication of Rh incompatibility, but the incidence has been greatly reduced by the use of antenatal and postnatal RhIG.

The goal of pretransfusion compatibility testing is to

TABLE 57–1			
ABO BLOOD GROUP SYSTEM			
ABO Group	**Red Cell Antigens**	**Naturally Occurring Antibodies In Plasma**	**Compatible Red Cells**
A	A	Anti-B	A,O
B	B	Anti-A	B,O
AB	AB	None	AB,O
O	None	Anti-A	A,B
		Anti-B	O

TABLE 57–2

RED BLOOD CELL COMPATIBILITY TESTING

	Indication	Advantage	Disadvantage
Nonemergent transfusion			
Type and Screen (T&S) (ABO and Rh of patient typed and serum screened against two red cells to detect clinically significant antibodies)	Red cell use possible	Blood not reserved unnecessarily	T&S takes 45–60 min
		Better use of personnel and resources	Time needed to select and crossmatch unit (approximately 10 min if negative antibody screen)
		Safety with uncrossmatched blood if patient's antibody screen is negative	
Type and crossmatch	Red cell use expected	Current standard of care for safe transfusion with optimal therapeutic effect	Red cells reserved from inventory; takes 60–90 min
Emergent transfusion			
Type specific, uncrossmatched	Red cells needed urgently	Patient receives ABO group–compatible red cells	Possible antibody in recipient (rare unless previously transfused or pregnant); takes 10–20 min
		Can use ABO group–specific whole blood	Typing error under pressure
Type unknown, uncrossmatched	Red cells needed desperately	O red cells rapidly available	Must use group O red cells (Rh-negative preferred); do not use group O whole blood
		Potentially lifesaving	Possible antibody in recipient (rare unless previously transfused or pregnant)

MAJOR CROSSMATCH

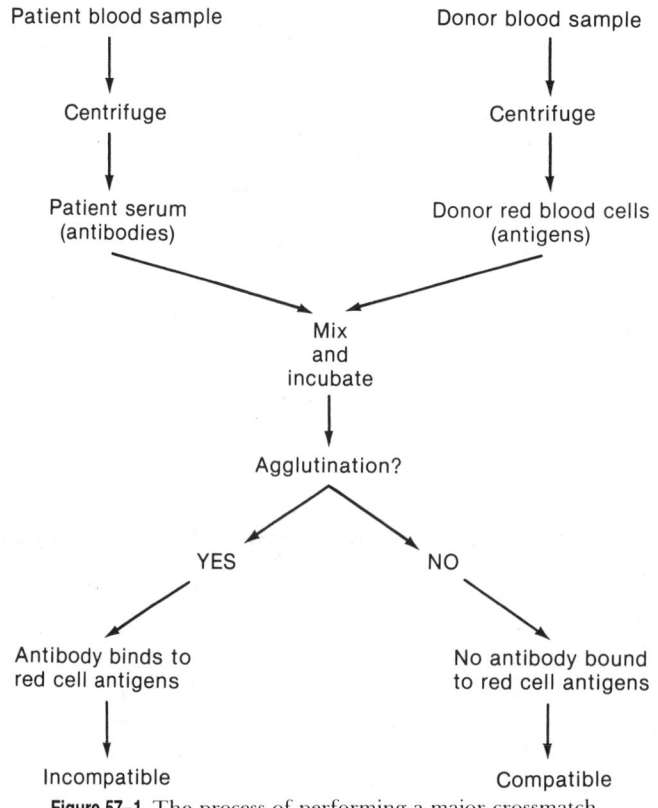

Figure 57–1. The process of performing a major crossmatch.

crossmatch donors and recipients so that transfused blood products have an acceptable survival time in the recipient and do not cause clinically significant destruction of the host's own red cells.[6] The completeness of the crossmatching process in the emergency setting is primarily time dependent (Table 57–2). The procedure to completely type and crossmatch red blood cells requires 60 to 90 minutes in the absence of complicated serologic problems. The recipient's cells are typed for ABO and Rh, and then the serum is screened for unexpected antibodies. Next, the donor cells are mixed with the recipient's serum to identify any major crossmatch incompatibility (Fig. 57–1). If the patient is stable enough to tolerate a 60- to 90-minute delay in transfusion, this is certainly the most desired approach. When a unit of blood is crossmatched for a patient, that unit is labeled and may not be used by another patient. Unfortunately, the ratio of crossmatched to transfused blood is approximately 2:1 to 3:1. If the patient is stable and the need for a blood product is possible but not absolutely determined, then a type and screen may be performed instead of a complete crossmatch.[7] With a type and screen, the recipient's cells are typed for ABO and Rh, and the serum is analyzed for unexpected antibodies, but there is no formal crossmatch with a specific donor unit until requested. The antibody screen is capable of detecting 99% of all blood incompatibilities in patients not previously transfused.

If a patient requires a blood product sooner than type, screen, and crossmatch allow, ABO-compatible (type-specific) blood can be available within 10 to 20 minutes. The recipient's blood is typed and ABO type-specific blood is released. A complete antibody screen and crossmatch are performed by the blood bank as soon as possible. Future crossmatches are not complicated by the administration of type-specific blood, and only one fatal reaction has been reported in the literature in reviews of more than 30 million transfusions of ABO-compatible blood. Uncrossmatched blood products are required when any transfusion delay cannot be tolerated by the patient.[8, 9] Type O is the so-called *universal donor*, because there are no blood group antigens for A and B. Type O packed RBCs should, therefore, be well tolerated by recipients of any blood type. Because type O, Rh-negative blood occurs in only 6% of the population, some blood banks may not store more than a few units. Blood samples must be obtained prior to all uncrossmatched transfusions so that crossmatching for specific units can proceed as soon as possible. Type O, Rh-positive blood is common (occurring in 37% of the population) and can be used quite safely in male patients with no transfusion history. Problems possibly encountered with transfusion of uncrossmatched blood include complications with future crossmatches and the possibility of transfusing incompatible blood as a result of the presence of a clinically significant, non-ABO antibody. These non-ABO antibodies occur with a rate of 0.04% in persons with no history of transfusion or pregnancy and a rate of 0.3% in previously transfused persons or multiparous women. Non-ABO antibody reactions are seldom life threatening.

BLOOD COMPONENTS
Transfusion Therapy

Blood components available for use in the emergency setting[10–13] are derived from the centrifugation and separation of whole blood. These products may be grouped according to the role they play in expanding circulating volume, increasing oxygen carrying capacity, or improving hemostasis (Fig. 57–2).

The use of component therapy instead of whole blood has several advantages. In fact, in some hospitals whole blood is not kept in inventory, whereas blood components are readily available. With component therapy, patients receive only the blood product needed for their particular clinical problem. Components are usually relatively concentrated and have greater biologic activity so that excess transfusion volume can be minimized. In massive transfusions, fresh frozen plasma and platelet concentrates can deliver labile clotting factors and viable platelets not adequately supplied by whole blood alone.

Shock is defined as a "generalized state of inadequate tissue perfusion, which results in impaired respiration at the cellular level".[14, 15] While the clinical causes of poor circulation (C) are being corrected, the effective blood volume may be augmented by the infusion of isotonic crystalloid fluids, keeping in mind that only one third of the infused volume stays in the vascular space. These infusions are given in boluses of 10 to 20 ml per kilogram body weight with ongoing clinical assessment.[16] Once a patient requires an excess of 40 to 50 ml per kilogram body weight of crystalloid to maintain adequate capillary perfusion and vital signs, transfusion with colloids or blood products should be considered.[17]

In cardiogenic, obstructive, or distributive shock that responds poorly to initial crystalloid infusion, the use of 5% albumin or plasma protein fraction (Plasmanate) for volume expansion is helpful, as the colloidal properties of these components allow them to remain almost entirely in the vascular space (Table 57–3). RBCs should not be used for volume expansion but should be considered in patients experiencing acute onset of decreased oxygen-carrying capacity (uncompensated anemia with hemoglobin < 8 gm/dl), as may occur in sepsis.

Hypovolemic shock in the pediatric trauma patient may be classified by degree of blood loss.[18] Classes I and II are usually manageable with isotonic crystalloid infusions. Class III hemorrhage requires the additional transfusion of volume expanders such as albumin or Plasmanate. Patients in severe class III or class IV hemorrhage need crystalloid infusions as well as colloidal volume expansion and transfusion of RBCs to restore adequate oxygen-carrying capacity. If whole blood is used, it should be given in a volume equivalent to the estimated blood loss. The indications for transfusion and the special features of particular products used to reestablish circulating volume are all to be considered when attempting to restore the circulating volume.[19, 20] The blood components are used to increase oxygen-carrying capacity (Table 57–4).[21, 22] In massive transfusions (classes III and IV hemorrhage) it is important to follow coagulation studies and platelet counts. Fresh frozen plasma and platelet concentrates may be required to stop bleeding caused by deficiencies of labile clotting factors (Factors V and VIII) and decreased numbers of viable platelets not supplied by whole blood or other components.[23]

Many chronically ill patients are in a compensated state of cardiac or respiratory insufficiency or have physiologically adapted to long-standing degrees of anemia. In these situations, the decision to transfuse blood products must be made judiciously, and infusions must proceed very slowly, accompanied by close monitoring of the patient's clinical status.

Problems with hemostasis may result from hereditary or acquired coagulopathies. Blood components are also used to improve hemostasis (Table 57–5).[24–30]

Artificial Blood Substitutes

Blood substitutes are potentially useful in patients with acute trauma or hemorrhage who need greater oxygen-carrying capacity when blood is not readily available; for

BLOOD COMPONENTS

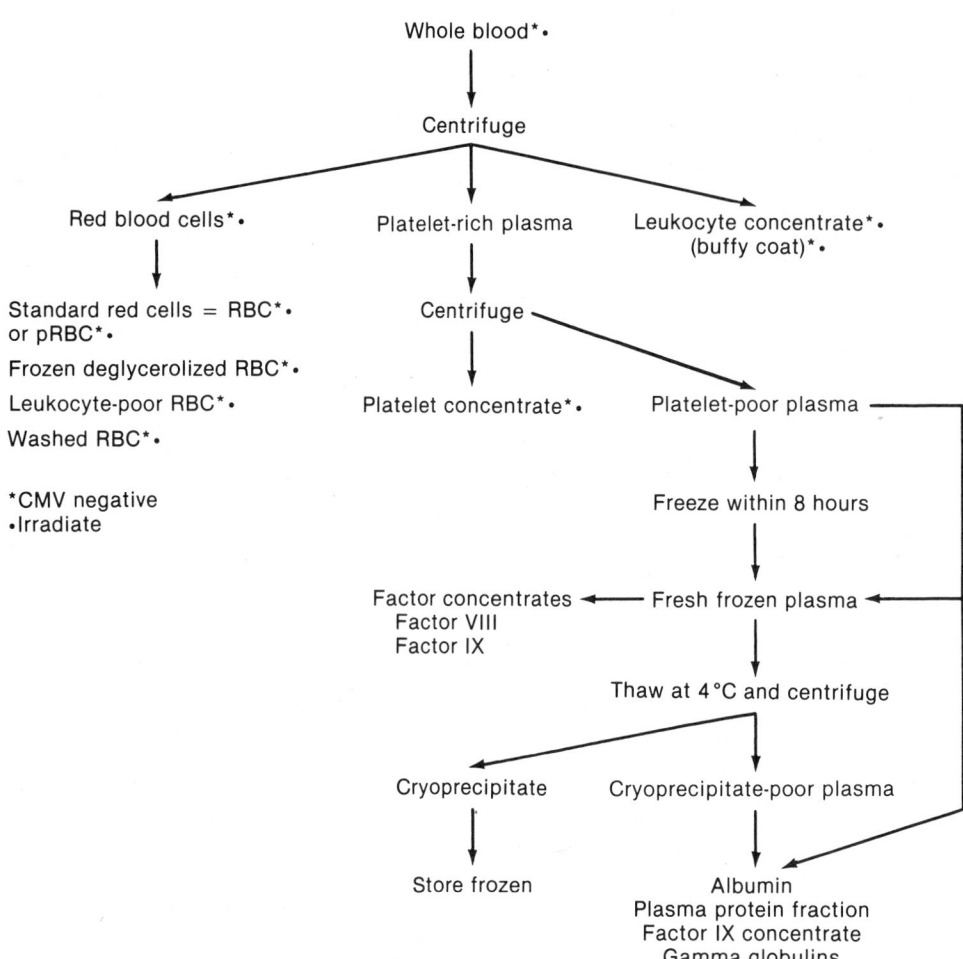

Figure 57–2. The derivation of various blood products.

patients refusing blood transfusion on religious grounds; and for patients who are difficult to crossmatch because of rare blood type, multiple alloantibodies, or autoantibodies. However, despite research for more than 50 years, blood substitutes are currently unavailable for clinical use.[31]

Fluosol-DA 20% is a hydroxyethyl starch that can be used for volume expansion as well as improving oxygen-carrying capacity. However, the solution has limited oxygen-carrying capacity, a short half-life of 24 hours, and severe cardiopulmonary side effects; is unstable at room temperature, requiring frozen storage; and has the potential to cause oxygen toxicity, as therapy with Fluosol-DA requires concurrent administration of 60% to 100% oxygen in order to release oxygen to the tissues.[32] Licensure was denied by the Food and Drug Administration in 1983.

Hemoglobin solutions show potential as blood substitutes.[33, 34] The early hemoglobin solutions had a high affinity for oxygen but were excreted rapidly and caused renal failure with repeated infusions. Renal toxicity was caused by red cell stroma. As a result, efforts have been directed toward developing stroma-free hemoglobin solutions. However, these products are not avaialble for clinical trials in humans.

Salvaged Autologous Blood

Intraoperative blood salvage has reduced the use of banked blood by 50% to 90%.[35] Several centers have used salvaged autologous blood in trauma patients, with generally favorable results.[36, 37] However, blood salvage in the emergency situation poses unique problems in (1) predicting which patients will benefit from the procedure, (2) collecting blood efficiently without contamination, and (3) scheduling the service to be available when needed. The main contraindication to salvage of shed blood is contamination with either bacteria or malignant tumor cells.

Granulocytes

Ordering transfusions of granulocytes is not often the responsibility of the emergency department physician. Granulocyte transfusions may be indicated for neonates with bacterial sepsis; patients with infections and documented functional defects of granulocytes, as in chronic granulomatous disease; and neutropenic patients ($<0.5 \times 10^9$ granulocytes/L) with fevers and suspected or documented sepsis who have not responded to appropriate antibiotic therapy.[38]

Gamma Globulin Preparations

Gamma globulin therapy is the replacement of antibody with pooled human immunoglobulin.[39] The gamma globulin preparation known as immune globulin (IG) is prepared by cold ethanol fractionation of large pools of human blood donor plasma. This preparation is available for intramuscular use only and does not transmit infectious diseases. Side

TABLE 57–3

BLOOD COMPONENTS AND SYNTHETIC COLLOIDS USED TO REESTABLISH CIRCULATING VOLUME

Colloid	Description	Volume/Dose	Indications	Crossmatch?	Adverse Effects	Special Features
Albumin 5%, 25%	96% albumin, 4% globulin 5% iso-oncotic and iso-osmotic with plasma 25% is hyperoncotic Cold alcohol fractionation, heated 10 hr at 60°C to inactivate HBV and HIV 25% usually diluted to 5% prior to infusion	250-, 500-ml bottles	For albumin and PPF: Shock Burns Adult respiratory distress syndrome Ascites Peritonitis Hemodialysis-associated hypotension Plasma exchange replacement Nephrotic syndrome	No	For albumin and PPF: Rare: Volume overload Bacterial contamination Febrile reactions Urticaria Headache Decreased synthesis of globulins with massive doses of albumin	For albumin and PPF: Stable storage No blood group antibodies No fibrinogen No filter needed No disease transmission
Plasma protein fraction (PPF) (Plasmanate) 5%	83% albumin and 17% globulins Cold alcohol fractionation, heated 10 hr at 60°C to inactivate HBV and HIV			No	Hypotensive episodes with rapid infusion of PPF, because of prekallekrein activator	For PPF: Contraindicated during cardiopulmonary bypass
Hetastarch 6%	Made from waxy starch composed of amylopectin		Volume expansion Leukapheresis	No	Pruritus Long PT, PTT Short TT	For dextran and hetastarch:
Dextran 40 (low molecular weight) Dextran 70 (high molecular weight)	Branched chain polysaccharide composed of glucose units		Volume expansion Used to prevent thrombosis	No	Anaphylactic reactions Bleeding Short TT Renal failure	Stable storage No compatibility testing No disease transmission No blood filter

HBV = Hepatitis B virus; HIV = human immunodeficiency virus; PT = prothrombin time; PTT = partial thromboplastin time; TT = thrombin time.

TABLE 57–4

BLOOD COMPONENTS USED TO IMPROVE OXYGEN-CARRYING CAPACITY

Component	Description	Volume/Dose	Indications	Crossmatch?	Adverse Effects	Special Features
Red blood cells packed in CPD or CPDA-1 (RBC)	Whole blood unit spun and most of plasma removed; contains RBCs, few nonviable WBCs and platelets, some plasma	250 ml Child: 3 ml/kg increases Hb 1 gm/dl Adult: 1 U increases Hb 1 gm/dl and Hct 3%–4% in non-bleeding patient	RBC components transfused to increase oxygen-carrying capacity	Yes	All red cell components have similar adverse effects, including: Transfusion reactions Disease transmission Graft-versus-host disease Iron overload Alloimmunization Hemolysis if hypotonic solutions are administered	Hct 70%–80% so may need to add 50–100 ml normal saline per unit to decrease viscosity No medications can be added to any blood component
Red blood cells with additive solution (RBC-AS)	100 ml of additive solution added to red cells after most of plasma is removed	350 ml	Longer shelf life with additive solutions	Yes		Hct 50%–60%; can remove additive solution and plasma to decrease K or plasma Hb
Saline-washed red blood cells (washed RBCs)	Red cells washed with normal saline; plasma and >70% WBCs and platelets removed	Some RBCs lost with washing	Prevent anaphylaxis in IgA-deficient patients with anti-IgA antibodies	Yes		Allow 1 hour for washing 24-hour outdate after washing
Leukocyte-poor red blood cells (leuko-poor RBCs)	Red cells after most of WBCs removed; AABB standards specify that at least 70% of WBCs must be removed with loss of <30% red cells; in-line filtration removes up to 99.9% of WBCs	Some RBCs lost in filtration	Prevention of severe recurrent febrile nonhemolytic transfusion reactions Reduced risk of sensitization to HLA antigens May be useful for reducing CMV transmission	Yes		Washed RBCs and FDC used previously for leuko-poor RBCs; two febrile nonhemolytic transfusion reactions should be documented before leukocyte-poor cellular components (RBCs and platelets) are provided
Frozen deglycerol-ized red blood cells (FDC)	Red cells frozen with glycerol to prevent hemolysis and stored frozen; thawed and washed when needed	Some RBCs lost in making FDC	Rare RBC storage PNH Prevent anaphylaxis in IgA-deficient patients Decrease WBCs	Yes		Expensive Allow 3 hours for preparation 24-hour outdate
Whole blood	Unmodified unit; no viable platelets or WBCs; decrease in Factors V and VIII over time	450 ml blood + anticoagulant Child: 8–10 ml/kg increases Hb 1 gm/dl Adult: 1 U increases Hb 1 gm/dl	Increase oxygen-carrying capacity and volume in actively bleeding patients with loss of >25% blood volume	Yes; cannot use as "universal donor" in non-O recipient because of anti-A and anti-B in plasma	All those listed above plus: Volume overload Higher rate of allergic and febrile nonhemolytic transfusion reactions	Not always available Advantage is single donor exposure in bleeding patient

AABB = American Association of Blood Banks; CMV = cytomegalovirus; CPD = citrate-phosphate-dextrose; CPDA-1 = citrate-phosphate-dextrose-adenine-1; Hb = hemoglobin; Hct = hematocrit; PNH = paroxysmal nocturnal hemoglobinuria; WBC = white blood cells.

TABLE 57–5

BLOOD COMPONENTS USED TO IMPROVE HEMOSTASIS

Component	Description	Volume	Indications/Dose	Crossmatch?	Adverse Effects	Special Features
Platelet concentrate (random donor unit)	Made from one unit of whole blood Contains few WBCs and plasma	5.5×10^{10} platelets in 40–50 ml plasma	Decreased or dysfunctional platelets with bleeding Prophylactic dose if platelets <20,000 Dose = 1 U/10 kg	No ABO-compatible platelets preferred	Transfusion reactions Disease transmission Alloimmunization	1 U expected to increase count 5,000–10,000 in adult CMV-negative, volume-reduced, leukocyte-depleted, and gamma-irradiated transfusions may be indicated; these manipulations take extra time in the laboratory
Plateletpheresis (single donor unit)	Collected from a single donor during a 2–3-hr apheresis procedure Contains fewer WBCs, few RBCs, and plasma	3×10^{11} platelets in 200 ml plasma	HLA-matched provided to refractory patients; non-HLA–matched may be provided to reduce donor exposures Dose = 1 U/adult	No Same as platelet concentrates	Same as platelet concentrate	
Fresh frozen plasma (FFP)	Plasma frozen within 8 hr of collection Contains all coagulation factors and complement	Pediatric size, 75–125 ml; adult size, 200 ml	Documented coagulopathy with bleeding Dose = 10–20 ml/kg	No ABO-compatible plasma preferred	Same as platelet concentrate Allergic reactions common	Call laboratory to start thawing 1 hr before anticipated time of transfusion
Cryoprecipitate (Cryo)	FFP is thawed at 4°C, then spun Cryo contains Factor VIII (80–100 U), fibrinogen (250 mg), von Willebrand antigen, Factor XIII, and fibronectin	5–10 ml per donor unit	Factor VIII deficiency (hemophilia A) Von Willebrand's disease Fibrinogen decrease or dysfunction Dose dependent on indication	No	Same as platelet concentrate	Allow time for thawing and pooling of units prior to transfusion
Factor VIII concentrate (lyophilized)	Factor concentrate made from large pools of plasma	Vials contain from 250–1000 Factor VIII units, reconstituted with 5–30 ml Lot and number of units on vial	Factor VIII deficiency Dose dependent on severity of bleed	No	Same as platelet concentrate	Monoclonal VIII in use Recombinant VIII in trials
Factor IX concentrate (lyophilized)	Contains vitamin K–dependent factors (II, VII, IX, X; protein C, S)	#units on vial (500–1000 units), reconstituted with diluent provided	Factor IX deficiency Factor VIII antibodies	No	Same as platelet concentrate Thrombotic events have been reported	Risk of thrombosis, viral transmission

effects of the IG intramuscular preparations include fever, allergic reactions, and pain at the site of injection. Intramuscular preparations cannot be given intravenously because of anaphylactic reactions.

IG is used in patients with immunodeficiency syndromes and for immune prophylaxis against hepatitis A. RhIG is a special hyperimmune globulin used to prevent hemolytic disease of the newborn.

The intravenous preparations of immune globulin (IVIG) are approved for use in humoral immune deficiency states and for treatment of idiopathic thrombocytopenic purpura. Adverse reactions occur in 1% to 15% of patients undergoing transfusion and generally are mild, consisting of fever, headache, nausea, and vomiting.[40] Anaphylaxis may occur in immunoglobulin A (IgA)–deficient patients with antibody to IgA.

Cytomegalovirus-Negative Blood Products

Cellular blood components (whole blood, red cells, platelets) can transmit cytomegalovirus (CMV); fresh frozen plasma and cryoprecipitate have not been shown to transmit CMV.[41] CMV disease from transfusion can be prevented by transfusing cellular products that are negative for antibody to CMV. CMV antibody–negative (CMV-negative) cellular products should be provided to certain high-risk groups, including low-birth-weight neonates, pregnant women, CMV-negative patients with solid organ or bone marrow transplants from CMV-negative donors, CMV-negative acquired immunodeficiency syndrome (AIDS) patients, and patients with severe combined immunodeficiency; it should also be provided during intrauterine transfusion in the fetus. Antibody to CMV in blood donors varies regionally from 40% to 100%, so provision of cellular products negative for anti-CMV is difficult in certain areas of the country.

Irradiation of Blood Products

Transfusion-associated graft-versus-host disease (TA-GVHD) is caused when viable lymphocytes in blood components are transfused into susceptible patients.[42, 43] Gamma irradiation at 1500 to 3000 rads interferes with the lymphocytes' ability to proliferate and can prevent TA-GVHD.[44, 45] Patients who are at high risk for TA-GVHD are those with

congenital immunodeficiency syndromes, those undergoing intrauterine transfusion or bone marrow transplant, and those with certain hematologic malignancies.

Volume Reduction

Reduction in the amount of plasma remaining in platelet concentrates and plateletpheresis are performed by the laboratory[46] when circulatory overload is a critical clinical problem. For neonatal transfusion, the total volume of stored platelet concentrates can be reduced to less than 50 ml and still provide acceptable platelet recovery and laboratory studies.[47, 48] For older children, the volume of several units of pooled platelets can be reduced to about 50 ml. The laboratory procedure for volume reduction takes about 2 hours, so this may not be practical in the emergency situation. Additive solutions can be removed from red cells to decrease the volume by about 100 ml while increasing the hematocrit concentration. Fresh frozen plasma and cryoprecipitate cannot be volume reduced.

TRANSFUSION COMPLICATIONS
Transfusion Reactions

Transfusion reactions may be classified as immediate (acute) or delayed, hemolytic or nonhemolytic, immunologic or nonimmunologic, or a combination of these (Table 57–6).[49] Immediate reactions usually occur within 2 to 4 hours of the transfusion, whereas delayed complications may become evident days to years later. Some reactions are life threatening and must be recognized promptly so that appropriate management can be initiated. Early symptoms such as fever and chills may signal the beginning of a life-threatening hemolytic transfusion reaction or a less serious febrile reaction.[50] It is important to closely monitor patients who develop any alteration in physical signs or symptoms during blood product transfusion. The transfusion should be stopped immediately and the intravenous line kept open with an isotonic solution (normal saline or lactated Ringer's solution). Emergent medical intervention is instituted if signs of shock, anaphylaxis, pulmonary edema, or circulatory overload are present. All labels on the blood product are checked with the patient's identification to ensure that the patient received the correct unit. The discontinued bag of

---

	TABLE 57–6			
	IMMEDIATE AND DELAYED ADVERSE EFFECTS OF TRANSFUSION			
	Immediate Effects	**Usual Cause**	**Delayed Effects**	**Usual Cause**
Immunologic effects	Hemolysis with symptoms	Red cell incompatibility	Hemolysis	Anamnestic antibody to red cell antigens
	Febrile nonhemolytic reaction	Donor's granulocytes	Graft-vs.-host disease	
		Antibody to IgA	Posttransfusion purpura	Engraftment of transfused functional lymphocytes
	Anaphylaxis	Antibody to plasma proteins	Alloimmunization to RBC or WBC antigens, platelets or plasma proteins	
	Urticaria			Development of antiplatelet antibody (usually Pl^A1)
	Noncardiac pulmonary edema	Antibody to leukocytes or complement activation		
				Exposure to antigens of donor origin
Nonimmunologic effects	Marked fever with shock	Bacterial contamination	Iron overload	Multiple transfusions (100+)
	Congestive heart failure	Volume overload	Hepatitis	
	Hemolysis with symptoms	Physical destruction of blood (e.g., freezing or overheating)	Acquired immunodeficiency syndrome	Non-A, non-B; occasionally B (rarely A)
		Mixing nonisotonic solutions with red blood cells	Protozoal infection	Human immunodeficiency virus type 1
				Malaria parasites, babesia

Adapted from RH Walker (ed). AABB Technical Manual. 10th ed. Arlington, VA, American Association of Blood Banks, 1990.

TABLE 57-7

LABORATORY EVALUATION OF SUSPECTED TRANSFUSION REACTIONS

1. Clerical check of patient and unit identification
2. Inspection for hemolysis of postreaction specimen
3. Direct antiglobulin (Coombs') test on postreaction specimen
4. Inspection of unit for discoloration, clots, gas
5. If fever or hypotension is present or unit is abnormal on inspection: perform Gram stain and culture on unit
6. If hemolysis occurs: recrossmatch, check for unexpected antibodies; order urine, hemoglobin, bilirubin, and haptoglobin tests

blood component, the entire infusion set, and all forms and labels should be sent to the blood bank immediately to determine whether a hemolytic transfusion reaction occurred (Table 57-7).

Immediate hemolytic transfusion reactions occur by immune and nonimmune mechanisms. Acute hemolysis resulting from ABO incompatibility accounted for 51% of transfusion-associated deaths reported to the Food and Drug Administration from 1976 through 1985.[51] Red cell antigens bind circulating IgM anti-A or anti-B antibodies and activate the kinin, complement, and coagulation systems. Immediate hemolysis of RBCs can result in shock, acute renal failure (acute tubular necrosis), and disseminated intravascular coagulation. Fever is the most common initial manifestation of a hemolytic transfusion reaction and is present about 75% of the time.[50] Hemolysis must always be considered when fever is associated with transfusion. In the unconscious patient, hemoglobinuria is often the first indication of a hemolytic reaction. Other signs and symptoms of immediate hemolysis include chills; chest, back, or flank pain; nausea; vomiting; tachypnea; tachycardia; and hypotension. Transfusion must be discontinued immediately once a reaction is suspected. The intravenous line must be kept in place and the vital signs monitored. Medical intervention includes treatment of shock, if present, and maintenance of urine flow. The risk of fatal hemolytic transfusion reaction is estimated to be 1 per 100,000 transfusions. This is largely caused by ABO incompatibility resulting from clerical or human error in patient identification or blood product labeling.[52] Nonimmune hemolysis of red cells occurs less often and may result from infusion of hypotonic or hypertonic solutions, mechanical damage, overwarming, or bacterial contamination.[53-56]

The most common immediate transfusion reactions are febrile nonhemolytic and allergic reactions. Febrile nonhemolytic reactions occur with 1% to 2% of transfusions. These reactions are caused by antibodies in the patient's plasma to HLA or leukocyte-specific antigens in the transfused component and occur most often in multiply transfused or previously pregnant patients. However, an increase in temperature of 1°C or more, associated with transfusion, cannot be assumed to be a febrile nonhemolytic reaction, and the transfusion must be stopped so that a hemolytic transfusion reaction or bacterial contamination of the unit can be excluded. The transfusion cannot be restarted. Febrile nonhemolytic reactions recur in 10% to 12% of patients, and leukocyte-poor components are recommended when a patient has had two or more febrile nonhemolytic reactions.

Allergic reactions to donor plasma proteins occur in 1% to 4% of transfusions.[57] If urticaria is the only sign of an adverse reaction, the transfusion can be restarted after an antihistamine is given and the hives have faded. Anaphylactic reactions may occur in IgA-deficient individuals with antibodies to IgA.[58] Washed or frozen deglycerolized red cells and plasma products from IgA-deficient donors must be transfused to prevent further reactions.

Transfusion-related acute lung injury (TRALI), or noncardiogenic pulmonary edema, is a rare but life-threatening reaction caused by passive transfer of donor antibody directed against the patient's leukocytes.[59] This results in leukoagglutination and stasis in the pulmonary microvasculature. Aggressive management includes intubation, positive-pressure ventilation, and fluid resuscitation.

Delayed hemolytic transfusion reactions present with hemolysis 1 to 10 days after transfusion and are rarely life threatening. RBCs are coated with IgG antibody and complement, and extravascular destruction occurs in the reticuloendothelial system. These reactions are not commonly seen in the emergency department but should be considered in a recently transfused patient with fever, jaundice, anemia, and a positive direct antiglobulin (Coombs') test.[60] Other delayed adverse effects of transfusion are rarely seen by the emergency department physician (see Table 57-6).

Complications of Massive Transfusion

Massive transfusion is generally defined as the transfusion of one or more blood volumes within a 24-hour period.[61] Complications associated with massive transfusion include hypothermia, metabolic abnormalities, and citrate toxicity (Table 57-8).[62-65] Disseminated intravascular coagulation (DIC) may be present and usually results from tissue damage, poor perfusion, and the clinical situation requiring massive transfusion, rather than from the transfusion itself.[66]

Adverse effects of massive transfusion are related to the length and temperature of red cell storage and the antico-

TABLE 57-8

ADVERSE EFFECTS OF MASSIVE TRANSFUSION

Effect	Cause
Effects caused by blood storage	
Hypothermia	Blood stored at 4°C
Hyperkalemia	Potassium leak during storage
Metabolic acidosis	pH fell during storage
Pulmonary dysfunction	Possibly microaggregates
Anticoagulant-preservative solution effects	
Citrate toxicity	Citrate in anticoagulant-preservative solution
Metabolic alkalosis	Citrate metabolized to bicarbonate
Hypokalemia	Associated with metabolic alkalosis
Hypocalcemia	Citrate binds ionized calcium
Dilutional effects	
Dilutional thrombocytopenia	No viable platelets in RBCs or whole blood
Dilutional coagulopathy	Decreased Factors V and VIII (labile factors) in RBCs and whole blood
Immunologic effects Hemolysis, immune	Incompatible plasma or red cells
Effects caused by mechanical administration of blood Hemolysis, nonimmune	Overwarming of blood Trauma to red cells from rapid infusion Incompatible hypotonic solutions

agulant-preservative solution. Packed RBCs and whole blood are stored at 4°C for up to 35 days if collected with citrate-phosphate-dextrose-adenine-1 (CPDA-1). Several biochemical changes have been reported with red cells stored in CPDA-1, including potassium leaks from the red cells that increase plasma potassium levels at a rate of 0.5 to 1.0 mEq/L/day of storage in citrate-phosphate-dextrose (CPD)–preserved whole blood;[67] plasma pH that becomes increasingly acidic as the cells metabolize glucose to pyruvate and lactate, so that a 35-day-old unit of red cells has a pH of 6.7; and hemoglobin released from senescent red cells in the unit, resulting in an increase of plasma hemoglobin from 8 mg/dl at collection to 658 mg/dl at 35 days of storage. The levels of 2,3-diphosphoglycerate (2,3-DPG) and adenosine triphosphate (ATP) fall in stored red cells. Optimal oxygen release to the tissues does not take place immediately after transfusion because of decreased levels of 2,3-DPG. This "storage lesion" is reversible, and normal tissue oxygenation takes place within 24 hours of transfusion.[68]

The anticoagulant solution for blood collection contains sodium citrate and citric acid. Citrate is present in excessive amounts to prevent coagulation during storage and acts by binding ionized calcium. This accounts for its anticoagulant effect. Side effects caused by citrate toxicity when banked blood is rapidly infused can include decreased ionized calcium with hypotension and arrhythmia, perioral and peripheral tingling, nausea and vomiting, chills, chest pain, and tetany.[69] The routine administration of calcium is discouraged, as it has been associated with myocardial hyperexcitability.[70] Citrate is metabolized in vivo to bicarbonate, which can result in significant metabolic alkalosis and hypokalemia. Potassium levels need to be monitored periodically during massive transfusion.

Coagulation disorders occur frequently with massive transfusion. Mannucci et al. reported that 93% of patients undergoing massive transfusion had one or more abnormal coagulation tests, with thrombocytopenia being the most frequent abnormality seen.[71] Some have recommended the routine administration of platelets and fresh frozen plasma after a certain number of units of RBCs or whole blood have been transfused.[72] However, because of the risks of transfusing unnecessary blood components, even in the massive transfusion setting, it is recommended that platelet counts, coagulation screening tests, and fibrinogen levels be checked at specified intervals during massive transfusion before routinely ordering platelets, fresh frozen plasma, or cryoprecipitate. If the platelet count is greater than 50,000/μl, it is unlikely, on the basis of thrombocytopenia alone, that abnormal bleeding is occurring.[73] If the platelet count is less than 50,000/μl and there is continued significant hemorrhage, platelet transfusion is appropriate. Platelets are stored in donor plasma, so 50 ml of plasma containing coagulation factors is transfused with each unit of platelets ordered.[74] If coagulopathy is present requiring fresh frozen plasma transfusion, 10 to 20 ml/kg is an appropriate dose. Bleeding may also be caused by decreased fibrinogen levels, either from hemodilution or DIC. A fibrinogen level less than 100 mg/dl may be associated with abnormal bleeding. Cryoprecipitate, at a dose of 1 U/100 ml plasma volume or 3 to 4 U/10 kg will increase the fibrinogen from 0 to 200–250 mg/dl.[75]

Ideally, blood should be warmed prior to transfusion to prevent hypothermia[76, 77]; however, rapid warming in an unlicensed microwave or overwarming with a standard blood warmer may result in hemolysis of the unit.[55] Blood flow at high pressure or through small-gauge needles may damage RBCs, causing hemolysis or shortened intravascular survival.[78] Finally, red cells must be infused with normal saline.[79] Simultaneous infusion of hypotonic or hypertonic solutions may lead to hemolysis,[80] whereas infusion with lactated Ringer's solution, which contains ionized calcium (3 mEq/L), may result in clotting of the blood.

Transmission of Infection

Several infectious agents are transmitted by transfusion (Table 57–9). To decrease the risk of disease transmission, healthy volunteer donors are screened for risk factors by a confidential medical history and for evidence of infection by laboratory testing. Units of donated blood are tested for syphilis, hepatitis B surface antigen, antibodies to human immunodeficiency virus type 1 (HIV-1), hepatitis C virus (HCV), and human T-cell lymphotropic virus type I (HTLV-I) and for two nonspecific surrogate markers for non-A, non-B hepatitis: hepatitis B core antibody and alanine aminotransferase (ALT).[81] Units that are negative for all these tests are labeled for transfusion. Despite improved donor selection and laboratory testing, transmission of infectious diseases continues to occur.

Viral hepatitis is the disease most commonly transmitted by transfusion. Ten percent of cases of transfusion-transmitted hepatitis are a result of the hepatitis B virus, despite sensitive screening tests for hepatitis B surface antigen.[82] The other 90% are non-A, non-B hepatitis, with about 85% of these now thought to be HCV.[83] Infection with non-A, non-B hepatitis may not be clinically apparent in the months following transfusion, as 75% of those infected are anicteric. However, 30% to 50% of infected recipients develop chronic active hepatitis, and 10% to 20% of these develop cirrhosis.[84] Antibody testing for HCV was initiated in 1990. With the introduction of this new screening test, the risk of transfusion-transmitted hepatitis is expected to decrease from 1%–4% per transfusion recipient to 0.5%–2.5%.[85]

AIDS transmission by transfusion has a current estimated risk of infection ranging from 1 in 40,000 to 1 in 1,000,000.[52] For transfusion recipients, the risk of HIV-1 infection is related to the "window" period, the time between infection

---

TABLE 57–9

INFECTIOUS DISEASES TRANSMITTED BY TRANSFUSION

Viral infections
  Posttransfusion Hepatitis
    Hepatitis C virus (HCV)
    Hepatitis B virus (HBV)
  Acquired immunodeficiency syndrome (AIDS)
    Human immunodeficiency virus (HIV-1, HIV-2)
  Human T-cell lymphotropic viruses (HTLV-I, HTLV-II)
  Cytomegalovirus
  Epstein-Barr virus
  Parvoviruses

Protozoal infections
  Malaria
  Toxoplasmosis
  Trypanosomiasis (Chagas' disease)
  Babesiosis

Bacterial infections
  Syphilis
  Brucellosis
  Gram-negative sepsis
    Pseudomonas
    Citrobacter
    Escherichia
    Yersinia
  Gram-positive organisms
    Staphylococcus aureus
    Normal skin flora

and when the donor's blood begins to test positive for the antibody.

Transmission of protozoal diseases by transfusion is rare in the United States but it is a significant problem in endemic areas.[86-88] Bacterial contamination of units is a rare complication of transfusion therapy, but the consequences of transfusing a contaminated unit are often life threatening. Deaths related to bacterial contamination of blood components increased from 4% of transfusion-associated deaths in 1976–1978 to 10% from 1986–1988.[89] Bacterial contamination of platelet concentrates ranges from 0% to 10%.[89] This high rate is due to storage at room temperature and increased numbers of platelets being transfused. Contamination of RBCs is most often by gram-negative organisms that are able to grow and proliferate at 4°C. Gram stain examination of donor blood immediately prior to transfusion is possible, but bacteria are not always seen with Gram stain, even in cases of significant contamination. It must be remembered that the units usually appear normal despite contamination with *Yersinia enterocolitica*. Bacteria cannot be cultured from segments attached to red cell units, so the bags must be entered for Gram stain and culture prior to transfusion of the unit. This automatically gives the unit a 24-hour outdating period, which may complicate inventory management. The best approach is to suspect bacterial contamination whenever a transfusion reaction consists of fever, chills, or hypotension. If bacterial contamination is suspected, the patient's blood and the donor blood remaining in the bag are cultured, and antibiotics are given until transfusion-associated sepsis has been excluded.

References

1. Bhatia HM, Sathe MS. Incidence of "Bombay" (O_h) phenotype and weaker variants of A and B antigens in Bombay (India). Vox Sang 1974;27:524.
2. Davey RJ, Touralt MA, Holland PV. The clinical significance of anti-H in an individual with the O_h (Bombay) phenotype. Transfusion 1978;18:738.
3. The Rh blood group system. *In* Mollison PL, Englefreit CP, Contreras M (eds). Blood Transfusion in Clinical Medicine. 8th ed. Oxford, England, Blackwell Scientific, 1987, pp 328–372.
4. Pollack W, Ascari WQ, Crispen JF, et al. Studies on Rh prophylaxis. II. Rh immune prophylaxis after transfusion with Rh-positive blood. Transfusion 1971;11:340.
5. Woodrow JC, Donohue WTA. Rh-immunization by pregnancy; results of a survey and their relevance to prophylactic therapy. Br Med J 1968;4:139.
6. Holland PV, ed. Standards for Blood Banks and Transfusion Services. 13th ed. Arlington, VA, American Association of Blood Banks, 1989.
7. Mintz PD, Nordine RB, Henry JB, Webb WR. Expected hemotherapy in elective surgery. NY State J Med 1976;76:532.
8. Barnes A. The blood bank in hemotherapy for trauma and surgery. *In* Barnes A, Umlas J (eds). Hemotherapy in Trauma and Surgery. Washington, DC: American Association of Blood Banks, 1979, pp 77–87.
9. Blumberg N, Bove J. Un-cross-matched blood for emergency transfusion. JAMA 1978;240:2057.
10. Coffin CM. Current issues in transfusion therapy: Indications for use of blood components. Postgrad Med 1987;81:343.
11. Propp DA. Blood component therapy. J Emerg Med 1988;6:151.
12. Hogman CF, Bagge L, Thorer L. The use of blood components in surgical transfusion therapy. World J Surg 1987;11:2.
13. Snyder EL, ed. Blood Transfusion Therapy: A Physician's Handbook. 2nd ed. Arlington, VA, American Association of Blood Banks, 1987.
14. Mayer TA. Initial evaluation and management of the injured child. *In* Mayer TA (ed). Emergency Management of Pediatric Trauma. Philadelphia, WB Saunders, 1985, p 12.
15. Rutherford RB, Buerk CA. The pathophysiology of trauma and shock. *In* Zuidema GD, Rutherford RB, Ballinger WF (eds). The Management of Trauma. Philadelphia, WB Saunders, 1979, pp 38–79.
16. Perkins RM, Levin DL. Shock in the pediatric patient. Part II. Therapy. J Pediatr 1982;101:319.
17. Shock. *In* Barkin RM, Rosen P (eds). Emergency Pediatrics: A guide to Ambulatory Care. St Louis, CV Mosby, 1986, pp 20–32.
18. Ziegler MM. Major trauma. *In* Fleisher G, Ludwig S (eds). Textbook of Pediatric Emergency Medicine. 2nd ed. Baltimore, Williams & Wilkins, 1988, pp 896–918.
19. Snyder EL. Clinical use of albumin, plasma protein fraction and isoimmune globulin products. *In* Kolins J, Britten AFH, Silvergleid AJ (eds). Plasma Products: Use and Management. Arlington, VA, American Association of Blood Banks, 1982, pp 87–107.
20. Alving BM, Hojima Y, Pisano JJ, et al. Hypotension associated with prekallikrein activator (Hageman-factor fragments) in plasma protein fraction. N Engl J Med 1978;299:66.
21. Leikola J, Myllyla G. The clinical use of red blood cell components. *In* Summers SH, Smith DM, Agranenko VA (eds). Transfusion Therapy: Guidelines for Practice. Arlington, VA, American Association of Blood Banks, 1990, pp 1–25.
22. Snyder EL. Clinical use of white cell-poor blood components. Transfusion 1989;29:568.
23. Counts RB, Haisch C, Simon TL, et al. Hemostasis in massively transfused trauma patients. Ann Surg 1979;190:91.
24. NIH Consensus Conference. Platelet transfusion therapy. JAMA 1987;257:1777.
25. Murphy S. ABO blood groups and platelet transfusion. Transfusion 1988;28:401.
26. Lee EJ, Schiffer CA. ABO compatibility can influence the results of platelet transfusion. Results of a randomized trial. Transfusion 1989;29:384.
27. Kickler TS. The challenge of platelet alloimmunization: Management and prevention. Transfusion Med Rev 1990;4:8.
28. NIH Consensus Conference. Fresh frozen plasma: Indications and risks. JAMA 1985;253:551.
29. Ness PM, Perkins HA. Cryoprecipitate as a reliable source of fibrinogen replacement. JAMA 1979;241:1690.
30. Factor IX complex and hepatitis. Food and Drug Administration Drug Bulletin 1976;6:22.
31. Winslow RM. Blood substitutes: Current status. Transfusion 1989;29:753.
32. Gould SA, Rosen AL, Sehgal LR, et al. Fluosol-DA as a red-cell substitute in acute anemia. N Engl J Med 1986;314:1653.
33. Keipert PE, Adeniran AJ, Kwong S, Benesch RE. Functional properties of a new crosslinked hemoglobin designed for use as a red cell substitute. Transfusion 1989;29:768.
34. Gould SA, Sehgal LR, Rosen AL, et al. The development of polymerized pyridoxylated hemoglobin solution as a red cell substitute. Ann Emerg Med 1986;15:1416.
35. Williamson KR, Taswell HF. Indications for intraoperative blood salvage. J Clin Apheresis 1990;5:100.
36. Jurkovich GJ, Moore EE, Medina G. Autotransfusion in trauma: A pragmatic analysis. Am J Surg 1984;148:782.
37. Mattox KL. Autotransfusion in an emergency department. J Am Coll Emerg Phys 1975;4:218.
38. McCullough J, Quie PG. Granulocyte transfusions: A current appraisal. *In* Allen JC (ed). Infection and the Compromised Host: Clinical Correlations and Therapeutic Approaches. 2nd ed. Baltimore: Williams & Wilkins, 1980, pp 1–35.
39. Kaufman DB, Roifman CM. Immunoglobulins: Newer concepts in immunoglobulin therapy and altered host defense states. *In* Petz LD, Swisher SN (eds). Clinical Practice of Transfusion Medicine. New York, Churchill Livingstone, 1989, pp 737–763.
40. NIH Consensus Conference. Intravenous immunoglobulin: Prevention and treatment of disease. JAMA 1990;264:3189.
41. Bowden R, Sayers M. The risk of transmitting cytomegalovirus infection by fresh frozen plasma. Transfusion 1990;30:762.
42. Anderson KC, Weinstein HJ. Transfusion-associated graft-versus-host disease. N Engl J Med 1990;323:315.
43. Sanders MR, Graeber JE. Posttransfusion graft-versus-host disease in infancy. J Pediatr 1990;117:159.
44. Holland PV. Prevention of transfusion-associated graft-vs-host disease. Arch Pathol Lab Med 1989;113:285.
45. Leitman SF, Holland PV. Irradiation of blood products: Indications and guidelines. Transfusion 1985;25:293.
46. Walker RH (ed). Technical Manual. 10th ed. Arlington, VA, American Association of Blood Banks, 1990, pp 640–641.
47. Moroff G, Friedman A, Robkin-Kline L, et al. Reduction of the volume of stored platelet concentrates for use in neonatal patients. Transfusion 1984;24:144.
48. Simon TL, Sierra ER. Concentration of platelet units into small volumes. Transfusion 1984;24:173.
49. Walker RH (ed). Technical Manual. 10th ed. Arlington, VA, American Association of Blood Banks, 1990, pp 411–432.
50. Pineda AA, Brzica SM, Taswell JG. Hemolytic transfusion reaction: Recent experience in a large blood bank. Mayo Clin Proc 1978;53:378.
51. Sazama K. Reports of 355 transfusion-associated deaths: 1976 through 1985. Transfusion 1990;30:583.
52. NIH Consensus Conference. Perioperative red blood cell transfusion. JAMA 1988;260:2700.
53. Davey R, Lee B, Coles S. Acute intraoperative hemolysis following rapid infusion of hypotonic solution. Lab Med 1986;17:282.
54. Wilcox GJ, Barnes A, Modanlou H. Does transfusion using a syringe infusion pump and small-gauge needle cause hemolysis? Transfusion 1981;21:750.
55. Staples PJ, Griner PF. Extracorporeal hemolysis of blood in a microwave blood warmer. Transfusion 1971;285:317.

56. Braude AI. Transfusion reactions from contaminated blood: Their recognition and treatment. N Engl J Med 1958;258:1289.

57. Stephen CR, Martin RC, Bourgeois-Gavardin M. Antihistaminic drugs in treatment of nonhemolytic transfusion reactions. JAMA 1955;158:525.

58. Pineda AA, Taswell HF. Transfusion reactions associated with anti-IgA antibodies: Report of four cases and review of the literature. Transfusion 1975;15:10.

59. Eastlund T, McGrath PC, Britten A, Propp R. Fatal pulmonary transfusion reaction to plasma containing donor HLA antibody. Vox Sang 1989;57:63.

60. Pineda AA, Taswell HF, Brzica SM. Delayed hemolytic transfusion reaction: An immunologic hazard of blood transfusion. Transfusion 1978;18:1.

61. Wilson RF, Dulchavsky SA, Soullier G, Beckman B. Problems with 20 or more blood transfusions in 24 hours. Am Surg 1987;53:410.

62. Collins JA. Problems associated with massive transfusion of stored blood. Surgery 1974;75:74.

63. Counts RB, Haisch C, Simon TL, et al. Hemostasis in massively transfused trauma patients. Ann Surg 1979;190:91.

64. Moore SB. Management of transfusion in the massively bleeding patient. Hum Pathol 1983;14:267.

65. Kruskall MS, Mintz PD, Bergin JJ, et al. Transfusion therapy in emergency medicine. Ann Emerg Med 1988;17:327.

66. Hewson JR, Neame PB, Kumar N, et al. Coagulopathy related to dilution and hypotension during massive transfusion. Crit Care Med 1985;13:387.

67. Bailey DN, Bove JR. Chemical and hematological changes in stored CPD blood. Transfusion 1975;15:244.

68. Beutler E, Muel A, Wood LA. Depletion and regeneration of 2,3 diphosphoglyceric acid in stored red blood cells. Transfusion 1969;9:109.

69. Dzik WH, Kirkley SA. Citrate toxicity during massive blood transfusion. Transfusion Med Rev 1988;2:76.

70. Wolf PC, McCarthy LJ, Hafleigh V. Extreme hypercalcemia following blood transfusion combined with intravenous calcium. Vox Sang 1970;19:544.

71. Mannucci PM, Federici AB, Sirchia G. Hemostasis during massive blood replacement. Vox Sang 1982;42:113.

72. Reed LR, Heimbach DM, Counts RB, et al. Prophylactic platelet administration during massive transfusion. Ann Surg 1986;203:40.

73. McCullough J, Steeper TA, Connelly DP, et al. Platelet utilization in a university hospital JAMA 1988;259:2414.

74. Simon TL, Henderson R. Coagulation factor activity in platelet concentrates. Transfusion 1979;19:186.

75. Corrigan JJ. Consumption coagulopathy and the disseminated intravascular coagulation syndrome. In Corrigan JJ (ed). Hemorrhagic and Thrombotic Disease in Childhood and Adolescence. New York, Churchill Livingstone, 1985, pp 177–206.

76. Boyan CP, Howland WS. Cardiac arrest and temperature of bank blood. JAMA 1963;183:58.

77. Boyan CP. Cold or warmed blood for massive transfusion. Ann Surg 1964;160:282.

78. Herrera AJ, Corless J. Blood transfusions: Effect of speed of infusion and of needle gauge on hemolysis. J Pediatr 1981;99:757.

79. Holland PV (ed). Standards for Blood Banks and Transfusion Services. 13th ed. Arlington, VA, American Association of Blood Banks, 1989, p 35.

80. Ryden SE, Oberman HA. Compatibility of common intravenous solutions with CPD blood. Transfusion 1975;15:250.

81. Holland PV (ed). Standards for Blood Banks and Transfusion Services. 13th ed. Arlington, VA, American Association of Blood Banks, 1989, p 15.

82. Polesky HF, Hanson MR. Transfusion-associated hepatitis C virus (non-A,non-B) infection. Arch Pathol Lab Med 1989;113:232.

83. Alter HJ, Purcell RH, Shih JW, et al. Detection of antibody to hepatitis C virus in prospectively followed transfusion recipients with acute and chronic non-A, non-B hepatitis. N Engl J Med 1989;321:1494.

84. Alter HJ. Chronic consequences of non-A, non-B hepatitis. In Seeff LB, Lewis JH (eds). Current Perspectives in Hepatology. New York, Plenum Medical, 1989, pp 83–97.

85. Centers for Disease Control. Public Health Service Inter-Agency guidelines for screening donors of blood, plasma, organs, tissues, and semen for evidence of hepatitis B and hepatitis C. MMWR 1991;40(RR-4):1–17.

86. Guerrero IC, Weniger BC, Schultz MG. Transfusion malaria in the United States, 1972–1981. Ann Intern Med 1983;99:221.

87. Smith RP, Evans AT, Popovsky M, et al. Transfusion-acquired babesiosis and failure of antibiotic treatment. JAMA 1986;256:2726.

88. Schmunis GA. Chagas' disease and blood transfusion. In Dodd RY, Barker LF (eds). Infection, Immunity and Blood Transfusion. New York, Alan R Liss, 1985, pp 127–145.

89. Goldman M, Blajchman MA. Blood product-associated bacterial sepsis. Transfusion Med Rev 1991;5:73.

CHAPTER 58

Hereditary Bleeding

Elizabeth H. Perry
M. Lois Hall

Hereditary bleeding disorders can be best evaluated and appropriately treated by understanding how they interfere with the normal blood clotting process. For clarity, the hemostatic mechanism can be separated into defects in the formation of a platelet plug (including disorders of blood vessels, connective tissue, and platelets), and defects in formation of a fibrin clot (including coagulation factor deficiencies); however, it must be remembered that these processes are closely interrelated and inseparable. Table 58–1 summarizes the points at which these disorders interrupt normal physiology and outlines the disease entities discussed in this chapter. Hemophilia A, hemophilia B, and von Willebrand's disease will be considered in the greatest depth, as they are by far the most frequently encountered of all the hereditary bleeding disorders.

When any inherited bleeding disorder is suspected, a detailed medical history, including a complete family history, is taken. The history includes pertinent details of bleeding episodes, including the patient's age at the onset of bleeding, sites of bleeding, duration of bleeding episodes, and manipulations necessary to stop bleeding; previous hemostatic challenges such as operations (circumcision, tonsillectomy), trauma, and eruption of dentition and dental extractions; and a history of epistaxis, easy bruising, menorrhagia, or prolonged menses. A thorough review of medications may uncover the use of drugs that inhibit platelet function. The family history may indicate a pattern of autosomal dominant, autosomal recessive, or X-linked recessive inheritance. If the history and physical examination strongly suggest a bleeding disorder, laboratory tests are performed to further evaluate the clotting process.

CLOTTING PROCESS

The normal blood clotting process is highly integrated and includes interaction among blood vessels, platelets, and plasma coagulation factors. While hemostasis is occurring, naturally occurring inhibitors in the plasma prevent clot extension, and the fibrinolytic system is activated for eventual lysis of the thrombus.

The first step in normal hemostasis is the formation of the platelet plug by interaction of the injured blood vessels and platelets. Steps include vessel constriction, followed by adhesion and aggregation of platelets at the injured areas. Coagulation occurs when the plasma clotting factors that are present in precursor forms are converted in sequential reactions to active enzymatic or cofactor forms, and a fibrin clot is formed. The coagulation factors that are responsible for significant inherited bleeding disorders are listed in Table 58–1. The molecular biology and complex interactions of these factors are currently being studied. For practical purposes, however, the in vitro clotting tests serve as a basis for our understanding of the process of blood coagulation. The fibrin clot is formed when thrombin (factor IIa) is generated from its inactive precursor prothrombin (factor II) and converts fibrinogen (factor I) to insoluble fibrin.

TABLE 58-1

INHERITED BLEEDING DISORDERS

Disorder	Inheritance
Defects in Formation of Platelet Plug (Primary Hemostasis)	
Vascular and connective tissue disorders	
Marfan's syndrome	AD
Ehlers-Danlos syndrome	AD/AR/XR
Hereditary hemorrhagic telangiectasia	AD
Osteogenesis imperfecta	AD/AR
Platelet disorders	
Thrombocytopenic disorders	
Abnormal platelet size	
May-Hegglin anomaly	AD
Bernard-Soulier syndrome	AR
Hereditary macrothrombocytopenia, deafness, and renal disease	AD
Wiskott-Aldrich syndrome	XR
Associated with congenital anomalies	
Fanconi's aplastic anemia	AR
Thrombocytopenia–absent radius (TAR) syndrome	AR
Dyskeratosis congenita	XR
Other	
Megakaryocytic hypoplasia	AR
Familial thrombocytopenia	AD
Thrombopoietin deficiency	?
Platelet function disorders	
von Willebrand's disease	AD
Glanzmann's thrombasthenia	AR
Bernard Soulier giant platelet syndrome	AR
Afibrinogenemia	AR
Storage pool deficiency	
Hermansky-Pudiak syndrome	AR
Chediak-Higashi syndrome	AR
Wiskott-Aldrich syndrome	XR
Thrombocytopenia–absent radius (TAR) syndrome	AR
Familial disorders	AD
Platelet release defects	
Ehlers-Danlos syndrome	AD/AR/XR
Osteogenesis imperfecta	AD/AR
Familial disorders	AD
Type I glycogen storage disease	AR
Cyclooxygenase deficiency	AR
Thromboxane synthetase deficiency	AR
Defects in Formation of Fibrin Clot (Secondary Hemostasis)	
Factor deficiencies	
Factor VIII deficiency	
Hemophilia A (classic hemophilia)	XR
von Willebrand's disease	AD
Factor IX deficiency	
Hemophilia B (Christmas disease)	XR
Afibrinogenemia (factor I)	AR
Hypofibrinogenemia (factor I)	AR/AD
Prothrombin deficiency (II)	AR
Factor V deficiency	AR
Factor VII deficiency	AR
Factor X deficiency	AR
Factor XI deficiency	AR
Factor XIII deficiency	AR
Combined deficiency of factors V and VIII	AR
Other	
Dysfibrinogenemia	AD
Dysprothrombinemia	AR
alpha$_2$-antiplasmin deficiency	AR

AD = Autosomal dominant; AR = autosomal recessive; XR = sex-linked recessive.

Thrombin is generated by two pathways: the extrinsic pathway, which is activated by tissue thromboplastin, normally "extrinsic" to the circulation; and the intrinsic pathway, in which all the factors necessary for clot formation are present in liquid blood and coagulation is initiated by surface contact (Fig. 58–1). The extrinsic system is activated following injury when tissue factor is released and comes into contact with blood; this is measured in the laboratory by the prothrombin time (PT). The intrinsic system is measured in vitro by the partial thromboplastin time (PTT) or activated partial thromboplastin time (aPTT). The PTT is performed by adding a partial thromboplastin (phospholipid without tissue factor) to a sample of citrated plasma, adding calcium, and measuring the time to formation of a fibrin clot. Most laboratories use the aPTT, in which a surface activator (e.g., kaolin, ellagic acid) is added to the basic PTT assay. In vivo, exposed collagen fibers in the subendothelium of the injured blood vessels initiate the reactions. Formation of the fibrin clot involves interaction of the extrinsic system with the intrinsic system. Integrity of both systems is necessary for normal hemostasis, and there is interaction between the two systems. The thrombin time (TT) measures the thrombin-induced conversion of fibrinogen to fibrin.

When a detailed medical history, family history, and physical examination suggest a bleeding disorder, a laboratory assessment consisting of a battery of screening tests is used to help determine the cause of the abnormal bleeding. Screening tests for adequate platelet plug formation include a platelet count, a blood smear for platelet morphology, and measurement of bleeding time. Screening tests for formation of the fibrin clot include the PT, PTT (or aPTT), and TT. The need for further laboratory testing, including tests of platelet function and coagulation factor assays, is based on the results of these screening tests. The clinical history often dictates which additional laboratory tests are indicated. Specific tests for hemophilia A and B and von Willebrand's disease will be discussed in the next sections.

Normal values for the screening tests are generally established in all laboratories for adult patients; however, pediatric hospitals often have established normal values for preterm newborns, term newborns, and young infants. Examples of normal values for neonates and adults are listed in Table 58–2. Neonates have a normal number of platelets and normal platelet morphology. Platelet function has been described by some to be abnormal in neonates, with abnormal bleeding times and aggregation. The PT and TT values are similar to adult values, as are levels of fibrinogen and the cofactors V, VIII, and XIII. Levels of the vitamin K–dependent factors II, VII, IX, and X and the contact system factors XI and XII are decreased in newborns and reach adult levels at between 6 and 12 months of life. The prolonged PTT in newborns is explained by decreased levels of the vitamin K–dependent and contact system factors. If the PTT is prolonged beyond the normal values for newborns or if there is clinical bleeding in an otherwise healthy newborn male or a newborn male with a family history of hemophilia, specific assays for factors VIII and IX should be done.

HEMOPHILIA A AND B

The hemophilias are a group of inherited bleeding disorders caused by deficiency of any of the plasma clotting factors necessary for normal hemostasis. Hemophilia A and hemophilia B are inherited bleeding disorders caused by the deficiency or absence in the plasma of clotting factor VIII (hemophilia A, or classic hemophilia) or plasma clotting factor IX (hemophilia B, or Christmas disease). These two diseases are the most common of the hemophilias and account for 90% to 95% of all patients with clotting factor deficiencies other than von Willebrand's disease.

Seventy per cent of hemophilia A and B is transmitted as a sex-linked recessive disorder on the X chromosome. The sons of a carrier mother have a 50% chance of having

Factors Measured in the Coagulation Screening Tests

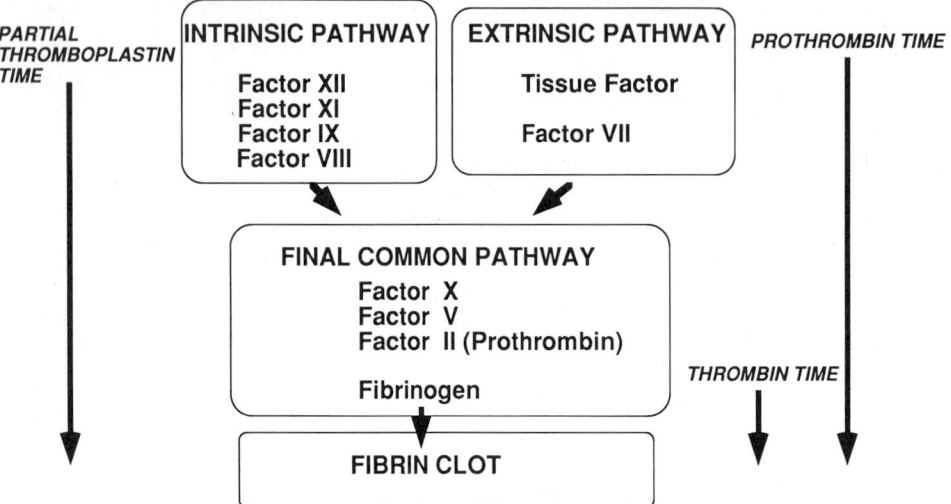

Figure 58–1. Factors measured in coagulation screening tests.

hemophilia, and her daughters have a 50% chance of being carriers. All daughters of a man with hemophilia are carriers, and his sons do not inherit the trait. Thirty per cent of hemophiliacs have no previous family history of the disease. This is an extremely high mutation rate for a genetic disorder. A small proportion of hemophiliacs are female. The incidence of hemophilia worldwide is fairly constant. Approximately 1 in 10,000 males is affected with severe X-linked hemophilia. The number of those with mild to moderate hemophilia is probably greater than this, as they often remain undiagnosed. Roughly 80% of hemophiliacs have factor VIII deficiency, and 20% have factor IX deficiency.

Hemophilia A and B are both classified by measurable factor activity in the plasma. Whereas a normal person has factor VIII or IX levels of 100% (range, 75% to 135%), a severe hemophiliac has factor VIII or IX levels of <1%. Moderately severe hemophiliacs have levels of 1% to 5%, and mild hemophiliacs have levels of 6% to 40% of factor VIII or IX. Clinical manifestations of the disease relate to

the degree of factor deficiency in most cases. Patients with severe hemophilia have severe bleeding episodes, including hemarthroses, soft tissue and muscle bleeds, gastrointestinal and genitourinary hemorrhages, and central nervous system bleeding without apparent trauma. Patients with moderate hemophilia bleed with mild trauma, having less frequent and less severe bleeding episodes than those with severe hemophilia, and those with mild hemophilia usually do not bleed except with dental extractions, surgery, or major trauma. Bleeding in hemophiliacs is typically delayed in onset, usually occurring hours following the hemostatic challenge.

In hemophilia A and B, factor VIII or IX levels less than 40% are reflected by a prolonged PTT. In severe hemophilia the PTT is in the range of 70 to 90 seconds. With both hemophilia A and B, the patient has a normal PT, TT, fibrinogen level, platelet count, platelet function, and bleeding time. Clinically hemophilia A and hemophilia B are indistinguishable, so clinical manifestations cannot be relied

	TABLE 58–2			
	COAGULATION STUDIES ON CORD BLOOD OF NORMAL NEONATES			
Laboratory Test	**Term Neonate (N = 40)** **Mean (Range)**	**Adult Normal**	**Age When Adult Normals Are Reached**	
Prothrombin time	11.4 (10.0–13.2)	10–13	Birth	
Partial thromboplastin time	59.9 (40.0–83.7)	35–45	3 mo	
Thrombin time	20.2 (16.1–24.6)	13–20	Birth–days after birth	
Fibrinogen	0.24 (0.09–0.39)	0.2–0.4 gm/dl	Birth	
Factor II	50% (28%–78%)	70%–130%	6 mo	
Factor V	126.6% (91%–190%)	70%–130%	Birth	
Factor VII	78.4% (25%–150%)	70%–130%	Day 5 after birth	
Factor VIII	109.6% (61%–194%)	70%–130%	Birth	
Factor IX	32.6% (14%–53%)	70%–130%	6 mo	
Factor X	47% (22%–72%)	70%–130%	6 mo	
Factor XI	36.9% (21%–72%)	70%–130%	6 mo	
Factor XII	65% (34%–112%)	60%–200%	6 mo	
Factor XIII	Present	Present	Birth	
Platelet count	358 (222.5–665)	$150–200 \times 10^9$L	Birth	

Adapted from Swinehart CD. Coagulation studies on cord blood of normal newborns. MS thesis, University of Minnesota, 1973; and Andrew M, Paes B, Milner R, et al. Development of the human coagulation system in the full-term infant. Blood 1987;70:165.

on to make the diagnosis. Either type may be suspected in an otherwise healthy male newborn, child, or adult with clinical bleeding. Because the PTT is prolonged in both hemophilia A and B, specific assays for factor VIII and IX must be performed using mixing studies or factor VIII– or IX–deficient substrates in order to make the diagnosis. Within families, all affected members are affected to the same degree and bleeding patterns are similar, with some families having predominantly soft tissue bleeding episodes and other families having a preponderance of hemarthroses. A tendency toward inhibitor (antibody) formation is also seen in some families.

The day-to-day management of the hemophilic patient requires coordinated comprehensive care and is generally provided by the patient's physician in conjunction with a regional hemophilia center. Annual appointments in a hemophilia center are indicated for all patients with severe hemophilia. At that time the patient is evaluated by specialists in pediatrics, orthopedics, and dentistry, and social, financial, and educational issues are addressed. A laboratory evaluation is done annually, including tests for inhibitor formation.

Emergency Medical Service Considerations

If a patient is known to have hemophilia A or B and is followed by a comprehensive hemophilia center, the center places a record of the patient's name, birth date, blood type, weight at annual evaluation, type of factor deficiency, and hospital number in a prominently placed notebook in the emergency department. Treatment recommendations for life-threatening, serious but not life-threatening, and less serious bleeding episodes are detailed in this record. This record is reviewed annually by the nurse coordinator and medical director of the hemophilia center. When hemophiliacs travel and the hemophilia center is aware of this travel, a record can be sent to the emergency department in the city where the patient is visiting. Guidelines for treatment of clinical bleeding episodes in patients with hemophilia A and B are listed in Table 58–3.

Prompt aggressive treatment is mandated if a patient with hemophilia complains of a headache or has altered mental status, difficulty breathing, or injury to the neck or airway. In these cases, or if any other life-threatening bleed is suspected, *treat first* and *evaluate second*. If an intracranial bleed is suspected, treat the patient and then send him or her for a computed tomography (CT) scan or other assessment. Coagulation studies do not need to be performed each time a patient comes into the emergency department. Any patient documented to have hemophilia by a long PTT and specific factor assay will always have those laboratory results in the baseline state. However, if bleeding does not respond to the appropriate treatment, a platelet count and factor assay should be ordered, as thrombocytopenia or a factor inhibitor may be present. If a venipuncture is performed for treatment or laboratory tests, a pressure dressing must be applied to the site. Delayed bleeding is characteristic of hemophilia, and the patient may return with a serious hematoma, possibly requiring treatment, following venipuncture. No intramuscular injections should be given. Aspirin and other medications that cause platelet dysfunction are contraindicated in patients with bleeding disorders.

Therapeutic Intervention

Treatment of bleeding episodes in a hemophiliac depends on the age of the patient, the difficulty of vascular access, and the severity of the bleeding episode. In small children, a visit to the pediatrician, hemophilia center, or emergency department may be indicated for each bleeding episode. At

that time a decision can be made whether to treat the bleed conservatively, with pharmacologic agents, or with factor replacement.

The treatment of bleeding episodes is different for hemophilia A and B, as one consists of factor VIII deficiency and the other consists of factor IX deficiency. Home therapy is an option for patients with either type of hemophilia. The decision as to what product to use for replacement varies from center to center. Some centers use cryoprecipitate and fresh frozen plasma for replacement in small children to cut down on donor exposures. Concerns about factor concentrates include transmission of viral infections, immunosuppression, induction of inhibitors, and cost.

The components available for treatment of hemophilia A and B are listed in Table 58–4. In an emergency, or if the type of hemophilia is not immediately known, fresh frozen plasma can be used, as it contains 1 U/ml (100%) of all the coagulation factors.

Hemophilia A

The treatment of bleeding episodes in patients with hemophilia A (factor VIII deficiency) depends on the severity of the bleeding episode and the severity of hemophilia. In mild hemophiliacs, non–life-threatening bleeds can be treated conservatively with splinting, immobilization, or bed rest or with 1-deamino-(8-D-arginine)-vasopressin (desmopressin, or DDAVP) (Table 58–5). In moderate to severe hemophilia, conservative measures may be useful; however, treatment with factor replacement is generally necessary (Table 58–6). Either factor VIII concentrate or cryoprecipitate can be infused.

Viral inactivation methods have improved since the 1980s. For factor VIII preparations, the best method for viral inactivation seems to be solvent/detergent treatment, followed by immunoaffinity chromatography. The ultrapure recombinant factor VIII preparations do not transmit viruses; however, there is a concern about cost and a possible increase in the incidence of inhibitors. Single-donor cryoprecipitate from a dedicated donor, usually the father of a hemophiliac, is also available at some centers.

The management of patients with inhibitors (antibodies to factor VIII) is extremely difficult and must be supervised by a hematologist. It is much more difficult to achieve hemostasis in the presence of inhibitors, and hemostasis may be impossible in some patients. Treatment alternatives for patients with factor VIII inhibitors are factor VIII from other species and prothrombin complex concentrates (PCCs), which "bypass" the need for factor VIII. In some cases, plasma exchange for antibody removal, immunosuppression to prevent antibody rebound, and treatment with high doses of factor VIII concentrate may be necessary. If a patient with an inhibitor presents in the emergency department with a life-threatening bleed, a hematologist must be contacted immediately.

Hemophilia B

Hemophilia B can be treated with conservative measures, fresh frozen plasma, or factor IX concentrate. Guidelines for treatment of bleeding problems are detailed in Table 58–3. The high-purity factor IX concentrates contain minimal factor X and no factor II or VII. These preparations are less thrombogenic and less likely to transmit viruses than the previously used PCCs.

Patients with factor IX inhibitors are treated with PCC or recombinant factor VIIa under the direct supervision of a hematologist or director of a hemophilia center. PCC carries a significant risk of thrombosis and disseminated intravas-

TABLE 58–3

GUIDELINES FOR TREATMENT OF CLINICAL BLEEDING PROBLEMS IN PATIENTS WITH HEMOPHILIA A, HEMOPHILIA B, AND VON WILLEBRAND'S DISEASE

Clinical Problem	Hemophilia A*†‡ (Factor VIII Deficiency)	Hemophilia B*§ (Factor IX Deficiency)	Von Willebrand's Disease	Special Considerations
Head/CNS injury	Concentrate 100%	Concentrate 40%	Cryoprecipitate (1–2 bags/10 kg)	Immediately replace factor; evaluate Some factor VIII concentrate contains vWF
Neck/airway bleeds	Concentrate 100%	Concentrate 40%	Cryoprecipitate	Immediately replace factor; evaluate
Major trauma or surgery	Concentrate 100%	Concentrate 40%	Cryoprecipitate/DDAVP	Immediately replace factor; evaluate
Abdominal pain	Concentrate 40%–80%	Concentrate 40%	Cryoprecipitate	Immediately replace factor; evaluate
Gastrointestinal bleeds	Concentrate 40%–80%	Concentrate 40%	Cryoprecipitate DDAVP	Immediately replace factor; evaluate
Soft tissue/muscle bleeds	Local measures; if no response, factor VIII 40%–60% (concentrate or cryoprecipitate)	Local measures; if no response, concentrate or infuse FFP to 30%	Local measures DDAVP Cryoprecipitate	Local measures include ice, rest, analgesia
Hematuria Traumatic Spontaneous	Infuse factor VIII to 40%–50% Bed rest, fluids	Concentrate or FFP to 30% Bed rest, fluids	Cryoprecipitate Bed rest, fluids	Corticosteroids/factor replacement may be used
Mouth/tongue bleeds	Infuse single dose factor VIII to 40%, then EACA or AMCA for 5–6 days	Infuse single dose factor IX to 30%, then EACA or AMCA for 5–6 days	DDAVP plus EACA or AMCA	Sedation; npo then liquid diet × 48 hr; no foreign objects in mouth
Joint bleeds	Infuse factor VIII to 40% once, then local measures	Infuse factor IX to 30% once, then local measures	Rare except in type III vWD	Local measures include ice, splints, rest
Nose bleeds	Local measures	Local measures	Local measures DDAVP	
Dental care Routine	None	None	None	Requires careful dental technique
Extractions, deep cleaning	Infuse factor VIII to 40%; EACA or AMCA 1 day preop then 7–10 days	Infuse factor IX to 30%; EACA or AMCA 1 day preop then 7–10 days	DDAVP, EACA, or AMCA	
Menorrhagia	—	—	Hormonal therapy; cryoprecipitate	Oral contraceptives to control menses; short-term EACA or AMCA has been used
Lacerations Minor Major	Local measures Local measures/infusion to 50%	Local measures Local measures + infusion to 30%	Local measures DDAVP	Treat before suturing and before suture removal

*Hemophilia A and hemophilia B patients with the presence of inhibitors (antibodies) require different treatment than listed here.
†In mild hemophilia A, DDAVP should be used before cryoprecipitate or concentrate.
‡1 unit of factor VIII per kilogram raises the factor VIII activity by 2% (2% = 2 U/dl = 0.02 U/ml)
§1 unit of factor IX per kilogram raises the factor IX activity by 1% (1% = 1 U/dl = 0.01 U/ml)
AMCA = Tranexamic acid; DDAVP = 1-deamino-(8-D-arginine)-vasopressin; EACA = epsilon-aminocaproic acid; FFP = fresh frozen plasma; vWD = von Willebrand's disease; vWF = von Willebrand factor.

TABLE 58-4

THERAPEUTIC PLASMA PRODUCTS

Product	Contents	Use/Dose	Special Considerations
Fresh frozen plasma	All clotting factors (1 U/ml)	Replace any stable or labile clotting factor; 10–20 ml/kg	Transfusion reactions, disease transmission, circulatory overload
Cryoprecipitate	Factor VIII and vWF (80 U/bag); Fibrinogen (250 mg/bag); Factor XIII Fibronectin	Hemophilia A (see Table 58–3 for dose); vWD (dose = 2–4 bags/10kg); fibrinogen deficiency or abnormality (4 bags/10 kg)	Transfusion reactions, disease transmission
Human factor VIII concentrates Intermediate purity High purity Ultra pure	Factor VIII (U/vial on label)	Severe hemophilia A, life-threatening bleed in mild or moderate hemophilia A (see Table 58–3 for dose)	Transfusion reaction, disease transmission, inhibitor formation cost
Recombinant factor VIII	r-factor VIII	Hemophilia A	High cost, availability, and increase in inhibitor formation are concerns
Purified factor IX concentrates	Factor IX (U/vial on label); <5 U factors II, VII, <20 U factor X per 100 U factor IX	Severe hemophilia B, life-threatening bleed in mild or moderate hemophilia B (see Table 58–3 for dose)	Transfusion reaction, disease transmission, high cost
Prothrombin complex concentrates (PCC)	Factors II, VII, IX, X	Hemophilia A with inhibitor; hemophilia B; factors II, VII, X deficiency with life-threatening bleed	Consult hematologist when treating inhibitor patients; risks include disease transmission and thrombosis
Porcine factor VIII	Porcine factors VIII	Hemophilia A inhibitor patients responsive to porcine factor VIII	Reserved for management of patients with inhibitors

vWD = von Willebrand's disease; vWF = von Willebrand factor.

TABLE 58-5

PHARMACOLOGIC AGENTS

Agent	Activity	Use	Dose	Special Considerations
Desmopressin (DDAVP)	Increases factor VIII and vWF	Mild or moderate hemophilia A and type I vWD	0.3 µg/kg over 30 min	Facial flushing and warmth, hyponatremia, thrombotic potential tachyphylaxis
Epsilon-aminocaproic acid (EACA)	Antifibrinolytic	Hemostasis after dental work or oral injury or surgery	75 mg/kg IV or po q 6 hr; maximum dose, 6 gm q 6 hr	Side effects: nausea, vomiting, diarrhea, dizziness, impotence
Tranexamic acid (AMCA)	Antifibrinolytic	Same as EACA	20–25 mg/kg IV or po q 8 hr	Better tolerated and more potent than EACA; 4.8% mouthwash used to reduce oral bleeding
Vitamin K$_1$	Synthesis of coagulation factors (II, VII, IX, X)	Prevent vitamin K deficiency	Children, 2–5 mg/day po; adults, 5–25 mg/day po	Use when prescribing antibiotics to patients with bleeding disorders
Oral contraceptives	Increase factor VIII and vWF	Supress menstrual bleeding	Per package insert	Begin in anticipation of menarche in patients with severe bleeding disorders
Analgesics (acetaminophen, codeine, meperidine)	Pain control	Acute and chronic pain relief	As directed	All aspirin-containing medications are contraindicated; no IM injections
Nonsteroidal anti-inflammatory agents	Control pain and reduce inflammation	Chronic pain caused by arthropathy	As directed	Consult hematologist before prescribing; may need to infuse factor concurrently

vWD = von Willebrand's disease; vWF = von Willebrand factor.

TABLE 58–6

DOSE CALCULATIONS FOR REPLACEMENT

Factor VIII replacement in hemophilia A (classic hemophilia)
  1 U factor VIII per kilogram raises the factor VIII activity
    2% (0.02 U/ml).*†
  For rapid calculation of replacement of factor VIII to 100%
    (1.0 U/ml), assume a plasma volume of 40 ml/kg.
    (40 ml/kg) × (patient's weight in kg) = number of factor
    VIII units to infuse
Factor IX replacement in hemophilia B (Christmas disease)
  1 U factor IX per kilogram raises the factor IX activity by
    1% (0.01 U/ml).*‡

---

*Factor content of each vial of lyophilized concentrate of factor VIII or IX is indicated on the label.
†Cryoprecipitate contains 80 U factor VIII activity per bag.
‡Fresh frozen plasma contains 1 U factor IX activity per milliliter of plasma.

cular coagulation (DIC). The recombinant VIIa must be given every 2 hours, and patients must have laboratory evidence of overcompensated DIC without evidence of clinical DIC. Treatment for serious bleeds is generally provided on an inpatient basis. Neither PCC nor recombinant factor VIIa produces prompt hemostasis, and it might take 1 to 2 days to get a bleeding episode under temporary control.

VON WILLEBRAND'S DISEASE

Von Willebrand's disease (vWD) is the most common inherited bleeding disorder, estimated to occur in 1 in 200 persons if mild, moderate, and severe vWD are included. vWD is not a single disease, but rather is a group of qualitative and quantitative disorders that result in decreased levels of von Willebrand factor (vWF) in the plasma. vWD is classified as a disorder of platelet function, as the platelets have abnormal adhesion to exposed subendothelial collagen at the sites of vascular injury because of the lack of plasma vWF. Von Willebrand factor also serves as a carrier protein and stabilizes coagulant factor VIII in the circulation. Consequently, a deficiency in vWF results in a mixture of clinical and laboratory findings that reflect impaired platelet function, impaired coagulation, or both. In vWD, bleeding symptoms may be mild and variable, so not all patients are referred for evaluation.

The first step in making the diagnosis is a high index of suspicion on the part of the physician, based on medical history, family history and type of bleeding episodes. vWD presents most often with skin and mucosal bleeding. There may be easy bruising, epistaxis, gum bleeding, prolonged bleeding from cuts, and prolonged or heavy menses. Hemarthroses are unusual. The symptoms disappear during pregnancy, but postpartum bleeding is common. There are several subtypes of vWD. Most commonly, vWD is inherited as an autosomal dominant trait (types I and II) and presents with a mild to moderate bleeding tendency. Types I and II vWD are clinically indistinguishable. The bleeding episodes vary in severity and frequency, both within individual patients and from patient to patient. Type I vWD has a quantitative deficiency in normal vWF, whereas in type II vWD, the size of the multimers of vWF are abnormal, with absence of the large and intermediate size multimers. Type III vWD is rare, probably inherited as an autosomal recessive trait, and is characterized by absence of vWF. Patients have frequent severe bleeding episodes and may even have hemarthroses. Type III vWD may be clinically confused with hemophilia A.

To diagnose vWD, a full battery of tests aimed specifically at making this diagnosis should be performed and carefully interpreted. It is often necessary to repeat the battery of tests on several different occasions to document sufficient abnormal results to establish the diagnosis. Tests for vWD include the screening tests previously described and assessment of the factor VIII complex, including factor VIII clotting activity (VIII:C), von Willebrand factor antigen (vWF:Ag, or VIIIR:Ag), ristocetin cofactor and evaluation of multimer size of vWF by agarose gel electrophoresis or crossed immunoelectrophoresis. Other tests, such as platelet adhesion and agglutination with ristocetin, can also be performed to help make the diagnosis.

Management of bleeding episodes depends on the severity. Mild bleeding may be controlled by direct local measures. In more severe bleeds, DDAVP may be used for patients with type I vWD. DDAVP is contraindicated in patients with type IIB vWD, because abnormal platelet aggregation and thrombosis have been reported. Oral contraceptives may be used to control menses. Replacement therapy with cryoprecipitate is indicated in life-threatening bleeding episodes or bleeds that are unresponsive to DDAVP. Some of the newer factor VIII concentrates contain significant amounts of vWF and may be used for bleeding in vWD, under the direction of a hematologist or the hemophilia center. As with hemophilia A and B, any patient with vWD who arrives for emergent care with injury to the head, chest, abdomen, or neck should be treated with cryoprecipitate before any diagnostic tests are performed.

OTHER DEFECTS IN PLATELET PLUG FORMATION

Hereditary vascular, connective tissue, and platelet disorders may result in abnormal hemostasis because of defective platelet plug formation (see Table 58–1). Hereditary hemorrhagic telangiectasia (Osler-Weber-Rendu disease) is the most common vascular disorder associated with bleeding. Bleeding occurs from telangiectases, which are the size of small veins but lack smooth muscle. The lesions are not prominent in childhood. Epistaxis, gastrointestinal and genitourinary bleeding, and menorrhagia are the most frequent bleeding manifestations. Coagulation studies are usually normal. Operative bleeding may be life threatening in Marfan's and Ehlers-Danlos syndromes.

Platelet disorders associated with defects in platelet plug formation may be divided into thrombocytopenic and functional disorders (Table 58–7). All of these disorders, except for von Willebrand's disease, are rare to very rare. As with the rare coagulation factor deficiencies, most major hemophilia centers have at least one patient with each disorder.

OTHER DEFECTS IN FIBRIN CLOT FORMATION

Although hemophilia A and B are low-prevalence disorders, the rest of the inherited factor deficiencies are rare, with approximately 1000 cases or families reported (see Table 58–1). The large hemophilia centers may have one or two patients with each of the factor deficiencies. The rarest is prothrombin (factor II) deficiency, with fewer than 50 cases reported in the literature. Factor deficiencies are inherited as autosomal recessive traits, except for dysfibrinogenemia, which is autosomal dominant. Bleeding may be mild to severe depending on the degree of factor deficiency. Soft tissue bleeding is prominent. Factor XIII deficiency is characterized by bleeding from the umbilical stump and abnormal wound healing. These patients also have a high frequency of intracranial hemorrhage, often resulting in death. Factor XIII is not measured in the plasma screening tests, and presumptive diagnosis is made by clot solubility in urea or monochloroacetic acid. Prophylactic treatment for

TABLE 58–7

RARE HEREDITARY PLATELET DISORDERS

Disorder	Characteristics	Laboratory Findings	Treatment	Special Considerations
Bernard-Soulier syndrome	Thrombocytopenia in 30%; functional disorder caused by abnormal platelet adhesion; severe bleeding	Giant platelets on smear; absent platelet adhesion; no agglutination with ristocetin; absent, decreased, or abnormal platelet membrane glycoprotein Ib; normal vWF	DDAVP Platelets	Alloimmunization possible with frequent platelet transfusions. Low or abnormal glycoprotein Ib causes decreased platelet adhesion
Glanzmann's thrombasthenia	Severe bleeding; normal platelet count and morphology	Absent clot retraction; absent aggregation; platelet membrane glycoprotein IIb-IIIa decreased or abnormal; normal agglutination with ristocetin	DDAVP Platelets	Alloimmunization. Abnormal glycoprotein IIb-IIIa causes decreased platelet aggregation during primary hemostasis
May-Hegglin anomaly	Thrombocytopenia in 30%; mild to very mild bleeding	Giant platelets; granulocytes have inclusions resembling Dohle bodies	DDAVP	
Wiskott-Aldrich syndrome	Thrombocytopenia; severe bleeding early in life	Small platelets	Platelets	Immunodeficiency
Storage pool disease	Normal platelet count; mild bleeding	Prolonged bleeding time; abnormal secondary aggregation	DDAVP	Associated with other hereditary disorders such as TAR, Chédiak-Higashi syndrome
Platelet release defects	Mild bleeding	Abnormal secondary aggregation	DDAVP	

DDAVP = 1-Deamino-(8-D-arginine)-vasopressin; TAR = thrombocytopenia–absent radius; vWF = von Willebrand factor.

factor XIII deficiency is possible because of the low concentration of factor necessary for hemostasis (5%) and its long half-life of 6 to 10 days.

COMPLICATIONS OF HEREDITARY BLEEDING DISORDERS

Serious complications of inherited bleeding disorders are related to bleeding as well as the treatment of bleeding episodes. Acute bleeding in patients without inhibitors can generally be stopped with treatment. Intracranial bleeding continues to be a common cause of morbidity and mortality. Death occurs in 30% to 40% of patients with intracranial hemorrhage, and permanent neurologic sequellae occur in about 50%. In older hemophiliacs and some children, chronic problems are a major source of concern. Among those encountered are chronic degenerative arthritis, flexion contractures, peripheral nerve compression injuries, hemophilic blood cysts (pseudotumors), and chronic synovitis. Acute and chronic pain may result in drug addiction and abuse.

The complications related to treatment of bleeding episodes have become a major concern to those taking care of patients with hemophilia. Transfusion reactions are discussed in Chapter 57. Allergic reactions are common, as the components used for treatment are made from plasma. Some of the concentrates contain alloantibodies, and anti-A and anti-B in the concentrates may result in a hemolytic anemia. Hypervolemia and hyperproteinemia may be problems if hemophilia B is managed with fresh frozen plasma infusions. Thrombotic complications such as deep vein thrombosis, pulmonary embolism, and DIC have been reported with the use of prothrombin complex concentrates for treatment of hemophilia B or inhibitor patients.

The major complication of treatment is transmission of infection. Human immunodeficiency virus type 1 (HIV-1) and hepatitis have been transmitted to a large percent of hemophiliacs treated with concentrate, cryoprecipitate, and fresh frozen plasma. The leading cause of death in hemophiliacs is acquired immunodeficiency syndrome (AIDS), not bleeding. Approximately 80% to 90% of patients with severe hemophilia A are seropositive for HIV-1. Approximately 7% to 9% of infected patients have developed AIDS, and more than 50% of these have died.

Hemophiliacs are routinely immunized against hepatitis B; however, chronic hepatitis C and non-A, non-B hepatitis cause significant morbidity. Eighty-five percent of posttransfusion hepatitis consists of hepatitis C. Hepatitis C may be clinically inapparent in the months following infection, as three fourths of these patients are anicteric. However, 30% to 50% of those infected develop chronic active hepatitis, and of these, 10% to 20% develop cirrhosis.

Selected References

Abildgaard CF, Suzuki Z, Harrison J, et al. Serial studies in von Willebrand's disease: Variability versus "variants." Blood 1980;56:712.

Aledort LM, Levine PH, Hilgartner M, et al. A study of liver biopsies and liver disease among hemophiliacs. Blood 1985;66:367.

Andrew M. Transfusion in the newborn: Plasma products. In Kennedy MS, Wilson SM, Kelton JG (eds). Perinatal Transfusion Medicine. Arlington, VA, American Association of Blood Banks, 1990, pp 145–177.

Andrew M, Paes B, Milner R, et al. Development of the human coagulation system in the full-term infant. Blood 1987;70:165.

Aronson DL. The development of the technology and capacity for the production of factor VIII for the treatment of hemophilia A. Transfusion 1990;30:748.

Berliner SH, Lusky A, Zilvelin A, et al. Hereditary factor XIII deficiency: Report of four families and definition of the carrier state. Br J Haematol 1984;56:495.

Bolan CD, Alving BM. Pharmacologic agents in the management of bleeding disorders. Transfusion 1990;30:541.

Bray GL. Recent advances in the preparation of plasma-derived and recombinant coagulation factor VIII. J Pediatr 1990;117:503.

Caen JP, Castaldi PA, Leclerc JC, et al. Congenital bleeding disorders with long bleeding time and normal platelet count. I. Glanzmann's thrombasthenia (report of fifteen patients). Am J Med 1966;41:4.

Colman RW, Hirsh J, Marder VJ, Salzman EW (eds). Hemostasis and Thrombosis. 2nd ed. Philadelphia, JB Lippincott, 1987.

Corrigan JJ. Hemorrhagic and thrombotic diseases in childhood and adolescence. New York, Churchill Livingstone, 1985, pp 1–71.

DeChristopher PJ. Adverse effects of blood transfusion. In Summers SH, Smith DM, Agranenko VA (eds). Transfusion Therapy: Guidelines for Practice. Arlington, VA, American Association of Blood Banks, 1990, pp 113–155.

Dietrich SL, Mosley JW, Lusher JM, et al. Transmission of human immunodeficiency virus type 1 by dry-heated clotting factor concentrates. Vox Sang 1990;59:129.

Forbes CD, Madhok R. Genetic disorders of blood coagulation: Clinical presentation and management. In Ratnoff OD, Forbes CD (eds). Disorders of Hemostasis. 2nd ed. Philadelphia, WB Saunders, 1991, pp 141–202.

Gatti L, Mannucci PM. Use of porcine factor VIII in the management of seventeen patients with factor VIII antibodies. Thromb Haemostas (Stuttgart) 1984;51:379.

Gootenberg JE, Buchanan GR, Holtkamp CA, Casey CS. Severe hemorrhage in a patient with gray platelet syndrome. J Pediatr 1986;109:1017.

Gralnick HR. Von Willebrand's disease. In Ratnoff OD, Forbes CD (eds). Disorders of Hemostasis. 2nd ed. Philadelphia, WB Saunders, 1991, pp 203–244.

Harker LA, Slichter SJ. The bleeding time as a screening test for evaluation of platelet function. N Engl J Med 1972;287:155.

Hedner U, Glazer S, Pingel K, et al. Successful use of recombinant factor VIIa in patient with severe haemophilia A during synovectomy. Lancet 1988;2:1193.

Heisel MA, Gomperts ED, McComb JG, Hilgartner M. Use of activated prothrombin complex concentrate over multiple surgical episodes in a hemophilic child with an inhibitor. J Pediatr 1983;102:951.

Holmberg L, Nilsson IM, Borge L, et al. Platelet aggregation induced by 1-desamino-8-D-arginine vasopressin (DDAVP) in type IIB von Willebrand's disease. N Engl J Med 1983;309:816.

Jackson JB, Sannerud KJ, Hopsicker JS, et al. Hemophiliacs with HIV antibody are actively infected. JAMA 1988;260:2236.

Kobrinsky NL, Gerrard JM, Watson CM, et al. Shortening of the bleeding time by 1-deamino-8-D-arginine vasopressin in various bleeding disorders. Lancet 1984;1:1145.

Kobrinsky NL, Tulloch H. Treatment of refractory thrombocytopenic bleeding with 1-deamino-8-D-arginine vasopressin (desmopressin). J Pediatr 1988;112:993.

Lind SE. Prolonged bleeding time. Am J Med 1984;77:305.

Lusher JM, Schneider J, Mizukami I, Evans RK. The May-Hegglin anomaly: Platelet function, ultrastructure and chromosome studies. Blood 1968;32:950.

Lusher JM, Shapiro SS, Palascak JE, et al and the Hemophilia Study Group. Efficacy of prothrombin-complex concentrates in hemophiliacs with antibodies to factor VIII: A multicenter therapeutic trial. N Engl J Med 1980;303:421.

Mannucci PM. Desmopressin (DDAVP) for treatment of disorders of hemostasis. Prog Hemost Thromb 1987;8:19.

Mannucci PM, Canciani MT, Rota L, Donovan BS. Response of factor VIII/von Willebrand factor to DDAVP in healthy subjects and patients with haemophilia A and von Willebrand's disease. Br J Haematol 1981;47:283.

Marcus AJ. Platelets and their disorders. In Ratnoff OD, Forbes CD (eds). Disorders of Hemostasis. 2nd ed. Philadelphia, WB Saunders, 1991, pp 75–140.

McLeod BC, McKenna R, Sassetti RJ. Treatment of von Willebrand's disease and hypofibrinogenemia with single donor cryoprecipitate from plasma exchange donation. Am J Hematol 1989;32:112.

O'Brien RT, Ater JL. Injuries to children with hematologic disorders. In Mayer TA (ed). Emergency Management of Pediatric Trauma. Philadelphia, WB Saunders, 1985, pp 216–225.

Pierce GF, Lusher JM, Brownstein AP, Goldsmith JC, Kessler CM. The use of purified clotting factor concentrates in hemophilia: Influence of viral safety, cost, and supply on therapy. JAMA 1989;261:3434.

Reese EP, McCullough JJ, Craddock PR. An adverse pulmonary reaction to cryoprecipitate in a hemophiliac. Transfusion 1975;15:583.

Rousell RH, Kasper CK, Schwartz RS. The pharmacology of a new pasteurized antihemophilic factor concentrate derived from human blood plasma. Transfusion 1989;29:208.

Seeler RA, Telischi M, Langehennig PL, Ashenhurst JB. Comparison of anti-A and anti-B titers in factor VIII and IX concentrates. J Pediatr 1976;89:87.

Smith KJ. Review of hemostasis. In Dixon MR, Brubaker DB, Blomback B (eds). New Advances in Hemostasis for Transfusion Medicine. Arlington, VA, American Association of Blood Banks, 1990, pp 1–16.

Sussman II, Spivack M. Indications and use of fresh frozen plasma, cryoprecipitate, and individual coagulation factors. In Dutcher JP (ed). Modern Transfusion Therapy. Boca Raton, FL, CRC Press, 1990, pp 206–227.

Swinehart CD. Coagulation studies on cord blood of normal newborns. MS thesis, University of Minnesota, 1973.

Triplett DA, Brandt JT, Batard MAM, et al. Hereditary factor VII deficiency: Heterogeneity defined by combined functional and immunochemical analysis. Blood 1985;66:1284.

Walker RH (ed). Technical Manual. 10th ed. Arlington, VA, American Association of Blood Banks, 1990, pp 354–359.

Warrier AI, Lusher JM. DDAVP: A useful alternative to blood components

in moderate hemophilia A and von Willebrand disease. J Pediatr 1983;102:228.

Weiss AE. The hemophilias. In Corriveau DM, Fritsma GA (eds). Hemostasis and Thrombosis in the Clinical Laboratory. Philadelphia, JB Lippincott, 1988, pp 128–168.

Weiss HJ. Congenital disorders of platelet function. Semin Hematol 1980;17:228.

Williams MD, Cohen BJ, Beddall AC, et al. Transmission of human parvovirus B19 by coagulation factor concentrates. Vox Sang 1990;58:177.

Yawn DH. Hemostatic agents. In Dixon MR, Brubaker DB, Blomback B (eds). New Advances in Hemostasis for Transfusion Medicine. Arlington, VA, American Association of Blood Banks, 1990, pp 39–51.

Anemia

Patrick L. Carolan

INTRODUCTION

Hemoglobin is a tetramer composed of four polypeptide chains: two alpha and two non-alpha. Each polypeptide chain is covalently linked to one heme group (protoporphyrin IX).

During the evolution of the fetal to the adult erythrocyte, sequential changes in hemoglobin components occur (Fig. 59–1). Minor structural variations result in important differences in the physicochemical properties of fetal and adult hemoglobins and the abnormal hemoglobin variants.

The primary function of the red blood cell (RBC) is to deliver adequate quantities of oxygen to the tissues. Factors that regulate oxygen binding by the RBC and unloading to the tissues do so by modifying the characteristics of the oxyhemoglobin dissociation curve (Fig. 59–2). The sigmoid shape of this dissociation curve and its relative position are governed by two important properties: cooperativity and oxygen affinity. *Cooperativity* refers to an interaction between globin moieties in which oxygen binding by one globin molecule facilitates binding of additional oxygen molecules to the remaining heme groups of the hemoglobin tetramer. The sigmoid shape of the dissociation curve ensures the release of a considerable amount of oxygen from hemoglobin following a relatively small change in oxygen tension. *Affinity* refers to the tendency of heme groups to bind or release oxygen and is governed primarily by temperature, intracellular pH, and 2,3-diphosphaglycerate (2,3-DPG) concentration. A shift of the dissociation curve to the right lowers oxygen affinity, favoring release of oxygen to the tissues. Conversely, factors directing a leftward shift of the curve are associated with more avid binding of oxygen by hemoglobin and decreased tissue oxygen delivery. Various clinical disorders are associated with changes in oxyhemoglobin affinity (Table 59–1).

Tissue oxygen delivery is a dynamic process. Tissue oxygen consumption is expressed by the following equation:

$$Vo_2 = 1.34 \times Q \times Hgb \times (Sao_2 - Svo_2),$$

where Vo_2 = oxygen consumption, 1.34 = ml of O_2 bound to 1 gm Hgb, Hgb = hemoglobin concentration (gm/dl), Q

The contributions of Theresa M. Haynes, S.E., to manuscript preparation and Mitchell J. Einzig, M.D., to manuscript review are gratefully acknowledged.

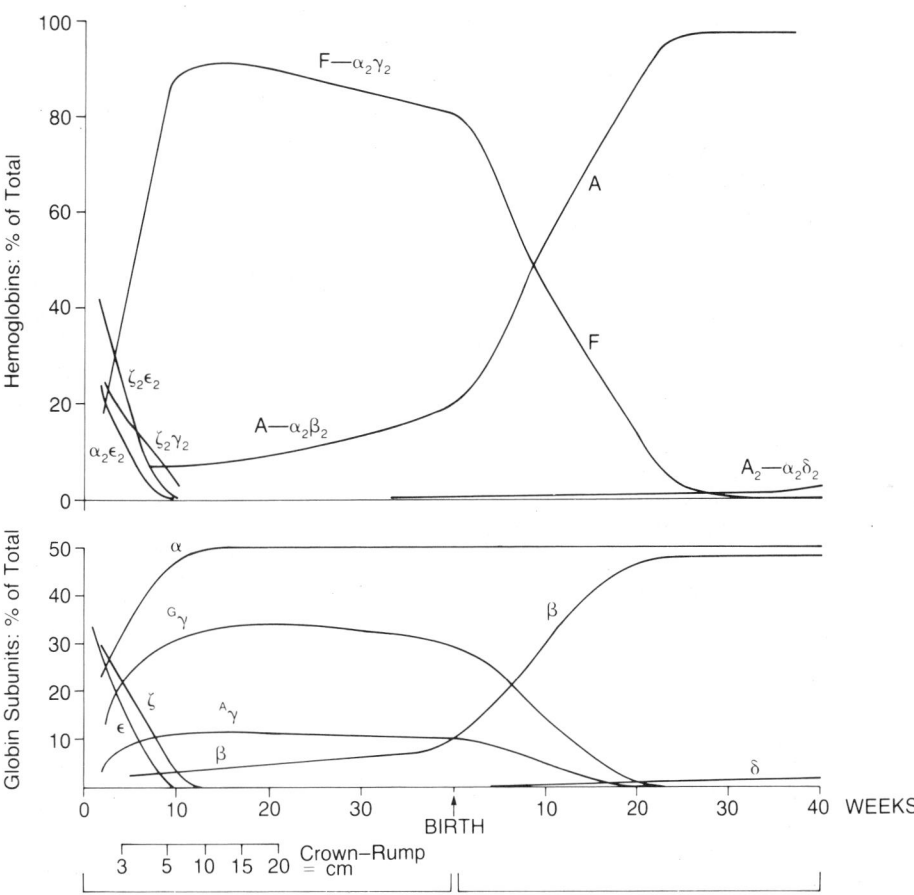

Figure 59–1. Changes in hemoglobin tetramers (*top*) and in globin subunits (*bottom*) during human development from embryo to early infancy. (From Bunn HF, Forget BG. Hemoglobin: Molecular, Genetic and Clinical Aspects. Philadelphia, WB Saunders, 1986.)

= blood flow (ml/min), SaO_2 = percent oxygen saturation of arterial blood, and SvO_2 = percent oxygen saturation of venous blood.

The quantity of oxygen that is ultimately delivered to the tissues is determined not only by the hemoglobin concentration, but also by factors regulating blood flow and oxyhemoglobin binding. The clinical significance of an anemia must therefore be viewed within the context of the complex interplay of these variables.

CLINICAL EVALUATION

Anemia evident in the neonatal period is generally the result of blood loss, isoimmunization, or congenital hemolytic anemia. Anemia first detected at 3 to 6 months of age suggests a congenital disorder of hemoglobin synthesis (thalassemia) or structure (hemoglobinopathy). Nutritional iron deficiency is rarely responsible for anemia in term infants prior to 6 months of age or in healthy preterm infants prior to the time they have doubled their birth weight. Between 6 months and 2 years of age, nutritional iron deficiency becomes most prevalent, especially when associated with a history of early or excessive cow's milk intake. Other important historical features include the patient's race and ethnicity, diet, use of medications, and symptoms of systemic illness. A family history of anemia, jaundice, gallstones, or splenectomy may suggest an hereditary hemolytic anemia (spherocytosis, hemoglobinopathy, or red cell enzyme deficiency).

Symptoms and signs that parents may note include pallor, poor appetite, excessive tiredness, or irritability. Older children may exhibit shortness of breath, reduced exercise or activity tolerance, or, less commonly, palpitations or syncope.

Signs and symptoms suggesting anemia are generally seen once hemoglobin values fall below 7 to 8 gm/dl. These findings may include generalized pallor, especially evident

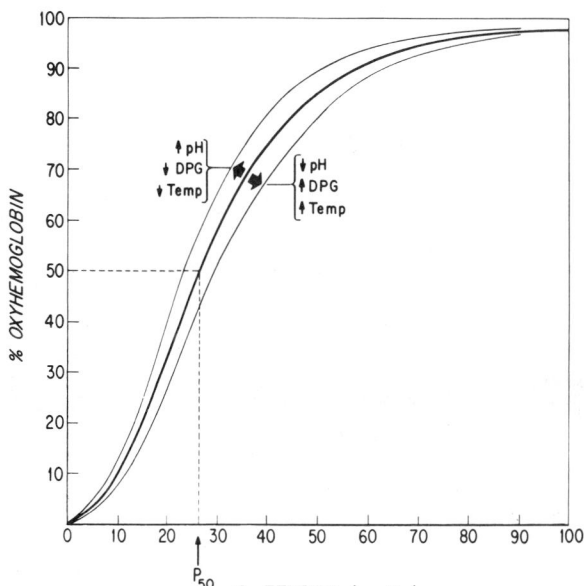

Figure 59–2. The principal factors that influence the position of the oxyhemoglobin dissociation curve. (From Bunn FH, Forget BG. Hemoglobin: Molecular, Genetic and Clinical Aspects. Philadelphia, WB Saunders, 1986.)

TABLE 59-1

DISPLACEMENT OF THE OXYHEMOGLOBIN DISSOCIATION CURVE IN VARIOUS CLINICAL DISORDERS*

I. Shift to the right
 A. Increase in red cell 2,3-diphosphoglycerate
  1. High-altitude adaptation
  2. Pulmonary hypoxemia
  3. Cardiac right-to-left shunt
  4. Severe anemia; decrease in red cell mass
  5. Congestive heart failure
  6. Decompensated hepatic cirrhosis
 B. Functionally abnormal hemoglobin variants
II. Shift to the left
 A. Decrease in red cell 2,3-diphosphoglycerate
  1. Septic shock
  2. Severe acidosis
  3. Following transfusion of stored blood
  4. Hypophosphatemia
  5. Panhypopituitarism
 B. Functionally abnormal hemoglobin variants
 C. Methemoglobinemia
 D. Carbon monoxide intoxication

*Corrected to pH 7.4.

From Oski FA. Human hemoglobins: Normal and abnormal. *In* Nathan DG, Oski FA (eds). Hematology in Infancy and Childhood. Philadelphia, WB Saunders, 1987, p 621.

in the conjunctival and oral mucous membranes. Pallor of the palmar and digital creases corresponds to a hemoglobin value of 5 gm/dl or less. Tachycardia, a hemic cardiac murmur, and bounding central and peripheral pulses may also be noted. As the anemia worsens and compensatory mechanisms fail, signs of congestive heart failure such as tachypnea, tachycardia, gallop rhythm, rales, or hepatomegaly may be present.

Other associated examination findings may include tortuosity of retinal vessels (hemoglobinopathy), glossitis with diminished vibratory and position senses (vitamin B_{12} deficiency), generalized lymphadenopathy (infection, malignancy), maxillary and frontal bone overgrowth (thalassemia syndromes), or splenomegaly (immune or hereditary hemolytic anemia).

DIAGNOSTIC EVALUATION
Electronic RBC Counting

The electronic red cell counter provides direct measurements of Hgb concentration, total RBC count, and mean corpuscular volume (MCV). The hematocrit (Hct), mean corpuscular hemoglobin (MCH), and mean corpuscular hemoglobin concentration (MCHC) are derived from the following calculations:

$$Hct = MCV \times RBC$$
$$MCH = Hgb/RBC \text{ or } MCHC \times Hgb$$
$$MCHC = Hgb/Hct$$

The red cell distribution width (RDW) has also been added to the automated blood count. The RDW reflects the heterogeneity of red cell size and is the equivalent of "anisocytosis" that is noted on the peripheral blood smear. Lower RDW values reflect homogeneous red cell populations. Conditions associated with variable RBC sizes, such as hemolysis or reticulocytosis, have larger RDW values. Age-appropriate values for RDW have been established for pediatric patients.

Alterations in blood osmolality or turbidity may result in errors in electronic cell counting. The presence of cold agglutinins may result in microaggregation of red cells, which electronic cell counters will detect as single cells. Falsely low RBC counts with falsely elevated MCVs result. Marked elevations of white blood cell (WBC) counts produce several alterations as well. First, because WBCs and RBCs are counted together (accounting for a negligible error of 0.1% in RBC determinations normally), marked leukocytosis will elevate the RBC count. This error can rise to more than 10% when WBC counts are greater than 300,000. Hyperleukocytosis also increases blood turbidity, which results in an overestimation of hemoglobin content. For similar reasons, marked changes in blood glucose, sodium, and triglyceride concentrations may alter automated red cell values (Table 59-2).

DEFINITION OF ANEMIA

Definitions of anemia are derived from normative population-based survey data (Table 59-3). The limits for differentiating normal from abnormal values are set at two standard deviations above or below the mean of values for the normal population. Determinations of normal or abnormal should be interpreted in conjunction with preexisting hematologic values. As an example, the normal values for healthy individuals without cardiopulmonary disease (Table 59-3) may not apply to patients with cyanotic congenital heart disease or bronchopulmonary dysplasia. Both of these conditions are marked by chronic arterial desaturation and, as a result, a secondary polycythemia.

CLASSIFICATION OF ANEMIAS

A number of schemes have been devised for classification of the anemias. Using information derived from the peripheral blood smear and automated blood indices, the anemia may be classified as microcytic and hypochromic, normocytic and normochromic, or macrocytic (Fig. 59-3).

A review of the peripheral blood smear remains an important first step in the laboratory evaluation of an anemia. Features to be noted on the peripheral blood smear include RBC size, degree of central red cell pallor, uniformity of size, abnormalities of shape, basophilic stippling, and presence of inclusions. Normally the RBC diameter should approximate the size of the nucleus of a small lymphocyte. When identification of a small lymphocyte is difficult, size relationships may be established by reference to central red cell pallor. If the central pallor of the RBC exceeds one third of the diameter of the total cell, the cells are likely to be hypochromic, and therefore microcytic.

MICROCYTIC ANEMIAS

Approximately 98% of anemias associated with microcytosis are caused by iron deficiency or thalassemia syndromes. Thalassemia-associated anemia is manifested by a uniform

TABLE 59-2
ARTIFACTS IN ELECTRONIC CELL COUNTING

Cause	Hgb	Hct	RBC	MCV	MCH	MCHC
Cold agglutinins	—	—	↓	↑	↑	—
Hyperleukocytosis	↑	↑	↑	—	—	—
Hyperglycemia	—	↑	—	↑	—	↓
Hypernatremia	—	↑	—	↑	—	↓
Hypertriglyceridemia	↑	—	—	—	↑	↑

From Stockman JA. Using electronic RBC counts to diagnose anemia. Contemp Pediatr 1989;6:112.

TABLE 59–3

RED BLOOD CELL VALUES AT VARIOUS AGES: MEAN AND LOWER LIMIT OF NORMAL (–2 SD)*

Age	Hemoglobin (gm/dl)		Hematocrit (%)		Red Cell Count (10¹²/L)		MCV (fl)		MCH (pg)		MCHC (gm/dl)	
	Mean	*–2 SD*	*Mean*	*–2 SD*	*Mean*	*–2 SD*	*Mean*	*–2 SD*	*Mean*	*–2 SD*	*Mean*	*–2 SD*
Birth (cord blood)	16.5	13.5	51	42	4.7	3.9	108	98	34	31	33	30
1 to 3 days (capillary)	18.5	14.5	56	45	5.3	4.0	108	95	34	31	33	29
1 wk	17.5	13.5	54	42	5.1	3.9	107	88	34	28	33	28
2 wk	16.5	12.5	51	39	4.9	3.6	105	86	34	28	33	28
1 mo	14.0	10.0	43	31	4.2	3.0	104	85	34	28	33	29
2 mo	11.5	9.0	35	28	3.8	2.7	96	77	30	26	33	29
3 to 6 mo	11.5	9.5	35	29	3.8	3.1	91	74	30	25	33	30
0.5 to 2 yr	12.0	10.5	36	33	4.5	3.7	78	70	27	23	33	30
2 to 6 yr	12.5	11.5	37	34	4.6	3.9	81	75	27	24	34	31
6 to 12 yr	13.5	11.5	40	35	4.6	4.0	86	77	29	25	34	31
12 to 18 yr—female	14.0	12.0	41	36	4.6	4.1	90	78	30	25	34	31
male	14.5	13.0	43	37	4.9	4.5	88	78	30	25	34	31
18 to 49 yr—female	14.0	12.0	41	36	4.6	4.0	90	80	30	26	34	31
male	15.5	13.5	47	41	5.2	4.5	90	80	30	26	34	31

*These data have been compiled from several sources. Emphasis is given to studies employing electronic counters and to the selection of populations that are likely to exclude individuals with iron deficiency. The mean ± 2 SD can be expected to include 95% of the observations in a normal population.
From Dallman PR. Fetal and adult hemoglobin. *In* Rudolph A (ed). Pediatrics. 16th ed. New York, Appleton-Century-Crofts, 1977, p 1111.

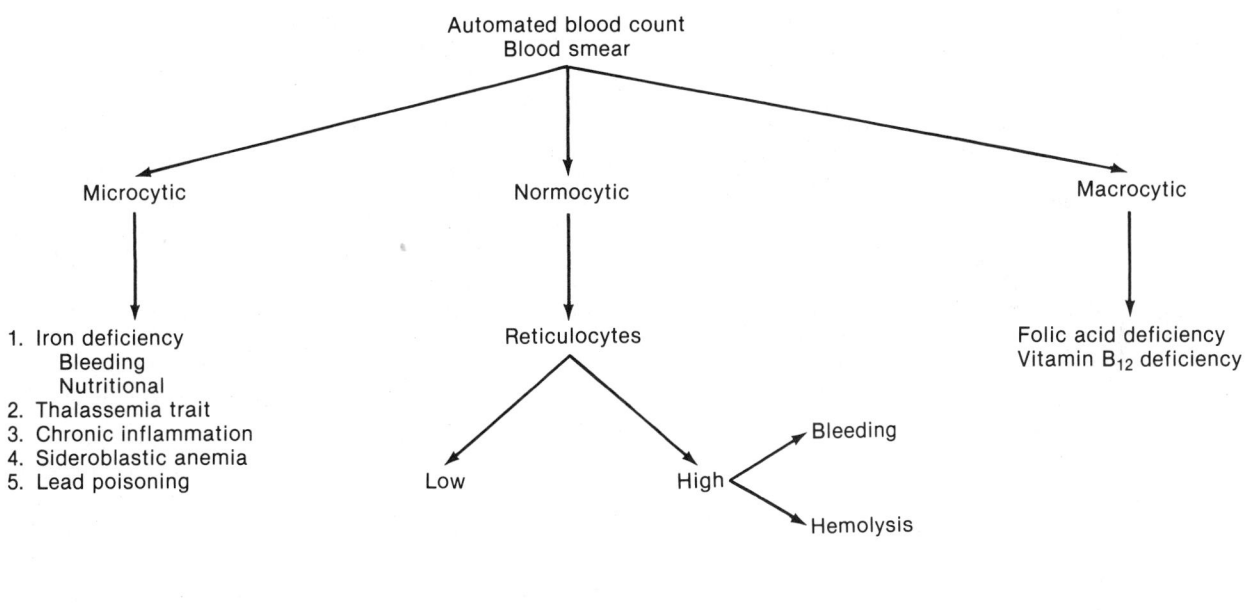

Figure 59–3. Morphologic classification and differential diagnosis of the anemias. (Adapted from Segel GB. Anemia. Pediatr Rev 1988;10:79. Reproduced by permission of Pediatrics.)

TABLE 59–4

SCREENING METHODS IN EVALUATING MICROCYTOSIS

Method	Formula	Thalassemia	Iron Deficiency
Discriminant function	MCV – (5 × Hgb) – RBC – 8.4	<1	>1
	MCV ÷ RBC	<3.8	>3.8
	MCV ÷ RBC	<13	>13
RBC count		>5.0 × 10^{12}/L	<5.0 × 10^{12}/L
RDW	$\sigma/\mu \times 100$	<14%	>14%

μ = Median cell volume; σ = standard deviation.

Adapted from Johnson CS, Tegos C, Butler E. Routine erythrocyte measurements and differentiation from iron deficiency. Am J Clin Pathol 1983;80:31.

decrease in RBC size. This is contrasted with iron deficiency anemia, which is associated with notable red cell size variations caused by erythropoietin-induced marrow stimulation secondary to systemic iron deficiency (Table 59–4). Use of the RDW will permit identification of 88% to 92% of iron deficiency anemias and approximately 79% to 84% of thalassemia-related anemias. Patterns of laboratory test results for the disorders producing microcytosis and hypochromia also assist in the diagnosis (Table 59–5).

Iron Deficiency Anemia

Iron deficiency anemia is the single most common hematologic abnormality in children between the ages of 6 months and 2 years. As many as 30% of infants 10 to 15 months of age manifest iron deficiency anemia and approximately 30% to 70% of infants in the same age group have been found to be iron deficient but not anemic.

Factors contributing to the development of iron deficiency in infants include the variable iron content and bioavailability in the normal infant diet in light of the substantial amounts of dietary iron needed to support normal growth; the effect of mild intercurrent illness on iron absorption and metabolism; and finally, circumstances in which blood loss may contribute to a reduction of endogenous iron stores.

During pregnancy, placental iron transport is negligible until the latter portion of the third trimester. As a result, the infant's initial iron endowment will be greatly altered by premature birth and low birth weight. There is also a wide variation in hemoglobin mass and, hence, iron endowment in term infants. During the minutes following delivery, uterine contractions send placental blood through umbilical veins, resulting in a 20 ml/kg increase in the infant's blood volume. Clamping the cord too early after delivery may reduce the newborn's body iron content by 15% to 30%. Any additional perinatal blood loss will further alter body iron stores. A dietary history of early or excessive cow's milk intake, early solid food intake, or breast-feeding beyond 6 months of age without the use of iron supplements are additional factors predisposing to iron deficiency. Frequent infections appear to exert a separate additional effect on iron absorption and therefore contribute to iron deficiency.

Signs and symptoms suggesting anemia may appear late or go unnoticed until the iron deficiency anemia is severe. At this stage, pallor, listlessness, irritability, and anorexia will be evident. Nonhematologic manifestations of iron deficiency include gastrointestinal bleeding, malabsorption with intestinal mucosal atrophy, reduced skeletal muscle work capacity, growth retardation, abnormal leukocyte function, and behavioral alterations such as reduced attentiveness or irritability.

Iron deficiency anemia evolves slowly. The earliest stage is marked by iron storage depletion and is indicated by a reduction in stainable iron stores in the bone marrow and reticuloendothelial systems; a reduction in serum ferritin is also noted. In the second stage, iron-deficient erythropoiesis occurs as a result of a reduction in circulating iron, as evidenced by decreased serum iron and total iron-binding capacity (TIBC). This stage is also marked by a reduction in transferrin saturation (Fe/TIBC) and an elevation of free erythrocyte protoporphyrin (FEP) in the blood. The third and final stage is overt iron deficiency anemia.

The cause of microcytic anemias in many patients will be suggested by analysis of automated cell counts and indices referenced against discriminate function calculations and RDW (see Table 59–4). RDW increases with progressive iron deficiency. An RDW value greater than 20 is seen exclusively in iron deficiency. In such patients, a therapeutic trial of iron (6 mg/kg/day of elemental iron) may be undertaken (Table 59–6). This therapeutic trial of iron remains the "gold standard" for the diagnosis of iron deficiency. A response to iron is indicated by reticulocytosis beginning 2 to 3 days after treatment. The peak elevation in reticulocyte count is seen at 7 to 10 days. Initially the hemoglobin will increase at a rate of 0.25 to 0.40 gm/dl/day. Subsequently, this rate will level off to an increase of 0.15 gm/dl/day. Once a normal hemoglobin level has been obtained, supplemental iron should be continued for an additional 2 to 3 months.

Thalassemias

The thalassemias are disorders of globin chain production. Alpha-thalassemia and beta-thalassemia refer to various de-

TABLE 59–5

LABORATORY TEST RESULTS IN DISORDERS PRODUCING HYPOCHROMIA AND MICROCYTOSIS

Disorder	Serum Iron	Iron-Binding Capacity	Ferritin	FEP	Hemoglobin Electrophoresis	Marrow Iron Stores
Iron deficiency	↓	↑	↓	↑	—	↓
Chronic disease anemia	↓	↓	↑	↑	—	↑
Sideroblastic anemia	↑	—	↑	↓	—	Ring sideroblasts
Beta-thalassemia trait	—	—	—	—	↑ Hemoglobin A_2	—
Alpha-thalassemia trait	—	—	—	—	—	—

*FEP = Free erythrocyte protoporphyrin.

Adapted from Steinberg MH, Dreiling BJ. Microcytosis. Its significance and evaluation. JAMA 1983;249:85. Copyright 1983, American Medical Association.

TABLE 59–6

ANEMIA: THERAPY AT A GLANCE

Medication	Dose	Route	Frequency
Ferrous sulfate	6 mg/kg/day*	PO	tid
Folic acid	1 gm/day	IM	q day
Vitamin B$_{12}$	500 μg/day†	IM	q day × 10 days
	500 μg‡	IM	q mo × 2 mo

*Dosage expressed as mg/kg/day of elemental iron. Nonanemic iron-deficient patients may be supplemented at 3 mg/kg/day.
†Initial replacement dose to restore tissue levels.
‡Maintenance replacement dose.

grees of impairment of alpha and beta chain synthesis, respectively. Beta-thalassemia trait is the primary differential consideration in patients suspected of having iron deficiency anemia. Beta-thalassemia trait is carried by approximately 4% of persons of Mediterranean heritage, and by smaller percentages of blacks and Asians.

The heterozygous beta-thalassemia trait results in a mild hypochromic, microcytic anemia. The RDW is normal and serves as an important feature distinguishing this anemia from iron deficiency anemia. Hemoglobin electrophoresis reveals an elevation in the minor adult hemoglobin, Hgb A$_2$, to greater than 4%. Homozygous beta-thalassemias (beta-thalassemia major, or Cooley's anemia) are characterized by much greater degrees of anemia.

The alpha-thalassemias occur in Asians and blacks. The clinical syndrome seen is determined by the number of alpha globin genes that are expressed. A *four-gene deletion* occurs only in Asians and results in the production of Bart's hemoglobin, leading to severe fetal hydrops and fetal death. A *three-gene deletion* results in a moderately severe chronic hemolytic anemia known as *hemoglobin H disease*. In hemoglobin H disease, precipitation of unpaired beta chains in the red cell produces the characteristic Heinz body RBC inclusion. A *two-gene deletion* results in alpha-thalassemia trait. Microcytic, hypochromic cells are noted, but anemia is generally absent. As in the case of beta-thalassemia trait, the RDW is normal. Alpha-thalassemia trait is distinguished from beta-thalassemia trait by a normal hemoglobin A$_2$ value on hemoglobin electrophoresis.

Anemia of Chronic Inflammation

Anemias associated with chronic inflammatory diseases, such as juvenile rheumatoid arthritis, or infections may be normochromic or hypochromic. It is thought that an internal block in iron utilization occurs in combination with an insensitivity of erythroid precursors to erythropoietin.

Sideroblastic Anemia

The sideroblastic anemias are seen most commonly in older patients as a preneoplastic condition leading frequently to leukemia. Sideroblasts form when iron accumulates in the mitochondria of developing erythroblasts as a result of a failure to incorporate iron into the heme molecule. This accumulation of iron within the mitochondrion produces the characteristic ring sideroblasts identified by Prussian blue staining of bone marrow preparations.

Lead Toxicity Anemia

Blood lead levels greater than 15 to 18 μg/dl will inhibit critical enzymes involved in heme synthesis, resulting in an elevation of FEP concentration in blood. Additional effects on vitamin D and cortisol metabolism, renal function, and behavior have been reported at venous blood lead levels of less than 25 μg/dl.

NORMOCYTIC, NORMOCHROMIC ANEMIAS

The normocytic, normochromic anemias may be caused by acute blood loss, RBC destruction, or a failure in marrow RBC production. Examples of occult sources of blood loss include intracranial, intra-abdominal, or intrathoracic bleeding or hemorrhage associated with long-bone fractures. In the newborn, blood loss associated with fetoplacental, feto-maternal, or twin-to-twin transfusion must be considered as well. Chronic blood loss is associated with iron deficiency and, therefore, with microcytic and hypochromic blood indices.

The reticulocyte count differentiates the various normochromic anemias. Reticulocytes are young RBCs containing residual RNA. The normal reticulocyte percentage is 1.0, representing approximately 50,000 cells/μL of blood. A normal bone marrow response to anemia results in an elevation of the reticulocyte count to six to eight times the resting level. Any response less than this is considered an inadequate bone marrow response to the anemia. The differential diagnosis of the normocytic anemias is characterized by the presence or absence of reticulocytosis (see Fig. 59–3).

Blackfan-Diamond Anemia

Blackfan-Diamond anemia (congenital hypoplastic anemia) and transient erythroblastopenia of childhood (TEC) are the most common causes of reticulocytopenic, normochromic anemias in children.

Patients with Blackfan-Diamond anemia present during the first year of life with severe, progressive anemia. Pallor in an otherwise normal-appearing infant is the usual presenting sign. Some infants manifest anemia at birth. Approximately 75% of affected infants present prior to 4 months of age. One third of all patients exhibit short stature or associated congenital anomalies such as cleft palate, eye defects, abnormalities of the thumb, congenital heart disease, or mental retardation. The cause of this anemia is unclear.

Minimal diagnostic criteria for Blackfan-Diamond anemia include moderate to severe anemia beginning in early infancy, reticulocytopenia, and normal WBC and platelet counts.

Although anemia may be severe, necessitating repeated transfusions, most patients with Blackfan-Diamond anemia will show reticulocytosis and an elevation in the hemoglobin concentration following treatment with corticosteroids. In many cases, prednisone is administered in doses of 2 mg/kg/day and tapered to the lowest dose necessary for maintenance of an acceptable hemoglobin. Many patients require prolonged corticosteroid therapy. However, approximately 20% of patients will experience a complete spontaneous remission of their disease.

Transient Erythroblastopenia of Childhood

TEC is a disorder marked by an acquired defect of bone marrow red cell production. When available, hemoglobin values are normal prior to the onset of the anemia. TEC occurs at a mean age of 18 to 24 months, and its precise cause is unknown. Seasonal clustering of TEC has been observed in several studies, suggesting a common viral origin. However, a common viral association has not been demonstrated. Patients with TEC do not have congenital anomalies or exhibit growth retardation. Like patients with Blackfan-Diamond anemia, patients with TEC have a normochromic anemia with reticulocytopenia. Hemoglobin values of 4 to 5 gm/dl are not unusual. However, unlike Blackfan-Diamond anemia, TEC spontaneously remits in the majority of patients within a few weeks to months from the time of diagnosis. Corticosteroids are not beneficial in this disorder. Treatment is generally supportive, but patients with severe anemia may require RBC transfusion.

Hemolytic Anemias

The hemolytic anemias are defined by the combination of normocytic red cell indices and reticulocytosis in the absence of bleeding. RBC destruction may be caused by factors extrinsic to the red cell (antibody-mediated hemolysis or mechanical red cell fragmentation) or factors intrinsic to the red cell (membranopathy, enzymopathy, or hemoglobinopathy). Extrinsic factors producing hemolysis are generally acquired, whereas intrinsic red cell abnormalities are typically inherited. Antibody-mediated anemia, or immune hemolytic anemia (IHA), results from the production of antibodies by the patient against RBC surface antigens directly or against viral antigens, medications, or other factors; these antibodies are then bound to the red cell. These antibodies may be of the immunoglobulin G (IgG) or M (IgM) classes. IgG antibodies usually interact better with RBCs at 37°C than at lower temperatures and are therefore referred to as *warm-reacting antibodies*. IgM antibody is generally directed against the I antigen on the RBC membrane. Cold temperatures favor the interaction of the IgM antibody with the I-group RBC antigen and hence the designation *cold agglutinin*. The IgG (warm) IHA is seen in 70% to 90% of patients with antibody-mediated hemolysis, whereas the IgM (cold) IHA accounts for the remaining 10% to 30%. Acute forms of both the warm and cold IHAs generally follow acute viral infections or are idiopathic in nature. Chronic IHAs are frequently associated with collagen vascular disease, immunodeficiency, or lymphoreticular malignancy.

The Coombs' test will be positive in most patients with IHA. A direct Coombs' test is a measure of red cell agglutination that occurs following addition of anti-human gamma globulin (Coombs' reagent). A positive Coombs' test indicates the presence of auto-antibody bound to the red cell membrane. This is true for both IgG and IgM types of IHA.

The clinical severity of antibody-mediated hemolysis is highly variable. In addition to varying degrees of anemia and reticulocytosis, spherocytes may be present on the peripheral blood smear. Spherocytes are RBCs that have lost membrane function, resulting in an alteration of the RBC surface volume. Red cells therefore appear rounder and somewhat more dense on the peripheral blood smear.

Patients with IgG IHA will generally respond to corticosteroids. Prednisone in a dosage of 2 mg/kg/day is generally effective and should be continued until the hemoglobin and reticulocyte counts approach normal. Alternative therapies for patients who do not respond to steroid therapy include splenectomy, immunosuppressive therapies, intravenous gamma globulin, or plasmapheresis.

RBC destruction may also occur in association with systemic diseases, leading to fibrin deposition within small blood vessels. These microangiopathic hemolytic anemias are notable for the presence of schistocytes or fragmented RBCs on the peripheral blood smear. Disseminated intravascular coagulation, the hemolytic-uremic syndrome, and thrombotic thrombocytopenic purpura are examples of diseases causing microangiopathic hemolytic anemias. The severity and duration of the hemolytic component frequently correspond to the severity of the underlying disease process. Treatment is focused on the underlying disease process.

Hereditary Erythrocyte Membrane Disorders

Intrinsic RBC abnormalities resulting in hemolytic anemia include disorders of hemoglobin structure, membrane structure, or enzyme function. Examples of RBC membrane disorders resulting in hemolytic anemia include hereditary spherocytosis and hereditary elliptocytosis. Episodic pallor, jaundice, splenomegaly, and anemia (negative direct Coombs' test) with reticulocytosis are seen to varying degrees in each of these membrane defects.

Spherocytosis. Hereditary spherocytosis is the most common form of the red cell membrane defect. It is estimated to be present in approximately 1 per 5000 persons. Although it is especially common in persons of Northern European ancestry, it has been reported in all population groups. It is inherited in an autosomal dominant pattern. A history of episodic anemia, jaundice, cholelithiasis, or splenectomy will be evident in approximately 75% of first-degree relatives. More than half of those affected will present in the neonatal period with a hemolytic crisis and severe hyperbilirubinemia.

In this disorder, the spherocyte is believed to result from a deficiency of spectrin, a protein component of the RBC membrane skeleton. This in turn produces a loss of surface membrane and a reduction in RBC surface volume. Sphered RBCs are smaller than normal red cells, stain more densely, and lack the normal central pallor. An incubated osmotic fragility test (hypotonic lysis) confirms the presence of spherocytes, suggesting hereditary spherocytosis, although spherocytes associated with the IHAs may produce a positive result as well. The Coombs' test will aid in distinguishing these two conditions. Spherocytes function normally but are selectively trapped in the spleen because of their abnormal shape. As a result, splenectomy will correct the anemia, reticulocytosis, and jaundice, although the morphologic abnormality will persist. Splenectomy is usually reserved for patients with severe anemia and splenomegaly or those who have repeated aplastic crises.

Elliptocytosis. The clinical features of hereditary elliptocytosis (ovalocytosis) are highly variable. Many patients have a mild subclinical condition that escapes detection, making estimates of prevalence difficult. It is inherited in an autosomal dominant fashion. The precise cause of the membrane defect is unknown. There is no confirmatory test for hereditary elliptocytosis, but the presence of more than 25% elliptical RBCs on the peripheral blood smear of the affected patient and the parent is diagnositc. Splenectomy is reserved for the small percentage of patients with severe anemia.

Red Cell Enzyme Deficiencies. More than 20 different RBC enzyme deficiencies have been characterized. These enzyme deficiencies may result in reduced RBC survival because of an abnormality in RBC glucose metabolism or an enhanced susceptibility of the RBC to oxidative stresses. The most common of these disorders are represented by deficiencies of the enzymes glucose-6-phosphate dehydrogenase (G6PD) and pyruvate kinase (PK).

G6PD Deficiency. G6PD deficiency is an X-linked disorder. A number of variants possess normal enzyme activity and stability and therefore cause no clinical symptoms. Other mutations, however, possess little activity and are very unstable. The A⁻ variant (G6PDA⁻), which is seen in approximately 10% of black males, functions normally but is unstable. Hemolysis occurs only after severe oxidative stresses such as that posed by antimalarial medications. Normal dosages of other oxidant medications such as salicylates or sulfonamides generally do not cause problems. In contrast, the Mediterranean G6PD variant, G6PDB⁺, possesses less than 5% of normal activity and is very unstable. In this variant, potentially life-threatening hemolysis may follow exposure to an oxidative stress. Agents posing such an oxidant stress include phenacetin, sulfonamides, nitrofurans, antimalarials, and salicylates. Acute episodes of hemolysis are marked by pallor, anemia, reticulocytosis, hyperbilirubinemia, and hemoglobinuria. Heinz body RBC inclusions may be apparent on the peripheral blood smear. The diagnosis is confirmed by G6PD assay. Proper management includes identification of the G6PD deficiency and withdrawal or avoidance of oxidant medications.

Pyruvate Kinase Deficiency. Although relatively rare, pyruvate kinase deficiency is the most common abnormality of the Embden-Meyerhof glycolytic pathway. It is inherited in an autosomal recessive manner and is most frequently seen in people of Northern European ancestry. The clinical manifestations vary greatly from death in utero associated with severe fetal hydrops to low-grade chronic hemolysis. Splenomegaly generally develops in infancy. Diagnosis is confirmed by direct assay of pyruvate kinase activity.

MACROCYTIC ANEMIAS

Red cells are considered to be macrocytic when the MCV exceeds the mean MCV plus two standard deviations. Macrocytosis can be seen in conditions producing reticulocytosis, as well as in aplastic anemias. These conditions are contrasted with the macrocytic anemias associated with folate and vitamin B_{12} deficiency. The peripheral blood smear in folate and vitamin B_{12} deficiencies reveals macro-ovalocytes, nucleated RBCs, Howell-Jolly bodies, and hypersegmented polymorphonuclear leukocytes.

Folic Acid Deficiency

Folic acid deficiency rarely occurs because of the widespread use of vitamin-fortified infant formulas and vitamin supplements. Situations that may predispose to folate deficiency include poor dietary intake and malabsorption. Folate is present in a wide variety of foods including meats (liver), eggs, green vegetables, and whole-grain cereals. A diet that is poor in these items may lead to folate deficiency and anemia. A proper diet is especially important at times of increased need for folate, such as during periods of rapid growth, or in patients with chronic hemolytic anemias.

Folate deficiency may also occur from malabsorption associated with small-bowel disease. Inhibition of folate absorption may occur in patients taking phenytoin, oral contraceptives, or trimethoprim. Chemotherapeutic agents, especially methotrexate, may interfere with metabolic activation of folate. The diagnosis of folate deficiency is established in patients with macrocytic anemia by measurement of the serum folic acid concentration. Treatment should include 1 mg/day of folic acid until hematologic parameters normalize (see Table 59–6).

Vitamin B_{12} Deficiency

Vitamin B_{12} deficiency occurs rarely in children but may be associated with pernicious anemia, congenital absence of intrinsic factor, or malabsorption associated with ileal disease. In addition to the characteristic findings on the peripheral blood smear and bone marrow, neurologic symptoms associated with diminished position and vibratory sensation (posterior column dysfunction) may be present.

Diagnosis is confirmed by measurement of serum vitamin B_{12} concentrations. Treatment requires the use of parenteral vitamin B_{12} initially at 500 μg/day intramuscularly for 10 days to restore tissue levels. Maintenance injections of 500 μg of vitamin B_{12} should subsequently be administered every 2 months. The anemia generally resolves 1 to 2 months after the start of parenteral treatment.

DISPOSITION

Asymptomatic patients with mild anemia (hemoglobin concentration greater than 8 to 10 gm/dl) may be evaluated and treated as outpatients in most cases. However, hospitalization should be considered for newly diagnosed patients with moderate to severe anemia (hemoglobin concentration less than 8 gm/dl); patients with an acute or chronic anemia who demonstrate irritability, fatigue, dizziness, weakness, shortness of breath, or signs of congestive heart failure; patients with a chronic anemia and a hemoglobin concentration less than 5 gm/dl; patients with a transfusion-dependent anemia; and patients with significant underlying systemic illness. The duration of hospitalization and the timing of posthospitalization follow-up will be directed by the cause and severity of the anemia and the initial response to therapy.

Selected References

Burstein Y, Berns L. Acquired immune hemolytic anemia in children. Pediatr Ann 1982;11:310.

Cartwright GE, Lee GR. The anaemia of chronic disorders. Br J Haematol 1971;21:147.

Crowley C, Necheles TF. Hereditary disorders of the erythrocyte. Clin Perinatol 1976;3:161.

Dessypris EN, Krantz SB, Roloff JS, et al. Mode of action of the IgG inhibitor of erythropoiesis in transient erythroblastopenia of childhood. Blood 1982;59:114.

Diamond LK, Wang WC, Alter BP. Congenital hypoplastic anemia. Adv Pediatr 1976;22:349.

Gilman PA. Hemolysis in the newborn infant resulting from deficiencies of red blood cell enzymes: Diagnosis and management. J Pediatr 1974;84:625.

Glader BE. Diagnosis and management of red cell aplasia in children. Hematol Oncol Clin North Am 1987;1:431.

Glader BE. Screening for anemia and erythrocyte disorders in children. Pediatrics 1986;78:368.

Habibi B, Homberg JC, Schaison G, et al. Autoimmune hemolytic anemia in children. Am J Med 1974;56:61.

Jansson LT, Kling S, Dallman PR. Anemia in children with acute infections seen in a primary care setting. Pediatr Infect Dis 1986;5:424.

Johnson CS, Tegos C, Beutler E. Routine erythrocyte measurements and differentiation from iron deficiency. Am J Clin Pathol 1983;80:31.

Labotka RJ, Mauer HS, Honig GR. Transient erythroblastopenia of childhood. Am J Dis Child 1981;135:937.

Monson CM, Beaver DB, Ditton TB. Evaluation of erythrocyte disorders with mean corpuscular volume (MCV) and red cell distribution width (RDW). Clin Pediatr 1987;26:632.

Novak RW. Red blood cell distribution width in pediatric microcytic anemias. Pediatrics 1987;80:251.

Oski FA, Sardowitz PO, Helm B. The red cell volume distribution (RDW) and the diagnosis of iron deficiency. Pediatr Res 1985;19:265A.

Reeves JD. Iron supplementation in infancy. Pediatr Rev 1986;8:177.

Reeves JD, Vichinsky E, Addrego J, et al. Iron deficiency in health and disease. Adv Pediatr 1983;30:281.

Segel GB. Anemia. Pediatr Rev 1988;10:77.

Stockman JA. Using electronic RBC counts to diagnose anemia. Contemp Pediatr 1989;6:99.

Zupanska B. Autoimmune hemolytic anaemia in children. Br J Haematol 1976;34:511.

CHAPTER 60

Sickle Cell Hemoglobinopathy

Earl J. Reisdorff

INTRODUCTION

Sickle cell anemia is an autosomal recessive hemoglobinopathy caused by a single amino acid substitution: valine for glutamic acid in the sixth position of the globin beta chain.[1] The resulting abnormal hemoglobin polymerizes or "crystallizes" in the presence of relative hypoxemia (Fig. 60–1). When the hemoglobin polymerizes within the erythrocyte, the cell changes from a biconcave disc into a sickle-shaped cell. This causes the cell to lose its flexibility. The fragile sickled cells are prone to fragmentation and produce sludging in capillary beds.

The heterozygous sickle cell *trait* (hemoglobin AS) is found in 8% to 10 % of North American blacks. The homozygous state, sickle cell *disease* (hemoglobin SS), occurs in 1 in 400 to 600 black newborns. Sickle cell hemoglobinopathies are also found in other races originating from malaria-endemic regions.[2] In the United States, more than 50,000 people are affected, and 1500 infants with sickle cell hemoglobinopathies are born annually.[3, 4]

Children with sickle cell disease (Hb SS) develop chronic

anemia, episodic pain, and both structural and physiologic organ dysfunction and have an increased susceptibility to infections. An anemia is present by 6 to 9 months of age. Those with sickle cell trait have both the abnormal hemoglobin S (35% to 45% of the total hemoglobin) and the normal hemoglobin A (55% to 65% of the total hemoglobin). Though hematuria, splenic infarction, and vaso-occlusive crises have been reported in patients with sickle cell trait, these occurrences are rare.[6] Patients with sickle cell trait have a normal life expectancy.

Sickle cell disease is associated with considerable mortality; 20% to 30% of deaths occur before the age of 5 years, with a median age at death of 14 years. Current survival is much improved as a result of infection prophylaxis and advances in therapy. However, the highest mortality rate occurs in children between 1 and 3 years old, with bacterial infection being the leading cause of death (Fig. 60–2, Table 60–1).[7]

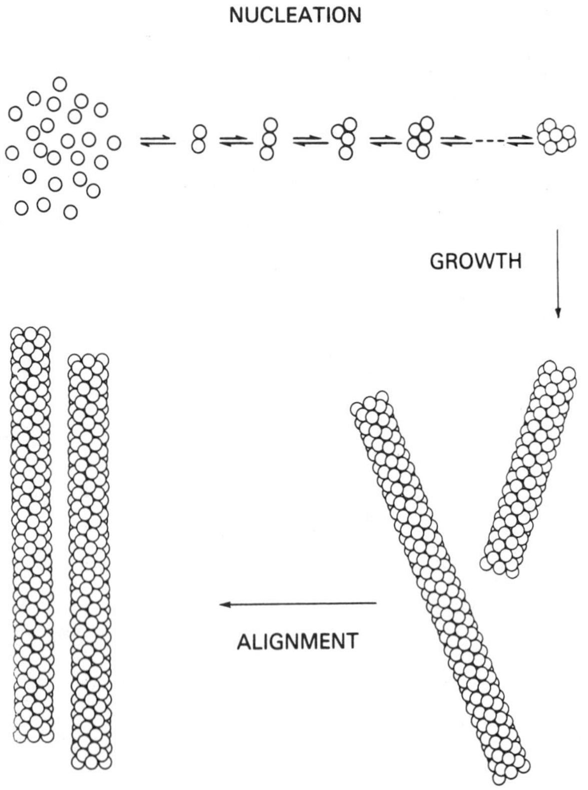

MICROSCOPIC PHYSIOLOGY

Hemoglobin S contains two normal alpha chains and two abnormal beta chains as a consequence of the valine–glutamic acid substitution. Hemoglobin S functions similarly to hemoglobin A in the presence of oxygen. In the hypoxemic state, the deoxygenated hemoglobin S responds differently. The hemoglobin tetramers form long strands of crystallized hemoglobin. Similar polymerization occurs with low pH or elevated 2,3-diphosphoglyceric concentrations. Sickling is inhibited by hemoglobin F. The process of crystallization is usually reversed with reoxygenation of the hemoglobin molecule.

With hemoglobin crystallization and the formation of the flexible sickled shape, red cell transit time is increased, producing sludging in the capillary bed. This leads to occlusion of small blood vessels and decreased flow. Ultimately, localized tissue ischemia occurs. The microcirculatory hypoxia may be severe enough to cause tissue infarction and necrosis.

As cells containing hemoglobin S circulate, they undergo many cycles of sickling and unsickling as they pass through the capillary beds. During these cycles, some part of the membrane may fragment and become lost. These cells are permanently deformed and are at risk for rupture because of their extreme fragility. In addition, some cells remain irreversibly sickled (4% to 44%) despite high oxygen tensions.[5, 8]

NUCLEATION

GROWTH

ALIGNMENT

Figure 60–1. Possible mechanism for deoxyhemoglobin S polymerization. (From Dean J, Schechter AN. Sickle-cell anemia: Molecular and cellular bases of therapeutic approach. N Engl J Med 1978;299:761. Reprinted by permission of The New England Journal of Medicine.)

TABLE 60–1

DEATHS IN PATIENTS WITH SICKLE HEMOGLOBINOPATHIES (COOPERATIVE STUDY OF SICKLE CELL DISEASE [CSSCD] ENTRANCE WHEN YOUNGER THAN 20 YEARS OF AGE)

Cause	No. of Patients (%)
Bacterial infection	28 (38.4)
Cerebrovascular accident	9 (12.3)
Other	
Sickle cell disease related	8 (11.0)
Non–sickle cell disease related	
Trauma	5 (6.8)
Other	4 (5.5)
Unknown	
Died outside CSSCD center	14 (19.2)
Died at CSSCD center	
Autopsy not performed	3 (4.1)
Autopsy performed	2 (2.7)

From Leiken SL, Gallagher D, Kinney TR, et al. Mortality in children and adolescents with sickle cell disease. Pediatrics 1989;84:504. Reproduced by permission of Pediatrics.

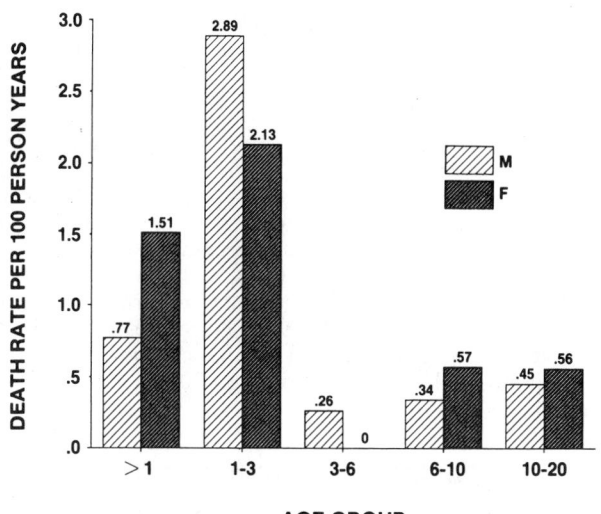

Figure 60–2. Death rates in patients with Hb SS by sex who were entered in the Cooperative Study of Sickle Cell Disease at less than 20 years of age. (From Leiken SL, Gallagher D, Kinney TR, et al. Mortality in children and adolescents with sickle cell disease. Pediatrics 1989;84:503. Reproduced by permission of Pediatrics.)

Patterns of pain during vaso-occlusive crises vary among patients. About 20% of patients with sickle cell disease have frequent and severe vaso-occlusive episodes, with about 10% to 15% of all sickle cell patients requiring frequent hospitalization because of pain crises. Thirty percent of patients rarely have vaso-occlusive pain, and the remaining 50% with sickle cell disease may have one severe crisis each year or multiple mild crises.[9]

PATHOPHYSIOLOGY
Vaso-occlusive Crisis

The vaso-occlusive crisis ("pain crisis") is a frequent problem that brings patients with sickle cell disease to the emergency department. A vaso-occlusive crisis is precipitated by capillary sludging and, ultimately, tissue ischemia. Pain is the characteristic feature of a vaso-occlusive episode. Although it frequently starts in an extremity, it can be felt in any part of the body.

A vaso-occlusive crisis may be precipitated by high-altitude exposure or other forms of hypoxia, cold exposure (especially swimming in cold water), dehydration, acidosis, fatigue, stress, menses, or infections. In children, an acute viral illness precedes more than 80% of vaso-occlusive crises. Some patients wake from sleep with pain, though they were pain free when they went to bed. There are also conflicting reports regarding the influence of seasonal and weather changes in precipating vaso-occlusive crises. Despite these precipitating factors, however, in many cases, an obvious precipitant may not be determined.

Young children tend to have pain in the limbs during a vaso-occlusive crisis, whereas adolescents more commonly develop pain in the abdomen.[10] When the musculoskeletal system is involved in a vaso-occlusive crisis, the pain is usually constant, following a pattern similar to previous episodes. Infants commonly present with *sickle dactylitis*, or hand-foot syndrome, which occurs from ischemia in the bone marrow in the extremities.

The severity of pain may vary from a barely discernible ache to an intense, debilitating pain. The severity of pain tends to worsen with age in males until the age of 30 years,

when there is a decline in the number of vaso-occlusive episodes.[11] The duration of pain for a given episode ranges from hours to weeks and follows a variable pattern of temporal clustering.

Because infections can precipitate vaso-occlusive crises, determining the presence of an infection is critical. Pain crises are often accompanied by a low-grade fever and leukocytosis. However, a temperature above 38.4°C (101°F) or an absolute band cell count greater than 300 cells/mm^3 is more likely to be associated with an infection than with tissue ischemia.

Aplastic Crisis

The average hemoglobin in a child with sickle cell anemia is 7.5 gm/dl with a range of 5.5 to 9.5 gm/dl. (Table 60–2). A chronic hemolytic anemia exists because of the fragility of the red blood cells (RBC). A precipitous fall in hemoglobin is usually the result of an aplastic crisis or a splenic sequestration crisis.

The most common cause of an acute aplastic (anemic) crisis is infection-induced bone marrow depression of erythropoiesis (e.g., parvovirus infection). Other causes include folate deficiency and drug toxicity (phenylbutazone). The period of diminished RBC production usually lasts from days to several weeks. Even a brief period of aplasia can be life threatening, as the RBC life span for a sickling cell is already shortened from a normal of 120 days to 20 days. The hallmark of an aplastic crisis is a reticulocyte count below 3% (usually the reticulocyte count is about 12%).

An aplastic crisis can occur at any age. A patient with an aplastic crisis requires close monitoring, even if the hemoglobin appears to be adequate, because the hemoglobin may fall precipitously within a few days.

Infections

Bacterial infection poses a serious threat to the child with sickle cell anemia.[12] In the first 10 years of life, the most common infections are bacteremia, pneumonia, osteomyelitis, meningitis, and urinary tract infections.[13] The primary pathogens are the encapsulated organisms: *Streptococcus pneumoniae, Haemophilus influenzae, Escherichia coli,* and *Staphylococcus aureus. Mycoplasma* pulmonary infections are also seen.

The increased risk of infection results from splenic infarction. Splenic infarction may occur as early as 5 months of age and is routine by 5 years of age. The susceptibility to bacterial infections results from deficient antibody formation and impaired phagocytosis.[14, 15] In addition, serum IgM levels are decreased and the complement activation system is defective.

An infectious crisis can be rapidly overwhelming, especially in children younger than 5 years. During the first 5

TABLE 60–2

MEAN LABORATORY VALUES AND RANGES FOR PATIENTS WITH SICKLE CELL ANEMIA

	Mean	Range
Hemoglobin	7.5 gm/dl	5.5–9.5 mg/dl
Hematocrit	22%	17.0–29.0 gm/dl
Reticulocyte count	12.0%	5.0–30.0%
White blood cell count	13,000/mm^3	12,000–15,000/mm^3

From Zurcher RL, Hamilton GC. Sickle cell disease. *In* Hamilton GC, Sanders AB, Strange GR, Trott AT (eds). Emergency Medicine: An Approach to Clinical Problem-Solving. Philadelphia, WB Saunders, 1991, p 462.

years of life, *Streptococcus pneumoniae* is the primary pathogen, and sepsis from this organism is the most common cause of death. The middle ear and lungs are frequent primary sites of infection. After 5 years of age, gram-negative organisms cause infections more frequently.

H. influenzae infections, which are more common in sickle cell patients compared with other children,[16] tend to have a more insidious course than *S. pneumoniae*.

Bacterial pneumonia is 100 times more common in sickle cell patients than in the general population, and hypoxia, often caused by pneumonia, exacerbates sickling. Though the most common organisms causing pneumonia are *S. pneumoniae* and *H. influenzae*, *Mycoplasma* infections are also common, especially in patients who fail empiric antibiotic therapy. Viral infections can also occur.

Patients with sickle cell anemia have an increased incidence of osteomyelitis, often caused by *Salmonella* (50%).[17, 18] Osteomyelitis may also be caused by staphylococcal infections.[13] Sickle cell patients are also at increased risk for meningitis and urinary tract infections. In fact, bacterial meningitis and septicemia are 600 times more common in sickle cell patients than in other children.[19]

Splenic Sequestration

Splenic sequestration is characterized by a decrease in the hematocrit of 30%, ongoing erythropoiesis, and an enlarging spleen.[20] With splenic sequestration, the spleen becomes suddenly engorged with RBCs. This rapid engorgement of the spleen creates a relative deficiency of circulating RBCs. Given the preexisting state of anemia in children with sickle cell disease, a sequestration episode may be severe enough to cause shock and death. Though the exact mechanism of splenic sequestration is unknown, it is thought to result from vaso-occlusion of the splenic vein. The accompanying splenomegaly is often dramatic. Clinical signs include pallor, weakness, tachycardia, dyspnea, and massive splenomegaly.

Splenic sequestration is usually seen in children less than 5 years because after that age the spleen is frequently too scarred to accommodate this phenomenon. A frequent cause of death in patients less than 5 years old with sickle cell disease, acute splenic sequestration may be the initial presenting condition.[21, 22] Parents should be taught to palpate the spleen to assist in identifying initial splenic enlargement during early sequestration.

A major sequestration crisis is defined by an absolute hemoglobin value of less than 6 gm/dl or a drop in the hemoglobin of greater than 3 gm/dl. A minor sequestration crisis still results in a decrease in the hemoglobin level, but the child has an absolute hemoglobin greater than 6 gm/dl. Because splenic sequestration can be recurrent, splenectomy is often advised for survivors.[23]

Dactylitis

Sickle dactylitis, also known as the *hand-foot syndrome*, is rare after the age of 5 years. It results from vaso-occlusive sludging in the marrow of the bones of the hands and feet. Dactylitis is the most common presentation of sickle cell anemia in children 6 to 24 months of age. The hands and feet become tender, with nonpitting edema resulting from symmetric infarction of the metacarpals and metatarsals. Children often develop a low-grade fever (less than 38.6°C [101.5°F]). There is no decrease in the patient's baseline hemoglobin level. If symptoms of tenderness persist, radiographic signs of osteolytic activity may be seen in 2 to 3 weeks as a result of microinfarction of the bone. One or all four extremities may be affected.

Neurologic Complications

Complications involving the central nervous system occur in 10% to 26% of children with sickle cell disease.[6, 24] Of patients less than 20 years of age who have died from sickle cell–related causes, 12.3% died from a cerebrovascular accident (CVA).[7] Although a vaso-occlusive crisis involving the brain can be painless, the patient may complain of a headache, hemiparesis, or cranial nerve palsy. In addition, the patient may present with an altered mental status or seizures. The mean age at onset of a CVA is 10 years. CVAs in younger children are usually ischemic; intercranial bleeding is more common in older patients. Nevertheless, the vaso-occlusive events that occur in young children may later predispose the adolescent and young adult to subarachnoid hemorrhage.

Cardiovascular Complications

Because the child with sickle cell disease has chronic anemia, the cardiovascular system compensates with an increased cardiac output. Therefore patients with sickle cell disease may have a chronically elevated cardiac output without congestive heart failure. However, patients are prone to eventual development of congestive heart failure.

Genitourinary Complications

Priapism is a painful, prolonged, involuntary penile erection. In sickle cell disease, it is associated with sludging within the penile cavernous sinuses, thereby diminishing the outflow of blood from the penis. Episodes lasting more than 3 hours are unlikely to resolve spontaneously.

Priapism can result in impotence and decreased fertility.[25] Impotence results from chronic scarring of erectile tissue and occurs in as many as 80% of patients.

Renal complications from sickle cell disease include the inability to concentrate the urine (isosthenuria), painless hematuria, and renal papillary necrosis. Other complications that occur with increased frequency include urinary tract infections, hyperuricemia, and chronic renal failure.

Abdominal Complications

Abdominal pain is a common presentation of sickle cell disease, especially during a vaso-occlusive crisis. It can be extremely difficult to discern whether the abdominal pain is caused by the vaso-occlusive crisis or by a surgically correctible condition. Liver, splenic, and mesenteric infarctions occur. Abdominal guarding and rebound can be present in a vaso-occlusive crisis. However, bowel sounds are typically present with a vaso-occlusive crisis and absent with an acute abdomen.

Because of increased RBC turnover, bilirubin gallstones commonly form. This can lead to biliary colic or a gallstone ileus. Acute cholecystitis can occur at any age. Although 30% of children have pigmented gallstones, less than 10% are symptomatic.[4] However, some authors have challenged the notion that most gallstones in sickle cell disease are silent.[26]

EMS CONSIDERATIONS

The major task of EMS personnel in caring for the patient with sickle cell disease is to identify serious complications such as sepsis, a CVA, or an acute abdomen. Oxygen therapy is not required in the field for a routine vaso-occlusive crisis. However, in patients with respiratory distress, oxygen given at 4 to 6 L/min by nasal cannula is indicated. Intravenous fluid, although important in the emergency department, is not essential in the prehospital setting unless hypovolemia is suspected. Cardiac monitoring should be performed if the patient is having chest pain. Analgesics should not be routinely given. The use of prehospital analgesia may alter the critical initial physical examination by the emergency department physician.

DIFFERENTIAL DIAGNOSIS

The most critical part of the differential diagnosis in a patient with known sickle cell disease is determining what type of sickle crisis is occurring (aplastic, vaso-occlusive, or splenic sequestration). The rest of the differential diagnosis is symptom oriented. For example, the differential diagnosis for a fever may include an infection. Abdominal pain has a number of causes, some of which are surgically correctible (e.g., appendicitis, biliary colic, pancreatitis). Chest pain can be caused by conditions such as pulmonary infection, myocardial infarction, and pulmonary infarction.

In the child not yet diagnosed with sickle cell disease who presents with painful hands and feet, conditions such as leukemia, osteomyelitis, septic arthritis, Lyme disease, and rheumatologic entities such as juvenile rheumatoid arthritis and rheumatic fever must be excluded. In addition, causes of anemia other than sickle cell disease must be considered (e.g., glucose-6-phosphate dehydrogenase deficiency, thalassemia, congenital hypoplastic anemia).

CLINICAL EVALUATION
History

Most patients with sickle cell disease who come to the emergency department have already been diagnosed. The exception is the infant who first presents with dactylitis, sepsis, or pneumonia. The primary task of the history is to determine whether a life-threatening condition exists and to identify a precipitant, especially if there is an infectious cause. A vaso-occlusive crisis often has a characteristic pain pattern, and deviations from this pattern may indicate a complication such as pulmonary infarction or osteomyelitis. The patient should be questioned regarding any change in mentation or muscle weakness.

The past medical history is significant for determining normal patterns of pain crisis. A surgical history is important in the diagnosis of the sickle cell patient with abdominal pain. In the infant with suspected dactylitis, a family history of sickle cell disease should be explored. The physician should also ask whether a pneumococcal vaccination has been given. In addition, some patients may know their baseline hemoglobin concentration, reticulocyte count, and the most advantageous therapeutic intervention. The patient should also be asked for the presence or absence of headaches, acute joint swelling, or back pain (pyelonephritis). The physician should also obtain the history and pattern of blood transfusions.

Physical Examination

The physical examination should look for evidence of respiratory distress, meningitis, sepsis, splenomegaly, jaundice, localized bone pain, an acute abdomen, costovertebral angle tenderness, and a localized neurologic defect. A temperature greater than 38.4°C (101°F) is indicative of an infection. Hypotension can occur because of splenic sequestration or septic shock. Tachycardia may indicate fever, sepsis, or hypovolemic shock. Tachypnea may indicate pulmonary disease, pulmonary infarction or infection, or acute anemia.

Mucous membranes and conjunctiva should be inspected for pallor, which is suggestive of anemia. Fundoscopy should be performed to assess retinal damage. The physician should inspect for signs of upper respiratory tract infection, especially otitis media. The neck is assessed for meningeal signs, and the heart is examined for a cardiac rub as well as an S_3 gallop resulting from congestive heart failure. The lungs are auscultated for rales, a pleural friction rub, or decreased breath sounds suggesting an infiltrate. The abdomen should be carefully evaluated; active bowel sounds, lack of fever, and absent peritoneal signs suggest a vaso-occlusive crisis. In the preschooler, the spleen should be carefully palpated to determine its size when evaluating for a splenic sequestration crisis.

In the toddler who is not yet diagnosed as having sickle cell disease, the only physical finding may be tenderness and edema in the hands and feet. Limping may suggest aseptic necrosis of the femoral head, which is a relatively common ischemic complication of sickling in late adolescence or adulthood but is rare in younger children. A thorough neurologic examination should be performed to detect focal or generalized neurologic findings.

DIAGNOSTIC EVALUATION
Newborn Screening

Newborn screening programs are dramatically effective in reducing mortality. Cord blood can be used for blood specimens from newborns in the delivery room.[27] Patients who are diagnosed through programs such as these are then enrolled in comprehensive treatment programs. Early detection of patients with sickle cell disease permits prophylactic penicillin therapy, which markedly reduces the incidence of *S. pneumoniae* septicemia and death.[28]

Hemoglobin electrophoresis is the most accurate diagnostic study to determine sickle cell anemia, sickle cell trait, and sickle cell thalassemia. The erythrocytes of individuals who are homozygous for sickle cell disease contain at least 90% hemoglobin S. Patients who are heterozygous for sickle cell gene (sickle cell trait) have both hemoglobin A (50% to 60%) and hemoglobin S.

Sickle Prep

In undiagnosed cases, the emergency physician may need a rapid assay for determining whether sickle cell disease is present. The sickle prep is a peripheral blood smear specially prepared to induce RBC sickling. Although it can be a useful test, it is limited in its ability to diagnose sickle cell disease in infants younger than 4 to 6 months of age, and it cannot diagnose sickle cell trait.

Hemoglobin Measurement

All patients who present to the emergency department with a complaint referrable to sickle cell disease must have their hemoglobin level measured. Patients with sickle cell trait have normal hematologic values. A drop in hemoglobin value of 3 gm/dl suggests major acute splenic sequestration crisis, an uncompensated aplastic crisis, or another possibly unrelated condition (e.g., gastrointestinal hemorrhage).

Reticulocyte Count

Because of the accelerated RBC turnover, reticulocytes appear in the peripheral blood smear. The mean reticulocyte count is 12% in a patient with sickle cell disease. If the reticulocyte count is less than 3%, an aplastic crisis should be considered. An extremely high reticulocyte count can indicate a hemolytic process.

Urinalysis

Urinalysis should be obtained in any patient with a fever or dysuria. RBCs or tissue in the urine may be seen with papillary necrosis. Isosthenuria, the inability to concentrate the urine, is typically present; the urine specific gravity is usually about 1.010. The specific gravity can be relatively low in patients with sickle cell disease, even when they are dehydrated. Urine cultures should be obtained in children with evidence of urinary tract infection.

Arterial Blood Gas Measurement

An arterial blood gas measurement should be obtained in all sickle cell patients with chest pain not following a typical vaso-occlusive crisis pattern.[5] In addition, the patient who is markedly dyspneic should have a blood gas determination. A large arterioalveolar gradient suggests either pulmonary infection or pulmonary infarction. A ventilation-perfusion scan should be considered in these cases, although interpretation can be extremely difficult.

Blood Cultures

Blood cultures should be obtained in patients with a temperature higher than 38.4°C (101°F) and in those patients suspected of being bacteremic or septic. The child with radiographic evidence of a pulmonary infection should also have blood cultures drawn.

Radiologic Studies

Patients with chest pain, dyspnea, or suspected pneumonia should have a chest radiograph performed. Extremity radiographs should be obtained in patients in whom ischemic necrosis of the femoral or humeral heads is suspected.

Avascular necrosis of the femoral head occurs in 12% of patients. Small lytic lesions can also be seen on plain radiographs in patients with sickle dactylitis. A bone scan can determine the presence of osteomyelitis and should be considered in patients with bony pain that does not resolve after other symptoms of vaso-occlusive crisis abate or in patients with joint or bone discomfort that is atypical for their vaso-occlusive crisis.

A lumbar puncture should be obtained when meningitis is a consideration. Patients with sickle cell disease are at much greater risk for developing meningitis. A computed tomographic (CT) or magnetic resonance imaging (MRI) scan should be considered in patients with lateralizing neurologic signs or new neurologic deficits.

Abdominal radiographs should be obtained in the patient with abdominal pain that does not resolve with rehydration and analgesia, is accompanied by leukocytosis, or is without bowel sounds when a surgically correctable cause is suspected. In patients with right upper quadrant pain, an ultrasound of the gallbladder is indicated to exclude the possibility of biliary obstruction from bilirubin gallstones.

THERAPEUTIC INTERVENTION
Intravenous Fluids

Sickle cell patients are frequently dehydrated as a result of poor fluid intake, inability to produce hyperosmotic urine, and elevated insensible fluid losses when a fever is present. Intravenous fluid therapy is essential for the treatment of vaso-occlusive crisis. Fluids should be promptly administered. A 10-ml/kg intravenous bolus of isotonic crystalloid solution (normal saline [NS] or lactated Ringer's [LR]) should be given. Fluids are then maintained at 1.5 to 2.0 times the usual maintenance therapy using D5/.2NS. Slightly hyponatremic fluids can decrease the mean corpuscular hemoglobin concentration, which interferes with the ability of hemoglobin S to polymerize. If the patient is in shock from an aplastic crisis or splenic sequestration, fluid resuscitation should be aggressive.

TABLE 60–3

RECOMMENDED INITIAL DOSE AND INTERVAL OF ANALGESICS NECESSARY TO OBTAIN ADEQUATE PAIN CONTROL IN SICKLE CELL DISEASE

	Max Dose (mg)	Route*	Interval	Comments
Severe pain				
Morphine	0.10–0.15 mg/kg/dose (max 10 mg)	SC, IM	q 3 hr	Drug of choice
Merperidine	1.5 mg/kg/dose (max 100 mg)	IM	q 3 hr	Increased incidence of seizures; avoid in patients with renal or neurologic disease
Moderate pain				
Oxycodone (Percocet or Percodan)	1 to 2 tabs/dose (1 tab = 5 mg)	po	q 4 hr	Patients over age 5
Methadone	0.15 mg/kg/dose	po	q 6 hr	Effective in patients usually requiring parenteral narcotics. NOT FOR ROUTINE USE.
Meperidine	1.5 mg/kg/dose (max 100 mg/dose)	po	q 3½ hr	
Mild pain				
Codeine	0.75 mg/kg/dose	po	q 4 hr	May be effective up to 6 hr
Aspirin	1.5 gm/m²/24 hr divided into six doses	po	q 4 hr	May be given with a narcotic for added analgesia
Acetaminophen	1.5 gm/m²/24 hr divided into six doses	po	q 4 hr	May be given with a narcotic for added analgesia
Ibuprofen (Motrin)	300 to 600 mg/dose	po	q 6 hr	

*Continuous intravenous infusion of narcotic provides excellent pain control but should be performed only by institutions familiar with its use.
IM = Intramuscular; po = per os (by mouth); SC = subcutaneous.
From Vichinsky E, Lubin BH: Sickle cell anemia. Hematol Oncol Clin North Am 1987; 1:492.

Oxygen

Oxygen is commonly given to patients with vaso-occlusive crises. The effectiveness of oxygen in this setting is unclear, but for the brief time that the patient is in the emergency department 2 to 4 L of oxygen delivered by nasal cannula is unlikely to have any untoward effect. Prolonged oxygen therapy, however, can decrease erythropoiesis.[29]

Patients who are in shock, septic, or having a splenic sequestration crisis require oxygen therapy. Any patient who has chest pain, respiratory distress, or confirmed hypoxia (especially with $PaO_2 < 70$ mm Hg) should be given oxygen. Oxygen saturations can be followed by pulse oximetry.

Analgesia

Drug addiction is an infrequent problem among sickle cell patients, but physicians tend to be concerned about drug addiction in sickle cell patients who are given narcotic analgesics. More often, however, analgesia therapy given for the vaso-occlusive crisis is inadequate. Because analgesics can mask other conditions, it is important to exclude such conditions before diagnosing a patient as having a vaso-occlusive crisis and administering narcotic analgesics.

The preferred parenteral narcotic for a vaso-occlusive crisis is morphine (0.10 to 0.15 mg/kg given every 3 hours) (Table 60–3). Multiple doses of meperidine are generally avoided because of its short duration of action and seizures associated with the metabolic by-product normeperidine.[30] Normeperidine has poor analgesic activity and has been associated with CNS excitation.[31, 32] In addition, in one study, despite receiving equal amounts of meperidine intramuscularly, sickle cell patients had lower serum concentrations of the drug than control patients.[33]

Oral analgesics can be extremely effective in controlling pain and potentially decreasing hospital admission rates.[34, 35] For mild pain, oral aspirin, acetaminophen, or codeine may be appropriate. When drug abuse is a concern, the physician can contract with patients to limit narcotic use during pain crises. Alternative regimens include using the narcotic agonist-antagonist butorphanol or a long-acting narcotic such as methadone. Some painful vaso-occlusive crises can be managed on an outpatient basis using oral opiates such as hydromorphone, oxycodone, and methadone.[34, 36]

Antibiotics

Meningitis is 600 times more likely in a patient with sickle cell disease than in the general population.[19] Bacterial pneumonia is 100 times more common in sickle cell patients. A child with a temperature of 38.4°C (101°F) or greater needs to have blood cultures obtained immediately, and as soon as this has been done, antibiotics to cover for *S. pneumoniae* and *H. influenzae* are given. Initial choices of antibiotics include amoxicillin, cefotaxime, and cefuroxime. If a specific site of infection can be identified (e.g., osteomyelitis, urinary tract infection), the antibiotic therapy plan should address the particular organ system.

Pneumococcal sepsis in children with sickle cell disease has a 14% mortality rate. Penicillin prophylaxis is one of the most effective interventions to decrease the incidence of sepsis and death in children 6 months to 5 years old. Prophylactic penicillin therapy is started at age 3 to 4 months and continued until at least age 5 years. The beginning oral dose is 125 mg twice daily,[29] and from age 3 years to 5 years the oral dose is 250 mg twice daily. If the child is febrile, the parents should be asked about compliance to prophylactic antibiotics.

Because *S. pneumoniae* and *H. influenzae* are the primary pathogens involved in infections among sickle cell patients, an excellent drug choice is cefuroxime at a dose of 150 mg/kg/day. For meningitis, as much as 200 to 240 mg/kg/day of cefuroxime can be given intravenously in divided doses every 6 to 8 hours. Generally, cefuroxime (50 mg/kg intravenous piggyback) can be given in the emergency department; for the child who appears to be markedly septic, a dose of 75 mg/kg intravenous piggyback can be given. For outpatient management of mild infections, oral antibiotic alternatives include cefaclor or amoxicillin-clavulanate.

Salmonella osteomyelitis can be treated with intravenous trimethoprim-sulfamethoxazole (2.5 mg/kg, based on the trimethoprim component given every 6 hours). As an alternative, ceftriaxone (25.0 to 37.5 mg/kg every 12 hours), which gives better coverage for *S. aureus*, can be given.

Transfusion Therapy

Blood transfusions are given to children undergoing splenic sequestration crises and severe aplastic crises (Table 60–4). In addition, transfusions may be required in the management of a CVA or priapism or for perioperative management prior to surgery. Blood transfusion carries the risk of alloimmunization, human immunodeficiency virus (HIV) and hepatitis infection, volume overload, and, with multiple transfusions, iron overload. Transfusion may also markedly decrease erythropoiesis.

Transfusion therapy can be a difficult decision. Clearly, in the case of acute sequestration crisis with hypotension, blood should be transfused; a hematologist should be consulted emergently to best direct therapy. An initial transfusion of 10 ml/kg of packed RBCs can be started in the emergency department.[37]

Patients with an aplastic crisis may also require a packed RBC transfusion. When aplastic, splenic sequestration, or hemolytic crises occur, exchange transfusion is preferred. Priapism may also require exchange transfusion. For patients with a hemoglobin level greater than 6 gm/dl, transfusion is rarely indicated.

Symptom-Specific Therapy

Priapism

The physician should provide intravenous hydration and pain relief. If priapism is not relieved after 2 to 3 hours, the patient should receive an exchange transfusion. Surgical therapy may be required if an exchange transfusion does not relieve the priapism. The patient must also empty the bladder frequently. Sitting in a tub of warm water may assist in voiding, but a urinary catheter may be required.

TABLE 60–4

INDICATIONS FOR TRANSFUSION IN SICKLE CELL ANEMIA

Severe anemic crises (aplastic, sequestration, hemolytic)
Life-threatening events
Acute, impending, or suspected cerebrovascular accident
Acute progression of lung disease
Preparation for major surgery
Acute priapism with no response to intravenous hydration
Recalcitrant leg ulcers
Pregnancy
Chronic organ failure (cardiac, renal, pulmonary, hepatic)

From Lubin BH, Vichinsky E. Current Therapy in Hematology-Oncology. 3rd ed. Philadelphia, BC Decker, 1988, p 36.

CVA

With an ischemic cerebral infarct the patient may require an exchange transfusion to decrease the level of hemoglobin S to about 30%. This should be done in urgent consultation with the hematologist. For an ischemic CVA, intravenous hydration is also required.

Immunizations

Because infections are commonly associated with sickle cell crises, immunization against infection is a major part of the comprehensive care of the sickle cell patient. The patient should receive all routine childhood immunizations (oral poliovirus vaccine, diphtheria-tetanus-pertussis vaccine, measles-mumps-rubella vaccine, and boosters), as well as the pneumococcal vaccine, the *H. influenzae* vaccine, the hepatitis B vaccine series, and an annual influenza vaccine. In addition, the patient should receive prophylactic penicillin. Antibody response against certain strains of *S. pneumoniae* is minimal in some children. Therefore children who have been immunized are still at some risk for pneumococcal sepsis.[38–40]

DISPOSITION

Patients with sickle cell disease who present to the emergency department must be admitted if myocardial or cerebral ischemia, an acute abdomen (appendicitis), a serious infection (38.4°C temperature), splenic sequestration, or an aplastic crisis is suspected; prolonged priapism exists; or vaso-occlusive crisis does not respond to rehydration and analgesia. Patients with hypoxia and pulmonary infarction also require admission. Those patients with vaso-occlusive crises who do respond to intravenous rehydration and analgesia may be discharged with close follow-up and defined parameters regarding analgesia regimens.

If a patient with vaso-occlusive crisis is discharged home, he or she should be advised to maintain adequate oral hydration, take pain medication (following a 3-day protocol), and return immediately if a fever over 38°C (100.4°F) occurs. (Table 60–5). The patient should also return if the pain worsens, the pattern of pain changes, or the patient starts vomiting. Preschool children should be reevaluated in 24 hours by the emergency physician, private pediatrician, or

---

TABLE 60–6
DOCUMENTATION

1. Chief complaint.
2. Vital signs, including orthostatic blood pressures and accurate temperature.
3. Description of the chief complaint, especially the pattern of pain. Patient should describe whether there are any similarities to or differences from previous vaso-occlusive crises and whether there was any precipitating event (weather changes, activities, presumed infections).
4. Thorough physical examination focusing on chest, abdominal, and neurologic findings. Musculoskeletal examination should also be comprehensive.
5. Hemoglobin and reticulocyte count levels, along with results of other studies deemed necessary (e.g., a chest radiograph should have the interpretation recorded).
6. Therapy administered: intravenous fluids or blood products, bolus volumes and infusion rates, and type of fluid; analgesics given, the type, and dose.
7. The patient's response to therapy.
8. Discharge instructions and follow-up arrangements (date- and time-specific).
9. Discussion with consultants.
10. Indications for admission (if applicable).

hematologist. Careful follow-up instructions must be documented (Table 60–6).

References

1. Ingram VM. Gene mutations in human hemoglobin: The chemical difference between normal and sickle cell hemoglobin. Nature 1957;180:326.
2. Vichinsky EP, Lubin BH. Sickle cell anemia and related hemoglobinopathies. Pediatr Clin North Am 1980;27:429.
3. Kolata G. Panel urges newborn sickle cell screening. News. Science 1987;236:259.
4. Lessin LS, Jensen WN. Sickle cell anemia 1910–1973: An overview. Arch Intern Med 1974;133:529.
5. Lukens JN. Sickle cell disease. Disease Month 1981;27:1.
6. Galloway SJ, Harwood-Nuss AL. Sickle-cell anemia: A review. J Emerg Med 1988;6:213.
7. Leikin SL, Gallagher D, Kinney TR, et al. Mortality in children and adolescents with sickle cell disease. Pediatrics 1989;84:500.
8. Charache S. Advances in the understanding of sickle cell anemia. Hosp Pract 1986;21:173.
9. Greenberg J, Ohene-Frempong K, Halus J, et al. Trial of low doses of aspirin as prophylaxis in sickle cell disease. J Pediatr 1983;102:781.
10. Brozovic M, Anionwu E. Sickle cell disease in Britain. J Clin Pathol 1984;37:1321.
11. Baum KF, Dunn DT, Maude GH, et al. The painful crisis in homozygous sickle cell disease. A study of the risk factors. Arch Intern Med 1987;147:1231.
12. Pegelow C, Powars D, Overturf G. Sickle cell disease. Am J Dis Child 1979;133:448.
13. Zarkowsky H, Gallagher D, Gill F, et al. Bacteremia in sickle cell hemoglobinopathies. J Pediatr 1986;109:579.
14. Pearson HA, Cornelius RA, Schwartz AD, et al. Transfusion-reversible functional asplenia in young children with sickle cell anemia. N Engl J Med 1970;283:334.
15. Pearson HA, Spencer RD, Cornelius EA. Functional asplenia in sickle cell anemia. N Engl J Med 1969;281:923.
16. Powars D, Overturf FG, Turner E. Is there an increased risk of *Haemophilus influenzae* septicemia in children with sickle cell anemia? Pediatrics 1983;71:927.
17. Adeyokunnu AA, Hendrickse RG. Salmonella osteomyelitis in childhood. A report of 63 cases in Nigerian children of whom 57 had sickle cell anemia. Arch Dis Child 1980;55:175.
18. Landesman SH, Rao SP, Ahonkhai VI. Infections in children with sickle cell anemia. Special reference to pneumococcal and salmonella infections. Am J Pediatr Hematol Oncol 1982;4:407.
19. Pitel PA, Harper JL. Sickling syndromes in children. In Harwood-Nuss A, Linden C, Luten RC, et al (eds). The Clinical Practice of Emergency Medicine. Philadelphia, JB Lippincott, 1990, p 724.
20. Solanki DL, Kletter GG, Casto O. Acute splenic sequestration crisis in adults with sickle cell disease. Am J Med 1986;80:985.

TABLE 60–5
DISCHARGE INSTRUCTIONS

1. You have had a vaso-occlusive crisis (pain crisis) caused by your sickle cell disease. It is important that you drink increased amounts of fluids so that you do not become dehydrated.
2. You will receive a prescription for a pain medicine. You should take it as instructed for the next 3 days. If, at the end of 3 days, you are still having pain, you need to see your private pediatrician, call your hematologist, or return to the emergency department.
3. Your temperature must be taken four times a day and any additional time that you feel warm. If your temperature is greater than 100.4°F, you must return to the emergency department immediately.
4. If your pattern of pain changes, the pain increases, you start having new symptoms, or you begin to vomit, you should return to the emergency department promptly.
5. You should call your pediatrician or hematologist tomorrow either to be reevaluated or to schedule a follow-up appointment soon.

21. Johnson FL, Look AT, Cockerman J, et al. Bone marrow transplantation in a patient with sickle cell anemia. N Engl J Med 1984;311:780.
22. Topley AM, Rogers DW, Stevens CG, et al. Acute splenic sequestrations and hypersplenism in the first five years in homozygous sickle cell disease. Arch Dis Child 1981;56:765.
23. Charache SL, Lubin B, Reid CD (eds). Management and Therapy of Sickle Cell Disease. National Institutes of Health publication no 85-2117. Bethesda; MD, US Department of Health and Human Services, 1985.
24. Vichinsky E, Lubin BH. Suggested guidelines for the treatment of children with sickle cell anemia. Hematol Oncol Clin North Am 1978;1:483.
25. Emond A, Holman R, Hayes R, et al. Priapism and impotence in homozygous sickle-cell disease. Arch Intern Med 1980;140:1434.
26. Alexander-Reindorf C, Nwaneri RU, Worrell RG, et al. The significance of gallstones in children with sickle cell anemia. J Natl Med Assoc 1990;82:645.
27. NIH Consensus Development Conference Statement. Newborn screening for sickle cell disease and other hemoglobinopathies, Bethesda, MD, US Government Printing Office, 1987.
28. Gaston MH, Verter JI, Woods G, et al. Prophylaxis with oral penicillin in children with sickle cell anemia. A randomized trial. N Engl J Med 1986;314:1593.
29. Embury SH, Garcia JF, Mohandas N, et al. Effects of oxygen inhalation on endogenous erythropoietin kinetics, erythropoiesis and properties of blood cells in sickle cell anemia. N Engl J Med 1984;311:291.
30. Tang R, Shimomura S, Rotblatt M. Meperidine-induced seizures in sickle-cell patients. Hospital Formulary 1980;15:764.
31. Mather LE, Meffin PJ. Clinical pharmacokinetics of pethidine. Clin Pharmacokinet 1978;3:352.
32. Szeto HH, Inturrisi CE, Houde R, et al. Accumulation of normeperidine, an active metabolite of meperidine, in patients with renal failure of cancer. Ann Intern Med 1977;86:738.
33. Abbuhl S, Jacobson S, Gibson JG. Serum concentration of meperidine in patients with sickle cell crisis. Ann Emerg Med 1986;15:433.
34. Friedman EW, Webber AB, Osborn HH. Oral analgesias for treatment of painful crisis in sickle cell anemia. Ann Emerg Med 1986;15:787.
35. Powers RD. Management protocol for sickle-cell disease patients with acute pain: Impact on emergency department and narcotic use. Am J Emerg Med 1986;4:267.
36. Holman GH. Use of narcotics in sickle cell disease. Letter. Am J Dis Child 1988;142:483.
37. Rao S, Gooden S. Splenic sequestration in sickle-cell disease: Role of transfusion therapy. Am J Pediatr Hematol Oncol 1985;7:298.
38. Ahonkhai VI, Landesman SH, Fikrig SM, et al. Failure of pneumococcal vaccine in children with sickle-cell disease. N Engl J Med 1979;301:26.
39. Broome CV, Facklam RR, Fraser DW. Pneumococcal disease after pneumococcal vaccination: An alternative method to estimate the efficacy of pneumococcal vaccine. N Engl J Med 1980;303:549.
40. Overturf GD, Field R, Edmonds R. Death for type 6 pneumococcal septicemia in vaccinated child with sickle-cell disease. N Engl J Med 1979;300:143.

CHAPTER 61

Pediatric Malignancies

Gert-Paul Walter

ONCOLOGIC EMERGENCIES

Pathologic Fractures (Spontaneous Fractures)

Almost any cancer can metastasize to bone and cause pathologic fractures. In fact, most pathologic fractures are from metastatic lesions, not primary tumors. Even death can occur as a result of acute hypercalcemia from bony metastases.

Vertebrae are the most common site of metastases, followed by ribs, skull, femur, and pelvis. Vertebrae have a rich vascular supply, and the venous drainage is valveless. Most metastases develop in the marrow of the vertebral body.

Pathologic fractures occur when 30% to 50% of the bone is replaced with tumor. Only 50% to 80% of patients complain of pain prior to fracture. Swelling and tenderness is less common. Biopsy of large lesions in which the primary tumor is unknown is important for diagnosis but may cause seeding of the tumor.

Radiographic Evaluation

Radiographs and scintiscans are useful tests to evaluate skeletal metastases. Classic pathologic fractures present with a lytic, blastic, or mixed radiographic appearance.

Three different types of bony destruction are described: (1) large, solitary, well-defined lytic areas, grater than 1 cm, with sharp geographic borders; (2) bone with the moth-eaten appearance of multiple small lytic areas and with ill-defined margins (Fig. 61–1); and (3) multiple small lytic areas, usually less than 1 mm and representing an aggressive tumor. Before the lesion can be seen on radiographs of spongy bone, 40% to 50% of the bone must be destroyed, but less destruction is needed in cortical bone to visualize tumor (Fig. 61–2).

Computed tomography (CT) is useful in assessing the size and extent of a known lesion and is especially helpful for

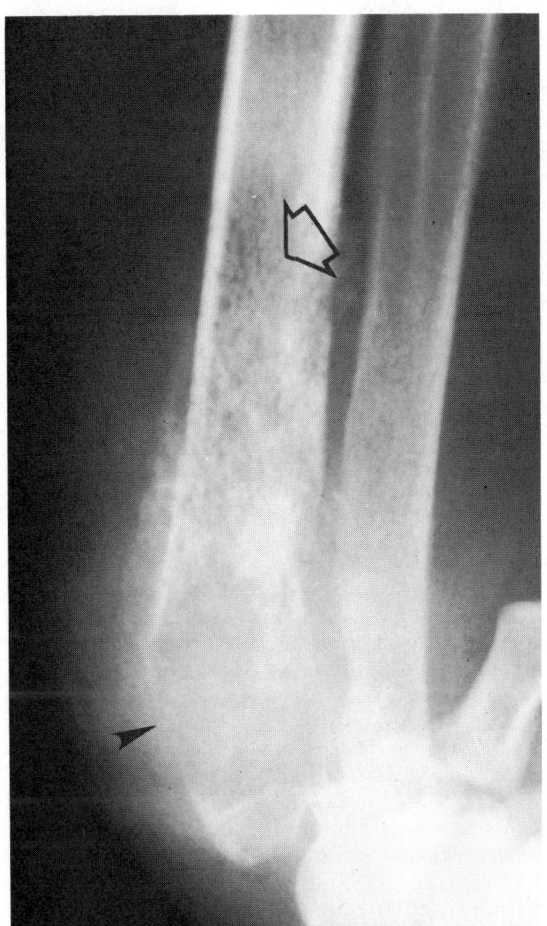

Figure 61–1. Malignant/aggressive characteristics of this canine osteosarcoma that strongly point toward malignant tumor include the *moth-eaten* bone destruction *(open arrow)*, soft tissue tumor bone, poorly defined proximal margin, and the break through the cortex *(arrowhead)*. (Courtesy of A. Oestreich, M.D., Cincinnati, OH.)

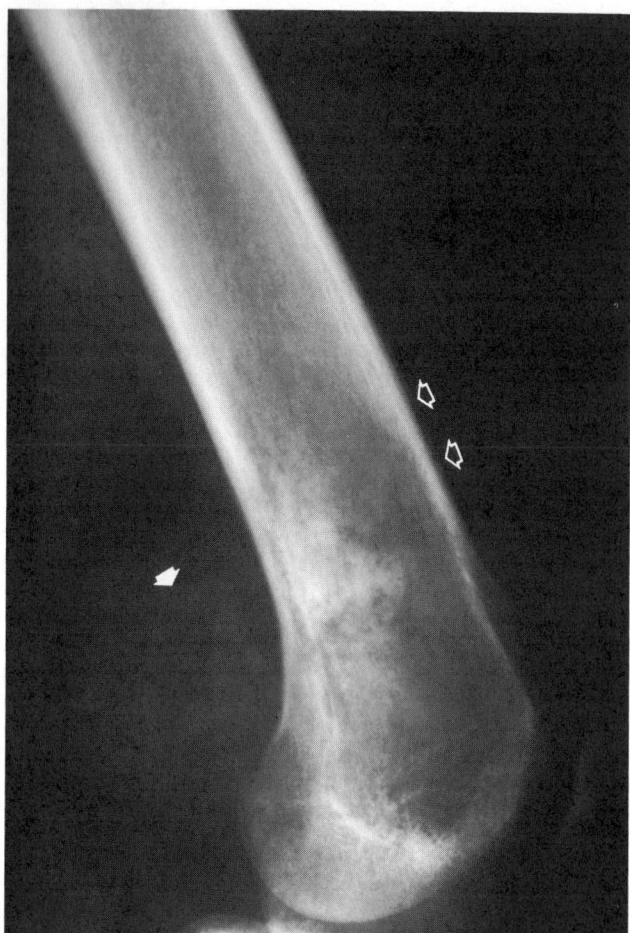

Figure 61–2. Characteristics of the radiograph of this teenager's osteosarcoma that strongly point toward malignant tumor or another highly aggressive lesion include the lack of any well-defined upper margin to the *permeative* bone destruction, the large soft tissue mass with unsharp tumor-bone *(white arrow)*, and the relatively thin periosteal reaction *(open arrows)*. (Courtesy of A. Oestreich, M.D., Cincinnati. Reprinted by permission of the publisher from Oestreich AE. Pediatric Radiology—Medical Outline Series. 3rd ed. New Hyde Park, NY, Medical Examination, 1984. Copyright 1984 by Elsevier Science Publishing Co., Inc.)

fication of the tumor matrix in the medullary cavity and in surrounding soft tissue.

Treatment

In recent years surgical treatment has moved from amputation to prostheses and internal fixation with methylmethacrylate glue. After surgery, irradiation inhibits further tumor growth.

In children up to age 14, periosteal rebuilding of the donor site occurs if autografts (fibula, clavicle, ribs) are used. The autograft itself becomes incorporated into the recipient site.

Ewing's sarcoma and osteosarcoma are the most common primary bone tumors. Pathologic fractures occur in only 2% to 5% of patients with Ewing's sarcoma and osteosarcoma.

Bony changes seen with childhood acute leukemia consist most commonly of osteoporosis, followed by focal osteolytic lesions, periosteal reactions, transverse metaphyseal lucencies, and transverse alternating bands of density. Spontaneous fractures are rare.

Superior Vena Cava Syndrome

Superior vena cava syndrome (SVCS) is an emergency but is rare in children and adolescents. In patients of all ages,

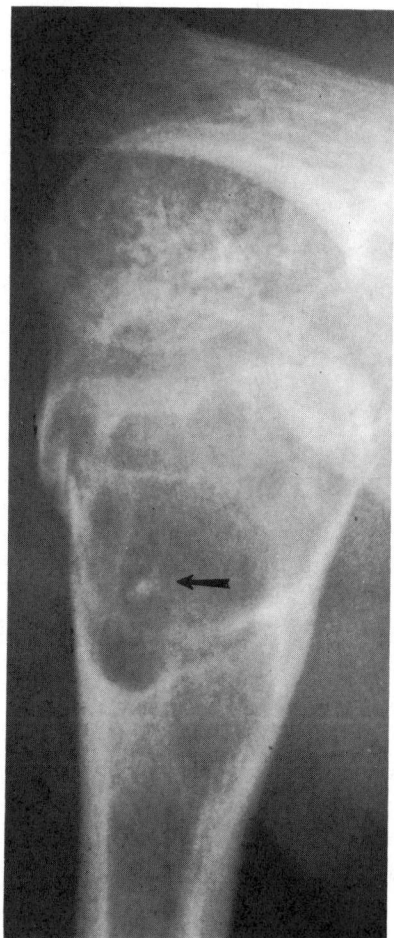

Figure 61–3. The fact that the pathologic fracture through this 5-year-old patient's humerus is through a unicameral bone cyst is indicated by the dense chip in the lucent lesion, a "fallen fragment sign," which had not been present previously. The well-defined geographic margins of the lesion itself are a sign of the benign nature. (Courtesy of A. Oestreich, M.D., Cincinnati, OH.)

evaluating the spine. The potential for magnetic resonance imaging (MRI) is uncertain, but it is useful for identifying intramedullary lesions and delineating soft tissue involvement. MRI can accurately differentiate benign from malignant fractures of vertebrae in 94% of cases. Most vertebral metastases cause compression fractures only when the entire vertebral body is infiltrated by tumor with complete replacement of marrow. Disk disruption and vertebral body fragmentation occur in only 4% of metastatic lesions.

The *fallen fragment sign* is associated with pathologic fractures resulting from benign (unicameral) bone cysts (Fig. 61–3). These are nonsolid, whereas malignant lesions are solid (Table 61–1). The classic radiographic image is caused by fracture of the cyst and dislodgement of fragments into the cystic cavity. If the radiographs are taken in different planes, movement of the fragment in the cyst may be seen.

Radiographic differential diagnosis includes osteomyelitis, eosinophilic granuloma, histiocytic lymphoma, osteosarcoma, and metastatic neuroblastoma. In osteomyelitis, formation of a sheath of new bone is usually seen around the infection site, which is usually located in the metaphysis. Osteosarcoma usually presents in the metaphysis with ossi-

TABLE 61–1

DISTINGUISHING CHARACTERISTICS OF BENIGN AND MALIGNANT BONE TUMORS

	Benign	Malignant
Signs and symptoms	Almost always painless No swelling	Painful Local swelling Possible: fever, weight loss
Laboratory characteristics		Possible: anemia, elevated erythrocyte sedimentation rate, high alkaline phosphatase level
Radiologic characteristics	Sharp, well-defined margins	No distinct border tumor Periosteal reaction Onion peel or sunburst pattern

Note: Usually a biopsy must be performed for the diagnosis to be certain.

SVCS is most often iatrogenic, usually secondary to cardiac surgery. Mediastinal tumors are the major cause of primary SVCS. Half of the tumors are primary, and the other half are metastatic. The most common malignancies are lymph node tumors (70%), especially lymphosarcomas (35%).

Only 1.5% of children who have mediastinal masses caused by tumors develop SVCS. The lesion is better tolerated if it develops slowly, as collateral circulatory drainage develops. Rapid malignant obstruction is poorly tolerated. Occlusion is usually secondary to thrombosis of the narrowed superior vena cava, not to mass effect or direct tumor blockage.

Early in the course of the illness, there are few signs and symptoms. Symptoms commonly include headache, nausea, hoarseness, stridor, respiratory distress (as a result of tracheal edema), and, occasionally, chest pain. Lethargy and dizziness may occur because of increased intracranial pressure. Signs include dilatation of the head, neck, and upper extremity veins. The skin may be cyanotic or flushed (plethora). Often conjunctival edema is present, possibly with proptosis. Seizures may occur from increased intracranial pressure. The condition is worsened by bending over, and patients may have to sleep sitting upright. Most patients have symptoms for less than 1 month.

Diagnosis

The chest radiograph usually reveals a mass; 75% of these appear on the right of the superior mediastinum. The chest radiograph may also reveal a pleural effusion or infiltrate or cardiomegaly, or it may be entirely normal.

CT and MRI scans are useful to delineate the extent of the tumor and thrombus. The CT scan may yield the only positive result. If contrast CT is used, two criteria are required to diagnose SVCS: decreased opacification of central venous structures inferior to the site of obstruction and opacification of collateral venous routes.

Treatment

The first priority is to establish airway patency and supply oxygen. The physician should assess for airway obstruction, stridor, cyanosis, intercostal retractions, accessory muscle use, and tachypnea. The goal of treatment is to cause rapid shrinking of tumor mass. Initial surgery should be limited to getting enough tissue to establish the diagnosis.

The traditional view is that rapid initial treatment should not be delayed to establish a definite diagnosis. More recent views support establishing a definitive diagnosis. Because the tumor's histologic appearance determines treatment, rapid establishment of the diagnosis before treatment is initiated may affect the course of therapy. However, these patients are poor anesthesia risks and often do not tolerate open thoracotomy for biopsy.

Radiation therapy is the treatment of choice for all tumors except lymphomas. High-dose radiation can provide symptomatic relief within 24 to 72 hours. SVCS caused by Hodgkin's or non-Hodgkin's lymphoma may be treated just as effectively with chemotherapy.

Diuretics may improve or worsen symptoms. Exacerbation of symptoms is from decreased venous return to heart.

Electrolyte Abnormalities
Tumor Lysis Syndrome

The tumor lysis syndrome (TLS) occurs during aggressive chemotherapy in patients with large tumor burdens and inadequate urinary output. Rapid cell lysis results in derangements of uric acid, calcium, potassium, and phosphate. The tumors most commonly causing the syndrome are advanced leukemia and non-Hodgkin's lymphoma.

Elevated serum uric acid levels, serum lactate dehydrogenase levels greater than 600 IU/L, and renal failure are risk factors. A serum uric acid level greater than 10 mg/dl; a serum potassium level greater than 6.0 mEq/L; a serum phosphorus level greater than 6.0 mg/dl; and a serum calcium level less than 8.0 mg/dl all require treatment.

Imaging of the urinary tract should be limited to renal ultrasonography or CT during the initial diagnostic evaluation, as radiocontrast media may cause hyperuricosuria.

Alkaline diuresis (40 mmol/L of $NaHCO_3$ at a rate of 3 to 5 L/m^2/day or 0.5 to 1.0 mmol/kg/dose to keep urine pH >6.5) should be started as soon as possible, preferably before chemotherapy, as it minimizes deposition of uric acid and phosphate in the kidney. High plasma urate levels (greater than 10 mg/dl) can precipitate uric acid crystals in the renal collecting ducts, causing renal failure. Diuresis with intravenous mannitol (0.5 to 1.0 gm/kg/dose) or furosemide (1.0 to 2.0 mg/kg/dose) may be needed. Low-dose dopamine (5 μg/kg/min) may be needed to promote renal perfusion. Diuresis is stopped as soon as uric acid levels return to normal.

Acute hyperkalemia occurs as potassium leaks out of lysed cells. The risk of life-threatening hyperkalemia is greatest during the 24 hours after chemotherapy. The serum potassium level rises before there are characteristic electrocardiographic (EKG) changes. Hyperkalemia has resulted in cardiac arrest. Pseudohyperkalemia (falsely elevated serum potassium) may occur if a serum sample is taken during the cell lysis phase in a patient with a greatly elevated platelet or white cell count.

Treatment of hyperkalemia consists of 3 gm/kg of glucose intravenously and 0.3 U/kg of regular insulin intravenously over 10 minutes. Calcium resonium (1 gm/kg) is given rectally, and calcium gluconate 10% is infused intravenously to protect the myocardium (Table 61–2).

Acute hyperphosphatemia from leakage of cell contents can result in calcium phosphate deposits in the renal tubules, causing renal failure and hypocalcemia. This is treated with oral aluminum hydroxide and maintenance of adequate urine output.

Renal failure with direct invasion of the tumor into the kidneys or the ureters may require short-term dialysis. Hyponatremic encephalopathy may develop with resultant cerebral edema. Coma and seizures may occur with apnea and an altered respiratory drive.

TABLE 61–2

PEDIATRIC MALIGNANCIES: THERAPY AT A GLANCE

Condition	Therapy
Hyperuricemia	1. Alkaline diuresis (IV 40 mmol/L $NaHCO_3$ at 3 to 5 L/m²/day or 0.5 to 1.0 mmol/kg per dose to keep urine pH > 6.5).
	2. Diuresis with IV mannitol (0.5 to 1.0 gm/kg/dose) and/or furosemide (1.0 to 2.0 mg/kg/dose).
	3. Low-dose dopamine (5 µg/kg/min IV).
	4. Allopurinol (200 mg/m² IV initial dose, then half that dose every 8 hr).
Hyperkalemia	1. 3 gm/kg of glucose and 0.3 U/kg of regular insulin IV over 10 minutes.
	2. Calcium resonium 1 gm/kg rectally and calcium gluconate 10% IV (0.5 mEq/kg).
	3. Aluminum hydroxide po.
Hypercalcemia	1. Etidronate (Didronel) IV 7.5 mg/kg/day with normal saline for at least 3 days.
	2. Calcitonin (4 IU/kg q 12 hr IV/IM).
	3. Glucocorticoids (2 mg/kg hydrocortisone hemisuccinate q 8 hr).

Hypercalcemia

The most common cause of hypercalcemia in malignancy is direct bony invasion by tumor cells with resultant release of calcium by osteoclastic activity. Another significant source is humorally mediated interposition of tumor-produced humoral and paracrine factors on the normal regulatory process, the exact mechanism of which is poorly understood.

The most common tumors seen in children with calcium derangement are T-cell lymphomas and leukemias. Hypercalcemia is also reported with rhabdomyosarcoma, neuroblastoma, and renal carcinoma.

Signs of hypercalcemia include thirst, polyuria, and constipation. The patient may have nonspecific complaints of bloating, abdominal pain, mild confusion, constipation, and anorexia. Severe hypercalcemia may present with bone pain, pronounced confusion, and coma. Severe hypercalcemia in patients with known malignancy is a poor prognostic factor.

All patients with a malignancy who feel ill should have serum calcium, albumin, chloride, blood urea nitrogen (BUN)/creatinine, bicarbonate, and total protein levels assayed. A high serum calcium level usually indicates aggressive disease but may also signal renal failure. Hypoalbuminemia is common in cancer patients; if present, the degree of hypercalcemia will be underestimated by the serum calcium level. Most patients with hypercalcemia of malignancy have a serum chloride concentration less than 98 mEq/L and a mild metabolic alkalosis. Many patients with hypercalcemia of malignancy are confined to bed (malaise, mental status changes, bone pain, or fracture), and their immobility exacerbates the bone resorption caused by malignancy.

Intravenous saline hydration will lower the serum calcium level by expanding the intravascular volume, increasing the glomerular filtration rate, and enhancing fractional excretion.

In the vast majority of patients with cancer, hypercalcemia is caused by osteoclastic bone resorption. Drugs that specifically inhibit osteoclastic bone resorption are usually effective in the treatment of hypercalcemia of malignancy. These include calcitonin, mithramycin, glucocorticoids, phosphate, and the diphosphonates.

Etidronate (Didronel) is a diphosphonate given as an infusion of 7.5 mg/kg/day with normal saline for at least 3 days. Etidronate brings serum calcium levels into the normal range in 80% of patients. However, nausea can occur, and caution must be used in patients with an elevated serum creatinine level greater than 2.5 mg/dl. Calcitonin should be used in the first 24 to 72 hours, because etidronate takes several days to show an effect.

Calcitonin (4 IU/kg q 12 hours intravenously) and glucocorticoids (2 mg/kg hydrocortisone hemisuccinate q 8 hours) can be used in patients with renal failure. Calcitonin inhibits bone resorption but lasts only 24 to 72 hours. The combination of parenteral calcitonin and glucocorticoids can lower serum calcium more rapidly than either one alone, but most patients still remain somewhat hypercalcemic.

Mithramycin is also effective. Side effects include nausea and vomiting, bone marrow suppression, platelet dysfunction, and liver and renal toxicity.

Furosemide (which increases excretion of sodium and calcium) should be used only in volume overload, as maintenance of the contracted state will offset any small beneficial effect of volume diuresis. High doses must be given and carry the danger of dehydration and electrolyte abnormalities.

Acute Infection

Infections are the leading cause of death in cancer patients. Many cancer survivors have a high risk of infection because of immunosuppressive medication, bone marrow transplantation, irradiation, and immunosuppression secondary to the cancer. Children have a lower overall mortality rate compared with adults (3% versus 19%) and a lower infection mortality rate (2% versus 8%).

Bacteria

Gram-positive bacterial infections are the most common pathogens, occurring in 78% of infections. This is largely because of the more frequent use of indwelling catheters (the source of infection in 27% of cases); the use of prophylactic antibiotics directed mostly against gram-negative bacteria; and the use of more advanced cephalosporins with greater gram-negative coverage. Also, children have gram-positive oral flora, which are becoming more resistant to methicillin and oxacillin.

Of infections associated with an absolute granulocyte count (AGC) below 500 cells/mm³, 85% are caused by bacteria, with *Staphylococcus aureus*, *Staphylococcus epidermidis*, and *Streptococcus viridans* being most prevalent. The most serious infections are caused by gram-negative aerobes, including *Escherichia coli*, *Klebsiella*, and *Pseudomonas aeruginosa*. *Haemophilus influenzae* can cause infection in patients with a normal AGC.

Viruses

More than half of children with acute lymphocytic leukemia who die during remission are found to have disseminated viral infection. The most common agents are varicella zoster, cytomegalovirus, herpes simplex virus, and measles in children with leukemia. Varicella zoster and measles are the most serious.

Fungi

Fungal infections are a serious cause of mortality in the patient with an AGC of 100/mm³ for a duration of more than 2 weeks. The infectious agent is commonly *Aspergillus* or *Candida*, with *Mucor* and *Rhizopus* also prevalent. Up to

64% of patients with prolonged granulocytopenia have disseminated fungal infections at autopsy.

Neutropenia

The development of granulocytopenia is the most important factor affecting the outcome of infections. The duration of granulocytopenia is also an important predictor. As the AGC falls below 500/mm³, there is an increase in the infection rate of 5% to 30%.

Diagnosis. It is often difficult to identify the source of infection in the granulocytopenic patient, and therefore all possible sites must be cultured. In granulocytopenic cancer patients, 30% of fevers are caused by bacteremia, 20% are caused by bacteria from a specific source, and 10% are caused by fungi. In 40% of cases a source is never identified and may be noninfectious. Fever may be the only sign, as up to 55% of children with bacteremia may be asymptomatic.

The lung is the most common source of infection in children with cancer. Retrosternal pain and odynophagia in a febrile, neutropenic patient already on a broad-spectrum antibiotic is most likely a result of esophagitis, commonly from *Candida albicans*. Pseudomembranous colitis from *Clostridium difficile* is a common cause of intractable diarrhea and abdominal pain in patients on antibiotic therapy. Necrotizing enterocolitis is caused by ischemia of the bowel resulting from hemorrhagic or bacteremic shock and allows entrance of bacteria into the bowel wall. Perirectal cellulitis can occur in the immunocompromised patient. Predisposing factors are anal fissures, constipation, local radiotherapy, and rectal manipulation such as rectal temperature measurement, digital examinations, and barium enemas.

The evaluation must include a thorough clinical history, physical examination, chest radiograph, complete blood cell count, three blood cultures obtained at 15-minute intervals, urinalysis, and cultures of urine, stool, sputum, the perineum, the pharynx, aspirated body fluids, and drainage from lesions. A lumbar puncture, a CT scan of the suspected site, and a bone marrow aspiration are additional considerations.

Noninfectious sources of fever are allergic reactions, blood product reactions, high-dose chemotherapy (methotrexate or cytosine arabinoside), and the tumor itself, particularly in lymphomas and other solid tumors. Neoplastic fevers are often intermittent, with a relatively low heart rate, and the patient may appear less toxic than would be expected from the magnitude of the fever.

Therapeutic Intervention. Empiric therapy for the febrile agranulocytic patient is begun immediately, commonly with double or triple antibiotic therapy. A typical regimen includes an aminoglycoside and an antipseudomonal penicillin, unless *S. aureus* or a fungus is suspected. Monotherapy with third-generation cephalosporins and imipenum antibiotics has also become an alternative. Specific pathogen–directed therapy often results in secondary infections if granulocytopenia and fever last more than 1 week. Amphotericin B is still the antifungal agent of choice.

Children with acute leukemia and lymphoma have a higher rate of infection than patients with other neoplasms (9.1 per 100 patients years, compared with 0.6 per 100 patient years, respectively). Patients with lymphomas have a defect in cellular immunity that predisposes them to viral and fungal infections. Polymicrobial infections occur in 15% to 21% of leukemia and lymphoma patients.

Pneumocystis carinii causes infection after chemotherapy is finished, often after corticosteroid withdrawal. Infection usually presents with 4 to 5 days of upper respiratory tract symptoms and fever. A chest roentgenogram shows hazy, bilateral alveolar infiltrates that begin at the hila. The treatment of choice is trimethoprim-sulfamethoxazole (20 mg/kg/day of trimethoprim given intravenously in three divided doses).

Meningitis

It is often difficult to discern whether meningeal signs and symptoms are the result of central spread of the malignancy or of an infection. Laboratory analysis of the cerebral spinal fluid in meningeal carcinomatosis typically reveals sterile fluid with an increased protein content, decreased glucose concentration, moderately increased numbers of mononuclear cells, and, occasionally, tumor cells. The most useful test when tumor cells or bacteria are found is the Gram stain.

Lyme disease can present as meningitis without a history of tick bite. CSF cells appear as markedly atypical plasmacytoid mononuclear cells, consistent with non-Hodgkin's malignant lymphoma. Patients display significant increases in immature immunoblasts, mature plasma cells, and mature lymphocytes. Nuclear pleomorphism and significant numbers of mitotic figures are present. Antibody titers for *Borrelia burgdorferi* antigen confirm Lyme disease.

Spinal Cord Compression

Spinal cord compression (SCC) occurs in 5% to 10% of all patients with cancer. Bone is the second most common site of tumor metastases; the lung is first. The most common site of secondary bony tumor is the vertebral column, with two thirds of cases involving the thoracic spine. The metastases are usually extradural.

The most common tumor to cause SCC in children is lymphoma. Though lymphomas metastasize to the cord by the lymphatic route with contiguous spread, other tumors spread hematogenously. The most common cause of cord compression is pressure from an extradural mass. Other causes are pathologic fractures, intradural metastases, occlusion of the radicular arteries, and severe angulation following vertebral collapse. The body of the vertebrae, located anterior to the cord, is involved in 85% of all metastases to the cord.

The most common complaint, and usually the first symptom, is back pain, occurring in 96% of cases. The pain is constant and worse with lying down and often causes patients to wake several times at night. Coughing or straining worsens the pain. Radicular pain occurs in 60% of cases. Advanced disease is evidenced by autonomic dysfunction such as loss of bladder or bowel control, sensory loss, or weakness.

Physical findings include tenderness of the spine, and a positive result on the straight leg raise test, weakness, a positive Babinski's sign, a palpable bladder, a change in deep tendon reflexes, and a decrease in anal sphincter tone. Once these signs appear, progression to paraplegia can be rapid.

Radiologic Evaluation

Plain spine roentgenograms demonstrate lesions in 85% of cases of SCC documented by myelography and show destruction of vertebral bodies, loss of pedicles, and vertebral collapse. Myelography is the current diagnostic standard but provides only indirect evidence of compression; it may soon be replaced by MRI. The main advantage of both techniques over CT is that they visualize the entire cord. The disadvantages of myelography are patient discomfort, the lack of visualization of soft tissue detail, the need to do two or more punctures if there is a complete block of the cord at a particular level, and occasional complications from the use of contrast material.

MRI demonstrates the nature and extent of cord compression and provides information on the presence of bone marrow metastases and paravertebral soft tissue masses. However, MRI images are more likely to be technically poor than are myelograms. Patient motion is a major difficulty, particularly in pediatric patients. MRI is as sensitive as myelography in detecting epidural metastases that cause cord compression, but MRI tends to be more sensitive than myelography when cord compromise has not yet developed. It is also more sensitive for detecting vertebral body metastases.

The primary disadvantage of MRI is the long scan times of up to 30 minutes. The requirement to remain motionless is difficult for young children.

CT is excellent at visualizing the surrounding soft tissue details, which is important in determining the surgical approach. Silent metastases are present in up to 17% of cases and are missed by CT in 10%. Radionuclide bone scanning is sensitive for diagnosing vertebral body metastases, but it cannot predict the presence or absence of cord compression.

Therapeutic Intervention

The most important prognostic factor in SCC is the physical condition of the patient at initiation of treatment. Radiotherapy is the treatment of choice in ambulatory patients with SCC, but anterior laminectomy is being used more frequently. Chemotherapy is an alternative in select cases (i.e., Ewing's sarcoma, neuroblastoma) and may become more common in the future.

Except for patients with lymphoma, children who are paraplegic at onset rarely walk again, and for these, radiation therapy alone is used. The anterior approach laminectomy, followed by radiation therapy, may allow a return of ambulation in up to 85% of patients, but the operative mortality rate is as high as 7%.

The long-term prognosis is poor. Patients with limited neurologic dysfunction and pain do well; patients who are paraplegic at presentation often remain so unless aggressively treated.

Seizures

A seizure is the first presenting sign in 6% to 29% of patients with intracerebral metastases. Metastases in the frontal lobes are most frequently associated with initial presentation of seizures.

Tumor is present clinically (seizures or focal neurologic deficits) before it is demonstrable on CT scans in only 0.5% to 1.5% of cases. MRI scans may reveal lesions in another 25% of these patients. MRI is the most sensitive technique, though cost, the patient's condition, and availability limit its use.

Long-Term Effects of Treatment

Long-term effects of treatment are becoming increasingly important. There are three major areas of concern: second malignancies, endocrine effects, and structural changes.

Short stature is common in children previously treated for brain tumors, most of which do not directly involve the hypothalamic-pituitary axis. Final height may be adversely affected by malnutrition, occult tumor, chemotherapy, precocious puberty, growth hormone (GH) deficiency, and spinal growth impairment. Gonadal dysfunction can occur with chemotherapy and with direct irradiation. Spinal irradiation causes short stature directly by impairment of vertebral growth. The younger the patient during treatment, the greater the loss of height.

The risk of developing a second malignancy within 20 years after the first ranges from 3% to 12%. Immunosuppressive therapy, ionizing radiation, and alkylating agents (such as cyclophosphamide) are associated with an increased incidence of second malignancies. In acute lymphocytic leukemia, there is a bimodal distribution of second malignancies. Median time to development of hematopoietic or lymphatic malignancies is 22 months. The second peak occurs with solid tumors at 77 months (5 to 15 years). One third of these are multifocal brain tumors.

In children with successfully treated Hodgkin's disease, acute nonlymphocytic leukemia or bone sarcomas are predominant in the first decade, and tumors of the breast and colon are most common after that.

Psychological testing indicates the two most important risk factors for mental impairment are cranial radiation treatment and the child's age at time of treatment; the younger the patient, the more noticeable the effects. There are intelligence quotient (IQ) differences, and mild but significant visual-spatial and verbal memory deficits.

Other long-term effects are less frequent and universal. SVCS secondary to fibrosing mediastinitis may occur from prior irradiation. Children treated with bone marrow transplants may develop a graft-versus-host reaction. This can result in scleroderma, dry eyes and mouth, pulmonary insufficiency, and cataracts. Studies of long-term effects in patients with Hodgkin's disease seem to show early atherosclerosis and myocardial infarctions in some people if the chest has been irradiated. Dose-related cardiomyopathy can occur with anthracycline, used in some protocols for Hodgkin's disease. Patients with Hodgkin's disease also have impaired T lymphocyte–mediated immunity. This results in viral infections being common before, during, and long after treatment. Staging of Hodgkin's disease often involves splenectomy. When combined with aggressive radiation and chemotherapy, subsequent serious infections by encapsulated bacteria may result. Head and neck irradiation may result in thyroid dysfunction within 5 years, particularly in children with Hodgkin's. Osteoradionecrosis may occur and is believed to be related to high-dose radiation.

COMMON PEDIATRIC TUMORS
Hodgkin's Lymphoma

The most common malignancies in children are leukemia (20%), CNS tumors (15%), lymphoma (equally divided between Hodgkin's and non-Hodgkin's) (10%), neuroblastoma (7%), soft tissue tumors (5%), Wilms' tumors (4%), and bony tumors (3.4%).

Hodgkin's lymphoma is a neoplasm of the lymphoid tissue that originates from one lymph node. In children, the lymphocyte-predominant type is most common. Histologically, an abundance of lymphocytes are present with few abnormal cells. Diagnosis is made by finding neoplastic reticulum cells, usually by incisional or excisional biopsy of a lymph node or affected tissue. The multinucleated Reed-Sternberg cell is the most common malignant cell found.

Ten percent of patients with Hodgkin's lymphoma are younger than 10 years, and it rarely occurs before age 5. The male-to-female ratio is 4:1. The most frequent presenting complaint is painless cervical adenopathy, with no identifiable infectious source, which persists beyond 6 weeks. One third of children present with night sweats, fever, and weight loss. Laboratory studies reflect anemia, altered lymphocyte and platelet counts, elevated erythrocyte sedimentation rate, and elevated serum alkaline phosphatase.

Survival in children is equal or better than that in adults. Therapy usually consists of radiation alone or in combination with chemotherapy. Hodgkin's disease is responsive to a large variety of chemotherapeutic agents.

Non-Hodgkin's Lymphoma

Malignant non-Hodgkin's lymphoma is a neoplasm of the immune system. It is different from most cancers that start in one organ in that it spreads by following the circulation of the normal cellular components. For this reason, on discovery non-Hodgkin's lymphoma is usually widespread and scattered in lymphoid tissue. Lymphomas in children usually occur in the bone marrow and the thymus.

Patients present with one of two "classic" syndromes, depending on the type of lymphoma. Lymphoblastic lymphomas present with chest pain, dysphagia, dyspnea, and SVCS. It is typically an intrathoracic tumor with a mediastinal mass. Nonlymphoblastic lymphomas (undifferentiated or large cell) present with abdominal swelling and pain, nausea and vomiting, change in bowel habits, and possibly gastrointestinal bleeding. Intussusception may occur and is caused by ileocecal lymphoma. This tumor progresses rapidly, often with remarkable day-to-day increases in size.

Initial emergency department evaluation should include a chest roentgenogram, abdominal or chest CT scan (depending on the clinical presentation), a complete blood cell count, liver and renal studies, and determinations of serum uric acid and lactate dehydrogenase levels.

In patients presenting with SVCS, the tumor responds to emergency irradiation but is equally as responsive to emergent initiation of chemotherapy. Chemotherapy is preferred, because the serious long-term consequences of mediastinal irradiation (esophagitis, cardiac damage, and damage to growth plates in bones) are avoided. The treatment of nonlymphoblastic lymphomas may result in tumor lysis syndrome, the severity of which is directly correlated to the bulk of the tumor.

Therapy consisting of surgery and radiation alone resulted in a survival rate of less than 50%. Management with combination chemotherapy alone has a better than 90% survival rate.

Rhabdomyosarcoma

Sarcomas are primary malignancies of soft tissue, bone, and cartilage. Soft tissue tumors in children commonly originate in skeletal muscle (rhabdomyosarcoma) or interfascial planes (undifferentiated sarcomas).

Whites develop rhabdomyosarcoma three times more frequently than blacks. Incidence is bimodal, occurring up to age 5 years and again in late adolescence. Major sites of involvement are the head (40%), genitourinary tract (20%), limbs (20%), and trunk (15%). The tumor is composed of rhabdomyoblasts, which are of mesenchymal origin. Differential diagnosis includes other small round cell tumors of children, including Ewing's sarcoma, lymphoma, and neuroblastoma.

With combined-modality treatment, more than 50% of children survive. Radiation therapy is effective in local disease. Surgery is useful both for the initial biopsy and for evaluation of the extent of disease. Total resection is feasible in only 15% of patients. Combination chemotherapy helps to control micrometastases and shrink the primary site.

Tumors in Bone
Ewing's Sarcoma

Ewing's sarcoma represents 10% to 30% of primary malignant bone tumors in children. The age at onset is typically between 5 and 30 years. Patients usually present with pain, soft tissue swelling, fever, leukocytosis, and an elevated erythrocyte sedimentation rate. The tumor commonly occurs in long bones of the extremities, pelvis, and ribs.

Roentgenography reveals permeative, radiolucent destructive lesions with little osteosclerosis and frequent extension of tumor into adjacent soft tissue. The lesions usually appear in "onion peel" or "sunburst" patterns (Fig. 61–4). The onion peel appearance is the result of subperiosteal new bone formation in multiple concentric layers. Lesions that have the sunburst pattern show perpendicular spicules of reactive periosteal new bone. Pathologic fractures occur in only 2% to 5% of cases.

Radiographic differential diagnosis includes osteomyelitis, eosinophilic granuloma, histiocytic lymphoma, osteosarcoma, metastatic neuroblastoma, and malignant lymphoma. Evaluation for osteomyelitis usually reveals formation of an involucrum, as well as a metaphyseal location. Osteosarcoma usually presents in the metaphysis with ossification of tumor matrix in the medullary cavity and in affected soft tissue.

The final diagnosis of Ewing's sarcoma is made by satisfying radiologic and histopathologic criteria and is often made by excluding other small, round cell tumors.

Osteosarcoma

Osteosarcoma (osteogenic sarcoma) originates in mesenchymal tissue and forms neoplastic osteoid and osseous

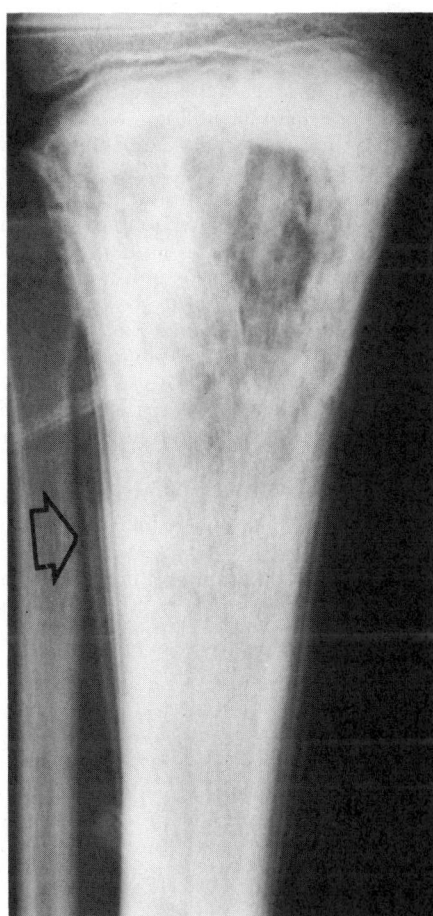

Figure 61–4. Among the malignant tumor characteristics of this tibial Ewing's sarcoma are the onion-skin layers of periosteal reactions *(arrow)*, some interrupted. (Courtesy of A. Oestreich, M.D., Cincinnati, OH.)

tissue. Average age at time of discovery is 15 years, with 65% of patients between 10 and 20 years of age. Osteosarcoma usually arises in the metaphyseal portion of long bones, most frequently around the knee. However, it may arise in any bone and even in soft tissue (extraosseous osteosarcoma).

The clinical presentation may be subtle, but most often there is pain and soft tissue swelling. Pathologic fractures may occur. Patients may relate onset of symptoms to trauma, but trauma has not been implicated as a cause. Biopsy helps to differentiate osteosarcoma from Ewing's sarcoma, chondrosarcoma, osteomyelitis, cortical defects, bony abnormalities associated with metabolic disease, and benign tumors.

Radiographically, osteosarcoma can present with all types of bony change, from nearly normal to extremely dense or almost total destruction. There is almost always a highly irregular and interrupted periosteal response; the sunburst and onion peel patterns are classic types. Benign lesions often have a uniform, homogenous, and solid periosteal reaction that appears to represent a response to a single event. Calcified tumor cartilage often resembles small nests of bone infarcts seeded throughout the spongy portion of bone and appears extremely dense. It can metastasize to lung, bone, lymph nodes, liver, soft tissues, and brain.

Wilms' Tumor

Wilms' tumor (nephroblastoma) is the second most common childhood tumor of the abdomen and accounts for about 5% of all pediatric malignancies. The incidence is about 0.75 per 100,000. The mean age at discovery is 3 years, with a range of 2 to 5 years. The tumor arises from varying combinations of embryonic tissue (epithelium, stroma, and kidney) and is bilateral in 10% of cases.

The most common presentation is a painless flank mass or swelling. Hypertension occurs in about 10% to 30% of patients and hematuria in about 25%. The patient may have anemia from bleeding into the tumor. Congenital anomalies are fairly frequent, especially with bilateral tumors.

The diagnosis is suggested by finding a painless abdominal mass, combined with an abnormal abdominal ultrasound or intravenous pyelogram. The differential diagnosis includes renal abscess, multilocular cysts, or polycystic kidney disease. A chest roentgenogram is useful to exclude pulmonary metastases, as the lung is the primary area of spread.

The cure rate is greater than 80% in patients with unilateral disease and about 50% in those presenting with metastatic tumor. The treatment is surgical nephrectomy, followed by local irradiation or combination chemotherapy.

Neuroblastoma

Neuroblastoma is a relatively frequent pediatric tumor, accounting for about 500 new cases annually in the United States, or 8% of childhood tumors. It is derived from neural crest progenitor cells that normally give rise to the sympathetic nervous system and adrenal medulla. The median age at diagnosis is 2 years.

Sixty-five percent of the tumors originate in the retroperitoneum; most are in an adrenal gland. They are usually quite large at presentation. Metastases to bone and marrow, lymph nodes, liver, and subcutaneous tissue are found in 70% of newly diagnosed patients. Signs and symptoms are usually from mass effects of the tumor or metastases but may include diarrhea, hypertension, ataxia, and ocular abnormalities. Weight loss, fever, anemia, and bone pain usually indicate metastatic spread.

Brain Tumors

Brain tumors are the most common type of solid childhood tumors. About 1500 new cases are diagnosed annually in the United States. The most common brain tumors are glial cell tumors (astrocytoma and ependymomas), followed by primitive neuroectodermal tumors such as medulloblastomas and pinealoblastomas. Metastases are uncommon.

Signs and symptoms may be generalized or localized. Local effects depend on where the tumor is located in the brain. General effects include headache, vomiting, lethargy, irritability, and signs of increased intracranial pressure.

Treatment goals consist of relief of intracranial pressure and neurologic dysfunction; the diagnosis is determined by tissue sampling. Children who survive brain tumors often suffer severe consequences of treatment, especially growth retardation and endocrine deficiencies.

Primary CNS lymphomas are extremely rare in immunocompetent patients, but in children with the acquired immunodeficiency syndrome (AIDS), non-Hodgkin's lymphoma is being seen with increasing frequency.

Retinoblastoma

Retinoblastoma is a potentially fatal neoplasm of childhood that arises from the retina. It occurs in about 1 in 15,000 live births. Ninety percent occur before the age of 5 years, and 50% to 65% occur unilaterally.

If the tumor is still contained within the globe, the most common finding is leukocoria, or the "white pupil." This is caused by reflection of the examination light off the tumor itself. The patient may still have normal vision and pupillary response. Children with tumor confined to one globe have a 90% survival rate. Patients who present with metastatic disease usually present with focal neurologic impairment or a mass near the orbit. The child may present with an apparent orbital cellulitis that is actually an inflammatory reaction to glaucoma or tumor necrosis. Unlike with a periorbital cellulitis, the white blood cell count is normal, and there is no fever.

Because diagnosis is made on clinical grounds in the majority of cases, most ancillary testing is of little benefit. CT scans enable detection, particularly if calcium is present, as it is in 90% of cases.

The mainstay of therapy for bilateral retinoblastoma is enucleation of the worst eye and irradiation of the other eye to preserve vision. Irradiation is also used in unilateral disease when less than 50% of the retina is affected. Combination chemotherapy is used in patients at risk for metastatic spread. The average age at onset of the second neoplasms is 12.4 years.

Histiocytosis X (Langerhans Cell Histiocytosis)

The origin of Langerhans cell histiocytosis is poorly understood. It is currently thought to be a group of diseases and not a truly malignant neoplasm; eosinophilic granuloma, Hand-Schüller-Christian disease, and Letterer-Siwe disease are included. These are characterized by proliferation of benign-appearing histiocytes with surrounding eosinophils. Lesions appear as "punched-out" areas of bone or as skin infiltrates that appear similar to seborrheic dermatitis. Lesions can be localized or diffusely spread and occur with or without organ dysfunction. The survival rate is virtually 100% in patients with local disease, nearly 100% in those with no organ dysfunction, and 30% in those with abnormal blood cell counts and organ dysfunction (abnormal liver functions or pulmonary infiltrates on chest roentgenograms). The age at onset is the most important prognostic factor, with younger patients less likely to survive. The median age at onset is 3 years.

Selected References

Adelstein D, Hines J, Carter S, et al. Thromboembolic events in patients with malignant superior vena cava syndrome and the role of anticoagulation. Cancer 1988;62:2258.

Albano E, Pizzo P. Infectious complications in childhood acute leukemias. Pediatr Clin North Am 1988;35:873.

Benz G, Brandeis W, Willich E. Radiological aspects of leukemia in childhood: An analysis of 89 children. Pediatr Radiol 1976;4:206.

Cohen L, Balow J, Magrath I, et al. Acute tumor lysis syndrome: A review of 37 patients with Burkitt's lymphoma. Am J Med 1980;68:486.

Conrad E. Pitfalls in diagnosis: Pediatric musculoskeletal tumors. Pediatr Ann 1989;18:45.

Craft A, Reed M, Gardner P, et al. Virus infections in children with ALL. Arch Dis Child 1979;54:755.

Dhingra K, Newcom S. Acute tumor lysis syndrome in non-Hodgkin lymphoma induced by dexamethasone. Am J Hematol 1988;29:115.

Fidler M. Incidence of fracture through metastases in long bones. Acta Orthop Scand 1981;52:623.

Ganick D. Wilms' tumor. Hematol Oncol Clin North Am 1987;1:696.

Habermann E, Lopez R. Metastatic disease of bone and treatment of pathological fractures. Orthop Clin North Am 1989;20:469.

Harrington KD. Current concepts review. Metastatic disease of the spine. J Bone Joint Surg 1986;68A:1110.

Hohl R, Schilsky R. Nonmalignant complications of therapy for Hodgkin's disease. Hematol Oncol Clin North Am 1989;3:331.

Janin Y, Becker J, Wise L, et al. Superior vena cava syndrome in childhood and adolescence: A review of the literature and report of three cases. J Pediatr Surg 1982;17:290.

Jenkin R, Anderson J, Chilcote R, et al. The treatment of localized non-Hodgkin's lymphoma in children: A report from the children's cancer study group. J Clin Oncol 1984;2:88.

Kadota R, Allen J, Hartman G. Brain tumors in children. J Pediatr 1989;114:511.

Karp J, Dick J, Angelopulos C, et al. Empiric use of vancomycin during prolonged treatment induced granulocytopenia. Am J Med 1986;81:237.

Kelly P, Eisman J. Hypercalcaemia of malignancy. Cancer Metastasis Rev 1989;8:23.

Klastersky J, Daneau D, Verhest A. Causes of death in patients with cancer. Eur J Cancer 1972;8:149.

Li F, Cassady J, Jaffe N. Risk of second tumors in survivors of childhood cancer. Cancer 1975;35:1230.

Lokich J, Goodman R. Superior vena cava syndrome. Clinical management. JAMA 1975;231:58.

Magrath I. Malignant non-Hodgkin's lymphomas in children. Hematol Oncol Clin North Am 1987;1:577.

Miser J, Miser A, Bleyer W, et al. Septicemia in childhood malignancy. Analysis of 101 consecutive episodes. Clin Pediatr 1981;20:320.

Mundy G, Yates A. Recent advances in pathophysiology and treatment of hypercalcemia of malignancy. Am J Kidney Dis 1989;14:2.

Ochs J, Mulhern R. Late effects of antileukemic treatment. Pediatr Clin North Am 1988;35:815.

Pao W, Kun L. Hodgkin's disease in children. Hematol Oncol Clin North Am 1989;3:345.

Pizzo P, Robichaud K, Wesley R, et al. Fever in the pediatric and young adult patient with cancer. A prospective study of 1001 episodes. Medicine 1982;61:153.

Shalet S, Clayton P, Price D. Growth impairment following treatment for childhood brain tumours. Acta Pediatr Scand 1988;343:137.

Siegel S, Wolff L, Baehner R, et al. Treatment of Pneumocystis carinii pneumonitis. A comparative trial of sulfamethoxazole-trimethoprim versus pentamidine in pediatric patients with cancer: Report from the Children's Cancer Study Group. Am J Dis Child 1984;138:1051.

Stokes D. The tumour lysis syndrome. Anaesthesia 1989;44:133.

Struhl S, Edelson C, Pritzker H, et al. Solitary (unicameral) bone cyst. Skeletal Radiol 1989;18:261.

Viscoli C. Aspects of infections in children with cancer. Recent Results Cancer Res 1988;108:71.

Viscoli C, Perlino G, Moroni C, et al. Infections in children with cancer. Ital J Pediatr 1985;11:37.

Yedlicka J, Cormier M, Gray R, et al. Computed tomography of superior vena cava obstruction. J Thorac Imag 1987;2:72.

Yuh W, Zacher C, Barloon T, et al. Vertebral compression fractures: Distinction between benign and malignant causes with MR imaging. Radiology 1989;172:215.

CHAPTER 62

Leukemia

Stephen Penaskovic

INTRODUCTION

Acute leukemia is the most common malignancy in children.[1] It consists of a diverse group of hematologic malignancies characterized by leukemic cell infiltration of the bone marrow and widespread peripheral dissemination of leukemic blasts. The resulting complications are rapidly fatal and until relatively recently had a 100% mortality rate. The advent of chemotherapy and aggressive supportive care has resulted in long-term survival rates of 60% to 70%.[2]

The leukemias are classified into two broad groups: acute and chronic. Acute lymphoblastic leukemia (ALL) is the most common type, accounting for about 80% of cases, or 2000 new cases each year. The next most common type is acute nonlymphoblastic leukemia (ANLL), accounting for 17% of cases. Chronic myelogenous leukemia (CML) and its juvenile form account for the remaining 3%.[3]

ALL is a disease of both children and adults, with the initial peak incidence occurring from 3 to 5 years of age,[3] with greatest frequency in white males.[4] In contrast, ANLL has a relatively constant incidence in regard to age, sex, and race.[3]

Children with Down syndrome have at least an 11-fold risk of developing acute leukemia.[5] Association of ANLL with Kleinfelter's syndrome,[6] neurofibromatosis,[7] Fanconi's anemia,[8] and Bloom's syndrome[9] are well documented.

ANATOMY AND PHYSIOLOGY

The leukemias are believed to result from the malignant transformation and proliferation of primitive white blood cell precursors in the bone marrow. The resulting poorly differentiated derivatives, called *blasts*, replace their non-malignant cellular counterparts, causing severe disruption of normal hematopoiesis.[10] Peripheral blast invasion results in multiorgan manifestations.

Most children with acute leukemias are symptomatic for 2 to 4 weeks before being seen by a physician. The initial symptoms tend to be nonspecific and can be confused with a protracted viral illness. Complaints of weakness, irritability, weight loss, and fever are frequent. As the illness progresses, signs of bone marrow failure develop including granulocytopenia and thrombocytopenia. Easy bruising, nosebleeds, petechiae, purpura, lassitude, and fever are common. Peripheral invasion of blasts results in lymphadenopathy and hepatosplenomegaly (more pronounced in ALL)[11]; rarely, testicular involvement is an early finding. Evidence of elevated intracranial pressure at presentation as a result of central nervous system involvement is found in less that 5% of children with ALL[12] but is indicative of an extremely poor prognosis.[13] ANLL may present with myeloblastic chloromas (greenish tumors appearing around the orbits and skin) and gum hyperplasia.[11] Bone pain (i.e., sternal tenderness or a persistent limp) caused by subperiosteal infiltration of leukemic cells, hemorrhage, or metabolic changes may be the presenting complaint. Retinal examination may reveal leukemic retinopathy, which is characterized by intraretinal hemorrhages, white-centered hemorrhages, and cotton-wool spots.[14] Rare presentations include clitorism,[15] priapism,[16] pericarditis,[17] pericardial tamponade,[18] osteoporosis, vertebral compression fractures,[19] otomastoiditis,[20] and pyoderma gangrenosum, a painful ulcerating skin lesion.[21]

Elevated leukocyte counts greater than 100,000 cells/mm³ may cause sludging of the microvasculature resulting in cerebral or pulmonary leukostasis. Rapid tumor lysis may result in hyperuricemia, severe metabolic abnormalities, renal failure, and disseminated intravascular coagulation.

Chronic leukemias are massive overgrowths of mature cells and tend to be relatively indolent disorders in their initial stages. Initial presenting complaints are generally nonspecific. Physical signs include pallor, fever, ecchymosis, hepatosplenomegaly, and sternal tenderness. Symptoms are related to organ infiltration, particularly of the brain, lung, retina, and penis; hyperviscosity and metabolic consequences of cellular hyperproliferation.[22]

In about 5% of cases metamorphosis to a "blast crisis" leads to the clinical picture of de novo acute leukemia. This stage is characterized by progressive systemic symptoms, increased leukocyte counts with a high proportion of immature cells, basophilia, and increased resistance to chemotherapy. The blast crisis is associated with high mortality, with death generally occurring within 3 months of its onset.[22]

DIAGNOSTIC EVALUATION

The diagnosis of leukemia is suggested by the history, physical examination, and an abnormal complete blood cell (CBC) count (Table 62–1). Anemia and thrombocytopenia occur in more than two thirds of patients with ALL at initial presentation. Leukocyte counts are variable; more than 50% of patients have normal or low white cell counts, whereas 17% have counts of more than 50,000 cells/mm³. An increased leukocyte count at diagnosis is associated with a poor prognosis.[23] To confirm the diagnosis, a bone marrow aspirate showing greater than 25% blast forms is required.[22] Definitive classification depends on special staining and cellular analysis techniques.

In addition to the CBC count, serum electrolyte, uric acid, and serum calcium levels, and renal and liver function tests should be performed in newly diagnosed or known leukemic patients. Abnormal liver function test results at diagnosis are presumably a result of leukemic infiltration of the liver. Serum phosphate and lactate dehydrogenase (LDH) levels may be obtained if leukemic cell lysis occurs.[24] Blood gas measurements may be obtained to evaluate oxygenation and acid-base status. Blood and urine cultures are indicated in the febrile leukemic patient, especially those who are neutropenic.

Useful radiologic studies include a chest radiograph, which may show an anterior mediastinal mass in 10% of newly diagnosed patients with ALL.[24, 25] Bone lesions may be evident on the radiograph, even if there is no associated pain. These include radiolucent metaphyseal bands, osteolytic and osteosclerotic lesions, and periosteal new bone formation.[26] Vertebral compression fractures and spinal osteoporosis may also be early features.[19]

DIFFERENTIAL DIAGNOSIS

Acute leukemia may mimic a number of childhood illnesses, including the following:

Infectious mononucleosis
Juvenile rheumatoid arthritis
Acute infectious lymphocytosis
Idiopathic thrombocytopenic purpura
Pertussis, parapertussis
Aplastic anemia
Neuroblastoma
Lymphoma
Retinoblastoma
Rhabdomyosarcoma

The atypical lymphocytosis of infectious mononucleosis, viral hepatitis, cytomegalovirus infection, and *Toxoplasma gondii* infection may be mistaken for malignant cells, especially because these illnesses may also be associated with fever, lymphadenopathy, splenomegaly, anemia, and thrombocytopenia.[13] Specific serologic studies usually differentiate these disorders. Juvenile rheumatoid arthritis may present with bone pain, fever, arthralgia, and splenomegaly.[25] The extreme lymphocytosis associated with pertussis, parapertussis, and acute infectious lymphocytosis may be confused with acute leukemic proliferation,[25] but the distinction becomes clearer when interpreted in the context of coryza and the characteristic "whooping" cough seen in some of these patients. In idiopathic thrombocytopenic purpura, the hemoglobin and leukocyte counts are usually normal, and adenopathy and hepatosplenomegaly are absent.[13] Because ALL may rarely present with isolated thrombocytopenia,[27] a bone marrow aspirate is generally recommended in these patients and in other patients in whom the diagnosis is unclear.

THERAPEUTIC INTERVENTION

Life-threatening conditions such as severe anemia, hemorrhage, sepsis, hyperleukocytosis, rapid tumor lysis syndrome, metabolic derangements, and renal failure must be identified early and treated aggressively. Many of the complications associated with leukemia may be suspected on the basis of an abnormal CBC count. Packed red blood cell and platelet transfusions are required fairly frequently, especially when the patient presents with marked pancytopenia and is symptomatic. Febrile neutropenic patients require the initiation of broad-spectrum antibiotics after appropriate cultures are obtained.

Definitive treatment of leukemia is accomplished utilizing various combinations of chemotherapeutic agents and radiation for prolonged periods (2.5 to 3 years) under the

---

TABLE 62–1

SYMPTOMS, PHYSICAL FINDINGS, AND LABORATORY FEATURES IN CHILDREN WITH ALL

Clinical or Laboratory Feature	% of Patients
Symptoms and physical findings	
Fever	61
Bleeding (e.g., petechia or purpura)	48
Bone pain	23
Lymphadenopathy	50
Splenomegaly	63
Hepatosplenomegaly	68
Laboratory features	
Leukocyte count (per mm³)	
<10,000	53
10,000–49,000	30
>50,000	17
Hemoglobin (gm/dl)	
<7.0	43
7.0–11.0	45
>11.0	12
Platelet count (per mm³)	
<20,000	28
20,000–99,000	47
>100,000	25

From Miller DR. Acute lymphoblastic leukemia. Pediatr Clin North Am 1980;27:269.

supervision of a pediatric hematologist-oncologist. If chemotherapy fails, particularly in patients with ANLL or CML, bone marrow transplantation is an effective alternative.[10, 28] Because chemotherapeutic agents are quite toxic, some complications of leukemia may be drug related (Table 62–2).

HEMATOLOGIC COMPLICATIONS
Anemia

Anemia is a common problem in the leukemic patient. Of patients with ALL, 43% initially presented with a hemoglobin level of less than 7 gm/dl (see Table 62–1). Common causes include bone marrow failure secondary to leukemic infiltration, bone marrow suppression from radiation or chemotherapeutic agents, and hemorrhage resulting from underlying coagulation disorders or thrombocytopenia.[29]

Generally, a hemoglobin level greater than 8 to 9 gm/dl is tolerated well in the hemodynamically stable, nonbleeding patient and does not require transfusion in the emergency department. Compromised anemic patients without evidence of congestive heart failure may be transfused with 5 to 10 ml of packed red blood cells per kilogram over 3 to 4 hours while on a cardiac monitor.[29] Supplemental oxygen is recommended to maximize oxygen saturation of the transfused blood. Caution must be exercised to avoid overly rapid volume infusions, which increase cardiovascular stress.

Furosemide (1 mg/kg) may be given to avoid fluid overload but may exacerbate intravascular sludging if the patient has hyperleukocytosis (CBC count greater than 100,000 cells/mm³). The presence of congestive heart failure and severe anemia warrants further caution, and no more than 3 to 5 ml packed red blood cells per kilogram over 3 to 4 hours is initially advised. A partial exchange transfusion may be required in patients with congestive heart failure who require rapid correction of the anemia. In all cases of blood product transfusion, irradiated blood elements are preferred to avoid graft-versus-host problems in the future.

Hemorrhage

Severe hemorrhage is a common cause of death in leukemic patients and is usually associated with profound thrombocytopenia with platelet counts of less than 10,000/mm³. Other important factors that predispose leukemic patients to a bleeding diathesis include ulceration of mucosal surfaces, functional impairment of platelets, deficiency of plasma coagulation factors, and severe underlying infection.[29]

Disseminated intravascular coagulation (DIC) is suspected when life-threatening hemorrhage develops from multiple sites. Conditions associated with DIC include sepsis, hypoxia, hypotension, disseminated malignancy, and a subset of ANLL known as *acute promyelocytic leukemia*.[29] Although heparin therapy has been recommended for bleeding patients with acute promyelocytic patients in DIC, these patients can be successfully managed with intensive chemotherapy and blood products (platelets and fresh frozen plasma) without the routine use of heparin.[30]

Complications of thrombocytopenia include epistaxis, gastrointestinal bleeding, hematuria, and intracranial hemorrhage. Intra-abdominal hemorrhage related to thrombocytopenia and resulting in an acute abdomen has responded to platelet transfusions, obviating surgical intervention.[31] Treatment of coagulopathies related to coagulation factor defects consists of fresh frozen plasma (10 to 15 ml/kg) and heparin therapy in cases of thrombosis.

Because of the high risk of complications associated with low platelet counts, thrombocytopenia is aggressively treated to maintain the platelet count above 20,000/mm³.[13] All episodes of gross bleeding are treated with supplemental platelet infusions when the platelet count is less than 100,000/mm³.[32] This may be achieved by giving 4 to 6 U/m² body surface area, assuming that 1 U/m² of platelets raises the platelet count by 10,000 to 15,000/mm³.[29] Although platelets are generally given over 1 to 2 hours, they may also be given by intravenous push when necessary for uncontrollable bleeding caused by severe thrombocytopenia.

INFECTIOUS COMPLICATIONS
Fever in the Neutropenic Patient

Infectious complications are the leading cause of death in patients with hematologic malignancies.[33] The susceptibility to infections is a result of a combination of severe neutropenia, defects in cellular and humoral immunity, and disruption of the integrity of the skin and mucous membranes. Of these, the most important predictor of the incidence and severity of infection is the absolute neutrophil count (ANC), which represents the absolute number of polymorphonuclear leukocytes and band forms.[34] At levels below 500 cells/mm³ the risk of infection rises rapidly, especially when the cell count is depressed for extended periods of time.

The level of fever that should prompt therapy is arbitrarily defined.[29] In general, two or three low-grade elevations above 38°C (100.4° F) or a single elevation above 38.5°C (101.3°F) in concert with a granulocyte count of less than 500/mm³ are sufficient to begin empiric therapy. Fever should not be attributed to blood products, cancer, or medications. In addition, the patient may be receiving drugs that mask the febrile response (i.e., steroids, antipyretic-containing analgesics).[35]

Approximately 85% of the organisms isolated when the neutropenic patient first becomes febrile are bacterial.[33] The most commonly isolated organisms include gram-negative rods such as *Escherichia coli*, *Klebsiella*, *Enterobacter*, *Serratia*, and *Pseudomonas*.[36] Gram-positive isolates, however, are becoming increasingly common, particularly *Staphylococcus aureus* and *Streptococcus epidermidis*,[37, 38] especially in children with deep intravenous catheters.[39] Disseminated fungal infections are seldom a cause of infection in the newly febrile neutropenic patient, unless the patient has a history of being on a prolonged course of broad-spectrum antibiotics or steroids or has a protracted, profound neutropenia.

	TABLE 62–2	
TOXICITIES OF THE COMMONLY USED ANTILEUKEMIC DRUGS		
Drug	**Acute Toxicity**	**Long-term Toxicities**
Vincristine	Peripheral neuropathy, SIADH	Cardiomyopathy
Cyclophosphamide	Myelosuppression, hemorrhagic cystitis	Infertility
L-Asparaginase	Coagulopathy, pancreatitis, hepatitis	
Daunorubicin	Myelosuppression, mucositis	Cardiomyopathy, alopecia
Methotrexate	Myelosuppression, mucositis, hepatic fibrosis	Cirrhosis
6-Mercapto-purine	Myelosuppression, mucositis, cholestasis	
Cytosine arabinoside	Myelosuppression, mucositis, neurotoxicity	Neurotoxicity

SIADH = Syndrome of inappropriate antidiuretic hormone.

TABLE 62–3

BASIC LABORATORY EVALUATION OF THE FEBRILE NEUTROPENIC PATIENT

Complete blood cell count with differential
Blood urea nitrogen/creatinine
Liver function tests
Urinalysis
Chest radiograph
Sinus radiographs
Blood cultures (aerobic, anaerobic), two sets
Urine culture
Lumbar puncture

Because the lungs, soft tissue (especially the perirectal area), and mucosal surfaces are the most frequent sites of serious infection,[40] the history and physical examination should focus on these areas, although frequently signs of infection will be absent or muted because of the poor inflammatory response in neutropenic patients. Pertinent historical information includes the presence of sore throat, cough, dyspnea, dysphagia, chest pain, mental status changes, headaches, or pain on defecation.[33] The physical examination should give special attention to areas that may harbor occult infection, such as eye grounds (possibly harboring a fungal enophthalmitis), the perirectal area, lungs, sinuses, sites of invasive procedures, skin, oropharynx, muscles, bones, and joints.

Because infections of the central nervous system (CNS) are unusual in the leukemic patient, a lumbar puncture is not considered as part of the routine evaluation unless specific signs that suggest a CNS infection are present (e.g., headache, vomiting, photophobia, meningeal signs, seizure, change in mental status, or focal neurologic signs) (Table 62–3).[41] Caution should be exercised when performing a lumbar puncture in the leukemic patient, as bleeding complications may result. Mapstone et al. have described development of quadriplegia secondary to hematoma formation after a high neurosurgical spinal tap, despite aggressive platelet support prior to the procedure.[42] Finally, viral serologic tests for hepatitis, Epstein-Barr virus, and cytomegalovirus may be performed when viral causes are suspected, but these are seldom diagnostically helpful in the emergency department.

Empiric Antibiotic Therapy

Recommended empiric therapy utilizes a combination of antibiotics for broad-spectrum coverage (Table 62–4). Although monotherapy with third-generation cephalosporins has received much attention,[37, 38] conflicting results preclude its recommendation at this time.[43] Appropriate cultures should be obtained before antimicrobial therapy is begun.

Fever in the Non-neutropenic Patient

In addition to being susceptible to the same infections as their healthy pediatric counterparts, non-neutropenic patients are particularly prone to three other types of infections: *Pneumocystis carinii* pneumonia, catheter-related sepsis, and *Haemophilus influenzae* bacteremias. Children with central venous catheters and subcutaneously implanted venous access devices have increased susceptibility to fungemias and bacteremias from gram-positive coagulase-negative organisms and gram-negative rods.[44, 45] In these patients, antibiotic coverage should include an aminoglycoside and vancomycin after peripheral blood cultures and blood cultures from the

suspicious catheters themselves (i.e., "pullback" cultures) are obtained.[41]

H. influenzae bacteremia and sepsis typically occur when the patient is in remission on maintenance chemotherapy. It is caused by nontypable invasive strains and has been documented in children as old as 12 years. Clinical presentations vary, ranging from septic arthritis and interstitial infiltrates to fulminant sepsis. Therefore, empiric antibiotic regimens should include coverage for *H. influenzae*, with some possible choices being ticarcillin or carbenicillin.[46]

Pulmonary Infiltrate in the Neutropenic Patient

The lung is the most common site of serious infection in children with leukemia and may be associated with a mortality rate of as much as 80%.[47] Potential pathogens include bacteria, viruses, fungi, and protozoa, occurring singly or in combination. Definitive diagnosis is difficult in the emergency department, because sputum is frequently unobtainable in young children and invasive tests such as an open lung biopsy or fiberoptic bronchoscopy are often not available or practical. Noninfectious causes of pulmonary infiltrate must also be included in the differential diagnosis. These include drug reactions, pulmonary edema, pulmonary embolism, neoplasia, radiation pneumonitis, pulmonary hemorrhage, adult respiratory distress syndrome (ARDS), and oxygen toxicity.[41, 48]

Studies should include a CBC count with differential, chest radiograph, blood culture, and arterial blood gas measurement. Sputum, if available, should be sent for culture and Gram stain. Attempts to narrow down the differential diagnosis are based on the radiographic appearance of the infiltrate, the duration and extent of neutropenia, and the underlying disorder.[46, 48, 49] Nevertheless, most pa-

---

TABLE 62–4

EMPIRIC ANTIBIOTIC THERAPY FOR FEBRILE NEUTROPENIC PATIENTS

Agent	Dose
Semisynthetic antipseudomonal penicillin*	
Ticarcillin	300 mg/kg/day IV q 4 hr
Pipercillin	300 mg/kg/day IV q 4 hr
Carbenicillin	500 mg/kg/day IV q 4 hr
plus	
Aminoglycoside	
Tobramycin	8 mg/kg/day IV q 8 hr
Gentamicin	3–7.5 mg/kg/day IV q 8 hr
Amikacin	20 mg/kg/day IV q 6 hr
plus	
First-generation cephalosporin	
or	
Penicillinase-resistant penicillin (if gram-positive cocci are suspected)	
Cefazolin	140 mg/kg/day IV q 6 hr
Cephalothin	170 mg/kg/day IV q 4 hr
Oxacillin	100–200 mg/kg/day IV q 4 hr
Vancomycin†	40 mg/kg/day IV q 6 hr

*Third-generation cephalosporins such as ceftazidime (150 mg/kg/day IV q 6 hr) may be substituted for patients with a nonanaphylactic penicillin allergy.

†Vancomycin may be substituted in patients with deep in-dwelling catheter infections that are frequently caused by coagulation-negative *Staphylococcus*.

tients are admitted for diagnostic evaluation and are initially treated empirically.

Diffuse infiltrates in the non-neutropenic child are most likely caused by *P. carinii* infection, which is unique in that it commonly occurs when the child is in remission after completion of chemotherapy. Symptoms include dry cough, fever, and tachypnea. Hypoxia is characteristic, as is the absence of auscultatory signs.[50] Other causes of diffuse infiltrates include *Legionella, Mycoplasma*, viruses, and fungi.[48] Cytomegalovirus is especially common in bone marrow recipients.[49] A diffuse infiltrate presenting acutely may represent pulmonary edema and warrant a trial of diuretics.[49]

Treatment and disposition of patients with suspected pneumonia depends on the clinical appearance, immunologic status, and the most likely pathogens (Fig. 62–1). In most cases, admission for a diagnostic workup and broad-spectrum antibiotic therapy is warranted.

Viruses

Varicella zoster virus (VZV), the etiologic agent of chickenpox, may viscerally disseminate in as many as one third of severely neutropenic patients.[51] Although fatality rates of 7% have been primarily associated with pneumonia,[52] any organ system may be affected, particularly the lung, brain, and liver. Reactivation of VZV in the dorsal ganglia results in zoster (shingles) and is also more common in leukemic patients. Although cutaneous dissemination may occur, visceral dissemination is rare, except in bone marrow recipients, who have mortality rate of 5%.[53]

Prophylaxis with varicella zoster immune globulin (VZIG) within 72 hours of exposure to infection markedly decreases mortality in immunocompromised patients with varicella infection. The recommended dose is 1 vial per 10 kilograms of body weight, to a maximum of 5 vials.[48] Intravenous acyclovir is generally reserved for inpatient treatment of disseminated disease in neutropenic patients.[54]

Herpes simplex virus (HSV) may result in severe gingivostomatitis mimicking chemotherapy-induced mucositis, thereby increasing the risk of bleeding and secondary bacterial infection. Fortunately, visceral dissemination is rare,[52] even when cutaneous spread is extensive,[50] except in bone marrow recipients. Although topical acyclovir may be used to treat mild to moderate lesions,[55] intravenous acyclovir is warranted for disseminated infection or severe mucocutaneous involvement.[41]

Measles may also cause fulminant disease in patients with acute leukemia; this is associated with an increased incidence of bacterial pneumonia and otitis media. Dissemination can result in hepatitis, encephalitis, and nephritis, as well as complications of cutaneous and visceral bleeding.[52] Human serum immune globulin (0.5 ml/kg; maximal dose, 15 ml) provides some protection from measles and should be given for exposure.[50] Mumps,[56] infectious mononucleosis,[50] rubella, polio virus, and the common respiratory viruses are unusual causes of serious infection and generally do not require special treatment or prophylaxis, although each case must be evaluated individually.

Miscellaneous Infections

Mucositis is frequently a complication of chemotherapy (see Table 62–2).[41] It is an inflammation of the oral mucosa that renders the leukemic patient susceptible to both local and invasive infections caused by oropharyngeal flora.

Esophagitis is clinically characterized by dysphagia, retrosternal pain, and burning and may occur with or without accompanying oral lesions.[52] The most common causes are *Candida*, infection, cytomegalovirus, herpes simplex virus, and bacteria and may result in disseminated infection.[57] A barium swallow may suggest the diagnosis by exhibiting ragged or cobblestone appearance of the distal esophageal mucosa. Treatment is with amphotericin B and acyclovir when HSV is suspected.[41]

Typhlitis is a necrotizing lesion of the cecum and terminal ileum that typically occurs in the setting of cancer chemotherapy and neutropenia.[58] It often presents as an acute intra-abdominal emergency that has an associated mortality rate of more than 50%.[59] Common presenting signs are fever, right lower quadrant pain with a palpable mass, peritoneal signs, and sepsis often caused by gram-negative bacteria. *Pseudomonas* and fungi (i.e., *Candida*) are invariably present.[58] Besides a characteristic history and physical examination, radiographs may reveal a large soft tissue density in the right lower quadrant, local or diffuse "thumbprinting," and varying degrees of dilated loops of bowel.[60] Treatment is with broad-spectrum antibiotics and maximum supportive therapy.[59]

Perianal cellulitis is an important cause of occult sepsis.

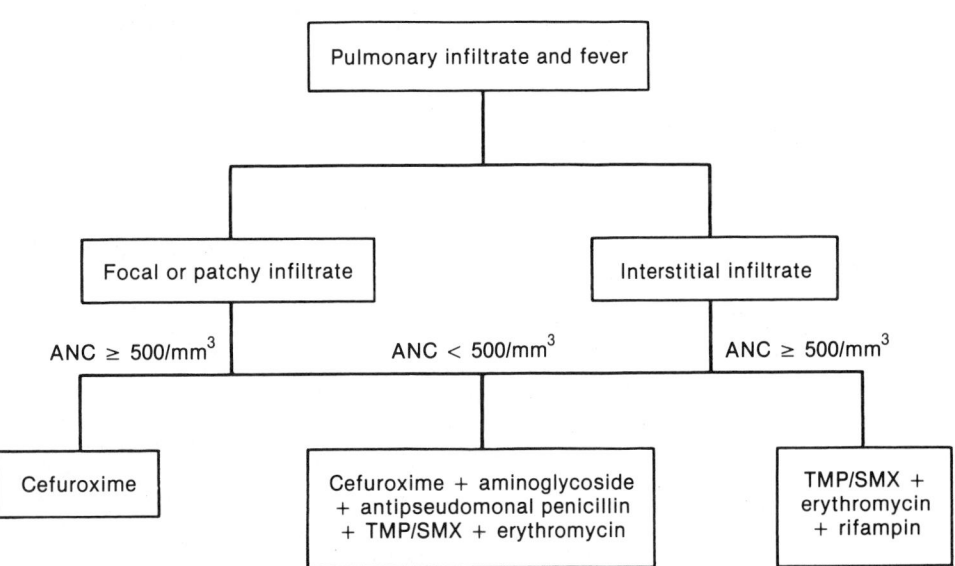

Figure 62–1. Approach to treatment of pneumonia in the child with cancer. Cefuroxime, 200 mg/kg/day IV q 8 hr; erythromycin, 50 mg/kg/day IV q 6 hr; TMP/SMX, 20 mg/kg/day trimethoprim component IV q 6 hr; rifampin, 20 mg/kg/day IV q 12 hr. (Adapted from Barston WJ, Brady MT. Management of infections in children with cancer. Hematol Oncol Clin North Am 1987;1:801.)

Most cases begin as small fissures at the anal opening, allowing the entrance of colonic gram-negative rods and anaerobes. Physical findings are limited to perianal tenderness without erythema and are easily overlooked. Although cellulitis is usually responsive to clindamycin, broad-spectrum gram-negative antibiotic coverage and supportive measures and surgical intervention may be required.[41]

In patients with acute leukemia, *Cryptosporidium* may cause a protracted, life-threatening diarrhea that is extremely resistant to treatment.[61, 62] Diagnosis is made by identifying the characteristic cysts in a fresh stool specimen.[63] Treatment is supportive.

Lastly, seemingly benign infections in the neutropenic patient (e.g., otitis media, pharyngitis, and sinusitis) may be associated with significant bacteremias and warrant tympanocentesis and sinus aspiration (with appropriate cultures) before intravenous antibiotics are begun. Non-neutropenic patients are generally treated with conventional antibiotic therapy.

HYPERLEUKOCYTOSIS

Hyperleukocytosis, defined as a white blood cell (WBC) count greater than 100,000/mm³, is associated with potentially life-threatening complications because of the large numbers of leukemic cells causing vascular sludging, hemorrhage, and hypoxia of major organ systems, particularly of the lung and brain.[64] Other complications include DIC, retinal hemorrhage, acute tumor lysis syndrome, lactic acidosis, priapism, and clitorism.[65] Patients with ANLL are most prone to develop hyperleukocytosis, followed by CML patients in a blast crisis.[66]

Cerebral leukostasis may be associated with sudden death from cerebral hemorrhage in patients with ALL and ANLL, despite a relatively normal platelet count in such patients. Because of the lethality of this condition, any leukemic patient with a rapidly rising WBC count exceeding 100,000/mm³ should be considered at risk for intracranial hemorrhage, and prophylactic measures should be rapidly instituted.[66] Treatment involves cranial irradiation (600 rads) to prevent CNS hemorrhage,[67] hydroxyurea, and leukopheresis, followed by definitive antileukemic therapy.[68] Associated thrombocytopenia may be corrected using platelet supplementation.

Pulmonary leukostasis typically presents with symptoms of respiratory insufficiency such as hypoxia and tachypnea and may mimic pneumonia. The chest radiograph may show patchy infiltrates or be completely normal. Pulmonary leukostasis is suggested when WBC counts are more than 150,000/mm³, especially if other manifestations of hyperleukocytosis are present (e.g., lethargy, retinal hemorrhage, or papilledema).[66] When vascular stasis is severe, pulmonary hemorrhage may occur; this is associated with a grave prognosis.[29] Treatment consists of aggressive supportive care, as well as rapid institution of definitive chemotherapy, hydroxyurea, and leukopheresis.[69]

CENTRAL NERVOUS SYSTEM LEUKEMIA

CNS leukemia may be classified as occult or overt. Occult involvement is asymptomatic and is usually diagnosed on routine surveillance lumbar punctures performed by the oncologist. This procedure identifies those patients who are candidates for preventive therapy (intrathecal methotrexate or cranial irradiation), as CNS leukemia is almost invariably followed by bone marrow relapse.[70]

In contrast, overt CNS leukemia frequently presents with signs and symptoms of increased intracranial pressure. Although headache is the single most common symptom,

TABLE 62–5
ADMISSION CRITERIA FOR LEUKEMIA PATIENTS
Unstable vital signs
Fever in neutropenic (ANL <500) patients
Relapse of primary disease
Severe or symptomatic electrolyte or acid-base abnormalities
Sepsis
Mental status changes
Severe anemia or thrombocytopenia

nausea, vomiting, nuchal rigidity, lethargy, irritability, incontinence, papilledema, cranial nerve palsies (third or seventh), and seizures may also be present.[71] Disturbances of visual and auditory function are common and may be presenting complaints.[72] In fact, any neurologic sign or symptom in a patient with acute leukemia requires evaluation to exclude CNS leukemia.[71]

Diagnosis of CNS leukemia requires cytologic confirmation of the presence of leukemic cells in the cerebrospinal fluid (CSF). Other findings include elevated CSF pressure and CSF protein levels and decreased CSF glucose levels.[71]

Treatment of overt CSF leukemia typically involves a combination of CNS radiation treatments and methotrexate.[72] Complications of therapy include leukoencephalopathy, postradiation somnolence syndrome, seizures, and neuropsychiatric problems.[10]

RELAPSE

Signs of relapse in extramedullary sites are important to identify, as they may herald resurgence of the primary disease.[71] The most common site of relapse in ALL patients is the bone marrow, whereas extramedullary recurrence is most often reported in the testis and CNS.[25] The anterior segment of the eye is a rare site of relapse, accounting for between 0.5% and 2.6% of cases.[73]

Overt testicular recurrence may occur in up to 15% of boys undergoing chemotherapy.[71] It typically presents as painless testicular swelling that may be unilateral or bilateral and may go unnoticed. For that reason, no physical examination in the leukemic child is complete without a thorough examination of the external genitalia. Treatment of testicular relapse is with local radiation and chemotherapy.[24]

The use of CNS preventive therapy has dramatically reduced the incidence of CNS relapse, which now occurs in less than 5% of children.[12] CNS relapse typically presents with signs and symptoms of increased intracranial pressure. Iritis and hypopyon are the most frequent clinical findings in patients with ocular anterior segment relapse.

TABLE 62–6
DISCHARGE INSTRUCTIONS
1. Return any child for reevaluation if flu-like symptoms are present for more than 1 week, especially if bruising, lymphadenopathy, or lethargy develop.
2. For known leukemic patients, return the child for reevaluation if fever exceeds 38°C (oral) three times in 24 hours or if one oral temperature exceeds 38.5°C.
3. For known leukemic patients, return the child for reevaluation if bruising, cough, sore throat, rectal pain, abdominal pain, vomiting, diarrhea, or mental status changes occur.

DISPOSITION

Leukemic patients may be quite ill despite benign-appearing presentations, and a liberal admission policy is warranted (Table 62–5). Although most parents of leukemic children develop a fairly sophisticated understanding of the child's disease process, this should not be assumed. Detailed, written instructions should be provided if the child is discharged (Table 62–6). Frequently, consultation with a hematologist-oncologist is necessary to arrange close follow-up.

References

1. Silverberg E, Lubera J. Cancer statistics 1986. Cancer 1986;36:9.
2. Poplack DG. Acute lymphoblastic leukemia. In Pizzo PA, Poplack DG (eds). Principles and Practice of Pediatric Oncology. Philadelphia, JB Lippincott, 1988.
3. Neglia JP, Robinson LL. Epidemiology of the childhood acute leukemias. Pediatr Clin North Am 1988;35:675.
4. Miller RW, Dalager NA. US childhood cancer deaths by cell type, 1960–68. J Pediatr 1974;85:664.
5. Mulvihill JJ. Persons at high risk of cancer. In An Approach to Cancer Etiology and Control. New York, Academic Press, 1975, p 3.
6. Muts-Homshma SJM, Muller HP, Geracost JPM. Kleinfelter's syndrome and acute non-lymphoblastic leukemia. Blut 1981;44:15.
7. Bader JL, Miller RW. Neurofibromatosis and childhood leukemia. J Pediatr 1978;92:925.
8. Schroeder TM, Pohler E, Hufnagl HD, et al. Fanconi's anemia, terminal leukemia and "forme fruste" in one family. Clin Genet 1979;16:260.
9. German J, Bloom D, Passarge E. Bloom's syndrome VII. Progress report for 1978. Clin Genet 1979;15:316.
10. Sallam SE, Weinstein HJ, Nathan DG. The childhood leukemias. J Pediatr 1981;99:676.
11. Hakami N, Monzon CM. Acute nonlymphoblastic leukemia in children. Hematol Oncol Clin North Am 1987;1:567.
12. Russell NH, Lewis IJ, Martin J. Acute lymphoblastic leukemia presenting with raised intracranial pressure. Arch Dis Child 1985;60:575.
13. Miller DR. Acute lymphoblastic leukemia. Pediatr Clin North Am 1980;27:269.
14. Schachat AP. The leukemias and lymphomas. In Ryan SJ (ed). Retina. Vol 2. Medical Retina. St Louis, CV Mosby, 1989.
15. Williams DL, Bell BA, Ragab AH. Clitorism at presentation of acute lymphocytic leukemia. J Pediatr 1985;107:754.
16. Vadakan V, Ortega J. Priapism in acute lymphoblastic leukemia. Cancer 1972;30:373.
17. Chu JY, Demello D, O'Connor DN, et al. Pericarditis as the presenting manifestation of acute nonlymphocytic leukemia in a young child. Cancer 1983;52:322.
18. Mancuso L, Marchi S, Giuliano P, Pitrols F. Cardiac tamponade as first manifestation of acute lymphoblastic leukemia in a patient with echocardiographic evidence of mediastinal lymph node enlargement. Am Heart J 1985;110:1303.
19. Blatt J, Martini ML, Penchansky L. Characteristics of acute lymphoblastic leukemia in children with osteopenia and vertebral compression fractures. J Pediatr 1984;05:281.
20. Nabors MW, Narayan RK, Poplack DG. Intracranial and otological presentation of acute lymphoblastic leukemia. Neurosurgery 1985;17:309.
21. Gilman AL, Cohen BA, Urbach AH, Blatt J. Pyoderma gangrenosum as a manifestation of leukemia in children. Pediatrics 1988;110:1303.
22. Altman A, Altman AJ. Chronic leukemias of childhood. Pediatr Clin North Am 1988;35:765.
23. Hammond GD, Sather H, Bleyer WA, et al. Stratification of prognostic factors in the design and analysis of clinical trials for acute lymphoblastic leukemia, hematology and blood transfusions. In Bochner, Schellong, Hiddemann (eds). Acute Leukemias. Berlin, Springer-Verlag, 1987.
24. Poplack D. Leukemias and lymphomas of childhood. In DeVita VT, Hellman S, Rosenberg SA (eds). Cancer Principles and Practice of Oncology. Vol 2. Philadelphia, JB Lippincott, 1989.
25. Poplack D, Reaman G. Acute lymphoblastic leukemia in childhood. Pediatr Clin North Am 1988;35:853.
26. Akber J, Gallagher M, Mathew L, et al. Destructive skeletal lesions as the primary initial manifestation of acute childhood leukemia. Am J Pediatr Hematol Oncol 1988;10:258.
27. Dubansky SA, Boyett JM, Falletta J, et al. Isolated thrombocytopenia in children with acute lymphoblastic leukemia: A rare event in a pediatric oncology study group. Pediatrics 1989;84:1068.
28. Sanders JE, Thomas ED, Buckner CD, et al. Marrow transplantation for children in first remission of acute non-lymphoblastic leukemia: An update. Blood 1985;66:460.
29. Dutcher JP, Wiernik PH (eds). Handbook of Hematologic and Oncologic Emergencies. New York, Plenum, 1987.
30. Goldberg MA, Ginsburg D, Mayer RJ, et al. Is heparin administration necessary during induction chemotherapy for patients with acute promyelocytic leukemia? Blood 1987;69:187.
31. Kornberg A, Eldor A. Acute surgical abdomen caused by thrombocytopenia in patients with acute leukemia and multiple myeloma. Israel J Med Sci 1983;19:1094.
32. Kobrinsky NL, Robinson LL, Nesbit ME. Acute non-lymphocytic leukemia. Pediatr Clin North Am 1980;27:345.
33. Wiernik PH. The management of infection in the cancer patient. JAMA 1980;244:185.
34. Bodey GP, Buckley M, Sathe YS, et al. Quantitative relationships between circulating leukocytes and infection in patients with acute leukemia. Ann Intern Med 1966;64:328.
35. Pizzo PA. Empiric therapy and precaution of infections in the immunocompromised host. In Mandell GL, Douglas RG, Bennett JB (eds). Principles and Practice of Infectious Disease. 2nd ed. New York, John Wiley & Sons, 1985.
36. Moellering RC. Principles of anti-infective therapy. In Mandell GL, Douglas RG, Bennett JB (eds). Principles and Practice of Infectious Diseases. 2nd ed. New York, John Wiley & Sons, 1985, p 153.
37. Pizzo PA, Hathorn JW, Hiemenz J, et al. A randomized trial comparing ceftazidime alone with combination antibiotic therapy in cancer patients with fever and neutropenia. N Engl J Med 1986;315:552.
38. de Pauw BE, Williams K, de Neeff J, et al. A randomized prospective study of ceftazidime versus ceftazidime plus flucloxacillin in the empiric treatment of febrile episodes in severely neutropenic patients. Antimicrob Agents Chemother 1985;28:824.
39. Johnson PR, Decker MD, Edwards KM, et al. Frequency of Broviac catheter infections in pediatric oncology patients. J Infect Dis 1986;154:570.
40. Pizzo PA. Infectious complications in the child with cancer: I. Pathophysiology of the compromised host and the initial evaluation and management of the febrile cancer patient. J Pediatr 1981;98:341.
41. Barson WJ, Brady MT. Management of infections in children with cancer. Hematol Oncol Clin North Am 1987;1:801.
42. Mapstone TB, Rekate HL, Shurin SB. Quadriplegia secondary to hematoma formation after lateral C-1, C-2 puncture in a leukemic child. Neurosurgery 1983;12:230.
43. Kramer BS, Rawphal R, Rand K. Antibiotic therapy in cancer patients with fever and neutropenia. N Engl J Med 1987;316:410.
44. Johnson PR, Decker MD, Edwards KM, et al. Frequency of Broviac catheter infections in pediatric oncology patients. J Infect Dis 1986;154:570.
45. Press OW, Ramsey PG, Larson EB, et al. Hickman catheter infections in patients with malignancies. Medicine 1984;63:189.
46. Bartlett AV, Zusman J, Daum RS. Unusual presentations of Haemophilus influenzae infections in immunocompromised patients. J Pediatr 1983;102:55.
47. Pizzo PA. Fever and infection in the child with cancer. In Nelson JD (ed). Current Therapy in Pediatric Infectious Disease. St Louis, CV Mosby, 1986, p 218.
48. Albano EA, Pizzo PA. Infectious complications in childhood acute leukemias. Pediatr Clin North Am 1988;35:873.
49. Ramsey PG, Rubin RH, Tolkoff-Rubin NE, et al. The renal transplant patient with fever and pulmonary infiltrate: Etiology, clinical manifestations and management. Medicine 1980;59:206.
50. Pizzo PA. Infectious complications in the child with cancer. II. management of specific infectious organisms. J Pediatr 1981;98:513.
51. Feldman S, Hughes WT, Daniel CB. Varicella in children with cancer: Seventy-seven cases. Pediatrics 1975;56:388.
52. Joshi JH, Schimpff SC. Infections in patients with acute leukemia. In Mandell GL, Douglas RG, Bennett JB (eds). Principles and Practice of Infectious Disease. 2nd ed. New York, John Wiley & Sons, 1985.
53. Novelli VM, Brunell PA, Geiser CF, et al. Herpes zoster in children with acute lymphocytic leukemia. Am J Dis Child 1988;142:71.
54. Shepp DH, Dandliker RN, Meyers JD. Treatment of varicella-zoster virus infection in severely immunocompromised patients. N Engl J Med 1986;314:208.
55. Whitley RJ, Levin M, Barton N, et al. Infections caused by herpes simplex virus in the immunocompromised host: Natural history and topical acyclovir therapy. J Infect Dis 1984;150:323.
56. deBoer AW, deVaan GAM. Mild course of mumps in patients with acute lymphoblastic leukemia. Eur J Pediatr 1989;148:618.
57. Walsh TJ, Belitsos NJ, Hamilton SR, et al. Bacterial esophagitis in immunocompromised patients. Arch Intern Med 1986;146:1345.
58. Koretz MJ, Neifeld JP. Emergency surgical treatment for patients with acute leukemia. Surg Gynecol Obstet 1985;161:149.
59. Shamberger RC, Weinstein HJ, Delory MJ, et al. The medical and surgical management of typhlitis in children with acute non-lymphoblastic (myelogenous) leukemia. Cancer 1986;57:603.
60. Abranson SJ, Berdon WE, Baker DH. Childhood typhlitis: Its increasing association with acute myelogenous leukemia. Radiology 1983;146:61.
61. Lewis IJ, Hart CA, Baxby D. Diarrhea due to Cryptosporidium in acute lymphoblastic leukemia. Arch Dis Child 1985;60:60.
62. Miller RA, Holmberg RE, Clausen CR. Life-threatening diarrhea caused by cryptosporidium in a child undergoing therapy for acute lymphocytic leukemia. J Pediatr 1983;103:256.

63. Baxby D, Blundell N. Sensitive, rapid, simple methods for detecting cryptosporidium in faeces. Lancet 1983;ii:1149.
64. Dearth JC, Fountain KS, Smithson WA, et al. Extreme leukemic leukocytosis (blast crisis) in childhood. Mayo Clin Proc 1978;53:207.
65. Maurer HS, Steinherz PG, Gaynon PS, et al. The effect of initial management of hyperleukocytosis or early complications and outcome of children with acute lymphoblastic leukemia. J Clin Oncol 1988;6:1425.
66. Dutcher JP. Hyperleukocytosis in leukemia—an emergency. In Dutcher JP, Wiernik PH (eds). Handbook of Hematologic and Oncologic Emergencies. New York, Plenum, 1987.
67. Gilchrist GS, Fountain KS, Dearth JC, et al. Cranial irradiation in the management of extreme leukocytosis complicating childhood acute lymphocytic leukemia. J Pediatr 1981;98:257.
68. Albinar AR. Managing the problem of hyperleukocytosis in acute leukemia. Am J Pediatr Hematol Oncol 1984;6:287.
69. Prakash VBS, Divertie MB, Banks PM. Aggressive therapy in acute respiratory failure from leukemic pulmonary infiltrates. Chest 1970;75:345.
70. Gribbon MA, Hardisty RM, Chessels IM. Long-term control of central nervous system leukemia. Arch Dis Child 1977;52:673.
71. Poplack DG, Kun LE, Cassady JR, Pizzo PA. Leukemias and lymphomas of childhood. In DeVita VT, Hellman S, Rosenberg SA (eds). Cancer Principles and Practice of Oncology. Vol 2. 3rd ed. Philadelphia, JB Lippincott, 1989.
72. Fuks JZ, Marcus S. Meningeal leukemia and carcinomatosis. In Dutcher JP, Wiernik PH (eds). Handbook of Hematologic and Oncologic Emergencies. New York, Plenum, 1987.
73. Novakovic P, Kellie SJ, Taylor D. Childhood leukemia: relapse in the anterior segment of the eye. Br J Ophthalmol 1989;73:354.

CHAPTER 63

Human Immunodeficiency Virus

Karen K. Smith
Ann Petru

INTRODUCTION

The human immunodeficiency virus (HIV) is responsible for what has rapidly become a global pandemic of acquired immunodeficiency syndrome (AIDS), the greatest public health threat of our time. The first adult cases of AIDS were reported in 1982,[1] and the first pediatric cases were reported the following year.[2, 3] Reported cases continue to increase exponentially. The first reported pediatric case was acquired through transfusion.[2] As the infection spread in the adult community to intravenous drug users, women of childbearing age were increasingly infected either directly through needle sharing or indirectly by sexual contact with an infected IV drug user. As a consequence of the increasing incidence of HIV infection in women, perinatal transmission is now the most common route of infection for children.

By November 1991, 3426 cases of AIDS in children under 13 years old had been reported in the United States.[4] This number is underestimated because of lack of recognition of the disease and because of delayed submission of case reports to health departments. Furthermore, this number reflects only those children who meet the Centers for Disease Control (CDC) criteria for pediatric AIDS, thus omitting the majority of HIV-infected children who may or may not have symptoms of HIV disease. Transmission occurred perina-

tally in 77% of reported cases and through transfused blood products in 18% of cases; the remaining cases have undocumented sources of infection.[5]

Fifty-three percent of infected children are black, 23% are Hispanic, and 23% are white (non-Hispanic). Boys and girls are nearly equally affected, unlike adult AIDS, which is predominantly a male disease. Estimates in 1986 suggesting that there would be over 3000 cases of pediatric AIDS were correct.[6] Current estimates predict 11,000 to 14,000 cases of pediatric AIDS by 1993.[4] There were between 10,000 and 20,000 children with symptomatic HIV infection in the United States as of 1991.[7] The numbers may climb even higher as more sensitive diagnostic tests are developed and as more treatment options for young infants lead to earlier and more widespread testing of pregnant women. However, there is currently no proven effective method for preventing perinatal transmission.

For physicians in emergency department settings, the child with HIV provides additional challenges above and beyond the medical problems. Certain factors have a major impact on the care for and treatment of infants and children with HIV. These include poverty; lack of regular medical care; insufficient food and transportation; and parental illness, drug use, and inability to access both medical and community resources.

PATHOPHYSIOLOGY

HIV is an RNA virus in the lentivirus family of retroviruses.[8] Retroviruses contain the enzyme, reverse transcriptase, which allows the virus to transcribe its RNA genome into DNA, which then is incorporated into the host cell genome. As a group, retroviruses typically cause slow, progressive disease, leading to the death of the host.

The term *HIV* refers to a group of viruses with similar structure and pathologic effects. Only one of these viruses, HIV-1, causes most of the recognized disease worldwide. HIV-2 is emerging as a new pathogen in some areas of the world and in certain populations, causing immunodeficiency that is clinically indistinguishable from HIV-1.[9] However, antibody testing for HIV-1 does not reliably detect antibody to HIV-2, making the diagnosis of the latter type of immunodeficiency difficult.[10] HIV-1 will be referred to in this context as HIV, as most scientific information currently available was obtained from studies of HIV-1.

The principal target cell of HIV in the human host is the T4 lymphocyte.[8] Most of the pathologic effects of HIV can be explained by a review of the pivotal role that T4 lymphocytes play in coordinating and modulating immune function. These cells are involved in nearly all aspects of the immune system, either directly or indirectly.

There are two structural categories of T cells: those that contain T8 antigen on the cell surface, and those that contain T4 antigen (also called CD4). These two categories can be further divided according to function.[11] The T8 cells include cytotoxic (or killer) cells and suppressor cells. Killer cells destroy foreign or infected cells; suppressor cells provide feedback to suppress immune function. The T4 lymphocytes include both helper cells and inducer cells. Helper T cells have multiple functions. They secrete lymphokines, which activate macrophages and T and B cells; they recognize foreign antigen; and they serve as a modulator for T8 cell functions. Finally, inducer T4 cells control the growth of the various T-cell subsets. Thus a significant depletion of the T4 cells has a widespread impact on immune function.

In pediatric HIV infection there is also impaired regulation of B-cell production of antibody, so that many children with HIV infection produce excessive amounts of nonspecific antibody, yet cannot make specific antibody to encountered antigens.[12] As a consequence, children with HIV become susceptible to infection with common bacterial pathogens.[13]

Additional problems are encountered when the host is an infant or young child. The immune responses of neonates and young infants are immature compared with those of older children and adults. In infants, complement level is low,[14] opsonin activity is poor,[15] neutrophil activity is below normal,[16] and T- and B-cell cooperation and immunologic memory formation are immature.[17]

EPIDEMIOLOGY

As stated earlier, in 77% of reported cases of pediatric AIDS, infection was acquired perinatally.[12] The timing of transmission from mother to infant is poorly understood. It has been shown that fetuses as young as 8 weeks of gestation can be infected.[18] It is likely, however, that a significant proportion of infants acquire HIV late in gestation or during labor and delivery, presumably as a result of exposure to infected blood and secretions.[19, 20] Current estimates are that 25% to 40% of infants born to infected mothers become infected with HIV.[21, 22]

Breast milk can also be a source of HIV infection. A few women (infected with HIV after delivery by receiving a blood transfusion) transmitted HIV to their infants through breast milk.[23, 24] As a consequence, infected mothers are discouraged from breast-feeding their infants in countries where infant formula is readily available.[25]

The risk of HIV infection from blood products has been substantially reduced as a result of the screening tests used.[26-28] However, in the early 1980s, blood products were a significant risk to recipients of transfusions and to patients who required factor concentrate for treatment of hemophilia and other bleeding diatheses. The risk of acquiring HIV varied with the type of blood component administered. Pooled blood products, such as factor concentrates, carried greater risks. More than 90% of hemophiliacs who received factor replacement therapy between 1981 and 1984 are probably now infected.[29] Recipients of a single transfusion of HIV-contaminated red blood cells or platelets acquired HIV infection at rates approaching 80% to 100%.[30, 31]

Other routes of infection, primarily in teenagers, are intravenous drug use and sexual intercourse.[32, 33] The rising incidence of other sexually transmitted diseases in this population suggests that current attempts to influence the behavior of young people are suboptimal and meet with limited success.[34, 35] Sexual abuse has also been shown to transmit HIV.

There is no evidence that immune globulin, insect bites, or contact with urine, tears, or saliva of infected individuals transmits HIV. Casual contact in family and school settings does not result in HIV infection.[36]

NATURAL HISTORY OF HIV

In adults, early infection with HIV may cause an acute clinical illness similar to infectious mononucleosis. The incubation period is generally 2 to 4 weeks.[37] This is followed by a latent phase that lasts months to many years.[38] The acute illness has not been documented in young children, and the latent phase is generally much shorter. Children who have contracted the virus perinatally or by neonatal transfusion often have symptoms within the first 2 years of life.[29, 39] Current statistics are based on cases reported to the CDC that meet the definition of AIDS (Table 63–1).[12] About one third of children diagnosed with AIDS are less than 1 year old at the time of diagnosis, and 50% are diagnosed by age 2 years. Although most children develop the disease early, some experience latent periods that are as long as 8

to 10 years. As HIV-infected patients are followed for longer periods of time, the potential duration of the latent phase is expected to increase.

Alterations in immune function often precede clinical illness but are highly variable in children.[40] The immunologic hallmark of adult HIV disease is depletion of the T lymphocytes, but this is not universally seen in infected children.[41] The decrease in T cells leads to a decreased T4-to-T8 cell ratio.[37] In addition, T- and B-cell function may be depressed, and impaired immune regulation typically leads to hypergammaglobulinemia and, less commonly, hypogammaglobulinemia.[13, 38]

Infants born to infected mothers are not all infected with HIV, yet virtually all have maternally derived antibody to HIV. This antibody may persist for up to 15 months and cannot be distinguished from endogenously produced antibody. For this reason, a specific definition of HIV infection in infants has been established by the CDC. There are separate definitions for children with perinatal infection who are less than 15 months old and for all other children (Table 63–2). To enable an accurate description of the clinical stage or severity of illness in children, a detailed classification schema has also been developed (Table 63–3). This system separates the children less than 15 months old who have maternal antibody but no clinical or laboratory evidence of infection (class P-O) from those with proven infection. The latter group is divided according to absence (class P-1) or presence (class P-2) of HIV-related symptoms.[42]

The clinical presentation of HIV disease in children varies widely.[12, 13, 43] Early in the course of HIV infection, the symptoms may be subtle. The diagnosis may be suggested only when the findings are clustered together (Table 63–4). In infants, the usual symptoms at presentation include failure to thrive, developmental delay, chronic diarrhea, and thrush. On examination, many of these children have hepatosplenomegaly and generalized lymphadenopathy. Other children do not have this constellation of symptoms but present with recurrent bacterial infections. Most of the infections are typical pediatric problems caused by usual childhood pathogens but occur more frequently and are less responsive to treatment.

Later in the course of their disease, children may develop more serious and even life-threatening bacterial infections, including sepsis, pneumonia, and meningitis. In others, clinical findings are insidious and include chronic parotid enlargement, HIV encephalopathy, and lymphocytic interstitial pneumonitis. In its advanced stage, the child may be found to have *Pneumocystis carinii* pneumonia or end-stage renal or cardiac disease. Although opportunistic infections (other than *P. carinii*) and malignancies such as B-cell lymphoma and Kaposi's sarcoma are typical presenting findings in adults with HIV, they are quite rare in children.[44]

DIAGNOSTIC EVALUATION

For the emergency department physician evaluating a child with possible HIV disease, a few nonspecific laboratory tests are sufficient for the initial evaluation. These include a complete blood cell (CBC) count, a chemistry panel (liver function tests, blood urea nitrogen, serum creatinine, total protein and albumin), and quantitative immunoglobulin determinations.[43] The CBC count may show no abnormalities, depending on the stage of the child's disease (see Table 63–4).[45, 46] In pediatric HIV infection, elevated quantitative immunoglobulin levels may be one of the first laboratory abnormalities noted. Although not specific for HIV disease, hypergammaglobulinemia in the presence of certain clinical findings is strongly suggestive of HIV infection.[38] In the

TABLE 63–1

CENTERS FOR DISEASE CONTROL CASE DEFINITION (SUMMARIZED) FOR PEDIATRIC AIDS, SUMMARY OF SEPTEMBER, 1987, REVISION

I. Without laboratory evidence of HIV infection (tests not done or inconclusive*), a patient with AIDS:
  A. Does not have another cause of immunodeficiency, such as the following:
    1. High-dose or long-term systemic corticosteroid therapy or other immunosuppressive-cytotoxic therapy ≤3 months before the onset of the indicator disease
    2. Hodgkin's disease, non-Hodgkin's lymphoma (other than primary brain lymphoma), lymphocytic leukemia, multiple myeloma, other cancer of lymphoreticular-histiocytic tissue, or angioimmunoblastic lymphadenopathy ≤3 months after diagnosis of the indicator disease
    3. A genetic (congenital) immunodeficiency syndrome or an acquired immunodeficiency syndrome atypical of HIV infection (such as one with hypogammaglobulinemia)

       and

  B. Has had one of the following AIDS indicator diseases definitively diagnosed:
    1. Candidiasis of the esophagus, trachea, bronchi, or lungs
    2. Extrapulmonary cryptococcosis
    3. Cryptosporidiosis with diarrhea persisting >1 mo
    4. Cytomegalovirus disease of an organ other than liver, spleen, or lymph nodes in a patient >1 mo old
    5. Herpes simplex virus infection causing a mucocutaneous ulcer persisting >1 mo or bronchitis, pneumonitis, or esophagitis in a patient >1 mo old
    6. Primary lymphoma of the brain in a patient <60 yr old
    7. Kaposi's sarcoma in a patient <60 yr old
    8. Lymphoid interstitial pneumonia and/or pulmonary lymphoid hyperplasia in a child <13 yr old
    9. *Mycobacterium avium* complex or *Mycobacterium kansasii* disease disseminated to a site other than the lungs, skin, or cervical or hilar lymph nodes
    10. *Pneumocystis carinii* pneumonia
    11. Progressive multifocal leukoencephalopathy
    12. Toxoplasmosis of the brain in a patient >1 mo old
II. With laboratory evidence of HIV infection, a patient with AIDS:
  A. Has had one of the already listed AIDS indicator diseases definitively diagnosed or one of the following AIDS indicator diseases definitively diagnosed:
    1. Multiple or recurrent bacterial infections (at least two within 2 years) in a child <13 yr old, including septicemia, pneumonia, meningitis, bone or joint infection, abscess of internal organ or body cavity (except otitis media or superficial skin or mucosal abscesses)
    2. Coccidioidomycosis disseminated to a site other than the lungs or cervical or hilar lymph nodes
    3. HIV encephalopathy
    4. Histoplasmosis disseminated to a site other than the lungs or cervical or hilar lymph nodes
    5. Isosporiasis with diarrhea persisting >1 mo
    6. Kaposi's sarcoma
    7. Primary lymphoma of brain
    8. Other non-Hodgkin's lymphoma of B-cell or unknown immunologic phenotype (small, noncleaved Burkitt's or non-Burkitt's lymphoma or immunoblastic sarcoma)
    9. Disseminated nontubercular mycobacterial disease involving a site other than the lungs, skin, or cervical or hilar lymph nodes
    10. Tuberculosis involving at least one site other than the lungs
    11. Recurrent nontyphoid *Salmonella* bacteremia
    12. HIV wasting syndrome

       or

  B. One of the following AIDS indicator diseases diagnosed presumptively:
    1. Esophageal candidiasis
    2. Cytomegalovirus retinitis with loss of vision
    3. Kaposi's sarcoma
    4. Lymphoid interstitial pneumonia or pulmonary lymphoid hyperplasia in a child <13 yr old
    5. Acid-fast infection (species not identified) disseminated to a site other than the lungs, skin, or cervical or hilar lymph nodes
    6. *Pneumocystis carinii* pneumonia
    7. Toxoplasmosis of the brain in a patient >1 mo old
III. With laboratory evidence against HIV infection (negative test results), a patient with AIDS:
  A. Does not have another cause of underlying immunodeficiency (listed in section I)

       and

  B. Has had *Pneumocystis carinii* pneumonia definitively diagnosed

       or

    Has had definitive diagnosis of one of the AIDS indicator diseases listed in section I, plus a T-helper lymphocyte count <400/mm³

*Includes children with seropositivity who are <15 mo old, have an HIV-infected mother, and do not have other evidence for immunodeficiency or for HIV infection.
From Falloon J, Eddy J, Wiener L, et al. Human immunodeficiency virus infection in children. J Pediatr 1989;114:1.)

TABLE 63–2

SUMMARY OF THE DEFINITION OF HIV INFECTION IN CHILDREN

Infants and children under 15 months of age with perinatal infection:

1. Virus in blood or tissues
    or
2. HIV antibody
    and
    evidence of both cellular and humoral immunodeficiency
    and
    one or more categories in class P-2
    or
3. Symptoms meeting Centers for Disease Control case definition for AIDS

Older children with perinatal infection and children with HIV infection acquired through other modes of transmission:

1. Virus in blood or tissues
    or
2. HIV antibody
    or
3. Symptoms meeting Centers for Disease Control case definition for AIDS

child with advanced disease, laboratory studies may show evidence of hepatitis or renal disease.

The HIV antibody is available through most facilities, but it may take 2 to 3 weeks before results are returned. Furthermore, pre- and post-test counseling regarding the implications of the test results are essential and are required by law in many states. In general, this test is best done by a physician who can have ongoing contact with the patient. Many tertiary care centers have access to additional specific tests for HIV. These include HIV antigen (P-24), HIV gene

TABLE 63–3

SUMMARY OF THE CLASSIFICATION OF HIV INFECTION IN CHILDREN UNDER 13 YEARS OF AGE

Classification	Definition
P-0	Indeterminate infection
P-1	Asymptomatic infection
	A Normal immune function
	B Abnormal immune function
	C Immune function not tested
P-2	Symptomatic infection
	A Nonspecific findings
	B Progressive neurologic disease
	C Lymphoid interstitial pneumonitis
	D Secondary infectious diseases
	D-1 Specified secondary infectious diseases listed in the Centers for Disease Control surveillance definition for AIDS
	D-2 Recurrent serious bacterial infections
	D-3 Other specified secondary infectious diseases
	E Secondary cancers
	E-1 Specified secondary cancers listed in the Centers for Disease Control surveillance definition for AIDS
	E-2 Other cancers possibly secondary to HIV infection
	F Other diseases possibly caused by HIV infection

amplification by polymerase chain reaction (PCR) technology, and HIV culture.[47–49] These tests are of particular value for the early identification of perinatally infected infants who may have maternal antibody present. The diagnosis of HIV infection is confirmed by a positive culture and is highly supported by a positive HIV antigen or PCR test result.

CLINICAL EVALUATION

Children known to have immunodeficiency who are seen in an emergency department setting are evaluated differently from those who are not yet diagnosed with HIV. The known infected child must be carefully assessed for typical complications in a systematic fashion. Even more challenging will be the undiagnosed child who presents with one, some, or many HIV complications but who has not been recognized as having HIV disease. Awareness of the clinical constellation of failure to thrive, chronic or recurrent thrush, recurrent minor or serious bacterial infections, and diarrhea should lead to suspicion of HIV and appropriate testing.

Uncommonly a child may present critically and acutely ill with respiratory failure caused by opportunistic pathogens or with overwhelming sepsis or meningitis. In this case, recognition of the severity of illness eventually leads to appropriate diagnostic tests, and only later is HIV proven to be the underlying problem. It must be remembered that HIV is not the only cause of these multisystem illnesses or of overwhelming opportunistic infections. Other congenital immunodeficiencies, such as severe combined immunodeficiency syndrome or DiGeorge's syndrome, can present with similar findings and must be considered in the initial evaluation.

Growth and Developmental Manifestations

Many children with HIV have problems growing and gaining weight, especially in the first few years of life and at the end stage of HIV disease. Some of the reasons for this failure to thrive include inadequate intake from thrush or encephalopathy; inadequate intake and excess metabolic demands from underlying pulmonary, cardiac, or other chronic disease and excessive losses from diarrhea or malabsorption.[50] In addition, infants of drug-using mothers may not be cared for in an optimally nurturing environment. They may not have access to enough or the proper food and may suffer from drug withdrawal and the long-term effects of prenatal drug exposure.

Developmental delays may be subtle and manifest themselves as minor motor dysfunction, delayed language ability, and cognitive deficits. Such delays can progress insidiously or may be quite dramatic and incapacitating.[51] Factors contributing to these delays may be the previously mentioned psychosocial effects, HIV encephalopathy, chronic illness, and neurostructural defects secondary to prenatal drug toxicity.

Pulmonary Manifestations

Most children with symptomatic HIV infection are at particular risk for bacterial and *P. carinii* pneumonia and for lymphocytic interstitial pneumonitis. Other pathogens including cytomegalovirus (CMV), fungi such as *Candida*, and atypical *Mycobacteria* organisms, can cause similar pulmonary findings. These disease processes combined account for the majority of the morbidity and mortality in patients with HIV.[52]

P. carinii pneumonia (PCP) is associated with fatality rates of up to 20% per episode in adults. The rate is perhaps higher in children.[53] Recurrences are common, and mortality

TABLE 63–4

HIV: STAGES OF DISEASE

	Asymptomatic Stage	Early Symptomatic Stage	Late Symptomatic Stage	End Stage

Clinical findings	None	Lymphadenopathy
		Hepatosplenomegaly
		Diarrhea
		Slow weight gain
		Developmental delay
		Thrush
		Recurrent mild infections
			Fever
			Failure to thrive
			Progressive CNS involvement
			Recurrent serious infections
			Parotid enlargement
			Lymphocytic interstitial
			  pneumonitis
				Pneumocystis carinii
				  pneumonia
				Nephropathy
				Cardiomyopathy
				Malignancies
				Opportunistic infections

HIV markers	Ab: + Cx: −/+ PCR: −/+	+ −/+ +	+ −/+ +	+ → − + +
Immunologic markers	T4: N T4/T8: N IgG IgA IgM: ↑	N to ↓ N to ↓ ↑ ↑	↓ ↓ ↑ ↑	↓ ↓ ↑ ↑ or ↓
Other laboratory results	WBC: N Hemoglobin: N LFTs: N	N N to ↓ N	↓ ↓ N to ↑	↓ ↓ ↓ N to ↑

Ab = Antibody; Cx = HIV culture; IgA = immunoglobulin A; IgG = immunoglobulin G; IgM = immunoglobulin M; LFT = liver function test; PCR = polymerase chain reaction; WBC = white blood cell count; ↑ = increased; ↓ = decreased; N = normal.

increases with each relapse. In adults and occasionally in children, PCP is often the presenting disease that leads to the diagnosis of AIDS.[37] Adults and teenagers typically have a prolonged prodrome of respiratory symptoms. Children, unlike adults, often present with an abrupt onset of tachypnea and hypoxemia with a rapidly deteriorating respiratory state. The chest radiograph shows bilateral mixed alveolar and interstitial infiltrates (Fig. 63–1). The diagnosis of PCP is confirmed by examination of stains of bronchial washings obtained by bronchoscopy.[54]

Even with a promptly made diagnosis of PCP and appropriate therapy, there may be significant deterioration. All of these patients should be hospitalized, evaluated thoroughly, and treated promptly. The two most commonly used medications for PCP in children are intravenous trimethoprim-sulfamethoxazole and pentamidine (Table 63–5).[55]

Although the risk for PCP in adults is clearly related to a low T₄ count,[56] this relationship is not as apparent in children. The numbers of children with PCP associated with HIV are so small that no large epidemiologic studies are available. Anecdotal experience from some of the larger centers treating children with HIV suggests that younger age is a more significant risk factor for PCP than a low T₄ count. Therefore current recommendations are to use PCP prophylaxis for children younger than 12 months with proven HIV infection; all HIV infected children with less than 20% T₄ cells; all children over 6 years with less than 200 T₄ cells; and based on a sliding scale of T₄ cells for children between 1 and 6 years old.[57] The usual prophylactic regimen is trimethoprim-sulfamethoxazole three times weekly; alternatives such as aerosolized or intravenous pentamidine or oral dapsone are available.

Bacterial pneumonias are also common in this population. The pathogens are generally the same as those seen in normal children and include *Haemophilus influenzae, Streptococcus pneumoniae,* and *Staphylococcus aureus.*[53, 58] Because of their underlying immunodeficiency, children with HIV may also present with tuberculosis, which may be inapparent and difficult to diagnose. Other rare and unusual bacterial pathogens can be seen, particularly if the child has been treated with multiple courses of antibiotics.

The approach to diagnosis should include a blood culture, a sputum culture when possible, a CBC count and chest radiograph, and tests for urinary bacterial antigens. Skin testing for tuberculosis should be routine and should include testing for cutaneous anergy. A negative skin test result does not eliminate the possibility of tuberculosis.

Treatment of suspected bacterial pneumonia in children with HIV should be guided by the predictable sensitivity patterns for the common pediatric pathogens in the community. Hospitalization is generally required for initial treatment.

Another common pulmonary manifestation of HIV in children is lymphocytic interstitial pneumonitis (LIP). Its cause is unknown. It is thought to be a direct consequence

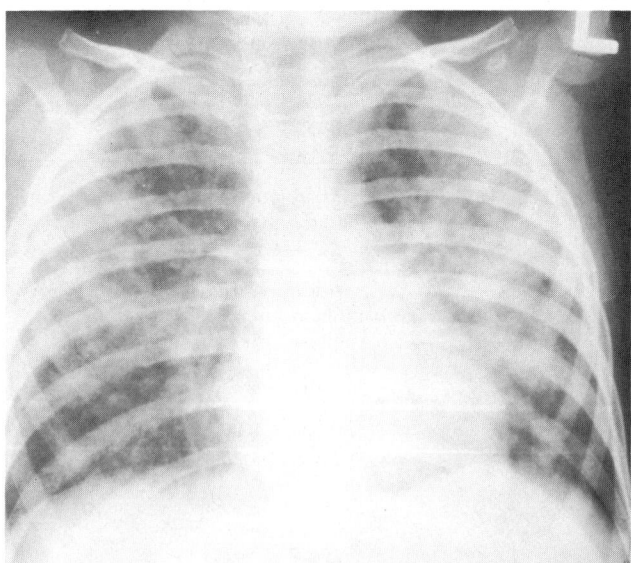

Figure 63–1. The diffuse, small to medium-sized, unsharp nodular infiltrate, relatively more severe near the hila and less severe superiorly, in this 3-year-old child is not specific, but strongly suggests the diagnosis of *Pneumocystis carinii* pneumonia, especially since he is immunocompromised (chemotherapy) and has rapidly deteriorating symptoms. As is typical, these densities first became more confluent, then improved with treatment for *Pneumocystis*. (Courtesy of A. Oestreich, M.D., Cincinnati, OH.)

TABLE 63–5

TREATMENT FOR *PNEUMOCYSTIS CARINII* PNEUMONIA

Drug	Dose	Comments
Trimethoprim-sulfamethoxazole	Trimethoprim, 20 mg/kg/day; sulfamethoxazole, 100 mg/kg/day IV divided q 6 hr and infused over 60–90 min	Must be diluted in large amounts of 5% dextrose Monitor renal function, fluid balance
Pentamidine	4 mg/kg/day IV single dose infused over a minimum of 60 min	May cause hypo- or hypertension, hypo- or hyperglycemia Monitor for thrombocytopenia

of HIV infection, although Epstein-Barr virus (EBV) may be an important cofactor. LIP is diagnosed definitively on the basis of histologic findings from a lung biopsy specimen but can be diagnosed presumptively when bilateral reticulonodular interstitial pulmonary infiltrates are present on the chest radiograph for 2 or more months with no pathogen identified and no response observed to antibiotic treatment.[59]

Unlike PCP, LIP usually has a gradual onset and may be first noted on a chest radiograph (Fig. 63–2). The child may lack symptoms at the time of diagnosis. Symptoms, when present, include tachypnea, hypoxia, and nonproductive cough. On examination, there is an absence of fever or adventitious breath sounds. Digital clubbing is a late finding.[60] In contrast to PCP, LIP is often associated with generalized lymphadenopathy and parotid enlargement.[61] Its clinical course is slow but may be progressive and eventually lead to respiratory failure. Spontaneous improvements have been seen. Treatment for LIP has included the use of oxygen for hypoxemia, chronic steroid therapy, and intravenous gamma globulin. The efficacy of these forms of treatment is undetermined.

Respiratory syncytial virus (RSV) can also be problematic for children with HIV. The diagnosis should be confirmed by testing tissue for RSV using a direct fluorescent antibody technique. Occasionally, bronchoscopy is required to confirm the diagnosis and differentiate this disease from CMV, PCP, and severe LIP. Ribavirin may be considered for symptomatic RSV pneumonia with respiratory compromise.

Cardiac Manifestations

Cardiac symptoms are uncommon but are of great concern when present in pediatric patients with HIV. Involvement of the pericardium, myocardium, and heart valves has been reported. Infections caused by CMV, coxsackievirus, EBV, tuberculosis, PCP, *Cryptococcus neoformans*, *Nocardia*, and *Toxoplasma gondii* have all been implicated as primary causes of cardiomyopathy. There is also some evidence that HIV may directly infect the heart. When symptoms are present, cardiomyopathy may be fatal. Signs and symptoms may reflect congestive heart failure, pericardial tamponade, endocarditis, or arrhythmias. Evaluation includes laboratory tests for the primary causative agent. Treatment is supportive and directed against the underlying cause when appropriate. Cardiac tumors including lymphoma and Kaposi's sarcoma have been reported in adults with HIV but have not been well described in children.[62, 63]

Gastrointestinal Manifestations

The gastrointestinal consequences of HIV infection and its subsequent immunodeficiency are tremendously varied and can involve any organ of the gastrointestinal tract.[64] Often multiple causes must be considered for each presenting complaint. Diarrhea is the most common gastrointestinal complaint found in symptomatic children with HIV. The causes of diarrhea are multiple, and the exact cause may be difficult to determine. The diarrhea may be so severe as to produce significant wasting and require prolonged treatment; occasionally it can be life threatening.[54, 65] The pathogens include all the usual organisms that produce diarrhea in children, as well as some unusual pathogens seen in the immunocompromised host (Table 63–6).[64, 66, 67] HIV itself has been implicated as a possible pathogen causing enteropathy.[68] The consequences of severe, prolonged diarrhea of any cause in children with HIV include nutritional deficiencies caused by inadequate intake, excessive losses, and malabsorption. Fluid and electrolyte imbalances and excoriated perineal skin need close attention. Admission to the hospital is indicated for fluid and electrolyte abnormalities or severe wasting, particularly in young infants.

The most common oral manifestation of HIV infection is candidiasis (thrush).[69] It typically appears as white plaques on an erythematous base that are usually discrete but sometimes confluent. Management consists of topical antifungal agents, usually administered for 3 to 5 days beyond resolution of visible lesions. Oral nystatin often fails. Thrush has been successfully treated by administering clotrimazole vaginal suppositories orally; this is done by placing a suppository inside a nipple and allowing the infant to suck formula

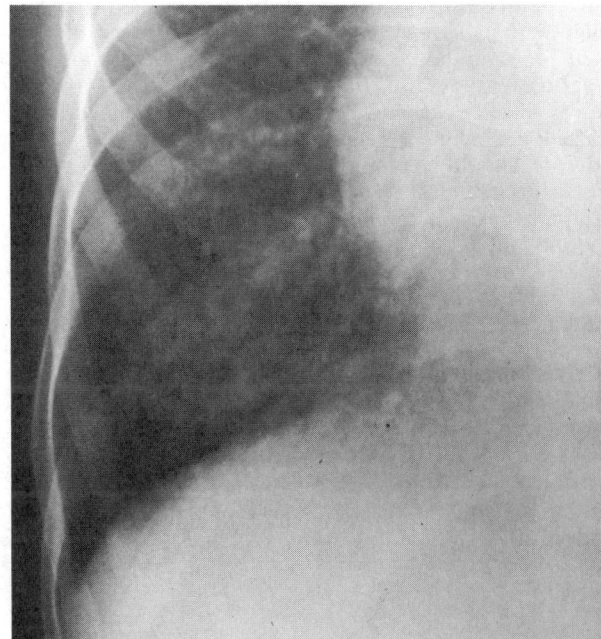

Figure 63–2. The small nodular densities in the lower lung of this 7-year-old patient, HIV positive with congenital AIDS and cardiomyopathy, are more characteristic of lymphocytic interstitial pneumonitis than of *Pneumocystis*. (Courtesy of A. Oestreich, M.D., Cincinnati, OH.)

TABLE 63–6

APPROACH TO EVALUATION OF DIARRHEA

Enteric Pathogen	Associated Symptoms	Diagnostic Tests	Recommended Treatment
Bacteria			
Salmonella	Abdominal pain, fever, chills	Stool, blood, urine cultures	Ceftriaxone, 50–75 mg/kg/day q 12–24 hr
Shigella	Bloody diarrhea, fever	Stool, blood cultures	Trimethoprim-sulfamethoxazole (TMP-SMZ), 8 mg TMP/kg/day q 12 hr
Campylobacter	Abdominal cramping, fever	Stool culture	Erythromycin, 40 mg/kg/day qid
Mycobacterium avium-intracellulare	Fever, malaise, weight loss, anorexia, night sweats	Blood culture, acid-fast examination of stool	No proven effective treatment; consider clarithromycin
Protozoa			
Cryptosporidium	Profuse watery diarrhea, severe wasting, weight loss	Examination of stool, duodenal aspirate or rectal biopsy	Spiramycin 8 mg/kg/day tid or qid
Isospora belli	Profuse watery diarrhea, severe wasting, weight loss	Examination of stool, duodenal aspirate or rectal biopsy	Trimethoprim-sulfamethoxazole (TMP/SMZ), 8 mg TMP/kg/day q 12 hr
Giardia lamblia	Nausea, abdominal cramping, malabsorption	Stool examination, enterotest (string test), duodenal biopsy	Furazolidone or quinacrine HCl, 6 mg/kg/day tid
Viruses			
Cytomegalovirus	Retinitis, colitis, hepatitis, encephalitis	Stool culture, tissue culture from biopsy	Ganciclovir (possibly)
Human immunodeficiency virus	Enteropathy without other proven cause	Biopsy, culture	None
Rotavirus	Watery diarrhea	Rotazyme	None
Adenovirus	Watery diarrhea, fever, conjunctivitis, hepatitis	Stool culture, tissue culture by biopsy	None

through the nipple (Table 63–7). The suppository dissolves as the formula is consumed. Long-term safety has not been evaluated, but short courses are well tolerated and are effective in young infants.[70]

Candidal esophagitis is also a common infection in HIV-infected patients. Symptoms in older children include dysphagia, odynophagia, and retrosternal pain.[71] If these symptoms are coupled with evidence of oral candidiasis, the diagnosis of candidal esophagitis should be strongly considered. Infants with feeding problems, thrush, failure to gain weight, irritability, and emesis should also be carefully evaluated for candidal esophagitis. The diagnosis is suggested by barium swallow and confirmed by endoscopy. Treatment consists of either oral ketoconazole or intravenous amphotericin B for about 2 weeks.[72] Herpes simplex virus (HSV) and CMV should be considered in the differential diagnosis if thrush is absent or treatment fails.[73]

Hepatitis, which can be chronic or fatal, has also been reported in HIV-infected patients.[74] Pathogens include CMV, *Cryptosporidium*, *Mycobacterium avium-intracellulare*, EBV, hepatitis B and C, and adenovirus.[75, 76] Biliary disease and pancreatitis (secondary to biliary obstruction) have been described in adults with HIV. These are caused by CMV or *Cryptosporidium*.[71]

Gastrointestinal bleeding can occur and may be caused by infectious agents at all levels of the gastrointestinal tract. Peptic ulcer disease, portal venous congestion with secondary esophageal varices, and thrombocytopenia have been reported in adults with HIV and should be suspected in children with gastrointestinal hemorrhage.[71] Young infants may also have gastrointestinal blood loss because of formula intolerance.

Renal Manifestations

HIV-associated nephropathy is a well-recognized entity in adults[77] and has been reported in pediatric patients. Nephrotic syndrome, glomerulonephritis, and renal tubular acidosis have all been reported in pediatric HIV patients.[78, 79] The clinical findings include persistent proteinuria, hematuria, hypoalbuminemia, hyponatremia, metabolic acidosis, edema, and progressive renal failure. In one pediatric HIV treatment program, 40% of symptomatic patients had intermittent abnormalities on urinalyses or electrolyte determinations.[79]

Central Nervous System Manifestations

Damage to the central nervous system (CNS) contributes substantially to morbidity and mortality in HIV-infected patients.[80, 81] These patients are at increased risk for a variety of CNS infections, as well as for the direct pathogenic effect of HIV in the CNS.[82] They are also at increased risk for CNS tumors, principally lymphomas.

In adults with HIV, the central nervous system is a common site for opportunistic infections. In children, however, bacterial meningitis from common pediatric pathogens (*H. influenzae*, *S. pneumoniae*) is much more frequently reported. Less commonly, group B streptococcal and gram-negative organisms are found. Immunodeficiency increases

TABLE 63–7

SUMMARY OF TREATMENT FOR THRUSH

Drug	Formulation	Dosage
Nystatin suspension	100,000 U/ml	1–5 ml po qid for 5–10 days
Clotrimazole	100-mg vaginal suppositories	One suppository orally (dissolved in mouth) or placed into nipple tid or qid for 5–7 days
Ketoconazole	200-mg tablet	200 mg daily (adults) 3.3–6.6 mg/kg/day (children over 2 years)

the risk for meningitis and may make its detection more difficult because of a lack of meningeal signs. Furthermore, spinal fluid findings may be difficult to interpret, because HIV encephalitis may cause mild pleocytosis. Finally, many of these children may be receiving antibiotics that may alter the cerebrospinal fluid (CSF) findings. Despite these limitations, a lumbar puncture remains the cornerstone for diagnosis of meningitis. Treatment should be instituted promptly with antibiotics that cover common pathogens.

HIV commonly infects the CNS and may be asymptomatic or may cause encephalopathy.[83, 84] Encephalopathy is present in up to 50% of HIV-infected children.[85] The CSF may show mild increases in protein, lymphocytic pleocytosis, and the presence of HIV antibody or positive HIV culture.[82] Encephalopathy is manifested by developmental delay, a loss of developmental milestones, microcephaly, and motor dysfunction. Seizures are rare. Computed tomography may demonstrate calcifications in the basal ganglia and cerebral atrophy with compensatory ventriculomegaly.[86] The clinical course may be progressive or static.[87] Zidovudine (formerly called azidothymidine, or AZT) may reverse the symptoms in some children.[88]

Uncommon CNS infections include neurosyphilis and encephalitis caused by CMV, HSV, or varicella. *Toxoplasma* encephalitis and cryptococcal meningitis are commonly reported in adults with HIV but are distinctly uncommon in children.

Rarely, these children will present with focal symptoms suggestive of an intracerebral mass lesion. Causative agents include bacterial, mycobacterial, viral, protozoal, and fungal pathogens, as well as noninfectious entities such as lymphoma or infarction. Computed tomography and magnetic resonance imaging are useful diagnostic tools.

Infectious Disease Manifestations

Recurrent bacterial infections are common in children with HIV and are noteworthy because of their increased frequency and severity.[89] The typical diagnoses are otitis media, sinusitis, purulent rhinitis, pneumonia, sepsis, urinary tract infections, and lymphadenitis. Osteomyelitis, septic arthritis, and meningitis also occur more frequently than in children without HIV disease. The pathogens are the same as in immunocompetent hosts, but specimens for culture should be obtained whenever possible to ensure appropriate antibiotic selection. Treatment failures are common, and culture results are essential in these situations. When a bacterial infection is suspected and the child looks toxic, regardless of whether fever is present, the physician must obtain cultures, give antibiotics, and arrange for hospital admission. If the child has a low-grade fever, looks well, and has mild focal findings, then obtaining appropriate cultures, giving selected antibiotics as indicated, and arranging careful follow-up may allow outpatient management. Drug-induced fever must be considered in certain settings but should be a diagnosis of exclusion.

Parasitic infections are commonly described in adults and typically occur in the gastrointestinal tract and less commonly in the lungs and CNS. They are less common in children but should be considered especially when evaluating adolescents and young adults.

Serious consequences may occur with common viral infections. Varicella can be life threatening and complicated by pneumonia, encephalitis, and hepatitis.[90] Known exposure to varicella should prompt the administration of varicella zoster immune globulin (VZIG), which should be given within 96 hours of exposure.[91] VZIG may not prevent the disease but usually attenuates it and extends the incubation period up to 28 days after exposure. If a child develops varicella, regardless of whether VZIG has been given, hospitalization is indicated for treatment with intravenous acyclovir (500 mg/m²/8 hours). Treatment should be continued until the lesions dry up and no new ones emerge, usually 5 to 7 days. Some of these children develop varicella zoster (shingles) after having varicella in early childhood. Shingles can be managed on an outpatient basis in children with reliable families. The child may require hospitalization if shingles are severe or oral therapy fails.[92] Oral acyclovir can help to minimize the severity of the illness. Pain medications may also be needed.

HSV infections also occur in these children.[90] The most common diagnoses are stomatitis and esophagitis. CNS and pulmonary infections are uncommon but must be considered in ill children without other obvious pathogens. The critical diagnostic tests are viral culture for HSV and direct fluorescent antibody (DFA) tests for HSV antigen in samples obtained from tissue or open lesions. DFA tests can distinguish HSV types 1 and 2 from varicella zoster virus and can enable quick selection of optimal therapy. Oral acyclovir is effective for mild cases (10 mg/kg, up to 200 mg/dose tid), but hospitalization and intravenous therapy are indicated if lesions are severe, if patients cannot take in adequate fluids, or if there is evidence of dissemination. Admission is absolutely indicated for all neonates, all children with suspected ocular involvement, and all children with eczema herpeticum. Treatment should include intravenous acyclovir in all these patients. Some may also benefit from the addition of topical antiviral agents for focal infections.[72]

Measles (rubeola) infection in HIV-infected children can be life threatening and can occur regardless of immunization status, as primary vaccine failure has been seen in some immunologically normal children.[93] Furthermore, many children with HIV either never mount a protective immune response or lose it earlier than might be expected. Many HIV-infected children older than 3 years are seronegative despite vaccine. Despite early warnings that live viral vaccines, including MMR, may be dangerous for children with HIV, there are no reports of serious adverse outcome when MMR was given.[94] All children should be given the measles-mumps-rubella vaccine at the age of 15 months, regardless of HIV status, and should be given a second dose at age 5 years or older.[91, 93, 95] If measles is prevalent in the community, the first vaccine dose may be given between the ages of 6 and 12 months.

When children with HIV are known to have been exposed to measles, regardless of vaccination history, they should be given immune globulin (IG), 0.5 ml/kg, up to 15 ml intramuscularly, within 6 days of exposure. Prophylaxis may be ineffective or may not be given if exposure is unrecognized. Hospitalization may be required for severe infections. No specific antiviral therapy has been proven effective, but some agents, such as intravenous ribavirin, have been used with varying success.

During epidemics, exposure to unrecognized measles (e.g., while waiting in physicians' offices and emergency departments) accounts for a large proportion of cases. It is imperative that emergency department staff members recognize measles and identify susceptible immunodeficient children who might have been exposed to allow for appropriate administration of immune globulin.

Poliomyelitis caused by the wild virus remains an extremely rare disease in the United States. However, vaccine-associated polio warrants comment, because most cases of polio occur in immunocompromised household contacts of children immunized with oral polio vaccine (OPV). As a consequence, the current recommendation is to immunize all HIV-positive children and their household contacts with inactivated polio vaccine (IPV).[95, 96]

Fungal diseases in HIV-infected children include candidiasis and cryptococcosis and, in certain geographic areas, histoplasmosis, coccidioidomycosis, and blastomycosis.[97] Focal disease can be found in the gastrointestinal tract, pulmonary tract, and central nervous system.

Syphilis is important in the context of non-transfusion–acquired HIV disease. It affects a significant proportion of HIV-infected adults, can be difficult to diagnose because of false-negative test results, and can cause congenital disease.[98]

Hematologic Abnormalities

Anemia is found in the majority of children with AIDS.[99] Depending on the severity, the condition may warrant multiple transfusions. Microcytic anemia suggests iron deficiency from poor intake, malabsorption, or excess metabolic demands. Normocytic anemia may reflect chronic disease from HIV or other secondary infections or may reflect a Coombs' test–positive autoimmune disease. Macrocytic anemias are found as a side effect of zidovudine[100] or as a result of vitamin B_{12} malabsorption. Workup should be guided by red blood cell indices and may include a reticulocyte count, iron studies, Coombs' test, and vitamin B_{12} measurements.

Thrombocytopenia is quite common in HIV infection and may be an early marker of disease.[99, 101] The cause is thought to be autoimmune in nature. Marked improvements have been noted in some patients when zidovudine therapy is begun. Conventional therapy for immune thrombocytopenic purpura (ITP), such as administration of steroids or intravenous immunoglobulin,[101] has also been effective. Treatment may require platelet transfusion to prevent serious bleeding. Concurrent liver disease may exacerbate the bleeding diathesis.

Neutropenia has also been commonly reported and can increase the risk of infection in these hosts. The cause is likely to be autoimmune or may be secondary to medications such as zidovudine or trimethoprim-sulfamethoxazole.[72] For severe neutropenia, granulocyte colony–stimulating factor (GCSF) has been used in adults with some success.

Lymphopenia is classically found in advanced HIV infection in adults. Its presence is variable in children. Zidovudine may improve the low lymphocyte count.[37]

Malignancies are reported with an increased frequency in children with HIV disease.[102] A few cases of Kaposi's sarcoma have been found in children, but the most common neoplasm reported is B-cell non-Hodgkin's lymphoma.[44] The most common primary sites are the CNS and the abdomen. Typical presenting symptoms include fever, weight loss, diffuse adenopathy, hepatomegaly, and neurologic findings. In children with HIV, symptoms of a CNS mass lesion suggest lymphoma until proven otherwise.

Ophthalmologic Manifestations

Opportunistic infections of the retina are common in adult AIDS patients but are less common in children.[103] CMV, varicella, and *T. gondii* are reported causative agents in children. Symptoms include loss of visual acuity, anisocoria, and photophobia. Physical examination may show loss of light reflex, cotton-wool spots secondary to necrotic retinitis, retinal hemorrhage, retinal thickening, and calcification. Secondary glaucoma may develop. Eye involvement may be more common in the presence of encephalopathy or concurrent opportunistic infections. CMV retinitis may be improved with ganciclovir.[104] Optic neuritis or papillitis may be seen with infections such as CMV, varicella, or zoster and may present with unilateral blindness.[105]

DISPOSITION

The indications for hospital admission are multiple (Table 63–8). A careful family assessment is essential in high-risk populations. Any concern about compliance or follow-up should prompt serious consideration of hospitalization. If the child has a primary care provider, this person should be contacted to discuss appropriate disposition. Some children need hospitalization for diagnostic procedures such as bronchial lavage, or they may need to be evaluated by subspecialists in a medical center equipped to address the special needs of this population.

If the decision has been made to manage the patient as an outpatient, follow-up with a primary care provider should be arranged. Medications, including possible anticipated side effects, should be reviewed. The symptomatic HIV-infected child is often on multiple medications, making medication errors by the parent or guardian more likely. The physician should review with the parent or guardian the indications for returning to the emergency department or for contacting the family physician.

INFECTION CONTROL

It is essential for health care workers to understand that many HIV-infected patients present with an unknown diagnosis, and therefore all health care workers should exercise standard precautions while in contact with all patients. Universal precautions consist of the use of appropriate barrier techniques to prevent exposure to a patient's blood or body fluids.[106–108]

Specific guidelines include wearing gloves while in contact with all blood and body fluids, while touching mucous membranes or nonintact skin, or while handling soiled items or surfaces. Masks and protective eyewear are recommended during procedures that may generate spurts, splashes, or aerosols of blood or body fluid. All protective gear, including gloves, should be changed between patients and should not replace standard meticulous hand washing.

Particular care should be taken to prevent needle-stick injuries. Needles should never be recapped or manipulated unless necessary for the procedure. Appropriate containers for needle disposal should be readily available. Although saliva has not been implicated in the spread of HIV, hand ventilation devices should be used instead of mouth-to-mouth resuscitation. Health care workers with weeping or exudative lesions should refrain from direct patient contact until their lesions are resolved.

TABLE 63–8
CLINICAL INDICATIONS FOR HOSPITALIZATION
Severe wasting
Severe diarrhea
Significant dehydration
Acute pneumonia
Acute hypoxemia or respiratory distress
Suspected sepsis or high fever
Meningitis
New focal neurologic findings
Significant gastrointestinal bleeding
Symptomatic thrombocytopenia
Neutropenia with fever
Abdominal mass
Varicella
Congestive heart failure
Renal failure
Significant metabolic imbalance
Failure of outpatient treatment

All needle-stick injuries should be reported promptly to the appropriate hospital personnel. All hospitals should have a mechanism to evaluate the risk to the health care worker with each particular injury. When it is known that the patient has HIV and the injury is considered significant, zidovudine can be used for the exposed health care worker.[109] The efficacy of prophylactic zidovudine is under study.

OTHER CONSIDERATIONS

Because of widespread discrimination against people with AIDS, there are federal and state laws that protect their rights of confidentiality regarding the diagnosis of an HIV-related condition.[110] The laws vary from state to state, and each hospital's interpretation may differ. The health care provider should be familiar with the hospital's suggested guidelines, especially in regard to what can be written in the medical record and to transmitting information to other physicians or agencies. Some states also have strict laws regarding documentation of informed consent for HIV testing.

Another medicolegal issue related to HIV disease that may arise in the emergency department is informed consent for administering blood transfusion. Blood transfusions are highly unlikely to transmit HIV infection,[111] but the physician who orders a transfusion should discuss this issue with the patient's family. Because of this small but present risk, transfusion of any blood product should be given only when absolutely necessary.

An additional medicolegal issue exists for those children in foster care. A court order may be necessary for consent for HIV testing in these children or for instituting any treatment that may be experimental or particularly invasive.

THERAPEUTIC INTERVENTION

Although there are limited data to support the widespread use of zidovudine for children with symptomatic HIV infection, the FDA has approved its use in children with AIDS. Research is under way to determine the ideal dose in the early stage of illness and in combination with intravenous immunoglobulin.

Most referral centers use zidovudine to treat children with moderate to severe HIV disease. Reported side effects from zidovudine, which include headaches, nausea, and rash, are uncommon in children. However, many children do experience significant hematologic side effects that may limit the dose they can receive and require close monitoring. The most commonly seen hematologic side effects are neutropenia and anemia.[88, 100] Intravenous immunoglobulin has a significant beneficial effect in reducing the incidence of serious bacterial infections in children with early and symptomatic HIV infection.[112, 113]

References

1. Gottlieb MS, Schroff R, Schanker HM, et al. Pneumocystis carinii pneumonia and mucosal candidiasis in previously healthy homosexual men. N Engl J Med 1981;305:1425.
2. Ammann AJ, Wara DW, Dritz S, et al. Acquired immunodeficiency in an infant: Possible transmission by means of blood products. Lancet 1983;1:956.
3. Oleske J, Minnefor A, Cooper R, et al. Immune deficiency syndrome in children. JAMA 1983;249:2345.
4. Centers for Disease Control. Division of AIDS/HIV information. Personal communication. February 7, 1992.
5. Curran JW, Jaffe HW, Hardy AM, et al. Epidemiology of HIV infection and AIDS in the United States. Science 1988;239:610.
6. Morgan WM, Curran JW. Acquired Immunodeficiency Syndrome: Current and future trends. Public Health Rep 1986;101:495.
7. Oleske JM, Connor EM, Boland MG. A perspective on pediatric AIDS. Pediatr Ann 1988;17:319.
8. Ho DD, Pomerantz RJ, Kaplan JC. Pathogenesis of infection with human immunodeficiency virus. N Engl J Med 1987;317:278.
9. Clavel F, Mansinho K, Chararet S, et al. Human immunodeficiency virus type 2 infection associated with AIDS in West Africa. N Engl J Med 1987;316:1180.
10. Denis F, Leonard G, Sangare A, et al. Comparison of 10 enzyme immunoassays for detection of antibody to human immunodeficiency virus type 2 in West African sera. J Clin Microbiol 1988;26:1000.
11. Selwyn P. AIDS: What is now known, I. History and immunovirology. Hosp Pract 1986;21:67.
12. Falloon J, Eddy J, Wiener L, et al. Human immunodeficiency virus infection in children. J Pediatr 1989;114:1.
13. Rubenstein A. Pediatric AIDS current problems. Curr Probl Pediatr 1986;16:364.
14. Adamkin D, Stitzel A, Urmson J, et al. Activity of the alternative pathway of complement in the newborn infant. J Pediatr 1978;93:604.
15. Miller ME. Natural defense mechanism: Development and characterization of innate immunity. In Stiehm R, Fulginitis VA (eds). Immunologic Disorders of Infants and Children. Philadelphia, WB Saunders, 1973, p 127.
16. Mills EL, Thompson T, Bjorksten B, et al. The chemiluminescence response and bactericidal activity of polymorphonuclear neutrophils from newborns and their mothers. Pediatrics 1979;63:429.
17. Pabst HF, Kreth HW. Ontogeny of the immune response as the basis of childhood disease. J Pediatr 1980;97:519.
18. Lewis SH, Reynolds-Kohler C, Fox HE, et al. HIV-1 in trophoblastic and villous Hofbauer cells and haematological cells and haematological precursors in eight-week fetuses. Lancet 1990;335:565.
19. Vogt MW, Witt DJ, Craven DE, et al. Isolation patterns of the human immunodeficiency virus from cervical secretions during the menstrual cycle of women at risk for the acquired immunodeficiency syndrome. Ann Intern Med 1987;106:380.
20. Pyun KH, Och HD, Dufford MTW, et al. Perinatal infection with human immunodeficiency virus: Specific antibody responses by the neonate. N Engl J Med 1987;317:611.
21. Blanche S, Rouzionx C, Moscato M, et al. Prospective study of infants born to women seropositive for human immunodeficiency virus type I. N Engl J Med 1989;320:1643.
22. Ryder RW, Nsa W, Hassig SE, et al. Perinatal transmission of the human immunodeficiency virus type I to infants of sero-positive women in Zaire. N Engl J Med 1989;320:1637.
23. Ziegler JB, Cooper DA, Johnson RO, et al. Postnatal transmission of AIDS-associated retrovirus from mother to infant. Lancet 1985;1:896.
24. Lepage P, Van dePerre P, Carael M, et al. Postnatal transmission of HIV from mother to child. Letter. Lancet 1987;2:400.
25. Centers for Disease Control. Recommendations for assisting in the prevention of perinatal transmission of human T-lymphotropic virus type III lymphadenopathy-associated virus and acquired immunodeficiency syndrome. MMWR 1985;34(suppl 48):721.
26. Cumming PD, Wallace EL, Schorr JB, et al. Exposure of patients to human immunodeficiency virus through the transfusion of blood components that test antibody negative. N Engl J Med 1989;321:941.
27. Leitman SF, Klein HG, Melpolder JJ, et al. Clinical implications of positive tests for antibodies to human immunodeficiency virus type I in asymptomatic blood donors. N Engl J Med 1989;321:917.
28. Centers for Disease Control. Safety of therapeutic products used in hemophilia patients. MMWR 1988;37:441.
29. Desposito F, McSherry GD, Oleske JM. Blood product acquired HIV infection in children. Pediatr Ann 1988;17:341.
30. Ward JW, Bush TJ, Perkins HA, et al. The natural history of transfusion-associated infection with human immunodeficiency virus. N Engl J Med 1989;321:947.
31. Ward JW, Deppe DA, Samson S, et al. Risk of human immunodeficiency virus infection from blood donors who later developed the acquired immunodeficiency syndrome. Ann Intern Med 1987;106:61.
32. Centers for Disease Control. Update: Acquired immunodeficiency syndrome—United States, 1981–1988. MMWR 1989;38:229.
33. Centers for Disease Control. Acquired immunodeficiency syndrome associated with intravenous drug use—United States, 1988. MMWR 1989;38:165.
34. Centers for Disease Control. Summary of notifiable diseases, United States, 1988. MMWR 1989;37:1.
35. Huszti HC, Clopton JR, Mason PJ. Acquired immunodeficiency syndrome educational program: Effects on adolescents' knowledge and attitudes. Pediatrics 1989;84:986.
36. Lifson AR. Do alternate modes for transmission of human immunodeficiency virus exist? JAMA 1988;259:1353.
37. Jenson HB. Retrovirus infections and the acquired immunodeficiency syndrome. Adv Pediatr Infect Dis 1990;5:93.
38. Kamani N, Lightman H, Leiderman R, et al. Pediatric acquired immunodeficiency syndrome related complex: Clinical and immunologic features. Pediatr Infect Dis J 1988;7:383.
39. Krasinski K, Borkowsky W, Holzman R. Prognosis of human immunodeficiency virus infection in children and adolescents. Pediatr Infect Dis J 1989;8:216.
40. Petersen J, Church J, Gomperts E, et al. Lymphocyte phenotype does

not predict immune function in pediatric patients infected with human immunodeficiency virus Type 1. J Pediatr 1989;115:944.

41. Grossman M. Human immunodeficiency virus infections in children: Public health and public policy issues. Pediatr Infect Dis J 1987;6:113.

42. Centers for Disease Control. Classification system for human immunodeficiency virus (HIV) infection in children under 13 years of age. MMWR 1987;36:225.

43. Barrett D. The clinician's guide to pediatric AIDS. Contemp Pediatr 1988;5:24.

44. Epstein L, DiCarlo F, Joshi V, et al. Primary lymphoma of the central nervous system in children with acquired immunodeficiency syndrome. Pediatrics 1988;82:355.

45. Ellaurie M, Burns E, Bernstein L. Thrombocytopenia and human immunodeficiency virus in children. Pediatrics 1988;82:905.

46. Hoots W, O'Brien N. Hematologic manifestations of pediatric HIV infection. Semin Pediatr Infect Dis 1990;1:77.

47. Petru A, Dunphy MG, Azimi P, et al. Reliability of polymerase chain reaction in the detection of human immunodeficiency virus infection in children. Pediatr Infect Dis J 1992;11:30.

48. Rogers M, Ou C, Rayfield M, et al. Use of the polymerase chain reaction for early detection of the proviral sequences of human immunodeficiency virus in infants born to seropositive mothers. N Engl J Med 1989;320:1649.

49. Epstein L, Boucher C, Morrison S, et al. Persistent human immunodeficiency virus type 1 antigenemia in children correlates with disease progression. Pediatrics 1988;82:919.

50. Prestridge L, Klish W. Pediatric HIV infection and AIDS. Nutrition and wasting. Semin Pediatr Infect Dis 1990;1:73.

51. Fishman M, Lifschitz M, Wilson G. Neurodevelopmental abnormalities. Semin Pediatr Infect Dis 1990;1:107.

52. Vernon D, Holzman B, Lewis P, et al. Respiratory failure in children with acquired immunodeficiency syndrome and acquired immunodeficiency syndrome-related complex. Pediatrics 1988;82:223.

53. Katkin J, Hansen T, Langston C, et al. Pulmonary manifestations of AIDS in children. Semin Pediatr Infect Dis 1990;1:40.

54. Berkowitz C. AIDS and parasitic infections including Pneumocystis carinii and cryptosporidiosis. Pediatr Clin North Am 1985;32:933.

55. Masur H, Lane C, Kovacs J, et al. Pneumocystis pneumonia: From bench to clinic. Ann Intern Med 1989;111:813.

56. Phair J, Munoz A, Detels R, et al. The risk of Pneumocystis carinii pneumonia among men infected with human immunodeficiency virus type 1. N Engl J Med 1990;322:161.

57. Husson RN, Pizzo PA. Lung disease in children with HIV, Part 1: Infections. J Crit Illness 1990;5:440.

58. Krasinski K, Borkowsky W, Bonk S, et al. Bacterial infections in human immunodeficiency virus infected children. Pediatr Infect Dis J 1988;7:323.

59. Centers for Disease Control. Revision of the CDC surveillance case definition for acquired immunodeficiency syndrome. MMWR 1987;36(suppl 1S):115.

60. Rubinstein A, Morecki R, Silverman B, et al. Pulmonary disease in children with acquired immune deficiency syndrome and AIDS-related complex. J Pediatr 1986;108:498.

61. Itescu S, Brancato LJ, Buxbaum J, et al. A diffuse infiltrative CD8 lymphocytosis syndrome in human immunodeficiency virus (HIV) infection: A host immune response associated with HLA-DR5. Ann Intern Med 1990;112:3.

62. Ludomirsky A, Garson A. Pediatric HIV infection and AIDS: Clinical expression of heart complications. Semin Pediatr Infect Dis 1990;1:59.

63. Lipshultz S, Chanock S, Sanders S, et al. Cardiovascular manifestations of human immunodeficiency virus infection in infants and children. Am J Cardiol 1989;63:1489.

64. Doyle MG, Pickering LK. Gastrointestinal tract infections in children with AIDS. Semin Pediatr Infect Dis 1990;1:64.

65. McLoughlin LC, Nord KS, Joshi VV, et al. Severe gastrointestinal involvement in children with the acquired immunodeficiency syndrome. J Pediatr Gastroenterol Nutr 1987;6:517.

66. Arbo A, Santos J. Diarrheal diseases in the immunocompromised host. Pediatr Infect Dis J 1987;6:894.

67. Williams EK, Lohr JA, Guerrant RL. Acute infectious diarrhea II. Diagnosis, treatment and prevention. Pediatr Infect Dis J 1986;5:458.

68. Ullrich R, Zeitz M, Heise W, et al. Small intestinal structure and function in patients infected with human immunodeficiency virus (HIV): Evidence for HIV-induced enteropathy. Ann Intern Med 1989;111:15.

69. Rodgers VD, Kagnoff MF. Gastrointestinal manifestations of the acquired immunodeficiency syndrome. West J Med 1987;146:57.

70. Mansour A, Gelfand EW. A new approach to the use of antifungal agents in infants with persistent oral candidiasis. J Pediatr 1981;93:161.

71. Cello JP. Gastrointestinal manifestations of HIV infection. Infect Dis Clin North Am 1988;2:387.

72. Kaplan LD, Wofsy CB, Volberding PA. Treatment of patients with acquired immunodeficiency syndrome and associated manifestations. JAMA 1987;257:1367.

73. Scott GB. Clinical manifestations of HIV infection in children. Pediatr Ann 1988;17:365.

74. Duffy LF, Daum F, Kahn E, et al. Hepatitis in children with acquired immune deficiency syndrome. Gastroenterology 1986;90:173.

75. Krilov LR, Rubin LG, Frogel M, et al. Disseminated adenovirus infection with hepatic necrosis in patients with human immunodeficiency virus infection and other immunodeficiency states. Rev Infect Dis 1990;12:303.

76. Janner D, Petru AM, Belchis D. Fatal adenovirus hepatitis in a child with AIDS. Pediatr Infect Dis J 1990;9:434.

77. Glascock RJ, Cohen AH, Danovitch G, et al. Human immunodeficiency virus (HIV) infection and the kidney. Ann Intern Med 1990;112:35.

78. Connor E, Gupta S, Joshi V, et al. Acquired immunodeficiency syndrome-associated renal disease in children. J Pediatr 1988;113:39.

79. Strauss J, Abitbol C, Zilleruelo G, et al. Renal disease in children with the acquired immunodeficiency syndrome. N Engl J Med 1989;331:625.

80. Belman AL, Diamond G, Dickson D, et al. Pediatric acquired immunodeficiency syndrome, neurologic syndromes. Am J Dis Child 1988;142:29.

81. Price RW, Brew B, Sidtis J, et al. The brain in AIDS: Central nervous system HIV-1 infection and AIDS dementia complex. Science 1988;239:586.

82. Ashkenazi S, Kohl S. Central nervous system abnormalities in pediatric HIV infection and AIDS. Semin Pediatr Infect Dis 1990;1:94.

83. Ho DD, Bredesen DE, Vinters HV, et al. The acquired immunodeficiency syndrome (AIDS) dementia complex. Ann Intern Med 1989;111:400.

84. Fauci AS. The human immunodeficiency virus: Infectivity and mechanisms of pathogenesis. Science 1988;239:617.

85. Dalakas M, Wichman A, Sever J. AIDS and the nervous system. JAMA 1989;261:2396.

86. Belman AL, Ultmann MH, Horoupian D, et al. Neurological complications of infants and children with acquired immune deficiency syndrome. Ann Neurol 1985;18:560.

87. Epstein LG, Sharer LR, Oleske JM, et al. Neurologic manifestations of human immunodeficiency virus infection in children. Pediatrics 1986;78:678.

88. Pizzo P, Eddy J, Falloon J, et al. Effect of continuous intravenous infusion of zidovudine (AZT) in children with symptomatic HIV infection. N Engl J Med 1988;319:889.

89. Pahwa S, Kaplan M, Fikrig S, et al. Spectrum of human T-cell lymphotropic virus type III infection in children. JAMA 1986;255:2299.

90. Hanson C, Kaplan SL. Opportunistic infections. Semin Pediatr Infect Dis 1990;1:31.

91. Thomas P. Immunization of children infected with HIV: A public health perspective. Pediatr Ann 1988;17:347.

92. Pahwa S, Biron K, Lim W, et al. Continuous varicella-zoster infection associated with acyclovir resistance in a child with AIDS. JAMA 1988;260:2879.

93. Centers for Disease Control. Measles prevention: Recommendations of the Immunization Practices Advisory Committee (ACIP). MMWR 1989;38:1.

94. Edwards MS, Baker CJ. Pediatric HIV infection and AIDS: Immunizations. Semin Pediatr Infect Dis 1990;1:150.

95. Centers for Disease Control. Immunization of children infected with the human T-lymphotropic virus III/lymphadenopathy associated virus. MMWR 1986;35:595.

96. Report of the Committee on Infectious Diseases. 1988 Redbook. Elk Grove Village, IL, American Academy of Pediatrics 1988, pp 336–338.

97. Glatt AE, Chirgwan K, Landesman SH. Treatment of infections associated with human immunodeficiency virus. N Engl J Med 1988;318:1439.

98. Centers for Disease Control. Recommendations for diagnosising and treating syphilis in HIV-infected patients. MMWR 1988;37:601.

99. Mitsuyasu RT, Miles SA, Yarchoan R. Hematologic and virologic issues in HIV disease. Hematology 1989, Education in Progress. New York, American Society of Hematology, p 87.

100. Englund JA, Baker CJ: Chemotherapeutic approaches to pediatric HIV infection. Semin Pediatr Infect Dis 1990;1:130.

101. Saulsbury FT, Boyle RJ, Wykoff RF, et al. Thrombocytopenia as the presenting manifestation of human T-lymphotropic virus type III infection in infants. J Pediatr 1986;109:30.

102. McClain KL, Rosenblatt H. Pediatric HIV infection and AIDS: Clinical expression of malignancy. Semin Pediatr Infect Dis 1990;1:124.

103. Dennehy PJ, Warman R, Flynn JT, et al. Ocular manifestations of pediatric patients with acquired immunodeficiency syndrome. Arch Ophthalmol 1989;107:978.

104. Levin AV, Zeichner S, Duker JS, et al. Cytomegalovirus retinitis in an infant with acquired immunodeficiency syndrome. Pediatrics 1989;84:683.

105. Litoff D, Catalano RA. Herpes optic neuritis in human immunodeficiency virus infections. Arch Ophthalmol 1990;108:782.

106. Task Force on Pediatric AIDS. Pediatric guidelines for infection control of human immunodeficiency virus (acquired immunodeficiency virus) in hospitals, medical offices, schools and other settings. Pediatrics 1988;82:801.

107. Centers for Disease Control. Recommendations for prevention of HIV transmission in health-care settings. MMWR 1987;288:1293.

108. Donowitz LG. Practical infection control for human immunodeficiency virus infection in children. Pediatr Infect Dis J 1989;8:133.

109. Centers for Disease Control. Public Health Service statement on management of occupational exposure to human immunodeficiency virus including considerations regarding zidovudine postexposure use. MMWR 1990;39:RR-1.

110. Blendon, RJ, Donelan K. Discrimination against people with AIDS. N Engl J Med 1988;319:1022.

111. Friedland GH, Klein RS. Transmission of the human immunodeficiency virus. N Engl J Med 1987;317:1125.

112. Rosenblatt HM, Englund JA, Shearer WT. Immunotherapeutic approaches to pediatric HIV infection. Semin Pediatr Infect Dis 1990;1:140.

113. National Institute Child Health and Human Development Intravenous Immunoglobulin Study Group. Intravenous immune globulin for the prevention of bacterial infections in children with symptomatic human immunodeficiency virus infection. N Engl J Med 1991;325:73.

SECTION NINE

Dermatologic Emergencies

CHAPTER 64

Dermatologic Emergencies

Bernard A. Cohen
Holly W. Davis

INTRODUCTION

Rashes account for a third of acute pediatric visits to the practitioner and a significant percentage of visits to emergency departments and urgent care centers. Although most dermatoses are mild and more irritating than serious, some may be associated with life-threatening complications or may provide diagnostic clues to underlying systemic disorders.

ANATOMY AND PHYSIOLOGY

The skin is actually the largest organ of the body and, given its many component parts and appendages, one of the more complex. The external layer of the epidermis is comprised largely of keratinocytes, which proliferate in its basal cell layer, differentiate, and then gradually migrate upward to the granular layer where they flatten out and lose their nuclei. Here their membranes thicken, and they become increasingly more tightly packed, forming the protective barrier of the stratum corneum from which the top one to two cell layers are shed each day. Total turnover time from basal layer to shedding is approximately 28 days.

The epidermis also contains melanocytes whose purpose is to protect nucleated cells in lower layers from the damaging effects of ultraviolet (UV) light. Exposure to UV light oxidizes preformed melanin, darkening its color, and stimulates increased melanin production and dispersal to nearby keratinocytes through dendritic extensions.

The dermal, or lower, layer of the skin provides strength and elasticity, creating a tough mechanical barrier. Although it is relatively acellular, being made up largely of collagen and elastin, it is nevertheless quite complex in that it contains cutaneous blood vessels, lymphatics and nerves, and mast cells and other inflammatory cells and provides structural support for the dermal appendages (i.e., hair follicles, sebaceous glands, apocrine and eccrine sweat glands, and the nails).

Finally, the underlying subcutaneous tissue, comprised mainly of fat cells, serves as a protective cushion and thermal insulator, as well as a source of stored energy. It also forms a conduit for vascular plexuses and is a site of hormonal metabolism.

The skin responds to insults, injury, or disease in a number of ways. Scaling occurs because of overproliferation of epidermal cells and premature shedding of the stratum corneum and is a common phenomenon. Breaks in the skin barrier caused by trauma, scratching and excoriation, excess drying, excess moisture, infection, or other processes trigger the complement cascade and immunoglobulin deposition, which in turn stimulates an inflammatory response consisting of vasodilatation (erythema) and migration of neutrophils, lymphocytes, mononuclear cells, and macrophages to the dermis and epidermis. This can result in elevated lesions and induration. Bacterial invasion also stimulates an immune response and, if the invading organism secretes an epidermolysin, can promote vesiculation and blister formation. Blistering is also a common response to thermal or chemical insults.

Antigenic or other stimulation of mast cells, which reside around cutaneous vessels, results in release of histamine, promoting formation of urticarial wheals or angioedema.

Following inflammation, pigmentary changes occur because of increased or decreased pigment production and abnormal transfer of pigment from melanocytes to keratinocytes.

EMERGENCY MEDICAL SERVICE CONSIDERATIONS

Most acute dermatologic problems are of mild severity, and affected patients are unlikely to seek emergency medical service (EMS) transport for medical care. However, on occasion, children with Stevens-Johnson syndrome, toxic epidermal necrolysis, and staphylococcal scalded skin syndrome can develop hypovolemia as a result of exudation of fluid into extensive skin lesions and can also have problems with thermoregulation. Initial assessment and stabilization efforts should thus be directed toward circulatory status and maintenance of temperature.

Of the disorders characterized by purpura, meningococcemia and other infections accompanied by septic shock and purpura fulminans are the ones most likely to be encountered by EMS personnel. In such cases, assessment of cardiovascular status, oxygen delivery to help combat tissue hypoxia, and establishment of vascular access followed by volume expansion are mainstays of initial management. EMS personnel should wear masks and implement precautions to prevent direct contact with the patient's secretions.

CLINICAL EVALUATION
Historical Data

The practitioner must obtain a detailed history of skin symptoms, including the date of onset, inciting factors, evolution of lesions and their distribution, and the presence or absence of pruritis. Recent immunizations; exposure to drugs, toxins, soaps, lotions and topical agents; allergies; and dietary changes may trigger a new skin eruption. The family history may suggest an hereditary or infectious disorder, and the clinician may find it necessary to interview and examine family members with similar complaints.

Skin Examination

Examination of the skin must be performed in a well-lit room. The clinician should inspect the entire skin surface, including the hair, nails, scalp, and mucous membranes. This may present a problem in infants and adolescents, in whom it may be necessary to examine the skin in small segments to prevent cold stress or embarrassment. Although no special equipment is required, a hand lens or otoscope and side lighting are helpful in the assessment of skin texture and lesion morphology.

Rash Assessment

First, the general health of the patient should be noted. Attention should then turn to the distribution and pattern of the rash. *Distribution* refers to the location of skin findings, whereas *pattern* defines a specific anatomic or physiologic arrangement. For instance, in atopic dermatitis, the distribution of the rash might include the arms, legs, buttocks, and neck. Identification of a flexural or intertriginous pattern in the same patient will help to further narrow differential diagnostic possibilities. Other patterns include sun-exposed sites, acrodermatitis, pityriasis rosea–like eruptions, and clothing-covered sites.

Next, the clinician should consider the local organization of the lesions. *Organization* refers to the relationship of primary and secondary lesions to one another in a given location. Are the lesions scattered or clustered (herpetiform)? Are they arciform, linear, or serpiginous?

Assessing the anatomic depth of the lesions in the skin is also helpful. Superficial lesions with little or no induration or firmness are characteristic of dermatitic processes, whereas indurated or deep-seated eruptions may suggest a cellulitis, angioedema, or panniculitis.

Finally, the practitioner may develop a working diagnosis using the morphology of the skin lesions. Primary lesions including macules, papules, plaques, vesicles, bullae, nodules, and tumors arise de novo. Secondary lesions such as pustules, erosions, ulcers, scars, and excoriations evolve from primary lesions or result from manipulation (especially scratching) of primary lesions by the patient.

DIAGNOSTIC EVALUATION

Several simple bench laboratory studies can be useful. These include Gram stains, potassium hydroxide (KOH) preparations, Tzanck smears, and scabies and lice preparations. In a minority of cases bacterial or viral cultures may be needed.

KOH Preparations

When fungal infections are suspected, a KOH preparation of skin scrapings, scalp scale, or hairs scraped off close to the scalp can be useful in confirming the presence of the causative organisms. Skin scrapings are obtained by vigorously scraping the active border of a lesion with a scalpel blade, pushing the scales onto a glass slide. Scales are then moved toward the center of the slide but kept in a thin layer. One drop of 20% KOH is placed over the scales, and a cover slip is applied and gently pressed down to crush the scales. The slide is then heated gently (but not to the boiling point), and again the cover slip is pressed down. The preparation is then viewed under the microscope at $10 \times$ power with the condenser set down to maximize contrast. On focusing slowly up and down, hyphae can be identified as long, branching septate rods crossing cell membranes. The same procedure is used for hairs, which should be carefully examined near their roots where hyphae and spores are most likely to be found.

Tzanck Smear

When herpes simplex or varicella zoster are suspected as the cause of vesicular lesions or when the origin of the lesion is unclear, a Tzanck smear can prove useful. To obtain a good specimen, a vesicle is gently unroofed using a scalpel blade or scissors, and the base is gently scraped. Scrapings are then spread thinly on a glass slide. Following air drying, the preparation is stained either with Giemsa or Wright's stain. In positive preparations, multinucleated giant cells are readily observed.

Scabies and Lice Preparations

A scabies preparation is particularly useful in confirming infestation when secondary eczematous changes may be masking the underlying cause, but the initial distribution of lesions is suspicious. A fresh burrow or papule with a small dark spot at one end (the mite) is most likely to yield the offender. Such lesions are often best located around the wrists, palms, or on the soles in young children. The black dot is lifted out with the end of a needle and placed on a glass slide. A drop of mineral oil is applied, followed by a cover slip, which is gently pressed down. If such an ideal site is not found, scrapings of a burrow or pustule may be obtained using a scalpel blade. To ensure adherence of the scrapings, it is useful to apply a drop of oil to the site prior to scraping. Scrapings are then transferred to a glass slide, a second drop of mineral oil is added, and a cover slip is pressed down over the preparation. Positive findings include the body of the eight-legged mite, smooth oval eggs, or feces (seen as tiny brown pellets that tend to be found in clusters).

In most patients with head lice, mobile adult lice can be found on close inspection of the scalp with the naked eye. However, in some cases adults are elusive, and only nits are seen adhering to hairs (especially above and behind the ears). A few such hairs should be clipped and placed on a glass slide with mineral oil, followed by a cover slip, which is gently pressed down. Microscopically the nit appears as a thick-walled oval egg case rounded at one end and tapered at the other.

PAPULOSQUAMOUS DISORDERS

Papular and scaly eruptions account for the majority of rashes that prompt visits to the emergency department (Table 64–1). In acute dermatitis, scale and red papules on an inflamed base may be associated with crusts and blisters. Scratching in response to intense pruritus can result in extensive excoriations. After several days to weeks, secondary chronic changes appear, including thickening of the skin (lichenification), alteration in pigmentation (hyper- and hypopigmentation), and increased scale formation.

TABLE 64–1

PAPULOSQUAMOUS DISORDERS

Disorder	Skin Lesions	Distribution	Diagnostic Studies	Admission Criteria
Irritant dermatitis	Papules, vesicles, scales, crusts	Face, trunk, extremities, especially convex surfaces		Severe bacterial superinfection
Contact dermatitis	Papules, vesicles, scales, crusts	Face, trunk, extremities, especially exposed sites	Patch testing	Severe bacterial superinfection
Atopic dermatitis	Papules, vesicles, scales, crusts, lichenification, pigmentary changes	Flexures, face; occasionally generalized	Serum immunoglobulin E	Severe bacterial superinfection, eczema herpeticum
Seborrheic dermatitis	Erythema, papules, scales, pigmentary changes	Face, scalp, perineum, axillae; rarely generalized		Severe bacterial superinfection
Ringworm	Erythema, scales, papules, pustules, vesicles	Scalp, trunk, extremities	KOH preparation	
Psoriasis	Erythematous plaques with silvery scale	Scalp, trunk, extremities, nail pits, dystrophy	Skin biopsy	Acute erythrodermic or pustular psoriasis
Pityriasis rosea	Papules, scaly patches, "Christmas tree" pattern	Trunk, proximal extremities	Syphilis serology	

Irritant Diaper Dermatitis

Irritant dermatitis is the most common dermatitis of childhood. In infants and toddlers, irritation from urine, stool, or topical preparations may produce diaper dermatitis. Infrequent diaper changing is a major predisposing factor. Erythema, scaling, and papules are prominent on the convex surfaces of the perineum, genitals, and anterior thighs but spare the skin creases (Fig. 64–1).

Differential Diagnosis

When secondary infection occurs with *Candida* or bacteria, erosive lesions and pustules spread to the inguinal and gluteal folds. Discrete satellite papules and pustules appear at the margins of the rash and may extend beyond the diaper area on the legs and abdomen. In *candidal diaper dermatitis* (a common sequela of antibiotic therapy), erythema is intense and the eruption has sharp borders with tiny pinpoint papules and pustules (Fig. 64–2), whereas with *staphylococcal diaper dermatitis*, larger thin-walled pustules and bullae are seen (Fig. 64–3). These rupture early, leaving a thin collarette of scale around the denuded erythematous base (see "Staphylococcal Pustulosis"). Budding yeast and pseudohyphae are readily demonstrated on KOH preparations from pustules and eroded patches in candidal diaper dermatitis. Gram stain preparations from the base of pustules or bullae demonstrate gram-positive cocci in clusters and neutrophils in staphylococcal diaper dermatitis.

Occasionally the first manifestation of psoriasis is a diaper dermatitis that is resistant to standard therapy for irritant diaper dermatitis and is negative for *Candida* and bacteria on smears, stains, and cultures.

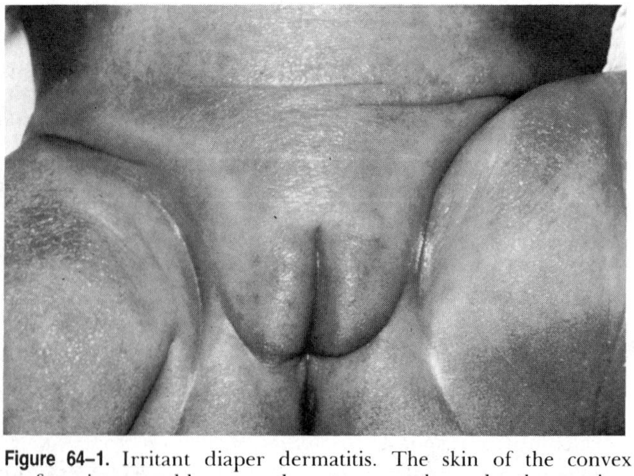

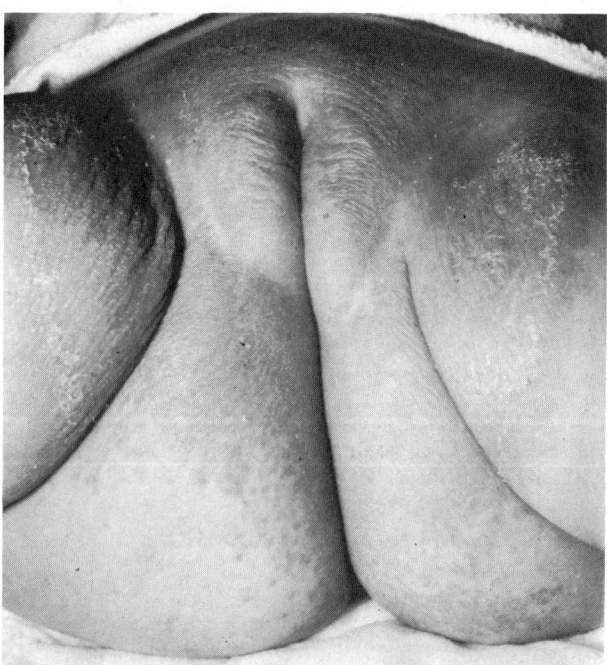

Figure 64–1. Irritant diaper dermatitis. The skin of the convex surfaces is covered by an erythematous papular and scaly eruption. Note that the skin creases are spared.

Figure 64–2. Candidal diaper dermatitis. The perineum is covered with an erythematous eruption consisting of coalescent papules and pustules. Tiny, discrete satellite lesions are seen at the margins, and intertriginous areas are involved.

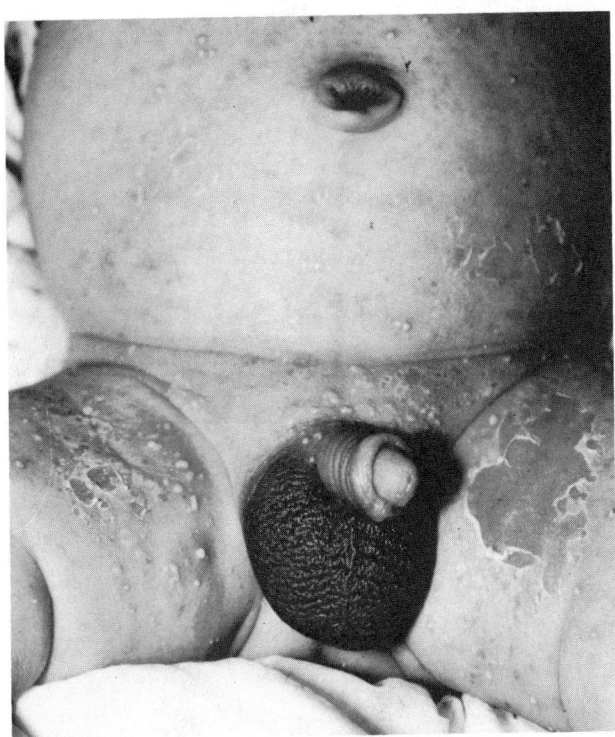

Figure 64–3. Staphylococcal diaper dermatitis. Staphylococci produce larger, thinner-walled pustules than those seen with *Candida*, and bullae may be seen as well. These rupture early, leaving a thin, peeling rim around a denuded erythematous base. (From Zitelli BJ, Davis HW (eds). Atlas of Pediatric Physical Diagnosis. 2nd ed. New York: Gower Medical Publishing, 1992.)

Therapeutic Intervention

Initial management of all forms of diaper dermatitis includes frequent diaper changes and thorough cleaning with tap water. Use of superabsorbent diapers that keep moisture away from the skin may also reduce the risk of irritant dermatitis. In uncomplicated irritant dermatitis, occlusive topical preparations such as zinc oxide paste (1-2-3 ointment, Balmex, or Desitin cream) will provide a protective barrier. A low-potency topical corticosteroid (Table 64–2) may be applied once or twice a day for the first 3 to 4 days to decrease inflammation and the associated burning and pruritus. However, high-potency topical corticosteroids (e.g., Lotrisone) should be avoided in the diaper area.

Candidal diaper dermatitis responds to topical antifungals (Table 64–3), which should be applied with each diaper change for up to 7 to 10 days. Infants with secondary staphylococcal impetigo or pustulosis may progress to deeper seated cellulitis and sepsis (see "Staphylococcal Pustulosis"). Hence, pustulosis requires treatment with oral cephalexin, erythromycin, cloxacillin, or dicloxacillin. Simultaneous use of topical mupirocin or bacitracin may hasten symptomatic relief and reduce spread to other family members. Infants with fever may require a full evaluation for sepsis and parenteral therapy.

Other Forms of Irritant Dermatitis

In infancy, a perioral irritant dermatitis is commonly seen secondary to irritation caused by milk, juices, and repeated wetting with saliva or water followed by drying. This may be a particular problem during periods of intense drooling in response to teething.

A generalized irritant dermatitis with particular involvement of skin folds may occur after exposure to soaps, detergents, or bleach in laundered clothing. In the latter cases, noncovered areas (hands, feet, face) are spared. Localized irritant reactions may result from limited contact with organic solvents, acids, and alkalis.

Therapeutic Intervention

Aggressive use of lubricants (Table 64–4) usually alleviates symptoms in infants with perioral irritant dermatitis. In managing generalized irritant dermatitis, tap water or aluminum acetate compresses (Burow's solution, Blueboro) and oral hydroxyzine or diphenhydramine help relieve itching. Although severe reactions may require systemic corticosteroids, most are safely managed with emollients and medium-strength topical corticosteroids. It should be noted that only low-potency preparations should be used on the face and intertriginous areas because of the risk of skin atrophy. Topical steroids should be tapered as lesions clear.

Contact Dermatitis

Allergic contact dermatitis is common in children, particularly in the summer. Poison ivy, or rhus dermatitis, typifies a type IV delayed hypersensitivity reaction, which requires a period of sensitization from 7 to 14 days before clinical signs appear. On reexposure to the antigen (whether leaves, stems or roots of the plant), erythematous papules and vesicles on an erythematous edematous base develop, often in a linear pattern along exposed areas of skin (Fig. 64–4). Involvement of the face, neck, and genitals tends to be characterized by patchy erythema (the surface of which has a microvesicular appearance) and moderate to severe swelling. Intense pruritus results in excoriations, crusting, and a risk of secondary bacterial infection.

Other common inciting agents of contact dermatitis are nickel in jewelry (bracelets, necklaces, earrings); hair care products, which produce dermatitis involving the scalp, face, neck, and periauricular areas; dyes and glues in shoes; elastic; ethylenediamine in topical lotions; neomycin; and topical anesthetics. Attention to the distribution of lesions and a detailed history of exposure help identify the offending agent.

Therapeutic Intervention

Topical corticosteroids (see Table 64–2) are adequate treatment for most forms of contact dermatitis and for localized eruptions of rhus dermatitis, but widespread poison ivy and cases of significant facial, hand, or genital involvement usually require oral corticosteroids to prevent or reverse severe swelling. Prompt relief occurs within 3 days of starting prednisone (0.5 to 1.0 mg/kg/day given in two divided doses). Steroids should be tapered over 2 to 3 weeks with close clinical monitoring. Shorter courses should be avoided, as symptom relapse occurs when steroids are tapered too quickly. Oral hydroxyzine or diphenhydramine is also helpful in relieving pruritus and reducing scratching.

Atopic Dermatitis

Atopic dermatitis, or eczema, rarely appears before 8 weeks of age, and months of observation may be necessary before the diagnosis is clearly established. In 75% of children there is a family history of atopic conditions such as allergic rhinitis, sinusitis, asthma, and food allergy. Although chronic changes, including lichenification, pigmentary alteration, and scale, are characteristic, acute exacerbations are associated with increased erythema, vesicles, crusts, and impetiginization. In infants, the rash is widespread, with involvement

TABLE 64–2

TOPICAL STEROIDS

Group	Generic Name	Trade Name	Potency
1	Betamethasone dipropionate augmented 0.05% Clobetasol propionate 0.05% Diflorasone diacetate 0.05%	Diprolene 0.05% Temovate 0.05% Psorcon 0.05%	Super high
2	Amcinonide Betamethasone dipropionate Diflorasone diacetate Halcinonide Fluocinonide Diflorasone diacetate Desoximetasone	Cyclocort ointment 0.1% Diprosone ointment 0.05% Florone ointment 0.05% Halog cream 0.1% Lidex cream 0.05% Lidex ointment 0.05% Maxiflor ointment 0.05% Topicort cream 0.25%	High
3	Betamethasone dipropionate Betamethasone benzoate Betamethasone valerate	Diprosone cream 0.05% Benisone gel 0.025% Valisone ointment 0.1%	
4	Triamcinolone acetonide Flurandrenolide Fluocinolone acetonide	Aristocort ointment 0.1% Kenalog ointment 0.1% Cordran ointment 0.05% Synalar cream 0.025%	
5	Triamcinolone acetonide Flurandrenolide Fluocinolone acetonide Triamcinolone acetonide Fluocinolone acetonide Betamethasone valerate Hydrocortisone valerate	Aristocort cream 0.1% Cordran SP cream 0.05% Fluonid cream 0.01% Kenalog cream 0.1% Synalar cream 0.01% Valisone cream 0.1% Westcort cream 0.2%	Mid
6	Hydrocortisone 1%, urea 10% Flumethasone pivalate Desonide	Alphaderm cream 1% Locorten cream 0.03% Tridesilon cream 0.05%	
7	Hydrocortisone 1% Dexamethasone Methylprednisolone acetate Prednisolone	Hytone cream 1% Hytone ointment 1% Hexadrol cream 0.04% Medrol ointment 0.25% Meti-Derm cream 0.5%	Low
8	Hydrocortisone 0.5%	Cortaid cream	

TABLE 64–3
TOPICAL ANTIFUNGALS

Generic Name	Trade Name	Indications
Nystatin	Mycostatin, Nilstat	*Candida*
Amphotericin B	Fungizone	*Candida*
Miconazole	Monistat-Derm	*Candida*, dermatophytes
Clotrimazole	Lotrimin, Mycelex	*Candida*, dermatophytes
Ciclopirox olamine	Loprox	*Candida*, dermatophytes
Tolnaftate	Tinactin	Dermatophytes
Econazole nitrate	Spectazole	*Candida*, dermatophytes
Naftine hydrochloride	Naftin	Dermatophytes
Ketoconazole	Nizoral	Yeast, dermatophytes
Oxiconazole nitrate	Oxistat	Dermatophytes

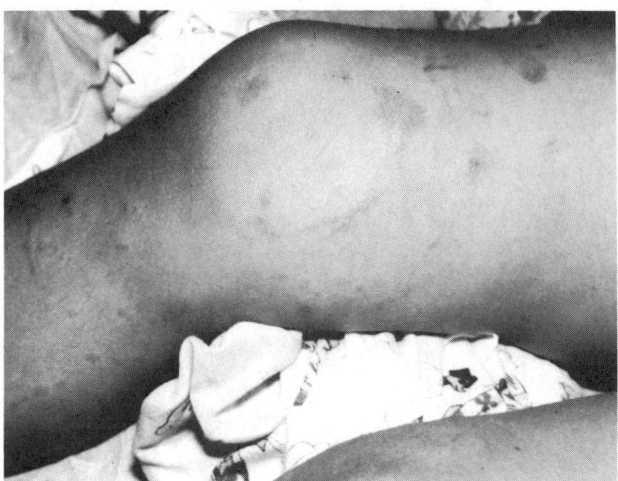

Figure 64–4. Poison ivy (rhus dermatitis). Contact with the plant oil by a sensitive individual results in formation of papules and vesicles on an erythematous edematous base, which often appear in linear patterns on exposed areas of skin.

of the cheeks, forehead, scalp, trunk, and extensor surfaces of the extremities (Fig. 64–5). The diaper area is invariably spared. Pruritus is severe, often resulting in significant irritability, and interferes with sleeping and eating, sometimes impeding weight gain. In older children, the flexures of the wrists, ankles, elbows, and knees tend to be involved (Fig. 64–6), whereas in adolescents and adults, lesions are usually restricted to the flexural creases of the arms, neck, legs, and hands.

Differential Diagnosis

Atopic dermatitis can be distinguished from seborrhea by its characteristic sparing of intertriginous areas. The distribution of lesions and exposure history help differentiate it from contact dermatitis. Atopic dermatitis lacks the thick, silvery scales of psoriasis, and the lesions are less discrete and different in distribution from those of pityriasis rosea (PR).

Complications

The major complication of atopic dermatitis is secondary infection. Because the skin barrier is compromised, lesions are vulnerable to invasion by streptococci and staphylococci, with resultant impetiginization or development of cellulitis. Infection may advance with frightening rapidity in patients on steroid therapy.

In patients with viral illnesses that produce exanthems, lesions may appear first and cluster heavily in sites of preexisting dermatitis. This is especially true of varicella and herpes simplex. In fact, primary herpes simplex infection in atopic dermatitis patients may result in a medical emergency, eczema herpeticum, or Kaposi's varicelliform eruption (see "Herpes Infections").

TABLE 64–4
RELATIVE GREASINESS OF COMMON SKIN LUBRICANTS

Lubricant	Relative Greasiness
Petrolatum	More greasy
Aquaphor ointment base	
Mineral oil	
Eucerin cream	
Acid mantle cream	
Keri lotion	
Lubriderm lotion	
Complex 15 phospholipid moisturizing cream and lotion	
Cetaphil lotion	
Carmol 10% lotion	
LactiCare lotion	
Moisturel skin lubricant-moisturizer	
Neutraderm lotion	
Shepard's skin cream	Less greasy

From Cohen BA. Common dermatoses of childhood. Am Fam Physician 1985;32:186–203. Published by the American Academy of Family Physicians.

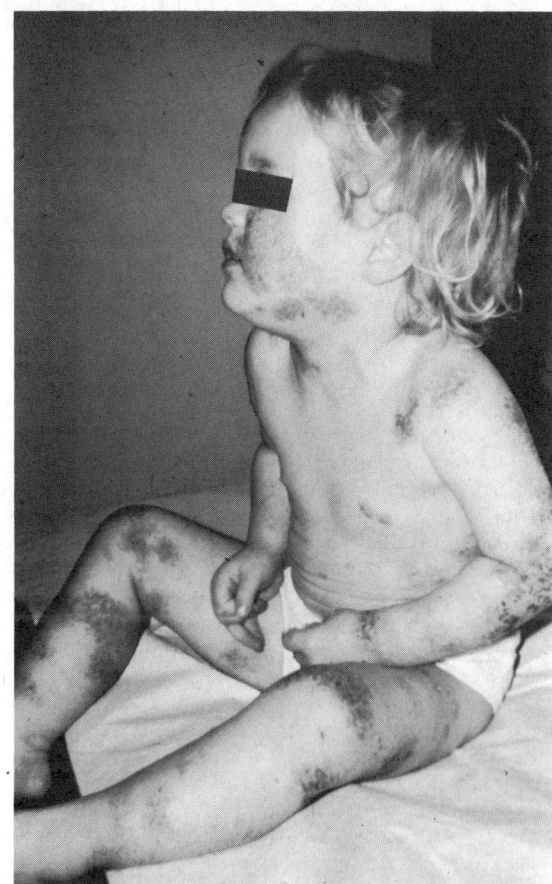

Figure 64–5. Infantile atopic dermatitis or eczema. This girl demonstrates the widespread involvement typical of infantile eczema. The cheeks, trunk, and extensor and flexor surfaces of the extremities are involved. (Courtesy of Dr. Michael Sherlock.)

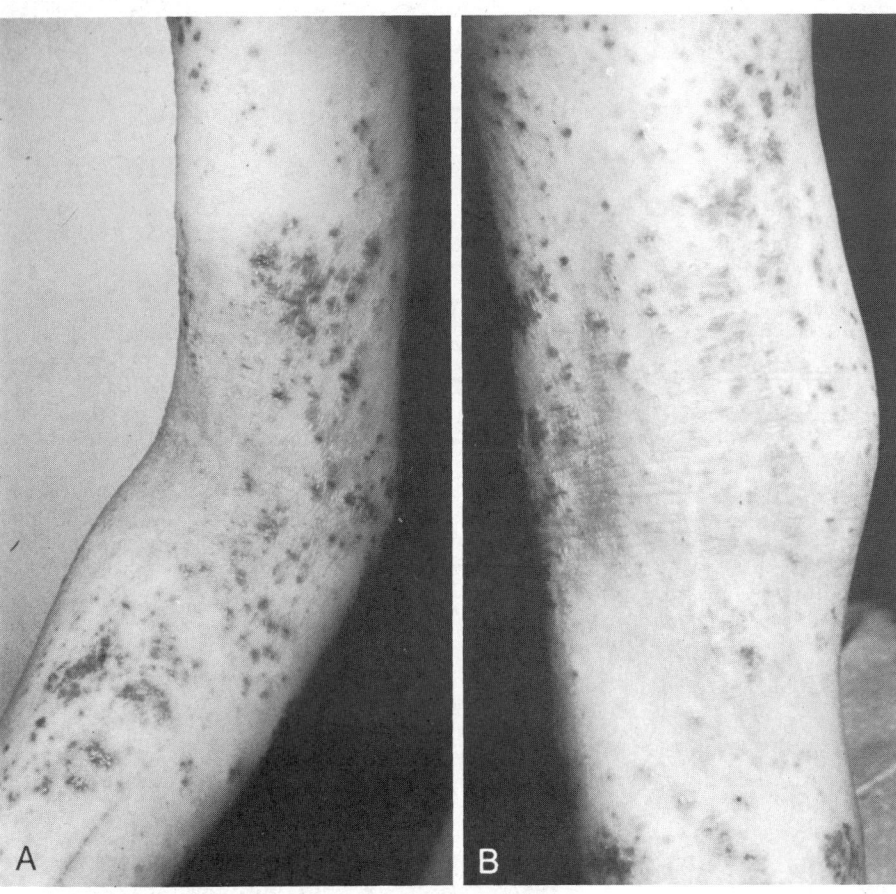

Figure 64–6. *A, B,* Childhood eczema. This 10-year-old boy had severe chronic eczema that primarily involved the flexures of the elbows, knees, and wrists. Note the lichenification. (Courtesy of Dr. Michael Sherlock.)

Therapeutic Intervention

Acute flares of eczema should be treated with cool tap water compresses or tepid tub baths two to three times a day, followed by liberal application of a bland emollient (Eucerin cream, Aquaphor, Acid Mantle cream, Vaseline, or vegetable shortening) to the entire skin surface. Medium-potency topical steroid ointment (see Table 64–2) should be applied twice a day to eczematous patches only. As the skin improves, the potency of the topical steroid may be reduced by mixing it with the emollient and decreasing the frequency of application. Lubricants should be continued on a regular schedule (once or twice daily), even during periods of remission and especially after bathing and swimming. Antipruritics such as hydroxyzine (2 mg/kg/day in four divided doses) or diphenhydramine (2 to 5 mg/kg/day in four divided doses) are important for relief of itching and because they help break the itch-scratch cycle that perpetuates the rash. However, round-the-clock use of antihistamines should be restricted to a few days because of the risk of sedation and behavioral changes, particularly in young children. A single bedtime dose may be safely used in chronic eczema.

Oral antimicrobial therapy is indicated if impetiginization has occurred, as this may progress with unusual rapidity in patients being treated with either topical or oral steroids. Development of cellulitis or spread of infection from the skin to contiguous joints and bones or by bacteremia requires appropriate culturing and hospitalization for parenteral therapy.

Seborrheic Dermatitis

Seborrheic dermatitis is an erythematous, scaly, greasy rash occurring in areas where sebaceous glands are most prominent (e.g., the hair-bearing areas of the face, the scalp, the axillae and inguinal areas, and the neck and postauricular areas). Although the cause is unclear, data support a role for *Pityrosporum* (a yeast) in some patients. The initial manifestation of seborrheic dermatitis is "cradle cap," a thick, tenacious, scaly eruption on the scalp that appears in the first few weeks of life. Red, scaly, greasy, hypopigmented patches may then spread to involve the postauricular areas, neck, axillae, and diaper area (Fig. 64–7). Occasionally, lesions become generalized to the trunk and proximal extremities. In adolescence, the primary manifestations tend to be dandruff, flaking of the eyebrows, and postauricular and flexural scaling. In contrast to atopic dermatitis, pruritis is mild or absent, there are no systemic symptoms, and affected infants continue to feed and grow normally. Most improve spontaneously by 6 months of age.

Differential Diagnosis

Widespread red, eroded patches in a seborrheic distribution in infants with poor growth should suggest *acrodermatitis enteropathica* (AEP). These children develop a rapidly progressive eruption that is associated with diarrhea, hair loss, and listlessness. A defect in gastrointestinal zinc absorption results in low serum and tissue zinc levels and accounts for the clinical findings in AEP. Affected children respond to high doses of oral zinc within 2 to 3 days. Similar findings occur in children with malabsorption from chronic diarrhea and diets deficient in zinc. Essential fatty acid and biotin deficiencies also produce an AEP-like reaction.

Seborrheic dermatitis with a petechial or purpuric component should suggest the diagnosis of *histiocytosis X.* This disease is associated with chronic draining ears, hepatosplenomegaly, chronic diarrhea, and poor growth. The lungs, bone marrow, and central nervous system may also be involved.

Therapeutic Intervention

In uncomplicated seborrheic dermatitis, cradle cap usually responds to antiseborrheic shampoos containing selenium, salicylic acid, or zinc pyrithione (Head & Shoulders, Sebulex). Tap water compresses (twice daily), low-potency topical steroids (see Table 64–2), and emollients (see Table 64–4) are required for treatment of intertriginous lesions, often for several weeks. Postinflammatory pigmentary changes last for several months, but eventually pigmentation returns to normal. Secondary candidiasis or bacterial infection should be considered when satellite lesions are found or when the dermatitis fails to respond to usual topical measures.

Fungal Infections (Ringworm)

Dermatophytes may infect the nonhairy, or glabrous, skin of the trunk, extremities, and face (tinea corporis); the feet, with particular involvement of the toe web spaces (tinea pedis); and the scalp (tinea capitis). Fomite spread of fungus is also a problem, particularly in cases of ringworm of the scalp.

Tinea Corporis

Dermatophyte infections of glabrous skin produce a localized dermatitic reaction. Patches typically begin as single red papules or pustules that expand outward with a red annular border and a scaly hyperpigmentated or violaceous center. Untreated, they can enlarge to as much as 5 cm. Lesions have an active inflammatory border comprised of 2- to 3-mm vesicles or pustules that rupture and then scale (Fig. 64–8). Pruritus is often intense, and autoinoculation after scratching may lead to multiple widespread lesions. The infecting organism may be acquired from an infected domestic animal (*Microsporum canis*) or by direct human contact (*Tricophyton tonsurans*).

Differential Diagnosis. Differential diagnoses include atopic dermatitis (which is more diffuse, symmetric, and chronic), nummular eczema (whose lesions have microvesicles throughout and do not clear centrally), the herald patch of PR (which is KOH negative and followed by the characteristic PR eruption), and granuloma annulare (in which the annular rim is firm and tends not to have overlying epidermal changes).

Tinea Cruris

Tinea cruris, or "jock itch," involves the perineum and upper thighs. *Epidermophyton* and *Trichophyton* species are

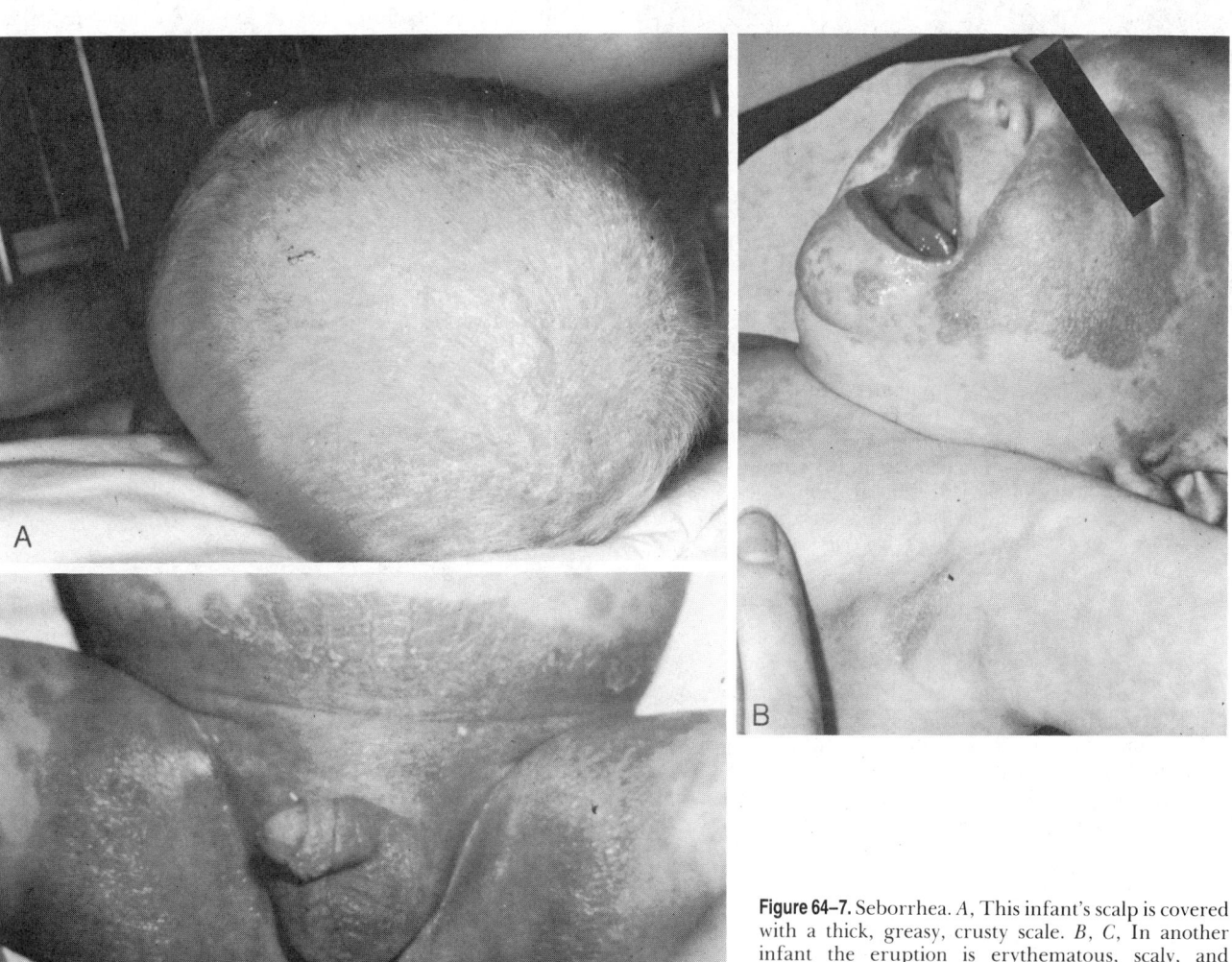

Figure 64–7. Seborrhea. *A,* This infant's scalp is covered with a thick, greasy, crusty scale. *B, C,* In another infant the eruption is erythematous, scaly, and slightly greasy and is prominent over the cheeks, axillae, and diaper area. (*B* and *C* Courtesy of Dr. Michael Sherlock; from Zitelli BJ, Davis HW (eds). Atlas of Pediatric Physical Diagnosis. 2nd ed. New York: Gower Medical Publishing, 1992.)

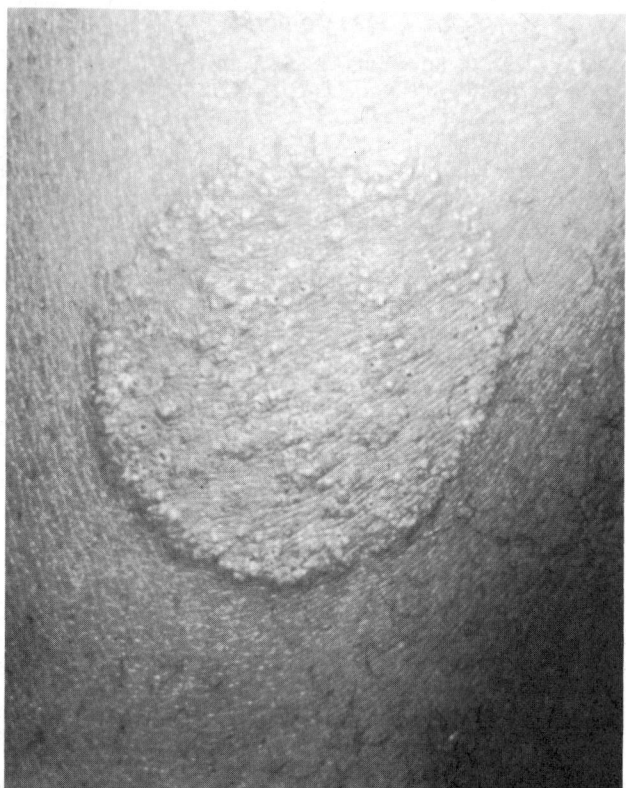

Figure 64–8. Tinea corporis. This pruritic annular lesion has an active erythematous vesicular border and a scaly, hyperpigmented center. (Courtesy of Dr. Michael Sherlock.)

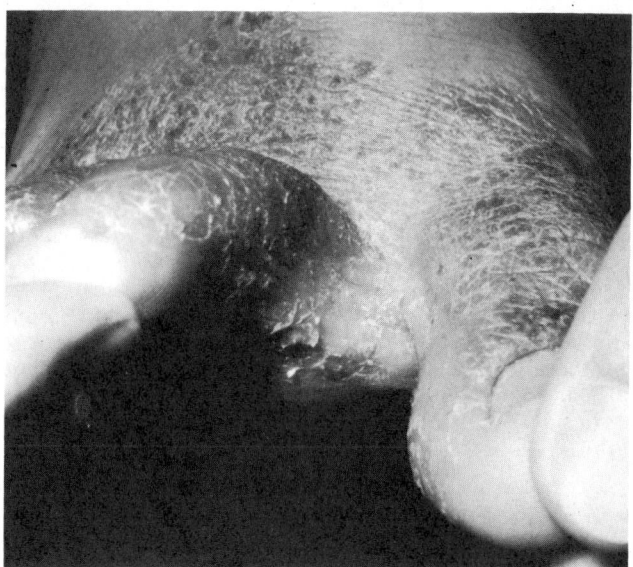

Figure 64–9. Tinea pedis. In this boy, scaling and fissuring began in the toe web spaces and has spread to involve the dorsum of the toes. (Courtesy of Dr. Michael Sherlock.)

causative. The problem is not seen until adolescence and predominantly affects boys. Obesity, wearing tight-fitting clothing or wet bathing suits (for prolonged periods), and chafing as a result of vigorous athletic activity are known predisposing factors. Shared clothing and towels in locker rooms and intimate contact are probable modes of acquisition.

The involved area is erythematous and scaly, and its borders are sharply demarcated from surrounding normal skin; occasionally the border has tiny active vesicles and pustules. The problem is embarrassingly pruritic.

Differential Diagnosis. Differential diagnostic considerations include seborrhea, psoriasis, irritant and contact dermatitis, and erythrasma (caused by *Corynebacterium*, which has a coral-colored fluorescence on Wood's lamp examination).

Tinea Pedis

Tinea pedis, or athlete's foot, is acquired from contact with infected desquamated skin scales on shower, bathroom, locker room, and gymnasium floors. Growth of the fungus is fostered by the warm, moist environment of shoes.

Lesions are first noted between the toes and can later spread to the dorsum and plantar surfaces. Scaling, fissuring, tiny vesiculopustular lesions, and maceration are seen and result in simultaneous itching and burning (Fig. 64–9).

Tinea Capitis

Tinea capitis is common in childhood and may become epidemic in schools and day-care centers. Fungal infection of the hair weakens the shafts, which then break, producing patches of partial alopecia. Typically, scalp ringworm begins

as subtle areas of minimal scale that are commonly misdiagnosed as seborrheic dermatitis or dandruff (Fig. 64–10). In other instances the residual hair stubs dot the surface of the involved scalp, creating a salt-and-pepper appearance. Occasionally, annular lesions similar to those of tinea corporis are seen. In other patients, pustules form on an erythematous base, rupture, weep, and form golden crusts simulating impetigo. In fact, whenever crusted lesions or pustules are seen involving the scalp, tinea capitis, not staphylococcal or streptococcal infection, should be suspected as the source. More intense inflammatory infections produce painful, edematous, exudative plaques or masses (kerions) that may heal with scarring and permanent hair loss.

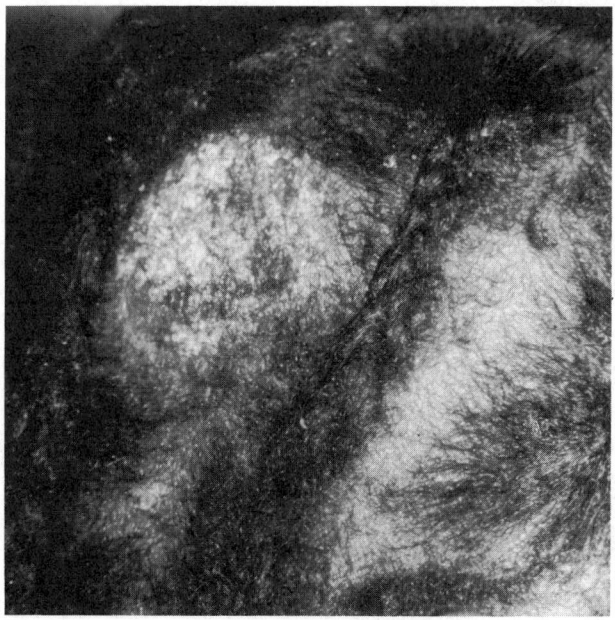

Figure 64–10. Tinea capitis. This child has a mildly pruritic, dry, scaling, circular scalp lesion with partial alopecia.

Diagnostic Evaluation

Prompt diagnosis of dermatophyte infections is necessary to initiate treatment and reduce the risk of spread to siblings and classmates. A KOH preparation may be made of scalp scale and hairs scraped off close to the scalp or from scrapings of scale from skin lesions on the trunk or extremities or scale under the nails. Fungal cultures should be obtained when the KOH preparation is negative but the clinical findings are highly suggestive of tinea infection.

Therapeutic Intervention

Topical antifungals are effective for tinea corporis, tinea cruris, and tinea pedis (See Table 64–3). Keeping the affected areas dry is important in treating both tinea pedis and tinea cruris. Hence, application of absorbent powders may be helpful, as are avoidance of shoes (which promote sweating) in the former instance and wearing loose-fitting cotton underwear in the latter. In constrast, tinea capitis must be treated with oral agents. Griseofulvin (Grifulvin V), 10 to 15 mg/kg/day, is the treatment of choice, but patients with a history of hypersensitivity to griseofulvin or with recalcitrant infection may be treated with oral ketoconazole. Corticosteroids are indicated as adjunctive treatment in managing kerions, as they significantly reduce the risk of scarring and permanent hair loss. Prednisone is begun at a dosage of 0.5 to 1.0 mg/kg/day, which is then tapered over 2 weeks. Twice-weekly shampooing with 2.5% selenium sulfide shampoo reduces spore formation and shedding and thus may also reduce the risk of spread of tinea capitis. Close contacts, including all family members of patients with any form of tinea, should be examined for evidence of infection, and all suspicious lesions should be treated or cultured.

Families should be instructed not to share towels, bed linens, hats, scarves, combs, brushes, or hair care products. Brushes, combs, and hats of affected patients should be washed at frequent intervals until the infection has been eradicated.

Psoriasis

More than 20% of patients with psoriasis experience their first episode before the age of 20 years, and about 2%

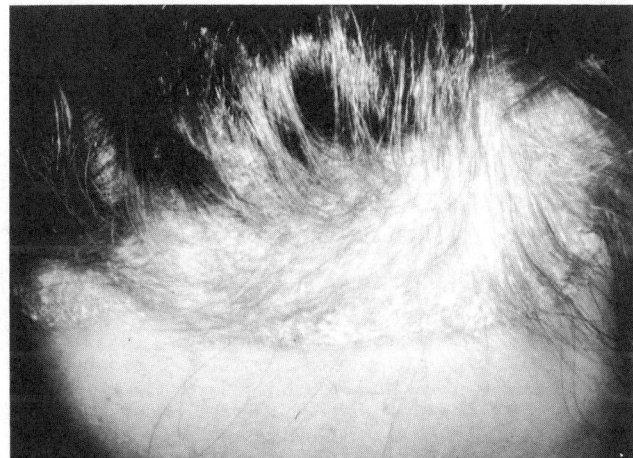

Figure 64–11. Psoriasis. Well-circumscribed, erythematous plaques covered by thick, silvery scale are typically found on the extensor surfaces of the elbows and knees and over the sacrum, scalp (shown here), and genital areas. (From Zitelli BJ, Davis HW (eds). Atlas of Pediatric Physical Diagnosis. 2nd ed. New York: Gower Medical Publishing, 1992.)

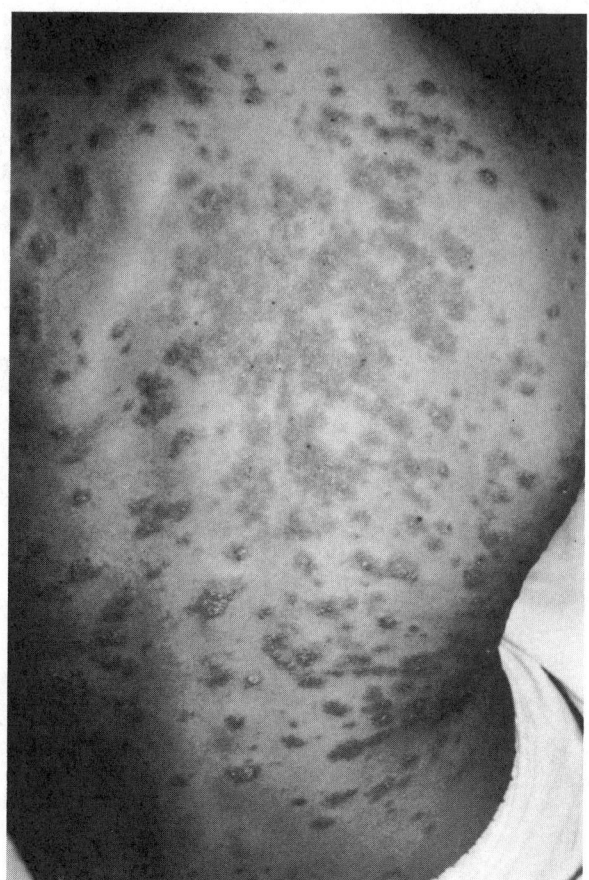

Figure 64–12. Guttate psoriasis. In some children, streptococcal or viral pharyngitis may precipitate the appearance of water droplet–like psoriatic patches.

become symptomatic in the first 2 years of life. Circumscribed round or oval red plaques with overlying thick, silvery scale typically appear on the extensor surfaces of the elbows and knees, over the sacrum, or on the scalp and genital areas (Fig. 64–11). Lesions are often induced in areas of local injury such as abrasions, surgical scars or burns, a response known as the *Koebner phenomenon*. Thickening and fissuring of the palms and soles may also be seen. Nail changes, including pitting, yellowing, onycholysis (separation of the nail plate from the underlying skin), and increased friability, are common. The rash may remain localized to extensor surfaces of the extremities or may slowly spread over the trunk. Children may develop eruptive water-droplet–like patches known as *guttate psoriasis* (Fig. 64–12) in association with acute streptococcal or viral pharyngitis. In infancy, psoriasis may masquerade as a recalcitrant diaper dermatitis. Patients with psoriasis often complain of pruritus, and scratching may lead to secondary bacterial infection.

Therapeutic Intervention

The rash and itching respond, at least temporarily, to topical emollients and medium-potency topical corticosteroids. Anthralin, a plant derivative with antipsoriatic properties; tar products; and keratolytics such as salicylic acid, lactic acid, and urea may also be useful. Localized disease (e.g., on the palms and soles) may require high-potency topical corticosteroids. Outpatient phototherapy with ultraviolet B light (sunburn wavelengths) or ultraviolet A light (long-wavelength ultraviolet light) combined with an oral photosensitizer (psoralen) is effective for widespread or recalcitrant psoriasis. This therapy, however, should be administered to children only by trained personnel in a closely supervised medical setting.

Occasionally, patients develop generalized *erythrodermic* or *pustular psoriasis* associated with fever, arthralgias, and fluid and electrolyte changes. Disease activity may become cyclical, with periodic relapses and remissions. Hospitalization is indicated for close monitoring until the acute episode settles down, which is usually accomplished with conservative measures such as tepid compresses, whirlpool baths, low-potency topical steroids, and lubricants. Patients may subsequently improve with traditional topical therapy and phototherapy. Treatment with methotrexate or synthetic retinoids (13-*cis*-retinoic acid [isotretinoin], etretinate, etretin) may be necessary in patients with severe recalcitrant disease.

Pityriasis Rosea

PR is a self-limited disorder characterized by 0.5- to 2.0-cm pink, oval, scaly dermatitic patches primarily involving the trunk and proximal extremities. Lesions begin as small round papules that enlarge to form ovals that tend to have their long axes oriented along skin tension lines, resulting in a characteristic "Christmas tree" pattern on the chest and back (Fig. 64–13). In about half of the patients, the appearance of a large (5- to 10-cm) "herald" patch on the trunk or proximal extremities precedes the onset of the more generalized rash by several days. On occasion, this may clear centrally, simulating tinea corporis. Lesions may be mildly pruritic in some patients.

PR can occur at any age but is more common in adolescents and young adults. Although the cause is unknown, the occasional report of associated prodromal flu-like symptoms and peak incidence in the winter and early spring suggest an infectious, probably viral, cause. The rash reaches its peak in several weeks and then gradually fades over another 4 to 6 weeks.

Differential Diagnosis

PR must be differentiated from secondary syphilis by obtaining a rapid plasma reagin (RPR) test or Venereal Disease Research Laboratory (VDRL) test in all sexually active adolescents. History of a chancre, lymphadenopathy,

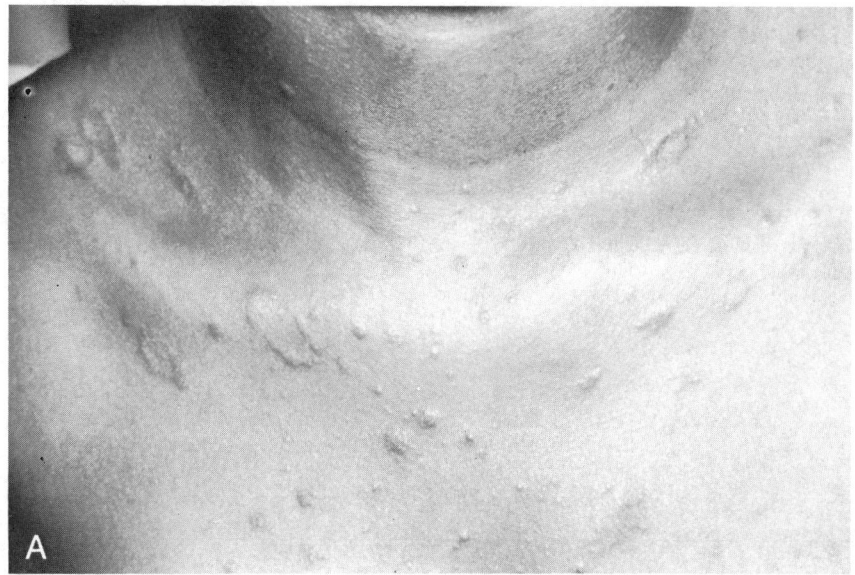

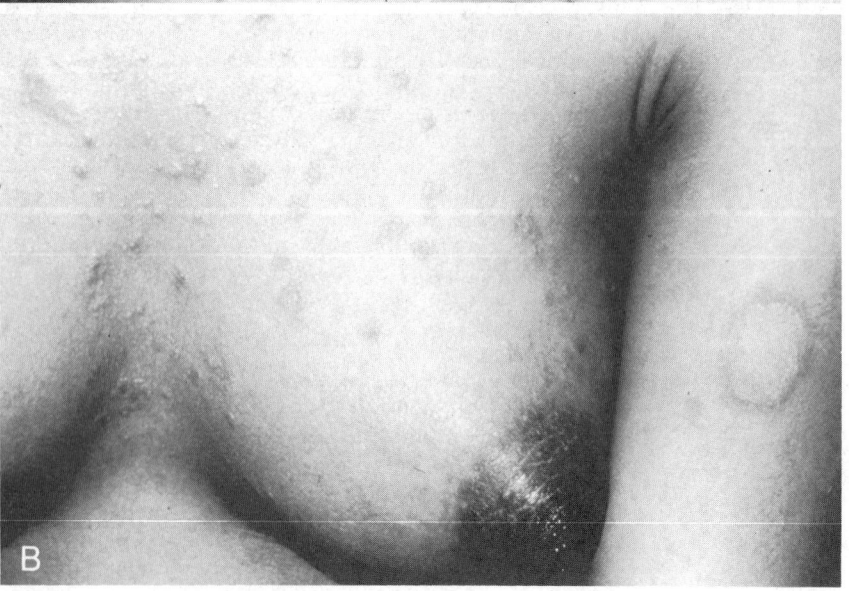

Figure 64–13. Pityriasis rosea. *A,* This exanthem is characterized by lesions that begin as small, round papules that enlarge to form ovals with their long axes oriented along skin tension lines. These may be raised or macular and usually are scaly. *B,* In about 50% of cases the rash is preceded by the appearance of a single large herald patch on the trunk or a proximal extremity. (Courtesy of Dr. Michael Sherlock; from Zitelli BJ, Davis HW (eds). Atlas of Pediatric Physical Diagnosis. 2nd ed. New York: Gower Medical Publishing, 1992.)

or hepatosplenomegaly suggests syphilis. Guttate psoriasis may be difficult to distinguish from PR without a skin biopsy, although the surface scale tends to be thicker and silvery in psoriasis. Other dermatitic processes such as seborrheic dermatitis and atopic dermatitis demonstrate distinctly different and characteristic distributions and clinical patterns. As noted, the herald patch is often mistaken for ringworm, but fungus can be quickly excluded by lack of pruritus and a negative KOH scraping.

Therapeutic Intervention

In most cases of pityriasis, education regarding the course of the disorder and reassurance are sufficient. When patients complain of pruritis, oral antihistamines (hydroxyzine or diphenhydramine) should be prescribed for symptomatic relief. Moisturizing creams or lotions may also be helpful.

VESICULOPUSTULAR ERUPTIONS

Vesiculopustular rashes may represent benign self-limited disorders or rapidly progressive fatal disease. Immediate diagnosis is mandatory, especially in infants and immunocompromised children. Thorough examination, identification of clinical patterns, and a few bedside diagnostic techniques permit differentiation of these disorders (Table 64–5).

Impetigo

Impetigo is a superficial infection of the epidermis caused by staphylococci, streptococci, or both. In recent years *Staphylococcus* has become the predominant causative organism. Exposed portions of the body—the forearms, lower legs, and face—are most commonly affected. Lesions are pruritic and teeming with organisms and thus can be a source of transmission to others, as well as to other sites as a result of scratching. The peak incidence occurs in summer and fall because of increased exposure of skin surface to injury and insect bites.

In streptococcal impetigo (now comprising a minority of cases), honey-colored crusts develop over abrasions, insect bites, and other breaks in the integument. Bullous impetigo is caused by strains of staphylococci that elaborate a soluble exotoxin known as *epidermolysin*, which produces a superficial blister by cleaving the skin high in the epidermis. Hence, bullous impetigo is characterized by superficial, flaccid, expanding bullae that rupture rapidly and crust over and around which new bullous rims form (Fig. 64–14). Untreated, blisters and crusts may expand to up to 5 cm in diameter, and multiple smaller satellite lesions commonly develop from inoculation by rubbing and scratching. Although in most cases lesions remain fairly localized, in children with preexisting dermatitis or varicella, the infection can spread rapidly to involve extensive portions of the skin surface.

TABLE 64–5
VESICULOPUSTULAR ERUPTIONS

Disorder	Skin Lesions	Distribution	Diagnostic Studies	Admission Criteria
Infections				
Bacterial				
Impetigo	Honey-colored crusts, flaccid bullae, collarettes of scale around denuded bases of ruptured bullae, satellite bullae	Face, trunk, extremities	Gram stain, bacterial culture	
Staphylococcal scalded skin syndrome	Generalized "sunburn" periorificial crusting, Nikolsky's sign	Total body; mucous membranes spared	Gram stain of skin (usually negative, but Gram stain and culture of nasopharynx or conjunctivae usually positive); skin biopsy	All newborns, extensive skin involvement, dehydration, serious underlying infection
Staphylococcal pustulosis	Papules, pustules	Trunk, diaper area	Gram stain	Cellulitis recalcitrant to outpatient therapy, systemic symptoms
Viral				
Herpes simplex	Grouped thick-walled vesicles, pustules, erosions	Face, trunk, extremities, perineum, mucous membranes	Tzanck smear, viral culture	Newborns, compromised hosts, urinary retention, dehydration, disseminated infection
Herpes zoster	Grouped papules, vesicles, pustules, erosions, crusts	Dermatomal	Tzanck smear	Disseminated infection (compromised host), severe superinfection, ocular involvement
Noninfectious disorders				
Erythema multiforme	Papules, wheals, target lesions, erosions	Generalized; palms, soles; mucous membranes in Stevens-Johnson syndrome	Skin biopsy	Stevens-Johnson syndrome
Toxic epidermal necrolysis	Generalized "sunburn," generalized sloughing, Nikolsky's sign	Generalized; mucous membranes	Skin biopsy	Dehydration, severe mucous membrane involvement, severe bacterial superinfection

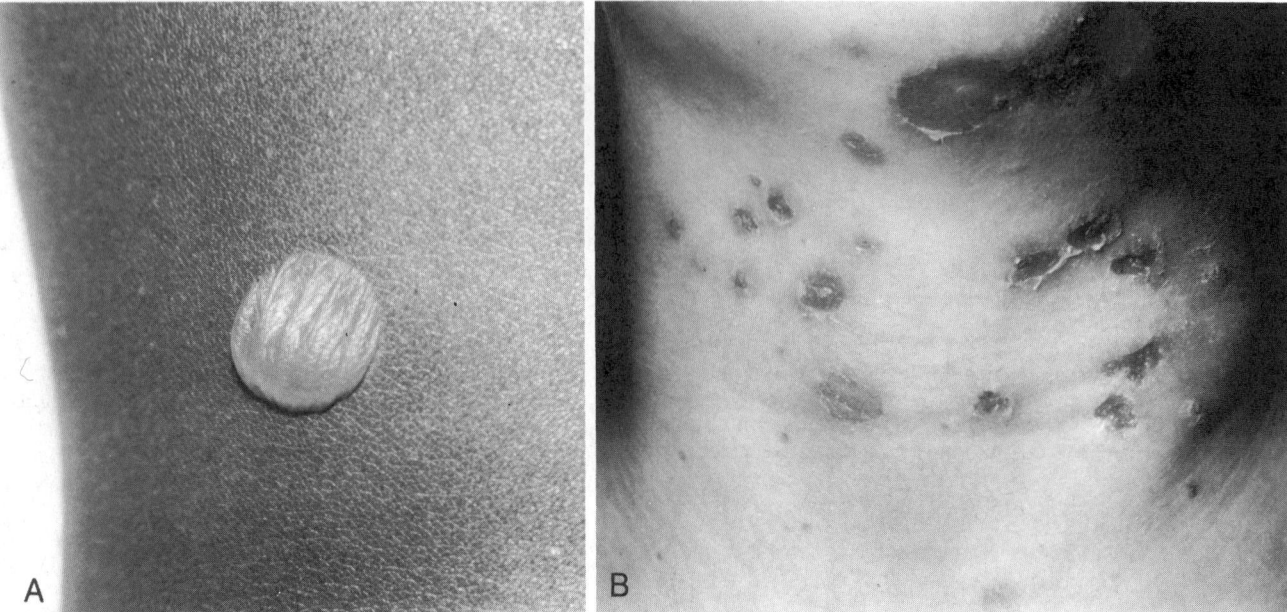

Figure 64–14. Bullous impetigo. *A*, A single, large, thin-walled flaccid bulla is seen on the thigh of this child. *B*, These lesions rupture rapidly and crust over, and new bullous rims form around their margins.

Therapeutic Intervention

Small, localized lesions on the extremities can be treated with a topical antibacterial ointment such as mupirocin (Bactroban), bacitracin, or bacitracin–polymixin B (Polysporin). Patients with more extensive involvement and those with facial lesions or associated nasopharyngitis require oral therapy with an agent directed at streptococci and staphylococci.

Staphylococcal Scalded Skin Syndrome (SSSS)

Staphylococcal infection with epidermolysin-elaborating strains, which occurs in infants, young children, and certain immunocompromised patients with low antibody titers against epidermolysin and decreased renal excretion of the toxin, can result in widespread blister formation termed SSSS. The appearance of bullae is preceded by development of a generalized tender, sunburn-like erythema (Fig. 64–15). Patients are febrile and irritable because of pain. The primary site of infection is usually the nasopharynx or conjunctivae. Intertriginous areas, the umbilical stump, the circumcision site, and other macerated areas are less frequent primary sites. In infants, particularly neonates, dissemination of bacteria from these sites may result in sepsis. Conversely, primary staphylococcal infections involving visceral sites such as the lungs, bones, joints, or deep soft tissues may produce SSSS. Consequently, seriously ill children should have a complete evaluation to exclude extracutaneous sources.

In patients with localized impetigo, Gram stains and cultures from skin lesions demonstrate the offending organism, but in patients with SSSS, the organism is only identified in specimens obtained from the primary site of infection, as it is absent at sites of denuded skin.

Therapeutic Intervention

Although most toddlers and older children have mild disease and respond quickly to oral antimicrobial therapy,

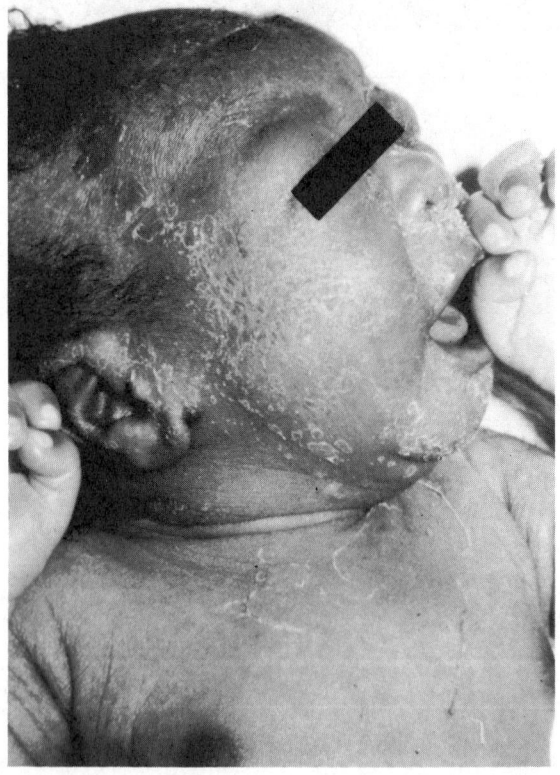

Figure 64–15. Staphylococcal scalded skin syndrome. In this disorder, patients develop fever and a diffuse intense erythroderma and irritability. Soon thereafter, the upper epidermis begins to separate, forming large bullae. Application of traction to the skin results in denudation of a sheet of epidermis, Nikolsky's sign. The nose, conjunctivae, umbilicus, and circumcision area are common sites of primary infection. (Courtesy of Dr. Michael Sherlock; from Zitelli BJ, Davis HW (eds). Atlas of Pediatric Physical Diagnosis. 2nd ed. New York: Gower Medical Publishing, 1992.)

newborns, infants, and children with extensive skin involvement, decreased oral intake, or systemic infection require hospitalization for parenteral antibiotics and for close monitoring and supportive measures, which include fluid replacement and pain medication. Patients with SSSS begin to improve within several days, as demonstrated by drying of blisters and erosions, generalized desquamation and occasionally postinflammatory hyperpigmentation.

Staphylococcal Pustulosis

In the newborn, staphylococcal pustulosis requires early diagnosis and treatment to reduce the risk of progression to sepsis or SSSS. Relatively large pustules (up to 5 mm) on a narrow red base appear most commonly in the diaper and periumbilical areas (see Fig. 64–3). The clinical diagnosis can be quickly confirmed by obtaining a Gram-stained smear, which shows neutrophils and numerous gram-positive cocci in clusters, and by culturing coagulase-positive staphylococci.

Therapeutic Intervention

If the infant is afebrile and feeding well, vigorous topical therapy, including compresses and antiseptics, and oral antibiotics may result in rapid clearing of the rash. However, close observation is necessary to detect early signs of systemic spread. Fever, lethargy, and poor feeding necessitate parenteral therapy.

Furuncles

In older children, pustulosis is a common complication of folliculitis, which typically involves the buttocks and thighs. Superficial follicular pustules may evolve into deep-seated furuncles (Fig. 64–16) or spread to neighboring follicles and soft tissue, creating an abscess or carbuncle. Ensuing painful cellulitis may be associated with fever, malaise, and sepsis.

Therapeutic Intervention

Localized folliculitis may improve with topical antibiotics or oral medications such as erythromycin, dicloxacillin, or

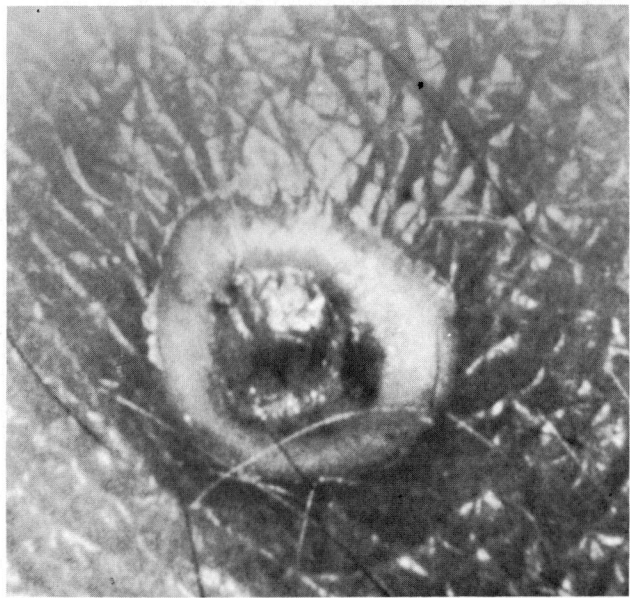

Figure 64–16. Furuncle. This child has developed a painful buttock abscess that has begun to spread through the adjacent soft tissues. (From Zitelli BJ, Davis HW (eds). Atlas of Pediatric Physical Diagnosis. 2nd ed. New York: Gower Medical Publishing, 1992.)

cephalexin. Abscesses should be incised and drained. Those lesions complicated by cellulitis may require parenteral therapy. Children with chronic folliculitis often have underlying keratosis pilaris (keratin plugging of hair follicles) and may benefit from the application of mild peeling agents with antiseptic activity, such as benzoyl peroxide, tretinoin (Retin A), lactic acid (Lachydrin), and urea (Carmol), and from the use of hydrating lotions or creams.

Varicella Zoster

Primary infection with the varicella zoster virus, or chickenpox, is discussed elsewhere; however, *herpes zoster,* or shingles, the disorder that results from reactivation of latent virus, will be reviewed here.

Following primary infection, the varicella zoster virus takes up residence in the genome of posterior spinal or cranial nerve cells and becomes dormant. Reactivation is not uncommon and may be caused in part by mechanical or thermal trauma, infection, or decreased host resistance. Lesions appear as grouped thin-walled vesicles on an erythematous base in a dermatomal distribution (Fig. 64–17). Pain or hyperesthesia may precede, develop concurrently with, or follow the appearance of lesions but is usually mild in children unless the cranial nerves are involved. The thoracic dermatomes are affected most often, followed by the cervical, trigeminal, lumbar, and facial dermatomes. Lesions generally crust over and heal within 14 days. In most cases the clinical course is mild; however, in immunocompromised children, particularly those with lymphoproliferative disorders, there is a significant risk of dissemination of infection.

Diagnosis can usually be made clinically based on the appearance and dermatomal distribution of the lesions. In questionable cases a Tzanck smear of scrapings from the base will reveal multinucleated giant cells, although this does not distinguish between herpes zoster and herpes simplex. Unfortunately, confirmation by viral culture is unreliable, and identification, when possible, may take 7 to 14 days.

Patients with herpes zoster can transmit the virus to susceptible others, resulting in varicella. However, communicability is lessened, as most lesions occur on clothing-covered sites and do not involve the nasopharynx.

Therapeutic Intervention

In otherwise healthy patients, symptomatic treatment with oral analgesics, if pain is a symptom, is the only therapy needed. However, when the eruption develops in an immunocompromised child, early intervention with parenteral antiviral agents is important. Furthermore, when the ophthalmic branch of the trigeminal nerve is involved, as signaled by lesions on the tip of the nose, urgent ophthalmologic consultation is indicated, and high-dose oral or parenteral acyclovir may be needed to reduce the risk of corneal scarring and permanent visual loss. Systemic corticosteroids have no place in the treatment of herpes zoster in children, in whom the risk of postherpetic neuralgia is negligible.

Herpes Simplex Infections

Herpes simplex virus infections usually result in development of lesions of the skin and mucous membranes. When symptomatic, primary infections are characterized by local lesions, regional adenopathy, fever, and malaise. The perioral skin and oral mucosa are the most common sites, although the hands and fingers and other portions of the face or the trunk may be involved. When the eyelids or periorbital tissues are affected, rubbing can result in spread

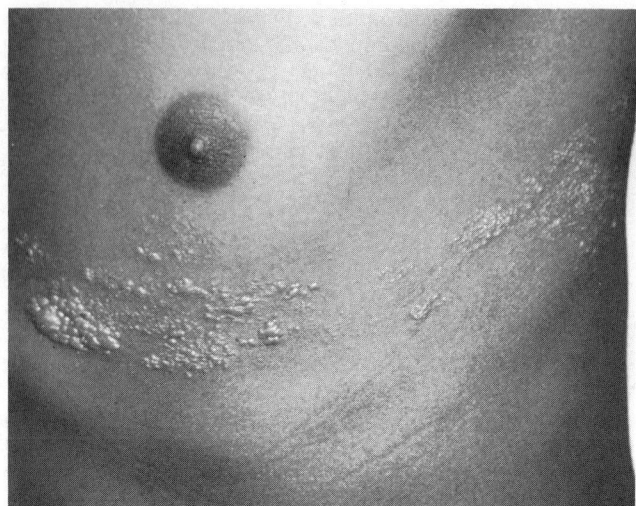

Figure 64–17. Herpes zoster. Reactivation of the varicella zoster virus has resulted in the appearance of grouped, thin-walled vesicles on an erythematous base in a dermatomal distribution. (Courtesy of Dr. Michael Sherlock; from Zitelli BJ, Davis HW (eds). Atlas of Pediatric Physical Diagnosis. 2nd ed. New York: Gower Medical Publishing, 1992.)

to the eye itself, causing keratoconjunctivitis. This produces characteristic dendritic ulcerations of the cornea and can result in permanent visual loss. Hence, urgent ophthalmologic consultation should be sought whenever there is any suspicion of ocular involvement. As is the case with other herpes viruses, after primary infection the virus becomes latent or dormant, taking up residence in local sensory ganglia, and can reactivate later, resulting in recurring infection.

Herpes Gingivostomatitis

The most common form of primary herpes simplex is herpes gingivostomatitis. Patients develop high fever, irritability, and extensive intraoral vesicles, pustules, and erosions (yellow ulcers with red halos) that involve gingival, labial, and buccal mucosae and the palate and tongue. The gingivae become swollen, intensely erythematous, and friable and bleed easily (Fig. 64–18). Yellowish debris rapidly builds up on mucosal surfaces, and halitosis is common. Anterior cervical nodes are enlarged and tender. Lesions are intensely painful and interfere with feeding and maintenance of oral hygiene. Infants and toddlers often drool copiously. Symptoms last from 5 to 10 days, and patients should be followed closely for signs of dehydration.

Differential Diagnosis. The intense gingivitis and gingival swelling, diffuseness of the inflammation, and ulcerations help distinguish herpes gingivostomatitis from coxsackie herpangina and other forms of aphthous ulcers and gingivitis.

Therapeutic Intervention. Treatment is generally supportive and symptomatic. Oral analgesics and topical application of a mixture of aluminum hydroxide–magnesium hydroxide (Maalox) and diphenhydramine elixir (which has topical anesthetic properties) prior to feedings help reduce pain in herpes gingivostomatitis. Use of a mixture of glycerine and peroxide facilitates oral cleansing until brushing can be resumed. Salty liquids and acidic fruit and vegetable juices should be avoided, as these exacerbate pain. In patients with severe oral involvement resulting in dehydration, administration of intravenous acyclovir will shorten the course of symptoms.

Primary Cutaneous Herpes Simplex

Primary cutaneous infections generally result from direct inoculation of previously traumatized sites and are associated with fever and regional adenopathy. Lesions consist of deep thick-walled vesicles on an erythematous base that rapidly become pustular (Fig. 64–19A). These are often grouped, tending to coalesce, but may occur singly. When seen on a thumb or finger, the lesion is called an *herpetic whitlow* (Fig. 64–19B). Over the ensuing 5 to 7 days, the pustules ulcerate and crust over, and drying and desquamation are complete in 10 to 14 days.

Differential Diagnosis. The thick-walled nature of the vesicles, their tendency to form clusters and coalesce, and the fact that they are more painful than pruritic help distinguish them clinically from impetiginous lesions. If clinical findings are uncertain, laboratory tests can be performed to establish the diagnosis. A Gram stain of vesicular or pustular fluid will reveal few, if any, bacteria, and a Giemsa stain of scrapings from the base of a fresh lesion will demonstrate multinucleated giant cells. If culture confirmation is necessary, viral cultures are positive in about 24 hours.

Therapeutic Intervention. Most cases of cutaneous herpes simplex infection are easily managed supportively with cool tap water compresses, lubricants, and oral analgesics as necessary.

Primary Genital Herpes Simplex

The majority of the previously described infections are caused by herpes simplex virus type 1. Herpes simplex virus type 2 is more commonly associated with genital lesions in adolescents and adults but can be a source of nongenital lesions as well. Genital herpes is seen in childhood and most commonly results from autoinoculation of virus from an oral lesion by the patient's own hands or from a parent with an active cold sore who fails to use good hand-washing technique before diaper changes or bathing young children. Less frequently, genital herpetic infections in young children

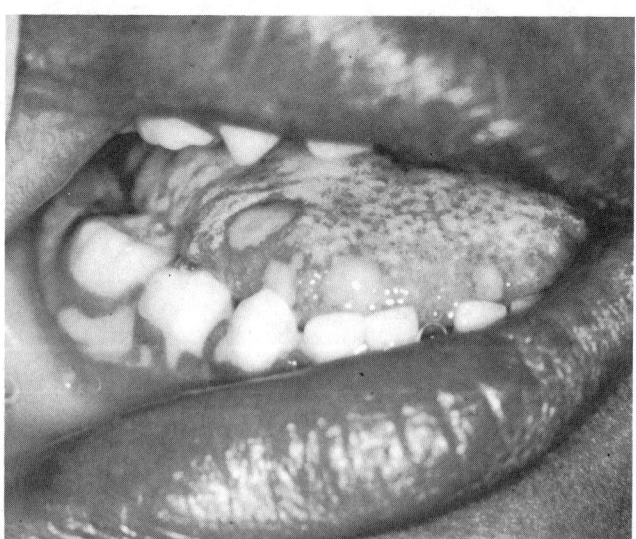

Figure 64–18. Herpetic gingivostomatitis. This child had high fever and intense oral pain. His tongue, gingivae, palate, and other mucosal surfaces were studded with shallow yellow ulcers surrounded by red halos. The gingivae were also diffusely edematous, markedly erythematous, and friable. (From Zitelli BJ, Davis HW (eds). Atlas of Pediatric Physical Diagnosis. 2nd ed. New York: Gower Medical Publishing, 1992.)

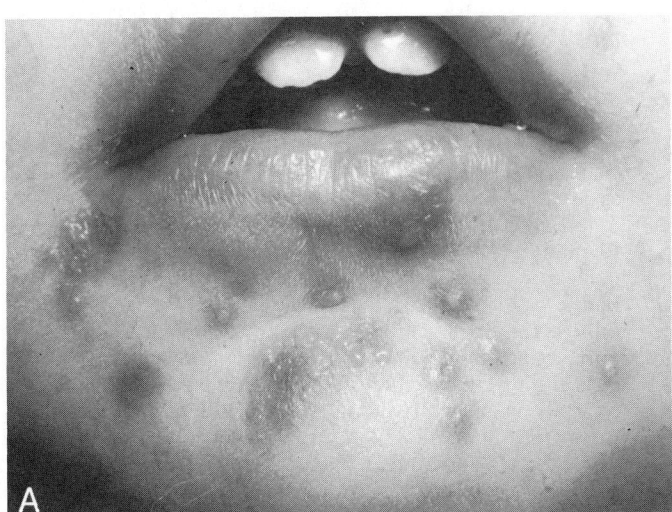 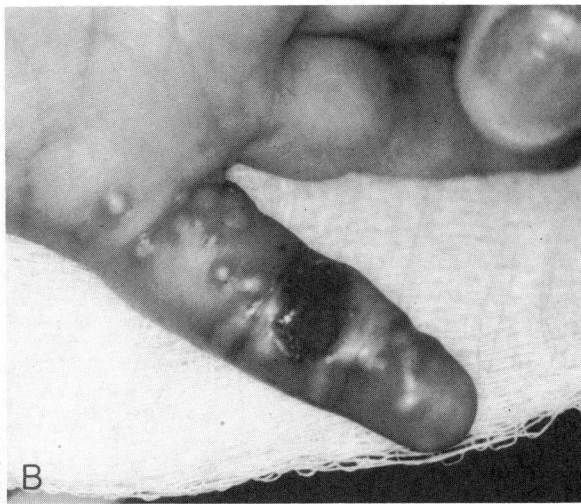

Figure 64–19. Primary cutaneous herpes simplex. *A*, Deep, thick-walled vesicles and pustules with red halos dot the chin and lip of this toddler. Some have coalesced, ruptured, and crusted. (Courtesy of Dr. Michael Sherlock.) *B*, This child has a herpetic whitlow consisting of thick-walled pustules that involve the finger. Some have coalesced and ulcerated. (From Zitelli BJ, Davis HW (eds). Atlas of Pediatric Physical Diagnosis. 2nd ed. New York: Gower Medical Publishing, 1992.)

are acquired as a result of sexual abuse. Lesions are similar in appearance to those of primary cutaneous herpes simplex but are localized to the perineal area (Fig. 64–20). They tend to ulcerate rapidly, resulting in intense dysuria. Tender inguinal adenopathy, fever, and malaise are prominent.

Therapeutic Intervention. Treatment is usually supportive and similar to that for other primary cutaneous lesions. However, in severe cases complicated by high fever and urinary retention, use of oral or parenteral acyclovir may be indicated.

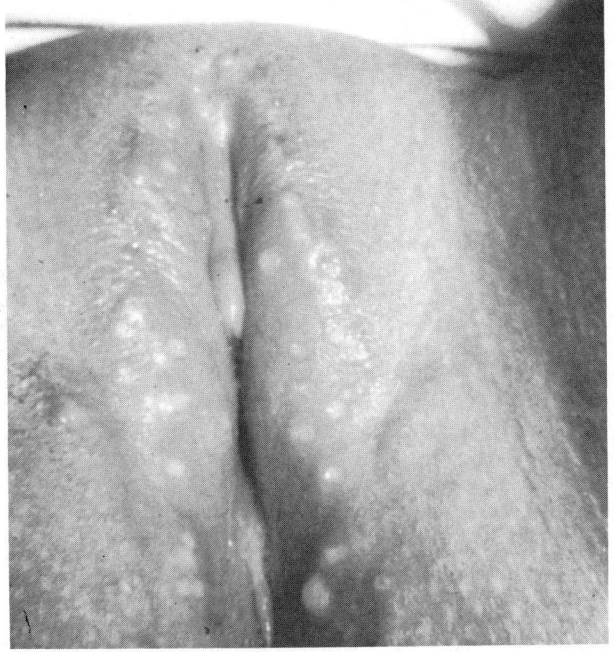

Figure 64–20. Genital herpes simplex. Thick-walled pustules and vesicles cover the perineum of this infant who had fever, irritability, and tender inguinal adenopathy. In this case the infection was transmitted by a parent with recurrent herpes labialis. (From Zitelli BJ, Davis HW (eds). Atlas of Pediatric Physical Diagnosis. 2nd ed. New York: Gower Medical Publishing, 1992.)

Disseminated Herpes Simplex

The majority of primary herpetic infections cause moderate misery but are not serious, but in the neonate or immunocompromised child, herpes may cause life-threatening disseminated disease involving the skin, lungs, abdominal viscera, and central nervous system. Whenever this is suspected, rapid confirmation should be sought using Tzanck preparations or cultures.

Children with diffuse atopic eczema and other forms of diffuse chronic dermatitis are also at risk for disseminated skin infection with herpes simplex; this is known as *eczema herpeticum*, or *Kaposi's varicelliform eruption*. Following a prodrome of high fever, discomfort, and irritability, herpetic lesions appear in multiple crops over a large portion of the skin surface, with clustering in sites of atopic dermatitis. These evolve to form pustules, which often become hemorrhagic, and then rupture and crust over (Fig. 64–21). Fever and systemic symptoms are prominent. Severity ranges from mild to severe and is, in part, dependent on the extent of the preceding dermatitis. When cutaneous involvement is extensive, fluid losses may be severe. In some cases, the virus spreads to involve the viscera, including the lungs, gastrointestinal tract, and central nervous system.

Therapeutic Intervention. Parenteral acyclovir (5 mg/kg every 8 hours), close monitoring, and fluid and electrolyte replacement are important in management of disseminated herpetic infections. Secondary infection is an ever-present risk and, when present, should be treated with systemic antibiotics. Hydroxyzine or diphenhydramine are helpful in combating pruritus, which is often intense.

Recurrent Herpes Simplex Infection

Following entry into its latent or dormant state, the herpes simplex virus can reactivate, causing localized recurrences at or near the site of the original primary infection. A prodrome of localized stinging, burning, or itching often precedes the eruption of a small patch of tiny grouped vesicles containing yellow serous fluid. Vesicles often have thinner walls than those seen in primary infection (Fig. 64–22). Vesicular fluid becomes cloudy in a few days, and then lesions gradually crust over. The lips and perioral area are the sites most commonly involved. Fever and constitutional

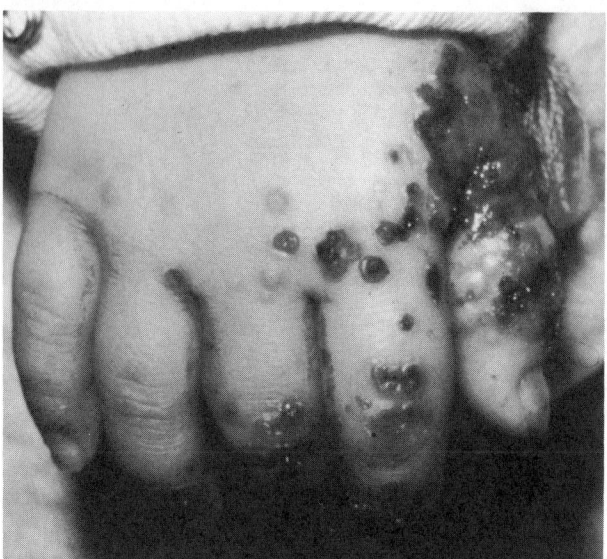

Figure 64–21. Eczema herpeticum (Kaposi's varicelliform eruption). This child with infantile eczema became infected with herpes simplex. Herpetic lesions appeared in crops, clustering in eczematous areas. These rapidly became hemorrhagic and later ulcerated. (Courtesy of Dr. Michael Sherlock; from Zitelli BJ, Davis HW (eds.) Atlas of Pediatric Physical Diagnosis. 2nd ed. New York: Gower Medical Publishing, 1992.)

symptoms are absent in recurrent infections, although regional adenopathy may be present. Precipitating factors may include a febrile illness, sunlight, local injury, emotional stress, and menses.

Differential Diagnosis. The presence of prodromal discomfort and the painful nature of the lesions help distinguish them from those of impetigo and contact dermatitis. Their small size differentiates the lesions of herpes simplex from those of herpes zoster.

Therapeutic Intervention. Treatment consists of application of tap water or aluminum acetate (Burow's solution)

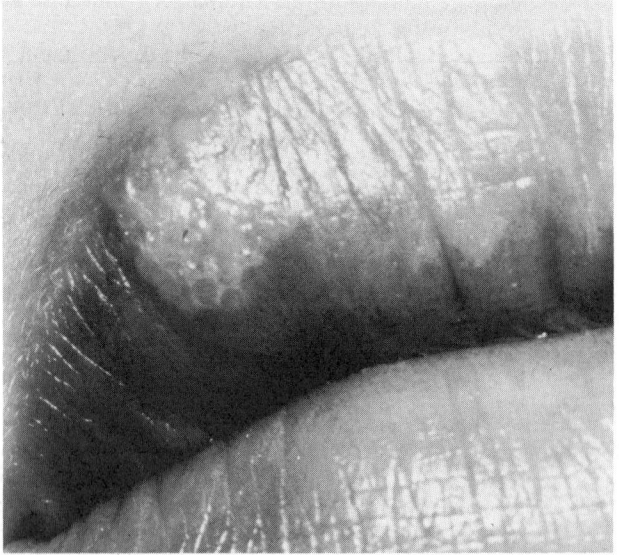

Figure 64–22. Recurrent herpes labialis. The appearance of this patch of tiny grouped vesicles was preceded by itching and burning. (From Zitelli BJ, Davis HW (eds). Atlas of Pediatric Physical Diagnosis. 2nd ed. New York: Gower Medical Publishing, 1992.)

compresses. Oral analgesics usually suffice to relieve symptoms.

Erythema Multiforme

Erythema multiforme (EM) is an acute reactive process that may be triggered by a number of factors, including drugs, vaccines, toxins, and viral and bacterial infections. The hallmark of EM is the "target," or "bull's-eye," lesion formed by a central dusky vesicle or macule with alternating pale and violaceous rings. Erythematous papules, annular plaques, and urticarial wheals are usually present. In EM minor, the most common variant, lesions frequently occur on the extremities and tend to be symmetric; however, the entire skin surface may become involved, and lesions are typically seen on the palms and soles (Fig. 64–23). In some cases, they may vesiculate either centrally or peripherally. Recurrent crops appear over 1 to 3 weeks and are accompanied by mild systemic symptoms consisting of low-grade fever, malaise, and myalgias. Although the rash usually heals without scarring, marked hyperpigmentation or hypopigmentation may result, particularly in dark-skinned individuals. Recurrent episodes of EM have been reported with barbiturates, streptococcal infections, and herpes simplex.

Rarely, EM lesions rapidly vesiculate, resulting in widespread cutaneous blistering (often hemorrhagic), accompanied by severe mucous membrane involvement; this is known as *Stevens-Johnson syndrome*, or EM major (Fig. 64–24). Common triggering agents include anticonvulsants, sulfonamides, allopurinol, herpes simplex, and *Mycoplasma pneumoniae* infections. In these children, the conjunctivae and the mucosae of the nose, mouth, urethra, and anus develop erosions and hemorrhagic crusts. Third spacing of fluids into skin lesions, decreased oral intake, and associated fever may result in dehydration. Systemic symptoms are prominent and include high fever, marked malaise, and arthralgias. Vomiting, diarrhea, sore throat, and chest pain are common as well. Progressive denudation of the skin may produce a clinical picture indistinguishable from that of toxic epidermal necrolysis (TEN).

Therapeutic Intervention

Treatment of EM is symptomatic and consists primarily of oral analgesics and rest. However, increased insensible water losses, high risk of secondary infection, and occasional involvement of the airway and lungs necessitates hospitalization for close monitoring and intensive supportive measures for patients with Stevens-Johnson syndrome. Early evaluation by an ophthalmologist is mandatory to reduce the risk of synechiae formation and permanent visual loss. Although mortality may exceed 40% in adults and immunocompromised children, most children recover without residua.

The role of systemic corticosteroids in the treatment of EM is controversial. Although they may be useful in patients with reactions induced by selected drugs, their safety and efficacy are unproven. Some investigators have demonstrated an increased risk of complications and prolongation of hospital stay in patients receiving steroids.

Toxic Epidermal Necrolysis

Although originally described in adults, TEN has been reported in children, particularly in association with drug hypersensitivity reactions. Other factors, including toxins and infections, may also trigger TEN. A brief, virus-like prodrome is followed by generalized erythema and sloughing of a large portion of the skin surface. Severe involvement

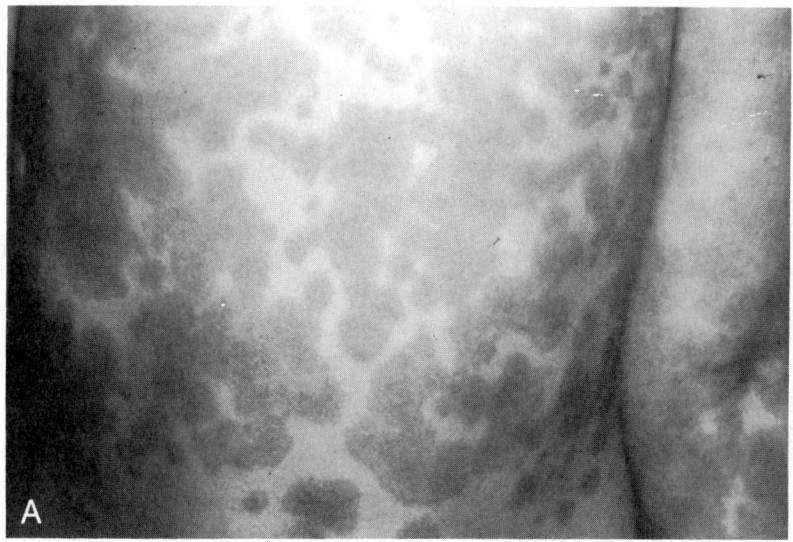

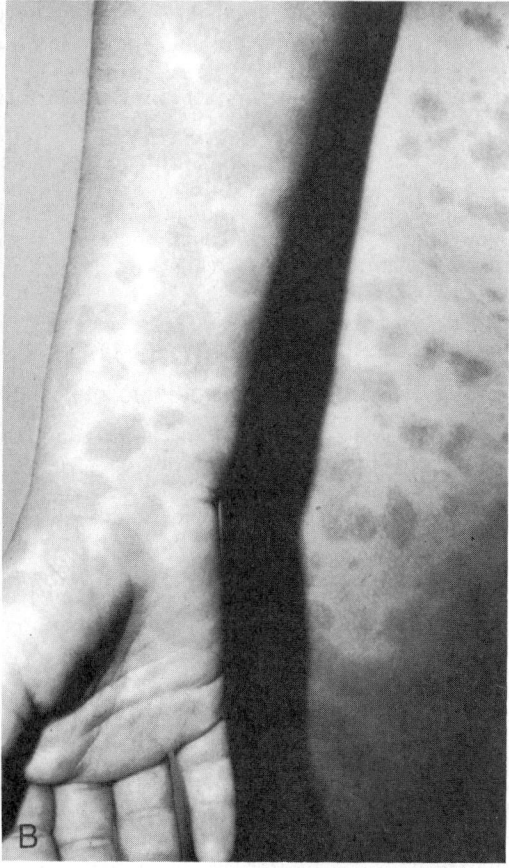

Figure 64–23. Erythema multiforme. *A,* This generalized erythematous eruption consists of numerous target lesions and wheals that have begun to coalesce into large plaques. *B,* Involvement of palms and soles is characteristic. (Courtesy of Dr. Michael Sherlock.)

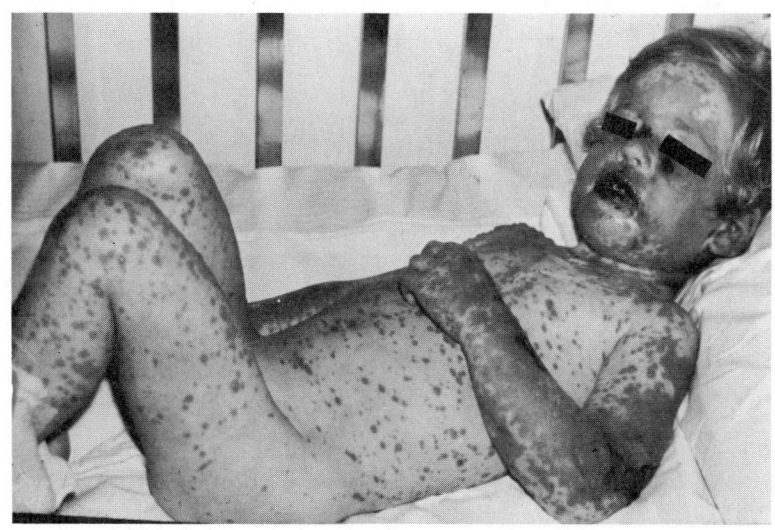

Figure 64–24. Stevens-Johnson syndrome. In this child, target lesions rapidly vesiculated, and inflammation and ulceration of mucous membranes were prominent in concert with severe systemic symptoms. (Courtesy of Dr. Michael Sherlock.)

of the mucous membranes results in a clinical picture similar to that of EM major, and progressive involvement of the airway may lead to adult respiratory distress syndrome. Although these children may be misdiagnosed with SSSS early in the course, it soon becomes apparent that the bullae have thicker walls and the erosions are deeper because they form by cleavage of the skin at the dermal-epidermal junction, with resultant full-thickness epidermal necrosis. Minor trauma by the examining finger produces an erosion or a positive Nikolsky sign anywhere on the skin surface.

Therapeutic Intervention

Management of TEN is similar to that for Stevens-Johnson syndrome. The hospital course may be protracted, and morbidity and mortality are high.

TOXIC ERYTHEMAS
Toxic Erythemas of Infectious Origin

Streptococcal and staphylococcal infections can be associated with diffuse erythroderma and characteristic exanthems when the inciting bacteria elaborate erythrogenic toxins. Knowledge of the clinical picture and course of evolution facilitate diagnosis, which can be confirmed by appropriate cultures.

Disorders include streptococcal and staphylococcal scarlet fevers, SSSS, and toxic shock syndrome. Findings in patients with scarlet fevers are reviewed here.

Streptococcal Scarlet Fever

Group A beta-hemolytic streptococci are responsible for streptococcal scarlet fever, a common childhood disease that has a peak incidence in winter and spring but can occur at any season. The organism is spread by close contact and shared utensils. Children are contagious during the period

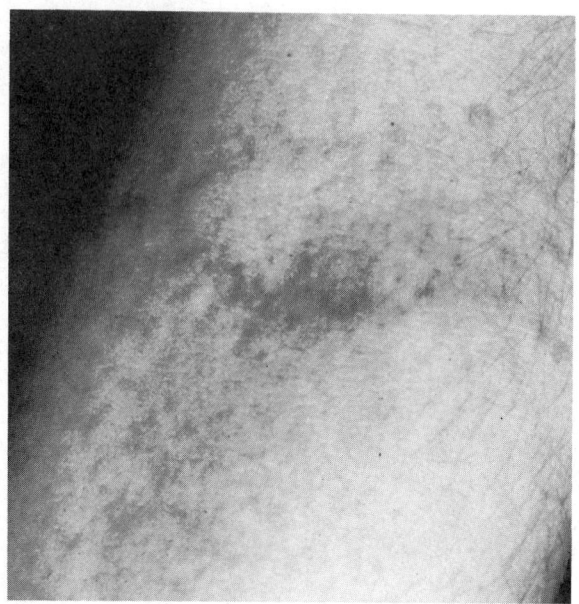

Figure 64–26. Pastia's lines. Within a few days of onset of scarlet fever, the rash becomes increasingly accentuated in skin creases, where petechiae may appear in a linear distribution. (From Zitelli BJ, Davis HW (eds). Atlas of Pediatric Physical Diagnosis. 2nd ed. New York: Gower Medical Publishing, 1992.)

of acute illness until they have been treated for at least 24 to 48 hours. Those with subclinical infection also serve as a major source of transmission. The incubation period is relatively brief, ranging from 12 hours to 7 days.

The classic case begins with abrupt onset of high fever and chills, headache, sore throat, vomiting, abdominal pain, and general malaise. The exanthem appears 12 to 48 hours later and quickly generalizes. Facial flushing with perioral pallor and diffuse, blanching erythema studded with pin-

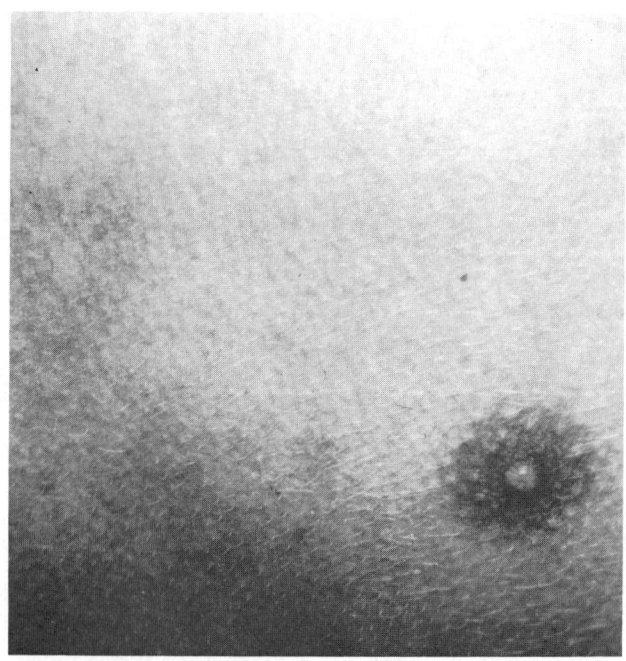

Figure 64–25. Streptococcal scarlet fever. This mildly pruritic, sandpaper-like rash that resembled a sunburn with goosebumps appeared in concert with a low-grade fever and sore throat. (Courtesy of Dr. Michael Sherlock.)

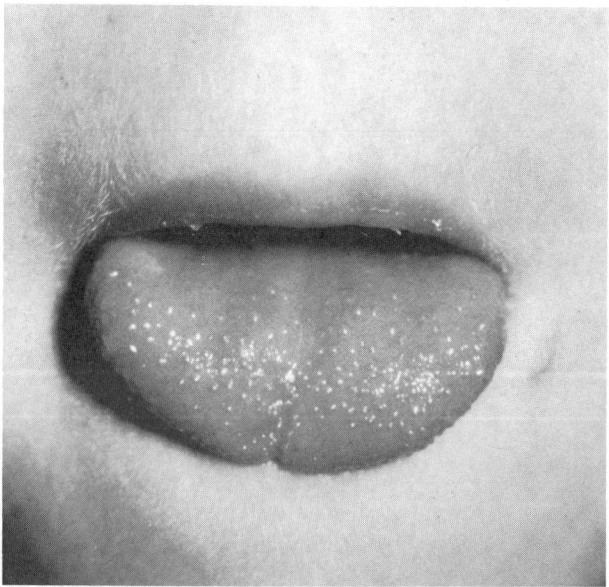

Figure 64–27. Strawberry tongue. The papillae are prominent and the tongue is a bright erythematous color. This phenomenon may be seen in streptococcal scarlet fever, staphylococcal toxic shock syndrome, and Kawasaki's disease. (From Zitelli BJ, Davis HW (eds). Atlas of Pediatric Physical Diagnosis. 2nd ed. New York: Gower Medical Publishing, 1992.)

head-sized papules that feel sandpapery on palpation are characteristic (Fig. 64–25). The rash tends to be pruritic, and some patients may manifest urticaria and dermographism. Over the ensuing few days, the rash becomes increasingly accentuated in skin creases, where petechiae may form in a linear distribution; this is known as *Pastia's lines* (Fig. 64–26). The pharynx and tonsils are erythematous, and palatal petechiae and tonsillar exudates are common. The papillae of the tongue become prominent, projecting through a white coating during the first day or two. This coating is then shed, leaving the characteristic red strawberry tongue (Fig. 64–27). Tender cervical adenopathy is commonly seen as well. Desquamation, which is directly proportional to the severity of the exanthem, begins about a week after onset, and shedding occurs in thin flakes.

Over the past several decades, the severity of scarlet fever has decreased considerably, and the spectrum of clinical findings has shifted to milder, less characteristic manifestations. Many patients are afebrile or have only low-grade fever, and malaise is usually mild. Pharyngitis may be absent or only mild erythema seen, and tongue changes may be subtle. In some patients, the rash is patchy rather than diffuse, although it is still accentuated around skin creases. In dark-skinned children, papules are often larger and rougher, and erythema may be difficult to detect. Some may have only pharyngitis and urticaria early on.

Even in children with a mild clinical picture, a throat culture will usually be positive for group A beta-hemolytic streptococci. However, in children younger than 3 years, a nasopharyngeal swab is more likely to yield the organism than a throat swab. On occasion, an infected wound or primary skin infection is the source, in which case the throat culture may be negative and oral findings absent.

Therapeutic Intervention. Scarlet fever, like streptococcal pharyngitis, is treated with a 10-day course of oral penicillin V in a dosage of 40 mg/kg/day, which results in clinical improvement in 24 to 48 hours. Erythromycin may be substituted in penicillin-allergic patients. Symptomatic treatment with oral analgesic and antipyretic agents is also useful to reduce malaise and discomfort. Oral hydroxyzine or diphenhydramine may be needed for patients with intense pruritus. Use of topical lubricants (see Table 64–4) can reduce pruritus as well and is especially helpful when desquamation begins. Despite early response to penicillin, the full 10-day course must be taken to prevent acute rheumatic fever and suppurative complications such as cervical adenitis and peritonsillar or retropharyngeal abscesses. Antimicrobial therapy does not prevent acute poststreptococcal glomerulonephritis.

Staphylococcal Scarlet Fever

In staphylococcal scarlet fever, the infecting agent (i.e., coagulase-positive *Staphylococcus*) elaborates an exotoxin that produces the exanthem. Transmission is by direct contact with other infected persons or carriers, by airborne particles, or by contaminated objects or food.

Most affected children have an antecedent skin or wound infection, purulent conjunctivitis, or nasopharyngitis with a purulent nasal discharge. They then abruptly develop fever with moderate malaise, followed rapidly by the appearance of a generalized erythematous exanthem that is often sandpapery in consistency and accentuated in skin folds (Fig. 64–28). The involved skin is usually tender but not pruritic, and secondary irritability is the rule. Within a few days, the involved skin begins to crack, fissure, and crust over. This is

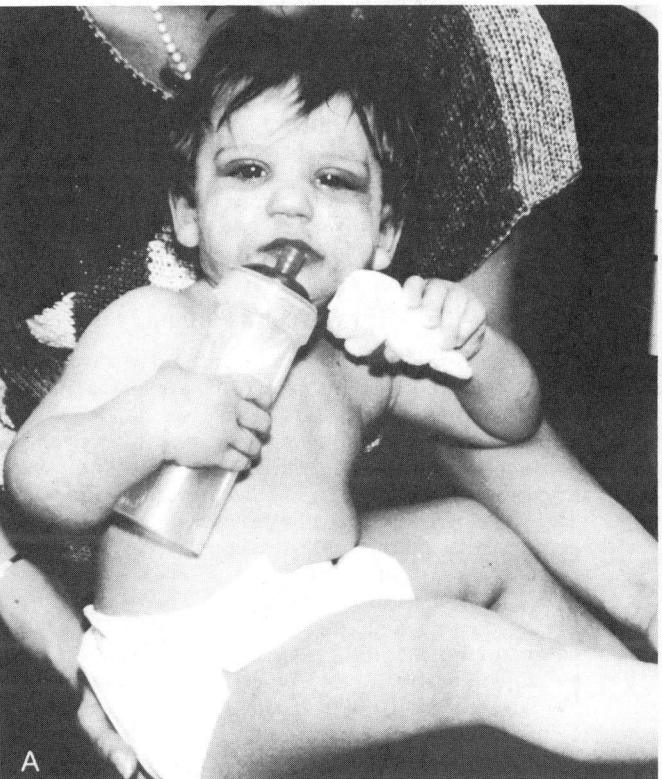
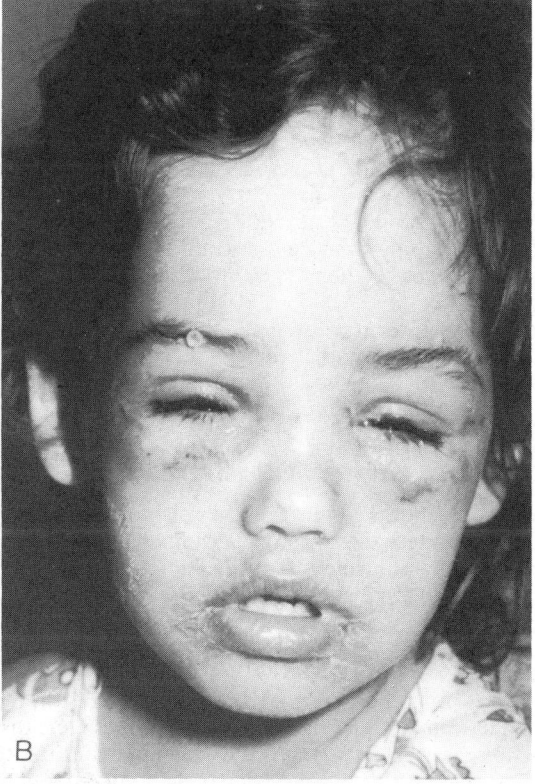

Figure 64–28. Staphylococcal scarlet fever. *A*, This child had moderate fever, irritability, and a generalized tender erythema. Inflammation was especially prominent around the eyes and mouth, where crusting, cracking, and fissuring developed the next day. He also had purulent conjunctival and nasal discharges and pharyngeal inflammation. *B*, The cracking, crusting, and fissuring typically found on day 2 or 3 are shown in another patient. This phenomenon is also seen in staphylococcal scalded skin syndrome. (*B*, Courtesy of Dr. Asphendiar Khorsandian, Daytona Beach, FL.)

especially prominent in perioral and periorbital areas and in skin creases. A Gram stain of purulent wound material or of ocular or nasal discharge is positive for gram-positive cocci in clusters. Cultures of these sites and of the pharynx in patients with antecedent nasopharyngitis will be positive for staphylococci.

Therapeutic Intervention. Oral antimicrobial therapy with cloxacillin, dicloxacillin, or cephalexin is sufficient in most cases. However, infants and toddlers with poor intake and severe systemic symptoms may require hospitalization for a few days of intravenous treatment. Administration of oral analgesics is important to relieve skin discomfort, which can be quite marked. Careful attention must also be given to ensuring adequate fluid intake.

Drug-Induced Eruptions

The majority of cutaneous drug reactions consist of morbilliform or maculopapular exanthems and thus simulate viral exanthems. The process begins between 5 and 14 days after the medication is started and is heralded by the appearance of erythematous macules and papules, which may be fine or blotchy. These usually begin on the face and trunk and spread peripherally over the ensuing few days. Most such eruptions are pruritic. With evolution, the lesions may become confluent. Resolution occurs within 1 or 2 weeks of discontinuing the offending agent.

Diagnosis is based on the history of medication intake, the appearance of the eruption, and absence of other signs of illness. Often diagnosis must be made empirically, which can result in misdiagnosis when the exanthem is actually of viral origin and develops coincidentally while the patient was on medication. Complete confirmation requires rechallenge with the suspected drug.

Another fairly common clinical picture is that of an urticarial/erythema multiforme–like reaction in which urticarial lesions, angioedema of the extremities, and periarticular swelling develop, usually during the course of therapy with cefaclor or sulfa-containing antimicrobial agents. This phenomenon can also be seen in children with upper respiratory tract infection who are not taking medication.

In contrast to true urticaria, lesions are usually only mildly pruritic, and many evolve into target lesions or gyrate plaques. They do not vesiculate (Fig. 64–29). The periarticular swelling is migratory and uncomfortable, and the overlying skin may be erythematous or bluish in color. The wrists and ankles are the sites most commonly involved. Painful migratory stocking-glove angioedema is also seen, and some patients develop facial angioedema as well. This serum sickness–like reaction waxes and wanes over 2 to 3 weeks and then gradually abates.

Therapeutic Intervention

Management of these disorders consists of discontinuation of the suspected drug and symptomatic care with oral analgesics and antihistamines as needed, as well as avoidance of the offending agent.

PURPURAS

Bleeding into the skin may be a self-limited finding in accidental trauma or the first sign of life-threatening disseminated disease (Table 64–6). Early diagnosis and treatment requires that the emergency department practitioner recognize purpura and evaluate the patient thoroughly and expeditiously.

Cutaneous hemorrhage can be distinguished from erythema caused by intravascular blood in dilated vessels by virtue of its failure to blanch when pressure is applied across

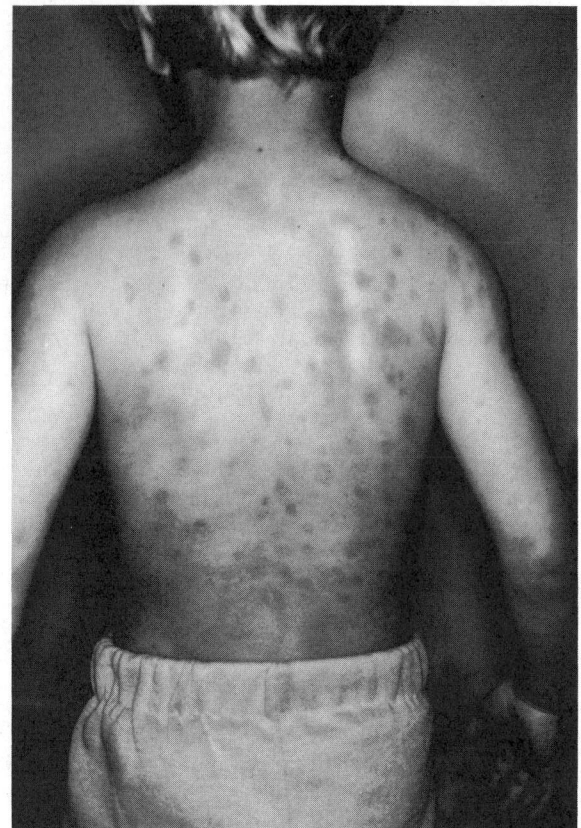

Figure 64–29. Urticarial/erythema multiforme–like reaction. This boy, who was taking cefaclor, presented with a mildly pruritic urticarial eruption in which many target lesions were noted. He also had angioedema of the forehead and periarticular swelling of the hands, wrists, and ankles.

the surface of the skin (diascopy). Diascopy can be performed by pressing the skin apart between the thumb and index finger or holding a glass or plastic slide over the area in question. Pinpoint areas of purpura are called *petechiae*; large confluent patches of purpura are referred to as *ecchymoses*. Purpura results from extravascular, intravascular, and vascular phenomena.

Extravascular Purpura

Trauma is the most common cause of extravascular purpura in children. Lesions caused by accidental trauma vary in size from less than 1 cm to many centimeters and are usually located over bony prominences such as the knees and elbows, the extensor surfaces of the lower legs and forearms, and exposed sites, including the chin and forehead. Hemorrhage is usually restricted to a discrete area of the skin. Petechiae are only occasionally present in otherwise normal patients, although they can occasionally be seen in children who have acute viral illnesses with normal platelet counts and repeated coughing or vomiting. In such cases, petechial lesions tend to be distributed over the face, neck, and upper chest. Extensive petechial lesions can also be seen over the head and upper body in children who are victims of major crushing blunt trauma to the chest or abdomen (Fig. 64–30).

Purpuric lesions or ecchymoses caused by nonaccidental or inflicted trauma are more likely to be located at less usual sites, including the hands, feet, thighs, buttocks, upper arms, trunk, back, cheeks, and ears (Fig. 64–31). In some cases, the pattern of bruising reflects the weapon used to inflict the injury.

TABLE 64–6

PURPURA

Disorder	Skin Lesions	Distribution	Diagnostic Studies	Admission Criteria
Extravascular purpura				
Accidental trauma	Hematoma, ecchymoses	Exposed sites, bony prominences	Usually not necessary	Other severe associated injuries
Child abuse	Bruises, welts, abrasions	Often over trunk, buttocks, thighs, upper arms, cheeks; may reflect pattern of weapon	CBC count, platelet count, coagulation studies, photographs, skeletal survey in children under 2 years	All injuries severe enough to require admission, other cases when safety cannot be ensured
Excessive coughing or vomiting with viral illness or crush injuries to chest and abdomen	Petechiae	Face, neck, upper trunk	CBC count, platelet count; other studies, radiographs, and CT scans as needed for crush injury	Crush injury
Intravascular purpura				
Idiopathic thrombocytopenic purpura	Petechiae, ecchymoses, hematomas	Exposed sites, bony prominences; possibly mucosal lesions	CBC count, platelet count, coagulation studies	Severe bleeding into central nervous system; bowel, lung, kidney involvement
Acute leukemia	Petechiae, purpura	May be anywhere, often generalized; often adenopathy, hepato-splenomegaly, sternal tenderness; possibly mucosal lesions	CBC count, differential, platelets, bone marrow	All new cases
Aplastic anemia	Petechiae, purpura, ecchymoses with thick, raised centers	May be generalized; increased at sites of trauma	CBC count, differential, platelets, bone marrow	All new cases, known cases with severe acute hemorrhage
Disseminated intravascular coagulation	Petechiae, purpura, areas of skin necrosis	Generalized	CBC count, differential, platelet count, coagulation studies, blood cultures	All cases
Clotting factor deficiencies	Ecchymoses with thick, raised centers	At sites of trauma, usually exposed surfaces	PT, PTT, coagulation profile	Depends on severity of injury
Vasculitis				
Henoch-Schönlein purpura	Palpable purpura	Extensor surfaces of arms, legs, buttocks	Skin biopsy, immunofluorescence	Severe abdominal pain, kidney involvement, dehydration

CBC = complete blood cell; CT = computed tomography; PT = prothrombin time; PTT = partial thromboplastin time.

Scars, sun damage, nutritional deficiency, and other factors that contribute to skin fragility may increase the risk of extravascular bruising, even after minor trauma.

Intravascular Purpura

Intravascular purpura results from any disorder that interferes with normal coagulation. Cutaneous purpura and petechiae are present, mucosal bleeding may be seen, and in severe cases, bleeding may occur in the kidneys, gastrointestinal tract, central nervous system, and other visceral sites. Causes include idiopathic thrombocytopenic purpura, acute leukemia with thrombocytopenia, aplastic anemia, sepsis with disseminated intravascular coagulation, and clotting factor deficiencies.

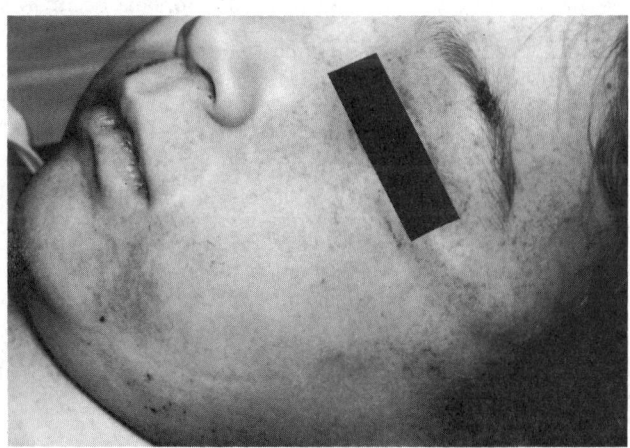

Figure 64–30. Petechial lesions are prominent in a child who was the victim of a crush injury to the chest and abdomen. (Courtesy of Dr. Don Nakayama, Children's Hospital of Pittsburgh, PA.)

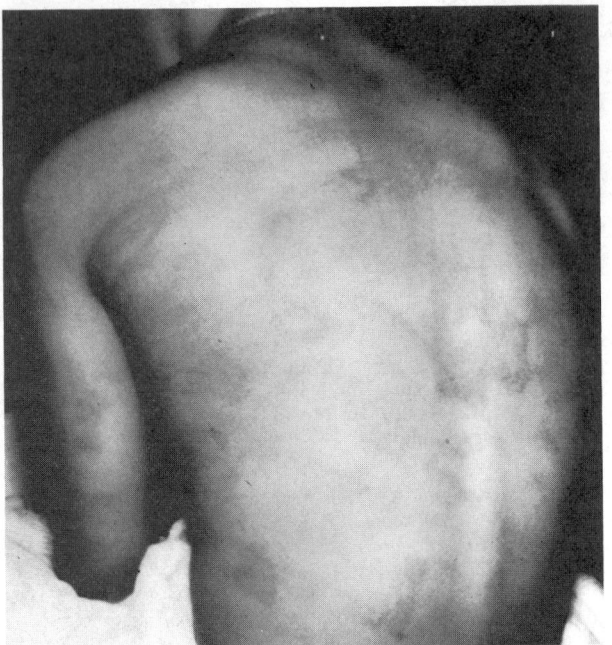

Figure 64–31. Inflicted bruises. Multiple linear ecchymoses are seen over the back of this adolescent, some showing the configuration of a looped electrical cord.

Idiopathic Thrombocytopenic Purpura

In children, idiopathic thrombocytopenic purpura (ITP) is the most common source of intravascular purpura. Patients typically present in winter and early spring, a few to several weeks after a viral illness, with petechiae, purpura, and ecchymoses and no history of trauma (Fig. 64–32). When injury has occurred, impressive ecchymoses may be seen. Many patients report gingival bleeding with brushing, and occult blood frequently is found in the stool and urine. Fortunately, severe hemorrhage is unusual. ITP is associated with the development of immunoglobulin G (IgG) antibodies that fix to platelets, resulting in increased destruction by the reticuloendothelial system. Platelet counts may dip below 10,000 cells/mm³ but usually return to normal within several weeks. Hemoglobin concentrations and white blood cell counts are usually normal, as is white blood cell morphology.

Therapeutic Intervention. Moderate and severe cases often benefit from intravenous gamma globulin therapy. Splenectomy is reserved for cases of life-threatening hemorrhage. Persistent cases may require treatment with systemic corticosteroids.

Antiplatelet antibodies and thrombocytopenia occur in a number of other disorders, including lupus erythematosus, leukemia, lymphomas, and drug reactions.

Acute Leukemia

Patients presenting with purpura and petechiae as early manifestations of acute leukemia often have an antecedent history of anorexia, weight loss, fatigue, or nonspecific "viral symptoms." Some complain of bone, back, or joint pain. Examination usually reveals hepatosplenomegaly and firm, nontender adenopathy. Sternal tenderness is also usually present. Hemoglobin tends to be decreased, and blast cells are often detected on differential white blood cell examination, although in some early cases a low white blood cell count and normal morphology are seen.

Aplastic Anemia

In aplastic anemia, bone marrow failure—whether idiopathic or caused by drugs, toxins, or radiation—results in depressed production of all cell lines. Purpura and petechiae may be the first signs noted and are accompanied by mucosal bleeding. When such patients incur contusions, the resulting ecchymoses often have thick, raised, indurated centers (Fig. 64–33). These patients are also vulnerable to serious bacterial infection.

Disseminated Intravascular Coagulation

Patients with sepsis and disseminated intravascular coagulation are severely, if not critically, ill and usually present in shock with some alteration in level of consciousness, thereby necessitating oxygen delivery, urgent volume expansion, and massive parenteral antimicrobial therapy. Rapid evolution of widespread purpura and petechiae are characteristic (Fig. 64–34). The petechiae tend to be palpable when the cause is meningococcemia. In many cases, large areas of skin may become necrotic, resulting in digit or limb loss or extensive scarring. Meningococci and *Haemophilus influenzae* type B are the most common causes of this condition.

Clotting Factor Deficiencies

Patients with inherited clotting factor deficiencies bruise easily but are less likely to have associated petechiae. Char-

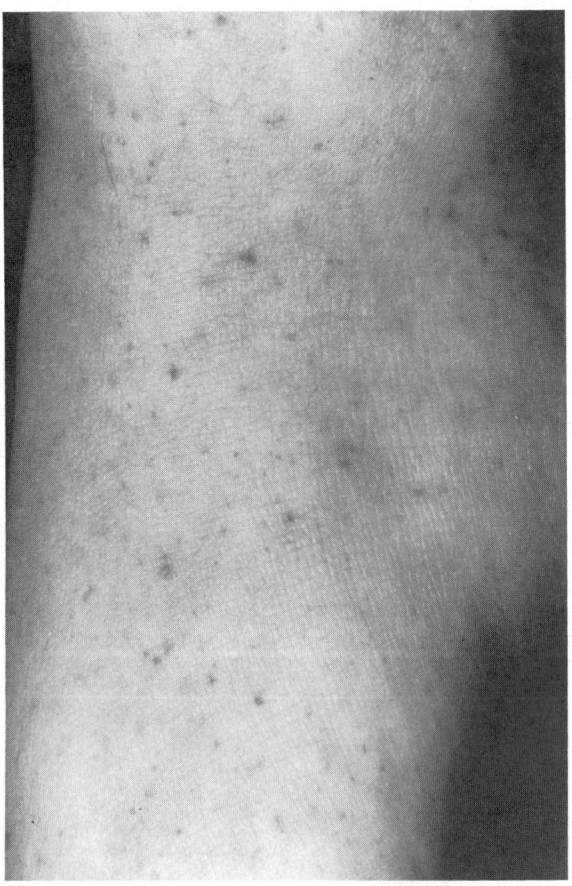

Figure 64–32. Idiopathic thrombocytopenic purpura. The sudden appearance of a generalized petechial rash prompted the presentation of this child, who had recently recovered from an upper respiratory infection. His platelet count was 13,000.

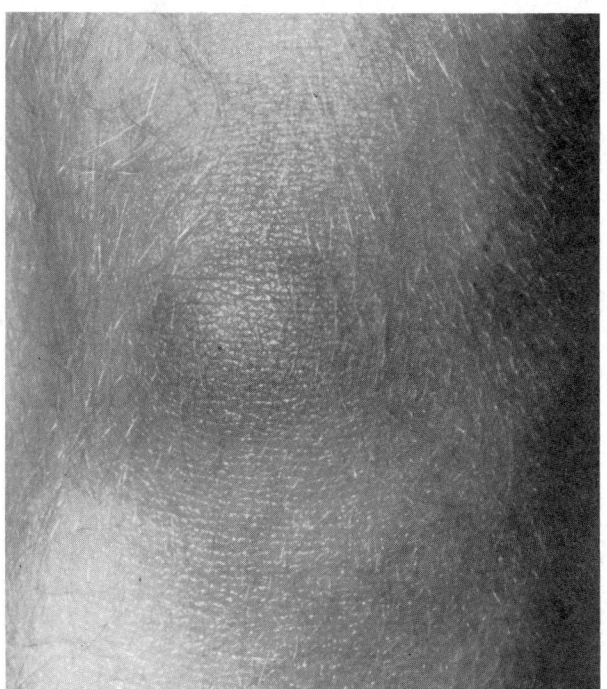

Figure 64–33. This patient with chronic idiopathic aplastic anemia demonstrates an ecchymosis with a thick, raised, indurated center. Patients with clotting factor deficiencies have similar bruises but tend not to have petechiae.

acteristically, their cutaneous ecchymoses have thick, raised centers (see Fig. 64–33). When there is a history of trauma, the mechanism fits the pattern found, although the bruise is more dramatic than would ordinarily be expected from the force applied. Males with factor VIII or IX deficiencies usually are diagnosed in infancy, but males and females with von Willebrand's disease may go undiagnosed until they have trouble with postoperative bleeding or present with an unusually severe bruise. Patients with von Willebrand's disease typically have a normal prothrombin time (PT), partial thromboplastin time (PTT), and platelet count, and diagnosis requires a full coagulation profile.

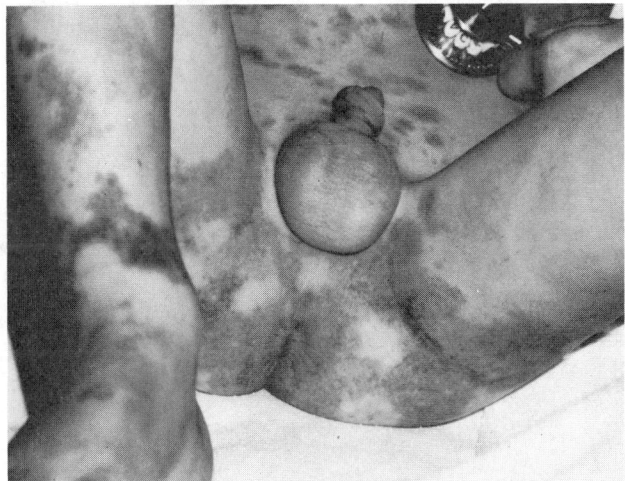

Figure 64–34. Disseminated intravascular coagulation. This child had generalized purpura and palpable petechiae with meningococcemia. The patient has also developed areas of cutaneous necrosis. (From Zitelli BJ, Davis HW (eds). Atlas of Pediatric Physical Diagnosis. 2nd ed. New York: Gower Medical Publishing, 1992.)

Vascular Purpura

Leukocytoclastic Vasculitis

Vascular purpura develops when an inflammatory process involves the vessel wall (vasculitis). Leukocytoclastic vasculitis is mediated by immune complex formation and deposition on the vascular basement membrane with subsequent activation of complement. Infectious agents, medications, autoimmune disorders, and malignancies may trigger vasculitis.

Henoch-Schönlein purpura (HSP) is a variant of leukocytoclastic vasculitis that occurs primarily in children and is in fact the most common form of vasculitis seen in the pediatric age group. The rash may begin with one to several days of urticaria. However, in time, mildly purpuric papules, urticarial plaques, and, rarely, hemorrhagic bullae appear. Purpuric lesions tend to appear in crops, the first being distributed below the waist, especially over the extensor surfaces of the legs and the buttocks (Fig. 64–35). Subsequent crops involve the extensor surfaces of the forearms, the cheeks, the ears, and at times the trunk. In rare cases, purpura may progress to form localized areas of cutaneous necrosis. Periarticular swelling, particularly of the hands and feet, and refusal to bear weight may occur at the peak of the rash. Most children develop some degree of crampy abdominal pain and hematuria.

When HSP is suspected, a thorough examination should be performed, with close attention to skin, abdominal, and joint findings. Laboratory evaluation should include stool and urine evaluation for occult blood. Normal results in the blood cell count, platelet count, and coagulation studies will exclude an intravascular etiology.

Therapeutic Intervention. Although many of these children may be observed at home, patients with severe abdominal pain, hematochezia, or progressive renal disease require hospitalization. Use of steroids may ameliorate gastrointestinal complications. Skin lesions usually resolve without scarring in several weeks, but recurrent rash may appear for several months.

PARASITIC INFESTATIONS

Scabies

Scabies is a highly contagious infestation by *Sarcoptes scabiei*, the itch mite that burrows under the skin and lays eggs. It is transmitted by direct contact with other infested humans. Scabies must be considered when any child with a generalized pruritic dermatitis fails to improve with therapy. Older children and adults typically develop papules, vesicles, pustules, and linear burrows on the hands, wrists, finger and toe webs, ankles, umbilicus, breasts, and intertriginous areas of the groin and axillae (Fig. 64–36). After the patient becomes sensitized to the mite, primary lesions are difficult to identify because of the development of a generalized acute dermatitis with extensive excoriations. Burrows are pathognomonic but evident in only 10% to 20% of cases. Unlike adolescents and adults, infants frequently have a more generalized eruption and demonstrate multiple burrows on involved areas, which include the palms and wrists; soles, dorsa, and instep of the feet; and trunk, head, and neck. They also are more likely to develop an intense nodular reaction to the mite. Because of intense pruritus, infested infants are irritable, sleep poorly, and eat poorly.

Scabies can often be diagnosed clinically, but definitive diagnosis is made by examination of a skin scraping. Mites, eggs, and fecal material are readily identified on low-power examination of scrapings obtained from a burrow or papule.

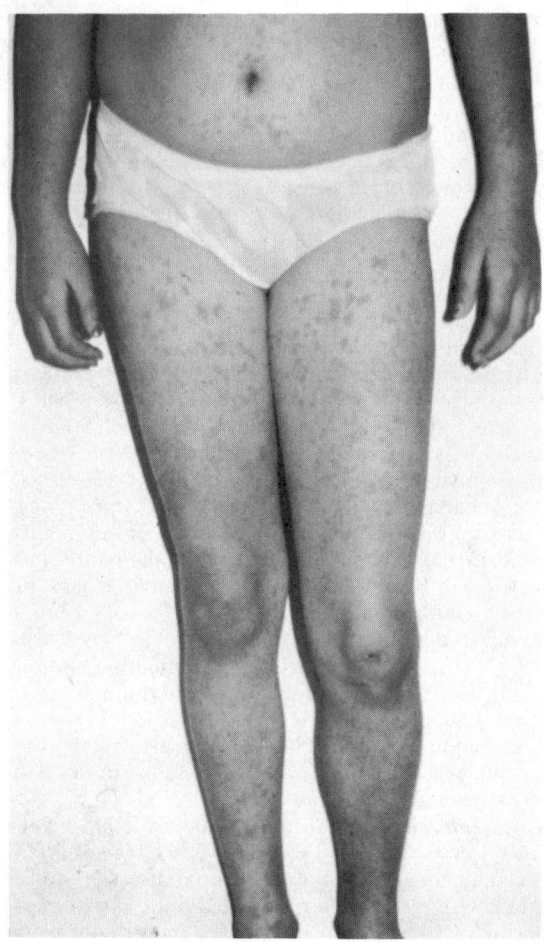

Figure 64–35. Henoch-Schönlein purpura. The sudden appearance of multiple purpuric lesions distributed from the waist down prompted this child to seek care. She later developed new crops of lesions over the extensor surfaces of the forearms and the cheeks and ears. Lesions may be macular, papular, or urticarial. Rarely, hemorrhagic bullae may form.

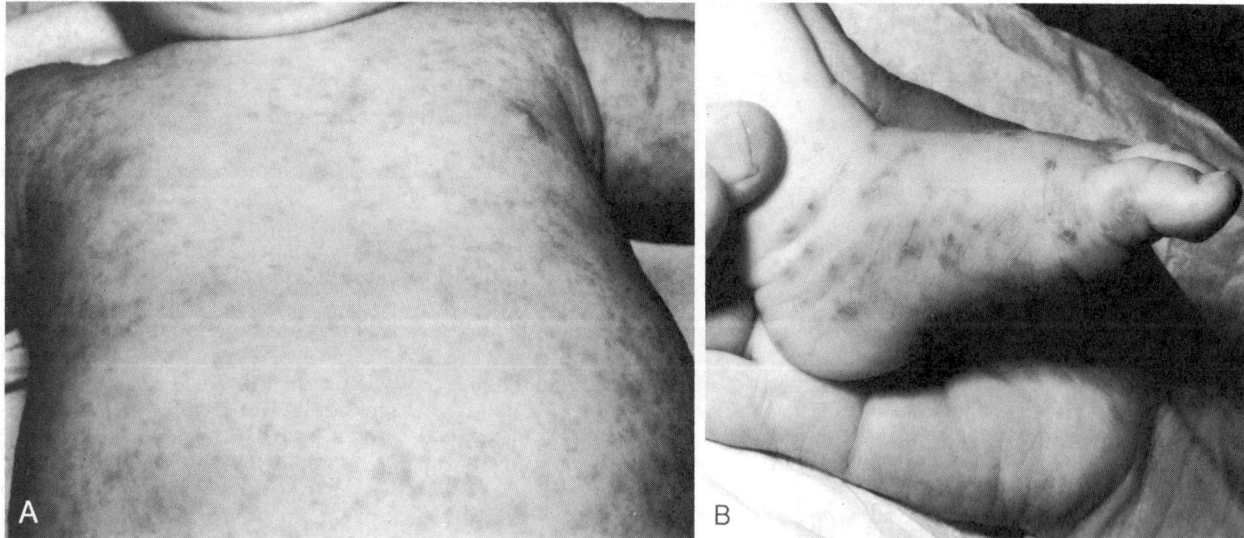

Figure 64–36. Scabies. *A, B,* In infants, pruritic papules, vesicles, pustules, and burrows are seen in a wide distribution over the trunk, axillae, and foot. The wrists are other prominent sites in infants. In older patients the web spaces of the fingers and toes, the axillae, and the groin are usual sites of involvement. (*B,* From Zitelli BJ, Davis HW (eds). Atlas of Pediatric Physical Diagnosis. 2nd ed. New York: Gower Medical Publishing, 1992.)

Therapeutic Intervention

Until 1990, the treatment of choice was gamma benzene hexachloride 1% lotion (Kwell), which was applied one time for a few to 12 hours, depending on the patient's age, and then washed off thoroughly. A second application 1 week later was often necessary. In 1990, 5% permethrin cream (Elimite) was approved by the Food and Drug Administration for scabies. This product is an effective scabicide with excellent ovicidal activity and has a better safety profile than Kwell. A single overnight treatment is usually sufficient. All members of the household should be treated, and all towels, bed linens, and any clothes that have been worn, even once, should be laundered in hot water or dry cleaned. Unfortunately, the use of these products in pregnancy is controversial. Five percent precipitated sulfur applied for 3 to 5 consecutive days is an alternative treatment in this setting.

Secondary bacterial infection should be treated with oral antibiotics that provide good coverage against gram-positive organisms (dicloxacillin, cephalosporins, amoxicillin–clavulanate potassium). Pruritus responds to cool compresses, lubricants, and oral antihistamines such as hydroxyzine or diphenhydramine but may take weeks to totally abate. Widespread pustules or cellulitis, particularly in infants, may require hospitalization for local skin care and parenteral antibiotics.

Lice

Humans may be infested with any of three different varieties of lice (head, body, and crab lice), all of which can involve the scalp hair in children.

The head louse (*Pediculus humanus capitis*) is by far the most common source of infestation in pediatric patients. Close physical contact with other infested humans; sharing combs, brushes, hats, or scarves; and shared use of towels and bed linens are all potential sources.

The lice take up residence on the scalp, and the females deposit their eggs in the form of nits, firmly cementing them to hair shafts near their point of exit from the scalp. As hairs grow, the nits move along with them.

Infested patients experience pruritus, and their scratching can result in excoriations of the scalp that are vulnerable to secondary bacterial infection accompanied by occipital and postauricular adenopathy. Careful inspection of the scalp usually reveals visible adults moving over the scalp surface. Nits appear as firmly adherent white dots or ovals that are most easily detected in the hair above and behind the ears (Fig. 64–37).

The body louse (*Pediculus humanus corporis*) can infest head hair in children but prefers the hair-bearing areas of the axilla and chest of adolescents and adults. It also inhabits bedding and clothing (especially seams), by which it is easily transmitted. Its bite causes formation of intensely pruritic urticarial papules that are distributed over the waist, axillae, neck, and shoulders. These are often obscured by excoriations caused by scratching and can easily become secondarily infected.

The crab louse (*Phthirus pubis*) is usually found inhabiting the hair of the pubic area and thus is primarily transmitted by sexual contact. It can, however, take up residence in eyelashes and other hair-bearing areas in adolescents and adults and in eyelashes and the scalp hair of children. Its bite produces pruritic papules that are often bluish in color and are localized to the lower abdomen and upper thighs of postpubertal patients.

Diagnosis is usually made by finding mobile adults on close inspection. When these are absent but nits are suspected, affected hairs can be examined microscopically.

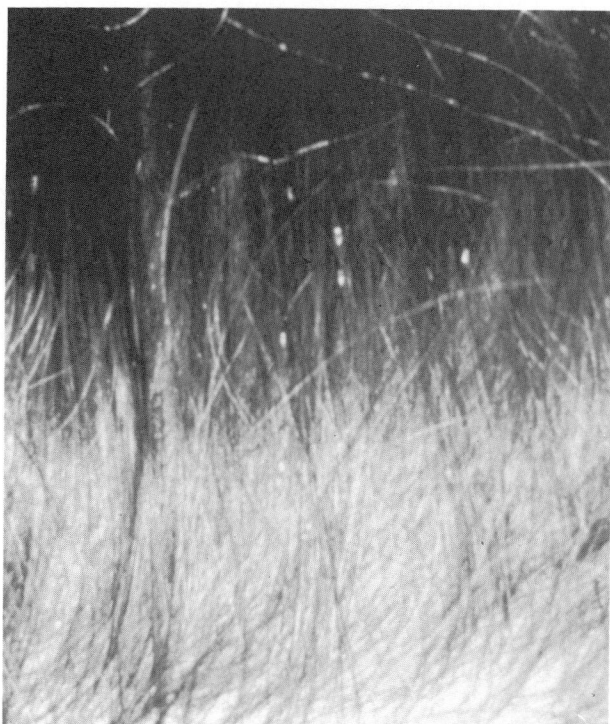

Figure 64–37. Lice. Nits dot the hairs of this child. They are tenaciously adherent and are usually found a few centimeters from the scalp, especially above and behind the ears. (Courtesy of Dr. Michael Sherlock; from Zitelli BJ, Davis HW (eds). Atlas of Pediatric Physical Diagnosis. 2nd ed. New York: Gower Medical Publishing, 1992.)

Therapeutic Intervention

Eradication of lice infestation is accomplished by application of permethrin lotion (Nix) or lindane shampoo to affected hair-bearing areas. All household members should be treated. Removal of nits on head hair is facilitated by applying a vinegar or formic acid (Step-2) rinse, which is left on for 20 minutes under a towel or shower cap. After a final rinse with water, careful combing with a fine-tooth comb completes removal.

Immediately after treatment, all towels, linen, and clothing and all hats, scarves, and coats should be washed or dry cleaned to rid the household of the insects.

Suggested References

Cohen BA, Davis HW, Mallory SB, Zitelli JA. Pediatric dermatology. *In* Zitelli BJ, Davis HW (eds). Atlas of Pediatric Physical Diagnosis. 2nd ed. New York, Gower Medical, 1992.

Davis HW, Carrasco M. Child abuse and neglect. *In* Zitelli BJ, Davis HW (eds). Atlas of Pediatric Physical Diagnosis. 2nd ed. New York, Gower Medical, 1992.

Davis HW, Karasic RB. Pediatric infectious disease. *In* Zitelli BJ, Davis HW (eds). Atlas of Pediatric Physical Diagnosis. 2nd ed. New York, Gower Medical, 1992.

Ellis D. Nephrology. *In* Zitelli BJ, Davis HW (eds). Atlas of Pediatric Physical Diagnosis. 2nd ed. New York, Gower Medical, 1992.

Hurwitz S. Clinical Pediatric Dermatology. Philadelphia, WB Saunders, 1981.

Malatack J, Blatt J, Penchansky L. Pediatric hematology and oncology. *In* Zitelli BJ, Davis HW (eds). Atlas of Pediatric Physical Diagnosis. 2nd ed. New York, Gower Medical, 1992.

Meneghini CL, Bonifazi E. An Atlas of Pediatric Dermatology. Chicago, Year Book, 1986.

Ruiz-Maldonado R, Parish LC, Beare JM. Textbook of Pediatric Dermatology. Philadelphia, Grune & Stratton, 1989.

Schachner LA, Hansen RC. Pediatric Dermatology. New York, Churchill Livingstone, 1988.

Weinberg S, Leider M, Shapiro L. Color Atlas of Pediatric Dermatology. 2nd ed. New York, McGraw-Hill, 1990.

Weston WL. Practical Pediatric Dermatology. Boston, Little, Brown, 1985.

Weston WL, Lane AT. Color Textbook of Pediatric Dermatology. St Louis, Mosby-Year Book, 1991.

SECTION TEN

Infectious Disease

CHAPTER 65

Immunizations

James P. Gillen

INTRODUCTION

Modern immunizations have made a greater impact on pediatric world health care than all other therapeutic interventions available to physicians. The emergency physician should be knowledgeable regarding the most current recommended schedules for active immunization of immunocompetent, unimmunized, immunodeficient, and immunosuppressed children as recommended by the Advisory Committee on Immunization Practices (ACIP) and the American Academy of Pediatrics.

DIPHTHERIA-TETANUS-PERTUSSIS VACCINE

The diphtheria-tetanus-pertussis (DTP) vaccine consists of diphtheria and tetanus toxoids adsorbed with pertussis vaccine and should be given intramuscularly at ages 2, 4, 6, and 18 months, along with a fifth dose given at or before school entry. (Tables 65–1 and 65–2). After age 7 years, a tetanus-diphtheria (Td) vaccine containing tetanus toxoid and a smaller amount of the diphtheria toxoid is given. Td should be given every 10 years except when contaminated wounds exist; then a 5-year interval is recommended (Table 65–3).[1–7]

Severe adverse reactions to the DTP immunization are allegedly caused by the whole-cell pertussis vaccine.[1, 4, 8–15] Many authors recommend pre- and posttreatment with acetaminophen to minimize reactions and febrile seizures.[1, 8]

Contraindications to administration of pertussis vaccine include encephalopathy occurring within 7 days of a previous DTP vaccination, convulsion with or without fever within 3 days of vaccination, persistent or unconsolable screaming or crying for 3 or more hours, collapse or shock-like state within 48 hours, temperature greater than 40.5°C (105°F) within 48 hours, or an immediate allergic reaction to the vaccine that is severe or anaphylactic. These patients can receive the Td vaccine, which has the usual concentration of toxoids without a pertussis component. The physician should also defer or omit the pertussis component if the child has progressive developmental delay or changing neurologic findings, a history of convulsions (unless they are well controlled), or a predisposition to seizures or neurologic deterioration.[1, 4, 6, 10, 12, 15]

Vaccines for tetanus and diphtheria are the only immunizations recommended during pregnancy in the United States.[5, 16, 17] Prevention of neonatal tetanus may be accomplished by antenatal immunization of the previously unimmunized mother.[1, 5, 6]

POLIOVIRUS VACCINES

There are two specific vaccines that prevent poliomyelitis: the trivalent live attenuated oral poliovirus vaccine (OPV) and the trivalent enhanced-potency formalin-inactivated (killed) poliovirus vaccine (IPV) which is given subcutaneously (see Table 65–1).[1–5, 9, 18, 19] OPV is the vaccine used most often in the United States, because it induces intestinal immunity, is simply administered, is well accepted by patients, results in immunization of some contacts of vaccinated patients, and has essentially eliminated infection associated with the wild poliovirus in this country[18]; it may also prevent simultaneous infection with wild polioviruses in epidemic areas.[18] OPV has, in rare cases, caused paralytic disease in vaccine recipients and their close contacts, especially in patients (vaccinees and contacts) who are immunocompromised.[1, 5, 18] Inadequately vaccinated or unvaccinated adults and household contacts of children given OPV should be treated with enhanced-potency IPV.[1, 18, 19]

The recommended schedule for both OPV and IPV consists of vaccination at 2 months, 4 months, 18 months, and just prior to school entry, although the 18-month vaccination may be given at age 15 months with the measles-mumps-rubella (MMR) and DTP vaccines (see Table 65–2).[1, 4, 5, 18, 19] The newer enhanced-potency IPV is produced in human diploid cells and produces an antibody response comparable to that of OPV.[1, 19] IPV should be used in all patients with compromised immunity or human immunodeficiency virus (HIV) infection, in household contacts of any patient who is immunodeficient, and in normal siblings of congenitally immunodeficient children (Table 65–4).[1, 3, 5, 19] IPV has trace amounts of streptomycin and neomycin, and therefore, patients truly allergic to these antibiotics could have a hypersensitivity reaction to this vaccine.[18, 19]

Pregnancy is a contraindication to administration of all live virus vaccines, except when contraction of the disease poses a greater threat to the mother or fetus than the vaccine itself.[1] OPV, however, has been given to pregnant women and to the children of pregnant women without any record of risk to the fetus.[1, 5, 18, 19] IPV is preferable if there is sufficient time to administer two doses of vaccine prior to anticipated exposure; otherwise OPV should be used.[1, 16, 17]

MEASLES-MUMPS-RUBELLA VACCINE

The MMR vaccine consists of three live attenuated viruses: measles and mumps are grown in chick embryo cell culture, and rubella is prepared in human diploid cell culture.[1, 4, 5, 20] Outbreaks of measles, especially in those older than 10 years of age, have led to the new recommendation of two doses

TABLE 65-1

VACCINES AVAILABLE IN THE UNITED STATES AND THEIR ROUTES OF ADMINISTRATION

Vaccine	Type	Route
BCG	Live bacteria	Intradermal (preferred) or subcutaneous
Cholera	Inactivated bacteria	Subcutaneous, intramuscular, or intradermal*
DTP	Toxoids and inactivated bacteria	Intramuscular
Hepatitis B	Inactivated viral antigen	Intramuscular
	Yeast recombinant-derived antigen	Intramuscular
Haemophilus influenzae b	Polysaccharide	Subcutaneous, intramuscular
	Polysaccharide-protein conjugate (PRP-D, HbOC, and PRP-OMP)	Intramuscular
Influenza	Inactivated virus	Intramuscular (preferred) or subcutaneous
Measles	Live virus	Subcutaneous
Meningococcal	Polysaccharide	Subcutaneous
MMR	Live viruses	Subcutaneous
Mumps	Live virus	Subcutaneous
Plague	Inactivated bacteria	Intramuscular
Pneumococcal	Polysaccharide	Intramuscular or subcutaneous
Poliomyelitis		
OPV	Live virus	Oral
IPV	Inactivated	Subcutaneous
Rabies	Inactivated virus	Intramuscular
Rubella	Live virus	Subcutaneous
Tetanus and Td, DT	Toxoids	Intramuscular
Typhoid	Inactivated bacteria	Subcutaneous (boosters may be intradermal)*
Yellow fever	Live virus	Subcutaneous

*Intradermal dose is lower.

BCG = Bacillus Calmette-Guérin vaccine (tuberculosis); DT = diphtheria and tetanus toxoids; DTP = diphtheria-tetanus-pertussis vaccine; IPV = inactivated poliovirus vaccine; MMR = measles, mumps, and rubella vaccine; OPV = oral poliovirus vaccine; PRP-D = *Haemophilus influenzae* type b diphtheria toxoid conjugate; HbOC = diphtheria CRM_{197} protein conjugate; PRP-OMP = meningococcal protein conjugate; Td = tetanus and diphtheria toxoids for adult ($\geq$7 years old) use.

Reprinted with permission from Report of the Committee on Infectious Diseases. 21st ed. Copyright © 1988, American Academy of Pediatrics.

of measles vaccine for all children after their first birthday (see Table 65-2).[20-22]

The first dose of measles-containing vaccine should be given at age 15 months unless the child lives in a high-risk area with recurrent measles transmission. Children in high-risk areas should receive their first dose of MMR at age 12 months, although efficacy may be slightly lower at this age. During outbreaks in these high-risk areas, monovalent measles vaccine or MMR may be given to children as young as 6 months of age. Children who receive the MMR vaccine

TABLE 65-2

RECOMMENDED SCHEDULE FOR ACTIVE IMMUNIZATION OF NORMAL INFANTS AND CHILDREN*

Recommended Age	Immunization(s)	Comments
2 mo	DTP, OPV, HbOC	Can be initiated as early as age 2 wk in areas of high endemicity or during epidemics. HbOC is the only approved vaccine for use in children younger than 15 mo as of October 1990.
4 mo	DTP, OPV, HbOC	2-mo interval desired for OPV to avoid interference from previous dose
6 mo	DTP, HbOC	A third dose of OPV is not indicated in the US but is desirable in geographic areas where polio is endemic
15 mo	Measles, mumps, rubella (MMR), HbOC	MMR preferred to individual vaccines; tuberculin testing may be done at the same visit
18 mo	DTP,†‡ OPV,§	See footnotes
4–6 yr	DTP,‖ OPV	At or before school entry
11–12 yr	MMR	Except where public health authorities require otherwise
14–16 yr	Td	Repeat every 10 yr throughout life

*For all products used, consult the manufacturer's package insert for instructions for storage, handling, dosage, and administration. Biologics prepared by different manufacturers may vary, and package inserts of the same manufacturer may change from time to time. Therefore, the physician should know the contents of the current package insert.

†Should be given 6 to 12 mo after the third dose.

‡May be given simultaneously with MMR (and HbOC) at age 15 mo.

§May be given simultaneously with MMR at 15 mo of age or at any time between 12 and 24 mo of age.

‖Up to 7 yr of age.

DTP = Diphtheria and tetanus toxoids with pertussis vaccine; MMR = measles-mumps-rubella vaccine (see text for discussion of single vaccines versus combination); OPV = oral poliovirus vaccine containing attenuated poliovirus types 1, 2, and 3; HbOC = *Haemophilus influenzae* b conjugate vaccine (diphtheria CRM_{197} protein conjugate); Td = Tetanus (full dose) and diphtheria (reduced dose) toxoids for adult use.

Reprinted but modified with permission from Report of the Committee on Infectious Diseases. 21st ed. Copyright © 1988, American Academy of Pediatrics. Modifications adapted with permission from "Immunization Protects Children." Copyright © 1990, American Academy of Pediatrics.

TABLE 65–3

GUIDE TO TETANUS PROPHYLAXIS IN WOUND MANAGEMENT*

History of Tetanus Immunization (Doses)	Clean, Minor Wounds		All Other Wounds†	
	Td	TIG	Td	TIG
Uncertain or fewer than three	Yes	No	Yes	Yes
3 or more‡	No§	No	No‖	No

*Td = adult type tetanus and diphtheria toxoids. If the patient is less than 7 yr old, diphtheria-tetanus or diphtheria-tetanus-pertussis vaccine is given (see text). TIG = tetanus immune globulin.

†Including, but not limited to, wounds contaminated with dirt, feces, soil, saliva, etc; puncture wounds and avulsions; and wounds resulting from missiles, crushing, burns, and frostbite.

‡If only three doses of fluid toxoid have been received, a fourth dose of toxoid, preferably an adsorbed toxoid, should be given.

§Yes, if more than 10 yr since the last dose.

‖Yes, if more than 5 yr since the last dose.

Reprinted with permission from the Report of the Committee on Infectious Diseases. 21st ed. Copyright © 1988, American Academy of Pediatrics.

before the age of 12 months need a repeat MMR vaccine at age 15 months and a third at school age.[1, 20–22]

Exposure to measles may be treated with measles vaccination in children older than age 12 months if given within 72 hours of exposure. Immune globulin (IG) or vaccine may be given in children younger than 12 months of age who are exposed. Immune globulin is preferred if measles exposure occurred more than 72 hours previously. Immune globulin may prevent or minimize measles if given within 6 days of exposure, especially in patients younger than 1 year, pregnant women, or immunocompromised patients. If immune globulin is given, immunization with measles vaccine should be delayed for 3 months.[1, 20, 21]

The timing of the second dose of MMR vaccine is debated. The ACIP recommends a second vaccine at the time of school entry (4 to 6 years of age), whereas the American Academy of Pediatrics (AAP) prefers waiting until entry to middle school or junior high school (age 11 to 12 years). Public health laws may mandate revaccination at school entry.[1, 20–22]

Contraindications to MMR vaccine include pregnancy, febrile illness, egg- or neomycin-induced anaphylaxis, IG administration less than 3 months previously, and altered immunocompetence, except in HIV-infected individuals.[1, 16, 17, 20, 21] Children with HIV infection (symptomatic and asymp-

TABLE 65–4

RECOMMENDATIONS FOR ROUTINE IMMUNIZATION OF HIV-INFECTED CHILDREN IN THE UNITED STATES*

Vaccine	Known Asymptomatic HIV Infection	Symptomatic HIV Infection
DTP	Yes	Yes
OPV	No	No
IPV	Yes	Yes
MMR	Yes	Yes
PRP-D	Yes	Yes
Pneumococcal	Yes	Yes
Influenza	Should be considered	Yes

*See text for age at which specific vaccines are indicated.

DTP = diphtheria-tetanus-pertussis vaccine; IPV = inactivated poliovirus vaccine; OPV = oral poliovirus vaccine; MMR = measles, mumps, and rubella vaccine; PRP-D = *Haemophilus influenzae* diphtheria toxoid conjugate vaccine.

Reprinted with permission from the Report of the Committee on Infectious Diseases. 21st ed. Copyright © 1988, American Academy of Pediatrics.

tomatic) should be given MMR vaccine at age 15 months and should be given IG if exposed to measles, regardless of vaccination status (see Table 65–4).[1, 3–5, 20, 21] A history of egg hypersensitivity may not necessarily preclude the use of MMR vaccination.[23]

Simultaneous administration of the DTP and OPV vaccines with the MMR vaccine does not alter antibody response or increase adverse reactions.[1, 4, 5, 9, 20] After age 12 months, trivalent MMR vaccine is the vaccine of choice, because mumps has risen in incidence, and rubella remains a threat to all first-trimester pregnancies.[24, 25]

HAEMOPHILUS INFLUENZAE TYPE B VACCINES

Haemophilus influenzae type b (Hib) is a major cause of meningitis, epiglottitis, bacteremia, cellulitis, pneumonia, empyema, septic arthritis, and otitis media in young children.[1, 26] The first vaccine used in the United States was a capsular polysaccharide preparation (PRP) in 1985. Antibody response was inadequate when the vaccine was given at less than 18 months of age, variable in the 18- to 23-month age group, and adequate when administered in children older than 24 months of age, when compared with the antibody response in children developing natural disease.[26–32] Covalently linking Hib capsular polysaccharide to diphtheria toxoid (PRP-D) resulted in a conjugate vaccine with an antibody response superior to that of PRP, especially in the 18- to 23-month age group.[27, 31] Two additional conjugated vaccines have been released, both of which have superior immunogenicity to PRP: the Hib conjugate vaccines diphtheria CRM$_{197}$ protein conjugate (HbOC), and the meningococcal protein conjugate (PRP-OMP).[28, 29] All three conjugated vaccines are now approved at age 15 months.[29] All children who received PRP at less than 24 months of age should be revaccinated with conjugated vaccine.[1, 27] Routine administration of HbOC at 2, 4, 6, and 15 months has been recommended[32, 33] (see Table 65–2). Recently, an alternative regimen using PRP-OMP at ages 2, 4, and 12 months has been approved.[33a] Children with sickle cell anemia or asplenia respond poorly to PRP and should receive conjugated vaccine.[34]

Chemoprophylaxis with rifampin (20 mg/kg/day, maximum 600 mg/day) should be given to all household contacts, including adults in those households with at least one contact younger than 48 months of age, regardless of immunization status. Day-care and nursery school contacts should be individually considered for immunization according to the degree of contact, unless two or more cases of invasive Hib occur. Infants younger than 1 month old should receive 10 mg/kg/day of rifampin.[1, 26, 27]

OPTIONAL VACCINES

Influenza Vaccines

The current influenza vaccines are multivalent, with various inactivated viruses changed annually according to predicted strains for that season.[1, 35] Split-virus, as opposed to whole-virus, vaccine is recommended for children 6 months to 12 years old in order to minimize febrile reactions. Two doses 4 weeks apart are recommended for children receiving influenza vaccine for the first time. Patients with severe hypersensitivity to chicken or egg protein who require the influenza vaccine should be skin tested.

Indications for influenza vaccine include children older than 6 months with chronic pulmonary diseases, including asthma, bronchopulmonary dysplasia, or cystic fibrosis, and patients with hemodynamically significant cardiac disease, immunosuppression, sickle cell anemia, HIV infection, diabetes mellitus, or chronic renal disorders. Household contacts and caregivers should also be vaccinated if the child is vaccinated. Children receiving long-term aspirin therapy, such as patients with rheumatoid arthritis or Kawasaki disease, should also be vaccinated.[1, 35]

There are no confirmed abnormalities induced by the influenza vaccine during pregnancy. Vaccination after consultation with public health authorities is recommended only for pregnant patients with serious underlying disease.[16, 17, 35] Immunization of the pregnant patient may protect the infant from influenza type A.[1, 35]

Pneumococcal Vaccine

The current pneumococcal vaccine consists of 23 types of purified *Streptococcus pneumoniae* capsular polysaccharide antigens protecting against the serotypes causing the majority of cases of bacteremia and meningitis in children.[1, 4, 36] Recommendations for the use of this vaccine include children older than 2 years with sickle cell disease, functional or anatomic asplenia, nephrotic syndrome, Hodgkin's disease (prechemotherapy), or HIV infection. Routine revaccination should not be performed at 3 to 5 years unless the patient is at high risk for overwhelming pneumococcal sepsis.[1, 36] The safety of pneumococcal vaccine for pregnant women has not been evaluated, and the vaccine should only be used for the high-risk pregnant patient.[16, 17, 36]

Varicella Vaccine

Varicella zoster immune globulin (VZIG) is the only commercially available product approved for general use against chickenpox.[1, 2, 37] Live attenuated Oka strain vaccine is safe and effective in normal subjects and in children with acute lymphoblastic leukemia.[38–41] Presently, this vaccine is not yet licensed by the United States Food and Drug Administration.

Hepatitis B Vaccines

There are two types of hepatitis B vaccine licensed in the United States. The original plasma-derived vaccine consists of alum-adsorbed hepatitis B surface antigen (HB$_s$Ag) particles that are purified, then inactivated with 8 mol urea, pepsin at pH of 2, and 1:4000 formalin.[42] This inactivation process kills all viruses found in human blood, including HIV. This vaccine is no longer made in the United States and is reserved for hemodialysis patients, immunocompromised hosts, and patients with yeast allergy.[1, 42] The recombinant hepatitis B vaccine is composed of HB$_s$Ag particles produced by yeast cells into which the plasmid for HB$_s$Ag has been genetically inserted, followed by lysis of these cells.[1, 42, 43] Both vaccines are given three times, at months 0, 1, and 6 after exposure.

Indications for hepatitis B vaccine include infants born to HB$_s$Ag-positive mothers, those at high risk of exposure to hepatitis B virus, household contacts, those with sexual exposure, and those with percutaneous or permucosal contact with the antigen. Use of the vaccine and hepatitis B immune globulin (HBIG) in the acute setting depends on the current vaccination and serologic status of the patient and the donor.[1, 42] Because hepatitis B vaccine is composed of HB$_s$Ag particles, there probably is little or no risk to the fetus, although this is presently unconfirmed. Pregnancy should not be a contraindication for high-risk seronegative women receiving recombinant hepatitis B vaccine.[17, 42, 44]

Rabies Vaccine

The rabies vaccine is the human diploid cell vaccine (HDCV) given on days 0, 3, 7, 14, and 28 after an animal bite. Human rabies immune globulin (HRIG) should be given on day 0 at a dose of 20 IU/kg, with half of the dose infiltrated into the wound and the remaining injected intramuscularly.[1, 45, 46] There are no reports of any risk to the fetus with HDCV or HRIG. Because rabies is essentially 100% fatal if contracted, both agents should be given regardless of pregnancy.[16, 17]

PASSIVE IMMUNIZATION
Human Immune Globulin

IG is obtained from pooled plasma of at least 1000 adults and treated with cold alcohol fractionation. IG is sterile, without the possibility of transmission of AIDS, hepatitis, or other viral illnesses.[1, 5, 42] It is given intramuscularly for antibody-deficient disorders, hepatitis A prophylaxis, and measles prophylaxis (especially in infants less than 1 year old).[1–3, 20–22]

Human Intravenous Immune Globulin

Intravenous immune globulin (IGIV) is similar to immune globulin but has been modified for intravenous use. Indications include antibody-deficient disorders, idiopathic thrombocytopenic purpura, and Kawasaki disease. Possible indications for IGIV are low birth weight, premature infants, and HIV-infected children.[1, 2, 5]

Human Specific Immune Globulins

Specific immune globulin is made from the pooled plasma of known donors with high titers of a specific antibody needed. Presently available "hyperimmune" globulins include tetanus immune globulin (TIG), VZIG, HBIG, and HRIG.[1–3, 7, 37, 42, 44, 45] There are no reported risks from administration of TIG, VZIG, HBIG, or HRIG to the pregnant patient.[16, 17] Pregnant women needing VZIG should be treated accordingly.[1, 37] TIG and HRIG should be used when indicated in the pregnant patient.[1, 16, 17]

CONCLUSIONS

Immunizations remain the cornerstone for prevention of infectious disease in infants and children. Emergency department physicians should update the immunization status of their pediatric patients, especially when a return visit to a private pediatrician seems unlikely. Physicians should not hesitate to combine immunizations (see Table 65–2) as immunogenicity is maintained and the frequency of adverse reactions is unchanged.[1, 4, 9, 27]

References

1. Peter G, Hall CB, Lepow ML, et al. Report of the Committee on Infectious Disease. Elk Grove Village, IL, American Academy of Pediatrics, 1988.
2. Advisory Committee on Immunization Practices. Immunization of children infected with human T-lymphotropic virus type III/lymphadenopathy-associated virus. MMWR 1986;35:595–598,603–606.
3. Advisory Committee on Immunization Practices. Immunization of children infected with human immunodeficiency virus—supplementary ACIP statement. MMWR 1988;37:181–182.
4. Smith DS. Immunization update: What, when, and how? Hosp Med 1990;5:89–107.
5. Advisory Committee on Immunization Practices. General recommendations on immunization. MMWR 1989;38:207–214,219–227.
6. Advisory Committee on Immunization Practices. Diphtheria, tetanus, and pertussis: Guidelines for vaccine prophylaxis and other preventive measures. MMWR 1985;34:405–414,419–426.
7. Centers for Disease Control. Tetanus—United States, 1987 and 1988. MMWR 1990;39:37–41.
8. Advisory Committee on Immunization Practices. Pertussis immunization;

family history of convulsions and use of antipyretics—supplementary ACIP statement. MMWR 1987;36:281–282.

9. Advisory Committee on Immunization Practices. New recommended schedule for active immunization of normal infants and children. MMWR 1986;35:577–579.

10. Long SS, DeForest A, Smith GS, et al. Longitudinal study of adverse reactions following diphtheria-tetanus-pertussis vaccine in infancy. Pediatrics 1990;85:294–302.

11. Gellis SS. Family history of convulsions and use of pertussis vaccine. Pediatr Notes 1989;13.

12. Gellis SS. Pertussis in neonates. Pediatr Notes 1989;13.

13. Gellis SS. The last of the studies of seizures and encephalopathy following DTP? Pediatr Notes 1990;14.

14. Centers for Disease Control. Pertussis surveillance—United States 1986–1988. MMWR 1990;39:57–66.

15. Pizza M, Covacci A, Bartoloni A, et al. Mutants of pertussis toxin suitable for vaccine development. Science 1989;246:497–500.

16. The American College of Obstetricians and Gynecologists. ACOG Tech Bull 1982;64:1–8.

17. Briggs GG, Freeman RK, Yaffe SJ. Drugs in pregnancy and lactation. 3rd ed. Baltimore, Williams & Wilkins, 1990.

18. Advisory Committee on Immunization Practices. Poliomyelitis prevention. MMWR 1982;31:22–26,31–34.

19. Advisory Committee on Immunization Practices. Poliomyelitis prevention: Enhanced-potency inactivated poliomyelitis vaccine—supplementary statement. MMWR 1987;36:795–798.

20. Advisory Committee on Immunization Practices. Measles prevention: Recommendations of the immunization practices advisory committee. MMWR 1989;38(S9):1–13.

21. Committee on Infectious Diseases. Measles: Reassessment of the current immunization policy. Pediatrics 1989;84:1110–1113.

22. Smith AL. Changes in the vaccine policy—a perspective. Pediatr Alert 1989;14:81–82.

23. Kemp A, Asperen PV, Mukhi A. Measles immunization in children with clinical reaction to egg protein. Am J Dis Child 1990;144:33–35.

24. Advisory Committee on Immunization Practices. Mumps prevention. MMWR 1989;38:388–400.

25. Advisory Committee on Immunization Practices. Rubella prevention. MMWR 1984;33:301–318.

26. Advisory Committee on Immunization Practices. Update: Prevention of Haemophilus influenzae type b disease. MMWR 1986;35:170–180.

27. Advisory Committee on Immunization Practices. Update: Prevention of Haemophilus influenzae type b disease. MMWR 1988;37:13–16.

28. Committee on Infectious Disease. Haemophilus influenzae type b conjugate vaccine: Update. Pediatrics 1989;84:386–387.

29. Advisory Committee on Immunization Practices. Supplementary statement: Change in administration schedule for Haemophilus b conjugate vaccines. MMWR 1990;39:232–233.

30. Harrison LH, Broome CV, Hightower AW, et al. Haemophilus influenzae type b polysaccharide vaccine: An efficacy study. Pediatrics 1989;84:255–261.

31. Berkowitz CD, Ward JI, Chiu CE, et al. Persistence of antibody and booster responses to re-immunization with Haemophilus influenzae type b polysaccharide and polysaccharide diphtheria toxoid conjugate vaccines in children initially immunized at 15 to 24 months of age. Pediatrics 1990;85:288–293.

32. Käyhty H, Peltola H, Eskola J, et al. Immunogenicity of Haemophilus influenzae oligosaccharide-protein and polysaccharide-protein conjugate vaccination of children at 4, 6, and 14 months of age. Pediatrics 1989;84:995–999.

33. American Academy of Pediatrics. Immunization Protects Children. November, 1990.

33a. Committee on Infectious Diseases. *Haemophilus influenzae* type b conjugate vaccines: Recommendation for immunization of infants and children 2 months of age and older: Update. Pediatrics 1991;88:169–172.

34. Rubin LG, Voulalas D, Carmody L. Immunization of children with sickle cell disease with Haemophilus influenzae type b polysaccharide vaccine. Pediatrics 1989;84:509–513.

35. Advisory Committee on Immunization Practices. Prevention and control of influenzae: Part I. Vaccines. MMWR 1989;38:297–298,303–311.

36. Centers for Disease Control. Pneumococcal polysaccharide vaccine. MMWR 1989;38:65–76.

37. Advisory Committee on Immunization Practices. Varicella-zoster immune globulin for the prevention of chicken pox. MMWR 1984;33:84–90,95–100.

38. Johnson C, Rome LP, Stancin T, et al. Humoral immunity and clinical reinfections following varicella vaccine in healthy children. Pediatrics 1989;84:418–421.

39. Starr SE. Status of varicella vaccine for healthy children. Pediatrics 1989;84:1097–1099.

40. Tselia M, Gershon AM, Steinberg SP, et al. Live attenuated varicella vaccine: Evidence that the virus is attenuated and the importance of skin lesions in transmission of varicella-zoster virus. J Pediatr 1990;116:184–189.

41. Arbeter AM, Ganometer L, Starr SE, et al. Immunization of children with acute lymphoblastic leukemia with live attenuated varicella vaccine

without complete suspension of chemotherapy. Pediatrics 1990;85:338–344.

42. Advisory Committee on Immunization Practices. Protection against viral hepatitis. MMWR 1990;39.

43. Flehmig B, Heinricy V, Pfisterer M. Simultaneous vaccination for hepatitis A and B. J Infect Dis 1990;161:865–868.

44. Routine Immunization for Adults. Med Lett 1990;32:54–56.

45. Advisory Committee on Immunization Practices. Rabies prevention—United States, 1984. MMWR 1984;33:393–402,407–408.

46. Advisory Committee on Immunization Practices. Rabies prevention: Supplementary statement on the pre-exposure use of human diploid cell rabies vaccine by the intradermal route. MMWR 1986;35.

CHAPTER 66

Fever and Sepsis

Jonathan I. Singer

INTRODUCTION

Fever is the single most common chief complaint made to physicians who evaluate ambulatory children. Febrile illnesses account for 30% of outpatient visits to clinics and 20% of emergency department encounters. The age distribution is skewed toward the first few years of life. Thus the assessment of preverbal, febrile infants and toddlers represents a common and most challenging diagnostic problem. The febrile episodes are usually short lived and uneventful and subside without specific therapeutic intervention.[1] However, the underlying cause of the febrile reaction may occasionally threaten life, especially when caused by an infectious disease.[2]

Fever is defined as an elevation of body temperature in response to a pathologic stimulus. Fever is defined by an oral body temperature of more than 37.7°C (99.8°F) or a rectal body temperature 38.3°C (101°F). Pediatric temperature assessments by palpation,[3] temperature-sensitive pacifiers,[4] axillary placement of mercury thermometers,[5] tympanic thermography,[6] or liquid crystal thermometer strips from any body location[7, 8] are unreliable.

For the purpose of this chapter discussion, the febrile patient is suspected to have an infectious disease and yet has no apparent focus of infection on examination. Based on observation scales or less formal subjective criteria, such a patient does not appear ill or toxic. Included are those patients who have invasion of their bloodstream by bacteria but do not exhibit signs and symptoms of serious systemic illness. By definition, these patients have occult bacteremia. Patients with occult bacteremia may have spontaneous resolution of their illness or may develop a variety of serious, and sometimes life-threatening, focal infections or generalized infection.

Septicemia is sharply differentiated from bacteremia. Septicemia represents a failure of the host's immune response to restrict invading microorganisms. The septic patient, in contrast to the bacteremic patient with no clinical findings, has a prostrating illness.[9] All septic patients are toxic appearing. They exhibit generalized signs of illness that are disproportionately severe for a localized disease. These manifestations include chills, gastrointestinal complaints, altered mental status, and abnormal vital signs.[10]

ANATOMY AND PHYSIOLOGY
Fever

The triggering stimulus for temperature elevation in infectious disease is the invading organism.[2] The host response to a pathogen, an endotoxin, or an exotoxin is the release of an endogenous pyrogen called *interleukin-1*. This low-molecular-weight protein is produced and released from circulating polymorphonuclear leukocytes and fixed activated mononuclear phagocytes.[11] Interleukin-1 acts on specialized receptors in the anterior hypothalamus to stimulate production of prostaglandins, thus increasing the level of cyclic adenosine monophosphate (AMP) and raising the hypothalamic set point. Information is then transmitted through the posterior hypothalamus to the vasomotor center, which directs sympathetic nerve fibers to constrict peripheral vessels and decrease heat dissipation.[12]

The likelihood of an individual child becoming febrile with an infectious disease is dependent on the age and underlying diseases of the patient. In the first month of life, temperature elevation with infectious disease is inconsistent. Only 50% of infants with infections of the skin, nail beds, eyes, nasal orifices, respiratory tract, or intestine become febrile. Pyrexia in excess of 38.9°C (102°F) may be a feature in less than three fourths of newborn infants with deep infection.[13] Children of all ages with chronic, debilitating diseases who may be taking steroids or antimetabolites may not consistently generate a febrile reaction with systemic infection.[14, 15]

Sepsis

Any intravascular infectious process has the potential to overcome the host defenses. In doing so, there may be activation of the coagulation system, activation of complement, and release of kinins, endorphins, prostaglandins, and other vasoactive substances. The net physiologic result may be decreased peripheral vascular resistance, diminished venous return to the heart, lowered cardiac output, and decreased systemic blood pressure. A febrile response may not occur. Hypothermia with temperatures less than 36.5°C (<97.6°F) may be seen with an equal or higher frequency than fever in the course of septicemia.[16]

Pathogens

The most common aerobic organisms associated with occult bacteremia in previously healthy children over 2 months of age, in descending order, are: *Streptococcus pneumoniae, Haemophilus influenzae, Neisseria meningitidis,* group A beta-hemolytic streptococci, *Salmonella* sp, and *Shigella* sp. The first three organisms account for more than 90% of bacteremic episodes. The organisms associated with septicemia in children beyond 8 weeks of age, in descending order, are: *H. influenzae, N. meningitidis, Staphylococcus aureus,* group A beta-hemolytic streptococci, *Streptococcus pneumoniae, Pseudomonas* sp, and other gram-negative rods.[9, 17]

In the first 2 months of life, group B streptococcus surpasses *Escherichia coli* as the most common cause of sepsis.[18] *Pseudomonas aeruginosa, Klebsiella* sp and other gram-negative enteric bacilli, *S. aureus, Staphylococcus epidermidis, H. influenzae,* and group A and group D streptococci are encountered less frequently.[19–21]

EMERGENCY MEDICAL SERVICE CONSIDERATIONS
Field and Hospital Triage

Regional protocols that define prehospital care of infants and children should address the chief complaint of fever. It is best to assume that a serious infectious disease exists in the febrile pediatric patient and to treat all such children cautiously. The pediatric patient with fever who is less than 3 months of age, a patient between 3 months and 24 months who has a temperature ≥40°C (104°F), a patient of any age with a temperature ≥41.1°C (106°F), all febrile immunoincompetent patients, and all patients who have a seizure associated with their febrile illness should be transported to the emergency department.

If decisions of transport are dependent more on physical examination rather than variations of temperature response, two factors are key. The febrile pediatric patient with a nonblanching eruption should be transported, as this may be an indication of overwhelming sepsis. Any febrile pediatric patient who looks sick, acts sick, or appears toxic should also be transported. The ability to recognize such a child is a necessary clinical skill for all individuals who provide a field or emergency department triage function. Experienced nonphysician examiners with mature clinical judgment can be proficient at this task. However, the observations need not be based on experience. Nelson prospectively studied large numbers of nontraumatized pediatric patients in the triage setting and developed a severity scoring system using five variables: respiratory effort, color, activity, temperature, and play (Table 66–1).[22]

Therapeutic Intervention

Patients with febrile seizures, hyperpyrexic patients with temperatures ≥41.2°C (106.1°F), and all patients with presumed sepsis should receive aggressive treatment for temperature elevation. Temperature reduction in these circumstances may reduce the risk of permanent neurologic damage. In all other circumstances, the argument for temperature reduction is one of patient comfort.

The logical therapy for pyrogen-induced fever is administration of a drug that lowers the physiologic set-point. This can be accomplished with comparable efficacy with acetaminophen, aspirin, and nonsteroidal anti-inflammatory drugs.[23, 24] These agents do not influence production of interleukin-1 but rather interfere with prostaglandin synthesis in the hypothalamus.[25] Acetaminophen appears to be the safest of the three drugs. The patient who receives 15 mg/kg of acetaminophen orally or rectally will often have temperature reduction within 15 to 30 minutes after antipyretic administration, with resultant subjective and objective clinical

TABLE 66–1

SEVERITY INDEX SCORING SYSTEM*

Variable	Point Value 0	Point Value 1	Point Value 2
Respiratory effort	Labored or absent	Some distress	No distress
Color	Cyanotic	Pale, flushed, mottled	Normal
Activity	Delirium, stupor, coma	Lethargy	Normal
Temperature‡	<97.4°F or >104°F	101.1°F–104°F	97.4°F–101°F
Play	Refuses to play	Decreased	Normal

*A patient's score is derived by summing the scores of the individual items. A score ≤7 identifies children who should receive rapid transportation to a health facility for immediate attention.

‡97.4°F = 36.3°C; 101.0° F = 38.3°C; 104.0°F = 40°C.

From Nelson KG. An index of severity for acute pediatric illness. Am J Public Health 1980;70:804.

improvement. The response to acetaminophen is not a clinically useful indicator by which to differentiate the causes of febrile illnesses in children[26] and cannot be used to discriminate between viral and bacterial infections.[27] It also cannot be used to distinguish children who are bacteremic from those who are not.[28]

CLINICAL EVALUATION
Patient Age

The risk for an inapparent, serious bacterial infection is inversely related to advancing age; the risk for bacterial sepsis is greatest for newborns. In the absence of dehydration and high environmental temperature, sepsis is one of the most common causes of fever in the first week of life.[29] In the first month of life, unsuspected bacterial infection plays a significant role in mortality, accounting for up to 50% of neonatal deaths.[30] Based on the history and physical examination, more than 75% of infected, febrile infants less than 60 days old may have no identifiable source of fever.[31] Although this group of febrile infants has a low risk of occult bacteremia (3.6%), those who are bacteremic tend to develop serious localized complications or septicemia.[32, 33] The incidence of transient bacteremia, persistent bacteremia, and occult life-threatening bacterial illness in infants between 2 and 3 months of age is lower than that in infants ≤2 months old.[34, 35] Fatal bacterial infections in the 3- to 6-month age group are uncommon. Death from bacterial illness in this age group occurs with one fourth of the frequency of that in infants ≤3 months old.[36] Distinctive symptoms of undeniably severe illness are the rule in infants 3 to 6 months old, and occult bacteremia is the exception.[37] The peak for febrile illnesses occurs in the 6- to 12-month age group.[38] Although life-threatening infection is seen in these patients, infants approaching 1 year of age are also likely to exhibit physical findings of serious infection.[39] However, nontoxic infants and children between 6 and 24 months old who have no apparent focus of infection but are bacteremic are an exception. Significantly, this occult bacteremia may be a precursor to sepsis in a small percentage of children in this age group.[40] Bacteremia without an apparent focus of infection is uncommon beyond the age of 2 to 3 years. Older children with serious bacterial illness are consistently recognized on the basis of clinical observations and infrequently have fevers of unknown origin.[41]

Degree of Temperature Elevation

The degree of temperature elevation beyond 38.3°C (101°F) is not significant in the first 8 weeks of life. What is significant, however, is a departure from the normal, as hypothermia may also indicate sepsis in this age group. Bacterial pathogens may be recovered from the blood of septic infants less than 8 weeks old when temperatures are less than 38.3°C.[33] Clinical studies have confirmed the familiar principle that bacteremia and septicemia may occur in infants younger than 8 weeks of age who have no fever or only low-grade fever.[32] Infants 2 to 3 months of age may also have serious infections in the absence of soaring temperatures. However, they are more likely to have focal bacterial infections with bacteremia or overwhelming sepsis when the temperature exceeds 40°C (104°F).[42, 43]

Beyond 3 months of age, the severity of illness and likelihood for bacteremia and septicemia with common organisms is proportional to the degree of temperature elevation. Children in this age group with or without an apparent focus of infection and with a rectal temperature less than 38.9°C (102°F) have a 1% rate of bacteremia.[37] With temperatures of 38.9°C to 39.4°C (102.9°F), the rate increases to 4%. With temperatures of 39.4°C to 40°C (104°F), the rate of bacteremia may exceed 8%. Patients with temperatures between 40°C and 41.1°C (106°F) may have rates of bacteremia of 11%.[41] At temperatures above 41.1°C, the rates of bacteremia may exceed 25%.[42, 44]

Duration of Fever

Most clinical data support the fact that a high fever identifies children with an increased risk of serious bacterial illness compared with the total population of febrile children. However, there is little information regarding the rapidity and onset of fever as the basis for recognizing serious illness. Rapid onset of hyperpyrexia without preceding complaints may be seen in 75% of children afflicted with *N. meningitidis*. Persistent bacteremia with this organism has been described in children with prolonged or less significant temperature elevations.[45, 46] Similarly, the other bacterial organisms that are responsible for most of the life-threatening illnesses of childhood have been isolated from the blood stream or other significant sites of immunologically competent children who have an indolent illness associated with prolonged fever.[47, 48] Therefore, a brief duration of fever cannot be used as a sole marker for the presence of occult bacteremia or sepsis.

Epidemiologic Clues

Beyond the first few months of life, the frequency of infectious disease in children may be influenced by association with other children, including day-care contacts and siblings. The secondary spread of invasive disease has been emphasized for contacts of those exposed to *H. influenzae*, *N. meningitidis*, and *S. pneumoniae*.[49, 50] More than a third of families with an infant infected with *Salmonella* sp or *Shigella* sp have at least one other family member with a recognized illness attributable to the same organism.[51, 52] These bacterial pathogens are generally responsible for disease in the young pediatric community at large. However, if epidemiologic data point to a specific pathogen, a contact who is ill should be suspected of infection with the same organism.

Epidemiologic clues are of less assistance in the diagnosis of serious bacterial infection during the first months of life. At this age, it may be difficult to determine whether bacterial pathogens were acquired at birth, on arrival in the nursery, or from household members.[53] Infants may not become symptomatic for weeks from an initial colonization with *H. influenzae*, *S. pneumoniae*, group B streptococcus, *Listeria monocytogenes*, or *E. coli*. Questions pertinent to the pregnancy, labor, birth, nursery experience, and potential communicable disease in the household may not distinguish the source, portal of entry, or the likely offending agent in a febrile infant less than 2 months of age.

Medical History

The specific immunologic impairment of the pediatric patient with malignant hematologic disorders, neoplasia, acquired immunodeficiency syndrome, granulocytopenia, hemoglobinopathy, dysgammaglobulinemia, diabetes mellitus, and asplenia may allow for an accurate prediction of an invading pathogen.[14] However, a bacterial pathogen may invade the blood stream of a compromised host and cause metastatic infection with a paucity of systemic manifestations.[15] It is essential to aggressively search for the source of the potentially life-threatening infection when fever accompanies an illness in the pediatric patient with compromised host defenses.

Identifying Occult Bacteremia

As a rule, clinical judgment is not predictive of occult bacteremia. The young patient with unsuspected *S. pneumoniae* bacteremia may appear well or to have a seemingly minor illness.[54] Only the presence of a cystic oral lesion predicts pneumococcemia. An isolated lesion first appears in the posterior maxillary tuberosity area, on the buccal surface of the alveolar ridge, or over the posterior hard palate. At first erythematous, it then becomes boggy, cystic, and fluid filled. The lesion may become ulcerative or necrotic. *S. pneumoniae* of identical serotype may be recovered from both the gingival lesion and the blood.[55] Transient gingival or cheek swelling may accompany it at the onset of the lesion.[56] This constellation of oral findings is pathognomonic of pneumococcemia. There are no pathognomonic physical findings of occult bacteremia caused by other organisms.

Identifying Sepsis

McCarthy et al. first reported that physicians should derive information about toxicity from observations of a febrile child's hydration, color, playfulness, alertness, and consolability.[37] He later showed that physician observation of the child's quality of vocalization, eye function, motor behavior, and response to various stimuli before the traditional physical examination aided in interpretation of the degree of illness.[58] From these initial studies, he proposed the six-item Yale Observation Scale as a predictive model for the presence of serious illness (Table 66–2).[59] This scale, though widely used, remained invalidated until McCarthy documented a relationship among a febrile child's overall appearance; the physical examination findings by auscultation, percussion, and palpation; and the presence of serious illness. The febrile child's appearance influences the positive predictive value of abnormal physical examination findings for serious illness.[60]

Because infants less than 6 weeks old inconsistently achieve sustained eye contact or a sociable smile, judging their degree of responsiveness and playfulness may make the decision about toxicity difficult. However, a presumptive diagnosis of sepsis can be made with confidence in older pediatric patients who appear toxic. Sepsis should also be suspected in the ill, febrile patient with changes in mentation, poor capillary filling, hypotension, tachypnea, tachycardia, oliguria, or evidence of coagulopathy.[61]

Clinical signs and symptoms of sepsis may not be as apparent in the neonatal period. The presenting complaints may be minimal, vague, nonspecific, and mimic noninfectious neonatal disorders. Behavioral changes, altered feeding, or altered stooling pattern are among the most common historical features in neonatal sepsis. The early complaint that the infant is "not doing well" typically indicates that the child is restless, not inclined to be handled, and responds listlessly to social contact. On examination, vital signs are often abnormal. Thermal instability with either fever or hypothermia is expected. Tachycardia consistently precedes hypotension and evidence of poor perfusion. Apnea or periodic breathing is as common as tachypnea.[62]

Neonatal sepsis and meningitis share common pathophysiology and pathogens and usually cannot be differentiated on clinical grounds. However, lethargy, obtundation, a high-pitched cry, a vacant stare, and seizures may reflect meningeal involvement.[63]

DIAGNOSTIC EVALUATION

The initial clinical impression of an experienced clinician based on the history and physical examination of the febrile child frequently provides dependable information with which to direct subsequent evaluation. If bacterial infection is a strong consideration, certain laboratory studies should be considered.

Blood Cell Count and Phase Reactants

The complete blood cell (CBC) count, serum C-reactive protein (CRP) determination, erythrocyte sedimentation rate (ESR), zeta sedimentation rate (ZSR), and determinations of fibrinonectin and elastase–alpha 1–proteinase inhibitor have been used to facilitate the initial evaluation of the pediatric patient with a febrile illness or suspected sepsis. None of these individual tests is sensitive enough to predict bacter-

---

TABLE 66–2

YALE OBSERVATION SCALE*

Observation Item	Point Value		
	1 (Normal)	**3** (Moderate Impairment)	**5** (Severe Impairment)
Quality of cry	Strong with normal tone *or* Content and not crying	Whimpering *or* Sobbing	Weak *or* Moaning *or* High pitched
Reaction to parent stimulation	Cries briefly, then stops *or* Content and not crying	Cries off and on	Continual cry *or* Hardly responds
State variation	If awake: stays awake *or* If asleep and stimulated: wakes up quickly	Eyes close briefly if awake *or* Awakes with prolonged stimulation	Falls to sleep *or* Will not rouse
Color	Pink	Pale extremities *or* Acrocyanosis	Pale *or* cyanotic *or* Mottled *or* ashen
Hydration	Skin normal, eyes normal *and* Mucous membranes moist	Skin and eyes normal *and* Mouth slightly dry	Skin doughy *or* Tented *and* Dry mucous membranes *or* Sunken eyes
Response (talk, smile) to social overtures	Smiles *or* Alert (≤2 mo)	Brief smile *or* Alert briefly (≤2 mo)	No smile; face anxious, dull, expressionless *or* No alerting (≤2 mo)

*A patient's score is derived by summing the scores of the individual items. Only 2.7% of patients with a score ≤10 have a serious illness; 92.3% with a score ≥16 have a serious illness.

From McCarthy PL, Sharpe MR, Spiesel SZ, et al. Observation scales to identify serious illness in febrile children. Pediatrics 1982;70:802. Reproduced by permission of Pediatrics.

emia or invasive bacterial infection, thereby limiting the use of any test as an isolated measure on which major management decisions can be safely based.[64] However, several tests can be obtained in a battery and interpreted together during the decision-making process.[65–68] Additional information may be gained if one or several of the tests are repeated.[69–71]

CBC Count

There are no uniformly accepted hematologic criteria for distinguishing the infected from the noninfected infant. Hence, the interpretation of the hematologic profile remains subjective. However, the CBC count analyzes both the quantitative and qualitative changes in the leukocyte series. These changes include total white blood cell count, absolute neutrophil count, percentage of bands, morphologic appearance, and platelet count.

There is a linear relationship between elevation of the total leukocyte count and the risk of bacteremia.[37] A fourfold risk of bacteremia exists in children ages 4 weeks to 2 years with a temperature of ≥38.8°C and a white blood cell count of ≥15,000 cells/mm³.[38] Another study found a threefold risk of bacteremia in children who had a temperature of ≥40°C when the leukocyte count was ≥15,000 cells/mm³ when compared with children without leukocytosis.[72] Depressed leukocyte counts are of equal importance, especially in the neonate. Leukopenia with total counts of <5000/mm³ may be observed late in the course of sepsis.[73] Neutropenia, defined as an absolute neutrophil count that falls below 2000/mm³, may also signify a septic process in the newborn.[74] Neutrophilia is considered a more reliable indicator of an infectious process after the neonatal period. An absolute neutrophil count of >10,000 cells/mm³ was found to be of greater use than the total leukocyte count in identifying bacterial illnesses in children. In previously healthy febrile children between 1 month and 2 years of age, those with >500 bands/mm³ had an 80% chance of having a bacterial illness.[75] The immature neutrophil–to–total neutrophil ratio may be a reliable indicator of bacterial infection, particularly in the neonatal period.[76, 77] The degenerative changes of vacuolization and toxic granulization in neutrophils have also been observed in bacteremic infants and children. Of the two, cytoplasmic vacuolization appears to be a more accurate indicator of bacteremia. Toxic granulization is thought to be invariably present in bacterial infection only in neonates.[66] In the first month of life, particularly in premature infants, thrombocytopenia may occur in the course of bacterial infection.[78] In term infants, the association of bacterial infection and thrombocytopenia is less striking.[66]

Serum C-Reactive Protein

Serum C-reactive protein (CRP) exists in trace amounts in the serum of pediatric patients when they are healthy. After tissue injury or destruction, CRP is one of several heterogeneous serum proteins (phase reactants) whose production is increased.[79] Beyond the newborn period, following an inflammatory reaction from any of several viral agents, concentrations of CRP may increase to 10 to 19 mg/L. Serum concentrations of >19 mg/L are regarded as suggestive of an invasive bacterial process or fungal septicemia.[80] Hyperpyrexic infants without a focus of infection and with a heightened CRP level have a higher prevalence of bacteremia.[72] One investigator found CRP levels ≥35 mg/L in five of seven bacteremic children evaluated in an emergency setting who had no identifiable primary source of infection.[65] In the newborn, an increase to 10 mg/L of serum CRP indicates a high likelihood of sepsis or meningitis. Such an

increase occurs consistently within a matter of hours after the onset of neonatal sepsis from common pathogens.[81–83]

ESR and ZSR

The ESR measures the free-fall of erythrocytes over either 1 hour (classic) or 30 minutes (shortened).[84] The ZSR measures the ability of red blood cells to pack under a standardized stress of alternating dispersion and compaction and is an alternative to the ESR. Both tests indirectly measure fibrinogen, another phase reactant. Either test may be used as a screening procedure to identify children with occult bacteremia or aid in the evaluation of potentially septic patients, particularly newborns. In separate studies, either the ZSR or the ESR was elevated in febrile, bacteremic children of all ages who presented to the emergency department.[41, 85] Another study found an elevated ESR in 80% of febrile bacteremic emergency department patients less than 8 weeks of age.[86] Adler and Denton demonstrated an elevated ESR in the course of proven systemic infection.[87]

Fibrinonectin

Plasma fibrinonectin is a glycoprotein found on many cell surfaces and in extracellular fluids. Fibrinonectin augments phagocytosis and promotes reticuloendothelial system clearance of particulate matter. Normal levels in the serum are 140 to 240 μg/ml. Quantitative levels can be measured within a 10-minute period with commercially available kits. Plasma concentrations decrease significantly from baseline several hours into septicemia in infants <3 months of age.[88, 89]

Elastase–Alpha 1–Proteinase Inhibitor

During phagocytosis, intracellular granules fuse with the newly formed phagocytic vacuole, and subsequent degranulation and exocytosis of various granule constituents occur. Elastase, a protease in the granules of neutrophils, is rapidly bound extracellularly and inactivated by alpha 1–proteinase inhibitor. This enzyme-inhibitor complex is stable and can be quantified by an assay in about 1 hour. Reference values are known for neonates, infants, and children. Elastase–alpha 1–proteinase inhibitor concentrations are increased in the course of invasive bacterial infections in the neonate and in infants beyond the neonatal period.[90, 91]

Blood Culture

Blood cultures are valuable for diagnosing the patient suspected to be bacteremic or septicemic. The traditional method of blood culturing involves the inoculation of blood into broth media, followed by manual subculture into solid media. New plating methods employ automated technology. The mean time to detection and presumptive identification of these isolates may vary according to plating method, size of the blood inoculum, and the quantity of bacteria in the blood stream.

In the absence of a fixed intravascular focus of infection, bacteria that enter the blood stream are removed by fixed macrophages. Thus bacteremia may be transient. However, the reticuloendothelial system can be overwhelmed, leading to septicemia with persistently high levels of intravascular bacterial growth. In the newborn, the actual colony counts in the course of bacteremia and septicemia vary greatly, ranging from <5 to >1000 organisms/mm. Culturing samples of blood as small as 0.2 to 0.5 ml should give positive results, although sample amounts of 1 to 3 ml are suggested.[92] In the older infant and child, 1 to 5 ml of blood are sufficient to yield isolates.[93]

False-negative blood culture results may be encountered in patients who are receiving antibiotic therapy at the time of blood sampling, as the antibiotics may inhibit bacterial growth. In addition, bacterial autolysis can occur, causing false-negative blood culture findings in some children with bacteremia.[94] Therefore, undue reliance must not be placed on a blood culture for documenting an invasive bacterial disease. Viable blood-borne bacterial organisms need not be necessary to substantiate systemic infection in the appropriate clinical setting.

Microbial Methods

The specific diagnosis of invasive disease may be facilitated by performing countercurrent immunoelectrophoresis (CIE), enzyme-linked immunosorbent assay (ELISA), latex particle agglutination, or centrifugation-augmented solid-phase immunoassay (CASPIA) to detect the presence of polysaccharide antigens elaborated by *H. influenzae, S. pneumoniae, N. meningitidis,* and group B streptococcus. These methods are most useful for patients who have been partially treated, as circulating capsular antigens may be detected in body fluids for several days even after bacterial cultures become sterile.[95] Various commercial antigen detection kits are currently available for detecting these common causes of bacteremia and septicemia. The kits differ in the serotypes covered and the specifics of technique. CIE is of limited utility in the evaluation of the febrile child with no apparent focus of infection, as CIE performed on blood and urine does not detect bacteremia in the first few hours of fever.[96] The various latex particle agglutination kits are not sensitive for diagnosing *H. influenzae, S. pneumoniae,* group B streptococcus, or *N. meningitidis* bacteremia in the absence of concurrent meningitis.[97–99] ELISA and CASPIA are more sensitive than CIE or particle agglutination for detecting antigens in body fluids.[100] ELISA and CASPIA are more likely to be useful in identifying invading organisms causing sepsis. However, their use in bacteremic patients needs further evaluation.

Other Cultures

Positive bacterial cultures from the skin, urine, pleural spaces, cerebrospinal fluid, joints, bones, and bone marrow substantiate systemic bacterial disease.[101] The recovery of pathogens from these sites implies a systemic infection in the patient who appears septic but has negative blood culture results. Cultures of body surfaces and orifices such as the nose, throat, external auditory canal, sinuses, and rectum are not helpful in identifying sepsis-causing pathogens.[102]

Lumbar Puncture

The physician evaluating the febrile child without an apparent focus of infection should consider performing a lumbar puncture when the likelihood of meningitis is increased and there are no contraindications. The decision to examine cerebrospinal fluid must be tailored to the clinical situation. Children at increased risk for intracranial infection include children less than 2 months of age; toxic-appearing children of all ages; children whose febrile illness is accompanied by a seizure, nuchal rigidity, a petechial rash, or an immuno-compromised state; and children with recently confirmed bacteremia.[103] A lumbar puncture is mandatory in the ill neonate, as there are no features to differentiate neonatal sepsis from neonatal meningitis. The organisms responsible for sepsis in the older infant or young child may also be isolated from cerebrospinal fluid.[104]

Cerebrospinal fluid examination can be postponed or withheld in the febrile patient who is unstable or when there is suspicion either of a central nervous system infection other than meningitis or of increased intracranial pressure associated with meningitis. Febrile patients at high risk for meningitis are considered unstable when there is an unprotected airway, generalized seizure activity, tenuously low or elevated blood pressure, or delayed capillary refill. Lumbar puncture should be delayed if a central nervous system syndrome is thought to be secondary to a subdural or epidural collection of fluid, cavernous sinus thrombosis, lateral sinus thrombosis, cerebral hemorrhage, brain tumor, spinal cord tumor, or brain abscess.[105] In these circumstances, the lumbar puncture may be followed by a decline in neurologic status.[106] Febrile patients suspected of meningitis and concurrent increased intracranial pressure are at risk of lethal post–lumbar puncture brain herniation. Lumbar puncture therefore should not be performed in those patients who exhibit cranial nerve palsies, absence of retinal venous pulsations, papilledema, focal seizures, or hemiparesis.[107]

Radiographic Evaluation

There are no widely accepted indications for obtaining a chest radiograph in the pediatric patient with fever. If febrile children of all ages were subjected to chest radiographs as a screen for pneumonia, the diagnostic yield would be exceedingly low. It is therefore suggested that chest radiographs be obtained only when there is clinical suspicion of pneumonia. The presence of rales is the single best clinical predictor of pneumonia in infants younger than 2 months[108] and in older children.[109] Tachypnea has also been found as another predictive physical finding for pneumonia in children of all ages.[110]

A chest radiograph should be obtained in the septic-appearing child without apparent focus of infection, as the radiograph may disclose an occult (pleural, parenchymal, or pericardial) focus of infection. In addition, a chest radiograph may exclude congenital or acquired cardiac disease as the cause of the child's moribund condition.

DIFFERENTIAL DIAGNOSIS

Fever

In the first few years of life, children experience at least three febrile episodes per year. These febrile events are often accompanied by signs and symptoms of upper respiratory tract disease.[111] Gastrointestinal or urinary tract infections are the next most frequent reasons for febrile illnesses in the young.[112, 113] Less frequently, the history has no pattern, and there are no abnormal findings on physical examination, thereby preventing specific diagnosis. Such undifferentiated febrile events are largely viral in origin,[114] with bacterial and rickettsial diseases accounting for the majority of the remaining undifferentiated febrile illnesses.[48]

Fever occurs in a number of less common, noninfectious diseases (Table 66–3). Fever may be found with collagen-vascular disorders, neoplastic conditions, central nervous system dysfunction, endocrine disturbances, or as a reaction to therapeutic agents. These noninfectious causes of fever are diagnosed infrequently in the emergency department.[115] Collagen and inflammatory disorders are generally found in older children. Collagen-vascular disease is also more likely when the fever has been prolonged.[47] Accurate interpretation of clinical findings will usually uncover even the most infrequent noninfectious causes of fever, such as central nervous system disorders, metabolic diseases, or tumors.[116]

TABLE 66–3

NONINFECTIOUS CAUSES OF FEVER

I. Toxic and traumatic
  A. Drugs
    1. Atropine
    2. Drug fever: antibiotics, iodides, barbiturates
  B. Anemia
    1. Aplastic anemia
  C. Hemorrhage into viscera
    1. Intracranial (subdural)
    2. Retroperitoneal
  D. Injury (tumor or infection, too)
    1. Hypothalamus
II. Metabolic
  A. Increased heat production
    1. Hyperthyroidism during toxic crisis
    2. High environmental temperature and humidity
    3. Dehydration
III. Immunologic-allergic
  A. Collagen group
    1. Rheumatic fever
    2. Disseminated lupus erythematosus
    3. Periarteritis nodosa
    4. Scleroderma
    5. Dermatomyosites
    6. Mixed collagen vascular disease
  B. Allergy
    1. Drug fever (see above)
    2. Serum sickness
IV. Neoplastic
  A. Localized
    1. Neuroblastoma
    2. Ewing's tumor
    3. Osteogenic sarcoma
    4. Pheochromocytoma
  B. Diffuse
    1. Leukemia
    2. Lymphoma
V. Idiopathic
    1. Ulcerative colitis
    2. Regional enteritis
    3. Sarcoid
    4. Infantile cortical hyperostosis
    5. Paroxysmal atrial tachycardia
    6. Weber-Christian disease
    7. Cyclic neutropenia

Sepsis

The most common cause of temperature instability, tachycardia, tachypnea, and inadequate organ perfusion manifested by altered mental status, hypoxia, acidosis, or oliguria is an overwhelming bacterial infection.[117] A primary focus of infection, such as meningitis, pyelonephritis, pericarditis, myocarditis, endocarditis, pneumonia, pyarthrosis, or osteomyelitis, may be demonstrable. These patients have a high-density bacteremia.[118] Not all infections characterized by a moribund appearance are bacterial in origin.[119] The "sepsis syndrome" has been reported with herpes simplex virus, enteroviruses, adenoviruses, influenza A and B viruses, respiratory syncytial virus, and parainfluenzae viruses.[63] Advanced cases of rickettsial disease also mimic bacterial sepsis.

Following infectious diseases, cardiac disease that leads to congestive heart failure accounts for clinical findings that are seen with sepsis. Tachycardia, tachypnea, pallor, cyanosis, and other signs of inadequate organ perfusion may occur with congenital heart defects such as anomalous coronary arteries, complex coarctations of the aorta, and hypoplastic left heart syndromes, as well as septal and valvular defects. Acquired structural disease such as Kawasaki syn-

drome with coronary artery aneurysms and infantile periarteritis may cause myocardial infarction, leading to a septic appearance. Rhythm disturbances such as a supraventricular tachycardia may also cause a septic appearance.[10]

Several metabolic derangements may simulate sepsis (Table 66–4). These include dehydration, uremia, hyponatremia, hypernatremia, hypoglycemia, and hyperammonemia. Children who have been poisoned from ingestion of many plants or medicine such as antipyretics, analgesics, anticonvulsants, antidepressants, and sedative-hypnotics may present with sepsis syndrome. Exposure to several insecticides, carbon monoxide, or oxidizing agents that alter oxygen affinity to hemoglobin can create metabolic stress, simulating sepsis. Of the gastrointestinal disorders that create sepsis syndrome, necrotizing enterocolitis or gastric perforation are encountered in the postnatal period, toxic megacolon of Hirschsprung's disease or intussusception present in the first few years of life, and enteric pathogens or perforated appendicitis are encountered at all ages. Children with spontaneous intracranial hemorrhage or infants who are abusively shaken may develop unexplained mental status changes and life-threatening alterations in vital signs. Children with endocrinopathies such as congenital adrenal hyperplasia, thyrotoxicosis, or unrecognized diabetic ketoacidosis may appear septic.[10]

THERAPEUTIC INTERVENTION

Patients Less Than 2 Months Old

Few infants develop fever in the first 2 months of life. Infants of this age constitute only 1% to 7% of all febrile children encountered in urban pediatric emergency departments.[33, 46] The prevalence of life-threatening infection in the postnatal period is difficult to assess. Some studies have actually documented a minimal risk of life-threatening infection,[43] whereas other studies have estimated the prevalence of life-threatening complications to be from 4% to 15%.[34, 120]

TABLE 66–4

DIFFERENTIAL DIAGNOSIS OF THE SEPTIC-APPEARING INFANT

Infectious diseases	Hematologic disorders
Bacterial sepsis	Severe anemia
Meningitis	Methemoglobinemia
Urinary tract infection	Gastrointestinal disorders
Virus infection	Gastroenteritis with
Congenital syphilis	dehydration
Cardiac diseases	Pyloric stenosis
Congenital heart disease	Intussusception
Paroxysmal atrial	Neurologic disease
tachycardia	Infant botulism
Myocardial infarction	Child abuse—intracranial
Pericarditis	bleeding
Myocarditis	
Endocrine disorders	
Congenital adrenal	
hyperplasia	
Metabolic disorders	
Hyponatremia	
Hypernatremia	
Inborn errors of metabolism	
Hypoglycemia	
Reye's syndrome	
Drug toxicity	

From Selbst SM. The septic-appearing infant. Pediatr Emerg Care 1985;1:160. © by Williams & Wilkins, 1985.

Diagnostics

All infants less than 60 days old who have a history of fever as measured by a rectal thermometer should undergo a complete sepsis evaluation. This includes infants who are actually afebrile on presentation to the emergency department.[121] The sepsis workup should include cultures of blood, urine, cerebrospinal fluid, and stool. In addition, a CBC count, urinalysis, and chest radiograph should be obtained.[33, 122] Submission of sera and various body fluids for virologic studies is advised during epidemics.[119]

Global Assessment: Nontoxic Patients

Because there are no clinical or laboratory criteria that reliably predict which non–toxic-appearing febrile infants less than 2 months old are likely to express a serious illness with a brief passage of time, conservative authorities advocate hospitalization.[34, 122–124] Others contend that such a restricted disposition should be reserved for patients in their first month of life.[125] Many private pediatricians and some academicians support home observation in the presence of a well appearance and negative laboratory investigations,[33] especially in females, and those more than 30 days old with temperatures less than 38.5°C (101.3°F) who have reliable and observant parents.[126] Until there are studies that address comparative outcomes of those infants admitted versus those discharged to home after emergency department evaluation, it is more prudent and less anxiety provoking for the physician to hospitalize all such infants. The inpatient physician may consider an infant at low risk for having serious bacterial infection and may choose to observe the clinical course rather than commit to parenteral antibiotics. The decision whether to treat all hospitalized infants or observe without antimicrobial therapy should be made by the physician responsible for inpatient care.

Global Assessment: Toxic Patients

The presence of toxicity on examination poses less of a dispositional dilemma for the emergency physician. Despite iatrogenic risks and financial costs, all ill-appearing children less than 2 months old should be hospitalized.[127] Empiric therapy should be initiated with ampicillin and an aminoglycoside or ampicillin and a third-generation cephalosporin (Table 66–5).[19, 21]

Patients 2 to 6 Months Old

Approximately 5% to 10% of the febrile pediatric emergency department patient population is between 2 and 6

TABLE 66–5	
SEPSIS: THERAPY AT A GLANCE*	
Agent	**Dose (mg/kg)**
Ampicillin	75–100
Ceftazidime	30–50
Cefotaxime	50
Cefuroxime	50–75
Ceftriaxone	100
Chloramphenicol	25–30
Gentamicin	2.5
Tobramycin	2.5
Amikacin	10

*First "stat" dose of antibiotic therapy for presumed bacterial sepsis or meningitis.

months of age. The risk for occult bacteremia is small.[36] There appears to be no correlation of the degree of fever with occult bacteremia unless the temperature exceeds 41°C.[37] At temperatures greater than 41°C, there is an increased incidence of meningitis and septicemia with a potential for a morbid outcome.[42, 128]

Diagnostics

Several surveys of febrile children report that a CBC count, ZSR, ESR, or CRP individually or as a group is beneficial in predicting bacterial illness.[72, 127] Others have not found a CBC count or tests for acute phase reactants useful in delineating the risk for serious bacterial infection.[128] Because of the low incidence of occult bacteremia in this age group, these blood tests are too costly to use as criteria for a decision on obtaining a blood culture. A chest radiograph may occasionally reveal infiltrates in the absence of objective findings in this age group, especially if the fever has been present for more than 12 hours. Regardless of symptomatology, urine cultures are a proven benefit in febrile infants in this age group, especially in females. This population has the highest incidence of occult urinary tract infections.[113]

Global Assessment: Nontoxic Patients

Clinical judgment is the best predictor of serious illness in this age group, as the physician's assessment of illness is more accurate than laboratory profiles.[129] Therefore, a well-appearing child without alarming historic features and a negative examination does not warrant a sepsis workup unless the temperature exceeds 41°C (105.8°F).

Global Assessment: Toxic Patients

Ill-appearing infants in this age group suspected to be septic should have a complete set of cultures obtained and should be admitted to an area that can closely monitor their progress for at least the first day of therapy. The development of hypoperfusion and hypotension may be delayed.[17] Cefuroxime, cefotaxime, or ceftriaxone are the agents of choice for presumed sepsis in this age group.[130, 131]

Patients 6 to 24 Months Old

Infants 6 to 24 months old pose the greatest diagnostic dilemma, as they constitute up to 50% of febrile episodes brought to the attention of the emergency physician, and the proportion of children with occult bacteremia is greatest in this group.[41] When recalled, one third of these patients found to be bacteremic at the initial encounter will have spontaneously recovered, while the remainder will have persistent bacteremia with or without a focus of infection. This focus includes the meninges in up to 7% of patients.[132] Studies have shown that bacteremic patients with no obvious source of infection, when treated with antibiotics at the initial encounter, have a better outcome that those who are bacteremic and do not receive antibiotics initially.[54, 133–135] Hence, developing an appropriate strategy involves discriminating between the child with bacteremia and the one without bacteremia. Laboratory adjuncts may be helpful in this regard.

Afebrile and slightly febrile 6- to 24-month-old children may have bacteremia.[136] The yield of positive cultures is low and the costs are high if blood cultures are obtained on all patients in this age group.[137] The percentage of positive cultures increases steadily in this age group when temperatures exceed 39.4°C (102.9°F) and is greatest when temperatures are ≥40°C. The yield of blood cultures may be increased by selectively acquiring them after positive screening laboratory investigations.[49]

Diagnostics

The superiority of a CBC count, ZSR, ESR, or CRP as a screening test for occult bacteremia has not been clearly demonstrated.[79] The most useful and cost effective of these studies in the febrile child without localized findings is a total white blood cell count. A count of more than 15,000/mm³ has reasonably good predictive value. An ESR accelerated over 30 mm/hour (Winthrobe) has a predictive value of similar magnitude. The two tests taken together are somewhat better than either alone. A child with a temperature ≥40°C, with a high white blood cell count, and an elevated sedimentation rate is an ideal candidate for a blood culture.[54, 138] Urinalysis, urine culture, and chest radiographs are optional studies. The decision to perform a lumbar puncture is based on the clinical assessment of the individual patient.

Global Assessment: Nontoxic Patients

Candidates for occult bacteremia may be treated expectantly with antibiotics, rather than withholding antimicrobial agents pending culture results. Prospectively investigated treatment regimens include penicillin (50,000 U/kg of intramuscular penicillin G benzathene–penicillin G procaine [Bicillin C-R], followed by penicillin V, 100 mg/kg/day, orally four times a day until culture results are known),[54] parenteral ceftriaxone (50 mg/kg/day for 2 days or until culture results are known),[139] and amoxicillin in doses exceeding 100 mg/kg/day, given orally in three divided doses.[135] Those treated with a standard amoxicillin dose of up to 50 mg/kg/day have no more rapid recovery or protection from major infectious morbidity than untreated patients.[140]

Global Assessment: Toxic Patients

Although fewer cases of septicemia occur in infants beyond the first year of life, the mortality in this age group of patients may parallel that found in the neonatal period. These deaths are usually caused by encapsulated bacterial pathogens (*H. influenzae, N. meningitidis, S. pneumoniae*) unless opportunistic pathogens are present in patients with compromised host defenses.[141] Empiric intravenous antimicrobial regimens as an in-patient should be tailored to the appropriate clinical scenario.

Patients More Than 2 Years Old

Children beyond the age of 2 years with fever constitute the second largest group of patients without a focus of infection that present to the emergency physician. They present the least problem in that they are often adequate historians who can relate the chief complaint and history of the present illness. They respond to contagion as young adults and exhibit classic physical findings during infection with virulent organisms. Mortality associated with community-acquired bacteremia in the normal host beyond 2 years of age is rare unless sepsis and meningitis coexist.[142]

Diagnostics

The clinician has no defined risk criteria or hard guidelines to shape the range of diagnostic testing in this age group. The diagnostic evaluation in the older pediatric patient must therefore be tailored to the clinical situation.

No diagnostic interventions may be indicated in many patients.

Global Assessment: Nontoxic Patients

If the patient does not have a predisposing illness or significant exposure and has a benign clinical appearance, no therapeutic intervention may be necessary.

Global Assessment: Toxic Patients

Invasive testing and hospitalization with prompt initiation of intravenous antibiotics is warranted for those patients beyond 2 years of age who appear septic.

DOCUMENTATION AND DISCHARGE INSTRUCTIONS

In discharging the febrile child without focus of infection from the emergency department, the physician must exclude historical factors that place the child at risk for serious infection. The child must not appear toxic, and the characteristics that define nontoxicity should be clearly noted in the chart. The child must not need a form of therapy that is hospital dependent, such as intravenous hydration or parenteral antibiotics. If a localized infectious disease is encountered, compliance to antibiotic therapy must be ensured. In all cases, the parents must be capable of observing their child closely and able to promptly return should their child's condition deteriorate. Although the specific instructions should be tailored to the characteristics of the specific patient encounter, parents of all febrile children should be encouraged to seek prompt attention if there is altered mental status, seizure, respiratory embarrassment, significant fluid loss, or petechial eruption.

Potential changes in clinical status must be observed, not only by the parents, but also by a vigilant physician. Children subsequently found to be bacteremic who are discharged home after an apparent trivial illness may deteriorate in a short period of time.[54, 139, 140] Regardless of whether they are treated expectantly, children at greatest risk for bacteremia (those age 3 to 24 months) should be reexamined within 24 hours from discharge from the emergency department.[54] Febrile patients without focus of infection who are younger than 3 months should be seen again 12 to 24 hours after discharge. Febrile patients beyond age 2 years, regardless of the specific evaluation and whether a focus of infection is apparent and the patient appears well, should also receive follow-up. A physician must maintain contact with the family during the subsequent 24 to 72 hours.[143] If the patient remains febrile, a second examination is warranted. A diagnosis that may not be readily apparent at the first event may be discovered at the second encounter.[144]

References

1. Marcinak JF. Evaluation of children with fever greater than or equal to 104°F in an emergency department. Pediatr Emerg Care 1988;4:92.
2. Atkins E. Fever—new perspectives on an old phenomenon. N Engl J Med 1983;308:958.
3. Banco L, Veltri D. Ability of mothers to subjectively assess the presence of fever in their children. Am J Dis Child 1984;138:976.
4. Banco L, Jayashekaramurthy S, Graffam J. The inability of temperature-sensitive pacifier to identify fevers in infants. Am J Dis Child 1988;142:171.
5. Treloar D, Muma B. Comparison of axillary, tympanic membrane, and rectal temperatures in young children. Ann Emerg Med 1988;17:435.
6. Rhoads FA, Grandner J. Assessment of an aural infrared sensor for body temperature measurement in children. Clin Pediatr 1989;29:112.
7. Scholefield JH, Gerber MA, Dwyer P. Liquid crystal forehead temperature strips: A clinical appraisal. Am J Dis Child 1982;136:198.

8. Ellis GL, Williamson B, White J. Liquid crystal thermometer strips. J Emerg Med 1989;7:675.

9. Johnston RB, Sell SH. Septicemia in infants and children. Pediatrics 1964;43:473.

10. Selbst SM. The septic appearing infant. Pediatr Emerg Care 1985;1:160.

11. Helminen M, Vesikari T. Spontaneous and inducible interleukin 1 production from peripheral blood monocytes in bacterial and viral infections in children. Pediatr Infect Dis 1987;6:1102.

12. Florman AL. Interleukin 1 and monitoring of acute infections. Pediatr Infect Dis 1985;4:450.

13. Craig WS. The early detection of pyrexia in the newborn. Arch Dis Child 1963;38:29.

14. Feigin RD, Shearer WT. Opportunistic infection in children. I. In the compromised host. J Pediatr 1975;87:507.

15. Lobel JS, Bove KE. Clinical pathologic characteristics of septicemia and sickle cell disease. Am J Dis Child 1982;136:453.

16. Berringer R, Harwood-Nuss AL. Septic shock (part 1). J Emerg Med 1985;3:475.

17. Jacobs RF, Sowell MK, Moss MM, et al. Septic shock in children: Bacterial etiologies and temporal relationships. Pediatr Infect Dis 1990;9:196.

18. Fischer GW. Immunoglobulin therapy of neonatal group B strep infection. An overview. Pediatr Infect Dis 1988;7:S13.

19. Odio CM, Saenz A, Salas JL, et al. Comparative efficacy of ceftriazidine versus carbenicillin and amikacin for treatment of neonatal septicemia. Pediatr Infect Dis 1987;6:371.

20. Eisenfeld L, Ermocilla R, Wirtschafter D, et al. Systemic bacterial infections in neonatal death. Am J Dis Child 1983;137:645.

21. Bradley JS. Neonatal infections. Pediatr Infect Dis 1985;4:315.

22. Nelson KG. An index of severity for acute pediatric illness. Am J Public Health 1980;70:804.

23. Harlan L, Landrigan P, Babineau R, et al. A comparison of antipyretic effect of acetaminophen and aspirin. Am J Dis Child 1972;124:880.

24. Similas P, Kouvalainen K, Keinanen S. Oral antipyretic therapy: Evaluation of ibuprofen. Scand J Rheumatol 1976;5:81.

25. Dinarello CA. Interleukin-1 in the pathogenesis of the acute-phase response. N Engl J Med 1984;311:1413.

26. Baker MD, Fosarelli PD, Carpenter RO. Childhood fever: Correlation of diagnosis with temperature response to acetaminophen. Pediatrics 1987;80:315.

27. Weisse ME, Miller G, Brien JH. Fever response to acetaminophen in viral versus bacterial infections. Pediatr Infect Dis 1987;6:1091.

28. Torrey SB, Henretig F, Fleisher G, et al. Temperature response to antipyretic therapy in children: Relationship to occult bacteremia. Am J Emerg Med 1985;3:190.

29. Gotoff S, Behrman R. Neonatal septicemia. J Pediatr 1970;76:142.

30. Speer CP, Hauptmann D, Stubbe P, et al. Neonatal septicemia and meningitis. Gottingen, West Germany. Pediatr Infect Dis 1985;4:36.

31. Crain EF, Shelov SP. Febrile infants: Predictors of bacteremia. J Pediatr 1982;101:686.

32. Caspe WB, Chamudes O, Louie B. The evaluation and treatment of the febrile infant. Pediatr Infect Dis 1983;2:131.

33. Rosenberg N, Vranesich P, Cohen S. Incidence of serious infection in infants under age two months with fever. Pediatr Emerg Care 1985;1:54.

34. Greene JW, Hara C, O'Connor S, Altemeier WA 3rd. Management of febrile outpatient neonates. Clin Pediatr 1981;20:375.

35. O'Shea JS. Assessing the significance of fever in young infants: The diagnostic and prognostic value of cerebrospinal fluid and other clinical and laboratory findings. Clin Pediatr 1978;17:854.

36. Pantell RH, Naber M, Lamar R, et al. Fever in the first six months of life: Risks of underlying serious infection. Clin Pediatr 1980;19:77.

37. McGowan JE, Bratton L, Klein JO, et al. Bacteremia in febrile children seen in a "walk-in" pediatric clinic. N Engl J Med 1973;228:1309.

38. Teele DW, Pelton FI, Grant MJA, et al. Bacteremia in febrile children under two years of age: Results of cultures of blood of 600 consecutive febrile children seen in a "walk-in" clinic. J Pediatr 1975;87:227.

39. Wright PF. Patterns of illness in the highly febrile young child: Epidemiologic, clinical, and laboratory correlates. Pediatrics 1981;67:694.

40. Meyers M, Wright P, Smith A, et al. Complications of occult pneumococcal bacteremia in children. J Pediatr 1974;84:656.

41. McCarthy PL, Grundy GW, Spiesel SZ, et al. Bacteremia in children: An outpatient clinical review. Pediatrics 1976;57:861.

42. McCarthy PL, Dolan TF. The serious implications of high fever in infants during the first three months. Clin Pediatr 1976;15:794.

43. Krober MS, Bass JW, Powell JM, et al. Bacterial and viral pathogens causing fever in infants less than three months old. Am J Dis Child 1985;139:889.

44. Press S, Fawcett NP. Association of temperature greater than 41.1°C (106°F) with serious illness. Clin Pediatr 1985;24:51.

45. Dashefsky B, Teele DW, Klein JO. Unsuspected meningococcemia. J Pediatr 1983;102:69.

46. Baltimore RS, Hammerschlag M. Meningococcal bacteremia: Clinical and serologic studies of infants with mild illness. Am J Dis Child 1977;131:1001.

47. McClung HJ. Prolonged fever of unknown origin in children. Am J Dis Child 1972;124:544.

48. Dechovitz AB, Moffet HL. Classification of acute febrile illnesses in childhood. Clin Pediatr 1968;7:649.

49. Child Day Care Infectious Disease Study Group. Public health considerations of infectious disease in child day care centers. J Pediatr 1984;105:250.

50. Singer JI, Berger OG. Simultaneous occult pneumococcal bacteremia in identical twins. J Pediatr 1981;98:250.

51. Weissman JB, Schmerler A, Weiler P, et al. The role of preschool children and day care centers in the spread of shigellosis in urban communities. J Pediatr 1974;84:797.

52. Wilson R, Feldman RA, Davis J, LaVenture M. Salmonellosis in infants: The importance of intrafamilial transmission. Pediatrics 1982;69:436.

53. Bryan CS, Reynolds KL, Derrick, CW Jr. Patterns of bacteremia in pediatric practice: Factors affecting mortality rates. Pediatr Infect Dis 1984;3:312.

54. Carroll WL, Farrell M, Singer JI, et al. Treatment of occult bacteremia: A prospective randomized clinical trial. Pediatrics 1983;72:608.

55. Burech DL, Koranyi K, Haynes RE, et al. Pneumococcal bacteremia associated with gingival lesions in infants. Am J Dis Child 1975;129:1283.

56. Yeager AM. Gingival lesions in infants with pneumococcal bacteremia. Am J Dis Child 1979;133:97.

57. McCarthy PL, Jekel JF, Stashwick CA, et al. History and observation variables in assessing febrile children. Pediatrics 1980;65:1090.

58. McCarthy PL, Jekel JF, Stashwick CA, et al. Further definition of history and observation variables in assessing febrile children. Pediatrics 1981;67:687.

59. McCarthy PL, Sharpe MR, Spiesel SZ, et al. Observation scales to identify serious illness in febrile children. Pediatrics 1982;70:802.

60. McCarthy PL, Sharpe MR, Spiesel SZ, et al. Predictive value of abnormal physical examination findings in ill appearing and well appearing febrile children. Pediatrics 1985;76:167.

61. Berringer R, Harwood-Nuss AL. Septic shock (part II). J Emerg Med 1986;4:49.

62. Graves GR, Rhodes PG. Tachycardia as a sign of early-onset neonatal sepsis. Pediatr Infect Dis 1984;3:404.

63. Glover DM, Wilson CB. Pediatric infections. Emerg Med Clin North Am 1985;3:25.

64. Squire EW Jr, Reich HM, Merenstein GB, et al. Criteria for the discontinuation of antibiotic therapy during presumptive treatment of suspected neonatal infection. Pediatr Dis 1982;1:85.

65. Bennish M, Beem MO, Ormiste V. C-reactive protein and zeta sedimentation ratio as indicators of bacteremia in pediatric patients. J Pediatr 1984;104:729.

66. Liu CH, Lehan C, Speer ME, et al. Degenerative changes in neutrophils: An indicator of bacterial infection. Pediatrics 1984;74:823.

67. McCarthy PL. Controversies in pediatrics: What tests are indicated for the child under three with fever. Pediatr Rev 1979;1:51.

68. Philip AGF. Response of C-reactive protein in neonatal group B streptococcal infection. Pediatr Inf Dis 1985;4:145.

69. Peltola H, Jaakkola M. C-reactive protein in early detection of bacteremic vs viral infections in immunocompetent and compromised children. J Pediatr 1988;113:641.

70. Christensen RD, Rothstein G, Hill HR, et al. Fatal early onset group B streptococcal sepsis with normal leukocyte counts. Pediatr Infect Dis 1985;4:242.

71. Rozyckih HJ, Stahl GE, Baumgart S. Impaired sensitivity of a single early leukocyte count in screening for neonatal sepsis. Pediatr Infect Dis 1987;6:440.

72. McCarthy PL, Jekel JK, Dolan TF. Comparison of acute phase reactants in the pediatric patient with fever. Pediatrics 1978;62:716.

73. Rodwell RL, Leslie AL, Tudehope DI. Early diagnosis of neonatal sepsis using a hematologic scoring system. J Pediatr 1988;112:761.

74. Wheeler JG, Chauvente AL, Johnson CA, et al. Neutrophil storage pool depletion in septic, neutropenic neonates. Pediatr Infect Dis 1984;3:407.

75. Todd JK. Childhood infections: Diagnostic value of peripheral white blood cell and differential cell counts. Am Dis Child 1974;127:810.

76. Manroe BL, Rosenfeld CR, Weinberg AG, et al. The differential leukocyte count in the assessment and outcome of early onset neonatal group B streptococcal disease. J Pediatr 1977;91:632.

77. Weitzman M. Diagnostic utility of white blood cell and differential cell counts. Am J Dis Child 1975;129:1183.

78. Zipursky A, Palko J, Milner R, et al. The hematology of bacterial infections in premature infants. Pediatrics 1976;57:839.

79. Singer JI, Buchino JJ, Chabali R. Selected laboratory and pediatric emergency care. Emerg Med Clin North Am 1986;4:377.

80. Peltola H, Holmberg C. Rapidity of C-reactive protein in detecting potential septicemia. Pediatr Infect Dis 1983;2:374.

81. Philip AGS, Baker CJ. Cerebrospinal fluid C-reactive protein in neonatal meningitis. J Pediatr 1983;102:715.

82. Sabel KG, Hanson LA. The clinical usefulness of C-reactive protein (CRP) determinations and bacterial meningitis and septicemia in infancy. Acta Paediatr Scand 1974;63:381.

83. Sabel KG, Wadsworth C. C-reactive protein (CRP) in early diagnosis of neonatal septicemia. Acta Paediatr Scand 1979;68:825.

84. Yagupsky P, Bearman JE. Shortened erythrocyte sedimentation rate. Pediatr Infect Dis 1987;6:494.

85. Bennish M, Vardiman J, Beem MO. The zeta sedimentation ratio in children. J Pediatr 1984;104:249.

86. Crain EF, Shelov SP. Febrile infants: Predictors of bacteremia. J Pediatr 1982;101:686.

87. Adler SM, Denton RL. The erythrocyte sedimentation rate in the newborn. J Pediatr 1975;86:942.

88. Koenig JM, Patterson LER, Rench MA, et al. Role of fibrinonectin in diagnosing bacterial infection. Am J Dis Child 1988;142:884.

89. Gerdes JS, Polin RA. Sepsis screen in neonates with an evaluation of plasma fibrinonectin. Pediatr Infect Dis 1987;6:443.

90. Speer CP, Ninjo A, Gahr M. Elastase-alpha 1-proteinase inhibitor in early diagnosis of neonatal septicemia. J Pediatr 1986;108:987.

91. Speer CP, Rethwilm M, Gahr M. Elastase-alpha 1-proteinase inhibitor: An early indicator of septicemia in bacterial meningitis in children. J Pediatr 1987;111:667.

92. Dietzman DE, Fischer GW, Schoenknecht FD. Neonatal *Escherichia coli* septicemia-bacterial counts in blood. J Pediatr 1974;85:128.

93. LaScalea LJ Jr, Dryja D, Sullivan TD, et al. Diagnosis of bacteremia in children by quantitative direct plating and radiometric procedure. J Clin Microbiol 1981;13:478.

94. Fischer GW, Smith P, Hemming VG, et al. Avoidance of false-negative blood culture results by rapid detection of pneumococcal antigen. JAMA 1984;253:1742.

95. Kaplan SL, Feigin RD. Rapid identification of the invading microorganism. Pediatr Clin North Am 1980;27:783.

96. Teele DW, Marshall R, Klein JO. Unsuspected bacteremia in young children: A common and important problem. Pediatr Clin North Am 1979;26:773.

97. Congeni BL, Igel HJ, Platt MS. Evaluation of a latex particle agglutination kit in pneumococcal disease. Pediatr Infect Dis 1984;3:417.

98. Ballard TL, Roe MH, Wheeler RC, et al. Comparison of three latex agglutination kits and countercurrent immunoelectrophoresis for the detection of bacterial antigens in the pediatric population. Pediatr Infect Dis 1987;6:630.

99. Blecker DL, Zimbro MJ, Erbe MB, et al. Polyclonal anti-group B streptococcus latex antigen detection test. Pediatr Infect Dis 1989;8:252.

100. Miotti PG, Viscidi RP, Eiden J, et al. Centrifugation-augmented solid-phase immunoassay (CASPIA) for the rapid diagnosis of infectious disease. J Infect Dis 1989;154:301.

101. Orlowski JP, Porembka DT, Gallagher JM, et al. The bone marrow as a source of laboratory studies. Ann Emerg Med 1989;18:1348.

102. Todd JK. Bacteriology and clinical relevance of nasopharyngeal and oropharyngeal cultures. Pediatr Infect Dis 1984;3:159.

103. Singer JI. Acute bacterial meningitis. *In* Rosen P, Baker FJ, Barkin RM (eds). Emergency Medicine: Concepts in Clinical Practice. 2nd ed. St Louis, CV Mosby, pp 2213–2222.

104. Glover DM, Wilson CB. Pediatric infections. Emerg Med Clin North Am 1985;3:25.

105. Yogev R. Suppurative intracranial complications of upper respiratory tract infections. Pediatr Infect Dis 1987;6:624.

106. Bonadio WA. Cerebral herniation syndrome as the presenting sign of Haemophilus influenzae meningitis. Pediatr Emerg Care 1987;3:253.

107. McGravey AR. A dilated, unreactive pupil in acute bacterial meningitis: Oculomotor nerve inflammation versus herniation. Pediatr Emerg Care 1989;5:187.

108. Losek JD, Kishaba G, Berens RJ, et al. Indications for chest roentgenogram in the febrile young infant. Pediatr Emerg Care 1989;5:149.

109. Zukin DD, Hoffman JR, Cleveland RH, et al. Correlations of pulmonary signs and symptoms with chest radiographs in the pediatric age group. Ann Emerg Med 1986;15:792.

110. Leventhal JM. Clinical predictors of pneumonia as a guide to ordering chest roentgenograms. Clin Pediatr 1982;21:730.

111. Fosarelli PD, Deangelis C, Winkelstein J, et al. Infectious illnesses in the first two years of life. Pediatr Infect Dis 1985;4:153.

112. Cone TE. Diagnosis and treatment: Children with fevers. Pediatrics 1969;43:290.

113. Bauchner H, Philipp B, Dashefsky B, et al. Prevalence of bacteriuria in febrile children. Pediatr Infect Dis 1987;6:239.

114. Murray DL, Zonana J, Seidel JS, et al. Relative importance of bacteremia and viremia in the course of acute fevers of unknown origin in outpatient children. Pediatrics 1981;68:157.

115. Jaffe D, Torrey SB. Diagnostic approach to febrile illnesses. In Ludwig S (ed). Pediatric Emergencies. Vol 7. New York, Churchill Livingstone, 1985.

116. Pizzo PA, Lovejoy FH Jr, Smith DH. Prolonged fever in children: Review of 100 cases. Pediatrics 1975;55:468.

117. Pryor RW, Kline MW, Matson JR. Septic shock: Principles of management in the emergency department. Pediatr Emerg Care 1989;5:193.

118. Bell LM, Alpert G, Campos JM, et al. Routine quantitative blood cultures in children with Haemophilus influenzae or Streptococcus pneumonia bacteremia. Pediatrics 1985;76:901.

119. Dagan R, Hall CB, Powell KR, et al. Epidemiology in laboratory diagnosis of infections with viral and bacterial pathogens in infants hospitalized for suspected sepsis. J Pediatr 1989;115:351.

120. Klein JO, Schlesinger PC, Karasic RB. Management of the febrile infant three months of age or younger. Pediatr Infect Dis 1984;3:75.

121. Bonadio WA, Heggenbarth M, Zachariason M. Correlating reported fever in young infants with subsequent temperature patterns and rate of serious bacterial infections. Pediatr Infect Dis 1990;9:158.

122. Powell KR. Evaluation and management of febrile infants younger than 60 days of age. Pediatr Infect Dis 1990;9:153.

123. Berkowitz CD, Orr DP, Uchiyama N, et al. Variability in the management of the febrile infant under two months of age. J Emerg Med 1985;3:345.

124. Wasserman GM, White CB. Evaluation of the necessity for hospitalization of the febrile infant less than three months of age. Pediatr Infect Dis 1990;9:163.

125. Crain EF, Gershel JC. Which febrile infants younger than two weeks of age are likely to have sepsis? A pilot study. Pediatr Infect Dis 1988;7:561.

126. DeAngelis C, Joffe A, Willis E, et al. Hospitalization vs outpatient treatment of young, febrile infants. Am J Dis Child 1983;137:1150.

127. DeAngelis C, Joffe A, Wilson M, et al. Iatrogenic risks and financial costs of hospitalizing febrile infants. Am J Dis Child 1983;137:1146.

128. Bonadio WA, Grunske L, Smith DS. Systemic bacterial infections in children with fever greater than 41°C. Pediatr Infect Dis 1989;8:120.

129. Soman M. Diagnostic workup of febrile children under 24 months of age—clinical review. West J Med 1982;137:1.

130. Word BM, Klein JO. Therapy of bacterial sepsis in meningitis in infants and children: 1989 poll of directors of programs in pediatric infectious diseases. Pediatr Infect Dis 1989;8:635.

131. Spritzer R, Kamp HJ, Dzoljic G, et al. Five years of cefotaxime use in a neonatal intensive care unit. Pediatr Infect Dis 1990;9:92.

132. Shapiro ED, Aaron NH, Wald ER, et al. Risk factors for development of bacterial meningitis among children with occult bacteremia. J Pediatr 1986;109:15.

133. Bratton L, Teele DW, Klein JO. Outcome of unsuspected pneumococcemia in children not initially admitted to the hospital. J Pediatr 1977;90:703.

134. Marshall R, Teele DW, Klein JO. Unsuspected bacteremia due to Haemophilus influenzae: Outcome in children not initially admitted to the hospital. Pediatrics 1979;95:690.

135. Baron MA, Fink HD, Cicchetti DV. Blood cultures in private pediatric practice: An eleven year experience. Pediatr Infect Dis 1989;8:2.

136. Kline MW, Lorin MI. Bacteremia in children afebrile at presentation to an emergency room. Pediatr Infect Dis 1987;6:197.

137. Dershewitz RA, Wigder HN, Wigder CM, et al. A comparative study of the prevalence, outcome and prediction of bacteremia in children. J Pediatr 1983;103:352.

138. Grossman M. Management of the febrile patient. Pediatr Infect Dis 1986;5:730.

139. Baskin MN, Fleisher GR, O'Rourke EJ. Outpatient management of febrile infants 28–90 days of age with intramuscular ceftriaxome (ABS). Ann Emerg Med 1990;19:4.

140. Jaffe DM, Tanz RR, Davis AT, et al. Antibiotic administration to treat possible occult bacteremia in febrile children. N Engl J Med 1987;317:1175.

141. Alario AJ, Nelson EW, Shapiro ED. Blood cultures in the management of febrile outpatients later found to have bacteremia. J Pediatr 1989;115:195.

142. Brian CS, Reynolds KL, Derrick W. Patterns of bacteremia in pediatric practice: Factors affecting mortality rates. Pediatr Infect Dis 1984;3:312.

143. Klein JO. The febrile child and occult bacteremia. N Engl J Med 1987;317:1219.

144. McLellan D, Giebink S. Perspectives on occult bacteremia in children. J Pediatr 1986;109:1.

CHAPTER 67

Diphtheria, Pertussis, and Tetanus

Carden Johnston

DIPHTHERIA

Five cases of diphtheria were reported to the Centers for Disease Control (CDC) in 1986; four of those were in children. The case fatality rate has remained about 5% since the advent of antibiotics and antitoxin therapy. Diphtheria is an uncommon diagnosis, and if it goes unrecognized or unsuspected, it can be fatal.

Corynebacterium diphtheriae is an irregularly staining gram-positive pleomorphic bacillus. Although three strains have been recognized by culture (*mitis, gravis,* and *intermedius*), only some of the bacteria produce toxins.

The only reservoir for *C. diphtheriae* is the human. The organism is primarily droplet spread (i.e., through coughing), although skin infections can predispose to respiratory colonization. Unimmunized children residing in crowded, poor conditions with limited access to health care are most likely to be infected with the organism.

Evidence from the Texas epidemic in the late 1960s suggests that an immunization rate of 90% or greater in the entire population could provide enough immunity to prevent diphtheria in any community. Clinical diphtheria reported in developed countries occurs in unimmunized children who have been exposed to a child from an underdeveloped country whose immunization status was unknown.

The disease state is protected by immunization, although fully immunized persons may be infected with the organism. Communicability usually lasts 2 weeks but has persisted several months. If the patient is treated, communicability lasts less than 4 days.

Pathophysiology

Most often *C. diphtheriae* enters the body through the respiratory tract. The organism localizes on the mucosal surface of the nose, pharynx, or upper respiratory tract. Less often, the skin, the eye, or the genital tract may be the area of colonization.

After the organism grows and a local inflammatory response occurs, a membrane may develop with associated edema, which may be marked. If colonization occurs on the skin, the lesion may be impetiginous or ulcerative with a sharp border. The membrane that develops contains fibrinoid material, red blood cells, and epithelial cells. The edema or the membrane may occlude the airway.

The toxin is distributed throughout by both lymphatics and blood. Although the toxin can affect any tissue, it most often causes lesions in the heart, nervous system, and kidney. Unlike tetanus, the diphtheria toxin can be neutralized if attached to the cell, but once intracellular, it cannot be neutralized by antitoxin.

Prevention

Antibody levels of 0.01 U/ml are protective against the disease-producing effect of *C. diphtheriae*. Often a health care worker is one of the first to be exposed to a patient with diphtheria. Immunizations are waning in 20- to 30-year-old U.S. adults, so it is essential for health care providers to maintain current immunizations.

If the patient has pharyngeal diphtheria, masks worn by the patient and health care worker will decrease droplet spread. If the infection is cutaneous, wearing of gloves, and, more importantly, hand washing will decrease the chances of infection. All close contacts should be cultured and observed for 7 days. A booster should be given to contacts if it has been 5 years or more since the last diphtheria toxoid injection.

Clinical Evaluation

Almost all of the cases of diphtheria can be suspected by history (Table 67–1). Young adults who are alcohol or drug abusers, poor, underimmunized, and undernourished are most likely to become infected, die, or sustain complications. The epidemics of the late 1960s, mostly seen in Texas, involved children who were unimmunized and lived in crowded, low-income areas. However, even middle-class children who are unimmunized may contract the disease and have serious complications after being exposed to an immunized infected person or carrier in a developed nation.

Common initial complaints are sore throat, dysphagia, nausea, headache, and chills. Vomiting is also common. These symptoms are the same in immunized or unimmunized patients and are often present before a pharyngeal lesion is extensive. The temperature is often low, with a mean of 38.5°C (101.3°F) for children younger than 5 years and 38.1°C (100.6°F) for those older than 15 years.

When seen, the membrane is helpful in prompting more definitive diagnostic techniques. The rare, classic membrane is dirty white to gray in color and progresses off of the tonsil area to surrounding soft tissue; when it is removed, the pharyngeal tissue bleeds. However, the membranes may also be small, white, localized, and indistinguishable from those caused by group A streptococcus. Parenthetically, a positive rapid streptococcal test does not exclude the diagnosis of diphtheria, as approximately 50% of the children found to have diphtheria also have laboratory indications of group A streptococcus in their pharynx. In one study, 54% of the patients diagnosed with diphtheria had a membrane located somewhere in the upper respiratory tract.

The membrane takes about 2 days to develop after symptoms start, but the average duration of symptoms before admission is 7 days. The longer the duration of symptoms, the more likely it is that the child will have a swollen neck. In one report, children less than 6 years old rarely had a

---

TABLE 67–1
DIPHTHERIA DIAGNOSIS

Definitive: By positive culture
Suggestive history:
    Young adults who are alcohol or drug abusers, poor, underimmunized, and undernourished
    Children living in crowded, low-income areas and who are unimmunized
    Unimmunized immigrants from underdeveloped countries
Initial complaint: Sore throat, dysphasia, nausea, headache, chills, vomiting
Physical findings:
    A membrane, classically dirty gray, progressing off the tonsil to surrounding soft tissue
    Membrane in larynx or nasopharynx
    Croup or runny nose
    Impetiginous lesions with gram-positive rods

swollen neck. Instead, an "erasure" edema was described that was brawny, warm, easily palpable, and erased the border of the sternocleidomastoid, mandible, and medial clavicle. The edema was pitting and found in about 30% of the patients.

Nasal diphtheria resembles a common cold and most often occurs in infants. Because the toxin is slowly absorbed by this route, signs of myocarditis or paralysis are delayed. A membrane on the nasal septum may be found only with diligent searching. The discharge, initially serosanguineous, becomes mucopurulent, often progressing to excoriation of the nares and upper lips.

Laryngeal diphtheria may be clinically indistinguishable from other types of infectious croup. Children with diphtheria isolated to the larynx do not appear as toxic as those with pharyngeal involvement; however, a membrane in the trachea can be massive and obstruct respiration.

Cutaneous diphtheria is more frequent in warmer climates and in late summer. The lesion is described as ulcerative, with a membranous base and sharply defined border.

Patients with diphtheritic myocarditis or neuropathy rarely present to the emergency department without upper airway disease or skin lesions. However, the physician must be aware that the diphtheria toxin may produce myocarditis. Arrhythmias, ST segment depression, and T wave inversion may develop early. Later, congestive heart failure occurs with a gallop rhythm and cardiac enlargement.

Another complication is involvement of the neurologic system by the toxin. A neuritis predominantly affecting the motor nerves occurs. Soft palate paralysis and ocular paralysis may occur. The phrenic nerve may also become paralyzed, but this usually occurs relatively late. A syndrome similar to Guillain-Barré with loss of deep tendon reflexes and elevation of the cerebral spinal fluid protein may also occur.

Diagnostic Evaluation

The physician should not wait for laboratory confirmation before initiating therapy. Direct stains, Gram stains, and even fluorescent antibody stains are nondiagnostic. Material from underneath the membrane or the membrane itself should be submitted to the laboratory for culture. The laboratory technician should be notified to look for diphtheria and to grow the specimen on special media.

Other laboratory studies are sensitive but not specific. The white blood cell count is usually elevated, and anemia may be present. Cerebrospinal fluid may have a mild pleocytosis when the patient has neurologic complications. The electrocardiogram shows ST segment and T wave changes or an arrhythmia, which may indicate a nonspecific myocarditis. Radiographs of the larynx and pharynx are not helpful in confirming the diagnosis.

Differential Diagnosis

Nasal diphtheria may resemble the common cold. Other diagnoses to consider include a foreign body, sinusitis, adenoiditis, and congenital syphilis (Table 67–2). Streptococci in the nose may mimic diphtheria closely.

Tonsilar or pharyngeal diphtheria must be differentiated from streptococcal pharyngitis. Streptococcal organisms were recovered from half the patients admitted with the diagnosis of diphtheria in one study. Patients with infectious mononucleosis present with large lymph nodes, a swollen neck, and pharyngitis. Other viral causes of pharyngitis should also be considered, including herpetic glossopharyngitis, which may be associated with large cervical lymph glands. Vincent's angina can cause upper airway obstruction

and a thick upper neck. Laryngeal diphtheria must be differentiated from epiglottitis, croup, foreign body aspiration, and bacterial tracheitis.

If a young patient has myocarditis, diphtheria must be considered as a cause. If a patient has bilateral absence of the deep tendon reflexes or paralysis of the soft palate, diphtheria should be considered, although local signs of infection should be apparent.

Therapeutic Intervention

As soon as diphtheria is suspected and before culture results are available, the equine antitoxin should be administered (Table 67–3). Twenty thousand to 40,000 units are given intravenously for pharyngeal and laryngeal disease of 48 hours duration or less. Forty thousand to 60,000 units are administered for nasopharyngeal lesions. If there is extensive disease with symptoms of 3 or more days duration, 80,000 to 100,000 units are given.

Because the antitoxin is of equine origin, a sensitivity test should be performed by applying a drop of 1:100 dilution of the serum in saline to a scratch on the volar surface of the forearm. On the other arm, a control drop of saline only is placed. A positive result consists of a wheal that is 3 mm or larger that forms on the serum side after 15 to 20 minutes.

If sensitivity exists, desensitization should then be carried out according to the package insert. Another method, if indicated because of disease severity, is to have two intravenous lines in place: one to administer equine antitoxin and the other to administer a 1:10,000 solution of epinephrine so that an allergic reaction can be controlled. The dose of antitoxin should be given intravenously to neutralize the toxin as rapidly as possible.

The second consideration is eradication of the organism. Penicillin G procaine in a dose of 25,000 to 50,000 U/kg/day divided every 12 hours is given intramuscularly for 14 days. Erythromycin, 40 mg/kg/day, is also effective.

Children with airway compromise should have the airway secured with nasotracheal intubation or tracheostomy. Hopefully, this procedure can be done under controlled conditions. However, the airway must ultimately be secured, especially if the child is to be transported to another facility and transport time is long.

Disposition

A patient who is considered to have diphtheria must be admitted and all close contacts cultured and immunized. A child with a fever, signs of respiratory obstruction, bull neck, erasure edema of the neck, or pharyngeal membrane should have antitoxin and antibiotic therapy initiated immediately and the child subsequently admitted. If there is a prolonged

TABLE 67–2
DIFFERENTIAL DIAGNOSIS FOR DIPHTHERIA

Pharyngitis	Paralysis
Croup	Tick paralysis
Pertussis	Botulism
Foreign body aspiration	Congenital syphilis
Retropharyngeal abscess	Adenoiditis
Bacterial tracheitis	Streptococcal pharyngitis
Epiglottitis	*Neisseria gonorrhea* pharyngitis
Myocarditis	Infectious mononucleosis
Infectious	Adenoviral infections
Metabolic	Herpetic dermatitis
Inflammatory	Vincent's angina
Myopathic	

TABLE 67-3

DIPHTHERIA, PERTUSSIS, AND TETANUS: THERAPY AT A GLANCE

Diphtheria
    Penicillin G procaine: 25,000 to 50,000 U/kg/day divided q
      12 hr IM
    Erythromycin: 40 mg/kg/day; maximum, 1.6 gm
Diphtheria antitoxin
    Pharyngeal and laryngeal disease of recent onset: 20,000 to
      40,000 U IV
    Nasopharyngeal disease: 40,000 to 60,000 U IV
    Extensive or prolonged disease: 80,000 to 100,000 U IV
Pertussis
    Erythromycin: 40 mg/kg/day po; maximum, 1.6 gm
Tetanus
    Tetanus immune globulin: 3000 to 6000 U IM, with half
      given locally at the site of infection
    Penicillin: 100,000 U/kg/day po or IV
    Diazepam: 0.2 mg/kg IV
    Lorazepam: 0.1 mg/kg IV
    Phenobarbital: 5 to 7 mg IV

fever with an upper respiratory tract infection in a child from an underdeveloped country, then the diagnosis should be considered.

Management of Contacts

A close contact is defined as someone residing in the residence of the source or a nonresident who has spent an accumulated total of 4 or more hours with the patient for 5 of the 7 days prior to recognition of illness. Any person who has had close contact with a patient with diphtheria and who has symptoms compatible with diphtheria (nausea, vomiting, headache, rhinorrhea, sore throat, or dysphasia) should receive antitoxin and antibiotic therapy and be admitted to the hospital.

All close patient contacts without symptoms should be cultured and treated with procaine penicillin or erythromycin.

All previously immunized, close patient contacts should have a booster dose of diphtheria toxoid if it has not been given in the previous 5 years. Close patient contacts who are unimmunized or in whom the current immunization status is unknown should receive antibiotic therapy, with cultures performed before and after treatment and should receive immunization. Contacts who cannot be observed closely or may be noncompliant should receive an initial dose of diphtheria toxoid and an injection of benzathine penicillin.

PERTUSSIS

Pertussis is both an epidemic and an endemic disease. There are 3000 to 4000 cases of pertussis reported in the United States annually, with five to ten deaths reported per year. The responsible organism, *Bordetella pertussis*, is a fastidious gram-negative pleomorphic bacilli. *B. pertussis*, *Bordetella parapertussis*, adenovirus, and *Chlamydia trachomatis* all can cause a whooping cough syndrome. Although these organisms cause clinically indistinguishable disease states, determining the causative organism is important for epidemiologic reasons.

Although pertussis can occur at any age, the disease is more easily recognized and more serious in the younger child. Seventy percent of the recorded cases are in children younger than 5 years; approximately 50% occur in those younger than 1 year, and 35% occur in infants younger than 6 months. The infection has been reported in the hospital nursery as a result of newborns contracting the disease from their ill adolescent parents. Nevertheless, it is rare in the newborn. Hospitalization rates are highest in the first 6 months of life because the trachea is smaller, increasing the potential for airway compromise.

Humans are the only host for *B. parapertussis*. Transmission is by droplet spread among close contacts. It is highly infectious, usually occurring among members of a household and in institutional care settings. Approximately 90% of unimmunized household contacts acquire the infection.

Communicability is highest in the early phase of the illness before coughing paroxysms occur. Although the degree of communicability decreases rapidly, it may last up to 3 weeks. Females are more commonly affected than males. There is no seasonal variation.

Pathophysiology

The *B. pertussis* organism spreads to the new patient through a droplet and then attaches to the cilia of epithelial cells in the respiratory tract. The capsule of the organism has antiphagocytic activity. Pertussis is believed to be a toxin-mediated disease.

Clinical Evaluation

Pertussis is characterized clinically by three progressive stages: catarrhal, paroxysmal, and convalescent (Table 67-4). The first stage, which lasts 1 to 2 weeks, is characterized by common cold symptoms: low-grade fever, malaise, rhinorrhea, lacrimation, cough, and conjunctival injection. At this stage, bacterial shedding and communicability is greatest.

In the classic paroxysmal stage, the parent describes the child as being more ill than the child demonstrates. The parent appears overly concerned, though the child does not appear severely ill by examination. Between coughing paroxysms the child usually shows symptoms only of a common cold.

Suddenly, with mild provocation, the child may cough repeatedly and be unable to complete inspiration for a prolonged time. During this episode, the child may develop cyanosis, bulging eyes, and protrusion of neck veins. This is followed by an inspiratory "whoop," which gives the disease its name. Vomiting may occur, and the patient will appear apathetic and exhausted. However, not all children whoop, making the diagnosis more difficult, and typical whoop is seldom heard in an older child or adult. This paroxysmal stage usually lasts 2 weeks but may last 4 weeks or more.

The convalescent stage is associated with a decrease in both the severity and the number of coughing paroxysms.

TABLE 67-4

PERTUSSIS DIAGNOSIS

Definitive: By positive culture or serum antibody rise
Suggestive: Direct immunofluorescent test
Clinical
    Catarrhal phase
      2 wk duration
      Upper respiratory or common cold symptoms
    Paroxysmal phase
      2 wk duration; paroxysms of coughing, followed by a
        "whoop" inspiration and maybe vomit; between
        paroxysms, the child may appear only mildly ill
    Convalescent stage
      2 to 12 wk duration; decrease in severity of paroxysms and
        whooping

However, the cough may last for months, which has given the disease the lay designation, "the 100-day cough."

In a school age child, and especially in the adolescent and young adult, the disease is difficult to distinguish from a persistent cough or lingering tracheobronchitis. It should be suspected in a child with delayed or no immunizations or in someone exposed to an inadequately immunized child. If the child lives in an area where the rate of pertussis immunization is low, the chance of having the disease increases. The younger the age, the more severe the disease and the more often pertussis is diagnosed and reported.

The physical findings vary from the classic description to the child with a prolonged "common cold." In the infant younger than 6 months, there may be findings of respiratory distress: tachypnea, grunting, retraction, or flaring of the nostrils.

Stimulating the gag reflex with a tongue blade will often initiate a series of paroxysmal coughs and an occasional whoop. This can dramatically change the impression of the severity of the illness. Unstimulated, the child appears to be mildly to moderately ill with a prolonged cold. During a provoked paroxysm, the child may be literally fighting for oxygen. Hypoxemia in young children with pertussis has been well documented.

Diagnostic Evaluation

Although many tests assist in diagnosing pertussis, culture of a specimen taken from the nasopharynx, not the oropharynx, is still the standard. The physician should use a Dacron or calcium alginate swab.

The laboratory should be advised to identify *B. pertussis* so a special medium can be prepared. There are many false-negative results when using the culture technique, so compulsive specimen collection is critical. The swab should be placed deep in the nasopharynx for at least 10 seconds before removing. Success in obtaining a positive culture is highest during the catarrhal phase.

The direct immunofluorescent test of nasopharyngeal secretion is sensitive but requires experienced personnel, as false-negative and false-positive results occur with some regularity. A serologic fourfold rise in pertussis antigen is diagnostic, but the sensitivity is poor. The enzyme-linked immunosorbent assay (ELISA) serologic test is promising but not yet commercially available. A countercurrent immune electrophoretic urine test has been developed with a sensitivity of 85% and specificity of 100%.

Supportive laboratory findings include a complete blood cell (CBC) count with absolute lymphocytosis. The degree of lymphocytosis usually parallels the degree of the patient's cough. Chest radiographs during the illness usually show perihilar infiltrates but may demonstrate atelectasis or hyperinflation, especially in the infant.

Differential Diagnosis

The following conditions must be considered in the differential diagnosis of pertussis:

Epiglottis
Foreign body aspiration
Bacterial tracheitis
Retropharyngeal abscess
Adenoviral infections
Parapertussis
Diphtheria

Because pertussis does not always appear in its classic form, a high index of suspicion must be maintained to eliminate further spread. Infant pneumonitis may be caused by pertussis but may be also caused by *Chlamydia*, *Mycoplasma*, cytomegalovirus, or other organisms. Bronchiolitis is most often caused by respiratory syncytial virus but has been found to be caused by *B. pertussis*. In patients with altered mental status and vomiting, Reye's syndrome and sepsis should be considered. Croup, epiglottitis, foreign body aspiration, congenital deformity causing stridor, and subglottic hemangioma should be considered in the child with respiratory distress.

Therapeutic Intervention

Children with pertussis should not need emergency tracheostomy although intubation and ventilation may be required. Humidified oxygen should be administered to the child with respiratory difficulty. The child's care should include comforting, decreased stimulation, careful fluid intake, pulmonary toilet, and maintenance of a patent airway. If the diagnosis of pertussis is suspected, a surgical mask should be placed on the child, the health care worker, and all visitors to prevent droplet spread.

Erythromycin (40 to 50 mg/kg/day) is the drug of choice. It will ameliorate symptoms in the catarrhal stage and decrease the spread of organism in the paroxysmal stage. In the paroxysmal stage, erythromycin decreases the number of coughing paroxysms when administered concurrently with albuterol. Albuterol and corticosteroids may possibly reduce paroxysms but have not been studied enough to receive a formal recommendation. Hyperimmune globulin is neither recommended nor commercially available in the United States.

Disposition

A child younger than 6 months diagnosed with whooping cough and having paroxysms of coughing or respiratory distress should be admitted to the hospital to a unit offering skilled nursing and careful monitoring. A child older than 6 months having cyanosis during coughing paroxysms should also be admitted. The child should be placed in isolation with respiratory precautions for 5 days after initiation of erythromycin therapy to decrease communicability.

When making the decision not to admit, the physician should consider the ability of the child's care provider to comply with instructions, clear the child's airway, prevent aspiration, and provide close attention to the child on a continuous basis. Distance from the emergency department, facilities for communication, and transportation time should all be considered.

A consultant should be freely used in making decisions regarding admission or medical therapy. A child admitted to the hospital should be under the care of a physician capable of recognizing and managing the complications of pertussis.

Discharge Criteria

Any child who is not immunocompromised and is in the catarrhal stage may be discharged from the emergency department if the provider can care for the child (Table 67–5). The provider must be instructed to return immediately if the child becomes worse and must have the means to do so. If the child has received more than two pertussis immunizations, the physician can feel more comfortable about sending the child home, although disease has been reported in children who have been completely immunized.

TABLE 67–5

PERTUSSIS: DISCHARGE INSTRUCTIONS AND DISPOSITION

Discharge Instructions

If vomiting is occurring, feed mostly liquids.
Keep the airway clear by having the child sleep on the stomach or side; help clear vomitus and secretions during coughing and vomiting episodes.
Administer erythromycin, 40 mg/kg/day.
Return or call if there are any questions.
Keep the patient away from unimmunized and preschool children, especially infants.

Disposition

Admit children less than 6 mo old and older patients with potentially severe disease.

Other Considerations
Household Contacts

Immunization with pertussis vaccine should be considered in household contacts younger than 7 years. If the child has received three immunizations and the last was given at least 6 months previously, if immunizations have been delayed, or if the child has received four immunizations but the last was more than 3 years previously, a booster diphtheria-tetanus-pertussis (DTP) vaccine should be administered.

Erythromycin (40 to 50 mg/kg/day) is recommended for all household and close contacts and should be administered for 14 days. The adult most likely will not have severe disease but may transmit the organism to household contacts.

Day-Care Centers

Children in day-care centers who are suspected to have pertussis should be excluded from attending. If the child has had close contact with a known case, erythromycin should be administered for 14 days and the child excluded from attending the center. After 5 days of antibiotic therapy, an asymptomatic child may return, as the risk of communicability is approximately zero.

Immunization records should be reviewed and the immunizations of every person in the center made as current as possible with respect to pertussis. Erythromycin should be given to classmates of every child with pertussis. All contacts should be monitored for respiratory symptoms during the 14-day incubation period.

Health Care Providers

A close contact may be defined as someone residing in the residence of the source or a nonresident who has spent an accumulated total of 4 or more hours with the patient for 5 of the 7 days prior to recognition of illness. A health care worker attending an inpatient with active disease, especially if the care worker has young children at home, should consider taking erythromycin.

Vaccination

In areas where pertussis has been excluded from routine vaccination in a significant percentage of children, the incidence of whooping cough syndrome has increased. Furthermore, as a result of costly litigious action, the cost of the vaccine has risen, making it more difficult for parents to provide immunizations for their children. Consequently, the percentage of immunized children may decrease and the disease incidence increase. The cost-to-benefit ratio of immunization, when compared with the risk of disease, dictates that immunization be routinely recommended. There is also a requirement to report pertussis to public health authorities.

TETANUS

The incidence of tetanus in the United States is low. Of the 60 reported cases in 1988, only two were in persons less than 20 years of age. More than 50% were older than 60 years. Unfortunately, this serious disease, which has a mortality rate of approximately 50%, is increasing in the young adult population of drug addicts, where the mortality rate approaches 100%.

The causative organism, *Clostridium tetani*, is a sporiform anaerobic gram-positive bacillus that produces a potent toxin, tetanospasmin, that binds to neurons. The organism is ubiquitous and is found in soil and feces.

Pathophysiology

The microbe does not elicit an inflammatory response, so colonization is difficult to recognize early. Up to 21% of wounds that cause tetanus are not readily recognized. Classically, the organism grows best and produces clinical tetanus in a necrotic, contaminated, unattended wound.

The exotoxin *tetanospasmin* is responsible for the clinical manifestations of tetanus. Effects of the toxin are noted in motor end plates of the skeletal muscle, spinal cord, brain, and, in some cases, autonomic nervous system. Spread of the toxin from the wound appears to be intraspinal from affected motor neurons and there is some hematogenous spread to distant neuromuscular junctions. A fragment of tetanus toxin may become attached to motor neurons in 6 hours.

Clinical Evaluation

Though the history is classically represented as someone stepping on a rusty nail, only 29% of tetanus cases come from such a lesion. A history of injury should be present, but the injury may be so minor that the patient or parent has a difficult time recalling it. Entry of the organisms to the body can occur from minor injuries such as sewing needles, insect bites, skin abscesses, and ulcers. Half of the wounds causing tetanus occur indoors, and no cause of entry can be found in about 10% of patients. However, 15% of tetanus patients in the United States were found to have had wounds severe enough to meet criteria for debridement. None of these patients underwent debridement or received tetanus immune globulin, and only one received a tetanus booster. The incubation period is 3 to 21 days.

A history of complete immunization is rarely present in a person with tetanus. Indeed, there have been few cases in patients who have been completely immunized. Only 8 of 140 cases reported to the Centers for Disease Control during a 2-year period had received the initial series of immunizations, and three of those had not had a booster in the previous ten years. The majority of children getting the disease had not received immunizations.

Generalized Tetanus

Generalized tetanus is the most common presentation of the disease. The initial finding is trismus, which occurs in about 50% of the cases. Although spasms may occur unilaterally in an extremity initially, they rapidly progress to become bilateral. Dysphagia is an early symptom in 10% of the cases but may be the only finding.

Headache, irritability, and restlessness may be early findings. Spasms of the cheek muscles draw the mouth up in the classic appearance known as *risus sardonicus* (sardonic smile). Spasms occur suddenly with minimal stimulation. Opisthotonos develops with back, extremity, and neck muscle spasms. The abdominal wall becomes rigid. The patient becomes apprehensive, although the sensorium remains clear. As the disease progresses, the muscle spasms become more severe and frequent.

Tetanospasms are painful tonic contractions that are unique to tetanus. A sudden spasm of all muscle groups leads to opisthotonos, flexion and abduction of the arms, clenching of the fists on the chest, and leg extension.

Glottic and laryngeal spasms, with the chest in full inspiration, may cause cyanosis, distention of neck veins, and a red face. This is a sustained, intense Valsalva maneuver. If the airway muscles do not relax or an artificial airway is not provided, hypoxia and death will result.

The child's temperature is expected to rise from the intense muscle activity. The spasms can be triggered by mild stimulation (e.g., sound, a cool breeze, or measuring temperature).

Local Tetanus

Local tetanus is manifested by muscle spasms occurring in the area of the initial contaminated wound. There is a persistent, painful rigidity. Symptoms may last for several weeks or months and disappear without residua. However, local tetanus may also progress to generalized tetanus.

Cephalic Tetanus

Cephalic tetanus is a variation of local tetanus occurring in a patient with a head wound. Probably because of the short distance from the site of the wound to the nervous system, the incubation period is often short in this form of the disease. The head wound is often minor, being a bump, bite, or even otitis media, and the prognosis is poor. Cranial nerves may be involved. Some patients progress to generalized tetanus.

Neonatal Tetanus

The history of a child with neonatal tetanus commonly reveals birth to an unimmunized mother and the practice of placing dried fecal material on the umbilical cord remnant. In such cases the setting of the birth is not clean, and the child is exposed to tetanus organisms in the first few hours of life. Because most of these children are not born in or near a clean hospital, the prognosis remains poor, and the mortality rate is as high as 99.5%. Initially, the child will have difficulty sucking, beginning as early as the third day of life. This will progress to the generalized form with trismus, opisthotonos, generalized seizures, and respiratory obstruction.

Diagnostic Evaluation

Laboratory studies are of little benefit except to exclude other diagnoses. An elevated peripheral white blood cell count may be seen on the complete blood cell count. The erythrocyte sedimentation rate is not elevated. Gram stain or culture of the wound has a low yield but should be attempted. The cerebral spinal fluid analysis is normal. Antibody titers to the organism will rise and confirm the diagnosis, but the results will take weeks to return (Table 67–6). A silent period following elicitation of a voluntary

TABLE 67–6
TETANUS DIAGNOSIS
Definitive
Rise in antibody titers
Positive culture
Electromyography is confirmatory
Suggestive
History
Unattended wound
Immunizations not current
Malnutrition
Drug abuse
Physical
Trismus
Risus sardonicus
Severe muscle spasms with clear sensorium

jaw jerk seen in normal patients is absent in patients with tetanus.

Differential Diagnosis

The most similar, confusing diagnosis is strychnine poisoning. Such patients appear afebrile and have similar spasms induced by stimuli. Strychnine poisoning, however, is less insidious in onset. Viral encephalitis, polio, and rabies are also considerations (Table 67–7). Hypocalcemia may also cause trismus and spasms. Hyperventilation causing respiratory alkalosis with subsequent shifts in ionized calcium must also be considered.

Extrapyramidal manifestations of phenothiazine ingestion may mimic some of the early signs of tetanus. Other diagnoses to be considered include dental or peritonsillar abscess, hysteria, a black widow spider bite, or hydrofluoric acid contamination of an extremity.

Therapeutic Intervention

All patients with suspected tetanus should be admitted to the hospital. If signs of respiratory compromise are present, the child must be admitted to a unit capable of providing skilled nursing and intensive care to children, as life-threatening spasms are apt to occur.

To neutralize the toxin that is not attached to tissues, human tetanus immune globulin is given. Although optimal doses are not established, 3000 to 6000 U are recommended (Table 67–3). Half of the dose is given intramuscularly around the wound, and the other half is given in muscle at a distant site. If tetanus immune globulin is not available, tetanus antitoxin made from horses is given (at least 20,000 U intravenously). The remaining amount (total dose is 50,000 to 100,000 U) is given intramuscularly, with half given near the wound. A test dose is given initially; desensitization should be performed according to the package insert if a reaction occurs.

To stop the production of more toxin, penicillin G (100,000 U/kg/day) is given intravenously every 6 hours for 10 to 14 days. Metronidazole may also be effective, although penicillin is still the drug of choice. The wound should be debrided to deprive the organism of a fertile area for growth.

Emergency airway management should be anticipated. Children may have a spasm during which they vomit and aspirate. During seizures, oxygen should be administered with gentle suctioning of the airway and rolling on the side so that vomitus does not interfere with respiration.

The patient should be sedated. The sedative should diminish pain and anxiety during a spasm, decrease the

TABLE 67–7

DIFFERENTIAL DIAGNOSIS FOR TETANUS

Tetanus
  Intoxications
    Phencyclidine hydrochloride
    Cocaine
    Strychnine
    Phenothiazine
    Hydrofluoric acid contamination
  Seizure disorder
  Hypocalcemia
  Hypomagnesemia
  Central nervous system trauma
  Central nervous system tumor
  Viral
    Encephalomyelitis
    Poliomyelitis
    Rabies
  Hysteria
  Black widow spider bites
  Neonatal tetanus
    Hypocalcemia
    Sepsis
    Hypoglycemia
    Hypomagnesemia
    Central nervous system trauma
    Pyridoxine deficiency
    Drug withdrawal

severity and frequency of spasms, act rapidly, and not interfere with respiration. Benzodiazepines work well. The dose of diazepam is 0.20 mg given intravenously slowly. The dose of lorazepam is 0.1 mg/kg given intravenously slowly. Phenobarbital (5 to 7 mg/kg given intravenously) may be also used.

Most children with generalized tetanus require neuromuscular blockade and mechanical ventilation. Pancuronium bromide (0.1 mg/kg given intravenously) should provide paralysis. Atricurium (average dose, 1.3 mg/kg/hour) has been used as a continuous infusion for 71 days to treat a patient with tetanus. It is imperative that sedation be given in these patients, as the disease and the neuromuscular blocking agents do not impair consciousness.

Disposition

All of the patients with tetanus as a consideration should be admitted to the hospital. There is no indication to discharge these patients from the emergency department except to transfer to another institution.

Management of contacts is not necessary. Hand washing and maintenance of current immunization status are required.

Other Considerations

Like other rare diseases, it is difficult to recognize this illness in its early stages. As the child develops generalized tetanus, the diagnosis becomes more obvious.

The tetanus vaccine is effective and inexpensive. If all people have current immunization, the incidence of this disease can be diminished, if not eradicated.

Selected References

American Academy of Pediatrics, Committee on Infectious Diseases. Diphtheria. *In* Report of the Committee on Infectious Diseases. 22nd ed. Elk Grove Village, IL, American Academy of Pediatrics, 1991, p 191.

American Academy of Pediatrics, Committee on Infectious Diseases. Pertussis (whooping cough). *In* Report of the Committee on Infectious Diseases. 22nd ed. Elk Grove Village, IL, American Academy of Pediatrics, 1991, p 358.

Bowler IC, Mandal BK, Schlecht B, et al. Diphtheria—the continuing hazard. Arch Dis Child 1988;63:194.

Brooks GF. Recent trends in diphtheria in the US. J Infect Dis 1969;120:500.

Cherry JD, Brunell PA, Golden GS, et al. Report of the task force on pertussis and pertussis immunization—1988. Pediatrics 1988;81:939.

Christie CD, Baltimore RS. Pertussis in neonates. Am J Dis Child 1989; 143:1199.

Fulginiti VA, Ray GC. Missed pertussis—still with us. Am J Dis Child 1985;139:656.

Onorato IM, Wassilak S. Laboratory diagnosis of pertussis: The state of the art. Pediatr Infect Dis J 1987;6:145.

Six killers of children. World Health 1987; Jan/Feb:87.

Sotomayor J, Weiner LB, McMillan JA. Inaccurate diagnosis in infants with pertussis: An 8 year experience. Am J Dis Child 1985;139:724.

Southall DP, Thomas MG, Lambert HP. Severe hypoxaemia in pertussis. Arch Dis Child 1988;63:598.

Summary of notifiable diseases, US 1988. MMWR 1989;37:20.

Tetanus—US, 1987–1988. MMWR 1990;39:37.

CHAPTER 68

Measles, Mumps, and Rubella

Raymond B. Karasic

MEASLES (RUBEOLA)

Measles (rubeola) remains an important illness in childhood. Despite the availability of an effective vaccine, the incidence of measles in the United States has risen virtually unabated since 1983, with more than 26,000 cases reported in 1990 alone. Outbreaks of measles have occurred in all pediatric age groups, including preschoolers, school-age children, and college students.

Prompt and accurate diagnosis of measles is essential for several reasons. First, measles is not a trivial illness; although the infection is seldom fatal in developed countries, serious complications can occur and should be anticipated. Second, the clinical features of measles overlap with, and must be differentiated from, those of other potentially serious diseases. Finally, the diagnosis of measles requires that specific control measures be initiated to prevent the spread of infection to susceptible individuals.

Pathophysiology

Measles is a highly contagious illness caused by infection with the measles virus. The virus is transmitted to susceptible individuals by airborne respiratory droplets or by direct contact with infected secretions. After multiplying in the host's respiratory epithelium and lymphoid tissue, the virus invades the blood stream and disseminates; this results in a generalized viral infection involving the skin, conjunctivae, respiratory tract, and occasionally other organs. During recovery from acute infection, there is a rise in serum and secretory antibodies, accompanied by production of interferon and a cell-mediated immune response to measles virus.

Although cell-mediated immunity appears to be the principal mechanism governing recovery from acute infection, circulating antibodies play a major role in preventing clinical measles. This observation provides the rationale for administering immune globulin to susceptible individuals who are exposed to measles.

Emergency Medical Service Considerations

It is essential that prehospital personnel be protected against this preventable infection. Preemployment screening is recommended for all emergency medical service (EMS) personnel to verify their immunity to measles. Nonimmune individuals should be immunized unless there is a specific contraindication to receiving measles vaccine.

On arrival at the hospital, patients with suspected or confirmed measles should be transferred promptly to an isolation room. Isolation is important, as some outbreaks of measles have been traced to hospital waiting areas.

Clinical Evaluation

Measles is an acute illness characterized by fever, conjunctivitis, cough, coryza, Koplik's spots on the buccal mucosa, and a generalized rash. After an incubation period (from exposure to onset of symptoms) of 8 to 12 days, the illness typically begins with fever and malaise. Fever gradually increases over 5 to 6 days, peaking at 40°C or higher when the rash is fully developed. Defervescence occurs by the second or third day of the rash; fever that persists beyond that time often indicates the presence of a complication.

Within the first 24 hours of the illness, patients develop conjunctivitis, cough, and coryza, which worsen over several days. The cough is prominent and often has a brassy, croup-like quality. Unlike the conjunctivitis and nasal symptoms, both of which subside as the temperature returns to normal, the cough tends to persist for about 10 days.

On the second or third day of illness, about 2 days before the onset of the rash, Koplik's spots may be seen. These pathognomonic lesions appear as whitish specks, 1 mm in size, on a bright red mucosal background. Initially few in number, Koplik's spots rapidly spread to involve the entire buccal and labial mucosal surface. These lesions generally disappear by the third day of the rash.

The hallmark of measles is the characteristic exanthem, which first appears 3 to 4 days after the onset of illness. It begins at the hairline as a discrete, erythematous, maculopapular rash and spreads downward, reaching the feet in 3 days. As the eruption becomes generalized, the older lesions on the face and upper parts of the body become confluent, while the newer lesions remain discrete. During its evolution, the rash changes in quality from red and blanching to brownish and nonblanching. The exanthem starts to fade on the third day, proceeding in a head-to-toe direction. Disappearance of the rash is often followed by a fine desquamation, which spares the hands and feet. Patients with measles are considered contagious from 4 days before to 4 days after the appearance of the rash.

Additional symptoms and signs that occur in some patients with measles include gastrointestinal complaints (anorexia, vomiting, diarrhea, abdominal pain), generalized or regional lymphadenopathy (cervical, postauricular, or suboccipital), and splenomegaly.

The severity of measles can vary considerably. Patients who have received immune globulin after exposure to measles tend to develop a mild form of the illness known as "modified measles"; this condition also occurs in infants who contract measles just as transplacental immunity is declining. In contrast, individuals with defective cell-mediated immunity (e.g., human immunodeficiency virus infection) are prone to develop severe, occasionally fatal, cases of measles.

Complications

The principal complications of measles involve the respiratory tract or central nervous system. Otitis media is a frequent minor complication, affecting approximately 5% of children with measles; it should be suspected in any patient who experiences ear pain or persistent fever during the course of the illness. Although mild laryngitis and tracheitis are usual features of uncomplicated measles, occasionally patients can develop severe upper airway inflammation. In such cases emergent intervention may be required to relieve the airway obstruction. Pneumonia is so common in patients with measles that it probably should be considered a regular manifestation rather than a complication. In one series, more than half of patients with measles had radiographically proven infiltrates. In general, pulmonary involvement represents an extension of the viral infection, especially when the pneumonia occurs early in the course of the disease. Nevertheless, bacterial superinfection should be considered in any patient with measles who develops moderate or severe pneumonia.

Acute encephalitis occurs in about 1 out of every 1000 cases of measles and usually has its onset when the rash is present. This complication appears to result from direct viral invasion of the central nervous system. The major symptoms and signs of encephalitis include seizures, lethargy, coma, and irritability. Examination of the cerebrospinal fluid reveals pleocytosis with predominantly mononuclear cells, mild protein elevation, and a normal glucose level. Approximately 10% to 15% of patients with measles encephalitis die, and 25% suffer long-term sequelae such as mental retardation, seizures, deafness, hemiplegia, or paraplegia.

Diagnostic Evaluation

In most cases of measles, a presumptive diagnosis can be made clinically based on the characteristic evolution of symptoms and signs. Nevertheless, laboratory confirmation is recommended in all suspected cases. Although measles virus can be grown in tissue culture, isolation of the virus is technically difficult and is not widely available. Instead, most laboratories use serologic methods to confirm the diagnosis of measles. Generally this involves measurement of antibody titers to measles virus in sequential (acute and convalescent) serum samples obtained 1 to 3 weeks apart; a fourfold or greater rise in titer is considered diagnostic. Alternatively the diagnosis can be made by demonstrating measles-specific immunoglobulin M (IgM) antibody in a single serum specimen collected during the acute illness. Physicians are required to report all cases of measles to the local health department.

Differential Diagnosis

Although the differential diagnosis of measles includes all illnesses that cause a maculopapular eruption, the intensity and brownish appearance of the measles rash help distinguish it from most other viral exanthems, including those of rubella, erythema infectiosum (fifth disease), roseola, and enteroviral infections. On the other hand, certain rashes can closely mimic measles (e.g., drug eruptions and exanthems caused by *Mycoplasma pneumoniae* and Epstein-Barr virus). Fortunately, in most cases the history and physical examination provide the clues needed to differentiate measles from its many imitators.

Patients who present with the constellation of fever, rash,

and conjunctival injection pose a particular diagnostic challenge because of the number of important illnesses other than measles that share these features. These include toxic shock syndrome, Kawasaki disease, Stevens-Johnson syndrome, adenoviral infections, and leptospirosis. The hallmark of toxic shock syndrome is hypotension, which can range in severity. Children with Kawasaki disease typically have marked oral mucous membrane involvement (diffuse hyperemia, strawberry tongue, cracked lips), lymphadenopathy, and swelling of the hands and feet. In Stevens-Johnson syndrome, the rash usually progresses to a generalized bullous eruption associated with severe inflammation of all mucous membranes. Patients with leptospirosis often have evidence of hepatitis and renal insufficiency as well as a history of swimming in potentially contaminated water.

Therapeutic Intervention

Because measles is a self-limited illness, treatment is primarily supportive. Antimicrobial agents are not indicated unless a bacterial complication is present or suspected. Headache or high fever can be treated with acetaminophen.

Most individuals with measles can be managed as outpatients. Hospitalization is generally reserved for treatment of serious complications.

Prevention

Although immunization has not been a traditional focus of emergency medicine, emergency physicians need to be familiar with the schedule of routine childhood immunizations. With regard to measles, individuals are considered immune if they (1) were born before 1957, (2) have documentation of physician-diagnosed measles, (3) have laboratory evidence of immunity, or (4) have documentation of adequate vaccination. The immunization schedule for measles vaccine, given as the combined measles-mumps-rubella (MMR) vaccine, has been changed from a one-dose to a two-dose regimen. The first dose of MMR vaccine is administered at 15 months of age and the second dose at 11 to 12 years of age or (if required by law) on entry to school. Individuals who are immunocompromised should not receive MMR or other live viral vaccines. An exception is patients with HIV infection; these should receive MMR vaccine according to the routine schedule.

Management of Exposed Individuals

There are two strategies for preventing infection in susceptible persons exposed to measles: passive immunization with immune globulin and active immunization with measles vaccine. Immune globulin is recommended for susceptible household contacts of patients with measles, especially children less than 1 year of age and immunocompromised individuals. Immune globulin can be administered within 6 days of exposure; the dose is 0.25 ml/kg (0.5 ml/kg in immunocompromised patients) given intramuscularly (maximum dose, 15 ml). Individuals who receive immune globulin should be immunized with measles vaccine about 3 months later, provided that they are at least 12 months of age.

An alternative strategy to prevent measles after exposure is active immunization of susceptible individuals with measles vaccine (preferably given as the MMR vaccine). This approach is recommended for immunocompetent individuals (or those with HIV infection) who are nonhousehold contacts of measles. To be effective, the vaccine must be administered within 72 hours of measles exposure.

MUMPS

Mumps is an acute systemic illness classically associated with parotitis. Additional manifestations that are relatively common include meningoencephalitis, orchitis, pancreatitis, and inflammation of other salivary glands.

Mumps virus is spread to susceptible individuals by the respiratory route. After it enters the pharynx, the virus multiplies in local tissues, and a viremic phase ensues. The resultant localization of the virus in glandular tissue or the central nervous system (CNS) is responsible for the clinical manifestations of mumps. A mumps virus infection is subclinical in approximately 30% to 40% of individuals. In general, both symptomatic and asymptomatic infections produce permanent immunity to mumps.

Clinical Evaluation

After an incubation period of 16 to 18 days (range, 12 to 25 days), mumps parotitis is heralded by a brief prodrome consisting of fever, headache, and malaise. Within about 24 hours patients develop localized pain over the parotid gland—frequently perceived as an earache—associated with progressive swelling and tenderness. The parotid swelling obliterates the angle of the mandible and often causes the earlobe to protrude outward. Examination of the oral cavity characteristically reveals inflammation around Stensen's duct. In most patients the parotitis begins unilaterally and then progresses over 2 to 3 days to involve the opposite gland; however, in about 25% of patients the disease remains unilateral. The total duration of parotid swelling is 7 to 10 days. Individuals with mumps are usually considered contagious from 1 to 2 days before the onset of parotid swelling until 5 days after onset, but on occasion the period of communicability is longer.

Complications

Involvement of the CNS in mumps, as evidenced by cerebrospinal fluid pleocytosis, is extremely common, occurring in more than 60% of all cases of mumps. However, symptomatic meningoencephalitis is seen in only 10% of mumps cases. Mumps meningoencephalitis generally occurs several days after the onset of parotitis, but it can precede or occur in the absence of parotitis and is clinically indistinguishable from other self-limited forms of viral meningitis. The illness presents with fever, headache, vomiting, nuchal rigidity, and, occasionally, delirium or seizures. Examination of the cerebrospinal fluid reveals a lymphocytic pleocytosis. The fever and other symptoms usually subside over several days, and patients recover without sequelae.

Orchitis is a common manifestation of mumps, affecting approximately one third of postpubertal males with mumps. The onset of orchitis, which is invariably accompanied by epididymitis, generally occurs during the first week of mumps infection. Though it characteristically follows parotitis, orchitis can precede or occur without parotid involvement. The illness begins with fever, chills, headache, nausea, and vomiting; abdominal pain may be prominent. As the fever appears, the testis becomes swollen, painful, and markedly tender. The duration of testicular involvement parallels the course of the fever, which lasts a median of 4 days. Fortunately, in 75% to 90% of patients with mumps orchitis, the process remains unilateral. As a result, although orchitis can lead to testicular atrophy, impotence or sterility are rarely sequelae of mumps.

Involvement of the pancreas is common during the course of mumps. Although pancreatitis can be severe, patients usually recover completely. Occasionally other glands are infected by mumps virus, resulting in a variety of unusual manifestations, including dacryoadenitis, thyroiditis, mastitis, oophoritis, and inflammation of Bartholin's gland.

Diagnostic Evaluation

A presumptive diagnosis of mumps can be made in patients with clinical evidence of nonsuppurative parotitis, especially during the late winter or spring months, and confirmatory tests are unnecessary. On the other hand, specific diagnostic tests should be considered in any atypical or severe illness (e.g., meningoencephalitis or orchitis) that is compatible with mumps. Although mumps virus can be isolated in tissue culture, serologic tests are the usual means of confirming mumps infection. If possible, paired (acute and convalescent) serum specimens should be obtained about 2 weeks apart for measurement of serum antibodies.

Differential Diagnosis

Other viruses that can cause acute parotitis include coxsackievirus, influenza virus, parainfluenza viruses, and cytomegalovirus. The most important entity to differentiate from mumps is suppurative parotitis, usually caused by *Staphylococcus aureus* or oral anaerobic bacteria. In this condition the parotid gland is extremely tender, and pus can be expressed from Stensen's duct; high fever and leukocytosis may be present. Noninfectious causes of acute parotid swelling include obstruction of Stensen's duct by calculi and insufflation of the gland caused by forceful blowing (e.g., into a balloon or wind instrument).

A variety of inflammatory processes can mimic parotitis; these include preauricular or cervical lymphadenitis, buccal cellulitis (caused by *Haemophilus influenzae* type b), odontogenic (dental) infection, osteomyelitis of the mandible (including actinomycosis), and Caffey's disease. In general these processes can be distinguished from parotitis by the distribution of the swelling and associated clinical features.

Therapeutic Intervention

As with measles, the treatment of mumps is supportive. Analgesic drugs are indicated for headache or pain associated with parotitis or orchitis. Patients who have severe or persistent vomiting as a result of meningoencephalitis may require intravenous administration of fluids. Mumps is generally a mild, self-limited illness, and thus hospitalization is seldom necessary.

Mumps vaccine is extremely effective in preventing mumps. It is given as a component of the MMR vaccine in a two-dose schedule as described earlier for measles.

There is no evidence that administration of mumps vaccine prevents infection in susceptible persons after exposure to mumps. On the other hand, immunization with mumps vaccine can protect against subsequent exposures and therefore should be considered in nonimmune individuals exposed to mumps infection.

RUBELLA

Rubella (German measles) is a mild, acute illness characterized by a 3-day rash and postauricular and suboccipital lymphadenopathy. Although rubella is a benign disease when acquired postnatally, infection during pregnancy can have severe consequences for the developing fetus, including spontaneous abortion, stillbirth, and congenital malformations. As with measles, there has been an increase in the incidence of rubella in the United States. Therefore an accurate diagnosis is essential to prevent the transmission of rubella, particularly to pregnant women.

Pathophysiology

Rubella virus is transmitted by the respiratory route. After infecting the respiratory epithelium, the virus replicates, enters the blood stream, and disseminates. Rubella infection is asymptomatic in 25% to 50% of cases. Infection with rubella virus induces both humoral and cell-mediated immune responses and usually results in permanent immunity.

Clinical Evaluation

After a typical incubation period of 16 to 18 days (range, 14 to 21 days), the first symptoms of rubella appear. In children there is no prodrome, and the first sign of rubella is the rash. In older patients the rash is usually preceded by a brief prodrome consisting of headache, malaise, anorexia, nausea, low-grade fever, conjunctivitis, coryza, sore throat, cough, and lymphadenopathy.

The exanthem of rubella is a pinkish-red maculopapular eruption that starts on the face and rapidly spreads downward to involve the neck, trunk, and extremities. The entire body is covered with discrete maculopapules by the end of the first day. The rash begins to fade on the second day, starting at the face, and usually by the end of the third day the entire rash has disappeared. Patients with postnatal rubella are considered contagious from a few days before until 5 to 7 days after the onset of the rash.

The temperature in rubella is characteristically normal, although low-grade fever can occur. During the prodrome or on the first day of the rash, an enanthem may be seen. The typical oral lesions are pinpoint reddish spots (Forschheimer spots) on the soft palate. Unlike Koplik's spots in measles, Forschheimer spots are not pathognomonic for rubella.

Lymphadenopathy in rubella is often detectable several days before the onset of the rash. Although generalized lymphadenopathy is usually present to some extent, involvement of the postauricular, suboccipital, and cervical lymph node chains is most characteristic of (but not pathognomonic for) rubella. Lymph node enlargement can persist for several weeks.

Joint involvement (arthralgias or arthritis) is uncommon in young children with rubella but occurs frequently in adolescent and adult patients. The process, which generally begins on the second or third day of the illness, can involve any number of large joints (knees, ankles, elbows) or small joints (hands). Treatment with nonsteroidal anti-inflammatory drugs is indicated in moderate or severe cases.

The most important complication of rubella infection is congenital rubella, which results from fetal infection during the first trimester of pregnancy. The congenital rubella syndrome, as originally described, was characterized by low birth weight, mental retardation, microcephaly, cataracts, deafness, and congenital heart disease. It is now recognized that intrauterine rubella infection can produce a much broader spectrum of abnormalities.

Thrombocytopenic purpura is an unusual complication of rubella, occurring in 1 out of every 3000 cases. The purpura usually follows the exanthem by several days. Although the problem is usually self-limited, the administration of intravenous immunoglobulin is of potential benefit. Encephalitis associated with rubella is rare, with an estimated incidence of 1 in 6000 cases. The clinical illness is similar to other postinfectious encephalitides. Most patients recover completely but may have residual electroencephalographic abnormalities.

Diagnostic Evaluation

The diagnosis of rubella should be considered in any patient who presents with a pinkish-red maculopapular rash, low-grade fever, and lymphadenopathy. Nevertheless, because of the similarity to other infectious exanthems and the epidemiologic importance of identifying rubella, laboratory confirmation is recommended in all suspected cases. The diagnosis of rubella can be confirmed by viral isolation or serologic testing. Although it is advisable to obtain sequential (acute and convalescent) serum samples for antibody determination, many laboratories can detect specific rubella IgM in a single specimen collected during the acute phase of the illness.

Differential Diagnosis

Most of the classic exanthematous diseases (measles, scarlet fever, erythema infectiosum, roseola infantum) can be differentiated from rubella on clinical grounds. However, several other infectious agents produce exanthems that closely mimic rubella, including enteroviruses, Epstein-Barr virus, and *M. pneumoniae*.

Therapeutic Intervention

Most cases of rubella are so mild that treatment is unnecessary. Hospitalization is rarely indicated. Headache can be treated with acetaminophen. Nonsteroidal anti-inflammatory drugs such as aspirin or ibuprofen can be used to treat arthritis. Patients with severe thrombocytopenia may require the administration of intravenous immunoglobulin.

Management of Exposed Individuals

When a pregnant woman is exposed to rubella, a blood sample should be obtained promptly and tested for rubella antibodies. If antibodies are detectable, then the woman is immune to rubella and the fetus is at no risk. If antibodies are not present, the test should be repeated about 3 weeks (and, if necessary, 6 weeks) later. If antibodies are detectable in the second (or third) specimen, it should be assumed that infection has occurred. Although the routine use of immune globin is not recommended for routine prophylaxis after exposure to rubella in early pregnancy, it may be considered if termination of pregnancy is not an option.

Administration of rubella vaccine does not prevent infection in susceptible persons after exposure to rubella. Nevertheless, immunization with rubella vaccine can protect against future exposures and therefore should be considered.

Selected References

Alpert G, Plotkin SA. A practical guide to the diagnosis of congenital infections in the newborn infant. Pediatr Clin North Am 1986;33(3):465.

Bakshi SS, Cooper LZ. Rubella. Clin Dermatol 1989;7(1):8.

Best JM, Banatvala JE, Morgan-Capner P, Miller E. Fetal infection after maternal reinfection with rubella: Criteria for defining reinfection. Br Med J 1989;299(6702):773.

Bligard CA, Millikan LE. Acute exanthems in children. Clues to differential diagnosis of viral disease. Postgrad Med 1986;79(5):150.

Boodley CA, Jaquis JL. Measles, mumps, rubella and chickenpox in the adult population. Nurse Pract 1989 Feb;14(2):12, 14, 16 passim.

Chaudary S, Jaski BE. Fulminant mumps myocarditis. Ann Intern Med 1989;110(7):569.

Cochi SL, Edmonds LE, Dyer K, Greaves WL, et al. Congenital rubella syndrome in the United States, 1980–1985. Am J Epidemiol 1989;129(2):349.

Freij BJ, South MA, Sever JL. Maternal rubella and the congenital rubella syndrome. Clin Perinatol 1988;15(2):247.

Fulginiti VA, Helfer RE. Atypical measles in adolescent siblings 16 years after killed measles virus vaccine. JAMA 1980;244(8):804.

Gordon SC, Lauter CB. Mumps arthritis: A review of the literature. Rev Infect Dis 1984;6(3):338.

Grattan-Smith PJ, Procopis PG, Wise GA, Grigor WG. Serious neurological complications of measles—a continuing preventable problem. Med J Aust 1985;143(9):385.

Hinman AR, Orenstein WA, Bloch AB, et al. Impact of measles in the United States. Rev Infect Dis 1983;5(3):439.

Hossain A, Bakir TM. Rubella and cytomegalovirus (CMV) infections: Laboratory aspects of investigation of antenatal, congenital, persistent, and subclinical infections. J Trop Pediatr 1989;35(5):225.

Istre GR, McKee PA, West GR, et al. Measles spread in medical settings: An important focus of disease transmission? Pediatrics 1987;79(3):356.

Khoury MJ, Erickson JD, Cordero JF, McCarthy BJ. Congenital malformations and intrauterine growth retardation: A population study. Pediatrics 1988;82(1):83.

Kinney JS, Kumar ML. Should we expand the TORCH complex? Clin Perinatol 1988;15(4):727.

Koskiniemi M, Donner M, Pettay O. Clinical appearance and outcome in mumps encephalitis in children. Acta Paediatr Scand 1983;72(4):603.

Labay MV, Ramos R, Hervas JA, et al. Membranous laryngotracheobronchitis, a complication of measles. Intensive Care Med 1985;11(6):326.

Leads from the MMWR. Rubella and congenital rubella—United States, 1984–1986. JAMA 1987;258(18):2491.

Manson AL. Mumps orchitis. Urology 1990;36(4):355.

Mast EE, Berg JL, Hanrahan LP, et al. Risk factors for measles in a previously vaccinated population and cost-effectiveness of revaccination strategies. JAMA 1990;264(19):2529.

McAnally T. Parotitis: Clinical presentations and management. Postgrad Med 1982;71(2):87.

Meyer HM Jr, Hopps HE, Parkman PD, Ennis FA. Control of measles and rubella through use of attenuated vaccines. Am J Clin Pathol 1978;70(suppl):128.

Miller CL. Surveillance after measles vaccination in children. Practitioner 1982;226(1365):535.

Murtagh J. Rubella. Aust Fam Physician 1987;16(11):1652.

Newton-John H, Murtagh J. Epidemic parotitis. Aust Fam Physician 1986;15(7):905.

Siegel MM, Walter TK, Ablin AR. Measles pneumonia in childhood leukemia. Pediatrics 1977;60(1):38.

Srugo I, Brunell PA. Measles vaccine. Pediatr Ann 1990;19(12):708.

Strome M. Non-neoplastic salivary gland diseases in children. Otolaryngol Clin North Am 1977;10(2):391.

Tarr RW, Edwards KM, Kessler RM, Kulkarni MV. MRI of mumps encephalitis: Comparison with CT evaluation. Pediatr Radiol 1987;17(1):59.

Wintermeyer L, Myers MG. Measles in a partially immunized community. Am J Public Health 1979;69(9):923.

Zilber N, Rannon L, Alter M, Kahana E. Measles, measles vaccination, and risk of subacute sclerosing panencephalitis. Neurology 1983;33(12):1558.

CHAPTER 69

Chickenpox

Raymond B. Karasic

INTRODUCTION

Chickenpox, also known as *varicella*, is a common, highly contagious disease characterized by a distinctive vesicular rash. Although the illness is generally associated with mild symptoms in otherwise healthy children, adults with chickenpox tend to have more severe manifestations. Varicella is of particular concern in immunocompromised individuals and pregnant women, whose offspring are at risk for developing congenital malformations or overwhelming infection.

Although a vaccine to prevent varicella has been available, it is not yet licensed for use in the United States. As a result, chickenpox remains one of the most common afflictions of childhood.

PATHOPHYSIOLOGY

Chickenpox results from primary infection with varicella zoster (VZ) virus, a member of the herpesvirus family. The virus is transmitted to susceptible individuals by direct contact with varicella or zoster skin lesions or by airborne droplets originating from such lesions. Although respiratory spread of VZ virus is also believed to occur, there is surprisingly little evidence to support this mechanism of transmission.

After entering the upper respiratory tract of the host, the virus multiplies in regional lymph nodes. Viremia ensues, which transports VZ virus to the skin and other organs. Acute infection leads to activation of both humoral and cell-mediated immune responses. Primary infection with VZ virus generally confers lifelong immunity, although second episodes of chickenpox have been reported.

Varicella zoster virus, like other herpesviruses, can produce a latent infection. After the primary infection (chickenpox), VZ virus enters a latent phase within the host's sensory ganglia. Subsequent reactivation of the latent virus results in zoster, or shingles. The development of zoster is associated with factors that depress cellular immunity to VZ virus, such as malignancy and the use of immunosuppressive medications.

CLINICAL EVALUATION

The symptoms and signs of varicella appear after an incubation period of 10 to 21 days. Although the rash is often the first indicator of illness, it is sometimes preceded by a prodrome consisting of low-grade fever, malaise, and headache.

In chickenpox the exanthem begins on the scalp or trunk and gradually becomes concentrated in the central portions of the body, especially the trunk and proximal extremities. In addition, varicella lesions tend to cluster at sites of preexisting skin inflammation (e.g., sunburn or atopic dermatitis). As a rule the rash is intensely pruritic. The lesions evolve rapidly from macules to papules to vesicles to crusts (scabs). A hallmark of chickenpox is the presence of lesions in all stages of development within a single area. The classical lesion in varicella is a thin-walled vesicle, 2 to 3 mm in diameter, sitting on an erythematous base, often described as a "dew drop on a rose petal."

The rash generally appears in several crops over 3 or more days; by the end of the first week, most lesions are crusted over. Patients with chickenpox are considered contagious from 1 to 2 days before the onset of the rash until all the lesions have crusted over (generally 5 to 7 days after the onset of the rash).

Mucous membrane involvement often occurs during the course of varicella. The most commonly affected site is the oral cavity, where the lesions appear as multiple vesicles or shallow ulcers.

Zoster represents the reactivation of latent VZ virus in a previously infected individual. Because the latent virus is localized in sensory nerve ganglia, the lesions of zoster have a characteristic unilateral dermatomal distribution that corresponds to the nerve roots affected. Although the trunk is the most common site of involvement, zoster can also occur on the face. Morphologically the lesions resemble those seen with varicella and evolve in a similar fashion. Marked neuralgia, which is a prominent symptom of zoster, is more common in adults than in children.

COMPLICATIONS

Although most patients with varicella or zoster recover uneventfully, immunocompromised individuals are prone to develop severe manifestations and complications. A distinctive hemorrhagic form of chickenpox occurs in some patients; others may exhibit less specific signs of disseminated or focal infection. Varicella tends to be more severe in adults than in children. Infected adults typically have high fever and a dense rash and also have a propensity to develop complications, especially pneumonia.

Varicella has been associated with congenital malformations (particularly limb scarring and atrophy) in infants whose mothers contracted the illness during early pregnancy. Fortunately this syndrome is extremely rare. Of greater concern is the neonate born to a woman who develops chickenpox within 5 days of delivery; such infants are at risk for disseminated, often fatal, varicella. The proposed reason for this complication is that pregnant women who have varicella for less than 5 days have not yet produced protective antibodies that can be passively transferred to their newborns.

The most frequent complication of varicella is bacterial superinfection of the skin lesions, usually by *Staphylococcus aureus* or group A beta-hemolytic streptococci. A wide spectrum of secondary infections can occur, including impetigo (usually bullous), erysipelas, cellulitis, and myositis.

Although pneumonia is a rare complication of chickenpox in healthy children, it is relatively common in adults and immunocompromised individuals with varicella. This complication, which can range in severity from mild to severe, is clinically similar to pneumonia caused by other viral agents.

Central nervous system involvement occurs in less than 1 of every 1000 cases of varicella. The most common manifestation is acute cerebellitis, which usually begins a week or more after the onset of varicella. Patients with this complication present with ataxia; examination of the cerebrospinal fluid typically reveals a lymphocytic pleocytosis with elevated protein and normal glucose levels. The illness lasts from several days to a few weeks and complete recovery is the rule. Rarely, varicella can cause a more severe form of encephalitis associated with cerebral edema and seizures. Additional neurologic complications of varicella include optic neuritis, transverse myelitis, and Guillain-Barré syndrome.

Reye's syndrome is a serious disorder characterized by encephalopathy and liver dysfunction. It generally has its onset during the recovery phase of certain viral infections, notably varicella and influenza type A or B. Reye's syndrome appears to be associated with the administration of salicylates during the antecedent viral infection. Fortunately this complication is now rare.

DIAGNOSTIC EVALUATION

Most cases of chickenpox or zoster can be diagnosed clinically by the characteristic rash; in such cases laboratory confirmation is unnecessary. When verification of the diagnosis is required, VZ virus can be cultivated from vesicular lesions, although viral isolation may take more than a week. Serologic methods can also be used to confirm the diagnosis; this involves measuring VZ antibody titers in acute and convalescent serum specimens collected 2 or more weeks apart. Another useful diagnostic technique is the Tzanck smear, which is prepared by scraping the base of a vesicle and staining the specimen obtained. The demonstration of multinucleate giant cells (with or without intranuclear inclusions) indicates the presence of a herpesvirus infection. Though not specific for VZ virus, this method has the advantage of providing rapid results.

DIFFERENTIAL DIAGNOSIS

Entities that can occasionally mimic chickenpox include disseminated herpes simplex infection, eczema herpeticum, impetigo, insect bites, and scabies. Herpes simplex virus infection can also produce a zoster-like eruption, particularly in neonates.

THERAPEUTIC INTERVENTION

Symptomatic treatment is generally sufficient for uncomplicated cases of chickenpox or zoster. Oral antihistamines can be used to relieve the pruritus. Drying agents, such as calamine lotion, may also be helpful; on the other hand, topically applied medications containing diphenhydramine should be avoided because of the risk of systemic absorption and consequent toxicity. Children should have their fingernails cut short to prevent the premature removal of scabs, which can lead to scarring. Acetaminophen is the preferred agent for treating fever or pain; aspirin should be avoided, as it may increase the risk of Reye's syndrome.

Immunocompromised patients who develop varicella or zoster and all patients with severe or disseminated varicella infection should be treated intravenously with acyclovir. For children less than 1 year old, the dosage of acyclovir is 30 mg/kg/day given intravenously in three divided doses for 7 to 10 days; in children 1 year old or older, the regimen is 1500 mg/m²/day in three divided doses given intravenously for 7 to 10 days. Although acyclovir has been used orally in patients with varicella and zoster, the indications for this route of administration have not been defined. Nevertheless, treatment with the oral form of acyclovir should be considered for certain high-risk patients, such as individuals 15 years of age or older who contract varicella.

DISPOSITION

Varicella is generally a mild, self-limited illness. Hospitalization is indicated primarily for the treatment of severe complications.

MANAGEMENT OF EXPOSED INDIVIDUALS

Susceptible individuals who are prone to develop progressive varicella after exposure should receive passive protection with varicella zoster immune globulin (VZIG). Candidates for VZIG administration after a significant exposure to varicella has occurred include immunocompromised, susceptible children; susceptible adolescents (>15 years old) and adults, especially pregnant women; neonates whose mothers have onset of varicella within 5 days before delivery or 2 days after delivery; and hospitalized premature infants. If possible, VZIG should be given within 48 hours of exposure and generally not more than 96 hours after exposure. The dose of VZIG is 125 U (one vial) for every 10 kg of body weight, given intramuscularly; the maximum dose is 625 U (five vials).

Selected References

American Academy of Pediatrics. Report of the Committee on Infectious Diseases. 22nd ed. Elk Grove Village, IL, American Academy of Pediatrics, 1991.

Asano Y, Itakura N, Kajita Y, et al. Severity of viremia and clinical findings in children with varicella. J Infect Dis 1990;161(6):1095.

Balfour HH Jr, Kelly JM, Suarez CS, et al. Acyclovir treatment of varicella in otherwise healthy children. J Pediatr 1990;116(4):633.

Brunell PA. Varicella-zoster infections. In Feigin RD, Cherry JD (eds). Textbook of Pediatric Infectious Diseases. 2nd ed. Philadelphia, WB Saunders, 1987.

DaSilva O, Hammerberg O, Chance GW. Fetal varicella syndrome. Pediatr Infect Dis J 1990;9(11):854.

Davis HW, Karasic RB. Pediatric infectious disease. In Zitelli B, Davis HW (eds). Atlas of Pediatric Physical Diagnosis. 2nd ed. New York, Gower Medical, 1992.

Feldman S, Moffitt JE. Varicella vaccine. Pediatr Ann 1990;19(12):721.

Krugman S, Katz SL, Gershon AA, Wilfert CM. Varicella-zoster infections. In Infectious Diseases of Children. 8th ed. St Louis, CV Mosby, 1985.

Moore DA, Hopkins RS. Assessment of a school exclusion policy during a chickenpox outbreak. Am J Epidemiol 1991;133(11):1161.

Prober CG, Gershon AA, Grose C, et al. Consensus: Varicella-zoster infections in pregnancy and the perinatal period. Pediatr Infect Dis J 1990;9(12):865.

Tsolia M, Gershon AA, Steinberg SP, Gelb L. Live attenuated varicella vaccine: Evidence that the virus is attenuated and the importance of skin lesions in transmission of varicella-zoster virus. J Pediatr 1990;116(2):184.

White CJ, Kuter BJ, Hildebrand CS, et al. Varicella vaccine (VARIVAX) in healthy children and adolescents: Results from clinical trials, 1987 to 1989. Pediatrics 1991;87(5):604.

CHAPTER 70

Toxic Shock Syndrome

Marsha D. Rappley
Sid M. Shah

INTRODUCTION

Toxic shock syndrome (TSS) is an acute febrile exanthematous illness associated with multisystem failure and profound, rapidly progressive shock. The mortality rate is 2.6% to 10% in menstruation-related disease and up to 50% in cases not associated with menstrual or vaginal sources of infection. The primary causative organism is *Staphylococcus aureus*. Streptococcal disease has also been implicated in a similar condition known as *toxic strep syndrome*.

TSS was first identified in 1978 in a series of seven children. A highly toxic disease was described, with affected individuals showing signs of only localized infection despite generalized multisystem involvement. Although uncommon in prepubertal children, TSS is a major consideration in the evaluation of toxic exanthematous disease in young people.

There is extensive documentation of nonmenstrual TSS. It has been associated with surgical wounds that do not appear inflamed, apparently minor wounds such as newly pierced ears, nasal surgery, nasal packing, surgical implants and splints, exit wounds of dialysis procedures, injection sites of insulin pumps, fasciitis, osteomyelitis, staphylococcal empyema, peritonsillar abscess, and cutaneous and subcutaneous abscesses. Vaginal sources of infection have occurred with the use of the contraceptive diaphragm and sponge, in the postpartum period, and after septic abortion. It has been described in burned children and adults, as well as in patients with human immunodeficiency virus (HIV) infection. TSS has occurred after influenza and influenza-like illness, most likely as a result of colonization of lower airways with *S. aureus*. It has also been described in association with bacterial tracheitis, croup, and sinusitis in children.

Approximately 60% to 80% of cases of TSS occur in menstruating women. One third of these cases occur in women between the ages of 15 and 19 years, with a mean age of 22 years and a range of 11 to 61 years. The mean age of cases not related to menstruation is 27 years. White women have been identified in 98% of menstruation-associated cases of TSS, but there is no significant difference in the sex or race of patients with nonmenstrual TSS. The incidence of menstruation-related cases appears to fluctuate, whereas the incidence of nonmenstrual cases remains more stable.

The peak onset of menstruation-associated TSS is the fourth menstrual day. It is less common in sexually active than in sexually inactive young women.

In 1980 an epidemiologic report of the association of TSS with a specific brand of highly absorbent tampon resulted in the removal of that brand from the market. Subsequent studies have continued to demonstrate an association among TSS, menstruation, and the use of highly absorbent tampons.

PATHOGENESIS

S. aureus associated with TSS is a phenotypically distinct organism. Isolates in TSS have been associated with the elaboration of toxic shock syndrome toxin-1 (TSST-1), staphylococcal enterotoxins A through E, gram-negative endotoxin, and endogenous host mediators. The precise mechanism of action, however, remains unclear.

TSST-1 is a potent T-cell mitogen in vitro and a potent stimulus for macrophage production of interleukin-1 (IL-1). TSST-1 has a significant immunosuppressive effect and may induce a state of hyperresponsiveness to endotoxin. Ninety per cent to 100% of S. aureus isolates of vaginal or cervical cultures obtained during menstruation produce TSST-1. However, only 40% to 64% of S. aureus isolates in nonmenstrual cases of TSS produce TSST-1. Both TSST-1–positive and TSST-1–negative isolates of TSS producing S. aureus induce morbidity and death in animal models in a manner that cannot be differentiated. Nonetheless, TSS associated with a nonmenstrual source of infection has a significantly higher fatality rate in humans.

Staphylococcal enterotoxins A through E have been associated with TSS. Enterotoxins A, B, C1, and D have been associated with TSST-1–negative strains. It appears these are capable of inducing TSS without the presence of TSST-1. Endotoxin from gram-negative bacteria has been associated with TSS but does not appear to be an essential mediator of the disease.

Several endogenous mediators, primarily IL-1 and tumor necrosis factor (TNF) appear to play a significant role in the pathogenesis of TSS. IL-1 is responsible for fever and other acute phase responses to inflammation. TSST-1 is an extremely potent stimuli for production of IL-1 by macrophages. TSST-1 also stimulates production of TNF, which directly stimulates production of IL-1, enhances the effects of endotoxin, and also inhibits migration of polymorphonuclear leukocytes. The latter effect may explain why an apparently innocuous wound may be associated with a highly toxic disease state.

TSST-1–producing strains of S. aureus frequently colonize nasal and vaginal mucosa. More than 90% of adults have circulating antibody to TSST-1 but have never had TSS. It is suggested that over time, women are likely to be colonized with TSST-1–producing staphylococci and that this may be episodic. Carrier states of vaginal and nasal colonization may be related. The carrier state exists in a similar distribution for both: 25% persistent, 50% intermittent, and 25% noncarriers.

Toxic Strep Syndrome

The clinical features of TSS produced by S. aureus are similar to those produced by group A streptococci in scarlet fever and sepsis. A severe toxic shock–like syndrome associated with streptococcal infection and scarlet fever toxin A has been described in a series of 20 patients. It is known that staphylococcal enterotoxin B and Streptococcus pyogenes exotoxin A share an extensive homology of primary molecular structure. Throughout history the exotoxin A of group A beta-hemolytic streptococcus (S. pyogenes) has been associated with virulent, highly toxic strains causing epidemics of scarlet fever, erysipelas, and sepsis. The reappearance of exotoxin A may indicate the resurgence of streptococcal strains that have increased potential to produce highly toxic disease. It is possible that preoccupation with staphylococcal TSS has resulted in a lack of recognition and underdiagnosis of the toxic strep syndrome. Toxic strep syndrome is more likely to be associated with an obvious soft tissue infection such as necrotizing fasciitis or empyema or a deep space infection such as osteomyelitis. This may not be associated with a scarlatiniform rash.

CLINICAL EVALUATION

The clinical presentation of TSS ranges from a relatively mild illness to a fulminant, rapidly fatal disease. The typical patient presents with a sudden onset of high fever associated with vomiting, diarrhea, headache, pharyngitis, profound myalgia, and profound hypotension, followed by tissue ischemia and multisystem organ failure.

The hypotension of TSS is profound and prolonged. It likely results from two mechanisms. There is a decrease in vasomotor tone as measured by a low systemic vascular resistance. This is compounded by the rapid onset of capillary vasodilation and nonhydrostatic leakage of fluid and colloid from the intravascular to the interstitial space. This is reflected in extensive generalized nonpitting edema that becomes apparent after fluid resuscitation.

Mental status changes include confusion, disorientation, and agitation. Other central nervous system (CNS) symptoms may include severe headaches and seizures. These may be caused by a toxic encephalopathy associated with TSS or the effect of hypotension. Typically there are no focal neurologic deficits. Diffuse cerebral edema is evident in histopathologic examination.

Intense conjunctival hyperemia is characteristic of TSS. The vascular dilation, pooling, and congestion of conjunctival vessels frequently cause subconjunctival and scleral hemorrhage.

Erythema and injection of the oropharyngeal mucosa, tongue, tympanic membranes, and vaginal mucosa is also common. The commonly described "strawberry tongue" or "raspberry tongue" appearance is caused by intense mucosal erythema.

The classic rash is a diffuse, fine maculopapular erythroderma often described as a scarlatiniform or sunburn rash. It appears early in the illness, first on the trunk and then spreading to the arms and legs, most prominently over the flexor surfaces. There may be marked erythema and edema of the palms and soles. Generalized desquamation of the hands and feet occurs 10 to 20 days into the illness. A pruritic, red, maculopapular rash has been reported 9 to 13 days after presentation in more than 50% of patients (Table 70–1).

Pulmonary complications are a leading cause of death in children with TSS. The child may present with difficulty breathing and progress rapidly to respiratory failure as a result of the development of noncardiogenic pulmonary edema (adult respiratory distress syndrome, or ARDS). In a hypotensive patient pulmonary involvement may not be immediately apparent until fluid resuscitation is well under way.

The decompensation of myocardial function is clearly the

TABLE 70-1

DERMATOLOGIC FEATURES IN TSS

Feature	Characteristics
Diffuse macular erythroderma (scarlatiniform rash)	Early and often transient; nonpruritic; initially over trunk, then spreading to arms and legs; flexural accentuation.
Petechiae, vesicles, and bullae	Uncommon.
Intense erythema of conjunctivae and all mucous membranes	Early and characteristic findings.
Subconjunctival or subscleral hemorrhage	
Strawberry or raspberry tongue	
Generalized nonpitting edema	Early and common. Edema particularly involves palms and soles.
Offending surgical or traumatic wound	Often noninflamed and nonpurulent.
Erythematous generalized urticarial maculopapular rash	Often pruritic; apparent at 7 to 14 days.
Desquamation of fingers, toes, palms, and soles	Apparent at 10 to 21 days.
Telogen effluvium (hair loss)	

Modified from Chesney PJ. Clinical aspects and spectrum of illness of toxic shock syndrome: Overview. Rev Infect Dis 1989;2(suppl 1):s3. Published by The University of Chicago Press.

most life-threatening event in TSS. Arrythmia may be the presenting sign. Postmortem examination of fatal TSS cases has confirmed the presence of cardiomyopathy, although the precise cause of this is unclear. The pathologic changes in myocardium may reflect toxin-mediated events. Alternatively, TNF may affect the transmembrane potential of myocardial fibers as it does skeletal muscle fibers.

Diffuse abdominal pain and tenderness can occur, but signs of peritoneal irritation are absent. Hepatomegaly may be present. The secretory, profuse diarrhea that develops at the onset of the illness is found in almost all patients with TSS. Fecal incontinence is common, and stool examination generally reveals an abnormally high number of neutrophils. Myalgias primarily involve the proximal limbs and the abdominal, lumbar, and cervical muscles. These muscles are frequently tender.

Acute renal failure is a common manifestation and appears to be the result of both toxin-mediated intrinsic renal damage and prerenal failure. Decreased urine output is common, particularly in patients in a hypotensive state. A foul-smelling cervical discharge may be present on pelvic examination, in addition to menstrual flow. Other findings may include tender external genitalia, vaginal ulcerations, and vaginal and vulvar hyperemia.

TSS can recur. The highest risk for recurrent disease is in untreated, menstruation-associated disease. TSS may recur repeatedly, with intensity and frequency varying with the menstrual cycle. The possibility of recurrent disease makes eradication of the organism a primary goal of treatment.

DIAGNOSTIC EVALUATION
Laboratory Studies

Leukocytosis with an increased number of immature neutrophils is common. Thrombocytopenia is generally present,

and if disseminated intravascular coagulation supervenes, marked thrombocytopenia, in addition to the presence of fibrinogen degradation products and abnormal bleeding and clotting times, will be present.

Diagnostic criteria for TSS include an elevated total bilirubin level and a hepatic transaminase level at least twice the upper limit of normal (see Table 70–1). When total bilirubin is elevated, the direct (conjugated) fraction is predominant.

Diagnostic criteria also include blood urea nitrogen (BUN) and creatinine levels of at least twice the upper limit of normal or urinary sediment with pyuria (>5 white blood cells [WBCs] per high power field [HPF] in the absence of a urinary tract infection [UTI]) (Table 70–2). Dramatically elevated serum concentration of creatinine phosphokinase usually accompanies generalized myalgias and severe muscle tenderness.

Laboratory evaluation should include appropriate cultures. Blood, throat, and cerebrospinal fluid (CSF) cultures are usually negative, but specimens obtained from a locally infected site, including vaginal cultures, may grow *S. aureus*. Bacteremia is not typically present.

More than 85% of all patients with TSS have hypocal-

TABLE 70-2

TOXIC SHOCK SYNDROME: CENTERS FOR DISEASE CONTROL CASE DEFINITION FOR PUBLIC HEALTH SURVEILLANCE

Clinical case definition
An illness with the following clinical manifestations:
1. Fever: temperature 38.9°C (102°F).
2. Rash: diffuse macular erythroderma.
3. Desquamation: 1–2 wk after the onset of illness, particularly palms and soles.
4. Hypotension: systolic blood pressure <90 mm Hg for adults or less than fifth percentile by age for children <16 yr of age; orthostatic drop in diastolic blood pressure >15 mm Hg from lying to sitting; orthostatic syncope or orthostatic dizziness.
5. Multisystem involvement: three or more of the following:
— Gastrointestinal: vomiting or diarrhea at onset of illness.
— Muscular: severe myalgia or creatinine phosphokinase level at least twice the upper limit of normal.
— Mucous membranes: vaginal, oropharyngeal, or conjunctival hyperemia.
— Renal: blood urea nitrogen or creatinine level at least twice the upper limit of normal for laboratory or urinary sediment with pyuria (>5 leukocytes per high power field) in the absence of urinary tract infection.
— Hepatic: total bilirubin, aspartate aminotransferase (AST), or alanine aminotransferase (ALT) level at least twice the upper limit of normal.
— Hematologic: platelets <100,000/mm.
— Central nervous system: disorientation or alterations in consciousness without focal neurologic signs when fever and hypotension are absent.
6. Negative results on the following tests, if obtained:
— Blood, throat, or cerebrospinal fluid cultures (blood culture may be positive for *Staphylococcus aureus*).
— Rise in titer to Rocky Mountain spotted fever, leptospirosis, or measles.
Case classification
Probable: a case with five of the six clinical findings described above.
Confirmed: a case with all six of the clinical findings described above, including desquamation, unless the patient died before desquamation could occur

From Centers for Disease Control. Case definitions for public health surveillance. MMWR 1990;39:38.

cemia; 20% to 80% have hypophosphatemia. The reason for this is unclear.

Ancillary Tests

A chest radiograph will show a reticular pattern of interstitial edema and pleural effusion in the presence of noncardiogenic pulmonary edema associated with TSS. Electrocardiographic (EKG) changes are predominantly nonspecific. Rhythm disturbances such as sinus tachycardia, first-degree atrioventricular block, premature ventricular beats on exertion, and aberrant conduction may be noted. Flattened T waves and nonspecific ST-T segment changes have been described.

DIFFERENTIAL DIAGNOSIS

The case definition for public health surveillance of the Centers for Disease Control is the basis for the diagnosis of TSS (see Table 70–2). As yet there is no confirmatory laboratory test. Isolation of *S. aureus* from a site not usually colonized by *S. aureus* supports the diagnosis of TSS. Isolation of TSST-1–producing *S. aureus* from a mucous membrane of a patient with symptoms and findings of TSS also supports but does not establish the diagnosis. These isolates may be found in the carrier state.

The differential diagnosis of TSS includes other febrile exanthematous illnesses and other causes of shock and sepsis. The exanthematous illnesses that resemble TSS are Kawasaki disease, staphylococcal scalded skin syndrome, scarlet fever, Rocky Mountain spotted fever, leptospirosis, and erythema multiforme major (Stevens-Johnson syndrome) (Table 70–3). Other exanthematous illnesses that may be mistaken for TSS are drug eruptions, enterovirus infections with myocarditis, and measles.

Fever and hypotension are prominent features of bacterial sepsis and meningococcemia. However, secretory, profuse diarrhea is atypical.

Nonmenstrual cases of TSS potentially pose a formidable diagnostic challenge to the emergency physician. A high index of suspicion will facilitate diagnosis when evaluating a patient in the postoperative period or a patient with a minor abrasion who has fever and hypotension out of proportion to the obvious infection. Again, recognition of profuse watery diarrhea and diffuse erythroderma may lead to the correct diagnosis. The median time lapse from a surgical

---

TABLE 70–3

MAJOR POINTS IN DIFFERENTIAL DIAGNOSIS OF TOXIC SHOCK SYNDROME IN CHILDREN

Disease	Incidence and Cause	Diagnostic Features
TSS	Most common in young women in association with menstruation, but nonmenstrual disease occurs in association with focal staphylococcal infections	*Hypotension, multiorgan involvement, thrombocytopenia,* fever, scarlatiniform rash with flexural accentuation, palmar erythema, mucous membrane erythema, "strawberry tongue" and conjunctival hyperemia, delayed desquamation (especially of hands and fingers), alopecia, and nail shedding
Kawasaki disease	Primarily occurs in children less than 5 yr of age; reported in some adults	*Nonpurulent cervical lymphadenopathy, thrombocytosis,* fever, polymorphic maculopapular erythema, mucous membrane erythema, "strawberry tongue" and conjunctival hyperemia, delayed desquamation of fingertips, cardiac sequelae
Staphylococcal scalded skin syndrome	Primarily occurs in children less than 5 years of age but seen in older children and adults; caused by epidermolytic toxins A and B, produced by strains of phage group II *Staphylococcus aureus*	Flexural or generalized erythema, fragile bullae and *extensive superficial desquamation, purulent conjunctivitis, rare oral and genital findings, characteristic cutaneous histopathologic features* with separation seen in granular layer
Scarlet fever	Occurs mostly in children 2 to 8 yr of age, resulting from infection by group A beta-hemolytic streptococci	Fever, characteristic macular erythema, flexural accentuation (Pastia lines), *sandpaper-like texture,* circumoral pallor, *pharyngitis,* postexanthematous desquamation of fingertips, *positive ASO titer*
Rocky Mountain spotted fever	Caused by *Rickettsia rickettsii,* acquired through exposure to ticks	Fever, *frontal headache,* followed by *characteristic eruption that begins on wrists and ankles and spreads centripetally,* with macular, papular, and characteristically *petechial* or *purpuric* components; conjunctival hyperemia may be prominent
Leptospirosis	Infecting organisms acquired through exposure to rats or their urine	Fever, *myalgia, petechial* or *purpuric skin lesions* characteristic but not invariably present, conjunctival hyperemia
Erythema multiforme major (Stevens-Johnson syndrome)	Associated most often with recurrent herpes simplex and drug reactions	*Target (iris) lesions,* palmoplantar lesions, crusted or inflammatory conjunctival lesions (or both), severe oral inflammation, crusted lips

ASO = Antistreptolysin O. Italics represent salient features of the disease.
From Resnick SD. Toxic shock syndrome: Recent developments in pathogenesis. J Pediatr 1990;116:321.

procedure to onset of TSS symptoms is 2 days, but TSS has occurred as many as 65 days postoperatively. It is important to examine all recent surgical wounds, abrasions, and lacerations for minor erythema, as the inflammatory response may be minimal at the site of infection. This may be a problem for surgeons who are reluctant to open wounds that do not appear to be severely inflamed.

THERAPEUTIC INTERVENTION

The severity of illness will determine the intensity and scope of management. Prompt correction of shock is essential, but prolonged resuscitation may be required. Multiple-organ failure is related to the severity of shock and may be reversible if the blood pressure can be effectively maintained. Hypotension associated with TSS is a high-output, low-peripheral-resistance process with capillary leakage similar to that seen in septic shock. Patients with TSS require large volumes of fluid and electrolytes to counteract the vascular volume loss to interstitial space. Patients who receive colloid solutions are more likely to have an abnormal chest radiograph than patients who receive only crystalloids. Inotropic agents and vasopressors may be required in patients unresponsive to fluid therapy. Invasive hemodynamic monitoring may also be required to assess the severity of volume depletion and the response to fluid therapy.

A comprehensive physical examination to detect any potential focus of *S. aureus* infection should be performed. Nasal packing, surgical drains, splints, other body packings, or a vaginal tampon or sponge should be promptly removed. Infected wounds such as abscesses should be identified and drained. Iodine-soaked gauze may be used to keep the wound open. Iodine vaginal douches have been advocated for vaginal tampon–associated TSS and may be of benefit if there is some doubt as to the focus of *S. aureus* colonization in the female patient.

In animal models the early use of intravenous immune globulin (IVIG) has reduced the mortality associated with TSS. No adverse reactions were noted in the IVIG-treated animals. Although there are no clinical studies to confirm the efficacy of IVIG in humans, administering IVIG to patients who are severely ill with TSS may be considered.

Appropriate antistaphylococcal antibiotics should be administered pending results of the cultures. The use of antibiotics has not been shown to alter the course of this toxin-mediated disease. However, a lower rate of recurrence has been noted following treatment with appropriate antibiotics. The use of beta-lactamase–resistant penicillins, vancomycin, or clindamycin is appropriate (Table 70–4).

The use of corticosteroids in the management of TSS is controversial. Reduction in severity of the illness and duration of fever was suggested by a retrospective study when corticosteroids were used early in the course of the disease.

Acute renal failure may develop requiring dialysis. Metabolic acidosis, electrolyte abnormalities, hypocalcemia, and hypophosphatemia may accompany renal disease in TSS. Cardiac arrythmias may develop acutely in the presence of cardiomyopathy associated with TSS. Treatment should be directed at specific arrythmias. Children are at greater risk for developing ARDS and may require ventilatory support more often than adults. Measures such as hyperventilation, mannitol, and dexamethasone may be needed to treat increased intracranial pressure associated with cerebral edema.

DISPOSITION

Milder forms of TSS occur more frequently than disease that meets the clinical case definition. Probable cases include those meeting five of the six major criteria (see Table 70–2). Adherence to the case definition allows identification of

TABLE 70–4
MANAGEMENT OF TOXIC SHOCK SYNDROME

Removal of potentially infected foreign bodies
Drainage and irrigation of infected sites
Intravenous administration of antibiotics
  Penicillinase-resistant penicillins
    Methicillin: 200–300 mg/kg/day in four to six doses; maximum adult dose, 12 gm/day.
    Oxacillin: 50–100 mg/kg/day in four doses up to 1.5–2.0 gm every 4–6 hours; maximum adult dose, 12 gm/day.
    Nafcillin: 100–200 mg/kg/day in four to six doses; maximum adult dose, 12 gm/day; 15- to 30-min infusion.
  Alternative antibiotics
    Vancomycin: 15–50 mg/kg/day in four doses; maximum adult dose, 2 gm/day.
    Clindamycin: 25–40 mg/kg/day in four doses; maximum adult dose, 4.8 gm/day.
Consider methylprednisolone for severe cases
Aggressive management and monitoring of:
  Hypovolemia and inadequate tissue perfusion
  Adult respiratory distress syndrome
  Myocardial dysfunction
  Acute renal failure
  Cerebral edema
  Hypocalcemia/hypophosphatemia
  Metabolic acidosis
  Disseminated intravascular coagulation
  Fluid and electrolyte abnormalities

Modified from Chesney PJ. Clinical aspects and spectrum of illness of toxic shock syndrome: Overview. Rev Infect Dis 1989; 2(suppl 1):s4. Published by The University of Chicago Press.

patients who need hospitalization and are most likely to benefit from aggressive therapy. The degree of hypotension is known to correlate with the severity of multiple-organ involvement. Mild cases of TSS may respond to early therapy and may not require hospital admission. These may include patients who appear to be well, have normal vital signs, and are able to comply with follow-up instructions.

Selected References

Bach MD. Dermatologic signs in toxic shock syndrome: Clues to diagnosis. J Am Acad Dermatol 1983;8:343.

Bartlett P, Reingold AL, Graham DR, et al. Toxic shock syndrome associated with surgical wound infections. JAMA 1982;247:1448.

Bartter T, Dascal A, Carroll K, et al. "Toxic strep syndrome"—a manifestation of group A streptococcal infection. Arch Intern Med 1988;148:1421.

Bass JW, Harden LB, Peixotto JH. Probable toxic shock syndrome without shock and multisystem involvement. Pediatrics 1982;70:279.

Bisno AL. Group A streptococcal infections and acute rheumatic fever. N Engl J Med 1991; 325:783.

Broome CV. Epidemiology of toxic shock syndrome in the United States; overview. Rev Infect Dis 1989;2(suppl):514.

Centers for Disease Control. Epidemiology of toxic shock syndrome, United States 1960–1984. MMWR 1985; 33:1955.

Chesney PJ. Clinical aspects and spectrum of illness of toxic shock syndrome: Overview. Rev Infect Dis 1989;2(suppl 1):s1.

Chesney PJ, Davis JP, Purdy WK, Chesney RW. Clinical manifestations of the toxic shock syndrome. JAMA 1981;246:741.

Chesney RW, Chesney PJ, Davis JP, Seger WE. Renal manifestations of staphylococcal toxic shock syndrome. Am J Med 1981;71:583.

Davis JP, Chesney PJ, Wand PJ, et al. Toxic shock syndrome: epidemiologic features, recurrence, risk factors and precautions. N Engl J Med 1980;303:1429.

Dinarello CA, Canno JG, Wolff SM, et al. Tumor necrosis factor (cachectin) is an endogenous pyrogen and induces production of interleukin-1. J Exp Med 1986;163:1433.

Faith G, Pearson K, Fleming D, et al. Toxic shock syndrome and vaginal contraceptive sponge. JAMA 1986;255:216.

Ferguson MA, Todd JK. Toxic shock syndrome associated with *Staphylococcus aureus* sinusitis in children. J Infect Dis 1990;161:953.

Frame JD, Eve MD, Hackett EJ, et al. Toxic shock syndrome in burned children. Burns 1985;11:234.

Gallo UG, Fontanarosa PB. Toxic streptococcal syndrome. Ann Emerg Med 1990;19:1332.

Garbe PL, Arko RJ, Reingold AL, et al. *Staphylococcus aureus* isolates from patients with nonmenstrual toxic shock syndrome. JAMA 1985;253:2538.

Ikejima T, Dinarello CA, Gill DM, et al. Induction of human interleukin-1 by a product of *Staphylococcus aureus* associated with toxic shock syndrome. J Clin Invest 1984;73:1312.

Jacobson JA, Kasworm EM. Toxic shock syndrome after nasal surgery: Case reports and analysis of risk factors. Arch Otolaryngol Head Neck Surg 1986;112:329.

Jacobson JA, Kasworm EM, Reiser RF, Bergdoll MS. Low incidence of toxic shock syndrome in children with staphylococcal infection. Am J Med Sci 1987;294:403.

Johnson LP, L'Italier JJ, Schlievert PM. Streptococcal pyrogenic exotoxin type A (scarlet fever toxin) is related to *Staphylococcus aureus* enterotoxin B. MGG 1986;203:354.

Kass EH, Parsonnet J. On the pathogenesis of toxic shock syndrome. Rev Infect Dis 1987;9(suppl):5482.

Kehrberg MW, Latham RH, Haslam BT, et al. Risk factors for staphylococcal toxic shock syndrome. Am J Epidemiol 1981;114:873.

Kline MW, Dunkle LM. Toxic shock syndrome and the acquired immunodeficiency syndrome. Pediatr Infect Dis J 1988;7:736.

Kniffen WD, Smith R, Stashwick CA. Toxic shock syndrome in three adolescent males. J Adolesc Health Care 1990;11:116.

McCarthy VP, Peoples WM, et al. Toxic shock syndrome after ear piercing. Pediatr Infect Dis J 1988;7:741.

Melish ME, Murata S, Fukunanaga C, et al. Endotoxin is not an essential mediator in toxic shock syndrome. Rev Infect Dis 1989;2(suppl 1):5219.

Nahass RG, Gocke DJ. Toxic shock syndrome associated with use of a nasal tampon. Am J Med 1988;84:629.

Notermans S, van Leeuwen WJ, Dufrenne J, et al. Serum antibodies to enterotoxins produced by *Staphylococcus aureus* with special reference to enterotoxin F and toxic shock syndrome. J Clin Microbiol 1983;18:1055.

Reingold AL, Hargrett NT, Dan BB, et al. Nonmenstrual toxic shock syndrome: A review of 130 cases. Ann Intern Med 1982;96:871.

Resnick SD. Toxic shock syndrome: Recent developments in pathogenesis. J Pediatr 1990;116:321.

Shands KN, Schmid GP, Dan BB, et al. Toxic shock syndrome in menstruating women: Association with tampon use and *Staphylococcus aureus* and clinical features in 52 cases. N Engl J Med 1980;303:1436.

Smith CB, Jacobson JA. Toxic shock syndrome. Dis Month 1986;32:82.

Smith DM, Gulinson J. Fatal cerebral edema complicating toxic shock syndrome. Neurosurgery 1988;22:598.

Solomon R, Truman T, Murray D. Toxic shock syndrome as a complication of bacterial tracheitis. Pediatr Infect Dis J 1985;4:298.

Sperber SJ, Francis JB. Toxic shock syndrome during an influenza outbreak. JAMA 1987;257:1086.

Stevens DL, Tanner MH, Winship J, et al. Severe group A streptococcal infections associated with a toxic shock–like syndrome and scarlet fever toxin A. N Engl J Med 1989;321:1.

Todd JK. Therapy of toxic shock syndrome. Drugs 1990;39:856.

Todd JK. Toxic shock syndrome. Clin Microbiol Rev 1988;1:432.

Todd JK, Todd BH, Franco-Buff A, et al. Influence of focal growth conditions on the pathogenesis of toxic shock syndrome. J Infect Dis 1987;155:673.

Tofte RW, Williams DN. Toxic shock syndrome: Evidence of a broad clinical spectrum. JAMA 1981;246:2163.

Wright SW, Trott AT. Toxic shock syndrome: A review. Ann Emerg Med 1988;17:268.

CHAPTER 71

Mononucleosis

William M. Maguire

INTRODUCTION

Mononucleosis ranks as the third most common reportable communicable disease in the United States. The incidence approaches 50 cases per 100,000 population. Certain subpopulations exhibit a higher incidence, notably college students and military recruits, where the incidence approaches 100 to 1000 cases per 100,000 population. No male-to-female preponderance has been reported, but females show a higher seroconversion rate for Epstein-Barr virus. No seasonal predominance has been indicated. Mononucleosis has long been known as "the kissing disease," and kissing has been substantiated as an important mode of transmission for the disease. Oral shedding of viral particles can occur up to 18 months following the outbreak of mononucleosis. Another documented but less frequent form of transmission is by blood product transfusion. There is no evidence for significant fecal or urinary shedding of the virus.

PATHOPHYSIOLOGY

The Epstein-Barr virus is a herpes type DNA virus that selectively infects bone marrow–derived B lymphocytes. The Epstein-Barr virus is unique in that it is not cytotoxic to its host cell. The infected cells, atypical mononuclear cells, infiltrate the normal lymphoid tissue, lymph nodes, spleen, and Waldeyer's ring. This infiltration results in a reactive hyperplasia. Some pathologic reports exist of severe cases of infectious mononucleosis showing infiltration of the heart, liver, adrenals, kidneys, and meninges. Histologically the lymph node architecture shows changes, but the nodal capsule is not invaded. Cells resembling Reed-Sternberg cells may also be seen.

CLINICAL EVALUATION

The most common presenting complaint of patients with mononucleosis is a severe sore throat, usually preceded by a 1- to 2-week prodromal phase marked by malaise, fatigue, retro-orbital headache, fever, nausea, and nonspecific abdominal complaints (Fig. 71–1). The incubation period for the disease is 30 to 50 days. The symptoms become prominent at the period of the most intense lymphocyte proliferation. The pharyngitis is remarkable for its severity and the degree of tonsillar enlargement. Grayish exudates on the tonsils and petechiae at the junction of the hard and soft palate are frequently seen; the petechiae are similar to those seen in measles. In rare cases the tonsillar enlargement can cause obstruction of the airway. Lymphadenopathy and hepatosplenomegaly are seen in at least 75% of patients with mononucleosis. Posterior cervical and epitrochlear nodes are commonly affected. Hepatomegaly is usually less impressive than splenomegaly. Approximately 20% of cases exhibit some viral exanthem. Supraorbital edema is reported in 10% of cases. Although liver enzyme abnormalities are reported in 83% to 100% of patients, only 5% to 10% of patients are ever icteric.

Mononucleosis usually follows a predictable course. After the initial prodrome, an acute phase lasting 2 to 3 weeks ensues, followed by a convalescent phase of 3 weeks to 4 months. This latter period is marked by lethargy.

It was previously thought that there were no true recurrences, and the lay press popularized the notion of a "chronic Epstein-Barr infection." The immunologic evidence tends to support the theory of a reactivation of the Epstein-Barr virus. The clinical syndrome is marked by fatigue, fevers, weight loss, arthritis, and depression. It is seen in both adult and pediatric populations. Although the incidence of mononucleosis has traditionally been thought to be highest in the young adult population (ages 15 to 22), subclinical cases are probably present in young children less than 4 years old. Previous studies on incidence have depended on the heterophile antibody test, but advances in Epstein-Barr–specific

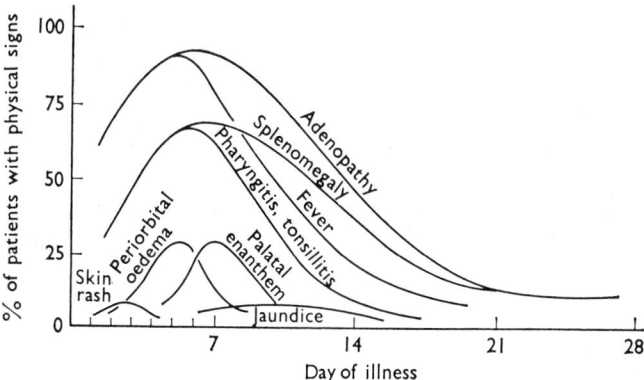

Figure 71–1. Usual frequency and duration of major physical signs in young adults with uncomplicated infectious mononucleosis. (From Rapp EC, Hewetson JF. Infectious mononucleosis and the Epstein-Barr virus. Am J Dis Child 1978;132:81. Copyright 1978, American Medical Association.)

antibody testing have shown that a large number of children younger than 6 years acquire the virus.

COMPLICATIONS

Complications associated with mononucleosis are numerous, but fatalities are rare. Airway obstruction is infrequent. Splenic rupture occurs in 0.2% of all cases of mononucleosis and is a potentially preventable cause of death. Hepatic enzyme elevations occur frequently, but cases of hepatic failure are rare. Pancreatitis associated with acute mononucleosis has also been reported, but no fatal cases have been reported. Cardiac complications, including myocarditis and pericarditis, have been reported in previous reviews of fatal mononucleosis. In one review of fatal mononucleosis, opportunistic infections and acute hemorrhage were cited as the major causes of death. Bone marrow damage secondary to Epstein-Barr virus infection was suspected as the underlying cause in these fatal cases. Increased splenic destruction of platelets, marrow suppression, and viral-induced antiplatelet antibodies have all been suspected of causing the thrombocytopenia seen in fatal cases of mononucleosis.

Neurologic involvement occurs in approximately 1% of patients diagnosed with mononucleosis. The spectrum includes subacute sclerosis, panencephalitis, Guillain-Barré syndrome, transverse myelitis, meningoencephalitis, and Reye's syndrome. Pulmonary complications of infectious mononucleosis are usually limited to pneumonitis. Bacterial superinfections are rare in children with mononucleosis, despite the neutropenia that accompanies the disease. It was previously believed that beta-hemolytic streptococcal infections usually accompanied episodes of mononucleosis, but recent evidence does not support this. Dermatologic complications are limited to a nonspecific viral exanthem and to iatrogenic rashes caused by treatment with amoxicillin.

DIAGNOSTIC EVALUATION

The complete blood cell (CBC) count has limited specificity. Of all patients with mononucleosis, 90% exhibit a lymphocytosis at some time during the course of the disease. The lymphocytes are described as atypical, and the number of atypical lymphocytes is generally highest in the early stages of the disease.

A more specific test to be considered in the evaluation of mononucleosis is the Monospot test. Unlike the heterophile antibody test, which is more time intensive for laboratory personnel, the Monospot test is rapid, simple, inexpensive, and generally available. False-positive results can occur, but false-negative results are rare. The Monospot test remains positive for up to 6 months after the onset of symptoms and then becomes negative again.

Another assay that may be useful in the diagnosis of infectious mononucleosis or in monitoring chronic Epstein-Barr syndrome involves specific Epstein-Barr virus serologic studies. Serologic tests specific for viral capsid antigen, nuclear antigen, early antigen, and others are available (Fig. 71–2).

Any child suspected of having mononucleosis warrants a CBC count and a Monospot test. If the initial tests do not confirm the diagnosis, the patient should have a repeat CBC count and Monospot test in 2 weeks. If the patient's condition is critical initially, or if the Monospot test and CBC count are still nondiagnostic at 2 weeks, immunoglobulin G (IgG) antibody tests should be performed. If the IgG test is negative, immunoglobulin M (IgM) tests should be performed and, if negative, repeated by the primary care physician in 2 weeks. For patients in whom chronic reacti-

Figure 71–2. Schematic representation of the evolution of various antibodies to various Epstein-Barr virus (EBV) antigens in children with infectious mononucleosis, the prototypic symptomatic EBV infection. The titers are geometric mean values expressed as reciprocals of the serum dilution. (Adapted from Sumaya CV, Ench Y. Epstein-Barr virus infectious mononucleosis in children. Pediatrics 1985;75:1011. Reproduced by permission of Pediatrics.)

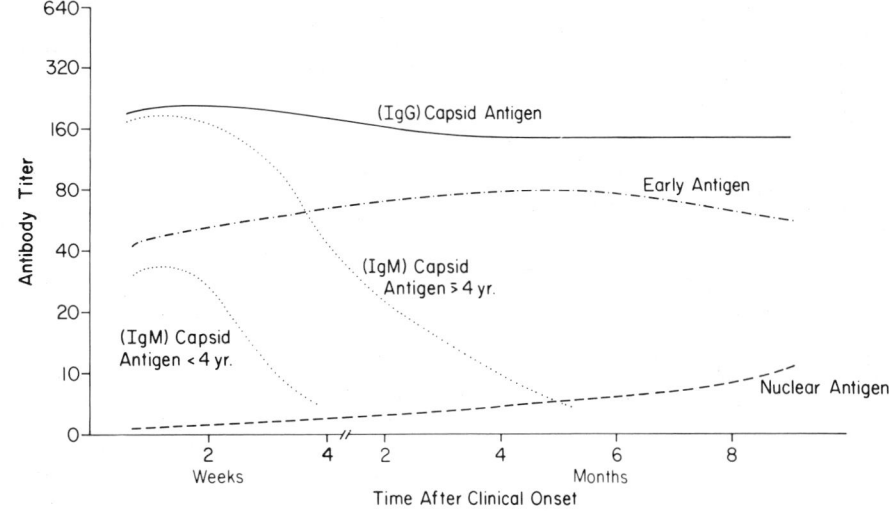

TABLE 71–1

DISCHARGE INSTRUCTIONS

General:	Increase hydration
	Follow up with private physician
Activity:	No participation in contact sports for at least 2 wk
	Rest
Fever:	Acetaminophen, 15 mg/kg every 4 hr
	Ibuprofen, 5 mg/kg every 6 to 8 hr for temperature <102°F
	Ibuprofen, 10 mg/kg every 6 to 8 hr for temperature >102°F
Pain:	Acetaminophen, 15 mg/kg every 4 hr
	Severe pain: codeine, 1 mg/kg up to 30 mg every 4 hr

vation of Epstein-Barr virus is suspected, IgM studies should be obtained.

DIFFERENTIAL DIAGNOSIS

If the CBC count, Monospot test, and serologic tests are inconclusive, then cytolomegalovirus (CMV) infection, toxoplasmosis, early hepatitis, or an atypical Epstein-Barr virus infection without antibody response should be considered. Clinically, mumps, streptococcal pharyngitis, diphtheria, adenovirus, rubella, and mycoplasmal, malarial, typhoid, and tuberculous infections might be considered, along with leukemia or lymphoma.

THERAPEUTIC INTERVENTION

The treatment for mononucleosis remains supportive. Saline gargles and analgesics are the mainstay therapies in mild cases. In some instances pain and tonsillar enlargement may lead to dehydration, and in these cases intravenous hydration may be indicated. Unless cultures or streptococcal screens show concomitant bacterial infection, antibiotic administration is not warranted. Anecdotal reports of the benefits of steroids exist, but no proof of efficacy has been shown in double-blind clinical trials. If the patient can maintain adequate hydration, he or she may be safely discharged. Specific discharge instructions should stress that the patient not participate in any contact sports because of the risks of splenic rupture (Table 71–1). An analgesic, either ibuprofen or acetaminophen, should be used for pain relief. In some cases the associated pain may be severe enough to warrant the use of codeine in the early stages of the infection. Bed rest and fluids are also recommended. Patients should follow up with their private physician in 2 weeks for a repeat CBC count and abdominal examination. Any complaints of increased abdominal pain or the inability to maintain adequate fluid intake warrant immediate return to the emergency department.

Selected References

Baehner RL, Shuler SE. Infectious mononucleosis in childhood. Clin Pediatr 1967;6:393.

Fleisher GR, Collins M, Fager S. Limitations of available tests for diagnosis of infectious mononucleosis. J Clin Microbiol 1983;17:619.

Fleisher G, Henle W, Henle G, et al. Primary infection with Epstein-Barr virus in infants in the United States: Clinical and serological observations. J Infect Dis 1979;139(5):533.

Rahal JJ, Henle G. Infectious mononucleosis and Reyes syndrome: A fatal case with studies for Epstein-Barr virus. Pediatrics 1970;46:776.

Rapp CE, Hewetson JF. Infectious mononucleosis and the Epstein-Barr virus. Am J Dis Child 1978;132:78.

Rutkow IM. Rupture of the spleen in infectious mononucleosis. Arch Surg 1978;113:718.

Sumaya CV. Epstein Barr virus infections in children. Curr Prob Pediatr 1987;XVII(12):685.

Sumaya CV, Ench Y. Epstein-Barr virus infectious mononucleosis in children: Clinical and general laboratory findings. Pediatrics 1985;75:1003.

Tamir D, Benderly A, Levy J, et al. Infectious mononucleosis and Epstein-Barr virus in childhood. Pediatrics 1974;53:330.

Timan L, Koller M, Budai J. Serologic follow-up of patients with infectious mononucleosis caused by EBV. Acta Pediatr 1981;22(3):243.

CHAPTER 72

Kawasaki Disease

Jeffrey Proudfoot

INTRODUCTION

Kawasaki disease is an acute vasculitis of unknown origin that affects children. It is similar in presentation to infantile polyarteritis nodosa. The disease is also referred to as *mucocutaneous lymph node syndrome* (MCLNS) and is characterized by fever, mucosal erythema, generalized rash, conjunctivitis, and cervical lymphadenopathy. Kawasaki disease is found most often in Asian children but has been found worldwide in all races and geographic regions. Epidemics usually occur in the winter and early spring, suggesting an infectious origin. The disease also has an increased incidence in children less than 5 years of age and in males. In the United States it is more common in Orientals and blacks than in whites. Kawasaki disease is important clinically because of its sequelae of myocarditis and coronary artery aneurysms, which may occur in up to 25% of children. The mortality rate for these sequelae is 1% to 2%. Kawasaki disease is the leading cause of acquired heart disease in children.

PATHOPHYSIOLOGY

The pathophysiology and cause of Kawasaki disease remain unknown. Epidemiologic data suggest that either infectious or toxic mechanisms may be responsible. Antecedent upper respiratory illness, rug cleaning, and proximity to open water have been linked with an increased incidence of the disease, and as noted earlier, seasonal epidemics occur in the winter and spring. Environmental or toxic agents are suspected because of the similarity of the disease to presentations of mercury poisoning and Stevens-Johnson syndrome. Cases associated with *Propionibacterium acnes* and the Epstein-Barr virus have been described. Immunoregulatory disturbances in Kawasaki patients have also been described, including deficiencies of T-suppressor lymphocytes and increased reverse transcriptase activity, raising the possibility of retroviruses as causative agents. These associations have not been found consistently in the various outbreaks of Kawasaki disease.

The disease is characterized by a vasculitis that affects small and medium arteries throughout the entire body, most significantly the coronary arteries. This involves destruction of the intima and media and perivascular infiltration with macrophages, lymphocytes, and mast cells, which ultimately leads to aneurysm formation. Coronary artery aneurysm and resultant thrombosis occur, resulting in myocardial infarction and sudden death in a minority of cases. Mortality in Kawasaki disease is directly attributable to the cardiac sequelae.

Classically the disease follows three distinct phases. The initial acute phase, which lasts up to 2 weeks, is characterized by sudden fever, rash, conjunctivitis, lymphadenopathy, and mucosal changes. Cardiac involvement in this stage involves tachycardia and, universally, myocarditis. As the fever and rash subside, the disease enters a second, or subacute, phase marked by arthritis and epidermal desquamation lasting 4 to 8 weeks. It is during this stage that cardiac and thrombotic vascular complications occur. Most fatalities caused by coronary thrombosis occur in this stage, as do congestive heart failure, pericardial effusion, and valvular involvement. Electrocardiographic changes in the form of nonspecific ST and T wave changes can be seen at this stage. The third, or convalescent, phase lasts up to 2 years and is characterized by a gradual return to normal. Cardiac involvement in this stage is related to formation of aneurysms.

Atypical presentations of Kawasaki disease have been reported. Clinical findings may be especially subtle in infants less than 6 months old. Nevertheless, this group is still at risk for coronary sequelae.

EMERGENCY MEDICAL SERVICE CONSIDERATIONS

Children with the presenting complaint of chest pain should be treated as a cardiac patient, receiving oxygen and cardiac monitoring. Intravenous morphine sulfate may be given for pain control. Any child with Kawasaki disease and hypotension or unresponsiveness should be treated as a patient with an acute myocardial infarction (MI) or ruptured aneurysm, with two large-bore intravenous lines, a fluid bolus, and rapid transport for definitive care.

CLINICAL EVALUATION

Diagnosis of Kawasaki disease is defined by established criteria from the Centers for Disease Control (Table 72–1). High fever in the 40°C (104°F) range, usually lasting up to 10 days, is the earliest sign in the typical presentation. This is followed by bilateral nonpurulent conjunctivitis, which has been associated with anterior uveitis. Most children also have mucosal involvement consisting of fissured or cracked lips with erythema of the pharynx and hypertrophy of the glossal papillae. These mucosal changes commonly develop 3 to 4 days after the development of fever. Characteristic extremity signs include brawny edema of the hands or feet with palmar and plantar erythema. About 2 weeks after the onset of fever, desquamation begins in the periungual regions and progresses to involve the entire palm or sole. The generalized exanthem is polymorphous in nature, usually morbilliform or urticarial and involving the diaper area and trunk. Vesicular or bullous lesions are uncommon. Tender and firm cervical lymphadenopathy occurs in approximately 50% of patients.

Other associated signs and symptoms present in children include extreme irritability and sleep disturbances in as many as 90% of patients; urethritis and sterile pyuria in 75%; and arthralgia and small joint arthritis in the acute phase, which can progress to involve weight-bearing joints, in approximately 30% of patients. Diarrhea, vomiting, and abdominal pain may also be present. Hydrops of the gallbladder can occur with or without obstructive jaundice. Hemolytic-

TABLE 72–1

DIAGNOSTIC CRITERIA FOR KAWASAKI DISEASE

Fever of at least 5 days or more without other explanation and at least four of the following criteria:

1. Bilateral conjunctival injection
2. One of the following mucous membrane changes:
   — Injected pharynx
   — Erythema, fissuring, crusting of the lips
   — Strawberry tongue
3. At least one of the following extremity changes:
   — Peripheral edema
   — Erythema of the palms and soles
   — Generalized or periungual desquamation
4. Rash, primarily truncal
5. Cervical lymphadenopathy (at least one node 1.5 cm or greater in diameter)

uremic syndrome is a rare complication that can occur early in the course of the disease.

Physical Examination

A thorough examination is required for any child with a high fever and no obvious source of infection. General inspection may reveal peripheral erythema or the diffuse rash that is present early in the course of the disease. A head and neck examination should detect conjunctivitis and mucosal or pharyngeal changes. Palpation for any cervical lymphadenopathy is necessary.

Chest examination requires close attention to signs of cardiac dysfunction. Murmurs, rubs, and tachycardia are all common to cardiac involvement with Kawasaki disease. Distant heart sounds or tachycardia out of proportion to fever signal the need for more extensive cardiac evaluation. Rales or jugular venous distention suggest compromised cardiac function and early congestive heart failure.

Examination of the extremities may reveal edema or desquamation characteristic of the second stage of the disease. Palmar or plantar erythema should be noted. See Table 72–2 for the differential diagnosis of Kawasaki disease.

TABLE 72–2

DIFFERENTIAL DIAGNOSIS OF KAWASAKI DISEASE

Infectious diseases
  Cervical adenitis
  Epstein-Barr virus
  Lyme disease
  Leptospirosis
  Meningitis (aseptic or bacterial)
  Rickettsial infections
  Scarlet fever
  Staphylococcal scalded skin syndrome
  Toxic shock syndrome
  Toxoplasmosis
  Viral infections (rubella, rubeola, echoviruses)
Drug-related disorders
  Drug reactions
  Stevens-Johnson syndrome
Rheumatologic diseases
  Infantile periarteritis nodosa
  Juvenile rheumatoid arthritis
Environmental diseases
  Heavy metal poisoning

DIAGNOSTIC EVALUATION
Laboratory Studies

All patients should have a complete blood cell (CBC) count, including platelet count; erythrocyte sedimentation rate determination; urinalysis; drug screen; blood and throat cultures; a chest radiograph; and an electrocardiogram (EKG). All children with a presumptive diagnosis of Kawasaki disease require echocardiographic evaluation within the first 2 weeks of illness.

Diagnosis depends on clinical acumen, as there is no single diagnostic test for this disease. There are few laboratory features that aid in the diagnosis. Most patients exhibit a leukocytosis with predominantly polymorphonuclear forms. Thrombocytosis is also common, with platelet counts into the millions. This usually peaks at 2 to 3 weeks after onset of the illness and coincides with the hypercoagulability seen clinically. The erythrocyte sedimentation rate and C-reactive protein level are frequently elevated in the acute phase.

Cardiac Evaluation

Because the most significant sequelae are cardiac related, a thorough cardiac evaluation of all patients with Kawasaki disease is necessary. The most common EKG findings are a prolonged PR interval, nonspecific ST and T wave changes, and tachycardia. Arrhythmias may be an indication of myocarditis. Echocardiography will help establish any evidence of aneurysm formation, hypertrophy, effusion of pericarditis, or valvular involvement. Angiography in selected instances may be necessary.

THERAPEUTIC INTERVENTION
Acute Therapy

Drug therapy is directed at limiting the inflammatory response and platelet aggregation to prevent the cardiac and thrombotic complications of Kawasaki disease (Table 72–3). Aspirin should be given in doses of 80 to 100 mg/kg in divided doses every 6 hours early in the acute phase. Although this has never been proven prospectively to reduce the incidence of aneurysms, the antipyretic and antiplatelet effect is important. As soon as the fever is controlled, the dose should be lowered to 3 to 5 mg/kg in one daily dose and continued for 6 to 8 weeks to help limit coronary thrombosis. Other dosage regimens have been used, and dipyridamole (3 to 6 mg/kg/day in three divided doses) may be substituted when aspirin is contraindicated.

Intravenous gamma globulin (IVGG) should be administered within the first 10 days of illness at a dosage of 400 mg/kg/day for at least 4 days. IVGG in conjunction with salicylates is the most effective therapy for prevention of coronary artery abnormalities and aneurysms. No significant adverse effects have been reported with IVGG treatment. A single 1-gm/kg dose of IVGG has been reported to be as efficacious as the 4-day regimen. The mechanism of IVGG therapy has been related to antitoxic or immunomodulating effects or to a direct anti–causative agent effect.

Use of thrombolytic agents (streptokinase or urokinase) to treat coronary artery thrombosis has been reported, with equivocal results. This has been most effective if initiated within 3 to 4 hours of onset of thrombotic symptoms.

Chronic Therapy

Patients with no coronary artery changes need reevaluation every 2 to 3 years. Those with small single coronary aneurysms must have long-term aspirin therapy at 3 to 5

TABLE 72–3
KAWASAKI DISEASE: THERAPY AT A GLANCE

Acute
  Aspirin: 80–100 mg/kg/day in four divided doses until 14th day of illness
  Intravenous gamma globulin: 400 mg/kg once daily for 4 days
Convalescent
  Aspirin: 3–5 mg/kg/day once daily; discontinue 6 to 8 weeks after onset of illness after verifying no coronary abnormalities on echocardiography
Chronic
  Aspirin: 3–5 mg/kg/day once daily. Dipyrimadole may be added in high-risk patients
  Coumadin or heparin combined with antiplatelet therapy if history of severe coronary involvement or prior coronary thrombosis
Acute coronary thrombosis
  Thrombolytic therapy with streptokinase, urokinase, or tissue plasminogen activator under supervision of cardiologist (controversial)

mg/kg once daily along with yearly cardiac evaluation until resolution of such lesions. The remainder of patients with multiple or large aneurysms (with or without obstruction) must have regulated physical activity and repeated ongoing cardiac evaluation in addition to salicylate therapy. This includes stress testing and evaluation for possible surgical intervention.

COMPLICATIONS
Cardiac Complications

Management of cardiac complications requires a thorough cardiac evaluation. Treatment of pericarditis should include prompt decompression of any tamponade. Myocardial infarction with or without cardiogenic shock can be treated as in the adult population with analgesics, oxygen, diuretics, pressors, and anticoagulants. Patients with symptomatic coronary aneurysms need hemodynamic monitoring and support until prompt surgical evaluation can be obtained.

Other Complications

Treatment of hemolytic-uremic syndrome is best done through supportive therapy aimed at maintaining renal function and treatment of acute renal failure. Hydrops of the gallbladder can be treated supportively with intravenous fluids, pain control, and general medical management.

DISPOSITION

All children with Kawasaki disease are at risk for cardiac complications (Table 72–4) and should be admitted to the

TABLE 72–4
RISK FACTORS FOR CORONARY ARTERY INVOLVEMENT

Male gender
Age <1 yr
Fever for at least 14 days or recrudescent fever
Hemoglobin less than 10 gm/dl
White blood cell count greater than 30,000/mm³
Westergren sedimentation rate greater than 101 mm/hr
Persistence of elevated C-reactive protein or sedimentation rate more than 30 days

hospital for prompt cardiac evaluation and intravenous pharmacologic therapy. Any child who exhibits evidence of cardiac involvement on the clinical evaluation or diagnostic studies should be admitted to a monitored unit and receive early pediatric cardiology consultation. Suspicion or evidence of coronary aneurysm mandates prompt surgical consultation.

Most cases are self-limited but require long-term monitoring because of the uncertainty of long-term sequelae. The main cause of death with Kawasaki disease is from myocardial infarction caused by coronary artery thrombosis. Patients with anerurysms greater than 8 mm in diameter are at highest risk for infarction. Care providers and families of patients diagnosed with Kawasaki disease should be trained in cardiopulmonary resuscitation.

PITFALLS

The major clinical pitfall with Kawasaki disease is the failure to consider the diagnosis in children less than 4 years old with unexplained fever. This is particularly important in the very young child at risk for coronary artery involvement who presents atypically. Although only 15% to 25% of these patients develop coronary artery aneurysms, the associated morbidity necessitates early discovery and close follow-up. Other critical actions include early electrocardiographic, echocardiographic, and possibly angiographic assessment of baseline cardiac function and prompt initiation of therapy with salicylates and gamma globulin.

Selected References

Burtt DM, Pollack P, Bianco JA. Intravenous streptokinase in an infant with Kawasaki's disease complicated by acute myocardial infarction. Pediatr Cardiol 1986;6:307.

Centers for Disease Control. Multiple outbreaks of Kawasaki syndrome—United States. MMWR 1985;34:33.

Enright T, Chua-Apolinario S, Lim DT. Kawasaki syndrome. Ann Allerg 1990;65:84.

Gersony WM. Diagnosis and management of Kawasaki disease. JAMA 1991;265:2699.

Kato H, Ichinose E, Inoue O, Akagi T. Intracoronary thrombolytic therapy in Kawasaki disease: Treatment and prevention of acute myocardial infarction. Prog Clin Biol Res 1987;250:445.

Kawasaki T. Acute febrile mucocutaneous syndrome with lymphoid involvement with specific desquamation of the fingers and toes in children. Jpn J Allergol 1967;16:178.

Levy M, Koren G. Atypical Kawasaki disease: Analysis of clinical presentation and diagnostic clues. Pediatr Infect Dis J 1990;9:122.

Marder VJ, Sherry S. Thrombolytic therapy: Current status. N Engl J Med 1988;318:1512.

Newburger JW, Burns JC. Kawasaki syndrome. Cardiol Clin 1989;7:453.

Newburger JW, Takahashi M, Burns JC, et al. The treatment of Kawasaki syndrome with intravenous gamma globulin. N Engl J Med 1986;315:341.

Rauch AM. Kawasaki syndrome: Review of new epidemiologic and laboratory developments. Pediatr Infect Dis J 1987;6:1016.

Shulman ST. IVGG therapy in Kawasaki disease: Mechanism(s) of action. Clin Immunol Immunopathol 1989;53:S141.

Shulman ST, Bass JL, Bierman F, et al. Management of Kawasaki syndrome: A consensus statement prepared by North American participants of The Third International Kawasaki Disease Symposium, Tokyo, Japan, December, 1988. Pediatr Infect Dis J 1989;8:663.

Suddleson EA, Reid B, Woolley MM, et al. Hydrops of the gallbladder associated with Kawasaki syndrome. J Pediatr Surg 1987;22:956.

Tatara K, Kusakawa S. Long term prognosis of giant coronary aneurysm in Kawasaki disease: An angiographic study. J Pediatr 1987;111:705.

CHAPTER 73

Infection-related Congenital Syndromes

Adrian Dana

INTRODUCTION

A number of biologic agents are known to infect the fetus either in utero or during birth. The classic agents are *T*oxoplasmosis, *R*ubella, *C*ytomegalovirus, and *H*erpes simplex (TORCH). Many other agents can also cause congenital infections, including syphilis, human immunodeficiency virus (HIV), hepatitis B, parvovirus B19, and enterovirus (Table 73–1). The incidence of some infections such as rubella has decreased markedly; the incidence of others, such as congenital syphilis or cytomegalovirus, is rising rapidly. The overall incidence of congenital infections is difficult to determine. However, 1% to 2% of all children born in the United States excrete cytomegalovirus. As many as 90% of infants born to mothers who test positive for hepatitis B antigen are infected with hepatitis B. In addition, about 30% of infants born to HIV-infected mothers will also be infected.

The infant's risk of acquiring a perinatal infection are directly related to the mother's risk of infection. Information regarding the outcome of previous pregnancies is important; a history of spontaneous abortions or neonatal death may indicate a risk to future pregnancies. A history of maternal illness during the pregnancy should be sought, especially in reference to febrile episodes or rashes. Many perinatal infections, including syphilis, herpes simplex, hepatitis B, and HIV, are related to the maternal risk for sexually transmitted diseases. Information regarding the history of venereal disease, genital lesions, number of sexual partners, and drug abuse should be sought. Drug abuse or transfusion may place mother and child at risk for blood-borne infections such as cytomegalovirus, hepatitis B, or HIV. Animal contacts or a history of ingesting raw or rare meats may raise the suspicion of toxoplasmosis. Results of serologic screening tests (e.g., syphilis or rubella serologies) performed on the mother are also valuable for diagnosis.

The infant may exhibit certain signs in the newborn period that should raise the clinician's suspicion of a congenital infection (Table 73–2). Infectious agents that can infect the fetus, especially during the third trimester, frequently cause premature delivery. Infectious agents may also interfere

---

TABLE 73–1

AGENTS KNOWN TO CAUSE CONGENITAL INFECTION

Cytomegalovirus
Enteroviruses
Hepatitis B
Herpes simplex virus
Human immunodeficiency virus
Parvovirus B19
Rubella
Toxoplasma gondii
Treponema pallidum
Varicella zoster virus

TABLE 73–2

CLINICAL FEATURES OF TORCH SYNDROMES

Clinical Features	Cytomegalovirus	Herpes Simplex	Rubella	Syphilis	Toxoplasmosis
Hepatomegaly	+	+	+	+	+
Jaundice	+	+	+	+	+
Skin lesions	Petechiae, purpura	Vesicles, petechiae	Petechiae, purpura, dermal erythroblastosis	Petechiae, vesicles, maculopapular	Petechiae, purpura
Bone lesions	—	—	Radiolucencies	Osteochondritis, periostitis	Radiolucencies
Eye lesions	Chorioretinitis	Keratoconjunctivitis, chorioretinitis	Retinopathy, cataracts	Chorioretinitis, interstitial keratitis	Chorioretinitis
Central nervous system lesions	Calcifications, microcephaly, hydrocephalus, hearing deficits	Encephalitis, hydrocephalus	Microcephaly, encephalitis, hearing deficits	Leptomeningitis, hydrocephalus	Hydrocephalus, calcifications, microcephaly

† = Frequently reported; — = not reported.

with fetal growth, causing infants to be small for their gestational age. Hepatosplenomegaly, jaundice, and hepatitis are commonly associated with the TORCH syndromes or other perinatal infections. A rash evident at birth or in the newborn period should also alert the physician to the possibility of congenital infection. Petechiae and purpura may be seen with any of the TORCH agents. Vesicular lesions may indicate herpes simplex or syphilis, and central nervous system lesions, including microcephaly, hydrocephalus, and intracranial calcifications, may indicate fetal infection.

It is important to understand the effect that the time at which the infection is acquired may have on the infant. Infectious agents that are acquired in utero are more likely to lead to stillbirth, abortion, intrauterine growth retardation, or fetal malformation. In general, the earlier in gestation that infection occurs, the more serious the sequelae. Infections acquired during the birth process are more likely to result in severe systemic disease. Syphilis, toxoplasmosis, and rubella usually cause in utero infection. Cytomegalovirus acquired in utero may result in severe congenital disease; however, this same virus may also be contracted during the birth process. Herpes simplex virus, on the other hand, is more likely to be acquired at the time of birth, only to result in severe illness a few days later.

CYTOMEGALOVIRUS

Cytomegalovirus (CMV) is a herpesvirus, a classification that also includes the herpes simplex viruses, varicella zoster virus, and Epstein-Barr virus. Herpesviruses have the ability to cause latent infections—that is, after initial infection, the virus continues to reside in certain host tissues in a quiescent state, only to be reactivated at some later date. The initial infection may be symptomatic or asymptomatic. Cytomegalovirus is ubiquitous, and most people residing in North America will contract CMV infection during their lifetimes. The annual incidence of intrauterine infection with CMV ranges from 0.4% to 2.2%. Congenital CMV infection is the most common congenital viral infection in the United States. In the United States it is estimated that each year more than 30,000 infants are born infected, and that 3000 to 4000 infants are born with symptomatic CMV disease. Many of these children die in infancy or are left with severe neurologic residua.

The acquisition and pathogenesis of congenital CMV infection is complex and incompletely understood. Intrauterine infection can occur whether maternal infection is primary or recurrent. That is, successive infants may be infected. In general, it appears that maternal recurrent infection leads most often to asymptomatically infected infants. The newborn is more likely to have a fulminant congenital CMV syndrome when the mother has had a primary CMV infection during pregnancy. However, it must be realized that not all infants of infected mothers are themselves infected, and an even smaller number show clinical evidence of disease. Primary maternal infection leads to transmission in about 40% of fetuses; about 11% of these exhibit symptoms of disease at birth. Severity of symptoms seems to be related to gestational age at the time of infection. Infants infected during the first or second trimester exhibit more severe disease, usually with neurologic complications; most infants infected in the third trimester are asymptomatic or minimally affected.

Clinical Evaluation

The signs of classic congenital CMV disease may be present at birth or shortly thereafter. The virus may infect many different organ systems. Typically the infants are small for gestational age and often are born prematurely. Hepatomegaly with or without splenomegaly is the most common abnormality. Jaundice may be a prominent feature, often persisting beyond the period characteristic of physiologic neonatal jaundice. Petechiae and purpura are also characteristic. The rash is usually caused by a depression of the platelet count. Thrombocytopenia may be severe and protracted.

CMV causes intrauterine encephalitis and periependymitis, which leads to gliosis and calcification. Although cerebral calcification may occur anywhere, paraventricular calcifications, when present, are pathognomonic. Microcephaly or hydrocephalus may result. Chorioretinitis is the principal eye abnormality associated with congenital CMV infection. If the characteristic central nervous system findings of calcifications, microcephaly, hydrocephalus, or chorioretinitis are present in the neonatal period, the prognosis for normal psychomotor development is poor.

Hearing loss may be the most frequent problem arising from congenital CMV infection. One prospective study indicated that as many as 6% of congenitally infected children have some degree of sensorineural deafness.

Diagnostic Evaluation

Diagnosis of congenital CMV infection is most often made either by detection of the virus itself or by serologic response.

CMV can easily be detected in the urine either by culture or by electron microscopy. To confirm congenital disease, virus isolation must be done in the first 2 weeks postnatally, because virus shed after this time may represent acquired infection.

There is no safe and effective treatment for congenital CMV infection. It seems unlikely that postnatally administered antiviral agents will reverse prenatal organ damage; prevention of congenital infection is the most productive strategy. Investigation into CMV vaccines is ongoing, but there have been no trials in pregnant women to date.

HERPES SIMPLEX

Herpes simplex virus (HSV) is another herpesvirus that can affect the neonate. Infection with herpes simplex is extremely common in humans and usually leads to a benign, self-limited disease. However, in the newborn, infection with herpes simplex can be devastating and carries a high morbidity. Herpes simplex is a double-stranded DNA virus. Type 1 has been most often associated with oral lesions. Type 2 is more often the cause of genital infections and neonatal disease.

Neonatal herpes infection is estimated to occur in 1 in 2000 to 1 in 5000 deliveries each year. There are an estimated 700 to 1000 cases of neonatal infection annually in the United States. As the rate of maternal genital infection rises, the incidence of neonatal disease will increase.

Acquisition of the infection by the newborn infant most often occurs intrapartum. Seventy percent to 90% of infants acquire HSV infection by this means. Infants come in close contact with HSV when the mother is shedding the virus in her genital tract, particularly the cervix; contact may occur in the birth canal or the virus may ascend from the cervix after rupture of the membranes has occurred. An increased risk of infection has been observed when rupture of the membranes precedes delivery by more than 6 hours. Cesarean delivery has been associated with a lower risk of infection. In utero infection may also occur but is a less common event. Early postnatal acquisition may ensue from exposure to care providers who are shedding the virus from labial lesions or a whitlow.

The risk to the infant appears to be highest when birth occurs by vaginal delivery to a mother with an active primary infection. In this setting, the risk to the infant may be greater than 50%. Recurrent maternal infection appears to decrease the chance of both acquisition of infection and dissemination. Women with recurrent genital infection shed virus for a shorter period of time and in lower concentrations than those with primary disease. Mothers with recurrent disease are likely to have higher antibody levels, which, when passed transplacentally, appear to protect the newborn from infection. Those infants who do acquire infection in the presence of high maternal or neonatal antiherpes antibody are more likely to have localized disease involving only the skin or mucous membranes.

Infants who contract HSV during labor or delivery are most likely to present with symptoms at between 4 and 16 days of age. Many of these infants will have been discharged home when symptoms occur and may present to the emergency department for treatment.

Clinical Evaluation

Disseminated infection with herpes simplex consists of disease affecting multiple organ systems and carries a dismal prognosis. Encephalitis is especially common, affecting about 70% of those with disseminated disease. Hepatitis is another principal manifestation, but organs other than the liver may also be involved, including the lungs, adrenal glands, and gastrointestinal tract. The vesicular rash of herpes simplex is pathognomonic when present but may be absent in as many as 20% of affected patients. Children with disseminated herpes infection usually present with constitutional symptoms, including fever, lethargy, irritability, and poor feeding. Jaundice, bleeding diatheses, and seizures may also occur. Without treatment, the mortality rate exceeds 80%.

Encephalitis without dissemination accounts for roughly one third of the patients presenting with neonatal herpes simplex. These infants tend to present somewhat later than those with disseminated infection. Clinical manifestations are those associated with central nervous system infection: irritability, temperature instability, lethargy, vomiting, or seizures. Skin vesicles occur in only 60% at any time during the illness, and therefore, vesicles are commonly absent at the time of presentation. Death occurs in half of these infants if they are untreated, and most survivors are significantly impaired.

Infection localized to superficial sites, including the skin, eye, or mucous membranes, carries a better prognosis but may still lead to significant morbidity. These children usually present with characteristic vesicular lesions on the skin or in the mouth. Eye disease usually presents as keratoconjunctivitis. Although mortality from localized infection is rare, long-term neurologic abnormalities have been reported in patients whose disease appeared localized.

Diagnostic Evaluation

The definitive diagnosis of neonatal herpes simplex infection is based on viral isolation. Viral cultures should be obtained from skin lesions, cerebrospinal fluid, oropharynx, rectum, and eye lesions. A presumptive diagnosis can be made by staining material obtained from skin lesions. A vesicle can be broken and a scraping of the base of the lesion smeared on a glass slide. Wright or Papanicolaou staining will reveal multinucleated giant cells. These multinucleated cells are characteristic of either herpes simplex or varicella zoster viral lesions. Smears may also be stained with fluorescent antibody that is specific for herpes simplex virus. Serologic testing is not especially useful in diagnosing herpes simplex during the acute infection.

All newborns diagnosed with HSV or suspected of having HSV infection should have a complete assessment to determine the extent of their disease. Liver function, hematologic parameters, and hemostasis should be measured. A chest radiograph may reveal viral pneumonitis. All infants should undergo examination of the cerebrospinal fluid to determine central nervous system involvement.

Therapeutic Intervention

Timely institution of specific antiviral therapy is essential to improve the outcome of this potentially devastating disease. The National Institute of Allergy and Infectious Diseases (NIAID) Collaborative Study Group showed that the use of vidarabine in infants with congenital herpes simplex infections improved the outcome regardless of the clinical presentation. Those children with disseminated disease who received treatment had an unacceptably high mortality rate of 70%; without treatment the mortality rate was 90%. Treatment improved the outcome substantially for those infants with encephalitis or skin and mucous membrane disease. Early treatment was also found to decrease the number of children who progressed to more serious disease. The recommended dosage of vidarabine was 30 mg/kg/day administered over 12 hours. Treatment should continue for at least 10 to 14 days.

Acyclovir, a newer antiviral agent, is effective against other herpes simplex infections. The NIAID Collaborative Study Group indicates the safety and efficacy to be about equal for vidarabine and acyclovir. Acyclovir is administered intravenously every 8 hours at a dose of 10 mg/kg. Duration of therapy is 10 days (Table 73–3).

Infants with ocular involvement should receive topical antiviral treatment in addition to the therapy outlined earlier. Few studies specifically address the treatment of ocular disease in newborns, but trifluorthymidine is considered the drug of choice. Ocular acyclovir has been successfully tried for acquired herpes keratoconjunctivitis but is not available in the United States.

CONGENITAL SYPHILIS

The incidence of syphilis in the United States has risen since 1978. Between 1978 and 1985, the reported cases of congenital syphilis rose from 108 to 268 cases per 100,000.

Syphilis is caused by the spirochete *Treponema pallidum*. *T. pallidum* is not easily cultured in the laboratory. The organism is too narrow to be seen by light microscopy, but it can be viewed by darkfield examination and appears as a fine, thready corkscrew. *T. pallidum* has the ability to cause chronic infection characterized by early clinical disease followed by latency and recrudescence.

Congenital syphilis is acquired transplacentally. Transmission is most likely to occur in the earlier stages of maternal infection, but vertical transmission has been reported to occur in succeeding pregnancies and over many years. Infection of the first-trimester embryo is rare, and syphilis is not a cause of first-trimester miscarriage. Vertical transmission after the fourth or fifth month of gestation results in hematogenous spread in the fetus, and therefore, infection is widespread. This results in stillbirth in 25% to 30% of cases of untreated maternal syphilis. Another 10% of infants die in early infancy. The neonatal death rate also remains higher in developing countries.

Clinical Evaluation

The clinical presentation of congenital syphilis is widely variable, and many infants are without symptoms at birth. The clinical presentation has been divided into two stages: early congenital and late congenital. Early disease presents clinically prior to 2 years of age; late congenital syphilis appears in children older than 2 years.

Infants with early congenital syphilis are often premature and are likely to be small for gestational age. Common findings include hepatosplenomegaly and osteochondritis of the long bones. Syphilitic rhinitis, known as *snuffles*, is somewhat less common but may be present in the first few weeks of life. Skin lesions may be variable. A diffuse desquamation of the skin, including the palms and soles, can occur. However, dermatologic manifestations may also take the form of papules, bullae (pemphigus syphiliticus), or wart-like lesions (condyloma lata). Hematologic abnormalities also vary. A Coombs'-negative hemolytic anemia may occur and may be associated with hydrops fetalis. Other manifestations may include thrombocytopenia, bleeding diathesis, or a leukemoid reaction. Other disease expressions include lymphadenopathy, pneumonia, and glomerulonephritis. Cerebrospinal fluid abnormalities occur in 60% of patients, but affected infants are often without neurologic symptoms at the time of birth.

The clinical manifestations of late congenital syphilis may represent scars of initial lesions or may result from ongoing inflammatory processes. Although not the most common feature of late disease, Hutchinson's triad is very specific for syphilis. Hutchinson's triad consists of peg-shaped upper central incisors (Hutchinson's teeth), interstitial keratitis, and deafness. Mulberry molars are more common, occurring in 65%, and are also specific for congenital syphilis. Abnormalities of facial appearance are among the most frequently seen stigmata; these include frontal bossing, high-arched palate, and saddle nose. Bony abnormalities result from periosteal reactions and occur characteristically in the tibia, leading to saber shins (Fig. 73–1) or in the clavicle (Higouménakis's sign). Central nervous system involvement may lead to mental retardation and seizure disorder. Rhagades, linear scars around the lips or other orifices, occur rarely.

Diagnostic Evaluation

Because the spirochetes cannot be isolated in the laboratory, the diagnosis relies on serologic tests. There are two general types of serologic tests available: the nontreponemal antibody tests and the treponemal antibody tests. The two nontreponemal tests in common use are the rapid plasma reagin (RPR) and the Venereal Disease Research Laboratory (VDRL) tests, both of which measure antibody to cardiolipin-lecithin. The disadvantage of these tests is the significant number of false-positive results. The treponemal tests in common usage include the fluorescent treponemal antibody absorption test (FTA-ABS) and the microhemagglutination–*T. pallidum* assay (MHA-TP). These two tests detect antibody specific for treponemes. As in the case of other congenital infections, the definitive diagnosis of congenital syphilis in the newborn is confounded by transplacental passage of maternal antibody. A fluorescent antibody test to detect specific immunoglobulin M (IgM) has been developed in order to diagnose disease in the newborn; a specific test for IgM detects only antibodies produced by the fetus or infant. However, this test is plagued by both false-positive and false-negative results.

Because of the difficulty in diagnosing congenital syphilis, the Centers for Disease Control have developed a diagnostic classification to aid clinicians. A "confirmed" case is one in which *T. pallidum* has been directly identified either by darkfield examination or other specific stains from lesions or tissue specimens. "Compatible" cases include those with (1) a positive serologic test for syphilis (STS) in a stillborn; (2) a reactive STS in an infant whose mother had untreated or inadequately treated syphilis during pregnancy; (3) a reactive VDRL test in cerebrospinal fluid; (4) a reactive STS in the presence of characteristic clinical manifestations, in-

---

TABLE 73–3

CONGENITAL INFECTIONS: THERAPY AT A GLANCE

Infection	Specific Therapy
Cytomegalovirus	None available, supportive only
Herpes simplex	Acyclovir, 30 mg/kg/day IV divided q 8 hr *or* Vidarabine, 30 mg/kg/day IV given over 12 hr
Syphilis	Penicillin G, 50,000 U/kg/dose every 8 to 12 hr IV *or* Penicillin G procaine 50,000 U/kg IM every day for 10 to 14 days
Toxoplasmosis	Pyrimethamine, 1 mg/kg/day divided q 12 hr (maximum dose, 25 mg per day) *and* sulfadiazine or trisulfapyrimidines, 85 mg/kg/day divided q 12 h

cluding skin and mucous membrane findings, bony lesions, nephritis, hemolytic anemia, hepatomegaly, or splenomegaly; (5) a fourfold rise in titers of nontreponemal tests (VDRL or RPR) and a confirmed treponemal test (FTA-ABS or MHA-TP) over 3 months; and (6) a reactive serologic test that does not revert to negative after 6 months. Congenital syphilis is considered unlikely if there is no reactive STS or the treponemal tests revert to negative by 6 months. Infection is also considered unlikely in an asymptomatic infant whose mother was treated during pregnancy if the mother's titers showed a fourfold decrease and the infant's STS is four times lower than mother's titer at the time of treatment.

All newborns at risk should have a complete blood cell (CBC) count, including a platelet and reticulocyte count. Long-bone radiographs may reveal the typical osteitis. All infants should undergo a spinal tap to check for neurosyphilis. A cerebrospinal fluid (CSF) VDRL test should be performed in addition to the routine CSF studies. Other studies, including a Coombs' test, liver function tests, or chest radiograph, should be considered.

Therapeutic Intervention

The treatment of choice for syphilis is penicillin. Treatment of the pregnant woman with penicillin is highly effective in preventing congenital syphilis in the newborn; alternate regimens with erythromycin have failed to treat the fetus adequately. Only penicillin regimens are recommended for neonatal congenital syphilis. The currently recommended regimens include aqueous penicillin G, 50,000 U/kg/dose every 8 to 12 hours intravenously for 10 to 14 days, or aqueous penicillin G procaine, 50,000 U/kg intramuscularly daily for 10 to 14 days.

TOXOPLASMOSIS

Toxoplasma gondii is a protozoan organism related to the coccidia. The definitive host for the organism is the cat. Only in cats does the *Toxoplasma* organism complete its life cycle to become an oocyst, which is then shed in the feces. Man becomes infected by ingestion or inhalation of oocysts in contaminated soil or by ingesting meat of infected animals that contains tissue cysts. The fetus may be infected transplacentally.

The presence of *Toxoplasma* antibodies in women of childbearing age has been documented to be as high as 72% in Paris and as low as 21% in London. Seroprevalence among pregnant women in New York City has been reported to be 32%, but in Denver antibody was detected in only 3% of prenatal patients. It is estimated that 3300 infants with congenital toxoplasmosis are born annually in the United States.

The *Toxoplasma* organism is transmitted when a pregnant woman becomes parasitemic and placental infection thereby occurs. Most often the mother is asymptomatic. Transmission of the parasite to the child is dependent on the time of acquisition of maternal infection. Infection occurring in the third trimester, especially late in the third trimester, carries a 90% chance that the infant will be born infected. If the mother is infected in the first trimester, the chance of transmission is much lower—about 20%. However, infants infected earlier in gestation are more likely to be severely symptomatic. Spontaneous abortion may also occur. It is primary infection occurring during pregnancy that carries a risk to the fetus. Mothers who have *Toxoplasma* antibodies before they become pregnant are extremely unlikely to have infected infants.

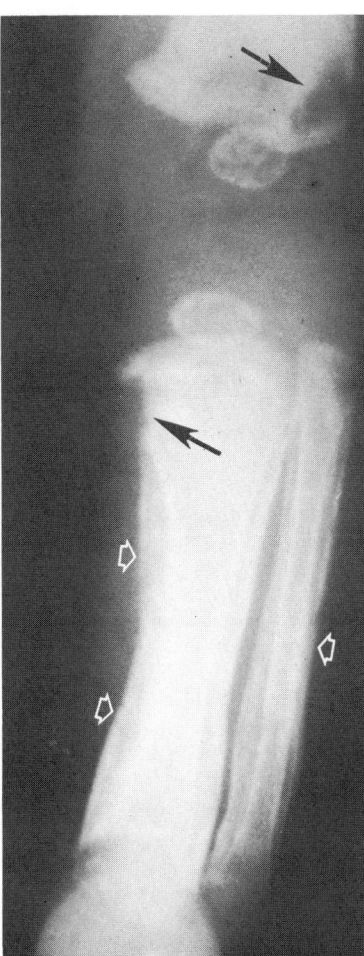

Figure 73–1. Typical destructive (metaphyseal: *black arrows*) and productive (diaphyseal: *open white arrows*) signs of congenital syphilis in a 2-year-old boy. The periosteal cloaking of the diaphyses may cause physical signs of "saber shin." The lucent Wimberger sign most typically spares the first few millimeters of metaphysis (i.e., membranous bone from the periphysis that also surrounds the physis), as in this example. (Modified from Oestreich AE, Crawford AH. Atlas of Pediatric Orthopedic Radiology. Stuttgart: Thieme, 1985. Courtesy of A. Oestreich, M.D., Cincinnati, OH.)

Clinical Evaluation

Symptoms in newborns with congenital *Toxoplasma* infection range from completely asymptomatic, subclinical infection to severe manifestations leading to early death. One third of infected newborns have some clinical indication of infection during the first few months of life; those with severe infection exhibit obvious signs at birth. Most infants, about 66%, appear completely normal at birth. However, a substantial number of those born with a subclinical infection eventually manifest the disease, some of them severely.

Infants born with apparent disease often have low birth weight. As is the case with many other congenital infections, jaundice, hepatosplenomegaly, and fever may occur. The most characteristic findings in congenital toxoplasmosis relate to the central nervous system and the eye. Intracranial calcifications occur in 11% to 36% of cases. The calcifications typically are scattered throughout the brain. Obstructive hydrocephalus is a common feature and may be present at birth or shortly thereafter; it is often progressive. Hydrocephalus may be the only central nervous system sign. However, some infants with congenital toxoplasmosis show signs of global central nervous system damage, including seizure disorder, abnormalities of muscle tone and posture, and psychomotor retardation. A smaller number of infants may exhibit microcephaly. Chorioretinitis is probably the most classic feature of congenital toxoplasmosis and is often bilateral. Newborns or young infants may present with strabismus, wandering eye movements, or leukocoria (white reflex) as indications of chorioretinitis. Retinal lesions are present in about 20% of patients at the time of birth. However, eye lesions resulting from congenital *Toxoplasma* infection can occur even years later.

Diagnostic Evaluation

Serologic testing is the most widely available method of diagnosis. There are a number of methods in common usage. Certain serologic methods, notably the complement fixation and indirect hemagglutination tests, have a high proportion of false-negative results in those with congenital disease. Because maternal immunoglobulin G (IgG) antibodies cross the placenta, specific IgM antibodies should also be measured.

Other laboratory workup in the infant suspected of congenital toxoplasmosis should include a CBC count with differential and platelet counts, as these infants may have anemia, eosinophilia, or thrombocytopenia. Liver function tests may be abnormal in those presenting with systemic symptoms. Cerebrospinal fluid abnormalities, including pleocytosis and elevated protein levels, have been reported even in subclinical cases. Infants may also require neurodiagnostic studies. Complete ophthalmologic examination is important.

Therapeutic Intervention

Specific chemotherapy directed against *T. gondii* is available and recommended for use in cases of congenital infection. Currently available antibiotic regimens are ineffective in the encysted stage, and therefore, the parasite is probably never completely eliminated by therapy.

The synergistic combination of pyrimethamine and sulfadiazine is recommended. Pyrimethamine is administered in a dose of 1 mg/kg/day in two divided doses (maximum dose, 25 mg/day). Sulfadiazine is administered in a dose of 85 mg/kg/day in two divided doses. Trisulfapyrimidines may be used instead of sulfadiazine. Spiramycin, a macrolide antibiotic, has also been found to be clinically effective against *T. gondii*. Currently there are no standard recommendations for the use of spiramycin in congenital toxoplasmosis; the drug is available in the United States only through the Centers for Disease Control.

In addition to specific antibiotics, supportive chemotherapy may also be required. Corticosteroids are recommended for those patients with evidence of persistent inflammation. These include patients with active chorioretinitis and those with signs of central nervous system inflammation (e.g., high cerebrospinal fluid protein levels).

INFECTION CONTROL CONSIDERATIONS

Presentation at the emergency department of an infant suspected of having a congenital infection demands consideration of proper infection control procedures to protect the staff members and other patients from exposure to infection. Most of the infections acquired transplacentally, such as syphilis, CMV, and hepatitis B, have the potential to be spread by contact with blood or other body fluids. Syphilis or herpes may be spread to personnel during contact with skin lesions. Generally standard universal precautions are adequate to prevent spread of congenital infection. Congen-

ital rubella is a special case, in that the virus can be isolated from the throat and nose, as well as from blood and urine, for as long as 1 year after birth. Infants suspected of having congenital rubella should be placed in contact isolation, and care should be taken to avoid exposure of susceptible persons. This includes avoidance of exposures in waiting rooms.

Selected References

Arven AM, Yeager AS, Bruhn LW, Grossman M. Neonatal herpes simplex infection in the absence of mucocutaneous lesions. J Pediatr 1982;100:715.

Beattie CP. Toxoplasmosis: With special reference to proposals for reducing congenital infection. Clin Exp Obstet Gynecol 1986;13:83.

Bryan EM, Nicholson E. Congenital syphilis. Clin Pediatr 1981;20:81.

Centers for Disease Control. Guidelines for the prevention and control of congenital syphilis. MMWR 1988;37:1.

Centers for Disease Control. 1989 sexually transmitted diseases treatment guidelines. MMWR 1989;38:11.

Chawla V, Pandit PB, Nkrumah FK. Congenital syphilis in the newborn. Arch Dis Child 1988;63:1393.

Conboy TJ, Pass RF, Stagno S, et al. Early clinical manifestations and intellectual outcome in children with symptomatic congenital cytomegalovirus infection. J Pediatr 1987;111:343.

Desmonts G, Couvreur J. Congenital toxoplasmosis: A prospective study of 378 pregnancies. N Engl J Med 1974; 290:1110.

Frenkel JK. Toxoplasmosis. Pediatr Clin North Am 1985;32:917.

Hurto C, Arvin A, Jacobs R, et al. Intrauterine herpes simplex virus infections. J Pediatr 1987;110:97.

Judge DM. Congenital syphilis. Prog Clin Biol Res 1988;281:87.

Kumar ML, Nankervis GA, Jacobs ID, et al. Congenital and postnatally acquired cytomegalovirus infection: Long-term follow-up. J Pediatr 1984;104:674.

MacDonald A, Tobin J. Congenital cytomegalovirus infection: A collaborative study on epidemiological, clinical and laboratory findings. Develop Med Child Neurol 1978;20:471.

Monif GR, Egan EA, Hold B, Eitzman DV. The correlation of maternal cytomegalovirus infection during varying stages in gestation with neonatal involvement. J Pediatr 1972;80:17.

Nankervis GA, Kumar ML, Cox FE, Gold E. A prospective study of maternal cytomegalovirus infection and its effect on the fetus. Am J Obstet Gynecol 1984;149:435.

Peckham CS. Cytomegalovirus in the neonate. J Antimicrob Chemother 1989;23:17.

Ricci JM, Fojaco RM, O'Sullivan MJ. Congenital syphilis: The University of Miami/Jackson Memorial Medical Center experience, 1986–1988. Obstet Gynecol 1989;75:687.

Stagno S, Pass RF, Cloud G, et al. Primary cytomegalovirus infection in pregnancy. JAMA 1986;256:1904.

Stagno S, Whitley RJ. Herpesvirus infections of pregnancy. N Engl J Med 1985;313:1270.

Whitley RJ. Neonatal herpes simplex virus infections. Clin Perinatol 1988;15:903.

Whitley R, Arvin A, Prober C, et al. A controlled trial comparing vidarabine with acyclovir in neonatal herpes simplex virus infection. N Engl J Med 1991;324:44.

Whitley R, Corey L, Arvin A, et al. Changing presentation of herpes simplex virus infection in neonates. J Infect Dis 1988;158:109.

Wilson CB, Remington JS, Stagno S, Reynolds DW. Sequelae in children born with subclinical congenital toxoplasma infection. Pediatrics 1980;66:767.

Yow MD, Williamson DW, Leeds LJ, et al. Epidemiologic characteristics of cytomegalovirus infection in mothers and their infants. Am J Obstet Gynecol 1988;158:1189.

CHAPTER 74

Parasitic Infections

Maria Jevitz Patterson

INTRODUCTION

Parasites comprise the top three infectious causes of worldwide mortality (malaria, schistosomiasis, and amoebiasis)

(Table 74–1). Among the most common parasites seen in the United States are *Enterobius, Ascaris, Strongyloides, Giardia,* and *Cryptosporidium.* In a 1976 survey by the Centers for Disease Control (CDC) of 414,820 stools submitted to state health laboratories for parasitic examination, 15.6% were positive (*Giardia,* 3.8%; *Trichuris,* 2.7%; *Ascaris,* 2.3%; *Enterobius,* which is not usually sought in stool, 1.7%; and *Entamoeba histolytica,* 0.6%).

Children are especially vulnerable to parasitic infestation because of lapses in personal hygiene and recreational habits (pica and close contact with pets and arthropod vectors). Children at increased risk for parasitic infection include children in day-care centers, immunocompromised children, and children who are travelers or refugees. Children are also at risk for zoonotic infection from their pets or from participating with their parents in eating exotic food.

It is estimated that more than 11 million U.S. children attend day care.[1] Day-care center attendance provides increased exposure to several infectious diseases, among them giardiasis, pinworm, and cryptosporidiosis.[1–11] Other disease-causing parasites include *Dientamoeba, Trichuris, Ascaris,* and *Strongyloides.*

An increasing number of U.S. children also travel internationally. A similar but distinct group are immigrants and refugees or, in certain locales in the United States, unregistered aliens.[12] Another group of U.S. children at risk are those who reside outside the U.S. for a time (e.g., those with military or missionary parents). One should review the duration of travel, conditions of travel, activities, and prophylaxis taken for infectious agents.

Parasitic infestations can also occur as a consequence of children's close interactions with pets. Common U.S. infestations include *Toxoplasma, Dipylidium caninum* (dog tapeworm), and *Dirofilaria immitis* (dog heartworm).

Clinical and Diagnostic Evaluation

It is important in the history and physical examination to define the organ systems affected (Table 74–2).[13] A travel history, including symptoms while traveling and immediately after traveling, any exposure to contaminated water or food or primitive sanitation, and insect exposure, should be elicited.

Laboratory evaluation should include a complete blood cell count, as peripheral eosinophilia (greater than 500 cells/mm³) suggests parasite infection.[14] The normal peripheral eosinophil count is 100 to 125 eosinophils/mm³ in adults and 225 eosinophils/mm³ in children younger than 12 years. Eosinophils are only moderately effective phagocytes; however, they are highly efficient cytotoxic cells against the helminths and tissue-invasive metazoan parasites. This response does not accompany protozoan infection, with the exception of *Pneumocystis* infection. Additional helpful laboratory evaluations include stool examination for fecal leukocytes (present in both bacterial and amoebic diarrheas, indicating inflammation of the intestinal mucosa from invasive pathogenesis) and for ova and parasites (definitive diagnosis requires identification of the parasite or its eggs by an experienced technologist). Ancillary studies include examination of duodenal aspirate, liver function testing, abdominal ultrasound, or specific parasitic serologic assays. Negative stool examinations obtained on three separate occasions, collected every other day, demonstrate a sufficient level of sensitivity to exclude parasitic infection.[15] Stool examinations may sometimes be negative even when eosinophilia is the presenting feature, as the eosinophilia might represent host response to a parasite migrating from the previous intestinal focus. Ideally, stools examined within 30 minutes of passing are examined for trophozoites, but fixed and stained stools are also useful to identify trophozoites. Formed stools, refrigerated or mixed with polyvinylalcohol or other fixatives, are suitable for detection of parasite eggs. Substances that compromise stool examination include barium, bismuth, antacids, and laxatives.

Stool samples are sometimes brought to the emergency department when the parents, after macroscopic examination, think that a child has "passed worms."[16] Confusing artifacts include remnants of partially digested capsules of oral medication, the jelly-like material in the lining of superabsorbent diapers, mucous threads, partially digested vegetable or fruit fibers, factitious seeding of diaper contents with annelids, or even maggot larvae–contaminated diaper contents.[17–21] In contrast, some contents resembling moving cucumber seeds or grains of rice are actually dog tapeworm proglottids.[22–24]

Management of parasitic disease encompasses both drug therapy and preventive approaches (Table 74–3). Preventive

---

TABLE 74–1

MEDICALLY IMPORTANT HUMAN PARASITES

Site of Infestation	Protozoa	Helminths		
		Nematodes	Trematodes	Cestodes
Blood/tissue	*Pneumocystis*	*Trichinella*	Schistosomes	*Echinococcus*
	Toxoplasma	Filaria	*Paragonimus*	*Taenia*
	Plasmodium	Cutaneous larva migrans:		
	Babesia	*Strongyloides,* hookworms		
	Leishmania	Visceral larva migrans:		
	Trypanosoma	*Toxocara*		
	Free-living amoeba	*Dirofilaria*		
Intestinal/urogenital tract	*Entamoeba histolytica*	*Enterobius*	*Fasciola*	*Taenia*
	Dientamoeba	*Ascaris*	*Clonorchis*	*Hymenolepis*
	Giardia	*Trichuris*		*Diphyllobothrium*
	Trichomonas	Hookworms		*Dipylidium*
	Cryptosporidium	*Strongyloides*		
	Isospora	*Anisakis*		
	Blastocystis			
Diseases Associated With Arthropod Parasites		Pediculosis		
		Scabies		
		Myiasis		

	TABLE 74–2				
	SYSTEMIC SIGNS AND SYMPTOMS ASSOCIATED WITH PARASITIC DISEASE				
Integumentary	**Cardiovascular**	**Respiratory**	**Gastrointestinal**	**Genitourinary**	**Central Nervous System**
Analgesia	Heart murmur	Cough	Abdominal pain	Cervicitis	Coma
Leishmaniasis	Chagas'	Ascariasis	Amoebiasis	Trichomoni-	Falciparum malaria
Perianal abscess/fistula	disease	Paragonimiasis	Anisakiasis	asis	Local lesion
Schistosomiasis	Myocarditis	Pneumonia	Giardiasis	Hematuria	Cysticercosis
Enterobiasis	Trichinosis	Ascariasis	Tapeworm infection	Schistoso-	Echinococcosis
Amoebiasis		Paragonimiasis	Strongyloidiasis	miasis	Free-living amoebiasis
Anal pruritus		Strongyloidiasis	Enterobiasis		Schistosomiasis
Enterobiasis		"Larva migrans"	Ascariasis		Toxoplasmosis
Pruritus		Pulmonary cyst/	Acute diarrhea		Meningoencephalitis
Onchocerciasis		mass	Trichuriasis		Free-living amoebiasis
Toxocariasis		Amoebiasis	Diarrhea/constipation		Ophthalmologic
Scabies		Echinococcosis	Tapeworm infection		changes
Swelling/erythematous			Chronic diarrhea		Free-living amoebiasis
lesions			Fluke infection		Chagas' disease
Chagas' disease			Cryptosporidiosis		Loiasis
Loiasis			Giardiasis		Onchocerciasis
Ulcer, abscess, eschar			Bloody diarrhea		Trichinosis
Chagas' disease			Amoebiasis		
Cutaneous leishman-			Intussusception		
iasis			Ascariasis		
Trypanosomiasis			Amoebiasis		
			Appendicitis		
			Enterobiasis		
			Amoebiasis		
			Tapeworm infection		
			Ascariasis		
			Trichuriasis		
			Hepatomegaly		
			Amoebic abscess		
			Chagas' disease		
			Fluke infection		
			Echinococcosis		
			Schistosomiasis		
			Visceral		
			leishmaniasis		
			Splenomegaly		
			Toxoplasmosis		
			Chagas' disease		
			Malaria		
			Schistosomiasis		
			Visceral		
			leishmaniasis		
			Bowel perforation/		
			obstruction:		
			Ascariasis		
			Amoebiasis		
			Passing worms/		
			proglottids:		
			Ascariasis		
			Tapeworm infection		

TABLE 74–3

COMMON PARASITIC INFECTIONS: THERAPY AT A GLANCE

Disease/Parasite	Drug of Choice	Dosage/Route
Amoebiasis		
Entamoeba histolytica		
Asymptomatic	Iodoquinol (diiodohydroxyquin)	30–40 mg/kg/day (maximum, 2 gm/day) po div q 8 hr × 20 days
Mild to moderate	Metronidazole	35–50 mg/kg/day po div q 8 hr × 10 days
		Then
	Iodoquinol	as above, × 20 days
Severe	Metronidazole	35–50 mg/kg/day po, IV div q 8 hr × 10 days
		Then
	Iodoquinol	as above, × 20 days
Ascariasis		
Ascaris lumbricoides	Pyrantel pamoate	11 mg/kg po × 1 dose
		or
	Mebendazole	100 mg bid × 3 days
Cryptosporidiosis		
Cryptosporidium spp.	No proved effective therapy	
Cutaneous larva migrans or creeping eruption (cutaneous hookworm)	Thiabendazole suspension	Topically bid × 2–5 days
		or
	Thiabendazole	50 mg/kg/day (maximum, 3 gm/day) po div q 12 hr × 3 days
Giardiasis		
Giardia lamblia	Furazolidone	6–8 mg/kg/day po div q 6 hr × 7–10 days
		or
	Quinacrine	6 mg/kg/day po div q 8 hr × 7 days (maximum, 300 mg/day)
		or
	Metronidazole	15 mg/kg/day div q 8 hr × 7 days (investigational)
Hookworm		
Necator americanus, Ancylostoma duodenale	Mebendazole	100 mg po bid × 3 days
Lice		
Pediculus capitis or *humanus, Phthirus pubis*	Pyrethrin *or* Permethrin *or* Lindane	Applied topically once; repeat in 1 week
	Petrolatum	For eyelashes
Malaria		
Prophylaxis		
For areas without resistant *Plasmodium falciparum*	Chloroquine phosphate	5 mg base/kg (maximum, 300 mg) po once weekly, beginning 1–2 wk before arrival in malarial zone and continuing for 6 wk after last exposure
For areas where chloroquine-resistant *P. falciparum* exist	Chloroquine phosphate	As above
		plus
	Pyrimethamine-sulfadoxine (Fansidar)	Have 500 mg tab available: 2–11 mo, ¼ tab; 1–2 yr, ½ tab
	Mefloquine (children > 15 kg)	15–19 kg, ¼ tab po; 20–30 kg, ½ tab po; 31–45 kg, ¾ tab po; > 45 kg, 1 tab po; tabs are 250 mg and are given once weekly beginning one week before travel, continued during travel, and given for 4 weeks after travel.

Table continued on following page

TABLE 74–3

COMMON PARASITIC INFECTIONS: THERAPY AT A GLANCE *Continued*

Disease/Parasite	Drug of Choice	Dosage/Route
Treatment of disease		
P. falciparum chloroquine-resistant	Quinine sulfate	25 mg/kg/day po div q 8 hr × 3 days *and*
	Pyrimethamine	0.5–1 mg/kg/day (maximum, 25 mg) po div q 12 hr × 3 days (supplemental folinic acid) *and*
	Sulfadiazine	120–150 mg/kg/day po div q 6 hr × 5 days
All *Plasmodium* except chloroquine-resistant *P. falciparum*	Chloroquine phosphate	10 mg base/kg (maximum, 600 mg) po stat, then 5 mg base/kg at 6 hr, 24 hr, and 48 hr after initial dose *then*
Plasmodium vivax, P. ovale, P. malariae, P. falciparum (chloroquine-susceptible)		exoerythrocytic stage of *P. vivax* and *ovale* requires primaquine
Pinworms		
Enterobius vermicularis	Pyrantel pamoate	11 mg/kg po × 1 dose *or*
	Mebendazole	100 mg po × 1 dose; repeat treatment in 2 wk
Pneumocystis pneumonia		
Pneumocystis carinii	Trimethoprim-sulfamethoxazole	20 mg trimethoprim–100 mg sulfamethoxazole/kg/day po, IV div q 6 hr × 14 days *or*
	Pentamidine isethionate	4 mg base/kg/day IM, IV daily × 14 days
Scabies		
Sarcoptes scabei	Permethrin *or*	Applied to all of body
	Lindane *or*	Applied to all of body below neck
	Crotamiton	
Tapeworms		
Taenia, Diphyllobothrium, Dipylidium	Niclosamide	Approximately 40 mg/kg po chewed thoroughly × 1 dose *or*
	Praziquantel	10–20 mg/kg × 1 dose
Cysticercus cellulosae (cysticercosis)	Surgical resection; Praziquantel	50 mg/kg/day div q 8 hr × 14 days
Echinococcus granulosus (hydatid cyst)	Surgical resection; Albendazole (investigational)	
Toxoplasmosis		
Toxoplasma gondii		
	Pyrimethamine	2 mg/kg/day po div q 12 hr × 3 days, then 1 mg/kg/day (maximum, 25 mg) po div q 12 hr × 4 wk (supplemental folinic acid) *and*
	Trisulfapyrimidines or Sulfadiazine	120 mg/kg/day po div q 6 hr × 4 wk after resolution of illness
Trichinosis		
Trichinella spiralis	Thiabendazole	50 mg/kg/day po div q 12 hr × 5 days
Trichomoniasis		
Trichomonas vaginalis	Metronidazole	15 mg/kg/day po div q 8 h (maximum, 1 gm/day) × 7–10 days; treat sexual partners
Trichuris trichiura (whip worm)	Mebendazole	100 mg po BID × 3 days
Visceral Larva Migrans		
Toxocara canis; T. cati	Thiabendazole	50 mg/kg/day (maximum, 3 gm/day) po div q 12 h × 5 days
	Diethylcarbamazine	6 mg/kg/day div q 8 h × 7 days
	Ivermectin (investigational)	

Verification of dosage and toxic side effects of the antiparasitic drugs requires review of the manufacturer's package insert. Many antiparasitic drugs, especially alternative drugs, must be obtained through the Parasitic Disease Drug Service, Centers for Disease Control, Atlanta (404) 639–3670. A consultation with a pediatric infectious disease specialist in these cases is appropriate.

efforts include good personal hygiene, vector control, proper environmental sanitation (e.g., not using untreated feces for fertilizer and appropriate disposal of human waste), strict food preparation, protection of skin from soil contamination, and protection of the water supply.[25]

PROTOZOA
Pneumocystis

Pneumocystis carinii is an opportunistic parasite brought to greater attention by the acquired immunodeficiency syndrome (AIDS) epidemic.[26, 27] Prior to 1980, *Pneumocystis* infections were recognized as sporadic pneumonias occurring in adults and children, usually those with decreased immune competence from leukemia or lymphoma, anticancer therapy, suppression associated with organ transplantation, prematurity, or congenitally acquired immunodeficiency.[28, 29]

These infections remain a leading cause of morbidity and mortality in children with hematologic or lymphoreticular cancer but now have become the most common life-threatening infection in patients with human immunodeficiency virus (HIV) infection.[30–33] In more than 60% of patients with HIV infection, *Pneumocystis* pneumonia is the AIDS-defining disease.[34] In children, the mortality rate associated with acute infection (resulting from extensive alveolar injury) approaches 40%.[35]

Pneumocystis is a protozoan parasite, although this classification is questioned by some. It is believed that most humans are latently infected with this opportunist of low virulence and that reactivation in the immunocompromised host results in acute disease. Both cyst and trophozoite stages are recognized, with the latter being more common in lung tissue in patients with acute pneumonia. The trophozoites actively replicate in alveolar spaces to massive numbers with hematologic or lymphatic dissemination.[36]

Clinical Evaluation

The clinical examination in all immunosuppressed patients must be scrupulous, as the usual signs and symptoms may be masked. Onset can range from a relatively long period of indolent insidious disease to abrupt fulminant pneumonitis.[37, 38] The classic presentation includes fever, tachypnea, dyspnea, mild or nonproductive cough, wheezing, rhonchi, and gradually progressive hypoxemia and respiratory distress.

Extrapulmonary manifestations include otitis media, lymphatic or splenic involvement, retroperitoneal infection, and widely disseminated disease.[36, 39–41] Radiologic manifestations can also vary from a normal roentgenogram, to hyperaeration, to the classic appearance of bilateral diffuse, interstitial, ground-glass infiltrates. Atypical radiologic findings include a unilateral infiltrate, lobar consolidation, pleural effusion, and nodular, cavitary, or pneumatocele lesions.[42] Once chest radiographic changes are present, the mortality rate for untreated non-AIDS patients approaches 100%.[37]

Diagnostic Evaluation

The laboratory diagnosis of *Pneumocystis* pneumonia is dependent on finding the characteristic cyst or trophozoite stages.[29, 43–45] In children with AIDS, the concentration of *Pneumocystis* is generally high enough that bronchoalveolar lavage, tracheal aspirates, or even induced sputum can establish the diagnosis.[46–49] However, in some children, more invasive procedures such as transthoracic needle aspiration or open lung biopsy may be required.

Therapeutic Intervention

Trimethoprim-sulfamethoxazole (TMP-SMZ) is considered the first-line therapy, with pentamidine reserved for patients who exhibit TMP-SMZ failure or drug intolerance. Drug-induced toxicity is common with both agents. Pentamidine can cause hypoglycemia, acute pancreatitis, and renal failure.

Continued prophylaxis is important for any patient who has had a previous *Pneumocystis* infection, as recurrence is common. In patients with AIDS, there is increased risk for *Pneumocystis* pneumonia when CD4 cells are fewer than 200/mm³, warranting empiric prophylaxis.[27, 50] TMP-SMZ is also the most commonly used suppressive agent.

Predictors of poor prognosis in adults with *Pneumocystis* pneumonia include recurrent infection, respiratory rate greater than 30 breaths/min, increased alveolar-arteriolar O_2 gradient, extensive bilateral infiltrates, concurrent pulmonary infection (often *Mycobacterium avium-intracellulare* or cytomegalovirus) and abnormal laboratory values (elevated lactate dehydrogenase (LDH), low albumin). Improved short-term survival in adult patients with AIDS and *P. carinii* pneumonia has accompanied the use of zidovudine.[51]

Toxoplasma gondii

Toxoplasma gondii, an obligate intracellular protozoan, is a member of the Coccidia subclass. There are three morphologic forms: trophozoites or tachyzoites (the acute infectious form), bradyzoites (the acute or latent encysted form), and oocysts (the sexual form in the intestinal tract of cats). Trophozoites can invade all nucleated cells but especially invade those of the brain, bone, and cardiac muscle.[52, 53] The cat is the definitive host. Children acquire the infection by ingesting either oocysts from cat feces or inadequately cooked meat containing tissue cysts (bradyzoites) (Fig. 74–1).

Transmission also occurs with primary maternal infection during pregnancy. Of infants with congenital infection, 90% are asymptomatic at birth (an estimated 2500 infants yearly in the United States). Symptomatic infants with the *Toxoplasma* triad present with hydrocephalus, chorioretinitis, and intracranial calcification.[54–56] The long-term prognosis for

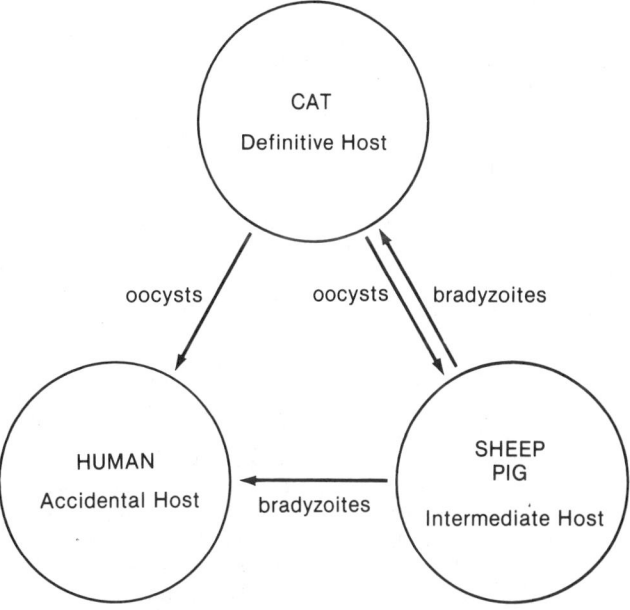

Figure 74–1. *Toxoplasma* life cycle.

children with even subclinical congenital infection is guarded.[57, 58] Additional human-to-human transmission has occurred through organ and bone marrow transplantation.[60]

Because mothers with primary infection and documented seroconversion are often asymptomatic, prevention of fetal transmission requires prospective screening during pregnancy.[59] Prompt diagnosis during pregnancy and the use of antiprotozoan therapy do not eliminate fetal infection but can greatly improve fetal outcome.[60, 61]

It is thought that only 10% of infected immunocompetent persons are symptomatic. Since the advent of AIDS, toxoplasmosis has become one of the most common causes of encephalitis (30% to 40% of patients with AIDS) and cerebral mass lesions.[33, 62]

Clinical Evaluation

Acute disease in older children and adults is characterized by cervical adenopathy, low-grade fever, malaise, and, rarely, extranodal disease.[63] In the immunodeficient patient, the disease is often a severe, fatal reactivation of a latent infection, with central nervous system involvement or widespread dissemination.[64]

Diagnostic Evaluation

Diagnosis is made by antigen detection and antibody response.[65] The differential diagnosis of toxoplasmosis in teenagers is generalized lymphoma or lymphosarcoma and in children with AIDS, central nervous system lymphoma or other mass lesions.[63, 66]

Therapeutic Intervention

The need for treatment of the acute lymphadenopathy form of toxoplasmosis in the immunocompetent, nonpregnant host is variable in that some people get better even without treatment.

Plasmodium (Malaria)

Malaria is the leading global parasitic disease and the most common febrile disease imported into the United States. Prevalence in the United States has been increasing since the 1970s among three groups: U.S. military personnel, foreign civilians, and U.S. civilians (an estimated 8000 imported cases in the United States in the period 1974–1983).[67, 68]

Malaria is caused by a protozoan parasite belonging to the genus *Plasmodium*. There are four species: *Plasmodium falciparum*, *Plasmodium ovale*, *Plasmodium vivax*, and *Plasmodium malariae*, all of which are transmitted from person to person by the bite of an Anopheles mosquito vector. The incubation period is 2 to 3 weeks after the bite but may be prolonged in patients who have received inadequate prophylaxis.

Importation of malaria from Mexico is associated with intramuscular injection of malaria parasites for putative treatment of Lyme disease.[69] The precedent for such therapy is the obsolete treatment of neurosyphilis in the pre-penicillin era by induction of malaria with its ensuing fever to kill the spirochetes. This practice is condemned because of high iatrogenic morbidity and mortality rates. Malaria (especially that caused by *P. falciparum*) is a life-threatening disease (4.2% mortality rate) that must be excluded in all returning, febrile U.S. travelers. The pathogenesis consists of mechanical obstruction caused by sequestration and sludging of parasitized erythrocytes in the vascular bed.

Clinical Evaluation

Any returning febrile traveler should be questioned regarding the compliant use of drug prophylaxis, including continuation for 4 to 6 weeks after leaving the endemic area. The likelihood of exposure to chloroquine-resistant organisms should be assessed. The clinical presentation includes recurring or sustained high fever, headache, diarrhea, abdominal pain, jaundice, cough, dyspnea, prostration, and altered consciousness progressing to coma. In children, fever is less often periodic.[67] Secondary infections are a significant complication, and increased mortality is associated with delayed diagnosis.

Physical examination may reveal hypotension, pulmonary edema, severe anemia, hepatosplenomegaly, or renal failure. The World Health Organization (WHO) criteria for severe or complicated malaria, most often associated with *P. falciparum*, are greater than 5% erythrocytes infected, encephalopathy/cerebral disease, acute respiratory distress syndrome, circulatory collapse, disseminated intravascular coagulation, hematocrit less than 20%, bilirubin level greater than 50 µmol/L (2.9 mg/dl), creatinine level greater than 265 µmol/L (3.0 mg/dl), and glucose level less than 2.2 mmol/L (40 mg/dl). Laboratory evaluation requires the examination of both thick and thin blood smears for intra- and exoerythrocytic forms by a microbiologist or a pathologist.

Therapeutic Intervention

The goal of therapy is to lower the parasitemia as promptly as possible. Treatment is based on suspicion of chloroquine-resistant *P. falciparum*.[70–72] Treatment for chloroquine-resistant *P. falciparum* includes quinine sulfate plus pyrimethamine sulfadoxine (Fansidar), tetracycline, or clindamycin; mefloquine; or parenteral treatment (for severe malaria) with quinine dihydrochloride or quinidine gluconate. Treatment for all other *Plasmodium* infections is chloroquine. Because *P. vivax* and *P. ovale* have exoerythrocytic tissue stages that can result in relapse, primaquine phosphate is recommended after initial therapy. Mefloquine is effective against all *Plasmodium* species, including chloroquine- or pyrimethamine sulfa–resistant strains.

Chloroquine has a small therapeutic window. Childhood chloroquine poisonings, with resultant cardiac and neurologic toxicity, have been reported when the dose range of 5 to 10 mg/kg of base is exceeded.[73, 74]

Prevention of infection requires mosquito eradication, use of insect repellents, netting or protective clothing, and chemoprophylaxis, which, for the pediatric patient, is chloroquine phosphate. Mefloquine prophylaxis has been approved for adults and the dosing guidelines revised.[75, 76] Mefloquine is the prophylactic drug of choice in adults and children (> 15 kg) traveling to chloroquine-resistant areas. If chloroquine phosphate is used for prophylaxis in children or adults traveling to chloroquine-resistant areas, a single dose of pyrimethamine sulfadoxine should be carried for initiation of presumptive treatment. Mefloquine should not be used for treatment once malaria is acquired; it is used only for prophylaxis.

Babesia

Babesiosis is a malaria-like illness caused by the protozoan parasite *Babesia microti*. Like malaria, it is transmitted by an arthropod vector. The deer tick *Ixodes dammini* that transmits *Babesia* also transmits Lyme disease.[77] Therefore, babesiosis has been reported in the same ecologic niches as Lyme disease—New England, Wisconsin, and Minnesota—and the geographic range of the tick is increasing. Rodents are the reservoir for *Babesia*. Person-to-person transmission has also been associated with transfusion of platelets and red blood cells[78, 79] but methods of screening blood donors for babesiosis are not yet available.

The clinical spectrum for babesiosis ranges from asymptomatic to fever, malaise, possible hemolytic anemia, and renal failure. Effective treatment has been inconsistent, but the malaria regimen of quinine plus clindamycin has most commonly been used.[70]

Free-Living Amoeba

Amoeba, free-living in water and soil world-wide, were originally thought to be harmless to humans and animals. However, two distinct human clinical associations have emerged: meningoencephalitis and keratitis.

Meningoencephalitis

The amoebic meningoencephalitides are divided into primary meningoencephalitis and granulomatous encephalitis.[80–83] The former is usually caused by infection with *Naegleria* species acquired by swimming in fresh or brackish water or swimming pools or using hot tubs by children and young adults in previously good health. The presumed portal of entry is the nasal cavity with inhalation of dust or aspiration of water. The clinical course is abrupt in onset, resembles acute bacterial meningitis, has a fulminant progression, and often leads to death within 1 week of onset of symptoms. Diagnostic suspicion is prompted by purulent meningitis in which specimens subjected to Gram stain, rapid antigen detection, and culture are negative and clinical deterioration continues despite treatment. Diagnosis is established by phase contrast microscopic examination of fresh spinal fluid for motile amoeba. Culture of the free-living amoeba on lawns of *Escherichia coli* is possible, but this method is not readily available. Serologic assays are not generally useful, because primary meningoencephalitis has a fulminant course, and granulomatous encephalitis is often unsuspected until autopsy.

The agent of granulomatous encephalitis is *Acanthamoeba* species, often associated with immunosuppression, including iatrogenic suppression or suppression from an underlying disease state. In contrast to infections by *Naegleria*, these often manifest as insidious chronic infections, usually fatal, mimicking a number of neurologic disorders with focal neurologic deficits and an altered mental status.[84] Entry into the central nervous system is thought to be by hematogenous spread from the skin or lungs. A brain computed tomography (CT) scan may reveal a ring-enhancing lesion. Cerebrospinal fluid (CSF) analysis shows lymphocytic pleocytosis. The diagnosis is established by brain biopsy.

Keratitis

Infectious keratitis associated with *Acanthamoeba* was first described in 1973 and originally thought to be associated with trauma. It is an increasing cause of corneal infection linked to ophthalmologic use of topical corticosteroids, increased use of soft contact lenses, or exposure to contaminated water in lens-cleaning solutions.[85–91] Presenting features are severe ocular pain and a progressive irregular epithelial lesion, often initially misdiagnosed as herpes and refractory to usual medication.[92] Diagnosis is made by examining corneal scrapings or lens fluid using phase contrast microscopy, Giemsa stain, or indirect fluorescent antibody staining.

Early keratoplastic surgery may be required to prevent partial or complete loss of vision. Prevention of amoebic keratitis entails cleaning and disinfection of lenses each time they are removed, disinfection of lenses at intervals suggested by the manufacturer, use of thermal rather than cold chemical disinfection, avoidance of homemade disinfection solutions, and avoidance of contact lens use while swimming.[87, 90–92]

Enteric Amoeba

In the United States, *Entamoeba histolytica* infections are most prevalent among immigrants, travelers, and Native American children.[93] Humans are at increased risk in endemic areas where there has been compromise of drinking water quality by heavy rain or flooding or use of human feces as fertilizer.[94]

Humans are the major reservoir, and transmission is fecal-oral. These infections are often acquired from contaminated water or vegetables. The cecum is the most common site of infestation; the most common extraintestinal site is the liver.

Clinical Evaluation

Symptomatic amoebiasis resembles severe giardiasis, with fever, colitis, and intussusception. Bloody diarrhea is more often seen with amoebiasis. Liver abscess is the most frequent extraintestinal manifestation; it is more common in children than in adults.

Intestinal amoebae may result in polymorphonuclear neutrophils in stools. Stools in amoebiasis should be inspected for trophozoites and cysts of *E. histolytica*, which must be distinguished from the commensal enteric amoebae: *Endolimax*, *Iodamoeba*, *Entamoeba coli*, and *Entamoeba hartmanni*. If proctoscopy is performed, superficial ulcers are characteristic, and histologic examination of the ulcer tissue aids in diagnosis. Serologic assays are also available. Radiologic examination is rarely needed, but imaging techniques such as ultrasound, a liver scan, or CT can help differentiate amoebomas from tumors and invasive amoebiasis from inflammatory bowel disease. Because intestinal amoebiasis can become worse with corticosteroid therapy, excluding amoebiasis prior to steroid treatment of suspected inflammatory bowel disease is required.[5]

Medical treatment is generally effective. Complications of intestinal amoebiasis include perforation; peritonitis; superficial amoebic abscess of the perianal skin in diapered children; migration to the appendix, resulting in appendicitis or amoeboma; and widely metastatic focal infection of the lungs or brain.[93–95]

Dientamoeba

Dientamoeba fragilis is a protozoan parasite capable of causing gastrointestinal symptoms.[96] It colonizes the cecum and proximal large bowel but is not invasive. It is not a true amoeba, but a flagellate; causes superficial mucosal irritation; and results in intermittent diarrhea, abdominal pain, anorexia, and peripheral eosinophilia. Children are more likely to be symptomatic than adults, and transmission among children in day-care centers is reported. Complications include appendiceal fibrosis and biliary infection.

Diagnosis is difficult, as there is no cyst form. Only the fragile trophozoites, which are not readily found on standard ova and parasite examination, are present. Stools should be examined promptly or placed in a preservative for stained examination. Treatment in the United States using diiodohydroxyquin is investigational.[70]

Giardia

Giardia lamblia is an enteric protozoan flagellate with worldwide distribution and associated with diarrhea. It is a common cause of diarrhea and malabsorption in children in day-care centers, immunocompromised children, and travelers.[30, 97–101] Children with cystic fibrosis are also at increased risk, as are adults with hepatic or pancreatic disease.[102, 103]

Infection can be acquired by ingestion of cysts from water or foods.[104, 105] Water-associated outbreaks have been reported with surface streams contaminated by beaver and other animal wildlife feces and with city water with sewage runoff, but not with well water without fecal contamination.[106–108] Outbreaks have also been associated with recreational water such as swimming pools and water slides.[109–111]

In day-care centers, fecal-oral transmission can occur from contaminated fomites (toys, bottles, utensils), especially among toddlers. Infected children serve as significant reservoirs in their families.[112]

The mechanism of diarrhea production is unclear. Trophozoites are found in the lumen of the proximal small bowel; cysts are found in the distal small bowel and colon.

Clinical Evaluation

The clinical presentation varies from no symptoms to acute diarrhea or even chronic diarrhea.[113] Frequently there are mild symptoms, abdominal discomfort, nonbloody diarrhea alternating with constipation, and flatulence. Protracted diarrhea in children may be associated with weight loss. Occasionally fat, carbohydrate, and vitamin malabsorption may result. Polyarthritis occurs in children and adults.[114] Rare complications include biliary infection, cholangitis, hepatitis, and chronic urticaria.[5]

Diagnostic Evaluation

Diagnosis involves identification of motile trophozoites or cysts (Fig. 74–2). Stool specimens and duodenal aspirates are most reliable.[115] The Enterotest (Hedeco, Palo Alto, CA) is easy to use and well tolerated by children.[116] A weighted gelatin capsule lined with a silicon rubber bag and absorbent string attached (90 cm for pediatric use) provides a sample of duodenal contents. The capsule is swallowed, then later retrieved for microscopic examination for duodenal para-

sites such as *Giardia*, *Strongyloides*, *Clonorchis*, *Fasciola*, and *Isospora*. Antigen detection systems have also been introduced for use with stool specimens or intestinal contents.[99]

Therapeutic Intervention

Treatment regimens include quinacrine, metronidazole, or furazolidone, with an efficacy rate of 80% to 90% after a single course.[5] Some treatment failures represent biologic variation in sensitivity.[117] Therefore, alternative drugs should be used if treatment failure occurs. Controversies in treatment of children relate to balancing the side effects of treatment against the anticipated cure rate and whether the goal should be parasitologic cure or freedom from symptoms in children in day-care centers. Recurrent infections are common among children in group settings, even with demonstrated negative results on stool examination.

Prevention is achieved by careful attention to hygiene and sanitation (i.e., frequent hand washing, especially after diaper changing or defecation, and before food preparation). Symptomatic carriers should not work in health care settings providing patient care or work in or attend day-care centers. Household and day-care center contacts should be tested for *Giardia*.

Trichomonas

Trichomoniasis is a common sexually transmitted disease with high prevalence and with high infectivity. It is estimated that millions of women and their generally asymptomatic male sexual partners are infected annually in the United States. *Trichomonas vaginalis* is a flagellated protozoan parasite whose nonsexual transmission is rare, and occurrence in prepubescent non-neonatal children raises the suspicion of sexual abuse.[118–120]

Vertical transmission from an infected mother to the newborn occurs during passage through an infected birth canal. Pathogenesis in the neonatal vagina appears to be influenced by maternal estrogen, which is metabolized by the age of 3 to 4 weeks. The infant's vaginal epithelium then becomes relatively resistant to *Trichomonas* and remains so until puberty.[121] The neonatal respiratory tract and eyes can also be colonized, resulting in respiratory distress or conjunctivitis.[122, 123]

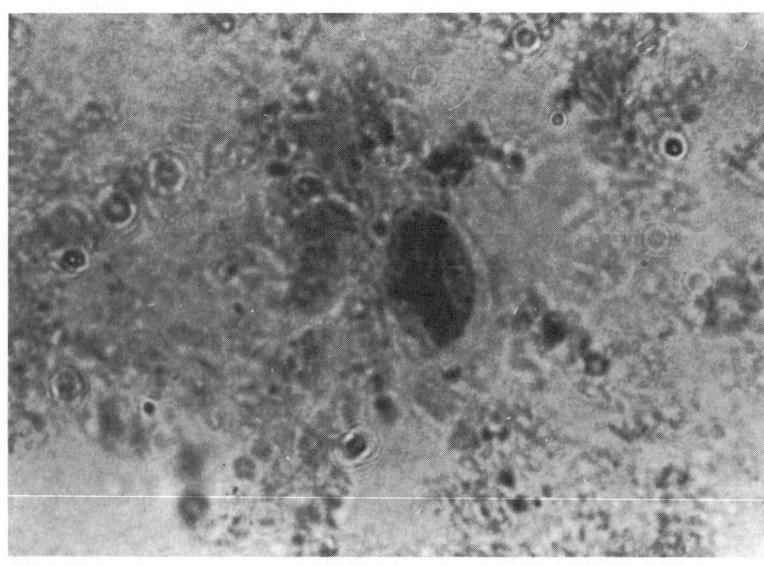

Figure 74–2. *Giardia* trophozoite (× 3500). (Courtesy of M. Kron, Tropical and Infectious Disease Laboratory, Departments of Pathology and Medicine, Michigan State University, East Lansing, MI.)

Clinical Evaluation

Vaginal trichomoniasis is associated with yellow purulent discharge, "strawberry spots" on the cervix, and erythema of the vulva and vagina.[124] The standard for diagnosis is the wet mount or hanging drop microscopic demonstration of motile protozoa in fresh vaginal secretions mixed with saline. More sensitive methods include culture or antigen-based detection systems. The direct examination of the vaginal sample by wet mount requires 10^4 to 10^5 *Trichomonas* organisms per milliliter. An alternative microscopic method to the wet mount is the Papanicolaou-stained cervical smear. A wet mount screen should accompany the examination of sexually active teens with purulent vaginal fluid or vaginal erythema.[125] Victims of sexual assault may have no *Trichomonas* detected on the initial wet mount and even on the culture but may subsequently develop an infection.

Therapeutic Intervention

Therapy for infants beyond the neonatal period and children is metronidazole. Metronidazole is contraindicated in the first trimester of pregnancy because of concerns about fetal malformation.

Cryptosporidium

The clinical spectrum for *Cryptosporidium* is broad: originally thought to be an incidental finding, then a recognized veterinary pathogen, a zoonosis, an opportunistic agent among immunocompromised patients, and finally a recognized common cause of diarrhea.[5, 6, 26, 126–131]

Cryptosporidium organisms are small, hardy protozoan parasites of the Coccidia subclass. In humans they have a predilection for the jejunum but are found throughout the entire gastrointestinal tract.

There are multiple important modes of transmission: zoonoses from mammalian hosts, including farm and companion animals; person-to-person in day-care centers; food- and water-borne; and environmental transmission of resistant cysts.[8, 10, 11, 127, 132–140] Mechanisms of pathogenesis remain unclear. No toxin has yet been identified in this cholera-like diarrhea. There is a higher prevalence in children than in adults.

Clinical Evaluation

Infection can range from an asymptomatic state to severe intractable diarrhea. Intractable diarrhea, insidious in onset, occurs in compromised hosts, but clinical infection is not confined to immunodeficient or malnourished patients. Infection is relatively common but self-limited, lasting about 20 days in immunocompetent children, although some normal children shed oocysts for up to 7 weeks.[7, 9, 128, 141–145]

The diarrhea is similar to that of giardiasis but generally with less bloating and less anorexia. Stools are voluminous, watery, nonbloody, and nonleukocytic and can be accompanied by dehydration. The diarrhea is secretory and followed by malabsorption of lactose and fat. Low-grade fever, malaise, weight loss, and crampy epigastric or, less commonly, right upper quadrant (biliary) pain may occur. Complications more common in immunocompromised children include cholecystitis, hepatitis, appendicitis, colitis, respiratory tract infection, and reactive arthritis.[145–148]

Diagnostic Evaluation

All patients with HIV infection and diarrhea require a comprehensive stool examination for routine enteric bacterial pathogens, mycobacterial species, protozoan parasites, and cytomegalovirus. Fecal blood or leukocytes are uncommon with *Cryptosporidium*. Direct stool examination with special techniques has replaced detection by intestinal biopsy.[149] The laboratory must receive a specific request to look for oocysts of *Cryptosporidium*, which are morphologically similar to *Candida* and *Blastocystis*.

Therapeutic Evaluation

There is no effective treatment for *Cryptosporidium*. Trials of spiramycin, a macrolide antibiotic, are ongoing but not promising.[150, 151] Nonspecific antidiarrheals have been associated with worsening symptoms. Remittance in patients with immunodeficiency is usually only brief. Supportive care with maintenance of fluid and electrolyte balance and avoidance of lactose is helpful, and oral rehydration is often adequate unless there is concurrent vomiting. When immunosuppression is associated with chemotherapy, discontinuing chemotherapy to allow restoration of the normal flora and function of the gut may result in resolution.[144, 152, 153]

Prevention is difficult, because the oocysts are remarkably environmentally resistant and are resistant to common disinfectants.[132, 154] Avoidance of soil contamination, especially of food and water, is important. Swimming pools employing rapid sand filter systems do not effectively clear the small 4- to 6-μ oocysts; outbreaks may require temporary closing of public pools.[155] Good hand washing and routine enteric precautions should be followed when caring for infected patients or children in day-care centers. Cryptosporidial infections do not require national notification but may need to be reported to local health departments.

Isospora

Isospora belli is a member of the protozoan Coccidia subclass. Its prevalence in the United States is not fully known. *Isospora* has become recognized as an enteric pathogen among the increasing number of patients with immune deficiency and chronic debilitation.[156]

Transmission is presumed to occur by ingestion of oocysts from fecally contaminated food or water. Malabsorption, especially of lactose and fat, accompanies an insidious chronic diarrhea. The disease is clinically indistinguishable from that of *Cryptosporidium*, with fever, headache, persistent watery diarrhea, colic, and weight loss.[157] Diarrhea is acute and self-limited in the immunocompetent host.

Diagnosis is made by examination of stools for cysts. When there is low parasitic infestation, duodenal aspiration or biopsy may be required.

Preliminary data suggest that TMP-SMZ may be effective, although relapse is common after the initial 7- to 10-day course.[157, 158]

Blastocystis

The clinical significance of *Blastocystis hominis* as a human pathogen is controversial.[159] If abundant and associated with chronic or recurrent diarrhea, it is treated with metronidazole.[159–161]

NEMATODES
Trichinella

Trichinella spiralis is a roundworm nematode. Areas of increased prevalence in the United States are the Northeast, the mid-Atlantic states, and any area with an influx of émigrés from southeast Asia.[13] This parasite infestation of swine and other animals is transmitted to humans through inadequately cooked meat containing encysted viable larvae. The most frequently incriminated meats are pork, wild boar, bear, and walrus. There are fewer than 100 cases reported annually in the United States.

Once ingested by humans, the encysted larvae lodge in the duodenum, and 1 to 2 weeks after ingestion they migrate to striated muscles, lung, myocardium, and brain tissue, where they are destroyed by the hosts' inflammatory process. Most infections are asymptomatic or are accompanied by self-limited symptoms related to the gastrointestinal tract. More extensive disease includes the triad of fever, myalgia, and periorbital edema.[162] Occasionally, myocarditis, dysphagia, cough, and focal seizures occur.[163] Heavy infestation can cause death.

Eosinophilia on the peripheral smear is supportive of the diagnosis. Muscle biopsy is confirmatory.[13] Serologic tests are also available, and a CT scan of the brain may document cysticercosis-like lesions.

Treatment is often supportive, with bed rest and salicylates. When drug therapy is instituted, mebendazole is the drug of choice, with consideration given to the use of adjunctive steroids to reduce inflammation.

Prevention requires proper food preparation for humans and swine. The incidence of trichinosis acquired from commercial pork in the United States is declining because of the Federal Swine Health Protection Act (1980) and other U.S. Department of Agriculture programs mandating that garbage fed to swine be heat treated to kill disease-causing organisms.[164]

Filaria

There are eight filarial nematodes (*Wuchereria*, *Brugia* sp., *Onchocerca*, *Loa loa*, and *Mansonella* sp.) that cause disease (filariasis) in humans. All have microscopic thread-like or filariform larvae that are usually found in the blood stream or lymphatic tissues. Transmission is by the bite of an arthropod vector. The adult filariae do not replicate in the human host, and maturation of micro-to-adult filariae is inefficient.

Disease is endemic in the tropics but is rare in North American children.[165] Many biting episodes are required to establish filarial infection.

Infection may be asymptomatic or result in fever, lymphadenitis, or lymphangitis. Classic elephantiasis presents only after many years of residence in an endemic area. *Loa loa* infection may occasionally present with ocular symptoms when there is subconjunctival migration of adult worms.

When appropriate (i.e., according to the history, peripheral eosinophilia, and elevated serum immunoglobulin E [IgE]), diagnosis is attempted with examination of a specially prepared blood smear. Diagnosis may also require examination of skin snips or a slit-lamp examination.

The decision regarding treatment is difficult, especially in children.[165] Diethylcarbamazine has been used for prophylaxis and for therapy.[166] Drug toxicity and host inflammatory response provoked by degenerating parasites can be expected. Complete cure is not ensured.

Toxocara

Toxocara canis is the dog roundworm.[167] Infections in humans are incidental to the life cycle of this zoonotic nematode. Incidence is increased in children who ingest ova from close contact with their pets, habits of pica, and relaxed personal hygiene.[168, 169] The risk from ingestion of soil contaminated with infected feces is greater than that from direct contact with infected dogs.[167]

After ingestion of ova, larvae hatch in the intestine, from which they enter the microvasculature and circulate ("migrans syndrome") to liver, lung, brain, and eye.[169–172] As a result of this life cycle, toxocariasis presents with two clinical manifestations: visceral and ocular larva migrans. The latter is one of the most frequent parasitic infections of the eye. Migration to cardiac and skeletal muscle has also been described. The larvae do not complete their life cycle in humans.

Visceral larva migrans may be characterized by a rash; adventitious lung sounds, especially wheezing; hepatosplenomegaly; lymphadenopathy; and fever. Ocular larva migrans usually is not marked by systemic signs, but examination of the fundi reveals chronic endophthalmitis, peripheral retinitis, or peripheral granuloma.

Peripheral eosinophilia is prominent in visceral larva migrans but not in ocular larva migrans. Because the larvae do not mature in humans, stool examination is negative. Serologic diagnosis (enzyme-linked immunosorbent assay [ELISA]) is available through the CDC, but definitive diagnosis is made by tissue biopsy. Tissue diagnosis is important in children in whom the differential diagnoses of leukocoria or retinoblastoma are being considered. Active larvae can persist for up to a decade in tissue.

Symptomatic infections are treated with diethylcarbamazine or thiabendazole. Thiabendazole treatment did not alter either eosinophil count or serologic titer in asymptomatic children.[168]

Dirofilaria immitis (Dog Heartworm)

Humans are only incidentally infected with the dog heartworm[173]; many species of mosquitoes serve as vectors. *Dirofilaria* cannot complete its life cycle in humans. In humans, the adult worm dies, degenerates, and can embolize to the pulmonary artery, where granuloma formation can ensue.[174]

Infections in humans range from asymptomatic to a pulmonary nodule. The latter appears on a chest radiograph as a coin-like lesion and must be differentiated from malignancy.[175] Diagnosis of the lung lesion requires thoracotomy.[174] Prevention is achieved by rigorous heartworm prophylaxis in dogs and control of the mosquito vector.

Enterobius (Pinworm)

Enterobius vermicularis (pinworm) is a small roundworm. Pinworm is the most prevalent and widely distributed helminth that infects humans in the United States.[176, 177] Humans are the only natural host, and prevalence is especially high in children, with peak occurrence at ages 5 to 14 years.[178]

The life cycle begins with ingestion of eggs or contaminated food or drink or inhalation from dust or sheets (Fig. 74–3). Within 6 weeks, the eggs hatch in the intestine, where the larvae mature to adult worms. Adults mate in the human cecum, and the female migrates nocturnally to the anus, where she deposits eggs and dies. Ovipositing is associated with anal pruritus, which results in reinfection and repetition of the life cycle in the same or another host.

Symptoms, which are usually mild, result from migration of the worms, mechanical irritation, or allergic reactions. Children or their parents report restless sleep. Migration of worms to ectopic sites may result in vulvovaginitis, urethritis, urinary tract infection, or appendicitis. Transfer to the conjunctival sac is also possible.

Clinical Evaluation

Physical examination may reveal small pieces of white thread-like material (adult worms) in the perianal area. The

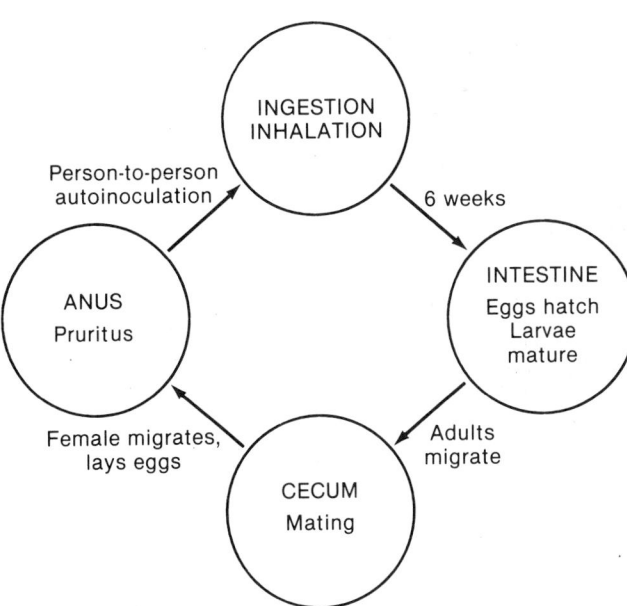

Figure 74–3. *Enterobius* (pinworm) life cycle.

adult male is 5 mm and the female 12 mm in length. Stool examination is of little value, as eggs are infrequently found there. The diagnostic method of choice is the tape test, best performed in the morning before defecation or bathing. Parents can be instructed in the use of a commercial applicator, tongue depressor, or glass slides secured with nonopaque tape. The sticky surface of the tape is applied to the perianal area and the tape then transferred sticky side down to the glass slide. Eggs are sought microscopically (Fig. 74–4). Pinworm infections are typically not accompanied by peripheral eosinophilia. Anal pruritus in children is also associated with beta-hemolytic streptococci, important in the differential diagnosis before antiparasitic therapy is started.[13, 179, 180]

Therapeutic Intervention

Treatment for pinworm is with single-dose mebendazole or pyrantel pamoate. Many recommend a repeat dose at 2 weeks.

The psychosocial issues (lack of association with uncleanliness or socioeconomic status) of pinworm infestation should also be addressed. Examination and treatment of household contacts should be considered. Children who are thumbsuckers may be refractory to treatment because of repeated autoinoculation. Children with urinary tract disease may have enuresis.

Complications of pinworm infestation can include excoriation and bacterial superinfection. Vulvovaginitis and, less commonly, ischiorectal abscess, tubo-ovarian abscess, foreign body granulomas, appendicitis ascribed to migration to the appendix, or even more wide migration have been reported.[181] Washing of bed linen and washable toys is advised since eggs are viable up to 2 weeks in the environment.

Ascaris

Ascaris lumbricoides is a soil-transmitted roundworm and is the most common intestinal parasite of humans. There is a special predilection for children. Worm infestation is also affected by age, sex, the degree of exposure, and genetic susceptibility.[182, 183] In the United States, prevalence is highest in the Southeast.

Ascaris is transmitted by the ingestion of infective eggs from fecally contaminated soil, food, or water. Larvae migrate from the intestine through capillary blood or lymphatics to the liver, heart, and lungs. Migration is completed by return to the large intestine, where infestation is often entirely asymptomatic.

Symptoms and signs of infection usually manifest at the stage of migration through the lungs (cough, fever). When worm infestation is significant, gastrointestinal obstruction may occur. In endemic areas obstruction may be subacute, resulting from an intertwined worm bolus and accompanying inflammation and spasm. Other gastrointestinal symptoms may include crampy diarrhea or colic and periumbilical pain. Most commonly, in the otherwise asymptomatic patient, passage of the adult worm brings the child to medical attention (Fig. 74–5). Children, especially young children, may have anorexia and show poor weight gain.

Diagnostic Evaluation

Diagnosis is achieved occasionally by demonstration of the adult worm in feces but more commonly by the presence of characteristic eggs (Fig. 74–6). Eosinophilia is generally absent. An abdominal plain film can sometimes delineate worms against the intestinal gas.

Therapeutic Intervention

Treatment requires mebendazole, which is given to the patient and all household contacts.[184] Treatment of the asymptomatic carrier should be carefully weighed against the risk of an increased chance for intestinal obstruction as a result of paralysis of a worm bolus, preventing spontaneous disentanglement.[185]

The most common abdominal complication is obstruction of the terminal ileum. When simple obstruction fails to improve with medical management, clinical and radiologic assessment for complication, especially volvulus, is imperative. The surgeon should be involved early in evaluation. In children with severe ascariasis the most common abdominal complications, in descending order, are intestinal obstruction, biliary disease, pancreatitis, appendicitis, and primary peritonitis.[186]

Trichuris

Trichuris trichiura, or whipworm, infestation peaks in endemic areas in school age children. Soil containing infective eggs is the vehicle for transmission, especially in children in whom geophagia is common. Flies may serve as disseminating agents to carry eggs from feces to food or other fomites. There are two major clinical expressions: dysentery and chronic colitis. The latter is often unrecognized.

The life cycle of *Trichuris* is incompletely understood. The adult is a tissue parasite localized to the large bowel and possibly the lower ileum, where inflammatory disease of the mucosa results.

Infections are often asymptomatic or chronic and are associated with poor nutritional status and poor growth. Gastrointestinal signs and symptoms may evolve, with loss of appetite, nausea, vomiting, and abdominal pain. Intestinal obstruction and perforation are uncommon, but the chronic effects of malnutrition, anemia, and growth retardation are significant. Sepsis-associated morbidity and mortality are underestimated. In massive infestation, rectal prolapse can occur.

Diagnosis is suggested by patient history, the presence of blood and mucus in the stool, striking anemia, and periph-

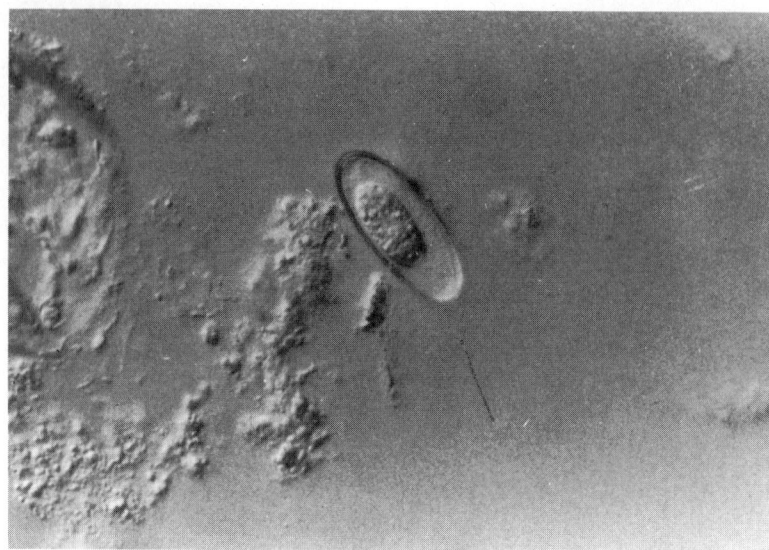

Figure 74–4. *Enterobius* egg (× 750). (Courtesy of M. Kron, Tropical and Infectious Disease Laboratory, Departments of Pathology and Medicine, Michigan State University, East Lansing, MI.)

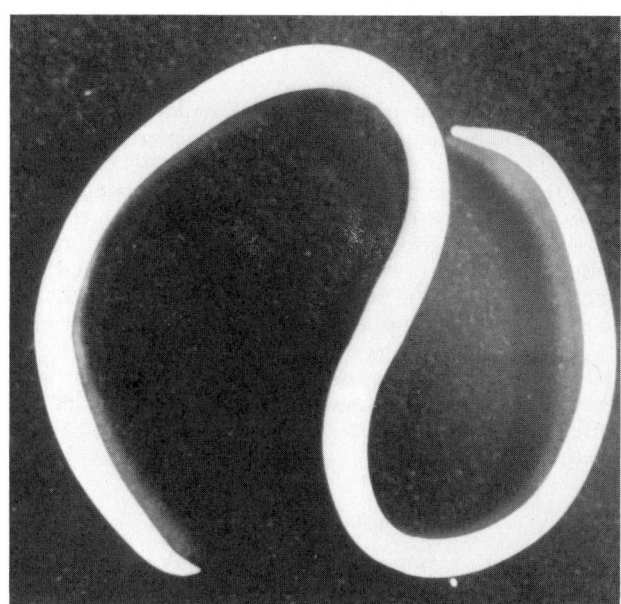

Figure 74–5. *Ascaris*, adult worm (adult range, 20 to 35 cm). (Courtesy of J. Dyke, Department of Microbiology, E.W. Sparrow Hospital, Lansing, MI.)

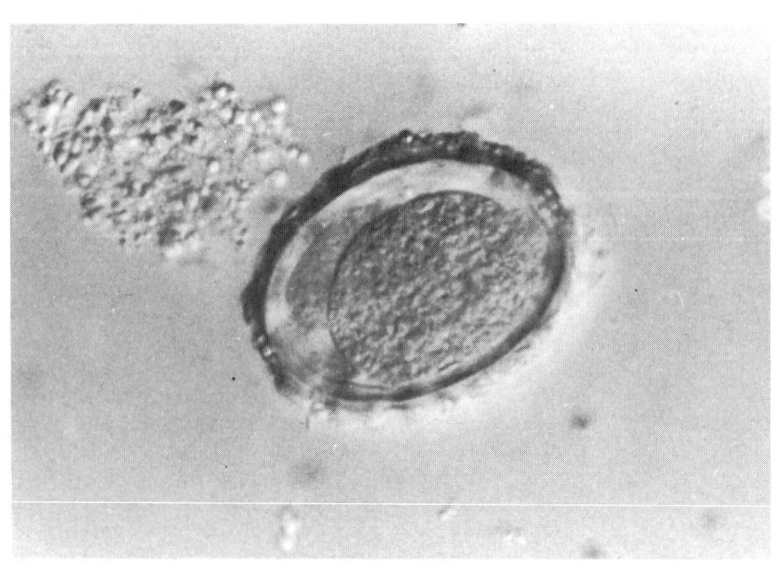

Figure 74–6. *Ascaris* egg (× 1500). (Courtesy of M. Kron, Tropical and Infectious Disease Laboratory, Departments of Pathology and Medicine, Michigan State University, East Lansing, MI.)

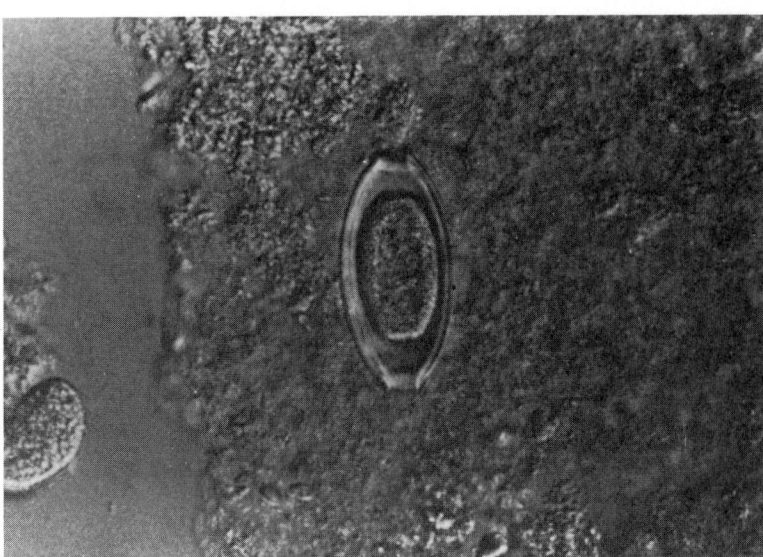

Figure 74–7. *Trichuris* egg (× 1000). (Courtesy of M. Kron, Tropical and Infectious Disease Laboratory, Departments of Pathology and Medicine, Michigan State University, East Lansing, MI.)

eral eosinophilia. Examination of stools for characteristic eggs is diagnostic (Fig. 74–7).

Trichuriasis colitis is similar to noninfectious inflammatory bowel disease (ulcerative colitis and Crohn's disease).[187] However, unlike ulcerative colitis and Crohn's disease, colitis associated with *Trichuris* infestation is reversible. Treatment with mebendazole may not effect cure, but may reduce the worm infestation sufficiently to achieve clinical improvement.

Hookworms

There are two principal species of hookworms: *Necator americanus* and *Ancylostoma duodenale*. These geohelminth infestations are associated with acute disease. Hookworms are endemic in nearly all tropical and subtropical areas.

Infection is transmitted through exposure of unprotected skin to soil contaminated with feces containing filariform larvae (Fig. 74–8). Skin penetration is generally required,

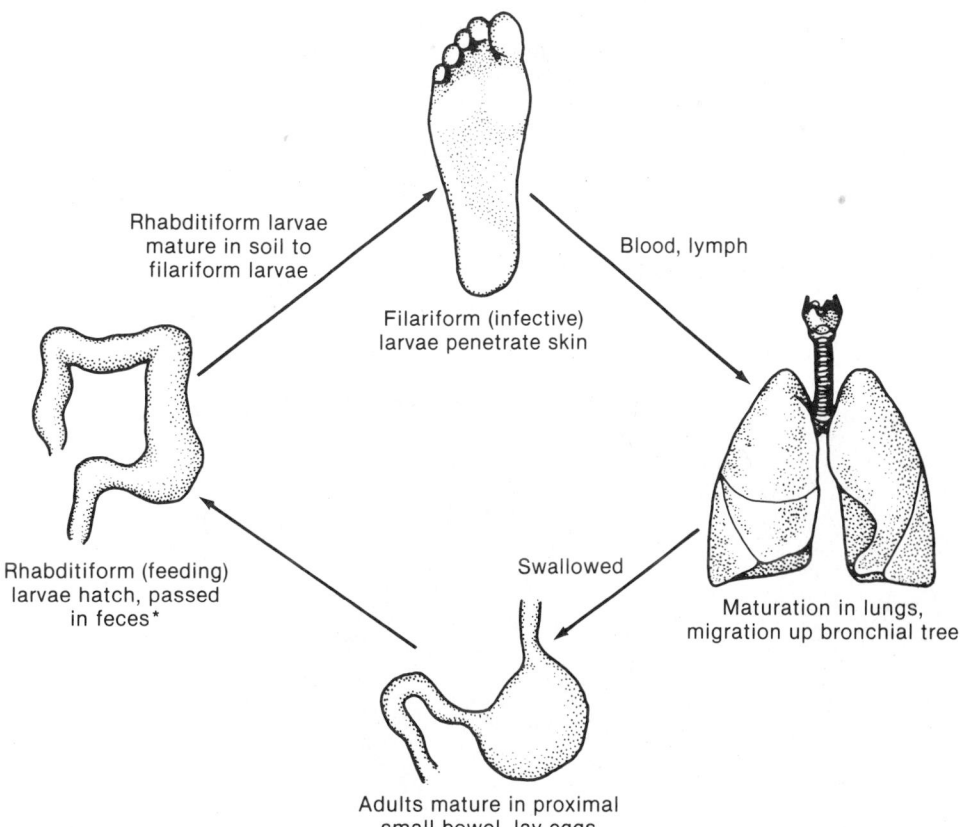

Rhabditiform larvae mature in soil to filariform larvae

Filariform (infective) larvae penetrate skin

Blood, lymph

Rhabditiform (feeding) larvae hatch, passed in feces*

Swallowed

Maturation in lungs, migration up bronchial tree

Adults mature in proximal small bowel, lay eggs

Life cycle: cutaneous larva migrans: *Strongyloides*/Hookworms

*In hyperinfection syndrome of *Strongyloides,* rhabditiform larvae disseminate and mature to filariform larvae in vivo

Figure 74–8. Hookworm life cycle.

although acquisition of *Ancylostoma* may be oral in children with a history of pica or may even occur with breast-feeding.[188] Skin exposure of 5 to 10 minutes is sufficient for transmission to the cutaneous blood vessels and then to the right heart. Within days of skin penetration, filariform larvae reach the lungs, where they ascend the respiratory tree to the epiglottis and from there descend to the proximal small intestine as young worms. They then attach to the mucosa and develop into adult worms. Time from penetration of the larvae to development of adult worms is about six weeks. After copulation, the females produce abundant eggs. The adult worms remain attached to the intestinal mucosa for many years, ingesting blood in amounts of approximately 0.05 ml/day for each worm.

Clinical Evaluation

Clinical signs are directly related to the life cycle and ultimately to the degree of worm infestation. Some patients are asymptomatic, whereas others manifest dermatitis, which is reflective of sensitivity to the secretions of the migrating larvae. Reinfection may elicit more severe dermatitis.[13] Dermatitis may be followed promptly by respiratory symptoms and then by laryngitis, pharyngitis, or dysphagia. Gastrointestinal manifestations can include epigastric pain, nausea, vomiting, anorexia, and flatulence.

The most common presenting feature, especially in children with protein malnutrition and poor body iron stores, is insidious anemia from persistent blood loss. It is estimated that blood loss worldwide directly related to hookworm infestation is equivalent to exsanguinating 1.5 million people per day.[188, 189] There is also a peripheral eosinophilia and occult blood in the stool. After the cutaneous and pulmonary phases of the life cycle, stools contain eggs and rhabditiform larvae (Fig. 74–9). A chest radiograph will reveal pneumonitis characterized by localized fluffy infiltrates.

Asymptomatic infested patients need not be treated. If worm infestation is associated with anemia, mebendazole therapy should be considered.

Complications of hookworm infections include bacterial superinfection and long-term growth and development deficits.

Cutaneous Larva Migrans

Skin penetration by any of the hookworm species can result in dermatitis. In particular, hookworms of animal species, most commonly dogs and cats, can cause serpentine tracks after penetrating human skin (Fig. 74–10). Hookworms of animal species represent a major zoonotic infection in the southeastern United States, especially along the Atlantic and Gulf coasts, but may also be present in other portions of the United States and Canada. Children are at increased risk because of noncompliance in wearing shoes and their propensity to expose all aspects of their skin to potential larvae (on beaches, in sandboxes, or on sandy soil).

There is a history of exposure with intensely pruritic, linear, erythematous, serpiginous tunnels and vesiculated areas on the dorsal and plantar aspects of the feet, interdigitally, or on the knees or buttocks. Peripheral eosinophilia is often present. Recovery of parasites from the advancing edge of the lesion is not practical, and serologic tests are unavailable.

If untreated, the larvae die in 2 to 8 weeks. Topical treatment with liquid nitrogen, dry ice, or ethylchloride has had mixed success. Thiabendazole may be used if the risk of toxicity is sufficiently low. Complications include secondary bacterial infection or eosinophilic papular folliculitis.

Strongyloides

Strongyloides is more common among adults. Although infestation with *Strongyloides stercoralis* is uncommon in the United States, its highest incidence is in southern Appalachia, Kentucky, and Tennessee.

This nematode helminth is similar to hookworms, with penetration into the skin and then migration of worms through the lungs to the gastrointestinal tract (see Fig. 74–10). However, the life cycle is unique, as it is completed in humans and is characterized by ongoing autoinfection, which is often low grade, moderated by the host immune response.

Clinical Evaluation

Many infestations with *Strongyloides* are asymptomatic, even chronic infections in immunocompetent hosts. Acute infection is marked by epigastric abdominal pain, weight loss, and nonbloody diarrhea. Occasionally there are signs and symptoms referable to the pulmonary system. Serpentine cutaneous manifestations (a form of cutaneous larva migrans) are also expected.[190] Acute strongyloidiasis is often self-limited.

Patients at increased risk of massive invasion are immu-

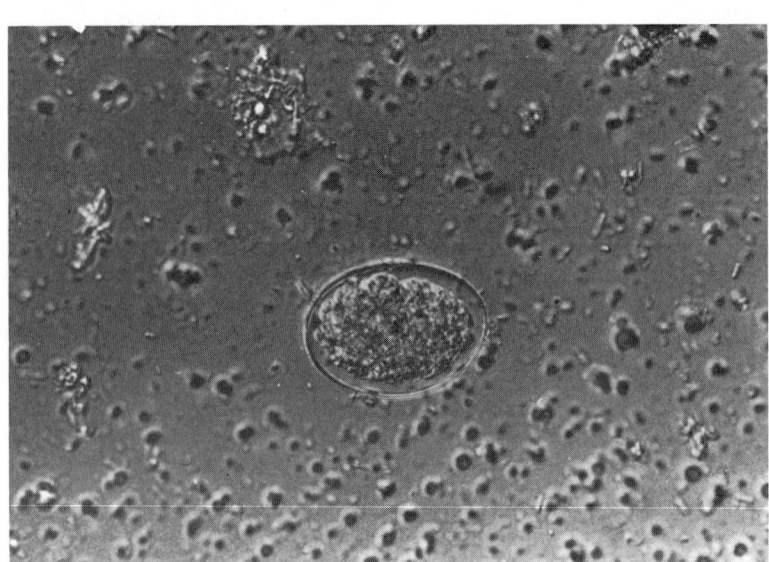

Figure 74–9. Hookworm egg (× 750). (Courtesy of M. Kron, Tropical and Infectious Disease Laboratory, Departments of Pathology and Medicine, Michigan State University, East Lansing, MI.)

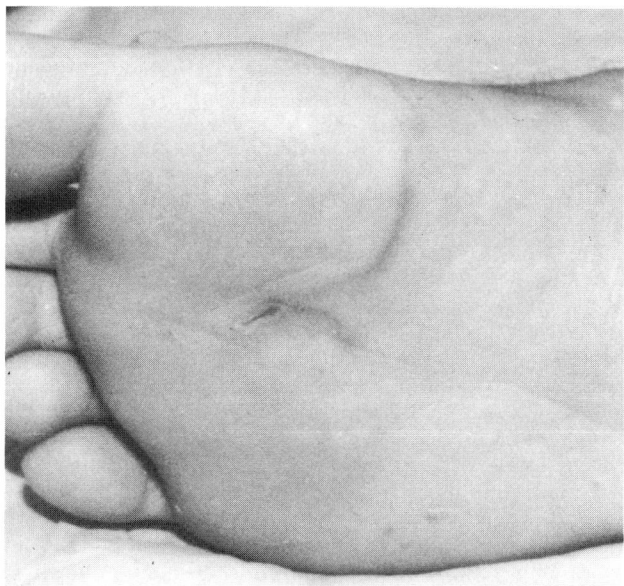

Figure 74–10. Cutaneous larva migrans. (Courtesy of R. Koup, Departments of Pediatrics and Medicine, University of Massachusetts, Worcester, MA.)

nocompromised hosts whose host-parasite balance is altered. Severe infections by *Strongyloides* are divided by some into hyperinfection (unchecked autoinfection of the lungs and gastrointestinal tract) and disseminated infection, in which spread to organs not ordinarily part of the life cycle is found.[190] Fulminant infection in these settings is associated with fever, vomiting, diarrhea, cough, dyspnea, and shock. Disseminated strongyloidiasis results in multisystem involvement leading to meningitis, hepatitis, pneumonia, and myocarditis.

Diagnostic Evaluation

Peripheral eosinophilia is present in acute and disseminated strongyloidiasis and less frequently in hyperinfection. Stool examination reveals rhabditiform larvae but rarely eggs. A duodenal aspirate or the less invasive Enterotest should be evaluated for fertile adult *Strongyloides* females or larvae.[191] Larvae may be found in sputum. Patchy infiltrates may be found on chest radiograph during pulmonary migration.

Therapeutic Intervention

Treatment of the immunocompetent host with thiabendazole is highly effective and can be monitored with repeat duodenal aspiration. Severe life-threatening strongyloidiasis may require monthly prophylactic drug administration.[190]

Anisakis

Among the growing list of common indigenous parasites of fish are the cestode tapeworm *Diphyllobothrium*, several nematode genera (*Anisakis*, *Eustrongyloides*, and *Phocanema*), and miscellaneous helminths in the trematode class. Most fish are parasitized and increasing reports of human infection have accompanied the emerging popularity of fish in the diets of health-conscious Americans and of sushi as a delicacy.[192–196]

Anisakis species do not develop to maturity in humans.

Infection is linked to eating raw or inadequately prepared (cooked, smoked, salted or marinated) seafood.

Many human infections are transient and confined to the intestinal lumen. Signs, symptoms, and time of presentation depend on where the infection is in the gastrointestinal tract: acute gastritis with epigastric pain, nausea, and vomiting occurs within hours of ingestion; acute small intestinal disease occurs about a week after ingestion; and chronic infestation presents months to years later. Infestation with *Phocanema*, which are less invasive nematodes, is often asymptomatic until the patient reports extracting a live roundworm from the throat.[195, 196] Tissue invasion or intestinal perforation are rare complications.

Diagnosis is suggested by the diet history and the presence of eosinophilia. Stool examination for eggs is not helpful, and serologic methods of diagnosis are unavailable. Early fiberoptic endoscopy in suspicious cases may aid in diagnosis and prevent the need for surgical treatment.[197] Microscopic lesions of eosinophilic infiltrates or abscesses and epithelioid granulomas occur.[192] A medical parasitologist should be consulted for identification of worms found on endoscopy. Depending on the symptoms, acute appendicitis, regional enteritis, or gastric carcinoma may need to be excluded. No effective anthelmintic drug therapy is available, and surgical management may be necessary.

TREMATODES

Schistosoma

The trematode helminths infecting humans include the blood flukes (*Schistosoma mansoni*, *Schistosoma haematobium*, and *Schistosoma japonicum*), the lung fluke *Paragonimus westermani*, and, in the intestinal and biliary tracts the flukes *Fasciola* sp. and *Opisthorchis* (formerly *Clonorchis*) *sinensis*. All have complex life cycles, and none are endemic to the United States. The blood flukes are a continuing risk for U.S. travelers to endemic areas.[198]

Infection with the blood flukes is referred to as *bilharziasis*. In the complex life cycle, the intermediate host, fresh-water snails, acquire the parasite in waters contaminated by human excrement (feces or urine) containing ova. The ova hatch in the water to form miracidia, which infect snails and develop to cercariae. Snails release the free-swimming cercariae, which can penetrate intact skin of humans. Transmission to humans is associated with fresh waters used for bathing, washing, wading, swimming, and boating. Infection may not be evident until years after leaving an endemic area. After penetrating human skin, the cercariae migrate to hepatic sinusoids where they mature into adult worms. Eggs are deposited in vasculature associated with the worms' final migration, either in the liver or surrounding the urinary bladder.

Clinical Evaluation

There are three presentations of disease: cercarial dermatitis (swimmer's itch), acute schistosomiasis (Katayama fever), and a chronic granulomatous disease.[199] Swimmer's itch is a transient papular and pruritic dermatitis occurring within hours of exposure and thought to be caused by interleukins or by the mediators of immediate hypersensitivity. Acute schistosomiasis is the most common presentation in travelers to endemic areas. It is a serum sickness–like syndrome associated with eosinophilia, headache, fever, chills, fatigue, and gastrointestinal discomfort, which is thought to be caused by an immune complex abnormality. In patients with long-standing infection, cell-mediated immune mechanisms result, with granuloma formation in the liver and abnormalities related to host response to ova trapped in tissue.

Complications of acute schistosomiasis include bloody diarrhea; those of chronic schistosomiasis include portal hypertension and fibrosis. In addition, urinary schistosomiasis is associated with frequency, dysuria, hematuria, and possibly obstructive uropathy. A rare but serious complication of acute schistosomiasis is a rapidly progressive transverse myelitis, which must be differentiated from spinal cord tumors.[200, 201] Other ectopic localizations include the rectum, heart, lung, brain, eye, and joints.[199]

Diagnostic Evaluation

Diagnosis is suggested by geographic history. Eosinophilia provides supportive evidence. Direct microscopic examination of stools (or urine) for eggs may provide definitive diagnosis, but egg excretion may be scanty. Therefore, serologic tests (ELISA) are important. When symptoms are related to the urinary bladder, hematuria, proteinuria, and leukocyturia (eosinophils) are noted.

A major clinical advance in therapy for acute schistosomiasis is praziquantel in a single oral dose; this is effective against all adult schistosomes, with a cure rate of 90% to 95% in children, accompanied by a reversal of the disease process. When a single member of a travel group is diagnosed, all should be evaluated.[199] Prudent advice for prevention for travelers includes avoidance of all fresh water in endemic areas. If fresh water is unavoidable, bath water should be heated to 50°C (122°F) for 5 minutes or treated with iodine or chlorine. Alternatively, vigorous towel drying or use of rubbing alcohol on exposed skin immediately after contact may prevent cercarial penetration.[198]

CESTODES
Taenia
Echinococcus and Hymenolepis

Tapeworms that commonly parasitize humans include *Taenia saginata*, *Taenia solium*, *Hymenolepis nana*, *Hymenolepis diminuta*, *Diphyllobothrium latum*, and *Dipylidium caninum*. The intermediate hosts of these include, respectively, cattle, hogs, arthropods, arthropods and rodents, fish, and dog or cat fleas. All these tapeworms parasitize humans in the small intestine in their adult stage.

T. solium infection has been the most frequent parasitic infection of the human nervous system (brain, eye, and cord) in the clinical presentation of neurocysticercosis.[202, 203] It is especially prevalent in Mexico, Latin America, and portions of the southwestern United States.[204, 205] *Echinococcus* cysts of liver, lung, and brain are most common in children (peak age, 5 to 12 years), who usually acquire infection by playing with dogs who harbor the adult worm. *D. caninum* shows a steadily increasing geographic spread linked to the expanding licensed canine population. Children less than 8 years of age are at increased risk. *Hymenolepis* and *Diphyllobothrium* are the most common intestinal tapeworms. *Taenia* sp. may elongate to several meters in the small intestine (Fig. 74–11).

Infection is generally acquired by the consumption of food and water contaminated with viable encysted larvae or eggs, by person-to-person transmission of eggs, or by autoinoculation.[202, 206] Children acquire the dog tapeworm by the accidental crushing and ingesting of fleas or by being licked on the face by dogs who have bitten and crushed egg-bearing fleas. The hatching of eggs and maturation of worms is followed by scolex attachment to the small intestinal

mucosa and the development and release of proglottids (egg-containing segments).

The clinical course is variable. Bowel infestation is generally asymptomatic but may be associated with loss of appetite and poor weight gain. Passage of proglottids often brings a patient to medical attention. With cerebral cysticercosis, localizing signs and symptoms indicate intraparenchymal lesions, most commonly presenting approximately 5 years after infestation. Careful skin examination in cerebral cysticercosis may reveal subcutaneous nodules. In the United States, seizure is the major presenting symptom.[207] The next most common presentations, as determined in a large retrospective study of children and adults, are acute increased intracranial pressure, meningitis, focal deficits, and acute psychosis.[207] Children more commonly develop cerebral edema, whereas adults develop obstructive hydrocephalus from cysticercosis.

Diagnosis is supported by strong clinical suspicion.[207] Peripheral eosinophilia is unreliable. Stool examinations for ova and proglottids provide definitive diagnosis of intestinal disease, but less often of cerebral disease. Antibody assays are variably helpful.[202, 208, 209] A surgical consultation for tissue diagnosis may be required in patients with cerebral disease,[84, 181] especially to exclude tumor (glioma), abscess, tuberculosis, and sarcoidosis. CT or magnetic resonance imaging (MRI) evaluation for suspected infections by the larval stages of *T. solium* or *Echinococcus* reveals a range of findings.[208, 210] A ring-shaped enhancing lesion is thought to represent active infection and diffuse cerebral calcification to be indicative of larvae degeneration.[211]

Infestation can resolve spontaneously, with the scolex dying about 18 months after infection. Neurocysticercosis, especially single cysts accompanied by acute inflammation, can also resolve without treatment. Seizures may be a major cause of long-term morbidity, and at least short-term anticonvulsant therapy for seizure control is often necessary. The treatment of choice for active neurocysticercosis is praziquantel; concurrent steroid therapy may be employed to prevent inflammation and cerebral edema.[202, 203, 211, 212] Before the availability of praziquantel, surgical resection was often needed to remove isolated large cysts or to establish a ventriculoperitoneal shunt for relief of hydrocephalus.[204] Niclosamide can be used to treat dog tapeworm infection in humans.[24, 70]

LICE

The causative ectoparasites of pediculosis are the head louse *Pediculus humanus* var. *capitis*, the body louse *Pediculus humanus* var. *corporis*, and the pubic louse *Phthirus pubis*. Adult head and body lice are 1 to 2 mm in length; eggs (nits) are 0.8 mm and resemble grains of sand. Adult pubic lice are smaller (0.8 to 1.2mm) and have large heavy claws. Transmission occurs from close personal contact and sharing of personal objects.

The most common form of pediculosis in children is caused by head lice. Adult head lice are viable for only 48 hours off the scalp; the eggs are viable for 10 days. The pubic louse (crab louse) is next most common in children and deposits eggs on the scalp hair, lashes, axillary hair, and pubic hair.

Itching is the principal complaint with an established infestation. Physical examination requires close inspection of the hair-bearing areas for adult lice or ovoid adherent nits. Laboratory confirmation is sometimes necessary to distinguish nits from the concretions associated with *Corynebacterium*.

Sexual or physical child abuse must be considered in the differential diagnosis. Eyelash involvement in prepubertal

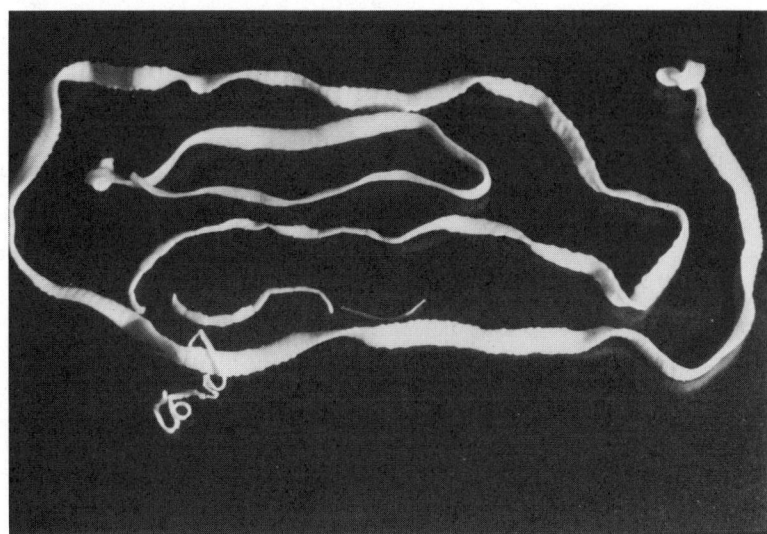

Figure 74–11. Adult tapeworm (*Diphyllobothrium*) (adult range is 10 to 15 m.) (Courtesy of J. Dyke, Department of Microbiology, E.W. Sparrow Hospital, Lansing, MI.)

children should raise the suspicion of sexual abuse.[213] The slate blue–colored macules (maculae ceruleae) associated with *Phthirus pubis* may be confused with purpura or traumatic bruising.[214] Pubic lice may coexist with other sexually transmitted disease.

Treatment of choice is the parent compound pyrethrin, now available over the counter as permethrin, (permethrin 1% creme rinse), a synthetic pyrethroid that is both pediculocidal and ovicidal (Table 74–4).[215–218] This product kills more rapidly than lindane, a chlorinated hydrocarbon, to which some lice may be resistant. Permethrin has no associated anemia and neurotoxicity, as reported for lindane, and has good selective toxicity. Residual activity remains on the hair for about 2 weeks to prevent reinfection but is only minimally absorbed through the skin. Pediculocides are too toxic for eyelash treatment, and therefore petrolatum is employed, which presumably works by suffocating the lice. Although many pediculocides are obtained without a prescription, these medications must be used in a specific way.

It is important to treat both the child and the environment. A spray preparation of pyrethrin and piperonyl butoxide is available for use on furniture, bedding, and other household objects. Other approaches include machine washing (hot water, hot dryer) of all bedding used in the previous 48 hours. Nonwashable stuffed toys should be placed in a hot dryer for 20 minutes, dry cleaned, or sealed in plastic for 14 days. Frequent vacuuming is also important.

Treatment of all family members may be considered, although some evidence shows that adults and even siblings may not be infected.[219] Children should not share accessories such as combs, brushes, hats, or head phones. Complications (which are not treatment failures) include secondary bacterial infection and transient (7 to 10 days) exacerbation of erythema and pruritus caused by the medication.

The National Pediculosis Association advocates a "no nits policy" for return to school or day care, as no pediculocide kills nits with 100% efficacy. However, the "no nit policy" is counterproductive, and a return to school 24 hours after shampoo treatment is appropriate.[219] Dead nit cases can cling to hair shafts in spite of a complete cure.

Lice infestation does not represent poor hygiene, and it is important to dispel this common psychosocial stigma.[220] Another misconception is that lice are transmitted to pets.

SCABIES

The scabies mite (*Sarcoptes scabiei*) is an ectoparasite of worldwide distribution. The scabies mite is rarely shed from the human body and survives only briefly (24 hours) in the environment. The incubation period is 3 to 6 weeks, which should prompt treatment of the entire family. Close personal contact (e.g., intercourse or, in the case of infants and their caregivers, prolonged holding, carrying, or hugging) is required for transmission. The incubation period for scabies is about 3 to 6 weeks.

Severe itching that is worse at night is characteristic of scabies. This is associated with hypersensitivity to the parasite. Infants sleep fitfully, are cranky, and have periods in which they rub their hands or feet together. This occurs in the setting of no preexisting skin lesions, which is unlike eczematous dermatitis. Often others at home or at day care are also itching. Other differential diagnoses include poison ivy, contact dermatitis, insect bites, and papular urticaria.[221].

The characteristic lesions are small, red, slightly elevated papules that can progress to vesicles and pustules, not unlike varicella, in an uneven distribution. Excoriations are easily found. In children, the small, wavy, thread-like burrows are less common. In infants, the lesions are distributed to the palms, soles, scalp, and face. In older children and adults,

TABLE 74–4
DISCHARGE INSTRUCTIONS FOR TREATMENT OF LICE (PEDICULOSIS)
General information: Transmission occurs by close personal contact and sharing personal objects. Infestation usually involves the head.
Medication use: Use a 1% permethrin liquid (Nix). It comes in a 2-ounce bottle and can be bought without a prescription. Make the hair slightly damp; then apply the shampoo (undiluted) to the hair and let it remain for 10 minutes, but no longer than 10 minutes. Wash thoroughly with soap and warm water. Dead lice and eggs can be removed with a fine comb. The treatment may be repeated in 1 week.
Other treatment: Petroleum jelly should be applied to the eyelashes to suffocate the lice in that area.
Environmental control: Machine wash all bedding used in the previous 48 hours in hot water and dry in a hot dryer. All nonwashable stuffed toys should be put in the dryer on a hot setting for 20 minutes, dry cleaned, or put in a sealed plastic bag for 14 days. Children should not share combs, brushes, hats, or head phones and may return to school 24 hours after shampoo with the permethrin.
Other information: Infestation by lice does not represent poor hygiene. Pets are not affected and do not need to be treated.

TABLE 74–5

DISCHARGE INSTRUCTIONS FOR TREATMENT OF SCABIES

General information: Transmission occurs by close personal contact. Family members may also require treatment.

Medication use: Use 1% permethrin (Nix). It comes as a cream (60-gm) and as a 10% lotion (2 or 6 ounce). *The drug should not be swallowed.* A thin layer of cream or lotion should be applied to all skin areas below the neck, avoiding the face and eyes. A second layer should be applied 24 hours after the first. The child should bathe 48 hours after the last application of the drug to remove the medication completely.

Contact treatment: All family members should be treated at the same time to prevent the spread of scabies.

Environmental control: Machine wash all bedding used in the previous 48 hours in hot water and dry in a hot dryer. All nonwashable stuffed toys should be put in the dryer on a hot setting for 20 minutes, dry cleaned, or put in a sealed plastic bag for 7 days.

---

the distribution more commonly spares the face but includes the webs of the fingers, the axillae, the flexural lines, and the genitalia.

Diagnosis is often made on the basis of clinical signs and symptoms. However, laboratory confirmation can be achieved by scraping a burrow or five to six nonexcoriated papules, overlaid with mineral oil, with a scalpel. The scrapings are examined for mites, eggs, and feces (scybala).

The treatment of choice is pyrethrin. This is safe for infants more than 2 months old and is available as a 5% cream used in a single application.[222, 223] Alternative treatments include crotamiton, 4% to 6% precipitated sulfur in petrolatum, or lindane. Some questions have been raised regarding the safety of lindane in children younger than 6 months and pregnant women, but such problems are thought to be attributed to improper use (Table 74–5).[213] Patients may also need an oral antihistamine, a topical antipruritic agent, or even a corticosteroid.

Treatment failure may be associated with inadequate application to all body sites, which should include subungual regions.[224] The lag before pruritus ceases, which is 1 to 3 weeks, should not be construed as treatment failure. It is important to advise against overuse of scabicides.

Because of the long incubation period during which the patient is infectious, the entire family and other intimate contacts should be treated. The necessity for decontaminating the household bedding, clothing, and toys is questionable, as survival rates for the parasite are low.[213] Normal laundering of bedding and clothing worn in the last several days appears to be sufficient. Toys placed in plastic for a week may be used without concern.

There is no nonhuman reservoir, so pets need not be treated or evaluated. However, the agent of canine scabies (sarcoptic mange) is able to feed on and irritate human skin, although it is unable to reproduce in humans. In this case the dog, not the child, should be treated.

MYIASIS

Myiasis is the unusual invasion of human body tissue by fly larvae. Eggs may hatch and larvae penetrate and develop (maggots) as they do in decaying organic matter. Reported sites of human infection include the eye or nasal mucosa; the skin port of ventilated patients; the diaper area, including the penis; and exposed areas of skin of the face, scalp, neck, and extremities.[225–227]

Recognition results in surgical consultation for excision with probing to ensure that no portions of the larvae are left behind.[226, 228, 229]

References

1. Crawford FG, Vermund SH. Parasitic infections in day care centers. Pediatr Infect Dis J 1987;6:744.
2. Klein JO. Infectious diseases and day care. Rev Infect Dis 1986;8:521.
3. Pickering LK, Bartlett AV, Woodward WE. Acute infectious diarrhea among children in day care: Epidemiology and control. Rev Infect Dis 1986;8:539.
4. Aronson SS, Gilsdorf JR. Prevention and management of infectious diseases in day care. Pediatr Rev 1986;7:259.
5. Panosian CB. Parasitic diarrhea. Infect Dis Clin North Am 1988;2:685.
6. Soave R, Johnson WD. Cryptosporidiosis and *Isospora belli* infections. J Infect Dis 1988;157:225.
7. Scully RE, Mark EJ, McNeeley BU. Case records of the Massachusetts General Hospital—case 39-1985. N Engl J Med 1985;313:805.
8. Alpert G, Bell LM, Kirkpatrick CE, et al. Outbreak of cryptosporidiosis in a day care center. Pediatrics 1986;77:152.
9. Combee CL, Collinge ML, Britt EM. Cryptosporidiosis in a hospital-associated day care center. Pediatr Infect Dis J 1986;5:528.
10. Centers for Disease Control. Cryptosporidiosis among children attending day care centers—Georgia, Pennsylvania, Michigan, California, New Mexico. MMWR 1984;33:599.
11. Diers J, McCallister GL. Occurrence of *Cryptosporidium* in home day care centers in west-central Colorado. J Parasitol 1989;75:637.
12. Gove S, Slutkin G. Infectious diseases of travelers and immigrants. Emerg Med Clin North Am 1984;2:587.
13. Chaudhry AZ, Longworth DL. Cutaneous manifestations of intestinal helminthic infections. Dermatol Clin 1989;7:275.
14. Wykoff HF. Eosinophilia. South Med J 1986;79:608.
15. Thomson RB, Haas RA. Intestinal parasites: The necessity of examining multiple stool specimens. Mayo Clin Proc 1984;59:641.
16. Borowitz SM, Hayden GF. In plain sight: The macroscopic stool examination. Contemp Pediatr 1990;7:115.
17. Ruttner N. Worms in diaper. Pediatrics 1983;71:466.
18. Weinberg AG. Worms in diaper. Pediatrics 1983;72:579.
19. Williams DG, Richmond S, Massam M. Disposable nappies—a cautionary tale. Arch Dis Child 1988;63:997.
20. Walterspiel JN, Dean P. Maggot on board. Pediatr Infect Dis J 1988;7:209.
21. Tunnessen WW. Scatologist's delight. Contemp Pediatr 1986;3:69.
22. Tunnessen WW. The strange tumor and the suspicious stool. Contemp Pediatr 1985;2:33.
23. Margolis B. Dog tapeworm infestation in an infant. Am J Dis Child 1983;137:702.
24. Chappell CL, Enos JP, Penn HM. *Dipylidium caninum*, an under-recognized infection in infants and children. Pediatr Infect Dis J 1990;9:745.
25. Warren KS. The present impossibility of eradicating the omnipresent worm. Rev Infect Dis 1982;4:955.
26. Lauzon D, Delage G, Brochu P, et al. Pathogens in children with severe combined immune deficiency disease or AIDS. Can Med Assoc J 1986;135:33.
27. Phair J, Munoz A, Detels R, et al. The risk of *Pneumocystis carinii* pneumonia among men infected with human immunodeficiency virus type 1. N Engl J Med 1990;322:161.
28. Pifer LL, Hughes WT, Stagno S, et al. *Pneumocystis carinii* infection: Evidence for high prevalence in normal and immunosuppressed children. Pediatrics 1978;61:35.
29. Cruickshank B. Pulmonary granulomatous pneumocystosis following renal transplantation. Am J Clin Pathol 1975;63:384.
30. Skinner R, Finlay JL, Sondel PM, et al. Infectious complications in pediatric patients undergoing transplantation with T lymphocyte-depleted bone marrow. Pediatr Infect Dis 1986;5:319.
31. Barson WJ, Brady MT. Management of infections in children with cancer. Hematol Oncol Clin North Am 1987;1:801.
32. Pizzo PA. Diagnosis and management of infectious disease problems in the child with malignant disease. *In* Rubin RH, Young LS (eds). Clinical Approach to Infection in the Compromised Host. 2nd ed. New York, Plenum, 1988, pp 439–466.
33. Masur H. Problems in the management of opportunistic infections in patients infected with human immunodeficiency virus. J Infect Dis 1990;161:858.
34. Glatt AE, Chirgwin K, Landesman SH. Treatment of infections associated with human immunodeficiency virus. N Engl J Med 1988;318:1439.
35. Bernstein LJ, Bye MR, Rubinstein A. Prognostic factors and life expectancy in children with acquired immunodeficiency syndrome and *Pneumocystis carinii* pneumonia. Am J Dis Child 1989;143:775.
36. Le Golvan DP, Heidelberger KP. Disseminated, granulomatous *Pneumocystis carinii* pneumonia. Arch Pathol 1973;95:344.
37. Hughes WT. *Pneumocystis carinii* pneumonitis. N Engl J Med 1987;317:1021.
38. Llibre JM, Tor J, Milla F. Acute eosinophilic pneumonia. N Engl J Med 1990;322:634.

39. Gherman CR, Ward RR, Bassis ML. *Pneumocystis carinii* otitis media and mastoiditis as the initial manifestation of acquired immunodeficiency syndrome. Am J Med 1988;85:250.

40. Barnett RN, Hull JG, Vortel V, et al. *Pneumocystis carinii* in lymph nodes and spleen. Arch Pathol 1969;88:175.

41. Telzak EE, Cote RJ, Gold JWM, et al. Extrapulmonary *Pneumocystis carinii* infections. Rev Infect Dis 1990;12:380.

42. Hopewell PC. *Pneumocystis carinii* pneumonia: Diagnosis. J Infect Dis 1988;157:1115.

43. Walzer P. Diagnosis of *Pneumocystis carinii* pneumonia. J Infect Dis 1988;157:629.

44. Weber WR, Askin FB, Dehner LP. Lung biopsy in *Pneumocystis carinii* pneumonia. Am J Clin Pathol 1977;67:11.

45. Scully RE, Mark EJ, McNeely WF, et al. Case records of Massachusetts General Hospital—case 9-1989. N Engl J Med 1989;320:582.

46. Gill VJ, Nelson NA, Stock F, et al. Optimal use of the cytocentrifuge for recovery and diagnosis of *Pneumocystis carinii* in bronchoalveolar lavage and sputum specimens. J Clin Microbiol 1988;26:1641.

47. Kovacs JA, Ng VL, Masur H, et al. Diagnosis of *Pneumocystis carinii* pneumonia: Improved detection in sputum with use of monoclonal antibodies. N Engl J Med 1988;318:589.

48. Rorat E, Garcia RL, Skolom J. Diagnosis of *Pneumocystis carinii* pneumonia by cytologic examination of bronchial washings. JAMA 1985;254:1950.

49. Ruffolo JJ, Cushion MT, Walzer PD. Techniques for examining *Pneumocystis carinii* in fresh specimens. J Clin Microbiol 1986;23:17.

50. Centers for Disease Control. Guidelines for prophylaxis against *Pneumocystis carinii* pneumonia for persons infected with human immunodeficiency virus. MMWR 1989;38:S5.

51. Harris JE. Improved short-term survival of AIDS patients initially diagnosed with *Pneumocystis carinii* pneumonia, 1984 through 1987. JAMA 1990;263:397.

52. McCabe RE, Remington JS. *Toxoplasma gondii*. *In* Mandell GL, Douglas RG, Bennett JE (eds). Principles and Practice of Infectious Diseases. 3rd ed. New York, Churchill Livingstone, 1990, pp 2090–2103.

53. Wilson CB, Remington JS. Toxoplasmosis. *In* Feigin RD, Cherry JD (eds). Textbook of Pediatric Infectious Diseases. 2nd ed. Philadelphia, WB Saunders, 1987, pp 2067–2078.

54. Diebler C, Dusser A, Dulac O. Congenital toxoplasmosis: Clinical and neuroradiological evaluation of the cerebral lesions. Neuroradiology 1985;27:125.

55. Collins AT, Cromwell LD. Computed tomography in the evaluation of congenital cerebral toxoplasmosis. J Comput Assist Tomogr 1980;4:326.

56. Dunn D, Weisberg LA. Serial changes in a patient with congenital CNS toxoplasmosis as observed with CT. Comput Radiol 1984;8:133.

57. Wilson CB, Remington JS, Stagno S, et al. Development of adverse sequelae in children born with subclinical congenital *Toxoplasma* infection. Pediatrics 1980;66:767.

58. Koppe JG, Loewer-Sieger DH, de Roever-Bonnet H. Results of 20-year follow-up of congenital toxoplasmosis. Lancet 1986;1:254.

59. McDonald JC, Gyorkos TW, Alberton B, et al. An outbreak of toxoplasmosis in pregnant women in Northern Quebec. J Infect Dis 1990;161:769.

60. McCabe R, Remington JS. Toxoplasmosis: The time has come. N Engl J Med 1988;318:313.

61. Daffos F, Forestier F, Capella-Pavlovsky M, et al. Prenatal management of 746 pregnancies at risk for congenital toxoplasmosis. N Engl J Med 1988;318:271.

62. Luft BJ, Remington JS. Toxoplasmic encephalitis. J Infect Dis 1988;157:1.

63. McCabe RE, Brooks RG, Dorfman RF, et al. Clinical spectrum in 107 cases of toxoplasmic lymphadenopathy. Rev Infect Dis 1987;9:754.

64. Koskiniemi M, Lappalainen M, Hedman K. Toxoplasmosis needs evaluation: an overview and proposals. Am J Dis Child 1989;143:724.

65. Brooks RG, McCabe RE, Remington JS. Role of serology in the diagnosis of toxoplasmic lymphadenopathy. Rev Infect Dis 1987;9:1055.

66. Remington JS, Gentry LO. Acquired toxoplasmosis: Infection versus disease. Ann NY Acad Sci 1970;174:1006.

67. Randall G, Seidel JS. Malaria. Pediatr Clin North Am 1985;32:893.

68. Centers for Disease Control. Summary of notifiable diseases, US, 1988. MMWR 1989;37:29.

69. Centers for Disease Control. Imported malaria associated with malariotherapy of Lyme disease—New Jersey. MMWR 1990;39:373.

70. Abramowicz M. Drugs for parasitic infections. Med Lett 1990;32:23.

71. Miller KD, Greenberg AE, Campbell CC. Treatment of severe malaria in the United States with a continuous infusion of quinidine gluconate and exchange transfusion. N Engl J Med 1989;321:65.

72. White NJ, Miller KD, Churchill FC, et al. Chloroquine treatment of severe malaria in children: Pharmacokinetics, toxicity, and new dosage recommendations. N Engl J Med 1988;319:1493.

73. Centers for Disease Control. Childhood chloroquine poisonings—Wisconsin and Washington. MMWR 1988;37:437.

74. Loney PD, Walling AD. Chloroquine overdosage in infancy: A case report. Am Fam Phys 1989;40:164

75. Centers for Disease Control. Recommendations for the prevention of malaria among travelers. MMWR 1990;39:RR3.

76. Centers for Disease Control. Change of dosing regimen for malaria prophylaxis with mefloquine. MMWR 1991;40:72.

77. Krause PJ, Telford SR III, Ryan R, et al. Geographical and temporal distribution of babesial infection in Connecticut. J Clin Microbiol 1991;29:1.

78. Smith RP, Evans AT, Popovsky M, et al. Transfusion-acquired babesiosis and failure of antibiotic treatment. JAMA 1986;256:2726.

79. Jacoby GA, Hunt JV, Kosinski KS, et al. Treatment of transfusion-transmitted babesiosis by exchange transfusion. N Engl J Med 1980;303:1098.

80. Ma P, Visvesvara GS, Martinez AJ, et al. *Naegleria* and *Acanthamoeba* infections: Review. Rev Infect Dis 1990;12:490.

81. Simon MW, Wilson HD. The amebic meningoencephalitides. Pediatr Infect Dis 1986;5:562.

82. Visvesvara GS, Martinez AJ, Schuster FL, et al. Leptomyxid ameba, a new agent of amebic meningoencephalitis in humans and animals. J Clin Microbiol 1990;28:2750.

83. McLaughin GL, Vodkin MH, Huizinga HW. Amplification of repetitive DNA for the specific detection of *Naegleria fowleri*. J Clin Microbiol 1991;29:227.

84. Matson DO, Rouah E, Lee RT, et al. *Acanthameba* meningoencephalitis masquerading as neurocysticercosis. Pediatr Infect Dis J 1988;7:121.

85. Robin JB, Chan R, Rao NA, et al. Fluorescein-conjugated lectin visualization of fungi and acanthamoebae in infectious keratitis. Ophthalmology 1989;96:1198.

86. Margo CE, Brinser JH, Groden L. Exfoliated cytopathology of *Acanthamoeba* keratitis. JAMA 1986;255:2216.

87. Kilvington S, Larkin DFP, White DG, et al. Laboratory investigation of *Acanthamoeba* keratitis. J Clin Microbiol 1990;28:2722.

88. Kilvington S, Beeching JR, White DG. Differentiation of *Acanthamoeba* strains from infected corneas and the environment by using restriction endonuclease digestion of whole-cell DNA. J Clin Microbiol 1991;29:310.

89. Centers for Disease Control. *Acanthamoeba* keratitis in soft-contact-lens wearers. MMWR 1987;36:397.

90. Stehr-Green JK, Bailey TM, Brandt FH, et al. *Acanthamoeba* keratitis in soft contact lens wearers: A case-control study. JAMA 1987;258:57.

91. Kirn TF. As number of contact lens users increases, research seeks to determine risk factors, how best to prevent potential eye infections. JAMA 1987;258:17.

92. Centers for Disease Control. *Acanthamoeba* keratitis associated with contact lenses—United States. MMWR 1986;35:405.

93. Richman TB, Kerdel FA. Amebiasis and trypanosomiasis. Dermatol Clin 1989;7:301.

94. Sotelo-Avila C, Kline MW, Silberstein MJ, et al. Bloody diarrhea and pneumoperitoneum in a 10-month-old girl. J Pediatr 1988;113:1098.

95. Rimsza ME, Berg RA. Cutaneous amebiasis. Pediatrics 1983;71:595.

96. Spencer MJ, Garcia LS, Chapin MR. *Dientamoeba fragilis*. Am J Dis Child 1979;133:390.

97. Wolf MS. Giardiasis. JAMA 1975;233:1362.

98. Burke JA. Giardiasis in childhood. Am J Dis Child 1975;129:1304.

99. Pickering LK, Engelkirk PG. *Giardia lamblia*. Pediatr Clin North Am 1988;35:565.

100. Steketee RW, Reid S, Cheng T, et al. Recurrent outbreaks of giardiasis in a child day care center, Wisconsin. Am J Public Health 1989;79:485.

101. Korman SH, Granot E, Ramu N. Severe giardiasis in a child during cancer therapy. Am J Gastroenterol 1989;84:450.

102. Roberts DM, Craft JC, Mather FJ, et al. Prevalence of giardiasis in patients with cystic fibrosis. J Pediatr 1988;112:555.

103. Baxter PS, Dickson JAS, Variend S, et al. Intestinal disease in cystic fibrosis. Arch Dis Child 1988;63:1496.

104. Birkhead G, Vogt RI. Epidemiologic surveillance for endemic *Giardia lamblia* infection in Vermont. Am J Epidemiol 1989;129:762.

105. Centers for Disease Control. Common-source outbreak of giardiasis—New Mexico. MMWR 1989;38:405.

106. Kappus K, Juranek D. *Giardia* in the well. JAMA 1988;259:1810.

107. Smith SA. *Giardia* in the well. JAMA 1988;259:1810.

108. Dykes AC, Juranek DD, Lorenz RA, et al. Municipal waterborne giardiasis: An epidemiologic investigation—beavers implicated as a possible reservoir. Ann Intern Med 1980;92:165.

109. Porter JD, Ragazzoni HP, Buchanon JD, et al. *Giardia* transmission in a swimming pool. Am J Public Health 1988;78:659.

110. Harter L, Frost F, Grunenfelder G, et al. Giardiasis in an infant and toddler swim class. Am J Public Health 1984;74:155.

111. Greensmith CT, Stanwick RS, Elliot BE, et al. Giardiasis associated with the use of a water slide. Pediatr Infect Dis J 1988;7:91.

112. DuPont HL, Sullivan PS. Giardiasis: The clinical spectrum, diagnosis and therapy. Pediatr Infect Dis J 1986;5:S131.

113. Ish-Horowicz M, Korman SH, Shapiro M, et al. Asymptomatic giardiasis in children. Pediatr Infect Dis J 1989;8:773.

114. Shaw RA, Stevens MB. The reactive arthritis of giardiasis. A case report. JAMA 1987;258:2734.

115. Paerregaard A, Hjelt K. Comparative study of four methods for detecting giardiasis in children. Pediatr Infect Dis J 1988;7:807.

116. Korman SH. The duodenal string test. Am J Dis Child 1990;144:803.

117. McIntyre P, Boreham PFL, Phillips RE, et al. Chemotherapy in giardi-

asis: Clinical responses and in vitro drug sensitivity of human isolates in axenic culture. J Pediatr 1986;108:1005.

118. Neinstein LS, Goldenring J, Carpenter S. Nonsexual transmission of sexually transmitted diseases: An infrequent occurrence. Pediatrics 1984;74:67.

119. Glaser JB. Hammerschlag MR, McCormack WM. Epidemiology of sexually transmitted diseases in rape victims. Rev Infect Dis 1989;11:246.

120. Jones JG, Yamauchi T, Lambert B. *Trichomonas vaginalis* infestation in sexually abused girls. Am J Dis Child 1985;139:846.

121. Al-Salihi FL, Curran JP, Wang J-S. Neonatal *Trichomonas vaginalis*: Report of three cases and review of the literature. Pediatrics 1974;53:196.

122. McLaren LC, Davis LE, Healy GR, et al. Isolation of *Trichomonas vaginalis* from the respiratory tract of infants with respiratory disease. Pediatrics 1983;71:888.

123. D'Auria A. *Trichomonas* conjunctivitis. Clin Microbiol Newslett 1984;6:96.

124. Wolner-Hanssen P, Krieger JN, Stevens CE, et al. Clinical manifesations of vaginal trichomoniasis. JAMA 1989;261:571.

125. Gilchrist MJR, Rauh JL. Office microscopy: Low-cost screening for STDs. Contemp Pediatr 1987;4:50.

126. Tzipori S. Cryptosporidiosis in animals and humans. Microbiol Rev 1983;47:84.

127. Janoff EN, Reller LB. *Cryptosporidium* species, a protean protozoan. J Clin Microbiol 1987;25:967.

128. Fayer R, Ungar BLP. *Cryptosporidium* spp. and cryptosporidiosis. Microbiol Rev 1986;50:458.

129. Neidich GA, Ohrt DW. Cryptosporidiosis: A pathogen more common than appreciated. S Dakota J Med 1989;42:5.

130. Hira PR, Al-Ali F, Zaki M, et al. Human cryptosporidiosis in the Arabian Gulf: First report of infections in children in Kuwait. J Trop Med Hyg 1989;92:249.

131. Forgacs P, Tarshis A, Ma P, et al. Intestinal and bronchial cryptosporidiosis in an immunodeficient homosexual man. Ann Intern Med 1983;99:793.

132. Current WL. The biology of *Cryptosporidium*. ASM News 1988;54:605.

133. D'Antonio RG, Winn RE, Taylor JP, et al. A waterborne outbreak of cryptosporidiosis in normal hosts. Ann Intern Med 1986;103:886.

134. Hayes EB, Matte TD, O'Brien TR, et al. Large community outbreak of cryptosporidiosis due to contamination of a filtered public water supply. N Engl J Med 1989;320:1372.

135. Rose JB. Occurrence and significance of *Cryptosporidium* in water. J Am Water Works Assoc 1988;80:53.

136. Jokipii L, Pohjola S, Jokipii AMM. Cryptosporidiosis associated with traveling and giardiasis. Gastroenterology 1985;89:838.

137. Ma P, Kaufman DL, Helmick CG, et al. Cryptosporidiosis in tourists returning from the Caribbean. N Engl J Med 1985;312:647.

138. Crawford FG, Vermund SH, Ma JY, et al. Asymptomatic cryptosporidiosis in a New York City day care center. Pediatr Infect Dis J 1988;7:806.

139. Centers for Disease Control. Cryptosporidiosis—New Mexico, 1986. MMWR 1987;36:561.

140. Taylor JP, Perdue JN, Dingley D, et al. Cryptosporidiosis outbreak in a day-care center. Am J Dis Child 1985;139:1023.

141. Macfarlane DE, Horner-Bryce J. Cryptosporidiosis in well-nourished and malnourished children. Acta Paediatr Scand 1987;76:474.

142. Sallon S, Deckelbaum RJ, Schmid II, et al. *Cryptosporidium*, malnutrition, and chronic diarrhea in children. Am J Dis Child 1988;142:312.

143. Miller RA, Holmberg RE, Clausen CR. Life-threatening diarrhea caused by *Cryptosporidium* in a child undergoing therapy for acute lymphocytic leukemia. J Pediatr 1983;103:256.

144. Lewis IJ, Hart CA, Baxby D. Diarrhoea due to *Cryptosporidium* in acute lymphoblastic leukemia. Arch Dis Child 1985;60:60.

145. Hart MH, Kruger R, Nielsen S, et al. Acute self-limited colitis associated with *Cryptosporidium* in an immunocompetent patient. J Pediatr Gastroenterol Nutr 1989;8:401.

146. Ramsden K, Freeth M. Cryptosporidial infection presenting as an acute appendicitis. Histopathology 1989;14:209.

147. Shepherd RC, Smail PJ, Sinha GP. Reactive arthritis complicating cryptosporidial infection. Arch Dis Child 1989;64:743.

148. Blumberg RS, Kelsey P, Perrone T, et al. Cytomegalovirus- and *Cryptosporidium*-associated acalculous gangrenous cholecystitis. Am J Med 1984;76:1118.

149. Tzipori S, Angus KW, Gray EW, et al. Vomiting and diarrhea associated with cryptosporidial infection. N Engl J Med 1980;303:818.

150. Saez-Llorens X, Odio CM, Umana MA, et al. Spiramycin vs. placebo for the treatment of acute diarrhea caused by *Cryptosporidium*. Pediatr Infect Dis J 1989;8:136.

151. Wittenberg DF, Miller NM, van den Ende J. Spiramycin is not effective in treating *Cryptosporidium* diarrhea in infants: Results of a double-blind randomized trial. J Infect Dis 1989;159:131.

152. Meisel JL, Perera DR, Meligro C, et al. Overwhelming watery diarrhea associated with a *Cryptosporidium* in an immuno-suppressed patient. Gastroenterology 1976;70:1156.

153. Oh SH, Jaffe N, Fainstein V, et al. Cryptosporidiosis and anticancer chemotherapy. J Pediatr 1984;104:963.

154. Madore MS, Rose JB, Gerba CP, et al. Occurrence of *Cryptosporidium*

oocysts in sewage effluents and selected surface waters. J Parasitol 1987;73:702.

155. Centers for Disease Control. Swimming-associated cryptosporidiosis—Los Angeles County. MMWR 1990;39:343.

156. Liebman WM, Thaler MM, DeLorimer A, et al. Intractable diarrhea of infancy due to intestinal coccidiosis. Gastroenterology 1980;78:579.

157. DeHovitz JA, Pape JW, Boncy M, et al. Clinical manifestations and therapy of *Isospora belli* infection in patients with the acquired immunodeficiency syndrome. N Engl J Med 1986;315:87.

158. Pape JW, Verdier R-I, Johnson WD. Treatment and prophylaxis of *Isospora belli* infection in patients with the acquired immunodeficiency syndrome. N Engl J Med 1989;320:1044.

159. Miller RA, Minshew BH. *Blastocystis hominis*: An organism in search of a disease. Rev Infect Dis 1988;10:930.

160. Senay H, MacPherson D. *Blastocystis hominis*: Epidemiology and natural history. J Infect Dis 1990;162:987.

161. Zierdt CH. *Blastocystis hominis*—past and future. Clin Microbiol Rev 1991;4:61.

162. Kasper DL, Kass EH. Infectious disease rounds: Headache, fever, and periorbital edema. Rev Infect Dis 1987;9:804.

163. Kreel L, Poon WS, Nainby-Luxmoore JC. Trichinosis diagnosed by computed tomography. Postgrad Med J 1988;64:626.

164. Bailey TM, Schantz PM. Trichinosis surveillance, United States, 1986. MMWR 1988;37:SS5.

165. Olness K, Franciosi RA, Johnson MM, et al. Loiasis in an expatriate American child: Diagnostic and treatment difficulties. Pediatrics 1987;80:943.

166. Nutman TB, Miller KD, Mulligan M, et al. Diethylcarbamazine prophylaxis for human loiasis. N Engl J Med 1988;319:752.

167. Embil JA, Tanner CE, Pereira LH, et al. Seroepidemiologic survey of *Toxocara canis* infection in urban and rural children. Public Health 1988;102:129.

168. Bass JL, Mehta KA, Glickman LT, et al. Asymptomatic toxocariasis in children: A prospective study and treatment trial. Clin Pediatr 1987;26:441.

169. Taylor MRH, Keane CT, O'Connor P, et al. The expanded spectrum of toxocaral disease. Lancet 1988;1:692.

170. Walsh SS, Robson WJ, Hart CA. Acute transient myositis due to *Toxocara*. Arch Dis Child 1988;63:1087.

171. Friedman S, Hervada AR. Severe myocarditis with recovery in a child with visceral larva migrans. J Pediatr 1960;56:91.

172. Gould IM, Newell S, Green SH, et al. Toxocariasis and eosinophilic meningitis. Br Med J 1985;291:1239.

173. Dayal Y, Neafie RC: Human pulmonary dirofilariasis: A case report and review of the literature. Am Rev Respir Dis 1975;112:437.

174. Merrill JR, Otis J, Logan WD Jr, et al. The dog heartworm *Dirofilaria immitis* in man: An epidemic pending or in progress? JAMA 1980;243:1066.

175. Ciferri F. Human pulmonary dirofilariasis in the west. West J Med 1981;134:158.

176. Katzman EM. What's the most common helminth infection in the US? MCN 1989;14:193.

177. Jones JE. Pinworms. Am Fam Phys 1988;38:159.

178. Vermund SH, MacLeod S. Is pinworm a vanishing infection? Am J Dis Child 1988;142:566.

179. Spear RM, Rothbaum RJ, Keating JP, et al. Perianal streptococcal cellulitis. J Pediatr 1985;107:557.

180. Kokx NP, Comstock JA, Facklam RR. Streptococcal perianal disease in children. Pediatrics 1987;50:659.

181. Nagar H. Surgical aspects of parasitic disease in childhood. J Pediatr Surg 1987;22:325.

182. Haswell-Elkins M, Elkins D, Anderson RM. The influence of individual, social group and household factors on the distribution of *Ascaris lumbricoides* within a community and implications for control strategies. Parasitology 1989;98:125.

183. Forrester JE, Scott ME, Bundy DAP, et al. Clustering of *Ascaris lumbricoides* and *Trichuris trichiura* infections within households. Trans R Soc Trop Med Hyg 1988;82:282.

184. Williams D, Burke G, Hendley JO. Ascariasis: A family disease. J Pediatr 1974;84:853.

185. Wiersma R, Hadley GP. Small bowel volvulus complicating intestinal ascariasis in children. Br J Surg 1988;75:86.

186. Louw JH. Abdominal complications of *Ascaris lumbricoides* infestation in children. Br J Surg 1966;53:510.

187. Bundy DAP, Cooper ES. *Trichuris* and trichuriasis in humans. Adv Parasitol 1989;28:107.

188. Hotez PJ. Hookworm disease in children. Pediatr Infect Dis J 1989;8:516.

189. Stoll NR. On endemic hookworm, where do we stand today? Exp Parasitol 1962;12:241.

190. Scowden EB, Schaffner W, Stone WJ. Overwhelming strongyloidiasis. An unappreciated opportunistic infection. Medicine 1987;57:527.

191. Beal CB, Viens P, Grant RGL, et al. A new technique for sampling duodenal contents: Demonstration of upper small-bowel pathogens. Am J Trop Med Hyg 1970;19:349.

192. Wittner M, Turner JW, Jacquette G, et al. Eustrongylidiasis—a parasitic infection acquired by eating sushi. N Engl J Med 1989;320:1124.
193. Schantz PR. The dangers of eating raw fish. N Engl J Med 1989;320:1143.
194. Fontaine RE. Anisakiasis from the American perspective. JAMA 1985;253:1024.
195. Kliks MM. Anisakiasis in the western United States: Four new case reports from California. Am J Trop Med Hyg 1983;32:526.
196. Valdiserri RO. Intestinal anisakiasis. Report of a case and recovery of larvae from market fish. Am J Clin Pathol 1981;76:329.
197. Sugimachi K, Inokuchi K, Ooiwa T, et al. Acute gastric anisakiasis. Analysis of 178 cases. JAMA 1985;253:1012.
198. Centers for Disease Control. Acute schistosomiasis in US travelers returning from Africa. MMWR 1990;39:141.
199. Doehring E. Schistosomiasis in childhood. Eur J Pediatr 1988;147:2.
200. Boyce TG. Acute transverse myelitis in a 6-year-old girl with schistosomiasis. Pediatr Infect Dis J 1990;9:279.
201. Centers for Disease Control. Acute schistosomiasis with transverse myelitis in American students returning from Kenya. MMWR 1984;33:445.
202. Binstock PD, Azimi PH, Williams RA. Cerebral cysticercosis in a 22-month-old infant. Am J Clin Pathol 1987;88:655
203. Mitchell WG, Crawford TO. Intraparenchymal cerebral cysticercosis in children: Diagnosis and treatment. Pediatrics 1988;82:76.
204. Brown WJ, Voge M. Cysticercosis. A modern day plague. Pediatr Clin North Am 1985;32:953.
205. Richards FO Jr, Schantz PM, Ruiz-Tiben E, et al. Cysticercosis in Los Angeles County. JAMA 1985;254:3444.
206. Richards F, Schantz PM. Cysticercosis and taeniasis. N Engl J Med 1985;312:787.
207. Scharf D. Neurocysticercosis. Two hundred thirty-eight cases from a California hospital. Arch Neurol 1988;45:777.
208. Schantz PM. Circulating antigen and antibody in hydatid disease. N Engl J Med 1988;318:1469.
209. Scully RE, Mark EJ, McNeely WF, et al. Case records of the Massachusetts General Hospital—case 45-1987. N Engl J Med 1987;317:1209.
210. Scully RE, Mark EJ, McNeely WF, et al. Case records of the Massachusetts General Hospital—case 20-1990. N Engl J Med 1990;322:1446.
211. Norman RM, Kapadia C. Cerebral cysticercosis: Treatment with praziquantel. Pediatrics 1986;78:291.
212. Levin JA, Smith JG Jr. Praziquantel in the treatment of cysticercosis. JAMA 1986;256:349.
213. Birmhall CL, Esterly NB. Uninvited guests: Skin infestations of childhood. Contemp Pediatr 1990;7:18.
214. Ragosta K. Pediculosis masquerades as child abuse. Pediatr Emerg Care 1989;5:253.
215. Bowerman JG, Gomez MP, Austin RD, et al. Comparative study of permethrin 1% creme rinse and lindane shampoo for the treatment of head lice. Pediatr Infect Dis J 1987;6:252.
216. Carson DS, Tribble PW, Weart CW. Pyrethrins combined with piperonyl butoxide (RID) vs 1% permethrin (NIX) in the treatment of head lice. Am J Dis Child 1988;142:768.
217. Abramowicz A. Permethrin for head lice. Med Lett 1986;28:89.
218. Meinking TL, Taplin D, Kalter DC, et al. Comparative efficacy of treatments for pediculosis capitis infestations. Arch Dermatol 1986;122:267.
219. Reeves JRT. Head lice and scabies in children. Pediatr Infect Dis J 1987;6:598.
220. Sarov B, Neumann L, Herman Y, et al. Evaluation of an intervention program for head lice infestation in school children. Pediatr Infect Dis J 1988;7:176.
221. Tunnessen WW. A summertime itch. Contemp Pediatr 1986;3:43.
222. Abramowicz A. Permethrin for scabies. Med Lett 1990;32:21.
223. Schultz MW, Gomez M, Hansen RC, et al. Comparative study of 5% permethrin cream and 1% lindane lotion for treatment of scabies. Arch Dermatol 1990;126:167.
224. Witkowski JA, Parish LC. Scabies: Subungual areas harbor mites. JAMA 1984;252:1318.
225. Kleeman FJ. *Dermatobia hominis* comes to Boston. N Engl J Med 1983;308:847.
226. Cogen MS, Hays SJ, Dixon JM. Cutaneous myiasis of the eyelid due to *Cuterebra* larva. JAMA 1987;258:1795.
227. Savino MF, Margo CE, McCoy ED, et al. Dermal myiasis of the eyelid. Ophthalmology 1986;93:1225.
228. Lane RP, Lovell CR, Griffiths WAD, et al. Human cutaneous myiasis—a review and report of three cases due to *Dermatobia hominis*. Clin Exp Dermatol 1987;12:40.
229. File TM Jr, Thomson RB, Tan JS. *Dermatobia hominis* dermal myiasis. Arch Dermatol 1985;121:1195.

Selected References

Addiiss DG, Juranek DD, Spencer HC. Treatment of children with asymptomatic and nondiarrheal Giardia infection. Pediatr Infect Dis J 1991;10:843.
Blondell R. Parasites of the skin and hair. Primary Care Clin Office Practice 1991;18:167.
Grossman M, Azimi P. New onset night eye blindness in a young girl. Pediatr Infect Dis J 1992;11:55.
Hughes W. *Pneumocystis carinii* pneumonia: New approaches to diagnosis, treatment and prevention. Pediatr Infect Dis J 1991;10:391.
Jones JE. Signs and symptoms of parasitic diseases. Primary Care Clin Office Practice 1991;18:1.
Kappus KK, Juranek DD, Roberts JM. CDC Surveillance Summaries. Results of testing for intestinal parasites by state diagnostic laboratories, United States, 1987. MMWR 1991;40(no. SS-4):145.
Locally acquired neurocysticercosis—North Carolina, Massachusetts, and South Carolina, 1989–1991. MMWR 1992;41:1.
Marx MB. Parasites, pets, and people. Primary Care Clin Office Practice, 1991;18:153.
Nahlen BL, Parsonnet J, Preblud SR, et al. International travel and the child younger than two years: II. Recommendations for prevention of travelers' diarrhea and malaria chemoprophylaxis. Pediatr Infect Dis J 1989;8:735.
Russell L. The pinworm, *Enterobius vermiculari*. Primary Care Clin Office Practice 1991;18:13.
Rutstein R. Predicting risk of *Pneumocystis carinii* pneumonia in human immunodeficiency virus-infected children. Am J Dis Child 1991;145:922.
Vuorio A, Jokipii A, Jokipii L. *Cryptosporidium* in asymptomatic children. Rev Infect Dis 1991;12:261.
Ware BR, Jones JE. The office diagnosis of common intestinal parasitic diseases. Primary Care Clin Office Practice 1991;18:185.
Wolfe M. Giardiasis. Clin Microbiol Rev 1992;5:93.

SECTION ELEVEN

Eyes, Ears, Nose, and Throat

CHAPTER 75

Otitis

Lisa Cahill
Dietrich Jehle

OTITIS MEDIA

Acute otitis media (OM) is the most common bacterial infection in the pediatric age group. Underdiagnosis can result in significant morbidity, including intratemporal and intracranial complications. Overdiagnosis can result in needless antimicrobial therapy. Improper diagnosis might also lead the examiner away from detection of other, more life-threatening conditions that also present with nonspecific symptoms such as fever and irritability.

Definition and Classification

Multiple terms have been employed to describe the various types of inflammatory disorders of the middle ear. Bluestone[1] has proposed the terminology in widest use.

Otitis media: An inflammation of the middle ear, without reference to cause or pathogenesis.
Middle ear effusion: The liquid resulting from otitis media. The effusion may be *serous* (thin, watery), *mucoid* (thick, viscid, mucus-like), or *purulent* (pus-like).
Otorrhea: A discharge from the ear.

Bluestone has also classified the various clinical patterns of middle ear inflammation into (1) otitis media without effusion, (2) acute otitis media, (3) otitis media with effusion, and (4) atelectasis of the tympanic membrane.

OM without effusion usually represents the early stage of acute otitis media. In this instance, the tympanic membrane (TM) is erythematous and opacified but demonstrates normal mobility by pneumatic otoscopy. This appearance may also be seen in the terminal stages of an acute OM. Simple erythema of the tympanic membrane does not indicate OM, as crying and fever can also cause symmetric erythema of the TMs. Significant asymmetry in color along with opacification of the tympanic membrane is more suggestive of OM.

Acute OM is defined by the rapid onset of signs and symptoms of middle ear inflammation. Sudden fever, otalgia, pulling at the ear, irritability, and otorrhea may be presenting complaints. The TM will appear bulging and opaque with markedly decreased mobility during pneumatic otoscopy.

The presence of middle ear fluid of unknown duration with minimal or no clinical symptoms is classified as OM with effusion. The TM usually is opaque with decreased mobility. Bubbles or an air-fluid level may be seen behind the TM. Terms such as *serous* and *mucoid* are often used to describe the type of middle ear effusion. In fact, the true nature of the fluid behind the TM is difficult to determine without tympanocentesis, and the general term *otitis media with effusion* best characterizes this variety of middle ear disease. The duration of effusions within the middle ear is classified as *acute* (less than 3 weeks duration), *subacute* (3 weeks to 3 months), and *chronic* (greater than 3 months).

Atelectasis of the middle ear is not a type of OM. This condition occurs most commonly when negative pressure within the middle ear, caused by eustachian tube dysfunction, results in retraction of the TM.

Epidemiology

OM is one of the most prevalent infectious diseases of childhood. Approximately two thirds of all children have at least one episode of OM by their second birthday.[2] The incidence of OM is highest during the latter half of the first year of life and declines thereafter.[3] However, a slight increase in incidence is seen around age 5, corresponding to initial exposure to school.

Some children are prone to develop infections of the middle ear, and others are not. This may be the result of factors inherent to the individual child, such as an abnormality in eustachian tube function or anatomy. The incidence of OM peaks in winter, corresponding to the peak season of concomitant viral infections in children. Inflammation caused by viral infections is of major importance in the pathogenesis of OM. It might be expected that children in day-care centers should experience a greater frequency of middle ear infections. However, it is uncertain that exposure to a day-care center is a definite risk factor for OM.

Breast-feeding is a protective factor against the development of OM in infancy.[4] It is unclear whether this protection is the result of immunologic factors present in breast milk or of mechanical factors such as a different type of sucking mechanism used by the infant for breast-feeding compared with bottle feeding. Frequent episodes of OM are seen in a small number of children with abnormal host defenses. Maternal cigarette smoking during pregnancy is a risk factor for OM in the child. Anatomic abnormalities such as a cleft palate can predispose a child to frequent infections of the middle ear. Defects in the immune system such as (e.g., immunoglobulin A [IgA] deficiency), chemotherapy, or ciliary dyskinesia may result in frequent episodes of OM.

Anatomy and Pathophysiology

The middle ear is an air space that lies within the petrous portion of the temporal bone. The roof of the middle ear separates it from the middle cranial fossae; the mastoid air space lies posteriorly. The middle ear and the mastoid air space communicate directly through the mastoid antrum. The lateral boundary of the middle ear is the tympanic membrane, and the anterior border is made up of the carotid artery and the eustachian tube. The inner ear is medial to the middle ear.

Dysfunction of the eustachian tube is central to the pathogenesis of OM. The eustachian tube is a conical structure lined with pseudostratified, columnar, ciliated epithelium that connects the middle ear to the nasopharynx. It equilibrates pressure between the middle ear and the internal auditory canal and allows drainage of middle ear secretions into the nasopharynx while simultaneously preventing reflux of nasopharyngeal secretions into the middle ear. The eustachian tube is usually closed but opens during yawning and swallowing as a result of contraction of the tensor veli palatini muscle.

Anatomic differences between the infant and adult eustachian tube explain the greater incidence of OM in infancy. The infant eustachian tube is approximately half as long as that of the adult. It also lies nearly horizonal, whereas in the adult it lies at about 45° to the horizonal plane. The cartilage that lines the adult eustachian tube is stiffer than that of the infant, and this helps to maintain patency of the tube and allow for more effective active opening by the tensor veli palatini muscle.

Obstruction of the eustachian tube is the most frequent initiating event in the development of OM. Infections of the middle ear are frequently preceded by signs of upper respiratory tract infection. Inflammation caused by upper respiratory tract infection causes functional obstruction of the eustachian tube, thereby leading to eustachian tube dysfunction.[5] Absorption of gas within the middle ear by its mucosal lining results in negative middle ear pressure. If the eustachian tube opens while there is negative pressure within the middle ear, infectious secretions from the nasopharynx may be drawn into the middle ear, resulting in acute OM. If the eustachian tube remains persistently closed, middle ear mucosal secretions may accumulate to form a middle ear effusion.

Allergy is frequently mentioned as a causative factor for OM. However, studies have not been able to establish this.

Significant nasal obstruction resulting from adenoidal hypertrophy or nasal inflammation may also result in OM. Pressure changes within the obstructed nasopharynx that occur during swallowing may result in propulsion of infected nasopharyngeal secretions into the middle ear, with subsequent development of OM.[6]

In addition to obstruction of the eustachian tube, abnormal patency of the eustachian tube may also result in OM. If the eustachian tube remains persistently open, any event that causes positive nasopharyngeal pressure, such as sneezing, can force nasopharyngeal secretions into the middle ear.

Microbiology

Bacterial pathogens can be isolated by needle aspiration of middle ear fluid in the majority of cases of acute OM.

Streptococcus pneumoniae and nontypable *Haemophilus influenzae* are the most frequent pathogens. *Branhamella (Moraxella) catarrhalis* has also been frequently isolated. Pathogens less frequently isolated include *Streptococcus pyogenes, Staphylococcus aureus*, gram-negative enterics, and *H. influenzae* type B. No bacterial pathogen is isolated in one third of middle ear aspirates in acute OM.[7] Gram-negative organisms are seen occasionally in OM in neonates but are rarely seen in older children except in those with chronic suppurative OM. Fluid aspirated from chronic middle ear effusions often contains *Pseudomonas aeruginosa*. The role of anaerobic bacteria in the pathogenesis of acute OM appears to be limited.[8] *Mycoplasma pneumoniae* plays a minor role in causing acute OM but is isolated more frequently during outbreaks of mycoplasmal respiratory disease.[9]

Although viral upper respiratory infections may be the major initiating event in the pathogenesis of acute OM, viruses are rarely grown from aspirates of middle ear fluid.[10] However, detection of viral antigens by enzyme-linked immunosorbent assay (ELISA) has demonstrated viral antigens in one fourth of aspirates from children with acute OM. Respiratory syncytial virus is the virus most commonly detected by this method.[11]

Clinical Evaluation
Signs and Symptoms

The clinical presentation of acute OM varies with age. The infant or young child with OM may present with nonspecific signs such as fever, irritability, poor feeding, vomiting, diarrhea, or otorrhea. Unable to verbalize ear pain, the child may pull the affected ear. Parents often describe fitful sleep with frequent wakening.

The child older than 2 to 3 years is able to give a history of ear pain. However, pain is not universally present in children with acute OM.[12] The pain associated with otitis may be brief, often resolving within a few hours without any therapy. Parents often assume that because the pain has resolved, the child's problem has also resolved and may mistakenly fail to seek medical attention. It is also important to note that otalgia is not always caused by middle ear infection.

Fever occurs in approximately 50% of children with acute OM. Caution must be exercised in attributing the fever to OM, because fever itself can cause symmetric erythema of the tympanic membranes. The presence of OM in a febrile child does not preclude the coexistence of a more serious infectious illness, and the diagnosis of OM in any child with a temperature of greater than 39.8°C should be made with caution (Table 75–1).[13]

The older child may complain of various unusual sensations in the affected ear such as "clogging," "popping," or "buzzing." Hearing loss is also a common complaint. Vertigo, nystagmus, and tinnitus can be symptoms of OM but are infrequent. Inflammation within the middle ear may cause

TABLE 75–1		
DIFFERENTIAL DIAGNOSIS FOR OTITIS MEDIA	
Infants/Children	**Older Children**
Sepsis	Pharyngitis
Meningitis	Otitis externa
Gastroenteritis	Cerumen obstruction
Viral upper respiratory tract infection	Viral upper respiratory tract infection
Urinary tract infection	

dysfunction of the facial nerve as it courses through the temporal bone. However, facial paralysis is rarely observed as a symptom of OM.

Physical Examination

A thorough physical examination is required to exclude other diseases with signs and symptoms similar to OM yet with the potential to cause greater morbidity or mortality. When examining the ear, certain physical findings suggest a specific diagnosis. Following perforation of the TM caused by acute OM, a discharge from the ear may be present. The discharge is usually gray, purulent material but may be blood tinged. Swelling or displacement of the external ear and the postauricular region suggests acute mastoiditis. Manipulation of the tragus should be performed; significant pain on manipulation suggests otitis externa.

There are two primary methods of otoscopic examination. A cooperative child may be examined in the parent's arms. However, young children who cannot cooperate must be adequately restrained and immobilized. This is done by placing the child supine on the examining table with one assistant restraining the child at the thighs and another assistant restraining the arms at the elbows about the head. This second assistant immobilizes the head between the child's arms. The examiner can hold the pinna with a free hand and gently pull up and out to straighten the external auditory canal. Visualization of the TM is frequently impossible in children because of obstruction by cerumen. Removal of cerumen can be accomplished with a cerumen curette under otoscopic visualization. An otoscope equipped with a surgical head is the optimal instrument for this procedure. Other options include suction or irrigation of the external auditory canal with lukewarm water using a dental irrigation device (e.g., Water Pik).

A necessary piece of equipment for examining children is a pneumatic otoscope with a rubber bulb attached. Any air leak from the otoscope head will render assessment of TM mobility impossible.

Prior to assessment of TM mobility, the appearance of the membrane should be noted. The tympanic membrane is normally translucent, and the malleus should be visible through it. In patients with acute OM, the membrane is often intensely erythematous and the landmarks obscured. There may be an outward bulging of the membrane caused by purulent fluid under pressure within the middle ear. Occasionally bubbles or an air-fluid level may be noted behind the TM.

Following inspection, the examiner should then gently apply positive and negative pressure within the external canal by means of the rubber insufflator bulb. To accomplish this, the ear speculum must be the largest one that will fit into the external auditory canal in order to obtain an adequate seal between the speculum and the canal. The TM is normally in a neutral position. It should move away from the examiner when subjected to positive pressure and toward the examiner when subjected to negative pressure. A tympanic membrane that is retracted moves only when negative pressure is applied within the external canal. In contrast, a TM that is bulging and moves only with positive pressure suggests fluid under pressure within the middle ear. A TM in neutral position that is poorly mobile is consistent with either thickening of the TM or the presence of fluid behind it. A complete lack of mobility suggests perforation of the TM, the presence of a functioning tympanotomy tube, or a malfunctioning pneumatic otoscope. In patients with acute OM, pneumatic otoscopy will reveal a TM that is either bulging or in the neutral position and poorly mobile.

Diagnostic Evaluation
Tympanometry

Tympanometry is another method available for the detection of middle ear fluid. This requires the use of an instrument known as the *electroacoustic impedance bridge*. The instrument measures the ability of the TM to reflect sound energy as the pressure within the external auditory canal ranges from negative to positive. The presence of fluid behind the TM increases the amount of sound energy reflected back toward the probe placed in the ear canal. Conversely, a normal TM "absorbs" much of the sound energy that strikes it. Although tympanometry has been shown to be a reliable method for detection of middle ear fluid,[14] it is somewhat cumbersome for frequent use in the emergency department. It also requires the patient's cooperation, which limits its use in acutely ill and frightened children.

Acoustic Otoscope

A related instrument with greater potential for widespread use in the acute care setting is the acoustic otoscope. This instrument emits sound from a probe tip held at the external auditory meatus and records the amount of sound that is reflected by the TM. The acoustic otoscope has the advantage of being a small hand-held device and, unlike tympanometry, does not require a seal between the probe and the external auditory canal. The instrument has been evaluated in the clinical setting and is a reasonably sensitive and highly specific test for the presence of fluid within the middle ear.[15] Unfortunately, neither tympanometry nor the acoustic otoscope can distinguish an acute from a chronic middle ear effusion.

Tympanocentesis

The most definitive method for determination of the presence of middle ear fluid is tympanocentesis. Although aspiration of fluid from the middle ear is rarely necessary, there are certain indications.[16] In the emergency department setting, these might include OM in critically ill patients, the presence of a suppurative complication of OM such as mastoiditis or intracranial abscess, OM in the immunocompromised host, or for pain relief. Tympanocentesis does not require specialized equipment but is usually performed in consultation with an otolaryngologist.

Therapeutic Intervention
Antibiotic Therapy

Amoxicillin is the most commonly employed antibiotic for the initial treatment of acute OM (Table 75–2). Excellent antimicrobial activity against the majority of middle ear pathogens and low cost justify its popularity.[17, 18] For the penicillin-allergic child, trimethoprim-sulfamethoxazole or erythromycin-sulfisoxazole are acceptable alternatives. These two combinations can also be used as second-line agents in cases of suspected failure of amoxicillin therapy caused by beta-lastamase–producing pathogens. Cefaclor and amoxicillin-clavulanic acid are also effective against β-lactamase producers. A 10-day course of antibiotic therapy is most commonly prescribed, although this duration is somewhat arbitrary. Longer or shorter courses may prove to be appropriate.

After the proper antibiotic therapy is instituted, the patient should demonstrate marked clinical improvement within 3 days. If improvement is not seen by this time, the patient

TABLE 75–2

OTITIS MEDIA: THERAPY AT A GLANCE

Antibiotics Frequently Used in OM		
Drug	Form	Dose
Amoxicillin	Chewable tabs: 125 mg Susp: 125, 250 mg/5 ml Caps: 250, 500 mg	40 mg/kg/day q 8 hr po
Trimethoprim-sulfamethoxazole	Tabs (reg strength): 80 mg TMP/400 mg SMZ Tabs (double strength): 160 mg TMP/800 mg SMZ Susp: 40 mg TMP/200 mg SMZ per 5 ml	8–10 mg/kg TMP or 40–50 mg/kg SMZ per day divided q 12 hr
Erythromycin-sulfisoxazole	Susp: 200 mg erythromycin and 600 mg sulfisoxazole/5 ml	50 mg/kg/day (as erythromycin) and 150 mg/kg/day divided q 6 hr
Cefaclor	Caps: 250, 500 mg Susp: 125, 250 mg/5 ml	40 mg/kg/day q 8 hr Maximum dose, 1 gm/day
Amoxicillin-clavulinate	Same as amoxicillin	Same as amoxicillin

should be reexamined and the antibiotic changed. In this case, the physician should select an antibiotic that is effective against beta-lactamase–producing pathogens.

Adjunctive Therapy

Supportive therapy includes the use of antipyretics and analgesics (including narcotics). Anesthetic ear drops can be administered by the emergency physician once perforation of the TM has been excluded by otoscopy. Oral antihistamines and decongestants have no documented efficacy in the treatment of acute OM. The use of systemic steroids or topical nasal steroid sprays is unproved in the management of either acute OM or OM with effusion.

Surgical incision of the TM, known as *myringotomy*, for the treatment of OM was the primary treatment in the preantibiotic era but currently is infrequently performed. Severe earache is one possible indication (although the efficacy for relieving pain is unclear). This is a procedure best reserved for the otolaryngologist. The primary care physician is prudent to instill anesthetic ear drops and to prescribe an oral analgesic (including narcotics) for pain management. Another indication for myringotomy is the presence of a significant complication of OM such as mastoiditis or meningitis. In this case, an otolaryngologist should be consulted for surgical drainage of the middle ear for pathogen identification.

Treatment of Chronic Disease

Most clinicians suggest a follow-up examination 2 to 3 weeks after a diagnosis of acute OM. If an effusion is still present, periodic examinations are performed and one or more additional courses of antimicrobial therapy prescribed. If an effusion still persists, surgical drainage is generally recommended. The optimal length of observation before

referring the patient for surgery is uncertain, as the long-term effects of persistent middle ear fluid are unknown. Children with middle ear effusions suffer temporary hearing loss while the effusion is present, and there is good evidence that hearing improves after surgical drainage.[19] In addition, persistent middle ear fluid may permanently damage middle ear structures. Despite these uncertainties, it is generally agreed that fluid persisting for more than 3 to 6 months should be drained.

Although myringotomy alone is a drainage option, myringotomy followed by tympanostomy tube insertion is the most successful approach. Tympanostomy tubes provide a long-lasting means of drainage of middle ear fluid. Tubes also prevent the buildup of negative pressure within the middle ear and may promote drainage of secretions down the eustachian tube and into the nasopharynx.

Another problematic patient is the individual who suffers frequent acute OM with clearing of effusion between episodes. For these patients, certain management options may decrease the risk of further middle ear infections. These include the use of prophylactic antibiotics, insertion of tympanostomy tubes following myringotomy, and adenoidectomy with and without tonsillectomy.

Antimicrobial prophylaxis decreases the incidence of OM in children.[20–22] The antibiotics best studied are ampicillin and sulfisoxazole. Generally the medication is given once daily at half the usual daily therapeutic dose throughout the winter months, when the frequency of OM is the greatest. Complications of long-term use of an antibiotic are minimal. Intermittent use of antibiotics for several days at a time starting with the first sign of upper respiratory tract infection may also be effective but has been inadequately studied. Criteria for selecting children that may benefit from long-term antimicrobial prophylaxis are not established. Prophylaxis is recommended for children with three episodes of OM in the previous 3 months or four episodes within the previous year.[23]

Myringotomy with insertion of tympanostomy tubes can also decrease the number of future middle ear infections. This is both an alternative to antimicrobial prophylaxis and an adjunct to prophylactic medication when a child continues to suffer episodes of OM. Although data to support this use of tympanostomy tubes are lacking, most physicians and most parents relate a marked decrease in the number of middle ear infections following tympanostomy tube insertion. Criteria for selecting children for this procedure are nebulous.

A third management option for the OM-prone child is adenoidectomy with or without tonsillectomy. Although this has been practiced for many years, studies demonstrating its efficacy are lacking. A large clinical study of adenoidectomy at the Children's Hospital of Pittsburgh suggests that adenoidectomy does lessen middle ear disease in some children.[24] However, determining which subset of children could benefit from adenoidectomy is undefined. The addition of tonsillectomy to adenoidectomy has not been shown to be of benefit for prevention of OM.

Complications

There are a large number of potential complications of OM, but their frequency has markedly decreased in the postantibiotic era. Complications of OM can generally be divided into intracranial complications, such as brain abscess and meningitis, and intratemporal complications, which involve the middle ear itself and adjacent temporal bone.

Intracranial Complications

Intracranial disease as a sequela of OM is a dreaded occurrence but is fortunately quite rare. Meningitis can arise from OM by direct invasion through the bone and dura. Meningitis and OM may also be concurrent infections and not causally related. A virulent pathogen in the nasopharynx may spread to both the middle ear, causing otitis, and the cerebrospinal fluid following bacteremia. Bacteria that cause meningitis associated with OM are usually the same microbes that cause meningitis alone, and therefore, the initial empiric antimicrobial therapy for meningitis should be unaltered in the presence of concomitant OM. Ampicillin and chloramphenicol or an acceptable third-generation cephalosporin would be reasonable choices in children older than 2 months. Neonates and immunocompromised children with meningitis-otitis of unclear origin should undergo tympanocentesis for identification of the organism infecting the middle ear.

Another intracranial complication of OM is an epidural abscess resulting from the spread of purulent material through bone to dura. Patients with this complication may have fever, headache, and severe ear pain. Further spread of purulent material through the dura will result in a subdural empyema. These children are markedly ill with fever, a stiff neck, a change in sensorium, seizures, and focal neurologic signs. Treatment involves antimicrobial therapy and surgical drainage with mastoidectomy.

Because the mastoid and lateral venous sinuses are adjacent structures, inflammation of the mastoid can result in lateral sinus thrombosis. Clinical signs and symptoms of sinus thrombosis include fever, headache, a change in mental status, papilledema, and seizures. When lateral sinus thrombosis or an intracranial abscess is suspected, a computed tomography (CT) scan should be obtained prior to lumbar puncture. Treatment includes antimicrobial therapy along with surgical intervention.[25]

Intratemporal Complications

The intratemporal complications of OM are more common and fortunately less serious, as they are localized to the middle ear and adjacent temporal bone. The most common complication of OM is transient hearing loss. This is so common that it might be better considered as part of the illness, rather than a complication. There is generally a conductive hearing loss because of the presence of fluid within the middle ear. Once the fluid resolves, hearing usually returns to baseline. Rarely, permanent conductive hearing loss results from numerous episodes of acute OM or a longstanding effusion. Temporary or permanent sensorineural hearing loss can occur but is even less common than conductive loss. Sensorineural loss presumably is caused by involvement of the round window. In addition to hearing loss, concern exists over the effect that frequent episodes of temporary hearing loss might have on a young child's neurologic development. Unfortunately, it is simply not known whether temporary hearing loss has any long-term detrimental effects on children.

Following hearing loss, the next most common complication of OM is perforation of the tympanic membrane. Perforation is commonly seen with acute OM and is not of major concern. The majority of perforations heal spontaneously over several days. Purulent discharge from the tympanic membrane may cause eczematoid external otitis. Topical ear drops consisting of a steroid-antibiotic mixture are often prescribed for this condition. However, there is no evidence that antibiotic ear drops penetrate the perforation and reach the infected middle ear, and if the drops reach the middle ear, there is concern over potential ototox-

icity from the medication. Because of these confusing issues, there is no consensus regarding the use of ear drops in patients with OM accompanied by perforation. Discharge from the ear caused by acute OM generally lasts less than 1 week; and any discharge lasting more than 2 weeks warrants consultation with an otolaryngologist.

Another intratemporal complication of OM is the development of a cholesteatoma, a cyst-like structure lined by stratified squamous epithelium. Growth of a cholesteatoma is caused by accumulation of keratin debris within the cyst and can result in invasive destruction of adjacent structures. Although the pathogenesis of cholesteatoma formation is not completely understood, eustachian tube dysfunction with negative middle ear pressure and retraction pocket formation most likely plays a central role. Symptoms of a cholesteatoma may include hearing loss, persistent ear discharge, tinnitus, and vertigo. However, young children are frequently asymptomatic. Diagnosis is made by careful otoscopic examination, with the classic appearance being a pearly white mass in the pars flaccid, located in the superior and posterior aspect of the TM. Because treatment for this disorder is surgical excision, any child with a suspected cholesteatoma should be evaluated by an otolaryngologist.

Inflammation of the mastoid air cells occurs in all patients with acute suppurative OM. The inflammation is usually mild and asymptomatic and resolves with resolution of the middle ear infection. Occasionally the inflammation is severe, with accumulation of purulent material in the mastoid air cell system and destruction of the thin septa that separate the air cells. Infection may spread to the periosteum covering the mastoid, causing postauricular erythema, swelling, and tenderness. There is often outward, inferior, and anterior displacement of the pinna. Further spread can result in a subperiosteal abscess behind the pinna or a soft tissue abscess in the neck just inferior to it. Diagnosis can be confirmed by a CT scan of the mastoid region. Treatment includes systemic antimicrobial therapy directed at the usual pathogens of OM. Prompt consultation with an otolaryngologist is indicated.

Patients with OM accompanied by vertigo and nystagmus are suffering from labyrinthitis. This complication of middle ear infections may require surgical drainage, along with antimicrobial therapy and possibly steroids.

Facial paralysis is another possible complication of OM. The paralysis occurs from inflammation and edema of the facial nerve as it courses through the middle ear. Standard therapy consists of myringotomy and parenteral antibiotics. Facial nerve decompression is rarely needed.

Disposition

The majority of patients with OM can be managed as outpatients. Treatment includes appropriate antimicrobial therapy along with measures to control fever and pain as necessary for each individual patient. All patients with acute OM should be instructed to contact a physician if there is any deterioration of their clinical status or failure to improve by the third day of therapy. Those who respond well to therapy should have a follow-up examination within 3 weeks to detect any persistent effusion (Table 75–3).

Infants younger than 1 month with OM who have fever or appear ill should be promptly hospitalized. Samples of middle ear fluid, blood, spinal fluid, and urine should be obtained for culture and antibiotic therapy urgently initiated. Those febrile infants between 4 and 12 weeks old with OM who appear well may be managed as outpatients provided other sources of infection, especially meningitis, have been excluded.[26]

Tympanocentesis should also be strongly considered for

TABLE 75–3

DOCUMENTATION AND DISCHARGE INSTRUCTIONS FOR PATIENTS WITH OTITIS MEDIA

Documentation
General appearance
State of hydration
Lack of nuchal rigidity
Description of tympanic membrane

Discharge Instructions
Take Antibiotics ± pain medications as directed
Schedule a follow-up examination within 3 weeks
Return if listless, lethargic, vomiting medications,
   or no improvement within 3 days

the immunocompromised patient with OM in order to detect unusual pathogens. Hospital admission for parenteral antibiotics would be appropriate for these patients if they have fevers or appear toxic. Suspicion of any intracranial or intratemporal complication of OM mandates prompt consultation for surgical drainage, as well as urgent intravenous antimicrobial therapy.

OTITIS EXTERNA

Otitis externa (OE) is an inflammation of the external auditory canal often referred to as *swimmer's ear*. Infectious organisms predominate as the cause of inflammation. The external auditory canal extends from the pinna to the tympanic membrane and is protected from invasion by microorganisms by a water-resistant, waxy coating. However, the integrity of this coating is frequently disrupted by trauma, excessive "wetness" within the canal, or, in young children, a foreign body. These will eventually cause local defenses in the canal to fail, with subsequent invasion by bacterial pathogens.

The causative organisms of OE include *Pseudomonas aeruginosa*, *Staphylococcus*, and mixtures of gram-positive and gram-negative organisms. Occasionally herpes viruses and fungi may be seen.

The spectrum of clinical disease from OE ranges from mild itching, irritation, or fullness to excruciating pain with severe swelling and purulent discharge with systemic signs and symptoms. The diagnosis is made by inspection of the ear and visualization with an otoscope. On physical examination there may be purulent, foul-smelling discharge from the canal, which is red, boggy, and swollen. There is severe pain with manipulation of the tragus. It is often impossible to visualize the TM because of external canal swelling and purulent discharge within. Less frequently, there may be a local cellulitis involving the auricle and surrounding skin with associated cervical adenopathy. In the debilitated or immunocompromised host, deep tissue invasion with necrosis may occur (known as malignant OE) with marked systemic toxicity. This can be rapidly fatal if not treated aggressively.

Therapeutic Intervention

The treatment of uncomplicated OE initially involves clearing away purulent discharge to be certain that a foreign body is not present and to allow for placement of antibiotic drops into the canal. This is done most effectively by suctioning but can also be performed with a curette or a cotton-tipped applicator. If there is intense edema of the canal, a cotton wick with antibiotic drops applied may be placed with forceps and left in the canal for 24 to 48 hours. Gauze (¼-in width) rolled in a spiral and soaked with antibiotic drops

is also appropriate. Antibiotic ear drops are instilled at a dosage of two to four drops four times a day for 7 to 10 days. The most frequently used antibiotic drops contain a combination of polymyxin, neomycin and hydrocortisone. These allow for coverage against both gram-negative and gram-positive organisms, with the addition of a steroid to reduce edema.

In toxic patients (those with systemic symptoms or a significant local cellulitis), a broad-spectrum systemic antibiotic is indicated. Patients suspected of having malignant OE need urgent intravenous antibiotic therapy with prompt consultation for surgical drainage. Appropriate antibiotics in this situation must include one with specific anti-pseudomonal coverage.

All patients should avoid getting water into the external canal for at least 10 days to 2 weeks. This may be accomplished by an ear plug or by utilizing a cotton ball in the canal sealed by petroleum jelly. Further episodes of OE may be prevented by keeping the canal dry. This can be accomplished by equal mixtures of white vinegar and water applied after swimming and at bedtime.

References

1. Bluestone CD. State of the art: Definitions and classification. *In* Lim DJ, Bluestone CD, Klein JO, Nelson JD (eds). Recent Advances in Otitis Media with Effusion. Toronto, BC Decker, 1984, pp 1–4.
2. Howie VM. Natural history of otitis media: Ann Otol Rhinol Laryngol 1975;84:67.
3. Wright PF, McConnell MB, Thompson JM, et al. A longitudinal study of the detection of otitis media in the first two years of life. Int J Pediatr Otorhinolaryngol 1985;10:245.
4. Tecle DW, Klein JO, Rosner B. Otitis media with effusion during the first three years of life and development of speech and language. Pediatrics 1984;74:282.
5. Bluestone CD, Cantekin EI, Berry QC. Effect of inflammation on the ventilatory function of the eustachian tube. Laryngoscope 1977;87:493.
6. Bluestone CD, Beery QC, Andrua W. Mechanics of the eustachian tube as it influences susceptibility to and persistence of middle ear effusions in children. Ann Otol Rhinol Laryngol 1974;83:27.
7. Bluestone CD, Klein JO. Otitis Media in Infants and Children. Philadelphia, WB Saunders, 1988, p. 45.
8. Luatney J, Jokipü AMM, Vayrynen J, et al. Aerobic and anaerobic bacteria in the middle ear and ear canal in acute otitis media. Acta Otolaryngol (Stockh) 1982;386:100.
9. Jensen KJ, Senterfit LB, Scully WE, et al. Mycoplasma pneumonia infections in children. An epidemiologic appraisal in families treated with oxytetracycline. Am J Epidemiol 1967;86:419.
10. Klein JO, Teele DW. Isolation of viruses and mycoplasma from middle ear effusions: A review. Ann Otol Rhinol Laryngol 1976;85:140
11. Kelin BX, Dollette FR, Yolken RH. The role of respiratory syncytial virus and other viral pathogens in acute otitis media. J Pediatr 1982;101:16.
12. Hayden GF, Schwartz RH. Characteristics of earache among children with acute otitis media. Am J Dis Child 1985;139:721.13.
13. Long SS. Approach to the febrile patient with no obvious focus of infection. Pediatr Rev 1984;5:305.
14. Paradise JL, Smith CG, Bluestone CD. Tympanometric detection of middle ear effusion in infants and young children. Pediatrics 1976;58:198.
15. Jehle D, Cottington E. Acoustic otoscopy in the diagnosis of otitis media. Ann Emerg Med 1989;18:396.
16. Bluestone CD, Klein JO. Otitis Media in Infants and Children. Philadelphia, WB Saunders, 1988.
17. Mandel EM, Bluestone CD, Rocketto JE, et al. Duration of effusion after antibiotic treatment for otitis media: Comparison of cefaclor and amoxicillin. Pediatr Infect Dis 1982;1:310.
18. Johnson CE, Carlin SA, Super DM, et al. A randomized controlled trial of cefaclor compared with amoxicillin for treatment of acute otitis media. Abstract. Am J Dis Child 1990;144:421.
19. Mandel EM, Bluestone CD, Paradise JL, et al. Efficacy of myringotomy with and without tympanostomy tube insertion in the treatment of chronic otitis media with effusion in infants and children: Results for the first year of a randomized clinical trial. *In* Lim DJ, Bluestone CD, Klein JO, Nelson JD (eds). Recent Advances in Otitis Media With Effusion. Toronto, BC Decker, 1984, pp. 308–311.
20. Perin JM, Charney E, MacWhinney JB, et al. Sulfisoxazole as chemoprophylaxis for recurrent otitis media. N Engl J Med 1974;291:664.
21. Liston TE, Foskee WS, Pierson WD. Sulfisoxazole chemoprophylaxis for frequent otitis media. Pediatrics 1974;71:524.

22. Varsano I, Volovitz B, Mimouni F. Sulfisoxazole chemoprophylaxis for frequent otitis media. Am J Dis Child 1985;139:632.
23. Bluestone CD, Klein JO. Otitis Media in Infants and Children. Philadelphia, WB Saunders, 1988, p 163.
24. Paradise JL, Bluestone CD, Rogers KD, et al. Efficacy of adenoidectomy for recurrent otitis media: Results from parallel random and nonrandom trials. Pediatr Res 1987;21:286A.
25. Bluestone CD, Klein JO. Otitis Media in Infants and Children. Philadelphia, WB Saunders, 1988, p 256.
26. Fleisher G, Ludwig S. Textbook of Pediatric Emergency Medicine. Baltimore, Williams & Wilkins, 1983, p 370.

CHAPTER 76

Pharyngeal Disease

Bertha Koomson
David M. Jaffe

PHARYNGITIS

Pharyngitis, an inflammatory disease of the mucous membranes and structures of the throat, is a common and potentially serious pediatric problem. Approximately 11% of all school-age children seek medical care for pharyngitis, which accounts for 5% of visits to pediatric offices.[1]

Anatomy and Physiology

Waldeyer's ring consists of lymphoid tissue that drains the oral and pharyngeal cavity. Therefore, it is the defense mechanism against infection in the mouth and throat. Many organisms can induce inflammation in Waldeyer's ring. Some are part of the normal oropharyngeal flora that became virulent, and others are external pathogens, but only a few are of clinical significance (Table 76–1).

Of the bacterial pathogens, streptococci, *Neisseria gonorrhoeae*, and *Corynebacterium diphtheriae* are the most frequently encountered, whereas adenovirus, Epstein-Barr virus, and coxsackievirus are the most common viral pathogens associated with viral pharyngitis.[2]

Viral Pharyngitis

It is estimated that viral causes account for about 37% of cases of nonstreptococcal pharyngitis. Management is generally symptomatic and is aimed at maintaining hydration, alleviating pain with local and systemic analgesics, ensuring adequate oral hygiene, and observing for complications.

Adenovirus

Adenovirus is the most common viral etiologic agent in young children.[2] It is often difficult to clinically distinguish adenoviral pharyngotonsillitis from streptococcal pharyngitis.

Epstein-Barr Virus

Epstein-Barr virus (EBV), a DNA herpesvirus, has been associated with a variety of clinical syndromes that frequently go unrecognized in young infants and children. EBV can cause fever without apparent focal infection. EBV pharyngitis may occur as part of the infectious mononucleosis syndrome with concomitant fever, lymphadenopathy, hepatosplenomegaly, and atypical lymphocytes in peripheral blood, or it may also present as a simple pharyngotonsillitis without exudate. Diagnosis depends on serologic testing; the heterophile antibody can be demonstrated by the Paul-Bunnell test or the rapid slide agglutination (Monospot) test. These tests will identify 90% of cases in older children but only 75% in children who are 2 to 4 years of age, and less than 30% in children under 2 years.[3] Multiple EBV-specific serologic antibody tests are available. The most commonly performed test is for antibody against the viral capsid antigen (VCA). Immunoglobulin G (IgG) and immunoglobulin M (IgM) anti-VCA antibodies are useful for identifying recent infections, as is the antibody against early antigen (EA). Antibody against EBV nuclear antigen (EBNA) occurs several weeks to months after the onset of the infection.

Therapeutic Intervention. Treatment of EBV infection is supportive. The infectious mononucleosis syndrome is self-limited and requires antipyretics, analgesics, fluids, and bed rest. The associated complication of airway obstruction secondary to tonsillar swelling can be treated effectively with steroids (prednisone, 2.5 mg/kg/day and tapered over 5 days, or dexamethasone, 1 mg/kg to 10 mg maximum, then 0.5 mg/kg every 6 hours).

Other complications such as splenic rupture, encephalitis, Guillain-Barré syndrome, myocarditis, hemolytic anemia, and thrombocytopenia, although rare, need to be recognized, as some have the potential of being fatal.

Coxsackievirus

The common clinical picture associated with coxsackievirus type A infection is herpangina, a painful condition characterized by small vesicles and ulcers over the anterior tonsillar pillars, palate, and posterior pharynx. Young infants with herpangina may appear ill with fever, irritability, and dehydration from refusal to eat or drink.[4] Treatment is aimed at temperature control, pain control, and rehydration.

Other clinical illnesses produced by coxsackievirus include hand-foot-and-mouth disease and acute lymphonodular pharyngitis, in which the lesions are less ulcerated and more nodular.

Herpes Simplex Pharyngitis

Herpes simplex, known commonly for the cold sore, may also cause an exudative pharyngitis in older children, although in younger children it produces gingivostomatitis. Treatment is symptomatic.[5]

Chlamydial Pharyngitis

Chlamydia trachomatis has been implicated in the origin of pharyngitis in adults.[6] However, in infants, although associated with nasopharyngeal infections and pneumonia, its role as a causative agent of pharyngitis remains unclear.[7]

Non–Group A Beta-hemolytic Streptococcal Bacterial Pharyngitis

The pathogenicity of *non–group A beta-hemolytic streptococcus* in respiratory infections is well established, but its significance in pharyngitis is unclear. Group B streptococci have been recovered in young adults with pharyngitis,[8] and group

TABLE 76–1			
DIFFERENTIAL DIAGNOSIS			
Bacteria	**Mycoplasmas**	**Viruses and Chlamydiae**	**Fungi**
Aerobic	*Mycoplasma pneumoniae*	Adenovirus*	*Candida* sp.
Grp A,B,C,G		Enteroviruses (poliovirus,	
Streptococci*		echovirus, coxsackievirus*)	
Streptococcus		Parainfluenza types 1 through 4	
pneumoniae		Epstein-Barr virus*	
Staphylococcus aureus		Herpes simplex	
Branhamella (Moraxella)		Respiratory syncytial virus	
catarrhalis		Influenza types A and B	
*Neisseria gonorrhoeae**		Cytomegalovirus	
Neisseria meningitidis		Rhinovirus	
Corynebacterium		*Chlamydia trachomatis*	
*diphtheriae**			
Corynebacterium			
hemolyticum			
Bordetella pertussis			
Haemophilus influenzae			
Salmonella typhi			
Treponema pallidum			
Mycobacterium sp.			
Anaerobic			
Peptococcus sp.			
Peptostreptococcus sp.			
Bacteroides sp.			

*Commonly encountered organisms in pharyngitis.
Adapted from Brook I. The Clinical Microbiology of Waldeyer's Ring. Otolaryngol Clin North Am 1987; 20:2.

C streptococci accounted for 2% of isolates in an outbreak of pharyngitis.[9] Both group B and group C streptococci have been recovered in large numbers from patients with clinical pharyngitis.[10] Hayden and Thomas found that non–group A beta-hemolytic streptococcus was isolated as often from the throats of age- and season-matched controls as from children with sporadic symptomatic pharyngitis. They have suggested that non–group A beta-hemolytic streptococcus may be more significant in epidemics of pharyngitis than in nonepidemic pharyngitis in children.[11]

Streptococcus pneumoniae has been found to cause local pharyngotonsillar infection and may spread to other body sites. *S. pneumoniae* much more commonly causes pneumonia, meningitis, bacteremia, and otitis media in children.

Mycoplasma pneumoniae can cause pharyngitis but usually only as part of a generalized infection. It was found in only 3% of children and adolescents with pharyngitis,[4] whereas 32% of children with *Mycoplasma* lower respiratory tract infection had clinical pharyngitis.[12] *Mycoplasma* pharyngitis is usually a self-limited illness that requires no specific antimicrobial therapy unless symptoms or signs of illness persist[13] or generalized infection is present. Erythromycin is the drug of choice and is given at a dose of 30 to 50 mg/kg/day for 7 to 10 days. Tetracycline (40 mg/kg/day) is a suitable alternative in children older than 8 years.

The incidence of diphtheria has markedly declined since the introduction of the diphtheria-tetanus-pertussis (DTP) vaccine but still occurs in unimmunized individuals, usually of low socioeconomic status. *Corynebacterium diphtheriae* causes an exudative pharyngotonsillitis with a thick pseudomembrane that can spread to involve the throat, tonsils, palate, and larynx, causing airway obstruction. The organism can also produce a lethal exotoxin that can cause distant organ disease such as myocarditis, cardiac arrhythmias, bulbar paralysis, peripheral neuritis, hepatitis, nephritis, and adrenal hemorrhages. *Corynebacterium hemolyticum* causes a membranous pharyngitis similar to that found in clinical diph-

theria. Although diagnosis can be made by culturing part of the membrane or material collected from beneath the membrane, the diagnosis must be made clinically, as unnecessary delays in therapy may harm the patient. Treatment must be prompt and consists of both killing the bacteria with penicillin G or erythromycin (Table 76–2) and neutralizing the exotoxin with equine serum antitoxin after sensitivity testing. Close contacts should be cultured and, if found to be positive, treated with antibiotics and given a booster dose of DTP or diphtheria-tetanus (DT) vaccine if they have not received a booster dose of diphtheria toxoid during the preceding 5 years.

Pharyngitis caused by *Neisseria gonorrhoeae* occurs in sexually active adolescents, and its presence in younger children should always raise the suspicion of sexual abuse. Although the infection is usually asymptomatic, it may cause mild symptoms or, rarely, acute exudative tonsillitis. Diagnosis is by culture of throat swabs in Thayer-Martin medium. It is important to obtain rectal and vaginal or urethral cultures, as well as a serum test for syphilis, whenever gonorrhea is suspected. Gonococcal pharyngitis in children should be treated with ceftriaxone (125 mg intramuscularly in a single dose). Children who cannot tolerate ceftriaxone may be treated with spectinomycin (40 mg/kg intramuscularly in a single dose). Children 8 years or older should also receive oral doxycycline (100 mg bid for 7 days). Children weighing more than 45 kg should be treated with adult regimens (ceftriaxone, 250 mg intramuscularly in a single dose, or ciprofloxacin, 500 mg in a single oral dose) and cultures repeated in 4 to 7 days. For penicillin-sensitive children, spectinomycin (40 mg/kg; maximum, 2 gm) or tetracycline (40 mg/kg/day for 5 days if older than 8 years) can be used.

Anaerobic bacteria commonly occur in polymicrobial infections of the pharynx and orofacial region and in tonsillar and peritonsillar abscesses, as well as in acute necrotizing ulcerating gingivostomatitis. Anaerobic bacteria are important, because they can produce capsular material that pro-

TABLE 76–2

PHARYNGEAL DISEASE: THERAPY AT A GLANCE

Agent	Dosage
Analgesics	
Acetaminophen	15 mg/kg/dose po q 4 hr
Acetaminophen with codeine	
Codeine	0.5–1 mg/kg/dose po q 4 hr
Steroids	
Prednisone (for obstructive Epstein-Barr virus tonsillitis)	2.5 mg/kg/day (maximum, 60 mg)
Dexamethasone	1 mg/kg to 10 mg maximum, then 0.5 mg/kg q 6 hr
Antibiotics	
Ceftriaxone	125 mg IM for patients weighing <45 kg
	250 mg IM for patients weighing >45 kg or older than 12 yr
Erythromycin	30–50 mg/kg/day po
Spectinomycin	40 mg/kg IM (maximum, 2 gm)
Tetracycline	40 mg/kg po (patients older than 8 yr)
Penicillin V	125–250 mg tid po
Agents for streptococcal pharyngitis	
Penicillin G benzathine	600,000 U IM for patients weighing <27 kg
	1.2 million U IM for patients weighing >27 kg
Penicillin G benzathine + penicillin procaine (also called Bicillin C-R 900/300)	900,000 U 300,000 U IM
Agents for peritonsillar abscess	
Penicillin G	100,000 U/kg/day IV q 16 hr

motes their virulence. They can be resistant to penicillins and first-generation cephalosporins through production of beta-lactamase.[2]

Group A Beta-hemolytic Streptococcal Pharyngitis

Group A beta-hemolytic streptococcal pharyngitis is the most common nonviral cause of pharyngitis.[14] The most common ages of occurrence are from 4 to 11 years; group A beta-hemolytic streptococcus infection in children younger than 3 years is rare and poorly understood. It presents with pharyngitis, other upper respiratory tract symptoms, or both. In addition, there is sometimes an associated acute otitis media, otitis media with effusion, or impetigo.[15]

Clinical Evaluation

Patients may present with a mild or unapparent infection or with signs and symptoms including fever and sore throat. Vomiting, headaches, malaise, abdominal pain, and meningismus may also be present. The presence of a scarlatiniform rash should be considered diagnostic of a group A beta-hemolytic streptococcal infection.[16] The pharynx is red and sometimes edematous, and the tonsils are enlarged, red, and often covered with patches of exudate. The soft palate and uvula may have petechiae, and the tongue may be red and edematous, giving it the appearance of a "strawberry

tongue." Swollen, tender cervical lymph nodes are common (Table 76–3).

Different combinations of these signs and symptoms have been used as clinical aids in the diagnosis of group A beta-hemolytic streptococcal infections, but even though these clinical signs and symptoms may strongly suggest group A beta-hemolytic streptococcus, laboratory tests are needed to achieve a high degree of diagnostic precision.

Diagnostic Evaluation

The gold standard of laboratory diagnosis is the throat culture. Careful swabbing of the tonsil or posterior pharyngeal wall with direct visualization gives the best results.

Group A streptococci are distinguished from other groups of beta-hemolytic streptococci by the use of the Bacitracin disk, latex agglutination, or fluorescent antibody staining. Unfortunately, culture results are unavailable for 24 to 48 hours. Rapid antigen diagnostic tests have become available for office and emergency department use. These tests involve extraction of group A streptococcus–specific carbohydrate antigen from the throat swab, then restoring the sample to optimal pH to enhance optimal antibody binding. Latex agglutination and enzyme-linked immunosorbent assay (ELISA) have been used, but the latter method is preferred, because the results are less subjective, are more easily interpretable, and have greater sensitivity.[17] These tests take only 10 minutes to perform. Sensitivity under ideal laboratory conditions ranges from 85% to 95%, and specificity ranges from 93% to 100%.[18] However, under less ideal conditions and in the hands of untrained personnel, sensitivity may be 58% or lower.[18] Therefore, any emergency department or clinic planning to use the rapid diagnostic test must obtain its own sensitivity and specificity figures by comparison with cultures, and testing should be done by designated staff who are trained and monitored by laboratory personnel.

Therapeutic Intervention

The objectives of treatment of streptococcal pharyngitis are (1) relief of symptoms, (2) promotion of clinical recovery, (3) prevention of suppurative complications, and (4) prevention of acute rheumatic fever. Antibiotics are the mainstay of treatment. Fortunately, penicillin, the antibiotic of choice,

TABLE 76–3

FREQUENCY OF SYMPTOMS AND SIGNS OF STREPTOCOCCAL PHARYNGITIS

	% of Patients
Symptoms	
Fever	90.5
Sore throat	77.0
Headache	48.5
Anorexia	36.6
Abdominal pain	26.2
Chills	22.3
Signs	
Red pharynx	100
Fever	90.5
Cervical adenopathy	75.8
Scarlatiniform rash	32.9
Pharyngeal or tonsillar exudate	25.5
Petechiae on palate	9.7

Adapted from Stillerman M, Bernstein SH. Streptococcal pharyngitis. Am J Dis Child 1961;101:476. Copyright 1961, American Medical Association.

remains highly effective against group A beta-hemolytic streptococci.[19] Alternative choices for penicillin-sensitive individuals are the cephalosporins, erythromycin, lincomycin, and clindamycin. Intramuscular benzathine penicillin G (600,000 U if the patient weighs less than 27 kg or 1.2 million U if the patient weighs more than 27 kg) ensures compliance, but oral penicillin V (125 to 250 mg three times daily for 10 days) is a suitable alternative. The combination of 900,000 U penicillin G benzathine and 300,000 U penicillin G procaine (Bicillin C-R 900/300) is effective and causes fewer and less severe local reactions. Symptomatic treatment with throat lozenges, antiseptics, mouthwashes, and oral analgesics may provide temporary relief of pain.

Some issues regarding the early treatment of streptococcal pharyngitis remain controversial. Studies have shown that pharyngeal injection and tender lymph nodes are significantly and more quickly improved when patients are treated with antibiotics instead of placebo. Whether this justifies early treatment of all children with sore throats is uncertain, especially because children treated early for streptococcal pharyngitis have a higher rate of reinfection.[15, 20, 21] Several studies have looked at the cost effectiveness of various treatment strategies. Factors such as the prevalence of group A beta-hemolytic streptococcus, the availability and accuracy of rapid antigen testing, and the costs involved need to be considered prior to developing a strategy for diagnosis and treatment. One practical strategy is to perform rapid antigen detection screening on all children with pharyngitis and to treat all who test positive. All children with "classic" clinical findings are also treated promptly, even though the screening tests may be negative, and those with negative screening tests or atypical findings are cultured. Treatment is instituted if culture results are positive.

A contact phone number for the patient or the family physician should be obtained to ensure the provision of follow-up for children with positive cultures. Children should not return to school until at least 24 hours after beginning antimicrobial therapy and until they are afebrile. Reculturing is reserved for children with recurrence or persistence of symptoms or those with previously documented rheumatic fever. Those with a persisting positive culture should be treated with an alternate antibiotic. Asymptomatic carriers need not be treated, as they appear to be at little risk of spreading infection or developing complications. However, a penicillin and rifampin combination is effective in eradicating group A beta-hemolytic streptococcus carriage.[22]

Complications

Complications of group A beta-hemolytic streptococcal pharyngitis such as dehydration, suppuration, and rheumatic fever are quite rare. Although acute dehydration is the most common complication, acute rheumatic fever remains the most serious. Incidence rates of rheumatic fever in the United States have declined for several decades and are presently 0.5 per 100,000.[23] However, more recent outbreaks of rheumatic fever show that it is still a threat and justify the use of antibiotics for documented group A beta-hemolytic streptococcal pharyngitis.[22] Antibiotic therapy is most effective in preventing rheumatic fever if begun within 9 days of the onset of pharyngitis. Acute glomerulonephritis may occur following streptococcal pharyngitis caused by nephritogenic strains of group A beta-hemolytic streptococcus. Unfortunately, this complication is not preventable.

Suppurative complications such as peritonsillar abscess and suppurative cervical lymphadenitis do occur in streptococcal infections but are quite unusual. Complaints of difficulty speaking and trismus differentiate a peritonsillar abscess from pharyngitis. Peritonsillar abscess may also be associated with drooling. The affected tonsil is enlarged and may push the uvula to the opposite side of the pharynx. In the event of respiratory compromise, emergency aspiration may be lifesaving. A child with a peritonsillar abscess should be admitted to the hospital for antibiotic therapy to ensure adequate treatment and observation. Penicillin G (100,000 U/kg/day IV) is used initially, but the final choice of antibiotic should be determined by throat culture results. Admission for pharyngitis depends on the presence of acute dehydration, airway obstruction, the need for intravenous antibiotic therapy, or the presence of other complications (Table 76–4).

OTHER PHARYNGEAL INFECTIONS

Stomatitis

Both specific and nonspecific mucosal defenses exist in the oral cavity and contribute to the maintenance of a healthy and intact oral mucosa. Systemic diseases such as leukemia and other debilitating or immunocompromising diseases increase the risk for oral infection. Radiation and chemotherapy can be toxic to the oral mucous membrane.

The differential diagnosis of lesions in the mouth is based on the clinical appearance (Table 76–5). Herpetic lesions have a propensity to occur on oral mucosa such as the gingiva, palate, or lateral aspect of the tongue. These lesions are initially vesicular and then rupture to become ulcers, which resolve in 7 to 14 days. Coxsackie lesions are also vesicular but have a propensity for the soft palate, uvula, and anterior tonsillar pillars. Aphthous ulcers, which usually affect nonkeratinized mucosa, are painful ulcers surrounded by a red halo. There is usually a history of recurrence or a positive family history of aphthous ulcers.

Therapeutic Intervention

Good oral hygiene is helpful in reducing the development of stomatitis especially in the immunocompromised patient. Symptomatic treatment to reduce discomfort in the mouth includes frequent rinses with normal saline or bicarbonate and the use of ice chips. Topical agents that produce an anesthetic effect include lidocaine, benzocaine, and diphenhydramine. In the young infant, lidocaine should be used cautiously, as it may suppress the gag reflex, with a subsequent risk of aspiration. Systemic acyclovir is reserved for immunodeficient patients who develop both oral and systemic herpes simplex virus infection.[24] Analgesics such as acetaminophen with codeine may be required for temporary symptomatic relief.

TABLE 76–4

ADMISSION CRITERIA FOR PATIENTS WITH STREPTOCOCCAL PHARYNGITIS

Acute dehydration
Airway obstruction
Need for intravenous antibiotic
  therapy
Complications
  Peritonsillar abscess
  Acute rheumatic fever

Note: All of the above are exceptional occurrences in patients with acute streptococcal pharyngitis.

TABLE 76–5

DIAGNOSTIC FEATURES OF STOMATITIS

Clinical Description	Differential Diagnosis	Presenting Symptoms	Distinguishing Features
White lesions	Pseudomembranous candidiasis	Burning	Plaques wipe off easily
	Hyperplastic candidiasis	—	Adherent plaques
	Trauma—physical, chemical, electrical	Pain	History, sloughing
	Bacterial—staphylococcal, streptococcal, diphtheria, *Treponema pallidum*	Pain	Erythema sloughing
Red lesions	Mucositis	Burning	Chemotherapy or irradiation
	Bacterial	Burning, pain	Erythema
	Viral (cytomegalovirus)	Burning	Mucosal erythema
Vesicular lesions	Herpes simplex virus, primary	Pain, malaise	Lymphadenopathy, fever, gingival lesions
	Herpes simplex virus, recurrent	Pain	Lip, gingiva
	Coxsackievirus	Pain	Oropharynx
	Varicella zoster virus (chickenpox)	Variable	Skin, oral mucosa
Ulcerative lesions	Viral	Pain	Round, 1–2-mm ulcers in clusters
	Aphthous	Pain	Nonkeratinized mucosa, family history, regular borders
	Trauma	Pain	History, irregular borders
	Fungal—*Candida, Aspergillus,* others	Variable	Indurated ulcer

List includes only the more common causes.
Adapted from Epstein JB. The painful mouth. Infect Dis Clin North Am 1988;2:1.

Oral Candidiasis

Oral candidiasis commonly occurs in infants, in immuno-compromised hosts, and in patients who are receiving broad-spectrum antibiotics. It may be self-limited. Numerous raised discrete or confluent cream-colored patches are seen on all mucous surfaces, including the tonsils. These lesions may be wiped off, leaving an erythematous or bleeding surface. Symptoms such as burning discomfort or dysphagia may be present, and other sites of candidal involvement, especially the perineum, may be seen. Topical antifungals such as nystatin and clotrimazole are the treatment of choice.[25]

Ludwig's Angina

Ludwig's angina, a cellulitis of the submandibular space, is a rare condition. Prompt recognition is important, as it is a rapidly progressive and sometimes fatal disease. Cases have been documented in children, and in one series, three out of four children had immunologic deficiencies.[24] Common predisposing factors include dental infections, oral cavity injuries, and fractures of the mandible. Streptococci are the most frequently isolated pathogens, but mixed isolates of gram-negative, gram-positive, and anaerobic organisms have also been documented.[24] Dysphagia, dysphonia, drooling, and a brawny, tense, painful swelling of the suprahyoid region of the neck are seen. Respiratory compromise rapidly occurs. The goals in management are airway maintenance and control of the infection. Prompt initiation of broad-spectrum antibiotics is mandatory.

Acute Necrotizing Ulcerative Gingivostomatitis

Acute necrotizing ulcerative gingivostomatitis (ANUG), also known as "trench mouth," is caused by *Borrelia vincenti* and by fusiform bacteria. A disease of teenagers and young adults, it causes severe point tenderness of the gum, gingival hyperemia, a "punched-out" appearance to the gum between the teeth, and sometimes a gray pseudomembrane over the gums. It is similar in appearance to herpetic gingivostomatitis, but ANUG is unusual in young children. Oral hygiene is important in the treatment of ANUG, and frequent hydrogen peroxide mouth rinses (diluted 1:1 with water)

are used. A 7-day course of penicillin helps eradicate the organisms. Dental follow-up is recommended.[26]

Retropharyngeal Abscess

Retropharyngeal abscess is a rare, deep neck infection extending from the anterior border of the cervical vertebrae to the posterior wall of the esophagus. Although group A streptococcus is the common etiologic pathogen, anaerobes, *Staphylococcus aureus, Escherichia coli, Haemophilus influenzae, Neisseria* sp., and *Klebsiella* sp. also cause retropharyngeal abscess.[27] The relatively higher larynx and narrow airway in children make airway obstruction a significant early complication. Other clinical features such as fever, neck swelling, anorexia, drooling, throat pain, and a toxic appearance are common.

The presence of cervical adenopathy with meningismus should raise the suspicion of retropharyngeal abscess. A lateral radiograph of the neck characteristically shows an increase in the width of the soft tissues anterior to the vertebrae of greater than half the width of the adjacent vertebral body, and on occasion, an air-fluid level is seen (Fig. 76–1).

The mortality rate for retropharyngeal abscess has fallen dramatically since the 1970s, but complications still occur. Airway obstruction remains the most serious complication, but pneumonia, sepsis, spontaneous perforation, and reformation of the retropharyngeal abscess also occur.[27]

Patients with retropharyngeal abscess should be admitted to the hospital. Intravenous antibiotics should be instituted in the emergency department. Use of antibiotics early in the disease frequently obviates the need for surgical drainage. Penicillin (100,000 U/kg/day IV) and cephalosporins are suitable antibiotic choices. Cardiorespiratory monitoring is essential, and intubation may be necessary.

PHARYNGEAL TRAUMA

Injuries to the pharynx and parapharyngeal region have the potential of becoming serious and sometimes life threatening if the airway is compromised. Sharp objects such as pins, pieces of plastic, and fish bones may get stuck in the oral mucosa, tonsils, or pharynx. Pencil-point injuries occur

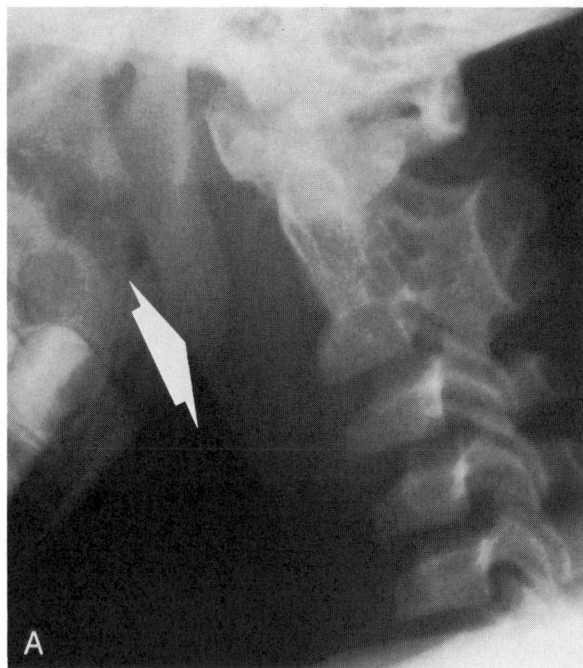 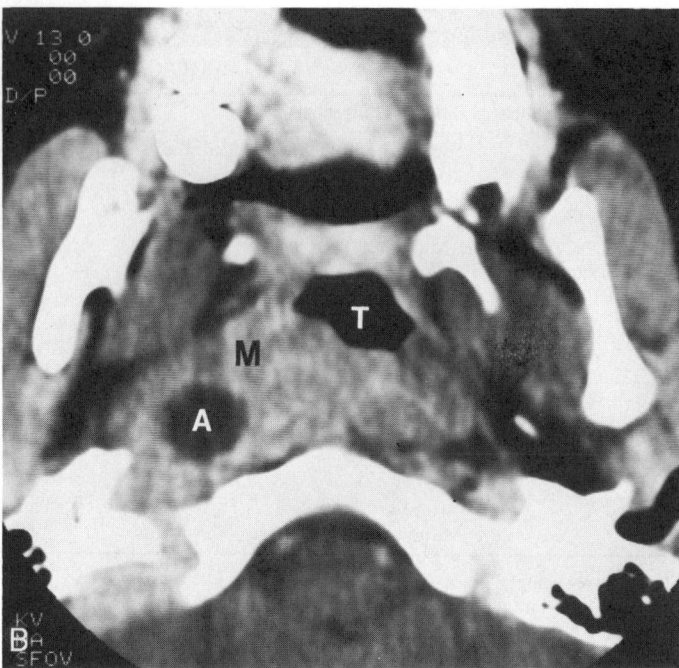

Figure 76–1. Retropharyngeal abscess in an 8-year-old child. *A*, Plain film shows considerably increased soft tissue *(arrow)* between upper airway air and cervical spine. *B*, A few days later, axial CT nicely shows the lower attenuation center of the abscess (A), the anterior and leftward shift of the trachea (T), and the soft tissue mass (M) of abscess and surrounding edema. (Courtesy of A. Oestreich, M.D., Cincinnati, OH.)

when there is accidental impalement of a pencil or pointed object into the palate. Most commonly a V-shaped tear at the junction of the hard and soft palate occurs, but trauma to the tonsillar pillar may also occur with laceration of the jugular, carotid, and palatine vessels, leading to loss of blood and occlusion of the airway.[28] Injury to the retromolar (parapharyngeal) region may cause vascular injury to the internal carotid artery, but fortunately this is a rare occurrence. Although a careful history is important, the injury may have been unobserved by an adult. Dysphagia and drooling in a young, well-looking child should raise the suspicion of pharyngeal trauma. Lateral neck radiographs will demonstrate radiopaque foreign bodies, but plastic objects will not be seen. A chest radiograph will identify mediastinal widening in a patient with respiratory distress secondary to pneumomediastinum. The presence of respiratory distress indicates the need for emergency intubation or tracheotomy. If the child can breathe or talk, no attempt should be made to remove the object in the emergency department. An otolaryngologist should be consulted immediately for endoscopic removal under general anesthesia.[26]

References

1. Palumbo FM. Pediatric considerations of infections and inflammations of Waldeyer's ring. Otolaryngol Clin 1987;20:311.
2. Brook I. The clinical microbiology of Waldeyer's ring. Otolaryngol Clin 1987;20:259.
3. Grose C. The many faces of infectious mononucleosis: The spectrum of Epstein-Barr virus infection in children. Pediatr Rev 1985;7:35.
4. Nakayama T, Takashi U. Outbreak of herpangina associated with coxsackie virus B3 infection. Pediatr Infect Dis 1989;8:495.
5. Glezen WP, Clyde WA. Group A streptococci, mycoplasmas, and viruses associated with acute pharyngitis. JAMA 1967;202:455.
6. Komaroff AL, Aronson MD. Serologic evidence of chlamydial and mycoplasmal pharyngitis in adults. Science 1983;222:927.
7. Huss H, Jungkind D. Frequency of chlamydia trachomatis as a cause of pharyngitis. J Clin Microbiol 1985;22:858.
8. Forr CB, Ellner PD. Distribution of hemolytic streptococci in respiratory specimens. Clin Microbiol 1979;10:69.
9. Rantz LA, Boisvert PJ. Hemolytic streptococcal and non-streptococcal diseases of the respiratory tract. Arch Intern Med 1946;78:369.
10. Quinn RW, Lowny PN. The anatomical area of involvement in streptococcal infections and the carrier state. Yale J Biol Med 1970;43:10.
11. Hayden GF, Thomas MF. Non-group A streptococci in the pharynx. Am J Dis Child 1989;143:794.
12. Stevens D, Swift PGF. *Mycoplasma pneumoniae* infections in children. Arch Dis Child 1978;53:38.
13. Broughton RA. Infections due to Mycoplasma pneumonias in childhood. Pediatr Infect Dis 1986;5:71.
14. Stillerman M, Bernstein SH. Streptococcal pharyngitis. Am J Dis Child 1961;101:476.
15. Levin RM, Grossman M. Group A streptococcal infection in children younger than three years of age. Pediatr Infect Dis 1988;7:581.
16. Shulman ST. Streptococcal pharyngitis: Clinical and epidemiologic factors. Pediatr Infect Dis 1989;8:816.
17. Berke CM: Development of rapid strept test technology. Pediatr Infect Dis 1989;8:825.
18. Mackenzie A, Li M. Evaluation of a kit for rapid detection of group A streptococci in a pediatric emergency department. Carn Med Assoc J 1988;138:917.
19. Nelson JD. The effect of penicillin therapy on the symptoms and signs of streptococcal pharyngitis. Pediatr Infect Dis 1984;3:10.
20. Pichichero M, Disney F. Adverse and beneficial effects of immediate treatment of group A β-hemolytic streptococcal pharyngitis with penicillin. Pediatr Infect Dis 1987;6:635.
21. Shulman ST. Streptococcal pharyngitis: Clinical and epidemiologic factors. Pediatr Infect Dis 1989;8:816.
22. Tanz RR, Shulman ST. Penicillin plus rifampin eradicates pharyngeal carriage of group A streptococci. J Pediatr 1985;106:876.
23. Lance MA, Bismo AL. Acute rheumatic fever: A vanishing disease in suburbia. JAMA 1983;249:895.
24. Barkin RM, Bonis SL. Ludwig angina in children. J Pediatr 1985;87:563.
25. Epstein JB. The painful mouth. Infect Dis Clin North Am 1988;2:1.
26. Fleisher G, Ludwig S. Textbook of Pediatric Emergency Medicine. Baltimore, Williams & Wilkins, 1988, pp 294–295, 426–427, 1020–1022, 1110–1111.
27. Thompson JW, Cohen SR. Retropharyngeal abscess in children: A retrospective and historical analysis. Laryngoscope 1988;98:589.
28. Singer JI. Management strategy for penetrating oropharyngeal injury. Pediatr Emerg Care 1989;5:4 250.

CHAPTER 77

Epistaxis

Laurie Wallace
Michael R. Clark

INTRODUCTION

Epistaxis (nosebleed) can be serious but fortunately is rarely fatal. The fatalities that have been reported occurred primarily in adults who suffered myocardial ischemia brought on by blood loss. Nosebleeds in children produce parental concern out of proportion to the actual danger to the child.

The majority of nosebleeds are self-treated by the patient and never require the assistance of a physician. If the epistaxis does not stop spontaneously, an emergency physician may be required to provide assistance. Only 5% to 10% of patients with epistaxis require an otolaryngologist to control the epistaxis.

Epistaxis in children is common. It is most often noted in patients between 2 and 10 years of age, is rarely encountered during infancy, and becomes decreasingly prevalent after puberty. From birth to 5 years of age, 30% of children have at least one nosebleed; the frequency increases to 56% in children 6 to 10 years of age. Epistaxis requiring hospitalization is rare.

The incidence of epistaxis peaks during the winter months. This increased incidence is attributed to the greater prevalence of upper respiratory tract infections and use of nonhumidified furnaces during the winter months.

ANATOMY AND PHYSIOLOGY

The arterial supply to the nose comes from two major sources: the external and the internal carotid artery systems. The major arterial branch to the nose from the external carotid artery is the internal maxillary artery. The major arterial branch to the nose from the internal carotid artery system is the ophthalmic artery.

The two major branches of the ophthalmic artery that supply the nose are the anterior and posterior ethmoidal arteries (Fig. 77–1). These arteries enter the nasal cavity by penetrating the cribiform plate. The two major branches of the internal maxillary artery that supply the nose are the sphenopalatine and descending palatine artery. The sphenopalatine artery enters the nasal cavity through the sphenopalatine foramen and divides into the nasopalatine artery as it emerges from the sphenopalatine foramen. The descending palatine artery enters the nasal cavity through the incisive foramen.

The blood supply to the nasal septum originates from branches of the sphenopalatine, anterior ethmoidal, and posterior ethmoidal arteries. The superior portion of the septum is supplied by the anterior and posterior ethmoidal arteries. The posterior portion of the septum is supplied by the nasopalatine artery. The anteroinferior portion of the septum receives its blood supply from all vessels supplying the nose, including the anterior and posterior ethmoidals, descending palatine, nasopalatine, and septal branches of the superior labial artery. This portion of the nasal septum is also referred to as *Little's area* or *Kiesselbach's plexus*.

Epistaxis can be classified as anterior or posterior based on the anatomic site of bleeding. This classification can be useful in determining both the cause and the management of epistaxis. Epistaxis from the anterior portion of the septum originates primarily in the area of Kiesselbach's plexus. Posterior epistaxis usually originates from the turbinate or lateral nasal wall. Up to 90% of epistaxes arise from the anterior part of the septum.

Anterior epistaxis from Kiesselbach's plexus is the most common site of epistaxis for several reasons. In this portion of the septum the mucosa is thin and friable, making it susceptible to the drying effects of inspired air. Second, this area is vulnerable to trauma from insertion of a foreign body, usually the finger. "Nose picking" is the most common cause of anterior nose bleeds.

Posterior epistaxis can present a significant challenge to the emergency physician. Posterior epistaxis is more common in older adults following an upper respiratory tract infection and is associated with hypertension and arteriosclerosis. Posterior epistaxis commonly occurs under the posterior wall of the inferior turbinate, in the inferior meatus, or from the nasopalatine plexus of Woodruff located at the posterior margin of the septum. With posterior nasal bleeding, the source of bleeding often cannot be visualized, and the bleeding can be significant, even causing hypovolemic shock.

DIFFERENTIAL DIAGNOSIS

Epistaxis in children is usually benign; however, it may be a manifestation of serious illness (Table 77–I). A thorough evaluation of epistaxis must include consideration of both local and systemic causes. The most common local causes of epistaxis include trauma, infections, and inflammatory disorders. Less common local causes of epistaxis include anatomic abnormalities, neoplasms, and topical medications. Systemic diseases that may cause epistaxis include inherited and acquired coagulopathies, hypertension, and, rarely, endometriosis from ectopic endometrial implants in the nose.

Trauma, especially digital trauma and foreign body insertion, is the most common cause of epistaxis. Repeated nose picking (epistaxis digitorum) leads to formation of granulation tissue within the nasal mucosa. This granulation tissue is friable and can be traumatized, leading to recurrent bleeding. Epistaxis from foreign body insertion is caused directly from traumatic placement of the foreign body or from pressure necrosis on the mucosal vessels.

Epistaxis is commonly seen with nasal fractures. The

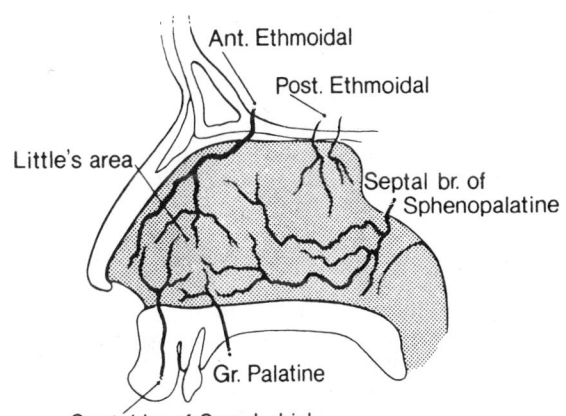

Figure 77–1. Nasal vessels supplying the septum. Little's area contains Kiesselbach's plexus of arterioles and is the most common site of epistaxis. (From Roberts JR, Hedges JR (eds). Clinical Procedures in Emergency Medicine. 2nd ed. Philadelphia, WB Saunders, 1991, p 1029.)

TABLE 77–1

DIFFERENTIAL DIAGNOSIS FOR EPISTAXIS

Local
  Trauma
    Epistaxis digitorum
    Fractures
  Inflammatory disorders
    Allergic rhinitis
    Rhinitis sicca
  Infectious disorders
    Upper respiratory tract infections
    Sinusitis
  Anatomic abnormalities
    Nasal septal deviation
    Choanal atresia
    Meningocele
  Benign and malignant neoplasms
    Polyps
    Angiofibromas
    Inverting papillomas
  Topical nasal medication
    Phenylephrine hydrochloride
    Cocaine
Systemic
  Inherited coagulopathies
    Factor XI deficiency
    Von Willebrand's disease
    Hemophilia A or B
    Glanzmann's thrombasthenia
  Acquired Coagulopathies
    Idiopathic thrombocytopenic purpura
    Vitamin K deficiency
    Malabsorption syndromes
  Hereditary hemorrhagic disorders
  Drugs
    Aspirin
    Chloramphenicol
    Chemotherapeutics
    Anticoagulants
  Hypertension
  Liver or bone marrow disease
  Idiopathic inflammatory diseases
  Endometriosis

---

bleeding may initially be profuse but usually stops spontaneously. Rarely, a nasal fracture will need to be reduced to control epistaxis. Blows to the nose that produce contusion without fracture may tear the nasal mucosa, leading to epistaxis. Mucosal tears occur commonly along the septum at the lateral recess of the piriform aperture and at the junction of the upper lateral cartilages with the nasal bones. With trauma, bleeding that persists and gradually becomes more serious suggests cerebral spinal fluid rhinorrhea.

Inflammatory disorders are common causes of epistaxis. The most prevalent inflammatory disorders include allergic rhinitis and rhinitis sicca (dry nose). Allergic rhinitis leads to mucosal inflammation, which predisposes the patient to bleeding. Vigorous nose blowing and frequent sneezing may precipitate epistaxis by increasing venous pressure, which causes disruption of the vessels. Rhinitis sicca results from inhaling dry air during the winter months. Over-the-counter decongestants further contribute to mucosal inflammation. The dry, crusted mucosa overlying the vessels becomes friable and can bleed spontaneously.

Infectious diseases involving the nose, sinuses, and adenoids also commonly contribute to epistaxis. Up to 62% of children have an upper respiratory tract infection during the week before epistaxis occurs. Rare infectious diseases causing epistaxis include tuberculosis and fungal infections such as rhinosporidiosis.

Neoplasms may also cause epistaxis in children. Benign neoplasms include polyps, inverting papillomas, and angiofibromas. The juvenile angiofibroma of the nasopharynx is the classic example of a tumor causing epistaxis in children. This tumor is seen almost exclusively in adolescent males. The patient may present with epistaxis and a history of intermittent nasal obstruction. On physical examination, bulging of the face or eyes may be evident. Examination of the nasopharynx typically shows a pale, bluish, smooth mass. These patients should be referred for surgical evaluation and excision. Malignant neoplasms of the nose, sinuses, or nasopharynx are rare causes of epistaxis, with squamous cell carcinoma and rhabdomyosarcoma being the most prevalent.

Systemic illnesses must be considered in patients with recurrent nasal bleeding and in patients who have other signs or symptoms suggested by the history or physical examination. Children with recurrent epistaxis have an increased incidence of clinically significant coagulation disorders. Von Willebrand's disease is one of the most common inherited coagulation disorders causing epistaxis. Von Willebrand's disease is an autosomal dominant disorder characterized by reduced factor VIII activity. It is typified by a prolonged bleeding time and decreased platelet adhesiveness. Factor VIII deficiency (classical hemophilia A) can also present with epistaxis. With hemophilia A, there is a reduced quantitative assay of factor VIII activity. Factor XI (plasma thromboplastin antecedent) deficiency, and factor IX (Christmas factor) deficiency are less common inherited coagulopathies that may contribute to epistaxis. Severe vitamin K deficiency or malabsorption syndromes may lead to an acquired coagulopathy. Epistaxis in association with these coagulopathies may require transfusion of fresh frozen plasma or cryoprecipitate to control bleeding.

Idiopathic thrombocytopenic purpura (ITP) is the most common acquired purpuric disorder that may present as epistaxis. ITP is characterized by a low platelet count (usually less than 20,000/mm^3) and abnormal clot retraction and bleeding time. ITP occurs most commonly in children between the ages of 2 and 6 years and commonly follows a viral illness. Glanzmann's thrombasthenia is a rare autosomal recessive hemorrhagic disorder that causes epistaxis and is characterized by chronic nonthrombocytopenic purpura, a prolonged bleeding time, and deficient platelet aggregation and clot retraction. Severe epistaxis in the thrombocytopenic patient may require platelet transfusion to control bleeding.

Hereditary and acquired blood vessel disorders can contribute to epistaxis. Hereditary hemorrhagic telangiectasia (Osler-Weber-Rendu disease) is an autosomal dominant blood vessel disease that commonly causes epistaxis. Coagulation studies in these patients are entirely normal; however, there is a defect in the contractile elements in the muscular and connective tissue elements in the walls of the blood vessels, which enables the vessels to become dilated, forming telangiectasias. These lesions are found in the skin or mucosal linings of the respiratory and gastrointestinal systems. These telangiectasias are prone to recurrent epistaxis and gastrointestinal hemorrhage. Vitamin C deficiency is an acquired blood vessel disorder that may cause epistaxis.

Drugs that may contribute to epistaxis include aspirin (by inhibition of platelet function) and anticoagulants such as warfarin and heparin, which inhibit the extrinsic and intrinsic clotting factors, respectively. Cocaine abuse can cause nasal septal perforation and epistaxis. Chemotherapeutic agents may contribute to epistaxis by causing thrombocytopenia. Nonsteroidal anti-inflammatory medications have also been implicated in causing epistaxis by interfering with platelet function.

Hypertension in association with coarctation of the aorta and renal failure may contribute to nosebleeds. Endometriosis has been reported as a cause of epistaxis during menstruation as a result of ectopic endometrial tissue implants in the nasal cavity. Idiopathic inflammatory diseases such as Wegener's granulomatosis and lethal midline granuloma are rare disorders that may lead to epistaxis.

EMERGENCY MEDICAL SERVICE CONSIDERATIONS

The patient should be positioned sitting up with the head flexed slightly forward so that the blood runs out of the nose instead of into the posterior pharynx, thereby avoiding obstruction of the airway with a clot. The patient should be instructed to pinch the nose with the index finger and thumb to compress the septum. Firm pressure on the nostrils for 10 to 15 minutes will stop most nosebleeds. Oxygen should be supplied orally if the patient is in respiratory distress. An intravenous line of 5% dextrose in lactated Ringer's solution (LR) or normal saline (NS) is indicated if the patient is hypotensive or blood loss appears significant.

CLINICAL EVALUATION
History

The history should determine the patient's general physical condition, the amount of blood lost, and the possibility of a coagulopathy from disease or drug therapy. Previous bleeding episodes and methods of control should be elicited. A history of trauma, surgery, allergy, or recent upper respiratory tract infection should also be elicited. In children, the possibility of a nasal foreign body should be explored. The patient should be asked which naris the bleeding originated from, as this may direct the physician to the most probable site of bleeding.

Physical Examination

The physical examination should focus on determining the source of bleeding. During the examination any evidence of an underlying illness that may contribute to the epistaxis should be noted. The vital signs should be assessed, with special attention to orthostatic changes.

The integument and mucous membranes should be inspected for any evidence of a coagulopathy (e.g., ecchymosis, petechiae, or purpura). Examination of the oropharynx and mucous membranes should note any telangiectasia occurring with Osler-Weber-Rendu syndrome. Any masses of the oropharynx or nasopharynx should also be noted. The nasal cavity should then be examined for the source of bleeding.

DIAGNOSTIC EVALUATION

Laboratory studies and radiographs are rarely necessary in the child with uncomplicated epistaxis. Coagulation studies or a complete blood cell count may be indicated in specific instances where the history or physical examination suggests a coagulopathy. If a sinus disease is suspected as the source of bleeding, sinus radiographs or a computed tomography (CT) scan may assist in the diagnosis.

THERAPEUTIC INTERVENTION

Before beginning the examination, all of the equipment that will be required in managing the patient should be assembled (Table 77–2). The patient should be positioned sitting upright with the head tilted forward. The physician should provide a large basin and tissue paper. Prior to examination the patient should be instructed to blow the

---

TABLE 77–2

EQUIPMENT REQUIRED FOR MANAGEMENT OF EPISTAXIS

Headlight
Nasal speculum
Fraser suction catheter
Cotton
Topical agent that combines vasoconstrictive and anesthesia properties (cocaine 5%–10% or 1% lidocaine mixed 2:1 with 1:100,000 epinephrine)
Antibiotic ointment (neomycin, bacitracin)
½-inch gauze
Bayonet forceps
Silver nitrate sticks

If a posterior source of bleeding is suspected, the following additional equipment may be required:

4 × 4 inch gauze
Silk suture
Foley catheter or Nasostat (posterior pharynx balloon)

---

nose in order to clear the nasal passages of blood and clots. Residual blood can be removed from the nares using a suction device. Following removal of clots and blood, the nasal speculum should be placed into the nares and the nasal cavity inspected for a bleeding source. The physician should begin with the naris from which the blood first originated. The nasal cavity should be inspected from anterior to posterior.

If persistent bleeding obscures visualization, a small piece of cotton dipped in a solution of cocaine and epinephrine can be placed in each naris and firm pressure applied for another 3 to 5 minutes (Table 77–3). Following removal of the cotton, adequate visualization usually reveals a small vessel located in the anterior septum in the area of Kesselbach's plexus as the bleeding source. Once the vessel is located, silver nitrate can be applied to the vessel and is usually successful in controlling bleeding. If bleeding is profuse, it may be difficult to apply silver nitrate directly to the vessel. In such instances bleeding can sometimes be controlled by first cauterizing the area around the bleeding source. This will slow the bleeding and prevent the silver nitrate from being washed away. A small eschar will remain following cautery and should be left in place. The eschar and surrounding mucosa should be covered with surgical lubricant or petroleum jelly daily to minimize drying and prevent rebleeding.

Heat cautery or electrocautery is discouraged because of the risk of septal perforation. For the same reason, cauteri-

---

TABLE 77–3

EPISTAXIS: THERAPY AT A GLANCE

1. Antibiotics: broad-spectrum cephalosporin or penicillin (amoxicillin, 40 mg/kg; trimethoprim, 8 mg/kg/day; sulfamethoxazole, 40 mg/kg/day; erythromycin, 40 mg/kg)
2. Decongestants (chlorpheniramine maleate–phenylephrine hydrochloride–phenylpropanolamine hydrochloride [Naldecon], pseudoephedrine hydrochloride [Sudafed])
3. Antibiotic ointment (bacitracin or neomycin)
4. Cocaine* 5%–10% or 4% topical lidocaine† with 1:100,000 epinephrine

*The maximum cocaine dose has not been established for pediatric patients. Up to 3 ml have been used in dermal lacerations without adverse effects. Death was reported in a 7.5-month-old girl who received 10 ml of tetracaine, adrenaline, cocaine containing 1:180 mg cocaine for an upper lip laceration.
†The maximum lidocaine dose is 3 mg/kg.

zation of both sides of the septum with silver nitrate should be avoided. If the bleeding source is visible but cannot be controlled with silver nitrate or if a coagulopathy is suspected, the an oxidized cellulous material such as Gelfoam or Avitene may control the bleeding by forming an artificial clot.

Most nosebleeds in children can be controlled with firm pressure or silver nitrate cautery. If these measures fail or the source of bleeding cannot be visualized, an anterior nasal pack can be applied. To place an anterior nasal pack, antibiotic-impregnated gauze should be placed in the nasal cavity using a bayonet forceps. The gauze should be placed in horizontal layered loops, beginning along the floor of the nose and working up to the roof (Fig. 77–2). Both ends of the nasal pack should remain outside the nasal cavity and should be secured to the external cheek to prevent the ends from falling into the nasopharynx. An anterior nasal pack will block drainage of the sinuses. If an anterior pack is necessary to control bleeding, the patient should be placed on antibiotics and decongestants to prevent sinusitis.

When the bleeding site cannot be identified in the anterior part of the nose but examination of the oropharynx demonstrates persistent bleeding, the nosebleed is classified as a posterior nosebleed. Posterior nosebleeds or anterior nose-

bleeds that persist despite an adequately placed anterior pack require insertion of a posterior nasal pack. A posterior nasal pack exerts direct pressure on the posterior nasal vessels and provides a buttress against which an anterior pack can be placed.

The simple posterior nasal pack is constructed out of a 4×4 gauze pad that is rolled up and tied with three silk sutures (Fig. 77–3). The gauze should be cut to the size of the distal phalanx of the patient's thumb. A Foley catheter is passed into the bleeding nostril and pulled out through the mouth with bayonet forceps. Two of the sutures are tied to the Foley catheter, which is then withdrawn from the nostril. The sutures are then untied from the catheter. Next, the sutures are pulled gently with one hand as the pack is advanced into the nasopharynx and the choana with the other hand. Prior to placement the posterior pack is impregnated with an antibiotic ointment to minimize bacterial colonization. Following placement of the posterior pack, an assistant should firmly hold the strings of the posterior pack while an anterior nasal pack is placed. The two strings can then be tied around a dental roll or roll of gauze just outside the nares to secure the pack in place. The third string should be cut just below the level of the soft palate or taped to the external cheek for later removal of the pack.

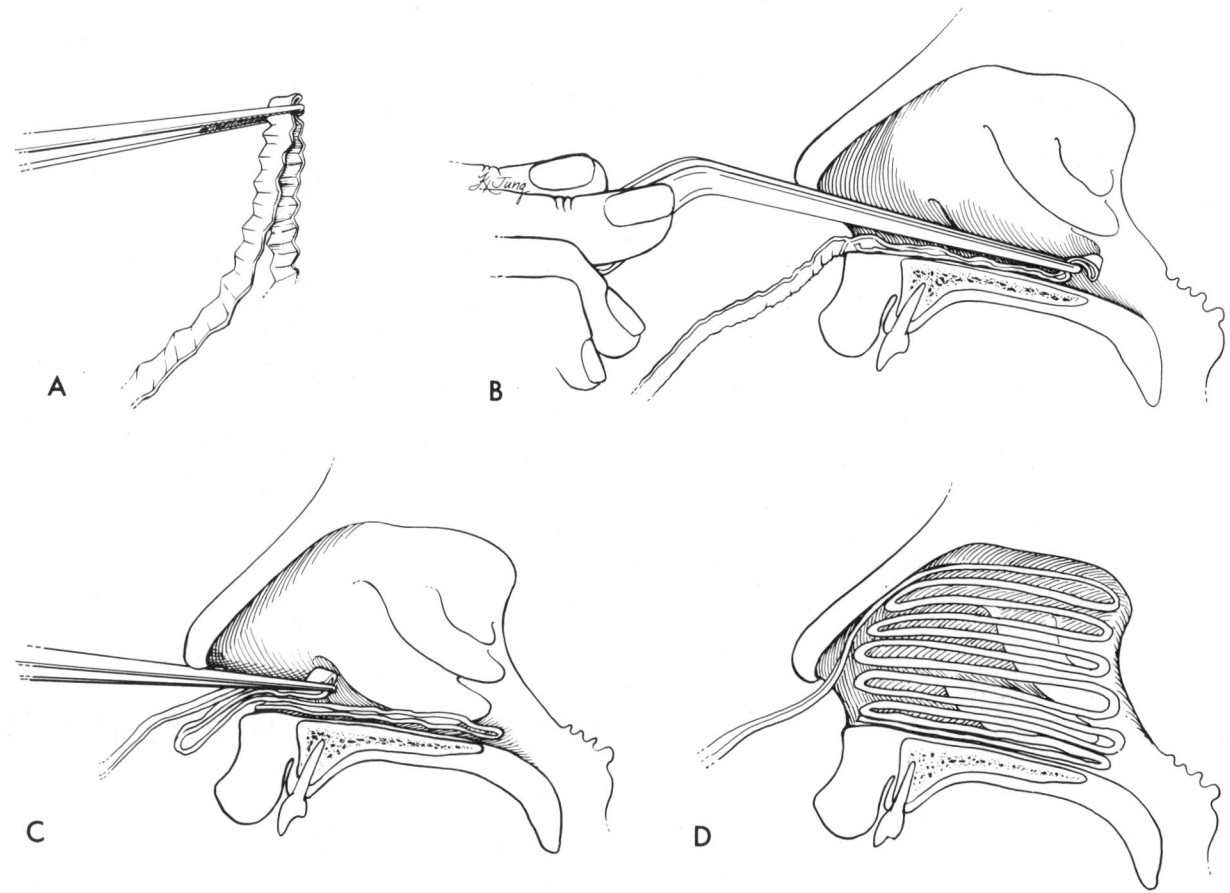

Figure 77–2. The key to placement of an anterior nasal pack that will control epistaxis adequately and stay in place is to lay the packing into the nasal cavity in an "accordion" manner, so that part of each layer of packing lies anteriorly, preventing the gauze from falling posteriorly into the nasopharynx. *A*, The first layer of ¼-inch Vaseline gauze strip is grasped approximately 2 to 3 cm from its end. *B*, This first layer is then placed on the floor of the nose through the nasal speculum *(not pictured here)*. The bayonet forceps and nasal speculum are then withdrawn. *C*, The nasal speculum is reintroduced on top of the first layer of packing, and a second layer is placed in an identical manner. After several layers have been placed, it is often useful to reintroduce the bayonet forceps to push the previously placed packing down onto the floor of the nose, making it tighter and more secure. *D*, A complete anterior nasal pack can tamponade a bleeding point anywhere in the anterior nasal cavities and will stay in place until removed by the physician or patient. (From Abelson TI, Witt WJ. Otolaryngologic procedures. *In* Roberts JR, Hedges JR (eds). Clinical Procedures in Emergency Medicine. 2nd ed. Philadelphia, WB Saunders, 1991, p 1034.)

A posterior nasal pack can also be constructed using a Foley catheter. The Foley catheter is inserted through the nares into the nasopharynx. The Foley balloon can then be inflated with 5 to 10 ml of water and traction applied to place the catheter in the nasopharynx. Following placement of the catheter, an anterior nasal pack can be applied; following which the catheter can be secured with an umbilical clip or a hemostat outside the nares to secure it in place. The columella is susceptible to pressure, and therefore, direct pressure should not be applied to the columella while securing the pack.

A third option for control of posterior nasal bleeding is the use of an intranasal balloon device. Many intranasal balloons are available (e.g., Nasostat, Epistat). These devices are inserted into the nares in a fashion similar to that used for placing a Foley catheter into the nasopharynx. Once the posterior balloon is inflated, there is a second anterior balloon that can be inflated to take the place of an anterior pack. The biggest advantage of these intranasal balloons is the ease and speed with which they can be placed.

Posterior packs should be left in place for 2 to 5 days. Patients with posterior nasal packs should also be placed on

TABLE 77–4
DISCHARGE INSTRUCTIONS FOR EPISTAXIS PATIENTS

1. Return in 24 to 48 hours for anterior pack removal.
2. Avoid bending, straining, sneezing, or picking nose.
3. Apply petroleum jelly or antibiotic ointment to nares when dry.
4. Use a humidifier to increase home humidity.
5. If epistaxis recurs, pinch nose for 15 minutes.
6. If epistaxis continues after pinching nose 15 minutes, return to the emergency department.
7. Use decongestants and antibiotics as directed.
8. Avoid aspirin and alcohol.

antibiotics and decongestants to prevent sinusitis. The antibiotic should be designed to be effective against a wide spectrum of nasal bacteria, including *Staphylococcus aureus*, *Staphylococcus epidermidis*, *Streptococcus viridans*, *Enterobacter* species, and gram-negative bacteria.

In rare instances (e.g., bleeding from tumors, surgical procedures, or trauma), treatment of epistaxis may require surgical control. Arterial ligation of the external carotid artery, internal maxillary artery, and anterior or posterior ethmoidal arteries has rarely been used in children to control epistaxis. Septal dermoplasty has been used in children with recurrent epistaxis secondary to hereditary telangiectasia and von Willebrand's disease.

DISPOSITION

Most epistaxes can be controlled in the emergency department with simple measures such as local nasal pressure, silver nitrate cautery, or anterior nasal packing, and the patients can usually be discharged home with appropriate discharge instructions (Table 77–4). Discharge instructions should include preventing the child from picking the nose or eschar. The patient should also be instructed to use humidified air, apply petroleum jelly to the nares daily, avoid sneezing or strenuous physical activity, and avoid aspirin and ethanol use, as this may increase the risk of rebleeding.

Patients with anterior nasal packing should be instructed to return for removal of the pack in 24 to 48 hours and should be given decongestants and antibiotics to minimize the risk of sinusitis. A broad-spectrum penicillin or cephalosporin is recommended.

If a posterior nasal pack is necessary to control epistaxis, consultation with an otolaryngologist is indicated. Patients with posterior nasal packs usually require hospital admission because of the risk of sudden airway obstruction if the pack becomes dislodged. Patients with bilateral anterior nasal packs may also require hospital admission. Other patients who may require admission include patients with a coagulopathy, underlying chronic illness, hypovolemic shock, or epistaxis secondary to trauma that is associated with other significant injuries.

Selected References

Beran M, Petruson B. Changes in the nasal mucosa of habitual nose bleeders. Acta Otolaryngol 1986;102:308.

Beran M, Petrusen B. Occurrence of epistaxis in habitual nose bleeders. J Otorhinolaryngol 1986;48:297.

Derkay SS, Hirsh BE, Johnson JT. Posterior nasal packing. Arch Otolaryngol Head Neck Surg 1989;115:439.

Guarisco JL, Graham HD III. Epistaxis in children: Causes, diagnosis, and treatment. Ear Nose Throat J 1989;68:522.

Jackson KR, Jackson RT. Factors associated with active, refractory epistaxis. Arch Otolaryngol Head Neck Surg 1988;114:862.

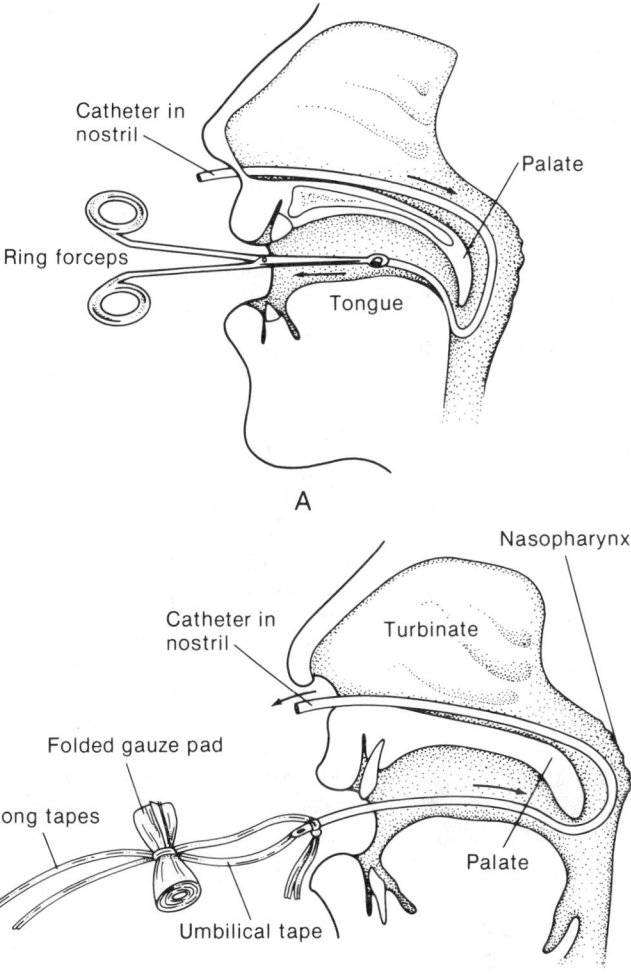

Figure 77–3. Posterior nasal pack. *A*, A rubber catheter is passed through the nose, grasped with a ringed forceps, and brought out through the mouth. *B*, A gauze pad is rolled into a cylinder and tied with two strings, which are used to tie the pack to the tip of the catheter. The pack is guided into the posterior pharynx with the finger, as the catheter is withdrawn through the nose. An interior pack is then placed.

Katsanis E, Luke KH, Hsu E. Prevalence and significance of mild bleeding disorders in children with recurrent epistaxis. J Pediatr 1988;113:73.

Koltai PJ. Nose bleeds in the hematologically and immunologically compromised child. Laryngoscope 1984;94:1114.

Mabry RL. Management of epistaxis by packing. Otolaryngol Head Neck Surg 1986;94:401.

McDonald TJ. Nosebleed in children. Background and techniques to stop the flow. Postgrad Med 1987;81:217.

Perretta LJ, Denslow BL, Brown CG. Emergency evaluation and management of epistaxis. Emerg Med Clin North Am 1987;5:265.

Petruzzelli GJ, Johnson JT. How to stop a nosebleed. Postgrad Med 1989;86:44.

Schaitkin B, Shauss M, Houch JR, et al. Epistaxis: Medical versus surgical therapy: A comparison of efficacy, complications, and economic considerations. Laryngoscope 1987;97:1392.

CHAPTER 78

Post-Tonsillectomy Hemorrhage

Laurie Wallace

INTRODUCTION

Hemorrhage is the most serious complication of tonsillectomy and adenoidectomy procedures and may lead to airway obstruction and cardiopulmonary arrest. The reported incidence of hemorrhage following adenotonsillectomy ranges from 0.1% to 8.1%. The frequency of major post-tonsillectomy hemorrhage requiring hemostatic surgery under general anesthesia is estimated to be 2.8%.

Post-tonsillectomy hemorrhage can be classified as primary (occurring within the first 24 hours) or secondary (occurring after 24 hours). Primary postadenotonsillectomy hemorrhage is thought to be related to surgical technique and difficulty obtaining intraoperative hemostasis. Secondary postadenotonsillectomy hemorrhage most commonly occurs 5 to 10 days after surgery and often coincides with sloughing of the surgical eschar from the tonsillar bed.

ANATOMY

The tonsils lie on each side of the oropharynx in the tonsillar bed between the diverging palatoglossal and palatopharyngeal arches. The tonsillar bed, also between these arches, is composed of two muscles: the palatopharyngeus and the superior constrictor muscle.

The major blood supply to the tonsil is from the tonsillar artery. The tonsillar artery passes through the superior constrictor muscle and enters the lower pole of the tonsil. The tonsillar artery is a branch of the facial artery, which is derived from the external carotid artery. The tonsillar bed also receives small arterial contributions from the lingual, descending palatine, and ascending pharyngeal arteries. Although these vessels originate primarily from the ipsilateral external carotid artery, they also receive small contributions from the internal carotid artery, vertebral arteries, and the contralateral vessels by collateral flow.

The venous supply of the tonsil arises from small vessels at its lower pole that pierce the superior constrictor muscle to join the external palatine veins.

Hemorrhage during tonsil surgery may originate from the tonsillar artery or its small arterial contributions. The most common source of bleeding during tonsil surgery is venous, from the external palatine vein. Rarely, hemorrhage during tonsil surgery may originate from the internal carotid artery, which lies directly lateral to the tonsil, if it is damaged while removing the tonsil.

The adenoids, also known as the *pharyngeal tonsils*, are a collection of lymphoid tissue located in the mucous membranes of the roof and posterior wall of the nasopharynx. The blood supply of the adenoids arises from bilateral contributions from the external and internal carotid arteries.

EMERGENCY MEDICAL SERVICE CONSIDERATIONS

The patient should be positioned sitting up with the head flexed slightly forward so that the blood will run out of the nose or mouth instead of into the posterior pharynx. This helps to avoid obstruction of the airway. Suction should be available to assist in clearing the airway, and oxygen should be supplied by nasal cannula or orally if the patient is in respiratory distress. An intravenous line of 5% dextrose in lactated Ringer's solution (D5LR) or normal saline (D5/.9NS) is indicated if the patient is hypotensive or blood loss appears to be significant.

CLINICAL EVALUATION

The history should determine the patient's general condition, the amount of blood lost, and whether there is a possibility of coagulopathy from disease or drug therapy (Table 78–1). The use of salicylates for pain control has been shown to significantly increase the incidence of postoperative hemorrhage. The time of the surgery in relation to the onset of hemorrhage should be elicited. As stated earlier, primary postoperative hemorrhage occurs within 24 hours of surgery, and secondary postoperative hemorrhage usually occurs between the fifth and tenth postoperative day. Secondary hemorrhages are usually less severe than primary hemorrhages but can be life threatening. Postoperative infection and poor eating habits may contribute to secondary postoperative hemorrhage.

After obtaining a brief history, a physical examination should be conducted. The vital signs should be assessed, with special attention to orthostatic changes. Skin color, distal pulses, and capillary refill should be assessed for evidence of hypovolemic shock. Any evidence of an underlying coagulopathy that may contribute to postoperative hemorrhage

TABLE 78–1
DOCUMENTATION FOR POST-TONSILLECTOMY HEMORRHAGE

1. History
   a. Amount of blood loss
   b. Past medical history: underlying coagulopathy
2. Physical examination
   a. Vital signs—orthostatic blood pressure
   b. Site of bleeding
   c. Evidence of underlying coagulopathy
3. Management
   a. Method of hemorrhage control
   b. Patient tolerance of procedure
   c. Condition following procedure
4. Discharge instructions—disposition

should be noted. The oropharynx should then be examined for the source of bleeding.

DIAGNOSTIC EVALUATION

In the child with a mild, uncomplicated postadenotonsillectomy hemorrhage, laboratory studies and radiographs are rarely indicated. In specific instances where the history or physical examination suggests a coagulopathy, coagulation studies and a complete blood cell count may be indicated. A complete blood cell count and determination of blood type and crossmatch may be indicated in cases of severe hemorrhage.

DIFFERENTIAL DIAGNOSIS

In the child who presents with a postadenotonsillectomy hemorrhage, a brief history and physical examination should establish whether the hemorrhage is a primary or secondary postoperative hemorrhage. Local nasopharyngeal and sinus disease must be considered in the child who presents with hemorrhage from the oropharynx or nose. Inherited and acquired coagulopathies must also be considered in the child who presents with an oropharyngeal hemorrhage.

THERAPEUTIC INTERVENTION

The management of a child with a postadenotonsillectomy hemorrhage should begin with ensuring a patent airway. Suction should be available to assist in clearing blood and clots from the oropharynx. In most children, an intravenous line should be established using D5LR or D5/.9NS. If the child appears to have lost a significant amount of blood, a fluid bolus of 20 ml/kg should be given and blood drawn for a complete blood cell count and a type and crossmatch. If the child has swallowed a large amount of blood, the placement of a nasogastric tube may prevent vomiting and the risk of aspiration.

Children who present to the emergency department with postadenotonsillectomy hemorrhage usually have a secondary hemorrhage from premature separation of the surgical eschar. Examination of the oropharynx may reveal a small clot in the tonsillar fossa. This clot should be removed from the fossa; this may be all that is necessary to stop the bleeding. If bleeding continues, local pressure using a sponge moistened with a solution of equal volumes of 1:1000 epinephrine and 4% topical lidocaine or 5% cocaine on a ring forceps may stop the bleeding (Table 78–2). Local pressure using four to five silver nitrate sticks may also be

successful in coagulating the bleeding vessels. Local pressure using thrombin packs or oxidized cellulous material (e.g., Gelfoam or Avitene) has also been successful in controlling hemorrhage.

If bleeding persists, the tonsillar fossa can be directly infiltrated with 1 to 3 ml of 1:1000 epinephrine, followed by local pressure using a sponge on a ring forceps. Care must be taken to aspirate prior to injecting into the tonsillar fossa to avoid injecting into the internal carotid artery, which lies just lateral to the tonsillar fossa.

In a child with massive post-tonsillectomy hemorrhage that persists despite local measures to control hemorrhage, an intramuscular injection of 0.2 U/kg of oxytocin has been successfully used to control bleeding by causing systemic vasoconstriction. Nevertheless, oxytocin use in children has not been approved by the U.S. Food and Drug Administration, and its use should be reserved for those patients in whom other measures have failed and shock is imminent. If hemorrhage persists despite the previously mentioned methods of hemostatic control, the intravascular volume should be supported with intravenous fluids and blood components while preparation is made for the child to return to the operating room. Surgical control of massive post-tonsillectomy hemorrhage may include ligation of the external carotid artery. Hemorrhage from the adenoid area may be successfully controlled with placement of a posterior nasal pack for 2 to 3 days.

DISPOSITION

Most postadenotonsillectomy hemorrhages are minor or have stopped prior to arrival at the emergency department. Patients can be managed in the emergency department with local measures such as clot removal, topical vasoconstriction, thrombin packs, or silver nitrate cautery. After consultation with an otolaryngologist, these patients may be discharged home with appropriate discharge instructions (Table 78–3) or admitted for observation.

Patients should be instructed to use humidified air, maintain a liquid diet for 24 to 48 hours, and avoid vigorous coughing and the use of aspirin, as this may increase the risk of bleeding. Patients should be given an antibiotic such as penicillin, as postoperative infection has been implicated as a cause of post-tonsillectomy hemorrhage.

Patients with postadenoidectomy hemorrhage who require

TABLE 78–2

POST-TONSILLECTOMY HEMORRHAGE: THERAPY AT A GLANCE

Hemorrhage control
  Local
    1:1000 epinephrine mixed 1:1 with 4% lidocaine or
    Cocaine 5% applied topically
  Systemic
    Pitocin,* 10 U/ml
    Oxytocin, 0.2 U/kg IM
  Oral antibiotics
    Penicillin, 40 mg/kg/day q 6 hr
    Amoxicillin, 40 mg/kg/day q 8 hr
    Erythromycin, 40 mg/kg/day q 8 hr

*Oxytocin (Pitocin) use in this setting has not been approved by the U.S. Food and Drug Administration. It should be used when other means of hemorrhage control have failed, shock is imminent, and the physician feels that oxytocin therapy may be lifesaving.

TABLE 78–3

DISCHARGE INSTRUCTIONS FOR POST-TONSILLECTOMY HEMORRHAGE PATIENTS

1. Use a humidifier to increase home humidity
2. Maintain a liquid diet for 24 to 48 hours
3. Avoid vigorous coughing
4. Avoid aspirin
5. Use antibiotics as directed (if prescribed)
6. Return to the emergency department immediately if bleeding should recur

---

TABLE 78–4

ADMISSION CONSIDERATIONS IN POST-TONSILLECTOMY HEMORRHAGE PATIENTS

1. Hypovolemic shock or a history of significant hemorrhage
2. Underlying coagulopathy or chronic illness
3. Posterior nasal pack (postadenoidectomy hemorrhage)

a posterior nasal pack often require admission because of the risk of sudden airway obstruction if the pack should become dislodged (Table 78–4). A small percentage of patients with postadenotonsillectomy present with massive bleeding and hypovolemic shock, which can lead to exsanguination and cardiopulmonary arrest. These patients represent a significant challenge to the emergency physician and require immediate consultation with an otolaryngologist. Following stabilization, these patients should be admitted to a surgical or critical care unit.

Selected References

Carithers JS, Gebhart DE, Williams JA. Postoperative risks of pediatric tonsilloadenoidectomy. Laryngoscope. 1987;97:422.

Chowdhury K, Tewfik TL, Schloss MD. Post tonsillectomy and adenoidectomy hemorrhage. J Otolaryngol 1988;17:46.

Copper JW, Randall C. Post-operative hemorrhage in tonsillectomy and adenoidectomy in children. J Laryngol Otol 1984;98:363.

Crysdale WS. Complications of tonsillectomy and adenoidectomy in 9409 children observed overnight. Can Med Assoc J 1986;135:1139.

Franco KL, Wallace RB. Management of postoperative bleeding after tonsillectomy. Otolaryngol Clin North Am 1987;20:391.

Kristensen S, Tveteras K. Post tonsillectomy hemorrhage: A retrospective study of 1150 operations. Clin Otolaryngol 1984;9:347.

Rasmussen N. Complications of tonsillectomy and adenoidectomy. Otolaryngol Clin North Am 1987;20:383.

Siodlak MZ, Gleeson MJ, Wengraf CL. Post tonsillectomy secondary hemorrhage. Ann R Coll Surg Engl 1985;67:167.

CHAPTER 79

Neck Masses

Kathleen M. Smith
Barbara M. Malone

INTRODUCTION

Neck masses include any visible swelling that disturbs the normal contour of the neck between the shoulder and the angle of the jaw. Neck masses arise as a result of inflammation, trauma, or antigenic or mitotic stimulation. They can be divided into two categories: cystic lesions, which consist mainly of pharyngeal cleft remnants and vascular malformations, and solid lesions, which are generally inflammatory or neoplastic. The most common causes of neck masses in childhood are reactive adenopathy and adenitis secondary to bacterial or viral infections (Table 79–1). Other common causes include hematomas, benign tumors, and congenital cysts. Children with congenital anatomic defects of the neck can develop neck masses if these defects are injured or infected. Neoplasms of the neck can be either primary or metastatic tumors.

Life-threatening situations arise when rapidly enlarging neck masses compromise vital structures such as the airway, carotid blood vessels, or cervical spinal cord. Enlarging neck masses can cause laryngeal and tracheal compression, because the child's airway is relatively compliant. Systemic toxicity caused by septicemia or thyroid storm is rare (Table 79–2).

TABLE 79–1

DIFFERENTIAL DIAGNOSIS OF NECK MASSES

I. Inflammatory causes
  A. Infection
    1. Cervical adenitis (viral or bacterial)
    2. Adenopathy secondary to local head and neck infection
  B. Immunologic causes
    1. Local hypersensitivity reactions
    2. Serum sickness reaction
    3. Lymphoid hyperplasia secondary to phenytoin
    4. Kawasaki disease
    5. Sarcoidosis
    6. Human immunodeficiency virus infection
II. Trauma
  A. Subcutaneous emphysema
  B. Hematoma secondary to trauma
    1. Hematoma of a major neck vessel adjacent to the airway
    2. Arteriovenous fistula
    3. Hematoma associated with a cervical spine injury
III. Tumors
  A. Benign
    1. Sternocleidomastoid tumor of infancy
    2. Epidermoid, keloid
    3. Lipoma, fibroma, neurofibroma
    4. Goiter
    5. Ranula
  B. Malignant
    1. Lymphosarcoma
    2. Hodgkin's disease
    3. Non-Hodgkin's lymphoma
    4. Leukemia
    5. Neuroblastoma, rhabdomyosarcoma, salivary gland carcinoma, epidermoid carcinoma, teratoma, nasopharyngeal squamous cell carcinoma, and thyroid malignancies
IV. Congenital causes
  A. Hemangioma
  B. Cystic hygroma
  C. Thyroglossal duct cyst
  D. Branchial cleft cyst
  E. Laryngocele
  F. Dermoid cyst
  G. Cervical rib
  H. Esophageal diverticulum

CERVICAL ANATOMY

The sternocleidomastoid muscle extends diagonally from the mastoid process of the skull to the superior sternum and clavicle and divides the neck into the anterior and posterior triangles. The anterior triangle is bounded by the sternocleidomastoid muscle, the midline, and the mandible. It contains most of the major vascular and visceral structures, including the airway. The posterior triangle is bounded by the sternocleidomastoid muscle, the trapezius, and the clavicle. The major contents of the posterior triangle are the accessory nerve, the lymph nodes, the external jugular vein, the brachial plexus, and the third part of the subclavian artery.

CLINICAL EVALUATION

In the acutely ill child with a neck mass, a rapid assessment must be made to look for airway or cervical vessel compromise and cervical spine injuries. The physician must examine the child for stridor, dysphagia, hoarseness, drooling, tachypnea retractions, accessory muscle use, air entry, and cy-

TABLE 79–2

LIFE-THREATENING CAUSES OF NECK MASSES

I. Infectious causes
   A. Adenopathy associated with epiglottitis, peritonsillar abscess, retropharyngeal abscess, Ludwig's angina
   B. Infection of brachial cleft cysts and laryngocoeles
II. Trauma
   A. Subcutaneous emphysema with associated airway or pulmonary injury
   B. Hematoma secondary to trauma
     1. Hematoma compressing the airway or causing vascular compromise
     2. Hematoma associated with cervical spine injury
III. Local hypersensitivity reaction with airway edema
IV. Tumor
   A. Mediastinal mass and airway compromise secondary to lymphoma, leukemia, teratoma, or rhabdomyosarcoma
V. Endocrine causes
   A. Thyroid storm
VI. Cardiovascular causes
   A. Coronary vasculitis associated with Kawasaki syndrome

and cause of the upper airway obstruction. Pulse oximetry is a noninvasive aid in determining the severity of airway obstruction in the child with respiratory distress.

Cervical spine immobilization and cervical spine radiographs are indicated in a child with a neck mass caused by trauma, particularly if there is neck pain, neurologic deficits, or hematoma. Cervical spine radiographs can identify abnormal soft tissue densities in addition to fractures or dislocations. Any abnormalities on the cervical spine radiographs or any cervical neurologic deficits can be further evaluated with a computed tomography (CT) scan of the cervical spine. Surgical consultation should be obtained for expanding hematomas caused by penetrating or blunt neck trauma. The airway should be protected until definitive treatment is obtained. Bleeding from minor trauma resulting in a neck mass should be evaluated with determinations of hemoglobin level, platelet count, prothrombin time, and activated partial thromboplastin time to look for an underlying coagulopathy.

A chest radiograph should be obtained in patients in respiratory distress whose histories and physical examinations suggest a tumor, infection, or air leak, checking for a

anosis. Mental status must be assessed by evaluating the child for agitation, anxiety, and lethargy, as well as noting how the child interacts with the parents and the environment.

Following the initial screening history and physical examination, the physician may more thoroughly evaluate the stable patient. The history relevant to the neck mass should include questions about trauma, age at onset, duration, progression, pain, wound discharge, and whether the mass changes with respirations, speech, or swallowing. Recurrent unilateral masses in children are suggestive of a congenital cyst. The most common congenital cysts are cystic hygromas, hemangiomas, branchial cleft cysts, and laryngoceles. Painless progressive enlargement of firm lymph nodes in the neck during a several-week period can be an ominous sign. Masses that are greater than 3 cm in diameter, fixed to adjacent tissue, or located in the posterior triangle of the neck are suggestive of a malignancy.

A detailed physical examination should be performed, noting the size, location, shape, contour, attachment to underlying tissue, crepitance, and presence of tenderness or fluctuance of the neck mass. The location of the neck mass is important in determining the diagnosis (Fig. 79–1). The entire neck should be palpated for other masses and a careful examination of the cervical spine, thyroid gland, and trachea performed. The chest should be auscultated to assess breath sounds, air entry, and the presence of stridor. Inspiratory stridor suggests an upper airway lesion, whereas expiratory stridor suggests a lower airway lesion. Biphasic stridor usually indicates a midtracheal lesion.

Because the leading causes of neck masses are reactive adenopathy and acute adenitis from a viral or bacterial infection, the patient should be examined carefully for local infections of the scalp, middle ear, pharynx, paranasal sinuses, teeth, and salivary glands. In children suspected of having a malignancy or human immunodeficiency virus (HIV) infection, the abdomen should be carefully examined for hepatosplenomegaly. Fever, rash, and generalized adenopathy are signs of systemic diseases such as Kawasaki disease, HIV infection, or infectious mononucleosis.

DIAGNOSTIC EVALUATION

A portable lateral neck radiograph obtained in the emergency department may be helpful in looking for the location

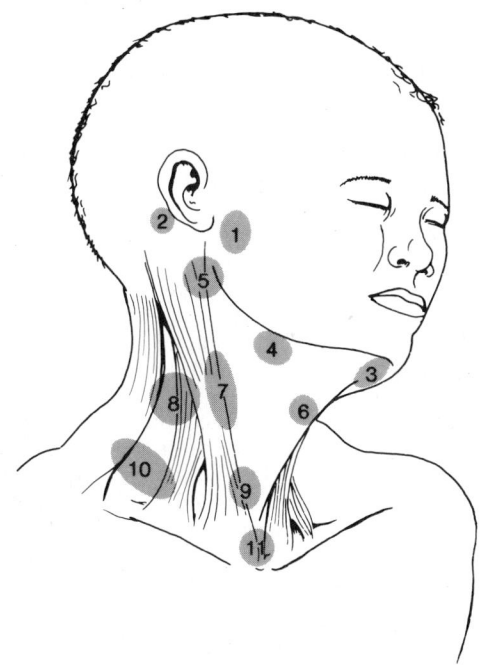

Figure 79–1. Area 1, parotid (preauricular): cystic hygroma, hemangioma, lymphadenitis, parotitis, granuloma, tuberculosis, sarcoidosis, Sjögren's syndrome, Caffey-Silverman syndrome, pleomorphic adenoma, mucoepidermoid carcinoma, lymphoma. Area 2, postauricular: lymphadenitis, brachial cleft cyst (first). Area 3, submental: lymphadenitis, cystic hygroma, thyroglossal duct cyst, dermoid cyst, sialadenitis. Area 4, submandibular: lymphadenitis, cystic hygroma, sialadenitis, cystic fibrosis, tumor. Area 5, jugulodigastric (tonsil node): lymphadenitis, brachial cleft cyst (first), parotid tumor, transverse process of C2, styloid process. Area 6, midline neck: hyoid, thyroid, lymphadenitis, thyroglossal duct cyst, dermoid cyst, laryngocele. Area 7, anterior border of sternocleidomastoid muscle: hyoid, thyroid cartilages, lymphadenitis, brachial cleft cyst (second, third, rarely fourth), carotid body tumor. Area 8, spinal accessory: inflammatory, lymphoma, metastatic carcinoma. Area 9, paratracheal: thyroid, parathyroid, esophageal diverticulum. Area 10, supraclavicular: fat pad, pneumatocele from apical lobes, cystic hygroma, lipoma, lymphoma, metastasis. Area 11, suprasternal: thyroid, lipoma, dermoid, thymus, mediastinal mass. (Modified from May M. Neck masses in children: Diagnosis and treatment. Pediatr Ann 1976; 93:519.)

mediastinal mass, pneumonia, or pneumomediastinum or pneumothorax, respectively.

In patients with life-threatening neck masses caused by infection, needle aspiration is used to determine the presence of fluid in the mass and the need for incision and drainage. Ultrasound is helpful in distinguishing cystic from solid lesions. Antibiotic therapy, although important in halting the local spread of infection and preventing hematogenous dissemination, cannot substitute for evacuation of pus by incision and drainage.

A complete septic evaluation should be performed in the neonate with a suspected infectious neck mass regardless of whether fever is present. A blood culture should be performed in older infants and children who appear septic. The fluid aspirated from the neck mass should be evaluated with Gram stain and cultured. Parenteral antibiotic therapy should be directed at the organisms that cause the various infectious neck masses. Adenitis in a neonate should alert the clinician to the possibility of a *Staphylococcus aureus* or group B streptococcal infection. *Haemophilus influenzae* is present in approximately 90% of the cases of epiglottitis, but other organisms should also be considered, including group A streptococcus, *S. aureus*, *Streptococcus pneumoniae*, and *Branhamella (Moraxella) catarrhalis*. Peritonsillar, retropharyngeal, and lateral pharyngeal abscesses and Ludwig's angina are caused by group A streptococcus, anaerobes, and *S. aureus*.

In most children, the lymph nodes are only slightly enlarged with minimal tenderness. Most of these lymph nodes regress without therapy within 2 to 3 weeks, but occasionally the lymphadenopathy may require several months for complete resolution. The patient should be periodically examined by the pediatrician until the lymph nodes return to their normal size.

Stable patients without life-threatening neck masses can be evaluated and treated more conservatively. Because infectious lymphadenitis is the most common benign cause of neck masses in children, it is not necessary to establish a cause in every case. Frequently the primary source of the adenitis is obvious (e.g., acute pharyngitis or otitis), but occasionally the primary infectious process is not apparent.

A more extensive evaluation is indicated in children who present with fever, large nodes (more than 3 cm in diameter), fluctuant nodes, toxicity, or failed antibiotic therapy. A complete blood cell count with differential can provide useful information when evaluating inflammatory masses and is essential in evaluating neoplasms. A throat culture for group A streptococci, testing for serum antibodies to streptococcal antigens, or serologic tests for infectious mononucleosis may aid in establishing a diagnosis. Such patients should also have a chest radiograph and an intradermal test for tuberculosis. A blood culture should be obtained if the patient appears septic. Needle aspiration should be performed on the largest or most fluctuant node. The fluid obtained should be sent for Gram stain and culture and for acid-fast stain if indicated. Serologic tests for Epstein-Barr virus, toxoplasmosis, cytomegalovirus, coccidioidomycosis, tularemia, histoplasmosis, and syphilis can be of value if the diagnosis remains uncertain. Intradermal testing for cat-scratch disease and atypical *Mycobacteria* infection is sometimes hampered by the lack of standardized commercial antigens. An excisional biopsy for histologic examination and culture should be performed if there is no decrease in the size of the node by 8 weeks after enlargement is first noted.

THERAPEUTIC INTERVENTION

In the child who presents with a neck mass and respiratory distress, oxygenation and airway management are the main priorities. The child should be kept upright, and oxygen should be administered.

The emergency department physician should consult an otolaryngologist or anesthesiologist when children with acute upper airway obstruction are difficult to intubate or, in rare instances, require a cricothyroidotomy or tracheostomy. If the patient's condition permits, controlled intubation with anesthetic induction is preferred.

Heliox is a helium and oxygen mixture that can be used as a temporizing measure prior to intubation. When helium is added to oxygen, it reduces the density of the inhaled gases and decreases the work of breathing associated with an upper airway obstruction.

Anaphylactic reactions should be treated with subcutaneous epinephrine (0.01 ml/kg, up to 0.3 ml of a 1:1000 solution), oxygen, diphenhydramine (1 to 2 mg/kg IV), and isotonic intravenous fluids for hypotension or poor perfusion. The beneficial effects of intravenous steroids are not noted until 8 to 12 hours after they are administered, but they should be administered immediately (hydrocortisone, 4 to 5 mg/kg IV, or methylprednisolone, 1 to 2 mg/kg IV).

Older infants and children with localized cervical adenitis and no evidence of sepsis can be managed with empiric oral antibiotic therapy, based on the perceived primary source of infection, after a careful physical examination has been performed. Penicillin V, dicloxacillin, amoxicillin-clavulanate, cephazolin, or erythromycin in dosages of 25 to 50 mg/kg divided into 6-hour doses are reasonable antibiotic choices when the primary source of infection is unclear.

An electrocardiogram (EKG) and chest radiograph are valuable in the management of the child with a neck mass and thyroid storm. Thyroid function tests should be obtained, but it is unlikely that the results will be available before therapy is initiated. The initial management is directed toward lowering the metabolic rate and reducing the cardiac work load through the use of acetaminophen and a beta blocker (propranolol, 30 to 100 µg/kg IV over 10 to 15 minutes). Intravenous fluids should be given to compensate for the increased insensible losses due to fever and an accelerated metabolic rate.

DIFFERENTIAL DIAGNOSIS
Infections

The majority of neck masses caused by infection consist of primary lymphadenitis or secondary lymphadenopathy. Patients with clinical findings consistent with peritonsillar, retropharyngeal, or lateral pharyngeal abscesses must be evaluated for airway compromise and carotid artery erosion. The warning sign of an impending carotid artery erosion and hemorrhage is hematemesis. Patients with epiglottitis may rarely present with a neck mass, and patients with infectious mononucleosis can present with neck masses and airway compromise caused by massive tonsillar hypertrophy.

Ludwig's angina is a dental infection that causes a bilateral board-like swelling and induration of the floor of the mouth and the submandibular and submental spaces of the neck. Chills, fever, dysphagia, stiffness of tongue movements, and trismus are common presenting signs. Airway compromise is the result of progressive pharyngeal and laryngeal edema; mediastinitis is also a complication.

Neck masses of congenital origin can become infected and cause airway compromise. Infections of branchial cleft cysts can progress to mediastinitis. This infection usually presents as an erythematous, tender, fluctuant mass over the area anterior to the sternocleidomastoid muscle. A laryngocele is an air-containing cyst that arises from the mucosa between the true and false vocal cords. With a Valsalva maneuver, a soft cystic mass can be noted to extend out of the larynx through the thyroid membrane. If the laryngocele becomes infected, it can obstruct the upper airway.

Trauma

Patients with a cervical spine injury may present with a hematoma over the fractured vertebrae. Penetrating neck trauma usually results in vascular injuries and hematomas, but central nervous system and peripheral nerve injury also frequently occur. Penetrating trauma to the lower neck can result in brachial plexus injuries. Arteriovenous fistulas may appear weeks after cervical trauma.

Blunt neck trauma can also present as a neck mass in children. Common mechanisms of injury include steering wheel injuries, direct blows to the neck occurring during sports, "clothesline" injuries sustained while driving recreational vehicles, and strangulation. Airway injury is most common with blunt neck trauma, but vascular injury also occurs. Perforation of the esophagus and larynx has also been reported.

Barotrauma in children with obstructive lung diseases may produce a pneumomediastinum and a crepitant neck mass. A child who presents with a pneumomediastinum should be carefully assessed and closely monitored for the development of a pneumothorax.

Local Hypersensitivity Reactions

Anaphylactic reactions are the result of immunoglobulin E (IgE)-mediated sensitivity to foreign substances such as bee stings, drugs, and other sensitizing antigens. Neck masses may arise as a result of tissue edema that obstructs the upper airway.

Tumors

Tumors of the neck may enlarge and compromise vital structures. Benign tumors such as cystic hygromas and hemangiomas can enlarge sufficiently to obstruct the airway or cause dysphagia. Approximately 27% of malignant tumors in childhood originate in the head and neck area. In order of frequency, these are lymphoid tumors (Hodgkin's disease, non-Hodgkin's lymphoma, leukemia, and lymphosarcoma), rhabdomyosarcoma, fibrosarcoma, thyroid malignancies, neuroblastoma, salivary gland carcinomas, epidermoid carcinoma, and teratoma. Patients with lymphoma, leukemia, teratoma, and rhabdomyosarcoma may present with mediastinal masses that obstruct the intrathoracic trachea.

Endocrine Disorders

Patients with Graves' disease present with an enlarged thyroid; bruits may be audible over the thyroid gland. Tachycardia, palpitations, dyspnea, cardiac enlargement, and cardiac insufficiency cause discomfort and may endanger the patient's life.

Cardiovascular Disorders

Kawasaki disease, or mucocutaneous lymph node syndrome, is characterized by a prolonged high fever, bilateral conjunctival injection, changes in the mucous membranes of the upper respiratory tract, edema and desquamation of the distal extremities, a polymorphous truncal rash, and an enlarged cervical lymph node. Infants less than 1 year of age may present with an atypical form of the disease. The primary threat to life is coronary artery vasculitis and its sequelae.

DISPOSITION

Neck masses in children most often represent benign lymphadenitis or secondary lymphadenopathy caused by infections. The majority of children require antibiotics, local care, and a repeat evaluation within 1 to 2 weeks. Those with tumors should be referred promptly to a surgeon and an oncologist for definitive diagnosis and treatment. Hospitalization is required for patients with neck masses who have severe local disease, systemic toxicity, or airway or vascular compromise.

Selected References

Barton LL, Feigin R. Childhood cervical lymphadenitis: A reappraisal. J Pediatr 1974;84:846.

Friedberg J. Clinical diagnosis of neck lumps: A practical guide. Pediatr Ann 1988;17:620.

Jaffe BF. Pediatric head and neck tumors: A study of 178 cases. Laryngoscope 1973;83:1644.

Knight PK, Reiner CB. Superficial lumps in children: What, when and why? Pediatrics 1983;72:147.

May M. Neck masses in children: Diagnosis and treatment. Pediatr Ann 1976;93:517.

Pounds LA. Neck masses of congenital origin. Pediatr Clin North Am 1981;28:841.

CHAPTER 80

Dental Emergencies

Carolyn R. Burt

DENTAL ANATOMY

In a healthy mouth the soft tissues are moist, firm, and an even, pale pink color. The teeth are made up of three main hard tissues: enamel, dentin, and pulp. The enamel, or outer surface, is whitish and consists of the hardest substance in the body. The underlying dentin is made up of a microporous structure that surrounds and communicates with the inner pulp, the neurovascular component. The crown of the tooth is the visible portion, above the gingiva. The root is covered by a thin layer known as the cementum to which the fibrous periodontal ligament attaches. These periodontal fibers in turn attach the tooth to the alveolar bone and suspend the tooth in its socket (Fig. 80–1).

In the permanent dentition, beginning from the midline and moving toward the posterior, the teeth consist of a central incisor, a lateral incisor, a canine or "eye" tooth, two bicuspids or premolars, and three molars in each quadrant, a total of 32 teeth. The third molar is often referred to as the "wisdom tooth." The primary dentition differs in that there are no premolars and only two molars in each quadrant for a total of 20 teeth. Some useful terms for describing teeth follow:

Facial: The part of the tooth that faces the oral vestibule

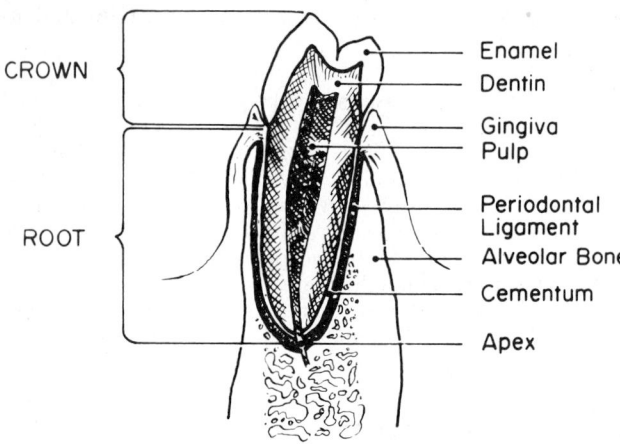

Figure 80–1. The dental anatomic unit. (From Amsterdam JT, Hendler BH, Rose LF. *In* Roberts JR, Hedges JR (eds). Clinical Procedures in Emergency Medicine. Philadelphia, WB Saunders, 1985, p 947.)

(incisors to canines: labial, and premolars to molars: buccal).

Lingual: The part of the tooth that faces the tongue.

Proximal: Refers to the contact surfaces of the teeth. Those closest to the midline are mesial; those toward the posterior, distal.

Incisal: Refers to the biting surfaces of the incisors and canines.

Occlusal: Refers to the biting surfaces of the premolars and molars.

Apical: Refers to the tip of the root.

Coronal: Refers to the visible portion or crown of the tooth.

Primary Dentition

The primary dentition consists of 20 teeth, 10 maxillary and 10 mandibular, that normally erupt between the ages of 4 and 30 months (Table 80–1). The timing of eruption may vary slightly, but the sequence and the symmetry of eruption are consistent. Retarded dental development occurs in hypothyroidism, hypopituitarism, and trisomy 21; accelerated eruption may be found in the adrenogenital syndrome and cerebral giantism.

Mixed Dentition

The stage known as mixed dentition is characterized by resorption of the roots of the primary teeth, exfoliation or shedding of the primary teeth, and the appearance of the permanent teeth. This stage begins at about age 6 years with the eruption of the first permanent tooth (usually the first molar) and continues until about age 12 when the last primary tooth is shed. This is often referred to as the "ugly duckling" stage since the teeth often appear spaced, uneven, and splayed during the various stages of exfoliation and eruption. In normal development these spaces gradually close as the full complement of permanent teeth assume their respective positions.

Permanent Dentition

Permanent dentition is the stage marked by the loss of the last primary tooth at about age 12 years. It is not complete until ages 18 to 20 with the eruption of the last permanent teeth, the third molars. The normal permanent dentition consists of 32 teeth, 16 in the maxillary jaw and 16 in the mandibular jaw (Table 80–1).

DENTAL ANOMALIES
Altered Number of Teeth

Anodontia, the congenital absence of teeth, may be partial or, in rare cases, total. The most frequently missing teeth are the third molars, maxillary lateral incisors, and mandibular second premolars. If extra teeth form, they are referred to as supernumerary teeth. They occur most often in the maxillary central incisor and third molar areas.

Altered Shape of Teeth (Morphology)

These may be alterations in the shape of the teeth, such as macrodontia (large teeth) or microdontia (small teeth). The maxillary lateral incisors may appear as slender, tapered teeth, referred to as "peg laterals." Twinning occurs by several mechanisms but is clinically observed as two teeth joined together. This is usually seen in the mandibular incisors. Congenital syphilis results in abnormally shaped teeth, referred to as "screwdriver" teeth or Hutchinson's incisors, and "mulberry molars" or molars whose biting surface appears lobular.

Genetic Disturbances

Disturbances may occur in the formation of the enamel or dentin. Amelogenesis imperfecta is a genetic trait that causes faulty production of enamel matrix and results in thin, defective enamel, giving the tooth a yellow discoloration. Dentinogenesis imperfecta is an analogous condition in which the teeth have abnormal dentin. These teeth appear bluish-brown and opalescent, fracture easily, and are subject to extreme wear.

Altered Calcification

Localized disturbances of calcification may appear that correlate with such insults as febrile illness, malnutrition, and drug ingestion. Discoloration is referred to as hypocalcification, whereas a more severe disturbance, hypoplasia, may cause pitting or areas devoid of enamel. Mottled enamel can result from excessive fluoride ingestion. Tetracycline stain is caused by ingestion of tetracycline during tooth development. It causes enamel hypoplasia, with discoloration ranging from yellow to brown or gray. Exposure to tetracycline from about the 4th month in utero to the 10th month of life for the primary teeth, and the 4th month of life to the 16th year for the permanent dentition, can potentially cause this type of permanent defect. Since all the enamel is completely formed on all the permanent teeth except the third molars by age 8 years, the tetracyclines should not be prescribed for pregnant women or children under 8 years of age. Doxycycline appears to cause no discoloration; oxytetracycline causes a light yellow color, and chlortetracycline, demethylchlortetracycline, and tetracycline cause stronger yellow or gray-brown discolorations. Other conditions may cause alterations in calcification such as porphyria, which is associated with reddish-brown teeth, and Rh incompatibility, which causes a generalized bluish tinge to the teeth.

ORAL LESIONS
Papillomas

Papillomas are benign, raised lesions in the mouth that are sometimes pedunculated. They are often caused by local

TABLE 80–1

CHRONOLOGY OF HUMAN DENTITION

Tooth	Hard Tissue Formation Begins	Amount of Enamel Formed at Birth	Enamel Completed	Eruption	Root Completed
Primary Dentition					
Maxillary					
Central incisor	4 mo in utero	Five sixths	1½ mo	7½ mo	1½ yr
Lateral incisor	4½ mo in utero	Two thirds	2½ mo	9 mo	2 yr
Cuspid	5 mo in utero	One third	9 mo	18 mo	3¼ yr
First molar	5 mo in utero	Cusps united	6 mo	14 mo	2½ yr
Second molar	6 mo in utero	Cusp tips still isolated	11 mo	24 mo	3 yr
Mandibular					
Central incisor	4½ mo in utero	Three fifths	2½ mo	6 mo	1½ yr
Lateral incisor	4½ mo in utero	Three fifths	3 mo	7 mo	1½ yr
Cuspid	5 mo in utero	One third	9 mo	16 mo	3¼ yr
First molar	5 mo in utero	Cusps united	5½ mo	12 mo	2¼ yr
Second molar	6 mo in utero	Cusp tips still isolated	10 mo	20 mo	3 yr
Permanent Dentition					
Maxillary					
Central incisor	3–4 mo		4–5 yr	7–8 yr	10 yr
Lateral incisor	10–12 mo		4–5 yr	8–9 yr	11 yr
Cuspid	4–5 mo		6–7 yr	11–12 yr	13–15 yr
First bicuspid	1½–1¾ yr		5–6 yr	10–11 yr	12–13 yr
Second bicuspid	2–2¼ yr		6–7 yr	10–12 yr	12–14 yr
First molar	At birth	Sometimes a trace	2½–3 yr	6–7 yr	9–10 yr
Second molar	2½–3 yr		7–8 yr	12–13 yr	14–16 yr
Mandibular					
Central incisor	3–4 mo		4–5 yr	6–7 yr	9 yr
Lateral incisor	3–4 mo		4–5 yr	7–8 yr	10 yr
Cuspid	4–5 mo		6–7 yr	9–10 yr	12–14 yr
First bicuspid	1¾–2 yr		5–6 yr	10–12 yr	12–13 yr
Second bicuspid	2¼–2½ yr		6–7 yr	11–12 yr	13–14 yr
First molar	At birth	Sometimes a trace	2½–3 yr	6–7 yr	9–10 yr
Second molar	2½–3 yr		7–8 yr	11–13 yr	14–15 yr

Adapted from Logan and Kronfeld. JADA 1933;20. Copyright by the American Dental Association.

irritation such as a sharp edge of a filling, a broken tooth, or an orthodontic appliance. If applicable, alteration or removal of the offending irritant is in order. The papilloma may require excision.

Aphthous Stomatitis (Canker Sores)

Aphthous stomatitis is a common type of recurrent ulcer in the mouth. The sores appear initially as small erythematous spots that develop into painful, shallow, yellowish ulcers. The lesions heal spontaneously in 7 to 14 days without scarring. The usual location of these lesions is the buccal mucosa, tongue, soft palate, and pharynx, in contrast to the lesions of recurrent herpes, which tend to be on the bound mucosal surfaces. The lesions may be precipitated by such factors as menses, allergies, trauma, or stress. Topical application of an anesthetic solution (viscous lidocaine) may provide symptomatic relief. For children over the age of 8 years, a tetracycline mouth rinse (250 mg/ml four times a day) produces good results and prevents secondary infection.

Herpes Simplex Virus

Herpes simplex virus type 1 (HSV-1) causes painful oral and perioral lesions. The herpes simplex virus type 2 (HSV-2) is generally found in the genital area. The herpetic lesions usually begin as clustered vesicles on an erythematous base that quickly rupture and leave irregularly shaped, crusted lesions. The vesicles are often preceded by burning or tingling. The severity of this type of stomatitis varies from a few small, painful ulcers to extensive ulceration involving the entire oral mucous membrane and lips, accompanied by fever and lymphadenopathy. Spontaneous healing without scarring typically takes 7 to 14 days. Symptomatic relief may be achieved with topical viscous lidocaine, gargles with Benadryl Elixir (diphenhydramine), or application of a topical steroid (Orabase with hydrocortisone ointment) two or three times daily.

Varicella Virus (Chickenpox)

The oral lesions of the varicella virus (chickenpox) appear initially as single, small, fluid-filled vesicles that rupture and form shallow ulcers. Symptomatic treatment is helpful in young children. The virus is considered contagious until the skin lesions are crusted and new ones are no longer appearing.

Scarlet Fever

Scarlet fever is caused by a group A beta-hemolytic streptococcal infection. It has an abrupt onset, generally accompanied by fever, malaise and sore throat, which may be followed in 12 to 48 hours by a distinctive rash. The rash consists of a generalized hyperemic papular eruption that may spare the perioral region. It has a characteristic sandpaper texture. The oral pharynx appears injected and may have soft palate petechiae and tonsillar exudates. Occasionally the oral manifestations are the only initial presenting features. Oral treatment consists of penicillin or erythromycin for 10 days.

Rubeola (Measles)

Rubeola (measles) is a highly contagious viral infection. On the second day of the illness, Koplik's spots appear on the buccal mucosa as small, irregular, bright red spots with bluish-white centers. Beginning opposite the molars, Koplik's spots spread to involve other portions of the oropharynx. The characteristic erythematous maculopapular skin rash typically does not appear until the third to fifth days of the illness. Koplik's spots begin to disappear with the appearance of the skin rash. Treatment is supportive.

Hand-Foot-and-Mouth Disease

Hand-foot-and-mouth disease is caused by the Coxsackie virus group A, type 16. This virus causes a distinctive syndrome of vesicular stomatitis and an exanthem involving the dorsa of the hands and feet. The rash is usually maculopapular, beginning on the face or trunk and spreading to the extremities. A vesicular eruption similar to varicella may occur. Treatment is symptomatic.

DISEASES OF ORAL MUCOSA AND GINGIVA
Mucocele (Mucous Cysts)

Small mucus-containing cysts may appear at any age in minor salivary gland areas of the oral cavity, primarily the lower lip and buccal mucosa. Superficial mucoceles appear translucent and round. Deeper mucoceles have a bluish appearance. They tend to recur even when ruptured. The treatment of choice is excision. The patient should be referred to a dentist or maxillofacial surgeon.

Fordyce's Granules or Spots

Fordyce's spots are ectopic sebaceous glands that appear as yellowish granules under oral mucosa, primarily that of buccal mucosa. The glands are present at birth, but they hypertrophy and first appear during preadolescence in approximately 50% of children. No treatment is required.

"Geographic Tongue"

A benign condition of the dorsum of the tongue that appears patchy or map-like is called "geographic tongue" or "migrating glossitis." The patchy appearance represents atrophic filiform papillae. The cause is unknown. Reassurance is all that is required.

Gingival Hyperplasia

Hyperplasia of the gingiva may be drug induced. Phenytoin therapy causes gingival hyperplasia in 40% of patients, particularly in younger children. The presence of local irritants seems to exacerbate the tissue response. Treatment in mild cases consists of good oral hygiene. In severe cases, surgical removal of the excessive tissue may be necessary. A similar lesion may be seen in patients on nifedipine therapy.

ORAL MANIFESTATIONS OF SYSTEMIC DISEASE
Diabetes Mellitus

Children with diabetes mellitus are more prone to periodontal disease. The degree of control of the diabetes correlates with its manifestations involving the oral cavity. In a brittle diabetic, the presence of a periodontal abscess may be sufficient to trigger ketoacidosis. Advanced periodontal disease in a young patient should prompt the emergency physician to exclude a diagnosis of diabetes.

Erythema Multiforme (Stevens-Johnson Syndrome)

Erythema multiforme is an acute, usually self-limiting disease precipitated by a variety of factors. Typically the lesions, referred to as "target lesions," are surrounded by a zone of normal skin and a halo of erythema.

Stevens-Johnson syndrome is a severe form characterized by bullae, mucous membrane lesions, and multisystem involvement that may be fatal, usually due to overwhelming infection and dehydration. Blistering of the mucous membranes may represent the sole expression of the disease in about 25% of cases. Treatment should be aimed at the underlying cause. Severe cases require admission for hydration and systemic corticosteroid treatment.

Blood Dyscrasias

Two types of blood dyscrasias, anemia and leukemia, have dramatic oral manifestations. In anemia the gingiva appear pale and bleed easily. A prolonged clotting time is also seen with pernicious anemia, and the tongue may be atrophic, beefy-red, and painful. In sickle cell disease and thalassemia an increase in the size of the jaw bones, particularly the premaxilla, may occur because of the increased demand for hematopoietic space. The gingiva may be massively infiltrated with leukemic cells in acute leukemic states, especially with acute granulocytic leukemia. The gingiva appear edematous, bluish-red, and hypertrophic and may have spontaneous gingival bleeding. Thrombocytopenic purpura and von Willebrand's disease may also present with spontaneous gingival bleeding.

Addison's Disease

In Addison's disease, any areas of surface epithelium that are under pressure (by watch bands, restrictive clothing, or masticatory forces on oral mucosa) may darken. This darkening is caused by an increase of melanin and is called *melanosis*. Orally, melanosis is seen primarily over the prominent portions of the gingivae, on the tongue, buccal mucosa, and lips.

DENTAL INFECTIONS
Dental Caries

Dental caries, or tooth decay, is a progressive disease that destroys the teeth. Caries is primarily a disease of childhood and adolescence, with peak periods of activity at 4 to 8 and 12 to 18 years of age. Children living in communities with adequately fluoridated water have an average of 60% fewer carious lesions owing to the increased surface resistance to acid breakdown. Eating between meals and diets high in sugars or sticky foods promote decay.

The most common cause of severe decay in children under age 3 years is called "milkbottle caries." Putting a child to bed with a bottle of milk or other sweetened liquid may result in rampant decay, characteristically to the maxillary anterior teeth. Caries in children usually occurs in the deep pits and fissures on the chewing surfaces and in between the teeth where they contact. Decay is rapidly invasive in children.

With penetration into dentin, there may be sensitivity to temperature changes or sweets. With progression of decay and irritation of the pulp, reversible pulpitis occurs. This usually causes intermittent pain and sensitivity to cold. Emergency treatment for reversible pulpitis consists of analgesia and dental referral. Progressive carious invasion into dental pulp causes irreversible pulpitis characterized by increased pain, often exquisite and constant. Immediate referral to a dentist is recommended. If this is not possible, relief is often obtained through local injection with a long-acting anesthetic such as bupivacaine and a prescription for an analgesic.

Untreated irreversible pulpitis may progress to involve infection of the periapical (root) area and the surrounding structures. The infection may drain by a fistula or cause an abscess. Pain from this type of infection is exacerbated by percussion or the pressure of biting or chewing. In addition, periapical infections in primary teeth may cause defects in underlying permanent teeth. Systemic symptoms such as fever and leukocytosis may accompany dental infection and should be treated according to the severity of symptoms. Patients with minimal nonfluctuant swelling of the gingiva should be given penicillin, analgesia, and dental referral within 24 hours. Small fluctuant swelling of the alveolar area may be incised and drained emergently.

Fascial Space Infection

Any patient with swelling involving the fascial planes should be admitted and placed on intravenous antibiotics together with an urgent consultation with an oral maxillofacial surgeon or otolaryngologist. A maxillary canine space infection can progress to infraorbital involvement rapidly and may lead to infection of the cavernous sinus and subsequent lethal thrombosis. Submandibular swelling may result from infection of any mandibular tooth and can dissect the neck fascial planes (Ludwig's angina), causing elevation of the tongue, potential respiratory difficulty, and even infection in the mediastinum. Trismus, or inability to open the mouth, may also occur. Small children may not present with the usual pain associated with a dental infection of the primary dentition. High fever, malaise, irritability, and poor feeding are often the presenting symptoms with dental infection.

Periodontal Disease

Progressive inflammation that involves the supporting structures of the teeth (periodontal fibers and alveolar bone) is called periodontitis. Early periodontal disease is limited to inflammation of the gingiva and is called gingivitis. The inflamed tissue appears red and swollen and may become ulcerated and bleed easily. The usual cause is invading bacteria and is associated with poor dental hygiene.

As with gingivitis, local causative factors are generally responsible for periodontitis. Poor oral hygiene results in accumulation of bacterial plaque. An inflammatory response results from the plaque and the toxic products of bacterial growth. With breakdown in the epithelial barrier, more severe infection destroys the supporting structures. Good oral hygiene with adequate tooth brushing and flossing may prevent this continuum. Occasionally food or pus can become trapped in a gingival pocket, causing a periodontal abscess. In the emergency department, treatment consists of a small incision to allow for drainage, a prescription for antibiotics, and saline rinses. The patient should be referred to a dentist for definitive care.

Maxillary Sinusitis

A diagnosis of maxillary sinusitis should be considered in the differential diagnosis of dental pain in the maxillary teeth. The apices of the maxillary teeth are in close proximity to the floor of the maxillary sinus. Inflamed sinuses may cause referred pain to the teeth and vice versa. The pain referred from the sinuses is generally described as throbbing in nature and usually exacerbated by bending over or lying down. There may be tenderness over the maxillary sinuses or nasal discharge without apparent dental cause. Sinus x-rays or a panorex radiograph may be useful. Management includes appropriate antibiotics, decongestants, and referral to an otolaryngologist.

Teething

Children may become irritable, with significantly increased salivation, and may have minor local gingival inflammation at the time of newly erupting teeth. Physicians frequently see teething children with transient systemic complaints such as low-grade fever, rhinorrhea, and mild diarrhea and no other apparent illness. Parental reassurance and symptomatic care are generally all that is required.

Pericoronitis

Acute infection around the soft tissue of an erupting molar, usually the wisdom tooth, is called pericoronitis. It results from an accumulation of bacteria under the flap of tissue known as the operculum. The tissue becomes erythematous, edematous, and painful. Additional trauma may occur from the opposing tooth and make chewing very painful. In severe cases there may be fever, malaise, lymphadenopathy, trismus, and pain radiating to the ear, throat, or floor of the mouth. Treatment consists of irrigation under the tissue flap using a flexible No. 18 gauge intravenous catheter, antibiotics, and dental referral. Occasionally excision of the operculum may be needed, but this is generally best done by the dentist.

Bacterial Endocarditis Prophylaxis

Bacterial endocarditis is a microbial infection of the endocardium of the heart caused by bacterial seeding of the blood stream. Certain patients with immunocompromised states, congenital heart conditions, prosthetic valves, or acquired cardiac lesions may be at risk for developing this condition after a dental procedure or manipulation of the soft tissue, which allows the entrance of blood-borne bacteria. Antibiotic prophylaxis is recommended for all dental procedures likely to cause gingival bleeding in susceptible patients. The most common causative organisms associated with bacteria after dental procedures are alpha-hemolytic streptococci. Recommendations for antibiotic prophylaxis are provided by the American Medical Association (Table 80–2).

DENTAL TRAUMA

Most injuries involve the anterior teeth, particularly the four maxillary incisors. Traumatic injuries to the teeth occur most frequently when children learn to become more independent: e.g., when they begin to walk, start school, learn to ride a bike or rollerskate, or engage in contact sports. Treatment is usually determined by age, extent of injury, and time lapsed since the accident. In cases of total tooth avulsion, time is of the essence and special care needs to be taken to preserve the vitality of the tooth. Once more serious injuries have been managed, any teeth suspected of injury should be examined. If intraoral radiographs are unavailable, a panoramic view is helpful in evaluating the extent of the injury and for detecting possible embedded foreign bodies or fragments of teeth. Even teeth that have been traumatized without apparent injury may have delayed complications and should be referred for dental follow-up within 24 hours.

TABLE 80–2

RECOMMENDED ANTIBIOTIC REGIMENS FOR DENTAL/RESPIRATORY TRACT PROCEDURES		
Conditions	**Drug**	**Dose**
Oral route	Amoxicillin	50 mg/kg up to 3.0 g 1 hr before procedure, then half that dose q6hr
Penicillin-allergic (oral)	Erythromycin	20 mg/kg up to 800–1000 mg 2 hr before procedure, then half that dose q6hr
	or	
	Clindamycin	10 mg/kg up to 300 mg 1 hr before procedure, then half that dose q6hr
Parenteral	Ampicillin	50 mg/kg IV or IM up to 2 g 30 min before procedure, then half that dose q6hr
Penicillin-allergic (parenteral)	Clindamycin	10 mg/kg IV up to 300 mg 30 min before procedure, then half that dose q6hr

Modified from Dajani AS, Bisno AL, Chung KJ, et al. Prevention of bacterial endocarditis: Recommendations by the American Heart Association. JAMA 1990; 264:2920, 2921. Copyright 1990, American Medical Association.

Tooth Fracture

The extent of fracture to the teeth, the age of the child, and the time since the injury will dictate the prognosis and appropriate treatment (Fig. 80–2).

Ellis Class I Fractures. Ellis class I injuries are fractures involving enamel only. Incomplete fractures or cracks of the enamel without loss of tooth structure are known as craze lines. They are common findings and generally do not require immediate treatment.

Cracked Tooth Syndrome. Patients who have repeated complaints of a toothache without apparent decay or periodontal involvement may be suffering from the cracked tooth syndrome. These patients often have a history of trauma or multiple dental restorations. The pain from this syndrome is exacerbated by chewing and by temperature changes. Symptomatic care and dental referral are appropriate emergency care. If the fracture involves only enamel but is complete (i.e., chipped or fragmented), smoothing of the rough edges with an abrasive disk or emery board usually suffices. If the tooth is especially sensitive, a few coats of Copalite varnish or clear nail polish may help temporarily, before dental referral. Enamel fractures generally carry a good prognosis.

Ellis Class II Fractures. Fractures extending into the dentin appear yellow or light brown in contrast to white enamel. Because of the vital microtubular structure, dentin needs protection from environmental exposure and to alleviate extreme sensitivity. Management of class II fractures depends on the age of the patient. In those less than 12 years old, the exposed dentin should be gently cleansed with warm saline and dried, and a thin layer of calcium hydroxide paste (Dycal) should be applied followed by several coats of varnish (Copalite) or clear nail polish. Older patients can be given analgesics and be told to avoid extreme temperatures while eating and follow up within 24 hours with their family dentist. For definitive management, one should obtain dental consultation for all instances of Ellis class II injuries in children. About 7% of teeth with fractures into the dentin become necrotic. Prognosis varies with the length of time before definitive treatment, the extent of dentinal exposure, and the age of the patient.

Ellis Class III Fractures. Fractures into the pulp are dental emergencies and need urgent referral and management by a dentist. Teeth with class III fractures show a pink or red blush or even blood at the center of the fracture. Emergency treatment should focus on smoothing rough edges, searching for tooth fragments that may be embedded in injured tissue or even aspirated, and providing analgesia and prophylactic antibiotics. A chest radiograph should be taken in all infants and children with a history of trauma in whom there are missing teeth or fragments that may have been aspirated.

Root Fractures

Fractures involving the root are less common in primary teeth and in permanent teeth with incomplete root formation. These injuries are seen mostly in maxillary incisors at two peak ages, 3 to 4 years and 11 to 20 years. Clinically, palpation may reveal a lack of coordination in movement of the crown and root. Painful or altered occlusion may be noted. Extraction is usually the treatment of choice in primary teeth. Depending on the level of fracture, the treatment in permanent teeth varies. Emergency care should be directed at providing prophylactic antibiotics and immediate referral.

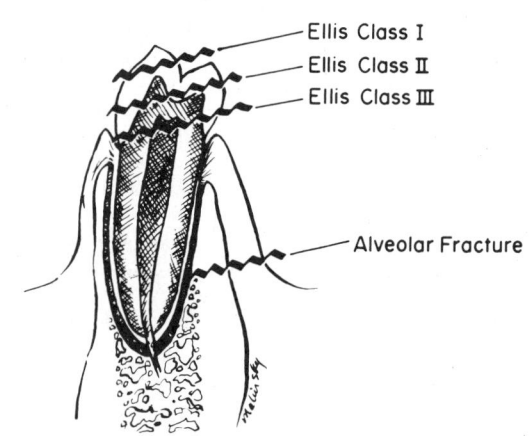

Ellis Class I
Ellis Class II
Ellis Class III

Alveolar Fracture

Figure 80–2. The Ellis classification for fractured alveolar teeth. (From Amsterdam JT. Emergency dental procedures. *In* Roberts JR, Hedges JR (eds). Clinical Procedures in Emergency Medicine. 2nd ed. Philadelphia, WB Saunders, 1991, p 1048.)

Displacement Injuries

Displaced teeth, luxated teeth, and complete avulsions are frequently seen in the emergency department. All require analgesia, prophylactic antibiotics, and dental referral. Specific intervention is required in some cases. The extruded primary tooth usually should not be repositioned because of the potential damage to the developing permanent tooth follicle. The patient should be referred for extraction. Significantly displaced and extruded permanent teeth should be repositioned after adequate analgesia. If definitive dental care is available immediately, the patient can simply bite gently on moist gauze while en route. If there will be a delay in definitive treatment, it may be necessary to provide a temporary splint for stabilization.

When injury involves total avulsion (total dislocation of the tooth from the socket), time is a critical factor. Retention of reimplanted teeth may vary from a few weeks to a lifetime. The success diminishes inversely with the time out of the mouth; good success is usually achieved if the teeth are replanted within 30 minutes. Root resorption and failure occur in teeth replanted after 2 hours. Parents or Emergency Medical Service personnel should be instructed to put the tooth back in place as soon as possible.

Before implantation, the tooth should be examined for debris. It can be gently rinsed if necessary, but one must avoid handling the root if possible. The child can then bite gently on a cloth or gauze while en route to the office or emergency department. If reimplantation is too traumatic at home, the tooth should be transported in the mouth of the patient under the tongue or in a cup of milk. The tooth should be replanted as soon as possible. A small amount of local anesthetic may be required. Once replanted, the tooth should be splinted and the patient referred to a dentist immediately. Prophylactic antibiotics, analgesics, and tetanus toxoid if needed should be given.

Splinting Techniques

Tooth stabilization is best done by a dentist, but if definitive dental care is unavailable for 24 hours, a temporary splint can be made in the emergency department. Soft wax can be gently molded over the injured tooth and two or three adjacent teeth on each side, on both the lingual and labial surfaces (Fig. 80–3). The patient should be told to have a soft diet and avoid hot foods (Table 80–3).

Premixed periodontal packs or a powder mix such as Ward's Wonder Pak may be used. These are easily molded to the teeth and can be applied to a wet or bloodied area. The material hardens to a thin, plaster-like consistency that adheres to the teeth and gums. It should be applied as with the wax splint, to encompass adjacent teeth.

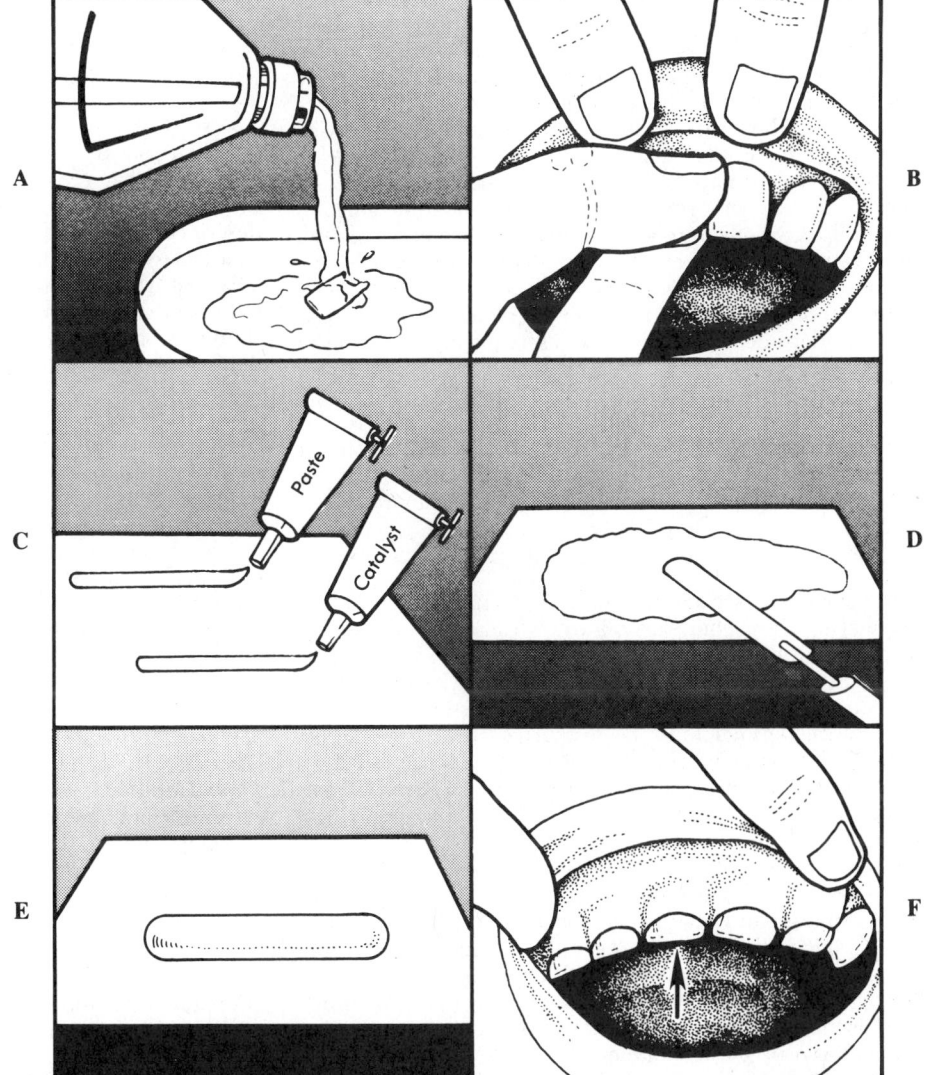

Figure 80–3. Reimplantation and stabilization of an avulsed tooth. *A,* The tooth is rinsed. *B,* The tooth is placed back into the socket. *C, D,* The periodontal pack is mixed. *E,* Splint material is ready for application. *F,* Packing is molded over the reimplanted tooth and two adjacent teeth to either side. (From Amsterdam JT. Dental emergencies. *In* Rosen PR, Baker FJ III, Dailey RH, et al (eds). Emergency Medicine: Concepts and Clinical Practice. 2nd ed. St Louis, CV Mosby, 1988, p 1063.)

TABLE 80–3
GENERAL DISCHARGE INSTRUCTIONS FOR TRAUMATIC DENTAL INJURIES
1. Follow-up with dentist within 24 hours
2. Stay on a soft diet for at least 3 days
3. Elevate the head 30–45 degrees
4. Avoid extremely hot or cold foods
5. Avoid straws and sucking
6. Use caution to avoid biting a "numb" lip or tongue
7. If bleeding continues, apply direct pressure
8. If bleeding persists in spite of above, return to dentist or emergency room

Soft Tissue Injuries

Blunt trauma to the mouth may initially seem worse than it actually is because of the amount of bleeding. The injury may involve only maceration and bruising and not require any suturing. A frequent injury seen in small children is small laceration of the maxillary labial frenum. Unless the laceration is severe or there is arterial bleeding, no treatment is required. These injuries heal nicely without complications. Reassurance to the family and prophylactic antibiotics are all that is necessary.

Lip and tongue lacerations larger than 1 cm or that are gaping should be repaired. The tissue needs to be well approximated in small, superficial intraoral lacerations. Deep tissues may be apposed with absorbable sutures (4–0, 5–0). Mucosal edges may be closed with either 4–0 chromic or silk sutures. When approximating tissues near the mucocutaneous junction of the lip, meticulous detail should be given to apposing the edges. Skin suturing should be done with 5–0 or 6–0 nylon monofilament sutures.

Tongue lacerations are sometimes difficult to suture, especially in the very young. In these children an alligator towel clip or a silk retention suture may be necessary for stabilization. In older children an assistant can usually immobilize the tongue adequately with a 2 × 2–inch gauze. Sufficient anesthesia can generally be obtained with topical viscous lidocaine, especially in cases requiring only one or two sutures.

For deep or difficult unilateral lacerations requiring more dense anesthesia, a lingual nerve block works well. Prophylactic antibiotics and a soft diet should be advised. Discharge instructions should be given regarding potential injury to the lip and tongue, which will be temporarily numb.

Burns

Burns may be seen in the form of electrical, chemical, or thermal injuries. One classic burn is caused by an aspirin placed adjacent to a tooth in an attempt to relieve pain from a toothache. The mucosa will appear white where the tissue is necrotic, and underneath will be red and ulcerated. In such cases, parents are instructed to give analgesics systemically for pain relief. Irrigation and topical ointment such as Orabase may provide some relief. Thermal burns from foods such as hot pizza are usually minor and heal spontaneously in a few days. Electrical burns occur most often in younger children 3 to 6 years of age, usually when they bite on an extension or appliance cord. The severity of these wounds can range from superficial to extensive third-degree burns that involve not only the lips but also the corners of the mouth and tongue. Often the extent of the damage is not immediately obvious and may not cause much pain owing to nerve damage. Immediate consultation with a maxillofacial or plastic surgeon should be obtained. Treatment depends on the extent of the burn. Tetanus immuni-

zation should be updated as necessary. Prophylactic antibiotics and analgesics should be given.

POSTPROCEDURE COMPLICATIONS

Small children may chew their lip while anesthetized and present to the emergency department with a macerated lip or cheek. Salt-water rinses, analgesia, and antibiotics usually suffice.

Patients may complain of persistent localized numbness after dental anesthesia. Occasionally the nerve sheath sustains minor trauma from the procedure and can cause transient paresthesia lasting up to 4 to 8 weeks. Treatment consists of reassurance.

Spasms in the masticator muscles, or trismus, may occur as a result of infection or hemorrhage. Treatment consists of local heat, analgesia, and a muscle relaxant. The patient should also be instructed to chew actively 3 to 4 minutes every hour. Any infection should be treated with antibiotics.

Occasionally the local anesthetic gets into the parotid gland and causes a temporary facial nerve paralysis resembling Bell's palsy. Patients' mouths may droop and they may be unable to close the eyelid on the affected side. The problem is self-limiting, but protection with an eye patch will prevent drying of the cornea.

Occasionally a blood vessel is nicked during a local anesthetic procedure, and a hematoma results. If this is large, a prophylactic antibiotic should be prescribed in addition to local pressure, initially ice, then heat. Hematomas generally resolve in 7 to 14 days.

Alveolitis

Postextraction pain is usually related to alveolitis. The term "dry socket" is sometimes used to describe this condition, since the removal of tooth and blood clot from the socket exposes the alveolar bone to the air. The pain is described as throbbing and may radiate to the ear. It is exacerbated by cold liquids and inhaling through the mouth. The best treatment is to irrigate with warm saline and place iodoform gauze soaked with eugenol in the socket. Patients should be given adequate analgesics and referred to their dentist for recheck in 24 hours.

Bleeding

Postextraction bleeding can usually be controlled by biting on a moist 2 × 2–inch gauze for 15 to 20 minutes. Biting on a moist teabag can also be helpful, since the tannic acid assists hemostasis. If bleeding persists after direct pressure, local anesthetic (1% lidocaine with 1:100,000 epinephrine) should be given. The anesthetic is injected into the socket area until it blanches, and then a small piece of Gelfoam is placed in the socket and sutured closed with 3–0 silk or chromic sutures. If bleeding persists, the patient should be evaluated for systemic problems. Patients whose postextraction bleeding responds to emergency treatment should be instructed to follow up with their dentist within 24 hours. They should not eat or drink for 2 hours, and then avoid extremely hot or cold foods, smoking, spitting, sucking, or drinking with a straw. Hemorrhage that is spontaneous should alert the physician to look for underlying coagulopathies or disorders such as leukemia.

Orthodontic Complications

Because the numbers of patients wearing orthodontic appliances are growing, the emergency physician should be prepared to handle problems that arise when the orthodontist is unavailable. Most orthodontic emergencies occur in

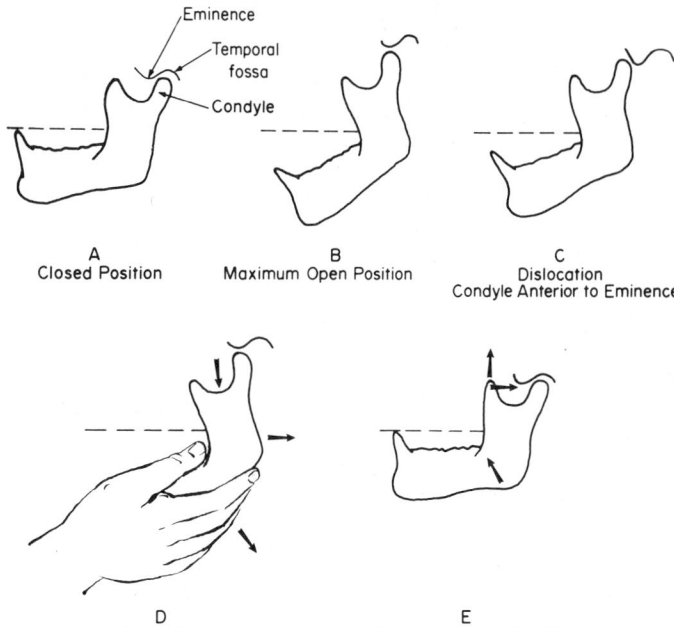

Figure 80–4. Technique for reducing mandibular dislocation. (From Amsterdam JT, Hendler BH, Rose LF. Dental emergencies. *In* Schwartz GR, Safar P, Stone JH, et al (eds). Principles and Practice of Emergency Medicine. 2nd ed. Philadelphia, WB Saunders, 1988, p 1562.)

children. Injuries may arise from broken wires after a punch in the mouth, sports activities, or motor vehicle accidents. Upon initial examination these injuries usually look worse than they are because of the bleeding. Once the area is irrigated and cleaned, they can be better assessed.

Often the lips or cheeks have become impaled by the hook-like attachments (ligature wires) that hold the arch wire in place. A local anesthetic may be required to release the tissue. Pulling on the lip may actually exacerbate the problem, and pushing may be preferable. Sometimes the injury is caused by a broken wire that is now digging into the soft tissue. Bending the wire with needle-nosed pliers or a hemostat may provide relief. An application of soft wax may be a temporary solution until the child can see an orthodontist. In any case, "less is better." The orthodontist will prefer minimal alteration of the intricate wiring.

TEMPOROMANDIBULAR JOINT (TMJ) DYSFUNCTION

The TMJ is complex, being both a hinge and a sliding joint. It is subject to significant forces when chewing. The syndrome results from disharmony in the joint or disturbances in the biting surfaces of the teeth and may be aggravated by trauma, stress, or habits such as cheek biting, lip chewing, clenching, or bruxing. The condition is generally seen in older patients, past the teen years. Patients usually complain of pain, often unilateral in the area of the TMJ. Pain may also be referred to the ear. It is usually exacerbated by chewing. The pain may be sharp or dull and often worsens during the course of the day. In extreme cases, trismus may occur secondary to spasm in the masticatory muscles. Emergency department treatment consists of moist heat four to six times daily, analgesia, a soft diet, a nonsteroidal anti-inflammatory agent, and occasionally muscle relaxants. Patients should be told to strictly avoid chewing gum and firm or sticky foods such as tough meat, bagels, and caramel candies. A dental referral is appropriate.

TEMPOROMANDIBULAR JOINT DISLOCATION

A TMJ dislocation may occur in conjunction with a traumatic injury, but more often than not it follows extreme opening of the jaws, as with yawning or laughter. It may be bilateral or unilateral. The sequence of muscle contraction and spasm causes the condyles to lock and the patient is unable to close the mouth completely. If there is suspicion of trauma, a radiograph should be taken to exclude an accompanying fracture before reduction. To rearticulate a dislocation, one should stand in front of a seated patient and place the thumbs on the outer surfaces of the mandibular molars, pressing downward and backward to guide the condyles back into place (Fig. 80–4). If the dislocation is fairly long-standing (hours or days), a muscle relaxant may be required before the procedure. A dental referral should be obtained and the patient instructed to eat a liquid or soft diet and avoid extreme opening of the mouth and chewing gum.

Selected References

Braham RL, Roberts MW, Morris ME. Management of dental trauma in children and adolescents. J Trauma 1977;17:857.

Capitano P. Dental emergencies for the non-dentist. Emerg Med 1986;18:16.

Dungy AF. Hospital aspects of dental trauma. Dent Clin North Am 1982;26:555.

Gibson DE, Verno AA. Dentistry in the emergency department. J Emerg Med 1987;5:35–44.

Grossman LI, Ship II. Survival rate of reimplanted teeth. Oral Surg 1970;29:899.

Hendler BH, Wagner D. Injury to the lip and oral mucosa—trauma rounds. Emerg Med 1974;6:278.

Johnson WT, Goodrich JL, James GA. Reimplantation of avulsed teeth with immature root development. Oral Surg 1985;60:420.

Klokkevold P. Common dental emergencies—evaluation and management for emergency physicians. Emerg Med Clin North Am 1989;7:29.

Laskin D. The role of the dentist in the emergency room. Dental Clin North Am 1975;19(4):675.

Levine N. Injury to the primary dentition; symposium on dentofacial trauma. Dent Clin North Am 1982;26:461.

Medford HM. Acute care of avulsed teeth. Ann Emerg Med 1982;11:559.

Mueller WA. Emergency dental care. Pediatrician 1989;16:147.

Pulver F. Treatment of trauma to the young permanent dentition. Dental Clin North Am 1982;26:525

Wright TM, Taylor PP, Allen EP, et al. A review of the oral manifestations of infections in pediatric patients. Pediatr Infect Dis J 1984;3:80.

CHAPTER 81

Ophthalmologic Emergencies

Roland B. Clark

ANATOMY
Bony Orbit

The walls of the bony orbit comprise the rigid eye socket. The orbital floor shares a common wall with the roof of the maxillary antrum. The infraorbital nerve courses on the orbital floor to its midpoint, where it enters the bony orbital floor to exit through the infraorbital foramen at the midportion of the inferior orbital rim. It supplies sensory innervation to the lower lid, cheek, and lateral nose. The orbital floor and medial orbital wall (the lamina papyracea) are the principal weak points of the bony orbit. These areas are commonly involved in blowout fractures.

Eyelids

The skin of the eyelids is thin, mobile, and loosely attached to the subcutaneous tissue, creating considerable potential subcutaneous space. Blunt injuries may produce dramatic lid swelling when the potential subcutaneous space is filled with blood or extracellular fluid.

The *tarsal plates* are two semilunar cartilaginous structures located deep in the substance of both lids. Their tarsal surfaces are covered only by tarsal conjunctiva. The tarsal plates are responsible for the rigidity and shape of the lids and the integrity of the lid margin. Lacerations of the lid margin that involve the tarsal plates require meticulous repair to reestablish the smooth contour of the lid.

The orbital space is sequestered from the subcutaneous lid tissues by the orbital septum. This connective tissue membrane arises from the margins of the tarsal plates and attaches at the orbital rim, where it is continuous with the periosteum. The resulting barrier protects the orbital space from local infections of the eyelids. Lacerations that violate the orbital septum may expose the orbital contents to infectious material and result in orbital cellulitis.

The *lacrimal puncta* are located on the lid margins of the upper and lower lids approximately 6 mm lateral to the medial canthus. They are the entry point for the tear collection system. The lacrimal canaliculi are minute tubular conduits connecting the lacrimal puncta with the lacrimal sac medially. The canaliculi are located approximately 1 mm beneath the lid margin. Tears enter the canaliculi at the puncta and course medially to enter the lacrimal sac and nasolacrimal duct. Lacerations involving the medial portion of the lid margins may involve the lacrimal canaliculi.

Conjunctiva

The conjunctiva, a densely vascularized thin mucous membrane, completely lines the interior surface of the lids from the lid margins to the superior and inferior cul-de-sacs. From the cul-de-sacs it reflects forward to cover the anterior surface of the globe, where it attaches at the limbus. The tarsal conjunctiva is attached firmly to the lids, but the bulbar conjunctiva is attached only loosely. The large potential bulbar subconjunctival space may fill with blood or tissue fluid.

Globe

The scleral shell of the globe is a semirigid connective tissue sphere upon which the extraocular muscles insert; it contains the complex and delicate intraocular structures. The eyeball is tough and remarkably resistant to injury and penetration. However, mechanical distortion of the globe may damage inner structures while doing no apparent harm to the outer surface.

Cornea

The cornea is the transparent disk at the anterior pole of the globe. The corneal stroma is a specialized lamellar connective tissue extension of the globe that forms the bulk of the corneal thickness. Overlying the anterior surface of the cornea is the corneal epithelium, and immediately beneath the epithelium lies Bowman's membrane. Whereas the corneal epithelium is fragile and easily injured, Bowman's membrane is quite resistant to mechanical injury and acts as a protective barrier for the inner layers of the cornea.

Anterior Segment

The important structures of the anterior segment are the *iris, trabecular meshwork, canal of Schlemm, ciliary body,* and *crystalline lens* (Fig. 81–1). The circumferential ciliary body lies posterior to the iris root. Within it lie muscle fibers which act on the lens through the zonular fibers to accomplish accommodation. Aqueous humor is elaborated by the ciliary body and flows through the posterior chamber and into the anterior chamber through the pupil. Aqueous exits the anterior chamber through the trabecular meshwork, enters the canal of Schlemm, and exits the globe.

Posterior Segment

The elements of the posterior segment of greatest interest are the *vitreous body, retina,* and *optic nerve.* The vitreous body is a transparent gel that fills the entire space of the globe from the posterior surface of the iris to the retina. In youth it remains relatively firm, but at about middle age it softens and becomes more fluid.

The retina lines the inner surface of the globe from the ora serrata anteriorly to the optic nerve head at the posterior pole. The visual sensory elements of the retina give rise to approximately 1 million nerve fibers; these aggregate at the optic disk to form the optic nerve.

OPHTHALMIA NEONATORUM

Inflammatory disorders of the eye that present during the neonatal period are collectively termed ophthalmia neona-

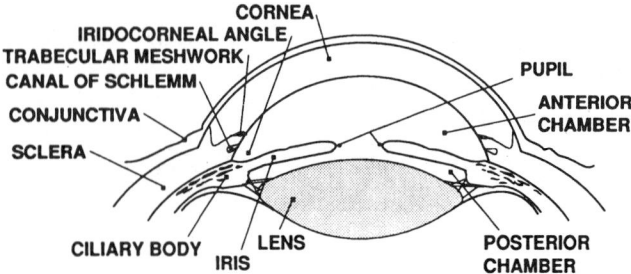

Figure 81–1. Normal anatomy of the anterior segment. (From Rosenberg CA, Adams SL. Narrow-angle glaucoma presenting as acute, painless visual impairment. Ann Emerg Med 1991;20:1021.)

torum. These infections are usually acquired from the mother's genital tract during birth.

Silver Nitrate. Silver nitrate as a 1% solution is instilled at birth in Credé prophylaxis to prevent gonococcal infection. During the first 24 hours of life silver nitrate is the most likely cause of acute conjunctivitis. No specific treatment is necessary, and the inflammation will subside spontaneously in a few days. Prevention of gonococcal ophthalmia neonatorum by instillation of silver nitrate is effective, although it does not prevent inclusion blennorrhea or herpes infection.

Gonococcal Conjunctivitis

Conjunctivitis due to *Neisseria gonorrhoeae* produces a profuse, purulent discharge beginning during the second to the fourth day of life. Prompt diagnosis and treatment are necessary, as a gonococcal infection may penetrate the intact cornea within 24 to 48 hours. Although incubation periods vary widely, they are helpful in distinguishing between gonococcal conjunctivitis and inclusion blennorrhea (Table 81–1). The diagnosis of gonococcal conjunctivitis may be confirmed by conjunctival smears. If it is not known whether the infecting organism is beta-lactamase producing, therapy should begin with parenteral cefotaxime in addition to topical therapy. If previous maternal cultures indicate that the organism is not beta-lactamase producing, both systemic therapy with parenteral aqueous crystalline penicillin G and topical erythromycin are indicated (Table 81–2).

Bacterial Conjunctivitis

Other types of bacterial conjunctivitis also occur from the second through the seventh days of life. The most common agents are *Staphylococcus aureus*, *Haemophilus* spp., *Streptococcus pneumoniae*, enterococci, and *Pseudomonas* spp., the last causing the most serious infections. Conjunctival smears and cultures confirm the diagnosis.

Inclusion Blennorrhea

Inclusion blennorrhea due to chlamydial infection has an incubation period of between 5 and 14 days, which is of help in distinguishing it from bacterial conjunctivitis. Giemsa stains of conjunctival scrapings reveal typical inclusion bodies in chlamydial conjunctivitis. Topical erythromycin or tetracycline ointment and systemic erythromycin should be given for 21 days. Inclusion blennorrhea is the most common cause of ophthalmia neonatorum in the United States.

TABLE 81–1

OPHTHALMIA NEONATORUM—COMPARATIVE INCUBATION PERIODS BASED ON THE PRINCIPAL CAUSES*

Etiology	Day 1	Day 2	Day 3	Day 4	Day 5	Day 6	Day 7	Day 8	Day 9	Day 10
Silver nitrate	●	●								
N. gonorrhoeae		●	●	●	●					
Other bacteria					●	●	●			
Chlamydia						●	●	●	●	●
Herpes simplex 2							●	●	●	

*Incubation periods may vary widely.

TABLE 81–2

THERAPY AT A GLANCE

Newborn Gonococcal Conjunctivitis (<7 days old)
Ceftriaxone (Rocephin): 50 mg/kg as a single dose. (If organism is known not to be beta-lactamase producing, may treat patient with aqueous penicillin G, 50,000–100,000 units/day divided into two doses.)
or
Cefotaxime (Claforan): 100 mg/kg/day divided into two doses
Preseptal Cellulitis (>3 mo)
Cefuroxime (Zinacef): 50–100 mg/kg/day divided into three or four doses
or
If associated with a facial lesion suggesting streptococcus or staphylococcus, use nafcillin, 100–150 mg/kg/day divided into q 4–6 hr doses and given over 15–30 min
Orbital Cellulitis
Nafcillin: 100–150 mg/kg/day divided into q 4–6 hr doses and given over 15–30 min
and
Cefuroxime (Zinacef): 75 mg/kg/day in three divided doses
Ceftriaxone (Rocephin): 50 mg/kg/day as single daily dose

Herpetic Keratoconjunctivitis

Herpetic keratoconjunctivitis usually appears about the seventh day, although it may occur earlier. Herpes simplex virus (type II) is the causative organism. Conjunctival scrapings demonstrate giant cells and diagnostic inclusion bodies on cytologic examination. Although the majority of cases of herpetic keratoconjunctivitis will subside spontaneously, topical antiviral medication is indicated. The examiner should be alert for the signs of systemic herpes infection. In the event of acute genital herpes, cesarean section may be indicated.

OCULAR INFECTIONS
Preseptal Cellulitis

By definition, infection of the lid anterior to the orbital septum is preseptal cellulitis. It presents with swelling, redness, and pain in the involved lid. There is no proptosis, chemosis, or restriction of ocular movement. Nasopharyngeal and sinus flora are usually the causative organisms, typically *H. influenzae*, *S. pneumoniae*, and staphylococci.

Management consists of obtaining swabs for culture and sensitivity testing from any visible wound site as well as from the conjunctival sac and nasopharynx. Because of the danger that preseptal cellulitis may be an early manifestation of orbital cellulitis, an MRI or CT scan may be necessary to exclude an orbital abscess or infection.

Once assured that there is no orbital involvement, the examiner may initiate treatment with oral antibiotics while awaiting culture results. Warm compresses may localize the infection and relieve swelling. Close outpatient follow-up is necessary. If inpatient treatment is chosen, intravenous cefuroxime is given; nafcillin should be considered for patients who have an associated skin lesion suggestive of *Streptococcus* or *Staphylococcus* (see Table 81–2).

Orbital Cellulitis

Orbital cellulitis is the most common cause of proptosis in childhood. The principal route of infection is spread from neighboring paranasal sinuses. Eyelid swelling and redness, severe orbital pain, proptosis, restriction of eye movement, and decreased visual acuity all occur commonly. Onset may be very rapid, and the child will be febrile and appear toxic. Local extension to the cavernous sinus may lead to involvement of cranial nerves II through VI.

Conjunctival and nasopharyngeal cultures should be obtained promptly. The child must be hospitalized and started immediately on parenteral antibiotics (nafcillin and chloramphenicol). Until cultures are available, antibiotic therapy should include both a beta-lactamase-resistant antibiotic for staphylococcal infection and an amoxicillin/clavulanate combination (oral) for *H. influenzae* infection resistant to ampicillin (see Table 81–2).

Acute Conjunctivitis

Conjunctival infection may result from a large number of potential bacterial and viral agents. Bacterial infections are often initially uniocular, with a purulent or mucopurulent discharge and no preauricular adenopathy. Viral conjunctivitis is commonly bilateral, with a thin or watery discharge and preauricular adenopathy. Unfortunately there are many exceptions to the general rule, and clinical diagnosis of a specific conjunctivitis is not always possible. Conjunctival swabs should be obtained for culture and sensitivity testing. Scrapings stained with Gram or Giemsa stain will often identify the organism.

Topical antibiotic therapy should begin while culture results are pending. A broad-spectrum antibiotic such as tobramycin or 10% sodium sulfacetamide should be administered every one or two hours. Antibiotic ointment may be applied at bedtime. Warm, moist compresses are comforting and reduce swelling.

A profuse purulent exudate, while not specific, should raise immediate concern about infection with *N. gonorrhoeae* or *N. meningitidis*. Gonococcus is locally invasive, whereas *N. meningitidis* may spread hematogenously and cause meningitis. Immediate diagnosis and treatment are mandatory.

LEUKOCORIA

By definition leukocoria means "white pupil." The finding of a white pupillary reflex does not fit the strict definition of an ocular emergency. Nevertheless, the examiner who first notes loss of the red reflex is confronted with one of the most important presentations of eye disease in childhood. The differential diagnosis includes congenital cataract, retinoblastoma, retinopathy of prematurity, persistent primary hyperplastic vitreous, retinal detachment, retinal dysplasia, and Coats disease.

Because of the very significant differential diagnosis, the finding of a white pupil in childhood demands immediate specialty referral.

PREHOSPITAL CARE OF THE INJURED EYE

Mechanical injuries of the eye are usually best left untouched by prehospital caregivers. The injured globe must be protected from any pressure to avoid extruding the contents of a potentially lacerated globe. For this reason eye pads must be completely avoided. A rigid eye shield, such as the Fox eye shield, vaults the anterior surface of the eye and offers the best protection. If a metal shield is unavailable, a paper cup or a cone fashioned from x-ray film will serve equally well. Finally, children must be restrained from rubbing or pressing on the injured eye.

Chemical eye injuries are the exception to the "hands-off" rule for eye injuries. If an eye has been exposed to chemical injury, prompt irrigation at the scene may prevent disastrous consequences. The eye should be gently irrigated with at least 1000 ml of a sterile solution prior to transport to the hospital. If a sterile solution is not immediately available, any temporary substitute is acceptable.

NONPENETRATING OCULAR TRAUMA

Adequate examination of the child with an injured eye may be difficult. The examiner may find it necessary to sedate the child or even resort to general anesthesia for adequate examination in the face of serious injury.

Lid Contusion

Contusion of the lids is extremely common in all age groups. Localized swelling often occurs within a few minutes of injury, and ecchymosis may follow in a few hours. Extravasated blood may migrate subcutaneously to produce ecchymosis of the lower lid even though the upper lid is the site of injury. Similarly, blood may migrate subcutaneously across the nasal bridge to appear on the lid of the uninjured eye. Lid swelling may be severe enough to prevent adequate examination of the underlying globe. It may be necessary to use a lid speculum to elevate the injured lid in order to inspect it. Early application of ice compresses will reduce swelling and may limit ecchymosis. As an isolated event, a lid contusion produces few complications other than the obvious cosmetic defect.

Subconjunctival Hemorrhage

Blood may accumulate in the subconjunctival space as a result of trivial or even unnoticed injury. The child is often unaware of the injury, and it is the parent who will be alarmed by the startling appearance of the red conjunctiva.

Subconjunctival hemorrhage may involve part or all of the bulbar conjunctiva. There are no complications to the isolated hemorrhage, and the blood is usually absorbed in about 2 weeks. Occasionally, subconjunctival hemorrhage may be a manifestation of systemic disease; recurring episodes should therefore be investigated.

Conjunctival Foreign Bodies

Foreign bodies of the conjunctiva invariably present with pain and tearing. Slit-lamp examination is invaluable for exact foreign body localization. If approached calmly, small children often can be examined on the parent's lap. Once the particle has been localized, it can usually be dislodged by topical anesthesia and gentle irrigation. If simple irrigation fails to dislodge the foreign body, gentle wiping with a moistened cotton-tipped applicator may be required.

Eversion of the upper lid and examination of the tarsal conjunctiva should be performed whenever possible. Foreign bodies of the upper tarsus may produce a corneal abrasion with each blink. These multiple linear abrasions of the upper corneal surface are often referred to as the "ice rink sign" because of their resemblance to the marred surface of an ice skating rink.

Corneal Abrasion

Abrasions of the cornea are invariably painful, and the younger child may resist any attempt at examination. Topical anesthesia with a drop of ophthalmic anesthetic may gain the necessary cooperation.

Most corneal abrasions are linear and result from grazing injuries. Slit-lamp examination is indicated whenever possible, although a simple hand-held magnifier may suffice. A sterile fluorescein-impregnated paper strip may be touched to the conjunctiva and the eye examined under cobalt blue illumination. Damaged corneal epithelial cells will fluoresce a brilliant green and render minute abrasions visible with magnification.

Once the diagnosis of corneal abrasion is established, a small amount of antibiotic ointment such as sodium sulfacetamide 10% should be placed in the inferior cul-de-sac. Larger abrasions may require a double patch for comfort, although children often tolerate abrasions remarkably well without patching. Follow-up examination should be done within 24 hours. Healing is usually complete in 1 to 3 days.

Corneal Foreign Bodies

Corneal foreign bodies are painful, and blepharospasm may prevent examination. Topical anesthesia is almost always necessary for examination and foreign body removal. If the foreign body is at the limbus, however, topical drops usually do not produce sufficient anesthesia for its removal. Improved anesthesia may be obtained by holding a cotton-tipped applicator saturated with topical anesthetic directly against the area of the foreign body for about 10 seconds.

Once pain is relieved a well-illuminated examination with some type of magnification should be performed; the slit-lamp examination is optimal. The foreign object may require a moistened cotton-tipped applicator for removal, but caution must be exercised to avoid injury to the surrounding corneal epithelium. Removal should be done under magnification.

If a cotton-tipped applicator fails to remove the foreign body, a sterile needle or corneal spud may be used to gently dislodge the particle in the cooperative adolescent. Removal of a corneal foreign body in the younger child must be deferred to an ophthalmologist. If the foreign body contains iron, a rust ring will often remain after it is removed. Usually the rust ring can be quickly removed with an electric corneal burr. However, if difficulty is encountered, antibiotics may be instilled, the eye firmly double-patched, and the patient referred for reexamination on the following day. By that time softening of the corneal epithelium may have occurred, making removal much simpler. In any case, a topical antibiotic, such as 10% sodium sulfacetamide, should be instilled. A firm double patch will do much to relieve pain during the healing process.

If there is significant photophobia, a drop of cycloplegic, such as 1% cyclopentolate, will relieve the pain caused by ciliary spasm. Reexamination should be performed within 24 hours.

Corneal Thermal Burn

Corneal burns in childhood are often the result of localized thermal injury from items such as curling irons or cigarettes. Such injuries are usually self-limited, as the tear film acts as a buffer between the cornea and the offending object. The corneal epithelium becomes edematous and opaque after injury, giving an alarming white irregular appearance to the anterior corneal surface. However, when the injured epithelium is shed, the underlying cornea is usually crystal clear.

Instillation of antibiotic drops or ointment in addition to patching is usually sufficient treatment. A follow-up examination should be performed within 24 hours.

Hyphema

Bleeding into the anterior chamber, or hyphema, is usually a result of blunt ocular trauma causing injury to an iris vessel. Hyphemas may be particularly difficult to observe against a dark iris. Small hyphemas may go unnoticed, although large hyphemas can fill the entire anterior cham-

ber. Rebleeding occurs in 16% to 20% of cases, and the second hemorrhage is frequently more severe than the initial bleeding. Notably, children with hyphemas often become markedly lethargic. The mechanism for this is unknown.

Treatment of hyphemas is somewhat controversial, although bed rest is always indicated. Many believe that when a hyphema involves greater than 5% of the anterior chamber the patient should be hospitalized. Other treatment options include topical cycloplegia, sedation, and topical steroids. Frequent reevaluation is necessary and is ideally performed by an ophthalmologist.

Complications of hyphema include glaucoma and corneal blood staining. Fibrin and other breakdown products of blood may obstruct the trabecular meshwork, leading to an increase in intraocular pressure. Administration of topical timolol drops 0.25% twice a day, oral acetazolamide, and a hyperosmotic agent such as glycerol, sorbitol, or mannitol will control elevated intraocular pressure. If glaucoma is persistent or severe, surgical removal of the anterior chamber clot may be indicated.

Corneal blood staining may occur, although it is more likely in the presence of glaucoma or large hyphemas. There is no specific treatment, and the staining usually absorbs over time.

Vitreous Hemorrhage

Vitreous hemorrhage in children is probably due to trauma for the most part, although diabetic retinopathy is by far the most common cause in adults. Blunt trauma produces a tear of a retinal vessel, resulting in intraocular bleeding. The injury may also cause a tear in the retina, which can lead to a retinal detachment.

Following a large vitreous hemorrhage the red reflex is lost, and details of the fundus examination may be obscured completely by the dark cloud of blood. When the retina cannot be directly observed, ultrasonography is indicated to determine the intraocular status. If a retinal tear or detachment has occurred, early surgical intervention is indicated.

Preretinal (Subhyaloid) Hemorrhage

Blood accumulation in the potential space between the sensory retina and the vitreous body is termed a preretinal hemorrhage. These hemorrhages have sharp curving margins and often assume the shape of a meniscus or boat. Retinal and preretinal hemorrhages occur in 15% of adults and almost 70% of children with subarachnoid and subdural hemorrhage. Moreover, mortality in patients with intraocular hemorrhages is markedly increased in comparison with mortality without hemorrhages. Treatment is directed at the underlying cause of the hemorrhage; there is no specific treatment for the hemorrhage itself.

Retinal Hemorrhage

Blood in the substance of the retina can result from traumatic deformation of the globe leading to direct mechanical damage to retinal vessels. Additionally, blunt trauma causes violent movement of the vitreous body, which may damage the retina indirectly.

Diagnosis of retinal hemorrhage is based upon awareness of the mechanism of injury, a high level of suspicion, and a detailed fundus examination. The appearance of the retinal hemorrhage varies with the layer of retinal involvement. Flame-shaped hemorrhages occur in the nerve fiber layer, while round hemorrhages arise from deeper layers.

No specific treatment is required, and the blood is absorbed over time. However, the presence of a retinal hemorrhage suggests significant ocular injury and mandates prompt ophthalmologic consultation.

Commotio Retinae

Commotio retinae results from blunt trauma producing a contrecoup injury to the posterior pole. There is marked edema of the sensory retina, giving it a milky appearance in which the retinal pigment epithelium and choroid are obscured. There is marked reduction of vision, and the visual prognosis is uncertain. There is no specific treatment.

Orbital Blowout Fracture

Forces directly impacting the globe and orbit are distributed to the orbital walls, resulting in fracture at the weakest point. The thin medial orbital wall, the lamina papyracea, overlies the posterior ethmoid air cells. Fracture of the medial wall permits air to enter the orbit, where it migrates subcutaneously, resulting in crepitus of the eyelids. Nose-blowing may produce sudden dramatic swelling of the lids.

Clinical findings in orbital blowout fractures include the following: (1) restriction of upward movement of globe with diplopia on upward gaze; (2) enophthalmos; (3) ptosis due to narrowing of the palpebral fissure; and (4) infraorbital hypesthesia. No specific treatment is required, and the fractures heal spontaneously. Many believe that antibiotics are indicated because of potential contamination of the orbital contents by nasal flora.

Blowout fractures of the orbital floor allow orbital fat and the inferior rectus and oblique muscles to herniate downward into the maxillary sinus, where they may become trapped by the fracture margins. The muscle trapping results in restriction of ocular movement in an upward direction and diplopia on attempted upward gaze. Loss of orbital volume results in enophthalmos and narrowing of the palpebral fissure, and injury to the infraorbital nerve on the orbital floor causes infraorbital anesthesia. Surgical repair is indicated on an elective basis if muscle trapping, diplopia, or a cosmetic deformity persists.

PENETRATING AND PERFORATING INJURIES

Eyelid Lacerations

Lacerations that are horizontally oriented and superficial enough to spare the orbital septum may be managed like any other laceration. However, if the orbital septum is lacerated, repair involves wound exploration and multilayered closure. Specialty referral is indicated.

Vertical lacerations of the lid surface must be approached differently. Wound healing and scarring cause contracture in the axis of the laceration. Simple closure of a vertical laceration may result in a prominent puckered scar that crosses the normal lid folds. A cosmetically acceptable outcome may require a complex repair.

Wounds that cross the eyelid margin are a special case. Because the tarsal plates lie immediately beneath the skin surface, lacerations over a few millimeters in length require complex multilayered closure that includes separate repair of the tarsal plate. Moreover, the lid margins must be aligned precisely or the result will be a cosmetically unacceptable notch or step-off of the lid margin.

Laceration of the lid margin between the lacrimal puncta and the medial canthus is another special case. The lacrimal canaliculi lie just 1 mm beneath the lid margin. Transection of a canaliculus requires a complex repair that is usually performed under the operating microscope.

Corneal Lacerations

Lacerations of the cornea are usually self-evident. Great caution must be taken to prevent any pressure on the lids, lest the contents of the globe be forced out between the margins of the wound. No effort should be made to force the eyelids apart to examine the eye, since this may exert pressure on the underlying globe.

Commonly, a knuckle of iris will prolapse through the wound and will be seen as a filamentous black extrusion. However, small perforations of the cornea may not be evident even on slit-lamp examination. Application of sterile fluorescein to the area, Seidel's test, will stain leaking aqueous a bright green under cobalt blue illumination. As with other intraocular injuries, children are often markedly lethargic after sustaining a corneal laceration.

Treatment consists of protecting the eye from pressure with a rigid shield, administration of systemic antibiotics, and definitive surgical repair.

Intraocular Foreign Bodies

Small, high-speed projectiles may enter the eye with little or no pain, and the actual injury may pass unnoticed. In childhood the foreign body is often a BB or pellet fired from an air rifle. A history of dull eye pain and blurred vision occurring hours or even days after the incident may be the only indication of injury.

Examination under magnification with bright illumination will usually locate the site of entry. Slit-lamp or funduscopic examination may reveal the location of the foreign body, although radiographs of the orbit using Sweet's method or the Comberg contact lens may be necessary to localize the foreign body. Precise localization is best accomplished with a CT scan or ultrasonography of the orbit.

Treatment is determined by the composition of the foreign body. Copper and iron foreign bodies decompose and must be removed, as they later produce intraocular inflammation (chalcosis and siderosis, respectively). Inert material (glass, porcelain, and so forth) is usually well tolerated and is best left untreated.

CHEMICAL EYE INJURIES

Alkali Burns

Lye burns are the most serious chemical eye injuries. The initial injury is immediately painful. Untreated, the alkali penetrates deep into ocular tissues, where it remains as a constant source of alkali, producing a liquefaction necrosis as it progresses. Epithelium is destroyed, blood vessels are coagulated, and mucus- and lipid-secreting elements of the conjunctiva and skin are lost. Glaucoma and uveitis develop rapidly. The end result is deep scarring of the conjunctiva and cornea and a blind eye.

Early copious irrigation is the treatment. Sedation, topical anesthesia, and even local anesthetic injections (to paralyze the eyelids to eliminate blepharospasm) may be necessary for adequate irrigation.

Irrigation can be performed with sterile normal saline solution and intravenous tubing. Once irrigation has begun, cotton-tipped applicators and forceps may be used to remove particulate matter. As irrigation progresses, the conjunctival pH should be checked with indicator paper. Even when a pH of approximately 7 has been attained, the pH should be rechecked frequently, as alkali may continue to leach from the ocular tissues. These same irrigation principles apply to other chemical eye injuries.

Once irrigation is well under way, emergency consultation

and hospital admission are indicated. Treatment consists of cycloplegia, topical steroids, and glaucoma medications.

Acid Burns

Acid burns of the eye, while potentially serious, are usually less severe than alkali burns. Acid burns produce local coagulation that limits penetration and buffers the pH of the acid.

Like alkali burns, acid burns are immediately painful, and prompt copious irrigation is required. Once the conjunctival pH has stabilized, reassessment will often reveal only superficial injury. These patients may require only topical antibiotics and reevaluation within 24 hours.

Hydrocarbon and Perfume Injury

Hydrocarbons and perfumes produce prompt irritation and deep injection of the conjunctival vessels. Prompt irrigation is indicated. Although these injuries are generally self-limiting, inflammation may persist for several days. Topical antibiotics and steroids may be required to reduce inflammation.

Selected References

Cinotti AA. Handbook of Ophthalmologic Emergencies. 3rd ed. New York, Elsevier, 1985, p 167.

Duke-Elder S. System of Ophthalmology, The Anatomy of the Visual System. Vol. II. St. Louis, C. V. Mosby, 1961.

Newell FW. Ophthalmology: Principles and Concepts. 6th ed. St. Louis, C. V. Mosby, 1986, p 215.

Ragge NK, Easty DL. Immediate Eye Care: An Illustrated Manual. St. Louis, Mosby–Year Book, 1991, p 231.

Read JE. Blunt trauma to the eye. *In* Wilensky JT, Read JE (eds): Primary Ophthalmology. Orlando, Grune & Stratton, 1984, p 68.

Scheie HG, Albert DM. Textbook of Ophthalmology. 9th ed. Philadelphia, WB Saunders, 1977, p 571.

Vaughan D, Asbury T, Tabbara KF: General Ophthalmology. 12th ed. East Norwalk, CT, Appleton & Lange, 1989, p 333.

SECTION TWELVE

Toxicology

CHAPTER 82

Poisoning in Children

Mark A. Kirk
Christian Tomaszewski
Ken Kulig

INTRODUCTION

Children under the age of 6 years represented 60% of the 1.6 million poisonings reported to the American Association of Poison Control Centers (AAPCC) in 1989.[1] The majority occurred in toddlers. There were 24 deaths and 6168 cases, resulting in moderate to major adverse medical outcomes.[1]

Most poisonings in children occur in the home and involve ingestions of common household products (Table 82–1). Less common are exposures to toxins by inhalation or by the dermal and ocular routes. In adolescents, intravenous drugs should be considered as a source of poisoning. Although most exposures are accidental before the age of 6 years, suicidal ingestions have been reported in children as young as 5 years.[1–4] Because a history of exposure to toxins is often absent or unclear, one should suspect poisoning in any case of psychosis, coma, seizures, dysrhythmias, metabolic acidosis, fire, or trauma.

Appropriate medical intervention in childhood toxic exposures requires identification of the products involved and determination of their toxicity. Children often respond differently than adults respond to the same toxin. For example, young children are relatively resistant to acute acetamino-

phen toxicity[5] but are more susceptible to lead intoxication than are adults.[6]

EMERGENCY MEDICAL SERVICE (EMS)

A poisoned child's outcome may be strongly influenced by the Emergency Medical Service (EMS) response. Assessment and treatment of poisoned patients can be difficult; asymptomatic patients require treatment decisions based on anticipation of toxicity. The safest approach to a poisoned patient is to assume the worst; deterioration may occur rapidly.

Naloxone and glucose are administered to all patients with altered mental status. Rapid identification and correction of hypoxia, hypovolemia, hypoglycemia, and hypothermia decrease morbidity. A rapid evaluation of the patient includes assessment of vital signs, pupil size and reactivity, and level of consciousness. The scene is searched for important historical evidence, such as pill bottles and empty containers. Any suspicious containers are brought to the emergency department (ED).

Preventing toxin absorption may involve skin decontamination, oral dilution, or administration of ipecac. For example, organophosphates will continue to be absorbed through the skin if allowed to remain in contact. In addition, contamination of health care providers may result in toxicity. Decontamination, including removal of all clothing and irrigation with soap and water, must be performed prior to transport. In the case of caustic ingestions, dilution therapy may be instituted with small amounts of milk or water given orally. The ideal prehospital procedure for gastrointestinal decontamination is controversial. Prehospital care providers need to be familiar with common antidotes and specific therapy for common toxins. Protocols are especially useful for toxin-induced seizures, hypotension, hypertension, cardiac arrhythmias, and coma. Decisions not to treat or transport a patient for ED evaluation need to be made with the assistance of a regional poison center or the medical control hospital. All suicidal patients, regardless of how trivial the ingestion, need to be transported to the hospital for both medical and psychiatric evaluation.

INITIAL EMERGENCY MANAGEMENT

Failure to appreciate the potential for serious toxicity is a major error in the management of the poisoned patient. The emergency physician should initially assume the worst-case scenario and anticipate rapid deterioration. In an acute toxic ingestion there is a variable amount of time that one can expect before symptoms of toxicity occur. An important goal of therapy in this asymptomatic period is to reduce or prevent toxicity by gastrointestinal decontamination.[7] One must anticipate potential complications and develop an early treatment plan. Once toxicity develops, supportive care is provided with careful attention to correcting hypoxia, hy-

---

TABLE 82–1
MOST COMMON TOXIC EXPOSURES REPORTED IN CHILDREN IN DECREASING ORDER OF FREQUENCY

1. Analgesics (acetaminophen, aspirin, ibuprofen, narcotics)
2. Cleaning agents
3. Plants
4. Cough and cold preparations
5. Vitamins
6. Alcohols (ethanol, isopropanol)
7. Hydrocarbons (gasoline)
8. Lead
9. Carbon monoxide

povolemia, hypoglycemia, and hypothermia. Prevention of further absorption of toxin should be continuously addressed.

Airway. Securing a patent airway and ensuring oxygenation take precedence in patient management. Because toxins may rapidly alter mental status, early endotracheal intubation may be performed to prevent aspiration. Patients requiring intubation may be lethargic yet responsive, making an atraumatic intubation difficult. The use of pharmacologic agents for rapid-sequence induction is generally safe. However, prolonged paralysis was reported when succinylcholine was administered to an organophosphate-poisoned patient.[8] Atropine, used commonly in rapid-sequence intubation in children, may have an additive effect in anticholinergic poisoning. Long-acting paralytic agents eliminate the ability to identify motor seizure activity; therefore, these agents are avoided in patients poisoned with seizure-inducing toxins. The endotracheal tube can be used for emergent administration of several drugs: *Naloxone, Atropine, Valium, Epinephrine,* and *Lidocaine* (NAVEL).[9] However, diazepam (Valium) can increase the incidence of bronchopneumonia when administered endotracheally.[10]

Hypotension. Virtually any toxin can affect cardiovascular function. All patients with a history of potentially serious ingestion should be placed on a cardiac monitor. Vascular access should be obtained early by peripheral intravenous, central intravenous, or intraosseous lines.[11, 12] The mechanism of toxin-induced hypotension may be any combination of decreased myocardial contractility, dysrhythmias, or peripheral vasodilatation.[13] Contractility is optimized by correcting acidosis and ensuring oxygen delivery. Dysrhythmias are treated with standard ACLS drugs. Volume replacement begins with 10 to 20 ml/kg boluses of crystalloid solution.[14] Large volumes of fluid may be required in poisonings by iron and rattlesnake envenomation. After fluid boluses, vasopressors may be required to treat hypotension. The usual agent in these cases is dopamine; however, norepinephrine (Levophed) is more appropriate for toxins that block the reuptake of norepinephrine, such as amphetamines and cyclic antidepressants.[13]

Central Nervous System (CNS) Abnormalities. Coma and seizures are common CNS manifestations of serious toxicity. Naloxone should be given. Though some references recommend 0.1 mg/kg, an initial dose of 2 mg intravenous, intraosseous, or endotracheal is safe. In fact, some opiates require much higher doses.[15, 16] Dextrose (2 to 4 ml/kg of 25% dextrose if <3 years and 1 to 2 ml/kg of 50% dextrose if >3 years) should be administered empirically to any patient with an altered mental status. Administration of benzodiazepines, phenytoin, and barbiturates should be considered in toxin-induced seizures. Additionally, early paralysis in status epilepticus may prevent complications such as hyperthermia, rhabdomyolysis, metabolic acidosis, and cardiovascular collapse.

PREVENTING ABSORPTION

Preventing further toxin absorption is an essential part of early management of both symptomatic and asymptomatic poisoned patients. One should irrigate with copious amounts of water to decontaminate the skin and eyes. Early gastrointestinal decontamination may prevent systemic absorption of ingested toxins. Gastric decontamination may be accomplished by gastric evacuation, administration of activated charcoal, cathartic administration, or a combination of the above.

Ipecac. Ipecac is effective in inducing emesis, although it is not always effective in preventing further toxin absorption. Ipecac induces vomiting by direct gastric irritation and by stimulating the chemoreceptor trigger zone of the CNS.[17] The mean time to emesis is 15 to 30 minutes after ipecac administration.[18–23] Corby demonstrated the recovery of 0% to 78% (mean 28%) of a magnesium hydroxide marker given prior to ipecac administration in children.[19] Several studies have reported variable results in the efficacy of ipecac in preventing toxin absorption.[24–29] There is extensive experience with syrup of ipecac, and it has a low risk of adverse effects. These effects include drowsiness, protracted vomiting, and diarrhea.[30, 31] Rarely reported severe complications include aspiration pneumonitis, pneumomediastinum, Mallory-Weiss tear, and gastric rupture.[32–36] Ipecac administration is contraindicated in obtunded or seizing patients and for ingestion of seizure-producing toxins (e.g., camphor, cyclic antidepressants, strychnine) and of caustics or hydrocarbons.

Gastric Lavage. Gastric lavage is an alternative to ipecac for gastric emptying. To effectively remove toxins, it is important to place the largest lavage tube that is safely possible. In children this may be a 24 to 28 French tube. Tap water or normal saline should be instilled in 15 ml/kg/cycle aliquots with careful attention to the output of fluid from the tube. Close monitoring of input and output may prevent the development of electrolyte aberrations.[37] Placing the patient in the left lateral decubitus Trendelenburg position may help prevent aspiration. Anyone with altered or rapidly changing mental status should have the airway protected by endotracheal intubation prior to lavage. Complications of gastric lavage include aspiration pneumonia, esophageal perforation, laryngospasm, arrhythmias, and charcoal empyema.[38–40] An unprotected airway in a patient with an altered mental status or ingestion of caustics is a contraindication to gastric lavage.

The limiting factor in the efficacy of gastric lavage, especially in children, is the size of the orogastric tube, because many ingested pills may be too large to pass through the tube's opening.[41, 42] Watson demonstrated less than 10% recovery of the estimated ingested drug when looking at adult patients who had overdosed on cyclic antidepressants and been treated with aggressive gastric lavage techniques.[43] Older studies in animals and humans have shown lavage to have limited efficacy when compared with ipecac,[25, 44, 45] but these studies have been criticized for the use of small nasogastric tubes or failure to report the technique utilized.[46, 47] Later studies with large orogastric tubes have shown lavage to be superior to ipecac for gastric emptying in human adult volunteers.[48–50] The majority of investigators have not studied the efficacy of lavage in children. Gastric lavage is labor-intensive and may delay the administration of activated charcoal.[43] The procedure should not be viewed as the standard of care for all poisoned patients; it should be utilized only in selected patients, such as those presenting early after an ingestion of potentially life-threatening toxins.

Activated Charcoal. Activated charcoal (AC) has a large adsorptive surface area and has been demonstrated to bind a wide variety of substances.[51, 52] It is usually administered as a slurry in a dose of 1 gm/kg. Several additives, such as milk and flavored syrup, have been used in an attempt to make AC more palatable, with variable effects on flavor and adsorptive capacity.[53, 54]

Activated charcoal has been demonstrated to be superior to gastric emptying in preventing drug absorption. Volunteer studies using salicylate, ampicillin, cimetidine, pindolol, tilidine, acetaminophen, tetracycline, and aminophylline have demonstrated the superiority of AC in preventing drug absorption when compared with ipecac or lavage.[26, 27, 50, 55–57] In a simulated overdose of aspirin by adult volunteers, AC decreased absorption significantly more than did ipecac when each was given 60 minutes after drug ingestion.[27] In this study, ipecac followed by AC was less effective than AC alone. The latter is ineffective in binding acids and alkaline corrosives, lithium, iron, ethanol, and possibly petroleum distillates.[51] Although rare, adverse effects of AC administration include vomiting and gastrointestinal obstruction.[58, 59] Although AC has been implicated in aspiration pneumonitis, AC aspiration does not appear to be any worse than aspiration of the gastric content itself.[60-63]

Clinical Comparisons. Gastric evacuation procedures are not essential for the management of all poisoned patients.[32, 64, 65] In awake overdose patients, the administration of AC alone was found to be as effective as ipecac followed by AC when clinical outcomes only were examined. Activated charcoal alone was also found to be as effective as gastric lavage followed by AC in obtunded patients, except in those presenting within 1 hour of ingestion.[64] An additional series of 476 patients showed no difference in clinical outcome between groups receiving gastric emptying procedures prior to AC administration versus AC alone.[65] A prospective evaluation of 200 acute oral ingestions showed an increased incidence of complications in the ipecac-charcoal group (5.4%) as compared with the AC-only group (0.9%). The authors concluded that AC alone was the treatment of choice in the majority of acutely poisoned patients.[32] Both the administration of ipecac, resulting in prolonged emesis, and the labor-intensive procedure of gastric lavage have been demonstrated to delay AC administration.[43, 64]

Recommendations. The approach to preventing toxin absorption in the poisoned child remains a clinical decision based on multiple factors. Ipecac may have a role in the home treatment of poisonings, especially when AC is not immediately available. When faced with a life-threatening overdose in either a symptomatic or an asymptomatic patient, AC should be considered the treatment of choice. The decision to use gastric lavage should take into account the time since ingestion, toxicity of the ingestant, and risks versus benefits of the procedure.

Although sorbitol and magnesium cathartics are a part of poisoning management and have been for many years, clinical studies have not demonstrated that these agents prevent toxin absorption.[66] Multiple cases of adverse effects, especially fluid and electrolyte abnormalities in infants, have resulted from cathartic administration in poisoned patients.[67-73] Therefore, cathartics should be limited to the first dose of AC.

Considerations in Gastrointestinal Decontamination. Occasionally, routine gastrointestinal decontamination procedures may be ineffective or even dangerous. Lithium and iron are examples of toxins not readily absorbed by AC. By mechanical cleansing of the bowel with polyethylene glycol solutions, whole bowel irrigation (WBI) may prevent absorption. This method may be considered for ingestion of iron and lithium and for certain sustained-release preparations. No adverse effect, such as weight gain or electrolyte imbalance, has been reported when WBI is used for bowel cleansing prior to operative or endoscopic procedures.[74-77] Typical dose of a polyethylene glycol electrolyte solution (Golytely) for a child is 25 ml/kg/hour until the effluent is clear.[74] Data supporting its use in poisoned patients are derived from case reports and volunteer studies comparing it with AC.[76, 78, 79] Until further studies in the poisoned patient can be analyzed, this technique should be used with caution.

In addition, routine gastrointestinal procedures are dangerous in the treatment of corrosive ingestions. In this case, dilution therapy with cold milk or water has been recommended. Treatment of caustic ingestions should avoid the accidental induction of vomiting; therefore, only small volumes of fluid (no more than 4 ounces) should be administered.[80] Neutralization should not be attempted, as this may produce an exothermic reaction resulting in further tissue damage.[81-83]

CLINICAL EVALUATION

History. Once initial stabilization and decontamination of the patient have been completed, one must obtain a relevant toxicology history. Identification of the ingestant by examining the label is essential. Identifying the toxin involved may be as simple as examining the container brought with the patient or as involved as sending someone to the scene for an intensive search. If the container is unlabeled, noting the typical use of the product may help in determining the potential toxins ingested. A large proportion of inadvertently ingested prescription drugs belong to someone other than the immediate family. These are often located outside their usual storage location in non–child-resistant containers.[84] Because of this, the family should give an inventory of all medications (prescription and over-the-counter) and chemicals stored in the home. Additionally, a detailed history with respect to parental employment and hobbies may reveal access to industrial hazards, such as heavy metals or solvents.

Once the substance to which the child has been exposed is identified, along with its toxicity, one must assess the potential amount ingested. For most toxins, it is the degree of exposure that determines whether one will manifest toxicity. Although it is best to assume a worst-case scenario, an attempt to accurately assess the amount may prevent unnecessary treatment or hospitalization. For any medication or toxin for which the volume of distribution (V_d) is known, the theoretical peak plasma concentration can be calculated with the following equation:

$$\text{Peak plasma concentration (mg/L or } \mu\text{g/ml)} = \frac{\text{Amount ingested (mg)}}{V_d \text{ (L/kg)} \times \text{child's weight (kg)}}$$

The amount ingested can often be gauged from the amount of liquid or number of pills missing from the container. This equation may overestimate final plasma levels because it assumes instantaneous absorption, but it may underestimate if the history of the amount of toxin ingested is inaccurately low. For drugs and toxins with known toxic levels, this calculation can be used to predict toxicity from the ingestion.

Additional useful history includes the time and events since the exposure to the toxin. For most toxins, a child will manifest symptoms of toxicity within several hours after ingestion. The delay can be up to 24 hours in the case of colchicine or oral hypoglycemic agents and up to days in the case of thyroxin or long-acting anticoagulants. The time of ingestion may also be important in determining the urgency of treatment.

Physical Examination. A directed examination focusing on vital signs (including core temperature) as well as the respiratory, cardiovascular, nervous, and dermal systems may provide the most important clues. A complete set of vital signs is essential in every case. Abnormal vital signs may be the only clue that the child is beginning to show toxic effects as well as the only clue suggesting the nature of the exposure (Table 82–2). Beyond simple changes in heart rate, dysrhythmias can result from medications such as cyclic antidepressants, cardiac medications, and sympathomimetics. The odors on the patient's skin, breath, and vomit may also provide helpful clues. Even the skin provides clues of toxicity, such as cyanosis in methemoglobinemia and a dry, flushed appearance in anticholinergic poisoning.

Another most useful aspect of the physical examination in poisoned patients is the neurologic assessment. A variety of toxins can cause characteristic changes in the pupils (Table

TABLE 82-2

EXAMPLES OF THE VITAL SIGN CHANGES COMMONLY ASSOCIATED WITH VARIOUS TOXINS

Temperature

Hypothermia	*Hyperthermia*
Barbiturates	Anticholinergics
Ethanol	Hallucinogens
Narcotics	MAO inhibitors
Phenothiazines	Salicylates
Sedative-hypnotics	Sympathomimetics

Heart Rate

Bradycardia	*Tachycardia*
Beta blockers	Anticholinergics
Calcium channel blockers	Ethanol
Clonidine	Methylxanthines
Cyanide	Sympathomimetics
Digitalis	Cyclic antidepressants
Organophosphates	Organophosphates
Sedative-hypnotics	

Blood Pressure

Hypotension	*Hypertension*
Antihypertensives	Amphetamines
Beta blockers	Anticholinergics
Calcium channel blockers	Methylxanthines
Iron	Phencyclidine
Narcotics	Sympathomimetics
Sedative-hypnotics	
Tricyclic antidepressants	

Respiratory Rate

Hypoventilation	*Hyperventilation*
Clonidine	Acidosis-inducing drugs (e.g., methanol, ethylene glycol)
Narcotics	
Organophosphates	Carbon monoxide
Sedative-hypnotics	Cyanide
Cyclic antidepressants	Methylxanthines
	Salicylates
	Sympathomimetics

TABLE 82-3

PUPIL CHANGES ASSOCIATED WITH SOME TOXINS AND DRUGS

Miosis	Mydriasis
Barbiturates	Antihistamines
Benzodiazepines	Atropine
Clonidine	Belladonna alkaloids
Ethanol	Glutethimide
Narcotics	LSD
Nicotine	Meperidine
Organophosphates	Phenothiazines
	Cyclic antidepressants

82–3). Additionally, nystagmus can be seen with sedative-hypnotics, ethanol, phencyclidine, and anticonvulsants such as phenytoin and carbamazepine. A large number of drugs can cause seizures or a decline in mental status (Table 82–4). Seizures from theophylline or isoniazid may be severe and resistant to conventional treatment.

The positive findings of the physical examination may form a classic toxidrome (Table 82–5). However, children may have different presentations from the toxidromes traditionally described in adults. For example, young children exposed to organophosphates present with CNS depression more frequently than with the classic peripheral muscarinic effects seen in adults.[85] Additionally, during the physical examination potential complications such as aspiration pneumonia or a paralytic ileus must be excluded.

DIAGNOSTIC EVALUATION

General Laboratory Studies. The laboratory's main role in the management of poisoned patients is to confirm the suspected diagnosis. Measurement of electrolytes and arterial blood gas can confirm the acidosis seen with salicylates, iron, methanol, ethylene glycol, carbon monoxide, or cyanide. Additionally, a blood gas value can help one assess the adequacy of ventilation in a comatose patient. With a co-oximeter, the blood gas value can also provide carboxyhemoglobin levels in smoke inhalation victims and methemoglobin levels in patients exposed to oxidizing agents (e.g., volatile nitrites, naphthalene, local anesthetics, or antimalarials).

In addition to aiding in the detection of a metabolic

acidosis, measuring electrolytes, glucose, and blood urea nitrogen (BUN) can provide other useful information. For example, an acute digoxin overdose can result in hyperkalemia; theophylline, in hypokalemia. Oral hypoglycemic agents and ethanol can cause hypoglycemia; isoniazid and calcium channel blockers can cause hyperglycemia. A serum osmolality can also be calculated: $2(Na) + glucose/18 + BUN/2.8$. This is compared with the measured serum osmolality, performed by the more accurate freezing point depression rather than vapor pressure change.[86] A measured osmolality greater than a calculated osmolality implies the presence of another osmotically active agent, such as ethylene glycol, methanol, isopropanol, or acetone.[87, 88]

Another useful measurement is the anion gap, which can alert the physician to the presence of unmeasured anions. A gap, $[Na - (Cl + HCO_3)]$, greater than 12 mEq/L can suggest poisoning by such agents as ethylene glycol, methanol, salicylates, or iron.[87, 89, 90] Although an elevated anion gap can be a useful clue, its absence does not exclude a significant ingestion, especially if the patient presents early. Additionally, a severe toxic acidosis can exist without the presence of an anion gap.

Renal and liver function tests are less useful acutely, serving more as a baseline. Any of the nonsteroidal agents can cause delayed, but usually temporary, renal dysfunction.[91] Furthermore, there are a variety of substances that cause delayed hepatotoxicity, including acetaminophen, carbon tetrachloride, and amatoxin.

Hematologic tests are rarely useful acutely. A blood count may aid diagnosis after exposure to toxins known to cause acute hemolysis, such as arsine and rattlesnake venom, or chronic anemia as in lead poisoning. As a baseline, a complete blood count (CBC) can be useful in identifying toxins known to cause bone marrow suppression, such as benzene and chloramphenicol. The coagulation profile can be helpful after exposure to known anticoagulants or direct liver toxins, e.g., salicylates and acetaminophen.

TABLE 82-4

SOME TOXINS THAT COMMONLY CAUSE SEIZURES

C	A	P
Caffeine and theophylline	Amphetamines and sympathomimetics	Phencyclidine (PCP)
Camphor	Anticholinergics	Phenol
Cicutoxin (water hemlock)	Antidepressants, cyclic	Propoxyphene
Also beta-blockers, hypoglycemic agents, isoniazid, lead, lithium, local anesthetics, methylxanthines, and others.		

Modified with permission from Barkin RM, Kulig K, Rumack BH. Poisoning and overdose. In Barkin RM, Rosen P (eds). Emergency Pediatrics. 3rd ed. St. Louis, CV Mosby, 1990.

			TABLE 82–5			
			TOXIDROMES			
Syndrome	Example	Vital Sign Changes	Pupils	CNS	Skin	Other
Opiate	Narcotics	↓ R, ↓ BP	C	Coma	—	—
Cholinergic	Organophosphates	↑ HR	C	Delirium Coma	Diaphoresis	Salivation Lacrimation Urination Diarrhea GI upset Emesis Fasciculations Weakness
Anticholinergic	Antihistamines Cyclic antidepressants Plants (belladonna alkaloids)	↑ HR, ↑ T ↑ BP	D	Delirium Coma	Dry, flushed	Decreased bowel sounds Urinary retention Decreased vision
Sympathomimetic	Cocaine Methylxanthines	↑ BP, ↑ HR	D	Agitation Hallucinations	—	May have reflex bradycardia with pure alpha effect

Key
Vital Signs: ↓, decreased; ↑, increased; R, respirations; HR, heart rate; BP, blood pressure; T, temperature.
Pupils: C, constricted; D, dilated.

Urinalysis may be helpful in the diagnosis as well as treatment of a poisoned patient. The presence of hemoglobin in the urine suggests drug-induced hemolysis, which can be more common in someone with glucose-6-phosphate dehydrogenase (G6PD) deficiency. Myoglobin in the urine from rhabdomyolysis, such as in poisoning by cocaine or LSD, requires more than adequate hydration and renal output.[92] The presence of calcium oxalate crystals in the urine may confirm an ethylene glycol ingestion.[93] Finally, the pH of the urine is important if one plans urine alkalinization to enhance removal of salicylates or long-acting barbiturates.

An EKG can be extremely useful, especially after ingestions of cardiac medications. Toxin-induced heart block, such as from digoxin or calcium channel blockers, may be manifested first in the EKG. Also, by examining the QRS axis and duration and checking for other conduction disturbances, one can diagnose and assess cardiotoxicity from cyclic antidepressants.[94, 95]

A variety of toxins are known to be radiopaque (Table 82–6). Thus, an abdominal radiograph is a useful tool in confirming the toxic exposure and assessing the efficacy of gastric decontamination procedures (Fig. 82–1). Additionally, radiographs of the chest are useful for diagnosing other poisoning complications: aspiration pneumonia from hydrocarbon ingestions, or pulmonary edema from an irritant gas such as chlorine.

Toxicology Screens. Toxicology screens can be a useful adjunct in confirming an ingestion of a particular toxin or in resolving discrepancies between history, physical examination, and laboratory data. Rarely will the screen identify a toxin that was not initially suspected on the basis of a careful history and physical examination such that changes in treatment are made. The most commonly used qualitative screen involves testing urine for several commonly found drugs.[96] However, the absence of a drug may simply reflect its absence from the testing battery. In contrast to qualitative urine screens, quantification of a drug or toxin usually requires serum rather than urine for analysis. Such quantification is essential when the level may influence subsequent treatment. This would include acetaminophen, salicylates, carbon monoxide, digoxin, ethylene glycol, iron, methanol, lithium, and theophylline. In contrast to urine and serum screens, gastric samples are no longer routinely used because of their poor sensitivity.[97] Unfortunately, in less than 5% of poisoning cases do the results of a "comprehensive," and therefore nonspecific, toxicology screen influence patient management.[97–99] However, one might still want to consider comprehensive screens, urine or serum, or both, in seriously ill patients (e.g., comatose or seizing) or confusing cases that do not fit any particular toxidrome. Serum tests should be considered for those toxins whose levels influence subsequent treatment. Nonetheless, regardless of what drug testing is available, toxicology screens cannot replace a good history and physical examination and rarely, if ever, alter the treatment plan for the patient.

ENHANCED ELIMINATION AND ANTIDOTES
Enhanced Elimination

After stabilization and decontamination, additional treatment may be directed at enhanced elimination of some toxins. The safest and most easily performed method is the administration of multiple doses of AC, which can remove agents even after they are absorbed into the blood stream. This is through the phenomenon called gastrointestinal dialysis.[51] The agents are bound to the charcoal in the gut lumen, making them unavailable for reabsorption into the circulation (Table 82–7). Such treatment has been used safely and efficaciously in infants as young as 6 weeks.[100] One should avoid repetitive doses of AC premixed with sorbitol because of the dangers of inducing electrolyte imbalances, especially in infants.[68, 101]

Another method for increased elimination in the case of

TABLE 82–6
COMMON RADIOPAQUE INGESTANTS
Chloral hydrate
Chlorinated hydrocarbons
Heavy metals (e.g., arsenic, lead, mercury)
Iodides, iron
Potassium
Some psychotropics (e.g., phenothiazines, cyclic antidepressants)

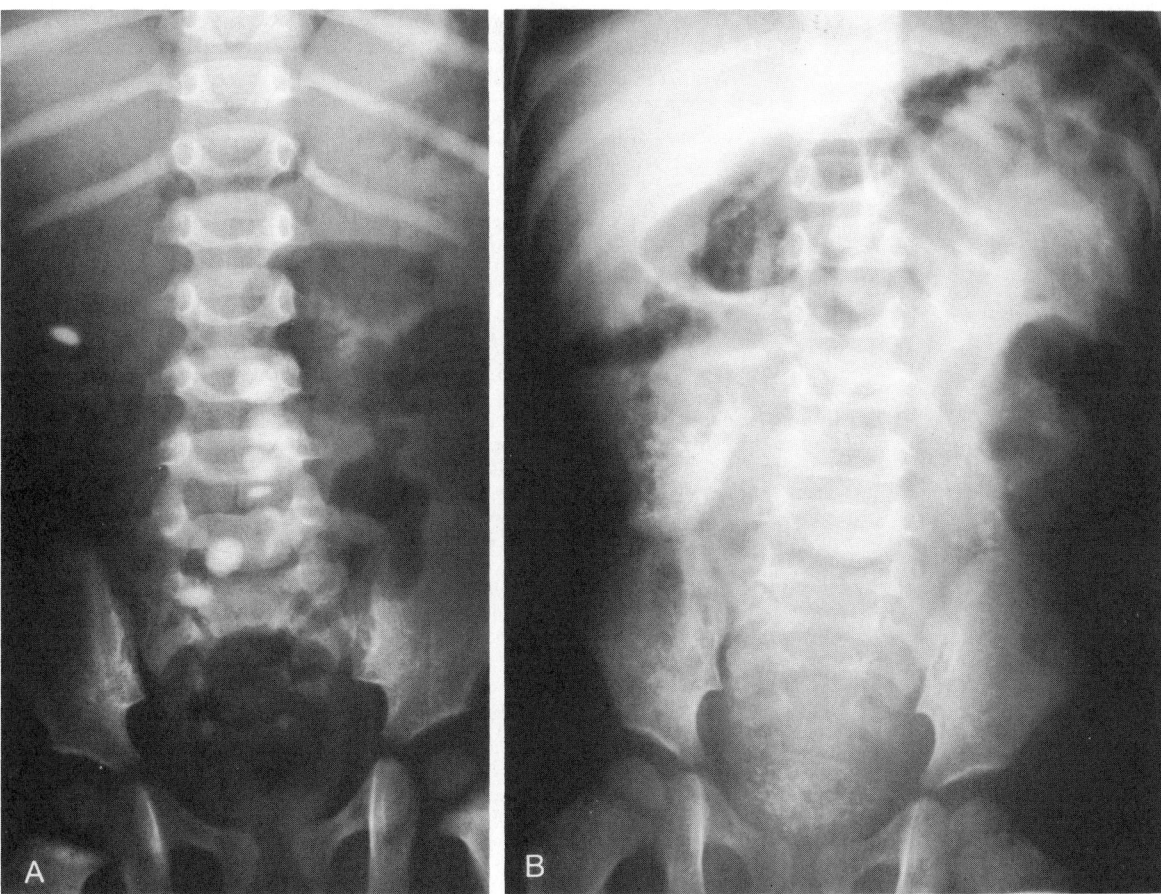

Figure 82–1. *A,* This 1½-year-old infant ingested iron pills (from the kitchen), seen as multiple dense tablets in various orientations in the bowel. *B,* This 2-year-old shows multiple speckled densities of dissolved iron-containing tablets throughout the colon (from a bottle of vitamins). Fortunately, neither child had more severe effects than vomiting from the single event. (Courtesy of A. Oestreich, M.D., Cincinnati, OH.)

phenobarbital and salicylates is alkalinization of the urine, typically to a pH of 7.5 or greater. Acidification of the urine, in the case of amphetamines or phencyclidine, is no longer recommended because of the danger of myoglobin-mediated renal toxicity.[102] Finally, an invasive way to enhance drug removal is with dialysis. This is very effective in the case of alcohols, ethylene glycol, salicylates, lithium, and theophylline.[103] Dialysis should be based on the total clinical picture rather than drug levels alone. However, dialysis is not entirely risk-free. In addition, it may be difficult to perform in neonates. Unfortunately, peritoneal dialysis is not as efficacious. A more controversial procedure indicated in some of the same poisons is charcoal hemoperfusion, which is rarely used in children.

Antidotes. Antidotes, although extremely useful when indicated, are usually an adjunct and not a replacement for good supportive care. Compared with the number of potential toxins to which a child might be exposed, there are few antidotes (Table 82–8). Some, like oxygen, naloxone, and atropine, are available on most prehospital vehicles and in physicians' offices. Others, like crotalid antivenin and intravenous 10% ethanol, may be more difficult to locate in adequate amounts. One problem with some antidotes is that they may improve the clinical picture temporarily, providing false assurance without correcting the underlying problem.

DISPOSITION

Any symptomatic poisoned patient is considered for admission to the intensive care unit (ICU). One study showed that poisoned pediatric patients who were seriously ill and were admitted to a pediatric ICU usually recovered without permanent sequelae and had a mortality of less than 1%.[104] Although this is not true in every case, patients who have ingested certain potentially serious toxins without exhibiting any symptoms may be observed for 6 hours and then discharged. Certain toxins have delayed toxicity, and in some cases the toxicity is not well established in humans; therefore, a longer observation period may be necessary to assure the absence of toxicity. Poison prevention educational materials should be presented prior to discharge, as parents may be more receptive to instruction after a child has been brought to the emergency department with an accidental ingestion.

TABLE 82–7	
METHODS OF ENHANCED ELIMINATION WITH EXAMPLES	
Multiple-Dose Activated Charcoal	**Urine Alkalinization**
Amitriptyline	Phenobarbital
Carbamazepine	Salicylates
Digoxin	**Hemoperfusion/Hemodialysis**
Phenobarbital	Methanol/ethylene glycol
Phenytoin	Salicylates
Salicylates	Lithium
Theophylline	Phenobarbital
	Theophylline

TABLE 82–8

ANTIDOTES USED IN TOXICOLOGY

Toxin	Antidote	Pediatric Dosage
Acetaminophen	N-Acetylcysteine	*Load:* 140 mg/kg (po or IV*)
		Main: 70 mg/kg × 17 doses
Anticholinergic	Physostigmine	0.02–0.06 mg/kg up to 0.5 mg slowly IV (over 5–10 min)
Alcohols	Ethanol	*Load:* 10 ml/kg of 10% ethanol in glucose solution
Methanol		*Main:* 1.5 ml/kg/hr of 10% ethanol to obtain blood ethanol
Ethylene glycol		level of 100 mg/dl
	4-Methylpyrazole*	Not established in children
Benzodiazepines	Flumazenil	Not established in children
Carbon monoxide	Oxygen	100% by tight-fitting mask or hyperbaric oxygen
Cyanide	Sodium nitrite	0.33 ml/kg of 3% IV
	Sodium thiosulfate	1.65 ml/kg of 25% IV
	Hydroxycobalamin*	Not established in children
Digoxin	Digoxin-specific antibodies (Fab) fragments	Dose determined by estimating body burden—one vial of Fab (40 mg) neutralizes 0.6 mg digoxin
Envenomation	Antivenin	
Rattlesnake		Dose based on degree of envenomation: administered in five-vial increments
Coral snake		
Black widow spider		
Iron	Deferoxamine	Begin at 15 mg/kg/hr; monitor for hypotension during infusion
Isoniazid (INH)	Pyridoxine (vitamin B$_6$)	1 mg per 1 mg of INH ingested
Methemoglobin inducers (e.g., nitrites)	Methylene blue	1–2 mg/kg of 1% solution IV (10 mg/ml)
Narcotics	Naloxone	2 mg given by IV, ET, SC, or intraosseous route
Organophosphates	Atropine	0.05 mg/kg; may repeat until dried secretions or full atropinization
	Pralidoxime (2-PAM)	25–50 mg/kg IV up to 2 gm q 6 hours

*Drug currently under investigation for clinical use.

An accidental ingestion also raises suspicion of child abuse or child neglect and, if suspected, necessitates a social service referral.[105–108] All patients with intentional suicidal ingestions are referred for psychiatric evaluation.[109, 110]

References

1. Litovitz TL, Schmitz BF, Bailey KM. 1989 Annual Report of the American Association of Poison Control Centers National Data Collection System. Am J Emerg Med 1990;8:394.
2. Toolan JM. Suicide in children and adolescents. Am J Psychother 1975;29:339.
3. Copeland AR. Childhood suicide: A report of four cases. J Forensic Sci 1985;30:965.
4. McIntyre MS, Angle CR. The adolescent overdose. Evaluation and referral. Emerg Med Clin North Am 1984;2:175.
5. Rumack BH. Acetaminophen overdose in young children. Am J Dis Child 1984;238:428.
6. Needleman HL, Schell A, Bellinger A, et al. The long-term effects of exposure to low doses of lead in childhood: An 11-year follow-up report. N Engl J Med 1990;322:83.
7. Spyker DA, Minocha A. Toxicodynamic approach to management of the poisoned patient. J Emerg Med 1988;6:117.
8. Selden BS, Curry SC. Prolonged succinylcholine-induced paralysis in organophosphate insecticide poisoning. Ann Emerg Med 1987;16:215.
9. Ward JT. Endotracheal drug therapy. Am J Emerg Med 1983;1:71.
10. Rusli M, Spivey WH, Bonner H, et al. Pathologic effects of endotracheal diazepam in cats. Ann Emerg Med 1986;15:644.
11. McNamara RM, Spivey WH, Unger HD, Malone DR. Emergency applications of intraosseous infusion. J Emerg Med 1987;5:97.
12. Orlowski JP, Porembka DT, Gallagher JM, et al. Comparison study of intraosseous, central intravenous, and peripheral intravenous infusions of emergency drugs. Am J Dis Child 1990;144:112.
13. Benowitz NL, Rosenberg J, Becker CE. Cardiopulmonary catastrophes in drug-overdosed patients. Med Clin North Am 1979;63:267.
14. Perkin RM, Levin DL. Shock in the pediatric patient. Part II. Therapy. J Pediatr 1982;101:319.
15. Goldfrank L. Opioids/opioid antagonist. *In* Rumack BH (ed). POISINDEX Information System. Denver, Micromedex, Inc., 1990 (edition expires 5/31/90).
16. American Academy of Pediatrics, Committee on Drugs. Emergency drug doses for infants and children and naloxone use in newborns: Clarification. Pediatrics 1989;83:803.
17. Moran DM, Crouch DJ, Finkle BS. Absorption of ipecac alkaloids in emergency patients. Ann Emerg Med 1984;13:1100.
18. Rodgers GC, Matyunas NJ. Gastrointestinal decontamination for acute poisoning. Pediatr Clin North Am 1986;33:261.
19. Corby DG, Decker WJ, Moran MJ, Payne CE. Clinical comparison of pharmacologic emetics in children. Pediatrics 1968;42:361.
20. Robertson WO. Syrup of ipecac—a slow or fast emetic? Am J Dis Child 1962;103:136.
21. Litovitz TL, Klein-Schwartz W, Oderda GM, et al. Ipecac administration in children under one year of age. Pediatrics 1985;76:761.
22. Manoguerra AS, Krenzelok EP. Rapid emesis from high-dose ipecac syrup in adults and children intoxicated with antiemetics or other drugs. Am J Hosp Pharm 1978;35:1360.
23. Krenzelok EP, Dean BS. Syrup of ipecac failures: A two-year review of 4306 patients (abstract). Vet Hum Toxicol 1984;26:413.
24. Levy G, Yaffe SJ. The study of salicylate pharmacokinetics in intoxicated infants and children. Clin Toxicol 1969;1:409.
25. Abdallah AH, Tye A. A comparison of the efficacy of emetic drugs and stomach lavage. Am J Dis Child 1967;113:571.
26. Neuvonen PJ, Vartiainen M, Tokola O. Comparison of activated charcoal and ipecac syrup in prevention of drug absorption. Eur J Clin Pharmacol 1983;24:557.
27. Curtis RA, Barone J, Giacona N. Efficacy of ipecac and activated charcoal/cathartic: Prevention of salicylate absorption in a simulated overdose. Arch Intern Med 1984;144:48.
28. Amitai Y, Mitchell AA, McGuigan MA, Lovejoy FH. Ipecac-induced emesis and reduction of plasma concentrations of drugs following accidental overdose in children. Pediatrics 1987;80:364.
29. Bond GR, Norman SA, Tendler JD, et al. Influence of time until emesis on the efficacy of decontamination using acetaminophen as a marker in a pediatric population (abstract). Vet Hum Toxicol 1989;31:336.
30. Czajka PA, Russell SL. Nonemetic effects of ipecac syrup. Pediatrics 1985;75:1101.
31. Gaudreault P, McCormick MA, Lacouture PG, et al. Poisoning exposures and use of ipecac in children less than 1 year old. Ann Emerg Med 1986;15:808.
32. Albertson TE, Derlet RW, Foulke GE, et al. Superiority of activated charcoal alone compared with ipecac and activated charcoal in the treatment of acute toxic ingestions. Ann Emerg Med 1989;18:56.
33. Robertson WO. Syrup of ipecac associated fatality: A case report. Vet Hum Toxicol 1979;21:87.
34. Tandberg D, Liechty EJ, Fishbein D. Mallory-Weiss syndrome: An unusual complication of ipecac-induced emesis. Ann Emerg Med 1981;10:521.

35. Klein-Schwartz W, Gorman RL, Oderda GM, et al. Ipecac use in the elderly: The unanswered question. Ann Emerg Med 1984;13:1152.

36. Wolowodiuk LJ, McMicken DB, O'Brien P. Pneumomediastinum and retropneumoperitoneum: An unusual complication of syrup-of-ipecac-induced emesis. Ann Emerg Med 1984;13:1148.

37. Rudolph JP. Automated gastric lavage and a comparison of 0.9% normal saline solution and tap water irrigant. Ann Emerg Med 1985;14:1156.

38. Wald P, Stern J, Weiner B, Goldfrank L. Esophageal tear following forceful removal of an impacted oral-gastric lavage tube. Ann Emerg Med 1986;15:80.

39. Comstock EG, Faulker TP, Boisaubin EV, et al. Studies on the efficacy of gastric lavage as practiced in a large metropolitan hospital. Clin Toxicol 1981;18:581.

40. Thompson AM, Robins JB, Prescott LF. Changes in cardiorespiratory function during gastric lavage for drug overdose. Hum Toxicol 1987;6:215.

41. Fane LR, Combs HF, Decker WJ. Physical parameters in gastric lavage. Clin Toxicol 1971;4:389.

42. Agocha A, Reyman L, Longmore W, et al. Can pills really fit through the lavage tubes? (abstract). Vet Hum Toxicol 1986;28:494.

43. Watson WA, Leighton J, Guy J, et al. Recovery of cyclic antidepressants with gastric lavage. J Emerg Med 1989;7:373.

44. Boxer L, Anderson FP, Rowe DS. Comparison of ipecac-induced emesis with gastric lavage in the treatment of acute salicylate ingestion. J Pediatr 1969;74:800.

45. Arnold FJ, Hodges JB, Barta RA, et al. Evaluation of the efficacy of lavage and induced emesis in treatment of salicylate poisonings. Pediatrics 1959;23:286.

46. Kulig K. Interpreting gastric emptying studies. J Emerg Med 1984;1:447.

47. Litovitz TL. Emesis versus lavage for poisoning victims. Am J Emerg Med 1986;4:294.

48. Auerbach PS, Osterloh J, Braun O, et al. Efficacy of gastric emptying: gastric lavage versus emesis induced with ipecac. Ann Emerg Med 1986;15:692.

49. Tandberg D, Diven BG, McLeon JW. Ipecac-induced emesis versus gastric lavage. Am J Emerg Med 1986;4:205.

50. Tenenbein M, Cohen S, Sitar DS. Efficacy of ipecac-induced emesis, orogastric lavage, and activated charcoal for acute drug overdose. Ann Emerg Med 1987;16:838.

51. Neuvonen PJ, Olkkola KT. Oral activated charcoal in the treatment of intoxications: Role of single and repeated doses. Med Toxicol 1988;3:33.

52. Picchioni AL. Efficacy of activated charcoal. Vet Hum Toxicol 1983;25:452.

53. Navarro RP, Navarro KR, Krenzelok EP. Relative efficacy and palatability of three activated charcoal mixtures. Vet Hum Toxicol 1980;22:6.

54. Scholtz EC, Jaffe JM, Colaizzi JL. Evaluation of five activated charcoal formulations for inhibition of aspirin absorption and palatability in man. Am J Hosp Pharm 1978;35:1355.

55. McNamara RM, Aaron CK, Gemborys M, Davidheiser S. Efficacy of charcoal cathartic versus ipecac in reducing serum acetaminophen in a simulated overdose. Ann Emerg Med 1989;18:934.

56. Neuvonen PJ, Olkkola KT. Activated charcoal and syrup of ipecac in prevention of cimetidine and pindolol absorption in man after administration of metoclopramide as an antiemetic. Clin Toxicol 1984;22:103.

57. Cordonnier J, Van den Heede M, Hendricks A. Activated charcoal and ipecac syrup in prevention of tilidine absorption in man. Vet Hum Toxicol 1987;29:105.

58. Watson WA, Cremer KF, Chapman JA. Gastrointestinal obstruction associated with multiple-dose activated charcoal. J Emerg Med 1986;4:401.

59. Ray MJ, Padin DR, Condie JD, Halls JM. Charcoal bezoar: Small bowel obstruction secondary to amitryptyline overdose therapy. Dig Dis Sci 1988;33:106.

60. Pollack MM, Dunbar BS, Holbrook PR, Fields AI. Aspiration of activated charcoal and gastric contents. Ann Emerg Med 1981;10:528.

61. Menzies DG, Busuttil A, Prescott LF. Fatal pulmonary aspiration of oral activated charcoal. Br Med J 1988;297:459.

62. Harsch HH. Aspiration of activated charcoal. N Engl J Med 1986;314:318.

63. Elliot CG, Colby TV, Kelly TM, et al. Charcoal lung: Bronchiolitis obliterans after aspiration of activated charcoal. Chest 1989;96:672.

64. Kulig K, Bar-Or D, Cantrill SV, et al. Management of acutely poisoned patients without gastric emptying. Ann Emerg Med 1985;14:562.

65. Merigian KS, Woodard M, Hedges JR, et al. Prospective evaluation of gastric emptying in the self-poisoned patient. Am J Emerg Med 1990;8:479.

66. Riegel JM, Becker CE. Use of cathartics in toxic ingestions. Ann Emerg Med 1981;10:254.

67. Brent J, Kulig K, Rumack BH. Iatrogenic death from sorbitol and magnesium sulfate during treatment for salicylism (abstract). Vet Hum Toxicol 1989;31:334.

68. Farley TA. Severe hypernatremic dehydration after use of an activated charcoal–sorbitol suspension. J Pediatr 1986;109:719.

69. Jones J, Heiselman D, Dougherty J, Eddy A. Cathartic-induced magnesium toxicity during overdose management. Ann Emerg Med 1986;15:1214.

70. Smilkstein MJ, Smolinske SC, Kulig KW, Rumack BH. Severe hypermagnesemia due to multiple-dose cathartic therapy. Vet Hum Toxicol 1986;28:494.

71. Caldwell JW, Nava AJ, Haas DD. Hypernatremia associated with cathartics in overdose management. West J Med 1987;147:593.

72. Zwanger ML. Hypermagnesemia and perforated viscus. Ann Emerg Med 1986;15:1219.

73. Shannon M, Fish SS, Lovejoy FH. Cathartics and laxatives: Do they still have a place in management of the poisoned patient? Med Toxicol 1986;1:247.

74. Tuggle DW, Hoelzer DJ, Tunell WP, et al. The safety and cost-effectiveness of polyethylene glycol electrolyte solution bowel preparation in infants and children. J Pediatr Surg 1987;22:513.

75. Tenenbein M. Whole bowel irrigation in iron poisoning. J Pediatr 1987;111:142.

76. Tenenbein M, Cohen S, Sitar DS. Whole bowel irrigation as a decontamination procedure after acute drug overdose. Arch Intern Med 1987;147:905.

77. Tenenbein M. Whole bowel irrigation as a gastrointestinal decontamination after acute poisoning. Med Toxicol 1988;3:77.

78. Brown CR, Becker CE, Olson KR, et al. Whole gut lavage in a simulated drug overdose. Vet Hum Toxicol 1987;29:492.

79. Rosenberg PJ, Livingstone DJ, McLellan BA. Effect of whole-bowel irrigation on the antidotal efficacy of oral activated charcoal. Ann Emerg Med 1988;17:681.

80. Temple AR, Wason S. Corrosives-alkaline. In Rumack BH (ed). POISINDEX Information System. Denver, Micromedix, Inc., 1990 (edition expires 5/31/90).

81. Rumack BH, Burrington JD. Caustic ingestions: A rational look at diluents. Clin Toxicol 1977; 11:27.

82. Wason S, Karkal SS. Coping swiftly and effectively with caustic ingestions. Emerg Med Rep 1989; 10:25.

83. Maull KI, Osmand AP, Maull CD. Liquid caustic ingestions: An in vitro study of the effects of buffer, neutralization, and dilution. Ann Emerg Med 1985; 14:1160.

84. Jacobson BJ, Rock AR, Cohn MS, Litovitz T. Accidental ingestions of oral prescription drugs: A multicenter survey. Am J Public Health 1989; 79:853.

85. Sofer S, Asher T, Shahak E. Carbamate and organophosphate poisoning in early childhood. Pediatr Emerg Care 1989; 5:222.

86. Hilborne LH, Howanitz PJ, Howanitz JH. Serum osmolality. N Engl J Med 1984; 310:102.

87. Smithline N, Gardner KD Jr. Gaps—anionic and osmolal. JAMA 1976; 236:1594.

88. Glasser L, Sternglanz PD, Combie J, et al. Serum osmolality and its applicability to drug overdose. Am J Clin Pathol 1973; 60:695.

89. Oh MS, Carroll HJ. The anion gap. N Engl J Med 1977; 297:814.

90. Oster JR, Perez GO, Materson BJ. Use of the anion gap in clinical medicine. South Med J 1988;81:229.

91. Court H, Volans GN. Poisoning after overdose with non-steroidal anti-inflammatory drugs. Adverse Drug React Acute Poisoning Rev 1984;3:1.

92. Curry SC, Chang D, Connor D. Drug- and toxin-induced rhabdomyolysis. Ann Emerg Med 1989; 18:1068.

93. Turk J, Morrell L, Avioli LV. Ethylene glycol intoxication. Arch Intern Med 1986; 146:1601.

94. Niemann JT, Bessen HA, Rothstein RJ, et al. Electrocardiographic criteria for tricyclic antidepressant cardiotoxicity. Am J Cardiol 1986; 57:1154.

95. Foulke GE, Albertson TE. QRS interval in tricyclic antidepressant overdosage: inaccuracy as a toxicity indicator in emergency settings. Ann Emerg Med 1987;16:160.

96. Hepler BR, Sutheimer CA, Sunshine I. Role of the toxicology laboratory in the treatment of acute poisoning. Med Toxicol 1986;1:61.

97. Kellerman AL, Fihn SD, LoGerfo JP, et al. Impact of drug screening in suspected overdose. Ann Emerg Med 1987;16:1206.

98. Brett AS. Implications of discordance between clinical impression and toxicology analysis in drug overdose. Arch Intern Med 1988;148:437.

99. Mahoney JD, Gross PL, Stern TA, et al. Quantitative serum toxic screening in the management of suspected drug overdose. Am J Emerg Med 1990;8:16.

100. Bronstein AC, Sawyer DR, Rumack BH, et al. Theophylline intoxication in a premature infant: multiple dose activated charcoal therapy (abstract). Vet Hum Toxicol 1984;26:404.

101. McCord MM. Toxicity of sorbitol-charcoal suspension. J Pediatr 1987;111:307.

102. McCarron MM, Schulze BW, Thompson GA, et al. Acute phencyclidine intoxication: Clinical patterns, complications and treatment. Ann Emerg Med 1981;10:290.

103. Garella S. Extracorporeal techniques in the treatment of exogenous intoxications. Kidney Int 1988; 33:735.

104. Lacroix J, Gaudreault P, Gauthier M. Admission to a pediatric intensive care unit for poisoning: A review of 105 cases. Crit Care Med 1989; 17:748.

105. Shnaps Y, Frand M, Rotem Y, Tirosh M. The chemically abused child. Pediatrics 1981; 68:119.
106. Dine MS, McGovern ME. Intentional poisoning of children—An overlooked category of child abuse: Report of seven cases and review of the literature. Pediatrics 1982; 70:32.
107. Rogers D, Tripp J, Bentovim A, et al. Non-accidental poisoning: an extended syndrome of child abuse. Br Med J 1976; 1:793.
108. Sutphen JL, Saulsbury FT. Intentional ipecac poisoning: Munchausen syndrome by proxy. Pediatrics 1988; 82:453.
109. Griglak MJ, Bucci RL. Medicolegal management of the organically impaired patient in the emergency department. Ann Emerg Med 1985; 14:685.
110. Murphy GE. The physician's responsibility for suicide. II. Errors of omission. Ann Intern Med 1975; 82:305.

CHAPTER 83

Acetaminophen

John G. Benitez
Donna L. Seger

INTRODUCTION

Acetaminophen (acetyl-p-aminophenol, APAP) has been available for over 100 years. After 1950, APAP became available as a prescription drug in the United States and in 1955 as an over-the-counter medication.[1]

APAP is as effective as acetylsalicylic acid (ASA) in its analgesic and antipyretic properties. APAP is a safe alternative to aspirin because of noncumulative kinetics and stable serum levels in dehydration states.[2, 3] It may be administered orally or rectally at a dosage of 10 to 15 mg/kg.[4] It is available in many formulations: tablets and capsules (80, 120, 160, 325, 500, and 650 mg), suppositories (120, 125, 325, 500 and 650 mg), drops (48 and 100 mg/ml), liquid (160 mg/5 ml), and elixirs (80, 120, 160 and 325 mg/5 ml). APAP is also a common ingredient in many products (Table 83–1).[1]

APAP is frequently administered to ameliorate symptoms after vaccination and during viral illness. It is effective in reducing the incidence of pain, fussiness, and fever after vaccination for diphtheria, pertussis, and tetanus (DPT) in children.[5, 6] However, in a study in patients with varicella, no relief of pruritus, anorexia, decreased activity, abdominal pain, vomiting, fussiness, insomnia, or headache was noted. A slight prolongation in time to total scabbing of lesions occurred when APAP was administered, theoretically owing to an increased time of viral shedding.[7] APAP is therefore useful for fever and as an analgesic but may not help the overall malaise in some viral diseases.

TOXICITY

APAP causes few adverse reactions in therapeutic doses.[2, 8] Rash and agranulocytosis occurred in a single patient after its administration. Methemoglobinemia does not occur after APAP administration, even with massive overdoses or in patients chronically receiving large amounts of this agent.[9] APAP does not affect coagulation and does not interact with anticoagulant drugs.[10]

In 1978 the first two pediatric cases of APAP overdose occurred in the U.S.; one was fatal.[3, 11] In 1988 three fatalities and 4.8% of reported poisonings were due to APAP or APAP combination products.

Liver toxicity secondary to APAP overdose was first reported in 1966.[12] However, children with levels in the hepatotoxic range have a decreased incidence of hepatotoxicity and death compared with adults.[2, 13] When hepatotoxicity occurs in children, the rise of serum transaminase levels is not as high as in adults.[2, 14] This increased protection is lost between the ages of 9 and 12 years, and in adolescents the incidence of hepatotoxicity is similar to that in adults.[2, 8, 13, 15] Protection from hepatotoxicity in the young may result from the frequency of spontaneous vomiting after an ingestion or the different rates of metabolism through each metabolic pathway. The fatality rate also may be low because of the effective treatment now available.[16]

PHARMACOLOGY

Acetaminophen contains a central benzene ring with two side chains, a hydroxyl group and an acetylated amino group. This latter group gives APAP its antipyretic activity.[17] This antipyretic action results from a direct action on the hypothalamic heat-regulating center. The site and mechanism of analgesic action is unexplained. The anti-inflammatory effects of APAP are small, as peripheral prostaglandin synthesis is not affected.[10]

APAP is a weakly ionized drug with a pKa of 9.5, and therefore absorption occurs in both the stomach and small intestine. Food delays absorption.[18] Peak serum levels occur 40 to 120 minutes after ingestion. Absorption of suspensions and elixirs is faster than that of tablets.[1, 19, 20] Distribution of acetaminophen is wide throughout most body fluids, and protein binding is small and variable. Tissue binding does not occur with therapeutic doses.[10] APAP is excreted primarily as sulfate and glucuronate conjugates. Eighty-four percent of an administered dose is renally excreted as conjugates within 12 hours, and an additional 6% is excreted in the next 12 hours. A small fraction (2%) is excreted as free APAP.[19, 21, 22]

Although APAP metabolic pathways are similar in children and adults, the activity of each pathway changes with age. Metabolism and elimination proceed through four parallel pathways. A small amount of APAP is excreted directly into the urine, and 80% to 90% of orally administered APAP is conjugated with sulfate and glucuronic acid. The cytochrome P-450 system conjugates APAP with mercapturic acid; the latter conjugates account for less than 4% of an administered dose. This pathway is not rate-limiting at therapeutic doses

TABLE 83–1

ACETAMINOPHEN-CONTAINING PRODUCTS

Over-the-Counter	Prescription
Tylenol	Tylenol with codeine
Tempra	Esgic
St. Joseph Aspirin-Free	Lortab
Anacin-3	Vicodin
Phenaphen	Percocet
Triaminicin	Tylox
Alka-Seltzer Plus Cold	Darvocet
Allerest Sinus	Lortab
Tylenol Cold Liquid	Phenaphen with Codeine
Benadryl Plus	
Comtrex	
Nyquil	
Contac Jr Liquid	

(Fig. 83–1).[23, 24] Rates of the conjugation pathways vary with age. Sulfate conjugation is the primary metabolic pathway in children. A gradual increase in the activity of the glucuronic acid pathway occurs with age; this pathway is poorly developed in neonates, and glucuronic acid conjugates are not detected in fetal liver cells. At 7 to 12 years of age, glucuronic acid conjugation reaches adult levels.[8, 21, 25]

The cytochrome P-450 system produces a toxic metabolite.[16, 23, 26, 27] The toxic moiety is believed to be *N*-acetyl-*p*-benzoquinoneimine (NAPQI).[26] Glutathione (GSH) reduces NAPQI to a nontoxic intermediate.[26, 28] At toxic APAP serum levels, the enzymes responsible for APAP conjugation become saturated in both the sulfate and glucuronide pathways. Consequently, an increased amount of APAP is metabolized through the cytochrome P-450 pathway.[28] With depletion of glutathione stores, NAPQI binds covalently to tissue proteins through two different mechanisms: as an electrophile and as an oxidizing agent.[24, 26, 29] Glutathione is an essential protein in the protection of cellular proteins from such toxic intermediaries.

Differences in drug metabolism in humans are age related. The ability to oxidize drugs through the P-450 pathway has been demonstrated in the liver cells of abortuses and in neonates. Therefore an infant may produce the toxic metabolite.[25] The activity of glutathione-*S*-transferase, the enzyme that catalyzes the reaction between glutathione and NAPQI, declines with age, which increases the availability of glutathione in the young.[28] This may explain the decreased toxicity observed in children.[2, 8] In addition, neonates

have only one tenth the amount of GSH as adults, which may put this population at risk.

How NAPQI exerts its toxic effect is not completely understood. It selectively binds to tissue proteins, and there are differences in the pattern of protein binding with age.

Whether induction of the cytochrome P-450 pathway increases the formation of NAPQI, and therefore increases hepatotoxicity, has not been determined. In animals the incidence and severity of hepatotoxicity was increased with phenobarbital, 3-methylcholanthrene, and alcohol.[27, 30] However, chronic ingestion of medications known to be hepatic inducers does not induce the cytochrome P-450 but induces the glucuronide pathway. Therapeutic doses of APAP and concomitant administration of hepatic inducers do not increase the risk of hepatotoxicity.[31] There is no agreement on whether chronic alcohol consumption worsens APAP-induced hepatotoxicity.[30, 32, 33] In addition, different substances may selectively induce different isoenzymes of cytochrome P-450. Selective induction of one specific isoenzyme of the cytochrome system may not increase hepatoxicity.[30, 31, 34]

The APAP plasma half-life is not age dependent, except in neonates. Children and adults have a plasma half-life ranging from 1.0 to 3.5 hours. Neonates have a slightly more prolonged half-life of 2.2 to 5.0 hours.[8, 19, 21] After an overdose, a prolonged half-life occurs because the enzymes for each metabolic pathway become saturated and cannot metabolize APAP any faster.[23] A half-life greater than 4 hours is associated with an increased risk of toxicity.[35] Cal-

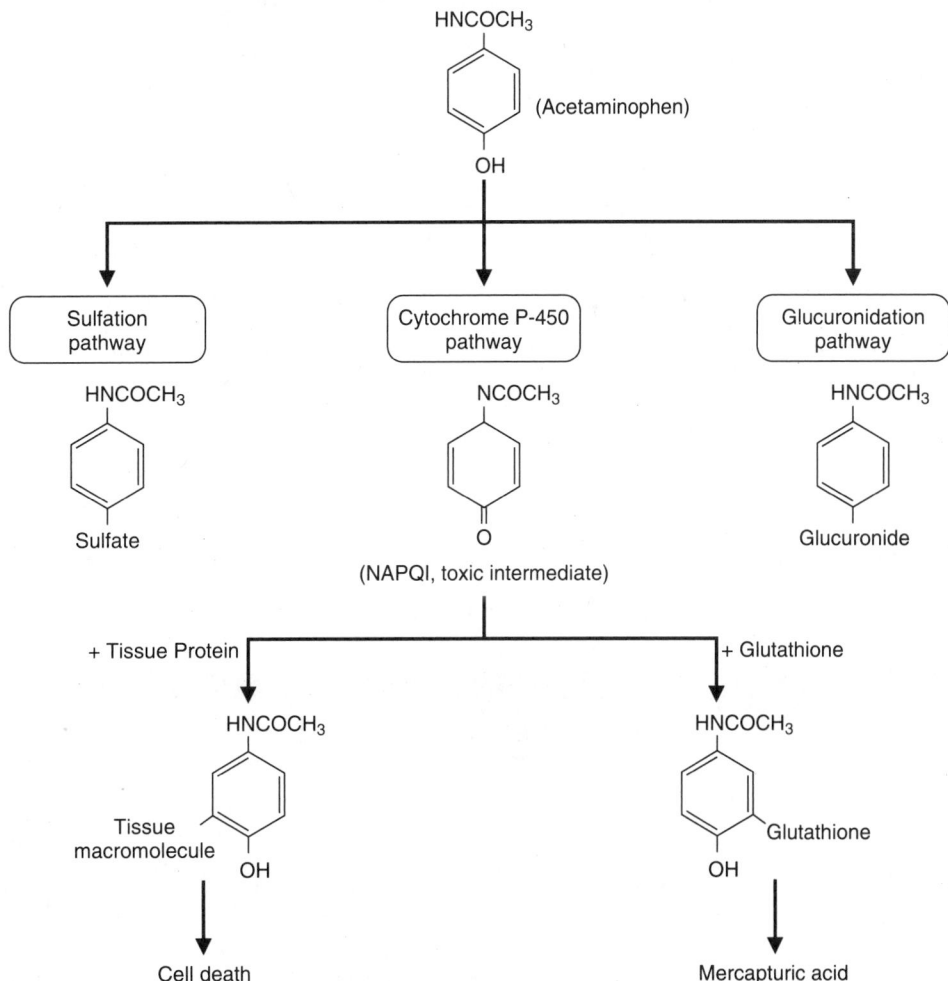

Figure 83–1. Acetaminophen metabolic pathways.

culation of the plasma half-life is therefore beneficial, especially if the time of ingestion is unknown.

CLINICAL EVALUATION

Patients presenting after toxic ingestions of APAP may show varied clinical pictures. A decreasing level of consciousness is not seen unless a coingestant is present. The patient may feel completely well and lack any signs of toxicity.[3, 16, 36, 37] As history is often unreliable or unobtainable, other methods of determining toxicity must be employed.[3, 38] Typically, the patient taking a large ingestion will progress through four clinical stages (Table 83–2).

Stage 1. Anorexia, nausea, and vomiting may occur and the patient appears pale during the initial 12 to 24 hours after ingestion.

Stage 2. Within 24 to 48 hours after ingestion, gastrointestinal symptoms from stage 1 disappear. Slight right upper quadrant tenderness may be noted. There may be decreased urinary output due to dehydration from vomiting, the antidiuretic effect of APAP, or acute tubular necrosis (ATN). Hepatic toxicity is manifested by increasing serum levels of transaminases and bilirubin and an increased prothrombin time.[3, 16, 36, 37]

Stage 3. Approximately 72 to 96 hours after ingestion, hepatic necrosis occurs. Jaundice, coagulopathy, hypoglycemia, encephalopathy, and renal failure may be present. Hepatotoxicity after APAP overdose carries a mortality rate of 2.4% to 14%.[39] Death is secondary to hepatic failure and is dependent on the degree of hepatic necrosis.[3, 16, 36, 37]

Stage 4. During the ensuing 7 to 8 days a rapid resolution of symptoms occurs. Hepatic regeneration, with complete return to normal of liver function test results, occurs over 1 to 3 weeks.[3, 16, 36, 37]

Acute renal toxicity is well described, often in association with liver toxicity. The mechanism may be similar to that of liver toxicity with binding of the active metabolite to cellular macromolecules.[40, 41] It is difficult to attribute the ATN directly to APAP toxicity because the incidence of ATN after APAP overdose is no higher than that of ATN in the general population.[42]

Pathology

The characteristic APAP-induced liver disorder is centrilobular necrosis with reticulin cell collapse. Patients who progress to death have massive and confluent necrosis of all lobules.[9, 36, 39]

Diagnostic Evaluation

Elevations in liver function test results are impressive, with serum glutamic-oxaloacetic transaminase (SGOT) and serum glutamate-pyruvic transaminase (SGPT) greater than 10,000

IU/L.[2, 3, 11, 16] The prothrombin time increases in severe intoxications. Although increased serum bilirubin does not correlate with liver damage, elevation of both the bilirubin and prothrombin time is a poor prognostic sign. A bilirubin greater than 4 mg/dl and a prothrombin time 2.2 times greater than normal implies a higher mortality rate (63%), and most patients develop encephalopathy. Only two patients with an elevated serum bilirubin and prothrombin time who did not develop encephalopathy have been described.[36]

Hypoglycemia and lactic acidosis may be present. Hypoglycemia may be a reflection of the inhibition of gluconeogenesis by an unknown mechanism. The lactic acidosis may be attributed to impaired hepatic clearance of lactate and to abnormal lactate metabolism in the liver.[43]

APAP Levels

An inaccurate history and lack of early symptomatology encumber the clinical diagnosis of APAP toxicity.[37, 38] Simple and rapid methods to assay free unchanged serum APAP are available. Single plasma level determinations are not as reliable as calculation of plasma half-life.[44] After ingestion, there is an extension in plasma half-life as patients develop a decreased capacity to conjugate APAP. Extension of plasma-half life to greater than twice normal signifies hepatic necrosis. If the half-life is less than 4 hours, there is no potential for hepatic damage.[35] However, calculation of plasma half-life is not readily accessible because at least two separate APAP serum levels, preferably more than 2 to 3 hours apart, are needed. On the basis of patient data, a nomogram for single plasma APAP levels has been constructed to predict the risk of hepatotoxicity (Fig. 83–2). Levels measured before the elapse of 4 hours are insignificant, as absorption is still occurring.[9, 32, 45, 46]

Additional laboratory tests to be obtained in patients with possible APAP ingestion include a complete blood count, platelets, electrolytes, blood urea nitrogen, liver function tests, a prothrombin time, and glucose level.[2, 32]

THERAPEUTIC INTERVENTION

Activated charcoal has been shown to decrease the absorption of orally administered APAP if given within one-half hour of the ingestion.[1, 20, 47] Unfortunately, most patients enter emergency care 1 hour or longer after ingestion, thereby decreasing the chances of inhibiting absorption.[9, 48, 49] Charcoal may inhibit absorption even after 1 hour, however, since food and other coingestants may delay gastric motility and APAP absorption. Controversy surrounds the administration of activated charcoal when N-acetyl-L-cysteine (NAC) treatment is being considered. Activated charcoal may bind to NAC and decrease its absorption.[50–52] Nevertheless, the serum concentration of NAC needed to prevent

TABLE 83–2			
SIGNS AND SYMPTOMS OF ACETAMINOPHEN OVERDOSE			
First Stage: 0–24 hr	Second Stage: 24–48 hr	Third Stage: 72–96 hr	Fourth Stage: 7–8 Days
None	May feel better	Jaundice	Hepatic regeneration
Anorexia	Right upper quadrant tenderness	Coagulation abnormality	Resolution of signs and symptoms
Nausea	Dehydration	Hypoglycemia	
Vomiting	Rising hepatic enzymes	Encephalopathy	
		Hepatic necrosis	
		Death	

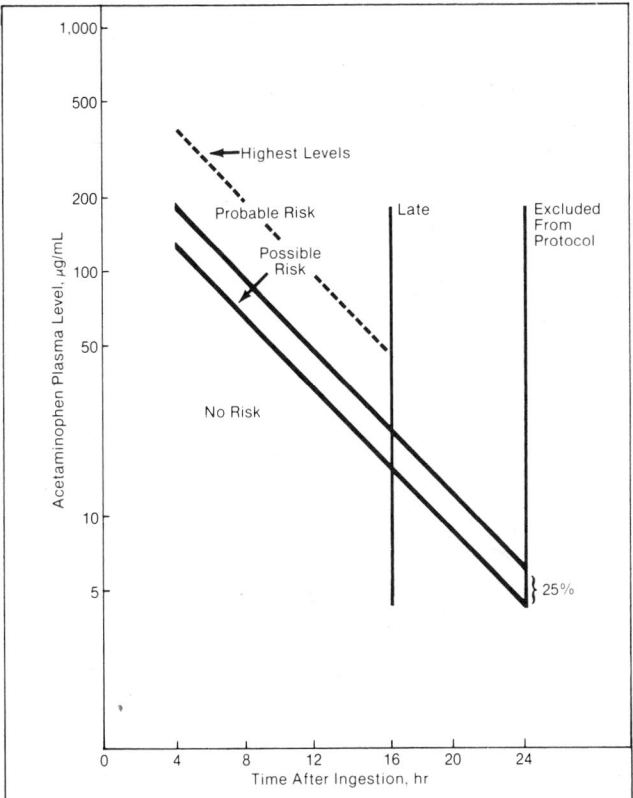

Figure 83–2. Nomogram for risk of hepatotoxicity from acetaminophen. The *possible risk line* is 25% below the established known risk line to ensure safety. (From Rumack BH, Peterson RC, Koch GG, et al. Acetaminophen overdose. Arch Intern Med 1981;141:380. Copyright 1981, American Medical Association.)

hepatotoxicity is unknown. Therefore, even if a statistically significant decrease in NAC absorption occurred, it would not necessarily be clinically significant. Given these considerations, the following guidelines are recommended:

1. In a mixed ingestion (APAP plus other coingestant), gastric evacuation may be performed if ingestion occurred within the previous hour. Charcoal should be administered if indicated by the toxicity of the coingestant. If NAC is subsequently indicated, relavage of the stomach contents should be performed to remove as much of the charcoal as possible. The initial dose of NAC should be increased by 20% to 30%, from 140 mg/kg to 180 mg/kg.[53]

2. In an unknown ingestion, gastric evacuation (if ingestion occurred within the previous hour) followed by charcoal administration should be performed. Charcoal alone may be administered if the time since ingestion is unknown. Laboratory investigation should be performed simultaneously with a physical examination to try to find the specific toxin ingested. If the serum APAP level is in the toxic range, the modified NAC loading regimen follows.

3. If APAP is the only drug ingested, charcoal may be administered within 1 hour of ingestion. APAP absorption is decreased by charcoal administration, although the clinical significance is still undetermined. If treatment begins more than 1 hour after ingestion, administration of NAC may begin immediately (Table 83–3).

Methods to enhance the elimination of APAP have been attempted. Ionic trapping of APAP in the urine is ineffective, because APAP is not primarily renally excreted and its excretion is not pH dependent. Also, forced diuresis is ineffective, as the percentage of free APAP excreted in the urine is insignificant. Charcoal hemoperfusion and hemodialysis have been attempted in humans to remove APAP and prevent the further formation of NAPQI. Hemoperfusion is not justified at this time in the management of APAP overdose.[1, 3, 54, 55]

ANTIDOTES

Several different agents to prevent hepatotoxicity have been evaluated. Since inhibitors of the cytochrome P-450 pathway, such as cimetidine, did not prevent hepatotoxicity, attempts were made to replenish glutathione stores.[53, 56, 57]

Glutathione is necessary to conjugate NAPQI and prevent hepatotoxicity. Therefore, sulfhydryl compounds such as cysteamine, methionine, and NAC have been evaluated as

---

TABLE 83–3

THERAPY AT A GLANCE: VANDERBILT UNIVERSITY APAP PROTOCOL

I. Children <1yr of age
  A. Amount ingested <66 mg/kg
    1. Give fluids
    2. Observe at home
    3. No specific treatment necessary
  B. Amount ingested 66–143 mg/kg
    1. Less than 15 min from ingestion and ipecac available
      a. Ipecac
      b. Observe at home
    2. More than 15 min since ingestion and ipecac available
      a. Ipecac
      b. Notify private pediatrician
  C. Amount ingested >143 mg/kg
    1. Ipecac
    2. Emergency department evaluation
    3. APAP level
  D. Poor or questionable history
    1. Ipecac
    2. Physician or hospital contact
II. Age >1 yr
  A. Amount ingested <100 mg/kg
    1. Fluids
    2. Observe
  B. Amount ingested 100–125 mg/kg
    1. Ipecac
    2. Observe at home
  C. Amount ingested >125 mg/kg
    1. Ingestion <2 hr
      a. Ipecac
      b. Hospital evaluation
    2. Ingestion >2 hr
      a. Hospital evaluation
III. Other considerations
  A. Possible increased toxicity
    1. Chronic liver disease
    2. Chronic medications: phenobarbital
  B. Charcoal
    1. Avoid if possible
    2. May be used if necessary
      a. Lavage prior to NAC use
      b. Do not delay NAC to give charcoal
IV. Administer NAC if:
  A. Unknown when ingestion occurred
  B. Substantial ingestion
    1. >125 mg/kg
    2. >10 gm adult weight
    3. and >7 hr since ingestion

NAC = *N*-acetyl-L-cysteine.

TABLE 83–4

ACETAMINOPHEN OVERDOSE CHECKLIST

History
- ☐ Time from ingestion
- ☐ Consider other coingestants
- ☐ Amount ingested

Laboratory
- ☐ APAP level (1 or more hr after ingestion)
- ☐ Baseline liver function tests, electrolytes, glucose

N-Acetyl-L-cysteine administration
- ☐ No charcoal in stomach
- ☐ Loading dose 140 mg/kg po
- ☐ Maintenance dose 70 mg/kg po for 17 doses

glutathione substitutes or precursors.[24] Oral or intravenous glutathione is not absorbed by hepatocytes and therefore cannot be used as an antidote.[58] Other sulfhydryl compounds such as dimercaprol and D-penicillamine offer little or no hepatic protection.[37, 46] Animal experiments revealed that cysteamine reduced the extent of arylation of proteins, the severity of hepatic necrosis, and mortality. Although cysteamine is effective in reducing hepatotoxicity, it has many side effects. Flushing, nausea, vomiting, drowsiness, and a feeling of "misery" accompany its administration. One episode of ventricular tachycardia has occurred following cysteamine administration.[46, 59, 60] Owing to cysteamine's side effects, methionine, an oral and intravenous preparation, has been investigated. Methionine is effective if given within 10 hours of ingestion; however, late in treatment it may enhance the development of hepatic encephalopathy as it is metabolized by the liver. No studies have confirmed this theoretical effect. Methionine has milder gastrointestinal and central nervous system effects than does cysteamine. Rashes, nausea, and vomiting also may occur.[37, 46, 60–62]

NAC is deacetylated in vivo to cysteine. NAC directly or indirectly conjugates and detoxifies NAPQI. NAC may also restore the activity of the intracellular proteolytic systems, and detoxify even after covalent binding has occurred. These proteolytic systems help eliminate the damaged arylated proteins. In vivo studies revealed that irreversible damage occurs if NAC is not administered within 16 hours.[26, 63] Intravenous administration is effective during a critical interval from ingestion to administration. Administration within 8 to 10 hours of ingestion provides almost complete protection. After 10 hours, this declines, although there is still some protection in patients treated up to 24 hours after ingestion.[45, 49, 63–67] Intravenous NAC is unavailable in the U.S. except as an investigational drug; oral NAC is available. NAC is safe even when administered late (12 to 36 hours) after serum transaminase levels start rising.[17, 67] The advantages of NAC are that it is effective in protecting against hepatotoxicity, its protective effect extends to later time intervals than other drugs, and it produces fewer side effects than other sulfhydryl compounds. Mortality is reduced from 5% to 10% with supportive therapy to 0.68% with NAC administration, while the incidence of hepatotoxicity is reduced from 40% to 60% to 1.4%. Side effects include the development of severe bronchospasm with intravenous administration.[68–70]

Administration of NAC is indicated when an APAP level is not obtainable immediately and the ingestion is greater than 150 mg/kg, or when the 4-hour (or later) serum APAP level falls on or above the line in the Rumack-Matthew nomogram. If the APAP level is in the nontoxic range, discontinuing the NAC is appropriate. NAC is given as a bolus of 140 mg/kg, followed by 70 mg/kg every 4 hours for 17 doses. If a patient vomits a dose within 1 hour of administration, that dose should be repeated (Table 83–4).[32]

The value of NAC in chronic APAP ingestion is undetermined. Once liver damage has occurred, NAC is of limited value. Its role in acute and chronic poisoning needs further investigation.

References

1. Ameer B, Greenblatt DJ. Acetaminophen. Ann Intern Med 1977;87:202.
2. Rumack BH. Acetaminophen overdose in young children. Am J Dis Child 1984;138:428.
3. Arena JM, Rourck MH, Sibrack CD. Acetaminophen: Report of an unusual poisoning. Pediatrics 1978;61:68.
4. Temple AR. Pediatric dosing of acetaminophen. Pediatr Pharmacol 1983;3:321.
5. Ipp MM, Gold R, Greenberg S, et al. Acetaminophen prophylaxis of adverse reactions following vaccination of infants with diphtheria-pertussis-tetanus toxoids-polio vaccine. Pediatr Infect Dis J 1987;6:721.
6. Lewis K, Cherry JD, Sachs MH, et al. The effect of prophylactic acetaminophen administration on reactions to DTP vaccination. Am J Dis Child 1988;142:62.
7. Dorna TF, DeAngelis C, Baumgardner RA, et al. Acetaminophen: More harm than good for chickenpox? J Pediatr 1989;114:1045.
8. Peterson RG, Rumack BH. Age as a variable in acetaminophen overdose. Arch Intern Med 1981;141:390.
9. Rumack BH, Matthew H. Acetaminophen poisoning and toxicity. Pediatrics 1975;55:871.
10. Koch-Weser J. Medical intelligence; drug therapy. N Engl J Med 1976;295:1297.
11. Nogen AG, Bremner, JE. Fatal acetaminophen over-dosage in a young child. J Pediatr. 1978;92:832.
12. Davidson DGD, Eastham WN. Acute liver necrosis following overdose of paracetamol. Br Med J 1966;2:497.
13. Meredity TJ, Newman B, Goulding R. Paracetamol poisoning in children. Br Med J 1978;2:478.
14. Green JW, Craft L, Ghishan F. Acetaminophen poisoning in infancy. Am J Dis Child 1983;137:386.
15. Rumack BH, Peterson RG. Acetaminophen overdose: Incidence, diagnosis and management in 416 patients. Pediatrics 1978;62(Suppl):898.
16. Rumack BH. Acetaminophen overdose. Am J Med 1983;11:1104.
17. Insel PA. Analgesic-antipyretics and anti-inflammatory agents; drugs employed in the treatment of rheumatoid arthritis and gout. In Gilman AG, Rall TW, Nies AS, Taylor P, (eds). Goodman and Gilman's The Pharmacological Basis of Therapeutics. 8th ed. Elmsford, NY, Pergamon Press, 1990, p 656.
18. Klotz U. Interactions of analgesics with other drugs. Am J Med 1983;75:113.
19. Peterson RG, Rumack BH. Pharmacokinetics of acetaminophen ingestions. JAMA 1977;238:500.
20. Levy G, Houston JB. Effect of activated charcoal on acetaminophen absorption. Pediatrics 1976;58:432.
21. Alam SN, Roberts RJ, Fischer LJ. Age-related differences in salicylamide and acetaminophen conjugation in man. J Pediatr 1977;90:130.
22. Levy G, Khanna NR, Soda DM, et al. Pharmacokinetics of acetaminophen in the human neonate: Formation of acetaminophen glucuronide and sulfate in relation to plasma bilirubin concentration of D-glucaric acid excretion. Pediatrics 1975;55:818.
23. Slattery JT, Levy G. Acetaminophen kinetics in acutely poisoned patients. Clin Pharmacol Ther 1979;25:184.
24. Mitchell JR, Thorgeirsson SS, Potter WZ, et al. Acetaminophen-induced hepatic injury: Protective role of glutathione in man and rationale for therapy. Clin Pharmacol Ther 1974;16:676.
25. Byer AJ, Traylor TR, Semmer JR. Acetaminophen overdose in the third trimester of pregnancy. JAMA 1982;247:3114.
26. Bruno MK, Cohen SD, Khairallah EA. Antidotal effectiveness of N-acetylcysteine in reversing acetaminophen-induced hepatotoxicity. Biochem Pharmacol 1988;37:4319.
27. Mitchell JR, Jollow DJ, Potter WZ, et al. Acetaminophen-induced hepatic necrosis. 1. Role of drug metabolism. J Pharmacol Exp Ther 1973;187:185.
28. Beierschmitt WP, Brady JT, Bartolone JB, et al. Selective protein arylation and the age dependency of acetaminophen hepatotoxicity in mice. Toxicol Appl Pharmacol 1989;98:517.
29. Mitchell JR, Potter WZ. Drug metabolism in the production of liver injury. Med Clin North Am 1975;59:877.
30. McClain CJ, Kromhout JP, Peterson FJ, et al. Potentiation of acetaminophen hepatotoxicity by alcohol. JAMA 1980;244:251.
31. Prescott LF, Critchley JAJH, Balali-Mood M, et al. Effects of microsomal enzyme induction on paracetamol metabolism in man. Br J Clin Pharmacol 1981;12:149.
32. Rumack BG, Peterson RC, Koch GG, et al. Acetaminophen overdose. Arch Intern Med 1981;141:380.

33. Benson GD. Hepatotoxicity following the therapeutic use of antipyretic analgesics. Am J Med 1983;75:85.
34. Prescott LF, Critchley JA. Drug interactions affecting analgesic toxicity. Am J Med 1983;75:133.
35. Prescott LF, Roscoe P, Wright N, et al. Plasma-paracetamol half-life and hepatic necrosis in patients with paracetamol overdosage. Lancet 1971;1:519.
36. Clark R, Borirakchanyavat V, Davidson AR, et al. Hepatic damage and death from overdose of paracetamol. Lancet 1973;1:66.
37. Prescott LF, Critchley JA. The treatment of acetaminophen poisoning. Ann Rev Pharmacol Toxicol 1983;23:87.
38. Ashbourne JF, Olson KR, Khayam-Bashi H. Value of rapid screening of acetaminophen in all patients with intentional drug overdose. Ann Emerg Med 1989;18:1035.
39. Proudfoot AT, Wright N. Acute paracetamol poisoning. Br Med J 1970;3:447.
40. Jeffery WH, Lafferty WE. Acute renal failure after acetaminophen overdose: Report of two cases. Am J Hosp Pharm 1981;38:1355.
41. Curry RW Jr, Robinson JD, Sughrue MJ. Acute renal failure after acetaminophen ingestion. JAMA 1982;247:1012.
42. Gabriel R, Caldwell J, Hartley RB. Acute tubular necrosis, caused by therapeutic doses of paracetamol? Clin Nephrol 1982;18:269.
43. Zabrodski RM, Schnurr LP. Anion gap acidosis with hypoglycemia in acetaminophen toxicity. Ann Emerg Med 1984;13:135.
44. Ambre J, Alexander M. Liver toxicity after acetaminophen ingestions. JAMA 1977;238:500.
45. Prescott LF, Illingworth RN, Critchley JA, et al. Intravenous N-acetylcysteine: The treatment of choice for paracetamol poisoning. Br Med J 1979;2:1097.
46. Prescott LF, Park J, Sutherland GR, et al. Cysteamine, methionine, and penicillamine in the treatment of paracetamol poisoning. Lancet 1976;2:109.
47. Van deGraff WB, Thompson WL, Sunshine I, et al. Adsorbent and cathartic inhibition of external drug absorption. J Pharmacol Exp Ther 1982;221:656.
48. Prescott LF. Paracetamol overdosage. Drugs 1983;25:290.
49. Harrison PM, Keays R, Bray GP, et al. Imposed outcome of paracetamol-induced fulminant hepatic failure by late administration of acetylcysteine. Lancet 1990;335:1572.
50. Elkins BR, Ford DC, Thompson MIB, et al. The effect of activated charcoal on N-acetylcysteine absorption in normal subjects. Am J Emerg Med 1987;5:483.
51. Renzi FP, Donovan JW, Martin TG, et al. Concomitant use of activated charcoal and N-acetylcysteine. Ann Emerg Med 1985;14:71.
52. North DS, Peterson RG, Krenzelok EP. Effect of activated charcoal administration of acetylcysteine serum levels in humans. Am J Hosp Pharm 1981;38:1022.
53. Ruffalo RL, Thompson JF. Cimetidine and acetylcysteine as antidote for acetaminophen overdose. South Med J 1982;75:954.
54. Helliwell M, Vale A, Goulding R. Haemoperfusion in "late" paracetamol poisoning. Hum Toxicol 1981;1:31.
55. Winchester JF, Gelfand MC, Helliwell J, et al. Extracorporeal treatment of salicylate or acetaminophen poisoning—is there a role? Arch Intern Med 1981;141:370.
56. Critchley JA, Scott AW, Dyson EH, et al. Is there a place for cimetidine or ethanol in the treatment of paracetamol poisoning? Lancet 1983;1:1375.
57. Mitchell MC, Scheneker S, Avant GR, et al. Cimetidine protects against acetaminophen hepatotoxicity in rats. Gastroenterology 1981;81:1052.
58. Black M. Acetaminophen hepatotoxicity. Gastroenterology 1980;78:382.
59. Smith JM, Roberts WO, Hall SM, et al. Late treatment of paracetamol poisoning with mercaptamine. Br Med J 1978;1:331.
60. Crome P, Volans GN, Vale JA, et al. Preliminary communications: Oral methionine in the treatment of severe paracetamol (acetaminophen) overdose. Lancet 1976;2:829.
61. Vale JA, Meredith TJ, Goulding R. Treatment of acetaminophen poisoning. Arch Intern Med 1981;141:394.
62. Piperno E, Mosher AH, Berssenbruegge DA, et al. Pathophysiology of acetaminophen overdosage toxicity: Implications for management. Pediatrics 1978;62(Suppl):880.
63. Smilkstein MJ, Knapp GL, Kulig KW, et al. Efficacy of oral N-acetylcysteine in the treatment of acetaminophen overdose. N Engl J Med 1988;319:1557.
64. Prescott LF. Treatment of severe acetaminophen poisoning with intravenous acetylcysteine. Arch Intern Med 1981;151:386.
65. Oh TE, Shenfield GM. Intravenous N-acetylcysteine for paracetamol poisoning. Med J Aust 1980;1:664.
66. Prescott LF, Park J, Ballantyne A, et al. Treatment of paracetamol (acetaminophen) poisoning with N-acetylcysteine. Lancet 1977;2:432.
67. Parker D, White JP, Paton D, et al. Safety of late acetylcysteine treatment in paracetamol poisoning. Hum Exp Toxicol 1990;9:25.
68. Peterson RG, Rumack BH. Toxicity of acetaminophen overdose. JACEP 1978;7:202.
69. Ho SW, Beilin LJ. Asthma associated with N-acetylcysteine infusion and paracetamol poisoning: Report of two cases. Br Med J 1983;287:876.
70. Vale JA, Buckley BM. Asthma associated with N-acetylcysteine infusion and paracetamol poisoning. Br Med J 1983;287:1223.

CHAPTER 84

Salicylates

Steven C. Curry

INTRODUCTION

Salicylate poisoning was the leading cause of accidental fatal poisonings in children in the United States for several decades but has declined in recent years. Since 1955 the number of flavored aspirin tablets for children allowed per container has been decreased, and child-proof caps are commonly used. Furthermore, the association of Reye's syndrome with the use of salicylates has caused pediatricians to recommend acetaminophen instead of aspirin, thus limiting the access of children to aspirin.

Serious salicylate intoxication carries high morbidity and mortality, especially when the seriousness of the condition is not recognized by the treating physician.[1] For example, progressive central nervous system (CNS) depression demands several immediate aggressive actions, not just endotracheal intubation and ventilation. A mild fall in arterial pH to 7.3 may have little consequence for children with most medical conditions but may result in major morbidity in those suffering from salicylate poisoning. In most cases of intoxication, declining blood levels are associated with recovery, but this is not necessarily true for salicylate poisoning. Therefore, physicians must become familiar with the pathophysiology, pharmacokinetics, clinical course, and treatment of salicylate intoxication.

Sources

All products capable of producing salicylate toxicity, including aspirin, are converted to salicylate during or after absorption, and it is salicylate that accounts for the clinical findings of salicylate toxicity. Aspirin (acetylsalicylic acid) is the most commonly ingested salicylate. However, a plethora of prescription and over-the-counter pharmaceuticals may produce salicylate poisoning:

Salsalate (salicylsalicylic acid)
Aspirin (acetylsalicylic acid)
Triethanolamine salicylate
Sodium thiosalicylate
Choline salicylate
Magnesium salicylate
Methyl salicylate
Sodium salicylate
Salicylic acid

Salicylic acid itself is used as a keratolytic agent, and systemic salicylate toxicity and death have resulted from dermal applications.[2, 3] Methyl salicylate (oil of wintergreen) is found in candy flavoring and numerous liniments. Death has resulted in children who have ingested relatively pure methyl salicylate or have ingested products containing it (e.g., Ben-Gay).[4]

PATHOPHYSIOLOGY
General and Metabolic

Salicylate directly stimulates the respiratory center in the brain stem to produce tachypnea, hyperpnea, and respiratory alkalosis.[5] However, alkalemia is not always present because of the ability of salicylate to produce metabolic acidosis.[5] Furthermore, the coingestion of CNS depressants may blunt or prevent hyperventilation and respiratory alkalosis.[6] At very toxic concentrations, salicylate causes both CNS and respiratory depression.[5]

One of the major toxic effects of salicylate is impaired production of adenosine triphosphate (ATP), the major immediate energy source for living cells. ATP is mainly produced either in cytoplasm through glycolysis or through oxidative phosphorylation in mitochondria. In glycolysis, each mole of glucose converted to pyruvate results in the net production of 2 moles ATP. Glycolysis can proceed in the absence of oxygen as long as pyruvate is converted to lactate. Unfortunately, the small amount of ATP produced by glycolysis is not adequate to support life except in selected tissues (e.g., erythrocytes).

In mitochondria, pyruvate from glycolysis undergoes a series of decarboxylations in Krebs' cycle mainly to yield CO_2, H_2O, reduced nicotinamide adenine dinucleotide (NADH), and reduced flavin adenine dinucleotide (FADH). The major source of the cell's ATP production then occurs via oxidative phosphorylation in the inner mitochondrial membrane as electrons from NADH and FADH are transported among various cytochromes before combining with oxygen to form water. With the addition of oxidative phosphorylation to glycolysis, a total of 36 to 38 moles ATP can be generated from each mole glucose.

Normally, ATP production is "coupled" to electron transport and oxygen consumption. That is, every time electrons are transported down the cytochrome system to combine with oxygen, the released energy is used to generate ATP. Salicylate "uncouples" oxidative phosphorylation.[7] Salicylate allows electron transport to continue, and in fact electron transport and oxygen consumption are accelerated to above-normal levels. However, the energy released from the transport of electrons down the cytochrome system is not used to generate ATP. Rather, much of the energy is wasted as heat.[5] The result of this uncoupling is impaired ATP production, increased oxygen consumption, and heat generation.

Salicylate also impairs ATP production by inhibiting various dehydrogenases in Krebs' cycle.[8, 9] Such inhibition prevents synthesis of NADH and FADH, energy-rich compounds that fuel oxidative phosphorylation.

The metabolic acidosis accompanying serious salicylate poisoning is poorly understood. While glycolysis and the anaerobic conversion of glucose to lactate are accelerated in salicylate poisoning in an attempt to meet ATP requirements, the conversion of glucose to lactate does not result in the production of hydrogen ions.[10–13]

$$Glucose + 2\,ADP^{3-} + 2\,HPO_4^{2-} + 10H^+ \rightarrow$$
$$2\,lactate^- + 2\,ATP^{4-} + 2\,H_2O + 10H^+$$

Cellular pH and concentrations of substrates influence the amounts of ATP and hydrogen ions produced in glycolysis. However, the fact that glycolytic production of lactate and ATP is not acidifying holds true regardless of pH.[12, 14, 15] Rather, a large portion of the acidosis of salicylate poisoning

is most likely due to hydrolysis of ATP produced in glycolysis and other pathways. The hydrolysis of ATP to ADP and phosphate results in the net production of hydrogen ions.[11]

$$ATP^{4-} + 4H^+ + H_2O \rightarrow ADP^{3-} + HPO_4^{2-} + 5H^+$$

Again, pH and substrate concentrations influence the dissociation of hydrogen ions from ATP, ADP, and phosphate. However, a net increase in hydrogen ion concentration will always occur from the hydrolysis of ATP. The production of ATP in oxidative phosphorylation results in the consumption of hydrogen ions through the opposite reaction:

$$ADP^{3-} + HPO_4^{2-} + 5H^+ \rightarrow ATP^{4-} + H_2O + 4H^+$$

During normal cellular metabolism, cells generally are hydrolyzing ATP and generating hydrogen ions at the same rate at which they are synthesizing ATP and consuming hydrogen ions in oxidative phosphorylation.[14] Uncoupling oxidative phosphorylation and inhibition of Krebs' cycle results in a state in which hydrogen ion production from the hydrolysis of ATP generated in glycolysis is not buffered by hydrogen ion consumption in oxidative phosphorylation. The result is an increase in hydrogen ion concentration and a fall in pH. Enhanced ATPase activity in uncoupled mitochondria[16] may contribute to acidosis.

Circulating lactate concentrations are normal in most patients with salicylate poisoning.[17] A rise in lactate concentration in some patients with salicylate poisoning may serve as a marker of increased activity in glycolysis, but lactate levels are also influenced by the ability of the liver to extract lactate and by the equilibrium of lactate with pyruvate.[14] Salicylate stimulates lipolysis, resulting in the ketosis often seen in salicylate poisoning.[5] Some patients with salicylate poisoning have, in part, a ketoacidosis.[17]

Salicylate has variable effects on glucose homeostasis that affect both blood glucose concentrations and acid-base balance. Stimulation of epinephrine and glucagon secretion in salicylate poisoning results in mobilization of amino acids and glycogen stores as well as stimulation of gluconeogenesis.[5, 18] These effects commonly prevail early in salicylate poisoning, producing hyperglycemia.

However, impaired ATP production from inhibition of Krebs' cycle dehydrogenases and uncoupling of oxidative phosphorylation increase glucose demand as glycolysis is accelerated to increase anaerobic ATP production. During times of increased glucose demand, alanine is the major substrate for gluconeogenesis. Unfortunately, salicylate is a potent inhibitor of alanine transaminase, preventing alanine's conversion to pyruvate to fuel gluconeogenesis.[19] Therefore, during times of increased glucose utilization, hypoglycemia may result from depletion of glycogen stores and impaired gluconeogenesis, especially in young children.[20, 21] Also, hypoglycorrhachia (a low cerebrospinal fluid [CSF] glucose level) has been noted in the presence of normal blood glucose concentrations.[22] It has been suggested that part of the CNS toxicity produced by salicylate is secondary to disordered glucose metabolism in the brain.

Many patients with salicylate intoxication suffer from hypokalemia if severe dehydration and impaired renal function have not caused hyperkalemia. The hypokalemia is due in part to gastrointestinal losses and obligatory urinary excretion of potassium with organic acids that have accumulated from the metabolic effects of salicylate.[5]

Gastrointestinal

Aspirin has a local corrosive effect on the GI tract. Acute intoxications are frequently accompanied by abdominal pain, vomiting, and hematemesis. Gastric perforations after acute aspirin ingestions have been reported.[23, 24] These GI effects contribute to dehydration and the occasional onset of bleeding severe enough to require transfusion. Methyl salicylate is also irritating, and the ingestion of salicylic acid, a keratolytic agent, can produce significant oropharyngeal burns as well as corrosive injury more distally.[25]

In patients chronically ingesting salicylates, there may be asymptomatic elevation of hepatocellular enzymes.[26–28] The acute ingestion of salicylate is not generally associated with hepatotoxicity.

Pulmonary

Noncardiogenic pulmonary edema (adult respiratory distress syndrome [ARDS]) is sometimes seen in adults suffering large, acute overdoses of salicylates[29] and is commonly seen in adults with chronic salicylate poisoning.[29, 30] Some authors have noted the rarity of ARDS in children with salicylate poisoning,[29] but ARDS can occur, especially in those with chronic intoxications.[21]

Fluid overload and hydrostatic pulmonary edema also can occur in patients who retain the large volumes of fluids administered in attempts at instituting an alkaline diuresis. Inappropriate secretion of antidiuretic hormone, hyponatremia, and hypervolemia have complicated salicylate poisoning in children.[31]

Cardiovascular

Acid-base and electrolyte abnormalities, occasional significant hyperthermia, and (most important) impaired ATP production in myocardial tissue may result in deleterious myocardial effects. Heart failure can occur[32] but usually is not a major problem except in patients near death and suffering from significant CNS depression. Both supraventricular and ventricular arrhythmias are possible. Two unexpected episodes of ventricular fibrillation have been witnessed in a severely poisoned patient who went on to make a complete recovery.

Coagulation and Platelets

Salicylate impairs activation of vitamin K–dependent coagulation factors.[33] Both acute and chronic salicylate intoxication may be accompanied by prolonged prothrombin times. A single dose of aspirin, but not other salicylates, inhibits platelet function for 8 to 12 days.

Despite these effects on platelet function and blood coagulation, bleeding disorders are rarely a cause of major morbidity in salicylate poisoning. Salicylate-induced coagulopathy is rapidly reversed by administration of parenteral vitamin K.[33]

Central Nervous System

The brain consumes large amounts of energy, and impairment of ATP production by salicylate can result in serious neurotoxicity. Agitation, confusion, hallucinations, and lethargy are noted in severe poisonings.[34] Even more severe cases are accompanied by coma, respiratory arrest, malignant cerebral edema, and brain death.[1, 32, 34–36]

Animal data indicate a critical CNS salicylate concentration at which malignant cerebral edema and death occur,[37] and this is consistent with clinical experience. Patients who die from salicylate poisoning despite supportive care frequently suffer a cerebral death. Those dying from heart failure and shock almost uniformly have developed serious CNS depression before severe cardiovascular toxicity, reiterating the ominous implications of progressive lethargy and coma in salicylate-poisoned patients.[32, 34, 36, 37]

Miscellaneous

Both hypocalcemia and hypercalcemia have been rarely reported after salicylate poisoning.[38, 39] Like all metabolic poisoning, serious salicylate poisoning may be accompanied by rhabdomyolysis[40, 41] and attendant complications, including hyperkalemia, disseminated intravascular coagulation, and myoglobinuric renal failure. However, renal failure has been reported in the absence of rhabdomyolysis.[42] Tinnitus almost always accompanies serious ingestions. Although salicylate toxicity is classically associated with hyperthermia, most patients with salicylate poisoning do not have significant elevations in body temperature.[32]

PHARMACOKINETICS

Absorption

During and after ingestion, various salicylate products, including aspirin, are rapidly converted to salicylate.[43] Salicylate impairs gastric emptying and may form a concretion in the stomach, allowing serum salicylate concentrations to rise for more than 24 hours after ingestion,[44] although toxic serum levels are usually reached within 6 hours. Liquid preparations are absorbed more rapidly. Enteric-coated salicylate tablets produce a delayed absorption, and toxic serum salicylate concentrations may not be achieved until many hours after ingestion.[45, 46]

The topical application of salicylic acid as a keratolytic agent can result in absorption of toxic amounts of salicylate.[2, 3, 47] The lack of a normal epidermal barrier allows 60% of salicylate applied to psoriatic skin under an occlusive dressing to be absorbed.[47] At least ten pediatric deaths from percutaneous salicylate intoxication have been reported.[2]

Distribution

Salicylate is widely distributed throughout body tissue. Much is protein bound and it is the free, unbound fraction of salicylate that is in equilibrium with tissue stores.[48] Salicylate also exists in blood and tissue as an equilibrium between un-ionized salicylic acid and the negatively charged salicylate ion.[49] At physiologic pH in blood and tissue, the great majority of salicylate exists in the ionized form. However, it is un-ionized salicylate that easily moves from blood across cell membranes into tissue to produce systemic toxicity.[44]

Any condition that decreases protein binding (increasing the free fraction of salicylate) or decreases pH (increasing the un-ionized fraction of salicylate) will raise the apparent volume of distribution (V_d) of salicylate. That is, decreased protein binding or a fall in pH is accompanied by a movement of salicylate from blood into tissue, raising the tissue burden of salicylate and worsening systemic toxicity while decreasing serum salicylate concentration. A decreased fraction of protein-bound drug is seen at toxic salicylate concentrations as well as in patients with hypoalbuminemia or uremia.[50–52] A drop in pH from 7.4 to only 7.2 almost *doubles* the amount of un-ionized drug that is able to leave blood and move into tissue. A healthy patient with low salicylate concentrations may have a V_d of 0.16 L/kg, while the same patient with elevated salicylate concentrations and acidosis may have a V_d greater than 0.34 L/kg.[53] Neonates and infants have higher V_d than older children.[44]

The changing V_d of salicylate makes interpretation of serum salicylate levels difficult. Patients with similar serum salicylate concentrations may have marked differences in tissue salicylate burdens and severity of toxicity. Serum salicylate concentrations in a poisoned patient may be falling not only because of metabolism and renal elimination of salicylate, but also because salicylate is moving into tissue and worsening toxicity. Therefore, patients can continue to deteriorate and even die while serum salicylate levels are stable or decreasing,[32, 35] especially if the blood pH is allowed to fall. For these reasons, it is important to treat the patient and not simply the serum salicylate concentration. This is especially important in patients with chronic salicylate poisoning who always have large V_d and large tissue burdens of salicylate for a given salicylate level.

Elimination

Salicylate undergoes hepatic metabolism by several routes, the two main ones being glucuronidation and conjugation to glycine to form salicyluric acid.[43] Both of these pathways are saturable, leading to zero-order elimination kinetics at low therapeutic salicylate concentrations. This results in a set amount of drug being metabolized per unit time, regardless how high serum salicylate concentrations may reach.

Such a shift to zero-order elimination kinetics allows serum salicylate concentrations to rise out of proportion to changes in dosage.[44] For example, doubling a patient's salicylate dose may result in three- or fourfold elevations in plasma salicylate concentrations. Second, as drug concentrations rise, renal excretion of salicylate becomes increasingly important as a route of drug elimination.[54] The decreased fraction of protein-bound drug also probably contributes to enhanced renal excretion at elevated serum salicylate concentrations. Un-ionized salicylate is reabsorbed by renal tubules, prolonging elimination. Alkaline urine favors the formation of ionized salicylate, preventing reabsorption and enhancing elimination.[44] Third, the elimination of salicylate becomes markedly prolonged as serum drug concentrations rise, because only a set amount of drug can be metabolized per unit time. Zero-order elimination kinetics, a larger than normal V_d, dehydration or renal insufficiency, and aciduria act together to markedly prolong the elimination of salicylate. It may take more than 1 or 2 days for serum salicylate levels to decrease by one half in untreated patients suffering from salicylate toxicity.

TOXIC DOSES

The acute ingestion of 150 mg/kg aspirin is not expected to produce toxicity other than GI irritation and vomiting. An acute ingestion of 150 to 300 mg/kg aspirin produces mild to moderate toxicity with abdominal pain, vomiting, dehydration, hyperpnea, tinnitus, mild CNS dysfunction, and acid-base disturbances. Ingestion of more than 300 mg/kg aspirin can produce moderate to severe toxicity and death. Patients with medical conditions that predispose them to a large V_d (e.g., chronic acidemia, renal failure, hypoalbuminemia) or patients who have ingested salicylate previously within the last 12 to 24 hours will become more toxic for a given ingestion.

The Done nomogram[55] is used only to assist in predicting the degree of toxicity after an acute, single ingestion of a non–enteric-coated salicylate (Fig. 84–1). A serum level should not be plotted on the nomogram if obtained less than 6 hours after ingestion; nontoxic levels drawn before 6 hours do not rule out impending toxicity. Furthermore, the Done nomogram assumes that absorption of salicylate is complete. However, as noted above, salicylate levels may rise for more than 24 hours after ingestion. Symptomatic patients

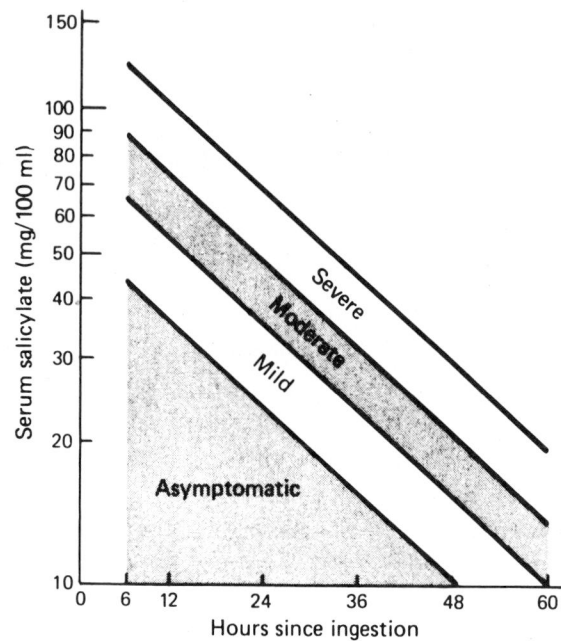

Figure 84–1. The Done nomogram. See text for a discussion of the interpretation of salicylate concentrations and the nomogram. (From Done AK. Salicylate intoxication. Significance of measurements of salicylate in blood in cases of acute ingestion. Pediatrics 1960; 26:800. Reproduced by permission of Pediatrics, copyright 1960.)

should be treated regardless of where they fall on the nomogram.

CLINICAL EVALUATION
Acute Salicylate Poisoning

Patients with acute salicylate poisoning usually appear and feel miserable. Presenting complaints and clinical findings include abdominal pain, persistent vomiting and hematemesis, tinnitus, tachypnea and hyperpnea, diaphoresis, tachycardia, dehydration, leukocytosis, and ketonuria. If dehydration has not limited potassium excretion, many patients will be hypokalemic. Older children usually present with respiratory alkalosis, mild metabolic acidosis, and alkalemia.[56] Young children are usually acidemic from metabolic acidosis by time of presentation, although a respiratory alkalosis is usually present.[56]

Serum glucose concentrations are frequently normal or elevated early in acute poisoning. Young children are more likely to develop hypoglycemia as glycogen stores are depleted in the face of impaired gluconeogenesis.

As the severity of poisoning progresses, acidemia and progressive CNS dysfunction (agitation, lethargy, seizures, coma) dominate as cerebral edema develops. Although uncommon in children, ARDS may develop. When CNS depression becomes significant, respiratory depression or apnea is possible. An elevated prothrombin time typically appears hours after ingestion but usually is not a cause of significant morbidity.

Children who die from salicylate poisoning usually develop CNS dysfunction and then die from cerebral failure or refractory shock. Acidemia is usually present by this time, and the combination of acidemia and CNS depression is ominous.[32, 34, 36, 37] Clinical deterioration can be rapid: patients who are awake and alert when admitted to the hospital can die within 6 hours.[1] Because of the rising V_d in severely poisoned patients, many children die while serum salicylate concentrations are falling or have fallen to relatively low levels.

Chronic Salicylate Poisoning

Chronic salicylate toxicity is best described as a syndrome rather than a specific dose of salicylate over a particular time. For example, a patient who is dehydrated and has impaired renal salicylate excretion may develop chronic toxicity while taking doses that otherwise would cause no problems. On the other hand, regular ingestion of excessive salicylate doses causes toxicity in an otherwise healthy person.

Although dehydration is common, gastroenteritis usually does not dominate the clinical picture as in acute poisoning. Rather, patients with chronic salicylate poisoning usually are brought in by family members because of changes in mentation, including lethargy, irritability, agitation, hallucinations, seizures, and coma.[21, 57, 58] Most children, regardless of age, will be acidemic. Tinnitus is common. ARDS is more common than in acute poisoning. An elevated prothrombin time is frequently noted. Elevated hepatic enzyme levels are commonly noted in patients chronically ingesting salicylate and are not specific for toxicity. Because of a large V_d, patients with chronic salicylate toxicity are much sicker for a given salicylate level than patients with acute poisoning.[57] In fact, a patient suffering from chronic salicylate toxicity can have what the laboratory reports to be a therapeutic serum salicylate concentration.

Patients taking carbonic anhydrase inhibitors such as acetazolamide are markedly predisposed to chronic salicylate toxicity, even while ingesting relatively small amounts of salicylate.[59, 60] Carbonic anhydrase inhibitors acidify blood and alkalinize CSF, increasing the un-ionized fraction of salicylate in blood that is able to move into the CNS where it is then trapped and concentrated at the higher pH.[37, 61] Furthermore, salicylate markedly increases the free fraction of acetazolamide in blood,[60] enhancing the effect of the carbonic anhydrase inhibitor on salicylate.

The difference between acute and chronic salicylate poisoning is not always distinct. The longer the time after an acute ingestion, the more the patient behaves like one suffering from chronic intoxication.

DIFFERENTIAL DIAGNOSIS

The differential diagnosis of salicylate poisoning is extensive and includes any disorder or poisoning that can produce metabolic acidosis, gastroenteritis, or CNS dysfunction. A convulsion from any cause (e.g., trauma, isoniazid, cocaine) is accompanied by a metabolic acidosis for 30 to 60 minutes after the seizure is terminated. In general, however, the differential diagnosis includes poisoning by theophylline, caffeine, iron, ethylene glycol, methanol, arsenic, or inorganic mercury salts; Reye's syndrome; diabetic ketoacidosis; sepsis; encephalitis; and meningitis. Most direct or indirect beta-adrenergic agonists (e.g., terbutaline, albuterol, sympathomimetics) can produce tachypnea, hypokalemia, hyperglycemia, leukocytosis, and metabolic acidosis, although the acidosis is usually mild in the absence of seizures or shock.

Diflunisal, a nonsteroidal anti-inflammatory agent, is a derivative of salicylic acid that is not hydrolyzed to salicylate and does not produce salicylate poisoning. However, serum salicylate concentrations determined colorimetrically are falsely positive in patients who have ingested diflunisal.

THERAPEUTIC INTERVENTION
Decontamination, Evaluation, and Disposition

Numerous studies have examined the effect of various decontamination techniques on absorption of salicylate. Charcoal alone appears to be superior to induction of vomiting with ipecac.[62, 63] Activated charcoal (1 gm/kg) should be administered to patients who have ingested potentially toxic amounts of salicylate. Saline cathartics do not appear to be helpful in models of aspirin poisoning.[64, 65] Repeated-dose (pulse) charcoal has been claimed to be effective in a small, historically controlled patient series.[66] However, a prospective controlled study in human volunteers ingesting nontoxic amounts of salicylate suggests that repeated doses of charcoal have little to offer.[67]

Initial laboratory work in symptomatic patients should include determinations of serum electrolytes, glucose, BUN, creatinine, salicylate concentration, prothrombin time, hemoglobin and hematocrit, and urinary ketones. Arterial blood gases should be measured to determine the type and degree of acid-base imbalance. Chest radiography should be performed in moderately or severely ill patients or those with respiratory distress or hypoxemia.

All patients with CNS depression or seizures should be presumed to be hypoglycemic and should receive appropriate doses of intravenous glucose if a serum glucose concentration cannot be quickly determined at the bedside. A patient who appears ill from salicylate poisoning should be treated, regardless of where salicylate concentrations fall on the Done nomogram. Although a 1989 study suggested that the Done nomogram may overestimate the severity of poisoning,[68] the nomogram may also underestimate some cases of poisoning. Mild dehydration and aciduria from persistent nausea and vomiting can lead to dehydration, impaired salicylate clearance, acidemia, an increased V_d, and worsening toxicity over several hours, even in those with early "mild" intoxications. Therefore, the patient who is asymptomatic or has only mild symptoms and whose 6-hour serum salicylate level falls in the mild range on the nomogram can be discharged home if nausea and vomiting have resolved, if adequate follow-up is ensured, and if a second serum salicylate level has been obtained to document that these levels are falling. All other patients should be admitted to the hospital.

The acute ingestion of enteric-coated salicylate may result in nontoxic serum salicylate concentrations 6 hours after ingestion, but still result in severe salicylate poisoning hours later because of delayed absorption. Considering the inaccurate histories that frequently accompany overdose victims, anyone who may have ingested more than 150 mg/kg of enteric-coated aspirin should be admitted for observation and serial measurement of salicylate levels.

Fluids and Alkalinization

Almost all symptomatic patients with salicylate poisoning are dehydrated. Fluid challenges using 0.9 normal saline or Ringer's lactate should be given rapidly to replenish intravascular volume and produce good urinary flow. After hydration, intravenous fluids should include adequate amounts of sodium and potassium to replenish depleted body stores.[5]

All efforts should be made to keep arterial pH at 7.4 or greater. Alkalinization of urine is performed to trap ionized salicylate in urine and prevent its absorption. Alkaline urine is more important in enhancing salicylate excretion than is diuresis.[69] However, a urinary output of 2 to 3 ml/kg/hr is desirable if the patient can tolerate a fluid load. If only maintenance intravenous fluid rates will be used, 10% glucose should be present in the infusions unless dangerous hyperglycemia is present.

Two important means by which sodium is reabsorbed from the renal distal and collecting tubules are (1) sodium reabsorption in exchange for secretion of potassium ions into the tubular lumen and (2) sodium reabsorption in exchange for secretion of hydrogen ions into the tubular lumen. Both bicarbonate and potassium are required to produce alkaline urine. Even during alkalemia, alkaluria will not occur if the body is preferentially secreting hydrogen ions rather than potassium ions into tubular lumens while reabsorbing sodium.

A recommended method to produce an alkaline diuresis is to rapidly hydrate the patient with normal saline until an adequate urinary output is obtained. Sodium bicarbonate is given intravenously in 1 mEq/kg boluses until the blood pH is 7.5, to prevent the V_d of salicylate from continuing to increase. A continuous infusion of 1 L D5W to which is added 50 to 100 mEq sodium bicarbonate and 40 mEq potassium chloride is started at 2 to 3 times the maintenance rate. Arterial blood gases, serum electrolyte and glucose levels, and urine pH are monitored every 2 to 4 hours in moderately ill patients and every 1 to 2 hours in those severely ill. Indwelling arterial and urinary catheters facilitate monitoring and blood sampling. A fall in urine pH despite alkalemia is treated by increasing the amount of potassium in the infusion as long as dangerous hyperkalemia is not present. Falls in arterial pH are treated with boluses of sodium bicarbonate and then by increasing the bicarbonate in the intravenous infusion. Tremendous amounts of potassium may be required (>100 mmol/L IV fluid) in the bicarbonate infusion to produce alkaluria. If evidence of fluid overload develops, or if urinary output does not approach the rate of IV infusion despite adequate hydration, IV furosemide may be given.

Carbonic anhydrase inhibitors such as acetazolamide should not be used to alkalinize urine. This agent alkalinizes urine but also alkalinizes CSF,[37, 61, 70] trapping salicylate in the CNS.

Neurotoxicity

Severe lethargy, seizures, coma, or continued deterioration in level of consciousness despite supportive care is an ominous sign and an indication for immediate dialysis and treatment for cerebral edema, even if serum salicylate concentrations are falling. Mannitol has been effective in reversing cerebral edema and coma from salicylate poisoning.[35]

Dialysis

Hemodialysis markedly enhances the clearance of salicylate and also allows for correction of acid-base and electrolyte disorders.[71] Hemodialysis is indicated for patients

1. Who are deteriorating despite supportive care and alkaline blood and urine.
2. Who are deteriorating and in whom an alkaline urine cannot be produced (aciduria in spite of alkalemia and high normal serum potassium concentrations).
3. With acute or chronic renal failure.
4. With severe lethargy, seizures, coma, convulsions, or progressively worsening CNS toxicity.
5. With ARDS in whom salicylate levels are not rapidly falling.

It was once believed that all patients with a serum salicylate concentration greater than 100 mg/dl (1000 mg/L) should undergo emergent hemodialysis. However, patients with decreasing serum salicylate levels greater than 100 mg/dl

who are awake and alert, with only moderate electrolyte and acid-base disorders, can do well with intensive supportive care as long as dialysis is instituted at the first sign of neurologic deterioration or other major complications. However, most patients with serum salicylate concentrations greater than 100 mg/dl require dialysis, especially if serum salicylate concentrations are rising. Peritoneal dialysis is not as effective as hemodialysis and should not be used if the latter is available. If peritoneal dialysis is the only option, the dialysate should contain 5% albumin to enhance salicylate clearance through protein binding.

General

Serial measurements of serum salicylate concentrations should be taken in all patients admitted to the hospital to detect rising serum levels that may result in delayed toxicity. If salicylate concentrations rise for more than 18 to 24 hours, endoscopy or a limited upper GI radiocontrast examination should be performed to seek evidence of a concretion of salicylate that may be endoscopically removed.

Parenteral vitamin K is effective in reversing a prolonged prothrombin time. Occasionally, GI bleeding is severe enough to require transfusions. Therefore, serial measurements of hemoglobin concentrations or hematocrits should be performed. The use of antacids to treat corrosive injury to the GI tract produced by salicylates seems rational, although there are no studies examining their efficacy in salicylate poisoning. Patients who have ingested salicylic acid and who complain of throat, chest, or severe epigastric pain may have suffered significant corrosive injury and should undergo endoscopic examination. Serial serum creatine kinase activity should be followed to detect rhabdomyolysis in patients with severe salicylate toxicity or evidence of renal insufficiency.[72]

Pulmonary edema is usually noncardiac in nature.[29, 30, 73–76] Treatment of significant ARDS consists of positive-pressure ventilation, continuous positive airway pressure (CPAP), and ensuring that salicylate concentrations are rapidly falling (e.g., dialysis).

Finally, the need for frequent and compulsive monitoring of arterial blood gases, serum electrolytes, serum glucose, and urine pH along with repeated neurologic and cardiopulmonary examinations cannot be overemphasized. The acid-base status and electrolyte levels of seriously poisoned patients are constantly changing. Small changes in serum potassium concentrations or arterial pH can have dramatic effects on the degree of toxicity and salicylate clearance.

References

1. McGuigan MA. A two-year review of salicylate deaths in Ontario. Arch Intern Med 1987;147:510.
2. von Weiss JF, Lever WF. Percutaneous salicylic acid intoxication in psoriasis. Arch Dermatol 1964;90:614.
3. Aspinall JB, Goel RM. Salicylate poisoning in dermatological therapy (letter). Br Med J 1978;2:1373.
4. Howrie DL, Moriarty R, Breit R. Candy flavoring as a source of salicylate poisoning. Pediatrics 1985;75:869.
5. Temple AR. Pathophysiology of aspirin overdosage toxicity, with implications for management. Pediatrics 1978;62(Suppl):873.
6. Gabow PA, Anderson RJ, Potts DE, et al. Acid-base disturbances in the salicylate-intoxicated adult. Arch Intern Med 1978;138:1481.
7. Cunarro J, Weiner MW. Mechanism of action of agents which uncouple oxidative phosphorylation: Direct correlation between proton-carrying and respiratory-releasing properties using rat liver mitochondria. Biochim Biophys Acta 1975;387:234.
8. Kaplan E, Kennedy J, David J. Effects of salicylate and other benzoates on oxidative enzymes of the tricarboxylic acid cycle in rat tissue homogenates. Arch Biochem Biophys 1954;51:47.
9. Dawkins P, Gould B, Sturman J, et al. The mechanism of the inhibition of dehydrogenases by salicylate. J Pharm Pharmacol 1967;19:355.

10. Krebs HG, Woods HG, Alberti KG. Hyperlactataemia and lactic acidosis. Essays Med Biochem 1975;1:81.
11. Mizock BA. Lactic acidosis. DM 1989;35:233.
12. Zilva JF. The origin of acidosis in hyperlactataemia. Ann Clin Biochem 1978;15:40.
13. Gevers W. Generation of protons by metabolic processes in heart cells. J Mol Cell Cardiol 1977;9:867.
14. Mizock BA. Controversies in lactic acidosis. JAMA 1987;258:497.
15. Johnston DG, Alberti KG. Acid-base balance in metabolic acidoses. Clin Endocrinol Metab 1983;12:267.
16. Lehninger AL. Biochemistry. 2nd ed. New York, Worth Publishers, 1975, p 519.
17. Bartels PD, Lund-Jacobsen H. Blood lactate and ketone body concentrations in salicylate intoxication. Hum Toxicol 1986;5:363.
18. Gilman A, Goodman L, Rall T, Murad F (eds). Goodman and Gilman's The Pharmacological Basis of Therapeutics. 7th ed. New York, Macmillan, 1985, p 684.
19. Gould B, Dawkins P, Smith M, et al. The mechanism of the inhibition of aminotransferases by salicylate. Mol Pharmacol 1966;2:526.
20. Limbeck GA, Ruvalcaba RHA, Samols E, et al. Salicylates and hypoglycemia. Am J Dis Child 1965;109:165.
21. Snodgrass W, Rumack BH, Peterson RG, et al. Salicylate toxicity following therapeutic doses in young children. Clin Toxicol 1981;18:247.
22. Thruston JH, Pollock PG, Warren S, et al. Reduced brain glucose with normal plasma glucose in salicylate poisoning. J Clin Invest 1970;49:2139.
23. Gumpel JM. Enteric-coated aspirin overdose and gastric perforation (letter). Br Med J 1975;4:287.
24. Robins JB, Turnbull JA, Robertson C. Gastric perforation after acute aspirin overdose. Hum Toxicol 1985;4:527.
25. Sacchetti A, Ramoska E. Ingestion of Compound W, an unusual caustic. Am J Emerg Med 1986;4:554.
26. Everson GW, Krenzelok EP. Chronic salicylism in a patient with juvenile rheumatoid arthritis. Clin Pharm 1986;5:334.
27. Ulshen MH, Grand RJ, Crain JD, et al. Hepatotoxicity with encephalopathy associated with aspirin therapy in rheumatoid arthritis. J Pediatr 1978;93:1034.
28. Doughty RA, Glesecke L, Athreya B. Salicylate therapy in juvenile rheumatoid arthritis. Am J Dis Child 1980;134:461.
29. Walters JS, Woodring JH, Stelling CB, et al. Salicylate-induced pulmonary edema. Radiology 1983;146:289.
30. Heffner JE, Sahn SA. Salicylate-induced pulmonary edema. Clinical features and prognosis. Ann Intern Med 1981;95:405.
31. Temple AR, George DJ, Done AK, et al. Salicylate poisoning complicated by fluid retention. Clin Toxicol 1976;9:61.
32. Thisted B, Krantz T, Strom J, Sorensen MB. Acute salicylate self-poisoning in 177 consecutive patients treated in ICU. Acta Anaesthesiol Scand 1987;31:312.
33. Hildebrandt EF, Suttie JW. The effects of salicylate on enzymes of vitamin K metabolism. J Pharm Pharmacol 1983;35:421.
34. Proudfoot AT. Toxicity of salicylates. Am J Med 1983;75:99.
35. Dove DJ, Jones T. Delayed coma associated with salicylate intoxication. J Pediatr 1982;100:493.
36. Proudfoot AT, Brown SS. Acidaemia and salicylate poisoning in adults. Br Med J 1969;2:547.
37. Hill JB. Salicylate intoxication. N Engl J Med 1973;288:1110.
38. Fox GN. Hypocalcemia complicating bicarbonate therapy for salicylate poisoning. West J Med 1984;141:108.
39. Reid IR. Transient hypercalcemia following overdoses of soluble aspirin tablets (letter). Aust NZ J Med 1985;15:364.
40. Skjoto J, Reikvam A. Hyperthermia and rhabdomyolysis in self-poisoning with paracetamol and salicylates. Acta Med Scand 1979;205:473.
41. Leventhal LJ, Kuritsky L, Ginsburg R, Bomalaski JS. Salicylate-induced rhabdomyolysis. Am J Emerg Med 1989;7:409.
42. Rupp DJ, Seaton RD, Wiegmann TB. Acute polyuric renal failure after aspirin intoxication. Arch Intern Med 1983;143:1237.
43. Dromgoole SH, Furst DE. Salicylates. In Evans WE, Schentag JJ, Jusko WJ (eds). Applied Pharmacokinetics. Principles of Therapeutic Drug Monitoring. 2nd ed. Spokane, WA, Applied Therapeutics, 1986, p 944.
44. Levy G. Clinical pharmacokinetics of aspirin. Pediatrics 1978;62:867.
45. Kwong TC, Laczin J, Baum J. Self-poisoning with enteric-coated aspirin. Am J Clin Pathol 1983;80:888.
46. Henry AF. Overdoses of Entrophen (letter). Can Med Assoc J 1983;128:1142.
47. Taylor J, Halprin K. Percutaneous absorption of salicylic acid. Arch Dermatol 1975;111:740.
48. Reynolds RC, Cluff LE. Interaction of serum and sodium salicylate: Changes during acute infection and its influence on pharmacological activity. Bull Johns Hopkins Hosp 1960;105:278.
49. Done AK. Aspirin overdosage: Incidence, diagnosis, and management. Pediatrics 1978;62(Suppl):890.
50. Alvan G, Bergman U, Gustafsson LL. High unbound fraction of salicylate in plasma during intoxication. Br J Clin Pharmacol 1981;11:625.
51. Perez-Matao M, Erill S. Protein binding of salicylate and quinidine in plasma from patients with renal failure, chronic liver disease and chronic respiratory insufficiency. Eur J Clin Pharmacol 1977;11:225.
52. Borga O, Cederlof IO, Ringberger VA, et al. Protein binding of salicylate in uremic and normal plasma. Clin Pharmacol Ther 1976;20:464.
53. Levy G, Yaffe J. Relationship between dose and apparent volume of distribution of salicylate in children. Pediatrics 1974;54:713.
54. Needs CJ. Clinical pharmacokinetics of the salicylates. Clin Pharmacokinet 1985;10:164.
55. Done AK. Salicylate intoxication. Significance of measurements of salicylate in blood in cases of acute ingestion. Pediatrics 1960;26:800.
56. Winters RW, White JS, Hughes MC, Ordway MC. Disturbance of acid-base equilibrium in salicylate intoxication. Pediatrics 1959;23:260.
57. Gaudreault P, Temple AR, Lovejoy FH. The relative severity of acute versus chronic salicylate poisoning in children: A clinical comparison. Pediatrics 1982;70:566.
58. Erganian JA, Forbes GB, Case DM. Salicylate intoxication in the infant and young child. J Pediatr 1947;30:129.
59. Anderson CJ, Kaufman PL, Sturm RJ. Toxicity of combined therapy with carbonic anhydrase inhibitors and aspirin. Am J Ophthalmol 1978;86:516.
60. Sweeney KR, Chapron DJ, Brandt JL, et al. Toxic interaction between acetazolamide and salicylate: Case reports and a pharmacokinetic explanation. Clin Pharmacol Ther 1986;40:518.
61. Rollins DE, Withrow DM. Tissue acid-base balance in acetazolamide-treated rats. J Pharmacol Exp Ther 1970;174:535.
62. Danel V, Henry JA, Glucksman E. Activated charcoal, emesis, and gastric lavage in aspirin overdose. Br Med J 1988;296:1507.
63. Curtis RA, Barone J, Giacona N. Efficacy of ipecac and activated charcoal/cathartic. Prevention of salicylate absorption in a simulated overdose. Arch Intern Med 1984;144:48.
64. Easom JM, Caraccio TR, Lovejoy FH Jr. Evaluation of activated charcoal and magnesium citrate in the prevention of aspirin absorption in humans. Clin Pharm 1982;1:154.
65. Sketris IS, Mowry JB, Czajka PA, et al. Saline catharsis: Effect on aspirin bioavailability in combination with activated charcoal. J Clin Pharmacol 1982;22:59.
66. Hillman RJ, Prescott LF. Treatment of salicylate poisoning with repeated oral charcoal. Br Med J 1985;291:1472.
67. Kirshenbaum LA, Mathews SC, Sitar DS, et al. Does multiple-dose charcoal therapy enhance salicylate excretion? Arch Intern Med 1990;150:1281.
68. Dugandzic RM, Tierney MG, Dickinson GE, et al. Evaluation of the validity of the Done nomogram in the management of acute salicylate intoxication. Ann Emerg Med 1989;18:1186.
69. Prescott LF, Balali-Mood M, Critchley JH, et al. Diuresis or urinary alkalinization for salicylate poisoning? Br Med J 1982;285:1383.
70. Javaheri S. Effects of acetazolamide on cerebrospinal fluid ions in metabolic alkalosis in dogs. J Appl Physiol 1987;62:1582.
71. Jacobsen D, Wilk-Larsen E, Bredesen JE. Haemodialysis or haemoperfusion in severe salicylate poisoning? Hum Toxicol 1988;7:161.
72. Curry SC, Chang D, Connor D. Drug- and toxin-induced rhabdomyolysis. Ann Emerg Med 1989;18:1068.
73. Hrnicek G, Skelton J, Miller WC. Pulmonary edema and salicylate intoxication. JAMA 1974;230:866.
74. Heffner JE, Starkey T, Anthony P. Salicylate-induced noncardiogenic pulmonary edema. West J Med 1979;130:263.
75. Davis PR, Burch RE. Pulmonary edema and salicylate intoxication (letter). Ann Intern Med 1974;80:553.
76. Zimmerman GA, Clemmer TP. Acute respiratory failure during therapy for salicylate intoxication. Ann Emerg Med 1981;10:104.

CHAPTER 85

Iron

Steven C. Curry

INTRODUCTION

Prenatal iron supplements are commonly found in young households. Many of these preparations are identical in appearance to candy; some are even sugar-coated. Many colorful and flavored chewable vitamin tablets for children are supplemented with iron, making their ingestion attractive.

PATHOPHYSIOLOGY

About 10% of dietary iron is absorbed each day, mainly in the duodenum. Iron is absorbed in the ferrous (Fe^{2+}) state. Free, unbound iron is extremely toxic to living cells, and the body has extensive mechanisms to keep iron bound to protein or other macromolecules at all times. After absorption, iron rapidly converts to the ferric state (Fe^{3+}) and is stored as ferritin in the intestinal mucosa. Ferric iron is transported in blood to other ferritin storage sites or to areas of iron incorporation while bound to the protein, transferrin. The total amount of iron that transferrin can bind is called the total iron binding capacity (TIBC). The TIBC usually far exceeds serum iron concentrations and ranges from about 300 to 435 µg/dl. Serum iron concentrations vary diurnally and normally range from 50 to 150 µg/dl.

Iron is directly corrosive to the gastrointestinal tract. Acute ingestions can be accompanied by abdominal pain, nausea, vomiting, hematemesis, melena, and intestinal perforations and infarctions.[1-7] The aspiration of an iron tablet has produced bronchial stenosis.[8]

The absorption of excessive quantities of iron results in systemic iron poisoning. Iron poisoning is accompanied by venous pooling and significant third-spacing of fluids,[3, 9-11] possibly secondary to elevated circulating ferritin levels. After absorption, iron is rapidly taken up by the liver and concentrated within hepatocytes.[12-14] In hepatocytes, iron is further concentrated within mitochondria, where it impairs oxidative phosphorylation by disrupting electron transport and destroying the structural integrity of mitochondrial membranes through generation of oxygen free radicals and lipid peroxidation.[3, 15-17] The ability of iron to impair adenosine triphosphate (ATP) production while stimulating oxygen consumption in the generation of oxygen free radicals can be confused with the action of an uncoupler of oxidative phosphorylation and is better described as *pseudouncoupling*.

The consequence of mitochondrial dysfunction and impaired oxidative phosphorylation is cell death. Because the liver is the first organ after the gut to encounter excessive quantities of iron, and because the liver takes up and concentrates iron from the portal circulation, hepatic necrosis is the most common organ dysfunction seen outside the GI tract. However, almost any organ can suffer mitochondrial damage, dysfunction, and necrosis in the face of large iron burdens. Severe acute iron poisoning can result in renal failure, myocardial degeneration and heart failure, adult respiratory distress syndrome, convulsions, coma, shock, and death.[7, 18, 19]

Metabolic acidosis is seen in significant iron poisoning. Hypovolemia from GI losses, GI bleeding, third-spacing of fluids, and venodilation results in hypoperfusion of tissue and acidosis. Anemia can at times be severe enough to contribute to impaired oxygen delivery. The hydration of absorbed ferric iron also may generate hydrogen ions.[3]

$$Fe^{3+} + 3\ H_2O = 3\ Fe(OH)_3 + 3H^+$$

Oxidative phosphorylation is a major buffer of hydrogen ions, consuming them in the generation of ATP.[20, 21] Impaired oxidative phosphorylation from iron-induced disruption of electron transport and mitochondrial structural damage hinders this buffering capacity, resulting in metabolic acidosis. Circulating lactate concentrations may be elevated,

reflecting an increased reliance on glycolysis for ATP production in the face of mitochondrial dysfunction.

Serious hepatic necrosis is accompanied by impaired gluconeogenesis and hypoglycemia. As gluconeogenesis is also an important buffer of hydrogen ions,[21, 22] such dysfunction also contributes to metabolic acidosis.

Coagulopathy can be seen early in iron poisoning in the absence of hepatic dysfunction.[22, 23] Elevated serum iron concentrations directly inhibit proteases such as thrombin, resulting in prolonged coagulation times. This initial coagulopathy resolves as serum iron concentrations fall. However, coagulopathy may reappear if hepatic necrosis develops over the next 24 to 72 hours.[23]

PHARMACOKINETICS AND TOXIC DOSES

In order to determine the amount of iron ingested, the amount of elemental iron must be calculated (Table 85–1). Reported toxic doses of elemental iron vary, mainly because of the extremely unreliable histories of amounts ingested. Patients become symptomatic after ingestions of only 20 mg elemental iron per kg body weight. The ingestion of more than 40 mg elemental iron per kg commonly results in moderate to severe poisoning. Because of unreliable histories surrounding most iron ingestions, any symptomatic patient or any patient with a history of ingesting more than 20 mg elemental iron per kg requires evaluation for iron poisoning.

After iron overdose, most of the iron is not absorbed but excreted in the stool. Although iron is normally absorbed in the duodenum, iron absorption may occur throughout the GI tract, including the colon, after overdose.[10]

Serum iron concentrations generally peak between 2 and 6 hours after overdose. The rapid clearance of iron from plasma with deposition in liver and other tissues can result in deceptively low serum iron concentrations within a few hours of a large ingestion.[3, 24] Unpredictable absorption during the first few hours coupled with relatively rapid clearance from blood can make a single determination of a serum iron concentration of little help, and perhaps misleading, when the reading is normal. Levels drawn early after ingestion may falsely reassure the physician that toxic serum iron concentrations will not occur. Because it is iron in tissue, not in blood, that produces systemic toxicity, many children have normal or low serum iron concentrations[3, 19, 24] by the time of onset of shock, coma, and death if several hours have elapsed since the time of ingestion.

CLINICAL EVALUATION

The first stage of iron poisoning occurs within the first few hours of ingestion and is due to the corrosive action of iron on the GI tract. Stage 1 is characterized by vomiting, hematemesis, abdominal pain, and diarrhea.[1-3, 6, 7] Pallor,

TABLE 85–1

ELEMENTAL IRON CONTENT OF COMMON IRON PREPARATIONS

Compound	Elemental Iron (%)
Ferrous sulfate	16
Ferrous gluconate	12
Ferrous fumarate	33
Ferrous phosphate	37
Ferrous pyrophosphate	12
Ferrocholinate	12
Ferric pyrophosphate	12
Ferroglycine sulfate	16
Ferrous carbonate, anhydrous	48

hypotension, and acidosis during stage 1 are secondary to hypovolemia and hypoperfusion from GI fluid and blood losses. Hypovolemia can be severe enough to cause death. Many children have hyperglycemia and leukocytosis as a reflection of stress.[25]

The second stage of iron poisoning is not always seen and can continue up to about the 12th to 24th hour after ingestion.[6, 7, 18] In stage 2, GI symptoms resolve. However, toxic quantities of iron are being or have been absorbed into the body, albeit not yet producing marked systemic symptoms. Many children lie quietly or sleep during this stage. If arterial blood gases are measured, metabolic acidosis is frequently seen. Coagulopathy in this stage is mainly due to elevated serum iron concentrations rather than to hepatic necrosis. Hypotension is due to unreplaced GI fluid losses, venodilation, and third-spacing of fluids. The resolution of GI symptoms can be falsely reassuring.[26] Physicians must be careful not to discharge a stage 2 patient from the emergency department.

Stage 3 may appear early in those with severe poisoning (often without stage 2) or may appear several hours after the onset of stage 2. Systemic effects of iron prevail with venous pooling of blood, third-spacing of fluid, multiple organ failure, hepatic necrosis, and possible involvement of other organ systems (e.g., coma, convulsions, renal failure, heart failure).[1, 6, 7, 18] Hypoglycemia and coagulopathy reflect hepatic dysfunction. Shock in this stage is due to hypovolemia from venous pooling, third-spacing of fluids, any unreplaced GI losses, and myocardial dysfunction secondary to toxic effects of iron on the heart.[1, 9, 11, 19] In addition to hypoperfusion, metabolic acidosis in this stage reflects impaired oxidative phosphorylation, hepatic necrosis, and possibly the failure of other organ systems (e.g., kidneys). Bowel infarctions may become apparent during stage 3 or several days later.[4, 5]

Stage 4 occurs days to weeks after acute poisoning and is uncommon. It is characterized by gastric outlet or small bowel obstruction from scarring produced by the corrosive effect of iron in the GI tract.

DIAGNOSTIC EVALUATION

In symptomatic patients with a history of ingesting iron, the diagnosis is straightforward. The presence of radiopacities on an abdominal radiograph is suggestive of iron poisoning, but their lack does not exclude this possibility.[25, 27]

Measurement of elevated serum iron concentration confirms the ingestion of iron, but these concentrations may be misleadingly low if measured early after ingestion or if measured after iron levels have peaked and have fallen back into the normal range, leaving an unrecognized toxic burden of iron in tissue.

Severe poisoning can be seen in children whose peak serum iron concentrations exceed 300 to 350 $\mu g/dl$. Hepatotoxicity is usually not seen unless these concentrations exceed 500 $\mu g/dl$. Again, patients may die in early stages of iron poisoning from hypovolemia or acidosis before developing hepatotoxicity or other organ system involvement.

Serum iron concentrations can be accurately measured by atomic absorption spectrometry in the presence of deferoxamine.[28] However, deferoxamine causes falsely low serum iron concentration readings by most colorimetric methods.[28, 29] Deferoxamine's interference is corrected by adding sodium hydrosulfite (sodium dithionite) during measurement.[29] Centers that do not take this precaution report falsely low serum iron concentrations in patients receiving deferoxamine.

It is presumed that deferoxamine also causes falsely low serum iron concentrations as measured by radioimmunoassay (RIA). More important, most RIA methods cannot measure serum iron concentrations greater than the TIBC. Therefore, serum iron concentrations reported as being nearly the same as the TIBC may be much higher in reality.

McGuigan and colleagues[30] described a rapid screening test to identify patients who have ingested toxic doses of iron within the previous 2 hours. Two test tubes, each containing 2 ml gastric fluid and two drops 30% hydrogen peroxide, are prepared; 2 ml of distilled water containing 250 mg deferoxamine mesylate (125 mg deferoxamine mesylate/ml) are added to one tube and the colors of the tubes are compared. The formation of ferrioxamine from deferoxamine and iron is accompanied by a color change that may vary from light orange to dark red. Care must be taken to ensure that laboratory ware is free of iron. Serum iron levels were elevated in eight of nine patients with a positive color test.[30] It is not known how to interpret a negative result because of the small number of patients in the study.

DIFFERENTIAL DIAGNOSIS

The differential diagnosis of iron poisoning includes poisoning by salicylate, acetaminophen, hepatotoxic mushrooms, copper salts, phosphorus, caustics, theophylline, caffeine, arsenic, and mercurial salts. Gastrointestinal disturbances are common in children with almost any infectious disease. Vomiting and diarrhea followed by acidosis and shock may be confused with sepsis or invasive GI infections. In the absence of secondary causes (e.g., aspiration, bowel infarction, infection), iron poisoning is not accompanied by fever.

EVALUATION AND DISPOSITION

Patients arriving in the emergency department who have remained completely asymptomatic (including no lethargy) for 6 hours after ingestion of iron and whose physical examinations are completely normal do not need further evaluation or treatment for iron poisoning. Those who have intentionally ingested iron in a suicide attempt may require psychiatric evaluation and treatment.

Symptomatic patients should have blood drawn for determination of serum electrolyte, glucose, blood urea nitrogen, and creatinine concentrations; baseline serum liver enzymes; complete blood count; prothrombin time; and serum iron concentration. An abdominal radiograph should be obtained for evidence of radiopacities, a factor that strongly suggests significantly elevated serum iron concentrations.

Moderately to severely ill patients (e.g., more than one episode of vomiting or diarrhea, hypovolemia, acidosis, lethargy) require treatment and admission to the hospital. Measurement of arterial blood gases may also be necessary.

In asymptomatic patients who have ingested iron less than 6 hours previously or in mildly symptomatic patients, the major diagnostic challenge is to predict which individuals have a significant risk of proceeding to systemic iron poisoning. Several investigators have performed retrospective studies examining the usefulness of symptoms, common laboratory values, and abdominal radiography in predicting which patients will develop serum iron concentrations of 300 $\mu g/dl$ or more.

Thus, most children with vomiting, diarrhea, a serum glucose concentration greater than 300 mg/dl, a white blood cell count greater than 15,000/m^3, or radiopacities seen on an abdominal film will have (or will have had) a serum iron concentration of 300 mg/dl or more.[25, 31] One should not wait for results of serum iron concentration tests to begin treatment with deferoxamine in these patients.

There are pitfalls in using these common indicators to predict who has elevated serum iron levels. First, the absence of these indicators cannot be used to exclude iron poisoning. Children may be severely poisoned with iron, yet have normal serum glucose concentration, normal WBC count, a normal abdominal film, and minimal vomiting or diarrhea. Second, these indicators are meant to detect (not exclude) patients with elevated serum iron concentrations when iron concentrations are not yet available. Normal indicators in a patient with an elevated serum iron concentration do not mean that therapy is not necessary.

Normal serum iron concentrations may be seen in seriously poisoned patients if drawn before or after peak serum iron concentrations have occurred (2 to 6 hours). The measurement of a normal serum iron concentration in an asymptomatic patient within 1 to 2 hours of ingestion is reassuring only if a second level drawn 1 to 2 hours later demonstrates that the concentration is not rising. An isolated normal or low serum iron concentration is reassuring several hours after ingestion only if the patient is asymptomatic, was never or only mildly symptomatic previously (e.g., a single emesis), has not received deferoxamine, has a completely normal physical examination, has no evidence of GI bleeding, has a negative abdominal radiograph, and has no acidosis or evidence of hypovolemia.

THERAPEUTIC INTERVENTION

General

Children who have ingested more than 20 mg elemental iron per kg should undergo gastric lavage if spontaneous vomiting has not occurred. Ipecac should be avoided since the ensuing vomiting can be confused with symptoms of iron poisoning. There are no data suggesting that gastric emptying procedures are of benefit in the patient who is already vomiting. Activated charcoal does not adsorb iron and need not be given for isolated ingestions of iron or vitamins with iron.

There are no data supporting out-of-date recommendations for enteral administration of bicarbonate or phosphate solutions in attempts to prevent iron absorption.[32, 33] In fact, enteral administration of phosphate solutions to iron-poisoned children has caused hypocalcemia, shock, and major morbidity.[34, 35]

In vitro and in vivo animal studies argue for administration of magnesium oxide (or hydroxide) to prevent iron absorption.[36, 37] It appears that 120 ml Milk of Magnesia is adequate for most ingestions,[37] but this dosage may be excessive for young children. Magnesium levels may rise with large doses of magnesium oxide. Serial magnesium levels should therefore be checked or the patient closely watched for evidence of magnesium toxicity. No human studies have been performed addressing the efficacy of magnesium oxide in preventing iron absorption after overdose.

All symptomatic children (with vomiting, diarrhea, or lethargy) are hypovolemic and should rapidly receive 20 ml/kg of 0.9 normal saline intravenously until volume resuscitated. This dose is repeated as needed in those who continue to show evidence of hypovolemia (e.g., tachycardia, hypotension, pallor, oliguria). There may be myocardial dysfunction in some stage 3 patients.[19] However, hypovolemia from third-spacing of fluids, venodilation, and GI losses is commonly underestimated and is the most important factor in causing hypotension, hypoperfusion, and shock. It is common for children to require 40 to 60 ml/kg normal saline until adequate urinary output returns. The ability of iron to induce pronounced relative and absolute hypovole-

mia has been reiterated after studies in an animal model of acute iron poisoning.[9]

Several reports described emergency gastrotomy for removal of iron tablets remaining in the stomach (as detected by abdominal radiography) after gastric lavage.[38–41] However, there are no controlled studies in humans or animals demonstrating that these children would not have done well with intensive supportive care and chelation with deferoxamine. It is not uncommon to note intact or partially dissolved tablets remaining in the stomach after gastric lavage. These patients almost always do well with intravenous deferoxamine and supportive care, and radiographic opacities disappear within 24 hours.

Seriously ill patients who develop signs of peritonitis or who have evidence of free air on abdominal films require abdominal exploration for infarcted or perforated bowel. Unfortunately, such patients are usually critically ill from the ingestion (e.g., shock, coagulopathy, hepatic necrosis, adult respiratory distress syndrome [ARDS], anemia), making the decision to operate more difficult.

The growth of *Yersinia* is dependent on iron.[42] Patients with chronic iron overload,[43] those with acute iron poisoning,[44] and those receiving deferoxamine[45] (making iron more available to the bacteria) are predisposed to infections by *Y. enterocolitica* and related species. Patients with acute iron poisoning who are suspected of having infection should therefore receive antibiotics active against *Yersinia* (e.g., trimethoprim-sulfamethoxazole).

Deferoxamine

Indications and Dosage. The introduction of the iron chelator deferoxamine mesylate has revolutionized the treatment of iron poisoning and markedly decreased morbidity and mortality (Table 85–2). At physiologic pH, deferoxamine complexes almost exclusively with ferric iron.[46] It complexes with non–protein-bound iron as well as with ferric iron from ferritin, hemosiderin, and to a lesser extent transferrin[47–51] to form ferrioxamine, a dark red-orange compound that is excreted in the urine.[3, 52] Deferoxamine does not remove significant amounts of iron from hemoglobin.[53]

TABLE 85–2

GUIDELINES FOR USE OF DEFEROXAMINE MESYLATE

Indications for therapy (any one of the following)
  Any moderately to severely symptomatic patient (e.g., more than one emesis, diarrhea, abdominal pain, lethargy, hypovolemia, acidosis) regardless of serum iron concentration
  Any patient with radiopacities from iron on an abdominal radiograph
  Any patient with a serum iron concentration greater than 300–350 µg/dl, regardless of total iron-binding capacity

Administration (after rapid and adequate fluid resuscitation)
  30 mg/kg IV over 1-hr loading dose optional
  15 mg/kg/hr IV as a continuous drip
  May be mixed in crystalloid fluid of choice

Halting deferoxamine (all the following conditions must be met)
  Patient has no further signs and symptoms of systemic iron poisoning (e.g., no acidosis, normal vital signs, liver function stable)

and

  Serum iron concentration is well within normal range or is low (deferoxamine causes falsely low serum iron concentrations [see text]).

and

  Vin-rose urine color is absent

Deferoxamine binds to and inactivates iron in cytoplasm and mitochondria to prevent iron from interfering with mitochondrial function and to prevent further mitochondrial damage.[3, 54–57] Deferoxamine can even reverse organ dysfunction in patients with chronic iron overload.[58] Therefore, an important (if not the most important) reason for giving deferoxamine is to remove iron from tissue, not just to remove iron from blood.

The preferred route of administration of deferoxamine mesylate is a continuous intravenous infusion at a rate of 15 mg/kg/hr[55] after rapid fluid resuscitation is complete. Most toxicologists do not give a loading dose of deferoxamine because of reported short elimination half-lives for the drug (about 1 hour). However, reported pharmacokinetic data regarding deferoxamine's distribution and elimination vary[59–62]; one investigator suggested that although the initial half-life of deferoxamine is 60 to 70 minutes, the terminal elimination half-life may be as long as 6 hours.[61] Therefore, final steady state deferoxamine concentrations might not be achieved for many hours after the onset of a continuous infusion. Indeed, while some investigators report steady-state plasma deferoxamine concentrations within 2 to 3 hours of initiation of a continuous infusion, others note that 12 hours may be required to reach steady state. Therefore, patients can receive an initial load of 30 mg/kg deferoxamine mesylate intravenously over 1 hour while starting a continuous intravenous infusion.

Deferoxamine mesylate can be given intramuscularly, suggested doses ranging from 45 mg/kg every 4 hours to 90 mg/kg every 6 hours. However, intramuscular administration has three disadvantages. First, studies in patients with chronic iron overload show that a continuous intravenous infusion of deferoxamine removes severalfold more iron than the same dose given intramuscularly.[51] Second, intermittent IM injections of deferoxamine result in much higher peak plasma concentrations than continuous IV infusions. These high concentrations may be more likely to result in deferoxamine-induced hypotension.[1, 24] Finally, the volume of deferoxamine mesylate required for IM injections is ridiculously large for many children and would have to be divided into multiple injections for each dose.

It is controversial whether the administration of large quantities of deferoxamine orally is beneficial in the treatment of acute iron poisoning.[3, 63, 64] In any event, such therapy is impractical in most instances: 100 mg deferoxamine mesylate binds 8.5 mg elemental iron[53]; if a 20-kg child has ingested 80 mg/kg elemental iron, almost 19,000 mg deferoxamine mesylate is required for a minimal metal:chelate ratio of 1:1.

A mistake made in the treatment of iron poisoning is to withhold deferoxamine therapy from symptomatic patients until results of serum iron concentrations are available. An important reason to give deferoxamine is to remove iron from tissue. A normal serum iron concentration may be seen early after ingestion, but serum iron levels may have risen far above normal by the time results return. A normal serum iron concentration a few hours after ingestion does not mean that it was not markedly elevated earlier and does not exclude elevated tissue burdens of iron. Published reports[19] and personal experience in noting vin-rose urine in iron-poisoned patients after serum iron concentrations have fallen well into the normal range illustrate the ability of deferoxamine to chelate elevated tissue burdens of iron in acutely poisoned patients. Because deferoxamine would be indicated in such patients regardless of serum iron concentration, immediate deferoxamine therapy after rapid hydration is indicated in any child with moderate to severe symptoms (e.g., diarrhea, more than one emesis, lethargy,

abdominal pain, evidence of hypovolemia, acidosis) regardless of results of serum iron concentrations.

Another laboratory value commonly misused in making a decision to administer or withdraw deferoxamine therapy is the TIBC. It seems rational that acute systemic iron poisoning should not result if the serum iron concentration never exceeds the TIBC. However, the assumption that serum iron concentrations must exceed the TIBC to produce systemic toxicity has never been proved. Patients with chronic iron overload suffer major organ dysfunction from systemic iron poisoning, but do not have serum iron concentrations greater than the TIBC. In addition, serum iron concentrations are constantly changing, and significant tissue burdens of iron may be present in the face of a serum iron concentration below the TIBC. Finally, and most important, methods used by most laboratories in measuring TIBC give falsely elevated TIBC values at toxic iron concentrations.[65] Higher serum iron levels are associated with falsely elevated TIBCs, making interpretation of the TIBC meaningless. Therefore, in addition to deferoxamine treatment for any moderate to severely symptomatic patient (regardless of the serum iron concentration), this agent should be given to any patient with an iron concentration equal to or greater than 300 to 350 µg/dl, regardless of the laboratory TIBC report. If the physician does obtain a TIBC, and if the serum iron concentration is reported to be higher than the TIBC, deferoxamine also should be administered.

The final parameter that is frequently misused in deciding to institute or withdraw deferoxamine therapy is the color of the urine. Deferoxamine combines with iron to form ferrioxamine, which is dark orange-red and is excreted in the urine. Past literature recommended a "deferoxamine challenge" that consisted of giving a single IM injection of deferoxamine and observing the color of the urine. The presence of vin-rose urine was taken to indicate the need for deferoxamine; its absence was regarded as evidence that deferoxamine was not required. This concept was further expanded to a recommendation that deferoxamine could be discontinued as soon as urine color became normal. In fact, the relationship between urine color and urine iron or ferrioxamine concentration is unpredictable. Cases have been documented in which serum iron and urine iron (ferrioxamine) concentrations were markedly elevated, yet vin-rose urine was not seen.[1, 66] While the presence of vin-rose urine probably indicates that deferoxamine is required and should be continued, the absence of vin-rose urine after administration of deferoxamine cannot be taken as evidence that deferoxamine is not required and should not be used alone to justify the discontinuation of deferoxamine in patients who are receiving chelation therapy.

Deferoxamine should be continued until all the following criteria are met: (1) the serum iron concentration is well within the normal range (or low), (2) vin-rose urine is absent, (3) the patient is free from evidence of systemic iron toxicity (e.g., normal vital signs, no acidosis, liver function stable). Most children with peak serum iron concentrations less than 400 to 500 µg/dl do well with 16 to 24 hours of a deferoxamine mesylate infusion. Patients suffering massive iron overdoses may require such an infusion for several days.

Dosage in Renal and Hepatic Dysfunction. Although deferoxamine enhances urinary iron excretion as ferrioxamine, increasing urinary elimination of ferrioxamine is not the main mechanism by which deferoxamine counteracts iron poisoning.[1, 2, 67, 68] Urinary iron excretion (ferrioxamine) may be acutely elevated after the administration of deferoxamine, but much of the ferrioxamine is not excreted for days afterward.[1] The most important protective action of deferoxamine is to combine with and inactivate iron by forming ferrioxamine, regardless of how quickly ferrioxamine may be excreted in urine. Therefore, deferoxamine infusion should be continued during acute iron poisoning, even if there is renal failure.

Dialysis and hemoperfusion can remove some ferrioxamine as well as deferoxamine.[69, 70] Recommendations have been made to continue deferoxamine and institute dialysis to remove ferrioxamine in the presence of renal failure.[3, 71] However, since the excretion of ferrioxamine may not be essential for deferoxamine's ability to prevent death from iron poisoning, it is not established that these procedures should be instituted only to enhance ferrioxamine clearance.

Numerous authors state that deferoxamine is extensively metabolized in the liver and other tissue, while ferrioxamine is excreted unchanged in the urine.[3, 52, 55, 72] However, Stivelman and colleagues[69] reported that deferoxamine's plasma half-life in patients with renal failure averaged 25.6 hours between dialysis sessions compared with only 2 hours during hemodialysis. Reported half-lives in patients with normal renal and hepatic function vary from about 1 to 6 hours. Therefore, despite claims of deferoxamine's extensive metabolic clearance, the infusion dose should be markedly decreased after the onset of renal failure. There are no data suggesting how to adjust deferoxamine mesylate doses in the face of hepatic dysfunction.

Toxicity. Deferoxamine mesylate produces hypotension at high infusion rates (probably greater than about 45 mg/kg/hr) or after large IM injections, and it has been suggested that this is due to pharmacologic histamine release.[1] The administration of deferoxamine mesylate at 15 mg/kg/hr to treat acute iron poisoning is rarely associated with hypotension.

Blake and colleagues[73] described two patients receiving deferoxamine for rheumatoid arthritis who became unconscious for 2 to 3 days after receiving one or two therapeutic doses of prochlorperazine for nausea. The ability of a combination of deferoxamine mesylate and prochlorperazine (but not each agent alone) to produce coma was confirmed in animals.[73] The cause of this interaction is unknown. On the basis of this report, patients receiving deferoxamine should not receive prochlorperazine.

There are no data with regard to acute iron poisoning supporting the manufacturer's recommendation that the total daily dose of deferoxamine mesylate be restricted to 6 gm or less. Relatively large doses or infusion rates of deferoxamine mesylate have been used safely to treat acute iron poisoning. Peck and colleagues[72] described a 19-year-old woman who received 37.1 gm deferoxamine mesylate over 52 hours for severe iron poisoning without adverse effect. Boehnert and colleagues[74] reported a 10-kg child who received 14.2 gm of this agent over 7 days at a rate of 35 mg/kg/hr (serum iron concentration 12,000 μg/dl) without developing evidence of deferoxamine toxicity.

Acute renal failure has been described after initiation of deferoxamine therapy in patients with acute iron poisoning.[75] The fact that iron poisoning itself may produce renal failure makes causal effect indefinite. However, animal studies and the occurrence of acute renal failure in patients with chronic iron overload receiving deferoxamine warrant concern.[75] In one study the infusion of deferoxamine mesylate (10 mg/kg/hr) to normovolemic mongrel dogs was accompanied by a significant fall in both glomerular filtration rate (GFR) and renal blood flow along with tubular dysfunction.[75] Fluid challenges prevented the decrease in GFR but not that in renal blood flow. The ability of deferoxamine to cause vasodilation, hypotension, and adverse renal effects illustrates the importance of adequate fluid resuscitation before and during deferoxamine therapy in patients with acute iron poisoning.

Four of eight patients who received 4 to 9 days of intensive IV deferoxamine therapy for chronic iron overload developed pulmonary interstitial and alveolar infiltrates and, in some cases, fibrosis.[76] Four cases of unexpected and rapidly fatal ARDS in adults with acute iron poisoning have been reported.[77] All had received deferoxamine for 65 to 106 hours before the onset of respiratory distress. Although severe acute iron poisoning itself can produce ARDS, these patients were not in shock or suffering from acidosis before respiratory failure. If deferoxamine-induced pneumonitis or ARDS is a real entity, it must be uncommon and appears to be limited to patients who receive IV deferoxamine for several days.

Anaphylactoid reactions induced by deferoxamine have been rarely reported[78, 79] and are probably the extreme of pharmacologic histamine release that is responsible for dose-dependent vasodilation. Deferoxamine-induced thrombocytopenia was reported in a patient with aluminum toxicity who had received repeated doses of deferoxamine.[80]

Patients with chronic iron overload (e.g., thalassemia, renal failure) or with aluminum toxicity commonly receive intermittent IV or subcutaneous infusions of deferoxamine for days, months, or years. Numerous reports document that deferoxamine therapy in these patients is associated with neurotoxicity characterized by neurosensory hearing loss and retinal changes leading to decreased visual acuity and changes in color vision.[45, 73, 81–88] Auditory and visual functions commonly improve after deferoxamine is discontinued.

These neurotoxic effects appear to be dose related[88] and usually do not appear until the patient has received deferoxamine for more than 1 week; most authors describe toxicity after several weeks or months of therapy. Nevertheless, a patient with end-stage renal disease developed ocular toxicity after a single dose of deferoxamine, suggesting that such an occurrence may be possible in a person with acute iron poisoning.[86]

Despite the proved or suspected adverse effects of deferoxamine described above, the medical literature contains almost no reports of toxicity resulting from short-term IV administration of deferoxamine mesylate at 15 mg/kg/hr to patients with acute iron poisoning. Considering what some authors estimate to be a 50-fold reduction in mortality from acute iron poisoning associated with the introduction of deferoxamine, there is no doubt that the benefits of this drug far outweigh any potential adverse effects in the treatment of acute iron poisoning.

References

1. Proudfoot AT, Simpson D, Dyson EH. Management of acute iron poisoning. Med Toxicol 1986;1:83.
2. McEnry JT, Greengard J. Treatment of acute iron ingestion with deferoxamine in 20 children. J Pediatr 1966;68:773.
3. Robotham JL, Lietman PS. Acute iron poisoning. Am J Dis Child 1980;134:875.
4. Knott LH, Miller RC. Acute iron intoxication with intestinal infarction. J Pediatr Surg 1978;13:720.
5. Roberts RJ, Mayfield S, Soper R, et al. Acute iron intoxication with intestinal infarction managed in part by small bowel resection. Clin Toxicol 1975;8:3.
6. Covey TJ. Ferrous sulfate poisoning: A review, case summaries and therapeutic regimen. J Pediatr 1964;64:218.
7. Jacobs J, Greene H, Gendel BR. Acute iron intoxication. N Engl J Med 1965;273:1124.
8. Tarkka M, Anttila S, Sutinen S. Bronchial stenosis after aspiration of an iron tablet. Chest 1988;93:439.
9. Vernon DD, Banner W Jr, Dean JM. Hemodynamic effects of experimental iron poisoning. Ann Emerg Med 1989;18:863.
10. Reissmann KR, Coleman TJ, Budai BS, et al. Acute intestinal iron intoxication. I. Iron absorption, serum iron and autopsy findings. Blood 1955;10:35.
11. Reissmann KR, Coleman TJ. Acute intestinal iron intoxication. II. Metabolic, respiratory and circulating effects of absorbed iron salts. Blood 1955;10:46.

12. Witzleben CL, Chaffey NJ. Acute ferrous sulfate poisoning: A histochemical study of its effect on the liver. Arch Pathol Lab Med 1966;82:454.

13. Witzleben CL. An electron microscopic study of ferrous sulfate–induced liver damage. Am J Pathol 1966;49:1053.

14. Ganote CE, Nahara G. Acute ferrous sulfate hepatotoxicity in rats: An electron microscopic and biochemical study. Lab Invest 1973;28:426.

15. Robotham JL, Troxler RF, Lietman PS. Iron poisoning: Another energy crisis. Lancet 1974;2:664.

16. Hunter FE, Gebicki JM, Hoffsten PE, et al. Swelling and lysis of rat liver mitochondria induced by ferrous ions. J Biol Chem 1963;238:828.

17. Gruger EH, Tappel AL. Reactions of biological antioxidants I. Fe(II)-catalysed reactions of lipid hydroperoxides with alpha-tocopherol. Lipids 1970;5:326.

18. Henretig FM, Temple AR. Acute iron poisoning in children. Clin Lab Med 1984;4:575.

19. Tenenbein M, Kopelow ML, deSa DJ. Myocardial failure and shock in iron poisoning. Hum Toxicol 1988;7:281.

20. Mizock BA. Controversies in lactic acidosis. JAMA 1987;258:497.

21. Mizock BA. Lactic acidosis. DM 1989;35:233.

22. Evensen SA, Forde R, Opedal I, et al. Acute iron intoxication with abruptly reduced levels of vitamin K–dependent coagulation factors. Scand J Haematol 1982;29:25.

23. Tenenbein M, Israels SJ. Early coagulopathy in severe iron poisoning. J Pediatr 1988;113:697.

24. Fischer DS, Parkman R, Finch SC. Acute iron poisoning in children: The problem of appropriate therapy. JAMA 1971;218:1179.

25. Lacouture PG, Wason S, Temple AR, et al. Emergency assessment of severity in iron overdose by clinical and laboratory methods. J Pediatr 1981;99:89.

26. Spencer IOB. Ferrous sulphate poisoning in children. Br Med J 1951;2:1112.

27. Ng RCW, Perry K, Martin DJ. Iron poisoning. Assessment of radiography in diagnosis and management. Clin Pediatr 1979;18:614.

28. Helfer RE, Rodgerson DO. The effect of deferoxamine on the determination of serum iron and iron-binding capacity. J Pediatr 1966;68:804.

29. Gevirtz NR, Wasserman LR. The measurement of iron and iron-binding capacity in plasma containing deferoxamine. J Pediatr 1966;68:802.

30. McGuigan MA, Lovejoy FH, Marino SK, et al. Qualitative deferoxamine color test for iron ingestion. J Pediatr 1979;94:940.

31. Knasel AL, Collins-Barrow MD. Applicability of early indicators of iron toxicity. J Natl Med Assoc 1986;78:1037.

32. Czajka PA, Konrad JD, Duffy JP. Iron poisoning: An in vitro comparison of bicarbonate and phosphate lavage solutions. J Pediatr 1981;98:491.

33. Dean BS, Krenzelok EP. In vivo effectiveness of oral complexation agents in the management of iron poisoning. Clin Toxicol 1987;25:221.

34. Geffner ME, Opas LM. Phosphate poisoning complicating treatment for iron ingestion. Am J Dis Child 1980;134:509.

35. Bachrach L, Correa A, Levin R, et al. Iron poisoning: Complications of hypertonic phosphate lavage therapy. J Pediatr 1979;94:147.

36. Decker WJ, Shafik HN, Corby DC, et al. Sequestration of iron by magnesium oxide: An in vitro study. Vet Hum Toxicol 1981;23:33.

37. Corby DG, McCullen AH, Chadwick EW, et al. Effect of orally administered magnesium hydroxide in experimental iron intoxication. Clin Toxicol 1986;23:489.

38. Venturelli J, Kwee Y, Morris N, et al. Gastrotomy in the management of acute iron poisoning. J Pediatr 1982;100:768.

39. Peterson CD, Fifield GC. Emergency gastrotomy for acute iron poisoning. Ann Emerg Med 1980;9:262.

40. Landsman I, Bricker JT, Reid BS, Bloss RS. Emergency gastrotomy: Treatment of choice for iron bezoar. J Pediatr Surg 1987;22:184.

41. Foxford R, Goldfrank L. Gastrotomy—a surgical approach to iron overdose. Ann Emerg Med 1985;14:1223.

42. Robins-Browne RM, Rabson AR, Koornhof HJ. Generalised infection with *Yersinia enterocolitica* and the role of iron. Contrib Microbiol Immunol 1979;5:277.

43. Robins-Browne RM, Prpic JK, Stuart SJ. *Yersiniae* and iron. A study in host-parasite relationships. Contrib Microbiol Immunol 1987;9:254.

44. Melby K, Slordahl S, Guttberg TJ, et al. Septicaemia due to *Yersinia enterocolitica* after oral overdoses of iron. Br Med J 1982;285:467.

45. Porter JB, Huehns ER. The toxic effects of desferrioxamine. Baillieres Clin Haematol 1989;2:459.

46. Goodwin JF, Whitten CF. Chelation of ferrous sulfate solution by deferoxamine B. Nature 1965;205:281.

47. Nielsen JB. Influence of desferrioxamine on renal excretion of iron: Preliminary report. Acta Med Scand 1963;173:499.

48. Wöhler F. Treatment of haemochromatosis with desferrioxamine. Acta Haematol 1963;30:65.

49. Bannerman RM, Callender ST, Williams DL. Effect of desferrioxamine and D.T.P.A. in iron overload. Br Med J 1962;2:1573.

50. Williams DR, Holstead BW. Chelating agents in medicine. J Toxicol Clin Toxicol 1983;19:1081.

51. Propper RD, Shurin SB, Nathan DG. Reassessment of the use of deferoxamine B in iron overload. N Engl J Med 1976;294:1421.

52. Meyer-Brunot HG, Keberle H. The metabolism of deferrioxamine-B and ferrioxamine-B. Biochem Pharmacol 1967;16:527.

53. Keberle H. The biochemistry of desferrioxamine and its relation to iron metabolism. Ann NY Acad Sci 1964;119:758.

54. Hershko C, Link G, Pinson A. Effects of iron loading and chelation on rat myocardial cells in culture. Blood 1984;64(Suppl 1):39a (abstract).

55. Lovejoy FH. Chelation therapy in iron poisoning. J Toxicol Clin Toxicol 1983;19:871.

56. Lipschitz DA, Dugard J, Simon MO, et al. The site of action of desferrioxamine. Br J Haematol 1971;20:395.

57. Karabus CD, Fielding J. Desferrioxamine chelatable iron in hemolytic megaloblastic and sideroblastic anaemias. Br J Haematol 1967;13:924.

58. Freeman AP, Giles RW, Berdoukas VA, et al. Early left ventricular dysfunction and chelation therapy in thalassemia major. Ann Intern Med 1983;99:450.

59. Summers MR, Jacobs A, Tudway D, et al. Studies in desferrioxamine and ferrioxamine metabolism in normal and iron-loaded subjects. Br J Haematol 1979;42:547.

60. Peters G, Keberle H, Schmid K, et al. Distribution and renal excretion of desferrioxamine and ferrioxamine in the dog and in the rat. Biochem Pharmacol 1966;15:93.

61. Allain P, Mauras Y, Chaleil D, et al. Pharmacokinetics and renal elimination of desferrioxamine and ferrioxamine in healthy subjects and patients with haemochromatosis. Br J Clin Pharmacol 1987;24:207.

62. Bentur Y, Koren G, Tesoro A, et al. Comparison of deferoxamine pharmacokinetics between asymptomatic thalassemic children and those exhibiting severe neurotoxicity. Clin Pharmacol Ther 1990;47:478.

63. Banner W Jr, Czajka P. Iron poisoning (letter). Am J Dis Child 1981;135:484.

64. Lietman PS, Robotham JL. Iron poisoning (letter). Am J Dis Child 1981;135:485.

65. Tenenbein M, Yatscoff RW. The total iron-binding capacity in iron poisoning. It is useful? Am J Dis Child 1991;145:437.

66. McEnery JT. Deferoxamine as a chelating agent. J Pediatr 1968;72:147.

67. Leikin S, Vossough P, Mochir-Fatemi F. Chelation therapy in acute iron poisoning. J Pediatr 1967;71:425.

68. Movassaghi N, Purugganan GG, Leikin S. Comparison of exchange transfusion and deferoxamine in the treatment of acute iron poisoning. J Pediatr 1969;75:604.

69. Stivelman J, Schulman G, Fosburg M, et al. Kinetics and efficacy of deferoxamine in iron-overloaded hemodialysis patients. Kidney Int 1989;36:1125.

70. Chang TMS, Barre P. Effect of desferrioxamine on removal of aluminium and iron by coated charcoal haemoperfusion and haemodialysis. Lancet 1983;2:1051.

71. Whitten CF, Chen YC, Gibson GW. Studies in acute iron poisoning. II. Further observations on deferoxamine in the treatment of acute iron poisoning. Pediatrics 1966;38:102.

72. Peck MG, Rogers JF, Rivenbark JF. Use of high doses of deferoxamine (Desferal) in an adult patient with acute iron overdosage. J Toxicol Clin Toxicol 1983;19:865.

73. Blake DR, Winyard P, Lunec J, et al. Cerebral and ocular toxicity induced by desferrioxamine. Q J Med 1985;56:345.

74. Boehnert M, Lacouture PG, Guttmacher A, et al. Massive iron overdose treated with high-dose deferoxamine infusion. Vet Hum Toxicol 1985;28:291(abstract).

75. Koren G, Bentur Y, Strong D, et al. Acute changes in renal function associated with deferoxamine therapy. Am J Dis Child 1989;143;1077.

76. Freedman MH, Grisaru D, Olivieri N, et al. Pulmonary syndrome in patients with thalassemia major receiving intravenous deferoxamine infusions. Am J Dis Child 1990;144:565.

77. Tenenbein M, Kowalskis S, Roberts D. Pulmonary toxicity in iron poisoning: Deferoxamine induced? Vet Hum Toxicol 1990;32:349(abstract).

78. Miller KB, Rosenwasser LJ, Bessette JM, et al. Rapid desensitisation for deferoxamine anaphylactic reaction (letter). Lancet 1981;1:1059.

79. Bousquet J, Navarro M, Robert G, et al. Rapid desensitisation for desferrioxamine anaphylactoid reactions (letter). Lancet 1983;2:859.

80. Walker JA, Sherman RA, Eisinger RP. Thrombocytopenia associated with intravenous desferrioxamine. Am J Kidney Dis 1985;6:254.

81. Wonke B, Hoffbrand AV, Aldouri M, et al. Reversal of desferrioxamine induced auditory neurotoxicity during treatment with Ca-DTPA. Arch Dis Child 1989;64:77.

82. Bene C, Manzler A, Bene D, Kranias G. Irreversible ocular toxicity from single "challenge" dose of deferoxamine. Clin Nephrol 1989;31:45.

83. Guerin A, London G, Marchais S, et al. Acute deafness and desferrioxamine (letter). Lancet 1985;2:39.

84. Davies S, Hungerford JL, Arden GB, et al. Ocular toxicity of high-dose intravenous desferrioxamine. Lancet 1983;2:181.

85. Barratt PS, Toogood IRG. Hearing loss attributed to desferrioxamine in patients with beta-thalassaemia major. Med J Aust 1987;147:177.

86. Pengloan J, Dantal J, Rossazza C, et al. Ocular toxicity after a single intravenous dose of desferrioxamine in two hemodialyzed patients (letter). Nephron 1987;46:211.

87. Cases A, Campistol JM, Sabater M, et al. Desferrioxamine-induced acute neurosensorial deafness (letter). Nephron 1988;48:326.

88. Olivieri NF, Buncic JR, Chew E, et al. Visual and auditory neurotoxicity in patients receiving subcutaneous deferoxamine infusions. N Engl J Med 1986;314:869.

CHAPTER 86

Caustic Ingestions

Michele K. Holloway-Nichols
Suman Wason

INTRODUCTION

The term *caustic* applies to both alkali- and acid-containing chemicals (Table 86–1). Between 5000 and 18,000 caustic ingestions are reported in the United States each year, alkali ingestions occurring more frequently than those of acids.[1, 2] However, the number of caustic ingestions has declined over the past two decades because of increased public awareness, child-resistant caps, and decreased concentration of caustics in household products.[1, 3]

Severe tissue injury can occur in seconds. Two peaks occur with regard to age distribution: children less than 5 years old and adults 20 to 30 years old. Children usually accidentally ingest a caustic substance amounting, in most cases, to only a "lick or a taste" exposure, compared with deliberate ingestions by adolescents or adults.[4]

PHYSIOLOGIC EFFECTS
Alkalis

In the solid state the alkali adheres to the mucous membranes of the oropharynx and esophagus; in the liquid state the injury is usually more localized to the esophagus.[5] Since the esophagus has an alkaline pH, it provides no buffering action.[3] Alkalis with a pH of 12 or greater are usually associated with significant tissue injury.[6] Esophageal burns most commonly occur in areas where the esophagus is narrow, such as at the levels of the cricopharyngeus muscle, aortic arch, left main stem bronchus, and diaphragmatic hiatus.[7] The incidence of gastric burns after alkali ingestions is unknown because endoscopy is rarely performed past an esophageal burn, in order to avoid perforation.

Alkaline substances cause liquefaction necrosis, which results in deep mucosal injury penetrating into smooth muscle in the esophagus.[4] Initially, an area of erythema is seen at the site of injury. In moderate to severe exposures, ulceration follows within 24 hours, associated with edema and narrowing 48 to 72 hours after ingestion. Saponification, thrombosis, necrosis, and infiltration of bacteria also occur.[3] Ten days after exposure, granulation tissue replaces the necrotic areas, forming scar tissue.[7] Within 3 to 6 weeks, strictures occur, at which time the patient experiences dysphagia, vomiting, and weight loss (Table 86–2).[4, 8]

Esophageal burns are endoscopically classified as follows: first degree, injury to mucosa only with superficial hyperemia, edema, and sloughing; second degree, injury penetrating the musculature with exudate formation, ulceration, and erosion; third degree, deep ulcers into muscle, with possible full-thickness erosion into the pleura or mediastinum.[4, 5]

Acids

Acids cause injury by a coagulation necrosis with eschar formation.[4] The eschar forms a physical barrier to deeper penetrating injury, and thus the esophagus is spared in more than 80% of acid ingestions.[6] Instead, acids cause injury to the stomach and small intestine, often resulting in acute gastric perforation most commonly affecting the antrum of the stomach.[7] In the healing phase after acid ingestion, pyloric stenosis is more common than esophageal strictures.

The effect of acid is enhanced in the antral area because of the acid pooling created by pyloric spasm.[5] Also, "skip" injuries occur with acids because of their relatively low viscosity and specific gravity, thereby sparing areas traversed quickly.[9] Although alkalis are more likely to cause esophageal burns, the site of injury caused by acids and alkalis may overlap.

EMERGENCY MEDICAL SERVICES CONSIDERATIONS

Airway compromise may occur after caustic ingestion. Oral endotracheal intubation or even tracheostomy may be necessary. Administration of oxygen, establishment of intravenous access, and cardiac monitoring are indicated. If there are no airway complications or obvious evidence of perforation, dilution with a maximal amount of 4 to 6 oz of water or milk is appropriate. If there are solid caustic crystals in the mouth, the patient should rinse and expectorate to prevent more crystals from being swallowed.[10, 11] Induction of emesis and administration of activated charcoal are contraindicated. Emesis may reintroduce the caustic into the airway, causing more damage or even obstruction.[9] Activated charcoal does not adsorb alkalis and its administration might place the patient at risk of respiratory aspiration and might obscure subsequent endoscopic evaluation. Neutralization with alkalis or acids is not recommended because this may cause thermal injury and delay treatment. The substance container should be brought to the hospital to facilitate accurate identification.

TABLE 86–1
COMMONLY AVAILABLE CAUSTIC PRODUCTS

Alkalis	Acids
Ammonia (ammonia)	Battery acid (sulfuric acid)
Bleaches (sodium hypochlorite)	Metal cleaners (hydrofluoric acid, zinc chloride)
Button (disk) batteries (potassium hydroxide)	Solder flux (hydrochloric acid)
Clinitest tablets (sodium hydroxide)	Swimming pool cleaners (hydrochloric acid)
Dairy pipeline cleaner (sodium hydroxide)	Toilet bowl cleaners (hydrochloric acid)
Detergents (sodium carbonate and silicate)	
Drain cleaners (sodium hydroxide)	
Lye (sodium hydroxide)	

TABLE 86–2

ACUTE AND CHRONIC FINDINGS AFTER CAUSTIC INGESTION

	Alkalis	Acids
Necrosis	Liquefaction	Coagulation
Common sites of injury	Esophagus	Stomach/small intestines
Depth of injury	Very deep	Superficial to deep
Airway edema	Less likely	More common
Complications:		
Perforation	Esophagus	Stomach
Stricture	Esophagus	Stomach
Carcinoma	Esophagus	Stomach

CLINICAL EVALUATION
Alkalis

The patient who has ingested an alkali may present with no clinical findings or with burns to the lips, oral mucosa, tongue, or pharynx, resulting in drooling, mouth pain, excessive salivation, or refusal to swallow (Table 86–3). With alkalis the oral burns are brown to yellow in color. Approximately 30% of patients who have oral burns also reveal esophageal burns on endoscopic examination. The absence of oral burns, however, does not exclude the presence of a significant esophageal burn: 10% to 30% of patients with an esophageal burn have been reported not to have an oropharyngeal burn.[1] One study, however, reported that all patients with significant esophageal burns on endoscopic evaluation had burns to the mouth or pharynx.[12]

Gaudreault and colleagues found no significant correlation between endoscopically confirmed esophageal injury and signs or symptoms in children who ingested a caustic substance, but there was a strong association among esophageal burns and vomiting, dysphagia, drooling, and abdominal pain.[13, 14] Tewfik and Schloss reported that with esophageal burns there was erythema of the lip or tongue in 87% and dysphagia or drooling in 70% of patients.[20] One review found that 50% of those with two or more of the signs or symptoms of drooling, vomiting, or stridor had serious burns. All children with fewer than two symptoms or signs had negative endoscopic results.[14]

Acids

Respiratory compromise from edema of the larynx or epiglottis may occur after acid ingestion and is reportedly more common than after alkali ingestion. Patients may present with hoarseness, stridor, or dyspnea. Since infants and younger children have a smaller laryngeal diameter than older children and adults, any narrowing of the airway may lead to severe compromise.[15] Although less likely to

TABLE 86–3

SIGNS AND SYMPTOMS AFTER CAUSTIC INGESTION

	Alkalis	Acids
Drooling	+ + +	+ +
Excessive salivation	+ + +	+ +
Mouth pain	+ + +	+ +
Oral burns	+ + +	+ +
Refusal to swallow	+ + +	+ +
Stridor	+ +	+ + +
Vomiting	+ + +	+ + +

+ = Lowest incidence; + + + = highest incidence.

cause esophageal injury, acids can also produce oral injury resulting in white to gray necrotic areas that are eventually replaced by a black eschar.[1, 4]

Pain (abdominal, back, or substernal) should alert the physician to the possibility of gastric perforation or necrosis, which can occur shortly after acid ingestion. Hematemesis or recurrent emesis may also signal perforation.[5, 8]

DIAGNOSTIC EVALUATION
Endoscopy

Endoscopic examination is the only reliable way to evaluate the esophagus for burns.[13] No specific guidelines exist as to which patients should be examined or at what time endoscopy should be performed. It can be performed selectively on the basis of several factors. Endoscopy exposes patients to the risk of general anesthesia along with the risks of aspiration of gastric contents and perforation of the esophagus or stomach. Flexible endoscopes offer less risk of viscous rupture than the rigid variety.[16]

Routine endoscopy after "caustic" ingestion in all patients is probably unnecessary. For instance, asymptomatic patients who have ingested ammonia, bleach, or household detergents need not undergo endoscopy. Rather, it is reserved for patients who have significant ingestions of true acids or alkalis (i.e., an acid pH <2 or alkali pH >13 in quantities exceeding a "lick or taste") regardless of symptoms. Patients with persistent symptoms such as vomiting, drooling, dysphagia, and stridor regardless of the product ingested should also undergo endoscopy.[17]

The presence of oral burns should raise suspicion of esophageal burns. Endoscopic examination should be done emergently in patients who are severely symptomatic.[8] They must be stable before endoscopy, regardless of whether one uses the guidelines of 24 hours, 24 to 48 hours, or 2 to 7 days after ingestion.[10] If possible, most clinicians avoid manipulation of the esophagus 7 to 21 days after caustic ingestion because this is the period when the esophageal wall is weakest as collagen is being deposited to repair injured tissue.[3] Most clinicians recommend examination only to the level of the first significant burn to avoid the possibility of further complications; others traverse superficial injuries for a more complete examination.[3, 9]

Laboratory

The laboratory adds little to the management of these ingestions. Determination of arterial blood gas, electrolytes including blood urea nitrogen and creatinine, and a complete blood count may be useful to monitor complications such as shock, hemorrhage, or renal failure.[1, 5] If there is evidence of hemorrhage or perforation, blood for type and crossmatching should be sent.

Radiology

A chest and abdominal film should be obtained in patients who have had more than a "lick or taste" exposure to strong acids or alkalis. Free intra-abdominal air, pneumomediastinum, or evidence of aspiration are serious complications in patients who initially may be asymptomatic. Upper gastrointestinal contrast studies often underestimate the extent of injury. Endoscopic examination is therefore far superior in this setting.[1, 13]

COMPLICATIONS
Alkalis

Pulmonary aspiration can occur at the time of ingestion, leading to early respiratory compromise. With strong alkalis, there may be acute erosion through the esophagus resulting in mediastinitis, or erosion through the aorta or bronchial arteries causing exsanguination.[4]

Esophageal strictures are the major concern after initial healing of the burn. First-degree burns do not cause strictures, second-degree burns may progress to strictures in 15% to 30% of patients, and third-degree burns result in strictures in up to 90% of reported cases.[1] If a stricture is developing, symptoms of dysphagia, vomiting, and weight loss usually occur 3 or 4 weeks after ingestion. However, strictures may present many years after the event. Squamous cell carcinoma of the esophagus (occurring at the site of a caustic burn) is 1000 times more common after caustic ingestion than in the general population.[1]

Acids

Respiratory complications and gastrointestinal perforation leading to peritonitis can occur after acid ingestion. Gastric scarring and pyloric stenosis may develop weeks to months later.[5, 10] The stenosis is believed to be due to prolonged exposure of the pyloric region to acid because of irritative pylorospasm at the time of ingestion. Gastric outlet obstruction presents with symptoms of vomiting and weight loss. Surgery is the usual treatment. These patients, too, are at increased risk of developing carcinoma at the site of the stricture.[8] Achlorhydria and protein-losing enteropathy have also been reported as late sequelae.[10]

THERAPEUTIC INTERVENTION

Dilution with water or milk is indicated only if there are no signs of perforation or respiratory compromise (Table 86–4). Ipecac-induced emesis and activated charcoal are contraindicated.[4] Charcoal is ineffective in adsorption of alkali and does not slow down tissue injury; it may also

---

TABLE 86–4

MANAGEMENT CHECKLIST

1. Ensure airway, breathing, and circulation
2. Dilute with small amounts of water or milk if no airway compromise or signs of perforation
3. Consult ENT services is significant airway compromise
4. Consult surgical services if clinical evidence of viscus perforation
5. Do not administer ipecac or activated charcoal
6. Refer all patients with greater than "lick or taste" of alkali pH >13; acids pH <2 for elective endoscopy within 24–48 hr
7. If "lick or taste" ingestion, observe for 4 to 6 hr; if no symptoms after observation period, discharge
8. If clinitest tablets ingested, refer for emergency endoscopy
9. If disk battery ingested, obtain chest film immediately; remove battery if above diaphragm
10. If deep esophageal or circumferential burns documented on endoscopic examination
    Admit
    NPO/intravenous fluids
    Antibiotics: Ampicillin 100 mg/kg/day × 10–14 days
    Consult surgical services
    Consider nasogastric intubation for nutrition or stenting, or gastrostomy for nutrition and subsequent retrograde dilatations
11. Follow-up:
    3–6 wk after ingestion: Monitor for strictures
    10–70 yr after esophageal stricture: Monitor for carcinoma

---

hinder the endoscopist's accurate assessment of the extent of injury.[1]

Children presenting to the emergency department most often experience only a "lick or taste" and exhibit no oral burns or symptoms. In these cases, cautious dilution with water or milk is recommended along with observation in the emergency department for 4 to 6 hours. The major risk of dilution is that emesis may occur if fluids are encouraged overzealously.[14] Dilution itself has not proved beneficial in preventing long-term sequelae. In addition, milk may possibly hinder subsequent endoscopic examination.[1, 7, 11, 18] If patients remain asymptomatic and are able to drink liquids without difficulty, they can be discharged after an observation period.

If clinical signs or symptoms of esophageal or gastric perforation are present, an emergent surgical evaluation should be sought. Patients ingesting acids are at particularly high risk of developing gastric and intestinal perforation and peritonitis.

If a significant ingestion has occurred and the product is an acid of pH <2 or alkali >13, the patient should be admitted and electively endoscoped to establish the severity of injury regardless of symptoms.[4] In a case of a severe third-degree esophageal burn, the patient may require a nasogastric tube or gastrostomy for nutrition or stenting. The tube is best placed during endoscopy to avoid additional trauma.[3, 8]

Antibiotics should be instituted for third-degree burns. Ampicillin, 100 mg/kg/day for 10 to 14 days, is recommended.[1, 7, 10] A cephalosporin or erythromycin is an acceptable alternative. Treatment with antibiotics appears to shorten the repair stages of injury but has little effect on prevention of late strictures.[3]

Long-term follow-up should consist of esophagography 1 month after ingestion in all patients with documented second- and third-degree burns, to seek evidence of stricture formation. When present, esophageal strictures may need to be dilated.

Lathyrogens, including beta-aminopropionitrile and D-penicillamine, have been discussed as therapeutic agents. They interfere with the covalent crosslinks during collagen synthesis, thus decreasing tensile strength. Their effectiveness in humans is unknown.[1, 10]

CONTROVERSIES

The importance of preventing strictures is obvious. Steroids are believed by some to decrease the granulation tissue formation, thus decreasing stricture formation, but others see no real benefit from their use. One review concluded that corticosteroids are of questionable benefit on the basis of three studies involving 344 patients that showed a decrease in the incidence of strictures in steroid-treated individuals, three studies involving 414 patients that revealed no benefit from steroids, and three further studies involving 165 patients that actually suggested a deleterious effect of steroids.[4] A controlled clinical trial conducted over 18 years and involving 60 patients showed no benefit from steroids in the prevention of caustic-induced strictures.[12] Steroids are therefore not routinely recommended after caustic esophageal burns, including third-degree burns, in view of the belief that they have no proved benefit and in fact may lead to serious complications.[4, 8, 10] Steroids are also contraindicated after acid ingestions because of the high risk of gastric perforation. Steroids might easily mask the devastating findings of an evolving gastric or intestinal perforation.[10, 15, 19]

Since third-degree and circumferential burns are prone to stricture in a large number of cases, corticosteroids may be considered in this specific setting.[4, 8, 10] When steroids have been used, the dosage has been 0.8 to 1.6 mg/kg/day of prednisolone parenterally or 1 to 2 mg/kg/day of prednisone orally for 2 to 3 weeks, followed by a tapering dose over 14 to 21 days.[7, 10] Active infections, peptic ulcer disease, or perforation are absolute contraindications to the use of steroids.[20]

SPECIFIC CAUSTICS

Clinitest Tablets. These contain copper sulfate, citric acid, anhydrous sodium hydroxide, and sodium carbonate. Ingestions of these tablets result in caustic and thermal burns to the larynx, esophagus, and stomach. Of nine children reported to have ingested Clinitest tablets, all developed esophageal strictures. However, of 18 adults ingesting Clinitest tablets, two died from laryngeal edema or intestinal perforation, six had esophageal strictures, and one had gastric perforation. Although not used in the current management of diabetes, these tablets are still commercially available.[4]

Detergents. Nonphosphate detergents with "balance builders" replaced phosphate-containing detergents in the 1970s, and as a rule have relatively low toxicity. However, these "balance builders" consisting of sodium carbonate and silicate can result in severe airway edema or laryngospasm. Symptoms of respiratory distress appear within 1 or 2 hours of ingestion. Granular automatic dishwashing detergents appear to have a higher propensity than liquid automatic dishwashing agents to cause caustic burns.[21, 22]

Cleaning Agents. Household bleaches and swimming pool cleaners contain sodium hypochlorite. Household bleach, accounting for approximately 5% of ingestions in children under 5 years of age, generally contains 4% to 6% sodium hypochlorite with a pH of 11 and represents a low risk of toxicity. The only therapy indicated is dilution with water or milk. Swimming pool cleaners, however, contain up to 20% sodium hypochlorite and should be treated in the same way as other stronger caustics.[1, 4]

Button Batteries. Button (or disk) batteries contain silver, mercury, manganese salts, and 40% to 45% potassium hydroxide or sodium hydroxide.[6] These batteries are commonly used in watches, hearing aids, calculators, and cameras. Damage is caused by pressure necrosis, electric current, and the corrosive effect of potassium hydroxide.[1] While most of the batteries traverse the gastrointestinal tract without any problem, severe complications can occur, especially if the battery becomes lodged in the esophagus. There may be perforation of the esophagus, tracheoesophageal fistula, and subsequent perforation of the aorta or bronchial arteries.[4, 23, 24] Any patient who has ingested a button battery should undergo radiography to locate the battery. If it is lodged in the esophagus, the Foley catheter technique of removal should be avoided. Endoscopic removal is preferred because inspection of the esophagus can be performed at the same time.[8] If the battery is in the stomach or lower GI tract and the patient is asymptomatic, no active intervention is necessary. However, if such a patient is or becomes symptomatic with abdominal pain or vomiting, an urgent surgical consultation should be obtained. Some physicians recommend endoscopic or surgical removal if the battery has not passed through the GI tract in 1 week, regardless of symptoms. Since it may take up to 14 days for a battery to traverse the tract, many physicians do not recommend removal in asymptomatic patients.[8]

Hydrofluoric Acid. Commonly used in pottery glazing, photography, metal cleaning, and microchip etching, this agent is highly toxic. Even topical exposure has lead to systemic toxicity owing to the fluoride ion. To decrease penetration and tissue damage due to fluoride ions, dermal burns are treated with topical or subcutaneous calcium salts. For significant hand and finger burns, arterial intravenous calcium may be indicated.[8]

Household Ammonia. This is generally considered to be relatively nontoxic. However, several cases of supraglottic edema and three reported cases of esophageal burns suggest that vigilance is necessary.[8, 25] Endoscopic evaluation is recommended only in patients with persistent symptoms.

A further source of ammonia is "smelling salts" capsules, which contain aromatic ammonia (18%) and alcohol (36%) in a 0.33-ml mixture. The vapors can be irritating and may result in pulmonary edema.[3] Their ingestion poses little risk of esophageal injury.[25]

References

1. Howell JM. Alkaline ingestions. Ann Emerg Med 1986;15:820.
2. Lovejoy FH Jr. Corrosive injury of the esophagus in children: Failure of corticosteroid treatment reemphasizes prevention. N Engl J Med 1990;323:668.
3. Range DR, Hirokawa RH, Bryarly RC Jr. Caustic ingestion. Ear Nose Throat J 1983;62:88.
4. Wason S. The emergency management of caustic ingestions. J Emerg Med 1985;2:175.
5. Goldman LP, Weigert JM. Corrosive substance ingestion: A review. Am J Gastroenterol 1984;79:85.
6. Kunkel DB. The toxic emergency: Burning issues; acids and alkalis. Part 1: Ingestion. Emerg Med 1984;16:167.
7. Moore WR. Caustic ingestions: Pathophysiology, diagnosis and treatment. Clin Pediatr 1986;25:192.
8. Wason S, Hanenson IB. Emergency management of caustic ingestion. Hosp Phys 1989;25:29.
9. Wasserman RL, Ginsburg CM. Caustic substance injuries. J Pediatr 1985;107:169.
10. Nelson R, Walson P, Kelley M. Caustic ingestion. Ann Emerg Med 1983;12:559.
11. Maull KI, Osmand AP, Maull CD. Liquid caustic ingestions: An in vitro study of the effects of buffer, neutralization, and dilution. Ann Emerg Med 1985;14:1160.
12. Anderson KD, Rouse TM, Randolph JG. A controlled trial of corticosteroids in children with corrosive injury of the esophagus. N Engl J Med 1990;323:637.
13. Gaudreault P, Parent M, McGuigan MA, et al. Predictability of esophageal injury from signs and symptoms: A study of caustic ingestion in 378 children. Pediatrics 1983;71:767.
14. Crain EF, Gershel JC, Mezey AP. Caustic ingestions. Am J Dis Child 1984;138:863.
15. Moulin D, Bertrand JM, Buts JP, et al. Upper airway lesions in children after accidental ingestion of caustic substances. J Pediatr 1985;106:408.
16. Cello JP, Fogel RP, Boland CR. Liquid caustic ingestion. Arch Intern Med 1980;140:501.
17. Wason S, Stephan M. Corticosteroids in children with corrosive injury of the esophagus. N Engl J Med 1991;324:418.
18. Rumack BH, Burrington JD. Caustic ingestions: A rational look at diluents. Clin Toxicol 1977;11:27.
19. Chodak GW, Passaro E Jr. Acid ingestion: Need for gastric resection. JAMA 1978;239:225.
20. Tewfik TL, Schloss MD. Ingestion of lye and other corrosive agents—a study of 86 infant and child cases. J Otolaryngol 1980;9:72.
21. Krenzelok EP. Liquid automatic dishwashing detergents: A profile of toxicity. Ann Emerg Med 1989;18:60.
22. Einhorn A, Horton L, Altieri M, et al. Serious respiratory consequences of detergent ingestions in children. Pediatrics 1989;84:472.
23. Litovitz TL. Battery ingestions: Product accessibility and clinical course. Pediatrics 1985;75:469.
24. Litovitz TL. Button battery ingestions. JAMA 1983;249:2495.
25. Wason S, Stephan M, Breide C. Ingestion of aromatic ammonia "smelling salts" capsules (letter). Am J Dis Child 1990;144:139.

CHAPTER 87

Organophosphates and Carbamates

Richard F. Clark
Steven C. Curry

INTRODUCTION

Organophosphate and carbamate insecticides (Tables 87–1 and 87–2) are the two groups of anticholinesterase pesticides that produce human toxicity. Poisoning from these agents is accompanied by a rise in the concentration of acetylcholine (ACh) at muscarinic and nicotinic cholinergic receptors, which in turn leads to cholinergic poisoning syndrome.

Seventy-seven thousand pesticide exposures were reported in the United States in 1983; 33,000 of these were attributed to organophosphates.[1] There were 4744 isolated carbamate exposures reported by the American Association of Poison Control Centers in 1988.[2] Children under 7 years of age composed 66% of those exposed to organophosphates and 36% of those exposed to carbamates in 1988.

PATHOPHYSIOLOGY

ACh is a neurotransmitter found at parasympathetic and sympathetic ganglia, skeletal neuromuscular junctions, terminal junctions of all postganglionic parasympathetic nerves, postganglionic sympathetic fibers to most sweat glands, and some nerve endings within the central nervous system (Fig. 87–1).[3] As the axon terminal is depolarized, vesicles containing ACh rupture, releasing ACh into the synapse or neuromuscular junction. ACh then binds to appropriate receptors on the post-synaptic side.[3]

Acetylcholinesterase (AChE), an enzyme found in both neuronal tissue and erythrocytes, hydrolyzes ACh into two inert fragments: acetic acid and choline.[4] Under normal circumstances, virtually all ACh released by the axon is hydrolyzed almost immediately.[3] Organophosphate and car-bamate insecticides form covalent bonds with the active site on AChE, rendering it enzymatically inactive[3–6] and causing accumulation of ACh within synapses and neuromuscular junctions.

Structure

Organophosphates

The basic formula for organophosphates is shown in Figure 87–2. The "X" or "leaving group" determines many characteristics of the compound and provides a means of classifying organophosphates into four main groups. The X in group I compounds is a quaternary nitrogen. In addition to being powerful cholinesterase inhibitors, group I substances also can directly stimulate cholinergic receptors. Group II compounds have a fluorine molecule as the leaving group. Like group I, the highly toxic and volatile nature of these compounds is well suited for chemical warfare. The leaving group of the third category is a cyanide molecule or a halogen other than fluorine. The fourth group is the broadest and comprises various subgroups based on the configuration of the R_1 and R_2 groups. Most of the insecticides currently in use fall into this class.[3]

"Direct" organophosphate compounds are able to inhibit AChE without being structurally altered by the body. Many of the more popular pesticides such as parathion and malathion are "indirect" inhibitors and require partial metabolism within the body to become active inhibitors. Most of the indirect inhibitors undergo oxygenation in the intestinal mucosa and liver after absorption to form more toxic "oxone" metabolites.[4, 7] Once the active form is achieved, it is free to combine with AChE. The bonding is completed as the leaving group of the organophosphate is cleaved by AChE, similar to the hydrolysis of choline from ACh, resulting in a stable bond between the remaining substituted phosphate of the organophosphate and AChE (Fig. 87–3). Although the splitting of the choline-enzyme bond in normal ACh metabolism is completed within microseconds, the severing of the organophosphate-enzyme bond can require up to 1000 hours.[3, 4, 8] The extended occupation of the active site on the AChE molecule inactivates the enzyme. In organophosphate poisoning, the complex becomes irreversibly bound during the next 24 to 72 hours, when one of the R groups (see Fig. 87–2) leaves the phosphate molecule. This step is termed *aging*. De novo synthesis of AChE is required to replenish its supply once aging has occurred.[4] Cholines-

TABLE 87–1
GENERIC NAMES OF COMMERCIALLY AVAILABLE ORGANOPHOSPHATE INSECTICIDES

Acephate	Demeton	Fenitrothion	Phosalone
Akton	Demeton-methyl	Fensulfothion	Phosfon
Aspon	Dialifor	Fenthion	Phosmet
Azinphos-methyl	Diamidfos	Fonofos	Phosphamidon
Bensulide	Diazinon	Isofenphos	Pirimiphos-ethyl
Bomyl	Dicapthon	Malathion	Profenofos
Bromophos	Dichlofenthion	Methamidophos	Propetamphos
Butonate	Dicrotophos	Methidathion	Ronne
Carbophenothion	Dimethoate	Methylparathion	Sulfotep
Chlorfenvinphos	Dioxathion	Methyltrithion	Sulprofos
Chlorpyrifos	Disulfoton	Mevinphos	Temephos
Coumaphos	EPN	Monocrotophos	TEPP (tetraethyl
Crotoxyphos	Ethephon	Naled	pyrophosphate)
Crufomate	Ethion	Oxydemeton-methyl	Terbufos
Cythioate	Ethoprop	Parathion	Tetrachlorvinphos
DDVP (dichlorvos)	Famphur	Phorate	Trichlorfon
DEF	Fenamiphos		

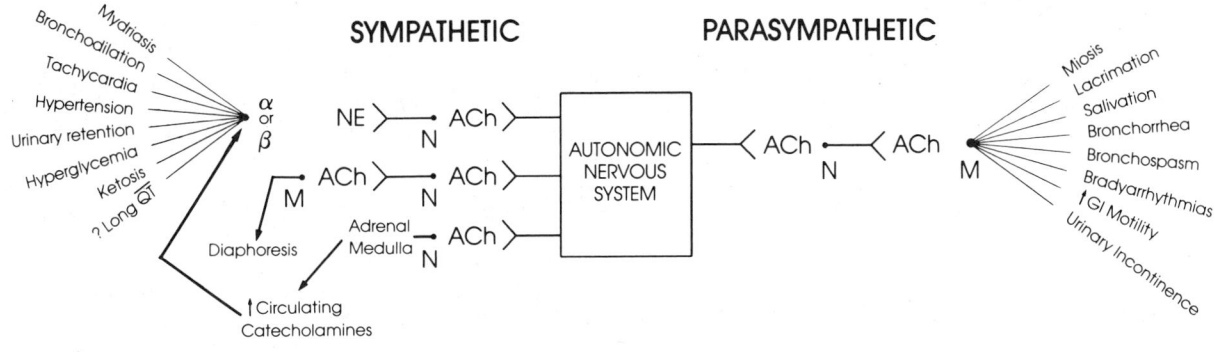

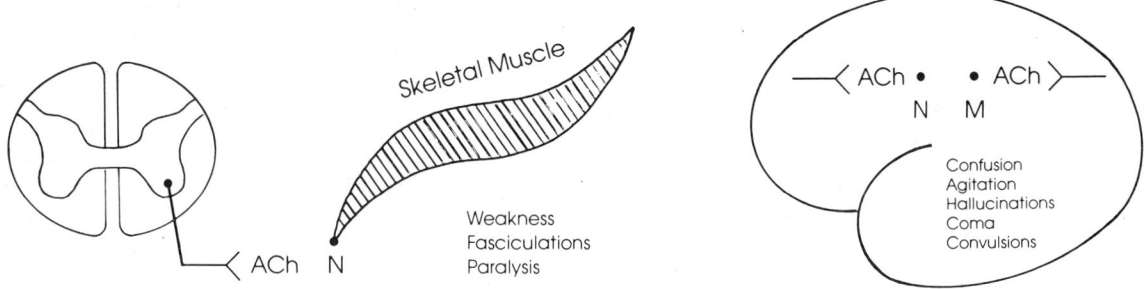

Figure 87–1. Pathophysiology of cholinergic poisoning syndrome affecting central, autonomic, and somatic motor nervous systems.

terase rejuvenators such as pralidoxime chloride have no effect on aged phosphorylated enzyme.

Carbamates

Carbamate insecticides are *N*-methyl carbamates derived from carbamic acid (Fig. 87–4). Medicinal carbamate anticholinesterases include physostigmine, pyridostigmine, and neostigmine. Other medications such as meprobamate and various urethanes are carbamate derivatives, but their toxicity is not associated with cholinesterase inhibition.[9] Thiocarbamate fungicides and herbicides (e.g., maneb, zineb, nabam, mancozeb) also do not inhibit AChE and do not produce cholinergic poisoning syndrome.

When exposed to carbamate compounds, AChE under-

goes carbamylation in a manner similar to phosphorylation by organophosphates, allowing ACh to accumulate in synapses.[10] With carbamate toxicity, there is no aging process, and the carbamate-AChE bond is rapidly hydrolyzed, reactivating the enzyme. The duration of toxic symptoms in carbamate poisoning generally is less than 24 hours.[11]

Pharmacokinetics
Organophosphates

Organophosphates are extremely well absorbed from the skin, lungs, gastrointestinal tract, mucous membranes, and

TABLE 87–2
GENERIC NAMES OF COMMERCIALLY AVAILABLE CARBAMATE INSECTICIDES

Aldicarb	Isolan
Aminocarb	Isoprocarb
Bendiocarb	Methiocarb
Bufencarb	Methomyl
Carbaryl	Oxamyl
Carbofuran	Pirimicarb
Cloethocarb	Promecarb
Dimetan	Propoxur
Dioxacarb	Trimethacarb
Formetanate	

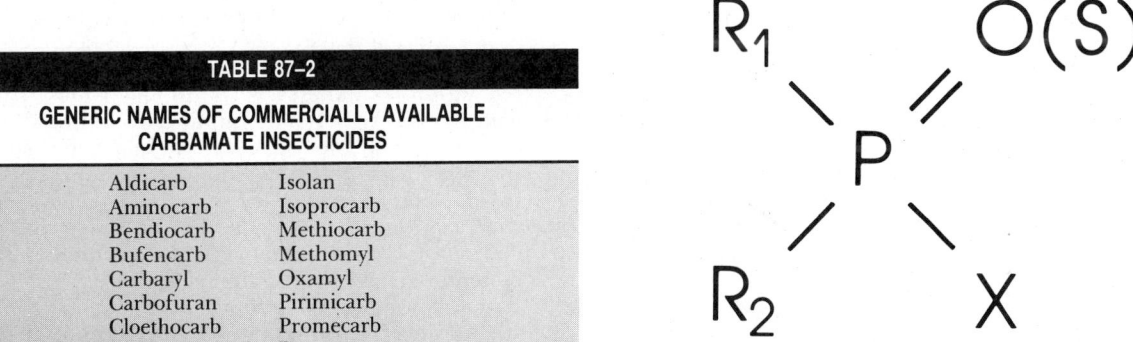

Figure 87–2. General structure of an organophosphate insecticide. X represents the leaving group. R_1 and R_2 may be aliphatic or aromatic groups that sometimes are identical.

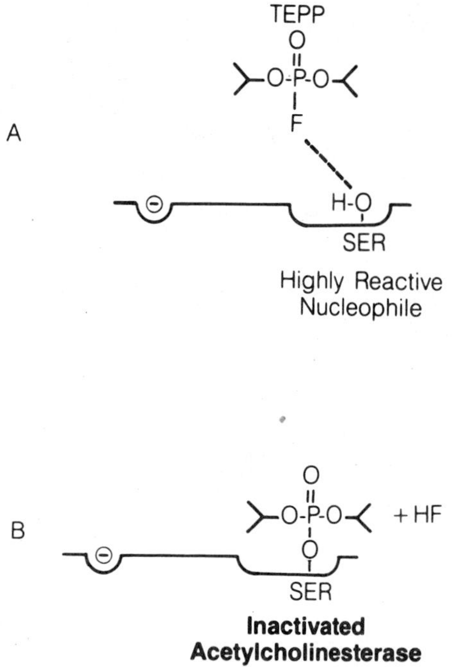

Figure 87–3. Mechanisms of inhibition of acetylcholinesterase by a representative organophosphate, TEPP. A fluorine atom (F) is the leaving group. R_1 and R_2 are only schematically shown through their oxygen linkages. A serine residue at the active site gives up a hydrogen atom to combine with the leaving group while the active site undergoes phosphorylation and inhibition. This initial inhibition is reversible with pralidoxime. However, as the inhibited phosphorylated enzyme "ages," one of the R groups is lost. The aged phosphorylated enzyme is unable to be rejuvenated by pralidoxime. (From Tafuri J, Roberts J. Organophosphate poisoning. Ann Emerg Med 1987; 16:193.)

conjunctiva following inhalation, ingestion, or topical contact.[3, 4, 6, 12] Intravenous and subcutaneous injections have also been reported.[13–15]

Poisonings can be chronic or acute. The difficulty in removing these compounds from the skin and clothing may account for many chronic poisonings. One report found that three individuals were symptomatic after wearing the same pair of parathion-contaminated trousers, with significant pesticide levels still detected in the garment after three washings.[16]

Most organophosphates are lipophilic.[3] When radiolabeled parathion was injected into mice, the greatest concentration one-half hour later was in the cervical brown fat and salivary glands, with high levels also measured in the liver, kidneys, and ordinary adipose tissue.[17]

Peak levels of organophosphates have been measured 6

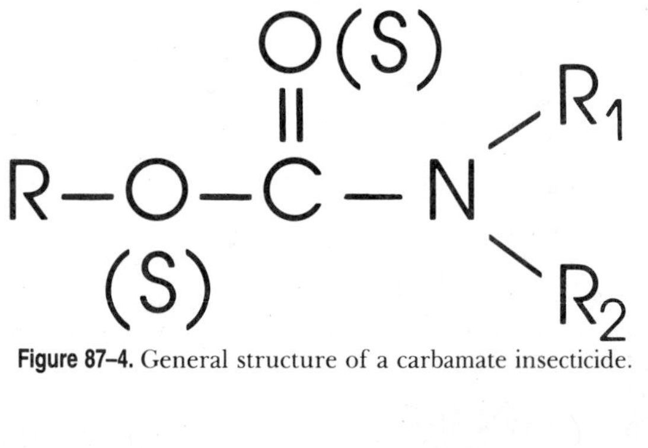

Figure 87–4. General structure of a carbamate insecticide.

hours after oral ingestion.[18] Although the plasma half-lives of these compounds range from minutes to hours,[19] prolonged absorption or redistribution from fat stores may allow for measurement of circulating insecticide concentrations for up to 48 days.[19–22] Delayed cholinergic crisis may recur in patients when fat stores of unmetabolized organophosphates are mobilized.[3, 23]

Organophosphates are metabolized by mixed function oxidases in the liver and intestinal wall.[3, 7, 11, 24] Although a more toxic compound is produced by the initial metabolism of some indirect AChE inhibitors, the phosphorylating ability of these substances is lost when any of the side chains are hydrolyzed. Inactive metabolites are excreted in urine.[3]

Carbamates

Carbamates are also absorbed across skin and mucous membranes as well as by inhalation and ingestion. Peak serum levels of some compounds have been measured 30 to 40 minutes following ingestion.[25] Most carbamates undergo hydrolysis, hydroxylation, and conjugation in the liver and intestinal wall, with 90% excreted in the urine within 3 days.[11, 26] There are two main pharmacokinetic characteristics distinguishing carbamates from organophosphates. First, carbamate insecticides do not easily cross into the central nervous system (CNS).[3, 11] CNS effects of carbamates are thus limited, although CNS dysfunction may be seen in massive poisonings or may result from hypoxemia secondary to pulmonary toxicity and paralysis. Secondly, the carbamate-cholinesterase bond does not "age" as in organophosphate poisoning and is therefore reversible, with spontaneous hydrolysis occurring over several hours.[11]

CLINICAL EVALUATION
Organophosphates

Patients may present following accidental or suicidal ingestion of organophosphate insecticides[27] or after working in areas recently treated with organophosphates.[28] Children can develop toxicity while playing in a residence recently sprayed or fogged by an exterminator.[29] Direct dermal contact with insecticide may be rapidly toxic. Organophosphates have been used for homicide.[5, 30]

Inhibition of neuronal AChE results in elevated synaptic concentrations of ACh. Clinical findings in organophosphate poisoning result from excessive stimulation of muscarinic and nicotinic cholinergic receptors by ACh in the central and autonomic nervous systems, as well as at skeletal neuromuscular junctions (see Fig. 87–1). The patient with classic organophosphate intoxication is unresponsive, with pinpoint pupils, muscle fasciculations, diaphoresis, emesis, diarrhea, salivation, lacrimation, urinary incontinence, and an odor of garlic; however, most presentations are not so typical.

Patients suffering massive ingestions have become symptomatic as soon as 5 minutes after ingestion, and deaths have occurred within 15 minutes.[3, 11, 31] Although most patients with acute poisoning become symptomatic within 12 hours of exposure, virtually every patient with significant ingestion will be symptomatic within 24 hours.[5] Most patients who become ill after ingesting an organophosphate become symptomatic within 8 hours and can be symptomatic for variable lengths of time. Highly lipophilic compounds such as dichlofenthion have caused cholinergic effects for as long as 48 days following oral ingestion.[20]

A wide variety of CNS findings have been reported. Many patients are awake and alert, complaining of anxiety, restlessness, insomnia, headache, dizziness, blurred vision, depression, tremors, or other nonspecific symptoms.[4, 5, 11]

Level of consciousness may deteriorate rapidly to confusion, lethargy, inappropriate behavior, coma, and convulsions.[4, 5, 11] Respiratory depression is, in part, centrally mediated.[5] Cholinergic extrapyramidal rigidity has been noted in severe cases. Choreoathetosis that has lasted several days after cholinergic features have resolved has also been reported.[32]

The effects of excessive ACh on the autonomic nervous system are mixed because cholinergic receptors are found in both the sympathetic and parasympathetic nervous systems (see Fig. 87–1). Excessive muscarinic activity has been characterized by various mnemonics, including SLUD (*s*alivation, *l*acrimation, *u*rination, *d*efecation) and DUMBELS (*d*efecation, *u*rination, *m*iosis, *b*ronchospasm or *b*ronchorrhea, *e*mesis, *l*acrimation, *s*alivation). Of these, miosis is the most commonly encountered sign. Bronchorrhea can be so profuse that it mimics pulmonary edema.[5] Nausea and diaphoresis are also extremely common.

Although muscarinic findings are emphasized in these mnemonics, they are not prevalent except in severe poisonings. In many cases excessive autonomic activity from stimulation of nicotinic adrenal receptors[9] (resulting in catecholamine release) and postganglionic sympathetic fibers offset parasympathetic findings. Mydriasis has been reported in as many as 13% of cases.[33] Bronchodilation and urinary retention can occur as a result of sympathetic activity on smooth muscle.[9] Excessive adrenergic influences on metabolism result in glycogenolysis with hyperglycemia and ketosis that is occasionally mistaken for diabetic ketoacidosis.[34, 35] Hypoglycemia has also been noted.[36]

The cardiovascular manifestations of organophosphate toxicity also reflect mixed effects on the autonomic nervous system.[37] Increased sympathetic tone usually initially prevails, with most patients presenting with sinus tachycardia,[5, 37] sometimes with hypertension. As toxicity becomes more severe, bradycardia with a widened PR interval and various atrioventricular blocks (sometimes with hypotension) resulting from excessive parasympathetic tone are seen.[5, 11, 37–40] Unequal sympathetic stimulation of myocardial cells is thought to be responsible for a third cardiac effect, a widened QT interval.[37, 41, 42] Although a long QT interval in organophosphate-poisoned patients is routinely noted, ventricular arrhythmias associated with this abnormality are rarely reported in the United States. Nevertheless, a long QT interval has been associated with polymorphous ventricular tachycardia ('torsades de pointes') in other countries.[4, 11, 37, 43, 44]

ACh stimulation of nicotinic receptors governs skeletal muscle activity. Excessive cholinergic stimulation at these sites behaves like a depolarizing neuromuscular blocking agent (e.g., succinylcholine) and initially results in fasciculations or weakness.[11, 30] Even patients who have little or no objective evidence of toxicity frequently complain of feeling weak. As the severity of poisoning progresses, paralysis ensues.[4] Paralysis of the respiratory muscles in combination with bronchorrhea, bronchoconstriction, and CNS depression leads to hypoxemia and respiratory arrest, the most common cause of death in organophosphate poisoning.[5]

In summary, the early clinical picture in organophosphate poisoning may be mixed,[45] with findings and complaints that may include weakness, fasciculations, tachycardia, hypertension, vomiting, diaphoresis, diarrhea, salivation, small or large pupils, and possibly urinary retention. As ACh concentrations continue to rise, the clinical picture begins to reflect muscarinic, skeletal muscle, CNS, and metabolic abnormalities, with bradycardia, heart blocks, hypotension, bronchorrhea, bronchospasm, salivation, diaphoresis, lacrimation, vomiting, diarrhea, urinary incontinence, miosis, fasciculations and paralysis, hyperglycemia, and ketosis.[3–5, 11] The patient is often lethargic and may rapidly become comatose

or convulse, although early seizures may be related to hypoxia. Secretions may become copious from every orifice, often hindering resuscitation efforts. The appearance of bradycardia, heart blocks, and hypotension carries a higher mortality rate.[5] There are rare case reports of patients presenting with only paralysis from nicotinic effects without other signs and symptoms suggestive of organophosphate toxicity.[46, 47]

Liquid preparations of organophosphates are usually dissolved in a hydrocarbon. Pulmonary aspiration following ingestion is extremely common in severe toxicity, and hydrocarbon pneumonitis may complicate the clinical picture.[11] Elevations in hepatic enzyme levels have been reported after ingestion in patients with severe parathion poisoning.[3, 48, 49] Although pancreatitis may result,[50, 51] elevated amylase concentrations are usually those of the salivary isoenzyme and do not reflect pancreatic inflammation.

With supportive care, some patients improve rapidly and are well within 2 or 3 days. In other cases, continuing redistribution and absorption of organophosphates may continue for days, leading to prolonged cholinergic symptoms and lengthy hospitalizations.

Carbamates

Poisoning from carbamate insecticides appears identical to that of organophosphate poisoning except for two main factors. First, carbamate insecticides cross into the CNS poorly, but CNS abnormalities may be seen in severe poisonings or may result from hypoxia resulting from respiratory embarrassment. Second, because the carbamate-AChE bond is easily hydrolyzed, even severe intoxications are usually limited to 1 to 2 days after absorption is complete.

DIAGNOSTIC EVALUATION
Cholinesterase Levels
Organophosphates

Plasma cholinesterase, or "pseudocholinesterase," is a nonspecific cholinesterase made in the liver that is able to metabolize various compounds, including succinylcholine and cocaine. Erythrocytes contain true AChE, the same enzyme found in neuronal tissue, that is specific for ACh.[52] Although inhibition of erythrocytic and plasma cholinesterases serves as a marker for anticholinesterase poisoning, such inhibition does not contribute to signs and symptoms of insecticide poisoning.

Following exposure to an anticholinesterase insecticide, plasma cholinesterase activity usually falls first.[4] This is rapidly followed by a decrease in red cell cholinesterase activity. By the time patients present with acute symptoms, both erythrocytic and plasma cholinesterase activities have usually fallen below baseline values.[5]

Plasma cholinesterase activity usually recovers before red blood cell cholinesterase activity, often returning to normal within a few days without repeat exposure to the inciting agent.[53] However, plasma cholinesterase activity is less specific for exposure to an anticholinesterase agent than red cell cholinesterase activity.[3] Low plasma cholinesterase levels are frequently found in patients with hereditary deficiency of the enzyme, malnutrition, hepatic parenchymal disorders, chronic debilitating diseases or some anemias.[3] Drugs such as morphine, codeine, and succinylcholine may cause plasma cholinesterase levels to fluctuate.[11] High plasma cholinesterase activity is seen in those with nephrotic syndrome.[3] Day-to-day variation in enzyme activity in healthy individuals may be as high as 20%.[3]

Erythrocytic cholinesterase activity has been thought to

more accurately reflect nervous tissue AChE activity than plasma cholinesterase because of the presence of true AChE in red cells. Organophosphate poisoning is said to be possible when red blood cell cholinesterase levels fall 50% below baseline values.[5, 11, 54] Although these statements are generally true, there are potential pitfalls in interpreting cholinesterase levels. First, it is AChE inhibition in nervous tissue that causes toxicity, and erythrocytic and plasma cholinesterase activity may not always reflect neuronal enzyme activity. In fact, organophosphate insecticides even vary in their ability to inhibit plasma or red cell cholinesterase to a greater extent. Therefore, some patients are symptomatic after moderate reductions in red blood cell cholinesterase, whereas others may be asymptomatic after losing 50% activity. The wide normal range of red cell and plasma cholinesterase activity (mean ± 2SD) also allows for patients with high-normal values to suffer significant falls in cholinesterase activity, yet still have "normal" cholinesterase activity.[28, 53, 55]

Red blood cell cholinesterase regenerates more slowly than AChE found in neurons.[5, 11] In order to completely replenish the supply, red blood cells in the circulation must be replaced. An average of 66 days are necessary for red blood cell cholinesterase to stabilize following severe inhibition[53] (assuming no treatment with pralidoxime), and levels may take up to 120 days to return to normal.[4] The patient may have completely recovered neuronal activity of AChE and be in no danger of suffering excessive cholinergic symptoms, yet still have low red cell cholinesterase levels. For this reason, in subacute organophosphate poisoning, it is difficult to accurately predict the time or length of exposure from red blood cell cholinesterase activity alone.

Carbamates

Carbamates also inhibit neuronal and erythrocytic AChE as well as plasma cholinesterase. However, the carbamate-AChE bond is much less stable than the organophosphate-AChE bond, with carbamate symptoms generally lasting no longer than 24 to 48 hours. The relative ease with which decarbamylation of cholinesterase takes place may result in the measurement of relatively normal red cell cholinesterase activity despite severe cholinergic symptoms if the assay is not performed within several hours of sampling.[56] Just as in organophosphate poisoning, the wide "normal" range of cholinesterase values may make interpretation of cholinesterase levels difficult at times without knowing the patient's baseline activity. Unlike organophosphates, carbamates do not produce depressed erythrocytic and plasma cholinesterase activities that persist for long periods of time after resolution of symptoms.

Atropine Challenge

An atropine sulfate challenge may be helpful in diagnosing cholinergic poisoning syndrome in the patient who presents with findings suggestive of this disorder but in whom no history is available to suggest excessive exposure to an organophosphate or carbamate insecticide. A test dose of 2 to 5 mg of atropine sulfate in adolescents or adults, or 0.05 mg/kg in children should produce classic anticholinergic findings such as mydriasis, tachycardia, and dry mucous membranes. The persistence of cholinergic findings after an atropine sulfate challenge strongly suggests the presence of organophosphate or carbamate anticholinesterase poisoning.[5] However, some patients suffering from mild to moderate anticholinesterase poisoning may also respond to these doses of atropine sulfate and become anticholinergic.

DIFFERENTIAL DIAGNOSIS

The first category of differential diagnoses for cholinergic poisoning syndrome comprises anticholinesterase agents (Table 87–3). In addition to organophosphate and carbamate insecticides, this category includes the medicinal anticholinesterases neostigmine, pyridostigmine, physostigmine (a carbamate that crosses the blood-brain barrier well), and echothiophate iodide. Probably the most common population to suffer cholinergic poisoning syndrome from medicinal anticholinesterases are patients with myasthenia gravis whose dosage of pyridostigmine is too large. Poisonings from agents in this group should have low plasma pseudo-cholinesterase or erythrocyte AChE activity.

The second category of substances producing cholinergic poisoning syndrome includes agents with cholinomimetic activity. These compounds directly stimulate muscarinic or nicotinic cholinergic receptors but do not inhibit AChE. Therefore, serum and erythrocytic cholinesterase activity should be normal. The ingestion of pilocarpine eye drops has produced mass poisonings and deaths.[57] Other cholinomimetic medicinal agents include preparations of carbachol, aceclidine, methacholine, and bethanecol. Muscarine-containing mushrooms are cholinomimetic, and patients ingesting them may present with salivation, diaphoresis, and vomiting. Finally, poisoning from nicotine alkaloids (e.g., nicotine, lobeline, and coniine) causes CNS, autonomic, and skeletal muscle symptoms similar to those seen in organophosphate and carbamate toxicity.[11] Nicotine alkaloid poisoning may result from the ingestion of tobacco products; from dermal and mucous membrane contact with or ingestion of nicotine-containing pesticides; or from the ingestion of various plants containing nicotine alkaloids (*Nicotiana attenuata* [wild tobacco], *N. glauca* [tree tobacco], and *N. trigonophylla* [desert tobacco]).[4]

The third category comprises miscellaneous drugs or toxins that can produce clinical pictures similar to that of cholinergic poisoning syndrome. Intoxications in this group also should be accompanied by normal erythrocytic and plasma cholinesterase activity. Water hemlock contains cicutoxin that can produce many symptoms also found in cholinergic poisoning syndrome.[11] Ingestions of chlorphenoxy herbicides can cause diaphoresis, fasciculations, CNS abnormalities, and weakness.[4, 11] Poisonings by chlorinated

---

TABLE 87–3

GENERAL DIFFERENTIAL DIAGNOSIS OF CHOLINERGIC POISONING SYNDROME

Anticholinesterase agents
  Organophosphate insecticides
  Organophosphate ophthlamic preparations
  Carbamate insecticides
  Carbate medicinal preparations
Cholinomimetics
  Pilocarpine
  Carbachol
  Aceclidine
  Methacholine
  Bethanecol
  Muscarine-containing mushrooms
  Nicotine alkaloids
Miscellaneous drugs or toxins
  Water hemlock
  Chlorphenoxy herbicides
  Chlorinated hydrocarbon insecticides
  Phencyclidine
  Diabetic ketoacidosis
  Hypoglycemia

hydrocarbon insecticides (e.g., DDT, lindane, heptachlor) can also produce convulsions, which may be accompanied by diaphoresis, incontinence, and drooling. The presentation of phencyclidine toxicity is extremely variable, but can include miosis, salivation, bronchospasm, coma, convulsions, and vomiting. Hyperglycemia and ketosis from organophosphate poisoning has been mistaken for diabetic ketoacidosis. Although miosis is a common finding in poisonings from opiates, phenothiazines, and alpha$_2$ agonists (e.g., clonidine), other cholinergic findings are notably absent. Finally, hypoglycemia from any cause may present with virtually any neurologic finding, diaphoresis, vomiting, and tachycardia.

THERAPEUTIC INTERVENTION
Organophosphates
Airway Management and Atropine Therapy

Death occurring in the emergency department results from respiratory failure and hypoxemia caused by CNS toxicity (coma, convulsions), nicotinic effects on skeletal muscle (weakness, paralysis), and excessive muscarinic effects on the cardiovascular and pulmonary systems (bronchospasm, bronchorrhea, aspiration, bradyarrhythmias and hypotension).

Maintenance of the airway is best assured by endotracheal intubation and positive-pressure ventilation in comatose victims, those with significant weakness, or those unable to handle copious secretions that may accompany the poisoning. The insidious and rapid onset of seizures and coma may also require emergent airway support. Only a nondepolarizing neuromuscular blocking agent should be used to induce pharmacologic paralysis. Metabolism of succinylcholine, a depolarizing agent, is extended in the presence of low plasma cholinesterase activity, resulting in markedly prolonged paralysis.[58]

The second priority is to control excessive muscarinic activity. Atropine sulfate competitively antagonizes ACh at muscarinic receptors to reverse excessive secretions, miosis, bronchospasm, vomiting, diarrhea, diaphoresis, and urinary incontinence.[5, 19] Intravenous doses should begin at 2 to 5 mg in adolescents and adults or 0.05 mg/kg in children and should be given every 2 to 3 minutes until atropinization occurs.[3-5, 11, 29] Tachycardia is not a contraindication to atropine sulfate therapy. Although the appearance of the pupils is often helpful in gauging the need for atropine, the miosis encountered in severe ingestions and by direct ocular exposure to organophosphates may respond only to topical ophthalmic atropine.[59] Furthermore, patients do not die from miosis; physicians should not use the onset of pupillary dilation as the single indicator that enough atropine sulfate has been given. If mydriasis is accompanied by bronchospasm, bronchorrhea, bradyarrhythmias, or other cholinergic signs, more atropine is needed.

Large doses of atropine sulfate can be required.[3-6, 11, 27, 30] Some patients with mild symptoms need only 1 or 2 mg of atropine sulfate for reversal of cholinergic toxicity, but the moderately poisoned adolescent or adult often requires daily doses up to 40 mg.[32, 45] Severe poisonings may require much higher doses. In acutely ill adolescents or adults, 5-mg boluses can be repeated every 2 to 3 minutes for stabilization. Adults have received more than 1000 mg atropine sulfate in 24 hours without producing atropinization,[45, 60] and total doses as high as 11,000 mg during the course of treatment have been reported.[61] Organophosphate toxicity in a 2-year-old boy was successfully treated with 707 mg of atropine sulfate given over 19 days.[62] Children have been managed with continuous infusions of atropine sulfate starting at .025 mg/kg/hr.[63, 64] Continuous infusions of atropine sulfate have

been utilized for as long as 32 days in severely poisoned patients.[21]

Atropine will do nothing for excessive nicotinic effects. While administration of adequate amounts of atropine will dramatically reverse bradycardia and bronchospasm, dry excessive secretions, and stop vomiting and diarrhea, atropine will not prevent weakness, paralysis, and respiratory arrest. Therefore, the patient who markedly improves after receiving atropine still must be closely monitored in an intensive care setting for impending respiratory failure.

Pralidoxime Therapy

Phosphorylated AChE undergoes hydrolytic regeneration at a slow rate, but this process can be markedly enhanced by using pralidoxime chloride, thus regenerating active enzyme (Fig. 87-5).[65] In addition to rejuvenating AChE, pralidoxime can reverse organophosphate toxicity by directly inactivating free organophosphate molecules and by exhibiting an atropine-like effect on nervous tissue.[3] Such regeneration of AChE lowers ACh concentrations to normal levels, reversing both muscarinic and nicotinic effects. An immediate rise in red blood cell cholinesterase activity, presumably paralleling a rise in neuronal AChE activity, is often noted after the administration of pralidoxime.[11]

Pralidoxime is unable to rejuvenate active enzyme from the organophosphate-AChE complex that has undergone aging.[11, 45, 66] Therefore, pralidoxime therapy is most effective if started early in the course of intoxication.

Historically it has been assumed that most phosphorylated AChE is aged within 24 to 48 hours of exposure, thereby explaining past recommendations that pralidoxime would only be effective if administered within the first 1 to 2 days.[3, 9] However, the rate of aging varies significantly for

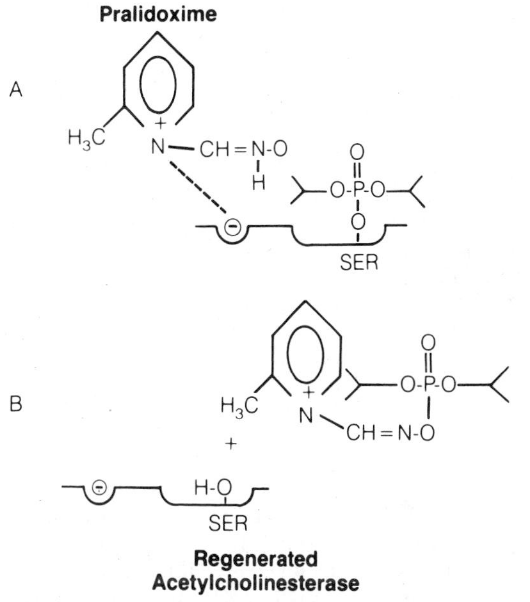

Pralidoxime

Regenerated Acetylcholinesterase

Figure 87-5. Mechanisms of acetylcholinesterase rejuvenation by pralidoxime. R$_1$ and R$_2$ are only schematically shown through their oxygen linkages. *A*, The positively charged aromatic nitrogen of pralidoxime is attracted to the "anionic" site of acetylcholinesterase, allowing the reactive oxime portion of the molecule to be placed over the phosphorylated active site of the enzyme. *B*, Pralidoxime then becomes phosphorylated, rejuvenating acetylcholinesterase. Pralidoxime has little or no effect on pseudocholinesterase because this enzyme lacks an anionic site to attract the drug. (Modified from Tafuri J, Roberts J. Organophosphate poisoning. Ann Emerg Med 1987; 16:193.)

various organophosphate insecticides, and some AChE may still be undergoing new inhibition as long as 7 weeks after ingestion in symptomatic patients. Dramatic reversal of paralysis, weakness, and cholinergic symptoms has occurred after late administration[5, 67] of the antidote.

The initial dose of pralidoxime chloride in adolescents and adults is 1 to 2 gm intravenously over 10 to 15 minutes (25 mg/kg IV over 10 to 15 minutes in children).[4, 19] Minimal plasma concentrations of 4 μg/ml are necessary to maintain enzyme reactivation.[68] Bolus dosing of pralidoxime chloride every 4 to 8 hours is not effective in maintaining these levels, and a constant infusion is more rational than intermittent bolusing. The present recommendation in adolescents and adults is an infusion of 250 to 500 mg/hour, titrating to symptoms.[19] The pharmacokinetics of pralidoxime chloride is not established in children, but loading children with 25 mg/kg of pralidoxime chloride intravenously over 15 to 30 minutes, followed by a continuous infusion of 10 to 20 mg/kg/hr is efficacious in treating symptoms associated with organophosphate poisoning and does not result in pralidoxime-associated toxicity.[69]

The side effects of pralidoxime chloride are minimal at normal doses.[70, 71] Severely poisoned patients have received 0.5 gm/hr for weeks without adverse effects.[5, 21] Rapid infusion can cause tachycardia or muscle rigidity,[5, 11] but patients rarely suffer adverse effects, and these are usually limited to light-headedness and nausea. High doses of pralidoxime have caused neuromuscular blockade or central respiratory depression,[9, 19] and apnea has been seen in an infant after the second dose.

Pralidoxime is not equally effective in reversing cholinergic symptoms in all types of organophosphate poisonings.[5, 19] It is particularly efficacious in reversing toxicity from parathion, diazinon, methyl parathion, EPN, TEPP, dimethoate, and dichlorvos.[3] Dimethoxy compounds such as malathion and methyl demeton can be more refractory to reversal.[3]

Decontamination

Rapid cutaneous absorption necessitates removal of all clothing. Medical personnel should avoid self-contamination by wearing gloves. The skin should be triple washed with water, soap and water, and again with water. Some sources recommend an alcohol wash,[72] but care should be taken to keep alcohol away from the eyes. Small amounts of insecticide remaining in areas such as the navel or gluteal folds are potentially enough to cause toxicity. Cutaneous absorption can also occur as a result of contact with vomitus and diarrhea if the initial exposure was through ingestion. It is difficult to remove oily pesticides from thick or long hair, even with repeated shampooing. Shaving scalp hair may be the only reasonable option in these instances.

In acute ingestions, if emesis has not occurred, evacuation of stomach contents is recommended. Because the onset of coma, seizures, and paralysis can be rapid, lavage is suggested. Although activated charcoal may adsorb some organophosphate insecticides, there are no studies demonstrating that activated charcoal changes the clinical course of organophosphate poisoning. Furthermore, there are no data suggesting that repeated-dose charcoal is efficacious.

Overall Strategy

The patient is first examined to ensure the presence of an adequate airway and ventilation (Table 87–4). If necessary, the patient is intubated and ventilated. Convulsions are treated with a benzodiazepine or phenobarbital.

Second, 2 to 5 mg atropine sulfate (0.05 mg/kg in young children) is given intravenously every 2 to 3 minutes until

---

TABLE 87–4

CHOLINERGIC POISONING SYNDROME: THERAPY AT A GLANCE*

1. Airway management and oxygen therapy
2. Atropine sulfate therapy
   Teenagers and adults: 2 to 5 mg IV push every 2–3 min until atropinization occurs
   Children: 0.05 mg/kg IV push every 2–3 min until atropinization occurs
3. Pralidoxime chloride therapy
   Teenagers and adults: 1 to 2 gm IV over 10–15 min followed by IV drip of 250 to 500 mg/hr
   Children: 25 mg/kg IV over 10–15 min followed by IV drip of 10 to 20 mg/kg/hr
4. Decontamination
   Remove all clothing
   Thorough water rinse
   Water and soap wash
   Final water rinse
   Protect rescuers from contamination
5. Gastrointestinal decontamination
   Gastric lavage if no vomiting and good airway ensured
   1 gm/kg activated charcoal without cathartic

*Initial management of a patient with cholinergic poisoning syndrome from unknown insecticide or from organophosphate insecticide. The initial management of known carbamate poisonings is identical except that pralidoxime probably is not indicated (see text).

---

the patient is atropinized. This may require as little as a single dose of atropine sulfate to as much as several hundred milligrams. Even after atropinization, the patient is constantly observed for evidence of impending paralysis. It is common for patients to become confused and agitated with large doses of atropine sulfate because of central anticholinergic effects. When central anticholinergic effects become evident but peripheral cholinergic findings (e.g., bradycardia, bronchorrhea, vomiting) necessitate the administration of more atropine, glycopyrrolate bromide, an antimuscarinic agent that does not cross the blood-brain barrier can also be used. The dose of glycopyrrolate bromide is 1 to 2 mg every 3 minutes in adolescents and adults, or 0.025 mg/kg every 3 minutes in children.

After atropinization, 2 gm pralidoxime chloride (25 to 30 mg/kg in young children) are given intravenously over 10 to 15 minutes. The adolescent or adult patient is immediately started on a pralidoxime chloride drip at a rate of 500 mg/hr (10 to 20 mg/kg/hr in children).

Hypotension in the absence of severe bradycardia is usually caused by hypovolemia secondary to vomiting, diarrhea, and diaphoresis. Adolescents and adults are treated with 500 to 1000 ml IV fluid challenges with 0.9 normal saline (NS) until adequate rehydration has occurred. Hypotensive children are treated with IV boluses of 30 ml/kg 0.9 NS. Hypotension refractory to fluid challenges (and not secondary to bradycardia or severe hypoxemia) is treated with dopamine or another vasopressor.

All of the patient's clothing is then removed, and the entire skin surface is thoroughly rinsed with water, scrubbed with soap and water, and then rinsed with water again. Care is taken to ensure decontamination of skin folds, particularly in the umbilicus and in and around the ears. When confronted with a severely symptomatic patient whose hair is filled with insecticide, the hair is cut short, and the hair and scalp are washed with shampoo two to three times. If a garlic odor or greasy texture remains in the hair, the scalp is shaved bald and washed with soap and water.

Any recurrence of muscarinic symptoms is treated with further doses of atropine sulfate or glycopyrrolate. Frequent recurrences are treated with an atropine sulfate drip. If pralidoxime is effective, marked anticholinergic findings may be noted after ACh concentrations have returned to normal if large amounts of atropine have been given previously. In this instance, the recurrence of vomiting may be from an ileus rather than from excessive gut motility. Most patients have a difficult time voiding after adequate atropinization, and therefore, a urinary catheter is placed in all atropinized patients.

After the patient has been completely asymptomatic and has not required atropine for 24 hours (anywhere from 1 day to several weeks after the onset of symptoms), the pralidoxime chloride infusion is halted, and the patient is closely observed for any recurrence of symptoms for another 24 hours. Pralidoxime chloride is restarted (and atropine sulfate used as needed) for recurrence of symptoms or for recurrent falls in cholinesterase activity.

Red cell and plasma cholinesterase activities are measured on admission and after the institution of pralidoxime therapy to document anticholinesterase poisoning and to note changes in red cell cholinesterase activity following pralidoxime therapy. Plasma cholinesterase may not rise with pralidoxime therapy, as this cholinesterase does not have an anionic site to attract the compound.

Red cell cholinesterase activity may be markedly depressed long after neuronal AChE levels have returned to normal. Therefore, it is not unusual to send a patient home with subnormal cholinesterase activity. However, cholinesterase activity is monitored immediately before and daily for 1 to 2 days after pralidoxime is stopped. A significant fall in cholinesterase activity may reflect redistribution of insecticide from fat stores or prolonged absorption.[3, 45, 67] Exacerbation of cholinergic symptoms accompanied by a sudden fall in cholinesterase activity 3 to 4 days after resolution of symptoms is not rare, and relapse up to 1 month after discharge from the hospital has been noted.[27, 45, 67] Therefore, late falls in cholinesterase activity are treated by reinstituting a pralidoxime chloride drip, even though the patient may still be asymptomatic. After another 24 hours of pralidoxime, assuming the patient is asymptomatic, pralidoxime is halted again, the patient is closely watched, and red cell and plasma cholinesterase activities are monitored daily for 1 to 2 days to detect another drop in activity that may require reinstitution of pralidoxime chloride and, possibly, atropine.

After the patient is asymptomatic and off of pralidoxime and atropine for one to two days, and after cholinesterase activities are documented to be stable off of medications, the patient may be discharged. Patients are generally not discharged in less than three days after the onset of poisoning since this is when a recurrent fall in cholinesterase activity is commonly detected.

Carbamates

The treatment of carbamate poisoning is identical to that of organophosphate poisoning, with two exceptions. First, most carbamate insecticides are monomethylcarbamates, and the use of pralidoxime in poisonings from monomethylcarbamates may increase AChE inactivation in carbaryl poisoning.[3, 4, 73–75] However, some data suggest that pralidoxime is useful in treating intoxications with the less common dimethylcarbamates such as isolan.[3] Fortunately, because of the rapid hydrolysis of the carbamate-AChE complex, symptoms, including weakness and paralysis, usually resolve within 24 to 48 hours without pralidoxime therapy. Nevertheless, the physician should not hesitate to administer pralidoxime to a poisoned patient in a cholinergic crisis if it is not known whether the patient is suffering from an organophosphate or carbamate poisoning.

Second, significant inhibition of red cell and plasma cho-

linesterase by carbamates generally does not last for more than 1 to 2 days, assuming absorption is complete. Patients usually have normal red cell and plasma cholinesterase levels by the time of discharge.

CHRONIC TOXICITY

Illness may also result from chronic exposure to excessive amounts of organophosphate insecticides. Chronic organophosphate poisoning is most common in workers who regularly come in contact with these substances, but is also possible in children who have repeated exposures to excessive amounts of organophosphate insecticides in their living environments. Although tolerance may be observed with long-term exposure to these chemicals,[3] persons undergoing such exposures may become symptomatic after variable lengths of time. Symptoms can range from vague neurologic complaints such as weakness and blurred vision to cholinergic findings such as miosis, nausea, vomiting, diarrhea, and diaphoresis.[76, 77] Erythrocyte cholinesterase levels are the most sensitive measure of chronic poisoning.[3, 78]

DELAYED SYNDROMES
Organophosphates
Intermediate Syndrome

Delayed muscle weakness without fasciculations or cholinergic features has been noted in patients 24 to 96 hours after acute organophosphate poisoning.[19, 79–81] This phenomenon has been termed the *intermediate syndrome*. A redistribution of the lipophilic pesticide from adipose tissue has been suggested as a cause,[23] but there are no data suggesting that the syndrome results from anticholinesterase activity. The muscle weakness in these patients can progress to respiratory distress and paralysis.[79–81] The most commonly affected muscles are the facial, extraocular, palatal, respiratory, and proximal limbs.[79, 80] There are no substantial data demonstrating that pralidoxime chloride or atropine sulfate are effective in the treatment of this disorder, although patients may be on these medications for control of cholinergic symptoms. The weakness and paralysis commonly resolve in 5 to 18 days.[19, 79]

Encephalopathy and Peripheral Neuropathies

Peripheral neuropathies have occurred after chronic organophosphate exposures and 2 to 3 weeks after acute exposures and appear to result from inhibition of the enzyme neurotoxic esterase (NTE).[19, 82] Such neuropathies may result from exposure to organophosphates that do not inhibit cholinesterase.[83]

The onset and clinical course of these symptoms is not altered by the administration of atropine sulfate or pralidoxime chloride.[5, 46, 84] Pyramidal tract signs may appear weeks to months after exposure.[19, 84] Recovery in these patients is variable over months to years, and residual deficits are common.[85–87]

Behavioral Toxicity

Behavioral changes may also be seen after acute and chronic exposure to organophosphate-containing compounds.[19] Symptoms include confusion, psychosis, anxiety, drowsiness, depression, fatigue, and irritability.[3, 11, 58, 67, 88] Changes may be noted on the electroencephalograms of these patients and can last for weeks.[19, 78, 89] Even though no specific treatment has been effective, most psychological abnormalities resolve within a year.[90]

Carbamates

If delayed neurologic symptoms follow carbamate insecticide poisoning, they must be very rare. In fact, because carbamates do not cause prolonged inhibition of neurotoxic esterase, they actually protect against the development of peripheral neuropathies after exposure to organophosphates.

References

1. Economic and Social Commission of Asia and the Pacific (ECSAP). Development/Environmental Trends in Asia and the Pacific: A Regional Overview. Bangkok, ESCAP, 1983.
2. Litovitz TL, Schimitz BF, Holm KC: 1988 Annual report of the American Association of Poison Control Centers national data collection system. Am J Emerg Med 1989;7:494.
3. Hayes WJ. Pesticides Studied in Man. Baltimore, Williams & Wilkins, 1982.
4. Haddad L, Winchester J. Clinical Management of Poisoning and Overdose. Philadelphia, WB Saunders, 1983.
5. Namba T, Nolte CT, Jackrel J, Grob D. Poisoning due to organophosphate insecticides. Am J Med 1971;50:475.
6. Mackey CL. Anticholinesterase insecticide poisoning. Heart Lung 1982;11:479.
7. Kubistova J. Parathion metabolism in female rat. Arch Int Pharmacodyn Ther 1959;118:308.
8. Smith PW. Bulletin: Medical problems in aerial applications. Washington, DC, Office of Aviation Medicine, Federal Aviation Administration, Dept of Transportation, 1982.
9. Gilman AG, Goodman LS, Rall TW, Murad F (eds). The Pharmacogical Basis of Therapeutics. 7th ed. New York, Macmillan, 1985.
10. Winteringham FW, Fowler KS. Substrate and dilutional effects on the inhibition of acetylcholinesterase by carbamates. Biochem J 1966;101:127.
11. Ellenhorne MJ, Barceloux DG. Medical Toxicology. New York, Elsevier, 1988.
12. Kipling RM, Cruickshank AN. Organophosphate insecticide poisoning. Anaesthesia 1985;40:281.
13. Rao AVR. An unusual case of diazinon poisoning. Indian J Med Sci 1965;19:768.
14. Wulfsohn NL, Smith JC, Foldes FF. Acute phospholine intoxication after intracutaneous injection. Clin Pharmacol Ther 1966;7:44.
15. Moody SB, Terp DK. Dystonic reaction possibly induced by cholinesterase inhibitor insecticides. Drug Intell Clin Pharm 1988;22:311.
16. Clifford NJ, Nies AS. Organophosphate poisoning from wearing a laundered uniform previously contaminated with parathion. JAMA 1989;262:3035.
17. Fredricksson T, Bigelow JK. Tissue distribution of P32-labeled parathion. Arch Environ Health 1961;2:663.
18. Nolan RJ, Rick DL, Freshour NL, Saunders JH. Chlorpyrifos: Pharmacokinetics in human volunteers. Toxicol Appl Pharmacol 1984;73:8.
19. Karalliedde L, Senanayake N. Organophosphorus insecticide poisoning. Br J Anaesth 1989;63:736.
20. Davies JE, Barquet A, Freed VH, et al. Human pesticide poisonings by a fat-soluble organophosphate insecticide. Arch Environ Health 1975;30:608.
21. Gerkin R, Curry S. Persistently elevated plasma insecticide levels in severe methylparathion poisoning. Abstract. Vet Hum Toxicol 1987;29:483.
22. Sakamoto T, Sawada Y, Nishide K, et al. Delayed neurotoxicity produced by an organophosphorous compound (Sumithion). Arch Toxicol 1984;56:136.
23. Gadoth N, Fisher A. Late onset of neuromuscular block in organophosphorus poisoning. Ann Intern Med 1978;88:654.
24. Sultatos LG, Shao M, Murphy SD. The role of hepatic biotransformation in mediating the acute toxicity of the phosphorthionate insecticide chlorpyrifos. Toxicol Appl Pharmacol 1984;73:60.
25. Casper HH, Pekas JC. Absorption and excretion of radiolabeled 1-naphthyl-N-methylcarbamate (cabaryl) by the rat. N D Acad Sci 1971;24:160.
26. Nye DE, Dorough HW. Fate of insecticides administered endotracheally to rats. Bull Environ Contam Toxicol 1976;15:291.
27. Hayes MM, Van Der Westhuizen NG, Gelfan M. Organophosphate poisoning in Rhodesia. S Afr Med J 1978;54:230.
28. Hodgson M, Parkinson D. Diagnosis of organophosphate poisoning. Letter. N Engl J Med 1985;313:329.
29. Zwiener RJ, Ginsburg CM. Organophosphate and carbamate poisoning in infants and children. Pediatrics 1988;81:121.
30. Namba T. Diagnosis and treatment of organophosphate poisoning. Med Times 1972;100:100.
31. Lokan H, Ross J. Rapid death by mevinphos poisoning while under observation. Forensic Sci Int 1981;23:179.
32. Joubert J, Joubert PH. Chorea and psychiatric changes in organophosphate poisoning. S Afr Med J 1988;74:32.
33. Etzel RA, Forthal DN, Hill RH, Demby A. Fatal parathion poisoning in Sierra Leone. Bull WHO 1987;65:645.
34. Durrant W. Massive glycosuroa and ketonuria in organophosphorous poisoning. Central Afr J Med 1978;24:253.
35. Meller D, Fraser I, Kryger M. Hyperglycemia in anticholinergic poisoning. Can Med Assoc J 1981;124:745.
36. Hruban Z, Schulman S, Warner NE, et al. Hypoglycemia resulting from insecticide poisoning. JAMA 1963;184:590.
37. Ludomirsky A, Klein HO, Sarelli P, et al. Q-T prolongation and polymorphous ("torsades de pointes") ventricular arrythmias associated with organophosphorus insecticide poisoning. Am J Cardiol 1982;49:1654.
38. Dekker M. Organophosphate insecticide poisoning. Clin Toxicol 1979;15:189.
39. Namba T, Greenfield M, Grob D. Malathion poisoning: A fatal case with cardiac manifestations. Arch Environ Health 1970;21:533.
40. Krop S, Kunkel AM. Observations on pharmacology of the anticholinesterases Sarin and Tabun. Proc Soc Exp Biol Med 1954;86:530.
41. Moss AJ, McDonald J. Unilateral cervicothoracic sympathetic ganglionectomy for the treatment of long QT interval syndrome. N Engl J Med 1971;285:903.
42. Schwartz PJ. Cardiac sympathetic innervation and the sudden infant death syndrome: A possible pathogenic link. Am J Med 1976;60:167.
43. Kiss Z, Fazekas T. Organophosphates and torsades de pointes ventricular tachycardia. J R Soc Med 1983;76:984.
44. Brill DM, Maisel AS, Prabhu R. Polymorphic ventricular tachycardia and other complex arrythmias in organophosphate insecticide poisoning. J Electrocardiol 1984;17:97.
45. Du Toit PW, Muller FO, Van Tonder WM, Ungerer MJ. Experience with intensive care management of organophosphate insecticide poisoning. S Afr Med J 1981;60:227.
46. Fisher JR. Guillain-Barré syndrome following organophosphate poisoning. JAMA 1977;238:1950.
47. Goldman H, Teitel M. Malathion poisoning in a 34 month old child following accidental ingestion. J Pediatr 1958;52:76.
48. Lutterotti A. Leberschadigung bei Vergiftung mit Insektiziden aus der Reine der Cholinesterase-Blocker. Med Welt 1961;46:2430.
49. Prellwitz W, Schuster HP, Schylla G, et al. Differential diagnosis of organ involvement in exogenous intoxications with the aid of clinical and clinical-chemical examinations. Klin Wochenschr 1970;48:51.
50. Dressel TD, Goodale RL, Arneson MA, Borner JW. Pancreatitis as a complication of anticholinesterase insecticide intoxication. Ann Surg 1979;189:199.
51. Marsh WA, Vukov GA, Conradi EC. Acute pancreatitis after cutaneous exposure to an organophosphate insecticide. Am J Gastroenterol 1988;83:1158.
52. Clay C, Stewart GO. Two unusual presentations of organophosphate poisoning. Anaesth Intensive Care 1982;10:279.
53. Coye MJ, Barnett PG, Midtling JE, et al. Clinical confirmation of organophosphate poisoning by serial cholinesterase analyses. Arch Intern Med 1987;147:438.
54. Milby TH. Prevention and management of organophosphate poisoning. JAMA 1971;216:2131.
55. Midtling JE, Barnett PG, Coye MJ, et al. Clinical management of field worker organophosphate poisoning. West J Med 1985;142:514.
56. Ecobichon DJ, Joy RM. Pesticides and Neurological Diseases. Boca Raton, FL, CRC Press, 1982.
57. Cordner SM, Fysh RR, Gordon H, et al. Deaths of two hospital inpatients poisoned by pilocarpine. Br Med J 1986;293:1285.
58. Selden BS, Curry SC. Prolonged succinylcholine-induced paralysis in organophosphate insecticide poisoning. Ann Emerg Med 1987;16:215.
59. Sachs A, Cameron GR, Cruikshank JD, et al. Medical Manual of Chemical Warfare. New York, Chem Publ Co, 1956.
60. Warriner RA, Nies AS, Hayes WJ. Severe organophosphate poisoning complicated by alcohol and turpentine ingestion. Arch Environ Health 1977;32:203.
61. Hopmann G, Wanke H. Maximum dose atropine treatment in severe organophosphate poisoning. Dtsch Med Wochenschr 1974;99:2106.
62. Worrell CL. The management of organophosphate intoxication. South Med J 1975;68:335.
63. Borowitz SM. Prolonged organophosphate toxicity in a twenty-six-month-old child. J Pediatr 1988;112:302.
64. LeBlanc FN, Benson BE, Gilg AD. A severe organophosphate poisoning requiring the use of an atropine drip. J Toxicol Clin Toxicol 1986;24:69.
65. Wilson IB. Molecular complementarity and antidotes for alkylphosphate poisoning. Fed Proc 1959;18:752.
66. Hobbiger F. Protection against the lethal effects of organophosphates by pyridine-2-aldoxime methiodide. Br J Pharmacol 1957;12:438.
67. Merrill DG, Mihm FG. Prolonged toxicity of organophosphate poisoning. Crit Care Med 1982;10:550.
68. Sundwall A. Minimum concentrations of N-methylpyridinium-2-aldoxime methane sulphonate (P2S) which reverse neuromuscular block. Biochem Pharmacol 1961;8:413.
69. Farrar HC, Wells TG, Kearns GI. Use of continuous infusion of pralidoxime for treatment of organophosphate poisoning in children. J Pediatr 1990;116:658.

70. Grob D, Johns RJ. Use of oximes in the treatment of intoxication by anticholinesterase compounds in normal subjects. Am J Med 1958;24:497.
71. Namba T, Okazaki S, Taniguchi Y, et al. Toxicity of PAM (pyridine-2-aldoxime methiodide). Naika Ryoiki 1958;6:437.
72. Fredricksson T. Percutaneous absorption of parathion and paraoxon, IV: Decontamination of human skin from parathion. Arch Environ Health 1961;3:185.
73. Morgan DP. Recognition and Management of Pesticide Poisonings. 3rd ed. Washington, DC, US Environmental Protection Agency, 1982.
74. Gosselin RE, Hodge HC, Smith RP, Gleason MN. Clinical Toxicology of Commercial Products. 4th ed. Baltimore, Williams & Wilkins, 1975.
75. Kurtz PH. Pralidoxime in the treatment of carbamate intoxication. Am J Emerg Med 1990;8:68.
76. Metcalf RL, Swift TR, Sikes RK. Neurological findings among workers exposed to fenthion in a veterinary hospital: Georgia. MMWR 1985;34:402.
77. Rosenberg J, Quenon SG. Organophosphate toxicity associated with flea-dip products—California. MMWR 1988;37:329.
78. Holmes JH. Organophosphorus insecticides in Colorado. Arch Environ Health 1964;9:445.
79. Senanayake N, Karalliedde L. Neurotoxic effects of organophosphate insecticides: An intermediate syndrome. N Engl J Med 1987;316:761.
80. Routier RJ, Lipman J, Brown K. Difficulty in weaning from respiratory support in a patient with the intermediate syndrome of organophosphate poisoning. Crit Care Med 1989;17:1075.
81. Parker PE, Brown FW. Organophosphate intoxication: Hidden hazards. South Med J 1989;82:1408.
82. Johnson MK. The delayed neurotoxic effect of some organophosphorus compounds: Identification of the phosphorylation site as an esterase. Biochem J 1969;114:711.
83. Cavanagh JB, Davies DR, Holland P, Lancaster M. Comparison of the functional effects of dyflos, tri-o-cresyl phosphate and tri-p-ethylphenyl phosphate in chickens. Br J Pharmacol 1961;17:21.
84. Vasilescu C, Alexianu M, Dan A. Delayed neuropathy after organophosphorus insecticide (Dipterex) poisoning: A clinical, electrophysiological and nerve biopsy study. J Neurol Neurosurg Psychiatry 1984;47:543.
85. Morgan JP, Penovich P. Jamaica ginger paralysis: Forty-seven year follow-up. Arch Neurol 1978;35:530.
86. Senanayake N. Tri-cresyl phosphate neuropathy in Sri Lanka, a clinical and neurophysiological study with a three year follow up. J Neurol Neurosurg Psychiatry 1981;44:775.
87. Barrett DS, Oehme FW. A review of organophosphorus ester-induced delayed neurotoxicity. Vet Hum Toxicol 1985;27:22.
88. Tabershaw IR, Cooper C. Sequelae of acute organic phosphate poisoning. J Occup Med 1966;8:5.
89. Grob D, Harvey AM, Langworthy OR, Lilienthal JL. The administration of diisopropyl fluorophosphate (DFP) to man: Effect on the central nervous system with special reference to the electrical activity of the brain. Bull Johns Hopkins Hosp 1947;81:257.
90. Gershon S, Shaw FH. Psychiatric sequelae of chronic exposure to organophosphate insecticides. Lancet 1961;1:1371.

CHAPTER 88

Anticholinergics

Brad S. Selden
Steven C. Curry

INTRODUCTION

Anticholinergic poisoning syndrome is a commonly occurring but frequently unrecognized disorder. It may be seen with use of medications intended to have anticholinergic effects or, more commonly, as an unsuspected adverse effect of a variety of drugs. The word *anticholinergic*, when used in the toxicologic sense, describes drugs or toxins that are competitive inhibitors of acetylcholine at muscarinic cholinergic receptors. Because these effects are the same as those of atropine, they are also described as *atropine-like, atropinic,* or *antimuscarinic*. Anticholinergic poisoning syndrome is the clinical illness resulting from muscarinic receptor blockade in the central and peripheral nervous system.

Because of the multitude of over-the-counter and prescription drugs with anticholinergic effects, anticholinergic poisoning is a common cause of tachycardia, central nervous system (CNS) depression, hallucinations, and coma in overdose patients, as well as in children receiving therapeutic doses of medications.

Children are sensitive to anticholinergic agents and are at increased risk for accidental anticholinergic poisoning. It has been suggested that receptor sensitivity of affected organs for atropinic agents is greatest in children and diminishes with increasing age.[1] In addition, the elimination half-life of many antimuscarinics is increased in children up to age 2 or 3 years because of an increased volume of distribution.[1] Interestingly, children with Down syndrome commonly exhibit a genetically determined and sometimes fatal hypersensitivity to atropine and atropinic drugs.[2–4]

Children may be at increased risk for anticholinergic toxicity from well-intentioned therapeutic overdosing of over-the-counter medications by their parents, or they may idiosyncratically develop anticholinergic signs after a single therapeutic dose. Pediatric and adolescent patients, historically lacking access to more efficacious mind-altering drugs, are the ones most likely to try anticholinergic plants (e.g., jimsonweed) as substances of abuse.

PHARMACOLOGY AND PATHOPHYSIOLOGY

There are two general classes of receptors for acetylcholine released from cholinergic nerve endings: muscarinic and nicotinic receptors. Muscarinic receptors are the postganglionic receptors for the parasympathetic nervous system and for most sweat glands of the sympathetic nervous system and are found in many organs, as well as in smooth muscle tissue lacking direct cholinergic innervation.[5] The peripheral signs of the anticholinergic poisoning syndrome result almost entirely from blockade of these receptors. CNS muscarinic receptors are located in the spinal cord, extrapyramidal system, reticular activating system, vestibular system, and cerebral cortex, and most CNS effects of anticholinergic drugs are from blockade of these receptors.[5, 6]

Nicotinic receptors are found in autonomic ganglia (including the adrenal medulla), brain, and spinal cord and are the effector receptor at skeletal neuromuscular junctions. They are much less sensitive to anticholinergic (antimuscarinic) drugs and do not play a significant role in anticholinergic poisoning. Partial blockade of nicotinic receptors is only seen with extremely high doses of atropinic drugs, and motor end-plate receptors remain almost unaffected.[5] However, paralysis has been reported in some patients with overdoses of anticholinergic quaternary ammonium compounds that resemble the nondepolarizing neuromuscular blockers.[7, 8]

The relative degree of central and peripheral anticholinergic effects varies depending on the drug involved. Those anticholinergic drugs with quaternary amine groups (e.g., glycopyrrolate, propantheline, and other gastrointestinal antispasmodics) cross the blood-brain barrier very poorly and therefore have little central effect. Most anticholinergic drugs (atropine, scopolamine, homatropine) possess a tertiary amine group and rapidly cross the blood-brain barrier. These drugs can have significant central effects.

CLINICAL EVALUATION
General

Patients with anticholinergic poisoning syndrome may not have all of the typical associated findings. There may be marked inter-individual variation in response to the same substance. Persons who become anticholinergic after a therapeutic dose of medication (e.g., promethazine hydrochloride [Phenergan]) may have marked central signs without many peripheral findings.

Patients with anticholinergic poisoning commonly have prolonged and widely fluctuating clinical courses. Absorption of anticholinergic drugs can be delayed, prolonged, and erratic because of decreased gastrointestinal motility.[9] Some anticholinergics, including cyclic antidepressants and carbamazepine, demonstrate an enterohepatic or enteroenteric circulation that may extend the period of intoxication.

Central Anticholinergic Poisoning Syndrome

Central anticholinergic poisoning syndrome results from muscarinic receptor blockade in the brain. The usual clinical course is one of CNS stimulation followed by depression.[5, 10] The central syndrome usually begins as slight disorientation and cognitive impairment in its mildest form and may progress through agitation, muscular hyperactivity, and hallucinations to seizures and coma[6] (Table 88–1).

The child with central anticholinergic poisoning may be alert or lethargic. Initially, patients commonly are confused, disoriented, and agitated. They may demonstrate constant movement and are difficult to physically control, sometimes to the point of combativeness.

Patients with central anticholinergic syndrome have a distinctive mumbling, fragmented speech pattern, although this is less easily discernible in younger children. They are usually slow to respond to questions, then begin speaking somewhat clearly, only to trail off into unintelligible words or syllables. Lucid sentences may be followed or interrupted by completely inappropriate verbalizations. Dysarthria and pressured speech are also reported.[11]

Children who become anticholinergic after therapeutic or toxic doses of antihistamines may become hyperactive and run about the house, continuously babbling incoherent words and sounds. As disorientation progresses, undressing is typical anticholinergic behavior.

Anticholinergic hallucinations are usually visual but may be auditory or tactile.[10, 11] When visual anticholinergic hallucinations occur, they usually consist of objects that are seen undistorted but out of place. In contrast, lysergide (LSD) or other indole-induced hallucinations frequently involve distorted images or wildly unusual and vivid colors. An inordinate number of anticholinergic-poisoned children see animals in their bedrooms, closets, or dresser drawers, as well as Lilliputian hallucinations of tiny animals or people.[11] These patients often speak to pets, friends or relatives that are not present. "Picking" at clothes, bed sheets, and imaginary insects or objects is also a classic central anticholinergic motor sign.[10-12]

Ataxia, tremor, and clonic movements are common as the central anticholinergic syndrome progresses. These are anticholinergic effects that will respond to physostigmine and must be differentiated from true seizure activity which, as in cyclic antidepressants, may be an independent, nonanticholinergic effect of the drug involved. For example, amoxapine, a mildly anticholinergic cyclic antidepressant, is known to produce prolonged, refractory seizures that are sometimes fatal in cases of overdose.[13]

Although dystonic medication reactions are commonly treated with anticholinergic drugs, dystonia and rigidity have been reported as a result of anticholinergic medication ingestion, perhaps in part because of their interaction with central monoaminergic systems.[14-16] This is universally associated with the development of hyperthermia when accompanied by coexisting anticholinergic inhibition of normal heat loss by perspiration. Tachypnea may be present as a result of agitation and fever. If anticholinergic toxicity progresses untreated, medullary respiratory depression and cardiorespiratory arrest can eventually occur.[17]

Sedation occurs early in the clinical course with the centrally acting anticholinergic agents or with those drugs primarily developed as or combined with sedatives (cyclic antidepressants, glutethimide, antihistamines). Later, depressed mental status may be caused by drug effects, exhaustion from excessive motor activity, or hyperthermia. Most anticholinergic seizures are generally of short duration and easily controlled; more prolonged activity should mandate an evaluation for other causes. Coma is also seen as a complication of anticholinergic poisoning and may have a prolonged, cyclical course, with the patient partially awakening to periods of severe agitation and hallucinations. All of the signs of central anticholinergic poisoning can also be seen as the patient emerges from coma. Following treatment and recovery, the amnesic effects of atropinic agents frequently cause the patient to be unaware of any combative or bizarre behavior that occurred during the intoxication.[10]

Peripheral Anticholinergic Poisoning Syndrome

Peripheral anticholinergic poisoning syndrome results from blockade of postganglionic muscarinic receptors in the parasympathetic nervous system and in those sweat glands with cholinergic sympathetic innervation. First affected are the functions of salivation, sweating, and bronchial secretion, followed by pupillary function, ocular accommodation, and

---

TABLE 88–1

CENTRAL AND PERIPHERAL ANTICHOLINERGIC POISONING SYNDROME: SIGNS AND SYMPTOMS

Central
  Agitation
  Disorientation
  Cognitive impairment
  Lethargy, sedation
  Muscular hyperactivity
  Mumbling, fragmented, dysarthric speech
  Undressing behavior
  "Picking" movements
  Hallucinations (visual, tactile, or auditory)
  Ataxia, tremor, myoclonic movements
  Dystonia and rigidity
  Seizures
  Coma (may be fluctuating or cyclical)
  Medullary respiratory depression and arrest
  Amnesia on recovery
Peripheral
  Hyperthermia
  Dry mouth
  Anhydrosis (dry axillae)
  Mydriasis and cycloplegia (variable)
  Supraventricular tachycardias (sinus or other)
  Flushed appearance
  Mild hypertension
  Hypotension with dysrhythmias in severe poisoning
  Urinary retention
  Hypoactive bowel sounds (variable)

Note: All signs need not be present for the diagnosis of anticholinergic poisoning syndrome (see text).

heart rate. At higher doses, bladder and intestinal motility are altered, with gastric motility and secretion affected last.[5]

Because saliva secretion is sensitive to antimuscarinic agents, dry mouth is usually an initial finding. This may add to dysphasia.[5]

Inability to lose heat through perspiration is the major cause of hyperthermia in patients with anticholinergic poisoning, especially when ambient temperature is high or agitation and increased muscular activity are present. Temperature may become dangerously elevated (up to 40°C to 43°C) in those with marked agitation, rigidity, and tremor.[18] Hyperthermia may persist for days until normal thermoregulation returns. Core temperature must be closely monitored to avoid heat-related complications.

Perspiration is also sensitive to anticholinergic blockade. Although adolescents usually become hyperpyrexic only with overdose, infants and young children are especially prone to develop "atropine fever" with even small doses of anticholinergic drugs.[5] Dry axillae are suggestive of atropinic effect in older children and adolescents, and this finding can be followed to assess recovery of normal sweating function and thermoregulation after poisoning. Young children may have dry axillae as a normal finding, making other peripheral signs of atropinism more important in this age group.

Although anticholinergic toxicity classically causes mydriasis and cycloplegia, effects on pupil size vary as a function of the drug involved and other pathologic processes (e.g., seizures or hypoxia). Because both cyclic antidepressants and phenothiazines also block alpha-adrenergic receptors responsible for pupillary dilation, pupil size is frequently normal in cyclic antidepressant overdose patients and may even be small in patients poisoned with some phenothiazines. Benztropine overdose patients may be severely anticholinergic but have normal-sized pupils. Similarly, diphenhydramine overdose may not be accompanied by pupillary dilation until up to 24 hours after other symptoms present, sometimes appearing only as the patient is awakening. Unilateral mydriasis has been frequently reported as a result of monocular contamination after handling scopolamine transdermal patches[19] or after topical ocular contamination with jimsonweed.[20]

Tachycardia is a universal cardiovascular finding in significant peripheral anticholinergic toxicity.[21] Mild bradycardia may be seen with low doses of anticholinergic drugs and is thought to be caused by central vagal stimulation.[5] Increased peripheral presynaptic release of acetylcholine (also increasing vagal effect) and blockade of high-affinity sympathetic ganglion receptors responsible for cardioacceleration may also be involved.[21] Anticholinergic vagolytic effects are pronounced in older children, but less so in young infants.[5] Focal peripheral vasodilation sometimes causes a flushed appearance in the cheeks and chest, but this is not responsible for hypotension. Conversely, mild hypertension is commonly present because of sinus tachycardia. Significant hypotension may be seen with volume depletion, rare unstable supraventricular dysrhythmias, or circulatory collapse in severe poisoning.[22]

Anticholinergic agents relax urinary bladder muscle; this is the primary reason agents such as imipramine have been used in the treatment of nocturnal enuresis.[23] Acute urinary retention with a palpable bladder may be found on physical examination. This effect also makes assessing response to fluid therapy by urine output unreliable (if not dangerous), unless a urinary catheter is in place.[22]

Although usually diminished, bowel sounds are commonly present in anticholinergic overdoses. Atropine-like drugs block cholinergic impulses from the intramural nerve plexuses responsible for gut motility, but not vagal impulses

from the CNS that also maintain some degree of intestinal tone.[5] However, ileus remains possible.

ETIOLOGIC AGENTS

The most commonly ingested prescription drugs to cause anticholinergic poisoning syndrome are cyclic antidepressants (Table 88–2). The most commonly ingested over-the-counter agents producing anticholinergic findings are sleeping aids containing diphenhydramine or doxylamine. Anticholinergic poisoning may arise from accidental or intentional misuse of medications employed primarily for their anticholinergic effects (e.g., antispasmodics or antiparkinsonian agents) or from drugs not widely known for these properties (e.g., antihistamines or centrally acting "muscle relaxants").

Antihistamines are probably the most frequent cause of acute anticholinergic poisoning in children. Pediatric patients are highly sensitive to anticholinergic effects of anti-

TABLE 88–2

A PARTIAL LIST OF COMPOUNDS POSSESSING ANTIMUSCARINIC PROPERTIES

Acetophenazine	Amitriptyline
Amoxapine	Anisotropine
Atropine	Azatadine
Belladonna alkaloids	Benztropine
Biperiden	Brompheniramine
Buclizine	Butaperazine
Carbamazepine	Carbinoxamine
Chlorpheniramine	Chlorphenoxamine
Chlorpromazine	Chlorprothixine
Clemastine	Clidinium
Cyclizine	Cyclobenzaprine
Cycrimine	Cyclopentolate
Cyproheptadine	Desipramine
Dexbrompheniramine	Dexchlorpheniramine
Dicyclomine	Dimethindene
Diphemanil	Diphenylpyraline
Dimenhydrinate	Diphenhydramine
Disopyramide	Doxepin
Doxylamine	Ethopropazine
Eucatropine	Flavoxate
Fluphenazine	Glutethimide
Glycopyrrolate	Hexocyclium
Homatropine	Hydroxyzine
Hyoscyamine	Imipramine
Isopropramide	Loxapine
Maprotiline	Meclizine
Mepenzolate	Methantheline
Methdilazine	Methixene
Methylscopolamine	Mesoridazine
Molindone	Nortriptyline
Orphenadrine	Oxybutynin
Oxyphencyclimine	Oxyphenonium
Perphenazine	Pheniramine
Phenyltoloxamine	Piperolate
Piperacetazine	Procainamide
Prochlorperazine	Procyclidine
Promethazine	Propantheline
Protriptyline	Pyrilamine
Quinidine	Quinine
Scopolamine	Terfenadine
Thioridazine	Thiothixine
Thiphenamil	Tridihexethyl
Trifluoperazine	Triflupromazine
Trihexyphenidyl	Trimeprazine
Trimethobenzamide	Trimipramine
Tripelennamine	Tropicamide
Triprolidine	

histamines and may present with agitation, tremor, hyperthermia, and convulsions.[10] Doxylamine (Bendectin, Nyquil) has caused severe anticholinergic toxicity and fatalities in children.[24] Seizures have been reported after pediatric ingestions of as little as 150 mg of diphenhydramine and death after a 500-mg ingestion.[25] Poisoning from topical application of antihistamine-containing lotions is also reported, and absorption may be enhanced in the child with a disrupted skin barrier from dermatitis or infection.[26] Children with encephalopathy who are suspected to have Reye's syndrome may actually be suffering from anticholinergic poisoning from topical application of diphenhydramine lotion (Caladryl) for the treatment of varicella.

Diphenhydramine has also been found to block reuptake of norepinephrine and dopamine in the CNS. Central stimulant effect from blockade of catecholamine reuptake also may help explain the agitation, increased muscular activity, rigidity, and hyperthermia sometimes seen in these and other anticholinergic overdoses.

Phenothiazines, especially promethazine (Phenergan) and prochlorperazine (Compazine), are commonly prescribed antitussive, antiemetic, and sedative agents. They are mildly anticholinergic but suppress nausea and vomiting by their depressant effect on the chemoreceptor trigger zone.[27] Although extrapyramidal dystonic reactions are more common, typical anticholinergic poisoning with hyperthermia and psychosis has been reported with therapeutic dosing of promethazine syrup in children and with topical application of promethazine cream.[28, 29]

Agents used primarily for their anticholinergic effects include gastrointestinal, genitourinary, and bronchial antispasmodics; mydriatic eye drops; some antiparkinsonian agents; antidiarrheals; and antivertigo and motion sickness medications. Both therapeutic and excessive doses of dicyclomine (Bentyl), widely used to treat infantile colic, have been reported to cause lethargy, agitation, seizures, respiratory arrest, and death in infants.[30]

Treatment with atropine, scopolamine, and cyclopentolate ophthalmic drops has caused anticholinergic poisoning and death in children.[31–33] These agents are well absorbed through the conjunctiva and by the nasal mucosa and gastrointestinal tract as they drain through the nasolacrimal duct into the nose and pharynx.[31] One drop of 1% atropine solution contains 0.5 mg of drug and has caused acute anticholinergic toxicity and death in young children undergoing ophthalmologic examination.[3, 32–34] Death has also occurred with therapeutic administration of atropine ophthalmic ointment,[33] which allows for more prolonged drug exposure and absorption than drops. Atropine may also cause mild anticholinergic symptoms when used as an inhaled bronchodilator.[35]

Atropine is also combined with the narcotic diphenoxylate as an antidiarrheal agent, creating a mixed clinical picture in overdose patients. Initially, anticholinergic signs may be seen, including typical mydriasis, flushing, hyperthermia, and seizures.[36] Diphenoxylate overdose may progress to miosis, unresponsiveness, hypoxic seizures, and cardiorespiratory arrest.[36] A prolonged narcosis requiring extended treatment with naloxone is commonly seen.[2] Onset of narcotism may be rapid or delayed because of the effects of both drugs on gastric emptying. Cardiac arrest has been reported up to 12 hours after ingestion, and intact tablets were recovered with gastric lavage 27 hours after ingestion of atropine sulfate–diphenoxylate hydrochloride (Lomotil).[2, 36]

In addition to eye drops, antispasmodics, and over-the-counter hypnotics, scopolamine is also found in transdermal patches for prophylaxis against motion sickness. This source of acute mydriasis or other anticholinergic effects will be missed unless the postauricular area is examined for the patch.[37]

Ingestions of the antimuscarinic antiparkinsonian drugs benztropine (Cogentin), amantidine (Symmetrel), biperidin (Akineton), and trihexyphenidyl (Artane, benzhexol HCl) are usually accidental causes of anticholinergic poisoning in the pediatric population. However, benztropine and trihexyphenidyl have been discovered to have potent amphetamine-like effects on central monoaminergic systems,[15, 16] as well as gamma-aminobutyric acid (GABA)–mediated, benzodiazepine-like anxiolytic effects,[16] and have been used as drugs of abuse by adolescents.[15, 16, 38, 39] One patient who chronically smoked diphenhydramine and benztropine stated they "caused him to feel 'speeded up,' see fires erupting in his room, feel invisible, and have blurred vision."[40]

Cyclic antidepressants possess varying degrees of anticholinergic effect, with amitriptyline, nortriptyline, desipramine, and doxepin having the greatest effects.[41, 42] Trazodone (Desyrel) and bupropion are essentially without anticholinergic effect.[41, 42] Amitriptyline is also used as a drug of abuse,[43] probably because of its central anticholinergic effects.

Among the antidysrhythmic agents, disopyramide[6] and quinidine have strong anticholinergic effects, with procainamide having somewhat less.[44] However, patients suffering large overdoses of drugs with quinidine-like membrane-stabilizing effects (e.g., disopyramide, cyclic antidepressants, and phenothiazines) may present with bradycardia and cardiac conduction delays instead of typical anticholinergic tachycardia.

Two of the centrally acting muscle relaxants have substantial anticholinergic properties.[45–47] Cyclobenzaprine (Flexeril) was intended to be an antidepressant and is structurally and pharmacologically similar to amitriptyline.[46] Its anticholinergic, sedative, and antihistaminic properties far exceeded its antidepressant effect.[46, 47] Seizures and quinidine-like cardiotoxic effects have been reported in cyclobenzaprine overdose but have not caused death.[46, 47] The muscle relaxant orphenadrine is also used as an antimuscarinic antiparkinsonian agent and structurally resembles diphenhydramine. It rapidly produces coma in overdose and has been shown to have strong quinidine-like, myocardial depressant effects.[48, 49] Orphenadrine, alone or in combination with other drugs, has been responsible for at least 50 reported deaths.[48, 49]

Children taking the anticonvulsant carbamazepine may develop anticholinergic signs after acute overdose or from rising drug levels with chronic use. A prolonged, cyclic pattern of ataxia, dysarthria, and hallucinations alternating with coma is seen in acute ingestions.[50] This extended intoxication after overdose is caused in part by prolonged absorption of carbamazepine (levels may rise for up to 72 hours) and the equally strong anticholinergic activity of its major metabolite.[51]

Glutethimide is a sedative-hypnotic medication with strong anticholinergic properties.[6, 52] Its lipophilic properties lead to a rapid distribution phase and onset of anticholinergic signs with convulsions, apnea, and shock in overdose.[52] It is imperative to closely observe patients after glutethimide overdose, as intoxication occasionally demonstrates a markedly cyclical course.

Meperidine use may result in an anticholinergic delirium.[52] These anticholinergic effects are seen as part of the psychosis, tremors, myoclonus, and seizures that occur with accumulation of the metabolite normeperidine in chronic dosing.[52]

Anticholinergic plant poisoning is most common from jimsonweed (*Datura stramonium*) abuse in adolescents but is also seen after ingestion of mandrake (*Mandragora officinarum*), henbane (*Hyoscyamus niger*), and deadly nightshade (*Atropa belladonna*).[53] Anticholinergic poisoning has been reported after consumption of burdock (*Arctium lappa*) root tea as a health food.[55]

Accidental mushroom ingestions remain very common among young children, whereas adolescents deliberately ingest them as mind-altering substances. Anticholinergic mushrooms include the fly agaric (*Amanita muscaria*) and the panther mushroom (*A. pantherina*), both producing either anticholinergic or cholinergic signs.[55] Symptomatology is usually brief and does not require intervention. Physostigmine may exacerbate cholinergic effects in some ingestions.[56]

DIAGNOSTIC EVALUATION

Important initial measures in the emergency department evaluation of possible anticholinergic poisoning include assessment of the airway and respirations, cardiac rhythm and blood pressure monitoring, and an immediate and accurate measurement of core temperature. An electrocardiogram should be obtained to evaluate supraventricular dysrhythmias and quinidine-like cardiotoxic effects of the group I antidysrhythmics, cyclic antidepressants, phenothiazines, and antihistamines.[57, 58] Measurement of total serum creatine kinase activity; urine dipstick testing for pH, heme pigments, and red blood cells; and a serum myoglobin determination should be ordered from the emergency department to assess for possible rhabdomyolysis. Because none of these tests may be abnormal early in the course of severe rhabdomyolysis, they should be followed at intervals throughout the acute symptomatic stage while the patient is at risk for rhabdomyolysis. Measurement of serum electrolytes helps assess possible hyperkalemia and hypocalcemia from rhabdomyolysis, whereas blood urea nitrogen (BUN) and creatinine determinations provide baseline evaluation of renal function and may also indicate muscle damage.[59] A rapid test for blood glucose should be performed in the child with seizures. An acetaminophen level should be obtained, especially because several over-the-counter preparations with anticholinergic effects (e.g., Sominex pain reliever) contain this drug. Establishing the absence of salicylates in blood will rule out the differential diagnosis of salicylate poisoning. Arterial blood gas determination and measurement of tidal volume should be used to assess respiratory and acid-base status, especially in the severely poisoned patient. Abdominal radiographs have been shown to reveal several types of phenothiazine, cyclic antidepressant, and antihistamine tablets in a cadaver model,[60] but this has not been found to be clinically useful in ruling out poisoning with these agents. As many patients with sedative intoxication develop aspiration pneumonitis, a chest radiograph may be indicated. Routine urine drug screens may assist in confirming the presence of a specific anticholinergic drug or reveal other coingestants but will miss many causes of anticholinergic poisoning. Examination of gastric contents (in cases of ingestion) may reveal drug concentrations several orders of magnitude greater than those in blood or urine and will provide the highest diagnostic yield. Sufficient doses of naloxone (4 to 10 mg IV push in the pediatric patient) may serve as a diagnostic as well as therapeutic intervention in patients with narcotic overdose and associated anticholinergic signs (e.g., diphenoxylate with atropine, meperidine). However, naloxone may precipitate seizures in patients taking meperidine if toxic concentrations of normeperidine, a toxic metabolite, are present.

DIFFERENTIAL DIAGNOSIS

The most frequently occurring toxic syndrome in the pediatric population that closely resembles anticholinergic toxicity is sympathomimetic poisoning (Table 88–3). Children may overdose on over-the-counter decongestant preparations, phenylpropanolamine or caffeine (alone or in combination), or their own sympathomimetic medication (e.g., methylphenidate [Ritalin] or pemoline [Cylert]).

Sympathomimetic overdose resembles anticholinergic toxicity in several ways, producing dilated pupils, hypertension, tachycardia, agitation, and tremor. Hyperthermia from increased muscular activity is also common, as are hallucinations. Like patients with anticholinergic poisoning, sympathomimetic overdose patients may progress to coma and rigidity, with resultant rhabdomyolysis.[59] Sympathomimetic poisoning differs from anticholinergic toxicity in that diaphoresis, rather than dry axillae, is usually present. Severe hypertension is more common in patients with sympathomimetic overdose and sometimes occurs with reflex bradycardia, as seen in pediatric ingestions of phenylpropanolamine.[61] Although they may hallucinate, patients with sympathomimetic intoxication usually exhibit normal speech, rather than the mumbling dysarthria seen in anticholinergic syndrome. Paranoid psychosis with persecutory delusions and episodes of acute terror predominate in stimulant overdose, unlike the simple, nonthreatening visual images common with anticholinergic toxicity. Although auditory and visual hallucinations occur in both syndromes, sympathomimetic hallucinations are also usually threatening in nature.[62] Whereas patients with central anticholinergic syndrome "pick" nonexistent insects off of their clothes and bed sheets, those with sympathetic psychosis commonly excoriate their arms and trunks while attempting to dig out deeply embedded imaginary parasites.[62]

Phencyclidine (PCP) intoxication is usually a differential diagnosis in the adolescent patient, but accidental ingestion by young children has also been reported.[63] PCP intoxication resembles anticholinergic poisoning in that tachycardia, hypertension, tachypnea, myoclonus, rigidity, and hallucinations and seizures may be present.[64] However, profound ataxia, bizarre behavior, staring spells, vertical and horizontal nystagmus, hyperreflexia, and diaphoresis are consistent with PCP's anesthetic and sympathomimetic effects.[63, 64]

Patients with heat stroke may have a clinical picture similar to that of patients with severe anticholinergic poisoning; this is complicated by the fact that the anhydrotic effect of anticholinergic medications is a known precipitant of heat illness.[65] Because the sequelae of uncontrolled hyperthermia is the same for both, aggressive cooling is mandated. Anticholinergic medication use or toxicity should be considered as a potentially treatable etiologic factor.

Neuroleptic malignant syndrome may be seen in pediatric patients taking antipsychotic agents (many of which are

---

TABLE 88–3

DIFFERENTIAL DIAGNOSIS OF ANTICHOLINERGIC POISONING SYNDROME

Sympathomimetic poisoning
Theophylline poisoning
Phencyclidine intoxication
Neuroleptic malignant syndrome
Late or chronic salicylate poisoning
Thyroid hormone ingestion
Meningitis or sepsis
Sedative or ethanol withdrawal
Nutmeg or other hallucinogen ingestion

anticholinergic) or receiving even a single dose of antiemetic phenothiazines.[65] The classic findings include anticholinergic signs of hyperthermia, altered mental status, and altered vital signs, but these patients frequently have profuse diaphoresis and pronounced muscular rigidity.

Salicylate intoxication may also mimic some anticholinergic signs. Children with chronic salicylism or those suffering from severe acute poisonings may be tachypneic, hyperthermic, agitated, confused, or hallucinating.

The spice nutmeg (Myristica fragans) is occasionally abused by adolescents and contains hallucinogenic amphetamines,[67] terpenes,[67, 68] and indoles.[68] Acute poisoning resembles anticholinergic toxicity, with flushing, tachycardia, dry mouth, hypertension, and delirium, but miosis may occur instead of mydriasis.[67–69]

Pediatric ingestion of thyroid hormone may cause fever, tachycardia, lethargy, and, rarely, seizures, but these patients usually manifest hyperthyroid signs of diaphoresis and diarrhea.[70]

The possibility of meningitis or sepsis must be addressed in the pediatric patient with altered vital signs and mental status. Less commonly, in older adolescents, the hyperadrenergic signs associated with sedative or ethanol withdrawal may also be considered in the differential diagnosis of anticholinergic poisoning.

THERAPEUTIC INTERVENTION

Important supportive care measures in the hospital include monitoring cardiac rhythm, core temperature, and fluid status (Table 88–4). A urinary catheter allows reliable monitoring of urine output and pH and is usually required because of relaxed bladder musculature. External cooling should be continued for the hyperthermic patient. If rhabdomyolysis is suspected or seems likely from the patient's antecedent course, it is treated with crystalloid infusion, mannitol, and urinary alkalinization.[59]

Administration of activated charcoal to those who present late (24 to 48 hours) after ingestion may be indicated for symptomatic patients because of delayed drug absorption from slowed gastric emptying and decreased intestinal motility. Large or serial doses of activated charcoal have been recommended for some patients with anticholinergic poisoning, especially those with enterohepatic drug circulation.[21] However, serial doses of activated charcoal in anticholinergic poisoning patients are discouraged; there are no data demonstrating that such therapy alters clinical course, and the decreased gut motility present in serious anticholinergic poisonings can allow for the formation of charcoal concretions that may produce intestinal obstruction.[71]

Physostigmine

Physostigmine is a cholinesterase inhibitor that increases the amount of acetylcholine at cholinergic nerve endings, thereby reversing the effects of anticholinergic drugs.[72] When used alone or in excessive amounts, physostigmine causes cholinergic effects of salivation, miosis, lacrimation, bradycardia, vomiting, abdominal cramps, diarrhea, diaphoresis, incontinence, and increased airway resistance and secretions.[73] Physostigmine is the only reversible anticholinesterase that crosses the blood-brain barrier well, reversing central as well as peripheral anticholinergic effects.[74] However, it is indicated only for those patients with severe agitation or combativeness or for patients suffering from seizures refractory to other anticonvulsants and should only be administered to patients who are clearly anticholinergic (i.e., those with tachycardia or dry axillae).

Anticholinergic-induced tachycardia usually does not

TABLE 88–4
ANTICHOLINERGIC POISONING SYNDROME: THERAPY AT A GLANCE

Prehospital
  Airway management with endotracheal intubation as needed
  IV access
  Assess core temperature and begin cooling if indicated
  Skin decontamination if topical agent
  Activated charcoal, 1 gm/kg body weight, po or by nasogastric tube (if ingested substance)
  Gastric lavage if appropriate setting
Emergency department and intensive care unit
  Airway stabilization (if not managed in field) or reassessment
  Cardiac, blood pressure, and core temperature monitoring
  Urinary catheter
  Consider gastric lavage and activated charcoal if not done in field
  As indicated:
  External cooling
  Phenobarbital, 10–20 mg/kg IV, for seizures (observe for respiratory depression)
  Succinylcholine, 1–2 mg/kg IV, for immediate pharmacoparalysis for intubation (may have extended effect if given after physostigmine)
  Pancuronium, 0.1 mg/kg IV; atracurium, 0.5 mg/kg IV; or vecuronium, 0.1 mg/kg IV for extended pharmacoparalysis
  Physostigmine salicylate, 0.02 mg/kg IV, up to 2 mg per dose, over 5–10 minutes
  If rhabdomyolysis is suspected:
  Replace fluid deficits with balanced crystalloid infusion, then infuse 2–3 times maintenance rate unless fluid restriction required
  Mannitol, 20% solution, 5 ml/kg (1 gm/kg) IV, over 10–20 minutes
  Sodium bicarbonate and potassium as needed to keep urine pH >6.0
  Monitor arterial blood gases, serum electrolytes, serum Ca^{++}, urine pH, and urine myoglobin

cause hemodynamic compromise, but physostigmine may be indicated in those rare instances in which supraventricular tachycardia with hypotension is not reversed by conservative measures such as intravenous fluids. Physostigmine should not be used in patients exhibiting bradydysrhythmias or conduction delays. Physostigmine should be administered only in the emergency department or intensive care unit with full resuscitation capability. Continuous cardiac and blood pressure monitoring is required.

A urinary catheter should be in place to allow bladder emptying. The action of succinylcholine is prolonged by anticholinesterases, and this effect should be anticipated if this drug is used for pharmacoparalysis.[74] Other contraindications to physostigmine pertinent to the pediatric patient include asthma and intestinal or urinary outlet obstruction.[76]

The pediatric dose of physostigmine salicylate is 0.02 mg/kg, up to 2 mg given intravenously over 5 to 10 minutes. Beneficial effects may take up to 20 minutes to occur, and a common pitfall in the use of this drug is repeating the dose too soon. If the patient clearly remains anticholinergic for 20 minutes after intravenous administration of physostigmine salicylate, the dose may be repeated until the desired end point is achieved (or until adverse effects limit further doses). The short duration of action of physostigmine salicylate (45 to 60 min)[76] may necessitate frequent repeat doses. Although continuous intravenous infusions have been used effectively,[77] they are usually unnecessary and less safe than physician-directed bolus therapy. If excessive cholinergic effects occur, atropine sulfate (0.01 mg/kg IV up to 2.0 mg total) or glycopyrrolate bromide (Robinul) (0.004 mg/kg to 0.008 mg/kg IV every 2 to 3 min) may be given as needed.[78] Glycopyrrolate may be preferable to atropine, as its charged quaternary amine group does not cross the blood-brain barrier well, thereby maintaining physostigmine's reversal of anticholinergic delirium while treating excessive peripheral cholinergic activity.

Adverse effects of physostigmine include excessive peripheral cholinergic activity as noted earlier, with bradydysrhythmias, heart block, and respiratory complications being most significant.[79, 80] Whether asystole is caused directly by physostigmine is debated.[79, 80] An increased incidence of seizures has been shown when large doses of physostigmine salicylate (0.3 mg/kg, or more than 20 mg for an average adult) were given simultaneously with cyclic antidepressant overdoses in mice.[81] Whether seizures in humans following physostigmine use are caused by the drug or the underlying poisoning is not clear.[82–86]

DISPOSITION

It is difficult to make specific recommendations regarding patient disposition, as this group of drugs varies widely in effect. It also may be difficult to accurately assess and interpret normal heart rate, blood pressure, and mental status in children, especially infants, when evaluating them for anticholinergic poisoning. Although onset of anticholinergic toxicity is usually rapid, drugs such as atropine and diphenoxylate or benztropine may demonstrate markedly delayed onset of effect or other severe nonanticholinergic complications. These exceptions make it difficult to determine a safe observation period for patients with suspected anticholinergic poisoning. In general, patients who remain completely asymptomatic and without alteration in mental status, vital signs, electrocardiogram, or pertinent physical examination for 6 hours may be safely discharged to the care of responsible guardians. Discharge instructions should include some signs of the anticholinergic syndrome, and parents should be instructed to return the child to the emergency department should these signs occur. All children who may have ingested toxic amounts of atropine sulfate–diphenoxylate hydrochloride (Lomotil) are admitted because of well-documented delayed onset of CNS depression that may accompany serious ingestions.

Any patient with anticholinergic poisoning requiring admission should be placed in a monitored intensive care setting or transferred to such a setting by advanced life support level medical personnel if such facilities are not available at the initial receiving hospital. These patients may be safely transferred to an unmonitored pediatric or psychiatric ward when anticholinergic signs and other toxic pharmacologic effects have completely resolved. Psychiatric evaluation is warranted in cases of intentional ingestion with the intent of suicide or self-injury, and in cases of possible nonaccidental ingestion or exposure, child protection services should be notified.

References

1. Kanto J, Klotz U. Pharmacokinetic implications for the clinical use of atropine, scopolamine and glycopyrrolate. Acta Anesthesiol Scand 1988;32:69.
2. Rumack BH, Temple AR. Lomotil poisoning. Pediatrics 1974;53:495.
3. Walsh FB, Hoyt WF. Neurotoxic substances. In Clinical Neuro-ophthalmology. 3rd ed. Baltimore, Williams & Wilkins, 1969, p 2661.
4. Harris WS, Goodman RM. Hyper-reactivity to atropine in Down's syndrome. N Engl J Med 1968;279:407.
5. Weiner N. Atropine, scopolamine and related antimuscarinic drugs. In Gilman AG, Goodman LS, Gilman A (eds). The Pharmacological Basis of Therapeutics. 7th ed. New York, Macmillan, 1985, p 130.
6. Spady GP, Guidry JR. Anticholinergic medications: Classification and potency. Samaritan Med 1987;5:29.
7. Ferguson A, Baker DA. Neuromuscular paralysis caused by an overdose of emepronium bromide (Cetiprin). Arch Emerg Med 1985;2:79.
8. Albuquerque EX, Eldefrawi AT, Eldefrawi ME, et al. Amantadine: Neuromuscular blockade by suppression of ionic conductance of the acetylcholine receptor. Science 1978;199:788.
9. Fahy P, Arnold P, Curry SC, et al. Serial serum drug concentrations and prolonged anticholinergic toxicity after benztropine (Cogentin) overdose. Am J Emerg Med 1989;7:199.
10. Jones J, Dougherty J, Cannon L. Diphenhydramine-induced toxic psychosis. Am J Emerg Med 1986;4:369.
11. Perry PJ, Wilding DC, Juhl RP. Anticholinergic psychosis. Am J Hosp Pharm 1978;35:725.
12. Woo OF. Acute intoxication with nonprescription antihistamines. Contemp Pharm Practice 1981;4:257.
13. Litovitz TL, Troutman WG. Amoxapine overdose: Seizures and fatalities. JAMA 1983;250:1069.
14. Howrie DL, Rowley AH, Krenzelok EP. Benztropine-induced acute dystonic reaction. Ann Emerg Med 1986;15:594.
15. Modell JG, Tandon R, Beresford TP. Dopaminergic activity of the antimuscarinic antiparkinsonian agents. J Clin Psychopharmacol 1989;9:347.
16. Dilsaver SC. Antimuscarinic agents as substances of abuse: A review. J Clin Psychopharmacol 1988;8:14.
17. Rumack BH. Anticholinergic poisoning: Treatment with physostigmine. Pediatrics 1973;52:449.
18. Goldstein MR, Kasper R. Hyperpyrexia and coma due to overdose of benztropine. South Med J 1968;61:984.
19. Mcrary JA, Webb NR. Anisocoria from scopolamine patches. JAMA 1982;248:353.
20. Savitt DL, Roberts JR, Siegel EG. Anisocoria from jimsonweed. JAMA 1986;255:1439.
21. Callaham M. Tricyclic antidepressant overdose. JACEP 1979;8:413.
22. Banner W. Toxic polypharmaceutical problems from south of the border. Arizona Poison Control System Newsletter 1983;5:1.
23. Rushton G. Nocturnal enuresis: Epidemiology, evaluation, and currently available treatment options. J Pediatr 1989;114:691.
24. Köppel C, Tenczer J, Ibe K. Poisoning with over-the-counter doxylamine preparations: An evaluation of 109 cases. Hum Toxicol 1987;6:355.
25. Hestand HE, Teske DW. Diphenhydramine hydrochloride intoxication. J Pediatr 1977;90:1017.
26. Woodward GA, Baldassano RN. Topical diphenhydramine toxicity in a five year old with varicella. Pediatr Emerg Care 1988;4:18.
27. Baldessarini RJ. Drugs and the treatment of psychiatric disorders. In Gilman AG, Goodman LS, Gilman A (eds). The Pharmacological Basis of Therapeutics. 7th ed. New York, Macmillan, 1985, p 387.
28. Dollberg S, Hurvitz H, Kerem E, et al. Hallucinations and hyperthermia after promethazine ingestion. Acta Pediatr Scand 1989;78:131.
29. Shawn DH, McGuigan MA. Poisoning from dermal absorption of promethazine. Can Med Assoc J 1984;130:1460.
30. Garriott JC, Norton LE. Two cases of death involving dicyclomine in infants. Clin Toxicol 1984;22:455.
31. Adler AG, McElwain GE, Merli GJ, et al. Systemic effects of eye drops. Arch Intern Med 1982;142:2293.
32. Hoefnagel D. Toxic effects of atropine and homatropine eyedrops in children. N Engl J Med 1961;264:168.
33. Heath WE. Death from atropine poisoning. Br Med J 1950;2:608.
34. Selvin BL. Systemic effects of topical ophthalmic medications. South Med J 1983;76:349.
35. Massey KL, Gotz VP. Ipratropium bromide. Drug Intell Clin Pharm 1985;19:5.
36. Cutler EA, Barrett GA, Craven PW, et al. Delayed cardiopulmonary arrest after Lomotil ingestion. Pediatrics 1980;65:157.
37. Klein BL, Ashenburg CA, Reed MD. Transdermal scopolamine intoxication in a child. Pediatr Emerg Care 1985;1:208.
38. Craig DH, Rosen P. Abuse of antiparkinsonian drugs. Ann Emerg Med 1981;10:98.
39. Crawshaw JA, Mullen PE. A study of benzhexol abuse. Br J Psychiatry 1984;145:300.
40. Brower KJ. Smoking of prescription anticholinergic drugs. Am J Psychiatry 1987;144:383.
41. Brogden RN, Heel RC, Speight TM, et al. Trazodone: A review of its pharmacological properties and therapeutic use in depression and anxiety. Drugs 1981;21:401.
42. Stark P, Fuller RW, Wong DT. The pharmacologic profile of fluoxetine. J Clin Psychiatry 1985;46:7.
43. Cohen MJ, Hanbury R, Stimmel B. Abuse of amitriptyline. JAMA 1978;240:1372.
44. Bigger JT, Hoffman BH. Antiarrhythmic drugs. In Gilman AG, Goodman LS, Gilman A (eds). The Pharmacological Basis of Therapeutics. 7th ed. New York, Macmillan, 1985, pp 748–783.
45. Clarke B, Mair J, Rudolf M. Acute poisoning with orphenadrine. Lancet 1985;2:1386.
46. Linden CH, Mitchiner JC, Lindzon RD, et al. Cyclobenzaprine overdosage. J Toxicol Clin Toxicol 1983;20:281.

47. O'Riordan W, Gillette, Calderon J, et al. Overdose of cyclobenzaprine, the tricyclic muscle relaxant. Ann Emerg Med 1986;15:137.
48. Sangster B, Van Heijst ANP, Zimmerman ANE, et al. Intoxication by orphenadrine HCl; mechanism and therapy. Acta Pharmacol Toxicol 1977;41(suppl 2):129.
49. Bozza-Marrubini M, Frigerio A, Ghezzi R, et al. Two cases of severe orphenadrine poisoning with atypical features. Acta Pharmacol Toxicol 1977;41(suppl 2):137.
50. Durelli L, Massazza U, Cavallo R. Carbamazepine toxicity and poisoning. Med Toxicol Adv Drug Exp 1989;4:95.
51. May DC. Acute carbamazepine intoxication: clinical spectrum and management. South Med J 1984;77:24.
52. Bertino JS, Reed MD. Barbiturate and nonbarbiturate sedative hypnotic intoxication in children. Pediatr Clin North Am 1986;33:703.
53. Eisendrath SJ, Goldman B, Douglas J, et al. Meperidine-induced delirium. Am J Psychiatry 1987;144:1062.
54. Heiser CB. Nightshades. San Francisco, WH Freeman, 1969, p 129.
55. Rhoads PM, Tong TG, Banner W. Anticholinergic poisonings associated with burdock root tea. Clin Toxicol 1984–85;22:581.
56. Hall AH, Spoerke DG, Rumack BH. Mushroom poisoning: Identification, diagnosis, and treatment. Pediatr Rev 1987;8:291.
57. Huxtable RF, Landwirth J. Diphenhydramine poisoning treated by exchange transfusion. Am J Dis Child 1963;106:496.
58. Craft TM. Torsades de pointes after astemizole overdose. Br Med J 1986;292:660.
59. Curry SC, Chang D, Connor D. Drug and toxin-induced rhabdomyolysis. Ann Emerg Med 1989;18:1068.
60. Savitt DL, Hawkins HH, Roberts JR. The radiopacity of ingested medications. Ann Emerg Med 1987;16:331.
61. Brown CR. Phenylpropanolamine—an ongoing problem. Clinical Toxicol Update, San Francisco Bay Poison Center 1987;9:1.
62. Gay GR. Clinical management of acute and chronic cocaine poisoning. Ann Emerg Med 1982;11:562.
63. Welch MJ, Correa GA. PCP intoxication in young children and infants. Clin Pediatr 1980;19:510.
64. McCarron MM, Schulze BW, Thompson GA, et al. Acute phencyclidine intoxication: incidence of clinical findings in 1,000 cases. Ann Emerg Med 1981;10:237.
65. Olson KR, Benowitz NL. Environmental and drug-induced hyperthermia. Emerg Clin North Am 1984;2:459.
66. Pearlman CA. Neuroleptic malignant syndrome: A review of the literature. J Clin Psychopharmacol 1986;6:257.
67. Ellenhorn MJ, Barceloux DG (eds).Nutmeg. In Medical Toxicology. New York, Elsevier, 1988, p 1286.
68. Payne RB. Nutmeg intoxication. N Engl J Med 1968;269:36.
69. Emboden W. Narcotic Plants. New York, Collier Books, 1979, p 47.
70. Litovitz TL, White JD. Levothyroxine ingestion in children: An analysis of 78 cases. Am J Emerg Med 1985;3:297.
71. Flores F, Battle WS. Intestinal obstruction secondary to activated charcoal. Contemp Surg 1987;30:57.
72. Manoguerra AS, Ruiz E. Physostigmine treatment of anticholinergic poisoning. JACEP 1976;5:125.
73. Granacher RP, Baldessarini RJ. Physostigmine: Its use in acute anticholinergic syndrome with antidepressant and antiparkinsonian drugs. Arch Gen Psychiatry 1975;32:375.
74. Goldfrank LR, Lewin NA, Flomenbaum NE, et al. Antidepressants: Tricyclics, tetracyclics, monoamine oxidase inhibitors, and others. In Goldfrank LR, Flomenbaun NE, Lewin NA, et al (eds): Goldfrank's Toxicologic Emergencies. 3rd ed. Norwalk, CT, Appleton-Century-Crofts, 1986, p 351.
75. Selden BS, Curry SC. Prolonged succinylcholine-induced paralysis in organophosphate insecticide poisoning. Ann Emerg Med 1987;16:215.
76. Physician's Desk Reference. Oradell, NJ, Medical Economics Co., Inc., 1988, p 967.
77. Stern TA. Continuous infusion of physostigmine in anticholinergic delirium: Case report. J Clin Psychiatry 1983;44:463.
78. Physician's Desk Reference. Oradell, NJ, Medical Economics Co., Inc., 1988, p 1700.
79. Pentel P, Peterson CD. Asystole complicating physostigmine treatment of tricyclic antidepressant overdose. Ann Emerg Med 1980;9:588.
80. Kulig K, Rumack BH. Physostigmine and asystole. Letter. Ann Emerg Med 1981;10:228.
81. Vance MA, Ross SM, Millington WR. Potentiation of tricyclic toxicity by physostigmine in mice. Clin Toxicol 1977;11:413.
82. Rumack BH. Anticholinergic poisoning: Treatment with physostigmine. Pediatrics 1973;52:449.
83. Stewart GO. Convulsions after physostigmine. Letter. Anaesth Intensive Care 1979;7:283.
84. Ordiway MV. Treating tricyclic overdose with physostigmine. Letter. Am J Psychiatry 1973;135:1114.
85. Newton RW. Physostigmine salicylate in the treatment of tricyclic antidepressant overdosage. JAMA 1975;231:941.
86. Aquilonius SM, Hedstrand U. The use of physostigmine as an antidote in tricyclic antidepressant intoxication. Acta Anaesthiol Scand 1978;22:40.

CHAPTER 89

Hallucinogens

Gloria J. Kuhn

CANNABIS

Cannabis sativa grows wild in most tropical areas of the world. The Arabic name for the cannabis extract is *hashish,* which means "grass."

Cannabis is the most widely used illicit drug in the world today.[1] Its frequency of use ranks below only that of alcohol, cigarettes, and caffeine.[2] In 1962 marijuana was used almost exclusively by the 18- to 25-year-old age group. Approximately 4 of every 100 people in that group admitted to use of the drug.[3] A survey completed in January 1980 revealed the number had risen. Sixty-eight of every 100 people in the same age group had used the drug, for a total involvement of approximately 21 million Americans. Forty percent of these people had used the drug a minimum of 100 times. More than 50 million people had used marijuana at least once. Unlike the users of the 1960s, most of whom were college students in large coastal cities, users of the 1980s represent all age groups, all geographic locations, and all socioeconomic classes.[4,6]

Since the 1980s, the use of marijuana has been declining. All types of usage among young people have decreased, and daily users, presumably the group most at risk, have declined from 10.7% of those surveyed in 1978 to 5% in 1984. Rates of use in older age groups have remained stable.

The reasons for the decrease in marijuana use are not evident. The drug is still widely available, and higher quality marijuana products are relatively easily procured. In 1978, 35% of high school seniors felt regular marijuana smokers ran a risk of hurting themselves physically, and 68% disapproved of regular use. By 1983, 63% of seniors felt that the drug might be physically harmful, and 83% disapproved of regular use.[7]

Cannabis is available in three forms: marijuana, hashish, and hashish oil. Marijuana is prepared from the ground dried leaves and flowers of the plant. Marijuana is frequently sold in 4- to 5-gm packets, which have enough material to make five to six joints or cigarettes, each containing 500 to 750 mg of marijuana. Prior to use, marijuana must be cleaned of seeds and small woody stems, which may comprise up to 50% or more of the packet that was purchased. A marijuana cigarette or joint is then made by rolling 500 to 750 mg of the material in a thin paper.

Marijuana smoke has a pungent smell that resembles the smell of burning wet hay or leaves and clings to the hair and wool garments. Smoking implements such as hollow smoking stones, minature smoking pipes, or air- or water-cooled smoking chambers may be used to cool and sweeten the highly irritating marijuana smoke; this permits the user to inhale and retain in the lungs a larger quantity of drug. In order to obtain maximal effect, marijuana users must master a smoking technique that is different from that used in smoking tobacco cigarettes. Experienced users inhale the smoke as deeply into the lungs as possible and hold their breath for 20 or 30 seconds or more in an effort to extract all the delta-9-tetrahydrocannabinol (delta-9-THC) into the capillary rich pulmonary circulation. (Delta-9-THC is the active ingredient of marijuana and comprises from 1% to up to 14% of the total marijuana amount.) With this technique, 50% of the delta-9-THC contained in the crude marijuana is delivered to the blood stream, with almost no delta-9-THC remaining in the exhaled breath.

Hashish may be prepared by either collecting the resin secreted by the leaves of high-quality cannabis plants or by boiling the plant to obtain an extract. This extract is dried and then pressed into bricks or cakes. The potency of this material is greater than ground marijuana, containing up to a 5% to 15% concentration of delta-9-THC.

The most potent of all the cannabis preparations is hashish oil, which is prepared by distilling the plant in organic solvents. The amount of delta-9-THC in this preparation ranges from 15% to 30%.

Pharmacology

The common name *marijuana* is derived from the Mexican/Spanish word *marijuana*, which refers to a mixture of cut, dried, and ground leaves and stems of the leafy green hemp plant. Marijuana is a unique psychoactive agent. The chemistry and pharmacology of marijuana do not resemble those of any other class of mind-altering drugs. Biochemists have identified more than 400 constituents in the plant's resin; approximately 60 are known collectively as *cannabinoids*, and these are the compounds responsible for the pharmacologic effects of the drug. Cannabinol, cannabidiol, and delta-9-THC are the major psychoactive compounds. The cannabinoid acids, which are psychotropically inactive and unstable, rapidly decarboxylate into neutral cannabinoids.[8]

Delta-9-THC is the main psychoactive agent in marijuana. Selective breeding now yields marijuana with a much higher concentration of delta-9-THC than was previously available. The most potent type of marijuana is sensemilla, which is prepared from unpollinated female hemp plants.[9]

There has been some controversy as to exactly how much delta-9-THC is contained in the marijuana sold on the street. Canadian laboratories analyzing street samples of both marijuana and hashish in 1971 showed a range of 0.02% to 3.46% delta-9-THC in marijuana and 1.0% to 14.4% delta-9-THC in hashish. Samples of marijuana analyzed by the Drug Enforcement Administration (DEA) showed increases in delta-9-THC concentration from 0.5% in 1974 to 3.5% in 1985 and 1988.

Route of Administration and Metabolism

Oral and inhalation routes of administration are those most commonly used and produce distinctly different plasma concentration curves as a result of the difference of absorption. Inhalation of ground marijuana in cigarette form is the most popular method of ingestion. The "average" joint in the United States is composed of about 500 mg of marijuana containing 1% delta-9-THC, 50% of which (2.5 mg) is bioavailable. Hashish or cannabis resin contains 5% to 15% delta-9-THC, and cannabis oil contains 28% delta-9-THC.[10]

When marijuana is smoked, 50% of the delta-9-THC is rapidly absorbed into the blood stream, producing peak plasma concentrations in less than 10 minutes. In one study, typical peak plasma concentrations ranged from 33 to 118 ng/ml in subjects who smoked an average of 13 mg of delta-9-THC.[11] After 1 hour the concentration had fallen to about 10% of the peak level, and after 4 hours the concentration was approximately 1 ng/ml.[11]

After oral administration, a slow and erratic absorption of delta-9-THC occurs. Peak plasma levels are reached in 1 to 2 hours. In one group of cancer patients a single 50-mg oral dose produced a mean peak plasma level of 3.9 ng/ml at 2

hours.[12] The rapid decline in plasma concentrations is a result of both the efficient tissue uptake of delta-9-THC and its metabolism. Delta-9-THC is highly lipid soluble and highly protein bound. It has a biphasic pattern in the plasma, with a high level during intoxication, dispersion throughout the body tissues, and then a slow graded release back into the blood.[13] Onset of action is in 10 to 30 minutes, and the duration of action is 2 to 4 hours. The half-life of delta-9-THC is 7 days, but it has been found in the urine in measurable quantities up to 6 weeks after abstinence in those who chronically ingest the drug.[14]

The primary metabolic pathways occur in the liver. Initially, delta-9-THC is converted to 11-hydroxy-delta-9-THC (11-OH-THC), with psychomimetic activity equal to that of delta-9-THC. Further oxidation results in the formation of 11-*nor*-delta-9-tetrahydrocannabinol-9-carboxylic acid (THC-COOH), an inactive metabolite. Free and conjugated THC-COOH represent the predominant urinary metabolite.[15]

Mechanism of Action

The actual mechanism of action by which marijuana produces its effects is unknown. Whether the drug produces its effects through specific receptors analogous to opiate and other receptors, or whether it acts through nonspecific membrane alterations, or even by some other mechanism, is uncertain.[16] The membrane-lipid interaction hypotheses are best supported at this time. The lipid microenvironment around membrane-bound receptors can affect receptor activity, receptor sensitivity, and specificity. It is postulated that delta-9-THC and other cannabinoids may directly and indirectly moderate the activity of these receptors by nonspecific lipid interactions.[17] This mechanism of action could explain the interactions between cannabis and other drugs, such as opiates, that have specific receptors or drugs such as alcohol and cocaine that share membrane-altering properties.[18]

Clinical Evaluation

Marijuana affects the reproductive, immune, cardiovascular, pulmonary, and central nervous systems. The intensity and duration of all effects are dependent on dose and frequency of dose.[15, 19, 20] The actual physical effects of marijuana ingestion are few, and none are specific to ingestion of cannabis.[13] There is conjunctival injection. Cardiovascular side effects include sinus tachycardia and nonspecific ST-T wave changes that are unrelated and not life threatening. Increased supine blood pressure, decreased standing blood pressure, impaired balance, peripheral vasoconstriction, and increased appetite have all been described.

Marijuana has gained wide use because of its psychological effects. In low doses, the drug has paradoxical effects, acting both as a stimulant and a depressant.[21] The user appears to be in a high, dream-like state. What an individual user experiences is dependent on and varies with the dose of delta-9-THC, the psychological "set" of the user (i.e., personality of the user and expectations of what the drug will do), and the setting (environmental and social situation).[22] Most users experience a pleasurable effect from the drug. About half of those who try the drug on an experimental basis continue to use it. Studies have shown that of those who used the drug daily in high school, 90% continued to use it 4 years after graduation, and half of them did so on a daily basis.[23, 24] Low doses of delta-9-THC produce euphoria, a sense of relaxation, passivity, and increased auditory, visual, and gustatory perceptions. The person may feel an unusually strong interest in what would ordinarily be mundane objects. Moderate doses intensify these effects and may also produce impaired short-term memory, disturbed thought patterns, lapses of attention, and decreased learning ability. Large doses cause distortion of body image, depersonalization, disorientation, paranoia, and marked sensory distortion.[25] Mood changes vary considerably, with a sense of increased well-being frequently felt, but anxiety and depression may also be enhanced by the drug. Drowsiness or hyperactivity and hilarity may occur. Passivity and apathy can be present. Ideas are disconnected, free-flowing, and altered in importance and emphasis. The individual may be withdrawn or talkative. There is a distortion of time sense, with individuals spending long periods reading, listening to music, or thinking. Users describe a sensation of enhanced concentration and the ability to experience sensations more fully. The larger the dose of delta-9-THC, the more distorted reality becomes.

First-time marijuana users who are unfamiliar with the drug's effect and who may use the drug in an unfamiliar or even frightening setting may have a panic attack.[26] Psychologically disposed individuals are more susceptible to these adverse reactions. Although prolonged or chronic psychotic disorders indistinguishable from functional disorders appear to have been precipitated by the use of marijuana, a premorbid psychopathology or vulnerability also seems to have been present.[27–30] Not all experts agree that cannabis causes a psychosis that persists after cessation of use of the drug.[31] Flashbacks have been described in some individuals, and like flashbacks occurring with other drugs, the actual mechanism by which this occurs is unknown.

There has been a great deal of discussion as to whether marijuana leads to use of stronger drugs.[9, 32, 33] Demonstration of prior use does not prove causality, but it is likely that someone who has made the decision to use illicit drugs such as marijuana is more likely to use other illicit drugs than an individual who does not use drugs. In addition, the process of procuring marijuana may lead the individual into contact with those who have used other drugs and may encourage use of these.

There is some evidence to suggest that both physical and psychological dependence and tolerance do occur with prolonged and continued use of the drug. A minority of regular users develop a growing inability to abstain from use, although the factors accounting for such selectivity are unknown.[34] Tolerance does result for several physiologic effects, and withdrawal phenomena, although mild, do occur.[28] In those who have been long-term heavy users, irritability, restlessness, and insomnia have been reported when the drug is abruptly discontinued.[27]

Two separate tomography studies have failed to confirm the existence of brain atrophy in chronic users[35, 36] that had been reported in an earlier study.[37] One study showed differences in the size of the ventricles of the brain of monkeys that were given delta-9-THC daily when compared with drug-free controls.[38] Whether brain damage occurs after long-term usage of marijuana is uncertain.

An amotivational syndrome has been described in chronic heavy users of marijuana and has been used to explain poor school performance, apathy, personality deterioration, and other signs of deterioration in such individuals. However, a panel of experts convened by the World Health Organization and the Addiction Research Foundation in Canada concluded that this is not a clinical state, but rather a manifestation of ongoing intoxication in frequent and heavy users.[30]

Cannabis is a bronchodilator. However, smoking the drug has been found to negatively affect the bronchopulmonary system.[39] This occurs most probably because of contaminants and other materials ingested during smoking. The smoke contains more tar than tobacco and is hotter on contact with the respiratory tree, because cannabis preparations burn at a higher temperature.[30] This may have severe consequences for those with underlying pulmonary problems such as asthma. Herbicides may also cause a problem. In the late 1970s, paraquat was sprayed on plants growing in Mexico. Lung damage did not appear to result from inhalation of these plants,[40] although skin and eye irritation have been noted on contact with paraquat.

Use of hashish has been associated with bronchitis, sinusitis, asthma, and rhinopharyngitis. Sputum-producing cough, difficulty in breathing, and wheezing were found after 15 months of use. Chest radiographs and sputum cultures were negative, and symptoms resolved after stopping the drug.[41]

The neoplastic effects of marijuana on the lung are not known at this time. Marijuana smoke contains more carcinogens and more tar than tobacco.[18] As noted previously, marijuana cigarettes burn at a higher temperature than do tobacco cigarettes, and marijuana cigarettes are smoked down to the very end of the material, which contains more delta-9-THC and polyaromatic hydrocarbons than does the rest of the cigarette. For these reasons, it is felt that marijuana cigarettes may have significant carcinogenic potential, but this has not been proven.

Marijuana is anti-androgenic and in males diminishes testosterone production and inhibits reproductive function.[41, 42] The magnitude of duration, and therefore the significance of these findings, is not known. In females, marijuana use shortens the menstrual cycle because of shorter luteal phases. In a study of women using marijuana three times a week or more for a 6-month period, there was a statistically higher incidence of abnormal menstrual cycles in which the women failed to ovulate and showed lowered prolactin levels.[43]

Delta-9-THC passes through the placental barrier and accumulates in the fatty tissues of the fetus. Pregnant rhesus monkeys given delta-9-THC had death, abortion, and fetal reabsorption rates that were four times those of drug-free controls.[44] Animal studies have shown that chronic exposure to marijuana during pregnancy causes growth retardation of the fetus. Infants born to mothers using marijuana had a higher number of nervous system abnormalities (e.g., tremors, high-pitched cries, and diminished response to visual stimuli) and small birth weight when compared with infants born to mothers who did not use marijuana.[45] Mothers using 2 to 14 joints per day had a statistically higher incidence of children with growth retardation and facial dysmorphogenesis, with rates that paralleled those found with fetal alcohol syndrome. The neurologic symptoms usually subsided in a few weeks, however, and infants tended to show catch-up growth in the first year of life.[46]

Cannabinoids appear to have a mild immunosuppressive effect on the immune system, but these symptoms are transient.[47]

Diagnostic Evaluation

Testing for Marijuana

The physical effects of marijuana used alone are usually so mild that extensive laboratory tests such as a complete blood cell count or electrolyte studies are not needed in the emergency department unless other drugs have been ingested or the patient has been involved in trauma. Urinalysis is the test of choice for detection of the drug itself, as plasma concentrations fall rapidly to one tenth of the peak concentration within 1 hour.[48] Metabolites in urine are present in detectable quantities (>20 ng/ml) within 1 hour of smoking marijuana and a slightly longer period after orally ingesting the drug. Those who use the drug only occasionally have detectable levels of the metabolites for up to 2 to 5 days and as long as 10 days after last use.[48] Users who are heavy chronic smokers have detectable levels of the cannabinoid metabolites for up to 4 weeks and possibly for 6 weeks after the last usage, as delta-9-THC, which is highly lipophilic, is stored in the soft tissues and slowly released back into the blood stream and metabolized.[14, 48]

It is possible for nonsmokers to ingest enough marijuana for a drug test to be positive. In one study, it was shown that four out of five individuals in a 6 × 8–foot room had positive drug tests when exposed to four marijuana cigarettes smoked over 1 hour once daily for 5 days.[49]

Drug Testing

The indications for drug testing in the pediatric population usually involve either unexplained changes in behavior or level of consciousness and include the following:

Acute confusion
Bizarre behavior
Unexplained seizures
Coma
Trauma where drug use is suspected
Intended commitment for psychiatric evaluation

Drug tests are also indicated in cases of trauma when it is suspected that drugs are present as this has an impact on the care given. Patients who have attempted suicide or are being committed for psychiatric care for any reason should also be tested for the presence of drugs. Drug screening tests have become quite popular and are used frequently by employers, insurance companies, and the armed forces. In these cases, the patient is best referred to a clinic for testing.

Effects on Psychomotor Skills

Studies have found that marijuana degrades attention, short-term memory, tracking, and coordination. Driving simulation tests and on-road studies have detected adverse effects on lane position variability, emergency response, and performance of subsidiary tasks needed in driving. Marijuana decreases speeding and risk-taking behavior, in contrast to alcohol, which has been found to increase these behaviors.[50]

A study of 1023 trauma victims found that 34.7% had used marijuana, and their serum levels were 2 ng/ml or higher. Of these patients, 32.6% had positive blood alcohol levels, and three fourths of these had levels of 100 mg/dl or more. In addition, 16.5% had consumed both alcohol and marijuana, which is highly significant, as these drugs have been found to have a cumulative effect.[51]

PSYCHEDELIC DRUGS

Approximately 14% of adolescents have been found to use hallucinogens.[52–55] In 1980, approximately 21% of Americans aged 18 to 25 years had used such drugs at some point, but only 1.2% had used these drugs in the preceding 30 days.[7]

Many drugs, when used under certain conditions or in toxic doses, can induce hallucinations, delusions, paranoid ideation, and mood alteration. These drugs include anticholinergic agents, bromides, antimalarials, cocaine, and steroids. Thus, there is no sharp line that divides psychedelics from other classes of centrally acting drugs. Drugs that are generally included in the psychedelics are related to the indoleamines, the phenylethylamines, or the phenylisoprophylamines (Table 89–1). Phencyclidine (PCP), often used for its psychedelic effect, is an arylcyclohexylamine. The effects of PCP can be differentiated both pharmacologically and clinically from those of true psychedelic drugs.

Lysergic Acid Diethylamide

Lysergic acid diethylamide (LSD) is the most potent psychoactive drug known.[53, 55] Although it can be found in naturally occurring ergot and in the seeds of the morning glory plant, most LSD is synthetically made.

Pharmacology

LSD and related compounds act at multiple sites in the central nervous system from the cortex to the spinal cord, but the actual mechanism by which the subjective effects of the drug are produced are uncertain, although there seems to be some interaction with serotonin synapses.[53]

LSD is manufactured in the form of tiny cylindrical tablets called *microdots* or tiny gelatin squares called *windowpane*. It may be produced in the form of a liquid that is placed on thin paper, which is then chewed; these papers are called *blotters*. The drug is usually taken orally but can be absorbed from intramuscular injection sites as well as the nasal mucosa. It is rapidly absorbed through the gastrointestinal tract and

	Derivation	Average Dose	Popular Name
Drugs with an indole nucleus			
LSD	Ergot fungus	0.1 mg	Acid
Psilocybin	Psilocybe mushroom	10 mg	Mushrooms
DMT	Cohaba snuff, synthetic	50 mg (smoked)	
Drugs with a phenylethylamine nucleus			
Mescaline	Peyote cactus	400 mg	Mesc, buttons
DOM	Amphetamine derivative	5 mg	STP
MDA	Amphetamine derivative	100 mg	
Atypical hallucinogens			
PCP	Synthetic	5 mg	Angel dust
Ketamine	Synthetic	500 mg (intramuscularly)	Green
THC	Cannabis	30 mg	Pot, hash

TABLE 89–1

CLASSIFICATION OF THE MAJOR HALLUCINOGENIC DRUGS

DMT = N,N-dimethyltryptamine; DOM = dimethoxymethylamphetamine; LSD = lysergide; MDA = 3-4-methylenedioxyamphetamine; PCP = phencyclidine; THC = tetrahydrocannabinol.
From Cohen S. The hallucinogens and the inhalants. Psychiatr Clin North Am 1984;7:681.

diffuses to all tissues. A majority of the drug is metabolized within the liver, and conjugated products are excreted in the bile and in the feces.[54] LSD used in doses as small as 15 μg/70 kg can produce alterations in mood and perceptions but as much as 10,000 μg has been ingested without producing a fatality. At an average dose of 1 to 2 μg/kg onset of physical symptomatology is between 30 and 60 minutes, and psychological effects occur between 60 and 90 minutes of ingestion. These effects usually last 6 to 12 hours.[54, 55]

Clinical Evaluation

Most of the physical effects of LSD are sympathomimetic. These include pupillary dilatation, increased blood pressure and heart rate, hyperreflexia, tremors, muscular weakness, and increased body temperature. Subjective symptoms are weakness, dizziness, drowsiness, nausea, and paresthesias. The majority of symptoms relate to mood and perceptual changes, and it is precisely for these reasons that the drug has been popular. A number of moods may coexist, but euphoria tends to be predominant. The patient experiences visual illusions, distortion of sensory perception, and synesthesias. A blending or overflow of one sensory modality to another may occur. Auditory hallucinations are rare. Preceding and present perceptions blend together so that time sense becomes subjective, and time appears to pass extremely slowly. Colors are heard, and some sounds may be seen. There is a loss of boundaries so that the sense of self-image becomes blurred, and the patient may have a sense of "oneness with the universe" or a feeling of being lost.[55] Depending on the individual, the experience can be pleasurable or produce profound fear. Paranoid thought disturbances can occur in which the individual has megalomaniacal feelings of omnipotence or illusions of suspicion and persecution. Emotional response to the drug is varied, ranging from a feeling of bliss to an intense feeling of hopelessness or depression and fear. The former is called a chemical "transcendental state" or a "good trip," whereas the latter is called a "bummer" or "bad trip." Prior pleasurable experiences do not preclude a bad trip on subsequent usage of the drug.

Diagnostic Evaluation

Diagnosis is based on a history of recent ingestion in a patient with appropriate symptoms. At this time, laboratory analysis for LSD is only done in experimental laboratories. The drug has a low toxicity, and no deaths from overdose have been reported. Mortality and morbidity have been caused either by trauma incurred when users attempted unreasonable acts or by attempts to "escape" perceived dangers during a bad trip.

Unless other, more toxic drugs have been ingested with the LSD, there is no place for the use of lavage, ipecac, or activated charcoal, as LSD is totally absorbed within 2 hours of ingestion. If there is no other medical or traumatic condition, the patient should be placed in a quiet, nonthreatening environment with minimal stimuli. Psychological support by trained personnel or friends who are familiar with how to "talk down" the patient is the most valuable form of treatment. The patient needs continual orientation and reassurance that nothing bad is happening, that the perceptions and feelings are a result of the drug, and the effects are time limited. If this is not effective, diazepam can be used as a last resort. Normally the entire syndrome clears in 12 hours.

Chronic Effects

Tolerance to LSD develops after 3 or 4 days of daily usage, but sensitivity returns after a comparable drug-free interval.[52] Withdrawal does not occur. Adverse psychological reactions that are prolonged for days or months or that require hospitalization are referred to as *LSD psychosis*. It appears that those with poor premorbid psychological adjustment, greater exposure to psychedelic drugs, and a history of poly-drug abuse are at higher risk for these complications.

A recurrence of the drug's effects without use of the drug is called a *flashback*; the mechanism by which this occurs is not known. A flashback may occur in up to 15% to 77% of users. These episodes may be precipitated by any of a number of stimuli, including the use of other drugs or stress. At times there is no apparent precipitating event.

Phencyclidine

Phencyclidine (PCP) is a member of the arylcyclohexylamines. It is related to ketamine, which is still in use as an anesthetic agent. The drug was discarded after a number of undesirable side effects were discovered, including postoperative psychosis, muscular rigidity, hallucinations, and delusions.[56, 57] It is frequently misrepresented by sellers as tetrahydrocannabinol (THC), mescaline, peyote, psilocybin, LSD, cocaine, or other psychoactive drugs. Federal reporting of the sale of piperidine, which is necessary for the manufacture of PCP, became mandatory in 1978.

Patterns of Use

PCP can be found in the form of tablets, capsules, paper squares, powder, and joints. The drug may be smoked, ingested orally, and snorted but is rarely used intravenously. It is known by a number of street names, including angel dust, peace pills, horse tranquilizer, cadillac, crystal joints, and DOA. The drug is most frequently smoked in a manner similar to marijuana after it has been mixed with dried leaf material such as tobacco, parsley, or even marijuana itself. There is a considerable variation in concentration. Studies have shown that joints ranging in weight from 100 to 400 mg contained an average of 1 mg PCP per 150 mg of weight.[58, 59] When sold as a powder, purity ranged from 88% to 100%; the amount of actual PCP varied from 0.5 to 31 mg but usually fell in the range of 2 to 6 mg.[60] Half of those admitting to abuse use the drug once a week, but "runs" occur in which the drug is used for 2 to 3 consecutive days. During this time, the patient will eat and sleep very little. This is followed by prolonged sleep, after which there is depression and sometimes disorientation. The amount of PCP in joints varies from 1 to 100 mg, and chronic users may smoke up to 1 gm in 24 hours.[59] PCP appears to alter associative pathways in the brain, which interferes with the ability to process and react appropriately to sensory stimuli. PCP is believed to affect multiple neurotransmitter receptors in the brain. The noradrenergic, dopaminergic, cholinergic, and serotinergic systems, as well as opiate receptors and endorphins, are all thought to be involved, perhaps explaining the variable clinical picture after ingestion. The drug inhibits the reuptake of dopamine, serotonin, and norepinephrine by synoptosomes. Evidence indicates that there is a PCP receptor that may be related to the gamma opioid receptor, the binding site for *N*-allyl-normetazocine.[52, 53]

Absorption, Metabolism, and Excretion

The drug is well absorbed from all routes. Most of the parent compound is hydroxylated, and the metabolites are conjugated with glucuronic acid in the liver. Most of the pharmacologic effects are from PCP itself, although some of the metabolites are active. There is considerable enterohepatic recirculation of the drug, which has implications for treatment of ingestion. The effects of PCP are noted immediately if it is given parenterally and in 2 to 5 minutes when it is smoked. Onset of symptoms is slower after oral ingestion, taking up to 15 minutes for manifestation. The half-life of the drug in overdose cases is 3 days. PCP is a weak base, and lowering urinary pH below 5 hastens excretion. Decreases in plasma pH cause decreases in concentration of the drug in the cerebrospinal fluid, producing a decrease in signs of intoxication. Although the high may only last 4 to 6 hours, the user usually requires 24 to 48 hours to return to normal. This is thought to be secondary to some binding of the drug in the nervous system.

Clinical Presentation

Effects of the drug are seen in the neurologic, cardiovascular, renal, gastrointestinal, and behavioral systems. The features are dose dependent, with low doses being 5 to 10 mg; moderate doses, 10 to 20 mg; and high doses, greater than 20 mg.[61] Of all the drugs discussed in this chapter, PCP is by far the most dangerous, with more than 300 deaths attributed to the drug as a result of behavioral toxicity. There have also been a number of deaths attributed to the physical effects of the drug itself.[62, 63] Minimal doses of the drug cause a vestibulocerebellar syndrome characterized by the sensation of weightlessness, nystagmus, and muscular incoordination.[52] This can result in death caused by trauma, with the drug undetectable as a result of the small quantities ingested.

The physical effects of PCP are characteristic, with nystagmus and hypertension being hallmarks of the drug.[63] The nystagmus is irregular, with jerky eye movements in any direction. Blood pressure may go up to 160/105 mm Hg or higher. Stroke and cerebral hemorrhage have occurred after ingestion. Sinus tachycardia, tachypnea, and hyperthermia with body temperatures as high as 42.0°C (108.0°F) occur.[64] Respiratory and cardiac arrest are possible sequelae of high doses of PCP. Those exposed to high doses are seen in a comatose state. The eyes remain open, with nystagmus appearing at rest.[65, 66] The most characteristic feature of massive or high-dose ingestion is prolonged coma.[66] Muscular rigidity and immobility are commonly reported with low to moderate doses of the drug. Patients exhibit bizarre posturing, tremors, writhing, and jerking movements. Higher doses can induce tonic-clonic seizures and even status epilepticus. Hyperreflexia is also frequent. The autonomic nervous system is stimulated, with resultant diaphoresis, salivation, lacrimation, urinary retention, and bronchorrhea. Bronchospasm may be severe enough to compromise respiratory function. A transient anticholinergic effect is thought to be present, but this is mild, as anticholinergic effects are less severe than those seen with atropine. Pupillary responses vary. Death is caused by respiratory depression, status epilepticus, or cardiovascular collapse.[67] Ataxia and slurred speech are common. Sinus bradycardia, occasional arrhythmias, and hypotension have also been reported, making the physical response to the drug unpredictable.[84] A major problem seen with PCP is rhabdomyolysis.[68] The mechanism of this is thought to be secondary to excessive isometric motor activity, generalized hypertonicity, and, finally, muscular activity as a result of severe agitation. Grand mal seizures may also contribute to the problem. PCP itself is not directly toxic to muscle tissue, although myoglobinuria and acute renal failure have been reported. PCP can also cause nausea and vomiting. Crampy abdominal pain and hematemesis have been seen but are thought to be secondary to by-products produced during synthesis of the drug.

The sensory and psychological manifestations of the drug are varied and bizarre and can induce a state resembling schizophrenia.[69, 70] The effects at low doses include euphoria, a pleasurable "high," amnesia, anxiety, agitation, disordered thought processes, and hallucinations. There is some controversy as to whether true hallucinations occur. Some researchers have used the absence of hallucinations to distinguish the effects of this drug from those of LSD and mescaline.[58, 63]

PCP ingestion may mimic schizophrenia after the acute toxic effects have subsided.[52, 71–73] PCP psychosis resembles acute paranoid schizophrenia and cannot be distinguished from the functional disease state without drug testing. Depersonalization, distortions of body image, and altered perceptions involving all sensations are the effects most frequently reported by users. The passage of time is distorted. A feeling of superhuman strength and invulnerability is present. Immobility, numbness, and detachment are reported desired effects. Psychosis has been reported to last longer than 30 days and has required hospitalization.[74] Homicide and self-mutilation have also been reported.[75]

A report of six pediatric patients aged 5 years or younger who had ingested the drug documented bizarre behavior, ataxia, and nystagmus as the most frequent findings.[76] One infant had symptoms after passive ingestion of smoke. All patients recovered within 72 hours, with most showing marked improvement within 24 hours. In contrast to adults, hypertension, hyperreflexia, and increased muscle tone were not as common. A literature review of 10 cases of PCP ingestion in children under the age of 6 years found that lethargy occurred in 90%, ataxia in 75%, nystagmus in 50%, and opisthotonos in 40%.[76, 77]

Diagnostic Evaluation

The diagnosis may be suspected in any individual with bizarre behavior or altered mental status. Hypertension, nystagmus, muscle rigidity, and tachycardia are supportive evidence. The diagnosis is established when the drug is found in urine or gastric contents. Analysis of blood is unreliable, as serum concentrations may be unrecoverable several hours after ingestion. Qualitative drug tests are accurate and reliable, but quantitative measures of PCP levels are not clinically useful.

Therapeutic Intervention

Monitoring of vital signs is especially important with ingestion of this drug. Treatment is supportive and aimed at normalizing vital signs, should that become necessary. There is no specific antidote or treatment. Emesis and gastric lavage are only necessary if other drugs are thought to have been ingested, as the drug is usually not taken orally. Ventilatory assistance and protection of the airway may be necessary in cases of massive ingestion, as prolonged or delayed hypoventilation and apnea have been reported. Intubation may be difficult because of muscle rigidity. Nasal gastric suctioning and multiple doses of activated charcoal have been advocated to interrupt the enterohepatic pathway.[78] Small doses of diazepam followed by intravenous phenytoin are used as necessary to control seizures. If seizures continue in spite of treatment, neuromuscular agents should be considered. Although acidification of urine has been shown to enhance excretion, this is not used because of the possibility of decreased myoglobin excretion and the development of acute tubular necrosis.[78, 79] Hypertension, if severe, can be treated with nifedipine, nitroprusside, or labetalol.

Violent and combative patients may need sedation, as "talking the patient down" is not as effective as with other drugs and may indeed make the patient worse.[80] Haloperidol is the recommended agent for chemical sedation. Dosage of haloperidol is not completely established, and the drug is not recommended for patients younger than 3 years. The initial dose in patients older than 3 years is 0.01 to 0.03 mg/kg in two or three divided doses. The maintenance dose is 0.05 to 0.15 mg/kg/day in two or three divided doses; the maximum dose is 6 mg per day.[81]

Hemodialysis is ineffective in removing the drug from the body. All patients ingesting PCP should be tested for myoglobinuria. Psychotic patients should have psychiatric evaluation and treatment as necessary, and patients requiring hospitalization should be admitted to an intensive care unit so that their vital signs may be closely monitored.

Effects on the Fetus

PCP crosses the placenta and can be detected in the urine of neonates whose mothers have used the drug. In two cases of newborn infants with positive urine tests for the drug, the infants were tremulous and had hypertonicity, vomiting, and diarrhea. They were successfully treated with phenobarbital. The symptoms described were similar to those of narcotic withdrawal.[82] Neonatal manifestations of maternal PCP are controversial, as there have been no controlled studies on the effects of PCP or its propensity as a teratogenic drug. In addition, many of the women utilizing PCP are polydrug abusers.[83]

Psilocybin and Psilocin

Both psilocybin and psilocin belong to the class of indoleamines and are derived from several species of mushrooms. Native Americans have used these drugs for centuries in various ceremonies. Chemically, the drugs are related to LSD, but LSD is 100 to 200 times more potent than these drugs. Psilocybin is the phosphorylated ester of psilocin. After ingestion of psilocybin, the phosphoric acid is removed, producing psilocin. The actions of the drugs are similar to that of LSD, but the duration of action is only 2 to 4 hours. Usually one or two dried mushrooms are ingested, which gives the abuser 20 to 60 mg of the drug and produces the desired psychedelic experience. Common street terms for the drug include "magic Mexican mushroom" or "silly putty." Treatment is similar to that for LSD ingestion.

Mescaline and Peyote

Mescaline and peyote, which belong to the phenylethylamine group, are derived from the Mexican peyote cactus and were once used by the Aztecs in religious ceremonies. The peyote cactus, which grows in the southwestern United States and Mexico, has a small crown, which when dried forms a small hard disk, thereby giving mescaline the street name "button." The effects of mescaline are identical to those of LSD, but LSD is 4000 to 5000 times more potent.

Mescaline is usually ingested orally in doses of 300 to 500 mg, and effects appear approximately 1 to 2 hours after ingestion, peak at 5 to 6 hours, and last 8 to 12 hours. In addition to the psychedelic effects, the drug produces physical effects, including nausea, vomiting, mydriasis, nystagmus, ataxia, tremors, and hyperreflexia. Treatment is similar to that for patients ingesting LSD.

Synthetic Drugs

A number of synthetic drugs can produce psychedelic experiences. These are chemically related to LSD and peyote. They are occasionally seen in the emergency department

and should be treated on a symptomatic basis. Dimethoxymethylamphetamine (DOM) is 100 times more potent than mescaline and has a long duration of action (i.e., up to 3 days). It is rarely abused because of this long duration of action. Methylenedioxyamphetamine (MDA) is thought to produce positive feelings without the perceptual distortions of LSD. This may be dose related, as LSD produces similar feelings at low doses. MDA is three to four times more potent than mescaline, and treatment is similar to that for patients who have used LSD.

References

1. Smart R, Arif A. The extent of drug abuse in the world: Prevention of drug abuse in 36 countries. World Health Stat Q 1984;37.
2. Millman RB, Sbriglio R. Patterns of use and psychopathology in chronic marijuana abusers. Psychiatr Clin North Am 1986;9:533.
3. Fishburne PM, Abelson HI, Cisin I. National survey on drug abuse: Main findings 1979. DHHS publication no (ADM) 80–976. Washington, DC, Dept of Health and Human Sciences, 1980.
4. Committee to Study the Health Related Effects of Cannabis and Its Derivatives. Marijuana and health. Washington, DC, National Academy Press, 1982.
5. Marijuana and health: Ninth annual report to the United States Congress for the Secretary of Health and Human Services. DHHS publication no (ADM) 82–1216. Rockville, MD, National Institute for Drug Abuse, 1982.
6. A drug retrospective: 1962 to 1980. Rockville, MD, National Institute on Drug Abuse, 1980.
7. Johnston LD, Bachman JG, O'Malley PM. 1983 highlights: Drugs and the nation's high school students. Washington, DC, US Government Printing Office, 1984.
8. Vollner L, Bieniek D, Korte F. Review of analytical methods for identification and quantification of cannabis products. Regul Toxicol Pharmacol 1986;6:348.
9. Schwartz RH. Marijuana: A crude drug with a spectrum of underappreciated toxicity. Pediatrics 1984;73:455.
10. McGuigan MA. Toxicology of drug abuse. Emerg Med Clin North Am 1984;2:87.
11. Ohlsson A, Lindgren J, Wahlen A. Plasma delta-9-tetrahydrocannabinol concentrations and clinical effects after oral and intravenous administration and smoking. Clin Pharmacol Ther 1980;28:409.
12. Frytak S. Metabolic studies of delta-9-tetrahydrocannabinol in cancer patients. Cancer Treatment Rep 1984;68:1427.
13. Jones RT. Drug of abuse profile. Cannabis Clin Chemistry 1987;33(suppl 11):72B.
14. Nahas G. Current statistics of marijuana research. JAMA 1982;242:585.
15. Dewey WL. Cannabinoid pharmacology. Pharmacol Rev 1986;38:171.
16. Bloom AS, Hillard CJ. Cannabinoids neurotransmitter receptors and brain membranes in cannabis. *In* Harvey DJ (ed). Marijuana Proceeding, Oxford Symposium on Cannabis. 1985, pp 217–231.
17. Martin BR. Cellular effects of cannabinoids. Pharmacol Rev 1986;38:45.
18. Bloodworth RC. Medical problems associated with marijuana abuse. Psychiatr Med 1987;3:173.
19. Fehr KO. Addiction Research Center/World Health Organization. *In* Fehr KO, Kalant H (eds). Cannabis and Health Hazards. Proceedings of the ARF/WHO Scientific Meeting on Adverse Health and Behavioral Consequences of Cannabis Use. Toronto, Addiction Research Foundation, 1983.
20. National Academy of Science, Institute of Medicine. Marijuana and health: Report of a study by a committee of the Institute of Medicine. Washington, DC, National Academy Press, 1982.
21. Turner CE. Cannabis: The plant, its drugs and their effects. Aviation Space Environ Med 1983;54:363.
22. Goldfrank LR, Mellinck M. Marijuana. *In* Goldfrank LR (ed). Toxic Emergencies: A Clinical Approach to Problem Solving. 2nd ed. Norwalk, CT, Appleton-Century-Crofts, 1981.
23. Marijuana and health: Ninth annual report to the United States Congress from the Secretary of Health and Human Services. DHHS publication no (ADM) 82–1216. Rockville, MD, National Institute on Drug Abuse, 1982.
24. Johnston LD, Bachman JG, O'Malley PM. Highlights from student drug use in America, 1975–1981. DHHS publication no (ADM) 82–1208. Rockville, MD, National Institute on Drug Abuse, 1981.
25. Kulberg A. Substance abuse: Clinical identification and management. Pediatr Clin North Am 1986;33:325.
26. Khantzian EJ, McKenna GJ. Acute toxic and withdrawal reactions associated with drug use and abuse. Ann Intern Med 1979;90:361.
27. Nahas GG. Keep Off the Grass. New York, Pergamon, 1979.
28. O'Brien, Fehr K, Kalant H (eds). Cannabis and Health Hazards. Proceedings of an ARF/WHO Scientific Meeting on Adverse Health and Behavioral Consequences of Cannabis Use. Toronto, Addiction Research Foundation, 1983.

29. Carney MW, Bacelle L. Psychosis after cannabis use. Br Med J 1984;288:1047.
30. Negrete JC. What's happened to the cannabis debate? Br J Add 1988;83:359.
31. Kandel DB. Marijuana users in young adulthood. Arch Gen Psychiatry 1984;41:200.
32. O'Donnell JA, Clayton RR. Determinants of early marijuana use. *In* Bechner GM, Freidman AS (eds). Youth Drug Abuse. Lexington, MA, Lexington Books, 1979.
33. O'Donnell JA, Voss HL, Clayton RR, et al. Young men and drugs: A nationwide survey. NIDA research monograph no 5. DHEW publication no (ADM)76–311. Washington, DC, US Government Printing Office, 1976.
34. Weller RA, Halikas JA, Morse C. Alcohol and marijuana: Comparison of use and abuse in regular marijuana users. J Clin Psychiatry 1984;45:377.
35. Hannerz J, Hindmarsh T. Neurological and neuroradiological examination of chronic cannabis smokers. Ann Neurol 1983;13:207.
36. Co RT, Goodwin DN, Gado N. Absence of cerebral atrophy in chronic cannabis users. JAMA 1977;237:1229.
37. Campbell AM, Evans M, Thompson JL, et al. Cerebral atrophy in young cannabis smokers. Lancet 1971;2:1219.
38. McGahan JP, Dublin AB, Sassenrath E. Long term delta-9-tetrahydrocannabinol treatment: Computed tomography of the brains of rhesus monkeys. Am J Dis Child 1984;138:1109.
39. Maykut MO. Health consequences of acute and chronic marijuana use. Prog Neuropsychopharmacol Biol Psychiatry 1985;9:209.
40. Landrigan P, Powell K, James L. Paraquat and marijuana: Epidemiologic risk assessment. Am J Public Health 1983;73:784.
41. Hollister LE. Health aspects of cannabis. Pharmacol Rev 1986;38:10.
42. Kolodny RC, Masters WH, Kolodner RM. Depression of plasma testosterone levels after chronic intensive marijuana use. New Engl J Med 1974;290:872.
43. Smith CG, Smith MT, Cesch NF, Effect of delta-9-tetrahydrocannabinol (THC) on female reproductive function. *In* Nahas GG, Paton WD (eds). Marijuana: Biological Effect. New York, Pergamon, 1979.
44. Hingson R, Alpert J, Day N. Effects of maternal drinking and marijuana use on fetal growth and development. Pediatrics 1982;70:538.
45. Qazi QH, Mariano E, Beller E. Abnormalities of offspring associated with prenatal marijuana exposure. Pediatr Res 1983;17:153A.
46. Tennes K. Effects of marijuana on pregnancy and fetal development in the human. Natl Inst Drug Abuse Res Mono Rev 1984;44:115.
47. Hollister LE. Marijuana and immunity. J Psychoactive Drugs 1988;20:3.
48. Schwartz RH, Hawks RL. Laboratory detection of marijuana use. JAMA 1985;254:788.
49. Cone EJ, Johnson RE. Contact highs and using cannabinoid excretion after passive exposure to marijuana smoke. Clin Pharmacol Ther 1986;40:247.
50. Gieringer D. Marijuana, driving and accident safety. J Psychoactive Drugs 1988;20:93.
51. Soderstrom CA, Trifillis AL, Belavadi SS. Marijuana and alcohol use among 1023 trauma patients. Arch Surg Sruv 1988;123:733.
52. Goodman LS, Gilman A. The Pharmacological Basis of Therapeutics. New York, Macmillan, 1985, p 561.
53. Freedman DX. Mode of action of hallucinogenic drugs. *In* Van Praag HM (ed). Handbook of Biological Psychiatry. New York, Marcel Dekker, 1981.
54. Caldwell J, Sever PS. The biochemical pharmacology of abused drugs: Amphetamines, cocaine and LSD. Clin Pharmacol Ther 1974;16:625.
55. Brown RT, Braden NJ. Hallucinogens. Pediatr Clin North Am 1987;34:341.
56. Luby ED, Cohen BD, Rosenbaum G, et al. Study of a new schizophrenomimetic drug—Sernyl. Arch Neurol Psychiatry 1959;81:363.
57. Davies BM, Beech HR. The effect of 1-arylcyclo-helyl-amine (Sernal) on twelve normal volunteers. J Mental Sci 1960;106:912.
58. Showalter CV, Thornton WE. Clinical pharmacology of phencyclidine toxicity. Am J Psychiatry 1977;134:1234.
59. Lundberg GC, Gupta RC, Montgomery SH. Phencyclidine: Patterns seen in street drug analysis. Clin Toxicol 1976;9:503.
60. Brecher EM. Licit and Illicit Drugs: The Consumer Union Report on Narcotics, Stimulants, Depressants, Inhalants, Hallucinogens, and Marijuana—Including Caffeine, Nicotine and Alcohol. Boston, Little, Brown, 1972.
61. Sioris LJ, Krenzelok ED. Phencyclidine intoxication: A literature review. Am J Hosp Pharm 1978;35:1362.
62. PCP: Update on Abuse. Rockville, MD, National Institute on Drug Abuse, 1980.
63. Miller NS, Gold MS, Millman R. PCP: A dangerous drug. Am Fam Physician 1988;38:215.
64. Kline NS, Lindenmayer JP. Psychotropic Drugs: A Manual for Emergency Management of Overdosage. 2nd ed. Oradell, NJ, Medical Economics, 1981.
65. Liden CB, Lovejoy FH, Costello CE. Phencyclidine: Nine cases of poisoning. JAMA 1975;234:513.
66. Burns RS, Lerner SE. Perspectives: Acute phencyclidine intoxication, Clin Toxicol 1976;9:477.
67. Johnstone M, Evans V, Baigel S. Sernyl (C1–395) in clinical anaesthesia. Br J Anaesth 1959;31:433.
68. Done AK, Aronow R, Miceli JN. The pharmakinetics of phencyclidine in overdose and its treatment. *In* Petersen RC, Stillman RC (eds). Phencyclidine (PCP) Abuse: An Appraisal. Rockville, MD, National Institute on Drug Abuse, 1978, p 210.
69. Fauman B, Aloinger G, Fauman M, et al. Psychiatric sequelae of phencylidine abuse. Clin Toxicol 1976;9:529.
70. McGuigan M. Toxicology of drug abuse. Emerg Clin North Am 1984;2:87.
71. Rainey JM, Crowder MK. Prolonged psychosis attributed to phencyclidine: Report of three cases. Am J Psychiatry 1975;132:1076.
72. Ban TA, Lohrenz JJ, Lehmann HE. Observations on the actions of Sernyl—a new psychotropic drug. Can Psychiatr Assoc J 1961;6:150.
73. Cohen BD, Rosenbaum G, Luby ED, et al. Comparison of phencyclidine hydrochloride (Sernyl) with other drugs. Stimulation of schizophrenic performance with phencyclidine hydrochloride (Sernyl), lysergic acid diethylamide (LSD-25), and amobarbital (Amytal) sodium: II. Symbolic and sequential thinking. Arch Gen Psychiatry 1962;6:395.
74. Allen M, Young J. Phencyclidine induced psychosis. Am J Psychiatry 1978;153:1081.
75. Fauman MA, Fauman BJ. Violence associated with phencyclidine abuse. Am J Psychiatry 1979;136:1584.
76. Welch MJ, Correa GA. PCP intoxication in young children and infants. Clin Pediatr 1980;19:510.
77. Linden CB, Lovejoy FH, Costello CE. Phencyclidine (Sernylon) poisoning. J Pediatr 1973;83:844.
78. Aronow R, Miceli J, Done A. A therapeutic approach to the acutely overdosed PCP patient. J Psychedelic Drugs 1980;12:259.
79. Hartness C, Buchan J, Bayer M. Phencyclidine. Top Emerg Med 1985;7:33.
80. Stein J. Phencyclidine induced psychosis: The need to avoid unnecessary influx. Milit Med 1973;138:590.
81. Fleisher G, Ludwig S. Textbook of Pediatric Emergency Medicine. 2nd ed. Baltimore, Williams & Wilkins, 1988.
82. Strauss A, Modanlou A. Neonatal manifestations of maternal phencyclidine abuse. Pediatrics 1981;68:550.
83. Smith C, Osch R. Drug abuse and reproduction. Fertil Steril 1987;48:355.

CHAPTER 90

Hydrocarbons and Inhalants

Maureen C. Prendergast

INTRODUCTION

Hydrocarbon compounds can be found in any home in a wide variety of cleaning agents, paints and varnishes, solvents, adhesives, fuels, lubricants, hobby and craft materials, cosmetics, and pesticides. Accidental hydrocarbon ingestion accounts for 5% to 7% of pediatric poisonings in children younger than 5 years.

"Sniffing" or "huffing" volatile hydrocarbons is popular among preteens and adolescents as a readily available, legal, and inexpensive means of intoxication. Systemic toxicity and sudden death are seen with this form of hydrocarbon ingestion more often than the predominantly pulmonary injury seen with oral ingestion. There are also reports of intravenous hydrocarbon abuse and toxicity from dermal exposure when diesel fuel is used as shampoo.

Hydrocarbons are organic compounds derived from crude oil, coal, or plant sources. Petroleum distillates are a subset of hydrocarbons, though the terms are used interchangeably, albeit incorrectly, in the medical literature. There are three major classes of hydrocarbons: aliphatic, or open-chain com-

---

TABLE 90–1

HYDROCARBON CLASSES

Aliphatic (open-chain) compounds:
   Petroleum ether or benzene
   Gasoline
   Naphtha
   Mineral seal oil, mineral spirits
   Kerosene
   Fuel oil
   Lubricating oils
   Paraffin wax
   Asphalt, tar
Cyclic (closed-chain) compounds:
   Alicyclic compounds: Three or more carbon rings; act more
   like aliphatic compounds than the more toxic aromatic
   compounds:
      Naphthenes
      Cyclohexane
      Cyclopentene
      Cyclopentadiene
   Aromatic compounds: Unsaturated hexagonal rings:
      Benzene
      Toluene
      Xylene
   Cyclic terpenes:
      Turpentine
      Pine oil
Halogenated hydrocarbons:
   Trichloroethane
   Trichloroethylene
   Tetrachloroethylene
   Carbon tetrachloride
   Methylene chloride

---

pounds; cyclic, or closed-chain compounds; and halogenated compounds (Table 90–1).

In general, hydrocarbons with the lowest viscosity and surface tension carry the greatest risk for aspiration following ingestion. Those with the greatest volatility carry the greatest risk for asphyxia. Terpenes, in addition to causing aspiration, may also produce a mild central nervous system (CNS) depression. Aromatics have a high potential for CNS depression and mild cardiac irritability and only a small risk of aspiration. The halogenated hydrocarbons carry a high risk for cardiac arrhythmias and produce CNS euphoria, but have only a small risk of aspiration. The toxic potential of each hydrocarbon compound varies tremendously with the unique properties of its class, the concentration in the product consumed, the total amount of ingestant involved, the route of exposure, and any other chemicals (organophosphates) that may be present in the same product (Table 90–2).

HYDROCARBON INGESTION

The National Data Collection System of the American Association of Poison Control Centers cited 11,000 reports

---

TABLE 90–2

TOXIC ADDITIVES

C =	Camphor
H =	Halogenated hydrocarbons
A =	Aromatics
M =	Metals
P =	Pesticides

---

of hydrocarbon ingestion, 95% of which were accidental, and only two of which were fatalities. Furniture polishes, gasoline, and lighter fluid accounted for the majority of cases of accidental ingestion in one study, representing 69% of ingested substances.

Pathophysiology

The most significant cause of morbidity and mortality in oral ingestion of hydrocarbons is chemical pneumonitis resulting from pulmonary aspiration. Early studies reported pulmonary complication as high as 25% to 68%, but a later study reported that only 12% of 950 children developed clinical or radiographic evidence of pneumonitis.

Once aspiration has occurred, an immediate chemical inflammatory response is initiated. Hydrocarbons solubilize surfactant, which produces alveolar collapse, ventilation-perfusion mismatch, and production of hyaline membranes. An initial acute alveolitis in the first 3 to 10 days leads to a chronic proliferative process in children who survive. The necrotizing pneumonia induced by hydrocarbons is predominantly nonbacterial. Severe hemorrhagic pulmonary edema with hepatization of the lungs is generally the cause of death. Pneumatoceles have been reported as a late complication. Pneumatoceles usually are not associated with impairment of respiratory function and generally resolve in 1 to 3 months.

Viscosity is measured as the speed at which a substance moves across a calibrated orifice in Saybolt Seconds Universal (SSU). The risk of aspiration is inversely proportional to the viscosity of the compound. In other words, low-viscosity hydrocarbons more easily "creep" from the pharynx and esophagus into the tracheobronchial tree. High-viscosity compounds (>100 SSU) are generally considered to pose minimal to no risk of aspiration (Table 90–3), whereas low-viscosity substances (<60 SSU) present a significant hazard of aspiration. Those compounds at less than 35 SSU pose the greatest risk for severe aspiration at even small volumes.

Once a hydrocarbon is ingested without concurrent aspiration, it poses minimal risk by resecretion from the blood stream into the lungs. However, a 10-kg child need aspirate only 2.5 ml of kerosene to produce fatal pneumonitis.

Systemic absorption contributes little to the CNS depres-

TABLE 90–3

TOXICITY BASED ON VISCOSITY

Nontoxic (>100 SSU): Low risk of aspiration; no systemic
   toxicity
   Asphalt, tar
   Lubricants (motor oil, transmission oil)
   Mineral oil, baby oil, suntan oil
Moderately toxic (<60 SSU): High risk of aspiration; systemic
   toxicity only in massive ingestions; gastric removal only if large
   volume ingested:
   Gasoline
   Kerosene
   Charcoal lighter fluid
   Petroleum ether (benzene)
   Turpentine
   Mineral spirits
   Toluene
   Xylene
Highly toxic (<35 SSU): Highest risk of aspiration; no systemic
   toxicity; never attempt gastric removal:
   Mineral seal oil
   Signal oil
   Oil furniture polish

sion associated with hydrocarbons toxicity. CNS toxicity in kerosene poisoning results from hypoxia secondary to aspiration pneumonia. This could be enhanced by the volatility of kerosene at body temperature, causing toxicity through inhalation and asphyxia by vapors. No CNS depression occurs in the absence of pulmonary complications with aliphatic hydrocarbons; however, aromatic hydrocarbons can cause CNS excitation, delirium, and coma, without hypoxia.

Generally all hydrocarbons cause some degree of nausea, vomiting, and diarrhea as a result of direct mucosal irritation, which may contribute to aspiration. Usually this does not require treatment.

Cardiac, renal, hepatic, metabolic, and hematologic toxicities are generally limited to the toxic hydrocarbons and to inhalation poisoning. However, there have been a few case reports of systemic toxicity produced by massive ingestion of gasoline and refined petrol, presumably overwhelming the high first-pass detoxification in the liver.

Volatile aliphatic hydrocarbons—methane, propane, and butane—exist solely in gaseous form at room temperature and normal atmospheric pressure. They are also the most flammable. These gases act as simple asphyxiants by displacing alveolar oxygen, thus causing hypoxia. They produce no direct toxic effects on the lung. This class of hydrocarbons is also readily absorbed through the capillary network of the lungs, thereby causing CNS depression.

Gasoline and naphtha fuels are also highly volatile and may cause CNS depression by inhalation of the fumes, without producing any signs of pulmonary toxicity. In the United States, gasoline contains up to 2% benzene, an amount that is usually inconsequential in the average accidental pediatric ingestion (which rarely exceeds a swallow) and does not warrant removal from the stomach.

Mineral spirits, kerosene, and mineral seal oil have very low volatility, which makes it easier for a child to swallow larger amounts. These compounds are responsible for a high percentage of cases of hydrocarbon aspiration. There is virtually no gastrointestinal absorption seen with ingestion of this class of compounds. Light gas oil, used in diesel fuel, has the same properties but may also contain up to 35% aromatic hydrocarbons, which can produce systemic toxicity.

Turpentine and pine oil are readily absorbed from the gastrointestinal tract and can cause CNS intoxication. Turpentine has a low viscosity similar to that of kerosene and does cause aspiration pneumonitis. It also causes some renal toxicity with proteinuria and hematuria, but only transiently.

Camphor is a cyclic ketone widely used topically as an antipruritic-analgesic in over-the-counter medications (e.g., camphorated oil [20%], Campho-Phenique [10%], and Vicks Vaporub [4.8%]). Camphor oil can be interchanged accidentally with castor oil and fed to children by the spoonful by well-meaning parents. Camphor poisoning is more common in children younger than 6 years of age, comprising 6% of accidental poisonings. Camphor is rapidly absorbed and causes severe CNS toxicity, with seizures and coma occurring in 20% to 42% of cases. Onset of symptoms occurs in as little as 5 minutes. The human lethal dose is 50 to 500 mg/kg, which can be as little as 1 teaspoon of camphor oil in a toddler.

Toxic metabolites may enhance systemic toxicity of the parent hydrocarbon. This is true for methylene chloride, found in paint stripping agents, and carbon tetrachloride, a common dry-cleaning solvent; both produce carbon monoxide when metabolized by liver enzymes. Aniline dyes and nitrobenzene produce methemoglobin when metabolized. The specific chemical properties of the individual hydrocarbon ingested must be ascertained in order to effectively manage the patient.

Clinical Evaluation

The vast majority of children (65% to 88%) who have ingested hydrocarbons are asymptomatic on presentation to the emergency department. Patients who develop aspiration pneumonitis will most likely have respiratory or CNS symptoms almost immediately after ingestion. Children who develop pneumonitis are symptomatic within 10 minutes of ingestion in 88% of cases. Manifestations of pulmonary complications may range from mild cough, wheezing, grunting, and tachypnea to severe respiratory distress, cyanosis, intercostal retractions, hemoptysis, and pulmonary edema. Any child with initial choking, coughing, or vomiting at the time of ingestion should be considered to have aspirated until proven otherwise, even if he or she appears asymptomatic in the emergency department.

The predominant CNS manifestation following nontoxic hydrocarbon ingestion is a decreased level of consciousness, seen in approximately 4% of ingestions; it is always associated with respiratory complications and hypoxia. In toxic hydrocarbon poisonings, CNS excitation, intoxication, seizures, and hyper-reflexia usually precede obtundation and coma. Persistent altered mental status in spite of adequate oxygenation suggests a toxic ingestion.

Tachycardia is a common finding and usually correlates with the degree of respiratory distress. Dysrhythmias can occur with hypoxia but may also result from myocardial sensitization by aromatic or halogenated hydrocarbons. Severe aspiration may also progress to shock and cardiorespiratory arrest. Disseminated intravascular coagulation and hemolysis may complicate a massive or toxic ingestion. Approximately 30% of patients develop fever and a mild leukocytosis within 1 hour of aspiration as a result of an inflammatory response.

Hydrocarbons act as an irritant to mucous membranes and produce an intense burning sensation in the mouth, throat, and eyes. Vomiting occurs in approximately 43% of patients, and diarrhea usually continues until the petroleum distillate has cleared the gastrointestinal tract.

Topical exposure to the eyes causes chemical conjunctivitis, which may produce severe dessication and burns of the cornea. Skin contamination can range from mild burning, erythema, and a contact dermatitis to frank second-degree burns. Fatal systemic absorption from topical exposure has occurred, and immediate decontamination of the skin and clothing should be part of initial management to prevent further absorption or inhalation.

Diagnostic Evaluation

Radiography

The most common radiographic finding in hydrocarbon pneumonitis is an increase in bronchovascular markings, which usually precedes the development of an infiltrate. Infiltrates are usually patchy and multilobar and predominantly basilar or perihilar in location. The least common area of involvement is the upper lobes. Lobar consolidations are rarely seen. Segmental atelectasis and evidence of air trapping are commonly seen, progressing to pneumothorax and pneumomediastinum only in the most severe cases.

In cases of severe aspiration, there is a progression of radiographic findings over 5 to 15 days, occasionally with the development of pneumatoceles, which usually resolve over several months.

An upright chest and abdominal radiograph may also be useful in the child who has ingested an unknown amount of hydrocarbons, as a double gastric bubble can sometimes be demonstrated. In addition, chlorinated hydrocarbons are radio-opaque and may give at least a visual estimate of the volume of hydrocarbon in the gastrointestinal tract.

Early chest radiograph findings correlate poorly with the clinical course of hydrocarbon ingestions and do not predict severity or outcome. Approximately 90% of patients who are symptomatic on presentation to the emergency department have an abnormal chest radiograph initially. Of patients who actually develop radiographic evidence of pneumonitis, approximately 88% have an abnormal chest radiograph at 2 hours, and 98% have an abnormal radiograph at 12 hours (Fig 90–1).

The most consistent finding associated with severe clinical deterioration was a rapid evolution of the radiographic abnormalities over repeated examinations. Overall, symptoms and physical findings in the first 6 hours are far more predictive of morbidity than later findings and should determine triage and management strategy. Repeated chest radiographs are unnecessary in the patient who remains asymptomatic over a 6-hour observation period.

Laboratory Studies

Laboratory studies, other than initial pulse oximetry, are not routinely necessary and should be mandated by the individual clinical picture and the type of hydrocarbon involved. Toxic hydrocarbons require extensive blood testing, including a complete blood cell count and measurement

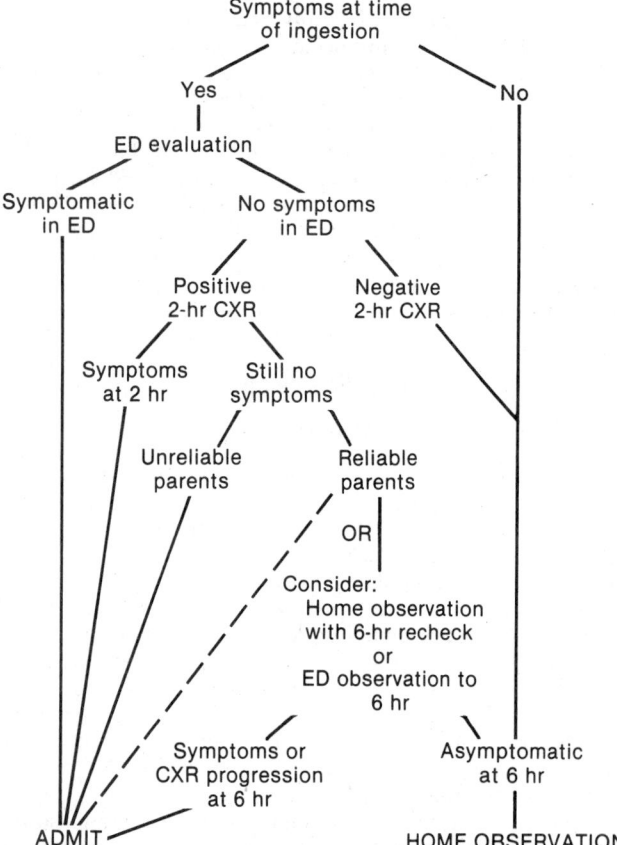

DISPOSITION

Protocol for Ingestion of Hydrocarbons

Figure 90–1. Emergency department evaluation for determining disposition with hydrocarbon ingestion.

of hepatic transaminases, coagulation profile, blood urea nitrogen (BUN), creatinine, and electrolytes. Baseline arterial blood gas determinations are not required in children who have no respiratory distress and normal results on pulse oximetry.

Emergency Medical Service Considerations

The patient should be moved to a safe environment if fume exposure persists or there is a risk of fire or explosion. Noxious fumes may cause asphyxia and toxicity to rescue personnel as well as the patient.

Oxygen and respiratory support should be provided for symptomatic patients. Agitating the young child with unnecessary procedures should be avoided to prevent vomiting from crying.

Decontamination of the skin and removal of contaminated clothing avoid continued dermal absorption. More adhesive substances can be removed with petrolatum or polyoxyethylene sorbitan (found in bacitracin-neomycin-polymyxin B [Neosporin] cream and polysorbate 80 [Tween 80]) or with Medi-Sol, which contains 70% base oil. All have been found effective in removing even tar and asphalt. After softening and removal, the area should be washed with soap and water and irrigated.

Milk, olive oil, and mineral oil have previously been recommended to increase the viscosity of the ingested hydrocarbons and to reduce the risk of aspiration. These measures are not currently recommended, as they may delay gastric emptying and promote vomiting. Prehospital induction of vomiting with syrup of ipecac should only be performed if instructed by medical control for significant ingestion of a known toxic hydrocarbon and with Advanced Cardiac Life Support (ACLS) intervention available. This should never be recommended for parents to attempt at home.

Completely asymptomatic children with nontoxic ingestions may be observed at home as long as adequate supervision can be ensured and specific instructions are given to return to the emergency department if any symptoms develop. Children with initial choking or vomiting should be observed in the emergency department even if symptoms have resolved after the first few minutes, as aspiration is likely to have already occurred.

Therapeutic Intervention

Asymptomatic children with nontoxic hydrocarbon ingestion may be observed at home by reliable parents. If reliable care cannot be ensured, the child should be observed in the emergency department for 6 hours after ingestion. The child who is still asymptomatic after that time may be safely discharged. All children who are symptomatic on emergency department presentation should be admitted for observation (see Fig. 90–1). If the parents are reliable, the asymptomatic child can be observed at home, with a re-examination performed at the emergency department or at the family doctor's office in 6 hours (Table 90–4).

Airway Management

Oxygen should be administered in hypoxic patients, and endotracheal intubation and artificial ventilation may be required in the compromised patient. Continuous positive airway pressure (CPAP) or positive end-expiratory pressure (PEEP) may be helpful in patients with pulmonary edema and high FIO_2 requirements. Intravenous hydration with crystalloid solutions should be performed and carefully

TABLE 90–4

**DISCHARGE INSTRUCTIONS FOLLOWING
HYDROCARBON INGESTION**

1. General: Return to the emergency department immediately if the child develops any of the following:
   Frequent cough
   Wheezing
   Difficulty breathing
   Lethargy
   Repeated vomiting
2. If the patient is discharged following an abnormal 2-hour chest radiograph, return for recheck in 6 hours.
3. If 2-hour chest radiograph is normal, recheck in 12 to 24 hours in office.

balanced to avoid fluid overload and exacerbation of pulmonary edema.

Gastric Emptying

Indications for gastric evacuation remain controversial. The physician should remove any amount of petroleum distillates containing toxic additives and any amount of halogenated aromatic or aliphatic hydrocarbon because of their inherent systemic toxic effects on the central nervous, cardiac, renal, hepatic, and hematopoietic systems (see Table 90–2). Other hydrocarbons, including kerosene and gasoline, demonstrate systemic toxicity only when large volumes are ingested, as in a suicide attempt (see Table 90–3). A "large volume" has been defined in some texts as greater than 2 ml/kg. However, several studies have demonstrated that as much as 20 ml/kg of kerosene can be safely ingested without signs of systemic toxicity. This information suggests that this class of hydrocarbons need not be removed, regardless of the volume ingested. There have been three case reports of severe systemic toxicity with large ingestions of gasoline (>100 ml). All of these patients were immediately symptomatic and critically ill on arrival at the emergency department. The clinical condition of the child on presentation should affect the decision regarding gastric evacuation of this class of hydrocarbon. Substances that do not produce systemic toxicity but carry a high risk of severe aspiration pneumonia should not be removed from the stomach, regardless of the amount ingested (see Table 90–3). Substances that are generally considered nontoxic, and even with frank aspiration cause at most a low-grade pneumonitis, need not be removed (see Table 90–3).

Once it has been determined that gastric evacuation should be performed, syrup of ipecac can be given. The incidence of pneumonitis was found to be 56% with lavage, but only 28% with induced emesis. Contraindications to the use of syrup of ipecac include unprovoked emesis, depressed mental status, seizures, or coma. Syrup of ipecac is also contraindicated for the ingestion of camphor, as the onset of seizures and coma may be so abrupt that obtundation may occur before the emesis is completed, thus compromising the airway. With any significant alteration of mental status, endotracheal intubation should precede nasogastric evacuation and lavage. Orogastric lavage is the method of choice if a concomitant poisoning has occurred with large particles or pill fragments.

Activated Charcoal and Cathartics

Activated charcoal absorbs benzene, kerosene, and turpentine in vitro and in animal models. However, charcoal is recommended only for benzene ingestion or for co-ingestions of toxic substances.

Saline cathartics such as sodium sulfate increase absorption of solvents to charcoal but are only recommended in conjunction with charcoal. Oil cathartics are not recommended. An increased incidence of pneumonitis was found in patients to whom mineral or olive oil was administered, compared with those not given oil (72% vs. 45%). In addition, oil cathartics may increase systemic absorption of hydrocarbons. Increased blood levels of solvents were found in rats treated with liquid paraffin as an oil cathartic.

Corticosteroids

Chemical pneumonitis secondary to hydrocarbon aspiration is caused by a profound inflammatory response. Clinical reports prior to 1964 attested to the value of corticosteroids in this setting, but later studies have failed to demonstrate a therapeutic benefit. Therefore, corticosteroids are not routinely recommended in the treatment of hydrocarbon ingestions. An exception to this is discretionary use if shock lung develops.

Additional Considerations

Methemoglobinemia should be considered if cyanosis is refractory to oxygen therapy; this occurs with hydrocarbons containing nitrobenzene or aniline dyes. Hyperbaric oxygen may be required in patients who have ingested methylchloride or carbon tetrachloride, which are metabolized to carbon monoxide. Lead levels should be measured in children ingesting gasoline.

Prognosis

There are few data available on long-term prognosis for children who survive hydrocarbon aspiration pneumonitis. A 1978 study found the majority of such children to be asymptomatic and to have normal chest radiographs 8 to 14 years later, although 75% had minor pulmonary function test abnormalities suggestive of small airway disease. Residual renal, hepatic, neurologic, and hematologic abnormalities may persist chronically in toxic poisonings or following solvent inhalation.

HYDROCARBON INHALATION

The more volatile inhalants exert their toxic effects through inhalation of psychoactive vapors released at room temperature, producing an inebriated state similar to that seen with alcohol intoxication. Although accidental exposures occur in the home or the industrial setting, the majority of cases involve the deliberate abuse of solvents by adolescents to achieve a state of euphoria. One study reported that 7% to 12% of high school students in the United States sniff glue, and 4% are habitual abusers. Substances abused by inhalation include the aromatic and halogenated hydrocarbons, alcohols, esters, ketones, volatile alkyl nitrites, anesthetic agents, and propellants. Solvents abused by adolescents include model glue, acrylic spray paints, paint thinner, nail polish remover, gasoline and other fuels, and many aerosol propellants such as hair spray, room deodorizers, insecticides, and deodorants. Most habitual abusers prefer toluene-based solvents for the higher degree of euphoria they produce. This is especially true of gold acrylic spray paint, which has been found to produce unique psychoactive effects not found with other colors of paint. Typewriter correction fluid (White-Out) is one of the most popular substances of abuse among adolescents.

Habitual hydrocarbon inhalation may lead to continued solvent abuse, often into adulthood. Intensive psychotherapy and family counseling is warranted whenever a child is found to be a solvent abuser.

There are three principal methods of abuse: sniffing, bagging, and huffing. Sniffing is simply inhaling the solvent directly from its container. Bagging is pouring the substance into a plastic bag, shaking it to vaporize the solvent, and then placing the bag over the mouth and nose and inhaling deeply. This is the most dangerous method of inhalation; many "baggers" have suffocated as a result of the bag adhering to the face when consciousness is lost or vomiting and aspiration occur. However, it is also the preferred method of abuse, as the highest concentrations of vapor may be achieved in this manner.

Huffing is placing a cloth soaked with solvent over the mouth and nose and inhaling the vapor from it. To counter the rising epidemic of solvent abuse, many manufacturers add oil of mustard (allyl isocyanate), a potent mucosal irritant, to deter abusers.

Mortality is rising in parallel with the increasing incidence of abuse. One British report listed 282 inhalation deaths between 1971 and 1983, rising to 385 between 1981 and 1985. Of these deaths, 51% were caused by direct toxic effects (presumably cardiac arrhythmias), 21% by plastic bag asphyxia, 18% by aspiration, and 10% by trauma, including autoerotic strangulation.

Physiology

Volatile hydrocarbons possess a high vapor pressure and lipid solubility and are rapidly absorbed into the blood stream across the alveolar-capillary membrane. The substances are then distributed to adipose tissues, where a drug reservoir may accumulate. The immediate pulmonary absorption bypasses the first-pass detoxification process by the liver, resulting in heightened CNS effects not seen with oral ingestions. Excretion is predominantly through the lungs, with a smaller amount excreted through the liver and kidneys.

Clinical Evaluation

Abusers present to the emergency department in some degree of intoxication ranging from mild euphoria to frank psychosis. They may have gold paint or white typewriter correction fluid around the mouth and nose or smell of chemical solvents. Some patients may also develop a perioral erythematous "glue-sniffer's rash."

Central Nervous System

Because of the rapid uptake of solvents by the lungs, the onset of intoxication is immediate but short in duration, usually lasting 30 minutes to 3 hours, depending on the substances involved and dose absorbed. For example, a toluene exposure at 12,000 ppm for 5 minutes will clear in 10 minutes, whereas the same exposure to acetone may require as much as 9 hours to clear. The earliest manifestations are those of central nervous system excitation comparable to that seen in ethanol intoxication (i.e., euphoria, restlessness, poor coordination, and ataxia). Some psychomimetic features have been reported with gasoline, lighter fluid, and toluene inhalation, producing both visual and auditory hallucinations. Central nervous system depression follows shortly, with continued inhalation marked by confusion, stupor, disorientation, blurred vision, tinnitus, and headache, progressing to coma, respiratory depression, and death. General anesthesia can be induced in humans with toluene after 1 minute of steady inhalation in high concentrations such as those obtained with bagging. Hypoxia and hypercarbia from rebreathing in a plastic bag will enhance the CNS depressive effect at lower concentrations of vapor. Cerebral infarction with hemiplegia has been reported as an acute complication of glue sniffing and with trichlorethylene secondary to cerebral vasospasm.

Cardiovascular System

Fatal cardiac arrhythmias were first reported in 1966 as causing "sudden sniffing death" with inhalation of solvents. The fluorinated hydrocarbons have been implicated most frequently, but sudden death has also been reported with inhalation of gasoline, cyclopropane, bromochromofluoromethane (yellow fire extinguishers), and toluene. Of the fluorinated hydrocarbons, trichloroethane (TCE), found in typewriter correction fluid, is the most notorious for precipitating fatal arrhythmias. It was previously thought that ventricular fibrillation was induced by hypoxia, but autopsy studies have in many cases revealed no evidence of suffocation or aspiration. It seems apparent that the solvent sensitizes myocardium to endogenous epinephrine. Typically, the sniffer suddenly acts startled, jumps up, and runs around for a moment before collapsing in ventricular fibrillation. This theory is supported by evidence of similar sudden death syndrome in asthmatic patients who use metered-dose inhalers excessively; these inhalers contain fluoroalkane propellants with isoproterenol or epinephrine. In one study in which dogs were exposed to fluorinated aerosol propellants followed by epinephrine, cardiac arrhythmias resulted, even though Po_2 and Pco_2 were in the normal range. This suggests a direct myocardial toxicity. Even when the propellant was stopped and normal ventilation resumed as soon as sinus slowing occurred, a fatal arrhythmia always followed. This suggests that a sniffer cannot depend on subjective warning sensations to stop "in time." Other studies suggest that a more complex mechanism involving direct myocardial toxicity as well as sensitization of the myocardium to epinephrine is responsible for sudden sniffing death.

Acute anterior wall myocardial infarction and ventricular fibrillation have been reported secondary to coronary vasospasm in a 16-year-old male who sniffed toluene. "Gluesniffer's heart," a dilated cardiomyopathy, may also occur in more chronic abusers.

Diagnostic Evaluation

Because most of the solvents abused contain toluene, blood chemistry analysis, including a complete blood cell count and measurement of serum electrolytes, calcium, magnesium, phosphate, glucose, BUN, and creatinine and arterial blood gases, should be performed (Table 90–5). If the substance cannot be identified or a chlorinated hydrocarbon or benzene is suspected, liver function tests should be included. Urinalysis should also be done to evaluate nephrotoxicity. Because toxicology screens do not routinely test for solvents, the laboratory analysis must be directed for hydrocarbons. Urine is more useful to analyze than blood, as the solvent rapidly diffuses out of the blood into fatty tissues and may not be recovered in detectable amounts. The blood alcohol level should also be determined, as most cases of abuse involve more than one substance. Determination of carbon monoxide, methemoglobin, and methanol levels may be necessary if methylene chloride, carbon tetrachloride, organonitrites, or alcohol additives are suspected. Lead levels should be measured in gasoline sniffers who have persistent neurologic abnormalities.

TABLE 90-5

DIAGNOSTIC EVALUATION OF SOLVENT ABUSE

1. Complete blood cell count
2. Urinalysis
3. Determination of electrolyte and glucose levels
4. Arterial blood gas measurement
5. Determination of BUN and creatinine levels
6. Measurement of calcium, magnesium, and phosphorous levels, if acidosis is present
7. Liver function tests if a chlorinated hydrocarbon, benzene, or anesthetic was ingested
8. Urine toxicology screen (if substance unknown or for legal purposes)
9. Determination of serum ethanol level
10. Consider a CT scan if there is persistent neurologic abnormality
11. Electrocardiogram
12. If indicated, determination of the following:
    Carboxyhemoglobin level
    Methemoglobin level
    Lead level
    Methanol level

TABLE 90-6

EMERGENCY DEPARTMENT MANAGEMENT OF SOLVENT INHALATION ABUSE

If the patient is intoxicated but alert, the following are needed:
1. Removal of offending solvent and any contaminated clothing
2. Oxygen, pulse oximetry
3. Intravenous 0.9% normal saline
4. Cardiac monitoring
5. Laboratory evaluation, including arterial blood gas measurements
6. Observation
7. Psychiatric evaluation

If the patient is obtunded or comatose, the following are also needed:
8. Intubation, oxygen
9. Thiamine, glucose
10. Naloxone
11. Fluid resuscitation
12. Intravenous bicarbonate if pH < 7.2
13. Electrolyte replacement as indicated
14. Consider nasogastric lavage and charcoal if abuse of other drugs is suspected
15. ICU admission

Therapeutic Intervention

Treatment for inhalation solvent toxicity is symptomatic (Table 90–6). Most patients recover rapidly from their intoxication with simple removal of the solvent source and administration of oxygen. Airway support and mechanical ventilation may be needed in the patient who remains obtunded. Cardiac monitoring should be instituted. Glucose, thiamine, and naloxone should be given in the comatose patient. Fluid resuscitation and electrolyte replacement are needed for the patient presenting with weakness and dehydration caused by renal tubular acidosis. Epinephrine and other catecholamines should be avoided to prevent cardiac arrhythmias.

The metabolic acidosis and electrolyte derangement seen when renal tubular acidosis complicates toluene abuse may be life threatening. Parenteral fluids, phosphorous, and potassium replacement should be aggressive. Both hyperchloremic non–anion gap metabolic acidosis with bicarbonate wasting and an elevated anion gap form have been reported. If serum bicarbonate is less than 10 mEq/L with a pH less than 7.2, intravenous bicarbonate should be given to restore the bicarbonate level to 10 to 12 mEq/L. If the bicarbonate is greater than 10 mEq/L, the acidosis will generally resolve with hydration alone in 2 to 3 days. Rhabdomyolysis with myoglobinuria has been reported with high concentrations of toluene and requires aggressive hydration and forced diuresis to avoid acute tubular necrosis.

Patients abusing trichloroethylene, especially in combination with alcohol, may present with a marked cutaneous vasodilation or "degreaser's flush" as a result of inhibition of acetaldehyde dehydrogenase. Propranolol may provide symptomatic relief.

Disposition

Patients rarely require hospitalization after acute intoxication unless evidence of systemic toxicity is found. Indications for admission include persistent obtundation or focal neurologic abnormality, metabolic acidosis or rhabdomyolysis, and cardiac arrhythmias.

In addition to medical therapy, immediate evaluation by a psychiatric crisis counselor to initiate intensive outpatient psychotherapy and family counseling is a mandatory minimum intervention.

Long-Term Effects

Prolonged solvent abuse or chronic industrial exposure may cause a broad spectrum of neurologic abnormalities (Table 90–7). The most common problems include a "stocking-glove" peripheral neuropathy ("huffer's neuropathy") and cerebellar degeneration with ataxia. Symptoms may actually progress for up to 3 months after cessation of abuse. Neurologic abnormalities are generally multifocal and may be permanent, although some improvement may be seen with abstinence. Severe cerebrocortical, cerebellar, and brain stem atrophy may be seen on computed tomographic (CT) scan.

Even short-term exposures to neurotoxic hydrocarbons may lead to long-term CNS abnormalities. Lead toxicity should be excluded, as it may occur with gasoline sniffing

---

TABLE 90-7

LONG-TERM EFFECTS OF SOLVENT INHALATION ABUSE

Cardiovascular-hematologic
  Aplastic anemia
  Leukemia
  Dilated cardiomyopathy ("glue-sniffer's heart")
Renal
  Glomerulonephritis/Goodpasture's syndrome
  Renal tubular acidosis
  Tubulointerstitial nephritis
  Nephrotic syndrome
Hepatic
  Hepatic necrosis
  Hepatic carcinoma
Central nervous system
  Peripheral neuropathies
  Dementia (organic brain syndrome)
  Cerebellar degeneration, ataxia
  Cranial nerve damage (oculomotor palsies, optic atrophy, deafness)
  Parkinson-like syndrome, tremors, choreiform movements
  Diffuse motor weakness, flaccid paralysis
  Vestibular dysfunction, dizziness
  Lead encephalopathy

and is a treatable cause of encephalopathy. In several cases of toluene habituation, a withdrawal syndrome similar to severe alcohol withdrawal has been noted.

Renal toxicity and electrolyte abnormalities have been observed in both the chronic and acute setting. Although acute tubular necrosis with renal failure is rare, it has been seen with massive exposures. Autoimmune glomerulonephritis and Goodpasture's syndrome are most commonly observed and may occur months to years after a single large exposure. There is a 2.8- to 8.9-fold increased risk for glomerulonephritis among solvent-exposed individuals. Nephrotoxicity is most common with the chlorinated hydrocarbons but has been reported with all types. Tubulointerstitial nephritis and nephrotic syndrome have also been reported.

Toluene may cause renal tubular acidosis with life-threatening metabolic derangement. Severe metabolic acidosis and both high and normal anion gap acidosis have been reported with associated hypokalemia, hypophosphatemia, bicarbonate wasting, and hyperchloremia. Non–anion gap acidosis may reflect the relative bicarbonate wasting rather than the accumulation of metabolites as seen in the high anion gap form. Toluene is metabolized in the liver to hippuric acid, which is excreted by the kidney and is toxic to the renal tubules. Recovery of renal function after renal tubular acidosis is generally complete.

Aplastic anemia and leukemia have been noted particularly with benzene exposure, which inhibits DNA synthesis in the bone marrow. A case of aplastic anemia was reported in a 12-year-old male who slept in a room treated 48 hours previously with an organochlorine pesticide, lindane.

Chromosomal aberrations may also occur. Intrauterine exposure to chlorinated biphenyl may result in cleft palate, bone abnormalities, low birth weight, and poor cognitive function in infants.

Selected References

Anas NV, Namasonthi C, Ginsburg CM. Criteria for hospitalizing children who have ingested products containing hydrocarbons. JAMA 1981;246:840.

Banner W, Walson P. Systemic toxicity following gasoline aspiration. Am J Emerg Med 1983;3:292.

Beamon RF, Siegel CJ, Landers G, et al. Hydrocarbon ingestion in children: A six year retrospective study. JACEP 1976;5:771.

Bergson P, Hales S, Lustgarten M, et al. Pneumatoceles following hydrocarbon ingestion. Am J Dis Child 1975;129:49.

Boon N. Solvent abuse and the heart. Br Med J 1987;294:722.

Bruckner J, Peterson R. Evaluation of toluene and acetone inhalant abuse. Toxicol Appl Pharmacol 1981;61:27.

Clark D, Tinston D. Acute inhalation toxicity of some halogenated and non-halogenated hydrocarbons. Hum Toxicol 1982;1:239.

Dally S, Garnier R, Bismuth C. Diagnosis of chlorinated hydrocarbon poisoning by x-ray examination. Br J Ind Med 1987;44:424.

Decker W. Absorption of solvents by activated charcoal polymers, and mineral sorbents. Vet Hum Toxicol 1981;23:44.

Dice W, Ward G, Kelley J, Kilpatrick WR. Pulmonary toxicity following gastrointestinal ingestion of kerosene. Ann Emerg Med 1982;11:138.

Eade NR, Taussig LM, Marks MI. Hydrocarbon pneumonitis. Pediatrics 1974;54:351.

Ehrenreich T. Renal disease from exposure to solvents. Ann Clin Lab Sci 1977;7:6.

Gibson DE, Moore GP, Pfaff GA. Camphor ingestion. Am J Emerg Med 1989;7:41.

Greer J. Adolescent abuse of typewriter correction fluid. South Med J 1984;77:297.

Hansbrough JF, Zapata-Sirvent R, Dominic W, et al. Hydrocarbon contact injuries. J Trauma 1985;25:250.

Hayden J, Comstock E. Clinical toxicology of solvent abuse. Clin Toxicol 1976;9:169.

King M. Neurologic sequelae of toluene abuse. Hum Toxicol 1982;1:281.

Kirk LM, Anderson RJ, Martin K. Sudden death from toluene abuse (letter). Ann Emerg Med 1984;13:68.

Laass W. Therapy of acute oral poisonings by organic solvents: Treatment by activated charcoal in combination with laxatives. Arch Toxicol 1980;4:406.

Lazar RB, Ho SU, Melen O, Daghestani AN. Multifocal central nervous system damage caused by toluene abuse. Neurology 1983;33:1337.

Litovitz TL, Normann SA, Veltri JC. 1985 Annual Report of the American Association of Poison Control Centers National Data Collection System. Am J Emerg Med 1986;4:427.

McCormick MJ, Mogabgab E, Adams SL. Methanol poisoning as a result of inhalational solvent abuse. Ann Emerg Med 1990;19:639.

Mizutani T, Oohashi N, Naito H. Myoglobinemia and renal failure in toluene poisoning: A case report. Vet Hum Toxicol 1989;31:448.

Ng RC, Darwish H, Stewart DA. Emergency treatment of petroleum distillate and turpentine ingestion. Can Med Assoc J 1974;111:537.

Parker MJ, Tarlow MJ, Milne Anderson J. Glue sniffing and cerebral infarction. Arch Dis Child 1984;59:675.

Phelan W. Camphor poisoning: Over-the-counter dangers. Pediatrics 1976;57:428.

Polkis A, Burkett C. Gasoline sniffing: A review. Clin Toxicol 1977;11:35.

Press E. Cooperative kerosene poisoning study: Evaluation of gastric lavage and other factors in the treatment of accidental ingestion of petroleum distillate products. Pediatrics 1962; 29:648.

Prockop L. Neurotoxic volatile substances. Neurology 1979;29:862.

Raunskov U. Acute glomerulonephritis and exposure to organic solvents in fathers and daughters. Acta Med Scand 1979;205:581.

Rugman F, Cosstick R. Aplastic anemia associated with organochlorine pesticide: Case reports and review of evidence. J Clin Pathol 1990;43:98.

Scott P. Hydrocarbon ingestion: An unusual case of multiple pulmonary pseudotumors. South Med J 1989;82:1032.

Streicher H, et al. Syndromes of toluene sniffing in adults. Ann Intern Med 1981;94:758.

Taher S, et al. Renal tubular acidosis associated with toluene 'sniffing.' N Engl J Med 1974;290:765.

Taylor G, Harris W. Cardiac toxicity of aerosol propellants. JAMA 1970;214:81.

Voigts A, Kaufman C. Acidosis and other metabolic abnormalities associated with glue sniffing. South Med J 1983;76:443.

Wiseman M, Banim S. Glue-sniffer's heart? Br Med J 1987;294:739.

Wolsdorf J. Kerosene intoxication: An experimental approach to the etiology of CNS manifestations in primates. J Pediatr 1976;88:1037.

Young R, et al. Recurrent cerebellar dysfunction as related to chronic gasoline sniffing in an adolescent girl. Clin Pediatr 1977;16:706.

Zimmerman S, et al. Hydrocarbon exposure and chronic glomerulonephritis. Lancet 1975;2:199.

CHAPTER 91

Narcotics and Sedative-Hypnotics

Barbara A. Murphy

INTRODUCTION

The word *narcotic*, derived from the Greek word for "stupor," originally applied to any sleep-inducing drug, whereas *opioid* referred specifically to drugs derived from the poppy *Papaver somniferum*. After development of synthetic forms, *opioid* became a generic term for substances binding to any of the opioid receptors found throughout the central nervous system.[1, 2]

The opioids are classified into three basic groups. The agonists produce analgesia and have other actions similar to those of morphine. The second group is represented by naloxone, a nearly pure competitive antagonist. The third group, mixed agonists-antagonists, have agonistic activity at some receptors and antagonistic activity at others.[3]

Indications for pediatric opioid use include pain control postoperatively, for cancer patients, and for sickle cell crises. Opioids are also used for sedation for burn care, decreasing discomfort during mechanical ventilation, and minimizing the risk of self-extubation.[4]

The sedative-hypnotics are a large group of unrelated compounds, all of which are central nervous system depressants. The term *sedative* refers to the capacity to allay anxiety and lessen irritability. The name *hypnotic*, derived from the Greek *hypnos* ("sleep") and *hypnosia* ("drowsiness"), is applied to drugs that induce sleep.[1]

Modern sedative-hypnotics can be classified into three categories. The *barbiturates* are derivatives of barbituric acid. The *benzodiazepines* are a group of three-ring, multiply substituted compounds with similar pharmacologic properties. The third group is comprised of a number of miscellaneous unrelated compounds that have enjoyed past popularity but have been largely replaced in use by the benzodiazepines.[5]

SOURCES AND ROUTES OF EXPOSURE

The majority of pediatric poisonings with these drugs occur in toddlers who escape the watchful eye of careproviders. At highest risk are children at home with elderly careproviders. Other accidental exposures occur when drug-using pregnant women deliver transplacentally drugged infants or when nursing mothers secrete drugs into breast milk. Iatrogenic poisoning occurs when a child is given adult preparations or doses or even the wrong drug. Even more rare are cases in which children are deliberately poisoned.[6-10]

After age 12, the profile of poisonings changes from accidental to intentional use by the child. In this age group most exposures occur through suicide gestures or attempts.

INCIDENCE AND PREVALENCE OF PEDIATRIC POISONINGS

The child ingests what is available, with benzodiazepines being the most available sedative-hypnotics. The most common narcotics involved in home poisonings are those most commonly prescribed: codeine and antidiarrheals.[11-13] Although heroin is the most popular street narcotic, an annual poll of high school students indicates that propoxyphene, oxycodone, and hydromorphone (more available at home) are more often chosen for experimentation and recreational use.[14, 15]

In a report of 1,368,748 human exposures, 61% were in children younger than 6 years, and 11% were in those age 6 to 19 years. There were no reported deaths caused by narcotics or sedative-hypnotics in those younger than 6. The four reported deaths from these drugs, all in the 15- to 17-year-old age group, were all attributed to suicide or drug abuse. Narcotic poisonings in those younger than 6 years and in the 6- to 17-year-old age groups were 0.4% and 1.6%, respectively, of the total, with more than half of the cases in both groups caused by codeine. Poisonings by sedative-hypnotics in these same age groups were 0.67% and 1.68%, respectively, of the total, with benzodiazepines being most commonly involved.

Relevance to Human Health

Although few pediatric deaths are attributable to narcotics and sedative-hypnotics, there is considerable associated morbidity. Immediate death is caused by respiratory depression. Other early complications may have resulting in-hospital mortality. Complications of prolonged coma, intubation, and mechanical ventilation include aspiration pneumonia, pulmonary abscess, sepsis, pneumothorax, pneumomediastinum, and pulmonary fibrosis.[16] The shock state, caused in part by hypotension, depressed cardiac contractility, and

increased venous capacitance, may result in acute renal failure and myocardial dysfunction.

Pulmonary edema, present in nearly all narcotic fatalities, may also occur with sedative-hypnotics. It is probably related to direct pulmonary capillary damage from pulmonary vasoconstriction during hypoxia. Cardiac dysrhythmias associated with the miscellaneous sedative-hypnotics may also be involved.[17-23]

Other acute complications include acute tubular necrosis associated with chloral hydrate and glutethimide, hepatocellular degeneration associated with chloral hydrate, and acute renal failure secondary to rhabdomyolysis in narcotic poisoning. Paraldehyde and chloral hydrate have a corrosive effect on the gastric mucosa, and overdoses may result in hemorrhage, perforations, and strictures.[24-27]

Hypoxic encephalopathy, prolonged seizures, and cerebral edema can result in long-term neurologic dysfunction, vegetative states, and coma. Peripheral motor and sensory neuropathies have been attributed to methaqualone effects.

PHARMACOLOGY AND PHYSIOLOGY
Narcotics

Narcotics are rapidly absorbed from the nasal mucosa, gastrointestinal tract, and lung; the effect and time of onset vary with the route of administration. Plasma proteins bind 30% of the drug. The free portion rapidly leaves the circulation and accumulates in solid organs and skeletal muscle. Most of a narcotic dose is conjugated with glucuronic acid, with minor amounts undergoing *N*-methylation. Conjugated and free drug are filtered by the glomeruli and excreted in urine, where trace amounts are detectable for up to 48 hours.

The opioids attach to specific saturable central nervous system binding sites. These same sites are receptors for the endogenous peptides: the enkephalins, which serve as neurotransmitters, and the endorphins, which act as neurohormones or modulators of synaptic activity. These endogenous peptides also produce some opioid effects. The opioids in turn may mimic some actions of the endogenous peptides.[3, 28-30]

The primary clinical effects of opioids are on the central nervous system. They produce drowsiness, mental clouding, and mood changes ranging from euphoria to apathy and decrease the perceived discomfort of continuous dull pain. They induce nausea and vomiting by stimulating the medullary emetic center. In some individuals the effect is excitatory, producing anxiety, agitation, and even convulsions with therapeutic doses.

Significant respiratory depression results from altered responsiveness to carbon dioxide and direct neuronal effects on respiratory rate, rhythm and volumes. Cardiovascular effects vary, but generally heart rate and diastolic blood pressure decrease, and mean arterial pressure increases.

Gastrointestinal effects include decreased gastric, biliary, and pancreatic secretions; sphincter of Oddi spasm; and decreased intestinal motility. In the urinary tract, detrusor and sphincter muscle tone increase, resulting in urgency with retention. Skeletal muscle effects include increased tone, rigidity, and rhabdomyolysis. Dilation of cutaneous blood vessels results in flushing, pruritus, histamine release, and urticaria.[3, 31, 32]

Barbiturates

Barbiturates are dependably absorbed orally and rectally. Lipid solubility enhances transmucosal uptake, but the prime rate-limiting factors are the solubility and distribution of the drug in intestinal contents. Intramuscular absorption is erratic, and the alkalinity of the drug causes tissue necrosis. Intravenous use provides immediate blood levels, but central nervous system effect requires time for passage across the blood-brain barrier.

Barbiturates distribute to all body tissues, including the fetus and breast milk. The three factors controlling distribution and excretion are lipid solubility, protein binding, and degree of ionization. More lipid-soluble forms cross membranes more rapidly, resulting in prompt central nervous system penetration with rapid onset of action, metabolism, and excretion and shorter duration of action. Part of a barbiturate dose binds reversibly to plasma proteins, with the degree of binding being directly proportional to lipid solubility. Because a barbiturate is a weak acid, with its pKa near the physiologic pH, tissue permeability is highly influenced by changes in body pH. Acidosis decreases ionization and increases tissue permeability, whereas therapeutic alkalinization increases ionization and decreases tissue permeability.

Metabolism occurs primarily in the liver, with minor contributions by the kidney. Most barbiturates are oxidized to inactive metabolites. Some undergo desulfuration, N-methylation, H-hydroxylation, or N-dealkylation to form new, active barbiturates (e.g., primidone). Excretion of metabolites is through the kidney. Non–protein-bound and ionized forms are filtered by the glomeruli and excreted unchanged.

Barbiturates depress all excitable tissue. Activity most probably occurs at the synapse (presynaptically by inhibiting transmitter release and postsynaptically by depressing responsiveness to repetitive impulses). Presynaptically, barbiturates may have a gamma-aminobutyric acid (GABA)–like effect or cause GABA release. They may also exert a non-adrenergic effect by inhibiting release of or sensitivity to acetylcholine. These depressive effects elevate the threshold of afterdischarges and suppress seizure activity.

Central nervous system depression ranges from mild sedation to deep coma, with children being especially subject to the effects of drowsiness and decreased mental acuity even at therapeutic levels. Rapid barbiturate withdrawal may induce seizures.

Barbiturates may increase response to pain. Respiratory neurogenic drive, hypoxic drive, and chemoreceptor response to carbon dioxide are depressed. Blood pressure, heart rate, cardiac output, renal plasma flow, and gastrointestinal secretions and motility are decreased. Barbiturate stimulation of hepatic microsomal enzymes results in an increased rate of metabolism of other drugs, as well as of the barbiturates themselves.[33–37]

Benzodiazepines

It is assumed that benzodiazepines all have the same mechanism of action and the same qualitative clinical effects. Oral absorption approaches 100%, although rates vary widely for individual drugs. Water-soluble forms are well absorbed intramuscularly, but for the lipid-soluble drugs, diazepam and lorazepam, absorption by this route is poor.

The drugs are distributed first to the fluid compartment and highly perfused organs, then to the central nervous system, and finally to adipose tissue. They cross the placenta and are secreted into breast milk. There is also significant biliary secretion and enterohepatic circulation. Major metabolism occurs in the liver by oxidation, hydroxylation, and formation of glucuronide complexes, which are eliminated through the kidney.[5, 38]

Benzodiazepine receptors scattered throughout the brain facilitate the action of GABA. The benzodiazepines may act presynaptically to increase GABA release or to make GABA-ergic interneurons more sensitive to excitation. A postsynaptic effect increasing the activity of GABA has also been postulated.

Clinical effects of benzodiazepines are almost totally in the central nervous system. All forms cause drowsiness progressing to stupor and coma with increased doses. Symptoms are more pronounced in children with deep or cyclic coma, and transient apnea has been reported. All result in some anxiolytic effect, muscle relaxation, and suppression of seizure activity, but the drugs vary in clinical usefulness for a given clinical effect. They have little or no gastrointestinal or cardiovascular effects, and observed effects on these systems are probably caused by other drugs used in combination.[38–40]

Miscellaneous Sedative-Hypnotics

The miscellaneous group of unrelated sedative-hypnotics have many features in common. All are readily absorbed from the gut and are used mainly in oral form, although paraldehyde and ethchlorvynol may also be used parenterally. They are distributed throughout the central nervous system, in all body fluids, across the placenta, and in breast milk. All are metabolized primarily in the liver, with metabolic products being excreted in the urine. All can cause excitement, euphoria, delirium or irrational behavior, and global central nervous system depression related to dose.[41]

CLINICAL EVALUATION
History

An objective history can be elusive. Young children rarely ingest poisons under direct observation. Distraught careproviders do not document time or remember the amount of drug that was available. When illegal or street drugs are involved, fear of reprisal and mixture of drugs with unknown substances makes accurate history taking impossible.

The history should attempt to identify the drugs, amount, time, route of exposure, and possibility of associated trauma. An awake, accidentally poisoned older child can often give helpful information, but frequently the patient is young or stuporous. Suicidal and drug-abusing children often give deliberately false histories. Pills and capsules should be absolutely identified; labels on containers may be inaccurate. If drugs or containers were not brought in, a friend or family member should be sent back for them.

The physician should briefly determine the social setting of the exposure. For the suicidal child, the physician should ask about a recent disappointment or disagreement, a warning threat, or a note. When applicable, any history of previous adjustment or psychiatric disorders, previous suicide attempts, drug abuse, or admission to treatment programs should be obtained. Because many pediatric adjustment and psychiatric disorders and drug abuse problems are linked to family dynamics, careproviders may be reluctant to discuss these problems, particularly with a stranger in an emergency setting. The minimum requirement is to identify that the child has suicidal ideation or a drug abuse problem in order to ensure appropriate admission and counseling.[42]

A past medical history, because it is less emotionally charged, is usually easier to obtain. This should focus on any preexisting pulmonary, cardiovascular, hepatic, or renal diseases that could potentiate drug effects or be exacerbated by the toxin itself or the treatment.

Physical Examination

Neurologic status can be quickly assessed by the AVPU method (i.e., whether the patient is *Alert*, responds to *Verbal* or *Painful* stimuli, or is *Unresponsive*). The child must be fully undressed to look for signs of trauma. Blood pressure should be measured in all patients, using the Doppler technique if necessary. Rectal or tympanic, but not oral, temperature should be measured in children who are unconscious, younger than 4 years, or suspected to be hypothermic.

The secondary survey, a complete head-to-toe examination, may reveal evidence of trauma or underlying disease. Some specific physical findings are typically associated with specific poisonings, but these can be confusing with mixed poisonings, secondary metabolic derangements, and preexisting medical conditions.

The level of consciousness, altered by all narcotics and sedative-hypnotics, can be accurately evaluated by the standard Glasgow Coma Scale or a modification of it for children younger than 5 (Table 91–1). High level responses cannot be assessed in the preverbal child, but state of arousability can be determined. The modified scale adjusts normal scores for the expected verbal and comprehensive ability of the young child.[43-45]

Chloral hydrate and heroin usually constrict the pupils, whereas benzodiazepines, glutethimide, and most other narcotics may dilate them. Oculocephalic reflexes may be absent in patients with barbiturate poisoning. Barbiturates, benzodiazepines, and narcotics blunt pain perception, whereas other sedative-hypnotics may increase it. Subtle sensory findings are unimportant in this setting. Ataxia, dysarthria, and incoordination, common to all sedative-hypnotic use, may be found in any poisoning case involving simultaneous alcohol use. Barbiturates diminish deep tendon reflexes, whereas meprobamate and methaqualone cause hyperreflexia. Flexor or extensor posturing may be caused by nonbenzodiazepine sedative-hypnotics. Gluthethimide, which causes cerebral edema, produces changing focal deficits.

TABLE 91–2

REED'S CLASSIFICATION OF COMA

Grade 0	Asleep but arousable to verbal responsiveness
Grade I	Responds to painful stimuli
Grade II	No response to painful stimuli
Grade III	Deep tendon and gag reflexes absent + grade II
Grade IV	Vital signs and respirations unstable + grade III

Reproduced, with permission, from Reed CE, Driggs MF, Foote CC. Acute barbiturate intoxication: A study of 300 cases based on a physiologic system of classification of the severity of the intoxication. Ann Intern Med 1952;37:290.

All narcotic- or sedative-hypnotic–poisoned patients require serial evaluations for changing level of consciousness. If the patient scores below normal on the Glasgow Coma Scale, repeated assessments should include Reed's Classification of Coma, which considers adequacy of circulation, respiration, and airway protective reflexes (Table 91–2). Depth of coma correlates with level of toxicity, unless head trauma or hypoxia are also present.[46]

DIAGNOSTIC EVALUATION

Most narcotic- and sedative-hypnotic poisonings cause no specific laboratory abnormalities. No testing is indicated for the asymptomatic or transiently affected patient. Toxicology screens usually take too long to influence acute management and often detect substances of little clinical importance.

For the symptomatic patient, determinations of glucose, electrolytes (with calculation of anion gap), blood urea nitrogen (BUN), and creatinine levels and arterial blood gases and urinalysis will guide fluid and oxygen therapy and exclude other causes of altered mental status. Determination of acetaminophen, salicylate, phenobarbital, and ethanol levels, readily available in most centers, assists in diagnosing mixed intoxications and may significantly affect treatment. Discolored urine should be examined for myoglobin, especially in the presence of seizure activity or opioid and barbiturate poisonings.

An electroencephalogram can give a reliable measurement of depth of coma, showing predictable and progressive changes as coma depth increases. An isoelectric tracing in severe barbiturate poisoning does not imply irreversible brain damage; full neurologic recovery has been documented in patients after drug-induced isoelectric studies.[47]

DIFFERENTIAL DIAGNOSIS

The differential diagnosis of narcotic or sedative-hypnotic intoxication is the differential diagnosis of coma (Table 91–3). Drug exposure may not be immediately suspected in a child found with altered mental status, and other disorders are so frequently associated with poisonings that trauma and underlying illness must be disproven. Laboratory tests (aside from toxicologic analyses) are not specific. Poisoning with mixed agents adds to the confusion.

THERAPEUTIC INTERVENTION

The child with absent gag reflex or inadequate air exchange should be endotracheally intubated and mechanically ventilated. Venous access for fluid and drug administration should be established. In hypotension, 20 ml/kg normal saline (NS) or lactated Ringer's (LR) solution is given over 10 minutes (Table 91–4). A second bolus of crystalloid should be given if required. When volume expansion greater

TABLE 91–1

GLASGOW COMA SCALE

Standard	Score	Modified for Children
Eyes open		Same as standard
Spontaneously	4	
To speech	3	
To pain	2	
None	1	
Best motor responses		Same as standard
Obeys	6	
Localizes pain	5	
Withdraws to pain	4	
Flexes to pain	3	
Extends to pain	2	
None	1	
Best verbal response		
Oriented	5	Oriented
Confused	4	Words
Inappropriate words	3	Vocal sounds
Incomprehensible	2	Cries
None	1	None
Normal scores		
Birth to 6 mo	9	
6–12 mo	11	
1–2 yr	12	
2–5 yr	13	
5 yr	14	
Over 5 yr	15	

(Modified from Simpson D, Reilly P. Paediatric coma scale. Lancet 1982;2:450.)

DIFFERENTIAL DIAGNOSIS

Etiology	Clues to Diagnosis
Nonstructural disorders	Nonfocal, dissociated examination
Intoxications	Diagnosis of exclusion, response to naloxone, specific toxicology screens
Single agents	
Mixed agents	
Infections	Fever, leucocytosis, stiff neck, CSF examination after normal brain CT scan, tachycardia, hypotension, respiratory alkalosis, metabolic acidosis, cultures for confirmation
Meningitis, encephalitis	
Sepsis	
Metabolic disorders	Medical history, response to O_2 and glucose, electrolytes, BUN, creatinine, liver functions, calcium, thyroid function, arterial blood gas
Circulatory disorders	Vital signs
Shock	Vital signs
Hypertensive encephalopathy	
Hyperthermia/hypothermia	Core temperature
Seizure—postictal phase	Medical history, increasing level of consciousness, incontinence, tongue biting
Psychogenic disorders	Normal examination, forced eye closure
Structural disorders	
Traumatic intracranial contusion or hemorrhage	Physical evidence of trauma, brain CT scan, focal neurologic examination
Intracerebral or brain stem hemorrhage	CSF examination after normal brain CT scan
Subarachnoid hemorrhage	CSF examination after normal brain CT scan

than 40 to 50 ml/kg is required, invasive monitoring and use of pressors should be considered. Cardiac monitoring for dysrhythmias should be established and a Foley catheter inserted to decompress the bladder and measure urine output. In the comatose child, skin necrosis should be avoided by frequent turning and padding of pressure points.

Dextrose 25% (2 ml/kg) and naloxone (0.01 mg/kg) are given intravenously. Naloxone can be repeated at 2- to 3-minute intervals, giving a minimum total dose of 0.2 mg/kg before excluding narcotics as an intoxicant. Thiamine is not routinely used in children, but 100 mg given intravenously should be considered in adolescents with possible ethanol abuse.

Gastric emptying should be performed regardless of time since ingestion. Drugs that delay gastric emptying or form gastric concretions can be removed in substantial quantities as long as 24 hours after ingestion. Ipecac should not be used in a child who is comatose or becoming less responsive or in one who is at risk for seizures, but it may be given orally to a fully awake child with a history of ingestion.

Gastric lavage should be done only in the presence of a gag reflex or after the child is endotracheally intubated. Lavage is done through the largest possible orotracheal tube with the child lying on the left side and with the head down.

After gastric emptying, activated charcoal (1 gm/kg) is given orally or through the lavage tube. Cathartics speed gut transit of charcoal and absorbed drug, but their efficacy has been questioned. Magnesium cathartics should be avoided in the presence of renal disease or when there is the potential for myoglobinuria (e.g., in the presence of high fever, seizures, or associated muscle trauma).[48-52]

Narcotics

Because naloxone rapidly reverses the respiratory depression of narcotic intoxication and is completely nontoxic, it is part of the initial management protocol for all coma of uncertain origin. Intravenous naloxone acts within 1 to 3 minutes, reaches peak effect in 5 to 10 minutes, and has a 12- to 20-minute half-life, with little detectable 45 minutes after a single dose. Because naloxone has variable affinity for different receptors, larger amounts are required to antagonize certain opioids. Codeine, buprenorphine, methadone, pentazocine, and propoxyphene may require large doses for reversal. The depressant effect of most narcotics lasts longer than the effect of naloxone, necessitating repeated doses.[53-56]

A continuous infusion is safer and more convenient than repeated boluses. After an initial effective dose is given, an infusion is started that delivers two thirds of the initial dose per hour. Fifteen minutes after the initial dose, a second bolus of one half the loading dose is given. This combination of boluses and infusion should maintain the initial reversal. If rapid intravenous access cannot be obtained, naloxone can be given subcutaneously, intramuscularly, endotracheally, intraosseously, or by sublingual injection. If the patient fails to respond to maximal naloxone dose, a nonnarcotic, mixed-intoxication, or nontoxic cause of coma is likely.[57-59]

Pulmonary edema, which can occur up to 12 hours after poisoning, is treated with oxygen, positive end-expiratory pressure, avoidance of fluid overload, and continued naloxone infusion. Diuretics and digitalis are not useful.

The antidiarrheal atropine sulfate–diphenoxylate hydrochloride (Lomotil), a morphine congener, is used in combination with atropine. Adults tolerate large doses without adverse effect, because the antidiarrheal effect is significantly greater than the central respiratory depressive effect. For children, however, there is a very narrow range between therapeutic and depressive dosage. For some children, the depressive effects are not dose related. According to the United States Food and Drug Administration (FDA), use in children younger than 2 years is contraindicated, and cautious use is recommended in children age 2 to 12 years.

Early effects, occurring within 2 to 3 hours, consist of classic anticholinergic symptoms: tachycardia, tachypnea, flushing, mydriasis, lethargy, and confusion. The late effect, beginning 2 to 36 hours after administration, is miosis, respiratory depression, and coma. Onset of symptoms may be delayed by decreased gastric motility, incomplete gastrointestinal decontamination, redistribution of drug from tissue compartments, and enterohepatic circulation.

All children with a history of diphenoxylate ingestion require admission with 36-hour observation for symptoms after routine gastric lavage and charcoal dosing. Symptomatic children require repeated charcoal dosing and naloxone infusion for a minimum of 12 hours.[60-63]

Barbiturates

Fluid therapy is important in barbiturate intoxication. After correction of hypotension, forced diuresis can be used to significantly increase the elimination of all barbiturates, especially phenobarbital. Forced diuresis can be achieved

TABLE 91–4

SEDATIVE-HYPNOTIC POISONING: THERAPY AT A GLANCE

Drug	Indication	Dose
Dextrose 25%	Hypoglycemia	2 ml/kg IV
Naloxone	Narcotic antagonist	1st bolus: 0.01 to 0.02 mg/kg IV 2nd bolus: ½ loading dose Infusion: ⅔ loading dose/hr
Ipecac	Induction of emesis	Older than 12 yr: 30 ml po 1 to 12 yr: 15 ml po 6 mo to 1 yr: 10 ml po Younger than 6 mo: not advised
Activated charcoal	Drug absorption in gut	1 gm/kg/dose po; repeated as required
Magnesium citrate	Cathartic	4 ml/kg po; maximum, 200 ml
Magnesium sulfate	Cathartic	250 mg/kg po; maximum, 30 gm
Furosemide	Diuresis	1 mg/kg IV
Sodium bicarbonate	Alkalinization of urine	2 mEq/kg IV bolus Infusion: 2 to 4 mEq/kg q 6–12 hr to maintain desired urine pH
Aminophylline	Reversal of benzodiazepine induced respiratory depression	1 mg/kg IV
Mannitol	Reduction of cerebral edema	0.25 mg/kg IV push, repeated q 5 min as needed
Propranolol	Control of ventricular dysrhythmias	0.01 to 0.1 mg/kg/dose IV; maximum, 1 mg/dose; repeat q 5 min; maximum total dose, 5 mg
Lidocaine	Control of ventricular dysrhythmias	1 mg/kg/dose IV, repeated q 8 min to maximum 3 mg/kg
Normal saline or lactated Ringer's solution	Fluid replacement	20-ml/kg boluses, repeated to correct hypotension

with furosemide (1 mg/kg IV) and D5/0.2 NS administered at a rate sufficient to achieve urine output of 0.1 ml/kg/min (two to five times the maintenance rate).[64, 65]

Alkaline diuresis is effective only with long-acting barbiturates and should be reserved for severe intoxication in which serum levels are above 80 μg/ml. This is achieved by using NaHCO₃. An initial bolus of 2 mEq/kg is followed by an infusion of 2 to 4 mEq/kg over the next 6 to 12 hours to maintain urine pH above 7.0. All children must be carefully monitored to avoid fluid overload.[33, 66]

Forced diuresis should be stopped when drug levels are still above the therapeutic range, and levels should then be allowed to decline by endogenous metabolism to protect against withdrawal seizures. If a seizure should occur, it should be treated acutely with a benzodiazepine. The patient should be reloaded with phenobarbital to a therapeutic level and the level then permitted to decrease by approximately 10% every 3 days until negligible.[67]

Hemodialysis and hemoperfusion have been shown to be effective in decreasing the duration of barbiturate coma and should be considered when conservative measures fail in patients with hepatic or renal impairment and in those in grade IV coma. Charcoal hemoperfusion is most effective for removing short-acting forms and should be used with drug levels greater than 50 μg/ml. Hemodialysis is effective for long-acting forms and should be used with drug levels greater than 100 μg/ml. Peritoneal dialysis is not effective.[68–70]

Because hypothermia is a frequent complication of barbiturate overdose, core temperature should be monitored. Barbiturate classification by action time is shown in Table 91–5.

Benzodiazepines

The treatment of pure benzodiazepine intoxication is supportive. More specific measures have been investigated, but because supportive therapy is so effective, no other therapy is recommended. Benzodiazepines are highly protein bound, so hemodialysis and diuresis are not effective.[71, 72] Physostigmine reverses central nervous system depression, but its risks outweigh its benefits.[73] Aminophylline in an intravenous dose of 1 mg/kg has been shown to rapidly reverse depressive effects in neonates.[74] Flumazenil (Mazicon), a specific antagonist, has shown effectiveness but is not yet recommended for use in children.[75, 76]

Diagnosis and patient monitoring in benzodiazepine intoxication is clinical. Toxicology screens do not detect some benzodiazepines but recognize a variety of active and inactive metabolites with highly variable elimination kinetics.

Chloral Hydrate

Most children tolerate a dose of 50 mg/kg to a maximum total dose of 1 gm without toxicity. The actual toxic dose range is undefined, as gastric irritative effects cause vomiting after ingestion in nearly 50% of children. If coma is to develop, mental status will be altered within 30 minutes. The child who remains asymptomatic after three hours of observation can be medically discharged.

TABLE 91–5

BARBITURATE CLASSIFICATION

Action Time	Generic Name	Onset of Action
Long	Phenobarbital	1 hr
	Mephobarbital	1 hr
	Primidone	1 hr
Intermediate	Amobarbital	3–30 min
	Butalbital	3–30 min
	Butabarbital	3–30 min
Short	Hexobarbital	3–30 min
	Pentobarbital	3–30 min
	Secobarbital	3–30 min

The symptomatic child requires monitoring for dysrhythmias, which include atrial and ventricular premature contractions and tachycardias, atrioventricular blocks, and asystole. The treatment of choice for ventricular dysrhythmias is propranolol (0.01 to 0.10 mg/kg IV per dose to a maximum of 1 mg per dose). This may be repeated every five minutes to a maximum dose of 5 mg. Ventricular dysrhythmias refractory to propranolol may respond to lidocaine (1 mg/kg/dose IV to a maximum of 3 mg/kg). Hemodynamically unstable patients require direct current synchronized cardioversion. Temporary pacing is required for high-grade atrioventricular block and torsades de pointes.[77–81]

Close observation for gastrointestinal hemorrhage and perforation includes repeated abdominal examinations, serial hematocrit measurements, and examination of stool and gastric lavage fluid for occult blood. Regular instillation of antacids through a nasogastric tube may protect gastric mucosa. A drip is prepared to deliver 1 ml/kg/hr or 60 to 80 ml per 1.73 m² per hr, adjusting the proportions of magnesium or aluminum antacids to control diarrhea or constipation. Children with evidence of hemorrhage may require endoscopy and transfusion.[26, 27, 82]

Patients with Reed's grade I or II coma show good recovery in 24 to 48 hours with support and monitoring. For patients with grade III or IV coma, charcoal hemoperfusion should be considered. Hemodialysis and peritoneal dialysis are ineffective because of high lipid solubility and binding to adipose tissue. Children younger than 2 years may be best treated by exchange transfusion. Recovery from grade III or IV coma with support and hemoperfusion or exchange should be expected in 3 to 5 days, with a less than 5% mortality rate.[83–86]

Ethchlorvynol

Ethchlorvynol, a highly lipid-soluble drug, is rapidly stored in adipose and neural tissue. The elimination pattern is biphasic, with levels declining rapidly at first, then rising in 7 to 14 hours with drug redistribution from lipids to plasma. This explains the large variations in length of coma (50 to ≥ 300 hours) and the difficulty in determining a drug's half-life.[33]

Aggressive support is the standard therapy, as measures to increase elimination rates produce variable results. Forced diuresis, hemodialysis, and peritoneal dialysis are not effective. Charcoal hemoperfusion can increase clearance rates, removing up to 30% of an ingested dose, but must be repeated at 4- to 6-hour intervals because of rebounding drug levels. Ion exchange resin hemoperfusion has been reported to remove up to 50% of drug in a single pass. Indications for hemoperfusion include ingestion of more than 100 mg/kg, serum levels greater than 10 mg/dl in the first 12 hours or greater than 7 mg/dl in the second 12 hours, or prolonged coma with life-threatening complications unresponsive to general support. In the child younger than 2 years, these are indications for exchange transfusion.[87–92]

Seizures may occur as serum levels decline and should be treated with phenytoin or benzodiazepines, avoiding barbiturates. Because hypothermia is common, core temperature should be monitored.[87]

Patients with Reed's grade I or II coma can be expected to recover in 24 to 48 hours with support. Patients with grade III or IV coma can be expected to recover in 3 to 5 days with support and hemoperfusion, with a mortality rate of less than 5%.

Glutethimide

All patients with a history of ingestion of glutethimide should be admitted even if asymptomatic. This highly lipid-soluble drug concentrates in adipose and neural tissue. Coma may be deep, prolonged, and cyclical as a result of slow redistribution from lipid stores, enterohepatic circulation, and production of active metabolites. Decreased intestinal motility, enterohepatic circulation, and formation of gastric concretions make repeated gastric lavage and charcoal dosing effective as long as 24 hours after ingestion.[5, 93–96]

The basis of treatment is support. Forced diuresis is ineffective, as less than 2% of the drug is excreted unchanged in urine, and is contraindicated because of the frequency of associated pulmonary edema. If seizures occur, diazepam is the drug of first choice, followed by phenytoin if seizures are recurrent or unresponsive to diazepam. Patients should be monitored for signs of cerebral edema and treated with mannitol (0.25 mg/kg IV push) at 5-minute intervals as needed to control intracranial hypertension.[97]

Hemodialysis and peritoneal dialysis are generally ineffective, but charcoal and resin hemoperfusion remain controversial. Hemoperfusion, although it increases clearance, does not appear to alter depth and duration of coma. When used, hemoperfusion must be repeated often because of cyclic redistribution of drug from tissue compartments. Possible indications for hemoperfusion are grade III or IV coma unresponsive to support, progressive deterioration despite aggressive support, and a flat line reading on the electroencephalogram.[70, 98] Other important considerations in glutethemide intoxication are metabolic acidosis, problems with body temperature regulation, and barbiturate-type skin lesions.[97]

Patients with grade I or II coma can be expected to recover in 24 to 48 hours. Patients with grade III or IV coma should recover in 3 to 5 days, with a less than 5% mortality rate. The major causes of mortality are pulmonary complications.

Meprobamate

Endoscopy may be required in meprobamate overdose to remove gastric concretions that prolong drug absorption. Beyond decontamination, support and monitoring of cardiovascular status are all that is usually required.[99–102] Hypotension may be profound, rapid, and unresponsive to volume expansion. Vasopressors should be used early to avoid commonly associated pulmonary edema. Dysrhythmias, primarily sinus bradycardia or tachycardia, are common and probably are caused by venous dilation and hypotension. Frequent suctioning and close attention to pulmonary toilet are important because of increased oral and nasal secretions.[103]

Symptoms, if they occur, should be apparent within 3 hours of ingestion. Quantitative meprobamate levels have some relationship to clinical effect, with levels of 5 mg/dl causing central nervous system depression and coma usually occurring at levels of 10 mg/dl.[103, 104]

Forced diuresis, although theoretically useful, is contraindicated because of the dangers of fluid overload. Peritoneal dialysis and hemodialysis have been shown to be of little value. Charcoal or ion exchange resin hemoperfusion are reported to be effective and should be considered in the patient who continues to deteriorate despite aggressive support or in those with grade III or IV coma unresponsive to support therapy.[105]

Methaqualone

Symptoms of methaqualone ingestion, which should be apparent within two hours, can be managed with supportive care in most patients. Hypotension and respiratory depression are less frequent than with other sedative-hypnotics.

Methaqualone, unlike other sedative-hypnotics, causes severe muscle hyperactivity, hyperreflexia, and muscle twitching severe enough to require pharmacologic paralysis and mechanical ventilation in some patients. Seizures, which are relatively frequent, should be treated with diazepam or phenytoin. Other considerations include management of bullous skin lesions, monitoring for pyrexia and thrombocytopenia, and rigorous pulmonary care to control excessive tracheobronchial secretions.[33]

Forced diuresis is ineffective, as less than 1% of the drug is excreted unchanged in urine, and contraindicated because of the danger of fluid overload. Hemodialysis and peritoneal dialysis are minimally effective. Charcoal and ion exchange resin hemoperfusion should be considered in severe poisonings in which plasma levels are greater than 40 μg/ml.[106, 107]

In patients with grade I or II coma, recovery is expected in 24 to 48 hours. In patients with grade III or IV coma, recovery should occur in 3 to 5 days with less than 5% mortality.

Paraldehyde

Paraldehyde has a very narrow margin of safety, and most toxic exposures are iatrogenic. The suggested therapeutic doses for children are 0.15 ml/kg (150 mg/kg) for sedation and 0.30 ml/kg (300 mg/kg) given every 4 to 6 hours for seizure control, but deaths have been reported with doses as low as 12 ml given rectally. All children with paraldehyde exposures should be admitted, as onset of action, rate of elimination, and toxic dose have high individual variation, and late complications are common.[108]

A prominent feature of poisoning with paraldehyde is increased anion gap metabolic acidosis from metabolism of paraldehyde to acetaldehyde and acetic acid. Toxic hepatitis with fatty liver changes may seriously slow metabolism. The corrosive effect on the lung from alveolar elimination may result in pulmonary hemorrhage and edema. Direct corrosive effect on the intestinal mucosa may result in esophagitis, gastritis, or proctitis.[109]

Central venous pressure or Swan-Ganz monitoring is often necessary to avoid overhydration. Positive end-expiratory pressure or constant positive airway pressure may be necessary to maintain adequate oxygenation in pulmonary edema. Metabolic acidosis should be managed by administering $NaHCO_3$ to keep the pH above 7.25. Hemodialysis or peritoneal dialysis should be used for patients developing acute renal failure or those with acidosis unresponsive to bicarbonate administration.[110, 111]

PATIENT DISPOSITION

When a pediatric patient is poisoned by narcotics or sedative-hypnotic drugs, the possibility of child abuse or neglect should be considered. Problems in locating parents or guardians, inconsistent histories, history of repeated poisonings, and observations at the scene by emergency medical service (EMS) personnel may raise suspicions about inadequate supervision or an unsafe home situation. No child should be discharged until these suspicions are satisfactorily addressed. All pediatric patients at risk for suicide require admission as long as there is continued risk. Most children require close post-discharge observation, and many require definite follow-up care. No child should be discharged until these can be ensured. Medical criteria for admission and consultation are summarized in Table 91–6.

OTHER CONSIDERATIONS

Beyond the responsibilities of medical care, the physician has legal responsibilities to maintain the safety of the child, the rights of the family, and the defense of the medical staff involved in the child's care. There must be thorough, accurate, and legible documentation of the entire medical encounter (Table 91–7).

Permission to treat the child should be obtained whenever possible from the parent or guardian, but lifesaving treatment should not be withheld if timely permission cannot be obtained. If for any reason permission to treat a minor is denied and the child is judged to be in imminent danger, treatment must be instituted and the immediate risk of morbidity or mortality documented. Appropriate judicial authority should be obtained as soon as possible to secure a court-appointed guardian for the child.[112]

TABLE 91–7

DOCUMENTATION

Substances involved or suspected, with amounts and times (when known)
History and physical examination
Results of all diagnostic studies
Notes on all invasive procedures
Times of repeated neurologic evaluations and vital signs
Nature and time of all therapeutic interventions both in the field and in the emergency department or physician's office
Requested consultations and time of request
Discharge instructions and evidence that the caretaker received and understood the instructions

TABLE 91–6

SEDATIVE-HYPNOTIC POISONING: CRITERIA FOR ADMISSION AND CONSULTATION

Ingestion of long-acting opioids, paraldehyde, or glutethemide
Ingestion of known or suspected toxic doses even if asymptomatic
Underlying illness potentiating or potentiated by drug effect
Unconsciousness, hypotension, hypoglycemia, seizure, dysrhythmia, or respiratory insufficiency at any time during the acute situation
Abnormal vital signs
Persistent altered mental status
Need for airway support or intervention
Cardiac dysrhythmias
Acid-base disorders
Recurrent seizures
Unstable vital signs
Pediatrics and pediatric or general intensivist for complications or altered mental status more than 30 min
Social services for suspected child abuse, neglect, unsafe home
Psychiatry for children with suicide potential or poisoning caused by drug abuse or experimentation
Nephrologist when hemodialysis, peritoneal dialysis, or hemoperfusion are required

References

1. Dorland's Illustrated Medical Dictionary. 26th ed. Philadelphia, WB Saunders, 1981, pp 687, 868, 1185.
2. Gerard J. The Herbal or General History of Plants. New York, Dover, 1975, pp 284, 310, 369.

3. Jaffe JH, Martin WR. Opioid Analgesics and Antagonists. *In* Gilman AG, Goodman LS, Gilman A (eds). The Pharmacological Basis of Therapeutics. 6th ed. New York, Macmillan, 1980, p 494.

4. Koren G, Levy M. Pediatric uses of opioids. Pediatr Clin North Am 1989;36:1141.

5. Harvey SC. Hypnotics and sedatives. *In* Gilman AG, Goodman LS, Gilman A (eds). The Pharmacological Basis of Therapeutics. 6th ed. New York, Macmillan, 1980, p 339.

6. Wezorek C, Dean B, Krenzelok E. Accidental childhood poisoning—influence of type of caretaker on etiology and risk. Vet Hum Toxicol 1988;30(6):574.

7. O'Brien TE. Excretion of drugs in human milk. Am J Hosp Pharm 1974;31:844.

8. Heckson GB, Altemeier WA, Martin ED, Campbell PW. Parental administration of chemical agents—a cause of apparent life threatening events. Pediatrics 1989;83:772.

9. Naumburg EG, Meny RG. Breast milk opioids and neonatal apnea. Am J Dis Child 1988;142:11.

10. Ramabadran K, Moore BE. SIDS and opioid peptides from milk. Am J Dis Child 1988;142:12.

11. Litovitz TL, Schmitz BF, Holm KC. 1988 annual report of the American Association of Poison Control Centers National Data Collection System. Am J Emerg Med 1989;7:495.

12. Aronow R, Puil SD, Wooley PV. Childhood poisoning, an unfortunate consequence of methadone availability. JAMA 1972;219:321.

13. Committee on Drugs. Use of codeine and dextromethorphan containing cough syrups in pediatrics. Pediatrics 1978;65:118.

14. National Trends 1975–1982. DHHS publication no ADM 83-1260. Washington, DC, US Government Printing Office, 1983, p 2.

15. National Institute for Drug Abuse. Annual Survey 1989—Student Drug Use, Attitudes and Beliefs. DHHS publication no ADM 89-1327. Washington, DC, US Government Printing Office, 1989, p 3.

16. Glassroth J, Adams GD, Schnall S. The impact of substance abuse in the respiratory system. Chest 1987;91:596.

17. Rice TB. Paregoric intoxication with pulmonary edema in infancy. Clin Pediatr 1984;23:101.

18. Benowitz NK, Rosenberg J, Becker CE. Cardiopulmonary catastrophies in drug overdose patients. Med Clin North Am 1979;63:278.

19. Overland ES, Severinghaus JW. Non cardiac pulmonary edema. Adv Intern Med 1978;23:307.

20. Prough DS, Roy R, Baumgarner J, Shannon G. Acute pulmonary edema in healthy teenagers following conservative doses of naloxone. Anesthesia 1984;60:485.

21. Verma RS. Pentazocine induced pulmonary edema. Anesthesia 1983;38:505.

22. Katz S, Aberman A, Frand UI, et al. Heroin pulmonary edema—evidence for increased pulmonary capillary permeability. Am Rev Respir Dis 1972;106:472.

23. Sklar J, Timms RM. Codeine induced pulmonary edema. Chest 1977;72:230.

24. Miller AB, Diamant M. Muscle damage and acute renal failure associated with heroin use. Med Ann DC 1972;41:571.

25. Rao TKS, Nicastri AD, Friedman EA. Renal consequences of narcotic abuse. Adv Nephrol 1978;7:261.

26. Gleich GJ, Mongan ES, Vaules DW. Esophageal stricture following chloral hydrate poisoning. JAMA 1967;201:266.

27. Veller ID, Richardson JP, Doyle JC, et al. Gastric necrosis: A rare complication of chloral hydrate intoxication. Br J Surg 1972;59:317.

28. Brunk BF, Delle M. Morphine metabolism in man. Clin Pharmacol Ther 1974;16:51.

29. Snyder SH. Drug and neurotransmitter receptors in the brain. Science 1984;224:22.

30. Martin WB. Pharmacology of opioids. Pharmacol Rev 1983;35:283.

31. Opioids/opioid antagonists. Poisondex, vol 63. Micromedex Inc, New York, 1990.

32. Iwamoto ET, Fudala PJ, Mundy WR. Opioids. *In* Ho IK (ed). Toxicology of CNS Depressants. Boca Raton, FL, CRC Press, 1987, p 145.

33. Bertino JS, Reed MD. Barbiturate and nonbarbiturate sedative-hypnotic intoxication in children. Pediatr Clin North Am 1986;33(3):703.

34. Harvey SC. Hypnotics and sedatives—the barbiturates. *In* Goodman LS, Gilman G (eds). The Pharmacological Basis of Therapeutics. 5th ed. New York, Macmillan, 1975, p 102.

35. Mark LC. Metabolism of barbiturates in man. Clin Pharmacol Ther 1963;4:504.

36. Arena JM. Poisoning: Toxicology-Symptoms-Treatments. 4th ed. Springfield, IL, Charles C Thomas, 1979, p 378.

37. Lehninger AL. Principles of Biochemistry. New York, Worth Publishers, 1982, p 78.

38. Chiu TH, Tietz EI, Rosenberg HC. Benzodiazepines. *In* Ho IK (ed). Toxicology of CNS Depressants. Boca Raton, FL, CRC Press, 1987, p 1.

39. Mohler H, Okata T. Benzodiazepine receptor: Demonstration in the central nervous system. Science 1977;198:849.

40. Shader RI, Greenblatt DJ. The use of benzodiazepines in clinical practice. Br J Clin Pharmacol 1981;11:55.

41. Hoskins B. Non barbiturate sedative-hypnotic agents. *In* Ho IK (ed). Toxicology of Depressants. Boca Raton, FL, CRC Press, 1987, p 57.

42. Kulberg A. Substance abuse: Clinical identification and management. Pediatr Clin North Am 1986;33:325.

43. Nass R. Rapid assessment of mental status in the infant and young child. Emerg Med Clin North Am 1987;5:739.

44. Teasdale G, Jennet B. Assessment of coma and impaired consciousness. Lancet 1974;2:81.

45. Simpson D, Reilly P. Pediatric coma scale. Lancet 1982;2:450.

46. Reed CF, Driggs MF, Foote CC. Acute barbiturate intoxication: A study of 300 cases based on a physiologic system of classification of the severity of the intoxication. Ann Intern Med 1952;37:290.

47. Bird TD, Plum F. Recovery from barbiturate overdose coma with a prolonged isoelectric encephalogram. Neurology 1968;18:456.

48. Corby DG, Decker WJ. Management of acute poisoning with activated charcoal. Pediatr 1974;54:324.

49. Levy G. Gastrointestinal clearance of drugs with activated charcoal. N Engl J Med 1982;307:676.

50. Picchioni AL. Activated charcoal: A neglected antidote. Pediatr Clin North Am 1970;17:535.

51. Picchioni AL. Activated charcoal products for medicinal (antidotal) use. Vet Hum Toxicol 1983;25:293.

52. Riegel JM, Becker CE. Use of cathartics in toxic ingestions. Ann Emerg Med 1981;10:254.

53. Handal KA, Schauben JL, Salamone FR. Naloxone. Ann Emerg Med 1983;12:438.

54. Rumack BH (ed). The Treatment of Poisoning: A Systemic Approach. Denver, Rocky Mountain Poison Center, 1978, p 326.

55. Moore RA, Rumack BH, Connor CS, et al. Naloxone: Underdosage after narcotic poisoning. Am J Dis Child 1980;134:156.

56. Stahl SM, Kasser IS. Pentazocine overdose. Ann Emerg Med 1983;12:28.

57. Tandberg ·D, Abercrombie D. Treatment of heroin overdose with endotracheal naloxone. Ann Emerg Med 1982;11:443.

58. Rosetti VA, Thompson BM, Miller J, et al. Intraosseous infusion: An alternative route of pediatric intravascular access. Ann Emerg Med 1985;14:885.

59. Maio RF, Gaukel B, Freeman B. Intralingual naloxone injection for narcotic induced respiratory depression. Ann Emerg Med 1987;16:572.

60. Wasserman CS, Green VA, Wise GW. Lomotil ingestions in children. Am Fam Phys 1975;11:93.

61. Curtis JA, Goel KM. Lomotil poisoning in children. Arch Dis Child 1979;54:222.

62. Rumack BH, Temple AP. Lomotil poisoning. Pediatrics 1974;53:495.

63. Mack RB. Toxic encounters of the dangerous kind. N C Med J 1981;42:858.

64. Mann JB, Sandberg DH. Therapy of sedative overdosage. Pediatr Clin North Am 1970;17:617.

65. Mawer GE, Lee HA. Value of forced diuresis in acute barbiturate poisoning. Br Med J 1968;2:790.

66. Lessen NA. Treatment of severe acute barbiturate poisoning by forced diuresis and alkalinization of the urine. Lancet 1960;2:338.

67. Smith DE, Wesson DA. A new method for treatment of barbiturate dependence. JAMA 1970;213:294.

68. Zawada ET Jr, Nappi J, Done G, Rollins D. Advances in the hemodialysis management of phenobarbital overdose. South Med J 1983;76:6.

69. DeBroe ME, Bismuth C, DeGroot G, et al. Haemoperfusion: A useful therapy for a severely poisoned patient. Hum Toxicol 1986;5:11.

70. Pond SM. Diuresis, dialysis and hemoperfusion. Emerg Med Clin North Am 1984;2:29.

71. Benzodiazepines. Poisondex, vol 63. Micromedex Inc, Denver, CO, 1990.

72. Haddad LM, Winchester JF. Clinical Management of Poisoning and Drug Overdose. Philadelphia, WB Saunders, 1983, p 475.

73. Kulig K, Rumack BH. Physostigmine and asystole. Ann Emerg Med 1981;10:228.

74. Kumer A, Motien MS, Amand NH. Aminophylline in neonatal diazepam intoxication. Ind Pediatr 1987;24:602.

75. Ashton CH. Benzodiazepine overdose: Are specific agonists useful? Br Med J 1985;290:805.

76. Hofer P, Scollo-Lavizzari G. Benzodiazepine antagonist RO 15–1788 in self poisoning. Diagnostic and therapeutic use. Arch Intern Med 1985;145:663.

77. Chloral hydrate. Poisondex, vol 63. Micromedex Inc, Denver, CO, 1990.

78. Bowyer K, Glasser S. Chloral hydrate overdose and cardiac arrhythmias. Chest 1980;77:232.

79. DiGiovanni A. Reversal of chloral hydrate associated cardiac arrhythmias by a beta-adrenergic blocking agent. Anesthesiology 1969;3:93.

80. Nordenberg A, Delisle G, Izukawa T. Cardiac arrhythmias in a child due to chloral hydrate ingestion. Pediatrics 1971;47:134.

81. Young JB, Vandermolen LA, Pratt CH. Torsades de pointes: An unusual manifestation of chloral hydrate poisoning. Am Heart J 1985;118:181.

82. Motil KJ. Peptic ulcer disease. *In* Oski FA, DeAngelis CD, Feigen RD. Pediatrics. Philadelphia, JB Lippincott, 1990, p 1693.

83. Heath A, Delin K, Eden E, et al. Hemoperfusion with Amberlite resin in the treatment of self-poisoning. Acta Med Scand 1980;207:455.

84. Vaziri ND, Kumar KP, Mirahmadi K, et al. Hemodialysis in the treatment of acute chloral hydrate poisoning. South Med J 1977;70:377.
85. Papadopoulou ZL, Novello AC. The use of hemoperfusion in children. Pediatr Clin North Am 1982;29:1039.
86. Mowry JB, Wilson GA. Effect of exchange transfusion in chloral hydrate overdose. Vet Hum Toxicol 1983;25(suppl):15.
87. Ethchlorvynol. Poisondex, vol 63. Micromedex Inc, Denver, CO, 1990.
88. Seyffart G. Ethchlorvynol. In Haddad LM, Winchester JF (eds). Clinical Management of Poisoning and Drug Overdose. Philadelphia, WB Saunders, 1983, p 516.
89. Benowitz N, Abolin C, Tozer T, et al. Resin hemoperfusion in ethchlorvynol overdose. Clin Pharmacol Ther 1980;27:236.
90. Due SL, Nagrawala I, Thompson A. Hemoperfusion with charcoal and resin cartridges. Ann Intern Med 1980;98:436.
91. Kathpalia SC, Haslitt JH, Lim VS. Charcoal hemoperfusion for treatment of ethchlorvynol overdose. Artif Organs 1983;7:248.
92. Hyde JB, Lawrence AG, Moles JB. Ethchlorvynol intoxication. Successful treatment by exchange transfusion and peritoneal dialysis. Clin Pediatr 1968;7:738.
93. Hansen AR, Kennedy KA, Ambre JJ, et al. Glutethimide poisoning: A metabolite contributes to morbidity and mortality. N Engl J Med 1975;292:250.
94. Orfanakis MG, Galloway WB. Glutethemide poisoning. Rock Mt Med J 1977;74:34.
95. Comstock EG. Glutethimide intoxication. JAMA 1971;215:1668.
96. Hayden JW, Comstod EG. Use of activated charcoal in acute poisoning. Clin Toxicol 1975;8:515.
97. Glutethimide. Poisondex, vol 63. Micromedex Inc, Denver, CO, 1990.
98. Seyffart G. Glutethimide. In Haddad IM, Winchester JF (eds). Clinical Management of Poisoning and Drug Overdose. Philadelphia, WB Saunders, 1983, p 531.
99. Schwartz HS. Acute meprobamate poisoning with gastrotomy and removal of a drug containing mass. N Engl J Med 1976;295:1177.
100. North DS. Meprobamate and bezoar formation. Letter. Ann Emerg Med 1987;16:471.
101. North DS, Krenzolek EP. Death associated with an acute meprobamate ingestion. Vet Hum Toxicol 1982;24(suppl):79.
102. Hassan E. Treatment of meprobamate overdose with repeated oral doses of activated charcoal. Ann Emerg Med 1986;15:73.
103. Meprobamate. Poisondex, vol 63. Micromedex Inc, Denver, CO, 1990.
104. Dennison J, Edwards JN, Volene GN. Meprobamate overdosage. Hum Toxicol 1985;4:215.
105. Maddock RK, Bloomer HA. Meprobamate overdosage: Evaluation of its severity and methods of treatment. JAMA 1967;201:99.
106. Methaqualone. Poisondex, vol 63. Micromedex Inc, Denver, CO, 1990.
107. Baggish D, Grey B, Jetlow P, et al. Treatment of methaqualone overdose with resin hemoperfusion. Yale J Biol Med 1981;54:147.
108. Paraldehyde. Poisondex, vol 63. Micromedex Inc, Denver, CO, 1990.
109. Burstein OL. The hazard of paraldehyde administration. JAMA 1943;110:187.
110. Hayward JN, Boshell BR. Paraldehyde intoxication with metabolic acidosis. Am J Med 1957;23:965.
111. Beier LS, Pitt WH, Gonick HC. Metabolic acidosis occurring during paraldehyde intoxication. Ann Intern Med 1963;58:155.
112. George JE. Law and Emergency Care. St Louis, CV Mosby, 1980, pp 35, 151, 179.

CHAPTER 92

Cocaine

Martin Harris

INTRODUCTION

Estimates based on a national survey on drug abuse indicate that there are 6 million current cocaine users in the United States and that some 22 million persons have admitted to trying cocaine.[1] Reports concerning complications of exposure to cocaine in the pediatric population generally reveal a bimodal distribution—neonates and young infants at one peak and adolescents at the other.[2] Estimates from various urban centers report that 10% to 15% of pregnant mothers use cocaine during pregnancy, and complications of transplacental exposure have become apparent.[2, 3] Infants and neonates have also been exposed through breast milk, and both accidental and intentional environmental exposures have been reported.[2, 4–6] At the other end of the pediatric spectrum, according to a recent National Institute on Drug Abuse (NIDA) survey, 50% of high school seniors view cocaine as readily available, 15.2% report that they have tried cocaine, and 0.8% report cocaine dependency.[7, 8] It is likely that 1 million adolescents have tried cocaine and that 400,000 others are current users, having tried cocaine in the previous month.[9] Cocaine abuse among adolescents begins early; 5% of eighth graders and 10% of tenth graders report having tried cocaine. In those adolescents identified as cocaine dependent, 21% report having tried cocaine by age 14.[10] According to data from the Drug Abuse Warning Network (DAWN), since 1986 cocaine has become the most frequent cause of drug-related emergency department visits, surpassing both ethanol and narcotics, with over 62,000 visits reported in cooperating facilities in 1989 alone. In addition, some 4200 of those visits involved patients 6 to 19 years old. During the last decade there has been a threefold increase in deaths related to cocaine abuse.

PHARMACOLOGY

Cocaine is a benzoic acid ester with an amino acid base. It is highly water and lipid soluble, is readily absorbed by all mucous membranes, and crosses the placenta by simple diffusion.[3, 11] Cocaine has two fundamental properties. By blocking the sodium channel and inhibiting the depolarizing sodium current, cocaine acts as a highly efficacious anesthetic that limits its own absorption by producing vasoconstriction.[11–14] In addition, through complex effects on dopamine, serotonin, and norepinephrine, cocaine is a centrally acting euphoriant with sympathomimetic properties. Initially cocaine stimulates release of dopamine and norepinephrine and blocks reuptake, resulting in acutely increased synaptic concentrations in the central and peripheral nervous system. The effect of cocaine on the inhibitory serotoninergic system is more complex. Generally production of serotonin is decreased by inhibiting uptake of its precursor tryptophan and inhibiting the enzyme tryptophan hydroxylase used in its production.[9, 15, 16] It is believed that dopaminergic system activation and serotonin inhibition are responsible for the euphoriant effects of cocaine. Dopaminergic system activation is critical in maintaining self-administrative and positive reinforcement behaviors.[7, 9, 13, 17] Activation of postsynaptic receptors by norepinephrine results in the adrenergic effects of cocaine, including tremor, mydriasis, tachycardia, and elevated blood pressure. Chronic cocaine use eventually results in depletion of dopamine, norepinephrine, and serotonin, as well as in increased neuroreceptor density and receptor supersensitivity, which may be responsible for the withdrawal symptoms and drug craving associated with its use.[15, 16]

Cocaine exists in multiple forms, including a paste, a powder (cocaine hydrochloride), and a free base alkaloid also known as "crack." The paste is smoked with tobacco or marijuana, and its use is generally confined to South America. Cocaine hydrochloride is a water-soluble, colorless, odorless, flaky powder that is injected intravenously as a solution or insufflated intranasally. The pharmacokinetics of cocaine vary widely from subject to subject and depend on the dose and route of administration.[3, 18–20] Intravenous use results in the onset of physiologic and subjective effects within minutes, with a duration of less than 60 minutes.[3, 18] Intravenous cocaine is often used with an opioid to decrease side effects; opioids are commonly found at autopsy after intravenous cocaine deaths.[3, 21, 22] Intranasal insufflation of cocaine results in a slightly delayed onset of symptoms (5 to 10 minutes) and a prolonged duration of action of approximately 90 minutes.[23] Cocaine powder is commonly adulterated with a number of substances during illicit distribution, which leads to unpredictable toxicity. Sugars, including mannitol and lactose, stimulants such as caffeine and amphetamine, local anesthetics, including benzocaine, procaine, and lidocaine, and toxins such as strychnine and quinine have all been isolated.[24, 25] Smoking free base or crack cocaine results in the most intense cocaine "highs." Its rapid onset of action, within seconds, is coupled with a brief duration of action, approximately 15 minutes.[11] In addition, at 70% pure cocaine, crack is relatively less contaminated with street adulterants. These factors, coupled with a relatively low cost—about $10 for each high—have resulted in an epidemic of cocaine use. Though morbidity can result regardless of route of administration, crack appears to be more rapidly addicting, associated with more complications, and abused by younger individuals than is cocaine powder.[7, 12, 26]

Reported routes of administration in infants and neonates include transplacental diffusion, transfer through breast milk, and exposure from the breast skin itself on which cocaine has been applied topically as an anesthetic for nipple soreness. Cocaine may remain in breast milk up to 60 hours after the mother's last use.[4, 27] Accidental cocaine ingestion, as well as passive crack smoke inhalation, by infants and toddlers present during heavy use by caregivers has been reported.[5] Cocaine has also been actively administered as a form of child abuse.

Cocaine is primarily metabolized by plasma cholinesterases in the blood and liver to the inactive metabolites benzoylecognine and ecgonine methyl ester, which are excreted in the urine.[3, 9, 28] A small amount, 2% to 6%, is metabolized in the liver to the active metabolite norcocaine. Plasma cholinesterase activity is relatively diminished in pregnant women, the fetus, and the neonate, resulting in prolonged detectable levels of 4 to 7 days in neonatal urine and possible prolonged effects in the newborn.[19, 27, 29–31]

Thin-layer chromatography and enzyme immunoassay are frequently used as screening methods, with confirmation done by gas chromatography or mass spectroscopy. Cocaine metabolites are readily detected 48 hours after a single use and may be detected up to 3 weeks after last use in long-term heavy users.[3, 32]

CLINICAL EVALUATION
Perinatal Effects

Along with the increase in cocaine use in the general population has been an increase in its use by pregnant women.[2, 33–36] Cocaine exposure in laboratory animals is associated with maternal hypertension, decreased uterine blood flow, and uteroplacental insufficiency, resulting in fetal hypoxemia, hypertension, and tachycardia.[33, 35] These effects are theoretically associated with the reported increase in spontaneous abortion in the first trimester in women who abuse cocaine, as well as with placental abruption and stillbirth in the third trimester. Maternal cocaine use has also been associated with increased rates of intrauterine growth retardation, low birth weight, and preterm delivery.[29, 31, 35–38] Congenital abnormalities have been reported in children born to cocaine-abusing mothers, including urogenital anomalies,[34] microcephalgia and other central nervous system abnormalities,[31, 39, 40] and retinal abnormalities.[41] The

exact teratogenic potential of cocaine remains unclear.[9, 35, 42] Newborns exposed in utero exhibit increased irritability, tremulousness, hypertonicity, brisk deep tendon reflexes, and abnormal sleep patterns.[36, 43, 44] Approximately 45% of newborns exposed to cocaine antenatally will have abnormal electroencephalograms in the first week.[44]

Infants exposed to cocaine in utero have been reported to have depressed interactive abilities and significant impairment in organizational ability as measured by the Brazelton score.[17] These symptoms are thought to be direct drug effects. This view is substantiated by prolonged detection of cocaine metabolites in neonates, although a neonatal withdrawal syndrome has not been entirely excluded.[17] Neurobehavioral abnormalities in the newborn are usually self-limited and rarely require treatment.[44] The long-term neurobehavioral consequences of intrauterine exposure to cocaine remain unknown.

Conflicting information exists as to the risk of sudden infant death syndrome (SIDS) in neonates after intrauterine exposure to cocaine. Cocaine exposure has been reported to increase the risk of SIDS by up to a factor of 10.[36, 45] Conversely, a recent large prospective study has failed to substantiate any increased risk of SIDS in infants exposed to cocaine in utero.[46]

Pulmonary Effects

Pulmonary dysfunction is common in cocaine smokers. Cough productive of black or bloody sputum and shortness of breath are frequently noted.[47] A syndrome known as "crack lung," resulting in fever, bronchospasm, pulmonary infiltrates, and eosinophilia, has been described.[48] Pneumomediastinum, pneumopericardium, and pneumothorax presumably secondary to Valsalva's maneuver or mouth-to-mouth cocaine vapor exchange used to increase drug absorption have been reported.[47, 49] Pulmonary gas exchange abnormality as indicated by diminished carbon monoxide diffusing capacity has been documented even after brief periods of cocaine alkaloid abuse.[47] Cardiogenic and noncardiogenic pulmonary edema have been reported, and pulmonary edema is frequently found at autopsy following fatal cocaine overdose.[22, 50, 51]

Cardiovascular Effects

Cocaine's major pathophysiologic effect on the cardiovascular system appears to be secondary to blocking the reuptake of norepinephrine, resulting in activation of sympathetic neurons. A direct cardiotoxic effect has been postulated but has yet to be confirmed. At doses typically used by cocaine abusers, stimulation of postsynaptic alpha receptors and beta$_1$ cardiac receptors results in increased heart rate, myocardial contractility, peripheral vascular resistance, coronary vascular resistance, and automaticity. After insufflation of 100 mg of cocaine, systolic blood pressure increases by approximately 20 mm Hg and heart rate increases by 20 beats/minute. Intravenous injection of cocaine hydrochloride or inhalation of cocaine alkaloid or free base can produce an increase in systolic blood pressure of 25 mm Hg and an increase in heart rate of approximately 30 beats/minute.[52] Although such effects undoubtedly result in increased myocardial oxygen demand, cocaine use is attended by a loss of autoregulation and an inappropriate increase in coronary vascular resistance, decreased coronary sinus blood flow, and diffuse coronary artery vasoconstriction.[53, 54] Myocardial infarction constitutes the primary cardiovascular complication of cocaine abuse. Angiography in many cases has revealed no coronary vascular abnormality. In many cases ergonovine challenge failed to provoke coronary spasm.[55-58] Increased myocardial oxygen demand and generalized reduction in coronary blood flow, possibly coupled with areas of focal vasoconstriction, may be sufficient to result in myocardial ischemia and infarction. Such effects would be expected to be especially deleterious to those with preexisting coronary vascular disease, yet myocardial infarction has been reported in patients as young as 16 years of age and in those with no evidence of preexisting heart disease.[14, 55, 56, 58] Cardiac complications are not related to the route of administration of cocaine and are not limited to massive overdoses of this drug.

Cardiac arrhythmias, including asystole, accelerated idioventricular rhythm, ventricular tachycardia, ventricular fibrillation, and sudden cardiac death associated with cocaine use, have been reported.[56, 59, 60] The contribution of ischemia, hyperthermia, and acidosis to the generation of these arrhythmias is probably considerable; however, the exact arrhythmogenic potential of cocaine remains unclear.

Cardiomyopathy as a result of multiple ischemic events has been reported as a consequence of cocaine abuse.[56, 61] A case of acute reversible "toxic" cardiomyopathy secondary to prolonged crack smoking has been reported.[62] This cardiomyopathy exhibited similarities to that which results from prolonged exposure to excessive levels of catecholamines, as seen in patients with pheochromocytoma. "Contraction band necrosis," a common biopsy finding in toxic cardiomyopathy from high levels of catecholamines, has been reported at biopsy and postmortem examination of cocaine abusers.[62]

Neurologic Effects

The acute neurologic complications of cocaine abuse constitute a major cause of morbidity and mortality. Many neuropsychiatric sequelae have been reported, including headache, confusion, psychosis, dystonic reaction, transient ischemic attacks, stroke, and convulsions.[63, 64] Seizures are frequently reported in both first-time and chronic users. Seizures are usually single, generalized, tonic-clonic, and of short duration, although status epilepticus and complex partial seizures have been reported.[64, 65] Prolonged, generalized convulsions appear to be a frequent preterminal event in adult cocaine abusers and are perhaps the most serious of the noncardiac complications of cocaine abuse.[64, 66] Tonic-clonic seizures have been reported as the presenting symptom in infants and toddlers with unsuspected cocaine ingestions.[6] Seizures in infants have also been reported after passive inhalation of crack smoke and after direct ingestion of cocaine used as an anesthetic for nipple soreness.[4, 5]

Adolescents may be more susceptible to development of seizures subsequent to heavy cocaine use than other age groups.[67] Cocaine lowers the seizure threshold, and the convulsant properties may be due to anesthetic effects similar to those of lidocaine.[12, 68] There is no pattern of abuse or route of administration of cocaine that may predispose a person to develop seizures or any other neurologic complication associated with its use.

A multitude of transient neurologic deficits have been reported, including sudden loss of consciousness, hemiparesis, paresthesias, aphasia, dizziness, vertigo, and ataxia.[64] The etiology of these events is unclear and probably multifactorial, including direct vasospasm, thrombosis, and hypotension associated with decreased cardiac output secondary to cardiac ischemia or arrhythmias.

Hemorrhagic and ischemic stroke are devastating complications associated with cocaine use. Intraventricular, intraparenchymal, and subarachnoid hemorrhage, as well as ischemic stroke involving nearly every vascular region of the brain and spinal cord, has been reported.[12, 69-74] Hemorrhage appears to occur with much greater frequency in cocaine-induced strokes than in strokes found in the general population; however, the incidence of ischemic stroke from cocaine may be underreported.[69, 70, 72, 75] The incidence of cocaine-induced stroke was found to be highest in young patients. It occurs most commonly in the third decade and decreases in each subsequent decade, which is a marked contrast to the incidence of stroke in the general population.[70]

Perinatal cerebral hemorrhage, hemorrhagic infarction, and ischemic infarction have all been reported in full-term infants born to cocaine-abusing mothers.[30, 74] An ultrasound study found that 39% of neonates exposed to cocaine antenatally had major brain abnormalities at birth, including hemorrhage and hemorrhagic infarctions, most of which occurred in neonatally "silent areas" of the brain.[76] Acute neurologic sequelae may also occur regardless of the route of administration of cocaine.[70] The etiology of stroke resulting from cocaine abuse, although unproved, most likely relates to its sympathomimetic effects. Transient hypertensive episodes may result in hemorrhage from previously existing vascular abnormalities. In patients with cerebral hemorrhage subsequent to cocaine exposure, occult aneurysms or arteriovenous malformations are frequently found.[12, 69, 70] Interestingly, 67% of those examined angiographically after an acute neurologic episode exhibited no detectable vascular abnormalities.[69] Spontaneous hemorrhage from normal intracerebral vessels is thought to occur as a consequence of exposure to cocaine.[70] Cerebral vasoconstriction secondary to increased levels of dopamine and norepinephrine, similar to that which occurs in the coronary vessels, may also contribute to the pathogenesis of cocaine-induced stroke. Cocaine also increases platelet aggregation through alterations in thromboxane production, although the contribution of increased platelet aggregation to cocaine-induced stroke is unknown.[77] Biopsy-proved vasculitis of small cerebral vessels has been reported as a consequence of crack smoking.[78] This vasculitis is not thought to contribute greatly to acute neurologic sequelae of cocaine use.[69, 78]

Psychological Effects

Acute alterations in mental status constitute the single most common reason for presentation to the emergency department following cocaine abuse, constituting about 30% of all such visits.[79] Use of small amounts of cocaine results in early central nervous system stimulation, characterized by euphoria, increased motor activity, enhanced feelings of self-esteem and self-confidence, emotional lability, and insomnia.[9, 16, 80] Continued use results in cocaine dysphoria, possibly as a result of dopamine depletion and neuroreceptor changes.[15, 16] Depression, apathy, agitation, social withdrawal, and suicidal ideation are hallmarks of this phase of cocaine abuse. Depression may also result from acute cocaine abstinence, particularly in the "crash" that follows a cocaine binge.[80] Depression is the reason most commonly related to hospital presentation in adolescents subsequently found to be positive for cocaine on drug abuse screens.[2] As cocaine abuse continues, a syndrome similar to paranoid schizophrenia may develop. Marked agitation, psychosis, paranoia, violent behavior, and hallucinations have all occurred. An acute syndrome of "agitated delirium," characterized by acute uncontrollable violent behavior and excessive strength, has been described in fatal cocaine intoxications.[81]

Other Considerations

Hyperpyrexia contributes significantly to the mortality associated with cocaine abuse. Hyperthermia is directly associated with death from cocaine, and hypothermia alone is sufficient to prevent death in some cases.[66] Cocaine's propensity to produce hyperpyrexia is well documented.[82, 83] The resetting of hypothalamic thermoregulatory centers by alterations in dopamine and its receptors and vasoconstriction resulting in diminished heat loss contribute to hyperthermia. Marked muscle activity, associated with agitative, combative behavior or convulsions, may also be responsible for heat generation. Hyperpyrexia, increased muscle activity, and possibly vasoconstriction resulting in muscle necrosis may cause rhabdomyolysis, myoglobinuria, and subsequent renal failure. Rhabdomyolysis presenting with back, flank, extremity, and chest pain mimicking myocardial infarction has been reported as a consequence of cocaine use.[83] Stimulation of central dopaminergic receptors followed by acute withdrawal may result in muscle destruction similar to that found in the neuroleptic malignant syndrome.[83, 84]

EMS CONSIDERATIONS

Prehospital personnel may be called on to deal with an agitated, delirious patient who is uncontrollably violent and who may suddenly convulse or develop apnea and cardiac arrest. In addition, struggling with such patients may aggravate hyperpyrexia and acidosis, further complicating an already grave situation. Patients should be transported in as controlled a manner as possible with careful attention to the possibility of sudden cardiopulmonary arrest and the need to establish and maintain a stable airway. Sudden convulsion is always a possibility in cocaine-intoxicated patients, and adequate precautions must be maintained. The potential for myocardial ischemia and infarction mandates cardiac monitoring and administration of supplemental oxygen. Intravenous access should be obtained, and agitation may be treated with careful administration of a titratable intravenous or intramuscular benzodiazepine (diazepam or midazolam). Chest pain suggestive of myocardial ischemia may be treated with sublingual nitroglycerin. Immediate cooling should begin during transport if hyperpyrexia is identified.

DIAGNOSTIC EVALUATION

The diagnosis of acute cocaine intoxication generally depends on the findings of sympathetic and central nervous system stimulation coupled with a history of cocaine use. Tachycardia, hypertension, mydriasis, tremor, diaphoresis, increased body temperature, agitation, and paranoia give rise to acidosis, cardiac ischemia, seizures, pulmonary edema, and death. Diagnosis is confirmed by laboratory analysis consisting of the identification of cocaine and its metabolites from a qualitative urine assay. Blood concentrations at death average 6.2 mg/L but exhibit a wide range, from 0.1 to 20.9 mg/L, and are independent of the route of administration.[22] The rate of increase of drug level rather than the absolute level of cocaine may be the most important factor in determining the lethality, although many lethal idiosyncratic reactions occur.[18, 85] Acute cocaine intoxication may result in several different clinicopathologic presentations, each requiring extensive evaluation. Acute chest pain in the setting of cocaine use requires cardiac monitoring for cardiac arrhythmias and serial serum creatinine kinase (CK) measurements with MB isoenzyme fractionation to exclude myocardial infarction. Serum CK may be markedly elevated with rhabdomyolysis, which can present with acute chest pain.

A chest radiograph must be performed in all patients presenting to the emergency department with chest pain to exclude pneumothorax, pneumopericardium, and pneumomediastinum. Pulmonary infiltrates may be found in the setting of "crack lung." Abdominal radiographs may be performed in those suspected of ingesting packets of cocaine

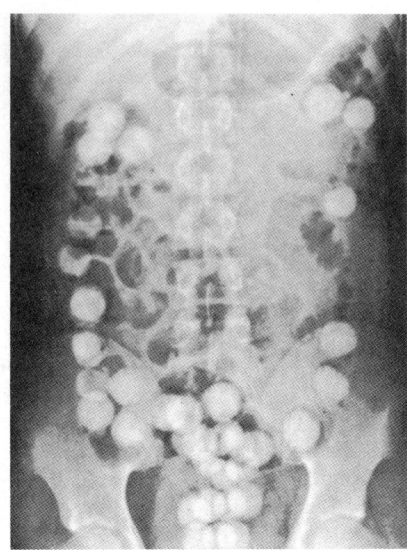

Figure 92–1. Abdominal radiograph shows radiopaque cocaine packages. (From McCarron MM, Wood JD. The cocaine "body packer" syndrome. JAMA 1983;250:1418. Copyright 1983, American Medical Association.)

or "body packing" (performed by cocaine smugglers) (Fig. 92–1). Generally these packets appear as rounded or sausage-shaped densities with an occasional air interface, although a negative radiograph does exclude gastrointestinal packing of cocaine.[86] Any patient presenting with persistent headache, seizure, or focal neurologic deficits must have a full neurologic evaluation, including computed tomography scan and lumbar puncture, to exclude intracranial hemorrhage and infarction. The serum glucose should be measured to exclude hypoglycemia as a cause of symptoms. A complete blood count may show a nonspecific leukocytosis.

DIFFERENTIAL DIAGNOSIS

The differential diagnosis of acute cocaine intoxication is broad and includes several medical conditions, acute psychiatric illness, and intoxication from other drugs with primary sympathomimetic effects (Table 92–1). Generalized sepsis and infection of the central nervous system, including meningitis and encephalitis, may present with fever, tachycardia, confusion, and seizures, quite similar to presentation with cocaine poisoning. Acute cocaine intoxication should be excluded in any child in whom the diagnosis of "benign" febrile convulsion is considered. Heat-related illness and heat stroke, thyrotoxicosis, and acute hypertensive emergencies with hypertensive encephalopathy from pheochromocytoma may present in a manner similar to that of cocaine poisoning. Acute intoxication from many stimulants, includ-

TABLE 92–1	
DIFFERENTIAL DIAGNOSIS OF ACUTE COCAINE INTOXICATION	
Medical Illness	**Drug Related**
Sepsis	Amphetamines
Meningitis	Anticholinergics
Heat-related illness	Caffeine
Thyrotoxicosis	Phenylpropranolamine
Pheochromocytoma	Phencyclidine
	Ethanol withdrawal
Psychiatric Illness	
Acute paranoid schizophrenia	
Acute mania	

ing caffeine, phenylpropanolamine, and amphetamines, produces a symptom complex similar to that of cocaine intoxication but generally produces symptoms for a duration longer than those normally expected from cocaine. Phencyclidine (PCP) poisoning may also present in a similar manner but is distinguished by marked horizontal and vertical nystagmus. Dry flushed skin, fixed and dilated pupils, and decreased or absent bowel sounds help to distinguish anticholinergic poisoning from that of cocaine. Withdrawal from ethanol may produce tachycardia, hypertension, seizures, and hallucinations, similar to the effects of cocaine intoxication. The differential diagnosis of cocaine poisoning is further clouded in that cocaine is frequently used with other drugs such as ethanol, marijuana, or opiates and is commonly diluted with adulterants such as anesthetics and stimulants, which may alter its presentation and therapy.

THERAPEUTIC INTERVENTION

Cocaine is rapidly absorbed from all mucous membranes and rapidly metabolized in patients with normal plasma cholinesterase activity, and symptoms are relatively short-lived. Decontamination from nasal mucosa may be accomplished with a petroleum-covered cotton-tipped applicator. Flushing the nose with water is not recommended since solubilization of cocaine and increased absorption may occur.[3] Except in the cases of massive packet or vial ingestion to prevent police arrest, or in "body packers" who ingest cocaine-filled condoms or latex bags during smuggling attempts, gastrointestinal decontamination is not indicated. In cases of body packing, psyllium hydrophilic mucilloid, repeated doses of activated charcoal with 20% sorbitol, or whole bowel irrigation with GoLYTELY solution orally or through a nasogastric tube should be administered to facilitate gastrointestinal passage.[85, 86] Because of the risk of seizures, ipecac should be avoided. Patients must be monitored closely until all material has passed. Any overt sign of toxicity or bowel obstruction may require emergency laparotomy.[51, 85, 86]

Patients presenting with signs of mild intoxication such as agitation and dysphoria, with no evidence of end-organ involvement, may be treated with simple reassurance and observation, preferably in a quiet environment, until symptoms subside. Occasionally intravenous sedation may be required. Careful titration of intravenous doses of diazepam, 0.1 to 0.2 mg/kg over 3 to 5 minutes, may be used to treat agitation (Table 92–2). Midazolam, 0.08 to 0.3 mg/kg, is rapidly absorbed (within 5 minutes) after intramuscular administration and may offer an alternative in patients in whom it is impossible to establish intravenous access.[51] Haloperidol, 0.01 to 0.03 mg/kg as an intramuscular or intravenous dose, may be effective in treating acute hallucinosis and psychosis. Chlorpromazine and other phenothiazines may lower the seizure threshold and should be avoided until of proven benefit.

Diazepam is also effective in treating symptoms resulting from cocaine-induced hyperadrenergic states. Mild hypertension and tachycardia should be treated with careful titration of intravenous diazepam. Controversy exists over the role of propranolol in treating hypertension secondary to cocaine, which is unresponsive to diazepam. Although recommended as therapy for cocaine-induced hypertension,[87] at least one case of hypertensive emergency requiring nitroprusside administration has been reported after beta blockade to treat cocaine toxicity resulted in unopposed alpha-adrenergic stimulation.[88] Combined alpha and beta blockade with labetalol has been recommended as the treatment of choice for hypertensive emergencies resulting from cocaine abuse.[85, 89, 90] Supraventricular tachycardias unresponsive to diazepam should be treated with parenteral beta blockade with propranolol (0.01 mg/kg/dose, maximum 1 mg) or combined alpha and beta blockade with labetalol. The short-acting beta blocker esmolol has theoretical advantages for treatment of cocaine-induced supraventricular tachyarrhythmias, but these potential benefits remain unproved.[51, 85]

Ventricular tachycardia secondary to cocaine abuse should be treated with phenytoin. Lidocaine is theoretically ineffective, may aggravate seizures,[12] and has been shown to increase significantly overall cocaine toxicity in laboratory rats.[91, 92]

Because coronary artery constriction and decreased coronary blood flow are thought to occur in the setting of cocaine-

TABLE 92–2		
THERAPY AT A GLANCE		
Mild Intoxication		
Agitation, mild hypertension, mild tachycardia	Diazepam	0.1–0.2 mg/kg IV slowly every 3–5 minutes up to 5 mg
	Midazolam	0.08–0.2 mg/kg IM*
Severe Intoxication		
Psychosis	Haloperidol	2–5 mg IM q 1–8 hr (adult) as needed 0.25-mg dose IM then 0.01–0.03-mg/ kg dose IM q 2 hr*
Supraventricular tachyarrhythmia	Propranolol	0.01 mg/kg 1 dose, max. 1 mg
	Esmolol	500 mg/kg/min ×1 min followed by constant infusion 50–100 mg/kg/ min*
Hypertension	Labatelol	20 mg (0.25 mg/kg) slow IV push over 2–5 min followed by 40 or 80 mg at 10-min intervals, max. 300 mg*
Seizures	Diazepam	0.1–0.2 mg/kg IV slowly every 3–5 min up to 5 mg
	Phenobarbital	10–20 mg/kg IV
	Phenytoin	10–15 mg/kg IV
	Thiopental, general anesthesia	
Hypothermia (malignant)	Evaporative cooling Dantralone 1 mg/kg	

*Safe and effective doses in children not established.

induced myocardial ischemia, sublingual and intravenous nitroglycerin should be used in the setting of acute unstable angina or suspected myocardial infarction due to cocaine abuse.[85, 91, 93] Documented myocardial infarction should be treated with thrombolysis.[55, 85] One study[54] demonstrated that alpha-adrenergic blockade in the cardiac catheterization laboratory with intracoronary phentolamine (0.4 mg/minute for a total dose of 2 mg) was highly effective in alleviating cocaine-induced vasoconstriction. Clinical applicability of phentolamine treatment to the setting of acute cocaine-induced cardiac disease has yet to be demonstrated.

Treatment of seizures should be empiric and based on presentation.[66, 68] In a study in dogs, pretreatment with diazepam prevented hyperthermia, acidosis, seizures, and death in animals administered cocaine. Barbiturates are effective in treating cocaine-induced seizures, but phenytoin is reported to be ineffective in laboratory animals.[12] Although controlling seizures and hyperpyrexia is of utmost importance in treating patients with acute cocaine poisoning,[66, 68] a single uncomplicated seizure in a nonintoxicated patient requires only observation; no further treatment is indicated if other possible causes of convulsion have been excluded. Patients with a prolonged convulsion or severe intoxication require aggressive management. Seizure control begins with diazepam and may be followed with phenytoin (10 to 15 mg/kg) or phenobarbital (10 to 20 mg/kg), although phenobarbital should be used in the setting of status epilepticus. If seizures prove refractory to this treatment, general anesthesia with thiopental or pentobarbital should be initiated.[12, 51, 85]

Hyperpyrexia should be managed by immediate attempts to lower body temperature. It contributes to brain injury and rhabdomyolysis and has a direct correlation to cocaine lethality in laboratory animals.[66] Evaporative cooling measures should be initiated upon recognition of hyperpyrexia, although cooling blankets and ice packs to axilla and groin may be helpful.[82, 85] Dantrolene (1 mg/kg) should be considered in patients who fail to respond to normal cooling measures.[83, 85] Rhabdomyolysis and myoglobinuric renal failure may be prevented with aggressive intravenous fluid administration, maintenance of adequate urine output, and rapid control of seizures and hyperpyrexia.

DISPOSITION

Patients manifesting signs of uncomplicated mild cocaine intoxication may be discharged after a period of observation in the emergency department (Table 92–3). Usually symptoms resolve and vital signs return to normal within 6 to 8 hours. Toddlers with accidental oral ingestion of cocaine warrant a prolonged period of observation because of delayed onset of symptoms after ingestion.[18] Cocaine is extremely addicting, and depression, chronic anxiety, paranoia, and sleep disorders are common manifestations of chronic cocaine abuse in adolescents.[9] Early psychiatric evaluation and close outpatient treatment is indicated. In cases of severe psychosocial dysfunction, inpatient treatment is warranted. A critical care setting is indicated for any patient

with manifestations of severe cocaine intoxication, including hyperthermia, acidosis, cardiac arrhythmias, status epilepticus, or chest pain suggestive of cardiac ischemia.

References

1. NIDA National Household Survey on Drug Abuse: Population estimates 1985. Rockville MD, DHHS Pub No (ADM) 1987;87–1539.
2. Shannon M, Lacouture P. Cocaine exposure among children seen at a pediatric hospital. Pediatrics 1989;83:337.
3. Mofenson H, Caraccio T. Cocaine. Pediatr Ann 1987;16:864.
4. Chandy N, Franks J, Wadlington W. Cocaine convulsions in a breast feeding baby. J Pediatr 1988;112:134.
5. Bateman D, Heagarty M. Passive freebase cocaine inhalation by infants and toddlers. Am J Dis Child 1989;143:25.
6. Ernst A, Sanders W. Unexpected cocaine intoxication presenting as seizures in children. Ann Emerg Med 1989;18:774.
7. NIDA Monograph Series: Mechanisms of cocaine abuse and toxicity (preface). Rockville MD, DHHS Pub No. (ADM) 1988;88-1585.
8. Johnston L, O'Malley P, Bachman J. National trends in drug use and related factors among American high school students and young adults, 1975–1986. Rockville, MD, NIDA, 1987.
9. Krug S. Cocaine abuse: Historical, epidemiologic and clinical perspectives for pediatricians. Adv Pediatr 1989;36:369.
10. Smith D, Schwartz R, Martin D. Heavy cocaine use by adolescents. Pediatrics 1989;83:539.
11. Jaffe J. Drug addiction and drug abuse. In Goodman LS, Gilman A (eds). The Pharmacologic Basis of Therapeutics. 8th ed. New York, Pergamon Press, 1990, pp 539–545.
12. Ritchie J, Greene N. Local anesthetics. In Goodman LS, Gilman A (eds). The Pharmacologic Basis of Therapeutics. 8th ed. New York, Pergamon Press, 1990, pp 319–320.
13. Grinspoon L, Bakalar JB. Drug dependence: Non-narcotic agents. In Kaplan HI, Freedman AM, Sadock BJ (eds). Comprehensive Textbook of Psychiatry. 3rd ed. Baltimore, William & Wilkins, 1980, p 13.
14. Mathias D. Cocaine associated myocardial ischemias. Am J Med 1986;81:675.
15. Daigle R, Clark H, Landry M. A primer on neurotransmitters and cocaine. J Psychoactive Drugs 1988;20:283.
16. Gawin F, Kleber H. Evolving conceptualizations of cocaine dependence. Yale J Biol Med 1988;61:123.
17. Dewit R, Wise R. Blockade of cocaine reinforcement in rats with the dopamine reception pimozide, but not with the noradrenergic blockers phentolamine or phenoxybenzamine. Can J Psychol 1977;31:195.
18. Van Dyke C, Byck R. Cocaine. Sci Am 1982;246:128.
19. Van Dyke C, Barash P, Jatlow P, et al. Plasma concentration after intranasal application. Science 1976;191:859.
20. Gawin F, Ellinwood E. Cocaine and other stimulants: Actions, abuse, and treatment. N Engl J Med 1988;318:1173.
21. NIDA Statistical Series: Data from the drug abuse warning network, annual data 1988. Washington DC, DHHS, Pub. No. (ADM) 1989;89-1634.
22. Mittleman R, Welti C. Death caused by recreational cocaine use. JAMA 1984;252:1889.
23. Javaid J, Fischman M, Schuster C, et al. Cocaine plasma concentration: Relation to physiological and subjective effects in humans. Science 1978;202:227.
24. Shannon M. Clinical toxity of cocaine adulterants. Ann Emerg Med 1988;17:1243.
25. Krenzelok E. Cocaine: Unusual aspects of acute exposure. Clinical Tox Forum 1989;1:1.
26. Gold M. Crack abuse: Its implications and outcomes. Resident and Staff Physician 1987;33:45.
27. Chasnoff I. Perinatal effects of cocaine. Contemp OB/GYN 1987; May:163.
28. Inaba T, Stewart D, Kalon W. Metabolism of cocaine in man. Clin Pharmacol Ther 1978;23:547.
29. Oro A, Dixon S. Perinatal cocaine and methamphetamine exposure: Maternal and neonatal correlates. J Pediatr 1987;111:571.
30. Chasnoff, I Bussey M, Savich R, et al. Perinatal cerebrum infarction and maternal cocaine use. J Pediatr 1986;108:456.
31. Bingol N, Fuchs M, Diaz V, et al. Teratogenicity of cocaine in humans. J Pediatr 1987;110:93.
32. Weiss R. Protracted elimination of cocaine metabolites in long term high dose cocaine abusers. Am J Med 1988;85:879.
33. Woods J, Plessinger M, Clark K. Effects of cocaine on uterine blood flow and fetal oxygenation. JAMA 1987;257:957.
34. Chavez G, Mulinare J, Cordero J. Maternal cocaine use during early pregnancy as a risk factor for congenital urogenital anomalies. JAMA 1989;262:795.
35. MacGregor S, Keith L, Chasnoff I, et al. Cocaine use during pregnancy: Adverse perinatal outcome. Am J Obstet Gynecol 1987;157:686.
36. Chasnoff I, Burns W, Schnoll S, et al. Cocaine use in pregnancy. N Engl J Med 1985;313:666.

TABLE 92–3
DISPOSITION

Mild intoxication	Close observation
	Psychiatric referral
Chronic impairment	Inpatient psychiatric
(psychosocial dysfunction)	hospitalization
Severe intoxication	Critical care hospitalization

37. Zuckerman B, Frank D, Hingson R, et al. Effects of maternal marijuana and cocaine on fetal growth. N Engl J Med 1989;320:762.

38. Chasnoff I, Griffith D, MacGregor S, et al. Temporal patterns of cocaine use in pregnancy. JAMA 1989;261:1741.

39. Mast J, Carpanzano C, Heir L. Cocaine as a teratogen: A controlled retrospective review. Ann Neurol 1989;26:106.

40. Ferriero D, Partridge C, Wong D. Congenital defects and stroke in cocaine exposed neonates. Ann Neurol 1989;26:154.

41. Ferriero D, Kabori J, Good W, et al. Retinal defects in cocaine exposed infants. Ann Neurol 1989;26:105.

42. Madden J, Payne T, Miller S. Maternal cocaine abuse and effect on the newborn. Pediatrics 1986;77:209.

43. LeBlanc P, Parekh A, Naso B, et al. Effects of intrauterine exposure to alkaloidal cocaine. Am J Dis Child 1987;141:937.

44. Doberczak T, Shanzer S, Senie R, et al. Neonatal neurologic and electro-encephalographic effects of intrauterine cocaine exposure. J Pediatr 1988;113:354.

45. Chasnoff I, Hunt C, Klette R, et al. Prenatal cocaine exposure is associated with respiratory pattern abnormalities. Am J Dis Child 1989;143:583.

46. Bauchner H, Zuckerman B, McClain M, et al. Risk of sudden infant death syndrome among infants with in utero exposure to cocaine. J Pediatr 1988;113:831.

47. Itkonow J, Schnoll S, Glassroth J. Pulmonary dysfunction in "freebase" cocaine abusers. Arch Intern Med 1984;144:2195.

48. Kissner D, Lawrence WD, Selis J, et al. Crack lung: Pulmonary disease caused by cocaine abuse. Am Rev Respir Dis 1987;136:1250.

49. Weiner MD, Putnam C. Pain in the chest in a user of cocaine. JAMA 1987;258:2087.

50. Karch S, Billingham M. The pathology and etiology of cocaine-induced heart disease. Arch Pathol Lab Med 1988;112:225.

51. Mueller P, Benowitz N, Olson K. Cocaine: Emergency aspects of drug abuse. Emerg Med Clin North 1990;481.

52. Resnick R, Kestenbaum R. Acute systemic effects of cocaine in man: A controlled study by intranasal and intravenous routes. Science 1976;195:696.

53. Hale S, Alker K, Rezkalla S. Adverse effects of cocaine on cardiovascular dynamics. Myocardial blood flow and coronary artery diameter in an experimental model. Am Heart J 1989;118:927.

54. Lange RA, Cigarroa RG, Yancy CW Jr, et al. Cocaine-induced coronary-artery vasoconstriction. N Engl J Med 1989;321:1557.

55. Frishman W, Karpenos A, Molloy T. Cocaine-induced coronary artery disease: Recognition and treatment. Med Clin North Am 1989;73:475.

56. Isner J, Estes NA, Thompson P. Acute cardiac events temporally related to cocaine abuse. N Engl J Med 1986;315:1438.

57. Cregler L, Mark H. Relation of acute myocardial infarction to cocaine abuse. Am J Cardiol 1985;56:794.

58. Pasternack P, Colvin S, Baumann F. Cocaine induced angina pectoris and acute myocardial infarction in patients younger than 40 years. Am J Cardiol 1985;56:847.

59. Benchimel A, Bartall H, Desser KB. Accelerated ventricular rhythm and cocaine abuse. Ann Intern Med 1978;88:519.

60. Nanji A, Filipenko JD. Asystole and ventricular fibrillation associated with cocaine intoxication. Chest 1984;85:132.

61. Weiss RJ. Recurrent myocardial infarction caused by cocaine abuse. Am Heart J 1986;111:793.

62. Chokshi S, Moore R, Pandian N, et al. Reversible cardiomyopathy associated with cocaine intoxication. Ann Intern Med 1989;111:1039.

63. Mody CK, Miller BL, McIntyre HB, et al. Neurologic complications of cocaine abuse. Neurology 1988;38:1189.

64. Lowenstein D, Massa S, Rowbotham M, et al. Acute neurologic and psychiatric complications associated with cocaine abuse. Am J Med 1987;83:841.

65. Ogunyomi A, Lodie G, Kramer L, et al. Complex partial status epilepticus provided by "crack" cocaine. Ann Neurol 1989;26:785.

66. Catravas J, Waters IW. Acute cocaine intoxication in the conscious dog: Studies in the mechanism of lethality. J Pharmacol Exp Ther 1981;217:350.

67. Schwartz K, Estroff T, Hoffman N. Seizures and syncope in adolescent cocaine abusers. Am J Med 1988;85:462.

68. Jonsson S, Omeara M, Young J. Acute cocaine poisoning: Importance of treating seizures and acidosis. Am J Med 1983;75:1061.

69. Levine S, Brust J, Futrell N, et al. Cerebrovascular complications of the use of the "crack" form of alkaloidal cocaine. N Engl J Med 1990;323:699.

70. Klonoff DC, Andrews BT, Obana WG. Stroke associated with cocaine use. Arch Neurol 1989;46:989.

71. Mercado A, Johnson G, Calver D, et al. Cocaine, pregnancy, and post-partum intracerebral hemorrhage. Obstet Gynecol 1989;73:467.

72. Engstrand B, Paras M, Tuchman A, et al. Cocaine related ischemic strokes. Neurology 1989;39(Suppl):106.

73. Peterson P, Moore P. Hemorrhagic cerebrovascular complications of crack cocaine abuse. Neurology 1989;39(Suppl 1):302.

74. Spires M, Gordon E, Choudhuri M, et al. Intracranial hemorrhage in a neonate following prenatal cocaine exposure. Pediatr Neurol 1989;5:324.

75. Moore P, Peterson P. Nonhemorrhagic cerebrovascular complications of cocaine abuse. Neurology 1989;39(Suppl 1):302.

76. Dixon S, Bejar R. Brain lesions in cocaine and methamphetamine-exposed neonates. Pediatr Res 1988;23:405A.

77. Togna G, Tempesta E, Togna AR, et al. Platelet responsiveness and biosynthesis of thromboxane and prostacycline in response to in vitro cocaine treatment. Haemostasis 1985;15:100.

78. Krendel D, Ditter S, Frankel M, et al. Biopsy proven cerebral vasculitis associated with cocaine abuse. Neurology 1990;40:1092.

79. Derlet R, Albertson T. Emergency department presentation of cocaine intoxication. Ann Emerg Med 1989;18:182.

80. Gawin F. Cocaine abuse and addiction. J Fam Pract 1989;29:193.

81. Welti C, Fishbain D. Cocaine induced psychosis and sudden death in recreational cocaine users. J Forensic Sci 1985;30:873.

82. Menashe P, Gottlieb J. Hyperthermia, rhabdomyolysis, and myoglobi-nuric renal failure after recreational use of cocaine. South Med J 1988;81:379.

83. Kosten T, Kleber H. Sudden death in cocaine abusers: Relation to neuroleptic malignant syndrome. Lancet 1987; May 23:1198.

84. Herzlich B, Arsura E, Pagala M, et al. Rhabdomyolysis related to cocaine abuse. Ann Intern Med 1988;15:335.

85. Brody S, Slovis C. Recognition and management of complications related to cocaine abuse. Emergency Medicine Reports 1988;9:1.

86. McCarron M, Wood J. The cocaine "body packer" syndrome. JAMA 1983;250:1417.

87. Gay G. Clinical management of acute and chronic cocaine poisoning. Ann Emerg Med 1982;11:562.

88. Ramoska E, Sacchetti A. Propranolol-induced hypertension in treatment of cocaine intoxication. Ann Emerg Med 1985;14:1112.

89. Gay G, Loper K. The use of labetalol in the management of cocaine crisis. Ann Emerg Med 1988;17:282.

90. Dusinberry S, Hicks M, Mariani P. Labatalol treatment of cocaine toxicity. Ann Emerg Med 1987;16:235.

91. Gradman A. Cardiac effects of cocaine: A review. Yale J Biol Med 1988;61:137.

92. Derlet R, Albertson T. Potentiation of cocaine toxicity with lidocaine. Society for Academic Emergency Medicine, Abstract 65, May 1990.

93. Blumenthal R, Flaherty J. Recognizing cardiac crisis in cocaine abusers. Journal of Critical Illness 1990;5:225.

CHAPTER 93

Phenothiazines

Javier A. Gonzalez del Rey
Suman Wason

INTRODUCTION

The phenothiazines are a group of drugs used mainly in the treatment of psychotic disorders. In the pediatric patient these drugs are used to control nausea and vomiting and to treat Tourette's disease and psychiatric problems. Because of their increasing use, especially in children receiving chemotherapy, the practitioner should be aware of their side effects and the management of overdose.

PHARMACOLOGY

The phenothiazines have been divided into three major groups based on substitutions in a basic three-ring structure: aliphatic, piperidine, and piperazine derivatives. The actions of these three groups are generally similar but vary according to dosage and chemical structure (Table 93–1).

The phenothiazines can be administered orally, intramuscularly, or intravenously. Gastrointestinal absorption is diminished owing in large part to increased presystemic metabolism in the gastrointestinal lumen or intestinal wall.

TABLE 93–1		
PHENOTHIAZINE ACTIVITY BY CHEMICAL CLASS		
	Aliphatic	**Piperidine**	**Piperazine**
	Chlorpromazine Promethazine Promazine	Mesoridazine Thioridazine	Perphenazine Fluphenazine Prochlorperazine Trifluoperazine
Extrapyramidal reactions	+	+	+ + +
Cardiovascular effects	+ + +	+ + +	+
Sedation	+ + +	+ + +	+
Antipsychotic effects	+	+ +	+ +

+ = Lowest incidence; + + + = highest incidence.

Intramuscular absorption is variable. The apparent volumes of distribution (Vd) of the phenothiazines are large (chlorpromazine Vd = 20 L/kg) after a therapeutic dose. Phenothiazines are highly protein bound. Because of the tissue distribution and storage, phenothiazine metabolites, some of which are active, may be found in urine months after the last dose.

Most phenothiazine elimination occurs through hepatic metabolism. Approximately one half of the absorbed drug is excreted by the kidneys after conjugation with sulfates or glucuronide; the other half is excreted through the enterohepatic system. Only about 1% of the absorbed drug is excreted unchanged through the kidneys.

Most of the therapeutic and toxic effects of the phenothiazines are based on their anticholinergic and antidopaminergic properties. Their antipsychotic and extrapyramidal activity is believed to be due to a combination of a postsynaptic blockade of dopamine receptors and anticholinergic activity in the central nervous system. Phenothiazines also lower the seizure threshold, especially in patients with previous seizure disorders or abnormal electroencephalographic patterns.

The cardiovascular effects of phenothiazines are the result of their quinidine-like action, local anesthetic effect, and direct depressant action on the myocardium. Hypotension (mostly postural) is the result of myocardial depression and peripheral alpha-adrenergic blockade, which results in vasodilation.

CLINICAL EVALUATION

The clinical findings after phenothiazine administration have no clear dose-response relationship. Hypotension and lethargy have been reported in toddlers after 100 to 375 mg of chlorpromazine (Table 93–2). Significant central nervous system depression has occurred after the ingestion of 200 to 1200 mg of chlorpromazine in pediatric patients. Among adults, central nervous system depression has been reported after ingestions of chlorpromazine exceeding 5 gm.

Although phenothiazines exhibit anticholinergic properties, miosis has been noted in 72% of children who were comatose after ingestion of phenothiazines. Other central nervous system manifestations of acute phenothiazine overdose range from mild sedation to coma. Children seem to be more susceptible to effects such as sedation and ataxia than are adults. Obtundation has been reported in as many as 60% of patients with acute overdose; it may appear within 1 to 2 hours after ingestion. The depth of phenothiazine obtundation rarely leads to respiratory depression requiring endotracheal intubation.

Because phenothiazines lower the seizure threshold, convulsions may occur following phenothiazine overdose, especially in those patients already prone to seizures. Although infrequent in children, convulsions may be multiple and prolonged.

The other component of the nervous system usually affected by phenothiazines is the autonomic nervous system. Central temperature control is disturbed, and hypothermia may occur in up to 40% of overdose patients. Other autonomic nervous system manifestations include skin flushing, dry mucous membranes, constipation, urinary retention, paralytic ileus, and hypotension.

The extrapyramidal reactions include a variety of syndromes that may present within hours after acute overdose or as side effects of chronic use of phenothiazines. Acute dystonic reactions may occur in up to 10% of phenothiazine overdoses. In children these usually present as confusion, slurred speech, dysarthria, dysphagia, lethargy, painless spasms, tremors, hypertonicity, or muscle restlessness. These reactions may appear between 5 and 30 hours after ingestion or may be delayed for up to 72 hours after the initial exposure to the drug. Extrapyramidal dyskinetic manifestations may also include opisthotonos, spasmodic torticollis, aimless movements of the tongue (rabbit syndrome), facial tics, lip smacking, and, rarely, laryngeal or pharyngeal spasm, which may cause severe respiratory distress. Akasthesias (hyperkinesia, agitation, anxiety) and parkinsonian reactions ("cogwheel" rigidity upon passive movement of neck, biceps, or quadriceps; pill-rolling tremor; immobility of facies; and slow speech) may present within the first few days of therapeutic treatment with phenothiazines. However, after moderate to severe overdose, these syndromes may appear within hours. The most serious central nervous system–mediated movement side effect of phenothiazines is tardive dyskinesia. This is characterized by involuntary and repetitive movements of the face, tongue, and lips. Tardive dyskinesia occurs more frequently in females who have been on phenothiazine therapy for years. The incidence of tardive dyskinesia after phenothiazine overdose is unknown.

TABLE 93–2	
SYMPTOMS AND SIGNS	
Central Nervous System	**Cardiovascular System**
Sedation	Hypotension
Coma	Dysrhythmias
Ataxia	Sudden death
Dystonia	
Seizures	
Temperature dysregulation	
Neuroleptic malignant syndrome	

The cardiovascular system is another target of phenothiazine toxicity. Diastolic hypotension commonly occurs after phenothiazine overdose, with an incidence as high as 25%. Dysrhythmias are also common after phenothiazine overdose. Sinus tachycardia has been present in 40% of reported overdose cases. Other rhythm disturbances include ventricular tachycardia, ventricular fibrillation, torsade de pointes (QT prolongation with atypical ventricular tachycardia), and cardiac arrest. Sudden death due to dysrhythmias has been reported as early as 3 to 5 hours after overdose. However, the majority of the ventricular arrhythmias have occurred in patients on continuous regimens of phenothiazines as opposed to in overdose patients. Electrocardiographic changes caused by phenothiazines include prolonged PR, QRS, and QT intervals; complete heart and bundle branch block; and U- and T-wave abnormalities.

The neuroleptic malignant syndrome (NMS) is another, albeit uncommon, complication of phenothiazine use, characterized by profound hyperthermia, tachycardia, hypotension, and severe extrapyramidal dysfunction. Massive rhabdomyolysis with subsequent renal failure has been reported after phenothiazine overdose NMS. In young infants the therapeutic use of phenothiazines has been associated with sudden infant death syndrome (SIDS).

DIAGNOSTIC EVALUATION

In emergency situations the ferric chloride test on urine has been used to confirm the diagnosis of an overdose. In this test, 1 ml of the patient's urine is added to 10 to 15 drops of 10% ferric chloride; a deep burgundy color confirms the presence of the phenothiazines. Since the specificity and sensitivity of this test are unknown, where ingestion of phenothiazines is suspected, a negative test should not change the approach to management of the patient. Treatment should be based on the patient's history, symptoms, and signs. Blood levels are difficult to obtain and do not correlate with symptoms or prognosis.

Some phenothiazines are radiopaque; therefore abdominal radiographs may be useful to confirm the diagnosis and evaluate the efficacy of the gastrointestinal decontamination (Fig. 93–1). The absence of pill fragments on radiograph should not preclude the use of ipecac syrup, gastric lavage, or activated charcoal in the initial management of these patients.

THERAPEUTIC INTERVENTION

Initial treatment should always include rapid assessment and management of the airway, breathing, and circulation (Table 93–3).

Induced emesis with syrup of ipecac is usually indicated within 30 minutes of the ingestion, provided that the patient does not have impaired consciousness. Despite the antiemetic effects of the phenothiazines, syrup of ipecac has been demonstrated to be effective in inducing emesis in these patients. In cases where an extremely large ingestion is suspected or when there are changes in the patient's level of consciousness, activated charcoal or gastric lavage is preferred. Gastric lavage may be effectively performed many hours after the ingestion owing to the slow absorption of the phenothiazines in the gastrointestinal system. Obtunded patients may theoretically benefit from lavage as late as 12 hours after ingestion. Because some phenothiazines are radiopaque, an abdominal radiograph may be helpful in the evaluation of the decontamination procedures. Multiple doses of activated charcoal (1 gm/kg administered every 6

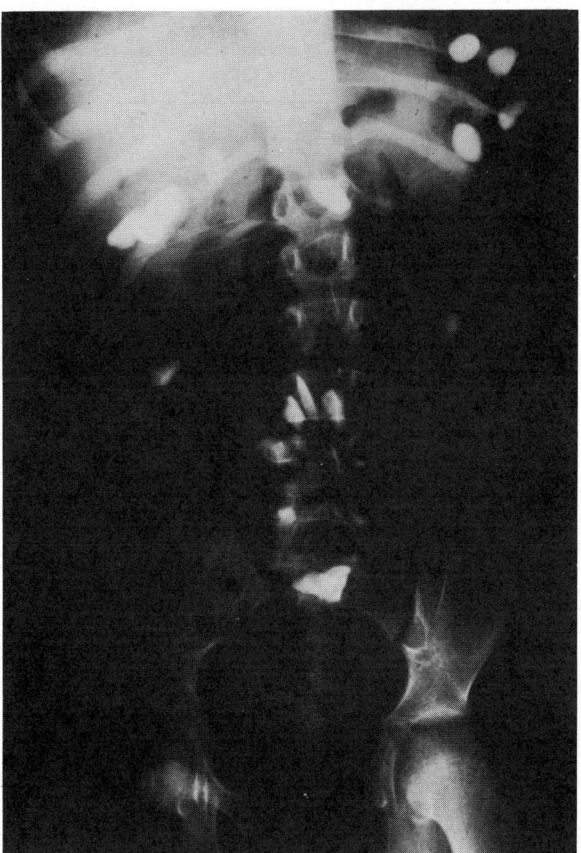

Figure 93–1. Radiograph showing the radiopaque appearance of phenothiazine tablets. Other ingestants that can give this appearance include chloral hydrate, iron tablets, tricyclic antidepressants, and enteric-coated tablets.

hours for 18 to 24 hours) may further increase phenothiazine clearance from the body after overdose (Table 93–4).

Diuresis, dialysis, and hemoperfusion are ineffective in removing significant quantities of phenothiazines. Exchange transfusion has been life-saving in an infant.

Convulsions should be treated in the usual fashion with intravenous diazepam (0.1 to 0.2 mg/kg/dose) or lorazepam (0.05 to 0.1 mg/kg/dose). It is important to evaluate constantly the ventilatory status of the patient because of the possibility of respiratory depression due to the additive effects of the benzodiazepine. Phenytoin and phenobarbital

TABLE 93–3
MANAGEMENT CHECKLIST

1. Ensure airway, breathing, and circulation
2. Gastrointestinal decontamination
     Avoid ipecac if central nervous system symptoms
     Avoid ipecac in patients with seizure disorder
     Activated charcoal (1 gm/kg); repeat every 6 hr for 18–24 hr if patient symptomatic
3. Special therapeutic notes
     Hypotension: if crystalloids do not restore blood pressure, consider levarterenol
     Acute dystonia: treat with intravenous diphenhydramine; discharge patients on 48–72-hr treatment of oral diphenhydramine
     Dysrhythmias: avoid quinidine, procainamide, and disopyramide

TABLE 93–4

THERAPY AT A GLANCE

	Dose	Frequency
Gastric Decontamination		
Activated charcoal	1 gm/kg	Most ingestions × 1
		Consider multiple doses in carbamazepine, digoxin, theophylline, tricyclic antidepressants
Ipecac	6–12 mo, 10 ml + fluids	Repeat × 1 in 20 min if no emesis
	1–12 yr, 15–30 ml + fluids	Repeat × 1 in 20 min if no emesis
	>12 yr, 30–60 ml + fluids	Repeat × 1 in 20 min if no emesis
Blood Pressure Support		
Lactated Ringer's solution	20 cc/kg	May repeat bolus once
0.9 Normal saline	20 cc/kg	May repeat bolus once
Norepinephrine	0.1–0.2 μg/kg/min	Continuous infusion
Dystonia		
Diphenhydramine	0.5–1.5 mg/kg dose (max. 5 mg/kg daily)	q 6 hr
Benztropine	2 mg/dose	Adolescents and adults
Hyperthermia		
Dantrolene	1 mg/kg (max. 50 mg)	q 12 hr
Bromocriptine	5 mg/kg	q 8 hr

have also been successfully used in the treatment of phenothiazine-induced seizures.

Acute dystonic reactions usually respond within 5 minutes to the administration of intravenous diphenhydramine (1 mg/kg/dose to a maximum of 50 mg). In the adolescent or young adult, benztropine mesylate may be used as an alternative (2 mg/dose). There is no documentation of the use or safety of this drug in infants and younger children. A maintenance dose of diphenhydramine should be given three to four times a day for 48 to 72 hours to avoid recurrences of dystonic reactions due to the prolonged half-life of some of the phenothiazines and their metabolites.

The initial management of hypotension should consist of administration of crystalloid fluid boluses (20 ml/kg/bolus). If after the infusion of 40 to 60 ml/kg there is no restoration of blood pressure, vasoactive drugs must be used. It has been postulated that because of their mixed alpha and beta effects, epinephrine and dopamine may worsen hypotension owing to an unopposed beta vasodilation. Norepinephrine may be used in dosages of 0.1 to 0.2 μg/kg/minute and slowly titrated to maintain an adequate blood pressure. Methoxamine is an alternative.

Like the tricyclic antidepressants, phenothiazines may produce prolongation of the QRS and QT intervals in association with ventricular tachyarrhythmias. Stable supraventricular tachycardia requires no treatment. When ventricular arrhythmias occur, alkalinization with sodium bicarbonate may be tried as an initial measure as is recommended for tricyclic-induced dysrhythmias. Lidocaine and phenytoin are the recommended drugs for persistent ventricular dysrhythmias. Because of the quinidine-like effects of the phenothiazines on the myocardium, quinidine, procainamide, and disopyramide should be avoided. In severe cases transvenous pacing and direct-current countershock may be necessary.

In the pediatric patient the thermal dysregulation caused by phenothiazines should receive special attention. Mild hypothermia is common and usually responds to passive external rewarming and supportive measures. In cases of malignant hyperthermia, dantrolene sodium (1 mg/kg every 12 hours to a maximum of 50 mg) orally, as well as bromocriptine mesylate (5 mg/kg given three times a day), may be used.

DISPOSITION

Hospitalization is recommended for all patients exhibiting central nervous system or cardiovascular symptoms. Asymptomatic patients may be released after 4 to 6 hours of observation. It is important to inform parents that dystonic reactions may occur for up to 72 hours after the ingestion of some phenothiazines.

Selected References

Barry D, Meyskens FL Jr, Becker CE. Phenothiazine poisoning: Review of 48 cases. Calif Med 1973;118:1.

Gupta J, Lovejoy FH Jr. Acute phenothiazine toxicity in childhood: A five year study. Pediatrics 1967;39:771.

Khan A, Blum D. Phenothiazines and sudden death syndrome. Pediatrics 1982;70:75.

Knight ME, Roberts RJ. Phenothiazine and butyrophenone intoxication in children. Pediatr Clin North Am 1986;33:299.

May DC, Morris SW, Stewart RM, et al. Neuroleptic malignant syndrome: Response to dantrolene sodium. Ann Intern Med 1983;98:183.

Mitchell AA, Lovejoy FH, Goldman P. Drug ingestions associated with miosis in comatose children. J Pediatr 1976;89:303.

Mueller PS, Vestter JW, Fermaglich J. Neuroleptic malignant syndrome: Successful treatment with bromocriptine. JAMA 1983;249:386.

Sinaniotis CA, Spyrides P, Vlachos P, et al. Acute haloperidol poisoning in children. J Pediatr 1978;93:1038.

CHAPTER 94

Theophylline

William Hardwick Jr.
Suman Wason

INTRODUCTION

Theophylline is an important drug in the management of asthma, although its role in acute management is questioned. Since the early 1970s theophylline has also been used as a respiratory stimulant in the treatment of apnea of prematurity. Widespread use combined with the drug's low therapeutic index makes theophylline a prominent toxicology problem.

PHARMACOLOGY

Theophylline (1,3-dimethylxanthine) is a methylxanthine structurally similar to caffeine (1,3,7-trimethylxanthine) (Fig. 94–1). The methylxanthines competitively inhibit phosphodiesterase, the enzyme involved in the breakdown of cyclic 3'5'-AMP. Increasing intracellular concentrations of cyclic AMP lead to relaxation of bronchial smooth muscles. Recent investigations have created doubt about this hypothesis. Several other mechanisms have been proposed to explain the beneficial effects of theophylline in asthma.

Adenosine has been shown to induce bronchoconstriction. Theophylline is structurally similar to adenosine and may act as an adenosine receptor antagonist. Other beneficial actions of theophylline in asthma include its ability to inhibit intracellular release of calcium, its prostaglandin antagonist

Caffeine
(1, 3, 7-Trimethylxanthine)

Theophylline
(1, 3-Dimethylxanthine)

Figure 94–1. Notice the similarity in structure of the caffeine and the theophylline molecule.

activity, and its induction of endogenous catecholamine release. The usefulness of theophylline in the treatment of apnea of prematurity is due to its ability to stimulate directly the central nervous system respiratory drive.

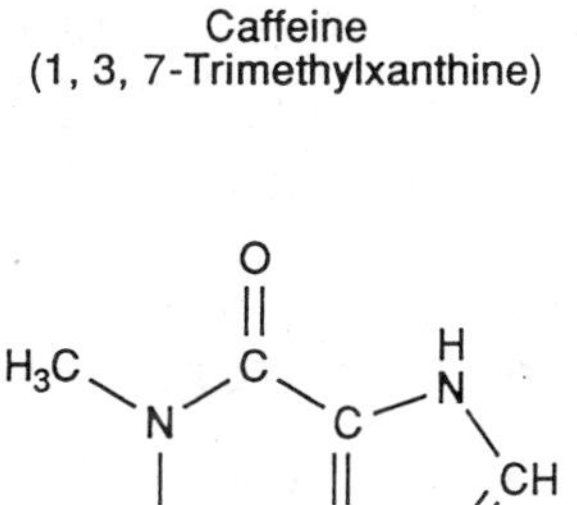

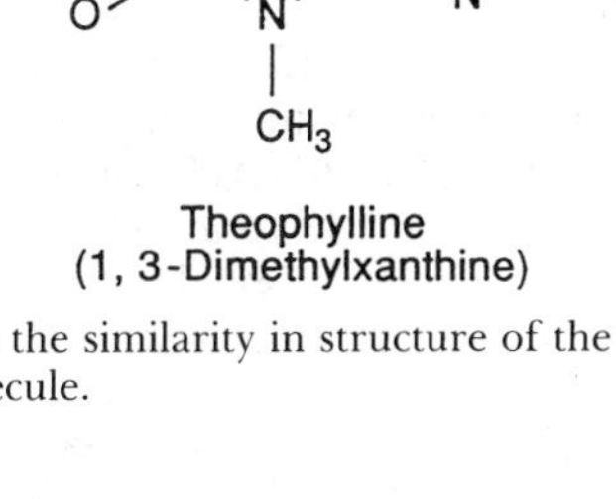

Theophylline is available for oral and intravenous use. When given orally, approximately 96% absorption of a plain, uncoated theophylline tablet occurs, with peak blood levels at 2 hours. Sustained-release preparations result in peak concentrations 4 to 8 hours after oral administration. Concurrent food intake delays absorption of sustained-release theophylline, although the percentage absorbed is not altered. In an overdose the time to peak concentration for nonsustained-release preparations remains about the same, whereas sustained preparations may have a delay to peak concentration of up to 18 to 24 hours.

Theophylline is largely protein bound in serum, approximately 85% to 90% of absorbed drug undergoing hepatic metabolism. Major metabolites are excreted by the kidneys. The volume of distribution of theophylline is relatively constant in adults and children, at approximately 0.5 L/kg. Therefore theophylline elimination is largely a function of clearance. At therapeutic doses theophylline elimination is subject to first-order kinetics (i.e., metabolism of a constant percentage of drug regardless of blood concentrations). At higher doses theophylline elimination is subject to Michaelis-Menten or dose-dependent kinetics (i.e., saturation of metabolic pathways results in decreased clearance at higher blood concentrations). Therefore in overdose the elimination half-life of theophylline may be much longer than at therapeutic doses.

Clearance of theophylline has been shown to vary with age, and wide fluctuations exist even in the pediatric age groups (Table 94–1). Clearance is reduced in newborns and infants. The half-life of theophylline in a premature neonate may be eight to nine times longer than that in a child 1 to 4 years of age. Throughout childhood, clearance progressively increases and half-life progressively decreases, with maximal clearance achieved between the ages of 1 and 9 years. By adolescence clearance has decreased to values similar to those in adults.

Other than age, one of the most readily identifiable influences on theophylline clearance is hepatic disease. The decreased clearance associated with impaired hepatic function is expected with a drug that is so completely metabolized in the liver; however, this decrease has been described only in certain types of hepatic dysfunction. In a study of patients with cirrhosis, a decreasing theophylline clearance accompanied an increase in the serum bilirubin. A significant decrease in theophylline clearance in patients with "decompensated cirrhosis" and in patients with acute hepatitis was also reported. However, patients with milder cirrhosis or cholestasis showed no difference in clearance from controls.

Decreased theophylline clearance has also been associated with acute viral infection. Prolonged theophylline half-lives can occur in asthmatic children with influenza or adenoviral infections. Influenza vaccination has also been implicated as a cause of decreased theophylline clearance.

The list of drugs that affect theophylline metabolism continues to increase. Erythromycin in all its forms (base,

TABLE 94–1		
THEOPHYLLINE PLASMA HALF-LIFE IN RELATION TO AGE		
Newborn	24 hr	
1–6 mo	6 hr	
6 mo to 18 yr	4 hr	
Adult	6–8 hr	

estolate, and ethylsuccinate) decreases theophylline clearance. Cimetidine markedly decreases theophylline clearance within 24 hours of administration of the first dose. Allopurinol may also be responsible for increased half-life when administered in high doses. Caffeine and other xanthines may act as competitive substrates and interfere with theophylline metabolism, but the data are not definitive.

On the other hand, phenobarbital, a known hepatic inducer, may increase the clearance of theophylline and decrease the half-life with prolonged use. Smoking cigarettes and marijuana increases clearance of theophylline also by induction of enzymes. Dietary tars in charcoal-broiled beef have produced similar results.

Theophylline crosses the placental barrier, with serum level in the newborn approaching that of the mother. Theophylline is also found in breast milk but at much lower concentrations than in blood. Usually no dosage adjustment is necessary in the nursing mother.

EMS CONSIDERATIONS

One of the concerns after significant theophylline overdose is the possibility of seizures. Therefore the routine use of ipecac is not recommended after theophylline overdose. During transport patients should be monitored for cardiac and central nervous system toxicity. Establishment of intravenous access is recommended.

CLINICAL EVALUATION

The toxic effects of theophylline can be viewed as an extension of the pharmacologic properties of the drug (Table 94–2). The incidence of theophylline toxicity clearly increases with increasing serum drug concentrations, but a predictable relationship has not been adequately documented. Although minor side effects such as vomiting start to occur at lower serum levels, they do not always precede the more life-threatening abnormalities such as arrhythmias and seizures. In general, the adverse symptoms and side effects of theophylline can be divided into three categories: gastrointestinal, neurologic, and cardiovascular.

Gastrointestinal symptoms include nausea, vomiting, and abdominal pain. In a retrospective study of theophylline-toxic children, 97% had vomiting. Similar studies have also reported vomiting as a major symptom in the majority of theophylline-toxic children. Hematemesis has been reported more frequently in children than in adults. Most of these gastrointestinal symptoms appear to be centrally mediated and can occur with either oral, intravenous, or rectal administration. Other adverse effects of theophylline on the gastrointestinal tract include relaxation of the gastroesophageal smooth muscle, leading to reflux. Additionally, hypersecre-

tion of gastric acids, even at therapeutic concentrations of theophylline, has been demonstrated. Diarrhea has been noted with serum theophylline concentrations greater than 20 µg/ml.

The stimulatory effect of theophylline on the central nervous system is poorly understood. Adverse effects of theophylline on the central nervous system include headache, irritability, agitation, and obtundation. Hallucinations have been reported. Some studies have suggested that children on theophylline may be predisposed to learning and behavioral problems secondary to hyperactivity and inattentiveness. A more serious neurologic effect of theophylline overdose is seizures. In children and adults, theophylline-induced seizures are most often generalized tonic-clonic convulsions, but focal seizures have been described. Seizures have been reported with concentrations as low as 25 µg/ml. In contrast, individuals have tolerated theophylline levels greater than 120 µg/ml with only minor central nervous system symptoms. In the adult literature seizures appear to be ominous. One report (four of eight patients) associated with theophylline-induced convulsions showed a 50% mortality. In adults theophylline-induced convulsions have been reported to be refractory to anticonvulsant therapy. But in two large pediatric series of theophylline toxicity, seizures responded promptly to intravenous diazepam alone and did not portend an ominous outcome.

The cardiac toxicity of theophylline is well known. Theophylline has inotropic and chronotropic effects, which appear to be due to several components, including a direct action on pacemaker tissue, a local release of norepinephrine, and a peripheral vagolytic effect. Clinically sinus tachycardia is the most consistent cardiac manifestation of theophylline toxicity. In adults tachycardia appears to be the most universal indicator of theophylline toxicity, with studies reporting increased heart rate in as many as 89% of toxic individuals. In two pediatric studies, tachycardia occurred in 82% and 61% of the children. Cardiac arrhythmias such as supraventricular and ventricular tachycardia, atrial fibrillation, ventricular fibrillation, and asystole have been reported with theophylline toxicity, particularly after bolus infusions. Rhythm disturbances have been reported with theophylline serum concentrations of around 40 µg/ml in adults and with somewhat higher levels in children. Other cardiovascular findings include hypertension or, less frequently, hypotension in the more severe cases.

Specific metabolic abnormalities are frequently seen with theophylline overdose, including hyperglycemia, hypokalemia, and metabolic acidosis.

Death with theophylline overdose is usually associated with prolonged, intractable seizures or cardiovascular collapse. The frequency of these life-threatening complications is less in children than in adults. The reported mortality rate with theophylline toxicity ranges from 14% to 33% in adults.

Chronic Versus Acute Ingestion

In recent studies a distinction has been drawn between theophylline toxicity occurring after an acute single ingestion and toxicity occurring from chronic overmedication. Olsen's study of theophylline-toxic adults and children reported few serious complications in acute overdose patients unless serum concentrations exceeded 100 µg/ml. In contrast, patients with chronic overmedication had increased seizures and arrhythmias at serum theophylline levels of only 40 to 70 µg/ml. A review of the English literature by Paloucek and Rodvold supports these findings.

TABLE 94–2

SIGNS AND SYMPTOMS

Gastrointestinal	Cardiovascular
Nausea/vomiting	Tachycardia
Abdominal pain	Tachyarrhythmias
Hematemesis	High output failure
Diarrhea	
Gastric acid hypersecretion	**Metabolic**
	Hyperglycemia
Central Nervous System	Hypokalemia
Headache	Hypophosphatemia
Agitation	Metabolic acidosis
Hallucinations	
Seizures	

DIFFERENTIAL DIAGNOSIS

Many toxins can produce signs and symptoms similar to the findings in theophylline overdose and should be considered in the differential diagnosis. The gastrointestinal symptoms of nausea, vomiting, and even hematemesis are common with ingestion of iron, salicylates, nonsteroidal anti-inflammatories, acetaminophen, and caustics. Central nervous system symptoms, particularly seizures, may occur with overdoses of cyclic antidepressants, other anticholinergics, and sympathomimetics, including cocaine, amphetamines, ephedrine, and phenylpropanolamine. Tachyarrhythmias and other cardiac dysrhythmias may also result from the cyclic antidepressants, sympathomimetics, caffeine, and digitalis.

DIAGNOSTIC EVALUATION

Theophylline has a relatively narrow therapeutic range, with therapeutic serum concentrations for bronchodilation defined as 5 to 20 μg/ml; greater than 10 μg/ml is thought optimal in the majority of patients. Serum concentrations somewhat lower are considered effective for apnea of prematurity.

There are several methods for measuring serum concentrations of theophylline, the most common being high-pressure liquid chromatography and spectrophotometric assay. Of these, high-pressure liquid chromatography is more sensitive, requires less serum, and has less interference from other drugs. Radioimmunoassay and enzyme immunoassay are more easily performed but tend to be less accurate. There is also recent evidence that salivary theophylline concentration may reliably predict serum levels. In studies with asthmatic children and healthy adults, the plasma:saliva ratio was found to be constant. However, in adults with chronic obstructive pulmonary disease, Hendeles found no correlation between salivary and serum theophylline levels.

THERAPEUTIC INTERVENTION

Any patient reporting an overdose of theophylline (i.e., >10 mg/kg) or showing symptoms or signs compatible with theophylline intoxication should be closely evaluated (Table 94–3). This evaluation may consist of only simple observation in an emergency setting with serum theophylline concentrations obtained at the appropriate times, such as 1 to 2 hours after ingestion of nonsustained-release forms or between 4 and 24 hours after ingestion of sustained-release preparations. Patients with serum theophylline levels greater than 20 μg/ml are at increased risk for toxicity.

Decontamination

The initial step in all cases of significant toxicity is discontinuation of the drug, followed by gastrointestinal decontamination when appropriate. Activated charcoal administration has two benefits in theophylline toxicity. First, the ability of activated charcoal to prevent further absorption of theophylline is well known. The addition of a cathartic will decrease transit time of the charcoal-theophylline complex as well as any unabsorbed theophylline. Second, multiple doses of activated charcoal dosed at 1 gm/kg given every 6 hours for 18 to 24 hours have been shown to increase the clearance and decrease the elimination half-life of theophylline even when the drug has been administered intravenously. This phenomenon, termed "gastrointestinal dialysis," is thought to result from the drug diffusing from the vascular space into the gut lumen. Some have recommended multiple doses of activated charcoal whenever serum the-

TABLE 94–3
THERAPY AT A GLANCE

1. Ensure airway, breathing, and circulation
2. Discontinue theophylline
3. Differentiate chronic from acute
4. Estimate serum concentration by determining mg/kg of body weight ingested. Estimated serum concentration = 2 (mg/kg ingested).
5. Determine serum concentrations
   2–4 hr postingestion after regular theophylline
   4–24 hr postingestion after sustained-release theophylline
   Determine serum concentrations every 2 hr, especially after sustained-release medication overdose, until concentrations decreasing
6. Gastrointestinal decontamination
   Avoid ipecac
   Activated charcoal (1 gm/kg); repeat every 6 hr for 18–24 hr until theophylline concentrations in therapeutic range
7. Observe for symptoms/signs
   Continue ABCs
   Cardiac monitoring
   Electrolyte monitoring
   Do not treat hyperglycemia
   Do not treat hypokalemia overzealously
   Consult nephrology service for possible hemoperfusion if serum concentration >50 μg/ml (chronic overdose) or >80 μg/ml (acute overdose)
8. Special therapeutic notes
   If vomiting hinders the administration of activated charcoal, consider ranitidine, droperidol, or placement of nasojejunal tube
   If volume replacement or pressors unsuccessful in treating hypotension, consider administration of propranolol

ophylline concentrations exceed 40 μg/ml. However, patients with significant theophylline ingestion often have pervasive vomiting, making it difficult for them to tolerate oral activated charcoal. Several modalities have been tried in these situations. Intravenous ranitidine, an H_2 antagonist, can be administered to control the excess gastric secretions caused by theophylline. Cimetidine, another H_2 blocker, may interfere with theophylline clearance and should be avoided. Other studies have used droperidol for its antiemetic effect. Occasionally a nasojejunal tube will need to be placed under fluoroscopic guidance in order to be able to administer activated charcoal.

Dialysis

More aggressive means of enhancing elimination may be indicated in cases of severe theophylline intoxication or in the face of life-threatening manifestations of toxicity. Since only a small percentage of unchanged theophylline is eliminated by the kidneys, fluid diuresis is ineffective in enhancing drug elimination. Exchange transfusion has not been valuable either. Some clearance of theophylline occurs through peritoneal dialysis, but not enough to be useful in an emergency situation. Hemodialysis, on the other hand, has been shown to increase clearance of the drug in anephric and uremic adults to levels comparable to metabolic clearance and may serve as a reasonable therapy in some situations. The most effective method for active removal of theophylline from serum is charcoal or resin hemoperfusion. Hemoperfusion involves the extracorporeal percolation of blood over an activated charcoal– or resin-impregnated filter. Using charcoal hemoperfusion, Chang et al. reported removal of 75% of an ingested theophylline dose in a 3-year-old girl. There are no definitive guidelines for the use of hemoperfusion, but previous recommendations using serum theophylline concentrations alone do not appear appropriate. Instead, a number of factors, including age, symptoms, underlying disease, and type of ingestion (acute versus chronic), should be considered. Suggested indications for hemoperfusion in theophylline toxicity include (1) any patient with serum theophylline level greater than 80 μg/ml after an acute overdose, (2) any patient with serum theophylline level greater than 50 μg/ml after a chronic overdose, (3) any patient with suspected prolonged half-life (i.e., neonates, adults with liver disease), and (4) any patient with life-threatening manifestations, such as refractory seizures or cardiovascular compromise.

Seizure Control

The treatment of theophylline-induced seizures is the same as with any other seizure. Most pediatric studies have shown satisfactory control with diazepam. In the face of truly refractory seizure activity, general anesthesia with neuromuscular blockade may be necessary.

Cardiovascular Therapy

The cardiac arrhythmias and cardiovascular collapse associated with theophylline intoxication should initially be treated the same as in any other patient with hemodynamic compromise. If inadequate perfusion or hypotension is present, administration of a fluid bolus and placement in Trendelenburg position is recommended. If perfusion or hypotension is unresponsive to volume replacement, pressors may be tried. Theophylline-induced cardiovascular collapse may be refractory to these standard interventions. The cardiac effects of theophylline toxicity may in part result from elevated plasma catecholamines, which lead to excessive adrenergic stimulation causing tachycardia, arrhythmias, and hypotension. Biberstein et al. reported a case of theophylline toxicity with shock and tachycardia that was unresponsive to pressors but resolved after the administration of propranolol, a beta blocker. It was postulated that excessive catecholamines resulted in unopposed beta stimulation of the peripheral vascular smooth muscle, resulting in vasodilation. Propranolol was thought to reverse this peripheral effect. In dogs intoxicated with theophylline, esmolol, a short-acting selective beta$_1$ antagonist, has shown similar effects. Similarly, propranolol and other beta blockers have been successfully used to treat the supraventricular tachycardia associated with theophylline toxicity. Lidocaine appears effective for the ventricular arrhythmias associated with theophylline.

Metabolic abnormalities, including hypokalemia, hyperglycemia, and acidosis, are associated with significant theophylline toxicity. These do not usually require specific therapy. These changes are reversed as theophylline is cleared from the body.

DISPOSITION

Asymptomatic patients with stable or decreasing theophylline concentration levels (drawn at appropriate peak times) can be followed on an outpatient basis with observation for symptoms of toxicity. Any patient with symptoms of theophylline toxicity or any patient with increasing serum theophylline levels should be considered for hospital admission (Table 94–4).

TABLE 94–4

ADMISSION CRITERIA

Theophylline concentrations >40 μg/ml
Cardiovascular and central nervous system symptoms
Those at risk for prolonged half-life (neonates, liver disease, concomitant medication)

Selected References

Amitai Y, Yeung AC, Moye J, et al. Repetitive oral activated charcoal and control of emesis in severe theophylline toxicity. Ann Intern Med 1986;105:386.
Arwood LL, Dasta JF, Friedman C. Placental transfer of theophylline: Two case reports. Pediatrics 1979;63:844.
Baker MD. Theophylline toxicity in children. J Pediatr 1986;109:538.
Bednarek FJ, Roloff DW. Treatment of apnea of prematurity with aminophylline. Pediatrics 1976;58:335.
Biberstein MP, Ziegler MG, Ward DM. Use of beta-blockade and hemoperfusion for acute theophylline poisoning. West J Med 1984;141:485.
Bukowskyj M, Nakatsu K, Munt PW. Theophylline reassessed. Ann Intern Med 1984;101:63.
Chang KC, Bell TD, Lauer BA, Chair H. Altered theophylline pharmacokinetics during acute respiratory viral illness. Lancet 1978;1:1132.
Chang TM, Espinosa-Melendez E, Francoeur TE, Eade NR. Albumin-collodion activated charcoal hemoperfusion in the treatment of severe theophylline intoxication in a three-year-old patient. Pediatrics 1980;65:811.
Cohen RM: A pharmacokinetic approach to the use of theophylline in status asthmaticus. Ann Allergy 1985;54:1.
Cushley MJ, Tattersfield AE, Holgate ST. Inhaled adenosine and guanosine on airway resistance in normal and asthmatic subjects. Br J Clin Pharmacol 1983;15:161.
Dietrich J, Krauss AN, Reidenberg M, et al. Alterations in state in apneic pre-term infants receiving theophylline. Clin Pharmacol Ther 1978;24:474.
Ehlers SM, Zaske DE, Sawchuk RJ. Massive theophylline overdose: Rapid elimination by charcoal hemoperfusion. JAMA 1978;240:474.
Fleetham JA, Ginsburg JC, Nakatsu K, et al. Resin hemoperfusion as treatment for theophylline-induced seizures. Chest 1979;75:741.
Furukawa CT, Shapiro GG, DuHamel T, et al. Learning and behavior problems associated with theophylline therapy. Lancet 1984;1:621.
Gaudreault P, Wason S, Lovejoy FH Jr. Acute pediatric theophylline overdose. A summary of 28 cases. J Pediatr 1983;102:474.
Jenne JW, Wyze MS, Rood FS, MacDonald FM. Pharmacokinetics of theophylline: Application to adjustment of the clinical dose of aminophylline. Clin Pharmacol Ther 1972;13:344.
Kappas A, Alvares AP, Anderson KE, et al. Effect of charcoal-broiled beef on antipyrine and theophylline metabolism. Clin Pharmacol Ther 1978;23:445.
Landay RA, Gonzalez MA, Taylor JC: Effect of phenobarbital on theophylline disposition. J Allergy Clin Immunol 1978;62:27.
Olson KR, Benowitz NL, Woo OF, Pond SM. Theophylline overdose: Acute single ingestion versus chronic repeated overmedication. Am J Emerg Med 1985;3:386.
Orange RP, Austen WG, Austen KF. Immunological release of histamine and slow-reacting substance of anaphylaxis from human lung. I. Modulation by agents influencing cellular levels of cyclic 3'-5' AMP. J Exp Med 1971;134 (P Suppl):136S.
Paloucek FP, Rodvold KA. Evaluation of theophylline overdoses and toxicities. Ann Emerg Med 1988;17:135.
Sarrazin E, Hendeles L, Weinberger M, et al. Dose-dependent kinetics for theophylline: Observations among ambulatory asthmatic children. J Pediatr 1980;97:825.
Sawyer WT, Caravati EM, Ellison MJ, Krueger KA. Hypokalemia, hyperglycemia and acidosis after intentional theophylline overdose. Am J Emerg Med 1985;3:408.
Shannon DC, Gotay F, Stein IM, et al. Prevention of apnea and bradycardia in low-birthweight infants. Pediatrics 1975;55:589.
Sintek C, Hendeles L, Weinberger M: Inhibition of theophylline absorption by activated charcoal. J Pediatr 1979;94:314.
Soifer H: Aminophylline toxicity. J Pediatr 1957;50:657.
Weinberger M. The pharmacology and therapeutic use of theophylline. J Allergy Clin Immunol 1984;73:525.
Weinberger M, Ginchansky E. Dose-dependent kinetics of theophylline disposition in asthmatic children. J Pediatr 1977;91:820.
Wells DH, Ferlauto JJ. Survival after massive aminophylline overdose in a premature infant. Pediatrics 1979;64:252.
Yarnell PR, Chu NS. Focal seizures and aminophylline. Neurology 1975;25:819.
Zwillich CW, Sutton FD, Neff TA, et al. Theophylline-induced seizures in adults: Correlation with serum concentrations. Ann Intern Med 1975;82:784.

CHAPTER 95

Cardiovascular Drug Ingestions

Kathryn Weise

INTRODUCTION

Of 1.58 million drug exposures reported to the American Association of Poison Control Centers during 1989,[1] 11,447 (0.72%) involved the ingestion of cardiovascular drugs by children under the age of 18 years. Cardiovascular drug ingestions represented the drug category with the third highest death rate following exposure when all age groups were considered. Most cardiovascular drug ingestions involved multiple drugs, regardless of the age of the patient, and resulted in mild to absent symptoms in the vast majority of patients. Only three deaths in children were reported. While pediatric death due to ingestion of drugs in this category is infrequent, the potential for morbidity and mortality may be high if prompt supportive care is unavailable.

CARDIAC GLYCOSIDES
Physiology

Digoxin and digitoxin, the two orally administered cardiac glycosides, exert their clinical effects on cardiac contractility through inhibition of the sodium-potassium ATPase pump in the myocardial sarcolemma. This inhibition of sodium efflux and potassium influx results in slight elevation of intracellular sodium, which leads to a net gain in intracellular calcium through a sodium-calcium exchange mechanism. Increased calcium is thus available for binding to troponin and subsequent muscle contraction.[2-4] Other effects of cardiac glycosides include augmentation of vagal tone, natriuresis through inhibition of the sodium-potassium ATPase pump in the renal tubules, and effects on sympathetic tone and plasma renin activity.[2]

The cardiotoxic effects of digitalis are related to ion shifts and their impact on automaticity and conduction. Automaticity is increased in atrial and ventricular tissue, while the refractory period is shortened. Automaticity is decreased in the sinoatrial node, resulting in a slowed sinus rate. The refractory period of the His-Purkinje system in the atrioventricular node is increased. The balance of these effects favors new pacemakers in atrial, junctional, or ventricular tissue, with or without blocks in atrioventricular conduction. Conduction may be slowed further by the vagal effects of digitalis.[5]

Acute and chronic toxicity may lead to similar dysrhythmias, although chronic toxicity may be complicated by underlying electrolyte abnormalities such as hypokalemia due to concurrent diuretic use. Hypokalemia, hypomagnesemia, and hypercalcemia may all potentiate digitalis toxicity.[5]

EMS Considerations

Cardiac monitoring and frequent evaluation of vital signs should be initiated en route to the receiving facility to reveal rhythm disturbances or inadequate blood pressure. Supplemental oxygen should be provided to any symptomatic patient. Intravenous access should be established. Since many digitalis ingestions are in combination with other drugs, information about possible coingested agents should be communicated.

Clinical Evaluation

Acute and chronic digitalis toxicity share many but not all clinical characteristics (Table 95-1). Patients suffering from chronic toxicity have cardiovascular disease for which they are receiving a cardiac glycoside, and symptoms may mimic those of the underlying cardiac dysfunction. Although cardiovascular symptoms are frequent, gastrointestinal complaints and central nervous system manifestations may occur in the absence of rhythm disturbances, and rhythm changes may be delayed up to 6 hours after acute exposure.[6] This delay following an acute ingestion may merely reflect the time necessary for digoxin to distribute to tissue sites.

Underlying heart disease, renal disease, risk of electrolyte abnormalities (hypokalemia, hypomagnesemia) through concurrent diuretic use or poor nutrition, and drug interactions[6,7] contribute to the risk of toxicity (Table 95-2).

Physical examination should be complete, with special attention paid to vital signs, capillary refill, and the strength of central and peripheral pulses, all of which reflect adequacy of circulation.

Diagnostic Evaluation

Rhythm disturbances should be documented by a 12-lead electrocardiogram (EKG) and followed continuously by cardiac monitoring. An arterial blood gas should be obtained to evaluate the acid-base status as a reflection of adequate cardiac output and oxygen delivery. Laboratory determination of serum electrolytes, including potassium, calcium, and magnesium, should be obtained. Hyperkalemia may result from acute digitalis poisoning owing to interference with the sodium-potassium ATPase pump and is a sign of serious acute toxicity. Hypokalemia, hypercalcemia, and hypomagnesemia may all potentiate the arrhythmogenic potential of cardiac glycosides.[6]

Plasma digoxin levels will document presence of the drug in the case of acute overdose and can help gauge the potential for toxicity in both acute and chronic ingestion. The utility of plasma digoxin concentrations has been disputed since plasma concentrations do not correlate well with tissue concentrations.[8,9] Levels measured in infants 6 months of age or younger may be falsely elevated by an endogenous substance that cross-reacts with digoxin in many digoxin radioimmunoassays.[10]

Differential Diagnosis

Other causes of malaise, gastrointestinal complaints, and cardiac arrhythmias should be considered. These include cardiomyopathies, infectious illnesses with myocardial involvement, electrolyte disturbances, and ingestion of other toxins, including phenothiazines, cyclic antidepressants, other cardiovascular drugs, hydrocarbons, organophosphates, cocaine, and phenytoin.

Therapeutic Intervention

Determination of the approximate time of ingestion is important since peak effects after oral or intravenous exposure to digoxin and digitoxin are delayed (Table 95-3). The magnitude of ingestion is best documented by serum digoxin concentrations obtained at least 4 hours after intravenous dosing or 6 hours after oral exposure. Serum concentrations between 0.8 and 2.0 ng/ml are generally consid-

TABLE 95–1

SIGNS AND SYMPTOMS OF DIGITALIS TOXICITY

Parameter	Chronic Toxicity	Acute Toxicity
History	Underlying cardiac disease	± Underlying cardiac disease
Symptoms	Frequently nonspecific	Frequently nonspecific
	GI: nausea, vomiting, anorexia	GI: nausea, vomiting, diarrhea
	Neurologic: confusion, visual changes, paresthesias, headache	Neurologic: mental status changes
	Cardiac: reflect diseased heart; atrial and ventricular ectopy common	Cardiac: ectopy uncommon; AV conduction disturbances predominate
Laboratory findings	Digoxin level: generally elevated; may be borderline	Digoxin level: expected to be high
	Potassium: normal or decreased	Potassium: normal or increased

ered within a therapeutic range; concentrations above 2.0 ng/ml may be toxic, with the degree of toxicity depending on the amount of digoxin in the body and on complicating factors such as underlying electrolyte abnormalities, coingestions, and baseline myocardial function. Serum digoxin concentrations that are only mildly elevated may be toxic if such complicating factors are present, especially in the case of chronic toxicity. Serum digoxin concentrations in excess of 6 ng/ml are associated with an increased risk of mortality.[11]

All digoxin-intoxicated patients require cardiac monitoring and intravenous access during the initial phase of evaluation while the extent of intoxication is being determined. Initial gut decontamination with gastric emptying, activated charcoal, and cathartic administration may decrease the total amount absorbed and should be considered if no contraindications exist (Fig. 95–1). Repeated doses of activated charcoal have been shown to accelerate drug clearance.[12] In patients with heart block or sinus bradycardia, it may be dangerous to attempt gastric emptying without atropine pretreatment since these maneuvers cause vagal stimulation with subsequent worsening of the rhythm or precipitation of asystole.[5, 13]

The use of digoxin-specific Fab fragments (Digibind) should be considered for the treatment of ingestions resulting in severe symptoms of toxicity. Criteria for severe toxicity include hyperkalemia, which occurs owing to poisoning of the sodium-potassium ATPase pump, and symptomatic arrhythmias. Fab fragments, which have a high affinity for digoxin, create a new equilibrium between digoxin and reversible digoxin binding sites on myocardial cells. This favors the removal of drug from tissue and tight binding to circulating Fab fragments, where digoxin is inactive. This antidote should be administered as soon as severe toxicity is determined, with dosing based on the total amount presumed to have been absorbed into the systemic circulation (Fig. 95–2). Clinical response, including reversal of arrhythmias and decrease in serum potassium concentrations, will begin within 30 to 40 minutes of administration.

Numerous studies have documented the efficacy and safety of Fab fragment administration in children and infants.[14–19] After this drug has been given, total serum digoxin levels will acutely rise, reflecting the release of digoxin from tissue binding sites. However, measured free digoxin levels will fall since most of the circulating digoxin is tightly bound to the Fab fragments.[6, 14, 20] This renders serum digoxin concentrations of limited value for monitoring the probability of positive inotropic effects of digoxin in this setting. Patients who are dependent on cardiac glycosides for adequate cardiac output may require the use of alternative inotropic support until the Fab fragments have been eliminated. Total digoxin concentrations in the serum may remain elevated for days while Fab fragments are being cleared by the kidneys.[20]

Supportive care in the compromised patient while waiting for the effects of Fab fragments to occur include all measures that both minimize arrhythmias and support cardiac output. These include oxygen administration, correction of observed electrolyte abnormalities, and pharmacologic treatment of specific arrhythmias (Table 95–4). After Fab administration, potassium will move back into cells, lowering serum potassium levels. Electrolytes must be reevaluated frequently to avoid hypokalemia.

Disposition

All patients who are at risk for symptomatic toxicity or in whom coingestions may exacerbate digoxin toxicity should be admitted for monitoring. Asymptomatic patients with elevated serum digoxin concentrations may have monitoring discontinued when adequate gastrointestinal decontamina-

TABLE 95–2

DRUGS POTENTIATING DIGITALIS TOXICITY IN CHILDREN

Drug	Action	Result
Quinidine	Decreased renal clearance and volume of distribution of digoxin	Increased serum digoxin levels; increased cardiac glycoside effect on heart
Verapamil	Decreased renal clearance of digoxin in adults and animals	Increased serum digoxin levels (not yet documented in children)
Indomethacin	Impairment of renal function with decreased digoxin filtration rate	Increased serum digoxin levels
Amiodarone	Decreased renal clearance of digoxin	Increased serum digoxin levels; may occur late

TABLE 95–3

DIGITALIS LEVELS

Parameter	Digoxin	Digitoxin
Peak effect		
Oral	4–6 hr	4–12 hr
Intravenous	1.5–3 hr	4–6 hr
Potentially toxic serum concentrations	>2 ng/ml	>40 ng/ml

Management of Digitalis Ingestion

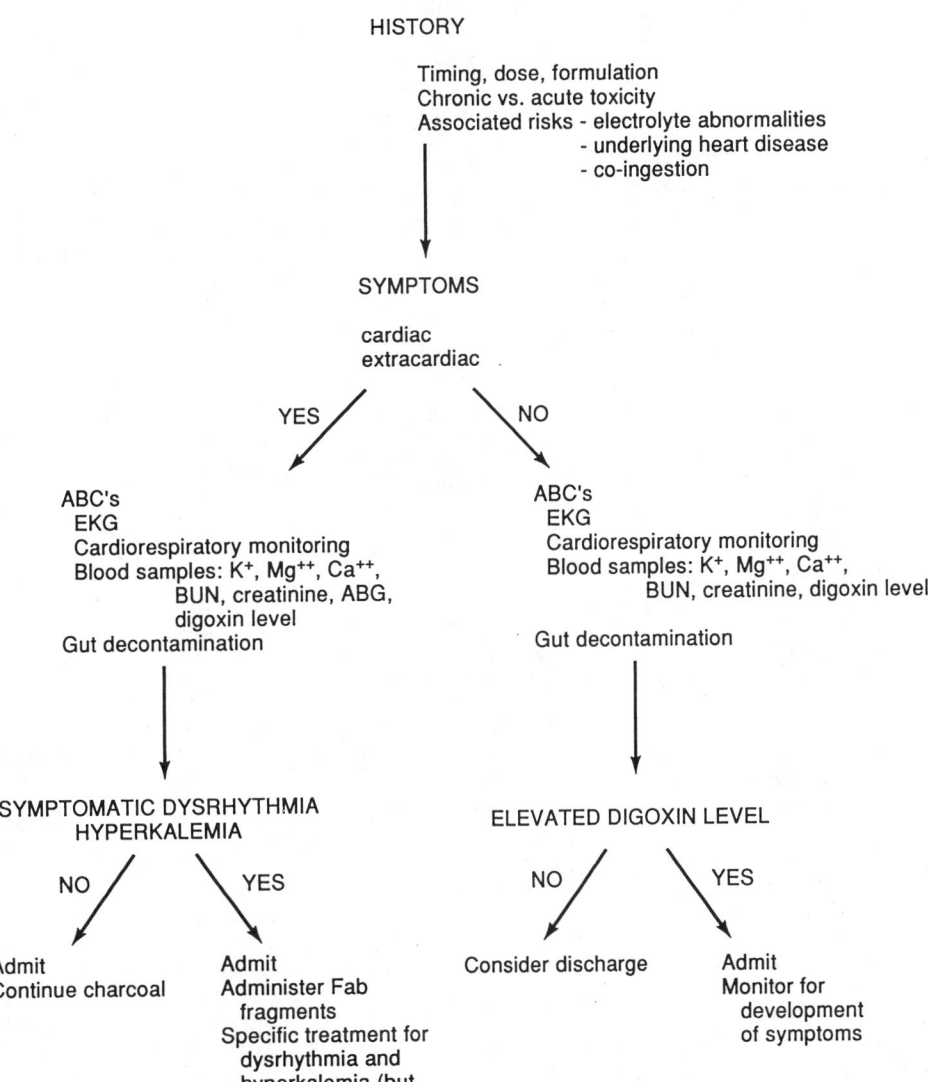

Figure 95–1. Successful management of digitalis intoxication requires complete historical data, frequent physical examination, appropriate assessment of laboratory values, gut decontamination, supportive care, and (in severe toxicity) administration of Fab fragments.

tion has been performed and serum digoxin levels are falling. Symptomatic patients must be closely monitored and managed until dysrhythmias and electrolyte abnormalities have been corrected. The recurrence of toxicity after Fab fragment treatment is rare and has been reported only when less than a full neutralizing dose was administered.[21]

ADRENERGIC AGENTS
Physiology

Alpha- and beta-adrenergic agents available for use in ambulatory patients may be divided into categories based on their mechanisms of action and therapeutic uses (Table 95–

	TABLE 95–4	
	PHARMACOLOGIC TREATMENT OF ARRHYTHMIAS IN DIGITALIS TOXICITY	
Arrhythmia	**Treatment**	**Comments**
Bradydysrhythmia	Oxygen	
	Fab fragments	See Figure 95–2
	Atropine, 0.03 mg/kg	Repeat at 0.06 mg/kg if unsuccessful
	Cardiac pacing	May result in tachydysrhythmia
Tachydysrhythmia	Oxygen	
	Fab fragments	See Figure 95–2
	Phenytoin, 15 mg/kg IV over 20 min	Drug of choice; may reverse AV nodal suppression
	Lidocaine, 1 mg/kg bolus, then 30–50 µg/kg/min drip	Therapeutic serum lidocaine: 1.5–5.0 µg/ml
	Overdrive cardiac pacing	May initiate fibrillation

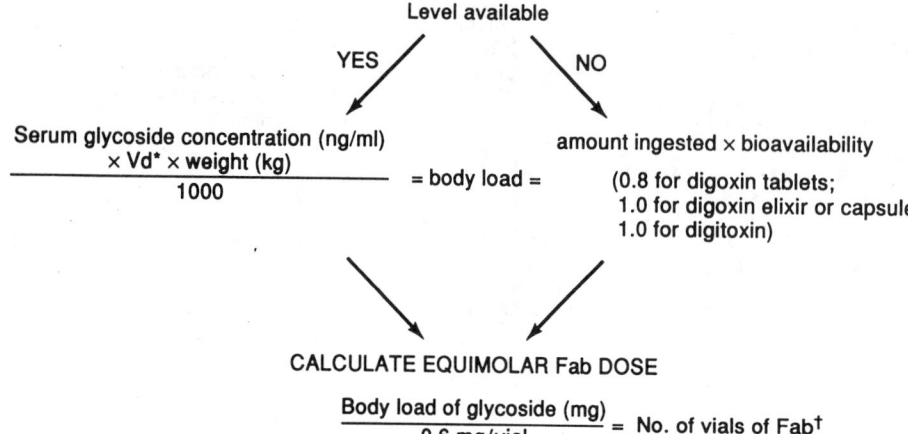

Fab Fragment Dosing

DETERMINE GLYCOSIDE BODY LOAD

Level available

YES / NO \

$$\frac{\text{Serum glycoside concentration (ng/ml)} \times \text{Vd*} \times \text{weight (kg)}}{1000} = \text{body load} = \quad \text{amount ingested} \times \text{bioavailability}$$

(0.8 for digoxin tablets;
1.0 for digoxin elixir or capsules;
1.0 for digitoxin)

CALCULATE EQUIMOLAR Fab DOSE

$$\frac{\text{Body load of glycoside (mg)}}{0.6 \text{ mg/vial}} = \text{No. of vials of Fab}^{†}$$

* Vd for digoxin = 5.6 L/kg
Vd for digitoxin = 0.56 L/kg

† If amount ingested is unknown and level is unavailable in severely toxic patient, empirically administer up to 20 vials in an adult.

Figure 95–2. The appropriate dose of Fab fragment to be administered in cases of severe digitalis toxicity may be approximated using an estimation of the body load of glycoside, calculated either from a serum glycoside concentration or from knowledge of the amount and formulation of drug ingested. (Adapted from Martiny SS, Phelps SJ, Massery KL. Treatment of severe digitalis intoxication with digoxin-specific antibody fragments: A clinical review. Crit Care Med 1988; 16:629. © Williams & Wilkins, 1988.)

5). *Sympathomimetics* stimulate alpha- or beta-adrenergic receptors with varying degrees of specificity depending on the drug; in supratherapeutic doses, many will result in both alpha- and beta-receptor stimulation. *Alpha- and beta-adrenergic blocking agents* interfere with receptor stimulation, generally causing symptoms opposite from their agonist counterparts, but they may possess some intrinsic sympathomimetic effects following large doses.

Alpha agonists and the related imidazolines, found in eye and nose drops, are used for their vasoconstrictor effects and may lead to toxic effects, including severe central nervous system depression and branch retinal artery occlusion.[22, 23] Phenylpropanolamine administered orally as a decongestant or for appetite suppression has been associated with the development of atrioventricular block, hypertensive crisis, intracerebral hemorrhage, seizures, and arrhythmias.[24–26] Decongestants such as ephedrine and pseudoephedrine possess mixed alpha- and beta-agonist activity, as do racemic and nonracemic epinephrine. Intoxication with these agents may result in tremulousness, diaphoresis, and hypertension.[27]

The orally administered, peripherally acting alpha-adrenergic blocking agents are used primarily as antihypertensives; toxic ingestion frequently results in hypotension. Yohimbine hydrochloride, an alpha$_2$ antagonist sometimes used in the treatment of impotence in diabetes, may lead to hypertension by norepinephrine release.[28–30] Ingestion of clonidine, a centrally acting alpha antagonist, may cause hypotension or a paradoxical severe hypertension. The *beta-adrenoreceptor blocking agents* are widely used for their antihypertensive and antiarrhythmic effects and for the treatment of angina. Nonselective beta-receptor antagonists (i.e., beta$_1$ and beta$_2$) possess both negative inotropic and negative chronotropic action, leading to hypotension and bradycardia when taken in excessive amounts, and may predispose to bronchospasm. The hyperglycemic response to epinephrine is blocked, leading to hypoglycemia in some patients.[31, 32] Presenting symptoms of nonselective beta blockade frequently include bradycardia, hypotension, seizures, and peripheral cyanosis.[31, 33] While most exposures to beta-blocking agents are through ingestion of tablets, toxic ingestion of atenolol through breast milk has been described.[34]

Clinical Evaluation

History should include factors that will affect the degree and possible extent of toxicity, such as underlying heart, renal, or hepatic disease. The time and amount of ingestion is estimated, and the drug formulation and any coingested agents are determined.

Physical examination is directed toward identification of signs of adrenergic stimulation or antagonism (Table 95–5). This includes assessment of adequacy of perfusion, blood pressure, heart rate, cardiac rhythm, respiratory drive, bronchospasm, adequacy of air movement, and mental status.

Diagnostic Evaluation

Continuous electrocardiographic monitoring should be initiated, and blood pressure should be evaluated frequently. Serum drug levels may confirm the suspicion of ingestion but will not alter treatment. If arrhythmias occur, serum electrolytes may aid in correction of abnormalities that exacerbate toxicity (e.g., potassium, calcium). Underlying clinical conditions such as renal and hepatic disease can be identified by the serum BUN, creatinine, and liver enzymes. A rapid glucose test, confirmed by laboratory analysis, should be performed to detect hypoglycemia or hyperglycemia.

Differential Diagnosis

All drug ingestions causing tachycardia, hypertension, hyperglycemia, and mental status changes (either agitation or obtundation) must be differentiated from adrenergic agonist ingestions. Cocaine toxicity leads to adrenergic stimulation through blockade of norepinephrine reuptake, resulting in primarily alpha-adrenergic symptoms.[6] Pheochromocytoma, although uncommon in children, must also be considered. Psychiatric causes of agitation may lead to increased adrenergic outflow but do not usually create life-

TABLE 95–5

PHYSIOLOGIC ACTIONS AND TOXICITIES OF ADRENERGIC AGENTS

Classification	Clinical Effects of Receptor Stimulation	Examples	Receptor Stimulation		
			α	β₁	β₂
Alpha agonists	Mydriasis	Methoxamine	+ + + +	− −	− −
	Vasoconstriction	Norepinephrine	+ + +	+ +	+
	Coronary dilatation	Epinephrine	+ +	+ +	+ + +
		Dopamine	+	+	+
Alpha antagonists	Miosis	Yohimbine	− −	0	0
	Postural hypotension	Clonidine	− −	0	0
	Reflex tachycardia				
Beta₁ agonists	Miosis	Isoproterenol	0	+ + +	+ + + +
	Tachycardia	Norepinephrine	+ + +	+ +	+
	↑ Cardiac contractility	Epinephrine	+ +	+ +	+ + +
	Accelerated AV conduction	Dopamine	+	+	+
	Renin release	Dobutamine	0 or +	+	0 or +
Beta₁ antagonists	± Hypotension	Esmolol	0	− −	0
	Cardiac dysrrhythmias	Propranolol	0	− −	− − −
	± Bradycardia	Nadolol	0	− −	− − −
	± Hyperkalemia	Metaprolol	0	− −	0/−
		Atenolol	0	− −	0/−
Beta₂ agonists	Miosis	Epinephrine	+ +	+ +	+ + +
	Vasodilatation	Isoproterenol	0	+ + +	+ + + +
	Bronchodilation	Norepinephrine	+ + +	+ +	+
	Hyperglycemia	Albuterol	0	+	+ + +
	Hypokalemia	Isoetharine	0	+	+ + +
		Metaproterenol	0	+ +	+ + +
		Terbutaline	0	+	+ + +
Beta₂ antagonists	Hypoglycemia with hypertension	Propranolol	0	− −	− −
	Bronchospasm	Nadolol	0	− −	− −
	Hyperkalemia (uncommon)				

Adapted from Ellenhorn MJ, Baraloux DG (eds). Medical Toxicology. Diagnosis and Treatment of Human Poisoning. New York, Elsevier, 1988, p 28.
− = inhibitory effect; 0 = no effect; + = stimulatory effect. Copyright 1988 by Elsevier Science Publishing Co., Inc.

threatening conditions. Increased intracranial pressure may cause hypertension and tachycardia, followed by bradycardia as herniation occurs.

Alpha-adrenergic blockade, with hypotension and reflex tachycardia, may mimic other systemic conditions, including volume loss and sepsis. Beta-adrenergic blockade must be primarily differentiated from other agents causing bradycardia, including cardiac glycosides and other antiarrhythmics, and from other causes of bronchospasm.

Therapeutic Intervention

Gut decontamination using lavage, charcoal, and cathartics may be useful in limiting the amount of absorption of orally ingested drugs but may not be effective in the case of mucosally absorbed agents such as eye drops, nose drops, or sprays.[6] Caution must be observed in using syrup of ipecac when the patient is at risk for apnea or seizures.

Specific therapy is chosen to compete with the offending

TABLE 95–6

MANAGEMENT OF ADRENERGIC AGENT TOXICITY

Drug Class	Symptom	Treatment
Alpha agonists	Hypertension and reflex bradycardia	Nitroprusside, 0.5–1.0 μg/kg/min and up
	Hypertension with tachycardia	Propranolol or labetalol
Alpha antagonists	Hypotension	Fluid administration; norepinephrine or dopamine
Beta agonists	Tachycardia	Propranolol, labetalol, esmolol; caution for hypotension
	Vasodilatation and hypotension	Fluid administration, alpha agonists (epinephrine, norepinephrine; caution for tachycardia)
Beta antagonists	Hypotension	Fluid administration; alpha agonists (norepinephrine, epinephrine); glucagon 50–100 μg/kg followed by infusion of 70 μg/kg/hr
	Bradycardia	Beta agonist (isoproterenol; caution for hypotension due to vasodilatation); epinephrine; pacing
	Bronchospasm	Beta₂ agonist (terbutaline; albuterol; epinephrine)

drug at the receptor level or to counteract symptoms through other mechanisms (Table 95–6). Severe hypertension with reflex bradycardia caused by adrenergic stimulation may be initially treated in the emergency setting with nitroprusside infusion or nifedipine.[26] Tachycardia and hypertension may respond to beta blockade with propranolol[35] or labetalol.[27] Ventricular ectopy may be managed with lidocaine; an initial bolus dose of 1 mg/kg is followed by a continuous intravenous infusion of 30 to 50 μg/kg/minute. Seizures may respond to diazepam, 0.2 mg/kg administered by slow intravenous push over several minutes, or rectally as a solution if intravenous access is difficult or unavailable.

Beta blockade sufficient to cause hypotension and bradycardia is treated with atropine and beta agonists such as isoproterenol; large doses of the beta agonist may be required depending on the severity of the antagonist intoxication.[33, 36, 37] Blood pressure must be continuously monitored since the peripheral vasodilating effects of isoproterenol may exacerbate the hypotension observed with beta-blocker toxicity.[6] In intoxications where hypotension limits the therapeutic effectiveness of isoproterenol, the addition of norepinephrine, beginning at 0.05 to 0.1 μg/kg/minute and titrating rapidly upward to achieve the desired effect, may be useful; dopamine and epinephrine can also be used. One may also consider the use of glucagon,[33, 38–40] which through a nonreceptor mechanism increases cyclic AMP, enhancing inotropy and chronotropy.[41] The recommended initial dose for glucagon is 50 to 100 μg/kg, followed by an infusion of 70 μg/kg/hour.[39, 40] The blood glucose should be monitored in all cases of beta-blocker toxicity since the ingestion may cause hypoglycemia,[32] whereas treatment may cause hyperglycemia.[31, 33] Glucagon administration may also be associated with the development of hypokalemia and hypocalcemia.[6] Bradycardia secondary to beta blockade unresponsive to pharmacologic measures may require external cardiac pacing.[42]

Alpha-antagonist–induced hypotension should be treated initially with fluid resuscitation. If hypotension persists after volume expansion, dopamine (5 to 20 μg/kg/minute) or norepinephrine (beginning at 0.05 to 0.1 μg/kg/minute) may be effective.

Disposition

Patients with mild symptoms and a reliable history of recent exposure may be discharged after several hours of observation. Those with ingestion of an unknown quantity or with coingestions may be at risk for delayed or severe symptoms and should be admitted for careful monitoring. Patients with airway compromise, those requiring blood pressure management, and those with dysrhythmias (including significant bradycardia or tachycardia) warrant direct admission to an intensive care unit, where continuous monitoring of blood pressure and cardiac rhythm may be performed.

CALCIUM CHANNEL BLOCKERS
Physiology

Calcium channel blockers fall into the category of class IV antiarrhythmic agents and are widely used for treatment of arrhythmias (verapamil) or angina (verapamil, diltiazem, nifedipine). These drugs inhibit calcium and sodium influx through the slow calcium channel, altering impulse conduction through slow-channel dependent tissue in the sinoatrial and atrioventricular nodes, altering coupling of myocardial excitation and contraction, and decreasing vascular smooth muscle tone.[6] Many differences exist in the molecular structure of these drugs, leading to varying degrees of inhibition of calcium influx and a wide range of clinical effects after ingestion of toxic quantities of drug (Table 95–7).[43, 44] Signs of overdose common to all three drugs are conduction abnormalities and hypotension. Overdose with verapamil has been associated with cerebral infarction in an adult, possibly due to severe hypotension,[45] as well as with hyperglycemia,[46, 47] thought to be due to impaired insulin release and altered peripheral glucose utilization. While reports of severe toxicity from pediatric ingestions of verapamil are rare, such ingestions may be fatal.[48] Diltiazem overdose rarely causes toxicity but has been associated with arrhythmias, neurologic symptoms, hypotension, and noncardiogenic pulmonary edema.[49–51] Nifedipine poisoning in a child resulted in tachycardia, mental status changes, pulmonary edema, seizures, and cortical infarction.[52]

EMS Considerations

Patients who have ingested toxic quantities of calcium channel blockers are at risk for dysrhythmias, hypotension, mental status changes due to poor central nervous system perfusion, and seizures.

Clinical Evaluation

A complete history will elicit underlying illnesses that might lead to exacerbation of arrhythmias or hypotension, approximate time of ingestion, the amount and formulation ingested, any possible coingested agents, and current symptoms. Sustained-release formulations of verapamil are available and may lead to prolonged effects owing to continued absorption; onset of symptoms may begin several hours after ingestion,[48, 53, 54] with peak serum concentrations occurring 5 hours after ingestion. Verapamil ingestions less than 25 mg/kg involving children were nontoxic in one retrospective study[49]; in this study the smallest toxic pediatric dose of nifedipine in a 1-year-old child was 200 mg, while the largest nontoxic ingestion of diltiazem was 120 mg in an 18-month-old child.

The physical examination is focused on the cardiovascular system, principally the cardiac rhythm and clinical signs of decreased cardiac output or inadequate blood pressure. Signs or symptoms of other organ involvement from inadequate perfusion must be sought, such as altered mental status and poor respiratory effort. Clinical evaluation must be repeated at frequent intervals since the onset of signs may be gradual or acute and the time of onset may be delayed by several hours after ingestion.

Diagnostic Evaluation

Continuous electrocardiographic monitoring should be maintained if a significant ingestion is documented or strongly suspected. Intermittent rhythm strips may be obtained if the level of suspicion is low. Frequent blood pressure monitoring by noninvasive means is adequate in the stable patient. Laboratory studies are directed at monitoring adequate oxygenation and tissue perfusion; thus include intermittent blood gas evaluation to evaluate oxygen tension and acid-base status. Concentrations of drug in blood may be obtained to document intoxication but are not useful in guiding patient management.

Differential Diagnosis

All other causes of hypotension and dysrhythmias in children must be considered. These include cardiomyopathy,

		TABLE 95-7		
		CALCIUM CHANNEL BLOCKER TOXICITY		
Drug	Mechanism of Action	Onset of Action (min)	Toxic Effects	Management
Verapamil	Nonselective inhibitor of slow Ca^{++} channels Prolonged AV nodal conduction	<30	Conduction defects Bradycardia Hypotension Decreased cardiac output Altered mental status Seizures Vomiting	Cardiac monitoring; oxygen, fluid administration, calcium gluconate 10% solution: give 0.2–0.5 ml/kg up to 10 ml over 5–10 min; may repeat in 15 min Isoproterenol, dopamine, or epinephrine infusion Gut decontamination Pacemaker if needed
Nifedipine	Selective inhibition of some slow Ca^{++} channels Increased AV nodal conduction and shortened AV node refractoriness	<20	Flushing Hypotension Palpitations	Same as above
Diltiazem	Slow channel inhibition at low concentrations; fast channel inhibition at high concentrations Prolonged AV nodal conduction Intermediate prolongation of AV node refractoriness	<30	Conduction abnormalities Hypotension	Same as above

myocarditis, and ingestion of other cardiotoxic drugs, including digoxin or other antiarrhythmic agents.

Therapeutic Intervention

Initial stabilization efforts are directed at preventing morbidity from conduction abnormalities, decreased cardiac output, or hypotension. A high concentration of inspired oxygen is administered as required to maintain adequate tissue oxygenation. The cardiac rhythm is monitored frequently, either by continuous cardiorespiratory impedance monitoring or by obtaining intermittent rhythm strips. Peripheral intravenous access should be secured initially, followed by central access if indicated by cardiovascular instability, a need for inotropic drug infusions, or a need for assessment of central pressures to aid in management decisions.

Gut decontamination may be useful in limiting total body load of drug if performed within the first few hours after ingestion of prompt-release preparations and possibly up to 8 to 10 hours following ingestion of time-release tablets. Verapamil, nifedipine, and diltiazem are all highly protein bound and thus are not believed to be effectively removed by dialysis or hemoperfusion,[6] although hemoperfusion may be useful in decreasing serum concentrations of verapamil in patients with decreased hepatic clearance.[55] One author[48] reported decreased serum concentrations of verapamil, with concomitant improvement in cardiac function, in a child maintained transiently on cardiopulmonary bypass.

Volume expansion with rapid infusion of an isotonic crystalloid solution may reverse hypotension caused by vasodilation.[46] Bolus infusion of calcium chloride (10 mg/kg)[56, 57] may be an effective antagonist to several adverse effects of verapamil, including bradycardia, hypotension, and seizures. If calcium administration is effective but short-lived, repeated bolus infusions or constant infusion of calcium chloride or calcium gluconate may be useful.[56, 58, 59]

Continuous infusion of isoproterenol may increase the heart rate in patients with calcium channel blocker overdose but may do little to support blood pressure. Epinephrine or dopamine infusion may improve vascular tone and cardiac output, resulting in improved blood pressure and vital organ perfusion,[56] but must be used with caution if ectopy is present. Repeated doses of calcium and multiple inotropic agents are frequently needed.[60–62] Insertion of a pacemaker may be needed to manage bradycardia in cases unresponsive to chronotropic drugs or in patients with ectopy.[62]

Disposition

Toxic effects of calcium channel blocking agents usually occur within several hours of ingestion. Toxic effects may remain significant for several days after ingestion; thus symptomatic patients must be monitored in a facility that is equipped to manage dysrhythmias and cardiogenic shock. Monitoring and treatment should be maintained until cardiac rhythm and cardiac output have returned to normal.

OTHER ANTIHYPERTENSIVE AGENTS
Physiology

Other oral antihypertensive agents can be divided into several groups based on mechanism of action (Table 95-8). These include diuretics, angiotensin converting enzyme (ACE) inhibitors, direct-acting vascular smooth muscle vasodilators, and centrally acting agents.

Diuretics may be further divided based on their diverse actions (Table 95-9). Thiazide diuretics, including chlorothiazide, hydrochlorothiazide, metolazone, and chlorthalidone, act at the cortical diluting segment or the early distal tubule, increasing sodium, chloride, magnesium, and potassium excretion. Overdose results in diuresis, lethargy, electrolyte changes, and sometimes coma by an unknown central nervous system mechanism. Hypotension may result from volume depletion, while electrolyte changes may induce dysrhythmias. Loop diuretics, including furosemide, bumetanide, ethacrynic acid, and xipamide, act at the thick ascending limb of the nephron, causing water, sodium, and potassium loss. Symptomatic volume depletion and severe electrolyte abnormalities may result. The potassium-sparing

		TABLE 95-8		
		ACTIONS, TOXICITY, AND MANAGEMENT OF ANTIHYPERTENSIVE AGENT OVERDOSE		
Class	**Drug**	**Action**	**Toxicity**	**Treatment**
Diuretics	See Table 9	Diverse	Volume depletion; hypotension electrolyte abnormalities; dysrhythmias	Volume replacement Correct electrolytes Gut decontamination
ACE inhibitors	Captopril Enalapril	Decrease conversion of angiotensin I to angiotensin II Potentiate hypotensive effects of bradykinin Reduce aldosterone secretion	Potential for hypotension and mental status changes Serious toxicity not documented in children	Fluid administration Pressor catecholamines (norepinephrine, dopamine, epinephrine) Gut decontamination
Direct-acting vasodilators	Hydralazine Diazoxide Minoxidil	Vascular smooth muscle relaxation Inhibition of insulin secretion (diazoxide) Increased catecholamine release (diazoxide)	Hypotension Reflex tachycardia Nonketotic hyperosmolar coma (diazoxide) Dysrhythmias	Fluid administration Pressor catecholamines with caution; may induce dysrhythmias Gut decontamination
Centrally acting agents	Clonidine HCl Guanabenz Methyldopa Reserpine	Central alpha$_2$ adrenergic stimulation results in ↓ sympathetic outflow Peripheral alpha-agonist activity at high doses (clonidine) resulting in vasoconstriction Depletion of norepinephrine in postganglionic neurons (reserpine)	Hypotension Bradycardia CNS depression Seizures Hypertension (clonidine) at high doses	Fluid administration Pressor catecholamines Atropine for bradycardia Naloxone or vasodilators for hypertension (clonidine) Gut decontamination

diuretics amiloride hydrochloride, spironolactone, and triamterene are weak diuretics that may lead to life-threatening hyperkalemia. Gastrointestinal symptoms of overdose of these diuretics include nausea, vomiting, abdominal pain, and gastrointestinal bleeding.[6]

ACE inhibitors lower systolic, mean, and diastolic blood pressures by decreasing conversion of angiotensin I to angiotensin II, potentiating the hypotensive action of bradykinin and inhibiting its degradation and slightly reducing the secretion of aldosterone. The major acute side effect from these drugs is hypotension, especially in patients who are depleted of salt and water.[6, 63] Renal function may be decreased after captopril therapy.[64, 65] Ingestion of toxic doses of enalapril in two adults resulted in hypotension and stupor responsive to fluid replacement.[66, 67] A recent report of 48 pediatric ingestions of captopril (12.5 to 100 mg) and

enalapril (5 to 15 mg) revealed no serious toxicity within these relatively low dose ranges; no patients required hospitalization.[68]

Oral direct-acting vascular smooth muscle relaxants act as vasodilators of venous or arterial beds. Few reports of poisoning with diazoxide or hydralazine are available. Diazoxide ingestion may be associated with prolonged hypotension and with hyperglycemia and hyperosmolar, nonketotic coma. Hydralazine poisoning may result in hypotension, shock, flushing, and tachycardia. Minoxidil, a long-lasting arteriolar vasodilator used primarily for treatment of hypertension, has recently become available as a topical preparation to enhance hair growth. Reports of ingestion reveal that tachycardia is common, while not all patients become hypotensive.[69] Hypotension may be severe and persistent, however, requiring prolonged pressor support.[70]

		TABLE 95-9		
		ACTIONS, TOXICITY, AND MANAGEMENT OF DIURETIC OVERDOSE		
Class	**Drug**	**Action**	**Toxicity**	**Treatment**
Thiazide	Chlorothiazide Hydrochlorothiazide Metolazone Chlorthalidone	Increased sodium, chloride, magnesium, potassium excretion	Diuresis Lethargy; coma	Airway management Fluid replacement Electrolyte replacement Gut decontamination
Loop diuretics	Furosemide Bumetanide Ethacrynic acid Xipamide	Water, sodium, and potassium loss	Diuresis Hypokalemia	Fluid replacement Electrolyte replacement Gut decontamination
Potassium-sparing diuretics	Amiloride HCl Spironolactone Triamterene	Weak diuresis Potassium retention	Hyperkalemia Dysrhythmias Nausea, vomiting Abdominal pain	Stop potassium intake Treat hyperkalemia with glucose (0.5–1.0 gm/kg) and insulin (0.25–0.5 units regular insulin per gram glucose given); repeat as needed Gut decontamination

Pediatric ingestions of the centrally acting antihypertensive agents clonidine, guanabenz, and reserpine have been reported.[71-80] Initial toxic effects of all three drugs include hypotension, bradycardia, and central nervous system depression. Reserpine, and most notably clonidine, have also been associated with severe hypertension after poisoning. Hypertension secondary to clonidine ingestion may respond to treatment with naloxone.[74, 81] Clonidine poisoning after ingestion of clonidine transdermal patches has been reported with some frequency since their release for use in management of hypertension and as an aid to stop smoking.[82-84]

Clinical Evaluation

History will include drugs ingested, formulation, time of ingestion, any underlying disease, and current symptoms. The physical examination is directed toward identification of cardiovascular instability and involvement of other vital organ systems affected by circulatory compromise or direct nervous system depression.

Diagnostic Evaluation

Electrocardiography may be useful in documenting dysrhythmias associated with electrolyte abnormalities or conduction disturbances. Serum concentrations of several of these agents may be available but will not be clinically useful in management. Electrolyte measurement will alert the physician to possible complications and appropriate interventions. Arterial blood gas evaluation in symptomatic patients will aid in assessment of adequacy of oxygenation, ventilation, and tissue perfusion.

Differential Diagnosis

Hypotension, dysrhythmias, and mental status changes may be caused by ingestion of many other toxins, including digoxin, class IA antiarrhythmic agents, ethchlorvynol, methadone, narcotics, tricyclic antidepressants, and alpha- and beta-adrenergic agents. Electrolyte disturbances from fluid losses, fluid shifts, or specific electrolyte ingestion may mimic antihypertensive drug ingestion if of sufficient severity to cause cardiac compromise. Myocarditis or cardiomyopathy may result in poor cardiac output, hypotension, rhythm disturbances, and mental status changes if central nervous system perfusion is inadequate.

Therapeutic Intervention

Intervention will be guided by the symptom complex observed; most will be supportive since no antidotes exist for this group of drugs. Careful and frequent monitoring of vital signs, mental status, and circulatory status is imperative, except perhaps in the case of ACE inhibitor ingestion, where toxicity has not been reported in children. In symptomatic patients management is directed toward maintenance of adequate tissue perfusion and oxygen. Thus peripheral intravenous access is obtained early and may be followed by central venous and arterial access if cardiovascular instability is seen or considered to be imminent.

Gut decontamination will decrease total load of drug if initiated within several hours of ingestion. Airway protection may be needed during this procedure if mental status changes appear likely or have occurred.

Hypotension may be initially treated with the administration of crystalloid or colloid as fluid boluses of 10 to 20 ml/kg. Since most agents discussed in this section exhibit vasodilating actions, fluid administration may be sufficient to maintain blood pressure. If this approach is unsuccessful

owing to bradycardia or poor myocardial function, pressor agents such as dopamine may be needed to reverse hypotension and bradycardia. Hypertension due to clonidine toxicity has been successfully reversed in some cases with the use of naloxone, but this drug has not always been effective[74, 81] and may require upward dose titration by constant intravenous infusion.

Disposition

Asymptomatic patients with a clear history of ingestion should receive gut decontamination with induced emesis or administration of activated charcoal and should be observed for signs of toxicity for up to 4 to 6 hours. Any symptomatic patient should be admitted for monitoring. Patients with rhythm disturbances, hypotension unresponsive to minimal fluid replacement, hypertension, or mental status changes are candidates for management in an intensive care setting.

OTHER ANTIARRHYTHMIC AGENTS
Physiology

The antiarrhythmic agents are often divided into four major classes based on mechanism of action (Table 95–10). Class II drugs (beta-adrenergic blockers) and class IV drugs (calcium channel blockers) have already been discussed.

Class IA antiarrhythmics available as oral preparations include disopyramide phosphate, quinine, and procainamide hydrochloride. All of these drugs act upon sodium-dependent conduction tissue, slowing conduction velocity, prolonging refractory period, and decreasing automaticity by inhibiting the fast sodium channel.[85] Toxicity results in a prolonged QT interval, bradycardia, asystole, and central nervous system depression.[6]

Commonly used class IB drugs include lidocaine hydrochloride, phenytoin, mexiletine, and tocainide; in contrast to class IA agents these drugs suppress automaticity but also shorten the refractory period. Elevated serum concentrations of lidocaine (>3.5 μg/ml) may result in conduction delay and heart block, depress myocardial contractility, and be associated with central nervous system symptoms ranging from mild lightheadedness to seizures, apnea, and coma.[6] Bioavailability of lidocaine by the enteral route is poor, but large oral doses may result in toxicity. Fewer reports of mexiletine and tocainide toxicity exist owing to their relatively recent approval for use, but both would be expected to share the central nervous system and myocardial toxicity seen with lidocaine.

Class IC drugs such as flecainide and encainide also inhibit the fast sodium channel but do not affect action potential duration. A recent report of findings in 120 cases of class IC antiarrhythmic overdose showed a high mortality rate (22.5%).[86] Nausea occurred within 30 minutes after ingestion, followed by bradycardia or tachyrhythmia between 30 minutes and 2 hours. Deaths were usually attributable to conduction disturbances progressing to electromechanical dissociation or asystole.

Class III antiarrhythmic agents include amiodarone and bretylium tosylate. These drugs specifically prolong refractoriness in atrial and ventricular fibers by a mechanism of action that remains unclear.[85] A case report of an amiodarone overdose (3.4 gm) described an unremarkable examination and no cardiovascular symptoms other than a short, self-limited run of ventricular tachycardia.[87] In other cases in adults, patients remained asymptomatic with either no EKG changes after ingestion of 6 gm[88] or EKG changes simulating an anteroseptal infarct after ingestion of 2.6 gm.[89] Temporary pacing was required for 2 weeks to treat first-

TABLE 95–10

CLASSES OF ANTIARRHYTHMIC AGENTS

Class	Mechanism of Action	Drug	Cardiac Action
I	Inhibit fast sodium channel	IA: Quinidine Procainamide Disopyramide HCl	Slowed depolarization ↓ Conduction velocity Lengthened action potential (↑ refractoriness)
		IB: Lidocaine HCl Mexiletine Tocainide Phenytoin	Slowed depolarization ↓ Conduction velocity Shortened action potential (↓ refractoriness) Slowed depolarization
		IC: Flecainide Encainide	↓ Conduction velocity No change in action potential
II	Beta-adrenergic blockade; variable cardioselectivity	Propranolol Labetalol Metoprolol Atenolol Others	Reduced membrane-bound adenylate cyclase and cAMP Decreased myocardial contractility Widened QRS complex
III	Variable	Amiodarone	Altered repolarization (QT prolongation) *without* affecting spontaneous phase IV depolarization
IV	Calcium channel blockade	Verapamil Diltiazem Nifedipine	Inhibit calcium and sodium influx across slow channels Altered SA and AV conduction, myocardial contractility and vasodilatation

degree atrioventricular block after ingestion of 15 gm of amiodarone and 4 mg of digoxin.[90] Overdose of bretylium tosylate, available only in parenteral form but frequently used during acute management of ventricular dysrhythmias refractory to lidocaine, resulted in hypotension and neuromuscular blockade suggestive of ganglionic blockade in an infant.[91]

EMS Considerations

Neurologic changes, dysrhythmias, and cardiovascular collapse may occur after ingestion of class I antiarrhythmic agents. Intravenous access should be obtained. Electrocardiographic monitoring should be performed throughout transport.

Amiodarone ingestion appears to offer little immediate risk in adults and adolescents; data on children do not exist. Thus careful monitoring of vital signs and cardiac rhythm should be maintained during transport.

Clinical Evaluation

Pertinent history includes underlying disease that may contribute to the development of rhythm disturbances and information about coingested agents. Physical examination is directed toward evaluation of cardiovascular compromise and thus should include vital signs and attention to peripheral perfusion, pulses, and rhythm.

Diagnostic Evaluation

Electrocardiographic monitoring will reveal rhythm disturbances, if present. No immediate electrolyte derangements are expected. In symptomatic patients, arterial blood gas evaluation will reflect adequacy of tissue perfusion.

Serum concentrations of quinidine (>8 μg/ml), procainamide (>16 μg/ml), and disopyramide (>9 μg/ml) may be associated with toxicity. Lidocaine toxicity may occur if concentrations exceed 3.5 μg/ml. Serum amiodarone con-

TABLE 95–11

MANAGEMENT OF ARRHYTHMIAS FROM CLASS I AND CLASS III ANTIARRHYTHMIC AGENTS

Class	Agent	Rhythm Disturbance	Management
IA	Disopyramide	QT prolongation Ventricular and supraventricular dysrhythmias	Avoid other class IA drugs Lidocaine; phenytoin; overdrive pacing
	Procainamide	Conduction disturbances Ventricular arrhythmias	Avoid other class IA drugs Lidocaine; phenytoin
	Quinidine	Delayed conduction Myocardial depression	Avoid other class IA drugs Lidocaine; phenytoin Avoid lidocaine and phenytoin if atypical ventricular tachycardia present; use isoproterenol or pacing
IB	Lidocaine	Heart block; sinus arrest	Avoid phenytoin, catecholamine support, cardiac pacing
	Tocainide: mexiletine	Heart block	Same
IC	Flecainide Encainide	Multiple QT prolongation; bradycardia	Little data available; supportive
III	Amiodarone	Torsades de pointes QT prolongation Bradycardia	Supportive Cardiac pacing

centrations greater than 2.5 µg/ml are considered toxic; the drug's elimination half-life is quite long (25 ± 12 days),[92] resulting in the potential for delayed or prolonged symptoms.

Differential Diagnosis

All causes of rhythm disturbances, including those drugs mentioned above under antihypertensive agents as well as myocarditis and cardiomyopathy, must be considered.

Therapeutic Intervention

Management of overdose with class I drugs is supportive, and management of dysrhythmias varies with the drug ingested (Table 95–11). Gut decontamination should be attempted, blood pressure supported, and rhythm disturbances vigorously treated.

Recommendations for management of amiodarone poisoning are provisional since few cases of severe toxicity have been reported. Gastric decontamination with lavage or emesis should be attempted. There is some evidence that cholestyramine may reduce the elimination half-life of amiodarone if administered hourly for 4 to 12 hours.[87, 93] Cardiac monitoring for 1 to 2 days has been suggested[87] in order to document any late symptomatic dysrhythmias. Cardiac pacing may be considered if symptomatic bradycardia ensues.[93]

Disposition

Any patient displaying cardiovascular instability or rhythm disturbances following class I antiarrhythmic poisoning should be admitted to a hospital unit capable of closely monitoring cardiac rhythm and cardiac performance. In light of the information relating to pediatric amiodarone overdose, the potential for dysrhythmias, and the long half-life of the drug, in-hospital monitoring of cardiac rhythm for several days is advisable at this time.

References

1. Litovitz TL, Schmitz BF, Bailey KM. 1989 Annual report of the American Association of Poison Control Centers National Data Collection System. Am J Emerg Med 1990;8:394.
2. Covinsky JO, Willett MS. Congestive heart failure. In DePiro JT, Talbert RL, Hayes PE, et al (eds). Pharmacotherapy: A Pathophysiologic Approach. New York, Elsevier, 1989, pp 127–132.
3. Fozzard HA, Sheets MF. Cellular mechanism of action of cardiac glycosides. J Am Coll Cardiol 1985;5:10A.
4. Katz M. Effects of digitalis on cell biochemistry: Sodium pump inhibition. J Am Coll Cardiol 1985;5:16A.
5. Sharff JA, Bayer MJ. Acute and chronic digitalis toxicity: Presentation and treatment. Ann Emerg Med 1982;11:327.
6. Ellenhorn MJ, Barceloux DG. Medical Toxicology: Diagnosis and Treatment of Human Poisoning. New York, Elsevier, 1988.
7. Koren G. Interaction between digoxin and commonly coadministered drugs in children. Pediatrics 1985;75:1032.
8. Ingelfinger JA, Goodman P. The serum digoxin concentration—does it diagnose digitalis toxicity? N Engl J Med 1976;274:867.
9. Lasagna L. How useful are serum digitalis measurements? N Engl J Med 1976;294:898.
10. Valdes R, Graves SW, Brown BA, Landt M. Endogenous substance in newborn infants causing false positive digoxin measurements. J Pediatr 1983;102:947.
11. Ordog GJ, Benaron S, Bhasin V, et al. Serum digoxin levels and mortality in 5100 patients. Ann Emerg Med 1987;16:32.
12. Lalonde RL, Deshpande R, Hamilton PP, et al. Acceleration of digoxin clearance by activated charcoal. Clin Pharmacol Ther 1985;37:367.
13. Hobson JD, Zettner A. Digoxin serum half-life following suicidal digoxin poisoning. JAMA 1973;223:147.
14. Kearns GL, Moss M, Clayton BD, Hewett DD. Pharmacokinetics and efficacy of digoxin specific Fab fragments in a child following massive digoxin overdose. J Clin Pharmacol 1989;29:901.
15. Kaufman J, Leikin J, Kendzierski D, Polin K. Use of digoxin Fab immune fragments in a seven-day-old infant. Pediatr Emerg Care 1990;6:118.
16. Zucker A, Lacina SJ, DasGupta DS, et al. Fab fragments of digoxin-specific antibodies used to reverse ventricular fibrillation induced by digoxin ingestion in a child. Pediatrics 1982;70:468.
17. Presti S, Friedman D, Saslow J, et al. Digoxin toxicity in a premature infant: Treatment with Fab fragments of digoxin-specific antibodies. Pediatr Cardiol 1985;6:91.
18. Martiny SS, Phelps SJ, Massey KL. Treatment of severe digitalis intoxication with digoxin-specific antibody fragments: A clinical review. Crit Care Med 1988;16:629.
19. Fazio A. Fab fragments in the treatment of digoxin overdose: Pediatric considerations. South Med J 1987;80:1553.
20. Wenger TL, Butler VP, Haber E, Smith TS. Treatment of 63 severely digitalis-toxic patients with digoxin-specific antibody fragments. J Am Coll Cardiol 1985;5:118A.
21. Antman EM, Wenger TL, Butler VP, et al. Treatment of 150 cases of life-threatening digitalis intoxication with digoxin-specific Fab antibody fragments. Final report of a multicenter study. Circulation 1990;81:1744.
22. Klein-Schwartz W, Gorman R, Oderda GM, Baig A. Central nervous system depression from ingestion of nonprescription eyedrops. Am J Emerg Med 1984;2:217.
23. Margargal LE, Samborn GE, Donoso LA, Gonder JR. Branch retinal artery occlusion after excessive use of nasal spray. Ann Ophthalmol 1985;17:500.
24. Burton BT, Rice M, Schmertzler LE. Atrioventricular block following overdose of decongestant cold medication. J Emerg Med 1985;2:415.
25. Maertens P, Lum G, Williams JP, White J. Intracranial hemorrhage and angiopathic changes in a suicidal phenylpropanolamine poisoning. South Med J 1987;80:1584.
26. Gibson RC, Oliver JA, Leak U. Nifedipine therapy of phenylpropanolamine induced hypertension. Am Heart J 1987;113:406.
27. Mariani PJ. Pseudoephedrine-induced hypertensive emergency: Treatment with labetalol. Am J Emerg Med 1986;4:141.
28. Linden CH, Vellman PW, Rumack B. Yohimbine: A new street drug. Ann Emerg Med 1985;14:1002.
29. Morales A, Surridge DH, Marshall PG. Yohimbine for treatment of impotence in diabetes (letter). N Engl J Med 1981;305:1221.
30. Goldberg MR, Hollister AS, Robertson D. Influence of Yohimbine on blood pressure, autonomic reflexes, and plasma catecholamines in humans. Hypertension 1983;5:772.
31. Weinstein RS. Recognition and management of poisoning with beta-adrenergic blocking agents. Ann Emerg Med 1984;13:1123.
32. Hesse B, Pedersen JT. Hypoglycaemia after propranolol in children. Acta Med Scand 1973;193:551.
33. Heath A. Beta-adrenergic blocker toxicity: Clinical features and therapy. Am J Emerg Med 1984;2:518.
34. Schmimmel MS, Eidelman AJ, Wilschanski MA, et al. Toxic effects of atenolol consumed during breast feeding. J Pediatr 1989;114:476.
35. Pentel PR, Asinger RW, Benowitz NL. Propranolol antagonism of phenylpropanolamine-induced hypertension. Clin Pharmacol Ther 1985;37:488.
36. Agura ED, Wexler LF, Witzburg RA. Massive propranolol overdose. Successful treatment with high dose isoproterenol and glucagon. Am J Med 1986;180:755.
37. Hurwitz MD, Kallenbach JM, Pincus PS. Massive propranolol overdose (letter). Am J Med 1986;81:1118.
38. Ehrgartner GR, Zelinka MA. Hemodynamic instability following intentional nadolol overdose. Arch Int Med 1988;148:801.
39. Smith RC, Wilkinson J, Hull RL. Glucagon for propranolol overdose. JAMA 1985;254:2412.
40. Jacobsen D, Helgeland A, Koss A. Treatment of beta-blocker poisoning (letter). Lancet 1980;1:1031.
41. Kahn CR, Shehter Y. Insulin, oral hypoglycemic agents, and the pharmacology of the endocrine pancreas. In Gilman AF, Rall TW, Nies AS, Taylor P (eds). The Pharmacologic Basis of Therapeutics. 8th ed. New York, Pergamon Press, 1990, p 1479.
42. Kenyon CJ, Aldinger GE, Joshipura P, Zaid GJ. Successful resuscitation using external cardiac pacing in beta adrenergic antagonist-induced bradysystolic arrest. Ann Emerg Med 1988;17:711.
43. Snyder S, Reynolds IJ. Calcium-antagonist drugs: Receptor interactions that clarify therapeutic effects. N Engl J Med 1985;313:995.
44. Braunwald E. Mechanism of action of calcium channel blocking agents. N Engl J Med 1982;307:1618.
45. Samniah N, Schlaeffer F. Cerebral infarction associated with oral verapamil overdose. Clin Toxicol 1988;26:365.
46. McMillan R. Management of acute severe verapamil intoxication. J Emerg Med 1988;6:193.
47. Heyman SN. Verapamil intoxication and hyperglycemia. J Emerg Med 1989;7:407.
48. Hendren WG, Scheiber RS, Garrettson LK. Extracorporeal bypass for the treatment of verapamil poisoning. Ann Emerg Med 1989;18:984.
49. Ramoska EA, Spiller HA, Myers A. Calcium channel blocker toxicity. Ann Emerg Med 1990;19:649.
50. Jakubowski AT, Mizgala HF. Effect of diltiazem overdose. Am J Cardiol 1987;60:932.
51. Humbert VH, Munn NJ, Hawkins RF. Noncardiogenic pulmonary edema complicating massive diltiazem overdose. Chest 1991;99:258.

52. Wells TG, Graham CJ, Moss M, Kearns GL. Nifedipine poisoning in a child. Pediatrics 1990;86:91.
53. Krick SE, Gums JG, Grauer K, Cooper GR. Severe verapamil (sustained release) overdose. DICP 1990;24:705.
54. Kozlowski JH, Kozlowski JA, Schuller D. Poisoning with sustained-release verapamil. Am J Med 1988;85:127.
55. Rosansky SJ. Verapamil toxicity-treatment with hemoperfusion. Ann Intern Med 1991;114:340.
56. Passal DB, Crespin FH. Verapamil poisoning in an infant. Pediatrics 1984;73:543.
57. Hattori VT, Mandel WJ, Peter T. Calcium for myocardial depression from verapamil. N Engl J Med 1982;306:238.
58. Moroni F, Mannaioni PF. Calcium gluconate and hypertonic sodium chloride in a case of massive verapamil poisoning. Clin Toxicol 1980;17:395.
59. Perkins CM. Serious verapamil poisoning: Treatment with intravenous calcium gluconate. Br Med J 1978;2:1127.
60. Horowitz BZ, Rhee KJ. Massive verapamil ingestion: A report of two cases and a review of the literature. Am J Emerg Med 1989;7:624.
61. Boisvert SC. Case review: A 27-year-old woman with verapamil overdose. J Emerg Nurs 1990;16:317.
62. Pentel PR, Salerno DM. Cardiac drug toxicity: Digitalis glycosides and calcium-channel and β-blocking agents. Med J Aust 1990;152:88.
63. Garrison JC, Peach MJ. Renin and angiotensin. In Goodman AG, Rall TW, Nies AS, Taylor P (eds). The Pharmacological Basis of Therapeutics. New York, Pergamon Press, 1990, pp 756–761.
64. Sturgill BC, Shearlock KT. Membranous glomerulopathy and nephrotic syndrome after captopril therapy. JAMA 1983;250:2343.
65. Harvelka J, Vetter H, Studer A, et al. Acute and chronic effects of the angiotensin converting enzyme inhibitor captopril in severe hypertension. Am J Cardiol 1982;49:1467.
66. Waeber B, Nussberger J, Brunner HR. Self poisoning with enalapril. Br J Med 1984;288:287.
67. Lau CP. Attempted suicide with enalapril. N Engl J Med 1986;315:197.
68. Spiller HA, Udicious TM, Muir S. Angiotensin converting enzyme inhibitor ingestion in children. Clin Toxicol 1989;27:345.
69. Isles C, Mackay A, Barton PJM, et al. Accidental overdose of minoxidil in a child. Lancet 1981;1:97.
70. McCormick MA, Forman MH, Manoguerra AS. Severe toxicity from ingestion of a topical minoxidil preparation. Am J Emerg Med 1989;7:419.
71. Artman M, Boerth RC. Clonidine poisoning. A complex problem. Am J Dis Child 1983;137:171.
72. Neuvonen PJ, Vilska J, Keranen A. Severe poisoning in a child caused by a small dose of clonidine. Clin Toxicol 1979;14:369.
73. Mendoza JE, Medalie M. Clonidine poisoning with marked hypotension in a 2 year old child. Clin Pediatr 1979;18:123.
74. Wiley JF, Wiley CC, Torrey SB, Henretig FM. Clonidine poisoning in young children. J Pediatr 1990;116:654.
75. Heidemann S, Sarnaik AP. Clonidine poisoning in children. Crit Care Med 1990;18:618.
76. Wedin GP, Richardson SL. Clonidine poisoning in children (letter). Am J Dis Child 1990;144:853.
77. Physician's Desk Reference. 41st ed. Oradell, NJ, Medical Economics, 1987, pp 2216–2217.
78. Hubbard BA Jr. Reserpine. JAMA 1955;157:468.
79. McKown CH, Verhulst HL, Crotty JJ. Overdosage effects and danger from tranquilizing drugs. JAMA 1973;185:425.
80. Loggie JMH, Saita H, Kahn I, et al. Accidental reserpine poisoning: Clinical and metabolic effects. Clin Pharmacol Ther 1967;8:692.
81. Wedin GP, Edwards JL. Clonidine poisoning treated with naloxone (letter). Am J Emerg Med 1989;7:343.
82. Corneli HM, Banner WW, Vernon DD, Swenson PH. Toddler eats clonidine patch and nearly quits smoking for life (letter). JAMA 1989;261:42.
83. Caraveti EM, Bennett DL. Clonidine transdermal patch poisoning. Ann Emerg Med 1988;17:175.
84. Hamblin JE, Martin CA. Transdermal patch poisoning (letter). Pediatrics 1987;79:161.
85. Bauman JL. The arrhythmias. In DePiro JT, Talbert RL, Hayes PE, et al (eds). Pharmacotherapy. A Pathophysiologic Approach. New York, Elsevier, 1989, pp 150–172.
86. Koppel C, Oberdisse U, Heinemeyer G. Clinical course and outcome in class IC antiarrhythmic overdose. Clin Toxicol 1990;28:433.
87. Goddard CJR, Whorwell PJ. Amiodarone overdose and its management. Br J Clin Pract 1989;43:184.
88. Bouffard Y, Berger Y, Dellafos B, et al. Acute poisoning with amiodarone, a clinical and pharmacologic study. Arch Mal Coeur 1985;78:130.
89. Oreto G, Lapresa A, Melluso C, et al. Intoxication aigue par l'amiodarone. Arch Mal Coeur 1980;73:857.
90. Garson A, Gillette PC, McVey P, et al. Amiodarone treatment of critical arrhythmias in children and young adults. J Am Coll Cardiol 1984;4:749.
91. Thompson AE, Sussmane JB. Bretylium intoxication resembling clinical brain death. Crit Care Med 1989;17:194.
92. Goodman AG, Rall TW, Nies AS, Taylor P (eds). The Pharmacological Basis of Therapeutics. New York, Pergamon Press, 1990, p 1657.
93. Nitsch J, Luderitz B. Enhanced elimination of amrinone by cholestyramine. Dtsch Med Wochenschr 1986;111:1241.

CHAPTER 96

Alcohols

G. Randall Bond

INTRODUCTION

Ethanol, isopropanol, ethylene glycol, and methanol are found in almost every American home. Alcohols are present in liquor, rubbing alcohol, perfumes, mouthwash, paint strippers, and automotive products (Table 96–1). In 1988 the American Association of Poison Control Centers recorded over 6000 childhood exposures to ethanol, over 10,000 to isopropanol, over 2400 to glycols (primarily ethylene glycol), and over 750 to methanol. Since most exposures are never reported to a poison center, these numbers represent only a portion of the problem. Fortunately most exposures are to small quantities and result in only minor or no symptoms.

ETHANOL
Pathophysiology

Ethanol is a particularly ubiquitous substance, present not only in most home liquor cabinets but also in many home cleaning products, aftershaves, colognes, mouthwashes, and other toiletries. Despite recent product reformulations, alcohol is found in many liquid medications.

Ethanol is rapidly and almost completely absorbed. The time to peak serum level varies with the stomach contents but generally occurs before 2 hours following ingestion. Ethanol is excreted unchanged in the breath, sweat, and urine, but the majority is metabolized in the liver prior to excretion. At low concentrations ethanol is oxidized by alcohol dehydrogenase to acetaldehyde. Acetaldehyde is further oxidized to acetate by aldehyde dehydrogenase. At higher concentrations the microsomal ethanol oxidase system (MEOS) also metabolizes ethanol. Both enzyme systems, but particularly the MEOS, are induced by exposure to ethanol, so the rate of elimination of ethanol is increased in those who consume alcohol. Children may metabolize ethanol twice as rapidly as nondrinking adults.

EMS Considerations

Alcohol toxicity should always be considered when a household product has been ingested or when a child presents with central nervous system (CNS) depression, seizure, or the smell of alcohol on the breath. EMS providers should bring the container of any product ingested by the child.

The EMS provider should evaluate the airway, monitor breathing, and check for hypoglycemia. Hypoglycemia is frequently found in association with alcohol ingestion in children. If the child is comatose or convulsing, empiric

---

TABLE 96-1

USUAL CONCENTRATION RANGE OF ALCOHOLS AND GLYCOLS IN COMMON PRODUCTS

	Ethanol	Ethylene Glycol*	Isopropanol	Methanol
Aftershave	14–79			
Antifreeze/coolant (for automobile radiators)		94–95		
Brake fluid		70–85		4
Canned heat (Sterno)	60			
Carburetor fluid				99
Cements (china, electronic, film, gasket, model)	7–30		5–20	0–1
Cleaners				
Liquid hand-dishwashing detergents	1–9			
Glass cleaners	9–10		3–14	1–38
Denatured ethanol†			2–5	
Duplicator fluid				60–99
Elixirs/cough and cold preparations	2–10			
Gasohol	10			10
Gas-line antifreeze (dry gas)				100
Hair tonics	25–66			
Model engine (airplane) fuel				43–77
Mouthwash	14–27			
Paint stripper/remover	25		2–11	3–28
Perfume/cologne	25–95			
Pipe sweetener				75
Rubbing alcohol	70		70–91	
Windshield de-icer		50	58–80	4–89
Windshield washing solution				17–99

Adapted from Litovitz T. The alcohols: Ethanol, methanol, isopropanol, ethylene glycol. Pediatr Clin North Am 1986;33:311. Used with permission.
*Also glycol ethers.
†Nonmethanol denaturants are more common.
Concentration range in percent is listed for ingredients when present; individual components may be absent from a product.

glucose therapy (2 ml/kg intravenous slow push of D25W) is given.

Clinical Evaluation

Important historical elements are the timing, quantity, and product composition associated with the ingestion. The quantity ingested and the alcohol content of the product can be used to estimate the maximum serum alcohol level (Table 96–2).

The symptoms of ethanol toxicity in children are similar to those in adults. Ataxia and CNS depression are frequently seen. Nausea and vomiting are also common. Coma may occur. Unlike in adults, in children hypoglycemia and seizures occur following ethanol intoxication. The exact frequency of this finding is poorly described, but in one retrospective study 24% of children ingesting ethanol were

hypoglycemic. Hypoglycemia has been associated with low levels of serum ethanol concentrations. Hypokalemia and metabolic acidosis have been reported.

Diagnostic Evaluation

Serum glucose and ethanol level are important in all ingestions of alcohol in childhood. Serum electrolytes should also be measured. Other laboratory studies are determined by possible coingested substances or the need to pursue alternative explanations for the patient's symptoms.

Differential Diagnosis

Differential diagnosis includes all causes of CNS depression. Trauma, CNS infection, hypertensive encephalopathy, postictal state, hypoglycemia of another etiology, and inges-

---

TABLE 96-2

ESTIMATING SERUM ALCOHOL LEVELS

$$\text{Est. level (mg/dl)} = \frac{\text{osm gap (mOsm/L)}}{10 \text{ (dl/L)}} \times \text{M.W. (mg/mOsm)}$$

$$\text{Est. level (mg/dl)} = \frac{\% \times \text{S.G. (gm/ml)} \times \text{vol ingested (ml)}}{\text{wt (kg)} \times V_d \text{ (L/kg)}}$$

		M.W. (mg/mOsm)	S.G.	V_d
$H_3C - H_2COH$	Ethanol	46	0.79	0.6
H_3COH	Methanol	32	0.79	0.6
$HOCH_2 - CH_2OH$	Ethylene glycol	62	1.11	0.6
$H_3C - HCOH - CH_3$	Isopropyl alcohol	60	0.79	0.6

M.W. = molecular weight; S.G. = specific gravity; V_d = volume of distribution.

tion of other CNS depressants should be considered. Primary hypoglycemia or hypoglycemia due to ingestion of aspirin, beta-adrenergic blockers, or oral hypoglycemic agents may produce similar symptoms. Head trauma must be considered when an adolescent has CNS depression beyond that expected from the serum ethanol level.

Therapeutic Intervention

An asymptomatic child whose maximum possible ingestion is calculated to raise the blood alcohol no higher than 25 mg/dl will not require further observation for ethanol toxicity. Because of the rapid absorption of alcohol, attempts to decontaminate the patient are rarely helpful unless initiated within the first hour or following massive ingestion. CNS depression may progress rapidly and contraindicate use of syrup of ipecac. Ethanol is not bound by activated charcoal, but it may be used if other potentially toxic substances have been ingested.

When the maximum possible amount of alcohol ingested is sufficient to result in toxicity, the patient must be observed until past the time of peak effect. Only supportive care is required following most ethanol ingestions. Maintenance of a patent airway and adequate ventilation through the period of ethanol toxicity are generally sufficient. Because ethanol is a peripheral vasodilator and a mild diuretic, fluid support may be necessary to maintain adequate blood pressure. If hypoglycemia is present, glucose, 0.5 gm/kg, should be given intravenous slow push. This is done with either 2 ml/kg of D25W or 5 ml/kg of D10W. A D10W and electrolyte infusion may be required through the period of toxicity. Glucose levels should be monitored until the patient is asymptomatic.

Disposition

Relapse following recovery is unexpected. Patients may be discharged when they are fully alert and ethanol levels have declined to less than 25 mg/dl. The social situation surrounding the ingestion of the alcohol-containing product should always be considered when preparing for discharge. Children may become intoxicated following sips of alcohol given by well-meaning adults. The possibility of child abuse or neglect should always be considered. Infants who present with alcohol intoxication may be victims of parents attempting to sedate their children with a "whiskey nipple."

ISOPROPYL ALCOHOL
Pathophysiology

Isopropyl alcohol (isopropanol) is found in glues, glass cleaners, spot removers, paint thinners, and automobile windshield cleansers and de-icers. It is most widely found as 70% rubbing alcohol. Rubbing alcohol is involved in the majority of exposures to isopropyl alcohol. Although most exposures today are oral, in the past many were due to "alcohol sponge baths" for fever reduction.

Isopropanol is a clear, colorless, slightly bitter tasting liquid with a characteristic odor. It is rapidly absorbed from the intestinal tract—80% in the first 30 minutes. Massive overdoses may delay absorption. Significant absorption may occur by dermal exposure and to a lesser extent by inhalation. Isopropanol is metabolized to acetone by hepatic alcohol dehydrogenase. It is eliminated in the urine as acetone (80%) and as parent isopropyl alcohol (20%).

The primary effect of isopropyl alcohol is CNS depression. Acetone contributes to the CNS depression, and its slow renal elimination prolongs the intoxicated state. In high concentrations isopropyl alcohol has a myocardial depressant effect, which may result in hypotension.

Clinical Evaluation

Important historical elements include the exact product composition, timing, and amount ingested. To a child, 1 ml/kg of 70% alcohol is an intoxicating amount. As little as 20 ml of rubbing alcohol can cause inebriation in an adult. In adults, 5 to 8 oz have been fatal.

Since isopropanol is a gastrointestinal irritant, patients may have nausea, vomiting, abdominal pain, and hematemesis. CNS depression is the most frequent significant symptom. Patients may have symptoms ranging from mild ataxia and inebriation to deep coma. The pupils are usually small. Depressed or absent deep tendon reflexes are common. Frequently acetone is noted on the breath. In severe cases myocardial depression and hypotension may be present. Hypothermia has been reported in severe cases. There are rare reports of renal tubular necrosis, acute myopathy, and hemolytic anemia. The occurrence of hypoglycemia following isopropyl alcohol ingestion in children is unsubstantiated by any case reports.

Diagnostic Evaluation

Laboratory evaluation should include measuring serum concentrations of isopropyl alcohol, acetone, ethanol, glucose, and electrolytes and a serum osmolality. A complete blood count, urinalysis, and renal function studies should be obtained. Since both isopropyl alcohol and acetone are osmotically active, the osmolar gap will reflect the isopropanol and acetone concentration.

Differential Diagnosis

The differential diagnosis of isopropyl alcohol ingestion includes methanol, ethylene glycol, ethanol, acetone, and sedative hypnotic agent ingestions, as well as hypoglycemia, head trauma, and CNS infection. The likelihood of one of the alcohols causing the symptoms can be determined by the presence of an osmolar gap. The osmolar gap is the difference between the measured osmolality and the calculated osmolality (Table 96–3). The "normal" osmolar gap of up to 10 mOsm/L is due to osmotically measured physiologic molecules not included in the calculated osmolality. Agents with osmolar activity include electrolytes, glucose, urea, ethanol, isopropyl alcohol, methanol, ethylene glycol, ketones, and mannitol. In the absence of an acetone ingestion (fingernail polish remover), diabetes, or the pharmacologic administration of mannitol, an osmolar gap suggests the presence of one of the alcohols. The presence of acetone on the breath, in urine, or in serum suggests isopropyl alcohol ingestion. A significant anion gap metabolic acidosis is uncommon with isopropyl alcohol or ethanol ingestion, suggesting the coingestion of ethylene glycol or methanol.

Therapeutic Intervention

Delayed gastrointestinal decontamination is unlikely to be helpful, and syrup of ipecac may be harmful. Gastric lavage should be performed if the patient presents early or after a large ingestion. Isopropyl alcohol is not bound by activated charcoal, but charcoal should be given if a coingestant is suspected.

The only management required for the majority of these patients is supportive care. Since respiratory depression is frequently associated with coma, adequate airway protection and ventilation should be assured. Adequate warming should be provided as needed. Isopropyl alcohol is a myocardial depressant. Hypotension, although infrequently present, is associated with poor outcome. In one series, 45% of hypo-

---

TABLE 96–3

OSMOLAR GAP

Osmolar gap = measured serum osmolality − calculated osmolality

$$\text{Calculated osmolality} = 2 \times \text{Na (mOsm/L)} + \frac{\text{BUN (mg/dl)}}{2.8} + \frac{\text{glucose (mg/dl)}}{18} + \frac{\text{ethanol (mg/dl)}}{4.6}$$

Serum osmolality must be measured by **freezing point depression.**

The range of the osmolar gap is large. Up to **10 mOsm/L** is within physiologic variation. An osmolar gap less than this does not guarantee the absence of a toxic serum alcohol concentration.

Check all units. Use of this formula requires that units be expressed as above. Some laboratories have changed to mg/L (mmol).

---

tensive patients died. When hypotension fails to respond to initial fluid resuscitation, extracorporeal removal of isopropyl alcohol is indicated. When gastrointestinal hemorrhage contributes to hypotension, appropriate blood component replacement is required.

Hemodialysis and peritoneal dialysis have been used for the removal of isopropyl alcohol; however, hemodialysis is more effective. In one report hemodialysis removed isopropyl alcohol 50 times more rapidly than hepatic and urinary elimination; hemodialysis removed acetone 40 times more rapidly than urinary elimination. The presence of deep coma without hypotension does not predict morbidity or mortality in the presence of adequate supportive care. Elevated isopropyl alcohol levels, even above 400 mg/dl, have not been associated with poor outcome in the absence of other complicating factors. Hemodialysis should be reserved for those patients with hypotension, particularly those unresponsive to initial fluid bolus.

Disposition

Although isopropyl alcohol has a serum half-life of 2.5 to 3.0 hours, that of acetone is much longer. Support should be continued until the patient is awake, alert, and neurologically normal. Because of the rapid and complete absorption of isopropyl alcohol, relapse following recovery is not expected. The patient may be discharged when recovery is complete.

METHANOL
Pathophysiology

Methanol is found in numerous commercial products, especially automotive products. It is used frequently in de-icers and windshield wiper solvents. Also known as wood alcohol, methanol has been the cause of multiple victim incidents from contaminated alcoholic beverages.

Methanol, by itself, is nontoxic and is only mildly inebriating. It is oxidized successively to formaldehyde, then formic acid, and finally carbon dioxide. The oxidation of methanol to formaldehyde is catalyzed by alcohol dehydrogenase. The metabolism from formaldehyde to formic acid is rapid, but the conversion of formic acid to carbon dioxide is delayed. This results in the accumulation of formic acid, the primary metabolic acid in methanol toxicity. Formic acid is also the direct ocular toxin causing the blindness associated with methanol toxicity.

A number of neurologic injuries have been associated with methanol poisoning. Formic acid is directly toxic to the optic nerve. Methanol intoxication may also produce retinal and cerebral hemorrhages, particularly in the basal ganglia. Patchy cerebral necrosis can also occur. The toxic mechanism

of these findings is unknown. Heparinization associated with hemodialysis may contribute to the risk of these injuries occurring. Permanent sequelae include parkinsonism, pseudobulbar palsy, transverse myelitis, seizures, and intellectual deterioration.

Clinical Evaluation

Methanol-intoxicated patients frequently do not experience any symptoms for 12 to 24 hours. This period may be even longer if ethanol has been ingested with the methanol. The earliest symptoms are nausea, vomiting, abdominal pain, headache, dizziness, and weakness. As the toxicity progresses, the patient may experience increasing CNS depression from confusion to coma. Seizures are rare. The most characteristic finding associated with methanol toxicity is that of visual changes. Complaints include blurred or dimmed vision and seeing spots before the eyes. Tunnel vision or central visual scotoma may be noted. Visual changes may progress to total blindness with loss of the pupillary reflex. Optic disk edema is common. Retinal hemorrhages may occur. Severely poisoned or untreated patients develop progressive acidosis, myocardial depression, shock, cerebral edema, and death.

Diagnostic Evaluation

Serum methanol level and arterial blood gases are the most useful laboratory parameters. Significantly elevated methanol levels predict significant toxicity even in the absence of symptoms, unless the methanol is removed or its metabolism is blocked. Metabolic acidosis reflects accumulation of the toxic metabolic formic acid. Without a serum methanol level, the osmolar gap may be used to estimate the methanol level (see Table 96–2). Because of the large physiologic variation in the "normal" osmolar gap, an osmolar gap less than 10 mOsm/L does not exclude a toxic serum methanol concentration. It is important when calculating the osmolar gap that osmolality is determined using the freezing point depression method. Methanol is extremely volatile; attempts to use vapor pressure elevation for determining osmolality lead to falsely low measurements.

Differential Diagnosis

Differential diagnosis is similar to that described for isopropyl alcohol. The particular distinguishing features of methanol intoxication include anion gap metabolic acidosis, osmolar gap, presence of visual changes, and absence of calcium oxalate crystals in the urine (Table 96–4).

Therapeutic Intervention

The approach to the methanol-intoxicated patient consists of restoring normal physiology, blocking further formation

TABLE 96–4

ALCOHOLS: DIFFERENTIAL DIAGNOSIS

	Increased Serum Osmolality	Anion Gap Metabolic Acidosis	Serum/Urine Acetone	Urinary Oxalate Crystals	Visual Changes
Ethanol	+	−	−	−	−
Isopropanol	+	−	+	−	−
Methanol	+	+	−	−	+
Ethylene glycol	+	+	−	+	−

of toxic metabolites, and enhancing elimination of methanol and its toxic metabolites. Large volumes of sodium bicarbonate may be required to restore normal pH. Fluids and inotropes should be used to restore physiologic circulating volume and enhance myocardial function.

Therapeutic Ethanol

Patients who are symptomatic, have a serum methanol level greater than 20 mg/dl, or have ingested more than 1 ml/kg should be treated with an inhibitor of methanol metabolism. Ethanol is administered intravenously as a 10% alcohol solution in D5W to competitively inhibit alcohol dehydrogenase from metabolizing methanol to formaldehyde (Table 96–5). Dosage recommendations are derived from adults, and, because of a slightly higher endogenous metabolism, children may require higher maintenance doses. Frequent monitoring of the serum ethanol and glucose concentrations is required. The continuous infusion of ethanol should be adjusted to achieve a serum ethanol level of 100 mg/dl. A 10% ethanol solution is not commercially available and must be made in the pharmacy. A 5% ethanol solution in D5W is commercially available, but the use of this product requires extremely large fluid volumes, particularly during dialysis. Oral administration of alcohol is an alternative but is less reliable for maintaining consistent levels, particularly if emesis is occurring. During dialysis, fluid volumes may be minimized by adding ethanol to the dialysis bath. An alternate alcohol dehydrogenase inhibitor is 4-methyl-pyrazole. Although 4-methyl-pyrazole has been used in Europe, it is not commercially available in the United States.

Folic Acid

Since formic acid is the ophthalmic toxin and the major cause of acidosis in methanol poisoning, aggressive efforts to enhance its elimination are warranted. Correction of the metabolic acidosis does not eliminate formate, although it

may increase the rate of elimination. Administration of activated folic acid (leucovorin) followed by folic acid at regular intervals increases the rate of metabolism of formate to carbon dioxide and decreases the toxicity. An initial dose of 50 mg leucovorin intravenously followed by 50 mg of folic acid every 4 hours for 3 days has been recommended (Table 96–6). The use of folic acid is an adjunctive therapy and does not alter the need for hemodialysis.

Dialysis

Although the metabolism of methanol to toxic metabolites can be effectively inhibited by ethanol, urinary elimination of methanol may take several days. During this time the patient must be kept intoxicated in a critical care unit. Hemodialysis has the advantage of lower risk, of lower cost, and of removing toxic metabolites of methanol. A serum methanol level greater than 50 mg/dl, visual changes, significant metabolic acidosis, or renal failure indicates the need for hemodialysis. Peritoneal dialysis should be avoided since it is not as effective as hemodialysis. New techniques have made hemodialysis available for even small infants. Hemodialysis should be continued until the serum methanol level is below 20 mg/dl. Ethanol may be used as the sole therapy if the initial methanol level is less than 50 mg/dl and there is no significant acidosis or visual change. In this situation,

TABLE 96–6

THERAPY AT A GLANCE
Ethanol
Support ventilation, hydration as needed
Monitor glucose and support as needed
Isopropyl Alcohol
Support ventilation as needed
Hemodynamic support
Hemodialysis if severe CNS depression and hypotension
Methanol
Correct acidosis
Hemodynamic support
Block metabolism of methanol using ethanol (Table 96–5) or 4-methyl-pyrazole
Administer leucovorin (50 mg IV) followed by folic acid (50 mg q 4 hr × 16 doses)
Hemodialysis if visual changes, acidosis, or methanol level >50 mg/dl
Ethylene Glycol
Correct acidosis
Correct hypocalcemia
Hemodynamic support
Ventilatory support
Block metabolism of ethylene glycol (Table 96–5) using ethanol or 4-methyl-pyrazole
Administer thiamine (2 mg/kg IV or IM) and pyridoxine (2 mg/kg IV or IM)
Hemodialysis if acidosis, hemodynamic instability, respiratory failure, renal failure, or ethylene glycol level >50 mg/dl

TABLE 96–5

ESTIMATED ETHANOL REQUIREMENTS TO ACHIEVE AND MAINTAIN A SERUM ETHANOL CONCENTRATION OF 100 mg/dl

	Loading Dose (ml/kg)	Maintenance (ml/kg/hr)	Maintenance During Hemodialysis (ml/kg/hr)
D5W/10% Ethanol (IV)	8.5*	1.4	3.3
43% Ethanol (oral)	2†	0.3	0.7
95% Ethanol (oral)	1†	0.15	0.35

*Deliver over ½ hour.
†Including first-hour maintenance.

as with patients after hemodialysis, ethanol infusion is continued until the serum methanol level is less than 20 mg/dl. At that point the infusion may be discontinued, but the patient should be observed for the recurrence of acidosis.

Disposition

When the patient has clinically recovered, the serum methanol level is less than 20 mg/dl, and observation for several hours following the discontinuation of ethanol therapy demonstrates no recurrence of acidosis, the patient may leave the hospital. Severely poisoned patients who present prior to extremis may survive if appropriately and aggressively treated. The pupillary light reflex can predict recovery of visual function. Patients who have no loss of the reflex may be expected to recover complete visual function. Those with total loss of the light reflex have a poor prognosis for recovery of vision.

Other Considerations

Decisions regarding ethanol therapy should never wait for a methanol level to return. A patient with an anion gap metabolic acidosis and an osmolar gap should receive ethanol therapy. A patient with known methanol ingestion and visual changes should begin ethanol therapy.

ETHYLENE GLYCOL
Pathophysiology

Ethylene glycol is found in a variety of detergents, paints, lacquers, polishes, cosmetics, and automotive antifreeze and de-icers. Ethylene glycol is clear, colorless, and odorless but has a sweet taste. Frequently, when it is used as an antifreeze, a yellow-green dye is added to aid in finding the source of automobile fluid leaks. The majority of ethylene glycol exposures, even in older children and adults, are accidental.

Ethylene glycol, by itself, is not a potent toxin; however, its products of oxidation are. Ethylene glycol is rapidly absorbed, with CNS depression frequently occurring within 1 to 12 hours of ingestion. The onset of acidosis may be delayed 12 hours or longer depending on the coingestion of ethanol. Ethylene glycol is oxidized in the liver and kidney to glycoaldehyde, glycolate, glyoxylate, and a variety of final metabolites, including oxalic acid (Fig. 96–1). The first step is catalyzed by ethanol dehydrogenase, which has 100 times greater affinity for ethanol. Conversion to glycolate is rapid, but subsequent oxidation to glyoxylate is slow. Glycolate is therefore the predominant metabolic acid in ethylene glycol poisoning. Lactic acid is also found in significant amounts in many patients. It has been suggested that acetaldehyde intermediates are the primary cause of CNS depression since maximal CNS depression occurs at the time of the serum peak levels, 6 to 8 hours after ingestion.

The pathologic changes are also related to the toxic products of ethylene glycol metabolism. Cerebrospinal fluid (CSF) findings of an elevated protein and cell count are common. Computed tomography, biopsy, and autopsy reports demonstrate cerebral and renal edema; focal petechiae in heart, lung, brain, and kidney; perivascular inflammation; degenerative myocardial changes; and acute tubular necrosis in severe poisonings. Calcium oxalate crystals in renal biopsy specimens and in the brain at autopsy have led many to attribute the inflammatory CNS response and acute renal failure to this oxalate. Others argue that since oxalate crystal deposition is not always associated with the presence or location of injury, other metabolites may be more important toxins. Hypocalcemia may result when production of oxalate leads to the formation of calcium oxalate crystals. Cardio-

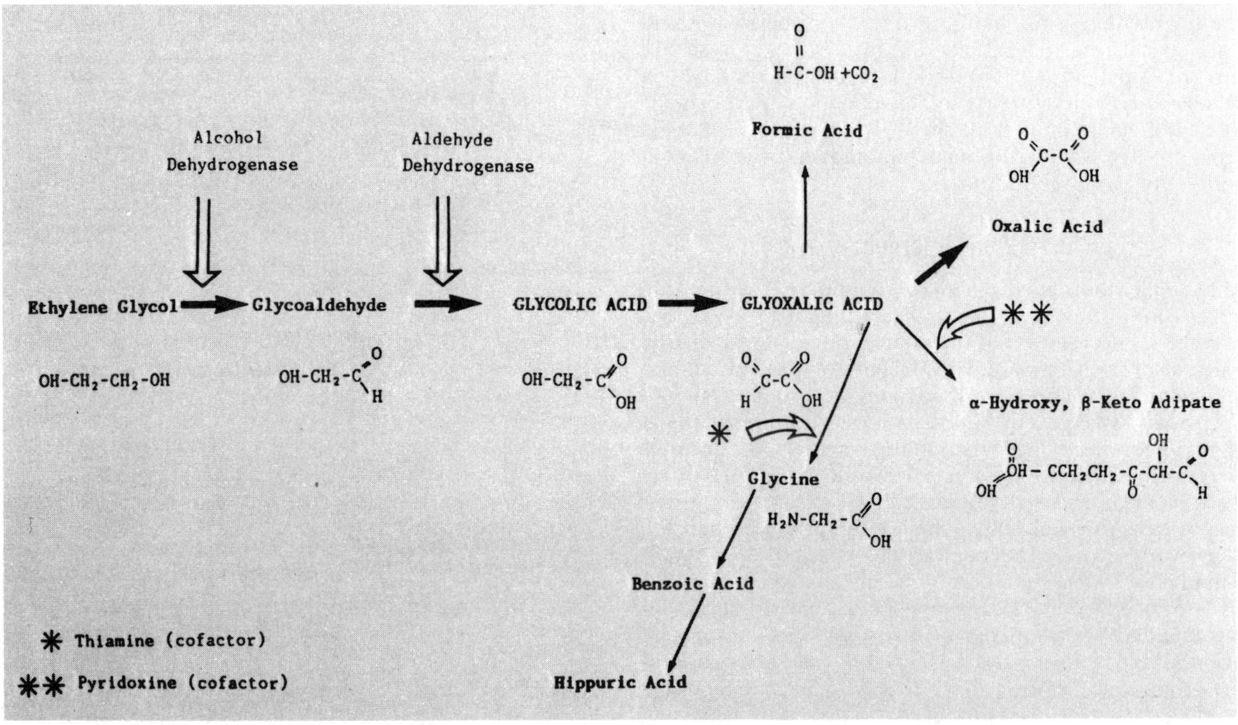

Figure 96–1. Ethylene glycol metabolism. (From Sabatini S, Morris R, Kurtzman N, Newsom G. Severe metabolic acidosis in an intoxicated patient. Am J Nephrol 1988;8:323. Basel, S Karger AG.)

pulmonary failure is the result of the direct cytotoxic effects of ethylene glycol metabolites as well as acidosis, hypotension, and hypocalcemia.

EMS Considerations

Since absorption is rapid, delayed gastrointestinal decontamination is probably of no value. The ability of activated charcoal to adsorb ethylene glycol is unproved. If EMS transportation will be prolonged, consideration may be given to the initiation of oral ethanol treatment using a high "proof" alcoholic beverage (see Table 96–5).

Clinical Evaluation

The toxicity of ethylene glycol has been divided into three phases: (1) CNS depression and metabolic acidosis, (2) cardiovascular collapse and pulmonary failure, and (3) renal failure. A fourth phase, consisting of facial diplegia, has been suggested. The most common presentation of ethylene glycol poisoning is drunkenness without the odor of ethanol on the breath. Other early signs include nausea, vomiting, depressed deep tendon reflexes, CNS depression, myoclonic jerks, and convulsions. Nystagmus and ophthalmoplegia are frequent. Low-grade fever has been described. Since the ethylene glycol metabolite oxalate binds calcium, hypocalcemic tetany may occur. Progressive symptomatology includes tachypnea and tachycardia associated with congestive heart failure and pulmonary edema. Without early aggressive intervention, renal failure frequently occurs.

Diagnostic Evaluation

The hallmark of ethylene glycol poisoning is the triad of anion gap metabolic acidosis, osmolar gap, and calcium oxalate crystalluria (see Table 96–4). Hypocalcemia can occur. Calcium oxalate crystals may be missed if only the classic tetrahedral form is sought. The elongated monohydrate form is also common and may be mistaken for hippurate crystals. Peripheral blood and CSF leukocytosis are common. As patients enter renal failure, blood urea nitrogen and serum creatinine will rise. Examination of the urine under ultraviolet light may show fluorescence because a fluorescent dye is added to many automotive products containing ethylene glycol.

Therapeutic Intervention

Management of ethylene glycol poisoning requires aggressive supportive care, blockade of metabolism to toxic metabolites, and removal of the toxin. Immediate correction of any acidosis is imperative. Mechanical ventilation and hemodynamic support with fluids and vasopressors should be provided as required. Minor pathways require thiamine and pyridoxine (see Fig. 96–1). Thiamine 2 mg/kg intravenously or intramuscularly and pyridoxine 2 mg/kg intravenously or intramuscularly should be given. In those patients who progress to renal failure, hemodialysis will be needed, but recovery of renal function can be expected.

Ethanol is effective in blocking the metabolism of ethylene glycol to the more toxic metabolites. Ethanol therapy is recommended for all patients with signs or symptoms of ethylene glycol toxicity and for children with a serum ethylene glycol concentration above 20 mg/dl. Enzyme blockade should be initiated when ethylene glycol toxicity is suspected, even before confirmatory levels are available. The ethylene glycol concentration can be estimated from the osmolar gap (see Table 96–2). The dosage and administration of ethanol are the same as for methanol intoxication (see Table 96–5).

When symptoms of hypocalcemia or a low serum calcium concentration are present, calcium replacement starting with calcium chloride, 10 to 20 mg/kg intravenously, should be given. Empiric calcium therapy is not recommended since it may increase crystal deposition.

Hemodialysis is recommended for those patients who have hemodynamic instability, respiratory failure, renal failure, acidosis, or serum ethylene glycol levels greater than 50 mg/dl. Hemodialysis should continue until the serum ethylene glycol level is less than 10 mg/dl.

Disposition

The acute metabolic toxicity may be considered resolved when ethylene glycol concentration is below 10 mg/dl and sufficient time has elapsed following the discontinuation of enzyme blockade for acidosis to have recurred. Once these criteria are met, the child may safely return home.

Selected References

Adelson L. Fatal intoxication with isopropyl alcohol (rubbing alcohol). Am J Clin Pathol 1962;38:144.

Adinoff B, Bone GHA, Linnoila M. Acute ethanol poisoning and the ethanol withdrawal syndrome. Med Toxicol 1988;3:172.

American Academy of Pediatrics, Committee on Drugs. Ethanol in liquid preparations intended for children. Pediatrics 1984;73:405.

Anderson TJ, Shuaib A, Becker WJ. Neurologic sequelae of methanol poisoning. Can Med Assoc J 1987;136:1177.

Arditi M, Killner MS. Coma following use of rubbing alcohol for fever control. Am J Dis Child 1987;141:237.

Berendt RC, Passerini L, LeGatt D, et al. Severe methanol intoxication: Methanol pharmacokinetics and serum osmolality. J Crit Care 1987;2:181.

Bove KE. Ethylene glycol toxicity. Am J Clin Pathol 1966;45:46.

Cummins LH. Hypoglycemia and convulsions in children following alcohol ingestion. J Pediatr 1961;58:23.

DaRoza R, Henning RJ, Sunshine I, et al. Acute ethylene glycol poisoning. Crit Care Med 1984;12:1003.

Denning DW, Berendt A, Chia Y, et al. Myocarditis complicating ethylene glycol poisoning in the absence of neurological features. Postgrad Med J 1988;64:867.

Dethlefs R, Naraqi S. Ocular manifestations and complications of acute methyl alcohol intoxication. Med J Aust 1978;2:483.

Ekins BR, Rollins DE, Duffy DP, et al. Standardized treatment of severe methanol poisoning with ethanol and hemodialysis. West J Med 1985;12:337.

Gabow PA. Ethylene glycol intoxication. Am J Kidney Dis 1988;XI:277.

Gibson PJ, Cant AJ, Mant TGK. Ethanol poisoning. Acta Paediatr Scand 1985;74:977.

Godolphin W, Meagher EP, Sanders HD, et al. Unusual calcium oxalate crystals in ethylene glycol poisoning. Clin Toxicol 1980;16:479.

Gonda A, Gault H, Churchill D, et al. Hemodialysis for methanol intoxication. Am J Med 1978;64:749.

Jacobsen D, Bredesen JE, Eide I, et al. Anion and osmolal gaps in the diagnosis of methanol and ethylene glycol poisoning. Acta Med Scand 1982;212:17.

Lacouture PG, Wason S, Abrams A, et al. Acute isopropyl alcohol intoxication. Am J Med 1983;75:680.

Leung AKC. Ethanol-induced hypoglycemia from mouthwash. Drug Intell Clin Pharm 1985;19:480.

Leung AKC. Ethyl alcohol ingestion in children. Clin Pediatr 1986;25:617.

Litovitz T. The alcohols: Ethanol, methanol, isopropanol, ethylene glycol. Pediatr Clin North Am 1986;33:311.

Litovitz TL, Schmitz BF, Holm KC. 1988 Annual report of the American Association of Poison Control Centers National Data Collection System. Am J Emerg Med 1989;7:495.

Lomaestro BM. Ethylene glycol toxicity—misinterpretation of laboratory data. Drug Intell Clin Pharm 1988;22:915.

MacLaren NK, Valman HB, Levin B. Alcohol-induced hypoglycemia in childhood. Br Med J 1970;1:278.

McCoy HG, Cipolle RJ, Ehlers SM, et al. Severe methanol poisoning. Am J Med 1979;67:804.

McLean DR, Jacobs H, Mielke BW. Methanol poisoning: A clinical and pathological study. Ann Neurol 1980;8:161.

McMartin K, Ambre J, Tephly T. Methanol poisoning in human subjects. Am J Med 1980;68:414.

Parry MF, Wallach R. Ethylene glycol poisoning. Am J Med 1974;57:143.

Peterson CD, Collins AJ, Himes JM, et al. Ethylene glycol poisoning—pharmacokinetics during therapy with methanol and hemodialysis. N Engl J Med 1981;304:21.

Phang PT, Passerini L, Mielke B, et al. Brain hemorrhage associated with methanol poisoning. Crit Care Med 1988;16:137.

Pons CA, Custer RP. Acute ethylene glycol poisoning. A clinico-pathologic report of eighteen fatal cases. Am J Med Sci 1946;211:544.

Ragan FA, Samuels MS, Hite SA. Ethanol ingestion in children. A five-year review. JAMA 1979;242:2787.

Rosansky SJ. Isopropyl alcohol poisoning treated with hemodialysis: Kinetics of isopropyl alcohol and acetone removal. J Toxicol Clin Toxicol 1982;19:265.

Selbst SM, DeMaio JG, Boenning D. Mouthwash poisoning. Clin Pediatr 1985;24:162.

Terlinsky AS, Grochowski J, Geoly KL, et al. Identification of atypical calcium oxalate crystalluria following ethylene glycol ingestion. Am J Clin Pathol 1981;76:223.

Turk J, Morrell L. Ethylene glycol intoxication. Grand rounds. Arch Intern Med 1986;146:1601.

Winter ML, Ellis MD, Snodgrass WR. Urine fluorescence using a Wood's lamp to detect the antifreeze additive sodium fluorescein: A qualitative adjunctive test in suspected ethylene glycol ingestions. Ann Emerg Med 1990;19:663.

CHAPTER 97

Heavy Metals

Margaret Boyer
Robert W. Lasek

LEAD

Lead poisoning remains prevalent in children despite the change to unleaded gasoline and the banning of lead-based paint. Lead is present in low concentrations in the air, drinking water, and food supply. This low-level exposure accounts for blood lead levels in children in the range of 4 to 6 μg/dl.

Higher lead levels occur in children who live in close proximity to major highways or in older housing, where leaded paints contain up to 50% lead by dry weight. The use of lead-based paint was banned in the United States in 1972. Currently paints can contain no more than 0.06% lead. Nevertheless, millions of houses built prior to the ban serve as sources of lead exposure. Paint chips may be directly ingested, or lead may be indirectly introduced into food and water as lead-laden dust settles.

Toxicity

Lead exerts its toxic effects primarily by binding to the sulfhydryl groups of various enzymes throughout the body. Cellular respiration is inhibited, and membrane transport can be disrupted because of inhibition of the sodium-potassium ATPase pump.

Hematologic manifestations of lead poisoning can be a sensitive indicator of increased lead levels. The complete blood count and peripheral blood smear may show a normocytic, hypochromic anemia and basophilic stippling of erythrocytes. Neither finding is sensitive; however, the presence of basophilic stippling is highly suggestive of lead poisoning.

Lead exerts profound effects on the synthesis of the heme moiety. First, lead inhibits delta-aminolevulinic acid dehy-

dratase, the enzyme responsible for the synthesis of porphobilinogen from precursors. Second, the mitochondrial enzyme ferrochelatase is inhibited. Ferrochelatase transports Fe^{3+} from ferritin and inserts it into protoporphyrin, forming the heme molecule. Inhibition of this enzyme results in an accumulation of protoporphyrin and serves as the basis for a simple screening test for lead poisoning. When iron integration into the heme molecule is disrupted, zinc may be inserted into the molecule, forming zinc protoporphyrin. The presence of this abnormal compound serves as another screening test for lead intoxication.

Central nervous system manifestations of lead poisoning are commonly the presenting complaint in children. At low levels of intoxication, subtle personality changes, behavioral problems, and cognitive impairments predominate. More dramatic presentations, with coma or seizures, are usually associated with higher-level exposures. The peripheral nerves may show segmental demyelination, presenting as foot or wrist drop.

Lead affects the kidney at the level of the proximal tubule and the loop of Henle. Long-term poisoning can result in interstitial fibrosis and end-stage renal failure. Acute poisoning is generally not associated with permanent renal damage.

Clinical Manifestations

Symptoms of acute intoxication include malaise, anorexia, nausea, vomiting, and abdominal pain. Irritability, apathy, loss of recently acquired psychomotor skills, and incoordination may be early signs of impending encephalopathy. Chronic intoxication symptoms are primarily neurologic and include decreased intelligence or behavioral and learning disorders.

Diagnostic Evaluation

The most useful indication of acute lead exposure is the whole-blood lead level. Whole-blood lead levels greater than 25 μg/dl are considered toxic.

The red blood cell zinc protoporphyrin test is useful in the diagnosis of chronic lead poisoning because it reflects the body's lead exposure over the life-span of an erythrocyte (120 days). Zinc protoporphyrin production begins when blood lead levels reach 15 to 25 μg/dl.

The measurement of free erythrocyte protoporphyrin (FEP) provides another means to aid in the diagnosis of chronic lead poisoning. Since this test samples the existing population of erythrocytes, which may be up to 4 months old, it is not useful for acute poisoning. The FEP can also be elevated in iron deficiency anemia, so it is necessary to concurrently measure whole-blood lead levels. In the presence of elevated whole-blood lead levels, a FEP level of greater than 35 μg/dl supports chronic exposure and is an indication for therapy. The child with FEP levels of 25 to 34 μg/dl should receive follow-up.

The calcium disodium EDTA ($CaNa_2EDTA$) lead mobilization test is reflective of total body lead burden and is useful when making decisions about therapy in children who have persistently elevated FEP levels and normal whole-blood lead levels. Care should be taken not to administer the test in patients with whole-blood levels greater than 55 μg/dl, as therapy is already indicated in these children, and the mobilization of the body's lead burden may precipitate encephalopathy.

The abdominal flat plate can be helpful if radiopaque material is seen in the acute ingestion. The diagnosis of chronic lead poisoning is suggested by the finding of "lead lines" or areas of increased density in the rapidly growing regions of the long bones of children (Fig. 97–1). Lead lines, commonly seen at the metaphyseal plates in the bones constituting the knee, are composed of calcium, the deposition of which was stimulated by the presence of lead. Radiographs of the extremities are not indicated when looking for evidence of suspected lead poisoning.

Therapeutic Intervention

The goal of treatment is to separate the child promptly from the source of lead and to support the child while reducing whole-blood lead levels through chelation therapy. Supportive care includes adequate fluid resuscitation and the monitoring and maintenance of renal function, since chelation therapy may induce renal failure. Close attention to fluid status is needed in the encephalopathic patient to minimize cerebral edema.

Specific treatment depends on the clinical presentation of the child. It is convenient to divide lead poisoning into three treatment categories: (1) encephalopathic, (2) symptomatic, and (3) asymptomatic. The child with a whole-blood lead level greater than 70 μg/dl constitutes a true medical emergency, requiring immediate intervention. Such a child would present with anorexia, lethargy, abdominal pain, or, rarely, with signs of encephalopathy ranging from subtle personality changes to incoordination, vomiting, and seizures.

In acute encephalopathy, treatment begins with the che-

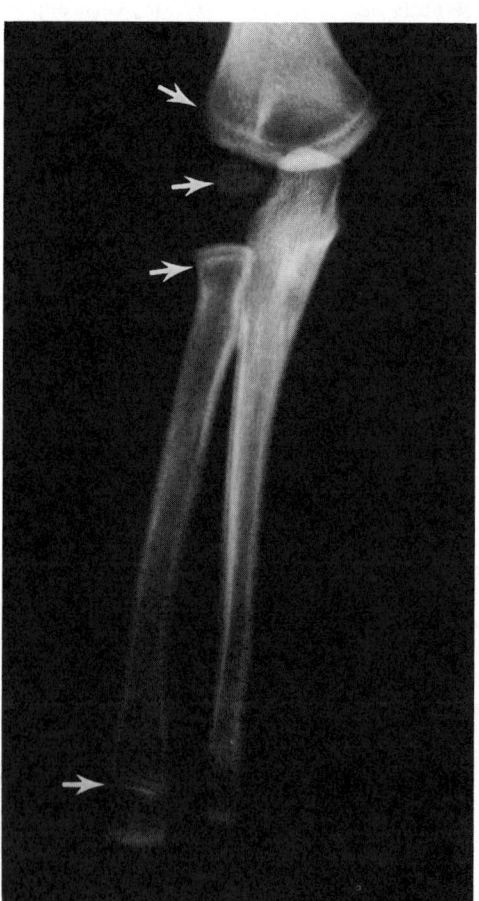

Figure 97–1. Ten months after this 2½-year-old girl's major episode of lead intoxication, the "lead lines" *(arrows)* have advanced away from the growth plates, as new normal bone has been laid down behind them. Such dense lines are found at the physeal margin of the metaphysis during active lead poisoning, and represent more tightly packed bone than normal. (Courtesy of A. Oestreich, Cincinnati, OH.)

TABLE 97–1
THERAPY AT A GLANCE

Lead
Acute Encephalopathy
Dimercaprol: 75 mg/m² IM q 4 hr or 12–24 mg/kg/day IM in divided doses. Contraindicated in hepatic failure and glucose-6-phosphate dehydrogenase deficiency.

Calcium disodium EDTA: 1500 mg/m²/day continuous IV infusion of 0.05% solution. At least one dose of dimercaprol should be given prior to initiation of infusion to prevent rise in blood levels from lead mobilization.

Symptomatic Without Encephalopathy
Dimercaprol: 50 mg/m² IM q 4 hr. May discontinue day 3 of therapy if blood lead <50 μg/dl.

Calcium disodium EDTA: 1000 mg/m²/day continuous IV infusion of 0.05% solution. Continue therapy for 5 days.

Arsenic
Dimercaprol: 3–5 mg/kg IM q 4 hr. Not to exceed 1 gm/day. Continue until urinary arsenic excretion <50 μg/day.

D-Penicillamine: 100 mg/kg/day orally in four divided doses. Duration of therapy is 5 days.

Mercury
Dimercaprol: 3–5 mg/kg IM q 4 hr for 2 days, then decrease to 2.5–3.0 mg/kg IM q 6 hr for 2 days, then further reduce to 2.5–3.0 mg/kg IM every 12 hr.

D-Penicillamine 100 mg/kg/day in four divided doses.

lating agent dimercaprol (or BAL for British anti-lewisite) (Table 97–1). Dimercaprol forms a stable complex with a number of metals, including lead, and is eliminated in the bile and urine. The dose is 75 mg/m² administered intramuscularly every 4 hours. An alternative dosing regimen is 12 to 24 mg/kg/day administered in 4 to 6 divided doses. Dimercaprol is contraindicated in the presence of hepatic failure or glucose-6-phosphate dehydrogenase deficiency. Dimercaprol can cause hemolysis in patients with this deficiency. Once the initial dose of dimercaprol has been given, therapy with intravenous CaNa₂EDTA begins. The dose of 1500 mg/m²/day is administered as a 0.05% solution by continuous intravenous infusion. CaNa₂EDTA so effectively mobilizes soft tissue lead stores that the blood lead level may rise initially, worsening an encephalopathy. Therefore CaNa₂EDTA should be given only after dimercaprol is administered. CaNa₂EDTA can be given by intramuscular injection; however, this is painful, even when mixed with procaine. Intramuscular CaNa₂EDTA could have a role when fluid restriction is necessary, as in cerebral edema. Chelation therapy is usually continued with dimercaprol and CaNa₂EDTA for a total of 5 days. In the event that further chelation therapy is needed, a 2-day hiatus is recommended.

In symptomatic patients without frank encephalopathy, both dimercaprol and CaNa₂EDTA are used, but the dosing schedule differs. Dimercaprol is given in doses of 50 mg/m² intramuscularly every 4 hours. CaNa₂EDTA is given (after the first dose of dimercaprol) by intravenous infusion at the rate of 1000 mg/m²/day. Dimercaprol may be discontinued on day 3 if the blood lead level falls below 50 μg/dl, with CaNa₂EDTA continued for 2 days more.

After chelation therapy and the return of safe blood lead levels (<25 μg/dl) the child no longer requires hospitalization. However, the child's environment must be inspected for possible lead hazards.

Asymptomatic children with increased body lead burdens may require chelation therapy. One author suggests that whole-blood lead levels between 56 and 69 μg/dl require treatment with CaNa$_2$EDTA, given at 1000 mg/m^2/day for 5 days and repeated until the whole-blood lead level remains below 50 μg/dl. The CaNa$_2$EDTA mobilization test is useful when the whole-blood level is between 25 and 55 μg/dl and the erythrocyte protoporphyrin level exceeds 35 μg/dl. Interval follow-up is necessary to monitor for repeat exposures.

ARSENIC

Arsenic is a tasteless, odorless, colorless element having many industrial applications. Arsenic-containing compounds have been used in wood preservatives, dyes, dessicants, defoliants, and even some homeopathic medicines. Arsenic is included in agricultural-use pesticides, herbicides, and rodenticides.

Arsenic poisoning is a common cause of heavy metal–related deaths, second only to lead. Insecticides account for most accidental arsenic ingestions involving children.

Arsenic exists in a trivalent state (As^{3+}) and in a pentavalent state (As^{5+}). Both forms disrupt oxidative phosphorylation, although As^{3+} is more toxic. Arsenic binds to and inhibits key sulfhydryl-containing enzymes involved with cellular respiration. As^{5+} competes with phosphate groups involved with oxidative phosphorylation, resulting in the loss of high-energy phosphate bonds.

Arsenic is almost completely absorbed in the gastrointestinal (GI) tract and penetrates the skin well. Once absorbed, arsenic first binds to hemoglobin, but within 24 hours is concentrated in the liver, lungs, kidneys, spleen, and nervous system, where it binds to sulfhydryl groups of tissue proteins. Arsenic is excreted in the urine. It is first detectable in urine 2 to 8 hours after ingestion, and may be found in detectable quantities for up to 10 days. At 2 to 4 weeks, arsenic can be found in areas of high sulfhydryl-containing tissues such as hair, skin, and nails.

Clinical Manifestations

During acute exposure, symptoms may develop in as little as 30 minutes or be delayed for several hours. The patient may complain of a metallic taste. A garlic-like odor on the breath is sometimes noted. In oral exposures there may be mild pharyngeal or esophageal irritation. Abdominal pain, nausea, vomiting, and diarrhea are usually the first symptoms of poisoning. In severe exposures, vasodilation and shock, encephalopathy, acute tubular necrosis, seizures, and death may occur.

In chronic exposures, symptoms are more insidious and affect various organ systems. A painful distal neuropathy is common, the feet being a common site. Other neurologic manifestations range from personality changes to frank encephalopathy. Dermatologic manifestations include hyperkeratosis, desquamation, and brittle nails. Mees' lines are white bands that occasionally develop across the nails. After chronic exposure the patient is at risk for developing aplastic anemia, leukemia, anemia, and thrombocytopenia. Malabsorption can be seen with long-term exposure.

Diagnostic Evaluation

When arsenic ingestion is suspected, a 24-hour urine collection for arsenic content is required. The accuracy of this test depends on the time of ingestion; those specimens collected within the first 3 days following ingestion are optimal. The half-life of arsenic in the blood is 10 hours, making serum levels less useful than urinary excretion. Hair arsenic levels provide another means for detecting arsenic, and may be positive for months after exposure. The analysis of hair for arsenic is unable to differentiate between endogenous and exogenous exposure.

Gutzeit's test provides a quick, reliable, qualitative test for arsenic exposure. Several drops of sulfuric acid and a few granules of zinc are added to a test tube containing 5 ml of fresh urine. The test tube is then covered with filter paper impregnated with silver nitrate. A dark discoloration of the filter paper confirms arsenic exposure.

Although arsenic is radiopaque, it is usually rapidly absorbed from the GI tract, rendering abdominal radiographs of limited diagnostic value.

Therapeutic Intervention

Following GI emptying, activated charcoal may be given. Nevertheless, activated charcoal absorbs arsenic to a very limited degree. Supportive therapy includes aggressive fluid management, as arsenic can cause hypotension through vasodilation or fluid losses into the extravascular space.

Dimercaprol remains the treatment of choice for severe arsenic poisoning (see Table 97–1). Dimercaprol is given in 3- to 5-mg/kg intramuscular doses every 4 hours to a maximum of 1 gm/day. Side effects include nausea, vomiting, headache, tachycardia, hypotension, and a burning sensation in the mouth. Dimercaprol therapy is continued until urinary arsenic excretion is less than 50 μg/day. In chronic arsenic poisoning the benefit from dimercaprol chelation therapy is less certain. While it reverses the hematologic manifestations, it may not completely reverse the neuropathy.

D-Penicillamine may be given after initial treatment with dimercaprol. The dose for D-penicillamine is 100 mg/kg/day given in four divided doses, up to a maximum of 1 gm/day, and continued for 5 days. Unlike dimercaprol, D-penicillamine may be given orally, and is less toxic. Adverse effects of D-penicillamine include fever, leukopenia, rash, and thrombocytopenia. If symptoms of arsenic intoxication persist after completion of D-penicillamine chelation therapy, it may be repeated.

MERCURY

Mercury poisoning in children still occurs because of its widespread use in industry and agriculture. Organic mercury salts are found in pesticides, weed killers, wood preservatives, and fungicides. The inorganic salts are found mainly in industrial and occupational poisonings. Elemental mercury vapor is toxic when inhaled.

The mercury ion has a high affinity for sulfhydryl groups present on enzymes and other tissue proteins, disrupting cellular functions. Mercury vapor is extremely toxic to the respiratory system and when inhaled is nearly completely absorbed. Toxic effects include pulmonary edema, necrotizing bronchiolitis, pneumonitis, and neuronal degeneration. Metallic mercury (quicksilver), which is in thermometers, is relatively nontoxic when ingested. Toxicity also depends on the chemical composition of the mercury compound. Organic mercury (methyl and alkyl mercurials) are more toxic than the inorganic salts. Organic mercury is better absorbed in the GI tract than are inorganic compounds. Inorganic mercurials are corrosive to the GI tract and may precipitate oliguric renal failure.

Clinical Manifestations

The ingestion of large amounts of mercury results in stomatitis, abdominal pain, bloody diarrhea, shock, and encephalopathy. In chronic exposure the symptoms are more insidious. Symptoms include irritability, lethargy, dermal erythema with desquamation, photophobia, insomnia, apathy, hypertension, sweating, and loss of hair, nails, and terminal phalanges.

Laboratory Evaluation

The diagnosis of mercury poisoning is often difficult because few tests correlate with body mercury burden. Whole-blood mercury content provides the best indicator of recent exposure to inorganic mercury. Expired air levels and spot urine assay do not always correlate with symptoms.

Therapeutic Intervention

Supportive therapy includes intravenous hydration, correction of fluid and electrolyte imbalances, and oxygen therapy when the lungs are involved. Vital signs, fluid intake and output, and renal function should be monitored.

Chelation therapy is indicated in symptomatic mercury poisoning (see Table 97–1). In severe poisoning dimercaprol, 3 to 5 mg/kg intramuscularly every 4 hours, is given for the first 2 days. The dose is then reduced to 2.5 to 3 mg/kg every 6 hours for 2 days, then every 12 hours for up to 7 days.

In less severe or chronic cases treatment is instituted with dimercaprol, with subsequent therapy utilizing D-penicillamine, 100 mg/kg/day for 5 days. Urine mercury levels are used to gauge the success of chelation. In chronic mercury poisoning, clinical improvement may not occur following chelation therapy.

Selected References

Centers for Disease Control. Preventing lead poisoning in young children. Monograph, 1985, pp 1–35.

Chisholm JJ. Poisoning due to heavy metals. Pediatr Clin North Am 1970;17:591.

Chouchair AK, Ajax ET. Hair and nails in arsenical neuropathy. Ann Neurol 1988;23:628.

Committee on Environmental Hazards and Committee on Accident and Poison Prevention. Statement on childhood lead poisoning. Pediatrics 1987;79:457.

Fuortes L. Arsenic poisoning. Postgrad Med 1983;83:233.

Gorby MS. Arsenic poisoning. West J Med 1988;149:308.

Hutton JT, Bonna L. Sources, symptoms, and signs of arsenic poisoning. J Fam Pract 1983;17:423.

Moel M, Sachs H. Renal function in 9–17 year olds after childhood lead poisoning. J Pediatr 1985;106:729.

Moutinho ME, Tompkins AL, Rowland TW, et al. Acute mercury vapor poisoning. Fatality in an infant. Am J Dis Child 1981;135:42.

Peterson RG, Rumack BH. D-Penicillamine therapy for acute arsenic poisoning. J Pediatr 1977;91:661.

Schoolmeister WL, White DR. Arsenic poisoning. South Med J 1980;73:198.

Sunderman FW. Perils of mercury. Ann Clin Lab Sci 1988;18:89.

Tiomelli S, Rosen JF, Chisholm JJ. Management of childhood lead poisoning. J Pediatr 1984;105:523.

CHAPTER 98

Tricyclic Antidepressants

Rodney L. Baker
Suman Wason

INTRODUCTION

The term *tricyclic antidepressant* (TCA) is a misnomer since a new antidepressant, maprotiline, which contains a four-ring structure but has therapeutic uses and toxic effects similar to those of TCAs, is now available. Also, fluoxetine, a bicyclic compound, is available for the treatment of depression. So although the term *cyclic antidepressant* is more appropriate, for the purpose of this discussion the more familiar term, *tricyclic antidepressant*, will be used.

TCAs are a group of drugs that are primarily used for the treatment of endogenous depression (Table 98–1). They are also used in the therapy of nocturnal enuresis in children, migraine headaches, trigeminal neuralgia, and peripheral neuropathies. The annual incidence of TCA overdose in the United States has been estimated to be 500,000. TCA overdose is probably the most common life-threatening overdose because of its narrow margin of safety, high mortality: exposure ratio, and availability in households of individuals with psychiatric illness.

PHARMACOLOGY

The term *tricyclic* refers to the three-ring structure of the central portion of the drug molecule. TCAs vary from each other by a different radical attached to the central ring (Fig. 98–1). The active agents, both therapeutically and in their toxic effects, are the parent compound, a tertiary amine, and the metabolites, which are usually secondary amines (see Table 98–1).

TCAs are rapidly absorbed from the gastrointestinal tract, although after large ingestion their anticholinergic effects may delay absorption. They are highly lipid soluble, resulting in large apparent volumes of distribution. Tissue concentrations are up to 40 times those attained in the serum. In the serum, up to 95% of TCAs are protein bound. Acidosis decreases protein binding of TCAs, whereas alkalosis increases it, thereby lowering the amount of active drug available to tissues.

Hepatic metabolism is the major route of elimination of TCAs, which involves demethylation, hydroxylation, and glucuronidation. The therapeutic half-life of TCAs is highly variable and ranges from 10 to 80 hours.

The mechanism of action of TCAs seems to be the result of central inhibition of biogenic amine reuptake. TCAs also demonstrate central and peripheral anticholinergic effects and are competitive antagonists of histamine receptors.

CLINICAL EVALUATION

The usual therapeutic dose of TCAs is between 2 and 4 mg/kg. The ingestion of as little as 10 to 20 mg/kg of most TCAs can result in serious toxicity. As little as 200 mg, four 50-mg tablets, in a toddler may be life-threatening.

The manifestations of TCA overdose are the result of their effects on the central and parasympathetic nervous systems and cardiovascular system (Table 98–2). Signs of toxicity usually appear within 4 hours of ingestion.

The early signs and symptoms following a TCA overdose are for the most part anticholinergic in nature. They include mydriasis, blurred vision, dry mouth, tachycardia, fever, flushed skin, decreased bowel sounds, urinary retention, and central nervous system excitation.

At therapeutic doses TCAs have a quinidine-like effect on the heart, resulting in altered repolarization and conduction. In an overdose this results in conduction abnormalities and supraventricular and ventricular dysrhythmias. The most common cause of death after TCA overdose is cardiotoxicity secondary to intractable myocardial depression, ventricular tachycardia, or ventricular fibrillation. Sinus tachycardia is the result of the anticholinergic effects of TCAs. However, it is not a sensitive predictor of serious cardiotoxicity. Malig-

TABLE 98–1

PHARMACOKINETICS OF SOME COMMONLY AVAILABLE TRICYCLIC ANTIDEPRESSANTS

	Doxepine	Imipramine	Desipramine	Amitriptyline	Nortriptyline
Absorption	Rapid	Rapid	Rapid	Slow	Slow
Peak concentration (hr)	2–4	1–2	4–6	2–12	7–8
Volume of distribution (L/kg)	20	5–20	28–60	8–10	21–57
Protein binding (%)	95	90	90	95	95
Hepatic metabolism (%)	90–100	90–100	90	95	90–100
Active metabolites	Yes	Yes	No	Yes	No
Half-life (hr)	8–24	8–16	22	10–20	16–90
Therapeutic concentration (ng/ml)	30–150	100–300	40–160	60–220	50–150
Toxic concentration (ng/ml)	>1000	>1000	>1000	>1000	>500

nant ventricular arrhythmias have developed without prior tachycardia.

Hypotension, another potential complication of TCA overdose, is the result of peripheral vasodilation due to alpha-receptor blockage and myocardial depression. Initially TCA overdose may cause hypertension secondary to the blocked reuptake of biogenic amines. This hypertension is usually short-lived and should not be treated, since the subsequent hypotensive effects are more sustained and critical.

The nervous system effects of TCA overdose result in ataxia, confusion, agitation, hallucinations, coma, myoclonus, and seizures. Mental status can deteriorate rapidly from mild sedation to coma with respiratory arrest. Mortality following an overdose of TCAs is increased if generalized seizures occur. This is most likely the result of an increased concentration of free TCAs in the serum due to the metabolic acidosis resulting from seizure activity.

The incidence of cardiotoxicity of amoxipine and loxapine is much lower than that encountered with the other TCAs. On the other hand, these TCAs have a potential for serious neurotoxic effects such as intractable status epilepticus. Reports of fluoxetine overdose indicate that it does not produce neurotoxicity or cardiotoxicity similar to the TCAs.

DIAGNOSTIC EVALUATION

Although some studies suggest that serum TCA concentrations exceeding 1000 ng/ml correlate well with toxicity, others show poor correlation between serum levels and clinical findings. The explanations for this may be that the serum represents only a small portion of the total body TCA load; metabolites that may have significant toxic effects are sometimes not measured, and serum concentrations are affected by protein binding and can change rapidly. In general, determination of quantitative TCA levels in an overdose situation is not recommended. However, a qualitative assay can be useful in documentation of a TCA ingestion.

On electrocardiography, a prolonged QRS interval in the limb leads exceeding 0.10 second is the most accurate predictor of subsequent dysrhythmias as well as seizures. If the QRS duration exceeds 0.10 second there is a 14% chance that ventricular arrhythmias will follow and a 34% chance that seizures will occur. The value of the EKG axis deviation in predicting TCA toxicity is still unclear, although some have reported that a terminal 40-msec axis of the QRS complex of greater than 120 degrees may be a more sensitive marker of severe toxicity.

THERAPEUTIC INTERVENTION

All patients with a history of potentially toxic ingestion of TCAs should be carefully observed with continuous cardiorespiratory monitoring (Table 98–3). The clinical status of patients with a TCA overdose at initial presentation can give one a false sense of security. Some patients may exhibit only mild sedation, which can rapidly progress to status epilepticus and cardiorespiratory arrest.

Decontamination

Gastrointestinal decontamination should be performed after every significant ingestion. The possibility of rapid

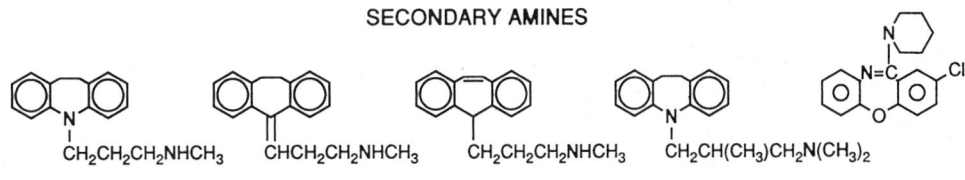

Figure 98–1. Chemical structure of tricyclics.

TABLE 98–2

SIGNS AND SYMPTOMS

Central Nervous System
Sedation
Coma
Confusion
Agitation
Myoclonus
Hallucinations
Seizures
Anticholinergic Findings
Mydriasis
Blurred vision
Dry mouth
Tachycardia
Fever
Flushed skin
Decreased bowel sounds
Urinary retention
Cardiovascular
Transient hypertension
Hypotension
Sinus tachycardia
Supraventricular arrhythmias
Ventricular arrhythmias
Conduction block

mental status deterioration and seizures makes induction of emesis by administration of syrup of ipecac potentially hazardous. Therefore in cases of significant ingestion the stomach should be lavaged, following which activated charcoal should be instilled. Repetitive charcoal administration, 1 gm/kg given every 3 to 4 hours for 18 to 24 hours, increases the elimination of TCAs from the vascular compartment. However, this increased elimination may not be clinically important, and there may be an increased risk of aspiration of charcoal following TCA ingestion, perhaps because of the combination of decreased mental status and decreased gastric emptying. Therefore activated charcoal must be administered with careful attention paid to protection of the airway. It is also advisable to withhold repetitive dosing of activated charcoal if bowel sounds are decreased.

TABLE 98–3

THERAPEUTIC INTERVENTION

1. Ensure airway, breathing, and circulation
2. Gastrointestinal decontamination
   Avoid ipecac
   Activated charcoal (1 gm/kg); repeat q 4–6 hr for 18–24 hr
   Do not administer repetitive charcoal if no bowel sounds present
   Protect airway if repetitive charcoal is used
3. Monitor
   Continue ABCs
   Obtain EKG: if QRS > 0.10 msec, treat with sodium bicarbonate, admit
   Continuous cardiac monitoring
4. Special therapeutic notes
   Do not treat hypertension
   Treat hypotension in following sequence with (a) fluids, (b) alkalinization, (c) norepinephrine, (d) dobutamine
   DO NOT USE quinidine, procainamide, or disopyramide for arrhythmia
   Treat ventricular arrhythmias in the following sequence with (a) alkalinization, (b) lidocaine, (c) phenytoin
   DO NOT USE physostigmine

Central Nervous System Treatment

The serious central nervous system toxicity of TCA overdose is manifested by seizures and coma. Coma is usually short-lived, resolving within 24 hours, but it may be severe enough to require support of the airway. Physostigmine can reverse the anticholinergic effects and improve the mental status of patients with organic brain syndrome secondary to TCA overdose. However, since it has the potential for serious complications, including bradycardia, asystole, and seizures, and since most TCA overdose patients do well with supportive care for these symptoms, physostigmine should not be used. Physostigmine is not effective in treating the cardiotoxicity of TCAs.

Generalized seizures have been associated with increased mortality from TCA overdose and therefore should be treated aggressively. Benzodiazepines, either diazepam or lorazepam, should be used because they are effective in TCA-induced seizures and their onset of action is rapid (Table 98–4). However, because of their relatively short duration of action, especially that of diazepam, they should be followed by a longer-acting anticonvulsant. Phenytoin, 15 mg/kg intravenously not to exceed a rate of 0.5 mg/kg/minute, is recommended as the drug of choice because of its efficacy in seizures secondary to TCA intoxication and its antiarrhythmic properties.

Cardiac Therapy

Cardioversion should be delivered to any hemodynamically compromised patient with tachyarrhythmia. Cardiac arrest secondary to TCA ingestion does not carry as poor a prognosis as that of a myocardial infarction or the more usual pediatric cardiac arrest that follows respiratory arrest. There have been reports of full neurologic recovery even after prolonged cardiorespiratory resuscitation after TCA overdose.

Alkalinization can temporarily reverse TCA cardiotoxicity whether done by administration of intravenous sodium bicarbonate or hyperventilation. Alkalinization has been shown to be effective in treating widened QRS complexes, hypotension, and arrhythmias (Fig. 98–2). Sodium bicarbonate should be administered at an initial dose of 1 to 2 mEq/kg intravenously, and arterial blood gases should be monitored; additional sodium bicarbonate should be administered to maintain the arterial pH between 7.45 and 7.50.

If alkalinization does not reverse the dysrhythmias, quinidine, procainamide, and disopyramide are contraindicated since they enhance the cardiac toxicity from TCAs. Lidocaine, which does not significantly depress conduction or contractility, should be used in the therapy of ventricular arrhythmias secondary to TCA overdose. Phenytoin may aid the control of TCA-induced arrhythmias since it improves intraventricular conduction. However, its use remains controversial, and it requires a longer period of time for safe administration. Currently it is recommended only if alkalinization and lidocaine fail to control the arrhythmia. The conduction delays caused by TCA overdose occur primarily distal to the atrioventricular node; therefore atropine has been generally ineffective. Isoproterenol may be helpful in controlling bradyarrhythmias while a pacemaker is being inserted for overdrive cardiac pacing.

TCA overdose can cause hypotension by direct vasodilation, alpha-receptor blockade, or myocardial depression. Initial therapy for hypotension is the administration of crystalloid fluid boluses (20 ml/kg/bolus of lactated Ringer's or 0.9 normal saline). Concurrently, alkalinization to a pH greater than 7.45 should be attempted with sodium bicarbonate. Persistent hypotension after fluid administration and

TABLE 98–4

THERAPY AT A GLANCE

	Dose	Frequency
Gastric Decontamination		
Activated charcoal	1 gm/kg in 70% sorbitol	Most ingestions ×1
		Consider multiple doses in carbazepine, digoxin, theophylline, tricyclic antidepressants
Ipecac	6–12 mo, 10 ml + fluids	×1 in 20 min if no emesis
	1–12 yr, 15–30 ml + fluids	×1 in 20 min if no emesis
	>12 yr, 30–60 ml + fluids	×1 in 20 min if no emesis
Initial Therapy		
Sodium bicarbonate	1–2 mEq/kg	As needed to keep pH ≥ 7.45
Antiarrhythmic Therapy		
Phenytoin	15 mg/kg	Loading dose
Lidocaine	1 mg/kg/dose	q 5–10 min PRN (max. 5 mg/kg) (maintenance 20–50 µg/kg/min
Cardiovascular Support		
Dobutamine	1–15 µg/kg/min	Continuous infusion
Norepinephrine	0.1–0.2 µg/kg/min	Continuous infusion
Seizure Control		
Diazepam	0.2 mg/kg	×1
Lorazepam	0.1 mg/kg	×1

alkalinization should be treated with vasopressors. Since TCAs block the reuptake of norepinephrine at nerve endings, pressors such as dopamine, which in part rely on norepinephrine release from storage vesicles, may be ineffective. Therefore norepinephrine or phenylephrine are preferred. If hypotension is still uncorrected, an inotropic agent like dobutamine may aid in reversing the myocardial depression.

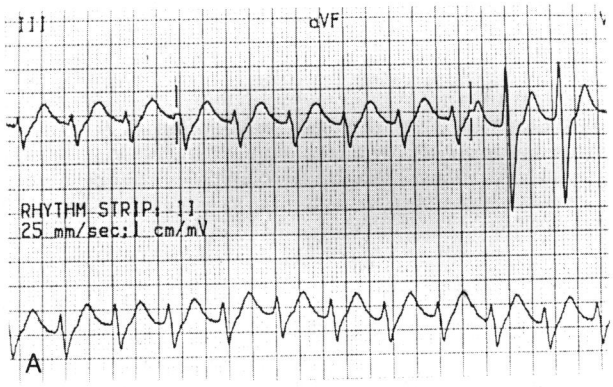

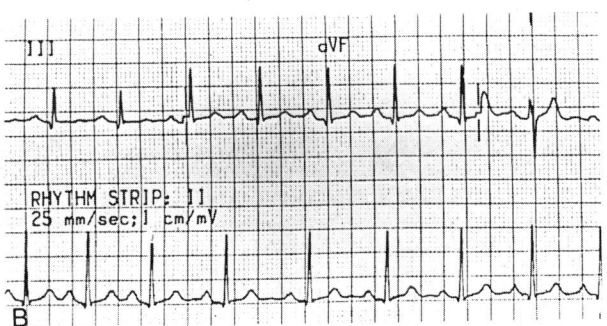

Figure 98–2. Cardiotoxicity from a tricyclic ingestion is manifested in this child by a prolonged QRS duration of > 0.10 seconds *(A)*. After bicarbonate administration *(B)*, the QRS interval shortens.

DISPOSITION

The patient with serious TCA intoxication, after stabilization and gastrointestinal decontamination, should be admitted to the intensive care unit for continued monitoring and therapy.

The patient without signs or symptoms following ingestion of a TCA should be closely observed in the emergency department for 6 hours. If after the period of observation the patient remains asymptomatic, he or she may be discharged. If neurologic or cardiac findings of intoxication develop during the observation period, the patient should be admitted to the hospital.

Selected References

Boehnert MT, Lovejoy FH. Value of the QRS duration versus the serum drug level in predicting seizures and ventricular arrhythmias after an acute overdose of tricyclic antidepressants. N Engl J Med 1985; 313:474.

Callahan M. Admission criteria for tricyclic antidepressant ingestion. West J Med 1982; 137:425.

Crome P, Newman B. Fatal tricyclic antidepressant poisoning. J R Soc Med 1979; 72:649.

Finnegan KT, Gabiola JM. Fluoxetine overdose. Am J Psychiatry 1988; 145:12.

Frommer DA, Kulig KW, Marx JA, et al. Tricyclic antidepressant overdose. JAMA 1987; 257:521.

Goldgerger AL, Curtis GP. Immediate effects of physostigmine on amitriptyline-induced QRS prolongation. J Toxicol Clin Toxicol 1982; 19:445.

Hoffman JR, McElroy CR. Bicarbonate therapy for dysrhythmia and hypotension in tricyclic antidepressant overdose. West J Med 1981; 134:60.

Kulig KW, Rumack BH, Sullivan JB, et al. Amoxapine overdose: Coma and seizures without cardiotoxic effects. JAMA 1982; 248:1092.

Levit A, Sullivan J, Owens M, et al. Change in amitriptyline plasma protein binding with increase in pH over 7.4. Vet Hum Toxicol 1984; 26:42.

Litovitz TL, Schmitz BF, Bailey KM. 1989 Annual report of the American Association of Poison Control Centers National Data Collection System. Am J Emerg Med 1990; 8:394.

Manoguerra AS. Tricyclic antidepressants. Crit Care Q 1982; 4:43.

Niemann JT, Bessen HA, Rothstein RJ, et al: Electrocardiographic criteria for tricyclic antidepressant cardiotoxicity. Am J Cardiol 1986; 57:1154.

Noble J, Mathew H. Acute poisoning by tricyclic antidepressants: Clinical features and management of 100 patients. Clin Toxicol 1969; 2:403.

Peterson CD. Seizures induced by acute loxapine overdose. Am J Psychiatry 1981; 138:1089.

Preskorn SH, Irwin HA. Toxicity of tricyclic antidepressants: Kinetics, mechanisms, interventions: A review. J Clin Psychiatry 1982; 43:151.

Spiker DG, Biggs JT. Tricyclic antidepressants: Prolonged plasma levels after overdose. JAMA 1976; 236:1711.

Swartz CM, Sherman A. The treatment of tricyclic antidepressant overdose with repeated charcoal. J Clin Psychopharmacol 1984; 4:336.

Thorstrand C. Clinical features in poisoning by tricyclic antidepressants with special reference to the ECG. Acta Med Scand 1976; 199:337.

Uhl JA. Phenytoin: The drug of choice in tricyclic antidepressant overdose? Ann Emerg Med 1981; 10:270.

CHAPTER 99

Mushroom and Plant Ingestions

Marion Hoelzer

MUSHROOM POISONING

Introduction

Mushrooms are fungi; they lack chlorophyll and the ability to manufacture their own nutrients. Mushrooms must absorb nutrients from decaying organic matter. The mushroom is actually a subterranean network of hyphae called the mycelium. The reproductive fruit that forms above ground is what is recognized as a mushroom.

There are certain characteristics of mushrooms that aid in identification (Fig. 99–1). These include the substrate where the mushroom was found and the mushroom stem (stipe), cap, and gill characteristics. The stem of the deadly *Amanita* species has distinguishing structural characteristics:

the presence of an annulus or death ring, and a volva or cup-like structure (death cup) at the base of the stem. Absence of these features does not exclude *Amanita* poisoning since handling may obscure the anatomy of a specimen. The cap should be inspected closely for color, shape, and size. Red or orange caps are characteristic of *Amanita muscaria*, while white caps are seen with *A. vera*. *Coprinus* mushrooms have caps that stain blue-black when bruised. Important gill characteristics include color, spacing, and attachment to the stem. Gill colors include white, yellow, red, green, brown, or black. Gill spacing may be close and crowded or distant. *Amanita* species have free attachment of the gills, meaning that there is a gap between the stem and gills. Twisting the stem of the *Amanita* mushroom causes no damage to the gills because of this free attachment.

Clinical Evaluation

Mushroom poisoning can mimic many other medical problems, and the history of ingestion can be lifesaving. Unfortunately the primary victims of poisoning are most often preschool children, who are unreliable historians. If able to talk, children often deny having ingested the mushroom when questioned.

An estimated 5000 mushroom species grow in the United States, yet few species cause poisonings. The *Amanita* mushrooms, specifically *A. phalloides*, account for the majority of fatalities. Individual mushrooms may vary in toxicity, depending on the age of the mushroom, season, and growing conditions. In addition, people vary in their response to mushroom toxins. Large quantities of mushrooms may be consumed by some family members without effect, yet cause severe symptoms in others. Toxicity in the pediatric age group may be related to consumption of the raw specimen. Adults often cook or boil mushrooms, which reduces or destroys some toxins.

Most of the initial symptoms will be gastrointestinal (GI) complaints and may mimic food poisoning. The chronology of symptoms is important (Table 99–1). Any GI symptoms occurring more than 6 hours after ingestion suggest *Gyromitra* toxicity or *Amanita* poisoning, the most lethal mushroom poisoning. With symptoms beginning early (within 20 to 120 minutes), one needs to consider muscarinic or ibotenic acid poisoning. Muscarinic poisoning resembles cholinergic toxicity, with perspiration, lacrimation, salivation, bradycardia, and pinpoint pupils. Ibotenic acid poisoning from *A. muscaria* should be considered if the patient appears intoxicated, confused, euphoric, and hyperkinetic and then lapses into a deep sleep.

Diagnostic Evaluation

Mushroom identification is mandatory. GI decontamination should not await identification.

Ideally an intact whole specimen is best. Optimally one should contact a local mycologist, usually through local

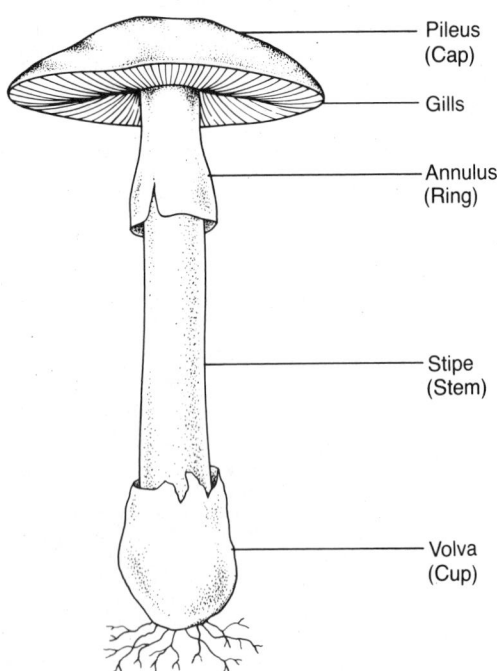

Figure 99–1. *Amanita virosa.* Note the annulus encircling the stipe (stem), and the volva or "cup."

Labels on figure:
- Pileus (Cap)
- Gills
- Annulus (Ring)
- Stipe (Stem)
- Volva (Cup)

TABLE 99–1
IMPORTANT MUSHROOM POISONING HISTORY
How many types of mushrooms were ingested?
What was approximate time of ingestion?
When did first symptoms occur?
What were first symptoms?
Was any alcohol consumed within 72 hr of meal?
Did anyone else eat the mushrooms, and are they sick?
Is anyone sick who did not eat mushrooms?

poison control centers, university botany departments, or botanical gardens, for immediate identification.

When an intact specimen is available, certain characteristics of the structure aid identification, as mentioned. A ring around the stem or a cup on the bottom of the stem are characteristic of *Amanita* mushrooms. White spores and white gills not attached to the stem also suggest *Amanita*. If *Amanita* poisoning is suspected, treatment for cyclopeptide poisoning is initiated. One must distinguish between *A. phalloides* and *A. virosa*, which cause cyclopeptide poisoning, and *A. muscaria* and *A. pantherina*, which cause ibotenic acid poisoning.

Meixner's Test

The Meixner test is simple and reliable and can be performed by the physician in the emergency department to determine the presence of amatoxin. A drop of juice from the mushroom is squeezed onto newspaper. The location of the spot is circled with a pencil and air dried, and a drop of concentrated hydrochloric acid is added. If a large quantity of amatoxin is present, a blue color develops in 1 to 2 minutes. For trace amounts it may take up to 20 minutes. The test should not be performed near heat or direct sunlight because hydrochloric acid on newsprint turns blue when exposed to high heat or sunlight (Table 99–2).

Therapeutic Intervention

Reduction of absorption is accomplished by gastric emptying and activated charcoal administration. Gastric contents

---

TABLE 99–2

MUSHROOM POISONING—CLINICAL SUMMARY

Group I   Cyclopeptides
Mushrooms: *Amanita, Galerina*
Stage 1: 6–24 hr postingestion: onset of nausea, vomiting, cholera-like diarrhea, abdominal pain
Stage 2: 12–48 hr postingestion: apparent recovery; rising hepatic enzymes
Stage 3: 24–72 hr postingestion: progressive hepatic and renal failure, coagulopathy, cardiomyopathy, encephalopathy, convulsions, coma, death

Group IA   Orellanine
Mushroom: *Cortinarius*
3–14 days postingestion: GI symptoms nephritis, oliguric renal failure

Group II   Monomethylhydrazine
Mushrooms: *Gyromitra, Helvella*
6–24 hr postingestion: GI symptoms, muscle cramps, delirium, convulsions, coma hemolysis, and methemoglobinemia may occur

Group III   Coprine
Mushrooms: *Coprinus, Boletus*
30 min after alcohol ingestion (up to 1 wk after mushroom ingestion): disulfiram-like reaction

Group IV   Muscarine
Mushrooms: *Clitocybe, Inocybe*
1–2 hr postingestion: cholinergic syndrome convulsions, coma

Group V   Muscimol, Ibotenic Acid
Mushrooms: *Amanita muscaria* and *A. pantherina*
1–2 hr postingestion: anticholinergic syndrome, altered perception

Group VI   Psilocybin
Mushrooms: *Psilocybe, Panaeolus*
1–3 hr postingestion: hallucinations, euphoria, paresthesias, mydriasis

Group VII   Gastrointestinal Irritants
Mushrooms: numerous
1–2 hr postingestion: nausea, vomiting, diarrhea

---

should be saved for spore analysis by a mycologist. Activated charcoal absorbs toxins well. The charcoal may be administered with a cathartic. Forced diuresis and charcoal hemoperfusion enhance excretion of toxins. With forced diuresis one needs to maintain urine output at 3 to 6 ml/kg/hour. This may be accomplished with oral or intravenous fluids. Furosemide, 1 mg/kg intravenously, will augment low urine output. The efficacy of hemodialysis in mushroom poisoning is controversial. The *Amanita* toxin is too large for hemodialysis. Supportive interventions include ensuring airway, breathing, and circulation; monitoring electrolyte and glucose levels; following hepatic and renal function; and using sedatives cautiously for anxiety or hallucinations. Thorazine, 1.0 mg/kg intramuscularly, is recommended for children.

MUSHROOM TOXINS
Cyclopeptides (Group I)

Group I includes the species *A. phalloides, A. virosa, Galerina marginata,* and *G. autumnalis* (see Table 99–2). Cyclopeptides are composed of two chains of amino acids bridged by a sulfur atom to form a two-ring structure. The cyclopeptides comprise two groups of toxins: amatoxins and phallotoxins. Amatoxins, primarily amanitin, constitute the only group responsible for human poisoning. They are heat stable and are not destroyed by drying, boiling, or other methods of cooking.

Amanitin is an intracellular toxin whose target is the liver cell nucleolus. Amanitin inhibits RNA polymerase, preventing transcription and causing a decrease in protein synthesis. This toxic effect manifests clinically as increasing liver transaminase levels. This mechanism accounts for the appearance of liver failure 3 to 4 days after ingestion.

Enterohepatic circulation of amanitin subjects the liver to repetitive toxic exposure. Serum amanitin is filtered by the kidneys, and a large portion is excreted in the urine. However, amanitin can damage the renal tubules, causing subsequent renal failure.

Initial symptoms occur after a latent period, usually 6 to 10 hours. However, *Amanita* toxicity is not excluded if symptoms occur earlier since several types of toxins may have been ingested. Amanitin causes irritation of the GI lining, producing severe colicky abdominal pain, nausea, vomiting, and a cholera-type diarrhea that is often bloody. A short-lived period of improvement follows. On the second to fourth day postingestion, abdominal pains return with severe liver damage, jaundice, and renal failure. Finally circulatory collapse, convulsions, coma, and ultimately death ensue.

Aggressive treatment of *Amanita* poisoning results in a 75% to 80% survival rate. Children less than 10 years old have a higher mortality rate, related to a larger absorbed dose of toxin per kilogram of body weight. The prothrombin time reliably predicts the severity of intoxication. Serum amanitin levels confirm the diagnosis of *Amanita* poisoning but do not correlate with the severity of intoxication nor patient outcome.

Penicillin prevents penetration of amanitin into hepatocytes and displaces the toxin from plasma proteins, providing for increased renal excretion. Penicillin also sterilizes intestinal flora, killing enteric bacteria that produce gamma-aminobutyric acid (GABA), a neurotransmitter responsible for the severe encephalopathy seen in the final stage of poisoning. The recommended dose of penicillin G is 300,000 to 1,000,000 U/kg/day (Table 99–3). Electrolyte abnormalities can occur with high-dose penicillin infusions.

Silymarin is the active principle in the milk thistle, *Silybum marianum*. This substance inhibits binding of amanitin to the

TABLE 99-3		
ANTIDOTES FOR MUSHROOM POISONING		
Group	Toxin	Antidote
I	Amatoxin	Penicillin 300,000–1,000,000 u/ kg/day; silibinin 20–50 mg/kg/ day; steroids?; dialysis
II	Monomethylhydrazine	Pyridoxine 25 mg/kg IV; methylene blue 1–2 mg/kg IV for methemoglobinemia > 30%
III	Coprine	None, supportive
IV	Muscarine	Atropine: adults 0.5–1.0 mg IV, children 0.01 mg/kg IV; repeat as necessary
V	Muscimol, ibotenic acid	Physostigmine: adults 1–2 mg IV, children 0.5 mg IV only for severe anticholinergic symptoms
VI	Psilocybin	None, supportive
VII	GI irritant	None, supportive

hepatic cell membrane, competes with the toxin for transmembrane transport, and prevents penetration of amanitin into the cell. Silymarin also interrupts enterohepatic circulation. The dose of silibinin, a water-soluble preparation of silymarin, is 20 to 50 mg/kg/day. Silibinin is not available in the United States.

Thiotic acid was initially believed to improve outcome in *Amanita* poisoning. In well-controlled animal experiments, thiotic acid was ineffective. A retrospective analysis of 205 poisonings showed a higher mortality rate associated with administration of thiotic acid.

Amatoxins are readily dialyzable and have a high affinity for charcoal. However, most of the toxin is tissue bound in the hepatocytes, the serum concentration has little correlation with clinical outcome, and there is no evidence that significant quantities of amatoxin are removed by either dialysis or charcoal hemoperfusion.

Case reports indicate that patients in fulminant hepatic failure have survived after liver transplant. Liver transplantation is still a controversial treatment, and success is based on a small number of case reports.

Supportive therapy and GI decontamination are helpful if begun early. Most patients present for treatment 6 to 12 hours after ingestion, limiting the effectiveness of decontamination procedures. Adequate fluid replacement should be guided by vital signs, electrolytes, and glucose determinations.

Orellanine (Group IA)

Cortinarius mushrooms are bright orange-brown and bell shaped and contain the toxin orellanine. Though found in Europe and North American coniferous forests, most of the poisonings have been reported in northern Europe. Those most commonly involved in poisonings include *Cortinarius orellanus*, *C. speciosissimus*, and *C. rainierensis*. Orellanine is a heat-stable toxin unaffected by cooking or drying. The toxin inhibits the enzyme alkaline phosphatase, interrupting ATP production and causing an interstitial nephritis and tubular necrosis.

Symptoms do not appear until 36 hours after ingestion. Initial complaints of thirst, nausea, and vomiting may be mild and do not compel the patient to seek medical attention. One to three weeks later patients develop back and flank pain, chills, night sweats, and polyuria, which progresses to oliguria and renal failure. Because of the lengthy delay to presentation, gastric decontamination is ineffective. The emphasis of therapy is toward correcting fluid and electrolyte imbalances. Fluid administration should be judicious to prevent fluid overload. Baseline urinalysis and liver and renal function should be documented. Hemodialysis is often necessary to treat the ensuing oliguric renal failure.

Monomethylhydrazine (Group II)

Some of the most succulent mushrooms are the morels. False morels, *Gyromitra esculenta*, are often collected in spring with true morels. Only a small number of people who eat false morels become sick. If someone does become ill, it is usually because the mushrooms were eaten raw or were incorrectly prepared. Gyromitrin is the toxin present in *Gyromitra* mushrooms. Gyromitrin is an unstable molecule easily hydrolyzed to monomethylhydrazine by moderate cooking temperatures.

Only 20 cases of *Gyromitra* poisoning have been reported in North America since 1900, but 50% of these were fatal. Not all species of *Gyromitra* contain gyromitrin. The most common toxigenic morel is *G. esculenta* (Fig. 99–2). Parboiling, then discarding the liquid, is the traditional method of detoxifying the mushrooms, but this is not foolproof. Monomethylhydrazine has a low boiling point and easily vaporizes. Cooks can easily be poisoned just by inhaling the cooking fumes.

Monomethylhydrazine is a principal ingredient in jet rocket fuel. Workers in aerospace centers exposed to monomethylhydrazine and other rocket propellants developed symptoms identical to gyromitrin poisoning. This led to research proving that monomethylhydrazine could be produced from gyromitrin by hydrolysis.

Monomethylhydrazine is toxic to the central nervous system (CNS) and causes liver damage. It interferes with enzyme reactions, requiring pyridoxal phosphate as a cofactor. Monomethylhydrazine binds pyridoxal phosphate and inhibits amino acid synthesis. GABA is an important neurotransmitter whose synthesis is catalyzed by pyridoxal phosphate. Monomethylhydrazine causes seizures by inhibiting the production of GABA.

There is a latent period of 6 to 12 hours before the onset of symptoms. Bloating and then nausea, vomiting, severe crampy abdominal pain, and watery or bloody diarrhea predominate. Severe cases can lead to jaundice, high fever, liver failure, ataxia, convulsions, and ultimately death. The mortality rate from monomethylhydrazine poisoning is approximately 14.5%.

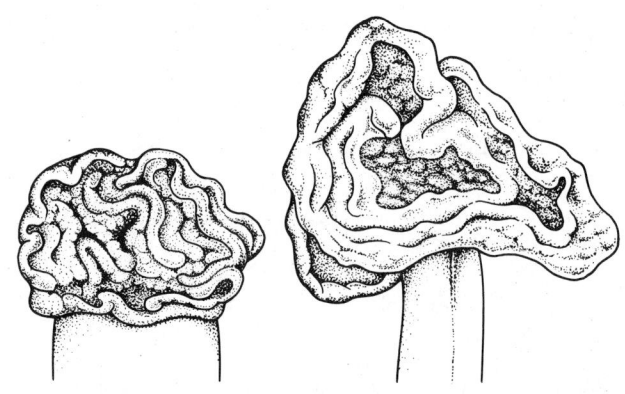

Gyromitra gigas   *Gyromitra esculenta*

Figure 99–2. *Gyromitra* contains the toxin monomethylhydrazine. *Gyromitra esculenta* (false morel) is named for its "brain-like" appearance.

Because monomethylhydrazine is a hemolytic toxin, methemoglobin and free hemoglobin are indicators of exposure as well as of progression of intoxication. This toxin is also hepatotoxic, and bilirubin and hepatic transaminases need to be monitored. Hypoglycemia also results from toxicity. Hydration status and electrolytes should be monitored.

Pyridoxine (vitamin B_6) protects against seizures. The dose is 25 mg/kg intravenously. Intravenous glucose should be given based on serum levels. Free hemoglobin levels should be monitored. Forced diuresis is used to prevent renal damage if levels continue to rise. If renal failure ensues, dialysis may be indicated. Hepatic failure may develop over 24 to 48 hours. If methemoglobin levels exceed 30%, methylene blue can be given. GI decontamination is also important to prevent continued absorption of toxin.

Coprine Poisoning (Group III)

Mushrooms responsible for coprine poisoning include *Coprinus atramentarius* (inky cap) and *Clitocybe* species. *Coprinus* mushrooms are called inky caps because the flesh of the caps dissolves by a process of autolysis into inky fluid at maturity.

Coprine is an amino acid derivative of glutamine. It has properties similar to disulfiram (Antabuse). The symptoms of coprine poisoning result from blocking the enzyme acetaldehyde dehydrogenase. Ethanol metabolism is halted and acetaldehyde accumulates, causing vasomotor effects through the beta receptors of the autonomic nervous system. The reaction to the toxin is dependent on the quantity of alcohol consumed.

The onset of symptoms is usually within 30 to 60 minutes after drinking alcohol, even if the mushrooms were consumed 4 to 5 days before. Flushing of the face, elevated blood pressure, a feeling of swelling in the extremities, paresthesia, pounding headache, a metallic taste, rapid breathing, and tachycardia ensue. Following these symptoms the patient experiences nausea, vomiting, sweating, and hypotension. Recovery is usually complete within 2 to 4 hours.

Supportive therapy is the mainstay of treatment. One should avoid elixirs, tinctures, or any medications with an alcohol base. Propranolol in low doses may help cardiac arrhythmias. Hypotension usually responds to isotonic fluids but occasionally requires vasopressors.

Muscarine Poisoning (Group IV)

This group of mushrooms includes *Clitocybe dealbata*, *Inocybe fastigiata*, and some species of *Boletus*. Muscarine was the first toxin to be isolated from the mushroom *A. muscaria*. However, the concentration of muscarine in *A. muscaria* is low. Ibotenic acid, not muscarine, is responsible for the predominant symptoms associated with *A. muscaria* poisoning. *Inocybe* mushrooms contain more than 100 times the concentration of muscarine as *A. muscaria*. Over 30 species of *Inocybe* have been shown to contain measurable levels of muscarine.

Muscarine affects parasympathetic cholinergic receptors of smooth muscle and glands. Muscarine, because of its quaternary amine configuration, cannot diffuse through the blood-brain barrier. Therefore toxic symptoms are primarily peripheral manifestations. Muscarine binds competitively to the acetylcholine receptors, causing excitation. Acetylcholinesterase degrades acetylcholine, thus terminating neurotransmission. It is unable to chemically modify muscarine; action on the receptor is terminated when the concentration of muscarine drops below necessary levels to maintain excitation (usually by passive diffusion). Atropine, the antidote

for muscarine poisoning, binds to but does not activate the receptor and is resistant to acetylcholinesterase degradation.

Symptoms occur 15 to 30 minutes after ingestion. The toxin is thermostable, so any method of preparation will not degrade the toxin. The sine qua non of muscarine poisoning is its organophosphate-like toxicity, with perspiration, salivation, and lacrimation. No other mushroom poisoning has this complex of symptoms. Myosis and bradycardia help distinguish muscarine toxicity from acute anxiety. Other symptoms include nausea, vomiting, and increased peristalsis with subsequent diarrhea. Vomiting removes much of the toxin. Dyspnea secondary to bronchospasm and increased bronchial secretions can also occur. Patients should be closely monitored for hypotension from fluid loss and dehydration.

GI decontamination often occurs as a consequence of the toxin since vomiting and diarrhea are prominent. Intravenous hydration is necessary to replace fluid loss. Often the symptoms are mild and self-limiting and are rarely as severe as organophosphate poisoning. The treatment for severe toxicity is atropine to counteract the effects of muscarine. Atropine should be titrated to cessation of secretions, not dilation of pupils. Atropine toxicity may result when dilation of pupils is used as the end point of therapy, particularly in children. Initial test doses are 0.5 to 1.0 mg intravenously in adults and 0.01 mg/kg in children, and may be repeated.

Ibotenic Acid—Muscimol Poisoning (Group V)

This group of mushrooms includes *A. muscaria* (fly agaric) and *A. pantherina* (the panther). Poisonings in North America became prevalent as individuals deliberately ingested these hallucinogenic mushrooms.

A. muscaria was used as an insecticide for flies. (*Muscaria* is a derivation of musta, Latin for fly.) The toxin muscarine was isolated from these mushrooms. Muscarine, however, is found in physiologically insignificant amounts. Rarely do *A. muscaria* or *A. pantherina* poisonings present with muscarinic symptoms. Rather, atropine worsens symptoms of fly agaric poisoning. The toxins responsible for symptomatology are ibotenic acid and muscimol. Ibotenic acid is found in greatest concentration in the bright red to orange-yellow cap of the fly agaric. Muscimol is 10 times more potent than ibotenic acid and is the decarboxylation product of this acid. Ibotenic acid and muscimol anticholinergic syndrome with primarily central and some peripheral manifestations. Ibotenic acid is a derivative of glutamic acid, and muscimol is a derivative of GABA. Unlike their biologic counterparts, these toxins cross the blood-brain barrier by an active transport mechanism. Muscimol and ibotenic acid are false neurotransmitters. Neither toxin is effectively removed from the receptors by the GABA or glutamate uptake system, and this contributes to their CNS effects.

Death from *A. muscaria* and *A. pantherina* is rare, less than 1%. Symptoms occur within 30 to 120 minutes of ingestion. There is an initial slowdown in performing tasks, progressing to incoordination of voluntary movements. Patients appear intoxicated. In severe poisonings this ataxia may progress to muscle twitchings, spasms, and cramps. Dizziness, visual distortions or illusions, elation, and an out-of-body experience follow. The visual illusions are a misinterpretation of sensory stimuli; for example, near objects appear far away and small objects seem enormous. Despite general incoordination, speech and articulation are spared, in contradistinction to alcohol intoxication. There is no alteration of blood pressure or pulse. Patients experience mild GI upset but seldom vomit, since muscimol is an effective antiemetic.

Despite the severity of the symptoms, they are usually transient and rarely persist beyond 6 hours. Death is rare.

GI symptoms are not prevalent in this type of poisoning.

Thus preventing toxin absorption and enhancing excretion constitute the cornerstone of therapy. The patient must be protected from self-destructive behavior that may occur during hallucinations. Diazepam may help to control seizures (0.1 mg/kg in children, up to 10 mg in adults). If life-threatening anticholinergic symptoms occur, physostigmine may be considered. If the patient manifests cholinergic symptoms, one should consider atropine, 0.01 mg/kg intravenously in children and 1 mg intravenously in adults as a test dose, which may be repeated as needed to control symptoms.

Psilocybin (Group VI)

The majority of the hallucinogenic mushrooms belong to the *Psilocybe* and *Panaeolus* species. The most common mushrooms responsible for intoxications are *Psilocybe cubensis* and *Panaeolus papillionaceus*. These mushrooms have been part of religious rites of the inhabitants of Mexico and Central America for generations. In the 1970s they became part of the North American pop culture and were popularized as "majic mushrooms." Most people who hunt these mushrooms do so for the hallucinogenic effect. *Psilocybe* are inconspicuous small brown mushrooms. Mushroom hunters rely on *Psilocybe* being found near dung in pastures and the stems staining blue with handling. Many poisonings go unreported because possession and use of *Psilocybe* is illegal.

The toxins implicated with the mushroom's hallucinogenic properties are the indole alkaloids psilocybin and psylocin. Psilocybin is chemically related to serotonin, the neurotransmitter, and is rapidly hydrolyzed to psylocin. The hallucinogenic activity of the toxin is unaltered by drying, cooking, or boiling. An oral dose of 4 mg of psilocybin in an adult causes relaxation, dysphoria, and intellectual detachment. At higher doses profound hallucinations and perceptual distortions occur. The effects are similar to those of LSD or mescaline. Psilocybe toxins are chemically related to LSD, have similar CNS effects, and produce cross-tolerance. The rate of decline in brain concentration of psilocybin correlates well with the length of hallucinogenic effect.

Symptoms begin within 30 minutes of ingestion. The patient becomes giddy, dizzy, nauseated, and restless. For the next 2 to 4 hours, visual hallucinations and perceptual distortions predominate. The potency of intoxication depends on how the mushrooms were prepared. The most pronounced effects occur when eaten raw on an empty stomach.

The duration of action is so short that specific medical therapy is rarely required. The fatality rate is low, less than 1%. Nevertheless, there are a few case reports of deaths in children, but the syndrome described was more characteristic of muscarine poisoning, and it has been disputed whether these were true psilocybin poisonings.

GI tract detoxification is important since vomiting and diarrhea are uncommon. The patient should be protected from self-destructive behavior. Diazepam may help control seizures. Hyperpyrexia may occur in children and should be treated with sponge baths, avoiding salicylates. Chlorpromazine, 50 to 100 mg intramuscularly in adults and 1.0 mg/kg intramuscularly in children, will control hallucinations.

Gastrointestinal Irritants (Group VII)

These mushrooms are a large heterogeneous group whose toxins have yet to be identified. They induce GI distress regardless of how they are prepared. The most common mushrooms involved in this poisoning are *Boletus luridus*, *Chlorophyllum molybdites*, and *Entoloma lividum*. These poisonings are characterized by what they do not involve: no liver damage, no central or peripheral nervous system stimulation, and no hallucinations. It is postulated that the toxins act as local irritants on the intestinal mucosa. *C. molybdites* is most often involved in severe gastroenteritis, requiring admission.

Nausea, vomiting, abdominal cramps, and severe diarrhea begin within 30 to 120 minutes after ingestion. In most cases symptoms are self-limiting and resolve within 3 to 4 hours. Persistent vomiting and diarrhea in children may lead to severe dehydration, requiring intravenous hydration. The biggest problem is in underestimating fluid losses.

Specific identification of the mushroom is not required, and may not be feasible, provided that the clinical picture is that of a GI irritant and not that of a more lethal mushroom. General supportive measures and close attention to hydration constitute the cornerstone of therapy. Electrolytes and fluid balance should be monitored closely. Antiemetics, antispasmodics, and antidiarrheals should be avoided since they slow elimination of the toxin from the GI tract.

PLANT POISONINGS
Introduction

Plant ingestions constitute 10% of calls to poison control centers. Houseplants are the most common toxic plant exposures, constituting approximately 9% of calls reported to the American Association of Poison Control Centers (AAPCC) in 1984 (Table 99–4). Most of these ingestions are nontoxic or cause self-limited gastric irritation. Children less than 1 year of age usually confine their ingestions to houseplants.

There are certain key questions in any toxic exposure that need to be asked: When was the plant ingested? What was consumed and how much? How long after ingestion did the symptoms begin, and what were the initial complaints? How was the plant prepared? Did anyone else eat the plant, and are they sick?

TABLE 99–4

TWENTY MOST FREQUENTLY REPORTED HUMAN PLANT EXPOSURES

Scientific Name	Common Name	Number of Exposures
Philodendron spp.	Philodendron	5657
Dieffenbachia spp.	Dumb cane	2776
Euphorbia pulcherrima	Poinsettia	2048
*Crassula argentea**	Jade plant	2015
*Brassaia actinophylla**	Schefflera	1756
Ilex spp.	Holly	1657
Pyracantha spp.	Firethorn	1071
Phytolacca americana or *rigida*	Pokeweed	949
Rhododendron spp.	Rhododendron, azalea	803
Scindapsus aureus or *pictus**	Pothos	785
*Anthericum** and *Chlorophytum*	Spider plant	784
Capsicum annuum conoides	"Fiesta" pepper	780
Sorbus spp.	Mountain ash	685
Lonicera spp.	Honeysuckle	656
Solanum dulcamara	Climbing nightshade	623
Aloe spp.	Medicine aloe	622
Toxicodendron radicans	Poison ivy	600
*Ficus elastica**	Rubber plant	578
*Ficus benjamina**	Weeping fig tree	533
Taxus spp.	Yew	

Adapted from Litovitz TL, Veltri JC. 1984 Annual report of the American Association of Poison Control Centers National Data Collection System. Am J Emerg Med 1985;3:429.
*Practically nontoxic.

Most plant poisonings begin with GI complaints. Specific syndromes or clustering of symptoms, such as anticholinergic or cholinergic toxicity, should be treated with the appropriate antidote. There are no specific antidotes available for most plant poisonings. Symptomatic treatment is required. Attention to airway is important, particularly with certain toxins, such as *Dieffenbachia*, that cause oropharyngeal swelling. Activated charcoal absorbs toxins well, and if diarrhea is not prominent, cathartics are given. Aggressive fluid management with attention to urine output and hydration status is important. Dialysis is ineffective in removing the toxins and becomes necessary only if renal failure ensues.

Emesis or gastric aspirate should be sent for toxin analysis. A complete blood count, electrolytes, and urinalysis will aid in assessing hydration. In certain poisonings hypoglycemia may be present. Blood urea nitrogen (BUN) and creatinine should be monitored for renal involvement. If the plant is hepatotoxic, liver functions are measured.

PLANT TOXINS
Alkaloids

Alkaloid toxins are nitrogen-containing organic compounds that act as bases and form salts with acids. There are eight types of alkaloids present in poisonous plants: pyridine, tropane, isoquinoline, indole, pyrrolizidine, quinolizidine, steroid, and amine.

Pyridine-Piperidine Alkaloids

Nicotine is representative of the alkaloid toxins in this group. It is a ganglionic stimulant that produces initial excitation followed by depression of transmission. Nicotine affects central and peripheral autonomic receptors. Respiratory arrest occurs from a combination of CNS depression and peripheral neuromuscular paralysis of the respiratory muscles.

A common source of nicotine-like poisoning is the poison hemlock *(Conium maculatum)*. This plant grows as a weed along roadsides throughout the United States. Poisonings occur when the plant is mistaken for wild carrot or parsley. Coniine is the toxic piperidine alkaloid, which is structurally related to nicotine. It also causes initial autonomic receptor stimulation followed by profound depression.

Initial excitatory symptoms begin with abdominal pain, nausea, and vomiting, followed by confusion, dizziness, and ataxia. Parasympathetic stimulation causes bradycardia, bowel hyperperistalsis, salivation, diarrhea, tachypnea, and myosis. The latter stages of poisoning are heralded by tachycardia, arrhythmias, hypotension, mydriasis, and respiratory depression leading to respiratory arrest.

Death results from respiratory failure. Intubation and mechanically assisted ventilation may be necessary. Supportive measures and gastric decontamination are important. Treating bradycardia with atropine may compound the subsequent tachycardia produced by the toxin. Dialysis is ineffective in removing the toxin.

Tropane Alkaloids

Tropane alkaloids are also called the belladonna alkaloids and include atropine, scopolamine, and hyoscyamine. These toxins produce an anticholinergic poisoning characterized by the phrase "mad as a hatter, hot as a hare, dry as a bone, red as a beet, blind as a bat."

The most common plant sources include *Datura stramonium* (jimson weed), *Hyoscyamus niger* (henbane), *Mandragora officinarum* (mandrake), and *Atropa belladonna* (deadly night-shade). Jimson weed poisoning is characteristic of toxicity seen with tropane alkaloids. The plant is a weed commonly found in the rich soil of fields and barn yards. The most frequent poisoning victim is a teenager who ingests the seeds for hallucinogenic effects. Intoxication occurs by ingesting the seeds, drinking a brewed tea, or smoking the plant. Toxins are rapidly absorbed from the GI tract or mucous membranes, detoxified in the liver, and excreted in the urine. Symptoms begin 2 to 6 hours after ingestion. The classic presentation begins with dry mouth and mydriasis, followed by fever, flushing, blurred vision, dry skin, tachycardia, confusion, delirium, and hallucinations. There is also decreased GI motility, which aids toxin absorption. Symptoms usually resolve in 24 hours.

If patients are seen early after ingestion, within 4 to 6 hours, they should receive gastric decontamination to prevent further absorption of the toxin. However, the toxin is so rapidly absorbed that these measures may not prevent toxicity.

Physostigmine is a specific antidote for anticholinergic poisoning. The initial dose is 0.01 to 0.03 mg/kg slow intravenous push; improvement should be evident within 15 minutes. The dose may be repeated every 20 to 30 minutes until there is clinical improvement or signs of cholinergic excess. Physostigmine has been associated with significant morbidity, such as hypotension, asystole, bronchospasm, and seizures. Some clinicians recommend supportive therapy alone. Medications containing anticholinergic effects should not be used. Hypertension usually resolves spontaneously. Hyperthermia should be treated with cooling blankets. Patients with mild symptoms may be discharged after 4 to 6 hours of observation if symptoms improve. Patients who require physostigmine or exhibit CNS symptoms should be admitted.

Indole Alkaloids

Indole alkaloids include such disparate toxins as ergotamine, strychnine, gelsemine (a neuromuscular blocking toxin), and potent psychoactive plants. Commercial grains, prior to mandatory inspection codes, harbored the fungus *Claviceps purpurea*. This fungus was a source of ergotamine and often infected rye and other grains. Accidental ingestion of the grain caused a burning in the extremities called St. Anthony's fire. Strychnine can be found in seeds from the *Strychnos nux vomica* tree; however, strychnine poisoning by seed ingestion is rare.

Gelsemium sempervirens, or yellow jessamine, contains gelsemine and sempervine indole alkaloid toxins. These toxins are potent neuromuscular blockers that bind to acetylcholine receptors. Within 15 to 30 minutes of ingestion, headache, dizziness, ptosis, dry mouth, and blurry vision begin. With more severe ingestions, muscle spasms, respiratory paralysis, and death ensue. Honey is sometimes made from jessamine blossoms, or children eat blossoms for the nectar with subsequent poisoning. Treatment is supportive and GI decontamination is essential.

Pyrrolizidine Alkaloids

Pyrrolizidine alkaloids are present in several plant species, most commonly *Senecio longilobus* (groundsel), *Amsinckia* (fiddle neck tarweed), and *Crotolaria* (rattlebox). The principal toxins responsible for poisonings are heliotrine, lasiocarpine, and retrorsine; they may be accidentally consumed in herbal teas or medicines. An infant fed *S. longilobus* tea developed severe hepatic necrosis presenting as a Reye's-like syndrome. *Crotolaria* seeds may contaminate bread or cereal and produce hepatic failure. Small young leaves have the greatest concentration of pyrrolizidine alkaloid toxin.

Pyrrolizidine toxins target the liver, causing hemorrhagic necrosis with hepatic venule occlusion. Patients present with symptoms of acute hepatic failure. Initially patients develop vomiting, jaundice, ascites, and hepatomegaly, which may progress to hepatic encephalopathy. Treatment is supportive, with close attention to impending liver failure. Profound hypoglycemia and massive elevation of liver transaminase levels are common. Patients who are obtunded should receive intravenous glucose after blood samples are drawn.

Steroid Alkaloids

The toxic components of steroid alkaloids are glycoalkaloids, which hydrolyze into a sugar and an alkamine. There are three important toxic alkamines, named for the plant families in which they are found. Solanine is the major toxin responsible for symptoms in the *Solanum* species. Plants common to this species include the potato, tomato, *Solanum nigrum* (black nightshade), and *S. pseudocapsicum* (Jerusalem cherry). Solanine is concentrated in the sprouts and stems of the plant. Ripe fruit contains the least amount of toxin. Aconitine is the potent alkamine toxin found in plants of the *Aconitum* species, such as the monkshood plant. All parts of the plant contain the toxin, but the concentration varies with the season. *Veratrum viride* (American hellebore) and *Zigadenus* species (death camas). These toxins causes local irritation to mucous membranes and the stomach lining. Once hydrolyzed, the alkamine targets the other organ systems, with preference to heart and brain. *Veratrum* toxins produce cardiac parasympathetic stimulation, which results in hypotension and bradycardia. Massive overdoses cause a digitalis-like cardiotoxicity.

GI and neurologic symptoms predominate. Burning of the mouth and throat are followed by nausea, vomiting, abdominal pain, and diarrhea. Bradycardia and hypotension are secondary to the alkamine effects (parasympathetic) on cardiac nerves. The bradycardia is responsive to atropine. Death camas and monkshood are highly cardiotoxic and may cause rapid death from arrhythmias. The cardiac arrhythmias resemble digitalis toxicity.

GI decontamination is recommended for those patients seen early (within 4 hours). General supportive care and attention to hydration status are the cornerstone of therapy. Seizures usually respond to diazepam. Bradycardia responds to atropine. Hypotension may require fluids and vasopressors. Procainamide and phenytoin may suppress ventricular arrhythmias.

Amine Alkaloids

The most notable amine alkaloid is colchicine, found in the autumn crocus (*Colchicum autumnale*), an ornamental garden plant, and the glory lily (*Gloriosa superba*). Accidental poisoning is rare but deadly. The most serious poisonings occur with ingestion of colchicine tablets. Toxic effects occur with plant ingestions, but large quantities of plant material must be consumed to achieve the severity of poisoning seen with tablet ingestion. Occasionaly the roots (tubers) of the glory lily are mistaken for sweet potatoes and eaten. Colchicine is a cellular poison, binding to tubulin and preventing the formation of tubules. This disrupts spindle formation, arresting cellular division. Thus cells with a high metabolic rate (bone marrow, intestinal epithelium) are primarily affected.

Symptoms occur after a 2- to 3-hour latent period and are primarily gastrointestinal: abdominal pain, nausea, vomiting, and diarrhea. Severe dehydration and hypovolemic shock may result from fluid loss and sequestration. Later, multisystem failure may begin. Hypoxia may result from interstitial edema and acute respiratory distress from respiratory muscle weakness and ascending paralysis. Rhabdomyolysis and myoglobinuria occur as a result of toxic effects on skeletal muscle. Renal dysfunction may be due to myoglobinuria, hypotension, and hypoxia and is temporary. Colchicine exerts its effects on rapidly dividing cells and can cause bone marrow suppression.

Initial aggressive fluid management may be lifesaving. Pulmonary function testing may predict early respiratory fatigue. Acute respiratory distress syndrome often presents within the first 24 to 36 hours. A consumptive coagulopathy may also occur a few days postingestion. An EKG may show signs of myocardial damage with elevation of cardiac enzymes. Cardiogenic shock portends a poor prognosis. GI decontamination should be done and may still remove toxins even 24 hours postingestion because of enterohepatic circulation.

Glycosides

Glycosides are another toxin found in poisonous plants. Hydrolysis of the glycoside produces a sugar and a toxic aglycone compound. There are four types of glycosides: cardiac, cyanogenic, saponin, and coumarin.

Cardiac Glycosides

The most notable plants containing cardiac glycosides include *Digitalis purpurea* (foxglove), *D. lantana*, *Nerium oleander* (oleander), *Thevetia periviana* (yellow oleander), and *Convellaria majalis* (lily of the valley). Many of these plants grow wild along highways or are used in gardens as ornamentals. Lily of the valley has caused the most poisonings, but cardiotoxicity is not a prominent manifestation. The most toxic of these plants is the oleander, which contains at least five potent cardiac glycosides. The cardiac glycosides produce a digitoxin-like toxicity and inhibit the sodium-potassium-ATPase cellular transport mechanism. (See Chapter 95.) Hyperkalemia is a prominent feature of oleander poisoning. Digoxin assays are helpful in establishing the diagnosis in patients not on digitalis medication. Clinical toxicity does not correlate with peak plasma levels because myocardial receptor concentration of digitalis varies widely with identical serum levels. Digitalis antibodies have been used successfully to treat plant cardiac glycoside poisoning.

Cyanogenic Glycosides

Amygdalin is the toxic moiety in this group of poisonous plants, which include cherry, peach, plum, and apricot pits as well as apple seeds. Mastication releases the amygdalin from the seed pit, which is hydrolyzed to hydrocyanic acid. The reaction liberating cyanide proceeds faster in an alkaline medium. Therefore the delay in onset of symptoms may be explained by the transit time from stomach (acid medium) to duodenum (more alkaline).

Cyanide poisons the cellular cytochrome oxidase system of the mitochondria, producing depressed cellular respiration. The body is capable of detoxifying the cytochrome oxidase system. Endogenous thiosulfate provides a substrate for cyanide, releasing cytochrome oxidase. The thiocyanide compound is nontoxic and is eliminated in the urine. However, this system may be rapidly overwhelmed owing to a limited supply of endogenous thiosulfate.

Symptoms of cyanide poisoning occur rapidly, within minutes of ingestion. There may be the characteristic odor of bitter almonds on the breath. Patients present agitated, diaphoretic, dyspneic, and with cyanosis and vomiting. This is followed rapidly by stupor, disorientation, convulsions, and coma. Death usually occurs within an hour of ingestion. Mortality may be as high as 95%.

Treatment of mild to moderate ingestions may require only GI decontamination, supportive care, and observation. Any progression of symptoms, CNS manifestations (mental status changes, seizures), or refractory hypotension may require immediate administration of the antidote for cyanide poisoning. The antidote works on the principle that cyanide has a higher affinity for methemoglobin than for cytochrome oxidase. Administration of sodium nitrite produces methemoglobin, which combines with cyanide to produce cyanomethemoglobin. The dose of sodium nitrite for children with a hemoglobin of 12 g/dL is 10 mg/kg (0.3 ml/kg of a 3% solution) immediately, followed by 5 mg/kg in 30 minutes if necessary. The dose must be adjusted based on the hemoglobin to prevent fatal methemoglobinemia. Methemoglobin levels must be monitored and maintained below 30%. Supplemental oxygen should be administered to offset the cellular hypoxia and iatrogenic methemoglobinemia. Should methemoglobin levels exceed 30%, a solution of 1% methylene blue should be infused slowly at 0.2 ml/kg.

Saponin Glycosides

Saponin glycosides are commonly found in pokeweed (*Phytolacca americana*), English ivy (*Hedera helix*), and ginseng (*Panex ginseng*). Pokeweed poisoning is most commonly seen in the eastern United States, where it grows abundantly in open fields and along roadways. The leaves are often boiled and used in "poke-salit," though this does not guarantee complete elimination of the toxin. Children often eat the purple berries; green berries are more toxic than mature purple ones. Phytolaccine is the toxin responsible for symptoms, causing GI irritation. The root is the most toxic part of the plant and is mistakenly eaten like horseradish or potato.

GI symptoms predominate, with severe abdominal cramps, persistent emesis, and diarrhea. Symptoms are self-limited and resolve within 48 hours.

There is no antidote. GI decontamination procedures and supportive therapy are important. Attention to hydration status and fluid administration will prevent hypotension.

Oxalates

There are two types of oxalate toxins: soluble (sodium and potassium salts) and insoluble (calcium salts). The insoluble calcium oxalate crystals are found in leaves of the *Dieffenbachia* (dumb cane) and *Calladium* plants and are called raphides. These needle-shaped raphides are contained within ideoblasts, which are specialized cells that extrude the crystals in response to biting or chewing the leaves. This produces salivation, burning, and swelling of the lips and tongue. As the swelling progresses, difficulty handling secretions and upper airway obstruction may occur.

Leaves of the rhubarb plant contain the soluble oxalates. Absorption from the GI tract is rapid and produces a profound hypocalcemia. The hypocalcemia manifests as weakness, tetany, hypotension, and may progress to seizures. Calcium oxalate crystals may form renal calculi or obstruct the renal tubules, causing renal failure.

Treatment of *Dieffenbachia* ingestion requires symptomatic care with topical anesthetics, cold packs, and demulcents. Severe cases may require narcotic analgesics. Any signs of respiratory obstruction or edema warrant admission for observation. The airway edema may present up to 6 hours

postingestion, and discharged patients must be cautioned about symptoms.

Patients with rhubarb poisoning who are seen within 4 to 6 hours of ingestion should have gastric decontamination performed. However, symptoms may be delayed up to 24 hours. Aggressive fluid administration will enhance renal excretion of calcium oxalate crystals. Oxalate-induced hypocalcemia may be refractory to therapy, but intravenous calcium gluconate is indicated for tetany, prolonged QT interval, or decreased serum calcium levels. A 10% solution of calcium gluconate is administered intravenously (10 ml in adults, 0.3 to 0.6 ml/kg in children) over 10 to 15 minutes and titrated until asymptomatic. Serum calcium levels are followed closely. Aggressive diuresis may prevent deposition of calcium oxalate crystals. Viscous xylocaine or diphenhydramine elixir may help oral mucosal irritation and burning.

Resins

The water hemlock (*Cicuta maculata*) and chinaberry (*Melia azedarach*) are the two most toxic of the resin-containing plants. Most poisonings occur when these plants are mistaken for edible wild carrots. Though all parts are toxic, the root has the highest concentration of toxins. Cicutoxin is the poison responsible for symptomatology. It is a CNS stimulant of cholinergic receptors in the basal ganglia and brain stem. Coniine, the toxin found in poison hemlock, produces CNS depression.

Symptoms begin within 15 to 90 minutes of ingestion. Nausea, vomiting, and abdominal pain may be suddenly followed by seizures and coma. Victims may also complain of salivation, dizziness, flushing, and diaphoresis. The overall mortality rate approaches 30%.

Because of the rapid onset of seizures, gastric lavage is recommended. Meticulous attention to airway management and immediate intravenous access are also necessary. Rhabdomyolysis with subsequent renal failure has been reported, requiring dialysis.

There is no antidote; supportive care is paramount for patient survival. Ventilatory support may be necessary. One should follow acid-base parameters and electrolytes and maintain adequate hydration. If creatine kinase levels are high, forced diuresis may be indicated. Diazepam should be used to control seizures initially. Phenytoin may be added if seizures persist.

Phytotoxins

Abrin and ricin are phytotoxins, the most lethal plant toxins known. They are found primarily in the jequirty bean (*Abrus precatorius*) and castor bean (*Ricinus communis*). The jequirty bean is an ornamental vine that flourishes in southern Florida. Its seeds contain abrin and are often strung into necklaces or rosaries. The castor bean is the commercial source of castor oil. Ricin is found in the fibrous seed residue after removal of the castor oil. Poisonings occur when the seeds or beans are chewed, thus releasing the toxins. The mature bean, if swallowed whole, is nontoxic because of the protective coating.

Both abrin and ricin are potent inhibitors of protein synthesis and are structurally related compounds. Initial symptoms are the result of local irritation and begin with burning of the mouth and throat and abdominal pain. A few hours later, nausea, vomiting, and bloody diarrhea ensue. Dehydration is a serious consequence, sometimes with massive fluid loss. After a few days the toxins produce systemic symptoms, primarily involving the heart, liver, kidneys, and CNS. Arrhythmias, hypotension, hepatic necrosis, and liver failure followed by renal failure may occur.

Changes in mentation, from confusion to seizures and coma, ensue.

There is no antidote, and treatment is supportive. Careful monitoring of fluid balance is important in patient management. Laboratory evaluation should include a complete blood count, electrolytes, renal function, glucose, and liver enzymes. Seeds should be removed from the stomach to prevent further absorption of toxin. Charcoal will help eliminate the toxin from the intestines. Cathartics may be unnecessary with the massive diarrhea that occurs.

Children are most often the victims of these poisons. Predicting the severity of poisoning is difficult. However, it is safe to discharge asymptomatic patients after a 4- to 6-hour period of observation, provided that there is reliable daily follow-up for 2 to 3 days. If any symptoms occur, the patient must return immediately. Symptomatic patients must be hospitalized.

Ornamental Plants

Mistletoe

Mistletoe (*Phoradindron flavescens*) is a semiparasitic plant that grows primarily on oak trees. The whole berries and leaves are used as Christmas ornaments. The berries, a common source of poisoning, contain phoratoxin, which is a gastrointestinal irritant and cardiotoxin. The mistletoe toxin acts as an acetylcholine agonist, causing vasoconstriction and bradycardia and producing depolarization by displacing calcium and altering cell membrane permeability.

There is no specific antidote. Routine GI decontamination should be followed. Patients should be monitored for arrhythmias for several hours and if asymptomatic may be discharged. Patients with electrolyte imbalances or cardiac arrhythmias should be hospitalized overnight. Patients at risk for arrhythmias include those with cardiac disease and those taking monoamine oxidase inhibitors.

Poinsettia

The toxic reputation of the poinsettia (*Euphorbia pulcherrima*) was founded on a single case report in Hawaii in 1919 from ingestion of a wild plant. There have been reports of ingestions and mild reactions but no other fatalities. Of 332 ingestions (usually leaves), only 7 cases had symptoms, consisting of local irritation and vomiting. Dermal contact with leaves can produce a contact dermatitis that may progress to painful vesicles. Chewing the leaves results in mucosal burns. Ingestion produces a self-limited vomiting. Treatment is symptomatic. GI decontamination should be done when spontaneous vomiting has not occurred. Though fluid loss is usually minor, initial evaluation of hydration status is important. Intravenous hydration may be required.

Selected References

Bain RJI. Accidental digitalis poisoning due to drinking herbal tea. Br Med J 1985;290:1624.

Boehnort M, McGuigan MA. Colchicine. Clin Toxicol Rev 1983;5:1.

Carlton BE, Tufts E, Girard DE. Water hemlock poisoning complicated by rhabdomyolysis and renal failure. Clin Toxicol 1979;14:87.

Dickstein ES, Kunkel FW. Foxglove tea poisoning Am J Med 1980;69:167.

Edwards N. Local toxicity from poinsettia plant: A case report. J Pediatr 1983;102:404.

Fiddes FS. Poisoning by aconitine: Report of two cases. Br Med J 1958;2:779.

Floersheim GL, Eberhard M, Tschumi P, et al. Effects of penicillin and silymarin on liver enzymes and clotting factors in dogs given boiled preparation of *Amanita phalloides*. Toxicol Appl Pharmacol 1978;46:455.

Floersheim GL, Weber O, Tschumi P, et al. Die Klinishe Knollenblatterpilzvergiftung (*Amanita phalloides*) prognostische Faktoren und therapeutische Massnahmen. Schweiz Med Wochenschr 1982;112:1164.

Fogh A, Kulling P, Wickstrom E. Veratrum alkaloids in sneezing powder. A potential danger. J Toxicol Clin Toxicol 1983;20:175.

Giusti G, Carnevali A. A case of fatal poisoning by *Gyromitra esculenta*. Arch Toxicol 1974;33:49.

Hall AH, Spoerke DG, Rumack BH. Mushroom poisoning: Identification, diagnosis, and treatment. Pediatr Rev 1987;8:291.

Heaney D, Derghazarain CB, Pines GF, et al. Massive colchicine overdose: A report on the toxicity. Am J Med Sci 1976;271:233.

Hruby K, Csomos G, Fuhrmann M, et al. Chemotherapy of *Amanita phalloides* poisoning with intravenous silibinin. Hum Toxicol 1983;2:183.

Ingle VN, Kale VG, Talwalker YB. Accidental poisoning in children with particular reference to castor beans. Indian J Pediatr 1966;33:237.

Iwatsuki S, Esquivel CO, Gordon RD, et al. Liver transplantation for fulminant hepatic failure. Semin Liver Dis 1985;5:325.

Kinamore PA, Jaeger RW, deCastro FJ. Abrus and ricinus ingestion: Management on three cases. Clin Toxicol 1980;17:401.

Klein AS, Hart J, Brems JJ, et al. Amanita poisoning: Treatment and the role of liver transplantation. Am J Med 1989;86:187.

Kröncke KD, Fricker G, Meier PJ, et al. Alpha-Amanitin uptake into hepatocytes. J Biol Chem 1986;261:12562.

Lampe KF. Mushroom poisoning in children updated. Paediatrician 1977;6:289.

Lampke K, McCann MA. Differential diagnosis of poisoning by North American mushrooms, with particular emphasis on *Amanita phalloides*-like intoxication. Ann Emerg Med 1987;16:956.

Levy R. Jimson weed poisoning—new hallucinogen on the horizon. JACEP 1977;6:58.

McMillan M, Thompson JC. An outbreak of suspected solanine poisoning in school boys: An examination of criteria of solanine poisoning. Q J Med 1979;190:227.

Merchant HC, Choksi ND, Ramamourthy K, et al. Aconite poisoning and cardiac arrhythmias. Indian J Med Sci 1963;17:857.

Mikolich JR, Paulson GW, Cross CJ. Acute anticholinergic syndrome due to Jimson seed ingestion. Ann Intern Med 1975;83:321.

Naidus RM, Rodiuen R, Mielke H. Colchicine toxicity: A multisystem disease. Arch Intern Med 1977;137:394.

Nelson DA. Accidental poisoning by *Veratrum japonicum*. JAMA 1954;156:33.

Olsnes S, Refsnes K, Pihl A. Mechanism of action of the toxic lectins abrin and ricin. Nature 1974;249:627.

Raubner A. Observations on the idioblasts of Dieffenbachia. Clin Toxicol 1985;23:79.

Rumack BH. Anticholinergic poisoning: Treatment with physostigmine. Pediatrics 1973;52:449.

Schumacher T, Hoiland K. Mushroom poisoning caused by species of the genus *Cortinarius fries*. Arch Toxicol 1983;53:87.

Short AIK, Watling R, MacDonald MK. Poisoning by *Cortinarius speciosissimus*. Lancet 1980;2:942.

Shumack GM, Wu AW, Ping AC. Oleander poisoning: Treatment with digoxin-specific Fab antibody fragments. Ann Emerg Med 1988;17:732.

Stapczynski JS, Rothstein RJ, Gaye WA. Colchicine overdose: Report of two cases and review of the literature. Ann Emerg Med 1981;10:364.

Starreveld E, Hope CE. Cicutoxin poisoning (water hemlock). Neurology 1975;25:730.

Tallqvist H, Vaananen I. Death of a child from oxalic acid poisoning due to eating rhubarb leaves. Ann Paediatr Fenn 1960;6:144.

Weden GP, Neal JS, Everson EP. Castor bean poisoning. Am J Emerg Med 1986;4:259.

Winek CL, Butala J, Shanon SP, et al. Toxicology of poinsettia. Clin Toxicol 1978;13:27.

SECTION THIRTEEN

Environmental Emergencies

CHAPTER 100

Mammal Bites

Richard C. Hunt

INTRODUCTION

The true incidence of mammal bites is unknown because many bitten patients never seek medical attention. In the United States estimates of mammal bites each year range from 500,000 to 2 million, and approximately 1% of emergency department visits are due to bite wounds.[1-4] A dog inflicts the wound in 80% to 90% of bites, a cat in 10%, a human in 3%, and a rodent in 2%.[2, 5] Children are at greatest risk for mammalian bites, with 40% of all bites occurring between the ages of 5 and 14 years.[1, 6]

Soft tissues, tendons, joint spaces, and bones may all be damaged from bite wounds.[1] Local and systemic infections, deformity, and amputation are all possible sequelae of bites.[4, 7, 8] Infections of bite wounds to the hand are particularly common complications and potentially cause long-term morbidity. While cosmetic deformity may occur from bite wounds on any part of the body, facial bites are notorious for causing disfiguring wounds.[9] Bites in children may be the first sign of child abuse.[10, 11]

A review of dog bites from 1979 through 1988 identified 157 dog bite–related fatalities during that period. Of the 157 deaths, 70% occurred among children who were less than 10 years of age. Pit bulls were involved in 42 (42%) of 101 deaths where a dog breed was reported, almost three times more than German shepherds, the next most commonly reported breed.[12]

ANATOMY AND PHYSIOLOGY

Human Bite Location and Mechanism of Injury

Human bites are most commonly located on the scalp and dorsum of the hand, with scalp bites being particularly common in children. Human bites on the hand often result from contact of a closed fist of one person with the open mouth of another. Other common locations of human bites include the penis, scrotum, vulva, breasts, ear, nose, and forearm.[8]

In a review of human bites to the face, the most commonly involved areas included, in decreasing order of frequency, the lower lip, ear, cheek, nose, and upper lip.[9] In a study of 322 human bites in children, the upper extremities (42%), face and neck (33%), and trunk (22%) were most commonly bitten.[7]

Five types of activities are engaged in while being bitten: fights (62%), play (26%), sexual activity (7%), sports events (5%), and abuse (1%). During play, 22% resulted from the patient inadvertently "running into another child's teeth." Most of the wounds encountered (73%) were abrasions, 13% were punctures, and 11.8% were lacerations.[7]

In human hand bites, the victim's fist striking the opponent's mouth causes an impact injury, an irregular laceration over the dorsal surface of the metacarpophalangeal joint. The impact injury has an increased propensity for infection compared with a shearing force injury. With a clenched fist, the teeth have easy entry into joint spaces, which are 10 times more prone to infection.[4]

Bite Location and Mechanism of Injury

Bite wounds from animals most commonly involve shear forces and have better outcomes than those involving impact forces. When an animal's teeth tear the human skin, the resulting linear lacerations are resistant to infection. Additionally, animal bites are usually superficial, not extending into the deep structures.[4]

Dog and cat bite wounds include tears, avulsions, punctures, and scratches. Crush injury with swelling, ecchymosis, and devitalized tissue may be present. A dog's teeth can exert a pressure of 200 to 450 lb/inch^2. Attack dogs can exert more than 450 lb/inch^2 with their jaws, enough to penetrate light sheet metal. In children, dogs strike the head in 60% to 70% of victims less than 5 years of age and in 50% of victims less than 10 years of age.[2, 3, 8]

Feline bites are frequently puncture wounds that are notoriously difficult to irrigate or cleanse, usually located on the upper extremities. Cat scratches are most frequently located on the upper extremities or in the periorbital region.[2, 3]

Bacteriology

The bacteriology of human and animal bites is complicated. The mammalian mouth supports the growth of 200 species of facultative organisms and obligate anaerobes. The largest numbers of organisms are in the gingival crevices and in plaque on teeth and are composed of bacteria in the range of 10^{11}/gm of tissue. This is 100,000 times greater than that required to produce infection in soft tissue.[4] Cultures of fresh wounds before clinical infection reflect the variety of anaerobic and aerobic organisms but are not predictive of the causative organism in later infections. Estimates of the percentage of patients who develop infection from bite wounds vary from 2% to 30%.[3]

In a study of open dog-bite wounds, on initial presentation 48% evidenced no bacterial growth. *Staphylococcus epidermidis* was the most common isolate, and multiple bacteria were isolated in 15.5% of patients. In clinically infected wounds, 50% showed multiple pathogenic organisms. The predominant pathogenic bacteria isolated from clinically infected wounds were, in order from highest to lowest frequency, *Enterobacteria, Pseudomonas, Staphylococcus aureus, Bacillus subtilis,* and beta *Streptococcus.* (*Pasteurella multocida* was not recovered as a contaminant or infectious organism in this study.[13]) Another study of 35 dog bites in children found that on initial presentation 40% of the cultures yielded potential wound pathogens, most notably *S. aureus, Streptococcus pyogenes, Clostridium* species, and various gram-negative rods.[6] The presence of *P. multocida* has been noted in only 20% to 25% of dog bite wounds and in 50% of cat bite wounds.[3]

Most studies of human bites are of the hand, and this may not accurately represent human bites elsewhere. Additionally, which of the organism present actually caused the infection remains unknown. The most frequent aerobic organism is *Streptococcus,* and the next most frequent is *S. aureus.* Other organisms seen in smaller numbers in human bites are *Eikenella corrodens, Bacteroides,* anaerobic cocci, *Fusobacterium* species, and *Peptostreptococcus.* Mixed aerobic and anaerobic infections may be more virulent.[14]

The microbiology of human and animal bite wounds, specifically in children with cellulitis, erythema, and tenderness, has been studied. Aspirates from bite wounds in children were cultured for aerobic and anaerobic bacteria. Aerobic bacteria were recovered in 18% of wounds, anaerobic bacteria in only 8%, and mixed aerobic and anaerobic bacteria in 74%. The most frequent pathogens in both human and animal bite wounds were *S. aureus,* anaerobic cocci, and *Bacteroides* species. *P. multocida, Pseudomonas fluorescens,* and M-5 were present only in animal bites.[15]

EMS CONSIDERATIONS

Because of the high frequency of facial bites, airway monitoring and control are important. External bleeding is usually easily managed.

If the victim is farther than 1 hour from medical care, the wound should be gently cleansed and irrigated with a non-irritant soap and gently debrided of foreign objects.[1] All wounds should be covered with saline-soaked gauze to prevent further contamination and drying of tissues. Splinting and elevation of extremities are important in cases of possible orthopedic injuries.

Each prehospital care provider should be knowledgeable of local regulations and laws regarding management of the animal that bit the victim. The need for observation for rabies is an important consideration.

CLINICAL EVALUATION

The time from injury to evaluation frequently correlates with infection rates. One group of patients presents within 8 to 12 hours of injury and has concerns about wound management and rabies. A second group presents after 12 hours with signs and symptoms of infection.[16] The type of animal inflicting the wound, the animal's immunization status, and whether the animal is domestic or feral should be determined. The location of the injury is usually obvious. However, with multiple bites patients may be unaware of some wounds, and a careful examination is necessary. Complaints of abnormal motor and sensory function distal to the wound should be elicited. The patient's age, antimicrobial and analgesic allergies, alcohol use, and diabetic history and the presence of immunosuppression are important historical factors. Prior splenectomy may increase the chance of infection.[3] Tetanus status should be ascertained. Rabies immunization status should be determined, particularly in zoo workers and veterinarians, who may have been immunized because they are at high risk for animal bites.

Physical examination should certainly include vital signs and a routine primary examination in all patients. A more comprehensive head to toe examination is necessary if major trauma has occurred.

An extended examination should focus on the wound itself. Location, extent, and depth of the wound should be noted; this may be aided with diagrams or with a camera.[3] If infection is evident, the extent of cellulitis, adenopathy, fever, systemic signs, or abscess formation should be documented. The wound should be carefully examined for nerve, vascular, or tendon compromise. Careful examination requires good lighting, local anesthesia, and assistance to retract tissue during exploration of deep structures. Sensation and motor strength distal to the wound should be tested. Foreign bodies, which may include dirt, gravel, or teeth, should be removed.

Hand bites require meticulous examination. Most involve the dorsum of the hand over the metacarpophalangeal points and are the result of punching an antagonist in the mouth. A small puncture wound on the dorsum of the hand can pierce the fascia, penetrate a joint capsule, and damage the articular surface of the metacarpophalangeal joint. When the fist is opened, the lacerated skin retracts proximally and the injury to the deeper structures is hidden. Flexion and extension of the hand while the wound is being explored may reveal far more damage to tendon or joint structures than initially suspected.

Child abuse may be manifested by human bites. Human bites produce a crushing injury, as opposed to the typical puncture wound of the skin seen with animal bites. Bites inflicted by adults can be identified by the width of the dental arch, which is greater than 4 cm. The source of human bite marks must be identified as adult or child since the healthy toddler may have numerous bite marks from a peer.[10]

DIAGNOSTIC EVALUATION

Cultures, aerobic and anaerobic, should be obtained from any infected wound before irrigation or debridement. Cultures should sample the depth of the wound; in the case of cellulitis the culture specimen should be aspirated by needle from the leading edge of the wound. Gram stains may be helpful in grossly purulent wounds. Uninfected wounds or fresh wounds need not be cultured since most show no growth.[2–5] In cases of established localized infection, a complete blood count and sedimentation rate may assist in the evaluation of systemic involvement.

Radiologic studies should be performed when deep structures are involved and in all hand bite wounds (Fig. 100–1). Closed-fist injuries may have positive radiologic findings in as many as 70% of patients.[14] In infected wounds radiographs may identify foreign bodies or osteomyelitis.

DIFFERENTIAL DIAGNOSIS

The differential diagnosis of late manifestations of bite wounds includes zoonotic infections. Tularemia is an ulceroglandular disease, usually caused by contact with rabbits;

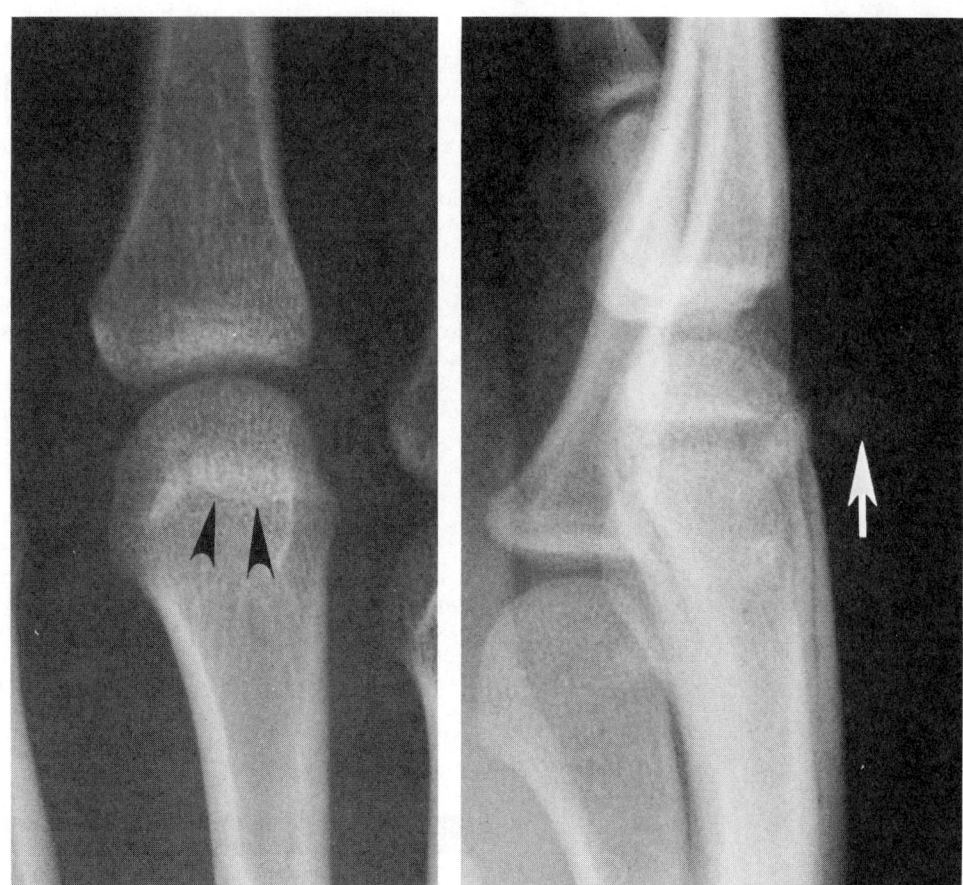

Figure 100–1. Subtle radiographic diagnosis of a human bite fracture. On the lateral, the fragment *(arrow)* dorsally displaced from the third metacarpal is obvious, but it is quite easily overlooked *(arrowheads)* on the frontal film. (Courtesy of A. Oestreich, M.D., Cincinnati, OH. Modified from Oestreich AE, Crawford AH. Atlas of Pediatric Orthopedic Radiology. Stuttgart, Thieme, 1985.

TABLE 100–1

FACTORS INFLUENCING INFECTION

High Risk
Location
  Hand, wrist, or foot
  Scalp or face in infants (high risk of cranial perforation;
    skull radiograph studies mandatory)
  Over a major joint (possibility of perforation)
Type of wound
  Punctures (impossible to irrigate)
  Tissue crushing that cannot be debrided (typical of
    herbivores such as cows, horses)
Patient
  Older than 50 yr
  Asplenic
  Chronic alcoholic
  Altered immune status
  Diabetic
  Peripheral vascular insufficiency
  Chronic corticosteroid therapy
Species
  Human (in hand wounds only)
  Primates (anecdotal evidence only)
  Pigs (anecdotal evidence only)
Low Risk
Location
  Face, scalp, ear, and mouth (all facial wounds should be
    sutured)
Wound type
  Large clean lacerations that can be thoroughly cleansed; the
    larger the laceration and the better the cleansing, the
    lower the infection rate
Species
  Rodents

From Callaham M. Animal bites. *In* Callaham M (ed). Current Therapy in Emergency Medicine. Toronto, BC Decker, 1987, p 896. Used with permission.

its first manifestation occurs approximately 2 days after inoculation. Bubonic plague outbreaks occur as a consequence of widespread infection of wild rodents by *Yersinia pestis*. It is characterized by lymphadenitis, which evolves into a characteristic bubo; the incubation period extends from 2 to 10 days. Cat-scratch fever is usually a self-limited solitary or regional lymphadenitis commonly preceded by a cat scratch or other injury to the skin. The period between scratch and appearance of primary lesion is 3 to 14 days.[17]

Another late manifestation is rat-bite fever, a systemic infection caused by either *Streptobacillus moniliformis* or *Spirillum minus*. In *S. moniliformis* the bite site is healed by the time systemic manifestations of chills, fever, and joint symptoms appear, less than 10 days after inoculation. In *S. minus*, which has an incubation time of 1 to 4 weeks, the bite site is inflamed with lymphangitis and regional lymphadenitis. Fever occurs without joint symptoms.[18]

THERAPEUTIC INTERVENTION
General Care

Fundamental principles of bite wound management are good surgical toilet with cleansing, irrigation, and debridement; consideration of sutures; consideration of antibiotic prophylaxis or treatment of established infection; and consideration of tetanus or rabies prophylaxis.

After administering local anesthesia to the bite wound, cleansing with a fine-mesh sponge with povidone-iodine solution should be gently performed to remove debris. Povidone-iodine solution has an excellent antibacterial and antiviral spectrum.[19]

Possibly the most important prophylaxis for infection is adequate high-pressure irrigation of the wound with sterile saline using maximal pressure against the barrel of a 35-ml syringe attached to a 19-gauge needle. This method is superior to soaking the wound or irrigation with low-pressure bulb-type syringes in reducing bacterial counts in contaminated wounds.[19] High volumes of irrigant are required, and recommendations range from a minimum of 200 to 1000 ml of saline.[2, 4] During irrigation the physician should wear gloves, goggles, and a mask in compliance with universal precautions.

Debridement should include all visible devitalized dermis and subcutaneous tissue. Excision of a thin margin of dermis from viable wound margins is thought to improve outcome. After debridement the wound is better exposed; therefore irrigation should be repeated.[5, 19]

Decisions about suturing bite wounds involve consideration of risk factors for infection. Those wounds with low risk of infection can be sutured. All facial wounds should be sutured because of their extensive vascular supply and potential for long-term disfigurement. Wound closure tapes are possible alternatives to sutures in selected cases.[2, 4, 8, 19]

Wounds already infected or greater than 12 hours old should not be sutured. Those wounds at high risk for infection also should not be sutured (Table 100–1). High risk factors include wounds on the hand, wrist, or foot, puncture wounds less than 5 mm, crushing wounds difficult to debride, age greater than 50 years, asplenism, chronic alcoholism, altered immune status, diabetes, steroid therapy, and cat or human bites.[20]

The wound should be dressed and immobilized in a position of function with a bulky dressing and elevated. This is particularly important in hand injuries, where bulky mitten hand dressings and a sling are appropriate.[2, 19]

Antibiotics

The use of antibiotic therapy in bite wounds is extremely controversial. Most authorities agree that wounds at high risk for infection should be treated with prophylactic antibiotics. Factors that support this approach include the following: (1) the rate of infection following a bite wound is still poorly defined; (2) many patients in the emergency department setting do not have or do not comply with

TABLE 100–2

GUIDE TO TETANUS PROPHYLAXIS IN WOUND MANAGEMENT

History of Absorbed Tetanus Toxoid (Tt)	Nontetanus-Prone Wounds		Tetanus-Prone Wounds	
	Td* (0.5 ml IM)	TIG (250 U IM)	Td* (0.5 ml IM)	TIG (250 U IM)
Unknown or less than three doses	Yes+	No	Yes+	Yes
Three or more doses	No=	No	No#	No

From Immunization Practices Advisory Committee (ACIP). Diphtheria, tetanus and pertussis. Guidelines for vaccine prophylaxis and other preventative measures—US 1985. MMWR 1985;34:405,419.

*Use DTP for children less than 7 years old (DT if pertussis vaccine is contraindicated); Td is preferred to Tt if patient 7 years or older.
+The primary immunization series should be completed.
=Yes, if more than 10 years since last dose.
#Yes, if more than 5 years since last dose. (More frequent boosters are unnecessary and many accentuate side effects.)
If three doses of *fluid* rather than absorbed toxoid are used, give a fourth dose, preferably absorbed.

TABLE 100-3

RABIES POSTEXPOSURE PROPHYLAXIS GUIDE*

	Animal Species	Condition of Animal At Time of Attack	Treatment of Exposed Person**
Domestic	Dog and cat	Healthy and available for 10 days of observation	None, unless animal develops rabies[+]
		Rabid or suspected rabid	RIG[#] and HDCV
		Unknown (escaped)	Consult public health officials. If treatment is indicated, give RIG[#] and HDCV.
Wild	Skunk, bat, fox, coyote, raccoon, bobcat, and other carnivores	Regard as rabid unless proven negative by laboratory tests[=]	RIG[#] and HDCV
Other	Livestock, rodents, and lagomorphs (rabbits and hares)	Consider individually. Local and state public health officials should be consulted on questions about the need for rabies prophylaxis. Bites of squirrels, hamsters, guinea pigs, gerbils, chipmunks, rats, mice, other rodents, rabbits, and hares almost never call for antirabies prophylaxis.	

From Immunization Practices Advisory Committee (ACIP). Rabies prevention—United States, 1984. MMWR 1984;33:393,407.

*These recommendations are only a guide. In applying them, take into account the animal species involved, circumstances of the bite or other exposure, vaccination status of the animal, and presence of rabies in the region. Local or state public health officials should be consulted if questions arise about the need for rabies prophylaxis.

**All bites and wounds should immediately be thoroughly cleansed with soap and water. If antirabies treatment is indicated, both rabies immune globulin (RIG) and human diploid cell rabies vaccine (HDCV) should be given as soon as possible, regardless of the interval from exposure. Local reactions to vaccines are common and do not contraindicate continuing treatment. Discontinue vaccine if fluorescent antibody tests of the animal are negative.

[+]During the usual holding period of 10 days, begin treatment with RIG and HDCV at first sign of rabies in a dog or cat that has bitten someone. The symptomatic animal should be killed immediately and tested.

[#]If RIG is not available, use antirabies serum, equine (ARS). Do not use more than the recommended dosage.

[=]The animal should be killed and tested as soon as possible. Holding for observation is not recommended.

adequate follow-up; and (3) the cost of routine early antibiotic therapy seems to be less than that resulting from an infection.[2, 3, 5, 19]

The recommended choice of antibiotic prophylaxis is diverse. Authors argue that amoxicillin–clavulanic acid controls almost all potential anaerobic and aerobic bacterial pathogens found in animal bite wounds and is therefore a reasonable choice for antibiotic prophylaxis.[3, 19] The usual adult dose is one 250-mg tablet, containing 250 mg of amoxicillin and 125 mg of clavulanic acid, every 8 hours. In children less than 40 kg, the usual oral dose of amoxicillin and clavulanic potassium is 20 to 40 mg/kg of amoxicillin given in divided doses every 8 hours.[21] For established infections, antibiotic therapy should be guided by culture results.[3]

Tetanus

Animal and human bites are tetanus-prone wounds. Tetanus prophylaxis should be based on guidelines from the American College of Emergency Physicians (Table 100–2).[22]

Rabies

Rabies is the most dreaded complication of animal bites and is frequently the reason patients seek medical attention. The incidence of rabies is only zero to five human cases each year in the United States; about 25,000 individuals receive prophylaxis annually. Survival is rare in patients with rabies. Recommendations for postexposure prophylaxis are based on recommendations from the Centers for Disease Control (Table 100–3).[23]

All wounds should be cleansed immediately and thoroughly with soap and water. When indicated, postexposure prophylaxis for rabies should proceed immediately. Five 1-ml doses of human diploid cell vaccine (HDCV) or absorbed rabies vaccine (RVA) should be administered intramuscularly on days 0, 3, 7, 14, and 28. The vaccine should be administered in the deltoid region for adults and children, and in the anterolateral thigh in infants. Rabies immune globulin (RIG) is also important. The recommended dose is 20 IU/kg; half the dose should be administered in the area

of the wound and half intramuscularly. Rabies vaccine and RIG should be administered in different limbs. When persons previously vaccinated with HDCV or RVA are exposed to rabies, RIG is not necessary. In this instance, two 1-ml doses of HDCV or RVA should be administered on days 0 and 3.[24]

DISPOSITION

Patients with any degree of infection beyond local wound cellulitis require admission for local wound care and intravenous antibiotics. Redness, swelling, or tenderness over large areas of the hand; lymphangitis; purulent drainage; or pain on passive range of motion are indications for admission in hand bite injuries.[1]

Specialty consultation and admission should be considered for certain patients. These include all hand bites except those that are superficial and less than 8 hours old; extensive infection at any site; damage of tendon, joint capsule, bone, or facial cartilage; severe disfigurement requiring plastic repair; tissue loss potentially requiring grafting; and potential poor compliance (Table 100–4).[19]

TABLE 100-4

ADMISSION CRITERIA

Admission
Infection beyond local cellulitis
Redness, swelling, or tenderness over large areas of the hand
Lymphangitis
Purulent drainage
Pain on passive range of motion of involved or adjacent joints

Specialty Consultation and Admission
All hand bites except superficial and <8 hr old
Extensive infection, any site
Damage of tendon, joint capsule, bone, or facial cartilage
Severe disfigurement requiring plastics repair
Tissue loss potentially requiring grafting
Potential poor compliance

TABLE 100–5

DOCUMENTATION AND DISCHARGE INSTRUCTIONS

Documentation

Diagram or photograph of wound with any associated cellulitis

Method and amount of irrigation

Exam for nerve, vascular, or tendon damage and foreign bodies

Wound closure if performed

Tetanus prophylaxis

Consideration of rabies prophylaxis

Notification of appropriate legal and health department officials

Discharge Instructions

Keep bandage clean and dry

Elevate affected extremity as much as possible

Take acetaminophen as directed on bottle for pain

Take antibiotics as directed if prescribed

Return to family or emergency physician in 48 hr for scheduled recheck, or sooner if fever, increased redness, swelling, pain, or pus occur

If sutures were placed, they should be removed by a family or emergency physician in _____ days. Please schedule an appointment.

Wounds that are not infected or only superficially infected can be followed up on an outpatient basis. Discharge instructions should include wound care, extremity elevation, pain control, antibiotic administration if indicated, and follow-up in 48 hours or sooner if signs of infection occur (Table 100–5).

References

1. Doan-Wiggins L. Animal bites and rabies. *In* Rosen P, Baker FJ, Barkin RM, et al (eds). Emergency Medicine: Concepts and Clinical Practice. 2nd ed. St. Louis, CV Mosby, 1988, pp 965–979.
2. Hodge D III, Fecklenburg FW. Bites and stings. *In* Fleischer GR, Ludwig S (eds). Textbook of Pediatric Emergency Medicine. 2nd ed. Baltimore, Williams & Wilkins, 1988, pp 627–647.
3. Goldstein EJC. Management of human and animal bite wounds. J Am Acad Dermatol 1989;21:1275.
4. Edlich RF, Spengler MD, Rodeheaver GT, et al. Emergency department management of mammalian bites. Emerg Med Clin North Am 1986;4:595.
5. Galloway RE. Mammalian bites. J Emerg Med 1988;6:325.
6. Boenning DA, Fleisher GR, Campos JM. Dog bites in children: Epidemiology, microbiology and penicillin prophylactic therapy. Am J Emerg Med 1983;1:17.
7. Baker MD, Moore SE: Human bites in children. Am J Dis Child 1987;141:1285.
8. Podgorny G. Human and mammalian bites. *In* Tintinalli JE, Krome RL, Ruiz E (eds). Emergency Medicine: A Comprehensive Study Guide. 2nd ed. New York, McGraw-Hill, 1988, pp 757–759.
9. Venter THJ. Human bites of the face: Early surgical management. S Afr Med J 1988;74:277.
10. Raimer BG, Raimer SS, Hebeler JR. Cutaneous signs of child abuse. J Am Acad Dermatol 1981;5:203.
11. Rosenberg NM, Meyers S, Shackleton N. Prediction of child abuse in an ambulatory setting. Pediatrics 1982;70:879.
12. Sacks JJ, Satten RW, Bonzo SE. Dog bite–related fatalities from 1979 through 1988. JAMA 1989;262:1489.
13. Ordog GJ. The bacteriology of dog bite wounds on initial presentation. Ann Emerg Med 1986;15:1324.
14. Callaham M. Controversies in antibiotic choices for bite wounds. Ann Emerg Med 1988;17:1321.
15. Brook I. Microbiology of human and animal bite wounds in children. Pediatr Infect Dis J 1987;6:29.
16. Rest JG, Goldstein EJC. Management of human and animal bite wounds. Emerg Med Clin North Am 1985;3:117.
17. O'Hanley P. Infections due to gram-negative bacilli. *In* Rubenstein C, Federman DD (eds). Scientific American Medicine. New York, Scientific American, 1990, Section 7, Chapter VII, pp 33–36.
18. Relman DA, Schoolnik GK, Swartz MN. Leptospirosis, relapsing fever, rat bite fever and lyme disease. *In* Rubenstein C, Federman DD (eds). Scientific American Medicine. New York, Scientific American, 1990, Section 7, Chapter VII, pp 5–6.
19. Trott A. Care of mammalian bites. Pediatr Infect Dis 1987;6:8.
20. Callaham M. Animal bites. *In* Callaham M (ed). Current Therapy in Emergency Medicine. Toronto, BC Decker, 1987, p 896.
21. McEvoy GK. AFHS Drug Information 90. Bethesda, MD, American Society of Hospital Pharmacists, 1990, pp 257–262.
22. American College of Emergency Physicians: Tetanus immunization recommendations for persons seven years of age or older. Ann Emerg Med 1986;15:1111.
23. Immunization Practices Advisory Committee (ACIP). Rabies Prevention—United States, 1984. MMWR 1984;33:393, 407.
24. Simon HB. Immunizations and chemotherapy for viral infections. *In* Rubenstein C, Federman DD (eds). Scientific American Medicine. New York, Scientific American, 1990, Section 7, Chapter XXXIII, p 12.

CHAPTER 101

Arthropod Envenomation

Leslie V. Boyer Hassen
Richard C. Dart

INTRODUCTION

Arthropods are protostome eucoelomates. The phylum Arthropoda includes crustaceans, horseshoe crabs, millipedes, and trilobites (extinct) in addition to the venomous species of interest here. Insect bites and stings that more commonly result in hypersensitivity reactions are discussed elsewhere (Chapter 32). This chapter will focus on those arthropods responsible for clinically significant envenomations, namely spiders, scorpions, and centipedes.

Venom has three essential purposes for the survival of the animal involved. The first of these, defense, is readily apparent in any bite or sting that causes immediate local pain. Examples include a scorpion sting and centipede bite, both of which usually cause enough pain to discourage the advances of even the largest human or animal attacker. The second purpose, prey immobilization, is vital to the survival of small predators, whose prospective meal might otherwise be prone to successful flight. Examples of this include the black widow spider bite and bark scorpion sting, both of which provide neurotoxins adequate for the neuromuscular impairment of victims. Third, many venoms contain enzymes analogous to mammalian pancreatic secretions, which begin the digestive process before the meal is consumed.

Although accidental and deliberate importation of exotic species occasionally result in envenomation, the vast majority of patients presenting to emergency departments have been bitten or stung by local fauna. Both the differential diagnosis (Table 101–1) and the approach to treatment of envenomation (Table 101–2) may thus be targeted specifically toward a small group of animals in most cases.

Mortality from arthropod envenomation is fortunately very low in the United States. Many mild cases can be cared for at home, and moderate reactions can often be managed without hospital admission. Severe local and systemic consequences are possible, however, and special concern must be afforded the very young.

Envenomation by arthropod species is of special interest

TABLE 101–1

SUMMARY OF CLINICAL FEATURES OF VARIOUS ARTHROPOD ENVENOMATIONS

Arthropod	Wound	Local Signs	Systemic Signs*
Widow spider	Bite	May have initial pain, mild erythema and edema. Two tiny punctae sometimes noted.	Spasm of large muscle groups, which may mimic acute abdomen; weakness; hypertension; rarely death
Brown spiders	Bite	Progression from tiny mark to target lesion to eschar to necrotic ulcer over several weeks	Rash, fever, chills, nausea, vomiting, leukocytosis, DIC, hemolysis, hemoglobinuria, renal failure, rarely death
Jumping spider	Bite	Pain, erythema, pruritus, and sometimes extensive edema	Minimal
Hobo spider, northern brown spider	Bite	May cause necrosis; similar to brown spider bite	Headache, lethargy, visual disturbances, weakness, hallucinations
Orb weaver	Bite	Pain, erythema, vesicles; usually resolving in 24 hr	Minimal
Running spider	Bite	Pruritic wheal with central petechiae	Nausea, abdominal cramps, headache, anxiety
Tarantulas	Bite; urticating hairs	Bite causes mild to moderate local pain and swelling; some species may cause numbness, lymphangitis. Urticating hairs cause dermatitis.	Minimal in most cases
Funnel-web spiders	Bite	Pain	Fasciculations, restlessness, diaphoresis, vomiting, borborygmi, pulmonary edema, rarely death
Wolf spiders	Bite	Mild to moderate inflammation; South American species may cause necrosis	Minimal
Phoneutria	Bite	Pain	Tachycardia, hypertension, diaphoresis, salivation, vertigo, nausea, vomiting, priapism, respiratory paralysis
Bark scorpion	Sting	Local pain, positive "tap test"	Neuromotor hyperactivity, roving eye movements, delirium, pulmonary edema
Other scorpions	Sting	Local pain, edema, erythema; may mimic hymenoptera sting	Generally none
Giant desert centipede	Bite	Edema, erythema, severe pain, mild local necrosis possible	Rare
Insects	Bite, sting, or simple contact	Variable, local inflammatory changes; stinger or urticating hairs may be present	Usually none; ingestion of blister beetle secretions may cause hemorrhagic gastroenteritis

*Allergic manifestations, including anaphylaxis, may occur with any bite or sting.
DIC = Disseminated intravascular coagulation.

to the pediatrician for several reasons. Children living in endemic areas are more likely than adults to spend time outdoors, poking around in woodpiles and dark corners, and thus receiving any number of different minor injuries, bites, and stings. Once injured, a young child may be unable to communicate how an injury occurred, hindering the recognition of specific envenomation. Unnecessary procedures may then contribute to morbidity, such as when meningitis is sought following a scorpion sting or appendicitis is suspected after a black widow spider bite. Furthermore, since similar envenomations deliver higher doses per kilogram to children than to adults, children are prone to more severe reactions. Complicating this is the additional factor of the infant's pattern of decompensation following respiratory depression; the net effect is a much greater risk of morbidity and mortality in the infant.

CLINICAL EVALUATION
History

Assessment of the unknown bite may prove challenging. The history should be as specific as possible regarding timing, location, and nature of the event. Symptoms of envenomation are most commonly sudden in onset, with crying and pain followed within minutes to hours by advancing local or systemic signs. Direct inquiry should be made regarding the child's play or sleep area at the time symptoms began. Questions should garner information as to any deep undergrowth in the yard; any nearby spider webs; any scorpions previously found in the home; whether anyone is home at that time who can pull back the crib blanket and look for an arthropod. If a specimen has been brought in, it should be carefully examined and, if necessary, preserved for consultative review.

Examination

Physical examination should include a full survey of the skin, with special attention to hands, feet, and, particularly among users of outhouses, the buttocks and genital region. The absence of cutaneous findings does not exclude either spider bite or *Centruroides* scorpion sting, but diagnosis may be aided by the discovery of tiny marks, erythema, edema, or local tenderness. Vital signs, the pulmonary condition, and the neurologic status should be considered fully. Repeated evaluation over several hours is often necessary to differentiate envenomation from other causes of wound or illness.

TABLE 101–2

SUMMARY OF MANAGEMENT OF ENVENOMATIONS

Arthropod	Therapy*	Admission Criteria	Discharge Criteria
Black widow spider	Calcium gluconate, methocarbamol, antivenin, diazepam, narcotics	Pain management, respiratory compromise, inability to rule out acute abdomen; pregnancy; severe hypertension	Resolution of severe pain; respiratory stabilization
Brown spiders	Routine wound care, consider dapsone	Systemic signs, necrotic wound requiring intensive management, hematuria	Resolution of systemic signs, stable wound
Jumping spider	Routine wound care		
Hobo spider, northern brown spider	Similar to brown spider	Severe neurologic signs; coagulopathy	Resolution of systemic signs, stable wound
Orb weaver	Routine wound care		
Running spider	Routine wound care		
Tarantulas	Routine wound care; steroid ointment and antihistamine for dermatitis		
Funnel-web spiders	First aid: pressure and immobilization, antivenom; supportive care	Systemic signs	Neurologic and respiratory stability
Wolf spiders	Routine wound care		
Phoneutria	Antivenom, local anesthesia, barbiturates	Observe for 6 hr; admit for systemic signs	Resolution of systemic instability
Bark scorpion	Benzodiazepines, barbiturates, observation; consider antivenin beta blockade	Progressive or severe neurologic or respiratory compromise; symptoms intolerable after ED observation (for at least 4 hr in children under 5)	Resolution of respiratory and neurologic impairment
Other scorpions	Routine wound care		
Giant desert centipede	Elevation, local anesthetic infiltration, supportive care	Severe pain and swelling; inability to rule out cellulitis	Improvement in local symptoms; stable renal function
Insects	Routine wound care	Systemic reaction to cantharidin ingestion; severe allergic signs	Cardiovascular and GI stability

*Routine wound care includes cleaning, tetanus prophylaxis if indicated, and possibly local application of an ice cube during initial period of inflammation.
ED = Emergency department; GI = gastrointestinal.

North American spider, scorpion, and centipede injuries vary greatly in their clinical presentation and sequelae (see Table 101–1). Not every arthropod bite or sting will result in envenomation. Anaphylaxis or other hypersensitivity response may occur alone or in combination with more specific envenomation reactions. Local infection, most often by skin contaminants but occasionally with less well known arthropod flora, may be introduced by a bite and may be difficult to distinguish from the underlying inflammatory response. Finally, although the effects may not be evident acutely, certain arthropods serve as vectors for spirochetes, rickettsia, and protozoa that may later cause systemic disease.

In most cases arthropod envenomations are readily distinguished from those of larger animals; deep, paired fang marks or embedded teeth suggest that the offending animal was larger than a spider. However, particularly in the case of minimally verbal young children, the differential diagnosis must always include those nonarthropod creatures endemic to the local ecology. Small, unpaired fang marks and clustered shallow lacerations are easily confused with arthropod bites and excoriations. Trauma from nontoxic sources may mimic envenomation. All envenomation sites should be inspected carefully for evidence of cactus spines, splinters, or other foreign bodies, as well as for signs of local infection.

DIFFERENTIAL DIAGNOSIS

Systemic and large local reactions to envenomation may mimic a variety of medical disorders. Black widow spider envenomations may cause dramatic abdominal rigidity and tenderness, suggesting an acute abdomen or intussusception. The movement disorder accompanying severe bark scorpion envenomation is commonly mistaken for seizure. Ataxia and lethargy from scorpion envenomation may suggest brain tumor or meningoencephalitis. Tissue injury from spider or centipede envenomation can result in local swelling, erythema, warmth, tenderness, and lymphangitis, which is indistinguishable from cellulitis.

WIDOW SPIDER

The black widow spider, *Lactrodectus mactans*, is found in every state of the United States except Alaska. The female, responsible for all human envenomations, is shiny black with a characteristic red or orange hourglass marking on the ventral aspect of a large globular abdomen (Fig. 101–1). She typically spins an irregular web in sheltered corners of fields, gardens, barns, garages, and outbuildings. She is most likely to bite when the web is disturbed by the unwary child or gardener. In regions where outdoor privies are in common use, human envenomations are likely to involve the buttocks or genital area.

Unlike many other arthropod venoms, that of the widow spider appears to lack toxins capable of provoking a local reaction (see Table 101–1). It does have several toxic components, including a potent neurotoxin that induces neurotransmitter release from nerve terminals.

The initial bite may be sharply painful or may be unrecognized. Local reaction is commonly trivial, with only a tiny papule or punctum visible on exam; the surrounding skin may be slightly erythematous and slightly indurated. Within 30 to 60 minutes of the bite, neuromuscular symptoms can become dramatic as involuntary spasm and rigidity affect the large muscle groups of the abdomen and limbs. Abdominal pain and rigidity may closely mimic an acute abdomen. Associated signs may include fasciculations, weakness, ptosis, priapism, vomiting, fever, salivation, perspiration, and bronchorrhea. Respiratory muscle weakness, combined with pain, may lead to respiratory arrest, particularly in young children. Hypertension with or without seizures may complicate management in elderly or previously hypertensive patients. Pregnancy may be complicated by uterine contractions.

Local management consists of routine cleansing, intermittent application of ice, and tetanus prophylaxis. Local incision and suction are not recommended. Pain and other neurologic symptoms may be managed initially with slow intravenous infusion of calcium gluconate 10% solution, 0.5 ml/kg/dose in children, to a maximum of 10 ml/dose in adults; however, the effects of this are often fleeting. An alternative muscle relaxant is methocarbamol, 15 mg/kg intravenously over 5 minutes followed by a similar dose in drip form over 4 hours (Table 101–3). Spasms and pain unrelieved by these measures may respond to diazepam (0.1 mg/kg) or to meperidine hydrochloride (1 mg/kg) every 3 to 4 hours. Careful observation of respiratory status is vital when using benzodiazepines or narcotics.

Antivenin against *Lactrodectus* venom may be used in severe cases involving respiratory arrest, seizures, uncontrolled hypertension, or pregnancy. It should not be used routinely in less severe settings because of the risks of allergic reaction or delayed serum sickness to the equine product. When antivenin is used, preliminary skin testing is advised to minimize the chance of unanticipated severe allergic reac-

TABLE 101–3

THERAPY AT A GLANCE

Drug	Dosing Suggestions
Black widow antivenin	1–2 vials diluted in 100 ml/vial IV over 10–20 min
Calcium gluconate	50 mg/kg/dose IV over 15 min, may repeat twice
Dapsone	25–100 mg by mouth daily for adults for 1 to 3 wk. Dosing not well established for children.
Diazepam	1.0–5.0 mg intravenously, titrate to effect
Diphenhydramine	1.25 mg/kg/dose, IV or orally, q 6 hr
Lidocaine	1% solution without epinephrine, injected locally
Methocarbamol	15 mg/kg/dose q 6 hr as needed
Morphine	0.05–1.0 mg/kg IV, titrate to effect. Use with caution with CNS toxins.
Phenobarbital	5–10 mg/kg/dose IV up to 20 mg/kg total. Use with caution with CNS toxins.
Scorpion antivenin	Guidelines not established, available only in Arizona. Contact poison control for assistance.

tion; even after a negative skin test the patient should remain under direct observation during treatment. The usual therapeutic antivenin dose is one to two vials by intravenous infusion.

Although the worst pain usually occurs during the first 8 to 12 hours following a bite, symptoms may remain severe for several days. All symptomatic children, pregnant women, and patients with a history of hypertension should be admitted to the hospital. Discharge is usually possible within 1 to 3 days, when hypertension and muscle spasm have subsided.

Prevention of subsequent envenomations involves destruction or removal of all widow spiders and egg sacs in close proximity to living and play areas. New spiders have a tendency to appear in past spiders' "favorite corners," and these areas should be watched for the new appearance of characteristically disorganized black widow webs.

BROWN OR VIOLIN SPIDERS

Thirteen species of spider in the genus *Loxosceles* are native to the United States, and at least five have been associated with necrotic arachnidism: *Loxosceles reclusa* (the true brown recluse spider), *L. laeta*, *L. refuscens*, *L. arizonica*, and *L. unicolor*. The brown spiders are about 1 cm in body length, 2 to 3 cm in leg length, and light or dark brown in color. They are marked with a dark violin-shaped spot centered anteriorly, such that the neck of the violin extends backward across the cephalothorax (Fig. 101–2).

Loxosceles spiders are most active at night from April to October, emerging from woodpiles and closets to hunt insects and other spiders. Naturally shy, they are not prone to bite humans unless threatened or trapped among bedsheets or clothing.

Loxosceles venom is a hemolysin and cytotoxin with a variety of enzymatic activities, including hyaluronidase, esterase, alkaline phosphatase, lipase, and protease. Pathogenesis is poorly understood but is known to be dependent on the function of both complement and polymorphonuclear leukocytes.

The clinical spectrum of loxoscelism runs from mild and transient skin irritation to severe local necrosis accompanied

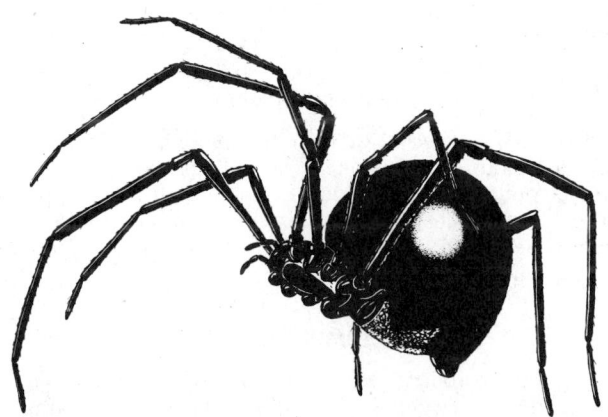

Figure 101–1. Adult female "black widow" spider, *Latrodectus hesperus.* Body length is 15 mm. (From Smith RL. Venomous Animals of Arizona. Tucson, University of Arizona, 1982.)

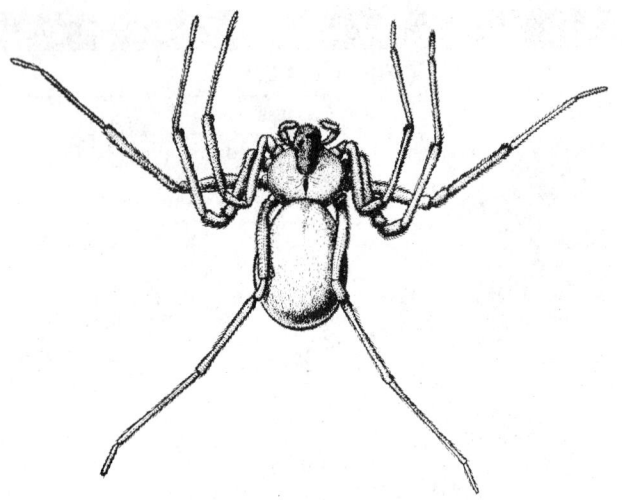

Figure 101–2. "Brown recluse" spider, *Loxosceles* sp. Body length is 9 mm. (From Smith RL. Venomous Animals of Arizona. Tucson, University of Arizona, 1982.)

by dramatic hematologic and renal injury. Isolated cutaneous lesions are the most common presentation; many bites resolve spontaneously without medical care.

Local symptoms usually begin at the moment of the bite itself, with a sharp stinging sensation, although some patients report no awareness of having been bitten at all. The stinging usually subsides over 6 to 8 hours, being replaced by aching and pruritus as the lesion becomes ischemic from local vasospasm. The site often becomes edematous, with an erythematous halo surrounding an irregular violaceous center. In more serious cases serous or hemorrhagic bullae may arise at the center, and a black eschar forms over several days. After 2 to 5 weeks this eschar sloughs, leaving an ulcer of variable size and depth that extends through skin and adipose tissue. The ulcer may heal over many months, leaving a deep scar.

Systemic involvement is less common but may occur with all *Loxosceles* species. Fever, chills, scarlatiniform rash, weakness, leukocytosis, arthralgias, nausea, and vomiting may all occur. In children in particular, hemolytic anemia with hemoglobinuria may accompany loxoscelism, usually beginning within 24 hours of envenomation and resolving within a week. The anemia is usually Coombs' negative and may be severe. Thrombocytopenia and disseminated intravascular coagulation have been reported. In severe cases hemoglobinuria and proteinuria have led to renal failure and even to death.

Treatment of loxoscelism depends on the severity of the lesion. Most mild envenomations will respond to application of local ice compresses, elevation of the affected extremity, and loose immobilization of the part. Necrotic lesions may need debridement after erythema has subsided around the central eschar; this can be followed with skin grafting when the wound is stable. In the past, efforts have been made to treat brown spider bites with corticosteroids, antihistamines, immediate surgical excision, and prophylactic antibiotics, none of which has shown clinical effectiveness. Recently, dapsone (a leukocyte inhibitor used in the treatment of leprosy) has gained popularity for the prevention of lesion progression. Clinical efficacy has been reported, although animal studies generally have not demonstrated efficacy. Dapsone may be administered in an oral dose of 25 to 100 mg daily divided every 12 hours. Dapsone should not be used in patients with glucose-6-phosphate dehydrogenase

deficiency. Potential side effects include methemoglobinemia, hemolysis, and idiosyncratic bone marrow suppression.

A basic laboratory evaluation should be performed for patients with moderate to severe local signs or any systemic signs of envenomation. This should include peripheral blood count, basic coagulation screening, and routine urinalysis in all cases; liver and renal function tests may be indicated in severe poisonings.

Cutaneous loxoscelism is usually treatable on an outpatient basis; severe necrotic or infected lesions may require hospitalization. Patients with systemic symptoms should be considered for admission when there is evidence of coagulopathy, hemolysis, and hemoglobinuria or rapid progression of other systemic signs. Discharge is appropriate when renal and hematologic status is stable.

OTHER SPIDERS

Nearly all spiders have venom glands, although most lack either the strong chelicerae ("fangs") or the large venom reservoir necessary to envenomate humans. Approximately 50 species of spiders in the United States have been implicated in medically significant bites.

Jumping Spider

One of the most common biting spiders in the United States is the jumping spider, of genus *Phidippus*. The bite produces pain, erythema, pruritus, and sometimes extensive swelling. Swelling has been reported to last up to 9 days.

Hobo Spider

The hobo spider, also called northwestern brown spider or *Tegenaria agrestis*, is a 10 to 15 mm, nondescript brown spider of Idaho, Oregon, and Washington that has recently been implicated in several cases of necrotic arachnidism similar to that seen in *Loxosceles* envenomation. Systemic effects reported include headache, visual disturbances, hallucinations, weakness, and lethargy. Hemorrhagic complications are reported in experimental animals. Since there has been relatively little documented experience with this bite, treatment is uncertain. It has been suggested that these be treated in a fashion similar to *Loxosceles* envenomations.

Orb Weaver

The golden orb weaver or black and yellow garden spider, *Argiope aurantia*, common in California, Oregon, and the eastern United States, is a large, brightly colored spider with a large orb web. Bites may cause local pain, swelling, erythema, and vesicle formation, which resolve within 24 hours.

Running Spider

Chiracanthium species, or running spiders, are known for their tenacious, painful bite from which the spider must often be pulled free. A pruritic, erythematous wheal appears within 30 minutes. Local necrosis, nausea, abdominal cramps, headache, and anxiety have been reported. Treatment is symptomatic.

Tarantulas

Tarantulas (suborder Mygalomorphae of the family Theraphosidae) are large, slow spiders capable of inflicting a painful bite when threatened. Although most genera inflict a bite no more dramatic than most hymenoptera stings, a few cause more severe pain and swelling, numbness, or lymphangitis. Several Latin American varieties possess urticating hairs, which the spider may flick by the thousands through the air into an attacker's skin and eyes; these cause an intense inflammation that may remain pruritic for weeks.

Funnel-Web Spiders

Funnel-web spiders, such as *Atrax robustus* of Australia, are a particularly venomous subgroup of the tarantulas. These have tough fangs, capable of piercing a human fingernail, and they are very aggressive. *Atrax* venom is a neurotoxin believed to cause release of various neurotransmitters. Immediately following a bite, patients complain of intense local pain; this may be followed by fasciculations, restlessness, borborygmi, diaphoresis, vomiting, and pulmonary edema. As these symptoms may occur in rapid sequence, first-aid recommendations have included limb immobilization and pressure wrapping to minimize lymphatic return prior to emergency medical treatment. Antivenom specific to *Atrax* envenomation has been developed and successfully used in Australia.

Wolf Spiders

The Lycosidae or wolf spider family includes various mid- to large-sized spiders (body length 3 to 35 mm) with mildly cytotoxic venom capable of provoking transient inflammation in humans. A South American species is somewhat more dangerous, provoking necrosis at the bite site. The most famous wolf spider species is *Lycosa tarantula*, to which the term tarantula was first applied. Its bite was once believed to cause tarantism, a syndrome of stupor, the desire to dance, and sometimes death; but this bite is now known to cause little more than stinging pain.

Banana Spider

The *Phoneutria* genus of South America includes the banana spider *Phoneutria nigriventer*, a large, aggressive spider with body length of 35 mm and leg length of 45 to 60 mm. Nocturnal hunters, these spiders may hide indoors during the daytime. Rarely, a specimen is accidentally imported with a banana shipment to the United States. Humans bitten by *P. nigriventer* may experience pain, tachycardia, hypertension, diaphoresis, salivation, vertigo, nausea, vomiting, priapism, and occasionally death from respiratory paralysis within 2 to 6 hours. Children under the age of 10 years are particularly susceptible.

A polyvalent antivenin effective against *Phoneutria*, *Loxosceles*, and *Lycosa* venoms is available from the Instituto Butantan in São Paolo, Brazil; local anesthesia and barbiturates may be used for pain relief.

BARK SCORPION

The only scorpion native to the United States whose venom is potentially life-threatening is the bark scorpion, *Centruroides exilicauda* (also called *C. sculpturatus* or *C. gertschi*). It may be straw-colored, yellow, or light brown in color; and it ranges in length from 48 to 68 mm (Fig. 101–3). Called the bark scorpion because of its predilection for hiding in the bark of trees, it may also be found in cracks and crevices, under rocks, or in woodpiles. Indoors it may hide in cool shady spots such as undersurfaces of chairs or between bedsheets. It is a nocturnal predator, feeding mostly on other small arthropods. It tends to sting humans only in self-defense.

C. exilicauda venom contains at least five neurotoxins. The resulting derangement of sodium flow causes spontaneous,

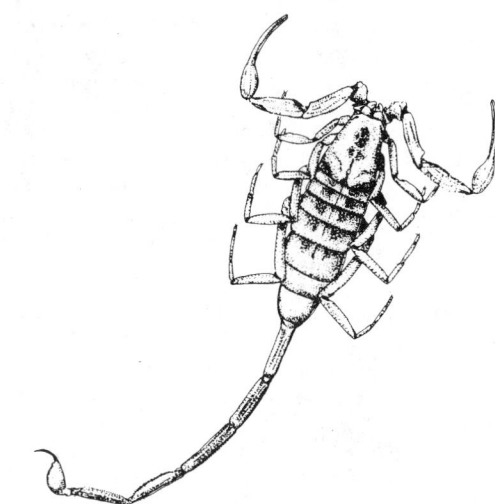

Figure 101–3. Bark scorpion. Body length is 70 mm. (From Smith RL. Venomous Animals of Arizona. Tucson, University of Arizona, 1982.)

repetitive, and prolonged axonal action potentials throughout the nervous system.

Clinical effects of these neurotoxins are the result of aberrant nerve conduction within the sympathetic, parasympathetic, and neuromotor systems. Sympathomimetic effects include tachycardia, hypertension, hyperthermia, mydriasis, and diaphoresis. Parasympathomimetic effects include salivation, lacrimation, bradycardia, urination, and vomiting; in rare cases there may also be clinically significant pulmonary edema. Neuromotor effects include muscle fasciculations, opisthotonos, roving eye movements, nystagmus, and generalized hyperactivity. Lethargy, confusion, and occasionally seizures occur; these may be a result of direct central nervous system toxicity, hypoxia, or both.

Young children are particularly prone to develop the more serious cardiorespiratory and neuromotor manifestations of scorpion envenomation. Whereas only 5% of adults stung by bark scorpions show these signs, 80% of those under age 2 years have significant neuromuscular involvement.

Although mild inflammation is common, local erythema and edema following *Centruroides* sting are usually trivial, and the point of envenomation itself may be indistinguishable from surrounding skin. This complicates diagnosis, particularly in children too young to give a clear history. In such cases a positive "tap test" may prove diagnostic: a sharp finger tap directly over the site of envenomation will often elicit sudden withdrawal of the extremity combined with an expression of pain.

Immediate local treatment of a scorpion sting is best limited to routine wound care. The site should be cleaned, and an ice cube may be briefly applied to minimize pain; but no procedures such as wound incision, prolonged cryotherapy, or tourniquet application should be undertaken. All children under the age of 5 years, and adults with significant systemic symptoms, should be evaluated by a physician.

Pain in the majority of cases can be managed effectively with brief local applications of ice and simple analgesics such as acetaminophen; in the majority of cases involving adults, no further intervention is necessary. Caution is urged in the use of opiates, as these may exacerbate neurologic symptoms and hypoventilation.

Respiratory compromise is generally the most significant risk following a serious envenomation, and it is most common in infants. This usually results from hypersecretion by upper airway mucosa and neuromotor paralysis or incoordination; pulmonary edema may be a complicating factor. Judicious use of benzodiazepines may improve the motor defect, but increased respiratory depression is a potentially serious drawback. Atropine may be useful for treatment of edema. Antivenin treatment should be considered in cases of severe respiratory compromise.

Cardiovascular effects are usually transient, and in healthy children specific intervention is rarely necessary. Parasympathetic effects of *C. exilicauda* envenomation are particularly transient, and atropine is seldom necessary. Tachyarrhythmias, when they occur, may be managed with beta blockers. Severe hypertension, particularly in healthy children, is rare; but this may be treated with nitroprusside, diazoxide, or hydralazine.

The area of greatest controversy in treatment of bark scorpion envenomation surrounds the issue of neuromuscular manifestations. Respiratory depression is risked with any of the common pharmaceutical interventions, and the outcome of envenomation with intensive care observation alone is unlikely to involve serious long-term morbidity. In the past, large doses of narcotics may have contributed to high mortality, particularly in children. Nevertheless, some form of symptomatic treatment is often strongly desired, and in settings where careful monitoring is possible, this may be undertaken with relative safety. Benzodiazepines in conservative doses may prove helpful in reducing neuromotor hyperactivity; phenobarbital in moderate doses (5 to 10 mg/kg intravenously) may be administered for what is commonly minimal therapeutic benefit. Narcotics, in general, should be avoided.

An antivenin specific to *C. exilicauda* has been developed but is not approved by the Food and Drug Administration; it is available only within the state of Arizona. It has been used with efficacy and minimal incidence of severe side effects, and it may find more general application, particularly in the treatment of seriously ill children. At this time, however, its use remains controversial owing to allergy and serum sickness that may follow serum administration, and it is considered an experimental treatment.

Children under the age of 5 years and adults with systemic symptoms should be observed for a minimum of 4 hours. Vital signs should be checked frequently during this time. Those with respiratory compromise, severe tachycardia or hypertension, pain or neurologic symptoms requiring use of ongoing parenteral medication should be admitted to the hospital for medical management and intensive monitoring. In most cases clinical signs will begin to abate by 6 to 12 hours postenvenomation and will reach a tolerably minimal level by 16 to 24 hours; mild symptoms may be noted by the patient for several days. Hospital discharge is appropriate when neurologic and cardiorespiratory stability have returned and when drug treatment is no longer necessary. This is usually possible by 24 hours after admission.

Control measures for indoor scorpions consist mainly of their individual removal from the home; they are notoriously resistant to chemical eradication. *Centruroides* scorpions fluoresce under near-ultraviolet light (such as a Wood's lamp) and may be located this way from distances of 20 feet during their nighttime activity. Crib legs in the nursery may be inserted in glass tumblers with smooth vertical walls to discourage climbing.

OTHER SCORPIONS

Other scorpions commonly implicated in envenomations in the United States include species of *Vejovis*, *Hadrurus*, and *Androctonus*. Although many of these species appear outwardly more threatening than do bark scorpions (e.g., the giant hairy scorpion of the southwestern United States), their stings rarely produce symptoms of serious medical importance. Likewise, stings of the other *Centruroides* species of the southeastern United States, such as *C. vittatus, C. hentzi, C. keysi,* and *C. gracilis,* evidently produce only local pain.

Medical management consists of cleaning, tetanus prophylaxis if needed, analgesia, and perhaps local application of ice to reduce inflammation. Hospital admission is rarely necessary.

Eight species of *Centruroides* native to Mexico have been implicated in human toxicity, often reported to involve dramatic pulmonary edema. Mortality from envenomation is reportedly high in many Mexican centers, and specific antivenom is commonly used in treatment.

Tityus species of South America produce severe local pain and erythema, accompanied by prominent parasympathetic symptoms; increased gastric acid secretion and acute pancreatitis have also been reported.

The genuses *Buthus* and *Parabuthus* of South Africa and India are reported to cause severe muscle spasms combined with parasympathetic and sympathetic effects; respiratory failure and, in the case of *Buthus,* cardiac abnormalities suggestive of ischemia may follow. Renal failure associated with hemolysis and hemoglobinuria has occasionally been reported with *Buthus* envenomations. *Leiurus* and *Buthus* species of the Middle East and North Africa have an envenomation pattern similar to that reported for the Indian *Buthus* species.

Treatment for these envenomations is similar to that for *Centruroides* species, but the more severe parasympathetic effects are more likely to require atropine treatment. Beta-receptor blockade has been suggested for prevention of myocardial damage and arrhythmias.

CENTIPEDES

Centipedes are long, multisegmented arthropods possessing one pair of legs for each segment (millipedes have two pairs per segment). They use venom, injected through a pair of hollow fangs, primarily to kill invertebrate and small vertebrate prey. The largest centipede species approaches 35 cm in length, but most are considerably smaller. The only United States species of particular medical significance is the giant desert centipede, *Scolopendra heros.* Centipede venom contains acid and alkaline phosphatase and amino acid naphthylamidase, lipoproteins, histamine, and serotonin.

Burning pain, edema, erythema, lymphangitis, and lymphadenopathy are common after a centipede bite. Following the initial presentation, envenomation by *Scolopendra* species may be slow to evolve, with local pain, edema, erythema, and lymphangitis persisting for 1 to 3 weeks. During this phase it is sometimes impossible to distinguish uncomplicated envenomation from cellulitis, and antibiotics may be administered. Careful observation of tightly swollen extremities should include repeated examination for potential compartment syndrome; intracompartmental pressure monitoring may be indicated. Laboratory evaluation is unnecessary in cases of mild envenomation, but should include urinalysis, complete blood count, and electrolyte and renal function testing in more serious cases.

Medical management is restricted to routine wound care; local infiltration with lidocaine may be used for immediate pain relief. There is not an antivenin available. Antihistamines and steroids have been suggested for more severe reactions.

INSECTS

Caterpillars

Many varieties of caterpillar, such as the larval forms of the puss moth and buck moth, possess spiny urticating hairs, or setae. Unicellular venom glands equip the bases of the setae. Direct injection of the venom into human skin occurs when the hairs are contacted. The hairs break off and penetrate the epidermis. Symptoms include an immediate burning sensation at the site, which may be followed by local erythema and papular or vesicular eruption that may persist for days. Contact with eyes or respiratory tract may trigger an irritant conjunctivitis or bronchitis. Treatment consists of removal of hairs with cellophane tape or irrigation, followed by supportive measures, including antihistamines.

Fire Ants

Fire ants, of genus *Solenopsis*, derive their name from the pain associated with their stings. Their venom contains necrotizing alkaloids. These insects will attack readily, in large groups. The ant first bites the skin with its strong mandibles, then curls and repeatedly stings the surrounding skin. A wheal forms at each site within minutes, which by 24 hours becomes a pustule 2 to 3 mm in diameter. Days later the site may slough, leaving a tiny scar. Dermal injuries from fire ant stings usually require no specific treatment beyond careful cleaning and antipruritics. Systemic reactions are usually due to hypersensitivity.

Blister Beetles

The blister beetles, of the family *Meloidae*, include dozens of United States species in addition to the infamous European *Lytta vesicatoria*, or "Spanish fly." When a blister beetle is restrained or otherwise threatened, its intersegmental membranes rupture and it secretes hemolymph, which contains cantharidin, a potent irritant sometimes used in the treatment of warts. Cantharidin may contact human skin either directly, while handling a beetle, or more remotely, during contact with contaminated plant material. Gastrointestinal toxicity is associated with its unfortunate reputation as an aphrodisiac. Ingestion may be followed by fever, hemorrhagic gastroenteritis, and urethral and genital inflammation. Treatment is symptomatic, with prompt, thorough irrigation of local lesions and admission for intravenous fluid support of ingestions.

MEDICOLEGAL CONSIDERATIONS

The indications for use of antivenin in the treatment of scorpion sting and black widow bite remain unsettled; risks of immediate hypersensitivity and delayed serum sickness response inherent in administration of serum products must be taken into consideration whenever antivenin use is contemplated. Risks involved should be presented to the patient's parents, and intensive care monitoring should accompany drug administration.

Selected References

Alario A, Price G, Stahl R, Bancroft P. Cutaneous necrosis following a spider bite: A case report and review. Pediatrics 1987;79:618.

Babcock JL, Marner DJ, Steele RW. Immunotoxicology of brown recluse spider (*Loxosceles reclusa*) venom. Toxicon 1986;24:783.

Banner WJ. Bites and stings in the pediatric patient. Curr Probl Pediatr 1988;Jan:8.

Burnett JW, Calton GJ, Morgan RJ. Blister beetles: "Spanish Fly." Cutis 1986;22.

Burnett JW, Calton GJ, Morgan RJ. Centipedes. Cutis 1986;37:241.

Butz WC. Envenomation by the brown recluse spider (Aranae, Scytodidae) and related species. A public health problem in the United States. Clin Toxicol 1971; 4:515.

Cooke JA, Miller FH, Grover RW, et al. Urticaria caused by tarantula hairs. Am J Trop Med Hyg 1973;22:130.

Curry SC, Vance MV, Ryan PJ, et al. Envenomation by the scorpion *Centruroides sculpturatus*. J Toxicol Clin Toxicol 1984;21:417.

Gayer KD, Burnett JW. Hymenoptera stings. Cutis 1988;41:93.

Gendron BP. *Loxosceles reclusa* envenomation. Am J Emerg Med 1990;8:51.

Ginsburg CM, Weinberg AG. Hemolytic anemia and multiorgan failure associated with localized cutaneous lesion. J Pediatr 1988;112:496.

Hobbs GD, Harrell RE Jr. Brown recluse spider bites: A common cause of necrotic arachnidism. J Emerg Med 1989; 7:309.

Iserson KV. Methemoglobinemia from dapsone therapy for a suspected brown spider bite. J Emerg Med 1985;3:285.

Key GF. A comparison of calcium gluconate and methocarbamol (Robaxin) in the treatment of latrodectism (black widow spider envenomation). Am J Trop Med Hyg 1981;30:273.

King LE Jr, Rees RS. Dapsone treatment of a brown recluse bite. JAMA 1983;250:648.

Lehmann CF, Pipkin JL, Ressmann AC. Blister beetle dermatosis. Arch Dermatol 1900;36.

Likes K, Banner WJ, Chavez M. *Centruroides exilicauda* envenomation in Arizona. West J Med 1984;141:634.

Maretic Z. Latrodectism: Variations in clinical manifestations provoked by *Latrodectus* species of spiders. Toxicon 1983;21:457.

Perry WJ. The brown recluse spider in Alabama: A report of five cases. J Med Assoc State of Alabama 1975; 44:551.

Presto AJ, Muecke EC. A dose of Spanish fly. JAMA 1970;214:591.

Rachesky IJ, Banner WJ, Dansky J, et al. Treatments for *Centruroides exilicauda* envenomation. Am J Dis Child 1984;138:1136.

Rees RS, O'Leary JP, King LE Jr. The pathogenesis of systemic loxoscelism following brown recluse spider bites. J Surg Res 1983;35:1.

Rimsza ME, Zimmerman DR, Bergeson PS. Scorpion envenomation. Pediatrics 1980;66:298.

Russell FE, Marcus P, Streng JA. Black widow spider envenomation during pregnancy. Report of a case. Toxicon 1979;7:188.

Schnur L, Schnur P. A case of allergy to scorpion antivenin. Ariz Med 1968;25:413.

Spielman A, Levi HW. Probable envenomation by *Chiracanthium mildei*: A spider found in houses. Am J Trop Med Hyg 1970;19:729.

Vest DK. Necrotic arachnidism in the northwest United States and its probable relationship to *Tegenaria agrestis* (Walckenaer) spiders. Toxicon 1987;25:175.

Wasserman GS, Anderson PC. Loxoscelism and necrotic arachnidism. J Toxicol Clin Toxicol 1983;21:451.

Wong RC, Hughes SE, Voorhees JJ. Spider bites. Arch Dermatol 1987;123:98.

CHAPTER 102

Reptile Bites

G. Randall Bond

INTRODUCTION

Poisonous reptiles fall into two groups: venomous snakes and venomous lizards. Venomous snakes are divided into five families: Colubridae, Elapidae, Hydrophidae, Viperidae, and Crotalidae. Most Colubridae are nonpoisonous, the primary exceptions being the African boomslang and the vine snake. The family Elapidae includes cobras, mambas, and coral snakes. Three species of coral snakes are indigenous to North America. The Hydrophidae (sea snakes) are closely related to the Elapidae in both venom and envenomation apparatus. Hydrophidae are found only in the warm waters of the Indian and Pacific oceans. Viperidae (Old World vipers) include asps, vipers, and adders; they are found in Africa, Asia, and Europe. Crotalidae or pit vipers are found in Asia but are most widely represented throughout North and South America as rattlesnakes, moccasins, and copperheads. Pit vipers have a triangular-shaped head, an elliptic pupil, and a unique heat-sensing organ located in a pit between the eye and the nostril on each side.

Poisonous lizards are native only to North America. The Mexican beaded lizard is found on the west coast of Mexico. The Gila monster inhabits the northern Mexican desert and parts of Arizona and surrounding states.

More than 8000 Americans suffer poisonous snakebites each year; of these, 10 to 15 may die. Approximately 30% of victims are children less than 18 years of age. In the United States, small children represent only 10% of poisonous snakebite victims but are disproportionately represented in mortality statistics. When bites occur to small children, they generally involve the lower extremities. Preteens and teenagers make up the majority of childhood snakebite victims; males are represented overwhelmingly. Many of these follow the adult pattern of being bitten on the upper extremity while attempting to catch or handle the snake. In the United States, the Crotalidae family, including rattlesnakes, moccasins, and copperheads, account for 95% of bites by poisonous snakes. Coral snakes account for 2%, and exotic snakes the remaining 3% of bites. Gila monsters are shy, and bites occur only when they are handled. Children have not been represented in recent reports of Gila monster bites.

ANATOMY AND PHYSIOLOGY

Most colubrids are considered nonpoisonous. Elapidae and Hydrophidae have front teeth modified into fixed fangs. Some cobras have a further modification of these fangs that allow them to "spit" venom accurately up to 3 m. The venom of Elapidae has a variety of effects, but neurotoxic weakness is the most prominent. This is particularly true of the three species of coral snake found in the southern United States. Sea snakes have the most potent venom, gram for gram. It is primarily neurotoxic with some myotoxic features. Because of their inefficient envenomation apparatus, elapid and sea snake bites result in envenomation only about 50% of the time.

Old World vipers and pit vipers have a pair of long, hinged, replaceable forward fangs for efficient envenomation. The heat-sensing organ of the pit viper makes this family very accurate in striking at prey. Nonetheless, as many as 20% to 25% of human victims may suffer only "dry" bites.

Snake venoms have a complex composition, including enzymes, proteins, polypeptides, metals, and other mediators. Tissue effect is both direct and through activation of host systems. Tissue-destructive snake enzymes include proteases, phospholipases, and hyaluronidases. The extent of swelling and necrosis is augmented by local tissue release of mediators, which contribute to venom-mediated capillary leak and loss of local vasoregulation. Although massive local edema is common following snakebite to the extremity, this is almost always edema of subcutaneous tissue and only rarely represents elevated intracompartmental pressure. This knowledge frequently obviates the need for "prophylactic" fasciotomies. Techniques to measure intracompartmental pressure should be used to identify those patients who require a fasciotomy.

Coagulopathy

Coagulopathy frequently occurs following crotalid envenomation. Evidence suggests that fibrinogenolysis and fibri-

nolysis are due to snake venom activation of plasminogen and direct fibrinolysis rather than being thrombin-induced, which would be related to disseminated intravascular coagulation (DIC). Fibrin degradation products are often elevated, with prothrombin time (PT) and partial thromboplastin time (PTT) prolongation. Clinically significant bleeding is uncommon. Investigations into the frequently associated thrombocytopenia suggest that it is consumptive either in association with local tissue damage, or fibrinogenolysis, or as a direct venom effect. The significance of a direct venom anticoagulation mechanism is that it is reversible with adequate administration of specific antivenin. Hemolysis may occur as a result of direct red cell injury or in association with a true DIC syndrome.

Neurotoxin

Most venom neurotoxins act at the myoneural junction. Where postsynaptic acetylcholine receptor blockade is the primary mechanism, anticholinesterase medications have a therapeutic role. Coral snake venom appears electrophysiologically to act postsynaptically, but victims do not respond to anticholinesterases. The Mojave rattlesnake neurotoxin acts presynaptically.

Allergy- and Venom-Mediated Effects

Angioedema, urticaria, and anaphylactic shock have resulted from snakebite and Gila monster bite. In almost all cases victims have had a prior exposure to venom, suggesting the role of immunoglobulin E–specific mediators, but venom components may produce a similar picture. Patients who die of rattlesnake envenomation frequently show massive systemic effects early or present late for care. In at least three death reports, it is suggested that venom was injected into a vein. Hypotension as a result of intravascular volume loss to tissues and bleeding is frequently noted. Anaphylaxis may play a role in some deaths.

Gila Monsters

Gila monsters have powerful jaws. Venom is pooled in the labial folds and enters the tissue of the victim by capillary action as the reptile inflicts a crushing, tearing wound. They may cling to the victim for a matter of minutes, increasing total envenomation. Venom causes intense pain, local swelling, and hypotension. Tissue destruction is primarily the result of the bite itself. Coagulopathy has been reported only once. Single case reports also document anaphylaxis and myocardial infarction.

EMS CONSIDERATIONS

The subject of prehospital care for victims of reptile envenomation has undergone significant debate. Techniques such as tourniquet application and incision and suction of the bite site, first described 2500 years ago, have been increasingly questioned and abandoned. Rational therapy is that which minimizes systemic effects without increasing the risk of local tissue damage.

Tourniquet Application

The placement of a tourniquet or constricting band to impede lymphatic return of venom to the systemic circulation has been advocated. Nevertheless, no good data support tourniquet use, particularly following crotalid envenomation. It is likely that if venous return is not restricted in addition to lymphatic return, little will be done to impede systemization of venom. When tourniquets are applied or when loose constricting bands become tourniquets as tissue edema spreads, venom-induced edema may be compounded and perfusion of injured tissue may be impaired. Constricting bands properly applied may be recommended for victims at extreme distance from definitive medical care, but they probably have little place in prehospital management by trained emergency medical technicians in urban systems.

Incision and Suction

The incision and suction technique is also of questionable value. Early animal studies using hypodermically injected venom suggested the potential recovery of 50% of venom when procedures are initiated within 3 minutes of envenomation. A more recent animal study using a new suction device yielded 23% to 34% recovery. No animal studies have demonstrated increased survival. It is unlikely that field application following natural envenomation could approach these results. Incision has the potential to damage deeper structures and increase local damage, especially if a cruciform incision is utilized. Oral suction increases the risk of infection. Even proponents of the technique do not recommend it unless the transportation time to definitive care is greater than 30 to 40 minutes and suction is initiated within 15 minutes of the bite. It should have no place in current emergency medical technician management of venomous snake bites.

Cryotherapy

In the 1950s many practitioners advocated prolonged submersion of the bitten extremity in an ice bath. This technique is not supported by animal data. Cooling, even briefly, has been almost universally condemned by current experts.

Electroshock

High-voltage electroshock therapy is the newest therapeutic suggestion. Three rodent studies failed to demonstrate any beneficial effect. This technique cannot be recommended at this time.

Summary

A reasonable prehospital protocol involves minimizing patient activity, removing potentially constrictive clothing and jewelry, splinting the affected extremity in a position of comfort, and traveling to the hospital at a safe speed. Analgesia and supportive care, including intravenous fluids, should be provided as required. This protocol is applicable to crotalid, coral snake, and Gila monster bites.

CLINICAL EVALUATION
Crotalid Bites

Pit viper bites usually cause significant pain from the moment of envenomation. Swelling occurs at the site of the bite and progresses at a variable rate depending on the amount and potency of the venom injected (Table 102–1). Local areas may become extremely swollen and tense. Ecchymosis may be noted. Fluid-filled or hemorrhagic bullae may form at the site of the bite. In time an area of necrosis may become apparent, which may include the site of envenomation.

The severity of the local edema should be assessed using repeated circumferential measurements taken every 15 min-

TABLE 102–1
FACTORS IN THE ASSESSMENT OF CROTALID ENVENOMATION SEVERITY
Degree of swelling
Rapidity of swelling advancement
Distal perfusion deficit
Regional lymph node tenderness
Bleeding from IV sites
Weakness, ptosis
Hypotension
Coagulopathy
Defibrination
Thrombocytopenia
Hemolysis
Rhabdomyolysis/myoglobinuria
Intracompartmental pressure elevation

utes at three sites on the affected extremity. Rapid proximal progression of swelling or the presence of systemic findings indicates a more significant envenomation and the need for aggressive early intervention with antivenin.

Frequently the first sign of systemic envenomation is tender regional lymph nodes. Other signs include nausea, a metallic taste, muscle fasciculations, bleeding from intravenous puncture sites, and, less commonly, hypotension and shock. Ptosis and weakness may be common signs following envenomation by some subspecies of the Mojave rattlesnake. Hypertension is often noted in association with extreme pain. When hypotension is present, it is almost always the result of diffuse capillary leak and hypovolemia.

Elapid Bites

Coral snake bites may not evoke a significant local reaction. Other than the bite injury itself, minimal or no swelling or pain may be noted. Patients may experience nausea, vomiting, excess salivation, euphoria, and dizziness. Neurologic findings include paresthesia at the bitten extremity, weakness, ptosis, diplopia, dyspnea, fasciculations, and respiratory muscle paralysis. Onset of neurologic symptoms may be delayed up to 12 hours and then symptoms may progress rapidly. No early findings predict patients with a severe neurologic course.

Gila Monster Bites

The severe crush injury and venom of the Gila monster bite produces immediate severe pain, frequently involving the entire extremity. Systemic signs of envenomation include weakness and dizziness associated with hypotension. Coagulopathy and myocardial infarction have been described once. An anaphylactoid presentation has been reported.

DIAGNOSTIC EVALUATION

A number of antibody-based venom identification tests are available. In North America, the ease of recognition of a crotalid envenomation, the lack of specific crotalid species detection, and the polyvalent nature of antivenin make the tests less useful. The role of the laboratory in snake venom poisoning is to better define systemic effects and monitor the success of therapy.

A complete blood count, platelet count, urinalysis, serum creatine kinase, PT, PTT, and fibrinogen and fibrin degradation products are useful in the management of crotalid envenomation. Serum fibrinogen and platelet count are the two most useful parameters to follow when a coagulopathy is present; either one or both may be decreased. When adequate antivenin has been given, the fall in fibrinogen and platelets will stop and begin to reverse. It is difficult to tell true DIC from the combination of thrombocytopenia and defibrination. When hemolysis is occurring, the urine will demonstrate hemoglobin without red blood cells. Creatine kinase may be elevated from direct venom-induced muscle injury or secondarily from a muscle compartment syndrome.

DIFFERENTIAL DIAGNOSIS

There is rarely any question of the occurrence of a snakebite. Occasionally a preverbal child living or camping in an area with a significant Crotalidae presence will present with an ecchymotic, painful limb swelling without a history of a bite. The presence of fang marks, blebs, ptosis, or coagulopathy will help to differentiate the injury from an acute fracture or sprain. More often, the issue is differentiating the bite of a poisonous snake from that of a nonpoisonous snake. When the snake is available, a triangular head, elliptic pupil, and paranasal pits will confirm the snake as a pit viper (Fig. 102–1). Rattles on the tail are another helpful feature but will not be present on a copperhead or

moccasin. Many common nonpoisonous snakes have colored stripes like the coral snake. Only a coral snake has red and yellow stripes next to each other. A helpful mnemonic is "red on black venom lack, red on yellow kill a fellow." The stripes of the coral snake are also unique in that they completely encircle the snake (including the ventral portion). Coral snakes have a black nose. Nonpoisonous striped snakes have a red nose.

THERAPEUTIC INTERVENTION
General Care

Local wound care starts with cleansing of the bite site. Exploration of the puncture wound is rarely needed unless aggressive first responders have incised into deep tissues. The status of tetanus immunization should be checked and updated. All rings and jewelry should be removed. The affected extremity should be elevated to minimize edema. The hand and forearm in bites to the upper extremities should be splinted in a position of function. Perfusion of the distal extremity should be assessed frequently. Decreased skin temperature reflects increased risk for distal ischemia. Even in this subgroup the majority did not have distal ischemia. The recommendation for prophylactic antibiotics following envenomation has been based on the argument that potentially decreased perfusion and local necrosis in association with an unsterile puncture wound put these victims at increased risk of cellulitis. No studies establishing the risk of infection or the benefit of prophylactic antibiotics have been published.

Concurrent with local wound care, severe pain and systemic symptoms, including hypovolemia, bleeding, respiratory muscle weakness, and anaphylaxis, must be addressed. Pain control may require large doses of intravenous narcotics. Fluids lost to third spaces should be rapidly replaced with a crystalloid or colloid solution. Coagulopathy and serious thrombocytopenia will be most rapidly corrected with antivenin. Since crotalid venom does not activate thrombin, heparin has no role in therapy. Transfusion of clotting components will result in their rapid consumption, so they should be used only to temporize when severe bleeding and shock are present. Blood loss should be replaced when significant. Occasionally with Mojave rattlesnake envenomation and frequently with coral snake envenomation, respiratory failure secondary to neuromuscular blockade will occur. Artificial ventilation may be required. When anaphylaxis occurs, therapy with epinephrine, fluids, histamine antagonists, and corticosteroids may be required. In the absence of hypersensitivity reactions, steroids are not beneficial.

The therapy of Gila monster bites is exclusively supportive. In addition to local wound care, narcotics and intravenous fluids are frequently required.

Antivenin

The decision to use antivenin is based on the clinical risks versus the therapeutic benefits. Gradation serves to help assess risk and anticipate antivenin requirements (Table 102–2). Higher grades have an increased risk of complications, including amputation, permanent deformity, and death.

Patients with grade 0 envenomation should not receive antivenin (Table 102–3). Initial recommendations for antivenin vary from 0 to 5 vials for grade 1, to 10 vials for grade 2, to 15 to 20 vials for grade 3. Many grade 1 envenomations may be managed without antivenin. Grade 2 and 3 envenomations should be managed with antivenin unless the risks

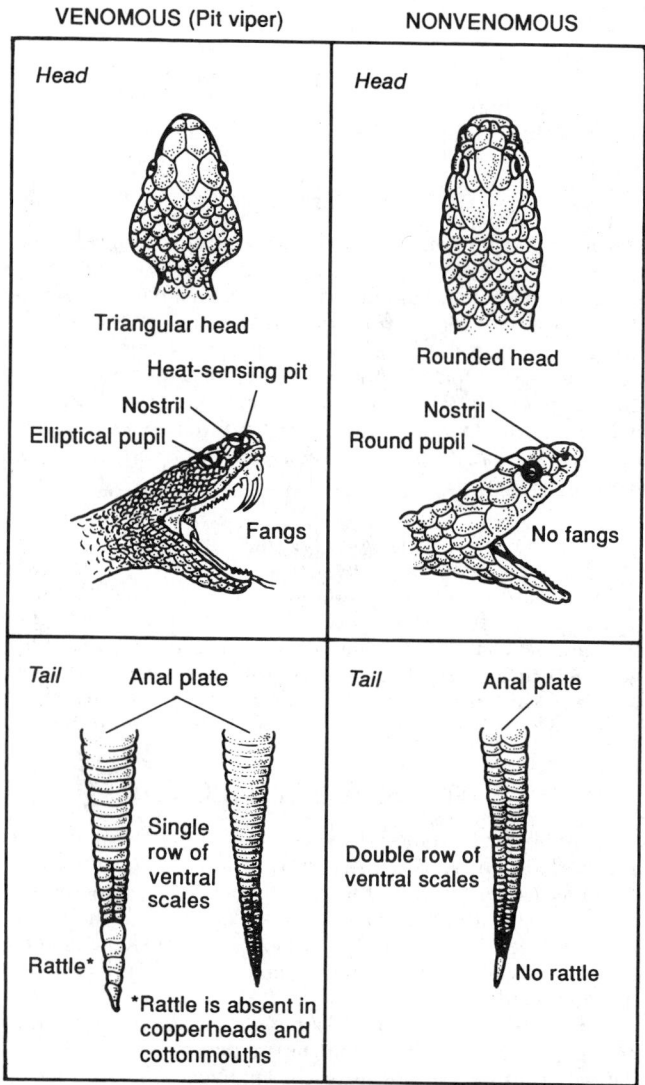

Figure 102–1. Identification of venomous and nonvenomous snakes.

TABLE 102–2

GRADATION OF CROTALID ENVENOMATION SEVERITY

Grade 0	No local or systemic reaction
Grade 1	Minimal local swelling
Grade 2	Moderate local swelling, regional lymphadenopathy
Grade 3	Severe local reaction or systemic signs

TABLE 102–4

SKIN TESTING AND ANTIVENIN ADMINISTRATION

Contraindications	Horse serum hypersensitivity, concurrent beta-blocker therapy
Skin testing	Administer 0.02 ml of 1:10 diluted horse serum (provided with the antivenin) intradermally. Read in 15 min. Any wheal, flare, urticaria, or anaphylactic reaction is a positive reaction.
Antivenom preparation	Add 10 ml bacteriostatic water to lyophilized antivenin. Mix until no undissolved particles remain. Remove a volume equal to that of the antivenin to be given from a 125- or 250-ml bag of normal saline and replace with antivenin.
Antivenom administration	Cardiac and frequent hemodynamic monitoring is required. Start infusion very slowly and double administration rate every 2 min, observing for a reaction (rash, urticaria, hypotension, respiratory distress). Administer over 30–90 min.
Hypersensitivity reaction	Stop antivenom administration. Reassess need for antivenom administration. Consider H_1, H_2 blocking agents, slower infusion rate, concurrent low-dose epinephrine administration, and corticosteroids if continued antivenom therapy is justified.

of therapy are high or the patient or parent refuses antivenin therapy (Table 102–4).

Because no early signs predict neurotoxicity and because response to antivenin may be limited once symptoms have begun, prophylactic antivenin (four to six vials) is recommended as soon as the occurrence of a bite by a coral snake has been established. More antivenin may be required in bites suffered by children or in those who present with neurologic symptoms.

Following the decision to use antivenin, skin testing should be conducted while the antivenin is being prepared. Skin testing may help in assessing the risk of immediate hypersensitivity reaction. The use of antivenin carries a 0% to 33% risk of an acute hypersensitivity reaction (itch, urticaria, anaphylaxis), a dose-related risk of delayed hypersensitivity (serum sickness), and a high rate of sensitization to horse serum. The risk of an immediate hypersensitivity reaction is probably somewhat less in children. For testing, 0.02 ml of a 1:10 dilution of horse serum provided with the antivenin is injected intradermally. A positive test is any wheal, erythema, or urticaria noted in 15 to 30 minutes. Reactions to antivenin occur even following a negative skin test 10% to 28% of the time. Reactions to antivenin following positive skin tests occur 50% to 100% of the time. Skin testing and antivenin administration should always occur in a monitored environment. Physicians should be prepared to treat an immediate hypersensitivity reaction. Patients receiving beta-blocker therapy may not respond to adrenergic therapy should anaphylaxis occur.

If a reaction occurs, the infusion should be stopped at once, the patient treated appropriately for the reaction, and the need for antivenin reassessed in view of the reaction. Patients with reaction to horse serum or to antivenin are frequently managed with antivenin using slower infusion rates, antihistamines, intermittent subcutaneous epinephrine (0.01 ml/kg of 1:1000, maximum 0.3 ml/dose), or continuous low-dose intravenous epinephrine (0.05 μg/kg/minute) and corticosteroids. If it is decided to continue the antivenin, the infusion should be restarted at a slow rate and advanced cautiously. A less immunologically reactive antivenin is being developed.

Surgical Intervention

Because of their experience in the 1950s and 1960s, several authors have argued that aggressive surgical therapy minimizes the need for amputation and improves functional outcome. Other reports have suggested that consumption of coagulation factors is local at the tissue site and have recommended surgical removal of venom and injured tissue. In contradiction, several recent series of large numbers of patients bitten by a variety of rattlesnakes in a variety of geographic locations treated with early adequate intravenous antivenin have demonstrated good functional outcome without surgical intervention. Others have demonstrated good functional outcome without the use of either surgery or antivenin in a series of patients bitten primarily by nonrattlesnake pit vipers. The incidence of compartment syndrome following snakebite appears to be much less than was previously perceived. Modern techniques allow the measurement of intracompartmental pressure and distal extremity blood flow before the decision to perform fasciotomy or digital dermotomy must be made. It is therefore appropriate to limit acute surgical intervention to treatment of a defined compartment syndrome or an avascular digit. As a local area of necrosis becomes defined, it may require debridement and occasionally skin grafting.

DISPOSITION

Patients who have no signs or symptoms and have no evidence of coagulopathy in the first 4 hours are unlikely to develop any bleeding diathesis. These patients may be treated as outpatients (Table 102–5). Symptomatic patients may be discharged to home when systemic symptoms have resolved, progression of swelling has ceased, perfusion to the distal extremity is good, and the patient's pain is manageable with oral analgesics. Patients who have grade 0 envenomation may be discharged from the emergency de-

TABLE 102–3

CROTALID ENVENOMATION: THERAPEUTICS AT A GLANCE

Analgesia
Local wound care
Update tetanus prophylaxis
Splint, elevate affected extremity
Fluid support
Antivenin administration (initial guideline)

Grade 0	0 vials
Grade 1	0–5 vials
Grade 2	10 vials
Grade 3	15–20 vials

TABLE 102–5

DISPOSITION

Discharge when	Progression of swelling has ceased; systemic symptoms are absent; pain is adequately controlled with oral analgesics
Follow-up care	Support affected limb (sling, crutches); receive local wound follow-up; return to physician if signs of serum sickness occur (rash, hives, fever, myalgia, joint swelling)

---

partment following a 4- to 6-hour observation period and appropriate wound care. All patients require close follow-up for wound complications and residual disability. They should receive further debridement of blebs or necrotic tissue as needed. Local swelling may persist for days to weeks.

Patients should also be warned of the likelihood of serum sickness if they have received antivenin. Symptoms of rash, itch, joint swelling, and low-grade fever usually start 5 to 10 days following the administration of antivenin. All symptomatic patients should receive corticosteroids and antihistamines for symptom control. The usual duration of serum sickness is 5 to 7 days, but this is variable. Patients who receive antivenin should be aware that they have probably acquired a sensitivity to horse serum. Caution should be used if they require horse serum–containing products in the future. This is particularly relevant to those whose bites are a result of intentional handling of a snake and who may again engage in high risk activities.

OTHER CONSIDERATIONS

The American Association of Zoologic Parks and Aquariums and the American Association of Poison Control Centers (AAPCC) attempt to maintain an up-to-date location database for exotic antivenin. Access to this information is available through AAPCC-designated regional poison centers or the Arizona Poison and Drug Information Center, at (602) 626–6016.

Selected References

Arnold RE. Treatment of venomous snakebites in the western hemisphere. Milit Med 1984;149:361.

Banner W, Russell F, Barton B, et al. Fatal rattlesnake bite in a child (abstract). Vet Hum Toxicol 1984;26(Suppl 2):43.

Bronstein AC, Russell FE, Sullivan JB, et al. Negative pressure suction in field treatment of rattlesnake bite (abstract). Vet Hum Toxicol 1985;28:297.

Budzynski AZ, Pandya BV, Rubin RN, et al. Fibrinogenolytic afibrinogenemia after envenomation by western diamondback rattlesnake (Crotalus atrox). Blood 1984;63:1.

Burch JM, Agarwal R, Mattox KL, et al. The treatment of crotalid envenomation without antivenin. J Trauma 1988;28:35.

Cable D, McGehee W, Wingert WA, et al. Prolonged defibrination after a bite from a "nonvenomous" snake. JAMA 1984;251:925.

Curry S, Gerkin R, Riffer E, et al. Successful treatment with antivenin of marked thrombocytopenia without significant coagulopathy following rattlesnake bites (abstract). Vet Hum Toxicol 1987;29:493.

Curry SC, Horning D, Brady P, et al. The legitimacy of rattlesnake bites in Central Arizona. Ann Emerg Med 1989;18:658.

Curry SC, Kraner JC, Kunkel DB, et al. Noninvasive vascular studies in management of rattlesnake envenomations to extremities. Ann Emerg Med 1985;14:1081.

Curry SC, Kunkel DB. Death from a rattlesnake bite. Am J Emerg Med 1985;3:227.

Garfin SR. Rattlesnake bites: Current hospital therapy. West J Med 1982;137:411.

Garfin SR, Castilonia RR, Mubarak SJ, et al. Rattlesnake bites and surgical decompression: Results using a laboratory model. Toxicon 1984;22:177.

Glass TG. Early debridement in pit viper bites. JAMA 1976;235:2513.

Glenn JL, Straight RC, Wolfe MC, et al. Geographical variation in Crotalus scutulatus scutulatus (Mojave rattlesnake) venom properties. Toxicon 1983;21:119.

Grace TG, Omer GE. The management of upper extremity pit viper wounds. J Hand Surg 1980;5:168.

Guderian RH, Mackenzie CD, Williams JF. High voltage shock treatment for snake bite (letter). Lancet 1986;2:229.

Hardy DL. Envenomation by the Mojave rattlesnake (Crotalus scutulatus scutulatus) in Southern Arizona, U.S.A. Toxicon 1983;2:111.

Hardy DL. Fatal rattlesnake envenomation in Arizona: 1969–1984. Clin Toxicol 1986;24:1.

Hardy DL, Jeter M, Corrigan JJ. Envenomation by the northern blacktail rattlesnake (Crotalus molossus molossus): Report of two cases and the in vitro effects of the venom on fibrinolysis and platelet aggregation. Toxicon 1982;20:487.

Ho CL, Lee CY. Presynaptic actions of Mojave toxin isolated from Mojave rattlesnake (Crotalus scutulatus) venom. Toxicon 1981;19:889.

Howe NR, Meisenheimer JL Jr. Electric shock does not save snakebitten rats. Ann Emerg Med 1988;17:254.

Jamieson R, Pearn J. An epidemiological and clinical study of snake bites in childhood. Med J Aust 1989;150:698.

Johnson EK, Kardong KV, Mackessy SP. Electric shocks are ineffective in treatment of lethal effects of rattlesnake envenomation in mice. Toxicon 1987;25:1347.

Jurkovich GJ, Luterman A, McCullar K, et al. Complications of Crotalidae antivenin therapy. J Trauma 1988;28:1032.

Kitchens CS, Van Mierop HS. Envenomation by the eastern coral snake (Micrurus fulvius fulvius). JAMA 1987;258:1615.

Kunkel DB, Curry SC, Vance MV, et al. Reptile envenomations. J Toxicol Clin Toxicol 1984;21:503.

Mandell F, Bates, J, Mittleman MB, et al. Major coagulopathy and "nonpoisonous" snake bites. Pediatrics 1980;65:314.

McCollough NC, Gennaro JF. Treatment of venomous snakebite in the United States. Clin Toxicol 1970;3:483.

Nelson BK. Snake envenomation. Med Toxicol 1989;4:17.

Parrish HM, Khan MS. Bites by coral snakes: Report of 11 representative cases. Am J Med Sci 1967;253:561.

Pearn J, Morrison J, Charles N, et al. First-aid for snake bite. Med J Aust 1981;68:293.

Pennell TC, Babu SS, Meredith JW. The management of snake and spider bites in the Southeastern United States. Am Surg 1987;53:198.

Pettigrew LC, Glass JP. Neurologic complications of a coral snake bite. Neurology 1985;35:589.

Piacentine J, Curry SC, Ryan PJ. Life-threatening anaphylaxis following gila monster bite. Ann Emerg Med 1986;15:959.

Russell FE, Bogert CM. Gila monster: Its biology, venom and bite—a review. Toxicon 1981;19:341.

Russell FE, Carlson RW, Wainschel J, et al. Snake venom poisoning in the United States. JAMA 1975;233:341.

Russell FE, Picchioni AL. Snake venom poisoning. Clin Toxicol Consult 1983;5:73.

Simon, TL, Grace TG. Envenomation cogaulopathy in wounds from pit vipers. N Engl J Med 1981;305:443.

Stewart ME, Greenland S, Hoffman JR. First-aid treatment of poisonous snakebite: Are currently recommended procedures justified? Ann Emerg Med 1981;10:331.

Sullivan JB Jr. Past, present and future immunotherapy of snake venom poisoning. Ann Emerg Med 1987;16:938.

Tu AT. Biotoxicology of sea snake venoms. Ann Emerg Med 1987;16:1023.

Wingert WA, Chan L. Rattlesnake bites in southern California and rationale for recommended treatment. West J Med 1988;148:37.

Wingert WA, Sullivan JB, Sinkinson CA. Snakebite management: Which approach to use. Emerg Med Rep 1984;5:37.

CHAPTER 103

Marine Animal Envenomation

N. Heramba Prasad

INTRODUCTION

It is estimated that worldwide approximately 40,000 to 50,000 marine envenomations occur annually. The majority of these envenomations do not pose any actual threat to life. Frequently the result is simply a minor form of contact dermatitis.

Water-related dermatoses and other illnesses may not manifest for days or even months, thereby challenging the diagnostic ability of inland physicians. Although children are frequently the victims of envenomations, limited information is available regarding the specific problems of children.

Most encounters with harmful marine animals are accidental. These encounters are classified into (1) traumatic, such as shark bites; (2) toxic, such as from ingestion of ciguatera or toxic shellfish; and (3) venomous, such as bites, stings, and contacts with *crinotoxic* animals, which produce poisons in specialized venom glands but do not possess an injecting device, or *acanthotoxic* animals, which have specialized venom glands and possess a traumatogenic organ.

Zoologically, marine animals are classified into invertebrates and vertebrates. Invertebrates are further divided into the following phyla: Protozoa (dinoflagellates); Porifera (sponges); Coelenterata (jellyfish, hydroids, sea anemones, corals); Echinodermata (starfish, sea urchins, sea cucumber); and Mollusca (snails, bivalves, octopus) (Table 103–1). In addition, phyla Platyhelminthes (flat worms), Rhynchocoela (ribbon worms), Anneledia (segmented worms), Arthropoda (joint-footed animals), Ectoprocta (moss animals), and Sipunculida (peanut worms) are also found in the ocean and can cause poisoning and various forms of dermatoses. The phylum Chordata contains all the animals possessing a notochord (Table 103–2).

TOXICOLOGY

Most marine venoms have a defensive function. They are made of mixtures of large-molecular-weight proteins and other compounds such as indole, histamine, serotonin, and kinins. They act by denaturing cell membranes, destroying mast cells, releasing histamine, releasing bradykinin, and causing differing degrees of cardiovascular damage and neurologic toxicity.

Protozoan Poisons

Dinoflagellates (phylum Protozoa; class Mastigophora) are the primary food suppliers of the sea. Exorbitant growth of these organisms tends to occur near coastal waters. Plankton blooms are also known to appear with weather disturbances that result in water upswellings, causing a phenomenon called "red tide," a massive overgrowth of various algae. This overgrowth may have other discolorations, but red is the most common. The red tide is poisonous to fish. It is estimated that the excessive proliferation of red algae can kill 100 tons of fish per day. Certain dinoflagellates found in French Polynesia are capable of producing ciguatoxin in fish. Eating mollusks contaminated by some dinoflagellates causes paralytic shellfish poisoning in humans.

Coelenterate Poisons

The phylum Coelenterata contains some of the most venomous creatures in the ocean. One of the most painful coelenterate stings is that of the Portuguese man-of-war

		TABLE 103–1		
		INVERTEBRATES		
Phylum	**Subgroup**	**Zoologic Name**	**Distribution**	**Common Name**
Protozoa	Order Dinoflagellata	*Gymnodinium breve*	Gulf of Mexico; Florida	Red algae
Coelenterata	Class Hydrozoa	*Millipora alcicornis*	Caribbean Sea	Stinging coral; fire coral
		Physalia physalis	Tropical Atlantic	Portuguese man-of-war; blue bottle
	Class Scyphozoa	*Chironex fleckeri*	Northern Australia	Sea wasp; box jellyfish
		Cyanea capillata	North Atlantic and Pacific	Sea nettle; hair jellyfish; sea blubber
	Class Anthozoa	*Acropora palmata*	Florida Keys; Bahamas; West Indies	Elk horn coral
		Anthopleura elegantissima	California coast	Sea anemone
Echinodermata	Class Asteroidea	*Acanthaster planci*	Indo-Pacific; Red Sea	Venomous starfish
	Class Echinoidea	*Diadema antillarum*	West Indies	Sea needle; cobbler; black sea urchin
	Class Hollothuroidea	*Actinopyga agassizi*	West Indies	Sea cucumber
Mollusca	Class Gastropoda	*Conus aulicus*	Polynesia	Court cone
		Conus gloria maris	Philippines	Glory-of-the-sea
		Conus textile	Indo-Pacific; Polynesia	Cloth of gold cone; woven cone
	Class Cephalopoda	*Octopus maculosus*	Indo-Pacific; Australia	Spotted octopus; blue-ringed octopus
		Octopus apollyon	Alaska to Baja California	Octopus
Porifera	Class Desmospongia	*Fibula nolitangere*	West Indies	Poison bun; sponge
		Microciona prolifera	Cape Cod to South Carolina	Red moss; oyster sponge

TABLE 103–2

VERTEBRATES

Phylum	Subgroup	Zoologic Name	Distribution	Common Name
Chordata	Order Rajiformes	*Dasyatis sayi*	Atlantic: Brazil to New Jersey	Blunt nose stingray
		Aetobatus narinari	Tropical seas	Spotted eagleray
		Dasyalis diptirurus	San Diego Bay	Diamond stingray
		Torpedo marmorata	Atlantic; Indian; Mediterranean	Marbled electric ray
	Class Osteichthyes	*Arius bendeloti*	West Africa	Sea catfish
		Noturus furiosus	Eastern North Carolina: Tar and Neuse rivers	Carolina madtom
		Bagre marinus	Cape Cod to Brazil	Sea catfish
		Trachinus aranius	Portugal; Mediterranean	Dragonfish; weeverfish
	Class Scorpaenidae	*Scorpaena guttata*	Gulf of California	Sculpin
		Synanceja norrida	Indo-Pacific; Australia	Stonefish
		Pterois russelli	Indo-Pacific; Australia	Zebrafish; lionfish
		Apistus carinatus	Indo-Pacific	Scorpionfish

(Physalia physalis). Its venom is a polypeptide and is believed to affect the sodium-potassium pump, causing damage to cell membranes. It is also noted to have hemolytic action, and it impedes the binding of calcium with the skeletal muscle tissues. The venom of the sea wasp, *Chironex fleckeri*, is known to have cardiotoxic, hemolytic, and dermatonecrotic properties. It can cause lethal ventricular fibrillation. In some cases it has produced sustained contractions of skeletal, respiratory, and vascular muscles.

Toxins from coelenterates are heat labile, nondialyzable, and degradable by proteolytic agents. Numerous fractions possessing individual characteristics have been identified. Thalassin (first isolated from the tentacles of *Anemonea sulcata*) causes severe anaphylaxis. Congestin (from sea anemones) produces intense vasodilatation and respiratory paralysis. Hypnotoxin (from *Physalia*) is known to cause central nervous system depression, resulting in coma and death. The excruciating pain that is characteristic of coelenterate stings is thought to be due to the release of serotonin (5-hydroxytryptamine).

INVERTEBRATES

Coelenterates

Coelenterates (Cnidariae) contain a single gastrovascular cavity. Two morphologic features are usually described: the polyp and the medusa. Many species go through both stages during their life cycle. The nutritive polyps have a crown of tentacles and a central mouth, giving them a characteristic cup shape. They reproduce by budding, giving rise to free-floating medusae (like an "umbrella with a tiny handle"). Many medusae join together to form colonies that exhibit commensalism with other animals.

Coelenterates are divided into three classes: Hydrozoa (hydroids, fire corals, and the Portuguese man-of-war), Schyphozoa (sea wasps, sea nettles, and other jellyfish), and Anthozoa (sea anemones). The venom-containing cells found in the tentacles of coelenterates are known as cnidocytes.

Nematocysts are found in cnidocytes. They contain a venom-filled capsule (cnidoblast) with a coiled, harpoon-like, eversible hollow tube. The tube, when uncoiled, is several hundred times longer than the cnidoblast, and it contains numerous barbs and spines. The cnidocil is a trigger situated on top of the cnidoblast. This trigger is sensitive to both chemical and pressure changes in the environment. When threatened, a Portuguese man-of-war can discharge thousands or even millions of nematocysts.

Hydrozoa

Hydroid stings usually produce mild, transient discomfort. However, some species, such as *Leptomedusa*, can inflict severe contact dermatitis. Repeated exposure to hydroid stings can cause sensitization and anaphylaxis. Erythema multiforme and desquamative eruptions have been reported.

Stinging corals *(Millipora)* are widely distributed in the tropical seas. They have an exoskeleton made of lime that contains numerous pores. The larger ones (gastropores) ensheathe feeding tubes equipped with stoma (gastrozooids). The smaller pores are known as dactylopores, and they house the tentacles with the nematocysts.

The most dangerous of the hydrozoans is the Portuguese man-of-war. The only portion of the animal that is usually seen is the purple float (pneumatophore), shaped like an inverted bell, which propels it through the water. Many polypoid and medusal forms attach together to a floating stem, forming a colony. Although the organism is only about 10 to 30 cm in diameter, the tentacles (dactylozooids) that hang from its underside can be as long as 30 m. Each tentacle contains thousands of nematocysts. When stung by a Portuguese man-of-war, the victim experiences intense pain. This is followed by the appearance of a rash. Linear red papules, beaded streaks, or erythematous welts develop. The rash may be accompanied by systemic reactions such as myalgias, nausea, vomiting, headache, and respiratory distress, leading to cardiovascular collapse and death.

A dead Portuguese man-of-war is not benign. The nematocysts are still capable of discharging when touched. Accidental envenomation of children walking along the seashore can occur. This is especially true after a heavy storm when numerous tentacles are washed ashore.

Schyphozoa

The jellyfish include a number of dangerous species. The box jellyfish or sea wasp *(Chironex)*, found in the waters near Australia, is perhaps the most venomous of all sea creatures. Schyphozoa are medusoid, free floating, and vary in size from a few millimeters to 2 m in length. The tentacles of *Cyanea capillata* are more than 36 m in length. *Chironex*, *Chiropsalmus*, and *Chirodropus*, all belonging to the class Cubomedusae, are sometimes seen hovering in large numbers near the sandy bottoms off the coasts of the Indo-Pacific region. The manifestations of their stings are similar to those of *P. physalis* but are much more serious and sometimes fatal within 30 seconds of envenomation. Stings by various other species of jellyfish have been known to cause symptoms ranging from mild stinging to severe burning, throbbing, or shooting pain that may render the victim unconscious (Table 103–3). Sea nettles, especially the *Chrysaora* and *Cyanea* species in the mid-Atlantic region, produce distinctive rash patterns. The effects of their envenomation are milder than those of the box jellyfish.

Irukandji Sting Syndrome. There are two types of jellyfish stings: type a stings, which lack local dermatoses but manifest severe systemic reactions, and type b stings, which form local weals but have no systemic reactions. Type a stings are referred to as Irukandji stings, named after an Australian tribe.

Anthozoa

Sea anemones can sometimes be seen in abundance near seashores. Their sting tends to cause localized burning, accompanied by erythema and swelling. Abscess formation has been reported. In general, the effects of anthozoan stings are quite mild.

Therapeutic Intervention

If the diagnosis is in doubt, the nematocysts can be obtained for microscopic examination by gentle scraping of the affected area with a glass slide or by pressing a piece of adhesive tape over the weal.

Treatment is directed toward preventing further envenomation by rinsing the affected area with sea water (see Table 103–3). Fresh water should *not* be used because the change in osmolarity will trigger the undischarged nematocysts. Use of normal saline is not advisable, as it does not have the same osmolality as sea water. In the unlikely event that the victim is seen away from the coastal region, use of commercially available sea-water preparations for aquarium use (e.g., Instant Ocean) may be appropriate. Topically applied alcohol in any form (although isopropyl alcohol is usually recommended), diluted vinegar, and papain (meat tenderizer or papaya latex) have also been used to neutralize the venom. Salt water should be heated, if possible, to enhance destruction of the heat-labile enzymes. After rinsing the area, a paste of sea water and baking soda should be used to coalesce the tentacles. If baking soda is not available, flour or talcum powder can be used. Anecdotes of successful removal of tentacles using shaving cream, toothpaste, and other household compounds abound in the folklore of coastal regions. The coalesced tentacles can then be scraped off with a knife or a sharp object such as a clean clam shell, a credit card, or a piece of thick cardboard. Gloves should be worn while attempting to remove the tentacles to prevent additional envenomation; however, the tentacles have been known to penetrate surgical gloves. If gloves are not available, thick rags or a handful of seaweed may be used. In the hospital, local symptoms such as itching can be treated with antihistamines, and steroids or epinephrine should be administered as indicated. Successful treatment of severe muscle spasms by intravenous calcium gluconate is reported. Narcotic analgesics are usually required. Intravenous fluid resuscitation to treat shock may be necessary. Tetanus immunization and local wound care should be performed when indicated.

Porifera

Approximately 4000 species of sponges are known to exist. Noteworthy among them are the North American red sponge (*Microciona prolifera*) and the poison bun sponge (*Fibula nolitangere*) (see Table 103–1). Sponge poisoning generally occurs from handling certain species, manifesting as local itching and burning and leading to vesiculation, joint effusion, and occasional pustules. The dermatitis has been known to spread to other areas of the body as well. Development of erythema multiforme and anaphylactic reactions has also been described.

Treatment consists of application of soothing lotions, antihistamines, and systemic corticosteroids if indicated. Anecdotally, diluted vinegar (2 tablespoons in 1 L of water) seems to effectively soothe the affected areas. Limited information on the value of antibiotics and antiseptics is available.

Echinoderms

The sea urchin, the sea cucumber, and the starfish are radially symmetric organisms that are usually passive. Approximately 5300 species are described in the phylum. Sea urchins are globule shaped and contain sharp, movable, and brittle spines that tend to break off after puncturing a victim's skin. The spines are usually of varying sizes. Some species do not possess venom sacs in the spines. A few species also possess pincer-like organs known as pedicellariae. These are small, delicate, seizing organs consisting of a conical head and a supporting stalk. The head contains three or four fangs surrounded by sensory hair. Contact with the sensory hair causes the "jaw" to close. Pedicellariae cause a more severe reaction than the spines. The larger the pedicellariae, the more venomous the organism. Sea urchin

---

TABLE 103–3

CLINICAL FEATURES AND TREATMENT OF SOME COMMON INVERTEBRATE STINGS AND BITES

Animal	Injury	Treatment
Portuguese man-of-war (nematocyst)	Electric shock–like sensation; multiple linear welts; headache, muscle cramps, nausea, vomiting, shock, cardiovascular collapse	Avoid fresh water; sea-water rinse; apply alcohol/vinegar; apply baking soda + sea-water paste to tentacles; scrape off; nematocyst precautions
Fire coral (nematocyst)	Redness, urticaria hemorrhage, zosteriform rash, abdominal pain	Same as above
Jellyfish (nematocyst)	Painful welts with characteristic pattern, muscle spasms, respiratory distress with sea wasp and sea nettle	Same as above; antivenin for sea wasp
Elkhorn coral	Intense stinging, weeping ulcers, septic sloughing, ulcer if untreated	Same as above; debridement/antibiotics
Sea urchins	Intense pain, redness, swelling, partial motor paralysis, irregular pulse, delayed granulomas	Prompt removal of spines—surgically if necessary; immersion in hot water (45°C) for 30–90 min
Sea cucumbers	Contact dermatitis, corneal injury	Nematocyst precautions; thorough eye exam
Coneshells	Local reaction, pain, paresthesia, respiratory paralysis, death	Loose tourniquet; direct compression; naloxone; neostigmine
Octopus	Minimal local reaction; occasionally neurotoxic symptoms	Symptomatic; direct compression with gauze and bandage

venom consists of serotonin and parasympathomimetic substances.

Sea urchins cause two types of reactions. The immediate local allergic reaction is characterized by a rash and local swelling. Spines contain a purple or black dye that may stain the puncture site. The wound may bleed profusely. Syncope, paresthesia, ataxia, cramps, and respiratory distress have occurred in some instances. The second type of reaction is a delayed one. This manifests in the form of a granuloma or a diffuse local swelling and inflammatory reaction. The cause of this delayed reaction is unclear.

Treatment usually consists of immersing the affected area in hot water until the pain subsides. The spines should be removed only if they are easily visible. If not, radiographs should be obtained and the removal attempted in a controlled environment with proper equipment, such as an operating microscope. Antibiotics are usually not necessary. If an infection develops, a third-generation cephalosporin and an aminoglycoside are appropriate.

Delayed-reaction granulomas can sometimes undergo spontaneous resolution. Occasionally, intralesional steroids may be indicated. Surgical exploration may be necessary if a retained spine is suspected.

Many species of starfish are toxic if ingested. *Acanthaster planci*, found mostly in the Indo-Pacific and Polynesian regions, is a well-known venomous starfish. It grows to a size of about 60 cm and possesses 14 or 16 rays. The venom, asterotoxin, is thought to be a saponin. Toxin isolated from *Asteria vulgaris* has severe cytolytic properties. Starfish envenomation may cause extreme pain, pruritus, protracted vomiting, and paralysis. Treatment is primarily symptomatic.

Sea cucumbers produce holothurin, a toxin that can cause contact dermatitis and eye irritation, sometimes resulting in blindness. Some sea cucumbers have been known to ingest coelenterate nematocysts, retaining these in an intact state for possible future use in defense.

Mollusca

Most mollusk poisoning results from the ingestion of toxic pelecypods such as oysters, clams, and scallops. Very few actual envenomations occur. The proboscis of cone shells contains a single radicular tooth possessing a venom sac. The venom may have curare-like action, causing skeletal muscle paralysis. Ataxia, convulsions, and paralysis may ensue early in severe envenomation, resulting in drowning. Various degrees of allergic and anaphylactic reactions, cardiac failure, coma, and death have been described. Use of neostigmine or edrophonium has been suggested to counteract muscle weakness. Severe hypotension may be treated empirically with naloxone to block the beta-endorphin vasodepressor response. Artificial ventilation may become nec-

essary. *Conus gloria maris* (glory-of-the-sea), found near the Philippines and considered to be extremely rare and thus valuable by collectors, is believed to cause lethal injuries.

The octopus is a shy and docile creature that usually does not pose any threat to humans. It belongs to the class Cephalopoda. The small, blue-ringed octopus, *Octopus maculosa*, found near Australia, is the only one known to cause severe envenomation. Death has been reported following its bite. The venom causes hypotension, bradycardia, and respiratory paralysis. Treatment is primarily supportive. Hot-water immersion does not seem to neutralize the venom. Some authorities recommend wide excision of the wound site.

VERTEBRATES

There are approximately 200 species of venomous fish in the world. Their venom apparatus is usually found in the spines in the gill covers and fins. The venom apparatus of the stingray is located on the dorsum of a whip-like caudal appendage. The catfish venom organ consists of one dorsal and two pectoral fin spines. Weeverfish contain venom in five to seven needle-sharp dorsal spines and two dagger-like dentinal spines.

Stingrays

Stingrays are peaceful bottom dwellers that may cause envenomation when swimmers step on them inadvertently. Eleven species of rays are identified along the coasts of the United States. They range in size from a few inches to a width of 4 to 5 feet. While wading along beaches, children may encounter a stingray, a diamond-shaped creature, half-buried in the sand. Playfully they may kick the animal. The animal retaliates by hurling its barbed tail. The barb is serrated and retropointed, and can inflict deep and irregular lacerations that are contaminated by debris from the barb. The immediate symptom is intense pain, usually out of proportion to what might be expected in nonvenomous injuries of similar intensity, developing in a matter of a few minutes and reaching maximum intensity in 90 minutes (Table 103–4). A 5-mm sting can inflict a wound of about 3 to 4 cm in length. Systemic symptoms such as muscle cramps, weakness, nausea, vomiting, paresthesia, lymphadenopathy, hypotension, and cardiac dysrhythmias can occur. Occasionally death has been reported. Crude venom extracts containing serotonin, nucleotidase, and phosphodiesterase have been shown to cause vasoconstriction, respiratory depression, and marked central nervous system changes.

Treatment is directed toward pain control, venom neutralization, and prevention of wound infection. The primary treatment is thorough irrigation of the wound with hot water

TABLE 103–4		
CLINICAL FEATURES AND TREATMENT OF SOME COMMON VERTEBRATE STINGS AND BITES		
Animal	**Injury**	**Treatment**
Stingrays	Intense pain, edema, syncope, paralysis, muscle spasms, seizures, vomiting, diarrhea	Thorough wound irrigation and wound care; local suction antibiotics
Catfish	Local pain, edema leading to gangrene; occasionally systemic signs	Hot-water immersion; wound care
Weeverfish	Pain, swelling, ischemia, gangrene	Hot-water immersion; wound exploration; antibiotics
Scorpionfish	Intense pain, rash vesicles, severe GI symptoms, respiratory distress, seizure, cardiac dysrhythmias	Hot-water immersion; wound irrigation; wound exploration; antivenin

to neutralize and remove as much toxin as possible. The wound is debrided and explored thoroughly to remove remnants of the sheath. The injured area is then again soaked in hot water. One author recommends using magnesium sulfate in the water because of its mild anesthetic properties. The wound is then treated as any contaminated wound. Tetanus immunization should be administered. Prophylactic antibiotics are recommended. A third-generation cephalosporin and an aminoglycoside for in-patient therapy, or trimethoprim-sulfamethoxazole for out-patient therapy, as initial treatment are appropriate.

Scorpaenidae

Scorpaenidae can be divided into three groups according to their venom apparatus: *Pterois* (lionfish, zebrafish), *Scorpaena* (scorpionfish, bullrout), and *Synanceja* (stonefish). The stonefish is the most dangerous, and its venom can be life-threatening.

Scorpaenidae have a bony plate extending from the eye to the gill cover, giving them the nickname "mailcheeked fishes." They generally inhabit shallow waters around coral reefs and sandy beaches. Many of these have become popular in aquarium collections, thereby increasing the risk of envenomation. The venom of *Synanceja verrucosa* is likened to cobra venom in its neurotoxicity. Although less venomous, scorpionfishes found near the Florida Keys, the Caribbean, the Gulf of Mexico, and the coast of southern California (commonly called "sculpin," see Table 103–2) are capable of producing severe systemic and cutaneous reactions. The venom is a nondialyzable, heat-labile protein. It causes vasodilatation, hypotension, and respiratory paralysis.

The initial manifestation of stonefish envenomation is excruciating pain that rapidly extends to proximal areas. Ecchymosis, erythema, induration, paresthesia, and regional lymphadenopathy occur to varying degrees. Necrosis of the wound site over several days has been reported. Systemic manifestations may include cardiac dysrhythmias, myocardial ischemia, hypotension, pulmonary edema, nausea, vomiting, seizures, and paralysis.

The treatment of venomous stonefish stings is similar to that of snakebites. Because the venom is extremely heat labile, immediate immersion of the affected areas in hot water for 30 to 90 minutes or until the symptoms subside is very effective. In addition, appropriate wound management and treatment of systemic manifestations should be undertaken.

Catfish

Both fresh-water and salt-water catfish are capable of producing venomous stings. The venom apparatus consists of axillary venom glands and dorsal and pectoral spines. Catfish venom has vasoconstrictive and dermatonecrotic factors. Intense pain following stings by certain tropical catfish, such as *Plotosus* and *Pterodoras*, can last up to 48 hours. In extreme cases the involved limb may develop massive edema, leading to gangrene. Stings by North American fresh-water and salt-water catfish produce mild and transient symptoms. Treatment consists of hot-water immersion of the stung area, adequate analgesia, wound irrigation, and debridement.

Weeverfish

The weeverfish, a short, stout-bodied fish, is found in temperate waters. Weeverfish can inflict extremely painful and fatal wounds. The venom apparatus consists of five dorsal spines and two opercular spines. The severity of the pain may cause the victim to lose consciousness. Cases have been cited (Halstead, 1988) where "the pain was so violent that the individual finally amputated his finger and thereby obtained prompt relief," and there are reports of fishermen "hammering their fingers with a thole pin, and others wrapping their fingers with vinegar-soaked paper and lighting it in [the] desperate hope of deadening pain." The venom possesses cardiotoxic, hemolytic, and neurotoxic properties. Serotonin in the dialyzable fraction of the venom is thought to be the cause of severe pain. The lethal portion seems to be in the nondialyzable portion. The manifestations and treatment of envenomation are similar to those for stingrays.

Sea Snakes

Fifty-two species of the family Hydrophiidae are known to be venomous, their venom being more neurotoxic than their terrestrial cousins, the cobra and krait. They are usually found in the warm waters of the Indo-Australian region. The only sea snake in the Atlantic ocean is the venomous *Pelamis platurus*, found off the eastern coasts of South America. Most sea snakes are said to be docile. Their fangs are short and tend to break off easily; thus many bites do not result in envenomation.

Symptoms of envenomation usually evolve slowly over a few hours. The bites are tiny puncture marks, usually 1 to 4 in number but sometimes as many as 10 to 20, and are not painful. The symptoms are gradually progressive, beginning as malaise, aching, and stiffness and leading to painful muscle spasms, hemoglobinuria, myoglobinuria, and progressive bulbar paralysis. Death is due to respiratory arrest, hyperkalemia, or delayed profound renal failure.

An equine polyvalent sea snake antivenin is available. Polyvalent Elapidae antivenin is an acceptable alternative if the Enhydrina antivenin is not available.

Selected References

Baden HP, Burnett JW. Injuries from sea urchins. South Med J 1977;70:459.

Bitseff EL, Garoni WJ, Hardison CD, et al. The management of stingray injuries of the extremities. South Med J 1970;62:417.

Burnett JW, Calton GJ, Burnett HW. Jellyfish envenomation syndromes. J Am Acad Dermatol 1986;14:100.

Cain D. Weeverfish sting: An unusual problem. Br Med J 1983;287:406.

Cross TB. An unusual stingray injury—the skin diver at risk. Med J Aust 1976;2:947.

Flecker H. Fatal stings to North Queensland bathers. Med J Aust 1952;1:35.

Halstead BW. Poisonous and Venomous Marine Animals of the World. Princeton, NJ, Darwin Press, 1988, p 727.

Halstead BW. Coelenterate (cnidarian) stings and wounds. Clin Dermatol 1987;5:8.

Halstead BW. Current status of marine biotoxicology—an overview. Clin Toxicol 1981;18:1.

Kizer KW. Marine envenomations. J Toxicol Clin Toxicol 1983–84;21:527.

Loder JS. Treatment of jellyfish stings. JAMA 1973;226:1228.

Soppe GG. Marine envenomations and aquatic dermatology. Am Fam Physician 1989; August:97.

Southcott RV. Australian venomous and poisonous fishes. Clin Toxicol 1977;10:291.

Southcott RV. Human injuries from invertebrate animals in the Australian seas. Clin Tox 1970;3:617.

Sutherland SK, Lane WR. Toxins and mode of envenomation of the common ringed or blue ringed octopus. Med J Aust 1969;1:893.

Weiner S. Stonefish sting and its treatment. Med J Aust 1958;3:218.

Williamson JA, Le Ray LE, Wohlfahrt M, Fenner PJ. Acute management of serious envenomation by box-jellyfish (*Chironex fleckeri*). Med J Aust 1984;141:851.

Yaffee HS, Stargartner F. Erythema multiforme from *Tedania ignis*. Arch Derm (Chicago) 1963;87:601.

Burns

Daniel W. Ochsenschlager

INTRODUCTION
Epidemiology and Prevention

Thermal injuries are the second most common cause of accidental death in children[1] and the most common cause of accidental death in the home environment. In fact, 94% of burns occur at home.[2] Approximately 600,000 children are burned annually and about 30,000 require hospitalization.[3] Death is related to the percentage of surface area involved and the degree of burn. When death occurs, it is typically within 16 to 18 days after the injury. Sepsis and respiratory complications are the two most frequent causes of death. Children under the age of 3 years and those with smoke inhalation are particularly at risk.

Not all burns are accidental: some are due to child abuse.[4, 5] The most common mechanism for this form of child abuse is intentional scalding,[6] the child's hands or feet usually being dunked in hot water with a characteristic "sock and glove" distribution.[7] In one series, 28% of scald burns in children were nonaccidental.[8]

Scalding is the most common cause of thermal injuries in children. Usually these burns are caused by spills when young children reach for pots or bump into adults who are carrying hot liquids. In some homes, tap water is hot enough to cause serious burns. In one study, 80% of homes had bathtub water temperatures greater than 54°C (130°F).[8] At that temperature, a child can suffer a full-thickness burn within 30 seconds (Fig. 104–1). Hot water heaters can be adjusted to a lower temperature (preferably about 120°F) without sacrificing comfort and also saving heating costs.[8, 9]

Infants can sustain significant burns to the mouth from formulas heated in microwave ovens.[10, 11] Any formula so warmed must be tested before use.

Classification

Burns are classified in terms of both degree and percentage. The degree is determined by the depth of skin injured.[12] A first-degree burn, such as sunburn, involves only the epidermis; it is fiery red in appearance, is painful to touch, and heals without scarring in 3 to 5 days.

Partial-thickness burns (second degree) involve the entire epidermis and part of the dermis, and may be superficial or deep. Superficial partial-thickness burns destroy the epidermis and the outer half of the dermis. In these burns the skin is blistered, red, and moist; blanches; contains hair; and is painful. These burns heal in 10 to 18 days, usually without scarring. Deep partial-thickness burns cause damage to the lower half of the dermis; the skin is usually pale white and may have blisters. There is sensitivity to pressure and pain. Healing occurs slowly in 21 to 28 days with some scarring.

Full-thickness third-degree burns cause complete destruction of the epidermis, the entire dermis, and some of the subcutaneous tissue. The skin appendages (hair, hair follicles, sweat glands, and neuroreceptors) are destroyed. The skin appears dry, white, and leathery. Full-thickness burns are insensitive to pain and touch. Healing can occur only by epithelial migration and contracture, which often makes grafting necessary. The classification of fourth-degree burn sometimes implies significant damage to the subcutaneous fat, muscles, and fascia. Fourth-degree burns are usually associated with molten metal, electrical burns, or flame burns in an unconscious patient (Table 104–1).[13]

It is important to be circumspect when assessing the depth of the burn on initial presentation, particularly when advising parents of the likely cosmetic results. The degree of burn is difficult to assess initially; it may change over the first few days, usually becoming deeper than originally appreciated.

Burns are also classified by percentage of total body surface area (BSA) involved. It is important in assessing burns to use the correct nomograms. Infants' and children's body proportions are quite different from those of adults

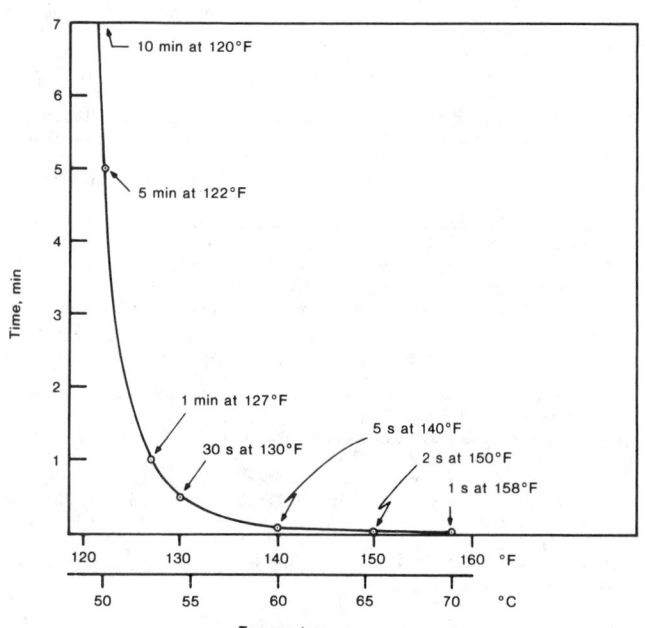

Figure 104–1. Duration of exposure to hot water to cause full-thickness epidermal burns of adult skin at various water temperatures. (From Katcher ML. Scald burns from hot tap water. JAMA 1981; 246:1219. Modified from Moritz AR, Henriques FC Jr. Studies of thermal injury. Am J Pathol 1947;23:695. Copyright 1981, American Medical Association.)

TABLE 104–1

DEGREE BURNS

Severity	Clinical Presentation	Healing
First degree	Red, blanching, pain	3–5 days
Partial thickness		
Superficial	Blisters, moist pain	10–18 days
Deep	Pale white, pain	21–28 days
Full thickness	Dry white, leathery to touch	Grafting necessary
Fourth degree	Damage to fat, fascia, muscle	Does not heal

and change as they mature. The infant's and child's head is proportionally larger and the extremities smaller in surface area than those of adults. The Lund and Browder chart gives accurate estimates of the BSA involved (Fig. 104–2).[14] First-degree burns are not usually included in the calculation of fluid requirements.

Pathophysiology

Pathophysiologic determinants of the depth of burn include (1) temperature, (2) time of exposure, and (3) tissue conductance of the skin.[15] The relationship of temperature and time is logarithmic (Table 104–2). The child's skin is thinner than that of the adult and therefore allows greater conductance of heat. It follows that children are more sensitive to thermal injury than adults.[16]

The concept of "concentric zones of thermal injury"[17] furthers an understanding of the pathophysiology of burns. The innermost zone, the zone of coagulation, is the central area where the cells are destroyed by coagulation necrosis. The next zone is the zone of stasis, which may survive or die depending on the various vascular and vasoactive factors occurring during the next 24 to 48 hours. The zone of stasis can be affected by resuscitative efforts. In the third and outermost zone, the zone of hyperemia, the cells sustain minimal injury and recover completely in 7 to 14 days. These zones are not static but can change with time. For example, a zone of stasis can become a zone of coagulation if the burn becomes infected or desiccated, or is improperly treated.

Causes

Scald burns are the most common cause of thermal injuries in children. Spills, usually involving coffee or tea, can result in superficial partial-thickness burns with irregular margins that heal in 10 to 14 days with minimal scarring. Hot grease retains more heat and can cause full-thickness burns.

Immersion burns, usually caused by hot tap water, are

TABLE 104–2

SCALD BURNS

Time	Temperature (F)
10 min	120°
5 min	122°
1 min	127°
30 sec	130°
5 sec	140°
1 sec	158°

These times reflect the duration of exposure to varied water temperatures to cause full-thickness scald burns in adults.

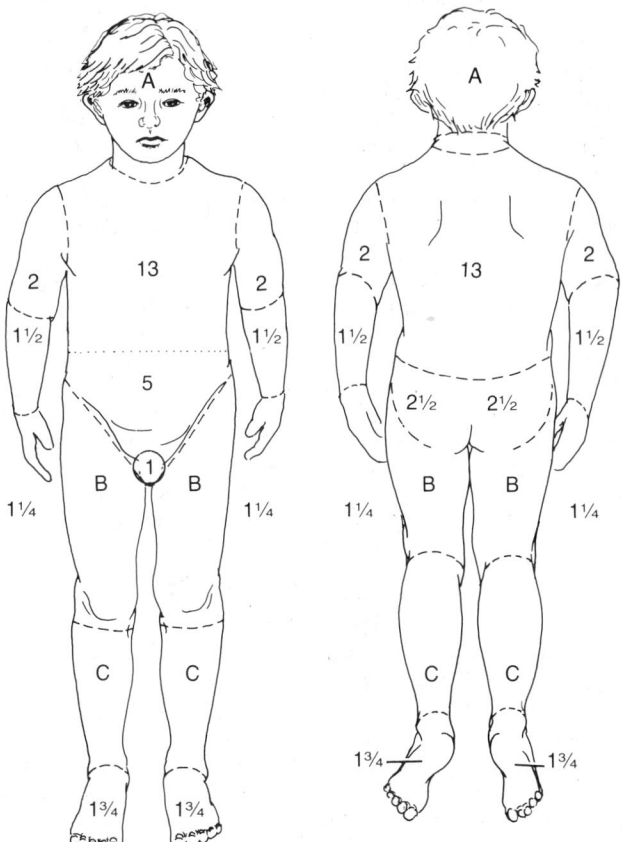

LUND AND BROWDER CHART

Age (years):	0	1	5	10	15	Adult
A: Half of head	9½	8½	6½	5½	4½	3½
B: Half of thigh	2¾	3¼	4	4¼	4½	4¾
C: Half of leg	2½	2½	2¾	3	3¼	3½

Total area burned = second-degree surface area and third-degree surface area

Initial fluid maintenance: Ringer's lactate solution* given at:

$$\frac{\text{Surface area burned} \times \text{weight (kg)}}{4} = * \text{ml/hr}$$

*Some authors recommend adding sodium bicarbonate or 5% albumin to the solution.

Figure 104–2. Lund and Browder charts are somewhat more accurate in estimating percentage of body surface burn than the rule of nines. Compared with adults, children have larger heads and smaller legs. Other areas are not relatively equivalent throughout life. The rule of nines is not accurate in determining the percentage of surface area burns in children. (From Roberts JR, Hedges JR. Clinical Procedures in Emergency Medicine. 2nd ed. Philadelphia, WB Saunders, 1991, pp 614–615.)

commonly deep partial thickness or full thickness with straight margins. These can be nonaccidental. They usually heal with scarring. Steam generally causes prompt and severe burns to the respiratory tract. Intense laryngospasm may occur; steam burns involving the larynx are usually fatal. Flash burns are caused by ignition of gases. Contact burns are often the result of an infant touching a hot iron, curling iron, or radiator. Older children frequently burn their inner legs on moped exhaust pipes. Contact burns from molten metal are usually severe: full thickness or greater. Flame burns are caused by direct contact with a flame and are generally full thickness. Chemical burns result from exposure to acids or alkali. Acids cause burning by coagulation necrosis and precipitation of protein. Alkalis produce liquefaction necrosis and cause loosening of tissue matrix, thus increasing the spread of the agent,[18] and therefore are usually more serious. Immediate and continuous irrigation with water for at least half an hour is necessary to prevent continued further penetration of alkalis and to reduce the tissue pH.[19] This neutralizing effect can be demonstrated for up to 20 minutes with acid burns and up to 1 hour with alkali burns. Acids should not be neutralized with a base because the reactions are exothermic and can cause additional thermal injury. Electrical burns cause extensive damage to fascia and muscle that belies the often small entrance and exit wounds. Although serious injuries are usually caused by high voltage (more than 500 volts), even household current can produce morbidity, notably electric cord burns to the commissure of the mouth caused by an infant biting an electrical cord. It is important to realize that when the eschar separates (usually during the second week), there can be life-threatening bleeding from the labial artery. Explosive burns usually involve accidents with firecrackers, which can cause full-thickness injuries and may result in significant trauma, especially to the hands and eyes. Radiation burns, with the exception of sunburns, are uncommon.

EMERGENCY MEDICAL SERVICE (EMS) CONSIDERATIONS

The EMS responders can provide valuable historical information from the scene of a fire. It is important to know whether patients were exposed to a large amount of smoke or may have suffered trauma from falling, jumping, or having the roof fall on them. The initial assessment of the patient, particularly the level of consciousness and respiratory effort, is important. The initial treatment (cardiopulmonary resuscitation [CPR], oxygen therapy) is of prognostic value and can influence further treatment especially regarding smoke inhalation.

EMS resuscitative efforts may include basic airway management, CPR, immobilizing patients with suspected axial injuries, establishing vascular access for fluids and possible drug administration, removing clothing, cooling the area of burn, irrigating areas of chemical or radiation contamination, and providing clean, preferably sterile dressings.

THERAPEUTIC INTERVENTION
Initial Resuscitation

Maintaining the airway is the first priority and intubation should be considered early if there is airway compromise. The usual indications for intubating a burned patient include evidence of thermal injury to the airway such as stridor, hoarseness, carbonized sputum, singed nasal hairs, and blistering of the palate or tongue, all of which indicate upper airway damage. Additional indications for intubation include a depressed level of consciousness, respiratory distress, and serious burns or swelling of the neck. Nasal tracheal intubation is usually preferred because it is better tolerated. For many patients, extubation is possible in 3 to 5 days. The neck should be immobilized in the neutral position before intubation if there is a suggestion of cervical injury.

All patients involved in a house fire or any fire in which they were exposed to smoke should receive 100% humidified oxygen at the scene. All forms of smoke inhalation, especially carbon monoxide, are treated with 100% oxygen. Oxygen is also required for patients in shock.

Smoke inhalation may result in serious respiratory compromise. The patient may appear cyanotic. Rales, wheezing, or rhonchi can be heard on auscultation. The patient who sustains trauma either during the fire or during ventilatory resuscitative measures may develop a pneumothorax. If there are deep burns to the circumference of the chest, massive edema may cause restriction of respiratory efforts and respiratory compromise.

An intravenous line should be established in patients with 20% or more burn or with major electrical burns. Intravenous sites are preferably in noninvolved extremities. Sterile technique should be used to prevent infections. Medical providers should wear gowns, gloves, caps, and masks. Central lines should be avoided whenever possible because of the high complication rate of infection, including septic thrombophlebitis. Generally, central lines are used only for burns involving more than 50% of the surface area. It may be necessary, especially in young infants, to begin fluid resuscitation through an intraosseous needle, the preferred site being the proximal tibia with intact overlying skin.

Tissue Resuscitation

Immediately after a burn, there is cessation of blood flow to the zone of coagulation and the beginning of an inflammation reaction. There is vasodilation to the remaining microvascularity. Within minutes after the burn, gaps between the endothelial cells are noted on electromicroscopy, allowing permeability of macromolecules of 150 angstroms and smaller.[20] These gaps may be caused by the direct effect of heat or by certain vasoactive substances (leukotrenes, prostaglandins, oxygen radicals, and histamine), or by both. They cause a large fluid and protein movement from the vascular to the interstitial space, beginning within the first several hours and sometimes lasting several days. The result is edema at the burn site, which can have deleterious effects on skin healing.

With burns of more than 30% BSA, in addition to edema localized to the burn itself, there is generalized edema in nonburned tissues.[21] In a 50% burn, 50% of the resuscitative fluid enters nonburned tissue,[22] and this may include the lung, GI tract, and soft tissue. Edema in the lung can cause pulmonary congestion. Gastrointestinal ileus may be the result in part of edema of the elementary tract. There are at least two proposed mechanisms for edema in nonburned tissue. The first and probably most important is the migration of protein from the intravascular to the interstitial space. The second theoretical cause of nonburned tissue edema is a decrease in the cell transmembrane potential.

These changes help to explain the often prolonged decrease in plasma volume. The plasma loss has been estimated at over 4 ml/kg/hr in burns of over 30% BSA.[21] Sodium is lost both into the cells and into the burn eschar.

Cardiac output is significantly depressed in burns of more than 40% BSA, probably secondary to hypovolemia.[23] Although the theory is controversial, it is postulated that in large burns a circulating myocardial depressant factor is present that also contributes to decreased cardiac output.[22, 24]

Cardiac output has usually recovered before normal plasma volume is restored.[18] It is not uncommon to have adequate cardiac output and perfusion coexisting with low central venous pressure and pulmonary artery wedge pressure. Likewise, the release of catecholamines may preserve blood pressure during a hypovolemic state. Therefore, a drop in blood pressure may be a late, ominous finding.

Urinary output is considered to be a guide to the adequacy of circulatory resuscitation; the goal is 1 ml/kg/hr of urinary output.[25] With burns, however, this reading can be misleading: urine production varies hourly in children. In addition, vasoactive agents, catecholamines, antidiuretic hormone, and aldosterone can influence urinary output. Hypertonic resuscitation solutions or hyperglycemia can also produce inaccurate urine measurements. Urinary output should therefore be viewed in relation to the patient's total pathophysiologic condition: 0.5 ml/kg/hr or less may be acceptable for a short time.

Fluid Resuscitation

Fluid resuscitation has four ideal objectives: (1) to establish circulatory function to support organ functions, (2) to promote blood flow to the skin in order to maximize burn healing, (3) to correct acid-base abnormalities with adequate fluid resuscitation, and (4) to minimize both local and general edema.

The primary objective during the initial resuscitation is to restore perfusion, not necessarily return the plasma volume to normal. Capillary leaks are increased directly by the rate of infusion; attempts at rapid and total restoration of plasma volume can lead to rapid edema.

There are many different methods of fluid resuscitation in burn patients and there is no general agreement on a preferred method; all are probably successful in organ resuscitation. However, some regimens may minimize the morbidity associated with localized and generalized edema.

Initial resuscitative fluids need not contain potassium. Potassium is released from heat-damaged cells, and the addition of potassium is initially not required. Potassium also should not be given until adequate kidney function is confirmed.

Parkland Formula

The most commonly used formula is the Parkland: lactated Ringer's solution, 4 ml/kg/% BSA burn, in the first 24 hours.[26] Generally, half of the recommended amount is given during the first 8 hours and the remainder evenly over the next 16 hours. Since few patients stay in the emergency department longer than the first 8 hours, the Parkland formula for this early period is amended as follows:

$$\text{IV rate in ml/hr} = \frac{\text{Wgt (kg)} \times \% \text{ BSA burned}}{4}$$

The total amount infused, however, depends on the individual response. Maintenance fluids must be added to this formula. Although its effectiveness has been questioned,[18, 27] Ringer's lactate solution has the advantage of being inexpensive and readily available. However, a considerable portion of the solution ends up in tissue as edema, and patients tend to remain hypovolemic. This is an important consideration if early wound excision is planned. Also, severe hypoproteinemia can further aggravate edema formation.

Hypertonic Saline

Other formulas increasingly advocated are the various hypertonic saline solutions (240 to 300 mEq/L sodium) with or without albumin.[28] Patients receiving these solutions require less fluid volume.[28–30] Because sodium does not cross into the cell, intracellular water is drawn from the cell to the extravascular space. The hypertonicity therefore may decrease the influx of fluid into the burn site, thereby potentially minimizing edema location.[14] Hypertonic saline solutions also increase myocardial contractility, produce precapillary dilatation, and decrease vascular resistance. There is also a decrease in pulmonary vascular resistance and in pulmonary edema.

The natriuresis produced by hypertonic solutions makes monitoring of urinary output somewhat unreliable, so it is

TABLE 104–3

CARVAL'S FORMULA FOR ELECTROLYTE SOLUTIONS FOR BURN RESUSCITATION

	Children	Infants
Sodium	132 mEq/L	81 mEq/L
Chloride	109 mEq/L	61 mEq/L
Bicarbonate		20 mEq/L
Lactate	26.6 mEq/L	
Glucose	47.8 gm/L	46.5 gm/L
Albumin	12.5 gm/L	12.5 gm/L
Potassium	3.8 mEq/L	0

recommended that the serum sodium level not exceed 160 mEq/L. One such solution contains sodium (250 mEq/L), chloride (150 mEq/L), and racemic lactate (100 mEq/L). This solution is given at 2 ml/kg/% BSA for the first 24 hours.

Albumin

Another type of hydrating solution contains colloid. Unburned tissue regains normal permeability after 8 hours. Studies suggest that colloid or albumin resuscitation should begin within the first 12 to 18 hours. The protein helps preserve intravascular oncotic pressure.[31] The ideal dosage of protein infusate is unknown.

Colloid products have some disadvantages. Albumin is expensive. Plasma has the potential of transmitting infections, including human immunodeficiency virus (HIV) and causing allergic reactions.

A balanced electrolyte-albumin solution has been used in children with great success by Carvagal and Parks.[32, 33] Using the surface area rather than body weight in the calculations may give a more accurate estimate of fluid needs (Fig. 104–3). When weight rather than surface area is calculated, small children with a small burn and older children with extensive burns are overhydrated. Because infants need less sodium than school-age children, two different solutions are used (Table 104–3). The volume of fluid given is based on square meters of surface area (Table 104–4). With this resuscitation schedule, potassium phosphate (20 to 30 mEq/L) is added after 12 hours when kidney function has been demonstrated to be adequate to prevent hypophosphatemia.

Dextran

Dextran, a chain polymer of glucose, is prepared in three forms (40,000, 70,000, and 150,000 molecular weight). It is metabolized and excreted by the kidney, about 40% being excreted in the urine during the first 24 hours. Compared with lactated Ringer's, dextran more significantly increases cardiac output and requires only half as much fluid. Dextran also reduces nonburn edema, yet has no effect on the edema

TABLE 104–4

CARVAL'S FORMULA FOR VOLUME OF FLUID IN FIRST 24 HOURS

Total volume estimate
   5000 ml/m² of burn
      plus
   2000 ml/m² of total body surface area
Infusion rate
   One-half volume given first 8 hr
   Remaining half given next 16 hr

of the burn itself. Urinary output is also increased, probably as a result of clearance of dextran compounds. This can make urinary output measurements of limited value in assessing the success of volume restoration. Once the infusion of dextran is stopped and is cleared into the urine, fluid loss into unburned tissue markedly increases secondary to the resultant hypoproteinemia. Serious hypotension can ensue. Dextran can cause allergic reactions, although this is rare. There have also been reports of interference with blood typing, platelet dysfunction, and bleeding difficulties. Bleeding dyscrasias, however, do not seem to occur with the recommended dose of less than 2 ml/kg/% BSA.

There is considerable controversy over the best fluid resuscitation regimen. In fact, different solutions may be suitable for different circumstances. Children with smaller percentage BSA burns of less than 50% and without inhalation injuries can be successfully resuscitated initially with lactated Ringer's or a balanced electrolyte-albumin solution. Patients with larger burns where general edema and hypovolemia are a serious consideration may appropriately require hypertonic saline, colloid, or dextran solutions. Certainly, there is more experience with lactated Ringer's and balanced electrolyte solutions in pediatric patients.[34]

SECONDARY SURVEY

The secondary survey includes evaluation for associated conditions such as intra-abdominal injuries, head injuries, fractures, and vascular injuries. Burns involving extremities should be examined carefully for compartment syndrome. This is usually associated with full-thickness circumferential burns and can occur within a few hours after the burn. All rings and bracelets should be removed. Pulse, capillary refill, color changes, and sensory and motor function should be carefully assessed. Because of the smaller diameter of their digits, children are more prone to vascular compromise. Serial circumferential measurement should be obtained in serious burns to the extremity. Numbness or deep throbbing pain are early signs of ischemia. Doppler, ultrasonic flowmeter, and tissue pressure manometers can be helpful in determining the adequacy of blood flow.[35] If there is significant vascular compromise, an escharotomy should be performed. Small escharotomies can be performed in the emergency department and usually involve limited bleeding and pain. The incision should extend the entire length of the eschar in the midlateral and midmedial aspect of the extremity to a depth sufficient for the edges of the eschar to separate.[36] Occasionally, escharotomy is necessary for circumferential burns to the chest. Parallel incisions are made along the anterior axillary lines to the waist, and another incision connects the two parallel incisions at the xyphoid.[16]

Burned extremities should be elevated and wrapped, beginning distally and proceeding proximally, to help prevent vascular compromise. Evaluation of burns around the orbits, especially ignition burns, should include an examination of the eyes with fluorescein to exclude corneal damage. Contact lenses sometimes worn by older children should be removed. The patient's mental status should be assessed: restlessness, confusion, or lethargy may indicate hypoxemia or shock.

Generally, placement of a urinary catheter with hourly monitoring of urinary output is necessary in patients with burns involving more than 20% of BSA. An adequate hourly output is 0.5 to 1.0 ml/kg, although this can vary from hour to hour. The urine should be examined for blood and myoglobin; both are common after extensive burns, especially electrical burns (Table 104–5). If there is significant myoglobinuria or hemoglobinuria, the fluid administration

TABLE 104–5

DIAGNOSTIC EVALUATION

Several baseline laboratory studies should be obtained:

Complete blood count. Hematocrit is usually elevated from loss of intravascular fluid; this should decrease with successful fluid resuscitation. White blood cell count can be elevated secondary to stress. Platelet count is often elevated.

Electrolytes. Potassium can be elevated from cellular destruction. Serum bicarbonate should be normal. Persistent acidosis implies continuing hypovolemic shock.

Glucose. Release of catecholamines can result in hyperglycemia.

Blood urea nitrogen (BUN). Hypotension may elevate BUN. Increasing BUN may signal impending renal failure.

Urinalysis. Urine should be examined for red blood cells, myoglobin, and hemoglobin. Reagents in most dip tests react positively to both myoglobin and hemoglobin. Urine specific gravity reflects circulatory status.

Total protein. Preservation of adequate levels of intravascular protein is vital to maintain adequate vascular volume. Serial serum protein analysis can indicate need for additional protein infusion.

Prothrombin/partial thromboplastin time (PT/PTT). Disseminated intravascular coagulopathy (DIC) has been associated with burns and frequently results in abnormal PT/PTT.

Blood type and crossmatch. Blood is rarely required during initial resuscitation but may be needed later for grafting, which can cause significant blood loss.

Chest radiography. Usually helpful if there is exposure to smoke or trauma.

rate should be increased to encourage a brisk diuresis. Also, 0.5 to 1.0 gm/kg of mannitol or 1 mg/kg of furosemide can be administered intravenously and repeated until the urine is clear.

Since patients with more than a 20% burn often have an adynamic ileus, a nasogastric (NG) tube attached to suction is indicated. Some centers advocate the use of an antacid, 30 ml/m²/hr, through the NG tube to help prevent ulcers (Fig. 104–3).

INITIAL CARE

Cooling decreases the severity of the burn if administered within 30 minutes of the time of injury; it also helps to relieve pain.[37] However, hypothermia is a problem in the pediatric age group, and cooling is not recommended for burns of more than 10% BSA.[38] Unfortunately, no studies specify the optimal duration and degree of cooling in children. Generally, sterile dressings soaked in cool and preferably sterile water are used. Extremely cold temperatures are avoided to prevent tissue damage from freezing.

All devitalized tissue and broken blisters should be debrided. Necrotic tissue is prone to infection. Whether or not to break and debride intact blisters remains controversial. Some believe that blisters should remain intact to prevent the migration of bacteria into the burn; others feel that since most blisters will soon rupture spontaneously anyway and since the necrotic roof of the blister can encourage infection, intact blisters should be broken and debrided. A reasonable approach is to leave thick blisters on the palm or sole intact, but to debride thin blisters. Children are not likely to protect blisters from rupturing. Some physicians recommend shaving the hair around the burn, but this is controversial.

Infection is a major cause of increased morbidity and mortality. Burns cause infection in three major ways: destruction of the skin allows the entry of bacteria locally and

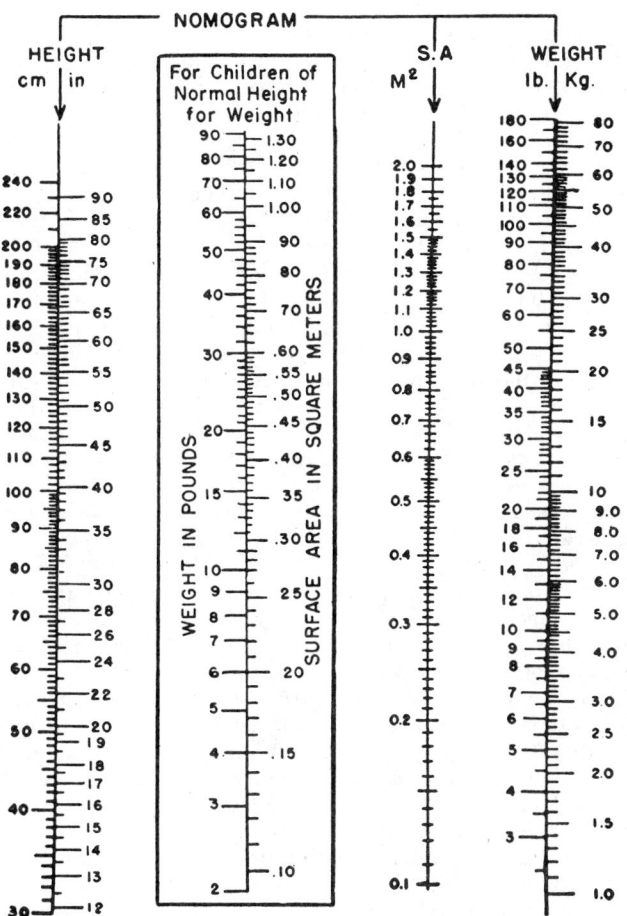

── NOMOGRAM ──

HEIGHT
cm | in

For Children of
Normal Height
for Weight

S.A
M²

WEIGHT
lb. | Kg.

Figure 104–3. Nomogram for estimation of surface area. The surface area is indicated where a straight line that connects the height and weight levels intersects the surface area column; or if the patient is roughly of average size, from the weight alone (*enclosed area*). (Nomogram modified from data of E. Boyd by C.D. West. From Behrman RE, Vaughan VC III. Nelson Textbook of Pediatrics. 13th ed. Philadelphia, WB Saunders, 1987, p 1521.)

into the blood, devitalized tissue and eschar are excellent media for bacterial growth, and major burns result in a profound systemic immunologic deficiency affecting humoral and cellular defense processes.

TREATMENT

Various biologic and synthetic dressings and antimicrobial agents are used to treat the injured skin. The goal for topical treatment is prevention of infection. Colonization of the patient's own staphylococcal organisms begins within a few hours after a burn; 3 to 5 days later, gram-negative organisms predominate. Because burned skin is ischemic, systemic antibiotics have little effect. Although various biologic dressings, allographs, xerographs, and homographs are of value in burn units, they are seldom used in the emergency department setting. The most commonly used burn therapy consists of topical antimicrobials; the mortality rate in burn patients has halved since their prevalent use. There is no ideal topical antimicrobial. In addition, all these agents impair reepithelization to varying degrees,[39] and bacterial resistance can develop, especially in burns of more than 50% BSA.

The most commonly used topical antimicrobial is silver sulfadiazine, a 1% white, water-soluble cream. It can be used open (without dressings) but is generally used either closed (covered with a dressing) or semiclosed (with impregnated mesh gauze) in children. The dressings are changed twice each day. The antimicrobial's mechanism of action seems to be primarily on the bacterial cell wall, but may also involve intracellular DNA replication. Silver sulfadiazine is relatively painless, easy to use, nonstaining, penetrating, and relatively effective. However, microbial resistance can occur, especially in large burns. The side effects are relatively rare. Four to nine percent of patients develop a mild rash, which is well tolerated and transient. Leukopenia can develop within the first 5 days but usually returns to normal even with continued use. Crystalluria and methemoglobinemia are rarely reported. A pseudoeschar or "peel" forms on the burn surface and may make it difficult to determine burn depth. There has been one report of an 8-month-old infant who developed hyperosmolarity from transdermal absorption of propylene glycol, a component of silver sulfadiazine. This hyperosmolarity may have contributed to the patient's death.

Silver nitrate (0.5% aqueous solution) has been used since 1965 for the treatment of burns. Its main advantages are that it is essentially painless and there is no hypersensitivity. However, it has several disadvantages. Because it is markedly hypotonic, significant leaching of sodium, potassium, and other solutes can occur. It has been estimated that 350 mEq or more of sodium can be lost for each square meter of burn surface per day. Silver nitrate also has minimal penetration into the eschar and therefore is less effective for infected burns. Some bacteria, particularly gram-negative organisms, can reduce nitrate to nitrite, resulting in rare cases of methemoglobinemia. Application is messy and time consuming: thick cotton dressings are soaked with silver nitrate every 2 hours. Virtually everything that silver nitrate touches turns brown or black. Silver salts become encrusted on newly healed skin and are difficult to remove.

Mafenide acetate 10%, a methylated sulfonamide, deeply penetrates eschar and is not appreciably bound by protein or inactivated by wound exudates. It therefore is particularly useful in the treatment of deep, electrical, or infected burns. One of mafenide's major disadvantages is that it is quite painful, probably because of its high osmolarity. It is a powerful carbonic anhydrase inhibitor and can cause a brisk alkaline diuresis. Metabolites of mafenide are acidotic and can lead to a hyperchloremic metabolic acidosis, especially in burns of more than 20% BSA. Discontinuing mafenide therapy usually reverses this side effect in 24 to 36 hours. Rarely, hemolytic anemia has been associated with mafenide. Because of the side effects, the use of this agent is restricted to selected situations and brief periods of treatment. Application is by the open method twice daily.

Monitoring

Patients with major burns should be carefully monitored, and vital signs taken every 15 minutes initially. Body temperature should be monitored. A slight fever is common, but pediatric patients with large burns are likely to suffer from hypothermia. Weight, pulse, urinary output, and central venous pressure should also be checked; Swan-Ganz monitoring may be necessary in large burns (Table 104–6). If there is any suggestion of smoke inhalation or respiratory compromise, serial arterial blood gases and pulse oximetry should be monitored. If carbon monoxide inhalation is suspected, a carboxyhemoglobin level should be obtained. Frequently, arterial blood gases, pulse oximetry, and even carboxyhemoglobin levels do not accurately reflect the degree of hypoxia or central nervous system insult resulting from carbon monoxide. Circumferential full-thickness extremity burns should be checked for vascular compromise, and circumferential chest burns for respiratory insufficiency.

TABLE 104–6

INDICATIONS OF SUCCESSFUL RESUSCITATION

1. Clear sensorium without restlessness
2. Controlled pain
3. Urinary output 0.5–1.0 ml/kg/hr
4. Normal to slightly elevated temperature
5. Adequate blood pressure and pulse
6. Good capillary refill
7. Normal central monitoring parameters (if done)

Antibiotics

Prophylactic penicillin is no longer used at most burn centers. Tetanus toxoid (0.5 ml intramuscularly) should be provided if the patient is immunosuppressed or has not received tetanus immunization in the previous 5 years.[40] Tetanus immune globulin (250 to 500 units) in addition to tetanus toxoid should be administered if the patient has had fewer than two tetanus immunizations, or if the last injection was given more than 10 years previously.

Analgesia

Burns are painful and intravenous morphine can be given (0.05 to 0.10 mg/kg). The IV route is preferred to the IM because the dosage can be more easily titrated, the duration of action is relatively short, and there is less danger of the drug being sequestered if there is inadequate circulatory resuscitation.[41]

Outpatient Burn Treatment

The physician must determine whether to admit the patient (Table 104–7). The most crucial and often the most difficult consideration is the ability of the parents to care for a burn at home. Burns in children and especially in infants are more difficult to treat than those in adults. Children are active, and burn dressings take a great deal of abuse. Also, many parents are reluctant to change dressings and debride burns in their own children. Children are usually uncooperative and there is almost always some pain involved.

The key to successful outpatient burn management is prevention of infection and close follow-up. The initial approach includes cleaning and debridement with mild soap and water. It is helpful in debridement of superficial partial-thickness burns to minimize contact with the damaged skin by using forceps or sterile gauze to pick up the edges of the dead skin and peel it off the base of the burn. For practical reasons, burns in outpatient children should be treated with closed or semiclosed technique, although minor burns to the face are often treated with open technique.[22]

A common method of treatment of burns on an outpatient basis uses silver sulfadiazine or a nonadherent impregnated gauze, and an outer layer of bulky gauze. The bulky gauze helps absorb the exudate. Elastic mesh often helps keep this dressing in place. The dressing is changed after 3 to 4 days or sometimes later.[37, 42]

TABLE 104–7

ADMISSION CRITERIA

1. 10% or greater body surface area partial thickness burn
2. 2% or greater body surface area full thickness burn
3. Burns to the hands, feet, face, or perineum
4. Social concerns (safety of the home environment)
5. Associated injuries such as smoke inhalation or major trauma
6. Chemical, explosive, or electrical burns

Another method is to use topical antimicrobial agents and frequent dressing changes. No single topical antimicrobial has proved superior, although several have been used. A common method is to clear the burn, apply silver sulfadiazine to the burn twice a day with a sterile tongue blade, and cover with a light layer of gauze.[43] This method has the advantage of a light semiclosed dressing and allows for frequent observation of the wound. However, it is time consuming and relatively expensive.

The last several years have seen a third technique for treating burns in outpatients: synthetic skin substitutes, i.e., Biobrane, Op-Site, Duroderm, and Epilock. These are constructed of various synthetics such as silicone polymers, polyvinylchloride, and polyurethane. Although all are different structurally, to some degree they share the properties of vapor and gas permeability in providing oxygen to the wound to prevent desiccation and excessive exudate formation, prevent infection, and promote reepithelialization.

It is necessary for these skin substitute dressings to be adherent to the burn and occlusive to prevent wound desiccation and migration of bacteria into the wound.[44] Large wounds require overlapping sheets. The dressings can be left in place for various periods, 1 day to several weeks.[45] Two disadvantages of these dressings are that it is difficult to keep them adherent for long periods to unusual contours of the body, and that some are not transparent, making access to check for infection difficult. The chief advantages are that dressing changes are infrequent, and application is easy. They also are relatively inexpensive and can be stored for prolonged periods. Studies suggest that the use of these dressings may result in decreased pain and improved reepithelialization compared with topical antimicrobials.[35, 46, 47]

Whichever method is used, it is often best to provide the necessary materials to the parents before discharge of the child. The dressing materials are expensive and often not covered by health plans and insurance carriers. It is helpful to demonstrate the dressing change technique. For mild analgesia, acetaminophen is helpful. For more painful burns in older children, codeine may be prescribed (0.5 to 1.0 mg/kg/dose every 4 to 6 hours). Later in the course of treatment, burns may become pruritic. An antihistamine usually is the only necessary treatment.[48] Initial follow-up to monitor for infection should be arranged for 1 to 2 days after discharge.

Some studies have used various antiprostaglandins and antithromboxane agents in the treatment of burns.[49] Such agents (e.g., steroids, indomethacin, aspirin) have been shown to decrease dermal ischemia in experimental animals.[45] Likewise, topical ibuprofen decreases early burn edema in sheep.[50] The extent of the role of anti-inflammatories in the management of burns in pediatric patients is unclear.

References

1. Durtschi MB, Kohler TR, Finley A, Helmbach DM. Burn injury in infants and young children. Surg Gynecol Obstet 1980;150:651.
2. Carvajal HF, Parks DH. Epidemiology. In Burns in Children: Pediatric Burn Management. Chicago: Year Book, 1988, pp 3–24.
3. O'Neil JA. Burns. Top Emerg Med 1982;4:28.
4. Libber S, Stayton M, Donelda J. Childhood burns reconsidered: The child, the family and the burn injury. J Trauma 1984;24:245.
5. Stair TO, Dorta J, Altieri MF, et al. Polyurethane and silver sulfadiazine dressing in the treatment of partial thickness burns and abrasions. Am J Emerg Med 1986;4:214.
6. Purdue G, Hunt JL, Prescott PR. Child abuse by burning, an index of suspicion. J Trauma 1988;28:221.
7. Antonacci AC. How do immunomodulators affect host defense in the burn patient? J Trauma 1984;24:101.
8. Feldman KW, Schaller RT, Feldman JA, et al. Tap water scald burns in children. Pediatrics 1978;62:1.
9. Heggers JP, Robson MC. Prostaglandins and thromboxane. Crit Care Clin 1985;1:59.

10. Thacker JC, Kenney JG, Stafford J, et al. Scald burns. Curr Concepts Trauma Care 1983;1:1.
11. Sando WC, Gallaher KJ, Rodgers BM. Risk factors for microwave scald injuries in infants. J Pediatr 1984;105:864.
12. Cohen CC. Burns in children. Pediatr Ann 1987;16:328.
13. Blank IH. What are the functions of skin lost in burn injury that affect short and long term recovery? J Trauma 1984;24:S10.
14. Bowser BH, Caldwell FT. The effects of resuscitation with hypertonic vs hypotonic vs colloid on wound and urine fluid and electrolyte losses in severely burned children. J Trauma 1983;23:916.
15. Boykin JV, Cruite SL. Mechanism of burn shock protection after severe scald injury by cold water treatment. J Trauma 1982;22:859.
16. Baxter CR. Emergency treatment of burn injury. Ann Emerg Med 1988;17:13.
17. Achauer BM, Martinez SE. Burn wound pathophysiology. Critical care clinic. 1985;1:47.
18. Mozingo DW, Smith AA, McManus WF, et al. Chemical burns. J Trauma 1988;28:642.
19. Luteman A, Fields C, Currier W. Treatment of chemical burns. Emerg Med Serv 1988;17:36.
20. Demling RH. Fluid resuscitation after major burns. JAMA 1983;250:1438.
21. Demling RH. Fluid and electrolyte management. Crit Care Clin 1985;1:27.
22. DeSantes D, Phillip P, Spotti HA, et al. Delayed appearance of a circulating myocardial depressant factor in burn patients. Ann Emerg Med 1981;10:22.
23. Cioffi WG, DeMeules JE, Gamelli RL. The effects of burn injury and fluid resuscitation on cardiac function in vitro. J Trauma 1986;26:638.
24. Goodwin CW, Jones D, Lam V, Pruitt BA Jr. Randomized trial of efficacy of crystalloid and colloid resuscitation on hemodynamic response and lung water following thermal injury. Ann Surg 1983;197:520.
25. Carvajal HF, Parks DH. Controversies in fluid resuscitation and their impact on the pediatric population. In Burns in Children: Pediatric Burn Management. Chicago: Year Book, 1988, pp 71–77.
26. Baxter CR. Controversies in the resuscitation of burn shock. Curr Concepts Trauma Care 1982;Spring:5.
27. Graves TA, Cioffi WG, McManus WF, et al. Fluid resuscitation of infants and children with massive thermal injury. J Trauma 1988;28:1659.
28. Katcher ML. Scald burns from hot tap water. JAMA 1981;246:1219.
29. Caldwell FT, Bowser B. Critical evaluation of hypertonic and hypotonic solution to resuscitate severely burned children. Ann Surg 1979;189:546.
30. Monafo WW, Halverson JD, Schechtman K. The role of concentrated sodium solutions in the resuscitation of patients with severe burns. Surgery 1984;95:129.
31. Goodwin CW, Long JW, Mason AD, et al. Paradoxical effect of hyperoncotic albumin in acutely burned children. J Trauma 1988;28:1656.
32. Carvajal HF, Parks DH. Optimal composition of burn resuscitation fluids. Crit Care Med 1988;16:695.
33. Carvajal HF. A physiologic approach to fluid therapy in severely burned children. Surg Gynecol Obstet 1980;150:379.
34. Baxter CR. Guidelines for fluid resuscitation. J Trauma 1981;21:687.
35. Solomon JB. Pediatric burns. Crit Care Clin 1985;1:159.
36. Wachtel TL. Epidemiology, classification, initial care and administrative consideration for critically burned patients. Crit Care Clin 1985;1:3.
37. Raine T, Heggers JP, Robson MC, et al. Cooling the burn wound to maintain microcirculation. J Trauma 1981;21:394.
38. Robinson MD, Seward PN. Thermal injury in children. Pediatr Emerg Care 1987;3:266.
39. Herndon DN, Thompson PB, Desai MH, Van Osten TJ. Treatment for burns in children. Pediatr Clin North Am 1985;32:1311.
40. Arturson MG. The pathophysiology of severe thermal injury. J Burn Care Rehabil 1985;6:129.
41. Perry S, Inturrisi CE. Analgesia and morphine deposition in burn patients. J Bone Care Rehabil 1983;4:276.
42. Shuck LW, Shunk JM. The outpatient burn. Curr Concepts Trauma Care 1982;Spring:15.
43. Monafo WW, Freedman B. Topical therapy for burns. Surg Clin North Am 1987;67:133.
44. Demling RH. Burns. N Engl J Med 1985;313:1389.
45. Robson MC, DelBeccarro EJ, Heggers JP, et al: Increasing dermal perfusion after burning by decreasing thromboxane production. J Trauma 1980;20:722.
46. Gerdling RL, Imbembo AL, Frationne RB. Synthetic skin substitute vs 1% silver sulfadiazine for treatment of inpatient partial-thickness thermal burns. J Trauma 1988;28:1265.
47. Wayne MA. Clinical evaluation of Epi-Lock: A semiocclusive dressing. Ann Emerg Med 1985;14:20.
48. Warden C. Outpatient care of thermal injuries. Surg Clin North Am 1987;67:147.
49. DelBeccarro EJ, Robson MC, Heggers JP, et al. The use of specific thromboxane inhibitors to preserve the dermal microcirculation after burning. Surgery 1980;87:137.
50. Demling RH, Lalonde C. Topical ibuprofen decreases early postburn edema. Surgery 1987;102:857.

CHAPTER 105

Drowning and Near-Drowning

Ray E. Keller

INTRODUCTION

Drowning is second only to motor vehicle accidents as the most common cause of accidental death in children. More than 7000 childhood deaths each year are attributable to drowning, and the incidence continues to rise.

Drowning is death from suffocation by submersion in a liquid. *Near-drowning* is survival, sometimes temporary, following asphyxia from a submersion episode. Children are at highest risk for drowning, with 40% of drownings occurring in children less than 4 years old. These drownings are mainly due to toddlers being left unattended in pools or bathtubs; 25% to 31% of toddler drownings occur while the children are unattended in bathtubs. Of all infant and toddler drownings investigated by the Cook County Medical Examiner's Office in Illinois from January 1985 to June 1989, 24% occurred in 5-gallon industrial buckets. The buckets are constructed of heavy plastic and are often used with mops in the home. Infants, because of their cephalad center of gravity, can easily fall head first into these buckets. The buckets often do not tip over, and the child remains upside down. Finally, child abuse and neglect should be considered as a possible cause for drowning in children.

A second peak in drowning incidence is seen in 15 to 24 year olds. These victims are usually male, with alcohol and drugs commonly involved. The increased incidence in males is attributable to their greater exposure to hazardous activities stemming from societal and biologic influences.

Hypoxic lap swimmers hyperventilate before swimming in order to become hypocarbic; this causes less stimulus to breathe. However, before their carbon dioxide rises, producing the stimulus to breathe, some swimmers lose consciousness from hypoxia. Two to three percent of drownings occur during rescue attempts. Epileptics and the mentally retarded are also more likely to drown, and they require constant supervision around water.

Scuba divers usually drown from inexperience or carelessness. Cerebral artery air embolism occurs when the lungs overinflate during too rapid an ascent, causing rupture of the alveolar-capillary basement membrane. The air travels through the arterial circulation and lodges in the brain. These divers present with sudden focal or global neurologic deficits. Decompression sickness, commonly referred to as "the bends," also results from rapid surfacing. Nitrogen bubbles form in blood vessels and tissues, producing slow onset of joint and muscle pain, pulmonary edema, acute respiratory disease syndrome, and neurologic deficits. These symptoms occur after diving to 80 feet or more and present minutes to hours after the dive. Both cerebral artery air embolism and decompression sickness are treated with hyperbaric oxygen.

PHYSIOLOGY

In animal studies, fresh water and salt water produce different physiologic changes in the lungs. However, the physiologic changes in humans who reach the hospital with fresh-water drowning are not significantly different from those with salt-water drowning. Most victims aspirate 3 to 4 ml/kg of fluid; 22 ml/kg is necessary to produce electrolyte changes, and 11 ml/kg to alter blood volume. Fresh water produces atelectasis by destroying surfactant. Salt water will draw fluid into the alveolar space, producing pulmonary edema; the surfactant may be diluted but not destroyed. The injury to the alveoli and pulmonary capillaries results in increased membrane permeability with exudation of proteinaceous material into the alveolar space and pulmonary edema. The final common pathway for both fresh- and salt-water drowning is hypoxia and intrapulmonary shunting.

An individual's response to submersion can be divided into three stages (Table 105–1). In stage I a small amount of fluid is aspirated during an initial struggle; this produces laryngospasm. In stage II further hypoxia and panic ensue and a large volume of water is swallowed. Stage III occurs when the laryngospasm relaxes. In 85% of victims a large volume of water is aspirated (wet drowning), while in 15% a small aspiration produces another episode of laryngospasm (dry drowning). This second episode of laryngospasm produces severe hypoxia, seizures, and death. Victims of dry drowning have no pulmonary damage from aspiration.

Vomiting with subsequent aspiration of stomach contents also contributes to morbidity. This occurs from the struggling and swallowing of large volumes of water. The composition of the immersion liquid will contribute to the type of pneumonia that may develop. Patients who survive hot-tub immersions are likely to develop *Pseudomonas aeruginosa* pneumonia.

The pulmonary effects of alveolar and pulmonary capillary destruction result in ventilation-perfusion mismatch and intrapulmonary shunting, producing hypoxia and hypercarbia. The pulmonary edema that develops may be a late manifestation, depending on the amount of initial damage to pulmonary structures and composition of fluid aspirated (Fig. 105–1).

The damage to the central nervous system (CNS) is related to the amount of time the brain is hypoxic and the severity of the hypoxia. A period of cerebral hypoperfusion may result following a hypoxic brain insult. This may result in further CNS damage. The reasons for this hypoperfusion are poorly understood.

Hypoxic CNS injury is certainly the most common neurologic insult, but traumatic injuries also occur. The most common of these is cervical spine trauma following diving injuries. The cardiovascular effects result from hypoxia and acidosis. These include arrhythmias, a decrease in contractility, and cardiogenic shock. Most patients are hypovolemic from increased permeability of pulmonary and systemic capillaries. A minority of patients will have an elevated central venous pressure from pulmonary hypertension. Renal failure is relatively uncommon but may occur from hypoxia or myoglobinuria. Coagulation disorders, hemolysis, and disseminated intravascular coagulation have been reported in drowning victims. Precipitating events may be hypoxia, acidosis, hypoperfusion, sepsis, or hemolysis.

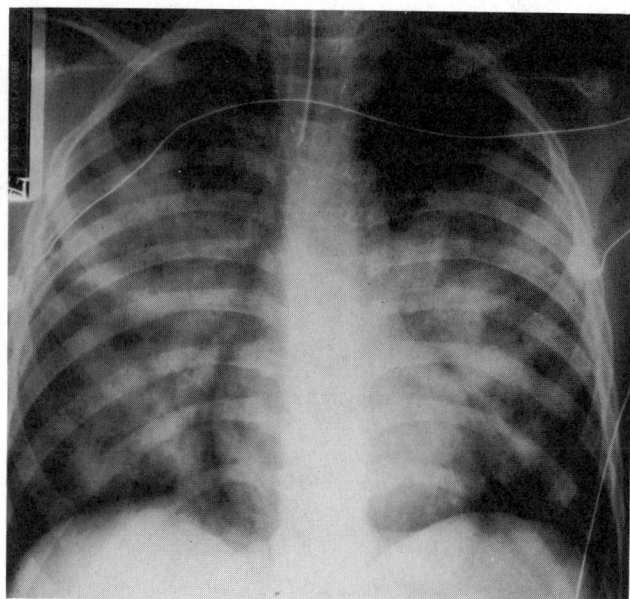

Figure 105–1. Two hours after an episode of near-drowning, this 8-year-old boy, now intubated, shows a characteristic bilateral "butterfly" configuration of unsharp parenchymal density representing acute pulmonary edema. Such edema may be delayed and therefore repeat films are often needed after a near-drowning event. (Courtesy of A. Oestreich, M.D., Cincinnati, OH.)

EMS CONSIDERATIONS

The initial management of emergent injuries begins with attention to airway, breathing, and circulation. The airway should be opened, and visible debris should be swept from the patient's mouth. These efforts can begin while the patient is still in the water. Attention must be paid to stabilizing the cervical spine if a spinal column injury is at all possible. Once removed from the water, chest compression should begin immediately, if necessary, and the airway suctioned. Spontaneously breathing patients should receive high-flow oxygen by a nonrebreather mask. If oxygenation by mask is in question, the patient should undergo endotracheal intubation. Indications for intubation include apnea, airway maintenance, excessive secretions, hypoxia, cyanosis, and hypercarbia. Cricoid pressure should be used during intubation to decrease the likelihood of aspiration. Postural drainage is not normally recommended, as this only delays restoration of oxygenation. Some advocate postural drainage only for salt-water drowning when water and pulmonary edema are interfering with effective ventilation. In no instance should time be wasted in attempting to drain fluid from the lungs in an apneic patient.

Most victims will be hypovolemic. A 20-ml/kg bolus of lactated Ringer's solution is recommended along with two large-bore intravenous lines.

Prehospital caveats include:

(1) Never withhold initial resuscitative efforts. Ten to twenty percent of patients who are initially comatose with fixed and dilated pupils experience full recovery.

(2) Do not prolong delay in transport in order to obtain intravenous access.

(3) Transport all patients to a hospital regardless of initial appearance.

(4) Remove wet clothing to prevent heat loss and to detect other injuries.

TABLE 105–1
INDIVIDUAL'S RESPONSE TO SUBMERSION

Stage I	Struggle → small aspiration → laryngospasm
Stage II	Increasing hypoxia and panic → larger volume of water swallowed
Stage III	Laryngospasm relaxes → large volume of water aspirated (85%)
	or
	Small aspiration → laryngospasm → severe hypoxia, seizure (dry drowning 15%)

THERAPEUTIC INTERVENTION
Initial Hospital Resuscitation

Evaluation begins with attention to airway with cervical spine control, breathing, and circulation. A history of events surrounding the immersion is helpful in influencing further diagnostic evaluation. Presentations range from asymptomatic individuals to those in cardiac arrest. All patients must have core temperatures measured to assess for hypothermia. Physical examination should be complete, with attention directed to the pulmonary, cardiac, and central nervous systems; signs of trauma should also be sought. Pulmonary examination may reveal rales, rhonchi, wheezing, or frothy sputum. Cardiac evaluation should focus on detection and treatment of arrhythmias. Neurologic examination includes the patient's level of consciousness, the Glasgow coma scale, and extremity movements.

Initial laboratory studies should include complete blood count with platelets, electrolytes, BUN, creatinine, prothrombin time, partial thromboplastin time, arterial blood gas, urinalysis, electrocardiogram (EKG), chest x-ray, and cervical spine radiograph. A head computed tomography scan and toxicology screen should be done in patients with an abnormal mental status. A nasogastric tube should be placed in patients who are artificially ventilated to decompress the stomach and reduce the likelihood of further aspiration.

Attention should be given to the possibility of barotrauma in patients receiving positive pressure ventilation. Resuscitation should continue for at least 30 minutes with patients in cardiac arrest. Longer efforts are required for hypothermic patients as well as those under the influence of barbiturates.

Treatment

Support of the pulmonary, cardiac, and central nervous systems is crucial. Alveolar gas exchange must be maintained and often requires continuous positive airway pressure or positive end-expiratory pressure. Positive pressure ventilation is the treatment for noncardiogenic pulmonary edema, which once instituted should be continued for at least 48 hours. This is necessary to permit adequate surfactant regeneration. Goals of ventilation continue to be maintaining a $PaCO_2$ less than 35 mm Hg and a PaO_2 greater than 100 mm Hg. Bronchospasm is common and should be treated with beta agonists and aminophylline. If aspiration has occurred, antibiotics should be started when signs of bacterial infection become evident. Initial choice of antibiotics should be based on sputum analysis. Clinical response combined with blood and sputum cultures will determine further antibiotic therapy. Effective pulmonary toilet is also important. Steroids should not be used for pulmonary aspiration, as no studies have shown them to be beneficial.

Definitive cardiac treatment is supportive with monitoring for arrhythmias. Treatment is according to advanced cardiac life support guidelines. Sodium bicarbonate should be given only for severe metabolic acidosis to improve myocardial contractility.

Cerebral damage produces the most devastating consequences of submersion injuries. Rapid restoration of oxygen delivery to the brain is most important for favorable outcome. Preventing the elevation of intracranial pressure is still attempted, although the efficacy is debated.

Victims who are comatose or who deteriorate neurologically should undergo intracranial pressure monitoring. If intracranial pressure is greater than 20 mm Hg or cerebral perfusion pressure is less than 60 mm Hg, intracranial pressure should be reduced. This is accomplished by (1)

maintaining the $PaCO_2$ between 25 and 30 mm Hg; (2) elevating the head 30 degrees; and (3) using furosemide or mannitol, which decreases extracellular fluid formation and subsequent cerebral edema. The use of furosemide or mannitol must be done with careful attention to vital signs, urinary output, and serum lactate levels to prevent shock. Cerebral oxygen requirements should also be kept at a minimum by preventing hyperpyrexia, using sedation including muscle paralysis, and inducing barbiturate coma. The use of hypothermia and steroids is generally not recommended for the control of cerebral edema. Both interfere with the body's immune response and have not been definitely shown to be beneficial.

No controlled prospective studies have shown that acutely lowering elevations in intracranial pressure affects outcome. It is possible that the initial period of hypoxia determines the future level of cerebral function. The late elevations of intracranial pressure seen in severely affected patients may be the result of the initial brain damage. Cerebral resuscitation represents a frontier in medicine, with the role of agents such as calcium channel blockers currently being investigated.

Late complications of immersion injuries are usually pulmonary. Pneumothorax or pneumomediastinum may develop from barotrauma. Pneumonia is common, and treatment should be based on sputum analysis; prophylactic antibiotics are not recommended. *P. aeruginosa* is a common cause of pneumonia following hot-tub immersion. Long-term survivors of near-drowning are predisposed to developing chronic lung disease. Large and small airway dysfunction as well as bronchial hyperactivity has been reported.

ICE-WATER DROWNING

Cases of survival following prolonged submersion in cold water have been reported. This dramatic event has been the subject of much debate and news media coverage. However, overall mortality is increased with hypothermia.

Survival after prolonged submersion occurs from a reduction in the basal metabolic rate (BMR). At 28°C the BMR is reduced by 50%. Infants are more likely to survive ice-water immersion, presumably on the basis of their large surface area. This allows for more rapid cooling. Another theory proposed is that infants have the primitive dive reflex that is seen in seals. This is thought to be augmented by submersion in cold water and by fear. Blood is shunted toward the heart, brain, and lungs and away from less oxygen-sensitive organs. However, some evidence suggests that this reflex is not operative in humans.

Hypothermia produces profound cardiovascular effects. Arrhythmias are common and include sinus bradycardia, atrial fibrillation, ventricular fibrillation at 28°C, and asystole at 22°C. The EKG may show inverted T waves or J (Osborn) waves. The oxygen-hemoglobin dissociation curve is shifted leftward, and arterial blood gases may have a falsely low pH with a falsely elevated $PaCO_2$ and PaO_2. Evidence has been reported that blood gas measurements may not have to be corrected for hypothermia.

Several points should be kept in mind when treating hypothermic patients: excessive manipulation may produce ventricular fibrillation; cardiac medications may be ineffective at low temperatures; toxicity may develop after rewarming; and resuscitation must continue until core temperature reaches 32°C.

PROGNOSIS

Patients who remain comatose for 2 to 6 hours after submersion do poorly. Patients showing any improvement

TABLE 105–2

ADMISSION CRITERIA

Submersion >1 min
History of cyanosis or apnea
Required artificial ventilation
Abnormal chest x-ray or arterial blood gas
Presence of any respiratory sign or symptom

in their neurologic examination during this period have a 50% chance of intact survival. Patients who respond to stimuli 2 to 6 hours after submersion will generally do well.

Allman et al. reported a series of 66 children who were victims of submersion episodes. All required cardiopulmonary resuscitation and had initial Glasgow coma scales of 3 upon arrival in the emergency department. Twenty-four percent of these survived neurologically intact. No patient with a Glasgow coma scale of 3 upon admission to the intensive care unit survived intact. Thus aggressive initial therapy is mandatory in all situations.

DISPOSITION

Anyone submerged for longer than 1 minute with a history of cyanosis or apnea, or requiring mouth-to-mouth resuscitation, should be admitted to the hospital and observed for at least 24 hours (Table 105–2). These victims are at risk for developing complications such as noncardiogenic pulmonary edema. Patients with an abnormal chest radiograph or arterial blood gas or who exhibit any respiratory symptoms should also be admitted. Discharged patients should be carefully observed for signs of respiratory compromise. The patient should be instructed to seek immediate medical care for any sign of breathing difficulty.

Selected References

Allman FD, Nelson WB, Pacentine GA, McComb G. Outcome following cardiopulmonary resuscitation in severe pediatric near-drowning. Am J Dis Child 1986;140:571.

Battaglia JD, Lockhart CH. Drowning and near-drowning. Pediatr Ann 1977;6:270.

Conn AW, Edmonds JF, Barker GA. Cerebral resuscitation in near-drowning. Pediatr Clin North Am 1979;26:691.

Dean JM, McComb JG. Intracranial pressure monitoring in severe pediatric near-drowning. Neurosurgery 1981;9:627.

Frewen TC, Sumabat WO, Han VK, et al. Cerebral resuscitation therapy in pediatric near-drowning. J Pediatr 1985;106:615.

Giammona ST. Drowning: Pathophysiology and management. Curr Probl Pediatr 1971;1:1.

Greensher J, Mofenson HC. Aspiration accidents: Choking and drowning. Pediatr Ann 1983;12:747.

Gulaid JA, Sattin RW. Drownings in the United States, 1978–1984. MMWR 1988;37:27.

Haward JS, Hay C, Matthews BR, et al. Temperature effect on the human dive response in relation to cold water near-drowning. J Appl Physiol 1984;56:202.

Heiser MS, Kettrick RG. Management of the drowning victim. Clin Sports Med 1982;1:409.

Jumbelic MI, Chambliss M. Accidental toddler drowning in 5-gallon buckets. JAMA 1990;263:1952.

Oakes DD, Sherck JP, Maloney JR, et al. Prognosis and management of victims of near-drowning. J Trauma 1982;22:544.

Orlowski JP. Adolescent drownings: Swimming, boating, diving, and scuba accidents. Pediatr Ann 1987;17:125.

Orlowski JP. Drowning, near-drowning, and ice water submersions. Pediatr Clin North Am 1987;34:75.

Orlowski JP, Abulleil MM, Phillips JM. The hemodynamic and cardiovascular effects of near-drowning in hypotonic, isotonic, or hypertonic solutions. Ann Emerg Med 1989;18:1044.

Reuler JB. Hypothermia: Pathophysiology, clinical settings and management. Ann Intern Med 1978;89:519.

Robinson MD, Seward PN. Submersion injury in children. Pediatr Emerg Care 1987;3:44.

Sarnaik AP, Preston G, Lieh-lai M, et al. Intracranial pressure and cerebral perfusion pressure in near-drowning. Crit Care Med 1985;13:224.

Tron VA, Baldwin VJ, Pirie GE. Hot tub drownings. Pediatrics 1985;75:789.

Wintemute GJ, Kraus JF, Teret SP, et al. Drowning in childhood and adolescence: A population-based study. Am J Public Health 1987;77:830.

CHAPTER 106

Electrical and Lightning Injuries

John J. Skiendzielewski
Kelly P. O'Keefe

ELECTRICAL INJURIES

Introduction

Greater than 2400 electrical injury victims require emergency treatment annually; approximately 1110 deaths occur. The populations at risk include power company workers, handyworkers, autoerotics, and children, who by themselves account for approximately one fifth of the deaths yearly. Pediatric electrical injury can be roughly grouped into two categories. Children under the age of 6 years are at greatest risk for suffering an electrical injury at home, from electrical outlets, extension cords, or bathtub accidents. Older children and adolescents, usually males, suffer injury from the use of power tools or from contact with high-tension lines.

Electrophysiology

The severity of electrical injury is predicated by several physical and physiologic variables, including voltage, current, resistance, type of current, duration of current flow, and pathway of current flow.

Voltage

Voltage is the measure of electromotive force in the system and can be related by Ohm's law to current and resistance:

$$I \text{ (current)} = \frac{V \text{ (voltage)}}{R \text{ (resistance)}} \quad or \quad Amps = \frac{Volts}{Ohms}$$

Most commonly voltage is the only variable of the equation that can be determined for electrical injuries since current flow depends on resistance, which is unknown. Injuries are commonly divided into low-voltage contacts (<1000 volts) and high-voltage contacts (>1000 volts), with the latter producing significantly greater amounts of tissue destruction. No fatalities have been reported from contact with long-distance communications lines (24 volts) or telephone lines (65 volts). Household current (120 or 220 volts) caused more than half of the 220 deaths in one study.

Current

Current or amperage is a measure of the rate of flow of electrons and is the most important single factor in electrocution. The following effects in humans of varying current flows are generally accepted:

0.001 amp: barely perceptible tingle
0.016 amp: "let go" current
0.020 amp: muscular paralysis
0.100 amp: ventricular fibrillation
2.000 amp: ventricular standstill

As the current flows through the skin, heat is generated, which causes blistering, a reduction in resistance, and subsequent greater current flow.

Type of Current

Alternating current (AC), which in the United States has a frequency of 60 Hertz, causes almost all nonlightning electrical deaths and is universally thought to be more dangerous than direct current (DC). Power companies use alternating current exclusively. Alternating current has remarkable capacity to depolarize cells owing to rapidly changing electron densities. Low-frequency electrical current produces tetanic muscle contractions that cause "freezing" to the circuit, allowing a longer duration of contact and subsequent current flows and tissue damage.

Duration of Contact

Heat production and subsequent tissue damage are directly proportional to the amount of time that the victim is in contact with the electrical source. However, death due to ventricular fibrillation may ensue from only momentary contact.

Resistance

Resistance is the measurement of difficulty of electron flow through a material. The primary source of resistance is the skin, but this can be altered significantly by sweating, blistering, and wetness (Table 106–1). Internal tissues vary considerably in resistance as well, with bone, fat, and tendon the most resistant, and nerves, blood vessels, and muscle the least. Previously it was thought that current flowed preferentially through the less resistant tissues, but studies have shown that except for bone, the volume of tissue traversed rather than the internal resistance of the individual tissues is more closely related to the extent of tissue injury. In other words, the internal milieu acts as a single uniform resistance, which is a function of volume or cross-sectional area. This suggests that, given equal voltage and skin resistance, the tissue destruction in an extremity would be greater than that of the torso.

Pathway of Current

The pathway of current has profound implications on tissue damage and survival. Current passing through the

TABLE 106–1

SKIN RESISTANCE

Site	Resistance (ohms/cm²)
Mucous membrane	100
Water immersion	1200
Sweaty skin	2500
Normal	30,000
Sole of foot	100,000–200,000
Calloused palm	1,000,000–2,000,000

head may produce brain or brain stem damage, while current traversing the chest is likely to cause cardiorespiratory events. In fact, current flow from the right to the left hand carries a 60% mortality rate. Hand-to-foot flows produce much less mortality, but the greater the distance between entry and exit points, the greater the opportunity for widespread organ damage owing to the dispersal of current.

Pathophysiology

The various clinical effects of electricity can be traced to heat production and cell membrane depolarization. Heat production is directly proportional to the current, the resistance, and the duration of contact. Although current traverses the body by the volume conductor mechanism described previously, the highest current flow passes through muscle, which occupies the largest cross-sectional area. Skeletal muscle thus suffers the highest temperature rise, and individual muscles of smaller cross-sectional diameter, such as those found in the wrist and elbow, achieve the highest temperatures. Coagulation necrosis and small arteriole and microarteriole thrombosis produce muscle destruction and myoglobin release. In some cases areas of muscle adjacent to bone suffer unexpectedly severe injury or progressive damage.

Total body heating is the usual mechanism of death in prolonged (>1 minute) high-voltage situations. Irreversible heat denaturation of the central nervous system occurs with a brief exposure to temperatures of 50°C (122°F), or slightly longer exposure at 45°C (113°F).

The skeletal muscle damage produced by heating may be intensified by electrical breakdown of cell membranes and subsequent cell lysis. Nerve muscle cells, because of their relatively large size, are especially vulnerable to the great transmembrane potentials applied during electric shock.

Conduction disturbances of the heart account for most of the deaths owing to low-voltage contact and some of the brief-duration high-voltage exposures. At current flows below the fibrillation threshold (<0.1 amp), muscle depolarization can cause tetany. With prolonged (>1 minute) exposure, tetany of the respiratory muscles may result in fatal hypoxia. Alternating current in the range of 0.1 to 2.0 amp produces ventricular fibrillation, exerting its effects during the vulnerable period of ventricular recovery (during the T wave). At current flows greater than 2 amp, the heart comes to a standstill and may spontaneously begin beating when the circuit is broken, but breathing often fails to restart and death occurs from hypoxia.

Cardiovascular Injury

The heart is susceptible to various forms of rhythm disturbance following electrical injury, including sinus tachycardia, atrial or ventricular ectopy, bundle branch blocks, first- and second-degree heart block, atrial fibrillation, and supraventricular tachycardia. Ventricular arrhythmias have occurred as late as 12 hours after injury, and endomyocardial biopsy of these patients showed focal myocardial fibrosis. Asystole has occurred during intravenous cannulations of a patient who was susceptible to mild vasovagal symptoms shortly after electric shock.

Although documented, true myocardial infarction is rare after electrical injury. Ischemic alterations of the electrocardiogram as evidenced by ST-T wave changes or abnormal thallium scan or echocardiogram may be present. Myocardial rupture following electrical injury has been described.

The peripheral vascular system also sustains significant morbidity from electrical injury, sometimes requiring amputation of an injured extremity. The mechanism of vessel injury is heat related, occurs from the intima outward, and results in thrombosis, which may be segmental. Although these changes occur most frequently with high-voltage injury, they may also be present after a low-voltage injury. Delayed hemorrhage, thrombophlebitis, and abdominal aortic aneurysms have also occurred.

Cutaneous Wounds

Victims of high-voltage electrical injury characteristically suffer combinations of different types of burns. *Contact* burns occur at the points of entry and exit of current. These have a charred central core of varying size and are surrounded by a gray-white leathery zone, which is surrounded by a blood-red zone of coagulation necrosis. Low-voltage contact may cause little or no burn, unless the duration of contact is relatively prolonged.

Localized *arc* burns may appear similar to contact burns and occur when electrical current jumps or arcs from a high-voltage source to a victim in close proximity. Arc-type burns may also be produced when current courses along a flexed extremity, bridging, for example, the flexed forearm and the upper arm. Noncontact *flash* burns occur when a victim is exposed to the intense heat of electricity arcing externally to the ground. Finally, *thermal* burns are secondary to the ignition of clothing and may be extensive and quite deep.

The most common electrical injury of children is a burn about the mouth caused by sucking on the end of an extension cord or biting through a live wire. The heat produced may reach 2500° to 3000°C. The most frequent sites of the burns are the commissure of the lips and both upper and lower lips. Associated tongue injuries are found in one third of the patients but are usually mild. Severe injuries typically progress to ischemia, coagulation necrosis, and eschar formation. Several weeks after injury the eschar sloughs, leaving a rather large defect with a potential for extensive scarring. A serious complication of this injury is delayed bleeding from the labial or occasionally the lingual artery. This typically occurs 1 to 2 weeks postburn.

Renal Injury

Electrical injury produces a hazard to the kidneys compared with a crush syndrome. Although renal damage from the blast effect of the initial shock or direct-current flow may occur, the primary pathologic process is acute tubular necrosis due to hemochromogen. Free hemoglobin is released by intravascular hemolysis, and large amounts of myoglobin are released into the circulation from heat-damaged skeletal muscle. Decreased glomerular filtration and renal cortical ischemia due to hypovolemia are thought to contribute to the severity of the insult.

Neurologic Injury

Immediate or delayed sequelae of electrical injury occur in both the central and the peripheral nervous systems. Current that traverses the brain through a scalp entry wound can cause respiratory center arrest or depression, coma, seizures, paresis, and amnesia. Unusual immediate brain injuries include intracerebral bleeding and explosion of the orbital roof with displacement of the brain into the orbits. Spinal cord manifestations of electrical injury can be either immediate or delayed, with the latter bearing a poorer prognosis. The symptoms of immediate injury usually occur within the first 24 hours and typically consist of transient weakness and paresthesia. Delayed sequelae of cord injury

can manifest themselves from a few days to 2 years after the event, are usually incomplete and predominantly motor, and have uncertain prognosis. Ascending paralysis, amyotrophic lateral sclerosis, transverse myelitis, and impotence have been reported. The postulated mechanism of these delayed sequelae is damage to the nutrient vessels of the cord either by thrombosis or by microvascular hemorrhage. Peripheral nerves can likewise be injured from direct passage of current, thermal injury, damage to their nutrient vessels, or the effects of a compartment syndrome.

Gastrointestinal Injury

The gastrointestinal tract can be damaged directly from passage of current through the abdominal wall or by the development of Curling's ulcerations of the stomach or duodenum, which occur more frequently with electrical burns than with thermal burns. Injuries that have recently been described include evisceration, large and small bowel perforation, stomach perforation, vesicoenteric fistula, esophageal stricture, and electrocoagulation of the liver and pancreas. Intraabdominal injuries should be suspected when postburn ileus persists for more than 1 or 2 days.

Skeletal Injury

Direct electrical trauma to bone, especially the skull, can result in full-layer necrosis of the scalp secondary to the large amount of heat production. Furthermore, tetanic contractions or secondary direct trauma from falls subsequent to shock are commonly encountered.

The immature skeleton may be even more at risk from the effects of electrical injury. The growth plate may be directly damaged by electrocoagulation, become ischemic owing to damage to the epiphyseal circulation, or become incapable of endochondral transformation by disruption of the metaphyseal circulation. These changes may profoundly retard longitudinal and latitudinal bone growth.

Ophthalmologic Injury

Significant structural damage to the eye due to electrical injury is unusual, unless the entry site is close to the eye. Generally the more superficial ocular structures are more severely injured, but coagulative injury to the posterior elements causing blindness and necessitating enucleation may occur. Cataract formation is a well-recognized, delayed complication of ophthalmologic electrical injury. Cataracts may occur from several days to 11 years after injury, may be due to impaired function of the sodium-potassium pump in the anterior lens capsule, and respond well to extraction or intraocular lens implantation.

Psychological Sequelae

The psychological sequelae of victims of electrical injury are often more severe than those of victims of thermal burns. Usually a pattern of generalized cerebral dysfunction emerges, with depression, post-traumatic flashbacks, avoidance behavior, and psychosocial deterioration.

EMS Considerations
Low-Voltage Accidents

In most low-voltage accidents, power to the circuit is easily terminated prior to EMS arrival. If, however, the child is still attached to a live circuit, the power must first be switched off to prevent injury to rescuers. If the child is unresponsive, usual advanced resuscitation procedures are immediately initiated, mindful of the possibility of cervical spine injury from secondary fall.

High-Voltage Accidents

The prehospital care of the victim of high-voltage injury presents a significant danger to the rescuer. Although various methods of wire extrication, including the use of wooden poles, ropes, gloves, rubber tools, or other nonconducting instruments, have been advocated, the rescuer should not approach or touch the victim until the power has been switched off. In some instances a power company may need to be notified to accomplish this. Once the power has been switched off, advanced resuscitation protocols are instituted, again with cervical spine precautions. Vigorous normal saline fluid resuscitation with large-bore intravenous lines and large-gauge tubing should be initiated, preferentially in an extremity that is unburned and avoiding the site of entry or exit wounds. If the patient remains unconscious, hyperventilation during transport may be effective in reducing intracranial pressure. After cervical spine immobilization and splinting of obvious fractures, monitored transport should ensue.

Therapeutic Intervention

A brief history of the event from the victim, rescuer, family members, or coworkers should include the voltage delivered, entry and exit points, duration of contact, and subsequent loss of consciousness or fall. A thorough physical examination should be performed, with special consideration given to neurologic assessment, the site of entry and exit, and hidden musculoskeletal injuries.

Initial diagnostic studies should include blood samples for arterial blood gas, complete blood count, serum electrolytes, glucose, BUN, creatinine, creatine kinase (CK), type and crossmatch for packed red blood cells, and urinalysis for myoglobin. Radiographs of the cervical spine, pelvis, chest, and other areas suspicious for injury should be obtained, as well as an electrocardiogram (EKG). CK-MB isoenzyme elevations, as an indication of myocardial injury, are not valid, as large amounts of CK-MB have been found in patients without other suggestion of cardiac injury. The source of enzyme has been traced to electrically damaged skeletal muscle. Total CK levels may be helpful as a therapeutic and prognostic indicator. If cardiac injury is suggested by the EKG, an echocardiogram or thallium scan may confirm the presence and extent of injury.

Continued therapeutic measures should include vigorous fluid resuscitation. In children, a bolus of 10 ml/kg of body weight of a balanced salt solution may be infused over a few minutes and repeated as needed. Surface burns are notoriously inadequate in determining the extent of injury, and the usual burn fluid resuscitation formulae are not valid in electrical injury. Rather, a child's resuscitation should be guided by urine output, and levels of 1.5 ml/kg/hour are sought to help prevent tubular necrosis. A Foley catheter should be inserted to assure accurate measurement of urine volume. Some authors have recommended the use of mannitol or furosemide to increase urine flow, but these must be used cautiously in children. Monitoring central venous pressure is essential in monitoring the circulatory blood volume. Alkalinization of the urine by adding 1 ampule of sodium bicarbonate to 1 L of intravenous fluid has been thought to facilitate myoglobin excretion but must be accomplished judiciously to avoid hypernatremia and cardiac failure. Nasogastric intubation should be performed to reduce the risk of aspiration of gastric contents due to ileus and rapid gastric dilatation, and antacid and cimetidine therapy should be instituted. Tetanus prophylaxis should be administered liberally.

Surgical consultation is necessary for wound exploration, debridement of devitalized muscle, and potential fasciotomy. Local burns may be treated with sulfadiazine or mafenide. Several authors suggest the use of parenteral antibiotics effective against anaerobic organisms in patients with obvious or suspected devitalized muscle.

The child with burns of the oral commissure should be seen promptly by a plastic or oral surgeon. Although surgical excision of the burn has been advocated, current consensus seems to favor a more conservative approach to this injury, consisting of local wound care and immediate splinting of the commissure with an appliance, with reconstructive surgery delayed for 9 to 12 months.

The child who suffers low-voltage injury and is seemingly asymptomatic presents a dilemma. At the very least a history and thorough physical examination should be followed by an EKG. Any EKG evidence of potential ischemia should be an indication for admission and further study. The disposition of patients without EKG abnormalities is controversial. One series with low-voltage injury found no major complications during 48 hours of monitoring and recommended that admission solely for cardiac monitoring is unnecessary. These recommendations were echoed in another series of patients with high-voltage injury. On the other hand, three patients with transthoracic low-voltage injury developed serious ventricular arrhythmias 8 to 12 hours after shock. It is prudent to admit those children with arm-to-arm passage of current for 48 hours of monitoring. Evidence does not exist to support admission and monitoring of asymptomatic patients with no EKG abnormalities and nontransthoracic pathway of current.

LIGHTNING INJURIES
Introduction

Over 2000 thunderstorms are brewing at any given moment, and lightning flashes occur at the rate of 8 million per year. From 77 to over 600 deaths in the United States are directly caused by lightning strikes each year, accounting for only one third of the number of people struck. Lightning is responsible for greater mortality than all other natural disasters.

Lightning strikes individuals most commonly, but 25% of lightning strike victims are injured simultaneously as part of a group. Although being outdoors increases the risk of being struck, injuries and deaths have occurred indoors. Injuries sustained while talking on the telephone when the wires are struck is an example of the latter. In one case a tree near a summer house was struck and the charge followed the root system under the home, killing a 13-year-old boy. Two thirds of all lightning victims survive.

Physics of Lightning

Lightning is the product of a tremendous difference in electrical potential between negatively and positively charged particles. These charges are formed when warm air at the surface of the earth rises and meets the cooler upper air, where cloud formation takes place. Water contained in the warm air changes form from vapor to liquid and then to solid if the temperature becomes even colder. This process is associated with the generation of an electric charge. An intense electric field is thereby created, with positive charges concentrated in the top layers of the cloud and negative charges in the lower portions. The ground, which is normally negatively charged with respect to the atmosphere, becomes positively charged as the thunderstorm with its negative base travels overhead. The difference in electrical potential between cloud and ground can reach 100 to 300 million volts. When this potential difference is enough to overcome the resistance of the intervening air, a lightning bolt emerges. Initially, small strokes extending small distances are emitted as leader strokes. With the progression of each leader stroke, the distance between the charged areas of the cloud and ground is shortened and the potential gradient is increased. Sparks are emitted from the ground structures until the spark from the ground, called the pilot stroke, and the leader from the cloud meet and a conducting pathway is constructed. A huge surge of electric current rapidly follows. Approximately 20 milliseconds is required for the leader to reach the ground, but only 20 microseconds or so is needed for the return stroke to be completed. This process may be repeated several times in the same channel. The strike may occur from cloud to cloud, cloud to ground, or even ground to cloud from tall skyscrapers or mountains.

Lightning may take various forms, described as streaked, forked, ribbon, sheet, or beaded. The most unusual form, ball lightning, is reported to appear as a globe that glows and hisses as it speeds from cloud to earth, rolling along whatever structures it encounters or passing through buildings, entering through an open door or window and leaving by means of another portal. Thunder is the tremendous pulse of sound that is created by the expansion and compression when the air around a lightning strike is rapidly heated and then cooled.

Mechanism of Injury

Lightning directly striking a person may produce the most serious injuries, but it is not the only or the most frequent mechanism of injury in lightning victims. Other methods of transferring the tremendous energy stored in the strike to the victim include side flash, contact voltage, ground voltage, heat production, and pressure waves. Secondary injuries may occur with fires produced by the lightning strike or by the falls that occur when the victim is struck.

A direct strike is most likely to occur when the victim is on open flat ground or on a hilltop, therefore becoming the tallest structure around. The chances of being directly hit are increased by carrying or wearing metal objects or other conductors. It should be remembered that while a direct hit may seem the most damaging type of injury, it is not always fatal.

Side flash, or splash injury, is probably more common than direct strike and occurs when the victim is in close proximity to an object such as a tree or light pole (or telephone or plumbing fixture when indoors) that has been struck by lightning. It occurs when the resistance of the object struck is greater than the resistance of the air between the object and the victim. The charge, following the path of least resistance, leaps from the structure to the victim. The flashes may occur within a radius of 30 m. Despite seeming less dangerous than direct strike, side flash, as all other mechanisms of strike, can be fatal. Indeed, lightning may directly strike one person and only stun the victim, but then splash off to another person, causing death.

Contact voltage injury occurs when the victim is in direct contact with an object that has been struck or splashed by lightning. Ground voltage injury occurs when the lightning charge is carried into the ground and then into the victim. The farther away from the actual strike, the less charge is transmitted. This has also been called step or stride voltage owing to the potential difference that may develop between

the victim's feet if one foot is closer to the point of contact than the other.

The high temperatures resulting from lightning are another source of injury. The contact temperature of lightning strike has been estimated to be between 8000° and 30,000°C, with a duration of contact from 0.001 to 0.010 second. These temperatures are responsible for the burns seen in lightning strikes, which are less severe than those seen with electrical injuries. The worst lightning burns occur from clothing on fire or on skin underlying a metal object that has been struck. These types of exposure increase the duration of contact and therefore the severity of injury. The same thermal forces are to some degree responsible for the tremendous pressure waves generated from the rapid expansion and cooling of air around the lightning strike. These electromechanical forces are powerful enough to cause the clothing and shoes to be ripped off the body, to cause blunt injury directly to the victim, and to cause the victim to be thrown in the air, leading to secondary blunt injury due to the resulting contact with the ground.

Pathophysiology
Cardiac

The most common cause of death in the lightning victim is cardiopulmonary arrest. It is widely held that lightning acts as a massive countershock, causing not only cardiac standstill but also respiratory arrest owing to its effects on the medullary respiratory center. The expected presenting rhythm is asystole. At some point the intrinsic pacemaker capability of the heart will lead to resumption of an organized rhythm. However, if the respiratory center has not been reactivated as well, hypoxia and resultant deterioration to ventricular fibrillation will ensue. A state of "suspended animation" and the "cessation of metabolism in all cells including the brain" have been hypothesized to account for cases of resuscitation after 10- to 15-minute periods of pulselessness and apnea after prolonged resuscitation.

Myocardial infarction either can result from direct damage by the lightning strike or may be secondary to hypoxia. Damage secondary to cardiopulmonary resuscitation may occur as well. Delayed myocardial infarction occurring 10 and 30 days after being struck by lightning has been reported in adults. A variety of dysrhythmias, both ventricular and atrial, have been reported. Congestive heart failure may accompany cardiac damage. Blunt injury may cause cardiac contusion. Rupture of the heart has occurred. A variety of EKG changes with gradual resolution and lack of sequelae have been reported (Table 106–2).

Neurologic

There is a wide variety of serious neurologic effects that may result from lightning strike. Apnea due to depression

---

TABLE 106–2

EKG CHANGES SEEN WITH LIGHTNING STRIKE

Q-T prolongation
Inverted T waves
Nonspecific ST segment changes
Flattening of T waves
Peaked T waves
Axis shift
Myocardial infarction pattern without cardiac sequelae— posterior, anterior, inferior
ST segment elevation

of the medullary respiratory center may persist for several hours. Skull fractures, intracerebral hematomas and hemorrhages, cerebral edema, and elevated intracranial pressure may occur from direct damage or from blunt trauma suffered after the strike.

The most common neurologic sequelae are transient loss of consciousness, which may accompany more than 75% of strikes, amnesia for the events, which may be permanent, and transient paralysis and paresthesia of the limbs. The phenomenon of keraunoparalysis is most interesting. The victim awakens while on the ground and is unable to move any of the limbs. This flaccid paralysis is usually accompanied by marked vasomotor changes and may last up to 24 hours. The lower extremities are more commonly involved than the upper extremities. The usual pattern is recovery over minutes to days.

Prolonged loss of consciousness may be due to trauma or hypoxia. Hypothermia should be considered as a cause if the victim has been outside in the rain for a prolonged period. Miraculous brain recovery has been seen despite prolonged arrest and apnea. One 10-year-old boy was even noted to have a higher I.Q. after returning to school following lightning strike, prolonged arrest, and resuscitation that included thoracotomy. Such events have promoted the theories of suspended animation and cessation of cellular metabolism and remain difficult to explain. On the other hand, death may come rapidly from massive brain swelling and herniation. Permanent peripheral nerve damage is possible but rarely seen; this may be because nerve tissue acts as a poor volume conductor. Permanent damage may more often result from microvascular damage.

Other neurologic problems include seizures. In general, lightning-induced seizures will respond to the usual anticonvulsant drugs. Cerebellar ataxia, Horner's syndrome, and cognitive dysfunction have been reported. Delayed sequelae include paralysis without bladder or bowel disturbance, paraplegia and hemiplegia, neuritis, and neuralgia.

Skin

The effects on the integument due to lightning are less severe than might be expected but can be dramatic. Despite the high voltages involved, the short duration of contact and level of skin resistance (lessened 100 times by rain or perspiration) prevent significant damage from occurring. The "flashover effect" is the term used to describe the phenomenon where current flows instantaneously over the surface of the body rather than through it, similar to the way electricity flows over a conducting wire. The result of this superficial pathway is the pathognomonic lesion of lightning strike on the skin—the arborescent, fern-like erythematous streaks (Fig. 106–1). These are similar to first-degree burns and may develop several hours after the strike. This condition resolves entirely within several days.

Deeper burns (second and third degree) may occur at the point of lightning strike or wherever metal such as a belt buckle or zipper is involved. These burns occur because of prolonged contact with the superheated metal. Exit wounds are, in general, not seen. The most severe burns may be sustained when the victim's clothing is set on fire. Deeper burns may follow a linear pattern or appear as multiple punctate lesions. Common burn sites are the trunk and legs, followed by the head and arms. Over 60% of lightning victims will have multiple burns, and approximately 10% will not be burned at all.

Ears

The most common injury suffered by the ear is rupture of the tympanic membrane, which may be seen bilaterally. This is felt to be a result of the tremendous shock wave caused by the rapid expansion of the air as it is heated. Hemorrhage or cerebrospinal fluid leak may be seen in conjunction with this injury. Other changes include rupture of Meissner's membrane, strial degeneration, decreased spiral ganglion cell population, basilar skull fracture, avulsion of the mastoid process, peripheral facial nerve palsy, and ossicle damage. Chronic otitis media may follow tympanic membrane rupture. Other otologic complications may include hearing loss, tinnitus, vertigo, and nystagmus.

Other

Damage to every part of the eye has been documented with lightning strike, but the most common lesions are cataracts. Developing immediately or over a prolonged time, cataracts may require surgery or resolve spontaneously. Fixed and dilated pupils seen immediately after lightning strike in the unconscious patient should not be taken as a prognostic sign. Resuscitative efforts should continue, as many victims have recovered completely despite having fixed and dilated pupils.

The lung has suffered all types of injury compatible with blunt trauma, including hemorrhage, contusion, and pneumothorax; hemoptysis and subcutaneous emphysema may also be noted. Pulmonary edema due to a variety of causes may occur and may resolve spontaneously within several days. Aspiration is commonly associated with alteration of consciousness.

Gastrointestinal hematoma secondary to blunt effect may occur. Gastric dilatation is common and may require nasogastric tube drainage.

Myoglobinuria may occur but is not seen to the extent it is with other electrical injures owing to the relative infrequency of deep burns and muscle injury. Blunt trauma to the kidneys and other portions of the genitourinary tract must be considered.

Vasoconstriction may be severe enough to cause mottling or cyanosis, and pulses may be absent. Vascular changes mimic those seen with compartment syndrome, but prophylactic fasciotomies are not indicated. In general, these changes are reversible, requiring only supportive care. Vascular thrombosis does occur, however, and amputation may be required.

The psychological effects of lightning in children can be severe and may linger for long periods. The most common reactions following a group strike are anxiety, particularly in relation to storms, and nightmares. Other sleep disturbances, separation anxiety, and nocturnal enuresis have been documented. Depression may last for several months. Hysterical paralysis, blindness, deafness, and muteness have been observed.

Effect of Lightning on the Fetus

There are numerous reports of lightning strikes occurring during pregnancy. Overall, roughly 50% of mothers go on to term with a normal delivery and healthy child, 25% of fetuses die prior to delivery, and 25% of cases result in neonatal death. The fetus is proposed to be at increased risk because it is surrounded by amniotic fluid. Obviously the prognosis for the fetus is much better if the mother is not seriously injured or killed. Should the mother suffer a cardiopulmonary arrest late in pregnancy, it is suggested that resuscitative efforts be continued at least long enough to perform a cesarean section. The chances of delivery of a normal infant are fair for those sections carried out within 15 minutes of maternal arrest. Survival of the fetus is unlikely if performed after 25 minutes.

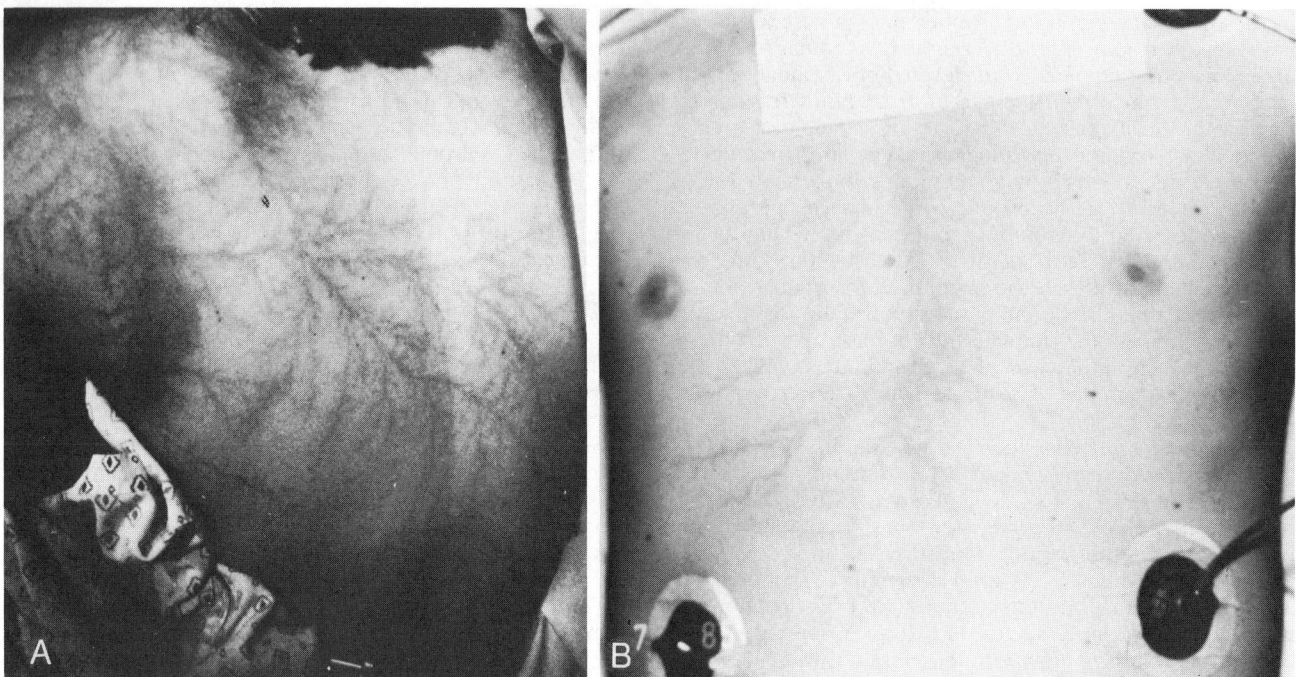

Figure 106–1. *A, B,* Arborescent burns due to lightning. (*B,* Courtesy of Michael R. Clark, M.D., Michigan State University, East Lansing, MI.)

EMS Considerations

For a group of children to be injured by a single bolt of lightning is not uncommon. Given multiple victims and limited medical resources, triage measures are mandated. Nevertheless, standard triage procedures must be ignored. The apparently dead lightning victim should be treated first, regardless of the absence of a heart rhythm or fixed and dilated pupils, which do not have the usual prognostic value. As mentioned above, the child may appear lifeless, without a pulse or spontaneous breathing, but at some point the heart will start again. The degree of damage incurred is due to the length of time that hypoxia is suffered after resuming a rhythm. Therefore the apparent dead must be treated first because often they will have complete recovery given appropriate care. Only one third of those struck by lightning die owing to their injuries, and the number would probably be significantly less if proper resuscitation were initiated as soon as possible. The patient who has a decreased level of consciousness but is able to moan can be assumed to have some degree of stability and will not suffer from a short delay in treatment.

Standard protocols for cardiac resuscitation and trauma care should be utilized and do not need to be modified. Unless the history of lightning strike is clear, standard protocol for alteration in mental status to include glucose and naloxone administration should be followed. Bystanders should be questioned regarding events, as the patient, even if awake, will generally suffer retrograde amnesia for the occurrence.

Diagnostic Evaluation

In the patient who appears to be minimally injured, blood for evaluation of hemoglobin, renal function, and muscle enzymes to include fractionation into isoenzymes should be drawn. Urine should be sent for routine analysis and for detection of myoglobin. In the sicker child who may be unstable or still unconscious, a more thorough trauma evaluation should be carried out to include arterial blood gas, serum chemistries (electrolytes, calcium, liver function, amylase, and lipase), and type and crossmatch as appropriate. Blood and urine should be sent for toxicologic screening.

All patients should have an EKG performed. They should remain on a cardiac monitor for the duration of their stay to detect any rhythm disturbance or other electrocardiographic abnormalities.

Radiographic studies are performed as necessary. The older child who is awake and alert without any signs of major trauma and without complaint may not need any studies. In the severely traumatized child, cervical spine films (lateral, anterior-posterior, and odontoid) and radiographs of the chest and pelvis are required as a minimum. The chest radiograph should be examined for evidence of trauma, aspiration, and pulmonary edema. The child with a decreased level of consciousness or focal neurologic deficit should have a computed tomography (CT) scan performed as soon as possible to exclude an injury that might be amenable to surgical treatment.

Intracranial pressure monitoring devices may be necessary to evaluate suspected elevated pressures and to guide therapy. An echocardiogram is helpful to evaluate suspected cardiac damage. Tests of visual acuity and hearing should be performed as necessary. The temperature should always be taken, especially in the child with altered mental status, to exclude hypothermia as a contributor.

Differential Diagnosis

The diagnosis of lightning strike is easy to make if a clear history of lightning bolt striking the patient or the surrounding area can be obtained from a bystander. It can be more difficult if the event is unwitnessed and the child is found unconscious in the rain with the clothes torn from the body (Table 106–3). Remember that lightning injury may occur without rain or indoors. In addition, other conditions can be confused with lightning strike (Table 106–4).

TABLE 106–3
CLUES TO DIAGNOSIS OF LIGHTNING STRIKE
History of recent thunderstorm Outdoor occurrence Younger age Multiple victims Partial or complete clothing disintegration Typical arborescent pattern of superficial erythema   or superficial linear or punctate burns Tympanic membrane injury/blood from ear Magnetization of metallic objects on body

Therapeutic Intervention (Table 106–5)

Airway/Breathing

Control of the airway is a priority. Premedication with lidocaine (1 to 2 mg/kg) and diazepam (0.1 to 0.2 mg/kg to a maximum of 10 mg) or thiopental (1 to 3 mg/kg) may help avoid abrupt elevation of intracranial pressure prior to intubation or suctioning. If the patient is more alert and able to protect the airway, more simple measures may be taken. At a minimum, pulse oximetry or arterial blood gases should be checked, and supplemental oxygen may be given as necessary. Lightning victims may be apneic for hours and hence will require mechanical ventilation. When securing the airway, the possibility of cervical spine trauma must always be considered. Positive end expiratory pressure should be avoided, if possible, as it may decrease venous return from the brain and thus increase intracranial pressure.

Circulation

Hypotension in the patient with altered mental status should be assumed to be due to blunt trauma until that possibility has been excluded. Fluid resuscitation should proceed with crystalloids given in 20-ml/kg boluses as necessary and with blood products (packed red blood cells) when major blood loss is present. Pressors should be avoided.

The presence of mottled, pulseless extremities with lightning strike may make the diagnosis of hypotension difficult to reach clinically, especially in the unconscious patient. Central monitoring lines may be necessary to assess the volume status. Dysrhythmias and cardiac damage might further complicate the issue. Central nervous system injuries should never be assumed to be the cause of the hypotension until all other possibilities have been eliminated. Fluids should not be withheld in the hypotensive patient because of concern of head injury.

Transient hypertension and generalized catecholamine excesses have been treated predominantly with beta-adre-

TABLE 106–4
DIFFERENTIAL DIAGNOSIS OF LIGHTNING STRIKE
Assault Seizure Subarachnoid or other intracranial   hemorrhage, cerebrovascular accident Cardiac dysrhythmia or other cardiac event Spinal cord or head injury Heavy metal poisoning or other toxic ingestion Hypothermia Electrolyte or glucose abnormality

TABLE 106–5	
THERAPY AT A GLANCE	
Unconsciousness	
Naloxone	0.01 mg/kg
Dysrhythmias	
Lidocaine	1 mg/kg IV bolus
Seizures	
Diazepam	0.1–0.2 mg/kg IV bolus
Lorazepam	0.03–0.05 mg/kg IV bolus up to 4 mg q 6 hr
Sedation	
Thiopental	1–3 mg/kg/dose IV
Phenobarbital	2–3 mg/kg/dose
Rhabdomyolysis	
Sodium bicarbonate	1 mEq/L IV
Mannitol	0.25 gm/kg IV push, then q 5 min prn

nergic blockers with variable results. Hydralazine has also been used.

Central Nervous System

The treatment of altered mental status will mandate the use of glucose and naloxone to exclude other etiologies for a decreased level of consciousness. Likewise, toxicologic causes and hypothermia should be sought. A CT scan should be done emergently in all unconscious patients. Management of elevated intracranial pressure is no different with lightning injury than with other etiologies.

Seizures should be treated aggressively. Lorazepam and diazepam should be the first-line drugs; Kandt et al. reported failure of phenytoin or phenobarbital to halt seizures in one patient, but others have had success with these agents. The child with transient loss of consciousness who becomes awake and alert should have a thorough neurologic examination performed and should be observed for several hours. If there is any focal defect or deterioration in mental status, a CT scan should be performed.

Burns

The typical arborescent pattern of erythema will resolve within hours to days and requires no specific treatment. Second-degree or third-degree burns should be treated as any other burns, with silver sulfadiazine cream or Biobrane and skin grafting as needed. Current tetanus status should be ensured. Massive fluid loading, escharotomy, and fasciotomy are rarely needed. The mottled, pulseless extremities sometimes seen may lead some to consider fasciotomy early, but the situation will usually resolve by itself over the course of several hours.

Myoglobinuria

In contrast to electrical injuries, myoglobinuria is rare in lightning strike. Nevertheless, urine output should be monitored. If myoglobinuria is present, treatment with fluids and bicarbonate is indicated.

Sequelae

One third of victims die from injuries directly attributable to the lightning strike. Survivors may have long-term sequelae, predominantly neurologic. These include permanent paralysis, dysesthesia, disturbances of mental function, psy-

TABLE 106–6
ADMISSION AND DISCHARGE CRITERIA

Electrical Injuries

Hospitalize all with EKG changes, arm-to-arm passage of current, high voltage injuries, serious burns, oral burns

May discharge the asymptomatic child with minor injury, no EKG abnormalities, and nontransthoracic pathway

Lightning Injuries

Hospitalize all victims except those children who are fully awake and alert, have no or minimal injury, a normal neurologic examination, and a normal EKG and lab studies

May discharge these children once head trauma has been ruled out after several hours of cardiac and neurologic monitoring in the emergency department and only if direct home supervision is available and close follow-up can be arranged

chiatric disorders, and personality changes. Neurologic problems may be delayed.

Cooper's analysis of lightning strike revealed a poor prognosis for victims suffering either leg burns or cranial burns. Patients with leg burns had a 30% mortality rate, which was five times greater than the death rate for patients without leg burns. Thirty-eight percent of victims with cranial burns died and had a four times greater mortality rate than patients without cranial burns. Seventy-seven percent of patients who suffered cardiopulmonary arrest at the time of the lightning strike died, accounting for all the deaths in the study.

Disposition

The majority of patients who are victims of lightning strike will be admitted to the hospital for treatment of their injuries and monitored for possible complications (Table 106–6). Children who are awake and alert and have no apparent injury, a normal neurologic examination, normal EKG, and normal lab studies may be discharged from the emergency room after several hours of monitoring and observation. Adequate home supervision and close follow-up must be assured. Consultation by ophthalmology and otolaryngology for development of delayed sequelae and by psychiatry, neurology, cardiology, surgery, and orthopedics may be needed. Appropriate documentation is summarized in Table 106–7.

Other Considerations

Basic measures that should be followed in order to prevent lightning strike are:

TABLE 106–7
DOCUMENTATION

Loss of consciousness
Pathway and source of current, voltage, and duration of contact
Neurologic examination
Extent of burns and oral involvement
Eye examination with visual acuity
Ear examination with hearing tests
EKG and rhythm abnormalities
Urinalysis and myoglobin
Serum abnormalities
Radiographic studies as appropriate
Appropriate consultation arranged
Appropriate discharge instructions

1. Take shelter in a building or automobile, if possible.
2. Avoid large, flat, open areas or hilltops.
3. Avoid direct contact with metal objects and remove metal objects such as jewelry or hairpins from the head and upper body.
4. Avoid trees, boats, and open water.
5. If caught on open ground, curl on ground on side with hands close together to reduce contact points or squat with feet together. If possible, lie or squat on a rubber raincoat or sheet, as it may give some protection from ground current.
6. If caught in a forest, seek shelter under a thick growth of short trees.
7. Avoid using the telephone.

Selected References

Electrical Injuries

Ahrenholz DH, Schubert W, Solem LD. Creatine kinase as a prognostic indicator in electrical injury. Surgery 1988;104:741.

Al Rabiah SM, Archer DB, Millar R. Electrical injury of the eye. Int Ophthalmol 1987;11:31.

Baker MD, Chiaviello C. Household electrical injuries in children. Am J Dis Child 1989;143:59.

Bingham H. Electrical burns. Clin Plast Surg 1986;13:75.

Budnick LD. Bathtub related electrocutions in the U.S. 1979–82. JAMA 1984;254:918.

Butler ED, Gant TD. Electrical injuries with special reference to upper extremities. Am J Surg 1977;134:95.

Cooper MA. Electrical and lightning injuries. Emerg Med Clin North Am 1984;2:489.

Daniel RK, Ballard PA, Heroux P, et al. High voltage electrical injury: Acute pathophysiology. J Hand Surg 1988;13A:44.

Dixon GF. The evaluation and management of electrical injuries. Crit Care Med 1983;11:384.

Donly KJ, Nowak AJ. Oral electrical burns: Etiology, manifestations, and treatment. General Dentistry 1988;36:103.

Esses SI, Peters WJ. Electrical burns: Pathophysiology and complications. Can J Surg 1981;24:11.

Flisak ME, Berman S. Electrical injury in the esophagus. AJR 1988;150:103.

Guinard JP, Chiolero R, Buchser E, et al. Myocardial injury after electrical burns: Short and long-term study. Scand J Plast Reconstr Surg Hand Surg 1987;21:301.

Hammond J, Ward CG. Myocardial damage and electrical injuries: Significance of early elevation of CPK-MB isoenzymes. South Med J 1986;79:414.

Hanumadass ML, Voora SB, Kagan RJ, et al. Acute electrical burns: A 10 year clinical experience. Burns 1986;12:427.

Hirschfeld JJ, Assael CA. Conservative management of electric burns to the lips of children. J Oral Maxillofac Surg 1984;42:197.

Hunt JL, Mason AD, Masterson TS, et al. The pathophysiology of acute electric injuries. J Trauma 1976;16:335.

Hunt JL, Sato RM, Baxter CR. Acute electric burns, current diagnostic and therapeutic approaches to management. Arch Surg 1980;115:434.

Jensen PJ, Thomsen PE, Bagger JP. Electrical injury causing ventricular arrhythmias. Br Heart J 1987;57:279.

Johnson EV, Kline LB, Skalka HW. Electrical cataracts: A case report and review of the literature. Ophthalmic Surg 1987;18:283.

Kinney TJ. Myocardial infarction following electrical injury. Ann Emerg Med 1982;11:622.

Kirchner JT, Larson DL, Tyson KR. Cardiac rupture following electrical injury. J Trauma 1977;17:389.

Kubernick M. Electrical injuries. Pathophysiology and emergency management. Ann Emerg Med 1982;11:633.

Leake JE, Curtin JW. Electrical burns of the mouth in children. Clin Plast Surg 1984;11:669.

Lewin RF, Arditti A, Sclarovsky S. Noninvasive evaluation of electrical cardiac injury. Br Heart J 1983;49:190.

Marchau M. Explosion of the orbital roof due to electric current. Neurosurgery 1988;23:769.

McBride JW, LaBrosse KR, McCoy HG, et al. Is serum creatine kinase-MB in electrically injured patients predictive of myocardial injury? JAMA 1986;255:764.

McLoughlin E, Joseph MP, Crawford JD. Epidemiology of high-tension electrical injuries in children. J Pediatr 1976;89:62.

Miller FE, Peterson D, Miller J. Abdominal visceral perforation secondary to electrical injury: Case report and review of the literature. Burns 1986;12:505.

Petty PG, Parkin G. Electrical injury to the central nervous system. Neurosurgery 1986;19:282.

Port RM, Cooley RO. Treatment of electrical burns of the oral and perioral tissues in children. J Am Dent Assoc 1986;112:352.

Salem MI. Bilateral anterior fracture-dislocation of the shoulder joints due to severe electric shock. Injury 1982;14:361.

Thompson JC, Ashwal SA. Electrical injuries in children. Am J Dis Child 1983;137:231.

Varghese G, Mani MM, Redford JB. Spinal cord injuries following electrical accidents. Paraplegia 1986;24:159.

Walton AS, Harper RW, Coggins GL. Myocardial infarction after electrocution. Med J Aust 1988;148:365.

Wright RK. Death or injury caused by electrocution. Clin Lab Med 1983;3:343.

Wright RK, Davis JH. The investigation of electrical deaths: A report of 220 fatalities. J Forensic Sci 1980;25:514.

Lightning Injuries

Amy BW, McMannis WF, Goodwin CW Jr, Pruit BA Jr. Lightning injury with survival in five patients. JAMA 1985;253:243.

Appelberg DB, Masters FW, Robinson DW. Pathophysiology and treatment of lightning injuries. J Trauma 1974;14:453.

Bartholomewe CW, Jacoby WD, Ramchand SC. Cutaneous manifestations of lightning injury. Arch Dermatol 1975;111:1466.

Bergstrom L, Neblegt LM, Sando I, et al. The lightning damaged ear. Arch Otolaryngol Head Neck Surg 1974;100:117.

Buechner H, Rothbaum J. Lightning strike injury: A report of multiple casualties resulting from a single lightning bolt. Milit Med 1961;126:755.

Castren JA, Kytilla J. Eye symptoms caused by lightning. Acta Ophthalmol 1964;42:139.

Cooper MA. Lightning Injuries: Prognostic signs for death. Ann Emerg Med 1980;9:134.

Cooper MA. Lightning strikes. Ann Emerg Med 1983;12:404.

Craig SR. When lightning strikes: Pathophysiology and treatment of lightning injuries. Postgrad Med 1986;79:109.

Dollinger SJ. Lightning strike disaster among children. Br J Med Psychol 1985;58:375.

Eriksson A, Ornehult L. Death by lightning. Am J Forensic Med Pathol 1988;9:295.

Flannery DB, Wiles H. Follow-up of a survivor of intrauterine lightning exposure. Am J Obstet Gynecol 1982;142:238.

Ghezzi KT. Lightning injuries: A unique treatment challenge. Postgrad Med 1989;85:197.

Kandt RS, Rossitch JC, Trippett TM, et al. Intracranial pressure (ICP) as a guide to prognosis in a lightning injured, comatose child. Childs Nerv Syst 1988;4:370.

Kotagel S, Rowlings CA, Chen S, et al. Neurologic, psychiatric, and cardiovascular complications in children struck by lightning. Pediatrics 1982;70:190.

McCrady-Kahn VL, Kahn AM. Lightning burns. West J Med 1981;134:215.

Moulson A. Blast injury of the lungs due to lightning. Br Med J 1984;289:1270.

Myers GJ, Colgan MT, VanDyke DH. Lightning strike disaster among children. JAMA 1977;238:1045.

Peters WJ. Lightning injury. Can Med Assoc J 1983;128:148.

Pierce MR, Harrison RA, Mitchell JM. Cardiopulmonary arrest secondary to lightning injury in a pregnant woman. Ann Emerg Med 1986;15:597.

Ravitch MM, Lane R, Safar P. Lightning strike: Report of a case with recovery after cardiac massage and prolonged artificial respiration. N Engl J Med 1961;264:36.

Rees WD. Pregnant women struck by lightning. Br Med J 1965;1:103.

Sharma M, Smith A. Paraplegia as a result of lightning injury. Br Med J 1978;61:1464.

Stanley LD, Suss RA. Intracerebral hematoma secondary to lightning stroke: Case report and review of the literature. Neurosurgery 1985;16:686.

Strasser EJ, Davis RM, Menchey JM. Lightning injuries. J Trauma 1977;17:315.

Taussig HB. Death from lightning and the possibility of living again. Ann Intern Med 1968;68:1345.

CHAPTER 107

Hypothermia and Frostbite

Daniel F. Danzl
Frank W. Lavoie

HYPOTHERMIA

Introduction

Accidental hypothermia is defined as a core temperature below 35°C without preoptic anterior hypothalamic dysfunction.[1, 2] Simple cold exposure or immersion is the usual cause. Core temperature depression secondary to other, miscellaneous factors is also common. These include infection, endocrinologic insufficiency, intracranial pathology, and intoxication. The incidence of each is to some degree age dependent. For example, serious infection as a cause for secondary hypothermia is seen more often in infants than in adolescents.[3]

During infancy and childhood, the behavioral and physiologic responses to local and systemic thermal stress differs from that in adulthood in many respects.[4] While newborn piglets instinctively huddle in the litter, human infants possess no behavioral defense mechanisms and are completely dependent on adults.[1, 5]

Generally all the thermoregulatory mechanisms active in adults are present in children but are far less efficient.[6] The relative importance of each heat conservation mechanism shifts from the day of birth through infancy and childhood. The reasons for these shifts include the infant's enlarged surface area, decreased subcutaneous layer, and inefficient neuromuscular and cardiovascular responses to cold.[7]

Anatomy and Physiology

Humans of all ages function optimally within a narrow 1°C range. At birth the infant exits from a warm, wet environment into a cold, dry atmosphere. Although the core temperature of the fetus exceeds that of the mother, the newborn rapidly loses heat.[6]

An infant's ability to control body temperature is limited by the exposed body surface area and the thermal insulation provided by subcutaneous fat. The degree of neuromuscular development present at birth determines the maximal rate of endogenous heat production and the hypothalamic setpoint.[8]

Infants and children vasoconstrict prior to initiation of nonshivering thermogenesis. Cold exposure initially stimulates skin receptors, which produces peripheral vasoconstriction and subsequent heat conservation. The internal core temperature will rapidly decline with a prolonged cold stress.[4, 5]

The thermoneutral environmental temperature in neonates and infants exceeds that present throughout life until senescence. The optimal critical temperature occupies a very narrow range. Deviations both above and below this temperature markedly increase oxygen consumption and metabolic requirements.[1]

Blood that is cooled below 37°C stimulates the preoptic anterior hypothalamus. This temperature regulatory center initially increases heat production by elevating the metabolic rate. This supplements heat production until stored glycogen and accessible adipose are depleted.[9]

There are five significant mechanisms of heat loss, and they can affect each pediatric age range differently. Except during immersion, *radiation* is the major cause of heat loss; approximately two thirds of heat is normally lost in this manner. The temperature gradient between the exposed body surface area and the environment is the major determinant. The greater surface area:mass ratio present in children increases radiative losses. Insulation by clothing or subcutaneous fat thickness decreases these losses.

Direct transfer of heat by *conduction* increases heat loss up to 5 times in wet clothing and 25 to 30 times in cold water. Wind and body motion increase heat loss through *convection*, which is commonly termed the windchill effect.[10]

Respiration and *evaporation* are the final two mechanisms of heat loss. These become more significant in dry, windy ambient conditions. Simply drying and swaddling infants restricts heat loss almost as effectively as a radiant heater.[1]

Physiologic circumstances vary with gestational age and weight. Preterm infants may lack the biochemical enzymatic development necessary to utilize available nutrients. They possess a lower metabolic rate, less insulation, and a proportionately greater surface area. In contrast, the small for gestational age infant has poor fuel storage despite more mature metabolic capabilities.[1]

Pathophysiology

Hypothermia has numerous effects on the various organ systems (Table 107–1). Clinically the most important pathophysiology involves the central nervous system (CNS) and the cardiovascular, respiratory, renal, and gastrointestinal systems.

Central Nervous System Effects

Cold progressively depresses the CNS.[11, 12] Cerebral enzyme systems are unable to function at temperatures that are well tolerated by the kidneys. As a result there is a linear decrease in cerebral metabolism with each degree drop in temperature. The electroencephalogram is silenced around 20°C. The ability to maintain cerebral perfusion by vascular autoregulation is lost around 25°C.[5, 13]

Cardiovascular Effects

As expected there is a progressive decrease in the heart rate after the initial tachycardia. The mean arterial pressure

and cardiac output also drop progressively. Vasoconstriction in the extremities increases the peripheral vascular resistance. This maintains the systemic blood pressure as the circulatory volume drops.

Direct heat application to the extremities can extinguish peripheral vasoconstriction. As a result, cold, hyperkalemic, acidotic blood pooled in the extremities returns to the "core." The resultant drop in temperature after initiating rewarming is termed core temperature afterdrop. Simple equilibration of the temperature gradient between the "shell" and the core also contributes to this afterdrop.[14] The clinical importance of core temperature afterdrop becomes more significant with increased extremity mass and surface area.[15]

Cold temperatures also depress electrical conduction through the His-Purkinje system. Conductive tissue is more sensitive to cold than is the myocardium. As conduction is rerouted through the myocardial fibers during cycle prolongation, arrhythmias develop.

Atrial arrhythmias are common below 32°C.[16] These rhythms should be considered innocent since the ventricular response will normally be slow. Below 30°C ventricular fibrillation and asystole are the major concerns.

The J (Osborn) wave may be present at the junction of the QRS complex and ST segment on the electrocardiogram (EKG) or rhythm strip.[17] Although not pathognomonic for hypothermia, its presence should suggest the diagnosis. The J wave may also be seen in young normal patients, in sepsis, and in association with CNS lesions or focal cardiac ischemia.[5, 18]

Respiratory Effects

Hypothermia initially stimulates the respiratory drive. After the metabolic rate eventually decreases, there is a progressive depression of the respiratory minute volume.[19] This occurs because of the 50% drop in carbon dioxide production for each 8°C fall in temperature.[1] In addition, cold-induced bronchorrhea mimics pulmonary edema. Protective airway reflexes become progressively ineffective.

Renal Effects

Renal blood flow drops progressively with temperature depression. Initially vasoconstriction in the extremities results in a relative central hypervolemia. As a result there is an acute large diuresis of dilute urine. This can be misleading clinically, and a deceptively "adequate" urinary output may be present despite hypovolemia.[20]

Gastrointestinal Effects

Hypothermia usually depresses the entire gastrointestinal tract. In neonates gastric dilatation is commonly reported.[21, 22] In older children this finding suggests myxedema. Ileus, vomiting, constipation, and poor rectal tone are commonly encountered.[5]

Predisposing Factors
Decreased Heat Production

At birth, thermogenesis is quite inefficient. Neonates lack neuromuscular development required for shivering during a period of decreased activity and poor adaptation to the cold. The physiologic options to thermoregulate are limited by the large surface area:mass ratio, relatively deficient subcutaneous layer, and absent behavioral defense mechanisms. Poorly adapted infants initially vasoconstrict and elevate metabolism. After 5 days of age, adapted infants

TABLE 107–1	
SYMPTOMS AND SIGNS	
Central Nervous System	**Renal**
Progressive depression	Polyuria
Apathy; irritability	Oliguria
Anorexia; poor suck	Anuria
Ataxia	Testicular torsion
Hyporeflexia	
Paradoxical undressing	**Gastrointestinal**
	Ileus, vomiting
Cardiovascular	Gastric dilatation in neonates
Initial tachycardia	Constipation
Bradycardia	Abdominal rigidity or
Dysrhythmias	distention
Peripheral vasoconstriction	Poor rectal tone
Respiratory	
Tachypnea	
Bronchorrhea	
Adventitious sounds	
Apnea	

increase lipolysis and can more effectively burn brown adipose tissue.[6, 23, 24]

Most acute neonatal hypothermia results from an emergent delivery and resuscitation. In more subacute cases, a weak cry, poor feeding, lethargy, and failure to thrive are noted.

Some infants will have paradoxical "rosy cheeks" while hypothermic. A delayed onset of hypothermia following the first several days of life should suggest septicemia.[9, 21, 22] Common associated findings reported in one series of 56 hypothermic infants age 4 to 113 days included malnutrition and low weight.[25]

Endocrinologic causes of decreased heat production include hypopituitarism, hypoadrenalism, and myxedema.[26] Of interest, congenital adrenal hyperplasia is more common in cold climates.[27]

The effect of malnutrition on thermostability varies with age and severity. Central neuroglycopenia directly impedes brain stem function.[28] In addition to hypoglycemia, marasmus and kwashiorkor are common causes of hypothermia in some settings. Kwashiorkor is less often associated with hypothermia because of the insulating effect of the hypoproteinemic edema.[29] In older children extreme exertion in cool climates can produce hypothermia.

Increased Heat Loss

A variety of dermatologic conditions increase heat loss. Associated erythrodermas include eczema, exfoliative dermatitis, and psoriasis.[30] Congenital lamellar ichthyosis also produces hypothermia.[31]

Burns usually result in some heat loss. Associated iatrogenic causes include overzealous burn treatment with topical cool liquids and cold intravenous infusions. Overcooling of heat stroke patients is another reported cause.[32]

Ethanol is the most common toxicologic agent that increases heat loss through cutaneous vasodilatation. Intoxication associated with paradoxical undressing has occasionally been reported in children. This is the removal of clothing in response to a cold stress.[33]

Accelerated conductive heat loss occurs in most drownings, especially in cold water. There are numerous survivors following prolonged submersion, including an 18 month old after submersion for 66 minutes.[34]

Impaired Thermoregulation

A variety of conditions impair thermoregulation centrally, peripherally, or metabolically. Hypothalamic function can also be disturbed by obstetric or other trauma, intracranial hemorrhage, or congenital lesions.

Newborn infants of mothers receiving medications that affect central thermoregulation may display an impaired metabolic response to cold for several days.[1] In therapeutic or toxic dose ranges, the phenothiazines, benzodiazepines, cyclic antidepressants, barbiturates, and general anesthetics are common offenders both pre- and postpartum.[35, 36] Acetaminophen and atropine have also been associated with hypothermia.[37–39]

Hypothermia has been observed in the shaken baby syndrome and may be a link in some cases of sudden infant death syndrome.[40, 41] Numerous other medical conditions, including Hodgkin's disease, anorexia nervosa, diabetic ketoacidosis, and uremia, contribute to hypothermia.[42, 43]

The most common cause of peripheral thermoregulatory failure is acute spinal cord transection.[44, 45] Victims are effectively poikilothermic and unable to conserve heat by vasoconstriction in the extremities. Associated trauma both causes and complicates hypothermia.[46] In older children diabetes and neuropathies are other peripheral causes.

Fetal and maternal hypothermia and bradycardia have occurred following magnesium sulfate infusion during preterm labor.[47] Fetal bradycardia also occurs during maternal hypothermia.[48]

Rare congenital anomalies associated with hypothermia include patients with agenesis of the corpus callosum and probable associated hypothalamic lesions. This is termed the Shapiro syndrome.[49–51] Spontaneous hypothermia has also been observed in one young boy with associated CNS lesions.[52]

EMS Considerations

In the prehospital setting the severity of hypothermia is often difficult to establish. There is no practical field thermistor probe. One should request documentation of the duration of exposure, obvious predisposing conditions, and circumstances of discovery.

Prehospital personnel should be guided by the axiom "no one is dead until warm and dead."[53] Initial field stabilization centers on prevention of further heat loss. A synopsis of medical control guidance is to rescue, examine, insulate, and transport gently.[54]

Patients with an extreme bradycardia and vasoconstriction may lack appreciable peripheral pulses. However, an extreme bradyarrhythmia may be metabolically sufficient to meet the depressed needs. Iatrogenic ventricular fibrillation can be easily precipitated by unnecessary closed chest compressions.[62]

Field rewarming options for pediatric patients are limited. Passive external rewarming with aluminum-coated foils or heated blankets should be initiated.[20] If available, active core rewarming with heated humidified oxygen can be coupled with active external rewarming of the trunk.

In immersion cases, gentle removal or cutting off of wet clothing limits further cooling by convection and evaporation. The child should not be allowed to exert, and a supine position should be maintained. One should consider administering heated intravenous fluids and the need for 25% or 50% dextrose and naloxone.

Advanced Life Support

The ideal advanced life support recommendations continue to evolve in hypothermia. While the optimal cardiopulmonary resuscitation (CPR) technique is unclear, closed chest compressions can maintain neurologic viability for hours in children.[5, 55, 62] In a hypothermic swine cardiac arrest model, the cardiac output, cerebral perfusion, and myocardial perfusion averaged 50%, 55%, and 31% of that generated with normothermic closed chest compressions.[55] However, flow did not decrease over time as it does at 37°C.

Intermittent flow may provide some neurologic support during evacuation.[57] In the field, initiate CPR unless no signs of life are present, chest-wall depression is impossible, obviously lethal injuries are present, or rescuers will be endangered.[62]

Clinical Evaluation

Historical circumstances of heat loss in children are often less helpful than in adults unless cold exposure is obvious. Subtle presentations dominate in younger age ranges. The severity of hypothermia is seldom appreciated initially. An insidious onset is common in infants. The paradoxical rosy cheeks often present are also misleading. In older children the circumstances of discovery and acuteness of temperature depression facilitate diagnosis.

Hypothermic infants are usually lethargic, drowsy, and apathetic to surroundings. Feeble attempts to cry or suck are associated with minimal spontaneous motion. Coldness to the touch is a common physical finding. Neonatal cold injury often produces edema and sclerema, a diffuse hardening of the skin.[1, 25, 29]

Alimentary function is depressed and can produce abdominal distention and bilious vomiting. This will mimic a surgical abdomen when coupled with cold-induced rectus spasm.

The neurologic evaluation will often be misleading.[13, 58] Absence of the Moro reflex does not necessarily imply CNS dysfunction. In older children hyporeflexia and areflexia predominate. This finding may mask a spinal cord injury if misattributed to hypothermia. Judgment is rapidly affected. Adolescents in particular are noted for failing to pursue preventive measures to avoid progressive hypothermia.

Diagnostic Evaluation
Acid-Base Balance

Reliable clinical prediction of acid-base status is impossible.[62, 59] Following an initial respiratory alkalosis from hyperventilation, a respiratory acidosis is caused by respiratory depression. Coexistent metabolic acidosis is produced by lactate generation, tissue hypoperfusion, and impaired lactic acid metabolism and excretion.

Correction of arterial blood gases was initially suggested to facilitate clinical interpretation.[60] Since arterial samples are always warmed in the machine to 37°C before electrode measurements are obtained, the in vitro correction factor for the change in pH per degree centigrade is 0.0147. That is, one would add 0.0147 pH units per degree centigrade below 37°C.

The accepted initial hypothesis was that 7.42 is the ideal "corrected" pH at all core temperatures. However, physiologic observations of ectotherms functioning in relatively alkaline states have led to reconsideration.[61, 63–65]

The neutral pH of water at 37°C is 6.8. There is experimental and clinical evidence that this 0.6 pH offset from 7.4 should be maintained at all temperatures (Fig. 107–1).[66] This maximizes enzymatic function, cellular integrity, and waste disposal. To achieve acid-base balance, simply maintain the uncorrected pH and P_{CO_2} at 7.4 and 40 mm Hg at all core temperatures.[67]

Optional ventilatory regimens, including the use of carbogen, are under study to help achieve homeostasis. A 1% to 2% versus 5% carbon dioxide concentration in one study of 28 children undergoing cardiac bypass with induced hypothermia facilitated acid-base balance.[68]

Clinical observations suggest that this approach maximizes cerebral and coronary blood flow and cardiac output while decreasing the incidence of lactic acidosis. In a study of cardiac bypass patients, those left with an ectothermically uncorrected pH of 7.4 developed ventricular fibrillation half as frequently.[69]

Hematologic Evaluation

Hematologic evaluation is necessary in all moderate or severe cases. One should obtain rapid bedside glucose, arterial blood gases uncorrected for temperature, complete blood count, electrolytes, blood sugar, BUN, creatinine, calcium, magnesium, amylase, lipase, and coagulation studies. If the level of consciousness is not consistent with the degree of hypothermia, consider toxicologic screening.

The hematocrit increases 2% per 1°C drop in temperature and may therefore be misleading. The significance of an elevated white cell count depends on the age of the infant or child and the maturity and predominance of the cell types.[70] Leukopenia is common during sepsis. Hypothermia induces hepatic, splenic, and splanchnic sequestration.

Serum electrolytes should be rechecked frequently during rewarming. There are no safe predictors of their values. For example, hypothermia will obscure premonitory EKG changes normally seen with hyperkalemia. Target cells are resistant to insulin, and hyperglycemia will persist briefly until glycogen storage is depleted.

Except in mild cases, a clotting screen should include a platelet count and fibrinogen level.[71] In one report of neonatal cold injury, thrombocytopenia was found in six of seven infants. Physiologic hypercoagulability is present, and resembles a disseminated intravascular coagulation–like syndrome.[72–75]

Infection and Cultures

Since fever, the classic sign of infection, is absent, comprehensive culturing is always indicated.[76] The only potential exception is obvious acute exposure. Hypothermia compromises host defenses.[77] The bone marrow release and circulation of neutrophils are impaired.[78] An acquired neutrophil dysfunction has been identified in children.[79] Because of the significant incidence of infectious complications, a prior recommendation to maintain hypothermia for control of cerebral edema after near-drowning has been abandoned.[80]

The incidence of infection varies with age and clinical circumstances. In five studies of hypothermic infants, 8% to 74% were septic.[3, 9, 21, 22, 29] The percentage drops with aging. In one study, 27 of the 51 hypothermic infants were septic.[3] Laboratory clues included anemia, uremia, glucose, and leukocyte abnormalities. The predominant organisms were streptococcus, staphylococcus, hemophilus, and Enterobacteriaceae. In another large series, 9 of 57 infants were septic.[81, 82] Right upper lobe lung infections were the predominant source in another report.[9, 22]

The physician should obtain comprehensive culturing (cerebrospinal fluid, blood, urine) and radiographic screening. In addition to a chest and abdominal film, a cervical spine radiograph in older children should be considered. Gastric aspiration was an additional diagnostic aid for one investigator.[21]

Empiric broad-spectrum antibiotic recommendations vary with age range. They usually include a parenteral aminoglycoside combined with ampicillin or a third-generation cephalosporin.[3]

Therapeutic Intervention

After the patient's arrival in the emergency department, one should confirm hypothermia and continuously monitor the cardiac rhythm and the core temperature. If obtained rectally, accurate probe placement must be verified to avoid cold stool. The tympanic temperature best reflects the hypothalamic temperature. Esophageal probes are reserved for endotracheally intubated patients. Administration of heated humidified oxygen can falsely elevate the esophageal reading.[83]

One should maintain vital signs on a flow chart while initiating basic life support and advanced life support as indicated. Airway management should not differ from normothermia. Hypothermia depresses protective airway reflexes, induces bronchorrhea, and predisposes to aspiration. Supplemental oxygen is helpful because of the adverse effects of hypothermia on tissue oxygenation. The oxyhe-

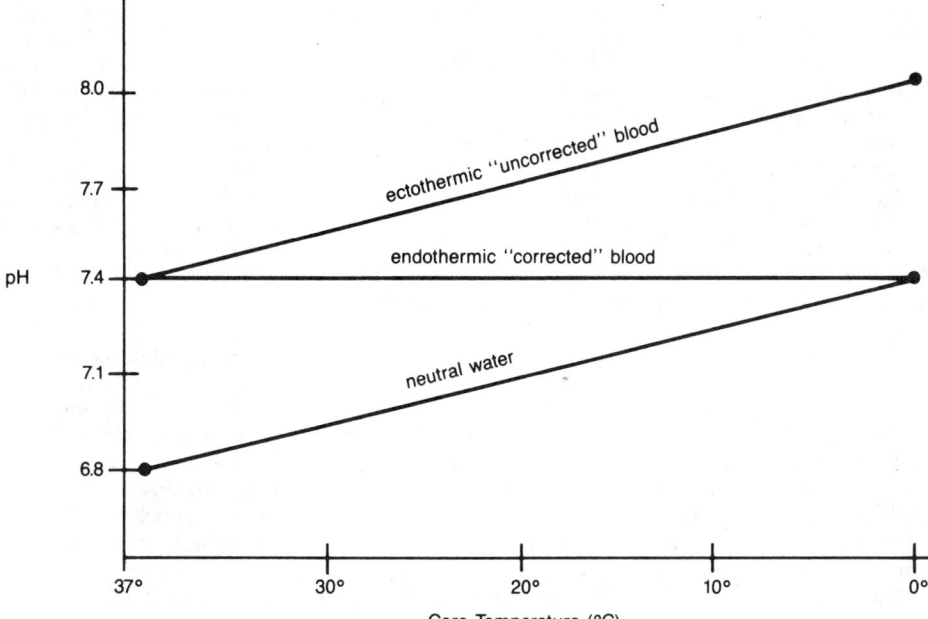

Figure 107–1. Ectotherm's physiologic 0.6 pH unit offset from neutral water progressively diminishes if arterial blood gases are temperature corrected. (From Danzl DF, Pozos RS, Hamlet MP. Accidental hypothermia. *In* Auerbach PS, Geehr EC (eds). Management of Wilderness and Environmental Emergencies. 2nd ed. St Louis, CV Mosby, 1989, p 45.)

moglobin dissociation curve shifts to the left. Gentle technique and preoxygenation will minimize the risk of ventricular arrhythmias during endotracheal intubation.

Most patients with chronic hypothermia will require volume resuscitation to maintain perfusion. In one series of hypothermic neonates, rapid volume expansion dramatically lowered mortality.[84]

The quantity of heat transfer with heated intravenous fluids in a child is usually negligible.[85] An entire liter of fluid at 42°C would be required to provide 12 Kcal to a 30-kg child at 30°C. This would only elevate a 30-kg child's core temperature approximately 0.67°C.

In hypovolemic children, heating intravenous fluids to 40° to 42°C is desirable. Consider 5% dextrose in 0.45 or 0.9 normal saline until laboratory studies are available. Rapid central venous administration of heated intravenous fluids produces myocardial thermal gradients. In addition, catheter tip contact with the right atrium can induce dysrhythmias.

In moderate and severe hypothermia, one should insert a nasogastric tube. Gastric dilatation and decreased enteric motility are to be expected. Indwelling bladder catheters facilitate monitoring of volume resuscitation and vascular fluid shifts.

Rewarming

The choice of passive versus active rewarming options varies with the patient's age and with multiple ancillary factors.[10, 86] Spontaneous passive external rewarming is noninvasive and ideal for mild hypothermia (>32.2°C) in older children. The patient is placed in a favorable atmosphere and insulated from further heat loss. The patient must be capable of sufficient endogenous thermogenesis to rewarm at an acceptable rate.[87]

Active rewarming, the direct transfer of exogenous heat to the patient, can be achieved externally or internally. Factors mandating active rewarming include infancy, cardiovascular instability, fuel depletion, endocrinologic insufficiency, severe hypothermia, and centrally or peripherally impaired thermoregulation.[84, 88–90] Aggressive rewarming of infants minimizes energy expenditures. During rewarming one should maintain vigorous monitoring for respiratory, hematologic, metabolic, and infectious complications.

Active External Rewarming

There are numerous sources of heat for external application: radiant heaters, electric blankets, thermal mattresses, heated containers, and warm baths.

The major cardiovascular objection to active external rewarming is core temperature afterdrop, which probably does not become significant until adolescence. Extinguishing peripheral vasoconstriction can induce adverse fluid and electrolyte fluxes if a significant quantity of blood is pooled in the extremities.[15]

Other rewarming techniques each present unique considerations. Topical heat application has been reported to cause thermal injury in hypoperfused vasoconstricted skin in children.[91] Immersion rewarming offers no advantages over the other techniques and greatly complicates monitoring.

Preterm infants have been successfully rewarmed on a heated water-filled mattress without complications.[92] In general, combining active external rewarming with active core rewarming techniques averts many of the complications clinically reported in adults.

Active Core Rewarming

Core rewarming techniques are effective, safe, and easily combined with selected active external rewarming modalities when desired. Heated humidified oxygen is always indicated. Advantages include assurance of adequate tissue oxygenation, reduction of cold-induced bronchorrhea, and decreased pulmonary secretion viscosity. Heated inhalation suppresses the amplitude of shivering, which minimizes energy expenditures. The quantity of heat exchanged is greater by endotracheal tube than by mask or mist.[59]

Heated Peritoneal Dialysis

Heat conduction is very efficient intraperitoneally. Heated peritoneal dialysis should be considered in severe cases, with persistent cardiovascular instability, and following major toxin ingestions.

Rewarming by peritoneal dialysis is an invasive option and usually not warranted in stable patients. This technique should be used in addition to all other available techniques while rewarming cardiac arrest patients.

Prelavage radiographs should exclude free intraperitoneal air or pneumatosis intestinalis. Gastric and bladder catheterization should be performed. One should infuse 10 ml/kg of isotonic dialysate (0.9 normal saline or Ringer's lactate heated to 40° to 42°C). Fluid should be retained for 15 to 20 minutes and then aspirated. Double catheter systems with outflow suction are more efficient.[93]

Rewarming rates in children usually far exceed the 1° to 2°C/hour observed in adults.[94] The serum potassium must also be monitored since dialysate supplementation may be necessary.

Heated Irrigation

The amount of heat transfer available from irrigation fluids is generally limited by the surface area available for heat exchange. Heated irrigation is inefficient and should not be chosen as the sole rewarming modality.

Closed irrigation systems through intragastric or intracolonic balloons are preferable but rarely available. Direct gastrointestinal irrigation can induce significant fluid and electrolyte fluxes.[95]

Afferent and efferent thoracostomy tube irrigation is another option that has been evaluated in a canine model and a few adults.[96] It offers a number of technical and theoretical advantages over mediastinal irrigation.

One potential clinical indication would be a pediatric hypothermic cardiac arrest victim presenting to an emergency department without cardiac bypass capability. The cardiac output generated during hypothermia with closed chest compressions may exceed that by open massage. The heart seems to function as a passive conduit during CPR with severe hypothermia.[62, 97] The wisdom of open massage of a cold, contracted, stone-hard heart has been questioned.[98]

Heated thoracostomy tube irrigation also does not interrupt CPR. This technique is experimental and may prove to have limitations. For example, left-sided thoracostomy tube insertion in perfusing patients could mechanically induce ventricular fibrillation. Right-sided irrigation could preferentially rewarm the conduction system.

Diathermy

Diathermy is the transmission of heat through the conversion of energy. Low-frequency and ultrasonic microwave radiation delivers heat to deep tissues.[99] Potential contraindications would include frostbite, edema, and the rare child with a metallic implant.

It has been evaluated both experimentally and clinically as a rewarming technique.[90, 94] Zhong et al. initially rewarmed 16 piglets with microwave radiation "until they squealed, suckled, and survived."[90] Subsequently, 20 of 28 human infants were successfully rewarmed with 90 to 100 watts microwave irradiation. The average infant required 45 minutes to reach 36°C. Ongoing research is addressing truncal application and dosimetry guidelines.

Extracorporeal Rewarming

Cardiopulmonary bypass and hemodialysis are the most efficient rewarming modalities during cardiac arrest.[100] They should also be considered for patients who fail to rewarm at a sufficient rate with less invasive techniques. Examples include patients with completely frozen extremities, rhabdomyolysis, and major electrolyte disturbances.[34, 98, 101]

An optional bypass technique in small children involves cannulation of the iliac vessels rather than the femoral artery and vein. With the warmer set at 38° to 40°C, heated oxygenated blood flow is generated.

Hemodialysis may prove to be a more versatile option in spontaneously perfusing patients in some settings. Development of smaller two-way flow catheters allows cannulation of a single vessel.[102]

One must watch for local vascular complications and hemorrhage following anticoagulation.[103] Additional concerns include hemolysis, DIC, pulmonary edema, and acute tubular necrosis.[100]

Pharmacology

During hypothermic conditions, one can expect abnormal physiologic responses to medications. Protein binding will increase. In addition, enterohepatic degradation and renal excretion are altered.

There will usually be a subtherapeutic response to a standard dose of a medication administered while a child is hypothermic.[104] This can progress to toxicity during rewarming. Oral and intramuscular administration should be avoided because of erratic absorption.[1]

Pharmacologic alteration of the pulse or blood pressure is rarely indicated. Hypoglycemia, hypovolemia, or sepsis should be considered if there is a relative tachycardia disproportionate to the temperature.[5]

Catecholamines should be reserved for patients failing to respond to volume resuscitation and rewarming. The vasculature is usually maximally vasoconstricted. Exceeding low-dose catecholamine support will not effectively support the blood pressure. If there is coexistent frostbite, catecholamines will increase tissue loss.[5, 105]

Atrial arrhythmias are commonly seen and usually innocent. Hypothermia slows the ventricular response. Thus atrial antiarrhythmics are not indicated. If there is a rapid ventricular response, recheck for fluid, electrolyte, and acid-base disturbances.

The ideal management of ventricular arrhythmias is unresolved. Bretylium tosylate is the agent of choice for ventricular fibrillation.[106, 107] This agent has been effective in numerous animal models.[108] In pediatric patients the optimal dosage, rate of infusion, and role of prophylaxis with bretylium are unknown.

Steroid administration should be withheld unless there is reason to suspect hypoadrenocorticism.[1] Since cold induces adrenal unresponsiveness to adrenocorticotropic hormone, it is possible to falsely diagnose decreased adrenal reserve.[109] Increased protein binding of cortisol will also decrease the free active fraction. Steroids should be reserved for patients who fail to rewarm, have proven hypoadrenocorticism, or have a previous history of steroid dependence. Routine thyroid hormone administration is also not indicated unless there is a strong reason to suspect myxedema.

Disposition

Early recognition of subtle symptoms facilitates the diagnosis of hypothermia in infancy and early childhood. In older children there is usually a history of exposure or participation in outdoor recreational activities (Table 107–2).

Disposition decisions depend on a variety of factors. A hypothermia outcome score (HOS) has been derived on a large database of 428 cases.[110] Predictors of outcome following multivariant analysis include prehospital cardiac arrest, a low or absent blood pressure, elevated BUN, and the need for endotracheal or nasogastric intubation in the emergency department. However, HOS is currently of limited application owing to the small number of pediatric cases in that series.

TABLE 107–2

DOCUMENTATION

Documentation
Details of exposure: site, duration
Predisposing factors: medications, illness, infection
Associated trauma: frostbite, immersion, submersion
Prehospital treatment
Description of clothing
Physical findings
Vital sign flow sheet: include hourly rate of rewarming, Glasgow coma score

Diagnostics
Laboratory studies, radiographs, EKG
Rewarming technique and response

Discharge Instructions
Remain in warm environment
Monitor child's temperature
Recheck within 24 hr

Unlike for near-drowning victims, there is no validated predictor of outcome for hypothermic patients. In-patient admission and culturing of all infants is required. Also, admission of those children without an obvious history of exposure and mild hypothermia should be considered.

All moderately and severely hypothermic (<32.3°C) children require admission and monitoring. They require further evaluation of predisposing factors and culturing.

FROSTBITE

Introduction

Peripheral cold injuries in children occur as a result of the failure to provide or maintain adequate protection from the environment. Adaptive behavioral reactions to a peripheral cold stress are often lacking in children.

Frostbite is a completely preventable injury that occurs independently or in conjunction with systemic hypothermia.[111] Much of the physiology and pathophysiology of hypothermia and frostbite overlap. However, the unique consideration in frostbite is the pathogenesis of the freezing cascade. Both the freeze-thaw insult and the subsequent progressive dermal ischemia damage tissue.[112]

The incidence and severity of pediatric frostbite correlate with the predisposing factors associated with the cold exposure.[113] In older children the increased participation in outdoor recreational activities results in unanticipated and often underestimated exposures.[101]

Pathophysiology

The cutaneous circulation is one of the physiologic keys to maintaining thermoneutrality. The baseline cutaneous circulation exceeds nutritional requirements, reflecting the "radiator" function of the skin. Cold-induced vasoconstriction will reduce this flow up to tenfold.[113] The skin structures most at risk (fingers, toes, ears, nose) contain arteriovenous anastomoses, which facilitate shunting. This "life-versus-limb" mechanism limits radiative heat loss.[114]

The pathologic phases of frostbite are initiated when the tissue temperature drops to below 0°C. Tissue is injured both by cellular architectural damage following ice crystal formation and by microvascular thrombosis. Prior to ice crystal formation, cutaneous sensation is lost. Radiation and conduction of heat from the deeper tissues prevent crystallization until the skin temperature drops below 0°C.[114]

The exposure circumstances determine the location and rate of ice crystal formation. Ice crystallization usually begins extracellularly. This induces diapedesis of water out of the cell to maintain osmotic equilibrium. Cellular dehydration increases the intracellular osmolarity, which results in cellular collapse. Only with extremely rapid cooling is there more initial intracellular crystallization (Table 107–3).[113]

Progressive microvascular collapse then develops. Red cells sludge and microthrombi develop during the first several hours after thawing. Anaerobic metabolic by-products extend the surrounding injury. Arteriovenous shunting produces thrombosis, increased tissue pressure, ischemia, and finally necrosis.[115]

Progressive dermal ischemia is also partially mediated by thromboxane.[112] Analysis of fluid in vesicles suggests prostaglandin involvement.[116] The arachidonic acid breakdown products released from damaged tissue include prostaglandin $F_2\alpha$ and thromboxane A_2. These mediators aggregate platelets, immobilize leukocytes, and result in vasoconstriction.[117]

Injury to the microvasculature is probably the ultimate determinant of progressive tissue damage.[118] Endothelial cells are as susceptible to freezing injury as are the epiphyses.[119]

After tissue has been thawed, edema will progress for 48 to 72 hours. Thrombosis and early necrosis become apparent after resolution of this edema. Final demarcation often requires more than 60 to 90 days.

Etiology

Common factors predisposing to pediatric frostbite are mainly environmental. Although there are some individuals with variable cold tolerance, there are no data to suggest that age affects susceptibility to frostbite. Any conditions or clothing that impairs peripheral circulation is associated with frostbite.

Although air itself is a poor thermal conductor, the associated cold and wind (windchill index) will markedly increase heat loss. Direct skin contact with good thermal conductors, including water, volatile liquids, and metal, also affects the extent and rapidity of tissue destruction.[120, 121]

TABLE 107–3

FREEZING INJURY CASCADE

Prefreeze Phase
Superficial tissue "cooling"
Increased viscosity of vascular contents
Microvascular constriction
Endothelial plasma leakage

Freeze-Thaw Phase
*Extra*cellular fluid ice crystal formation*
Water diapedesis across cell membrane
*Intra*cellular dehydration and hyperosmolality
Cell membrane denaturation/disruption
Cell shrinkage and collapse

Vascular Stasis and Progressive Ischemia
Vasospasticity and stasis coagulation
Arteriovenous shunting
Vascular endothelial cell damage/prostanoid release
Interstitial leakage/tissue hypertension
Necrosis/demarcation/mummification/slough

Reproduced by permission from Danzl DF. Frostbite. *In* Rosen P, Barkin R, Braen R, et al. (eds). Emergency Medicine: Concepts and Clinical Practice. 3rd ed. St. Louis, CV Mosby, 1992.
*Extremely rapid cooling produces more initial intracellular than extracellular ice crystallization.

Clinical Presentation
Symptoms

Intense vasoconstrictive ischemia and neuropraxia produce the most common presenting symptom, anesthesia. The distal extremities, ears, and nose are especially at risk. Reestablishment of perfusion causes significant pain. A dull, continuous ache progresses to a throbbing sensation in 48 to 72 hours.[114]

Signs

The initial presentation of frostbite can be deceptively benign. Frozen tissues do not always appear mottled and waxy. In severe cases the dermis will not roll over bony prominences. Soft, pliable subcutaneous tissues suggest a superficial injury.[113]

Favorable signs after thawing include normal sensation, warmth, and color. A residual violaceous hue is ominous. The delayed appearance of small hemorrhagic blebs reflects damage to the subdermal vascular plexi. Early clear vesicle formation is a more favorable predictor.

Therapeutic Intervention
Prehospital Treatment

It is rarely practical to attempt field rewarming of frozen tissue. The child's wet or constrictive clothing should be removed gently; the affected areas should be insulated and immobilized. Friction massage will increase tissue loss.

In severe cases frozen parts should be kept away from dry heat sources to prevent gradual, incomplete thawing. Field rewarming should not be initiated if there is any possibility for incomplete thawing. Tissue refreezing also markedly extends the injury.[122]

Emergency Department Treatment

Thaw. Partially thawed or frozen tissue should be *rapidly* rewarmed by immersion in gently circulating water.[123] The water temperature should be maintained at 40° to 41°C by thermometer measurement.[124] Marginal tissue will be thermally injured if the water temperature exceeds 42° to 43°C.

Rewarming should be continued until the part feels pliable and distal erythema is present. This often requires 10 to 30 minutes of submersion. Direct tissue massage should be strictly avoided. Since reperfusion is intensely painful, parenteral analgesia is often indicated. Premature termination of thawing will increase tissue loss.

Postthaw. If the extremities are involved, they should be kept elevated to minimize edema formation. Persistent cyanosis after a complete thaw may indicate increased fascial compartment pressures. Rhabdomyolysis can occur with full-thickness freezing.[125] Cold-induced anesthesia may minimize pain perception. There are no radiographic or diagnostic techniques that accurately predict tissue loss at presentation.[113, 118]

Secondary dermal ischemia is associated with the accumulation of arachidonic acid breakdown products.[112] Topical aloe vera (Dermaide) specifically inhibits thromboxane when applied topically to frostbitten areas. Systemic ibuprofen also inhibits this cascade while facilitating fibrinolysis.[117]

Frostbite blister management recommendations include leaving blisters intact, debridement, and aspiration. Some authors feel that all intact blisters should be debrided to avoid tissue contact with the chemical mediators of ischemia.[116, 117] Others initially leave clear bullae intact.[111] Hemorrhagic blisters should not be debrided. Desiccation of deep dermal layers will extend the injury.

Children should be hospitalized for 24 to 48 hours to assess the extent of injury. Superficial injuries, especially to facial structures, may be followed as an outpatient. Tetanus immunity should be updated and streptococcal prophylaxis provided for 48 to 72 hours.[126] Elevation and daily hydrotherapy should be continued until the eschar sloughs. Sterile precautions may then be discontinued.

Ancillary Treatment Modalities

A variety of experimental antithrombotic, vasodilatory, and anti-inflammatory treatment regimens have yielded inconsistent results. Low-molecular-weight dextran and heparinization fail to enhance tissue salvage convincingly. The long-acting alpha blocker phenoxybenzamine may be useful with persistent vasospasm. Calcium channel blockers are also under study.[113, 127]

Sympathectomy

Theoretical advantages of sympathectomy include relief of vasospasm and reduction of edema.[122, 128] Surgical sympathectomy provides no substantial long-term benefits. A "medical" sympathectomy can be achieved by injection of an agent such as reserpine directly into a terminal artery. This may prove most useful in patients with persistent pain after gradual thawing.[127] Hyperbaric oxygen therapy has yet to be adequately evaluated.

Sequelae

The most common symptomatic sequelae of frostbite result from direct neuronal damage and abnormal sympathetic tone.[129] Intermittent paresthesia and burning are common complaints. Thermal perception and hidrosis are also altered after deep frostbite.

Premature destruction, fragmentation, or fusion of epiphyses is a major concern.[130, 131] Distal phalanges will shorten, and, in addition, frostbite arthritis has been reported.[132–134]

Delayed cutaneous findings include pigmentation changes and nail deformities. Squamous and epidermoid cell carcinoma can develop years later.[135] Osseous reabsorption and subchondral lytic defects begin to appear months after the cold insult.[136]

Summary

Early prediction of the severity of frostbite in the emergency department is inaccurate. Although most patients do not present with completely frozen tissue, rapid rewarming is still initiated in 40° to 41°C circulating water. Analgesia should be administered as required while achieving a complete thaw.

Involved extremities should be elevated, and sterile isolation intitiated. One should consider systemic and topical prostaglandin inhibition. Unless the injury is superficial, patients should be hospitalized for 24 to 48 hours to assess the extent of damage. Frequent wound evaluation and daily whirlpool baths with active exercise are indicated. Surgical intervention should be extremely conservative and delayed until there is clear tissue demarcation.

References

1. Maclean D, Emslie-Smith D. Accidental Hypothermia. Philadelphia, JB Lippincott, 1977, p 133.
2. Reuler JB. Hypothermia: Pathophysiology, clinical settings, and management. Ann Intern Med 1978;89:519.
3. Dagan R, Gorodischer R. Infections in hypothermic infants younger than 3 months old. Am J Dis Child 1984;183:483.

4. Wagner JA, Robinson S, Marino RP. Age and temperature regulation of humans in neutral and cold environments. J Appl Physiol 1974;37:562.
5. Danzl DF, Pozos RS, Hamlet MP. Accidental hypothermia. *In* Auerbach P, Geehr E (eds). Management of Wilderness and Environmental Emergencies. 2nd ed. St. Louis, CV Mosby, 1989, pp 35–76.
6. Perlstein PH, Hersh C, Glueck CJ, et al. Adaptation to cold in the first three days of life. Pediatrics 1974;54:411.
7. Lamb FS, Rosner MS. Neonatal resuscitation. Emerg Med Clin North Am 1987;5:541.
8. Boulant JA, Dean JB. Temperature receptors in the central nervous system. Ann Rev Physiol 1986;48:639.
9. El-Radhi AS, Al-Kafaji N. Neonatal hypothermia in a developing country. Clin Pediatr 1980;19:401.
10. Harnett RM, Pruitt JR, Sias FR. A review of the literature concerning resuscitation from hypothermia. Part II. Selected rewarming protocols. Aviat Space Environ Med 1983;54:487.
11. Lafferty JJ, Keykhah MM, Shapiro HM, et al. Cerebral hypometabolism obtained with deep pentobarbital anesthesia and hypothermia (30°C). Anesthesiology 1978;49:159.
12. Orlowski JP, Erenberg G, Lueders H, et al. Hypothermia and barbiturate coma for refractory status epilepticus. Crit Care Med 1984;12:367.
13. Fishbeck KH, Simon RP. Neurological manifestations of accidental hypothermia. Ann Neurol 1981;10:384.
14. Webb P. Afterdrop of body temperature during rewarming: An alternative explanation. J Appl Physiol 1986;60:385.
15. Hayward JS, Eckerson JD, Kemna D. Thermal and cardiovascular changes during three methods of resuscitation from mild hypothermia. Resuscitation 1984;11:21.
16. Thompson R, Rich J, Chmelik F, et al. Evolutionary changes in the electrocardiogram of severe progressive hypothermia. Electrocardiology 1977;10:62.
17. Ilia R, Ovsyshcher I, Rudnik L, et al. Atypical ventricular tachycardia and alternating Osborn waves induced by spontaneous mild hypothermia. Pediatr Cardiol 1988;9:63.
18. Solomon A, Barish RA, Browne B, et al. The electrocardiographic features of hypothermia. J Emerg Med 1989;7:169.
19. Kiley JP, Eldridge FL, Millhorn DE. Respiration during hypothermia: Effect of rewarming intermediate areas of ventral medulla. J Appl Physiol 1985;59:1423.
20. Segar WE. Effect of hypothermia on tubular transport mechanisms. Am J Physiol 1958;195:91.
21. El-Radhi AS, Jawad M, Mansor N, et al. Sepsis and hypothermia in the newborn infant: Value of gastric aspirate examination. J Pediatr 1983;103:300.
22. El-Radhi AS, Jawad MH, Mansor N, et al. Infection in neonatal hypothermia. Arch Dis Child 1983;58:143.
23. Himms-Hagen J. Thermogenesis in brown adipose tissue as an energy buffer. N Engl J Med 1984;311:1549.
24. Robinson M, Seward PN. Environmental hypothermia in children. Pediatr Emerg Care 1986;2:254.
25. Sofer S, Yagupsky P, Hershkowits T, et al. Improved outcome of hypothermic infants. Pediatr Emerg Care 1986;2:211.
26. Georgitis WJ, Hofeldt FD. Myxedema coma and cardiac arrest. JAMA 1982;247:980.
27. Lyen KR. Cold stress and congenital adrenal hyperplasia in heterozygotes. Med Hypotheses 1983;12:77.
28. Strauch BS, Felig P, Baxter JD, et al. Hypothermia in hypoglycemia. JAMA 1969;210:345.
29. Sadikali F, Owor R. Hypothermia in the tropics: A review of 24 cases. Trop Geogr Med 1974;26:265.
30. Reuler JB, Jones SR, Girard DE. Hypothermia in the erythroderma syndrome. West J Med 1977;127:243.
31. Garty BZ, Wiseman Y, Metzker A, et al. Hypernatremic dehydration and hypothermia in congenital lamellar ichthyosis. Pediatr Dermatol 1985;3:65.
32. Livingston JH, Groggins RC. Clinical curio: Hypothermia caused by treatment of a scald. Br Med J 1984;228:771.
33. Sivaloganatham S. Paradoxical undressing due to hypothermia in a child. Med Sci Law 1985;25:176.
34. Bolte RG, Black PG, Bowers RS, et al. The use of extracorporeal rewarming in a child submerged for 66 minutes. JAMA 1988;260:377.
35. Drenck NE, Staffeldt HV. Repeated deep accidental hypothermia. Anaesthesia 1986;41:731.
36. Kallenback J, Bagg P, Feldman C, et al. Experience with acute poisoning in an intensive care unit. A review of 103 cases. S Afr Med J 1981;59:587.
37. Lacoutre PG, Lovejoy FH, Mitchell AA. Acute hypothermia associated with atropine. Am J Dis Child 1983;137:291.
38. Greene JW, Craft L, Ghishan F. Acetaminophen poisoning in infancy. Am J Dis Child 1983;137:386.
39. Lieh-Lai MW, Sarnaik AP, Newton JF, et al. Metabolism and pharmacokinetics of acetaminophen in a severely poisoned young child. J Pediatr 1984;105:125.
40. Ludwig S, Warman M. Shaken baby syndrome: A review of 20 cases. Ann Emerg Med 1984;13:104.
41. Dunne KP, Matthews TG. Hypothermia and sudden infant death syndrome. Arch Dis Child 1988;63:438.
42. Buccini RV. Hypothermia in Hodgkin's disease. N Engl J Med 1985;312:244.
43. Guerin JM, Meyer P, Segrestaa JM. Hypothermia in diabetic ketoacidosis. Diabetes Care 1987;10:801.
44. Ashworth M, Arthur M, Pye G, et al. Missed injuries of the spinal cord. Br Med J 1982;284:1334.
45. Altus P, Hickman JW, Nord HJ. Accidental hypothermia in a healthy quadriplegic patient. Neurology 1985;35:427.
46. Best R, Syverud S, Nowak RM. Trauma and hypothermia. Am J Emerg Med 1985;3:48.
47. Rodis JF, Vintzileos AM, Campbell WA, et al. Maternal hypothermia: An unusual complication of magnesium sulfate therapy. Am J Obstet Gynecol 1987;156:435.
48. Jadhon ME, Main EK. Fetal bradycardia associated with maternal hypothermia. Obstet Gynecol 1988;72:496.
49. Shapiro WR, Williams GH, Plum F. Spontaneous recurrent hypothermia accompanying agenesis of the corpus callosum. Brain 1969;92:423.
50. Pineda M, Gonzalez A, Fabreques I, et al. Familial agenesis of the corpus callosum with hypothermia and apneic spells. Neuropediatrics 1984;15:63.
51. Sanfield JA, Linares OA, Cahalan DD, et al. Altered norepinephrine metabolism in Shapiro's syndrome. Arch Neurol 1989;46:53.
52. Sander KB, Bommen M, Brook CG. Spontaneous hypothermia in a young boy. Arch Dis Child 1983;58:230.
53. Gregory RT, Patton JF. Treatment after exposure to cold. Lancet 1972;1:377.
54. Steinman A. Prehospital management of hypothermia. Response 1987;6:18.
55. Maningas PA, DeGuzman LR, Hollenbach SJ, et al. Regional blood flow during hypothermic arrest. Ann Emerg Med 1986;15:390.
56. Niemann JT, Rosborough J, Hausknecht M, et al. Pressure-synchronized cineangiography during experimental cardiopulmonary resuscitation. Circulation 1981;64:945.
57. Hochachka PW. Defense strategies against hypoxia and hypothermia. Science 1986;231:234.
58. Huet RCG, Harkliczek GF, Coad NR. Pupil size and light reactivity in hypothermic infants and adults. Intensive Care Med 1989;15:216.
59. Miller JW, Danzl DF, Thomas DM. Urban accidental hypothermia: 135 cases. Ann Emerg Med 1980;9:456.
60. Severinghaus JW, Astrup PB. History of blood gas analysis III. Carbon dioxide tension. J Clin Monit 1986;2:60.
61. Swain JA, White FN, Peters RM. The effect of pH on the hypothermic ventricular fibrillation threshold. J Thorac Cardiovasc Surg 1984;87:445.
62. Danzl DF, Pozos RS, Auerbach P, et al. Multicenter hypothermia survey. Ann Emerg Med 1987;16:1042.
63. Rahn H, Reeves RB, Howell BJ. Hydrogen ion regulation, temperature, and evolution. Am Rev Resp Dis 1975;112:165.
64. Swain JA. Hypothermia and blood pH. A review. Arch Intern Med 1988;148:1643.
65. White FN. Reassessing acid-base balance in hypothermia: A comparative point of view. West J Med 1983;138:255.
66. Becker H, Vinten-Johansen J, Buckberg GD, et al. Myocardial damage caused by keeping pH 7.40 during systemic deep hypothermia. J Thorac Cardiovasc Surg 1981;82:810.
67. Delaney KA, Howland MA, Vassallo S, et al. Assessment of acid-base disturbances in hypothermia and their physiologic consequences. Ann Emerg Med 1989;18:72.
68. Matthews AJ, Stead AL, Abbott TR. Acid-base control during hypothermia. Anaesthesia 1984;39:649.
69. Kroncke GM, Nichols PD, Mendenhall JT, et al. Ectothermic philosophy of acid-base balance to prevent fibrillation during hypothermia. Arch Surg 1986;121:303.
70. Shenaq SA, Yawn DH, Saleem A, et al. Effect of profound hypothermia on leukocytes and platelets. Ann Clin Lab Sci 1986;16:130.
71. Holm IA, McLaughlin JF, Feldman K, et al. Recurrent hypothermia and thrombocytopenia after severe neonatal brain infection. Clin Pediatr 1988;27:326.
72. Cohen IA, Amir J, Gedaliah A, et al. Thrombocytopenia of neonatal cold injury. J Pediatr 1984;104:620.
73. Mahajan AL, Myers TJ, Baldini MG. Disseminated intravascular coagulation during rewarming following hypothermia. JAMA 1981;245:2517.
74. Carden DL, Nowak RM. Disseminated intravascular coagulation in hypothermia. JAMA 1982;247:2099.
75. Patt A, McCroskey BL, Moore EE. Hypothermia-induced coagulopathies in trauma. Surg Clin North Am 1988;68:775.
76. Lewin S, Brettman LR, Holzman RS. Infections in hypothermic patients. Arch Intern Med 1981;141:920.
77. Sung Y, Akriotis V, Barker C, et al. Susceptibility of human and porcine neutrophils to hypothermia in vitro. Pediatr Res 1985;19:1044.
78. Biggar WD, Bohn D, Kent G. Neutrophil circulating and release from bone marrow during hypothermia. Infect Immun 1983;40:708.
79. Clardy CW, Edwards KM, Gay JC. Increased susceptibility to infection

in hypothermic children: Possible role of acquired neutrophil dysfunction. Pediatr Infect Dis 1985;4:379.

80. Bohn DJ, Biggar WD, Smith CR, et al. Influence of hypothermia, barbiturate therapy and intracranial pressure monitoring on morbidity and mortality after near-drowning. Crit Care Med 1986;14:529.

81. Yagupsky P, Sofer S. Infection in hypothermic infants. Pediatr Infect Dis 1986;5:112.

82. Yagupsky P, Mares AJ, Gorodischer R. Pyloric stenosis associated with hypothermia. J Trop Pediatr 1986;32:270.

83. White JD, Butterfield AB, Almquist TD, et al. Controlled comparison of humidified inhalation and peritoneal lavage in rewarming immersion hypothermia. Am J Emerg Med 1984;2:210.

84. Tafari N, Gentz J. Aspects on rewarming newborn infants with severe accidental hypothermia. Acta Paediatr Scand 1974;63:595.

85. Myers RA, Britten JS, Cowley RA. Hypothermia: Quantitative aspects of therapy. JACEP 1979;8:523.

86. Moss J. Accidental severe hypothermia. Surg Gynecol Obstet 1986;162:501.

87. Samuelson T, Doolittle W, Hayward J, et al. Hypothermia and cold water neardrowning: Treatment guidelines. Alaska Med 1982;24:106.

88. Stamm-Racine J, Ferrier PE. Management of neonatal hypothermia. J Pediatr 1985;106:532.

89. Kaplan M, Eidelman AI. Improved prognosis in severely hypothermic newborn infants treated by rapid rewarming. J Pediatr 1984;105:470.

90. Zhong H, Qinyi S, Mingjiang S. Rewarming with microwave irradiation in severe cold injury syndrome. Chin Med J 1980;93:119.

91. Feldman KW, Morray JP, Schaller RT. Thermal injury caused by hot pack application in hypothermic children. Am J Emerg Med 1985;3:38.

92. Sarman I, Can G, Tunell R. Rewarming preterm infants on a heated, water filled mattress. Arch Dis Child 1989;64:687.

93. Jessen K, Hagelsten JO. Peritoneal dialysis in the treatment of profound accidental hypothermia. Aviat Space Environ Med 1978;49:426.

94. White JD, Butterfield AB, Greer KA, et al. Controlled comparison of radiowave regional hyperthermia and peritoneal lavage-rewarming of immersion hypothermia. J Trauma 1985;25:101.

95. Kristensen G, Gravesen H, Benveniste D, et al. An oesophageal thermal tube for rewarming in hypothermia. Acta Anaesthesiol Scand 1985;29:846.

96. Brunette DD, Sterner S, Robinson EP, et al. Comparison of gastric lavage and thoracic cavity lavage in the treatment of severe hypothermia in dogs. Ann Emerg Med 1987;16:1222.

97. Niemann JT, Rosborough J, Hausknecht M, et al. Blood flow without cardiac compression during closed chest CPR. Crit Care Med 1981;9:380.

98. Althaus U, Aeberhard P, Schupbach P, et al. Management of profound accidental hypothermia with cardiorespiratory arrest. Ann Surg 1982;195:492.

99. White JD, Butterfield AB, Greer KA, et al. Comparison of rewarming by radio wave regional hyperthermia and warm humidified inhalation. Aviat Space Environ Med 1984;55:1103.

100. Splittgerber FH, Talbert JG, Sweezer WP, et al. Partial cardiopulmonary bypass for core rewarming in profound accidental hypothermia. Am Surg 1986;52:407.

101. Hauty MG, Esrig BC, Hill JG, et al. Prognostic factors in severe accidental hypothermia: Experience from the Mt. Hood tragedy. J Trauma 1987;27:1107.

102. O'Keeffe KM. Treatment of accidental hypothermia and rewarming techniques. In Roberts JR, Hedges JR (eds). Clinical Procedures in Emergency Medicine. Philadelphia, WB Saunders, 1985, p 1040.

103. Seuffert G. An Alaskan experience with cardiopulmonary bypass in resuscitating patients with profound hypothermia and cardiac arrest. Alaska Med 1984;26:31.

104. Wong KC. Physiology and pharmacology of hypothermia. West J Med 1983;138:227.

105. Chernow B, Lake CR, Zaritsky A, et al. Sympathetic nervous system "switchoff" with severe hypothermia. Crit Care Med 1983;11:677.

106. Danzl DF, Sowers MB, Vicario SJ, et al. Chemical ventricular defibrillation in severe accidental hypothermia. Ann Emerg Med 1982;11:698.

107. Kochar G, Kahn SE, Kotler MN. Bretylium tosylate and ventricular fibrillation in hypothermia. Ann Intern Med 1986;105:624.

108. Murphy K, Nowak RM, Tomlanovich MC. Use of bretylium tosylate as prophylaxis and treatment in hypothermic ventricular fibrillation in the canine model. Ann Emerg Med 1986;15:1160.

109. Felicetta JV, Green WL, Goodner CJ. Decreased adrenal responsiveness in hypothermic patients. J Clin Endocrinol Metab 1980;50:93.

110. Danzl DF, Hedges JR, Pozos RS, et al. Hypothermia outcome score: Development and implications. Crit Care Med 1989;17:227.

111. Mills WJ Jr. Frostbite. Alaska Med 1973;15:27.

112. McCauley RL, Hing DN, Robson MC, et al. Frostbite injuries: A rational approach based on the pathophysiology. J Trauma 1983;23:143.

113. Smith DJ, Robson MC, Heggers JP. Frostbite and other cold-induced injuries. In Auerbach PS, Geehr EC (eds). Management of Wilderness and Environmental Emergencies. 2nd ed. St. Louis, CV Mosby, 1989, pp 101–118.

114. Purdue GF, Hunt J. Cold injury: A collective review. J Burn Care Rehabil 1986;7:331.

115. Lazarus HM, Hutto W. Electric burns and frostbite: Patterns of vascular injury. J Trauma 1982;22:581.

116. Robson MC, Heggers JP. Evaluation of hand frostbite blister fluid as a clue to pathogenesis. J Hand Surg 1981;6:43.

117. Heggers JP, Robson MC. Frostbite: Experimental and clinical evaluations of treatment. J Wilderness Med 1990;1:27.

118. Schoning P, Hamlet MP. Experimental frost-bite in Hanford miniature swine. II. Vascular changes. Br J Exp Pathol 1989;70:51.

119. Marzella L, Jesudass RR, Manson PN, et al. Morphologic characterization of acute injury to vascular endothelium of skin after frostbite. Plast Reconstr Surg 1989;83:67.

120. Purdue GF, Layton TR, Copeland CE. Cold injury complicating burn therapy. J Trauma 1985;25:167.

121. Drez D, Faust DC, Evans JP. Cryotherapy and nerve palsy. Am J Sports Med 1981;9:256.

122. Kyosola K. Clinical experiences in the management of cold injuries: A study of 110 cases. J Trauma 1974;14:32.

123. Mills WJ, Whaley R, Fish W. Frostbite: Experience with rapid rewarming and ultrasonic therapy. Alaska Med 1961;3:28.

124. Malhotra MS, Matthew L. Effect of rewarming at various water bath temperatures in experimental frostbite. Aviat Space Environ Med 1978;49:874.

125. Raifman MA, Berant M, Lenarsky C. Cold weather and rhabdomyolysis. J Pediatr 1978;93:970.

126. Didlake RH, Kokokra JS. Tetanus following frostbite injury. Contemp Orthop 1985;10:69.

127. Hamlet MP. An overview of medically related problems in the cold environment. Milit Med 1987;152:393.

128. Arregui R, Morandeira JR, Martinez G, et al. Epidural neurostimulation in the treatment of frostbite. PACE 1989;12:713.

129. Kumar VN. Intractable foot pain following frostbite: Case report. Arch Phys Med Rehabil 1982;63:284.

130. Selke AC. Destruction of phalangeal epiphyses by frostbite. Radiology 1969;93:859.

131. Reed MH. Growth disturbances in the hands following thermal injuries in children. II. Frostbite. Can Assoc Radiol J 1988;39:95.

132. Leung AKC, Lai PCW. Digital deformities from frostbite. Can Med Assoc J 1985;132:14.

133. McKendry RJR. Frostbite arthritis. Can Med Assoc J 1981;125:1128.

134. Brown FE, Spiegel PK, Boyle WE Jr. Digital deformity: An effect of frostbite in children. Pediatrics 1983;71:955.

135. Rossis CG, Yiacoumettis AM, Elemenoglou J. Squamous cell carcinoma of the heel developing at a site of previous frostbite. J Royal Sci Med 1982;75:715.

136. Carrera GF, Kozin F, Flaherty L, et al. Radiographic changes in the hands following childhood frostbite injury. Skeletal Radiol 1981;6:33.

CHAPTER 108

Smoke Inhalation and Carbon Monoxide Poisoning

S. William Snover

INTRODUCTION

Approximately 10,000 people die annually in the United States as the result of fire. Less than half of these deaths are due to thermal injury; the majority of the deaths result from the inhalation of smoke and other toxic products of pyrolysis. Smoke inhalation is frequent and induces distinct patterns of injury and death. Carbon monoxide is the most commonly encountered toxin produced by fire that results in the death of the fire victim.

ANATOMY AND PATHOPHYSIOLOGY

Victims of fire suffer from three distinct but overlapping injuries, either singly or in combination. The first and most obvious injury is the thermal injury resulting from flame, superheated gases, or steam. The second injury results from the inhalation of the smoke produced by the fire. Smoke inhalation can result in immediate, early, or delayed death. The third injury results from the inhalation of toxins produced as products of pyrolysis. Carbon monoxide is the most common and most important of these toxins and is responsible for most of the immediate and early fire-related deaths. Most victims of smoke inhalation or early toxin-related death also have some degree of thermal injury.

Three distinct syndromes of death are recognized in fire-related inhalation injuries. The first is an asphyxia-obtundation syndrome, which is most responsible for immediate or early death. While total consumption of oxygen by the fire in an enclosed space can be encountered, the syndrome is more likely due to carbon monoxide or other toxic products of combustion. The second syndrome is that of airway obstruction, which produces early death, usually in less than 12 hours. This is due to the mechanical and noxious effects of smoke toxicity. Thermal injury to the upper airway plays a limited role in this syndrome. The third syndrome is recognized as the hypoxia-hypoventilation syndrome, most frequently seen in late deaths, occurring from 12 hours to several weeks postinjury. This produces adult respiratory distress syndrome with interstitial pulmonary edema. Sepsis plays a significant role. Pneumonia is seen in up to 71% of fire victims who die after more than 12 hours. Direct airway contamination and hematogenous spread of bacteria from contaminated surface wounds play a role.

Smoke refers to all products of combustion or pyrolysis and includes all of the gases and particulates that are normal products of combustion and those that are unique to a particular material being burned. Smoke carries the products of combustion, including carbonaceous particles, oxides of sulfur and nitrogen, and various aldehydes. Pyrolysis of synthetic polymers, which are frequently involved in structure fires, produces additional toxins and products of combustion, including hydrocyanic acid, hydrochloric acid, sulfuric acid, various halogenated by-products, benzene, phosgene, isocyanates, and others (Table 108–1). These products are all noxious when inhaled, producing airway injury. The chemical injury causes a reduction of lung bacterial clearance and mucociliary transport. Peribronchial edema and necrosis of mucosal tissue are seen. Bronchoconstriction is caused by stimulation of airway irritant receptors. Increased pulmonary vascular resistance is produced by a variety of mechanisms, including cerebral anoxia, epinephrine release, and interstitial edema. This resistance causes decreased cardiac output. Chemical tracheobronchitis with sloughing of airway mucosa causes occlusion of both central and peripheral airways. Inhalation of smoke-borne toxins

damages alveolar epithelium and capillary endothelium, producing increased permeability of the alveolar-capillary membrane and causing interstitial pulmonary edema. This can be immediate or delayed up to 1 week. These effects produce severe airway obstruction and ventilation perfusion mismatch.

Thermal injury to the upper airway can cause airway obstruction, but this is uncommon and is seen in less than 5% of victims. Inhalation of superheated steam, however, will exceed the upper airway's ability to protect itself and will more frequently cause a thermal injury.

Carbon monoxide is produced by the incomplete combustion of carbon-containing fuels. Carbon monoxide accounts for the greatest number of fire-related deaths and is also responsible for about one half of the over 3500 fatal poisonings reported in the United States each year. Thousands of additional nonfatal causes of carbon monoxide poisonings go unrecognized.

Carbon monoxide is a colorless, odorless, tasteless, nonirritating gas. It is the most common gaseous substance found in all types of fires regardless of the composition of the material that is being burned. It causes rapid death by producing tissue hypoxia.

Carbon monoxide combines with hemoglobin to form carboxyhemoglobin (COHb) and competes with oxygen for the available hemoglobin binding sites. The affinity of hemoglobin for carbon monoxide is approximately 250 times greater than for oxygen, so the COHb concentration is considerable even when the inspired concentration of carbon monoxide is small. Concentrations of 0.1% carbon monoxide in the inspired room air will produce a COHb level of up to 60% in a few minutes. With increased concentrations of carbon monoxide, the saturation of hemoglobin with carbon monoxide will become higher more rapidly. The carbon monoxide concentration in the smoke of a major fire may be as high as 10%. A firefighter or trapped victim exerting strenuously with an unprotected airway in such an environment will develop COHb concentrations as high as 75% in less than 1 minute. The result is usually fatal.

Hypoxia, resulting from the displacement of oxygen from hemoglobin by carbon monoxide, is the cause of most of the effects of carbon monoxide exposure. In addition, carbon monoxide causes myocardial depression and increases ventricular irritability. The resulting additional decrease in cardiac output due to hypotension and dysrhythmia adds to impaired tissue perfusion. Carbon monoxide, when transferred from hemoglobin to tissue, binds to cytochrome oxidase and is believed to interfere with cytochrome A_3- and P-450-based cellular metabolism, contributing to cellular asphyxia. This produces the immediate symptoms of unconsciousness, cardiac arrest, and death and may also be re-

TABLE 108–1

TOXINS PRODUCED BY COMBUSTION OF SPECIFIC MATERIALS

Material	Toxins Produced
Wood, cotton, paper	Acetaldehyde, formaldehyde, acrolein, formic acid, nitrous oxides, sulfur oxides, carbon monoxide, methane, acetic acid
Petroleum products	Acetic acid, formic acid, acrolein, sulfur oxides, carbon monoxide
Wool, silk, nylon	Phosgene, hydrogen cyanide, hydrogen sulfide, ammonia, carbon monoxide
Polyvinyl chloride (multiple manmade materials)	Hydrogen cyanide, hydrogen chloride, phosgene, chlorine, carbon monoxide
Nitrocellulose film, fabric	Nitrogen oxides, acetic acid, formic acid
Polyester resins	Hydrogen chloride, hydrogen fluoride, hydrogen bromide
Polyurethane	Isocyanates, hydrogen cyanide
Teflon	Hydrogen fluoride, octafluoroisobutylene
Rubber	Sulfur dioxide, hydrogen sulfide
Animal products	Hydrogen sulfide

sponsible for delayed symptoms and sequelae involving the heart and central nervous system (CNS). The heart and CNS are particularly sensitive to carbon monoxide poisoning owing to their higher metabolic rate. Finally, carbon monoxide causes the oxygen-hemoglobin dissociation curve to shift to the left (Fig. 108–1). This causes a further decrease in oxygen availability to tissues.

Cyanide has been implicated as an additional toxin present in the fire environment that causes cellular asphyxia. This is particularly true if synthetic polymers are fueling the fire. Like carbon monoxide, cyanide interferes with respiration at the cellular level by attaching to cytochrome. However, because cyanide and other toxic inhalants are difficult to detect and measure and treatment needs to be so immediate, it is best to focus on the need to treat carbon monoxide.

EMS CONSIDERATIONS

The successful management of victims of smoke inhalation is based on early recognition and vigorous therapy (Table 108–2). Thermal burns are present in 95% of cases. The presence of burns on the face or upper body is a sensitive indicator for the presence of an inhalation injury. Fires occurring in closed spaces such as structure fires result in a high incidence of inhalation injury. Nonproductive cough, hoarseness, singed nasal hair, eye irritation, soot in the oropharynx, bronchorrhea, carbonaceous sputum, and bronchospasm are clinical indicators of airway involvement. The presence of soot and the odor of smoke in association with headache, nausea, dyspnea, or chest pain should also provide strong clues to smoke inhalation injury.

Airway maintenance and administration of high-flow oxygen is mandatory. If the airway is compromised or spontaneous breathing is inadequate, early intubation is essential. Because airway compromise is frequently progressive in these injuries, any delay in providing airway access may result in the inability to intubate the victim when the situation deteriorates. Once intubated, ventilation should be assisted and initially maintained with 100% oxygen.

The mental status of the victim should be assessed. Mental

TABLE 108–2
SIGNS AND SYMPTOMS OF SMOKE INHALATION

Central nervous system	Dizziness
	Headache
	Seizure
	Confusion
	Coma
Pulmonary	Tachypnea
	Cough
	Hoarseness, sore throat
	Stridor
	Dyspnea
	Chest pain
	Wheezing
	Hemoptysis
	Carbonaceous sputum
Cardiac	Chest pain
	Cardiac dysrhythmias
Gastrointestinal	Nausea, vomiting
	Abdominal pain
Skin	Burns
	Bullae

confusion, dysequilibrium, or unconsciousness may be the only abnormalities present but may be the most sensitive indicators of impaired tissue oxygenation due to an inhalation injury. Other findings associated with carbon monoxide poisoning, such as "cherry red lips" or "ruddy complexion," are usually absent.

A severe upper airway obstruction that precludes successful endotracheal intubation requires a surgical airway. Intubation utilizing a fiberoptic laryngoscope is recommended and may successfully avoid the need to perform a surgical airway.

Fluid resuscitation can be initiated, but uninjured skin should be used to establish intravenous access. It is usually impossible to achieve venous access through burned skin, but if it cannot be obtained through other peripheral burn sites, these areas can be used. These sites need to be changed to unburned peripheral or central sites soon after arrival at the treating emergency department. Lactated Ringer's solution is the fluid of choice for early resuscitation. If trauma is involved, cervical spine precautions must be maintained throughout resuscitation. Preparation for transport to the receiving emergency department needs to be accomplished with as little delay as possible.

During transport, frequent suctioning of the airway to remove secretions, sloughed tissue, and aspirated debris will be required to maintain airway patency.

DIAGNOSTIC EVALUATION

The critical blood studies to obtain on victims of smoke inhalation include a complete blood count, arterial blood gases, and serum COHb level. If a thermal injury is also involved, the usual blood studies associated with the evaluation of burns are indicated. Hypoxemia needs to be corrected, and hypercapnea would indicate inadequate alveolar ventilation. Metabolic acidosis, if present, would indicate inadequate tissue perfusion or oxygenation, leading to anaerobic metabolism. This finding should be confirmed by measurement of blood lactate levels.

When interpreting arterial blood gases, one must know whether the oxygen saturation of hemoglobin is directly measured or a standard nomogram to calculate oxygen saturation based on measured PaO_2 is used. An early clue to the presence of carbon monoxide poisoning is a decreased

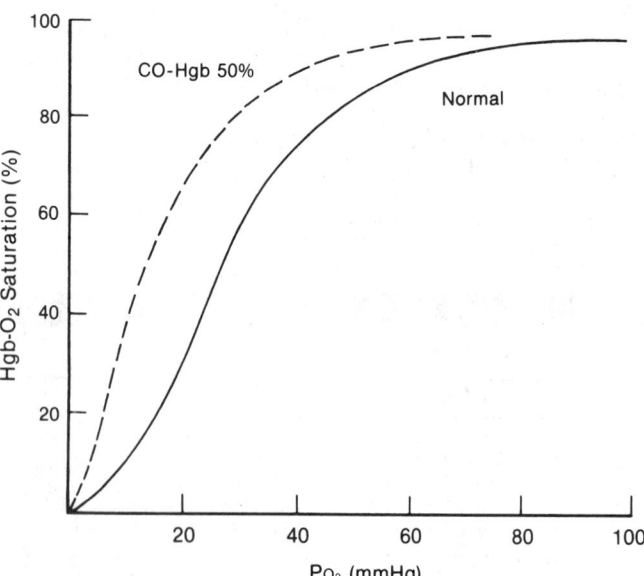

Figure 108–1. Normal oxygen-hemoglobin dissociation curve compared with oxyhemoglobin dissociation curve of 50% carboxyhemoglobinemia. (From Auerbach PS, Geehr EC. Management of Wilderness and Environmental Emergencies. 2nd ed. St Louis, CV Mosby, 1982, p 161.)

measured oxygen saturation in the presence of a high PaO$_2$. In the latter case the effects of carbon monoxide producing unsaturated hemoglobin will be missed in the presence of high dissolved PaO$_2$ from high concentrations of inhaled oxygen.

A measurement of the COHb concentration should be obtained. COHb levels, if obtained early, provide the best correlation with the amount of smoke inhaled. Even low concentrations of COHb can be responsible for significant symptoms and serious sequelae. This phenomenon is magnified if there has been any delay in evaluating arterial gases or measuring COHb concentration after the initial injury and if high-flow supplemental oxygen has been used.

Urinalysis should be obtained. Myoglobinuria may indicate significant muscle injury, which can lead to acute renal failure. The presence of urinary blood by dipstick in the relative absence of urine red blood cells is an indicator of this complication and should lead to urine myoglobin determination or blood creatine kinase levels.

A chest radiograph should be obtained. It is usually normal during the first hours or days after even a severe inhalation injury. The initial chest radiograph serves as a baseline for subsequent radiographic evaluation or for detecting preexisting lung disease.

Early fiberoptic bronchoscopy is indicated in any inhalation injury. This not only allows precise identification of the extent of large airway involvement but also permits bronchopulmonary lavage.

An electrocardiogram should be obtained. It can be useful in detecting myocardial ischemia or arrhythmia.

Early sputum Gram stain and culture offer little information. Serial daily sputum evaluations after admission are useful if a change in flora is detected.

THERAPEUTIC INTERVENTIONS
General Early Management

The initial findings described by rescue personnel may have changed significantly by the time the victim arrives in the emergency department (Table 108–3). Early management of fire-related inhalation injuries is directed toward the correction of hypoxemia and the relief of airway obstruction and bronchoconstriction. High-flow oxygen and early intubation are needed if the immediate or short-term patency of the airway is in question. Positive end expiratory pressure should be utilized in the intubated patient with persistent hypoxemia or atelectasis on chest radiograph.

TABLE 108–3
SIGNS, SYMPTOMS, AND CLINICAL FINDINGS IN INHALATION INJURIES RELATED TO TIME AFTER INJURY

Immediate (0–2 hr)	Unconsciousness, confusion, respiratory distress, bronchospasm, hypoxemia, hypercapnea, acidosis, low cardiac output, carbon monoxide poisoning
Early (2–24 hr)	Increasing hypoxemia, decreased lung compliance, pulmonary interstitial edema, respiratory distress, abnormal mental status, carbon monoxide poisoning
Late (12 hr to weeks)	Pulmonary failure or recovery, bacterial pneumonia → pulmonary failure, no pneumonia → chance of recovery

Humidification should be added to the inhaled air. Conscious victims should be encouraged to cough. Fiberoptic bronchoscopy should be performed as soon as possible. Fluid resuscitation of the burn victim should be based on the extent of the burn. Urine output is an indicator of the adequacy of fluid resuscitation, and catheterization of the bladder is usually necessary. Injury may occur at any level of the respiratory system, including the upper airway lying above the vocal cords, the proximal large airways of the tracheobronchial tree, and the distal small airways. There is no single diagnostic maneuver that effectively evaluates all levels, but all levels require evaluation.

The findings of soot, carbonaceous sputum, singed nasal hairs, facial burns, or burns of the oral or nasal cavities are sensitive indicators of smoke inhalation and associated airway injury. Examination of the lungs may reveal wheezes or rales that were previously absent or missed. Bronchodilating drugs are indicated if wheezes or rales are present. Funduscopic examination revealing venous hyperemia or flame hemorrhages of the retina are additional diagnostic clues to the presence of carbon monoxide poisoning. Cutaneous blisters are indicators of both thermal injury and severe carbon monoxide poisoning.

Continuous cardiac monitoring should be performed. If cardiac dysrhythmia is present, appropriate antidysrhythmic drug therapy should be instituted. If there is pulmonary edema or impaired cardiac output, appropriate vasoactive drugs should be utilized.

Bronchospasm due to stimulation of irritant receptors by the inhaled smoke may be present early and may require aggressive therapy. The effects of minimal bronchoconstriction will be magnified by the presence of lower airway edema and intrabronchial debris. Intravenous bronchodilators such as aminophylline or subcutaneous terbutaline should be administered. Inhaled bronchodilators as well as inhaled or intravenous mucolytic agents can be used.

While the use of corticosteroids in the treatment of inhalation injuries is controversial, most evidence indicates that steroid-treated patients have a high rate of delayed septic complications and increased mortality with little evidence of any benefit. Persistent life-threatening bronchospasm refractory to bronchodilator therapy may respond to one or two doses of intravenous steroids. If no response is seen after two steroid doses, no response to repeated doses is expected. Therefore steroids play no role in the management of inhalation injury unless used in the treatment of refractory bronchospasm. There is no evidence that the prophylactic use of antibiotics is beneficial.

Early Management of Carbon Monoxide Poisoning

The initial arterial blood gases may suggest carbon monoxide toxicity if a low oxygen saturation is measured in the presence of a high PaO$_2$. If high-flow oxygen has been given prior to obtaining the arterial blood gases, this finding may be lost even when significant carbon monoxide poisoning is present (Table 108–4).

The half-life of COHb when breathing room air is 300 to 330 minutes. Breathing 100% oxygen at ambient atmospheric pressure will reduce the half-life of COHb to approximately 90 minutes. If the patient has not been intubated it is difficult to achieve inspired oxygen concentrations of 100% unless aviator-type masks are used and a leak-proof seal between the mask and the face exists.

Hyperbaric oxygen can significantly shorten the half-life of COHb. The administration of 100% oxygen at 3.0 atmospheres absolute will reduce the half-life to 23 minutes. The most severe cases, treated with hyperbaric oxygen for

	TABLE 108–4	
	CARBOXYHEMOGLOBIN CONCENTRATION AND EXPECTED ASSOCIATED SYMPTOMS	

Carboxyhemoglobin Concentration* (%)	Severity	Expected Symptoms
10	Mild	Psychomotor impairment
10–20		Dyspnea, headache
20–30		Headache, nausea, lethargy, mild weakness
30–40	Moderate	Nausea, vomiting, syncope, severe generalized weakness
50	Severe	Loss of consciousness, seizures, dysrhythmia, cutaneous blisters
60	Potentially	Coma
70	lethal	Death

*These figures generally relate to acute carbon monoxide exposure. Victims of long-term, low-level exposure may be much more symptomatic at lower carboxyhemoglobin concentrations.

two half-lives (46 minutes), will have nontoxic COHb levels. Hyperbaric oxygen also reduces cerebral edema by producing cerebral vasoconstriction while preserving cerebral oxygenation.

Loss of consciousness at the time of admission or prior to admission and an elevated COHb level correlate with the development of delayed neurologic and cardiovascular sequelae. Referral to a hyperbaric facility should be considered. The exception to this is the patient who is too unstable for safe transport. Most multiplace hyperbaric chambers are located in comprehensive medical facilities capable of managing the spectrum of injuries.

If there is no loss of consciousness, referral to a hyperbaric facility is based on the symptomatology and measured COHb level. If there are any abnormal clinical findings particularly relating to the CNS or heart, the patient should be treated with hyperbaric oxygen when there is an elevated COHb concentration. If a COHb concentration of 40% or greater is measured, referral to a hyperbaric center is indicated, even if the patient has no clinical findings, has minimal symptoms, and distant transport will be required. A multiplace facility is preferred. At COHb concentrations of 25% to 39%, referral to a hyperbaric facility should be considered. Patients who have not been unconscious and have COHb concentrations of 24% or less can be treated with 100% oxygen by mask for 4 to 5 hours. Referral to a hyperbaric facility should be considered if the patient has any significant symptoms after the first 2 hours of treatment. The symptoms would include persistent headache, nausea, dysequilibrium, chest pain, shortness of breath, dysrhythmia, or abnormal neurologic findings. A brief psychometric battery has been developed that is a sensitive indicator of neurologic dysfunction caused by carbon monoxide and serves as an indictator for referral to a hyperbaric treatment facility.

The disadvantage in using hyperbaric oxygen relates to the incidence of barotrauma to the ears, sinuses, and lungs and to the potential for seizures resulting from CNS toxicity. While there are many considerations involved in making an early decision to refer victims of smoke inhalation to a hyperbaric facility, there has been successful litigation when hyperbaric oxygen was withheld in seriously poisoned patients.

The possibility of cyanide poisoning should also be considered. Sodium nitrite can be administered at a dosage of 0.33 ml/kg of a 3% solution up to a maximum of 10 ml, followed by sodium thiosulfate 1.65 ml/kg of a 25% solution. The sodium thiosulfate can be repeated at one half the initial dose in 30 minutes if inadequate response is noted and if cyanide toxicity is still being considered.

Late Management of Inhalation Injuries

Because inhalation injuries are dynamic, the patient must be continuously reevaluated for the development of an airway obstruction resulting from thermal and chemical injury, pulmonary edema, chemical or bacterial pneumonitis, and cardiorespiratory failure from direct injury or from systemic toxicity arising from inhaled toxins, including carbon monoxide. If respiratory insufficiency or respiratory failure persists, continuous mechanical ventilation must be maintained.

If an inhalation injury complicates a thermal burn, fluid resuscitation must be balanced by efforts to minimize the production of pulmonary edema, which results from direct injury to the lung and the cardiac depressant effects of the inhaled toxins. While there is fear that excessive fluid resuscitation may contribute to pulmonary edema in inhalation injuries, this has not been found to be a problem. Inadequate resuscitation poses a greater threat.

The most significant late complication that contributes to mortality is infection. Infection can result from inhalation of contaminants in the smoke, from aspiration, and from the hematogenous spread of organisms from burned areas of the body, or it can be iatrogenic due to invasive procedures, including intravascular lines, endotracheal tubes, and bladder catheters.

If any change in sputum flora is seen on Gram stain, cultures of blood and sputum should be obtained. Antimicrobial therapy should be based on the infecting organism and antibiotic sensitivity. If the infecting organism cannot be identified by noninvasive means, transtracheal aspiration, transbronchial biopsy, or open lung biopsy should be considered. There is no evidence that prophylactic antibiotics are beneficial; they only lead to overgrowth by resistant organisms.

Atelectasis commonly occurs. This may be related to shallow respiration, loss of alveolar surfactant, or airway occlusion by debris. Treatment is the same as for other causes of atelectasis.

Late Management of Carbon Monoxide Poisoning

Carbon monoxide poisoning, if overlooked during the early management, can be detected and treated during later phases of treatment. Children with carbon monoxide poisoning have presented with delayed neurologic sequelae, including headache, irritability, personality changes, confusion, memory loss, and cardiac dysrhythmia, and have been successfully treated with hyperbaric oxygen up to 21 days after exposure. Hyperbaric oxygen should be used for severe cases of carbon monoxide poisoning regardless of the time between exposure and presentation, especially when the delay is sufficient to preclude a diagnosis by laboratory measures.

DISPOSITION

Children who initially present with minimal or no symptoms may have a delayed onset of respiratory distress. Hospitalization for observation is recommended if there has been any exposure to thick smoke, especially if it involves combustion of synthetic polymers, a situation frequently encountered in dwelling fires. Any victim presenting with soot or burns on the face should be admitted, no matter how minimal the findings.

Carbon monoxide poisoning may also cause delayed neurologic symptoms, providing another indication for inpatient observation. Delayed symptoms have been seen in patients whose initial presentation was benign. The interval is usually only hours to a few days, but delays up to 40 days have been reported. These long delays are rare, and hospitalization beyond 3 or 4 days merely for observation with no evidence of airway or neurologic symptoms is not indicated.

Mental deterioration, incontinence, gait disturbance, mutism, memory impairment, personality alterations, parietal lobe dysfunction, motor symptoms including hemiplegia, hypotonus, extrapyramidal rigidity, and akinesia, as well as cortical blindness and chorea have all been reported in association with carbon monoxide poisoning. Carbon monoxide should be considered in any acute encephalopathic state. Seventy-five percent of all victims show recovery within 1 year.

OTHER CONSIDERATIONS
Nonfire-related Carbon Monoxide Poisoning

Carbon monoxide poisoning is encountered in situations not involving fire. Auto exhaust, which contains up to 9% carbon monoxide, and coal gas, which contains up to 18% carbon monoxide, are the frequent sources of accidental or intentional poisoning. Poorly maintained auto exhaust systems, improperly ventilated heating systems, nonventilated charcoal fires, and improperly ventilated industrial furnaces are common sources of carbon monoxide. A surge of cases of accidental carbon monoxide poisoning is encountered early in the heating season each year as people first use coal- or gas-fueled heating systems without proper annual maintenance of the furnace or chimney.

The most common misdiagnosis of subacute or low-level carbon monoxide poisoning is that of a flu-like viral illness. Headache, nausea, vomiting, dizziness, lethargy, syncope, diarrhea, and hyperventilation syndrome have all been seen in patients found to have chronic low-level carbon monoxide toxicity. The onset of symptoms may be insidious if the concentration of carbon monoxide is low.

Routine emergency department screening of patients presenting with flu-like symptoms has a low yield and is not recommended. The examining physician should routinely inquire about heating sources in the home. Carbon monoxide poisoning should always be considered when a person with coma or altered neurologic status is found in a confined area with poor ventilation. Children who become ill while traveling in an automobile should have auto exhaust suggested as an etiology of their symptoms. Gastrointestinal symptoms are common in children even at low COHb levels, suggesting an increased susceptibility. The urban population who seal windows with plastic and augment their heat with gas ovens or space heaters may be at particular risk. If the diagnosis is missed and these patients are sent home with an incorrect diagnosis, the outcome can be disastrous.

A blood COHb level should be obtained on all patients in whom there is suspicion of carbon monoxide poisoning. COHb levels should be done on all emergency department patients who require arterial blood gas determinations. A careful funduscopic examination needs to be performed. Bright-red retinal veins or retinal flame hemorrhages can be pathognomonic of carbon monoxide poisoning.

Many patients can be successfully treated without admission. It is important that the patient not return to the offending environment until the source of carbon monoxide has been eliminated (Table 108–5).

Carbon Monoxide Poisoning in Pregnancy

Carbon monoxide poisoning is potentially fatal to both the pregnant patient and her fetus. The fetus can die or suffer severe neurologic sequelae even when the mother survives intact. The severity of initial maternal symptoms seems to be the best predictor of the risk of morbidity for the fetus.

Unique properties of fetal hemoglobin cause it to have a slower uptake and much longer half-life than adult hemo-

---

TABLE 108–5

DISCHARGE INSTRUCTIONS FOR SMOKE INHALATION AND CARBON MONOXIDE EXPOSURE

You have experienced smoke inhalation, carbon monoxide exposure, or both. The smoke that you inhaled can be chemically irritating to your lungs and increases the chance of lung infection. Carbon monoxide is one of the gases in smoke that can affect your brain and heart. You were brought to the hospital to be checked for the effects of smoke inhalation and/or carbon monoxide on your body.

You have been evaluated and treated by our medical team, which now feels that the carbon monoxide and/or smoke has been sufficiently removed from your body and that you may return home.

Occasionally aftereffects of both smoke inhalation and carbon monoxide exposure may be seen or felt several days later. Therefore it is very important that you closely follow the instructions below:

Activity and Limitations
1. Rest at home for 24 hours. You are permitted normal activity.
2. Eat what you normally eat. Each day drink at least 6 to 8 glasses of liquid.
3. Take your temperature by mouth twice a day, once in the morning and once in the evening for 5 days. Record it on a temperature card.
4. You may return to work/school in _____ days.
5. If you smoke, it is strongly recommended that you do not smoke for _____ days after you leave the hospital.

Precautions
If any of the following symptoms occur, call your family doctor, the Department of Hyperbaric Medicine, or our Emergency Department.
1. Wheezing, shortness of breath.
2. Sudden cough that does not go away.
3. Coughing up large black flecks of sputum.
4. Temperature in excess of 100°F or above recorded two times in a row.

In case of isolated exposure to carbon monoxide only, these symptoms warrant attention as well:
1. Nausea and/or vomiting.
2. Severe headache not relieved by aspirin or Tylenol.
3. Unusual irritability, memory loss, or personality changes.

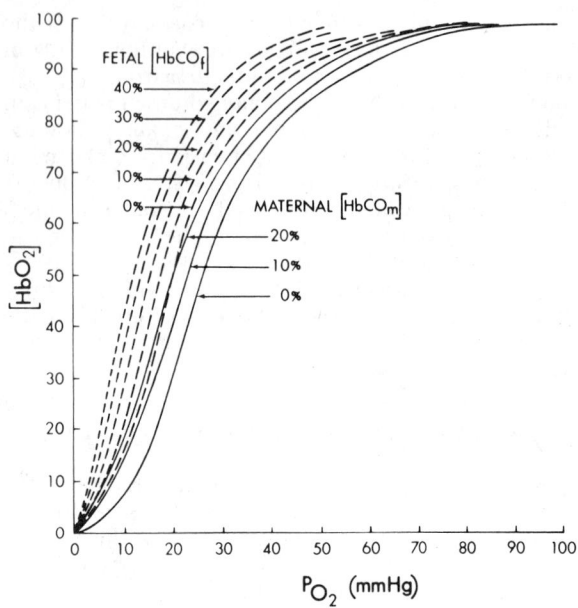

Figure 108–2. Human maternal and fetal oxyhemoglobin saturation curves showing carbon monoxide effect. The oxyhemoglobin saturation (HbO_2) is that percentage of hemoglobin not bound as carboxyhemoglobin. (From Longo LD. The biological effects of carbon monoxide on the pregnant woman, fetus, and newborn infant. Am J Obstet Gynecol 1977; 129:69.)

globin. At a steady state, fetal COHb concentrations can be 15% higher than those in the mother. Fetal hemoglobin has an oxygen-hemoglobin dissociation curve already to the left of the normal adult curve. A further shift to the left from carbon monoxide poisoning will increase tissue hypoxia in the fetus (Fig. 108–2).

Hyperbaric oxygen therapy poses no risk to the fetus. Hyperbaric oxygen should be considered for symptomatic carbon monoxide poisoning during pregnancy. It should be used in asymptomatic pregnant females with confirmed elevations of blood COHb concentrations, if there is evidence of fetal distress, or if the maternal COHb concentration is greater than 20%. If hyperbaric oxygen is not available, 100% oxygen by tight-fitting, nonrebreather mask for at least five times as long as was necessary to reduce maternal COHb to less than 5% is recommended. In severe poisoning, transfer to a hyperbaric facility should be sought.

Chronic Low-Level Smoke Inhalation in Children

Young children who live in homes heated by wood-burning stoves are more likely to develop symptoms of respiratory tract infection and otitis media. These children are more prone to the development of severe illness associated with persistent airway irritation, particularly asthma and bronchitis.

Cigarette smoke in the household environment has been associated with increased incidence of illness involving the upper airway and middle ear in children and can be considered a form of chronic low-level smoke inhalation. Smoking parents of children with these recurrent illnesses should be strongly encouraged and helped to cease cigarette consumption or be advised to confine their smoking to the outdoors. In northern climates this will limit cigarette consumption, particularly during the winter months. The concentration of carbon monoxide in second-hand smoke has been found to be two and a half times greater than the carbon monoxide inhaled by the smoker through a filtered cigarette.

Prevention

There are approximately 750,000 residential fires annually in the United States, which are responsible for the majority of fire deaths. Most occur at night while occupants are sleeping. Smoke detectors are valuable as early warning devices to alert occupants to the presence of a fire.

Carbon monoxide detectors are also available. Although not as important as smoke detectors for the general population, homes heated by coal or fuel oils are particularly vulnerable to carbon monoxide accumulation. Owners of such homes should be encouraged to use carbon monoxide detectors.

Selected References

Burke JF. The sequence of events following smoke inhalation. J Trauma 1981;21(Suppl):721.

Burney RE, Wu S, Nemiroff NJ. Mass carbon monoxide poisoning: Clinical effects and results of treatment of 184 victims. Ann Emerg Med 1982;11:394.

Caravate EM, Adams CJ, Joyce SM, et al. Fetal toxicity associated with maternal carbon monoxide poisoning. Ann Emerg Med 1988;17:714.

Choi HS. Delayed neurologic sequelae in carbon monoxide intoxication. Arch Neurol 1983;40:433.

Crocker PJ, Walker JS. Pediatric carbon monoxide toxicity. J Emerg Med 1984;3:443.

Dolan MC, Haltom TL, Barrows GH, et al. Carboxyhemoglobin levels in patients with flu-like symptoms. Ann Emerg Med 1987;16:782.

Fein A, Leff A, Hopewell PC. Pathophysiology and management of the complications resulting from fire and inhaled products of combustion: Review of the literature. Crit Care Med 1980;8:94.

Gemelli F, Cattani R. Carbon monoxide poisoning in childhood. Br Med J 1985;291:1197.

Ginsberg MD. Carbon monoxide intoxication: Clinical features, neuropathology, and mechanisms of injury. Clin Toxicol 1985;23:281.

Hart IK, Kennedy PGE, Adams JH, et al. Neurological manifestations of carbon monoxide poisoning. Postgrad Med J 1988;64:213.

Hollander DI, Nagey DA, Welch R, et al. Hyperbaric oxygen therapy for the treatment of acute carbon monoxide poisoning in pregnancy. J Reprod Med 1987;32:615.

Horovitz JH. Diagnostic tools for use in smoke inhalation. J Trauma 1981;21(Suppl):717.

Hunt JL, Agee RN, Pruitt BA. Fiberoptic bronchoscopy in acute inhalation injury. J Trauma 1975;15:641.

Lacey DJ. Neurologic sequelae of acute carbon monoxide intoxication. Am J Dis Child 1981;135:145.

Loke J, Matthay RA. Managing victims of smoke inhalation. J Resp Dis 1981;6:87.

Longo LD. The biological effects of carbon monoxide on the pregnant woman, fetus, and newborn infant. Am J Obstet Gynecol 1977;129:69.

Mathiew D, Nolf M, Durocher A, et al. Acute carbon monoxide poisoning: Risk of late sequelae and treatment of hyperbaric oxygen. Clin Toxicol 1985;23:315.

Mellins RB, Park S. Respiratory complications of smoke inhalation in victims of fires. J Pediatr 1975;87:1.

Moylan JA. Inhalation injury. J Trauma 1981;21(Suppl):720.

Moylan JA. Smoke inhalation and burn injury. Surg Clin North Am 1980;60:1533.

Myers RAM, Lindberg SE, Cowley RA. Carbon monoxide poisoning: The injury and its treatment. JACEP 1979;8:479.

Myers RAM, Messier LD, Jones DW, et al. New directions in the research and treatment of carbon monoxide exposure. Am J Emerg Med 1983;2:226.

Myers RAM, Snyder SK, Emhoff TA. Subacute sequelae of carbon monoxide poisoning. Ann Emerg Med 1985;14:1163.

Myers RAM, Snyder SK, Majerus TC. Cutaneous blisters and carbon monoxide poisoning. Ann Emerg Med 1985;16:603.

Norkool DM, Kirkpatrick JN. Treatment of acute carbon monoxide poisoning with hyperbaric oxygen: A review of 115 cases. Ann Emerg Med 1985;14:1168.

Olson KR. Carbon monoxide poisoning mechanisms, presentation, and controversies in management. J Emerg Med 1984;1:233.

Putnam CE, Loke J, Matthay RA, et al. Radiographic manifestations of acute smoke inhalation. Am J Roentgenol 1977;129:865.

Stephenson SF, Esrig BC, Polk HC, et al. The pathophysiology of smoke inhalation injury. Ann Surg 1975;182:652.

Turnbull TL, Hart RG, Strange GR, et al. Emergency department screening for unsuspected carbon monoxide exposure. Ann Emerg Med 1988;17:478.

Van Hoesen KB, Camporesi EM, Moon RE, et al. Should hyperbaric oxygen be used to treat the pregnant for acute carbon monoxide poisoning? JAMA 1989;261:1039.

Variend S, Forrest ARW. Carbon monoxide concentrations in infant deaths. Arch Dis Child 1987;62:417.

Venning H, Roberton D, Milner AD. Carbon monoxide poisoning in an infant. Br Med J 1982;284:651.

Watkins CG, Strope GL. Chronic carbon monoxide poisoning as a major contributing factor in the sudden infant death syndrome. Am J Dis Child 1986;140:619.

Zikria BA, Weston GC, Chodoff M, et al. Smoke and carbon monoxide poisoning in fire victims. J Trauma 1972;12:641.

SECTION FOURTEEN

Trauma

CHAPTER 109

Evaluation and Stabilization of the Injured Child

Ronald F. Maio

INTRODUCTION

Definition

Trauma is injury to an individual resulting from exposure to external agents. These include motor vehicle crashes, falls, assaults, penetrating injuries, fires, poisonings, and drownings. Pediatric trauma patients are not well defined. Some investigators have used age 15 years or under as a guideline[1]; some use age 14 years and under.[2] The National Pediatric Trauma Registry includes patients up to 20 years of age.[3] In this chapter patients 20 years or younger are designated as pediatric trauma patients. Furthermore, pediatric age groups are divided into seven categories, based on the variations in equipment and procedural difficulties encountered in treating these different groups: newborns (0 to 6 weeks), infants (6 weeks to 1 year), toddlers (1 to 3 years), preschoolers (3 to 5 years), young children (5 to 9 years), adolescents (9 to 12 years), and teenagers (13 to 20 years).

Morbidity and Mortality

Injuries are the major cause of death in persons under the age of 45 years; motor vehicles and firearms are the first and second most common mechanisms of injury.[4] Injuries are responsible for half the deaths of those age 1 to 4 years, more than half the deaths of those age 5 to 14 years, and nearly four fifths the deaths of those age 15 to 24 years.[5] The effects of long-term disability on children are also devastating: for every child that dies, 12 are permanently disabled.[6]

Blunt trauma is the most common type of injury in children, with motor vehicle injuries being the most frequent mechanism[7, 8]; the most common cause of death is central nervous system (CNS) injury. In urban areas, however, child abuse, drowning, and penetrating trauma can account for 40% of all trauma deaths.[7] In Michigan, penetrating trauma is the most common cause of death in black, urban teenagers.[10]

The Role of the Physician

Emergency physicians, pediatric emergentologists, general surgeons, pediatric surgeons, pediatricians, and radiologists are all important players on the pediatric trauma team. Pediatric trauma centers have reported between 30% and 50% of their patients arriving as interhospital transports.[7, 8] Therefore it is likely that the first physician to evaluate the pediatric trauma patient will be an emergency physician, not a general or pediatric surgeon. The emergency physician has the responsibility of not only initially stabilizing the patient, but also assuring that the patient is sent to the next most appropriate level of care in a safe and timely manner.

The decision to operate for wound repair and control of bleeding is a critical component of the resuscitation of the injured patient. Assuring that the patient is delivered to a facility with qualified surgeons, or obtaining expeditious surgical consultation in the emergency department, is the responsibility of the emergency physician.

Whether at a small rural hospital or a university center, it is the emergency physician who can most effectively interface with other institutions, prehospital care providers, or interhospital transport teams. The emergency physician knows how to marshal available resources most effectively to respond to the patient's needs.

ANATOMY AND PATHOPHYSIOLOGY

Airway

Significant differences are seen in the airways of toddlers and younger age groups when compared to adults (Fig. 109–1). By late adolescence these differences are almost completely resolved.

The infant's trachea is more anterior than the adult's and is funnel shaped, with the narrowest level being at the cricoid ring. In the infant the mucosa of the hypopharynx and periglottic areas are redundant and more prone to edema than in the adult. The adenoids are large and occupy a large part of the nasopharyngeal area, as does the tongue. The toddler and younger child are especially prone to airway obstruction from soft tissue. Probably the most significant airway difference is diameter. The diameter of the newborn's airway is 4 mm, while that of the adult is 16 mm. A decrease in diameter of 1 mm in an infant reduces the overall cross-sectional area of the airway by almost 50%. Multiple or rough attempts at procedures may cause mucosal or glossal edema and compromise the airway.

Oral endotracheal intubation is facilitated by placing the patient in the "sniffing" position. However, concern for cervical injuries may preclude use of this position. In younger patients, endotracheal tubes that fit snuggly in the cords will not pass safely through the cricoid narrowing.

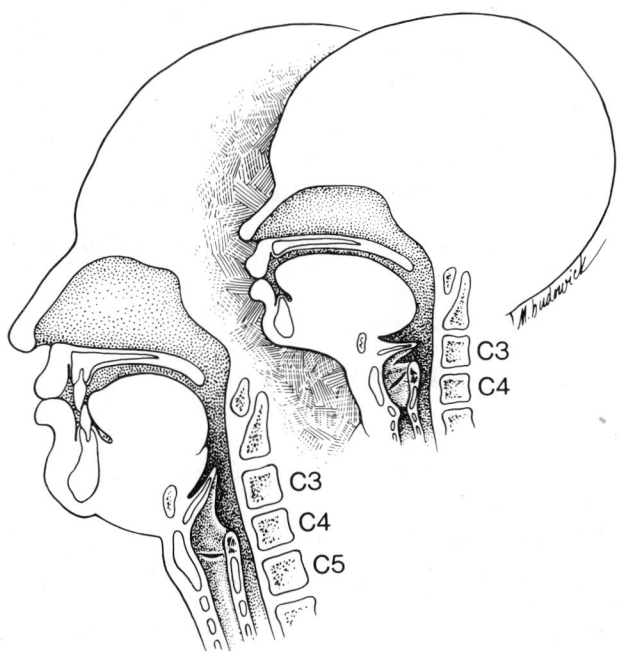

Figure 109–1. Comparison of adult and pediatric airways. (From Finucone BT, Santora AH. Principles of Airway Management. Philadelphia, FA Davis, 1988, p 222.)

Chest

The lower airways are smaller in toddlers and younger children than in adults and are especially prone to obstruction by mucus, blood, or active constriction. The tidal volume for these patients ranges from 5 to 7 ml/kg. The normal respiratory rate for the pediatric age groups is quite varied (Table 109–1). Air movement is much more dependent on diaphragmatic motion in young pediatric age groups. When this motion is impeded by pressure from the thoracic or abdominal cavity, respiration can quickly become compromised. Also, the thinness of the diaphragm in young pediatric age groups makes it vulnerable to rupture when strained by significant abdominal compression caused by blunt abdominal trauma.

The thin chest wall of young pediatric age groups allows the easy transmission of breath sounds throughout the chest and into both hemithoraces equally. Quality of breath sounds is best determined by listening high in the axillae. The compliant chest wall of adolescents and younger age groups allows for significant intrathoracic injuries with minimal external evidence of trauma. Therefore the presence of even a single rib fracture raises the concern of a significant intrathoracic injury. Frequently this intrathoracic injury will be a pulmonary contusion. Although single lobe contusions are usually well tolerated, blood from these injuries can plug small endotracheal tubes.

The mediastinum of an infant is very mobile. Small changes in intrapleural pressure result in major changes in the position of the mediastinum. This can lead to obstructed venous return and reduced cardiac output. Pneumothorax and tension pneumothorax are especially lethal problems in the young pediatric age groups.[11] Even small unilateral changes in intrathoracic pressure push the mediastinum into the opposite hemithorax and compromise venous return and right heart filling, with subsequent decrease in cardiac output.

Aortic injuries in the pediatric population are relatively rare. Cardiac contusions can occur in all pediatric age groups. Penetrating cardiac and lung injuries occur less frequently in younger children because of the relatively lower incidence of penetrating trauma in this age group compared to that in teenagers and adults. Esophageal injuries, although relatively rare in children, can occur from both blunt and penetrating injuries.

Hemodynamic

At birth the blood volume is 90 ml/kg and falls to 80 ml/kg at 1 year of age. By the teen years blood volume equals 70 ml/kg. Blood pressure and pulse also vary by age group (Table 109–2).

A major difference in the response to shock between children and adults is the way the blood vessels respond. As blood volume drops by 20% or more, the body responds with tachycardia and an increase in the peripheral vascular resistance. Young people can maintain a normal blood pressure despite profound hypovolemia. Once this compensation is overwhelmed, the blood pressure drops precipitously. In pediatric patients of all age groups, the compensation may be so effective that the first sign of significant shock may be an altered mental status as opposed to significant changes in blood pressure and pulse.

Abdomen

The relatively wide, short abdomen of younger children is poorly protected by the rib cage and pelvis. This results in less protection of the liver, spleen, rectum, and bladder. The lack of deep recesses in the young child's pelvis and the thin pelvic diaphragm permit blunt or penetrating superficial perineal injuries to result in bladder, rectal, or other abdominal injuries.

TABLE 109–1	
NORMAL RESPIRATORY RATES	
Age	**Rate (breaths/min)**
Newborn	30–60
Infant (1–6 mo)	30–40
Infant (6–12 mo)	24–30
1–4 yr	20–30
4–6 yr	20–25
6–12 yr	16–20
>12 yr	12–16

From American Academy of Pediatrics, American College of Emergency Physicians. Advanced Pediatric Life Support. Elk Grove Village, IL, 1989, p 20.

TABLE 109–2		
BLOOD PRESSURE AND PULSE		
Age and Weight	**Pulse Rate (beats/min)**	**Blood Pressure (mm Hg)**
Infant (≤10 kg, ≤1 yr)	160	80
Preschool child (<20 kg, <5 yr)	140	90
Adolescent (<50 kg, >10 yr)	120	100

Modified with permission from Ramenofsky ML. Pediatric trauma. *In* Moore EE, Ducker TB, Edlich RF, et al (eds). Early Care of the Injured Patient. 4th ed. Toronto, BC Decker, 1990, p 320.

Splenic injury is the most common organ injury in the abdomen. Both the spleen and the liver are vulnerable to injury. The first portion of the duodenum is not as well protected in adolescents and younger children as in adults, making an intramural hematoma more common in these younger age groups. This injury can occur from relatively mild trauma. Tears of the high jejunum and near the ileocecal valve can occur in children; this injury is extremely rare in adults.

By 2 years of age the glomerular filtration rate has reached adult levels. Normal urine output for infants is 2 ml/kg/hour; by adolescence the rate is 1 ml/kg/hour. As with other abdominal organs, the kidneys are also more vulnerable to injury. Renal injuries are most likely to be associated with direct trauma to the flank area. The force applied to this area may be underestimated because the compliance of the rib cage precludes lower rib fractures.

Central Nervous System
Brain Injury

In newborns and infants the cranial sutures have not fused and will expand when the intracranial pressure (ICP) increases. These open sutures, along with open fontanels, can result in hypovolemic shock from intracranial bleeding—a situation not seen in older children. Open fontanels and sutures can also preclude signs and symptoms of an expanding mass until rapid decompensation occurs.

In infants and young children the musculature of the neck is not strong enough to hold the relatively large head in a protective attitude. The head acts as a weighted end on the child's body, increasing the likelihood that the child will strike a surface headfirst.

Brain injury occurs by primary and secondary processes. Primary injuries occur at the time of trauma. Included in primary injuries are concussive injuries; these are relatively common compared with other primary CNS injuries, such as epidural and subdural hematomas and intracerebral hemorrhage. Secondary processes develop after the injury, when alterations in cerebral perfusion and oxygenation result in increased ICP with subsequent cellular ischemia and hypoxia, herniation, and brain death.

The most important factor affecting secondary brain injuries is the ICP. The cerebrospinal fluid, cerebral blood flow, and actual brain tissue interact to maintain normal ICP (≤ 15 mm Hg).

Cerebral blood flow decreases when the head is upright and in the midline. Cerebral blood flow increases with hypercarbia or hypoxia and decreases with hypocarbia secondary to hyperventilation. The brain will frequently show a hyperemic secondary response immediately after brain injury. Osmotic diuretics such as mannitol increase this reactive hyperemia and can transiently increase the secondary injury.[12]

When the limits of the buffer system are reached, the ICP rises sharply and cerebral perfusion decreases. The cardiovascular system attempts to compensate by increasing systemic blood pressure—Cushing's phenomenon—which can lead to a reflexive bradycardia in association with cerebral herniation.

Spinal Cord Injury

The spinal column of adolescents and younger age groups is softer and more flexible than that of adults. The relatively larger head of toddlers and younger age groups allows for greater momentum with cervical flexion and extension. Flexibility can be so extreme as to allow for significant cord injury without evidence of radiographic abnormalities.[13, 14] The lumbar spinal cord is at risk for damage from flexion injuries that occur when lap seatbelts in automobiles are improperly worn or are used without a shoulder harness.

Musculoskeletal Injury

Injuries to growing bones may result in bending of the bone and injuries through the growth plate. This can result in long-term disability.

EMS CONSIDERATIONS
Triage

In situations with multiple victims, field personnel may seek guidance as to which patients take priority for treatment and transport and where the patients must go. The decisions made in these situations will depend on the local EMS protocol, number of victims, availability of local resources, presence of a regionalized trauma system, operational environment, and availability of specialized transport services. The pediatric trauma score[15] and mechanism of injury[16] may be helpful criteria for triage decisions.

Prehospital Care and Transport

Prehospital therapeutic interventions and their impact on the timely transport of the trauma patient are controversial areas in trauma care.[17–23] Although the benefit of advanced life support in prehospital trauma care is heavily debated, this level of care is provided or desired by most EMS systems. Of greatest importance is that the patient's condition not be made worse by transport maneuvers. Therapeutic interventions should focus on airway, circulation, and CNS stabilization. Time spent evaluating and treating the patient at the scene must be weighed against the delay in the patient receiving definitive care. Thus on-scene time may vary depending on the severity of the patient's injuries and the time it will take to transport the patient to the hospital.

Mechanism of Injury

Knowing specifics about how an injury occurred or the forces involved can be valuable in identifying patients with potential life-threatening injuries who initially appear stable. Important areas of information regarding motor vehicle crash victims are the speed of the vehicle the patient was in or struck by; the degree of crush of the vehicle; the seating position of the patient; the type and proper application of a seatbelt, if used; and if the accident was a rollover or if the patient was ejected from the vehicle.[16] Information regarding mechanisms for penetrating trauma that should be obtained includes the type of firearm used and the range and direction from which it was fired; the length and width of any weapons used in a stabbing; and the handedness and sex of a stabbing victim's assailant. For a victim of blunt assault, information to be obtained is the position of the victim when assaulted; the assailant's weapon; and the sex and size of the assailant. If a patient has fallen, important data include how far the victim fell (e.g., number of building stories); how much of the fall was actually a free fall as opposed to a bounce off an object(s); and what was the position of the victim when hitting the ground or bouncing off an object(s).

EMERGENCY DEPARTMENT EVALUATION AND STABILIZATION

Overview

For the first 20 to 30 minutes after the patient's arrival, the emergency physician may be the only physician directing care. In many community hospitals, especially rural hospitals, the time to surgical evaluation may be much longer. It is usually only at trauma centers or large teaching hospitals that the patient will be awaited by the ideal multiphysician team.

In the evaluation and initial treatment of the pediatric trauma patient, certain mistakes must be avoided. One recent study on preventable trauma deaths found that most mistakes in the initial care of pediatric trauma patients involved airway control and ventilation and failure to recognize and appropriately treat visceral injuries causing significant hemorrhage.[1] A problem of lesser magnitude was the failure to recognize and expeditiously treat intracranial hematomas. Preventable deaths can be minimized by treatment strategies that include rapid transport to a definitive care facility.

Airway and Ventilation

Assuring a patent airway and adequate ventilation is the most important task in the stabilization period. Ideally, adequate ventilation should be obtained without completely removing cervical spine immobilization devices. On the other hand, the physician should not be afraid to remove these devices if they prevent critical access to the patient. If necessary, an assistant can provide gentle cervical spine immobilization while airway control and ventilation are being accomplished.

Initial attempts at airway control should concentrate on relieving soft tissue obstruction, clearing secretions, and providing supplementary oxygen. Caution must be practiced when using oral airways in young age groups. These devices can cause pharyngeal injury or obstruction when inappropriately placed. Nasal airways can be helpful in the obtunded patient who does not tolerate an oral airway. These airways also help to dilate the nasal passage and identify the naris to be used for subsequent nasotracheal intubation. In the younger age group these devices may cause damage and severe bleeding to the nasal mucosa and adenoids.

If the patient has spontaneous respirations, the above actions combined with high-flow oxygen by mask should suffice to assure adequate ventilation initially. If the patient does not have adequate respiratory effort, assistance with bag and mask is necessary.

If adequate ventilation is not obtained, the next step is endotracheal intubation. Orotracheal or nasotracheal routes can be used (Table 109–3). Blind nasotracheal intubation requires minimal movement of the cervical spine and precludes resistance to insertion of the laryngoscope by semicomatose patients. In younger age groups, blind nasotracheal intubation can be difficult to perform. The vocal cords are anterior, and the adenoids can become an obstacle. These conditions do not make nasotracheal intubation contraindicated in young age groups, but rather decrease the likelihood of its successful completion. Orotracheal intubation allows for direct visualization and placement of the endotracheal tube, but it has more potential for cervical spine movement and may be difficult in the semicomatose patient or patient with an intact gag reflex. When performed with manual stabilization of the cervical spine, orotracheal intubation has been found to be safe and effective in trauma patients.[24, 25]

Midface fractures are relative contraindications to naso-

tracheal intubation. However, this should not preclude the nasal route if the physician feels that this is the most appropriate method at the time. Any resistance to passage and increase in bleeding indicate that the nasal route should be abandoned. Even though there is an increased risk of sinusitis and meningitis with nasal intubation and midface fractures, the alternatives (a traumatic or struggling oral intubation or a surgical airway) may also prove risky.

If an airway cannot be established by endotracheal intubation, surgical procedures are necessary. A temporizing measure is needle cricothyroidotomy (Fig. 109–2). A 14-gauge catheter can be used. A 3.0- or 3.5-mm pediatric endotracheal tube adapter can be attached to the catheter hub and the patient can be ventilated using a bag-valve device. In adults, respiratory rates of 20/minute with a 1-second inhalation phase and a 2-second exhalation phase have been recommended.[26] In adolescents and younger age groups, respiratory rates and inspiratory:expiratory ratios will be determined by clinical and laboratory parameters.

Age	Endotracheal Tube (mm OD, mm ID)	Bronchoscope (mm)	Tracheostomy Tube (No.)
Newborn, <1 kg	3.8, 2.5	2.5	00
Newborn, >1 kg	4.5, 3.0	3	0
1–6 mo	5.2, 3.5	3	1
6–12 mo	5.8, 4.0	3.5	2
12–18 mo	6.5, 4.5	3.5	2
18–26 mo	7.2, 5.0	4	3
3–4 yr	7.8, 5.5	4	4

TABLE 109–3

SIZE SELECTION OF ENDOTRACHEAL TUBES, TRACHEOSTOMY TUBES, AND BRONCHOSCOPES

From Finucone BT, Santora AH. Principles of Airway Management. Philadelphia, FA Davis, 1988, p 254.

OD = outside diameter; ID = inside diameter.

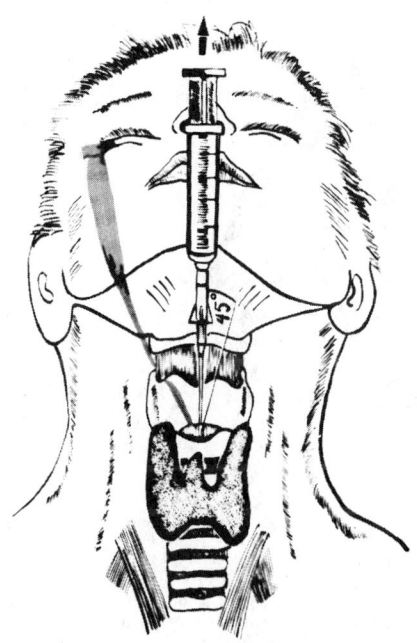

Figure 109–2. Needle cricothyroidotomy. (From Mayer T. Evaluation and general management of the injured child. *In* Mayer T, Matlak ME, Nixon GW, et al (eds). Emergency Management of Pediatric Trauma. Philadelphia, WB Saunders, 1985, p 6.)

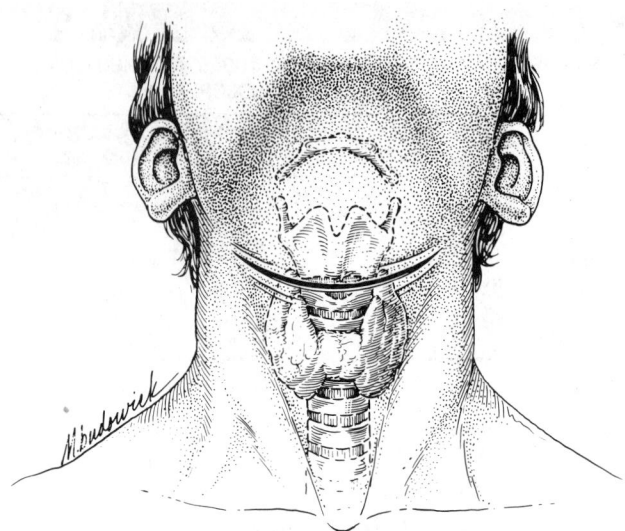

Figure 109–3. Transverse incision at the level of the cricothyroid ligament. (From Finucone BT, Santora AH. Principles of Airway Management. Philadelphia, FA Davis, 1988, p 214.)

Optimum pressures and ventilation ratios for all pediatric age groups have not been determined.

Catheter ventilation may permit careful repeated attempts at endotracheal intubation without the threat of hypoxia or may allow for transport to or arrival of personnel who can obtain airway control. If airway control is not adequate with needle ventilation, more aggressive surgical intervention is necessary. In teenagers cricothyroidotomy is the method of choice (Fig. 109–3). In younger age groups cricothyroidotomy has not been recommended. If appropriate-size tracheostomy tubes are not available, a well-lubricated endotracheal tube of similar diameter can be used (see Table 109–3). A wire-guided method for cricothyroidotomy and tracheostomy is now available,[27] although no studies have been

reported comparing its effectiveness or complication rate with standard methods of surgical control of the airway.

Once intubation has been accomplished, ventilation may still be difficult. One cause of difficulty, gastric dilatation, can be treated with nasogastric tube suction. A 1 year old will require a No. 12 French nasogastric tube and a teenager a No. 18 French. Pneumothorax may also interfere with ventilation. If awake, the patient may complain of chest, shoulder, or diaphragmatic pain, as well as shortness of breath. A tension pneumothorax occurs when the mediastinum is shifted away from the side of the pneumothorax. In situations in which the patient is rapidly decompensating, an intravenous catheter may be placed through the chest wall to "vent" the chest. The catheter should be placed ipsilateral to the pneumothorax in the midclavicular line of the second intercostal space. A needle placed too far medially can easily injure mediastinal vessels in younger patients. For adolescents and teenagers, a 14- or 16-gauge catheter can be used. In infants a 21-gauge catheter is adequate. Immediately after the chest is vented, a chest tube should be placed (Fig. 109–4). This should be placed in the anterior axillary or midclavicular line of the fourth intercostal space. In infants a No. 12 French chest tube should be used, while in teenagers a No. 26 or 28 French may be necessary. In teenagers, if a hemopneumothorax is suspected, a larger tube (No. 32 to 36 French) should be placed.

Another problem that can affect ventilation is an open pneumothorax. The first step in handling this problem is covering the wound with an occlusive dressing. Next a chest tube should be placed through a separate incision. If a tension pneumothorax develops prior to tube placement, the dressing can be temporarily removed to permit release of intrathoracic air. A flail chest can also adversely affect ventilation. Intubation and mechanical ventilation may be needed in severe cases of flail chest.

Special Considerations

Timing of Intubation. A difficult decision is when to intubate a spontaneously breathing patient prior to trans-

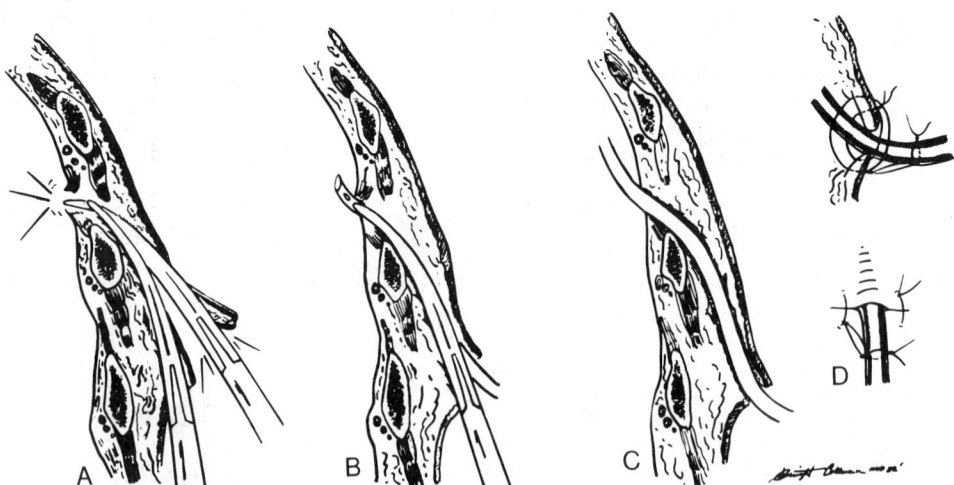

Figure 109–4. Chest tube placement in the pediatric patient. The patient is positioned rolled slightly on the side with the arm raised. The skin is anesthetized for a distance of 2 to 3 cm over the body of the sixth rib at the middle or anterior axillary line. *A,* After a 1.5-cm skin incision is made over the middle of the sixth rib in the middle or anterior axillary line, a subcutaneous tunnel is created bluntly with a curved hemostat; it extends slightly posteriorly and over the top of the fifth rib into the fourth intercostal space. The pleura is entered by firmly advancing the hemostat. *B,* The chest tube is then advanced into the pleural space with the hemostat. *C,* This creates a subcutaneous tunnel tract, which serves to anchor the chest tube. *D,* The chest tube is sutured to the skin, with the sutures tied around the chest tube to help secure it. (From Mayer T. Evaluation and general management of the injured child. *In* Mayer T, Matlak ME, Nixon GW, et al (eds). Emergency Management of Pediatric Trauma. Philadelphia, WB Saunders, 1985, p 21.)

	Early (<25% Blood Volume Loss)	Prehypotensive (25% Blood Volume Loss)	Hypotensive (40% Blood Volume Loss)
	TABLE 109–4		
	SYSTEM RESPONSES TO BLOOD VOLUME LOSS IN THE PEDIATRIC PATIENT		
Cardiac	Weak, thready pulse, increased heart rate	+ Tilt test, increased heart rate	Frank hypotension, tachycardia to bradycardia
CNS	Lethargic, irritable, confused, combative	Changes in level of conciousness, dulled response to pain	Comatose
Skin	Cool, clammy	Cyanotic, decreased capillary refill, cold extremities	Pale, cold
Kidneys	Decreased urinary output; increased specific	Increased BUN	No urinary output

Adapted with permission from the American College of Surgeons Committee on Trauma. Advanced Trauma Life Support (ATLS™) Student Manual. Chicago, American College of Surgeons, 1989, p 220.

port. Most often this will concern the unconscious patient or the patient with waxing and waning levels of consciousness. Multiple factors are involved in this decision-making process: mode of transportation, distance, weather, availability of hospital assistance along the route, and skill level of personnel. Unfortunately respiratory parameters, such as arterial blood gases, respiratory rate, or tidal volume, will not always identify those patients who might deteriorate in transport. As a general guideline it is always better to intubate the patient prior to transport if there are any concerns regarding compromise of ventilation during transport.

Suspected Elevated ICP. Intubation, no matter how efficiently accomplished, will increase the ICP. Short-acting barbiturates will help sedate the patient and decrease the ICP. The use of barbiturates is with some risk. Hypotension or laryngospasm may occur. Because of this, barbiturates should be avoided if hypovolemia is suspected or hypotension present.

Intravenous lidocaine also temporarily decreases the ICP.[28, 29] Using a lidocaine bolus along with a short-acting benzodiazepine (midazolam 0.1 mg/kg) is a good approach if the emergency physician decides that a patient with possible increased ICP needs to be sedated for intubation.

Nasogastric Tubes. The nasogastric tube can be crucial to maintaining adequate ventilation by decompressing a dilated stomach. However, it does not assure that the stomach is empty and that aspiration from vomiting is precluded. Placing a nasogastric tube in a conscious child may be difficult. An agitated child may dislodge intravenous lines, disrupt splints or pressure dressings, increase the ICP, and be difficult to transport. Once again the risks and benefits of doing a procedure must be weighed. If cribriform plate fractures are suspected, the gastric tube should be placed through the mouth.

Bleeding and Circulation

Most external bleeding sites can be controlled with direct pressure. It may be necessary to reach into the wound and digitally put pressure over briskly bleeding vessels. Younger pediatric age groups can have serious blood loss from scalp wounds. A continuous interlocking stitch, using size 3–0 nonabsorbable suture, is a rapid way to control scalp bleeding. The wound can be carefully explored and repaired once the patient is stabilized. For lower extremity amputations, bulky dressings along with a pneumatic antishock garment can be used to control bleeding.

Obtaining venous access is a critical action during the stabilization period and can be the limiting step in pediatric trauma resuscitations.[30, 31] The type of intravenous line chosen and the site used are functions of the patient's age and condition (Table 109–4) and the abilities of the individual starting the intravenous line. The infant's femoral vein can accept a No. 5 French catheter and provides a large and secure line during the resuscitation phase. Femoral cannulation is much less risky than cannulation of the internal jugular or subclavian vein. Intraosseous infusion is another option for obtaining venous access (Fig. 109–5).[32–37] Intraosseous lines should be placed proximal to any fracture sites. If all these attempts fail, internal jugular or subclavian vein cannulation should be attempted. However, these procedures can be extremely difficult to perform and are associated with a higher frequency of complications in infants than in older pediatric groups or adults.[38] Saphenous or median cubital vein cutdown can also be done (Fig. 109–6). In teenagers, venous access via the internal jugular or subclavian vein is more readily accomplished than in younger age groups; however, it should only be used when all other routes are unsuccessful.

Use of a pneumatic antishock garment (PASG) is a controversial issue in prehospital trauma care.[39–46] Proponents claim that the device may tamponade bleeding, facilitate venous access, and increase blood pressure. Opponents claim that the device is ineffective in tamponading bleeding, increases blood pressure by elevating the vascular resistance (which may adversely affect cardiac output), and is associated

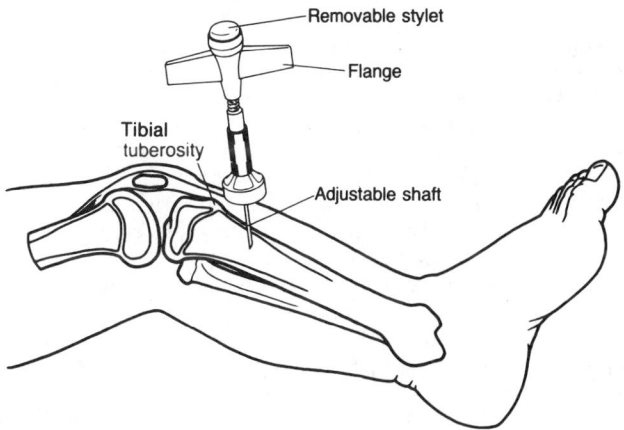

Figure 109–5. Placement of the Illinois sternal or iliac bone marrow–aspiration needle in the proximal tibial location. (From Fiser DH. Intraosseous infusion. N Engl J Med 1990;322:1580. Reprinted by permission of The New England Journal of Medicine.)

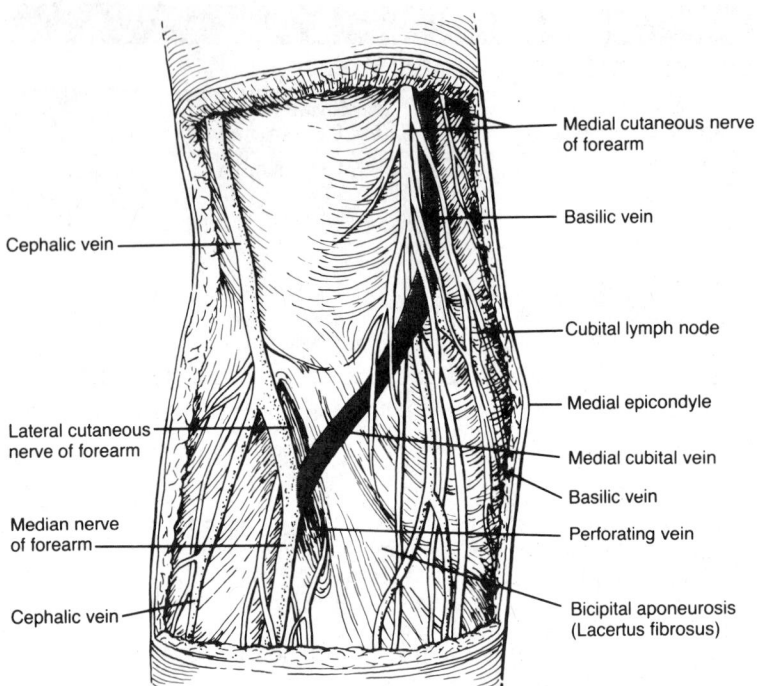

Cephalic vein

Lateral cutaneous
nerve of forearm

Median nerve
of forearm

Cephalic vein

Medial cutaneous nerve
of forearm

Basilic vein

Cubital lymph node

Medial epicondyle

Medial cubital vein

Basilic vein

Perforating vein

Bicipital aponeurosis
(Lacertus fibrosus)

Figure 109–6. Anatomy of the basilic vein at the antecubital fossa. (From Wax PM, Talan DA. Advances in cutdown techniques. Emerg Clin North Am 1989; 7:80.)

with serious complications. Although recommended by textbooks on pediatric trauma care,[47–49] few studies have evaluated the use of PASGs in children. PASGs come in two pediatric sizes: Toddler-mast and Pedi-mast.[50] The toddler type (Toddler-mast) is for children between ages 2 and 4 years. The larger type (Pedi-mast) will fit children between 46 and 58 inches in height and 40 and 100 lb in weight. Anecdotally, the leg compartment of adult PASGs has been used to treat toddlers and infants. PASGs should be used with caution in isolated chest injuries.[51] In these injuries the trousers can increase bleeding.

The patient's normal blood volume is 80 to 90 ml of blood per kilogram, or 8% of body weight. It will take 3 ml of crystalloid to replace 1 ml of blood. Lactated Ringer's or 0.9 normal saline are acceptable initial fluids. An initial fluid bolus is 20 ml/kg. Prompt surgical consultation should be sought if hemodynamic instability persists after the first fluid bolus is given. If the patient responds to the first or second bolus, a maintenance rate of 5 ml/kg/hour for 1 to 2 hours is continued while the patient is observed. Failure of the second bolus to improve vital signs indicates the need for blood. A volume of blood equaling one half the total blood volume should be typed and crossed. While blood is being obtained, a third bolus of 20 ml/kg should be given.

Packed red blood cells (RBCs) can be given at a 10 to 15 ml/kg dose. Usually a unit of packed cells contains approximately 250 ml of RBCs but only minimal amounts of plasma. This is the same red cell mass that is in two thirds of a unit of whole blood. As a general rule, if more than 25% of the blood volume is lost, half the volume replacement will be with packed RBCs and half with crystalloid. For example, a child weighing 20 kg with a 500-ml blood loss would require 250 ml of packed RBCs and 750 ml of crystalloid. Type-specific or O-negative blood is an acceptable choice of therapy when exsanguinating hemorrhage precludes waiting for fully matched blood.

Physicians need to consider other causes of hypotension, such as tension pneumothorax, pericardial tamponade, and neurogenic shock. For the treatment of pericardial tamponade in infants, an 18-gauge angiocatheter can be used to aspirate pericardial fluid (Fig. 109–7). The catheter can be

sewn in place if multiple aspirations are required. In teenagers, a long (5 cm) angiocatheter can be used and sewn in place. Neurogenic shock will often respond to the initial fluid boluses. With neurogenic shock, bradycardia is often present. Sometimes atropine or a sympathomimetic agent such as phenylephrine may be effective.

Myocardial injury is another cause of decreased perfusion. It is rarely the etiology of decreased perfusion in those patients who are hypotensive soon after an injury. Cardiac rhythm monitoring may show atrial or ventricular dysrhythmias when a contusion is present. Inotropic agents, such as dopamine, may be necessary to manage cardiac failure when a significant contusion occurs. Lidocaine or other antiarrhythmics can be used for rhythm disturbances.

Controlling metabolic acidosis will help maintain adequate cardiac output. If the arterial pH is less than 7.2 and the acidosis is metabolic, bicarbonate can be given at a dose of 1 mEq/kg. Younger age groups are susceptible to heat loss, which can adversely affect cardiac output. Infants are especially prone to hypothermia during resuscitation.

Special Considerations

Catheter Size. The size of the intravenous catheter selected depends on the size of the patient and the clinical situation. Also, multiple factors will affect the rate of flow. These factors include the fluid given, the length of the catheter, whether or not the catheter is tapered, the pressure on the fluid being transfused, and, most important, the internal diameter of the catheter (Table 109–5). A 20-kg child who has lost 50% of his or her blood volume will require replacement of 800 ml of blood volume. Using the recommendations previously discussed, 400 ml will be packed RBCs and 1200 ml crystalloids. A child with this type of hemorrhage needs immediate fluid and blood infusion. With an 18-gauge intravenous catheter and pressure cuff infusion, a flow rate of 200 ml/minute of crystalloid and 100 ml/minute of packed RBCs can be obtained. Using a single 18-gauge intravenous catheter, we could administer the appropriate quantity of fluids in 10 minutes. If the child is 40 kg, 800 ml of packed RBCs and 2400 ml of crystalloid must be given. This would take 20 minutes using a single 18-gauge catheter. If a 16-gauge catheter is used it would take 14 minutes. With two 18-gauge intravenous catheters it would take 10 minutes. With a No. 8 French introducer catheter, it could take as little as 5 to 6 minutes. If more than one physician is present, vascular access responsibilities should be distributed (Table 109–6).

Intraosseous Catheters. The intraosseous route (IO) is effective for the administration of fluid and medications in children. However, its value in the hypovolemic pediatric trauma patient may be limited by its flow rate. One recent study in sheep was able to infuse 200 ml of crystalloid over 2 minutes.[52] Syringes (60 ml) were used to administer the fluid. Rates of blood flow through the IO needle were not measured. A porcine study did measure the flow rate of whole blood using 13-gauge IO catheters and pressure infusion (300 mm Hg) in "large" and "small" swine.[53] In large swine, 45 ml/minute of blood could be delivered; in small swine 15 ml/minute. The bigger and more severely hypovolemic the patient is, the less ideal IO infusion becomes. Using the IO route for the case described previously for the 20-kg child, enough crystalloid could be given in 12 minutes to compensate for a 50% blood volume loss; to deliver 800 ml of whole blood, it would take almost another 18 minutes. This compares to a 10-minute total fluid/blood resuscitation time using an 18-gauge catheter and pressure infusion. For most pediatric trauma cases a single IO line will not be sufficient.

Blood Products. Platelets should be given to the trauma patient if the platelet count is less than 20,000/mm³, if the count is 30,000/mm³ or less and the patient is to have surgery, or if the count is 50,000/mm³ or less and the patient is bleeding. In a patient with a 5-L blood volume, one unit of platelets will raise the count by 5000/mm³; for a patient with a 1-L blood volume, one unit of platelets will raise the count by 25,000/mm³. Fresh frozen plasma (FFP) provides

coagulation factors and fibrinogen. Transfusion of FFP is indicated if the prothrombin time or partial thromboplastin time exceeds one and a half times the control. Some physicians have used the general rule that one unit of FFP should be given for every three or four units of packed RBCs. One unit of cryoprecipitate delivers 250 mg of fibrinogen and 80 units of Factors V and VIII. Cryoprecipitate is rarely needed in trauma except for patients with low fibrinogen, von Willebrand's disease, or hemophilia A.[54]

Traumatic Cardiopulmonary Arrest. The decision on what action to take for a traumatic arrest depends on the presence of organized electrical activity on the cardiac monitor, the mechanism of injury, and the time the arrest occurred. Thoracotomy in children 15 years of age and older is most successful when done on those patients who have penetrating chest injuries and arrest after arrival to the emergency department or while in transport.[55, 56] Thoracotomy for victims of blunt trauma is rarely successful and is recommended only for those patients who arrest after or immediately before arrival to the emergency department. Success rates for emergency department thoracotomy following blunt traumatic arrest in adolescents and older pediatric age groups vary from 0% to 12.5%.[54, 57] Patients with blunt trauma who benefit from this procedure are usually found to have pericardial tamponade. Using closed chest cardiopulmonary resuscitation and fluid therapy will almost never be sufficient to successfully resuscitate a traumatic

TABLE 109–5				
IN VITRO FLOW RATE VARIANCE OF INTRAVENOUS CATHETERS				
Catheter	Gravity	Pump	Syringe	Pressure Infusion Cuff
Flow Rates in ml/min (Tap Water–Plastic Bag)				
0.12-inch IV tubing	180	285	200	665
14 gauge	125	215	180	330
16 gauge	100	180	165	285
18 gauge	60	150	140	200
Flow Rates in ml/min (Whole Blood)				
0.12-inch tubing	140	335	125	400
14 gauge	90	200	120	200
16 gauge	65	125	100	180
18 gauge	35	80	100	100

From Dula DJ, Miller HA, Donovan JW. Flow rate variance of commonly used IV infusion techniques. J Trauma 1981; 26:481. © by Williams & Wilkins, 1981.

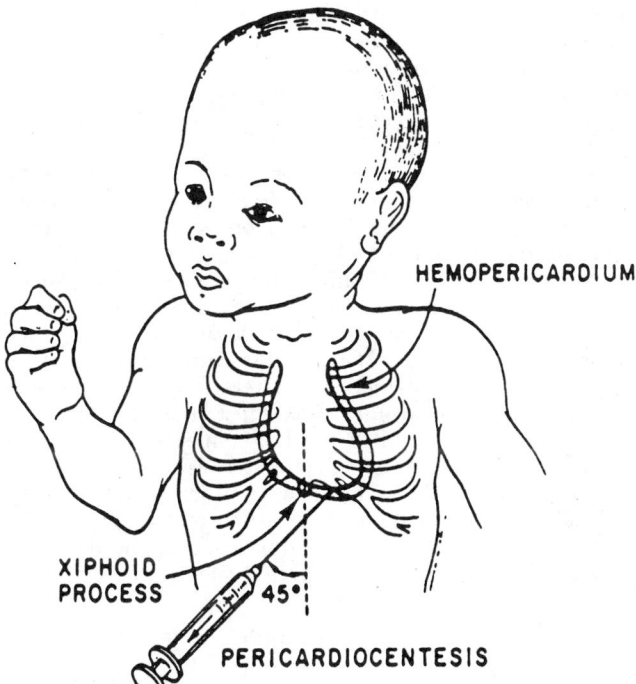

Figure 109–7. Pericardiocentesis. (From American Academy of Pediatrics, American College of Emergency Physicians. Advanced Pediatric Life Support. Elk Grove Village, IL, American Academy of Pediatrics; Dallas, American College of Emergency Physicians, 1989, p 91.)

TABLE 109–6		
SUGGESTED PRIORITIZATION OF RESPONSIBILITIES FOR AIRWAY AND IV ACCESS		
One Physician	Two Physicians	Three Physicians
A	**A**	**A**
Airway	Airway	Airway
Peripheral IV	Femoral IV	
Femoral IV	Internal jugular or subclavian IV	**B**
Tibial intraosseous infusion		Peripheral IV
	B	Tibial intraosseous fusion
Internal jugular or subclavian IV	Peripheral IV	Cutdown
	Tibial intraosseous fusion	
Cutdown	Cutdown	**C**
Femoral Saphenous		Femoral IV
		Internal jugular or subclavian IV

From American Academy of Pediatrics, American College of Emergency Physicians. Advanced Pediatric Life Support. Elk Grove Village, IL, 1989, p 3.

arrest. The appropriateness of closed chest cardiopulmonary resuscitation in hypovolemic arrest is questionable.[58-60] When withholding thoracotomy and administering a fluid bolus to patients with electrical activity but no pulse, the physician must assume that the patient has an extremely low blood pressure, causing cardiac activity to be clinically undetectable. Thoracotomy must be performed promptly if fluid therapy does not rapidly alter the clinical picture or if intravenous access cannot be immediately secured.

When faced with traumatic arrest, the physician should secure the airway and consider the three most likely causes: hypovolemia, tension pneumothorax, and pericardial tamponade. If intravenous lines are in, large amounts of fluid or blood can be given while the emergency physician "vents" each side of the chest with a 16- or 14-gauge catheter. If this does not dramatically change the vital signs, pericardiocentesis should be done. After securing the airway, if no intravenous lines are in place, the emergency physician can make a brief attempt at establishing intravenous lines and then proceed to venting the chest and doing a pericardiocentesis. If the patient is still in arrest, the physician must then decide on the benefit of a thoracotomy. If the emergency physician cannot get anyone to provide definitive care for the patient after emergency thoracotomy, and if he or she cannot find a transport service and receiving hospital to transfer the patient if the patient does respond to open thoracotomy, the procedure should not be done. However, protocols should be developed to transport patients who have had emergency department thoracotomies. For the vast majority of emergency departments, emergency thoracotomy of the pediatric trauma patient will be a rare event; however, it would be tragic to withhold this therapy from someone who would have survived simply because the logistics of transport had not been defined.

While pharmacologic and electrical therapy may be used as adjuncts, it is unlikely that they alone will successfully resuscitate the patient. The incidence of cardiac arrest from cardiac contusion, occurring immediately after the accident, has not been reported in the pediatric population. However, a recent study of pediatric patients with cardiac contusions did not demonstrate any rhythm disturbances or other electrocardiogram abnormalities.[61] Prolonged pharmacologic treatment of traumatic arrests is unwarranted. Patients who respond to prolonged pharmacologic therapy are rarely discharged alive from the hospital, and they almost invariably have severe brain stem or high cervical cord injuries or profound anoxic encephalopathy.

Cervical Spine Stabilization

Standard backboarding for young pediatric age groups may not maintain the spine in an appropriate position.[62] If a special board is unavailable, a pad may be placed under the back and the external auditory meatus aligned with the shoulders. Any collars that are used should be rigid in nature and should facilitate proper occiput placement. Although the cervical spine has been traditionally emphasized in discussions of trauma evaluation, concern must also be given to thoracic and vertebral fractures. Patients should remain on backboards until radiographic studies or physical examination excludes vertebral injuries.

One study recommends the use of methylprednisolone for treatment of spinal cord injuries.[63] The dosage of methylprednisolone used was 30 mg/kg as a loading dose, followed by an infusion of 5.4 mg/kg for 23 hours. Only patients receiving the first dose of medication within 8 hours of injury showed any benefit.

Maintaining a Stable ICP

Hyperventilation, head elevation, and vigilance against fluid overload are essential in the control of the ICP. A $PaCO_2$ in the range of 25 to 30 mm Hg should be maintained. With a backboarded patient, head elevation might only be accomplished by placing the patient in reverse Trendelenburg. Benzodiazepines (i.e., diazepam 0.20 mg/kg) can be used acutely to control seizures. The patient is loaded with phenytoin (10 to 20 mg/kg, maximum of 1 gm, infused at less than 1 mg/kg/minute up to 50 mg/minute). In the intubated patient, pancuronium at 0.1 mg/kg can be used for paralysis. Patients with a Glasgow coma score of 7 or less should usually be intubated. The Glasgow coma score for nonverbal patients such as infants has unfortunately not been standardized.

Special Considerations

Diuretics. Furosemide (0.5 to 1.0 mg/kg), a loop diuretic, and mannitol (0.25 to 1.0 gm/kg), an osmotic diuretic, can be used to decrease cerebral edema by reducing the cerebral blood volume by reducing intravascular volume. However, diuretics may not be prudent in the early care of the multiple trauma victim, who may have a reduced intravascular volume. Mannitol will also initially expand cerebral intravascular volume and accentuate the cerebral hyperemia seen acutely in pediatric head trauma. Diuretic use to decrease cerebral edema should occur only after discussion with the neurosurgical consultants or if the patient manifests rapid neurologic deterioration.

Fluid Volumes. Overly aggressive fluid resuscitation may contribute to the development of cerebral edema. Preschoolers are especially adversely affected by overly vigorous attempts at fluid resuscitation. Nonetheless, volume should never be withheld from the patient who is severely hypovolemic because of the fear of subsequent cerebral edema.

Nontraumatic Causes of Coma. It is possible for a pediatric trauma patient to present in coma secondary to hypoglycemia or drug or alcohol intoxication; the incidence of this is unknown. Some patients may have a head injury along with intoxication or hypoglycemia. Trauma patients in coma or with an altered sensorium should be assumed to have intracranial pathology until proven otherwise. Hyperglycemia in the head-injured patient may be harmful.[64] The routine administration of intravenous glucose should therefore be carefully considered. The blood glucose can now be rapidly estimated at the bedside. It is probably wise for the emergency physician to withhold the routine use of glucose in the pediatric trauma patient in coma unless hypoglycemia is suspected. Naloxone in the usual range of therapeutic doses is extremely safe. Giving this drug routinely to all pediatric trauma patients with altered sensorium would probably not be harmful. However, just because naloxone is safe does not justify unnecessarily administering thousands of doses of it a year. Emergency physicians should therefore not feel obligated to use this drug routinely on all pediatric trauma patients with altered sensorium, but should have no hesitation about administering it if narcotic intoxication (with or without head trauma) is suspected.

Extremity Injuries

The next step in the patient's stabilization is to identify extremity injuries that compromise circulation. Closed vascular injuries cannot be immediately treated, but orthopedic injuries may have vascular compromise resolved by immediate reduction of the fracture or dislocation. These injuries should usually be reduced only after consulting an orthopedist. Occasionally time constraints may require the emergency physician to take action before consultation. Reducing fractures or dislocations should not be done at the expense of more pressing concerns (i.e., airway and circulation). Open fractures should be covered with sterile dressings. Intravenous antibiotics should be considered, and the tetanus immunization of the patient ascertained. Choice of antibiotics can vary from single drug therapy using cefazolin to multiple drug therapy, which may include a penicillin and an aminoglycoside.

Amputated limbs should be wrapped in a sterile moist dressing, placed in a plastic bag, and placed on ice. Care must be taken to protect the limb from direct contact with the ice or water bath; failure to do this could result in damage to the limb from freezing. Blind clamping of vessels is discouraged. Routine use of tourniquets is also not advised. Direct pressure with bulky dressings or digitally is recommended. There may be rare instances when the physician does not have enough help to apply pressure to a hemorrhaging limb as well as control the patient's airway and begin fluid resuscitation. In these cases temporary use of a tourniquet may permit airway control and venous access without ongoing limb hemorrhage. The tourniquet should be removed as soon as possible and direct pressure applied.

Reevaluation

Having addressed areas of immediate therapeutic concern, the physician can now perform a thorough head-to-toe examination. The main purpose of this examination is to determine the extent of injuries, which in turn will be used to determine the need for transport, other therapeutic needs, and potential life-threatening injuries. The scalp should be palpated for any lacerations, deformities, or foreign bodies. The ear canals should be examined for blood or hemotympanum. The eyes should be examined for pupillary response, symmetry of pupils, ocular penetration, and presence of contact lenses. A funduscopic examination should be done to look for retinal injury or papilledema. Any disconjugate gaze should be noted. The orbital rims should be palpated for crepitus or deformity. The nasal septum should be examined for evidence of deformity, hematoma, or bleeding. The oropharynx should be examined for evidence of foreign bodies, loose teeth, or nasopharyngeal bleeding. The neck should be palpated posteriorly for evidence of cervical spine deformity or pain. Anteriorly, the trachea should be palpated to assure that it is not deviated. The neck should be palpated anteriorly for crepitus, and any jugular venous distension should be noted.

The chest wall should be palpated for evidence of crepitus, asymmetric movement, and deformity. The lungs and heart should be auscultated. The patient should be "log rolled" to examine the posterior trunk. At this time the thoracic and lumbar spine can be palpated for evidence of spine injury.

The abdomen should be gently palpated for evidence of tenderness, guarding, rebound, or distension. In the patient with altered sensorium or in the patient experiencing severe pain from extremity injuries, the abdominal examination may be unreliable. Evidence of bruising should be noted. The pelvis should be compressed to test for stability and tenderness. The femoral pulses should be palpated. A rectal examination should be done, paying particular attention in males to the position of the prostate gland. Sphincter tone should also be evaluated. The perineum should be examined for evidence of ecchymosis. When a pelvic fracture is suspected in females, a gentle digital vaginal examination should be done to make sure the fracture site does not open into the vaginal canal. In males, blood at the tip of the meatus indicates an injured urethra.

The extremities should be examined for evidence of adequate perfusion, swelling, and deformity. Spontaneous movement of limbs should also be noted. The Glasgow coma scale score should be calculated, and deep tendon reflexes of the upper and lower extremities should be tested.

If the patient has not spontaneously voided, the physician should consider placing a Foley catheter. For comatose patients or patients who are hemodynamically unstable, a urinary catheter is necessary. An infant will need a No. 8 French catheter, most younger children a No. 10, and older children a No. 12. Proper resuscitation should result in a urine output of 1 to 2 ml/kg/hour.

TRANSPORTATION TO A HIGHER LEVEL OF CARE

After the initial evaluation and stabilization of the patient, the emergency physician is faced with a critical decision regarding whether the patient needs to go to a higher level of care. Frequently this decision is unclear and may depend on laboratory or radiographic evaluation.

Criteria for Patient Selection

One triage tool that can be helpful in transport decisions is the pediatric trauma score (PTS).[15, 65] This scoring method can be used to identify rapidly pediatric patients who are in need of care at a trauma center (Fig. 109–8). A PTS of 8 or less indicates a need for trauma center care. This score must be interpreted by considering any therapy that the patient received prior to the score being calculated. Decisions to transport made in the emergency department must consider the PTSs that were taken or estimated upon arrival of prehospital care providers. For instance, a 10 year old who has a PTS of 10 upon arrival to the emergency department might have received 3 L of fluid in the field for a blood pressure of 50 mm Hg. The PTS can be done without any special equipment or laboratory tests. The weakness of this method is the inability to identify some significant head injury patients. Another difficulty is the method by which isolated cervical spine injuries are scored. An 8 year old, quadriplegic from a fall, may be conscious with normal vital signs and have a PTS much greater than 8 yet definitely require trauma center care. Consideration of the mechanism of injury can also be used in deciding who to transfer to a trauma center (Table 109–7).[66]

	+2	+1	-1
Size	>20 kg	10 - 20 kg	<10 kg
Airway	Normal	Maintainable	Nonmaintainable
CNS	Awake	Obtunded	Comatose
Systolic BP	>90 palpable at wrist	90 - 50 palpable at groin	<50 nonpalpable
Open wounds	None	Minor	Major or penetrating
Skeletal	None	Closed fracture	Open / multiple

Figure 109–8. (Based on Ramenofsky ML, Ramenofsky MB, Jurkovich GJ, et al. The predictive validity of the Pediatric Trauma Score. J Trauma 1988;28:1038. © by Williams & Wilkins, 1988.)

TABLE 109-7

MECHANISMS OF INJURY AND INJURIES TO BE CONSIDERED IN DECISION TO TRANSFER TO TRAUMA CENTER

Penetrating injury to chest, abdomen, head, neck, and groin
Two or more proximal long bone fractures
Combination with burns of ≥15%, face or airway
Flail chest
Evidence of high impact
   Falls 20 ft or more
   Crash speed (ΔV) 20 mph or more: 30-inch deformity of
      automobile
   Rearward displacement of front axle
   Passenger compartment intrusion 18 inches on patient side
      of car, 24 inches on opposite side of car
   Ejection of patient
   Rollover
   Death of same-car occupant
   Pedestrian hit at 20 mph or more

From American College of Surgeons. Hospital and Prehospital Resources for Optimal Care of the Injured Patient. Chicago, 1986, Appendix F.

Timing of the Transport

Once the emergency physician decides to transport, delay should be minimized. Delaying the transport for further testing is not beneficial to the patient nor cost efficient. Frequently the emergency physician at the smaller hospital faces a dilemma. If radiographic or laboratory studies are not performed, there is the risk of being criticized for an incomplete evaluation or for too quickly "dumping the patient" at the trauma center. On the other hand, a more in-depth evaluation might result in the physician being criticized for wasting valuable time or doing unnecessary tests.

Transfer protocols between institutions should be developed and frequently reviewed. Sending physicians should have ready access to medical advisers of transport services, emergency physicians at the receiving hospital, and senior housestaff at the receiving surgical service. Communication is the key to successfully handling the numerous difficult decisions that arise in trauma care and transport.

Mode of Transport

In general, helicopter transport should be considered when transport distances are between 50 and 150 miles, and fixed-wing aircraft when distances are greater than 150 miles.[67–71] Helicopters are also used to respond to the scene of the accident and to provide physician or trauma nurse support to patients who are undergoing prolonged extrication. However, more important than transport distance are the medical and environmental circumstances of the case and the purpose of the transport.[72]

An attribute of aeromedical transport is the flight crew. Members of these crews are trained in transporting patients with multiple intravenous lines, medication, splints, and ventilator support. Crews of ground ambulances may have limited experience or training in handling these types of treatments.

Making transport decisions can be a difficult task for the emergency physician. Early notification of a helicopter service will help decrease time to definitive care. The air ambulance service could be activated as soon as the community hospital is aware that it will be receiving a critically injured child.

Transport Personnel

The sending physician should be aware that not all air ambulance services offer physician crew members or have them available 24 hours a day. Only 20% of helicopter services provide physicians on their flight team.[73] One recent study has suggested that nurse transport teams can be just as effective as physician-nurse teams for interhospital transport.[73] Previous studies have concluded that the physician's presence in the flight crew is helpful, but that as flight nurses gained more experience, the benefit of a physician flight crew member could rapidly decrease.[74, 75] The main value of the physician may be in areas of judgment rather than procedural skills.[74] Quite possibly this benefit could be realized by radio communication between a physician and the nurse/paramedic flight team. In no way should emergency physicians feel they are advocating inferior care by transporting a patient without a physician in attendance.

DIAGNOSTIC EVALUATION

Radiographic Studies

The initial radiographic studies most frequently recommended are those of the chest, lateral cervical spine, and pelvis.[76–79] Of the three, the chest radiograph is the most likely to affect the treatment decisions of the physician during initial stabilization. A pneumothorax, a hemothorax, or evidence of an improperly placed endotracheal tube would indicate problems that need to be immediately addressed. Evidence of a pelvic fracture would alert the physician to a potential source of significant bleeding. The crosstable lateral cervical spine radiograph has often been emphasized as the most important radiograph in the initial stabilization of the trauma patient; the validity of this concept is questionable. First of all, a "normal" crosstable lateral radiograph does not exclude a cervical fracture.[80–82] Up to 15% of all C1–C3 fractures cannot be seen on the crosstable lateral radiograph. Thus even if the lateral cervical spine radiograph is "normal," the patient still has to be maintained in spinal immobilization. Endotracheal intubation must always be done in a manner that prevents cervical spine movement regardless of what the crosstable lateral radiograph shows. Therefore, a crosstable lateral cervical spine radiograph does little to alter what the sending physician will do.

Frequently copies of radiographs taken at the sending hospital accompany the patient. The quality of these copies may be poor and interpretation difficult. Most institutions have policies that prevent original films from being sent without interpretation by the institution's radiologists. The wisdom of such policies is questionable in light of the fact that these radiographs are often read the next day by physicians who play no role in the early care of the patient.

Although an abdominal or head computed tomography (CT) scan may be appropriate in the work-up of the patient, doing it before transport may be inappropriate. If the sending institution cannot deliver definitive care, the value of doing the evaluation is questioned. Even if the study will not delay transport, the emergency physician must consider the risk to the unstable patient in the radiology department; the patient must be appropriately monitored while these studies are being done. As with plain radiographs, the quality of copied CT scans can be a significant problem. Occasionally it may be possible to perform high-quality CT scans without delaying patient transport or putting the patient at risk through inappropriate monitoring. Such studies may make the care of the patient at the receiving hospital much more efficient.

Laboratory Studies

The utility of laboratory studies in the initial stabilization of the pediatric trauma patient is minimal.[83] An arterial blood gas can alert the physician to inadequate ventilation that may not be apparent on clinical examination; it can show if the head trauma patient is being appropriately hyperventilated. Significant acidemia will alert the physician of inadequate resuscitation even in the face of favorable changes in blood pressure and pulse. The primary value of the initial hematocrit is its use as a baseline. A normal initial hematocrit or hemoglobin in no way implies that significant hemorrhage has not or is not taking place. On the other hand, a low hemoglobin or hematocrit might indicate significant blood loss or an underlying preexisting anemia that has nothing to do with the injury. Typing and crossmatching blood should be done immediately if it is anticipated that blood will be needed. It is often useful to provide the transport team with a tube of blood that can be used by the receiving hospital for blood banking, even if it is not anticipated that blood will be needed during transport.

Obtaining a sample of blood for ethanol determination and of urine for toxicology screen can be valuable in the injured adolescent. Even if the results of these tests will be available after the patient is already transported, these data can be useful when reported to the receiving hospital, both for acute care and in the rehabilitation phase.

Peritoneal Lavage

Most surgeons use the abdominal CT scan to evaluate abdominal injuries in pediatric blunt trauma patients who appear hemodynamically stable.[84-86] Diagnostic peritoneal lavage is becoming extremely limited in the evaluation of the injured child. If imaging capabilities are unavailable or the patient is unstable, the emergency physician must consider how the results of a peritoneal lavage will influence the plan of action. If the physician will be sending the patient regardless of the results of the lavage, it makes little sense to perform it and could make evaluation and therapy decisions difficult at the receiving hospital. Fluid in the abdomen from lavage can make subsequent interpretation of CT scans difficult. Also, once a patient undergoes peritoneal lavage, it is almost impossible to use physical examination of the abdomen to monitor the patient. In some isolated hospitals with limited imaging capabilities and transport resources, a positive lavage is an indication for transport to a distant center. At these isolated hospitals, if the emergency physician feels lavage is necessary and alone bears responsibility for the transfer decision, he or she should lavage the patient (Fig. 109–9).

If the patient is hemodynamically unstable and immediate surgical evaluation is mandatory, the emergency physician must question the value of doing the lavage. Any surgeon faced with a hemodynamically unstable patient and a negative lavage, performed by another physician, will question the credibility of the lavage results. If the patient's vital signs have stabilized by the time the surgeon arrives, a positive lavage will also place the surgeon in a predicament. The positive lavage puts pressure on the surgeon to perform a laparotomy; he or she bears responsibility for the surgical decision but did not perform the test that has compelled the consideration of a surgical option. It is possible that a negative lavage in a hemodynamically unstable patient will force the emergency physician to reconsider other causes for hemodynamic instability (i.e., tension pneumothorax or pericardial tamponade) that have been overlooked or that have rapidly developed.

If the emergency physician feels obligated to lavage, the method of Lazarus is safe and effective. (Fig. 109–9).[87-89] This technique uses a percutaneous wire-guided approach and has less chances of complication than the open approach.[90] Ten to fifteen ml/kg of lavage fluid is used.

Diagnostic peritoneal lavage is not the preferred method of evaluation for hemodynamically stable younger pediatric blunt trauma patients and should rarely be done by the emergency physician without first consulting the surgeon who ultimately will be responsible for the case. Surgeons from both sending and receiving hospitals should be readily available for telephone consultation.

Summary

The three most important diagnostic tests to do when treating the pediatric trauma patient who is being transported to another facility for definitive care are a chest radiograph, arterial blood gases, and hemoglobin. A pelvis and crosstable lateral cervical spine are radiographs of secondary importance. A tube for blood banking should be drawn, and blood alcohol level and a urine toxicology screen should be performed or the samples sent with the patient. Diagnostic peritoneal lavage will often be of limited value in contrast with CT in the initial evaluation and stabilization of the pediatric trauma patient.

INTERACTING WITH THE PATIENT AND THE FAMILY

The emergency physician and emergency department staff must make every effort to be sensitive to the anxiety of the pediatric trauma patient. Efforts should be made to explain to the patient any procedures that will be done. Physician and staff should never lie to the patient; if a procedure or test is going to be painful or "scary," the patient should be gently informed. Being able to comfort the child not only treats the emotional suffering but also gains cooperation during treatment and evaluation. More important than what is said is how it is said as well as how the patient is touched. Even if the patient appears unconscious or is an infant, he or she should be spoken to and calmly touched.

Interaction with the parents and family of the injured pediatric patient should be approached with calmness and sensitivity. Frequently family members have no idea as to the specifics of an injury-producing event. When family members are asked what they know about the event, they might respond that "the school told me to come to the hospital and said Mary's been hurt" or "the police said Tom's been in an accident and that we should come here." The physician should briefly explain the specifics of what occurred, the estimate of the extent of injuries, and the current plan of action. These discussions should be carried out in an area that affords some degree of privacy. The emergency physician must be prepared for the spectrum of reactions from disbelief to hysteria, and one should let the family express some of these emotions. After several minutes of these expressions, family members will usually gradually return to a state where discussions can continue. The emergency physician can ask questions about the patient that have implications for the patient's care, such as allergy history or chronic medical problems. These types of questions will help the family focus on assisting the child instead of on their own anxiety. One report has suggested that it can be extremely comforting for family members to be in the resuscitation room with the child.[91] It is possible that the

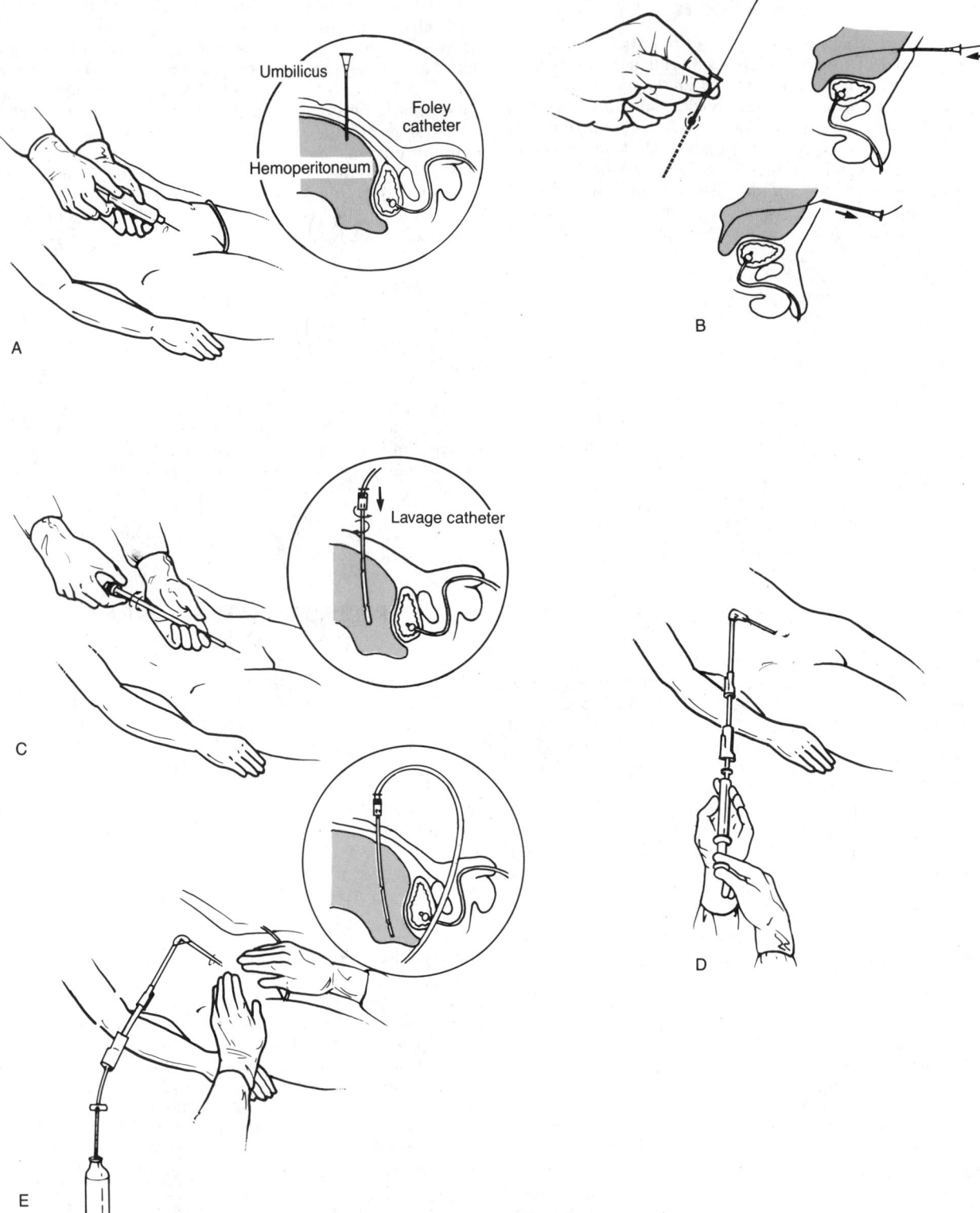

Figure 109–9. *A*, Peritoneal penetration. An 18-gauge, 2 3/4-inch needle is inserted through the fascia into the peritoneum. Note the mandatory Foley catheter in place. *B*, Guide wire insertion: the floppy end is inserted through the needle. (Easy passage suggests peritoneal entry.) The needle is then removed and the guide wire left in place. A portion of the guide wire should always be held during its use. *C*, Lavage catheter insertion. A standard No. 9 French catheter with multiple side holes is inserted over the guide wire in a twisting and turning fashion and advanced deeply into the pelvic gutter. The wire is then removed. *D*, Paracentesis (aspiration). The operator attaches the syringe and aspirates for blood. If more than 10 ml of blood is aspirated, the study is positive. *E*, Lavage. If no blood is aspirated, the operator attaches intravenous tubing to a connector and runs 1 L of normal saline (or Ringer's lactate) into the abdominal cavity (10 to 20 ml/kg in children). The operator should gently rock the abdomen to distribute the fluid before lowering the intravenous bottle below the level of the patient, in order to allow fluid to drain into the bottle from the abdominal cavity. Layered skin closure is preferred at the completion of the procedure when the lavage is negative; dressing without repair is preferred when the lavage is positive. (Modified from Honigman B, Marx J, Pons P, et al. Emergindex. Englewood, CO, Micromedex, 1983.)

presence of the parents may aid in comforting the patient and in lessening the parents' anxiety. It may also be extremely comforting to parents to have been with their child even if, unfortunately, the child expires in the resuscitation room.

Particular efforts should be made at the trauma center to inform and comfort parents of an injured child. Frequently parents will arrive several hours after the patient has arrived. The surgical team may be with the patient in surgery. The attending emergency physician should briefly discuss the case with the parents or family and attempt to contact members of the surgical team to talk with the parents. If the patient is in surgery, the family should be directed to the surgical waiting room. Families will never fail to appreciate the sensitivity and compassion given to them.

References

1. Dykes EH, Spence LJ, Bohn DJ, et al. Evaluation of pediatric care in Ontario. J Trauma 1989;29:724.
2. Kaufman CR, Rivara PR, Maier RV. Pediatric trauma: Need for surgical management. J Trauma 1989;29:1120.
3. Ramenofsky ML. National Pediatric Trauma Registry. *In* Harris BH (ed). Proceedings of the National Conference on Pediatric Trauma: Progress in Pediatric Trauma. Ped Emerg Care 1988;4:77.
4. Rice DP, MacKenzie EJ. Cost of Injury in the United States: A Report to Congress–1989. San Francisco, Institute for Health and Aging, University of California and Injury Prevention Center, The Johns Hopkins University, 1989, pp xx–xxiv.
5. Committee on Trauma Research, Commission on Life Sciences, National Research Council and the Institute of Medicine. Injury in America: A Continuing Public Health Problem. Washington, DC, National Academy Press, 1985, pp 18–20.
6. National Safety Council. Accident Facts. Chicago, 1988, pp 15–19.
7. Beaux CW, Smith GS, Georgeson KE. The first two years: Experience with major trauma at a pediatric trauma center. J Trauma 1990;30:37.
8. Pecelet MH, Newman KD, Eichelberger MR, et al. Patterns of injury in children. J Pediatr Surg 1990;25:85.
9. Tepas JJ III, DiScala C, Ramenofsky ML, et al. Mortality and head injury: The pediatric perpective. J Pediatr Surg 1990;25:92.
10. Michigan Department of Public Health Report. Lifelines for Children: Child Mortality in Michigan (Technical Report). 1989, pp 16, 40.
11. Polley TZ, Coran AG. Special problems in management of pediatric trauma. Crit Care Clin 1986;2:775.
12. Tyson GW. Head Injury Management for Providers of Emergency Care. Baltimore, Williams & Wilkins, 1987, p 228.
13. Pang D, Willberger JE. Spinal cord injury without radiological abnormalities in children. J Neurosurg 1982;57:114.
14. Ruge JR, Sinson GP, McLane DG, et al. Pediatric spinal injury: The very young. J Neurosurg 1988;68:25.
15. Ramenofsky ML, Ramenofsky MB, Jurkovich GJ, et al. The predictive validity of the pediatric trauma score. J Trauma 1988;28:1038.
16. Pepe PE, Copass MK. Prehospital care. *In* Moore EE, Ducker TB, Edlich RF, et al (eds). Early Care of the Injured Patient. Toronto, BC Decker, 1990, p 43.
17. Trunkey DD. Is ALS necessary for prehospital trauma care? (editorial). J Trauma 1984;24:86.
18. Hedges JR, Sacco WJ, Champion HR. An analysis of prehospital care of blunt trauma. J Trauma 1982;22:989.
19. Compton J, Little JM. Role of the intensive care ambulance in the transport of accident victims. Aust N Z J Surg 1983;53:435.
20. Jacobs LM, Sinclair A, Beiser A, et al. Prehospital advanced life support: Benefits in trauma. J Trauma 1984;24:8.
21. Smith P, Bodai BI, Hill AS, et al. Prehospital stabilization of critically injured patients: A failed concept. J Trauma 1985;25:65.
22. Potter D, Goldstein G, Fung SC, et al. A controlled trial of prehospital advanced life support in trauma. Ann Emerg Med 1988;17:582.
23. Cales RH. Advanced life support in prehospital trauma care: An intervention in search of an indication? (editorial). Ann Emerg Med 1988;17:651.
24. Stene JK. Anesthesia for the critically ill trauma patient. *In* Siegel J (ed). Trauma, Emergency Surgery and Critical Care. New York, Churchill Livingstone, 1987, pp 843–862.
25. Grande CM, Barton CR, Stene JK. Appropriate techniques for airway management of emergency patients with suspected spinal cord injuries. Anesth Anal 1988;67:710.
26. Stewart RD. Manual translaryngeal jet ventilation. Emerg Med Clin North Am 1989;7:155.
27. Emergency Cricothyrotomy Catheter Set. Cook Catheter Company, Bloomington, IN.
28. Stoelting RK. Circulating changes during direct laryngoscopy and tracheal intubation: Influence of duration of laryngoscope with and without prior lidocaine. Anesthesiology 1977;47:381.
29. Bedford RF, Parsing JF, Poberreskim L. Lidocaine or thiopental for rapid control of intracranial hypertension. Anesth Analg 1980;59:435.
30. Kettrick RG, Ludwig S. Resuscitation: Pediatric basic and advanced life support. *In* Fleisher GR, Ludwig S (eds). Textbook of Pediatric Emergency Medicine. Baltimore, Williams & Wilkins, 1983, pp 19–20.
31. Kanter RK, Zimmerman JJ, Strauss RH, et al. Pediatric emergency intravenous access: Evaluation of a protocol. Am J Dis Child 1986;140:132.
32. Fiser DH. Intraosseous infusion. N Engl J Med 1990;322:1579.
33. Harte FA, Chalmers PC, Walsh RF, et al. Intraosseous fluid administration: A parenteral alternative in pediatric resuscitation. Anesth Analg 1987;66:687.
34. Zimmerman JJ, Coyne M, Logsdon M. Implementation of intraosseous infusion technique by Aeromedical Transport Programs. J Trauma 1989;29:687.
35. Valdes MM. Intraosseous fluid administration in emergencies. Lancet 1977;1:1235.
36. Mayer TA. Emergency pediatric vascular access: Old solutions to an old problem. Am J Emerg Med 1986;4:98.
37. Spivey WH. Intraosseous infusions. J Pediatr 1987;111:639.
38. Graff DB, Ahmed N. Subclavian vein catheterization in the infant. J Pediatr Surg 1974;9:171.
39. Mattox K. Blind faith, poor judgement and patient jeopardy. Prehosp Disas Med 1989;4:39.
40. McSwain NE. Pneumatic anti-shock garment: Does it work. Prehosp Disas Med 1989;4:42.
41. Mackersie RC, Cristensen JM, Lewis FR. The prehospital use of external counterpressure: Does MAST make a difference? J Trauma 1984;24:882.
42. Bickwell WH, Pepe PE, Wyatt CH, et al. Effect of antishock trousers on the trauma score: A prospective analysis in the urban setting. Ann Emerg Med 1985;14:218.
43. Mattox KL, Bickell WH, Pepe PE, et al. Prospective MAST study in 911 patients. J Trauma 1989;29:1104.
44. Pepe PE, Bickell WH, Mattox KL. The effect of anti-shock garments on prehospital survival. J World Assoc Emerg Dis Med 1987;3:40.
45. Bourn S, Taigman M. Seeking approval for the antishock garment. JEMS 1989;14:35.
46. McSwain NE. Pneumatic anti-shock garment: State of the art. Ann Emerg Med 1988;17:506.
47. Ziegler MM. Major trauma. *In* Fleisher GR, Ludwig S (eds). Textbook of Pediatric Emergency Medicine. Baltimore, Williams & Wilkins, 1983, p 777.
48. American Academy of Pediatrics, American College of Emergency Physicians. Advanced Pediatric Life Support. 1989, pp 81–83.
49. Mayer TA. Transportation of the injured child in emergency. *In* Mayer TA, Matlak ME, Nixon GW, Walker ML (eds). Management of Pediatric Trauma. Philadelphia, WB Saunders, 1985, pp 510–511.
50. David Clark Company, Worcester, MA.
51. McSwain N, Mattox K. Deja vu all over again: The ultimate MAST duel. Presented at the 6th Annual Conference of the National Association of EMS Physicians, Houston, June 17, 1990.
52. Halvorsen L, Bay BK, Perron PR, et al. Evaluation of an intraosseous infusion device for resuscitation of hypovolemic shock. J Trauma 1990;30:652.
53. Schoffstall JM, Spivey WH, Davidheiser S, et al. Intraosseous crystalloid and blood infusion in a swine model. J Trauma 1989;29:384.
54. Borucki DT (ed). Blood Component Therapy. 3rd ed. Washington, DC, American Association of Blood Banks, 1981, pp 55–57.
55. Beaver BL, Colombani PM, Buck JR, et al. Efficacy of emergency room thoracotomy in pediatric trauma. J Pediatr Surg 1987;22:19.
56. Powell RW, Gill EA, Jurkovich GJ, et al. Resuscitative thoracotomy in children and adolescents. Am Surg 1988;54:188.
57. Mayer T. Evaluation and general management of the injured child. *In* Mayer T, Matlak ME, Nixon GW, et al (eds). Emergency Management of Pediatric Trauma. Philadelphia, WB Saunders, 1985, pp 9, 16, 45, 510–511.
58. Luna GK, Padlin EG, Kirkman C, et al. Hemodynamic effects of external cardiac massage in trauma shock. J Trauma 1989;29:1430.
59. Mattox KL. And the beat goes on (editorial). J Trauma 1989;29:1452.
60. Rothenberg SS, Moore EE, Moore FA, et al. Emergency department thoracotomy in children—a critical analysis. J Pediatr Surg 1989;29:1322.
61. Ildstad ST, Tollerud DJ, Weiss RG, et al. Cardiac contusion in pediatric patients with blunt thoracic trauma. J Pediatr Surg 1990;25:287.
62. Herzenberg JE, Hensinger RN, Dedrick DK. Emergency transport and positioning of young children who have an injury of the cervical spine: The standard backboard may be hazardous. J Bone Joint Surg 1989;71A:15.
63. Bracken MR, Shepard MJ, Collins WF, et al. A randomized controlled trial of methylprednisolone or naloxone in the treatment of acute spinal cord injury. N Engl J Med 1990;322:1405.
64. Tyson GW. Head Injury Management for Providers of Emergency Care. Baltimore, Williams & Wilkins, 1987, p 231.

65. Tepas JJ, Mollitt DL, Talbert JL, et al. The pediatric trauma score as a predictor of injury severity in the injured child. J Ped Surg 1987;22:14.
66. Pepe PE, Copass MK. Prehospital care. *In* Moore EE, Ducker TB, Edlich RF, et al (eds). Early Care of the Injured Patient. Toronto, BC Decker, 1990, p 43.
67. Rhee KJ, Burney RE, Mackenzie JR, et al. Predicting the utilization of helicopter emergency medical services: An approach based on need. Ann Emerg Med 1984;13:916.
68. Cordell W, Bock H. Lifeline: A physician staffed, helicopter-mediated emergency service in Indiana. J Indiana State Med Assoc 1980;73:660.
69. Cooper M, Klippel A. A hospital-based helicopter service: Will it fly? Ann Emerg Med 1980;9:451.
70. Harless K, Morris A, Cengil M, et al. Civilian ground and air transport of adults with acute respiratory failure. JAMA 1978;240:361.
71. Mayer TA. Transportation of the injured child. *In* Mayer TA, Matlak ME, Nixon GW, Walker ML (eds). Emergency Management of Pediatric Trauma. Philadelphia, WB Saunders, 1985, pp 320–322.
72. Burney RE, Fischer RP. Ground versus air transport of trauma victims: Medical and logistical considerations. Ann Emerg Med 1986;15:1491.
73. Schwartz RJ, Lenworth MJ, Lee ML. The role of the physician in a helicopter emergency medical service. Prehosp Disas Med 1990;5:31.
74. Rhee KJ, Strizeski M, Burney RE, et al. Is the flight physician needed for hospital emergency services? Ann Emerg Med 1986;15:174.
75. Baxt WG, Moody P. The impact of the physician as part of the aeromedical prehospital team in patients with blunt trauma. JAMA 1987;257:3246.
76. Maier RV. Evaluation and resuscitation. *In* Moore EE (ed). Early Care of the Injured Patient. Philadelphia, BC Decker, 1990, pp 68–69.
77. American Academy of Pediatrics, American College of Emergency Physicians. Advanced Pediatric Life Support, 1989, pp 68–69.
78. Templeton JM, O'Neill JA. Pediatric trauma. Emerg Med Clin 1984;2:906.
79. Jorden RC. Multiple trauma. *In* Rosen P (ed). Emergency Medicine Concepts and Clinical Practice. 1st ed. St. Louis, CV Mosby, 1983, pp 126–127.
80. Ross SE, Schwab CW, David ET, et al. Clearing the cervical spine: Initial radiologic evaluation. J Trauma 1987;27:1055.
81. Shaffer MA, Doris PE. Limitation of the cross table lateral view in detecting cervical spine injuries: A retrospective analysis. Ann Emerg Med 1981;10:508.
82. Streitweiser DR, Knapp R, Wales LR, et al. Accuracy of standard views in detecting cervical spine fractures. Ann Emerg Med 1981;10:508.
83. Bryant MS, Tepas JJ, Talbert JL, et al. Impact of emergency room laboratory studies on the ultimate triage and disposition of the injured child. Am Surg 1988;54:209.
84. Taylor GA, Fallat ME, Potter BM, et al. The role of computed tomography in blunt abdominal trauma in children. J Trauma 1988;28:1660.
85. Buntain WL, Gauld HP, Maull KR. Prediction of splenic salvage by computed tomography. J Trauma 1988;28:24.
86. Kuhn JP, Berger PE. Computed tomography in the evaluation of blunt abdominal trauma in children. Radiol Clin North Am 1981;19:503.
87. Matlak ME. Abdominal injuries. *In* Mayer TA, Matlak ME, Nixon GW, Walker ML (eds). Emergency Management of Pediatric Trauma. Philadelphia, WB Saunders, 1985, pp 333–334.
88. Lazarus HM, Nelson JA. A technique for peritoneal lavage without risk of complications. Surg Gynecol Obstet 1981;153:889.
89. Sherman JC, Delaurier GA, Hawkins ML, et al. Percutaneous peritoneal lavage in blunt trauma patients: A safe and accurate diagnostic method. J Trauma 1989;29:801.
90. Lazarus HM, Nelson JA. Peritoneal lavage with low morbidity. JACEP 1979;8:316.
91. Doyle CJ, Post H, Burney RE, et al. Family participation during resuscitation: An option. Ann Emerg Med 1987;16:673.

CHAPTER 110

Craniocerebral Trauma

Mary A. Letourneau

David M. Jaffe

INTRODUCTION

Epidemiology

Trauma remains the leading cause of death in children older than 1 year in North America. Each year, almost 16 million children are seen in emergency departments for their injuries, and an estimated 600,000 children are subsequently hospitalized.[1] Nearly 80% of deaths that occur in pediatric trauma victims are associated with a significant central nervous system (CNS) injury.[2] At least 30% of pediatric trauma deaths can be directly attributed to head injury.[3]

Head trauma can result from many different types of pediatric injury, including motor vehicle collisions, falls, sports and recreation mishaps, and child abuse (including the "shaken baby syndrome"). Blunt head injuries from motor vehicle collisions account for approximately 37% of all brain injuries in children but cause most of the morbidity and mortality.[1, 3–5] Head injury rates for male children are twice those for females. For infants and toddlers up to 4 years of age, head injury rates are high primarily because of an increased incidence of falls. Head injury rates increase dramatically for all children aged 15 to 19 years, with the majority of these injuries occurring secondary to motor vehicle collisions. However, an alarming 17% of head injuries in this age group are caused by assault, and penetrating injuries are becoming increasingly prevalent in large urban centers.[6, 7]

Approximately 150,000 children suffered a traumatic head injury in 1986 in the United States. An estimated 10 in 100,000 children aged 0 to 19 years die each year because of a head injury. Many are hospitalized, with the median length of hospital stay ranging from 5 to 8 days. Children occupy hospital beds for more than 550,000 days per year because of head injuries, with short-term hospital care costs exceeding $10,000 per patient (1981 dollars).[3] The hospital care costs alone exceed $1 billion per year. Each year an estimated 29,000 persons aged 0 to 19 years have a permanent disability from moderate or severe traumatic brain injury.[3]

Special Considerations in Children

Pediatric head injuries differ from adult head injuries in many aspects. Head injuries are much more common in children. Because a child's head is large relative to the trunk, it is often the leading contact point in deceleration impacts. The types of trauma that more commonly involve children (e.g., motor vehicle collisions, auto-pedestrian collisions, child abuse, and falls) are also more apt to cause head injury. There are also important anatomic differences between children and adults. The cranium is thinner and the brain less myelinated in children, allowing more severe injuries with milder forces.[2, 8] Overall, children develop relatively fewer intracranial mass lesions and relatively more intracranial hypertension than adults. Significantly increased intracranial pressure (ICP) is seen in almost 80% of children sustaining serious head injuries,[9, 10] compared with 40% to

50% of adult patients.[11, 12] Nearly 50% of children also develop an entity previously known as *malignant brain edema*, which consists of cerebral hyperemia in the immediate phase after head injury.[13] However, children with open sutures, larger subarachnoid spaces and cisterns, and greater brain extracellular space better tolerate an expanding intracranial mass or brain swelling. The tendency to develop diffuse brain swelling and cerebral hyperemia puts children at increased risk of secondary brain injury.

The outcome from head injuries in children is significantly better than that in adults.[14–16] Therefore, aggressive management in even severely head-injured children is warranted.

ANATOMY AND PHYSIOLOGY
Anatomy

The scalp, skull, brain, and surrounding structures are all susceptible to injury from head trauma, and numerous pathologic entities may occur secondary to head trauma (Fig. 110–1). The scalp is composed of five layers: skin with hair, the vascular subcutaneous tissue, the galea aponeurosis, the areolar tissue, and the pericranium (periosteum). The looseness of the tissue separating the galea and the pericranium creates a potential space and permits the occurrence of subgaleal hematomas, large flaps, and "scalping" injuries.[17] Immediately below the pericranium lies the skull, composed of the cranial vault (calvarium) and the base. The skull is a bony container for the brain and provides considerable protection. The base of the skull is irregular and rough with major buttresses. When the head encounters an impact, unequal forces of acceleration and deceleration may be set up between the skull and brain. This may result in the brain striking the irregular surfaces of the base of the skull or the side opposite the impact, producing a contrecoup injury.[17] The outer and inner tables of the skull are separated by the diploic space, which is traversed by small veins. The dura is firmly adherent to the internal table of the skull. In certain areas it splits into two surfaces and forms venous sinuses, which are usually located just beneath the suture lines. The midline sagittal sinus is especially vulnerable to injury. The meningeal artery is located between the dura and the inter- nal surface of the skull. After the dura is reflected, the second layer is the thin, transparent arachnoid. The third layer, the pia, is firmly attached to the brain cortex. The bridging veins from the cortex to the sagittal sinus are important, because rupture of these veins can produce a subdural hematoma. The brain itself is bathed in cerebrospinal fluid (CSF) within the subarachnoid space, which forms cisterns, ventricular cavities, interconnecting channels, and foramina.[18]

Normal Physiology

The volume of the cranial vault, except in infants with open fontanelles and sutures, remains constant and contains blood, brain tissue, cerebrospinal fluid, and other pathologic masses such as hematomas or tumors. This can be simplified as follows:

$$V_{intracranial} = V_{CSF} + V_{blood} + V_{brain} + V_{other}$$

where V_{other} represents any additional intracranial space-occupying lesions.[19]

The compartment made up of CSF accounts normally for approximately 10% of the total intracranial volume. It is the most elastic of the compartments, and with increases in the volume of the other compartments, it can decrease its volume, primarily by displacement into the relatively distensible subarachnoid space.[20] The rate of CSF absorption from the ventricular space can also be increased.

The regulation of cerebral blood flow (CBF) and cerebral blood volume is not fully understood. The cerebral blood volume (V_{blood}) comprises 8% of the total intracranial volume. As the volume of the other components increases, compression of the low-pressure venous system will first displace blood from the cranium into the systemic circulation.[19] As the ICP rises, cerebrovascular dilatation, combined with expulsion of venous blood as part of the compensatory process already referred to, causes a gradual shift of blood volume from the venous to the arterial side of the cranial circulation. This occurs because of autoregulation, the ability of the brain to alter the diameter of arterioles, allowing constant blood flow over a range of perfusion pressures. The normal range of autoregulation appears to be between

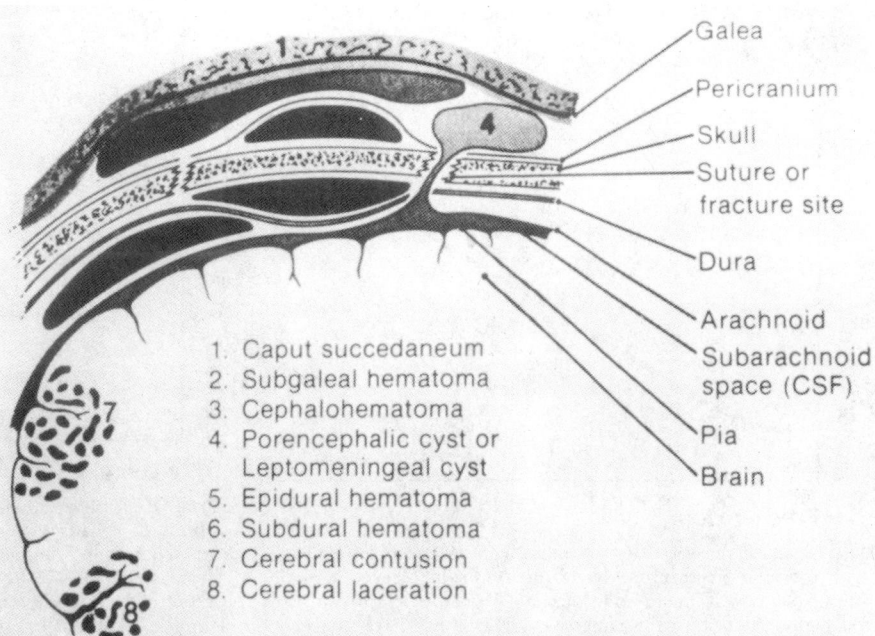

Figure 110–1. Brain, skull, surrounding structures, and pathologic entities secondary to trauma. (From Rosman NP, Herskowitz J, Caster AP, et al. Acute head trauma in infancy and childhood. Pediatr Clin North Am 1979;26:707.)

1. Caput succedaneum
2. Subgaleal hematoma
3. Cephalohematoma
4. Porencephalic cyst or Leptomeningeal cyst
5. Epidural hematoma
6. Subdural hematoma
7. Cerebral contusion
8. Cerebral laceration

Galea
Pericranium
Skull
Suture or fracture site
Dura
Arachnoid
Subarachnoid space (CSF)
Pia
Brain

45 and 160 mm Hg.[19] The most important factors controlling intracranial blood volume are the $PaCO_2$ and the local metabolic requirements of the brain. Cerebral blood flow increases linearly with increasing $PaCO_2$ within the physiologic range of 20 to 100 mm Hg (Fig. 110–2).[19] Hypoxemia also increases cerebral blood flow. In patients with normal hemoglobin levels, increasing CBF becomes evident at a PaO_2 of 50 to 60 mm Hg and increases exponentially below this value (Fig. 110–3).[19]

Pathophysiology

Brain injury, whether caused by penetrating or blunt trauma, occurs in two phases. Primary brain injury results from direct mechanical damage inflicted at the time of injury and may be diffuse or local. Such injuries include concussions, contusions, lacerations, and tearing and shearing injuries to vessels and nerves.

Secondary injury to CNS tissue occurs after the primary event and can be caused by hypoxia, ischemia, or elevated ICP and its consequences. It is a dynamic process evolving over a period of hours to days and involves loss of cerebral autoregulation, development of both extracellular and intracellular edema, and breakdown of the blood-brain barrier.[2] Secondary systemic injury, primarily involving the pulmonary and cardiovascular systems, may contribute to the dysfunction. Hypoxia, hypercarbia, hypertension, hypotension, decreased cardiac output, anemia, and seizures all may contribute to exacerbate the brain injury. Because little, except for prevention, can be done to alter the extent of primary injury, management is directed at preventing secondary injury.

Because increased ICP occurs frequently in children, children are very susceptible to secondary brain injury. Under normal circumstances, cerebral blood flow is regulated and depends in part on $PaCO_2$ and PaO_2. However, there is some evidence that CBF regulation may be impaired in head trauma patients.[21] As the normal compensatory mechanisms are exhausted in response to a brain injury, small additional increments in volume result in large increases in ICP (Fig. 110–4).[19] It is important for the emergency physician to understand this relationship between intracranial volume and pressure, because by the time patients show symptoms of increased ICP, they are already on the steep part of the ICP-volume curve (see Fig. 110–4) and are at risk for sudden increases in ICP. ICP may become sufficiently high to compromise CBF or cause herniation.

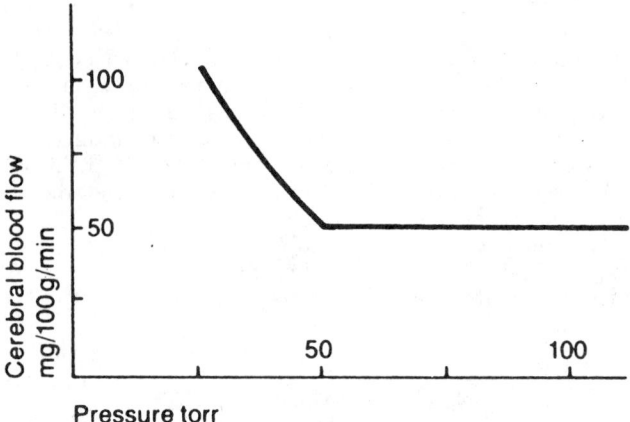

Figure 110–3. Lowering the PaO_2 below 50 mm Hg increases cerebral blood flow. (From Bruce DA. The pathophysiology of increased intracranial pressure. *In* Current Concepts Scope Publications. Kalamazoo, MI, Upjohn, 1978, p 15.)

The syndrome of malignant brain edema is seen frequently among children with head injury, presenting as a rapid deterioration of the neurologic status.[13] It consists of an increased vascular response to injury that results in an elevation of CBF with the development of "cerebral hyperemia," rather than true cerebral edema.[22, 23] It occurs in up to 50% of severely head-injured patients and is the most common cause of neurologic deterioration in the pediatric age group.[13] It is important to recognize, as it may be confused with an expanding intracranial hematoma; a computed tomographic (CT) scan will allow a distinction to be made and exclude a surgical mass lesion.[2]

True cerebral edema is another complication of head injury that may lead to significant secondary injury. It may be either focal or diffuse. It may present quickly following

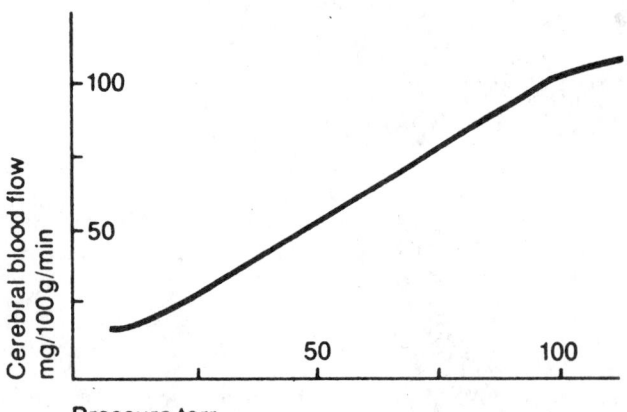

Figure 110–2. Increasing $PaCO_2$ from 20 to 100 mm Hg causes a linear increase in cerebral blood flow. (From Bruce DA. The pathophysiology of increased intracranial pressure. *In* Current Concepts Scope Publications. Kalamazoo, MI, Upjohn, 1978, p 15.)

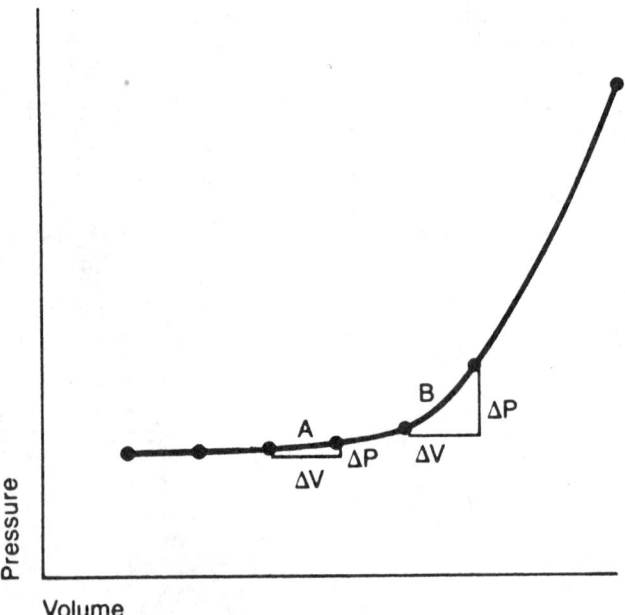

Figure 110–4. Intracranial pressure-volume curve. At A, a change in volume (ΔV) causes only a small change in pressure (ΔP). At B the same change in volume causes a much greater change in pressure. (From Bruce DA. The pathophysiology of increased intracranial pressure. *In* Current Concepts Scope Publications. Kalamazoo, MI, Upjohn, 1978, p 19.)

head injury but usually develops over the first 24 to 48 hours after injury. Prevention of the progression of cerebral edema requires early intervention with correction of hypoxia.

Herniation Syndromes

Diffusely or focally increased ICP can result in herniation of the brain at several locations. The least serious form of herniation is cingulate or subfalcial, occurring when one cerebral hemisphere is displaced underneath the falx cerebri into the opposite supratentorial space.[24] This is associated with a loss of leg function as a result of compression of one or both anterior cerebral arteries. However, this is rarely clinically diagnosed, as the symptoms may be lacking at the time of presentation, especially in patients in coma.

Transtentorial or uncal herniation is of major clinical importance in head injury. This type of herniation is usually the result of a focal mass lesion, diffuse brain swelling or edema, or acute hydrocephalus. The mass forces the ipsilateral uncus of the temporal lobe through the tentorial hiatus into the space between the cerebral peduncle and the tentorium. This results in compression of the third cranial nerve (oculomotor nerve) and parasympathetic paralysis of the pupil on the same side, causing it to become fixed and dilated. The cerebral peduncle is simultaneously compressed, resulting in a contralateral hemiparesis.[24] Progressive deterioration in the level of consciousness results from increased ICP and brain stem compression. The posterior cerebral artery can be compressed against the free edge of the tentorium, resulting in an infarction of the occipital lobe.[24] If the herniation continues untreated, brain stem deterioration occurs, progressing to hyperventilation and decerebration (extensor response) and finally to apnea and death. Alteration of respirations, with the development of bradycardia, systemic hypertension, and respiratory arrest, is a terminal event. The earliest symptoms include headache, and the earliest signs are pupillary changes associated with a decreased level of consciousness. In children younger than 4 years, bradycardia is a frequent early sign of elevated ICP and impending herniation. Recovery from transtentorial herniation seems to be dependent on the degree of neurologic function present at the time of cessation of herniation.[25] Children tolerate brain stem compression produced by the herniation syndrome better than adults, and an attempt should always be made to relieve the herniation, even at a late stage.[25]

Another herniation syndrome can occur when the herniation is upward to the supratentorial space from the infratentorial space. It usually occurs in cases of a posterior fossa mass lesion and significant hydrocephalus. With removal of supratentorial CSF, a pressure gradient develops with decompression and movement of the posterior fossa contents through the tentorial notch, resulting in the symptoms and signs of a transtentorial herniation. Although this is an uncommon syndrome, it is important to recognize it, as additional attempts to remove supratentorial CSF will only worsen the situation.[25]

Cerebellar tonsillar herniation through the foramen magnum occurs much less frequently in head trauma. This type of herniation produces compression of the medulla oblongata and upper cervical spinal cord. It usually occurs following chronic or subacute complaints and is most often caused by a posterior fossa tumor or diffuse brain swelling. It is difficult to diagnose on clinical examination and may be suspected when the history includes such symptoms as morning headache, vomiting, stiff neck, or head tilt. If herniation is complete, with compression of the medulla with its vital respiratory and cardiovascular centers, respiratory and cardiac arrest will occur, causing death.[25]

EMERGENCY MEDICAL SERVICE CONSIDERATIONS

Initial assessment in the field should include rapid patient immobilization and cervical spine stabilization before extrication or further manipulations are attempted. Vital signs should be obtained quickly. The vital signs are part of the neurologic as well as the cardiorespiratory assessment. Attention should also be paid to the patient's temperature, as the brain-injured patient may develop centrally mediated hyperthermia, which should be controlled to reduce excessive metabolic demands.

Initial assessment of airway, breathing, and circulation, with intervention as necessary, should proceed immediately. If intubation is indicated for airway control, the neck should be stabilized manually during laryngoscopy. Breathing should be assisted as necessary after the airway is controlled, and intravenous access should be obtained.

A brief neurologic examination is warranted, including pupillary size and response to light, and level of responsiveness (e.g., alert, responsive only to verbal or painful stimuli, or unresponsive). Prehospital personnel should question observers at the scene regarding the type of trauma and the patient's condition immediately after the incident. Severely injured children should be transported to institutions that can provide appropriate full-service facilities, including a pediatric intensive care unit.

CLINICAL EVALUATION
History

Information obtained from the patient or parents, emergency medical service (EMS) personnel, police, or any other witnesses should include a description of the mechanism of injury. This may allow anticipation of the type of injuries likely to be present. It is important to determine whether the injury was blunt or penetrating and to obtain a description of the forces and distances involved. It is also important to obtain history regarding the patient's level of consciousness immediately after the event and to document the presence and duration of loss of consciousness. Documentation of any changes in the level of consciousness since the injury and any other neurologic changes, particularly deterioration, is of the utmost importance. Postinjury observations, including the patient's respiratory effort, verbalization, and movement of extremities, should also be documented. A history of any other symptoms or signs of brain injury should also be elicited, including headache, vomiting, irritability or lethargy, disorientation, memory loss for the event, perseverative questioning, or visual disturbances. Any history of seizure activity or focal neurologic deficit should also be sought. At some point in the assessment of the patient, an attempt should be made to obtain information using the AMPLE mnemonic: *a*llergies, *m*edicines, *p*ast medical history (particularly the presence of any previous neurologic abnormality), *l*ast meal, and *e*vents leading to the injury.

Physical Examination

Initial assessment of the patient with a head injury is directed at prevention and treatment of secondary CNS injury. Therefore, it is important to assess the cardiorespiratory system prior to obtaining a detailed neurologic examination.[2] The assessment of the patient should occur concurrently with establishment of an adequate airway, assurance of adequate oxygenation and ventilation, and correction of hypovolemic shock. Although cervical spine injury is uncommon in surviving children,[26, 27] cervical spine stabilization should be maintained throughout the initial assessment and management of the patient until cervical spine injury can be excluded.

Airway Assessment

Adequate oxygenation and ventilation are essential to the head-injured patient, as hypoxia and hypercarbia can convert reversible brain injury to irreversible injury. Because airway obstruction is the most frequent source of ventilatory failure,[28] airway patency should be assured immediately. Because of the relatively large tongue and oropharynx, the mandibular block of tissue easily obstructs the airway in the unconscious child. Blood, vomitus, teeth, orthodontia, dirt, and other debris may also cause obstruction. An adequate airway should be established by positioning (jaw thrust), suctioning, or inserting an oropharyngeal airway or endotracheal tube.

Breathing Assessment

Once airway patency has been assured, all patients with moderate to severe head injury should be given supplemental oxygen while breathing is assessed. This should include assessment of respiratory rate, chest expansion, position of the trachea, signs of cyanosis, and auscultation of the chest to ensure adequate and equal aeration. Signs of respiratory distress include tachypnea, use of accessory muscles, and flaring of the alae nasae. Ventilation should be assisted when the injured child is unable to maintain an adequate airway or breathe independently or is in uncompensated shock, or to facilitate hyperventilation in a head-injured child with a Glasgow Coma Score (GCS) less than or equal to 8.[29]

Circulation Assessment

Circulation should be assessed by heart rate, blood pressure, skin color, and peripheral perfusion. Intravenous access should be obtained rapidly. If peripheral access cannot be obtained, tibial intraosseous infusion provides quick access for rapid fluid resuscitation and drug administration.[30] It is important to rapidly provide adequate circulatory volume for all severely injured children. In head-injured children with an altered level of consciousness and in shock, the depressed level of consciousness cannot be fully evaluated until the hypotension is reversed, as the shock itself may cause an altered level of consciousness.[2] Hypovolemic shock is rarely attributable to a head injury alone. If the patient is in shock, the physician should assume that the hypotension has a cause other than the head injury and should look actively for evidence of injuries such as intra-abdominal hemorrhage, intrathoracic hemorrhage, pelvic fracture, or other orthopedic injuries. However, small children may lose enough blood from scalp lacerations or hematomas to cause shock.[2] Therefore, all sites of bleeding should be controlled with direct pressure.

Neurologic Assessment

The neurologic examination is essential in establishing the severity of the head injury and its clinical course and must include assessment of cortical and brain stem function. The level of consciousness is the most important factor in neurologic assessment.[24] A brief, initial neurologic examination should include pupillary size and response to light and the level of responsiveness (e.g., alert, responsive only to verbal or painful stimuli, or unresponsive). Use of the 15-point Glasgow Coma Scale requires little extra time and provides better prognostic information than the general level of responsiveness for children older than 3 years (Table 110–1). The scale assesses three areas of patient responsiveness:

TABLE 110–1

GLASGOW COMA SCALE

Assessed Response	Score
Eyes open	
Spontaneously	4
To speech	3
To pain	2
No response	1
Best verbal response	
Oriented	5
Confused	4
Inappropriate words	3
Incomprehensible sounds	2
No response	1
Best motor response (upper limb)	
Obeys commands	6
Localizes pain	5
Withdraws	4
Abnormal flexion to pain	3
Abnormal extension to pain	2
No response	1

From Teasdale G, Jennett B. Assessment of coma and impaired consciousness. A practical scale. Lancet 1974;2:81–84.

eye opening, best verbal response, and best motor response. Modifications have been proposed for preverbal children,[31,32] although these changes have not been validated (Table 110–2). Repeat examinations are essential.

The vital signs can be observable indices of brain stem function. Changes in the vital signs can help define the patient's status neurologically, as well as give important information on the general status of the multiple trauma victim. Head injury can produce several types of abnormal respiratory patterns. Cheyne-Stokes respiration is a pattern of breathing in which there is a crescendo, decrescendo, and apnea phase, occurring in a regular, rhythmic pattern. It indicates diffuse diencephalic or upper midbrain involvement.[33] Central neurogenic hyperventilation is a sustained regular pattern of hyperventilation; causes include lesions in the lower midbrain and mid pons.[33] It may be an early sign of neurologic abnormality. As neurologic dysfunction progresses, the respirations may become ataxic, with a com-

TABLE 110–2

CHILDREN'S COMA SCORE*

Assessed response	Score
Ocular response	
Pursuit	4
Extraocular muscles (EOM) intact, reactive pupils	3
Fixed pupils or EOM impaired	2
Fixed pupils and EOM paralyzed	1
Verbal response	
Cries	3
Spontaneous respirations	2
Apneic	1
Motor response	
Flexes and extends	4
Withdraws from painful stimuli	3
Hypertonic	2
Flaccid	1

*The maximum score assignable is 11; the minimum score is 3.

From Raimondi AJ, Hirschauer J. Head injury in the infant and toddler: Coma scoring and outcome scale. Childs Brain 1984;11:12–35. Published by S. Karger AG, Basel.

pletely irregular pattern. Deep and shallow breaths occur at random, with unpredictable periods of apnea; the lesion with this pattern is at the level of the medulla or pons. Apnea represents a grave prognostic finding in the head-injured patient. However, resuscitation should still be initiated, as up to 15% of pediatric patients with apnea secondary to head injury survive.[34]

The pulse rate may also be related to the head injury. Elevations in ICP may produce bradycardia. Progressive bradycardia associated with progressive systemic hypertension is known as *Cushing's response* and suggests a surgical lesion.[24] However, this is usually a late response. A rapid pulse rate in a head-injured patient may be secondary to significantly increased ICP and is usually a preterminal sign. However, other sources of tachycardia should be sought, as it most often represents blood loss, and the site of the hemorrhage must be identified.

An elevated blood pressure may also reflect a rise in the ICP. The usual change seen with a rise in ICP is a rise in systolic blood pressure, often with a widening of the pulse pressure and an associated bradycardia. Hypotension should not be assumed to be caused by the head injury and most likely represents hypovolemia.

Quick evaluation of the brain stem is accomplished by observing pupillary size, contour, and response to light (cranial nerves II and III). More complete brain stem evaluation requires further cranial nerve examination, including assessment of the corneal reflex (cranial nerves V and VII) and determination of the presence of a gag reflex (cranial nerves IX and X). In addition, oculocephalic responses ("doll's eyes") or oculovestibular responses (cold calorics) are important in testing the integrity of the brain stem. The test for cold calorics can be performed without moving the neck but requires intact tympanic membranes. Oculocephalic reflexes should not be tested until the cervical spine has been evaluated for the presence of fractures.[24] The fundi should be examined for evidence of retinal hemorrhage or papilledema. Positive findings in the fundi may have specific implications as to the cause and type of head trauma. The presence of fresh retinal hemorrhages following head injury usually implies a significant degree of trauma[35] and may indicate the presence of an associated intracerebral hemorrhage. Retinal hemorrhages in infants younger than 1 year are usually a result of the shaken baby syndrome and represent child abuse.[36] In the older child, papilledema may begin to develop within a few hours of the onset of increased ICP, although it usually takes 12 to 24 hours for significant papilledema to develop following head trauma.[37] The absence of venous pulsations will be an earlier sign.

In addition to a complete neurologic examination, the head and neck should be thoroughly examined. The scalp should be inspected for any lacerations and palpated with a gloved finger to discover any fractures. The ear canals should be examined for evidence of a hemotympanum as an indicator of basilar skull fracture. The diagnosis of basilar skull fracture is primarily clinical; other signs include periorbital ecchymosis ("raccoon's eyes"), ecchymosis in the mastoid area (Battle's sign), and CSF rhinorrhea or otorrhea. The neck should be examined carefully because of possible cervical spine injury. Initial assessment may be limited by the method needed for cervical spine stabilization. Cervical spine pain, tenderness to palpation, or irregularities suggest cervical spine injury. Other signs of spinal cord injury are priapism, hypotension with relative bradycardia, decreased motor power and sensation below the level of the lesion, and decreased anal sphincter tone.[17]

The extent of examination of the motor system will depend on the level of consciousness of the child. The alert child should have muscle strength and gait examined. In the nonresponsive patient, intermittent flexor (decorticate) or extensor (decerebrate) posturing should be noted. Abnormal posturing should not be mistaken for seizure activity. These are ominous signs suggesting acutely raised ICP.[38] Any obvious paralysis or asymmetric extremity movement should be noted. The deep tendon reflexes and plantar responses should also be tested.

DIAGNOSTIC EVALUATION
Laboratory Studies

Laboratory studies are indicated in children with significant head injury or altered level of consciousness. Such studies may assist in identifying the degree of hemorrhage, the presence of preexisting disease, and the extent of additional injuries. They should include a complete blood cell count, platelet count, clotting studies, determination of serum electrolyte and glucose levels, urinalysis, and arterial blood gas measurements. Blood for type and crossmatch should be sent if significant blood loss has occurred or is suspected or if a surgical procedure is indicated. Ethanol levels and toxicologic screening tests on blood and urine should be obtained if the patient appears intoxicated or there is a concern about possible intoxication, particularly in older children and adolescents, or if the circumstances surrounding the injury are unknown.

Lumbar puncture should not be performed in the child with head injury unless complicating central nervous system infection is suspected. It is usually contraindicated in the presence of significantly elevated ICP and is absolutely contraindicated if there is evidence of a mass lesion.[18]

Diagnostic Imaging

The radiologic evaluation of a child with head injury may include obtaining cervical spine and skull radiographs, CT scanning, or magnetic resonance imaging (MRI). Although cervical spine injuries are rare in children who survive multiple trauma,[39] cervical spine radiographs should be obtained in all patients sustaining severe injury or with a significantly abnormal level of consciousness, as well as in those patients complaining of cervical pain, those with cervical tenderness to palpation, or those with neurologic deficits suggesting cervical cord injury. Almost half of children with traumatic spinal cord injury may have no associated radiographic abnormalities.[40] However, because most of these children will experience neurologic symptoms following injury (e.g., numbness, paresthesias, or paralysis), specific clinical assessment must be performed along with radiologic studies for a complete evaluation. Cervical spine radiographic assessment should include anteroposterior, lateral, and open-mouth views. However, additional views, including oblique, flexion, and extension views, and even CT examination may be necessary if the clinical examination suggests a cervical spine injury.

The value of obtaining skull radiographs in children with mild to moderate head injury remains controversial.[41–43] The rationale for obtaining radiographs in head-injured children has been to detect skull fractures. Because the skull is more elastic in younger children than in adults, a fracture may suggest a greater force of injury. Also, treatment may be of benefit in children who have depressed skull fractures. An early childhood fracture may lead to the formation of leptomeningeal cysts and a subsequent "growing fracture" of childhood. In the younger child, a skull fracture, if present, may also suggest child abuse. The presence of a skull fracture has been shown to be a poor predictor of underlying intracranial injury.[44, 45] There are no universally recognized, specific criteria that can be used in all circumstances to indicate when skull radiographs should be obtained. Therefore, it is necessary to combine the history, neurologic examination, and additional physical findings to identify the patients who may benefit from obtaining skull radiographs (Table 110–3).

Children with severe head injury urgently require a CT scan of the head to exclude a treatable intracranial hematoma. Major mortality reductions have been shown to result if certain intracranial lesions are evacuated within 4 hours of injury.[46, 47] CT scanning is safe, rapid, and noninvasive; can readily identify intracranial hematomas, intraparenchymal hemorrhage, cerebral edema, and shifts of midline structures; and can help to delineate depressed and basilar skull fractures.[48] It is the diagnostic procedure of choice if serious intracranial injury is suspected.[49] A CT scan should be obtained on all patients with a persistent decreased level of consciousness, those who undergo a deterioration of their level of consciousness, and those who have focal neurologic deficits, penetrating brain injuries, depressed skull fractures, or fractures in the vicinity of the middle meningeal artery. Neurosurgical consultation should be available to ensure proper benefit from the CT scan.

Magnetic resonance imaging has become an increasingly available diagnostic tool in the evaluation of patients with head trauma.[50-53] It has been shown to be superior to CT in detecting nonhemorrhagic lesions such as cortical contusions and white matter shearing lesions[50, 53] and in evaluating patients with subacute or chronic injury. Surgical management has been shown to be unaltered by the additional information provided by MRI.[52, 53] However, there are also logistical problems with MRI, including the longer time required to obtain the scans, difficulty in placing critically ill patients with supportive equipment in the magnet, and decreased access to these patients during the imaging process.[50] Therefore, CT remains the evaluation of choice for acute head injury.

DIFFERENTIAL DIAGNOSIS

In all children who present with a history of head trauma and a decreased level of consciousness, attention must be directed to the total patient to look for contributing factors (Table 110–4). In all patients, particularly multiple trauma

TABLE 110–3
INDICATIONS FOR OBTAINING SKULL RADIOGRAPHS

History
  Age <1 year
  Documented loss of consciousness
  Significant injury to temporal area
  Penetrating injury
  Previous craniotomy with shunt tube in place
Physical examination
  Depressed level of consciousness
  Palpable hematoma in temporal or parietal areas
  Palpable skull depression
  Open skull fractures
  CSF rhinorrhea or otorrhea
  Hemotympanum
  Battle's sign
  Raccoon's eyes
  Focal neurologic signs
  Suspected child abuse

Adapted from Leonidas JC, Ting W, Binkiewicz A, et al. Mild head trauma in children: When is a roentgenogram necessary. Pediatrics 1982;69:139–143. Reproduced by permission of Pediatrics.

TABLE 110–4
ASSOCIATED DIAGNOSTIC ISSUES IN HEAD-INJURED CHILDREN

Multiple trauma (hypoxia, hypercarbia, shock)
Intoxication or ingestion
Underlying medical problem (metabolic, neurologic, etc)
Cerebrovascular abnormalities (aneurysm, arteriovenous malformation)
Posttraumatic seizures
Suspected child abuse

cases, hypoxia, hypercarbia, and shock need to be excluded as possible causes of neurologic depression. A history of underlying medical conditions, including metabolic and neurologic disorders that may complicate the injury, should be obtained. In the older child and adolescent, intoxication with alcohol or drugs should also be considered. In patients with a suspected intoxication, it must be assumed that the intoxication could be masking an underlying significant head injury, and a CT scan should be obtained. In children presenting with a head injury associated with seizure activity, it may be difficult to distinguish the cause of the abnormal level of consciousness, and close observation is indicated along with possible evaluation by CT scan. Occult head trauma should be considered in the neurologically depressed or ill-appearing infant, and child abuse, particularly the shaken baby syndrome, should be suspected (Fig. 110–5).

THERAPEUTIC INTERVENTION

The principal goal in the initial management of head injury is prevention of secondary brain injury as a result of hypoxia, hypercarbia, and hypotension. This is accomplished

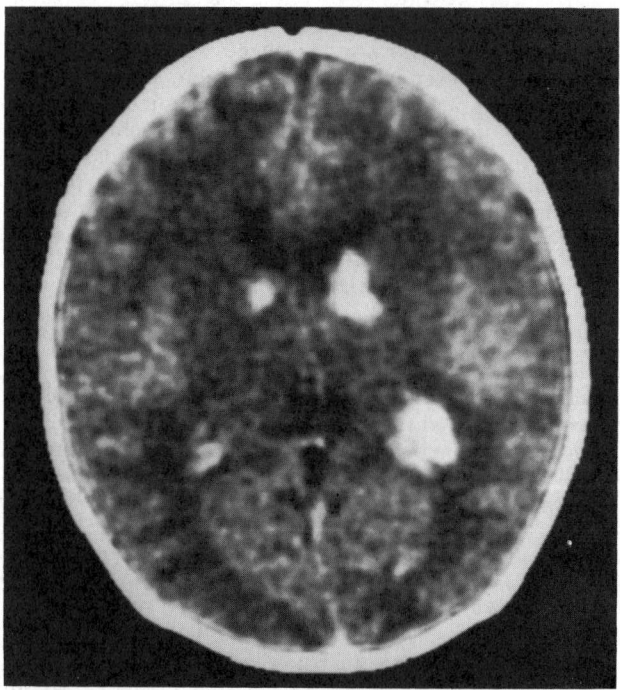

Figure 110–5. CT scan shows intraventricular and subarachnoid hemorrhages secondary to a shaking-type injury. This 2-month-old infant was comatose. Fresh hemorrhage is seen within the frontal horns and atria of the lateral ventricles, more severe on the left side. There is also blood in the interhemispheric fissure posteriorly, indicating acute subarachnoid hemorrhage. (Courtesy of Dr. Kenneth Thorp, Lansing, MI.)

by providing an adequate airway and adequate oxygenation, correcting hypovolemia, and preventing or controlling increased ICP (Table 110–5). Fortunately, meticulous trauma-oriented management also addresses most of the immediate needs for proper care of the patient with serious head injury. It is important during the first moments of airway assessment to immobilize the cervical spine in all injured children who are preverbal, have a reduced level of consciousness, are complaining of neck pain, have neurologic deficits, or have a mechanism of injury suggesting a high-energy transfer (e.g., a fall or motor vehicle collision). Reasonable immobilization can be achieved with appropriately sized, commercially available rigid collars or with tape and bolsters formed of sandbags, towel rolls, or bags of intravenous solutions.

Because hyperventilation with adequate oxygenation is often immediately effective in reducing ICP, children with a GCS of less than or equal to 8 and with signs of brain stem injury or posturing should receive orotracheal intubation to facilitate hyperventilation and oxygenation. Intubation is best accomplished by skilled personnel who can use rapid-acting anesthetic agents, thereby minimizing the tendency of laryngoscopy to cause an acute rise in ICP. When orotracheal intubation is indicated prior to full radiographic and clinical evaluation of the cervical spine, the neck and cervical spine should be stabilized manually during laryngoscopy. After intubation, noninvasive monitoring of end-tidal CO_2 permits immediate adjustments of respiratory therapy to keep the $Paco_2$ in the range of 25 to 30 mm Hg.

In addition to hyperventilation, intravenous mannitol (0.5 gm/kg) or furosemide (1 mg/kg) will reduce ICP rapidly and should be used if signs of herniation are present (Table 110–6). The head should be elevated to approximately 30 degrees and maintained straight with respect to the body to prevent impediments to cerebral venous drainage. It is important to keep the brain-injured child normotensive. Ultimately, a state of "euvolemic dehydration" is achieved by administering diuretics and restricting fluid input.[20] This approach presupposes adequate treatment of all hemodynamically significant hemorrhage. Dopamine at low to moderate doses (5 to 10 μg/kg/min) may be required to maintain adequate mean arterial blood pressure (MAP) and urine output.

The use of ICP monitoring in head-injured patients should be directed and managed by the consulting neurosurgeon. Direct ICP monitoring is rarely indicated in the emergency department. Clinical deterioration should be treated with the use of mannitol and furosemide until neurosurgical intervention is available.

Seizures occur frequently in children following head injury. One study found that approximately 10% of children developed posttraumatic seizures, with 98% of the seizures occurring within the first 7 days after injury. Severe head injury (GCS less than or equal to 8), diffuse cerebral edema, and acute subdural hematoma increase the likelihood of seizure development.[54] Electrical seizure activity increases both cerebral metabolic activity and blood flow and should be controlled.[20] True seizures should be treated with phenytoin (10 to 20 mg/kg infused slowly at 1 mg/kg/min). Phenytoin is preferred over phenobarbitol for treatment of posttraumatic seizures, as it enters the brain quickly and has little sedative effect. If the patient is in status epilepticus, intravenous lorazepam (0.05 to 0.10 mg/kg) or diazepam (0.1 to 0.3 mg/kg) should be given first, followed by phenytoin. Attention should be directed to the airway and respiratory status when using the benzodiazepines and a bag-mask setup should be readily available in case respiratory assistance is required. In cases of severe head injury, prophylactic phenytoin has been shown to reduce the incidence of seizures in the first week after injury and is currently recommended.[55]

The use of corticosteroids in head trauma has been controversial, with conflicting evidence presented from animal and human trials. Later studies have shown no benefit in ICP trends or clinical outcome in head-injured patients treated with high-dose steroids.[56, 57] There is also good evidence that the use of prophylactic barbiturate coma does not improve outcomes in patients with severe head injury.[58]

Intravenous antibiotics are indicated in the treatment of penetrating brain injuries, open depressed skull fractures, and pneumocephalus.[2] Broad-spectrum coverage directed at *Staphylococcus* species, *Streptococcus pneumoniae* and *Haemophilus influenzae* has been recommended. No benefit has been found with the use of prophylactic antibiotics in patients with routine basilar skull fractures.[59] Patients treated prophylactically have developed meningitis with organisms resistant to commonly used antibiotics.[60]

PROGNOSIS

The majority of children admitted to the hospital following mild head injury with loss of consciousness or skull fracture recover completely within 24 to 48 hours without recognized sequelae. However, some studies have shown neurobehavioral and cognitive sequelae in some children sustaining mild

---

TABLE 110–6

CRANIOCEREBRAL TRAUMA: THERAPY AT A GLANCE

Diuretics
  Mannitol, 0.5–1 gm/kg IV
  Furosemide, 1–2 mg/kg IV. or IM
Anticonvulsants
  Phenytoin, 10–20 mg/kg slow IV push (maximum rate of administration, 50 mg/min)
  Lorazepam, 0.05–0.1 mg/kg IV push (maximum total dose, 4 mg)
  Diazepam, 0.1–0.3 mg/kg IV push (maximum, 1 mg/min)
Antibiotics
  Ampicillin, 200 mg/kg/day IV, divided q 4–6 hr
  and
  Methicillin, 200 mg/kg/day IV, divided q 4–6 hr
  or
  Cefazolin, 100 mg/kg/day IV, divided q 6 hr

TABLE 110–5

INITIAL MANAGEMENT OF HEAD INJURY

1. Provide airway.
2. Immobilize cervical spine.
3. Oxygenate adequately (Pao_2 = 80–90 mm Hg).
4. Hyperventilate ($Paco_2$ = 25–30 mm Hg).
5. Maintain blood pressure.
6. Elevate head 30 to 45 degrees.
7. Place head and neck in midline position.
8. Minimize stimuli (pain, suctioning, movement).
9. Administer diuretics (for increased ICP or documented deterioration).
10. Treat seizures.
11. Administer antibiotics (penetrating injuries, open fractures).
12. Monitor ICP.

Adapted from Walker ML, Storrs BB, Mayer TA. Head injuries. *In* Mayer TA (ed). Emergency Management of Pediatric Trauma. Philadelphia, WB Saunders, 1985, p. 283.

head injury.[61, 62] Even children with mild injury not requiring hospitalization have shown some functional morbidity.[63]

The majority of children who sustain severe head injuries also do well. The prognosis for recovery is better in children than in adults. One study showed good outcomes at 1 year in 55% of pediatric patients, compared with 21% of adult patients.[64] The relatively low incidence of mass lesions and the high incidence of diffuse cerebral swelling suggest a different pathophysiologic response to injury in the child's brain, which may play a role in the improved survival of children following severe head injury.[14] The intact survivors often have minor physical, cognitive, and neurobehavioral deficits that require ongoing evaluation and therapy.

TYPES OF INJURY
Scalp Contusions and Lacerations

Contusions and lacerations of the scalp are the most frequent complications of head injury. In the older child, most scalp swellings following head trauma are the result of subgaleal hematomas.[18] In newborn infants, scalp swellings may be caused by other entities such as a caput succedaneum or cephalohematoma. Focal swelling with increased transillumination suggests a porencephalic or leptomeningeal cyst, either of which may be associated with a "growing" fracture of the skull.[65]

Scalp lacerations should be cleaned and irrigated thoroughly and closed as needed with sutures, staples, or hair ties. Open wounds should be palpated with a gloved finger to check for underlying fractures. The child's tetanus status should also be documented. No treatment is required for subgaleal hematoma, caput succedaneum, or cephalohematoma. Aspiration of the contents of these structures is contraindicated because of the risk of introducing infection.[18] A leptomeningeal cyst should be treated surgically by removing or replacing the protruding arachnoid and repairing the dural tear.[37]

Skull Fractures

Linear skull fractures comprise approximately 75% of all skull fractures in children.[18] The presence of a linear fracture does not in itself necessitate specific treatment, but it may indicate that significant intracranial injury has occurred. Linear skull fractures across the temporoparietal area may be associated with an injury to the underlying middle meningeal artery and may result in an epidural hemorrhage.[18] Linear fractures of the skull in an infant or young child should raise the possibility of child abuse or neglect.

Depressed skull fractures may involve either a disruption of the bony calvarium or, in a newborn, an indentation in the skull unaccompanied by a break in the cranial vault. Depressed fractures are classified as open or closed, depending on whether the overlying skin is lacerated or intact. If a laceration overlies the fracture site, treatment involves meticulous debridement of the wound, copious irrigation with a sterile solution, and administration of parenteral antibiotics to prevent complicating infection.[25] Depressed skull fractures may be palpable as an indentation or a "step-off" or diagnosed with the aid of tangential skull radiographs, which may demonstrate a characteristic double density. Depressed fractures are of particular concern, because the underlying brain may suffer contusion or laceration. Elevation of depressed fractures has been advocated if the depression is deeper than 5 mm, if the depressed fragment extends below the inner table of the skull,[18] if there is correlation of the fracture with underlying neurologic deficit, or if there is another reason for wound exploration (e.g., an open fracture, active hemorrhage, or a retained foreign body).[37]

Basilar skull fractures can occur at any point in the base of the skull and can involve the frontal, ethmoid, sphenoid, temporal, or occipital bones; the typical location is in the petrous portion of the temporal bone. These fractures can be difficult to recognize on skull radiographs because of the anatomic complexity of the base of the skull. The diagnosis is usually established by recognizing coexisting signs, including hemorrhage into the nose, nasopharynx, or middle ear (hemotympanum) and bleeding over the mastoid bone (Battle's sign) or around the eyes ("raccoon's eyes").[18] Traumatic injury to the cranial nerves, most frequently the first, seventh, and eighth, can also occur, producing cranial nerve palsies. Cerebrospinal fluid rhinorrhea and otorrhea reflect fractures of the cribriform plate or petrous temporal bone with tearing of the overlying meninges and subsequent leakage of CSF from the subarachnoid space through the fracture site.[18] This provides a route for meningeal infection, with *H. influenzae* type b and *S. pneumoniae* the usual pathogens. There is no clear evidence that prophylactic antibiotic therapy diminishes the frequency of meningeal infection.[59] Pneumocephaly or opacification of the maxillary or sphenoid sinuses may be seen as radiologic features of basilar skull fractures.

Diastatic fractures are traumatic separations of cranial bones at a suture site. They most frequently affect the lambdoidal suture and most often occur in the first 4 years of life. There is no specific therapy other than observation in children younger than 3 years of age, and such fractures can become the sites of "growing" fractures.[18]

"Growing" fractures indicate the development of a cyst at the site of either a linear or a diastatic skull fracture that prevents fusion of the fracture margins (Fig. 110–6). Such cysts are usually porencephalic, communicating with a lateral ventricle. They occur most often in the parietal bone and

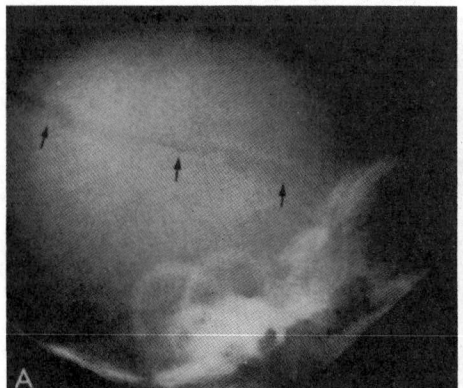
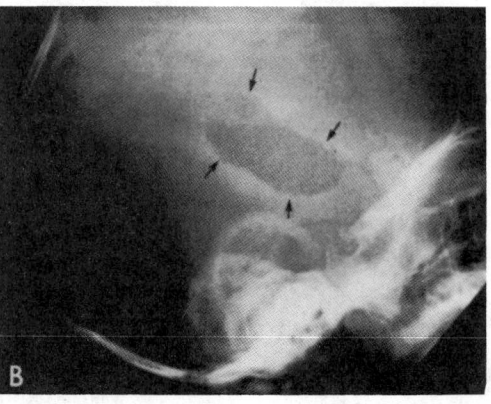

Figure 110–6. *A*, Lateral radiograph of a 2-month-old child shows a linear diastatic fracture. *B*, Two months after the injury there is healing of the posterior portion of the fracture with progressive bony erosion anteriorly. (From McLaurin RL, Towbin R. *In* Youmans JR (ed). Neurological Surgery. 3rd ed. Philadelphia, WB Saunders, 1990, p 2165.)

develop within 6 months of head injury, usually in children younger than 3 years of age. They must be surgically repaired.[18]

Intracranial Hemorrhage

Intracranial hemorrhages can be classified as extracerebral (epidural, subdural, subarachnoid) or intracerebral involving brain parenchyma. The availability of CT scanning has made the diagnosis and localization of intracranial hemorrhages more precise. Extracerebral hemorrhages are of special consideration in children, as they may occur following relatively mild head trauma and without associated skull fractures or loss of consciousness.[69]

An epidural hematoma is a collection of blood between the inner table of the skull and the dura (see Fig. 110–1). Epidural hematomas typically occur in the temporal region and are associated with fractures that cross and tear the middle meningeal artery. At least one fourth of epidural hematomas in children are of venous origin, with hemorrhage derived from the dural sinuses and diploic veins.[18] Acute epidural hematomas are rare in infants and young children. The age of presentation presumably reflects the close adherence of the dura to the inner table of the skull in infancy; also, the branches of the middle meningeal artery are not yet grooved within the inner table.[66] Epidural hematomas are usually unilateral, and seizures occur in less than 25% of patients. Retinal and preretinal hemorrhages are also found in less than 25% of children affected. The relatively large amount of extravasated blood that may be present can produce symptoms and signs of acutely increased ICP. Although an epidural hemorrhage is relatively rare (0.5% in unselected head injuries), it must be considered, as it may be rapidly fatal. The "biphasic course" described as characteristic of acute epidural hematoma (i.e., impairment of consciousness followed by a lucid interval, then return to lethargy or coma) is seldom seen in children.[18] It may also present clinically with a contralateral hemiparesis. A dilated and fixed pupil on the same side as the impact area is a hallmark of this injury. If an epidural hematoma is suspected clinically, the diagnosis should be confirmed by CT scan, which usually reveals a lenticular density (Fig. 110–7).

Epidural hematoma requires immediate surgical intervention. If treated early, prognosis is usually excellent, but secondary brain injury will occur rapidly if the hematoma is not quickly removed. The outcome for children with epidural hematomas is related to the neurologic state at the time of surgical decompression and the accompanying brain injuries. Survivors tend to be relatively free of neurologic sequelae, as the adjacent brain rarely sustains significant injury.[66]

Acute subdural hematomas occur five to ten times more frequently in children than do epidural hematomas.[18] Acute subdural hematomas characteristically are of venous origin, resulting from tearing of bridging meningeal veins, and there is an associated skull fracture in approximately 30% of cases.[44] Underlying contusion is frequently associated with it. A shaking injury without direct trauma to the head may also produce subdural hemorrhage (Fig. 110–8).[36] Acute subdural hemorrhages in children are usually seen in infancy, with a peak frequency at 6 months of age. Approximately 75% of subdural hematomas are bilateral.

Seizures occur in 75% of patients with subdural bleeding,[18] and retinal and preretinal hemorrhages are also frequently found. Symptoms and signs of increased ICP are also commonly present. Symptoms may be slower to appear with an acute subdural hematoma, as such a hematoma is usually caused by venous bleeding. If a subdural hemorrhage is

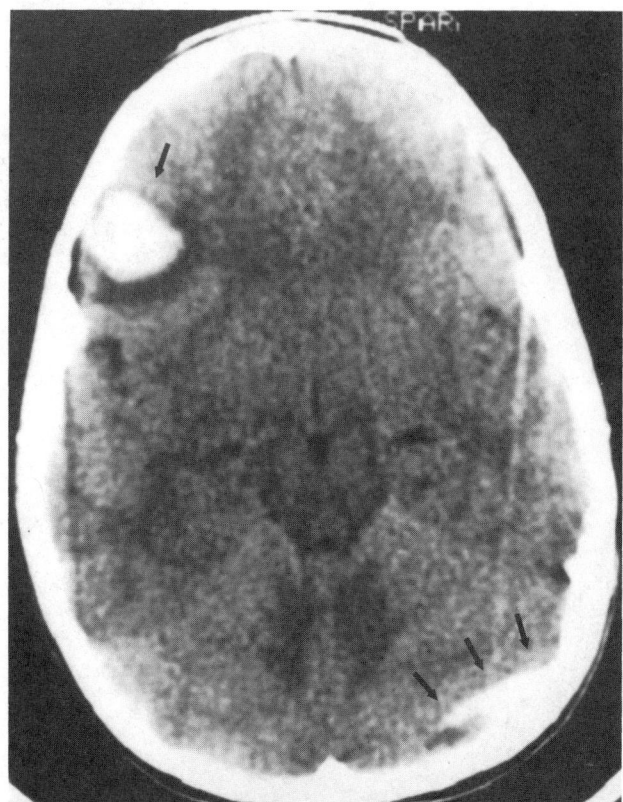

Figure 110–7. CT scan shows an epidural hematoma secondary to a coup-contre-coup injury. This 16-year-old patient was involved in a motor vehicle accident. There is intracerebral hemorrhage in the right frontal region near the site of impact with the windshield. The contre-coup force produced an epidural hematoma in the left occipital region *(arrows)*. (Courtesy of Dr. Kenneth Thorp, Lansing, MI.)

suspected clinically, the diagnosis usually can be confirmed by CT scan, which will show a crescentic configuration (Fig. 110–9). Underlying primary brain injury is often severe, and the prognosis is often dismal, even if the hematoma is evacuated early. The mortality in acute subdural hematoma is less than in acute epidural hematoma, but the morbidity is greater. Potential sequelae of subdural hematoma include motor deficits, seizures, hydrocephalus, and developmental delay.

Intracerebral hematomas are associated with bruising of the parenchyma of the brain. The majority occur in the frontal and temporal lobes and are usually contralateral to the site of skull impact. Traumatic subdural hematomas are also commonly present[66] but are poorly visualized on CT scan until 1 or 2 days after the injury.[2] Most of these hematomas require surgical removal if the hematoma is accessible. If the CT scan demonstrates a hemorrhagic contusion rather than an intracerebral hematoma, aggressive nonsurgical management is indicated.

Penetrating Injuries

Penetrating injuries to the brain are not uncommon in children.[25] All types of sharp objects can penetrate the immature skull or the orbit and enter the brain. Protruding foreign bodies should not be removed in the emergency department. Neurosurgical consultation is required for all patients with penetrating injuries. Emergency department management should include anticonvulsants, antibiotics, and tetanus prophylaxis.[25]

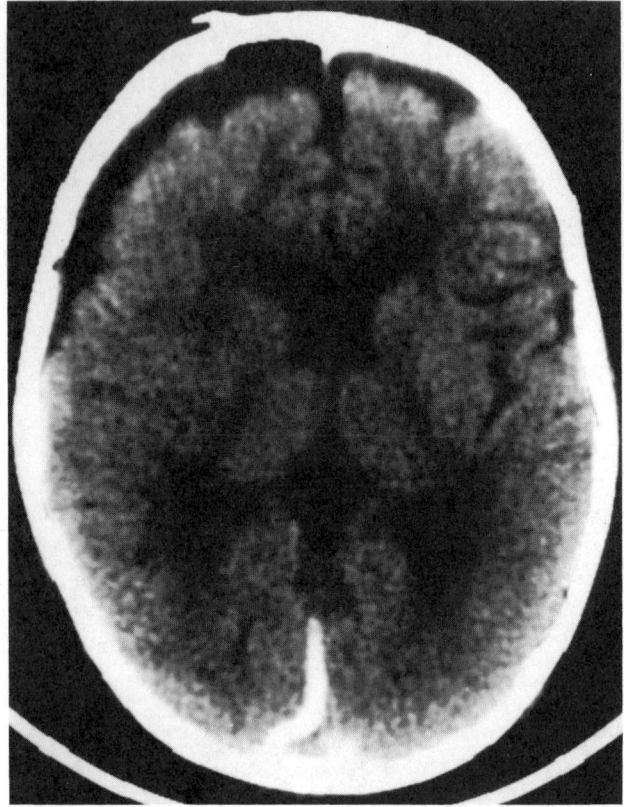

Figure 110–8. CT scan shows a parafalcine subdural hematoma. The acute subdural hematoma extends from the right occipital pole into the inner hemispheric fissure. This represents a "wrap-around" subdural hematoma, which can result from a "shaken-baby" injury. Also noted is a right frontal subdural hygroma and frontal atrophy due to a previous injury. (Courtesy of Dr. Kenneth Thorp, Lansing, MI.)

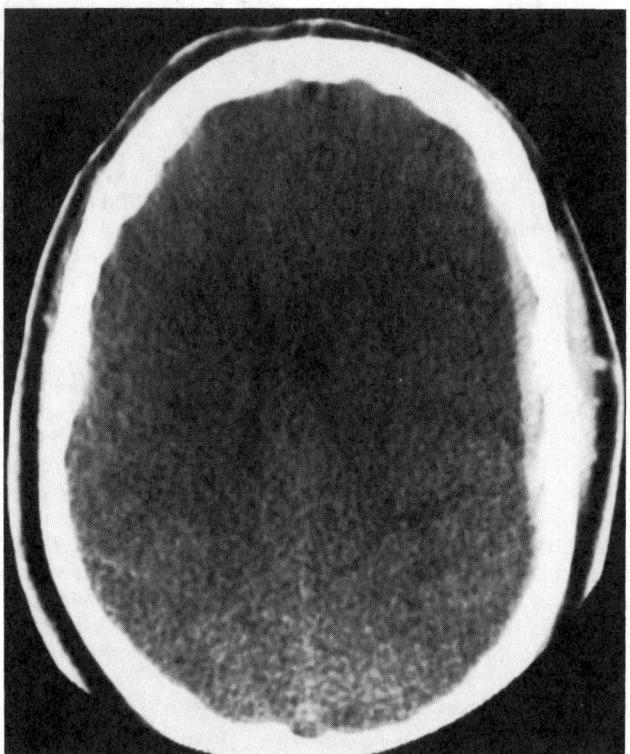

Figure 110–9. CT scan shows an acute subdural hematoma. A collection of blood lies in the subdural space adjacent to the left frontal parietal cortex and the adjacent skull. This produces medial displacement of underlying brain parenchyma. (Courtesy of Dr. Kenneth Thorp, Lansing, MI.)

Gunshot wounds inflict injury far beyond their direct penetration because of the amount of energy exerted on the brain, the trajectory of the missile, and the amount of scatter of bone and metallic fragments (Fig. 110–10).[24] The patient needs to be stabilized as with a closed head injury. An extensive search should be made for all entrance and exit sites. A CT scan will need to be obtained, along with neurosurgical consultation. Surgical debridement routinely is performed when the bullet has traversed the intracranial compartment.[25]

Cerebral Contusion

Cerebral contusion is a bruising or crushing injury to the brain and generally results from blunt trauma to the head. The area of the contusion is usually hemorrhagic and surrounded by edema. Overlying subarachnoid hemorrhage is frequently present.[24]

Contusions may occur anywhere, but typical locations are the frontal poles, the subfrontal cortex, and the anterior temporal lobes, as these portions of the brain impact forcefully against the fixed irregular surfaces of the surrounding skull.[18] Contusions may occur directly under the site of impact or on the contralateral side (a contrecoup lesion).

Patients with cerebral contusions usually present with significant alterations in their state of consciousness or focal neurologic signs. The CT scan provides radiologic confirmation of the suspected lesion. Patients sustaining cerebral contusion should be admitted to the hospital for a period of observation.

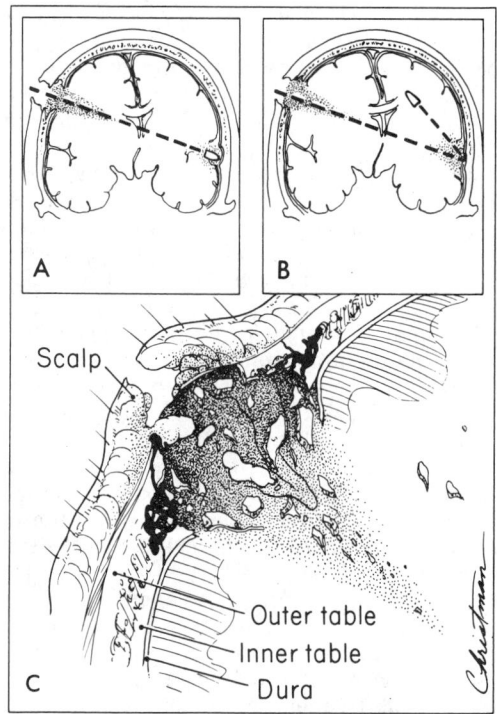

Scalp

Outer table
Inner table
Dura

Figure 110–10. Schematic of a gunshot missile wound. The brain injury may be complicated by inward passage of bone fragments and intracranial ricochet of the missile. *A*, Initial bullet track. *B*, Ricochet of the bullet within the brain. *C*, Bone fragments carried into the brain. (From Becker DP, Miller JD, Young HF, et al. Diagnosis and treatment of head injury in adults. *In* Youmans JR (ed). Neurological Surgery. 2nd ed. Philadelphia, WB Saunders, 1982, p 2055.)

TABLE 110-7

CRITERIA FOR HOME OBSERVATION AFTER MILD HEAD INJURY IN NEUROLOGICALLY NORMAL CHILDREN

1. No history of loss of consciousness, or
2. Unclear history of loss of consciousness, or
3. Loss of consciousness <5 min with normal CT scan, or
4. History of loss of consciousness >24 hours ago, and
5. Reliable caretakers, and
6. Access to EMS system, physician, or hospital

Concussion

Cerebral concussion is characterized by a transient impairment of consciousness with loss of awareness and responsiveness immediately following head injury.[18] It is usually caused by blunt trauma. Concussion is more likely to occur when the head moves freely after the impact, as in acceleration or deceleration injuries. The loss of consciousness has been attributed to an increase in ICP followed by a temporary shear strain on the upper brain stem.[18]

Minor head injury followed by a brief loss of consciousness is common in children of all ages. Symptoms and signs of a concussion may include pallor, headache, nausea and vomiting, somnolence or irritability, and amnesia. Posttraumatic amnesia consists of a failure to acquire or retain new information over the several minutes to hours after impact; it is typically manifested by perseverative questioning.[18] In the absence of a definite history of loss of consciousness, this technique can be helpful in establishing the diagnosis of concussion.

Children who have sustained a concussion should be admitted to the hospital for overnight observation. However, if a CT scan shows no abnormalities, the patient may be discharged home from the emergency department with appropriate discharge instructions.

DISPOSITION
Mild Head Injury

Mild head injury in children is a frequently encountered problem in the emergency department. Neurosurgical criteria for definition of a mild head injury include GCS of 13 to 15 on presentation, loss of consciousness of less than 20 minutes, and no evidence of intracranial hemorrhage.[67] The vast majority of these patients recover completely within 24 hours without recognized sequelae.

TABLE 110-8

ESSENTIAL DISCHARGE INSTRUCTIONS

Call or return to the emergency department if your child shows any of the following signs after leaving the hospital:
1. Persistent or increasing headache
2. Persistent vomiting 6 to 8 hours after injury
3. Drowsiness (wake your child at 4-hr intervals during the night)
4. Irritability or change in normal behavior
5. Weakness or clumsiness of an arm or leg
6. Neck pain or stiffness
7. Blurry vision or double vision
8. Poor balance when walking
9. Convulsions or seizures
10. Watery or bloody discharge from the nose or ears
11. Fever

TABLE 110-9

CRITERIA FOR SHORT-TERM HOSPITALIZATION

1. Decreased level of consciousness (GCS < 15)
2. Loss of consciousness > 5 min
3. Abnormal neurologic examination
4. Posttraumatic amnesia > 10 min
5. Labile physiologic responses (e.g., persistent vomiting, irritability, behavior changes)
6. Posttraumatic seizures
7. Linear, depressed, or basilar skull fracture
8. Unreliable caretakers
9. Suspected child abuse

For patients with mild head injuries, the single most important treatment is careful observation in the period following the injury so that neurologic deterioration can be identified. The patient's clinical status should direct whether this observation can take place at home or in the hospital. Criteria for home observation in patients with a normal neurologic examination include a history of no loss of consciousness, unclear history of loss of consciousness, loss of consciousness less than 5 minutes and a normal CT scan, or a history of loss of consciousness 24 hours or more earlier (Table 110-7). Patients must be discharged with appropriate discharge instructions to a reliable careprovider with access to the EMS system, a physician, or a hospital (Table 110-8).

Recommended criteria for short-term hospitalization include decreased level of consciousness (GCS < 15), loss of consciousness for greater than 5 minutes, abnormal neurologic findings, presence of posttraumatic amnesia, labile physiologic responses (including persistent vomiting 6 to 8 hours after injury or somnolence), seizures, and linear skull fractures. Patients should also be admitted to the hospital for observation if there is any suspicion of child abuse or if the careproviders do not appear able to adequately observe the child at home (Table 110-9).

All patients with more severe head injury, including those with a GCS of 12 or lower, rapid deterioration of consciousness, abnormal neurologic examination, open skull fractures, depressed or basilar skull fractures, penetrating injuries, or evidence of increased ICP need to be admitted to the hospital with ongoing management and neurosurgical evaluation.

References

1. Rodriguez JG, Brown ST. Childhood injuries in the United States. Am J Dis Child 1990;144:627.
2. Walker ML, Storrs BB, Mayer TA. Head injuries. In Mayer T (ed). Emergency Management of Pediatric Trauma. Philadelphia, WB Saunders, 1985, p 272.
3. Kraus JF, Rock A, Hemyari P. The causes, impact, and preventability of childhood injuries in the United States: Brain injuries among infants, children, adolescents, and young adults in the United States. Am J Dis Child 1990;144:684.
4. Chan BSH, Walker PJ, Cass DT. Urban trauma: An analysis of 1,116 pediatric cases. J Trauma 1989;29:1540.
5. Tepas JJ III, DiScala C, Ramenofsky ML, et al. Mortality and head injury: The pediatric perspective. J Pediatr Surg 1990;25:92.
6. Cooper A, Barlow B, Niemirska M, et al. Fifteen years' experience with penetrating trauma to the head and neck in children. J Pediatr Surg 1987;22:24.
7. Beaver BL, Moore VL, Peclet M, et al. Characteristics of pediatric firearm fatalities. J Pediatr Surg 1990;25:97.
8. Kissoon N, Dreyer J, Walia M. Pediatric trauma: Differences in pathophysiology, injury patterns and treatment compared with adult trauma. Can Med Assoc J 1990;142:27.
9. Mayer T, Walker ML. Emergency intracranial pressure monitoring in pediatrics: Management of the acute coma of brain insult. Clin Pediatr 1982;21:391.
10. Bruce DA, Raphaely RA, Swedlow D, et al. The effectiveness of iatrogenic barbiturate coma in controlling increased ICP in children. In Schulman

K, Maramou A, Miller JD, et al (eds). Intracranial Pressure IV. Berlin, Springer-Verlag, 1980, pp 630–632.

11. Marshall LF, Smith RW, Shapiro HM. The outcome with aggressive treatment in severe head injuries. Part 1: The significance of intracranial pressure monitoring. J Neurosurg 1979;50:20.

12. Miller JD, Becker DP, Ward JD, et al. Significance of intracranial hypertension in severe head injury. J Neurosurg 1977;47:503.

13. Bruce DA, Alavi A, Bilaniuk L, et al. Diffuse cerebral swelling following head injuries in children: The syndrome of "malignant brain edema". J Neurosurg 1981;54:170.

14. Bruce DA, Schut L, Bruno LA, et al. Outcome following severe head injuries in children. J Neurosurg 1978;48:679.

15. Gennarelli TA, Spielman GM, Langfitt TW, et al. Influence of the type of intracranial lesion on outcome from severe head injury. J Neurosurg 1982;56:26.

16. Becker DP, Miller JD, Ward JD, et al. The outcome from severe head injury with early diagnosis and intensive management. J Neurosurg 1977;47:491.

17. Subcommittee of Advanced Trauma Life Support of the American College of Surgeons Committee on Trauma. Advanced Trauma Life Support Student Manual. Chicago, American College of Surgeons, 1989, pp 109–121.

18. Rosman NP, Herskowitz J, Caster AP, et al. Acute head trauma in infancy and childhood. Pediatr Clin North Am 1979;26:707.

19. Bruce DA. The pathophysiology of increased intracranial pressure. *In* Current Concepts Scope Publications. Kalamazoo, MI, Upjohn, 1978.

20. Pascucci RC. Head trauma in the child. Intensive Care Med 1988;14:185.

21. Lewelt W, Jenkins LW, Miller JD. Effects of experimental fluid-percussion injury of the brain on cerebrovascular reactivity to hypoxia and to hypercapnia. J Neurosurg 1982;56:332.

22. Kuhl DE, Alavi A, Hoffman EJ, et al. Local cerebral blood volume in head-injured patients. Determination by emission computed tomography of 99mTc-labeled red cells. J Neurosurg 1980;52:309.

23. Obrist WD, Thompson HK Jr, Wans HS, et al. Regional cerebral blood flow estimated by 133 xenon inhalation. Stroke 1975;6:245.

24. Rockswold GL. Head injury. *In* Tintinalli JE, Krome RL, Ruiz E (eds). Emergency Medicine: A Comprehensive Study Guide. New York, McGraw-Hill, 1988, pp 829–839.

25. Bruce DA, Schut L, Sutton LN. Neurosurgical emergencies. *In* Fleisher GR, Ludwig S (eds). Textbook of Pediatric Emergency Medicine. Baltimore, Williams & Wilkins, 1988, pp 1112–1126.

26. Kewalramani LS, Draus JF, Sterling HM. Acute spinal-cord lesions in a pediatric population: Epidemiological and clinical features. Paraplegia 1980;18:206.

27. Hubbard DD. Injuries of the spine in children and adolescents. Clin Orthop 1974;100:56.

28. King DR. Trauma in infancy and childhood: Initial evaluation and management. Pediatr Clin North Am 1985;32:1299.

29. Nakayama DK, Gardner MJ, Rowe MI. Emergency endotracheal intubation in pediatric trauma. Ann Surg 1990;211:218.

30. Fiser DH. Intraosseous infusion. N Engl J Med 1990;322:1579.

31. Raimondi AJ, Hirschauer J. Head injury in the infant and toddler: Coma scoring and outcome scale. Childs Brain 1984;11:12.

32. Hahn YS, Chyung C, Barthel MJ, et al. Head injuries in children under 36 months of age. Childs Nerv Syst 1988;4:34.

33. Plum F, Posner JB. Diagnosis of Stupor and Coma. 3rd ed. Philadelphia, FA Davis, 1980.

34. Raphaely R, Swedlow D, Downes J, Bruce DA. Management of severe pediatric head trauma. Pediatr Clin North Am 1980;27:715.

35. McClelland CQ, Rekate H, Kaufman B, et al. Cerebral injury in child abuse: A changing profile. Childs Brain 1980;7:225.

36. Caffey J. The whiplash-shaken infant syndrome: Manual shaking by the extremities with whiplash-induced intracranial and intraocular bleeding. Pediatrics 1974;54:396.

37. McLaurin RL, McLennan JE. Diagnosis and treatment of head injury in children. *In* Youmans JR (ed). Neurological Surgery. Philadelphia, WB Saunders, 1982, pp 2084–2136.

38. Bushore M. Children with multiple injuries. Pediatr Rev 1988;10:49.

39. Henrys P, Lyne ED, Lifton C, et al. Clinical review of current spine injuries in children. Clin Orthop 1976;129:172.

40. Pang D, Pollack IF. Spinal cord injury without radiographic abnormality in children—the SCIWORA syndrome. J Trauma 1989;29:654.

41. Leonidas JC, Ting W, Binkiewicz A, et al. Mild head trauma in children: when is a roentgenogram necessary? Pediatrics 1982;69:139.

42. Bell RS, Loop JW. The utility and futility of radiographic skull examination for trauma. N Engl J Med 1971;284:236.

43. Ferry PC. Skull roentgenograms in pediatric head trauma: A vanishing necessity? Pediatrics 1982;69:237.

44. Harwood-Nash DC, Hendrick EB, Hudson AR. The significance of skull fractures in children. Radiology 1971;101:155.

45. Thornbury JR, Campbell JA, Masters SJ, Fryback DG. Skull fracture and the low risk of intracranial sequelae in minor head trauma. AJR 1984;143:661.

46. Seelig JM, Becker DP, Miller JD, et al. Traumatic acute subdural hematoma: Major mortality reduction in comatose patients treated within four hours. N Engl J Med 1981;304:1511.

47. Mayer T, Walker ML. Traumatic acute subdural hematoma. N Engl J Med 1982;306:355.

48. Peyster RG, Hoover ED. CT in head trauma. J Trauma 1982;22:25.

49. Thornbury JR, Masters SJ, Campbell JA. Imaging recommendations for head trauma: a new comprehensive strategy. Am J Rad 1987;149:781.

50. Gentry LR, Godersky JC, Thompson B, et al. Prospective comparative study of intermediate-field MR and CT in the evaluation of closed head trauma. Am J Rad 1988;150:673.

51. Hadley DM, Teasdale GM, Jenkins A, et al. Magnetic resonance imaging in acute head injury. Clin Rad 1988;39:131.

52. Kelly AB, Zimmerman RD, Snow RB, et al. Head trauma: comparison of MR and CT experience in 100 patients. Am J Neuro Rad 1988;9:699.

53. Zimmerman RA, Bilaniuk LT, Hackney DB, et al. Head injury: early results of comparing CT and high-field MR. AJR 1986;147:1215.

54. Hahn YS, Fuchs S, Flannery AM, et al. Factors influencing posttraumatic seizures in children. Neurosurgery 1988;22:864.

55. Temkin NR, Dikmen SS, Wilensky AJ, et al. A randomized, double-blind study of phenytoin for the prevention of post-traumatic seizures. N Engl J Med 1990;323:497.

56. Braakman R, Schouten HJA, Blaauw-van Dishoeck M, et al. Megadose steroids in severe head injury. Results of a prospective double-blind clinical trial. J Neurosurg 1983;58:326.

57. Dearden NM, Gibson JS, McDowall DG, et al. Effect of high-dose dexamethasone on outcome from severe head injury. J Neurosurg 1986;64:81.

58. Ward JD, Becker DP, Miller D, et al. Failure of prophylactic barbiturate coma in the treatment of severe head injury. J Neurosurg 1985;62:383.

59. Ingelzi RJ, VanderArk GD. Analysis of the treatment of basilar skull fractures with and without antibiotics. J Neurosurg 1975;43:721.

60. MacGee EE, Cauthen JC, Brackett CE. Meningitis following acute traumatic cerebrospinal fluid rhinorrhea. J Neurosurg 1970;33:312.

61. Barth JT, Macciocchi SN, Giordani B, et al. Neuropsychological sequelae of minor head injury. Neurosurgery 1983;13:529.

62. Gulbrandsen GB. Neuropsychological sequelae of light head injuries in older children 6 months after trauma. J Clin Neuropsychol 1984;6:257.

63. Casey R, Ludwig S, McCormick MC. Morbidity following minor head trauma in children. Pediatrics 1986;78:497.

64. Alberico AM, Ward JD, Choi SC, et al. Outcome after severe head injury: Relationship to mass lesions, diffuse injury, and ICP course in pediatric and adult patients. J Neurosurg 1987;67:648.

65. Kingsley D, Till K, Hoare R. Growing fractures of the skull. J Neurol Neurosurg Psychiatry 1978;41:312.

66. Edwards MS, Pitts LH. Brain and spinal cord trauma. *In* Berg BO (ed). Manual of Child Neurology. Greenbrae, CA, Jones Medical Publications, 1982, pp 135–145.

67. Levin HS, Mattis S, Ruff RM, et al. Neurobehavioral outcome following minor head injury: A three-center study. J Neurosurg 1987;66:234.

CHAPTER 111

Spine and Spinal Cord Trauma

R. N. Hensinger

INTRODUCTION

Incidence

Fractures of the spine in children are uncommon, comprising a reported incidence of 2% to 5% of all spinal injuries.[1-6] Most spine injuries involve the cervical spine; however, significant and disabling injuries also occur in the thoracic and lumbar regions. Neonates are more prone to cervical injuries than to dorsal or lumbar spine trauma.[7, 8] Occasionally, infant spine injuries are caused by child abuse or battering.[9] The young child in the first decade is more often a victum of pedestrian accidents, trauma as a passenger in a car, or a fall from a height.[10–13] In the second decade, spine injuries are often the result of sports and recreation-related activities (44%) (e.g., tobogganing, bicycling, motor-cycling)[14–16] and motor vehicle accidents (37%).[6] As many as 50% of children who have mild vertebral injuries are never admitted to the hospital, and thus reports are skewed toward the more severely injured.[6, 17]

Cervical injuries are often associated with trauma to other parts of the body, usually the head or the face. Evidence of head or facial trauma, particularly in the comatose patient, should alert the physician to the possibility of a less obvious cervical spine injury. Children are relatively more elastic than adults and any force is transmitted over many bony segments, with multiple vertebral fractures being the rule.[4, 12, 18, 19] In children, innocuous-appearing fractures of the lumbar or thoracic transverse processes are often associated with serious abdominal injury (21%), particularly to the spleen and liver.[20] Lumbar spine injuries can be associated with life-threatening vascular injuries requiring emboliza-tion.[21]

Injuries to the child's cervical spine are most commonly found in the upper cervical region above the C3 level, unlike adult injuries, which are more common in the lower cervical region.[4, 22–25] In most series of pediatric cervical fractures, there is a relatively low incidence of neurologic deficit. When neurologic injuries do occur, children have a better prognosis than adults.[4, 18, 26]

Neurologic Injury

Thirteen to fifteen percent of all spinal cord injuries occur in children, with males predominating 2:1.[6, 13] The vertebral column in the young child is more elastic than the spinal cord itself.[8] Pan and Wilberger have reported a condition known as "spinal cord injury without radiographic abnor-mality" (SCIWORA).[27] This has been most often reported in children younger than 10 years old.[28–31] Myelography is of limited assistance in the diagnosis, but magnetic resonance imaging (MRI) has been helpful in identifying the site and extent of the lesion.[31–34] Because few data are available on the value of MRI in prognosis and surgical planning,[35] the computed tomographic (CT) myelogram remains an essential study prior to spinal cord decompression.[32]

Spinal cord injury in children peaks in those younger than 10 years and again in teenagers. In the young child, the lesion is more often at the cervicothoracic junction, and the paraplegia is more likely to be permanent.[31] The teenager is more likely to have a transient or an incomplete neurologic deficit that improves with time. Patients with a delayed onset of paraplegia (2 hours to 4 days) may have sustained a vascular insult to the spinal cord.[33] This is typically located at the midportion of the thoracic spine (watershed area) and is usually associated with a blow to the chest or abdomen, resulting in shock or profound hypotension from a ruptured spleen or a retroperitoneal hematoma. Such an injury generally results in complete and permanent paraplegia. The MRI scan is helpful in defining the lesion.[32]

In older children, a vertebral fracture is the most common cause of neurologic injury, and in the majority (83%), a bony injury can be identified radiologically.[6] Fracture dislocations are more common than distraction or compression injuries and usually occur at the thoracolumbar junction (36%); the remainder of spinal cord injuries occur between the T4 and L2 levels.[36]

A randomized, controlled trial using methylprednisolone in patients with acute spinal cord injury demonstrated improved neurologic recovery if the drug was given within the first 8 hours.[37] However, none of those studied were younger than 13 years. Nevertheless, until contradictory data are presented, it would seem prudent to treat all children with spinal cord injury similarly. The methylprednisolone dose is a 30-mg/kg intravenous bolus, followed by an infusion of 5.4 mg/kg/hr for 23 hours.[37]

ANATOMY AND PHYSIOLOGY
General Development

Cervical growth plates, which lack complete ossification, and hypermobility cause confusion in the interpretation of cervical radiographs in children with neck pain or stiffness.[38] Cervical spine radiographs in trauma patients are often difficult to interpret and have a high rate of serious interpretation errors, especially in inexperienced physicians.[39] The problem is further compounded by the limited ability of the frightened child with a painful neck to cooperate during a physical examination. In addition, the child may struggle, making it difficult to obtain satisfactory and accurately positioned radiographs.

In general, children younger than 8 years have a higher incidence of injury to the upper cervical spine than do adolescents or adults. Such injuries tend to involve synchondroses, and, rarely, facet fractures or vertebral dislocations. After 8 years of age, the ligaments become more effective in restraining skeletal structures.[40, 41] By age 8 to 10 years, the bony cervical spine has approached adult configuration, and most of the cartilage lines have disappeared.[42, 43] The exceptions include the vertebral ring apophyses, which appear at the end of childhood and fuse to the vertebral bodies at about age 25 years.[42]

Injuries of the thoracic and lumbar spine are rare in the young child, and fractures in teenagers tend to have the adult pattern. Unlike the adult spine, the immature spine has the capacity to remodel the vertebral body, but not the posterior elements. Restoration of height of a compressed vertebra is a result of the hypervascularity of the reparative response with stimulation of the apophysis. This accounts for the infrequent occurrence of kyphosis in children with multiple compression fractures.

A knowledge of normal physical development is essential when interpreting a child's radiograph. Physeal plates are generally smooth, regular, and in predicted locations and have subchondral sclerotic lines. Fractures are irregular, without sclerosis, and usually in unpredictable locations. The dates of physeal appearances and disappearances may vary and are often expressed as averages.[44]

Upper Cervical Spine (C1–C2)

At birth the atlas is composed of three ossification centers: one for the body (anterior ring) and one for each of the two neural arches.[45] The anterior ring is occasionally bifid, is not usually present at birth, and appears during the first year of life (Fig. 111–1). On rare occasions, it is absent and may close by fusion of the neural arches anteriorly.[42, 46] The posterior arch of the first cervical vertebra is usually closed by the third year. Occasionally its development is incomplete or remains completely absent throughout life.[42, 45] Rarely, there may be an independent ossification center appearing in this region (posterior tubercle). The neurocentral synchondroses that link the neural arches of the atlas to the body are best seen in the open-mouth radiograph view (Fig. 111–2). They close by the seventh year and should not be mistaken for fractures.[42, 45]

The developing axis has three (occasionally four) ossification centers at birth: one for each neural arch, one (occasionally two) for the body, and a fourth for the

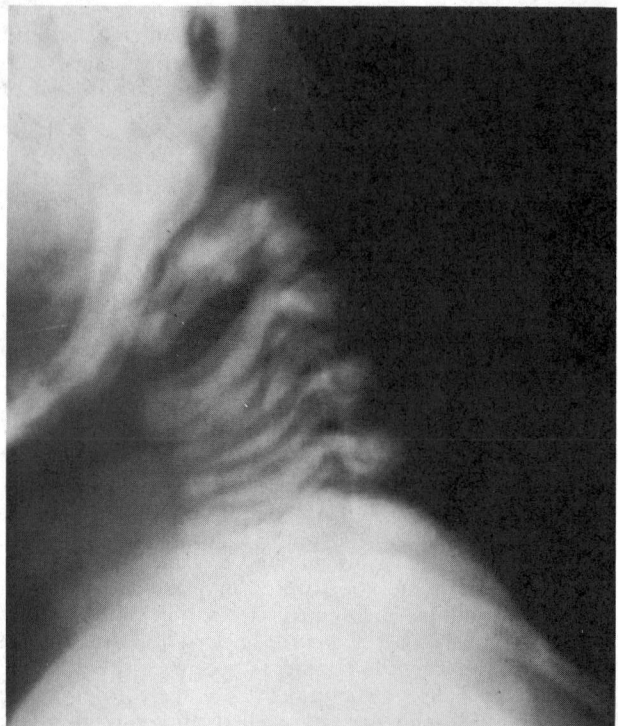

Figure 111–1. Extension radiograph of a 6-week-old child shows that the anterior arch of the atlas slides upward to protrude beyond the ossified part of the dens, giving the mistaken impression of odontoid hypoplasia. Note that the anterior portion of the ring of C1 is not yet ossified.

dens.[42, 46] In the anteroposterior open-mouthed view of a young child, the dens (odontoid process) is positioned between the neural arches. It surmounts the body of the axis and is separated from it by a synchondrosis; the vestigial disk space of the odontoid runs well below the level of articular processes of the axis.[46] This basilar epiphysis of the odontoid may persist up to 11 years of age as a narrow, sclerotic line and can resemble a nondisplaced fracture. Below this are the synchondroses between the body and the neural arches which together combine to form the letter "H" (see Fig. 111–2).

The odontoid fuses with the neural arches and the body of the axis between 3 and 6 years of age, essentially the same time that the remainder of the vertebral body joins the neural arches. Therefore, no epiphysis or synchondrosis should be present in the axis in the open-mouthed view of a child more than 6 years of age.[42, 46] The normal synchondrosis between the dens and the arch of C2 is not seen on the lateral view of the cervical spine but is easily visible on the oblique view and should not be mistaken for a fracture.[47] The tip of the odontoid is not ossified at birth and has a V-shaped appearance. A small ossification center, known as the *summit ossification center*, appears at its tip at age 3 to 6 years and fuses with the main portion of the odontoid by age 12 years.[42, 46]

Lower Cervical Spine (C3–C7)

The third to seventh cervical vertebrae ossify from three centers: one from the body and one from each neural arch. The neural arches close at the second or third year, and the neurocentral synchondroses between the neural arches and the vertebral body fuse between the third and the sixth years. In the lateral radiograph, the ossified portion of the vertebral body in the young child is wedge shaped and then becomes squared off at about 7 years of age.[42, 46, 47] The bodies, neural arches, and pedicles enlarge radially by periosteal apposition, similar to the periosteal growth seen in long bones.[47]

At birth, the vertebral bodies possess superior and inferior cartilage plates firmly bonded to the disk.[42, 47] The interface between vertebral body and end plate is similar to the physis of a long bone.[1] The vertebral body is analagous to the metaphysis, and the clear space between it and the end plate represents the physeal plate where longitudinal growth occurs.[47] Stress applied to the vertebral bodies results in splitting the cartilage end plate at the growth zone in the area of columnar and calcified cartilage, rather than at the stronger junction between it and the vertebral disk.[1] The apophyseal rings on the upper and lower surfaces of the vertebral body begin to ossify late in childhood and fuse to the vertebral body by age 25 years. Apophyseal fractures have been reported, usually in the lower cervical region.[48]

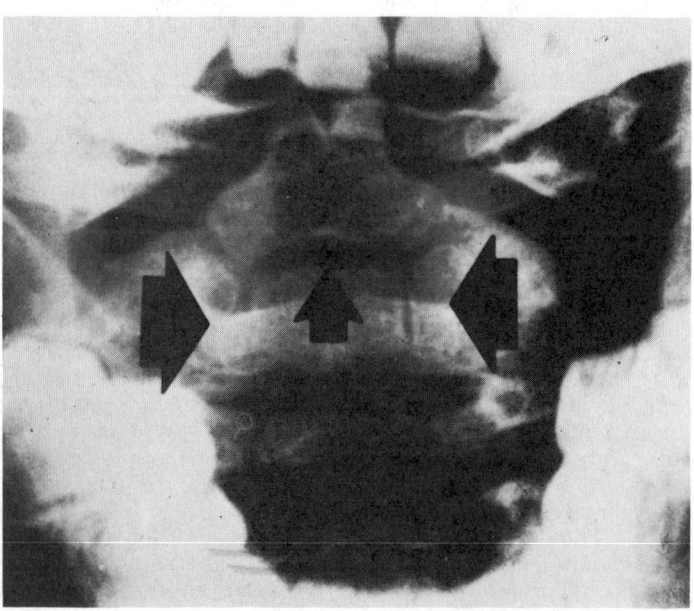

Figure 111–2. The epiphysis at the base of the odontoid process is shown *(small arrow)*, well below the level of the superior articular facet of the axis. The synchondroses between the body of the axis and the neural arches are also shown *(large arrows)*. Just above this are the synchondroses between the odontoid process and the neural arches. The odontoid process therefore surmounts the body of the axis and is sandwiched between the neural arches. The epiphyseal line and synchondroses combine to form the letter "H." (From Fielding JW. Selective observations on the cervical spine in the child. *In* Ahstrom JP Jr (ed). Current Practice in Orthopaedic Surgery. Vol 5. St Louis, CV Mosby, 1973, p 31.)

The inferior end plates are believed to be more susceptible to fracture than the superior end plates because of the mechanical protection provided the latter by the developing uncinate processes.[48]

Thoracic and Lumbar Spine

The development of the thoracolumbar spine in children is more straightforward than that of the cervical spine. In the thoracolumbar spine, there is an increased cartilage-to-bone ratio, a ring apophysis, and hyperelasticity. In newborns and young children, the vertebrae are largely cartilaginous, and radiographically the intervertebral spaces appear widened in relation to the vertebral bodies (Fig. 111–3). With aging, the ossification centers enlarge, and this cartilage-to-vertebra ratio gradually reverses. The vertebral apophyses are secondary centers of ossification that develop in the cartilaginous end plates located at the superior and inferior surfaces of the vertebral bodies. The apophyses are thicker at their periphery than at the center and thus appear as a ring with early ossification. These are seen initially between the ages of 8 and 12 years and normally fuse with the vertebral bodies by the 21st year. They may be confused with an avulsion fracture. The vertebral apophysis is equivalent to the epiphysis of a long bone and is separated from the vertebral body (the metaphysis) by a narrow cartilaginous physis. Vertical growth of the vertebrae occurs equally at the top and the bottom.

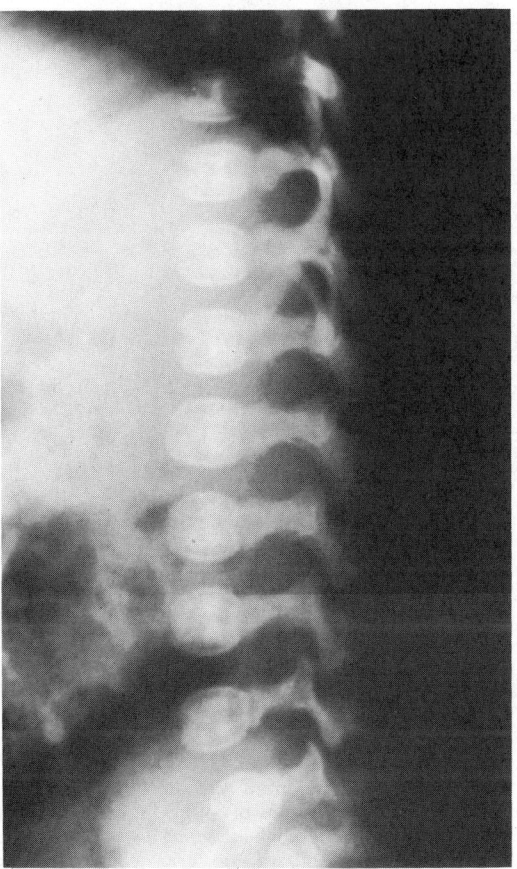

Figure 111–3. Radiograph of a normal spine in a 10-week-old infant. The superior and inferior vertebral end plates and vertebral apophyses are cartilaginous. Thus, there is apparent widening of the intervertebral spaces relative to the ossific portion of the vertebrae. The anterior and posterior notching of the walls of the vertebral body is due to normal vascular channels and may be confused with a fracture.

In the infant, lateral radiographs show horizontal conical shadows of lessened density extending inward from the anterior and posterior walls of the vertebral bodies that may be confused with fracture (see Fig. 111–3).[49] The posterior notch results from an actual indentation in the posterior vertebral wall at the point of entrance and emergence of the posterior arteries and veins. These indentations occur in all vertebrae and at all ages. In the infant, the anterior conical shadow is usually more obvious than the posterior and results from the presence in this area of a large sinusoidal space within the vertebra.[49] This anterior notch is not permanent and disappears with ossification of the anterior and lateral walls of the vertebral body, usually in the first year of life.

By 8 to 10 years of age, the biomechanical properties of the bony thoracolumbar spine have approached those of the adult, and the fracture patterns are similar, with the exception of the late development of progressive spinal deformity. Paralytic scoliosis occurs in essentially all children who sustain a complete spinal cord injury prior to the adolescent growth spurt age (less than 12 years in girls and 13 years in boys).[50] Disk space narrowing and spontaneous interbody fusion following injury is uncommon in children, as the healthy intervertebral disks typically transmit the force to the vertebral bodies.[19]

Mobility

The cervical region is normally the most flexible area of the spine, especially in children. It may be difficult to determine normal from abnormal mobility in a young child's neck. Little biomechanical testing of the immature spine has been performed, and most concepts are interpolated from testing adults.

The most mobile articulation in the cervical spine is between the atlas and axis. Half of all cervical rotation occurs here. Some side-to-side bending is also present, but hyperextension is limited by the dens. Subluxation is present if there is more than 10 degrees of forward flexion at C1–C2.[51] The child should be evaluated for instability if, at age 3 to 10 years, the distance between the spinous process of C1 and C2 is greater than 10 mm in the neutral recumbent radiograph. The atlanto-occipital joint allows some flexion and extension but little rotation. The C2–C3 joint is slightly mobile in flexion and extension, but not in rotation. The relatively mobile C1–C2 joint is therefore located between two relatively stiff joints. This concentrates forces at the atlantoaxial joint and partly explains the high percentage of cervical injuries at this level.

The anterior arch of the atlas is firmly held against the odontoid process by the transverse atlantal ligament. This space is called the *atlanto-dens interval (ADI)* and on the lateral radiograph is measured from the anterior edge of the dens to the posterior edge of the anterior arch of the atlas (Fig. 111–4). Further stability is provided by accessory ligaments such as the alar ligaments that connect the tip of the odontoid process with the occipital condyle and the capsular ligaments. In the adult, anterior displacement of the ring of C1 from the odontoid of up to 3 mm is within the range of normal. When the distance between the odontoid process and the anterior arch of C1 is 3 to 5 mm, the physician should suspect a transverse ligament rupture, and when the distance is 10 to 12 mm, all ligaments have failed.[52] Radiographic surveys of children suggest that an ADI of up to 4 mm may be normal.[38, 53, 54] If the space between the dens and anterior arch of C1 is asymmetric on the flexion view, the ADI should be measured at the midportion of the dens. A slight increase in the neutral ADI may indicate an injury of the transverse atlantal ligament. This can be a useful sign of acute injury when flexion-extension views would be potentially hazardous.

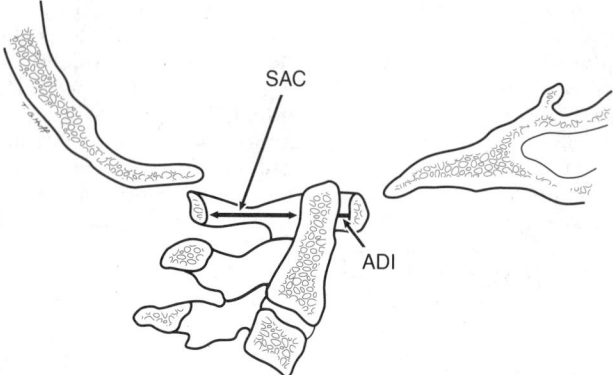

Figure 111–4. Sagittal views of the atlantoaxial joint demonstrate the atlantal-dens interval (ADI). The space available for the cord (SAC) is the distance between the posterior aspect of the odontoid and the posterior ring of C1. (From Hensinger RN, Fielding JW. The cervical spine. *In* Morrissy TR (ed). Lovell and Winter's Pediatric Orthopaedics. 3rd ed. Philadelphia, JB Lippincott, 1990, p 718.)

The ADI in children is slightly larger than in the adult; this is probably because of the greater ligamentous laxity thought to be present in children and the incompletely ossified structures. A lateral extension radiograph in a young child may give a mistaken impression of odontoid hypoplasia, because the anterior arch of the atlas slides upward and protrudes beyond the ossified portion of the dens to lie against the unossified tip.[38]

In the infant and young child, the cervical vertebral bodies are simply a series of elastic cartilages and can be stretched up to 2 inches without disruption, whereas the less elastic cervical spinal cord can only tolerate a stretch of 1/4 inch.[8] This elasticity probably accounts for the frequent occurrence in the young child of spinal cord damage without radiologic evidence of bony injury, both in the cervical and the thoracolumbar spines.[2, 6, 11, 31] The criteria for lower cervical instability in the adult have been defined[55] but may not be appropriate for the young child. In children, the intraspinous distance posteriorly can be helpful to diagnose traumatic ligamentous tears. At any given level, the intraspinous distance may be 1.5 times greater than the intraspinous distance on either one level above or one level below the area in question.[56, 57] Increased intraspinous distance, divergence of the articular processes, and widening of the posterior aspect of the disk space are indicative of instability in pediatric cervical spine injuries.[56, 57]

Pseudosubluxation of C2 on C3

One of the most frequently overinterpreted findings on pediatric cervical spine films is hypermobility of C2 on C3 in flexion. Although this injury pattern can indeed occur in children,[58] the most common explanation is C2–C3 pseudosubluxation (Fig. 111–5). Nine percent of children between the ages of 1 and 16 years have marked forward displacement of C2 on C3 in flexion, clearly resembling a subluxation.[38] Forty percent of normal children less than 8 years of age demonstrate a definite tendency toward excessive anterior displacement of C2 on C3 in flexion. Similar displacement occurs less frequently between C3 and C4, most often in younger patients.[38] Pseudosubluxation is a well-recognized phenomenon in small children but has also been reported in teenagers.[59]

Swischuk described the importance of the posterior cervical (spinolaminar) line (see Fig. 111–5) as a helpful guide to differentiate pathologic subluxation from normal pseudosubluxation.[60] On the posterior cervical line in flexion and extension, all three of the anterior edges of the spinous processes of C1, C2, and C3 should line up within 1 mm of each other.[56, 57] It is important for clinicians to be aware of the propensity of normal children to demonstrate pseudosubluxation, particularly at the C2–C3 level. A negative clinical history of injury and the absence of neck pain or limitation of motion are important clues to avoid inappropriate treatment.

The facet joint angles are shallow in children.[46] The C1–C2 angles range from 55 degrees in the newborn and progress to 80 degrees by age 8 years. In the lower cervical spine, the angle begins at 30 degrees in the newborn and progresses to 65 degrees in the adult. This relative flatness of the facet joints adds to the greater mobility and forward translational motion that children demonstrate in their cervical spine.[46]

Retropharyngeal Soft Tissues

The space between the cervical spine and the pharynx in the region of C3 has been estimated to be a maximum of 5 mm in adults. An increase in width after trauma is presumptive evidence of hemorrhage or edema secondary to fracture or dislocation.[61, 62] Weir suggests an average value of 3.5 mm for the retropharyngeal space (opposite the inferior base of C2) and 8.9 mm for the retrotracheal space (opposite the inferior base of C6) for normal children younger than 15 years.[62] Further investigation is needed if the retropharyngeal space is wider than 8 mm and the retrotracheal space is more than 22 mm.

In inspiration, the pharyngeal wall is close to the vertebra, whereas in forced expiration, there may be a marked physiologic increase in the width of the retropharyngeal soft tissue shadow.[63] Crying displaces both the hyoid bone and

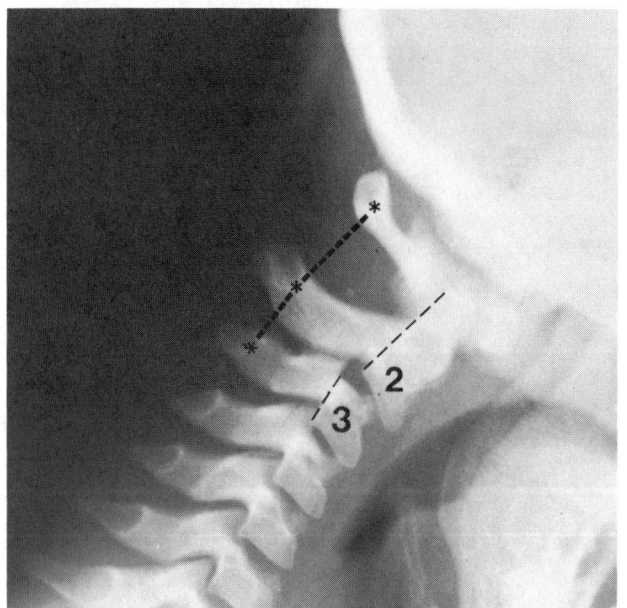

Figure 111–5. Pseudosubluxation of C2 on C3. Hypermobility is common in children under the age of 8 years. Specific measurements of the movement of the vertebral bodies *(thin dotted line)* is unreliable, whereas the relationship with the posterior elements *(thick dotted line)* is more consistent. In flexion the posterior arch of C2 normally aligns itself in a straight line with C1 and C3. Note the relative horizontal nature of the facet joints, which allows greater mobility. (From Swischuk LE. Anterior displacement of C2 in children: Physiologic or pathologic? A helpful differentiating line. Radiology 1977;122:759. © 1977, Williams & Wilkins Co., Baltimore.)

the larynx forward, increasing the width of this shadow. This should be considered when interpreting the films of a frightened, crying child.

CLINICAL EVALUATION

Several problems peculiar to children may result in diagnostic errors. Failure to recognize paralysis represents the most serious error. An unresponsive or comatose child should be considered to have a spinal injury until proven otherwise. Determining the presence or extent of paralysis may prove difficult in an uncooperative child. Gross flexion or reflex withdrawal of the limbs may mislead the physician into thinking that voluntary movement is present.

Stimulation and handling may produce crying and lead the physician to erroneously assume that sensation is intact. Serial observation over a period of time may be necessary to determine the true neurologic status of the patient (Table 111–1). The diagnosis of birth injuries of the spinal cord should be suspected in a floppy infant or child with a nonprogressive neurologic lesion following a difficult delivery. The single most important finding is the demonstration of a sensory level (Fig. 111–6). In the older child, as in the adult, pain and tenderness of the spine are usually present. Inability to walk and muscle spasm are often present with unstable injuries to the spine.

DIAGNOSTIC EVALUATION

When evaluating the injured child, the emergency physician must determine whether radiographic evaluation of the cervical spine is necessary. Indications for cervical spine radiographs in adult trauma patients include neck pain or tenderness, intoxication or decreased mentation, neurologic deficit, and distracting injuries (Table 111–2). For initial screening, lateral, anteroposterior, odontoid, and oblique radiographs are recommended.[54, 64] If the patient is medically unstable, then a simple cross-table lateral radiograph is sufficient until the patient's condition permits a complete evaluation. The false-negative rate for a single cross-table lateral radiograph is 23% to 26%. Therefore, the physician should always follow up with a complete cervical study.[54, 64]

Rachesky et al. attempted to identify which injured chil-

dren required cervical radiographs by reviewing 2133 children who had radiographs for a trauma-related event, 25 (1.2%) of whom had a documented cervical spine injury.[65] They concluded that cervical spine radiographs were indicated if the child had a complaint of neck pain or there was head or facial trauma associated with a motor vehicle accident. In this study, the prospective use of these criteria would have diminished the number of radiographic examinations by 32%. Whenever the diagnosis of a cervical spine injury is made, a careful examination should be made of the remaining cervical spine, as in children there is a high incidence (24%) of multiple-level injury in the cervical area (Fig. 111–7).[66]

Further imaging, particularly flexion-extension radio-

TABLE 111–1
TRAUMA MOTOR INDEX

Neurologic Level	Muscles
Cervical	
4	Diaphragm
5	Biceps
6	Wrist extensors
7	Triceps
8	Flexor profundus
Thoracic	
1	Hand intrinsics
2–9	Intercostals
10–12	Abdominals
Lumbar	
2	Iliopsoas
3	Quadriceps
4	Tibialis anterior
5	Extensor hallicus
Sacral	
1	Gastrocnemius
2	Bladder sphincter
3	Anal sphincter
	Bulbocavernous reflex

Adapted from Stauffer ES. Cervical spine trauma. Section 24. *In* Orthopaedic Knowledge Update 1: Home Study Syllabus. Chicago, AAOS, 1984, pp 199–208.

TABLE 111–2
RADIOLOGIC SCREENING FOR CERVICAL SPINE INJURIES IN THE TRAUMA PATIENT

Patient Status*	Initial Radiographs	Secondary Test
Physiologically stable		
Alert, asymptomatic	None	None
Symptomatic	Lateral, anteroposterior, odontoid, right and left oblique	CT scan, tomography, flexion-extension radiographs as indicated
Decreased mentation	Lateral, anteroposterior, odontoid, right and left oblique	CT scan, tomography, flexion-extension radiographs as indicated
Physiologically unstable		
Alert, asymptomatic	None	None
Symptomatic	Lateral†	Complete workup after resuscitation
Decreased mentation	Lateral†	Complete workup after resuscitation

*The terms used are defined as follows: *alert:* normal level of consciousness; *asymptomatic:* no neck pain or tenderness and no neurologic findings compatible with cervical origin; *symptomatic:* any complaint of neck pain, tenderness, or neurologic findings compatible with cervical origin; *decreased mentation:* Glasgow Coma Score of 13 or less; *physiologically stable:* blood pressure of 90 mm Hg or higher, respiratory rate of 13 to 29, pulse rate of 60 to 110; *physiologically unstable:* vital signs outside limits just mentioned.

†Apply Philadelphia collar and assume patient has an unstable cervical fracture if the lateral radiograph is normal.

From Bachullis BL, Long WB, Hynes GD, Johnson MC. Clinical indications for cervical spine radiographs in the traumatized patient. Am J Surg 1987;153:473.

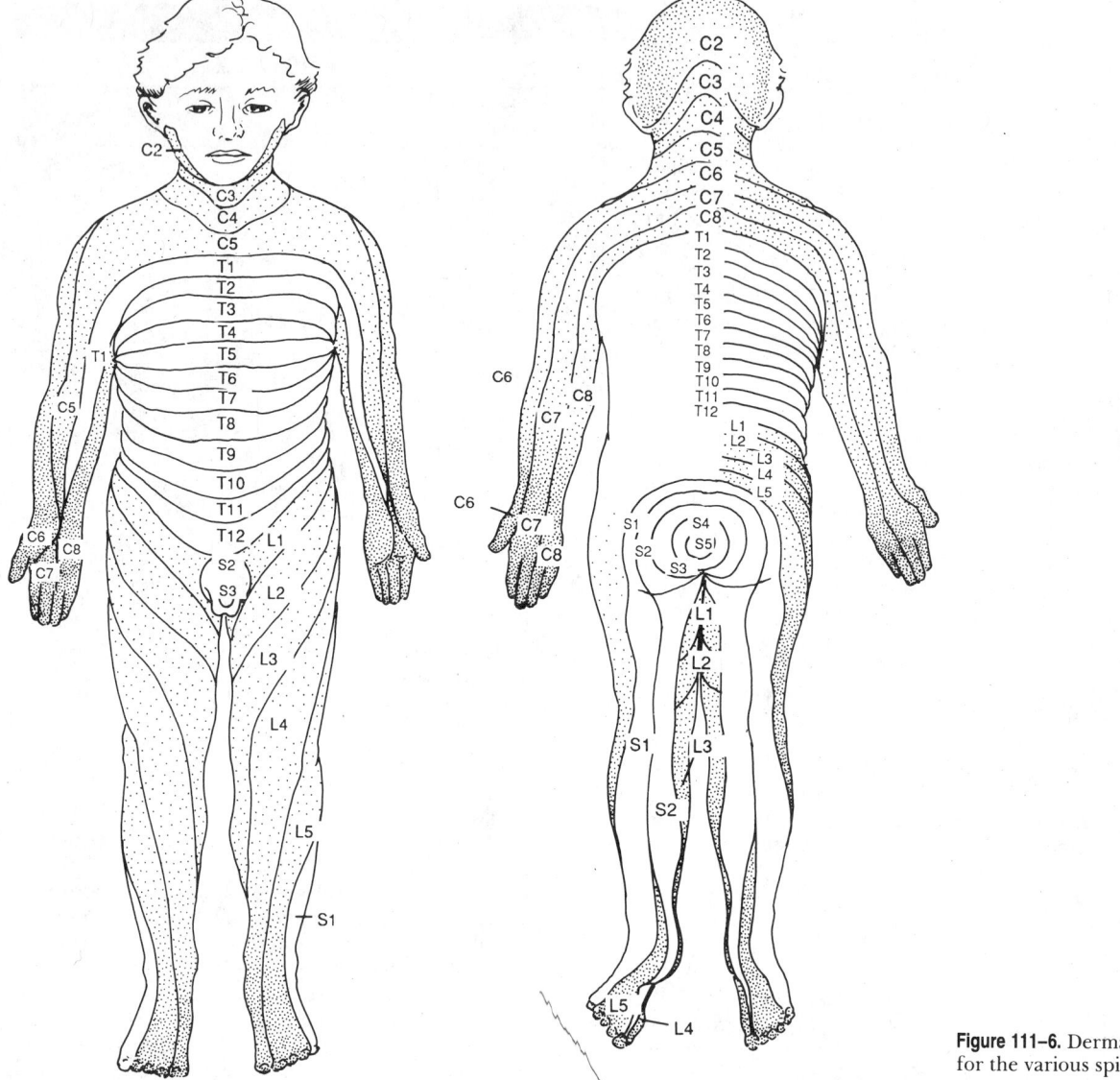

Figure 111–6. Dermatome patterns for the various spinal cord levels.

graphs, may be required to assess stability. Previously, tomograms were used to assess the extent of the bony injury, but these have been largely replaced by CT scans.[64] CT should be used not as a screening tool, but to more specifically characterize suspicious areas found on radiographs.[64] CT may identify occult fractures in the posterior elements that are not clearly seen on routine films. Thus, plain films may show a vertebral body fracture where CT would show an additional fracture through the posterior elements of the same vertebra. CT is recommended for all patients with C1 fractures and for treatment planning for those who have documented cervical injury.[67, 68]

EMERGENCY MEDICAL SERVICE CONSIDERATIONS

In one study, neurologic deficit or death occurred in 11 of 300 multiply injured patients with unrecognized cervical spine injury because their necks were moved during the course of emergency management; thus serious neck injury can be overlooked, especially in those with multiple injuries.

A large variety of pediatric-size cervical stabilization devices are available commercially. Although the rigid types perform better than soft foam in mechanical testing, even the best device allows 17 degrees of flexion, 19 degrees of extension, four degrees of rotation, and six degrees of lateral motion.[69] To gain more control following an acute injury, it is recommended that these devices be supplemented with tape, sand bags, and other supports.[70] Under these circumstances, spine motion can be limited to three degrees in any direction.[70]

The child with a cervical injury is at particular risk of further fracture displacement during resuscitation. One study of four patients with unstable cervical injuries who failed resuscitation in the emergency department showed that longitudinal axial traction during emergency intubation actually increased the spinal deformity.[71] Therefore, intubation prior to radiographic evaluation of those with suspected unstable cervical injuries should be attempted first by the nasotracheal route, rather than with axial traction and standard laryngoscopy.

Adults may be safely positioned supine on a flat backboard to immobilize the cervical spine, but small children are different. Young children have disproportionately larger heads and are at risk for developing kyphosis and anterior translation of the upper cervical segment when the fracture pattern is unstable (Fig. 111–8). In children less than 6 years of age, use of the split mattress technique is recommended

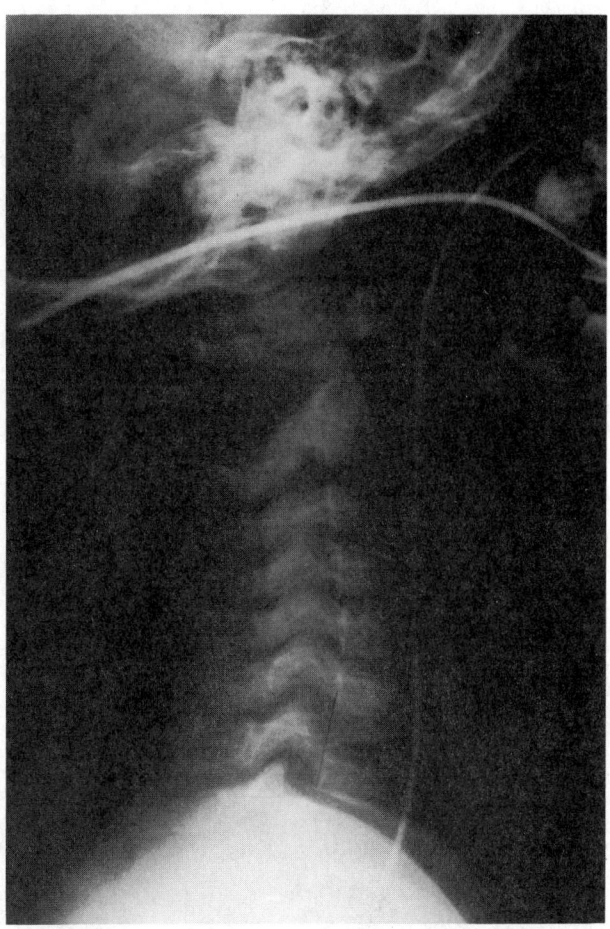

Figure 111–7. Cervical injury at C1 in a 3-year-old child. There are several levels of injury. Note the distraction at occiput–C1, C1–C2, and C6–C7.

to elevate the thorax 2 to 4 cm and lower the occiput (Fig. 111–9).[72] However, this immobilization protocol tends to reduce displaced fractures and makes their recognition and diagnosis more difficult.[73]

Advanced Immobilization

Skull tongs and halo devices can be used in the young child.[74–77] In children, the pins should be placed anterolaterally, posterolaterally, and perpendicular to the skull.[74, 75, 78] In the small child, a CT scan of the skull should be obtained to make sure there is sufficient bone for pin placement. A modified low-torque, multiple-pin technique will permit the use of the halo in children as young as 8 months.[76]

NEONATAL TRAUMA

Neuromuscular control of the cervical muscles in the newborn is undeveloped, and the normal infant is unable to adequately support the head until about 3 months of age. Infants, therefore, are incapable of protecting the cervical spine and spinal cord against the excessive torsion and traction forces that may occur during delivery and the months following birth. These forces may exceed the stretch capability of the neck. Bony injury usually involves the upper cervical spine, although lower cervical injuries have been reported.[79, 80] The normal ligaments of a child's neck may not be able to protect the less elastic spinal cord, possibly explaining the occurrence of severe cord injuries without skeletal injury.[81] Spinal cords removed from newborns dying from cervical trauma show changes over long segments, suggesting that longitudinal traction is a major factor.[43, 82]

Cervical injury is probably underreported, as the infantile spine, with its large percentage of cartilage, is difficult to evaluate radiologically, especially if the lesion occurs through cartilage or at the cartilage-bone interface.[1] Furthermore, the spine may appear normal following removal of the injuring force that produced the deformity. If routine radiographs are normal, then flexion-extension views are necessary. MRI is superior to CT in the diagnosis of upper cervical spinal cord compression.[83] For children, however, MRI has some minor disadvantages, including increased imaging time and decreased bony resolution. Sometimes it may be preferable to do both CT and MRI studies.[84] Ultrasound can be useful in the evaluation of parenchymal damage to the neonatal cervical spinal cord, in which the laminae are not yet ossified.[85] A cervical spine lesion should be considered in the differential diagnosis of infants who are found to be floppy at birth, particularly if the delivery was difficult. Complete flaccid paralysis with areflexia is usually followed by the typical pattern of hyperreflexia once spinal cord shock resolves. Brachial plexus birth palsies also warrant cervical spine radiography. If there is no devastating neurologic deficit, the prognosis is generally good.

OCCIPUT-C1 LESIONS

Atlanto-occipital injuries may occur during traumatic deliveries or major blunt trauma and imply an injury to the tectorial membrane and alar ligaments (Fig. 111–10).[86, 87] Occiput-C1 lesions are infrequently reported in surviving patients, as such lesions often result in lethal cervicomedullary cord damage.[86, 87] Also, many occiput-C1 dislocations may spontaneously reduce and are initially unrecognized.[88, 89]

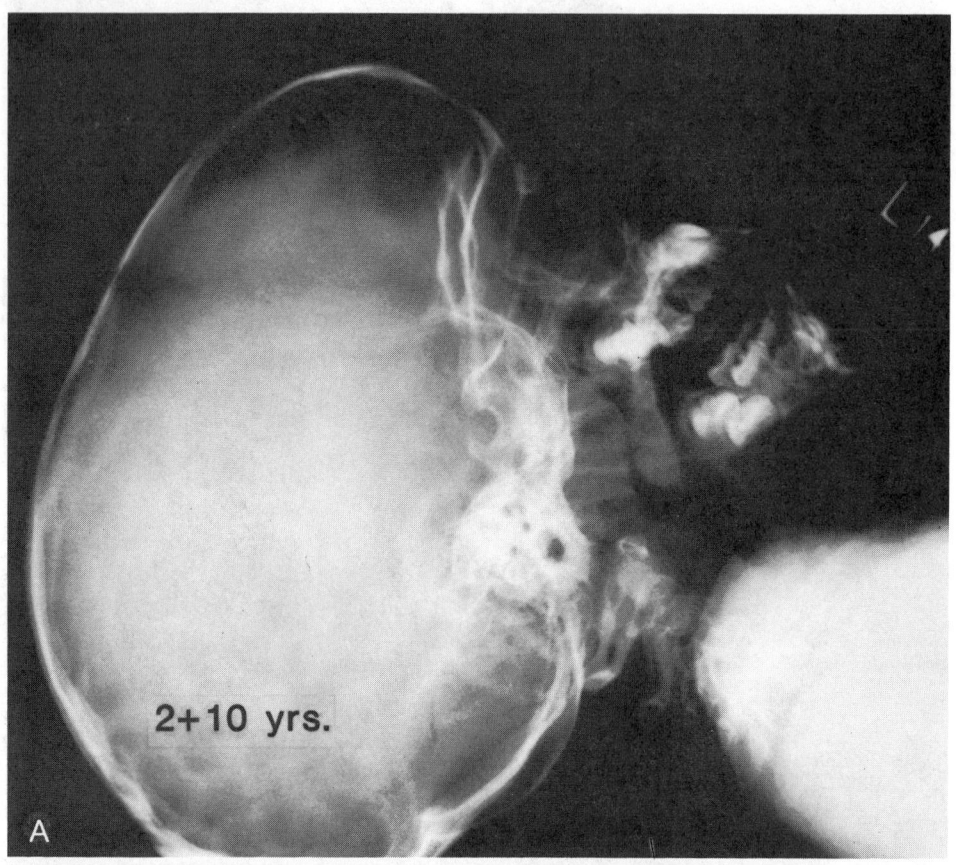

2+10 yrs.

A

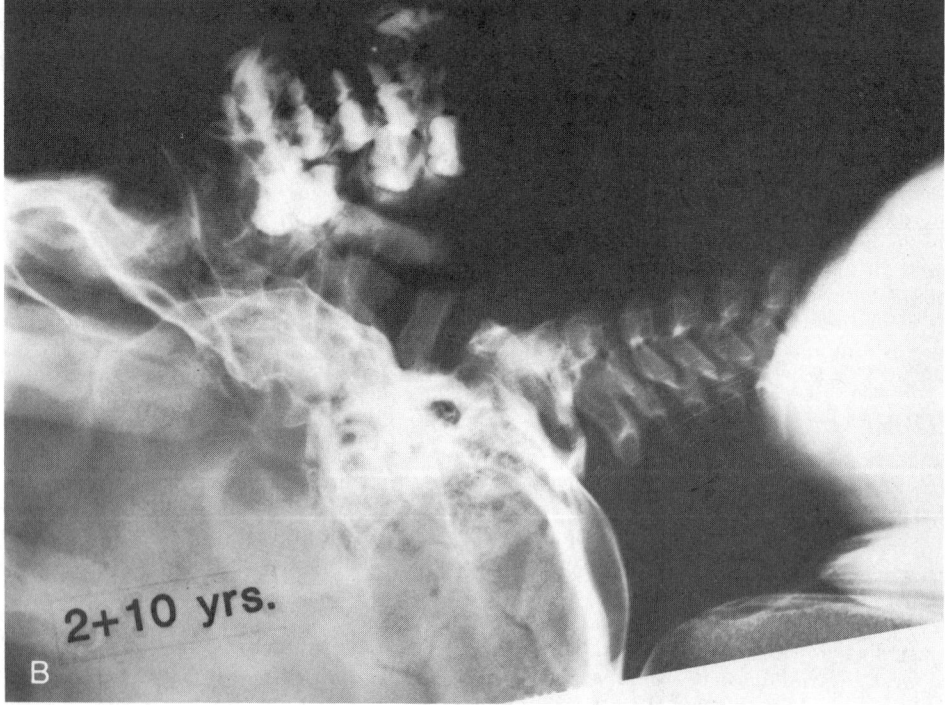

2+10 yrs.

B

Figure 111–8. Supine lateral radiograph of a child aged 2 years and 10 months on a backboard who had a fracture of the odontoid process. *A* demonstrates the anterior translation of the upper segment of the cervical spine, kyphosis at the site of the translation of the upper segment of the cervical spine, and kyphosis at the site of the fracture. The large cranium resting on the backboard forces the neck into flexion, accentuating the deformity. With a rolled sheet under the thorax *(B)*, there is considerable improvement in the reduction of the fracture at the odontoid. (From Herzenberg JE, Hensinger RN, Dedrick DK, et al. Emergency transport and positioning of young children who have an injury of the cervical spine: The standard backboard may be dangerous. J Bone Joint Surg 1989;71A:15.)

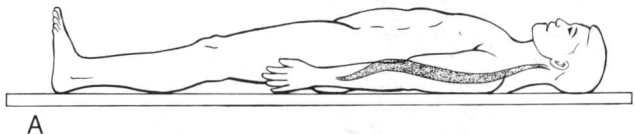

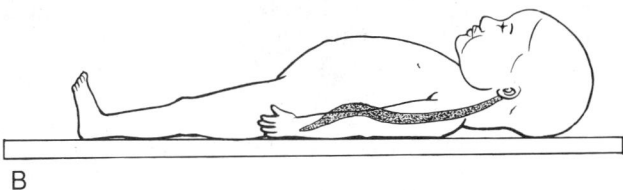

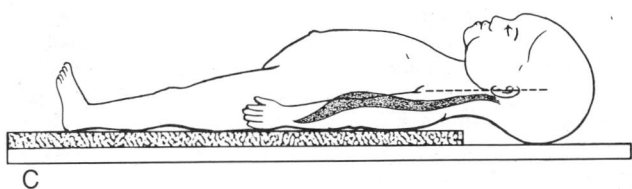

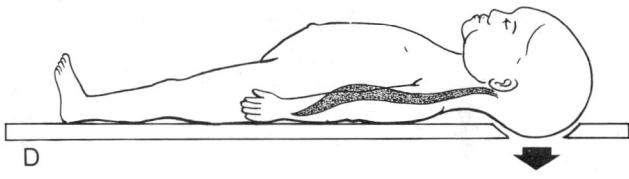

Figure 111–9. *A,* Adult immobilized on a standard backboard. *B,* Child on a standard backboard; the relatively large head flexes the neck into a kyphotic position. *C,* Child on a modified backboard that has a double-mattress pad to raise the thorax, providing safe cervical positioning. *D,* Child on a modified backboard that has a cut-out to recess the occiput, obtaining a safe cervical position. (From Herzenberg JE, Hensinger RN, Dedrick DK, et al. Emergency transport and positioning of young children who have an injury of the cervical spine: The standard backboard may be dangerous. J Bone Joint Surg 1989;71A:15.)

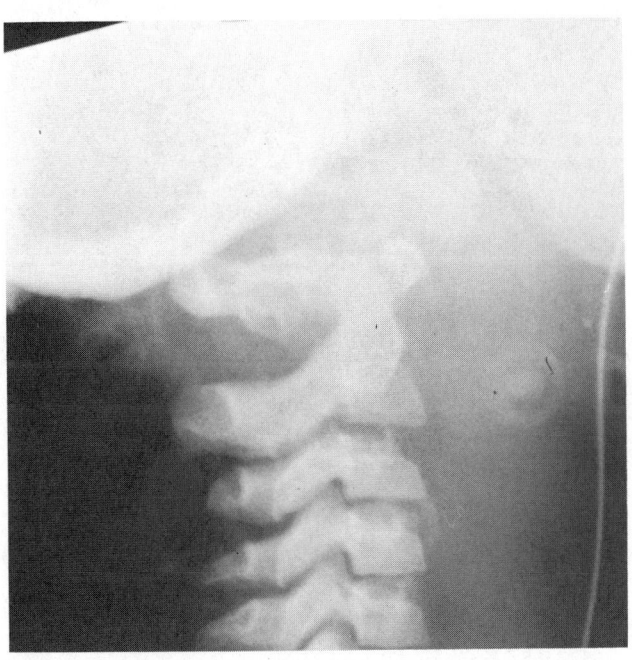

Figure 111–10. An 8-year-old child sustained an occiput–C1 dislocation in a motor vehicle accident. The lateral radiograph demonstrates vertical displacement between the occiput and ring of C1. The child has no neurologic function below C1 and is ventilator dependent.

These injuries are probably a result of sudden deceleration accidents, in which the head is carried forward, with a sudden craniovertebral dislocation and immediate spontaneous reduction, resulting in normal radiologic findings. Autopsy findings include disruption of the craniovertebral joints, spinal cord, and vertebral arteries.[90]

Treatment for the rare individual who survives this injury involves gentle reduction; minimal traction is recommended. Great care must be taken not to overdistract the injury site. Halo fixation followed by posterior occipital cervical fusion is the definitive treatment.[91] Chronic or late occiput-C1 instability can be difficult to diagnose.[91, 92] Carefully controlled flexion-extension lateral views or reconstructed CT scans are helpful.[93]

FRACTURES OF THE ATLAS

Fracture of the ring of C1, also known as the *Jefferson fracture*, is a rare pediatric cervical fracture.[94] The literature contains isolated case reports and small series.[95–97] The cause is an axial compression load applied to the head and transmitted through the lateral occipital condyles to the lateral masses of C1. The ring of C1 is usually broken in more than one location. In children, isolated single fractures, probably hinging on the synchondroses, have been described. Fractures through the synchondroses have also been reported.[97] As the lateral masses separate, the transverse atlantal ligament may rupture or be avulsed and result in C1–C2 instability.[97]

Although plain radiographs may show the fracture in certain cases, CT scans are far superior in visualizing the arch of C1 acutely and assessing healing in the follow-up period. Treatment consists of immobilization in a Minerva cast or halo.

ATLANTOAXIAL SEGMENT INJURY

The three most important lesions occurring at the C1–C2 level in children are traumatic ligament disruptions, rotatory displacement, and odontoid fractures. Stability at this joint is almost entirely dependent on ligaments that must simultaneously protect the articulation and allow for its extensive mobility. Approximately 50% of cervical rotation takes place between the first and second vertebrae around the anteriorly eccentric odontoid process. The spinal canal of C1 is large compared with that of the other cervical segments and safely accommodates this degree of rotation and some degree of pathologic displacement without compromise of the spinal cord. This has been expressed as the "Rule of Thirds": the spinal canal at C1 is occupied equally by the spinal cord, odontoid, and "free space."[98] The "free space" provides a buffer zone to prevent neurologic injury.[98] Anterior displacement of the atlas exceeding a distance equal to the width of the odontoid may place the adjacent segment of the spinal cord in jeopardy. The vertebral arteries, which supply the upper spinal cord and cerebellum, are fixed in the foramen transversarium of C1 and C2; they can be carried forward and compressed by an atlantoaxial shift, causing ischemic damage to the neural tissue.

Traumatic Ligament Disruptions

Displacement of C1 and C2 exceeding 3 mm in the adult and 4.5 mm in children suggests ligament damage at the atlantoaxial articulation. In children, it can be reasonably assumed that displacements of more than 5 mm in flexion are indicative of atlantoaxial ligament compromise, especially if there is a documented history of trauma.[99] Isolated traumatic rupture of the transverse atlantal ligament and acute atlantoaxial instability are rare in otherwise normal children.

Chronic atlantoaxial instability is frequently found in children with juvenile rheumatoid arthritis, Reiter's syndrome, Down syndrome (Fig. 111–11), Larson's syndrome, and bone dysplasias such as mucopolysaccharidosis, multiple epiphyseal dysplasia, achondroplasia, pseudoachondroplasia, and Kniest syndrome.[81, 100–106] Atlantoaxial instability and spinal cord compression are associated with upper cervical anomalies such as the Klippel-Feil syndrome and occipitalization of the atlas. Certain craniofacial malformations have a high incidence of associated anomalies of the cervical spine such as Apert's syndrome, hemifacial microsomia, and Goldenhar's syndrome.[107] In these conditions, atlantoaxial instability usually can be visualized with flexion-extension CT scans. When the head is flexed, the gantry must be tilted to remain parallel to the area of interest.[100]

Children with C1–C2 instability are at increased risk of developing neurologic compromise from relatively minor trauma. With forward displacement of C1 on C2, the spinal cord is compressed against the intact odontoid. Long-track signs, cranial nerve or sphincter dysfunction, or a change in physical tolerance should be investigated.

Studies of conservative treatment of acute ligament injuries in this area are infrequent. In acute cases, treatment involves reduction in extension, followed by surgical stabilization of C1–C2. For chronic instability, as in Down syndrome, minor degrees of C1–C2 instability can be ob-

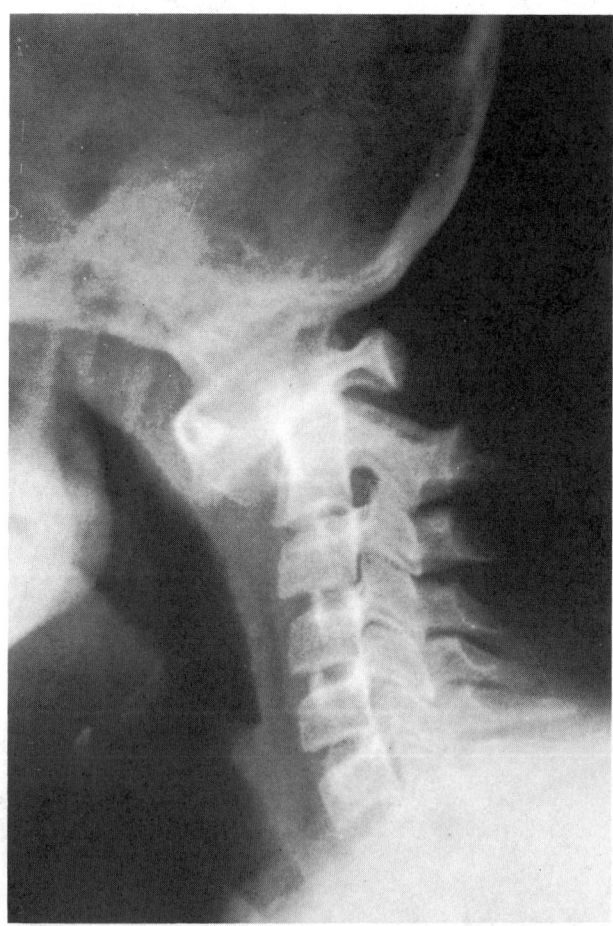

Figure 111–11. An 11-year-old with Down syndrome with severe atlantoaxial instability. The patient's gait was clumsy. Physical examination revealed poor coordination of the extremities; there was no other evidence of neurologic dysfunction. Two years after surgical stabilization, the patient had no symptoms referable to the cervical spine.

served.[81] However, those who develop translation of greater than 10 mm or have less than 10 mm of translation and neurologic deficit or a history of neurologic symptoms should be surgically stabilized.

Atlantoaxial Rotatory Displacement

The onset of atlantoaxial rotatory displacement may be spontaneous or associated with trivial trauma or may follow an upper respiratory tract infection. Typically, the child awakes with a "crick" in the neck, and with little or no treatment, this resolves within 1 week. Rarely, these deformities persist, and the patients present with a resistant, unresolving torticollis (atlantoaxial rotatory fixation).[108] This problem may occur within the normal range of motion or with an anterior shift of the atlas on the axis as a result of fractures of C1 or C2 or ligamentous deficiency and may lead to atlantoaxial instability. Although rare, neurologic deficits may be associated with rotatory displacements, particularly with associated anterior displacement.[109]

The origin of this type of displacement is still theoretical, as sufficient anatomic and autopsy evidence is unavailable. The obstruction is probably capsular and synovial interposition that produces pain in the initial stages, with resultant muscle spasm. In most cases this resolves in a few days, representing the common rotatory subluxation of childhood; occasionally it may persist, resulting in rotatory fixation. The condition is complicated by muscle spasm, which holds the neck in flexion and may aggravate the forward displacement of C1 on C2. The torticollis caused by atlantoaxial rotatory displacement may be similar to that seen with muscular torticollis, congenital anomalies of C1, or neurogenic problems such as posterior cranial fossa tumors or ocular dysfunction.

The torticollis position is typically likened to a robin listening for a worm, or the "cocked-robin" position. The head is tilted to one side and rotated to the opposite side with slight flexion. When torticollis is acute, the child resists attempts to move the head, complaining of marked pain with any passive attempts to do so. If the deformity becomes fixed, the pain subsides, but the torticollis deformity persists and is associated with a diminished range of neck motion.

In the acute stages, the diagnosis primarily is dependent on the history and clinical findings, as the findings on plain films are not diagnostic and can be seen in torticollis from other causes. In the open-mouth anteroposterior view, the lateral mass of C1 that has rotated forward appears wider and closer to the midline (medial offset), whereas the opposite lateral mass is narrower and away from the midline (lateral offset). One of the facet joints may be obscured because of apparent overlapping. The radiologic findings of rotatory displacements are sometimes difficult to demonstrate because of difficulty in positioning as a result of associated pain; occasionally there is difficulty in radiographic interpretation. CT has become the technique of choice for this condition.[109–111] CT scans with right and left stress images are helpful to confirm the diagnosis.[112]

Many cases of atlantoaxial rotatory displacement probably do not reach medical attention. A stiff neck with a slightly twisted head often resolves over a few days. If the complaints are mild and have been present for less than 1 week, a simple soft collar and analgesics are used. If there is no spontaneous improvement or the symptoms have been present for more than 1 week, more aggressive treatment should be instituted. If the condition has been present for less than 1 month, head halter traction and bed rest are usually sufficient to achieve remission of the clinical findings.[112] If no anterior displacement is demonstrated, a simple support such as a sternal occipital mandibular immobilization (SOMI)

brace or Philadelphia collar should be continued until symptoms have completely subsided. If the atlas is displaced anteriorly on the axis, then gradual reduction should be obtained, followed by immobilization in the corrected position. Careful follow-up is necessary in these patients to exclude continued atlantoaxial instability. If the condition has been present for 1 to 3 months, halo traction is often necessary. However, the C1–C2 articulation may remain unstable following immobilization and require surgical correction and fusion. If the condition has been present for more than 3 months, the deformity typically is fixed. In those whose spinal canal is compromised by anterior C1 displacement, additional insult could be catastrophic. In these patients, C1 to C2 fusion is indicated to achieve stability and maintain correction.

Odontoid Fractures

Odontoid fractures are one of the most common cervical injuries in children, occurring at an average age of 4 years.[44, 113] Fractures of the odontoid process in children are "growth plate" injuries of the synchondrosis (Fig. 111–12). The cartilage line at the base of the odontoid has the histologic appearance of a synchondrosis, rather than a physis, and closes much earlier than a normal physis.[43]

The odontoid fracture is frequently associated with head or facial trauma.[114] Severe falls or automobile accidents are the usual cause. There may be relatively few associated injuries and no neurologic deficits caused by the odontoid fracture.[44] This injury may follow trivial head trauma. Clinically, children often resist attempts to extend the neck.[113]

Anteroposterior radiographic evaluation may be of little value, as it may only show the normal synchondrotic line; the displacement or angulation may only be apparent on the lateral view. The displacement is usually anterior, with the dens tilted posteriorly.[115] Posterior angulation of the odontoid process is present in approximately 4% of normal children and suggests caution in the interpretation of this

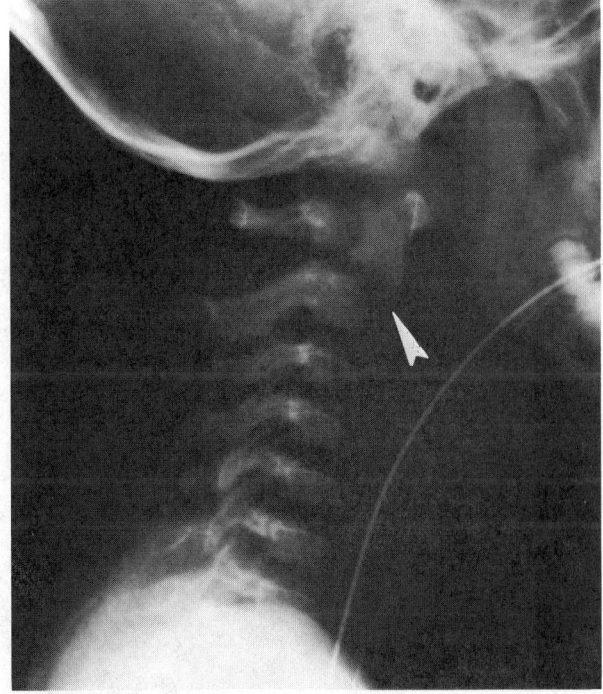

Figure 111–12. Young child (2 years old) with a fracture of the odontoid through the synchondrosis.

particular finding; lateral tomograms help differentiate fractures from this normal variant.[116] Dynamic CT views in flexion and extension with lateral sagittal reconstruction have largely replaced lateral tomograms for evaluating instability.[84, 100]

Diagnosis of odontoid injuries can be particularly difficult in children with underlying congenital and developmental cervical problems.[117] Morquio's syndrome, spondylo-epiphyseal dysplasia, neurofibromatosis, and osteogenesis imperfecta may have dysplastic appearances to the odontoid, making diagnosis of fracture of instability problematic.

Acute odontoid fractures should be reduced by recumbency in hyperextension followed by a Minerva jacket or halo vest.[44, 72] These injuries should heal in 6 weeks.[118]

SPONDYLOLISTHESIS OF C2 (HANGMAN'S FRACTURE)

Bilateral spondylolisthesis of C2 on been occasionally reported in children from 6 to 18 months of age.[119, 120] The mechanism of injury is usually hyperextension, and few patients are neurologically compromised. Reduction by gentle positioning and immobilization in a halo or Minerva cast is recommended.

LOWER CERVICAL INJURIES (C2–C7)

Subluxation of C2 on C3 is one of the more difficult diagnostic problems in the neck-injured child, as the radiographic findings may be similar to those found in pseudo-subluxation of C2 on C3. The true nature of the lesion may only become apparent with the passage of time. It is important to correlate the radiographic findings with the clinical history and examination. A significant subluxation is more likely if the child sustained sufficient trauma, followed by pain, spasm, limited motion, or tenderness. Persistence of symptoms after adequate conservative therapy is also suggestive of significant injury. Radiographically demonstrable abnormalities, such as ossification of the posterior longitudinal ligament, avulsion fractures of the tips of the spinous processes, compensatory lordosis, "swan neck," or failure to correct the subluxation when the spine is placed in extension, may be associated with the subluxation. Absent lordosis or reversal of lordosis may occur in normal subjects and is not always indicative of injury.

Injuries below the C3 level are less common in children than in adults. One study reported 19 lower cervical injuries from a group of 84 pediatric cervical injuries.[26] The mean age for lower cervical injuries was 13.6 years and for upper cervical injuries, 6.2 years.

Hyperextension injuries to the lower cervical spine in children may result in a physeal fracture through the vertebral end plate.[48, 88] Usually the inferior end plate is fractured, which may possibly be related to the protective effect of the developing uncinate processes of the superior end plate. These injuries are not generally recognized clinically but have been identified in autopsy studies.[1] The end plate may break completely through the cartilaginous portion or exit through the bony edge.[48]

Many serious injuries below the C3 level are associated with ligamentous disruption and initially are unrecognized (Fig. 111–13). With a ligamentous disruption, gradual displacement of one segment on the other, with secondary adaptive changes, occurs in the spine, making reduction difficult. If such lesions are suspected, periodic observation is recommended, along with protection in an extension orthosis if necessary. Posterior ligamentous disruption has limited potential for healing. If instability is documented, the injury should be stabilized by posterior fusion.

CHILD ABUSE

The "shaken baby syndrome," or "whiplash shaken infant syndrome,"[9, 121] has been associated with intracranial and intraocular hemorrhages resulting in death or latent cerebral injury, retardation, and permanent visual or hearing defects, in addition to fractures of the spine and spinal cord injuries. A spinal cord injury reported in a 2-year-old girl was caused by violent shaking, producing a cervical fracture-dislocation with spontaneous reduction.[9]

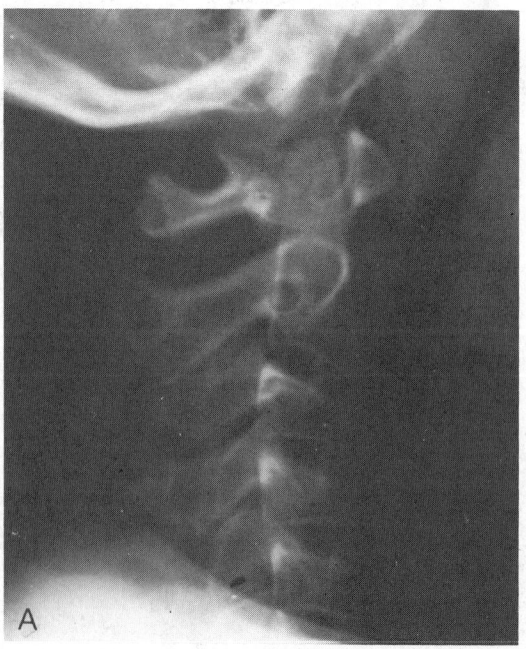
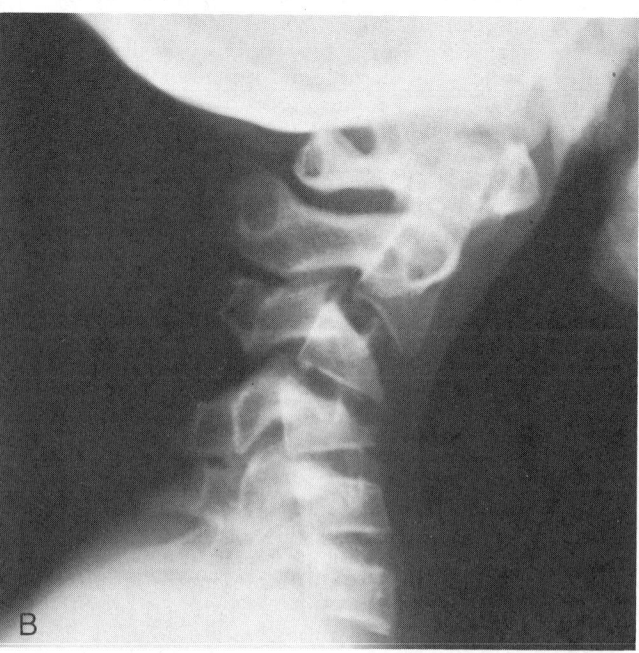

Figure 111–13. *A*, Lateral roetgenogram of a 14-year-old male who sustained a ligamentous injury of the cervical spine while playing football. *B*, Four weeks later, there is marked cervical kyphosis at C3–C4.

INJURIES TO THE THORACIC AND LUMBAR SPINE

Compression Fractures

Compression fractures caused by hyperflexion are more common than distraction, shear, or subluxation-dislocation injuries.[13] In the immature spine, the intact disk is more resistant to vertical compression than the vertebral body. With vertical pressure loading, the major distortion is a bulge in the vertebral end plate, with only a slight change in the annulus and no alteration in the shape of the nucleus pulposus.[122] It has been suggested that the blood in the spongiosa is a major shock-absorbing mechanism. With additional force increase, the end plate breaks and the nuclear material is ruptured into the vertebral body. Thus, in the child who is in a preflexed position (e.g., during tobogganing), the blood is squeezed from the vertebra, the shock-absorbing properties are decreased, and less force is required to cause a vertebral injury.[14, 15]

In older patients, the nucleus no longer consists of fluid, and compression forces are transmitted through the annulus.[122] This results in either tearing of the annulus, with general collapse of the vertebrae as a result of buckling of the sides, or a marginal plateau fracture.[82] Similarly, a greater and more rapidly applied force in the immature spine causes a bursting type injury, similar to that seen in adults. The vertebral disk of the child has a greater degree of turgor and is capable of transmitting the force of the injury through several levels.[6, 16, 18, 122] Clinically, multiple

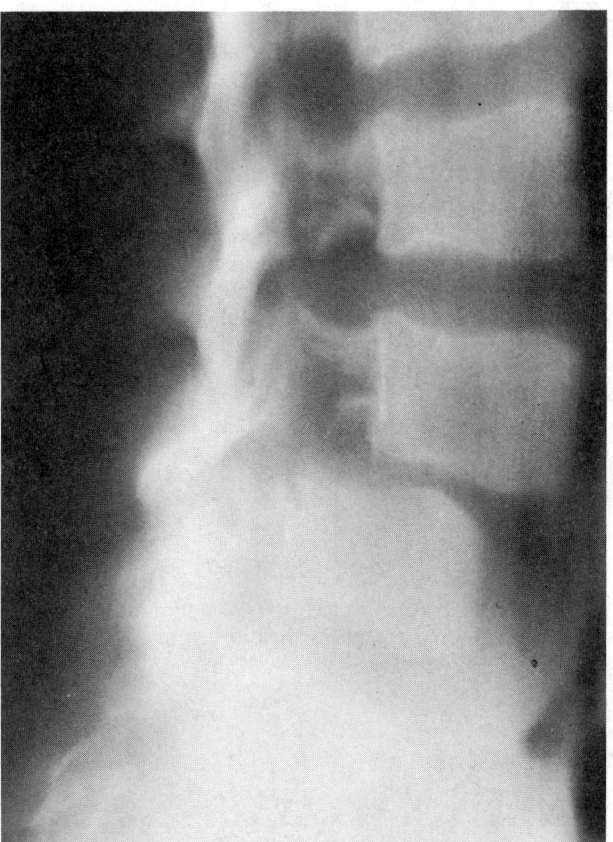

Figure 111–15. This 13-year-old Boy Scout was injured when a tree fell directly across his back during a storm. Lateral laminagraphic views demonstrate a traumatic spondylolysis at the L4–L5 level due to disruption of the pedicle and facet.

compression fractures (50% to 75%) are more common in children, usually occurring from the midthoracic to the midlumbar areas (Fig. 111–14).[4, 13]

During compression of the immature spine, the vertebral body always breaks before the normal disk gives way. This is supported clinically, as only a few cases of children with posterior herniated disks have been reported, and these followed significant load bearing, as in weight lifting and gymnastics.[123]

Distraction and Shear Injuries

Children killed by violent injuries (e.g., pedestrians hit by a car) sustain spinal fractures primarily of the shear type (Fig. 111–15).[1] Typically the injury does not cause rupture of the intervertebral disk; instead, the vertebra fractures through the cartilaginous end-plate apophysis. This mechanism is perhaps most applicable to the cervical spine, as stretching or shear injuries in children do not occur as often in the thoracic or lumbar spine. Infrequently, children may have a flexion-rotation mechanism combined with compression, which leads to a shearing injury and spondylolisthesis.

Chance Fractures in Children

The pathomechanics of Chance fractures were first described in a review of lumbar spine injuries associated with seat belts.[124] The mechanism is forward flexion over a lap belt, producing distraction of the posterior vertebral elements and anterior compression. This injury was uncommon in children[124] before the advent of mandatory seat belt

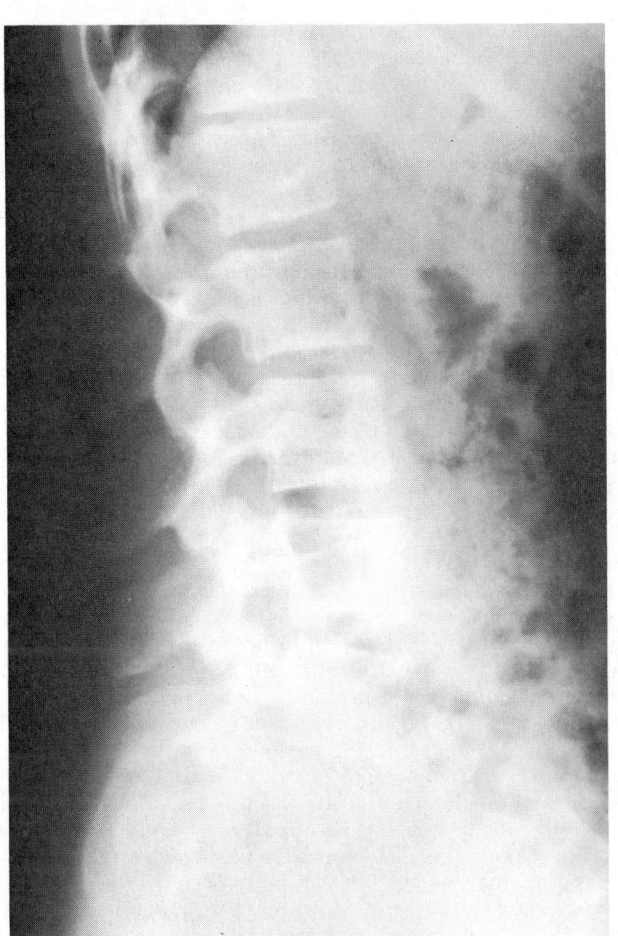

Figure 111–14. This 15-year-old female was in a motor vehicle accident, sustaining multiple compression fractures, wedging of L1, and anterior buckling of L4.

restraints. As rear seats continue to have lap belts without shoulder harnesses, this injury appears to be on the increase in children.[125] The fractures are primarily in the lumbar spine, usually between L1 and L3, but can also occur at L4 (Fig. 111–16). In children, the injury is more likely to occur in the midlumbar spine than in the usual adult location of the thoracolumbar junction, which may be related to children having a higher center of gravity.[126] There has been a high association with intraabdominal injury in children.[126] Ecchymosis occurring in a lap belt distribution should always alert the examiner to search for a Chance fracture. The abdominal injuries can dominate the early clinical picture, causing delay in detecting the spinal fracture.[127]

Bilateral facet dislocations are slightly more common than fracture through the lamina. Routine lateral views of the spine are the best means for making this diagnosis. The CT scan may not reveal the presence of this injury because of limitations in detecting horizontal fractures and dislocations in the axial plane.[128]

Radiologic Findings

The radiologic appearance of thoracolumbar injuries depends on the force and mechanism of injury. Compression resulting from hyperflexion is the most common injury and

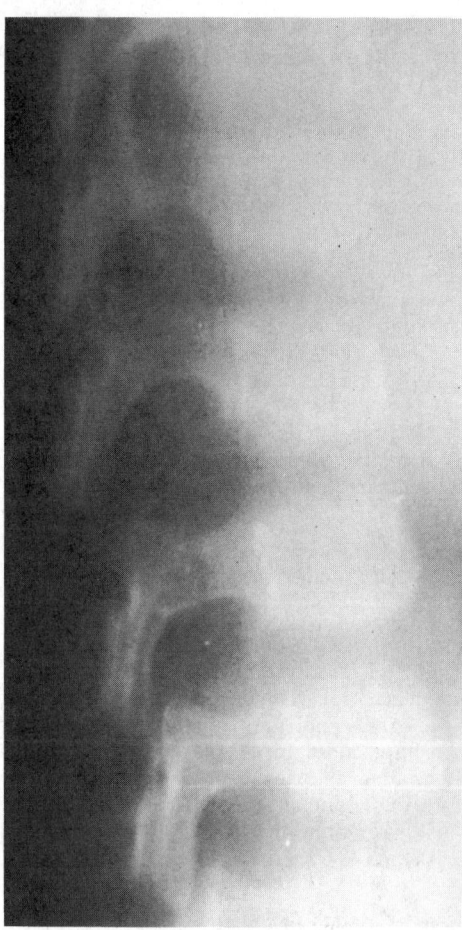

Figure 111–16. This 16-month-old female sustained traumatic paraplegia as a passenger in an automobile accident. Lateral laminagram demonstrates spreading and angulation of the spinous process and vertebral bodies, suggesting posterior ligamentous disruption similar to the Chance fracture in the adult. (Courtesy of Jesse C. DeLee, M.D., University of Texas Health Science Center, San Antonio, TX.)

can range from slight flattening of the normally convex end plates to frank wedging of the vertebrae.[3] Compression fractures in children can be classified according to appearance: (1) wedge shaped or (2) beak shaped, with upper or lower prominent anterior contours.[12] Both types may be asymmetric on the sagittal view as well as the frontal view. There may be a zone of increased density in the vertebral body as a result of compression and overlapping of the spongiosa.[12, 13] In the infant, anterior and posterior notching of the vertebral bodies caused by the normal vascular channels may be confused with a fracture (see Fig. 111–3).[49] Multiply damaged vertebrae are the rule; the highest number of fractured vertebrae reported in one patient is 11.[12] Clinically observable kyphosis is uncommon, unless there is a fracture-dislocation.[12] True fracture lines are seldom seen in children with compression fractures before puberty. Rarely is there an avulsed vertebral corner, as might be seen in the adult.[13] With greater force, the end plate ruptures, and the disk is extruded into the vertebral body, forming a Schmorl's node, commonly in the lower thoracic and upper lumbar vertebrae (Fig. 111–17). Typical adult fracture patterns, such as complete fracture of the vertebral body and fracture-dislocation and subluxation of the facets, are less commonly seen. As in the adult, CT and sagittal reconstruction scans are more accurate than plain radiographs in detecting posterior arch fractures and assessing bony fragments and narrowing of the spinal canal.[30, 129, 130] The tomographic cuts must be at right angles to the vertebrae or the lesion will be confused with a pseudofracture.[128] MRI is better than CT in detecting injuries to the soft tissues (e.g., ligaments, intervertebral disks, and spinal cord) and impingement of the spinal cord by the intervertebral disk or an epidural hematoma.[32, 131, 132]

Progression of the deformity is uncommon in children unless the injury is unstable (as in a fracture-dislocation) or a neurologic deficit is present. There is a great propensity for the vertebral body to restructure.[133] In the child younger than 10 years (but rarely after 12 years of age), the vertebral body tends to return to its normal shape, even with multiple compression fractures, and kyphosis is uncommon.[13, 18, 133] Complete restitution is possible, but only if there is no protrusion of the nucleus pulposus into the vertebra.[13] The vertebral end plate is the area of active growth, and if it is damaged, there will be little subsequent correction of the deformity, be it kyphosis or scoliosis. Asymmetric growth of a damaged vertebra, particularly in the dorsolumbar area, is usually compensated by the undamaged adjacent vertebrae and seldom results in significant scoliosis. Spontaneous interbody fusion is rare in children.

Treatment

Compression fractures heal quickly, with little tendency to further progression. Thus, for the mild injury, symptomatic treatment with a short period of bed rest or immobilization with a cast or corset is sufficient. Many children can be treated at home or require only a short period of hospitalization.[17] In reports comparing casts to bed rest, the specific treatment did not affect the outcome, and the children were generally asymptomatic in 1 to 2 weeks.[13, 18, 19] Posterior tenderness in the area of the fracture occasionally persists but does not pose a serious problem.[13] If the end plate is fractured and the disk herniates into the vertebral body, symptoms may persist but can be expected to resolve with nonoperative treatment. However, the kyphotic deformity caused by the damaged vertebral end plates may not resolve without specific management.

Children who sustain an unstable injury such as a vertebral subluxation or fracture-dislocation should be reduced in the

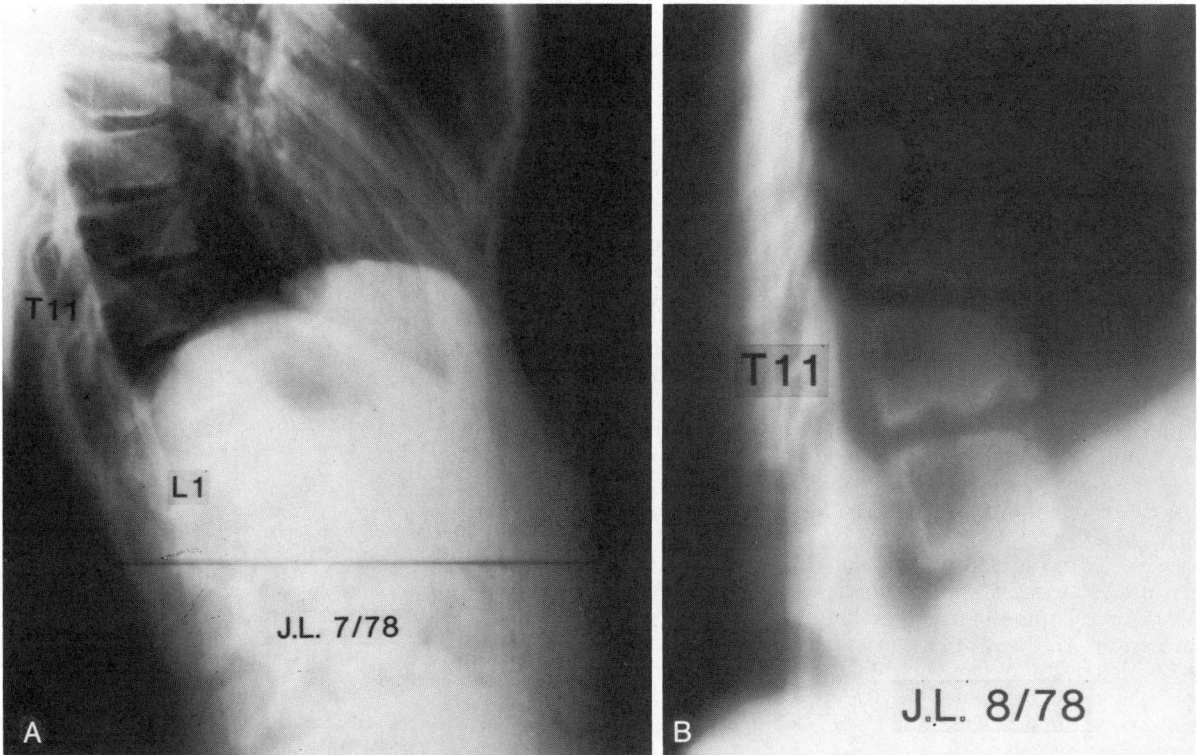

Figure 111-17. This 15-year-old male had persistent back pain after a weight-lifting program. *A*, Routine views suggest mild end-plate changes. *B*, Laminagraphic view demonstrates Schmorl's node formation and end-plate irregularity at T11. Subtle changes on plain radiographs may belie significant end-plate changes or disk protrusion into the vertebral body.

same manner as an adult with a similar injury.[134, 135] The child should be cared for on a turning frame or remain at complete bed rest with logrolling instituted until the acute symptoms subside. The dislocation should be reduced promptly in neurologically injured children, particularly those with a low lesion that involves the conus medullaris and nerve roots. Risk of neurologic injury increases with canal narrowing; the risk at T12 is 35%; at L1, 45%; and at L2 and below, 55%.[132] Children with burst fractures that result in spinal canal narrowing of more than 25% and kyphosis are at increased risk of further canal compromise and should be considered for early correction and decompression.[134] As in the adult, spinal instrumentation is helpful in reducing the deformity and stabilizing the fracture site.[29, 50] Open reduction must be accompanied by a posterior spine fusion at least one level both above and below the fracture site. Spontaneous interbody fusion seldom occurs and should not be depended on to provide long-term stability.[18, 19] Injuries that would be classified as stable in the adult may spontaneously progress in the child. This is common when there has been severe crushing in the vertebral body and end plate (burst fracture) and disruption of the posterior support ligaments[19] and may represent a Salter type IV injury to the vertebral epiphysis, with a growth arrest leading to progressive deformity.[19] Early recognition, reduction, and surgical stabilization will prevent late deformity and progressive kyphosis or late neurologic injury.[19, 135]

Neurologic Injury

The most devastating problem for the child with a thoracolumbar spine injury is paraplegia. The spinal cord–injured child can be expected to have increased susceptibility to long-bone fractures, hip dislocation, pressure sores, joint contractures, and genitourinary complications.[10, 136] In addition, the child can be expected to develop progressive spinal deformity (scoliosis, kyphosis, and lordosis). For many, the original injury is often overshadowed by the severity of these late spinal deformities. Scoliosis seriously erodes the child's ability to sit easily, and in the young child the pelvic obliquity leads to subluxation of the hip and ischial pressure sores.[29]

In immature children, usually girls younger than 12 years and boys younger than 14 years, the incidence of progressive spine deformity following traumatic paraplegia is 86% to 100%.[29, 50, 136] The onset of curvature has been reported as early as 3 years of age. Progressive lumbar lordosis is less common (18%) and is usually associated with hip flexion contractures, particularly in the ambulatory patient.[50]

PREVENTION OF SPINAL INJURIES

Infant and child car seats should be installed in a rear-facing position for greater protection or at least until the child can sit unsupported.[137] Facing the seat rearward may prevent cervical fractures that would otherwise occur with sudden deceleration. In this position the impact of a front-end collision is distributed over the entire back, pelvis, and head of the infant.[138] As children grow older, however, they want to see forward and out the window and therefore become less tolerant of the rear-facing position.

Car seats should be maintained and adjusted to fit the child correctly as they grow. Similarly, as the seasons change and children change from wearing lightweight, thin clothing to thick, heavy layers of clothing, necessary adjustments to the car seat restraint are needed.[139]

Sports-related cervical injuries are becoming more prominent as more children engage in physical activities. One Canadian study reported 42 spinal injuries between 1976 and 1983, predominantly in teen-age boys playing in organized ice hockey leagues.[140] The mechanism of injury was usually a blow to the head with the neck in slight flexion, resulting from a push from behind or check into the boards and producing a large strain on the cervical vertebrae. The identical mechanism may occur in football players from "spearing" and in shallow-water divers.

It has been suggested that the back of the football helmet exerts a guillotine-like action on the posterior aspect of the cervical spine.[141] However, most authors feel that helmet injuries are usually a result of axial loading and flexion rather than hyperextension.[78] Helmets have not been shown to contribute directly to cervical spine injuries; in the extremes of flexion and extension, the back edge of a football helmet does not impinge on the spine.[142] Studies of motorcycle accidents showed that minor spinal injuries and major head injuries were diminished in helmet wearers, but there was no significant reduction in the number of severe spinal injuries.[143] Similarly, with improved football helmets, head injuries decreased and neck injuries increased until the rules were changed.[144]

A review of trampoline injuries to the cervical spine, largely in teenagers and young adults, identified 114 catastrophic cervical spine injuries resulting in quadriplegia.[145] The American Academy of Pediatrics published a statement in 1977 calling for a ban on the use of trampolines in schools. They also stated that the trampoline should not be used in routine physical education classes, competitive sports, or home or recreational settings.

The decision regarding athletics after transient neuropraxia is a difficult one, and most orthopedists do not permit continued high-risk sports exposure. Children who sustain minor neurologic deficits without radiographic abnormality are apt to be treated with minimal immobilization and early return to activity. However, prudence dictates that all contact and noncontact sports be restricted for at least 3 months.

Children with Down syndrome are at particular risk of chronic C1–C2 instability and should have a screening lateral flexion-extension radiograph made prior to allowing participation in contact sports and in other vigorous sports that could result in head or neck trauma.[146, 147]

References

1. Aufdermaur M. Spinal injuries in juveniles necropsy findings in twelve cases. J Bone Joint Surg 1974;56B:513.
2. Babcock JL. Spinal injuries in children. Pediatr Clin North Am 1975;22:487.
3. Hachen HJ. Spinal cord injury in children and adolescents: Diagnostic pitfalls and therapeutic considerations in the acute stage. Paraplegia 1977;15:55.
4. Hadley MN, Zabramski JM, Bronner CM, et al. Pediatric spinal trauma. Review of 122 cases of spinal cord vertebral column injuries. J Neurosurg 1988;68:18.
5. Henrys P, Lyne ED, Lifton C, Salciccioli G. Clinical review of cervical spine injuries in children. Clin Orthop 1977;129:172.
6. Kewalramani LS, Tori JA. Spinal cord trauma in children: Neurologic patterns, radiologic features, and pathomechanics of injury. Spine 1980;5:11.
7. Koch BM, Eng GM. Neonatal spinal cord injury. Arch Phys Med Rehabil 1979;60:378.
8. Leventhal HR. Birth injuries of the spinal cord. J Pediatr 1960;56:447.
9. Swischuk LE. Spine and spinal cord trauma in the battered child syndrome. Radiology 1969;92:733.
10. Campbell J, Bonnett C. Spinal cord injury in children. Clin Orthop 1975;112:114.
11. Glasauer FE, Cares HL. Traumatic paraplegia in infancy. JAMA 1972;219:38.
12. Hegenbarth R, Ebel KD. Roentgen findings in fractures of the vertebral column in childhood examination of 35 patients and its results. Pediatr Radiol 1976;5:34.
13. Horal J, Nachemson A, Scheller S. Clinical and radiological long term follow-up of vertebral fractures in children. Acta Orthop Scand 1972;43:491.
14. Herkowitz HN, Samberg C. Vertebra column injuries associated with tobogganing. J Trauma 1978;18:806.
15. Odom JA, Brown CW, Messner DG. Tubing injuries. J Bone Joint Surg 1976;58A:733.
16. Shrosbree RD. Spinal cord injuries as a result of motorcycle accidents. Paraplegia 1978;16:102.
17. Anderson JM, Schutt AH. Spinal injury in children; a review of 156 cases seen from 1950 through 1978. Mayo Clin Proc 1980;55:499.
18. Hubbard DD. Injuries of the spine in children and adolescents. Clin Orthop 1974;100:56.
19. McPhee IB. Spinal fractures and dislocations in children and adolescents. Spine 1981;6:533.
20. Sturm JT, Perry JF. Injuries associated with fractures of the transverse processes of the thoracic and lumbar vertebrae. J Trauma 1984;24:597.
21. Sclafani SJA, Florence LO, Phillips TF, et al. Lumbar arterial injury: Radiologic diagnosis and management. Radiology 1987;165:709.
22. Gaufin LM, Goodman SJ. Cervical spine injuries in infants: Problems in management. J Neurosurg 1975;42:179.
23. Hause M, Hoshino R, Omata S, et al. Cervical spine injuries in children. Clin Orthop 1977;129:172.
24. Kewalramoni LS, Kraus JF, Sterling HM. Acute spinal cord lesions in a pediatric population: Epidemiological and clinical features. Paraplegia 1980;18:206.
25. Ruge JR, Sinson GP, McLone DG, et al. Pediatric spinal injury: The very young. J Neurosurg 1988;68:25.
26. Birney TJ, Hanley EN. Traumatic cervical spine injuries in childhood and adolescence. Spine 1989;14:1277.
27. Pang D, Wilberger JD. Spinal cord injury without radiologic abnormalities in children. J Neurosurg 1982;57:114.
28. Glasauer FE, Caves HC. Biomechanical fractures of traumatic paraplegia in infancy. J Trauma 1973;13:166.
29. Lancourt JE, Diskson JH, Carter RE. Paralytic spinal deformity following traumatic spinal cord injury in children and adolescents. J Bone Joint Surg 1981;63A:47.
30. Walsh JW, Stevens DB, Young AB. Traumatic paraplegia in children without contiguous spinal fracture or dislocation. Neurosurg 1983;12:439.
31. Yngve DA, Harris WP, Herndon WA, et al. Spinal cord injury without osseous spine fracture. J Pediatr Orthop 1988;8:153.
32. Betz RR, Gelman AJ, DeFilipp GJ, et al. Magnetic resonance imaging (MRI) in the evaluation of spinal cord injured children and adolescents. Paraplegia 1987;25:92.
33. Choi JU, Hoffman HJ, Hendrick EB, et al. Traumatic infarction of the spinal cord in children. J Neurosurg 1986;65:608.
34. Mirvis SE, Geisler FH, Jelinek JJ, et al. Acute cervical spine trauma: Evaluation with 1.5-T MR Imaging. Radiology 1988;166:807.
35. Cotler HB, Kulkarni MV, Bondurant FJ. Magnetic resonance imaging of acute spinal cord trauma: Preliminary report. J Orthop Trauma 1988;2:1.
36. Kolowich P, Phillips W. Seat belt lumbar fractures in children. Orthop Trans 1986;10:566.
37. Bracken MB, Shepard MJ, Collins W, et al. A randomized, controlled trial of methylprednisolone or naloxone in the treatment of acute spinal-cord injury. N Engl J Med 1990;322:1405.
38. Cattell HS, Filtzer DL. Pseudosubluxation and other normal variations in the cervical spine in children. J Bone Joint Surg 1965;47A:1295.
39. Annis JAD, Finlay DBL, Allen MJ, Barnes MR. A review of cervical radiographs in casualty patients. Br J Radiol 1987;60:1059.
40. Ehara S, El-Khoury GY, Sato Y. Cervical spine injury in children: Radiologic manifestations. AJR 1988;151:1175.
41. Townsend EH Jr, Rowe ML. Mobility of the upper cervical spine in health and disease. Pediatrics 1952;10:67.
42. Bailey DK. The normal cervical spine in infants and children. Radiology 1952;59:712.
43. Sherk HH, Schut L, Lane J. Fractures and dislocations of the cervical spine in children. Orthop Clin North Am 1976;7:593.
44. Sherk HH, Nicholson JT, Chung SMK. Fractures of the odontoid process in young children. J Bone Joint Surg 1978;60A:921.
45. Ogden JA. Radiology of postnatal skeletal development XI. The first cervical vertebra. Skeletal Radiol 1984;12:12.
46. Ogden JA. Radiology of postnatal skeletal development XII. The second cervical vertebra. Skeletal Radiol 1984;12:169.
47. Parke WW, Schiff DCM. The applied anatomy of the intervertebral disc. Orthop Clin North Am 1971;22:309.
48. Lawson JP, Ogden JA, Bucholz RW, Hughes SA. Physeal injuries of the cervical spine. J Pediatr Orthop 1987;7:428.
49. Wagoner G, Pendergrass EP. The anterior and posterior "notch" shadows seen in lateral roentgenograms of the vertebrae of infants: An anatomic explanation. AJR 1939;42:663.
50. Mayfield JK, Erkkila JC, Winter RB. Spine deformity subsequent to acquired childhood spinal cord injury. J Bone Joint Surg 1981;63A:1401.
51. Allington NJ, Zembo M, Nadell J, Bowen JR. C1-C2 posterior soft-tissue injuries with neurologic impairment in children. J Pediatr Orthop 1990;10:596.

52. Fielding JW, Cochran GVB, Lawsing JF III, Hohl M. Tears of the transverse ligament of the atlas: A clinical and biomechanical study. J Bone Joint Surg 1974;56A:1683.

53. Locke GR, Gardner JI, VanEpps EF. Atlas-dens interval (ADI) in children: A survey based on 200 normal cervical spines. Am J Roentgenol Ther Nucl Med 1966;97:135.

54. Shaffer MA, Doris PE. Limitation of the cross table lateral view in detecting cervical spine injuries: A retrospective review. Ann Emerg Med 1981;10:508.

55. White AA, Johnson DM, Penjab MM. Biomedical analysis of clinical stability in the cervical spine. Clin Orthop 1975;100:85.

56. Pennecot GF, Gouraud D, Hardy JR, Pouliquen JC. Roentgenographical study of the stability of the cervical spine in children. J Pediatr Orthop 1984;4:346.

57. Pennecot GF, Leonard P, Peyrot DGS, et al. Traumatic ligamentous instability of the cervical spine in children. J Pediatr Orthop 1984;4:339.

58. Jones ET, Hensinger RN. C2-C3 dislocation in a child. J Pediatr Orthop 1981;1:419.

59. Harrison RB, Keats TE, Winn HR, et al. Pseudosubluxation of the axis in young adults. J Can Assoc Radiol 1980;31:176.

60. Swischuk LE. Anterior displacement of C2 in children: Physiologic or pathologic? Radiology 1977;122:759.

61. Templeton PA, Young JWR, Mirvis SE, Budderneyer EU. The value of retropharyngeal soft tissue measurements in trauma of the adult cervical spine. Skeletal Radiol 1987;16:98.

62. Weir DC. Roentgenographic signs of cervical injury. Clin Orthop 1975;109:9.

63. Ardan GM, Kemp FH. The mechanisms of changes in form of the cervical airway in infancy. Med Radiogr Photogr 1968;44:26.

64. Bachulis BL, Long WB, Jumes GD, Johnson MC. Clinical indications for cervical spine radiographs in the traumatized patient. Am J Surg 1987;153:473.

65. Rachesky I, Boyce WT, Duncan B, et al. Clinical prediction of cervical spine injuries in children. Radiographic abnormalities. Am J Dis Child 1987;141:199.

66. Hadden WA, Gillespie WJ. Multiple level injuries of the cervical spine. Injury 1985;16:628.

67. Acheson MB, Livingston RR, Richardson ML, Stimac GK. High-resolution CT scanning in the evaluation of cervical spine fractures: Comparison with plain film examinations. AJR 1987;148:1179.

68. Clark CR, Igram CM, El-Khoury GY, Ehara S. Radiographic evaluation of cervical spine injuries. Spine 1988;13:742.

69. Millington PJ, Ellingsen JM, Hauswirth BE, Fabian PJ. Thermoplastic minerva body jacket—a practical alternative to current methods of cervical spine stabilization. Phys Ther 1987;67:223.

70. Huerta C, Griffin R, Joyce SM. Cervical spine stabilization in pediatric patients: Evaluation of current techniques. Ann Emerg Med 1987;16:1121.

71. Bivins HG, Bezmalinovic Z, Price HM, Williams JL. The effect of axial traction during orotracheal intubation of the trauma victim with an unstable cervical spine. Ann Emerg Med 1988;17:25.

72. Herzenberg JE, Hensinger RN, Dedrick DK, Phillips WA. Emergency transport and positioning of young children who have an injury of the cervical spine. The standard backboard may be hazardous. J Bone Joint Surg 1989;71A:15.

73. Herzenberg JE, Hensinger RN. Pediatric cervical spine injuries. Trauma Q 1989;5:73.

74. Garfin SR, Roux R, Botte MJ, et al. Skull osteology as it affects halo pin placement in children. J Pediatr Orthop 1986;6:434.

75. Letts M, Kaylor K, Goruw G. A biomechanical analysis of halo fixation in children. J Bone Joint Surg 1988;70B:277.

76. Mubarak SJ, Camp JF, Vuletich W, et al. Halo application in the infant. J Pediatr Orthop 1989;9:612.

77. Botte MJ, Byrne TP, Garfin SR. Application of the halo device for immobilization of the cervical spine utilizing an increased torque pressure. J Bone Joint Surg 1987;69A:850.

78. Ballock RT, Lee TQ, Triggs KJ, et al. The effect of pin location on the rigidity of the halo pin-bone interface. Neurosurgery 1990;26:238.

79. McLain RF, Clark CR, El-Khoury GY. C6-C7 dislocation in a neurologically intact neonate. Spine 1989;14:125.

80. Shulman ST, Madden JD, Esterly JR, Shanklin DR. Transection of spinal cord. A rare obstetrical complication of cephalic delivery. Arch Dis Child 1971;46:291.

81. Tredwell SJ, Newman DE, Lockitch G. Instability of the upper cervical spine in Down syndrome. J Pediatr Orthop 1990;10:602.

82. Stern WE, Rand RW. Birth injuries to the spinal cord: Report of 2 cases and review of the literature. Am J Obstet Gynecol 1959;78:498.

83. Lanska MJ, Roessmann U, Wiznitzer M. Magnetic resonance imaging in cervical cord birth injury. Pediatr 1990;85:760.

84. McAfee PC, Bohlman HH, Han JS, Salvagno RT. Comparison of nuclear magnetic resonance imaging and computed tomography in the diagnosis of upper cervical spinal cord compression. Spine 1986;11:295.

85. Babyn PS, Chuang SH, Daverman A, Davidson GS. Sonographic evaluation of spinal cord birth trauma with pathologic correlation. AJR 1988;151:763.

86. Collato PM, DeMuth WW, Schwentker EP, Boal DK. Traumatic atlanto-occipital dislocation. J Bone Joint Surg 1986;68A:1106.

87. Gillis FH, Binna J, Sotrel A. Infantile atlanto-occipital instability. Am J Dis Child 1979;133:30.

88. Davis D, Bohlman H, Walker AE, et al. The pathological findings in fatal cranio-spinal injuries. J Neurosurg 1971;34:603.

89. Bucholz RW, Burkhead WZ. The pathologic anatomy of fatal atlanto-occipital dislocations. J Bone Joint Surg 1979;61A:248.

90. Bohlman HH, Davis DD. The pathology of fatal craniospinal injuries. In Brinkhous KM (ed). Accident Pathology. 1968 Proceedings of an International Conference. Washington, DC, US Government Printing Office, pp 154–159.

91. Georgopoulos G, Pizzutillo PD, Lee MS. Occipito-atlantal instability in children. J Bone Joint Surg 1987;69A:429.

92. Gabrielson TO, Maxwell JA. Traumatic atlanto-occipital dislocation with case report of a patient who survived. Am J Roentgenol 1966;97:624.

93. Powers B, Milla MD, Kramer RS, et al. Traumatic anterior atlanto-occipital dislocation. Neurosurgery 1979;4:12.

94. Wirth RL, Zatz LM, Parker BR. CT detection of a Jefferson fracture in a child. AJR 1987;149:1001.

95. Marlin AE, Gayle RW, Lee JF. Jefferson fractures in children. J Neurosurg 1983;58:277.

96. Marlin AE, Williams GR, Lee JF. Jefferson fractures in children. J Neurol Neurosurg Psychiatr 1984;47:781.

97. Mikawa Y, Watanabe R, Yarmano Y, Ishii K. Fractures through a synchondrosis of the anterior arch of the atlas. J Bone Joint Surg 1987;69B:483.

98. Steel HH. Anatomical and mechanical consideration of the atlanto-axial articulation. Proceedings of the American Orthopaedic Association. J Bone Joint Surg 1968;50A:1481.

99. de V de Beer J, Hoffman EB, Kieck CF. Traumatic atlantoaxial subluxation in children. J Pediatr Orthop 1990;10:397.

100. Roach JW, Duncan D, Wenger DR, Maravilla A. Atlanto-axial instability and spinal cord compression in children. Diagnosis by computed tomography. J Bone Joint Surg 1984;66A:708.

101. Burke SW, French HG, Roberts JM, et al. Chronic atlanto-axial instability in Down syndrome. J Bone Joint Surg 1985;67A:1356.

102. Hammerschlag W, Ziv I, Wald U, et al. Cervical instability in an achondroplastic infant. J Pediatr Orthop 1988;8:481.

103. Hensinger RN, DeVito PD, Ragsdale CG. Changes in the cervical spine in juvenile rheumatoid arthritis. J Bone Joint Surg 1986;68A:189.

104. Kobori M, Takahashi H, Mikawa Y. Atlanto-axial dislocation in Down's syndrome. Report of two cases requiring surgical correction. Spine 1986;11:195.

105. Kransdorf MJ, Wherle PA, Moser RP Jr. Atlanto-axial subluxation in Reiter's syndrome. Spine 1988;13:12.

106. Miz GS, Engler GL. Atlanto-axial subluxation in Larsen's syndrome. A case report. Spine 1987;12:411.

107. Sherk HH, Whittaker LA, Pasquariello PS. Facial malformations and spinal anomalies: A predictable relationship. Spine 1982;7:526.

108. Fielding JW, Hawkins RJ. Atlanto-axial rotatory fixation. J Bone Joint Surg 1977;59A:37.

109. Jacobson G, Adler DC. Examination of the atlanto-axial joint following injury with particular emphasis on rotational subluxation. Am J Roentgenol Radium Ther Nucl Med 1956;76:1081.

110. Apple JJ, Kirks DR, Merten DF, Martinez S. Cervical spine fractures and dislocations in children. Pediatr Radiol 1987;17:45.

111. Geehr RB, Rothman SLG, Kier EL. The role of computed tomography in the evaluation of upper cervical spine pathology. Comput Tomogr 1978;2:79.

112. Phillips WA, Hensinger RN. The management of rotatory atlanto-axial subluxation in children. J Bone Joint Surg 1989;71A:664.

113. Seimon LP. Fracture of the odontoid process in young children. J Bone Joint Surg 1977;59A:943.

114. Nachemson A. Fracture of the odontoid process of the axis. A clinical study based on 26 cases. Acta Orthop Scand 1960;29:185.

115. Bhattacharyya SK. Fracture and displacement of the odontoid process in a child. J Bone Joint Surg 1974;56A:1071.

116. Swischuk LE, Hayden CK Jr, Sarwar M. The posteriorly tilted dens: A normal variation mimicking a fractured dens. Pediatr Radiol 1979;8:27.

117. Perovic NM, Kopits SE, Thompson RC. Radiologic evaluation of the spinal cord in congenital atlanto-axial dislocations. Radiology 1973;109:713.

118. Grogono BJS. Injuries of the atlas and axis. J Bone Joint Surg 1954;36B:397.

119. Pizzutillo PD, Rocha EF, D'Astous J, et al. Bilateral fractures of the pedicle of the second cervical vertebra in the young child. J Bone Joint Surg 1986;68A:892.

120. Weiss MH. Hangman's fracture in an infant. Am J Dis Child 1964;126:268.

121. Caffey J. The whiplash shaken infant syndrome. Pediatrics 1974;54:396.

122. Roaf R. A study of the mechanics of spinal injuries. J Bone Joint Surg 1960;42B:810.

123. Bulos S. Herniated intervertebral lumbar disc in the teenager. J Bone Joint Surg 1973;55B:273.

124. Blasier RD, LaMont RL. Chance fracture in a child: A case report with nonoperative treatment. J Pediatr Orthop 1985;5:92.
125. Koop SE, Winter RB, Lonstein JE. The surgical treatment of instability of the upper part of the cervical spine in children and adolescents. J Bone Joint Surg 1984;66A:403.
126. Smith WS, Kaufer H. Patterns and mechanisms of lumbar injuries associated with lap seat belts. J Bone Joint Surg 1969;51A:239.
127. Gumley G, Taylor TKF, Ryan MD. Distraction fractures of the lumbar spine. J Bone Joint Surg 1982;64B:520.
128. Taylor GA, Eggli KD. Lap-belt injuries of the lumbar spine in children. A pitfall in CT diagnosis. AJR 1988;150:1355.
129. Boechat MI. Spinal deformities and pseudofractures. AJR 1987;148:97.
130. Gellad FE, Levine AM, Joslyn JN, et al. Pure thoracolumbar facet dislocation: Clinical features and CT appearance. Radiology 1986;161:505.
131. Tarr RW, Drolshagen LF, Kerner TC, et al. MR imaging of recent spinal trauma. J Comput Assist Tomogr 1987;11:412.
132. McArdle CB, Crofford MJ, Mirfakhraee M, et al. Surface coil MR of spinal trauma: Preliminary experience. AJNR 1986;7:885.
133. Hubbard DD. Fractures of the dorsal and lumbar spine. Orthop Clin North Am 1976;7:605.
134. Bradford DS, McBride GG. Surgical management of thoracolumbar spine fractures with incomplete neurologic deficits. Clin Orthop 1987;218:201.
135. Jackson RW. Surgical stabilization of the spine. Paraplegia 1975;13:71.
136. Audic B, Maury M. Secondary vertebral deformities in childhood and adolescence. Paraplegia 1969;7:11.
137. Shelness A, Charles S. Children and car seats. Pediatrics 1986;77:256.
138. Diekema DS, Allen DB. Odontoid fracture in a child occupying a child restraint seat. Pediatrics 1988;82:117.
139. Connery BJ, Hall CM. Cervical spine fractures in rear car seat restraints. Arch Dis Child 1987;62:1267.
140. Tator CH, Edmonds VE. National survey of spinal injuries in hockey players. Can Med Assoc J 1984;130:875.
141. Schneider RC. Serious and fetal neurosurgical football injuries. Clin Neurosurg 1964;12:226.
142. Virgin H. Cineradiographic study of football helmets and the cervical spine. Am J Sports Med 1980;8:310.
143. Bachulis BL, Sangster W, Gorrell GW, Long WB. Patterns of injury in helmeted and nonhelmeted motorcyclists. Am J Surg 1988;155:708.
144. Torg JS, Vegso JJ, O'Neill J, Sennett B. The epidemiologic, pathologic, biomechanical, and cinematographic analysis of football-induced cervical spine trauma. Am J Sports Med 1990;18:50.
145. Torg JS, Das M. Trampoline and minitrampoline injuries to the cervical spine. Clin Sports Med 1985;4:45.
146. Committee on Sports Medicine. Atlantoaxial instability in Down syndrome. Pediatrics 1984;74:152.
147. Davidson RG. Atlantoaxial instability in individuals with Down's syndrome: A fresh look at the evidence. Pediatrics 1988;81:857.

CHAPTER 112

Maxillofacial Trauma

Susan L. Gin-Shaw

INTRODUCTION

Facial trauma in the pediatric age group is uncommon, accounting for less than 10% of all maxillofacial injuries. In one large series, only 6% of 1500 facial fractures were in children, and in another, only 4.8% of 500 facial fracture cases were in patients younger than 12 years.

ANATOMY

Anatomic differences affect the age-related distribution of different types of injuries. Orbital and skull fractures predominate in children younger than 5 years, whereas mandible fractures account for a large proportion of fractures in those 12 to 16 years old.

The child's skull is composed of the cranial vault, which protects the much smaller facial portion. The face-to-cranium ratio increases from 1:8 at birth to 1:2.5 in the adult as the midface grows. Most of this growth occurs around the ages of 6 to 7 years, which coincides with the eruption of permanent teeth. Therefore, midface fractures are rare in children younger than preschool age.

Pediatric facial bones are also protected by incompletely pneumatized sinuses, which provide additional structural support. This advantage is lost as the sinuses expand through puberty. Finally, the infant's mandible is relatively protected by fat pads, which enlarge from birth and reach their maximum thickness around 9 months. Protection afforded by these fat pads is offset, however, by the inherent weakness of the pediatric mandible caused by permanent teeth buds, which occupy most of the mandibular body.

CLINICAL EVALUATION

The evaluation of facial trauma begins with inspection of the face viewed straight on and from the top of the head, looking for asymmetry and cheekbone depression. The eyes should be examined for shape, pupillary alignment, light response, extraocular movements, and visual acuity.

Palpation of the face should be systematic; the periorbital ridges, zygomas, nose, maxilla, teeth, and mandible are palpated for displaced fractures. Intraoral inspection is performed, checking for lacerations, malocclusion, and difficulty in opening or closing the mouth. Intranasal inspection is performed with a speculum to determine displacement of the septum or nasal bones and to examine for a septal hematoma. Areas with subcutaneous emphysema should also be noted. Finally, in cooperative children, facial sensation testing of the trigeminal nerve should be performed. Facial nerve motor function is evaluated by having the child wrinkle the forehead, smile, and close the eyes tightly. Complete facial nerve paralysis in the absence of an obvious laceration or fracture should suggest a temporal bone fracture, especially in children younger than 5 years.

THERAPEUTIC INTERVENTION

Airway compromise is the most immediate problem associated with massive facial trauma. The pharynx should be manually cleared and suctioned, and the jaw-thrust maneuver performed. A comminuted mandibular fracture may destabilize the musculature of the tongue, causing the tongue to fall backward and occlude the airway. A large suture tie or towel clip can be used to protract the tongue in this case. Bag-mask ventilation and nasotracheal intubation may be impossible in the presence of massive facial trauma. Because up to 10% of facial injuries are associated with cervical spine injuries, the cervical spine should be radiographically cleared early in the course of evaluation. Oral intubation may also be difficult in the presence of massive facial trauma but is preferred over cricothyroidotomy in children younger than 3 years.

Facial bleeding, even if profuse, is seldom the sole source of hypotension in a child with multiple trauma. Most arterial bleeding arises from the superficial temporal, external maxillary, or angular arteries. Bleeding is controlled with direct pressure, rather than by blind clamping, which may injure branches of the facial nerve.

SPECIFIC FACIAL FRACTURES
Nasal Fractures

Nasal fractures are the most common type of facial fracture encountered in children. Although most of these fractures can be treated on an outpatient basis, damage to the nasoseptovomerine complex is associated with later hypoplasia of the midface and nose. In addition, childhood nasal fractures tend to have long-lasting cosmetic effects. Of patients with a history of childhood nasal fractures, 40% to 50% had some nasal deformity as compared with a control group without known trauma who had a nasal deformity in 10% to 20%.

The pediatric nasal bones are separated by an open suture in the midline. This suture predisposes children to splay or open-book type fractures with the nasal bones overriding the frontal processes of the maxilla. The immature nasal skeleton is largely cartilaginous and is subject to fracture and dislocation from the nasal bones.

The nose should be inspected and palpated, both full face and in profile, for deviations, dislocations, and flattening of the dorsum. Bony crepitus may be difficult to appreciate because of edema. Intranasal inspection with a speculum should be performed to exclude a septal hematoma, which appears as a dark purplish swelling over the septum. A septal hematoma may result in pressure necrosis of the septal cartilage with collapse of the dorsum of the nose. Any septal deviation should be gently palpated with a cotton-tipped applicator. An area of fluctuance may represent an early hematoma, and the diagnosis can be confirmed with needle aspiration.

Complications of nasal fractures include subcutaneous emphysema, traumatic telecanthus, and cerebrospinal fluid (CSF) rhinorrhea. Subcutaneous emphysema indicates involvement of the paranasal sinuses within the fracture line. Traumatic telecanthus occurs when a severe blow to the nose produces a comminuted nasal fracture with detachment of the medial palpebral ligaments. The eyes appear widely spaced with rounding of the medial canthi (Fig. 112–1). CSF rhinorrhea indicates a concomitant fracture of the cribriform plate and possible damage to the olfactory nerves. Because a large degree of force is necessary to produce traumatic telecanthus or a fracture of the cribriform plate, associated head injury should be excluded.

The utility of nasal radiographs in children is controversial and should not replace a thorough examination. Useful radiographic views for delineating nasal fractures are the lateral nasal projection (Fig. 112–2) and the exaggerated Waters view taken at 30 degrees to 45 degrees. The latter view demonstrates the midline relationship of the septum to both nasal bones.

Most children with uncomplicated nasal fractures can be sent home after control of epistaxis. Obvious nasal dislocations and splayed nasal bones may be reduced with firm digital pressure under local anesthesia in cooperative children. A plaster of paris or prefabricated splint is then applied over paper tape on the skin. Because of the rapidity of healing in children, a follow-up examination within 3 to 4 days with an otolaryngologist or plastic surgeon should be arranged. Most surgeons prefer closed reduction under general anesthesia within 5 to 7 days of injury.

Septal hematomas require immediate incision and drainage after consultation with an otolaryngologist. Anterior nasal packing is necessary to prevent reaccumulation of the hematoma. Nasal packing is a relative indication for admission for a young child. Prophylactic antibiotics with coverage for gram-positive aerobes and anaerobes should be instituted. Penicillin, amoxicillin, cephalexin, or erythromycin provide adequate coverage (Table 112–1).

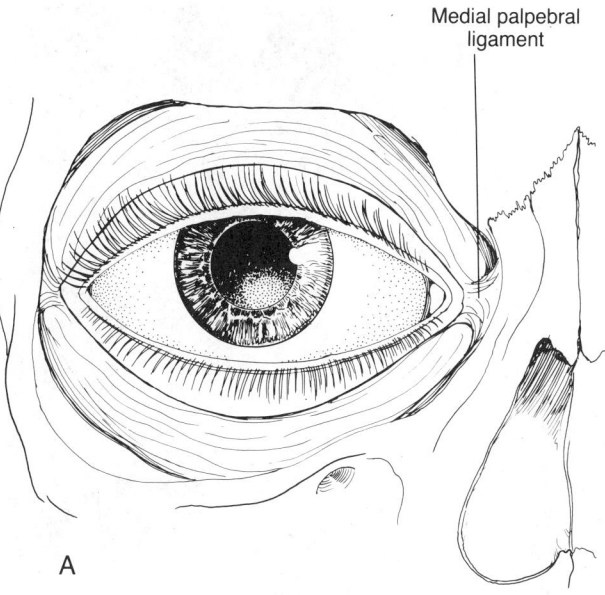

A

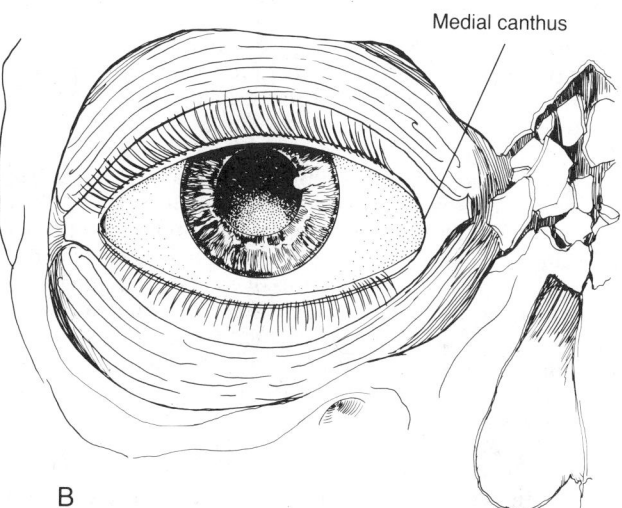

B

Figure 112–1. Telecanthus. With fracture of the nasal and orbital bones, the normal attachment of the medial palpebral ligament is disrupted. This results in a rounder appearance of the medial canthus and the illusion that the eyes are farther apart.

Fractures involving the paranasal sinuses also require prophylactic antibiotics to prevent sinusitis. These patients should receive a follow-up examination in 1 to 3 days.

Patients with nasal and cribriform plate fractures require admission and neurosurgical consultation. The use of antibiotics to prevent meningitis remains controversial, and the decision should be made in conjunction with the neurosurgeon. Similarly, a child with palpebral ligament detachment may require admission for neurologic observation and surgical correction.

Many nasal fractures, even when managed correctly, will heal with thickening over the dorsum. The potential for nasal and midface hypoplasia should be discussed and the importance of timely follow-up emphasized.

Malar Complex (Tripod) Fractures

Zygomatic fractures are uncommon in children younger than 6 years. These fractures result from direct blunt force

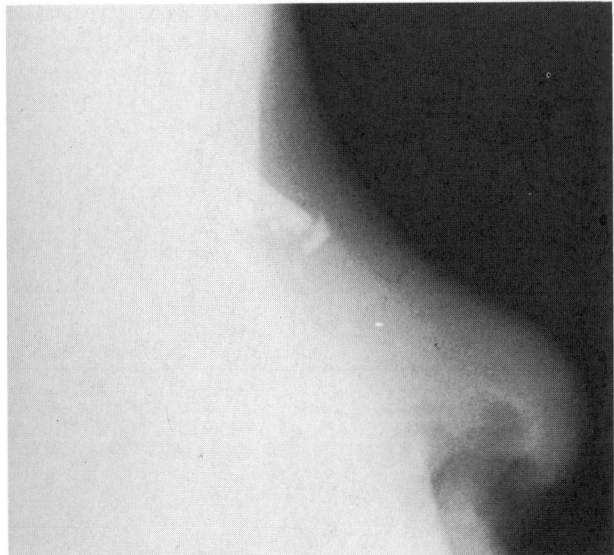

Figure 112–2. Lateral nasal projections clearly illustrate fractures of the nasal bones.

to the cheekbone. The zygomaticofrontal suture fracture is the most common malar fracture in the pediatric population. More severe force may result in a tripod or malar complex fracture involving the temporozygomatic, zygomaticofrontal, and zygomaticomaxillary sutures.

The child with a malar fracture typically presents with periorbital edema and subconjunctival hemorrhage. Bleeding into the maxillary sinus may cause unilateral epistaxis. Flattening of the cheekbone, which is best appreciated by viewing the patient from the top of the head, is apparent if the zygomatic arch has been depressed. Palpation may reveal a bony step-off along the infraorbital rim. Anesthesia of the inferior eyelid and lateral nose indicates injury to the infraorbital nerve as it exits the foramen near the zygomaticomaxillary suture line. Rarely, the patient may have difficulty opening the mouth as a result of impingement on the mandibular coronoid process by a rotated zygomatic arch. Finally, the eyelid may appear to be tethered laterally and downward from traction on the lateral palpebral ligament.

The best radiographic views to delineate malar complex fractures are the Waters, Caldwell, and submental vertex or bucket-handle views. The bucket-handle view demonstrates depressed zygomatic arch fractures well.

Most patients with tripod fractures do not require admission. Minimally displaced fractures do not require operative management, but patients with significant cosmetic deformities or functional debility require referral to a specialist. Such fractures may require open reduction within 7 days with interosseous wiring or minicompression plates designed for the zygoma. An ophthalmologic examination should be performed to exclude ocular trauma.

Orbital Fractures

Orbital blow-out fractures are increasingly common in school age and older children. Direct blunt trauma to the relatively noncompressible globe is the usual mechanism (Fig. 112–3). Most of the force is transmitted to the weakest points of the bony orbit, i.e., the floor or the medial wall. Orbital contents, including periorbital fat and, rarely, the inferior rectus muscle, herniate into the maxillary sinus below (Fig. 112–4). By strict definition, a blow-out fracture does not include the infraorbital rim.

Orbital roof fractures have been reported with increasing

TABLE 112–1
MAXILLOFACIAL TRAUMA: THERAPY AT A GLANCE

Penicillin V potassium
  Suspension: 125 mg or 250 mg/5 ml
  Tab: 125, 250, 500 mg
  Dosage: 25–50 mg/kg/24 hr q 6 hr po
Amoxicillin
  Suspension: 125 or 250 mg/5 ml
  Cap: 125, 250 mg
  Dosage: 20–40 mg/kg/24 hr q 8 hr po
Cephalexin
  Suspension: 125 or 250 mg/5 ml
  Cap: 250, 500 mg
  Dosage: 25–50 mg/kg/24 hr q 6 hr po
Erythromycin
  Suspension: 200 or 400 mg/5 ml
  Tab: 200 mg (chewable); 250, 400, 500 mg
  Dosage: 20–50 mg/kg/24 hr q 6 hr po
Dicloxacillin
  Suspension: 62.5 mg/5 ml
  Cap: 125, 250, 500 mg
  Dosage: 25–100 mg/kg/24 hr q 6 hr po
Amoxicillin (AMX)–Clavulanic acid (CLA) (Augmentin)
  Suspension: 125 mg AMX/31.25 CLA or 250 mg AMX/62.5 mg CLA/5 ml
  Tab: 250 AMX/125 mg CLA or 500 mg AMX/125 mg CLA
  Dosage: 30–50 mg AMX/kg/24 hr q 8 hr po
Fentanyl (Sublimaze)
  Suspension: 50 μg/1 ml
  Dosage: 1–2 μg/kg slow IVP
Meperidine (Demerol)
  Dosage: 1–2 mg/kg IM
Promethazine (Phenergan)
  Dosage: 1 mg/kg IM
Chloral hydrate
  Suspension: 500 mg/5 ml
  Cap: 250, 500 mg
  Dosage: 25–50 mg/kg po

frequency with advances in high-resolution computed tomographic (CT) imaging. These fractures are thought to be the result of blunt impact to the superior orbital rim that causes buckling of the orbital roof. Children younger than

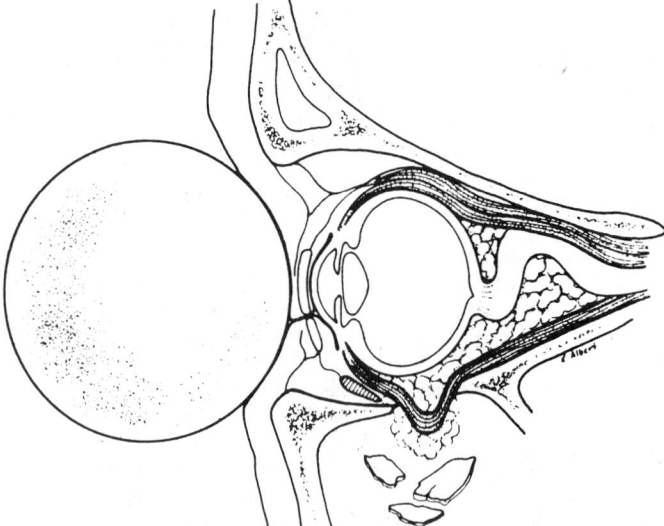

Figure 112–3. Orbital blow-out fractures. Pressure to the orbital contents results in a downward displacement of the orbital floor. Extraocular muscles and periorbital fat can extrude into the maxillary sinus, resulting in enophthalmos and restriction of upward gaze. (Courtesy of Ms. Karen Abbott.)

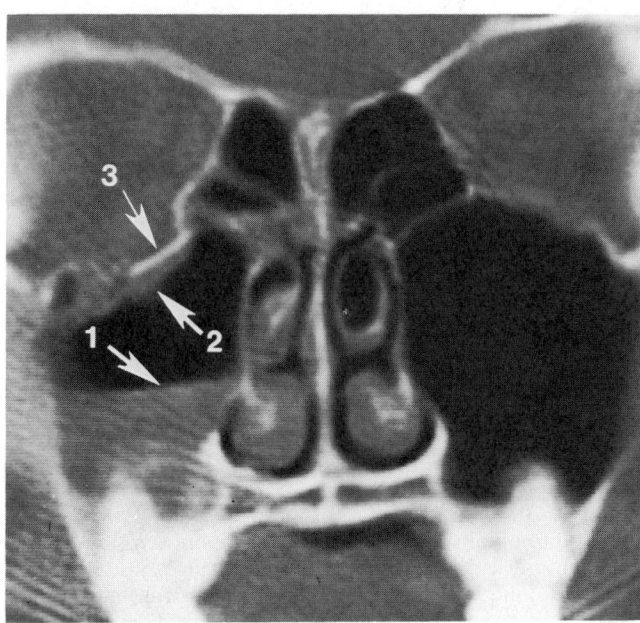

Figure 112–4. Coronal CT scan illustrates graphically the triad of radiographic findings on the upright Waters view plain radiograph of an orbital floor blow-out fracture: (1) gas-fluid level in the maxillary sinus; (2) teardrop of soft tissue (prolapsed muscle and/ or hematoma) in the upper sinus; (3) fracture fragment itself. (Courtesy of A. Oestreich, M.D., Cincinnati, OH.)

7 years may be prone to this type of injury because of the lack of pneumatization of the frontal sinus, which would dissipate the force in older children and adults. Orbital roof fractures may be nondisplaced, or the fragments may be superiorly or inferiorly displaced (a "blow-in" fracture). In more than half of the cases reported, such fractures are associated with more extensive skull fractures and neurologic injuries. Complications include ocular injuries, dural lacerations, and orbital encephaloceles.

Patients may present with marked periorbital edema, which makes examination difficult. The physician should check for enophthalmos (recession of the globe within the orbit) and horizontal pupil malalignment. Patients may complain of diplopia from limitation of upward gaze, which is attributed to entrapment of the inferior rectus muscle. Limitation of upward gaze is more commonly caused by injury to the third cranial nerve or by traction on the inferior rectus muscle by fibrous bands connecting it to the herniated fat pad below.

Subcutaneous emphysema indicates involvement of a sinus, usually through a medial wall fracture of the lamina papyracea of the ethmoid bone. Patients complain of marked periorbital swelling after blowing their nose.

The physician should document visual acuity and perform a funduscopic examination to exclude associated retinal detachment, lens dislocation, or hyphema.

Blow-out fractures are best demonstrated by the Waters view. Classic findings are opacification of the maxillary sinus or an air-fluid level in the involved sinus. The "hanging drop sign" is a soft tissue mass representing herniated orbital contents in the superior aspect of the maxillary sinus. Unfortunately, interpretation of sinus films in children is often difficult. Although the maxillary and ethmoid sinuses are present at birth, aeration does not begin for 4 or 5 months. Incomplete pneumatization of these sinuses accounts for the abnormal radiographs found in more than half of the films obtained in children less than 12 months old who have no history of trauma. Orbital CT scans are useful in equivocal

cases and will delineate the extent of the fracture. Medial blow-out fractures and orbital roof fractures are best demonstrated with coronal sections (Fig. 112–5).

Medial blow-out fractures are considered open fractures involving the ethmoid sinus; for this reason prophylactic antibiotics such as penicillin, amoxicillin, cephalexin, or erythromycin are indicated. All patients with blow-out fractures need referral to an otolaryngologist or plastic surgeon within 3 to 5 days. If diplopia or entrapment is present, next-day referral is indicated after intraocular injury has been excluded.

Nondisplaced orbital roof fractures may be managed conservatively and long-term ophthalmologic follow-up arranged. Displaced fractures, especially those with associated neurologic injury, usually require open reduction.

Maxillary Fractures

LeFort fractures are extremely rare before age 6 years but begin to increase in incidence in the 6- to 11-year-old age group. LeFort fractures are the result of violent deceleration forces such as those encountered in automobile-pedestrian and motor vehicle accidents. An associated head injury is common and should be treated first.

Children with LeFort fractures have edema and ecchymosis of the entire midface. Malocclusion and open-bite deformities are common. Bilateral epistaxis may occur secondary to bleeding into the maxillary sinuses.

LeFort I fractures (Fig. 112–6) involve the lower maxilla, inferior nasal septum, walls of the maxillary sinuses, and pterygoid plates. The diagnosis is made clinically when mobility of the maxillary segment is demonstrated when traction is applied to the upper incisors. Dentoalveolar injuries are commonly associated with this type of fracture.

LeFort II fractures (see Fig. 112–6) involve the roof of the nasal bones, ethmoid sinuses, pterygoid plates, medial orbital walls, orbital floors, and lateral walls of the maxillary sinuses. Midface instability may be demonstrated in the anteroposterior or inferosuperior plane. In the latter case, wrinkling in the skin above the nose when upward pressure is applied to the maxilla is diagnostic.

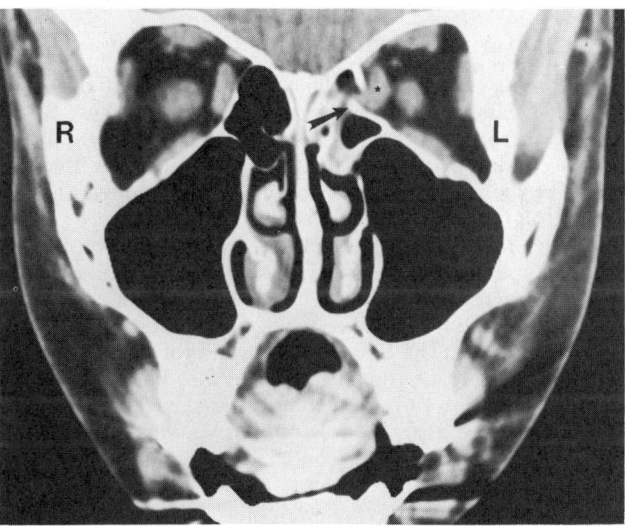

Figure 112–5. This 11-year-old boy was struck in the nose with a fist. He complained of diplopia. Coronal CT scan of the facial bones shows a depressed fracture of the medial wall of the left orbit (*arrow*) causing entrapment of the medial rectus muscle (*) resulting in paralysis of the left lateral gaze. Plain films showed no abnormality. (Courtesy of Bing Tai, M.D., Lansing, MI.)

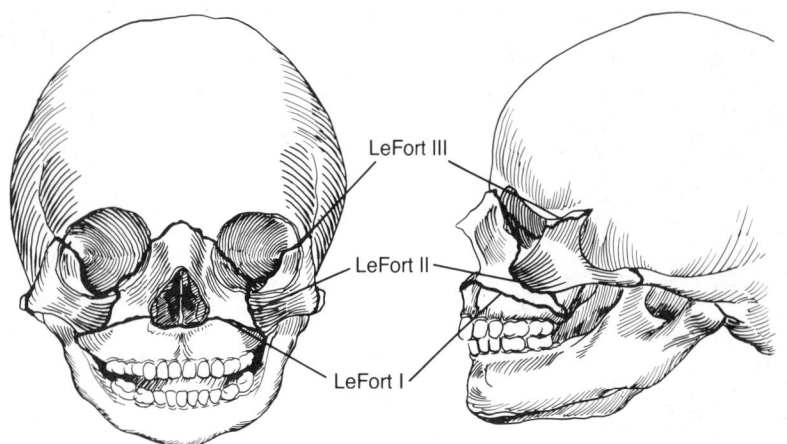

Figure 112–6. LeFort classification of fractures. Type I causes separation of the maxilla. Type II results in a mobile maxilla and nose. Type III produces craniofacial separation, often appearing as a sunken or depressed midface.

LeFort III fractures (see Fig. 112–6) involve the same fractures as those in LeFort II fractures except that the fracture line extends through the zygoma. All LeFort fractures may be unilateral, and it is possible to have a LeFort II fracture on one side with a LeFort III fracture on the other.

Facial films may demonstrate only a few of the fractures, and CT scanning is commonly performed in part to evaluate an accompanying head injury. Coronal sections as well as sagittal views may be necessary (Fig. 112–7).

Airway management is the primary concern. The cervical spine should be radiographically evaluated and the patient orally intubated if indicated. Nasal intubation is not recommended because of the additional risk of intracranial intubation if the cribriform plate is involved.

An ophthalmologic examination is necessary for patients with LeFort fractures. Nearly 10% of all periorbital fractures are associated with intraocular injuries.

Children with LeFort fractures require admission, usually for concomitant head injuries. Once stable, these patients require open reduction with interosseous wiring or compression plating and intermaxillary fixation. The goals of surgical treatment are to reestablish occlusion and to restore midfacial height.

Mandibular Fractures

The most common mandibular fracture in children less than 10 years old is the subcondylar fracture (Fig. 112–8). These fractures most often result from direct blows to the chin secondary to falls or motor vehicle accidents. Because of the resiliency of developing bone, the subcondylar area is prone to greenstick fractures.

The child with a mandibular fracture will complain of pain on opening or closing the mouth. Because many mandibular fractures also involve dentoalveolar injuries, the physician should check for malocclusion and step-offs in dentition, inspect the floor of the mouth for areas of ecchymosis, and palpate the lingual aspect of the gingiva for tenderness and deformities. Nondisplaced subcondylar fractures may have a subtle presentation. In small children, a chin laceration may be the only clinical sign. Patients with unilateral condylar fractures may demonstrate jaw deviation when the mouth is opened widely. Patients with bilateral condylar fractures may exhibit an open bite deformity. Bony crepitus may be palpable when the examiner's finger is placed in the auditory meatus as the mouth is opened and closed.

Dental panorex views demonstrate most mandibular fractures. Because of long exposure times, however, patient cooperation is required, and as a result, such views are

difficult to obtain with toddlers. In addition, symphyseal and parasymphyseal fractures may be difficult to visualize. Lateral and oblique mandibular views demonstrate most angle, body, and parasymphyseal fractures. The Towne's "horse face" view is particularly useful for subcondylar fractures.

Most children with displaced mandible fractures should be admitted for observation. Limitation in mouth opening places the airway at risk, especially if the child is vomiting. Feeding may be difficult in infants. Bilateral parasymphyseal fractures may cause detachment of the genioglossus muscle, which allows the tongue to fall backward and occlude the airway. The tongue can be protracted with a towel clip or a large suture.

Condylar and subcondylar fractures often heal well without immobilization or attempts to regain anatomic reduction. Early motion and a soft diet encourage remodeling of the fracture callus and reduce the incidence of bony ankylosis of the temporomandibular joint. Subcondylar fractures associated with parasymphyseal fractures have also been managed effectively with early functional use. The parasymphyseal fracture is reduced with a compression plate or prefabricated acrylic splint without intermaxillary fixation. This allows for early range of motion of the mandible. Because fractures of the condylar region are associated with growth disturbances, children with such fractures need long-term follow-up to monitor for adequate mandibular growth and functional recovery.

Fractures through the body of the mandible usually require immobilization, as the muscles of mastication and the opening muscles on the floor of the mouth tend to distract the fracture segments. Fixation should be accomplished within 5 to 7 days of injury. Consultation with an oral surgeon, otolaryngologist, or plastic surgeon familiar with pediatric mandibular fractures is mandatory.

Any fracture involving the alveolar ridge or the tooth root is considered an open fracture and should be treated with prophylactic antibiotics. Administration of penicillin or erythromycin for 5 days provides coverage for most oral flora.

Parents of a child with a condylar fracture should be advised of the potential adverse effect on future mandibular growth and of the possibility of bony ankylosis of the temporomandibular joint. In addition, mandibular fractures may damage permanent teeth.

SOFT TISSUE INJURIES OF THE FACE

Facial Lacerations

Children often require sedation as well as local anesthesia to adequately clean, debride, and explore wounds. Intra-

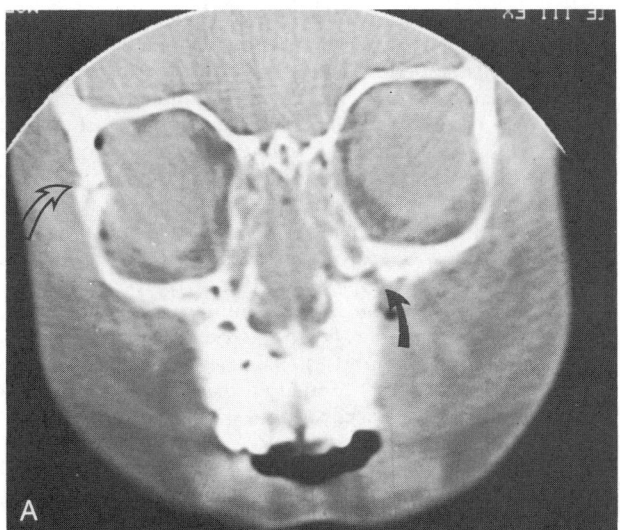

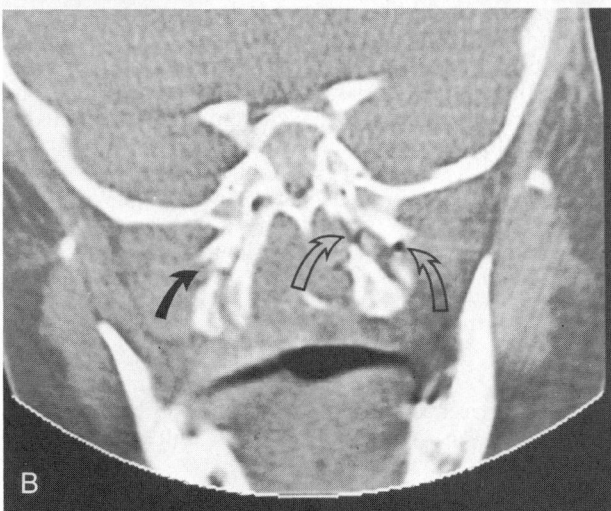

Figure 112–7. *A*, This patient had a LeFort II fracture on the right and a LeFort III fracture on the left. Coronal CT scan of the facial bones demonstrates a fracture through the left zygomaticofrontal suture (*open arrow*), a component of the LeFort III fracture. On the right, a maxillary fracture (*solid arrow*) is seen as part of the LeFort II fracture. *B*, The patient also had bilateral fractures of the pterygoid processes. One fracture is seen on the left (*solid arrow*) and two fractures through the pterygoid plate on the right (*open arrows*).

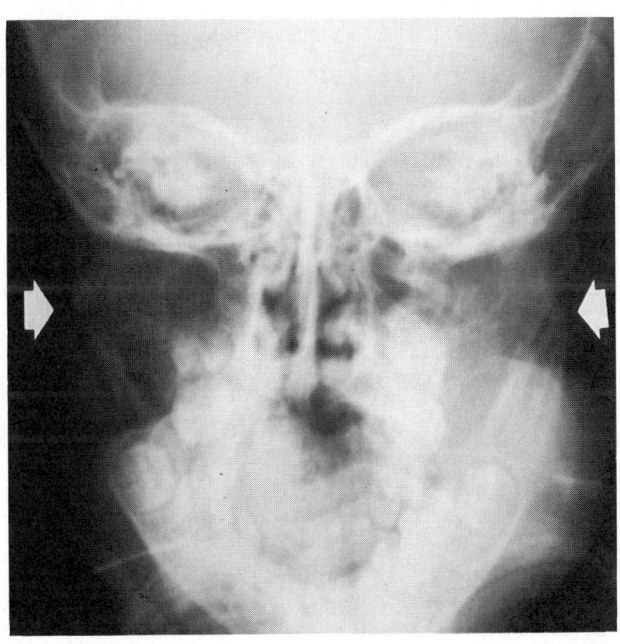

Figure 112–8. Mandible condyle fractures (*arrows*), as in this 2½-year-old boy, may be identified on an angled frontal facial film (Towne view) by careful examination of the film. In this case, the condyle heads are also dislocated, as better shown on CT. (Courtesy of A. Oestreich, M.D., Cincinnati, OH.)

muscular meperidine (Demerol) and promethazine (Phenergan), oral chloral hydrate, or intravenous fentanyl have been used for pediatric sedation.

Before wound closure, the face is examined for evidence of a sensory or motor deficit. Deep lacerations of the cheek may injure branches of the facial nerve or the parotid duct. Stenson's duct lies near the middle third of an imaginary line extending from the tragus to the midpoint of the upper lip. The intraoral papilla near the second maxillary molar should also be inspected for salivary flow.

Simple lacerations may be closed in a layered fashion as needed with 6–0 or 7–0 nylon. Round wounds are closed elliptically and placed parallel to skin creases. Crush injuries, V- or U-shaped flap wounds, stellate lacerations, and injuries with significant amounts of avulsed tissue may need plastic surgery consultation. Facial sutures should be removed in 4 to 5 days in children.

Eyelid Lacerations

Horizontal eyelid lacerations may be closed if the aponeurosis of the levator palpebrae muscle has not been violated. Unrepaired lacerations of this muscle result in ptosis, which may be inapparent initially because of periorbital edema. Lacerations involving the medial canthus need immediate ophthalmologic consultation to exclude injury to the lacrimal canaliculi. Acute repair of such injuries is preferred, as late repairs often result in inadequate tear drainage.

Vertical lacerations involving the lid margin also need an ophthalmologic consultation. Without meticulous closure and eversion of the lid margin, disconcerting notching commonly occurs.

Eyebrow Lacerations

Eyebrow lacerations may be closed in the emergency department. Care should be taken to maintain the hairline. Eyebrow hairs should never be shaved.

Nasal Lacerations

Through-and-through nasal lacerations are closed in layers using 5–0 or 6–0 absorbable sutures in the mucosa and cartilage and 5–0 or 6–0 nylon for skin. Local anesthesia should not contain epinephrine, as the nose contains terminal capillaries. Prophylactic antibiotics such as amoxicillin–clavulanic acid, dicloxacillin, or erythromycin are recommended for coverage of streptococci of the pharynx and staphylococci of the skin. Patients should be referred to an otolaryngologist to monitor for both skin infection and chondritis.

Ear Lacerations

Simple lacerations of the pinna are easily repaired, but complex lacerations and near avulsions need referral. Anesthesia of the pinna is accomplished by infiltrating around the entire base of the ear with 1% lidocaine without epinephrine. Through-and-through lacerations require a layered closure with 5–0 or 6–0 nylon for both skin layers. Closure of the cartilage with absorbable suture remains controversial. Some plastic surgeons prefer suturing the cartilage, whereas others simply close the skin on both sides. Injuries involving the cartilage should be splinted by packing the pinna anteriorly and posteriorly with petroleum jelly gauze and then applying a compression dressing to the ear.

Subperichondral hematomas should be evacuated to avoid chondritis and pressure necrosis, complications that lead to the development of a flattened pinna. Initially these hematomas may be aspirated and a pressure dressing applied. The ear should be rechecked in 24 hours for re-accumulation of the hematoma. If this occurs, the hematoma should be incised and drained under local anesthesia. The incision should extend through the perichondrium. Depending on the size of the hematoma, a drain can be placed below the perichondrium and a pressure dressing re-applied.

Lacerations of the Lips and Mouth

Accurate closure of lacerations involving the vermilion border is critical, because even a 1-mm step-off is quite noticeable. Both sides of the vermilion border can be marked with indelible ink before the area is prepped. The first cutaneous suture should align the two marks.

Through-and-through lacerations are closed in layers using absorbable suture in the deep tissue and the wet mucosa. The latter can often be left open if the laceration is superficial.

Full-thickness cheek lacerations are closed in layers, beginning with absorbable suture in the mucosa. The wound is then irrigated from the outside, prepped, and closed using deep absorbable sutures as needed. Tongue lacerations need only be closed if deep. A tight closure is unnecessary and may contribute to the development of infection. An assistant can aid by protracting the tongue with a piece of gauze.

The use of prophylactic antibiotics is controversial in lacerations of the lips and mouth. Older children should rinse the mouth with a 1:1 solution of peroxide and mouthwash twice daily to prevent food particles from accumulating in mucosal wounds. An infant's careprovider should swab the child's mouth with half-strength peroxide twice or three times daily.

Selected References

Altieri M, Brasch L. Antibiotic prophylaxis in intraoral wounds. Am J Emerg Med 1986;4:507.

Amaratunga NA. Mandibular fractures in children—study of clinical aspects, treatment needs and complications. J Oral Maxillofac Surg 1988;46:637.

Billmire DA, Neale HW, Gregory RO. Use of IV fentanyl in the outpatient treatment of pediatric facial trauma. J Trauma 1985;25:1079.

Converse JM, Smith B, Obear MF, Wood-Smith D. Orbital blowout fractures: A ten-year survey. Plast Reconstr Surg 1967;39:20.

Crockett DM, Mungo RP, Thompson RE. Maxillofacial trauma. Pediatr Clin North Am 1989;36:1471.

Glasier CM, Mallory GB Jr, Steele RW. Significance of opacification of the maxillary and ethmoid sinuses in infants. J Pediatr 1989;114:45.

Greenwald MJ, Boston D, Pensler JM, Radowski MA. Orbital roof fractures in childhood. Ophthalmology 1989;96:491.

Grymer LS, Gutierrez C, Stoksted P. Nasal fractures in children: Influence on the development of the nose. J Laryngol Otol 1985;199:735.

Helveston EM. Eye trauma in childhood. Pediatr Clin North Am 1975;22:501.

Hurt TL, Brock F, Peterson BM, Lynch F. Mandibular fractures in association with chin trauma in pediatric patients. Pediatr Emerg Care 1988;4:121.

Jones KM, Bauer BS, Pensler JM. Treatment of mandibular fractures in children. Ann Plast Surg 1989;23:280.

Leake D, Doykos J, Habal MB, Murray JE. Long-term follow-up of fractures of the mandibular condyle in children. Plast Reconstr Surg 1971;47:127.

Maniglia AJ, Kline SN. Maxillofacial trauma in the pediatric age group. Otolaryngol Clin North Am 1983;16:717.

McGraw BL, Cole RR. Pediatric maxillofacial trauma. Arch Otolaryngol Head Neck Surg 1990;116:41.

Messinger A, Radkowski MA, Greenwald MJ, Pensler JM. Orbital roof fractures in the pediatric population. Plast Reconstr Surg 1989;84:213.

Myall RW, Sandor GK, Gregory CE. Are you overlooking fractures of the mandibular condyle? Pediatrics 1987;79:639.

Raflo GT. Blow-in and blow-out fractures of the orbit: Clinical correlations and proposed mechanisms. Ophthal Surg 1984;15:114.

Stucker FJ, Bryarly RC, Shockley WW. Management of nasal trauma in children. Arch Otolaryngol 1984;110:190.

Walton RL, Hagan KF, Parry SH, Deluchi SF. Maxillofacial trauma. Surg Clin North Am 1982;62:73.

CHAPTER 113

Thoracic Trauma

Arnold G. Coran

INTRODUCTION

Blunt injuries account for 80% to 90% of all cases of chest trauma in the pediatric age group.[1] Although less than 15% of thoracic injuries in children and adults require a major operation, injuries to the cardiorespiratory system account for 25% of the deaths in children and more than half of the deaths in adults.[2, 3] Othersen has reported a mortality rate of 60% in children suffering chest injuries and major injuries to other organ systems simultaneously.[4]

Injured children differ from their adult counterparts anatomically, physiologically, and psychologically. Infants and children have more pliable chest walls, which results in a lower incidence of rib fractures in this age group, even with significant external trauma and forces. Significant pulmonary parenchymal injuries and cardiovascular injuries can occur without rib fractures in smaller children. Likewise, the younger the patient, the more mobile the mediastinum. As a result, blood or air under tension in one hemithorax can shift the mediastinum to the other side with resultant obstruction of the opposite main stem bronchus and vena cava, resulting in decreased venous return and decreased cardiac output. Most children hyperventilate when frightened or stressed; this results in air swallowing and rapid gastric dilatation. The acute gastric dilatation may mimic an acute abdomen in a child, impair respiration by elevating the diaphragms, and even obstruct flow through the abdominal vena cava, which can result in a decreased cardiac output.

Thoracic trauma includes the following injuries: rib fractures, sternal fractures, pneumothorax, hemothorax, traumatic asphyxia, pulmonary contusion, tracheal and bronchial injuries, cardiac injuries with cardiac contusion and tamponade, injuries to the thoracic aorta, diaphragmatic rupture, and esophageal perforation. Of these injuries, tension pneumothorax, massive hemothorax, cardiac tamponade, flail chest, open pneumothorax, tracheal or bronchial laceration, severe pulmonary parenchymal injury, aortic rupture, and esophageal perforation are life threatening or potentially life threatening.

The initial evaluation of the injured child requires a rapid sequential evaluation of the airway, breathing, and circulation. The airway should be cleared of all debris (e.g., mucus, blood, and vomitus), and endotracheal intubation should be performed if there is any question of adequate ventilation. In the unconscious patient, this should be done with cervical spine control and assuming a cervical fracture is present. The orotracheal route is preferred to nasotracheal intubation in small children. If there is massive facial trauma, a cricothyroidotomy may be required as a temporizing procedure until a tracheostomy can be performed in the operating room.

FRACTURES OF THE THORACIC CAGE

Rib fractures are far less common in children than they are in adults. Most children with fractures of the ribs or sternum can be treated with pain medication and bed rest, and recovery is rapid. An intercostal block is often effective in relieving the pain of a rib fracture. A flail chest can occur in the presence of multiple rib fractures. This usually results from severe trauma such as a high-speed automobile accident. A flail chest produces paradoxical motion of the chest wall such that, on inspiration, the chest retracts rather than expands, and on expiration, the chest expands rather than retracts. This causes inadequate gas exchange, which can lead to significant hypoxemia. In the younger child, flail chest is often associated with mediastinal shifts that can compress the bronchi and the vena cava. Immediate treatment consists of stabilization of the chest wall with sandbags or towel clips. Definitive treatment requires endotracheal intubation and mechanical ventilation for 7 to 10 days.[5]

PNEUMOTHORAX

The most common serious injury seen with thoracic trauma is a pneumothorax, either simple or tension (Fig. 113–1). A small, simple pneumothorax involving between 10% and 20% of the volume of the hemithorax may be treated conservatively with bed rest, observation, and supplemental oxygen. However, placement of a chest tube is appropriate for any type or any degree of traumatic pneumothorax. If air continues to accumulate in the pleural space after the initial injury, from a laceration in the lung parenchyma or the bronchus, then there is a tension pneumothorax, which can be life threatening if not treated immediately. An untreated tension pneumothorax leads to a mediastinal shift with vena caval obstruction and resultant decreased cardiac output and shock. Physical examination reveals decreased breath sounds and hyperresonance to percussion. A chest radiograph establishes the diagnosis, but in many cases a chest tube must be inserted before a confirmatory radiograph can be obtained. Rib fractures are often absent in children with pneumothoraces. Under emergent circumstances, the pneumothorax can be initially evacuated with a needle thoracotomy, followed shortly thereafter by a chest tube. However, in most circumstances, a chest tube should be inserted initially through the third or fourth

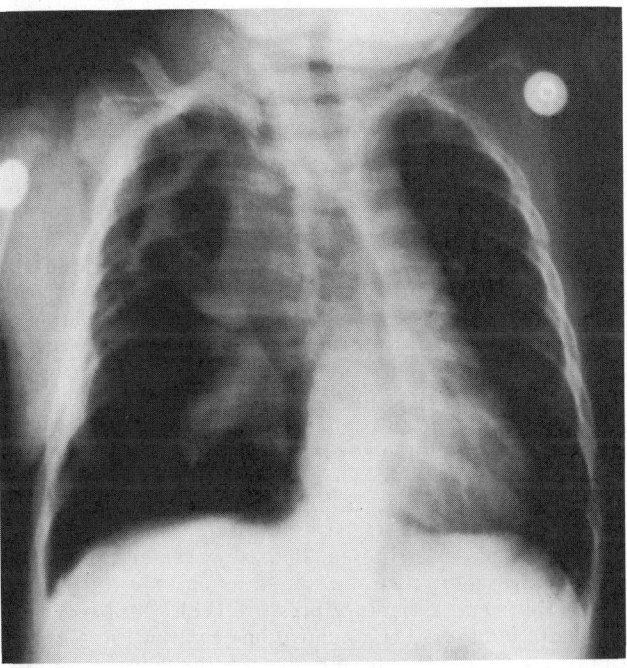

Figure 113–1. Right pneumothorax. Blunt trauma to the right chest in a 2-year-old child.

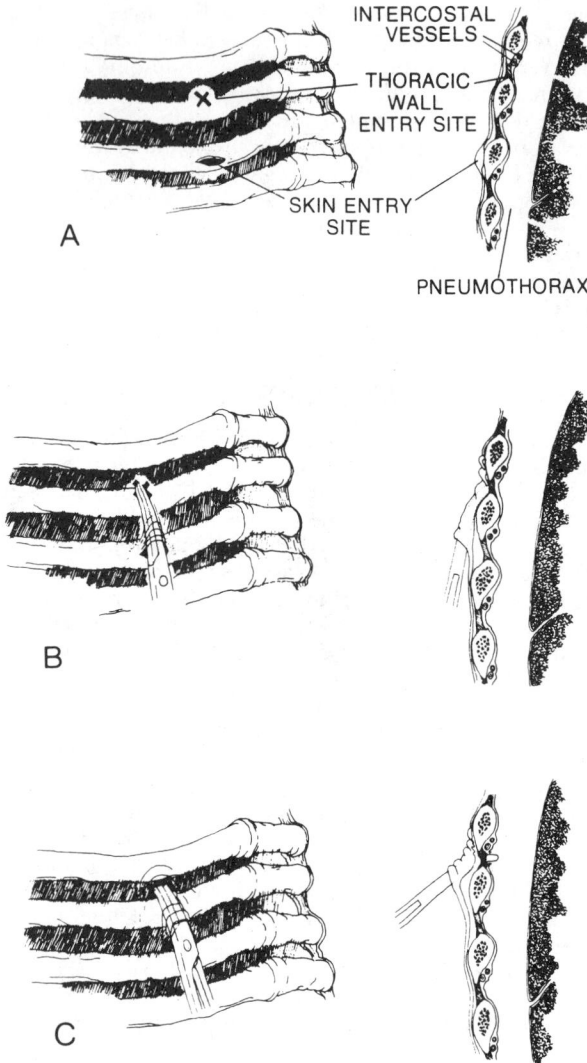

Figure 113–2. Chest tube placement. *A*, Topography. Blunt dissection subcutaneously *(B)* and into the pleural space *(C)*. (From Hughes WT, Buescher ES. Pediatric Procedures. 2nd ed. Philadelphia, WB Saunders, 1980, p 237.)

intercostal space in the midaxillary line (Fig. 113–2). In patients with an open pneumothorax with extensive damage to the soft tissues and bony tissues of the chest wall, the wound should be closed and a chest tube placed in order to adequately evacuate any air in the pleural cavity.

All children sustaining blunt or penetrating injuries to the chest that require tube thoracotomy should receive broad-spectrum antibiotics because of the risk of contamination of the pleural space with disruption of the pulmonary parenchyma. Pleural contamination can result in empyema formation if not treated with antibiotics. Most children who sustain a traumatic pneumothorax and are treated with a chest tube and antibiotic coverage do not develop an empyema.

If gas exchange is compromised in the child with a pneumothorax, endotracheal intubation and mechanical ventilation may be required. If there is evidence of a pulmonary laceration, then the amount of airway pressure and the positive end-expiratory pressure (PEEP) applied must be minimized to reduce continuation of the air leak through the pulmonary tear. The use of high-frequency jet ventilation with low airway pressures has been shown to be effective in allowing a traumatic pulmonary laceration to seal.

HEMOTHORAX

Massive hemothorax from blunt or penetrating trauma in childhood is relatively rare and is usually caused by a tear in an intercostal artery. A pulmonary parenchymal injury results in a significant hemothorax far less commonly (Fig. 113–3). Rarely, a massive hemothorax results from rupture of the heart or the thoracic aorta. Cardiac and aortic rupture require an immediate thoracotomy to control hemorrhage. The first priority in management of massive hemothorax in children is management of the blood loss and the resulting hemorrhagic shock with expeditious transfusion of blood. Simultaneously, the hemothorax is evacuated with a large-bore chest tube placed through the third or fourth intercostal space in the midaxillary line. In most cases, chest tube placement and blood transfusion stabilize the child, and thoracotomy is not required. Indications for thoracotomy include continuing drainage of blood from the chest tube with hemodynamic instability, which may indicate damage to a major cardiovascular structure in the mediastinum or inadequate drainage of blood by the chest tube, resulting in a pleural clot that cannot be evacuated.[6, 7]

CARDIAC TAMPONADE

Injuries to the heart can result from either penetrating or blunt trauma, but penetrating trauma is a more common cause of these injuries. Most patients who receive a gunshot wound to the heart experience exsanguination at the scene and seldom reach the emergency department. Blunt trauma and stab wounds to the heart often result in cardiac tamponade, with the patient reaching the hospital alive but in extremis. Although children rarely suffer gunshot wounds to the heart, which make up the majority of isolated cardiac injuries, they often have injuries to other structures in the chest.[8]

Patients with cardiac tamponade have a narrow pulse pressure, muffled heart sounds, and distended neck veins and are in shock. Heart size may be increased on chest radiograph (Fig. 113–4). A child in shock with suspected cardiac tamponade should undergo an immediate pericardiocentesis, using the subxiphoid technique. If unclotted blood is found, the plastic pericardiocentesis needle is left

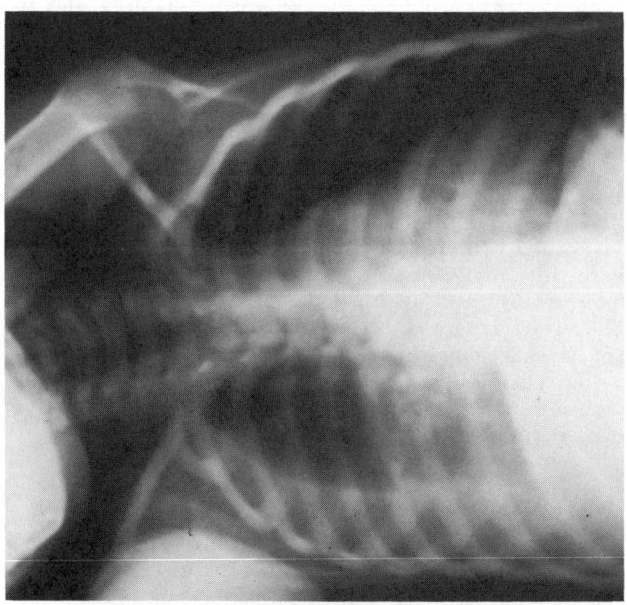

Figure 113–3. Right hemothorax from blunt trauma.

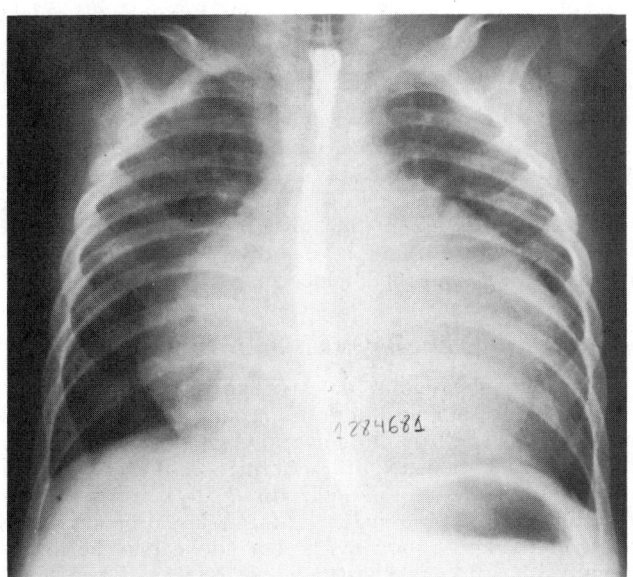

Figure 113–4. Cardiac tamponade from blunt trauma. A contrast study of the esophagus was taken to rule out esophageal perforation.

in place and the patient is immediately taken to the operating room for an emergency thoracotomy.

Less life-threatening injuries to the heart include myocardial contusion, which results exclusively from blunt chest trauma. These patients may demonstrate an injury pattern on the electrocardiogram and have elevated serum levels of creatine kinase–MB.

Sternal fractures are often associated with myocardial contusions. These patients are at risk for the development of major arrhythmias and for that reason must be monitored in an intensive care unit. The course of most of these children, however, is quite benign.[9]

Rarely, rupture of the ventricular septum or of the chordae tendinae of the mitral valve can occur, resulting in mitral regurgitation. Urgent repair of these lesions with cardiopulmonary bypass is indicated.

TRAUMATIC ASPHYXIA

Traumatic asphyxia occurs mostly in younger children with pliable chest walls. It is manifested by petechial hemorrhages in the sclerae and skin of the upper limbs and head and results from a sudden, severe crushing blow to the chest when the glottis is closed. This elevates intrathoracic pressure suddenly and forces venous blood in the chest back into the great veins in the head and arms, producing the petechial hemorrhages. These patients often have neurologic deficits from suffusion of the brain and often present in coma. However, almost all cases of traumatic asphyxia are self-limited and reversible.[10]

PULMONARY CONTUSION

Next to pneumothorax, the most common serious injury seen in children with chest trauma is pulmonary contusion (Fig. 113–5 and 113–6). This is seen primarily with blunt trauma and represents a blast injury to the lung parenchyma.[11] Extensive pulmonary contusion can lead to the adult respiratory distress syndrome (ARDS), which results in severe bilateral interstitial pulmonary infiltration with significant hypoxemia secondary to intrapulmonary shunting. In addition, superimposed pulmonary edema and pneu-

monia can occur, which aggravate the intrapulmonary shunting and hypoxemia.[12] The mainstay of treatment is mechanical ventilation with low airway pressures and PEEP. In addition, fluid restriction and diuresis are used to treat pulmonary edema and reduce the amount of fluid accumulated in the pulmonary interstitial space. Paralysis of these patients while on the ventilator allows the reduced airway pressures required to adequately oxygenate the child.

AORTIC RUPTURE

Rupture of the aorta at the level of the ligamentum arteriosus is extremely rare in children because of the marked elasticity of their arteries and the absence of atherosclerosis. In addition, this injury is usually associated with high-speed motor vehicle accidents in which the victim is crushed by the steering wheel.[13] Ninety percent of patients with traumatic aortic rupture die at the scene of the accident. The chest radiograph usually demonstrates widening of the mediastinum (Fig. 113–7), fracture of the left first rib, obliteration of the aortic knob, deviation of the trachea to the right, presence of a pleural cap of blood, depression of the left main stem bronchus, or a left pleural effusion. Definitive diagnosis is made by arteriography (Fig. 113–8). These patients require an emergent operation using left heart bypass or a vascular shunt.

TRACHEOBRONCHIAL INJURIES

Injury to the trachea or bronchi can result from either penetrating or blunt trauma. These injuries are unusual in childhood but can be fatal. The rarity of the injury is probably a result of the flexibility and mobility of the

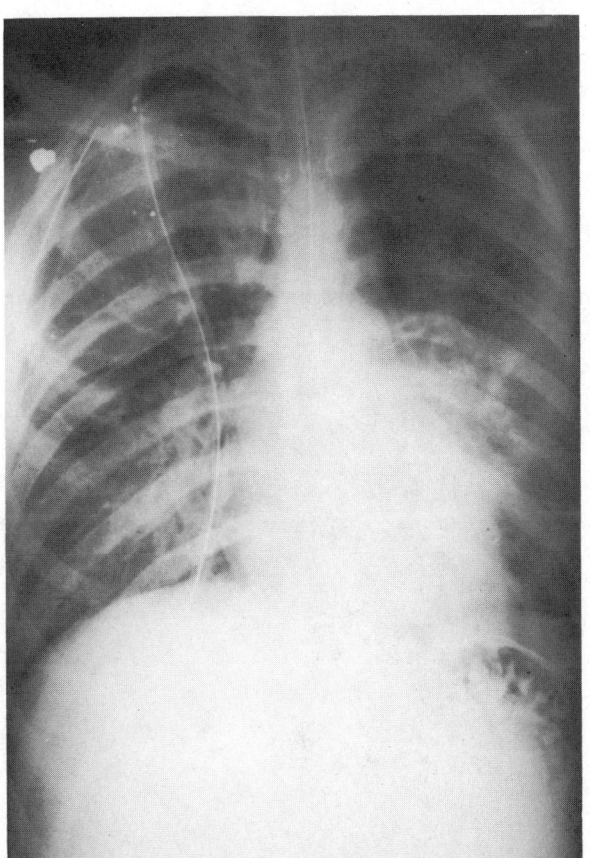

Figure 113–5. Right pulmonary contusion.

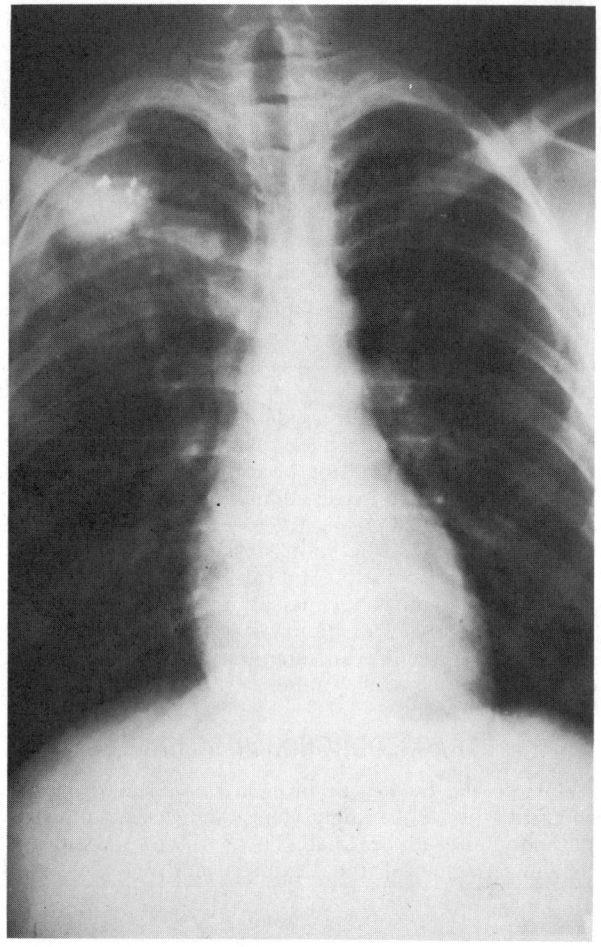

Figure 113–6. Resolving right pulmonary contusion with a small residual in the right upper lobe.

mediastinum in childhood. Most injuries occur close to the carina.

Bronchial injuries usually present with massive tension pneumothorax, subcutaneous emphysema, and hemoptysis.

A continuing massive air leak following chest tube placement signals the presence of this injury. Diagnosis is best determined with bronchoscopy. Bronchography may be needed for distal bronchial tears.

Distal bronchial tears may seal spontaneously and merely require chest tube drainage; more proximal injuries usually require direct repair.[14] Most of these injuries can be repaired electively, but if the air leak is uncontrollable with one or more chest tubes, emergency thoracotomy and repair of the bronchial tear are required. If a distal bronchial tear does not seal with a chest tube, a lobectomy may be needed.[14]

DIAPHRAGMATIC RUPTURE

Rupture of the diaphragm can occur from both penetrating and blunt trauma. Blunt trauma almost always produces rupture of the left diaphragm and creates radial tears that can result in immediate visceral herniation. It is not unusual for a diaphragmatic traumatic rupture to be missed, even for months.[15] Diaphragmatic ruptures should be suspected if the diaphragm, especially the left side, cannot be clearly identified on an initial chest radiograph taken after abdominal or chest trauma (Fig. 113–9). The diagnosis can be confirmed by passing a nasogastric tube and observing the stomach in the left chest. A barium swallow further confirms the injury. Traumatic tears of the diaphragm from either blunt or penetrating trauma should be repaired emergently to prevent respiratory embarrassment and strangulation of the gastrointestinal tract. Early emergent repair is best done through the abdomen to permit exploration for other associated injuries. Late elective repair can be done either through the chest or the abdomen, depending on the preference of the surgeon.

ESOPHAGEAL PERFORATION

Esophageal perforations occur from penetrating and blunt trauma. The most common cause of perforation of the esophagus is from a penetrating injury, usually a gunshot wound. Esophageal perforation secondary to blunt trauma is caused by the sudden passage of gastric contents into the esophagus. This results in a linear tear in the distal esophagus close to the gastroesophageal junction, as seen in adult patients with pernicious, forceful vomiting. Whatever the

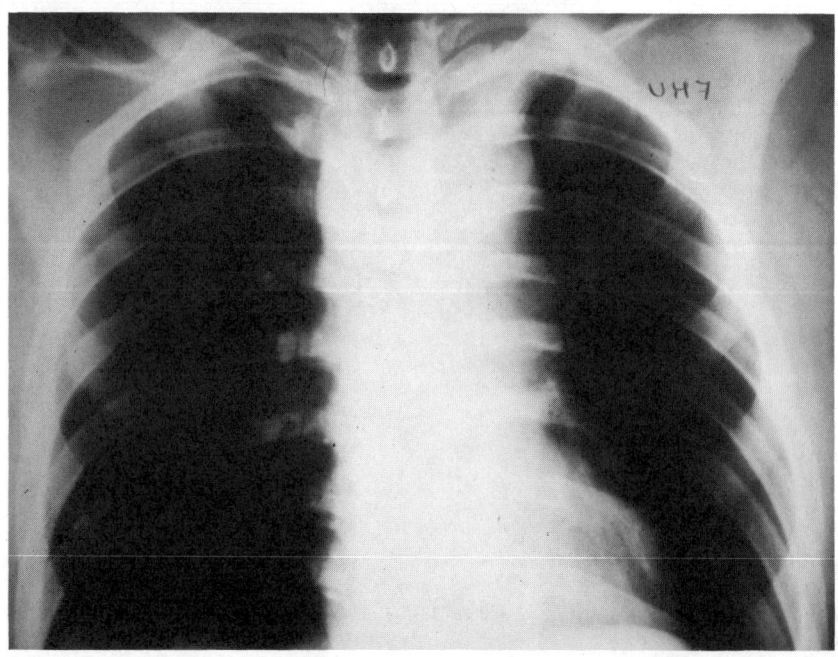

Figure 113–7. Traumatic rupture of the thoracic aorta from a steering wheel injury. Chest radiograph shows a widened mediastinum, obliteration of the aortic knob, and an apical cap of fluid.

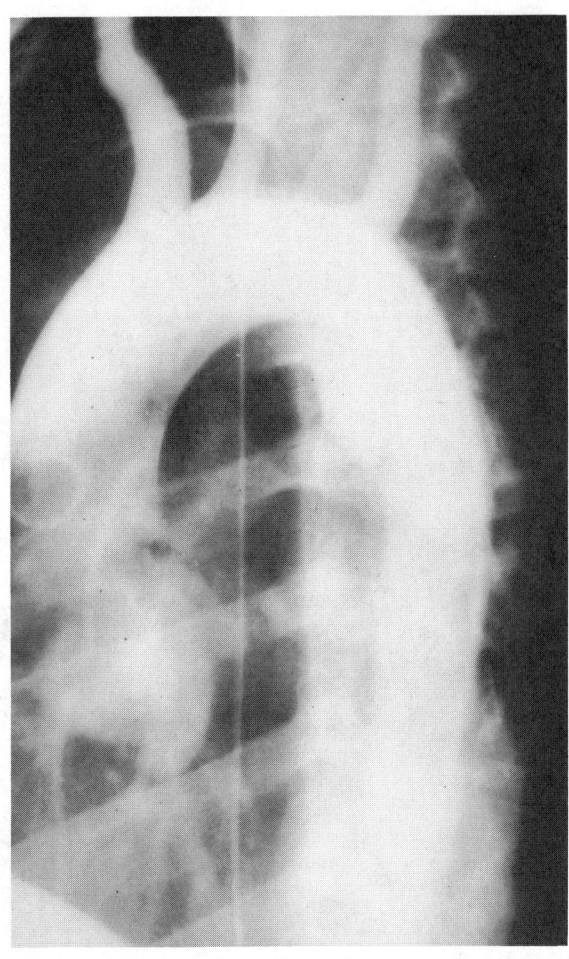

Figure 113–8. Aortogram shows an obvious tear in the aorta at the isthmus.

cause, esophageal perforation results in mediastinitis and spillage of esophageal contents into the pleural space. With distal perforations, rupture usually occurs into the left pleural cavity; with middle esophageal perforations, rupture of esophageal contents occurs in the right pleural cavity. Mediastinal and subcutaneous air should suggest the diagnosis, which can then be confirmed by a water-soluble contrast study showing the site of perforation (Fig. 113–10).

Treatment consists of thoracotomy, on the right for middle esophageal perforations and on the left for distal esoph-

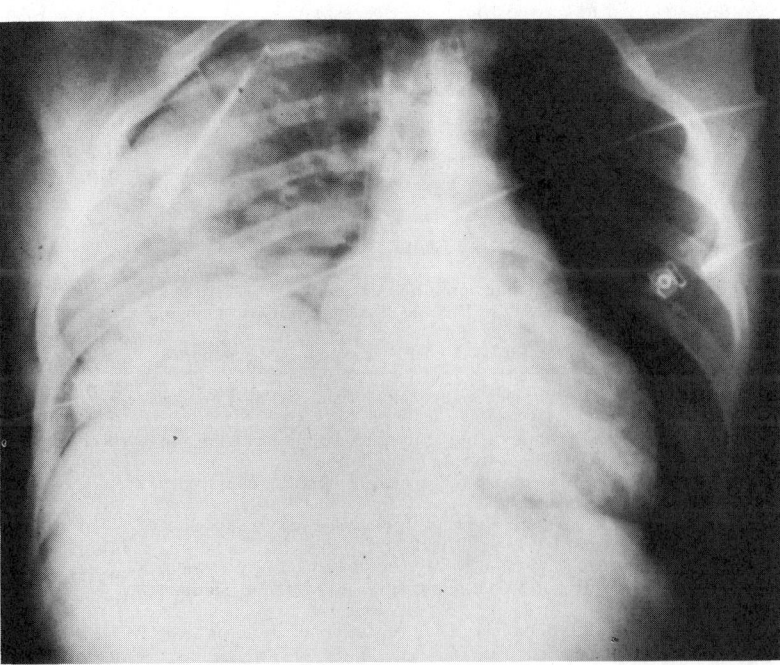

Figure 113–9. Right diaphragmatic rupture from blunt abdominal and thoracic trauma.

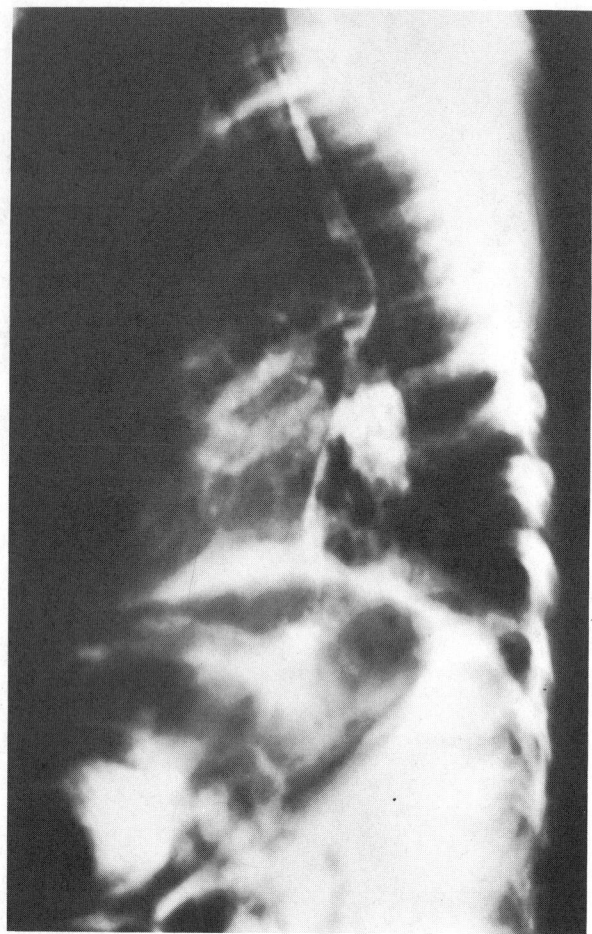

Figure 113–10. Esophageal perforation from blunt abdominal and thoracic trauma. Extravasation of contrast material from the lower esophagus into the right mediastinum is seen.

ageal perforations, with wide drainage of the mediastinum and, if possible, primary repair of the esophagus. If the perforation is extensive and associated with a large amount of devitalized esophageal tissue, then a diverting cervical esophagostomy and gastrostomy are necessary.[4]

References

1. Haller JA, Shermeta DW. Major thoracic trauma in children. Pediatr Clin North Am 1975;22:341.
2. Accident Facts. Chicago, National Safety Council, 1986.
3. Eichelberger MR, Randolph JG: Thoracic trauma in children. Surg Clin North Am 1981;61:1181.
4. Othersen HB. Cardiothoracic injuries. In Touloukian RH (ed). Pediatric Trauma. New York, John Wiley & Sons, 1978, pp 345–354.
5. Cullen P. Treatment of flail chest. Use of intermittent mandatory ventilation and positive end-expiratory pressure. Arch Surg 1975;100:1099.
6. Bodai V, Smith P, Blaisdell WF. The role of emergency thoacotomy in blunt trauma. J Trauma 1982;22:487.
7. Griffith GL, Todd EP, McMillan RD, et al. Acute traumatic hemothorax. Ann Thorac Surg 1978;26:204.
8. Golladay ES, Donaho JS, Haller JA. Special problems of cardiac injuries in infants and children. J Trauma 1979;19:526.
9. Miller FB, Shumate CR, Richardson JD. Myocardial contusion. When can the diagnosis be eliminated? Arch Surg 1989;124:805.
10. Haller JA, Donaho JS. Traumatic asphyxia in children: Pathophysiology and management. J Trauma 1971;11:453.
11. Fulton RL, Peter ET, Wilson JN. The pathophysiology and treatment of pulmonary contusions. J Trauma 1970;10:719.
12. Trinkel JK, Furman RW, Hinshaw MA, et al. Pulmonary contusion, pathogenesis and effect of various resuscitative measures. Ann Thoracic Surg 1973;16:568.
13. Castagna J, Nelson RJ. Blunt injuries to the branches of the aortic arch. J Thorac Cardiovasc Surg 1975;69:521.
14. Kirsch MM, Orringer MB, Behrendt DM, et al. Management of tracheobronchial disruption secondary to nonpenetrating trauma. Ann Thoracic Surg 1976;22:931.
15. McCun RP, Roda CP, Eckert C. Rupture of diaphragm caused by blunt trauma. J Trauma 1976;16:531.

CHAPTER 114

Abdominal Trauma

Arnold G. Coran

INTRODUCTION

Any child sustaining multiple trauma should be suspected of having an intra-abdominal injury. Blunt trauma accounts for 80% of all cases of abdominal trauma; the remaining are due to penetrating injuries, usually from gunshot wounds. Prompt diagnostic evaluation and expeditious operative or nonoperative management of intra-abdominal injuries in children results in low morbidity and mortality.[1–3]

Children differ from adults in their response to trauma, which may make initial evaluation more difficult. For example, a child may become severely depressed and regress developmentally following a major accident. This may make communication with the child difficult during physical examination. Children hyperventilate with stress and develop gastric dilatation. Gastric dilatation can mimic an acute abdomen and can lead to vomiting and aspiration pneumonia. Occasionally, severe gastric dilatation can compress the inferior vena cava and lead to a decrease in venous return and cardiac output. Therefore, a nasogastric tube should be placed to relieve gastric dilatation before examining the abdomen of an injured child.

The mechanisms of injury in children are also different than in adults. Most adults sustain blunt abdominal trauma in motor vehicle accidents, whereas the majority of children are subjected to blunt abdominal trauma from falls and bicycle accidents. In addition, a significant portion of blunt abdominal injuries in young children is secondary to child abuse.

DIAGNOSTIC EVALUATION

Penetrating injuries of the abdomen in childhood are treated with immediate laparotomy for gunshot wounds and selective laparotomy for stab wounds. In a child who has sustained a stab wound to the abdomen, is hemodynamically stable, and shows no signs of peritoneal irritation, careful observation is a reasonable approach. If peritoneal signs develop, immediate laparotomy is indicated.

Blunt abdominal trauma in childhood presents a more complex diagnostic problem. Children who are hemodynamically unstable following blunt abdominal trauma should be taken to the operating room immediately to control hemorrhage. Children who are hemodynamically stable following blunt abdominal trauma require a diagnostic evaluation.

The history is important, as the mechanism of injury provides clues to potential damage. Most children sustaining blunt abdominal trauma also suffer other injuries that may suggest the presence of an intra-abdominal injury. Lower chest trauma with or without rib fractures may suggest a splenic injury when on the left or a liver injury when on the right. In the unconscious child, the abdominal examination is unreliable. In fact, even in the conscious child who is frightened, the physical examination of the abdomen may not be reliable or reproducible. Therefore, further evaluation of the abdomen is necessary. Peritoneal lavage is used in adults who have sustained blunt abdominal trauma to determine the presence of intraperitoneal bleeding. In adults, the presence of blood is an indication for laparotomy. However, in the pediatric age group, hemoperitoneum is not by itself an indication for exploratory laparotomy, as the majority of liver and spleen injuries are managed nonoperatively. For this reason, peritoneal lavage is seldom used in the evaluation of blunt abdominal trauma in children. Instead, the abdominal computed tomography (CT) scan has replaced lavage as the main diagnostic tool. The CT scan will demonstrate injuries to the liver and spleen and indicate whether intraperitoneal fluid is present. The scans are usually done with oral and intravenous contrast and provide excellent evaluation of retroperitoneal structures and most of the gastrointestinal tract.[4–9]

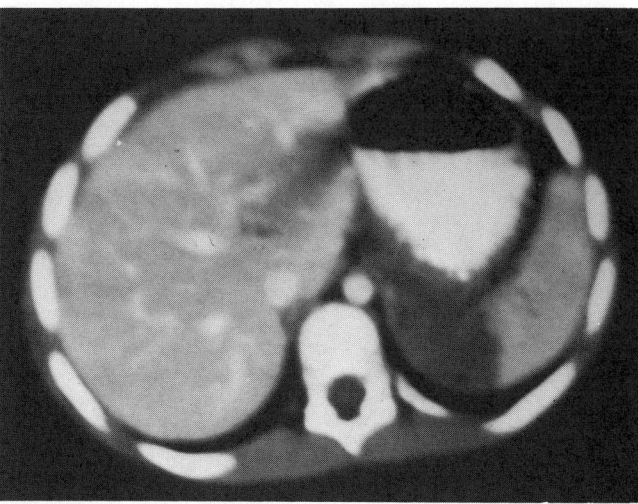

Figure 114–1. Fracture through the lower pole of the spleen from blunt trauma. The darker area represents devascularization of the lower pole of the spleen.

INJURIES TO THE SPLEEN

The spleen is the most commonly injured abdominal organ in children.[10, 11] Splenic injury usually results from a direct blow to the left upper quadrant of the abdomen or the left lower chest. Often there are ecchymoses over the left upper quadrant of the abdomen. Blood released from the splenic fracture may irritate the left diaphragm and cause shoulder pain. Rib fractures can occur with splenic injury in children but are much less frequent than in adults. Simultaneous injury to the left kidney is common and may present as microscopic or gross hematuria. The hemodynamically unstable child with a splenic injury should be taken to the operating room immediately to control hemorrhage. However, it is unusual for a child with an isolated splenic injury to be hemodynamically unstable after initial resuscitation. At our institution, which has a large volume of pediatric trauma, we have not seen a child with hemodynamic instability after initial resuscitation from an isolated splenic fracture since 1980. The hemodynamically stable child is evaluated with a CT scan, which is the most definitive diagnostic tool for delineating the splenic injury and for demonstrating the presence of blood in the peritoneal cavity (Fig. 114–1). Once the CT scan is completed, the child is admitted to a pediatric intensive care unit (ICU) with a nasogastric tube and Foley catheter in place and two intravenous lines in the upper extremities. The child is monitored closely and followed with serial hematocrit determinations until the abdominal tenderness is gone, which usually takes 2 to 4 days. It is extremely rare for splenic hemorrhage to occur after initial resuscitation and stability in the ICU. The child is then transferred to the floor and discharged on the seventh postinjury day. The nasogastric tube is removed once the ileus has resolved and feedings are started. Blood transfusions are given only for evidence of mild to moderate hemodynamic instability such as the development of tachycardia. Children tolerate a hematocrit level of 20% to 25% without much disability. Patients are usually not transfused unless the hematocrit falls below 20%. This is especially important in view of the present anxiety regarding transfusion-induced HIV infection and hepatitis. Following discharge from the hospital, moderate restriction on physical activity is maintained for about 2 months. At that time, a repeat CT scan is obtained to visualize complete resolution of the splenic injury.

Attempts should be made to preserve the spleen, either with suturing techniques or partial splenectomy. The radial and segmental blood supply to the spleen permits this type of surgical approach. One study has shown that the blood requirements for the operative management of splenic injuries are greater than those for the nonoperative management.[12]

The reason for this approach to splenic injury is the risk of postsplenectomy sepsis and death.[13, 14] The incidence of postsplenectomy sepsis is approximately 1% following splenectomy for trauma.[14, 15] *Pneumococcus* is the most common organism responsible but this syndrome can also be caused by infection with *Haemophilus influenzae* and meningococci. To reduce the incidence of this syndrome, all children undergoing splenectomy receive a polyvalent pneumococcal vaccine and the vaccine against *H. influenzae*.[16] In addition to vaccination, most children are kept on lifelong oral penicillin prophylaxis, although compliance may be imperfect with this approach. Clinical and experimental data have suggested that splenic autotransplantation may be helpful in diminishing the incidence of postsplenectomy sepsis; however, the available data are not convincing.[17–19]

INJURIES TO THE LIVER

After the spleen, the liver is the second most common intra-abdominal organ injured secondary to abdominal trauma. Most blunt injuries to the liver stop bleeding spontaneously without any significant hemodynamic instability. Nevertheless, liver injury can sometimes be the source of exsanguinating hemorrhage.[20–22]

Because of the large size of the liver within the abdominal cavity, penetrating injuries such as gunshot wounds result in a significant incidence of liver parenchymal injuries. Children with penetrating injuries to the liver should undergo emergency laparotomy.

There is often a history of a direct blow to the right upper quadrant of the abdomen or the lower right chest. There may be associated lower rib fractures on that side and evidence of injury to the right kidney with microscopic or gross hematuria. Children who present with blunt injuries to the liver and are hemodynamically unstable should undergo immediate laparotomy. However, most children suffering blunt injuries to the liver are usually hemodynamically stable and can be further evaluated before deciding

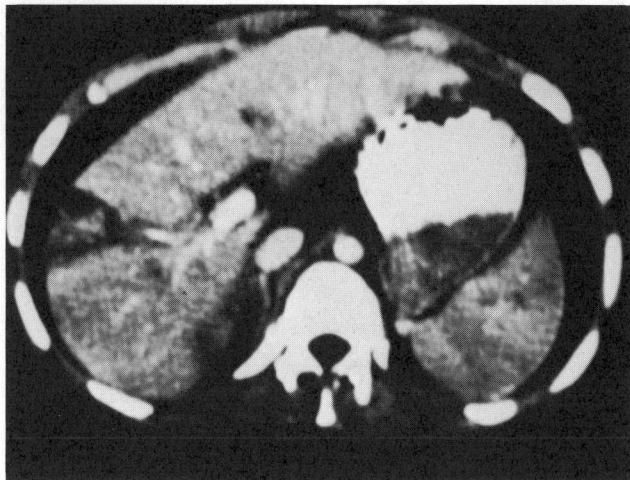

Figure 114–2. Fracture through the lateral border of the right lobe of the liver.

on therapy. The evaluation and management for a blunt liver injury are the same as those used for the hemodynamically stable child with a blunt splenic injury. Evaluation is performed with an abdominal CT scan using both oral and intravenous contrast.[7] The CT scan provides excellent anatomic detail of the liver injury and can be the sole diagnostic tool. In addition, fluid in the peritoneal cavity can be easily visualized with the CT scan (Fig. 114–2).

Although hemorrhage from severe liver injury is the most common cause of death attributable to intra-abdominal injury, the actual incidence of this type of hemorrhage is quite low, in both the pediatric and the adult population. In the past, it was not unusual to perform exploration for a liver injury, only to find that the bleeding had ceased at the time of laparotomy. Therefore, a conservative, nonoperative approach to liver injuries in children has been taken by most pediatric surgeons.[20, 23–26] However, there are still many who feel that the presence of hemoperitoneum with a liver injury is an indication for laparotomy.[27–31]

Once the decision for nonoperative management of the liver injury has been made, the child is admitted to the pediatric ICU, a nasogastric tube is placed, and two intravenous lines are started in the upper extremities. The child is observed for 24 to 48 hours. The patient is followed with serial hematocrit determinations and is discharged from the ICU to the floor when the abdominal tenderness and intestinal ileus have resolved. At that point, the nasogastric tube is removed, and feedings are started. The child is discharged from the hospital on the seventh postinjury day and kept on restricted activity for about 2 months. After 2 months, a CT scan is obtained to visualize resolution of the liver injury.

About 5% of children with blunt liver injuries suffer from exsanguinating hemorrhage with severe hemodynamic instability and require emergency laparotomy. In almost all of these cases, there is a significant liver injury associated with a tear in the retrohepatic vena cava or in a major hepatic vein. Surgical management of these children usually requires a major liver resection or even a formal lobectomy along with repair of the venous injury. These cases have an operative mortality rate as high as 50%.[27–29]

Late complications can occur from both the nonoperative and operative management of liver injuries in children and include bile peritonitis, extrahepatic biliary obstruction, and hemobilia.[20] Although the nonoperative approach to liver injury has been mainly adapted to the pediatric age group, there are several reports indicating the success of this approach in adults with liver injuries.[8, 12, 32, 33]

INJURY TO THE PANCREAS AND DUODENUM

Blunt trauma is more often the cause of pancreatic injury than penetrating trauma. Unlike liver and spleen injuries occurring after blunt abdominal trauma, the pancreas is injured in only 10% of patients of all age groups.[34] Blunt upper abdominal trauma can cause compression of the pancreas against the vertebral column at the junction of the body and tail. This is the usual mechanism of pancreatic injury from blunt abdominal trauma and can result in parenchymal disruption or, when more severe, disruption of the pancreatic duct.[35] The injury is usually caused by falls, bicycle handlebar injuries, child abuse, or motor vehicle accidents.

The CT scan is the primary diagnostic tool used to evaluate pancreatic injury. The scan is useful in detecting pancreatic edema secondary to trauma and in demonstrating fractures of the pancreas and fluid in the lesser sack resulting from traumatic pancreatitis. The false-negative rate for CT scans used to detect pancreatic trauma is less than 1%.[36] Ultrasonography is also useful in evaluating pancreatic trauma, although it is not as accurate in evaluating injuries to the liver and spleen.[37] Endoscopic retrograde cholangeopancreatography is not indicated for acute pancreatic injury. It is useful for evaluation of a persistent pseudocyst to determine whether a ductal injury is present. The serum amylase level is usually elevated in traumatic pancreatitis. However, elevated levels must be interrupted with caution, as other intra-abdominal injuries can also elevate serum amylase.[38]

The management of traumatic pancreatitis consists of nasogastric decompression of the stomach and intravenous nutrition. This is usually required for 1 to 2 weeks. Feedings can be started once the pancreatitis has resolved, as evidenced by decreased edema on CT scan or ultrasound, a return of the serum amylase to normal, and resolution of the intestinal ileus. The most common complication of pancreatitis is the formation of a pancreatic pseudocyst, which can occur with or without pancreatic duct disruption (Fig. 114–3). Most pseudocysts that develop following traumatic pancreatitis usually resolve spontaneously, unless the duct is disrupted. Many pseudocysts that do not disappear spontaneously can be drained percutaneously under CT or ultrasound guidance.[39–41]

Pancreatic duct disruption is quite rare in children and is seldom discovered at the time of the acute injury. If exploration is being performed for abdominal trauma and a

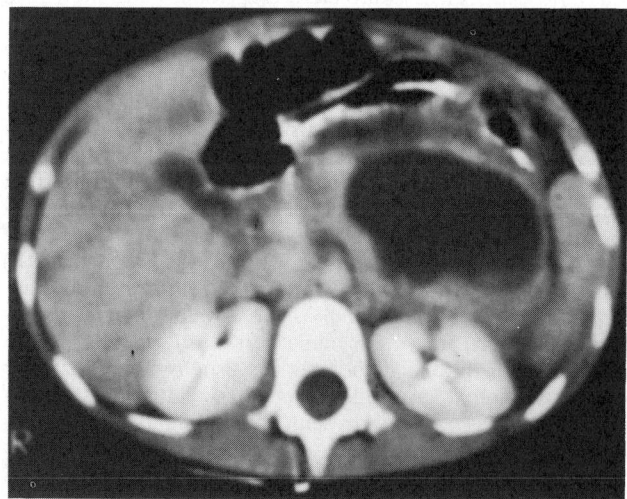

Figure 114–3. CT scan showing a large pseudocyst of the pancreas (*dark round area*).

transection of the pancreas and pancreatic duct is found between the body and tail of the gland, then this lesion is best managed by a distal pancreatectomy with ligation of the duct. If the patient is stable during the operation, then the spleen should be preserved, but in an unstable patient, the distal pancreatectomy should be combined with a splenectomy to expedite the procedure.[42]

Injury to the pancreatic head associated with perforation of the duodenum is extremely rare in children, occurring in less than 5% of cases of blunt pancreatic trauma.[39, 42–45] When the duodenal perforation and the pancreatic head injury are the result of blunt trauma, the best surgical approach is a duodenal diverticularization procedure.[46, 47] This involves closure of the duodenal perforation with effective drainage of the duodenum, usually through a duodenostomy tube, and closure of the gastric duodenal junction at the pylorus with bypass of the duodenum using a gastrojejunostomy. Severe rupture of the duodenum, usually from blunt trauma, without an associated pancreatic head injury should also be managed by duodenal diverticularization. Most duodenal perforations can be managed with simple primary closure, but occasionally, resection with primary anastomosis is required.[48–50]

Uncommon complications seen following operative and nonoperative management of pancreatic trauma include a persistent pancreatic fistula to the skin and a pancreatic abscess. A pancreatic fistula usually occurs following placement of a drain during the acute operative management of a pancreatic injury. Most pancreaticocutaneous fistulas close spontaneously with bowel rest and intravenous nutrition. Pancreatic abscesses usually require operative drainage with the placement of large drains.[51, 52]

The only other duodenal injury seen with abdominal trauma is intramural duodenal hematoma, which usually follows blunt trauma to the epigastrium. The fixed retroperitoneal location of the second portion of the duodenum allows a significant shearing force to tear the submucosal vessels, which results in the formation of a large intramural hematoma. This hematoma then compresses the duodenum and leads to upper intestinal obstruction with bilious vomiting and gastric dilatation. The hematoma is diagnosed by an upper gastrointestinal contrast study, which typically shows a coiled spring or a string sign in the second portion of the duodenum (Fig. 114–4). These hematomas are managed nonoperatively with nasogastric decompression and intravenous nutrition for 10 days to 3 weeks.[53, 54]

INJURIES TO THE GASTROINTESTINAL TRACT

Injury to the gastrointestinal tract is relatively common with penetrating abdominal trauma but rare with blunt trauma, occurring in less than 5% of blunt abdominal injuries in children.[20, 55] The low incidence of intestinal injuries secondary to blunt abdominal trauma in children contrasts with an incidence of up to 15% reported in adults.[56, 57] Because of this low incidence of intestinal injury with blunt abdominal trauma in children, the CT scan of the abdomen is still an excellent diagnostic tool for evaluating blunt abdominal trauma in children, although the CT scan can miss some intestinal perforations.

History and physical examination are usually not helpful in detecting an intestinal perforation following blunt abdominal trauma in the child. Likewise, there are no specific laboratory tests that are helpful in making the diagnosis. Although CT scanning is not as accurate in detecting hollow visceral injuries as in evaluating solid visceral injuries, the use of oral contrast significantly increases the accuracy rate for detecting intestinal perforation.[58–62] If CT evaluation is combined with periodic examination of the child's abdomen,

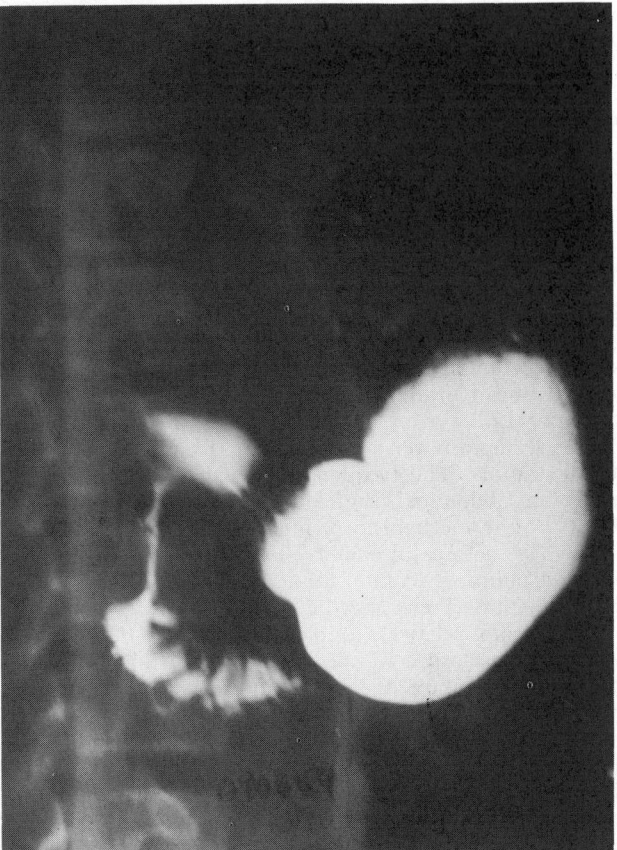

Figure 114–4. Traumatic duodenal hematoma. Note the string-like appearance of the second portion of the duodenum.

the risk of missing an intestinal perforation is significantly minimized.

When the physical findings are equivocal, a water-soluble contrast study of the gastrointestinal tract or diagnostic peritoneal lavage may be performed. A lavage is positive for intestinal perforation when more than 500 white blood cells per milliliter are present together with stool, bile, or bacteria.[63, 64]

Penetrating injuries to the abdomen in children are managed the same as those in adults; all gunshot wounds are explored and stab wounds are selectively explored. The controversy involves the management of blunt abdominal trauma with potential injuries to the gastrointestinal tract in children. Often the intestinal perforation is not obvious on initial examination and may not become apparent clinically until 48 to 72 hours after the injury, when the child develops an unexplained fever, an ileus, and an increase in abdominal pain. Frequently, pneumoperitoneum is not seen on repeated abdominal films, and even a water-soluble gastrointestinal study does not demonstrate the perforation. In this circumstance, a diagnostic peritoneal lavage may be helpful in diagnosing an intestinal perforation.

Stomach

Injury to the stomach from penetrating or blunt abdominal trauma is rare but is more common in children than in adults. Rupture following blunt trauma is usually caused by forceful compression of a dilated stomach.[65] This typically occurs following a meal, when the stomach is full and the child hits the handlebar of a bicycle with the upper abdomen. With a competent gastroesophageal sphincter and a closed pylorus, this compression can lead to gastric perforation. In penetrating trauma, the incidence of gastric perforation ranges from 7% to 13%[66-69]; in blunt abdominal trauma, the incidence is less than 2%.[70, 71] Gastric perforation is usually associated with bloody nasogastric drainage and the presence of free air on a plain upright radiograph of the abdomen. With blunt trauma, perforation usually occurs along the greater curvature.[72] Management consists of primary closure of the wound following debridement of the edges.

Small Intestine

Small bowel perforation secondary to penetrating trauma is more common than perforation of the stomach or the colon, with an incidence as high as 30% in adults.[69] This incidence is lower in children (18%).[68] Blunt abdominal trauma leads to fewer small bowel perforations than penetrating trauma. The frequency of small bowel perforation with blunt abdominal trauma in adults ranges from 9% to 25%.[69, 72] The mechanism of injury with blunt trauma appears to be a forceful compression of a distended loop of bowel at points of fixation to the retroperitoneum, such as the ligament of Treitz and the cecum.[73]

Treatment is relatively simple and consists of debridement and primary closure of the injury. If the injury involves more than one third of the circumference of the bowel or involves a mesenteric vascular injury, then a bowel resection and primary anastomosis are required. The morbidity rate following repair is low, provided there has not been a significant delay in diagnosis. There may be a significant injury to the superior mesenteric artery requiring primary vascular repair in addition to repair of the intestinal injury. Complete stripping of an extensive portion of the small bowel mesentery can occur with severe blunt trauma; this injury requires a massive bowel resection. Short bowel syndrome can result from this type of resection.

Colon

The incidence of colon injuries in children and adults is less than that of small bowel injuries. Blaisdell reported an incidence of between 4% and 9% in adults.[69] The incidence in children appears to be the same with both blunt and penetrating trauma.[74] Because of the low incidence of these injuries, perforation of the colon may be missed when CT scanning is the sole diagnostic tool used for the evaluation of blunt abdominal trauma.[75]

The management of colon injuries is controversial, ranging from primary repair to diverting colostomy.[76-81] Some surveys have suggested that morbidity is less with primary repair than with colostomy.[78-81] However, a severely injured patient who is unstable will have a lower morbidity and mortality with a diverting colostomy.[82, 83]

Anorectum

Most anorectal injuries result from direct blunt trauma or sexual abuse. The child with this type of injury is extremely frightened and difficult to examine. Therefore, most of these children are evaluated under anesthesia so that a proper digital examination, sigmoidoscopy, or vaginoscopy can be performed.[84]

Mucosal or partial-thickness injury to the rectal wall can be treated with primary repair following rectal cleansing. Full-thickness perforation is managed by direct repair, rectal cleansing, and proximal diverting colostomy. With extensive injuries, presacral drains should be placed.[85-87]

PELVIC FRACTURE

Fracture of the pelvis following blunt abdominal trauma can mimic a solid or hollow visceral injury in a child. Significant retroperitoneal bleeding occurs with this injury.[88, 89] Palpation of the pelvis can result in significant pain when a fracture is present, and a hematoma may be present in the labia or scrotum. Urethral injury is not infrequent with this type of fracture and is suggested by the presence of blood at the urethral meatus. A retrograde urethrogram is indicated to evaluate this injury. Pelvic fractures in children carry a low morbidity and mortality and are treated with bed rest and blood replacement.[89]

References

1. Holmes MJ, Reyes HM. A critical review of urban pediatric trauma. J Trauma 1984;24:253.
2. Mayer T, Matlak ME, Johnson DG, et al. The modified injury severity scale in pediatric multiple trauma patients. J Pediatr Surg 1980;15:719.
3. Wilt EM, Adkins RB. A ten-year experience with blunt trauma to the abdomen in children. Am Surg 1982;48:114.
4. Federle MP. Abdominal trauma: The role and impact of computed tomography. Invest Radiol 1981;16:260.
5. Federle MP, Crass RA, Jeffrey RB, Trunkey DD. Computed tomography in blunt abdominal trauma. Arch Surg 1982;117:645.
6. Jeffrey RB, Laing FC, Federle MP, Goodman PC. Computed tomography of splenic trauma. Radiology 1981;41:729.
7. Karp MP, Cooney DR, Berger PE, et al. The role of computed tomography in the evaluation of blunt abdominal trauma in children. J Pediatr Surg 1981;16:316.
8. Meredith JW, Trunkey DD. CT scanning in acute abdominal injuries. Surg Clin North Am 1988;68:255.
9. Toombs BD, Lester RG, Ben-Menachem Y, Sandler CM. Computed tomography in blunt trauma. Radiol Clin North Am 1981;19:17.
10. Drew R, Perry JF Jr, Fischer RP. The expediency of peritoneal lavage for blunt trauma in children. Surg Gynecol Obstet 1977;145:885.
11. Powell RW, Smith DE, Zarins CK, et al. Peritoneal lavage in children with blunt abdominal trauma. J Pediatr Surg 1976;11:973.
12. Delius RE, Frankel W, Coran AG. A comparison between operative and nonoperative management of adult and pediatric patients with blunt injuries to the liver and spleen. Surgery 1989;106:788.
13. King H, Shumacker HB. Splenic studies: Susceptibility to infection after splenectomy performed in infancy. Ann Surg 1952;136:239.
14. Singer DB. Postsplenectomy sepsis. In Rosenberg HS, Bolande RP (eds). Perspectives in Pediatric Pathology. Vol 1. Chicago, Year Book, 1973; pp 285–311.
15. Luna GK, Dellinger P. Nonoperative observation therapy for splenic injuries: A safe therapeutic option? Am J Surg 1987;153:462.
16. Appelbaum PC, Shaikh BS, Widome MD, et al. Fatal pneumococcal bacteremia in a vaccinated, splenectomized child. N Engl J Med 1979;300:203.
17. Pabst R, Kamran D. Autotransplantation of splenic tissue. J Pediatr Surg 1986;21:120.
18. Patel J, Williams JS, Shmigel B, Hinshaw JR. Preservation of splenic function by autotransplantation of traumatized spleen in man. Surgery 1981;39:683.
19. Traub A, Giebink GS, Smith C, et al. Splenic reticuloendothelial function after splenectomy, spleen repair, and spleen autotransplantation. N Engl J Med 1987;317:1559.
20. Oldham KT, Guice KS, Ryckman F, et al. Blunt liver injury in childhood: Evolution of therapy and current perspective. Surgery 1986;100:542.
21. Stone HH, Ansley JD. Management of liver trauma in children. J Pediatr Surg 1977;12:3.
22. Suson EM, Klotz D Jr, Kottmeier PK. Liver trauma in children. J Pediatr Surg 1975;10:411.
23. Cywes S, Rode H, Millar AJW. Blunt liver trauma in children: Nonoperative management. J Pediatr Surg 1985;20:14.
24. Giacomantonio M, Filler RM, Rich RH. Blunt hepatic trauma in children: Experience with operative and nonoperative management. J Pediatr Surg 1984;19:519.
25. Grisoni ER, Gauderer ML, Ferron J, Izant RJ. Nonoperative management of liver injuries following blunt abdominal trauma in children. J Pediatr Surg 1984;19:515.
26. Karp MP, Cooney DR, Pros GA, et al. The nonoperative management of pediatric hepatic trauma. J Pediatr Surg 1983;18:512.
27. Cogbil TH, Moore EE, Jurkovich GJ, et al. Severe hepatic trauma: A multi-center experience with 1,335 liver injuries. J Trauma 1988;28:1433.
28. Defore WW, Mattox KL, Jordan GL, Beall AC. Management of 1,590 consecutive cases of liver trauma. Arch Surg 1976;111:493.

29. Douglas RG, Holdaway CM, Shaw JH. Hepatic trauma in Auckland. Aust NZ J Surg 1988;58:307.
30. Feliciano DV, Mattox KL, Jordan GL, et al. Management of 1,000 consecutive cases of hepatic trauma (1979–1984). Ann Surg 1986;204:438.
31. Trunkey DD, Shires GT, McClelland R. Management of liver trauma in 811 consecutive patients. Ann Surg 1974;179:722.
32. Athey GN, Rahman SU. Hepatic hematoma following blunt injury: Non-operative management. Br J Accident Surgery 1986;13:302.
33. Farnell MB, Spencer MP, Thompson E, et al. Nonoperative management of blunt hepatic trauma in adults. Surgery 1988;104:748.
34. Nance FC. Management of injuries to the stomach, duodenum and pancreas. *In* Worth MH Jr (ed). Principles and Practice of Trauma Care. Baltimore, Williams & Wilkins, 1982.
35. Stone HH, Fabian TC, Satiani B, Turkleson M. Experiences in the management of pancreatic trauma. J Trauma 1981;21:257.
36. Jeffrey RB, Federle MP, Crass RA. Computed tomography in pancreatic trauma. Radiology 1983;147:491.
37. Gorenstein A, O'Halpin D, Wesson D, et al. Blunt injury to the pancreas in children: Selective management based on ultrasound. J Ped Surg 1987;22:1110.
38. Moretz JA, Campbell DP, Parker DE, et al. Significance of serum amylase level in evaluating pancreatic trauma. Am J Surg 1975;130:739.
39. Bass J, Dilorenz M, Desjardi M, et al. Blunt pancreatic injury in children— the role of percutaneous external drainage in the treatment of pancreatic pseudocysts. J Ped Surg 1988;23:721.
40. Windle R, Finlay D, Neoptolemos JP. Needle aspiration in the treatment of pancreatic pseudocyst in childhood. Ann R Coll Surg Engl 1983;65:331.
41. Arata JA, Jaffe ME, Matlak ME. Percutaneous drainage of traumatic pancreatic pseudocysts in childhood. AJR 1989;152:591.
42. Graham JM, Pokorny WJ, Mattox K, Jordon G. Surgical management of acute pancreatic injuries in children. J Pediatr Surg 1978;13:178.
43. Salonen IS, Aarnio P. Treatment of acute pancreatic injuries in childhood. Ann Chir Gynaecol 1985;74:167.
44. Grosfeld JL, Conney DR. Pancreactic and gastrointestinal trauma in children. Pediatr Clin North Am 1975;22:365.
45. Meier D, Gravier L, Votteler T, Coln D. Blunt trauma to the pancreas in children. South Med J 1978;71:895.
46. Berne CJ, Donovan AJ, White E. Duodenal diverticularization for duo- denal and pancreatic injury. Am J Surg 1974;127:503.
47. Vaughan GD, Frazier OH, Graham D, et al. The use of pyloric exclusion in the management of severe duodenal injuries. Am J Surg 1977;134:785.
48. Kashuk JL, Moore EE, Cogbill TH. Management of the intermediate severity duodenal injury. Surgery 1982;92:758.
49. Kelly G, Norton L, Moore G, et al. The continuing challenge of duodenal injuries. J Trauma 1978;18:160.
50. Stone HH, Fabian TC. Management of duodenal wounds. J Trauma 1979;19:334.
51. Owens BJ III, Hamit HF. Pancreatic abscess and pseudocyst. Arch Surg 1977;112:42.
52. Brandley EL III, Fulenwider JT. Open treatment of pancreatic abscess. Surg Gynecol Obstet 1984;159:509.
53. Holgersen LO, Bishop HC. Nonoperative treatment of duodenal hema- tomata in childhood. J Pediatr Surg 1977;12:11.
54. Touloukian RJ. Protocol for the nonoperative treatment of obstructing intramural duodenal hematoma during childhood. Am J Surg 1983;145:330.
55. Cywes S. Pediatric trauma in other countries. Proceedings of the Third National Conference on Pediatric Trauma. Coran AG, Harris BH (eds.): JB Lippincott, Philadelphia, 1990.
56. Cox EF. Blunt abdominal trauma: A 5-year analysis of 870 patients requiring celiotomy. Ann Surg 1984;199:467.
57. Dauterive AH, Flancbaum L, Cox EF. Blunt intestinal trauma: A modern- day review. Ann Surg 1985;201:198.
58. Peitzman AB, Makaroun MS, Slasky S, et al. Prospective study of com- puter tomography in initial management of blunt abdominal trauma. J Trauma 1986;26:585.
59. Kane NM, Cronan JJ, Dorfman GS, et al. Pediatric abdominal trauma: Evaluation by computed tomography. Pediatrics 1988;82:11.
60. Cook DE, Walsh JW, Vick CW, et al. Upper abdominal trauma: Pitfalls in CT diagnosis. Radiology 1986;159:65.
61. Donohue JH, Federle MP, Griffiths BG, et al. Computed tomography in the diagnosis of blunt intestinal and mesenteric injuries. J Trauma 1987;27:11.
62. Trunkey D, Federle MP. Computed tomography in perspective. J Trauma 1986;26:660.
63. Powell RW, Green JB, Ochsner MG, et al. Peritoneal lavage in pediatric patients sustaining blunt abdominal trauma: A reappraisal. J Trauma 1987;27:6.
64. Rothenberg S, Moore EE, Marx JA, et al. Selective management of blunt abdominal trauma in children—the triage role of peritoneal lavage. J Trauma 1987;27:1101.
65. Siemens RA, Fulton RL. Gastric rupture as a result of blunt trauma. Am Surg 1977;43:229.
66. Sinclair MC, Moore TC. Major surgery for abdominal and thoracic trauma in childhood and adolescence. J Pediatr Surg 1974;9:155.
67. Tunell WP, Knost J, Nance FC. Penetrating abdominal injuries in children and adolescents. J Trauma 1975;15:720.
68. Long JA, Philippart AI. Penetrating injuries in children. *In* Buntain WL (ed). Management of Pediatric Trauma. Philadelphia, WB Saunders, in press.
69. Blaisdell FW. General assessment, resuscitation and exploration of pen- etrating and blunt abdominal injury. *In* Trauma Management. Vol 1. Abdominal trauma. New York, Thieme-Stratton, 1982.
70. Pachter HL, Hofstetter SR. Open and percutaneous paracentesis and lavage for abdominal trauma. Arch Surg 1981;116:318.
71. Yajko RD, Seydel F, Trimble C. Rupture of the stomach from blunt abdominal trauma. J Trauma 1975;15:178.
72. Fischer RP, Miller-Crotchett P, Reed RL. Gastrointestinal disruption: The hazard of nonoperative management in adults with blunt abdominal injury. J Trauma 1988;28:1445.
73. Schenk WG, Lonchyna V, Moylan JA. Perforation of the jejunum from blunt abdominal trauma. J Trauma 1983;23:54.
74. Welch KJ. Abdominal injuries. *In* The Injured Child. Chicago, Year Book, 1979, p 155.
75. Kuhn JP. Diagnostic imaging for the evaluation of abdominal trauma in children. Pediatr Clin North Am 1985;32:1327.
76. Slim MS, Makaroun M, Shammai AR. Primary repair of colorectal injuries in childhood. J Pediatr Surg 1981;16:1008.
77. Thompson JS, Moore EE, Moore JB. Comparison of penetrating injuries of the right and left colon. Ann Surg 1981;193:414.
78. Stone HH, Fabian TC. Management of perforating colon trauma. Ann Surg 1979;190:431.
79. Burch JM, Gevirtzman BS, Jordan GL, et al. The injured colon. Ann Surg 1986;203:701.
80. Flint LM, Vitale GC, Richardson JD, et al. The injured colon. Ann Surg 1981;193:619.
81. Thompson JS, Moore EE, Moore JB. Comparison of penetrating injuries of the right and left colon. Ann Surg 1981;193:414.
82. Adkins RB, Zinkle PK, Waterhause G. Penetrating colon trauma. J Trauma 1984;24:491.
83. Cook A, Levine BA, Rusing T, et al. Traditional treatment of colon injuries. Arch Surg 1984;119:591.
84. Black CT, Pokorny WJ, McGill CW, et al. Ano-rectal trauma in children. J Pediatr Surg 1982;17:501.
85. Trunkey D, Hays RJ, Shires GT. Management of rectal trauma. J Trauma 1973;13:411.
86. Tuggle D, Huber PJ. Management of rectal trauma. Am J Surg 1984;148:806.
87. Robertson HD, Ray JE, Ferrari BT, et al. Management of rectal trauma. Surg Gynecol Obstet 1982;154:161.
88. Garcia V, Eichelberger MR, Ziegler M, et al. Use of military antishock trouser in a child. J Pediatr Surg 1981;16:544.
89. Reichard SA, Helikson MA, Shorter N, et al. Pelvic fractures in children— review of 120 patients with a new look at general management. J Pediatr Surg 1980;15:727.

CHAPTER 115

Genitourinary Trauma

Craig Marsden
Kenneth Jackimczyk

ANATOMIC CONSIDERATIONS

The increased relative frequency of genitourinary trauma in children compared with that in adults is explained by differences in the child's anatomy. The kidney, ureter, and bladder are disproportionately larger in children and have a more intraabdominal location that is unprotected by the bony pelvis and thorax. The kidney has less perinephric fat, and the abdominal musculature is less well developed. Fetal lobulation may persist in the kidney, making it more susceptible to blunt trauma. The thoracolumbar spine is more flexible in children, and extreme flexion, even without fracture, may result in the ureter stretching past its elastic limits, causing disruption.

Congenital abnormalities may increase the risk of injury, and there is a 10% incidence of preexisting anatomic abnormality present in children who sustain renal damage. Congenital abnormalities such as ureteropelvic obstruction, duplication of the upper collecting systems, cysts, and Wilms's tumors may predispose a child to injury and be first discovered at the time of trauma.

Renal Anatomy

The kidney is divided into four parts—parenchyma, capsule, collecting system, and major vessels—and is surrounded by Gerota's fascia and perirenal fat. Gerota's fascia can tamponade bleeding after capsule disruption. In children, this space is small, and therefore significant bleeding in this area is less likely.

There are three muscular borders about the kidney. The diaphragm lies superiorly. The psoas and quadratus lumborum muscles lie posteriorly and laterally, and the latissimus dorsi and serratus muscles lie posterior and inferiorly. The muscular and fascial protection for the kidney, however, is less developed in children than adults. Because the kidney is less fixed to the retroperitoneal structures, it is more mobile and more likely to sustain damage to the vascular pedicle.

Ureteral Anatomy

The ureters are mobile, sheathed tubes that run from the renal pelvis to the bladder. Congenital abnormalities such as a single ureter or duplicated ureters may be present. Blunt trauma usually causes injury at regions where mobile and fixed portions of the ureter meet, such as the ureteropelvic junction.

Bladder Anatomy

In children, the bladder is located more anteriorly and is almost completely intraabdominal. This makes the bladder more vulnerable to rupture from blunt trauma, with rupture usually occurring at the bladder dome. Infants also have a more broad area of peritonealization, and therefore, intraperitoneal rupture is more common in young children.

Urethral Anatomy

The urethra is divided into anterior and posterior sections. The posterior portion runs from the bladder neck to the inferior edge of the urogenital diaphragm. The anterior division begins at the inferior edge of the urogenital diaphragm and terminates at the external urinary meatus (Fig. 115–1). The urogenital diaphragm is a muscular and ligamentous structure attached anteriorly to the pubic arch and posteriorly to the transversus perinei muscle.

The bladder neck in males and the vaginal septum and bladder neck in females are points of relatively rigid fixation and can be avulsed or ruptured in blunt lower abdominal trauma. The suspensory ligament in males is also prone to injury with pelvic fractures.

CLINICAL EVALUATION
History

An accurate history will aid in the efficient radiographic evaluation of trauma. Blunt deceleration injuries from motor vehicle accidents, falls, or sports activities are common. Penetrating genitourinary injuries from gunshot or stab wounds are less common in children. Nevertheless, a gunshot injury, stab wound, or surgical procedure may result in penetrating trauma.

The location and pattern of pain should be determined. Colicky abdominal pain or flank pain is a possible indicator of genitourinary damage, but the pain is often nonspecific. It is important to realize that the patient with multiple trauma or altered mental status may not be able to localize pain, and significant injuries can be painless.

Urine color, hematuria, dysuria, and the timing and amount of the last void should be noted. A complete medical history, including preexisting urologic disease and prior surgery, should be obtained. Allergy to iodinated dyes is also important to ascertain.

Physical Examination

A thorough physical examination starts with inspection of the abdomen, back, and external genitalia. Complete exposure is essential, since ecchymosis, abrasions, or penetrating wounds may indicate possible urologic injury. Scrotal hematomas, localized areas of swelling, or blood at the external urethral meatus should be noted. Auscultation is of limited value, but an abdominal bruit may suggest a vascular pedicle injury.

Careful palpation of the abdomen, back, flank, penis, and testicles can often be useful in demonstrating an underlying injury. Localized tenderness or masses should be noted. Pain with pelvic compression is suggestive of a pelvic fracture. This is crucial, as 10% to 15% of pelvic fractures have associated genitourinary injuries. A rectal examination must be performed to check for a high-riding prostate secondary to urethral disruption.

DIAGNOSTIC EVALUATION
Urinalysis

Urinalysis is rapid and simple and should be performed on most children with suspected genitourinary trauma. Hematuria is the most common manifestation of urogenital

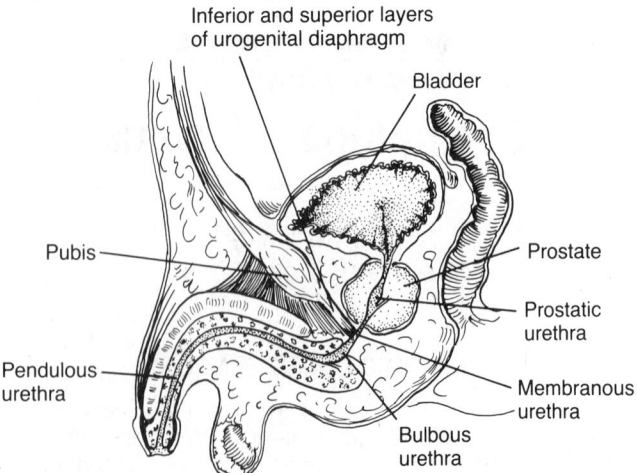

Figure 115–1. The anatomy of the male lower genitourinary system. (From Zbaraschuk I, Berger RE, Hedges JR. Emergency urologic procedures. *In* Roberts JR, Hedges JR (eds). Clinical Procedures in Emergency Medicine. 2nd ed. Philadelphia, WB Saunders, 1991, p 869.)

Figure labels: Inferior and superior layers of urogenital diaphragm; Bladder; Prostate; Prostatic urethra; Membranous urethra; Bulbous urethra; Pendulous urethra; Pubis

injury, and gross or microscopic hematuria is present in 85% to 90% of all genitourinary injuries. The correlation between the amount of hematuria and the severity of injury, however, is unclear, and with some serious entities such as vascular thrombosis, pedicle injuries, and urethral transection, hematuria may be absent. In the multiply traumatized child, once the presence of urethral injury has been excluded, a Foley catheter should be placed to obtain a urine specimen and monitor hourly urine output.

Penetrating trauma occurring in proximity to genitourinary structures, gross hematuria, and blunt trauma with accompanying microscopic hematuria and shock are indications for radiologic evaluation. Additionally, a significant mechanism of injury or positive findings on physical examination may warrant further radiologic evaluation.

Radiologic Evaluation

A chest radiograph may reveal lower rib fractures. Pelvic films may show bladder displacement or fractures. If a kidney, ureter, and bladder (KUB) view is obtained, it should be examined for vertebral body or transverse process fractures, paraspinal muscle spasm, free intraperitoneal or retroperitoneal air, psoas shadow obliteration, or elevation of a hemidiaphragm. Fractures occur less frequently in children than in adults because of the resilience of their skeletal system.

The intravenous pyelogram (IVP) is the study of choice for isolated urogenital trauma, because it allows visualization of all genitourinary structures and is readily available and relatively inexpensive. If isolated genitourinary trauma is suspected, an IVP should be obtained. When other intra-abdominal injuries are suspected, as with penetrating trauma, a one-view intraoperative IVP can be performed. A normal result may be reassuring, whereas an abnormal one may be useful in directing the laparotomy. The IVP can also assess the kidney function in the uninjured kidney.

An IVP is performed using 2 ml/kg of dilute sodium diatrizoate as a bolus, obtaining films at 0, 10, and 20 minutes. In a stable patient, a normal IVP may allow observation prior to considering further studies, and often no additional studies will be necessary.

Abdominal computed tomographic (CT) scanning is gaining acceptance as a primary form of evaluation after trauma, because it allows visualization of all solid organs in both intraperitoneal and retroperitoneal injuries. In the stable patient with multiple trauma who may have genitourinary injuries along with abdominal trauma, the CT allows the clinician to evaluate several systems simultaneously. However, it is relatively expensive, requires transport to the CT suite, and is more difficult to interpret than the IVP.

If IVP or CT do not lead to a definitive diagnosis, further evaluation may be warranted. Ureteral injury can be diagnosed on IVP alone, but retrograde pyelography may be more useful. Bladder and urethral injuries can best be delineated by a retrograde cystogram or urethrogram. Angiography, ultrasonography, and radionucleotide scanning may also be useful in cases in which CT or IVP are not definitive. Often, in patients with penetrating injuries, diagnosis is not made until the time of surgery.

RENAL INJURIES
Epidemiology

Renal injury is common in childhood, comprising 5% of all cases of childhood trauma. The kidney is second only to the brain in frequency of injury in the child, and renal trauma is four times more common than liver or intestinal injury.

Renal injury is not usually isolated. Associated trauma is found in almost half of patients with renal contusion, and the rate of associated injury rises when more significant renal damage occurs.

Etiology

The majority of pediatric renal injuries occur secondary to blunt trauma. Motor vehicle accidents, auto-pedestrian accidents, falls, and sports activities are the leading mechanisms. The availability of three- and four-wheel off-road vehicles has also led to accidents causing renal trauma.

Penetrating injuries are a much less common cause of renal trauma and account for less than 10% of cases. Operative renal procedures such as percutaneous biopsy or nephrostomy may result in iatrogenic injury to the kidney.

Signs and Symptoms

Cooperative children who are old enough to talk and are fully conscious may complain of abdominal, flank, or back pain. The parent or patient may note flank bruising or bloody urine.

Physical findings may alert the clinician to the presence of a renal injury. Shock occurring with trauma to the flank or upper abdomen or shock associated with hematuria mandate diagnostic genitourinary evaluation. Flank tenderness or ecchymosis may signify renal injury, whereas a flank mass implies disruption of the renal capsule. A penetrating injury located in the flank also warrants a genitourinary evaluation.

Diagnosis

Typically, hematuria alerts the emergency physician to the possibility of renal damage and has been considered the most reliable sign of injury. The urine is initially dipstick tested for blood, and it should be noted that false-negative dipstick tests do occur. The degree of hematuria does not necessarily correlate with the severity of injury, nor does the absence of hematuria exclude the possibility of renal injury. It is postulated that with renal contusion, parenchymal swelling might compress the vessels and the collecting system in the injured area, resulting in a normal urinalysis. About one third of pedicle injuries result in occlusion of the collecting system.

Because the extent of renal injury cannot be determined by hematuria alone, some guidelines are used to assess the need for further studies. Additional studies are recommended for the following:

Gross hematuria
Penetrating injuries overlying the kidney
Significant blunt deceleration injury with or without hematuria
Any microhematuria with shock
Blunt trauma with >20 red blood cells per high power field

In evaluating and managing children with renal injury, the goal should be to quickly and accurately assess the type, location, and extent of injury, as well as the level of function of the contralateral kidney. A normal IVP indicates no renal damage greater than contusion. If renal trauma is the only damage, an IVP with a tomogram will stage 80% to 85% of injuries. IVP still remains the primary imaging modality at most institutions.

Despite its usefulness, an IVP should not be performed indiscriminately. IVP dye may cause allergic reactions, and significant radiation exposure to the child may occur. The study requires 20 to 30 minutes to perform and potentially could delay identification or treatment of other significant injuries.

As stated earlier, most renal injuries may be staged by IVP (Fig. 115–2). A number of classification schemes have been devised, but the most widely used system, proposed by Nun in 1962, is presented in Table 115–1.

Classification

Class I injuries are a diagnosis of exclusion; patients with trauma and hematuria with a normal IVP are given this designation. Anatomically, this represents localized hemorrhage into the parenchyma without damage to the capsule, collecting system, or major vessels. Patients with subcapsular hematomas and superficial cortical lacerations are sometimes

Class	Injury	IVP Finding
I	Renal contusion	Normal
II	Cortical (capsular) laceration	Extrarenal dye extravasation
III	Caliceal laceration	Intrarenal dye extravasation
IV	Renal fracture	Intrarenal and extrarenal dye extravasation
V	Vascular pedicle injury	Unilateral renal nonvisualization

TABLE 115–1

CLASSIFICATION OF RENAL INJURY

placed in this group. Although the IVP is described as "normal," about 10% of patients with severe contusions have nonspecific findings such as decreased renal opacification, irregular cortical margins, delayed excretion, or renal enlargment.

Class II injuries are cortical lacerations in which there is extravasation of dye outside the normal renal silhouette on the IVP. *Class III* injuries are caliceal lacerations with extrarenal dye extravasation, and *class IV* injuries are complete renal fractures with both intrarenal and extrarenal dye extravasation.

Class V injuries are vascular pedicle injuries and are suspected when a kidney is not visualized on the IVP. Vascular injuries usually occur from blunt trauma, with rapid deceleration causing an intimal tear and thrombosis or, rarely, avulsion of the vessels. Because unilateral nonvisualization may also be caused by renal agenesis or hypoplasia, further studies are necessary after the IVP demonstrates nonvisualization. Most urologists utilize an angiogram or CT scan to define the problem. Patients with a mechanism of injury and physical findings consistent with the injury warrant IVP, as up to 40% of those with pedicle injury have no hematuria.

Diagnostic Evaluation
Computed Tomography

Intravenous contrast and nasogastric infusion of oral contrast (e.g., 2% Gastrografin) are used for CT unless contraindicated. Many physicians use an abdominal CT scan in lieu of IVP if multiple-system abdominal injury is suspected, so that other abdominal organs may be visualized.

The CT scan allows accurate staging of renal trauma. Small hematomas may be seen with class I renal contusions. Classes II to IV lacerations can be clearly demonstrated and staged, and class V vascular pedicle injuries can be seen in detail with CT.

CT scans may be superior to IVP in penetrating injuries of the back or flank, as CT allows good definition of retroperitoneal spaces. In some instances CT may allow nonoperative management in cases in which IVP may have resulted in exploration.

Renal Scan

Renal scans may be helpful in some instances, as they show the amount and location of vascularized renal tissue and can demonstrate congenital abnormalities and arterial injuries. If an IVP shows unilateral nonvisualization of a kidney, a renal scan can be used to confirm the presence of a kidney, and angiography may be avoided. A renal scan may be especially useful in the child with intravenous contrast allergy. Its sensitivity in detecting extravasation is excellent.

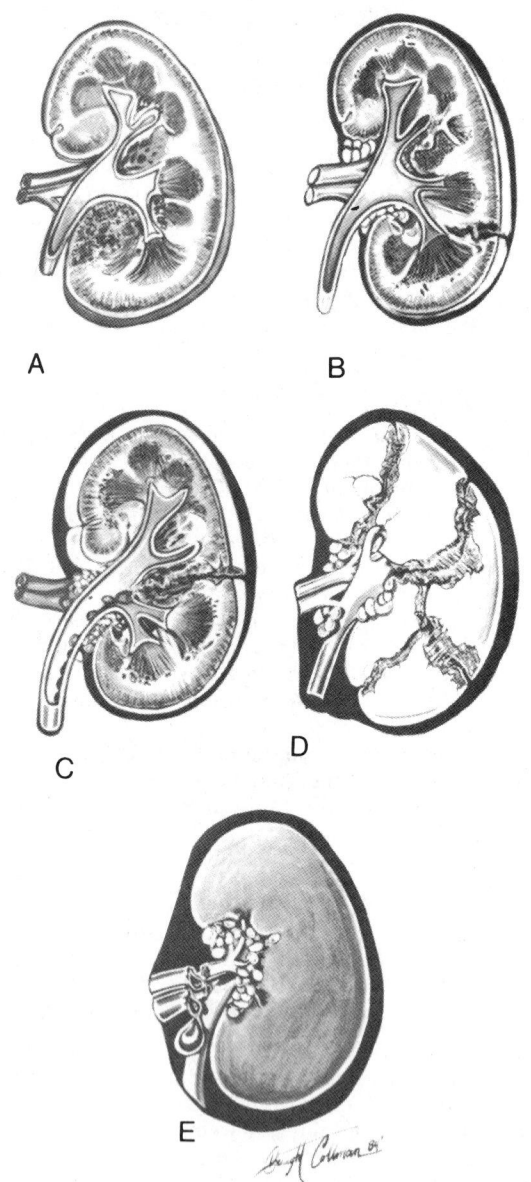

Figure 115–2. The five major types of renal injury. *A,* Renal contusion. *B,* Laceration of the cortex. *C,* Caliceal laceration. *D,* Fragmentation of the kidney. *E,* Renal pedicle injury, usually involving the renal blood vessels. (From Middleton RG, Matlak ME, Nixon GW, Mayer TA. Genitourinary injuries in children. *In* Mayer TA (ed). Emergency Management of Pediatric Trauma. Philadelphia, WB Saunders, 1985, p 346.)

Angiography

Angiography is technically difficult and has a high complication rate in children. Traditionally, angiography has been used to define the extent of injury if a unilateral, nonfunctioning kidney is seen on IVP. Currently it is used when CT scan findings are indeterminate for arterial injury or in consideration for therapeutic embolization for prolonged bleeding.

Retrograde Pyelography

The retrograde pyelogram can be used to evaluate unilateral nonvisualization, but other methods are more convenient. It is used mainly for evaluation of lower genitourinary injuries.

Ultrasound

Ultrasound is less specific than CT but can be useful in showing perirenal fluid accumulation. It may be used to confirm the absence of a kidney, but if a pedicle injury is suspected and a kidney is not visualized on IVP, further studies beyond ultrasound must still be done.

Diagnostic Protocols

A number of protocols have been devised for evaluation of blunt renal trauma; these are based on the mechanism of injury, urinalysis results, and CT or IVP results (Fig. 115–3). The protocol used in any particular institution may vary depending on the patient population, availability of various diagnostic studies, and experience of radiologic and urologic consultants. Hematuria alone may be an inaccurate parameter in assessing renal trauma and a high index of suspicion in renal trauma is necessary to ensure a timely diagnosis.

Treatment

The unstable patient must undergo fluid resuscitation to ensure adequate perfusion to the renal parenchyma. Renal contusions, which constitute about 85% of all renal injuries, are treated nonoperatively. Children with isolated renal contusions can be safely discharged home, with instructions to avoid contact sports for 4 to 6 weeks. The child should undergo a repeat urinalysis in 1 to 2 weeks.

Patients with minor cortical lacerations are admitted and placed on bed rest until microscopic hematuria clears. After hospital discharge, strenuous activity is avoided for several weeks after microscopic hematuria has resolved.

Patients with class III or IV renal injuries comprise about 15% of those with renal trauma. About one third of these patients will require immediate surgery. The management of the remaining two thirds of patients is controversial. Some urologists prefer observation and cite a lower nephrectomy rate in these patients as the reason for conservative management. Other urologists operate immediately, claiming there is a lower rate of delayed complications. Continued blood loss or an expanding flank mass requires operative intervention.

Renal pedicle injuries are uncommon, accounting for about 3% of renal injuries. Pedicle injuries require immediate surgery in order to salvage the kidney.

Other injuries may also require rapid surgical intervention. A shattered or nonfunctioning kidney, expanding or uncontained hematomas, pulsatile retroperitoneal hematomas, and major urinary extravasation all require operative repair.

Penetrating renal injuries are rare in children, but all patients except those with a superficial injury that does not demonstrate dye extravasation should be explored.

Prognosis

Contusions rarely cause permanent renal impairment. Hematuria usually resolves in 1 to 2 weeks, and short-term

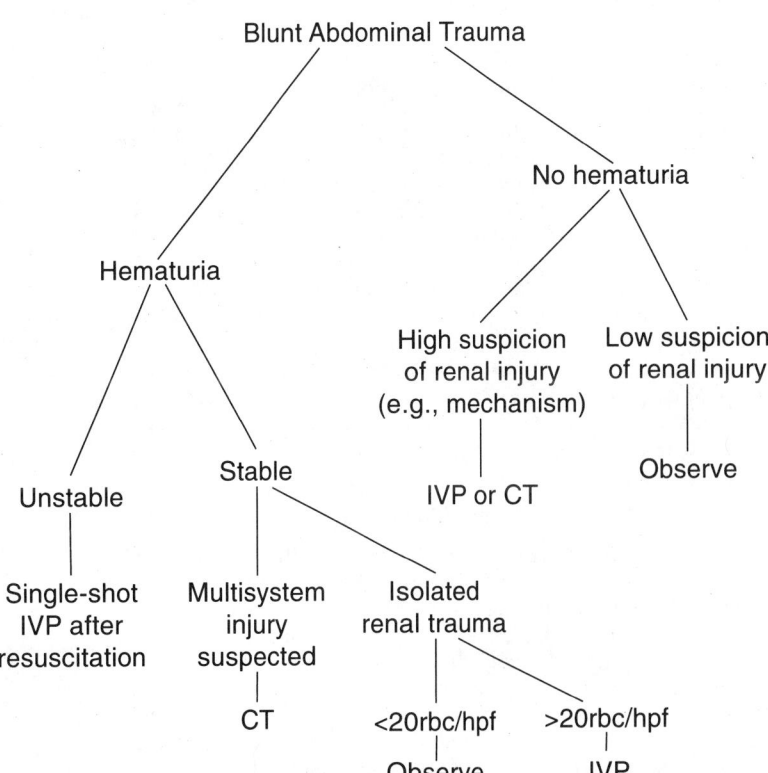

Figure 115–3. Diagnostic evaluation of renal injury with blunt abdominal trauma.

activity restriction minimizes scarring of the kidney parenchyma.

Minor cortical lacerations, even those that extend into the pyelocaliceal system, usually heal without sequelae. However, follow-up to check for the development of hypertension is important. Most urologists recommend a repeat CT scan or IVP 3 to 6 months after injury, as well as long-term blood pressure monitoring.

Class III and IV injuries are associated with short- and long-term complications. Infection or recurrent bleeding may occur in the first few days after injury, and any child presenting with fever or infection several days after blunt abdominal trauma should be evaluated for a missed renal injury. Late complications, such as arteriovenous fistulas, cysts, hydronephrosis, or renal insufficiency, may also occur. Delayed onset of renal vascular hypertension is a fairly common problem in patients with major renal injuries and may require nephrectomy. Most clinicians recommend serial renal scans for approximately 12 months after major renal surgery.

A severely fractured or shattered kidney usually requires a nephrectomy. Patient prognosis after a vascular injury is poor. Operative intervention must be undertaken within 4 to 6 hours after disruption of the renal vascular supply in order to save the kidney. Salvage rates are low, even with revascularization.

URETERAL INJURY
Etiology

Ureteral injury is uncommon, comprising only 2% of cases of genitourinary trauma. Penetrating injuries are usually iatrogenic and occur during abdominal operations. Because there is less periureteral fat in children than in adults, these injuries are relatively less common in children.

Ureteral injury caused by blunt trauma occurs more often in children than in adults. This is thought to be a result of the increased flexibility of the pediatric spine, allowing more pronounced hyperextension. When the ureter exceeds its normal limit of stretch, it ruptures at the ureteropelvic junction.

Signs and Symptoms

It is difficult to diagnose a ureteral injury, as the clinical signs and symptoms are nonspecific and may develop gradually. Penetrating iatrogenic injuries usually present with fever, flank pain, or abdominal pain. Drainage from a wound or flank swelling may occur.

Blunt trauma to the ureter may present as fever, pain, and flank swelling. The diagnosis of ureteral disruption must be considered in such cases to prevent delayed diagnosis.

Urinalysis may be helpful or misleading. More than half of patients have hematuria, and pyuria may also be present. Patients with complete transection, however, usually have clear urine.

Diagnosis

Diagnosis of ureteral injuries may be difficult, and less than 50% are discovered initially. IVP may show extravasation of dye but is nondiagnostic in up to one third of cases. IVP evaluation is difficult when a proximal ureteral injury is present, as the dye may dissect up into the renal pelvis. Ultrasound and CT scans are not usually diagnostic but may reveal associated hematoma, urinoma, or obstruction. When ureteral damage is suspected and the IVP is nondiagnostic, retrograde pyelography is used to visualize the injury.

Treatment

Ureteral injuries must be surgically repaired. A drainage procedure, stenting procedure, or direct anastomosis can be performed.

Prognosis

The complication rate with ureteral trauma is directly proportional to the length of time from injury to repair. Because the diagnosis is frequently delayed, complication rates are high.

Prompt diagnosis of minor injuries results in rapid healing without sequelae and a nephrectomy rate of less than 5%. Delayed repair leads to loss of kidney function in more than half of patients. Complications include urinoma, abscess, stricture, and fistula.

BLADDER INJURIES
Etiology

The bladder is the second most commonly injured genitourinary organ. In children, the bladder is an abdominal rather than a pelvic organ and is especially susceptible to trauma (Fig. 115–4). About 15% of patients with pelvic fractures have bladder injuries, and the possibility of a bladder injury should be considered in every patient with a pelvic fracture.

Most bladder injuries are the result of blunt trauma, but penetrating injuries from pelvic bone protrusion, gunshot wounds, or stab wounds may also occur. Iatrogenic injury from neonatal umbilical line placement, urethral catheter guide, cystoscopy, or laparoscopy is not uncommon.

Signs and Symptoms

Blunt trauma without rupture of the bladder results in bladder contusion. A child with a contusion has lower abdominal or suprapubic pain and tenderness. A feeling of urgency may be present, and voiding is possible. Lower abdominal guarding or bruising may be present, and hematuria is likely.

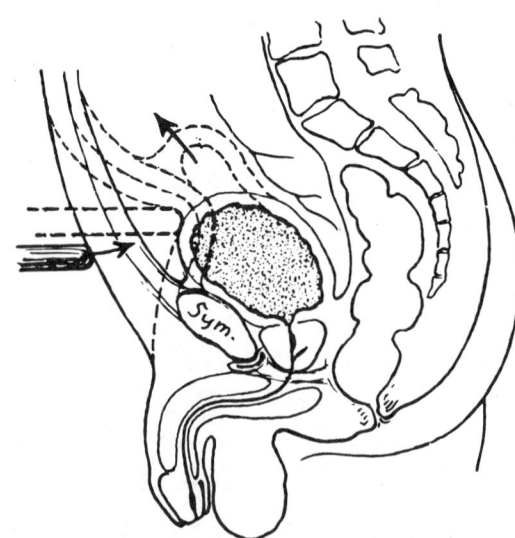

Figure 115–4. The bladder in the infant is more vulnerable to injury owing to the more abdominal location. A blunt force to the full bladder results in an intraperitoneal rupture of the bladder dome. (From Gonzales ET Jr, Guerriero WG. Genitourinary trauma in children. *In* Kelalis PP, King LR, Belman AB (eds). Clinical Pediatric Urology. 2nd ed. Philadelphia, WB Saunders, 1985, p 1144.)

Bladder rupture from blunt trauma may be either intraperitoneal or extraperitoneal. Younger children have an intraabdominal bladder, but as they grow, the bladder becomes more of a pelvic organ. As a result, rupture in a young child is usually intraperitoneal; as the child grows, extraperitoneal injury becomes more common.

Intraperitoneal rupture is suspected with lower abdominal pain and tenderness, hematuria, and difficulty voiding, but the clinical picture is variable, and a high level of suspicion must be maintained. Often, the injury is not diagnosed until abdominal pain, anuria, and signs of peritonitis have developed.

Signs of extraperitoneal rupture are variable and often subtle. Suprapubic pain and tenderness, along with dysuria or decreased urine output, suggest the possibility of bladder rupture. If the diagnosis is delayed, urine may dissect out into the surrounding tissues of the scrotum, buttocks, or thighs.

Hematuria is present in 95% of patients with bladder injury. Hematuria with a pelvic fracture mandates further investigation to exclude the possibility of a bladder injury.

Diagnosis

When a bladder injury is suspected, radiographic studies should be performed. An IVP is done first to evaluate the upper genitourinary structures, as dye extravasation from a ruptured bladder would obscure other IVP findings. Next, the urethra is evaluated. If a urethral injury is suspected, a retrograde urethrogram is done so that a catheter can be placed to facilitate a urinalysis and allow for further studies.

A cystogram is then obtained by instilling 5 ml/kg of iodinated contrast (e.g., 10% Renografin) through the catheter by gravity filling. Adequate bladder distention is necessary to avoid missing dye extravasation. A minimum of anteroposterior, left oblique, right oblique, and postevacuation views are required for adequate evaluation.

If there is no extravasation of dye on the cystogram, a diagnosis of contusion is made. Pelvic hematomas may often displace or deform the bladder outline, but the bladder remains intact. Extravasated dye from rupture may outline

the abdominal organs or loops of bowel, but findings may be more subtle.

Treatment

Bladder contusions are managed nonoperatively. Minor extraperitoneal lacerations may be treated by 7 to 14 days of drainage through a Foley or suprapubic catheter. More significant extraperitoneal lacerations and all intraperitoneal lacerations require operative repair and drainage.

Prognosis

Bladder injuries that are rapidly diagnosed and treated usually result in full recovery. When a problem is missed, however, complications can occur. These include abscess, sepsis, bladder dysfunction, strictures, and impotence.

URETHRAL INJURY
Etiology

Children are less likely to sustain urethral injuries than adults, because the pediatric urethra is more mobile and the pelvis is more flexible. However, children are very active and may sustain blunt urethral injuries during sports activities, while straddling bicycle handlebars, or when jumping fences (Fig. 115–5). Auto-pedestrian accidents resulting in pelvic fractures may also damage the urethra.

Signs and Symptoms

Classically, urethral injury presents with an inability to void and findings of blood at the urethral meatus. The findings on physical examination are related to the location and severity of the injury. Anterior injuries (those below the urogenital diaphragm) lead to more pronounced bleeding from the meatus, and blood or urine may extravasate into the penis, scrotum, perineum, or anterior abdominal wall. Posterior injuries (above the urogenital diaphragm) result in extravasation that is contained by Colle's fascia. Urine may migrate throughout the pelvis, retroperitoneum, and anterior thigh, but not in the genitalia or perineum.

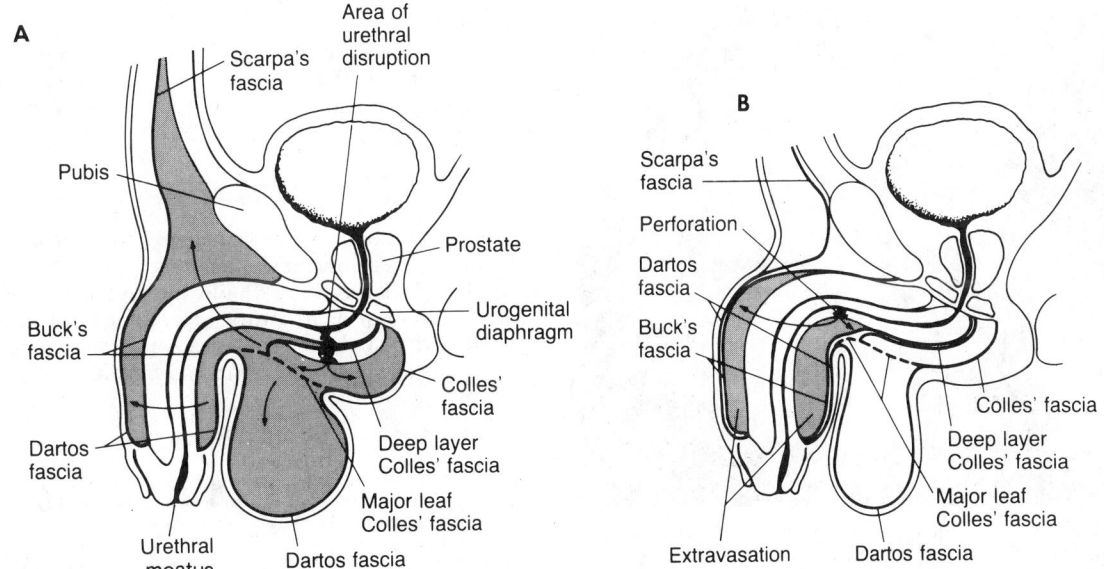

Figure 115–5. The male urethra is impinged against the symphysis pubis during a straddle injury. Usually the bulbous urethra is injured. This can result in a "butterfly" ecchymosis to the perineum. (From Guerriero WG. Problems in Urology: Genitourinary Trauma. Philadelphia, JB Lippincott, 1988; 2:252.)

A rectal examination must be performed in patients with suspected urethral injuries to evaluate for a high-riding prostate or the presence of bony spicules from a pelvic fracture.

Diagnosis

Diagnosis of a urethral tear is confirmed by retrograde urography (Fig. 115–6). Difficulty occurs, however, when the diagnosis is not considered, and attempts at Foley catheterization convert a partial urethral tear into a complete tear. Patients with signs or symptoms of urethral trauma should have a retrograde urethrogram performed prior to insertion of a Foley catheter.

A retrograde urethrogram is obtained by injecting 10 to 40 ml of a water-soluble iodinated dye (e.g., Renografin) into the urethra. The dye may be injected through a catheter-tip syringe or by placing a No. 8 to No. 18 French Foley catheter in the fossa navicularis about 2 cm proximal to the penile meatus and inflating the balloon with 1 to 2 ml of saline to keep the balloon in place. A Brodney-Knudson clamp may also be used to secure the syringe. Regardless of the technique used, it is important to prevent extravasation of the dye externally, which would make interpretation of the films difficult. When most of the dye has been injected, several views are obtained to check for extravasation.

Treatment

Contusions to the urethra do not require treatment unless the patient is unable to void, in which case a catheter is carefully placed. Minor tears may often be managed with suprapubic drainage for 10 to 14 days. Severe tears and complete disruption of the urethra require suprapubic drainage and surgical repair. The timing of the operative repair is controversial.

Prognosis

Contusions usually heal without sequelae, although some urologists recommend a follow-up urethrogram 4 to 6 months after injury to exclude stricture formation. Strictures, incontinence, and impotence are frequent complications of urethral tears. Because patient prognosis is worst with a complete tear, it is important to recognize an incomplete tear and avoid manipulation of the urethra resulting in complete disruption.

FEMALE EXTERNAL GENITALIA INJURIES
Etiology

Trauma to the labia, vulva, and clitoris is uncommon. When it occurs, child or sexual abuse should always be considered. Straddle injuries, falls, impalements, and motor vehicle accidents are other causes of injury.

Signs and Symptoms

Dysuria, discharge, or lower abdominal pain may lead a parent to examine a child and discover an injury. In most instances, a painful injury will bring the child immediately to the parent, and the problem will be readily seen. A careful physical examination allows the physician to determine the extent of most injuries. Vaginal inspection for a foreign body or internal injury may be required. The anal area should always be examined for signs of trauma.

Diagnosis

Inspection is the key to diagnosis of trauma to the external female genitalia. Diagnostic studies in addition to the physical examination are not required unless sexual or child abuse is suspected.

Treatment

Small lacerations may be allowed to heal by secondary intention. A near-normal appearance is usually restored with time. Larger lacerations should be copiously irrigated and closed with absorbable sutures. Hematomas are usually self-limited and respond to conservative treatment; attempts at drainage often result in protracted bleeding.

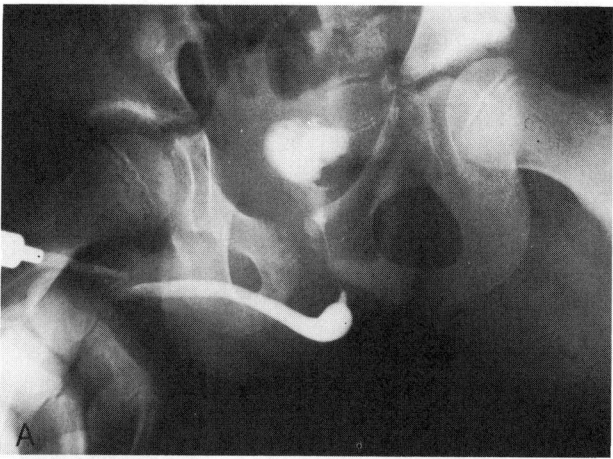
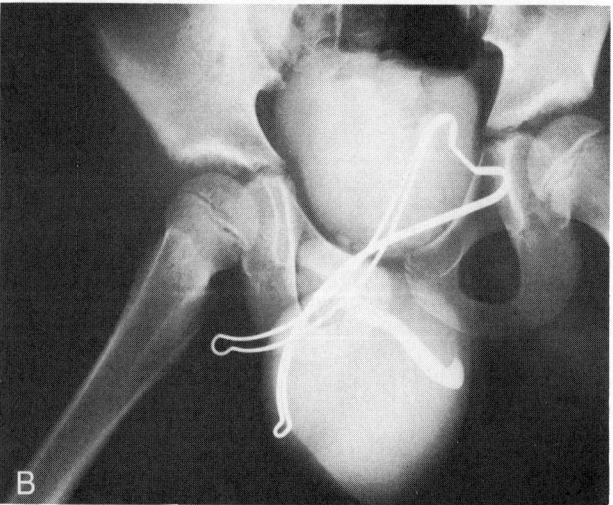

Figure 115–6. A urethrogram was performed in this boy after a straddle injury (A). The study shows diffuse extravasation of contrast material throughout the perineum and scrotum, which resulted from urethral disruption (B). After cystoscopy and suprapubic catheterization, the urethra healed and the patient suffered no long-term effects.

Selected References

Ahmed S, Morris LL. Renal paranchymal injuries secondary to blunt abdominal trauma in childhood: A 10 year review. Br J Urol 1982;54:470.
Carrol PR, McAninch JW. Staging of renal trauma. Urol Clin North Am 1989;16:193.
Cass AS. Blunt renal trauma in children. J Trauma 1983;23:123.
Cass AS. Diagnostic studies in bladder rupture. Urol Clin North Am 1989;16:267.
Cass AS, Gleich P, Smith C. Male genital injuries from external trauma. Br J Urol 1985;57:467.

Fleisher G. Prospective evaluation of selective criteria for imaging children with suspected blunt renal trauma. Pediatr Emerg Care 1989;5:8.

Guerriero WG. Ureteral injury. Urol Clin North Am 1989;16:237.

Javadpour N, Guinam P, Bush IM. Renal trauma in children. Surg Gynecol Obstet 1973;136:237.

Karp MP, Jeivett TC Jr, Kuhn JP, et al. The impact of computed tomography scanning on the child with renal trauma. J Pediatr Surg 1986;21:617.

Livine, PM, Gonzales ET. Genitourinary trauma in children. Urol Clin North Am 1985;12:53.

Mahboubi S. Abdominal trauma in childhood: Role of computed tomography. Pediatr Emerg Care 1985;1:37.

Mee SL, McAninch JW. Indication of radiographic assessment in suspected renal trauma. Urol Clin North Am 1989;16:187.

Morehouse DD. Emergency management of urethral trauma. Urol Clin North Am 1982;9:251.

Morse TS. Renal injuries. Pediatr Clin North Am 1975;22:379.

Peterson NE. Complications of renal trauma. Urol Clin North Am 1989;16:221.

Pierce JM. Disruptions of the anterior urethra. Urol Clin North Am 1989;16:329.

Sandler CM, Corriere JN. Urethrography in the diagnosis of acute urethral injuries. Urol Clin North Am 1987;16:283.

Tunberg T, Juda J. Review of multiple traumatic injuries in an urban pediatric population. Pediatr Emerg Care 1985;1:116.

CHAPTER 116

Soft Tissue Injury and Wound Repair

Vince Markovchick

INTRODUCTION

The skin is composed of two layers, the epidermis and the dermis (Fig. 116–1). The top layer, or epidermis, contains the epithelial cells and serves to protect deep tissue from desiccation and infection. The dermis contains blood vessels and nerve endings as well as fibroblasts, which produce the collagen that gives the skin its tensile strength. Beneath the dermis is the subcutaneous tissue through which blood vessels and nerves pass. Most subcutaneous tissue is made up of fat. Depending on the area of the body, the depth of subcutaneous tissue varies from almost nonexistent in the fingers to extensive in the abdomen.

The lines of static and dynamic skin tension (Fig. 116–2) are important factors in predicting and determining the ultimate cosmetic result. The static skin tensions commonly known as Langer's lines are the forces that stretch the skin over the underlying bony framework when the body remains motionless. Dynamic lines of skin tension are those that occur with contraction of underlying musculature. These can be tested by observing the direction and magnitude of tension on the laceration while the patient contracts the underlying musculature. In general, a linear scar intersecting the transverse axis of a joint or running perpendicular to these lines of skin tension will result in a more visible scar and has the potential for contracture and functional disability if it overlies a joint. The degree of wound tension (those forces that separate wound edges) can be estimated accurately by initial observation of the wound. If the wound edges are lying in close proximity, the tension is minimal

and the cosmetic results should be excellent. However, wounds with marked retraction of their edges (more than 5 mm) are subject to strong static skin tensions and heal with wide scars unless closed carefully in layers. Additional anatomy to be considered in the evaluation and repair of a wound includes underlying muscles, tendons, bones, joints, nerves, blood vessels, and ducts.

During the first few days after wounding, an inflammatory response results in an outpouring of tissue fluid cells and fibroblasts and an increase in blood supply to the wound. Leukocytes subsequently excrete proteolytic enzymes to dissolve damaged tissue and debris. Fibroblasts begin to form collagen fibers, which provide the tensile strength of a scar. Wound healing and scar revision are a continuous process occurring over a 6- to 12-month period, at which time the scar finally achieves maximal tensile strength. It is important to note that a wound achieves only 5% of its original tensile strength at 2 weeks and about 35% at 1 month (Fig. 116–3). It is for this reason that in a wound under tension the edges must be held in approximation by mechanical means for a period sufficient to allow the wound to gain tensile strength. This prevents subsequent widening of the scar after removal of the sutures, staples, or tape. The ideal way to achieve an excellent cosmetic closure in a wound under increased tension is to close it in layers with absorbable suture that will maintain the support of the wound for at least 4 weeks.

Wound healing occurs in specific stages (Fig. 116–4). The inflammatory phase represents maximal activity of the granulocytes. The granulation tissue phase, ensuing shortly after the onset of the inflammatory phase, includes both epithelial cell growth and neovascularization. The last phase of wound healing, wound contraction or remodeling, occurs over many months.

CLINICAL EVALUATION

History

It is important to ascertain whether the wound represents a cut or crush injury, blunt trauma, or a contaminated wound such as an animal bite. During triage, injuries caused by blunt or crushing forces should be given priority over those caused by sharp, shearing forces. The exact time of injury may assist in determining whether a wound should be closed primarily, allowed to heal by secondary intention, or receive a delayed primary closure. Any allergies to medications must be ascertained, particularly to antibiotics and local anesthetics, as well as the tetanus immunization history. If the latter is inadequate or if the patient has never been fully immunized, tetanus immune globulin as well as tetanus toxoid is indicated. It is important to obtain a history of current medications such as corticosteroid therapy, medical illnesses such as diabetes mellitus, immunodeficiency, or any other condition that would affect the immune system, since the normal wound healing process may be compromised in such situations.

Physical Examination

The exact location and length of the wound in centimeters should be recorded. Particular attention must be paid to the anatomy underlying the wound. Before infiltration with local anesthetics, appropriate sensory function must be tested in all full-thickness wounds. After the sensory status has been clearly determined, the wound may be anesthetized locally to facilitate examination. If there is a possibility of an underlying fracture, a radiograph should be obtained before attempting to move a joint through ranges of motion. Motor

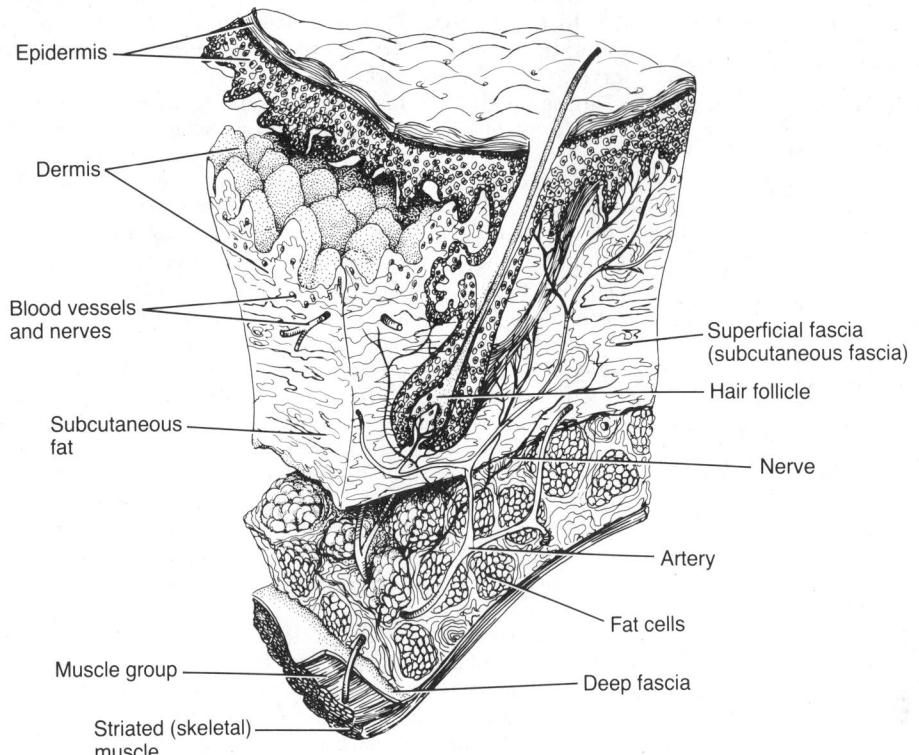

Epidermis

Dermis

Blood vessels
and nerves

Subcutaneous
fat

Muscle group

Striated (skeletal)
muscle

Superficial fascia
(subcutaneous fascia)

Hair follicle

Nerve

Artery

Fat cells

Deep fascia

Figure 116–1. The anatomy of the skin and subcutaneous tissue.

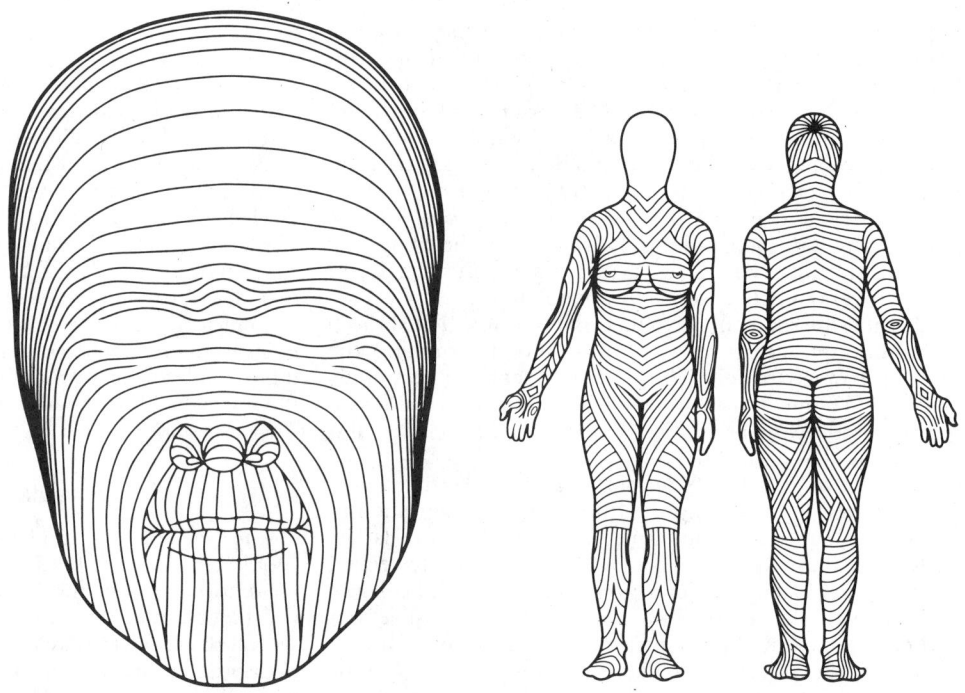

Figure 116–2. The skin tension lines of the face and body. Lacerations parallel to these lines tend to have less scarring. (From Simon RR, Brenner BE. Procedures and Techniques in Emergency Medicine. 2nd ed. Baltimore, Williams & Wilkins, 1987, pp 292, 293.

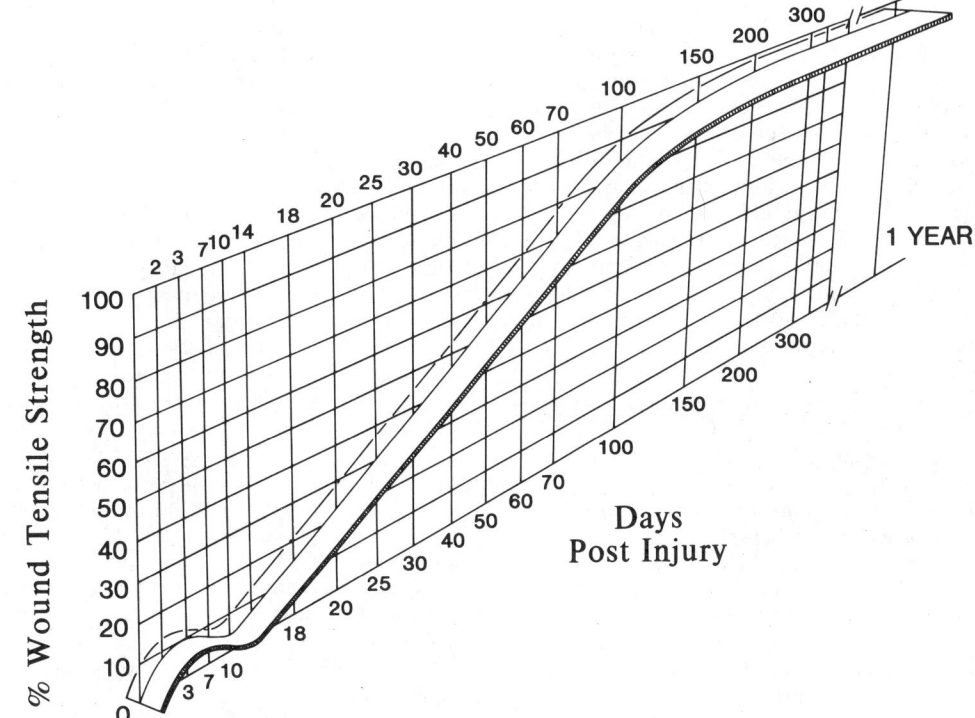

Figure 116–3. Graphic illustration of the percentage of tensile strength that develops in a wound in the days and months after injury. (From Trott A. Wounds and Lacerations: Emergency Care and Closure. St. Louis, MO, Mosby–Year Book, 1991, p 18.)

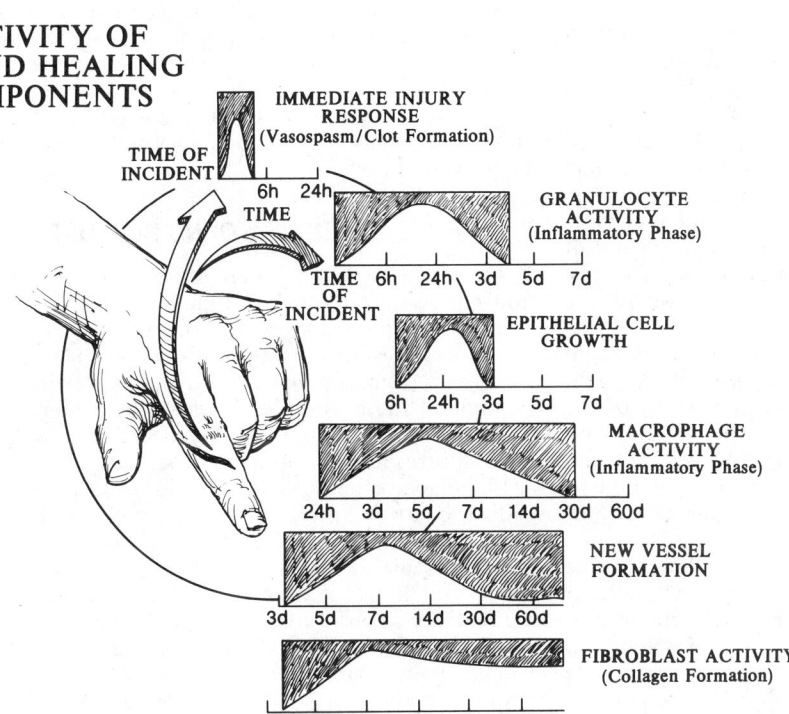

Figure 116–4. Graphic illustration of the various components of wound healing and their time frames. (From Trott A. Wounds and Lacerations: Emergency Care and Closure. St. Louis, MO, Mosby–Year Book, 1991, p 16.)

function testing should be performed to test the integrity of motor nerves, major muscle groups, and tendons. Distal pulses should be examined in any wound that overlies a major vessel. If the wound is over the course of a duct, such as Stensen's duct or the lacrimal ducts of the eye, the integrity of these structures must be determined. After this part of the examination is completed, every wound must be locally explored. Complete control of bleeding, as well as good anesthesia, is a prerequisite in order to explore a wound adequately. The exploration should be both visual and tactile, and the examiner must ascertain the presence or absence of foreign bodies and determine the extent of injury. This is most important in regard to tendons, since these may be 90% lacerated and yet the patient may still exhibit normal motor function. The exploration should also determine the ultimate depth of the wound and is necessary to plan properly the repair of the wound.

DIAGNOSTIC EVALUATION

Special diagnostic procedures are not indicated in the care of most wounds; the physical examination and local exploration are adequate in most instances. However, if there is a suspicion of a fracture or joint penetration, a radiograph should be obtained. When the wound is full thickness, and a foreign body cannot be completely ruled out by local exploration, radiographs may be helpful. If the history is such that the foreign body is unlikely to be visualized on routine radiography (e.g., a wood splinter), special studies such as ultrasound, xeroradiography, or computed tomography (CT) may be indicated. It is important to inform the patient in all instances in which small foreign bodies are present in a wound that although every effort has been made to localize and remove these, there is always a possibility of residual foreign material being left in the wound.

THERAPEUTIC INTERVENTION

Anesthesia

Several local anesthetic agents are available for routine use. Care must be taken to avoid exceeding the maximal safe dose of these agents. In addition, large wounds in certain areas of the body such as the forehead, hands, and feet may be amenable to regional nerve blocks rather than large amounts of local infiltrative anesthesia.

There are several methods of attaining wound anesthesia in children. Topical anesthesia is an effective means of obtaining good anesthesia for minor laceration repair. The agent most commonly used is tetracaine (0.5%), epinephrine (1:2000), and cocaine (11.8%). Studies have confirmed the efficacy and safety of this compound, which is an excellent means of achieving good anesthesia in selected wounds. Great care must be taken never to use this agent in the proximity of mucous membranes (conjunctiva or oral mucous membranes), since it can be rapidly absorbed and lead to status epilepticus and even death. The agent should be applied on cotton and held on the wound for at least 10 minutes before wound repair.

Local infiltration with as small a gauge of needle as possible (25 or 27 gauge) provides excellent anesthesia. The wound can be entered from the cut surface just below the dermis. Slow infiltration prevents unnecessary pain. In addition, buffering 1% lidocaine with 1 mEq/ml sodium bicarbonate in a ratio of ten parts lidocaine to one part bicarbonate will raise the pH to an approximately neutral level and decrease the burning discomfort that is felt secondary to the infiltration of this local anesthetic. The shelf life of this buffered solution is about 24 hours.

When possible, field nerve block anesthesia should be considered for wounds in the distribution of the median and ulnar nerves of the hand and the sural and posterior tibial nerves of the foot. In addition, facial wounds in the supraorbital and infraorbital distribution lend themselves well to field nerve block anesthesia. To reduce the discomfort of percutaneous injection, antecedent topical cryotherapy with an ice cube is helpful.

Analgesia

Systemic analgesia and sedation are occasionally desirable to ensure and enhance the quality of wound repair, especially in small children. Short-acting benzodiazepines or short-acting narcotics such as fentanyl provide a high margin of safety and efficacy if used properly. Fentanyl, injected in dosages of 2–4 μg/kg intravenously, provides excellent analgesia and sedation of the patient. Care must be taken to monitor the respiratory status of the child, observe respirations at all times, and if possible monitor the child with a pulse oximeter during the procedure. If there is any respiratory compromise secondary to the narcotic effect of fentanyl, it can be rapidly reversed with naloxone. Such analgesia is helpful in the repair of lacerations of the tongue or oral cavity, and of extensive wounds of the face that for cosmetic reasons require meticulous plastic surgical technique.

WOUND PREPARATION

The most important factor in the prevention of subsequent wound infections is meticulous wound preparation, copious irrigation, and debridement. Skin prepped with a 1% povidone-iodine solution has a substantially reduced bacterial count. The wound should not be exposed to a concentration of iodine greater than 1%, nor should any detergents be routinely used on open wounds. Contaminated wounds, such as bites, should be irrigated with normal saline solution. An 18-gauge catheter or needle attached to a 30-ml syringe provides approximately 10 pounds per square inch of irrigating pressure, which is the ideal pressure to dislodge bacteria and contaminants in a wound and yet not damage the tissue. Devitalized tissue and embedded foreign bodies should be removed by meticulous exploration and sharp debridement.

TYPES OF WOUND CLOSURE

There are two basic goals for wound closure: function and cosmesis. The goal in functional wound closure is to return the injured part to full function as soon as possible. It may be necessary to compromise the cosmetic results when the goal is primarily that of a functional closure. Therefore, in some of these wounds, there will be a more visible scar, since it is often necessary to close them in a single layer and leave sutures in for a prolonged period.

If the goal is one of cosmetic closure, the primary effort is directed toward minimizing the visibility of the subsequent scar. If the direction of the wound is perpendicular to the lines of normal skin tension, the ultimate cosmetic result will be poorer than if it were parallel. An example of this is a vertical laceration of the forehead. The lack of viability and tidiness of the wound edges, as well as the presence of a foreign body, will have an adverse effect on the ultimate result. It is therefore essential to remove all foreign bodies, particularly ground-in dirt within the dermis, since allowing debris to become part of the scar will result in permanent tattooing. Wound edges that are nonviable should be excised at the time of the repair. If there are large amounts of tension on a wound and it is not closed carefully in layers, the ultimate result will be a wide scar. If the wound is approximated but the edges are uneven, there will be magnification of the ultimate scar by the resultant shadows. If the wound edges are inverted, this will have a poorer cosmetic result. Suture marks cause an unsightly scar and can be avoided by a proper deep-layer closure and removal of the top layer of sutures within 5 or 6 days. Finally, if the wound becomes infected, the appropriate procedure is to remove all the sutures, open the wound, irrigate it, and allow it to heal by secondary intention. This will also have a poor cosmetic result and can be prevented in most instances by meticulous wound preparation.

The three types of wound closure are primary, secondary, and delayed primary. Primary closure is defined as surgical closure of a wound before the formation of granulation tissue. In general, this should be performed within 6 to 8 hours of wounding in all areas of the body with the exception of the face and scalp, which may be closed primarily with no increased incidence of infection up to 24 hours after injury. The contraindications to primary closure include old wounds, contaminated wounds, a debilitated host, or a compromised circulation in the area of the wound (particularly common with flap lacerations and crush injury lacerations).

Secondary closure is defined as healing by granulation without surgical repair. Indications for allowing a wound to heal by secondary intention are partial-thickness avulsions such as those found with fingertip injuries, contaminated small wounds such as stab wounds, and wounds that are infected. Meticulous cleansing, irrigation, debridement, and foreign body removal should be performed in all wounds, including those that will be allowed to heal by secondary intention.

Delayed primary closure is defined as surgical closure of a wound after 3 to 5 days. The indications for the use of this procedure are initially contaminated wounds, which should not be closed primarily because this may result in an increased incidence of infection. These wounds are closed subsequently to accelerate the time of wound healing and improve the cosmetic result. All wounds not closed primarily may be considered for delayed primary closure if they are clean and noninfected after 3 to 5 days. The technique for closure of these wounds is essentially the same as that for primary closure.

MATERIALS

Three types of materials used for wound closure are tape, staples, and sutures. Tape may be used on simple, small, linear lacerations that are made by shearing forces and are not expected to swell over time and increase the tension on the wound edges. The tape should be applied with benzoin for adhesiveness and should be left in place for as long as possible. Staples may be used in linear lacerations where cosmetic results are not a major consideration, such as scalp wounds and wounds of the trunk. The advantage of staples is that they can be applied rapidly and they greatly decrease the time of wound repair. Suturing is the most common form of wound repair and, in general, should be used in all full-thickness lacerations that are under any tension or in wounds in which an excellent cosmetic and functional result is deemed necessary. The type of suture material and needle size should be determined by the nature of the specific wound. In general, the smallest-diameter suture and smallest cutting needle size should be used. There has been an advance in needle design with the availability of a compound, curved needle, which enhances the ease of placement of deep intradermal sutures in the layered closure of lacerations.

TECHNIQUES OF WOUND CLOSURE

It should be decided whether to close the wounds in a single layer or in multiple layers (Table 116–1). In general, all wounds in which a functional result is the primary goal should be closed in a single layer to avoid the placement of deep sutures in areas with great sensitivity, such as fingertips. Facial wounds may be closed in a single layer if they are partial thickness, involve thin skin such as the eyelids, or have absolutely no tension and no potential for subsequent swelling and increased tension. Otherwise, most full-thickness wounds of the face should be closed with deep sutures to give the best possible cosmetic result.

Single-Layer Closure

There are two basic methods of placing interrupted percutaneous sutures for a single-layer closure, the simple interrupted and horizontal mattress methods. Both methods are useful when the goal is a single-layer closure of a wound under tension. Horizontal mattress sutures are superior for wounds under great tension or stress, including wounds over joint surfaces, the pretibial area, or the dorsum of the foot. The horizontal mattress suture is also excellent where skin edges tend to override if simple sutures are tied too tightly, e.g., in the eyelids and the dorsum of the hand. Simple interrupted sutures should be meticulously placed with the needle passed through the skin at an angle perpendicular to the skin surface and equidistant from the wound edges (Fig. 116–5). This prevents inversion of the wound edges with improperly placed simple interrupted sutures (Fig. 116–6). The horizontal mattress suture (Fig. 116–7), by nature, always results in eversion of the wound edges, and for this reason is also useful for hemostasis when there is active bleeding from the cut edges of the wounds.

In tidy, linear lacerations the percutaneous sutures may be placed in a running fashion. Techniques of running closures include simple (Fig. 116–8), locked (Fig. 116–9), horizontal mattress (Fig. 116–10), and subcuticular running sutures (Fig. 116–11). These sutures are useful for the final closure of a wound that has been closed in layers or in small, tidy linear lacerations under minimal tension. The disadvantage of this type of suture is that if one of the sutures breaks, the entire closure is affected. Running subcuticular sutures can be left in place for several weeks while the wound gains maximal tensile strength, with a resultant narrow scar with only two percutaneous suture marks at either end.

Layered Closure

If the goal of wound closure is cosmetic, strong consideration should be given to a layered closure in all full-thickness wounds under tension and those with the potential to develop tension over the first several days. Layered wound closure includes closure of muscle fascia with 3–0 or 4–0 simple or horizontal mattress sutures followed by closure of the dermis with interrupted, intradermal sutures in which the knot is buried below the dermis in the subcutaneous tissue (Fig. 116–12). Care must be taken to place these sutures so that the passage of the needle through the cut edge of the dermis is exactly the same depth and directly across on both sides of the wound edge. The number of intradermal sutures that need to be placed will be directly proportional to the amount of tension on the wound. After placement of the intradermal sutures, the surface may be closed with either tape or a running layer of fine 6–0 nonabsorbable suture. The top layer closure should prevent differential swelling of the wound edges. This is particularly important in areas where there is differential drainage from edges of the wound, such as in a transverse laceration of the

TABLE 116–1

SUTURE REPAIR OF SOFT TISSUE INJURIES

Location	Anesthetic	Suture Material	Technique of Closure and Dressing	Suture Removal
Scalp	Lidocaine 1% with epinephrine	3-0 or 4-0 nylon or polypropylene	Interrupted in galea; single tight layer in scalp: horizontal mattress if bleeding not well controlled by simple sutures	7–12 days
Pinna (ear)	Lidocaine 1% (field block)	6-0 nylon 5-0 Vicryl* or Dexon in perichondrium	Close perichondrium with 5-0 Vicryl interrupted; close skin with 6-0 nylon interrupted: stint dressing	4–6 days
Eyebrow	Lidocaine 1% with epinephrine	4-0 or 5-0 Vicryl and 6-0 nylon	Layered closure	4–5 days
Eyelid	Lidocaine 1%	6-0 nylon or silk	Single-layer horizontal mattress	3–5 days
Lip	Lidocaine 1% with epinephrine or field block	4-0 silk or Vicryl (mucosa) 5-0 Vicryl (SQ, muscle) 6-0 (skin)	Three layers (mucosa, muscle, and skin) if through and through, otherwise two layers	3–5 days
Oral cavity	Lidocaine 1% with epinephrine, or field block; sedation may be necessary in children	4-0 Vicryl	Simple interrupted or horizontal mattress: layered closure if muscularis of tongue involved	7–8 days or allow to dissolve
Face	Lidocaine 1% with epinephrine or field block	4-0 or 5-0 Vicryl (SQ) 6-0 nylon (skin)	If full-thickness laceration, layered closure desirable	3–5 days
Neck	Lidocaine 1% with epinephrine	4-0 Vicryl (SQ) 5-0 nylon (skin)	Two-layered closure for best cosmetic results	4–6 days
Trunk	Lidocaine 1% with epinephrine	4-0 Vicryl (SQ, fat) 4-0 or 5-0 nylon (skin)	Single or layered closure	7–12 days
Extremity	Lidocaine 1% with epinephrine	3-0 or 4-0 Vicryl (SQ, fat, muscle) 4-0 or 5-0 nylon (skin)	Single-layer closure is adequate, although layered or running SQ closure may give better cosmetic result; apply splint if wound over a joint	7–14 days
Hands and feet	Lidocaine 1% (if field block with 2% lidocaine or 0.25% bupivacaine)	4-0 or 5-0 nylon	Single-layer closure only with simple or horizontal mattress interrupted suture, at least 5 mm from cut wound edges; horizontal mattress sutures should be used if much tension on wound edges; apply splint if wound over a joint	7–12 days
Nailbeds	Lidocaine 2% or bupivacaine 0.25% digital nerve block	5-0 Vicryl	Gentle, meticulous placement to obtain even edges	Allow to dissolve

*Vicryl and Dexon suture can be interchanged throughout the table.

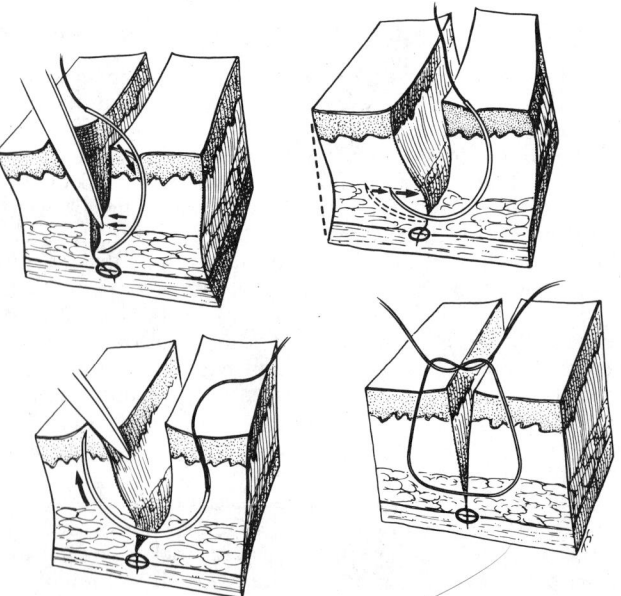

Figure 116–5. Skin eversion is accomplished with simple sutures that are deeper than they are wide and that include a wider bite of dermis than epidermis. (From Spicer TE. Facial and soft tissue trauma in childhood. *In* Mayer T (ed). Emergency Management of Pediatric Trauma. Philadelphia, WB Saunders, 1985, p 292.)

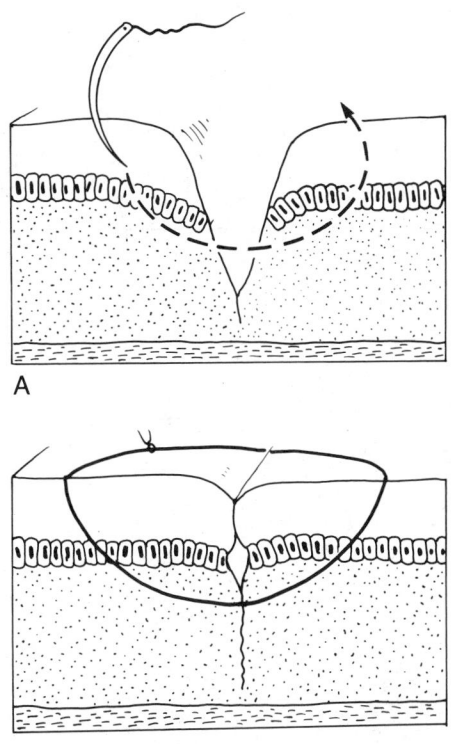

A

B

Figure 116–6. Skin edges are inverted when the stitch is shallow and wide. There is a risk of poor tissue healing and the wound reopening after suture removal.

forehead. In addition, meticulous placement of the sutures can be used to achieve the final evening of the wound edges in an effort to obtain the best cosmetic result.

Flaps and Stellate Lacerations

When closing a flap, great care must be taken not to compromise the venous and lymphatic drainage. Therefore, special consideration should be given to the placement of corner sutures that do not compromise circulation to the flap (Fig. 116–13). This can be accomplished by using a half-

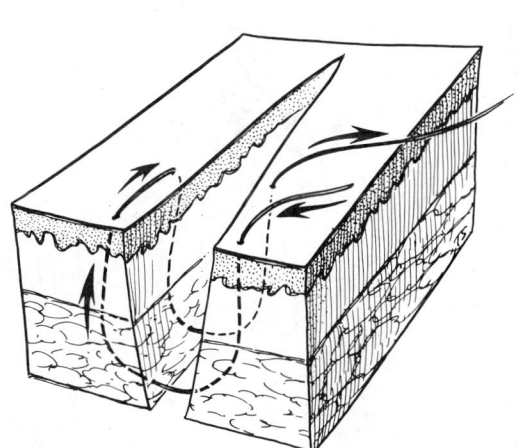

Figure 116–7. Horizontal mattress sutures guarantee eversion. Special care is required to avoid tight sutures with tissue strangulation. (From Spicer TE. Facial and soft tissue trauma in childhood. *In* Mayer T. Emergency Management of Pediatric Trauma. Philadelphia, WB Saunders, 1985, p 292.)

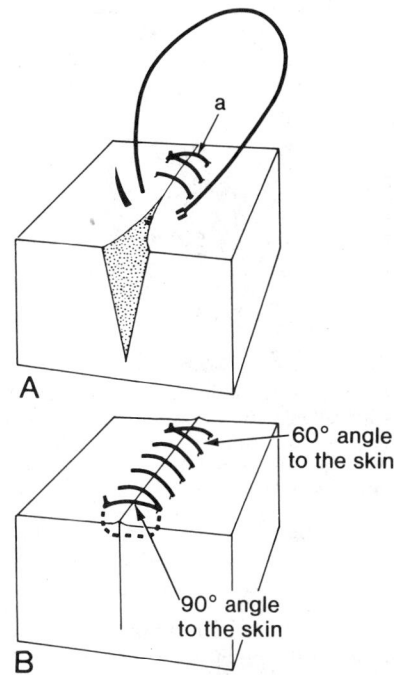

A

60° angle to the skin

90° angle to the skin

B

Figure 116–8. The running suture. A simple suture is started at one end and then "run" down the length of the laceration. The suture lies diagonally above the skin. (From Simon RR, Brenner BE. Procedures and Techniques in Emergency Medicine. 2nd ed. Baltimore, Williams & Wilkins, 1987, p 280.)

buried (Fig. 116–14) or completely buried horizontal mattress suture. After placement of this corner suture, it is important not to place percutaneous sutures in such a fashion that together they result in full-thickness compromise of circulation to and from the flap. A half-buried, buried, or pursestring suture is useful for closing stellate lacerations (see Fig. 116–13) bringing into approximation the cut edges of the flap. The remainder of the wound can then be closed with simple interrupted sutures.

PITFALLS IN WOUND MANAGEMENT

Scalp. Before closure of a scalp wound, it is important to carefully visualize and palpate the depths of the wound. Sometimes a skull fracture can be either directly visualized or palpated and yet not visualized on plain film radiography. This is especially important in wounds caused by large forces over a small area that may result in a depressed skull fracture. The wound edges must be tightly approximated with full-thickness sutures to prevent ongoing hemorrhage and subsequent hematoma formation.

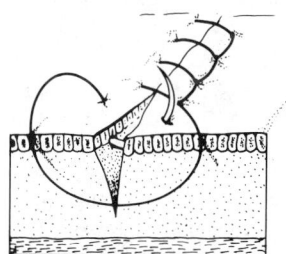

Figure 116–9. The running locking suture. This strong suture allows for good hemostatic control and is excellent for repair of the scalp.

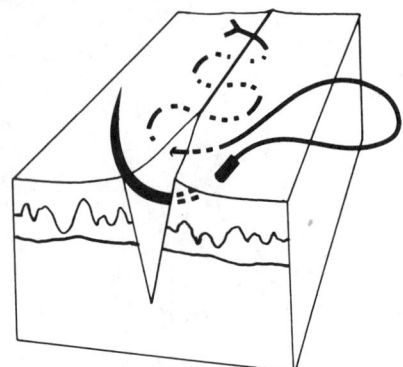

Figure 116–10. The running horizontal mattress suture. The technique is the same as for a conventional horizontal mattress suture except that the suture is not cut and tied with each stitch. (From Simon RR, Brenner BE: Procedures and Techniques in Emergency Medicine. 2nd ed. Baltimore, Williams & Wilkins, 1987, p 294.)

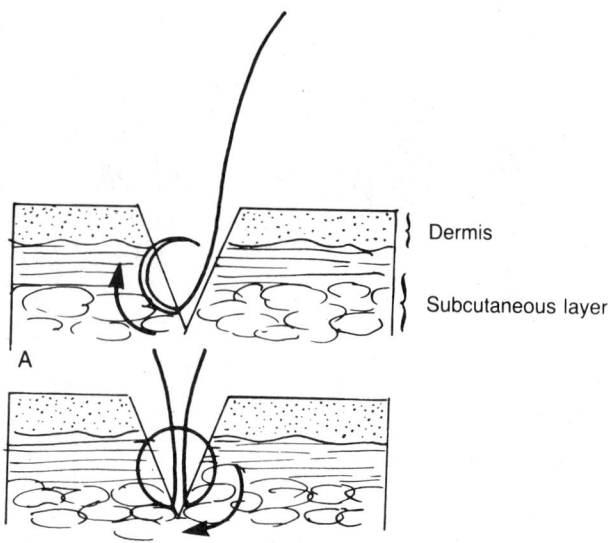

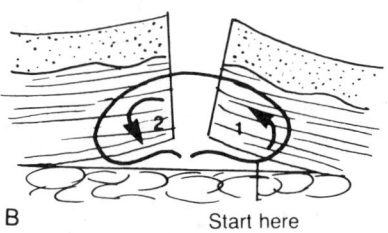

Figure 116–12. *A, B,* Inverted subcutaneous stitches. (From Lammers RL. Principles of wound management. *In* Roberts JR, Hedges JR (eds). Clinical Procedures in Emergency Medicine. 2nd ed. Philadelphia, WB Saunders, 1991, p 535.)

Pinna. Anesthesia should be by field block rather than by direct infiltrative filtration into the pinna. It is important not to use lidocaine with epinephrine to obtain anesthesia for repair of ear lacerations. Once the repair is complete, it is critical to dress the ear with a stint dressing of moistened cotton balls, which when dry will conform to the contours of the pinna. This stint dressing should be covered by several layers of gauze and a firm wrap and left in place for 24 to 48 hours. This is necessary to prevent formation of a painful subsequent hematoma between skin and perichondrium, requiring drainage.

Eyebrow. Wounds that extend into or through the eyebrow should generally be closed without excision. If excision is necessary in the eyebrow, it should not be done in a perpendicular fashion but rather parallel to the direction of the hair follicles. In addition, the eyebrow should never be shaved.

Eyelid. Careful examination must be made to make sure there is no penetration of the globe. In addition, if the wound is through the tarsal plate or into the area of the lacrimal apparatus, it should be referred to a consultant for

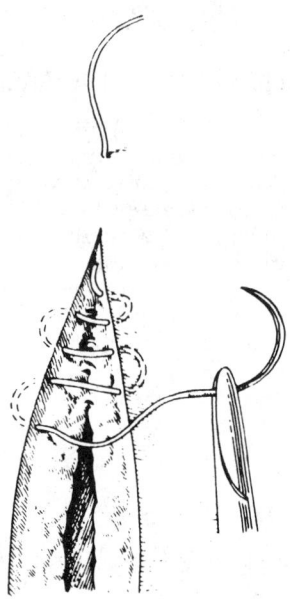

Figure 116–11. The subcuticular stitch. The suture is introduced into the skin in line with the incision, approximately 1 to 2 cm away. By backtracking each stitch slightly, one can produce a straight scar. (From Grimes DW, Garner RW. "Reliefs" in intracuticular sutures. Surg Rounds 1978; 1:46.)

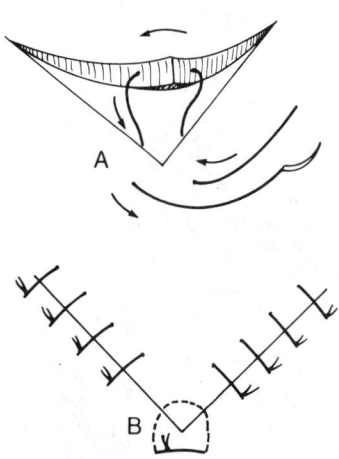

Figure 116–13. *A, B,* Approximation of a corner flap with a half-buried horizontal mattress stitch. Because of its applicability to this closure, this is often called a "corner stitch." (From Lammers RL. Principles of wound management. *In* Roberts JR, Hedges JR (eds). Clinical Procedures in Emergency Medicine. 2nd ed. Philadelphia, WB Saunders, 1991, p 543.)

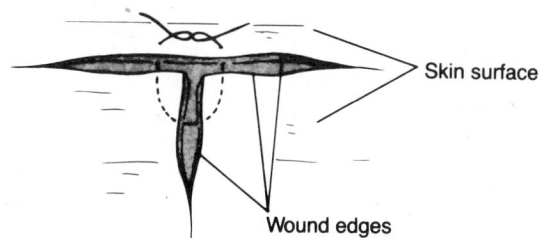

Figure 116–14. View from above a stellate laceration, showing closure with half-buried mattress stitches. (From Lammers RL. Principles of wound management. *In* Roberts JR, Hedges JR (eds). Clinical Procedures in Emergency Medicine. 2nd ed. Philadelphia, WB Saunders, 1991, p 546.)

proper closure, since improper repair of such a wound can result in permanent cosmetic or functional deformity.

Lip. Exact approximation of the vermilion border is vital to obtain the best cosmetic result. For this reason, it is advantageous to use field block rather than local infiltrative anesthesia, which may distort the vermilion border. Also, a watertight closure of the mucosa should be done before closure of the muscle and dermis. The closure can be checked by attempts to irrigate the wound and see whether any of the irrigation fluid leaks into the oral cavity after the mucosa has been sutured.

Oral Cavity and Mucous Membranes. Indications for closure of mucous membrane and tongue lacerations are when these are gaping or actively bleeding or are likely to result in a functional deformity: e.g., full-thickness wounds perpendicular through the tip of the tongue. It is often necessary to sedate children to obtain easy access to the oral cavity and perform the repair. In general, all lacerations of the oral cavity in children should be closed with an absorbable suture, eliminating the need for suture removal. These sutures generally dissolve with exposure to saliva in about 7 to 12 days.

Face. Careful attention must be paid to the underlying anatomy of the face, particularly with wounds that are over the parotid gland, Stensen's duct, or any of the major branches of the facial nerve. Before anesthesia of facial wounds, motor and sensory function of these major nerves should be carefully documented. If a major branch of the motor nerve or Stensen's duct appears to be involved, the patient is referred to a consultant for definitive repair.

Neck. Wounds of the neck that penetrate the platysma muscle cannot be visually explored to their full depth, and a surgical consultation should be obtained. Wounds that are gaping sufficiently to allow their entire depth to be explored may be closed as any other laceration, provided that no deep structures are injured.

Trunk. In wounds involving the chest wall, back, or abdominal cavity, the underlying anatomy is most important. If there is any question that the laceration may have penetrated the thorax or abdominal cavity, a surgical consultation should be obtained.

Extremities. Sensory function must be evaluated and documented before anesthesia of the wound. Meticulous control of hemorrhage and digital exploration of every wound is necessary to exclude a foreign body, partial lacerations of tendons, or penetration of joint space. If the wound is over a joint surface or will be under increased tension through normal range of motion, it should be splinted after the repair and the splint left in place for at least 1 or 2 weeks.

Hands and Feet. The same care must be taken to identify injury to underlying anatomic structures. Placement of in-

tradermal or subcuticular sutures on the hand and fingers is extremely hazardous and should be avoided; otherwise they may lead to damage to underlying structures such as digital nerves or subsequent suture granulomas in areas of great sensitivity such as fingertips. Sutures must be placed at least 5 mm from the cut edges of the wound. If the wound is under increased tension, horizontal mattress sutures should be used to prevent them from cutting through the wound edge. The need for proper splinting and strict elevation should be stressed to the patient.

Nailbeds. Wounds involving the nailbeds should be closed meticulously with absorbable sutures. Care must be taken when tying these sutures, since the tissue of the nailbed is friable; any suture that is tied too tightly will cut through the tissue. In painful wounds of the digits secondary to crush injuries, a longer-acting field block anesthetic such as bupivacaine is indicated. If grafts are placed (e.g., a full-thickness tidy laceration of a fingertip), a stint dressing must be carefully applied over the graft to prevent hematoma formation between graft and subcutaneous tissue. This dressing should be left in place for at least 1 week before removal and examination of the graft.

Bites. There is much controversy regarding the care of human and animal bites. In general, one should strongly consider secondary or delayed primary closure of all bites that have full-thickness penetration of the dermis, in all areas of the body except the face and scalp (Fig. 116–15). In addition, even though there are no current studies proving the efficacy of prophylactic antibiotics, it is common practice to prescribe these for 3 to 5 days after the injury. Cat bites carry a particularly high incidence of infection, and since these are puncture wounds, it is virtually impossible to locally explore and irrigate these wounds adequately. Therefore, full-thickness elliptical excision of tissue surrounding puncture wounds should be considered to improve irrigation.

Puncture Wounds. Puncture wounds of the foot, which usually are a result of a nail coming through the sole of a shoe or sneaker, may result in long-term morbidity. Several approaches have been advocated ranging from extensive excision, debridement, and irrigation to conservative therapy consisting simply of skin cleansing and soaks. A reasonable approach to puncture wounds of the foot would include local anesthesia surrounding the puncture wound, either by local infiltration or by a posterior tibial or sural nerve block. This should be followed by unroofing of the puncture wound, i.e., removal of what is usually thick and calloused epidermis. A blind probing of the wound with a fine splinter forceps can sometimes remove debris carried in with the injury, such as pieces of the sole of a sneaker or sock, or dirt. Although an attempt should be made to jet irrigate the wound, care must be taken to avoid injecting irrigation fluid that is not returned, and consequent increased swelling of the sole of the foot. Such irrigation may carry bacteria and debris deeper into the wound. It is appropriate to obtain a radiograph of the foot to exclude involvement of the bones and opaque foreign bodies. It is important to instruct the patient that these wounds have a high morbidity and potential for infection. Even if they do not become infected, there is often pain with weight bearing for several weeks. It is prudent to advise the patient to elevate the extremity and minimize weight bearing for at least 3 to 5 days. The efficacy of prophylactic antibiotics has not been proved, but if these are used a 3- to 5-day course is reasonable.

WOUND EXCISION

The best cosmetic results are often obtained by meticulous layered closure of a wound without excision. Wounds with edges that appear nonviable or are contaminated frequently

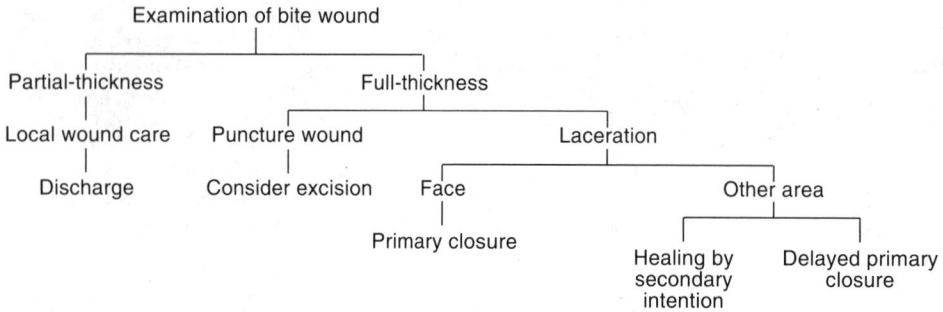

Figure 116–15. Approach to determining closure technique for bite wounds.

require sharp excision and debridement. Excision of tissue should be kept to a minimum and done in a linear and perpendicular fashion. Whenever wound edges are excised, the tension on a wound is increased. It may also be necessary to undermine tissue in order to mobilize and approximate the wound; such undermining can compromise the vascular supply. Relative contraindications to wound excision are in areas of the body where it is impossible or difficult to mobilize tissue and close the wound after the excision: e.g., the nose, hands and feet, and pretibial area of the leg.

SPECIALTY REFERRAL

Referral to a consultant should be considered when the primary care physician considers that definitive care of the wound is beyond his or her expertise, as in wounds with deep structure involvement such as those in tendons, nerves, joint capsules, eyelid tarsal plates, or lacerated ducts. If the patient or the family insists on referral to a specialist, it is appropriate to grant this request.

DRESSING AND SPLINTING

After repair of the wound, the area should be cleansed with sterile saline, the wound covered with antibiotic ointment, and a proper dressing applied. In general, a dressing should cover the wound for 24 to 48 hours and should be nonocclusive. If there is a potential for continued bleeding or hematoma formation, a compression bandage may be applied. If the wound is in an area where there will be tension, it should be splinted for 1 or 2 weeks.

AFTER-CARE INSTRUCTIONS

It is important to discuss with the patient expectations regarding normal wound healing and potential complications. The child and parents should be advised that all wounds will heal with a scar and be reminded that all efforts are directed toward minimizing the scarring and warned of the possibility of infection and hidden foreign bodies. Written instructions should cover the signs and symptoms of wound infection, and the need to return immediately should complications occur. An appointment should be made for suture removal, and the importance of returning in a timely fashion to avoid suture marks should be emphasized. Sunscreen (SPF 15 or greater) should be applied on the scar for at least 6 months after the injury to prevent ultraviolet hyperpigmentation.

DOCUMENTATION

The medical record should include all pertinent information obtained from the history and the physical examination, with careful attention to neuromuscular and motor function. It must be documented that all wounds have been explored prior to definitive care. A short surgical report should mention the type of anesthesia, the type of wound repair, the size and number of sutures, and the nature of the wound exploration. Specific after-care instructions should be documented. If the patient is concerned about the ultimate cosmetic results, documentation regarding the realistic expectations and degree of scarring should also be included in the medical record. Foreign bodies and wound contamination should be well documented, including confirmation that the patient has been informed of the possibility of a residual foreign body in this wound, despite careful management.

Selected References

Anderson AB, Colecchi C, Baronoski R, et al. Local anesthesia in pediatric patients: Topical TAC versus lidocaine. Ann Emerg Med 1990;19:519.

Billmire DA, Neale HW, Gregory RO. Use of IV fentanyl in the outpatient treatment of pediatric facial trauma. J Trauma 1985;25:1079.

Christoph RA, Buchanan L, Begalla K, Schwartz S. Pain reduction in local anesthetic administration through pH buffering. Ann Emerg Med 1988;17:117.

Dailey RH. Fatality secondary to misuse of TAC solution. Ann Emerg Med 1988;17:159.

Edlich RF, Rodeheaver GT, Morgan RF, et al. Principles of emergency wound management. Ann Emerg Med 1988;17:1284.

Ernst AA, Crabbe LH, Winsemius DK, et al. Comparison of tetracaine, adrenaline, and cocaine with cocaine alone for topical anesthesia. Ann Emerg Med 1990;19:51.

Hegenbarth MA, Altieri MF, Hawk WH, et al. Comparison of topical tetracaine, adrenaline, and cocaine anesthesia with lidocaine infiltration for repair of lacerations in children. Ann Emerg Med 1990;19:63.

Roettinger W, Edgerton MT, Kurtz LD, et al. Role of inoculation sites as a determinant of infection in soft tissue wounds. Am J Surg 1974;126:354.

Tandberg D. Glass in the hand and foot: Will an X-ray show it? JAMA 1982;248:1872.

CHAPTER 117

Pain Control in the Emergency Department

Bradford L. Walters

INTRODUCTION

Pain is a frequent complaint in the emergency department. There is no reliable means of measuring its severity. Many physicians tend to look at pain in a dose-related manner, meaning that one would expect the amount of pain perceived by a patient to correlate directly to the amount of tissue damage sustained or the severity of a disease. There is wide variance in the severity of reported pain in patients with similar injuries.

Anxiety and anticipation influence the perception of pain. This is an age-related phenomenon; older patients may be able to understand the importance of a painful procedure they are to undergo and therefore express less pain. Parental anxiety can significantly increase the distress of a child and thereby increase the perceived pain.

The expression of pain is influenced by various social and psychological factors. In certain cultures, stoicism is encouraged; in others, loud, vigorous expressions of pain are acceptable. These variations can complicate the physician's assessment of a given patient. Most physicians feel more positively toward a patient who is relatively stoic and uncomplaining. They therefore may undertreat the less vocal patient they feel most positive toward. A physician's personal biases also contribute considerably to the way pain is treated.

In children the assessment of pain can be more difficult than in adults. In the younger age groups communication is limited. Subjective and indirect means must be used to assess pain, and these are fraught with great imprecision. In the older age groups communication is easier, but fear of a strange place and intimidating people can discourage the expression of pain. However, just because children may not express pain does not mean that they are free of discomfort.

In neonates communication and reading body language in response to pain is the most difficult. Studies clearly show that pain is felt even in the first minutes of life. Behavioral and hormonal changes can be demonstrated in response to painful procedures being performed on neonates. However, such responses may be subtle, and it is impractical to use laboratory tests to ascertain whether a neonate is in pain.

The treatment of pain in pediatric patients has generally been poor. In a survey of burn units and their use of analgesics during dressing changes, far less medication was used in pediatric patients than in adult burn victims. Analgesic use in hospitals is frequently not based on the duration of action of the agent prescribed. In pediatric patients undergoing cardiac surgery, children received substantially less pain medication than adult patients; some children received none at all. Children undergoing general surgical procedures had a similar experience. A study of pediatric general surgical patients found that 16% received no analgesic medications postoperatively. Significant numbers of these patients reported severe pain even when they were provided with analgesics; undertreatment even was common.

Pain relief is rarely provided in such procedures as circumcision, lumbar puncture, arterial puncture, and intravenous cannulation. One author contends that children rarely need pain medications for procedures because they tolerate pain better than adults. Studies show that younger patients are more sensitive to pain and should receive more aggressive treatment for it.

Some physicians incorrectly believe that pediatric patients and adults metabolize narcotics in a different manner; children are more prone to respiratory side effects; and children simply require less pain medications than adults. In fact, all these axioms are false. After 1 month of age, children metabolize opioids in the same manner as adults. The incidence of respiratory complications is overstated and occurs no more frequently in the healthy child than in the adult.

Interestingly, physicians tend to advocate the use of analgesics for procedures they do not perform. General surgeons, unlike pediatricians, would use pain medications for lumbar punctures. Pediatricians advocate the use of analgesics more liberally in postoperative patients than their surgical colleagues do.

Joint relocations, fracture reductions, lumbar punctures, bone marrow aspirations, thoracentesis, and other invasive procedures are commonly performed in children without any premedication for pain. In adults the use of both sedatives and opioids is routine. Children with cancer express more fear and anxiety over the various procedures to which they are subjected, such as lumbar punctures and bone marrow aspirations, than over the pain of their disease. In spite of physicians' awareness of the discomfort involved in such procedures, premedication is underused.

PHYSIOLOGY OF PAIN

The perception of pain begins in the peripheral nervous system nociceptors. There are two types of pain receptors: myelinated small-diameter A-delta fibers and larger unmyelinated C fibers. The C fibers respond to a variety of stimuli such as heat, pressure, chemicals, and inflammation. The A-delta fibers tend to be more specific for a single type of outside stimulus. Repetitive stimuli increase activity in these nerves and may account for pain that persists long after the stimulus has stopped. This accounts for the phenomenon that pain intensity is increased with repeated noxious stimuli. Peripheral nerves enter the spinal cord through the dorsal horn and either synapse at that level or ascend several levels and then synapse. The ascending tracts go into the thalamus and brain-stem reticular formation before finally passing into the cortex. In addition to the ascending tracts, there are descending tracts that are believed to be able to modify the ascending impulses (Fig. 117–1).

Various mediators of pain activate the peripheral fibers. Substance P is a peptide thought to act as a neurotransmitter in both the spinal cord and the periphery. Other pain mediators include bradykinins, SRS-A, and a number of other chemicals that are elaborated when a specific tissue is injured. These chemicals influence and generally augment the transmission of pain impulses at both the tissue and central nervous system (CNS) levels.

In the CNS, pain perception becomes more complex and is poorly understood. One theory proposes that there are two types of nerve: a protopathic fiber that transmits a pain impulse and an epicritic fiber whose impulses block pain impulse transmission. The discernment of pain depends on the balance of the two inputs.

Modern theories have advanced this concept in the form of the gate theory, which proposes a "gate" within the spinal cord. This gate has not been identified anatomically but seems to account for the phenomenon that the ascending impulses can be modified by descending impulses. At the gate, both positive and negative inputs are processed. If positive inputs prevail, the gate opens, the impulse ascends to the brain, and pain is perceived. If negative impulses outweigh the positive ones, the gate remains closed and the effect is analgesia.

Endogenous opiates and opiate receptors are consistent with the gate theory. Various opiate receptors have been identified within the brain and spinal cord. This accumulation of receptors may represent the gate within the spinal cord. Stimulation of these receptors by an opiate results in various physiologic effects seen with opioid drugs.

A variety of endogenously secreted opioids called endorphins have also been identified. They are found in the same brain areas as the opiate receptors. Pain perception is modified by stimulation of these areas, releasing endorphins, which produces analgesia. An increase in the perception of pain is caused by the application of an opiate antagonist within these discrete areas to block the endorphin effect.

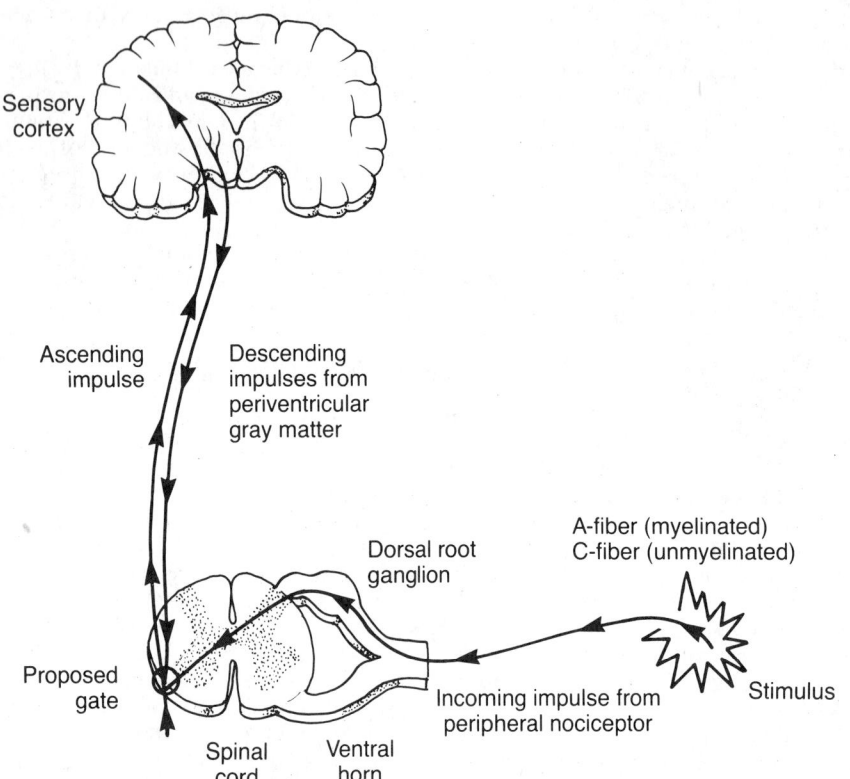

Figure 117–1. Diagram tracing the pain impulse along the peripheral nociceptor through the dorsal horn and up to the sensory cortex. Descending impulses can modify ascending impulses in an area of the spinal cord that represents the gate as proposed by the gate theory.

ROUTES OF ADMINISTRATION

Pain medications can be administered by a variety of routes. The oral route is the most common means of administration for most analgesics: it is simple, painless, and readily accessible. A disadvantage of this route is the long time required for sufficient levels of the drug to appear in the blood stream. In addition, there is virtually no way to titrate a drug given orally, since many variables influence absorption. Food in the stomach tends to delay absorption. In general, the oral route is best suited for patients in modest pain or in the outpatient setting. In this situation, the longer onset of action and erratic blood levels are less critical.

For more severe pain, the parenteral route is better. All opioids, and one nonsteroidal anti-inflamatory agent (ketorolac), can be administered intramuscularly (IM). The onset of action is faster for an IM agent than with oral administration. However, erratic absorption and inability to titrate an agent is problematic with the IM route. In a critically ill patient, decreased perfusion of peripheral tissues may add to the variability of absorption. A wide range of blood levels have been found in patients given the same dose of an IM analgesic agent. More side effects and greater respiratory depression have been observed with IM morphine than with its intravenous (IV) use. Some authors have condemned the IM route for pediatric patients in an emergency setting, considering it painful, less effective than the IV route, and one that carries the risk of greater complications. However, the IM route is certainly easy and remains a commonly used route despite its limitations.

The IV route allows greater control of the level of analgesia owing to the ability to titrate the effect of a given agent. In addition, with an IV line in place, it is easy to administer an opioid antagonist should a complication arise. The rapid onset of action of an analgesic given IV is accompanied by an equally fast recovery from the effects. In addition, absorption is more even and complete with direct administration into the blood stream. Repeated small doses of IV pain medications given slowly represent the safest, most rapid means of controlling significant pain in pediatric patients. The rapid onset of action of IV analgesics also lends itself more appropriately to the time constraints of the emergency department.

PHARMACOLOGIC INTERVENTION
Opioids

The most commonly used drugs for pain relief are the opioids. They are the most potent analgesics known and can produce serious side effects. Currently, they are the only analgesics that have a specific antagonist that reverses the agonist effects. This is a significant advantage over other analgesics.

The term *opioid* is used to classify drugs whose action closely parallels morphine and includes both natural and synthetic agents. Opiates are a specific group of phenanthrene alkaloids derived from an extract of the opium poppy. Examples include codeine and morphine. The various synthetic analgesics such as fentanyl, meperidine, and methadone have similar actions to morphine despite a dissimilar chemical structure.

These agents can be administered by many routes: IV, IM, subcutaneous (SQ), epidural, subarachnoid, transdermal, and transmucosal (nasal, buccal, and rectal). Continuous infusions of opioids, usually morphine, have been used successfully to control pain in children with cancer. Continuous administration is achieved by either an IV infusion or infusion through a fine needle in the SQ tissue of the thigh.

The IV route is the preferred means by which opioids should be administered in the emergency department in most cases of significant discomfort. Only by this route can the dose be easily titrated and quickly reversed. The onset of side effects is rapid, allowing them to be addressed more readily.

Adverse Effects. Along with a powerful analgesic effect, opioids possess a number of other physiologic effects that may be deleterious. These include sedation, euphoria, nausea, slowing of intestinal peristalsis, vomiting, biliary spasm, pruritus, miosis, urinary retention, vasodilatation, decreased cough, and respiratory depression. These side effects can also be beneficial. The patient with diarrhea who receives an opioid may have slowed intestinal activity. The antitussive effect is useful in cough preparations.

The greatest concern regarding opioids is respiratory depression, which is due to a blunting of the CNS response to both hypoxia and hypercarbia. In general, the dosage required for analgesia is less than that which will produce respiratory complications. Patients younger than 3 months of age who have a preexisting respiratory problem or airway compromise, or who have certain neurologic disorders, may be more sensitive to this effect. Healthy infants older than 3 months are no more sensitive to the respiratory depressive effects of opioids than an adult at equal plasma levels. Maximal respiratory depression occurs within approximately 7 minutes after IV administration of morphine, compared with 30 minutes after an IM dose and 90 minutes after SQ morphine. The emergency physician must be prepared to deal with respiratory depression by controlling the patient's airway and having an opioid antagonist available.

Tolerance, Addiction, Dependence. There is a great deal of misunderstanding concerning tolerance, addiction, and physical dependence. Tolerance refers to the lessening of the effect of a drug with repeated use. It varies for different physiologic properties of an opioid. For example, the tolerance of analgesia is similar to that of respiratory depression, while there will be less tolerance of the constipating effects. In general, the effects of tolerance are overcome by increasing the dose. Tolerance of respiratory depression occurs at about the same rate as that of analgesia, making dosage increases a safe practice in most cases.

Physical dependence and addiction are the most frequently misunderstood properties of opioids. Physical dependence occurs when continued administration of an agent is required to prevent the symptoms of withdrawal. Opiate withdrawal symptoms include dysphoria, agitation, piloerection, tachypnea, tachycardia, and diaphoresis. Dependence has been seen after 2 weeks of regular opioid administration in a hospital. It can be managed with a gradual reduction of the dose over 2 or 3 days, as opposed to sudden cessation. Dependence can occur with therapeutic use of opioid analgesics, although it rarely leads to addiction. Addiction involves a pathologic craving for opioids and compulsive drug-seeking behavior. It most often occurs with opioid use that is not under the supervision of a physician. Among adults, opioid addiction is highly unusual in a medical setting when given in a therapeutic regimen. In a study of 11,882 patients who received opioids for pain control, only four cases of addiction were noted. Many of the opinions regarding the addictive properties of opioids have been extrapolated from adult patients to children without any scientific support.

Agonists and Antagonists. Within the opioid group there are two general types, the pure agonists and partial agonists. The most commonly used are the pure agonists, which have essentially no ceiling to their analgesic, sedative, and respiratory depressive effects. They act in a purely dose-related manner with no limit to the level of respiratory depression that can be induced with increasing doses. The pure agonist group includes morphine, meperidine, fentanyl, and methadone. The second group includes many of the synthetic agents, generally partial agonists having mixed agonist-antagonist properties. Examples of the partial agonist opioids are pentazocine (Talwin), butorphanol (Stadol), and nalbuphine (Nubain). These drugs do have a ceiling effect, particularly to respiratory depression. Therefore, beyond a certain dose there will be no further respiratory depression. For this reason, they are suggested to be safer agents. However, the mixed agonist-antagonists can cause dysphoria and even precipitate withdrawal. Some practitioners feel there is little or no indication for the use of partial agonists in children.

One significant advantage of opioids is the ability to quickly reverse their effects. Naloxone is a direct competitive opioid antagonist that reverses the sedative, analgesic, and respiratory depressive effects of opioids. Naloxone (Narcan) is a pure antagonist with no agonist properties. Care must be taken to monitor the patient closely, as naloxone may have a shorter duration of action than the administered opioid. The patient may return to a stuporous state as the naloxone is cleared. This tends to occur in the setting of an overdose, not with therapeutic use of opioids.

Morphine. Morphine has been used for many years and is relatively inexpensive. The dosage of morphine for children is 0.10 mg/kg IV every 2 hours and 0.10 to 0.15 mg/kg IM or SQ every 3 to 4 hours (Table 117–1). Oral morphine has been used to control postoperative pain in children in doses of 0.20 to 0.40 mg/kg every 4 hours. Morphine can cause the release of histamine, which may produce a pruritic rash, hypotension, and bronchospasm in asthmatic patients.

Meperidine. Meperidine (Demerol) is the most commonly used parenteral pure agonist. Its actions and complications are nearly identical to those of morphine. With IM administration, serum levels of meperidine can vary widely. A serum concentration of 0.7 μg/ml is correlated with analgesia in 95% of patients. The most reliable means of achieving

TABLE 117–1

PAIN MEDICATIONS AND ADJUVANT DRUGS

Agent	Route	Dosage	Frequency
OPIOIDS			
Morphine	IV	0.1 mg/kg	q 2 hr
	IM/SQ	0.10–0.15 mg/kg	q 3–4 hr
	PO	0.2–0.4 mg/kg	q 4 hr
Meperidine	IV	0.8–1.0 mg/kg	q 2 hr
	IM	1.0–1.5 mg/kg	q 3–4 hr
Fentanyl	IV	1.0–2.0 μg/kg	q 1–2 hr
Codeine	PO	0.5–1.0 mg/kg	q 4 hr
NSAIDs			
Ibuprofen	PO	4.0–10.0 mg/kg	q 6–8 hr
Naproxen	PO	5.0–7.0 mg/kg	q 8–12 hr
Tolmetin	PO	5.0–7.0 mg/kg	q 6–8 hr
Aspirin	PO	10.0–15.0 mg/kg	q 4 hr
Acetaminophen	PO	10.0–15.0 mg/kg	q 4 hr
	PR	15.0–20.0 mg/kg	q 4 hr
SEDATIVES			
Diazepam	IV	0.2 mg/kg	q 2–4 hr
Midazolam	Intranasal or PO	0.2–0.3 mg/kg	Sedation for procedures
	IM	0.15 mg/kg	
	IV	0.07–0.10 mg/kg	
Hydroxyzine	IM	0.2 mg/kg	Sedation for procedures
	PO	0.25 mg/kg	
Methohexital	IM	10.0 mg/kg	Sedation for procedures
Pentobarbital	IM	5.0–6.0 mg/kg	Sedation for procedures
	IV	2.0–6.0 mg/kg	
Chloral hydrate	PR, PO	50–100 mg/kg	Sedation for procedures

this level is IV administration. The dosage of meperidine in children is 0.8 to 1.0 mg/kg IV every 2 hours and 1.0 to 1.5 mg/kg IM or SQ every 3 to 4 hours. The duration of action is shorter than that of morphine.

In general, opioids cause minimal decrease in cardiac function. However, meperidine may have a significant cardiac depressive effect. The metabolite of meperidine, normeperidine, may induce seizures. Dysphoria may occur with chronic meperidine administration.

Codeine. Codeine is the most commonly used oral opioid, generally reserved for less severe pain not requiring parenteral agents. Doses of codeine for children start at 0.5 to 1.0 mg/kg orally every 4 hours. It is commonly combined with acetaminophen in both tablet and elixir form.

Fentanyl. Fentanyl and the related agents, sufentanil and alfentanil, are opioids with short duration of action. Their effects are virtually identical to those of morphine, except that they are rapidly metabolized. In addition, fentanyl does not cause the release of histamine that can occur with morphine. Fentanyl is therefore the drug of choice for asthmatic patients. Short-acting agents are ideal for the emergency department where sedation and pain control can be achieved without having the patient subjected to a long recovery period. Fentanyl is the most commonly used short-acting agent in the emergency department and is quite safe. In a study of 2000 pediatric patients undergoing repair of facial lacerations, fentanyl was administered by plastic surgery residents intravenously to provide sedation and pain control. There were only three complications. In all three cases, the fentanyl was given too rapidly, resulting in rigidity of the chest wall. This complication is readily reversed with naloxone and is unusual if the drug is given over 2 or more minutes. The dosage of fentanyl is 1 to 2 µg/kg IV given slowly, with additional doses of 0.5 µg/kg every 1 to 2 minutes to achieve the desired effect. Children are no more sensitive to the respiratory depressant effect of fentanyl than adults at equal plasma levels. Nevertheless, a physician should be in attendance at all times during IV administration of fentanyl. The high lipophilic property of fentanyl and its related agents allows its administration mucosally (nasally or orally as a lollipop) as well as transdermally. The major impediment to the use of fentanyl in the emergency department is concern over its use by a physician other than an anesthesiologist. It is thought that many of the objections to the use of fentanyl outside the operating room are based on anecdotal opinion and not on clinical studies.

Nonsteroidal Anti-Inflammatory Drugs (NSAIDs)

NSAIDs are a large group of analgesics. They are the most commonly prescribed pain medication in the adult population and are gaining wider acceptance for use in children. The mode of action of NSAIDs is interference with the production of prostaglandins. They inhibit the enzyme prostaglandin synthetase, which results in a significant reduction of serum prostaglandin levels. These analgesics are useful in painful inflammatory conditions such as arthritis, sprains, bone pain, and rheumatoid disorders. NSAIDs have also been used effectively in children for pain after surgery.

Despite the popularity and over-the-counter availability of NSAIDs, there is limited research regarding their use in children. The most commonly used and available NSAID in children is ibuprofen (Motrin), which is available both on prescription and in over-the-counter preparations. The dosage in the pediatric age group is 4 to 10 mg/kg every 6 hours orally. Ibuprofen is the only NSAID that also is indicated as an antipyretic in children over 1 year old. It is available as a tablet, capsule, and suspension (100 mg/5 ml).

Naproxen (Naprosyn) and tolmetin (Tolectin) are FDA-approved NSAIDs for use in patients 2 to 12 years old, 5 to 7 mg/kg orally; naproxen is administered two to three times a day and tolmetin three to four times a day. Indomethacin (Indocin) is rarely used in pediatric patients because it has a high incidence of side effects. It should be given only after other NSAIDs have failed. The dosage of indomethacin is 0.5 to 2.0 mg/kg orally two or three times a day.

Ketorolac (Toradol) is a new NSAID that can be given parenterally. It has been approved for intramuscular use as an analgesic. Studies in adults have favorably compared 90 mg of ketorolac with 12 mg of morphine. At this time the drug is not approved for pediatric use, but it is likely that parenteral NSAIDs will eventually be so approved.

The side effects of NSAIDs are relatively few; the most common is gastrointestinal upset. The prostaglandin inhibition of NSAIDs limits the stomach's ability to protect itself from ulceration. GI bleeding can occur with chronic use. Nephrotoxicity can occur but is uncommon with short-term administration. Hepatoxicity can be a complication but again is rare with short-term use.

Acetaminophen and Salicylates. Acetaminophen is the most commonly used analgesic in children, 10 to 15 mg/kg orally every 4 hours. Rectal suppositories may be convenient in younger infants, although the absorption of acetaminophen can be erratic by this route. Short-term use of acetaminophen is safe without gastritis or bleeding problems. When acetaminophen is taken as an overdose, the resultant hepatotoxicity can be devastating. This is an unlikely complication in therapeutic doses.

Aspirin is also an effective analgesic for mild pain, 10 to 15 mg/kg orally every 4 hours. Salicylate use both as an analgesic and antipyretic has diminished since its association with Reye's syndrome. Gastritis is the most common side effect and occasionally leads to gastric hemorrhage. Generalized bleeding due to platelet function inhibition can be severe in aspirin-sensitive patients. Administration with food or antacids may reduce the incidence of gastritis and GI bleeding.

Sedative Agents

Sedatives reduce patient distress during painful procedures and serve as adjunctive agents to other analgesics.

Benzodiazepines. Benzodiazepines produce sedation, anxiolysis, hypnosis, amnesia, and muscle relaxation, but have little or no analgesic effect by themselves. They should not be used alone for painful procedures, but should be combined with some type of analgesic for pain relief. Sedatives are highly effective, and at appropriate doses usually do not interfere with cardiac and respiratory functions. They are frequently mixed with an opioid and can be given together IM, avoiding the need for two injections.

Diazepam. Diazepam (Valium) is one of the most common benzodiazepines used in the emergency department. It is well absorbed orally, but IM absorption is typically slow and unpredictable. IM administration is painful, and irritation of a vein is common with IV use because of the propylene glycol solvent. In general, the sedative effects of diazepam last longer than is desirable in the emergency department, and titration of effect is difficult owing to this long half-life. The IV dose is 0.2 mg/kg.

Midazolam. Midazolam (Versed) is a benzodiazepine approximately twice as potent as diazepam. As a water-soluble agent, it is less painful than the latter when given IM and does not cause the phlebitis common with diazepam. It has a short duration of action, making it better suited for emergency department use. Midazolam has a potent amnesic effect that is useful in painful procedures such as fracture and joint reduction.

The intranasal route for midazolam is particularly easy and effective in children, and 0.2 to 0.3 mg/kg instilled in the nose has been shown to have a potent sedative effect in preschool children. The onset of action is 5 to 10 minutes and respiratory or cardiac complications have not been reported. Midazolam can also be given orally, 0.2 to 0.3 mg/kg up to 5mg mixed in a flavored syrup. Satisfactory sedation in children undergoing laceration repair occurs within 30 minutes. Patients are sufficiently awake to be discharged approximately 15 minutes after completion of the procedure. IM doses of midazolam, 0.08 mg/kg, provide sedation about as quickly as an intranasal dose but are associated with the pain of an injection. Midazolam has been used IV for induction of anesthesia, 0.07 to 0.10 mg/kg slow IV push. Lower doses are generally satisfactory in providing short-term sedation for emergency department procedures. The drug can be titrated to the desired effect with a total dose of 0.5 to 1.0 mg. The respiratory depressant effect is of greater concern when midazolam is administered IV, especially with concomitant opioid use. Death has been reported from midazolam-induced hypoxia. The use of this agent must be confined to physicians who are comfortable with airway management. However, the advantages of short duration of action, potent sedative and amnesic effect, and less pain with administration make midazolam an effective adjunctive agent for controlling pain in children. When it is given IV in small incremental amounts, the desired actions can be titrated while potential respiratory complications are avoided.

Flumazenil. Flumazenil (Mazicon) is a competitive inhibitor at the benzodiazepine receptor. Flumazenil has no intrinsic agonist activity and quickly reverses the sedative and respiratory depressive effects of benzodiazepines. Flumazenil is not recommended for use in patients younger than 18 years owing to a lack of clinical studies. The recommended dose to reverse sedation in adults is 0.2 mg IV over 15 seconds, with repeated doses every 60 seconds until reversal of sedation occurs or 1.0 mg has been given.

Hydroxyzine. Hydroxyzine (Vistaril) is a mild sedative with antiemetic and antihistaminic properties. It is frequently added to either morphine or meperidine when given IM. It is well absorbed by both IM and oral routes. The oral preparation is typically used as a sedative or antipruritic. The antiemetic properties can counteract opioid-induced nausea. In adults the combination of hydroxyzine (100 mg) and morphine (10 mg) was found to be more effective than morphine alone. More drowsiness was reported in patients who received the combined preparation. In addition, the dose of hydroxyzine was much higher than that used in children. The hydroxyzine dosage is 0.2 mg/kg IM when given alone; a smaller dose is used when added to an opioid. Hydroxyzine has some respiratory depressive effect and potentiates that effect when combined with an opioid. Of the various adjuvants available, hydroxyzine seems to be effective and without any significant side effects. Its major disadvantage in children is that it can be given only IM or orally.

Barbiturates. Barbiturates are CNS depressants used for sedation. They have no intrinsic analgesic properties and should not be used alone. In doses that provide sedation there is minimal respiratory or cardiac depression. However, excessive doses can cause apnea, cardiovascular collapse, and coma. The onset of effect and duration of action varies with the lipid solubility of a particular barbiturate. The greater the lipid solubility, the more rapidly the drug enters the brain; this results in a faster onset and shorter duration of action. The ultrashort-acting barbiturates are highly lipid soluble, with a very rapid onset of action and rapid clearance. Thiopental (Pentothal) is an ultrashort-acting barbiturate. Pentobarbital (Nembutal), being less lipid soluble, takes longer to act and has a greater duration of action. Methohexital (Brevital) is a short-acting barbiturate that has provided sedation effective in children aged 2 months to 5 years undergoing computed tomography (CT). An IM dose of 10 mg/kg has a 4-minute onset of sedation, and by 90 minutes most patients are sufficiently awake to be discharged. Methohexital has been given rectally but can cause mucosal injury; it can also precipitate convulsions in patients with a seizure disorder. Thiopental can be given rectally, 25 to 45 mg/kg, and has been an effective sedative for CT. However, pentobarbital has also been reported to be an effective pediatric sedative, 5 to 6 mg/kg IM or 2 to 6 mg/kg IV, with recovery within 1 hour.

Chloral Hydrate. Chloral hydrate has effects similar as to those of the barbiturates, including a lack of analgesic effect. This drug is administered orally or rectally. It has a bad taste and the potential to cause gastric irritation. A dose of 50 to 100 mg/kg in healthy children older than 1 month has been used for sedation during radiologic studies. This dose should be reduced by half in younger infants or patients who are more ill. The onset of action is 30 to 60 minutes, and patient monitoring should continue for about 90 minutes after administration. Because a number of other drugs have a faster onset of action, are better tolerated, and have fewer side effects, the use of chloral hydrate is waning.

Ketamine. Ketamine is a dissociative anesthetic that has been used in subanesthetic doses for sedation and analgesia in children during emergency department procedures. In adults and older children, ketamine can cause an intense, postemergence delirium with bad dreams. The concomitant use of a benzodiazepine can prevent this unpleasant side effect in most patients. Respiratory depression is rare in subanesthetic doses of ketamine. The analgesic effect is intense, allowing procedures to be performed without additional local anesthetics or opioids. The patient enters a fugue-like state and can move or verbalize to some extent when stimulated, but remains anesthetized and amnesic. The recommended subanesthetic dose of ketamine is 2 mg/kg IM in the newborn to 6-month age group, 1 mg/kg in infants 6 months to 1 year old, and 0.5 mg/kg in those over 1 year old. One half of the dose can be repeated in 30 minutes if required. Ketamine causes an increase in oral secretions, and premedication with atropine, 0.01 mg/kg 15 minutes before its administration, is suggested. One author recommended an IV dose of 2 mg/kg, but noted that the desired effect of ketamine was usually reached before the full dose was administered. Pretreatment with diazepam was used to prevent unpleasant hallucinations. Another author supplemented local anesthesia with a combination of 0.4 mg/kg of ketamine and 0.08 mg/kg diazepam IV to patients already pretreated with morphine 0.2 mg/kg plus atropine 0.01 mg/kg. In 200 adult outpatient procedures this was found to be an effective and safe combination. The applicability of that regimen to pediatric patients appears to be limited, but ketamine's safety in subanesthetic doses was once again demonstrated.

Ketamine causes an increased heart rate, elevated blood pressure, and increased intracranial pressure. It therefore should not be used in patients with cardiac ischemia or a mass lesion of the brain. Approximately 30% of patients who receive ketamine experience postemergence hallucinations. However, this is less of a problem in patients under 15 years of age. Ketamine is effective and safe in subanesthetic doses in the emergency department, particularly in younger children.

DPT. A number of combination sedative and analgesic

cocktails have been used in pediatric patients. The DPT combination of Demerol (meperidine, 2.0 to 2.25 mg/kg), Phenergan (promethazine, 0.5 to 1.0 mg/kg), and Thorazine (chlorpromazine, 0.5 to 1.0 mg/kg) has been given as an IM injection since the 1950s. This combination has produced effective sedation in 20 to 30 minutes in most children. An additional half dose can be given 45 minutes later if the desired effect has not been achieved. The DPT combination has been criticized for a high incidence of side effects, including respiratory depression, seizures, and dystonic reactions; a slow onset of action; and a prolonged period of sedation after the procedure. However, other studies have found the combination safe and effective. In one such study of 487 pediatric patients there were three cases of respiratory depression requiring naloxone reversal. In this study, a dose of 2 mg/kg of meperidine was used. In a second prospective study by the same group, the safety of DPT was again confirmed. In 63 patients there were no clinically significant changes in vital signs or pulse oximetry. The average time for onset of action was 27 minutes, for duration of action 103 minutes, and for hours in the emergency department, 4.7. The biggest disadvantage of DPT is that it can only be administered IM.

Nitrous Oxide. Inhaled nitrous oxide is an effective sedative and analgesic with minimal cardiovascular and respiratory depressive effects. Nitrous oxide is commercially available in a 50% mixture with oxygen in a single tank or in an apparatus that will deliver a fixed concentration, with the two gases in separate containers. This inhaled analgesic has been used successfully for both dental and emergency department procedures in patients as young as 16 months. Administration is easy with either a nasal mask or a patient-held face mask. The complication rate is low. One caution about its use is that scavenging equipment is required to prevent leakage of the nitrous oxide into the air and the risk of exposing emergency department personnel to long-term effects.

Contraindications to the use of nitrous oxide are relatively few. It can cause an increase in the size of a pneumothorax and dilated bowel secondary to intestinal obstruction. It is contraindicated in patients suffering from decompression sickness. It should also be avoided in patients who have a decreased level of consciousness or are intoxicated. In most circumstances the drug can be self-administered. Younger children may not be able to hold on to a mask; a nasal mask has been used successfully. Close and frequent attention must be paid to the level of anesthesia.

LOCAL ANESTHETICS

All currently used local anesthetics have a similar structure: a lipophilic aromatic end coupled to an intermediate middle chain, which in turn is attached to a hydrophilic amine end. Differences in the pharmacologic properties of the various agents depend on changes in the structure of the three parts of the molecule. The linkage between the aromatic and middle chain allows local anesthetics to be classified into two basic groups, esters and amides (Table 117–2).

The exact mechanism of action of local anesthetics is unknown. Recent theories propose a slowing or blocking of the fast sodium channel of the nerve cell membrane.

The complication that occurs most frequently with local anesthetics is vasovagal syncope secondary to pain, fear, or anxiety. The most feared complication is an allergic reaction mediated by IgE antibodies, leading to anaphylaxis. This devastating event is rare, and overall these agents are extremely safe.

Any local anesthetic can produce a generalized systemic

TABLE 117–2	
LOCAL ANESTHETICS	
Name	Maximal Dose
Amides	
Lidocaine (Xylocaine)	5 mg/kg
Bupivacaine (Marcaine)	1.5 mg/kg
Mepivacaine (Carbocaine)	7 mg/kg
Etidocaine (Duranest)	3 mg/kg
Prilocaine (Citanest)	10 mg/kg
Esters	
Procaine (Novocain)	14 mg/kg
Chloroprocaine (Nesacaine)	14 mg/kg
Tetracaine (Pontocaine)	1.5 mg/kg
Benzocaine (Americaine)	Topical use only

reaction if given in a sufficient dose. Local anesthetics are labeled in multidose vials as a percentage solution rather than by milligrams per volume. Therefore, the physician may be unaware of the total dosage in milligrams. For example, infiltration of a small wound using 3 ml of 1% lidocaine results in a 30-mg lidocaine administration. With local anesthetics, a percentage solution by definition is the number of grams per 100 ml of solvent. Therefore, a 1% solution is 1 gm of lidocaine in 100 ml of water, making a final concentration of 10 mg/ml; a 2% solution represents a 20 mg/kg concentration. To avoid systemic toxicity, the actual dosage must be monitored in reference to the toxic level. For the two most commonly used agents, lidocaine and bupivacaine, the maximal recommended dose is 5 and 1.5 mg/kg, respectively. In a small child weighing 10 kg, this is a 50-mg maximal dose of lidocaine. With 2% lidocaine, that dose would represent a mere 2.5 ml, a typical volume used to repair a laceration.

A toxic reaction generally starts with CNS symptoms beginning with drowsiness, tinnitus, paresthesias, restlessness, tremors, anxiety, seizures, and finally coma with increasing doses. As the dosage reaches even higher levels there may be depression of cardiac function, arrhythmias, and hypotension, finally leading to shock and death.

The incidence of true allergy to local anesthetics mediated by IgE antibodies is actually rare. Anaphylactic reactions are limited to the ester local anesthetics, which are the only class that can stimulate IgE antibody production. The amide agents are unable to elicit such a response from the immune system. No true allergy has been demonstrated to the amide local anesthetics. Avoiding this extreme reaction is an advantage of amide anesthetics such as lidocaine or bupivacaine. Reported allergic reactions to an amide local anesthetic are vasovagal reactions, systemic toxicity, or cross sensitivity to the preservative used in multidose vials. Paraben, one such preservative, is structurally related to the ester class of local anesthetic and is a source of so-called lidocaine allergic reactions. There is no cross sensitivity between the ester and amide groups of drugs. In a patient who reports an allergy to an ester local anesthetic such as procaine, any of the amide agents can be used safely. However, in view of cross sensitivity to preservatives, one must use an agent that contains no such additive. A convenient source of preservative-free lidocaine is the preparation used for IV antiarrhythmic purposes. This formulation of lidocaine is packaged without any preservative. One can also avoid anesthetic allergies by using diphenhydramine (Benadryl), which has weak local anesthetic properties.

Lidocaine. Lidocaine (Xylocaine) is the most commonly used local anesthetic. It is effective when applied topically as well as by injection. Lidocaine is well tolerated by the tissues and causes little irritation or inflammation. It has relatively modest systemic toxicity, with a maximal dose of 5 mg/kg. It is packaged in a number of forms. Viscous lidocaine, 2%, is useful for topical anesthesia, particularly of mucosal surfaces. Injectable lidocaine is available in 0.5%, 1.0%, and 2.0% concentrations in multidose vials. No study has shown any greater clinical efficacy with the higher concentrations. There is therefore an increased risk of systemic toxicity without any clinical advantage from concentrations over 0.5% or 1.0%. To keep lidocaine stable and maintain a long shelf life, local anesthetics are packaged in an acidic solution. Commercial multidose preparations of 1% lidocaine have a pH of approximately 5.0. Buffering the lidocaine with sodium bicarbonate to a more physiologic pH of around 7.2 decreases the pain during administration. The exact mechanism behind this decrease in pain is undetermined, but it is known that the acidity of an agent does not cause the pain upon administration. Buffering does not compromise the anesthetic effect of the local anesthetic. Generally, 4 ml of 1% lidocaine with 1 ml of sodium bicarbonate (8.4%) will buffer the solution to near-physiologic pH. Only small amounts of the buffered lidocaine should be mixed, because the shelf life of the solution is reduced to about one week.

Bupivacaine. Bupivacaine (Marcaine), an amide type of local anesthetic, is more potent and longer lasting than lidocaine. However, it is also more toxic and the maximal dose should be no greater than 1.5 mg/kg. This agent is generally available in either a 0.25% or 0.50% solution. There is little advantage in the higher concentration. Bupivacaine also can be buffered to decrease the pain of infiltration. Its greater duration of action makes it an ideal drug for regional anesthesia and nerve blocks.

Procaine. Procaine (Novocain) is well tolerated and has low systemic toxicity. It is still used extensively in dentistry but less so in emergency medicine. As an ester agent it carries the risk of a rare anaphylactic reaction and offers no significant advantage over lidocaine or bupivacaine.

Tetracaine. Tetracaine (Pontocaine) is an ester local anesthetic approximately ten times as potent as procaine and ten times as toxic. It is still used as a topical anesthetic alone or in combination with other agents. Cetacaine is a commercial mixture of tetracaine and benzocaine used for topical anesthesia.

Benzocaine. Benzocaine (Americaine) is a highly toxic ester local anesthetic but is so poorly soluble in water that it is slowly absorbed. It is used exclusively as a topical agent and is one of the few agents capable of stopping itching. It can be combined with other local anesthetics, as in Cetacaine, or added to sunburn cream preparations.

Topical Anesthetics. TAC is a combination topical anesthetic (tetracaine 0.5%, adrenaline [epinephrine] 1:2000, and cocaine 11.8%) used to avoid the pain of local infiltration. In one report TAC was found to be equal in efficacy to and better tolerated than infiltrated lidocaine. In another study TAC increased the incidence of infection. This was believed to be a result of the intense vasoconstriction induced by TAC, which decreases the ability of the skin to withstand infection from bacteria applied to the wounds. There have also been fatalities in children treated with TAC. One report described a 7-month-old child who was found dead 3 hours after having had this agent applied to the oral mucosa; death was attributed to a cocaine induced arrhythmia. Cocaine is readily absorbed from the mucosal membranes, and the total dose administered in this case was too high for an infant.

Guidelines for the use of TAC include its avoidance on mucosal membranes, lacerations supplied by end arteries (i.e., fingertips, ear, and penis), and highly contaminated wounds at risk for infection. Its use in young infants should be approached with caution owing to the high concentration of cocaine. Absorption of cocaine occurs readily even with the use of TAC on skin wounds. Of children receiving TAC, cocaine metabolites were detectable in 56.5% 20 to 40 minutes after its application. A parent accompanying the patient can hold an applicator soaked with TAC to the wound for approximately 20 minutes. This frees emergency personnel to tend to other duties and makes the use of TAC more efficient. A safer combination is TLE (tetracaine, lidocaine, and epinephrine).

Epinephrine in Local Anesthetics. The addition of epinephrine to various local anesthetics is a common practice. Both lidocaine and bupivacaine are commercially available with epinephrine added to act as a vasoconstrictor. This actually does little to increase the level of anesthesia and bleeding control. The most common sites where epinephrine-induced vasoconstriction is encouraged are the face, scalp, and oral mucosa, where bleeding from wounds can be brisk. However, few physicians wait the necessary 10 minutes for epinephrine to exert its vasoconstrictive effect before repairing a wound. Use of vasoconstrictors results in a decrease in the ability of the skin to withstand infection, because of decreased blood flow to the skin. This effect is advantageous with large wounds in which a large amount of a local anesthetic would be required. The added epinephrine slows the absorption of the drug and reduces the risk of a systemic reaction. This preparation is also commonly used in peritoneal lavage incisions to reduce local bleeding, which could contaminate the lavage fluid. With the abundant vascular supply to the head and neck, nerve blocks tend to wear off quickly. Use of a local anesthetic with epinephrine can prolong such a block.

Selected References

Anand KJS, Phil D, Hickey PR. Pain and its effects in the human neonate and fetus. N Engl J Med 1987;317:1321.

Anderson AB, Colicchi C, Baronoski R, et al. Local anesthesia in pediatric patients: Topical TAC versus lidocaine. Ann Emerg Med 1990;19:519.

Bartfield JM, Gennis P, Barbera J, et al. Buffered versus plain lidocaine as a local anesthetic for simple laceration repair. Ann Emerg Med 1990;19:1387.

Beyer JE, DeGood DE, Ashley LC, et al. Pattern of postoperative analgesic use with adults and children following cardiac surgery. Pain 1983;17:71.

Billmire DA, Neale HW, Gregory RO. Use of IV fentanyl in the outpatient treatment of pediatric facial trauma. J Trauma 1985;25:1079.

Brogden RN. Nonsteroidal anti-inflammatory analgesics other than salicylates. Drugs 1986;4:27.

Brown DT, Beamish D, Wildsmith JAW. Allergic reaction to an amide local anaesthetic. Br J Anaesth 1981;53:435.

Burckart GJ, White TJ III, Siegle RL, et al. Rectal thiopental versus an intramuscular cocktail for sedating children before computerized tomography. Am J Hosp Pharm 1980;37:222.

Christoph RA, Buchanan L, Begalla K, et al. Pain reduction in local anesthetic administration through pH buffering. Ann Emerg Med 1988;17:117.

Chudnofsky CR, Wright SW, Dronen SC, et al. The safety of fentanyl use in the emergency department. Ann Emerg Med 1989;18:635.

Cohen FL. Postsurgical pain relief: Patient status and nurse's medication choices. Pain 1980;9:265.

Covino BG. Pharmacology of local anesthetics. Res Staff Phys 1982;28:60.

Dailey RH. Fatality secondary to misuse of TAC solution. Ann Emerg Med 1988;17:159.

de Jong RH. The toxic effects of local anesthetics. JAMA 1978;239:1166.

Dundee JW, Halliday NJ, Harper KW, Brogden RN. Midazolam. A review of its pharmacological properties and therapeutic uses. Drugs 1984;28:519.

Fitzmaurice LS, Wasserman GS, Knapp JF, et al. TAC use and absorption of cocaine in a pediatric emergency department. Ann Emerg Med 1990;19:515.

Gamis AS, Knapp JF, Glenski JA. Nitrous oxide analgesia in a pediatric emergency department. Ann Emerg Med 1989;18:177.

Goetting MG, Thirman MJ. Neurotoxicity of meperidine. Ann Emerg Med 1985;14:1007.

Haslam DR. Age and the perception of pain. Psychonomic Sci 1969;15:86.

Hennes HM, Wagner V, Bonadio WA, et al. The effect of oral midazolam on anxiety of preschool children during laceration repair. Ann Emerg Med 1990;19:1006.

Hupert C, Yacoub M, Turgeon LR. Effect of hydroxyzine on morphine analgesia for the treatment of postoperative pain. Anesth Analg 1980;59:690.

Koren G, Butt W, Chinyanga H, et al. Postoperative morphine infusion in newborn infants: Assessment of disposition characteristics and safety. J Pediatr 1985;107:963.

Levine J. Pain and analgesia: The outlook for more rational treatment. Ann Intern Med 1984;100:269.

Mather M, Mackie J. The incidence of postoperative pain in children. Pain 1983;15:271.

McKay W, Morris R, Mushlin P. Sodium bicarbonate attenuates pain on skin infiltration with lidocaine, with or without epinephrine. Anesth Analg 1987;66:572.

Miser AW, Cavis DM, Hughes CS, et al. Continuous subcutaneous infusion of morphine in children with cancer. Am J Dis Child 1983;137:383.

Miser AW, Chayt KJ, Sandlund JT. Narcotic withdrawal syndrome in young adults after the therapeutic use of opiates. Am J Dis Child 1986;140:603.

Miser AW, Miser JS, Clark BS. Continuous intravenous infusion of morphine sulfate for control of severe pain in children with terminal malignancy. J Pediatr 1980;96:930.

Nahata MC, Clotz MA, Krogg EA. Adverse effects of meperidine, promethazine, and chlorpromazine for sedation in pediatric patients. Clin Pediatr 1985;24:558.

Newberger PF, Sallan SE. Chronic pain: Principles of management. J Pediatr 1981;98:180.

Paris PM. Pain management in the child. Emerg Med Clin North Am 1987;5:699.

Perry S, Heidrich G. Management of pain during debridement: A survey of U.S. burn units. Pain 1982;13:267.

Pryor GJ, Kilpatrick WR, Opp DR. Local anesthesia in minor lacerations: Topical TAC vs lidocaine. Ann Emerg Med 1980;9:568.

Schecter NL. Pain and pain control in children. Curr Probl Pediatr 1985;15:1.

Schecter NL. The undertreatment of pain in children: An overview. Pediatr Clin North Am 1984;30:781.

Selbst SM, Henretig FM. The treatment of pain in the emergency department. Pediatr Clin North Am 1989;36:965.

Shannon M, Berde CB. Pharmacologic management of pain in children and adolescents. Pediatr Clin North Am 1989;36:855.

Stewart RD. Nitrous oxide sedation/analgesia in emergency medicine. Ann Emerg Med 1985;14:139.

Stiehm ER: Nonsteroidal anti-inflammatory drugs in pediatric patients. Am J Dis Child 1988;142:1281.

Strain JD, Harvey LA, Foley LC, et al. Intravenously administered pentobarbital sodium for sedation in pediatric CT. Radiology 1986;161:105.

Swafford LI, Allen D. Pain relief in the pediatric patient. Med Clin North Am 1968;52:131.

Terndrup TE, Dire DJ, Madden CM, et al. A prospective analysis of intramuscular meperidine, promethazine, and chlorpromazine in pediatric emergency department patients. Ann Emerg Med 1991;20:31.

Varner DTA, Ebert JP, McKay RD, et al. Methohexital sedation of children undergoing CT scan. Anesth Analg 1985;64:643.

Williamson PS, Williamson ML. Physiologic stress reduction by an anesthetic during newborn circumcision. Pediatrics 1983;71:36.

Wilton NCT, Leigh J, Rosen DR, et al. Preanesthetic sedation of preschool children using intranasal midazolam. Anesthesiology 1988;69:972.

Yaster M, Deshpande JK. Management of pediatric pain with opioid analgesics. J Pediatr 1988;113:421.

Zeltzer LK, Jay SM, Fisher DM. The management of pain associated with pediatric procedures. Pediatr Clin North Am 1989;36:941.

CHAPTER 118

Regional Anesthesia

Alice S. Yih
William M. Maguire

INTRODUCTION

Regional anesthesia is a valuable adjunct in the treatment of injured children (Table 118–1). Regional techniques offer the advantages of not distorting anatomic landmarks, leading to better cosmetic results; using lower doses of anesthetic agents, thereby minimizing toxicity; and enabling the anes-

---

TABLE 118–1

CONTENTS FOR A REGIONAL ANESTHESIA TRAY

Sterile prep components
  3 prep sponges
  3 gauze sponges
  4 towels
  1 antiseptic solution receptacle
Sterile procedure components
  1 1-ml tuberculin syringe (used to measure vasoconstrictors)
  1 3-ml syringe (used for skin wheal)
  1 10-ml syringe (used for local anesthetic injection)
  1 25- or 27-gauge, ⅝-inch (1.6-cm) skin wheal needle
  1 18-gauge, 1½-inch (3.8-cm) needle (used to withdraw local anesthetic solution from the vial)
  4 22-gauge block needles of various lengths (1½-, 2-, 3-, and 4-inch [3.8-, 5.1-, 7.7-, and 10.2-cm])
  1 25-gauge, 1½-inch (3.8-cm) block needle
  1 25-gauge, 1.5-cm block needle
  1 local anesthetic solution receptacle (30-ml capacity)
  1 narrow-bore anesthesia extension set
  1 three-way stopcock
Drugs
  1% lidocaine
  1% lidocaine with epinephrine
  0.25% bupivacaine
  2% lidocaine with epinephrine

---

thetization of difficult areas (e.g., palms, soles) when extensive repairs are required.

PREPARATION

Prior to any procedure, a brief history should be elicited from the patient or parents. Attention should be focused on drug allergies, current medications, and past medical problems. Although adults can usually tolerate regional nerve block procedures without sedation, children may not. Most regional techniques require precise placement of the anesthetic agent at a particular location, and a moving, uncooperative child minimizes the likelihood of a successful block. An adjunct (e.g., midazolam, fentanyl, hypnosis) may be used to calm the child prior to attempting a regional nerve block.

UPPER EXTREMITY BLOCKS
Wrist Blocks

Wrist blocks are commonly used and easily performed. A total wrist block can be achieved by blocking all three nerves: the median, the radial, and the ulnar.

Median Nerve Block

To perform a median nerve block, the dorsum of the hand is rested on the table (Fig. 118–1). The wrist is extended by placing a roll of gauze behind the wrist on the table. The nerve is located between the palmaris longus and flexor carpi radialis tendons, which are best located by having the patient actively flex the wrist and oppose the thumb and little finger. After antiseptic skin preparation, a 1.5-inch, 25-gauge needle is inserted perpendicularly into the skin at the level of the proximal wrist crease. Penetration of the flexor retinaculum is indicated by a "pop" sensation. Once paresthesia is obtained in the median nerve distribution, 2 to 5 ml of local anesthetic are instilled. If the palmaris longus is absent, the needle is inserted on the ulnar aspect of the flexor carpi radialis.

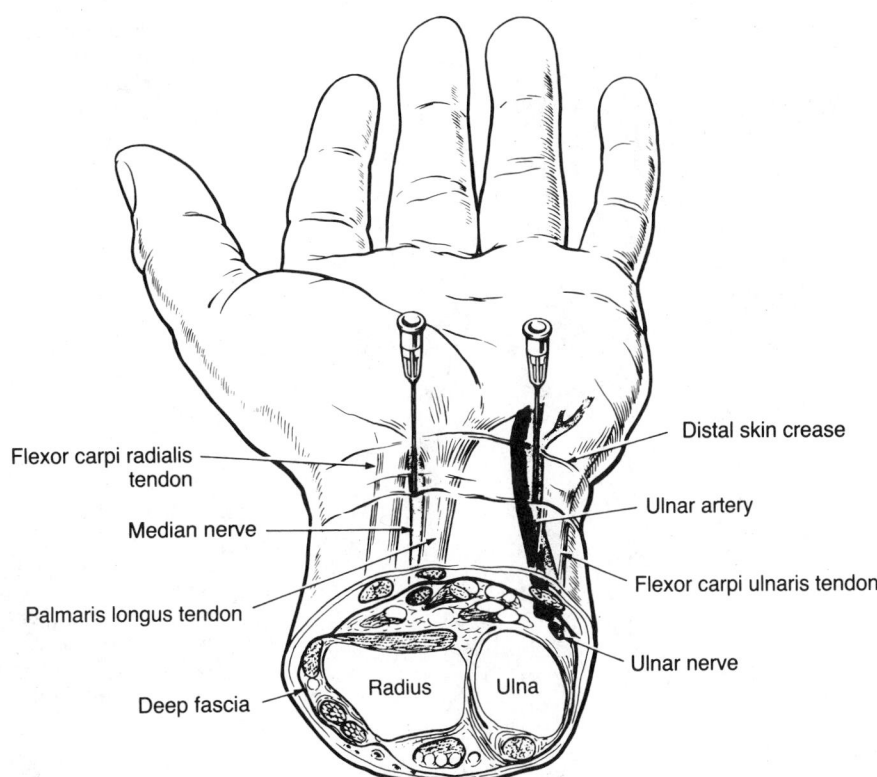

Figure 118–1. Landmarks and technique of needle insertion for median and ulnar nerve block at the wrist. (From Cousins MJ, Bridenbaugh PO. Neural Blockade in Clinical Anaesthesia and Management of Pain. 2nd ed. Philadelphia, JB Lippincott, 1987, p 409.)

Radial Nerve Block

The radial nerve is located superficially at the radial aspect of the wrist. A 1.5-inch, 25-gauge needle is inserted into the subcutaneous tissue lateral to the radial artery at the proximal flexor wrist crease (Fig. 118–2). The tissue is infiltrated in a semicircular fashion around to the midportion of the dorsum of the wrist. A total of 10 to 12 ml of anesthetic are used in the adolescent to block the sensory branches of this nerve.

Ulnar Nerve Block

Two major branches of the ulnar nerve at the level of the wrist—the palmar and the dorsal branches—must be blocked for successful ulnar anesthesia. The palmar branch is located between the ulnar artery and the flexor carpi ulnaris tendon (Fig. 118–3). The flexor carpi ulnaris, which inserts on the

pisiform bone, is easily located at the ulnar styloid process. The patient should flex and ulnarly deviate the wrist to locate this tendon. A 1.5-inch, 25-gauge needle is inserted perpendicularly between the flexor carpi ulnaris and ulnar artery at the level of the superior crease of the wrist. Paresthesia should be elicited and local anesthetic injected (3 ml).

The dorsal branch of the ulnar nerve is blocked by infiltrating 5 to 10 ml of anesthetic subcutaneously, starting at the site of the palmar branch block and continuing around to the mid-dorsum of the wrist.

DIGITAL NERVE BLOCKS

There are two sets of nerves that supply sensation to the fingers: the dorsal and volar digital nerves (Fig. 118–4). The volar digital nerve originates from the median nerve and innervates the entire palmar surface of the thumb and the

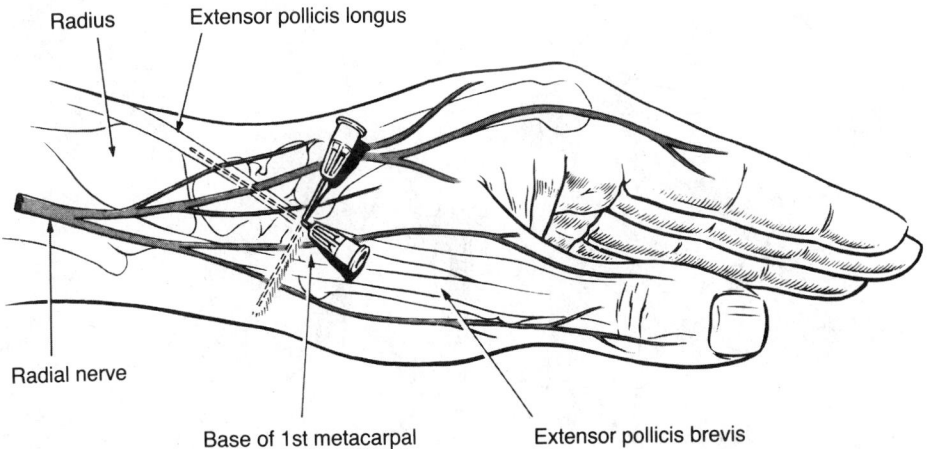

Figure 118–2. Landmarks and technique of needle insertion for radial nerve block at the wrist. (From Cousins MJ, Bridenbaugh PO. Neural Blockade in Clinical Anaesthesia and Management of Pain. 2nd ed. Philadelphia, JB Lippincott, 1987, p 411.)

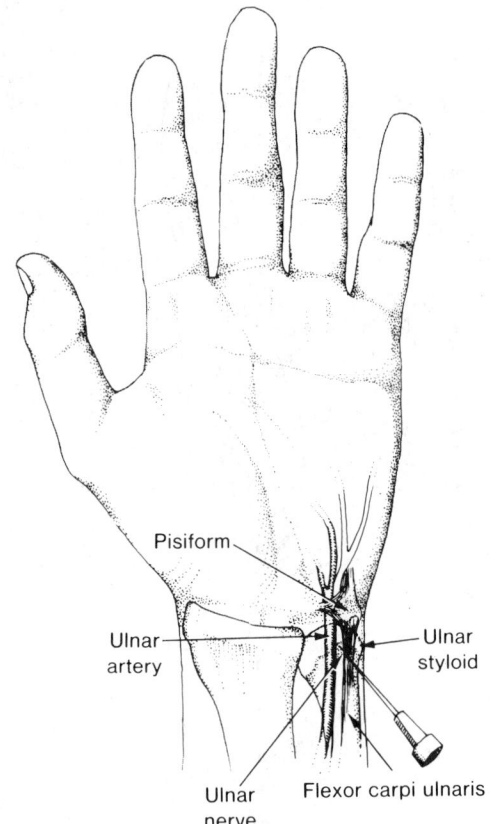

Figure 118–3. Ulnar nerve block at the wrist. The ulnar artery and ulnar nerve course beneath the flexor carpi ulnaris tendon. (From Simon RR, Brennan BE. Emergency Procedures and Techniques. 2nd ed. Baltimore, Williams & Wilkins, 1987, p 107. © 1987, the Williams & Wilkins Co.)

index, middle, and lateral half of the ring fingers. In addition, the volar digital nerve innervates the distal portion of the dorsum of the middle three fingers, including the subungual area.

The dorsal digital nerves originate either from the ulnar nerve or the superficial radial nerve. They supply only the proximal dorsum of the middle three fingers but innervate much of the distal dorsum and subungual areas of the thumb and fifth finger.

There are three different approaches to a digital block: the dorsal, the interdigital web space, and the volar approach. To use the dorsal approach for blocking all four digital nerves to each finger, use a 1-inch, 25-gauge needle inserted from the dorsum volarly until resistance by the palmar skin is felt; then 1 ml of lidocaine without epinephrine is instilled to block the palmar digital nerve. The needle is withdrawn, and 0.5 ml is injected just deep to the point of entry to block the dorsal nerve. The needle is then withdrawn and the procedure repeated on the other side.

The interdigital web space approach blocks primarily the palmar nerve, although the dorsal digital nerve is usually blocked by diffusion of the anesthetic solution. The patient's fingers are extended and widely abducted. A 1.5-cm, 25-gauge needle is inserted into the web space approximately 2 to 3 mm dorsal to the palm and advanced to the hub parallel to the fingers. Approximately 2 ml of local anesthetic are instilled, and the injection site is gently massaged to facilitate diffusion.

For the thumb and fifth fingers, both the palmar and the dorsal branches must be blocked separately to obtain complete anesthesia. The volar approach is more painful than the other approaches as it requires insertion of a needle in the palm between the metacarpal bones. It is generally not recommended, because it offers no advantages over the other two methods.

ANKLE NERVE BLOCKS

There are five nerve blocks possible at the level of the ankle: the posterior tibial, anterior tibial, superficial peroneal, saphenous, and sural (Fig. 118–5). These nerve blocks provide anesthesia to the foot.

Posterior Tibial Nerve Block

The posterior tibial nerve is located behind the posterior tibial artery (Fig. 118–6). This nerve block results in anesthesia in the area of the medial and lateral plantar nerves. Using a 1.5-inch, 25-gauge needle, a skin wheal is raised behind the posterior tibial artery, and the needle is advanced perpendicularly to the skin. Paresthesia in the sole of the foot indicates that the needle is in the vicinity of the nerve. About 5 to 10 ml of local anesthetic are instilled. If paresthesia is not elicited, up to 30 minutes may be required to achieve anesthesia. Injection of 10 ml of local anesthetic in

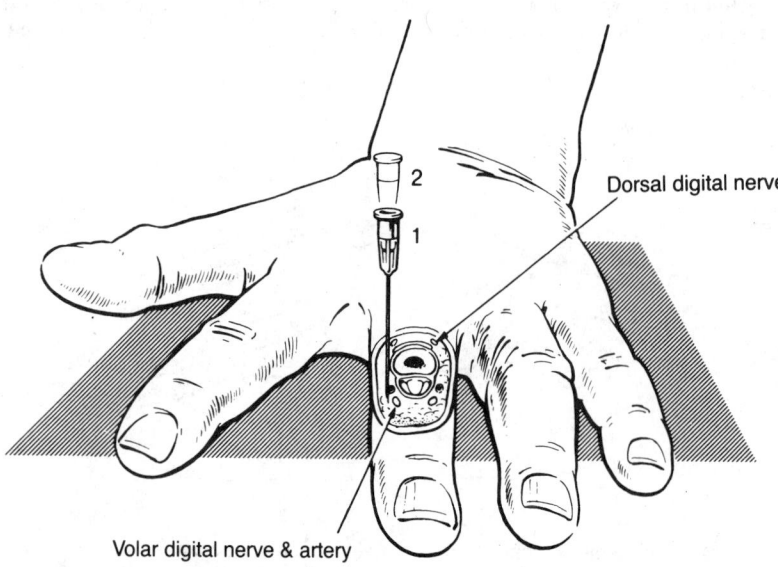

Figure 118–4. Technique of digital nerve block at the base of the finger. 1 = Position for anesthetizing the volar digital nerve; 2 = position for anesthetizing the dorsal digital nerve. (From Cousins MJ, Bridenbaugh PO. Neural Blockade in Clinical Anaesthesia and Management of Pain. 2nd ed. Philadelphia, JB Lippincott, 1987, p 414.)

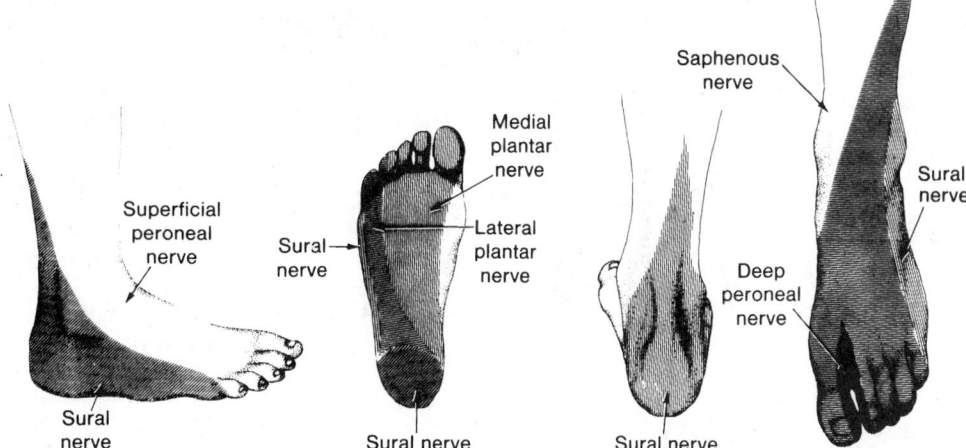

Figure 118–5. Sensory nerve supply to the foot. (From Simon RR, Brennan BE. Emergency Procedures and Techniques. 2nd ed. Baltimore, Williams & Wilkins, 1987, p 110. © 1987, the Williams & Wilkins Co.)

a fan-like manner may also provide nerve blockade without eliciting paresthesia.

Anterior Tibial (Deep Peroneal) Nerve Block

The anterior tibial nerve is located between the anterior tibial muscle and extensor hallucis longus muscle tendons at the level of the malleoli. The needle is inserted just medial to the extensor hallucis longus tendon, which is easily located by active dorsiflexion of the great toe. If paresthesia is elicited in the lateral aspect of the great toe and the medial

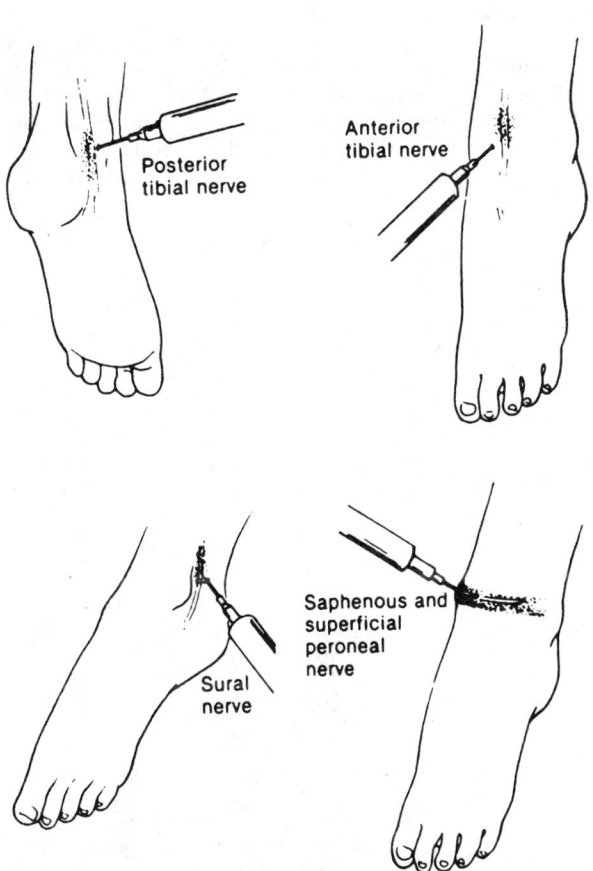

Figure 118–6. Technique used to perform ankle nerve blocks. (From Schurman DH. Ankle block anesthesia for foot surgery. Anesthesiology 1976;44:348.)

aspect of the second toe, 5 ml of local anesthetic is instilled. If no paresthesia is elicited, the needle is advanced until it touches the tibia and then withdrawn slightly; the anesthetic is then deposited.

Superficial Peroneal Nerve and Saphenous Nerve Blocks

To block the superficial peroneal nerve and saphenous nerve, a circumferential injection is made at the level of the superior border of the malleoli. Approximately 10 ml of local anesthetic is instilled subcutaneously. A successful block anesthetizes the dorsum and medial aspect of the foot and ankle.

Sural Nerve Block

The sural nerve is blocked by instilling 5 ml of anesthetic subcutaneously posterior to the distal fibula. An alternate method is to inject subcutaneously from the lateral aspect of the Achilles tendon to the posterior border of the lateral malleolus.

DENTAL BLOCKS

The bone in children is usually less dense and allows more rapid and complete diffusion of local anesthetic. The anesthetic agent most often used is 2% lidocaine with 1:100,000 epinephrine. Because of the rich vascularity of the oral cavity, vasoconstriction with epinephrine is important to increase the duration of anesthesia. Long-acting anesthetics such as bupivacaine should not be used in children because of the possibility of self-inflicted oral trauma (e.g., biting the tongue).

Dental blocks are performed more easily with the additional use of sedation. The patient can be pretreated with 100% oxygen for several minutes, followed by administration of a 40% to 50% nitrous oxide mixture. Using more than this level of nitrous oxide will induce nausea and vomiting. Use of other sedatives may also be helpful.

Supraperiosteal Technique

The supraperiosteal technique is the most common method for intraoral local anesthesia of individual teeth (Fig. 118–7). In case of severe dental pain, this technique provides useful non-narcotic analgesia. This technique is usually effective for maxillary teeth and the six lower anterior teeth

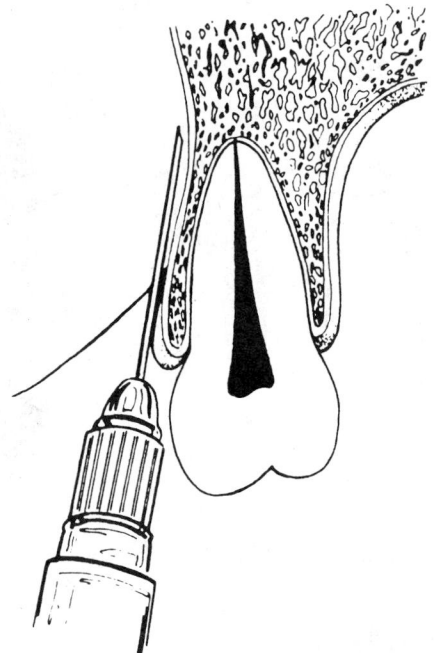

Figure 118–7. Technique for supraperiosteal injection. (From Manual of Local Anesthesia in Dentistry. New York, Cook-Waite Laboratories, Inc.)

(incisors and canines). Topical anesthesia is applied first to render the needle puncture painless. The lip is grasped and extended to delineate the mucobuccal fold. With the needle bevel facing the tooth, the mucobuccal fold is punctured, directing the tip of the needle toward the apex of the tooth and depositing up to 1 ml of local anesthesia. In children, anesthesia can be accomplished with shallower needle penetration than in adults.

The mental nerve infiltration technique is similar to the supraperiosteal injection. Its usefulness in pediatric dental pain is limited, as all anterior teeth are easily anesthetized supraperiosteally, but it is useful in situations requiring lower lip anesthesia. It is relatively painless when topical anesthetic is applied to the mucosa and injection is slow.

Inferior Alveolar Nerve Block

The inferior alveolar block has a high success rate in children because the mandibular foramen is located more inferiorly than in adults. However, the technique is similar to that used in adults. The mandibular ramus convexity is located by palpation with the index finger, and the pterygomandibular triangle is visualized. The needle and syringe are positioned on the primary molars on the opposite side of the mandible (Fig. 118–8). The skin over the triangle is punctured, and the needle is advanced until the needle tip reaches the bone. The needle is then pulled back slightly, and 1 to 2 ml of local anesthetic is instilled. To anesthetize the lingual nerve, anesthetic is injected as the needle is withdrawn (Fig. 118–9). The areas anesthetized are the ipsilateral mandibular teeth, the buccal mucosa anterior to the first molar, and the anterior two thirds of the tongue.

OPHTHALMIC NERVE BLOCK

The lateral and medial branches of the supraorbital nerve, the supratrochlear nerve, and the infratrochlear nerve may be blocked by a subcutaneous injection where the nerves exit the superior aspect of the orbit (Fig. 118–10). Anesthesia is achieved ipsilaterally to the lambdoid sutures. The supraorbital notch, which is aligned with the pupil along the supraorbital ridge, is palpated. This is the site of the supraorbital nerve; approximately 0.5 to 1.0 cm medial to it is the supratrochlear nerve.

The patient is placed in the recumbent position, and a skin wheal is raised over the supraorbital notch. Local anesthetic (3 ml) is instilled after eliciting paresthesia over the forehead. A finger or a roll of gauze can be held beneath the orbital rim to prevent diffusion down into the upper lid. Alternatively, placing a line of anesthetic subcutaneously

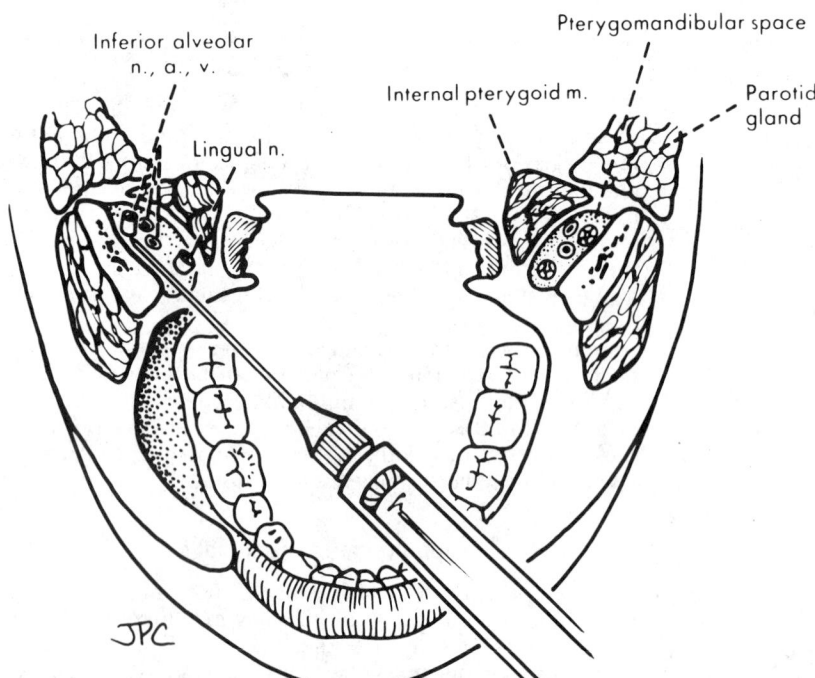

Figure 118–8. For the inferior alveolar nerve block, the needle is inserted parallel to the medial surface of the ramus. (From Cousins MJ, Bridenbaugh PO. Neural Blockade in Clinical Anaesthesia and Management of Pain. 2nd ed. Philadelphia, JB Lippincott, 1987, p 574.)

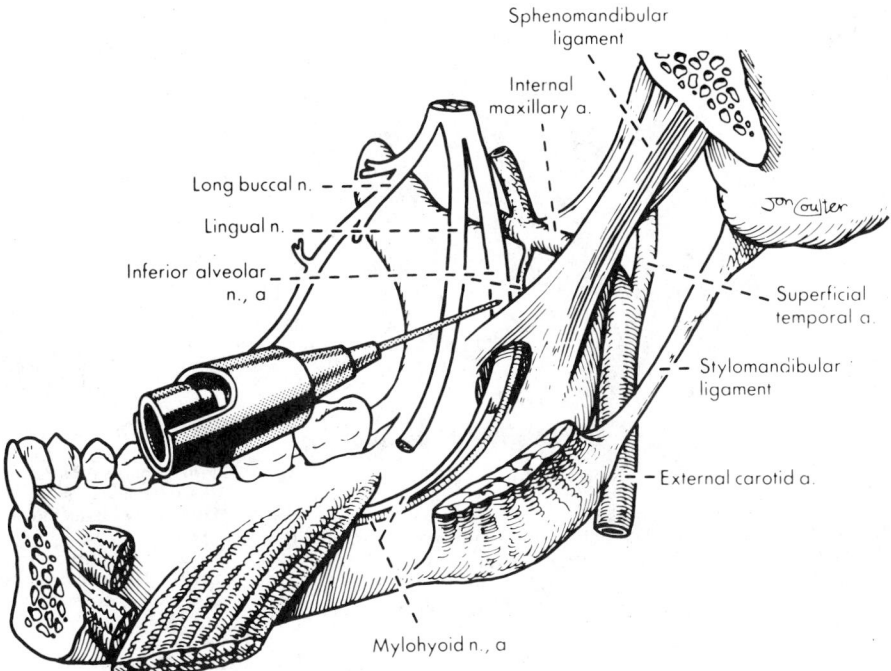

Figure 118-9. The coronoid notch is in a direct line with the point at which the inferior alveolar nerve enters the ramus of the mandible. (From Cousins MJ, Bridenbaugh PO. Neural Blockade in Clinical Anaesthesia and Management of Pain. 2nd ed. Philadelphia, JB Lippincott, 1987, p 573.)

from the lateral to the medial aspect of the orbital rim will usually ensure anesthesia.

Infraorbital Nerve Block

There are two approaches to the infraorbital nerve: intraoral and extraoral. The infraorbital nerve innervates the skin over the maxilla, nose, upper lip, and lower eyelid (Fig. 118-11). The nerve can be found by locating the infraorbital foramen, which is on the inferior orbital rim aligned with the pupil in a midgaze position (Fig. 118-12).

To perform the intraoral approach, the cheek is retracted and the mucosa punctured directly opposite the upper second bicuspid (premolar) tooth approximately 0.5 cm from the buccal surface. Directing the needle parallel to the long axis of the tooth, its tip can be palpated with the other hand in the foramen. The needle must not be aimed too posteriorly or superiorly, as it may enter the orbit. Aspiration for free-flowing blood should be performed, followed by injection of 1 to 2 ml of anesthetic. Pressure should be held over the inferior orbital rim to prevent expansion of the lower eyelid. If the exact position of the needle in the infraorbital foramen is uncertain, a field block can be achieved by instilling 5 ml of local anesthetic in a fan-like direction in the upper buccal fold.

When performing the extraoral approach, the same landmarks are used to locate the infraorbital foramen. This procedure is more difficult than the intraoral approach, especially when attempting to anesthetize the upper lip. Vasoconstrictors should not be used for the infraoral nerve block, as the facial artery and vein lie on either side of the nerve.

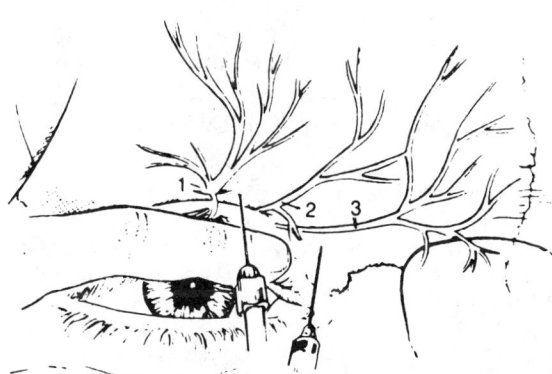

Figure 118-10. Local injection of the (1) lateral and (2) medial branch of the supraorbital nerve and the (3) supratrochlear nerve. A finger is placed on the inferior rim of the infraorbital rim to avoid swelling of the eyelid. (From Eriksson E. Illustrated Handbook in Local Anaesthesia. 2nd ed. Philadelphia, WB Saunders, 1980, p 970.)

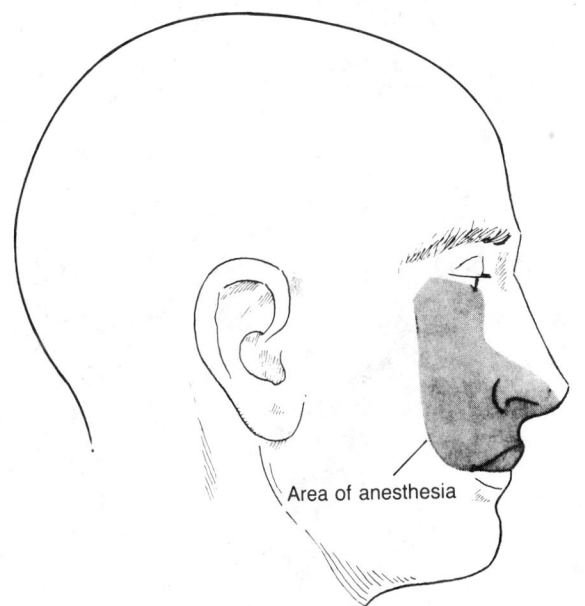

Figure 118-11. Area of anesthesia of a unilateral infraorbital nerve block. Anesthesia includes the lower eyelid and the upper lip. (From Moore D. Regional Block. 4th ed. Springfield, IL, Charles C Thomas, 1975.)

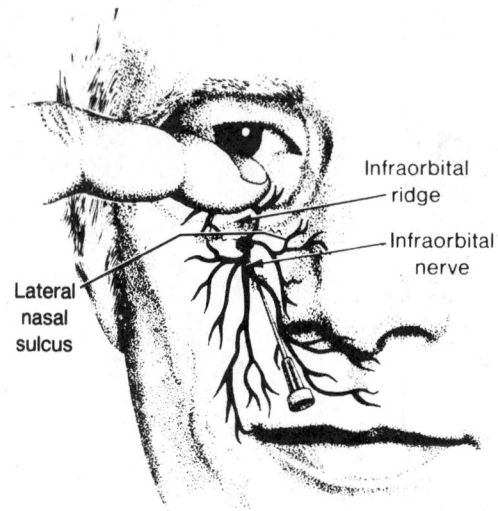

Figure 118–12. The infraorbital nerve courses through a foramen that lies inferior to the infraorbital ridge. (From Simon RR, Brennan BE. Emergency Procedures and Techniques. 2nd ed. Baltimore, Williams & Wilkins, 1987, p 96. © 1987, the Williams & Wilkins Co.)

REGIONAL BLOCK OF THE EXTERNAL EAR

Regional anesthesia of the external ear is easily accomplished. Sensory innervation to the external ear is derived from the auriculotemporal nerve, greater auricular nerve, mastoid branch of the occipital nerve, and the occipital nerves (Fig. 118–13). Injection of 1% lidocaine with epinephrine solution in a ring-like or crisscross fashion will achieve adequate analgesia. In the former method, a total of three punctures are made, starting at the most cephalic aspect of the skin just behind the ear. The needle is inserted subcutaneously, aiming toward the tragus; it is pulled back to just short of withdrawal from the skin while injecting the anesthetic and then redirected posteriorly. This is repeated

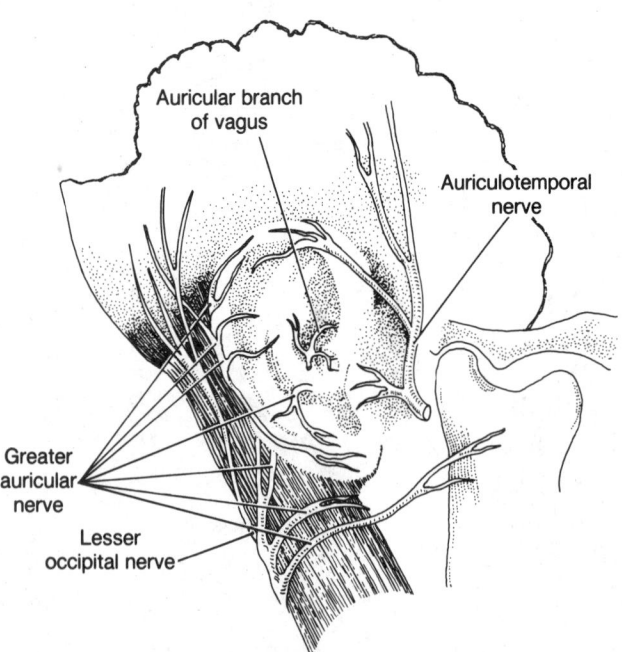

Figure 118–13. Sensory nerve supply to the ear. (From Simon RR, Brennan BE. Emergency Procedures and Techniques. 2nd ed. Baltimore, Williams & Wilkins, 1987, p 101. © 1987, the Williams & Wilkins Co.)

at two other sites: just behind the external ear and inferior to the pinna.

The second method requires a total of two punctures, starting at the same site as for the ring block except extending the needle further to reach in front of the tragus. The needle is pulled back while injecting the anesthetic and redirected toward the mid aspect of the skin behind the external ear. The needle is then withdrawn completely, and the procedure is repeated, starting at the most inferior aspect of the skin behind the ear.

Selected References

Amsterdam JT. Regional anesthesia of the head and neck. *In* Roberts JR, Hedges JR (eds). Clinical Procedures in Emergency Medicine. 2nd ed. Philadelphia, WB Saunders, 1991, pp 486–498.

Green DP. Operative Hand Surgery. 2nd ed. London, Churchill Livingstone, 1988.

Lloyd-Thomas AR. Pain management in paediatric patients. Br J Anesth 1990;64:85.

Malamed SF. Handbook of Local Anesthesia. 3rd ed. St Louis, CV Mosby, 1990.

McCarthy JG. Plastic Surgery. Vol 1. Philadelphia, WB Saunders, 1990.

Orlinsky M, Dean E. Local and topical anesthesia and nerve blocks of the thorax and extremities. *In* Roberts JR, Hedges JR (eds). Clinical Procedures in Emergency Medicine. 2nd ed. Philadelphia, WB Saunders, 1991, pp 450–486.

Yaster M, Maxwell LG. Pediatric regional anesthesia. Anesthesia 1989;70:324.

CHAPTER 119

Injury Prevention

Frederick P. Rivara

INTRODUCTION

In 1966, the National Academy of Sciences called injuries "the neglected disease of modern society."[1] Two decades and 2,500,000 trauma deaths later, the Academy issued a similar report stating, "Injury is the principal public health problem in America today; it affects primarily the young and will touch one of every three Americans this year."[2]

INJURIES AND ACCIDENTS

Throughout this chapter, the term *injury* refers to "damage resulting from acute exposure to physical or chemical agents." Use of this term focuses scientific attention on the problem (i.e., the damage to the person). The term *accident* will be avoided; it is an inaccurate anachronism reflecting unscientific attitudes toward injuries and connotes events occurring at random, without pattern or predictability. The term *accident* should also be abandoned because of its moral connotations; accidents have been viewed as rightful punishment for negligent and careless behavior.

This work was supported in part by grant no. CCR 002570 from the Centers for Disease Control.

In this chapter, injuries include homicides, suicides, and assault-related trauma, as well as the group of problems previously referred to as "accidents." Although the circumstances surrounding these types of injuries may be dissimilar, the actual mechanisms of injury, the agents involved, and the types of trauma produced are often identical. A firearm will produce the same type of damage whether it discharges unintentionally during mishandling or is used during an assault. In addition, prevention of these injuries may be the same (i.e., removing the gun from the environment of the child or adolescent).

Some of these episodes of homicides and "unintentional injuries" may actually represent disguised suicides or suicidal tendencies. Homicides may be victim precipitated; single vehicle motor vehicle fatalities may represent a suicide on the part of the driver.[3]

Scope of the Problem

About 57 million Americans require medical treatment for injuries every year, and approximately 143,000 die. From before the first birthday through age 44, injuries are the leading cause of death in the United States. In children from 1 to 4 years of age, injuries are responsible for nearly half of all deaths and cause three times more deaths than the next leading cause, congenital anomalies. Throughout the rest of childhood and adolescence, injuries cause more deaths than all other causes combined. In 1985 it was estimated that for children age 5 to 9 years, the risk of dying from injuries during the following 15 years is 2.6 times greater than the risk of dying from all other causes combined.[4]

The major causes of fatal injuries vary with age (Table 119–1). Motor vehicle injuries lead the list. Deaths from fires and burns are a particular problem in young children. Drowning, many cases of which occur in pools and not infrequently in bathtubs, also constitutes a major hazard for young children.

In 5- to 9-year-old children, pedestrian injuries are the most common cause of death from trauma and are second only to cancer among all causes of death in this age group. Drowning and deaths from fires and burns also take a major toll in this age group.

As children enter the teenage years, motor vehicles become increasingly important as a cause of serious and fatal injury. In these adolescent years, suicide and homicide take a large toll, with firearms playing an important role in these tragedies.

Nonfatal injuries constitute a large burden on the health care system. Population-based studies indicate that of 1000 children and adolescents 0 to 19 years of age, 247 receive medical care for an injury each year.[5] Of these 2.5% require

hospital admission for care, and 55% have at least short-term, temporary disability from their injuries. An estimated 317,000 children younger than 15 years were hospitalized for treatment of trauma in 1985.[6]

The cost of trauma in the United States is enormous, amounting to $157.6 billion dollars in 1985[6]; trauma in children accounted for $13.8 billion. The cost of injuries to children represents a relatively small proportion of the total, because the cost for care of an injured child is 15% to 20% of that of an injured older adult.

CAUSES OF INJURY AND PREVENTIVE OPTIONS

In order to cause an injury, energy, usually mechanical or thermal, is transferred to the body in a dose that exceeds the threshold for tissue damage. Most serious scientists involved with injury research have discounted the theory of "accident proneness."[7, 8] Although some persons in a given group have higher injury rates than others, the available evidence indicates that over a long period of observation, this is essentially a shifting group of persons, with new individuals constantly entering and leaving the group. The concept of "accident proneness" is in fact counterproductive in that it shifts attention away from potentially more modifiable factors such as the product or the environment.

In the child who appears to be at increased risk of injury, attention should be directed toward the child's physical, social, and cultural environment. Although factors such as young maternal age, single parenthood, high household stress, and low maternal education are associated with increased risk of childhood injury, the most likely common pathway for all of these factors is poverty.[9–12] An analysis of child and adolescent deaths found that poor children were 2.6 times more likely to die from trauma than non-poor children.[13] Death from motor vehicle injuries was more than twice as common among poor children, who were also four times more likely to die from drowning and five times more likely to die from fire. Similar high risks for the poor have been found for residential fires and pedestrian injuries.[14–17]

Poor children live in more hazardous environments with higher fire risks, higher traffic density, and fewer satisfactory play areas. Injury prevention devices such as infant restraints, smoke detectors, and bicycle helmets are less available. Family stress and a greater number of life changes also contribute to the problem.

Injury prevention efforts must be focused. Pediatricians must be specific when either giving advice about injury prevention or setting up an intervention. Only when parents are given specific advice such as "Buy and use a car seat," "Get a bicycle helmet for the child," and "Don't let young children cross streets alone" is the advice effective.

In general, injury prevention strategies that are passive

TABLE 119–1					
VIOLENT DEATHS IN CHILDREN AND ADOLESCENTS IN THE UNITED STATES, 1986					
	Age in Years				
	<5	**5–9**	**10–14**	**15–19**	**Total**
All injuries	4607	2133	2776	12,895	22,411
Motor vehicle injuries					
Occupant	658	397	643	5714	7412
Pedestrian	500	502	285	500	1787
Drownings	754	326	323	659	2062
Fire- and burn-related injuries	859	321	177	262	1619
Homicides	660	134	245	1838	2877
Suicides	0	5	250	1896	2151

(i.e., work automatically) are more effective than those that are active and require repeated behavior change on the part of the individual. For example, air bags are more effective than seat belts, because they work automatically; seat belts in turn are more effective than telling people to drive more carefully.

MOTOR VEHICLE INJURIES

Motor vehicle injuries are the leading cause of serious and fatal injuries in individuals of all ages. In the teenage years, motor vehicle crashes alone account for 40% of all deaths. On the positive side, a solid base of research and experience supports the conclusion that large and sustained reductions in motor vehicle crash injuries can be accomplished by using approaches that focus on the main components of these crashes. These components are the motor vehicle occupants, including drivers and passengers; bicycle–motor vehicle collisions; and pedestrian–motor vehicle collisions.

Occupants

Injuries to passenger vehicle occupants are the predominant cause of motor vehicle deaths among children and adolescents, with the exception of the 5 to 9-year-old age group, in which pedestrian injuries make up the largest proportion of the total. The peak injury and death rate for both males and females of all ages are the years 16 to 19.

Much attention has been given to child occupants younger than 4 years of age. Use of child restraint devices in this age group can be expected to reduce fatalities by 71% and the risk of serious injuries by 67%.[18] All 50 states and the District of Columbia have laws mandating the use of these devices. Overall, use in 1988 was up to 84%, an outstanding pediatric injury control success story.

Handouts given to parents by physicians emphasizing the positive benefits of the use of child seat restraints have been successful in improving parent acceptance. Careful studies have shown that toddlers who normally ride restrained behave better during car trips than children who ride unrestrained.

Films discussing the advantage of child seat restraint use can be shown to parents in waiting rooms or to mothers on postpartum hospital floors. Many hospitals and communities have adopted loaner programs, renting child seat restraints at low cost. This is especially important for low-income families, who have the lowest rate of restraint use.

Children weighing less than 20 pounds may use an infant seat or be placed in a "convertible" infant-toddler child restraint device. Infants weighing less than 20 pounds should be placed facing backward; older toddlers who weigh more than 20 pounds can be placed in a forward-facing convertible or toddler seat.

Unfortunately, child safety seat misuse is common. One study found a 65% misuse rate of child seats.[19] Common errors include seats facing in the wrong direction, safety belts improperly routed around the safety seat, and misuse of toddler seat harnesses and shields.

Older children, as they graduate from child safety seats, are often not adequately restrained. Many children ride in the back seat, restrained with lap belts only. Unfortunately, the increased use of lap belts has been associated with a marked rise in seat belt–related injuries, especially fractures of the lumbar spine and hollow viscus injuries of the abdomen.[20] Equipping rear seats with lap belts and shoulder harnesses will not entirely solve the problem; most children in the 4 to 8-year-old age group are too small to use the shoulder harness comfortably and safely. Redesign of these rear seat restraints is necessary.

Teenage Drivers

Drivers age 15 to 17 years have 2.5 times the rate of collisions per 1000 registered drivers as motorists 18 years of age and older.[21] One strategy used to decrease the rate of crashes, and presumably injuries, is driver education. The federal government has been contributing 10% of the more than $300 million spent annually for high school driver education courses. The premise underlying such expenditures has been that high school driver education courses promote higher levels of safety on the highway. However, well-designed studies in Connecticut have failed to find differences in the crash experience of drivers who had had driver education and otherwise similar drivers who had not.[22] In fact, it has been found that higher rates of driver education in schools correlate with higher percentages of 16- and 17-year-old licensed drivers on the road. Because driver education is not associated with lower crash fatality rates among those who take it, and because many states allow teenagers to drive a year earlier after taking driver's education, the net result is that as more driver education is provided, fatality rates in the 16- and 17-year-old population increase. In Connecticut, state funding for driver education in high schools was eliminated in 1976. In those communities dropping driver education, the licensing of 16- and 17-year-olds decreased by 57%, and the reported crashes in the overall 16- and 17-year-old population decreased by 63%.[23]

Research has also indicated a possible injury reduction advantage from restricting 16- and 17-year-olds to daytime driving. Almost half of the fatal crashes involving drivers under the age of 18 occur in the 4 hours before or the 4 hours after midnight.[21] In states imposing night-time driving curfews on teenagers under 18 years, there has been a significant decrease in crash involvement and fatalities.[24]

Finally, teen alcohol abuse associated with driving is a major problem. Approximately half of all deaths from motor vehicle crashes in this age group involve the use of alcohol. It is clear that impairment of driving occurs with blood alcohol concentrations as low as 0.05 gm/ml.[25] At present, all 50 states have raised the minimum age for purchase of alcohol to 21 years. Studies have estimated that this has resulted in a 13% reduction in night-time fatal crashes.[26]

Other interventions that have been successful include (1) implementing compulsory blood alcohol tests in traffic injury cases; (2) adopting legislation that mandates administrative licensing suspension (automatic suspension of licenses if the driver's blood alcohol concentration exceeds the legal limit)[27]; and (3) raising state and federal alcohol excise taxes to reduce alcohol availability, perhaps resulting in as much as a 15% reduction in fatalities.[28]

Bicycle–Motor Vehicle Injuries

Each year in the United States, approximately 600 children and adolescents die from injuries incurred from riding bicycles. Bicycles are one of the most common reasons children with trauma visit emergency rooms, accounting for some 300,000 visits annually in the United States.[29]

Several studies indicate that the majority of severe and fatal bicycle injuries involve head trauma.[30, 31] A logical step in the prevention of these head injuries is the use of helmets. As an analogy, motorcycle helmets can reduce the risk of fatal head injuries by 25% to 30%. A case-control study from Seattle indicated that bicycle helmets are far more effective for the prevention of bicycle injuries, reducing the risk of head injury by 85% and brain injury by 88%.[32] However, surveys show that only 1% to 5% of children and adolescents wear helmets when bicycling.[33]

Physicians can be an effective source of advice to parents

and children on the need for a bicycle helmet and should incorporate such advice into their anticipatory guidance schedules. Appropriate helmets have a firm polystyrene liner and bear a label indicating approval by the Snell or American National Standards Institute (ANSI) testing organizations.

Community education programs led by a coalition of physicians, educators, bicycle clubs, and community service organizations have been successful in promoting the use of bicycle helmets.[34] In Seattle, such a coalition increased helmet use from 5% to 16% in the first 2 years[35] and to 33% by the fourth year.

Consideration should also be given to other methods of prevention. Bicycle paths are a logical way to separate bicycles and motor vehicles. Safe riding training for children can be provided in the school and community; again, the evidence of effectiveness is limited.

Pedestrian–Motor Vehicle Injuries

Approximately 6600 pedestrians per year are killed and 100,000 are injured.[36] Children and the elderly are clearly the group at the greatest risk; in fact, for 5 to 9-year-old children, pedestrian injuries are the single most common cause of traumatic death. Fatality statistics also understate the childhood injury problem; injured children have much lower fatality rates than other age groups. In addition, poor children appear to be at much higher risk of pedestrian injury than non-poor children.[16]

Few children are injured at night; most injuries occur during the day, with peaks in the after-school period. Improved lighting or retroreflective clothing would therefore not be expected to prevent injuries. Most of the injuries occur on arterial roads, indicating that speed bumps on residential streets are not the answer. It is surprising that approximately 30% of pedestrian injuries occur while the individual is in a marked crosswalk. It appears children have a false sense of security when in a crosswalk, and few drivers routinely stop and look for children when approaching such crosswalks.

One important risk factor for childhood pedestrian injuries is simply the developmental level of the child. Careful studies indicate that few children younger than 9 or 10 years have the developmental skills to successfully negotiate traffic 100% of the time.[37–38] Children have a poor ability to judge the distance and speed of traffic and are easily distracted by playmates or other factors in the environment. Many parents, however, are unaware of this potential mismatch between the abilities of the young school age child and the skills needed to safely negotiate traffic.

Prevention of pedestrian injuries should consist of a multifaceted approach. Engineering changes in roadway designs are extremely important as passive prevention measures. These might include one-way street networks; proper placement of transit or school bus stops, sidewalks in urban and suburban areas, and edge striping in rural areas to delineate the edge of the road; and curb parking regulations.[39]

Legislation and police enforcement are important components of any campaign to reduce pedestrian injuries. Right-turn-on-red laws increase the hazard to pedestrians, and in many cities, few drivers stop for pedestrians in crosswalks.

Education of children in pedestrian safety has long been a mainstay of many programs. However, rigorous evaluations of these programs have produced conflicting and confusing results.[36] In addition, the children in most need of protection—those in the 5 to 7-year-old age group—are the least likely to benefit from this instruction.

FIRE- AND BURN-RELATED INJURIES

About 6000 burn injury deaths occur each year in the United States. For both injuries and deaths, the first decade of life is the period at highest risk. Burns are second only to motor vehicle crashes in the number of years of life lost per death, reflecting the relatively young population involved in serious burn injuries. The likelihood of burn injury is strongly related to socioeconomic status: the lower the family income, the higher the risk of fire- and burn-related injury and death.[13] Among children 10 to 14 years of age, burns involving flammable substances are eight times more frequent in males than in females.

One of the first effective prevention interventions involved inflammable fabrics. Burns resulting from ignition of clothing were a common, serious burn injury, especially in small children. At least one third of these injuries involved infant sleepwear. Such burns affected an average of 30% of the body surface, requiring hospitalization for an average of 70 days. In 1967 the Federal Flammable Fabrics Act was passed, requiring children's sleepwear to be flame retardant. As a result of this and similar state legislation, clothing ignition burns in small children now account for only a small fraction of burns in children.[40]

Another hazard is tap-water scalds. Scald burns account for 40% of the burn injuries in children requiring hospitalization. Unlike children with flame burns, children with scalds generally do not die; however, many such children face long hospitalizations, multiple surgical procedures, and severe disfigurement. At least 25% of these scald burns involve tap water. A study in Seattle found 80% of residences surveyed had hot tap water temperatures greater than 54.4°C (130°F).[41] The risk of full-thickness burns increases geometrically at temperatures above 54.4°C. At 62.2°C (150°F), a full-thickness burn will be produced in adult skin in 2 seconds. A simple and effective preventive maneuver is simply to turn down the water heater temperature to 51.7°C (125°F). At this setting, dishwashers and washing machines will still operate effectively, but the risk of serious scald injury is greatly reduced. In 1980, Florida became the first state requiring new water heaters to be preset at a temperature of 51.7°C.

Nearly 70% of all fire deaths in the United States occur in private dwellings. Of these deaths, 60% are caused by smoke asphyxiation and not flame burns. Smoke detectors provide an inexpensive but effective method of preventing the majority of these deaths. By offering information on smoke detectors in their offices, physicians can alter parental behavior and increase smoke detector use.[42]

Cigarettes are estimated to cause 45% of all fires and 22% to 56% of deaths from house fires.[43] Most cigarettes made in this country burn for as long as 28 minutes, even if left unattended. Studies indicate that fire-safe or self-extinguishing cigarettes are feasible. If such cigarettes replaced present types, nearly 2000 deaths and more than 6000 burns would be prevented annually.[44]

Other approaches have not proven effective. The Consumer Product Safety Commission supported a large study, Project Burn Prevention, in two Massachusetts communities.[45] There was a widespread mass media effort to educate the public about burn risks, numerous small community presentations, and educational programs in elementary and high schools. None of the programs brought about a statistically significant reduction in burn incidence or severity. The school program did result in increased knowledge about burn hazards, but this did not result in decreased frequency of burn injury. This and similar studies indicate that product modification, rather than education, is the most effective method of decreasing fire- and burn-related injuries.

POISONING

In 1970, 226 poisoning deaths occurred in children younger than 5 years, compared with only 55 such deaths in 1985. Poisoning prevention is one of the success stories of pediatrics and represents the effectiveness of passive strategies (i.e., child-resistant packaging and dose limits per container). The Poison Prevention Packaging Act has been remarkably effective in reducing poisoning deaths and hospitalizations.[46] However, compliance with the law by pharmacists is only 70% to 75% at present.[47] In addition, difficulty using child-resistant containers is an important cause of poisoning in young children. A survey by the Centers for Disease Control found that in 18.5% of households in which poisoning occurred in children younger than 5 years, parents had replaced the child-resistant closure, and 65% of the child-resistant closures used did not work properly.[48] Nearly one fifth of ingestions are of drugs owned by grandparents, an age group that has difficulty using traditional child-resistant containers.

Other poisoning interventions, such as "Mr. Yuk" stickers, are far less effective. They do not deter young children from ingesting labeled medications and may in fact be attractive to children younger than 3 years.[49]

DROWNING

In 1986, 2122 drownings, primarily associated with recreational activities, occurred in children and adolescents in the United States. In children, drowning ranks second only to motor vehicle injury as a cause of traumatic death. It is estimated that 140,000 water-related injuries occur annually from swimming activities alone. Diving and sliding head-first into the water, resulting in spinal cord damage, account for the most serious aquatic injuries. Of the estimated 700 spinal cord injuries resulting from aquatic activities each year, the majority cause permanent paralysis.

In Los Angeles, half of all drownings take place in residential pools. This rate is similar to that of other areas with pools, but is much higher than in areas without a large number of pools.[50] Children younger than 5 years do not understand the consequences of falling into deep water and usually do not call for help.[51]

The most effective way to prevent childhood pool drownings is through fencing. To be most protective, these barriers should restrict entry to the pool from the yard and residence, use self-closing and self-latching gates, be at least five feet high, and have no vertical openings more than four inches wide. Ordinances to require appropriate fencing have been demonstrated to be effective. Many people have advocated "water-babies" and other swimming instruction for young children, but the efficacy of such techniques is untested. The potential exists for both parent and child to become less vigilant around water, and the majority of child victims drown during lapses in adult supervision.[51]

Among adolescents and young adults, alcohol and drug use have been found to be involved in nearly half of all drowning deaths. The restriction of the sale and consumption of alcoholic beverages in boating, pool, harbor, marina, and beach areas may combat this dangerous combination of activities.

The use of personal flotation devices is also important. Coast Guard data show that although only 7% of boats involved with mishaps lacked available personal flotation devices, such boats accounted for 29% of all boating fatalities.

FIREARM INJURIES

Injuries to children and adolescents involving firearms occur in three different situations: nonintentional injury, suicide attempt, and assault. In children younger than 18 years, firearms are the fifth leading cause of death from nonintentional trauma in the United States. Five hundred children die each year from nonintentional gunshot wounds. An additional 8000 children and adolescents are left with permanent sequelae, not including emotional and psychological problems.[52]

Nonintentional firearm injuries generally occur in a family dwelling; 85% of firearm deaths occur in the home. In children younger than 16 years, poverty is more closely related to shooting deaths than race or population density. Urban white children have the lowest death rate, rural white children have an intermediate rate, and urban black children have the highest fatality rate.

Suicide is the third most common cause of death in teenage males and the fourth most common cause in females. From the 1950s to 1982, the suicide rates for children and adolescents more than doubled.[53] As with homicides, firearms are the most common means of suicide in males of all ages. The difference in the rate of suicide between males and females is related less to the number of attempts than to the method. Women die less often in suicide attempts, because they use less lethal means, mainly drugs. The use of firearms in a suicidal act usually converts an attempt into a fatality.

Homicides are second only to motor vehicle crashes as a cause of death in teenagers older than 15 years. In 1985, more than 2900 children and adolescents were homicide victims; nonwhite teenagers accounted for almost half the total, making homicides the most common cause of death among nonwhite teenagers. At present almost 95% of homicides among males involve firearms, 75% of which are handguns.

There are an estimated 210 to 220 million firearms in the United States. Since the 1960s, more than 6 million firearms have been sold in the United States each year. Handguns account for approximately 20% of the firearms in use but are involved in 90% of criminal and other firearm misuse.

For every firearm death resulting from self-defense, there were 1.3 nonintentional firearm deaths, 4.6 firearm homicides, and 37 firearm suicides involving guns kept in the home.[54] Comparison of Seattle to Vancouver, British Columbia, a similar city 140 miles away but in a country with restrictive gun control laws, indicates that homicides were 1.63 times more frequent in Seattle than in Vancouver, a difference resulting entirely from a 4.8-fold greater rate of handgun homicides in Seattle.[55] Similarly, among 15- to 24-year-olds, suicide rates were 1.38 times higher in the Seattle area, again a result of a tenfold greater rate of suicide by handguns.[56]

Of all firearms, handguns pose the greatest risk to the health of children and adolescents. Regulation and elimination of handguns, rather than of all firearms, would appear to be the most appropriate focus of efforts to reduce shooting injuries in children and adolescents.

Information and education campaigns in firearms safety have been tried in the past. No data exist to support the effectiveness of such programs in decreasing the number of gunshot wounds in children. Regardless of the merits of safety education, firearms around the home pose a risk to children and adolescents, who do not have adequate judgment to safely handle these weapons. Elimination of these weapons from the environment of children and adolescents is the necessary key to reduction in firearm fatalities and injuries. Furthermore, safety education has no effect on the use of firearms in homicides and suicides. Most homicides are perpetrated by relatives or acquaintances and are acts of rage. Eliminating handguns would certainly not eliminate arguments, but it would decrease the likelihood of a fatal conclusion. In an assault, the chance of death is five times greater with a firearm than with a knife.

References

1. National Academy of Sciences. Accidental Death and Disability: The Neglected Disease of Modern Society. Washington, DC, National Academy Press, 1966.
2. National Academy of Sciences. Injury in America: A Continuing Public Health Problem. Washington, DC, National Academy Press, 1985.
3. Holinger PC. Violent deaths among the young: Recent trends in suicide, homicide, and accidents. Am J Psychiatr 1979;136:1144.
4. Budnik LD, Chaiken BP. The probability of dying of injuries by the year 2000. JAMA 1985;254:3350.
5. Rivara FP, Calonge N, Thompson RS. Population based study of unintentional injury incidence and impact during childhood. Am J Public Health 1989;79:990.
6. Rice DP, MacKenzie EJ, et al. Cost of Injury in the United States: A Report to Congress. San Francisco, CA, Institute for Health and Aging, University of California, and Injury Prevention Center, The Johns Hopkins University, 1989.
7. Langley J. The "accident prone" child—the perpetuation of a myth. Austr Paediatr 1982;18:243.
8. Sass R, Cook G. Accident proneness: Science or nonscience. Int J Health Serv 1981;11:175.
9. Taylor B, Wadsworth J, Butler NE. Teenage mothering, admission to the hospital, and accidents during the first five years. Arch Dis Child 1983;58:6.
10. McCormick MC, Shapiro S, Starfield BH. Injury and its correlates among 1 year old children. Am J Dis Child 1981;135:159.
11. Daniels JH, Hampton RL, Newberger EH. Child abuse and accidents in black families. Am J Orthopsych 1983;48:595.
12. Beautris AL, Fergusson DM, Shannon DT. Childhood accidents in a New Zealand birth cohort. Austr Paediatr 1982;18:238.
13. Nersesian WS, Petit MR, Shaper R, et al. Childhood death and poverty: A study of all childhood deaths in Maine, 1976 to 1980. Pediatrics 1985;75:41.
14. Federal Emergency Management Agency. Fire in the US. Washington, DC, Federal Emergency Management Agency, 1982.
15. Mierley MC, Baker SP. Fatal house fires in an urban population. JAMA 1983;249:1466.
16. Rivara FP, Barber M. Sociodemographic determinants of childhood pedestrian injuries. Pediatrics 1985;76:375.
17. Pless IB, Verreault R, Arsenault L, et al. The epidemiology of road accidents in childhood. Am J Public Health 1987;77:358.
18. Kahane CJ. An evaluation of child passenger safety. The effectiveness and benefits of safety seats (summary). DOT publication no (DOT HS)806-889. Washington, DC, National Highway Traffic Safety Administration, 1986.
19. Ziegler PN. Child safety seat misuse. Research note. Washington, DC, National Highway Traffic Safety Administration, 1985.
20. Reid AB, Letts RM. Pediatric Chance fractures and intra-abdominal injuries. Abstract. J Trauma 1989;29:1303.
21. Robertson LS. Patterns of teenaged driver involvement in fatal MV crashes: Implications for policy choice. J Health Politics Policy Law 1981;6:303.
22. Robertson LS, Zador PL. Driver education and fatal crash involvement of teenaged drivers. Am J Public Health 1978;68:959.
23. Robertson LS. Crash involvement of teenaged drivers when driver education is eliminated from high schools. Am J Public Health 1980;70:599.
24. Preusser DF, Williams AF, Zador PL, Blomberg RD. The effect of curfew laws on motor vehicle crashes. Law Policy 1984;6:115.
25. AMA Council on Scientific Affairs. Alcohol and the Driver. JAMA 1986;255:522.
26. Dumochel W, Williams AF, Zador PL. Raising the alcohol purchase age: Its effects on fatal motor vehicle crashes in 26 states. J Legal Studies 1987;249:66.
27. Zador PL, Lund AK, Fields M, Weinberg K. Fatal crash involvement and laws against alcohol-impaired driving. Washington, DC, Insurance Institute for Highway Safety, 1988.
28. Phelps CE. Alcohol taxes and highway safety. In Graham J (ed). Preventing Automobile Injury: New Findings from Evaluation Research. Dover, MA, Auburn House, 1988.
29. Bicycle related injuries: Data from the National Electronic Injury Surveillance System. MMWR 1987;36:269.
30. Fife D, Davis J, Tate L, et al. Fatal injuries to bicyclists: The experience of Dade County, Florida. J Trauma 1983;23:745.
31. Guichon DMP, Myles ST. Bicycle injuries: One year sample in Calgary. J Trauma 1975;15:504.
32. Thompson RS, Rivara FP, Thompson DC. A case-control study of the effectiveness of bicycle safety helmets. N Engl J Med 1989;320:1361.
33. Weiss BD. Bicycle helmet use by children. Pediatrics 1986;77:677.
34. Bergman AB, Rivara FP, Richards DD, Rogers LW. Anatomy of a children's bicycle helmet campaign. Am J Dis Child 1990;144:727.
35. Diguiseppi CG, Rivara FP, Koepsell TD, Polissar L. Bicycle helmet use by children: Evaluation of a community-wide helmet campaign. JAMA 1989;262:2256.
36. Rivara FP. Child pedestrian injuries in the United States: Current status of the problem, potential interventions, and future research needs. Am J Dis Child 1990;144:692.
37. Young DS, Lee DN. Training children in road crossing skills using a roadside simulation. Accid Anal Prev 1987;19:327.
38. Rothengatter JH. A behavioral approach to improving traffic behavior of young children. Ergonomics 1984;27:147.
39. Zeeger CV. Feasibility of Roadway Countermeasures for Pedestrian Accident Experience. Warrendale, PA, Society of Automotive Engineers 1984, p 104.
40. McLoughlin E, Clarke N, Stahl K, et al. One pediatric burn unit's experience with sleepwear-related injuries. Pediatrics 1977;60:405.
41. Feldman KW, Schaller RT, Feldman JA, McMillon M. Tap water scald burns in children. Pediatrics 1978;62:1.
42. Reisinger KS, Blatter MM, Wacher F. Pediatric counseling and subsequent use of smoke detectors. Am J Public Health 1982;72:392.
43. Mierley MC, Baker SP. Fatal house fires in an urban population. JAMA 1983;249:1466.
44. Maguire A. There's death on the block, there's hope in Congress. J Public Health Policy 1987;8:451.
45. McLoughlin E, Vince CJ, Lee AM, Crawford JD. Project Burn Prevention: Outcome and implications. Am J Public Health 1982;72:241.
46. Walton W. An evaluation of the Poisoning Packaging Prevention Act. Pediatrics 1982;69:363.
47. Dole EJ, Czajka PA, Rivara FP. Evaluation of pharmacists' compliance with the Poison Packaging Prevention Act. Am J Public Health 1986;76:1335.
48. Centers for Disease Control. Unintentional ingestions of prescription drugs in children <5. MMWR 1987;36:125.
49. Fergusson DM, Horwood LJ, Beautris AL, Shannon FT. A controlled field trial of a poisoning prevention method. Pediatrics 1982;69:515.
50. O'Carroll P, Alkon E, Weiss B. Drowning mortality in Los Angeles county. JAMA 1988;100:380.
51. Directorate for Epidemiology. Swimming pool drownings. Washington, DC, Division of Hazard Analysis, US Consumer Product Safety Commission, 1987.
52. Jagger J, Dietz P. Deaths and injuries by firearms who cares. JAMA 1986;255:314.
53. Boyd JH, Mosciki EK. Firearms and youth suicide. Am J Public Health 1986;76:1240.
54. Kellermann AL, Reay DT. Protection or peril? An analysis of firearm related deaths in the home. N Engl J Med 1986;314:1557.
55. Sloan JH, Kellermann AL, Reay DT, et al. Handgun regulations, crime, assaults and homicide. A tale of two cities. N Engl J Med 1988;319:1256.
56. Sloan JH, Rivara FP, Reay DT, et al. Firearm regulations and rates of suicide: A comparison of two metropolitan areas. N Engl J Med 1990;322:369.

SECTION FIFTEEN

Orthopedics

CHAPTER 120

Bone Development and Pediatric Considerations

Wassam M. Rahman
Ira S. Landsman

INTRODUCTION

When managing musculoskeletal trauma, the physician must be aware of several differences between children and adults. Immature bone is more pliable because of an increased porosity and decreased density. This causes unique fracture patterns such as torus, greenstick, and bowing fractures. Injury to the growth region of bone, the physis, can result in significant growth malformation. Excellent bone remodeling in children allows malunited fragments to realign without significant deformity. This excludes physeal, rotational, and intra-articular fractures. The periosteum is stronger, thicker, and more loosely attached to the underlying immature bone. This contributes to remodeling and repair. Healing of fractures is quicker and nonunion is uncommon in children because of the thick, vascular, osteogenic periosteum. Injuries to joints and ligaments usually result in growth-plate tears or avulsions such as tibial spine avulsions, as opposed to anterior cruciate tears as seen in adults. Diagnosing fractures in children is often difficult because of equivocal clinical findings and radiolucent components of immature bone on radiographs. For these reasons, good bone alignment must be attempted whenever possible to minimize potential future deformity.

BONE ANATOMY

An understanding of the gross anatomy of bone permits accurate description of fractures (Fig. 120–1). The diaphysis makes up the main shaft of the bone and develops by an interaction between the periosteum and underlying developing cartilage, resulting in the cortex. As the cortex develops and matures, the bone loses its porosity and becomes harder and denser.

The metaphysis is characterized by its thinner cortex and more porous bone. In the metaphysis, osteoblastic, osteoclastic, and osteolytic activity occur, resulting in extensive remodeling and thus transforming cartilaginous bone to more porous bone. The increased porosity of the thinner, fenestrated cortex devoid of solid bone components contrib-

utes to the "buckle fracture" that commonly occurs in this region. The strong periosteal attachment to the metaphyseal area stabilizes the metaphyseoepiphyseal junction.

The epiphysis is a cartilaginous structure at either end of long bones. The physis is sandwiched between the epiphysis and the metaphysis. The process of ossification progresses until the epiphysis fuses with the metaphysis, marking the end of bone growth.

The physis, more commonly known as the "growth plate," is found between the epiphysis and metaphysis, with a contour following the metaphyseal surface. Injury to the physis is assumed if there is disruption of the epiphyseal or metaphyseal surfaces. The major function of the physis is its contribution to longitudinal bone growth. The physis contains various histologic zones, the most important being the zone of growth. This area is responsible for both longitudinal and circumferential bone growth. Disruption of this zone can result in growth failure and subsequent deformity. New cells formed in this layer form cartilage, which in turn ossifies.

The periosteum of immature bone is thicker, more loosely attached, and more vascular; it has muscle fiber attachments and surrounds the cortex. These features, along with an osteogenic potential, contribute to rapid callus formation, remodeling, and bone growth.

The diaphysis and metaphysis receive blood from branches of major vessels (Fig. 120–2). The blood supply of

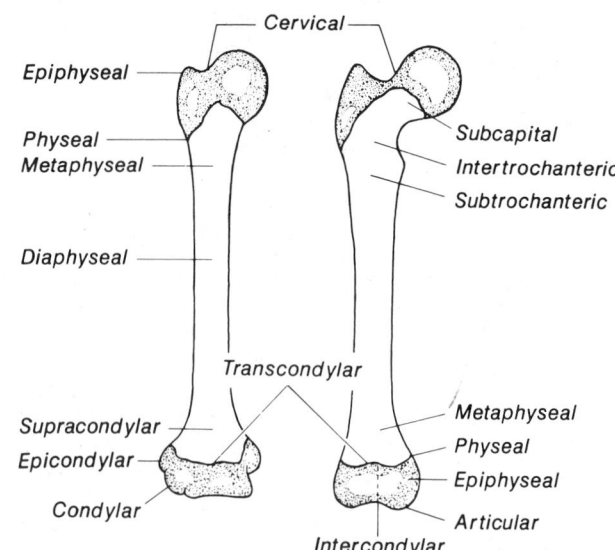

Figure 120–1. Schematic drawing of a humerus *(left)* and femur *(right)* from a 10-year-old child, showing various anatomic locations and definitions. (From Ogden JA. Skeletal Injury in the Child. 2nd ed. Philadelphia, WB Saunders, 1990, p 5.)

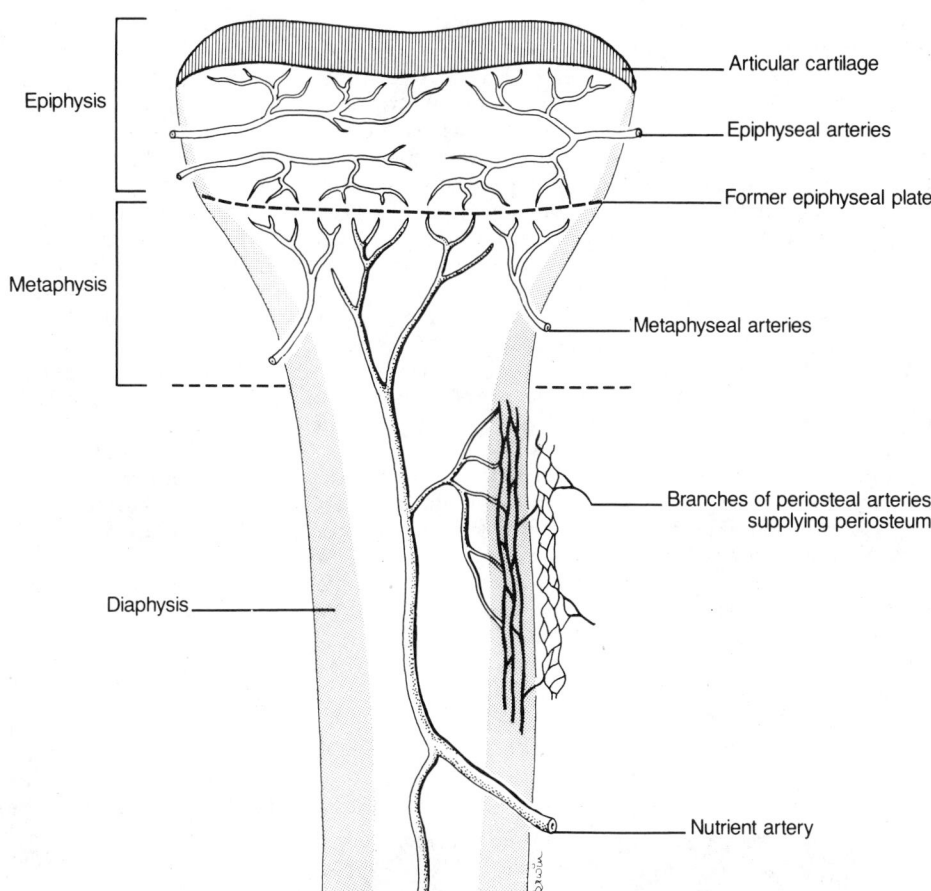

Epiphysis

Metaphysis

Diaphysis

Articular cartilage

Epiphyseal arteries

Former epiphyseal plate

Metaphyseal arteries

Branches of periosteal arteries supplying periosteum

Nutrient artery

Figure 120–2. Schematic diagram of blood supply to mature long bone. (From Cormack DH. Han's Histology. Philadelphia, JB Lippincott, 1982, p 314.)

the periosteum is supplied by small vessels that nourish bone formation and the bone matrix. The epiphysis receives its blood supply from penetrating vessels and canals. The blood supply to the physis is derived from epiphyseal, metaphyseal, and perichondrial vessels. Fractures can cause vascular compromise to the epiphysis and physis that hinder bone growth. When the metaphyseal circulation is compromised, there is no significant effect on chondrogenesis, although ossification may be delayed until circulation is resumed.

BIOMECHANICS OF FRACTURES

Fracture patterns are determined by the nature of the external forces, bone maturity, density, porosity, and elasticity (Fig. 120–3). All these factors are reflected in the bone's capacity to absorb kinetic energy. When the forces of shearing, compression, and tension exceed the physiologic internal resistance of bone and cartilage to deformation, a fracture occurs at the area of weakness. The increased porosity

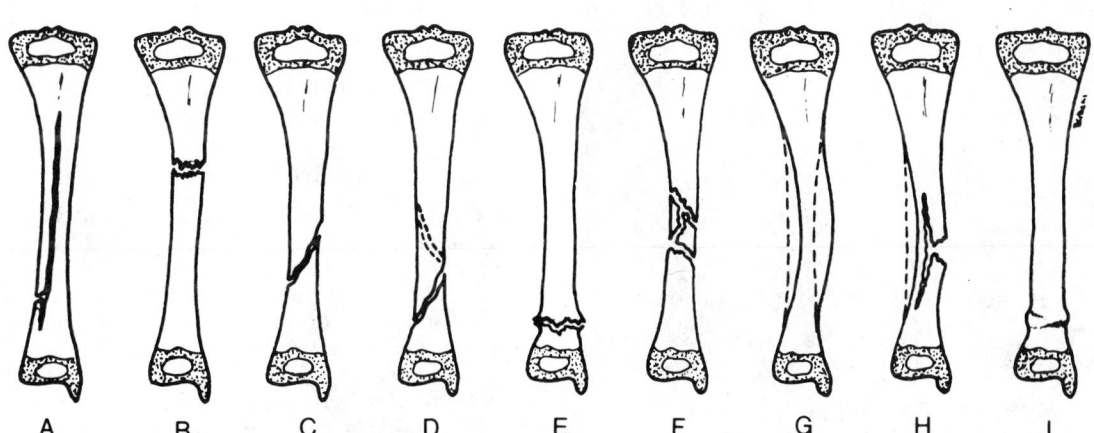

A   B   C   D   E   F   G   H   I

Figure 120–3. Schematic of a tibia from a 3-year-old child, showing various types of fractures: *A*, longitudinal; *B*, transverse; *C*, oblique; *D*, spiral; *E*, impacted; *F*, comminuted; *G*, bowing (plastic deformation); *H*, greenstick; and *I*, torus. (From Ogden JA. Skeletal Injury in the Child. 2nd ed. Philadelphia, WB Saunders, 1990, p 7.)

makes immature bone more pliable, causing deformity before breaking, unlike the shattering seen in more compact and dense mature bone. The metaphyseal porosity in immature bone makes it vulnerable to a compression stress, resulting in "buckle" (torus) fractures. The increased elasticity and decreased cortical width of immature bone allow more energy absorption, resulting in greenstick fractures rather than complete fractures as seen in more mature bone.

Axial load and a compression force result in torus bowing and oblique fractures. The torus or "buckle" fracture results from the increased porosity of bone at the metaphysis. A typical example of this occurs when a child lands on an outstretched hand, resulting in a "buckling" at the cortex of the distal ulna and radius (Fig. 120–4).

An oblique fracture is caused by axial overload and shearing of bone. The fracture is propagated at a 30-degree angle to the axis of load.

Traumatic bowing or "plastic deformity" is caused when the axial load causes bones like the ulna or fibula to bend with compression. The force is insufficient to cause a fracture, although there may be a fracture in an adjacent bone.

A lateral force on bone causes transverse or greenstick fractures. In transverse fractures the lateral force and resulting angulation may allow one of the bone fragments to pierce through the disrupted periosteum. The fracture line is perpendicular to the longitudinal axis of the bone.

A greenstick fracture occurs when bone is bent until a fracture is propagated and then recoils to its former position.

The fracture line does not traverse the whole width of the bone. The two ends recoil, with the help of muscle and the periosteum, almost to the original position.

Spiral fractures result from axial torsion in which the fracture line curves around the bone in an oblique fashion. This type of fracture in infancy should arouse the suspicion of child abuse.

Comminuted fractures are uncommon in early childhood but increase in frequency as the bone matures. This is thought to be due to the flexibility and porosity of young bone. When this occurs in more mature bone, the kinetic energy is dissipated in multiple directions, resulting in more than three fragments of bone.

Avulsion fractures occur when a bone fragment attached to a ligament is sheared off the axial skeleton. This type of injury is usually seen at the tibial spine, ulnar styloid, and bases of the phalanges.

Perichondrial ring avulsions are usually caused by shearing of bone at the site of the physis. Significant injury results in growth failure and subsequent deformity.

CLINICAL EVALUATION
History

A history of the injury is usually given by the parent of the injured child. The age, mechanism of injury, time interval, initial treatment, magnitude of disability, and significant medical history (e.g., chronic diseases, allergies, immunization status, previous injuries, medications) should be documented. If the explanation of the injury does not coincide with the physical and radiologic findings, the possibility of child abuse should be considered.

Physical Examination

The physical examination should be performed in a gentle and reassuring manner, with the child in a comfortable position. Younger children may prefer being examined on a parent's lap. On initial inspection the child's behavior, gait, interaction with parents, and hygiene should be noted. The uninjured extremity is first examined, then compared with the injured part. Obvious deformity, motor function, soft tissue injury, skin color, and swelling must be noted. Vascular integrity is assessed by palpating the character of distal pulses, skin color, skin temperature, and sensation. The stability of the joints and contiguous soft tissues is assessed, checking for crepitus, tenderness, and range of motion. The joints above and below the injury are always examined so that subtle fractures or dislocations are not missed. Deformity and point tenderness are good predictors of fractures. The finding of ecchymosis is a poor predictor of fractures in children. A compartment syndrome is suspected when there is palpable muscle tension, intractable pain, swelling, sensory deficit, or pain with muscle stretching.

DIAGNOSTIC EVALUATION

Radiographs should be obtained when the history and physical findings suggest the possibility of a fracture. An anteroposterior view, a lateral view, and radiographs of the joints distal and proximal to the injury are recommended. Comparison views of a contralateral bone or joint may be needed when there is doubt concerning the findings on the initial radiograph. Knowledge of the radiographic findings of bone development, especially in reference to the physis, can be useful in differentiating normal from abnormal findings (Figs. 120–5, 120–6). A reference text showing the normal age- and sex-related radiographs can aid in evaluating fractures.

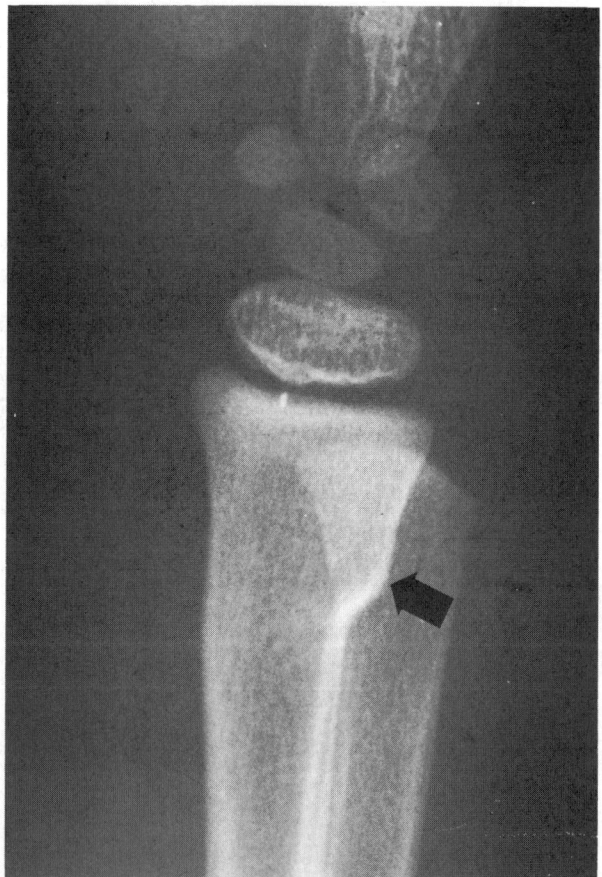

Figure 120–4. This 5-year-old girl fell on her outstretched hand, sustaining a torus fracture of the distal radius (*arrow*), recognized as an abrupt change in contour 1 cm proximal to the physis on this lateral radiograph. (Courtesy of A. Ostereich, M.D., Cincinnati, OH.)

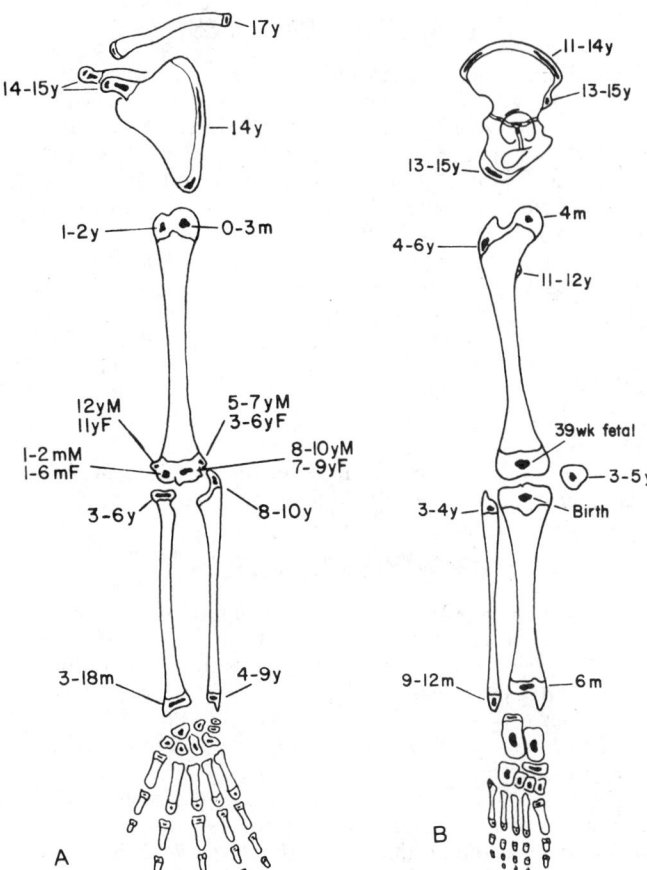

Figure 120–5. Schematic of ages of onset of secondary ossification of major long bones in the arm *(A)* and leg *(B)*. (From Ogden JA. Skeletal Injury in the Child. 2nd ed. Philadelphia, WB Saunders, 1990, p 84.)

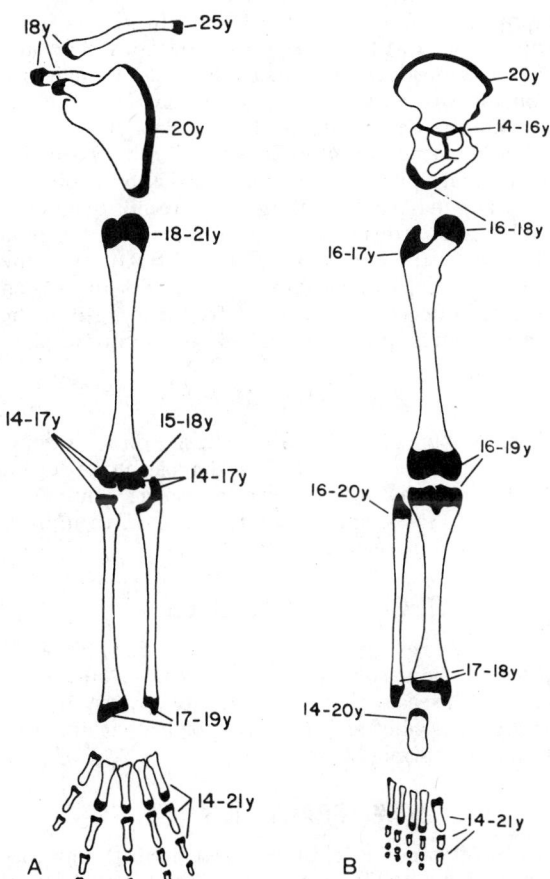

Figure 120–6. Schematic of ages of physeal closure (physiologic epiphysiodesis) in the major long bones of the arm *(A)* and leg *(B)*. (From Ogden JA. Skeletal Injury in the Child. 2nd ed. Philadelphia, WB Saunders, 1990, p 84.)

CLASSIFYING FRACTURES

It is important to characterize and classify fractures to ensure proper radiographic interpretation and communication. A complete fracture refers to a fracture line interrupting both cortices of bone. These fractures have many configurations depending on the intensity and angle of the stress applied. Complete fractures may be transverse, oblique, spiral, or comminuted. Incomplete fractures occur when the fracture line interrupts only one cortex, as seen in the greenstick type. In a closed fracture, the soft tissue and skin overlying the fracture are intact. An open fracture occurs when the overlying soft tissue and skin are disrupted. Displacement describes fragments that are not aligned with one another. Angulation describes the relationship of the fragments to the longitudinal axis (Fig. 120–7). A valgus deformity occurs when the distal fragment is angled *away* from the body's midline; a varus deformity, when the distal fragment is angled *toward* the body's midline.

GROWTH PLATE INJURIES

Approximately 15% of all pediatric bone injuries involve the growth plate. Males are more likely than females to sustain injuries owing to the different mechanisms of injury and the later closure of growth plates. The distal physes of long bones are more likely to be disrupted. The distal ulna, distal radius, and phalangeal physes are the most common sites of disruption.

The Salter-Harris classification system (types I to V) is used to describe the radiologic findings and kinetics of injury, and has implications regarding the management and potential growth deformity of the bone (Fig. 120–8). Disruption of growth may result from (1) malalignment and nonunion of the growth plate; (2) destruction of the plate by infection, crushing, or avascular necrosis; and (3) bony overgrowth and bridging between the epiphysis and metaphysis.

Type I injuries result from shearing, avulsion, and torsional forces. The epiphysis completely separates from the metaphysis. If the periosteum is intact, displacement may not occur and the radiographs may appear normal. However, this fracture may be seen as an apparent widening of the growth plate (Fig. 120–9). Stress films may be necessary to rule out a more serious injury. If there is tenderness and swelling over the growth plate, the injury should be treated as a type I injury based on the clinical findings. Type I injuries have an excellent prognosis.

Type II fractures result from a lateral displacement force that passes through the plate, tearing the periosteum on one side and leaving a triangular fragment on the metaphysis. Since the zone of proliferation remains intact, normal growth may continue.

Type III fractures are usually seen in more mature growth plates where the epiphysis is more developed and the growth plate partially fused. The fracture plane runs transversely through the physis then through the epiphysis. This fracture therefore has a worse prognosis.

Type IV fractures result in the fracture line extending from the articular surface of the epiphysis through the physis and metaphysis. These fractures are most commonly seen in the condyles of the humerus and the tibia. Bony bridging from the metaphysis to the epiphysis may occur during healing and cause premature closure of the growth plate.

Type V fractures are the result of damage to the growth plate by compression of the physis, with disruption of the germinal cells. These are difficult to diagnose radiologically. The prognosis is poor, as this injury commonly results in growth arrest. These injuries must be differentiated from type I fractures, since the outcome is much worse with a type V fracture.

FRACTURE DESCRIPTION

The important details of the clinical and radiologic findings must be clearly communicated to any consultant (Table 120–1).

CHILD ABUSE

It is documented that approximately 1% of children in the United States have been abused. In one study, 10% of children under 5 years of age seen for trauma had "nonaccidental" injuries. Estimates of skeletal injury resulting from child abuse range from 10% to 30% in all children under 3 years of age. During the evaluation of an injured child, the physician must suspect abuse when there is a history of multiple previous injuries, an inconsistent mechanism of injury, unexplainable soft tissue injuries, old fractures on routine radiographs, an unkempt physical presentation, and a poor nutritional status. Any fracture in a child under 1 year of age is even more suspicious.

Patterns of skeletal injury resulting from child abuse reflect the developmental characteristics of immature bone (Table 120–2). The periosteal reaction of new bone formation resulting from subperiosteal hemorrhage stems from indirect torsional, accelerational, and decelerational forces. The loosely adhering periosteum separates from the cortex along the metaphysis and diaphysis, allowing a blood clot to organize around the bone. These skeletal findings are commonly seen in newborns after traction during difficult breech presentation. Similar forces are applied when the extremities are used as a handle to shake the child. A series of microfractures result and traverse the weak, immature matrix of the metaphysis. Remodeling, periosteal thickening, and overgrowth are seen as lucencies on radiographs. The metaphyseal lesions produced by torsional, accelerational, and decelerational forces resulting from shaking a child by the extremities or thorax are considered diagnostic of child abuse.

Epiphyseal injuries tend to occur beyond infancy and are usually accidental. Spiral fractures of the diaphysis of long bones in infancy may suggest abuse, but are not diagnostic unless other factors arouse suspicion. Injuries to the scapula and small bones of the hands and feet, and fractures of the sternum and spine, are suspicious of abuse. Fractures seen in child abuse, in decreasing order of frequency, are of the ribs, humerus, femur, tibia, skull, hand, ulna, and radius.

BIRTH TRAUMA

Musculoskeletal birth injuries occur during difficult deliveries, such as breech deliveries. In decreasing order of incidence, the fractures seen involve the clavicle, humerus, femur, humeral physes, and femoral physes. Birth injuries can easily be misinterpreted as child abuse.

PATHOLOGIC FRACTURES

Pathologic fractures are caused by stress through weak areas of bone. Lesions such as tumors, cysts, fibromas, and metabolic bone diseases (e.g., rickets, osteogenesis imperfecta) provide areas where fractures may be propagated with less force than in normal bone.

OTHER FRACTURES

Many fractures occur in clusters based upon the mechanism of injury. Waddell's triad results from a pedestrian

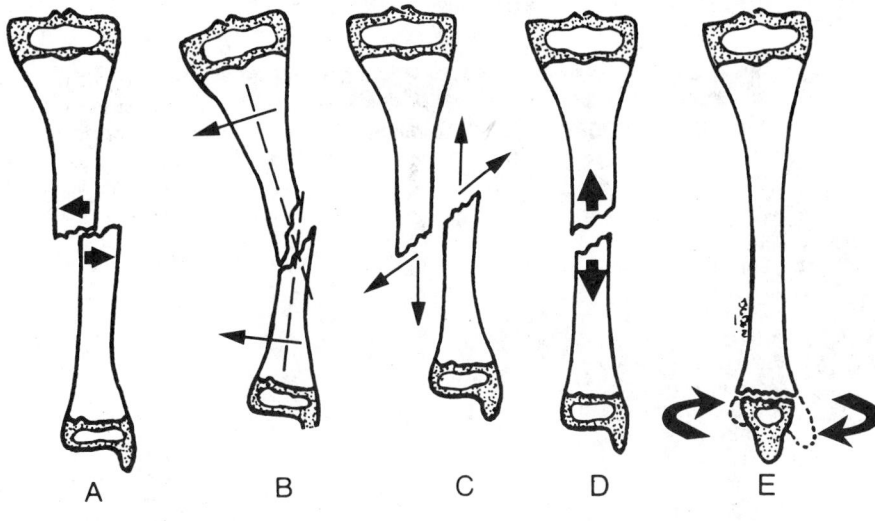

Figure 120–7. Schematic of the tibia from a 6-year-old child, showing the relationships of fracture fragments to each other. *A,* Translocation; *B,* angulation; *C,* overriding; *D,* distraction; *E,* rotation in a distal epiphyseal fracture. (From Ogden JA. Skeletal Injury in the Child. 2nd ed. Philadelphia, WB Saunders, 1990, p 9.)

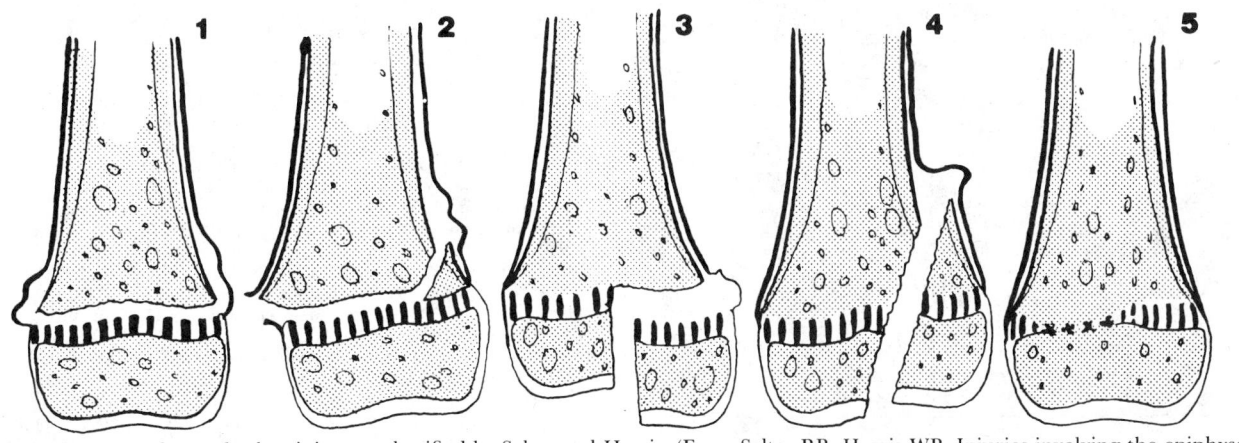

Figure 120–8. Types of growth-plate injury as classified by Salter and Harris. (From Salter RB, Harris WR. Injuries involving the epiphyseal plate. J Bone Joint Surg 1963; 45A:587.)

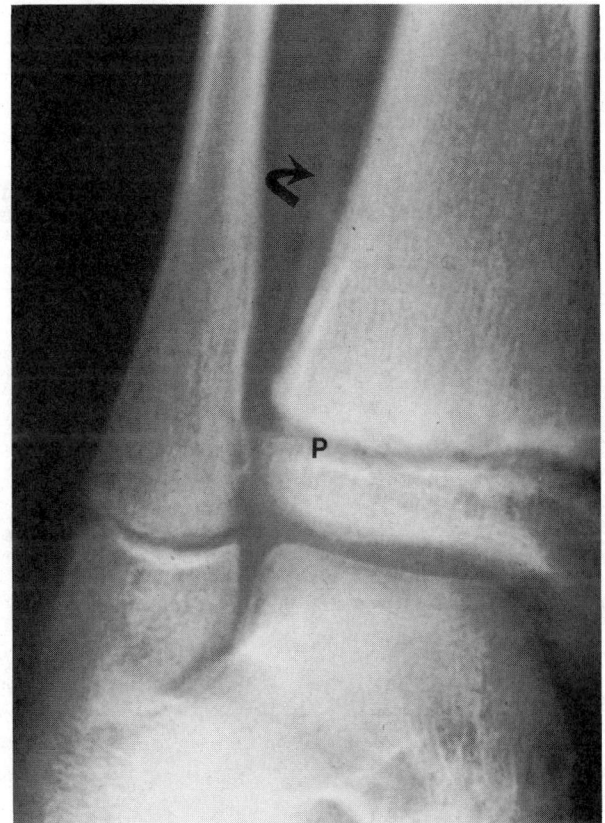

Figure 120–9. The best evidence of a Salter I fracture of the distal tibia physis (P) of this 13-year-old patient was the periosteal reaction *(arrow)* along the shaft a few weeks later. (Courtesy of A. Oestreich, M.D., Cincinnati, OH.)

TABLE 120–1

OUTLINE FOR REPORTING SKELETAL INJURIES

A. Brief history
  1. Age, sex, medical history
  2. Mechanism of injury with time interval
B. Clinical findings
  1. Disability
  2. Deformity
  3. Soft tissue injury
  4. Neurovascular status
C. Radiologic interpretation
  1. Anatomic location
  2. Type of fracture
    a. Buckle (torus)
    b. Transverse
    c. Oblique
    d. Spiral
    e. Greenstick
    f. Longitudinal
    g. Bowing (plastic deformation)
    h. Comminuted
    i. Pathologic
    j. Butterfly
    k. Avulsion
    l. Perichondrial ring
  3. Complete vs. incomplete
  4. Open vs. closed
  5. Relationship of fracture fragments
    a. Nondisplaced
    b. Displaced
      (i) Impacted
      (ii) Overriding (bayonet)
      (iii) Lateral shift
      (iv) Rotation
      (v) Distraction
    c. Angulation: direction of apex of fracture fragments

motor vehicle accident in which a school-age child's femur is fractured by the car's bumper contact at that level, the chest and abdomen hits the hood, and the child is then thrown back from the car, injuring the contralateral side of the skull.

TABLE 120–2

RADIOLOGIC FINDINGS OF CHILD ABUSE BY SPECIFICITY

High specificity
  Metaphyseal lesions
  Posterior rib fractures
  Scapular fractures
  Spinous process fractures
  Sternal fractures
Moderate specificity*
  Multiple fractures, especially bilateral
  Fractures of different ages
  Epiphyseal separations
  Vertebral body fractures and
    subluxations
  Digital fractures
  Complex skull fractures
Common, but low specificity*
  Clavicular fractures
  Long bone shaft fractures
  Linear skull fractures

*Moderate- and low-specificity lesions become high when a history of trauma is absent or inconsistent with injuries.
From Kleinman PK. Diagnostic Imaging of Child Abuse. Baltimore, Williams & Wilkins, 1987.

Stress fractures are common in early spring and summer as a result of increased activity after a period of relative inactivity and improper athletic training. The subtle cortical changes of periosteal thickening can be seen on the tibia, fibula, metatarsals, ribs, pelvis, femur, and humerus.

Toddlers' fractures occur between the ages of 9 months and 3 years. The first sign is when the child stops walking. Radiologically, there is soft tissue swelling soon after injury, and later a nondisplaced fracture line may appear. The mechanism is a compression stress force. The tibia and fibula are most commonly involved.

Selected References

Akbarnia BA, Akbarnia NO. The role of the orthopedist in child abuse and neglect. Orthop Clin North Am 1976;7:733.

Akbarnia B, Torg JS, Kirkpatric J, et al. Manifestations of the battered child syndrome. J Bone Joint Surg 1974;56A:1159.

Centers for Disease Control. Childhood injuries in the United States. Am J Dis Child 1990;114:627.

Chan RNW, Ainscow D, Sikorski JM. Diagnostic fractures in the multiply injured. J Trauma 1980;20:684.

Currey JD, Butler G. The mechanical properties of bone tissue in children. J Bone Joint Surg 1975;57A:810.

Devas MB. Stress fractures in children. J Bone Joint Surg 1963;45B:528.

Engh CA, Robinson RA, Milgram J. Stress fractures in children. J Trauma 1970;10:532.

Kleinman PK, Marko SC, Blackbourne B. The metaphyseal lesion in abused infants. A radiologic-histopathologic study. AJR 1986;146:895.

Mann DC, Rajmaira S. Distribution of physeal and nonphyseal fractures in 2,650 long-bone fractures in children aged 0–16 years. J Pediatr Orthop 1990;10:713.

Mizuta T, Benson WM, Foster BK, et al. Statistical analysis of the incidence of physeal injuries. J Pediatr Orthop 1987;7:518.

Ogden JA. Injury to the growth mechanisms of the immature skeleton. Skeletal Radiol 1981;6:237.

Peterson CA, Peterson HA. Analysis of the incidence of injuries to the epiphyseal growth plate. J Trauma 1972;12:275.

Rang W, Wright J. Pitfalls in fractures. Pediatr Ann 1989;18:53.

Salter RB, Harris WR. Injuries involving the epiphyseal plate. J Bone Surg 1963;45A:587.

CHAPTER 121

Management of Orthopedic Injuries

Deborah Lubitz

FRACTURE HEALING

Fracture healing occurs rapidly in children. A hematoma forms at the fracture site, followed by an intense inflammatory reaction. While the cells of the periosteum form the earliest new bone, granulation tissue and capillary buds invade the area from surrounding soft tissue, forming new cartilage. The formation of a callus by the active osteoblastic periosteum occurs quickly, and clinical union usually takes place within several days. Once union occurs, the fragments cannot be manipulated and their position will not change. As healing progresses, the bone organizes and is then resorbed, and new bone is laid down according to the forces or stresses applied to the bone. This process is called remodeling, and it proceeds rapidly in children. Future growth of the bone then provides for further remodeling. Remodeling can correct for some abnormalities of fracture angulation and displacement after fracture reduction.

CLASSIFICATION OF INJURY

The accurate description of an orthopedic injury requires precise terminology. The use of appropriate terms will assist in conveying the proper image of the injury to the orthopedist. Each of the following categories should always be used when characterizing a fracture: (1) type of fracture, (2) anatomic location, (3) direction of the fracture line(s), (4) position of the fragments (displacement), (5) alignment of the fragments (angulation), and (6) associated soft tissue injury. See Figs. 120–3 and 120–7.

Type of Fracture

Fractures in children differ from those in adults in the degree of cortical disruption. In a complete fracture (through-and-through) both cortices are interrupted. In an incomplete fracture (greenstick) only one cortex is interrupted. These fractures occur in children because their bones are soft and compliant. If an axial load (along the long axis of the bone) is applied, one or both cortices may wrinkle or buckle. This type of fracture, torus (buckle) fracture, occurs most commonly at the metaphysis. A bending deformity can occur in children's bones when the stress is not significant enough to cause failure and fracture but is severe enough that the bone cannot return to its original contour. An avulsion fracture results when a bone fragment is pulled away by the attached tendon or ligament. Epiphyseal (physeal) fractures are those that involve the growth plate (physis); they are therefore unique to children. These injuries are common in children because the cartilaginous growth plate is the weakest portion of the bone. The Salter-Harris classification of growth plate fractures provides an estimate of the prognosis for proper healing and the likelihood of future growth disturbances. The prognosis deteriorates from type I to type V. See Fig. 120–8.

Anatomic Location

The location of fracture should be noted as precisely as possible, including the name of the bone. Long bones may be divided into thirds—proximal, middle, and distal—to describe fracture location. Other terms, such as head (e.g., femoral head), neck, shaft, and base (e.g., the base of the proximal phalanx), may be used. If there is an exact designation for the area (e.g., ulnar styloid, distal humeral condyle), it should be used.

Direction of the Fracture Line

The direction of the fracture line is described in relation to the long axis of the bone. The fracture line in a transverse fracture occurs at a right angle to the long axis of the bone. The fracture line in an oblique fracture runs across the bone at other than a right angle. A spiral fracture results from a rotational force and encircles the shaft of the long bone in a spiral, oblique manner. This type of fracture is common in the long bones of toddlers. Any fracture in which there are more than two fragments is comminuted.

Position of the Fragments

If the ends of the fracture fragments are not in their normal position, they are displaced. If the fracture surfaces are still in contact for some distance along their length, there is partial displacement. The displacement is described as the position of the distal fragment in relation to the proximal. The displacement may be dorsal or volar, anterior or posterior, lateral or medial. Valgus may be used to describe a deformity that is shifted away from the midline of the body, while varus denotes a displacement toward the midline. If there is strong muscle spasm as a result of the injury, as often occurs with femur fractures, there may be complete displacement with overlapping of the fragments, also called bayonet apposition. If the fragments are separated along the long axis of the bone, the fragments are distracted.

Alignment of the Fragments

If the longitudinal axes of the fragments deviate from their normal alignment, there is angulation. Angulation is described both by the degrees of the angle and by the direction of the apex of the angle. The same terms used to describe the direction of displacement are used to describe the direction of angulation.

Associated Soft Tissue Injury

It is important to evaluate the extent of the injury to the surrounding tissue, often caused by the sharp fragments of bone. With a closed (simple) fracture, the overlying skin remains completely intact. An open (compound) fracture is one where the overlying skin is broken. The break may be as obscure as a puncture wound or laceration near the site of the fracture, or the bone fragments may be seen protruding through the skin. With an open fracture there is significant risk of infection to soft tissues or bone. A fracture where there is associated neurologic, vascular, ligamentous, or muscular injury is called complicated.

NONFRACTURE INJURIES

Sprain

A sprain is an injury to the supporting ligaments of a joint. In a first-degree sprain there is only minor tearing of ligamentous fibers. There is minimal hemorrhage, swelling, and point tenderness over the ligament. There is normal joint movement and no functional disability. A second-degree tear is more severe, yet is still partial. There will be more hemorrhage, swelling, and tenderness, with significant pain on motion and loss of function (e.g., inability to bear weight on an ankle). With a third-degree sprain there is complete tearing of the ligament, with abnormal movement of the joint when stresses are applied. When the joint is stressed, a second-degree sprain will usually be very painful. Conversely, with complete tears there will usually be little pain and abnormal movement of the joint when stressed.

Strain

A strain is an injury to a musculotendinous unit and is graded in a manner similar to a sprain. In a third-degree strain there is complete loss of function in addition to severe pain and spasm, hemorrhage, and swelling. Any force applied to the muscle will result in sharp pain at the site of injury. An apparent third-degree strain, however, may be an avulsion fracture at the tendon insertion.

Dislocation

In a dislocation abnormal forces applied to a joint cause damage to supporting ligaments and complete loss of continuity between the articular surfaces. These are relatively uncommon occurrences in young children because the growth plate and perichondrium are weaker than the ligaments of the joint, but they will be seen in adolescents. Dislocations should be described by which joint or bone is displaced and the direction of the displaced (or distal) bone relative to the normal structures. If an associated fracture is present, it is termed a fracture-dislocation. If the skin overlying a dislocation is broken, it is an open dislocation, which carries significant risk of joint infection.

Subluxation

In a subluxation there is an incomplete dislocation with partial continuity between the two bones that make up the joint. The most common subluxation seen in pediatrics is subluxation of the radial head, the so-called "nursemaid's elbow." In this injury there is a tear in the distal attachment of the annular ligament around the radial head. The radial head protrudes from under the ligament, which then becomes trapped in the radiohumeral joint. There is usually a history of a strong pull on the extended arm, pain, and refusal to use the arm. The child will hold the elbow slightly flexed and the forearm pronated. On physical examination the only finding may be pain with attempts to supinate the arm. Rapid supination with elbow flexion will usually reduce the injury.

Diastasis

A diastasis is a disruption of the interosseous membrane connecting two bones such as the radius and ulna or the tibia and fibula.

EMS CONSIDERATIONS

In a patient with multiple trauma, musculoskeletal injuries rarely take precedence. Following initial stabilization, the secondary survey will include examination of the musculoskeletal system. Local pressure should be used to control external hemorrhage, and unstable fractures should be splinted. Open fractures should be covered with a sterile dressing prior to splinting.

If the fracture is an isolated injury, a splint should be applied in the prehospital setting. Splinting avoids further damage to surrounding tissue and will relieve pain. Fractures should generally be splinted in the position in which they are found; manipulation should be avoided. The joints above and below the injury must be immobilized in order to decrease movement of the damaged bone. A neurovascular examination of the extremity distal to the injury must be documented prior to splinting.

There are numerous types of commercially available splinting devices, starting with simple cardboard or wooden splints. These should be padded and secured with gauze or elastic wrapping. Inflatable air splints are easy to apply (although clothing should be removed) and may help to control swelling and bleeding. These splints must be used carefully. When inflated to high pressures, they can reduce blood flow to the extremity and cause ischemia. Vacuum splints conform to the contours of the injured limb, immobilize well, and do not cause excessive pressure on the tissues. If none of these splints are available, many everyday items such as pillows, towels, canes, and umbrellas may be used. If they are applied correctly and allow penetration by radiographs, even these simple devices may be left in place after arrival at the hospital.

Femoral fractures should be immobilized with continuous traction. The half-ring splints applied posteriorly, such as the Thomas or Hare traction splints, are commonly used. The newer Sager traction splint is applied along the inner or outer side of the leg, eliminating the posterior half-ring. This eliminates the sciatic nerve compression and proximal femoral flexion that may occur with the half-ring. The Sager traction splint can be used for both adults and children; the actual weight of traction applied is measured to avoid overtraction and possible growth plate damage.

CLINICAL EVALUATION

A detailed description of the mechanism of injury should be obtained if possible. Specific information about the site and degree of pain and swelling, restriction of joint movement, and weakness or loss of sensation should be elicited.

If there is a history of injury and there is an obvious deformity of the extremity, making the diagnosis is easy. For those patients with badly deformed limbs, the initial examination should be limited so as to avoid causing unnecessary discomfort, and the extremity should be splinted before the patient is moved. The neurovascular status of the limb distal to the injury must be evaluated initially and serially, especially after any intervention or manipulation. Any evidence of ischemia to the limb should be treated emergently.

When the nature of the injury is not obvious, a more complete examination must be done. The severity of complaints and physical findings in the more common childhood fractures, such as buckle, greenstick, or growth plate fractures, may be markedly unimpressive. The injured area or extremity should be carefully inspected for swelling, hemorrhage (ecchymosis), erythema, abrasions, lacerations, or puncture wounds. Palpation of the entire extremity to elicit tenderness should begin at an area far from the identified site of pain. The range of motion of the joints above and below the injury should be evaluated, but movement should not be forced in the presence of pain. The physician will often be able to pinpoint the site of tenderness and swelling well enough to distinguish between bone or ligamentous injury. When a ligamentous injury is suspected in an older child, stability of the joint should be evaluated, especially the knee and ankle. Severe pain may lead the child to resist examination, and complete evaluation of the joint may be difficult.

DIAGNOSTIC EVALUATION

Radiographs should be obtained whenever a fracture is suspected. In many cases, such as when there is deformity of the limb or severe swelling and localized tenderness over the diaphysis, the radiograph merely confirms the diagnosis and allows for complete characterization of the fracture. In young children, radiographs are more often needed to make the diagnosis. Fractures involving the ends of the long bones (metaphysis, physeal growth plate, and epiphysis), which are common in children, often result in only minor physical findings.

It is necessary to obtain at least two views taken at right angles to each other. These are usually the frontal (anteroposterior) and lateral views. If it is impossible to obtain these views because of a deformity, a splint, or severely restricted motion, two oblique views at right angles should be obtained. Other oblique views or specialized views may be obtained if more information is needed.

It is generally recommended that radiographs also be taken of the joint areas proximal and distal to the suspected site of injury. This is particularly important with diaphyseal (shaft) injury, as there is occasionally an associated fracture or dislocation at the end of the injured bone. Missing a dislocation of the elbow or hip could be devastating to the future viability or function of the extremity.

There is continuing controversy regarding the routine use of comparison views of the normal side. These views may identify subtle abnormalities common in pediatric injuries and avoid over-reading normal anatomic features that may look like fractures. Most pediatric radiologists feel that they do not need comparison views, but these views may be helpful to nonradiologists who are often responsible for the initial radiologic interpretation and treatment of the patient. The physician must balance clinical suspicion for the presence of a fracture, experience in interpreting pediatric radiographs, availability of radiologic consultation, and potential ramifications for the patient if the fracture is missed. Perhaps the best suggestion is to obtain comparison views if the diagnosis remains questionable after radiographs of the injured side are seen (in the hand or foot, comparison may be made with other phalanges, metacarpals, or metatarsals on the same side).

There are several common pitfalls in the interpretation of pediatric extremity radiographs. Nondisplaced Salter I fractures are commonly missed because fracture lines through cartilage cannot be seen. Some injuries are not easily seen on standard views; this is particularly true around the elbow and ankle. Subtle abnormalities, such as buckle fractures or displacement of small epiphyses (the medial epicondyle of the humerus is the classic example), may be missed. Additionally, normal features and normal variants may be misinterpreted as fractures. Many of these problems can be avoided. Buckle or greenstick fractures may be more easily recognized by carefully following the smooth contours of the cortex, looking for any discontinuity. The physical examination must be correlated with the radiograph. If a possible abnormality is seen on the radiograph, but there is no clinical abnormality in that area, a fracture is unlikely. If, on the other hand, a strong clinical suspicion is present but radiographs fail to demonstrate a fracture, other views or comparisons should be considered. A radiologist may be helpful in deciding which additional views to obtain.

Evaluating the soft tissue changes on radiographs will often help to detect fractures. Significant localized soft tissue swelling and obliteration of the normal muscle-fat interfaces often indicate a fracture. In the context of trauma, fluid in a joint is usually indicative of an adjacent fracture. The effusion may be clinically apparent, but typically is not. In the elbow and ankle the fat pads around the joint should be evaluated on the lateral projection. The anterior fat pads are normally visible, but elevation or distortion of the anterior fat pad indicates the presence of an effusion and probable fracture. The presence of the posterior fat pad on a radiograph is always abnormal and signifies the presence of a fracture.

When a dislocation is suspected, radiographs should be obtained before attempting a reduction. It is important to know whether there is a fracture-dislocation because there is a risk of damaging soft tissues with sharp bone fragments or trapping articular fragments within the joint during the reduction. If one is convinced clinically that a toddler has a radial head subluxation (nursemaid's elbow), it is not usually necessary to obtain radiographs prior to reduction. If the attempted reduction is unsuccessful, radiographs should be obtained.

MANAGEMENT

Areas of possible injury should be identified for radiographic evaluation. The clinician should be generous in deciding which areas warrant radiography; children in pain (or with depressed consciousness) are often unable to identify every site that hurts or distinguish between superficial pain (a skin abrasion) and deep pain (a fracture). Sometimes the exact site of injury cannot be well localized, and radiographs of the entire extremity must be obtained. Although potentially life-threatening injuries must be addressed first, significant musculoskeletal injuries should be evaluated and treated as soon as it is feasible. Unstable fractures should be splinted, and open fractures should be cultured and covered with a sterile dressing prior to splinting.

An isolated musculoskeletal injury, limbs with obvious deformities, unstable fractures, and painful fractures should be splinted prior to radiography. Ice should be applied outside the splint; an icepack is never placed next to the skin inside a splint. If the injury was splinted in the prehospital setting, it is usually best to perform a limited examination (always including the neurovascular examination), leaving the splint in place until after radiographs are obtained.

Analgesia should be administered to patients who are in pain. Intramuscular or intravenous medication may be used (Table 121–1); it may be preferable to place an intravenous line in a patient who is likely to need other medications or further analgesia for fracture reduction.

Identical fractures are often treated differently in children and adults, so definitive treatment of most pediatric fractures should be performed in consultation with an orthopedist. Prompt union occurs in most children's fractures, so prolonged immobilization is usually unnecessary; for the same reason there is rarely a chance to correct initial errors in treatment easily. Healing and remodeling of immature bones can often correct imperfect alignment. Residual angulation that is in the plane of motion of the adjacent joint will remodel to some extent. Fractures close to the growth plate will correct more satisfactorily than midshaft fractures. Angulation that is not parallel to the plane of motion of the adjacent joint and rotational malalignment will not remodel; therefore these angulations must be corrected. Even though remodeling does occur, it should not be expected to remedy every problem. As a rule, any fracture with a visible limb deformity should be reduced prior to plaster immobilization.

In diaphyseal fractures, overriding with side-to-side contact of the fragments is often desirable. The disruption of the nutrient artery that occurs with a diaphyseal fracture results in an increase in blood flow to the epiphyses. The resultant acceleration of longitudinal growth compensates for residual shortening of the bone. This is especially true for femoral shaft fractures.

While the vast majority of pediatric fractures may safely be managed with closed reduction, certain fractures require open reduction to achieve correct anatomic alignment. Intra-articular fractures and type III and type IV growth plate fractures must be anatomically reduced to prevent later deformities of the bone or joint.

Not all fractures should have circumferential plaster immobilization applied at the time of presentation to the emergency department. When significant swelling has occurred, it may be desirable to immobilize the fracture with a splint for at least 24 hours while keeping the limb elevated and applying ice. The swelling will decrease, and the cast will fit better. Casting of fractures that do not need to be reduced may also be delayed 12 to 24 hours if casting in the emergency department is impractical. In these situations the splint should be one that conforms to the contours of the limb to provide proper immobilization, such as molded aluminum or plaster. Preformed plaster rolls covered with padding are convenient and easy to use. Casting is also usually delayed for an injury that has a high potential for developing vascular compromise or a compartment syndrome. Distal humeral fractures, such as supracondylar fractures, are usually treated in this manner because major blood vessels and nerves course close to the bone in this

TABLE 121–1

SUGGESTED ANALGESIC AGENTS FOR TREATMENT OF FRACTURES PRIOR TO REDUCTION AND CASTING

Medication	Dose	Route	Onset (min)	Peak Effect (min)	Duration (hr)	Comments
Morphine	0.05–0.1 mg/kg (max. = 10 mg)[a]	IV	10	30	1–2	The IV route may be preferable for narcotics because the effect
Meperidine (Demerol)	0.5–1.0 mg/kg (max. = 50 mg)[a]	IV	10	30	2–4	is more rapid and can be titrated to the desired effect.
	1.5–2.0 mg/kg (max. = 100 mg)[a]	IM	10–20	60	3–5	The respiratory depression secondary to morphine lasts much longer (>8 hr) than useful analgesia. Adverse effects (respiratory depression and hypotension) can be reversed with IV naloxone (Narcan).
Hydralazine (Vistaril)	1.0 mg/kg (max. = 50 mg)[a]	IM	15–30	30–60	4–6	Hydralazine is given with narcotics; reduces the anxiety associated with pain and potentiates the analgesia obtained with narcotics. Hydralazine should not be given IV because it may cause severe tissue necrosis.
Fentanyl	1–2 μg/kg[b]	IV	3–5	15	0.5–1	With short duration of action, may be more useful for short, painful procedures. Must be given slowly because rapid administration may cause chest wall rigidity. Respiratory depressant effects last several hours. Cardiorespiratory monitoring is suggested.
Ketorolac[c] (Toradol)	1–2 mg/kg (max. = 60 mg)	IV	30	60–120	Up to 6–8	Injectable nonsteroidal. Antiplatelet activity is major adverse effect. Use with caution in patients with renal dysfunction. Also may cause transient hyperkalemia.

[a]Maximum initial dose. When relatively higher doses are used, must consider higher level of monitoring. Assure adequate hydration to reduce the risk of orthostatic hypotension.

[b]Recommended initial dose. Some patients may need up to 5 μg/kg to achieve analgesia. The risk of adverse effects increases with increasing dose.

[c]Routine use in children has not been established.

area. The arm is elevated with slight traction for 12 to 24 hours prior to reduction (if necessary) and casting.

When a fracture is clinically suspected but not identified on the initial radiographs, the presence of a fracture should be assumed. The injured extremity should be immobilized with either a cast or splint, and the patient reevaluated in 5 to 10 days. A healing fracture should be apparent on repeat radiographs done at that time (Figure 121–1).

Joint dislocations should be reduced after radiographs show the absence of an associated fracture. Fracture-dislocations should be reduced by an orthopedist. After reduction, the joint must be stabilized and immobilized to prevent recurrent dislocation.

First-degree sprains cause minimal dysfunction. Treatment modalities include *r*est, *i*ce, *c*ompression (usually with an elastic wrap), and *e*levation (RICE). A second-degree sprain may require joint immobilization. Complete ligamentous tears (third-degree sprain) will usually require operative repair followed by prolonged immobilization.

SPECIAL CONSIDERATIONS

Open Fractures

A fracture is considered to be open whenever the overlying skin is broken. Whether it is a gaping wound with protruding bone fragments or a small laceration or puncture wound in the vicinity of the fracture, all open fractures must be considered contaminated.

Initially the wound should be cultured and covered with a sterile dressing and the extremity splinted. The neurovascular status of the distal extremity must be assessed. Radiographs should be carefully evaluated for the presence of foreign material in the wound. All patients should receive broad-spectrum antibiotics with activity against both gram-positive and gram-negative organisms. The combination of cefazolin and gentamicin will be adequate for most situations; penicillin should be added if there is a high risk of contamination with clostridial species (an injury occurring in a farm or field environment). If the patient's tetanus series is incomplete, or the last dose was received more than 5 years ago, tetanus immunization must be administered. Surgical debridement should be performed in the operating suite as soon as the patient's condition allows.

Vascular Compromise

The blood supply to the extremity distal to the site of a fracture or dislocation may be impeded in two ways. Arterial blood supply may be interrupted as a result of damage to, or occlusion of, the vessels. Alternately, a compartment syndrome occurs when swelling within a closed fascial com-

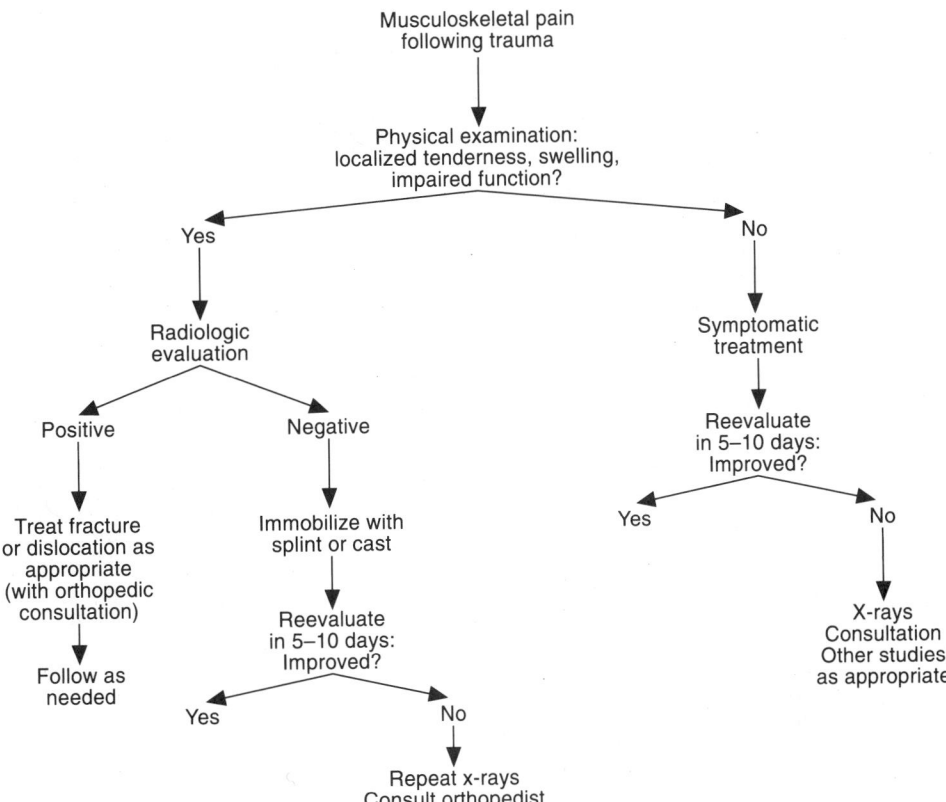

Figure 121–1. The clinical approach to an orthopedic injury.

partment gradually raises interstitial pressure and causes diminished tissue perfusion. Tissue perfusion may also be significantly decreased under a cast that is too tight.

The signs and symptoms of vascular compromise vary. Complete disruption of the arterial supply produces a cold, pulseless, and pale or cyanotic extremity. Decreased tissue perfusion due to compartment syndrome presents a more subtle picture. Distal pulses, skin color, and capillary refill are often unchanged. Pain is the most consistent sign of impending ischemia. The pain is progressive, deep, and poorly localized; one should suspect ischemia if a patient complains of increasing or unrelieved pain in an immobilized extremity. Characteristically the pain is exacerbated by movement of the fingers or toes. An expanding neurologic deficit with paresthesia and paralysis of the distal limb is a cardinal sign of ischemia.

Extremity ischemia is a surgical emergency; irreversible damage to nerves and muscles will begin within 6 to 8 hours of the onset of severe vascular compromise. Displaced fractures or dislocations must be immediately reduced; if circulation does not improve, prompt arteriography and surgical repair are essential. If the ischemia is the result of a compartment syndrome, decompressive fasciotomy must be performed.

Selected References

American Academy of Pediatrics Committee on Radiology. Comparison radiographs of extremities in childhood: Recommended usage. Pediatrics 1980;65:646.

Currey JB, Butler G. The mechanical properties of bone tissues in children. J Bone Joint Surg 1975;57:810.

Gustilo RB, Mendoza RM, Williams DN. Problems in the management of type III (severe) open fractures: A new classification of type III open fractures. J Bone Joint Surg 1984;24:742.

McCauley RGK, Schwartz AM, Leonidas JC, et al. Comparison views in extremity injury in childhood: An efficacy study. Radiology 1979;131:95.

Merten DF. Comparison radiographs in extremity injuries of childhood: Current application in radiological practice. Radiology 1978;126:209.

Rorabeck CH, Macnab I, Waddell JP. Anterior tibial compartment syndrome: A clinical and experimental review. Can J Surg 1972;15:249.

Salter RB, Harris WR. Injuries involving the epiphyseal plate. J Bone Joint Surg 1963;45A:587.

Shapiro F. Epiphyseal growth plate fractures-separations. A pathophysiologic approach. Orthopedics 1982;5:720.

Siffert RS. The effect of trauma to the epiphysis and growth plate. Skeletal Radiol 1977;2:21.

CHAPTER 122

Hand and Wrist Injuries

Robert A. Felter

INTRODUCTION

Hand injuries and infections are frequent causes of emergency visits by children. The constant exploration of their world combined with lack of experience and poor judgment places a child's hands at great risk. The human hand is a complex structure. Orthopedic hand injuries are challenging to diagnose and treat, especially in the skeletally immature child.

ANATOMY

The bony structure of the hand consists of the carpals, metacarpals, and phalanges. The carpals are arranged in two rows. Although carpals have their adult shape at birth, they form predominantly in cartilage and therefore in children appear radiolucent in a radiograph. The carpals ossify from the center to the periphery. While the main function of the cartilage is as a framework for later ossification, it also provides some protection to the ossified centers as well as to the growth centers. However, the lack of ossification makes injury difficult to detect. The scaphoid (navicular) is the largest and most frequently injured carpal bone. It is visible between ages 4 and 6 years and is completely ossified by age 13 to 16 years. The blood supply to the scaphoid flows oddly from the distal aspect of the bone to the proximal pole, directly in the path of many fractures. Disruption of the blood supply can result in avascular necrosis and nonunion, although this is less common in children.

The epiphyses of the metacarpals are located distally, with the exception of the thumb metacarpal, which is proximal. All epiphyses of the phalanges are proximal. So-called "pseudoepiphyses" (radiolucent areas on the opposite end of the epiphyses) can be found in metacarpals and phalanges and can be confused with fractures.

The arterial supply to the hand is provided by the radial and ulnar arteries. These anastomose in the superficial and deep palmar arches, which branch into digital arteries to each of the fingers and thumb. The Allen test demonstrates the contribution of the radial and ulnar artery to the blood flow of the hand. Up to 7% of the population have an incomplete arch.

Three nerves supply the motor and sensory function to the hand: the radial, median, and ulnar. The radial nerve supplies motor function to the extensors of the wrist and fingers. Motor function of the radial nerve can be tested by wrist extension or finger extension while the wrist is extended. Sensory function is best tested by two-point discrimination just proximal to the dorsal thumb web space.

The median nerve supplies motor function to both intrinsic and extrinsic muscles. The extrinsic muscles include finger flexors except those of the ring and little fingers. The intrinsic muscles include most of the thenar eminence muscles. The motor function of the median nerve is tested by abduction of the thumb during palpation of the thenar eminence. One should check for sensory innervation by two-point discrimination on the volar pad of the index finger.

The ulnar nerve supplies the flexors of the ring and little fingers as well as the interossei and hypothenar eminence muscles. Motor function is tested by spreading fingers against resistance. Sensory function is best tested by two-point discrimination on the volar pad of the little finger.

The joints of the hand include the immobile carpalmetacarpal joint and mobile intercarpal joints. These joints are rarely injured. The metacarpophalangeal joints are biaxial ball-and-socket joints. The collateral ligaments that cross these joints are at their maximum length with complete flexion of the joint. The interphalangeal joints are hinge joints that allow for movement in one plane only. The joint is held together by the collateral ligaments and the volar plate. During flexion the volar plate shortens. At 15 to 20 degrees of flexion, the collateral ligaments are at maximum length. The hand should be immobilized with the metacarpophalangeal joints at 90 degrees flexion and the interphalangeal joints at almost complete extension.

EXAMINATION OF THE HAND

A systematic approach to the examination of the hand is essential. The hand should be inspected for any swelling or deformity. This can be accomplished by watching the child spontaneously use the hand. The fingers should be observed in a partially and fully flexed position, looking for normal alignment. This is critical in determining any rotational deformity (Fig. 122–1).

The neurologic examination is best performed by testing motor function and two-point discrimination distal to the area of injury. In the younger child this is often difficult. Sweating and wrinkling of skin immersed in water can aid in the diagnosis of the young child who cannot cooperate with the examination, since these two responses require innervation.

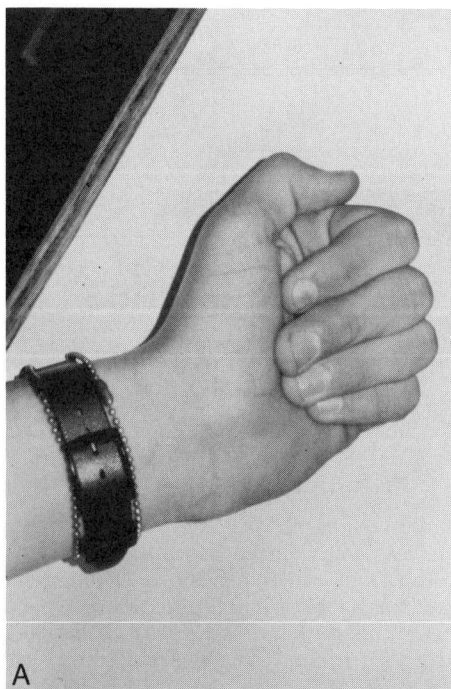

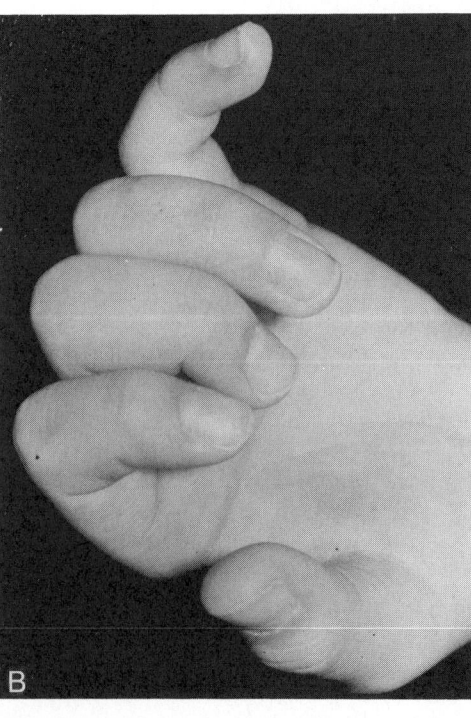

Figure 122–1. When the hand is examined, the fingers should be flexed to inspect for normal alignment *(A)*. With a rotational deformity due to a fracture, the finger may be misaligned *(B)*.

In the area of injury and distal to it, the hand should be examined for vascular integrity, tendon function, and joint stability. The skin should be examined for lacerations, puncture wounds, or discoloration.

GENERAL MANAGEMENT PRINCIPLES

Bleeding should be controlled by gentle direct pressure with sterile gauze. During examination a bloodless field is necessary and can be accomplished by a blood pressure cuff or appropriate tourniquet. The blood pressure cuff should not be left on for more than 15 minutes at a time. Bleeding vessels are never clamped, as this may inadvertently damage nearby nerves.

Edema is a serious problem in the hand and should be avoided. The physician should recommend elevation early and frequently and avoid constricting dressings during immobilization. Hand rest and immobilization are often required, but correct positioning is vital. The wrist should be kept in 20 to 30 degrees of extension, metacarpophalangeal joints at 75 to 90 degrees, and interphalangeal joints near full extension. The thumb should be abducted away from the palm.

Immobilization can be accomplished with a bulky dressing in the very young child or a plaster splint in the older child. However, universal splints should not be used in children, and immobilization of a single digit is usually not adequate. One exception is treatment of the mallet finger. Remodeling occurs along the plane of joint motion. Growth will not correct rotational deformities; therefore these must be recognized and treated.

DIAGNOSTIC EVALUATION

Radiologic evaluation is indicated in all but the most insignificant trauma to the hand and wrist. Liberal use of radiology for detection of foreign bodies, especially glass, is also prudent. Routine hand radiographs should include three views, one being a true lateral. Further views should be obtained if the diagnosis remains uncertain. Because of the multiple normal variations in the ossification of growth centers and changes accordant with growth, comparison views may be useful.

FRACTURES
Carpals

All of the carpal bones are present at birth. Their cartilaginous matrix ossifies from the center to the periphery. The radiologic appearance of the carpals changes with age, and radiographs do not show cartilaginous injuries. The cartilage absorbs shocks and therefore protects the growing carpal bones from injury. The most commonly injured of the carpal bones is the navicular, but fracture of this bone is rare before the age of 7 years. If there is any suspicion that the navicular is fractured, it should be treated as if it were fractured. Suspicion should be raised in wrist trauma with pain in the anatomic snuff box. The diagnosis of navicular fracture can often be made by radiograph. In addition to the three standard wrist views, one may need to obtain additional navicular views (Fig. 122–2).

When a fracture is present, a short-arm thumb spica cast should be applied and the child referred to an orthopedic surgeon for further evaluation. If the diagnosis is uncertain but there is some suspicion of fracture, the child's extremity can be placed in a thumb spica splint or cast for 10 to 14 days, at which time another radiograph should be taken.

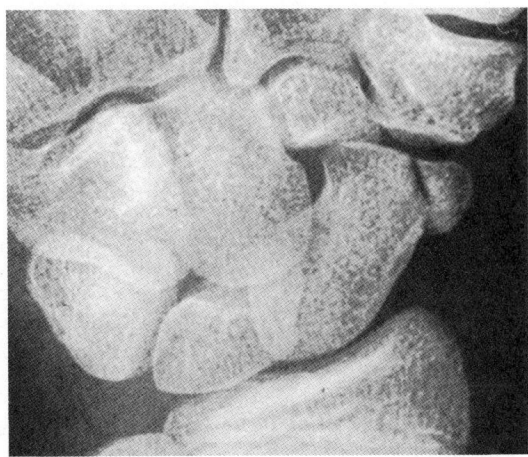

Figure 122–2. A distal navicular fractue in a 14-year-old patient. (From Ogden JA. Skeletal Injury in the Child. 2nd ed. Philadelphia, WB Saunders, 1990, p 533.)

Navicular fracture complications, including nonunion and avascular necrosis, occur but are less common in children.

Fractures of the other carpal bones are rare and easily missed. Suspicion of an intercarpal or carpometacarpal disruption warrants immediate orthopedic referral.

Metacarpals

Fractures of metacarpals can involve proximal, midshaft, or distal portions. Proximal fractures are usually due to crush injuries or direct trauma. They are uncommon. Midshaft fractures are less common in children than in adults, and the treatment is similar. Immobilization of these fractures is usually adequate. If there are multiple or unstable fractures, wire fixation may be required (Fig. 122–3).

Distal fractures, especially of the fifth metacarpal (boxer's fracture), are more common in adolescent males (Fig. 122–4). These often result from striking another person or a firm surface such as a wall. Careful inspection may reveal a laceration, which may be caused by the teeth of the person struck. These fractures can be either metaphyseal or physeal injuries. Any deformity that is rotational needs to be treated, as this will not correct spontaneously. A boxer's fracture is suspected on physical examination, with pain, swelling, and loss of the knuckle prominence over the injured joint. The diagnosis can be made by radiograph. Anteroposterior, lateral, and oblique views should be obtained. The radiographs must be evaluated for angulation and involvement of the growth plate. Metacarpal fractures of the fourth and fifth metacarpals with less than 30 degrees of angulation are generally managed by immobilization with an ulnar gutter splint and orthopedic follow-up. The more proximal the fracture, the less angulation acceptable. Angulation of greater than 40 degrees in the fourth and fifth metacarpals and 20 degrees in the second and third metacarpals generally requires more aggressive management, warranting an immediate orthopedic consultation. Increased morbidity and poor outcome exist for angulation that is not in the plane of motion or if there is a rotational deformity, involvement of the physis, or an unstable fracture. Complications of metacarpal fracture include increased angulation and rotation during therapy. In addition, rotational or angular deformity may accentuate during growth. If there is damage to the growth plate, a short, deformed metacarpal may

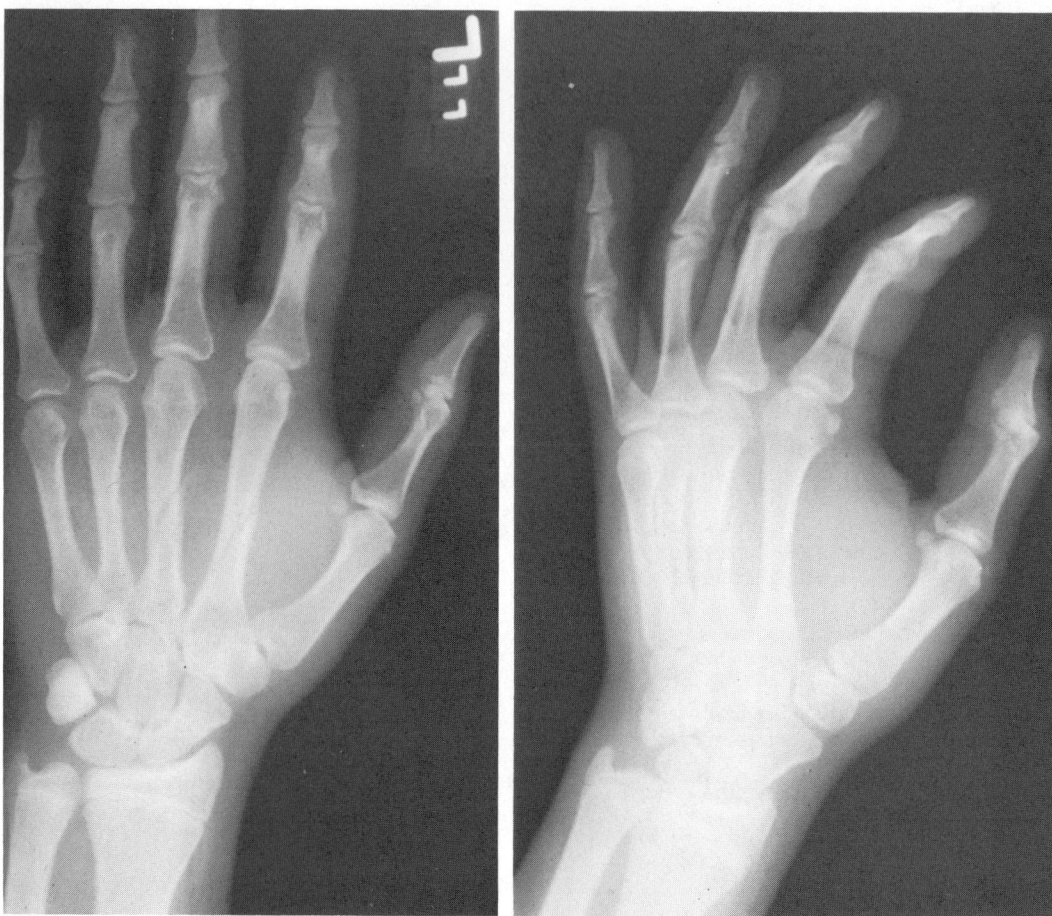

Figure 122–3. Spiral fractures of the left ring finger, middle finger, and index finger metacarpals.

result. In addition, there may be damage to surrounding structures such as tendons, ligaments, or nerves. In metacarpal fractures some loss of knuckle prominence may be unavoidable.

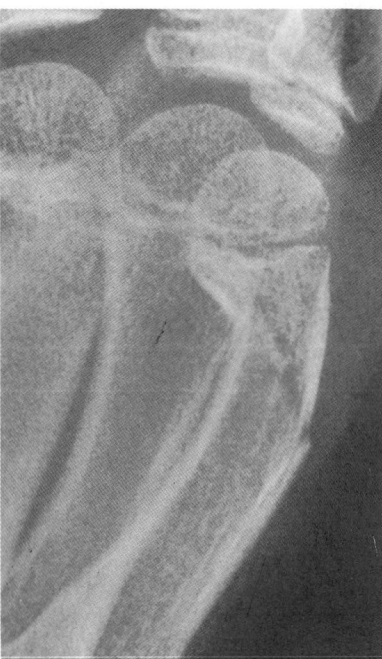

Figure 122–4. This "boxer's fracture" shows moderate angulation of the metaphyseal fracture of the fifth metacarpal. (From Ogden JA. Skeletal Injury in the Child. 2nd ed. Philadelphia, WB Saunders, 1990, p 546.)

Proximal Phalanx

Malalignment is the most common complication of fractures of both the proximal and the middle phalanx. Therefore the physical examination must include careful inspection for any angular deformity. Fractures of the proximal end of the proximal phalanx are often Salter II fractures. An exaggeration of this fracture is called the extraoctave fracture of the fifth proximal phalanx, which requires reduction (Fig. 122–5). Reduction may be accomplished by placing a pencil between the fourth and fifth digits and using it as a fulcrum to reduce the fracture.

Midshaft fractures tend to angulate more because of unbalanced muscle pull. This is due to the insertions of the flexor and extensor tendons into the base of the middle phalanx, the pull of the interosseous muscles on the base of the proximal phalanx, and the associated ligamentous attachments at the metacarpophalangeal and interphalangeal joints. Fractures of this type interrupt the normal longitudinal arch. Distal or neck fractures are often complicated because of rotation and usually require immediate referral (Fig. 122–6). Intracondylar fractures may require pinning, and oblique fractures tend to rotate and shorten during the healing process.

Spiral or comminuted fractures are unstable and may require open reduction and internal fixation. The proximal interphalangeal joint is the most frequently injured joint in the hand, and an injury here is often difficult to manage. Complications include the imposition of the volar plate into the joint, causing a 90-degree rotation of the condylar fragment, which becomes entrapped by the capsule and collateral ligament. This complication is difficult to diagnose clinically or radiographically. If undiagnosed it may lead to a permanent deformity.

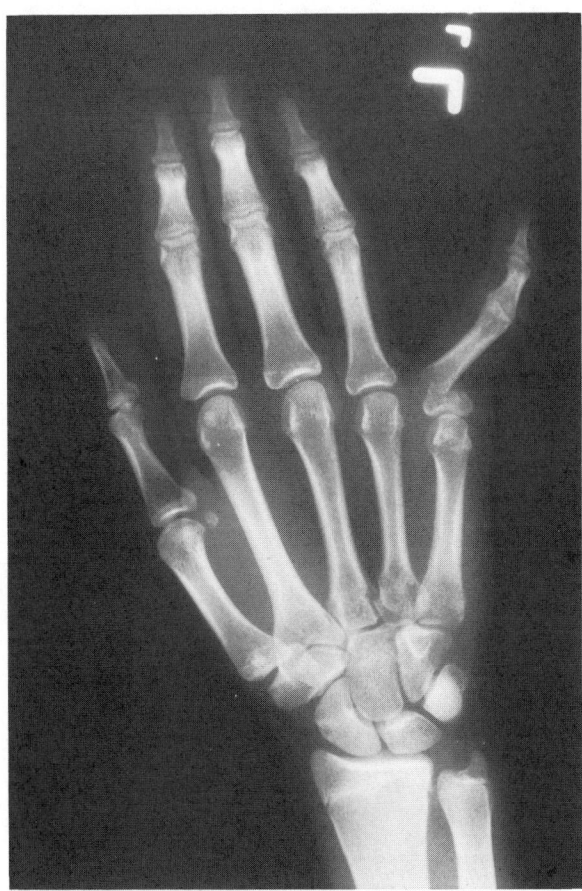

Figure 122–5. "Extra-octave" fracture of the proximal phalanx.

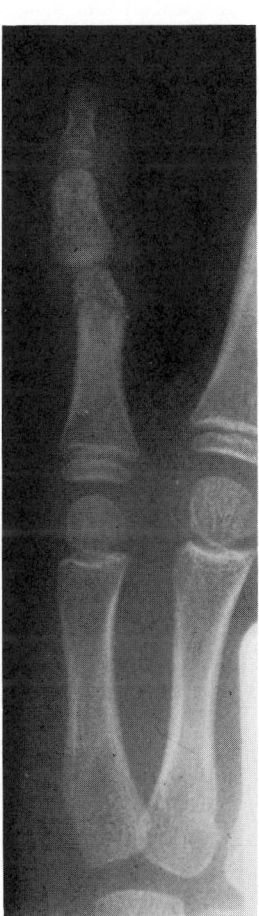

Figure 122–6. Fracture of the distal end of the proximal phalanx. This injury carries a high rate of angular deformity.

Middle Phalanx

Middle phalanx fractures are frequently complicated by angulation and rotation. Fractures of the proximal portion can involve the growth plate. Salter II fractures without angulation may be managed with a buddy taping or rotation splinting. The Salter III fracture is the analogue of a collateral ligament tear in an adult and may require internal fixation (Fig. 122–7). Fractures of the midshaft will angulate toward the palm if the fracture is distal to the insertion of the flexor superficialis tendon. If a fracture occurs proximal to the insertion, the reverse is true. This injury is usually treated by closed reduction and immobilization in complete extension. A fracture of the distal aspect of the middle phalanx is dangerous because the cartilage cap is not visible on radiograph. Therefore it may be displaced or not evident at the time of injury.

Distal Phalanx

Fractures of the distal interphalangeal joint may lead to a mallet finger deformity. In the adult the extensor tendon is pulled from its insertion on the distal phalanx; in the child one may see a Salter I or Salter II fracture (Fig. 122–8). In the older child a Salter III injury may be present, which may require open reduction and fixation. Closed Salter I and II fractures require a dorsal splint over the middle and proximal phalanx in full distal interphalangeal extension, which must be continuously worn for 6 weeks.

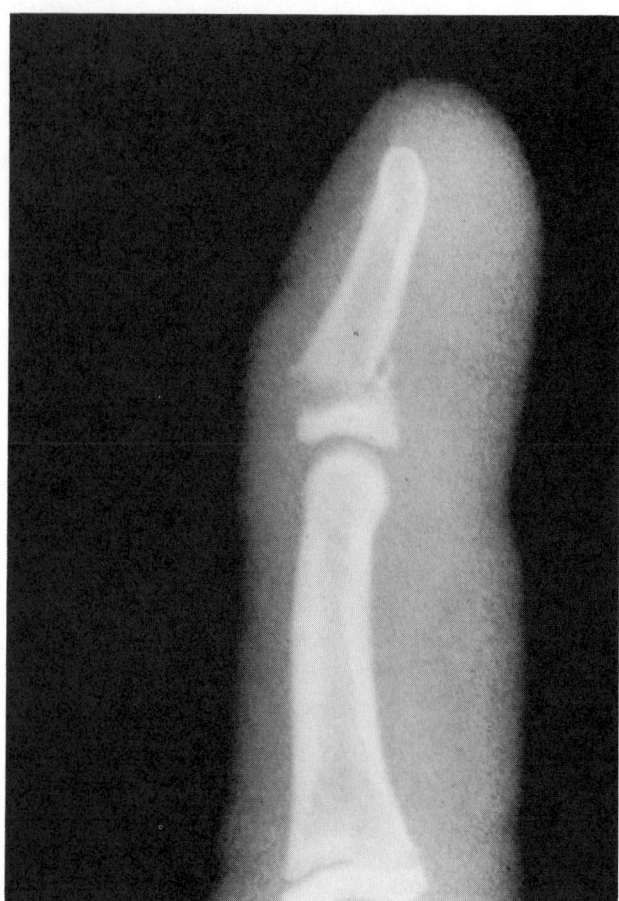

Figure 122–8. Salter II fracture of the distal phalanx in a child, presenting as a mallet deformity.

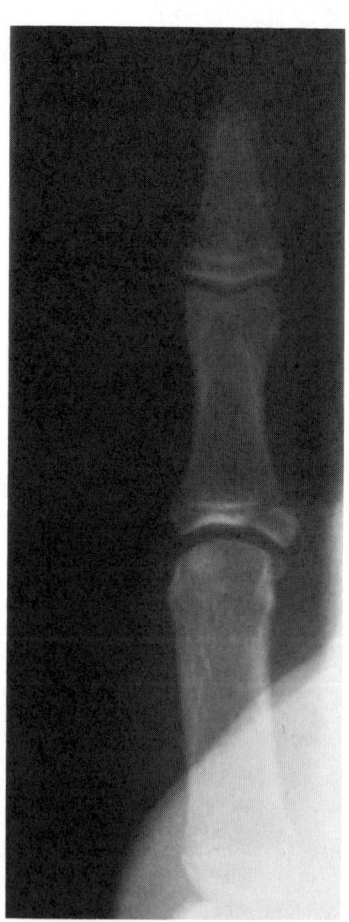

Figure 122–7. Salter III fracture of the middle phalanx. This intra-articular injury may require fixation.

Thumb

Injuries to the thumb include the proximal and distal phalanx as well as the metacarpal. Impaction injuries to the base of the thumb metacarpal may produce Bennett's fracture in adults, but they usually result in Salter II fractures in children. Less than 30 degrees of angulation usually does not require reduction. If there is more than 30 degrees of angulation with radial deviation, a closed reduction is usually adequate. If there is ulnar deviation, open fixation is often required.

The forces that produce a gamekeeper's thumb in an adult (a collateral ligament tear) usually result in a Salter III fracture of the proximal phalanx in a child. If there is any displacement of the joint surface, open fixation is required.

Fractures of the proximal phalanx and metacarpal base usually involve an epiphyseal injury. A closed injury at the middle phalanx joint with joint instability suggests an epiphyseal injury. However, stress radiographs may be necessary to make the diagnosis. Salter I and II fractures of the proximal phalanx can usually be managed with closed reduction to correct angulation. Salter III and IV fractures require open reduction. Distal or condylar fractures of the proximal phalanx may be unstable and are often more complicated than they initially appear. Little remodeling occurs at the end of the distal end of the phalanx. Fractures of the distal phalanx of the thumb are managed similarly to other digits. Management of tuft fractures depends on whether they are open or closed. Salter I and II fractures require immobilization. Salter III and IV fractures involve the interphalangeal joint and may require operative management.

DISLOCATIONS AND JOINT INJURIES

Dislocations occur in children but are frequently associated with fractures. All potential dislocations should be evaluated radiographically before attempting reduction. Metacarpophalangeal joint dislocations can be complicated by interposition of the volar plate into the joint space, making closed reduction impossible. The radiographic appearance of a "simple" metacarpophalangeal joint dislocation shows displacement of the phalanx on the metacarpal at 90 degrees. If the bones appear to be parallel on radiograph, a closed reduction is less likely to be successful and an open reduction is required. Complex dislocations may also show widening or lateralization of the joint space. Physical examination with a complex dislocation shows dimpling of the skin on the palmar surface. If there is no evidence of a complex dislocation, relocation may be achieved by applying longitudinal traction on the digit and then moving the joint into flexion with continued traction until reduction is achieved. After traction the joint is unstable and must be immobilized.

Proximal interphalangeal dislocations are more common than distal interphalangeal dislocations. Distal interphalangeal dislocations are more often open. If the radiograph demonstrates no epiphyseal injury, reduction may be achieved by hyperextending the joint and then pushing the distal bone into the reduced position in a dorsal-to-palmar direction. Again, after reduction the joint must be tested for stability. If the reduced joint is unstable, the patient should immediately be referred to an orthopedist. If it is stable, the digit is splinted in slight flexion (20 to 30 degrees) to allow for healing of the volar plate. The patient should follow up with an orthopedist. Suspicion of a volar plate injury should be high when a hyperextension injury leads to pain and swelling of the proximal interphalangeal joint. Even if radiographs are negative, immobilization and close follow-up are advisable.

FINGERTIP INJURIES

Fingertip avulsion varies from quite superficial to complete amputation at the distal interphalangeal joint. A frequent cause of minor avulsions is from clipping an infant's nails with clippers or scissors. These apparently minor injuries cause great parental anxiety and guilt. They tend to bleed for a long time, but blood loss is never significant in the absence of hematologic disease. Direct pressure for up to 10 minutes and simple dressing are usually adequate.

Avulsions of soft tissue that are not the result of a crush injury and do not involve bone may be managed by cleansing, a Xeroform gauze dressing, and a covering dry dressing (Fig. 122–9). Tetanus toxoid is given when indicated by the immunization history. Antibiotics are rarely indicated, but close follow-up is mandatory. Complete healing takes place in about 12 weeks.

Fingertip avulsions from crush injuries and those suspicious for bony involvement require radiologic evaluation. Avulsions with bone exposed can be managed similarly to more superficial avulsions with one exception. Exposed bone should be rongeured back so that no bone is exposed. Then the injury is dressed (Fig. 122–10). With a partial amputation, it is worthwhile to loosely reattach any remaining skin. Even tissue that appears severely contused will often regenerate. Skin grafts are rarely required before 12 years of age. If the bone is involved, the child is placed on broad-spectrum antibiotics with good staphylococcal coverage and close follow-up is arranged.

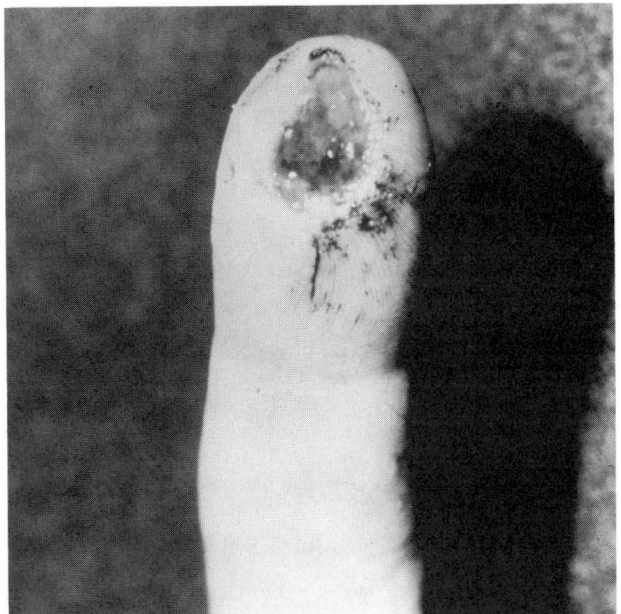

Figure 122–9. Avulsion of the soft tissue of the fingertip. This injury healed well without any surgical repair.

NAIL INJURIES

Subungual hematomas covering less than one third of the nailbed can be managed by trephination of the nail; a heated paper clip is usually adequate to perform the trephination. Radiographs should be obtained to exclude fractures. More extensive hematomas are usually associated with nailbed lacerations, which should be repaired. After local anesthesia the nail is carefully removed, the hematoma evacuated, and the nailbed laceration repaired with 6–0 to 7–0 chromic suture material. The nail may be replaced and loosely

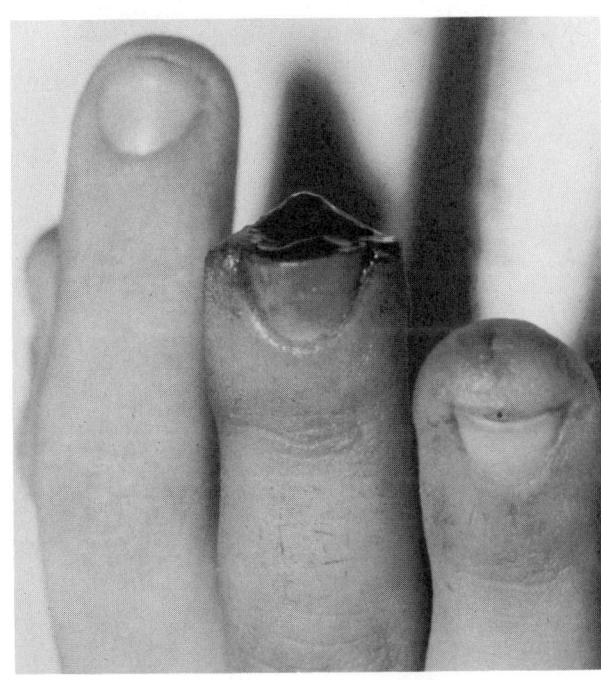

Figure 122–10. Fingertip avulsion with bone exposed.

sutured in place, or a nonadherent dressing may be placed under the eponychium. Close follow-up with dressing changes is mandatory. Nail avulsions are managed similarly, with repair of any nailbed lacerations and replacement of the nail to serve as a splint. If the nail is damaged, a nonadherent dressing can be placed under the eponychium and then dressed. Nail avulsions associated with a Salter I fracture of the distal phalanx (Seymour's lesion) may be complicated by osteomyelitis. This fracture may be difficult to detect. If this open fracture occurs, the patient should be placed on oral antibiotics. A fracture of the tuft without associated injuries can be managed symptomatically (Fig. 122–11).

Amputations at the distal interphalangeal joint or proximal to this joint will not regenerate. If the amputated part is available, it should be gently cleansed with normal saline, wrapped in a sterile gauze wet with normal saline, and placed in a container of ice. The patient is emergently referred to a hand specialist for possible replantation.

LACERATIONS

Lacerations are the most common hand injury. After bleeding has stopped, the neurovascular status distal to the wound should be assessed. After this, if pain or bleeding limits the examination, a regional block or tourniquet can be used to facilitate evaluation of the tendon integrity. The wound should be explored for tendon lacerations and foreign bodies, with minimal manipulation of the tissue.

Superficial lacerations are repaired with simple interrupted sutures after regional anesthesia. Subcutaneous sutures are unnecessary. For digital lacerations, anesthesia is best accomplished by a digital block in the distal palmar crease area. Circumferential ring blocks can compromise circulation, and fingers on a small hand should never be directly injected. The skin in most of the hand will not stretch; therefore if there is tissue loss, grafting may be

required. After suturing, the hand is immobilized and elevated.

Tendon lacerations are often difficult to diagnose in children. Partial tendon lacerations may maintain normal function. Therefore tendon lacerations can be diagnosed only by direct exploration. Extensor tendons have communications that can also confuse evaluation. To anticipate possible tendon involvement, one should determine the position of the hand at the time of injury. All tendon lacerations, especially flexor tendons, require specialist evaluation.

Puncture wounds are often deceptively benign in appearance early after an injury. Puncture wounds over the area of the flexor tendon sheath, especially over flexor creases, must be followed carefully because of the high incidence of infection. High-pressure injection injuries (e.g., paint spray gun) can cause significant morbidity and usually require open debridement.

If there is any possibility of a retained foreign body, a thorough evaluation is required. Metal and most glass foreign bodies can be seen on radiograph. Other material, especially plant matter (e.g., splinters), should be removed. Small foreign bodies not causing symptoms need not be removed emergently but should be followed for complications, especially infection.

Pencil lead may be removed by gentle debridement, but often some tattooing remains. Fish hooks should be removed carefully. Sometimes pushing the hook through the wound actually causes damage and should be avoided. After anesthesia, a string (silk suture) or umbilical tape is wrapped around the curve of the hook. A tongue is used to apply pressure over the area where the barb would be positioned, and a brisk tug dislodges the barb and removes the hook.

Nerve lacerations are difficult to diagnose on children and do not require immediate primary repair. Possible nerve lacerations are referred to an orthopedist or plastic surgeon.

HAND INFECTIONS
Paronychia

Paronychia account for the majority of hand infections seen in children. In the early stage there is cellulitis of the eponychium without visible pus. Treatment consists of warm moist compresses, elevation, and oral antibiotics directed against staphylococcus. As the process continues there is abscess formation under the eponychium. This abscess must be drained. After soaking in warm povidone-iodine solution, a No. 11 scalpel blade can be used to separate the eponychium from the nail until pus is released and the overlying dead skin can be debrided. This can sometimes be accomplished without anesthesia, as there is little pain. Warm compresses and oral antibiotics are utilized until the infection is clear.

In more advanced cases the abscess becomes subungual. This requires a regional nerve block and removal of at least part of the nail to obtain complete release of the abscess. Dressing with a Xeroform gauze under the eponychium is used, as well as splinting and oral antibiotics. The dressing should be changed in 3 to 5 days.

Felon

Felons are infections of the pulp at the tip of the finger. These are extremely painful injuries and often secondary to a puncture wound. The fingertip is swollen, red, and has throbbing pain. The area must be drained to avoid osteomyelitis or ischemic necrosis of the tactile tip of the finger. An incision is made on the dorsolateral aspect of the tip,

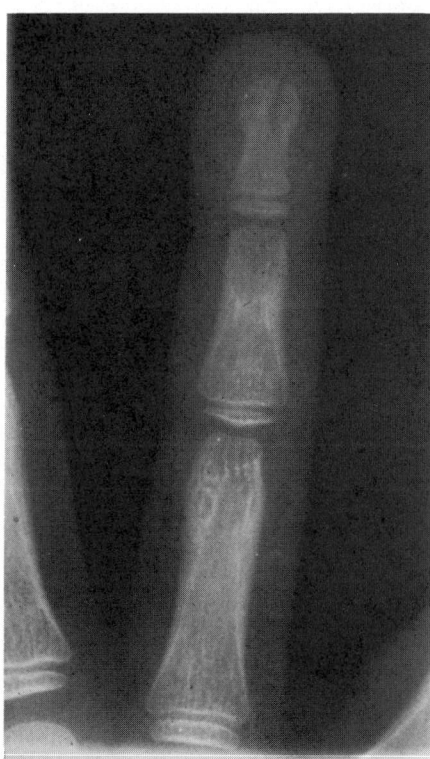

Figure 122–11. Tuft fracture of the distal phalanx.

although some recommend an anterior approach. A complete dissection is necessary, allowing the pulp to separate from the phalanx. This allows drainage by disrupting the septae attached to the phalanx. Extreme caution is necessary when making this incision to avoid injury to sensory nerves. A drain is inserted and the wound immobilized. The hand must be elevated. Analgesics and oral antibiotics are prescribed along with arrangement for close follow-up.

Whitlow

A herpetic whitlow is a viral infection of the fingertip that may mimic a felon. Prior to the appearance of the typical herpetic lesions, the fingertip may be painful. Analgesics and supportive care are all that is required.

Tenosynovitis

A flexor tenosynovitis is an uncommon infection in children but has a high morbidity rate. The infection is often secondary to a puncture wound over the flexor tendon sheath, especially in the area of flexor creases (Fig. 122–12). The cardinal signs of flexor tenosynovitis are (1) tenderness and swelling along the entire flexor sheath; (2) finger held in flexion; and (3) severe pain with passive finger extension. If this condition is suspected, the child should be admitted for intravenous antibiotics and immediate orthopedic consultation for potential surgery.

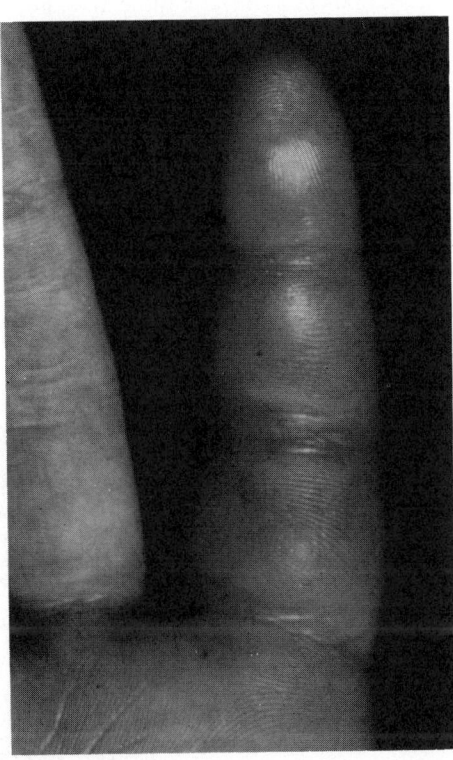

Figure 122–12. Flexor tenosynovitis of the index finger. Note the diffuse swelling.

Bites

Bite wounds are common in children. Human bite wounds can cause serious infection and should be suspected in all lacerations over the metacarpophalangeal joints. These should be referred for possible admission, intravenous antibiotics, and surgical debridement. Dog bite wounds have a lower rate of infection and can be managed by meticulous debridement, irrigation, oral antibiotics, and close follow-up. Cat bite wounds, often puncture wounds, are more frequently infected, often with *Pasteurella multocida*.

All bite wounds to the hand should receive antibiotics for staphylococcus, streptococcus, and anaerobes. Deep space infections are usually secondary to penetrating injury and are uncommon in childhood. The hand will be painful and swollen, with most of the swelling on the dorsal surface, even if the entry wound is on the flexor surface. These infections need immediate treatment, including admission to a hospital, intravenous antibiotics, and orthopedic or plastic surgery evaluation. Localized cellulitis of the hand can be initially managed on an outpatient basis with elevation, immobilization, oral antibiotics, and close follow-up. If improvement is not seen in 24 to 48 hours, intravenous therapy is required.

Selected References

Aghababian RV, Conte JE Jr. Mammalian bite wounds. Ann Emerg Med 1980;9:79.

Callaham M. Prophylactic antibiotics in common dog bite wounds: A controlled study. Ann Emerg Med 1980;9:410.

Carter PR. Injuries to the major nerves of the hand. Emerg Med Clin North Am 1985;3:351.

Goldstein EJ, Citron DM, Finegold SM. Dog bite wounds and infection: A prospective clinical study. Ann Emerg Med 1980;9:508.

Hamlin C. Diagnosis of wrist injuries. Emerg Med Clin North Am 1985;3:311.

Hentz V. Functional anatomy of the hand and arm. Emerg Med Clin North Am 1985;3:197.

Herndon J. Hand injuries—special considerations in children. Emerg Med Clin North Am 1985;3:405.

Herndon J. Tendon injuries—extensor surface. Emerg Med Clin North Am 1985;3:333.

Herndon J. Tendon injuries—flexor surface. Emerg Med Clin North Am 1985;3:341.

Kilgore ES. Hand infections. J Hand Surg 1983;8:723.

Lewis R. High-compression injection injuries to the hand. Emerg Med Clin North Am 1985;3:373.

Lewis RC. Infections of the hand. Emerg Med Clin North Am 1985;3:263.

Malinowski RW, Strate RG, Perry JF Jr. The management of human bite injuries of the hand. J Trauma 1979;19:655.

Margles SW. Principles of management of acute hand injuries. Surg Clin North Am 1980;60:655.

Melone C Jr. Joint injuries of the fingers and thumb. Emerg Med Clin North Am 1985;3:319.

Melone C Jr, Grad J. Primary care of fingernail injuries. Emerg Med Clin North Am 1985;3:255.

Melone C Jr, Isani A. Anesthesia for hand injuries. Emerg Med Clin North Am 1985;3:235.

Peeples E, Boswick JA Jr, Scott FA. Wounds of the hand contaminated by human or animal saliva. J Trauma 1980;20:383.

Southcott R, Rosman MA. Non-union of carpal scaphoid fractures in children. J Bone Joint Surg 1977;59B:20.

Stein F. Foreign body injuries of the hand. Emerg Med Clin North Am 1985;3:383.

Van Herpe LB. Fractures of the forearm and wrist. Orthop Clin North Am 1976;7:543.

Watson FM. Fractures in the hand: Metacarpals and phalanges. Emerg Med Clin North Am 1985;3:293.

Wood V. Fractures of the hand in children. Orthop Clin North Am 1976;7:527.

CHAPTER 123

Upper Extremity Injuries

Karen Villalba
Ken J. Kroger

SCAPULAR FRACTURE
Anatomy

Scapular ossification begins in the eighth week of gestation and is usually complete by 22 years of age. Ossification centers and growth plates are easily mistaken for fracture lines. The body of the scapula is a flat triangular bone with a bony spine projecting from its superior dorsal aspect. It is on this distal spine that the scapula makes its only connection with the axial skeleton, at the acromioclavicular joint.

Clinical Evaluation

Scapular fractures in children are rare and usually result from severe direct trauma. The greatest significance of a scapular fracture is its association with other life-threatening injuries. The examiner should always suspect coexistent thoracic, vertebral, upper extremity, vascular, and neuro-plexus injuries.

The patient will present with pain, swelling, and often ecchymosis over the injured scapula. The involved extremity is held in adduction, and the patient complains of pain with any movement of the shoulder, especially abduction.

Radiographic Evaluation

Scapular radiographs should include an anteroposterior and transscapular lateral view. The routine radiographic examination of the shoulder is inadequate to exclude a scapular fracture. The majority of fractures found in children involve nonarticular regions.

Therapeutic Intervention
Fractures of the Scapular Body

Fractures of the scapular body are usually the result of direct, crushing injuries. The infraspinous region is more commonly fractured than the supraspinous region. Because of the surrounding musculature, the fracture fragments are rarely displaced. Treatment is generally nonoperative. Patients are immobilized with a sling for comfort. As pain subsides, passive and eventually active range of motion should be increased. The fracture will heal within 4 weeks, and most bony irregularities will remodel with growth.

Fractures of the Scapular Neck

Fractures of the scapular neck usually extend from the suprascapular notch inferolaterally to the axillary border just beneath the glenohumeral joint. In addition to the anteroposterior and tangential views, axillary views may be helpful in delineating displaced fractures. Orthopedic consultation is advised for displaced neck fractures, which usually require reduction. Nondisplaced fractures are managed with immobilization and early limited range of motion.

Fractures of the Glenoid

Glenoid fractures can be divided into two types: type I are rim fractures, and type II are comminuted or stellate fractures. Rim fractures are often associated with shoulder dislocations. Displaced rim fractures associated with shoulder dislocations are often reduced simultaneously with a joint reduction. Conservative therapy is recommended for most simple rim fractures. Similarly, stellate fractures are managed conservatively with relatively good functional result despite a gross irregularity of the joint. Avulsed fragments can be excised at a later date.

CLAVICULAR INJURIES
Anatomy

Clavicular fractures are common fractures. They can be classified based on the area of injury: proximal (medial: 3%), middle (92%), and distal (lateral: 5%). Subluxation or dislocation of the acromioclavicular or sternoclavicular joint is unusual in children.

The clavicle is the first bone to ossify. Two centers of ossification are present in utero, at the junctions of the middle and lateral clavicle and at the junction of the middle and proximal end. The secondary ossification center on the sternal end of the clavicle develops much later and fuses with the shaft by age 25 years.

The clavicle is an S-shaped bone that lies subcutaneously throughout its entire length, making it susceptible to injury.

The weakest and most frequently fractured area of the clavicle is at the junction of the middle and lateral portions (Fig. 123–1). Fractures of the middle clavicle are typically displaced, with the distal segment being pulled inward by the pectoralis major and downward by the weight of the arm. The medial segment is typically pulled upward by the sternocleidomastoid muscle. Beneath the clavicle lies the brachial plexus, subclavian vessels, first rib, and lung parenchyma. Hence fractures of the clavicle may produce injuries to any of these structures.

The most frequent cause of clavicular fractures is by an indirect force when a child falls on an outstretched hand. Fractures can also occur with a direct blow to the clavicle. Pulmonary and neurovascular complications are more fre-

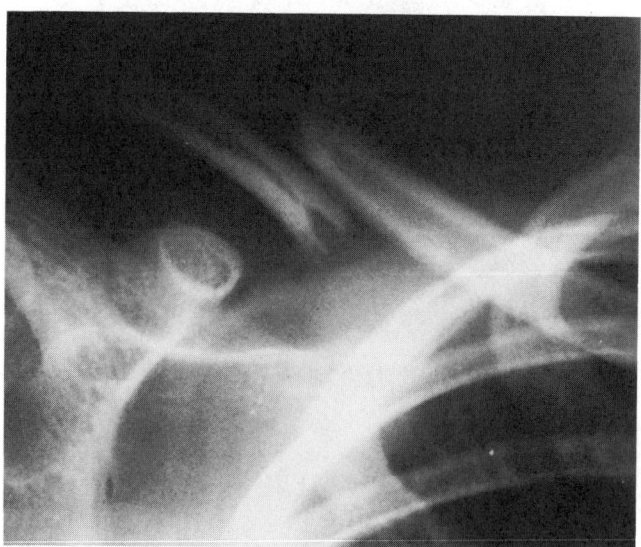

Figure 123–1. Radiograph demonstrates a displaced clavicle fracture.

quent with direct forces. Clavicle fractures can also result from birthing.

Birth-Related Trauma

Clavicular fractures associated with birthing are typically asymptomatic and are the most common birth-related fracture. About 1.7% of neonates sustain clavicular fractures; most go undetected initially. These fractures are usually greenstick fractures. With healing, a callus will form with a palpable deformity and the fracture will be apparent on radiograph. These fractures can also present with pseudoparalysis; the child fails to move the affected arm. One must be certain to exclude a brachial plexus injury, which can coexist with clavicular fracture.

Clavicular fracture does not require treatment other than care in handling the infant. A splint can be used if the extremity is painful or if there is pseudoparalysis for 3 weeks. Even if the fracture is displaced, the bone will rapidly form callus and remodel; the deformity will resolve within 6 to 9 months.

Therapeutic Intervention
Fracture of the Distal (Lateral) Clavicle

These fractures are uncommon. When they do occur, they usually involve the epiphysis. The epiphysis will be securely anchored by an intact inferior periosteal sleeve, which is still firmly attached to the scapula. If there is displacement, the medial metaphysis and shaft will be displaced superiorly and can be palpated. In addition to the anteroposterior radiograph, stress radiographs with the patient holding weights may better define the fracture. Treatment consists of a figure-of-eight strap and orthopedic referral. Owing to the intact periosteal tube, the bone will regenerate and remodeling will occur.

Fracture of the Middle Clavicle

Fractures involving the middle third of the clavicle can be asymptomatic without evidence of trauma until callus formation. These are usually greenstick fractures. If the fracture is displaced, the patient holds the affected arm with the shoulder drooped forward, inward, and downward.

On anteroposterior radiograph, the fracture may be obvious or may be suggested by loss of the soft tissue density above the superior border of the clavicle. Occasionally a lordotic view will show the injury.

Treatment consists of a figure-of-eight splint for 3 to 4 weeks. If the fracture is overriding or markedly displaced, an orthopedist may perform reduction using local anesthesia. An injury here rarely involves the brachial plexus and vascular structures. If there is damage to vascular structures, immediate open reduction is indicated to minimize hemorrhage.

Fracture of the Proximal (Medial) Clavicle

As a result of fracture, the medial clavicle is often driven inward or forward. The force produces a sternoclavicular dislocation in an adult but produces a Salter I or Salter II epiphyseal fracture in the child. Owing to the late ossification of this area, an epiphyseal injury can occur as late as 25 years of age.

Physical examination will demonstrate swelling and tenderness with either a palpable asymmetric protuberance of the medial end of the clavicle (anterior displacement) or a palpable depression (posterior displacement).

An anteriorly displaced fracture is treated simply with a sling. Since the posterior periosteal tube is intact, remodeling

will occur with correction of the defect. Nevertheless, some orthopedists advocate closed, manual reduction.

Posterior displacement may result in death due to tracheal laceration, massive hemothorax, great vessel injury, or damage to the esophagus. Other complications include mediastinitis, thoracic outlet syndrome, syncope from carotid artery compression, and arteriovenous fistula formation. Therefore the posteriorly displaced medial clavicle fracture can be a life-threatening event. If the airway is compromised, intubation is necessary. If there is cardiovascular collapse, immediate thoracotomy is indicated. Computed tomography has been recommended to ascertain the relationship of the clavicle to the mediastinal structures.

If the patient is stable, orthopedic consultation should occur before the child leaves the emergency department. The subsequent management is dependent on the orthopedist. Some argue that with an intact periosteal sleeve, the bone will regenerate and remodel. A sling and complete restriction from sports are required. Others advocate closed reduction in the operating room under general anesthesia or open reduction with internal fixation.

SHOULDER DISLOCATIONS
Introduction

Although shoulder (glenohumeral joint) dislocations are rare in children, they can result from trauma. These are classified according to the anatomic position of the displaced humeral head in relationship to the glenoid fossa (anterior or posterior).

Atraumatic dislocations of the glenohumeral joint occur in children who have excessive joint laxity caused by Ehlers-Danlos syndrome, congenital absence of the glenoid, or deformities of the proximal end of the humerus.

Clinical Evaluation

With a traumatic dislocation the child presents with a painful shoulder. In anterior dislocations the arm will be held in a slightly abducted and externally rotated position and the shoulder has a square rather than a rounded contour. The anterior humeral head can be palpated anteriorly. In posterior dislocations the arm will be held adducted and internally rotated, with the humeral head palpated posteriorly. In atraumatic dislocations the patient will present with a painless shoulder and can typically reduce the dislocation without manipulation by the physician. The integrity of the axillary nerve is tested by assessing the sensation over the deltoid muscle.

Radiographic Evaluation

Radiographs of the shoulder should include an anteroposterior view and a true scapular lateral view. On the true scapular lateral view the anterior or posterior location of the humerus in relationship to the glenoid fossa defines the type of dislocation. Associated fractures of the greater tuberosity, anterior glenoid rim, or compression fracture of the posterior lateral humeral head (Hill-Sachs deformity) must be sought.

Therapeutic Intervention

In children adequate relaxation for reduction can be accomplished with narcotics and muscle relaxants. Anterior dislocations can be reduced by the following methods:

1. *Stimson technique.* The patient is placed prone on the examining table and 5 lbs of weight is taped to the wrist of the affected extremity. Less weight may be sufficient if the

patient is smaller in size. After approximately 15 to 20 minutes, the shoulder should be reduced.

2. *Traction with countertraction.* The patient is placed supine on the examining table with a folded sheet passed across the chest into the axilla and then posteriorly across the back. An assistant pulls the sheet to produce the countertraction. Concomitantly the physician pulls the wrist of the affected extremity to produce steady longitudinal traction. Gentle internal and external rotational forces may be used to facilitate reduction.

3. *Lateral traction.* Lateral traction is applied by a folded sheet or towel across the proximal humerus while longitudinal traction is employed by the physician.

4. *Posterior dislocations.* Longitudinal traction coupled with pressure on the humeral head should reduce the dislocation into the glenoid fossa. Orthopedic referral should be instituted.

Regardless of the method employed, the patient should be placed in a sling and swathe immobilizer and referred to an orthopedic surgeon for follow-up.

PROXIMAL HUMERAL FRACTURES
Introduction

The proximal epiphysis accounts for 80% of the humeral length. Damage to the epiphyseal plate may cause a limb length discrepancy.

The mechanism of injury can be due to either direct or indirect forces. The child may either receive a direct blow to the posterior lateral aspect of the shoulder or fall backward onto an outstretched dorsiflexed hand with the elbow extended. Birth fractures can occur in this area secondary to shoulder-pelvic dystocia.

Pathologic fracture of the metaphysis secondary to a unicameral bone cyst is most common in the proximal humerus. Unicameral bone cysts are cavities filled with serous fluid and lined with a thin membrane of connective tissue. In proximal metaphyseal fractures, the radiographs should be carefully examined for evidence of a unicameral bone cyst.

The newborn who presents with a "floppy arm" or reluctance to move the upper extremity may have a humeral shaft fracture. Thorough radiographic evaluation of the clavicle, shoulder, humerus, and elbow must be performed prior to the diagnosis of a birth palsy. In the older child, pain, swelling, and tenderness of the humerus can be indicative of a fracture. However, greenstick fractures may present with minimal symptoms.

Radiographic Evaluation

On physical examination, swelling and tenderness will be present in the shoulder, and the upper part of the distal fragment may be palpable under the coracoid process. Radiographic examination must include two views of the humerus perpendicular to one another. If there are any doubts regarding a fracture, comparison radiographs of the uninjured shoulder should be obtained.

Therapeutic Intervention

Orthopedic consultation is necessary for management and disposition of proximal humerus fractures. Treatment of these fractures is dependent on the age of the patient, involvement of the physis, grade of displacement, and degree of angulation. In children less than 11 years old, the remodeling is efficient given any amount of apposition of the two bone surfaces. Therefore simple immobilization

using a sling, sling and swathe, hanging long-arm cast, or "salute position" shoulder spica are treatment options. In children 12 years and older, with less time for remodeling available, a more anatomic position is necessary to minimize the chance of limb length discrepancy. Manipulation may be necessary, depending on the degree of angulation. With severely displaced fractures or fractures associated with dislocation, open reduction and internal fixation may be required.

Complications

Fractures of the proximal humerus typically heal well with few complications because substantial remodeling potential exists. Complications are more likely to occur in adolescents and may include transient pain, restricted range of motion, muscle weakness, slight anterior or varus angulation, and humeral shaft thickening.

HUMERAL SHAFT FRACTURES
Introduction

Fractures of the humeral diaphysis (shaft) are rare in children. They usually result from a direct blow. Indirect forces such as falling on an outstretched arm can also cause these fractures. They are more frequent in children younger than 3 years or older than 12 years of age.

Anatomy

The important anatomic consideration with respect to injuries of the humeral shaft involves the location of the radial nerve and the presence of a supracondylar process. The radial nerve courses around the humerus from a posterior to an anterior position along the lateral aspect of the bone at the junction of the middle and distal thirds of the humerus. Therefore the radial nerve can be damaged from a humeral diaphyseal fracture.

A supracondylar (supracondyloid) process is present in 1% of individuals. It is a hook-shaped process of the distal humerus at the junction of the metaphysis and diaphysis anteromedially (Fig. 123–2). A fibrous band extends from the tip of the bone to the medial epicondyle. The median nerve and brachial artery may course beneath this fibrous band. Hence fractures of the humerus in this area may compress the brachial artery or median nerve.

Therapeutic Intervention

The treatment of a fracture of the humeral diaphysis is dependent on the age of the child. In neonates, closed reduction of any grossly displaced fracture should be followed with a small splint or by binding the arm to the chest with a soft bandage for 7 to 14 days. In older children any of the following methods may be employed:

1. *Collar and cuff.* The collar and cuff consists of a cotton-padded stockinette around the patient's neck that fastens at the patient's wrist. Traction is produced by the weight of the arm.

2. *Coaptive splints.* Coaptive splinting consists of medial and lateral splints secured with a roller bandage. In addition, a sling is applied.

3. *Sugar tong* or *U-shaped splint.* The U-shaped splint consists of a plaster splint applied from the axilla medially, around the elbow, then brought laterally to the anterior shoulder. A sling is used to support the upper extremity.

4. *Hanging cast.* The hanging cast involves the arm in a long-arm cast with the arm supported by an around-the-neck sling.

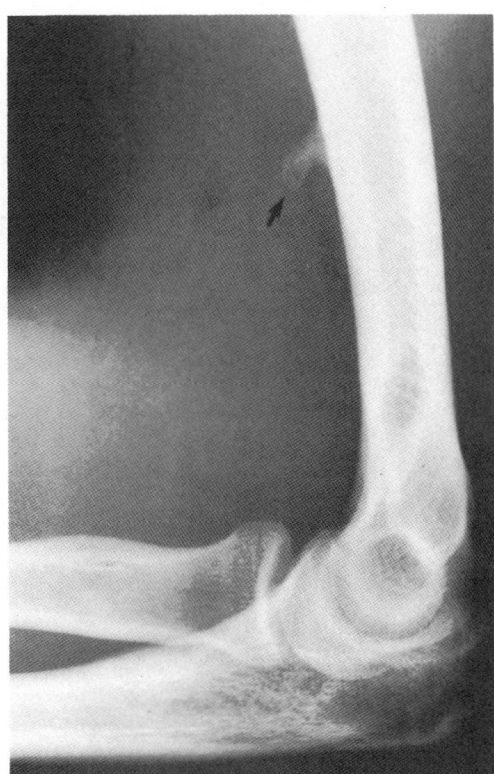

Figure 123–2. This well-defined bony excrescence *(arrow)* arises from the anterior, medial aspect of the humerus. It may rarely be associated with symptomatic median nerve compression. (From Weissman BN, Sledge CB. Orthopedic Radiology. Philadelphia, WB Saunders, 1986, p 172.)

In cases where correct positioning of the bony fragments cannot be maintained with the shoulder at the side, a shoulder spica cast may be used.

Complications

The prognosis for humeral shaft fractures is excellent when the fractured fragments maintain alignment during union. Angulation of up to 15 to 20 degrees can be accepted since there is appreciable remodeling capability.

Vascular injury is uncommon. When it does occur there is often a significant soft tissue injury. Radial nerve injuries are most frequently seen in fractures at the junction of the middle and distal third of the humerus. The prognosis is usually excellent. If the radial nerve is intact, initial recovery of function will occur within the first 8 to 12 weeks.

With the arm bound to the trunk, rotational deformities (usually <12 degrees) may occur. The distal fragment will be internally rotated in relationship to the proximal segment.

ELBOW INJURIES
Anatomy

The distal humerus consists of two columns of bone terminating in the condyles (Fig. 123–3). The thin bone connecting the two condyles is the *coronoid fossa.* The articular surfaces of the condyles are the *trochlea* medially and the *capitellum* laterally (Table 123–1). The *epicondyles* are the nonarticulating surfaces of the condyles where the forearm muscles attach. The relative exposure of the neurovascular structures at the elbow makes them susceptible to injury.

Radiographic Evaluation

The elbow should be evaluated with an anteroposterior and lateral view. The anteroposterior view should have the elbow as fully extended as possible; the lateral view should have the elbow flexed at 90 degrees. Additional oblique views may also be required to identify fractures of the radial head or coronoid fossa. Comparison radiographs of the unaffected elbow may be required to diagnose fractures.

On lateral radiograph the capitellum should appear as a teardrop. Additionally, the anterior humeral line should be drawn through the anterior humerus, which should intersect the middle of the capitellum (Fig. 123–4). With a supracondylar extension fracture, the anterior humeral line may completely miss the capitellum. Additionally, on the lateral elbow radiograph, occult radial neck fractures may be delineated by drawing the radiocapitellar line through the middle of the radial head (Fig. 123–5). The line should intersect the middle of the capitellum.

The lateral radiograph should also be evaluated for the "fat pad sign." The anterior fat pad is located in the coronoid

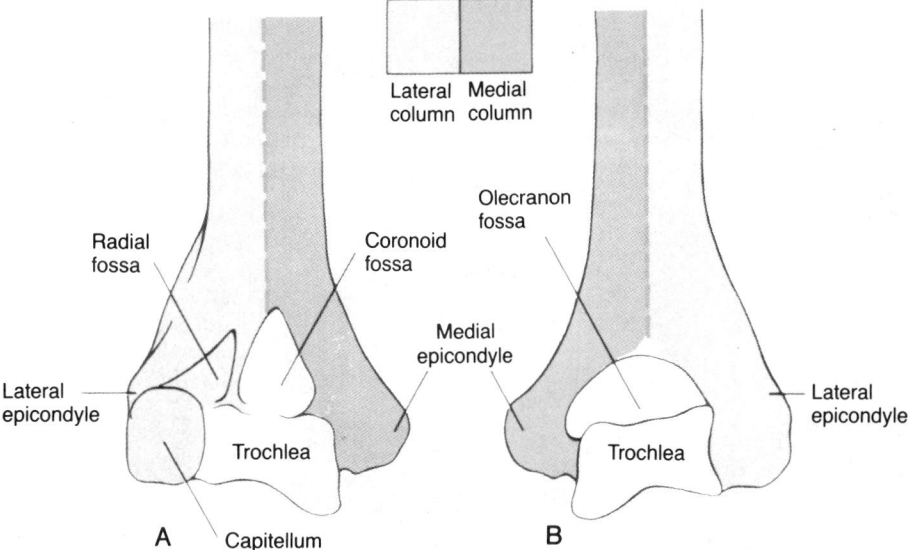

Figure 123–3. *A,* Anterior and *B,* posterior views of the medial and lateral columns of the distal humerus. (Modified with permission from Jupiter JB, Mehne DK. Trauma to the adult elbow and fractures of the distal humerus. *In* Browner BD, Jupiter JB, Levine AM, Trafton PG (eds). Skeletal Trauma. Vol 2. Philadelphia, WB Saunders, 1992, p 1148.)

TABLE 123–1		
DISTAL HUMERAL OSSIFICATION CENTERS		
Ossification Center	Age of Initial Appearance	Age of Fusion (yr)
Capitellum	3–6 mo	14–16
Medial epicondyle	5–7 yr	18–20
Trochlea	9–10 yr	14–16
Lateral epicondyle	9–13 yr	14–16

fossa and is seen as a lucency just anterior to the fossa on the lateral radiograph. With a fracture this anterior fat pad may be distended by capsular blood and may extend more anteriorly ("sail sign") (Fig. 123–6). The posterior fat pad lies in the deep olecranon fossa, which is not normally visible on the lateral radiograph. However, in occult elbow fractures, the capsule may be distended and the posterior fat pad will be visible.

SUPRACONDYLAR FRACTURES (EXTENSION TYPE)

Supracondylar fractures are usually seen with an immature skeleton, with a peak incidence in the first decade of life. The injured child has usually fallen on an outstretched, dorsiflexed hand with the elbow hyperextended. During the first decade of life the olecranon fossa is thin and weak. When the elbow is forced into hyperextension, the olecranon process is forced into the olecranon fossa, creating a lever that fractures the supracondylar region. The distal fragment of the fracture is displaced posteriorly.

Supracondylar fractures are often classified as nondisplaced; displaced with an intact posterior cortex; or displaced without cortical contact. In the fracture that is complete and displaced, the extremity will be S-shaped.

Radiographic Evaluation

In the displaced fracture the radiographic appearance is unmistakable (Fig. 123–7). Nevertheless, careful evaluation

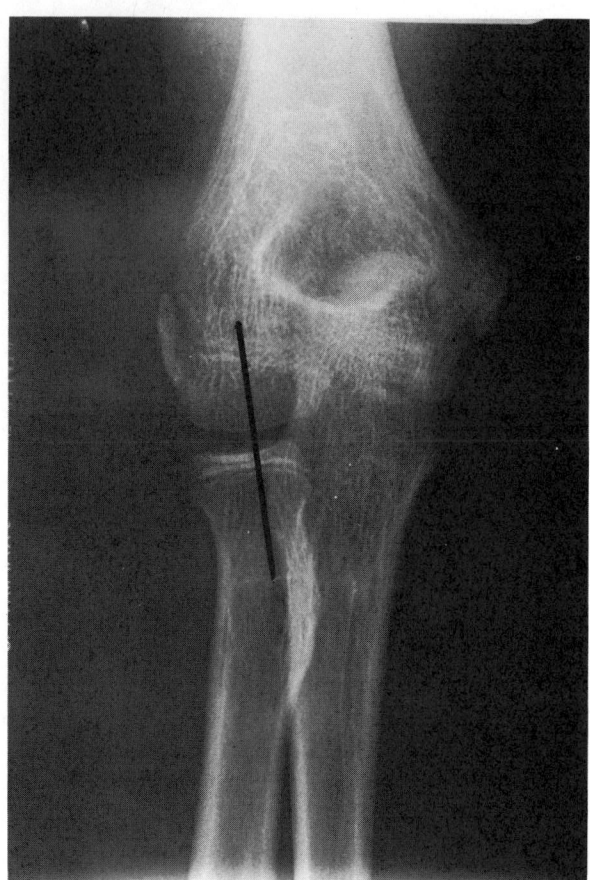

Figure 123–5. The radiocapitellar line. On the anteroposterior view, a line that bisects the proximal radial shaft passes through the capitellum.

of the relationship of the condyles to the radius and ulna must be ascertained to exclude an associated elbow dislocation.

The nondisplaced fracture may be difficult to diagnose by radiograph. Sometimes the only radiographic findings may be a fat pad sign or posterior displacement of the capitellum in relation to the anterior humeral line. Oblique views of the elbow may demonstrate the fracture.

Therapeutic Intervention

Orthopedic consultation is imperative. Vascular and neurologic function (motor and sensory) must be carefully evaluated. Displaced supracondylar extension fractures may require open reduction and internal fixation owing to the high incidence of complications.

Nondisplaced fractures are treated with immobilization; either a posterior splint or cylindric cast. The need for hospitalization is determined by the degree of soft tissue injury, severity of pain, and reliability of the parents.

Displaced fractures with an intact posterior cortex require reduction, which is usually done under general anesthesia. The elbow is then immobilized in a fixed position. Percutaneous pin fixation may be required to maintain the reduction.

A severely displaced fracture is managed by an orthopedist. The fracture fragments are reduced by manipulation or traction techniques. The reduction may be maintained with external stabilization, percutaneous pin fixation, or traction. Open reduction and internal fixation are considered for an open fracture or for severe vascular compromise.

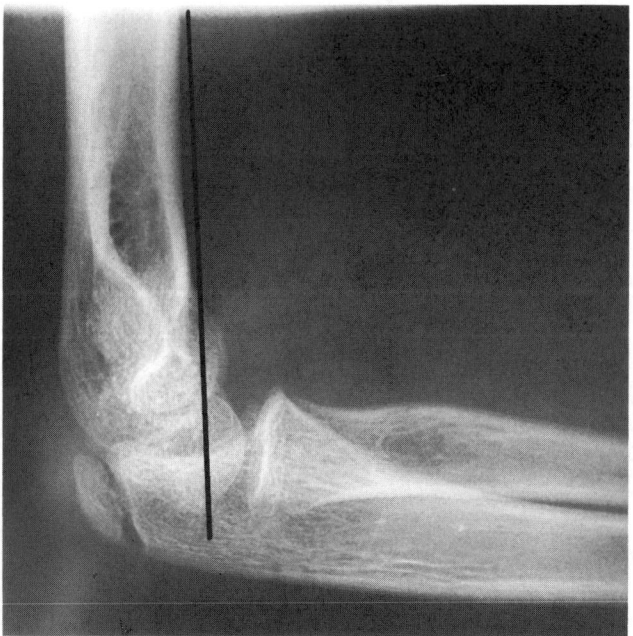

Figure 123–4. The anterior humeral line. A line drawn along the anterior humeral cortex normally passes through the capitellum.

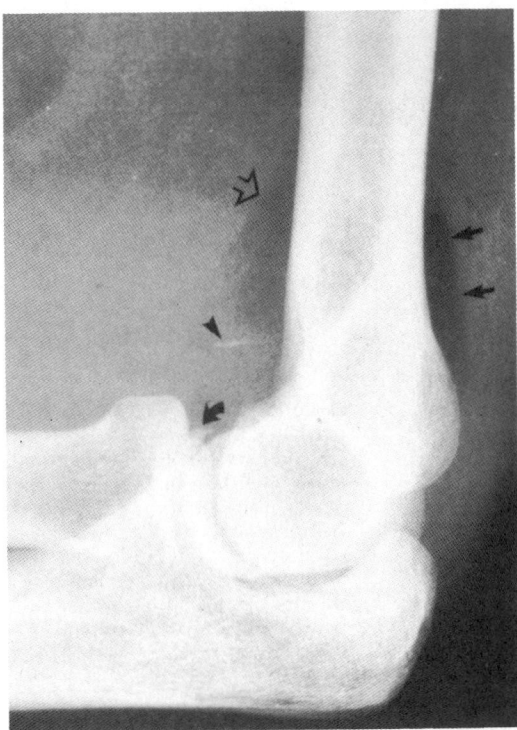

Figure 123–6. Coronoid process fracture with hemarthrosis. The posterior fat pad *(arrows)* is clearly seen on this lateral view with the arm flexed to 90 degrees, indicating joint effusion. The anterior fat pad *(open arrow)* is well seen. There is a fracture of the coronoid process *(curved arrow)*, and a loose body *(arrowhead)* is present. (From Weissman BN, Sledge CB. Orthopedic Radiology. Philadelphia, WB Saunders, 1986, p 179.)

posterior displacement seen in an extension-type supracondylar fracture. The child will give the history of falling on the flexed elbow.

The patient presents with the elbow flexed. The olecranon is less protuberant since it is displaced anteriorly. Radiographs of the elbow may reveal anterior angulation of the distal fragment.

Therapeutic Intervention

Complications include injury to the ulnar nerve and loss of range of motion. Treatment of these fractures is determined by the orthopedic consultant and includes pin fixation or open reduction and internal fixation.

LATERAL CONDYLAR PHYSIS FRACTURES
Introduction

Fractures of the lateral condylar physis can cause significant loss of mobility in the elbow. The lateral condylar physis can be fractured by two mechanisms. One involves the child falling forward on the palm with the elbow flexed, and the second is from forces created with the forearm adducted and supinated with the elbow extended.

Classification

The lateral condylar physis fracture can have two anatomic configurations (Fig. 123–8). In the Salter-Harris type IV fracture (Milch type I), the fracture begins in the metaphysis and transverses laterally to the trochlea through the capitellotrochlear groove. This fracture is relatively stable.

In the Salter-Harris type II fracture (Milch type II), the fracture begins in the metaphysis and transverses into the

Complications

Supracondylar fractures have a high incidence of complications. The incidence of nerve injuries is approximately 7%. The radial nerve is the most commonly injured. The most frequent direction of displacement is posteromedially, and in this fracture the proximal laterally displaced bony spike will injure the radial nerve. With posterolateral displacement, the median nerve and often the brachial artery will be tented by the displaced proximal spike and injured. Ulnar nerve deficits are due to pin fixation during treatment, and are not a direct result of the fracture. The prognosis of these nerve injuries is excellent; most resolve completely.

Vascular complications are the most serious sequelae. The incidence is approximately 0.5%, and they are usually associated with displaced supracondylar fractures. The brachial artery may be damaged by impingement, complete transection, spasm, or intimal tear. The resultant ischemia can cause intermittent claudication, compartment syndrome, Volkmann's contracture, gangrene of the extremity, and partial gangrene with muscle necrosis.

Therefore careful attention must be focused on the evaluation of the distal circulation, including checking the pulse, capillary refill, and dynamic movement of the distal musculature. The five Ps—*p*ain, *p*allor, *p*ulselessness, *p*aresthesia, and *p*aralysis—suggest Volkmann's ischemia. An early finding of Volkmann's ischemia is pain aggravated by passive extension of the fingers. If there is any question of vascular compromise, compartment pressures should be measured.

SUPRACONDYLAR FRACTURES (FLEXION TYPE)

The flexion-type supracondylar fracture produces anterior angulation of the distal fragment as opposed to the

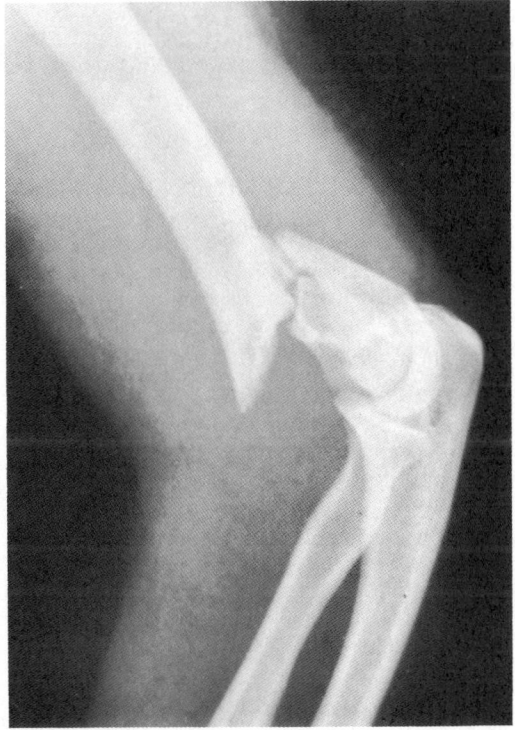

Figure 123–7. Supracondylar fracture, extension type. The lateral view shows an oblique fracture of the distal humerus with angular deformity. The distal fragment is displaced posteriorly. (From Weissman BN, Sledge CB. Orthopedic Radiology. Philadelphia, WB Saunders, 1986, p 186.)

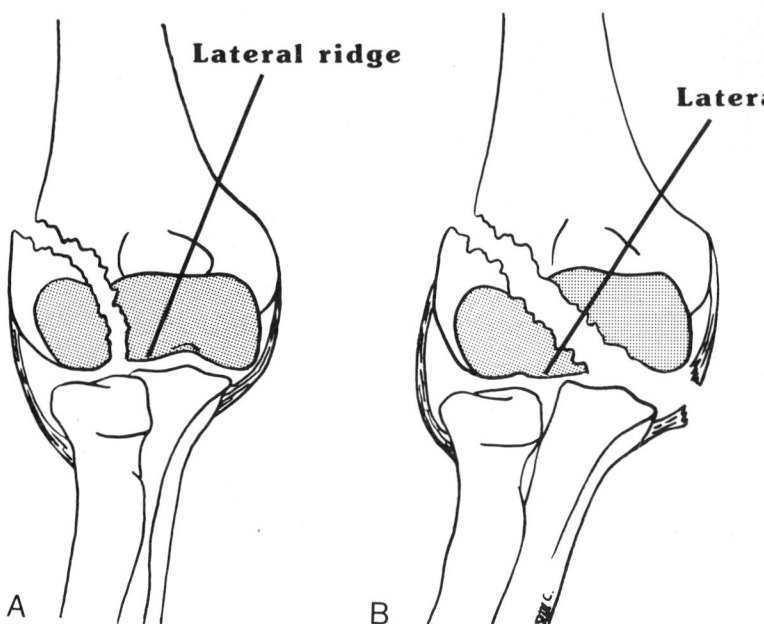

Figure 123–8. Milch classification of abduction lateral condylar fractures. *A*, Type I fractures involve only the lateral side of the elbow, and the joint is stable in the mediolateral plane. *B*, In type II fractures the fracture line is medial to the lateral ridge of the trochlea, and dislocation may occur. The ulnar collateral ligament may be torn. (From Weissman BN, Sledge CB. Orthopedic Radiology, Philadelphia, WB Saunders, 1986, p 188.)

apex of the trochlea, which can produce elbow instability (Fig. 123–9). The displaced fragment may have lateral rotatory displacement.

Therapeutic Intervention

Orthopedic consultation is required since these fractures are often treated aggressively. Treatment for nondisplaced fractures consists of simple immobilization.

Complications from this injury include lateral condylar overgrowth with spur formation; avascular necrosis of the fracture fragment; delayed union or nonunion; and residual deformity (valgus and varus). Tardive ulnar nerve palsy is a late complication of these fractures, occurring at a mean of 22 years after the injury. Both motor and sensory loss may be involved.

MEDIAL CONDYLAR PHYSIS FRACTURES
Introduction

Fractures involving the medial condylar physis are exceedingly rare. This fracture can be caused by falling on the flexed elbow or the outstretched hand. Fractures can extend into the trochlear apex or extend into the capitellotrochlear groove.

Therapeutic Intervention

Orthopedic consultation is necessary. For nondisplaced fractures, immobilization in a long-arm splint or cast is satisfactory. In displaced fractures, open reduction with internal fixation may be required. The most frequent complication is missing the fracture. Untreated cases may result in nonunion, cubitus varus, limitation of function, and ulnar nerve neuropathy.

DISTAL HUMERUS PHYSIS FRACTURES
Introduction

Fractures involving the entire distal humeral physis are relatively uncommon. The distal humeral physeal fractures

are due to rotatory shear forces and are most commonly seen with birth-related injuries and child abuse cases. The elbow of the child will be swollen, and there may be palpable crepitus.

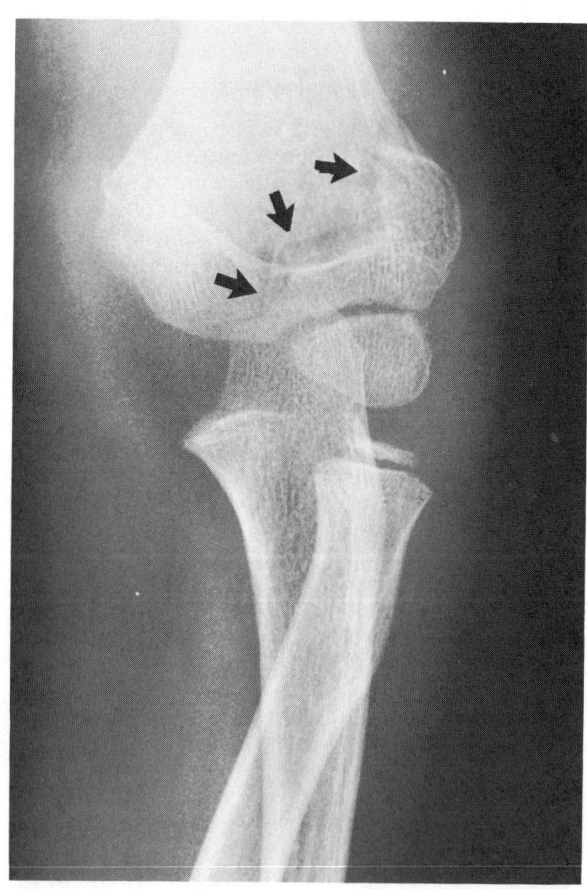

Figure 123–9. A subtle fracture *(arrows)* involving the lateral condyle (Milch type II).

Therapeutic Intervention

The treatment of these fractures is similar to other elbow fractures; orthopedic consultation is necessary. The fracture is reduced and then immobilized. Both closed and open techniques have been used.

Children do not usually incur the necessary rotatory forces that cause these fractures. Therefore child abuse should be considered. Avascular necrosis of the trochlea, nonunion, and cubitus varus can result.

MEDIAL EPICONDYLAR APOPHYSIS FRACTURES

Introduction

Medial epicondylar apophyseal fractures are typically seen in the age range from 9 years to 14 years. This fracture is associated with elbow dislocations in 50% of cases. Other associated injuries with this fracture include fractures of the radial neck, olecranon, or coronoid process.

Clinical Evaluation

The medial aspect of the elbow will be tender and swollen. In significantly displaced fractures, the bony fragment may be palpable and freely mobile. It is imperative to evaluate for ulnar nerve injury; an ulnar nerve deficit requires operative intervention.

Radiographic Evaluation

The radiographic evaluation should include measurement of the displacement of the fractured fragment. Comparison radiographs of the unaffected elbow will aid in this measurement. A displaced fragment of greater than 5 mm or displacement within the joint space constitutes a significantly displaced fracture (Fig. 123–10). Additionally, the associated injuries of elbow dislocation, radial neck fracture, olecranon fracture, or coronoid process must be excluded.

Therapeutic Intervention

In the nondisplaced or minimally displaced fracture (i.e., <5 mm), immobilization with a posterior splint is adequate. If the displaced fragment is intra-articular, greater than 5 mm, or has an ulnar nerve deficit, orthopedic consultation is imperative.

These fractures tend to heal well since they are not intra-articular. However, ulnar nerve dysfunction, loss of full extension, and nonunion can result.

Chronic Tension Stress Injuries

Chronic tension stress injury (also known as little league elbow syndrome) affects the medial epicondylar apophysis. This usually afflicts a young baseball pitcher who has repetitively thrown many balls and is just beginning to throw curve balls. There is local tenderness and swelling over the medial epicondyle, decreased extension of the elbow, and increased pain when the elbow is extended with a valgus stress. The radiographic appearance will reveal a widened and irregular physis. The bone will be hypertrophied with an increased bone density in comparison to the unaffected arm. The treatment is immobilization and a change in the throwing pattern to prevent a permanent disability.

PROXIMAL RADIUS FRACTURES

Introduction

Proximal radial fractures in children are uncommon. The age range of children with this fracture is 4 to 14 years old, with a mean of 9 to 10 years old. Two mechanisms of injury can produce these fractures: a valgus stress and an elbow dislocation. A valgus stress occurs when a child falls on an

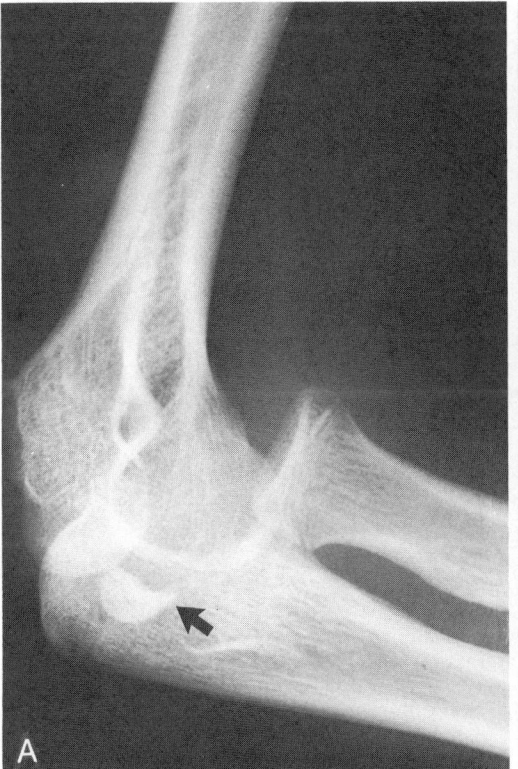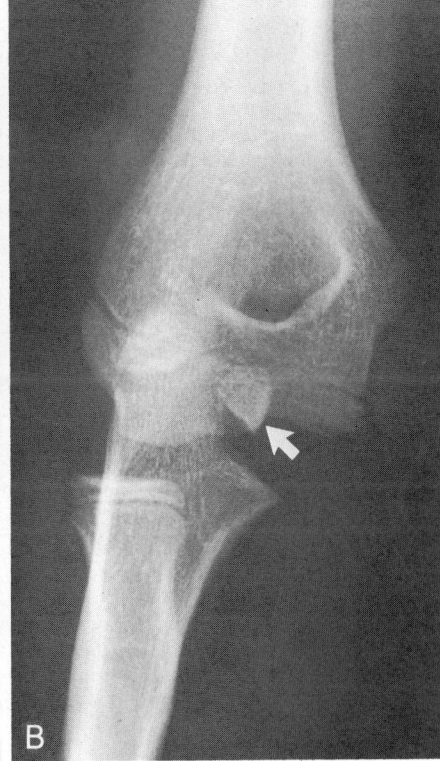

Figure 123–10. *A,* The avulsed medial epicondyle *(arrow)* is seen in this radiograph of an elbow dislocation. *B,* After reduction, the medial epicondyle *(arrow)* is entrapped in the elbow joint.

outstretched hand with the elbow hyperextended and the forearm sustains a valgus strain. Fractures of the medial epicondylar apophysis, olecranon, or coronoid process can be associated proximal radius fractures. Two patterns of fracture have been noted in association with an elbow dislocation. In the first pattern the radial head is displaced as a consequence of closed reduction; in the second pattern the radial head is displaced upon elbow dislocation.

In the skeletally immature, radial neck fractures are far more common than radial head fractures owing to the large amount of cartilage in the radial head and the narrower, weaker metaphysis in the neck.

Classification

The fractures can be classified according to the Salter-Harris classification of physeal fractures. Fractures of the proximal radius can be angulated, and the degree of angulation is important for treatment. Angulation of less than 30 degrees is mild. Angulation from 30 to 60 degrees is considered moderate and may require closed reduction to immobilization. Angulation greater than 60 degrees is severe and may require open reduction and internal fixation since closed reduction is difficult to obtain. Angulation should be measured on the anteroposterior view of the elbow.

Clinical Evaluation

The patient will present with a swollen, tender elbow. The injured elbow is often carried in a semiflexed position, with the forearm in neutral rotation. Much of the pain and swelling comes from intra-articular bleeding. The pain is increased with passive supination or pronation rather than with flexion or extension. Often the pain is referred to the wrist, but tenderness will be localized over the radial head and neck.

Radiographic Evaluation

If standard anteroposterior and lateral views are inconclusive but a fracture is still suspected, oblique views with the radius in various degrees of rotation may reveal subtle fracture lines. In the nondisplaced or minimally displaced radial neck fracture, a posterior fat pad sign may be the only radiographic finding. The posterior fat pad usually indicates elbow effusions or hemarthrosis. The anterior fat pad may also be prominently bowed in the traumatized elbow. A large part of the radial neck is extracapsular, and fractures involving this region may not produce an intra-articular effusion or subsequent posterior fat pad sign.

Therapeutic Intervention

In minimally displaced or nondisplaced fractures of the radial neck, immobilization with a posterior splint or long-arm cast is adequate. In patients with angulation greater than 30 but less than 60 degrees, closed reduction with subsequent immobilization is the treatment of choice. Open reduction and internal fixation are indicated in fractures that are nonreducible by closed methods, that have complete displacement, or that have angulation of greater than 60 degrees.

With minor fractures of the radial head, treatment with an elbow sling is sufficient. Radial head angulation of less than 30 degrees or translocation of 3 mm or less will spontaneously correct through remodeling, provided that the child is less than 10 years old.

Complications

Loss of pronation and supination may result from a proximal radius fracture. The blood supply to the radius courses the rim of the epiphyseal plate. If the vascular supply is interrupted from an epiphyseal plate injury, avascular necrosis may ensue.

Radial head overgrowth, premature physeal closure, nonunion of the radial neck, radioulnar synostosis, and myositis ossificans are possible complications. Vascular and nerve injuries are rare.

OLECRANON FRACTURES
Introduction

Olecranon fractures are uncommon in children. There are two mechanisms of injury: falling on an outstretched hand with a valgus or varus stress, or a direct blow to the posterior elbow. The patient has swelling over the olecranon. An abrasion or contusion overlying the olecranon may also be present.

Radiographic Evaluation

Radiographs may demonstrate a fracture line that may be between the epiphyseal-metaphyseal interface or may involve the metaphyseal fragment. There may also be a partial or total lateral dislocation of the radial head, as well as a radial neck fracture or a medial epicondyle fracture.

Therapeutic Evaluation

In epiphyseal olecranon fractures, immobilization is the treatment of choice unless there is significant displacement, which would require open reduction and internal fixation. In metaphyseal olecranon fractures, nondisplaced fractures require immobilization. Displaced fractures may require closed reduction or open reduction and internal fixation.

In coronoid process fractures, immobilization is adequate. Orthopedic consultation is necessary. Complications include overgrowth of the epiphysis, nonunion, and transient ulnar neuropraxia.

POSTERIOR ELBOW DISLOCATIONS
Introduction

Elbow dislocations are defined by the relationship of the proximal radius and ulna to the distal humerus. The elbow is markedly swollen, and the arm is held in a flexed position. The forearm is shortened, and the normal relationship of the olecranon to the radius and ulna is lost.

Radiographic Evaluation

On the lateral view the olecranon is posterior to the condyles. On the anteroposterior view the relationship of the condyles to the radius and ulna will be lost with superimposition of the distal humerus over the radius and ulna.

Therapeutic Intervention

Most elbow dislocations can be reduced by closed means. An orthopedist should be consulted prior to reduction. Two techniques are used: the "puller" or the "pusher." In the puller technique the patient is either seated or lying supine, with the elbow flexed approximately 60 to 70 degrees (Fig. 123–11). One of the physician's hands is placed at the wrist

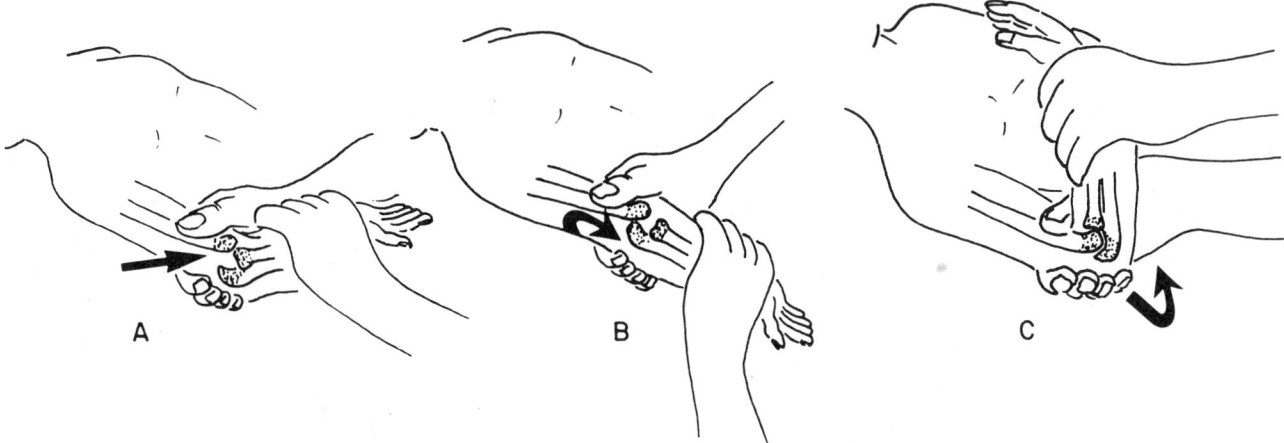

Figure 123–11. Schematic of reduction of a posterior elbow dislocation using elbow flexion. (From Ogden JA. Skeletal Injury in the Child. 2nd ed. Philadelphia, WB Saunders, 1990, p 434.)

and a distally directed longitudinal force is applied, while the other hand braces the proximal radius and ulna and pulls it anteriorly.

In the pusher technique the patient lies supine (Fig. 123–12). One of the physician's hands grasps the patient's wrist, pulling longitudinally and distally, while the other hand is placed over the distal humerus, pushing the olecranon with the thumb. Open reduction is sometimes required.

Complications

Fractures of the medial epicondylar apophysis, coronoid process, or radial neck can be associated with posterior elbow dislocations. Brachial artery injury as well as ulnar, radial, or median nerve injury can occur. In addition, owing to the reduction techniques, the radius and ulna can be translocated, with the resultant radius articulating with the trochlea and the ulna articulating with the capitellum.

ANTERIOR ELBOW DISLOCATIONS

Anterior dislocations are rare and result from a direct blow to the posterior aspect of the flexed elbow. In the

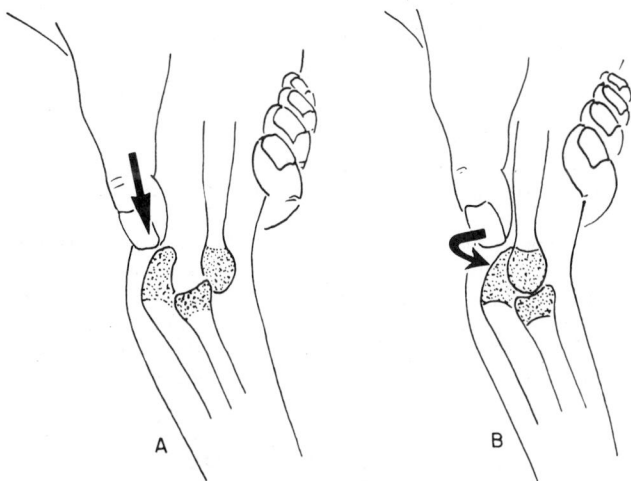

Figure 123–12. Schematic of reduction of an elbow dislocation using mild elbow hyperextension. (From Ogden JA. Skeletal Injury in the Child. 2nd ed. Philadelphia, WB Saunders, 1990, p 434.)

lateral radiograph the ulna and radius lie anterior to the humerus. On the anteroposterior radiograph the ulna and radius are superimposed on the proximal humerus anteriorly.

Therapeutic Intervention

For joint reduction the patient is positioned with the elbow flexed. The examiner will apply two forces concomitantly: one proximally and longitudinally to the humerus, and the second from the anterior to the posterior direction on the proximal radius and ulna. The forces applied are opposite to those applied with the posterior dislocation.

Complications from anterior elbow dislocation include brachial artery rupture, significant soft tissue disruption, and avulsion of the triceps insertion from the posterior olecranon.

RADIAL HEAD SUBLUXATION
Introduction

This condition is the most frequent elbow injury in the child. The condition is described by various terms, the most common being nursemaid's elbow, temper tantrum elbow, slipped elbow, pulled elbow, and subluxation of the radial head. This occurs when the child's elbow is extended and the forearm is pronated, and then a sudden pulling traction force is placed on the child's hand or wrist. Longitudinal distraction on the pronated radius results in a portion of the annular ligament slipping between the head of the radius and the capitellum. The annular ligament is a strong band of fibers that encircles the head of the radius and maintains the proximal radioulnar joint. Firm traction of the extended elbow with the forearm in pronation produces an annular ligament tear. When the traction is released, the annular ligament becomes caught between the radial head and the capitellum. The peak incidence is between 1 and 3 years of age, although cases involving adolescents have been reported.

Clinical Evaluation

The diagnosis is based largely on a history of sudden longitudinal traction on the child's hand or forearm such as a parent preventing a child's fall when the child stumbles. An audible snap may be noticed. The elbow will be held in a flexed and pronated position. The elbow will flex from 30 to 120 degrees; however, any attempts at passive supination will lead to resistance. There is no elbow effusion, but there is local tenderness over the radial head.

Radiographic Evaluation

Radiographs of the elbow are normal. Their only value is to exclude associated fractures, which are rare. The child may return from radiographic examination with a subluxation reduced owing to the forearm being supinated and extended by the radiology technician for the anteroposterior projection.

Therapeutic Intervention

If a typical history is obtained; the entire extremity is examined carefully; there is no elbow effusion; and the only point tenderness is limited to the radial head, the manipulative reduction can be performed. If there is any suspicion of other injury, radiographs should be viewed prior to manipulation.

The patient's forearm is held in two regions. One hand is placed at the elbow with the thumb directly over the radial head so that the snapping sensation of reduction can be felt. The other hand grasps the patient's forearm, firmly supinating it (Fig. 123–13). If the characteristic snapping sensation is not felt, then the elbow is flexed maximally until the palpable, sometimes audible click is perceived. There should be a snapping sensation perceived as the annular ligament reduces. One should reexamine the patient after 15 minutes. Occasionally several attempts at reduction are necessary. If the reduction was successful, the patient will be using both arms and will have full range of motion of the affected elbow. Rarely, symptoms persist beyond 2 to 3 days.

If reduction failures are suspected, or if it is the third injury, sling immobilization and orthopedic referral are recommended. After the reduction has been accomplished, it is important to explain to the parents the mechanism of injury and means of prevention.

Complications

Recurrent "pulled elbows" occur in 5 to 30% of children with an initial pull. Recurrences are common if sudden longitudinal forces on the extremity are repeated. After 5 years of age the annular ligament becomes stronger and

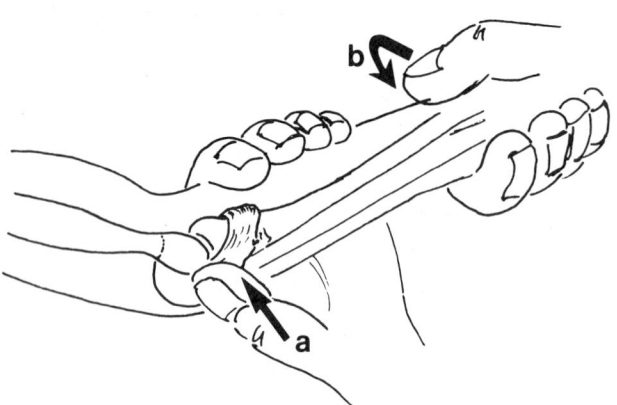

Figure 123–13. Mechanism of reduction of a pulled elbow. The thumb is placed directly over the radial head (a) while the forearm is rapidly supinated (b). (From Ogden JA. Skeletal Injury in the Child. 2nd ed. Philadelphia, WB Saunders, 1990, p 445.)

attaches firmly to the radial neck, thus preventing this condition.

FOREARM FRACTURES
Introduction

Forearm fractures in children usually result from a fall on an outstretched hand. According to Blount et al., 75% of fractures of the shaft of the radius and ulna are in the distal third, 18% in the middle third, and 7% in the proximal third. Because of the close proximity of the radius to the ulna, if one bone is found to be fractured, the other should be closely inspected for fracture or dislocation.

Most forearm fractures in children are distal compression fractures or nondisplaced, angulated greenstick fractures. Residual deformities in children tend to correct with subsequent remodeling and growth. Closed reduction and immobilization usually result in complete functional recovery, provided that rotational deformities do not exist at the fracture site after reduction.

Clinical Evaluation

The radius and ulna are two parallel bones connected by an intraosseous membrane. During pronation the radius lies across the ulna. Biomechanically the radius and ulna make up a ring, and therefore when one bone is found to be fractured, a second associated fracture, dislocation, or ligamentous injury should be suspected. Shaft fractures of the forearm are usually the result of a fall on the outstretched hand or a direct blow.

The diagnosis is usually obvious because of the pain, swelling, crepitation, and deformity. However, compression (buckle or torus) deformities are often subtle. The joint above and below must be evaluated, and the distal neurovascular status must be assessed.

Radiographic Evaluation

Anteroposterior and lateral radiographs, including both proximal and distal joints, are essential. To determine rotational defect, useful landmarks on lateral projection are the ulnar styloid (points down); the coronoid process of the ulna (points up); and the radial styloid (not visualized). On the anteroposterior view the radial styloid and radial tuberosity will be on opposite sides of the shaft, while the coronoid and styloid process of the ulna are hidden. When in doubt, the unaffected extremity can be used for comparison.

MONTEGGIA'S FRACTURE-DISLOCATION
Introduction

In 1814 Monteggia described an injury involving a fracture of the proximal third of the ulna and an associated radial head dislocation. A major oversight regarding this injury occurs because one becomes distracted by the obvious ulnar deformity and misses the radial head dislocation. When viewing a true lateral projection, an imaginary line along the anterior cortex of the humerus should intersect the middle third of the capitellum. A second imaginary line bisecting the radial shaft should pass through the center of the capitellum whether the elbow is flexed or extended (Fig. 123–14). Using these criteria, a Monteggia injury will unlikely be missed.

Therapeutic Intervention

Emergency department management of Monteggia's fractures include immobilization in a posterior long-arm splint and orthopedic referral.

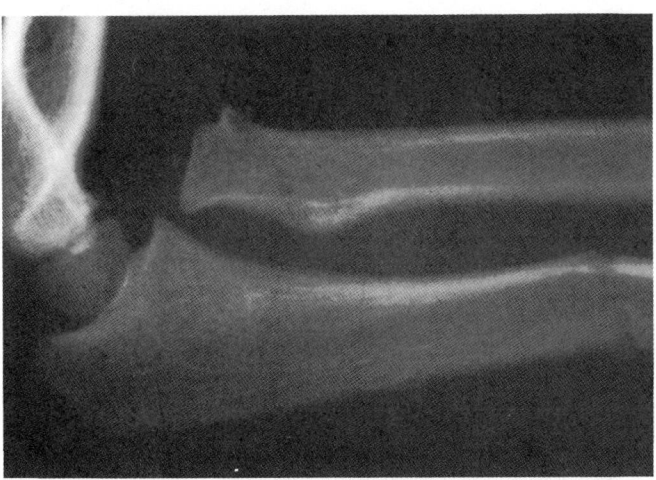

Figure 123–14. Acute Monteggia injury. Unfortunately, this radiograph was read as an "ulnar greenstick fracture"; the radial head dislocation was missed. (From Ogden JA. Skeletal Injury in the Child. 2nd ed. Philadelphia, WB Saunders, 1990, p 489.)

Unlike in adults, operative repair in children is implemented only when closed radial head reduction cannot be accomplished or maintained. Manipulative closed reduction of the ulnar fracture and radial head dislocation usually requires general anesthesia. Adequate radial head reduction is more critical than absolute anatomic realignment of the ulnar fracture.

If reduction of the radial head can be maintained, children have minimal sequelae from the Monteggia lesion. There are no significant problems with the healing ulnar fracture, and redislocation of the radial head is rare.

GALEAZZI'S FRACTURE-DISLOCATION
Introduction

In 1934 Galeazzi described a fracture of the distal shaft of the radius combined with dislocation of the distal radioulnar joint. The most likely mechanism of injury is a fall on the outstretched hand with the forearm in extreme pronation.

The Galeazzi lesion is an extremely uncommon injury in children. When present, the child complains of pain about the distal forearm and wrist with notable distal radial joint swelling and tenderness.

Therapeutic Intervention

The most common radial fracture site is at the junction of the middle and distal thirds. The fracture is usually of the greenstick type with angular displacement. The shaft fracture is always recognized, but the dislocation may be overlooked. Anteroposterior and lateral projections are generally adequate, but some authors recommend computed tomography or arthrography to verify associated triangular fibrocartilage disruption. Emergency department management consists of immobilization, ice, and analgesia until orthopedic reduction can be performed. Nonoperative closed manipulation and reduction under general anesthesia are usually performed.

DISTAL RADIUS AND ULNAR FRACTURES
Introduction

Of all the long bone fractures in children, the distal radius is by far the most common. This is due to the relative weakness of the metaphyseal bone. Fractures of the distal radius and ulna are of four general types: physeal (most commonly Salter-Harris type I or II); torus compression; complete (rare); and greenstick (common). Distal radial fractures in children are rarely intra-articular and therefore have few long-term complications.

The most common mechanism of injury is a fall on an outstretched hand. An extension-type fracture results in a dorsal angulation of the distal fragment from a fall with the wrist in extension. A flexion-type fracture results in opposite angulation as a result of a fall with the hand in dorsiflexion.

Clinical Evaluation

If there is a classic fork-like deformity, the diagnosis is obvious. However, with nondisplaced fractures or torus fractures, the examiner must often rely on reproducible localized bony tenderness. Neupraxias of either the median or the ulnar nerves may occur from stretching forces at the time of the acute deformity. Subsequent neural compromise may develop from soft tissue swelling.

Radiographic Evaluation

Routine anteroposterior and lateral projections identify most distal radial and ulnar fractures (Fig. 123–15). However, nondisplaced physeal fractures are often subtle, and the only radiographic findings may be anterior displacement of the normal fat pad that overlies the pronator quadratus muscle. This is evident on the lateral projection as a result of subperiosteal hemorrhage from the occult fracture.

Therapeutic Intervention

Closed reduction is the treatment of choice and can generally be performed using a hematoma block or regional anesthesia. General anesthesia may be necessary for the younger child.

Torus fractures usually occur approximately 2 to 3 cm proximal to the physis. The periosteum and cortex remain intact. Treatment is with a short-arm cast for 3 weeks to avoid reinjury.

With greenstick fractures, the periosteum and cortex disruption is limited to one side of the shaft at the apex of the angulation. Although these fractures are subtle and easily reduced, recurrent deformity can occur while in the cast. As a result of this complication, controversy exists regarding fracture management. Some authors feel that in the young child angulation less than 30 degrees will correct with remodeling and that manipulative reduction is unnecessary. However, others advise anatomic reduction for any angulation to limit the advancing deformity once in the cast. Most authors accept 10 degrees angulation with frequent reexamination while casted.

Complete fractures of the distal radius and ulna are often overriding, making reduction difficult and maintaining the reduction even more challenging.

FOREARM PLASTIC (BOWING) DEFORMATION
Introduction

Skeletally immature long bones in children are more porous owing to the greater number and size of the haversian canal systems. This makes the child's bones more flexible, leading to some degree of plastic deformation prior to fracture. If sufficient longitudinal forces are applied, microfractures along the concave border occur. Although no gross fracture is evident, the end result is a fixed bowing, called plastic deformation.

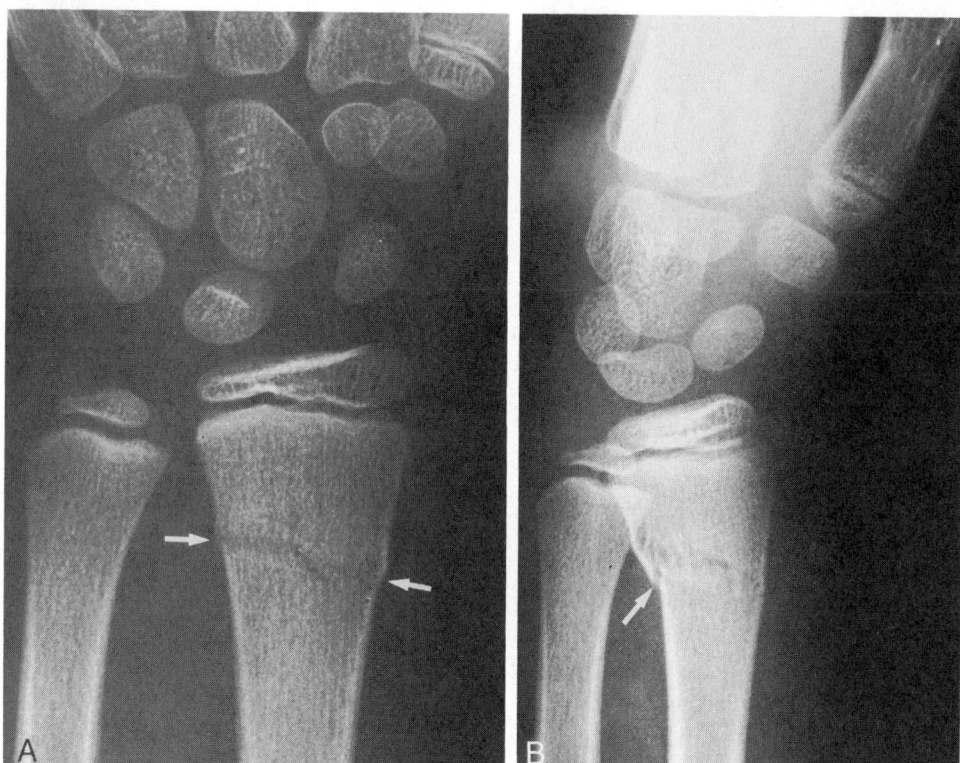

Figure 123–15. Fracture of the distal radius can be subtle. *A*, Note the slight buckling of cortex *(arrows)* on the anteroposterior view. *B*, On lateral projection, the fracture *(arrow)* is more obvious.

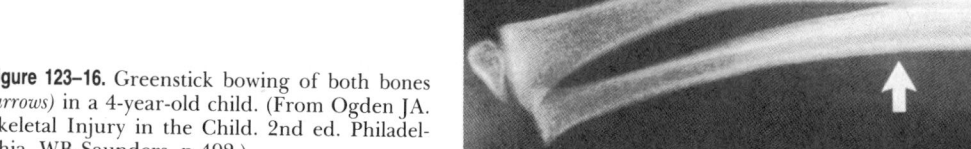

Figure 123–16. Greenstick bowing of both bones *(arrows)* in a 4-year-old child. (From Ogden JA. Skeletal Injury in the Child. 2nd ed. Philadelphia, WB Saunders, p 492.)

The forearm is the most common site for this deformity, and one or both bones may be involved. The injury is commonly demonstrated with a diaphyseal fracture of one bone and a bowing deformity of the other.

Clinical Evaluation

Clinically there will be deformity when compared with the unaffected extremity. The child will often complain with local tenderness and pain with palpation. If both bones are involved there may be a decrease in supination and pronation (Fig. 123–16).

The bowing deformity is best demonstrated on the lateral view. When in doubt, a view of the unaffected forearm should be used as a comparison. The proximal and distal joints should be evaluated. With healing there may be cortical thickening on the concave aspect, but periosteal new bone does not form. If clinical signs and plain radiographs are inconsistent, a bone scan will be diagnostic.

Therapeutic Intervention

Without proper treatment there can be a loss of full supination and pronation. In children younger than 4 years of age, remodeling will correct most of the deformity without significant long-term functional loss. However, manipulative reduction to within 85% correction under general anesthesia is advised in children older than 4 years of age.

Selected References

Allman FL. Fractures and ligamentous injuries of the clavicle and its articulation. J Bone Joint Surg 1967;49A:774.

Aponte JE, Ghiatas A. Acute plastic bowing deformity: A review of the literature. J Emerg Med 1989;7:181.

Blount WP, Shaefer AA, Johnson JH. Fractures of the forearm in children. JAMA 1942;120:111.

Bowen A. Plastic bowing of the clavicle in children. J Bone Joint Surg 1983;65A:403.

Farkas R, Levine S. X-ray incidence of fractured clavicle in vertex presentation. Am J Obstet Gynecol 1950;59:204.

Hall RH, Isaac F, Booth CR. Dislocations of the shoulder with special reference to accompanying small fractures. J Bone Joint Surg 1959;41A:489.

Mabrey JD, Fitch RD. Plastic deformation in pediatric fractures: Mechanism and treatment. J Pediatr Orthop 1989;9:310.

Mann DC, Rajmaira A. Distribution of physeal and nonphyseal fractures in 2,650 long-bone fractures in children aged 0–16 years. J Pediatr Orthop 1990;10:713.

Ogden JA, Conologue GJ, Bronson ML. Radiology of postnatal skeletal development. III. The clavicle. Skeletal Radiol 1979;4:196.

Post M. Current concepts in the treatment of fractures of the clavicle. Clin Orthop 1989;245:89.

Rockwood CA. Fractures of the outer clavicle in children and adults. J Bone Joint Surg 1982;64B:642.

Salter RB, Harris WR. Injuries involving the epiphyseal plate. J Bone Joint Surg 1963;45A:587.

Salter RB, Zaltz C. Anatomic investigations of the mechanism of injury and pathologic anatomy of "pulled elbow" in young children. Clin Orthop 1971;77:134.

CHAPTER 124

Pelvic and Lower Extremity Injuries

Oliver Hayes

INTRODUCTION

The incidence of serious pelvic and lower extremity injuries in children has increased in recent decades, mostly owing to an escalation of motor vehicle accidents involving children. Leading causes of pelvic and lower extremity trauma include traffic-related accidents (injuries to motor vehicle occupants, pedestrians, and cyclists), falls, child abuse, fires, and athletic injuries. Specific lower extremity injuries are age related; bumper injuries to pedestrian children result in trochanteric fractures in the 6- to 7-year-old age group, while older children sustain femoral shaft fractures (Fig. 124–1). A specific grouping of injuries—Waddell's triad—results from motor vehicle–pedestrian accidents in which the victim's femur is fractured by the bumper, the torso is injured at the level of the car's hood, and a head injury occurs when the victim strikes the ground.

EMS CONSIDERATIONS

After initial assessment and resuscitation of life-threatening conditions, immobilization should be completed prior to transport. Steps of immobilization include assessing distal motor, sensory, and vascular status; splinting the injured extremity; and immobilizing the entire patient. Repeat evaluation of distal neurovascular status should be done approximately every 15 to 20 minutes during prolonged transport. Backboard and immobilization should be provided in any patients suspected of having pelvic fractures.

Traction splint application is indicated whenever fracture of the distal or midshaft femur is clinically suspected. Some authors also advocate the use of traction splints for clinically suspected tibial fractures. Controversy exists regarding the benefits of traction splinting with open fractures because of possible retraction of exposed bone fragments into the wound without surgical debridement. A variety of traction splints with applications for the pediatric patient are available, including the Hare, Trac 3, and adjustable Sager splints.

If the neurovascular status is compromised after traction splinting, adjustments must be made. Splints with an adjustable bar should be positioned to provide a length sufficient to extend 10 to 15 cm beyond the heel. After slight elevation of the injured leg, the padded half-ring is placed against the ipsilateral ischial tuberosity (the Sager device is positioned against the ipsilateral pubic symphysis or laterally against the greater trochanter). The thigh strap is then secured. The ankle harness is secured first to the ankle and then to the distal end of the traction device. Traction is gradually applied to obtain fracture stabilization. Knee and support straps can then be secured. Size limitations of these devices preclude their use in infants and very small children. Such patients can be adequately splinted with armboards, vacuum splints, or conventional metallic splints.

Evidence supports both short- and long-term use of pneumatic antishock trousers in the management of pelvic frac-

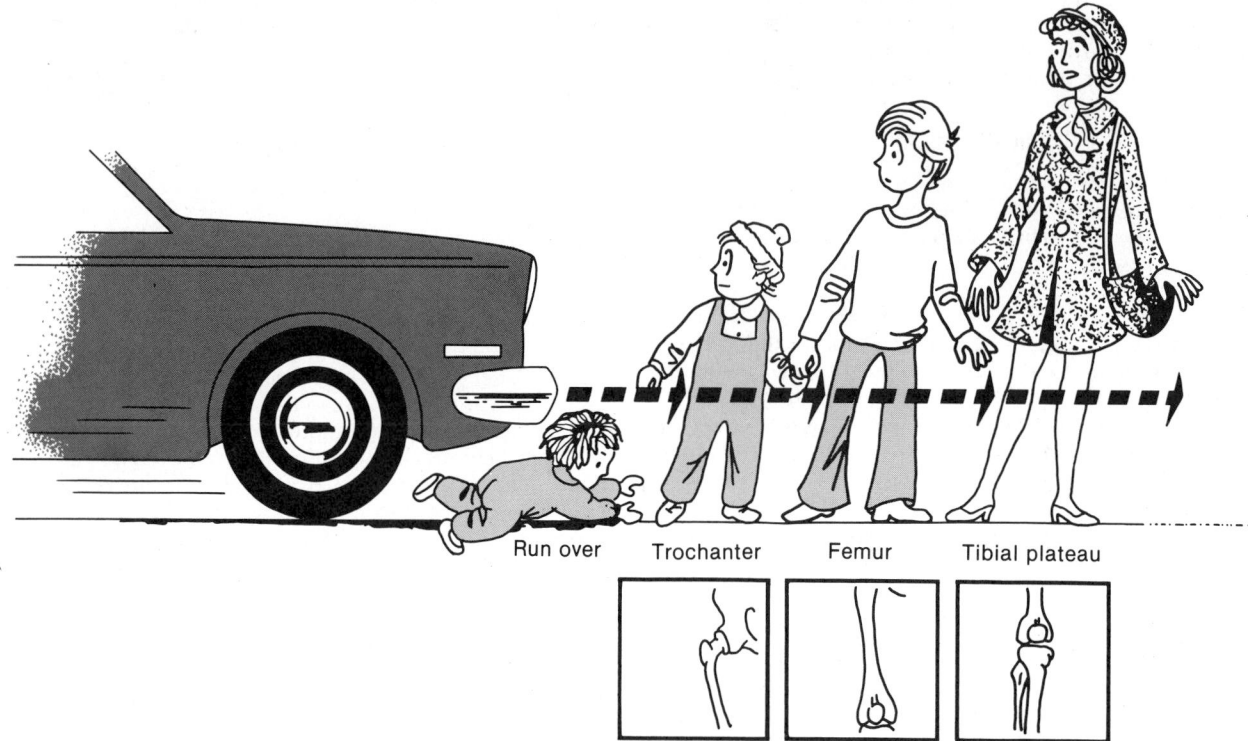

Figure 124–1. Age determines the site of a bumper fracture. (Redrawn from Rang M. Children's Fractures. 2nd ed. Philadelphia, JB Lippincott, 1983.)

tures. However, meticulous monitoring of adequate tissue perfusion in the lower extremities is necessary to prevent the complications of pressure necrosis or compartment syndrome. Pressure with the pneumatic suit should be maintained below the mean arterial pressure.

PELVIC INJURIES

Pelvic fractures may be associated with injuries of abdominal or pelvic contents, which may take precedence in the intitial treatment and resuscitation of the patient. Skeletal injuries of the pelvis may involve epiphyseal, apophyseal, or diaphyseal fractures, while soft tissue injuries are predominantly contusions, strains, and overuse syndromes. Additionally, growth plate injuries are much more common than ligamentous or musculotendinous injuries in the immature pelvis.

Anatomy

In the immature skeleton the pelvis is composed of three separate bones—the ilium, ischium, and pubis—which converge at the acetabulum to form the triradiate cartilage (Fig. 124–2). Undisturbed growth and ossification of the triradiate cartilage are critical for normal acetabular formation. The acetabulum forms within the triradiate cartilage at approximately 12 years of age and fuses at age 18 years.

The ischium and pubis have interposed cartilage, which is found at the inferior ramus of the pubis. This endochondral area eventually fuses and enlarges between 4 and 10 years of age (Fig. 124–3).

Secondary centers of ossification appear at various locations and ages within the pediatric pelvis. The ossification center of the iliac crest first appears laterally and anteriorly on the iliac crest and advances posteriorly until it reaches the posterior iliac spine. Fusion occurs between 14 and 17

years of age. The anterior superior iliac spine (ASIS) usually develops from the iliac crest apophysis and normally ossifies by age 15 years. Muscles of hip flexion attach at the ASIS (sartorius) and at the anterior inferior iliac spine (AIIS; rectus femoris). Radiographic demonstration of the ischial tuberosity often reveals an irregular surface owing to remodeling of the bone. Finally, the development of the cartilaginous region of the symphysis pubis represents an area of potential epiphyseal injury. The normal amount of widening of the symphysis is highly variable and dependent on the extent of ossification of the radiolucent cartilage.

Pelvic Fractures

For the purposes of this review pelvic fractures are divided into three groups: (1) fractures of the pelvic ring, stable and unstable; (2) intra-articular fractures of the acetabulum (described in the section on hip injuries); and (3) avulsion fractures and epiphysiolysis secondary to violent muscular contraction.

Avulsion fractures represent the most common type of pelvic fractures. Many cases probably remain undiagnosed. The most common pelvic ring fracture involves a ramus and is typically a unilateral superior pubic ramus fracture. Unstable fractures are relatively rare in children.

Fractures of the Pelvic Ring

The history of severe local pain and inability to stand and walk is normally present in patients with fractures of the pelvic ring. The physical examination should demonstrate local tenderness and swelling at the fracture site. With unstable fractures, a deformity of one or both of the hips as well as pelvic ring instability may be present. In the supine patient, posterior subluxation of the ilium at the sacroiliac (SI) joint may go unidentified. Physical examination should

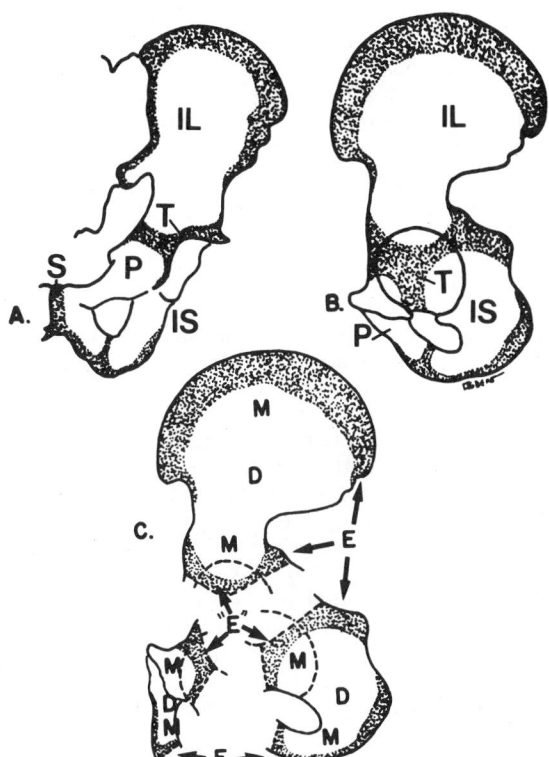

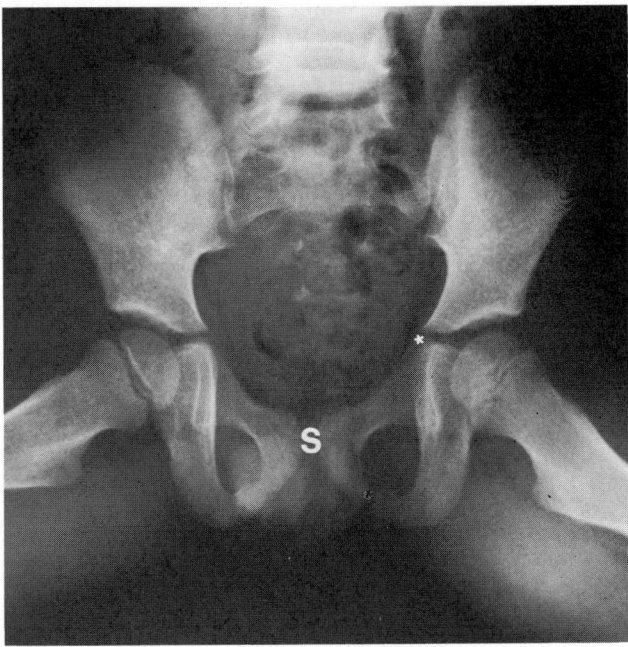

Figure 124–3. Radiograph shows the cartilage at the ischiopubic junction (*white circle*), the triradiate cartilage (*asterisk*), and the symphysis pubis (*S*).

Figure 124–2. Anterior (*A*) and lateral (*B*) schematics of the developing pelvis, showing relative areas of bone (*white*) and cartilage (*stippled*). IL = Ilium; IS = ischium; P = pubis; S = symphysis pubis; T = triradiate cartilage. *C,* Exploded view to emphasis the analogy of each component bone to a long bone and how several "epiphyses" fuse to form ischiopubic junctions and the symphysis pubis. E = Epiphysis; M = metaphysis; D = diaphysis. (From Ogden JA. Skeletal Injury in the Child. 2nd ed. Philadelphia, WB Saunders, 1990, p 627.)

include manual pelvic compression with elicitation of tenderness at fracture sites. Regional examinations of the abdomen, external genitalia, rectal and pelvic areas, and femoral and distal leg pulses should be performed. A complete neurologic examination should be done. The lumbosacral plexus lies near the SI joint and may be injured with SI joint disruption.

Radiologic examination is necessary to confirm suspected injuries. Gonadal shields should be avoided because of possible fracture concealment. Because of the position of the pelvis within the body, a standard anteroposterior radiograph actually provides a slightly oblique view of the pelvis and is not always adequate for fracture delineation. Two additional views may be helpful: the inlet view, which is 30 degrees cephalad off the vertical and demonstrates the extent of pelvic compression or expansion; and the tangential view, which is 40 degrees caudad off the vertical and demonstrates the extent to which disruptions have occurred in the vertical plane of the pelvis (Fig. 124–4).

Unstable Pelvic Ring Fractures. Unstable injuries are usually the result of direct crushing or compressive forces. Hypovolemic shock is a common occurrence secondary to hemorrhage from cancellous bone or severed blood vessels. Loss of greater than 50% of circulating blood volume may occur with pelvic fractures; hemorrhagic shock is the most serious life-threatening complication initially. Mortality from hemorrhage in the pediatric age group ranges from 0% to 15% in various series.

A separation of the pubic symphysis accompanied by

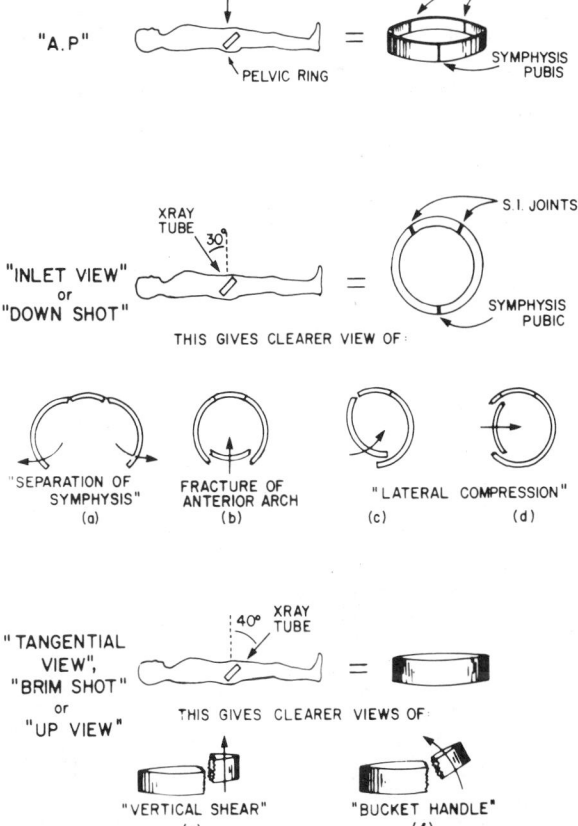

Figure 124–4. Radiologic evaluation and classification of pelvic ring fractures. (From Watts HG. Fractures of the pelvis. Orthop Clin North Am 1976;7:615.)

partial SI joint disruption is an unstable fracture (Fig. 124–4A). The pelvic ring is opened anteriorly at the pubic symphysis and posteriorly with separation at the SI joint secondary to either avulsion of the anterior capsule of the joint or fracture of the ilium or sacrum. Supine positioning of the patient aggravates the deformity, and the child may be made more comfortable by lying on his or her side.

Fractures of the anterior arch (Fig. 124–4B) result from crush injuries in the anteroposterior direction. These injuries yield bilateral pubic rami fractures and thus create a floating segment. This injury has a high association with urethral or bladder disruptions. If a urethral injury is suspected, a retrograde urethrogram should be performed.

Lateral compression fractures result from crushing forces at the lateral aspect of the pelvis, folding the ilium centrally (by fracture) with the pelvis hinged anteriorly at the pubic symphysis or posteriorly at the SI joint (Fig. 124–4C). If sufficient force is exerted on the lateral aspect of the pelvis, an entire free segment of the pelvis may be displaced medially, with disruptions both anteriorly and posteriorly (Fig. 124–4D). With vertical shear fractures, the pelvis is fractured both anteriorly and posteriorly, with superior displacement of the free pelvic segment often secondary to muscle spasm (Fig. 124–4E). The bucket-handle injury is a variation of the vertical shear injury in which pelvic ring disruptions occur anteriorly and posteriorly, resulting in a free pelvic segment that rotates toward the midline in a "bucket-handle fashion."

Hemorrhagic shock often accompanies severe pelvic fractures. Recent evidence suggests that laceration of small arterial branches at the fracture site is the major source of bleeding. Hemorrhage may be extraperitoneal, intraperitoneal, or retroperitoneal. The magnitude of blood loss, especially in the intraperitoneal region, may be massive. Retroperitoneal bleeding following pelvic fracture has a high mortality rate but is fortunately less common in children. Intraperitoneal bleeding will require laparotomy for definitive control. Retroperitoneal bleeding is much more difficult to control with exploratory surgery. Alternatively, angiographic evaluation with selective embolization has been proposed. Disruption of the ilium or SI joint separation is associated with injury to the common iliac vessels. Avulsion of the superior gluteal artery often accompanies posterior pelvic disruptions.

Urethral injury in children is infrequent, with partial tears being more common than complete disruption. Disruption of the urethra near the apex of the prostate results in rupture of the puboprostate ligament with subsequent displacement of the bladder superiorly (Fig. 124–5). Urethral injury should be suspected in patients with anterior pelvic fractures or pubic symphysis disruption, blood at the urethral meatus or on the undergarments, inability to avoid, displaced prostate on digital rectal examination, or in whom it is difficult to gently pass a Foley catheter.

In pediatric pelvic fractures, bladder injury is seen more often than urethral disruption. Signs of significant bladder injury include inability to void, suprapubic tenderness, and hematuria. Catheterization of the bladder is indicated unless resistance is met during initial passage. An excretory cystogram is helpful in finding small tears of the bladder.

An uncommon complication of pelvic fracture is bowel injury, occurring in less than 3% of cases. However, a reactive ileus is common. Entrapment of bowel between osseous fragments with subsequent obstruction has been described.

Stable Pelvic Ring Fractures. With a stable pelvic ring fracture, the pelvic ring remains intact and treatment is directed at correcting other injuries and providing comfort to the patient. Initial management consists of bedrest, early ambulation with crutches, and analgesics. If there is displacement of the fracture fragment off the margin of the ring, evaluation by an orthopedist is mandatory to determine if reduction is necessary.

A fracture of a wing of the ilium is the result of direct force against the lateral aspect of the pelvis, causing an infolding of the pliable wing of the ilium. Such fractures are uncommon in children.

The discovery of an isolated fracture in an ischiopubic ramus in one hemipelvis should lead to a search for a second fracture in the pelvic ring (Fig. 124–6). However, in the resilient pediatric pelvis, single ramus fractures have been reported. Straddle injury represents an important cause of inferior pubic rami fractures. If only one ramus or both rami on the same side are fractured, the patient may be treated symptomatically as an outpatient.

A minimal separation of the pubic symphysis is difficult to diagnose radiographically. Frequently the diagnosis must be made on physical examination alone. Treatment is symptomatic.

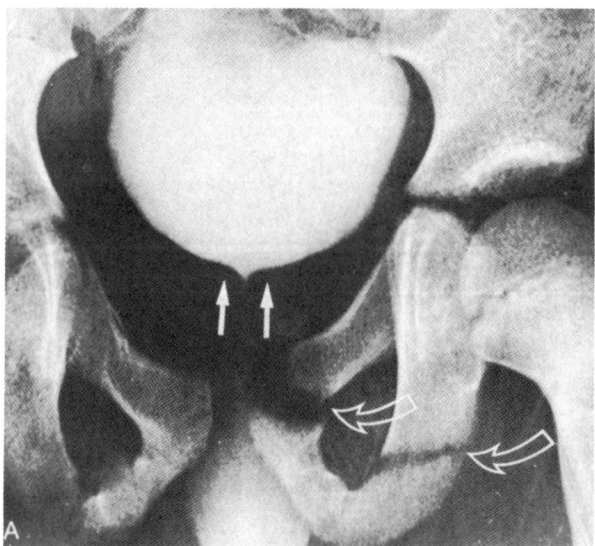 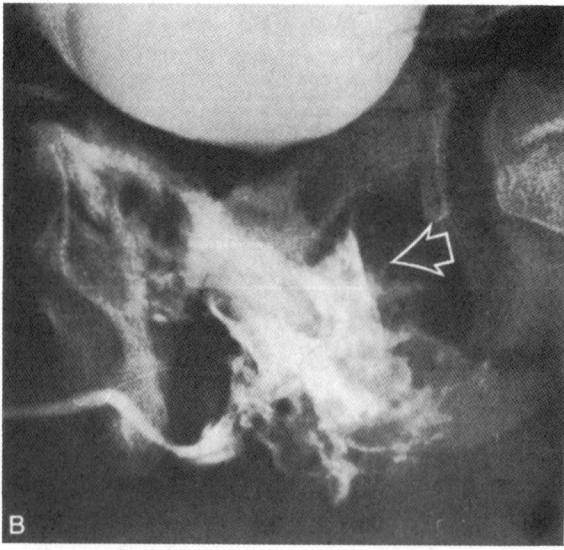

Figure 124–5. Multiple ramus injuries *(curved open arrow)* were associated with a bladder *(A, arrows)* and urethral *(B, arrow)* injury. (From Ogden JA. Skeletal Injury in the Child. 2nd ed. Philadelphia, WB Saunders, 1990, p 644.)

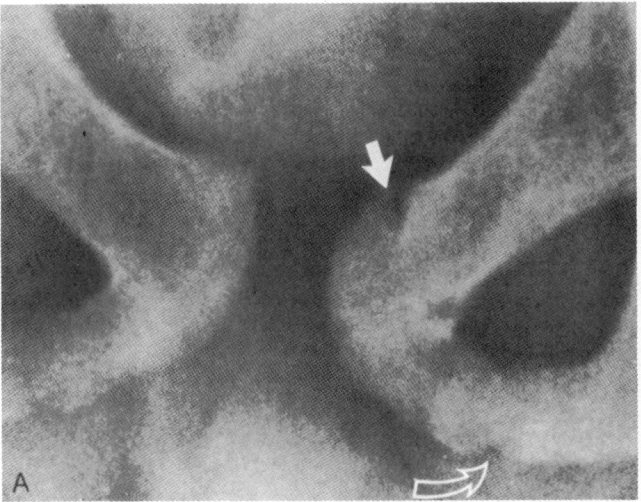
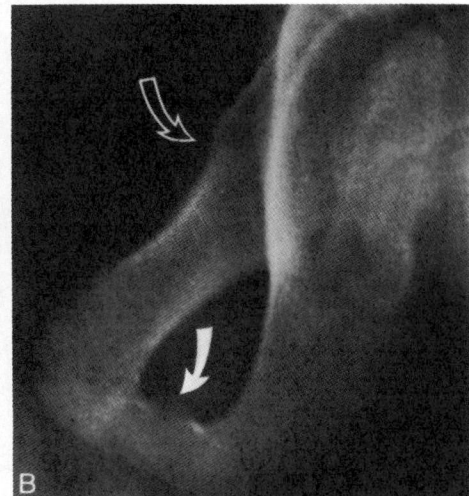
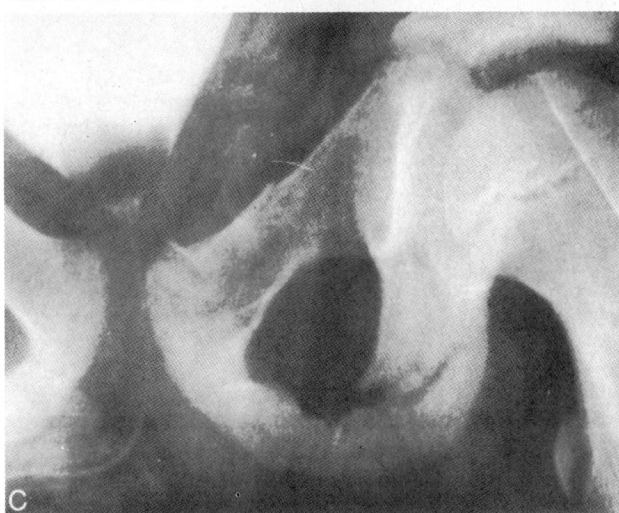

Figure 124–6. *A,* Minimally disrupted pubic ramus fracture *(solid arrow).* The ischial radiolucency *(open arrow)* is the normal synchondrosis, not a fracture. *B,* Fracture through the superior ramus in an 11-year-old child *(open arrow).* The apparent inferior ramus fracture *(solid arrow)* was really the closing ischiopubic synchondrosis. *C,* Multiple fractures of both rami. (From Odgen JA. Skeletal Injury in the Child. 2nd ed. Philadelphia, WB Saunders, 1990, p 636.)

Avulsion Fractures of the Pelvis

Pelvic avulsion fractures are a common type of pediatric pelvic fracture and are usually found in adolescent athletes between the ages of 14 and 17 years. Proposed mechanisms of injury are either violent muscular contraction or excessive amount of muscle stretch at an open apophysis. Common sites of pelvic avulsion fracture are the ASIS, AIIS, ischium, and iliac crest. Athletic modes of injury are usually involved with a history of extreme amount of effort in sprinters, jumpers, and soccer or football players (Fig. 124–7). Patients usually present with localized swelling, tenderness, and limitation of motion about the fracture site. Significant displacement of the avulsed fracture is uncommon; when present, reduction is necessary for optimal muscle function. Complications are unusual. Treatment consists of rest, relief from weight bearing with the use of crutches, muscle relaxants and analgesics, and discontinuation of the athletic activity.

Iliac spine avulsions are usually caused by activities involved with running and jumping. Common complaints are sudden onset of severe pain with the activity, severity of pain sufficient to result in discontinuation of the activity, and the feeling of a "snap" with the onset of pain. Swelling and tenderness are present. Ischial spine avulsions commonly occur with activities such as hurdling or gymnastics. Symptoms include sudden onset of pain, antalgic gait, and discomfort upon sitting. Referral to an orthopedic surgeon familiar with this injury is required. Avulsions of the iliac crest are an uncommon injury in children but may lead to

growth discrepancy. Symptoms may occur acutely or chronically such as with an apophysitis.

Soft Tissue Injuries

Soft tissue injuries constitute the majority of injuries found in young athletes. Usually these injuries are minor and can be treated with rest, ice, elevation, and return to regular activity with diminishment of pain.

Strain injuries in the pelvis commonly involve muscles arising in the symphysis pubis, such as the adductor longus, adductor brevis, and gracilis. Additionally, strains of the hamstrings and iliopsoas occur with some frequency. These injuries are associated with violent stretching or contraction of a musculotendinous unit. Treatment is supportive.

A particularly disabling (short-term) contusion is injury of the iliac crest (hip pointer). This injury occurs when a patient falls to the ground and strikes the iliac crest. Physical examination reveals difficulty in walking or standing upright secondary to the pain, local tenderness, and swelling, as well as local ecchymosis.

HIP INJURIES
Anatomy

The development of the acetabulum is chiefly determined by an aggregated growth plate of the triradiate cartilage, which is a confluence of the iliac, pubic, and ischial bones.

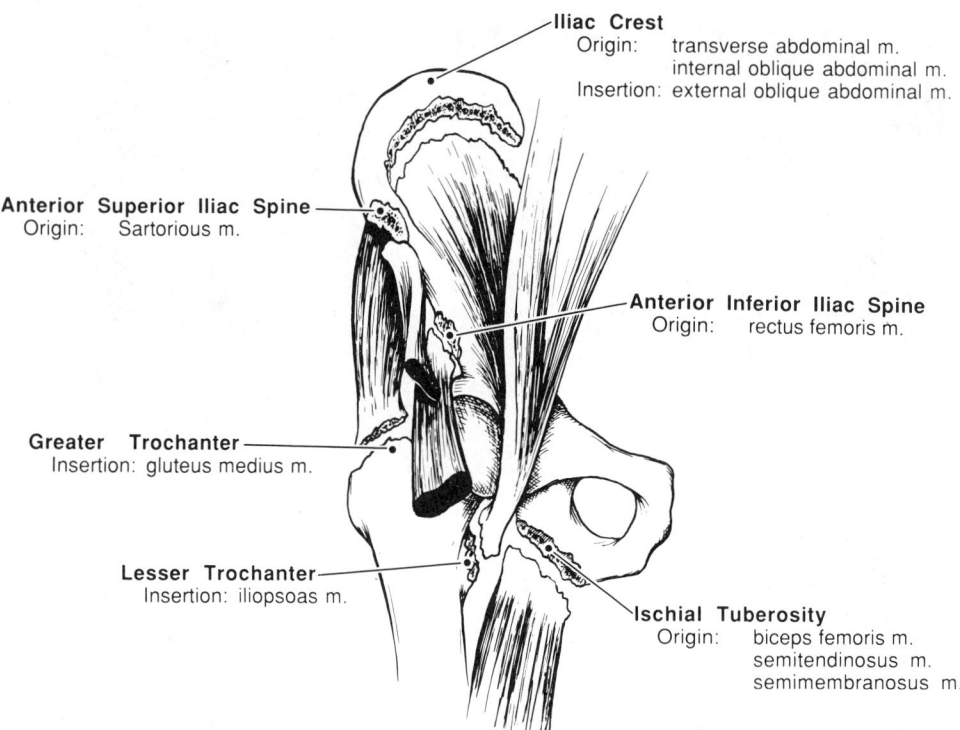

Iliac Crest
Origin: transverse abdominal m.
           internal oblique abdominal m.
Insertion: external oblique abdominal m.

Anterior Superior Iliac Spine
Origin: Sartorious m.

Anterior Inferior Iliac Spine
Origin: rectus femoris m.

Greater Trochanter
Insertion: gluteus medius m.

Lesser Trochanter
Insertion: iliopsoas m.

Ischial Tuberosity
Origin: biceps femoris m.
           semitendinosus m.
           semimembranosus m.

Figure 124–7. Muscle attachments about the pelvis and proximal femur. (From Wojtys EM. Sports injuries in the immature athlete. Orthop Clin North Am 1987; 18:700.)

At birth the capital epiphysis and greater trochanter are a single mass of cartilage, and no femoral neck is present. During the first year of life, capital femoral ossification centers appear, with subsequent development of the femoral head and appearance of the femoral neck. Ossification centers appear for the greater and lesser trochanter at ages 3 years and 8 years, respectively.

The vascular supply to the proximal femur is through the medial and lateral circumflex arteries, which originate from the femoral artery. Of lesser importance in the child is the artery of the round ligament, which provides a small complement of the blood supply to the femoral head. Injuries to the medial and lateral circumflex artery may result in significant hip problems.

Traumatic Hip Dislocation

Hip dislocation has a bimodal age distribution, with increased frequencies between the ages of 4 and 7 years and between 11 and 15 years.

When classifying traumatic hip dislocations, a line is drawn from the anterior superior iliac crest through the acetabulum to the ischial tuberosity; when the femoral head lies in front of this line it is referred to as an anterior dislocation; if it lies behind this line it is a posterior dislocation (Fig. 124–8).

Dislocations in children under the age of 6 years are often a result of minimal trauma such as falls or "doing splits." These dislocations are attributed to the laxity of the joint below the age of 6 years. In older children, usually severe trauma such as a motor vehicle accident or athletic injury is involved.

With a traumatic hip dislocation, the child is in pain and active movement of the affected hip is resisted. The child holds the painful thigh still and resists passive movement of the leg (Fig. 124–9).

Posterior dislocations make up approximately 80% of all pediatric traumatic hip dislocations; the femur is positioned between the sciatic notch and the acetabulum. The joint

capsule is torn posteriorly by the femoral head, and the involved lower limb is held in flexion, adduction, and internal rotation. The position is similar with the posterior ischiatic dislocation, with the exception that the leg may be in abduction or adduction (see Fig. 124–9). The femoral head may be palpable in the gluteal region in both injuries. The child is in severe pain and often resists active or passive motion at the hip.

Radiologic examination is essential to define the specific type of dislocation and to determine if a fracture is present. Gross displacement of the femoral head is usually visible on the anteroposterior view (Fig. 124–10). Additional views often required include that of the contralateral hip and a true crosstable lateral view of the hip joint. The standard

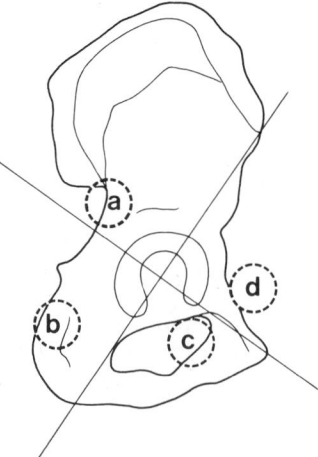

Figure 124–8. Types of hip dislocation. Posterior hip dislocations are (A) iliac and (B) ischiatic varieties; anterior hip dislocations are (C) obturator and (D) pubic varieties. (From Barquet A. Traumatic Hip Dislocation in Childhood. Berlin, Springer-Verlag, 1987, p 19.)

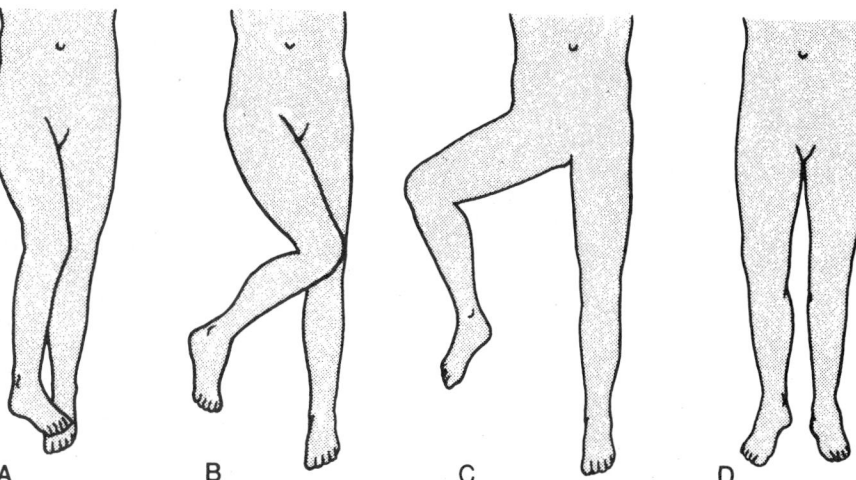

Figure 124–9. Typical deformity of the lower limb in the main varieties of traumatic hip dislocation: (A) iliac, (B) ischiatic, (C) obturator, (D) pubic. (From Barquet A. Traumatic Hip Dislocation in Childhood. Berlin, Springer-Verlag, 1987, p 50.)

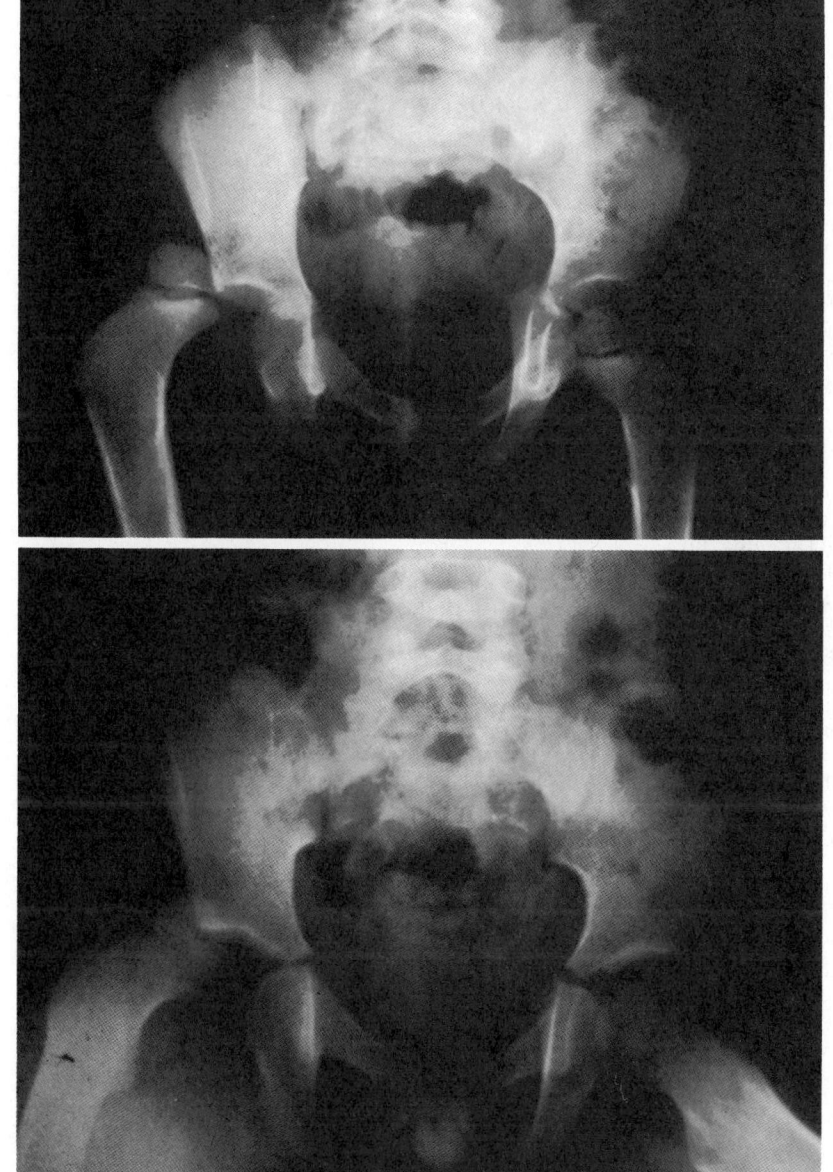

Figure 124–10. Traumatic posterior dislocation of right hip: iliac type. (From Tachdjian MO. Pediatric Orthopedics. 2nd ed. Vol 4. Philadelphia, WB Saunders, 1990, p 3219.)

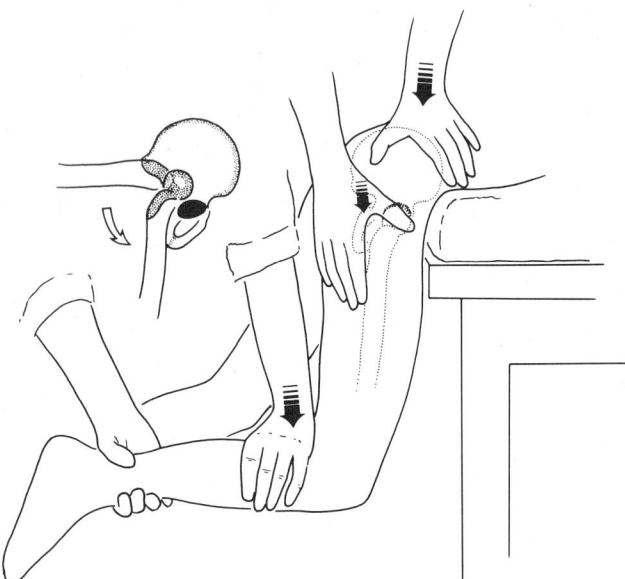

Figure 124–11. Closed reduction, method of Stimson. (From Ogden JA. Skeletal Injury in the Child. 2nd ed. Philadelphia, WB Saunders, p 667.)

anteroposterior view may demonstrate a seemingly normal appearance in retroacetabular dislocation. Computed tomography can define both the type of dislocation and whether associated fractures are present.

Early reduction (within 12 hours) is the recommended treatment of traumatic hip dislocations. General anesthesia is preferred unless associated injuries contraindicate its use. Closed reduction of acute uncomplicated posterior dislocations is usually possible, with the chief obstacle to reduction being the iliofemoral ligament. Three methods of closed reduction of posterior dislocations have been described: (1) the gravity method of Stimson (Fig. 124–11); (2) the direct method of Allis; and (3) the circumduction method of Bigelow. Reduction should be accomplished by physicians familiar with these procedures.

Anterior traumatic hip dislocations constitute approximately 10% of all pediatric dislocations. The anterior dislocations can be classified as either superior (pubic) or inferior (obturator). The affected limb is normally abducted, externally rotated, and shortened. These dislocations are often the result of a fall, with the impact being a direct blow on the posterior aspect of an abducted and externally rotated thigh. On physical examination, the femoral head is sometimes palpable in the groin (pubic dislocation). Avulsion fracture of the greater trochanter may accompany anterior dislocation. The diagnosis is confirmed with two-view radiographs of the anteroposterior hip and crosstable lateral hip.

Prompt closed reduction is usually possible with general anesthesia except with fracture-dislocation, for which open reduction is usually necessary. The procedure for reduction is best accomplished by an orthopedist.

Nerve and vascular injuries occur with total hip dislocation. Femoral shaft fractures may also occur and may not be appreciated acutely. Femoral head fractures associated with posterior dislocation have also been described. Acetabular fracture may occur with dislocation as in adults. Traumatic separation of the capital femoral epiphysis may occur either as a result of the dislocation or secondary to vigorous reduction. The major complications of traumatic hip dislocation are aseptic necrosis, sciatic nerve palsy, degenerative arthritis, and myositis ossificans.

Femoral Neck Fractures

Fractures of the femoral neck are rare in children. Because the vascular supply to the femoral head is distributed in the area of the femoral neck, such fractures can yield ischemic necrosis. A classification of four types of femoral neck fractures has been described based on anatomic locations: type 1, transepiphyseal; type 2, transcervical; type 3, cervical trochanter; and type 4, peritrochanteric (Fig. 124–12). Transepiphyseal fracture is the rarest type and has the worst prognosis. Transcervical and cervical trochanteric fractures are the most common. Peritrochanteric fractures have the overall best prognosis. Unfortunately, complications are common with femoral neck fractures, with avascular necrosis being the most frequent.

Stress fractures of the femoral neck secondary to chronic repetitive microtrauma may occur. The diagnosis should be suspected in a competitive athlete with persistent discomfort in the groin region. Local tenderness as well as limitation of motion may be seen. Plain radiographs may appear normal, and a bone scan may be necessary to demonstrate the lesion.

Acetabular Fractures

Fractures of the acetabulum are uncommon in children; they may be associated with hip dislocation but at a rate less than in adults. Long-term effects seem to be associated with the status of the superior dome of the acetabulum or the presence of loose fragments within the joints. All acetabular fractures should be referred to an orthopedic surgeon.

Trochanteric Fractures

Avulsion fractures of the greater trochanteric apophysis are seen most often in adolescents. The growth center

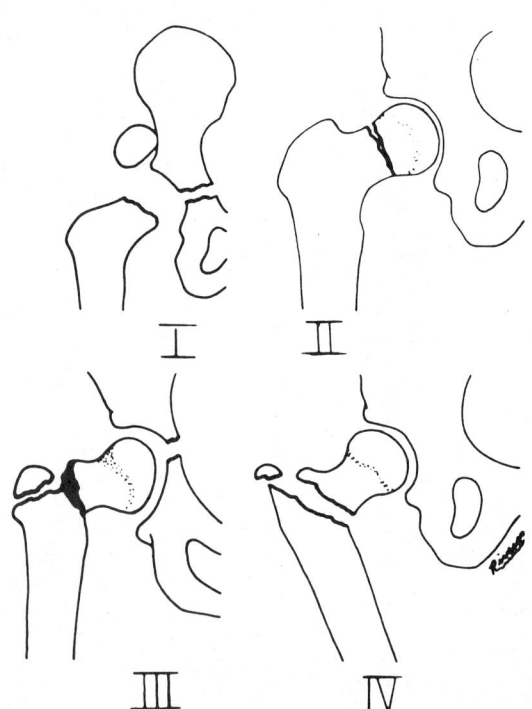

Figure 124–12. Classification of hip fractures in children: I, transepiphyseal, with or without dislocation from the acetabulum; II, transcervical; III, cervicotrochanteric; IV, trochanteric. (From Canale ST. Fracture of the hip in children and adolescents. Orthop Clin North Am 1990;21:341.)

appears initially at 4 years of age and does not completely fuse with the proximal femur until 18 years of age. Avulsion is usually the result of sudden vigorous contraction of the gluteus medius or minimus muscles against resistance or a direct blow to the hip. Complete avulsion is a serious injury that requires internal fixation. A small accessory ossification center at the tip of the greater trochanter is sometimes confused as a fracture. This finding is a normal variant in children between the ages of 7 and 10 years.

Usually the adolescent complains of experiencing a sudden sharp pain in the anterior hip while running, which resulted in immediate cessation of activity. Additionally, pain along the inner aspect of the thigh, a limp, an inability to flex the thigh, and tenderness in the region of the lesser trochanter are present. External rotation of the thigh may be seen. Radiographs must be taken with the thigh in external rotation for an adequate view of the lesser trochanter. Comparison views may be necessary. Most authors advocate nonoperative treatment.

Soft Tissue Injury

Contusions, abrasions, and muscular strains constitute the predominant forms of hip injuries that children will sustain. These injuries are frequently minimal and can be treated with a brief period of rest, ice, and gradual return to regular activities.

The iliopsoas is one of the most common muscles to be strained in children, often with involvement at the site of tendon attachment. The mechanism of injury involves a forced extension of the flexed hip, such as a sudden stop while sprinting. The leg is held in flexion and adduction, with marked resistance to movement. Specific therapy consists of bedrest with hip flexed and adducted, ice, analgesia, and early mobilization on crutches.

Snapping hip syndrome has been described as irritation of the iliotibial band of the greater trochanteric bursa associated with hip flexion and extension, especially in internal rotation. Patients will frequently describe a sensation of hip dislocation. Treatment consists of nonsteroidal anti-inflammatory medication and rest.

Femur Injuries

Fracture of the femur, especially in the middiaphyseal region, is a relatively frequent injury in children. The most common site of fracture is the middle third of the femur (Fig. 124–13). These fractures are generally a result of a violent injury. The peak age for femoral fractures is 3 years. Femoral fractures occurring in children younger than 3 years should evoke suspicion of child abuse.

Pediatric subtrochanteric fractures are usually due to direct trauma of the hip area. There is a tendency of the proximal fragment to be displaced superiorly and medially secondary to muscle forces, which creates an unstable fracture. Unfortunately bone remodeling and healing in this region of the femur are not as extensive as in other areas, and permanent disability may result.

Fractures of the Femoral Shaft

Fractures of the femoral shaft are common in childhood and are serious injuries. Extensive soft tissue damage accompanies such a fracture. Blood loss of 500 ml is common. The source of this bleeding is usually from the profunda femoris artery or from the vessels within the bone itself. Usually, distal fracture fragments are laterally rotated with variable amounts of overriding.

The fracture is often obvious from the clinical examina-

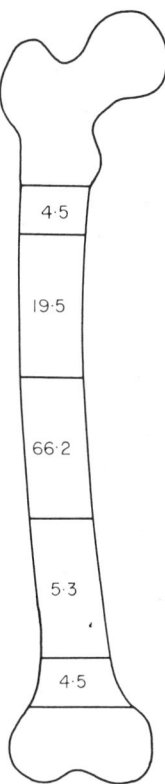

Figure 124–13. Incidence of femoral fracture by site from a large series. (From Burwell HN. Fractures of the femoral shaft in children. Postgrad Med J 1968;45:617.)

tion, with deformity, tenderness, and swelling of the fracture site, shortening of the limb, and external rotation. Gentle examination is important to minimize further soft tissue damage. The neurovascular status in the lower limb should be assessed for injury to the femoral or popliteal vessels or to the sciatic nerve (particularly with posterior displacement of the distal fragment). With femoral fractures, the physical examination should consider injury to the ipsilateral hip. In patients with a traumatic hip dislocation and femoral fracture, 45% of dislocations go unrecognized initially. Proper splinting should precede radiographs.

Complications such as hypotension are rare in the child who sustains a closed femoral fracture without vascular injury. Only one half of children with femoral fractures have a measurable drop in hematocrit. Children with hypotension or a falling hematocrit should be evaluated for other injuries.

Arterial injury can occur with a closed femoral shaft fracture. Distal arterial pulses are present in approximately one fourth of the patients with arterial injury. This is probably due to either partial arterial injury or significant collateral circulation. Characteristics that favor arterial injury are high-velocity or high-energy injuries, significant soft tissue damage, markedly displaced fracture fragments, absence of distal pulses on presentation, increasing limb girth, and progressive neurologic signs. The presence of such signs and symptoms indicates a need for prompt arteriography or exploration.

Fractures to the distal metaphyseal aspect of the femur are relatively uncommon in children. When these fractures occur they are often incomplete, such as a torus fracture, or, if complete, are transverse in orientation. These fractures usually heal without complication, with the possible exception of an angular deformity. Early referral to an orthopedic surgeon is recommended.

KNEE INJURIES

The pattern of injuries to the child's knee joint is significantly different from the adult pattern. More often severe injuries result in fractures of the bones that form the knee rather than in ligamentous injuries. Ligamentous injuries of the knee joint do occur in children; however, such injuries are less frequent than fractures and are extremely rare in children less than 14 years old. The paucity of injuries to ligaments is probably due to thick articular and growth cartilage, which absorbs impact energy, and the greater tensile strength differences of ligaments with respect to epiphyseal growth plates.

The area about the knee determines approximately 65% of the longitudinal growth of the lower extremity, with the distal femoral epiphysis consistently contributing two thirds of this growth, and the proximal tibial epiphysis one third. The ossification center of the distal femur is present at birth and fuses between the ages of 14 and 19 years. The cruciate ligaments blend into the epiphyseal cartilage of the distal femur (at the intercondylar notch) and the proximal tibial spines. The menisci assume their characteristic shape during prenatal development. At birth the patella is cartilaginous and therefore radiolucent. Central ossification begins at approximately 5 years of age and proceeds centrifugally, often resulting in irregular margins. The lateral and medial collateral ligaments firmly attach to the growth epiphysis. The tibial tuberosity is a distinct structure at birth; a secondary ossification center forms around 7 years of age and fuses between 13 and 19 years.

Hip disease or injury can cause knee pain. Legg-Calvé-Perthes disease and slipped capital femoral epiphysis may present as knee pain because the child may be unable to localize the discomfort. In a child who complains of knee pain after injury, the following conditions should be considered: (1) distal femoral epiphyseal separation; (2) tibial spine fracture; (3) patellar dislocation or fracture; (4) tibial tuberosity avulsion; (5) proximal tibial epiphyseal separations; and (6) knee dislocation.

Distal Femoral Epiphyseal Injuries

Epiphyseal separations and fractures of the distal femoral epiphysis are often described by the Salter-Harris system. The child will have severe pain and inability to bear weight on the affected leg. The knee joint will be swollen, and a joint effusion may be present. Circumferential tenderness is usually present around the entire epiphyseal plate. Examination should include careful assessment of the neurovascular status. This injury occasionally presents as an apparent ligament separation. All such injuries should be referred to an orthopedist.

Type I fractures may be difficult to diagnose because of subtle or no findings on radiographs. Standard radiographic views for knee evaluation, as well as valgus and varus stress and anteroposterior stress views, may be necessary to demonstrate the injury. Comparison films of the uninjured leg are often helpful. Type II fractures are often reported as the most frequent type of distal femoral injury in children and have the best prognosis. Types III, IV, and V fractures have a much poorer prognosis.

Proximal Tibial Injuries

A fracture or avulsion of the tibial spine is an injury usually found in 8- to 15-year-old children, often resulting from bicycle accidents or athletic injury. Because the anterior cruciate ligament attaches to the base of the tibial spine, such injuries usually have a component of anterior cruciate

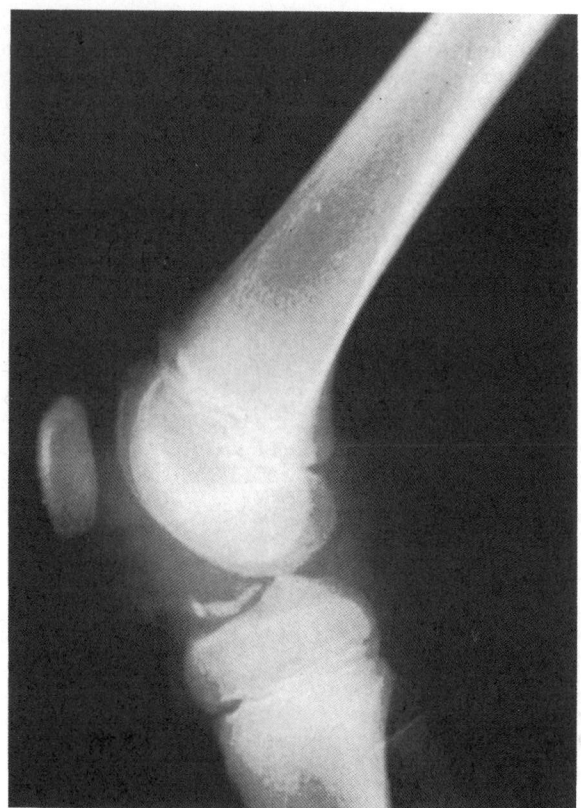

Figure 124–14. A minimally displaced fracture of the anterior tibial spine was treated conservatively by an above-knee cast with the knee in extension. (From Tachdjian MO. Pediatric Orthopedics. 2nd ed. Vol 4. Philadelphia, WB Saunders, 1990, p 3288.)

disruption owing to avulsion of the spine. Concomitant painful hemarthrosis often precludes diagnosis with an anterior drawer sign. Anteroposterior and lateral radiographs are essential to visualize the bone fragment and degree of displacement (Fig. 124–14). Emergency department treatment includes analgesia, splinting the knee, elevation, and possible knee aspiration for large, painful effusions. Open and closed treatment are both used depending on injury.

Tibial Tuberosity Injuries

The two major problems associated with the tibial tuberosity are those of acute avulsion injuries and the Osgood-Schlatter lesion. Avulsion fractures occur in boys between the ages of 14 and 16 years. The mechanism of the injury involves a violent active contraction of the quadriceps muscle or passive flexion of the knee with the quadriceps contracted. A preexisting Osgood-Schlatter lesion may predispose individuals to an acute avulsion. Type I fractures involve only the most distal portion of the tuberosity (Fig. 124–15). Type II fractures are those in which the fracture line extends into the joint and there is little or no displacement of the distal fragment. Type III injuries are those with significant joint involvement. Diagnosis is based on pain and swelling at the proximal end of the tibia as well as the inability to extend the knee against gravity or force. Radiographs are essential; the lateral view identifies fragment size and the extent of displacement. Emergency department treatment consists of splint immobilization, analgesia, ice, and referral to an orthopedist. Open reduction and surgical fixation are frequently used.

The Osgood-Schlatter lesion is a partial separation of the

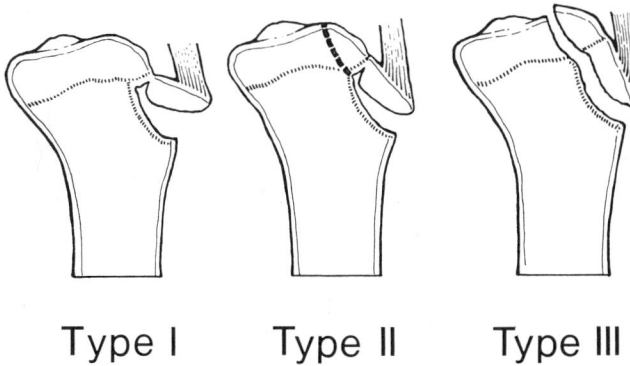

Type I   Type II   Type III

Figure 124–15. Classification of tibial tuberosity fractures. (From Singer KM, Henry J. Knee problems in children and adolescents. Clin Sports Med 1985;4:385.)

endochondral or osseous chondral portion of the tibial tuberosity. Chronic repetitive trauma is thought to be the most likely cause. It is seen bilaterally in 25% of patients. Treatment is generally supportive, with discontinuation of sports or activities that exacerbate the condition and immobilization with a splint.

Knee Dislocations

Dislocations of the knee are extremely rare in children. Because trauma sufficient to cause knee dislocation in the child is usually great, these injuries are frequently associated with distal femur or proximal tibial fracture as well as significant soft tissue damage, including blood vessel and nerve injury. Careful evaluation of the posterior tibialis and dorsalis pedis pulses should be performed in children with knee dislocation. If the pulses are absent, prompt reduction of the dislocation should be performed and the pulses reevaluated. Because collateral circulation of the knee is poor, such injuries may lead to Volkmann's ischemia in the lower extremity. The popliteal artery traverses the popliteal fossa and is anchored above the femur at the adductor hiatus and below the tibia by the fibrous arch over the soleus muscle. Anterior knee dislocation causes a stretch on the popliteal artery, which may yield internal damage, while posterior dislocation may cause complete disruption of the artery. Arteriography provides limited information and may delay the time interval between discovery of injury and surgical correction. Observation of a warm but pulseless leg after reduction of a dislocation of the knee is unwarranted and should prompt expedient surgical evaluation.

Floating Knee

The floating knee is a term applied to a flail knee segment resulting from fracture of the femur as well as ipsilateral tibia-fibula fracture (Fig. 124–16). This unusual fracture is associated with life-threatening injuries in children and, unlike in adults, appears not to be associated with fat embolis. It is usually caused when a child riding a bicycle collides with an automobile. The automobile bumper strikes the lower leg, resulting in the tibia-fibula fracture, and the hood of the car causes the femur fracture. Associated injuries are often missed on initial examination.

Injuries to the Extensor Mechanism of the Knee

The extensor mechanism of the knee—quadriceps tendon, patella, patellar ligament, and tibial tuberosity—is a common site of injury in the child. Although acute dislocation of the patella is seen in young, physically active people, it is an infrequent injury in the skeletally immature individual. Acute dislocation is often associated with a preexisting abnormality of the extensor mechanism, such as patellar-femoral dysplasia. Between 5% and 10% of acute dislocations are complicated by an osteochondral fracture, which is found as a small fragment off the lateral femoral condyle or medial aspect of the patella. The vast majority of acute dislocations are lateral. Medial dislocation is extremely rare and is usually associated with muscle disease or paralysis such as polio.

Acute dislocation may be caused by either a direct blow to the medial side of the patella or a twisting muscular contraction when there is valgus strain on the knee. Most dislocations reduce spontaneously or are reduced by the patient prior to arrival at the hospital. Therefore certain diagnosis is not always possible. The patient is often unsure the patellar dislocation has occurred, and it may sometimes be difficult to differentiate this injury from a meniscal tear or ligamentous disruption. There is often tenderness along the medial aspect of the patella and over the lateral femoral condyle. The patellar apprehension test is performed by gently pushing laterally on the patella; it is positive if it yields apprehension in patients who feel their patella is prone to dislocate.

Radiographs are taken of the knee to exclude other injuries and to determine if an osteochondral fracture has occurred. Splinting and immobilization, crutches, and referral to an orthopedist for evaluation of chronic underlying pathology or chronic subluxation are appropriate.

Intra-articular dislocation, although rare, may occur in children. There are two types: horizontal, where the superior or inferior pole of the patella is displaced into the femoral intercondylar notch (Fig. 124–17); and vertical, where the patella is rotated on its vertical axis and the edge is lying in the intercondylar notch. Closed reduction is usually not effective. Open reduction is the primary procedure for both reduction of the dislocation and injury repair of ligaments or tendons.

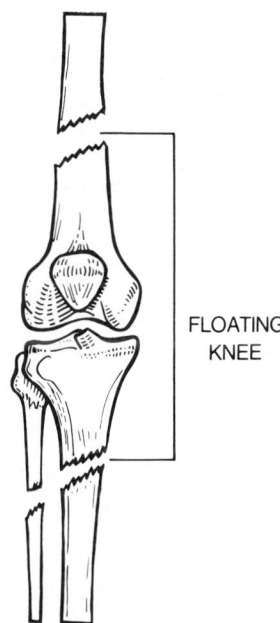

FLOATING KNEE

Figure 124–16. Diagram of the floating knee injury in children. (From Letts M, Vincent N, Gouw G. The "floating knee" in children. J Bone Joint Surg 1986;68B:442.)

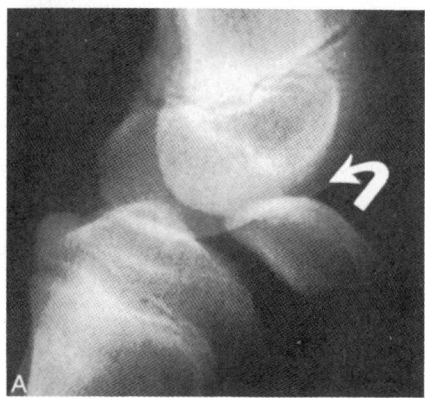

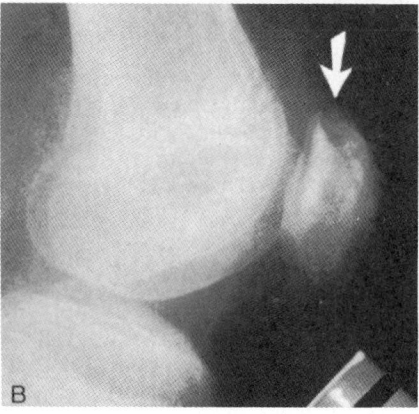

Figure 124–17. *A*, Lateral radiograph of intra-articular dislocation *(arrow)* of the patella. *B*, Postreduction film showing osteoporosis of the proximal pole where quadriceps avulsion occurred *(arrow)*. (From Ogden JA. Skeletal Injury in the Child. 2nd ed. Philadelphia, WB Saunders, 1990, p 754.)

Patellar Fractures

Patellar fractures may occur from a direct blow to the patella, a patellar dislocation, or an avulsion injury. These injuries are often difficult to diagnose in younger children owing to the minimal ossification of the patella. Predisposing factors to patellar fractures are neuromuscular disease (especially cerebral palsy) and sports activities involving jumping. A patellar injury that is rare yet unique to children is the "sleeve fracture," so named because the cartilaginous lower pole of the patella is often avulsed with little or no bone attached (Fig. 124–18).

The diagnosis is supported by the absence of direct trauma to the knee, instability to the knee, severe pain, and inability to bear weight or actively extend the knee. The patella assumes a higher than normal position on the affected side, and a palpable gap is present at the inferior pole of the patella. Lateral view radiographs usually demonstrate the fracture best. Referral to an orthopedic surgeon is necessary.

Direct blows to the patella may result in a stellate fracture in the older child and a crush fracture in the younger child. These fractures should be distinguished from the bipartite patella, which is a developmental anomaly. Differentiation is sometimes difficult. Patients with a bipartite patella are usually asymptomatic; this anomaly is found bilaterally in approximately 40% of patients and is more frequent in males. Chronic fractures may also simulate this appearance. Patellar fractures should be referred to an orthopedic surgeon.

Osteochondral fractures infrequently occur on the medial or lateral femoral chondylar articular surface or on the patellar surface in children. This type of fracture occurs almost exclusively in the adolescent. These fractures are usually caused by a direct blow to the knee or by rapid dislocation of the patella associated with spontaneous reduction. The clinical features include an adolescent-aged patient, a history of a direct blow to a flexed knee, an audible or felt snap in the knee, a bloody effusion with occasional fat droplets, and the inability to actively extend the knee joint. The fracture is often difficult to appreciate on radiograph, and additional views of the knee such as oblique, tunnel, and patellar may be necessary. Negative radiographs have been reported. Treatment consists of arthroscopic surgical removal of the loose fragment.

Proximal Tibial Injuries

Fracture of the intercondylar eminence of the tibia is an injury usually seen in 8- to 15-year-old children. The anterior cruciate ligament attaches to the base of the eminence (tibial spine) and is often injured as a part of this injury. The patient presents with a painful swollen knee with the inability to bear weight and reluctance to extend the knee. Anterior drawer sign is often present. Radiographs usually provide the diagnosis; the lateral view is often best. Treatment is immobilization and orthopedic referral.

Meniscal Injuries

Meniscal injuries are rare in skeletally immature individuals; adolescents experience this injury most frequently. Symptoms are often nonspecific, with pain being the most common, reported in approximately 84% of all patients. Pain and knee swelling and pain and knee instability are the most predictable symptom complexes, suggesting a significant meniscal injury. Thirty-six percent of patients describe some type of locking of the knee. Joint line tenderness is the most predictable sign, with McMurray's sign present in

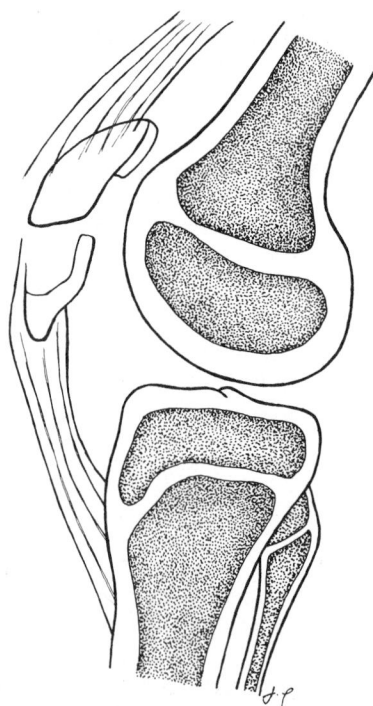

Figure 124–18. Sleeve fracture of the patella. (From Nicholas JA, Hershman EB. The Lower Extremity and Spine in Sports Medicine. Vol 2. St Louis, CV Mosby, 1986, p 127.)

approximately one half of patients. Accurate diagnosis within the emergency department is often difficult in the acutely injured patient. Once a fracture is excluded, immobilization with referral to an orthopedic surgeon is often warranted since arthroscopy is usually required for definitive diagnosis.

Ligamentous Injuries

The usual approach to ligamentous injuries of the knee in children is to diagnose aggressively but to treat conservatively. Although uncommon, ligament injury must be considered in all pediatric patients with acute knee pain after injury. The appearance of ligamentous injury and the time of physeal closure about the knee may be related, in that ligament injury is rare before 14 years of age. In addition, ligament damage may accompany chondro-osseous fracture and remain undiagnosed if the examiner is not alert to such lesions.

The examination should focus on a careful assessment of the knee, including examination for laxity of the unaffected knee. The examiner should focus on medial-lateral as well as anteroposterior instability of the knee. Stress radiographs in a relaxed patient may be helpful.

Few injuries to the collateral ligaments have been reported in children less than 14 years of age. In examining the child's knee, the medial structures are best tested with the knee in 30 degrees of flexion. The medial opening of the knee in extension indicates serious damage to medial structures. If there is medial stability in extension but not in flexion, the examiner must check for rotary instability owing to possible damage of the cruciate ligaments such as a positive anterior drawer sign, which demonstrates injury to the anterior cruciate. Lateral instability is less common than medial instability but is more disabling. The amount of laxity should be checked against the uninjured knee because of variable amounts of physiologic opening. Lateral instability should be evaluated in 0 degrees and 30 degrees of flexion. Instability at 0 degrees of flexion indicates major damage to the lateral collateral apparatus. Instability at 30 degrees is a less serious injury. Stress radiographs may be helpful. Careful examinations of radiographs may reveal avulsion fractures at the insertion of the collateral ligaments. Acute treatment is conservative, with immobilization, elevation, and the use of crutches.

Isolated cruciate ligament injuries are rare in children but are associated with tibial spine injuries. Anterior instability is more difficult to diagnose than medial or lateral instability. The anterior drawer sign should be tested in neutral, internal, and external rotation. Anterior laxity in the neutral position suggests injury to the anterior cruciate, while laxity in internal rotation suggests involvement of both the anterior and the posterior cruciate ligaments. Posterior instability is extremely rare in the child, with physical examination usually demonstrating a grossly positive posterior drawer sign. Routine as well as stress radiographs should be performed. Acute treatment of cruciate injuries should be conservative, with immobilization, use of crutches, and possible aspiration of hemarthrosis. Referral to an orthopedic surgeon is necessary.

LEG INJURIES

Fractures of the shaft of the tibia or fibula are common in infants and children. This region is especially susceptible to injury as the child is first learning to walk (the toddler fracture). Often these fractures present as minimally displaced spiral fractures, heal rapidly, and have a minimal effect on growth.

Metaphyseal fractures of the tibia are relatively uncommon in children, with the modal period being between 3 and 8 years of age. Twisting injuries rather than direct trauma are the most frequent cause. Distal fragments if displaced are in the lateral direction, but opposition is usually good. Torus fractures are common and not innocuous, in that such an injury may lead to valgus angulation with medial overgrowth owing to asymmetric development after the injury. Parents should be warned of this complication in advance. Significantly displaced metaphyseal fractures of the tibia (especially those from direct trauma) may result in vascular compromise to the distal extremity. This complication is related to the position of the trifurcation of the tibial artery in relation to the tibial metaphysis. Proximal tibial fractures with lateral displacement of the fracture fragments are associated with major arterial injury and possible development of compartment syndrome. Prompt orthopedic referral of metaphyseal fractures is recommended.

Fractures of the tibial and fibular diaphysis are the most common type of leg fractures in children. The most common mechanism of injury is twisting. Direct trauma secondary to motor vehicle accidents is also common. Tibial fractures in infants secondary to attempts at intraosseous infusion placement have been reported. Infants and young children up to the age of approximately 40 months demonstrate an isolated spiral fracture of the tibia, which has been termed the CAST (childhood accidental spiral tibial) fracture. Distal metaphyseal and diaphyseal spiral fractures are also well described as toddler fractures. Children between the ages of 3 and 6 years of age similarly experience spiral tibial fractures, often extending more proximally into the metaphysis and sometimes accompanied with greenstick fractures of the fibular metaphysis. In children between the ages of 5 and 10 years, transverse fractures of the tibia secondary to direct trauma predominate. Adolescents commonly experience midshaft tibial fractures, frequently with the formation of a butterfly fragment.

With the exception of the toddler fracture, tibial fractures usually do not present a diagnostic problem. A child who is first learning to walk may sustain a twisting injury and subsequently refuse to bear weight; such a child should be evaluated for the toddler fracture. Examination often reveals no deformity, but careful palpation may localize the tenderness. Fractures are not always evident on radiographs and must be splinted for 10 to 14 days for reexamination for evidence of callus formation on radiograph. In the older child, examination often reveals swelling, tenderness, deformity, and occasional crepitus. Radiographs should confirm the diagnosis. Careful evaluation of the nerve and vascular function should be completed. Undisplaced fractures may be treated on an outpatient basis; a more complicated fracture may require admission to the hospital. All of these injuries require a reduction of fractures, immobilization in a long-leg cast with the knee flexed, elevation, and analgesia. The most serious complication of lower leg fracture is the development of a compartment syndrome. A compartment syndrome is usually associated with leg fractures that involve crush injury, vascular injury, or severe soft tissue injuries such as those secondary to a ringer-type injury. Irreversible changes occur after 6 to 8 hours, related to vascular compromise. Significant pain on passive stretching of the involved compartment muscle is an early finding. Other later findings include paresthesia, pallor, pulselessness, and paralysis.

Selected References

Borquet A. Traumatic hip dislocations with fracture of the ipsilateral femoral shaft in childhood. Arch Orthop Trauma Surg 1981;98:69.

Brunette DD, Fifield G, Ruiz E, et al. Use of pneumatic antishock trousers in the management of pediatric pelvic hemorrhage. Pediatr Emerg Care 1987;3:86.

Buchan JR. Bowel entrapment by pelvic fracture fragments: A case report and review of the literature. Clin Orthop 1980;147:164.

Burnell HN. Fractures of the femoral shaft in children. Postgrad Med J 1969;45:617.

Canale ST. Fractures of the hip in children and adolescents. Orthop Clin North Am 1990;21:341.

Clancy WG, Foltz AS. Iliac apophysitis and stress fractures in adolescent runners. Am J Sports Med 1976;4:214.

Clanton TO, DeLee JC, Sanders B, et al. Knee ligament injuries in children. J Bone Joint Surg 1979;61A:1195.

Craig CL. Hip injuries in children and adolescents. Orthop Clin North Am 1980;11:743.

Crawford AH. Fractures about the knee in children. Orthop Clin North Am 1976;7:639.

Dalton HJ, Slovis T, Helfer RE, et al. Undiagnosed abuse in children younger than 3 years with femoral fracture. Am J Dis Child 1990;144:875.

Dick T. Traction splinting: A comparative look at the tools of the trade. J Emerg Med Serv 1981;6:26.

Donohue JP. Urethral and bladder injuries in children. Pediatr Clin North Am 1975;22:393.

Garnet RA. Pediatric urethral and perineal injuries. Pediatr Clin North Am 1975;22:401.

Gartland JJ, Brenner JH. Traumatic dislocations in the lower extremity in children. Orthop Clin North Am 1970;1:29.

Green NE, Allen BL. Vascular injuries associated with dislocation of the knee. J Bone Joint Surg 1977;59A:236.

Griffen PP, Anderson, Green WT. Fractures of the shaft of the femur in children. Orthop Clin North Am 1972;3:213.

Houghton GR, Ackroyd CE. Sleeve fractures of the patella in children. J Bone Joint Surg 1979;61B:165.

Isaacson J, Louis DS, Costenbader JM. Arterial injury associated with closed femoral shaft fracture. J Bone Joint Surg 1975;57A:1147.

Izant RJ, Hubay CA. The annual injury of fifteen million children. J Trauma 1966;6:65.

Izhar UH, Munkange L. Femoral fracture in children (a prospective study of 204 fractures). Med J Zambia 1982;16:51.

Letts M, Vincent N, Gouw G. The "floating knee" in children. J Bone Joint Surg 1986;688:4423.

Micheli LJ. Overuse injury in children's sports. Orthop Clin North Am 1983;14:337.

Nogi J. Common pediatric musculoskeletal emergencies. Emerg Med Clin North Am 1984;2:409.

Nolan RA. Tibial epiphyseal injuries. Contemp Orthop 1978;1:11.

Ogden JA, Tross RB, Murphy MJ. Fractures of the tibial tuberosity in adolescents. J Bone Joint Surg 1980;62A:205.

Peclet MH, Newman KD, Eichelberger MR, et al. Patterns of injury in children. J Pediatr Surg 1990;25:85.

Pennsylvania Orthopedic Society. Traumatic dislocation of the hip joint in children. Final report by the Scientific Research Society. J Bone Joint Surg 1968;50A:79.

Quinby WC. Fractures of the pelvis and associated injuries in children. J Pediatr Surg 1966;1:353.

Reed MH. Pelvic fractures in children. J Can Assoc Radiol 1976;27:255.

Reichard SA, Helikson MA, Shorter S, et al. Pelvic fractures in children—review of 120 patients with a new look at general management. J Pediatr Surg 1986;15:727.

Singer KM, Henry J. Knee problems in children and adolescents. Clin Sports Med, 1985;4:385.

Soren A, Felto JF: Pathology, clinic, and treatment of Osgood-Schlatter disease. Orthopedics 1984;7:230.

Torode I, Zieg D. Pelvic fractures in children. J Pediatr Orthop 1985;5:76.

Waters PM, Millis MB. Hip and pelvic injuries in the young athlete. Clin Sports Med 1988;7:513.

Wolfgang GL. Stress fracture of the femoral neck in a patient with open capital femoral epiphyses. J Bone Joint Surg 1977;59A:680.

Worsing RA. Principles of prehospital care of musculoskeletal injuries. Emerg Clin North Am 1984;2:205.

Young JWR, Burgess AR, Brumback RJ, et al. Lateral compression fractures of the pelvis: The importance of plain radiographs in the diagnosis and surgical management. Skeletal Radiol 1986;15:103.

CHAPTER 125

Ankle and Foot Injuries

Edward P. Sloan
T. J. Rittenberry

ANATOMY

Three bones form the ankle joint (Fig. 125–1): the weight-bearing tibia and non–weight-bearing fibula of the lower leg articulate with the talus, the most proximal tarsal bone. The tibia forms the ankle "plafond" (ceiling), as well as the medial malleolus. The fibula forms the lateral malleolus. These bones form the tibiofibular syndesmosis, or fibrous joint, at the ankle. The joint between the talus and tibia is called the talocrural or tibiotalar joint.

The ankle is a hinge joint that permits plantar flexion and dorsiflexion about a transverse axis. Excessive inversion and eversion are prevented by ligaments that connect the tibia, fibula, talus, and calcaneus. The strong deltoid ligament joins the tibia and talus medially. Three lateral collateral ligaments support the fibula laterally. Anterior and posterior ligaments, part of the syndesmosis, also support these bones.

Thirteen tendons, each wrapped by a fibrous retinaculum, cross the ankle joint external to the articular capsule. No muscles cross the ankle joint.

The bones of the foot are separated into the hindfoot, midfoot, and forefoot (Fig. 125–2). The hindfoot includes two tarsals, the talus and calcaneus, which form the subtalar joint. The hindfoot is separated from the midfoot by Chopart's joint. The midfoot includes five tarsals: the navicular, the cuboid, and three cuneiforms. The tarsal navicular articulates with the talus and cuneiforms on the medial side of the foot; the cuboid articulates with the calcaneus and metatarsals laterally. Lisfranc's joint separates the midfoot and forefoot. The forefoot includes the metatarsals and phalanges.

The nerves and muscles that direct ankle and foot movement can be divided into three compartments. The anterior crural muscles, which effect foot inversion and eversion, ankle dorsiflexion, and toe extension, are innervated by the deep peroneal nerve (L4–S1). This nerve provides sensory function to the web space between the great and the second toes. The posterior crural muscles, which effect ankle plantar flexion, foot inversion, and toe flexion, are innervated by the tibial nerve (L4–S3). This nerve provides sensory function to the heel of the foot. The lateral crural muscles effect ankle plantar flexion and foot eversion. The superficial peroneal nerve (L5–S2) provides motor function to these muscles as well as sensation to the dorsum of the foot. The medial and lateral plantar nerves (S1–S3), which are the terminal branches of the tibial nerve, provide motor innervation to the foot intrinsic muscles and sensation to the plantar surface of the foot. The saphenous and sural nerves provide sensation to the medial and lateral sides of the dorsal foot, respectively.

Although difficult to conceptualize, the numerous movements of the ankle and foot are essential to the understanding of ankle and foot injuries. Ankle plantar flexion (flexion) is the downward movement of the foot away from the leg. Dorsiflexion (extension) is the upward movement of the foot toward the leg. Inversion is the non–weight-bearing, inward movement of the plantar surface of the foot toward the

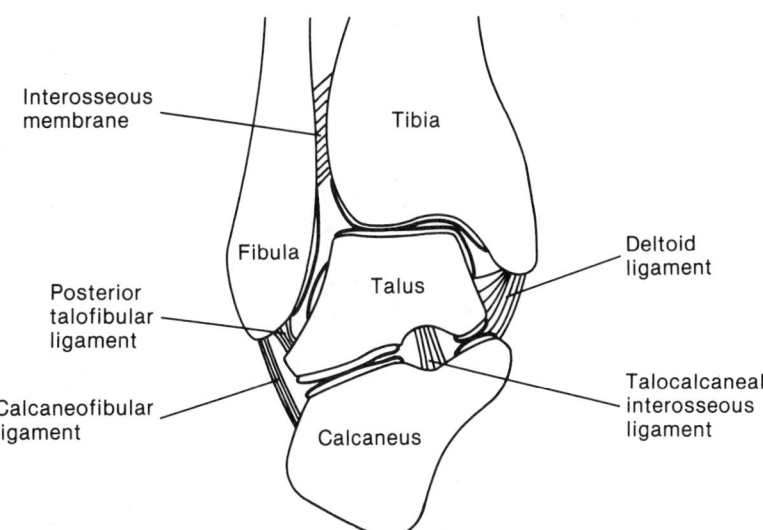

Figure 125–1. Frontal section through the talocrural and subtalar joints. The ankle is formed by the articulation of the tibia, fibula, and talus.

midline. Supination is the same as inversion, except that the lateral foot is load bearing on the ground. Eversion is the non–weight-bearing, outward movement of the plantar surface of the foot away from the midline. Pronation is the same as eversion, except that the medial foot is load bearing on the ground. External rotation is twisting that causes the forefoot to move away from the midline. Internal rotation is twisting that causes the forefoot to move toward the midline. Adduction is the medial displacement of only the forefoot relative to the leg, while abduction is the lateral displacement of the forefoot relative to the leg.

Plantar flexion, supination, adduction, and internal rotation occur together. Dorsiflexion, pronation, abduction, and external rotation occur together.

CLINICAL EVALUATION

The clinical evaluation of the ankle and foot involves a brief history, physical examination, radiographs, and a repeat physical examination following review of the radiographs. The physician must determine when and how the injury occurred and if the injury has resulted in altered function. The physical examination determines likely fractures or dislocations, ligament disruption, joint instability, neurovascular compromise, and soft tissue disruption.

Joint deformity readily suggests fracture or dislocation about the ankle and foot. When gross deformity is absent, determining which bones and ligaments are injured is made difficult by the soft tissue swelling and diffuse tenderness that follow injury. It is important to palpate the medial and lateral malleoli both at their distal tip (to detect fractures caused by ligamentous avulsion) and at their epiphyseal plates (to diagnose a nondisplaced Salter I injury). Salter I injuries are more likely in children less than 10 years of age since the ankle ligaments are relatively strong and the growth plate is the structure that is most likely to be disrupted. As children approach age 15 years, the growth plate strengthens, such that ligamentous injuries and fractures of the metaphysis occur with increasing frequency.

When a patient complains of ankle pain, careful palpation of the calcaneus, fifth metatarsal base, tarsals, proximal fibula, and Achilles tendon is necessary, since injury to any of these structures can cause generalized ankle pain. Palpation of the collateral ligaments often reveals sprained lateral collateral ligaments. Deltoid ligament disruption rarely occurs in isolation. When significant medial tenderness and swelling are detected, the examination should exclude joint instability and fractures of the posterior and lateral malleoli

and of the proximal fibula. Vascular function is assessed by posterior tibial and dorsalis pedis artery palpation, toe capillary refill, and the general appearance of the foot. Even when an ankle dislocation causes diminished pulses owing to vessel compression, adequate perfusion is verified if the foot is pink, warm, and has normal capillary refill. When a dislocation results in cyanosis, prevention of soft tissue destruction can be achieved only by prompt reduction.

Motor function is assessed by the presence of great toe flexion and extension; sensory function is assessed by light touch sensation in the great toe web space and on the dorsum and plantar surface of the foot.

The soft tissues must be examined for puncture wounds caused by the protrusion of a bone fragment through the skin as a fracture-dislocation occurs. While superficial abrasions do not increase the risk of osteomyelitis, the increased risk associated with a contaminated open fracture mandates wound cultures, antibiotics, and operative decontamination. Degloving injuries of the ankle, as with a lawnmower, can cause removal of the perichondrial ring, growth arrest, and a resultant deformity. With all degloving injuries, the physical examination and radiographs should determine physis involvement.

Ankle stress testing, which attempts to move the talus within the ankle mortise, can diagnose otherwise undetected ankle instability. Stress testing is usually not indicated acutely since splinting, non–weight bearing, and orthopedic referral will be recommended for severe sprains regardless of whether the ligaments have been completely disrupted. However, when mortise radiographs reveal asymmetry or when patient compliance and follow-up are unsure, confirmation of ankle instability may be preferred. The anterior drawer test, or sagittal stress testing, is performed with the knee flexed 45 degrees and the ankle plantar flexed. Anterior stress is applied to the heel while the lower leg is stabilized (Fig. 125–3). Excessive movement of the heel and foot indicates disruption of the lateral ankle ligaments.

The talar tilt test is performed with the knee flexed, the lower leg stabilized, and the ankle held at 90 degrees. Laxity with heel and foot inversion indicates lateral ligament disruption. Excessive movement with eversion stress confirms disruption of the deltoid ligament.

DIAGNOSTIC EVALUATION

The radiographic evaluation of the ankle includes three views: the anteroposterior (AP), lateral, and mortise. On the AP view the lateral malleolus extends 1 cm more distal than

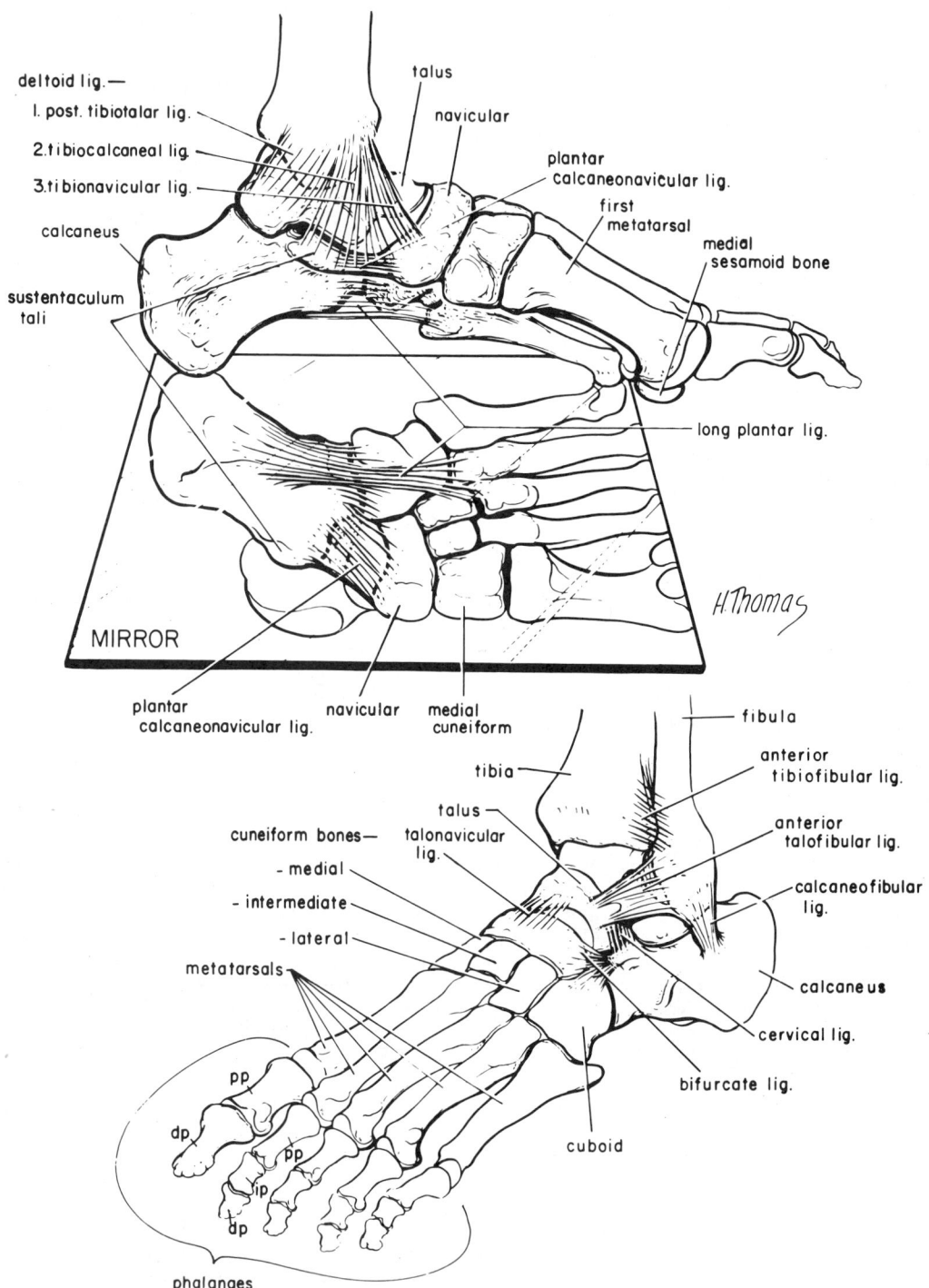

Figure 125–2. Skeleton of the foot showing ligamentous attachments. pp = Proximal phalanx; ip = intermediate phalanx; dp = distal phalanx. (From Jaffe WL, Gannon PJ, Laitman JT. Paleontology, embryology, and anatomy of the foot. *In* Jahss MH (ed). Disorders of the Foot and Ankle. 2nd ed. Philadelphia, WB Saunders, 1991, p 15.)

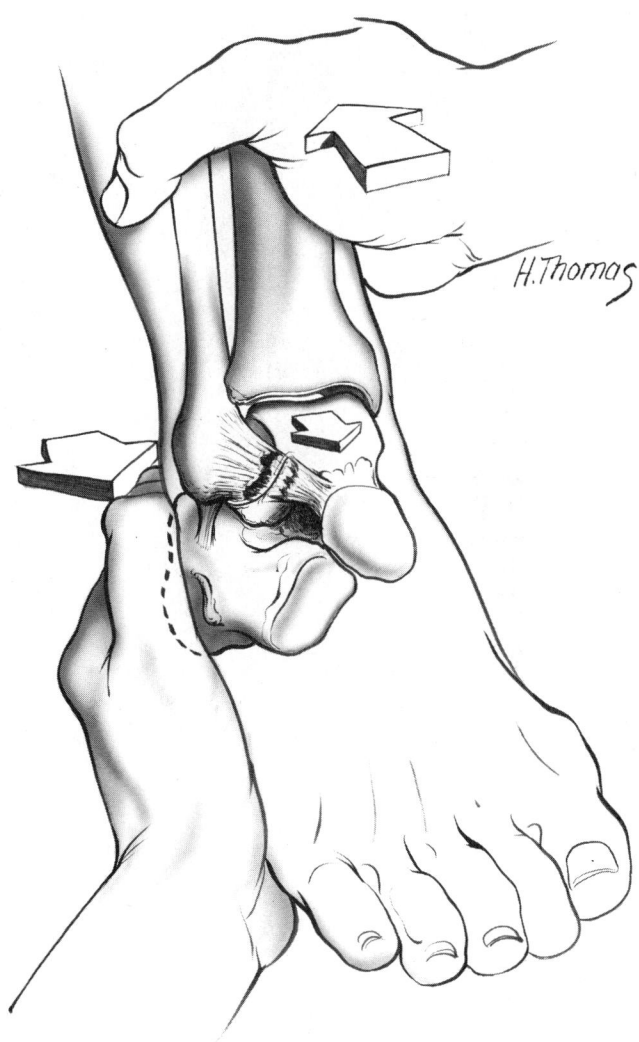

Figure 125–3. The anterior draw sign, a test of ankle stability. (From Hoppenfeld S. Physical examination of the foot by complaint. *In* Jahss MH (ed). Disorders of the Foot and Ankle. 2nd ed. Philadelphia, WB Saunders, 1991, p 56.)

the medial malleolus, and the physis of the fibula is located distal to the epiphysis of the tibia. There is overlap of the distal tibia and fibula as a result of the ankle joint syndesmosis.

The lateral view allows visualization of the posterior malleolus (the posterior tibial plafond), the talus, the calcaneus, and the base of the fifth metatarsal. A lateral film that does not include all of these bones (especially the fifth metatarsal) should be repeated.

The mortise view, obtained with 15 to 20 degrees of leg internal rotation, provides the best visulization of the ankle mortise. The lateral clear space, formed by the talofibular joint, the superior space between the tibial plafond and dome of the talus, and the medial clear space, which is part of the tibiotalar joint, should all uniformly measure 3 to 4 mm. A difference of 2 mm or more suggests mortise instability. This view also visualizes the talus dome, so osteochondral fractures can be detected.

Oblique views, obtained with the leg rotated 45 degrees, can be obtained when a highly suspected fracture is not visualized on the three-radiograph examination. The internal oblique radiograph provides another view of the distal fibula. The external oblique radiograph provides another view of the distal tibia.

Radiographs of the entire tibia and fibula should be obtained whenever a fracture is suspected proximal to the ankle mortise. Findings that suggest a proximal fibular

fracture due to ankle stress and syndesmosis disruption include point tenderness of the fibular shaft, external rotation deformity of the foot, isolated medial ankle tenderness, isolated posterior malleolus fracture, and loss of the normal overlap of the distal tibia and fibula on AP radiograph without a distal fibular fracture.

The tibial and fibular epiphyses appear at 1 to 2 years of age (Fig. 125–4). The medial malleolus appears at age 6 to 7 years. These epiphyses begin to fuse by age 15 years and fully fuse by age 20 years. Several normal variants may simulate fractures in the distal tibia and fibula. The metaphysis may have "bumps" that simulate a torus fracture, as well as accessory ossification centers. The physis may be angulated or depressed, have irregular mineralization at its edge, and leave a residual line once it is fused. The epiphysis may have radiolucent clefts, be slightly offset from the metaphysis, and have a separate ossification center. All of these findings should prompt reexamination for growth plate tenderness and comparison radiographs of the uninjured ankle, since many of these variants occur bilaterally.

The radiographic evaluation of the foot also includes three views. The AP view visualizes the talonavicular and calcaneocuboid joints and the tarsals, metatarsals, and phalanges. The lateral view visualizes the distal tibia and fibula, talus, calcaneus, and anterior tarsals (which may reveal small chip fractures). The 45-degree internal oblique view improves the visualization of the tarsals and their articulations and

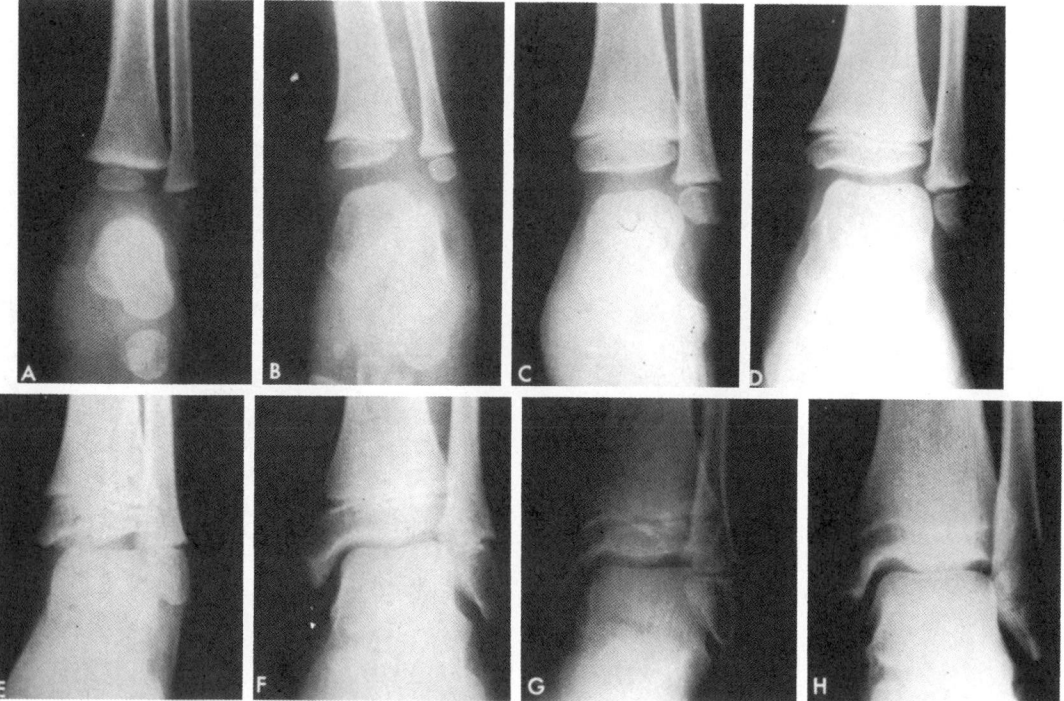

Figure 125–4. Ossification of the distal epiphyses of the tibia and fibula. *A,* One year of age; *B,* 2 years; *C,* 4 years; *D,* 6 years; *E,* 7 years; *F,* 10 years; *G,* 12 years; *H,* adult. (From Tachdjian MO. Pediatric Orthopedics. 2nd ed. Philadelphia, WB Saunders, 1990, p 3303.)

provides an additional view of the metatarsal and phalangeal shafts.

The numerous accessory bones of the foot require attention since each may simulate a fracture in the growing foot. The talus dome may have a lucent defect that simulates a fracture. The calcaneus may have a double ossification center as well as developmental spurs. The apophysis of the calcaneus, which appears at age 10 years and fuses by age 16 years, may simulate an avulsion fracture. The tarsal navicular may have multiple ossification centers and may remain bipartite. All of the tarsals may reveal irregular edges during development. The epiphyses of the metatarsals and phalanges appear at about age 3 years and fuse at about age 18 years. The epiphysis of the great toe metatarsal is located proximal to the metatarsal diaphysis, and the epiphyses of the other metatarsals are distal to the metatarsal shafts. Often there may be accessory growth centers distally on the great toe metaphysis and proximally on the metatarsal shafts. The fifth metatarsal may have numerous longitudinal ossification centers at its base. The phalangeal epiphyses may be split and have clefts and fissures. The tendency to have bilateral normal variants necessitates the inspection of comparison views when a fracture is suspected on the basis of these findings.

ANKLE INJURY

Ankle injuries occur as a result of forces that disrupt the circular support structure of the talus: the tibial plafond superiorly, the medial malleolus and deltoid ligament, the calcaneus interiorly, and the lateral malleolus and lateral collateral ligaments. In children the ankle ligaments are strong relative to the tibial and fibular growth plates. Although ligamentous sprains can occur with minor disruptive forces, severe forces will usually cause growth plate disruption before they cause complete ligamentous disruption. The growth plates of the distal tibia and fibula account for 15% to 25% of all physeal injuries, second only to distal radius

physis injuries. A Salter I fracture should always be considered in ankle injuries that result in pain or soft tissue swelling without radiographic evidence of a fracture.

The emergency physician must assess whether the ankle is stable following ankle injury. Although in adults ankle stability is judged only by mortise uniformity, the assessment of ankle stability in children must also consider physis alignment and Salter fracture occurrence. As in adults, loss of mortise integrity indicates ankle instability. In children, however, displacement of the tibial and fibular epiphyses due to a Salter fracture also renders the ankle unstable, even if the mortise remains uniform. Salter III and IV fractures, because they more often require operative intervention and result in complications, should be considered unstable injuries, even if the ankle mortise and physes remain well aligned. In the presence of a Salter I or Salter II fracture, as long as the physes are aligned and the mortise is uniform, the ankle is often assumed to be stable enough to allow splinting and non–weight-bearing therapy at home.

Anatomic injury is related to foot position (supination or pronation), forced movement of the foot (inversion and eversion), and whether the foot rotates relative to the lower leg. When the foot is supinated and excessive foot inversion occurs, stress will cause injury to the lateral ankle. Minor foot inversion will cause a lateral ankle sprain; stronger forces will cause a Salter fracture of the fibular epiphysis. Extreme foot inversion will cause the talus to strike the medial malleolus, resulting in an additional Salter fracture of the tibial epiphysis. When the foot is pronated and excessive foot eversion occurs, stress will cause a deltoid ligament sprain or disruption of the tibial epiphysis. Extreme foot eversion will cause the talus and tibial epiphysis to strike the lateral malleolus and cause a fracture of the fibular metaphysis. Forces that cause foot external rotation to occur in addition to foot inversion or eversion cause greater injury to the tibiofibular syndesmosis and to the growth plates. Forces that cause rotation therefore increase the risk of mortise disruption, physis displacement, ankle instability,

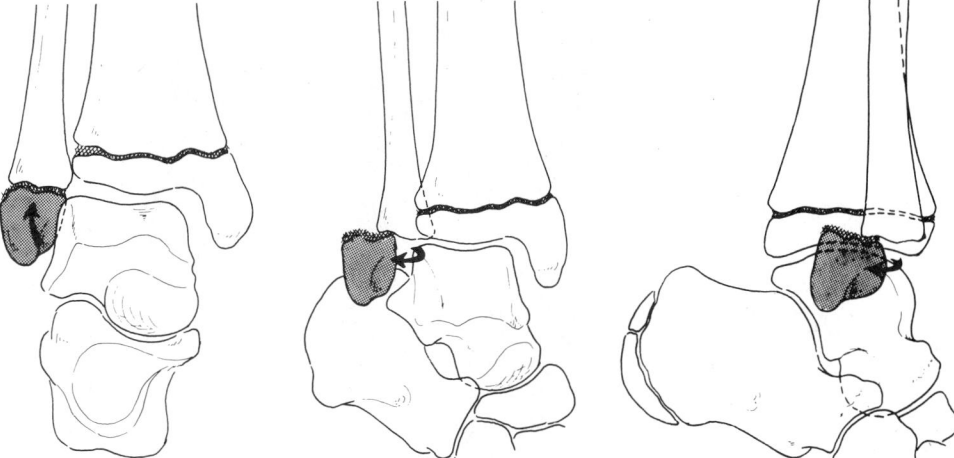

Figure 125–5. Salter type I injury to the distal epiphysis of the fibula. Anteroposterior, oblique, and lateral projections in an 11-year-old. (From Kelikian H, Kelikian AS. Disorders of the Ankle. Philadelphia, WB Saunders, 1985, p 235.)

and complications. Axial loading causes injury by forcing the calcaneus and talus into the distal tibia, causing comminution of the tibial plafond.

Distal Fibula Injuries

Supination and forced foot inversion will cause injury to the lateral ankle structures. Lateral ankle sprains are the most common injury, resulting from partial disruption of the lateral collateral ligaments. A small avulsion fracture of the lateral malleolus may accompany lateral ankle sprains when the physis has fused. This avulsion fracture can be treated as would a lateral ankle sprain, with immobilization, non–weight bearing, and follow-up with an orthopedist in 2 to 3 days.

Salter I and II fractures of the distal fibula are more likely to occur when foot external rotation accompanies supination and inversion. A Salter I fracture can be diagnosed either by tenderness of the fibular physis or by displacement of the fibular epiphysis. The fibular epiphysis should be closely examined on the ankle radiographs since it can rotate out of its normal alignment with the fibular metaphysis without being obviously displaced or causing any associated disruption of the ankle mortise (Fig. 125–5). A Salter I fracture should be suspected if the foot is externally rotated on physical examination and there is significant soft tissue swelling and point tenderness laterally. Fibular Salter II fractures are also seen but are less common than fibular Salter I injuries and tibial Salter II injuries. Except in unusual circumstances, fibular Salter III and IV fractures do not occur.

Rarely, the inferior tibiofibular ligament of the ankle syndesmosis will cause an avulsion fracture of the medial portion of the fibular epiphysis. This injury, when isolated, can be treated as an ankle sprain. Fibular metaphyseal injuries are seen with intercalary tibiofibular diastasis, in which the tibial epiphysis strikes the fibular metaphysis and causes disruption of the interosseous membrane and an oblique fibular metaphyseal fracture above the ankle mortise (Fig. 125–6). This injury is similar to the adult Maisonneuve fracture.

Complications are infrequent with fibular Salter I and II injuries. Because the growth plate germinal cells remain uninjured with these fractures, angular, rotational, and leg length deformities are rare. Complications are more likely, however, when fibular metaphyseal fractures occur with ankle mortise disruption.

Distal Tibia Injuries

Medial ankle sprains occur in the presence of foot pronation and forced foot eversion. Although isolated deltoid ligament sprains can occur, complete disruption of the medial ankle structures usually causes other ankle injuries. The strength of the deltoid ligament causes the tibial epiphysis to disrupt in the child. As the tibial growth plate closes, transverse avulsion fractures of the medial malleolus can be seen with forced eversion, as in adults.

Isolated Salter I fractures of the tibial physis are rare. As with the fibula, rotation of the tibial epiphysis can occur without displacement or fracture and should be suspected if the foot is fixed in the externally rotated position on exam-

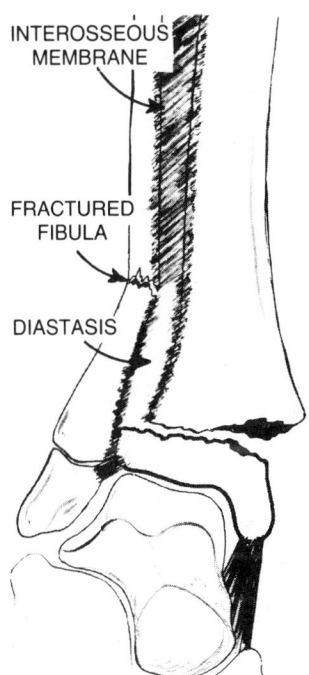

INTEROSSEOUS MEMBRANE

FRACTURED FIBULA

DIASTASIS

Figure 125–6. Schematic drawing of an intercalary tibiofibular diastasis in a patient with a Salter type I injury of the distal tibial epiphysis and a low suprasyndesmotic transverse fracture of the distal fibula. (From Kelikian H, Kelikian AS. Disorders of the Ankle. Philadelphia, WB Saunders, 1985, p 259.)

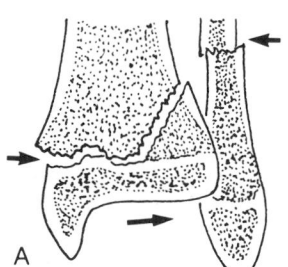

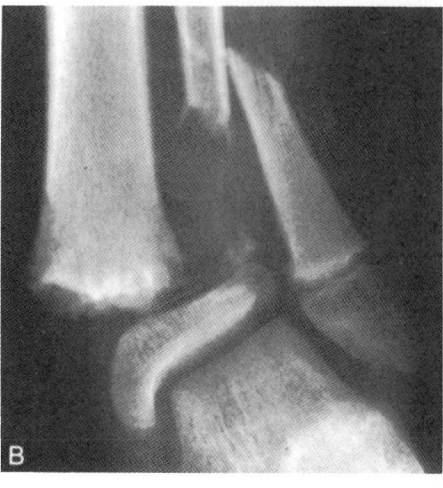

Figure 125–7. *A,* Schematic of Salter type II injury with posteriorly based metaphyseal fracture. The mechanism of injury appears to be pronation and eversion. *B,* Salter type II injury. (From Ogden JA. Skeletal Injury in the Child. 2nd ed. Philadelphia, WB Saunders, 1990, p 836.)

ination. Salter II fractures, which occur as a result of forced foot external rotation, are the most common tibial physis fracture (Fig. 125–7). Up to 15% of children who sustain a tibial Salter II fracture have some deformity due to growth arrest, even if there is only minimal (< 2 mm) fracture fragment displacement. This complication rate is felt to result from an associated Salter V (crush injury) of the tibial physis. Even though operative intervention is usually unnecessary for Salter I and II fractures, the risk of growth arrest warrants orthopedic consultation, immobilization, and absolute non–weight bearing. Intercalary tibiofibular diastasis is an injury to the syndesmosis due to a Salter I or II fracture of the tibial epiphysis. Despite the ankle deformity and fibular metaphysis fracture, the ankle mortise is maintained with this diastasis, often allowing for successful closed reduction.

Tibial Salter III fractures can occur as a result of two mechanisms. Foot supination and inversion will cause the talus to strike the medial malleolus, resulting in a fracture of the medial tibial epiphysis. Displacement can result in growth complication rates that approach 30% (that of Salter IV fractures), such that aggressive operative intervention is indicated if closed reduction is inadequate. The juvenile Tillaux fracture is a Salter III fracture of the lateral tibial epiphysis that occurs owing to forced foot external rotation (Fig. 125–8). This injury occurs late in childhood, when closure of the medial portion of the tibial physis allows the inferior tibiofibular ligament to pull away a portion of the unclosed lateral portion. Joint incongruity often requires operative intervention with this type of Salter III injury.

Tibial Salter IV fractures have the worst prognosis, with up to 30% resulting in growth deformities. Forced foot

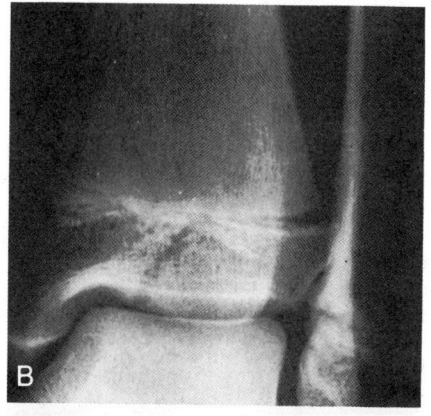

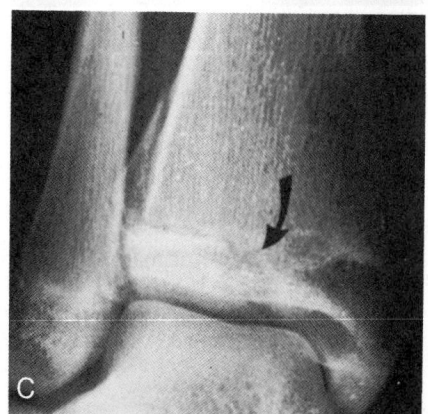

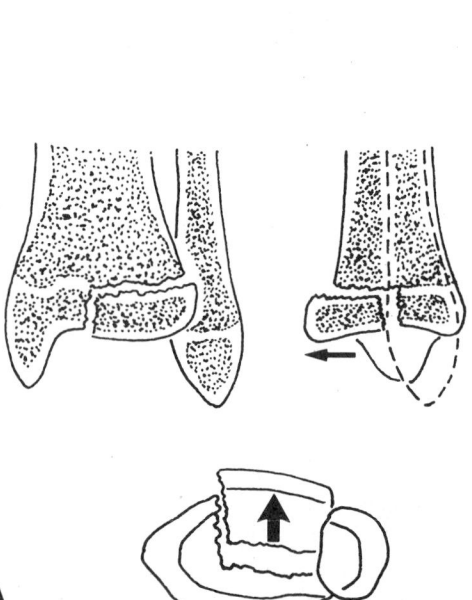

Figure 125–8. *A,* Schematic of a fracture of Tillaux, a Salter type III injury of the anterolateral tibial epiphysis. (Used with permission from Ogden JA: Skeletal Injury in the Child. 2nd ed. Philadelphia, WB Saunders, 1990, p 838.) *B,* Salter type III injury of the lateral tibia (Tillaux fracture). *C,* Comparable Salter type IV injury *(arrow).* (From Ogden JA. Skeletal Injury in the Child. 2nd ed. Philadelphia, WB Saunders, 1990, p 838.)

inversion and rotation, along with axial compression, cause the talus to strike and fracture both the medial tibial epiphysis and the metaphysis. The triplane fracture, a Salter IV fracture that has multiple tibial epiphysis and metaphysis fragments, results from extreme foot external rotation (Fig. 125–9). Joint incongruity and growth complications prompt aggressive operative intervention.

Axial loading injuries can drive the talus into the distal tibia, such that comminution of the tibial epiphysis and metaphysis occurs. This injury, called a pilon fracture in adults, is especially devastating if the distal fibula is also fractured and leg length cannot be maintained. The distal tibial metaphysis can also sustain a toddler's fracture, which is a longitudinal, nondisplaced tibial metaphysis fracture in children 1 year to 3 years of age that simulates an ankle sprain and prevents weight bearing.

General Treatment Principles

With all ankle sprains it is best to assume a Salter I or V fracture and possible growth arrest, such that non–weight bearing and orthopedic follow-up in 2 to 3 days are advised. It is important to assess for epiphyseal displacement and mortise disruption with Salter II to IV fractures, since these findings increase complication risk, mandate immediate orthopedic consultation, and may require hospitalization. Although outpatient therapy in selected cases is possible for unstable, high-risk fractures, admission for evaluation and possible reduction is more consistent with the complication rate seen with these fractures. Fractures that cause mortise derangement and fracture fragment displacement of greater than 2 mm, as well as Salter II to IV fractures, should be considered high risk.

The acute management of pediatric ankle fracture-dislocations centers on the management of a severely displaced tibial epiphyseal plate. Whereas in adults severe force disrupts the ankle mortise, in children the tibial epiphysis is often displaced with the ankle mortise remaining intact. The emergency management depends on the neurovascular status of the foot. If there is compromise, immediate reduction,

preferably under general anesthesia to allow for minimal trauma to the growth plate, is indicated. When immediate orthopedic consultation is not possible, gentle reduction can be attempted in the emergency department. With the knee flexed to relax the Achilles tendon, gentle traction need only reduce the tibial epiphysis enough to return adequate vascular supply to the foot. Unlike in adults, there should be no forced manipulation in children since the germinal cells of the growth plate may be damaged by the fracture fragments. If there is adequate neurovascular function, there is no absolute need to reduce the tibial epiphysis since the tibiotalar joint is intact. This injury can be splinted and the patient admitted, with frequent examinations to assure that the vascular status is maintained as swelling increases.

FOOT FRACTURES
Talus Fractures

The talus is most commonly fractured in its neck owing to forced dorsiflexion (Fig. 125–10). In adults this is seen with forceful braking in motor vehicle accidents. In children this injury is rare but important because of the risk of avascular necrosis associated with talus neck fractures. With nondisplaced talus neck fractures, immobilization in plantar flexion most often allows for healing without avascular necrosis or the need for operative reduction. If the fracture fragments are displaced but not dislocated from the subtalar and tibiotalar joints, closed reduction often allows for successful treatment. When the fracture fragments are dislocated or when closed reduction of displaced fracture fails, operative reduction provides improved results. Complete anatomic reduction is required since avascular necrosis, seen in up to 50% of talus fractures, often mandates secondary operative procedures to return the foot to adequate functioning.

Transchondral fractures, which occur at the cartilaginous surface of the talar dome, can occur in children over 10 years of age. These fractures are difficult to diagnose. The clinician must always look at the talar dome on the mortise view of the ankle in order to assure that there are no irregularities suggestive of a transchondral fracture. Operative repair of the articular surface is often required to remedy the chronic pain seen with this injury. Orthopedic consultation is recommended for all talus fractures.

Calcaneus Fractures

Although the calcaneus is the most commonly fractured tarsal, it occurs only rarely in children. The fact that only 5% of calcaneal fractures occur in children may be due to the elasticity of the calcaneus, which allows transmission of energy to the distal tibia. A fall with a direct axial load is the most common mechanism, but lawnmowers can also cause calcaneal injuries. There are three significant differences in pediatric calcaneal injuries as compared to adults. First, Böhler's angle will not reliably detect calcaneal fractures until the teenage years (Fig. 125–11). Second, intra-articular fractures are less likely to require operative reduction owing to less frequent comminution and successful nonoperative therapy. Third, associated injuries to the lumbar spine, contralateral calcaneus, and renal pedicle are less likely to be seen in children. For example, associated lumbar spine fractures are seen in 5% of children as compared to 10% in adults. Intra-articular calcaneal fractures may cause significant pain and soft tissue swelling. Pediatric extra-articular fractures, which can be treated nonoperatively, must be excluded clinically since many are undiagnosed by radiograph. Extra-articular fractures can be immobilized and

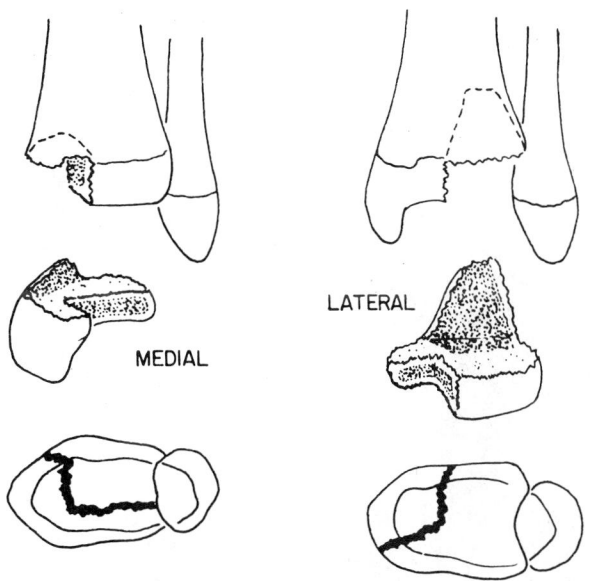

TRIPLANE FRACTURE

Figure 125–9. Schematic of medial and lateral triplane fractures. (From Ogden JA. Skeletal Injury in the Child. 2nd ed. Philadelphia, WB Saunders, 1990, p 840.)

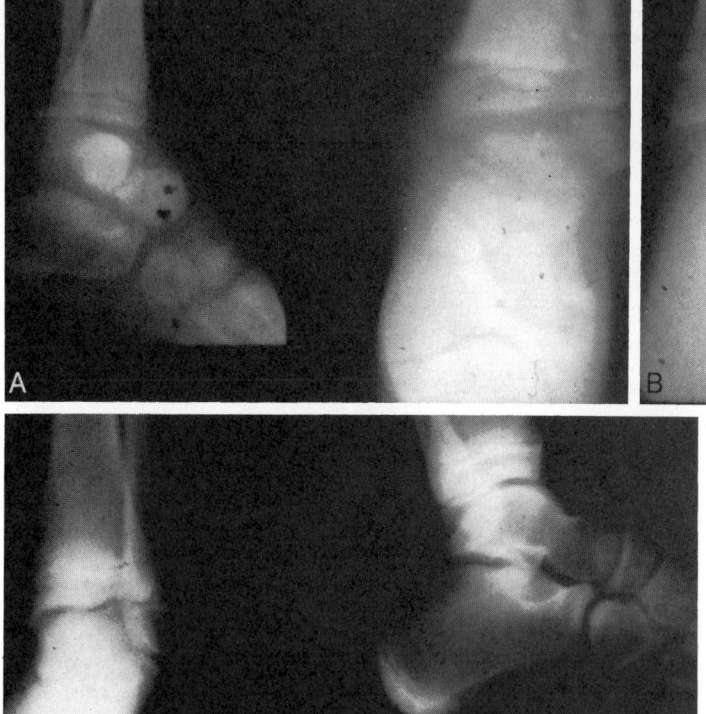

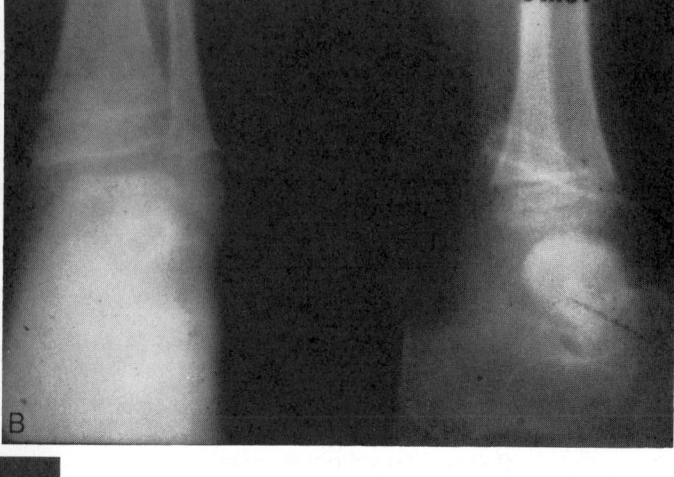

Figure 125–10. Salter type I fracture of the neck of the talus in a child. (From King RE, Powell DF. Injury to the talus. *In* Jahss MH. Disorders of the Foot and Ankle. 2nd ed. Philadelphia, WB Saunders, 1991, p 2308.)

treated on an outpatient basis. One example is a calcaneus apophyseal fracture, which can occur as a result of direct trauma or avulsion by the Achilles tendon. All children who sustain significant heel trauma should be immobilized and offered orthopedic follow-up because up to one third of calcaneus fractures will not be apparent on radiographs.

Midfoot Fractures

Fractures of the cuboid, navicular, and cuneiforms usually result from direct trauma to the midfoot. Irregularities of these bones during growth makes fracture exclusion difficult. Management for these injuries includes ice, elevation, avoidance of weight bearing, analgesic therapy, and orthopedic follow-up when a fracture is suspected.

Although they can occur owing to direct trauma, tarsometatarsal (Lisfranc's joint) fractures usually occur as a result

of forced abduction and plantar flexion, as with jumping in the tiptoe position (Fig. 125–12). To exclude this injury it is important to make sure that there is no fracture at the base of the second metatarsal, which is firmly anchored to the cuneiforms and metatarsals in a recess next to the first metatarsal. A fracture at this location should prompt inspection of the other metatarsal bases, where displaced fractures frequently occur. Nonoperative therapy can be attempted, but open reduction with Kirschner wire is often required. Orthopedic consultation is recommended since vascular compromise, although rare, is a possible complication.

Metatarsal Fractures

Metatarsal shaft fractures occur as a result of direct trauma, twisting, or an axial load on the forefoot. Metatarsal stress fractures are rare but can occur in children. Outpatient

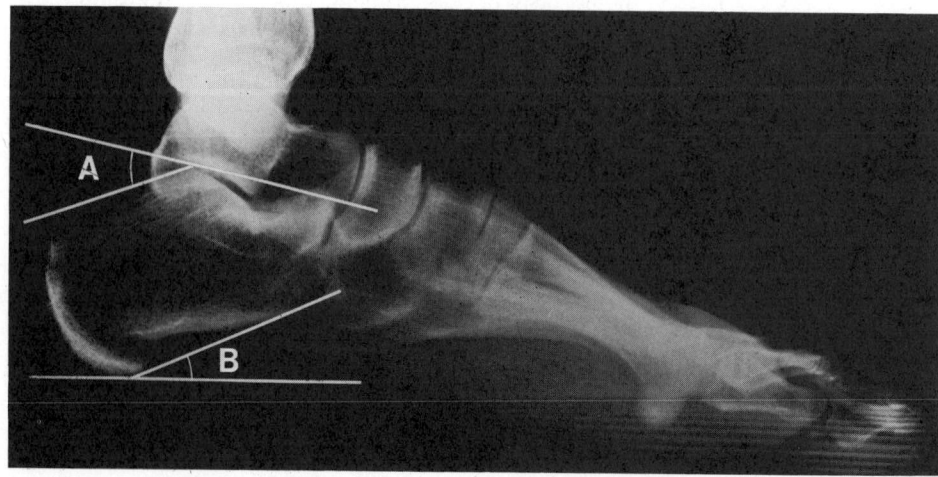

Figure 125–11. Radiographic parameters used to describe the inclination and structural configuration of the calcaneus. A = Böhler's angle; B = calcaneal pitch. (From Shereff MT. Radiographic analysis of the foot and ankle. *In* Jahss MH. Disorders of the Foot and Ankle. 2nd ed. Philadelphia, WB Saunders, 1991, p 104.)

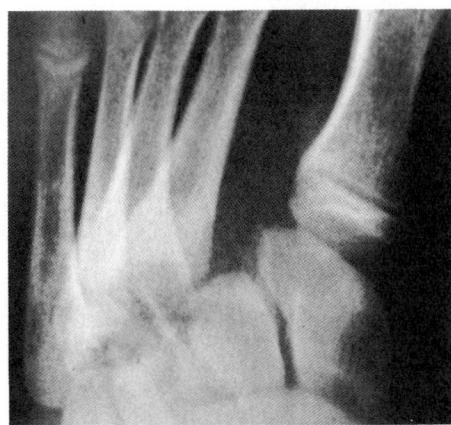

Figure 125–12. Lisfranc's dislocation. (From Ogden JA. Skeletal Injury in the Child. 2nd ed. Philadelphia, WB Saunders, 1990, p 887.)

therapy with immobilization and orthopedic follow-up is the rule, even for those shaft fractures that may require operative intervention. The presence of more than two metatarsal fractures, especially when associated with a crush injury, usually indicates a need for admission or elevation, observing for a possible compartment syndrome.

The Jones fracture is a metatarsal neck fracture that is distal to the apophysis at the base of the fifth metatarsal. This transverse diaphyseal fracture occurs especially in young athletes as a result of direct trauma, not inversion-induced avulsion by the peroneus brevis tendon. Nonunion is a significant complication of the Jones fracture, such that operative intervention is often necessary. Delay in diagnosis is also a problem owing to initially normal appearing radiographs. Small cortical defects in the lateral metatarsal diaphysis should raise the suspicion of a nondisplaced Jones fracture, even if a clear cortical break is not seen. Inversion injury and direct trauma can cause a fracture of the apophysis of the fifth metatarsal (see Fig. 125–10). This injury can be treated with immobilization and nonoperative therapy.

Phalangeal Fractures

Phalangeal injuries in children occur owing to direct trauma or axial trauma, as with kicking injuries. Fractures can most often be treated by buddy taping the fractured toe to the next toe, with interposed padding to prevent soft tissue breakdown. Rotational deformity of the toe should be noted since it may require closed reduction to prevent malunion. Metatarsophalangeal and interphalangeal dislocations can be reduced with gentle longitudinal traction; a twisting motion may facilitate reduction if straight traction cannot achieve reduction. These injuries can be treated as are toe fractures, with immobilization and non–weight-bearing therapy. As with all injuries that affect the lower extremity and impair gait, crutches should be offered if the injury causes painful ambulation. This is especially true with fracture of the great toe, which bears weight during the push-off phase of each step.

Finally, two preventable injuries can cause significant foot morbidity. Bicycle spoke injuries occur when the foot is caught in the spokes of a wheel and compressed against the frame of the bicycle. This injury should be viewed as is the washing machine wringer injury of the hand, one that causes significant soft tissue trauma. Documentation of a normal neurovascular examination and full skin integrity is necessary, as is giving clear instructions to the parents regarding the need to ice and elevate the foot to prevent massive swelling. Even if the injury appears trivial initially, this mechanism should prompt conservative therapy and orthopedic follow-up in case there is neurovascular compromise or the need for wound care or skin grafting. Lawnmower injuries also cause devastating pediatric foot morbidity. Children should never be allowed to ride on a riding mower with their parents, nor should teenagers be allowed to use walking mowers without adequate foot protection. With these injuries, prevention more effectively prevents morbidity than does therapy provided after the injury has occurred.

Selected References

Atken AP, Poulson D. Dislocations of the tarsometatarsal joint. J Bone Joint Surg 1963;45A:246.

Brook GJ, Greer RB. Traumatic rotational displacements of the distal tibial growth plate. J Bone Joint Surg 1970;52A:1666.

Canale ST, Kelly FB. Fractures of the neck of the talus. J Bone Joint Surg 1978;60A:143.

Cooperman DR, Spiegel PG, Laros GS. Tibial fractures involving the ankle in children. The so-called triplane epiphyseal fracture. J Bone Joint Surg 1978;60A:1040.

Dias LS, Giegerich CR. Fractures of the distal tibial epiphysis in adolescence. J Bone Joint Surg 1983;65A:438.

Dias LS, Tachdjian MO. Physeal injuries of the ankle in children. Clin Orthop 1978;136:230.

Dunbar JS, Owen HF, Nogrady MB, et al. Obscure tibial fracture of infants—the toddler's fracture. J Can Assoc Radiol 1964;25:136.

Goldberg VM, Aadalen R. Distal tibial epiphyseal injuries: The role of athletics in fifty-three cases. Am J Sports Med 1978;6:263.

Harty M. Anatomic considerations in injuries of the calcaneus. Orthop Clin North Am 1983;4:179.

Hawkins LG. Fractures of the neck of the talus. J Bone Joint Surg 1970;52A:991.

Izant RJ, Rothman BF, Frankel V. Bicycle spoke injuries of the foot and ankle in children: An underestimated "minor" injury. J Pediatr Surg 1969;4:654.

Kavanaugh JH, Brower TD, Mann RV. The Jones fracture revisited. J Bone Joint Surg 1978;60A:776.

Kleiger B, Mankin HJ. Fracture of the lateral portion of the distal tibial epiphysis. J Bone Joint Surg 1964;46A:25.

Marmor L. An unusual fracture of the tibial epiphysis. Clin Orthop 1970;73:132.

Ross PM, Schwentker EP, Bryan H. Mutilating lawn mower injuries in children. JAMA 1976;236:480.

Schmidt TL, Weiner DC. Calcaneal fractures in children. Clin Orthop 1982;171:150.

Spiegel MD, Cooperman DR, Laros GS. Epiphyseal fractures of the distal ends of the tibia and fibula. A retrospective study of 237 cases in children. J Bone Joint Surg 1978;60A:1046.

Wilson DW. Injuries of the tarso-metatarsal joints. J Bone Joint Surg 1972;54B:677.

CHAPTER 126

Back Pain

Steven E. Krug

INTRODUCTION

Back pain is an unusual complaint for children and adolescents and may indicate significant underlying pathology. The more benign functional and mechanical causes of back pain that are common in adults are uncommon in

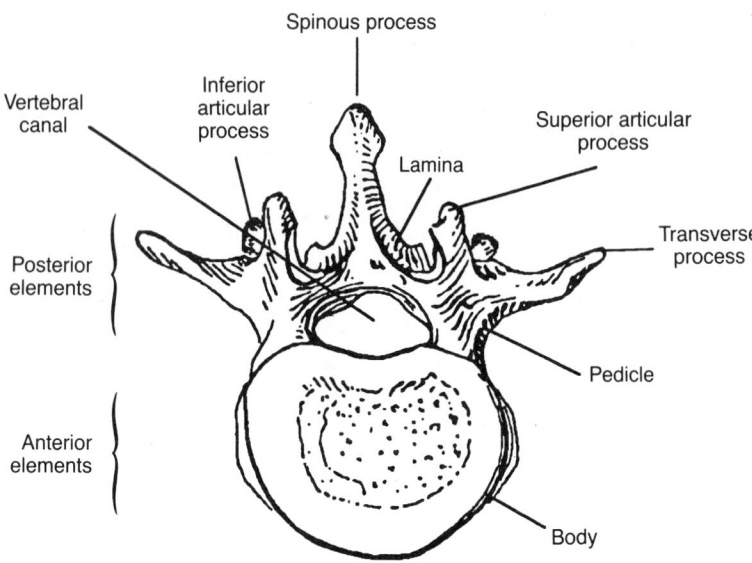

Figure 126–1. Vertebral anatomy.

children. It is therefore important that back pain be approached with a careful and complete evaluation to determine its cause.

ANATOMY AND BIOMECHANICS

The typical vertebra consists of an anterior or ventral portion, the body, and a posterior or dorsal vertebral arch (Fig. 126–1). This arch contains the foramen, which transmits the spinal cord, meninges, and associated blood vessels. Between the posterior elements of adjacent vertebrae, on either side, are intervertebral foramina, through which the spinal nerves and blood vessels pass. The vertebral arch has on each side a vertically narrow anterior part, the pedicle, and behind this the broader lamina. Projecting from this arch are seven processes, a paired transverse, superior and inferior processes, and a single posterior spinous process. The opposed surfaces of the vertebral bodies are bound to each other by fibrocartilaginous intervertebral disks and by anterior and posterior ligaments. Each disk consists of an outer fibrous layer, the annulus fibrosus, and an inner core, the nucleus pulposus.

The vertebrae articulate with one another by a series of cartilaginous joints between the vertebral bodies and a series of synovial joints between the vertebral arches. The joints between the vertebral arches are synovial. The spinous and transverse processes are connected by the supraspinous, interspinous, and intertransverse ligaments, while the laminae are connected by the ligamenta flava. The anterior portion of the spinal column bears weight and absorbs shock. In addition to protecting the spinal cord, the posterior elements direct the motion of the spine (anterior flexion, lateral flexion, extension, and rotation). The lumbar spine is much more mobile than either the thoracic or the sacral spine, and it provides for most of the flexibility and mobility of the back, as well as being the most common location of mechanical or trauma-related back pain disorders.

EMS CONSIDERATIONS

Children with back pain should be transported in a position that provides comfort, unless there has been significant trauma. With major trauma the patient should have the entire spine (cervical, thoracic, and lumbosacral) immobilized on a backboard with an appropriately sized collar device, tape, and sandbags.

CLINICAL EVALUATION
History

In addition to questions about the patient's past and present medical illnesses, the history should focus on the pain's mode of onset, nature, and severity; any change in the character of the patient's presenting symptoms; and any associated systemic complaints (Table 126–1).

The history should start with questions regarding the onset of the pain, including the actual time of onset and what the patient was doing at the time. Antecedent illnesses, changes in level of activity such as exercise or sports, and direct relationships to trauma are important. Investigation into the nature of the pain should include the location, radiation, frequency, and duration of the pain and whether it is constant or intermittent. Additionally, the presence of

TABLE 126–1
BACK PAIN—IMPORTANT HISTORICAL FINDINGS
Mode of Onset
Events surrounding first symptoms
Antecedent injury or illness
Nature of Pain
Frequency
Duration
Location
Radiation
Character—constant or intermittent
Aggravating or relieving factors
Severity of Pain
Response to medications
Activity limitation
Presence and character at night
Change in Symptoms
Changes in severity of pain
Changes in nature of pain
Systemic Complaints
Gait alteration
Bowel or bladder dysfunction
Headache
Fever, weight loss, malaise
Intercurrent illnesses

Adapted from Bunnell WP. Back pain in children. Pediatr Rev 1984;6:183. Reproduced by permission of Pediatrics.

any aggravating or relieving factors (positions, activities) should be documented.

Severity of pain is difficult to quantify objectively. However, pain that limits a patient's regular activity or that is present at night or awakens the patient from sleep is likely to be severe. The patient's response to reasonable dosing of analgesic medications may also help to determine the severity of pain.

A change in the patient's symptoms may also provide information about the causative process. Whether the pain and associated symptoms are improving or worsening is important, as are any associated changes in the patient's activities. Any changes in the character or location of the pain must also be elicited.

Systemic complaints may also help to narrow the differential diagnosis. Changes in bowel or bladder function or changes in gait patterns are indicators of potentially serious pathology. Fever, weight loss, malaise, or intercurrent illnesses are suggestive of nonfocal disease.

Physical Examination

The physical examination of the patient with back pain should be complete (Table 126–2). The key points to cover in the examination include general observation and inspection, local palpation and percussion, assessment of gait pattern and range of motion, examination of the adjacent body compartments (thorax and abdomen), a general musculoskeletal examination, and, finally, a careful neurologic examination.

Observation of the patient at rest may provide an overall assessment of the patient's illness severity and level of comfort. This portion of the examination should also include an assessment of the patient's standing posture and relative ease of motion. The patient should be observed from several

---

TABLE 126–2

BACK PAIN—IMPORTANT PHYSICAL FINDINGS

Observation
Standing posture
Spinal deformity
Ease of motion
Cutaneous markings
Palpation
Muscle spasm (paravertebral, hamstring)
Bony or soft tissue tenderness
Joint tenderness
Pelvic obliquity
Percussion
Bone pain
Joint pain
Range of Motion
Lumbar spine
Thoracic spine
Pelvis
Peripheral joints
Gait Pattern
Posture, rate, stride length, stance and swing phases
Neurologic Examination
Muscle bulk and tone
Spinal sensory examination
Deep tendon and superficial reflexes
Straight-leg raising test
Adjacent Body Compartments or Structures
Chest, abdomen, pelvis, retroperitoneum, perineum, genitalia, lower extremities

Adapted from Bunnell WP. Back pain in children. Pediatr Rev 1984;6:183. Reproduced by permission of Pediatrics.

---

vantage points, although posture is generally best observed from the side. While scoliosis by itself is not an acceptable explanation of back pain in children or adolescents, a visual examination of the back will detect obvious spinal deformity or asymmetry.

Each section of the spinal column should be inspected for deformity. The cervical spine should be examined for tilt or torticollis. The thoracic and lumbar spine should be assessed for kyphosis, lordosis, and scoliosis. The presence of certain "birthmarks" or lesions such as a hairy nevus, hemangioma, lipoma, or dermoid sinus, especially when present in the midline, can be indicative of spina bifida or other underlying skeletal abnormalities. The skin should also be carefully examined for the presence of cutaneous manifestations of systemic diseases such as café au lait spots or skin tags.

The forward bend test will assist in the identification of scoliosis. The child should be examined from both the back and the side in this position. This position may help to accentuate rotational asymmetry of the rib cage or the lumbar paraspinous muscle masses due to kyphosis or scoliosis. Attention should be given to the symmetry of the height of the iliac crests as evidence of a shortened limb. The ease and speed with which the patient moves from the erect to the forward bending position will provide some measure of the severity of pain and any associated muscle weakness.

The back should be carefully palpated to determine the presence of muscle spasm and to locate areas of vertebral tenderness. The spinous process of each vertebral body from the cervical through the sacral spine should be carefully palpated to determine accurately the location of tenderness. Likewise, each rib on both sides of the spinal column and each intervertebral disk should be palpated. The adjacent soft tissues must also be carefully palpated, with attention directed toward the supraspinous and interspinous ligaments and paraspinal muscles on either side of the vertebral column.

The iliosacral joints should be palpated and the iliac crests compressed to elicit tenderness. Additional stress can be applied to the sacroiliac joint by flexing the hip 90 degrees and adducting the leg across the midline. The posterior aspect of the coccyx, the posterior iliac spines and the iliac crests, the ischial tuberosities, and the greater trochanters should also be palpated. Percussion may help to elicit pain not noted during palpation or to induce radiation in areas of tenderness.

The range of motion of the spine may be difficult to assess accurately because patients may compensate for areas of diminished spine mobility by using the pelvis and nonpainful areas of the spine, especially in the lumbar spine. Placing a mark on the skin overlying the third or fourth lumbar vertebra and an additional mark over the sacrum may help to demonstrate true flexion of the lumbar spine as the patient bends over. In addition to flexion, the spine should be assessed for extension, lateral bending, and rotation.

The patient's gait pattern should be assessed, with attention paid to posture, rate, and stride length. Mechanically, gait is composed of two phases: stance and swing. The stance or weight-bearing component begins with the heel strike, progressing to midstance, and ending with metatarsal push-off. Abnormalities of this phase may help to identify muscle weakness or neurologic deficits, thereby localizing precipitating lesions affecting the spinal cord. Deficiencies of the swing phase, while perhaps not as easy to elicit, can likewise localize cord or vertebral column lesions. Attention should also be paid to the width of the base of the gait, any motion of the pelvis, and the patient's center of gravity.

A neuromuscular examination should include an assessment of muscle bulk, tone and strength, deep tendon reflexes, and a complete sensory examination (touch, pain, position). Careful examination of the extremities is important because lesions of the spinal cord or cauda equina, such as tumors or herniated disks, will manifest as altered sensation, reflexes, or muscle strength. Straight-leg raising tests, which serve to identify hamstring spasm, if positive, also suggest the presence of intraspinal pathology. As such, this neurologic examination should be conducted with attention toward levels of innervation. The superficial reflexes (cremasteric, abdominal, anal) also may help to identify the level of a spinal cord lesion. Careful examination of the pelvis, flanks, and genitalia and careful inspection, palpation, percussion, and auscultation of the abdomen and thorax should also occur.

DIAGNOSTIC EVALUATION

Children with unexplained back pain should have laboratory or radiologic studies performed as indicated to exclude systemic diseases or severe local pathology (Table 126–3). In the emergency department the goal is to identify those children in need of immediate medical or surgical intervention. In general, a complete blood cell count (CBC), erythrocyte sedimentation rate (ESR), and urinalysis should be performed on all patients. These tests will provide some insight into the presence of certain infectious or inflammatory disorders. Depending on the concern for rheumatologic disorders, additional testing for histocompatibility (HLA) antigens and for the presence of rheumatoid factor, antinuclear antibodies, complement subtypes, and a lupus erythematosus preparation may assist in that determination in follow-up care.

In addition to the suggested routine laboratory analyses, a standard evaluation should include anteroposterior, lateral, and oblique radiographs of the lumbosacral (and, if indicated, thoracic or cervical) spine. Tomograms, computed tomography (CT), or magnetic resonance imaging (MRI) may be necessary to better define areas of suspicion. CT and MRI can also provide a determination of pathology within the spinal canal. Similarly, radionuclide scanning may prove to be a valuable diagnostic aid in identifying infectious, neoplastic, and traumatic lesions.

DIFFERENTIAL DIAGNOSIS
Trauma-Related Disorders

Mechanical or trauma-related processes are uncommon in children. Most children and adolescents are physically active and are not prone to postexercise muscle strain or soreness.

TABLE 126–3

BACK PAIN—LABORATORY AND RADIOLOGIC EVALUATION

Acute Laboratory Analyses
CBC, ESR, urinalysis
Other Laboratory Analyses
HLA-B27, antinuclear antibodies, rheumatoid factor
Acute Radiographic Studies
Plain films (anteroposterior, lateral, oblique)
Tomograms
Computed tomography
Other Studies
Magnetic resonance imaging
Radionuclide scanning
Myelography
Electromyography

Adapted from Bunnell WP. Back pain in children. Pediatr Rev 1984;6:183. Reproduced by permission of Pediatrics.

TABLE 126–4

DIFFERENTIAL DIAGNOSIS OF BACK PAIN

Traumatic
Muscle strain
Herniated nucleus pulposus
Interspinous process ligament sprain
Vertebral fracture
Developmental Abnormalities
Posture
Limb length inequality
Scoliosis
Scheuermann's kyphosis
Spondylolysis/spondylolisthesis
Spina bifida occulta
Calcification of intervertebral disk
Diastematomyelia
Anomalous vertebral articulations
Infectious
Diskitis
Vertebral osteomyelitis
Sacroiliac arthritis
Spinal epidural abscess
Rheumatologic
Ankylosing spondylitis
Juvenile rheumatoid arthritis
Neoplastic
Benign bony tumors
  Osteoid osteoma, benign osteoblastoma
Malignant bony tumors
  Ewing's tumor, osteogenic sarcoma, bone cyst, granuloma
Spinal cord tumors
  Glioma, neurofibroma, teratoma, lipoma, neurenteric cyst,
    astrocytoma, ependymoma, arteriovenous malformation
Metastatic malignancies
  Neuroblastoma, Wilms' tumor, leukemia, lymphoma
Other
Hematologic
  Sickling hemoglobinopathies, chronic anemia
Cardiovascular
  Aortic aneurysm
Respiratory
  Pneumonia, pneumothorax, rib fracture
Gastrointestinal
  Pancreatitis, cholelithiasis, peptic ulcer, hepatitis
Genitourinary
  Pyelonephritis, urolithiasis, ectopic or intrauterine
    pregnancy, retroperitoneal abscess, pelvic inflammatory
    disease, testicular torsion or cancer
Metabolic
  Rickets, malnutrition, anorexia nervosa, Cushing's syndrome,
    muscular dystrophy
Psychogenic

While this can certainly occur in a child who begins a strenuous exercise or sports-related conditioning program, the history must confirm this suspicion. Younger athletes are in fact more likely to develop inflammation of the iliac apophysis than chronic muscle strains. Even with the history of an abrupt initiation of vigorous activity, one should still consider the other disorder classes, particularly the developmental abnormalities (Table 126–4).

Herniated Intervertebral Disks

Herniated intervertebral disks are uncommon in children, with less than 2% of all such lesions occurring in this population. Herniated disks are even rarer in children under the age of 10 years. Nearly two thirds of affected adolescents will complain of back pain as their chief complaint, with sciatica representing the chief concern of the other third. Unlike the typically acute onset of symptoms seen in the adult population, children are more likely to present with a more gradual onset of symptoms. Physical examination should demonstrate muscle spasm, decreased lumbar lordosis, diminished forward flexion, "sciatic scoliosis," gait alteration, and significant limitation of straight-leg raising. A positive straight-leg raising test on the side contralateral to the pain is strongly suggestive of nerve root compression. A careful neurologic examination of the lower extremities may help to localize the herniated disk with the finding of muscle atrophy or weakness and sensory or reflex deficits.

The evaluation of this lesion should include standard radiographs to determine the presence of vertebral lesions and disk-space narrowing. CT and MRI should better identify the lesion, although many still recommend myelography. Early treatment is conservative, including activity or sports limitation, bracing, and nonsteroidal anti-inflammatory drugs. Patients with extruded disk fragments or bladder or bowel dysfunction may warrant more aggressive surgical therapy.

Vertebral Fractures

Adolescents can occasionally injure the ligaments of the spine, with the interspinous ligaments being the most common site of injury. Fractures of the thoracic or lumbar vertebrae most commonly occur at the thoracolumbar junction. These injuries typically occur during activities with a potential for high impact and rapid deceleration, such as skiing. Motor vehicle–related injuries can also be the cause of spine injury. Children "appropriately" restrained in motor vehicles with a lap seatbelt are susceptible to fractures of the midlumbar spine (Fig. 126–2). In addition to fractures of the vertebral body itself, fractures of the posterior elements of the spine (pedicles; articular, transverse, and spinous processes; pars interarticularis) may be caused by repetitive stress or may be due to a direct blow. The inferior articular processes in the lumbar spine are the elements most frequently injured. While many fractures of the spine are benign, a careful orthopedic evaluation for potential instability should occur upon identification of these injuries.

Overuse Syndromes

While overuse syndromes are not commonly diagnosed in children, certain activities can cause mechanical or trauma-related back pain. Dancers and gymnasts engage in repetitive actions that place stress on the back. This may predispose them to mechanical problems such as muscle sprain, liga-

mentous strain, apophyseal compression fractures, and disk degeneration, as well as some of the developmental problems (spondylolysis, spondylolisthesis, Scheuermann's kyphosis). Even the seam from a tight pair of jeans has been suggested as a cause of back pain.

Developmental Disorders

Postural abnormalities and scoliosis are common findings in young children and adolescents. However, these rarely cause significant back pain and therefore are diagnoses of exclusion. If the evaluation of the patient's back pain fails to identify a pathologic cause, these patients can be approached with conservative and symptomatic care. Exercise and behavior modification may alleviate pain that is due to posture or mild scoliosis. It is probably advisable to refer children with severe scoliosis, or any degree of scoliosis that appears to provoke back pain, for an orthopedic evaluation (Fig. 126–3).

Dorsolumbar Kyphosis

Dorsolumbar kyphosis or Scheuermann's disease is a painful, fixed kyphotic deformity occurring at the thoracolumbar junction. It typically develops around the time of puberty (ages 14 to 18 years) in athletically active children. The estimated frequency of this disorder is reported to be anywhere between 4% and 88%, although a recent survey of healthy high school students demonstrated varying degrees of this disorder in nearly 60% of males and 30% of females. Scheuermann's disease is believed to result from repeated trauma and is characterized radiologically by irregular vertebral end plates, narrowing of the intervertebral disk space, wedging of one or more adjacent vertebral bodies, fragmentation of epiphyseal rings, sclerosis of the adjacent vertebral margins, and an increase of normal kyphosis beyond 40 degrees (Fig. 126–4). This disorder may also be characterized by the presence of Schmorl's node, a herniation of the intervertebral disk through the vertebral end plate into the vertebral body (Fig. 126–5).

The most common presenting complaint of Scheuermann's disease is back pain that is generally localized to the thoracolumbar junction. This pain is typically aggravated by physical activity, especially with forward flexion. Physical examination should demonstrate point tenderness of the involved vertebrae, flattening of normal lumbar lordosis with loss of lumbar mobility, and some associated paraspinous muscle spasm. Conservative therapy of activity limitation

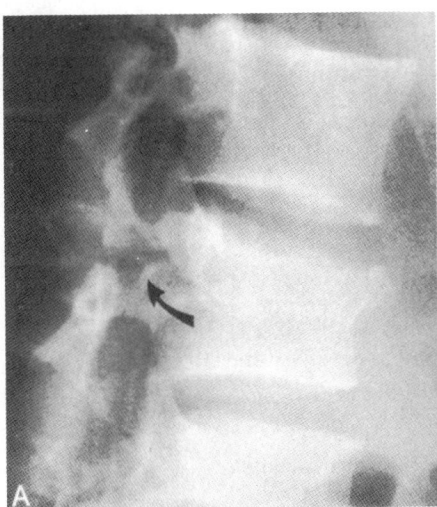
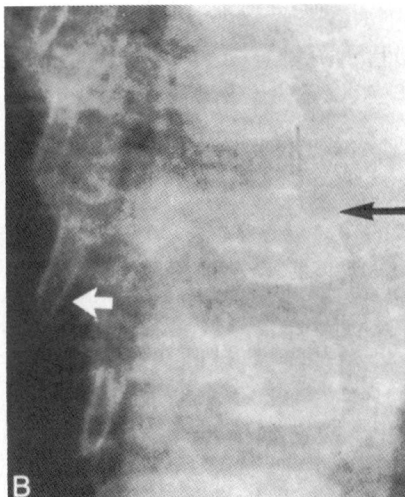

Figure 126–2. *A,* Moderate crush of L3 with posterior extension *(arrow).* This is a variation of a Chance fracture. *B,* Posterior displaced Chance fracture *(arrows)* in a 5-year-old child. (From Ogden JA. Skeletal Injury in the Child. 2nd ed. Philadelphia, WB Saunders, 1990, p. 608.)

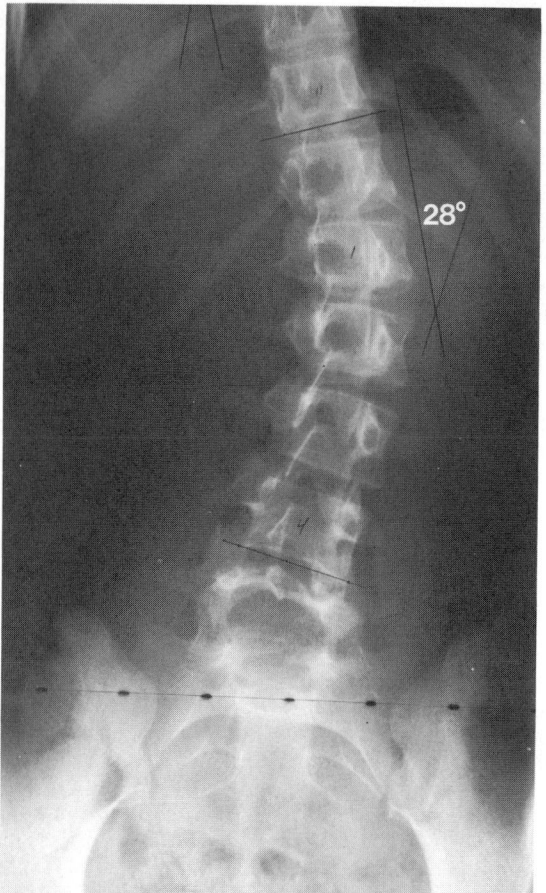

Figure 126–3. Anteroposterior radiograph shows mild to moderate lumbar scoliosis. The angle between the lower end plate of T-11 and that of L-4 measures 28 degrees, convex to the left. (Courtesy of A. Oestreich, Cincinnati, OH.)

and occasionally orthopedic bracing is sufficient to treat the majority of patients.

Spondylolysis

Spondylolysis specifically refers to a defect or fracture of the pars interarticularis, the part of the spinal column between the superior and the inferior articulations of the vertebrae (Fig. 126–6). The pars interarticularis defect occurs in 5% of males and up to 35% of females. This typically occurs at the level of L-5, most commonly in older children and teenagers, particularly those who are physically active. This disorder is especially common in female gymnasts, in whom the incidence has been estimated to be four times that in controls. These children will have back pain that is induced by strenuous activity and that is at least partially relieved by rest.

Spondylolisthesis

Children with spondylolysis may further develop spondylolisthesis, which is perhaps the single most common cause of back pain in older children. Spondylolisthesis is characterized by an anterior slippage of one vertebra on top of the other, typically L-5 on S-1. In addition to pain aggravated by activity and relieved by rest, these patients may complain of a spinal deformity that is reminiscent of lumbar lordosis. These children may experience some pain relief by leaning forward, a position that stabilizes the slipped vertebrae in a

forward-flexed position. On examination there may be a palpable step-off or shortening of the torso, with a crease between the costal margin and the iliac crest. Neurologic examination may demonstrate spasm of the hamstring muscles owing to involvement of the L-5 and S-1 nerve roots. This may also manifest as a gait disturbance characterized by a shortened stride length.

The diagnosis of spondylolysis and spondylolisthesis is made with routine lumbar spine radiographs, including oblique views. In addition to the forward slip of L-5 on S-1, secondary changes, such as a rounding off of the superior surface of the body of S-1 or a trapezoidal-shaped body of L-5, may be seen. CT and MRI can be helpful in confirming this diagnosis when routine radiographs are equivocal. Treatment is conservative and symptomatic, with restriction of painful activities. Occasionally, posterior spinal fusion is required.

Spina Bifida Occulta

Another condition associated with back pain is spina bifida occulta, or failure of the fusion of the two lateral halves of the vertebral arch. This common condition can result in hypermobility of the spine, back pain, and sciatica. Diastematomyelia, an abnormal cleft of the spinal cord, may be associated with spina bifida. This cleft is caused by a protruding bone spicule that projects into the cord anteriorly from a normal or abnormal vertebral body. In addition to back pain, these patients will present with progressive neurologic dysfunction, as this anomaly serves to fix the cord and prevent normal migration during growth. Anomalous articulations and other malformations of the spinal column can produce back pain; however, the hallmark symptoms or signs in these patients relate to cord compression and its associated neurologic dysfunction.

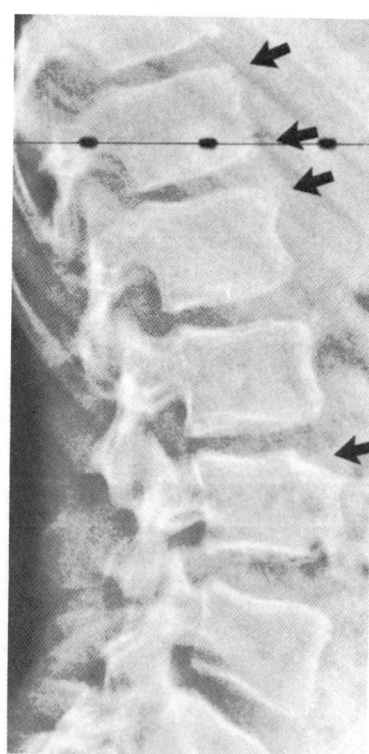

Figure 126–4. Radiographic appearance in Scheuermann's disease: deformity of multiple levels *(arrows)*, especially L-3. (From Ogden JA. Skeletal Injury in the Child. 2nd ed. Philadelphia, WB Saunders, 1990, p 604.)

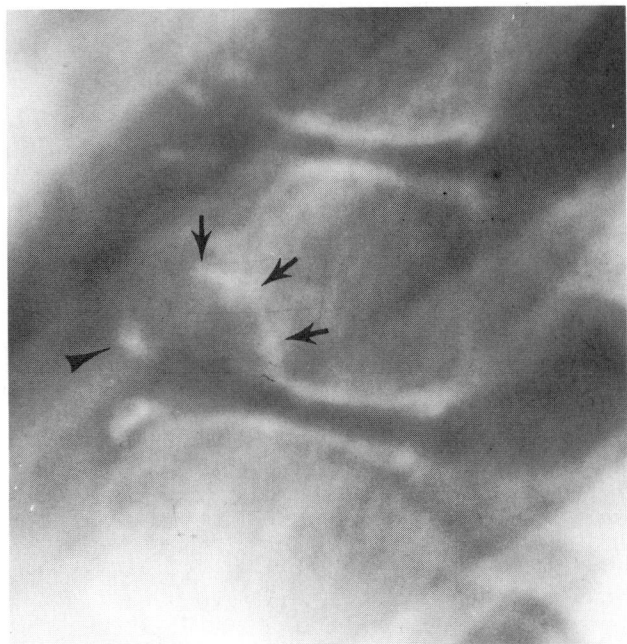

Figure 126–5. Arrows point to the dense margins of a Schmorl's node that represents disk material that had protruded through the weakened inferior plate of a lower thoracic vertebral body in this 11-year-old girl as a feature of Scheuermann's disease. Note the undisplaced ring apophysis *(arrowhead)* secondary growth center behind which the Schmorl's node developed. (Courtesy of A. Oestreich, M.D., Cincinnati, OH. Modified with permission from Oestreich AE. Pediatric Radiology—Medical Outline Series. 3rd ed. New Hyde Park, Medical Examination, 1984. Copyright 1984 by Elsevier Science Publishing Co., Inc.)

Infectious Disorders

Diskitis

Infection of the intervertebral disk space, or diskitis, occurs primarily in younger children, although it should be considered in the differential diagnosis of an adolescent with fever and localized back pain. It can be a complication of intravenous substance abuse. While presumed to be an infectious disease, there is still debate regarding the actual pathophysiology and causative organisms of this disorder.

The chief symptom is back pain, typically without radiation. In younger children this back pain may be manifested as irritability, with hip and abdominal pain as common accompaniments. Younger children will commonly present with a nonacute history of fever, malaise, irritability, limp, or refusal to walk. In one review the average length of symptoms prior to diagnosis was 5 weeks.

Physical findings are dependent on the age of the child and can range from minimal findings to point tenderness, paraspinal muscle spasm, loss of lumbar lordosis, and hamstring spasm. Children may complain of pain when they move about and may support their sitting posture with their arms extended posteriorly. This diagnosis may not be confirmed with laboratory tests; the white blood cell count (WBC) is usually normal, the ESR is elevated only 50% of the time, and blood cultures are almost always negative. While likely to be normal early in the course of the disease, plain films will eventually demonstrate the characteristic narrowing of the disk space, adjacent vertebral body erosions, and end-plate sclerosis. Treatment should include admission for bed rest and infection surveillance. Disk biopsies are culture positive only 25% of the time. If administered, antibiotics should treat *Staphylococcus aureus*. Antibiotic therapy remains controversial and is not indicated unless the host is immunologically compromised or the child's symptoms fail to resolve promptly.

Osteomyelitis

The presenting symptoms and signs of vertebral osteomyelitis can be identical to those of diskitis. The cause of vertebral osteomyelitis is usually *S. aureus*. Although tuberculous osteomyelitis is rare, all children with a suspected vertebral or disk infection should receive tuberculin skin testing. In contrast to diskitis, laboratory tests (CBC, ESR, blood cultures) are more likely to be abnormal in children with vertebral osteomyelitis. Radiographs are usually normal early in the illness but will demonstrate patchy osteoporosis of the affected vertebrae, narrowing of the disk space, or even vertebral collapse within 3 to 4 weeks. Radionuclide bone scanning should provide a definitive diagnosis and localize the site of infection. Treatment should include hospital admission for antibiotic therapy, which may last 6 to 8 weeks. It may be reasonable to delay the administration of antibiotics in the emergency department to allow for a needle biopsy of the affected vertebrae or an adjacent paraspinal abscess, which may provide culture material for

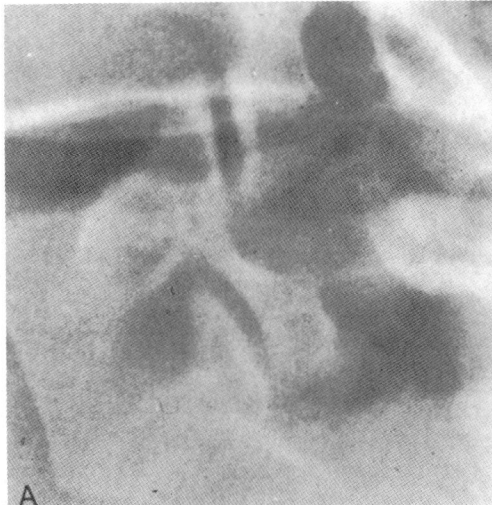
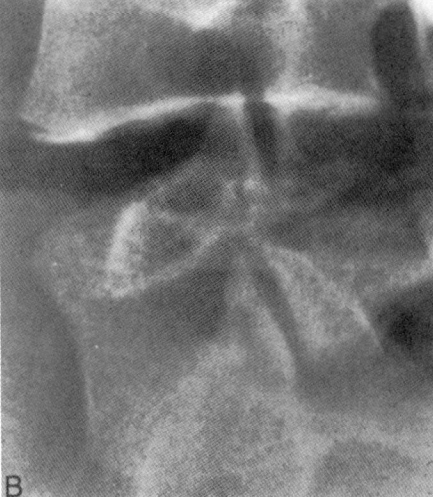

Figure 126–6. Spondylolysis. *A,* Radiograph shows an attenuated pars interarticularis. *B,* There is spondylolysis on the contralateral side in the same patient. (From Ogden JA. Skeletal Injury in the Child. 2nd ed. Philadelphia, WB Saunders, 1990, p 611.)

A   B

definitive characterization of the infecting organism and facilitate eventual ambulatory antibiotic therapy.

Epidural Abscess

Although uncommon, spinal epidural abscesses should be considered. If not diagnosed and treated in a timely fashion, these abscesses can result in permanent and devastating neurologic deficits. Spinal epidural abscesses most commonly involve the thoracic and lumbar spine. The clinical presentation is similar to that of diskitis, with severe back pain exacerbated by movement, local tenderness and muscle spasm, fever, and signs of systemic toxicity. Unfortunately many of these patients will already have developed signs of cord compression with sensory motor deficits or urinary retention. The vast majority of patients will have abnormal WBCs and elevated ESRs. Examination of the cerebrospinal fluid will show evidence of parameningeal infection. Plain radiographs may occasionally demonstrate vertebral changes; however, radionuclide scanning, myelography, and MRI are the best studies to define the abscess. These lesions require immediate surgical drainage followed by parenteral antibiotic therapy. *S. aureus* is the most commonly cultured organism.

Rheumatologic Disorders

The rheumatologic disorders are an uncommon cause of back pain in children. The inflammatory diseases that most frequently cause back pain include ankylosing spondylitis, juvenile rheumatoid arthritis (JRA), dermatomyositis, and rheumatic fever, although scleroderma, systemic lupus erythematosus, and the Henoch-Schönlein syndrome can occasionally cause back pain.

Ankylosing Spondylitis

Although a disease of adult males, ankylosing spondylitis may be seen in children as young as 6 years of age. The pain and stiffness experienced by these patients historically begin in the sacroiliac joints and gradually ascend the spinal column. Symptoms and findings include back pain, decreased chest expansion, and an asymmetric destruction of affected joints. Approximately half will have arthritic involvement of larger peripheral joints. These patients will also have signs of systemic illness with fever, anorexia, anemia, and growth retardation. While the presence of sacroiliitis is considered to be a hallmark of ankylosing spondylitis, most laboratory test results (ESR, C-reactive protein, immunoglobulin G [IgG], IgA, HLA-B27) are not specific for this disorder.

Juvenile Rheumatoid Arthritis

JRA may involve the back, although the most frequent location of spinous discomfort is in the cervical area. As many as one half of children with the polyarticular form of JRA will have neck stiffness and pain. These children will have systemic findings, such as fever, growth failure or weight loss, rashes, and arthritis of one or more larger peripheral joints. Examination will commonly reveal significant limitation of motion and atrophy of the paraspinous muscles. Laboratory tests may fail to confirm the diagnosis of JRA, as a significant number of affected children will be seronegative (i.e., negative antinuclear antibody and rheumatoid factor assays), with nonspecific findings of only mild to moderate anemia and a leukocytosis. Radiographic changes that may be seen include demineralization of articular structures, decreased joint spaces, and loss of cervical lordosis.

Neoplastic Disorders

Osteoid osteoma and osteoblastoma are benign bone tumors, typically occurring in adolescents and young adults. These tumors usually involve the posterior elements of the vertebral column—namely, the transverse and spinous processes, pedicles, and laminae. These present with back pain, with or without point tenderness, and scoliosis. In addition, these children may also experience leg pain, neck tilt, shoulder pain, and paraparesis.

On radiologic examination, osteoid osteoma and osteoblastoma appear as a lytic area surrounded by sclerosis or as sclerosis of one of the posterior elements. However, plain radiographs commonly fail to demonstrate these tumors. Radionuclide bone scanning, tomograms, or CT will help to identify those lesions not seen on routine radiographs. These studies are especially important in the examination of the child or adolescent with a persistently painful scoliosis to prevent worsening scoliosis or nerve compression. The only means of treatment that will provide consistent long-term pain relief and control of the lesion is total excision.

Other lesions may mimic the symptoms or signs of osteoid osteoma and osteoblastoma and may have a similar appearance. Osteogenic sarcoma is a malignant but extremely rare lesion of the spine that is clinically and radiologically indistinguishable from the commoner osteoblastoma. Ewing's tumor is a rare but malignant and extremely destructive tumor of the spine, typically involving the vertebral body. Ewing's tumor is also commonly confused with vertebral osteomyelitis, as it may also present with pain, fever, and a leukocytosis. Aneurysmal bone cysts are also associated with back pain and occasionally paraparesis. These lesions may have a radiologic appearance similar to osteoblastoma, although they will only involve the vertebral body.

The spine is a common site of metastasis for a number of malignancies, including neuroblastoma, Wilms' tumor, lymphoma, and leukemia. The child will present with signs of systemic illness in addition to the symptoms pertaining to the back. Back pain may also be the most commonly prominent symptom of tumors of the spinal cord and the cauda equina syndrome. Tumors of the cord occur most commonly in younger children, whereas lesions of the cauda equina are found most commonly in adults. The origin of many of these lesions may be developmental (intramedullary cyst, lipoma, teratoma), and 70% of the primary tumors are benign. In addition to back or neck pain, which may worsen with cough or physical activity, these children may have radiating extremity pain and eventually neurologic deficits. Sensory function is more commonly affected with lesions of the cauda equina, while motor dysfunction is most commonly seen in younger children with cord tumors. Bowel and bladder dysfunction are typically late findings in both. CT or MRI provides the best means to evaluate intraspinal masses.

Other Disorders

Numerous other disorders can result in pain that is referred to the back. Inflammation of posterior peritoneal or retroperitoneal structures (such as pancreas, duodenum, liver, spleen, kidneys, ovaries, and uterus) is perhaps the most common cause of pain referred to the back. Similarly, inflammation or disorders of the structures in the thorax can result in pain in the upper back. Children with sickle cell disease may have back pain secondary to infarction of the vertebral column or from infarction or inflammation of intra-abdominal or intrathoracic structures. Testicular pain due to torsion or malignancy can also refer pain to the back. Pregnancy, especially in the middle or third trimester, may result in posture change and back pain; nearly one third of women experience back pain during labor.

Disorders that potentiate osteoporosis or osteomalacia may significantly weaken bone structure and potentiate trauma-induced lesions. Osteoporosis and subsequent stress fractures may result from a number of causes, including malnutrition, disuse, Cushing's syndrome, rheumatoid arthritis, and anorexia nervosa. Osteomalacia can be the result of vitamin D–deficient states, renal disease, and hyperparathyroidism. Children who have been subjected to radiation therapy will develop asymmetry of the spine owing to abnormal bone growth. Diseases that promote muscle weakness, particularly those such as muscular dystrophy that affect the strength and support of the spinal column, result in mechanical back pain. Finally, while back pain is a much more frequent site of nonorganic or psychogenic pain in adults, it can also be the location of psychogenic pain in children.

THERAPEUTIC INTERVENTION

The management of back pain will be directed by the findings of clinical, laboratory, and radiologic evaluations. Children should be approached with a careful assessment for underlying pathology. The presence of significant pathology (fracture, tumor, inflammation, infection) of the spine or adjacent body compartments should prompt the appropriate medical or surgical referral for inpatient or ambulatory management. The decision to admit a child should be based on the suspected underlying cause, the severity and perceived manageability of the patient's pain, and the reliability of follow-up care.

The ambulatory management of the more benign mechanical, overuse, or trauma-related disorders is conservative and focused on symptom relief. Discharge instructions should include recommendations for analgesic or anti-inflammatory agents. Ibuprofen (5 to 10 mg/kg/dose) should provide mild to moderate pain relief as well as significant anti-inflammatory action. Patients who fail to obtain adequate pain relief with ibuprofen may require an opioid analgesic. Children with moderate to severe pain generally require ambulatory follow-up (or, for especially severe pain, inpatient care) to assure adequate pain management, and further evaluation to determine the cause. Adolescent patients with associated spasm of paravertebral muscles may benefit from a short course of a skeletal muscle relaxant such as methocarbamol (15 mg/kg/dose) or diazepam (0.25 mg/kg/dose). Finally, the patient and parents should be instructed regarding exercise and activity restrictions that may promote healing or pain relief. Perhaps the most important component of ambulatory management is the follow-up.

Selected References

Azouz EM, Kozlowski K, Marton D, et al. Osteoid osteoma and osteoblastoma of the spine in children. Pediatr Radiol 1986; 16:25.
Baker DR, McHollick W. Spondylolysis and spondylolisthesis in children. J Bone Joint Surg 1956; 38A:933.
Bradford DS, Garcia A. Lumbar disc intervertebral disc herniations in children and adolescents. Orthop Clin North Am 1971; 2:583.
Bunnell WP. Back pain in children. Orthop Clin North Am 1982; 13:587.
Bunnell WP. Back pain in children. Pediatr Rev 1984; 6:183.
Butt WP. Radiology for back pain. Clin Radiol 1989; 40:6.
Bywaters EGL. Ankylosis spondylitis in childhood. Clin Rheum Dis 1976; 2:387.
Carty H, Owen R. Role of radionuclide studies in pediatric orthopedic practice: A review. J R Soc Med 1985; 78:478.

Ciullo JV, Jackson DW. Pars interarticularis stress reaction, spondylolysis and spondylolisthesis in gymnasts. Clin Sports Med 1985; 4:95.
Cole R. Intraspinal tumours. Arch Dis Child 1988; 63:1007.
Fischer GW, Popich GA, Sullivan DE, et al. Discitis: A prospective diagnostic analysis. Pediatrics 1978; 62:543.
Fisk JW, Baigent ML, Hill PD. Scheuermann's disease: Clinical and radiological survey of 17 and 18 year olds. Am J Phys Med 1984; 63:18.
Gonzalez R, Marino RV. A diagnostic approach to childhood back pain. J Am Osteopath Assoc 1986; 86:454.
Hoppenfeld S. Back pain. Pediatr Clin North Am 1977; 24:881.
Jackson DW, Wiltse LL, Cirincione RJ. Spondylolysis in the female gymnast. Clin Orthop 1976; 117:68.
Johnson DL, Falci S. The diagnosis and treatment of pediatric lumbar spine injuries caused by rear seat lap belts. Neurosurgery 1990; 26:434.
King HA. Back pain in children. Pediatr Clin North Am 1984; 31:1083.
Merryweather R, Middlemiss JH, Sanerkin NG. Malignant transformation of osteoblastoma. J Bone Joint Surg 1980; 62:381.
Micheli LJ. Back injuries in gymnastics. Clin Sports Med 1985; 4:85.
Nelson CL, Janecki CF, Gildenberg P, et al. Disk protrusions in the young. Clin Orthop 1972; 88:142.
O'Brien TM, McManua F. Discitis: The irritable back of childhood. Ir J Med Sci 1983; 152:404.
Rothman SL. Computed tomography of the spine in older children and teenagers. Clin Sports Med 1986; 5:247.
Russwurm H, Bjerkreim I, Ronglan E. Lumbar intervertebral disc herniation in the young. Acta Orthop Scand 1978; 49:158.
Schaller JG. Juvenile rheumatoid arthritis. Pediatr Ann 1982; 11:375.
Statham P, Gentleman D. Importance of early diagnosis of acute spinal epidural abscess. J R Soc Med 1989; 82:584.
Tachdjian MO, Matson DD. Orthopedic aspects of intraspinal tumors in infants and children. J Bone Joint Surg 1965; 47:223.
Teitz CC. Sports medicine concerns in dance and gymnastics. Clin Sports Med 1983; 2:571.
Tertti M, Paajanen H, Kujala UM, et al. Disc degeneration in young gymnasts. Am J Sports Med 1990; 18:206.
Turner RH, Bianco AJ. Spondylolysis and spondylolisthesis in children and teenagers. J Bone Joint Surg 1971; 53:1298.
Wilcox PG, Spencer CW. Dorsolumbar kyphosis or Scheuermann's disease. Clin Sports Med 1986; 5:343.
Wiltse LL, Jackson DW. The treatment of spondylolisthesis and spondylolysis in children. Clin Orthop 1976; 117:92.
Wenger DR, Bobechko WP, Gilday DJ. The spectrum of intervertebral disc space infection in children. J Bone Joint Surg 1978; 60A:100.

CHAPTER 127

Limping, Arthritis, and Orthopedic Infections

Mont R. Roberts
Earl J. Reisdorff

THE LIMPING CHILD
Introduction
The Normal Gait

Walking is a complex skill, requiring a balance of coordination and strength. Integrity of the lumbar spine, pelvis, hip, knee, ankle, and foot is also essential. Children typically cruise (walk holding onto objects) at 10 months of age. They take their first independent steps from 10 to 18 months of age. Compared with the adult, the child walks at a faster cadence (steps per minute) but a slower velocity (distance traveled per minute). The child's hips, knees, and ankles are more flexed than the adult's, providing a lower center of gravity and greater balance. Children are usually unable to stand on one foot for 1 second until 2.5 to 3 years of age. By the age of 3 years children exhibit a mature walking pattern.

Types of Limp

Any alteration in a normal gait can be called a limp. An antalgic limp is caused by pain. Attempts to bear weight on a painful limb will activate reflexes that inhibit normal walking. In an effort to minimize discomfort, the child will decrease single-limb support time on the painful limb. With an antalgic limp the length of the stride on the opposite side is shortened to allow a shift of weight back to the normal leg as soon as possible. Other compensatory measures include walking on the heel if there is a splinter in the ball of the foot or walking stiff-legged to reduce any motion from a painful knee. The child with diskitis or vertebral osteomyelitis walks slowly to avoid jarring of the spine.

Neuromuscular disease can also affect gait. Hip girdle weakness, especially involving the hip extensors, due to muscular dystrophy results in a lordotic gait. The Trendelenburg limp of a child with a dislocated hip is due to the pelvic tilting away from the dislocated side. Children with Legg-Calvé-Perthes (LCP) disease or slipped capital femoral epiphysis (SCFE) also have a Trendelenburg gait.

Clinical Evaluation

History

Regarding a limp, the examiner should ask when and how it started as well as if it is painful, constant, worse in the morning (suggesting juvenile rheumatoid arthritis [JRA]), or worse at the end of the day (suggesting muscle fatigue). A history of recent or prior injury is important. Most children sustain minor trauma almost daily, and the significance of a history of trauma when there are no obvious objective findings is limited. If activity worsens a limp that is persistent, a stress fracture should be suspected. Although older children can localize the pain more precisely, pain from hip pathology is notorious for its radiation to the knee. Constitutional symptoms such as fever, weight loss, or malaise suggest infection, rheumatoid disease, or occult malignancy. One should review major developmental milestones; deterioration of walking ability suggests a central nervous system tumor or neuromuscular disease.

Gait Examination

The child should wear little clothing below the waist. Ideally the child's posture and stance while standing should be noted to detect pelvic tilt, scoliosis, compensatory knee flexion, or leg length discrepancy. The child should walk barefoot, allowing the physician to observe the feet and toes. Observation while running, squatting to pick up a toy, or, in the older child, hopping on one leg, heel walking, or toe walking is helpful. Children may concentrate more on the gait when they know they are being observed. Thus having a child run or walk up and down a hall several times may distract the child and produce a more representative gait. It is often helpful to have the parents point out what concerns them about the child's gait.

General Physical Examination

The feet, ankles, knees, hips, and back should be assessed through active and passive range of motion testing, with any pain or limitation recorded. The joints should be inspected for warmth, tenderness, effusion, or erythema; the extremities should be inspected for ecchymoses, erythema, puncture wounds, or deformities and palpated for tenderness, masses, or warmth. Muscle strength testing and a brief neurologic examination should be performed. The general physical examination should note the presence of fever, rash, or pallor.

Diagnostic Evaluation

The physical examination should determine the need for radiographic evaluation. Two views from perpendicular planes should be obtained for specific areas suspected of pathology. Comparison views are frequently needed. Skeletal radiographs, which include the pelvis to the toes on a single film, may be useful. These should be taken in the anteroposterior and "frog leg" positions with the patient supine. Follow-up radiographic studies in addition to the repeat clinical evaluation may be required. Nondisplaced fractures and stress fractures may become apparent only when a follow-up radiograph reveals the periosteal reaction or sclerotic margins of an earlier undetected fracture.

Bone scans may be helpful in detecting stress fractures and other conditions prior to their appearance on plain radiograph. Other diagnostic imaging studies that may be useful when used in conjunction with evaluation by an orthopedic specialist include computed tomography, magnetic resonance imaging, myelography, and arthrography.

The laboratory evaluation of the limping child in the emergency department must be tailored to the acuity of the condition. When obvious trauma has been excluded clinically or radiographically, most patients warrant a complete blood count (CBC) and erythrocyte sedimentation rate (ESR). Measurement of other acute-phase reactants such as C-reactive protein (CRP) may be useful. Testing for streptococcal infection can be performed by a throat swab or an antistreptolysin O titer or streptozyme. Selected cases may require testing for rheumatoid factor (RF), antinuclear antibodies (ANA), histocompatibility antigens (HLA-B27), creatine kinase, or hemoglobin electrophoresis. These studies are usually not indicated in the emergency department for the initial evaluation of most children with a limp. Arthrocentesis is essential in the management of the patient with suspected septic arthritis. When infection is considered, culture of the aspirate, Gram stain, and blood cultures should be obtained.

Differential Diagnosis

Toddlers Age 1 to 3 Years

It may be difficult to determine a limp in this age group. Rather than limp, a toddler may ask to be carried everywhere. In children under age 5 years with an acute limp of unknown etiology, up to 20% had a fracture. The majority of fractures involved the tibia-fibula in children in the 1- to 2-year age group.

A child who exhibits increased side-to-side tilting of the pelvis and marked lordosis of the lumbar spine may likely have congenital dislocation of the hip (Table 127-1). The child with bilateral congenital hip dislocation may be more difficult to diagnose since abnormalities are symmetric.

If a swollen knee appears to be the primary cause of the limp, one should consider JRA. The most common age of presentation is 2 years, and the knee is frequently the first joint involved. Persistent bowing of the legs may suggest a problem with calcium and phosphorus metabolism such as rickets. Persistent toe walking may indicate cerebral palsy. An antalgic gait in a young child may be due to a foreign

TABLE 127–1

DIFFERENTIAL DIAGNOSIS OF LIMB PAIN IN CHILDHOOD

Organic Conditions	Neoplastic
Traumatic	Leukemia
Stress fracture	Lymphoma
Myohematoma	Neuroblastoma
Myositis ossificans	Histiocytosis X
Orthopedic	Bony tumors
Chondromalacia patellae	Osteogenic sarcoma
Osteochrondritis dissecans	Ewing's sarcoma
Osgood-Schlatter disease	Chondrosarcoma
Slipped capital femoral	Soft tissue tumors
epiphysis	Rhabdomyosarcoma
Legg-Calvé-Perthes disease	Fibrosarcoma
Hypermobility syndromes	Synovial cell sarcoma
Collagen-Vascular	**Hematologic**
Juvenile rheumatoid arthritis	Sickle cell anemia
Systemic lupus	Hemophilia
erythematosus	**Endocrine**
Dermatomyositis	Hypercortisolism
Mixed connective tissue	Hyperparathyroidism
disease	Hypothyroidism
Henoch-Schönlein purpura	Osteoporosis
Familial Mediterranean fever	Myopathies
Palindromic rheumatism	**Nutritional**
Rheumatic fever	Scurvy (vitamin C)
Inflammatory bowel disease	Rickets (vitamin D)
Infectious	Hypervitaminosis A
Bacterial	Hypercholesterolemia
Osteomyelitis	**Miscellaneous**
Diskitis	Storage diseases
Septic	Mucopolysaccharidoses
Septic arthritis	Mucolipidoses
Pyogenic	Recurrent arthralgias/myalgias
Pyogenic myositis	associated with strep and
Viral	other infections
Toxic	**Syndromes of Unknown Origin**
"Toxic" synovitis	Fibromyalgia
"Transient" synovitis	Growing pains
Rubella vaccination	**Psychosomatic**
Viral myositis	Hysteria/conversion reactions
	Reflex neurovascular
	dystrophy
	School phobia

From Bowyer SL, Hollister JR. Limb pain in childhood. Pediatr Clin North Am 1984;31:1054.

body such as a splinter in the foot. A child who refuses to walk or has a slow, cautious gait may have diskitis or osteomyelitis.

Age 4 to 10 Years

Children 4 to 10 years of age have a mature gait pattern and should be able to run well. A common hip problem causing limp at this age is toxic or transient synovitis. This can usually be distinguished from septic arthritis; synovitis is associated with a normal temperature, normal white blood cell count (WBC), and a normal ESR. LCP disease is most prevalent in children of this age. Children with LCP disease develop a gradual Trendelenburg limp as well as groin, hip, or knee pain.

Age 11 to 16 Years

SCFE is a common hip problem in adolescence. The obese child with this condition may limp and complain only of knee pain. LCP disease occasionally occurs in this age group.

Participation in athletics results in an increased frequency of injuries such as stress fractures and overuse syndromes.

Stress fractures are most common in the tibia but can also occur in the pelvis, femoral neck, tarsal bones, and metatarsal bones. Osgood-Schlatter disease is osteochondritis of the anterior tibial tubercle caused by overuse of the quadriceps muscle. Secondary gain may cause one to minimize discomfort (to participate in sports) or to maximize symptoms (to be excused from gym classes). Septic arthritis from gonorrhea should be considered in addition to arthritis associated with the collagen-vascular diseases. Other orthopedic conditions causing an altered gait to consider in this group include idiopathic scoliosis, spondylolisthesis, and pathology of the knee, which includes patellar subluxation, chondromalacia patellae, osteochondrosis of the proximal patellar tendon, and osteochondritis dissecans. Adolescence is the peak age for osteogenic sarcoma, and its most common sites of occurrence are the distal femur and proximal tibia.

Specific Conditions

Trauma

Injuries are a common cause of limping in children. Since most children are active and are continuously sustaining minor trauma, the history of trauma is often unrelated to the true cause of a patient's limp.

The "toddler's fracture," a nondisplaced oblique fracture of the distal tibial shaft, along with other tibia-fibula fractures, is the cause of an acute limp in up to 10% of children under age 5 years. Child abuse should be considered in the child with a fracture of the femur or tibia. Puncture wounds, retained subcutaneous foreign bodies of the feet, insect bites, and irritation of the feet from poorly fitting shoes may cause a toddler to limp.

In athletic young children and adolescents, several sports-related injuries occur. Stress fractures are a process of fatigue failure of bones. The tibia and fibula are most commonly involved in adolescents. Other locations include the metatarsals, femurs, pelvis, and lumbar spine. Soft tissue injuries to any of the musculotendinous units may also develop chronically as sports-related overuse syndromes. Trauma may also result in contusions, sprains, and avulsion injuries of muscle attachments.

Congenital Dislocation of the Hip

A congenital dislocation of one or both hips (CDH) results from the pathologic development of the hip structures. Most children with CDH are firstborns, and the left hip is involved more frequently. The diagnosis of CDH should be made as soon as possible in the neonatal period. When CDH is diagnosed after 6 months of age, simple closed reduction and immobilization will usually not provide a satisfactory result. Traction may be required prior to manipulation under general anesthesia. Beyond 18 months of age, open reduction and complex surgical procedures are often necessary, and less satisfactory results are obtained.

The stability of the hip is classified according to whether the hip is dislocated, dislocatable, or subluxable. Dislocation is detected clinically by the Ortolani test. A relaxed, supine infant has each hip separately examined. One hand stabilizes the pelvis while the other hand positions the long finger on the posterior aspect of the hip over the greater trochanter (Fig. 127–1). The thumb is placed anteriorly over the region of the lesser trochanter. With the knee and hip flexed approximately 90 degrees, the thigh and leg are abducted gently while lifting the femoral head anteriorly. A positive Ortolani test results when this maneuver results in a palpable "clunk" with the reduction of the dislocated hip into the acetabulum. A dislocatable or subluxable hip is detected with

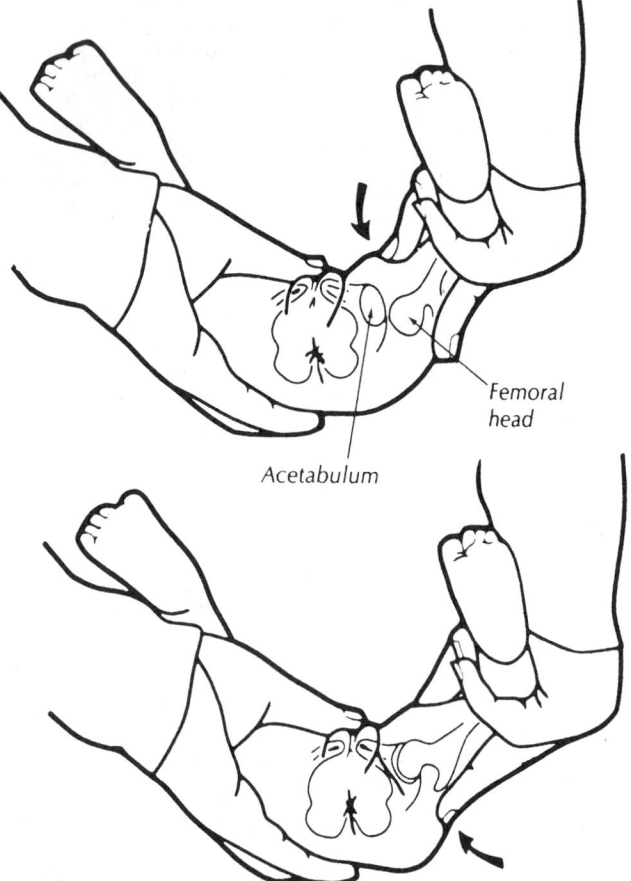

Femoral head

Acetabulum

Figure 127–1. Examination technique for congenital dislocation of the hip. (From Burnside JW. Physical Diagnosis: An Introduction to Clinical Medicine. 16th ed. Baltimore, Williams & Wilkins, 1981, p 246.)

the Barlow test. With the infant in the same position as for the Ortolani test, the thigh is gently adducted and pressure is applied posteriorly. A positive test results when the head of the femur is palpated to move partially or completely out of the acetabulum.

In the older child the proximal femur becomes more permanently fixed in the dislocated position, and the joint capsule and soft tissues mold to accommodate this position. Physical findings include bunching of the skin on the dislocated side owing to effective thigh shortening, a lower position of the knee when the patient is in the supine position, and free moving or "pistoning" of the femur up and down with respect to the pelvis. The patient has a limp. The patient with bilateral CDH will have a waddling lordotic gait, and the perineal space is widened.

The evaluation of radiographs in CDH is difficult. In the newborn period x-ray studies are unreliable. At 6 weeks of age and older, typical radiographic lines become apparent, which help to define the location of the head of the femur in an abnormally lateral and superior position. The patient with suspected or confirmed CDH should be immediately referred to an orthopedic specialist.

Transient Synovitis

Transient synovitis, also called toxic synovitis, is a common cause of limping in children from age 18 months to 12 years. Transient synovitis is primarily a diagnosis of exclu-

sion. The cause of transient synovitis remains unknown but has been attributed to infection, trauma, allergy, or an early presentation of LCP disease.

A child with transient synovitis presents to the emergency department with a history of a limp or a refusal to bear weight on a leg. There may be a history of recent minor trauma. There is frequently a history of an upper respiratory tract infection in the preceding 2 weeks or occasionally evidence of a recent streptococcal infection. The symptoms vary from mild hip pain to an inability to bear weight on the affected leg. Usually the symptoms are present for less than 2 weeks. The child has a normal or minimally elevated body temperature; pain in the knee, thigh, or hip with active or passive range of motion of the hip; and a limitation of abduction and rotation of the hip. Importantly, there is an absence of other clinical findings that would suggest another explanation for the condition. The WBC count and ESR may be normal or minimally elevated. A WBC count greater than 15,000/mm^3 is unusual with transient synovitis of the hip in one series. Radiographs are usually normal or may show an increased medial joint space in the hip owing to the presence of an effusion. Ultrasonography has detected an effusion in up to 95% of cases of transient synovitis involving the hip.

The clinical approach is directed at excluding potentially catastrophic conditions. Transient synovitis is clinically indistinguishable from LCP disease, and follow-up of patients with transient synovitis demonstrated that some cases were actually early presentations of LCP disease. The prognosis for transient synovitis is unclear, probably owing to differences in its definition. Opinions vary from no long-term sequelae to up to 60% abnormal radiographs after 15 years of follow-up.

Legg-Calvé-Perthes Disease

LCP disease is a self-limited disorder of the hip initiated by idiopathic avascular necrosis of the femoral head complicated by a subchondral stress fracture that heralds the clinical onset of the condition. This disorder occurs primarily in males, with an average age at onset of 6 years and the majority of patients present between the ages of 4 and 9 years.

Patients with LCP disease present most commonly with a limp and minimal to no pain in the hip. The pain may be referred to the knee or thigh and is usually aggravated by activity and relieved by rest. The symptoms may be acute or insidious. There is occasionally a history of trauma.

The physical examination will reveal a nontoxic child with a normal temperature. The gait will reveal an antalgic limp, internal rotation, and a limitation of hip abduction.

The CBC is usually normal, and the ESR is either normal or mildly elevated. The radiographic evaluation may appear normal early in the disease but subsequently undergoes classic changes, which provide a staging of the disease radiographically (Fig. 127–2). The *initial phase* reveals a smaller ossific nucleus of the femoral head caused by avascularity; this is associated with a widening of the medial joint space either from effusion or from hypertrophy of the epiphyseal cartilage. During this phase the subchondral radiolucent zone (crescent sign or "Caffey's sign") due to epiphyseal stress fracture appears. The extent of the fracture line determines the extent of the necrotic fragment of bone, and together with the age of the patient is a useful prognostic indicator for outcome. The femoral head will have a varying degree of increased radiodensity, partially from collapse and crowding of the avascular trabeculae by the new bone formation. In the second phase, called the *fragmentation phase*, the epiphysis begins to fragment and there are areas

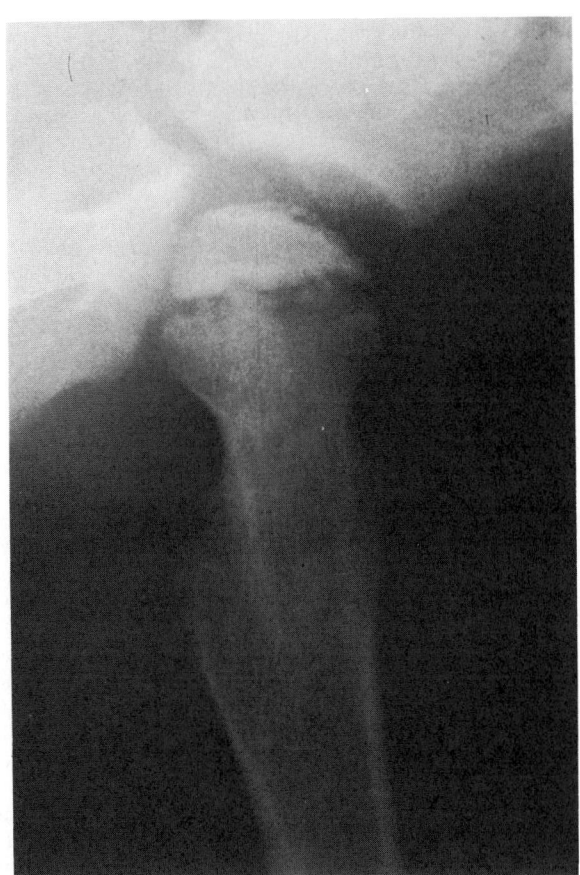

Figure 127–2. Radiograph demonstrates the early findings of Legg-Calvé-Perthes disease. There is a subchondral lucency of the subcortical margin of the femoral head. A slight collapse of the lateral margin of the epiphysis of the femoral head is noted.

of increased radiodensity and radiolucency. This may be related to new bone forming on old bone and ingrowth of fibrous vascular tissue from the periphery. In the *reparative* or *reossification phase*, normal bone density returns and alterations in the shape of the proximal femur become apparent. The final *healed phase* represents the hip joint after the disease and the repair process are complete. Technetium bone scanning is both sensitive and specific for LCP disease.

LCP disease can be clinically indistinguishable from transient synovitis, but the patient with LCP disease eventually has characteristic radiographic changes. A bone scan will discriminate between the two conditions. The child with a septic hip holds a posture of flexion and abduction of the hip, in contrast to the adduction seen in LCP disease. The child with rheumatoid disease may have a rash, evidence of systemic illness, and elevated acute-phase reactants in the serum. Radiographs will show the ossific nucleus of the femoral head to be larger rather than smaller as in LCP disease.

Treatment varies with the severity of disease. Most cases will require no treatment if they present in the early stages with minimal avascular necrosis and fracture. Those cases with involvement of most of the femoral head need treatment as directed by orthopedic referral, which focuses on containment of the femoral head within the acetabulum either with orthotics or with surgical procedures.

Slipped Capital Femoral Epiphysis

This uncommon condition is the most common hip disease causing limp in the adolescent, primarily obese males. SCFE occurs when the capital femoral epiphysis is displaced relative to the femoral neck (Fig. 127–3). The slippage usually results in the capital epiphysis becoming displaced posteriorly and inferiorly with respect to the femoral neck; the relationship of the femoral head to the acetabulum remains normal.

The condition can be classified as acute, chronic, or acute on chronic. An acute slip presents with symptoms for only a matter of a few weeks or less. A chronic slip is defined as greater than 3 weeks of symptoms. Acute on chronic slips have symptoms for longer periods of time with a definite recent increase in intensity of symptoms.

The obese adolescent male patient with SCFE will present with a dull, aching pain in the thigh, hip, groin, or knee. The pain is worse with physical activity. There is no fever or evidence of systemic illness. There is an antalgic, Trendelenburg gait. There may be tenderness anteriorly over the hip joint and limitation of the range of motion of the hip to flexion, internal rotation, and abduction. Classically the hip will externally rotate with flexion.

Radiography must include both anteroposterior and lateral views, as the slip may only be seen on the lateral film. A line drawn along the superior border of the femoral neck in the anteroposterior view should transect the epiphysis by at least 20%. The degree of slippage is graded as mild, moderate, or severe depending on the percentage of displacement. Severe slippage is defined as greater than 50% displacement.

Treatment of SCFE is an emergency since any further amount of weight bearing may result in conversion of a mild slip to a severe slip with an increased risk of multiple

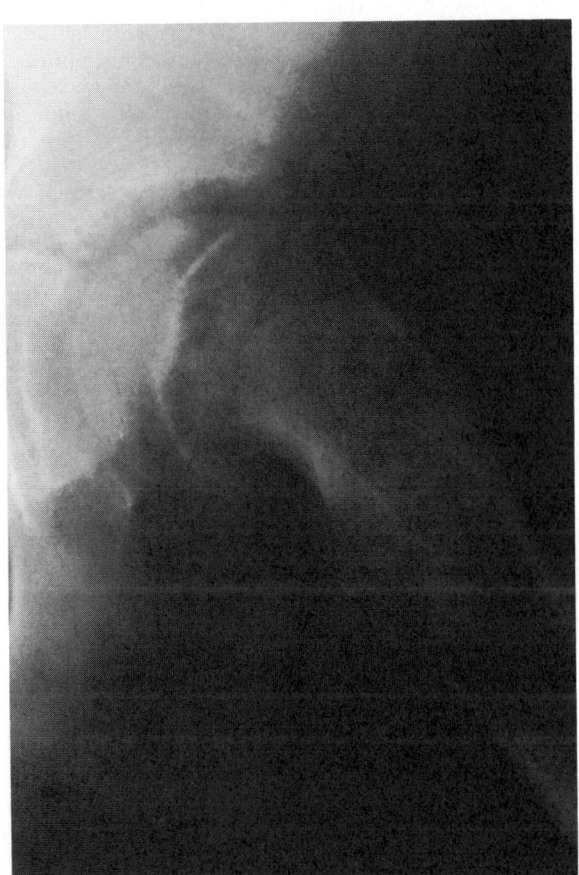

Figure 127–3. Typical radiographic view of a slipped capital femoral epiphysis, which is displaced posteriorly and inferiorly in relation to the femoral neck.

complications, including avascular necrosis. Patients must be admitted to the hospital for bed rest, traction, and orthopedic procedures that fix the femoral head on the neck until the physis has closed.

Osgood-Schlatter Disease

Osgood-Schlatter disease is osteochondrosis of the anterior tibial tubercle. The etiology is unclear, but it is thought to be caused by overuse of the quadriceps muscle, resulting in a traction injury to the apophysis of the tibial tuberosity where it is attached. Adolescents of both sexes are affected. Patients complain of pain in the anterior leg, which is made worse with leg extension. Tenderness is noted over the tibial tuberosity, which may be enlarged. Pain is made worse with resistance to leg extension. The diagnosis is clinical since radiographs may be normal or may show fragmentation of the tibial tuberosity, which may be a normal variant. Radiographs should be done to exclude tumors or stress fractures. The disease may be bilateral. The goal of treatment is restriction of activity over about 6 weeks to avoid pain. Immobilization is not usually needed. The condition resolves when the apophysis fuses to the metaphysis with maturity.

Neoplasms

Tumors may result in a limp from local pain in a lower extremity or the pelvis or from central neurologic weakness due to an intracranial mass. A gradually progressive deterioration in gait may indicate a central lesion. Bone tumors in childhood are uncommon. Osteosarcoma is the most common pediatric bone malignancy. It occurs most commonly in adolescents in the distal femur or the proximal tibia. Patients complain of knee pain that is worse at night and unrelated to activity. The physical examination should focus on the afflicted extremity and adjacent joints and extremities. It is important to discriminate between extremity tenderness and joint tenderness, as intraosseous tumors rarely extend into the adjacent joint.

The serum alkaline phosphatase can be elevated with osteosarcoma. Radiographs of all bones and adjacent joints in the affected extremity are needed. Malignant lesions of the bone will be rapidly growing, and the margin with normal bone will not be sclerotic. Benign bone tumors, being more slow growing, have the opportunity for normal bone to develop a sclerotic margin around the mass. A bone tumor destroying or replacing bone creates a radiolucent defect. If the tumor produces a matrix, it may produce an organized-appearing radiodense ossification or a radiodense disorganized calcification. Conditions that may mimic neoplasms include osteomyelitis, stress fractures, avulsion fractures, or myositis ossificans, all of which may cause focal bone abnormalities.

Leukemia is the most common malignancy of childhood. The patient may have nonspecific aching pain and a limp or refusal to walk. Radiographs may show osteolytic lesions or periosteal elevation but can be normal in 25% to 60% of patients.

Miscellaneous Conditions

There are numerous conditions that can be responsible for a limp in the child, including arthritic conditions and orthopedic infections, which are discussed later. Patients with hemophilia may develop hemarthrosis, which results in a limp when the foot, ankle, knee, or hip is involved. Sickle cell anemia may present with vasoocclusive episodes, which cause variably severe joint and limb pain. Infarction of long bones can occur, with the humerus, tibia, and femur most often affected. Patients may present with a limp when the infarction involves the lower extremities. The patient may have a fever with a normal or elevated WBC count and ESR. Radiographs may not be helpful acutely, but long-standing disease may result in sclerosis, periosteal reaction, and infarction. Osteomyelitis and septic arthritis need to be considered when fever is present.

Abdominal and genitourinary conditions may cause an alteration of gait. Inguinal adenitis, testicular torsion, or acute appendicitis can cause pain with movement of the lower extremities.

Therapeutic Intervention

For most conditions that cause a child to limp, a delay in diagnosis does not pose a threat to the child. Therefore without a readily discernible cause for the limp, the child should be referred to an orthopedist or neurologist for subsequent evaluation. Nevertheless, certain conditions must be excluded at the time of initial evaluation. These include fractures, SCFE, septic arthritis, osteomyelitis, CDH, tumors, and child abuse. The younger child unable to give a history may have an occult lower extremity fracture. If the history is inconsistent with the type of fracture, if there is evidence of old trauma in various stages of healing, or if any other part of the evaluation is suspicious, child abuse should be suspected. Fractures involving the physis may not be readily apparent on radiograph, especially Salter I or V fractures. A history of trauma with tenderness circumferentially around the physis suggests an undisplaced growth plate fracture. These injuries should be treated as fractures and referred to an orthopedist. A febrile child with an inability to bear weight on an extremity with decreased joint motion or bone tenderness should be considered to have septic arthritis. With a high fever and elevated WBC count and ESR, the child will need immediate orthopedic evaluation, hospital admission, and emergent arthrocentesis. The adolescent with a limp and clinical or radiographic findings suggestive of SCFE needs immediate hospitalization with bed rest, traction, and orthopedic consultation. The patient with CDH or a malignant tumor may not require emergency measures; however, the most important concern is identification of the problem and the assurance of timely specialist intervention and definitive care.

ARTHRITIS
Clinical Evaluation

The subjective complaint of pain in an extremity is termed arthralgia. Arthritis is the swelling of a joint or pain, tenderness, or warmth in a joint and is associated with a limitation of the range of motion.

The clinical assessment should focus on the primary joint affected. The duration of joint inflammation, the progression of any limitation of range of motion, and the past history of similar episodes should be determined. The involvement of a single joint as compared to multiple joints should be determined. One should ascertain if there is migratory joint inflammation. Other information should include recent trauma, recent exposure to known infectious diseases, recent rubella immunization, current medications, allergies, and a family history of rheumatic diseases.

The physical assessment should include a careful examination of all the joints. Infants and younger children should be offered a toy to evaluate active range of motion. Toddlers and older children should be observed while walking to evaluate the weight-bearing joints. Joints should be put through passive range of motion. Inspection should involve the opposite limb for comparison of any erythema, ecchymoses, swelling, or rash. Swelling of a joint may be caused by a serous, purulent, or bloody effusion. The joint swelling seen with rheumatoid arthritis caused by synovial hypertrophy or periarticular edema may be boggy compared with the fluctuance of an effusion. The joint should be assessed for warmth and tenderness. The extremities around inflamed joints should be examined for edema, atrophy, nodules, or lymphangitis. Limb atrophy may cause an adjacent joint to appear swollen when it is not.

Diagnostic Evaluation

A careful history and physical examination may be all that is necessary to diagnose a simple problem such as a local allergic reaction to an insect bite or a subluxed radial head (nursemaid's elbow). When the cause of the joint complaint is not readily apparent, or when serious pathology is suspected, determination of the ESR, CRP, and total and differential WBC count is indicated. A throat swab for streptococcal screening and a urinalysis should be done. In the presence of a fever or elevated acute-phase reactants, a blood culture should be done.

Arthrocentesis is the most critical procedure for acute monoarticular arthritis (Table 127–2). It is technically more difficult to perform in young children and infants because of poor cooperation; sedation or general anesthesia may be required. Ultrasound of the hip may be useful to detect small amounts of fluid prior to arthrocentesis. In the absence of a fever or elevated WBC count, ESR, or CRP determination, the diagnosis of septic arthritis is unlikely.

The majority of cases with monoarticular joint swelling should be examined radiographically since an orthopedic disorder may be present. When symptoms persist for greater than 2 weeks and the diagnosis is uncertain, further studies may be indicated, including ANA, serum immunoglobulins, RF, and streptozyme. Titers for antibodies to *Yersinia, Salmonella, Chlamydia, Mycoplasma,* viruses, and the Lyme disease spirochete, *Borrelia burgdorferi,* should be considered. Repeat radiographs may be indicated to detect stress fractures or evolving necrosis.

Differential Diagnosis

Acute single-joint inflammation is commonly seen with trauma or infections (Table 127–3). Migratory arthritis suggests acute rheumatic fever or gonococcal disease. When the single joint involved is the hip, the diagnoses reviewed in the preceding discussion on limping are most relevant; JRA of the hip is rare. The knee is the most commonly affected joint in monoarticular and pauciarticular JRA. The knee is also the most common site of musculoskeletal tumors in children. Lyme disease most commonly involves the knee joint. Hemophilia and leukemia should be considered with single-joint involvement in arthritis.

When multiple joints are involved asymmetrically, orthopedic and neoplastic conditions (except leukemia) are less likely. Symmetric involvement of joints usually suggests JRA.

The pain of JRA is typically mild. Gentle range of motion can be performed, and walking is usually possible when the lower extremities are involved. The joints affected with septic arthritis, acute rheumatic fever, and systemic lupus erythematosus (SLE) are extremely painful.

The presence of a rash in association with fever or elevated ESR is suggestive of connective tissue disease. The specific clinical findings of extraarticular pathology, in conjunction with tests for ANA, RF, serum complement assays, serum immunoglobulins, and HLA antigens, will aid in diagnosis. Connective tissue diseases other than JRA, including SLE, dermatomyositis, scleroderma, and mixed connective tissue disease, are seen less often.

The differential diagnosis of arthritis includes a broad range of conditions. At the initial presentation septic arthritis must be excluded. Unstable fractures, dislocations, SCFE, and neoplastic disease such as leukemia and osteogenic sarcoma should be identified.

Specific Conditions
Juvenile Rheumatoid Arthritis

JRA is the most common pediatric connective tissue disease. JRA encompasses a group of diseases characterized by chronic, nonsuppurative synovitis and associated with a number of extraarticular conditions. By definition persistent arthritis must be present for at least 6 weeks, and the age at presentation is under 16 years. This condition differs from adult rheumatoid arthritis. In JRA the joints involved are predominantly the larger joints, such as the knees, wrists, and ankles, rather than the hands. The etiology of JRA is unknown. An autoimmune response to unidentified antigens, possibly related to viral infection, is a hypothesized mechanism. Complete recovery is possible for the majority of children with JRA.

There are three primary subgroups of JRA (Table 127–4). The condition is termed pauciarticular (or oligoarticular) when four or less joints are involved; polyarticular when five or more joints are involved; and systemic when a variable number of joints are involved and systemic disease is present.

Pauciarticular JRA. The pauciarticular onset form is the most frequently encountered subgroup. Half of the time it

---

TABLE 127–2

SYNOVIAL FLUID ANALYSIS

	Normal	Traumatic (Hemorrhagic) Arthritis	Acute Rheumatic Fever	Juvenile Rheumatoid Arthritis	Septic Arthritis
Appearance	Clear, yellow to colorless	Bloody, xanthochromic or straw colored	Cloudy yellow	Cloudy yellow	Cloudy yellow to purulent
Mucin clot	Good	Variable	Variable	Fair to poor	Poor
WBC*	<200	<5000	5000–50,000	5000–80,000	50,000–200,000
PMNs†	<25%	<25%	50%	50–75%	75–100%
Comments	No fibrin clot	High number of RBCs	Large fibrin clot	Large fibrin clot	Bacterial culture positive

*White blood cell counts can vary greatly.
†Polymorphonuclear leukocytes can vary somewhat.
RBCs = red blood cells.

TABLE 127–3

DIFFERENTIAL DIAGNOSIS OF ARTHRITIS

Acute Onset	Insidious Onset
Toxic Child	**Toxic Child**
Systemic JRA	Systemic JRA
Infection: bacterial, viral	Infection: tuberculous, fungal
Leukemia	Sarcoidosis
SLE	Neuroblastoma
Reiter's syndrome	Other neoplasms
Reactive arthritis	
Sickle cell disease	
Serum sickness	
Acute rheumatic fever	
Vasculitis: Henoch-Schönlein purpura, Kawasaki's syndrome	
Inflammatory bowel disease	
Well Child	**Well Child**
Trauma	Pauciarticular JRA
Toxic synovitis	Polyarticular JRA
Reflex neurovascular dystrophy	Seronegative spondyloarthropathies
Hemophilia	Osteochondroses: Legg-Calvé-Perthes, Osgood-Schlatter disease
SCFE	SCFE
Pigmented villonodular synovitis	Lyme disease
	Mechanical derangement
	Diskitis
	Osteoid osteoma
	Foreign body synovitis
	Hypermobility
	Patellofemoral joint disease
	Synovial hemangioma

JRA = juvenile rheumatoid arthritis; SLE = systemic lupus erythematosus; SCFE = slipped capital femoral epiphysis.
From Morrissy RT (ed). Lovell and Winter's Pediatric Orthopaedics. 3rd ed. Philadelphia, JB Lippincott, 1990, p 305.

TABLE 127–4

SUBGROUPS OF JUVENILE RHEUMATOID ARTHRITIS

	Polyarticular Rheumatoid Factor Negative	Polyarticular Rheumatoid Factor Positive	Pauciarticular Type I	Pauciarticular Type II	Systemic Onset
Percent of JRA patients	20–25	5–10	35–40	10–15	20
Sex	90% girls	80% girls	80% girls	90% boys	60% boys
Age at onset	Throughout childhood	Late childhood	Early childhood	Late childhood	Throughout childhood
Joints	Any; multiple	Any; multiple	Few; large joints: knee, ankle, elbow	Few; large joints: hip girdle	Any; multiple
Sacroiliitis	No	Rare	No	Common	No
Iridocyclitis	Rare	No	30% chronic iridocyclitis	10–20% acute iridocyclitis	No
Rheumatoid factor	Negative	100%	Negative	Negative	Negative
Antinuclear antibodies	25%	75%	90%	Negative	Negative
HLA studies	?	HLA-DR4	HLA-DR5, -DRW6, -DRW8	HLA-B27	?
Ultimate morbidity	Severe arthritis, 10–15%	Severe arthritis, >50%	Ocular damage, 10%; polyarthritis, 20%	Subsequent spondyloarthropathy, ?%	Severe arthritis, 25%

From Behrman RS, Vaughan VC (eds). Nelson Textbook of Pediatrics. 13th ed. Philadelphia, WB Saunders, 1987, p 516.

begins in a single joint, usually the knee. It is further subdivided into types I and II disease. Type I disease usually occurs in girls before the age of 4 years and involves a few larger joints; the primary morbidity is ocular damage from chronic iridocyclitis. Serologic tests for RF are negative but ANA testing is positive 90% of the time; HLA-B27 is unrelated. Joint destruction is usually minimal. Iridocyclitis can lead to permanent visual impairment warranting early evaluation by an ophthalmologist. The type II form of the pauciarticular presentation primarily affects boys over the age of 8 years. The large joints of the lower extremities and the hip girdle are usually involved, and sacroiliitis is common. Serologic testing for RF and ANA are negative, but HLA-B27 is present in 75% of cases. Iridocyclitis can occur but is usually self-limiting. Early in the disease this form of JRA is similar to juvenile ankylosing spondylitis. Long-term morbidity is related to the development of ankylosing spondylitis, Reiter's syndrome, or inflammatory bowel disease.

Polyarticular JRA. The polyarticular form of JRA occurs in 25% to 35% of cases. It can be RF positive or negative. Testing for ANA is positive 25% of the time in RF-negative patients and 75% of the time in RF-positive patients. Girls are predominantly affected, and both large and small joints are affected. The joint involvement is frequently symmetric. The involvement of the temporomandibular joint is common, and the cervical spine is involved 50% of the time. Long-term morbidity is related to joint destruction, primarily in the hips, and is seen most frequently in RF-positive patients.

Systemic JRA. The systemic onset form of JRA is the least common form, occurring in 20% of cases. Its hallmark is the occurrence of fever and rash and prominent extra-articular manifestations. Intermittent high fever, over 39.4°C (103°F), in a quotidian or biquotidian pattern is seen with shaking chills. The rash is a pale, erythematous, macular eruption with coalescence and occasionally central pallor. The rash is primarily central but may occur anywhere on the body, including the palms and soles. Hepatosplenomegaly, pleuritis, and pericarditis are frequently seen. The serologic tests for RF and ANA are negative. The development of joint inflammation is minimal at the outset, but the ultimate morbidity is related to long-term disability related to joint destruction, which is seen in about one fourth of patients.

Diagnostic Evaluation. Laboratory studies may reveal elevated acute-phase reactants (ESR, CRP), especially in the systemic onset form of JRA. A low hematocrit may be seen owing to an anemia of chronic disease. Synovial fluid analysis, usually done to exclude septic arthritis, reveals from 5000 to 80,000 WBCs/mm³, predominantly polymorphonuclear cells, without bacteria. The synovial fluid glucose may be decreased and the protein elevated.

Radiographs show only soft tissue swelling early in the disease. Later findings reveal erosion, fusion, and bone destruction within the joint.

Therapeutic Intervention. Most patients with JRA do not suffer from significant long-term disability. The unpredictable course of the disease can be frustrating. The goal of medical therapy is to maintain joint function and manage extra-articular manifestations. Physical and occupational therapy is important to maintain joint motion and muscle strength. The first line of drug therapy is the nonsteroidal antiinflammatory drugs (NSAIDs); aspirin is the initial drug of choice (Table 127–5). Aspirin levels are followed with doses sufficient to maintain a therapeutic level of 20 to 30 mg/dl. The other NSAIDs are increasingly being used because of the association of salicylates with Reye's syndrome. Corticosteroids are used in JRA for severe systemic onset JRA unresponsive to salicylates, for decompensated pericarditis or myocarditis, and for iridocyclitis unresponsive to other ophthalmic drugs. The use of intraarticular steroid injections, orthopedic surgical treatment, and other drugs such as gold salts, chloroquine, and occasionally cytotoxic agents should be directed by a consulting specialist.

Aseptic Postinfectious Arthritis

Reactive arthritis or postinfectious arthritis refers to arthritis in one or more joints related to an infection in a site distant from the affected joints. In this condition no organisms are isolated from the joint fluid. Antigens or inactive microbial remnants may be present in the joint fluid with reactive arthritis. Nevertheless, the distinction between infectious and reactive arthritis is becoming less clear.

Reiter's syndrome, with the classic triad of arthritis, conjunctivitis, and urethritis, is often considered to be a reactive arthritis, with the presumed site of infection in the genital tract or gastrointestinal tract. The infectious agent is typically an enteric pathogen, including *Shigella*, *Salmonella*, *Yersinia*, and *Campylobacter*. This is most commonly seen in boys, and there is a strong correlation with HLA-B27. More than one joint is typically involved, with the large joints of the lower extremities predominating. The arthritis lasts from 1 month to 1 year and is self-limited; recurrences are uncommon. Other manifestations include oral and genital ulcers, anemia, and slightly elevated acute-phase reactants. Therapy is with aspirin or another NSAID, and physical therapy.

Other causes of aseptic postinfectious arthritis include *Mycoplasma* infection, *Chlamydia* infection, and poststreptococcal arthritis. The discrimination of rheumatic fever from poststreptococcal arthritis may be difficult. Carditis is seen in rheumatic fever; carditis is absent in poststreptococcal arthritis. Arthritis has also been associated with viral infections such as hepatitis, mononucleosis, rubella, and enteroviral infections.

TABLE 127–5

ANTI-INFLAMMATORY DRUG DOSES

	Dose (mg/kg)	Daily Maximum (mg)	Comments
Aspirin	80–130	4500	Monitor serum levels
Indomethacin	2.5	200	Liquid available
Indomethacin-SR	2.5	200	SR taken bid
Ibuprofen	20–40	3200	Liquid 20 mg/ml
Tolmetin	25	2000	
Fenoprofen	40	3200	
Naproxen	10–15	1000	Liquid taken bid
Prednisone	0.1–1.0		Use as low a dose as possible

Lyme Disease

The spirochete *B. burgdorferi* causes Lyme arthritis, which is an aseptic postinfectious arthritis. However, the response of the arthritis early in the disease to antibiotic therapy suggests that the condition may be an infectious arthritis. Late diagnosed cases, after failure of antibiotic therapy, suggests an associated immune complex mechanism for the arthritis.

The Lyme disease spirochete is transmitted by deer ticks of the *Ixodes* genus. This disease is now the most common vector-borne infection in the United States. In the early stage of infection, symptoms include arthralgias and erythema chronicum migrans lesions. Within days to weeks after the initial inoculation, the symptoms include the skin (recurrent rashes), nervous system (meningitis, neuritis), and musculoskeletal system (migratory arthritis) (Table 127–6). In the late infection stage, during the second and third year of illness, chronic arthritis begins. The knee is the joint most commonly involved. Serologic evidence of elevated antibody titers to *B. burgdorferi* is found after the first several weeks of infection.

Current treatment guidelines for children under age 8 years with early infection include amoxicillin or penicillin V (50 mg/kg/day in divided doses) for 10 to 30 days. In penicillin-allergic patients, erythromycin (30 to 50 mg/kg/day in divided doses) is substituted. High-dose parenteral penicillin G therapy (200,000 to 300,000 units/kg/day up to 20 million units) or ceftriaxone (75 to 100 mg/kg/day intrave-nously or intramuscularly, maximum 2 gm/day) for 14 days is indicated for patients with late infection with neurologic complications or arthritis unresponsive to oral therapy.

Preventive measures include avoiding high-risk grassy areas; wearing long pants, long-sleeved shirts, and high socks and shoes; using insect repellents; and checking for and removing ticks daily when potentially exposed.

SEPTIC ARTHRITIS
Introduction

Septic arthritis is an inflammation of the joint caused by pus-forming organisms. Bacteria gain entrance into the joint by hematogenous spread, direct extension (e.g., from osteomyelitis), and direct inoculation (e.g., during joint aspiration, penetrating wound).

Septic arthritis is most frequent in children 1 to 2 years of age. Joints of the lower extremities are involved in more than 90% of cases. The knee is the most commonly affected joint (40% of all cases).

Most cases of joint infection (93%) are monoarticular. The incidence of polyarticular septic joints is significantly increased if the infective agent is *Neisseria gonorrhoeae;* half of the patients infected by *N. gonorrhoeae* have multiple joint involvement. *Staphylococcus aureus, Streptococcus pneumoniae, Salmonella* (especially in sickle cell disease), *Haemophilus influenzae* (in children <2 years), and *N. gonorrhoeae* (especially in adolescents) are the common bacteria that cause septic arthritis.

TABLE 127–6

MANIFESTATIONS OF LYME DISEASE BY STAGE*			
	Early Infection		**Late Infection**
System†	**Localized (Stage 1)**	**Disseminated (Stage 2)**	**Persistent (Stage 3)**
Skin	Erythema migrans	Secondary annular lesions, malar rash, diffuse erythema or urticaria, evanescent lesions, lymphocytoma	Acrodermatitis chronica atrophicans, localized scleroderma-like lesions
Musculoskeletal system		Migratory pain in joints, tendons, bursae, muscle, bone; brief arthritis attacks; myositis‡; osteomyelitis‡; panniculitis‡	Prolonged arthritis attacks, chronic arthritis, peripheral enthesopathy, periostitis or joint subluxations below lesions of acrodermatitis
Neurologic system		Meningitis, cranial neuritis, Bell's palsy, motor or sensory radiculoneuritis, subtle encephalitis, mononeuritis multiplex, myelitis‡, chorea‡, cerebellar ataxia‡	Chronic encephalomyelitis, spastic parapareses, ataxic gait, subtle mental disorders, chronic axonal polyradiculopathy, dementia‡
Lymphatic system	Regional lymphadenopathy	Regional or generalized lymphadenopathy, splenomegaly	
Heart		Atrioventricular nodal block, myopericarditis, pancarditis	
Eyes		Conjunctivitis, iritis‡, choroiditis‡, retinal hemorrhage or detachment‡, panophthalmitis‡	Keratitis
Liver		Mild or recurrent hepatitis	
Respiratory system		Nonexudative sore throat, nonproductive cough, adult respiratory distress syndrome‡	
Kidney		Microscopic hematuria or proteinuria	
Genitourinary system		Orchitis‡	
Constitutional symptoms	Minor	Severe malaise and fatigue	Fatigue

*The classification by stages provides a guideline for the expected timing of the illness' manifestations, but this may vary from case to case.
†Systems are listed from the most to the least commonly affected.
‡The inclusion of this manifestation is based on one or a few cases.
From Steere AC. Lyme disease. N Engl J Med 1989;321:589. Reprinted by permission of The New England Journal of Medicine.

Neonates

In the neonate the leading pathogen is *S. aureus*, followed by *Streptococcus* sp. (Table 127–7). Although *S. aureus* is more common in children over 2 years of age, it can cause a significant number of cases of septic arthritis in children in the first month of life. *Candida albicans* is emerging as a more common pathogen and is typically a hospital-acquired infection. Hospital-acquired infections of the joint are associated with significant mortality (27%); the majority of survivors develop deformities of the musculoskeletal system.

Infants

H. influenzae type b and *S. pneumoniae* are the most common organisms in children younger than 2 years of age. It is unusual that *S. aureus* is the causative organism between 1 month and 18 months of age. In infants and children 1 month to 3 years old, *H. influenzae* is the leading cause of septic arthritis; it is unusual for *H. influenzae* to cause a joint infection after age 6 years. Extraarticular infection is common with *H. influenzae*. In one study of *H. influenzae* septic arthritis, 35% of children had an associated otitis media and 30% had concurrent meningitis. The hip was involved in 26% of cases, the ankle in 26%, and the knee in 19%. An overlying cellulitis was seen in 22% of cases. Osteomyelitis occurred concurrently in 26% of cases.

Children Over 2 Years

Group A streptococci and *S. aureus* predominate in children older than 2 years of age. In children over 3 years old the causes of septic arthritis are usually by the same organisms as those found in adults; 33% are due to *S. aureus*, followed by hemolytic streptococci (18%), *N. gonorrhoeae* (7%), and "unknown" (34%).

Pathophysiology

When infected, the synovial membrane becomes edematous and swollen. There is an increased amount of synovial fluid, which may be thin and cloudy, containing leukocytes that are predominantly neutrophilic. The WBC count is usually higher than 50,000/mm³. The pathogenic bacteria may be seen on Gram stain. The glucose content of synovial fluid is typically decreased, and the protein content is elevated. After a few days of persistent infection, pus accumulates in the joint cavity, leading to destructive and degenerative changes. The synovial membrane is eventually replaced by granulation tissue. The infection may then extend to underlying bone. Fibrin within the joint clots, producing loculations of pus and adhesions that restrict joint motion.

Clinical Evaluation

History

Most children with septic arthritis have an acute onset of fever. There is pain, swelling, and limitation of motion in the affected joint. In infants, septic arthritis of the hip may be difficult to diagnose and may result from an underlying osteomyelitis.

With *H. influenzae* type b septic arthritis in children, there are usually 3 days of fever and joint symptoms prior to hospitalization, often accompanied by or immediately preceded by a viral illness or otitis media.

Joint pain is the predominant complaint. If the lower limb is involved, the child walks with a limp; weight bearing ultimately becomes so painful that the child may not walk at all. The child may be anorexic, irritable, and feverish, with a temperature as high as 40° to 40.5°C (104° to 105°F). The infected joint may be warm and swollen; this reflects the excessive effusion and distention of the joint capsule. The joint will often be partially flexed, minimizing discomfort. Often the hip will be in 30 to 65 degrees of flexion and 15 degrees of abduction.

Septic arthritis of the hip in the neonate may not be accompanied by a fever or toxic appearance. The manifestations may be vague, such as poor feeding and irritability. The peripheral WBC count and differential may be normal. Nevertheless, there should be some tenderness to the hip and some limitation of the hip motion. This may be subtle; it may only be noticed that the baby cries when its diaper is changed.

Physical Examination

A fever is present in over 90% of patients with *H. influenzae* type b septic arthritis; tenderness occurs in 87% of patients; and there is decreased range of motion in 74% of patients. With septic arthritis of the hip, the joint capsule may become so distended that the femoral head is pushed laterally and eventually dislocates.

TABLE 127–7				
SEPTIC ARTHRITIS: ETIOLOGIC APPROACH TO THERAPY				
Age Group	**Common Pathogens**	**Uncommon Pathogens**	**Rare Pathogens**	**Parenteral Antibiotic Considerations**
Neonate–6 wk	*S. aureus* Group B streptococci	Enteric bacilli *Candida* *N. gonorrhoeae*	*H. influenzae*	Nafcillin or oxacillin + aminoglycoside Ceftriaxone Cefotaxime Cefuroxime
6 wk–3 yr	*S. aureus* *H. influenzae* Group B streptococci Group A streptococci	Gram-negative bacilli		Cefuroxime Ceftriaxone Cefotaxime
>3 yr	*S. aureus* Hemolytic streptococci	Gram-negative bacilli *N. gonorrhoeae*	*S. pneumoniae* *H. influenzae*	Nafcillin Oxacillin Cefazolin

Modified with permission from Tachdjian MO. Pediatric Orthopedics. 2nd ed. Philadelphia, WB Saunders, 1990, p 1417.

Diagnostic Evaluation

The diagnosis of septic arthritis can be confirmed by recovery of the organism from the affected joint. Also, clinical findings consistent with joint infection and recovery of organisms on blood culture suggest the diagnosis. Confirmatory findings on joint fluid analysis also suggest the diagnosis.

Radiology

Increased fluid of the joint capsule increases the opacity within the joint. Periarticular fat and muscle shadows are displaced by the distended capsule. In the hip the femoral head may be displaced laterally or even subluxed. Comparison views with the contralateral side may assist in demonstrating abnormalities. One should always inspect for osteomyelitis in the adjacent bone.

Laboratory Tests

Cultures should be taken of various specimens from differing sites. Joint cultures are positive in only 80% of patients. A blood culture can be positive despite a negative culture of joint fluid. There appears to be minimal change in blood culture yield if the patient has received antibiotics. One report had positive blood cultures in 47% of patients who had not received antibiotics and in 43% of those who had. However, prior antibiotic treatment reduced the synovial fluid yield from 80% to 38%.

The peripheral WBC count and the ESR are often elevated. Although the sedimentation rate can be helpful, it is less reliable in children with sickle cell anemia, children on steroids, and neonates.

Synovial Fluid Analysis

Any joint suspected of being infected should be promptly aspirated, especially the hip, where the blood supply to the physis and femoral head may be compromised early in the course of the infection. Since the hip is so difficult to aspirate, the technique should not be performed by the emergency physician. Aspiration of other joints should be performed under strict aseptic conditions. If attempted in the emergency department, the child should be appropriately sedated and restrained to minimize discomfort. An 18- or 20-gauge lumbar puncture needle is used. The needle is generally inserted into the joint through the easiest access route into the site of maximal fluctuation. Areas of cellulitis should be avoided to prevent introducing infection into a joint containing a sterile effusion.

The gross appearance of the joint fluid may be misleading. A clear-appearing fluid may be infected with a high bacterial count, whereas turbid fluid may be seen in inflammatory arthritis. Joint aspiration fluid should be cultured and a Gram stain prepared. Gram stain of purulent joint effusions suggests a causative organism in about one third of cases. Latex agglutination techniques can rapidly detect bacterial antigens for *H. influenzae, Neisseria meningitidis, S. pneumoniae,* and group B streptococci.

It can be difficult to distinguish a noninfectious from an infectious inflammatory process from the synovial fluid cell count alone. The synovial fluid cell count from an infected joint is usually between 15,000 and 250,000/mm^3, with a high proportion of polymorphonuclear leukocytes. The polymorphonuclear leukocyte count usually ranges from 80% to 100%. Griffin and Green report an average WBC count of 57,000/mm^3 (range 10,000 to 250,000). Some authors contend that in 55% of patients the joint fluid cell count is 50,000/mm^3 or less; 34% of patients have a joint fluid cell count less than 25,000/mm^3.

Joint fluid glucose levels are not a major help in separating septic from nonseptic disease. Although typically regarded as being reduced, the synovial fluid glucose can be normal or even elevated with septic arthritis. Synovial fluid protein is usually elevated.

Differential Diagnosis

The differential diagnosis includes osteomyelitis, acute rheumatoid arthritis, transient synovitis, tuberculosis arthritis, acute rheumatic fever, cellulitis, and hemarthrosis. Osteomyelitis is a difficult condition to distinguish from joint sepsis. In osteomyelitis the maximal point of tenderness is often over the metaphysis; in septic arthritis it is directly over the joint line. In general, the range of motion of the joint is less restricted and less tender with osteomyelitis when compared with septic arthritis. More limb swelling is associated with osteomyelitis; more joint swelling is seen with septic arthritis.

The red, hot, swollen, and painful joints and high temperatures associated with rheumatic fever may be mistaken for suppurative arthritis. Migratory joint involvement and cardiac manifestations are associated with acute rheumatic fever.

Septic arthritis of the knee is most likely to be confused with acute onset of monoarticular JRA and less frequently with acute rheumatic fever. With JRA the knee is usually less painful and the range of motion is greater. Differentiating between septic arthritis of the hip and transient synovitis is extremely difficult. Transient synovitis is usually not seen before the child walks.

Suppurative arthritis can also mimic joint sepsis. Suppurative bursitis, although common in adults, is generally a rare condition in children. Suppurative bursitis is caused by *S. aureus* in over 90% of cases.

Therapeutic Intervention
Antibiotic Therapy

The initial antibiotic choice is ideally based on Gram stain interpretation. When several organisms are considered in the differential diagnosis of etiology, treatment should be either a multiple antibiotic regimen or a single agent with a wide spectrum of efficacy.

Antibiotic therapy is also determined by the age of the patient. Infection in the newborn with no identifiable organism on Gram stain should be presumed to be due to staphylococci, group B streptococci, or coliforms. Nafcillin or oxacillin combination with an aminoglycoside provides excellent antimicrobial coverage.

In children less than 2 months of age, antibiotic coverage must be selected against staphylococci, streptococci, gonococci, and gram-negative organisms. *H. influenzae* is not a primary consideration. Therefore antibiotic regimens include nafcillin and an aminoglycoside; ceftriaxone; or cefuroxime.

In children 2 months to 3 years of age, therapy should include bactericidal agents for *H. influenzae*, staphylococci, and streptococci. Regimens include cefotaxime, or nafcillin combined with ampicillin. Cefuroxime (100 to 150 mg/kg/24 hours) is an excellent alternative choice (Table 127–8). Ceftriaxone (50 to 75 mg/kg/day divided in two doses) or ampicillin (100 to 200 mg/kg/day) with sulbactam (15 to 30 mg/kg/day) have also been used with good results.

In children greater than 3 to 4 years of age, *S. aureus* is a primary infecting organism. Therefore oxacillin (150

TABLE 127-8

INTRAVENOUS ANTIBIOTIC DOSES FOR BONE AND JOINT INFECTIONS IN INFANTS BEYOND THE NEWBORN PERIOD*

	Dose (mg/kg/day)	Maximum (gm/day)	Dosing Interval (hr)
Ampicillin	150–200	6–12	q 6
Nafcillin	150–200	4–12	q 6
Oxacillin	150	4–12	q 6
Gentamicin	6.0–7.5	†	q 8
Ceftriaxone	50–75	4	q 12–24
Cefuroxime	75–150	4–6	q 8
Cefotaxime	100–150	8–10	q 8
Cefazolin	75–100	4–6	q 8
Vancomycin	40	2–4	q 6
Clindamycin	25–30	1.2–2.7	q 8

*Orthopedic or infectious disease specialist should be consulted for antibiotic dosing.
†No maximum dose given; serum levels should be monitored.

mg/kg/24 hours) or cefazolin (100 mg/kg/24 hours) is a consideration.

When *H. influenzae* is the pathogen in children 2 years of age or younger, a lumbar puncture should be considered because 20% of children will also have meningitis. *Streptococcus* and *Haemophilus* are usually treated for 10 to 14 days, while *S. aureus* and coliforms usually require 21 days of therapy.

Drainage

The current management of acute suppurative joint infections includes adequate drainage of purulent material from the infected site in addition to antibiotic therapy. Patients may also require open surgical drainage, especially when the hip is involved or if a substantial amount of pus persists after initial needle aspiration.

Prognosis

Although death is a rare sequela of septic arthritis, severe complications such as joint destruction, limb shortening, and deformity can occur. The outcome is unsatisfactory in 40% to 43% of hip infections, 8% to 10% of knee infections, and 15% to 33% of ankle infections. The prognosis is worse for newborns with septic arthritis of the hip. Adverse outcome includes an absent or abnormal femoral head (deformed or small) and an absent femoral neck.

The prognosis is determined by several factors, including the length of time between the onset of symptoms and the initial treatment; the specific joint involved (the prognosis is poor if the hip is the affected site); the presence of associated osteomyelitis; and the age of the patient (infants do worse than older children).

OSTEOMYELITIS

Introduction

Osteomyelitis is a pyogenic infection of the bone. Although osteomyelitis can occur at any age, it most frequently occurs in infants and children. Osteomyelitis is most commonly caused by *S. aureus*, but it may also be caused by *S. pneumoniae*, *Salmonella*, or other pyogenic organisms (Table 127–9). Osteomyelitis usually results from hematogenous seeding, although it may be caused by direct extension of an adjacent infective process by an open fracture. Another cause is spread from a decubitus ulcer. A traumatic puncture of the foot can lead to osteomyelitis of the calcaneus caused by *Pseudomonas aeruginosa*. With nonhematogenous osteomyelitis, organisms vary greatly, including *S. aureus*, *Staphylococcus epidermidis*, *P. aeruginosa*, *Escherichia coli*, *Streptococcus faecalis*, *Enterobacter*, *Serratia*, *Klebsiella pneumoniae*, and *Aeromonas hydrophila*.

When infected, the bone becomes inflamed and may form an abscess. Irregular decalcification of the infected bone occurs in the early stages from absorption of dead bone. If osteomyelitis goes untreated in children, vascular thrombosis and elevation of the periosteum will deprive the affected denuded cortical bone of blood supply, causing bony necrosis. The most common sites of involvement are the metaphyses of the distal femur and proximal tibia. Complications from osteomyelitis can include pathologic fractures, growth plate disturbance, and joint destruction.

Salmonella osteomyelitis is associated with sickle cell disease. Although *S. aureus* is still a common etiology of osteomyelitis in the sickle cell patient, the incidence of salmonella osteomyelitis is several hundredfold higher than that of the general population. Salmonella osteomyelitis is characterized by the involvement of multiple sites. Multiple punched-out, destructive lesions throughout the metaphysis and diaphysis

TABLE 127-9

OSTEOMYELITIS: ETIOLOGIC APPROACH TO THERAPY

Age Group	Common Pathogens	Uncommon Pathogens	Rare Pathogens	Parenteral Antibiotic Considerations
Neonates–6 wk	*S. aureus* Group B streptococci Enteric bacilli	*H. influenzae*	*Candida*	Nafcillin or oxacillin + aminoglycoside Ceftriaxone Cefuroxime Cefotaxime
6 weeks–3 yr	*S. aureus* Streptococci	*H. influenzae* *Pseudomonas* sp.	*Candida* *M. tuberculosis*	Ceftriaxone Cefuroxime Cefotaxime Nafcillin + ampicillin
>3 yr	*S. aureus* Streptococci	*Pseudomonas* sp.	*M. tuberculosis* *Candida*	Nafcillin Oxacillin Cefazolin Clindamycin Vancomycin

Modified with permission from Tachdjian MO. Pediatric Orthopedics. 2nd ed. Philadelphia, WB Saunders, 1990, p 1094.

are seen on radiograph. Salmonella is sensitive to third-generation cephalosporins such as cefotaxime and ceftriaxone. Ampicillin, chloramphenicol, or trimethoprim-sulfamethoxazole are alternative antimicrobials. Surgical drainage of the bone abscesses is often indicated, and the recurrence rate of infection is high.

H. influenzae type b as a cause of osteomyelitis in infants and children is generally regarded as uncommon. However, in one review involving children 1 month to 24 months of age, *H. influenzae* type b caused 13.3% of all cases of osteomyelitis.

With *H. influenzae* osteomyelitis, fever is almost universal; 75% will have a preceding respiratory tract infection; 75% will have localized swelling; and 69% will have decreased range of motion. A concurrent suppurative arthritis (joint infection) is present in 75% of children, and meningitis can be concomitant in 19%.

Clinical Evaluation

History

The child with osteomyelitis may appear septic with a high fever, chills, vomiting, and dehydration. In the neonatal period these signs may be absent. Tenderness of the bone is the predominant local symptom. The pain is often severe, constant, and may be aggravated by motion. If a bone of the lower limb is involved, the child will often limp. On gentle palpation there is sharp tenderness over the metaphysis of the affected bone. The infant may cry constantly throughout the examination, but slight digital pressure over the point of tenderness may cause the cry to increase in intensity, thus localizing the infection. Localized swelling and warmth may be discernible; however, redness is unlikely in the early stages. Muscles of the adjacent joint are usually in protective spasm, as characterized by partial flexion.

Ninety-three percent of patients will have a single bone infected, and 65% of bones infected involve the lower extremities. Osteomyelitis involves the femur in 25% of cases, the tibia in 24%, and the fibula in 5%. The calcaneus is involved in 4% of cases of osteomyelitis. Thirty-one percent of children with osteomyelitis are less than 2 years of age; 41% are over age 5 years.

Osteomyelitis can present without an acute phase. This *subacute* osteomyelitis has an insidious onset with mild pain and little functional impairment. Subacute osteomyelitis usually develops because of an altered host-pathogen relationship. Systemic signs are mild to absent; the child usually appears healthy and afebrile.

Diagnostic Evaluation

Radiology

In the first few days of osteomyelitis, most changes are limited to the surrounding soft tissue. Comparison views of the contralateral limb are frequently necessary to discern subtle soft tissue changes. Alterations in radiographic density cannot be detected until there is at least a 35% to 50% decrease in bone mineral content. Therefore osseous changes are not seen until about 10 to 14 days after the onset of infection. The local inflammatory exudate that forms may give a hazy, smoky appearance to the medullary cavity of the metaphysis. In 7 to 12 days, irregular spotty areas of rarefaction represent absorption of trabeculae and necrosis. Subperiosteal new bone formation then occurs, indicating a spread of infection through the cortex. Sequestered dead bone appears as a dense area with a sharp outline.

Bone Scan

The diagnosis of acute osteomyelitis can be made in the first 24 to 48 hours of infection by a bone scan. A bone scan will show localized increased uptake of radionuclides corresponding to the site of osteomyelitis. A normal bone scan does not completely exclude acute osteomyelitis.

Laboratory Tests

Although leukocytosis and an elevated ESR are found in the majority of children, normal values are seen in enough children to render the tests nondiagnostic. The WBC count is often elevated, with a high percentage of neutrophils on peripheral smears. With osteomyelitis a bacterial diagnosis can be established in 78% of patients. The affected area of bone should be aspirated to obtain material for bacteriologic examination. The procedure is an extremely painful one and is performed with the child appropriately sedated and restrained. This procedure is best performed by the orthopedic consultant.

Differential Diagnosis

Differential diagnosis for acute osteomyelitis includes acute rheumatic fever, septic arthritis, acute rheumatoid arthritis, cellulitis, acute leukemia, poliomyelitis, infantile cortical hyperostosis, hypervitaminosis A, and malignant bone tumors such as Ewing's sarcoma. Other conditions that should be considered include stress fracture, myositis ossificans, Osgood-Schlatter disease, SCFE, transient synovitis, rheumatoid arthritis, SLE, Henoch-Schönlein purpura, rheumatic fever, pyogenic myositis, lymphoma, histiocytosis X, neoplasms, sickle cell disease, hemophilia, hyperparathyroidism, and rickets. In osteomyelitis the site of maximal tenderness is localized over the metaphysis, whereas in inflammatory joint disease the tenderness is found primarily over the joint. In addition, joint motion causes greater pain with an inflammatory joint disease than it does with osteomyelitis.

Therapeutic Intervention

The affected limb should be immobilized in a well-padded splint or bivalve cast with the joints in the functional position.

The treatment for osteomyelitis should include bactericidal antibiotics given parenterally in doses high enough to control the infection significantly. The bacteriology of osteomyelitis in neonates (< 2 months of age) is unique because group B beta-hemolytic streptococci and gram-negative enteric bacilli are frequent pathogens. Neonatal group B streptococcal osteomyelitis typically has a subacute, indolent course with a predilection for involving the proximal humerus. In children between 2 months and 3 years of age, the most common organism is staphylococcus. Antibiotic coverage should target *Staphylococcus* sp., *Streptococcus* sp., and *Haemophilus*.

In children over 3 years of age, *S. aureus* and streptococci are still the most common causes of osteomyelitis. Adolescents using intravenous drugs should have an aminoglycoside added to cover potential *Pseudomonas* or *Serratia marcescens*.

Selected References

Bowyer SL, Hollister JR. Limb pain in childhood. Pediatr Clin North Am 1984;31:1053.

Brewer EJ. Pitfalls in the diagnosis of juvenile rheumatoid arthritis. Pediatr Clin North Am 1986;33:1015.

Brower AC. The osteochondroses. Orthop Clin North Am 1983;14:99.

Busch MT, Morrissy RT. Slipped capital femoral epiphysis. Orthop Clin North Am 1987;18:637.

Chung SMK. Identifying the cause of acute limp in childhood. Clin Pediatr 1974;13:769.

Chung SMK, Pollis RE. Diagnostic pitfalls in septic arthritis of the hip in infants and children. Clin Pediatr 1975;14:758.

Conrad EU. Pitfalls in diagnosis: Pediatric musculoskeletal tumors. Pediatr Ann 1989;18:45.

Dubey L, Krasinski K, Hernanz-Schulman M. Osteomyelitis secondary to trauma or infected contiguous soft tissue. Pediatr Infect Dis J 1988;7:26.

Fink CF. Reactive arthritis. Pediatr Infect Dis J 1988;7:58.

Fink CW, Nelson JD. Septic arthritis and osteomyelitis in children. Rheum Dis Clin North Am 1986;12:423.

Fox L, Sprunt K. Neonatal osteomyelitis. Pediatrics 1978;62:535.

Galloway SJ, Harwood-Nuss AL. Sickle-cell anemia: A review. J Emerg Med 1988;6:213.

Goldings EA, Jericho J. Lyme disease. Rheum Dis Clin North Am 1986;12:343.

Goldstein HA. Bone scintigraphy. Orthop Clin North Am 1983;14:243.

Green NE, Edwards K. Bone and joint infections in children. Orthop Clin North Am 1987;18:555.

Griffin PP, Green WT Sr. Hip joint infections in infants and children. Orthop Clin North Am 1978;9:123.

Hensinger RN. Congenital dislocation of the hip: Treatment in infancy to walking age. Orthop Clin North Am 1987;18:597.

Illingworth CM. 128 limping children with no fracture, sprain, or obvious cause. Clin Pediatr 1978;17:139.

Illingworth CM. Recurrences of transient synovitis of the hip. Arch Dis Child 1983;58:620.

Keeley K, Buchanan GR. Acute infarction of long bones in children with sickle cell anemia. J Pediatr 1982;101:170.

Kulhanjian J, Dunphy MG, Hamstra S, et al. Randomized comparative study of ampicillin/sulbactam vs. ceftriaxone for treatment of soft tissue and skeletal infections in children. Pediatr Infect Dis J 1989;8:605.

Kunnamo I, Kallio P, Pelkonen P, Hovi T. Clinical signs and laboratory tests in the differential diagnosis of arthritis in children. Am J Dis Child 1987;141:34.

Lebel MH, Nelson JD. Haemophilus influenzae type B osteomyelitis in infants and children. Pediatr Infect Dis J 1988;7:250.

Marchal GJ, Van Holsbeeck MT, Raes M, et al. Transient synovitis of the hip in children: Role of US. Radiology 1987;162:825.

McCarthy PL, Wasserman D, Spiesel SZ, et al. Evaluation of arthritis and arthralgia in the pediatric patient. Clin Pediatr 1980;19:183.

Meyers S, Lonon W, Shannon K. Suppurative bursitis in early childhood. Pediatr Infect Dis J 1984;3:156.

Miller EH, Semian DW. Gram-negative osteomyelitis following puncture wounds of the foot. J Bone Joint Surg 1975;57:535.

Morrissy RT. Bone and joint infection in the neonate. Pediatr Ann 1989;18:33.

Mosca VS. Pitfalls in diagnosis: The hip. Pediatr Ann 1989;18:12.

Nade S. Choice of antibiotics in management of acute osteomyelitis and acute septic arthritis in children. Arch Dis Child 1977;52:679.

Ortiz-Neu C, Marr JS, Cherubin CE, et al. Bone and joint infections due to salmonella. J Infect Dis 1978;138:820.

Oudjhane K, Newman B, Oh KS, et al. Occult fractures in preschool children. J Trauma 1988;28:858.

Paterson D. Septic arthritis of the hip joint. Orthop Clin North Am 1978;9:135.

Phillips WA. The child with a limp. Orthop Clin North Am 1987;18:489.

Steere AC. Lyme disease. N Engl J Med 1989;321:586.

Thompson GH, Salter RB. Legg-Calvé-Perthes disease: Current concepts and controversies. Orthop Clin North Am 1987;18:617.

Waldvogel FA, Vasey H. Osteomyelitis: The past decade. N Engl J Med 1980;303:360.

Welkon CJ, Long SS, Fisher MC, Alburger PD. Pyogenic arthritis in infants and children: A review of 95 cases. Pediatr Infect Dis J 1986;5:669.

Wiley JJ, Fraser GA. Septic arthritis in childhood. Can J Surg 1979;22:326.

SECTION SIXTEEN

Neurology

CHAPTER 128

The Neurologic Examination

Douglas S. Smith

INTRODUCTION

Emergency physicians are called upon to evaluate children for a wide variety of neurologic complaints. Pediatric neurologic conditions can be placed into four categories. The *critically ill* patient with neurologic symptoms requires immediate assessment and intervention for life-threatening illness. The patient with *urgent* neurologic symptoms requires prompt recognition of disease and severity with timely intervention. As with the latter conditions, the patient with a *chronic* neurologic problem and an *acute related symptom* and the patient with a chronic neurologic problem and *unrelated symptoms* require a thorough neurologic examination.

Despite advances in neuroimaging, the clinical examination remains the simplest and most important tool in evaluating neurologic emergencies. A physician in the emergency department must acquire proficiency and confidence in the ability to assess accurately the patient's initial status as well as to determine progression of disease.

The emergency department does not lend itself to a quiet, methodic, in-depth neurologic examination. In addition, children are not simply "little adults" but rather are people in development. The neurologic capabilities and hence the examination varies for the infant, adolescent, and all stages in-between.

The physician must evaluate the emergent, critical patient to enable prompt recognition of life-threatening neurologic conditions. Furthermore, the physician must have a standard approach to the nonemergent neurologic examination, which is useful in the emergency department setting.

THE CRITICAL PATIENT
Essential Evaluation

The neurologic examination proceeds after the vital signs have been addressed and a physical examination assessing any life-threatening conditions has been completed. Any effort to maximize neurologic outcome will be undermined if these are neglected. The vital signs may also reveal the presence of Cushing's triad for increased intracranial pressure: elevated systolic blood pressure, bradycardia, and decreased respiratory rate.

Directed Neurologic Examination

A brief, directed neurologic examination is critical. The physician must initially obtain a quick but accurate assessment of level of consciousness; pupil size, symmetry, and reactivity; and presence of cerebral herniation.

Level of Consciousness

Consciousness is a continuum from the normal alert state to deep coma with various levels of stupor in-between. The normal alert state requires intact cerebral hemispheres and brain stem function. Coma occurs when both cerebral hemispheres or the brain stem are nonfunctional. Stupor occurs with partial dysfunction of one or both of these components. Many terms are employed to describe stuporous states, including but not limited to drowsy, listless, lethargic, and obtunded. Unfortunately these descriptive terms are not quantitative and definitions are not universal. The Glasgow Coma Scale (Table 128–1) provides a particularly useful means of assessing level of consciousness by allowing quantification and increased reliability between observers.

The Glasgow Coma Scale is both reproducible and reliable in evaluating the verbal child, as it is easily ascertained by nonphysician personnel such as paramedics and nurses. This scale serves at least three useful functions. First, it is an estimate of impairment, which aids in determining the urgency for intervention. Second, it has prognostic implications. Third, and perhaps most important, it can be used to follow the clinical course as a neurologic "vital sign," identifying either improvement or deterioration.

To use the Glasgow Coma Scale, the examiner records the best response in each category and assigns an overall score. Scores less than 9 suggest severe injury and demand aggressive intervention. Likewise, a decrease in the score of 3 or more should trigger immediate response regardless of the initial score. In addition, the motor responses can be observed for symmetry, with abnormal findings adding valuable information in localizing the injury.

Attempts to assess arousability (i.e., eye opening and verbal response) should follow stepwise stimulation beginning with voice, then touch, and finally pain. The child who arouses and remains awake is conscious, but impairment indicates either coma in the absence of response or some intermediate state of stupor. The stuporous or comatose patient must now have an immediate assessment of the cerebral hemisphere function using the best motor response. Pain should be elicited in deep soft tissue structures through subungual pressure in all extremities, and centrally by vigorous sternal rubbing or supraorbital pressure. The comatose or stuporous patient can respond to such stimulation in characteristic patterns that reflect the level of function of the cerebral hemispheres. For example, the child may vocalize (thus assessing best verbal response) and either withdraw the

TABLE 128–1					
THE GLASGOW COMA SCALE*					
1. Eye Opening		2. Best Motor Response		3. Best Verbal Response	
Spontaneously	4	Obeys command	6	Oriented/appropriate	5
Response to voice	3	Localizes pain	5	Disoriented conversation	4
Response to pain	2	Flexion withdrawal	4	Inappropriate words	3
No response	1	Decorticate posturing	3	Incomprehensible sounds	2
		Decerebrate posturing	2	No responses	1
		No response	1		

*Used for the verbal child.

stimulated limb or localize the central pain. This indicates considerable cerebral function since the patient has awareness of self and environment. Asymmetry of motor response is indicative of localized injury. Decorticate posturing is flexion of the arm, wrist, and fingers with lower extremity extension and occurs with cortical or hemispheric injury. Decerebrate posturing is extension of both upper and lower extremities and occurs with high pontine and midbrain destructive lesions. The examiner then records the best response in each category, assigning an overall score.

Pupil Size, Symmetry, and Reactivity

The presence or absence of pupillary reactivity is an important finding in distinguishing metabolic from structural etiologies in the comatose patient. Reactivity persists in most metabolic conditions, the exceptions being asphyxia, hypothermia, and the ingestion of glutethimide, barbiturates, atropine, and scopolamine. However, intravenous atropine given during resuscitation does not fix the pupils.

When examining for pupillary reactivity, it is critical to use a bright light that is rapidly presented to the pupil. One may need to diminish the light in the room. Many metabolic conditions result in relative decreases of the sympathetic innervation and cause small but reactive pupils; therefore an ophthalmoscope can be valuable in assessing the pinpoint pupil. Any reactivity implies intact pathways. Finally, symmetry of pupillary response must be assessed. A unilateral fixed and dilated pupil suggests early uncal herniation.

Cerebral Herniation

Cerebral herniation is a rapidly progressing, fatal development if not immediately recognized and aggressively treated. The two presentations to consider are uncal and transtentorial or central herniation.

Uncal Herniation. Uncal herniation is brought on by an enlarging, space-occupying mass lesion such as an intracranial hemorrhage in the lateral cranial vault or temporal lobe. The most important neurologic finding is due to compression of the oculomotor nerve as the uncus and hippocampal gyrus shift. Ipsilateral pupillary dilatation with or without reactivity and contralateral hemiparesis is the earliest sign of uncal herniation. It is critical to recognize this syndrome at the earliest stage since the effects can often be reversed with prompt intervention. Progressive pressure leads to increasing stupor, decorticate or decerebrate posturing, and abnormal respiratory pattern. Finally, prominent brain stem dysfunction occurs with dilatation of both pupils, loss of brain stem reflexes such as the doll's eye maneuver, and eventual death.

Other causes for anisocoria should be sought, especially congenital asymmetry and trauma. However, in the presence of altered consciousness, unequal pupils should be consid-

ered cerebral herniation. Conversely, the awake, alert, nontraumatic patient with unequal pupils does not have cerebral herniation, and another etiology should be sought.

Transtentorial or Central Herniation. Transtentorial or central herniation is more commonly seen with diffuse increased intracranial pressure such as with Reye's syndrome. It occurs when pressure is exerted centrally on the diencephalon rather than laterally as in the uncal herniation syndrome. The first sign is alteration in the level of consciousness, with decorticate posturing as the condition progresses. As the brain stem is compressed there is dilatation of both pupils with loss of brain stem reflexes. Finally, decerebrate posturing and ataxic to apneic respirations develop.

EMS CONSIDERATIONS

Regardless of the setting, it is mandatory that the prehospital provider communicate the level of consciousness, the pupillary size, and pupillary reactivity. The Glasgow coma scale serves as an excellent standard for reference. In addition to a simple number, comment should be made about each of the three categories in the scale: eye movements, motor response, and verbal response.

THE STABLE PATIENT

In addition to the patient with a catastrophic neurologic injury or condition, physicians are frequently called upon to evaluate stable patients for complaints that require a careful and complete neurologic examination. Examples of such conditions include headaches, seizures, and behavioral disorders.

The pediatric neurologic examination includes all of the elements of the adult examination with the additional need to assess development. This requires the examiner to evaluate mental status; cranial nerve function; motor, sensory, and cerebellar functions; and deep tendon reflexes. The emergency department neurologic examination in the stable child consists of three distinct components: the historical, the observational or "hands off," and the interactive or "hands on."

Historical

It is unrealistic to imagine that a practicing emergency department physician could hope to retain large quantities of information pertaining to normal and abnormal developmental findings. To assess the developmental status of the child, the physician may either refer to a development chart or simply ask the caregiver what the child's normal capabilities in the areas of motor, language, and social skills are. The physician can then make a comparison with the current status and can identify, for example, the child who normally ambulates independently but is not using the left side or who can no longer maintain balance sitting independently. In addition to information concerning the individual patient, often a parent will be able to use siblings for comparison. For example, during the history one can determine if the child's language or motor skills seem to be delayed in comparison to older children in the family.

The emergency department physician will greatly enhance the quality of evaluation by using the observations of the parent. Parents will notice subtle alterations in their child's normal functional status long before the clinician can detect an abnormality. A caregiver's concern about neurologic deterioration should never be minimized.

Observational

The observational component of the neurologic examination is unquestionably the most important. Mental status is determined by the interaction between the child and the parents or environment. Smiling and playing are reassuring findings. In contrast, the withdrawn, quiet, noninteractive patient should immediately alert the observer to underlying disease. Interaction with parents will often reveal asymmetry of movement of facial muscles as well as extremities.

Motor function will best be examined during this stage. The child should be allowed to perform to his or her maximal developmental ability. For example, the ambulating patient should be observed walking to a parent or down the hall for a cookie. The observant clinician can note muscle strength, symmetry of movement, and balance and coordination during walking. In the younger child, the parent should be asked if this represents the normal gait or if some abnormality is present. Playing with a toy can likewise provide information about motor control. Slightly older children (>4 years) can be surprisingly cooperative by walking on their toes and heels as well as performing a finger-to-nose test.

By the end of the historical and observational portions of the evaluation, the experienced clinician will have a strong inclination as to the presence or absence of abnormal neurologic findings.

Interactive

The interactive component of the neurologic examination includes the use of a light to assess symmetry and pupillary response and a funduscopic examination. This is rarely difficult in children over age 4 and can often be achieved with patience in younger children, especially the ill pediatric patient not resisting the examination. Extraocular movements can be determined by having the caregiver hold the head steady while a toy or light is moved in all positions.

Infant reflexes can be useful either by their absence at the appropriate time in development or by their abnormal persistence. The Moro reflex is present at birth and can usually be elicited until around 3 months of age. The baby is "startled" by supporting the head off the cart and suddenly moving the head backward 10 to 15 degrees. The reflex is extension of the trunk and extension and abduction of the arms followed by flexion and adduction. The involvement of the legs is variable. The grasp reflex is elicited by placing a finger on the palmar surface of the hand. A tight grip is the response seen normally in the child between ages 1 and 3 months. Finally, the Landau reflex is seen in the 3- to 18-month-old patient. It consists of supporting the infant horizontally in the prone position while the infant raises its head and arches its back. The presence, absence, or asymmetry of these reflexes should be noted.

Finally, deep tendon reflexes should be elicited. The technique is the same as in adults except that the reflex hammer should be avoided. Adequate examination can be performed by tapping the desired tendon with the fingertips.

Selected References

1. Dean JM, Hanley DF. Evaluation of the comatose child. *In* Rogers MC (ed). Textbook of Pediatric Intensive Care. Baltimore, Williams & Wilkins, 1987, pp 597–614.
2. Huttenlocher PR. The nervous system. *In* Behrman RE, Vaughan VC, Nelson WE (eds). Nelson Textbook of Pediatrics. 13th ed. Philadelphia, WB Saunders, 1987, pp 1274–1281.
3. Kennedy C. Neurologic examination. *In* Barness LA (ed). Manual of Pediatric Physical Diagnosis. 5th ed. Chicago, Year Book, 1981, pp 193–208.
4. Pitts LH. Neurological evaluation of the head injury patient. Clin Neurosurg 1982; 29:203.
5. Plum F, Posner JB. The Diagnosis of Stupor and Coma. 3rd ed. Philadelphia, FA Davis, 1982.

CHAPTER 129

Seizures and Status Epilepticus

Theodore M. Barnett
Gary S. Wasserman

INTRODUCTION

A seizure is "a sudden, involuntary, time-limited alteration in function secondary to an abnormal discharge of neurons in the central nervous system."[1] Epilepsy is a condition in which seizures are recurrent over time and has many causes. The incidence of epilepsy is from 11 to 49 cases per 100,000 population,[2] with the majority of cases beginning before the age of 20 years.

CLINICAL EVALUATION

Many conditions may mimic seizures.[3–11] The mimicry may manifest as an alteration of consciousness, abnormal movements, or both. Many children present to the emergency department after an "event." An accurate diagnosis and appropriate care plan depend on obtaining an adequate history and examination without the benefit of actually seeing the episode (Table 129–1). Conditions that can appear similar to seizures include breath holding, syncope, migraine headaches, and pseudoseizures (Table 129–2).

Although sometimes difficult, it is important to distinguish between seizures and other episodic phenomena. A paroxysmal event is likely to frighten a child's parents, and if the event appears life threatening, parental anxiety is especially high.[12] An accurate diagnosis may help relieve some of this anxiety and spare the child unnecessary testing. Inappropriate therapy is at best unhelpful and may be harmful to the child. Appropriate diagnosis and counseling of the patient and parents may be therapeutic in and of itself.[13, 14]

When evaluating the child who has had a "seizure," the physician should obtain as much information about the event

TABLE 129–1

CONDITIONS THAT CAN MIMIC SEIZURES

Event	Altered Consciousness	Abnormal Movements
Breath-holding spells*	+	±
Vasovagal syncope (fainting)*	+	−
Stretch syncope	+	−
Migraine	+	−
Pseudoseizures	±	−
Gastroesophageal reflux	+	−
Shuddering attacks	−	+
Cardiac dysrhythmias	+	−
Startle reaction	−	+
Tourette's syndrome	−	+
Movement disorders	−	+
Parasomnias	+	±
Vertigo	±	±
Rage attacks	±	±
Fugue states	+	−

*These entities may produce secondary generalized tonic-clonic seizures as a result of hypoxia or ischemia.

as possible. Important historical points include a careful description of events before, during, and after the seizure (Table 129–3). In most cases the history must be obtained from observers and not the patient.

A thorough general physical examination should be performed, with particular emphasis on the neurologic examination. Computed tomography and laboratory tests should be performed as indicated by the history and examination. An electroencephalogram (EEG) is rarely helpful or available in the acute setting.

It is important to reassure the parents if the child's condition is presently stable. Many parents believe that their child is dying during a seizure[12] and remain concerned even after it has stopped. If the child is still convulsing or otherwise unstable, it is still important to have someone speak with the parents and attempt to obtain a history. Not only is this discussion beneficial to them, but they may also be able to provide some clue as to the cause of the seizure. It is important to explain if you have arrived at a diagnosis and, if not, what else needs to be done (i.e., neurologic consultation, EEG, or other tests).

CLASSIFICATION OF SEIZURES

Seizures should be classified accurately to enhance communication with consultants, select appropriate diagnostic tests, choose appropriate therapy, and give an accurate prognosis (Table 129–4). This classification does not consider the cause of the seizure. Common causes of seizures include perinatal injuries, vascular insults, metabolic abnormalities, head injuries, central nervous system (CNS) infections, neoplasms, intoxication or drug withdrawal, and hereditary disorders. Many seizures have no definite cause determined.[1, 15] In addition to classification of seizure type and cause, epilepsies and epileptic syndromes may also be classified, but this is usually beyond the province of the emergency physician.[16]

THERAPEUTIC INTERVENTION

Immediate life support measures are first priority regardless of the cause of the seizure. Airway, breathing, and circulation should be quickly evaluated and maintained with oxygen, positioning, suctioning, intravenous access, and intubation as needed. Heart rate, respiratory rate and depth, blood pressure, and oxygen saturation should be monitored. Blood should be obtained for laboratory tests, which may include a complete blood cell count; measurement of serum electrolyte, calcium, magnesium, phosphorus, glucose (and bedside glucose determination), blood urea nitrogen (BUN), creatinine, and ammonia levels; liver function tests; and anticonvulsant drug levels. Both blood and urine may be sent for toxicologic screening. If hypoglycemia is suspected or documented, intravenous dextrose should be given. Thiamine should precede the dextrose if alcoholism is a possibility. Naloxone is indicated for any comatose patient and in suspected opioid overdose. Anticonvulsive therapy is initiated, and efforts are continued to determine the cause of the seizures (Table 129–5). Computed tomography of the head, electroencephalography, electrocardiography, and other procedures are performed as necessary.

The treatment of choice varies depending on the history, mechanism of CNS insult, clinical presentation, and resources available (Table 129–6). Most physicians initially choose a benzodiazepine such as diazepam (Valium), lorazepam (Ativan), or midazolam (Versed). These drugs are preferably given intravenously, but sometimes are given rectally when intravenous access is difficult (or intramuscularly, in the case of midazolam). Many practitioners use diazepam primarily because they are familiar with it and thus are more comfortable with its usage.

Diazepam has an 88% success rate of lysing seizures in status epilepticus.[17] Diazepam (undiluted) can be administered rectally in the same dose used intravenously. It is

TABLE 129–2

DIFFERENTIATING SEIZURES AND OTHER CONDITIONS

	Breath Holding	Syncope	Migraine	Pseudoseizures	Seizures
Precipitating factors	Amost always	Almost always	Sometimes	Frequently with stress	Occasionally
Family history	Often positive for breath holding	Often positive for syncope	Often positive for migraine	Often positive for psychiatric disturbance	Often positive for seizures
Description of attack	Upset or crying, then apnea, followed by loss of consciousness, then decreased tone	Pallor and dizziness, then loss of consciousness, then decreased tone	Varies	Varies, but often with violent or nonrhythmic movement	Loss of consciousness, followed by rigidity or rhythmic movement
Postictal state	Usually none	Usually none or mild	Occasionally	Usually none	Usually marked
Electroencephalogram	Usually normal	Usually normal	Occasionally abnormal	Usually normal	Often abnormal

TABLE 129–3

HISTORY TAKING IN PAROXYSMAL EVENTS

What were the circumstances leading up to the event?

Was there any warning, such as an aura, dizziness, etc?

How long did the episode last? (To get an accurate appraisal of the duration of the event, it may be helpful to say "now," start timing, and have the witness tell you to stop after what he or she feels is the correct amount of time.)

What was the exact sequence of events?

Did loss or alteration of consciousness occur? If so, describe the alteration and note if it occurred initially or later.

Were there any abnormal movements? If so, have the witness describe or demonstrate.

Did any of the following occur: incontinence, self-injury, apnea, or cyanosis?

Did there appear to be any postictal state (confusion, amnesia, somnolence)?

Obtain past medical history, specifically including previous similar events, developmental status, recent illnesses, and medications.

Obtain a family history, especially of neurologic, psychiatric, and social problems.

---

rapidly absorbed and achieves similar plasma levels.[18] Diazepam is administered rectally through a lubricated tuberculin syringe (without a needle) or by using butterfly intravenous tubing by cutting off the needle. The end is inserted 3 to 5 cm into the rectum, the medication is injected, and the patient is observed for 5 to 10 minutes. This dose may be repeated once. The intraosseous route is another alternative for administration.[19] The main disadvantages of diazepam are irritation to vessel lining, respiratory depression, and a short (10- to 30-minute) anticonvulsant half-life necessitating either repeated dosing or the addition of a second drug to prevent recurrence of seizures. Many physicians prefer lorazepam because its duration of action is longer, respiratory depression appears to be less, and it is less irritating to tissues.[20, 21] Lorazepam stops seizures within 10 minutes in 75% to 92% of children in large series.[22-24] Additional or higher doses of lorazepam have a diminishing chance of effectiveness after the first unsuccessful dose.[25] One shortcoming of storing lorazepam in the emergency department is that it requires refrigeration. The water solubility and reduced tissue irritation of midazolam allow absorption from intramuscular injection, but no controlled studies of seizures have been performed.[26] Nonconvulsive status epilepticus is often resistant to or made worse by benzodiazepines.[27]

The usual second-line therapy involves the use of phenytoin (Dilantin) or phenobarbital (Luminal). Phenytoin has been successful in 60% to 80% of seizures.[128-30] Phenytoin is advantageous, being nonsedative in patients in whom neurologic status must be followed closely. When mixed with many intravenous solutions, especially glucose, phenytoin precipitates as the pH is lowered during the dilution process. Thus, it is best administered when infused as close to the venous catheter as possible or in a specially prepared 30-minute infusion setup.[31] Phenytoin, when given too rapidly, may induce bradycardia, cardiac conduction defects, or hypotension. Therefore, the patient should be placed on a cardiac monitor, and the infusion rate should not exceed 25 to 50 mg/min or 0.7 mg/kg/min. Phenytoin cannot be given intramuscularly because of its alkalinity and crystallization in tissue.

Phenobarbital is long acting and sedative, but extremely effective when used in high doses for refractory status epilepticus.[25] The morbidity and mortality rates (8% and 19%, respectively) of status epilepticus are at least partly

---

related to episodes that last more than 3 hours,[32] therefore defining a time frame in which to start the very-high-dose phenobarbital protocol.[33] Pentobarbital (Nembutal; 3 to 6 mg/kg intravenously), a short-acting barbiturate, is an alter-

TABLE 129–4

CLASSIFICATION OF SEIZURES

I. *Partial (focal, local) seizures.* Partial seizures are those in which, in general, the first clinical and electroencephalographic changes indicate initial activation of a system of neurons limited to part of one cerebral hemisphere. A partial seizure is classified primarily on the basis of whether consciousness is impaired during the attack. Impaired consciousness is defined as the inability to respond normally to exogenous stimuli by virtue of altered awareness or responsiveness. When consciousness is not impaired, the seizure is classified as a *simple partial seizure.* When consciousness is impaired, the seizure is classified as a *complex partial seizure.* Impairment of consciousness may be the first sign, or simple partial seizures may evolve into complex partial seizures. In patients with impaired consciousness, aberrations of behavior (automatisms) may occur. A partial seizure may not terminate but instead progress to generalized motor seizures. There is considerable evidence that simple partial seizures usually have unilateral hemispheric involvement and only rarely have bilateral hemispheric involvement; complex partial seizures, however, frequently have bilateral hemispheric involvement. Partial seizures can be classified into one of the following three groups:
   A. Simple partial seizures (consciousness not impaired)
      1. With motor symptoms
      2. With somatosensory or special sensory symptoms
      3. With autonomic symptoms
      4. With psychic symptoms
   B. Complex partial seizures (with impairment of consciousness)
      1. Beginning as simple partial seizures and progressing to impairment of consciousness
         a. With no other features
         b. With features as in A.1–A.4
         c. With automatisms
      2. With impairment of consciousness at outset
         a. With no other features
         b. With features as in A.1–A.4
         c. With automatisms
   C. Partial seizures secondarily generalized
II. *Generalized seizures (convulsive or nonconvulsive).* Generalized seizures are those in which the first clinical changes indicate initial involvement of both hemispheres. Consciousness may be impaired, and this impairment may be the initial manifestation. Motor manifestations are bilateral. The ictal electroencephalographic patterns initially are bilateral and presumably reflect neuronal discharge that is widespread in both hemispheres.
   A. Absence seizures
      1. Typical absence seizures
      2. Atypical absence seizures
   B. Myoclonic seizures
   C. Clonic seizures
   D. Tonic seizures
   E. Tonic-clonic seizures
   F. Atonic seizures
III. *Unclassified epileptic seizures.* Unclassified epileptic seizures include all seizures that cannot be classified because of inadequate or incomplete data and some that defy classification. This includes some neonatal seizures (e.g., rhythmic eye movements, chewing, and swimming movements).

Modified from Dreifuss FE. Classification of epileptic seizures and the epilepsies. Pediatr Clin North Am 1989;36:265–279.

TABLE 129–5

SEIZURES: THERAPY AT A GLANCE

I. General medical management
  A. Ensure adequate airway and breathing. Give supplemental oxygen. Consider oxygen saturation monitoring. Protect the cervical spine in trauma patients.
  B. Provide circulatory support as needed. Monitor heart and blood pressure.
  C. Consider obtaining rapid glucose screen; arterial blood gas measurements; complete blood cell count; determination of electrolyte, calcium, magnesium, phosphorus, glucose, and anticonvulsant drug levels; toxicology screen; ammonia level; liver function tests; and measurement of blood urea nitrogen and creatinine levels.
  D. Start an IV line with D5NS or D5LR at a keep-open rate. If unable to establish IV, begin therapy with rectal agents or consider intraosseous line.
  E. If rapid glucose test < 60 or not known, give 0.5 to 1.0 gm/kg dextrose as D25W (2 to 4 ml/kg). If alcoholism is a consideration, give 100 mg of thiamine IV or IM prior to glucose.
  F. If patient is comatose or opioid ingestion is suspected, give 0.1 mg/kg initial dose (maximum, 2.0 mg) of naloxone.
  G. Consider sodium bicarbonate, 1 mEq/kg, if pH < 7.10 from a metabolic acidosis.
II. Pharmacotherapy of seizures
  A. Benzodiazepines (choose one):
    1. Diazepam, 0.1 to 0.5 mg/kg IV or 0.3 to 0.5 mg/kg rectally (maximum, 10 mg per dose). May be repeated once after 5 min if seizures persist.
    2. Lorazepam, 0.05 to 0.1 mg/kg IV (maximum, 2 to 4 mg per dose). May be repeated once after 5 min if seizures persist.
    3. Midazolam, 0.2 mg/kg IM (maximum, 5 mg per dose). May be repeated once after 5 min if seizures persist.
  B. If seizures persist, choose one of the following. If one is unsuccessful, use the other.
    1. Phenytoin, 15 to 20 mg/kg (maximum, 1200 mg per dose). Must be administered as a slow IV push at a rate of 0.7 mg/kg/min (maximum rate, 50 mg/min). Monitor cardiac status (rate, rhythm, and blood pressure) while phenytoin is infusing.
    2. Phenobarbital, 10 to 20 mg/kg (maximum, 1000 mg). Administer IV at 100 mg/min. Monitor closely for respiratory depression and hypotension.
  C. (Optional) Paraldehyde mixed 2:1 with peanut, cottonseed, or olive oil (dose: 0.3 ml/kg). Not available as a parenteral formulation, so must be given rectally. Repeat in 2 hours if needed. Not often used because of difficult administration and efficacy of barbiturates.
  D. If seizures still persist, choose one of the following. If not already intubated, the patient should probably be intubated at this point.
    1. Phenobarbital, 5 to 10 mg/kg/dose, repeated at 10- to 20-min intervals until seizures are controlled.
    2. Pentobarbital, 3 to 6 mg/kg/dose, given as an IV infusion at 50 mg/min to a maximum of 500 mg. Monitor for hypotension.
  E. Other drugs to consider
    1. Sodium valproate. Dilute syrup (250 mg/5 ml) 1:1 with water and give 20 mg/kg as a retention enema. May cause an increase in serum phenobarbital concentration or a decrease in serum phenytoin concentration. Peak serum levels occur in 3 to 5 hours.
    2. General anesthesia with inhalation agents can be used, but requires electroencephalogram monitoring and slow withdrawal.
    3. Carbamazepine solution for intravenous use. Dosage not yet established. Consult with a neurologist.

TABLE 129–6

PHARMACOKINETICS OF ANTICONVULSANTS USED IN THE EMERGENCY DEPARTMENT

Drug	Therapeutic Level (µg/ml)	Toxic Level (µg/ml)	Half-life (hr)	Time to Steady State (oral)	Dosage	Route	Comments
Carbamazepine (Tegretol)	4–12	>12	12–17	3–7 days	15–25 mg/kg/day	Oral	Maintenance therapy; dose varies with age
Diazepam (Valium)	20–50	NA	14–90	NA	0.1–0.5 mg/kg; max, 10–20 mg	IV	Duration may be only 10–30 min
					0.3–0.5 mg/kg	Rectal	
Lorazepam (Ativan)	NA	NA	4–16	NA	0.05–0.1 mg/kg; max, 2–4 mg	IV or rectal	Repeat only once
Midazolam (Versed)	NA	NA	NA	NA	0.1–0.3 mg/kg; max, 5–10 mg	IV or IM	Titrate slowly IV
Paraldehyde	NA	NA	NA	NA	50–200 mg/kg = 0.3 ml/kg	Rectal	Mix 2:1 with peanut or other oil
Pentobarbital (Nembutal)	NA	NA	NA	NA	3–6 mg/kg; max, 500 mg	IV	50 mg/min or less; titrate to induce coma
Phenobarbital (Luminal)	15–40	>40	15–60	2–3 wk	10–20 mg/kg; max, 1000 mg	IV or IM	IV push at 100 mg/min or less
					4–6 mg/kg/day	Oral	Maintenance therapy
Phenytoin (Dilantin)	10–20	>30	12–36	5 days	15–20 mg/kg; max, 1200 mg	IV	IV at ≤ 0.7 mg/kg/min or less; max, 25–50 mg/min
					4–8 mg/kg/day	Oral	Maintenance therapy
Sodium valproate (Depakene)	50–100	>100	12	3 days	20 mg/kg as enema	Rectal	250 mg/5 ml syrup diluted 1:1 with water
					15–30 mg/kg/day	Oral	Maintenance therapy

native to induce coma in an effort to control seizure activity. General anesthesia with inhalation agents is a less often used alternative.

Paraldehyde, another choice for refractory status, is currently not available in a parenteral form.[34, 35] It is sometimes successful when other drugs have failed. Sodium valproate (Depakene) is also effective in some refractory cases but must be given as a retention enema or through a gastric tube.[36–39]

Localized (focal) epileptic activity does not necessarily mean a localized pathologic lesion, as the phenomenon of partial or lateralized movements has been associated with diffuse cerebral insults such as drug intoxication, carbon monoxide poisoning, or metabolic abnormalities.[40] Tonic, atypical absence, and myoclonic status are difficult to control but may respond to sodium valproate.[41] Typical absence status is best treated with a benzodiazepine.[41] Simple and complex partial status and tonic-clonic status are treated as discussed previously. Excessive treatment of partial status epilepticus can be worse than the condition itself.

ADMISSION CRITERIA AND DISCHARGE INSTRUCTIONS

Admission criteria for patients suffering from seizures depend greatly on the cause of the seizure. Nevertheless, certain features should prompt admission. These include new-onset focal seizures, seizures lasting more than 15 minutes, continued impairment of consciousness, lack of a reliable caregiver, parental concern, and seizures with life-threatening complications such as apnea. The cause of the seizure may necessitate admission, as in cases of intoxication or CNS infection. Some physicians prefer to admit all patients with a first-time nonfebrile seizure.

If the patient is sent home, a competent careprovider should understand the risk of recurrence and what to do if seizures recur, any medications to be given, and plans for follow-up.

STATUS EPILEPTICUS

Status epilepticus has many variations. It is classically defined as a seizure, or repetitive seizures, without an intervening return of consciousness, lasting 30 minutes or more.[42–44] Convulsive (motor) status epilepticus may result in death in 10% to 12%[45] of victims or permanent neurologic impairment in up to 37%.[46] Nonconvulsive status epilepticus (nonmotor, or so-called *petit mal status*) does not present the same immediate problems, although it is still important as an emergency. The term *prolonged seizure activity* has been used to describe continuous generalized or focal seizures lasting 10 minutes or longer, as well as three or more separate seizures within a 30-minute period.[47]

Clinical Evaluation

Convulsive status epilepticus requires prompt therapy and simultaneous evaluation for its origin. In most series (of which large-case-number pediatric series are rare), the prognosis is grave in the symptomatic group when known epileptics are excluded.[48–50] Neuronal ischemic changes have been shown to occur in primates in 15 to 30 minutes and are irreversible within 60 to 90 minutes.[51] Status epilepticus may cause hypoglycemia, myoglobinemia, hyperkalemia, hyperpyrexia, dehydration, lactic acidosis, hypotension, increased intracranial pressure, and respiratory failure.[52]

Vascular, traumatic, and metabolic causes are frequent, and brain tumor is another common cause of "unheralded status," in which status epilepticus is the first occurrence of

seizures in a previously healthy patient.[53] Other frequent causes are intoxications, drug withdrawal, CNS infections, and encephalopathies such as Reye's syndrome or acute malignant hypertension. Unheralded status appears to be more common in young children than in adults, and accidental intoxication is a major cause. Poisoning is a common cause of seizures in children, and more than 100 substances may induce convulsions.[54] The five leading drug causes of seizures, in descending order, are cyclic antidepressants, stimulants (cocaine and amphetamines), antihistamines, theophylline, and isoniazid[55] (Table 129–7).

Therapeutic Intervention

The principles of therapy include addressing airway, breathing, and circulation (the ABCs); establishing vascular access; rapid serum glucose determination; and emergent pharmacotherapy. Individual physicians have their own drug of choice following the initial benzodiazepine. The cause of the seizure may influence the choice of anticonvulsant (e.g., phenobarbital for theophylline-induced seizures or phenytoin in the patient with closed head injury).

Admission Criteria and Discharge Instructions

Patients suffering from status epilepticus should be admitted to the hospital for further evaluation, observation, and treatment. If seizures persist, intensive care unit admission is warranted. Patients usually remain in the hospital until they have been seizure free for a minimum of 24 hours, allowing drug sedation to resolve.

FEBRILE SEIZURES

A febrile seizure is an event in infancy or childhood, usually occurring between 3 months and 5 years of age, that is associated with fever but without evidence of intracranial infection or defined cause. Seizures associated with fever in children who have suffered a previous nonfebrile seizure are excluded from this definition.[56, 57] Simple febrile seizures last less than 15 minutes, have no focal component, and do not occur in series with a total duration of more than 30

TABLE 129–7
AGENTS MOST LIKELY TO INDUCE STATUS EPILEPTICUS SEIZURES

Stimulants:	Cocaine, amphetamines and related compounds, camphor, monoamine oxidase inhibitors and related compounds, theophylline and related compounds, strychnine, phencyclidine (PCP)
Depressants:	Phenothiazines, haloperidol, chlorprothixene, anticholinergics, lithium, carbamazepine
Opioids:	Methyl morphine (codeine), propoxyphene hydrochloride
Miscellaneous:	Isoniazid, hydrazine, phenol, salicylates, halogenated hydrocarbon pesticides, quaternary ammonium compounds (benzalkonium chloride), boric acid and related compounds, ergot derivatives, organophosphate insecticides, cyanide, carbon monoxide, clonidine
Withdrawal:	Narcotics, alcohol, barbiturates, anticonvulsants

Modified from Wasserman GS. Poisoning leads to some status epilepticus cases. JAMA 1976;236:1927. Copyright 1976, American Medical Association.

minutes. Complex febrile seizures are focal, prolonged, and may occur in series.

From 2.2% to 5.0% of children suffer a febrile seizure.[58] Siblings of patients with febrile seizures are more likely to have febrile seizures,[59] as are children with higher temperatures, though this may be related to rate of rise instead of absolute temperature.[60] Boys are at a higher risk than girls.[61] Febrile seizures usually occur in the presence of a clinically recognizable infection, most commonly upper respiratory tract infections, otitis media, gastrointestinal infections, and roseola infantum.[62]

Clinical Evaluation

Simple febrile seizures are benign,[63–66] but all children who present with fever and a seizure deserve thorough evaluation to exclude more ominous etiologies.[67] A careful history and physical examination of the child who is alert and appropriate may be sufficient, but other patients may require further study. Routine seizure laboratory tests, such as electrolyte determinations, are rarely helpful.[68] The problem usually is determining which children need lumbar puncture to exclude meningitis or encephalitis. The following factors correlate with serious illness: duration of fever greater than 24 hours prior to onset of seizures;[69] age less than 6 months;[70] physician visit within 48 hours; occurrence of convulsions in the emergency department; focal seizures; and an abnormal neurologic or physical examination.[71] Ultimately, clinical judgment must determine which children require a lumbar puncture.[56, 68, 72]

Therapeutic Intervention

Preventing further febrile seizures begins with adequate temperature control. Acetaminophen, in doses of 15 mg/kg given every 4 hours (with a maximum of five doses in a 24-hour period), should be instituted promptly. If needed, ibuprofen, 10 mg/kg every 6 to 8 hours, may be given as well. Most febrile seizures do not recur after 24 hours.[73] Children who present with their first, simple febrile seizure are not candidates for anticonvulsant therapy.[56] In patients with complex or multiple febrile seizures, anticonvulsant use remains controversial. Factors to consider in initiating anticonvulsant therapy are risk of recurrence, parental anxiety, severity of the episode, and hazards of treatment.

Patients with seizures at lower temperatures, with more than three episodes in a year, who are less than 15 months old, or with epilepsy or febrile seizures in first-degree relatives are more likely to reconvulse than those with higher temperatures.[74–77] Children whose seizures had complex features are more likely to have both febrile and afebrile seizures, and the risk increases with increasing number of complex features.[78] Children older than 6 years and those younger than 6 months with febrile seizures also may be at increased risk for afebrile seizures.[65, 79, 80] Treatment may not alter the prevalence of epilepsy at a later time,[81–83] and the recurrence rate of febrile seizures has varied widely in published studies.[81–87]

A variety of agents have been tried for prophylaxis of febrile seizures. Phenytoin[88] and carbamazepine[89] are ineffective. Phenobarbital is effective in preventing recurrence of febrile seizures but must be given daily to maintain adequate blood levels.[87, 90] Intermittent dosing of phenobarbital when the child has a fever is of virtually no value.[87] Intermittent dosing of diazepam rectally when the child is febrile is effective,[81, 85, 91] but appropriate teaching of the parents regarding dose, administration, and hazards is essential.[85] Parents may not recognize the presence of fever prior to onset of febrile convulsions, making intermittent dosing of any medication valueless. Even if a drug is effective in preventing recurrences, its side effects must also be considered, particularly if it is given on a regular basis and not intermittently. Phenobarbital has been found to cause significant impairment of cognitive performance, even after it has been discontinued.[92] For most children, the decision to start a prophylactic drug regimen is best made by the child's regular physician in consultation with the parents.

Admission Criteria and Discharge Instructions

Patients who have suffered a simple febrile seizure may be discharged to the parents' care providing (1) there is no concomitant illness requiring admission, (2) the parents understand the diagnosis and treatment plan, and (3) they are comfortable taking the child home. A complex seizure, uncertain diagnosis, uncomfortable parents, or suspected lack of good home care should prompt admission.

Discharge instructions should include temperature control, returning for any recurrence of seizures, and treatment and follow-up of both the underlying illness and the seizure.

References

1. Holmes GL. Epidemiology and classification of epilepsy. In Diagnosis and Management of Seizures in Children. Philadelphia, WB Saunders, 1987, p 1.
2. Epilepsy Foundation of America. Basic Statistics on the Epilepsies. Philadelphia, FA Davis, 1975.
3. Aicardi J, Gastaut H, Misès J. Syncopal attacks compulsively self-induced by Valsalva's maneuver associated with typical absence seizures. A case report. Arch Neurol 1988;45:923.
4. DiMario FJ, Chee CM, Berman PH. Pallid breath-holding spells. Clin Pediatr 1990;29:17.
5. Holmes GL. Differential diagnosis of epilepsy: Nonepileptic episodic phenomena. In Diagnosis and Management of Seizures in Children. Philadelphia, WB Saunders, 1987, p 46.
6. Holmes GL. Breath-holding attacks in children. Postgrad Med 1988;84:191.
7. Lombroso CT, Lerman P. Breathholding spells (cyanotic and pallid infantile syncope). Pediatrics 1967;39:563.
8. Vining EP, Freeman JM. Paroxysmal events which are not seizures. Pediatr Ann 1985;14:726.
9. Ferry PC. 'Shuddering spells.' Seizures or not? Am J Dis Child 1986;140:19.
10. Haines SJ. Decerebrate posturing misinterpreted as seizure activity. Am J Emerg Med 1988;6:173.
11. Rothner AD. 'Not everything that shakes is epilepsy.' The differential diagnosis of paroxysmal nonepileptiform disorders. Cleve Clin J Med 1989;56:S206.
12. Baumer JH, David TJ, Valentine SJ, et al. Many parents think their child is dying when having a first febrile convulsion. Dev Med Child Neurol 1981;23:462.
13. Wyllie E, Friedman D, Rothner AD, et al. Psychogenic seizures in children and adolescents: Outcome after diagnosis by ictal video and electroencephalographic recording. Pediatrics 1990;85:480.
14. Lempert T, Schmidt D. Natural history and outcome of psychogenic seizures: A clinical study in 50 patients. J Neurol 1990;237:35.
15. Porter RJ. Etiology and classification of epileptic seizures. In Robb P (ed). Epilepsy Updated: Causes and Treatment. Chicago, Year Book, 1980, p 1.
16. Dreifuss FE. Classification of epileptic seizures and the epilepsies. Pediatr Clin North Am 1989;36:265.
17. Delgado-Escueta AV, Wasterlain C, Treiman DM, Porter RJ. Management of status epilepticus. N Engl J Med 1982;306:1337.
18. Dulac O, Aicardi J, Rey E, Olive G. Blood levels of diazepam after single rectal administration in infants and children. J Pediatr 1978;93:1039.
19. Spivey WH, Unger HD, Lathers CM, McNamara RM. Intraosseous diazepam suppression of pentyletetrazol-induced epileptogenic activity in pigs. Ann Emerg Med 1987;16:156.
20. Walker JE, Homan RW, Vasko MR, et al. Lorazepam in status epilepticus. Ann Neurol 1979;6:207.
21. Levy RJ, Krall RK. Treatment of status epilepticus with lorazepam. Arch Neurol 1984;41:605.
22. Lacey DJ, Singer WD, Horwitz SJ, Gilmore G. Lorazepam therapy of status epilepticus in children and adolescents. J Pediatr 1986;108:771.
23. Crawford TO, Mitchell WG. Lorazepam for status epilepticus and serial seizures in children: 218 consecutive doses. Ann Neurol 1985;18:412.
24. Crawford TO, Mitchell WG, Snodgrass SR. Lorazepam in childhood

status epilepticus and serial seizures: Effectiveness and tachyphylaxis. Neurology 1987;37:190.

25. Crawford TO, Mitchell WG, Fishman LS, Snodgrass SR. Very-high-dose phenobarbital for refractory status epilepticus in children. Neurology 1988;38:1035.
26. Mayhue FE. IM midazolam for status epilepticus in the emergency department. Ann Emerg Med 1988;17:643.
27. Livingston JH, Brown JK. Non-convulsive status epilepticus resistant to benzodiazepines. Arch Dis Child 1987;62:41.
28. Cranford RE, Leppik IE, Patrick B, et al. Intravenous phenytoin in acute treatment of seizures. Neurology 1979;29:1474.
29. Earnest MP, Marx JA, Drury LR. Complications of intravenous phenytoin for acute treatment of seizures. JAMA 1983;249:762.
30. Wilder BJ, Ramsay RE, Willmore LJ, et al. Efficacy of intravenous phenytoin in the treatment of status epilepticus: Kinetics of central nervous system penetration. Ann Neurol 1977;1:511.
31. Porter RJ. Therapy: Status Epilepticus. In Epilepsy. Philadelphia, WB Saunders, 1989, p 129.
32. Dunn DW. Status epilepticus in children: Etiology, clinical features, and outcome. J Child Neurol 1988;3:167.
33. Frost MD. Editorial comment: Status epilepticus. Pediatr Trauma Acute Care 1988;1:17.
34. Curless RG, Holzman BH, Ramsay RE. Paraldehyde therapy in childhood status epilepticus. Arch Neurol 1983;40:477.
35. Bostrom B. Paraldehyde toxicity during treatment of status epilepticus. Am J Dis Child 1982;136:414.
36. Manhire AR, Espir M. Treatment of status epilepticus with sodium valproate. Br Med J 1974;3:808.
37. Vajda FJ, Mihaly GW, Miles JL, et al. Rectal administration of sodium valproate in status epilepticus. Neurology 1978;28:897.
38. Thorpy MJ. Rectal valproate syrup and status epilepticus. Neurology 1980;30:1113.
39. Snead OC, Miles MV. Treatment of status epilepticus in children with rectal sodium valproate. J Pediatr 1985;106:323.
40. Aminoff MJ, Simon RP. Status epilepticus: Causes, clinical features, and consequences in 98 patients. Am J Med 1980;69:657.
41. Shields WD. Status epilepticus. Pediatr Clin North Am 1989;36:383.
42. Hauser WA. Status epilepticus: Frequency, etiology, and neurological sequelae. In Delgado-Escueta AV, Wasterlain CG, Treiman DM, et al (eds). Advances in Neurology. Vol 34. Status Epilepticus. New York, Raven Press, 1983, p 3.
43. Lederman RJ. Status epilepticus. Cleve Clin Q 1984;51:261.
44. Sawyer GT, Webster DD, Schut LJ. Treatment of uncontrolled seizure activity with diazepam. JAMA 1968;203:913.
45. Delgado-Escueta AV, Bojorek GJ. Status epilepticus: Mechanisms of brain damage and rational management. Epilepsia 1982;23:S29.
46. Aicardi J, Chevrie JJ. Convulsive status epilepticus in infants and children: A study of 239 cases. Epilepsia 1970;11:187.
47. Prensky AL, Raff MC, More MJ. Intravenous diazepam in the treatment of prolonged seizure activity. N Engl J Med 1967;276:779.
48. Celesia GG. Modern concepts of status epilepticus. JAMA 1976;235:1571.
49. Janz D. Conditions and causes of status epilepticus. Epilepsia 1961;2:170.
50. Oxbury JM, Whitty CW. Causes and consequences of status epilepticus in adults. Brain 1971;94:733.
51. Meldrum BS, Brierley JB. Prolonged epileptic seizures in primates. Arch Neurol 1973;28:10.
52. Plum F, Posner JB, Troy B. Cerebral metabolic and circulatory responses to induced convulsions in animals. Arch Neurol 1968;18:1.
53. Oxbury JM, Whitty CW. The syndrome of isolated epileptic status. J Neurol Neurosurg Psychiatr 1971;34:182.
54. Olson KR, Pentel PR, Kelley MT. Physical assessment and differential diagnosis of the poisoned patient. Med Toxicol 1987;2:52.
55. Olson KR, Kearney TE, Dye JE, Benowitz NL. Seizures associated with poisoning and drug overdose: Changing patterns of causes and poison center consultations. Abstract. Vet Hum Toxicol 1990;32:361.
56. Consensus Development Panel. Febrile seizures: Long-term management of children with fever-associated seizures. Pediatr Rev 1981;2:209.
57. Millichap JG. The definition of febrile seizures. In Nelson KB, Ellenberg JH (eds). Febrile Seizures. New York, Raven Press, 1981, p 1.
58. Hauser WA. The natural history of febrile seizures. In Nelson KB, Ellenberg JH (eds). Febrile Seizures. New York, Raven Press, 1981, p 5.
59. Hauser WA, Annegers JF, Anderson VE, Kurland LT. The risk of seizure disorders among relatives of children with febrile convulsions. Neurology 1985;35:1268.
60. Rosman NP. Febrile seizures. Emerg Med Clin North Am 1987;5:719.

61. Ouellette EM. The child who convulses with fever. Pediatr Clin North Am 1974;21:467.
62. Hirtz DG, Nelson KB. The natural history of febrile seizures. Annu Rev Med 1983;34:453.
63. Chamberlain JM, Gorman RL. Occult bacteremia in children with simple febrile seizures. Am J Dis Child 1988;142:1073.
64. Livingston JH, Brown JK, Harkness RA, et al. Cerebrospinal fluid nucleotide metabolites following short febrile convulsions. Dev Med Child Neurol 1989;31:161.
65. Nelson KB, Ellenberg JH. Prognosis in children with febrile seizures. Pediatrics 1978;61:720.
66. Verity CM, Butler NR, Golding J. Febrile convulsions in a national cohort followed up from birth. II—Medical history and intellectual ability at 5 years of age. Br Med J [Clin Res] 1985;290:1311.
67. Vining EP, Freeman JM. Seizures which are not epilepsy. Pediatr Ann 1985;14:711.
68. Bettis DB, Ater SB. Febrile seizures: Emergency department diagnosis and treatment. J Emerg Med 1985;2:341.
69. Anderson AB, Desisto MJ, Marshall PC, Dewitt TG. Duration of fever prior to onset of a simple febrile seizure: A predictor of significant illness and neurologic course. Pediatr Emerg Care 1989;5:12.
70. Rossi LN, Brunelli G, Duzioni N, Rossi G. Lumbar puncture and febrile convulsions. Helv Paediatr Acta 1986;41:19.
71. Joffe A, McCormick M, DeAngelis C. Which children with febrile seizures need lumbar puncture? Am J Dis Child 1983;137:1153.
72. Wears RL, Luten RC, Lyons RG. Which laboratory tests should be performed on children with apparent febrile convulsions? An analysis and review of the literature. Pediatr Emerg Care 1986;2:191.
73. Green AL, MacFaul R. Duration of admission for febrile convulsions? Arch Dis Child 1985;60:1182.
74. el-Radhi AS, Withana K, Banajeh S. Recurrence rate of febrile convulsions related to the degree of pyrexia during the first attack. Clin Pediatr 1986;25:311.
75. el-Radhi AS, Banajeh S. Effect of fever on recurrence rate of febrile convulsions. Arch Dis Child 1989;64:869.
76. Knudsen FU. Recurrence risk after first febrile seizure and effect of short term diazepam prophylaxis. Arch Dis Child 1985;60:1045.
77. Knudsen FU. Frequent febrile episodes and recurrent febrile convulsions. Acta Neurol Scand 1988;78:414.
78. Annegers JF, Hauser WA, Shirts SB, Kurland LT. Factors prognostic of unprovoked seizures after febrile convulsions. N Engl J Med 1987;316:493.
79. Pavone L, Cavazzuti GB, Incorpora G, et al. Late febrile convulsions: A clinical followup. Brain Dev 1989;11:183.
80. Verity CM, Butler NR, Golding J. Febrile convulsions in a national cohort followed up from birth. I—Prevalence and recurrence in the first five years of life. Br Med J [Clin Res] 1985;290:1307.
81. Knudsen FU. Effective short-term diazepam prophylaxis in febrile convulsions. J Pediatr 1985;106:487.
82. Knudsen FU. Optimum management of febrile seizures in childhood. Drugs 1988;36:111.
83. Wolf SM, Forsythe A. Epilepsy and mental retardation following febrile seizures in childhood. Acta Paediatr Scand 1989;78:291.
84. Berg AT, Shinnar S, Hauser WA, Leventhal JM. Predictors of recurrent febrile seizures: A metaanalytic review. J Pediatr 1990;116:329.
85. Camfield CS, Camfield PR, Smith E, Dooley JM. Home use of rectal diazepam to prevent status epilepticus in children with convulsive disorders. J Child Neurol 1989;4:125.
86. Gururaj VJ. Febrile seizures. Clin Pediatr 1980;19:731.
87. Wolf SM, Carr A, Davis DC, et al. The value of phenobarbital in the child who has had a single febrile seizure: A controlled prospective study. Pediatrics 1977;59:378.
88. Melchior JC, Buchthal F, Lennox-Buchthal M. The ineffectiveness of diphenylhydantoin in preventing febrile convulsions in the age of greatest risk, under three years. Epilepsia 1971;12:55.
89. Camfield PR, Camfield CS, Tibbles JAR. Carbamazepine does not prevent febrile seizures in phenobarbital failures. Neurology 1982;32:288.
90. Herranz JL, Armijo JA, Arteaga R. Effectiveness and toxicity of phenobarbital, primidone, and sodium valproate in the prevention of febrile convulsions, controlled by plasma levels. Epilepsia 1984;25:89.
91. Woody RC, Laney SM. Rectal anticonvulsants in pediatric practice. Pediatr Emerg Care 1988;4:112.
92. Farwell JR, Lee YJ, Hirtz DG, et al. Phenobarbital for febrile seizures—effects on intelligence and on seizure recurrence. N Engl J Med 1990;322:364.

CHAPTER 130

Coma

J. Stephen Huff
Jorge Montes

INTRODUCTION

Coma represents brain failure and is found in critically ill children in a variety of clinical situations. Not only is the comatose child critically ill, there is also the possibility of imminent death.

Some persistence of unresponsiveness is implied in the term *coma*. Brief interruption of consciousness is typically investigated as syncope or possibly seizure activity. This chapter focuses on enduring loss of consciousness and acute alteration of consciousness.

Gradations of consciousness exist between full alertness and coma. Even the term *alertness* does not fully convey the normal wakeful state, for consciousness has both alerting and content qualities.[1] Content properties include functions of the cerebral cortex such as speech and memory, whereas alerting functions reside throughout the brain stem in the reticular activating system.

A variety of terms are used to describe the altered states of consciousness between wakefulness and coma. *Coma* is best defined as an eyes-closed, unresponsive state. When the patient is stimulated, some arousal may occur, but the return to consciousness is not complete, and the patient's responses are inappropriate for the stimulus. *Light coma* implies that some fragment of normal responsiveness is present; yawning, a gag response, or some avoidance of noxious stimuli may be evident. With *deep coma* these fragmentary responses are lost. Abnormal respiratory patterns or reflex postures may be seen, or the patient may be flaccid without spontaneous respirations. *Stupor* is a state in which an unresponsive patient will briefly return to full alertness if vigorously stimulated, but will lapse into unconsciousness if stimulation is not continued. *Obtundation* refers to a state of blunted awareness with slowed arousal response. These terms are inexact for accurate and reliable clinical evaluation. Placing such a label on a patient is not a substitute for detailed, documented serial examinations. Numbered scoring systems decrease variability between observers but lack clinical detail.

The term *persistent vegetative state* describes the patient who fails to regain functional awareness of the environment after at least 1 month in coma. Such individuals have spontaneous respirations and may have wake-sleep cycles but show little motor movement other than chewing or swallowing. The *locked-in syndrome* is a different condition where the patient is immobile because of destruction of motor tract outflow. With careful testing, the patient is shown to be awake and alert.

ANATOMY AND PHYSIOLOGY

For a person to be fully conscious with both content and alerting properties intact, the brain stem and both cerebral hemispheres must be physically intact, functional, and interactive. The eyes-closed, unresponsive state implies that the brain stem, both cerebral hemispheres, or some combination of the two regions are impaired. Destruction or dysfunction of one hemisphere may impair the content of consciousness but should not of itself impair alertness. For example, aphasia may be present, but an eyes-closed, unresponsive state will not result unless the other hemisphere or the brain stem is also impaired.

The basic cellular unit of the nervous system is the neuron, which requires a continuous supply of glucose and oxygen. Interruption in supply of these substrates results in loss of consciousness in less than 20 seconds. Other alterations in the cellular environment may disrupt the physiology of neurons and their interactions. Neurons have electrical potentials that fluctuate in the course of their functioning. Seizures alter consciousness through disruption of normal neuronal electrophysiology. Abnormally low serum sodium levels cause alterations in consciousness by interfering with the normal electrical potentials of neurons. The activity of the blood-brain barrier and blood–cerebrospinal fluid (CSF) barriers are important in disorders of osmolality. Toxins may affect neurons diffusely or show a predilection for affecting certain neuronal systems.

Coma may result from either dysfunction on a cellular level or gross anatomic disruption. The numerous causes of coma may be coarsely grouped into metabolic, toxic, or structural processes. Destruction of areas of brain by a mass lesion is an example of a macroanatomic change. The impairment may result from direct physical destruction or from ischemia as a result of secondary vascular compression. However, even with a seemingly clear-cut cause such as a subdural hematoma, a complicated process is involved. The force required to produce the hematoma is distributed throughout the intracranial contents. Some lesions are remote from the site of major injury in the coup-contrecoup injury pattern. In addition, smaller injuries occur throughout the brain from diffuse shearing forces. Brain edema from blood-brain barrier disruption may complicate the injury further. Intracranial pressure (ICP) is yet another aggravating factor. An increase in ICP may be the final stage in severe head trauma, meningitis, anoxic injury, or Reye's syndrome. If ICP is greater than the mean arterial blood pressure, blood flow to the brain stops. Brain death occurs at that time.

EMERGENCY MEDICAL SERVICE CONSIDERATIONS

The cause of coma may be evident on the patient's arrival (e.g., in cases of trauma or near drowning). A brief survey of the scene and patient history obtained during stabilization are valuable. Key points include any medication use, toxin exposure, or suspected trauma.

Specific intervention may be directed by the history. For example, in the diabetic patient with coma, administration of intravenous glucose is indicated after a blood sample is obtained.

Contact with medical control concerning an impending arrival is imperative. Information concerning response to interventions, vascular access, and the airway techniques employed is valuable.

CLINICAL EVALUATION

Clinical evaluation and therapeutic management of the comatose patient commence simultaneously. In most instances, the patient presenting to the emergency department in a comatose state is undergoing rapid pathophysiologic changes. The diagnostic approach must be methodical, with the understanding that the primary goal is to maintain life during the diagnostic workup.

The authors would like to thank Ms. Regina Butt for assistance with the word processing of this manuscript.

The cause of coma is usually determined by the history. In the majority of cases, a careprovider or another observer will give a description of preceding events. Questioning should begin as soon as the patient arrives. Another physician or nurse may elicit the history while stabilization efforts are taking place.

An appreciation of age-related differences in clinical presentations is important. For example, the subtle manifestations of seizures in the neonate may be difficult to detect. These patients may be erroneously admitted to the hospital with a suspected diagnosis of sepsis. Initial questions should probe for any history of infection, infectious exposure, or trauma. A history of diarrhea, vomiting, or change in the feeding pattern should always be obtained. Emesis and progressive deterioration of consciousness in a patient with a recent history of upper respiratory tract infection or varicella raises the possibility of Reye's syndrome. Electrolyte imbalance, especially hyponatremia, is a cause of resistant seizures and unresponsiveness. In patients with medical conditions such as diabetes or asthma, the coma may reflect a complication of these processes. Any history of seizure disorder or previous surgical interventions (i.e., ventriculoperitoneal shunts, brain tumor) should be noted. A history of other medical conditions such as hepatic dysfunction, renal failure, pulmonary disease, or endocrine dysfunction should be sought from the caregivers or medical records. Any medication in the household should be noted. If the child is older, questions regarding drug use or suicidal ideation are appropriate.

Physical examination also proceeds during resuscitation efforts. The initial evaluation should assess the adequacy of respirations and circulation and verify unresponsiveness. The airway is the first priority in assessment and management. If spontaneous respirations are absent, ventilation is started immediately. Tremendous skill is necessary for appropriate airway management in a child. Therefore, the physician should assume responsibility for clearing and maintaining the airway. The presence of possible trauma should always be considered, and motion of the neck should be minimized. Simple basic maneuvers to ensure airway patency can be performed without any significant movement of the cervical spine. Extension or other manipulations of the neck should be avoided until radiographs have been obtained or there is certainty that no cervical spine injury is present. Simultaneously with airway management, the physician should assess the adequacy of the respiratory effort. Significant numbers of neurologically impaired pediatric patients may be hypoxic or hypercarbic. Either of these conditions may exacerbate the original neurologic injury and must be corrected.

Blind nasal intubation should not be attempted in the neurologically impaired patient less than seven years old, as the anterior position of the trachea in the younger patient makes this technique extremely difficult. In the older child, blind nasal intubation may be achieved but is not recommended for several reasons. Nasotracheal intubation is facilitated by the patient's spontaneous breathing; the severely comatose child may be apneic or have a poor or irregular respiratory effort. Nasal intubation is contraindicated in the presence of basilar skull fractures, which are almost impossible to exclude in the acute setting. A physician who does not intubate children on a regular basis will be more familiar with oral intubation techniques, which are recommended in the emergent setting. If the child is struggling or fighting the intubation, appropriate anesthetic agents may be used. The physician should be familiar with the use and complications of muscle relaxants prior to their use. Long-acting agents will preclude neurologic assessment of the patient for a prolonged period.

These patients should be closely monitored in the emergency department with pulse oximetry, transcutaneous P_{O_2} or P_{CO_2} monitoring, and capnography if available. The use of high mean airway pressures and high levels of positive end-expiratory pressure (PEEP) should be avoided when ventilating neurologically impaired children, because increases in the intrathoracic pressures may be transmitted to the intracranial vault. The only exception to this rule is when high levels of PEEP are needed to treat persistent hypoxemia. In select cases, the ICP should be monitored so that other techniques such as head elevation may be used to limit significant increases in ICP.

A major goal of therapy is to ensure adequate perfusion to the injured brain. The clinician should consider multiorgan failure, which is not unusual in the setting of brain failure, and should direct efforts to prevent any secondary injury to other organ systems. The ideal fluid for the initial resuscitation of the neurologically impaired child should be an isotonic solution such as lactated Ringer's (LR) or 0.9 normal saline (NS). If the child requires glucose in addition, D5NS or D5LR should be administered. The use of D5W or other hypotonic fluids may increase cerebral edema and worsen the neurologic outcome of the child. The use of hypertonic saline solutions for initial resuscitation and stabilization of the neurologically impaired child remains controversial.

The physical examination also proceeds during resuscitation efforts. The presence of fever is suggestive of meningitis, encephalitis, or a benign febrile seizure with prolonged postictal state. Nuchal rigidity suggests meningeal irritation from an infectious or inflammatory process (e.g., blood in the CSF). The development of meningismus may be blunted or absent in the comatose patient. The odor of alcohol suggests both ethanol intoxication and ethanol-induced hypoglycemia.

The general physical examination should focus on the skin and the nervous system. The presence of petechiae or purpura suggests vasculitis and the need for prompt therapy. The examiner should be alert to signs of trauma, as the suspicion of head injury may change the course of the evaluation.

The respiratory rate and pattern should be noted. Deep, rapid respirations may signal an underlying metabolic acidosis. A variety of respiratory patterns have little localizing value but should be identified (Fig. 130–1).

The optic disks should be carefully examined. Papilledema suggests increased ICP, usually of days' to weeks' duration. The combination of blurring of disk margins, disk swelling, and disk hyperemia are signs of early papilledema. Fully developed papilledema produces obvious disk swelling and flame-shaped retinal hemorrhages. Retinal venous pulsations probably indicate ICP of less than 190 mm H_2O in adults. However, these pulsations may be absent in 20% of normal individuals and are less studied in children. Retinal hemorrhages may indicate a recent rapid increase in ICP. Subhyaloid hemorrhages with layered blood on the retina are pathognomonic of subarachnoid hemorrhage from aneurysm or arteriovenous malformation rupture. Retinal hemorrhages may also be seen with carbon monoxide poisoning and Rocky Mountain spotted fever. Preretinal and retinal hemorrhages in infants are suggestive of child abuse.

In the infant, the anterior fontanelle, if open, is a crude but direct measure of ICP. A bulging fontanelle in a quiet infant suggests increased ICP.

Spontaneous movements of the patient should be noted. Light coma is signified by semipurposeful movements. Limb motion across the midline of the body or limb abduction is likely to represent purposeful movement. Brief flickering movements may be the only manifestation of seizure activity.

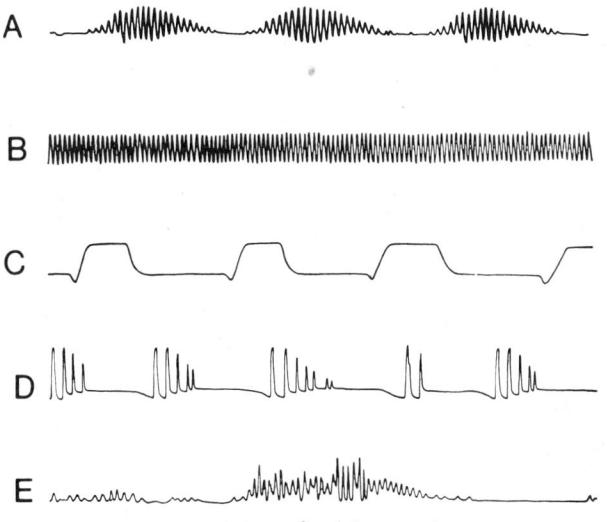

Figure 130–1. Abnormal respiratory patterns in comatose patients. *A,* Cheyne-Stokes respirations. *B,* Sustained hyperventilation. *C,* Apneustic breathing. *D,* Cluster breathing. *E,* Ataxic breathing. (From Plum F, Posner JB. The Diagnosis of Stupor and Coma. Philadelphia, FA Davis, 1980, p 34.)

Orofacial dyskinesia or rhythmic involuntary movements of the tongue, face, mouth, or jaw have been reported with metabolic encephalopathies. Response to painful stimulation should be noted. Flexor posturing, with flexion of the upper extremities and extension of the lower extremities, confirms deep coma. Extensor posturing, in which the upper extremities and lower extremities are in rigid extension, may be present spontaneously or occur in response to stimulation. Assessing these postures may provide evidence of one of the herniation syndromes. The abnormal posturing may also be present with diffuse brain injuries, drug-induced coma, and focal structural lesions. Repeated provocative stimulations should be consistent, because the location of the stimulus and limb position prior to testing may influence motor responses.

If full horizontal roving eye movements are spontaneously present, the function of a large part of the brain stem must be intact. Inspection for asymmetry of facial tone may reveal a cheek that puffs out with exhalation, indicating weak facial muscles consistent with a hemiplegia. Gentle opening of the eyelids, followed by release and observation for any asymmetry of closure, may suggest hemiparesis. The usual response in coma is a seemingly unhurried, steady closure of the lids. With a hemiplegia, the weaker orbicularis oculi causes lid closure to lag on the weaker side. This eyelid-opening maneuver is also useful in testing for pseudocoma. The patient feigning unconsciousness will resist eye opening or quickly clamp the eyelids shut when they are released.

Specific cranial nerves are tested for the presence of reflex arcs. A reflex arc demonstrates the integrity of the cranial nerves of the afferent and efferent paths, as well as the interneurons connecting these cranial nerve nuclei (Fig. 130–2). A bright light that produces pupillary constriction when directed into the eyes confirms the integrity of the cranial nerve II-III arc. The "swinging flashlight test" tests the afferent function of cranial nerve II and, more importantly, the relative efferent functions of the third cranial nerve bilaterally. Particularly worrisome in the comatose patient is a dilated pupil that is nonreactive to light. This suggests an acute lesion of cranial nerve III and may reflect impending herniation of the ipsilateral temporal lobe (Fig.

130–3). Unusual exceptions have been noted in which the third cranial nerve seemed to be directly affected by inflammation in bacterial meningitis; these patients had a dilated, unresponsive pupil but were not in coma.

Corneal sensation testing invokes the cranial nerve V-VII reflex arc. Repetitive testing with drops of water avoids corneal trauma. A direct and consensual response is present in patients in light coma with intact cranial nerves. A hand-clap that elicits a symmetric blink response shows an intact VIII-V arc and suggests light coma. Also useful in evaluating the comatose patient is testing of the vestibulo-ocular response. This is a persistently confusing element of the neurologic examination, particularly when the term *Doll's eyes* is used. In the comatose patient with functioning peripheral vestibular structures and intact cranial nerves III, VI, VIII, and interneurons, when the head is turned quickly to the left, the eyes will appear to lag behind briefly. Nystagmus will not be present. In this example, the left eye will fully adduct and the right eye fully abduct. A mirrored response should be present with head motion to the right. The absence of eye movement implies a diffuse suppression of the brain stem. The neck should never be moved when trauma or a cervical lesion is suspected.

Caloric testing involves instilling a small quantity of cold water into the ear canal after examination verifies that the canal is patent and the tympanic membrane is intact. Nystagmus is never present in the comatose patient. In the patient with an intact brain stem and cranial nerves, the response to cold water irrigation of the left ear canal is tonic deviation of both eyes symmetrically to the left. Irrigation of the right ear provokes a similar response, with slow deviation of the eyes to the right. Absence of a caloric response implies diffuse dysfunction. Fragmentary responses may be present. Precise description of the stimulus and response is urged. Failure of ocular adduction during vestibulo-ocular testing is consistent with an internuclear ophthalmoplegia or medial longitudinal fasciculus syndrome. Partial or complete ophthalmoplegia may be present with toxic coma, particularly coma produced by tricyclic antidepressants, carbamazepine, or narcotics. Rarely, it is also reported in trauma patients with brain stem compression. Cold caloric–induced symmetric downward ocular deviation suggests sedative-hypnotic drug overdose.

Some spontaneous conjugate eye movements may be present. Abrupt, spontaneous, arrhythmic, and conjugate downward jerks of both eyes, followed by slow return to midposition, define ocular bobbing; this response usually indicates pontine or cerebellar structural lesions, although it has also been reported with metabolic encephalopathies. Another disorder of vertical gaze in comatose patients has been called *ocular dipping.* This is characterized by repetitive slow, conjugate downward eye movements and a nadir at the extreme of downgaze, followed by rapid upward movements. Spontaneous roving eye movements are also present. This has been reported in patients with anoxic damage to the basal ganglia. Sustained upgaze in coma has also been reported with hypoxic encephalopathies. Rhythmic conjugate horizontal eye movements always suggest the possibility of partial seizures.

If spontaneous movements of the extremities are present, they should be tested for equal responses on both sides. One subtle sign of hemiparesis is facial asymmetry; the paralyzed buccal musculature allows the weak cheek to puff out during expiration. Gently opening the eyelids and allowing them to fall tests for symmetric tone of the orbicularis. Passive movements of the limbs assess motor tone. Holding the extremities slightly elevated and dropping them to the bed is a quick assessment for hemiparesis; the hypotonic side will fall faster.

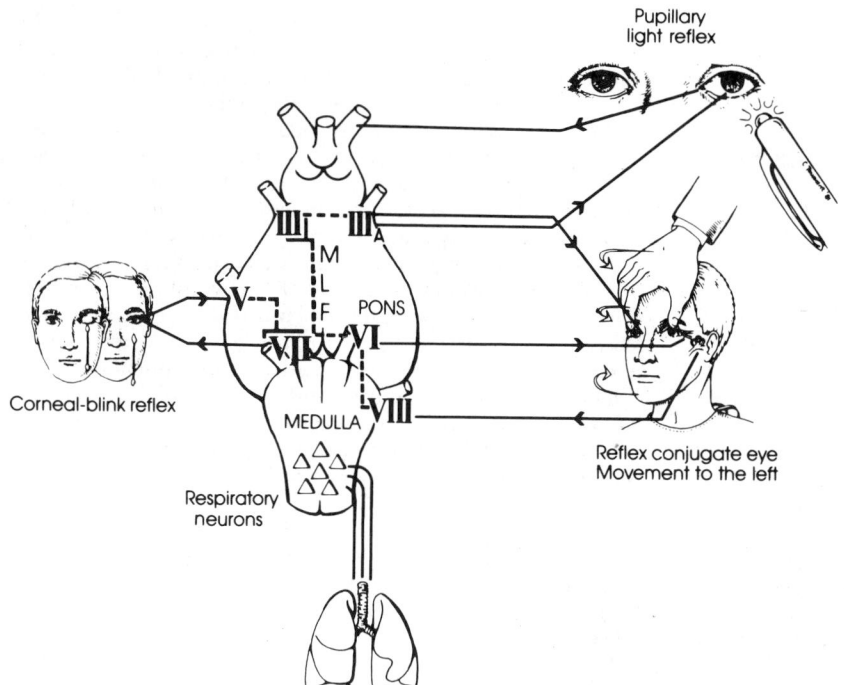

Figure 130–2. Brainstem reflexes for examination of the comatose patient. (From Ropper AH. Coma and other disorders of consciousness. *In* Braunwald E, et al. (eds). Harrison's Principles of Internal Medicine. New York, McGraw-Hill, 1987, p 115. Reproduced with permission of McGraw-Hill, Inc.)

Reflex testing is perhaps the least useful component of the neurologic examination in the acute setting. Asymmetry may be a valuable clue in lesion localization. Classically, increased muscle stretch reflexes reflect an upper motor neuron lesion of the involved pathway; however, with acute lesions this is frequently absent. The presence of extensor toe reflex movements, known as *Babinski's response*, suggests an upper motor lesion in the pathway tested, but again, with acute lesions, this may be absent. The isolated presence of Babinski's sign in a child with a head injury is not ominous and in fact may be transiently present in children with minor head injury.

Pseudocomas are usually easily distinguished from brain dysfunction. Allowing an arm to fall toward the face to see if avoidance of striking occurs is useful. The truly comatose patient will not resist passive elevation of the eyelids and will not avoid gaze contact, as occurs with fictitious coma. Caloric testing is the best procedure for confirming coma. If nystagmus is present, the cortex is physiologically awake and pseudocoma is diagnosed.

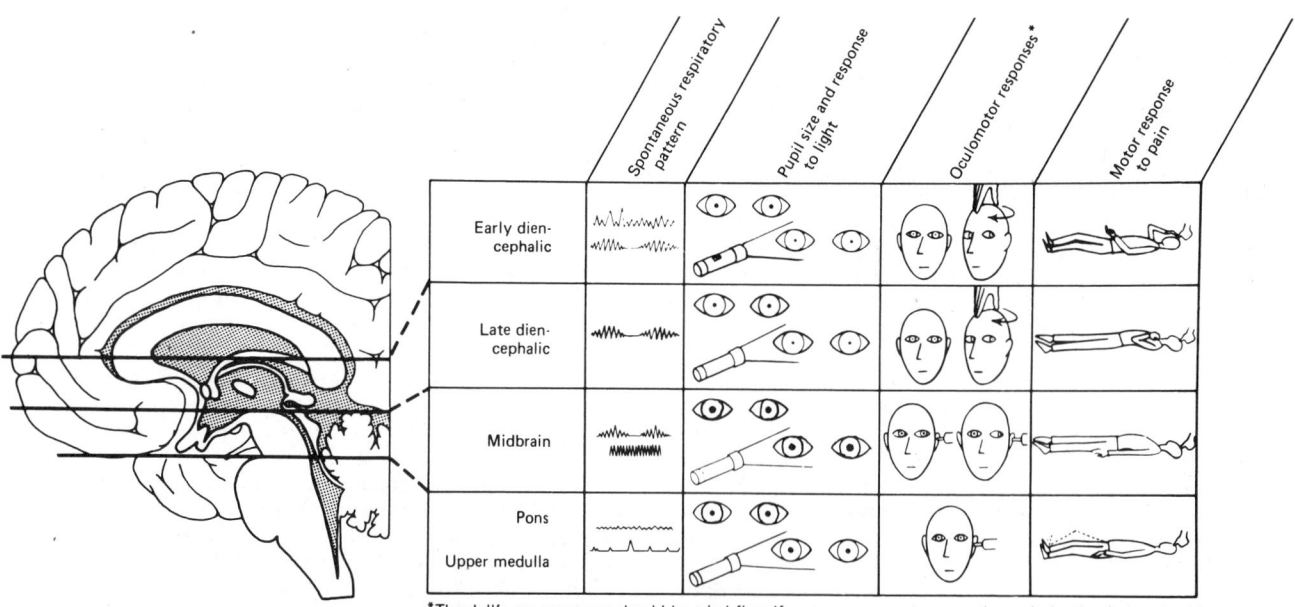

*The doll's eye maneuver should be tried first; if no eye movement occurs, then caloric stimulation should be performed by ice-water lavage of the external ear canal.

Figure 130–3. Summary of herniation syndromes. (From Simon R. Coma. *In* Mills J, et al. (eds). Current Emergency Diagnoses and Treatment. Los Altos, CA, Lange, 1985, p 87. Adapted from Plum F, Posner JB. The Diagnosis of Stupor and Coma. 3rd ed. Philadelphia, FA Davis, 1980.)

The herniation syndromes indicate the progressively destructive processes that may occur with enlarging intracranial mass lesions (see Fig. 130–3). The classic rostral-caudal progressive brain dysfunction of the herniation syndromes has been challenged. Computed tomographic (CT) scanning has shown that horizontal displacement of the brain correlates with decreased levels of consciousness more closely than actual tentorial herniation. With ICP monitoring, many patients demonstrate an abrupt rise in ICP that cannot be aborted; perfusion ceases at that time, and brain death occurs without the appearance of a classic herniation syndrome. Nevertheless, the herniation syndromes provide useful models of how mass lesions can progressively destroy the brain. The clinical course of herniation reflects complex interactions of increased ICP, ischemia, hemorrhage, and hydrocephalus.

The combination of particular signs and symptoms that occurs with certain toxic ingestions has been termed a *toxidrome*. The presence of a toxidrome may suggest a cause for the coma, as well as the appropriate therapy. For example, the combination of small pupils and coma suggests an opiate overdose, thus requiring naloxone. The anticholinergic pattern includes fever, tachycardia, urine retention, mydriasis, and perhaps seizures and coma. The cholinergic syndrome of salivation, lacrimation, urination, and defecation occurs with carbamate or organophosphate intoxication. However, in one study of children with acute organophosphate or carbamate intoxications, the classic findings of miosis, excessive salivation, and gastrointestinal syndromes were infrequent.

A ventriculoperitoneal shunt discovered by history or with physical examination raises the possibility of shunt failure or infection; either may cause coma. In this instance, urgent neurosurgical consultation is recommended. Forced pumping of the device may be attempted (Chapter 132).

DIAGNOSTIC EVALUATION

Laboratory studies may define the cause of coma or guide further interventions. Although administration of intravenous dextrose should never be delayed for laboratory test results, failure to obtain a blood sample before the dextrose is given may leave the final diagnosis in doubt. If peripheral circulation is poor as a result of shock, the results of the rapid glucose test may be misleading. Common laboratory studies indicated in patients with coma include measurement of serum electrolytes, blood urea nitrogen (BUN), glucose, and creatinine levels and a complete blood cell count. Unexpected abnormalities of the serum calcium may occasionally be detected. Arterial blood gas determination is indicated to ensure adequate oxygenation and carbon dioxide elimination. Unsuspected serum acidosis or alkalosis may be detected and may be a cause of coma. Co-oximetry may reveal the presence of an abnormal hemoglobin complex or carbon monoxide intoxication. Measurement of serum osmolality may be helpful in selected cases by detecting osmotically active substances.

More exotic laboratory work is indicated in patients with an undetermined diagnosis or when the patient's condition deteriorates. For example, abnormal results on liver function tests, a prolonged prothrombin time, and an elevated serum ammonia level may support the consideration of Reye's syndrome. Thrombocytopenia may suggest a coagulopathy. Peripheral blood smears or hemoglobin electrophoresis may detect sickle cell hemoglobinopathies, which only rarely are complicated by coma. Toxicologic screening is usually unrewarding; directed toxicologic testing is useful when clinical findings are consistent with a toxidrome.

A lumbar puncture should be performed if there is a suspicion of meningitis or encephalitis; therapy for suspected bacterial meningitis should not be delayed pending lumbar puncture or other diagnostic maneuvers. Specific testing for bacterial antigens may support the diagnosis of bacterial meningitis. The possibility of herpes simplex encephalitis deserves consideration in the comatose patient with seizures that are difficult to control.

Radiologic tests for the comatose patient include cervical spine radiography if trauma is suspected. A child may arrive in the emergency department apneic and flaccid from an upper spinal cord injury. Undiagnosed spinal cord injuries are sometimes discovered late in the clinical course.

Cranial computerized tomography is certainly the initial neuroimaging procedure of choice in the comatose child. Skull radiography has little place in management of the comatose patient except as a quick screening tool for skull fractures.

Other radiographic tests include a chest radiograph, looking specifically for correct endotracheal tube positioning or an infectious process. In patients with multiple trauma, an abdominal CT scan should be considered to exclude intra-abdominal injury. Neurologic impairment without abdominal signs is a low-yield indication for an abdominal CT scan in the uninjured child. Plain abdominal radiographs have aided the diagnosis in the uncommon patient with intussusception and altered mental status. Long-bone surveys may detect additional signs of trauma or abuse.

Electroencephalography is rarely employed in the emergency department but is the procedure of choice for diagnosis of patients with unusual seizures. Some patients, after having a "cardiac arrest," are flaccid and unresponsive, with fixed, dilated pupils. In several cases, such patients have been demonstrated to be in status epilepticus. Once the seizures were controlled, the findings that suggested brain death disappeared, and the patients made a full recovery.

DIFFERENTIAL DIAGNOSIS

The differential diagnosis of coma is extensive (Table 130–1). The majority of cases involve cranial trauma, toxic ingestion, hypoglycemia, or a seizure-related state. Unsuspected ingestion, seizures occurring with a postictal state, or trauma account for many of the cases in which initial diagnostic uncertainty exists. In a summary of 616 pediatric patients with coma or altered mental status who were admitted to a pediatric intensive care unit over a 10-year

TABLE 130–1
CAUSES OF COMA

Coma from central nervous system disease or trauma
  Trauma
  Vascular events
    Subarachnoid hemorrhage
    Hemorrhage
    Infarction
    Migrainous event
  Infections
  Neoplasms
  Seizures
Coma from systemic causes
  Hypoxia
  Metabolic encephalopathies
  Toxins
  Environmental causes
  Hypertensive encephalopathy
  Deficiency states
Psychogenic coma

TABLE 130-2

CAUSES OF ALTERED MENTAL STATUS*

Condition	Cases No.	Cases %
Status epilepticus or postictal	58	9
Hyponatremic seizures	32	5
Intracranial vascular lesions	10	2
Trauma		
Accidental	86	14
Nonaccidental	54	9
Neoplasms	6	1
Infection		
Encephalitis	56	9
Meningitis	100	16
Sepsis	50	8
Gastroenteritis	36	6
Encephalopathy		
Anoxic/ischemic	78	13
Toxic/Reye's syndrome/other	50	8

*Causes of coma or altered mental status in 616 children admitted to the Pediatric Intensive Care Unit, Children's Hospital of the King's Daughters, 1980–1989.

period, infections were the leading cause of coma (Table 130–2). An approach to the differential diagnosis is based on the physical examination, metabolic status, and structural lesions (Fig. 130–4).

A special consideration in children younger than 24 months is the shaken baby syndrome (SBS). SBS refers to injuries resulting from violent episodes of traumatic shaking; the abrupt acceleration and deceleration forces cause intracranial shearing forces with diffuse hemorrhages. Often some blunt traumatic event precipitates full development of this syndrome. The brain, retina, and cervical spinal cord are the target systems. Intracranial or retinal hemorrhages may be the only signs of injury; diffuse retinal hemorrhages are characteristic. The patient may present with cardiac arrest, respiratory distress or apnea, seizures, or coma. This diagnosis should be highly considered in the infant with altered mental status and respiratory distress. Frequently, additional historic or physical signs of abuse are present. Magnetic resonance imaging (MRI) of the brain may be diagnostic, even when CT scans are normal.

In infants younger than 2 years, a depressed level of consciousness or coma has been reported as an atypical presentation of intussusception. Rarely, migrainous events cause decreased responsiveness or coma. A history of prior headaches suggests the diagnosis, though other causes must be excluded.

Reye's syndrome is an encephalopathy occurring predominantly in children. The classic history is that of a prodromal viral illness followed by protracted emesis with deterioration in consciousness. Elevation of ICP is a central event in the progression of the syndrome. The diagnosis is suggested by hepatic dysfunction, with increased serum transaminase and serum ammonia levels and a prolonged prothrombin time. Liver biopsy is the definitive diagnostic test, and a range of histologic and ultrastructural abnormalities are possible. A spectrum of illness exists within this syndrome; noncomatose patients outnumber comatose patients by a 3:1 ratio. Glucose supplementation is essential early in the disease, whereas ICP monitoring is critical in advanced disease.

Hyponatremia in children younger than 2 years may result from water intoxication when formulas are excessively diluted. Seizures and unresponsiveness are the usual presentations. The serum sodium level should be checked in every first-time afebrile seizure patient. A clue to hyponatremia-induced seizures is the failure of conventional management to control the seizures. Once diagnosed, efforts should be aimed at raising the sodium level to at least 120 mEq/L, which usually will halt the seizure activity.

Unsuspected toxic ingestions are often the cause of unknown coma in toddlers and adolescents. For example, cocaine intoxication can be a cause of seizures in young children. In addition, children with carbon monoxide intoxication may present with altered mental status.

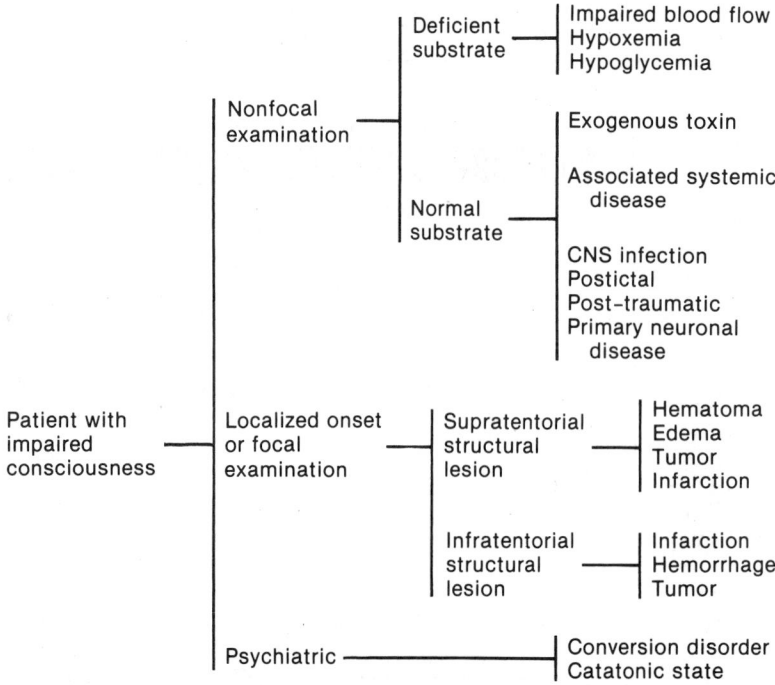

Figure 130–4. This approach has many exceptions and is intended as a guide only. Approach to differential diagnosis of the comatose patient.

TABLE 130-3
COMA: THERAPY AT A GLANCE

Nonspecific interventions
　Oxygen supplementation
　Dextrose, 0.5–1.0 gm/kg/IV (2–4 ml/kg D25W)
In select cases
　Naloxone, 0.10 mg/kg/dose; if no response, may repeat 0.1
　　mg/kg every 5 min based on clinical suspicion
Pharmacologic interventions in select cases with increased ICP
　Mannitol, initial dose, 0.25–1.0 gm/kg/dose; may repeat
　　q 3–4 hr
　　　　　　　　　or
　Furosemide, 1 mg/kg/dose
　Ethacrynic acid, 1 mg/kg/dose
Initial choice of anticonvulsant
　Lorazepam, 0.05–0.10 mg/kg up to 4 mg
　　　　　　　　　or
　Diazepam, 0.2–0.3 mg/kg/dose q 5–10 min

THERAPEUTIC INTERVENTION

Specific management depends on the specific diagnosis. For the patient in a deep coma without protective airway reflexes, endotracheal intubation is a necessity to decrease the possibility of aspiration. Endotracheal intubation also allows assisted ventilation to begin, controlling either respiratory rate or tidal volumes as clinically indicated. Gentle intubation, possibly with pharmacologic paralysis, is essential, particularly in the head-injured patient, because any pharyngeal or tracheal stimulation may trigger reflexes that further increase ICP. Protection of the cervical spine in trauma patients is axiomatic. Rapid intravenous access, with sampling of blood before any pharmacologic intervention, is the next step. The clinical setting dictates fluid choice and rate. Unless hypotension is present, a keep-open or maintenance fluid rate is sufficient. Intravenous access provides a route for drug administration.

Nonspecific pharmacologic intervention in pediatric coma patients is limited to intravenous dextrose. Accurate bedside testing techniques for glucose may replace the empiric administration of dextrose. Other nonspecific drugs for coma management—namely, naloxone and thiamine—should be used selectively when a possible benefit exists. In children, accidental overdose of diphenoxylate or propoxyphene may require large quantities of naloxone.

The pharmacologic management of head-injured patients with suspected increased ICP is controversial. Intubation with hyperventilation, achieving a $PaCO_2$ of 25 to 30 mm Hg, is recommended. The use of osmotic or loop diuretics when increased ICP is suspected is controversial, and recommendations vary with consultants. An initial dose of mannitol (0.25 to 0.5 gm/kg) may be given if markedly increased ICP is suspected or a herniation syndrome is evolving. The administration of a loop diuretic such as furosemide (1.0 mg/kg) or ethacrynic acid (1.0 mg/kg) enhances the response to mannitol. Head elevation to about 30 degrees is usually recommended as an easy, rapid measure to lower ICP, but individual response to head elevation is unpredictable. Steroid therapy is determined by consulting the neurosurgeon.

Generalized tonic-clonic status epilepticus is a true emergency and requires an aggressive approach. Rarely, a comatose patient is discovered to have nonconvulsive status epilepticus, which traditionally refers to partial seizures with complex symptomatology but may also include those seizures with minimal motor manifestations. Often these patients have a seizure history. Supplementing the patient's current anticonvulsant medication while rapidly determining the serum anticonvulsant levels will be adequate. When seizure activity is suspected, diazepam or lorazepam is used to terminate the seizures (Table 130–3).

Evaluation with a coma scale is part of the initial management. The scale in most common use is the Glasgow Coma Scale. However, this scale does not incorporate the presence or absence of hemiparesis. The Glasgow Coma Scale has been modified so that it may be easily adapted to children and give the clinical detail needed for the age variability in the neurologic examination (Table 130–4). The original scale was not applicable to patients younger than 5 but has now been modified, recognizing the variable age-related verbal and motor responses.

DISPOSITION

An enduring state of unresponsiveness dictates admission and consultation. When the cause of coma has been exactly determined, the coma has been reversed, and expectations are that the condition will not recur, the patient may be discharged with appropriate instructions. For example, a patient with a simple case of hypoglycemia involving either decreased food intake or a recent increase in insulin dose as the implicated cause of coma could be considered for discharge. A clear understanding of instructions by careproviders or the patient is another prerequisite for discharge. Obviously, new onset of coma or continued coma mandates admission. A period of unresponsiveness that has resolved may also warrant admission for observation and further investigation.

TABLE 130-4
MODIFIED GLASGOW COMA SCALE FOR PEDIATRIC PATIENTS

Adult Scale		Pediatric Scale	
Response	**Score**	**Response**	**Score**
Eyes open			
Spontaneously	4		
To speech	3	As in adult scale	
To pain	2		
None	1		
Best verbal response		Best verbal response	
Oriented	5	Oriented	5
Confused	4	Words	4
Inappropriate words	3	Vocal sounds	3
Incomprehensible sounds	2	Cries	2
None	1	None	1
Best motor response			
Obeys commands	6		
Withdraws to touch	5		
Withdraws to pain	4	As in adult scale	
Flexion to pain	3		
Extension to pain	2		
None	1		

Selected References

Alexander R, Crabbe L, Sato Y, et al. Serial abuse in children who are shaken. Am J Dis Child 1990;144:58.

Barret LG, Vincent FM, Arsac PL, et al. Internuclear ophthalmoplegia in patients with toxic coma: Frequency, prognostic value, diagnostic significance. J Toxicol Clin Toxicol 1983;20:373.

Beal MF. Amitriptyline ophthalmoplegia. Neurology 1982;32:1409.

Bleck TP, Smith MC. Diagnosing brain death and persistent vegetative states. J Crit Illness 1989;4:60.

Buettner UW, Zee DS. Vestibular testing in comatose patients. Arch Neurol 1989;46:561.

Cain DL. A useful eye sign in the apparently unconscious patient. Ann R Soc Surg Engl 1983;65:265.

Corneli HM, Gormley CJ, Baker RC. Hyponatremia and seizures presenting in the first life. Pediatr Emerg Care 1985;1:190.

Dezateux CA, Dinwiddie R, Helms P, et al. Recognition and early management of Reye's syndrome. Arch Dis Child 1986;61:647.

Drake ME, Erwin W, Massey EW. Ocular bobbing in metabolic encephalopathy: Clinical, pathologic, and electrophysiologic study. Neurology 1982;32:1029.

El-Mallakh RS. Internuclear ophthalmoplegia with narcotic overdosage. Ann Neurol 1986;20:107.

Ernst AA, Sanders WM. Unexpected cocaine intoxication presenting as seizures in children. Ann Emerg Med 1989;18:774.

Feinberg WM, Ferry PC. A fate worse than death: The persistent vegetative state in childhood. Am J Dis Child 1984;138:128.

Fisher CM. Acute brain herniation: A revised concept. Semin Neurol 1984;4:417.

Fisher CM. The neurological examination of the comatose patient. Acta Neurol Scand 1969;45(suppl 36):1.

Greenberg DA, Simon RP. Flexor and extensor postures in sedative drug-induced coma. Neurology 1982;32:448.

Hotson JR, Sachdev HS. Amitriptyline: Another cause of internuclear ophthalmoplegia with coma. Ann Neurol 1982;12:62.

Kleeman CR. Metabolic coma. Kidney Int 1989;36:1142.

Levin AV, Magnusson MR, Rafto SE, et al. Shaken baby syndrome diagnosed by magnetic resonance imaging. Pediatr Emerg Care 1989;5:181.

Levin BE. The clinical significance of spontaneous pulsations of the retinal vein. Arch Neurol 1978;35:37.

Madsen MA. Emergency department management of ventriculoperitoneal cerebrospinal fluid shunts. Ann Emerg Med 1986;15:1330.

McGravey AR. A dilated unreactive pupil in acute bacterial meningitis: Oculomotor nerve inflammation versus herniation. Pediatr Emerg Care 1989;5:187.

Mullally WJ. Carbamazepine-induced ophthalmoplegia. Arch Neurol 1982;39:64.

Parish RA, Woolf AR, Eichner M, et al. The significance of Babinski signs in children with head trauma. Ann Emerg Med 1985;14:329.

Plum F, Posner JB. The Diagnosis of Stupor and Coma. Philadelphia, FA Davis, 1980, pp 1–11.

Posner J. Coma and other states of consciousness: The differential diagnosis of brain death. Ann NY Acad Sci 1978;315:215.

Reilly PL, Simpson DA, Sprod R, Thomas L. Assessing the consciousness level in infants and young children: A paediatric version of the Glasgow Coma Scale. Childs Nerv Syst 1988;4:30.

Ricci LR, Hoffman SA. Ethanol-induced hypoglycemic coma in a child. Ann Emerg Med 1982;11:202.

Rizzo M, Corbett J. Bilateral internuclear ophthalmoplegia reversed by naloxone. Arch Neurol 1983;40:242.

Roberts TA, Jenkyn LR, Reeves AG. On the notion of doll's eyes. Arch Neurol 1984;41:1242.

Ropper AH. Lateral displacement of the brain and level of consciousness in patients with an acute hemispheral mass. N Engl J Med 1986;314:953.

Rosenberg ML. Spontaneous vertical eye movements in coma. Ann Neurol 1986;20:635.

Sneed RC, Stover SL. Undiagnosed spinal cord injuries in brain-injured children. Am J Dis Child 1988;142:965.

Spaide RF. Shaken baby syndrome: Ocular and computed tomographic findings. J Clin Neuro Ophthalmol 1987;7:108.

Tomasi LG, Rosman NP. Purtscher retinopathy in the battered child syndrome. Am J Dis Child 1975;129:1335.

CHAPTER 131

Cerebral Palsy

Eric A. Davis

INTRODUCTION

Cerebral palsy (CP) is defined as a nonprogressive central motor deficit related to events occurring in the prenatal and the perinatal periods. Its relation to cerebral anoxia was described in 1843. It is currently the single most widespread permanent physical disability in the United States.

Estimates of the total number of cases of cerebral palsy in the United States range from 300,000 to 700,000. The incidence ranges from 1.6 to 5 per 1000 live births, which, when combined with those who acquire the disorder postnatally, accounts for more than 10,000 new cases each year. Some studies have documented a recent rise in the number of cases, which is believed to be secondary to the development of neonatal intensive care and subsequent increases in the survival of both low-birth-weight infants (those weighing less than 2500 gm) and those with anoxic brain damage.

ANATOMY AND PHYSIOLOGY

The first concept basic to the understanding of CP is that it is a central disorder. The deficits in CP lie primarily in the pyramidal, extrapyramidal, and secondary motor pathways in the brain, as opposed to the peripheral disorder lesions of the anterior horn cells, nerves, neuromuscular junction, and muscle. CP is a nonprogressive motor deficit.

By definition, the damaging event occurs between conception and the first several years of life. Hemorrhagic causes usually occur in premature infants younger than 32 weeks old. This is a result of the fragility of the blood vessels, the larger proportion of total cerebral blood flow to the subependymal capillary bed, and the difficulties of autoregulation of cerebral blood flow in the neonate. Hypoxic-ischemic insults are more common in term and near-term infants. Severe hypoxia may lead to total necrosis of the brain; moderate hypoxia, to scarring and cyst formation; and mild hypoxia, to focal damage.

The specific neuroanatomic location may also be used to classify the type of CP. Lesions of the upper motor neurons (pyramidal system) are found between the penetrating branches of the major cerebral arteries. Hypoxic-ischemic insults most commonly injure areas that lead to spastic forms of CP. Spastic diplegia is associated with periventricular injury of the internal capsule; spastic quadriplegia occurs with lateral ventricular injury, frequently with cystic degeneration of the central white matter, often with cortical involvement. Spastic hemiplegia tends to be associated with atrophy of the opposite cerebral hemisphere.

Injury to the basal ganglia results in CP of the choreoathetotic form. In an anoxic insult, degeneration of the caudate nuclei and putamen occur, and with kernicterus (bilirubin encephalopathy) is seen pigmentary degeneration of the dentate and brain stem nuclei. Damage to the cerebellum and cerebellar pathways causes ataxic cerebral palsy.

This neurologic damage causes a lack of inhibition of less advanced motor areas of the central nervous system (CNS). This causes a persistence of primitive reflexes and reactions, the numerous protective and postural reflexes do not develop in the regular fashion, and cerebral palsy results.

CLASSIFICATION

The classification of CP is based on the most prominent clinical manifestations. Although the factors causing these disorders are multiple, they all result in a central, neuromuscular dysfunction caused by a static, nonprogressive injury or insult affecting the immature brain. There may be considerable overlap and disagreement in classifying an individual; patients do not always easily fit into any one of the following categories.

Spastic Cerebral Palsy

Spastic CP is the most common form and accounts for 50% to 70% of all cases. It involves lesions of the upper motor pathways (pyramidal system), which leads to spasticity, hypertonicity, exaggerated stretch reflexes, persistence of certain primitive reflexes (e.g., grasp and Moro), and the abnormal pyramidal reflexes (e.g., Babinski). There is increased and abnormally distributed muscle tone, delayed control of postural mechanisms, and the inability to coordinate movements. These findings become apparent between the ages of 6 months and 1 year. Contractures often form, along with skeletal deformities caused by the increased muscle tone exerted on growing bones and joints. Pseudobulbar palsy, in which there is paresis of the facial, lingual, and pharyngeal muscles, may be present and complicate the processes of speech, feeding, and control of secretions. Ocular involvement is common and consists of optic atrophy, nystagmus, and strabismus. Children with spastic palsy are also at significant risk for associated mental retardation and seizures.

Spastic CP may be further subclassified according to the area of the body most affected.

Spastic Quadriplegia. Spastic quadriplegia accounts for 20% to 30% of all cases of spastic CP. In this form, all four extremities are affected, each approximately to the same degree. It is associated with extensive cortical and hemispheric lesions, and some degree of mental retardation is common, as are seizures.

Spastic Diplegia. Spastic diplegia accounts for 30% to 50% of all cases of spastic CP. This classification refers to those children in whom all four limbs are affected, but with more pronounced spasticity and neuromuscular dysfunction in the legs. Involvement of the hands and arms may be minor. Intelligence may be normal or borderline.

Spastic Hemiplegia. Spastic hemiplegia occurs in 10% to 30% of children with spastic cerebral palsy. In this form of CP, one side of the body is affected. These children are at risk for developing focal seizures, visual field deficits, cortical sensory deficits, and scoliosis.

Spastic Paraplegia. In spastic paraplegia, a rare type, only the lower extremities are affected; the upper limbs are spared. Spinal cord lesions should always be excluded in these children.

Spastic Monoplegia. In spastic monoplegia, only one limb is affected. Usually a peripheral disorder or an asymmetric aplegia or hemiplegia with single limb predominance is actually present. This form is very rare.

Athetoid or Extrapyramidal Cerebral Palsy

Athetoid CP accounts for 25% of all cases of CP. It is caused by damage to the extrapyramidal system. The primary manifestations are hypotonia in early infancy, followed by the later development of choreoathetoid movement and dystonia, in most cases appearing between 18 months and 3 years of age. Abnormal dyskinetic movements of the tongue and facial, pharyngeal, and laryngeal muscles lead to facial grimacing, drooling, and speech difficulties.

Ataxic Cerebral Palsy

Accounting for less than 10% of children with CP, ataxic CP results from defects in the cerebellum and cerebellar pathways. It is characterized by loss of balance and position sense, intention tremor, ataxia, clumsiness (especially of the upper extremities), and overreaching for objects.

Atonic Diplegia

Atonic diplegia is a rare form, seen in less than 5% of those with CP. It consists of hypotonia and motor disability,

and a severe mental deficit is usually present. Some degree of spasticity may develop later.

CLINICAL EVALUATION
History

Many cases of CP are diagnosed as a result of neurodevelopmental examinations in the newborn period, but often the child goes undiagnosed, particularly if he or she has mild symptoms. Therefore, a child may first come to the attention of a physician when the parents note something in the child's activity that they feel is abnormal. Early signs include a poor sucking response, which may be associated with increased drooling, choking, and trouble swallowing. Aspiration along with the associated complaints is a common event in these infants. Hypotonia, or "floppiness," may be noted, as well as perceived "stiffness," especially during crying when the infant becomes opisthotonic. Persistent fisting with one hand while the other remains normal and precocious development of handedness (which should not occur prior to 1 year of age) may also be noticed. Complaints that the infant is not "cuddly" and becomes irritable with handling may also occur with CP.

The most obvious developmental abnormalities are manifested when the child begins locomotion. Asymmetric use of the left and right sides of the body or the use of the upper limbs to pull the legs along results in impaired crawling. Pulling to a standing position occurs or may be achieved by using the arms while the legs remain in extension, often with scissoring of the feet. Ambulation is commonly delayed and, when finally achieved, may result in a lurching gait, or one leg may be dragged.

It is important for the clinician to determine whether the disorder is progressive or nonprogressive, as well as central or peripheral. Careful attention should be given to eliciting a history of possible risk factors. Also, detailed questions should be directed to the parents to determine if the problem is getting worse or staying the same. Even with a detailed history, it may be difficult to determine this, and serial examinations may be needed.

Deep tendon reflexes tend to be increased with central lesions, even with central forms of hypotonia, and decreased with peripheral lesions. Contractures are more common with central lesions; muscle atrophy is common with peripheral myopathy or neuropathy. Delays in social and adaptive functions and language indicate central lesions. Increased muscle tone is more common with central lesions and decreased muscle tone with peripheral, although hypotonic CP is an exception. Fasciculations (especially in the tongue) are most common in peripheral disorders of the anterior horn cell.

The precise causes of CP are often obscure. It is extremely difficult to delineate specific causal factors, as 19% to 70% of children with CP have been shown to have no high risk factors, and up to 62% of all pregnancies have some complication at term or birth. Additionally, in many instances, it is impossible to determine which developed first, the anomaly or the risk factor.

There is also much disagreement as to when in the child's development CP occurs. With a better understanding of the disease, it is now estimated that 50% of cases are prenatal, 33% are perinatal, and 10% are postnatal, with 7% mixed, showing multiple possible causes.

Major Risk Factors

Studies focusing on neonatal intensive care found premature birth and low birth weight in 23% to 40% of cases

(Table 131–1). However, the converse does not hold true; 98.9% of children with birth weights less than 2500 gm are free of cerebral palsy. As the birth weight declines, the risk rises from 3.4 per 1000 in infants weighing more than 2500 gm, to 13.9 per 1000 in those weighing 1500 to 2500 gm, and 90.4 per 1000 in those weighing less than 1500 gm. CP in low-birth-weight infants is most typically the spastic type and often is associated with normal intelligence or mild mental retardation.

The second major risk factor is birth asphyxia. An Apgar score of 3 or less at 5 minutes was associated with a 5% (30-fold) increase in CP at 10 minutes, a 10% increase (60-fold) at 15 minutes, and a 40% (250-fold) increase at 20 minutes. Overall, 25% to 30% of children with CP have some history of asphyxia. In addition, many of the minor risk factors are only statistically significant when associated with a below normal Apgar score.

Minor Risk Factors

Mechanical trauma during birth has been postulated to be a significant cause of CP. One study reported a 25% incidence of trauma as a cause for hypoxic-ischemic injury in term infants. Breech presentation has also been associated with an increased risk of CP, even when other confounding factors have been taken into account. The precise role trauma plays in the genesis of CP is still unknown.

The effects of prenatal ischemic or hypoxic events that do not kill the fetus are impossible to detect, but their association with later development of CP is suggested by several factors. Events such as abnormal uterine bleeding, infarction of the placenta, and other disorders that interfere with fetal oxygenation (termed *prenatal deprivation of supply*) have a higher incidence of CP. Also, neuropathologic studies in children with CP show that some have cystic degenerative lesions. Such lesions are associated with ischemic or vascular events occurring during gestation after the formation of major cerebral structures.

Metabolic causes of CP are now seen less frequently. Bilirubin encephalopathy (kernicterus) has markedly decreased since the advent of Rh typing and immunization and advances in the management of hyperbilirubinemia (e.g., phototherapy and exchange transfusion). Despite this, kernicterus remains the second most important metabolic cause of CP after asphyxia. Severe hypoglycemia in the neonatal period may cause CP.

Seizures seem to be an important cofactor, and it is often difficult to determine whether the hypoglycemia or other coexisting factors are responsible. Severe acidosis, in any stage of labor or shortly after birth, and amino acid–urea cycle disorders are rare causes.

Lead exposure in the postnatal period (but not prenatally) has caused spastic forms of CP. Mercury as a causative factor was documented in Japanese children who developed spastic quadriplegia and mental retardation after their mothers had ingested contaminated fish during pregnancy. Finally, alcohol is possibly a risk factor, as suggested in a study in which three cases of ataxic CP and one of spastic hemiplegia were found among 48 children born to mothers who were alcoholic.

Congenital infections of bacterial meningitis, viral encephalitis, rubella (in one study, 71 out of 624 cases with a history of rubella), cytomegalovirus (up to 5% of all cases of CP), and toxoplasmosis have all been implicated as risk factors. Ataxic syndromes have been shown to be hereditary in an autosomal recessive pattern. In countries where iodine deficiency is prevalent, neurologic cretinism may be encountered. This condition consists of spastic diplegia, mental retardation, and deafness. Multiple other factors have been implicated, including third-trimester bleeding, intrauterine growth retardation, toxemia, meconium staining, chorioamnionitis, and polyhydramnios, although the exact mechanism is unclear.

Physical Examination

Hypotonia may be tested for by the anterior *scarf sign*, in which the infant is placed supine with both shoulders flat on the table. The arm is then adducted across the neck, and the elbow should not move past the chin when the head is held midline. If the elbow moves beyond the chin with the shoulders flat on the table, increased range of motion of the shoulder joint and hypotonia are indicated. Normal strength in the affected muscles suggests a central lesion.

The presence of hypertonia may be elicited by testing the primitive reflexes. Reflexes that are present to an exaggerated degree or remain for an unusual period of time may be indicative of cerebral insult or injury.

Primitive Reflexes Type I

Type I primitive reflexes occur and are suppressed during the interuterine period and are not present at the time of birth.

Primitive Reflexes Type II

Type II primitive reflexes appear in the interuterine period. They are normally suppressed by the age of 6 months with the development of upper motor neurons. A full-term to 2- to 3-month-old infant normally assumes a "flexor habitus" posture, in which flexion responses predominate. As the child matures, the flexion component becomes less pronounced.

The *Moro reflex* consists of upper extremity extension, followed by abduction, adduction, semiflexion of the elbows, and wrists held with the thumbs and index fingers in the C position. It can be elicited either by striking the side of the crib or bassinet, holding the infant in a supine position and along the forearm and causing sudden head and neck extension, or by elevating the infant by the upper extremities and suddenly releasing the arms.

The *tonic labyrinthine reflex* consists of shoulder retraction, upper extremity flexion, and lower extremity extension when the infant's neck is placed in extension. If the neck is flexed, a total body flexion habitus results. It is replaced by

TABLE 131–1

APPROXIMATE DISTRIBUTION OF CAUSES IN CEREBRAL PALSY

Cause	Incidence (%)
Low birth weight, preterm birth	35–40
Perinatal asphyxia in term infants	25–30
Congenital and perinatal infections (cytomegalovirus, rubella, toxoplasma, neonatal meningitis)	5–10
Intrauterine ischemic events	5–10
Congenital brain anomalies not evident on clinical examination	5–10
Perinatal metabolic conditions other than asphyxia (hyperbilirubinemia, hypoglycemia, hyperosmolarity, amino acid disorders)	5
Genetic causes	2–5

From Paneth N. Etiologic factors in cerebral palsy. Pediatr Ann 1986; 15:191.

the Landau reflex as the infant matures. It is also called *opisthotonic posturing* or *decorticate rigidity* and may be seen with head trauma, meningitis, and other conditions causing cerebral damage.

The *asymmetric tonic neck reflex* is characterized by chin extension and occipital flexion with rotation of the head to either side; the child assumes the "fencing position."

The *positive support reflex* consists of momentary lower extremity extension followed by flexion when the great toe region is stimulated while the infant is suspended by the axilla. This passes into the mature response of extension of the legs to support body weight around 2 months of age. Persistence of this response beyond 3 months is indicative of hypotonic cerebral palsy, whereas patients with spastic forms of CP show an exaggerated mature response.

The *symmetric tonic neck reflex* consists of head extension with arm extension and leg flexion or head flexion with upper extremity flexion and leg extension. This appears at 20 weeks of age and disappears when crawling begins.

The *plantar grasp* consists of plantar flexion grasp with stimulation of the great toe area. It becomes suppressed by 9 months of age.

The *Galant reflex* consists of inward truncal curvature when the paravertebral area from the thoracic to the sacral area is stimulated. It is difficult to determine when this reflex is suppressed and replaced by a voluntary withdrawal response and it should only be used when coupled with other reflexes.

Primitive Reflexes Type III

Type III primitive reflexes are the postural reactions of the righting and equilibrium responses that occur as the primitive type II reflexes become suppressed. These herald the beginning of the gross motor milestones.

The *Landau reaction* consists of truncal, hip, knee, and ankle extension with voluntary head extension. This occurs at 2 to 3 months of age and is replaced by the derotative righting response.

The *derotative righting response* consists of derotative axial responses of the shoulders, followed by the body, hips, and lower extremities when the head is rotated past 45 degrees. A second reflex consists of derotation of the body, followed by the hips and upper extremities, with crossing of the lower extremities. With the disappearance of this reflex, real voluntary movements (motor milestones) begin.

DIAGNOSTIC EVALUATION

Most children have strong evidence of CP on physical examination and history. However, because approximately 10% of cases may be acquired postnatally (and thus have some potential for intervention), and because the diagnosis and prognosis of the disease can be devastating, a comprehensive investigation may be desirable for a large proportion of those affected (Table 131–2).

Computed tomography (CT) of the brain is a useful adjunct. One study found that 63% of all those with CP had abnormalities; this figure rose to 88% in the preterm child. Possible findings consistent with CP include porencephalic cysts, infarction, hydrocephalus, ventriculomegaly, diffuse or focal atrophy, subdural effusions, and agenesis of the corpus callosum. Other rare diagnoses include congenital tumor, neurofibromatosis (aqueductal stenosis with dilatation of the ventricular system), tuberous sclerosis (subependymal calcifications), and congenital infections such as toxoplasmosis or cytomegalovirus (microcephaly with intracranial calcifications). Nevertheless, not all patients with CP demonstrate CT changes, and in those who do, the

TABLE 131–2
CEREBRAL PALSY: DIFFERENTIAL DIAGNOSES

Leukodystrophies (familial centrolobar sclerosis)
Hydrocephalus
Subdural effusions
Intracerebral tumor
Spinal cord lesions
Muscular dystrophy
Werdnig-Hoffman disease
Benign congenital hypotonia
Erb palsy (arm)
Sciatic or peroneal injury (leg)
Neurofibromatosis (von Recklinghausen's disease)
Tuberous sclerosis
Cerebelloretinal hemangioblastomatosis (von Hippel–Landau disease)
Encephalotrigeminal syndrome (Sturge-Weber syndrome)
Ataxia-telangiectasia
Spinocerebellar degenerations (Friedreich's ataxia)
Hereditary metabolic diseases (aminocodurias urea cycle)
Sphingolipidoses (GM$_1$ gangliosidosis, Tay-Sachs disease)
Niemann-Pick disease
Gaucher's disease
Postmeningitis and postencephalitis states
Congenital infections (cytomegalovirus, toxoplasmosis, congenital syphilis, rubella)
Lesch-Nyhan syndrome
Thyroid disorders (cretinism)
Hyperammonia syndrome
Heavy metal poisoning (mercury, lead)

severity of the condition does not always correlate with the clinical findings.

The value of laboratory tests in detecting a cause of CP is debated. However, certain conditions may be discovered through laboratory screening in some children. Amino acid screening; iodine screening; thyroid studies; tests for congenital infections; determination of ammonia, pyruvate, and lactate levels; measurement of copper and ceruloplasmin levels; heavy metal studies; and genetic assays may all be considered in certain cases.

The child with lower extremity weakness will need spinal radiographs to exclude a compressive lesion. A thorough eye examination may detect chorioretinitis seen with congenital infections, macular changes seen with certain degenerative disorders, or papilledema.

SPECIAL PROBLEMS
Associated Disabilities

The physical and mental handicaps associated with CP predispose these patients to a significantly higher incidence of medical problems. The most common associated condition is mental retardation, which occurs in 30% to 70% of those with CP. The more severe degrees of intellectual deficit are associated with more profound neuromuscular involvement, making these children difficult to evaluate. Speech is often involved, making communication problematic.

Seizures occur in 30% to 50% of patients, and although they may occur in infancy, the most common age at presentation is from 2 years to 6 years. Infantile spasms and minor motor forms producing massive severe activity have grave prognostic implications. Because of feeding difficulties, therapeutic anticonvulsant levels are difficult to maintain.

Ocular abnormalities are common. Strabismus is the most frequent abnormality, presenting in 20% to 69% of patients, with esotropia more prevalent then exotropia. Refractive errors are also a frequent finding, occurring in 25% to 75% of patients, and visual field deficits may occur in as many as 25%.

Behavioral problems, including attention deficit disorder and emotional lability, also occur. Restlessness, inability to concentrate, low frustration tolerance, and rapid shifts in emotion interfere with learning and adaptation. Frustration and depression, especially when accompanied by mental retardation, are serious problems among adolescent patients. These may manifest as physical aggression.

Acute Conditions

The pseudobulbar palsy and attendant swallowing disorders that accompany CP can lead to poor food intake, malnutrition, and failure to thrive. Maldevelopment of oropharyngeal structures and dental problems may further impair oral intake.

Drooling is a serious cosmetic problem. Aspiration, inability to clear secretions, and absent or inadequate cough lead to frequent pneumonias. CP patients frequently have attendant decreased vital capacity and restrictive lung disease. This makes pneumonia a serious disorder. It is a major cause of shortened life expectancy, and consideration for admission should be given to all CP patients with acute pneumonia.

Dental caries are especially troublesome in those with CP. Defects of the dental enamel may occur during tooth development, and abnormal muscle tone enhances malocclusion problems. Infections ranging from apical abscesses to more severe deep space infections occur.

Acute and chronic otitis media are common because of the pseudobulbar palsy and attendant loss of oral control. Use of routine antibiotic therapy is recommended.

Contractures may result from the constant increase in muscle tone. Acute long-bone fractures and especially hip dislocation are common orthopedic conditions. Severe spasticity, coxa valga, relative tightness of the hip adductors and flexors, and non–weight bearing of the legs all contribute to the development of hip dislocations. If the hips are allowed to dislocate and especially if the problem becomes chronic, the patient becomes predisposed to osteoarthritis and perineal hygiene problems. Scoliosis may also result, and immobility of the patient may lead to pressure sores and decubiti. Orthopedic consultation should be obtained as soon as possible.

Child abuse is a problem in young patients with CP. A study published in the mid 1980s reported that 20% of children with CP had suffered child abuse injuries severe enough to warrant their removal from their home by the state. Also, 43% were considered at risk for abuse to the point that some intervention had been undertaken.

Selected References

Allen M, Capute A. Neonatal neurodevelopmental examination as a predictor of neuromotor outcome in premature infants. Pediatrics 1989;83:498.

Barabus G, Taft L. The early signs and differential diagnosis of cerebral palsy. Pediatr Ann 1986;15:203.

Capute A. Early neuromotor reflexes in infancy. Pediatr Ann 1986;15:217.

Cohen M, Dottner P. Prognostic indicators in hemiparetic cerebral palsy. Ann Neurol 1981;9:353.

Davis G, Hill P. Cerebral palsy. Nursing Clin North Am 1980;5:35.

Erenberg G. Cerebral palsy: Current understanding of a complex problem. Postgrad Med 1984;75:87.

Erhardt R. Sequential levels in the visual-motor development of a child with cerebral palsy. Am J Occup Ther 1987;41:43.

Gillies F. Neuropathologic indicators of abnormal development. In Freeman JH (ed). Prenatal and Perinatal Factors Associated with Brain Disorders. Bethesda, MD, US Dept Health, Education and Welfare, 1984.

Graham M, Levine M, Trounce J, et al. Prediction of cerebral palsy in very low birthweight infants: Prospective ultrasound study. Lancet 1987;12:593.

Harris S. Early neuromotor predictors of cerebral palsy in low-birth weight infants. Dev Med Child Neurol 1987;29:508.

Matthews D. Controversial therapies in the management of cerebral palsy. Pediatr Ann 1988;17:762.

Miller G. Minor congenital anomalies and ataxic cerebral palsy. Arch Dis Child 1989;64:557.

Nelson K, Ellenberg J. The asymptomatic newborn and risk of cerebral palsy. Am J Dis Child 1987;141:1333.

Nelson K, Ellenberg J. Neonatal signs as predictors of cerebral palsy. Pediatrics 1979;64:225.

Nelson K, Ellenberg J. Obstetric complications as risk factors for cerebral palsy or seizure disorders. JAMA 1984;251:1843.

Newton E. The relationship between intrapartum obstetric care and chronic neurodevelopmental handicaps in children. NY State J Med 1988;10:531.

O'Reilly O, Walentynowicz J. Etiological factors in cerebral palsy: An historical review. Develop Med Child Devel 1981;23:633.

Paneth N. Etiologic factors in cerebral palsy. Pediatr Ann 1986;15:191.

Schouman-Claeys E, Picard A, Lalande G, et al. Contribution of computed tomography in the aetiology and prognosis of cerebral palsy in children. Br J Radiol 1989;62:248.

Stanley F. Prenatal risk factors in the study of the cerebral palsies. Clin Dev Med 1984;87:87.

Stanley F, Alberman E. Birthweight, gestational age and the cerebral palsies. Clin Dev Med 1984;87:57.

Sugita K, Iai M, Nakajimu H, et al. Consistency and changes in the development of extremely low birthweight infants. Brain Dev 1988;10:231.

Taft L. Cerebral palsy. Pediatr Rev 1984;6:35.

Tawdorf K, Melchior J. CT findings in spastic cerebral palsy. Neuropediatrics 1984;15:120.

Wing E, Rousseau S. A changing pattern of cerebral palsy and its implications for the early detection of motor disorders in children. Childcare Health Dev 1983;9:227.

CHAPTER 132

Hydrocephalus and Ventricular Shunts

Stephen R. Guertin

INTRODUCTION

Children shunted for hydrocephalus present to the emergency department for reasons ranging from a simple low-pressure headache to life-threatening impending herniation. Early shunt dysfunction with mild symptomatology can precipitously progress to a dangerous situation.[1] Children with preexisting visual impairment who are shunted for hydrocephalus are at risk for permanent blindness from a single episode of shunt dysfunction.[2] In this circumstance, elevated intracranial pressure can cause ischemia of the optic nerves and even infarction of an already stretched occipital cortex. Undiagnosed gradual ventricular dilation caused by partial shunt dysfunction results in permanent changes of the cerebral white matter.[3] It is imperative, therefore, that emergency medicine specialists become familiar with the signs and symptoms of cerebrospinal fluid (CSF) shunt dysfunction, be able to identify CSF shunt components, and develop a system for evaluating shunt function.

CHILDREN WITH CSF SHUNTS

Hydrocephalus requiring a CSF shunt is, by definition, obstructive.[4] CSF either cannot flow out of the ventricles or, once into the subarachnoid space, cannot flow around the brain and spinal cord and out the arachnoid villi. If the obstruction occurs at any place between the ventricles, communication is lost between the ventricles and the subarachnoid space. This is called *noncommunicating hydrocephalus*. When the obstruction is around the CSF cisterns or over the surfaces of the brain at the level of the arachnoid villi, the ventricles do communicate with each other and with the subarachnoid space. This is called *communicating hydrocephalus*.

A preexisting condition requiring a CSF shunt may influence the way shunted children present to the emergency department. Such conditions include X-linked congenital acqueductal stenosis, infection-related scar or web formation within the acqueduct of Sylvius,[4] a Dandy-Walker cyst of the fourth ventricle that occludes CSF passage through the acqueduct of Sylvius,[5] cysts along the central CSF pathways that obstruct outflow,[6] fibromata from neurofibromatosis,[7] tubers from tuberous sclerosis,[8] and arteriovenous malformations, especially those involving the great vein of Galen.[9]

Virtually any child with a brain tumor has some degree of hydrocephalus.[10] Shunts are necessary in those cases in which tumors on or near the midline cannot be extirpated. Communicating hydrocephalus results when tumor spreads over the meninges and convexities of the brain, obliterating the arachnoid granulations and the CSF cisterns.[11] Communicating hydrocephalus from fibrosed and obliterated arachnoid villi can also been seen after meningitis and after the chemical arachnoiditis associated with subarachnoid hemorrhage from either trauma or rupture of a vascular malformation.[12, 13]

The most common cause of hydrocephalus requiring a CSF shunt is myelomeningocele with the Arnold-Chiari malformation.[4] Eighty percent of children with myelomeningocele and 96% of those with lumbar myelocele and paraplegia require shunting. Another growing group of shunted children consists of those born prematurely weighing less than 1500 gm. Blood-induced inflammation in the acqueduct can cause noncommunicating hydrocephalus; similarly, blood disseminated throughout the subarachnoid space can cause communicating hydrocephalus. Of those infants who survive their initial germinal matrix-intraventricular hemorrhage, 2% to 10% will require shunting.[14, 15]

Essentially all CSF shunt systems will fail, at some point, requiring at least one revision. More than half of the children shunted for neutral tube defects require revision within 3 years; more than 20% of these require multiple revisions.[16] As many as 80% of the neonates shunted for posthemorrhagic hydrocephalus require revision within months of placement.[17]

SYMPTOMS AND SIGNS OF MECHANICAL DYSFUNCTION

After CSF shunt placement, reduction in ventricular volume is accompanied by a loss of the dilated hydrocephalic child's remarkable volume-buffering capacity.[18] Normal children, especially young children, have much steeper intracranial volume–pressure response curves than do adults. That is, in children, intracranial pressure (ICP) increases more sharply and more rapidly in response to increased intracranial volume. Children with dilated ventricles, on the other hand, have flat intracranial volume–pressure response dynamics. They accommodate much larger increases of intracranial volume before an accompanying pressure increase is felt, and the degree of pressure increase is less.[19] Once shunted, however, these children revert to normal ICP dynamics and reach the point of markedly altered compliance at much smaller volumes than do adults. As ICP increases, even moderately, resistance to CSF and venous outflow increases dramatically. Further volume retention, even of only small amounts, can suddenly result in a dangerously and symptomatically high ICP. This applies not only to moderate increases of CSF volume, but also to increases of intracranial blood volume. This is seen in situations where, despite small or normal-appearing ventricles and only moderately high ICP (5 to 15 cm H_2O), sudden clinical deterioration occurs.[20] The rapidity of onset and spontaneous return to baseline are consistent with sudden cerebral vasodilation.

On the other hand, CSF shunts can cause rapid or chronic overdrainage of spinal fluid as a result of body positional change or the effects of respirations.[21–24] Once overdrainage occurs, a low ICP results. With sudden overdrainage, even brain stem shifts can occur with intermittent traction of the medulla.[4, 22, 23]

Symptoms and signs of high ICP include headache, changes in sensorium (lethargy, irritability, disorientation, coma), nausea, and vomiting.[4, 25, 26] Especially ominous are a precipitous change in sensorium, decerebrate posturing, pupillary changes, and the components of Cushing's triad. Cushing's triad (i.e., systemic vascular hypertension, bradycardia, and respiratory ataxia) occurs when blood supply to the medulla is compromised. The presence of these changes suggests impending herniation at either the tentorial notch or the foramen magnum. Indications of increased ICP may be an enlarging head or bulging fontanel, fluid extravasation along the shunt tract, upward gaze palsy, diplopia, dilated scalp veins, and increased muscle tone. Any preexisting abnormality of movement or muscle tone will be accentuated when ICP is increased. Asymmetric ventricular dilation[23] and polycystic undrained areas can result in focal weakness and uncal herniation. Intermittent high pressure results in recurrent high-pressure signs and symptoms, including cyclic vomiting.[21]

Signs and symptoms of *gradual ventricular enlargement* caused by partial dysfunction include gait disturbance, urinary incontinence, worsening of cerebral palsy, deteriorating school performance, visual deterioration, and hypothalamic signs.[4, 26] Hypothalamic signs include either a voracious or an absent appetite, growth abnormalities, and pituitary insufficiency.[27]

Brain stem signs such as stridor, laryngospasm, syncope, disturbed consciousness, pallor, respiratory ataxia or arrest, and a vacillating heart rate can result from high pressure.[4] These phenomena, however, are most often seen with sudden overdrainage and *low pressure* causing upward traction on the brain stem.[22, 23] If suspected, especially in the presence of marked indentation of cranial defects or collapse of the fontanel, these life-threatening phenomena can be partly ameliorated by tipping the child into a 15- to 30-degree Trendelenburg position and providing supporting ventilation. Dispute exists about nausea, vomiting, and sensorium change in low-pressure states. Some authors believe that low-pressure headaches are not accompanied by marked changes in level of consciousness, are not associated with nausea and vomiting, are accentuated by being upright, and are relieved by recumbency.[24] In the emergency department, these features may help distinguish high- from low-pressure headache.

The relationship between seizures and CSF shunts is a complex one. Onset of new seizures after shunt insertion or an acute seizure in a known seizure patient with a CSF shunt do not alone indicate shunt dysfunction. However, because seizures are temporally related to shunt malfunction, seizures in a shunted child should prompt the emergency physician to evaluate the shunt system.[28] The electroencephalogram (EEG) is abnormal in up to 98% of children prior

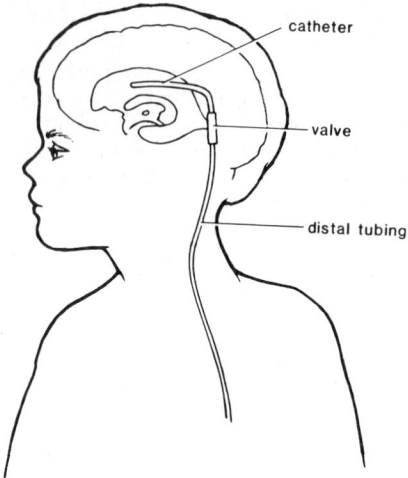

Figure 132–1. Basic ventriculoperitoneal shunt system showing the ventricular catheter, valve device, and distal tubing. Reservoirs are placed between the ventricular catheter and the valve device. Antisiphon and on-off devices are placed distal to the valve apparatus. (From Post EM. Currently available shunt systems: A review. Neurosurgery 1985;16:257.)

to shunting.[29] Spike and sharp wave activity, which is particularly predictive of epilepsy, is present preoperatively in more than 40% of children who require CSF shunting. At least 25% of children who require a shunt have preexisting seizures.[30] Even the ventricular configuration after shunting may influence seizure activity.[31] The incidence of new-onset seizures after a shunt operation ranges between 5% and 10%, with 80% of these occurring within the first postoperative year.[30] Again, seizures in a shunted patient, when anticonvulsant levels are therapeutic, should be considered to be related to mechanical dysfunction of the shunt system.

CSF SHUNT COMPONENTS

All CSF shunt systems must contain intraventricular tubing, a valve apparatus, and distal tubing (Fig. 132–1). An exception to this is the unishunt system, a molded shunt without connections and with an in-line double bubble reservoir and a slit valve located at the distal end.[32] Reservoirs, when included in the shunt system, must be placed between the ventricular tubing and the valve apparatus. Antisiphon devices and on-off valves are placed distal to the valve apparatus. Each component must be located, identified, and

followed. Often several of them are present in the same patient.

Intraventricular Tubing

Intraventricular tubing can be located anteriorly, pass anteriorly from a posterior insertion site, or be located posteriorly within the lateral ventricles or within the fourth ventricle. CSF enters the tubing through multiple small holes or through larger perforations protected by longitudinal slots. A unique variation is the flanged intraventricular tube, designed with the hope that the flanges would prevent envelopment by choroid plexus and thus reduce the incidence of proximal obstruction. Unfortunately, however, the presence of flanges allows for even firmer investiture of the tubing by choroid plexus, making removal especially hazardous.[32]

Valves

There are four valve types used in CSF shunts (Fig. 132–2).[32] *Slit valves* operate like a foramen ovale. CSF pressure opens the slit flap, and back pressure closes the flap, thus allowing only one-way flow. *Ball-in-cone valves* open when CSF pressure pushes a ball out of a cone, into which it is ordinarily wedged by a spring. Back pressure immediately wedges the ball back into the cone, again resulting in only one-way flow. *Miter valves* are made of folded siliconized rubber resembling a duck call whistle. CSF pressure opens the leaflets, allowing outflow, but any back pressure immediately apposes the leaflets, again allowing only one-way flow. *Diaphragm valves* are hinged over an aperture like a trap door. CSF pressure lifts the diaphragm off the aperture, allowing CSF outflow, and back pressure closes the trap door, thus allowing only one-way flow.

The most important aspect in identifying the valve type is to identify the means of pumping the system.[33, 34] To do this, one must simply recognize whether the system is tubular or domed. *Tubular systems* consist of two one-way valves (slit valves or ball-in-cone valves) encased in metal cylinders. Between the valves is a Silastic pumping chamber. When this chamber is depressed, spinal fluid is ejected distally out through the second (distal) valve. When the chamber is released, it refills with spinal fluid coming from the ventricle through the first (proximal) valve.

Domed systems can consist of one or two one-way valves of any variety. The dome is actually the pumping chamber. In one apparatus (the Heyer-Schulte system), the dome also functions as a reservoir when a distal occluder is manipulated.[33] In any domed system, once the dome has been

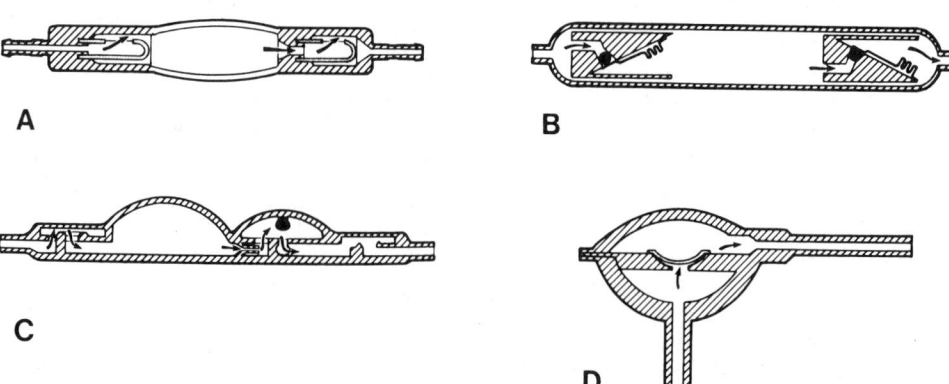

Figure 132–2. Valve types. *A,* Slit valve. *B,* Ball-in-cone valve. *C,* Miter valve. *D,* Diaphragm valve. (From Post EM. Currently available shunt systems: A review. Neurosurgery 1985;16:257.)

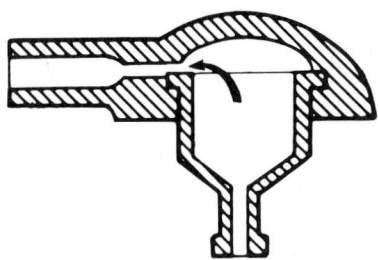

Figure 132–3. Rickham reservoir. Arrow indicates flow of cerebrospinal fluid. (From Post EM. Currently available shunt systems: A review. Neurosurgery 1985;16:257.)

located, a simple compression should propel CSF distally. Once released, the dome should refill with CSF drawn proximally from the ventricle. An interesting variation among domed systems is the double dome placed proximal to a distal slit valve (uni-shunt system).[32, 34] After first depressing the proximal dome, compression of the distal dome tests forward flow and refill. After first depressing the distal dome, compression of the proximal dome gives some assessment of proximal (ventricular) patency. If the distal dome is compressed, the proximal dome can act as a reservoir, allowing both sampling of CSF and instillation of dye or antibiotic into the ventricles.

Distal Tubing

Distal tubing is composed of siliconized rubber. The vast majority of distal tubes go into the peritoneal cavity. When the peritoneum cannot be used, the right atrium is commonly used. Although previously fraught with complications and a high rate of failure, the ventriculopleural shunt with an antisiphon device has been resurrected as an effective means of diverting CSF when the ventriculoperitoneal and ventriculoatrial routes cannot be used.[35] A last alternative that has been tried with some success is the ventricle-gallbladder shunt.[36]

Peritoneal tubing should be free floating and well within the abdominal cavity. Close attention should be paid for the presence of kinking or contour abnormalities of the distal tubing.[37]

Reservoirs

A reservoir is a device that allows access into the cerebral ventricle. For a reservoir to be effective, it must be located between the cerebral ventricle and the valve(s). The Rickham reservoir rests on the skull directly over the burr hole connecting it to the ventricular catheter (Figs. 132–3 and 132–4). Other reservoirs may be located further down the skull (Fig. 132–5). Because the reservoir is located before the one-way valves, aspiration through the reservoir establishes that the ventricular tubing is at least sufficiently open to allow CSF withdrawal. Because of this access to the ventricle, CSF from within the ventricle can be sampled through the reservoir for cell counts, cultures, Gram stains, and chemical analysis. After manually occluding the system downstream from the reservoir, infusion into the reservoir deposits the infused material (e.g., dye, antibiotics, radionuclide) into the cerebral ventricle. This is especially useful when instilling antibiotics for ventriculitis or when using dye to determine whether communication exists between intracranial CSF spaces. Easily identified by plain films, the reservoir should be seated firmly against the skull and connected to both proximal and distal shunt system components (see Fig. 132–4).

Antisiphon and On-Off Devices

Some valves directly incorporate an antisiphon device. The antisiphon device can also be added separately. The device is located distal to the actual valve. Respirations and standing create large pressure gradients between the head and the abdomen or chest. This results in excessive draining or *siphoning*, of CSF from the head. The antisiphon device is simply a diaphragm running parallel to the CSF flow that is sucked against the walls of the system when negative pressure exists, thus reducing the siphoning effect.[38, 39]

The on-off device is also placed distal to the valve apparatus.[34, 39] It allows the system to be occluded, theoretically allowing the patient to develop and maximize alterna-

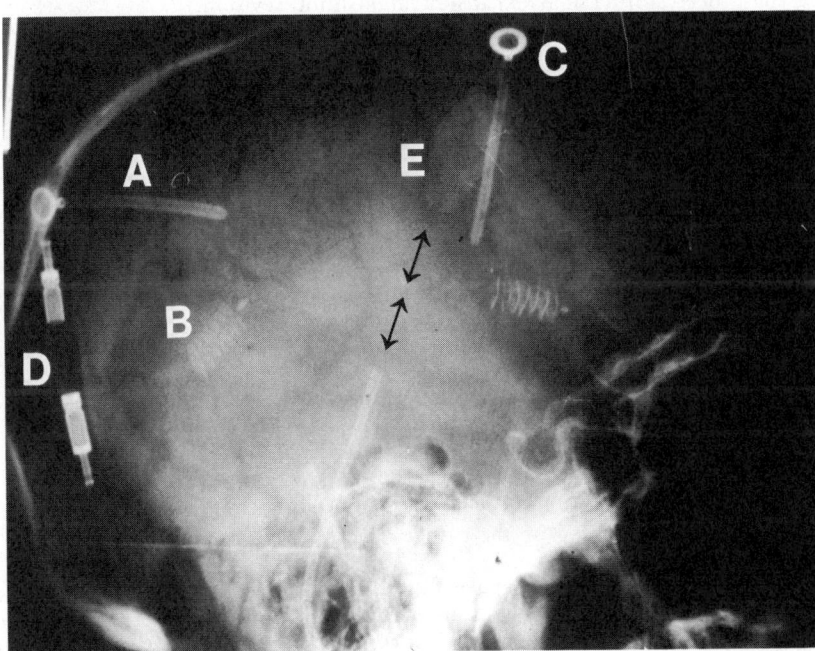

Figure 132–4. Advantages of the plain radiograph. A = Ventricular catheter; B = flanged isolated ventricular catheter; C = Rickham reservoir; D = tubular valve (slits) apparatus; E = domed valve apparatus. Notice the site of disconnection *(arrows)* between the domed valve and the distal tubing.

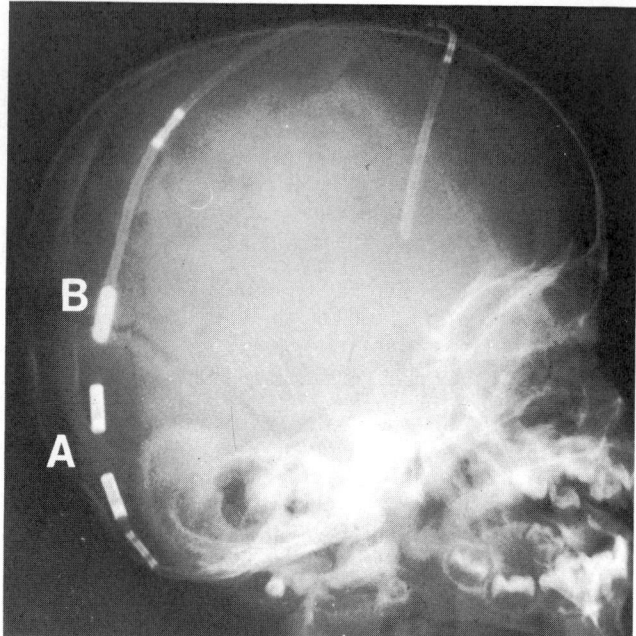

Figure 132–5. A = Tubular valve apparatus (ball-in-cone). The flat base proximally marks the location of the reservoir (B). Note the site of disconnection over the mastoid process. No distal tubing can be seen.

tive means of absorbing CSF and, at some point, to be shunt independent. The emergency physician must be aware of the presence of an on-off device. Even though the device is designed to open under high pressure, it can create considerable ICP problems if forgotten in the occluded position.

EVALUATING CSF SHUNTS
Identifying Shunts

The first step in identifying the components of the CSF shunt system and diagnosing problems with the system is **inspection.**[33] The number of craniotomy scars and the presence of skull defects indicate possible shunt locations and the past need for cranial expansion and shunt revision. Bulging of either the fontanel or the craniotomy sites indicates high ICP. A sunken fontanel or craniotomy sites imply low ICP. Distended scalp veins, sprung sutures, and "sunsetting" eyes are all indicators of high ICP. The external bumps associated with Rickham reservoirs, domed systems, tubular systems, and distal tubing allow for ready palpation of these elements of the system. Swelling over the shunt site should be considered diagnostic of shunt failure.[25] Palpation of a floating reservoir confirms that the Rickham reservoir has popped out of the skull and CSF is tracking outside of the skull and brain by passing around the reservoir and the ventricular tubing. Swelling over any portion of the system also implies an underlying disconnection or perforation. Cellulitis, frank pus, or erosion of the scalp is associated with a high incidence of ventriculitis leading to mechanical dysfunction, especially among infants.[4] The distal tubing can usually be visually tracked and palpated across the neck, chest, and abdomen en route to the peritoneum, heart, pleural space, or gallbladder. Swelling at the distal insertion site implies fluid tracking up the catheter because of distal loculation.

Disconnection can occur after trivial trauma. The fibrous sleeve around the shunt tubing often will still conduct CSF, but ICP is invariably elevated, and disconnection can be

rapidly fatal.[1, 40] If flow studies (e.g., technetium Tc 99m clearance) are done alone, because of the fibrous sleeve, as many as one third of the studies could be interpreted as normal. Therefore, skull films should always be part of the evaluation.

Plain radiographs clearly elucidate all components, their origins, their connections, and their ultimate destinations.[33, 34] Anteroposterior and lateral views of the skull and neck are necessary to evaluate the number and type of ventricular catheters and confirm that their connections are intact (see Figs. 132–4 and 132–5). Reservoirs can be localized for subsequent tapping and their connections confirmed. Valve configurations (i.e., tubular or domed) and the locations of the pumping chambers can be established and connections to the distal tubing confirmed. An anteroposterior chest radiograph demonstrates any valve devices located on the chest, confirms atrial or pleural destinations, and verifies intact connections (Fig. 132–6). Right and left lateral decubitus films of the abdomen demonstrate the final destination of the ventriculoperitoneal tubing. With changes in body position, the peritoneal catheter should also change position, indicating that the peritoneal catheter is free floating. Tube migration, fixed or stuck distal tubing, curling within the abdominal wall or within pseudocysts and kinking or defects of the tube itself are easily shown by plain film. Fusiform swelling of the distal tubing seen on plain radiograph is an excellent indication of distal shunt obstruction (Fig. 132–7).[37]

Manual Testing

Once the pumping chamber has been identified, the system can be tested.[33, 34] First the pumping chamber is compressed. Easy compression implies that the distal components are patent and that CSF is diffusing freely out of the distal tubing. Difficult compression or high resistance implies that the distal tubing is blocked or that CSF is

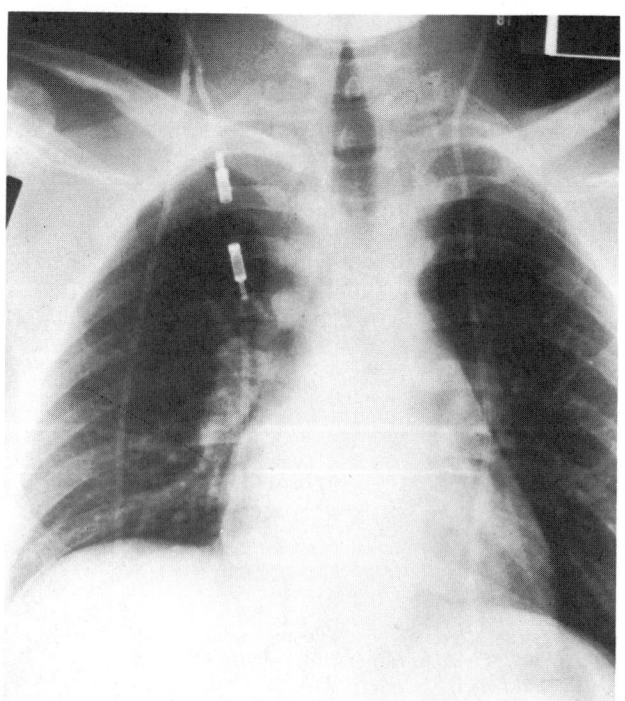

Figure 132–6. Following the tubing. The patient has three ventriculoperitoneal shunts. The tubular (slits) valve apparatus for one system is on the anterior chest wall.

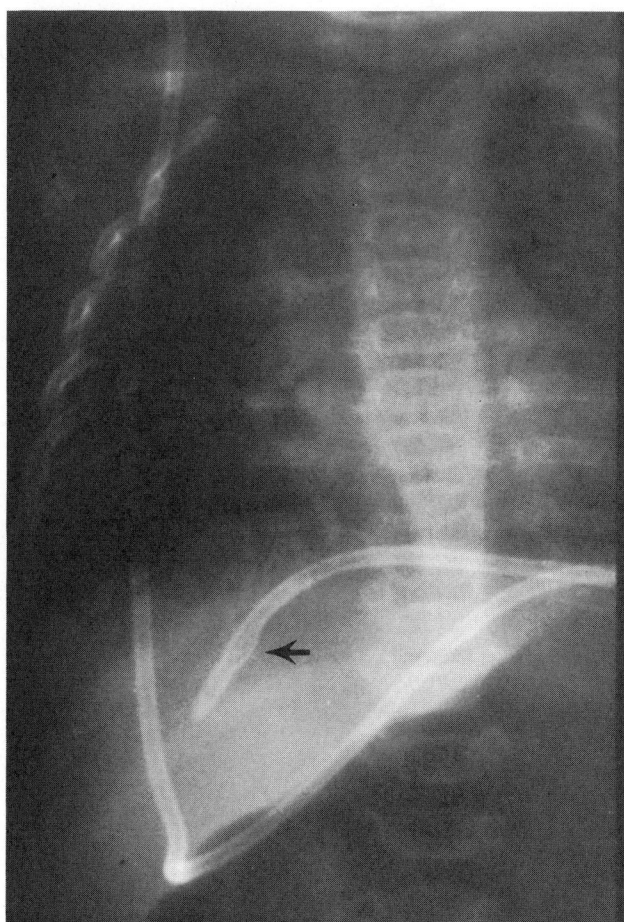

Figure 132–7. Distal tubing. Note the kink and also the "pantaloon" contour deformity *(arrow).*

loculated distally and under pressure. Refill of the pumping chamber should occur within seconds. If the chamber remains depressed or fills slowly, the proximal (ventricular) catheter must be at least partially occluded. Also, when pumping the system, the examiner should listen for a click during either compression or refill, implying incompetence of a valve.[41] Abnormal pumping results are helpful, and pumping is a most useful screen. However, it should not be relied on solely.[41, 42] With proximal obstruction, pumping is clearly abnormal in 60% of cases. In as many as 40% of cases in which obstruction exists, compression and refill of the pumping chamber indicate that the system is functioning properly.

Imaging

When shunt dysfunction is suspected, neuroimaging should be performed and the results compared with those of previous studies. This allows the assessment of relative changes in ventricular volume. Even though ventricle size may appear normal or only slightly enlarged, if the previous scan showed small ventricles, the system is likely to be obstructed and under high pressure. Markedly enlarged ventricles usually imply that the shunt system is not working properly. In some cases, however, the presence of obvious gyri and sulci peripherally on the scan and the presence of enlarged ventricles on previous studies may indicate that this appearance is normal. This is especially true in a child with minimal cortical mantle or porencephaly.

Computed tomography (CT) and magnetic resonance imaging (MRI) scans provide the emergency physician with additional clues to those provided by an assessment of ventricular volume alone.[41, 42] Asymmetric dilation and polycystic brain are easily visualized.[43, 44] Contrast CT may even allow the investigator to delineate whether isolated dilated areas communicate with the shunt system (Fig. 132–8). The CT scan is especially helpful in locating a proximal catheter that is obstructed because it has migrated outside the ventricle (Fig. 132–9). The presence of well-defined sulci and gyri, especially if surrounded by expansive subarachnoid fluid, is in sharp contrast to brain parenchyma flattened against the cranial vault by high ICP. Obliteration of the perimesencephalic cistern on the CT scan, in the presence of signs of high pressure, is a strong warning that life-threatening shunt malfunction has occurred and that structures are crowding together at the tentorial notch.[45] Periventricular hypodensity, especially around the anterior horns of the lateral ventricles, indicates transependymal flow of CSF from the ventricle into the parenchyma (Fig. 132–10).[46] This is a result of inadequate elimination of CSF either through the normal pathways or through the shunt system. The MRI scan of this phenomenon is highly sensitive, demonstrating a clearly demarcated periventricular rind of hyperintensity, seen most often around the anterior horns of the lateral ventricles.[46]

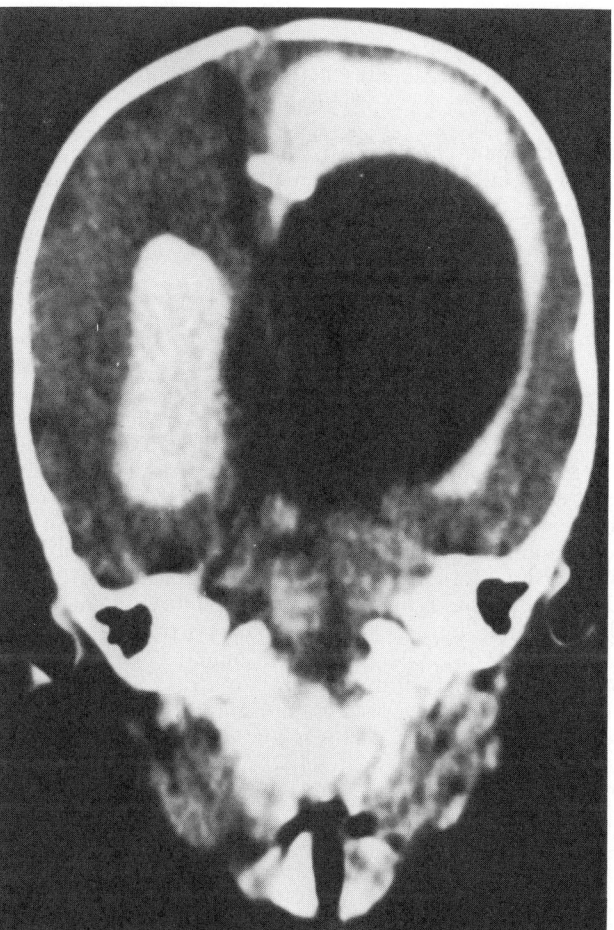

Figure 132–8. Contrast ventriculography through a Rickham reservoir. The lateral ventricles both contain dye and obviously communicate. The massive cyst, however, does not fill with contrast. Note the shunt tubing over the surface of the cyst.

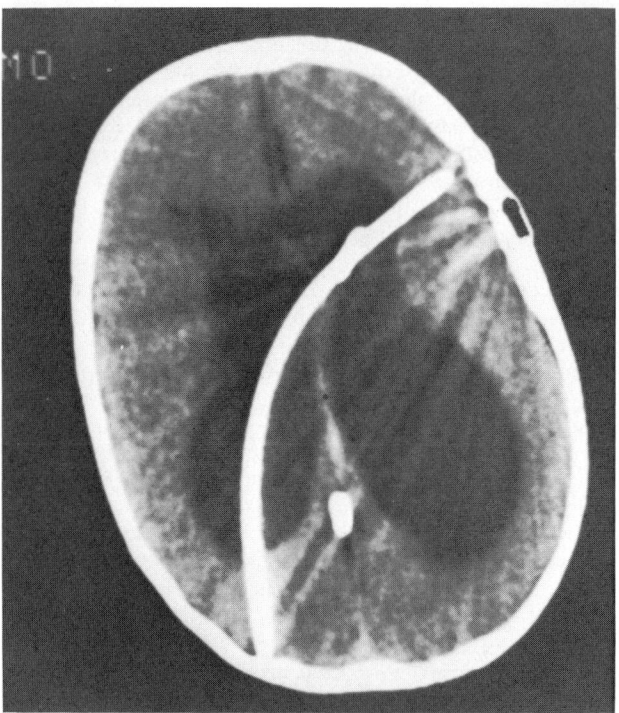

Figure 132–9. Proximal obstruction caused by catheter migration outside the ventricle and into the surrounding parenchyma.

Pressure Measurement and Radionuclide Clearance

The combination of pressure measurement obtained from a reservoir or pumping chamber and the rate of radionuclide clearance from the reservoir or pumping chamber is both highly sensitive and highly specific for shunt obstruction.[40, 42, 47] The study also allows the emergency physician to visualize the entire track and to evaluate the dissemination of nuclide after it has transversed the system.

In one method,[40] the reservoir is punctured, and pressure is measured. High pressure (>15 cm H_2O) implies distal obstruction. Normal pressure implies a normally functioning shunt or proximal obstruction. An attempt is made to gently aspirate CSF. If this can be done easily, the proximal catheter is patent. The spinal fluid is sent for analysis and cultures. Eighteen megabecquerels of technetium Tc 99m pertechnetate in 0.5 ml normal saline is then instilled. Reflux of technetium Tc 99m into the ipsilateral ventricle will occur if the proximal catheter is open or there is distal obstruction. Clearance of the technetium is then monitored. If no reflux of technetium into the ventricle has occurred, 50% of the radioactivity disappears within 5 minutes. If reflux has occurred, especially if there is gross ventriculomegaly, up to 20 minutes is allowed for 50% of the radioactivity to disappear. The technetium trail is followed to the distal catheter tip. Pooling or failure to freely disperse implies loculation or obstruction. Normal shunt function is determined by pressure of <15 cm H_2O, easy aspiration of CSF, reflux into the ipsilateral ventricle, spontaneous clearance of CSF, and free dispersal throughout the abdominal cavity.

A similar method utilizes 100 MCi technetium Tc 99m pertechnetate in 0.1 ml normal saline. The reservoir is accessed and pressure measured.[47] The technetium is injected and the rate of clearance monitored. Reflux of technetium into the ventricle without spontaneous clearance implies distal obstruction. Normally, 50% of the activity

clears within 5 minutes. The technetium trail is followed distally, observing for extravasation, loculation, or free dispersal. If pumping is required to visualize the distal tubing, proximal dysfunction must be suspected. Normal function is determined if ICP is < 20 cm H_2O, 50% of the technetium clears within 5 minutes, and there is good dissemination throughout the abdominal cavity.

During the evaluation of a CSF shunt system, even when infection is not suspected, there can be no doubt that accessing the system to measure pressure, to obtain fluid for analysis and culture, to inject radionuclide material, and even to decompress the system offers critical advantages that far outweigh the theoretic risks. Although there is concern that infection will be introduced or that mechanical dysfunction will be induced, these fears simply have not materialized.[48] Even if a technetium study is unavailable, pressure measurement rapidly distinguishes distal from proximal obstruction and, in the case of distal obstruction, allows for immediate gradual decompression through the reservoir.[33]

MECHANICAL DYSFUNCTION
Distal Obstruction

Distal obstruction of the CSF shunt is the easiest form of mechanical dysfunction to diagnose and treat. Common causes include disconnection, fibrosis or plugging with cel-

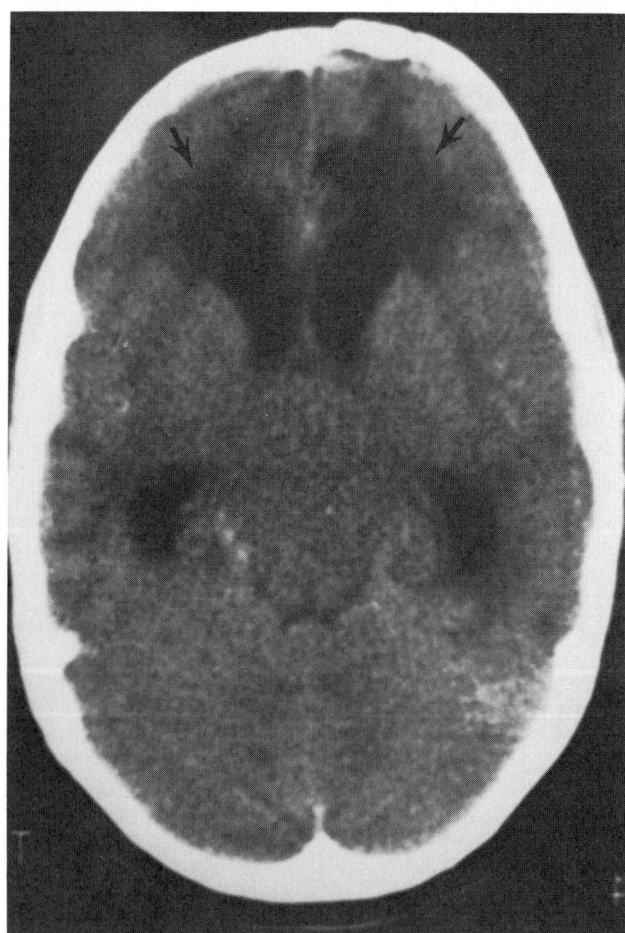

Figure 132–10. Periventricular transependymal cerebrospinal fluid flaring off the anterior horns (*arrows*) of the lateral ventricles. This indicates an obstructed shunt system. The perimesencephalic cistern shows satisfactory volume.

lular debris, kinking, catheter migration, and loculation of spinal fluid. Children with distal obstruction have signs and symptoms of high ICP. Plain radiographs may locate the cause. The pumping chamber may be difficult to compress, but refills promptly. The CT scan shows enlarging ventricles or the other "softer" signs of mechanical obstruction (e.g., flattened sulci and gyri and transependymal CSF accumulation). Puncturing the reservoir and measuring pressure with a manometer indicates high ICP. CSF analysis may be consistent with low-grade infection. If a technetium study is done, there is delayed or absent clearance and abnormal or absent distal dissemination.

Treatment includes notification of neurosurgery and close monitoring of the child until corrective surgery takes place. If signs and symptoms are relatively mild, medical therapy may be initiated. *Osmotic agents* given intravenously include isosorbide (2 gm/kg every 6 hours), glycerol (1 gm/kg every 6 hours), and mannitol (0.25 to 1.0 gm/kg every 6 hours) (Table 132–1). Osmotic agents may work primarily by pulling water from available brain parenchyma; thus their relative ineffectiveness when there is little cortical mantle from which to extract water.[3] However, experimentally, the use of osmotic agents demonstrates an inverse relationship between serum osmolarity and cerebrospinal fluid production. A 1% increase in serum osmolarity can result in as much as a 6% decrease in CSF production.[49]

The use of osmotic agents poses three dangers. Osmotic diuresis may further dehydrate a child who has been vomiting and not eating because of increased ICP. Second, if surgical intervention does not take place within 24 hours and the osmotic agents are stopped, rebound intracranial hypertension may occur. Finally, during the immediate 5 to 15 minutes after the osmotic agents have been given, water is drawn from the interstitial space of the entire body. The result is a markedly higher cardiac output and transiently elevated cerebral blood flow and blood volume. If ICP is already quite high when osmotic agents are given, ICP may actually increase further before it begins to come down.

Diuretic agents, such as acetazolamide (25 mg/kg/day) and furosemide (1 mg/kg/day) can also be used if the child's signs and symptoms do not require immediate manometric decompression.[50] At recommended doses, both agents decrease

---

TABLE 132–1

ICP AND VENTRICULITIS: THERAPY AT A GLANCE

Mildly elevated ICP
  Osmotic agents
    Isosorbide, 2 gm/kg q 6 hr
    Glycerol, 1 gm/kg q 6 hr
    Mannitol, 0.25–1.0 gm/kg q 6 hr
  Diuretic agents
    Acetazolamide, 25 mg/kg, first dose
    Furosemide, 1.0 mg/kg/dose
Extremely high ICP
  Lidocaine, 1.0 mg/kg IV push
  Thiamylal 2.0–5.0 mg/kg IV push
  Atropine, 0.02 mg/kg IV push
  Intubate and hyperventilate
  Manometry-guided decompression; consider a ventricular
    tap
Ventriculitis
  Gram-positive bacteria
    Vancomycin, 10 mg/kg IV
    Vancomycin, 20 mg via Rickham reservoir
    Rifampin, 10 mg/kg po
  Gram-negative bacteria
    Gentamicin, 5 mg via Rickham reservoir
    Ceftazidime, 50 mg/kg IV push

CSF production by 50% to 60%.[3] CSF reduction begins within 30 minutes after an intravenous injection, and peak effect occurs usually within 90 minutes. Duration of effect is up to 2.5 hours.

The use of diuretic agents also poses several dangers.[50, 51] Because they cause diuresis, they may compound the dehydrating effects of several days of poor oral intake and vomiting associated with the shunt dysfunction. If used chronically, acetazolamide causes a hypochloremic metabolic acidosis, dehydration, diarrhea, and tachypnea. Chronic furosemide therapy causes a contraction alkalosis, dehydration, and hypokalemia.

The greatest danger in the emergency department, however, is from acetazolamide.[51] After intravenous administration, there can be an immediate increase in ICP because of drug-induced cerebral acidosis. The result is subsequent vasodilation and an increase in cerebral blood volume. In response to this increased intracranial volume, the ICP may increase 75% to 150% above baseline and stay there for up to 3 hours. The agent should be used for milder cases or only after the intracranial space has been mechanically decompressed.

In children who are deeply comatose or posturing or have respiratory ataxia, two things must be done as rapidly as possible. Lidocaine (1 mg/kg) is given intravenously to reduce coughing and the Valsalva maneuver, both of which will markedly increase ICP. Thiopental or thiamylal (Surital) (2 to 5 mg/kg) is given intravenously to reduce ICP. Atropine is given for bradycardia, and a nondepolarizing muscle relaxant is administered. The child is then intubated and hyperventilated. Second, in cases of distal obstruction, the child can be mechanically decompressed. Mechanical decompression is accomplished by slowly removing CSF from the ventricular compartment. A 25-gauge butterfly needle is attached to a manometer with the three-way stopcock taken from a standard lumbar puncture tray. The child's reservoir or pumping chamber (if there is no separate reservoir) is needled at a 60-degree angle and the manometer allowed to passively fill. The stopcock is then turned, allowing only a manometric amount of CSF to be collected. This process of taking off only the amount of CSF contained within the manometer is repeated slowly and carefully until the ICP falls to between 10 and 15 cm H_2O.[33]

The complications of mechanical decompression occur only if the pressure is lowered too rapidly.[39, 52, 53] These complications include subdural and subarachnoid hemorrhage and pneumocranium (Fig. 132–11). Again, however, by slowly and passively allowing only manometric amounts of CSF out of the head, these complications are avoided.

Proximal Obstruction

Obstruction of the ventricular catheter most often occurs from cellular debris, fibrosis, and infection; envelopment by choroid plexus; and catheter migration.[25] The child has signs and symptoms of elevated ICP. Radiographic surveys show all connections intact and when the pumping chamber is tested, refill is absent or delayed in more than 60% of the cases. The CT scan may show enlarging ventricles, but regardless of the ventricular size, the emergency physician must look for the softer signs of shunt obstruction. The CT scan may also show that the catheter tip has migrated outside of the ventricular system (Fig. 132–9). Needling the reservoir or pumping chamber discloses normal pressure and CSF withdrawal may be difficult or impossible. If a technetium study is done, there will be delayed or absent clearance, or clearance will occur only when the system is pumped.

Because the ventricular catheter is blocked, the emergency physician cannot decompress the patient through the res-

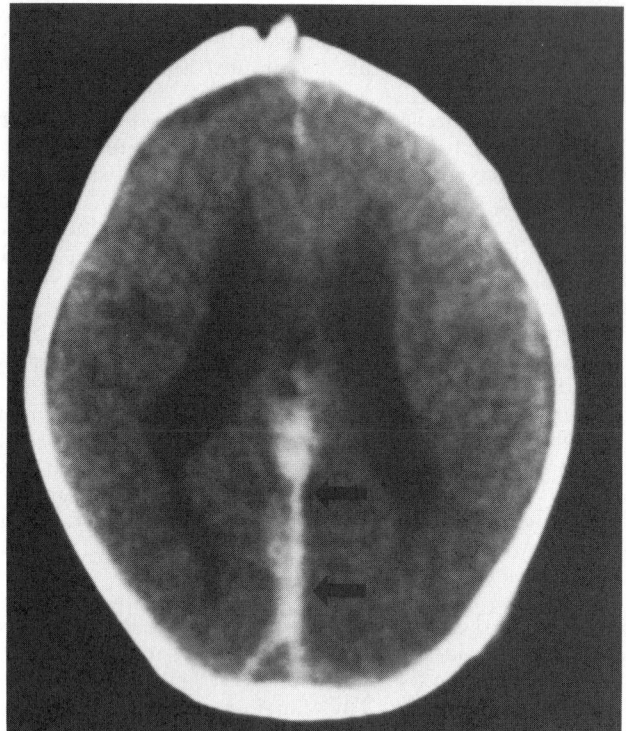

Figure 132–11. Excessively rapid decompression has resulted in a subdural hemorrhage *(arrows)*.

mittent high pressure from intermittent proximal catheter occlusion, and intermittent high pressure despite normal shunt function.

Rapid CSF clearance from the intracranial space results in sudden *intracranial hypotension,* often induced by postural change or exercise.[22, 23, 56] The best indication that this has occurred is the presence of cold sweats, a sunken fontanel, a slack encephalocele, or depressed craniotomy sites. An extreme form of this phenomenon results when there is sudden upward traction on the brain stem. The child may then faint, stop breathing, become pale and bradycardic, or even show cranial nerve signs such as laryngospasm. Immediately laying the child supine, or even tipping the child 15 to 30 degrees in the Trendelenburg position, helps alleviate the symptoms. The ultimate treatment for this is upgrading the shunt valve and using an antisiphon device.[24, 38, 57]

Another mechanism causing these recurrent episodes occurs despite apparently normal shunt function and ICP. This is the phenomenon of *secondary vasomotor pressure waves.*[20, 55] Once the hydrocephalic child has been shunted, the child's intracranial space will not tolerate volume expansion nearly as well. The intracranial volume pressure curve is steeper and markedly shifted to the left by comparison with the dynamics prior to shunting. Therefore, a situation is reached whereby, at relatively low volumes and ICPs, compliance markedly deteriorates, resistance to cerebrospinal fluid outflow rises markedly, and abrupt clinical deteri-

ervoir. Treatment is based on the child's condition. The child must be observed closely and neurosurgery notified immediately. If signs and symptoms are mild, a cautious attempt at osmotic or diuretic therapy can be initiated, preferably with low-dose mannitol and furosemide. If the child is in peril, the airway must be secured and hyperventilated until neurosurgery decompresses the intracranial space.

In an attempt to save the child's life, the emergency physician may have to attempt a *ventricular puncture.*[34] After preparing the scalp, a spinal needle is chosen based on the age and size of the child. A 1½-inch needle is used for newborns, a 2½-inch needle is used for children up to 4 years of age, and a 3½-inch needle is used for children older than 4 years. The intracranial space is entered through the coronal suture approximately 1 cm lateral to the midline and directed straight to the base of the skull on a plane parallel to the falx. After the dural pop is felt, the needle is then redirected toward the base of the skull in line with the inner canthus of the ipsilateral eye. As with decompression through a reservoir, only enough CSF compatible with lowering the ICP to 10 to 15 cm H$_2$O should be removed; that amount should be drained slowly and passively.

Slit Ventricle Syndrome

Small ventricles on the CT scan are a normal finding after shunting and do not themselves cause symptoms.[54] Many children, however, present with intermittent signs and symptoms of shunt dysfunction and small ventricles on CT scan (Fig. 132–12). This recurrent phenomenon, which most often symptomatically resolves by itself, is called the *slit ventricle syndrome.* A number of conditions exist to produce the syndrome.[21–24, 54–56] These include true low pressure from overdrainage, normal pressure and shunt function with secondary pressure waves from sudden vasodilation, inter-

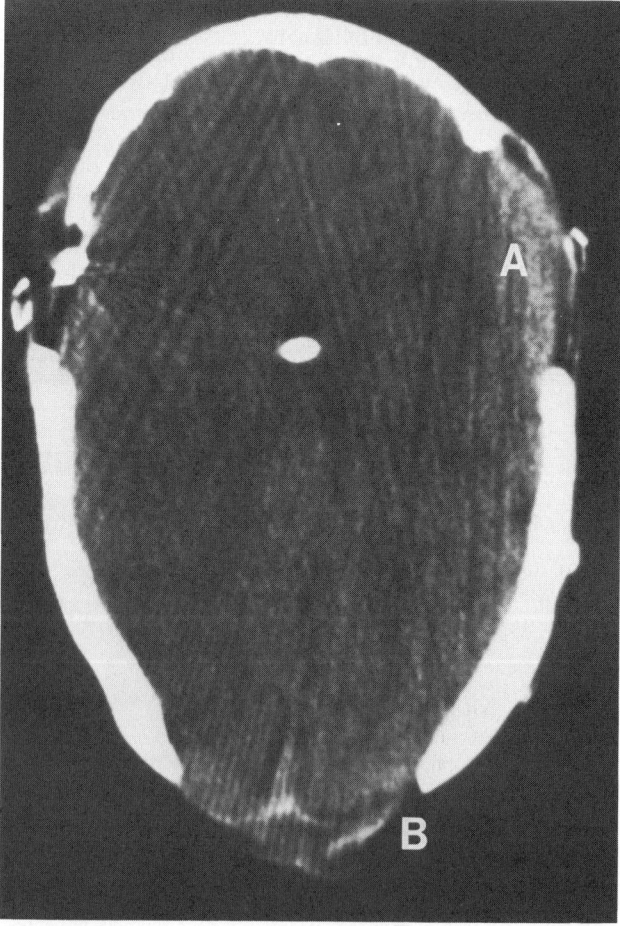

Figure 132–12. Slit ventricle syndrome. The ventricles are imperceptible. Note the sites of previous cranial expansion (A) and the encephalocele (B).

oration occurs in response to even minor alterations in cerebrovascular tone. In this group of patients, provided the physician is convinced that intermittent proximal occlusion is not the cause of the child's signs and symptoms, antimigraine therapy aimed at preventing the episodic vasodilation may be considered.[55]

Slit ventricle syndrome can also occur because of intermittent high pressure secondary to *intermittent proximal catheter occlusion.*[54–56] Especially with small ventricles, coaptation of the ventricular walls may contribute to transient obstruction of the ventricular catheter tip.[23] More often, the catheter is partially occluded or ball-valved with cellular debris, fibrotic reaction, or partial migration. On the CT scan, the ventricles may be enlarged by comparison. The pumping chamber refills slowly, if at all. Intracranial hypertension may not be measurable because of the obstruction, but technetium clearance is abnormal. Resumption of adequate shunt function ameliorates the child's symptoms, but the child still requires shunt revision and placement of an antisiphon device if recurrence is to be prevented.

A last type of abnormality in slit ventricle syndrome occurs when, after prolonged ventricular low volume, the child develops a thickened skull. When measured, the ICP is high, but technetium clearance is normal, indicating good CSF shunt function.[54, 56] When operated on, these children invariably exhibit venous engorgement until cranial expansion is accomplished. Venous outflow obstruction contributes to the pathophysiology, and these children are even more sensitive to secondary vasomotor pressure waves. With cranial morcellation, the venous outflow obstruction is relieved, and the child is given a new set of expansile "sutures" with which to adapt to episodes of increased intracranial blood volume.

VENTRICULITIS

Shunt infection must be considered to be the cause of fever when no other cause can be found in a shunted child, especially if there are accompanying signs of encephalopathy or shunt dysfunction.[33, 34, 55, 58] Two to five percent of all shunts become infected.[59] Although *Staphylococcus aureus* and gram-negative infections may present as fulminant life-threatening situations, more than half of all infections are from *Staphylococcus epidermidis* and present in an insidious fashion. Two thirds of all shunt infections occur within 1 month of shunt surgery, and 80% occur within 6 months of the previous shunt operation.[60] The presence of cellulitis, erosion, or frank pus over the insertion site are good predictors that the shunt system is infected.[5] Fever is present in two thirds of cases in which there is external evidence of wound infection. When there is no external evidence of wound infection, more than 90% of infected patients present with fever as part of the complaint. Shunt malfunction is present in 65% of infected cases when there is no obvious wound infection and in 86% of cases when there is clear evidence of wound infection.[61] Seeding the peritoneum with infection from above can result in peritonitis or localized collections of infected CSF.[62, 63]

In ventriculoatrial shunt infections, in contrast to ventriculoperitoneal shunt infections, blood cultures are positive more than 80% of the time. Pumping the shunt prior to obtaining the blood cultures will increase the yield.[58] Systems that do not terminate in the circulation, however, rarely have positive blood culture results. It is imperative, therefore, to obtain CSF.[58, 59] Infected patients typically have only mildly elevated cell counts of 50 to 200 cells/mm³, which is typical of the cellularity which can be induced by the presence of the shunt itself. Gram stain should be done on a centrifuge specimen to concentrate the cells and bacteria. Even so, the Gram stain may show no organisms.[59] This is especially true in cases of slime-producing *Staphylococcus*

species, which are tightly adherent to the shunt tubing. Cultures obtained from the shunt give a 96% yield and are the best test for ventriculitis.[58]

If CSF cannot be aspirated from the shunt system, a lumbar puncture can be cautiously considered. An attempt must be made to exclude elevated ICP prior to the lumbar puncture, lest the test end in herniation.[64] In noncommunicating hydrocephalus, the lumbar CSF is not contiguous with that in the lateral ventricles. In fact, in children with noncommunicating hydrocephalus, lumbar CSF routinely has elevated protein levels and monocytosis because of decreased CSF circulation. This can be mistakenly interpreted as being consistent with infection when none actually exists.[58]

Treatment varies to some extent based on Gram stain and final culture results. Infections with blood-borne organisms such as *Haemophilus influenzae, Streptococcus pneumoniae,* and *Neisseria meningitidis* will respond to intravenously administered antibiotics alone.[59, 65] In these cases, urine, CSF, and serum counterimmunoelectrophoresis is helpful during the early diagnostic process. Coliforms and mixed aerobic and anaerobic infections suggest perforation of bowel with an ascending infection and require externalization of the system, as well as intraventricular and systemic antibiotics.[62] In this circumstance, the first dose of gentamicin, 5 mg as a bolus, can be instilled directly into the lateral ventricle through the reservoir.

Intravenous and intraventricular vancomycin combined with oral rifampin, acting synergistically, provide the most effective combination against the *Staphylococcus* species.[58, 66–68] Treatment ultimately requires extirpation of the shunt system and externalization, but the first intraventricular dose of vancomycin (20 mg as a bolus, in a solution for intrathecal injection) can be given in the emergency department.[69]

MISCELLANEOUS COMPLICATIONS

Almost all non–central nervous system (CNS) complications of CSF shunt systems relate to the final destination of the distal tubing. For example, in *ventricle-gallbladder* shunts, the most common complication is gallbladder atony, which can be treated with cholecystokinin. Ascending infection from cholecystitis, obstructive jaundice, fistula formation to small bowel, and reflux biliary ventriculitis have also been described.[36]

With *ventriculopleural* shunts, symptomatic hydrothorax can occur at any time (Figs. 132–13 and 132–14). Pneumothorax and even pneumocranium secondary to erosion into the bronchiolar system have also been described.[35]

The non-CNS complications associated with *ventriculoatrial* shunts tend to be life threatening.[4] Descending infection causes endocarditis with potential valve incompetence and heart failure. Pulmonary embolus can occur when a thrombus generated at the distal shunt tubing, along the atrial wall, or on the heart valves breaks off and enters the pulmonary circulation. Cardiac tamponade results when the distal shunt tubing erodes through the right atrium. If the catheter becomes disconnected, it can embolize to the pulmonary artery and may also cause a dysrhythmia. Long-standing endocarditis causes prolonged deposition of immune complexes on the renal basement membrane. The resulting "shunt nephritis" is potentially reversible, provided the ventriculoatrial shunt is removed and the endocarditis treated.[70]

Ventriculoperitoneal systems are most commonly complicated by partial or complete obstruction of the peritoneal end.[63, 71, 72] This results from kinking or plugging, as well as from migration and loculation. Peritoneal catheters can migrate into the abdominal wall, out of the peritoneal cavity into the pleural space, into the vagina, into the retroperitoneal space, through the bladder, and into the rectum.[72] Hepatic abscess has occurred after the distal catheter has

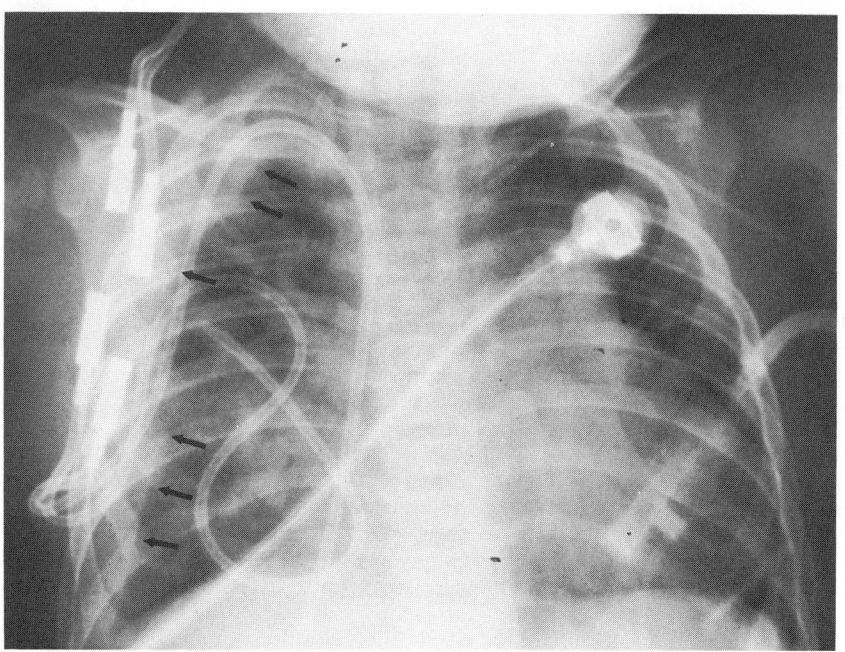

Figure 132–13. Ventriculopleural shunt with large pleural effusion *(arrows)*. The radiograph was taken in the lateral decubitus position.

become insinuated into the liver. Perforation of the gallbladder, small bowel, colon, and stomach has also occurred (Fig. 132–15).[72] Volvulus has occurred both with connected functional peritoneal catheters and with remnants left in the peritoneal cavity. Bowel has been strangulated by peritoneal tubing, causing obstruction and necrosis.[72] Peritonitis can result from both a descending infection (ventriculitis) and perforation of bowel by the distal tubing. Mixed organisms or coliforms found in CSF suggest an ascending infection secondary to perforation.[62] Interestingly, less than 25% of known cases of bowel perforation are associated with clinical peritonitis.[73] Intestinal perforation can present as an otherwise asymptomatic protrusion of shunt tubing from the anus (see Fig. 132–15).[73, 74]

Of special interest are loculations of CSF known as *pseudocysts* (Fig. 132–16).[63, 75, 76] Because pseudocysts usually present with abdominal distension, nausea, and vomiting, the emergency physician should be alerted to this possibility once it has been ascertained that the child has a CSF shunt. The diagnosis is readily made by abdominal ultrasound. A physical clue to the presence of a CSF pseudocyst is swelling around the abdominal insertion site and a palpable mass (Fig. 132–17). Because the loculation often prevents free diffusion of cerebrospinal fluid, it can also cause distal obstruction and symptoms of shunt malfunction. When the pseudocyst is opened, CSF cultures are positive in up to 36% of the cases. Cultures and appropriate antibiotics are essential in the treatment of pseudocysts.

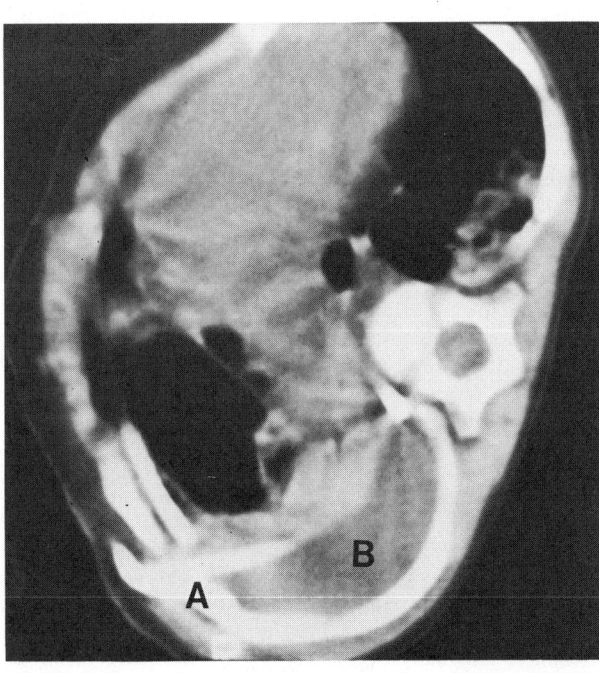

Figure 132–14. CT scan of the chest. Ventriculopleural shunt (A) with large pleural effusion (B).

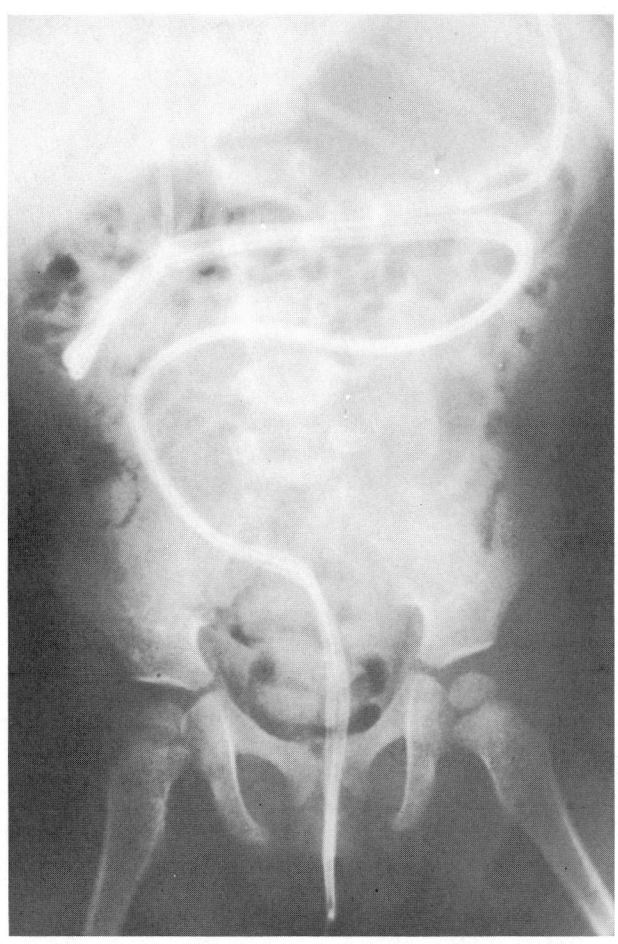

Figure 132–15. Anal protrusion of distal cerebrospinal fluid shunt catheters. This child had mixed gram-negative ventriculitis.

The most innocuous complication of a CSF ventriculoperitoneal shunt is the opening of the tunica vaginalis and the creation of a large inguinal hernia or migration of shunt tubing into the scrotum.[77] The ensuing hydrocele rapidly brings the child to the emergency department.

When children are shunted because of brain tumor, there is the potential for tumor cells to seed into the peritoneal cavity, creating *brain tumor metastasis* by CSF.[78] A child whose shunt system has been fitted with a filter precisely to prevent this complication is at risk for obstructing the system with tumor cells.[33] Chronic hydrocephalus can cause erosion of the base of the skull especially at the ethmoid plate. The siphoning effect inherent in shunt systems can then cause enough negative pressure to draw air into the cranium and

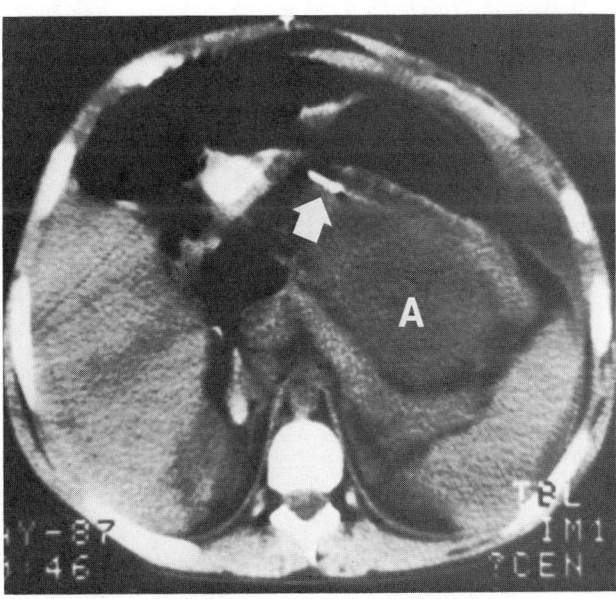

Figure 132–16. Massive abdominal loculation of cerebrospinal fluid (A). Note the peritoneal catheter entering the loculation cavity *(arrow)*.

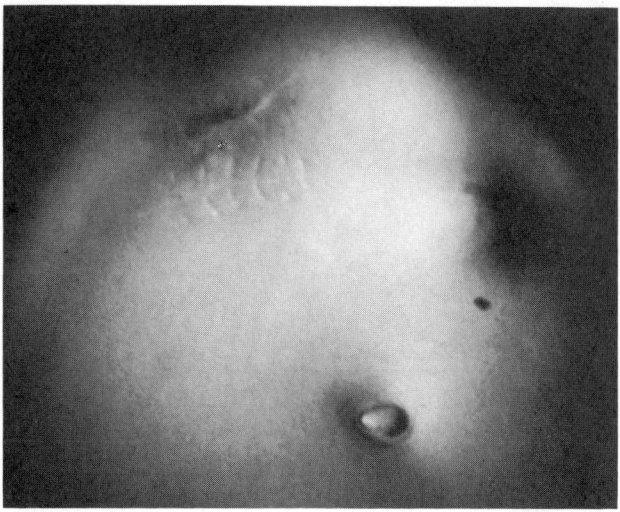

Figure 132–17. External bulge indicating an underlying cerebrospinal fluid pseudocyst.

create headache and mental status changes. This *pneumocranium* is readily diagnosed on CT scan.[53] Although extremely rare, *erosion of a blood vessel* by the proximal tube is a catastrophic complication of the cerebrospinal fluid shunt.[79] The erosion results in either intraventricular or intraparenchymal hemorrhage.

References

1. Neuren A, Ellison PH. Acute hydrocephalus and death following V-P shunt disconnection. Pediatrics 1979;64:90.
2. Arroyo HA, Jan JE, McCormick AQ, et al. Permanent visual loss after shunt malfunction. Neurology 1986;35:25.
3. Gilmore HE. Medical treatment of hydrocephalus. *In* Scott RM (ed). Hydrocephalus. Vol. 3. Concepts in Neurosurgery. Baltimore, Williams & Wilkins, 1990.
4. Bell WE, McCormick WF. Hydrocephalus. *In* Bell WE, McCormick WF (eds). Raised Intracranial Pressure in Children: Diagnosis and Treatment. Philadelphia, WB Saunders, 1978.
5. Hirsch J-F, Pierre-Kahn A, Renier D, et al. The Dandy-Walker malformation. J Neurosurg 1984;61:515.
6. Ryder JW, Kleinschmidt-DeMartens BK, Keller TS. Sudden deterioration and death in patients with benign tumors of the third ventricle areas. J Report of an unusual case. J Neurosurg 1986;64:216.
7. Afifi AK, Jacoby CG, Bell WE, et al. Aqueductal stenosis and neurofibromatosis: A rare association. J Child Neurol 1988;3:125.
8. McLaurin RL, Towbin RB. Tuberous sclerosis: Diagnostic and surgical considerations. Pediatric Neurosci 1985–86;12:43.
9. Godersky JC, Menezes AH. Intracranial arteriovenous anomalies of infancy: Modern concepts. Pediatric Neurosci 1987;13:242.
10. Cohen ME, Duffner PK. Brain Tumors in Children; Principles of Diagnosis and Treatment. New York, Raven Press, 1984.
11. Gamache FW, Posner JB, Patterson RH. Metastatic brain tumors. *In* Youman JF (ed). Neurological Surgery. Vol 5. Philadelphia, WB Saunders, 1982.
12. Beyerl B, Black PM. Posttraumatic hydrocephalus. Neurosurgery 1984;15:257.
13. Mohr JP, Kistler JP, Zabramski JM, et al. Intracranial aneurysms. *In* Barnett HJM, et al (ed). Stroke: Pathophysiology, Diagnosis and Management. Vol 2. New York, Churchill Livingstone, 1986, p 643.
14. Hawgood S, Spong J, Yu VYH. Intraventricular hemorrhage; incidence and outcome in a population of very-low-birth-weight infants. Am J Dis Child 1984;138:136.
15. Slabaugh RD, Smith JA, Lemons J, et al. Neonatal intracranial hemorrhage and complicating hydrocephalus. J Clin Ultrasound 1984;12:261.
16. Liptak GS, Masiulis BS, McDonald JV. Ventricular shunts survival in children with neural tube defects. Acta Neurochir 1985;74:113.
17. Dykes FD, Dunbar B, Lazarra A, et al. Posthemorrhagic hydrocephalus in high-risk preterm infants: Natural history, management, and long-term outcome. J Pediatr 1989;114:611.
18. Fried A, Shapiro K, Takei F, et al. A laboratory model of shunt-dependent hydrocephalus. J Neurosurgery 1987;66:734.
19. Shapiro K, Fried A, Marmarou A. Biomechanical and hydrodynamic characterization of the hydrocephalic infant. J Neurosurg 1985;63:69.
20. Shapiro K, Fried A. Pressure-volume relationships in shunt-dependent childhood hydrocephalus. J Neurosurg 1986;64:390.
21. Coker SB. Cyclic vomiting and the slit ventricle syndrome. Pediatr Neurol 1987;3:297.
22. Faulhauer K, Schmitz P. Overdrainage phenomena in shunt treated hydrocephalus. Acta Neurochir 1978;45:89.
23. Kiekens R, Mortier W, Pathmann R, et al. The slit-ventricle syndrome after shunting in hydrocephalic children. Neuropediatrics 1982;13:190.
24. McLaurin RL, Olivi A. Slit-ventricle syndrome: Review of 15 cases. Pediatr Neurosci 1987;13:118.
25. Sekhar LN, Moossy J, Guthkelch N. Malfunctioning ventriculoperitoneal shunts. J Neurosurg 1982;56:411.
26. Vassilouthis J. The syndrome of normal-pressure hydrocephalus. J Neurosurg 1984;61:501.
27. Carmel PW. Surgical syndromes of the hypothalamus. Clin Neurosurg 1980;27:133.
28. Hack CH, Enrile BG, Donat JF, et al. Seizures in relation to shunt dysfunction in children with meningomyelocele. J Pediatr 1990;116:57.
29. Saukkonen A-L. Electroencephalographic findings in hydrocephalic children prior to initial shunting. Childs Nerv Syst 1988;4:339.
30. Venes JL, Dauser RC. Epilepsy following ventricular shunt placement. J Neurosurg 1987;66:154.
31. Saukkonen AL, Serlo W, von Wendt L. Electroencephalographic findings and epilepsy in the slit ventricle syndrome of shunt-treated hydrocephalic children. Childs Nerv Syst 1988;4:344.
32. Post EM. Currently Available Shunt Systems: A review. Neurosurgery 1985;16:257.
33. Guertin SR. Cerebrospinal fluid shunts; evaluation, complications, and crisis management. Pediatr Clin North Am 1987;34:203.
34. Madsen MA. Emergency department management of ventriculoperitoneal cerebrospinal fluid shunts. Ann of Emerg Med 1986;15:1330.
35. Jones RFC, Currie BG, Kwok BCT. Ventriculopleural shunts for hydrocephalus: A useful alternative. Neurosurgery 1988;23:753.
36. West KW, Turner MK, Vane DW, et al. Ventricular gallbladder shunts: An alternative procedure in hydrocephalus. J Pediatr Surg 1987;22:609.
37. Le Roux P, Berger M, Benjamin D. Abdominal x-ray and pathological findings in distal unishunt obstruction. Neurosurgery 1988;23:749.
38. Gruber R, Jenny P, Herzog B. Experiences with the anti-siphon device (ASD) in shunt therapy of pediatric hydrocephalus. J Neurosurg 1984;61:156.
39. Portnoy HD, Schulte RR, Fox JL, et al. Antisiphon and reversible occlusion valves for shunting in hydrocephalus and preventing post-shunt subdural hematomas. J Neurosurg 1973;38:729.
40. Reilly PL, Savage JP, Doecke L. Isotope transport studies and shunt pressure measurements as a guide to shunt function. Br J Neurosurg 1989;3:681.
41. El-Gohary MA, Forrest DM, Starer F. The role of the CT scan in the management of blocked ventricular shunt. Pediatr Surg 1988;4:247.
42. Di Rocco C, Caldarelli M. Surveillance of CSF shunt function. *In* Di Rocco C (ed). The Treatment of Infantile Hydrocephalus. Vol II. Boca Raton, FL, CRC Press, 1987.
43. Kalsbeck JE, DeSousa AL, Kleiman MB, et al. Compartmentalization of the cerebral ventricles as a sequela of neonatal meningitis. J Neurosurg 1980;52:547.
44. Rahman N, Adam KAR. Congenital polycystic disease of the brain: Report of an unusual case. Dev Med Child Neurol 1988;28:62.
45. Johnson DL, Fitz L, McCullough DC, et al. Perimesencephalic cistern obliteration: A CT sign of life-threatening shunt failure. J Neurosurg 1986;64:386.
46. Wolpert SM. Radiological investigation of pediatric hydrocephalus. *In* Scott RM (ed). Hydrocephalus. Vol 3. Concepts in Neurosurgery. Baltimore, Williams & Wilkins, 1990.
47. Hayden PW, Rudd TG, Shurtleff DB. Combined pressure-radionuclide evaluation of suspected cerebrospinal fluid shunt malfunction: A seven-year clinical experience. Pediatrics 1980;66:679.
48. Noetzel MJ, Baker RP. Shunt fluid examination: Risks and benefits in the evaluation of shunt malfunction and infection. J Neurosurg 1984;61:328.
49. Volpe JJ. Mechanisms of brain injury. *In* Volpe JJ. Neurology of the Newborn. Philadelphia, WB Saunders, 1987.
50. Shinnar S, Gammon K, Bergman E Jr, et al. Management of hydrocephalus in infancy: Use of acetazolamide and furosemide to avoid cerebrospinal fluid shunts. J Pediatr 1985;107:31.
51. Di Rocco C. The medical treatment. *In* Di Rocco C (ed). The Treatment of Infantile Hydrocephalus. Boca Raton, FL, CRC Press, 1987.
52. Epstein F. How to keep shunts functioning or "the impossible dream." Clin Neurosurg 1985;32:608.
53. Ruge JR, Corullo LJ, McLone DG. Pneumocephalus in patients with CSF shunts. J Neurosurg 1985;63:532.
54. Epstein F, Lapras C, Wisoff JF. "Slit-ventricle syndrome": Etiology and treatment. Pediatr Neurosci 1988;14:5.
55. Obana WG, Raskin NH, Cogen PH, et al. Antimigraine treatment of slit ventricle syndrome. Neurosurgery 1990;27:760.
56. Wisoff JR, Epstein FJ. Diagnosis and treatment of the slit ventricle syndrome. *In* Scott RM (ed). Hydrocephalus. Vol 3. Concepts in Neurosurgery. Baltimore, Williams & Wilkins, 1990.
57. Hyde-Rowan MD, Rekate HL, Nulsen FE. Re-expansion of previously

collapsed ventricles: The slit ventricle syndrome. J Neurosurg 1982;56:536.

58. Venes JL. Infections of CSF shunt and intracranial pressure monitoring devices. Infect Dis Clin North Am 1989;3:289.
59. Klein DM. Shunt infections. *In* Scott RM (ed). Hydrocephalus. Vol 3. Concepts in Neurosurgery. Baltimore, Williams & Wilkins, 1990.
60. Schoenbaum SC, Gardner P, Shillito J. Infections of cerebrospinal fluid shunts: Epidemiology, clinical manifestations and therapy. J Infect Dis 1975;131:543.
61. Odio C, McCracken GH, Nelson JD. CSF shunt infections in pediatrics. Am J Dis Child 1984;138:1103.
62. Rush DS, Walsh JW, Belin RP, et al. Ventricular sepsis and abdominally related complications in children with cerebrospinal fluid shunts. Surgery 1985;97:420.
63. Bryant MS, Bremer AM, Tepas JJ, et al. Abdominal complications of ventriculoperitoneal shunts. Am Surg 1988;54:50.
64. Addy DP. When not to do a lumbar puncture. Arch Dis Child 1987;62:873.
65. Rennels, MB, Wald ER. Treatment of Haemophilus influenzae type b meningitis in children with cerebrospinal fluid shunts. J Pediatr 1980;97:424.
66. Gombert ME, Landesman SH, Corrado ML, et al. Vancomycin and rifampin therapy for Staphylococcus epidermidis meningitis associated with CSF shunts. J Neurosurg 1981;55:633.
67. McGee SM, Kaplan SL, Mason EO, et al. Ventricular fluid concentrations of vancomycin in children after intravenous and intraventricular administration. Pediatric Infect Dis J 1990;9:138.
68. Vichyanond P, Olson LC. Staphylococcal CNS infections treated with vancomycin and rifampin. Arch Neurol 1984;41:367.
69. Steele RW. Central nervous system infections. *In* Steele RW. A Clinical Manual of Pediatric Infectious Disease. Norwalk, CT, Appleton-Century-Crofts, 1990.
70. Zamora I, Lurbe A, Alvarez-Garijo A, et al. Shunt nephritis: A report on five children. Childs Brain 1984;11:183.
71. Agha FP, Amendola MA, Shimzi KK, et al. Abdominal complications of ventriculoperitoneal shunts with emphasis on the role of imaging methods. Surg Gynecol Obstet 1983;156:473.
72. Hlavin ML, Mapstone TB, Gauderer MWL. Small bowel obstruction secondary to incomplete removal of a ventriculoperitoneal shunt: Case report. Neurosurgery 1990;26:526.
73. Hornig, GW, Shillito J. Intestinal perforation by peritoneal shunt tubing: Report of two cases. Surg Neurol 1990;33:288.
74. Miserocchi G, Simi VA, Ravagnati L. Anal protrusion as a complication of ventriculo-peritoneal shunt. J Neurosurg Sci 1984;24:43.
75. Gaskill SJ, Marlin AE. Pseudocysts of the abdomen associated with ventriculoperitoneal shunts: A report of twelve cases and a review of the literature. Pediatr Neurosci 1989;15:23.
76. Hahn YS, Engelhard H, McClone DG. Abdominal CSF pseudocyst. Pediatr Neurosci 1985–86;12:75.
77. Moazam R, Glenn JD, Kaplan BJ, et al. Inguinal hernias after ventriculoperitoneal shunt procedures in pediatric patients. Surg Gynecol Obstet 1984;159:570.
78. Hoffman HJ, Hendrick EB, Humphreys RP. Metastasis via ventriculoperitoneal shunt in patients with medulloblastoma. J Neurosurg 1976;44:562.
79. Snow RB, Zimmerman RD, Derinsky O. Delayed intracerebral hemorrhage after ventriculoperitoneal shunting. Neurosurgery 1986;19:305.

CHAPTER 133

Syncope

Steven E. Krug

INTRODUCTION

Syncope is a sudden, reversible, and generally brief loss of consciousness and muscle tone. Up to 15% of children experience syncope before the end of adolescence.

EMERGENCY MEDICAL SERVICE CONSIDERATIONS

Although syncope is typically a benign complaint in children, the life-threatening cardiac or central nervous system disorders that can cause syncope mandate a compulsive prehospital approach. Most children will have regained consciousness prior to the arrival of the emergency medical service (EMS) unit. If they have normal mental status and vital signs, they may be transported in a recumbent position, preferably with supplemental oxygen delivered by a face mask or nasal cannula. No matter how well the child may appear, he or she should be monitored during transport. Vascular access should be obtained in patients with a persistent alteration of mental status and in those with evidence of circulatory insufficiency. An effort should be made to exclude any associated trauma, as such patients may require spine immobilization.

CLINICAL EVALUATION
History

A thorough history may identify the precipitating cause of syncope (Table 133–1). The events preceding or surrounding the syncopal episode and the environment in which it occurred should be well described. If the child is preverbal or otherwise unable to describe the event, witnesses should be questioned as to any abrupt changes in the child's posture and whether the child had been coughing, swallowing, defecating, or urinating at the time of the episode. The presence of significant psychophysiologic factors (anxiety, pain, fatigue, sight of blood, hunger, prolonged standing posture, excessively warm or crowded environment) is suggestive of vasovagal syncope. Abnormal behaviors such as hyperventilation or hallucinations suggest a psychiatric or toxicologic cause.

The presence of premonitory symptoms may help to determine the causative disorder. Patients with tachyarrhythmias, for example, may note palpitations, whereas hypoglycemic children may be aware of diaphoresis and tachycardia. Further evidence for vasovagal syncope is provided when a typical prodrome (pallor, diaphoresis, nausea, dizziness, blurred vision) is described. Older children may be able to describe the premonitory aura seen with migraine or epilepsy. Conversely, an abrupt loss of consciousness is more likely to be associated with a cardiac cause of syncope.

The appearance of the child during the event may also provide insight into the cause. Persistent or severe pallor or cyanosis suggests cardiac syncope. Abnormal motor activity or incontinence during the spell may indicate significant cerebral hypoxemia or primary epilepsy.

The duration of the syncopal spell and the nature of recovery are also important. If the child has a prolonged

TABLE 133–1
SYNCOPE: FACTS TO OBTAIN DURING HISTORY TAKING
Events preceding the syncopal episode
Environment where the episode occurred
Presence of premonitory symptoms
Child's position at onset of attack
Appearance of child during episode
Presence of associated symptoms
Duration of attack
Prior history of syncope, headache, epilepsy, migraine, blood loss, trauma, diabetes, arrhythmia
Family history of syncope, epilepsy, migraine, sudden death

loss of consciousness, true syncope is unlikely. Likewise, if recovery is slow, with abnormal mental status, speech, or motor function, or if there is a persistent focal deficit, then a migraine or seizure disorder should be suspected.

Finally, a complete medical and family history should be elicited. If the patient has had a previous similar episode, the physician should determine the similarities with previous syncopal events or the situations in which they occurred. Medication use and the possibility of substance abuse should be determined. The adolescent female patient may be pregnant or have heavy menstrual flow resulting in anemia. The family history should be examined for clues of one of the "long QT syndromes," specifically inquiring for a history of congenital hearing loss, arrhythmias, or sudden unexplained deaths.

Physical Examination

The patient's vital signs should include any postural changes (i.e., standing, sitting, supine). In an adolescent, a standing systolic blood pressure of less than 80 mm Hg or a 30 mm Hg or greater decrease in the systolic blood pressure on standing is diagnostic of orthostatic hypotension. Vagal maneuvers may be cautiously performed in an attempt to replicate the syncopal episode, with careful monitoring of blood pressure, heart rate, and cardiac rhythm.

A thorough physical examination should focus on the cardiovascular and neurologic systems. The cardiovascular examination may help to identify disorders that result in poor cardiac output or cerebral perfusion. The pulses should be assessed for quality and regularity, with careful auscultation for bruits over the carotids. The heart should be examined for murmurs, extra sounds, rubs, or irregularity. The neurologic examination should search for the presence of any focal deficits or persistent changes in mental status. In adolescent females, the examination should exclude the presence of pregnancy.

DIAGNOSTIC EVALUATION

Unless the patient's history and physical examination are absolutely confirmatory for a benign (i.e., vasovagal) cause of syncope, all children with syncope should have laboratory studies performed, including a complete blood cell count and measurement of serum electrolyte and glucose levels. A measurement of calcium and magnesium levels should also be considered. In older children, or in patients with a suspected toxic exposure, a toxicology panel is indicated. Finally, a urine pregnancy test should be strongly considered for postpubertal females (Table 133–2).

An electrocardiogram (EKG) is perhaps the single most important test in the evaluation of syncope. The EKG elucidates heart rate, rhythm, and conduction intervals, as well as chamber size and structural heart disease. The EKG may also identify children who need more sophisticated cardiovascular testing (echocardiography, maximal exercise testing, Holter monitoring, cardiac catheterization, and intracardiac electrophysiology study).

Roentgenographs are of limited benefit in the evaluation of the child with syncope. However, a child with a persistent or severe cough may need radiologic evaluation for pulmonary disease or sinusitis. The syncopal child with a persistent or focal neurologic deficit should be evaluated with computed tomography (CT) scanning, followed by an electroencephalogram (EEG).

Efforts to duplicate the syncopal event can be attempted. Vagal maneuvers or hyperventilation may be attempted but should only be performed with cardiac monitoring. Carotid sinus massage should never be attempted in a nonhospital

TABLE 133–2
SYNCOPE: DIAGNOSTIC EVALUATION
Acute studies for all patients:
Blood glucose determination
Serum electrolyte determination
Hematocrit determination
Toxicology panel
12-lead electrocardiogram
Acute studies for certain patients:
Arterial blood gas measurement
Urine pregnancy test
Chest radiograph
Head CT scan
Other studies to consider:
Electroencephalogram
Echocardiogram
Holter monitoring
Cardiac electrophysiology test
Exercise stress testing
Tilt table test

setting. In performing these maneuvers, attention should be directed toward changes in blood pressure, heart rate, and rhythm. Studies have shown the head-up tilt table test to be useful in stimulating vasovagal reactions believed to be responsible for syncopal events. Performance of the upright tilt test in conjunction with an isoproterenol infusion may increase the sensitivity of this test in identifying those susceptible to neurally mediated syncope. Such procedures are rarely performed in the emergency department.

DIFFERENTIAL DIAGNOSIS

The principal causes of syncope can be divided into eight broad pathophysiologic categories: vascular/reflex, cardiac, neurologic, respiratory, gastrointestinal, metabolic, toxic, and psychologic (Table 133–3). All causes of true syncope result in either significant decreases in cerebral blood flow below a critical perfusion threshold (30 ml per 100 gm of brain per minute) or inadequate delivery of metabolic substrates to the brain.

Vascular/Reflex Disorders

Vasovagal or *vasodepressor syncope,* the simple faint, is the most common cause of syncope. As many as 25% of young adults have experienced one or more episodes of vasodepressor syncope during adolescence. It is caused by a sudden loss of resistance in the peripheral circulation, resulting in decreased venous return and a lowered cardiac output. This fall in peripheral vascular resistance is not accompanied by an increase in cardiac output. In fact, there is generally a decrease in heart rate. These changes result in a profound and rapid fall in arterial pressure and cerebral hypoperfusion.

These episodes are likely to occur during or immediately following frightening, painful, or emotionally stressful experiences. They are also most likely to occur in certain environmental settings, such as a hot, crowded room, or in subjects who are fatigued or hungry. Typically, this form of syncope occurs with the patient either in an upright or sitting position.

These episodes are characterized by a decrease in arterial pressure with a loss or impairment of consciousness. These episodes are also typified by autonomic changes, including pallor, diaphoresis, mydriasis, nausea, hypotension, and

TABLE 133–3

TRANSIENT LOSS OF CONSCIOUSNESS: DIFFERENTIAL DIAGNOSIS

Vasovagal
  Common faint
  Swallow, cough, micturition, and defecation syncopes
  Carotid sinus syncope
Orthostatic hypotension
  Dehydration, hemorrhage, pregnancy, autonomic instability
Cardiovascular
  Impaired cardiac filling (tamponade, hypovolemia, myxoma)
  Decreased contractility (cardiomyopathy, congenital heart
    disease, myocardial infarction)
  Dysrhythmias (bradyarrhythmias, atrioventricular node
    block, sick sinus syndrome, asystole, tachyarrhythmias,
    long QT syndromes, fibrillation)
  Valvular obstruction (aortic stenosis, mitral prolapse)
  Pulmonary vascular obstruction (pulmonary hypertension,
    pulmonary embolism)
Neurologic
  Trauma
  Epilepsy
  Basilar artery migraine
  Vertigo
  Cerebrovascular insufficiency
  Space-occupying lesion
Respiratory
  Breath holding
  Tussive disorder
Gastrointestinal
  Gastroesophageal reflux
Hematologic
  Anemia
Metabolic/toxic
  Hypoxia
  Hypoglycemia
  Electrolyte disorders (Na^+, Ca^{2+}, Mg^{2+}, K^+)
  Toxins
Psychologic
  Hysteria
  Hyperventilation
  Self-induced Valsalva effect

bradycardia. Many patients may be able to describe a prodrome of these symptoms.

Vasovagal syncope is usually benign and self-limited. The episode may be aborted if, on recognition of prodromal symptoms, the patient is placed in a recumbent position with the legs elevated. This, combined with calm reassurance, is usually sufficient to manage the majority of episodes. If the syncopal event persists, treatment may be necessary with either atropine or other agents that increase systemic vascular resistance.

Carotid sinus syncope also stems from vagotonia. This may be induced by hyperextension or turning of the head, shaving, or pressure exerted from external devices such as tight collars or orthodontic appliances. Stimulation of the sinus in susceptible patients results in an exaggerated vagal response, causing either a drop in arterial pressure and or a slowing of the heart rate.

Orthostatic hypotension is another relatively common cause of syncope. This is a common problem in elderly or debilitated patients. The cause is a failure of normal physiologic compensatory mechanisms for postural changes. However, even in children, prolonged standing or bed rest can promote syncope with sudden changes in posture.

Any process that results in significant vascular volume loss (hemorrhage, dehydration) or venous pooling (pregnancy) may produce orthostatic syncope. Diseases or trauma of the spinal cord can produce reductions of peripheral vascular resistance and increased venous pooling, resulting in hypotension and syncope. Finally, certain medications such as vasodilators or beta blockers may compromise compensatory mechanisms and promote syncope.

Although generally uncommon in children, micturition, defecation, or swallowing may precipitate syncope. The micturition and defecation causes of syncope are hypothesized to be caused by the Valsalva maneuver and associated vasovagal reactions or orthostatic hypotension. Swallowing syncope is probably the result of unopposed glossopharyngeal reflex input to the central nervous system, resulting in excessive vagal stimulation of the cardiovascular system. The ingestion of hot food or liquids may precipitate syncope.

In patients with vascular or reflex syncope, induction of the Valsalva maneuver, carotid sinus massage, or ocular pressure may reproduce the causative arrhythmia and the syncopal episode. Severely affected children, such as those who develop asystole or profound episodes of bradycardia, may require medical or surgical vagolysis or even pacemaker insertion.

Cardiac Disorders

Any disorder that results in impaired cardiac filling, decreased cardiac ejection, or an obstruction to cardiac outflow will potentiate syncope. These generally more serious cardiac causes of syncope are uncommon in children.

Disorders that may result in impaired cardiac filling include hypovolemia or any cause of shock or hypotension. *Cardiac tamponade* secondary to a pericardial effusion, pneumopericardium, or a tension pneumothorax may result in decreased cardiac filling. Impairment of cardiac ejection may be caused by diminished contractility or arrhythmias.

Bradyarrhythmias that produce significant reductions in cardiac output can cause syncope. This is especially significant in newborns and small infants, as cardiac output in that population is highly dependent on heart rate. Although common in infants with congenital lesions, symptomatic sinus bradycardia can occur in infants with structurally normal hearts. These bradyarrhythmias may mimic apneic spells. They are believed to be caused by either the "sick sinus syndrome" or excessive vagal tone.

Bradyarrhythmias can be precipitated by defecation, yawning, or micturition in newborn infants. In addition to negative chronotropy, vagal stimulation can also produce vasodepressor effects and delay myocardial conduction (prolongation of the PR interval). In older children, bradyarrhythmias may be secondary to third-degree heart block.

Asystole can occur as a severe manifestation of the sick sinus syndrome. It has been proposed that syncope caused by asystole may occur as an extreme manifestation of a neurally mediated hypotension-bradycardia syndrome or as an uncommon manifestation of status epilepticus.

Tachyarrhythmias causing syncope can be of atrial or ventricular origin. Atrial arrhythmias include paroxysmal atrial tachycardia, atrial flutter, and atrial fibrillation. The presence of accessory conduction pathways, as in patients with Wolff-Parkinson-White syndrome, may result in excessive conduction or a rapid ventricular response to atrial flutter or fibrillation. In some patients, a rapid ventricular response can progress to ventricular tachycardia and fibrillation.

The prognosis of children with ventricular tachycardia is highly dependent on the finding of structural abnormalities, as sudden death typically occurs only in those children with structurally abnormal hearts. There are three different groups of children who are at risk for sudden cardiac death: the infant with a cardiac tumor, the older child with a prolonged QT interval, and the adolescent after surgical repair of congenital heart disease.

Although unexplained syncope in children with structurally normal hearts is generally considered to be benign, these life-threatening ventricular arrhythmias can occur in children with "normal" hearts. A thorough evaluation performed for occult arrhythmias with unexplained syncope may include 24-hour Holter monitoring, and maximal exercise testing and prompt consideration for electrophysiologic testing.

Another group of disorders to consider in the syncopal child are associated with delayed ventricular repolarization (i.e., the *long QT syndromes*). A long QT interval extends the myocardium's period of vulnerability and is thought to predispose the patient to ectopic beats, which can trigger ventricular tachycardia, ventricular fibrillation, or asystole and, hence, sudden cardiac death. International registries of these rare patients have identified three risk factors for sudden death: congenital deafness, female gender, and prior episodes of syncope.

The prolonged QT syndromes are believed to occur secondary to sympathetic imbalance. This pathogenetic mechanism is supported by the therapeutic success of beta blockade and high thoracic sympathectomy. Making the diagnosis and initiating treatment in children with QT syndromes is imperative, as the mortality rate for untreated patients is more than 70%. The mortality rate decreases to less than 10% for those patients treated with beta blockade. Approximately 20% of those treated with beta blockers continue to have syncopal events and may require left stellate sympathectomy, which is generally 100% palliative.

An EKG should serve to identify those children with a prolonged QT interval, but unfortunately, 25% of children with tachyarrhythmic syncope and structurally normal hearts have normal QT intervals. Commonly, these patients may have a resting bradycardia and their heart rate may fail to accelerate normally with exercise. Precise measurement of the QT interval is desirable but may be technically difficult, especially in patients with higher resting heart rates and inherently shorter QT intervals. Exercise or the induction of the Valsalva maneuver during the EKG may exacerbate QT prolongation.

Many drugs are also known to cause prolongation of the QT interval. These include tricyclic antidepressants, phenothiazines, some calcium channel blockers, and a number of anti-arrhythmics (e.g., quinidine, procainamide, beta blockers). Syncope is a complication of quinidine therapy in children. Hypokalemia, hypocalcemia, and, to a lesser extent, hypomagnesemia can also potentiate QT prolongation.

The final group of cardiac disorders that may cause syncope are those that result in valve or vessel obstruction. This outflow obstruction can be at the atrial (myxoma, mitral stenosis, or tricuspid stenosis), or ventricular system (aortic or pulmonic stenosis, tetralogy of Fallot) level, or within the pulmonary vascular system (right atrial or ventricular thromboembolism, pulmonary embolism, pulmonary hypertension).

Neurologic Disorders

Epilepsy, although not a true cause of syncope, is the most common cause of syncope-like episodes in children. Children of all ages may be affected by epilepsy, with between 6% and 7% having a convulsion in the first 7 years of life. Children may not experience a preseizure aura, and depending on the type of epilepsy, there may be no overt tonic or clonic activity. As a result, seizures and syncope may be difficult to distinguish clinically (Table 133–4).

The majority of seizures end spontaneously and often are followed by a postictal state characterized by mental or motor impairment. When present, the postictal phase can help to differentiate true syncope from epilepsy. In children younger than 5 years, the presence of a high fever may aid this differentiation, as up to 4% of young febrile children experience a febrile seizure. With the exception of an EEG, laboratory studies may not help to distinguish a seizure from syncope, as the two share numerous common precipitants. Finally, there may be an association between syncope and seizures, either with a syncopal episode followed by a convulsion or, as mentioned earlier, with seizures precipitating hypotension, cardiac dysrhythmias, or syncope.

Migraines, much like true epilepsy, may also mimic syncope. Although rare in children, involvement of the basal arterial system can cause a loss of consciousness lasting several minutes. Basilar artery migraine attacks may also include transient visual symptoms (transient blindness, scotoma, blurred vision), ataxia, or vertigo. This form of migraine can occur in all age groups and is more common in females. Typical migraine attacks may be easily diagnosed, but distinguishing them from focal epilepsy can be difficult.

Other neurologic precipitants of syncope include trauma, vertigo, mass lesions of the central nervous system, central autonomic dysfunction, and disorders that can cause cerebrovascular insufficiency (transient ischemic attacks, stroke, arteriovenous malformations, subclavian steal, carotid or vertebral artery stenosis, thrombotic or embolic diseases).

Respiratory Disorders

Breath holding is a common cause of syncope in infants, toddlers, and preschool children, occurring in as many as 5%. When crying, most children have a relative prolongation of the expiratory phase. In some, this may be severe enough to provoke desaturation and cyanosis. The child's back may arch, and the child may become sufficiently hypoxic to suffer a loss of consciousness. Occasionally, the hypoxia may precipitate a brief tonic-clonic convulsion.

Breath holding is often associated with precipitating emotional or benign physical trauma. In addition to these "cyanotic" spells, children may experience "pallid" breath-holding spells. *Pallid syncope*, or reflex anoxic seizure, is not caused by breath holding but instead represents the pediatric counterpart of adult vasovagal syncope. Typically, these spells are precipitated by minor trauma, with the child turning pale and falling to the ground. Like adult vasovagal syncope, these episodes are caused by vagally mediated bradycardias or even short runs of asystole. The occurrence of these spells in young children is explained either by excessive vagal tone or autonomic dysfunction and may be reproduced with ocular compression.

Tussive syncope is commonly associated with asthma, pertussis, or cystic fibrosis. Children with severe coughing paroxysms may also experience other neurologic symptoms, including dizziness, confusion, headache, vision and speech disturbances, and movement disorders. Proposed mechanisms include a reduction in cardiac output as a result of the associated Valsalva maneuver, a reduction in cardiac output secondary to high intrathoracic pressures and diminished venous return, hypoxia secondary to the precipitating bronchospasm and inadequate ventilation, or changes in neck positioning with compression of the basilar or carotid arteries.

Gastrointestinal Disorders

Gastroesophageal reflux can be confused with syncope or epilepsy. It is extremely common in infants, having an estimated incidence of 1 in 500. Although fluid aspiration

TABLE 133–4

CLINICAL DISTINCTION BETWEEN EPILEPSY AND SYNCOPE

Symptom	Epilepsy	Syncope
Precipitating event	Usually absent	Usually present
Loss of consciousness	Usually >2 min	Usually <2 min
Premonition	Aura	Nausea, dizziness, blurred vision
Incontinence	Common	Uncommon
Posture at onset	Any	Usually upright
Appearance	Rubor, cyanosis	Pallor, clammy
Motor activity	Usually prominent	Usually minimal
Pulse	Increased	Decreased or irregular
Resulting headache, lethargy, confusion	Common	Uncommon
Family history	+ for epilepsy	+ for syncope

Adapted from Oppenheimer EY, Rosman NP. Seizures and seizure-like states in the child: An approach to emergency management. Emerg Med Clin North Am 1983;1:125.

may be suspected as the cause of choking in an infant during or shortly after a feeding, esophageal reflux and tracheal aspiration can also occur between feedings. In especially young infants, gastroesophageal reflux may cause apnea, hypotonia, pallor, or cyanosis and may be the cause of as much as 10% of near-miss sudden infant death episodes.

Metabolic Disorders

Hypoxemia or severe *anemia* can affect the delivery of oxygen to the central nervous system, creating a syncopal episode. Likewise, systemic *hypoglycemia* results in inadequate tissue delivery of glucose and a possible transient loss of central nervous system function. Other electrolyte and metabolic disorders can provoke syncope-like events, especially those that can precipitate epilepsy (e.g., sodium, calcium, or magnesium deficiency) and, occasionally, those that precipitate arrhythmias (potassium deficiency).

Toxic Disorders

A number of medications and toxins can provoke a syncope-like reaction (Table 133–5). Drugs that result in decreased vascular tone, decreased cardiac filling pressures, or diminished cardiac output include barbiturates, phenothiazines, tricyclic antidepressants, calcium channel blockers, beta blockers, nitrates, arterial vasodilators, and other antihypertensive agents. Similarly, medications that reduce vascular volume, such as diuretics, may also provoke a syncopal reaction. In older children, cocaine ingestion is perhaps the most common toxic cause of acute loss of consciousness occurring secondary to either epilepsy or syncope. Finally, carbon monoxide may cause syncope by inducing hypoxemia.

Psychologic Disorders

Hysterical or *conversion syncope* can be remarkably convincing and can mimic organic disease. It occurs in adolescents or young adults, generally in the presence of others. These patients usually fall so that they do not injure themselves, and they may have an apparent mental status change for a prolonged period of time. These patients usually demonstrate an overall lack of concern and a calm emotional detachment.

Syncope can also be a primary symptom of epidemic or mass hysteria. These events typically occur in settings in which large numbers of children, usually preteens or teenagers, are clustered together. Unlike children with conversion reactions, who show indifference, these children are highly anxious. Reassurance and diffusion of the extreme anxiety generally promote resolution of symptoms.

Hyperventilation is another "psychologic" cause of syncope. When severe, the associated hypocapnia can result in a significant reduction in cerebral blood flow.

Finally, syncope may be self-induced, caused by utilizing a Valsalva maneuver. This is typically seen in moderate to severely retarded children and may be confused with absence seizures.

THERAPEUTIC INTERVENTION

A child with syncope requires immediate assessment of and appropriate interventions for airway, breathing, and circulation. Unless the child looks perfectly well, he or she should receive supplemental oxygen and remain in a recumbent position. Similarly, vascular access should be obtained in children with evidence of circulatory insufficiency, dysrhythmias, or persistent mental status changes. A rapid bedside glucose measurement will determine the presence of hypoglycemia and the need for supplemental dextrose.

All children with syncope should have a 12-lead EKG performed and, if they are still symptomatic, continuous cardiac monitoring. The treatment for arrhythmias depends on both the type of arrhythmia and whether the patient is hemodynamically stable with a normal mental status.

Treatment is urgent for symptomatic tachyarrhythmias, using either synchronized cardioversion, or rapidly acting medications such as adenosine (for supraventricular tachy-

TABLE 133–5

DRUGS AND TOXINS THAT CAUSE SYNCOPE

Adrenergic antagonists
Antidysrhythmics (quinidine, procainamide, lidocaine, phenytoin, beta blockers, digitalis)
Antihypertensives
Barbiturates
Benzodiazepines
Diuretics
Insulin
Phenothiazines
Substances of abuse (cocaine, alcohol, marijuana, opiates)
Toxins (carbon monoxide, heavy metals, hydrocarbons)
Tricyclic antidepressants
Vasodilators (nitrates, calcium channel blockers)
Vincristine

arrhythmias) or lidocaine (for ventricular tachycardia). Patients with "stable" supraventricular tachyarrhythmias may be treated less urgently. Because of the inherent risk of ventricular fibrillation in ventricular tachycardia, even hemodynamically stable children warrant rapid pharmacologic intervention.

The treatment for bradyarrhythmias, much like that for tachyarrhythmias, is dependent on the patient's hemodynamic status. Atropine, followed by epinephrine, is the initial medication used for symptomatic patients. Patients with severe and persistent bradyarrhythmias may require isoproterenol or epinephrine infusions or external or internal cardiac pacing.

Hypotension should be treated initially with large-bore vascular access and a 20-ml/kg bolus of an isotonic fluid. Additional fluid therapy depends on clinical response to the initial fluid push. It is not advisable to demonstrate orthostatic hypotension in patients who have baseline evidence of circulatory insufficiency.

Children with persistent alterations in mental status, focal deficits or findings on neurologic examination, or evidence of arrhythmias or cardiac disease require admission for monitoring and further diagnostic evaluation. Patients with persistent alterations in mental status need acute toxicologic screening and a cerebral CT scan. Children who have normal cardiac and neurologic examinations can usually be discharged from the emergency department and re-evaluated as outpatients. This is especially important for those with a family or medical history of syncope.

Selected References

Aicardi J. Epileptic syndromes in childhood. Epilepsia 1988;29(suppl 3):51.

Beder SD, Cohen MH, Riemenschneider TA. Occult arrhythmias as the etiology of unexplained syncope in children with structurally normal hearts. Am Heart J 1985;109:309.

Benatar A, Hill ID, Fraser CB, et al. Prolonged QT syndrome in childhood. S Afr Med J 1982;62:139.

DiMario FJ, Chee CM, Berman PH. Pallid breath-holding spells: Evaluation of the autonomic nervous system. Clin Pediatr 1990;29:17.

Garson A, Smith RT, Moak JP, et al. Ventricular arrhythmias and sudden death in children. J Am Coll Cardiol 1985;5:130B.

Gordon TA, Moodie DS, Passalacqua M, et al. A retrospective analysis of the cost-effective workup of syncope in children. Cleve Clin Q 1987;54:391.

Haslam RH, Freigang B. Cough syncope mimicking epilepsy in asthmatic children. Can J Neurol Sci 1985;12:45.

Kapoor WN. Diagnostic evaluation of syncope. Am J Med 1991;90:91.

Kapoor WN, Cha R, Peterson JR, et al. Prolonged electrocardiographic monitoring in patients with syncope. Am J Med 1987;82:20.

Kapoor WN, Peterson JR, Karpf M. Micturition sycope: A reappraisal. JAMA 1985;253:796.

Kenigsberg K. Treatment of swallowing syncope. Pediatrics 1987;80:459.

Krug SE. Cocaine abuse: Historical, epidemiological, and clinical perspectives for pediatricians. Curr Prob Pediatr 1989;19:447.

Kunis RL, Garfein OB, Pepe AJ, et al. Deglutition syncope and atrioventricular block selectively induced by hot food. Am J Cardiol 1985;55:613.

Lassiter HA. Recurrent asystole in a child. West J Med 1984;141:240.

Levine RJ. Epidemic faintness and syncope in a school marching band. JAMA 1977;238:2373.

Lloyd EA, Hauer RN, Zipes DP, et al. Syncope and ventricular tachycardia in patients with ventricular preexcitation. Am J Cardiol 1983;73:79.

Lombroso CT, Lerman P. Breathholding spells: Cyanotic and pallid infantile syncope. Pediatrics 1967;39:563.

Moss AJ, Schwartz PJ, Crampton RS, et al. The long QT syndrome: A prospective international study. Circulation 1985;71:17.

Oppenheimer EY, Rosman NP. Seizures and seizure-like states in the child: An approach to emergency management. Emerg Med Clin North Am 1983;1:125.

Papazian O. Common epileptic syndromes in children. Pediatr Ann 1991;20:15.

Paul T, Guccione P, Garson A. Relation of syncope in young patients with Wolff-Parkinson-White syndrome to rapid ventricular response during atrial fibrillation. Am J Cardiol 1990;65:318.

Pedley TA. Differential diagnosis of episodic symptoms. Epilepsia 1983;24(suppl 1):31.

Pratt JL, Fleisher GR. Syncope in children and adolescents. Pediatr Emerg Care 1989;5:80.

Rein AJ, Simcha A, Ludomirsky A, et al. Symptomatic bradycardia in infants with structurally normal hearts. J Pediatr 1985;107:724.

Ruckman RN. Cardiac causes of syncope. Pediatr Rev 1987;9:101.

Sapire DW, Casta A. Vagotonia in infants, children, adolescents and young adults. Int J Cardiol 1985;9:211.

Sapire DW, Casta A, Wolf WJ, et al. Vagotonia as a cause of syncope. J Pediatr 1986;109:394.

Schneider S, Rice DR. Neurologic manifestations of childhood hysteria. J Pediatr 1979;94:153.

Schwartz PJ. Idiopathic long QT syndrome: Progress and questions. Am Heart J 1985;109:399.

Schwartz RH, Estroff T, Hoffman NG. Seizures and syncope in adolescent cocaine abusers. Am J Med 1988;85:462.

Shinnar S, D'Souza B. Migraine in children and adolescents. Pediatr Rev 1982;3:257.

Smith W. The long Q-T syndrome. Aust NZ J Med 1984;14:700.

Strasberg B, Rechavia E, Sagie A, et al. The head-up tilt table test in patients with syncope of unknown origin. Am Heart J 1989;118:923.

Thilenius OG, Quinones JA, Husayni TS. Tilt test for diagnosis of unexplained syncope in pediatric patients. Pediatrics 1991;87:334.

Vining EP, Freeman JM. Paroxysmal events which are not seizures. Pediatr Ann 1985;19:726.

von Bernuth G, Bernsau U, Gutheil H, et al. Tachyarrhythmic syncopes in children with structurally normal hearts with and without QT-prolongation in the electrocardiogram. Eur J Pediatr 1982;138:206.

Webb CL, Dick M, Rocchini AP, et al. Quinidine syncope in children. J Am Coll Cardiol 1987;9:1031.

Woody RC, Kiel EA. Swallowing syncope in a child. Pediatrics 1986;78:507.

CHAPTER 134

Weakness

David H. Fagin

INTRODUCTION

Acute weakness may result from pathologic abnormality anywhere in the nervous system from the central nervous system (upper motor neuron unit) to the peripheral nervous system (lower motor neuron unit). The lower motor neuron unit consists of the spinal column and its anterior horn cells, as well as the peripheral nerve and muscle.

Weakness resulting from central nervous system (CNS) abnormality is usually acute and often life threatening. CNS abnormality usually results in an alternation in mental status, increased deep tendon reflexes, Babinski's sign, ankle clonus, and spasticity. CNS weakness is usually asymmetric and cranial nerve palsies may be present. Children with weakness from CNS abnormality are more likely to have an underlying medical condition such as sickle cell disease or congenital heart disease.

Weakness associated with lower motor unit disease often has an insidious onset and can present with a wide range of physical findings, as the abnormality may occur in the spinal column, the peripheral nerve, the neuromuscular junction, or in the muscle itself. Lower motor unit disease usually results in absent to diminished tendon reflexes, hypotonia, and possibly muscle fasciculations. Involvement of the spinal column often results in loss of bowel or bladder control. Children with spinal cord injuries present with a mixture of sensory and motor findings depending on the location of the injury.

CLINICAL EVALUATION

A thorough history and physical examination are essential. The possibility of spinal trauma should be addressed immediately. The family should be questioned as to the initial presentation of the weakness and how quickly it progressed. The physician should also ask about cranial nerve, sensory, or respiratory muscle involvement. The family should be questioned about the possibility of a toxin or drug exposure, and a family history of similar weakness should be elicited. The physician should ask about any underlying medical problems such as sickle cell disease, seizure disorder, congenital heart disease, or cancer. The family of an infant presenting with weakness should be questioned about honey ingestion, which can produce infantile botulism. The physician should also investigate the possibility of a tick bite.

The physical examination should concentrate on a thorough neurologic examination, with careful testing of the child's reflexes, cranial nerves, peripheral sensation, and motor strength. Rectal sphincter and bladder tone should also be checked. Additionally, careful attention should be given to the child's respiratory status. Any child with suspected infection should be checked for meningismus or rash, and the skin should be thoroughly checked for a tick.

DIFFERENTIAL DIAGNOSIS

Weakness caused by CNS abnormality usually has a vascular, infectious, or traumatic origin (Table 134–1). The term *acute hemiplegia of childhood* is used to describe a number of conditions and anatomic abnormalities that result in cerebral infarction. These children often present before the age of 3 years with seizures and hemiplegia, which may be accompanied by fever and vomiting. Children with congenital heart disease may develop a stroke from increased blood viscosity. They are also more prone to cerebral emboli from endocarditis or arrhythmias and may develop brain abscesses. Sickle cell disease may cause stroke from vascular occlusion induced by the sickling process. Children with leukemia can have intracranial bleeding from either thrombocytopenia or leukemic infiltration of blood vessels. Bleeding from arteriovenous malformations or aneurysms may cause childhood stroke, but both of these conditions are rare. Systemic lupus erythematosus, diabetes mellitus, and polyarteritis nodosa may also cause cerebral infarction from arterial thrombi. Severe dehydration from any cause may result in cerebral vein thrombosis and stroke.

TABLE 134–1

DIFFERENTIAL DIAGNOSIS OF ACUTE WEAKNESS

I. Upper motor neuron unit (CNS)
  A. Vascular disorders (arteriovenous malformation, aneurysm, sickle cell disease, leukemia)
  B. Infectious disorders (meningitis, encephalitis, brain abscess)
  C. Trauma (epidural and subdural hematoma, cerebral contusions and hemorrhage, intra-oral trauma)
  D. Other (drugs, systemic illness, dehydration)
II. Lower motor neuron unit
  A. Spinal column and anterior horn cells (spinal trauma, transverse myelitis, tumor, and epidural abscess)
  B. Peripheral neuromuscular apparatus
    1. Presynaptic (Guillain-Barré, tick paralysis)
    2. Neuromuscular junction (infant botulism, myasthenia gravis, organophosphates and other toxins)
    3. Myopathy (periodic paralysis, electrolytes, rhabdomyolysis)

Childhood strokes may be caused by a number of infectious processes. Meningitis and encephalitis may cause an arteritis or vasculitis that ultimately leads to vascular occlusion and stroke. A brain abscess may cause hemiplegia, but symptoms usually develop slowly. Infections of the throat, ears, and sinuses can lead to inflammation of the internal carotid artery and stroke. Diphtheria may also present with weakness. Other infections such as tuberculosis, malaria, and cat-scratch disease can also cause childhood strokes.

Childhood head trauma may also cause acute weakness and may result in cerebral contusions or lacerations or epidural, subdural, or intracerebral hemorrhage. Intra-oral trauma may result in cerebral infarction from occlusion of the internal carotid artery.

A number of other conditions affecting the CNS may cause acute weakness or strokes. Children with prolonged seizures often have a temporary hemiparesis. Those who have ingested phencyclidine (PCP) and lysergic acid (LSD) may present with focal seizures and hemiparesis. Adolescents have presented with strokes after ingesting stimulants containing phenylpropanolamine. These cerebrovascular manifestations are thought to result from severe hypertension. A complicated migraine may also present with acute weakness. Neoplasms, inflammatory bowel disease, nephrotic syndrome, and a number of rarer conditions have also been linked to childhood strokes.

Lower motor unit disease can occur in the spinal column, the anterior horn cells, and the peripheral nerve and muscle. Spinal cord injury is usually secondary to severe trauma. Transverse myelitis is an inflammatory process occurring at the thoracic level of the spinal cord. It develops quickly, with symptoms of weakness accompanied by back pain, fever, myalgias, and often paresthesias of the legs. Frequently, loss of bowel and bladder control develops, and there is often a cerebrospinal fluid (CSF) lymphocytosis. Transverse myelitis has been associated with numerous infectious causes, but it is uncertain whether the inflammation is from the infection itself or its vascular complications. The lesion of transverse myelitis may be identified by magnetic resonance imaging (MRI).

Patients with a spinal epidural abscess present with fever, back pain, and radicular pain. This condition can lead to spinal cord dysfunction and paralysis if it continues undiagnosed. The infection is usually spread hematogenously; *Staphylococcus aureus* is the most common agent. There may be significant vertebral tenderness or a fluctuant mass, which usually occurs at the midthoracic or lower lumbar area. CSF analysis usually shows increase CSF protein and a mild leukocytosis. A spinal epidural abscess is a surgical emergency.

Fortunately, poliomyelitis is currently more important historically than clinically. It usually appears as an asymmetric pattern of scattered weakness. Bulbar involvement can result in respiratory embarrassment, and a CSF mononuclear pleocytosis is usually present.

Weakness may also occur because of abnormality in the peripheral neuromuscular apparatus, which includes the peripheral nerves, the neuromuscular junction, and the muscles themselves. Acute inflammatory polyneuroradiculopathy (Guillain-Barré syndrome), an autoimmune demyelinating disease, is the most common neuromuscular condition requiring critical care management in children. Weakness is often ascending and symmetric, beginning distally and progressing to the proximal muscles. Facial weakness occurs in 50% of patients. Sensory involvement is variable, and autonomic dysfunction may result in cardiac arrhythmias. Spinal fluid analysis reveals an increased CSF protein level and a normal cell count. Respiratory failure is the most ominous symptom and must be closely monitored.

TABLE 134–2

ACUTE WEAKNESS: THERAPY AT A GLANCE

Condition	Therapy
Meningitis	Antibiotics, dexamethasone (Decadron)
Spinal trauma	Immobilization, methylprednisolone (Solu-Medrol)
Spinal epidural abscess	Surgical decompression
Organophosphate toxicity	Atropine, pralidoxine
Tick paralysis	Removal of the tick
Periodic paralysis	
Hypokalemia	Potassium, acetazolamide
Hyperkalemia	Hydrochlorthiozide, acetazolamide
Normokalemia	Increase salt, administer acetazolamide

Treatment is supportive, and many of these children regain complete neurologic function.

Heavy metal poisonings and various medications may cause peripheral neuropathy in a child. Children with lead poisoning often present with colic, pallor, and weakness and may present with encephalopathy. Mercury and arsenic poisoning are also associated with peripheral neuropathy. Antibiotics and chemotherapeutic agents (especially vincristine) may cause peripheral neuropathy.

Tick paralysis is the result of release of a neurotoxin from a tick. Interestingly, many children who suffer a tick bite also have cerebellar symptoms. Symptoms usually develop from 4 to 7 days after attachment and initially include restlessness and irritability, as well as an ascending flaccid paralysis. Respiratory paralysis and death may follow if the tick is not removed. Rapid recovery usually follows tick removal (Table 134–2).

Infant botulism results from the intestinal production of the botulism toxin by *Clostridium botulinum* spores. The toxin interferes with the release of acetylcholine at the neuromuscular junction. Symptoms include generalized weakness, constipation, poor feeding, and dysphagia. Decreased deep tendon reflexes occur over a period of time, and cranial nerve palsies also may develop. Electromyography is helpful in suggesting the diagnosis, which is confirmed by identification of *C. botulinum* toxin or isolation of the organism in the feces. Treatment is supportive; antibiotics and antitoxin are not indicated. Ingestion of honey containing *C. botulinum* spores has been linked to infant botulism in previously reported cases.

Several other conditions may affect the neuromuscular junction and cause acute weakness. Myasthenia gravis is caused by antibodies directed at the muscle end-plate receptor; it may be congenital, familial, or autoimmune. Usually there is fluctuating weakness, but acute decompensation may occur from intercurrent illness, certain medications, and electrolyte imbalances. Organophosphate poisoning can cause weakness because of its potent anticholinesterase activity. Hypomagnesemia can also cause acute weakness. Shellfish poisoning and the bite of a black widow spider can cause toxin-mediated weakness.

Acute myopathic weakness is usually the result of disordered potassium metabolism or rhabdomyolysis. Acquired hypokalemia or hyperkalemia may cause acute weakness. Periodic paralysis is a set of familial conditions that result in intermittent weakness. These conditions usually cause intermittent weakness, which may be precipitated by exercise or cold. The serum potassium level may be low, normal, or

high. Hyperthyroidism can also cause a similar condition. Rhabdomyolysis and myoglobinuria can cause weakness and may occur secondary to trauma, exertion, or heat stroke.

DIAGNOSTIC EVALUATION

It is usually apparent from the history and physical examination whether the weakness involves the central or peripheral nervous systems. A CT scan is often necessary in evaluating a child with acute CNS weakness. Evaluation of the spinal fluid is also necessary if an infectious origin is suspected. Angiography and other studies may be necessary if the diagnosis is still unclear.

The evaluation of the child with lower motor unit disease is more complex. If the findings suggest spinal cord involvement, emergent neurologic or neurosurgical consultation is imperative. If neuromuscular abnormality is suspected, determination of serum electrolyte, calcium, magnesium, and creatine kinase levels and a toxicology screen may also be indicated. The physician should always consider spinal trauma and thoroughly examine the child for a tick.

ADMISSION CRITERIA

Almost all children with acute weakness require admission, as the evaluation often cannot be completed in the emergency department, and admission is necessary to follow the progressions of the weakness. Particular attention should be paid to the child's respiratory status, as a number of the conditions mentioned earlier may affect the respiratory muscles.

Selected References

1. Enberg RN, Kaplan RJ. Spinal epidural abscess in children. Clin Pediatr 1974;13:247.
2. Fenichel GM. Clinical syndromes of myasthenia in infancy and childhood. Arch Neurol 1978;35:97.
3. Gold AP, Carter S. Acute hemiplegic of infancy and childhood. Pediatr Clin North Am 1976;23:413.
4. Gorman RJ, Snead C. Tick paralysis in three children. Clin Pediatr 1978;3:249.
5. Johnson RO, Clay SA, Arnon SB. Diagnosis and management of infant botulism. Am J Dis Child 1979;133:586.
6. Paine RS, Byers RK. Transverse myelopathy in childhood. Am J Dis Child 1953;85:151.

CHAPTER 135

Ataxia

Mananda S. Bhende

INTRODUCTION

Ataxia refers to incoordination of movement without loss of muscle strength and with or without disturbance of balance.

Coordination of movement is mediated by the cerebellum, which modifies muscle tone and contraction so that movements are smooth. Thus cerebellar dysfunction can cause ataxia, but ataxia may also result from dysfunction of a variety of anatomic structures, such as the cerebral cortex (frontal ataxia) and the spinal cord and peripheral sensory nerves (sensory ataxia), or from disturbances in the vestibular labyrinthine pathways (labyrinthine ataxia). Ataxia can also be caused by drugs and toxins, and, rarely, it is a manifestation of a psychiatric disorder.

Ataxia can be classified according to the temporal mode of presentation (e.g., acute, acute remitting, or chronic). Chronic ataxia can be progressive or nonprogressive. The physician encountering a patient with ataxia should focus on common causes such as infections, drug ingestion, and neoplasm of the posterior fossa.

ANATOMY AND PHYSIOLOGY

The anatomy of the cerebellum and its intricate afferent and efferent systems is complex. The cerebellum, or "little brain," is located in the posterior fossa. Its ventral surface forms the roof of the fourth ventricle. Therefore, a space-occupying lesion such as a tumor, hematoma, or abscess that involves the cerebellum can impede cerebrospinal fluid flow. Acute hydrocephalus leads to signs of increased intracranial tension such as headache, vomiting, papilledema, and cranial nerve palsies.

The cerebellum is called a "silent" area of the brain, because electrical excitation of this structure does not cause sensory or motor movement. Nevertheless, removal of the cerebellum does cause movement to be abnormal. The cerebellum helps sequence motor activities. It also monitors and makes adjustments in the motor activities elicited by other parts of the brain so that movements are smooth.

The cerebellum is connected to the brain stem by three large paired peduncles through which the afferent and efferent connections between the cerebellum and the rest of the nervous system pass. The inferior peduncle connects the cerebellum to the medulla oblongata and carries important sensory fibers from joints, tendons, and muscles by the dorsal spinocerebellar tract, and from the vestibular apparatus by the vestibulocerebellar tract. The middle peduncle connects the cerebellum to the pons and carries afferent fibers from the cerebral cortex. Efferent fibers mainly pass through the superior peduncle, which connects the cerebellum to the midbrain.

The cerebellum is made up of two parts: a midline structure called the *vermis* and two lateral masses called *cerebellar hemispheres*. The flocculonodular lobe of the hemispheres, along with the caudal part of the vermis, receives the bulk of the vestibular afferent systems and is responsible for the maintenance of equilibrium when sitting, standing, or walking. The cerebellar hemispheres regulate the movement of the ipsilateral limbs, the rostral and caudal portions of the cerebellar hemisphere near the midline regulate the ipsilateral lower limbs, and the lateral midportion of the hemisphere controls the movements of the ipsilateral upper limbs.

Dysfunction in the cerebellum can result in two different clinical entities: the syndrome of cerebellar hemispheres, which affects ipsilateral limb movements, and the syndrome of midline structures, which causes swaying of the trunk, or titubation, when sitting, standing, or walking.

CLINICAL EVALUATION
History

A detailed history should be obtained. Knowing whether the onset is acute, acute but remittent, or chronic helps to formulate diagnosis. Does the ataxia involve only the trunk or also the limbs and eyes? Headaches, nausea, early morning vomiting, lethargy, blurred vision, and a change in mental function or behavior suggest a tumor.

Systemic complaints such as fever, rash, photophobia, and nuchal rigidity could indicate encephalitis or meningitis as the cause of the ataxia. If the patient has a recent history of viral illness, especially influenza, varicella, mononucleosis, *Mycoplasma* infection, or measles, the physician should consider the possibility of postinfectious acute cerebellar ataxia. This is usually benign and is one of the most common causes of acute ataxia. A history of head trauma is extremely important to elicit, as the ataxia may be a result of brain edema or cerebellar hemorrhage, which may require immediate neurosurgical intervention. Rarely, chronic suppurative otitis can lead to the formation of a cerebellar abscess.

A history of drug ingestion is important, as this is a common cause of acute ataxia. An accidental overdose of anticonvulsants (especially phenytoin), sedatives, antihistamines, alcohol, and drugs of abuse (e.g., phencyclidine) can cause ataxia. If a bottle of alcohol or glasses partially filled with alcohol are left within reach, a child may accidentally consume the beverage and present with ataxia. Any relationship between the ataxia and meals may suggest a metabolic disorder. Any other neurologic symptoms, such as paresthesias, dysthesias, weaknesses, speech changes, or history of seizures, should also be elicited.

Physical Examination

Vital signs should be checked, and in the critically ill child, shock, meningitis, septicemia, and metabolic events such as hypoglycemia should be excluded, as all of these can have acute ataxia as a presenting sign. In the comatose child who is ataxic, increased intracranial tension may be present. A compatible history and physical findings of papilledema, sixth nerve palsy, abnormal pupillary size, decreased heart rate, and increased blood pressure lead to the diagnosis of increased intracranial pressure, which should be immediately treated. The skin should be checked for rashes. The examiner should be alert for viral exanthems, especially vesicular or crusted lesions of varicella. Postinfectious acute ataxia usually presents 1 to 3 weeks after the antecedent illness. The physician should also check for otitis, pharyngitis, and lymphadenitis. The presence of heart murmurs and arrhythmias on cardiac examination may suggest an embolism. Splenomegaly can be present in patients with infectious mononucleosis. The abdomen should be palpated for masses, as a child with ataxia may have a neuroblastoma.

The approach to the child with ataxia varies with the child's age. Observing the young infant's spontaneous activity at play and while sitting, standing, and walking gives an idea of motor coordination. When there is truncal ataxia, the child may not be able to sit without the support of the upper extremities. Observations should be made before approaching and performing the general examination. The child may look perfectly well while lying in a comfortable and secure position; difficulty in maintaining balance may be obvious only when sitting or standing.

In an older child, the physician can perform the standard neurologic examination. The child should be made to walk and observed for narrow gait base. Mild abnormalities can be elicited if the child is made to walk in a tandem fashion (heel to toe) and made to turn quickly. A toddler generally has a wide-based gait. Asynergy (the loss of coordinated action between muscle groups) and dysmetria (the ability to gauge the distance, speed, and power of movement) can be tested by finger-to-object, toe-to-object, or heel-to-knee-to-shin maneuvers. Dysdiadochokinesia, a disturbance in the coordination of agonist and antagonistic muscle groups, can be tested by asking the patient to perform rapidly alternating hand or foot movements. Weakness, spasticity, or rigidity of a limb can impair these movements as well and should be checked. Nystagmus is checked both on horizontal and vertical gaze. Chaotic conjugate eye movements are called *opsoclonus*. When opsoclonus is present with myoclonus and ataxia, the child may have occult neuroblastoma. Assessment for quality of speech and a thorough examination of the cranial nerves and motor system, looking for asymmetry in strength, tone, and deep tendon reflexes, should be performed. Deep tendon reflexes are absent in Guillain-Barré syndrome and Fisher's syndrome.

Pure cerebellar ataxia is not associated with mental function changes, weakness, or abnormal sensory examination. Midline cerebellar disease can lead to equilibrium problems. The patient presents with swaying or titubation of the head and trunk. Diseases of cerebellar hemispheres can affect ipsilateral limb function.

A thorough sensory examination is performed, testing for proprioception and sensitivity to vibration, pain, touch, and temperature. Romberg's test should be performed. When the patient is unable to stand erect with eyes closed, but can do so with them open, the test result is abnormal. Any impairment demonstrated on these tests is diagnostic of sensory ataxia. Labyrinthine ataxia is normally associated with nystagmus and hearing deficits.

Tick toxin is a known antecedent of acute ataxia, and ticks should be carefully sought, especially in endemic areas. The physician should also look for things that can simulate ataxia, such as joint disease, a foreign body in the foot, and weakness

caused by Guillain-Barré syndrome, spinal cord disorders, or spasticity.

DIAGNOSTIC EVALUATION

A careful history and physical examination assists in selecting appropriate laboratory studies for diagnosis (Fig. 135–1). A complete blood cell count may show atypical lymphocytes in infectious mononucleosis, and the Monospot test may be positive. Determination of serum glucose, sodium, and ammonia levels can exclude hypoglycemia, hyponatremia, and hyperammonemia, respectively, as causes of ataxia.

Blood and urine toxicology screens should be obtained in all patients with pure cerebellar ataxia. If the patient is on anticonvulsant medication, serum levels should be measured. The toxicology screen should check for ataxia-causing drugs (e.g., anticonvulsants, hypnotics, phenothiazines, alcohol, heavy metals, and drugs of abuse such as PCP).

If there is any sign of increased intracranial tension, such as a headache, vomiting, papilledema, or cranial nerve palsy, a computed tomographic (CT) scan should be obtained. Scans should be performed both with and without contrast. Cerebral angiography may be required to further clarify the diagnosis.

A lumbar puncture should be performed after obtaining a CT scan and tested for appropriate viral and bacterial pathogens. Cerebrospinal fluid protein is increased in Guillain-Barré syndrome, and pleocytosis is usually found in acute postinfectious cerebellar ataxia. Cerebrospinal fluid immunoglobulin and myelin basic protein are measured if a

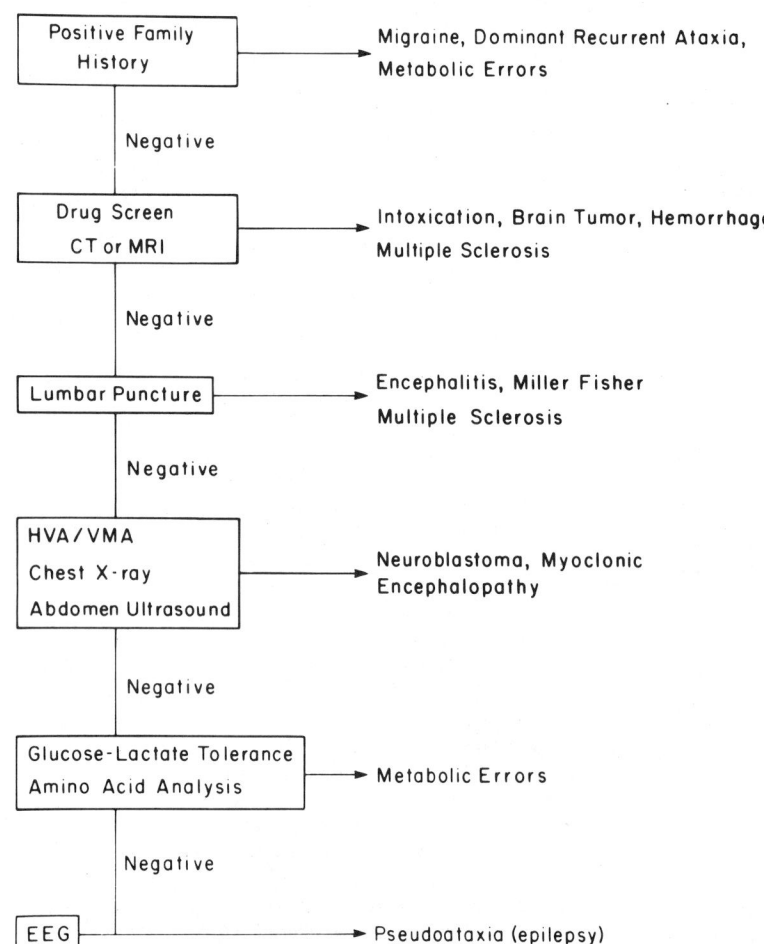

Figure 135–1. Diagnostic studies in acute cerebellar ataxia. (From Fenichel GM. Clinical Pediatric Neurology: A Signs and Symptoms Approach. Philadelphia, WB Saunders, 1988, p 225.)

demyelinating disease is suspected. Magnetic resonance imaging (MRI) is a more appropriate diagnostic evaluation than CT in those patients with elevated cerebrospinal fluid protein levels.

The triad of opsoclonus, ataxia, and myoclonus suggests an occult neuroblastoma. Chest and abdominal radiographs, ultrasonography, and 24-hour urine tests to determine homovanillic acid and vanillylmandelic acid levels are indicated in such cases.

Vestibular function tests such as electronystagmography and the Nylan-Bárány maneuver may be helpful in differentiating labyrinthine ataxia. Electromyography (EMG) and motor and sensory nerve conduction studies may be helpful in diagnosing sensory ataxias. Electroencephalography (EEG) may be helpful in patients with seizures presenting as ataxias.

Patients with chronic ataxia usually have been evaluated by a neurologist and do not present to the emergency department for further diagnostic evaluation. However, more sophisticated laboratory studies may be needed in these patients, including tests to measure blood and urine amino acid levels and blood pyruvate and lactate levels; a white blood cell count or fibroblast measurement may be needed to determine lipid metabolism. Serum immunoglobulin A (IgA) levels are decreased in patients with ataxia-telangiectasia.

DIFFERENTIAL DIAGNOSIS

As noted earlier, ataxia can be acute, acute remittent, and chronic (Table 135–1). Acute cerebellar ataxia, a common cause of acute ataxia, is characterized by the sudden onset of ataxia after a nonspecific infectious illness. The cause is usually heterogeneous (i.e., a number of infectious agents

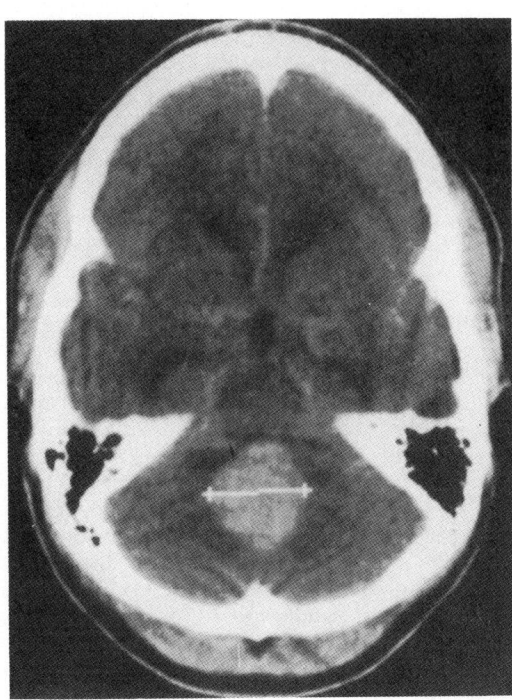

Figure 135–2. CT scan shows a midline infratentorial lesion in the vermis of the cerebellum. This enhancing tumor was a medulloblastoma. (From Fenichel GM. Clinical Pediatric Neurology: A Signs and Symptoms Approach. Philadelphia, WB Saunders, 1988, p 236.)

are directly or indirectly responsible for it). Cases have been reported after influenza, infectious mononucleosis, polio virus, coxsackievirus type B, echovirus type 6, herpes simplex virus, and infection with *Mycoplasma pneumoniae*, although they most commonly occur after varicella. The ataxia is often severe and of sudden onset. Children younger than 5 years are primarily affected, but older children can also present with ataxia. Nystagmus is present in about half of patients, and most have dysarthria. Patients may also complain of headache, dizziness, and photophobia. The cerebrospinal fluid usually shows a mild pleocytosis. Acute cerebellar ataxia usually has a benign course and resolves within a few weeks to 2 months. In about one third of cases, there can be residual symptoms.

Drug intoxication is a common cause of acute ataxia. Phenytoin, phenobarbital, carbamazepine, valproate, diazepam, alcohol, tricyclic antidepressants, PCP, hypnotics, sedatives, heavy metals (e.g., lead), insecticides (DDT), lindane, and organic solvents (e.g., carbon tetrachloride) can all cause ataxia. Toxicology screening tests of blood and urine should be performed in all children presenting with acute ataxia. The ingestion could be accidental, iatrogenic (as when trying to change doses of anticonvulsants), or suicidal.

Posterior fossa tumors usually present with slow onset but can be acutely recognized or actually have an acute presentation. The ataxia could result from dysfunction of the cerebellum or from hydrocephalus. Cardinal features are headache, vomiting, papilledema, neck stiffness, and sometimes a head tilt. About 50% of intracranial tumors in children occur in the posterior fossa. Astrocytomas, medulloblastomas, ependymomas of the fourth ventricle, and brain stem gliomas may all present in the posterior fossa. Medulloblastomas are usually midline tumors, and astrocytomas usually start in the cerebellar hemispheres (Fig. 135–2). A CT or MRI scan should be obtained. Steroids are often used

---

TABLE 135–1

ATAXIA: DIFFERENTIAL DIAGNOSIS

Acute ataxia
  Acute cerebellar ataxia (postinfectious, influenza, infectious mononucleosis, polio, coxsackievirus, echovirus, herpes simplex virus, *Mycoplasma* infection, varicella)
  Drug intoxication (anticonvulsants, alcohol, tricyclics, hypnotics, sedatives, phencyclidine, insecticides)
  Posterior fossa mass (tumor, abscess, hematoma)
  Head trauma (postconcussion trauma, subdural and parenchymal hematoma, hemorrhage, vertebrobasilar occlusion)
  Brain stem encephalitis
  Postinfectious encephalomyelitis
  Noncerebellar causes (labyrinthitis, hysteria, seizures)
  Hydrocephalus
  Weakness (Guillain-Barré syndrome, transverse myelitis, tick paralysis)
Acute remitting ataxia
  Inherited disorders (Hartnup disease, maple syrup urine disease, pyruvate decarboxylase deficiency, carnitine acetyltransferase deficiency)
  Basilar artery migraine
  Benign paroxysmal vertigo
Chronic ataxia
  Posterior fossa tumors (medulloblastoma, astrocytoma, ependymoma, cerebellar hemangioblastoma)
  Supratentorial tumors
  Hydrocephalus
  Hereditary ataxias (Friedreich's ataxia, Leigh's syndrome, ataxia-telangiectasia)
  Congenital malformations (aplasia, Arnold-Chiari malformation, Dandy-Walker malformation)

to reduce tumor size. Ventriculoperitoneal shunts are frequently placed by a neurosurgeon prior to tumor resection.

Ataxia may be present as a part of the postconcussion syndrome. A CT scan is necessary in this case to exclude bleeding, edema, cerebellar contusion, or cerebellar hematoma as causes. A rapidly expanding hematoma in the cerebellum can be lethal. Also, basilar skull fractures may occur as a result of head trauma, producing damage to the vestibular system; the patient may be ataxic as a result.

Weakness can produce ataxia, but this is a notorious diagnostic trap. Muscle strength should be checked. Guillain-Barré syndrome presents with ascending weakness, absence of deep tendon reflexes, and an increased cerebrospinal fluid protein level. Transverse myelitis has more prominent sensory changes, and such patients also have bowel and bladder problems. Tick paralysis, myositis, myasthenia gravis, poliomyelitis, and toxic neuritis can present with weakness and resultant ataxia. Careful observation is mandatory in these patients, as they may develop respiratory problems from muscle weakness and require ventilatory support.

Stroke resulting in acute ataxia is rare in children, but can occur. Vasculitis associated with lupus erythematosus can give rise to discrete pontine strokes and present with ataxia. Ataxia can also be a presenting symptom of multiple sclerosis in adolescents. Fisher's syndrome is characterized by ophthalmoplegia, ataxia, and areflexia; the clinical course is usually benign, with complete recovery. Ear disease as a cause of vertigo and ataxia is less common in children than in adults. Acute labyrinthitis can present with vertigo and ataxia, and ataxia can also develop as a consequence of heat stroke, a result of hyperthermia-induced cerebellar degeneration.

Basilar artery migraine and paroxysmal benign vertigo can present as recurrent acute ataxia. A family history and the paroxysmal nature of the ataxia is highly suggestive of the diagnosis. Prophylactic treatment is with propanolol.

Epilepsy may present as ataxia. A patient may have atypical petit mal seizures or be postictal, with no one witnessing the seizure. Metabolic conditions such as hypoglycemia, hyponatremia, and hyperammonemia may all result in acute ataxia. Rarely, thiamine deficiency, manifested as Wernicke's encephalopathy, may present as ataxia.

Metabolic disorders that cause acute intermittent ataxia include Hartnup's disease, pyruvate decarboxylase deficiency, maple syrup urine disease, argininosuccinicaciduria, and hypothyroidism.

Chronic ataxias are associated with congenital anomalies of the cerebellum, Friedreich's ataxia, ataxia-telangiectasia, Leigh's syndrome, hydrocephalus, and congenital anomalies such as the Arnold-Chiari and Dandy-Walker syndromes.

THERAPEUTIC INTERVENTION

There is no specific therapy for most ataxias (Table 135–2). Nevertheless, specific therapy, when available, is dependent on the cause of the ataxia.

Hypoglycemia should be diagnosed promptly and treated by giving 0.5 to 1.0 gm/kg of dextrose intravenously. A total dose of 2 to 4 ml/kg of D25W is given intravenously. If hyponatremia causes seizures, it must be promptly corrected with intravenous normal saline. Meningitis should be treated with antibiotics, and a cerebellar abscess requires neurosurgical intervention and antibiotics.

Acute cerebellar ataxia is self-limiting and usually a diagnosis of exclusion. Even if a cause such as varicella is obvious, a CT scan is normally obtained to exclude a space-occupying lesion. Toxicology screening tests for drugs and a lumbar puncture are performed. If everything else is excluded, the

TABLE 135–2
ATAXIA: THERAPY AT A GLANCE

No specific therapy for most ataxias
Acute cerebellar ataxia—diagnosis of exclusion; CT scan, lumbar puncture, toxicology screen
Treat treatable causes—hypoglycemia, hyponatremia, meningitis
Drug toxicity—treatment depends on drug; usually symptomatic
Increased intracranial tension
  Diagnose
  Hyperventilation, mannitol, CT scan
  Neurosurgical intervention
Opsoclonus, myoclonus, ataxia triad—exclude neuroblastoma
No sedatives—exacerbate symptoms
Conversion reaction, suicide attempt—obtain psychiatric consultation

physician is absolutely certain of the diagnosis, and the child has only mild ataxia, the child may be followed closely at home. The patient's case should be discussed with a neurologist who can later evaluate the child. The ataxic child may be vomiting and subsequently admitted for hydration. Care should be taken not to prescribe sedatives, as they exacerbate signs of ataxia.

Therapy for toxic ingestions depends on the drug and amount ingested and the presenting signs. Usually, if ataxia is caused by anticonvulsants and the serum level is only minimally higher than normal, withholding doses (after consulting with the neurologist) is all that is needed. If serum levels are quite high, the child may need therapy with activated charcoal along with further treatment, following the guidelines for the specific toxin ingested. If the toxic ingestion involves antihistamines and completely resolves during the workup of ataxia, the child may be discharged. If residual symptoms of ataxia are present or there are other indications (e.g., hypertension) for monitoring the child, the child should be admitted and treated appropriately.

Tick paralysis is effectively treated by removal of the tick. Patients with neuroblastoma may receive symptomatic relief with corticotropin. Therapy for posterior fossa tumors depends on the tumor type and is determined by the neurosurgeon. For conversion reactions presenting as ataxia and for suicidal patients, psychiatric consultation must be obtained.

DISPOSITION

Most patients with acute ataxia of unknown cause are admitted for diagnostic evaluation (Table 135–3). Patients may be discharged if, after extensive evaluation, the physician concludes that the patient has mild acute cerebellar ataxia and close follow-up is ensured. Patients who have

TABLE 135–3
ADMISSION AND DISCHARGE CRITERIA FOR ATAXIA PATIENTS

Most patients with new-onset acute ataxia are admitted to the hospital
Acute cerebellar ataxia—if workup is negative, patient may be sent home if ataxia is mild and close follow-up and good supervision are ensured. If any doubt, admit.
Drug toxicity—if very mild and patient improves while waiting in emergency department, patient may be discharged with close follow-up. Admit all others.

experienced a mild drug overdose with anticonvulsants are sometimes discharged if, by withholding doses, they improve markedly in the emergency department.

Selected References

Bell WE. Ataxia in childhood: Clinical approach and differential diagnosis. Lancet 1965;85:2.

Bennett HS, Selman JE, Rapin I, et al. Nonconvulsive epileptiform activity appearing as ataxia. Am J Dis Child 1982;136:30.

Donat JR, Auger R. Familial periodic ataxia. Arch Neurol 1979;36:568.

Fenichel GM. Ataxia. In Fenichel GM (ed). Clinical Pediatric Neurology: A Signs and Symptoms Approach. Philadelphia, WB Saunders, 1988, pp 233–247.

Kinast M, Levin HS, Rothner AD, et al. Cerebellar ataxia, opsoclonus, and occult neural crest tumor. Am J Dis Child 1980;134:1057.

King G, Schwarz GA, Slade HW. Acute cerebellar ataxia of childhood; report of nine cases. Pediatrics 1958;21:731.

Korobkin M, Clark RE, Palubinskas AJ. Occult neuroblastoma and acute cerebellar ataxia in childhood. Pediatr Radiol 1972;102:151.

Marks HG, Augustyn P, Allen RJ. Fisher's syndrome in children. Pediatrics 1977;60:726.

Peters ACB, Versteeg J, Lindeman J, et al. Varicella and acute cerebellar ataxia. Arch Neurol 1978;35:769.

Reilly PA, Johnston AW. Cerebellar ataxia in infectious mononucleosis. Scott Med J 1986;31:183.

Roberts KB, Freeman JM. Cerebellar ataxia and "occult neuroblastoma" without opsoclonus. Pediatrics 1975;56:464.

Solomon GE, Chutorian AM. Opsoclonus and occult neuroblastoma. N Engl J Med 1968;279:475.

Steele JC, Gladstone RM, Thanasophon S, et al. Acute cerebellar ataxia and concomitant infection with Mycoplasma pneumoniae. J Pediatr 1972;80:467.

Stumpf DA. Acute ataxia. Pediatr Rev 1987;8:303.

CHAPTER 136

Meningitis

Johanna Goldfarb

INTRODUCTION

About 20,000 cases of meningitis occur each year in the United States, and 70% are in children under 5 years of age. Most occur in the first year, with a peak incidence between 6 to 8 months of age, and 4% to 10% are fatal. Pneumococcal meningitis has the highest fatality rate, up to 20%. An even higher percentage of cases are associated with permanent neurologic damage, varying from hearing loss to devastating loss of cerebral function.

ANATOMY AND PHYSIOLOGY
Hematogenous Spread

Most cases of meningitis in childhood develop as the result of hematogenous seeding of the meninges. Bacteremia is almost always seen during the acute presentation of meningitis. The pathogens responsible for most episodes of meningitis in the pediatric age group are also responsible for most other serious pediatric infections (Table 136–1). The possibility of meningitis must be considered in every child under 2 years of age being evaluated for bacteremia or other serious bacterial infection. Empiric therapy in such

TABLE 136–1
BACTERIAL PATHOGENS CAUSING MENINGITIS IN CHILDREN

Newborns	*Streptococcus agalactiae* (group B streptococcus) *Escherichia coli* *Listeria monocytogenes* *Salmonella* sp.
After 6 wk of age	*Neisseria meningitidis* *Streptococcus pneumoniae* *Haemophilus influenzae* type b
After neurosurgery or open head trauma	*Klebsiella* sp. *Escherichia coli* *Pseudomonas aeruginosa* staphylococci, coagulase positive and negative

children must be effective against meningitis, even when there is another clear focus of infection. In particular, bacteremia with *Haemophilus influenzae* frequently causes focal infections in multiple sites simultaneously (Table 136–2).

Neisseria meningitidis, Streptococcus pneumoniae, and *H. influenzae* type b can colonize the respiratory tract of asymptomatic adults and children. There is often a history of an upper respiratory infection (URI) just before the onset of meningitis. A viral infection may interfere with local host defense mechanisms, allowing mucosal invasion in a previously well but colonized child.

The pathogens associated with neonatal sepsis and meningitis are different from those found in older children (Table 136–1). These organisms usually are introduced by exposure to vaginal flora at birth or to environmental flora (including that of caregivers) after birth. Often the newborn's gastrointestinal tract is the first site to be colonized with a potential pathogen such as the group B streptococcus. Breast feeding may be important in determining which organisms colonize the tract. Invasion and bacteremia do not occur in every colonized baby. With group B streptococci, the presence of passively acquired, organism-specific maternal antibodies increases protection from bacteremia in such infants.

Direct Extension

Other cases of meningitis are due to direct extension of infection from parameningeal sites. Sinusitis or a chronic otitis media may extend and spread directly to the central nervous system (CNS). In addition to meningitis, parameningeal infections may develop into brain abscesses or intracranial, extracerebral collections of pus (subdural or epidural empyema).

Head Trauma

Head trauma, even without cerebrospinal fluid (CSF) leak, is associated with an increased risk of meningitis. In most of

TABLE 136–2
BACTEREMIA-ASSOCIATED INFECTIONS IN CHILDREN

H. influenzae type b: Meningitis, pneumonia, otitis media, facial cellulitis, bone and joint infections, pericarditis, epiglottitis
N. meningitidis: Meningitis, bacteremia, arthritis
S. pneumoniae: Meningitis, pneumonia, otitis media, arthritis

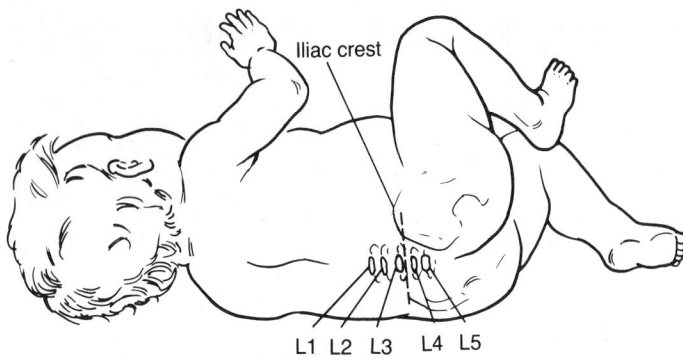

Figure 136–1. Lumbar punctures can be performed with patients either lying on their side or in a sitting position. Flexion of the lumbar spinal column facilitates entry into the subarachnoid space. The posterior superior iliac crest corresponds to the level of L4. Manometry is used to measure the opening pressure.

these cases, meningitis is caused by *S. pneumoniae*. A disruption of the sinuses allows direct seeding of the meninges by organisms that colonize the sinuses.

Postneurosurgery

Disruption of CNS integrity by surgical trauma is also associated with a risk of meningitis by direct seeding. The organisms responsible for these infections are different from those associated with bacteremia or sinusitis. Skin flora and hospital-acquired pathogens are more common. Staphylococci and gram-negative bacteria, including *Pseudomonas*, are regularly seen in this setting. Previous treatment with broad-spectrum antimicrobial agents may predispose the patient to have resistant organisms, including fungi.

CLINICAL EVALUATION

The Newborn

Irritability, poor feeding, hypothermia or hyperthermia, and increased sleepiness may be present in infected newborns. However, meningitis is often difficult to diagnose in these infants because of this nonspecific presentation. For this reason, a lumbar puncture is a routine part of the sepsis evaluation in newborns with fever or other nonspecific signs consistent with infection. Some series suggest that with a negative spinal tap, and no other risk factors for sepsis, newborns with fever can be managed as outpatients. The standard practice, however, is to admit and treat all infants up to the age of 4 weeks with fever for possible sepsis and meningitis until culture results are available. This is based on the small number of infants who, after presenting with nonspecific findings, develop apnea, seizures, or shock and have a fulminant course of sepsis or meningitis.

The Infant and Young Child (Older Than One Month)

Children with meningitis frequently have a recent history of a URI. A new fever in a child recovering from URI should suggest a secondary bacterial infection, including not only otitis media and pneumonia, but also sepsis and meningitis. A high fever, especially in a child under 2 years of age, must be evaluated with these diagnoses in mind. Classic signs of meningitis include neck stiffness, irritability, sleepiness, vomiting, and seizures. The presence of these signs with fever in any age group should suggest the possibility of meningitis.

Young children are often difficult to evaluate; examination is often incomplete. Nuchal rigidity may be absent in the very young, and also in comatose patients. In infants younger than 12 months with fever and nonspecific findings, it is appropriate to perform a lumbar puncture because it is difficult to carry out an adequate examination and the risks of a lumbar puncture are minimal. Some believe that a child who is ill enough to warrant a lumbar puncture should be admitted and treated empirically. Even if the CSF is normal, occult bacteremia may be present. Meningitis can follow bacteremia, even if oral or low-dose intravenous antimicrobial agents are given. Therefore, empiric antimicrobial agents used in this setting should have good CSF penetration and be given in doses effective against meningeal infection.

DIAGNOSTIC EVALUATION

Once the diagnosis of meningitis is under consideration, a lumbar puncture must be performed promptly (Figs. 136–1, 136–2). CSF should be collected for culture and chemistries (Table 136–3). A Gram stain may be useful in identifying organisms. If the fluid is grossly turbid, an unspun specimen can be used; if the fluid appears clear, spinning

TABLE 136–3					
CEREBROSPINAL FLUID FINDINGS					
Gram Stain	**Bacterial**	**Bacterial, Partially Treated**	**Tuberculosis**	**Viral**	**Parameningeal Focus**
Cells/ml	200–5000	200–5000	< 1000	< 1000	< 500
Cell type	Mostly PMN	Mostly PMN	Mostly L	PMN, L	Variable
Glucose	↓	↓ or normal	↓	Normal	Normal
Protein	↑	↑	↑	↑	↑
Gram stain	±	±	–	–	–
Bacterial culture	+	±	–	–	–

L = Lymphocyte; PMN = polymorphonuclear cell.

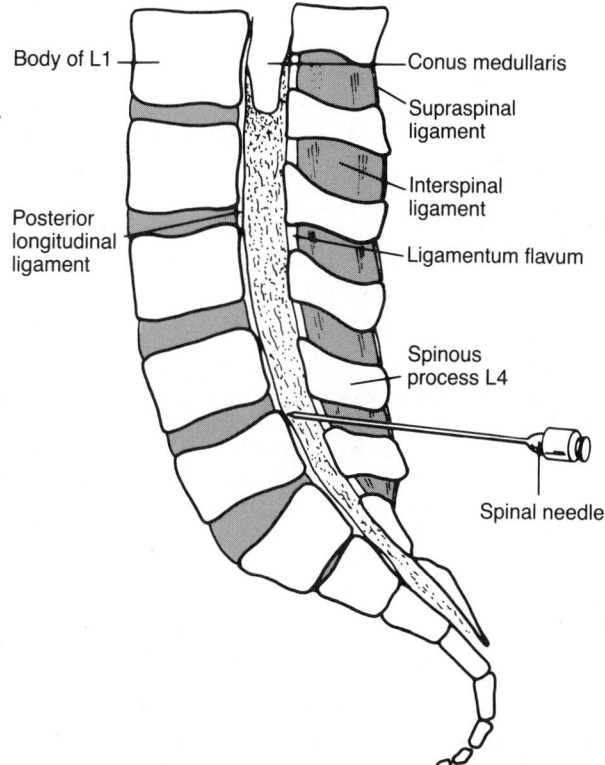

Figure 136–2. A spinal tap performed at the level of L4–L5 is far from the conus medullaris, which ends at the L1–L2 disk space. The needle should enter the subarachnoid space as it passes through the ligamentum flavum.

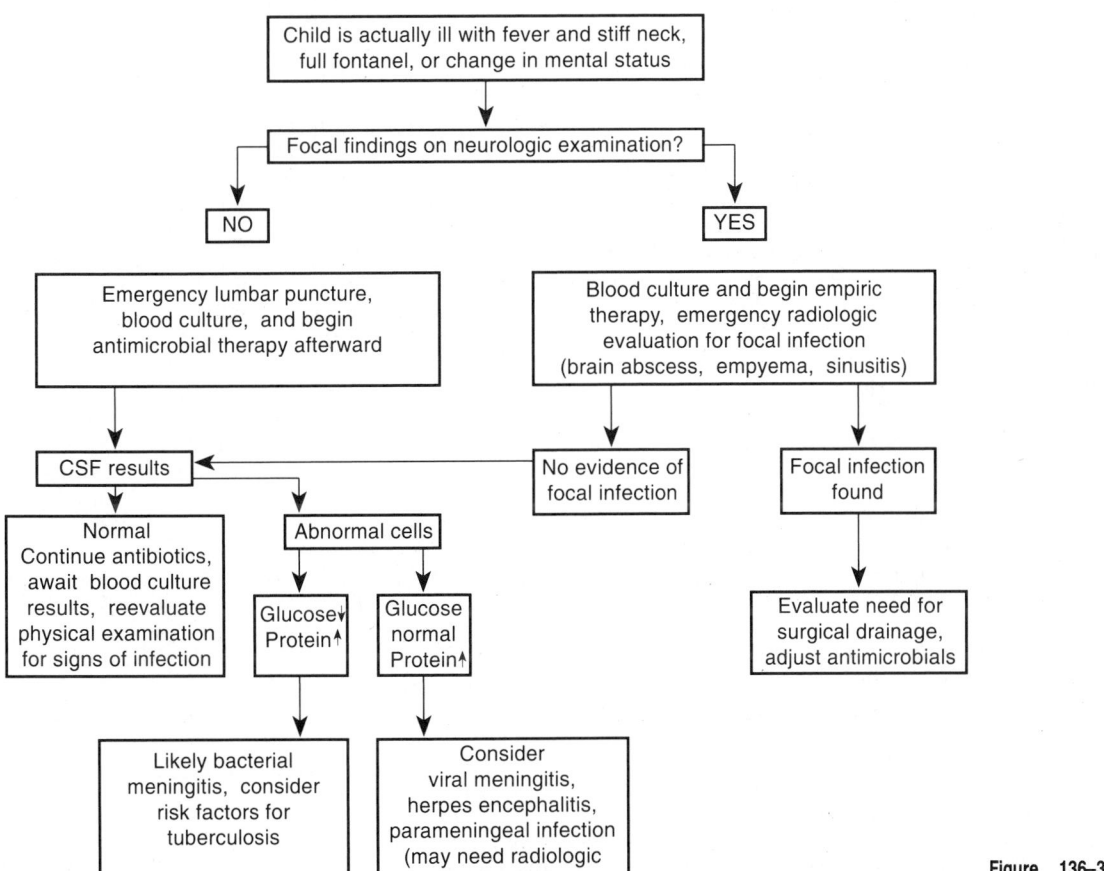

Figure 136–3. Management of acute meningitis.

the specimen and examining the sediment will increase the yield on Gram stain. A low CSF glucose level (less than half the serum glucose) suggests a bacterial etiology. Rarely, CSF glucose is low with viral infections, although this is seen frequently with mumps meningitis, occasionally with herpes simplex encephalitis, and sometimes with enteroviral meningitis. The child with partially treated bacterial meningitis may have a normal CSF glucose level, but the cellularity should still suggest a bacterial process; i.e., with bacteria there is usually a predominance of polymorphonuclear leukocytes. Early in the course of viral meningitis, polymorphonuclear cells may predominate. The cell type will change to a mononuclear predominance over the first hours of illness. The CSF protein is elevated with both viral and bacterial processes; extremely elevated protein should suggest the possibility of a CSF obstruction.

If the CSF reading is suggestive of acute bacterial meningitis (polymorphonuclear cells, low glucose, high protein), rapid antigen detection tests can be made. These may expedite the decision to give prophylaxis appropriately, but should never be used to limit treatment of a patient for all potential pathogens. The isolation and susceptibility patterns of the pathogen should be the gold standards used to narrow therapy.

When a space-occupying lesion is suspected, the lumbar puncture should be delayed pending emergency neuroimaging. However, therapy should not be delayed. After blood for culture is obtained, empiric antimicrobial therapy should be administered immediately (Table 136–4). A focal infection may be defined by use of contrast material and special views of the sinuses. Surgical intervention may be needed (drainage of focal intracranial infection). Lumbar puncture is contraindicated with a space-occupying lesion, as herniation may occur. If the study is normal, a lumbar puncture can be done. The CSF cell count is still useful in determining the presence of meningitis, even if the use of antimicrobials makes the culture results less accurate.

A baseline complete blood count is useful for following response to therapy. A low white blood cell count has prognostic significance, especially in newborns. Significant neutropenia correlates with a poor outcome in all age groups.

Many children presenting with mild dehydration and a history of abnormal fluid intake require measurement of electrolytes and blood urea nitrogen. Those who present in shock should be evaluated for disseminated intravascular coagulation (DIC).

DIFFERENTIAL DIAGNOSIS

Fever with neck stiffness in older children is highly suggestive of meningitis (Fig. 136–3). When this is accompanied by a change in mental status (lethargy, irritability, seizures), encephalitis or an encephalopathy, with or without concomitant meningitis, is likely. Other diagnoses, including brain abscess or intracranial collections of pus, should be considered when there are neurologic findings such as focal seizures or paralysis.

Nuchal rigidity is occasionally seen with a retropharyngeal abscess and severe cervical adenitis. In the absence of fever, but with altered sensorium or severe headache, a subarachnoid hemorrhage should be considered. The finding of CSF cells and negative culture results should prompt consideration of alternative diagnoses.

Epidemics of enteroviral infections occur during the summer months. Enteroviral infection in newborns often presents as fever and mild irritability, and meningitis is common. CSF shows pleocytosis with a lymphocytic predominance,

TABLE 136–4
BACTERIAL MENINGITIS IN CHILDREN: EMPIRIC THERAPY

Newborns

Ampicillin, 150–200 mg/kg/day	Divided every 6 hr
At 1 wk of age	Divided every 4 hr
and	
Gentamicin, 7.5 mg/kg/day*	Divided every 12 hr
or	
Amikacin, 22 mg/kg/day*	Divided every 8–12 hr
or	
Cefotaxime, 150–200 mg/kg/day†	Divided every 6–8 hr

Children over 6–8 wk

Ceftriaxone, 100 mg/kg/day	Divided every 12 hr
or	
Cefotaxime, 200 mg/kg/day	Divided every 6 hr
Chloramphenicol, 75–100 mg/kg/day*	Divided every 6 hr

Children After Neurosurgery or with Open CNS Wound‡

Vancomycin, 40–60 mg/kg/day*	Divided every 6 hr
and	
Ceftazadime, 200 mg/kg/day	Divided every 6 hr
and	
Gentamicin, 7.5 mg/kg/day*	Divided every 6–8 hr
or	
Amikacin, 22 mg/kg/day*	Divided every 8–12 hr

*Follow serum levels and adjust doses accordingly.
†Children beyond the immediate newborn period (> 4 wk) become more at risk for *H. influenzae* type b meningitis, and ampicillin and cefotaxime becomes the preferred empiric regimen, with ampicillin for *Listeria*.
‡Evaluate each child individually for a history of recent antimicrobial therapy and the presence of unusual colonizing agents such as fungus.

normal glucose, and moderately elevated protein. Young infants with CSF pleocytosis are usually admitted and treated empirically while negative bacterial cultures are awaited, in view of the serious consequences of missing bacterial meningitis. Viral cultures from rectal swabs and CSF are often positive. Herpes simplex infection is a possibility in ill-appearing newborns with a CSF reading suggestive of a viral process. Empiric acyclovir therapy is appropriate for such infants. Appropriate cultures should be sent; rectal swab, CSF, nasopharynx, and urine.

Herpes simplex infection also occurs in older children, usually in the form of severe encephalitis. Temporal lobe focal abnormalities on electroencephalography are specific for this presentation of herpes simplex. Empiric acyclovir therapy should be considered in older children with viral encephalitis. In this setting the CSF culture is most often negative. Other causes of the encephalitis should be sought while therapy is continued. An older child with mild viral meningitis during the enteroviral infection season, who looks well but who has nuchal rigidity, can be admitted and observed without therapy.

Encephalopathy from metabolic causes or drugs is usually not associated with fever, and there is usually no neck stiffness; the CSF is normal. In Reye's syndrome a low CSF glucose level often reflects a low serum glucose. This is most often seen in young children, CSF is otherwise normal in Reye's syndrome (Table 136–5).

THERAPEUTIC INTERVENTION

Once the diagnosis of meningitis is made or suspected, antibiotic therapy should be started immediately (see Table 136–4 and Table 136–6). Children with possible *H. influenzae* or *N. meningitidis* infections should be kept in respiratory

TABLE 136–5

DIFFERENTIAL DIAGNOSIS OF BACTERIAL MENINGITIS

Meningitis
Tuberculous meningitis
Cryptococcal meningitis
Viral meningitis:
    Enteroviruses
    Herpes simplex type 2
Viral encephalitis
    Herpes simplex type 1 or 2 (in newborn)
    Herpes simplex type 1 (older child, adult)
    Arboviruses
    Human immunodeficiency virus
    Epstein-Barr virus
Sepsis
Gram-negative bacteremia
Rocky Mountain spotted fever
Endocarditis
Parameningeal/Intracranial Foci
Brain abscess
Sinusitis
Epidural or subdural empyema
Noninfectious Conditions
Drug-induced encephalopathy
Epidermoid cyst of meninges
Cancerous meningitis
Subarachnoid bleed
Reye's syndrome

TABLE 136–7

MENINGITIS PROPHYLAXIS*

Meningococcal Infections
Household, day care center, nursery school contacts, and anyone with close, intimate contact with oral secretions should receive chemoprophylaxis: rifampin,† 20 mg/kg/day divided q 12 hr for 2 days (total 4 doses) (maximal dose, 600 mg/day)
Alternate therapy: if rifampin contraindicated and specific isolate is sensitive: sulfisoxazole, 500 mg daily for infants < 1 yr old and 1 gm every 12 hr for children > 12 yr and adults for a total of 2 days
H. influenzae Infections
Household contacts should receive chemoprophylaxis only if there is at least one child 4 years old or younger in household (all in household, adults, children, and patient, should receive therapy, including previously immunized children)
Day care contacts: Consider prophylaxis when two or more cases of serious *H. influenzae* infections have occurred within 2 mo. In small day care settings in which children under 2 yr old spend 25 hr/wk or more together, prophylaxis may be recommended even after a single case. However, unless most of the children and attendants participate, prophylaxis is unlikely to be useful.
Rifampin,† 20 mg/day in one daily dose for 4 days; maximal dose, 600 mg/day

*Remember, prophylaxis does not always prevent disease. Fever in a susceptible contact of a child with either *H. influenzae* or *N. meningitidis* infection should be promptly evaluated for possible early meningitis, even if prophylaxis was given.
†Pregnant women should not take rifampin. Rifampin causes orange urine, stool, and tears and it may stain soft contact lenses. Use with care in patients with significant liver dysfunction. (Adapted from Committee on Infectious Diseases. American Academy of Pediatrics: Report of the Committee on Infectious Disease, 1991. Elk Grove Village, IL, American Academy of Pediatrics, 1991.)

isolation until 24 hours after the start of effective antimicrobial therapy, to prevent secondary spread. Prophylaxis for close contacts should be considered (Table 136–7).

Controversy over the use of steroids continues. The American Academy of Pediatrics recommends that dexametha-

TABLE 136–6

BACTERIAL MENINGITIS IN CHILDREN: ORGANISM-SPECIFIC THERAPY

Specific therapy (when culture results are available)
H. influenzae type b
Ampicillin, 300–400 mg/kg/day divided every 4 hr
(if beta-lactamase–negative, sensitive organism isolated)
    or
Continue chloramphenicol, ceftriaxone, or cefotaxime for 10 days
Meningococcus
Penicillin G, 300,000 units/kg/day IV divided every 4 hr for 7–10 days
Pneumococcus
Penicillin-sensitive strains: Penicillin G, 300,000 units/kg/day IV divided every 4 hr for 10 days.
Relatively resistant strains: Ceftriaxone or cefotaxime for 10 days.
Truly resistant strains: Vancomycin, 60 mg/kg/day IV divided every 6 hr for 10 days.
Group B Streptococcus
Penicillin G, 300,000 mg/kg/day divided every 4 hr
    or
Ampicillin, 300–400 mg/kg/day divided every 4 hr
Continue an aminoglycoside (gentamicin or tobramycin) until child is stable and organism is identified as penicillin sensitive
Recurrence and relapse occur with this pathogen
Treat for 3 wk and follow CSF to be sure infection is clearing
E. coli, Salmonella
Use antibiotic sensitivities to guide therapy; treat for 3 wk or more; follow newborns with *Salmonella* closely for relapse; check CSF for response to therapy

sone (0.6 mg/kg/day divided in four doses for 4 days) be started immediately when the diagnosis of bacterial meningitis is certain and the child is over 2 months of age. This recommendation is made on preliminary data for *H. influenzae* meningitis. There may be a decreased risk of hearing loss when steroids are used. However, other authorities question these results and do not recommend steroids. When an organism other than *H. influenzae* is isolated or partially treated meningitis or aseptic meningitis is diagnosed, dexamethasone should be discontinued.

Supportive care is important, especially in the first 12 to 24 hours. Children with newly diagnosed meningitis must be regarded as critically ill and monitored intensively for life-threatening complications such as seizures with respiratory arrest, herniation with respiratory or cardiac arrest, septic shock, and DIC. Children admitted with dehydration should be hydrated promptly. If signs of shock are present or develop (poor perfusion, decreased capillary refill, decreased blood pressure), appropriate lines for arterial and venous pressure monitoring should be placed, and blood pressure supported with fluid and vasopressors. Platelets and clotting factors may be needed if DIC develops.

Seizures should be controlled acutely with diazepam and then with loading doses of phenytoin. Because of its sedating effect, phenobarbital should be avoided when possible. This is especially true during the early stages when assessment of mental status is most important. Most deaths and acute deteriorations occur in the first 24 hours of therapy. The child with rapidly progressing purpura is at great risk for rapid deterioration and death.

Newborns with true neutropenia have a poor prognosis. Neonates appear to have a smaller reserve pool of neutrophils, and their neutrophils are less effective than those of older children. White blood cell transfusions have been given in extremely neutropenic newborns for additional supportive therapy.

During the course of illness, the head circumference and neurologic findings must be followed closely. Complications of meningitis during the initial hospitalization include hydrocephalus and hearing loss. A return to normal mental status usually heralds survival. In the first days, prompt return to full alertness usually correlates with a good outcome. Hearing loss may be difficult to determine at first, especially in young infants. It sometimes presents as extreme irritability in infants who otherwise seem to be alert, awake, and improving. Hearing should be evaluated in all children before discharge, with follow-up in those who appear to have any deficit. There may be some improvement in hearing loss over time. An expanding head circumference, especially with full fontanel, sun-setting eyes, or other signs of increased intracranial pressure, should prompt an evaluation of the ventricular system. Shunting for hydrocephalus may be necessary. Since focal neurological deficits may occur, it is imperative that the neurologic examination be repeated several times each day initially and then daily.

Selected References

Barson WJ, Miller MA, Brady MT, Powell DA. Prospective comparative trial of ceftriaxone vs conventional therapy for treatment of bacterial meningitis in children. Pediatr Infect Dis 1985;4:362.

Baumgartner ET, Augustine A, Steel RW. Bacterial meningitis in older neonates. Am J Dis Child 1983;137:1052.

Broome CV, Mortimer EA, Katz SL, et al. Chemoprophylaxis to prevent the spread of *Haemophilus influenzae* B in day-care facilities. N Engl J Med 1987;316:1226.

Cherubin CE, Eng RHK, Norrby R, et al. Penetration of newer cephalosporins into cerebrospinal fluid. Rev Infect Dis 1989;11:526.

Committee on Infectious Diseases, American Academy of Pediatrics. Dexamethasone therapy for bacterial meningitis in infants and children. Pediatrics 1990;86:130.

Conly JM, Ronald AR. Cerebrospinal fluid as diagnostic body fluid. Am J Med 1983;75:102.

Enzenauer RW, Bass JW. Initial antibiotic treatment of purulent meningitis in infants 1 to 2 months of age. Am J Dis Child 1938;137:1055.

Feigin RD. Neonatal meningitis: Problems and prospects. Hosp Pract 1983;18:175.

Freedman RM, Ingram DL, Cross I, et al. A half century of neonatal sepsis at Yale. Am J Dis Child 1981;35:140.

Gold R. Bacterial meningitis—1982. Am J Med 1983;75:98.

Havens PL, Wendelberger KJ, Hoffman GM, et al. Corticosteroids as adjunctive therapy in bacterial meningitis. A metaanalysis of clinical trials. Am J Dis Child 1989;143:1051.

Jacobs RF, Wells TG, Steele RW. Yamuachi T. A prospective randomized comparison of cefotaxime vs ampicillin and chloramphenicol for bacterial meningitis in children. J Pediatr 1985;107:129.

Kaplan SL, Feigin RD. Treatment of meningitis in children. Pediatr Clin North Am 1983;30:259.

Lebel MH, Freij BJ, Syrogiannopoulos GA, et al. Dexamethasone therapy for bacterial meningitis. N Engl J Med 1988;319:964.

Mangi RJ, Quintiliani R, Andriole VT. Gram-negative meningitis. Am J Med 1975;59:829.

McCracken GH. Management of bacterial meningitis: Current status and future prospects. Am J Med 1984;76:S5A:215.

Naqvi SH, Maxwell MA, Dunkle LM. Cefotaxime therapy of neonatal gram-negative bacillary meningitis. Pediatr Infect Dis 1985;4:499.

Nelson JD. Emerging role of cephalosporins in bacterial meningitis. Am J Med 1985;79:S2A:47.

Osterholm MT, Pierson LM, White KE, et al. The risk of subsequent transmission of *Haemophilus influenzae* type B disease among children in day care. N Engl J Med 1987;316:1.

Smith AL: Neurologic sequelae of meningitis. N Engl J Med 1988;319:1012.

Stovring J, Snyder RD. Computed tomography in childhood bacterial meningitis. J Pediatr 1980;96:820.

Tauber MG, Sande MA. Principles in the treatment of bacterial meningitis. Am J Med 1984;76:S5A:224.

Tunkel AR, Ward JI, Band JD, et al. Bacterial meningitis: Recent advances in pathophysiology and treatment. Ann Intern Med 1990;112:610.

Yogev R. Advances in diagnosis and treatment of childhood meningitis. Pediatr Infect Dis 1985;4:321.

CHAPTER 137

Viral Encephalitis

Earl J. Reisdorff

INTRODUCTION

Viral encephalitis is an inflammatory process of the parenchyma of the brain. Encephalitis is characterized by an altered state of consciousness, impaired cognitive abilities, and a cerebrospinal fluid (CSF) pleocytosis. When the virus affects both the meninges and the brain, the term *meningoencephalitis* is used.

There are 1400 to 4300 cases of viral encephalitis reported annually to the Centers for Disease Control. The annual incidence of encephalitis is about 4.7 cases per 100,000. The overall mortality rate is 5% to 10%, but with some forms of encephalitis it can be as high as 70% to 80%.

ETIOLOGY

Viruses are the major cause of infectious encephalitis (Table 137–1). Thirteen percent of cases of encephalitis are arboviruses, 12% are herpes viruses, 10% are enteroviruses, 10% represent lymphocytic choriomeningitis, 5% are from other causes, and 48% are of unknown causes. Important nonviral causes of encephalitis include *Mycobacterium*, *Mycoplasma pneumoniae*, *Rickettsia rickettsii*, Lyme disease, *Leptospira interrogans*, *Treponema pallidum*, *Coccidioides immitis*, and *Naegleria* sp. In immunodeficient patients, *Toxoplasma gondii*, *Cryptococcus neoformans*, and *Listeria monocytogenes* can cause encephalitis.

Herpes Simplex Virus Type 1 (HSV-1)

Two strains of herpes simplex virus cause disease in humans. HSV-1 is associated with oral facial infections; HSV-2 with genital infections. HSV-1 is the important causative agent of acute postneonatal herpes simplex encephalitis; it is the single most common cause of nonepidemic encephalitis and accounts for 10% to 20% of all cases of encephalitis. Although individuals of all ages are susceptible to HSV-1 infection, 31% of cases of herpes simplex encephalitis occur in children. It can result from a primary infection (30%) or a reactivation of a previous infection (70%).

Arboviruses

No longer an official taxonomic term, *arbovirus* refers to more than 450 RNA viruses. The viruses are *ar*thropod-*bo*rne, forming the term *arbo*. This important class of RNA viruses includes St. Louis encephalitis (SLE), eastern equine encephalitis (EEE), western equine encephalitis (WEE), and California encephalitis (CE) viruses. Arboviruses account for about 10% of all cases of reported encephalitis, and can cause up to 50% of all cases of encephalitis in an endemic year.

Togaviruses are a group of arboviruses that cause eastern equine encephalitis, western equine encephalitis, Japanese B encephalitis, St. Louis encephalitis, Venezuelan equine encephalitis, and yellow fever. *Bunyaviruses* are another subset of arboviruses that cause the California and La Crosse encephalitides.

TABLE 137–1

COMMON INFECTIONS CAUSING ENCEPHALITIS

Togavirus (arbovirus)
  Eastern equine encephalitis
  Western equine encephalitis
  Venezuelan equine encephalitis
  St. Louis encephalitis
  Japanese encephalitis
  Powassan
Bunyavirus (arbovirus)
  California group
  La Crosse encephalitis
  California encephalitis
  Jamestown canyon
  Snowshoe hair
Arenavirus
  Lymphocytic choriomeningitis
Reovirus
  California tick fever
Rhabdovirus
  Rabies
Herpes virus
  Herpes simplex I and II
  Herpes varicella zoster
  Epstein-Barr virus
  Cytomegalovirus
Enterovirus
  Polioviruses 1–3
  Coxsackieviruses A2, 5, 6, 7, 9
  Coxsackieviruses B1–6
  Enteroviruses
  ECHO viruses 2–4, 6, 7, 9, 11, 14, 16, 18, 19, 30
Retrovirus
  HIV encephalitis
Myxovirus
  Measles encephalitis
Paramyxovirus
  Parainfluenza 3
Nonviral causes
  Mycoplasma pneumoniae
  Toxoplasma gondii
  Rickettsia rickettsii
  Naegleria fowleri

St. Louis Encephalitis (SLE)

SLE is the most common arbovirus (togavirus) disease in the United States. The annual incidence varies widely; the largest epidemic occurred in 1975 with 1815 reported cases and a mortality rate of 8%. SLE viruses are transmitted by mosquitoes.

Eastern Equine Encephalitis (EEE)

Infection by the EEE virus causes more serious illness, with a fatality rate of 74%. EEE occurs sporadically near freshwater marshes. Birds are the main reservoir and the virus is transmitted by mosquitoes.

Western Equine Encephalitis (WEE)

WEE occurs sporadically in irrigated rural areas of the western two-thirds of the United States. One of the highest attack rates of WEE occurs in infants under 1 year of age. Death is uncommon; the mortality rate is 2% to 3% but occasionally as high as 10%. Surviving children under 2 years of age infected by WEE can develop mental retardation, seizures, and spasticity. The WEE virus is also transmitted by mosquitoes. Garter snakes can also harbor the WEE virus after long periods of hibernation.

Japanese Encephalitis

Japanese encephalitis is the most widespread arbovirus-associated encephalitis internationally. It is most common in Asia, including India and southeast Asia.

California Encephalitis (CE)

CE has a wide geographic distribution and is most common in the upper Mississippi valley. The most important vector of the CE virus is the mosquito; the reservoir is a small rodent such as a squirrel. There is a predilection for woodland campers. The disease occurs primarily in children 5 to 9 years of age. Fatalities are rare, but personality changes and recurrent seizures are seen in up to 15% of affected children. Among ten types of CE virus, the most common is the La Crosse strain.

Enteroviruses

Enteroviral encephalitis occurs in children during warm summer months. Although enteroviruses cause 30% to 50% of all cases of viral meningitis, they cause only 2% to 10% of all cases of encephalitis. Children usually recover without sequelae.

Herpes Varicella

Herpes varicella encephalitis is rare. It most often affects immunocompromised patients. Varicella encephalitis has been reported to occur from 11 days before to 21 days after the onset of exanthema. The mortality rate in normal children with varicella encephalitis is 5.4 to 7.5 deaths per 10,000 reported cases.

Human Immunodeficiency Virus (HIV)

In addition to causing opportunistic infections, HIV attacks the brain, producing a form of encephalitis. The incidence of encephalitis has increased in parallel with the increase in HIV infections.

Other Viruses

Encephalitides due to the Epstein-Barr virus and cytomegalovirus also occur. Cytomegalovirus is exceedingly rare in previously healthy individuals but is more common in patients with immunodeficiency. Measles (rubeola) is a paramyxovirus that can also cause encephalitis. Immunization programs against measles have greatly diminished the incidence of measles encephalitis.

Mumps encephalitis is usually mild. In most cases there is fever, headache, nausea, vomiting, nuchal rigidity, and lethargy. The prognosis of mumps encephalitis is optimistic; the mortality rate is 1.5%.

The rabies virus causes encephalitis. Rabies is present in the saliva of infected dogs, cats, foxes, skunks, bats, and other domestic and wild animals. Lymphocytic choriomeningitis is a rare cause of encephalitis associated with exposure to certain rodents such as mice and hamsters.

Mycoplasma pneumoniae

Mycoplasma pneumoniae may be the cause of illness in up to 7% of patients treated for central nervous system (CNS) infection. The mortality rate in one report was 10%, with a morbidity of 24%.

Toxoplasmosis

Patients who develop toxoplasmic encephalitis are almost always immunodeficient and chronically infected with the protozoan. Almost one third of AIDS patients who are seropositive for *T. gondii* ultimately develop toxoplasmic encephalitis.

PATHOPHYSIOLOGY

Encephalitis is characterized by an inflammatory reaction involving both the meninges and blood vessels, with degenerative changes of the parenchymal nerve cells. The CNS is usually involved by hematogenous spread. Some forms of encephalitis can be contracted through direct neuronal spread such as herpes varicella zoster and rabies. Gross examination of the brain reveals edema and congestion. There may be small hemorrhages. Brain biopsy may show cellular inclusions suggesting herpes simplex, cytomegalovirus, measles, or rabies.

Herpes simplex encephalitis affects the frontal and temporal lobes. Rabies shows a predisposition for the brain stem and cortical gray matter. Herpes varicella virus is attracted to the cerebellum and may cause ataxia. Localized cerebritis may occur with other viruses, including the mumps, Epstein-Barr, polio, coxsackie, ECHO, enterovirus, and measles viruses. With EEE, lesions of the hippocampus can be pronounced.

Herpes Simplex Virus Type 1

HSV-1 encephalitis may be associated with bizarre behavior, olfactory or gustatory hallucinations, focal seizures, speech difficulties, memory loss, and anosmia. It accounts for 15% to 20% of all cases of viral encephalitis. There is no gender predominance, nor any seasonal predilection.

The course of herpes simplex encephalitis is progressive, with evolution from lethargy to deep coma. Terminally, brain stem herniation can occur. Common signs of HSV-1 encephalitis include an altered state of consciousness, abnormal behavior, and seizures. Focal neurologic deficits are evident in 60% of patients.

St. Louis Encephalitis (SLE)

The clinical presentation of SLE ranges from an aseptic, meningitis-like condition to a severe, fulminant encephalitis, leading to death within days. Headache, vomiting, and lethargy are typical. Meningeal signs and seizures are less common. The condition usually lasts 1 to 2 weeks. Children generally recover completely.

Eastern Equine Encephalitis (EEE)

EEE is both the most deadly and the least common arbovirus encephalitis in the United States. The onset is usually abrupt and characterized by a high fever, headache, and vomiting, followed by a decreased level of consciousness. Children generally show signs of meningismus. Mortality has been as high as 65% during some epidemics but is usually much lower; it is highest among younger children and children who develop coma. Mental impairment, seizures, and disturbed motor function are common among survivors.

Western Equine Encephalitis (WEE)

In infants, WEE is characterized by a septicemia-like picture and a bulging fontanelle. Older children may have a flu-like syndrome initially. Often, behavioral changes including delirium occur and may progress to coma. Symptoms usually last 1 to 2 weeks. The overall mortality rate of 3% to 10% usually involves infants; 37% to 64% of surviving infants have some permanent neurologic impairment.

California–La Crosse Encephalitis

California and La Crosse encephalitis usually occurs in children. The initial features of a flu-like syndrome last 2 or 3 days. The encephalitis is heralded by a headache, followed by seizures and a rapid progression to coma. Focal neurologic deficits develop in 20% of cases. Symptoms begin to resolve 3 to 5 days after onset, and most children recover without any neurologic sequelae. The peak incidence of California encephalitis is in the 5- to 9-year-old age group; 90% of the disease is seen in children under 15 years of age.

HIV Encephalitis

HIV encephalitis is characterized by loss of development milestones, dementia, weakness, and spasticity. Some children have involuntary movement disorders and seizures. HIV encephalitis causes a diffuse white matter disease with an inflammatory cell infiltrate.

Other Viruses

Lymphocytic choriomeningitis virus infection may be accompanied by arthritis, orchitis, parotitis, and cerebellar incoordination. With the measles virus, symptoms of encephalitis begin 1 to 8 days after the appearance of a rash, but it may be delayed for up to 3 weeks. The onset is usually abrupt and characterized by obtundation, which can rapidly progress to coma. Generalized seizures occur in 50% of patients. Neurologic morbidity (mental retardation, epilepsy, paralysis) is high. Measles encephalitis has occurred as a consequence of measles immunization; the incidence is estimated to be 1 per 1 million doses.

DIFFERENTIAL DIAGNOSIS

The differential diagnosis for the child with lethargy or seizures is extensive (Table 137–2). Trauma may be excluded by no history of injury, a physical examination showing no external injury or retinal hemorrhages, and a normal computed tomographic (CT) study.

Toxin-induced encephalopathy is supported by the presence of substances in the child's environment or a history of substance abuse. Toxins to consider include carbon monoxide, sedative-hypnotic agents, narcotic-opiates, and anticholinergics. A clinical response to naloxone suggests narcotic toxicity. Lead encephalopathy can also cause a viral encephalitis–like picture. Alcohols, including ethylene glycol and methanol, can also mimic viral encephalitis. Other possible diagnoses include endocrine disorders involving the metabolism of glucose, as well as syndrome of inappropriate antidiuretic hormone (SIADH). Uremic encephalopathy can be determined by measuring the serum BUN. Reye's disease is suggested by elevation of hepatic transaminase and serum ammonia. Other considerations involve testing for collagen vascular disease, neoplasms, or rare entities such as infantile botulism.

Alteration in cognitive function distinguishes viral encephalitis from aseptic meningitis. Other diagnoses to rule out are nonviral infectious encephalitis and bacterial meningitis; these distinctions can be difficult.

TABLE 137–2

DIFFERENTIAL DIAGNOSIS OF VIRAL ENCEPHALITIS

Infections
  Nonviral encephalitis
    Mycobacterium tuberculosis
    Mycoplasma pneumoniae
    Rickettsia rickettsii
    Lyme disease (*Borrelia burgdorferi*)
    Leptospira interrogans
    Treponema pallidum
    Coccidioides immitis
    Naegleria sp.
    *Toxoplasma gondii**
    *Cryptococcus neoformans**
    *Listeria monocytogenes**
  Meningitis
    Viral
    Bacterial (including *Mycoplasma,*
      Mycobacterium, Rickettsia)
    Fungal
    Protozoal
  Brain abscess
  Subdural, epidural empyema
  Sepsis
  Rabies
Trauma
  Epidural hematoma
  Subdural hematoma
  Subarachnoid hemorrhage
  Concussion, closed head injury
  Cerebral contusion
Toxins
  Carbon monoxide
  Lead
  Substances of abuse
  Sedative-hypnotic agents
  Opiates
  Anticholinergic agents
  Alcohols
Other Causes
  Tumors
  Leukemia
  Lymphoma
  Cerebrovascular event
  Hydrocephalus with shunt malfunction
  Postictal state
  Infantile botulism
  Reye's syndrome
  Cat-scratch disease
  SIADH
  Hypoglycemia
  Hyperglycemia, hyperosmolar coma
  Uremic encephalopathy
  Collagen vascular disease

*Seen more frequently in immunodeficient children.

CLINICAL EVALUATION

History

The onset of viral encephalitis may be sudden or gradual and is marked by fever, headache, vomiting, dizziness, and possibly a stiff neck. Ataxia, tremors, mental confusion, speech difficulties, stupor, hyperexcitability, delirium, convulsions, and coma may follow. There may be a prodrome lasting 1 to 4 days of fever and chills, headache, malaise, sore throat, conjunctivitis, and myalgias. For many of the arboviruses, the incubation period can last 5 to 15 days. A rapidly progressive clinical course without prodrome suggests HSV-1 or EEE.

A careful history must be obtained. The risk of drug or toxic exposure should be investigated. Any family history of migraine or epilepsy should be determined. One should ask about any recent or recurrent fever, infectious illness, or systemic condition and about headache, vomiting, stiff neck, seizures, irritability, or lethargy. Any travel history, animal or insect exposure, or prodromal illness should be investigated.

The time of year should be considered because the type of viral encephalitis varies according to the season. Arbovirus-induced encephalitis is a warm-weather disease. Sporadic cases of SLE, CE, EEE, and WEE begin during the hot summer months and subside during the autumn. Enteroviral encephalitis occurs predominantly during the summer and fall months. Mumps encephalitis occurs year round. Varicella encephalitis begins to rise in the winter months, peaks in the spring, and is lowest during summer and fall.

SLE, Japanese encephalitis, and WEE have a predilection for people in age extremes. The incidence of SLE is high in infants and lowest in children 5 to 12 years of age. WEE is not as common in children as in male adults. EEE attacks primarily the young; 70% of patients with EEE are under 10 years of age, and 25% below 1 year of age.

WEE and SLE are found throughout the United States. EEE is confined to the eastern seaboard. Powassan virus, a tick-borne virus, is found along the U.S.-Canadian border. California–La Crosse viruses have been isolated in states other than California and Wisconsin.

The physician should inquire about any bizarre behavior, olfactory or gustatory hallucinations, memory loss, or anosmia, because these are associated with HSV-1 (Table 137–3). With HSV-1, headache occurs in 80%, dysphasia in 76%, seizures in 67%, autonomic dysfunction in 60%, and ataxia in 40%. Focal paralysis, cranial nerve paralysis, and aphasia are also associated with HSV-1.

Physical Examination

The patient is usually drowsy, stuporous, or comatose. The body should be inspected for evidence of trauma, rash, needle marks to the limbs, meningismus, and cardiac disease. Drug or toxin exposure may be suggested by abnormal pupil

TABLE 137–3

CLINICAL FINDINGS IN PATIENTS WITH BIOPSY-PROVED HERPES SIMPLEX ENCEPHALITIS

Historical Findings	Percentage
Alteration of consciousness	97
Fever	90
Headache	81
Personality change	71
Seizures	67
Vomiting	46
Hemiparesis	33
Memory loss	24
Physical Findings	
Fever	92
Personality change	85
Dysphasia	76
Autonomic dysfunction	60
Ataxia	40
Hemiparesis	38
Seizures	38
Cranial nerve deficits	32
Visual field loss	14
Papilledema	14

Adapted with permission from Whitley RJ, Soong SJ, Linneman C Jr, et al. Herpes simplex encephalitis: clinical assessment. JAMA 1982; 247:312. Copyright 1982, American Medical Association.

size. The retinal examination should be performed to determine the presence of papilledema (increased intracranial pressure) and retinal hemorrhages (trauma, carbon monoxide toxicity). If there is fixed deviation of the eyes in a lateral direction, there may be focal seizures.

A physical examination should test the gag and cough response to determine patients' ability to protect their own airway. There may or may not be a stiff neck. With EEE, meningismus is usually present.

Neurologic disturbances may include hemiplegia, ataxia, and involuntary muscle movements. Focal neurologic disturbances are seen in 20% of patients with California–La Crosse encephalitis and 80% of those with HSV-1 encephalitis. Cranial palsies may be present, especially with HSV-1 encephalitis. Flaccid paralysis of the shoulder girdle muscles is consistent with tick-borne encephalitis.

Other features are more characteristic, albeit not diagnostic, of various forms of encephalitis. Lymphocytic choriomeningitis may be accompanied by arthritis, orchitis, or parotitis. Seizures occur in 50% of patients with rubella encephalitis.

DIAGNOSTIC EVALUATION

The definitive diagnosis of encephalitis is rarely made in the emergency department, but presumptive evidence of encephalitis can be obtained by lumbar puncture, neuroradiologic imaging, and blood tests.

Lumbar Puncture

A viral CNS infection is usually accompanied by cerebrospinal fluid (CSF) abnormalities, including pleocytosis with a lymphocytic predominance. There is usually a modest elevation of protein and a normal glucose level. However, these results may vary with different types of encephalitis. The CSF should also be tested for viruses and for bacteria (including *mycobacteria*) and fungi. A predominantly neutrophilic response in the CSF suggests a bacterial process. Nevertheless, early viral infection of the CNS can have a neutrophilic predominance. Normal CSF studies suggest a metabolic or toxic encephalopathy, although it does not entirely exclude early viral encephalitis. A lymphocytic pleocytosis may also be seen with a fungal or mycobacterial infection.

HSV-1

With herpes simplex encephalitis 90% to 95% of patients have abnormal CSF. The median white blood cell count is 130 WBCs/mm³. A characteristic CSF finding of HSV-1 in 75% to 85% of patients is red blood cells in the CSF due to necrotizing lesions; there may be up to 500 RBCs/mm³. The median protein concentration is 80 mg/dl, but 20% of patients have a normal protein concentration. The glucose concentration is usually normal. HSV-1 is rarely grown in the spinal fluid; cultures are negative in more than 95% of patients.

Arboviruses

SLE usually has a lymphocytic pleocytosis of 50 to 500 cells/mm³ and a protein concentration of 50 to 100 mg/dl. The glucose concentration is normal. Premortem isolation of the SLE virus is rare.

EEE usually shows an elevated CSF pressure with 200 to 2000 WBCs/mm³, half of which are neutrophils. The peripheral WBC count with EEE may be as high as 66,000 cells/mm³.

Western equine encephalitis CSF results show a mixture of neutrophils and lymphocytes; later in the course of the illness, only lymphocytes may be seen. Protein concentration is between 50 to 100 mg/dl.

California–La Crosse encephalitis shows pleocytosis, mainly of lymphocytes; the usual count is 50 to 200 cells/mm³.

Other Viruses

With measles encephalitis, CSF shows lymphocytic pleocytosis; the number of lymphocytes rarely exceeds 100 cells/mm³. The protein is generally 50 to 100 mg/dl and the glucose concentration is normal. With lymphocytic choriomeningitis, a high CSF lymphocyte count is present. With HIV infections, if a progressive encephalopathy is present, the HIV and antigen can usually be detected in the CSF.

Viral Detection

Some viruses can be detected in the CSF, but many are not. Togaviruses are rarely detected in the CSF. Enteroviruses, mumps, adenoviruses, herpes varicella zoster virus, and cytomegalovirus can be detected in the CSF. Viral antigens or antibodies may be detected in the CSF by enzyme-linked immunosorbent assays. St. Louis encephalitis virus, coxsackievirus, and echovirus have been cultured from the oropharynx.

Neuroradiology

CT scans of the head exclude cerebral trauma such as subdural hematoma, epidural hematoma, subarachnoid hemorrhage, or cerebral contusion. CT may also show signs of *Toxoplasma gondii* or cerebral edema, and can assist the neurosurgeon in selecting the site for brain biopsy.

No pathognomonic CT or magnetic resonance imaging (MRI) findings are noted with viral encephalitis. Nevertheless, signs of cerebral edema, obstructive hydrocephalus, and multifocal or disseminated lesions support the diagnosis of viral encephalitis.

With HSV-1 encephalitis, CT may show edema, mass effect, or hemorrhage. HSV-1 often shows hypodense enhancing lesions in the temporal or frontal lobes on CT. Early in the course of HSV-1 encephalitis, lesions may not be apparent; CT findings often are noted between the third and eleventh day of illness.

TABLE 137–4
VIRAL ENCEPHALITIS: THERAPY AT A GLANCE
Lethargy
D25W, 2–4 ml/kg
D50W, 1–2 ml/kg
Naloxone, 0.1 mg/kg
Intracranial Pressure
Hyperventilate, Pco₂ 25–30
Mannitol, 0.5 gm/kg 20% of solution
Furosemide, 1 mg/kg IV push
Seizure
Diazepam, 0.2 kg IV push
Midazolam, 0.15 mg/kg IV push
Phenytoin, 15 mg/kg at 1 mg/kg/min, not to exceed 50 mg/min
Antiviral Agent
Acyclovir, 10 mg/kg q8h over 1 hr

TABLE 137–5

EXPERIMENTAL SPECIFIC THERAPY FOR VIRAL CNS INFECTIONS

Virus	Agent	Dose	Comment
Cytomegalovirus	Ganciclovir	2.5–7.5 mg/kg IV q8h for 10 days, or longer if symptoms persist	Available on compassionate plea basis from Syntex Corporation; should have biopsy diagnosis before therapy; adjust dose for neutropenia and renal impairment Not yet used for congenital pediatric infections
Epstein-Barr	Ganciclovir	As above; duration uncertain	See above
Influenza A	Amantadine	5 mg/kg PO to a maximum of 150 mg if <10 yr old; 200 mg PO for >10 yr old; duration 7–10 days	Adjust dosage for renal impairment
Human immunodeficiency	3'-Azido-3'-deoxythymidine	250 mg PO q4h or 2.5–5.0 mg IV q4h	Available from Burroughs Wellcome Co. under protocol; important to exclude other concomitant CNS disease
Arenaviruses (hemorrhagic fevers)	Ribavirin	2 gm IV loading; then 1 gm q6h for 4 days, then 0.5 gm q8h for 6 days; or 2 gm PO loading and 1 gm q8h for 10 days may be adequate	Reported for Lassa fever only; hemolysis may result
Measles Acute	Ribavirin	2.5 mg/kg PO qid for 7 days	Dosage given has been used for uncomplicated measles; a dose three to five times greater might be considered for encephalitis
Subacute sclerosing panencephalitis	Ribavirin	10 mg/kg PO tid for 3 days, then 10 mg/kg bid for 6 wk	
Enterovirus Neonatal (high risk)	Human immunoglobulin for IV use	400 mg/kg IV as a single dose or divided over 2 days	High risk includes (1) concurrent maternal illness, (2) prematurity, (3) age <6 days at onset
Immunodeficiency disease	Human immunoglobulin for IV use	200–400 mg/kg IV q2–4 wk, based on response; intrathecal therapy may also be indicated	May want to screen lots for antibody against infecting virus; can check patient's serum and CSF for appearance of specific antibody

From Levin MJ, Rotbart HA. Current Therapy in Pediatric Infectious Disease–2. Toronto, BC Decker, 1988, p 145.

Routine Laboratory Studies

Other studies easily obtained through the emergency department are useful to exclude other causes of encephalopathy. Tests such as antibody titers, viral blood cultures, viral CSF cultures, or brain biopsy are not accessible to the emergency physician.

A drug screen and carboxyhemoglobin level test may be useful to eliminate toxic possibilities. A serum lead level test may be considered. A complete blood count may demonstrate basophilic stippling with lead toxicity. Sodium, glucose, and BUN testing may rule out metabolic causes for lethargy. WBC count and blood cultures may suggest bacteremia or sepsis. Hepatic transaminase and ammonia levels may be useful in excluding Reye's syndrome.

Ancillary Studies

Serial viral antibody titers can assist in diagnosing viral encephalitis, but this information is unavailable during emergent evaluation. One of the most definitive methods for diagnosing viral encephalitis is a brain biopsy, but is not accessible to the emergency physician.

The presumptive diagnosis of viral encephalitis is therefore based on the history, physical examination, and CSF evaluation. Neuroimaging studies may add weight to the presumptive diagnosis, and other more commonly used laboratory studies can be used to exclude other causes of lethargy.

THERAPEUTIC INTERVENTION
General Supportive Care

Most medical care for viral encephalitis is supportive (Table 137–4). Specific interventions require protection of the airway; the obtunded or comatose patient requires intubation. In addition, elevation of the head of the bed and hyperventilation decrease cerebral edema. Should seizures occur, diazepam may be given (0.2 mg/kg IV) followed by loading with phenytoin (15 to 20 mg/kg IV). The initial IV solution in the emergency department should be 0.9 normal saline at one half the maintenance rate.

If there is cerebral edema, hyperventilation, fluid restriction, and mannitol (0.5 gm/kg of 20% solution) should be considered. The use of dexamethasone is controversial.

Antiviral Therapy

Most viruses, particularly SLE, EEE, WEE, California–La Crosse, and Japanese B, have no specific therapy. Intraventricular immunoglobulin has been used to treat enterovirus encephalitis. The therapy with the greatest impact is that for HSV-1 encephalitis. Acyclovir is the treatment of choice, 10 mg/kg every 8 hours given over a 1-hour period for 10 to 14 days. The anticipated mortality rate for HSV-1 encephalitis treated without acyclovir is 30% to 70%. The rate for patients under 3 years of age whose HSV-1 encephalitis is treated with acyclovir is 6%. Acyclovir also significantly improves the outcome of surviving patients. Most children in whom early diagnosis is made can be expected to survive and resume near-normal functioning. Complications of acyclovir therapy are minor and may include rash, gastrointestinal upset, thrombophlebitis, and occasionally a mild azotemia.

Experimental treatment has been developed for other viral CNS infections (Table 137–5). The efficacy of such therapies is undetermined. The measles vaccine has decreased the incidence of measles encephalitis.

DISPOSITION

Any child in whom viral encephalitis is a possibility must be admitted to the hospital. All who show signs of obtundation require intensive care monitoring. Urgent consultation is required with a pediatric intensive care specialist, infectious disease specialist, and neurosurgeon. If the physician has enough presumptive evidence to suspect HSV-1 encephalitis, acyclovir therapy should be initiated urgently in the emergency department.

Selected References

Azimi PH, Cramblett HS, Haynes RE. Mumps meningocephalitis in children. JAMA 1969;207:509.

Brady MT, May R. Premortum isolation of St. Louis encephalitis virus: Case report on implications for hospital and laboratory personnel. Pediatr Infect Dis 1985; 4:548.

Chun RWM, Thompson WH, Grabow JD, et al. California arbovirus encephalitis in children. Neurology 1968;18:369.

Davis JM, Davis KR, Kleinman GM, et al. Computed tomography of herpes simplex encephalitis, with clinicopathological correlation. Radiology 1978; 129:409.

Dwyer JM, Erlendsson K. Intraventricular gamma-globulin for the management of enterovirus encephalitis. Pediatr Infect Dis J 1988;7:530.

Earnest MP, Goolishian HA, Calverley JR, et al. Neurologic, intellectual, and psychologic sequelae following Western encephalitis. Neurology 1971;21:969.

Greenburg SB, Taber L, Septimus E, et al. Computerized tomography in brain biopsy-proven herpes simplex encephalitis. Arch Neurol 1981;38:58.

Haverkos HW. Assessment of therapy for *Toxoplasma* encephalitis. The TE study group. Am J Med 1987;82:907.

Johnson KP. The pathogenesis of viral infections of the nervous system. Neurol Clin North Am 1984;2:179.

Johnson R, Milbourn PE. Central nervous system manifestations of chickenpox. Can Med Assoc J 1970;102:231.

Johnstone JA, Ross CAC, Dunn M. Meningitis and encephalitis associated with mumps infection: A 10-year survey. Arch Dis Child 1972;47:647.

Jubelt B. Enteroviral and mumps virus infections of the nervous system. Neurol Clin North Am 1984;2:187.

Kennard C, Swash M. Acute viral encephalitis: Its diagnosis and outcome. Brain 1981;104:129.

Kohl S. Herpes simplex viral encephalitis in children. Pediatr Clin North Am 1988;35:6465.

Kohl S, James AR. Herpes simplex virus encephalitis during childhood. Importance of brain biopsy diagnosis. J Pediatr 1985;107:212.

Koskiniemi M, Vaheri A. Acute encephalitis of viral origin. Scand J Infect Dis 1982;14:181.

Koskiniemi M, Vaheri A, Taskinen E. Cerebrospinal fluid alterations in herpes simplex virus encephalitis. Rev Infect Dis 1984;6:608.

Kumar R, Mathur A, Kumar A, et al. Clinical features and prognostic indicators of Japanese encephalitis in children at Lucknow (India). Indian J Med Res 1990;91:321.

Lehtokoski-Lehtiniemi E, Koskiniemi ML. *Mycoplasma pneumoniae* encephalitis: a severe entity in children. Pediatr Infect Dis J 1989;8:651.

Lind K, Zoffman H, Larssen SO. *Mycoplasma pneumoniae* infections associated with infection of the central nervous system. Acta Med Scand 1979;205:325.

Luft DJ, Brooks RJ, Conley FK, et al. Toxoplasmic encephalitis in patients with AIDS. JAMA 1984;252:913.

Menzies DW, Grocott HC, Huston AF, et al. Western equine encephalitis. Epidemiol Bull (Canada) 1986;12:27.

Michaels J, Sharer LR, Epstein LG. Human immunodeficiency virus type 1 (HIV-1) infection of the nervous system: A review. Immunodefic Rev 1988;1:71.

Przelomski MM, O'Rourke E, Grady GF, et al. Eastern equine encephalitis in Massachusetts: A report of 16 cases. Neurology 1988; 38:736.

Rantala H, Uhari M. Occurrence of childhood encephalitis: A population-based study. Pediatr Infect Dis J 1989;8:426.

Rennels MB. Arthropod-borne virus infections of the central nervous system. Neurol Clin 1984;2:241.

Schroth G, Gawehn J, Thron A, et al. Early diagnosis of herpes simplex encephalitis by MRI. Neurology 1987;37:179.

Selik RM, Starcher ET, Curran WJ. Opportunistic diseases reported in AIDS patients: Frequencies, associations and trends. AIDS 1987;1:175.

Taccone A, Gambaro G, Ghiorzi M, et al. Computerized tomography (CT) in children with herpes simplex encephalitis. Pediatr Radiol 1988;19:9.

Tenser RB. Herpes simplex and herpes zoster. Nervous system involvement. Neurol Clin 1984;2:215.

Whitley RJ, Arvin A, Corey L, et al. Vidarabine versus acyclovir therapy of neonatal herpes simplex virus. Pediatr Res 1986;20:323A.

Whitley RJ, Soong SJ, Linneman C Jr, et al. Herpes simplex encephalitis—clinical assessment. JAMA 1982;247:317.

CHAPTER 138

Cerebrovascular Syndrome

Margaret Orcutt Tuddenham
J. Stephen Huff

INTRODUCTION

Although arteriosclerotic vascular disease is the most common cause of stroke syndromes in adults, it is rarely associated with childhood stroke. Still, familial lipid abnormalities can cause early cerebrovascular disease. For children, the differential diagnosis includes such entities as arterial thrombosis, vasculitis, infection, emboli from a variety of causes, dural sinus thrombosis, cerebral vein thrombosis, cerebral hemorrhage, complex migraines, toxic ingestions, seizures, and metabolic derangements (Table 138–1). Unfortunately, the cause remains uncertain in many cases even after exhaustive evaluation.

ANATOMY AND PHYSIOLOGY

The major blood supply to the brain arrives from the carotid and vertebrobasilar circulations. Anastomoses found at the level of the circle of Willis are variable. All cerebrovascular disorders may be related to one of two mechanisms: either interruption of blood flow to part of the brain, or rupture of blood vessels with bleeding into the cerebral parenchyma (Fig. 138–1). The areas of cortex between distal portions of major arteries, the watershed areas, are particularly vulnerable to reductions in cerebral perfusion pressure.

Emboli interrupt blood flow to regions beyond the point of vessel obstruction, resulting in decreased oxygen and substrate supply to surrounding tissue, and in turn damage to neuronal tissue. This may progress to loss of the blood-brain barrier, leading to cerebral edema, which itself may be destructive. Emboli may originate in damaged vessels or

TABLE 138–1

DIFFERENTIAL DIAGNOSIS OF FOCAL NEUROLOGIC DEFECTS

Arterial thrombosis
　Moyamoya disease
　Aneurysm
　Fibromuscular dysplasia
　Periarteritis nodosa
　Other arteritis
　Vascular trauma
　Homocystinuria
Arterial embolus
　Cardiac defects
　Arrhythmias
　Endocarditis
　Fat emboli
Terminal arterial bed phenomenon (postarrest deficit)
Venous thrombosis or sinus thrombosis
　Cyanotic heart disease
　Malignancies
　Leukemias
　Disseminated intravascular coagulation
　Infection
　　Meningitis
　　Sinusitis
　　Orbital cellulitis
　　Mastoiditis
Hemorrhagic conditions
　Trauma
　Blood dyscrasias
　Arteriovenous malformations
　Interventricular hemorrhage (premature infants)
Toxic causes
　Chemotherapy
　Lactic acidosis syndromes
Seizures
　Todd's paralysis
Complex migraines

meningitis or to autoimmune entities such as systemic lupus erythematosus or Henoch-Schönlein purpura, may produce focal neurologic deficits. Varicella may produce an arteritis, giving rise to cerebral emboli.

Traumatic injury may predispose to occlusion of the middle cerebral artery, the internal carotid artery, or the dural venous sinus. Intraoral trauma may result in occlusion of the internal carotid in the tonsillar fossa. This injury occurs when a child falls with objects such as a pencil or toy in the mouth. The hallmark of a carotid artery tear is a latent period with slowly enlarging clots or delayed embolization. Focal hemiparesis, with or without seizures, may occur up to 24 hours after injury. Cervical trauma can also cause vertebrobasilar occlusion or the vessels may be directly injured, with intimal disruption leading to dissection; nontraumatic vascular dissections have also been reported. Long-bone fractures producing fat emboli may also associate with a latent period.

Migraines may mimic stroke, with hemiplegia or focal weakness, with or without headache. Hypoglycemic hemiplegia is another transient stroke-like syndrome. Moyamoya disease is a form of aneurysmal abnormality consisting of net-like vessels at the base of the brain. The most common presentation in children is recurrent hemiplegias. Children with cyanotic congenital heart disease are at risk for cerebral abscesses and aseptic infarctions. Unusual metabolic conditions such as homocystinuria and MELAS (mitochondrial encephalomyopathy with lactic acidosis and stroke) syndrome are rare causes of stroke in children.

EMS CONSIDERATIONS

A significant percentage of children present with seizures, making attention to the airway and ventilation imperative. A brief history of any trauma and any metabolic, toxicologic, or other reversible conditions should be obtained from

from abnormal cardiac valves. Paradoxic emboli may occur in children with cyanotic heart disease. Platelet aggregation abnormalities or coagulopathies are also risk factors for stroke.

Occlusion in a vein is likely to result in rupture of the vessel, with hemorrhage and an increase in intracranial pressure. Extravasated blood may act as a mass lesion. The presence of red blood cell components may produce vasospasm, which further compounds the ischemia.

An arteriovenous malformation (AVM) may occur in the cortex, cerebellum, or brain stem, with corresponding symptoms from mass effect. The admixture of normal and abnormal vessels commonly results in seizures. However, subarachnoid and intraparenchymal bleeds may originate from an AVM. Bruits heard over the head are a cardinal sign of AVM and should not be ignored, especially in an infant under 4 months of age. In older children, bruits are indicative of AVM only about 50% of the time. Aneurysms, rare in children under 10 years of age, may also present with focal findings if large enough to act as a mass lesion or lead to hemorrhage.

Cerebrovascular accidents occur in children with hemoglobinopathies such as sickle cell disease. Bleeding disorders, including the factor deficiencies and idiopathic thrombocytopenic purpura, may result in intracranial hemorrhage. Central nervous system (CNS) hemorrhage occurs in some patients with leukemia. Other causes of stroke in children with cancer include vascular thrombosis associated with disseminated intravascular coagulation, arterial or dural thrombosis associated with chemotherapy, and metastatic tumors. Vasculitis, whether secondary to infections such as

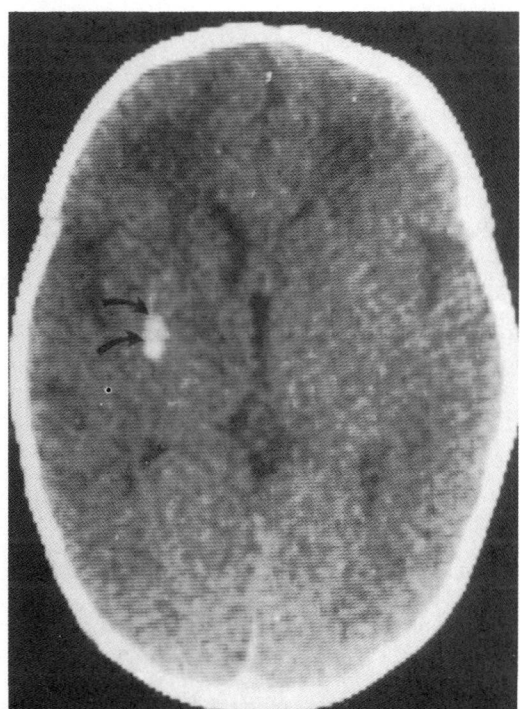

Figure 138–1. Cerebral hemorrhage. Arrows indicate a small hemorrhage. (From Fenichel GM. Clinical Pediatric Neurology: A Signs and Symptoms Approach. Philadelphia, WB Saunders, 1988, p 250.)

parents or care providers. Radio contact should be made to authorize intravenous access, obtain instructions for seizure management if necessary, and arrange transport to an appropriate facility.

CLINICAL EVALUATION
History

Once the patient is in the emergency department, ABCs must be addressed and a brief 30-second assessment performed. Intubation, ventilation, and vascular access should be accomplished with minimal delay. The search for a specific cause of stroke should then begin.

Initial inquiry should relate to the time and abruptness of onset of symptoms, the circumstances at time of onset, the presence or absence of seizures, alterations in level of consciousness, or ongoing systemic disorder of any kind. The history should be explored for diabetes, sickle cell disease, leukemia, or autoimmune or bleeding disorders. Any recent history of trauma should be explored; abuse may be a possibility when findings and history are not in agreement. A thorough family history may reveal migraines or hemophilia. Adolescents should be questioned, alone, about drug use. Ancillary personnel may be employed to question friends about recreational ingestions.

Physical Examination

The physical examination in the emergency department should aim to discover correctable causes as well as establish life-preserving and brain-preserving priorities. Neurologic findings are the central focus of the physical examination, but clues to systemic illness, occult trauma, old injury, or developmental delay will be found through a complete head-to-toe, clothes-off examination. Complete vital signs should be reviewed. Fever, if present, must be addressed. The examiner should pay close attention to unilateral findings or muscle atrophy.

The patient's general appearance and odor, the nature of the cry, the level of consciousness, and the state of anxiety should be observed. Cutaneous findings may indicate an infectious or autoimmune etiology, specifically meningitis or Henoch-Schönlein purpura. This should be followed by a detailed examination geared to reveal any deficits or abnormalities and any focal neurologic findings. The examiner should pay attention to age-related milestones and always use "pairs" (e.g., matching affected arm to unaffected arm) when attempting to determine focality. Many clues are offered by sick children apart from the verbal history; infants have fontanelles and expressive faces, toddlers do not stop "toddling" without grave provocation, and children with congenital cyanotic heart disease often have prominent clubbing and blue lips. Height, weight, and head circumference should be determined and compared with reference tables. Increased head circumference or decreased weight and height are excellent clues to CNS masses or any vascular abnormality, while height or weight deviation may signal metabolic, inherited, or even neglect-related disease processes. Ingestions must always be a consideration in any de novo CNS presentation from infancy to late adolescence.

Level of consciousness can be assessed at any age and should be part of the initial assessment. Signs of irritability, lethargy, or a "wandering" or worried gaze are cause for concern in infants, as is a bulging fontanelle. In neonates the Moro and suck reflexes should be evaluated. Children older than 4 months should have a good hand grasp, be able to bear weight, and be able to hold their head up when drawn forward from the supine position. Sidedness, reflexes,

tone, and sensory deficits can be assessed at all age levels, although a little ingenuity may be required in children under 2 years of age. Subtle signs of confusion, loss of developmental landmarks, tremors, cerebellar signs, and aphasia can provide insight into a lesion and its location.

DIAGNOSTIC EVALUATION
Laboratory Studies

Children are often hesitant to undergo phlebotomy for laboratory testing. The physician should carefully review the differential diagnosis before performing venipuncture so that repeat phlebotomy can be avoided. A rapid glucose test should be among the first taken—a drop of blood from the IV insertion catheter or venipuncture needle can be used. Children with juvenile-onset diabetes have been reported to sustain transient episodes of hemiparesis. Hypoglycemia must always be rapidly excluded as a cause of seizures.

Emergency department studies should include a complete blood count, platelet count, clotting studies, blood culture, and sickle test where appropriate. Sedimentation rate may be checked if autoimmune disease is a high consideration. Lumbar puncture should be considered in young febrile children with no focal findings on examination when meningitis is suspected, but this should wait until after neuroimaging in most other instances.

Radiology

Routine skull films in the context of minor head injury are not indicated but may still be useful in the context of cerebrovascular syndromes. Intracranial calcifications from tumor or AVM may be present. Spreading sutures and skull fractures are significant findings that may be apparent on plain films. A computed tomographic (CT) scan of the head is the neuroimaging procedure of choice in most instances and is essential in narrowing the differential diagnosis of stroke in children. CT reveals space-occupying lesions, midline shifts, and hemorrhage (Fig. 138–2). Further enhanced scans may provide evidence of vascular abnormalities. Mag-

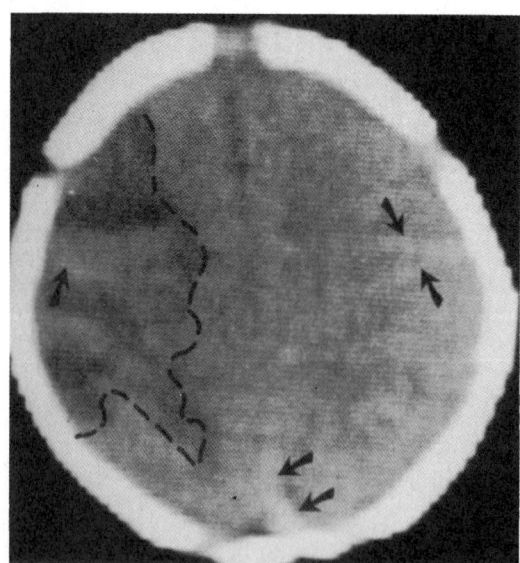

Figure 138–2. Cerebral infarction. An area is outlined that represents early changes resulting from infarction in the middle cerebral artery distribution. Arrows indicate hemorrhage. (From Fenichel GM. Clinical Pediatric Neurology: A Signs and Symptoms Approach. Philadelphia, WB Saunders, 1988, p 249.)

netic resonance imaging (MRI) arguably gives better CNS definition, but there is little need for MRI on an emergent basis. Angiography occasionally is the definitive study in cerebrovascular syndromes and should be undertaken under the direction of the neurologic consultant.

Electroencephalography

The electroencephalograph (EEG) is another test with limited usefulness in the emergency department setting. Valuable information may be gained from an EEG, but the test is rarely available at short notice.

DIFFERENTIAL DIAGNOSIS

Children presenting with signs of stroke (hemiplegia, aphasia, focal deficits, or coma) may be victims of a variety of calamities (Table 138–1). Identification of a focal brain lesion is by definition necessary to confirm a diagnosis of stroke. Localization of a lesion should be attempted. Defects in language production suggest a dominant hemispheral lesion. Unilateral motor weakness suggests a lesion in the motor pathways of the contralateral hemisphere. An increase in reflexes and tone support the diagnosis of an upper motor neuron lesion, although these findings may become abnormal only days later. Special attention should be paid to the possibility of trauma, especially in young "shaken" infants with no external evidence of violence. Relatively occult trauma after injuries such as intraoral lacerations must be considered, particularly when the event appeared to be minor and the initial pathologic condition is delayed 18 to 20 hours. A stroke may be the first sign of a blood dyscrasia such as sickle cell disease, or of congenital heart disease. The possibility of a process imitating ischemia should be considered: e.g., postictal paralysis, complicated migraine, and hypoglycemic hemiplegia. Sometimes, a cause is not identified, despite a thorough evaluation. Stroke in children generally has a better long-term outcome than in adults.

THERAPEUTIC INTERVENTION

Attendance to the ABCs is essential. Abnormal breathing patterns should be noted, because they may be clues to diagnosis as well as signs of worsening in the child's condition. Often the blood pressure is not taken in young children. Capillary refill, pulses, and blood pressure should all be used to assess circulatory status. Shock must be reversed.

Once the essentials have been taken care of, treatable or reversible causes of stroke may be addressed. Supportive care is the key factor in preventing further neurologic impairment. A child who is having seizures or who is metabolically deranged, hypotensive, or bleeding needs to have the specific etiology addressed in each instance. Confirming a diagnosis of stroke and finding the cause are essential factors, as the best therapy is often one that is specific to the identified cause. In general, cerebral edema is present in all infarcts; consequently, fluid replacement should be restricted in the first 24 to 72 hours. Steroid use in children is still controversial. These agents should be reserved for when the underlying problem may be responsive to steroids: e.g., arteritis or edema from tumors. Conditions that imitate strokes such as seizures, migraines, and toxicologic emergencies all have specific treatments. The importance of an etiologic diagnosis cannot be overemphasized. Children who have suffered cerebrovascular events require admission. If possible, pediatric neurologic consultation should be obtained.

Selected References

Daniels SR, Battes S, Lukin RR, et al. Cerebrovascular arteriopathy (arteriosclerosis) and ischemic childhood stroke. Stroke 1982; 13:360.
DiMario FJ, Packer RJ. Acute mental status changes in children with systemic cancer. Pediatrics 1990; 85:353.
Golden GS. Stroke syndromes in childhood. Neurol Clin 1985; 3:59.
Ichiyama T, Houdou S, Kisa T, et al. Varicella with delayed hemiplegia. Pediatr Neurol 1990; 6:279.
Lewis DW, Berman PH. Vertebral artery dissection and alternating hemiparesis in an adolescent. Pediatrics 1986; 78:610.
Mears GD, Leonard RB. Blunt carotid artery trauma: A case report. J Emerg Med 1988; 6:281.
Miller ST, Rieder RF, Rao SP, et al. Cerebrovascular accidents in children with sickle-cell disease and alpha-thalassemia. J Pediatr 1988; 113:847.
Mooney RP, Bessen HA. Delayed hemiparesis following nonpenetrating carotid artery trauma. Am J Emerg Med 1988; 6:341.
O'Connell BK, Towfighi J, Brennan RW, et al. Dissecting aneurysms of head and neck. Neurology 1985; 35:993.
Packer RJ, Rorke LB, Lange BJ, et al. Cerebrovascular accidents in children with cancer. Pediatrics 1985; 76:194.
Pearl PL. Childhood stroke following intraoral trauma. J Pediatr 1987; 110:574.

SECTION 17

Psychosocial Issues

Psychiatric Emergencies

Samuel M. Keim

INTRODUCTION

Recognizing the urgency of many pediatric psychiatric emergencies may be difficult. In contrast to an adolescent who presents after a suicidal gesture, a child with severe anxiety regarding a vague phobia may incite less sensitivity in the physician. Early psychiatric diagnosis and therapeutic intervention are critical.

The overall incidence of psychiatric emergencies among children is unclear. Mattsson and colleagues found that psychiatric patients represented 0.6% of the total pediatric emergency room population. The adult psychiatric incidence during that same period in the adult emergency room was found to be 3%.

Defining the Emergency

Pediatric psychiatric emergencies are often defined in reference to medical emergencies. One author noted that child psychiatric emergencies are often defined as "situations in which the life of the child or of someone else is in danger or the child is at high risk for a catastrophic trauma." Acknowledging the emotional dependence of children on adults, Morrison and Smith proposed that an emergency is "that situation in which the significant adults around the child can no longer help him master his anxiety and can no longer provide temporary ego support and controls." It is probable that "any dysfunction, pathology, or significant change in the body, individual, family, or other systems" that creates a crisis within the individual or his or her family constitutes an emergency. Others found that most pediatric psychiatric referrals "resulted from family crisis rather than intrapsychic crisis in the child."

Shafii and colleagues created a classification based on the most common presentations of psychopathology referred to a child psychiatric consultation service. Referrals secondary to suicidal, self-destructive, or markedly depressed behavior constituted 34% of the total. Behavior harmful or destructive to others added an additional 31%; 10% of the referrals were for abuse and neglect; another 10% were secondary to phobic or extreme anxiety; and the remainder were for psychotic behavior, runaway behavior, medical-psychiatric problems, and drug and alcohol abuse.

Crisis Intervention

Modern crisis intervention is derived from studies of bereaved and grieving patients. It was found that patients who developed psychiatric or psychosomatic complications of their grief appeared to be those individuals who were unsuccessful in venting that grief. A crisis situation resulted if a problem was great enough to exceed the individual's capability of maintaining emotional equilibrium.

Although the crisis state carries the risk of hazardous consequences for the individual, it is a time with great healing potential. Seemingly minuscule interventions from outside the individual can produce dramatic change quickly. Also, the outcome baseline may be healthier and more adaptive than the patient's state before the crisis.

In general, the unvented grief model is useful illustratively in teaching crisis intervention. The model contains (1) a stressor or precipitating event and (2) the individual's emotional blocking defenses. As Louis Paul wrote, "either or both stages may be blocked from awareness." He described four important steps: (1) practitioner identification of the major stressor, (2) practitioner discernment of the defense maneuvers employed by the patient, (3) revealing the major stressor to the patient, and (4) revealing to the patient the defenses being used to ward off recognizing the stressor.

The Family in Crisis

Because of the obvious emotional dependence children have on the significant adults in their lives, a breakdown of ego support from these adults—be it an emotional crisis or simply an absence from the environment—can produce a pediatric psychiatric emergency. In one study a family crisis was found to be the most common single precipitating factor for an adolescent seeking emergency psychiatric consultation.

The ability of the family to remain flexible and provide support in the face of new stressors determines to a great degree the individual child's crisis threshold. The family can be conceptualized to include school counselors and psychologists, family physicians and pediatricians, key religious figures, welfare workers, mental health workers, and any others involved in a significant way in the child's emotional support system. This obvious dependence led Morrison and Smith to define an emergency in child psychiatry as "that situation in which the significant adults around the child can no longer help him master his anxiety and can no longer provide temporary ego support and controls." This can lead to the child exhibiting coping maneuvers such as withdrawal (suicidal gestures, school phobia, conversion reactions, dissociation), projection (harmful or destructive behavior), or decompensation (extreme anxiety and psychosis).

Therapeutic crisis intervention must include a complete diagnostic evaluation of the family situation. Interviews must include both individual and conjoint sessions. Often the fundamental goal in family crisis intervention is the reestablishment of communication lines between the patient and the significant adults within the emotional support system. This goal is crucial to crisis intervention and is a mandatory first step if an outpatient disposition is to be achieved.

TEAM APPROACH

It is important and useful for the practitioner to perceive a mental health "team" when approaching child psychiatric emergencies (Fig. 139–1). The team should center around the child.

The physician first in contact with the crisis situation is considered to be the *emergency primary provider* (EPP), and this may be an emergency physician, a general pediatrician, or a family practice physician. EPPs must know the limits of their expertise and must accomplish a rapid but thorough assessment of the patient. This includes a responsibility to exclude organic disorders, since patients with existing psychiatric disorders may present to the emergency department with behavioral disturbance induced by organic illness.

The EPP must then identify which health care providers are already involved in the child's care. By doing this, the EPP can set the stage for the team approach to diagnosis and management of the crisis situation. The EPP must also know or determine which agencies and consultants are available in the community to assist as resources.

The role of the EPP includes coordination of the emergency clinical psychiatric evaluation. The entire team may be required simply to obtain a clear history of the presenting problem. Depending on the experience and time available to the EPP, this role also includes crisis intervention. It is certainly within the role of the EPP to identify all significant team members in the patient's environment and to contact them. If existing team members, such as a private primary care provider, are unavailable, the EPP must find adequate

temporary substitutes. Finally, the EPP must monitor the crisis intervention and ensure that proper disposition is made.

The emergency department or clinic nurse may be the first to encounter the patient in crisis. This person should be alert to statements made by the family or patient that may be helpful in the formulation of a history, and also watch for the potential of violence or elopement by the patient. The nursing staff should assess the vital signs and general condition of the patient, and always ensure the safety of the patient.

The role of the *primary care provider* (PCP) with the team varies, depending on any previous involvement with the patient. The PCP is often the physician to first encounter the crisis situation, and therefore he or she also takes the role of the EPP. If this is not the case, the PCP should be contacted soon after the patient's arrival in the emergency department. In all situations a PCP is an essential part of outpatient disposition.

The *child psychiatrist's* role within the team may depend upon his or her presence in the community. Owing to a nationwide shortage, rural and small communities may lack such resources. If the child has been under the care of a child psychiatrist, the latter or a substitute should come to the emergency department and play an integral role in the crisis intervention. If no child psychiatry involvement has taken place in the patient's past, this resource should be sought and implemented when available. For outpatients, nonurgent consultation or referral to a child psychiatrist should be made only if (1) the EPP is confident that the crisis has passed and (2) the family and social support unit is stable and functional, and outpatient referral is well understood by everyone on the team. Of course, the patient and family should also feel comfortable with this arrangement. When the child psychiatrist arrives at the emergency department, complete support should be given by the EPP and emergency department staff so that the crisis interview and intervention may be conducted without interruption. At disposition the child psychiatrist should explain, both in writing and verbally, the patient's diagnosis, current condition and prognosis, and disposition.

The *social worker* has become an important and fundamental team member in most emergency departments and may assist in all aspects of the crisis encounter. This team member is especially valuable in assisting difficult dispositions. The social worker can also help approach peripheral team members such as other social workers, clergy, and school contacts.

Child protective services should be involved if abuse is suspected and can work together with the social worker in finding temporary shelter services for the patient and family.

In summary, the EPP must have a self-perception as the coordinator of the crisis encounter and should identify, contact, and monitor all members of the intervention team during the patient's crisis encounter.

EMERGENCY CLINICAL PRESENTATION

The crisis interview and clinical evaluation are initiated by the patient's presentation (Table 139–1). Patients are frequently in unsafe situations when a crisis develops. The EPP is responsible for ensuring the patient's safety.

The child in crisis may initially contact the health care system by telephone. Often this takes the form of a phone call from a parent, teacher, counselor, or troubled youth inquiring, "What should I do?" The call is commonly directed at the PCP, an emergency department, or a crisis hotline. The person receiving this call must quickly estimate the nature and severity of the crisis. If it is life threatening, the emergency medical system (EMS-911) should be acti-

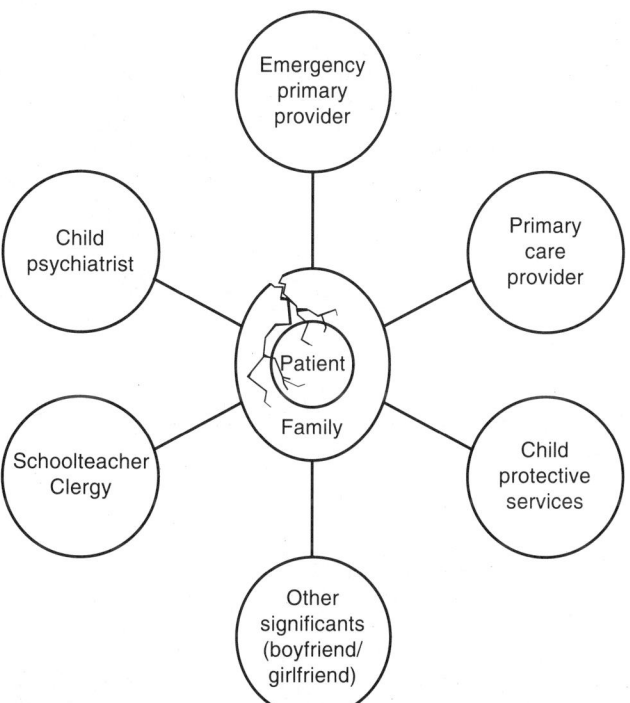

Figure 139–1. The dynamics of the team approach to psychiatric emergencies in children. All therapeutic efforts are focused on assisting the child in crisis.

vated. If patients are unwilling to volunteer the location, a clandestine activation of the EMS-911 should occur while they are still on the line, to help trace the call. The extent of diagnosis and management that occurs over the phone depends on the expertise of those receiving the call. Although it is common for an experienced crisis hotline to resolve approximately 50% of their calls over the phone, this is not recommended for the inexperienced. It is much safer to refer these individuals to their PCP, child psychiatrist, or nearest emergency department.

Interview

A thorough history and rapid but comprehensive differential diagnosis are crucial. A complete mental status examination, a family and social assessment, and a complete physical examination are mandatory. The interview should begin with a brief history of the presenting problem. This can be obtained from a variety of sources: the patient, family members, and the PCP. The history should aim at answering some key questions, oriented toward disposition as well as diagnosis (Table 139–2).

The interview should be conducted in a setting that optimizes patient comfort and minimizes anxiety for both patient and interviewer. This can be challenging in the emergency department setting. The room must be easy to monitor for prevention of elopement and violence. It may be necessary to involve hospital security.

The child in crisis often is accompanied by a family member. In nearly all of these cases the crisis is inextricably related to the family situation. Despite this, family members often are not interviewed and actually are somewhat feared by emergency department staff. Whether the patient is initially interviewed alone or with family members present, a brief social and family history should be obtained by the physician. This is necessary to ascertain which social support system has been functioning for the patient in the recent past, and any significant changes in that system. The physician must determine who are the significant adults in the child's environment and the current status of those relationships. From this information the physician should be able to identify any dysfunctional relationships that may have directly influenced the present crisis or could prevent resolution.

The physician should then inquire about any other significant relationships that may exist, e.g., boyfriend, girlfriend, best friend. These relationships are often perceived by children as the most significant in their environment. The physician should then assess how well the child is functioning in these relationships.

TABLE 139–1

EMERGENCY PEDIATRIC PSYCHIATRIC EVALUATION

1. Presentation
   a. Ensure patient's safety (activate EMS if necessary)
   b. Notify guardian/family members
2. Brief history of presenting problem
3. Brief social and family history
4. Brief mental status examination
5. Complete physical examination
6. Laboratory studies to rule out organicity
7. Consultation
   a. Child psychiatrist
   b. Social services
   c. Child protective services (if necessary)
8. Crisis intervention
9. Disposition

TABLE 139–2

KEY QUESTIONS IN CHILDHOOD PSYCHIATRIC EMERGENCIES

1. What is the presenting problem, behavior, or symptom?
2. What is the chronicity of the problem?
3. What is the severity of the problem?
4. What was the child's pre-crisis behavioral baseline?
5. What are the functions of the significant adults in the child's environment?
6. What is the child's prognosis for reestablishing meaningful communication with the social support system?
7. What is the suicidal or homicidal potential?
8. Is there an adequate disposition plan that includes a primary provider, the family, and the social support system to ensure the physical and mental safety of the patient?

An inquiry must be made regarding substance abuse by the patient, perhaps beginning with a question such as, "How many of your friends have used cocaine?" Family members may be questioned separately regarding this issue. This important information is necessary to exclude an organic basis of the present crisis. Finally, any psychiatric illness among family members should be determined.

A brief mental status examination should be conducted by the physician. Such an examination for the EPP should include the patient's appearance, mood, thoughts, and cognition.

The patient's outward appearance and general behavioral characteristics should be noted. For example, does the patient appear angry, anxious, tremulous, hyperactive, or warm and affable? Since the EPP has limited experience in child psychiatry, it is best to describe the child in common terms, avoiding psychiatric terminology unless it is clearly understood.

Mood or affect refers to the manner in which the child displays emotions. The EPP should be especially sensitive to depressed, euphoric, anxious, and fearful moods. The physician should also be able to determine whether the affect is flat or inappropriate.

The EPP should assess the quality of thoughts the patient has been having, including whether or not the child has paranoia, hallucinations, obsessions, or ambivalence. The EPP should note whether the child's thoughts appear to be tangential or loosely connected.

Finally, the physician should assess the patient's cognitive ability. This may be the best way to predict organicity. Is the patient oriented? Can he remember the name of a significant adult in his environment? A true concept of time in terms of weeks and months may not be developed until about the age of 8 or 9 years. Assessment of orientation requires an understanding of development milestones.

The physical examination should be performed, with special attention to the neurologic examination. Pupillary size, cerebellar signs, and fine motor function may be clues to organicity and substance abuse.

ORGANIC ILLNESS

Organic mental disorders are defined as transient or permanent disturbances of brain function attributable to specific physiologic factors and manifested as behavioral disturbances. In children the incidence of physical illness responsible for behavioral symptoms has been reported to be 1% to 4%. The Diagnostic and Statistical Manual of Mental Disorders lists ten classes of organic disorders: dementia, delirium, organic delusional disorder, organic hallucinosis, organic affective disorder, organic amnestic disorder, personality disorder, atypical or mixed organic mental

---

TABLE 139–3

DIAGNOSTIC EVALUATION TO EXCLUDE ORGANICITY

1. Electrolytes, BUN, and creatinine
2. Serum glucose
3. Serum calcium
4. Complete blood count
5. Urinalysis
6. Urine and serum drug screen
7. Electrocardiogram, chest radiograph, arterial blood gas
8. Cerebral CT or MRI scan
9. Lumbar puncture
10. Endocrine studies

---

disorder, intoxication, and withdrawal. In general the EPP should be alert to any acute or chronic medical condition that could contribute to the patient's behavioral state. In children, delirium and acute intoxication states will probably be most significant.

Delirium is defined as a clouding of consciousness or a reduced awareness of the environment. The DSM-III also requires the presence of disorientation, memory impairment, and two of the following: perceptual disturbance, incoherent speech, altered sleep-wake cycle, or altered psychomotor activity. It is crucial that the EPP not miss a diagnosis of an organic delirium by prematurely labeling a patient as having schizophrenia or brief reactive psychosis. If there is a doubt, an evaluation for organic, toxic, and metabolic causes is appropriate.

The physical examination can provide crucial data to assist in determining organicity. With uncooperative, disoriented, or combative patients, physical restraints may be necessary. Patients should be thoroughly examined for any head trauma. Clues to intoxication, increased intracranial pressure, cardiac dysfunction, infections, and endocrine disease should be compulsively sought.

If suspicious, the physician should proceed with laboratory studies to exclude suspected organic etiologies (Table 139–3). An initial battery should include an EKG, chest radiograph, BUN, creatinine, complete blood count, urinalysis, glucose, calcium, and toxicologic screen. If the latter screen for drugs of abuse is unavailable, the physician should test for those substances most likely consistent with the patient's presentation and history. In addition, an arterial blood gas, a lumbar puncture, and a head CT scan should be obtained in the emergency department if the history and physical examination suggest organicity but the cause is unclear. If there is a continuing suspicion of an organic etiology, but this cannot be proved, hospitalization is prudent. More thorough tests may then be pursued, and inpatient psychiatric consultation completed.

CLASSIFICATIONS

Pediatric psychiatric emergencies may be classified by diagnostic categories or by symptoms. Shafii and colleagues classified cases according to the major presenting problem or the most severe behavioral expression of psychopathology (Table 139–4). This method is especially useful for the EPP.

Another method of classification that modifies the ICD-9 system was developed by Turgay (Table 139–5). This modified system was developed with pediatric psychiatric emergencies in mind. Clinical syndromes such as mental retardation, learning disabilities, anorexia, enuresis, and encopresis are excluded in order to focus on emergency presentations. Suicide is not included in this classification system because the author felt it could be a part of any of

---

TABLE 139–4

SHAFII CLASSIFICATION OF PEDIATRIC PSYCHIATRIC EMERGENCIES

1. Suicidal, self-destructive, or marked depression
2. Harmful or destructive behavior toward others
3. Abuse or neglect
4. Phobic or extremely anxious behavior
5. Psychotic behavior
6. Runaways
7. Medical-psychiatric emergencies
8. Drug and alcohol abuse
9. Others: Severe family crisis, multiple-problem crisis

From Shafii M. The pediatric-psychiatric model for emergencies in child psychiatry: A study of 994 cases. Am J Psychiatry 1979; 136:1600. Copyright 1979, the American Psychiatric Association. Reprinted by permission.

---

the clinical categories. The system outlines the following psychiatric emergencies. All definitions are brief and, although adapted from the DSM-III-R Training Guide, should not be viewed as strict criteria for diagnosis.

Emotional Reactions to Physical Illness, Hospitalization, or Surgery

Children with or without chronic behavioral disturbances can experience extreme disequilibrium when placed in a health care facility. These acute crises can interfere with medical care, and nonpsychiatric hospital staff may be inexperienced or may feel ineffective in handling them. Often the staff's desire to complete a simple surgical procedure

---

TABLE 139–5

TURGAY CLASSIFICATION OF PSYCHIATRIC EMERGENCIES IN CHILDREN

I. Emotional reactions to physical illness, hospitalization, or surgery
II. Child abuse (physical, emotional, or sexual)
III. Adjustment reaction (including grief reaction)
IV. Organic psychotic conditions
   A. Alcoholic psychosis
   B. Drug withdrawal syndrome
   C. Drug-induced psychosis
   D. Pathologic drug intoxication
   E. Other organic psychotic conditions
V. Other psychoses
   A. Schizophrenic psychosis
      1. Early onset
      2. Late onset
      3. Adolescent schizophrenia
VI. Neurotic disorders
   A. Anxiety states
   B. Hysteria conversion reaction
   C. Phobic states
   D. Obsessive-compulsive disorders
   E. Neurotic depression
   F. Hypochondriasis
   G. Others
VII. Conduct disorders (including fire-setting, running away, aggressive behavior, school refusal)
VIII. Hyperkinetic syndrome (minimal brain dysfunction, attention deficit disorder)
IX. Psychophysiologic reactions (psychosomatic illnesses)
X. Complications of psychoactive drugs
XI. Others

From Turgay A. Psychiatric emergencies in children. Psychiatric J Univ Ottawa 1982; 7:255.

inhibits their ability to effectively prevent or curtail the emotional crisis.

The most common example in this classification is the intense anxiety reaction. This may be secondary to obvious stressors such as a surgical procedure. It may, however, have an occult etiology. The physician must recognize this destabilization. Frequently the child's accompanying family members are also involved in the disequilibrium and must be approached promptly to obtain their active involvement. Ignoring the parents can quickly lead to their destabilizing the situation further and possibly even removing the sick child from the facility.

Some of these crises could be averted if the physician would recognize the potential for anxiety reactions. Careful and thorough explanations of procedures to both the children and the parents and familiarizing them with the medical care environment are key to prevention. Prompt differentiation of an acute anxiety crisis as a maladaptive behavior from the psychological presentation of organic disease is crucial. The value of the mental status examination in this situation is clear. It is essential to document all medications the child has been given.

In most situations EPP can adequately coordinate crisis intervention without psychiatric consultation. If not, the psychiatrist should be quickly involved to avert a dangerous escalation of the problem. Admission is required only if the family is incapable of supporting the child as an outpatient.

Child Abuse

The management of child abuse requires a sensitivity to and awareness of the wide variety of clinical presentations. In addition to physical abuse, child abuse may take the form of neglect, emotional abuse, and Polle's syndrome (Munchausen's syndrome by proxy). Inpatient dispositions are nearly always required.

Adjustment Reaction

An adjustment reaction is a maladaptive reaction to an identifiable psychosocial stressor that occurs within 3 months of the onset of the stressor. The term adjustment reaction has been misused and overused by laypersons and mental health care providers alike. In the emergency clinical situation, it does retain some value. "Adjustment reaction" or "adjustment disorder" is understood by PCPs as being more descriptive of etiology than of the behavioral disturbance. The term is therefore useful as long as the physician recognizes that associated pathologic conditions, e.g., a depressed mood or a disturbance of conduct, may require very different treatments. The role of the EPP is to identify the stressors that led to the behavioral disturbance, ensuring proper consultation, and determining any suicidal risk. The differential diagnosis includes personality disorders exacerbated by stress and chronic mood disorders.

The symptoms of this disorder disappear when the stressor is removed or the individual develops a new coping mechanism. The physician should seek to define the stressors and their chronicity. Psychotherapy, both individual and group, usually promotes effective coping mechanisms. Temporary use of anxiolytics in the acute phase may be helpful, but chronic use is discouraged. Admission is warranted if family support is inadequate or suicide is a concern.

Organic Psychotic Conditions

Organic psychotic conditions are defined as transient or permanent disturbances of brain function that are attributable to specific physiologic factors and manifest as behavioral

disturbances. The presentation of a child with acute disorientation, clouded consciousness, or marked intellectual deficit should immediately arouse the physician's suspicion of organicity. The clinical history and constellation of symptoms may lead the physician to a specific and accurate organic syndrome or etiologic agent. Frequently, however, defining the cause requires inpatient admission and a medical consultation to further evaluate and manage the child. Consideration should be given to the functional syndromes that present in a similar fashion to their organic "look-alikes." Excluding organicity should always be given the first priority.

Alcoholic Psychosis. This is probably better referred to as alcoholic hallucinosis. This is fortunately rare in children, but it does occur. It is characterized by vivid auditory hallucinations developing shortly after cessation of, or reduction in, heavy alcohol ingestion in an individual with alcohol dependence. There is no clouding of consciousness. The alcoholic hallucinosis syndrome may occur simultaneously with the alcohol withdrawal delirium syndrome. In this clinical scenario, autonomic hyperactivity is also present. The differential diagnosis includes hypoglycemia, diabetic ketoacidosis, barbiturate withdrawal, head trauma, and schizophrenia. Acute management by the EPP should focus on excluding organic etiologies, controlling the hallucinations, and recognizing and addressing the reactive psychopathology, such as anxiety and agitation.

These patients will most likely need pharmacologic treatment in addition to reassurance and reality defining. Communications with the patient should be limited to repeated, simple, and concrete statements. Diazepam and chlordiazepoxide can be used orally or intravenously to control anxiety, agitation, and hallucinations. Short-acting barbiturates may also be effective but require intensive monitoring in view of the risk of respiratory depression. This acute phase may be followed by a chronic form with a prolonged course. Inpatient psychotherapy and a comprehensive rehabilitation program are mandatory.

Drug Withdrawal Syndrome. Like the alcohol withdrawal syndrome, other drug-dependent states may lead to psychopathology or behavioral disturbances upon cessation of use. These patients may also have "ego-dystonic hallucinations" similar to those in the alcoholic hallucinosis syndrome. Management should therefore be essentially the same as for the latter syndrome. Priority must be given to excluding the many other causes of organic hallucinosis.

Drug-Induced Psychosis. The use of hallucinogens, stimulants, or phencyclidine may produce profound hallucinations. Admission is suggested for intoxications that do not resolve in under 6 hours and for patients with inadequate family support.

Schizophrenia

Schizophrenia is a disorder characterized by the presence of one of the following for at least one week:

1. Two of the following:
   a. Delusions
   b. Prominent hallucinations
   c. Incoherence or marked loosening of associations
   d. Catatonic behavior
   e. Flat or grossly inappropriate affect
2. Bizarre delusions
3. Prominent hallucinations

The subtle distinctions among schizophrenic subtypes should be left to the child psychiatrist. It is important for the EPP to exclude organicity when considering the diagnosis of schizophrenia.

Psychotic clinical presentations are evident in many disorders. In the DSM-III-R, psychotic conditions include paranoid disorders, mood disorders and organic mental disorders, and psychotic disorders not elsewhere classified. Differentiation of these disorders is beyond the responsibility of the EPP or PCP. With adolescents, it is critical to exclude a substance abuse–induced organic delusional syndrome. Schizoaffective disorder, mood disorder with psychotic features, and autism may be especially similar in clinical presentation. There are no specific diagnostic criteria in the DSM-III for childhood schizophrenia, only for the adult form. The criteria involve no lower age limit, which may suggest that they are appropriate for children also.

After organic illnesses and other behavioral disturbances have been ruled out, drug management for schizophrenia in children may be valuable and at times essential. Sedatives, anxiolytics, stimulants, and antipsychotic agents have all been tried in childhood schizophrenia, and there appears to be general agreement that the antipsychotic drugs alone are of benefit. They should be used in the acute setting only after consultation with a child psychiatrist. In general, chlorpromazine is used for children under the age of 12 years and haloperidol for adolescents. It must be stressed that antipsychotic medications cannot be given in a therapeutic vacuum. The patient must be cared for in a structured, inpatient environment. Dispositions for exacerbations of chronic disease should be achieved with psychiatric consultation. These children should be sent home only if the family status is secure and functional.

Neurotic Disorders

Anxiety States. In children, separation anxiety and "stranger anxiety" are normal phases of development. If these anxiety states remain significant into adolescence, they may interfere with social relationships and normal development. These patients rarely are seen in the emergency department but may present to the primary pediatrician's clinic. Treatment of separation anxiety disorder usually focuses on improving the child's self-esteem and communication within the family. A few children appear to be negatively reinforced with each separation episode and become more anxious with each event. These children tend to be anxious all the time and manifest nearly constant signs, such as cold, sweaty hands, hyperreflexia, and psychophysiologic discomfort. Low doses of benzodiazepines may be used acutely, but chronic use should be avoided. Admission is required only for severe cases or for children with dysfunctional families.

Hysteria Conversion Reaction. In patients with a conversion disorder or hysterical neurosis, the predominant disturbance on presentation is a loss of or alteration in physical functioning suggesting a physical disorder. A thorough history should reveal the symptom to have a psychological basis. The alteration in physical function must also be found to be involuntary.

The physician should consider all physical disorders similar to the physical alteration in the patient. Schizophrenia, somatization disorder, hypochondriasis, a factitious disorder with physical symptoms, and malingering must also be considered.

In the acute clinical situation, psychiatric evaluation and therapeutic intervention are necessary. There is evidence that intensive psychotherapy is effective for patients with true hysterical neuroses. The EPP should be discouraged from using direct confrontation in an attempt to "break" the conversion. Admission may be required to ensure the accuracy of diagnosis and to implement psychotherapeutic intervention.

Phobic States. Phobias are disorders of intense anxiety produced when a specific stimulus is encountered. The anxiety is so severe that avoidance of the stimulus interferes with normal functioning and relationships. Although these are uncommon, the two main subtypes in children are simple phobia and social phobia. In social phobia (e.g., school phobia), children attempt to protect themselves from potentially embarrassing or humiliating social situations. In simple phobia, the reaction is usually attributable to an object, rather than to a social situation. The most common stimuli are animals, heights, or closed spaces. The differential diagnosis includes obsessive-compulsive disorder, schizophrenia, paranoid personality disorder, avoidance disorder of childhood, and major depression.

Anxiety generated from a phobic state can be thought of as "anticipatory fear or situational fear." Separation anxiety is a normal developmental response. When fears and anxieties interfere with normal functioning, they become pathologic. One should attempt to define the extent of social dysfunction caused by the anxiety. School refusal phobia should be watched with vigilance. Pharmacologic treatment for school refusal may include thioridazine, benzodiazepines, or imipramine. The behavioral therapy technique of exposure may be effective in childhood anxiety disorders, but such a technique should not be used in the emergency care setting. Benzodiazepines may be useful in relieving acute anxiety states. Admission is warranted when the etiology is unclear or when there is a severe crisis or an ineffective family situation.

Obsessive-Compulsive Disorders. Determination of an obsessive-compulsive disorder depends on recognition of either obsessions or compulsions, or both. Obsessions are disturbing thoughts that are recurrent even when patients make conscious attempts to prevent them. Compulsions are intentional, repetitive actions performed in an attempt to obtain an effect where no causal relationship exists. When patients try to prevent the compulsive activity, tension develops, which is relieved when they resume the activity. The disorder is characterized by an impairment of social functioning. The differential diagnosis includes organic mental disorder, schizophrenia, major depression, Tourette's disease, and other disorders of impulse control. It is now thought that the incidence in childhood is higher than previously thought. Substance abuse is also common in adolescents with this disorder.

These patients infrequently present to a PCP in an acute state. This disorder requires chronic therapy, probably in the form of "exposure-prevention of response behavioral" therapy. Pharmacologic agents used in this disorder have been of limited use, but include tricyclic antidepressants and low-dose neuroleptics.

Neurotic Depression (Dysthymic Disorder). This disorder is characterized by the child or adolescent having a depressive syndrome for the previous year that has not reached sufficient magnitude to meet the criteria of a major depressive episode. The patient has at least two of the following characteristics: poor appetite or overeating, insomnia or hypersomnia, low energy or fatigue, low self-esteem, poor concentration, and feelings of hopelessness. The differential diagnosis includes major depression, normal fluctuations of mood, obsessive-compulsive disorder, chronic substance abuse, attention deficit hyperactivity disorder, conduct disorder, oppositional defiant disorder, and mental retardation.

Dysthymic patients may present with worsening depression or acute states of anxiety. As in all depressed patients, the EPP must assess the suicidality of the patient. A thorough family interview should take place to ensure that functional communication exists within the family. Pharmacologic intervention is limited to symptomatic relief, such as therapy for acute anxiety states or insomnia. The absence of vegetative signs in dysthymic disorder suggests the limited value of antidepressants. Hospital admission is suggested when the diagnosis is unclear, suicide is a concern, or family support is inadequate.

Hypochondriasis. This disorder is characterized by an unrealistic interpretation of physical signs or symptoms as being abnormal. This interpretation leads the individual to become preoccupied with fears of having a serious disease. The differential diagnosis includes true organic disease, schizophrenia, dysthymic disorder, anxiety disorder, and major depression with psychotic features.

Patients may frequently have unrealistic fears about physical symptoms. However, when the negative results of the physician's examination and studies are carefully explained, their fears subside. In hypochondriasis, the fears do not abate and the patient may seek multiple medical opinions. Once organic etiologies have been excluded, traditional insight-oriented psychotherapy is indicated. Admission is indicated when the diagnosis is unclear and family functioning is inadequate.

Conduct Disorders

Children with disruptive behavioral disorders that are persistent and repetitive and tend to be more serious than commonly accepted "pranks" may have a conduct disorder. The characteristic behavior seriously violates other people's rights or societal norms: e.g., fire setting, running away, repetitive stealing or repetitive lying, vandalism, cruelty to animals, and repetitive violence. The differential diagnosis includes oppositional defiant disorder (which in many instances is a precursor of conduct disorder), dysthymic disorder, major depression, attention deficit hyperactivity disorder, and mental retardation.

The role of the EPP is to establish communication between family members and ensure psychiatric consultation. Behavioral therapy should be helpful. The behavioral characteristics that respond best to medication are hyperactivity and aggression. The child who lacks the hyperactivity component probably will not respond well to pharmacologic treatment. If a child does exhibit symptoms of an associated attention deficit disorder, a trial of stimulants may be warranted. If the child with a conduct disorder has aggression as a key associated feature, a trial of antipsychotics may be instituted.

Attention Deficit Hyperactivity Syndrome

A child with this disorder displays poor impulse control associated with difficulty maintaining attention and excessive motor restlessness. These children are typically identified in their early school years, but parents often describe an onset by age 3 years. Symptoms typically vary from situation to situation (school versus home) and therefore are often perceived differently by parents and teachers. Teachers are usually given primary consideration since their reports tend to be more objective than those of the parents. The differential diagnosis includes age-appropriate overactivity, conduct disorder, schizophrenia, affective disorders, and mental retardation.

The patients most often treated are those whose key feature is hyperactivity. Stimulant drugs are effective in reducing problems these children have in school situations, but the long-term results are disappointing. The best results are obtained if medication is joined with a comprehensive program of behavior modification. Methylphenidate is the medication most used. Hospital admission is required if the behavior exhibited is unmanageable at home or dangerous to other individuals.

Psychosomatic Illnesses

Somatization or psychosomatic illness is a disorder that technically requires the presence of 12 symptoms from a list of 37 (14 symptoms for women) for which the individual has sought attention. These symptoms, in the estimation of the physician, are inconsistent with the patient's actual health status. The physician should always remain suspicious that a true physical disorder may be exhibiting vague and confusing symptoms. Examples include hyperparathyroidism, porphyria, multiple sclerosis, and lupus. Psychiatric diseases to consider include schizophrenia, dysthymic disorder, anxiety disorder, major depression, conversion reaction, and hypochondriasis.

Once organicity has been ruled out, the EPP is often caught in a frustrating situation and must approach the patient with sympathy, open-mindedness, and thoroughness. The physician must first, and always, exclude organicity. Psychiatric diagnoses should be based on objectivity, not subjectivity, or the mere lack of evidence pointing to organicity. Physicians should show sympathy and honesty, explaining their confidence level, and should never tell the patient that organicity has been absolutely excluded. Simple concrete diagnoses should be avoided. The importance of time and follow-up in revealing the true nature of the disorder should be emphasized. The patient should be reassured that it is common and often normal for emotional problems to cause physical complaints. Functional symptoms are never treated with medications or procedures simply to appease the patient's desire for such.

The patient, and often family members, may be reluctant to accept a psychiatric etiology. Good communication between the EPP and the patient and family is essential; poor communication is probably the most common antecedent to litigation if organicity is missed. Admission is indicated only to exclude an organic cause or in situations of family dysfunction.

Complications of Psychoactive Drugs

Bizarre behavior in a child should be considered to have an organic cause until proved otherwise. If the child is on psychoactive medications, toxic side effects may be the cause. Methylphenidate may exacerbate psychotic symptoms if given to children with preexisting psychoses. The agitation component of the attention deficit–hyperactivity disorder may actually worsen. Withdrawal of the medication can also stimulate a disequilibrium as underlying behavioral disturbances are unmasked. Exacerbation of preexisting psychosis may also occur with imipramine. Substance abuse must also be considered in patients presenting with signs and symptoms of intoxication.

Others

Mood Disorders. There are two basic categories in this classification, bipolar disorders and depressive disorders. The essential difference between these two groups is that, in a bipolar disorder, there has been both a major depressive episode and a manic episode.

The major depressive episode is characterized by at least five of the following symptoms occurring simultaneously:

1. Depressed or irritable mood most of the day, and nearly every day.
2. Diminished interest or pleasure in activities.
3. Significant weight loss or gain.
4. Insomnia or hypersomnia.
5. Psychomotor agitation or retardation.
6. Fatigue.

7. Feelings of worthlessness.
8. Diminished ability to concentrate.
9. Recurrent thoughts of death or suicidal ideation.

A manic episode is briefly characterized by at least three of the following:

1. Inflated self-esteem or grandiosity.
2. Diminished need for sleep.
3. More talkativeness than usual.
4. Distractability.
5. Increase in goal-directed activity or psychomotor agitation.
6. Excessive involvement in high-risk activities.

These mood disturbances must be significant to alter social functioning or interfere with relationships with others. There must have been no delusions or hallucinations during this time. In childhood, many disorders and developmental disabilities produce mild depression. It is therefore important to distinguish between primary and secondary depression. The depressive episode must also be differentiated from a mere feeling of disappointment or unhappiness that is transient. In the preschool years, depression may present as a somatization disorder or a severe separation anxiety. In the early school-age years, school refusal, aggression, and somatizations may be associated with an underlying depression. In adolescents, symptoms more typical of adults emerge, such as depressed affect, vegetative signs, social isolation, and feelings of worthlessness. It is safe to say that, the younger the child, the more difficult it is to identify introspective symptoms.

It is important to assess the risk of suicide in all these patients. The EPP should then ensure that no organic disease process is present. Children with primary major depression should be referred to a child psychiatrist. The dexamethasone suppression test may be used by psychiatrists in children over the age of 6 years in an attempt to define which could benefit most from pharmacologic treatment. Tricyclic antidepressants such as imipramine have been most popular.

In bipolar disorder, lithium carbonate may be effective. The difficulty arises in the differentiation of bipolar disorders from attention deficit disorders with hyperactivity (for which lithium has no benefit), and conduct disorders with hyperactivity and aggressiveness (for which lithium has only minimal effect). Lithium may therefore have a role in defining the diagnosis. All mood disorders should be managed in close consultation with a child psychiatrist. Hospital admission is indicated for almost all new mood disorder patients. Assessment of suicidal potential is crucial.

DISPOSITION OF PSYCHIATRIC EMERGENCY PATIENTS

The EPP must be conservative and ensure the safety and well-being of the disturbed child. If hospitalization is required and organicity has been excluded, the EPP should work in concert with the child psychiatrist and social worker to determine the proper inpatient disposition. If an outpatient disposition is suggested by the consultant, the EPP should feel confident that this is a proper action and that the social support system is adequate to care for future crises.

The EPP must be aware of state regulations regarding the treatment of adolescents. Under no circumstances should unemancipated minors be released under their own recognizance after psychiatric consultation.

Selected References

Diagnostic and Statistical Manual of Mental Disorders (DSM-III). 3rd ed. Washington, DC, American Psychiatric Association, 1980.

DiSclafani A, Hall RCW, Gardner ER. Drug-induced psychosis: Emergency diagnosis and management. Psychosomatics 1981; 22:845.

Editorial. Stabilizing teens in crisis and fortifying their support network. Hosp Community Psychiatry 1987; 38:1211.

Hall RCW, Popkin MA, DeVaul RA, et al. Physical illness presenting as psychiatric disease. Arch Gen Psychiatry 1978; 35:1315.

Hillard JR, Slomowitz M, Levi LS. A retrospective study of adolescents' visits to a general hospital psychiatric emergency service. Am J Psychiatry 1987; 144:432.

Louis P. Crisis intervention. In Morrison GC (ed). Emergencies in Child Psychiatry. Springfield, IL, Charles C Thomas, 1975.

Mattsson A, Hawkins JW, Seese LR. Child psychiatric emergencies: Clinical characteristics and follow-up results. Arch Gen Psychiatry 1967; 17:584.

McDaniel KD. Pharmacologic treatment of psychiatric and neurodevelopmental disorders in children and adolescents (Parts 2 and 3). Clin Pediatr 1986; 25.

Morrison GC, Smith WR. Child psychiatric emergencies. In Morrison GC (ed). Emergencies in Child Psychiatry. Springfield, IL, Charles C Thomas, 1975.

Perlmutter RA. Family involvement in psychiatric emergencies. Hosp Community Psychiatry 1983; 3:255.

Rapoport JL, Ismond DR. DSM-III-R Training Guide for Diagnosis of Childhood Disorders. New York, Brunner/Mazel, 1990.

Shafii M, Whittinghill R, Healy MH. The pediatric-psychiatric model for emergencies in child psychiatry: A study of 994 cases. Am J Psychiatry 1979; 136:1600.

Tumulty PA. The approach to patients with functional disorders. N Engl J Med 1960; 263:123.

Turgay A. Psychiatric emergencies in children. Psychiatr J Univ Ottawa 1982; 7:254.

Visotsky HM. The Joint Commission on Mental Health of Children: Progress report. Psychiatr Ann 1975; 5:11.

CHAPTER 140

Drug Abuse

Marcus L. Martin

INTRODUCTION

A major problem facing youth in our society is drug abuse. The pediatric population, ranging from the neonate to the young adult, is subject to the untoward effects of drugs and other chemicals. Use of alcohol and other drugs is commonplace among teens and preadolescents, and dangerous patterns of multiple drug use are common. Reports show lifetime prevalence rates (drug use any time during life) as high as 93% for alcohol use, 70% for cigarette use, 55% for marijuana use, and 16% for cocaine use among high school seniors.[1] There is a 5% chemical dependency among adolescents, as evidenced by daily use of alcohol, marijuana, or both. As many as one third of ninth to twelfth grade students report the concurrent use of two or more drugs. Concurrent use of alcohol and marijuana is predominant, but cocaine use is rising.

The initiation of drug use typically occurs between the ages of 12 and 25 years, but alcohol and cigarette use may begin as early as age 10.[2-4] The earlier the age of starting a drug, the more likely addiction becomes. Ten percent of high school students using alcohol and 4% using marijuana started their use by the sixth grade.[1] Exposure to illicit drugs during pregnancy, predisposing to neonatal addiction, may occur in as many as one in ten newborns.[5]

More than 50% of fatal accidents and disabling injuries

involving youth, including motor vehicle accidents, suicide, and homicide, are associated with the use of alcohol or other drugs.[6-13] Adolescents account for 250,000 suicide attempts annually, the majority by drug ingestion.[14]

PATHOPHYSIOLOGY

Definitions and Patterns of Drug Abuse

Drug abuse (chemical abuse, substance abuse) refers to improper use of a substance or chemical with potential for injury or pathologic sequelae as a consequence.[15, 16] Persistent habitual indulgence in drug use is drug addiction. Addiction implies abuse, but abuse does not necessarily imply addiction. Early, controlled use gives way to compulsive use and subsequently to binges, in the typical pathway to addiction. The psychopathologic progression of drug use to addiction may include initial magnification of pleasure, euphoria, and increased awareness of emotions and self-esteem, as well as increased enthusiasm, heightened sexuality, and decreased social inhibitions.[17] Positive perception and absence of deleterious results lead to more frequent and compulsive use and larger drug doses to attain gratification. With lack of abstinence and with continued availability of supply, craving, tolerance, and psychological and physical dependence may develop. Personal deterioration and apathy are likely to ensue. Involvement in crime, abuse of friends and family members, and contraction of infectious diseases are some of the morbid consequences. Abstinence may lead to withdrawal, the symptoms of which may vary according to the dependent drug (Table 140-1). Abstinence, removal of

conditioning cues, psychological support, and physical detoxification aid in the extinction of addiction.

Behavioral and Risk Factors

Children may use alcohol, drugs, and various other chemical substances for a number of reasons. Initially, they may use a nonprescribed substance through curiosity and the desire to experiment, but probably most often because of factors relating to peer group and social pressures.[18-20] Close friends or relatives may influence their first experience with licit or illicit substances.[21] In the approach to any patient suspected of substance use, it is important to determine whether the degree of use is experimental, recreational, habitual, addictive, or for suicidal intent.[22]

Many factors influence substance use and abuse, including supply and demand, local unemployment levels, the number of one-person households, population density, psychological and social factors, family stability, and parental factors. Twenty-five percent of all school-age children have at least one alcoholic parent.[23] Illicit drug use has typically been a problem among young, low-income males. However, drug abuse among females has increased, with tendencies toward an earlier age of first use than that of males.[24-28] Early first use of drugs increases the risk of abuse.[29] A study of 4932 eighth grade students who regularly cared for themselves at home after school for 11 hours or more a week showed that these children were at twice as great a risk for substance use as students not left alone.[30]

Serious social, psychosocial, behavioral, academic, and family problems begin or worsen with drug use.[31] Adolescent substance abuse is associated with a higher incidence of stressful life events[32]; depression may coexist with substance abuse.[33] Having a major depressive disorder or anxiety disorder may double the risk of subsequent drug abuse and dependence.[34, 35] Adolescent girls with a history of bulimia or anorexia nervosa reportedly have substantially higher levels of substance abuse than those without major eating disorders.[36-39] There are correlates of school absenteeism, school grade retardation, school disciplinary problems, and increased school dropout rates among substance abusers.[21, 29, 40] Students who smoke are nearly three times more likely to report missing school through illness.[2] Family conflicts, running away, stealing, vandalism, and prostitution are cited problems for teens with heavy drug use.[40] The risk of acquiring human immunodeficiency virus (HIV), hepatitis, sexually transmitted diseases, and other infections is associated with drug abuse.[41] Drug abuse is also associated with sexual promiscuity, teenage pregnancies, and abortions. Morbidities related to children bearing children are poor nutrition, suicide, child abuse, and inadequate immunizations.[42, 43] Further risks and drug-related problems noted in adolescents are psychopathologic, medical, legal, and financial problems; school suspension or expulsion; low self-esteem; rejection of traditional values; lack of religiosity; divorce; boredom; sensation seeking; and violent behavior.[23, 44-47]

Organ System Toxicity

A large part of the national health care costs relates directly or indirectly to the effects of substance abuse. Drug and alcohol treatment, plus the more expensive medical and surgical care relating to the sequelae of drugs and alcohol, accounts for nearly $200 billion of the health care cost. Injuries, many of which are alcohol and drug related, account for $75 to $100 billion a year. Nearly half of all general hospital admissions are alcohol and drug related. Perinatal health care for one neonate suffering from drug-

---

TABLE 140-1	
DRUG WITHDRAWAL SIGNS AND SYMPTOMS	
Stimulants	
Anergia	Nausea and vomiting
(decreased energy)	Nervousness
Anhedonia	Personality changes
(limited ability to	Suicidal ideation
experience pleasure)	
Apathy	
Chills	
Depression	
Headaches	
Narcotics	
Craving	Fever
(marked and continuous)	Sneezing
Abdominal cramps	Yawning
Muscle aches	Diaphoresis
Diarrhea	Irritability
Nausea/vomiting	Tachycardia
Loss of appetite	Hypertension
Trembling	Piloerection
Weakness	Depression
Rhinorrhea	Suicidal ideation
Mydriasis	
Sedative-Hypnotics	
Weakness	Hallucinations
Tremors	Vomiting
Insomnia	Abdominal cramps
Diaphoresis	Orthostatic hypotension
Restlessness	Myoclonic seizures
	Status epilepticus
Alcohol	
Tremulousness	Seizures
Hallucinosis	Delirium tremens

Note: For cocaine, psychological and physical dependence may equal that seen in heroin.

related problems can cost over $100,000. The health care cost for one HIV-infected patient approximates $150,000 or more.[6, 48] Numerous deaths occur annually because of fatal arrhythmias and respiratory failure associated with drug abuse and overdose.

Neonates

The most common cause of teratogenic mental retardation is the fetal alcohol syndrome, seen in about 1 in 2000 births.[12, 49] Infants born to alcohol-abusing mothers tend to have low birth weight, microcephaly, irritability, hyperactivity, and maxillary hyperplasia.[12] Use of marijuana by pregnant mothers can result in lower infant birth weight and shorter infant length.[50] Neonates exposed to benzodiazepines in utero are prone to dysmorphism and central nervous system (CNS) dysfunction.[51] Infants born to opiate-abusing mothers have abnormal sleeping ventilatory patterns, with a five to ten times increased risk of sudden infant death syndrome (SIDS).[52] Fetal death in utero, spontaneous abortions, and placental abruptions due to cocaine use are reported.[53, 54] Both cocaine and amphetamines cause intrauterine growth retardation, preterm delivery, decreased head circumference, reduced brain growth, fetal distress, jitteriness, tachypnea, hypertonia, poor feeding, and depressed interactive behavior.[54–58] Perinatal cerebral infarction in infants is a devastating complication of maternal cocaine use.[59]

Signs of opiate withdrawal, including tremors, agitation, hyperreflexia, high-pitched cry, sneezing, poor feeding, yawning, nasal congestion, diaphoresis, vomiting, diarrhea, abnormal sleep patterns, abnormal suck-swallow coordination, convulsions, and respiratory distress may be seen from a few hours to a few days after birth.[25, 60] In a study of passively addicted full-term newborns of drug-dependent mothers who used either opiates, cocaine, amphetamines, benzodiazepines, alcohol, barbiturates, or other drugs, excessive weight loss was associated with abstinence symptoms during the first 3 weeks of life.[61] Pharmacologic treatment with phenobarbital, paregoric, or other agents to promote relaxation and prevent seizures may be needed during the neonatal abstinence syndrome. Infants of intravenous drug–abusing mothers are also reported to have impaired T-cell immunity predisposing them to infections during the first year of life.[62]

CLINICAL EVALUATION

Substances of abuse are commonly encountered in the practice of emergency medicine (Table 140–2). Some of these may not be as frequently abused as others, but physicians should be aware of them all.

Alcohol

There are more then 3 million teenage alcoholics in the United States.[7, 63] Many adults receiving alcohol and drug abuse treatment report abusing alcohol by age 18.[64] More than 50% of fatal accidents involving teens result from alcohol use. The primary alcohols resulting in patients presenting to the emergency department in an intoxicated state or with other health problems include ethyl alcohol (ethanol), isopropyl alcohol (isopropanol), methyl alcohol (methanol), and ethylene glycol.[65]

Ethanol is a CNS depressant. The lethal dose of ethanol ranges from 5 to 8 gm/kg in an adult and about 3 gm/kg in children.[66] Acute intoxication produces exhilaration initially. Slurred speech, a loss of coordination, staggering gait, and stupor are eventual toxic effects. The many different medical problems associated with chronic alcohol use include pancreatitis, hepatitis, cardiomyopathy, malnutrition, and vitamin deficiencies. With an absolute or relative decrease in alcohol consumption, withdrawal symptoms can develop in the chronic user.[67] Alcoholic hallucinosis, Wernicke's encephalopathy, Korsakoff's psychosis, and delirium tremens due to alcohol withdrawal are complications in chronic alcohol abusers. Death associated with ethanol use may occur as a result of trauma, suicide, and a combination of hypotension, myocardial dysrhythmias, seizures and respiratory depression.

Isopropanol is a more potent CNS depressant than ethanol and is commonly found in rubbing alcohol, dermatologic products, and antifreeze. The CNS effects are potentiated by the metabolite acetone. Methanol (wood alcohol) is used as a solvent and as antifreeze. Toxicity results from the formation of the metabolites formaldehyde and formic acid. Methanol ingestion can cause blindness, CNS toxicity, gastrointestinal symptoms, pancreatitis, renal failure, severe metabolic acidosis, shock, and death. Ethylene glycol is used as antifreeze and has intoxicating properties similar to those of ethanol. Severe metabolic acidosis, CNS depression, cerebral edema, circulatory collapse, renal failure, and death may occur with toxic ingestions. Intoxication in young children due to either isopropanol, methanol, or ethylene glycol is more likely to be the result of accidental ingestion than of intentional use.

Narcotics

Narcotics are considered as either opiates (products derived from opium poppy) or opioids (any compound, including synthetic drugs, the effects of which are antagonized by naloxone).[68, 69] The term *narcotic* is commonly extended to include any drug that can be substituted for heroin or morphine in abuse potential. The major use for narcotics is that of pain relief. Narcotics, however, are highly abusable and produce dependence. Some effects include euphoria, apathy, sedation, and constipation. Patients overdosing from narcotics present with miosis, respiratory depression, and CNS depression. Illicit administration of narcotics can be achieved by various means, including smoking, oral ingestion, nasal insufflation, subcutaneous injection ("skin popping"), intramuscular injection, or intravenous injection ("mainlining").[69]

Heroin has a rapid onset of action. Because heroin use results in an intense euphoria and a long-lasting effect (3 to 5 hours) and because it is absorbed by multiple routes into the human body, it has been one of the most popular drugs of abuse.[15, 70] Pure heroin is a white powder with a bitter taste. However, street heroin varies in color and taste because of impurities left from the manufacturing process and from the additives used during the marketing process. These additive "fillers" used to "cut" the heroin include mannitol, dextrose, lactose, brown sugar, talc, baking soda, quinine and quinidine, lidocaine, procaine, strychnine, caffeine, boric acid, mercurous salts, and dog manure.[15, 68, 69] Street heroin is usually only 2% to 5% pure heroin, the remainder being adulterants. In certain cases the presenting signs and symptoms of an acute heroin overdose may be just as much attributable to the adulterants as to the opiate effects of heroin, or to the home remedies initiated by the user's acquaintances.[15, 69, 71–77]

Quinine is a favorite cutting agent for two reasons: (1) its bitter taste is similar to that of heroin, thus preventing the buyer from accurately assessing the amount of cutting agent present; and (2) it produces a "flush" when injected intravenously because of its vasodilatory actions. This flush mimics the effect of heroin. Cinchonism is a toxic syndrome

TABLE 140–2

SUBSTANCES OF ABUSE

Classification	Common Name/Trade Name	Generic Drug/Chemical Substance	Derivation
Narcotics	Buprenex	Buprenorphine	Opium phenanthrene thebaine
	Codeine	Methylmorphine	Opium phenanthrene morphine
	Darvon	Propoxyphene	Synthetic narcotic
			Structurally related to methadone
	Demerol	Meperidine hydrochloride	Synthetic narcotic: Phenylpiperidine derivative
	Dilaudid	Hydromorphone (dihydromorphinone)	Hydrogenated ketone of morphine
	Fentanyl		
	(Sublimaze)	Fentanyl citrate	Synthetic narcotic:
	(Innovar)	Fentanyl & droperidol	Phenylpiperidine derivative
	(China white)	Alpha-methyl fentanyl	Illicit fentanyl analogues
		3-Methyl fentanyl	
	Heroin (Turkish, Mexican Tar/Brown, Malaysian Pink, Persian, Penang Pink, China white and others)	Diacetylmorphine	Acetylation of morphine
	Hycodan	Hydrocodone (dihydrocodeinone)	Modified codeine compound opium phenanthrene thebaine
	Lomotil	Diphenoxylate hydrochloride and atropine sulfate	Synthetic narcotic: Phenylpiperidine derivative
	Methadone (Dolophine hydrochloride)	(4,4-diphenyl-6-dimethylamino-heptanone-3-hydrochloride)	Synthetic narcotic
	Morphine	Morphine sulfate	Opium phenanthrene
	MPPP	1-Methyl-4-phenyl-4-propionoxypiperidine	Illicit meperidine analogue
	MPTP	1-Methyl-4-phenyl-1,2,3,6-tetrahydropyridine	By-product of MPPP
	Nubain	Nalbuphine hydrochloride	Synthetic narcotic chemically related to naloxone and oxymorphone
	Parapectolin/Paregoric	Parapectolin/Paregoric	Camphorated opium tincture
	Percocet	Oxycodone and acetaminophen	Modified codeine and acetaminophen
	Percodan	Oxycodone and aspirin	Modified codeine and aspirin
	Stadol	Butorphanol tartrate	Synthetic narcotic similar to pentazocine
	Talwin	Pentazocine hydrochloride	Synthetic narcotic benzomorphan derivative
	"T's and Blues"	Pentazocine and pyribenzamine (tripelennamine hydrochloride)	Synthetic narcotic and ethylenediamine antihistamine
	Tylox	Oxycodone and acetaminophen	Modified codeine compound opium phenanthrene thebaine and acetaminophen
	Vicodin	Hydrocodone (dihydrocodeinone)	Modified codeine compound opium phenanthrene thebaine
Depressant	Alcohol (ethanol)	Ethyl alcohol (hydroxylated, aliphatic hydrocarbon)	Fermentation/distillation
Sedative-Hypnotics (Barbiturates)		ULTRA-SHORT-ACTING	Barbituric acid
	Brevital	Methohexital	
	Pentothal	Thiopental	
		SHORT-INTERMEDIATE-ACTING	
	Amytal	Amobarbital	
	Butalbital	Butalbital	
	Butisol	Butabarbital	
	Nembutal	Pentobarbital	
	Seconal	Secobarbital	
	Tuinal	Amobarbital/secobarbital	
		LONG-ACTING	
	Gemonil	Metharbital	
	Phenobarbital (Luminal)	Phenobarbital	
	Mebaral	Mephobarbital	
Sedative-Hypnotics (Benzodiazepines)		ANXIOLYTIC	Benzodiazepine derivatives
	Ativan	Lorazepam	
	Centrax	Prazepam	
	Klonopin	Clonazepam	
	Librium	Chlordiazepoxide	
	Paxipam	Halazepam	
	Serax	Oxazepam	
	Tranxene	Clorazepate	
	Valium	Diazepam	
	Xanax	Alprazolam	
		HYPNOTIC	
	Dalmane	Flurazepam	
	Halcion	Triazolam	
	Restoril	Temazepam	
	Versed	Midazolam (sedative-anesthetic)	
Sedative-Hypnotics (Nonbarbiturates) (Nonbenzodiazepines)	Chloral hydrate (Noctec)	Trichloroethanol (active metabolite)	Chloral derivative
	Doriden	Glutethimide (3-ethyl-3-phenyl-2,6-piperidine-dione)	Piperidinedione derivative: Structurally related to barbiturates

TABLE 140–2

SUBSTANCES OF ABUSE Continued

Classification	Common Name/Trade Name	Generic Drug/Chemical Substance	Derivation
Sedative-Hypnotics (Nonbarbiturates) (Nonbenzodiazepines) (Continued)	Placidyl	Ethchlorvynol	Tertiary acetylenic alcohol
	Equanil	Meprobamate	Carbamic acid ester
	Meprospan		
	Miltown		
	Mandrax	Methaqualone plus diphen-hydramine	Quinazolone
	Quaaludes	Methaqualone	
	Sopor	Methaqualone	
	Noludar	Methyprylon (3,3-diethyl-5-methyl-2,4-piperidi-nedione	Piperidinedione derivative
Psychedelic-Hallucinogenics	Hashish*	Tetrahydrocannabinol	*Cannabis sativa*
	Jimson weed (locoweed)	Belladonna alkaloids	*Datura stramonium*
	LSD	D-Lysergic acid diethylamide	Ergot alkaloid fungus
		D-Lysergic acid amide	Morning glory seeds
	Marijuana*	Tetrahydrocannabinol	*Cannabis sativa*
	MDA	Methylene dioxyamphetamine	Synthetic amphetamine
	MDMA	3-4-Methylene dioxyamphetamine	Synthetic amphetamine
	MMDA	3-Methoxy-4,5-methylene dioxyamphetamine	Synthetic amphetamine
	Mescaline	3,4,5-Trimethoxyphenylethylam-ine	Peyote cactus/San Pedro cactus
	Nutmeg	Myristicin	*Myristica fragrans* tree
	PCP (phencyclidine)*	1-(1-Phencyclohexyl) piperidine	Synthetic anesthetic
	Psilocybin	Dimethyl-4-phosphoryltryptamine	Psilocybe mushroom
	STP	2,5-Dimethoxy-4-methylampheta-mine	Synthetic amphetamine
	Yohimbine	Indolealkylamine alkaloid	Corynanthe yohimbe tree (tree bark) from tropical Africa
Stimulants	Amphetamine sulfate (Benzedrine)	β-Phenylisopropylamine racemic amphetamine	Synthetic noncatecholamine sympathomimetic adrenergic compound
	Dextroamphetamine (Dexedrine)	β-Phenylisopropylamine Dextro isomer amphetamine	Amphetamine
	Methamphetamine (Desoxyn)	Methamphetamine hydrochloride	Amphetamine
	Amphetamine	Combinations of:	
	"Look-alikes"	Caffeine (1,3,7-trimethylxanthine)	Methylated xanthines
	"Street speed"	Ephedrine	Noncatecholamine sympathomimetic
		Phenylpropanolamine	Noncatecholamine sympathomimetic
	Cocaine hydrochloride	Benzoylmethylecgonine	*Erythroxylon coca*
	"Crack"	Benzoylmethylecgonine amino alcohol base	Free alkali Base cocaine
	Preludin	Phenmetrazine hydrochloride	Amphetamine analogue
	Ritalin	Methylphenidate	Amphetamine analogue
	Tenuate	Diethylpropion hydrochloride	Amphetamine analogue
	Tobacco	Nicotine	*Nicotiana tabacum*
Inhalants	Fingernail polish remover	Acetone	Hydrocarbon
	Model cement		
	Cleaning fluids	Benzene	Aromatic hydrocarbon
	Rubber cement		Coal tar
	Paint thinner		
	Cleaning fluid	Carbon tetrachloride	Halogenated hydrocarbon
	Aerosol propellant	Dichlorodifluoromethane/trichlorofluoromethane	Halogenated hydrocarbon
	Refrigerant		
	Fuel	Gasoline/kerosene	Aliphatic hydrocarbon petroleum distillate
	Solvent		
	Thinner		
	Lighter fluid	Naphtha	Aliphatic hydrocarbon Petroleum distillate
	Varnish thinner		
	Airplane glue	Toluene	Aromatic hydrocarbon Coal tar
	Lacquer thinner		
	Ink		
	Plastic cement		
	Liquid shoe polish		
	Dry cleaning fluid	Trichloroethane	Halogenated hydrocarbon
	Typewriter correction fluid		
	Spot remover		
	Anesthetic	Trichloroethylene	Halogenated hydrocarbon
	Degreaser		
	Dry cleaning fluid		
	Nitrites ("poppers," "locker room," "rush," "heart-on," "aroma of man," "jack aroma," "crypt tonight")	Amyl nitrite Butyl nitrite Isoamyl nitrite Isobutyl nitrite	Organic nitrites
	Nitrous oxide	Nitrous oxide	Dinitrogen oxide (inorganic gas)

*Some sources classify cannabinoids and phencyclidine into their own separate categories.

following prolonged exposure to cinchona alkaloids (quinidine, quinine). The syndrome may develop at relatively low levels of the alkaloid. Thus, chronic abuse of drugs mixed with these alkaloids can lead to the development of this syndrome, which includes headache, fever, mydriasis, visual defects, tinnitus, hearing loss, organic brain syndrome, rash, and vomiting.[78]

Fentanyl citrate is a synthetic narcotic analgesic and sedative used perioperatively and is commercially available as Sublimaze (fentanyl) and Innovar (fentanyl plus droperidol, a neuroleptic major tranquilizer).[79] A 100-μg (0.1-mg) dose of fentanyl is approximately equivalent in analgesic activity to 10 mg of morphine or 75 mg of meperidine.[79] It is suited for anesthesia because of its high potency, rapid onset, and short duration of action.[80] When it is given intravenously the onset of action is almost immediate. Fentanyl may produce signs of narcotism characteristic of and indistinguishable from natural opiates. The narcotic potency of fentanyl is reported to be 200 to 300 times that of morphine.[80, 81]

"China white" is a bogus name given to the family of the illicit potent analogues of fentanyl that first appeared on the streets of California in 1979.[82, 83] The term was originally used in reference to a pure form of heroin processed in southeast Asia.[84, 85] Drug dealers and addicts use the name "china white" or "synthetic heroin" to refer to illicit fentanyl.[86, 87] At least 10 different illicit fentanyl analogues have been identified, alpha-methyl fentanyl and 3-methyl fentanyl being the most commonly synthesized and abused; 3-methyl fentanyl may be more than 6000 times as potent as morphine and 1000 to 2000 times as potent as heroin.[18, 81, 82, 88] Abused primarily intravenously, 3-methyl fentanyl accounted for many deaths in the 1980s.[82, 87] A usual dose is a few micrograms compared with 8 to 16 mg per dose of street heroin.[85]

Other Narcotics. Drugs such as codeine (methylmorphine), meperidine, oxycodone, pentazocine, propoxyphene, and hydrocodone all have abuse potential, and their presence should be suspected in patients presenting with signs of narcotism.[68] Codeine is a natural ingredient in raw opium and is also produced from morphine and thebaine. Thebaine is a minor constituent of opium from which oxycodones and hydrocodone are produced. Propoxyphene (Darvon) has been one of the leading prescription drugs implicated in addiction and in both intentional and unintentional overdoses and death.[89]

Pentazocine (Talwin) combined with tripelennamine ("T's and Blues," "T's and B's") is commonly injected to produce euphoria and is associated with toxic and fatal reactions. Its abuse is less common now because in 1983 the pentazocine formula was changed to include naloxone.[18, 63] However, some abusers increase the dose of tripelennamine to 100 mg from the usual 50 mg to create "T's and Purples," and adjust to the short-term effects of naloxone in the Talwin formula.[63] After the change in Talwin formula, some users turned to codeine and glutethimide combinations.[18]

Buprenorphine (Buprenex) is a derivative of the opium phenanthrene thebaine. It has been used as a methadone substitute for heroin addicts and can produce dependence and withdrawal symptoms, as with other narcotics. Lomotil is an antidiarrheal agent containing diphenoxylate hydrochloride and atropine sulfate. Toxicity from Lomotil use includes the anticholinergic effects of atropine and the narcotic effects of diphenoxylate.

Butorphanol (Stadol), nalbuphine (Nubain), pentazocine, and buprenorphine all possess mixed opioid agonist-antagonist properties. Agonist-antagonist drugs produce varied effects depending on their CNS receptor site activity. They can all precipitate withdrawal symptoms.

Designer Drugs

The term *designer drug* is used to describe synthetic drugs of abuse that are similar in effect to the naturally acquired drugs they mimic. They include the fentanyl analogues (china white), meperidine analogues (MPPP, MPTP), and mescaline-amphetamine hybrids such as MDMA.[82, 90] Once synthesized, many novel drugs are legal until they are accurately described and placed under government control.[68] The term *designer drug* should be reserved for drugs with the following characteristics: (1) synthesized from common chemicals; (2) unique and original, being produced illicitly and exempt from DEA control; (3) skillfully marketed under attractive exotic names; and (4) selective pharmacologic activity and generally very potent.[82, 90]

Unfortunately, drug abusers unwittingly become investigational subjects for designer drugs. In 1982 MPPP (1-methyl-4-phenyl-4-propionoxypiperidine) was sold in California as "synthetic heroin" or "new heroin" and also referred to by some as china white.[68, 84, 91, 92] A by-product of the synthesis of MPPP is MPTP (1-methyl-4-phenyl-1, 2, 3, 6-tetrahydropyridine), which is selectively neurotoxic to the substantia nigra and has caused disastrous cases of Parkinson-like disease.[93, 94]

In recent years MDMA has been sold on the streets as MDMA, MDM, ADAM, Ecstasy, and XTC. It is a psychoactive drug.

Stimulants

Drugs of abuse classified as CNS stimulants include cocaine and crack cocaine, synthetic noncatecholamine sympathomimetics of the amphetamine type, amphetamine analogues, and amphetamine look-alikes that contain combinations of caffeine (methylated xanthine), anorexiants, and various other noncatecholamine sympathomimetics. Nicotine in tobacco and caffeine in coffee, tea, and soft drinks are the most socially acceptable and probably the most commonly abused stimulant substances.

Stimulants are introduced into the body by injection, ingestion, inhalation, and intravaginal and intrarectal insertion. Intense psychological dependence and severe social dysfunction may result from stimulant abuse. Clinically, the individual abusing stimulants may present with symptoms including euphoria, dysphoria, hyperactivity, insomnia, hypertension, tachycardia, cardiac dysrhythmia, impotence, personality and tic disorders, psychosis, and circulatory collapse.

Cocaine. Cocaine is the most potent naturally occurring CNS stimulant. It is absorbed via multiple routes. For recreational use it is usually snorted, smoked, or injected. The plasma half-life of cocaine is prolonged compared with heroin (60 minutes versus 5 minutes), but its subjective effects do not last as long as those of heroin. Cocaine does, however, have dependence-generating potential comparable with that of heroin.[95] Plasma and liver cholinesterase hydrolyze cocaine to the two major metabolites ecgonine methyl ester and benzoylecgonine, which account for 80% of the urinary metabolites.[96, 97] Benzoylecgonine has been detected in the urine up to 144 hours after cocaine use.[98]

Cocaine fatalities usually result from accidental overdose, although routine use predisposes the user to accidents and marked toxicity from sympathomimetic and CNS stimulation effects. The cocaine user may present with headache, tachycardia, hypertension, agitation, euphoria, giddiness, dilated pupils, tachypnea, apprehension, hallucinations, muscle twitches, seizures, paranoia, confusion, depression, psychosis, and violent behavior.[99–102] Nosebleeds relating to cocaine snorting and infection relating to intravenous abuse are common complications. Adolescent abusers who snort cocaine develop a spectrum of rhinitis problems that should not be dismissed as sinusitis or upper respiratory infection.[103] The greatest risk of death after cocaine use is attributed to cardiac arrhythmias, seizure, respiratory arrest, hyperthermia, and cerebrovascular accidents. A number of cocaine fatalities present with a neuroleptic malignant syndrome variant with hyperthermia, rigidity, agitation, and delirium.[104] Acute myocardial ischemia related to focal vasoconstriction of the coronary arteries, with or without thrombosis, and myocardial infarction may occur in young cocaine abusers with no known preexisting cardiac risk factors.[105–110]

For some drug users the immediate stimulant effects obtained from intravenous cocaine are moderated by drug combinations. Many prefer to combine cocaine with heroin for intravenous use ("speedball," "snowball").[111] The euphoric effects of heroin subdue the letdown when cocaine wears off. Procaine is a common cocaine cutting agent found in street samples. Other adulterants include mannitol, lactose, talc, lidocaine, tetracaine, strychnine, caffeine, phencyclidine, quinine, and phenylpropanolamine.[112–114] Intoxication from arsenic compounds used to cut cocaine is also reported.[115]

The most addicting form of cocaine is "crack," the popular term for the crystalline pieces of rocks of free-base cocaine that is smoked.[116–118] The 98-degree Centigrade melting point for "crack" is much lower than that for cocaine hydrochloride, thus allowing it to be smoked and inhaled.[119, 120] The rapid absorption by the lungs results in near-instantaneous psychoactive effects of euphoria and stimulation.[116] Depression and paranoid psychosis also occur with "crack" addiction.

"Crack lung" is a pulmonary disease caused by cocaine inhalation resulting in fever, bronchospasm, and transient pulmonary infiltrates.[121] Symptoms of chest pain, neck pain, and dysphagia may occur in "crack" smokers 1 to 6 hours after use. Pneumomediastinum, pneumopericardium, and pneumothorax have been reported.[122–125] Physical findings may include subcutaneous emphysema about the neck and mediastinal crunch (Hamman's sign) in the precordial area.

Cocaine use is reported to be as high as 10% to 17% in pregnant women in the United States, some of whom use it to reduce the pain of labor. The fetus may be adversely affected. Maternal cocaine use can result in cerebral infarctions in the newborn as well as neonatal withdrawal symptoms. Breast-fed infants of cocaine-dependent mothers may become irritable and tremulous, and develop tachycardia, tachypnea, and hypertension.

In children presenting with seizures of unknown etiology, cocaine intoxication should be considered until excluded. Cocaine-induced seizures may occur not only in children abusing the drug, but also by accidental ingestion, by passive inhalation of free-base cocaine, and in infants breast fed by cocaine-dependent mothers.[126]

Amphetamine. Amphetamine is a noncatecholamine compound that produces strong CNS stimulation.[127] The most common amphetamine compounds are amphetamine sulfate (Benzedrine), methamphetamine (Desoxyn), dextroamphetamine (Dexedrine), benzphetamine (Didrex), and the combination amphetamine plus dextroamphetamine (Biphetamine).[128] Phenmetrazine (Preludin) is an amphetamine variant. Amphetamines are generally taken orally, snorted, or injected. Street names for amphetamines include "bennies," "black beauties," "dexies," "speed," "crystal-meth," and "uppers." The street name may refer to the chemical name (e.g., "dexies" for dextroamphetamine).

Amphetamine and its analogues have been used therapeutically as general stimulants and appetite suppressants, as well as for narcolepsy and hyperactivity syndrome in chil-

dren. Intravenous abuse of amphetamine by teenagers led to the ban of Benzedrine inhalers in the late 1950s. In recent years stimulants, including amphetamines, have been commonly abused by high school students, with a nearly 28% prevalence.[1, 129] The CNS stimulant effects (mental alertness, high energy) made amphetamine use common among college students, athletes, and truck drivers. Abuse of amphetamines may result in sympathomimetic clinical effects as well as paranoia and psychosis. The amphetamine abuser may become anxious, restless, garrulous, suspicious, or tremulous. Long-term use leads to psychological dependence and tolerance. Intravenous use of amphetamines may produce an intense feeling of euphoria, heightened sexual awareness, and a sense of power.

Methamphetamine ("crank," "speed," "crystal") is popular for intravenous "mainlining."[63] Acute lead poisoning has been reported with intravenous methamphetamine adulterated with lead, owing to impurities in the illicit manufacturing process.[130] Synthetic amphetamine compounds such as MDA, MDMA, and STP may produce hallucinations in addition to the anxiety, dysphoria, tachycardia, hypertension, hyperthermia, and seizures that may be seen with amphetamine use. Rhabdomyolysis, coma, and death can also occur with amphetamine misuse.

Amphetamine "look-alikes" may contain various combinations of sympathomimetics, including ephedrine, pseudoephedrine, phenylpropanolamine, and caffeine. Unintentional misuse by teenagers of pills containing pure caffeine alone may result in overdose and cardiac failure.

A relatively new form of methamphetamine called crystal methamphetamine ("crystal-meth," "ice") is a smokeable street drug similar in concept to the "crack" form of cocaine.[5, 131–133] "Ice" is a pure form of methamphetamine hydrochloride. The "high" from "ice" lasts much longer than that from cocaine.[5, 134] Crystal methamphetamine can cause acute psychosis, violent behavior, auditory hallucinations, and extreme paranoia.[131, 134]

Other Stimulants. Methylphenidate hydrochloride (Ritalin) is a popular prescription drug of abuse; in large doses it mimics the effect of amphetamine.[135] Its structure is related to that of amphetamine and it is used medically to treat narcolepsy and attention deficit disorder in children. Chronic abuse of methylphenidate can lead to marked tolerance and psychic dependence with varying degrees of abnormal behavior.[136] Intravenous abuse of methylphenidate can lead to hepatic, renal, pancreatic, pulmonary, and CNS complications.[137]

Phenmetrazine is used medically to treat obesity by suppressing appetite. However, just as with the chemically related amphetamines, tolerance can quickly develop, and abuse of the drug can lead to intense psychological dependance and severe social dysfunction. Among older street-drug abusers, phenmetrazine used intravenously is a preferred stimulant.[63]

Nicotine is the toxic alkaloid of tobacco (*Nicotiana tabacum*) products. An estimated 350,000 deaths per year are attributed to tobacco smoking. These deaths are virtually preventable. Seventy percent of high school students have smoked cigarettes in their lifetime and as many as 20% smoke regularly.[1, 3, 138] Although all cultures are affected, adolescents who smoke regularly are more likely to come from single-parent families and to have lower socioeconomic status.[138] Nicotine toxicity can result from gastrointestinal, dermal, and pulmonary absorption. Catecholamine discharge is prompted by low doses of nicotine but suppressed by higher doses.[139] Systemic manifestations of nicotine use are variable and include weakness, dizziness, nausea, vomiting, abdominal pain, and headache. Nicotine toxicity may also result in hypertension, hypotension, confusion, arrhythmia, convulsion, coma, and respiratory failure.

Psychedelics-Hallucinogenics

Many of the drugs that are abused for their capacities to alter sensory perception (vivid illusions [distortion of perceived reality] and hallucinations [perceived experiences that do not truly occur]) are derived from plants, and some are synthetic.

Marijuana. Marijuana (Maria y Juana, Mary Jane) means intoxicant and is the common name used for the dried leaves and flowers of the *Cannabis sativa* plant. The names "pot," "grass," "weed," "joint," and "reefer" are also used in reference to marijuana. Smoking is the common method of marijuana abuse. Psychotoxins are found in the resins of the plant. Hashish is dried resin derived from flowering tops, and hashish or hash oil is the dark liquid obtained by repeated extractions of plant material, resulting in a high concentration of active drug.[140] The "buds" of marijuana plant prove more potent than the leaves for smoking.[141]

Although cocaine is gaining in popularity, marijuana is still probably the most commonly abused illicit substance in the United States, especially among the younger population, over 50% of high school seniors having tried it in their lifetime. The clinical effects of marijuana include increased heart rate, conjunctival vascular congestion, nystagmus, dry mouth, mucosal irritation, decreased coordination, tremors, anxiety, exhilaration, and lethargy.[31, 140–143]

The psychoactive effects of marijuana are distortion of time and space, social inhibitions, increased desire for sweet foods, increased acuteness of sensory perceptions (visual, auditory, gustatory, olfactory), distortion of abilities and limitations, euphoria, "flashbacks," erosion of ambition, hallucinations, mood alteration, paranoia, and psychosis. "Flashbacks" are spontaneous recurrences of the "trip" experienced with taking a drug, which may occur for months but generally decrease in frequency if the drug is not taken again. Metabolites leave the blood stream quickly. Urine testing can be a reliable indication of marijuana use because half-life in the urine of metabolites is about 3 days.[31, 143]

Lysergic Acid Diethylamide (LSD). LSD is the diethylamide derivative of the ergot alkaloid lysergic acid.[144] The ergot alkaloid occurs as a natural result of the parasitic fungus *Claviceps purpurea* infecting grains and also occurs in members of the morning glory family (*Ipomoea violacea* and *Rivea corymbosa*). The physiologic effects of LSD are mainly sympathomimetic. The psychoactive effects are hyperacusis, visual and auditory illusions and hallucinations, slowing of time, euphoria, and alterations in sound and in intensity of colors. Panic attacks, depersonalization, "flashbacks," mood swings, paranoia, violent behavior, and psychosis may also occur. LSD appears on the street as pills, liquid, powder or impregnated sugar cubes, gelatin capsules, and blotting paper.[144] A recent resurgence of LSD has occurred in high schools. A study of adolescents in a drug treatment program showed LSD to be the third most frequent drug abused.[146] Seventy percent of the boys and 47% of the girls had used LSD at least once. Liquid LSD placed on decorated blotting paper appears to be the most frequently used form.[63, 146]

Phencyclidine (PCP). PCP is a synthetic drug made in clandestine laboratories that is chemically related to the phenothiazines. Phencyclidine sprinkled on marijuana and smoked is the usual route of abuse. Its psychomimetic effects include amnesia, agitation, anxiety, delirium, dissociation, depersonalization, distortion of body image, hallucinations, catatonia, a feeling of increased physical strength, and psychosis. Many sources classify PCP into a category of its own rather than as a hallucinogenic, because of the multiple effects it can produce (CNS stimulation and depression, analgesia and anesthesia, psychedelic and cholinergic-like symptoms).[147] PCP is sold in the form of powder, liquid, granules, capsules, and tablets.

Other Hallucinogens. Seeds from the jimson weed plant (*Datura stramonium*), also known as "locoweed," have been commonly abused by adolescents for hallucinogenic effects.[148, 149] The leaves of jimson weed are odoriferous and the flowers are trumpet-like in appearance. The seeds, flowers, and leaves are all toxic and have been used to make psychedelic teas.[150] Contained in the spiny pods, the brown seeds become readily accessible during the fall months when the fruit matures, dries, and splits open. The principal alkaloid (hyoscyamine) of jimson weed has primarily anticholinergic effects but in high quantities may cause euphoria, confusion, hallucinations, paranoia, and toxic psychosis.[151]

Mescaline is naturally derived from the peyote cactus (*Lophophora williamsii*) and the San Pedro cactus (*Trichocereus pachanoi*) of the southwestern United States and Mexico but is also illicitly synthesized.[151, 152] The dried tops or "buttons" of the peyote cactus contain mescaline and have been used during Indian rituals. Persons chewing the mescal buttons may experience sensory alterations and psychic effects. Mescaline is 3000 times weaker than LSD and the mescaline "trip" is apparently "mellower" than LSD. However, in a study of adolescents taking mescaline, one-half reported experiences of intense headache, panic, and terrifying hallucinations.[152] The effects of LSD and mescaline can be indistinguishable. Mescaline is supplied in powder on the street and may be abused via multiple routes in the body.

Mushrooms that produce hallucinogenic effects are a form of substance abuse for adolescents that have become more popular. *Psilocybe mexicana*, *P. cubensis*, and various other members of the *Psilocybe* genus contain the hallucinogen psilocybin. Once ingested, psilocybin is converted to the active hallucinogenic agent psilocin.[151] Psilocybin and psilocin possess an indole structure similar to that of LSD.[141] Like *Psilocybe*, mushrooms of the *Paneolus* and *Conocybe* genera also contain the hallucinogen psilocybin. The hallucinogenic effects of psilocybin are similar to those of LSD. Individuals taking mushrooms that contain psilocybin report effects lasting up to 6 hours. Head trauma, loss of consciousness, other injuries associated with falls, and "flashbacks" have occurred during intoxication.[153] Muscle relaxation, pupillary dilatation, dry mouth, tachycardia, distortions of space and time, panic reaction, lassitude, pleasurable or frightening hallucinations, and acute psychosis are some effects associated with psilocybin ingestion. Certain members of the *Amanita* mushroom species (e.g., *A. muscaria*, *A. pantherina*) contain the substances ibotenic acid and muscimol, which can produce psychedelic symptoms.

Myristicin is derived from the fruit of the *Myristica fragrans* tree, which produces the spices of nutmeg and mace.[154] When abused, myristicin can cause hallucinations, elation, various anticholinergic symptoms, anxiety, and panic reactions.[155] The toxic chemical is metabolized to an amphetamine-like compound in the body.

Synthetic amphetamine compounds such as STP, MDA, MMDA, and MDMA have hallucinogenic and other psychoactive properties. In a random study of undergraduate students at one campus, 39% admitted to using MDMA ("ecstasy") at least once.[156]

Yohimbine, also called "yo-yo," is a presumed aphrodisiac in the form of a powdered plant substance.[63, 157] It can cause a dissociative reaction as well as generalized paresthesia, hypertension, and tachycardia. It is abused via the oral and intranasal routes and by smoking it.[18]

Sedative-Hypnotics

Compounds that cause behavioral depression, sedation, and hypnosis are included in this group of substances of abuse. These drugs cause a state of intoxication similar to that from ethanol and also produce varying degrees of anesthesia, sedation, tranquilization, and hypnosis. The types in this group can be generally categorized as the barbiturates, benzodiazepines, and nonbarbiturate-nonbenzodiazepines. Euphoria, sedation, sleep, coma, respiratory depression, pulmonary edema, hypothermia, and hemodynamic instability are main features of concern with sedative-hypnotic use.

Barbiturates. The barbiturates are derived from barbituric acid. The short- and intermediate-acting barbiturates such as amobarbital (Amytal), pentobarbital (Nembutal), secobarbital (Seconal), butabarbital (Butisol), and butalbital (contained in combination tablets such as Esgic and Fiorinal) are most widely abused.[158, 159] Tuinal, a combination of secobarbital and amobarbital, is a favored drug of abuse.[160] The long-acting barbiturates have an onset of action much longer than that of short- and intermediate-acting barbiturates and are less abused. Onset of withdrawal symptoms from barbiturates reflects the half-life of the drug used and generally occurs sooner after discontinuance of short-acting compounds than after that of longer-acting drugs abused.

Complications that may develop with barbiturate use include respiratory depression, pulmonary aspiration, pulmonary edema, pneumonia, cerebral edema, and coma. Barbiturate skin blisters (bullae) may also occur and appear as tense, erythematous lesions, generally in comatose patients.

Nonbarbiturate-nonbenzodiazepines. The nonbarbiturate-nonbenzodiazepine sedative hypnotics of abuse include glutethimide (Doriden), methaqualone (Quaalude, Mandrax, Sopor), ethchlorvynol (Placidyl), chloral hydrate (Noctec), meprobamates (Equanil, Miltown, Meprospan), and methyprylon (Noludar). Abuse of these drugs is a problem for the adult population and typically is not seen in children. Sudden apnea, acute laryngeal spasm, and respiratory depression may occur as well as hypotension, pulmonary edema, and seizures with severe glutethimide intoxication. Quaaludes and Sopor are trade names for methaqualone base products. Methaqualone has low-potency, sedative-hypnotic effects. It may cause euphoria and is abused for the popular notion of its aphrodisiac qualities. Methaqualone intoxication can cause anticholinergic symptoms, seizures, delirium, and coma. Legal production of methaqualone ceased in the United States in recent years. Ethchlorvynol can induce sleep in 15 minutes in the prescribed hypnotic dose and is also known to cause giddiness, hysteria, muscle weakness, ataxia, and hypotension. Drug dependence may develop with ethchlorvynol use and there may be severe withdrawal symptoms similar to those of barbiturate and alcohol withdrawal.[161] Chloral hydrate's hypnotic effect is due to its metabolite trichloroethanol. Hypotension, cardiac arrhythmias, respiratory depression, and coma may result from chloral hydrate intoxication. The meprobamates are minor tranquilizers used primarily to manage anxiety disorders. With drug abuse, physical and psychological dependence may occur. Euphoria, drowsiness, ataxia, arrhythmias, hypotension, respiratory depression, and coma may occur with meprobamate use. Methyprylon is a hypnotic drug that can cause hallucinations, mental confusion, and nightmares as well as hypotension, ataxia, and convulsions. Drug dependence may develop with methyprylon use, and withdrawal symptoms resemble those of barbiturates.

Benzodiazepines. Benzodiazepine abuse and intentional use for suicide attempts is common. When these agents are ingested alone, severe complications are unusual. About a dozen or more benzodiazepines are marketed for their anxiolytic or hypnotic effect. Alprazolam, chlordiazepoxide, clonazepam, chlorazepate, diazepam, halazepam, lorazepam, oxazepam, and prazepam are preferred to barbiturates as anxiolytics because of their less adverse CNS and cardiovascular effects. Dependence risks are higher with long-term use of high-potency, short half-life benzodiazepines such as lorazepam (Ativan), alprazolam (Xanax), and triazolam (Halcion); withdrawal symptoms are less likely with use of low-potency, long-acting drugs such as diazepam (Valium), chlorazepate (Tranxene), and flurazepam (Dalmane). Withdrawal symptoms include seizures, delirium, and most of the other symptoms similar to those of alcohol and barbiturate withdrawal. Because of the lower addiction potential, clonazepam (Klonopin) has been used to substitute for other benzodiazepines during withdrawal. Combined use of benzodiazepines with other sedative-hypnotic agents such as alcohol may synergistically enhance sedation, respiratory depression, and hemodynamic instability.

Inhalants

Inhalants, including the solvents, nitrites, and nitrous oxide, have been abused in the lifetime of about one fourth of high school seniors.[1] In most cases, inhalants such as airplane glue, spray paints, and typewriter correction fluid are inexpensive products easily obtained by adolescents to abuse for "highs."[63, 162]

Solvent abusers are typically young teenage males. "Sniffing" or "huffing" (inhaling through the mouth) solvent-soaked rags or cotton and "bagging" (material soaked with solvent and placed at the bottom of a bag and vapor inhaled) are the methods of solvent abuse.[162] Euphoria is the desired effect, but cerebral anoxia and neurologic damage, including mild cognitive impairment, severe dementia, and cerebellar ataxia, may occur with abuse.[162] However, with acute use toxicity for the most part involves the pulmonary and cardiovascular systems. Hypoxia, hypercarbia, and respiratory depression may result from inhalant abuse. Sudden death attributable to cardiac arrhythmias occur with fluorocarbon propellant, refrigerants, and cleaning fluid solvent abuse. Sniffing of toluene can cause profound bradycardia, which can lead to asystolic sudden death.[163] Spray paint (toluene) abusers have also been reported to develop life-threatening renal tubular acidosis.[164] Liver failure is another complication of solvent abuse.

The nitrites (amyl, butyl, isobutyl, and isoamyl nitrites), abused as supposed aphrodisiacs in toxic amounts, can cause methemoglobinemia, cyanosis, and hypotension. The nitrites are available across the counter at "head shops" and pornography stores and through mail order catalogs. These agents, also referred to as "room odorizer," "rush," "locker room," "poppers," "heart-on," "aroma of man," "jack aroma," and "crypt tonight," are widely used to produce a feeling of euphoria. Nitrites have been popular with homosexual men for their alleged ability to relax anal sphincter tone and prolong sexual orgasm,[165] and have become popular with heterosexual adolescents as a means of getting "high." Symptoms associated with nitrite use are light-headedness, dizziness, vasodilatory effects (pounding heart, blurred vision, warm feeling), and tracheobronchial irritation.

Nitrous oxide is best known for abuse by those in the dental and medical professions. Its abuse can cause hypoxia, anoxic encephalopathy, and death. Multiple cases of myeloneuropathy associated with nitrous oxide abuse have been reported.[166] Whipped cream dispensers, which are available in supermarkets, contain nitrous oxide as a propellant. Small cylinders containing nitrous oxide ("Whippets") are used by restaurants to make whipped cream. These are readily available products containing nitrous oxide and are abused by teenagers.[63, 166]

DIAGNOSTIC STUDIES

Specimen analysis by laboratories to determine drug content is complicated by the pressing problem of polydrug use, and more than one laboratory method may be required for accurate drug identification.[167] Routine screening is not recommended in all asymptomatic patients and may be considered unethical if not done for specific treatment purposes.[168, 169] All patients suspected of drug abuse who can verbally respond should be asked to describe their use of alcohol or other drugs during history taking or by using an appropriate questionnaire format.[170–172] The diagnosis can often be made on a clinical basis and thus obviate the need for laboratory testing. When drug testing is necessary, the methods generally used in toxicology laboratories include color spot tests, enzyme-multiplied immunoassay technique (EMIT), radioimmunoassay (RIA), thin-layer chromatography (TLC), gas-liquid chromatography (GLC), high-performance liquid chromatography (HPLC), and gas chromatograph–mass spectrometry (GC-MS).[173–175] Immunoassays are rapid, are easy to perform, and are often used as initial screens, later confirmed by a second method if needed. Some drugs of abuse detectable by urine immunoassays are opiates, barbiturates, amphetamines, marijuana, PCP, cocaine, and methaqualone.[174] Since the level of sensitivity for detection of most drugs by TLC is only in the low-microgram range, a negative screen for drugs detectable at lower concentrations may turn out to be positive by RIA or GC/MS. TLC false-negative results are more common than false-positive ones.[167] The level of sensitivity with RIA and GC-MS may be 50 to 100 times and 1000 times that of TLC, respectively. Drug identification by GC-MS is the more reliable and definitive method, and more expensive. However, even when laboratories use GC-MS for general screening, as one study showed, drug identification may be reliable only 50% to 70% of the time.[176] This may be due in part to technical limitations, laboratory error, or specimen inadequacies (e.g., not enough serum, no accompanying urine specimen, specimen mixups and mislabeling, contamination, or dilution).[173]

Plain radiographs may be used to detect radiopaque pills and concretions in the gastrointestinal tract, verify endotracheal and nasogastric tube placement, and detect pulmonary aspiration and obstruction. A computed tomography (CT) scan of the head should be obtained in selected patients with unexplainable CNS depression, seizure disorders, or head trauma resulting from drug abuse. Routine laboratory studies, including blood count, serum glucose, electrolytes, liver function studies, cardiac enzymes, urinalysis, and arterial blood gases or pulse oximetry, may be necessary to evaluate certain cases of drug abuse. An electrocardiogram and a lumbar puncture may also be needed to assist diagnosis and treatment, especially in patients with cardiovascular and CNS pathology.

THERAPEUTIC INTERVENTION

Drug abuse patients may present with toxic symptoms from acute use, chronic use, or overdose. The patient may also appear nontoxic, seeking counseling, detoxification, or treatment of withdrawal symptoms. Those presenting with toxic or withdrawal symptoms require immediate medical intervention and support.

The type of therapeutic intervention varies according to the problem (Table 140–3). The drug overdose patient may require airway management and oxygen, intravenous access and fluid administration, intravenous dextrose, gastric emptying (ipecac to induce emesis, or lavage), activated charcoal, cathartics, and skin decontamination. Specific treatment measures such as naloxone for narcotic toxicity should be used when appropriate. Alkaline diuresis for barbiturate overdose and alkalinizing the urine in cases of myoglobinuria may be useful. Dialysis may be required in certain overdose cases. New drugs such as flumazenil (a benzodiazepine antagonist) have been developed.[160] Continuous monitoring of vital signs and hemodynamic and respiratory supportive care are crucial measures in the management of toxic patients, who may be hypertensive, tachycardiac, or hyperthermic, particularly with stimulant use, and may require antihypertensive medication, heart rate reduction, and body cooling measures.

Drug abuse patients presenting with violent behavior require security measures—physical or chemical restraint. Agitated or violent patients are potentially dangerous to both themselves and staff. The cause of agitation is not always drug related and must be quickly recognized and effectively treated. Phencyclidine is a typical drug causing agitation, but a number of others, as previously discussed, can cause agitation and violence as a direct effect or result of withdrawal. The differential diagnosis for agitation and violence should also include organic mental disorders, functional psychosis, mood disorders, extrapyramidal drug effects, catatonia (neuroleptic malignant syndrome, lethal catatonia), personality disorders, mental retardation, autism, tic disorders, episodic behavioral dyscontrol, and attention deficit–hyperactivity disorders (Table 140–4). In addition to specific treatment of the toxic effects and withdrawal symptoms, creation of a safe and nonthreatening atmosphere, communication, and pacification are further measures that should be used for agitated patients. Chemical restraint with tranquilizers should be used when necessary. An anxiolytic may be effective in some cases, but in cases of severe agitation, rapid tranquilization with haloperidol or other antipsychotic agents may be required. However, a neuroleptic agent should be avoided when there is a possibility of neuroleptic malignant syndrome.[177]

Complete documentation in the medical record is important for medical and legal reasons. The time, amount, and routes of substance use and intentional as opposed to unintentional use should all be recorded. In all cases when restraint is used, a clear documentation of patient presentation and the reason for restraint is important. To avoid violation of individuals' civil liberties, use of the least restrictive measures necessary to manage them appropriately is suggested.

Drug abuse patients who are suicidal or have serious toxic or withdrawal symptoms require hospitalization. After medical stabilization in the emergency department or inpatient setting, social and psychiatric intervention is often necessary. The association of substance abuse and other psychiatric disorders (a combination often referred to as "dual disorder") is common.[178] "Bad trips" as a reaction to drug use are usually limited in duration, and when there are no accompanying medical or psychiatric problems, hospital admission is often unnecessary and may be contraindicated.[145] Voluntary and involuntary psychiatric commitment for treatment, and inpatient and outpatient drug abuse treatment and counseling programs, should be utilized as necessary for individual cases.

There are drug abuse programs for the underaged at federal, state, and local levels, and these are designed to halt the progression of alcohol and other chemical dependencies. The goal is accomplished through patient education, family

TABLE 140–3

THERAPY AT A GLANCE

Narcotics	Toxic Patient	Drug Withdrawal/Agitation (Adolescents)
	Protect airway, assist ventilation, provide oxygen therapy IV line Gut decontamination Syrup of ipecac, 5 ml orally for infants 6–8 mo of age (under medical supervision), 15 ml for infants 8–12 mo, 15–30 ml for infants 1 yr and older Activated charcoal, 1 gm/kg Cathartics (sorbitol, magnesium citrate) Cardiac monitor and electrocardiogram Naloxone, IV, IM, or SC; initial dose 0.1 mg/kg up to 2 mg, then repeat as needed to obtain opiate reversal Naloxone, adult dose 0.4–2 mg initially, additional doses if needed Children in coma, administer dextrose 20–25%, 0.5 gm/kg IV	Diazepam, 5–10 mg oral or IM dose q 6 hr until patient is comfortable or 3 days, then taper dose by 20% daily or Methadone, 10 mg oral or IM dose q 6 hr up to 40 mg for day 1 and day 2, then reduce daily dose by 20%; prolonged maintenance should be managed by a methadone maintenance program Clonidine, 0.1 mg q 8 hr po (requires close monitoring: watch for hypotension with usage, and rebound hypertension and withdrawal symptoms with discontinuation)

Alcohol	Toxic Patient	Drug Withdrawal/Psychosis/Agitation (Adolescents)
	Protect airway, assist ventilation, provide oxygen therapy IV line For comatose patients, administer glucose and naloxone; administer thiamine to chronic alcohol abusers IV fluids for volume depletion Multivitamins in IV fluids Rule out gastritis, pancreatitis, hepatitis, pneumonia, injuries, and other medical conditions Consider hemodialysis in patients with alcohol levels greater than 400 mg/dl	Calm the patient Provide relief from anxiety and hallucinations: Chlordiazepoxide, 25–50 mg orally up to q 6 hr PRN Diazepam, 2–10 mg orally daily in divided doses Diazepam, 5–10 mg IM or IV and repeat q 4 hr PRN Lorazepam, 2–6 mg orally daily in divided doses Haloperidol, 2–5 mg IM Paraldehyde, 0.15 gm/kg/dose orally or IM; paraldehyde corresponds to 0.15 ml/kg/dose of solutions containing 1 gm/ml Seizures: Diazepam, 0.1–0.3 mg/kg IV Phenobarbital, 5–10 mg/kg IV Phenytoin, 10–15 mg/kg IV Paraldehyde, 0.3 gm/kg per rectum; dilute in equal amounts of olive oil, 0.3 ml/kg/dose

Sedative-Hypnotics	Toxic Patient	Drug Withdrawal/Agitation
	Protect airway, assist ventilation, provide oxygen therapy IV line Fluid challenge for hypotension Cardiac monitor and EKG Administer glucose, and naloxone in patients with depressed mental status Gut decontamination Treat dysrhythmias in symptomatic patients Alkaline diuresis (urinary alkalinization) for phenobarbital Hemodialysis or hemoperfusion should be considered for individual cases of sedative-hypnotic overdose failing to respond to supportive therapy	Supportive therapy, anxiety modulation **Benzodiazepine Withdrawal** Diazepam, IV, IM, or orally, 0.04–0.2 mg/kg initially and repeat q 4 hr as needed, then taper up to 2.5 mg daily Alternative medications to treat withdrawal: Clonazepam Phenobarbital Propranolol, and clonidine may attenuate withdrawal symptoms **Barbiturate Withdrawal** Reinstitute usual barbiturate dose with gradual reduction, 10% every 3 days until discontinued *or* Utilize pentobarbital challenge (adolescents/adults) 1. When patient is no longer intoxicated, give 200 mg pentobarbital orally 2. If intoxication results (nystagmus, ataxia, dysarthria), patient's 6-hr pentobarbital requirement is 100–200 mg (if patient falls asleep, there is no evidence of tolerance) 3. If no intoxication occurs, give additional 100-mg oral doses q 2 hr until intoxication occurs 4. Total dose to produce intoxication is patient's 6-hr requirement; determine 24-hr requirement by multiplying 6-hr requirement by 4 5. Substitute 30 mg phenobarbital for each 100 mg pentobarbital; give this amount of phenobarbital in 3–4 divided doses for 2 days, then decrease phenobarbital by 30 mg daily **Nonbenzodiazepine-Nonbarbiturate Withdrawal** Supportive care Because of cross tolerance, phenobarbital or benzodiazepines may be used to treat withdrawal

Table continued on following page

TABLE 140–3

THERAPY AT A GLANCE *Continued*

Psychedelics-Hallucinogenics	Toxic Patient	Psychosis/Agitation

Supportive care	Calm, quiet room
	Reassurance
	Minimize sensory stimuli
	Gut decontamination when indicated
	For phencyclidine toxicity:
	  Treat hyperthermia (cooling measures)
	  Treat hypertension
	    Sublingual nifedipine (10-mg sublingual adult dose)
	    Hydralazine, 0.15 mg/kg/dose IM or IV (initial dose)
	  Treat seizures
	  Screen patient for myoglobulin and administer IV fluids as necessary to maintain good urinary output
	  Avoid urine acidification in presence of myoglobinuria
		Create safe, nonthreatening atmosphere
		Communicate, pacify
		Have adequate security personnel readily available
		Provide restraint
		  Avoid violation of civil liberties, but use physical or chemical restraint when necessary and document reasons
		Diazepam, 5–10 mg IV, IM orally (adolescent/adult)
		Haloperidol, 5–10 mg IM (adolescent/adult)
		Haloperidol, 3–5 mg orally (adolescent/adult)

Stimulants	**Toxic Patient**	**Drug Withdrawal/Agitation**

	Protect airway, assist ventilation, provide oxygen therapy
	IV line
	Cardiac monitor, EKG
	Gut decontamination
	Hypotension:
	  Fluid challenge/vasopressors
	Treat hyperthermia
	Treat hypertension
	Tachydysrhythmia in symptomatic patients:
	  Propranolol, 0.01–0.1 mg/kg dose IV slowly to a maximum of 1 mg.
	  For SVT consider verapamil (0.1–0.2 mg/kg up to 5 mg/dose), adenosine (0.05–0.15 mg/kg/dose), or cardioversion
	Seizures: Diazepam, phenobarbital, phenytoin
		Quiet, calm surroundings
		Diazepam, 0.1–0.3 mg/kg IV
		Haloperidol, 0.05–0.15 mg/kg/day orally (age 3–12 yr); 0.5–5.0 mg 2 or 3 times daily orally (adolescent/adult)
		Haloperidol, 2–5 mg IM initial dose (adolescent/adult); tranquilization may require repeated doses
		Suicide precautions

Inhalants	**Toxic Patient**	**Drug Withdrawal/Agitation**

	Supportive care
	Hyperventilation to enhance lung excretion of inhaled solvents
	Cardiac monitor, EKG
	IV line
	Screen for electrolyte disturbances
	Serum lead levels in patients sniffing gasoline
	Screen for acid-base disturbances
	Treat dysrhythmias in symptomatic patients
	For nitrites (treat methemoglobinemia):
	  Use Trendelenburg position and administer IV fluids to treat hypotension
	  Administer 100% oxygen
	  Administer methylene blue, 1–2 mg/kg IV over 5 min
	  Correct metabolic acidosis
	Administer naloxone, glucose, thiamine in cases of multiple ingestion
		Watch for agitation and withdrawal symptoms from other possible substances

Neonatal Abstinence Syndrome

Treat withdrawal symptoms, reduce irritability and prevent seizures:
  Swaddle in blankets
  Provide quiet, dark room; protect from noxious external stimuli
  Phenobarbital, 8–10 mg/kg/day in 4 divided doses orally, IM, or slow IV
  Paregoric, 3–5 drops q 3–6 hr and increase to 5–10 drops q 4 hr if necessary
IV fluids to prevent dehydration
Seizures:
  Correct treatable underlying abnormalities if they exist (e.g., hypoglycemia, hypocalcemia, hypomagnesemia, hyponatremia, meningitis, vitamin B_6 deficiency)
  Phenobarbital, 20 mg/kg loading dose slowly (not to exceed 20 mg/min)
  Diazepam, 0.1–0.3 mg/kg IV or 0.5 mg/kg rectal up to 10 mg/dose
  Lorazepam, 0.05–0.10 mg/kg slow IV push
  Phenytoin, 10–20 mg/kg loading dose IV, not to exceed 1 mg/kg/min or 50 mg/min

Chemical Dependency Treatment
(Inpatient or Outpatient Programs)
Patient assessment
Medical treatment/clearance
Patient education
Family intervention
Patient and family counseling
Social Services intervention
Psychiatric treatment
Detoxification
Relapse prevention
General Measures
Perform toxicology screens and consult toxicologist and psychiatrist as appropriate
Hospitalize unstable medical or psychiatric patients

TABLE 140-4

DIFFERENTIAL DIAGNOSIS OF AGITATED/VIOLENT PATIENTS

I. Organic mental disorders
  A. Psychoactive substance intoxication
  B. Substance withdrawal
  C. Delirium
  D. Dementia
II. Psychosis
  A. Organic
  B. Functional
III. Mood disorders
  A. Depression (psychotic)
  B. Mania
IV. Extrapyramidal conditions
  A. Acute dystonia
  B. Akathisia
V. Catatonic state
  A. Lethal catatonia
  B. Neuroleptic malignant syndrome
VI. Disorders usually first eminent in childhood
  A. Mental retardation
  B. Autism
  C. Tic disorders
  D. Attention deficit–hyperactivity disorders
  E. Episodic behavior dyscontrol
    1. Brain injury
    2. Infection
    3. Partial complex seizures
VII. Personality disorders
  A. Antisocial
  B. Border line
  C. Paranoid
  D. Histrionic
  E. Narcissistic
VIII. Homicidal patients
IX. Suicidal patients

intervention, counseling, medical and psychiatric treatment, and relapse prevention measures. Family involvement in treatment is vital and directly affects the recovery rates of adolescent drug abusers.[179] The typical course of treatment involves initial assessment, detoxification, inpatient and outpatient rehabilitation, after-care, and relapse prevention tracks. A multidisciplinary team in the treatment of drug abuse may include the patient and family, physician, psychologists and psychiatrists, nurses, social workers, counselors, teachers, and members of the clergy.[23, 172, 178–180] Community support groups and school-related student assistance programs should be used as determined by individual needs.[23, 46]

References

1. Johnston LD, O'Malley PM, Bachman JG. Use of Licit and Illicit Drugs by America's High School Students 1975–1984. National Institute on Drug Abuse. DHHS Publ No. (ADM) 85-1394. Washington DC, Government Printing Office, 1985.
2. Alexander CS, Klassen AC. Drug use and illnesses among eighth grade students in rural schools. Public Health Rep 1988; 103:394.
3. Macdonald DI. Prevention of adolescent smoking and drug use. Pediatr Clin North Am 1986; 33:995.
4. Kandel D, Logan J. Patterns of drug use from adolescence to young adulthood. I. Period of risk for initiation, continued use, and discontinuation. Am J Public Health 1984; 74:660.
5. America Drug Crisis. A war that's draining the life from America's health-care system. Medical essay. Mayo Clin Health Letter 1989; November:1.
6. Hoffman RS, Goldfrank LR. The impact of drug abuse and addiction on society. Emerg Med Clin North Am 1990; 8:467.
7. Macdonald DI. Patterns of alcohol and drug use among adolescents. Pediatr Clin North Am 1987; 34:275.
8. Schwartz RH. Alcohol, drugs and head injury. Pediatrics 1986; 78:1169.
9. Fowler RC, Rich CL, Young D. San Diego suicide study. Arch Gen Psychiatry 1986; 43:962.
10. Annual Summary of Births, Marriages, Divorces, and Deaths, United States, 1987. Hyattsville, MD Public Health Service, 1988, DHHS Publ No. (PHS) 88-1120, Vol 36, No. 13.
11. Williams AF, Peat MA, Crouch DJ, et al. Drugs in fatally injured young male drivers. Public Health Rep 1985; 100:19.
12. Rogers PD, Harris J, Jarmuskewicz J. Alcohol and adolescence. Pediatr Clin North Am 1987; 34:289.
13. Bernstein E, Woodall WG. Changing perceptions of riskiness in drinking, drugs, and driving: An emergency department–based alcohol and substance abuse prevention program. Ann Emerg Med 1987; 16:1350.
14. Bouknight RR. Suicide attempt by drug overdose. Am Fam Physician 1986; 33:137.
15. Kulberg A. Substance abuse: Clinical identification and management. Pediatr Clin North Am 1986; 33:325.
16. Devenyi P. Prescription drug abuse. Can Med Assoc J 1985; 132:242.
17. Gawin FH, Ellinwood EH. Cocaine and other stimulants. N Engl J Med 1988; 318:1173.
18. Siegel RK. New trends in drug use among youth in California. Bull Narcotics 1985; 37:7.
19. Wright JD, Pearl L. Knowledge and experience of young people of drug abuse 1969–84. Br Med J 1986; 292:179.
20. Beauvais F, Oetting ER, Wolf W, et al. American Indian youth and drugs, 1976–87: A continuing problem. Am J Public Health 1989; 79:634.
21. Robinson TN, Killen JD, Taylor CB, et al. Perspectives on adolescent substance use: A defined population study. JAMA 1987; 258:2072.
22. Hoffman AD. Drug and alcohol use and abuse: Medical and psychologic aspects. In Hofman AD (ed). Adolescent Medicine. Menlo Park, CA, Addison-Wesley, 1983, pp 328–349.
23. Anderson GL (ed). When Chemicals Come to School. Greenfield, WI, Community Recovery Press, 1987, pp 1–478.
24. Hser Y, Anglin MD, McGlothlin W. Sex differences in addict careers. 1. Initiation of use. Am J Drug Alcohol Abuse 1987; 13:33.
25. Klenka HM. Babies born in a district general hospital to mothers taking heroin. Br Med J 1986; 293:745.
26. Matteo S. The risk of multiple addictions: Guidelines for assessing a woman's alcohol and drug use. West J Med 1988; 149:741.
27. Buchta RM. Drug usage among adolescents: A survey from a pediatric/adolescent practice (letter to the editor). Am J Dis Child 1989; 143:765.
28. Johnson EM. Substance abuse and women's health. Public Health Rep 1987; July/Aug Suppl:42.
29. Zarek D, Hawkins D, Rogers PD. Risk factors for adolescent substance abuse. Pediatr Clin North Am 1987; 34:481.
30. Richardson JL, Dwyer K, McGuigan K, et al. Substance use among eighth-grade students who take care of themselves after school. Pediatrics 1989; 84:556.
31. Schwartz RH, Hoffman NG, Jones R. Behavioral, psychological, and academic correlates of marijuana usage in adolescents. Clin Pediatr 1987; 26:264.
32. Brown SA. Life events of adolescents in relation to personal and parental substance abuse. Am J Psychiatry 1989; 146:484.
33. Joshi NP, Scott M. Drug use, depression and adolescents. Pediatr Clin North Am 1988; 35:1349.
34. Deykin EY, Levy JC, Wells V. Adolescent depression, alcohol and drug abuse. Am J Public Health 1987; 77:178.
35. Christie KA, Burke JD, Regier DA, et al. Epidemiologic evidence for early onset of mental disorders and higher risk of drug abuse in young adults. Am J Psychiatry 1988; 145:971.
36. Lustick MJ. Bulimia in adolescents: A review. Pediatrics 1985, Sex, Drugs, Rock 'n' Roll Suppl: 685.
37. Palmer EP, Guay AT. Reversible myopathy secondary to abuse of ipecac in patients with major eating disorders. N Engl J Med 1985; 313:1457.
38. Killen JD, Taylor B, Telch MJ, et al. Depressive symptoms and substance use among adolescent binge eaters and purgers: A defined population study. Am J Public Health 1987; 77:1539.
39. Jonas JM, Gold MS. Cocaine abuse and eating disorders (letter to editor). Lancet 1986; 1:390.
40. Smith DE, Schwartz RH, Martin DM. Heavy cocaine use by adolescents. Pediatrics 1989; 83:539.
41. Goldsmith MF. Sex tied to drugs = STD spread. JAMA 1988; 260:2009.
42. News Reports. Times and mores exact morbid toll from youth. Hosp Pract 1987; 18:80E.
43. Press S. Crack and fatal child abuse (letter to editor). JAMA 1988; 260:3132.
44. Story M, York PVZ. Nutritional status of Native American adolescent substance users. J Am Diet Assoc 1987; 87:1680.
45. Kandel DB, Davies M, Karus D, et al. The consequences in young adulthood of adolescent drug involvement. Arch Gen Psychiatry 1986; 43:746.
46. Lopez C. Substance abuse prevention program—Albuquerque, New Mexico. JAMA 1987; 258:3231.
47. Newcomb MD, Maddahian E, Bentler PM. Risk factors for drug use

among adolescents: Concurrent and longitudinal analyses. Am J Public Health 1986; 76:525.

48. Lowe C. Maternal drug abuse—New York City. City Health Information 1989; 8:1.
49. Silverman MM, Denniston R. Status of the 1990 objectives on misuse of alcohol and drugs. Leads from the MMWR. JAMA 1987; 258:3367.
50. Zuckerman B, Frank DA, Hingson R, et al. Effects of maternal marijuana and cocaine use on fetal growth. N Engl J Med 1989; 320:762.
51. Laegreid L, Olegard R, Wahlstrom J, et al. Abnormalities in children exposed to benzodiazepines in utero (letter to editor). Lancet 1987; 1:108.
52. Ward SLD, Schuetz S, Krishna V. Abnormal sleeping ventilatory pattern in infants of substance-abusing mothers. Am J Dis Child 1986; 140:1015.
53. Critchley HOD, Woods SM, Barson AJ, et al. Fetal death in utero and cocaine abuse. Case report. Br J Obstet Gynaecol 1988; 95:195.
54. Chasnoff IJ, Burns WJ, Schnoll SH et al. Cocaine use in pregnancy. N Engl J Med 1985; 313:666.
55. Chouteau M, Namerow PB, Leppert P. The effect of cocaine abuse on birth weight and gestational age. Obstet Gynecol 1988; 72:351.
56. Hadeed AJ, Siegel SR. Maternal cocaine use during pregnancy: Effect on the newborn infant. Pediatrics 1989; 84:205.
57. Madden JD, Payne TF, Miller S. Maternal cocaine abuse and effect on the newborn. Pediatrics 1986; 77:209.
58. Oro AS, Dixon SD. Perinatal cocaine and methamphetamine exposure: Maternal and neonatal correlates. J Pediatr 1987; 111:571.
59. Chasnoff IJ, Bussey ME, Savich R, et al. Perinatal cerebral infarction and maternal cocaine use. J Pediatr 1986; 108:456.
60. Mathieu OR Jr. The drug-addicted newborn. In Reece RM (ed). Manual of Emergency Pediatrics. 3rd ed. Philadelphia, WB Saunders, 1984, pp 127–131.
61. Weinberger SM, Kandall SR, Doberczak TM, et al. Early weight-change patterns in neonatal abstinence. Am J Dis Child 1986; 140:829.
62. Culver KW, Ammann AJ, Partridge JC, et al. Lymphocyte abnormalities in infants born to drug-abusing mothers. J Pediatr 1987; 111:230.
63. The drugs on the street where you live. Emerg Med 1986; 18:128.
64. Kashani JH, Solomon NA, Dugan K, et al. Differences between early and late onset of substance abuse: An inpatient experience. South Med J 1987; 80:554.
65. Bryson PD. Alcohols. In Bryson PD (ed). Comprehensive Review In Toxicology. 1st ed. Rockville, MD, Aspen Systems Corp, 1986, pp 141–170.
66. Ellenhorn MJ, Barceloux DG. Alcohols and Glycols. In Ellenhorn MJ, Barceloux DG (eds). Medical Toxicology. New York, Elsevier Science Publishing, 1988, pp 781–812.
67. Elser BI. Alcohol withdrawal syndromes. In Gardner LB (ed). Textbook of Acute Internal Medicine. New York, Elsevier Sciences Publishing, 1986; pp 459–466.
68. Ellenhorn MJ, Barceloux DG. Opiates, opioids, and designer drugs. In Ellenhorn MJ, Barceloux DG (eds). Medical Toxicology. New York, Elsevier Science Publishing, 1988, pp 687–762.
69. Bryson PD. Drugs of abuse: Narcotics. In Bryson PD (ed). Comprehensive Review In Toxicology. 1st ed. Rockville, MD, Aspen Systems Corp, 1986, pp 181–197.
70. Stembach G, Morgan J, Eliastam M. Heroin addiction. Acute presentation of medical complications. Ann Emerg Med 1980; 9:16.
71. Joynt BP, Mikhael NZ. Sudden death of a heroin body packer. J Anal Toxicol 1985; 9:238.
72. Cuddy P. Management of acute opioid intoxication. Crit Care Q 1982; 4:65.
73. Khantzian E, McKeena G. Acute toxic and withdrawal reactions associated with drug use and abuse. Ann Intern Med 1979; 90:361.
74. Winek CL, Schweighardt FK, Fochtman FW, et al. Quinine in urinalysis for heroin. JAMA 1971; 217:1243.
75. Winek CL, Davis ER, Collom WD, et al. Quinine fatality. Case report. Clin Toxicol 1974; 7:129.
76. Lupovich P, Pilewski R, Sapira JD, et al. Cardiotoxicity of quinine as adulterant in drugs. JAMA 1970; 212:1216.
77. Drenik EJ, Younger KM. Heroin overdose complicated by intravenous injection of milk. JAMA 1970; 213:1687.
78. Ellenhorn MJ, Barceloux DG. Antiarrhythmic agents. In Ellenhorn MJ, Barceloux DG (eds). Medical Toxicology. New York, Elsevier Science Publishing, 1988, pp 169–207.
79. Barnhart ER. Fentanyl citrate, Innovar and Sublimaze. Physicians' Desk Reference. 43rd ed. Oradell, NJ, Medical Economics, 1989, pp 1049–1051, 1053–1055.
80. Gardocki JF, Yelnosky J. A study of the pharmacologic actions of fentanyl citrate. Toxicol Appl Pharmacol 1964; 6:48.
81. VanBever WFM, Niemeegers CJE, Janssen PAJ. Synthetic analgesics. Synthesis and pharmacology of the diasterioisomers of N-[3-methyl-1-(2-phenylethyl)-4-piperidyl]-N-phenylpropanamide and N-[3-methyl-1-(1-methyl-2-phenylethyl)-4-piperidyl]-N-phenylpropanamide. J Med Chem 1974; 17:1047.
82. Henderson GL. Designer drugs: Past history and future prospects. J Forensic Sci 1988; 33:569.
83. Stinson S. Structure of bogus china white solved. Chem Eng News 1981; 59:71.

84. Buchannan J. Opioids of abuse. CSHP Voice 1985; 12:47.
85. LaBarbera M, Wolfe T. Characteristics, attitudes, and implications of fentanyl use based on reports from self-identified fentanyl users. J Psychoactive Drugs 1983; 15:293.
86. Ayres WA, Starsiak MJ, Sokolay P. The bogus drug, three methyl and alpha methyl fentanyl sold as "china white." J Psychoactive Drugs 1981; 13:91.
87. Martin ML, Hecker J, Clark RF, et al. China white epidemic: An eastern United States emergency department experience (abstr). Ann Emerg Med 1989; 18:446.
88. Hicks Sl. Fentanyl (letter to editor). NC Med J 1984; 45:475.
89. Soumerai SB, Avorn J, Gortmaker S, et al. Effect of government and commercial warnings on reducing prescription misuse: The case of propoxyphene. Am J Public Health 1987; 77:1518.
90. Henderson G. Designer drugs: The new synthetic drugs of abuse. Clinical Update In Toxicology 1986; 1.
91. Baum RM. New variety of street drugs poses growing problem. Chem Eng News 1985; 9:7.
92. Shafer J. Designer drugs. Science 1985; March: 60.
93. Langston JW, Ballard P. Parkinsonism induced by 1-methyl-4-phenyl-1, 2, 3, 6-tetrahydropyridine (MPTP): Implications for treatment and the pathogenesis of Parkinson's disease. Can J Neurol Sci 1984; 11:160.
94. Langston JW, Ballard P. Chronic parkinsonism in humans due to a product of meperidine-analog synthesis. Science 1983; 219:979.
95. Hasin DS, Grant BF, Endicott J, et al. Cocaine and heroin dependence compared in poly-drug abusers. Am J Public Health 1988; 87:567.
96. Inaba T, Stewart DJ, Kalow W. Metabolism of cocaine in man. Clin Pharmacol Ther 1978; 23:547.
97. Ambre J. The urinary excretion of cocaine and metabolites in humans. A kinetic analysis of published data. J Anal Toxicol 1985; 9:241.
98. Hamilton HE, Wallace JE, Shimak EL, et al. Cocaine and benzoylecgonine excretions in humans. J Forensic Sci 1977; 22:697.
99. Mueller PD, Benowitz NL, Olson KR. Cocaine. Emerg Med Clin North Am 1990; 8:481.
100. Gold MS, Smith DE, Olden K. Cocaine: Helping patients avoid the end of the line. Emerg Med Rep 1985; 6:17.
101. Pearsall HR, Altesman RI. Cocaine abuse. Hosp Med 1987; 23:126.
102. Lowenstein DH, Massa SM, Rowbotham MC, et al. Acute neurologic and psychiatric complications associated with cocaine abuse. Am J Med 1987; 83:841.
103. Schwartz RH, Estroff T, Fairbanks DNF, et al. Nasal symptoms associated with cocaine abuse during adolescence. Arch Otolaryngol Head Neck Surg 1989; 115:63.
104. Kosten TR, Kleber HD. Sudden death in cocaine abusers: Relation to neuroleptic malignant syndrome (letter to editor). Lancet 1987; 1:1198.
105. Wehbie CS, Vidaillet HJ, Navetta FI, et al. Acute myocardial infarction associated with initial cocaine use. South Med J 1987; 80:933.
106. Rollingher IM, Belzberg AS, Macdonald IL. Cocaine-induced myocardial infarction. Can Med Assoc J 1986; 135:45.
107. Cregler LL, Mark H. Cardiovascular dangers of cocaine abuse. Am J Cardiol 1986; 57:1185.
108. Isner JM, Chokshi SK. Cocaine and vasospasm. N Engl J Med 1989; 321:1604.
109. Nademanee K, Gorelick DA, Josephson MA, et al. Myocardial ischemia during cocaine withdrawal. Ann Intern Med 1989; 111:876.
110. Tokarski GF, Paganussi P, Urbanski R, et al. An evaluation of cocaine-induced chest pain. Ann Emerg Med 1990; 19:1088.
111. Cohen S. Cocaine. JAMA 1975; 231:74.
112. Bryson PD. Drugs of abuse: Stimulants. In Bryson PD (ed). Comprehensive Review In Toxicology. 1st ed. Rockville, MD, Aspen Systems Corp, 1986, pp 219–237.
113. Lukas Z, Ewski T, Jeffrey WK. Impurities and artifacts of illicit cocaine. J Forensic Sci 1980; 25:499.
114. Siegel RK. Cocaine substitutes. Pharm Chem Newsletter 1982; 11:1.
115. Lombard J, Levin IH, Weiner WJ. Arsenic intoxication in a cocaine abuser (letter to editor). N Engl J Med 1989; 320:869.
116. Ellenhorn MJ, Barceloux DG. Cocaine. In Ellenhorn MJ, Barceloux DG (eds). Medical Toxicology. New York, Elsevier Science Publishing, 1988, pp 643–661.
117. Gold MS. Crack abuse: Its implications and outcomes. Resident and Staff Physician 1987; 33:45.
118. Washton AM, Gold MS, Pottash AC. "Crack": Early report on a new drug epidemic. Postgrad Med 1986; 80:52.
119. Smith DE. West coast and east coast drug abuse patterns, 1979–80. Ann NY Acad Sci 1981; 362:22.
120. Crack. Lancet 1987; 2:1061.
121. Kissner DG, Lawrence WD, Selis JE, et al. Crack lung: Pulmonary disease caused by cocaine abuse. Am Rev Respir Dis 1987; 136:1250.
122. Morris JB, Shuck JM. Pneumomediastinum in a young male cocaine user. Ann Emerg Med 1985; 14:194.
123. Shesser R, Davis C, Edelstein J. Pneumomediastinum and pneumothorax after inhaling alkaloidal cocaine. Ann Emerg Med 1981; 10:213.
124. Brody SL, Anderson GV, Gutman JBL. Pneumomediastinum as a complication of "crack" smoking. Am J Emerg Med 1988; 6:241.
125. Adrouny A, Magnusson P. Pneumopericardium from cocaine inhalation. N Engl J Med 1985; 313:48.

126. Ernst AA, Sanders WM. Unexpected cocaine intoxication presenting as seizures in children. Ann Emerg Med 1989; 18:774.

127. Ellenhorn MJ, Barceloux DG. Amphetamines. *In* Ellenhorn MJ, Barceloux DG (eds). Medical Toxicology. New York, Elsevier Science Publishing, 1988, pp 625–641.

128. King P, Coleman JH. Stimulants and narcotic drugs. Pediatr Clin North Am 1987; 34:349.

129. Johnston LD, Bachman JG, O'Malley PM. 1979 Highlights: Drugs and the Nation's High School Students: Five Year Trends. DHHS Publ No. (ADM) 81-930. Rockville, MD, National Institute on Drug Abuse, 1979.

130. Allcott JV, Barnhart RA, Mooney LA. Acute lead poisoning in two users of illicit methamphetamine. JAMA 1987; 258:510.

131. Jackson JG. Hazards of smokeable methamphetamine (letter to editor). N Engl J Med 1989; 321:907.

132. Cho AK. Ice: A new dosage form of an old drug. Science 1990; 249:631.

133. Sekine H, Nakahara Y. Abuse of smoking methamphetamine mixed with tobacco. I. Inhalation efficiency and pyrolysis products of methamphetamine. J Forensic Sci 1987; 32:1271.

134. Teng A. 1990's new designer drug invades EDs. Emerg Med News 1990; 12:1.

135. Fulton AI, Yates WR. Family abuse by methylphenidate. Am Fam Physician 1988; 38:143.

136. Barnhart ER. Ritalin. Physicians' Desk Reference. 43rd ed. Oradell, NJ, Medical Economics, 1989, pp 856–857.

137. Stecyk O, Loludice TA, Demeter S, et al. Multiple organ failure resulting from intravenous abuse of methylphenidate hydrochloride. Ann Emerg Med 1985; 14:597.

138. Boyle MH, Offord DR. Smoking, drinking and use of illicit drugs among adolescents in Ontario: Prevalence, patterns of use and sociodemographic correlates. Can Med Assoc J 1986; 135:1113.

139. Litovitz TL. Household products. Cigarettes and other tobacco products. *In* Hanson W (ed). Toxic Emergencies: Clinics In Emergency Medicine. Vol 5. New York, Churchill Livingstone, 1984, pp 254–256.

140. Selden BS, Clark RF, Curry SC. Marijuana. Emerg Med Clin North Am 1990; 8:527.

141. Yarbrough B. Plant poisoning: A comprehensive management guide. ER Reports 1983; 4:19.

142. Ellenhorn MJ, Barceloux DG. Marijuana. *In* Ellenhorn MJ, Barceloux DG (eds). Medical Toxicology. New York, Elsevier Science Publishing, 1988, pp 673–685.

143. Schwartz RH. Identifying and helping patients who use marijuana. Postgrad Med 1989; 86:91.

144. Ellenhorn MJ, Barceloux DG. Lysergic acid diethylamide. *In* Ellenhorn MJ, Barceloux DG (eds). Medical Toxicology. New York, Elsevier Science Publishing, 1988, pp 663–672.

145. Reece RM. Drug abuse, acute reactions. *In* Reece RM (ed). Manual of Emergency Pediatrics. 2nd ed. Philadelphia, WB Saunders, 1978, pp 109–131.

146. Schwartz RH, Comerci GD, Meeks JE. LSD: Patterns of use by chemically dependent adolescents. J Pediatr 1987; 111:936.

147. Bryson PD. Drugs of abuse: Phencyclidine. *In* Bryson PD (ed). Comprehensive Review In Toxicology. 1st ed. Rockville, MD, Aspen Systems Corp, 1986, pp 239–250.

148. Goldfrank L, Melinek M. Locoweed and other anticholinergics. Hosp Physician 1979; 8:18.

149. Klein-Schwartz W, Oderda GM. Jimsonweed intoxication in adolescents and young adults. Am J Dis Child 1984; 138:737.

150. Urich RW, Bowerman DL, Levisky JA, et al. *Datura stramomium*: A fatal poisoning. J Forensic Sci 1982; 27:948.

151. Tong TG, Pond SM. The underworld connection: Hallucinogens. *In* Hanson W (ed). Toxic Emergencies: Clinics In Emergency Medicine. Vol 5. New York, Churchill Livingstone, 1984, pp 104–109.

152. Schwartz RH. Mescaline: A survey. Am Fam Physician 1988; 37:122.

153. Schwartz RH, Smith DE. Hallucinogenic mushrooms. Clin Pediatr 1988; 27:70.

154. Brown RT, Braden NJ. Hallucinogens. Pediatr Clin North Am 1987; 34:341.

155. Goldfrank L, Lewin N, Flomenbaum N, et al. The pernicious panacea: Herbal medicine. Hosp Physician 1982; 18:64.

156. Peroutka SJ. Incidence of recreational use of 3, 4-methylenedimethoxymethamphetamine (MDMA, "ecstasy") on an undergraduate campus. N Engl J Med 1987; 317:1542.

157. Linden CH, Vellman WP, Rumack B. Yohimbine: A new street drug. Ann Emerg Med 1985; 14:1002.

158. Lewis DC, Gomolin IH. Drug overdose and withdrawal. *In* May HL (ed). Emergency Medicine. New York, John Wiley, 1984, pp 823–843.

159. Bryson PD. Drugs of abuse: Sedative-hypnotics. *In* Bryson PD (ed). Comprehensive Review In Toxicology. 1st ed. Rockville, MD, Aspen Systems Corp, 1986, pp 199–217.

160. Ellenhorn MJ, Barceloux DG. Sedative-hypnotics. *In* Ellenhorn MJ, Barceloux DG (eds). Medical Toxicology. New York, Elsevier Science Publishing, 1988, pp 575–603.

161. Barnhart ED. Placidyl. Physicians' Desk Reference. 43rd ed. Oradell, NJ, Medical Economics, 1989, pp 563–564.

162. Hormes JT, Filley CM, Rosenberg NL. Neurologic sequelae of chronic solvent vapor abuse. Neurology 1986; 36:698.

163. Zee-Cheng C, Mueller CE, Gibbs HR. Toluene sniffing and severe sinus bradycardia (letter to editor). Ann Intern Med 1985; 103:482.

164. Lavoie FW, Dolan MC, Danzl DF, et al. Recurrent resuscitation and "no code" orders in a 27-year-old spray paint abuser. Ann Emerg Med 1987; 16:1266.

165. Schwartz RH, Peary P. Abuse of isobutyl nitrite inhalation (Rush) by adolescents. Clin Pediatr 1986; 25:308.

166. Gillman MA. Nitrous oxide, an opioid addictive agent. Am J Med 1986; 81:97.

167. Gold MS, Verebey K, Dackis CA. Diagnosis of drug abuse, drug intoxication and withdrawal states. Fair Oaks Hospital Psychiatry Letter 1985; 3:23.

168. Schonberg SK, Beach RK, Brookman RR, et al. Screening for drugs of abuse in children and adolescents. Pediatrics 1989; 84:396.

169. King NMP, Cross AW. Moral and legal issues in screening for drug use in adolescents. J Pediatr 1987; 111:249.

170. US Preventive Services Task Force. Screening for alcohol and other drug abuse. Am Fam Physician 1989; 40:137.

171. Klitzner M, Schwartz RH, Gruenewald P, et al. Screening for risk factors for adolescent alcohol and drug use. Am J Dis Child 1987; 141:45.

172. Anglin TM. Interviewing guidelines for the clinical evaluation of adolescent substance abuse. Pediatr Clin North Am 1987; 34:381.

173. MacKenzie RG, Cheng M, Haftel AJ. The clinical utility and evaluation of drug screening techniques. Pediatr Clin North Am 1987; 34:423.

174. Osterloh JD. Utility and reliability of emergency toxicologic testing. Emerg Med Clin North Am 1990; 8:693.

175. Screening for drugs of abuse. Lancet 1987; 1:365.

176. Ingelfinger JA, Isakson G, Shine D, et al. Reliability of the toxic screen in drug overdose. Clin Pharmacol Ther 1981; 29:570.

177. Martin ML, Lucid EJ, Walker RW. Neuroleptic malignant syndrome. Ann Emerg Med 1985; 14:354.

178. Kofoed L, Kania J, Walsh T, et al. Outpatient treatment of patients with substance abuse and coexisting psychiatric disorders. Am J Psychiatry 1986; 143:867.

179. Macdonald DI. Drug abuse in adolescents: When to intervene, how to help. Postgrad Med 1985; 78:109.

180. Finley B. The role of the psychiatric nurse in a community substance abuse prevention program. Nursing Clin North Am 1989; 24:121.

CHAPTER 141

Medicolegal Considerations

Robert A. Felter

INTRODUCTION

The emergency department is the third most common area in the hospital to become involved in lawsuits. Only the operating room–recovery room and delivery room are more frequently so involved. Pediatrics ranks ninth among the medical specialties involved in litigation, but the unique aspects of emergency medicine make the emergency management of children more prone to litigation.

Not only has the incidence of malpractice suits increased, but the monetary value of the judgments has also risen. The national average is that one lawsuit occurs per 20,000 emergency department visits. With the rising number of emergency visits, emergency departments will become increasingly involved in litigation.

The increasing number of malpractice suits has many possible causes.[1,2] The rise in "consumerism" and the attitude that all wrongs must be punished lead many to take legal action. The medical profession may have contributed to this problem by fostering an omnipotent image.

A bad outcome is probably the most common problem

that leads to legal action.[3] Family members who feel guilty over the outcome that a child experiences may transfer that guilt to the treating physician. Diseases that are unexpected and sudden, and injuries that are severe, may prompt a desire for revenge or justice and thus precipitate legal action. Parents may refuse to accept the inevitable nature of certain diseases and injuries and assume that bad care must have been responsible. In all cases, whenever the rapport between the physician and the patient or family breaks down, the risk of legal action is increased.

Certain characteristics of the health care provider can lead to an increased risk of litigation. While good professional appearance is no guarantee of good care, patients and parents expect doctors to look professional with appropriate dress and demeanor. A disheveled or unprofessional appearance will raise doubt over whether the care given was adequate. Emergency physicians have such a brief time to establish rapport and create a confident atmosphere that appearance and demeanor are critical. The highly emotional nature of emergency department visits results in stressed parents who may be difficult to manage. Considerate and compassionate management of these parents is a required skill.

A physician with an all-knowing attitude increases the risk of medicolegal problems. When this extends to a reluctance to ask for consultations or help in challenging cases, the problem is accentuated. The emergency physician should use the patient's private physician as a frequent source of help.

Risks in Emergency Medicine

Emergency medicine has many unique aspects that put the practitioner at risk for legal action.[4, 5] Lack of an established doctor-patient relationship may be the most important contributor to litigation. Parents are more likely to accept a bad outcome as an "act of God" when treatment is rendered by a physician whom they trust. In addition, the private physician is more aware of the child's medical history and the family's reliability. In contrast, the emergency physician has only a brief time to establish rapport and trust. This period becomes briefer in the busy emergency department where the emergency physician must often manage several patients simultaneously. Furthermore, the emergency physician often relies on other health care personnel to deliver a portion of patient care while remaining responsible for their actions.[6]

Since emergency care is episodic, the emergency physician does not have the advantage of seeing the natural progression of a disease process. What may become clear in retrospect is often confusing early in the course. This "retrospecto-scope" is sometimes used by medical colleagues when criticizing the action of the emergency physician. The "fishbowl" nature of the emergency department allows others to review and observe the actions of the emergency physician, sometimes leading to unfortunate and inaccurate statements regarding care. Thus, the emergency physician is under added pressure to make the correct diagnosis during the initial visit.

Emergency visits are often highly emotional for parents and children. This accentuates both the good and bad experiences during the visit. Often, parents bring their children to the emergency department during inconvenient times. There may be a certain amount of associated guilt or anger. Most parents are unfamiliar with the hospital environment. The hectic nature of the emergency department adds to the confusion and may lead to the impression that emergency personnel are uncaring and unconcerned. All parents view their child's emergency as extremely serious; they frequently do not understand the triage process and are intolerant of other children being evaluated out of sequence.

The critical nature of many of the illnesses treated in the emergency departments also leads to more frequent complications and bad outcomes. The emergency physician must therefore be careful not to dismiss apparently minor complaints as minor illnesses.

The emergency physician is personally under a great deal of stress because of the need to manage critically ill patients, high volumes of patients, and often long hours. The frequent lack of positive feedback from patients and colleagues provides an additional burden. The 24-hour operation of an emergency department necessitates shift changes that lead to potential problems when the care of patients is assumed by the next shift.[7]

Risks in Pediatric Emergency Medicine

Certain aspects of pediatrics compound the problems inherent in emergency medicine. In the younger child the history may be sparse, absent, or misleading. The emergency physician must often rely completely on someone other than the patient for history. The history may reflect the parent's concerns rather than the child's disease.

The younger the child, the more unreliable is the physical assessment and the more subtle are the signs of disease and injury. If the child cannot or will not cooperate with the examination, the problem is compounded. The child may even attempt to mislead the physician because of fear or pain. Assessments must be based on the child's age and degree of cooperation. Many pediatric diseases progress rapidly, thus requiring close follow-up or extensive evaluation.

The emergency physician must depend on the child's care providers to ensure appropriate follow-up care; the parents must be involved and agree with the therapeutic and diagnostic plan. All instructions must be clear and simple, allowing for the parent to return if the child's condition changes or worsens.[8] It is advisable to involve the private physician when further evaluation is essential. Child abuse must always be a concern when unexplained or unusual injuries are noticed. The emergency physician must be the child's advocate, and every effort must be undertaken to ensure that the child receives appropriate care.

ANATOMY OF A LAWSUIT

Law can be divided into two major components, civil and criminal. Criminal law deals with offenses against the government or its citizens; prosecution is by the state. A statute defines these crimes and describes the intent necessary, the level of the crime, and the penalties. Civil law deals with private causes of action and is settled by negotiation or litigation. Settlement involves damages rather than penalties. Malpractice is a tort or civil wrong resulting from negligent management of a patient. Negligence is defined as a deviation from accepted standards of care. The standard of care has been defined as that level of skill and expertise possessed and exercised by the average, prudent practitioner in the same or similar circumstances practicing the same specialty.[9] Defining the accepted standard of care in a given situation can be difficult, especially in emergency medicine. Decisions in civil law are often based on previous decisions in similar or related cases. Since emergency medicine is a new specialty, there are fewer cases that can be used as reference. Decisions are often based on the testimony of expert witnesses and in difficult cases often depend on the credibility of these witnesses.[9]

Legal action against physicians can involve assault and battery or abandonment charges, but most involve negligence.[1] Malpractice is the basis for most legal action taken against emergency physicians. Assault and battery charges may be filed when appropriate consent to treat has not been obtained. A physician acting in good faith usually prevails in cases of assault and battery. Abandonment charges can be brought against an emergency physician if follow-up care or advice is refused or when inappropriate referral is made.

Four Elements

There are four necessary elements to the tort of malpractice. First, the physician must have a *duty* to treat the patient. In emergency medicine, this duty is recognized when a patient seeks care in an emergency department. Second, there must be a *breach in the standard of care* in the particular situation that resulted in the legal action. As mentioned, the definition of standard of care may be difficult, especially in an unusual or confusing case; it is what the ordinary and reasonably prudent physician would or would not do in a similar situation. Third, the plaintiff, the person initiating the lawsuit, must show that the action or inaction by the physician was the *proximate cause* of damages suffered. Fourth, it must be shown that *resultant damages* or injury occurred.[10]

Legal Process

When a person suffers damages, allegedly through the action or inaction of a physician, a complaint is commonly filed with the local court by the plaintiff's attorney. The complaint must state the cause of the action: it must state the alleged civil wrong and make a demand for compensation for the damage done. The complaint is then "served" on the defendant named in the lawsuit.

Usually, before making the formal complaint, the plaintiff's attorney has reviewed the medical records and consulted experts. The hospital risk manager should review all cases when medical records are requested by an attorney. This is often the first warning that legal action may follow.[10]

After the complaint has been served, there is a discovery period that may last from months to years. A subpoena is an order from the court requiring information or attendance at a hearing. This may take the form of a request for information, attendance at a deposition, or appearance in court. Medical records and related documents may also be subpoenaed.

During the discovery period, experts are consulted to render an opinion regarding the standard of care in the specific case. The testimony of these experts is usually obtained by deposition. Depositions are interviews taken under oath by the opposing counsel with the private counsel present.[11] Witnesses are also interviewed, or deposed, to obtain information regarding the particular events, statements made, and injuries sustained. Interrogatories are similar to depositions except that the questions and answers are provided in written form.

After the discovery period is completed, there is arbitration. This may be statutory, contractual, or voluntary and is directed toward resolution of the dispute. The results of arbitration may be binding or nonbinding. Up to 90% of litigation cases are settled out of court or voluntarily discontinued.[16] If negotiations between the opposing sides do not result in a settlement, the case proceeds to litigation, which may involve a bench trial, summary judgment, or jury trial. The results of trial may be later appealed by either side.

LEGAL ASPECTS OF PEDIATRIC EMERGENCY CARE

Certain legal issues are peculiar to the emergency care of children. The statute of limitation, the time after which a lawsuit can be filed after an event, is greatly extended in pediatrics. Although it varies from state to state, it may extend up to 3 years beyond the age of majority. Thus, the physician may be at risk for up to 20 years.[12]

The transfer of patients is another area of legal risk. As many hospitals are incapable of providing tertiary pediatric care, a protocol for transfer of pediatric patients should be available in all emergency departments. Patients should be transferred only if the original hospital is incapable of providing the required level of care. Recent federal legislation prohibits emergency transfer of patients for purely financial reasons.

The hospital to which the patient is to be transferred must be contacted and accept the transfer. Both emergency departments should keep clear records of all the information shared (Tables 141–1, 141–2). The child must be assured adequate care during transport. The responsibilities of the individual medical facilities during the transfer of a patient are sometimes unclear, and there is often a shared responsibility. A poor outcome during transport is likely to involve both hospitals in litigation, although the referring facility usually bears most of the responsibility. As much stabilization as possible should be provided before transport. The receiving facility should be consulted for treatment recommendations en route. Transfer should be timely but not at the expense of proper stabilization.

Physical and sexual abuse is another concern of the emer-

TABLE 141–1

MODEL CERTIFICATE OF TRANSFER

This is to certify that I, Dr. _____, provided emergency treatment for _____ at General Hospital on _____, 19____, at _____ (AM/PM). In addition (identify and check those sections that apply):

1. _____ I certify that the above-listed patient suffers from an emergency condition that is not yet stabilized. Nevertheless, based on the information available at this time, it is my judgment that the benefits to the patient that can reasonably be expected to occur by transferring this patient to another medical facility outweigh the increased risks to the patient's medical condition that may occur by effecting the transfer.

2. _____ I certify that the above-listed patient is in active labor. Nevertheless, based on the information available at this time, the benefits to the patient that can reasonably be expected to occur from transferring to another medical facility outweigh the increased risks to the patient's medical condition that may occur by effecting the transfer.

3. _____ I certify that the above-listed patient suffers from an emergency medical condition but was stabilized at the time of transfer.

4. _____ I certify that the above-listed patient did not suffer from an emergency medical condition and was not in active labor at the time of transfer.

5. _____ I certify that on behalf of the receiving hospital, Dr. _____ has agreed to accept the patient and ensure provision of appropriate medical treatment.

6. _____ I certify that the receiving facility will be provided with appropriate medical records of the examination and treatment of the patient.

7. _____ I certify that the patient will be transferred by qualified personnel and transportation equipment as required, including the use of necessary and medically appropriate life support measures.

Physician: _____ Date: _____

TABLE 141-2

BENEFITS AND RISKS OF TRANSFER: MODEL FORM

I certify that the following fetal and maternal risks and benefits of the transfer have been explained to the patient and/or family/legal representative, in addition to the information contained in the medical record:

RISKS:

[　] Precipitous delivery may occur en route endangering the life of the mother and/or fetus.
[　] Severe unexpected bleeding may occur.
[　] Other risks: ＿＿＿＿＿＿＿＿＿＿＿＿＿＿＿＿＿＿＿＿

＿＿＿＿＿＿＿＿＿＿＿＿＿＿＿＿＿＿＿＿＿＿＿＿＿＿＿

BENEFITS:

[　] Appropriate obstetric services available.
[　] Neonatal intensive care services available.
[　] Pediatric intensive care services available.
[　] Other benefits: ＿＿＿＿＿＿＿＿＿＿＿＿＿＿＿＿＿＿

＿＿＿＿＿＿＿＿＿＿＿＿＿＿＿＿＿＿＿＿＿＿＿＿＿＿＿

I certify that the following fetal and maternal risks and benefits of the transfer have been explained to the patient and/or family/legal representative, in addition to the information contained in the medical record:

RISKS:

[　] A cardiovascular/pulmonary event may occur en route and threaten the patient's life or further aggravate the patient's present condition.
[　] Other risks: ＿＿＿＿＿＿＿＿＿＿＿＿＿＿＿＿＿＿

＿＿＿＿＿＿＿＿＿＿＿＿＿＿＿＿＿＿＿＿＿＿＿＿＿＿＿

BENEFITS:

[　] Appropriate level of nursing care available.
[　] Appropriate specialist ＿＿＿＿＿＿＿＿＿＿＿＿＿＿ available.
[　] Appropriate specialty care unit ＿＿＿＿＿＿＿＿＿ available.
[　] Other benefits: ＿＿＿＿＿＿＿＿＿＿＿＿＿＿＿＿＿＿

＿＿＿＿＿＿＿＿＿＿＿＿＿＿＿＿＿＿＿＿＿＿＿＿＿＿＿

＿＿＿＿＿＿＿＿＿＿＿＿＿＿＿　＿＿＿＿＿＿＿＿＿＿＿

Physician　　　　　　　　　　　　　Date

gency physician. Statutory law requires the reporting of suspected child abuse to appropriate authorities. It is not the responsibility of the emergency physician to prove that abuse has occurred or to establish the identity of the perpetrator, but if there is a suspicion, appropriate steps must be taken. In addition to complete emergency department evaluation and testing, local authorities may need to remove the child immediately from the abusive environment.[13]

The emergency physician must recognize the risk of continued abuse. This is balanced against the obvious disruption caused by removal of the child from the family. Protection of the child must be the ultimate deciding factor in unclear cases. Laboratory tests should follow accepted chain of evidence procedures. A supportive approach to the parents or caregiver can often help diffuse an emotional situation, protect the child, and obtain social service assistance for the family.

CONSENT

Consent issues have received much attention in recent litigation. Physicians are also becoming more aware of the complexity of the consent problem. Special concerns include the presumed consent in an emergency; the difficulty of obtaining informed consent in an emergency; and consent for children, mature minors, and others. In general, it is always advisable to provide good and prudent medical intervention when dealing with children, even if the issue of consent remains uncertain.

Consent and informed consent are two different concepts.[1, 10] In order to render medical care legally, the physician must receive consent from all patients (or legal guardians in the case of children). Without this consent, the physician could be liable for charges of technical battery or nonconsensual touching. Informed consent goes beyond simple consent. Even if physicians have obtained consent to treat and are therefore not liable to battery charges, they may still be liable for not giving the patient sufficient additional information regarding the proposed medical intervention for the patient to make an informed decision. There has been much debate over what constitutes informed consent, but it is generally agreed that the information should reflect the nature of the patient's illness, the nature of the proposed therapy, reasonable alternative therapies, the chance of success with the proposed therapies, any substantial risks inherent in the therapies, and the risk of failing to undergo therapy for the illness.

It is generally recommended that the physician who will be providing the therapy should obtain the consent. Physicians who have referred a patient to another physician for treatment are generally not held liable for failure to obtain informed consent.

Competent adults may give consent for their own treatment. The age at which a child becomes an adult varies from state to state: from 18 to 21 years. Before this age, the child is considered incompetent to make decisions regarding medical care, with certain significant exceptions. These exceptions fall into two broad categories: one involves specific conditions such as child abuse, venereal disease, pregnancy, drug abuse, and emergencies; the other involves the individual child, who may be an emancipated or mature minor (Table 141-3).[12]

Children suffering from sensitive conditions must be assured medical care even if parental permission cannot be obtained (e.g., in circumstances of child abuse or pregnancy).

TABLE 141-3

CONSENT FOR TREATING MINORS

A minor is a person who by law has not attained an age at which he or she can give consent for treatment. The age of a minor can vary among states.

Ideally, a minor should not receive care in the emergency department without the signed consent of a parent or person legally responsible for the minor.

A minor can be treated without such consent under certain conditions.* Possible exceptions might include:

1. An emergency condition where any delay in treatment could jeopardize the health or welfare of the child.
2. The minor is on active duty in the armed services.
3. The minor is at least 12 years of age and requests treatment for possible venereal disease or pregnancy.
4. The minor is at least 15 years of age, lives away from home, and manages his or her own financial affairs. The minor must sign an "emancipated minor" form.
5. The minor is deserted or abandoned.
6. The minor is at least 12 years of age and presents for treatment relating to substance abuse.
7. The minor is married.
8. The minor is accompanied by a written consent for treatment to be used in the absence of parents or legal guardian.

*Conditions may vary among states. It is imperative that the treating physician consult legal and procedural guidelines for local standards.

The emergency physician should generally encourage the child to inform and involve the parent. If this is not possible, the appropriate local government agency should be involved. Clear documentation regarding the attempt to obtain consent should be on the emergency record.

Some states have enacted legislation that specifically addresses the need for consent in these sensitive conditions, the age at which a child can give consent for treatment without notification of the parents, and the issue of confidentiality. It is advisable for the emergency physician to become familiar with specific state laws regarding these issues. In some states no pertinent laws exist and the physician must do what is reasonable, prudent, and in the best interest of the child. It is better to be liable for giving the correct therapy without consent than to fail to treat a child who is likely to suffer from inaction. The emergency physician must remain the child's advocate.

In emergency conditions the minor may consent to treatment; if he or she is incompetent because of age, injury, or disease, consent can be assumed. Efforts should be made to reach parents or guardians, but emergency care should always be rendered if the delay could cause possible harm to the child. Attempts to reach the parents and the need for immediate intervention should be documented in the emergency record. Even after treatment has been initiated, emergency department personnel or designated hospital or local government personnel should continue to try to contact the parents. Consent may be given by telephone, but two emergency department personnel should listen to phone consent and document it on the emergency department record.[14]

Children living independently from the parents may sometimes be considered emancipated and therefore able to give consent for treatment. Most states have laws regarding emancipation in persons who are married or on military service. Others require judicial decisions. Mature minors may not be emancipated but are competent enough to understand the informed consent. Emancipated or mature minors may give consent for their own care. However, this is not a universally held concept and individual states have differing legal interpretations.

Frequently children are brought in by relatives, by a parent who is not their legal guardian, or by another care provider such as a schoolteacher or camp counselor. Written consent forms are often signed by the legal guardian; these forms can be used as consent for treatment, but the legal guardian should still be contacted.[12] In an emergency the nearest relative can give consent, but the legal guardian should be contacted as soon as possible.

What constitutes a true emergency, thereby relieving the physician of the need to obtain consent before treatment, continues to be debated.[12] The physician who acts in good faith and approaches the child as advocate, although not guaranteed to be free from litigation, will usually prevail if litigation follows.

The emergency physician may also employ the principle of therapeutic privilege when deciding to obtain informed consent. This principle is applied when a situation is so emotionally charged that full disclosure of therapeutic interventions may actually decrease the likelihood of a rational decision on the part of the guardian. For example, to detail every possible complication of a lumbar puncture to a distraught parent may cause that parent to refuse a medically indicated procedure that could have a significant beneficial impact on the child.

The opposite situation, refusal of consent, can be a significant concern to the emergency physician.[15] Most states have a provision to override the rights of parents in situations in which serious harm may befall the child if treatment is not rendered. The court may obtain temporary or permanent custody and allow the physician to perform medically indicated therapies. In conditions in which refusal of the recommended therapy does not definitely mean serious harm to the child, the parents should be encouraged to give consent. If they still refuse, this should be documented and the physician should attempt to arrange for an alternative therapy or arrange a follow-up visit to make sure the child's condition does not deteriorate. If, in the physician's opinion, harm could occur, and the parents or guardian refuse consent, appropriate authorities should be contacted immediately.

RISK MANAGEMENT AND QUALITY ASSURANCE

Risk management is rapidly becoming an important part of hospital operations. Most hospitals have a designated risk manager. It is imperative that each emergency department likewise have one individual designated as risk manager; this responsibility is usually assumed by the medical director. Excellent medical care does not make a physician or institution immune from legal action, especially if there is a bad outcome. Risk management aims at identifying, controlling, and preventing risks. It therefore seeks to avoid lawsuits, to provide successful defense, and to ensure adequate coverage for losses.

Quality assurance is intimately involved with risk management. In addition to being mandated by the Joint Commission on the Accreditation of Hospitals (JCAH) (Standard QA. 1, and Standard ER. 9, JCAH Manual 1990), efforts to ensure the best care of patients contribute to the avoidance of lawsuits. Quality assurance activities aim at setting standards of care for various areas of the hospital. Obviously, these standards must keep up to date with standards held nationally for similar institutions. Once standards are identified, activities should be monitored to ensure that they are maintained. When any deviation is noted, corrective action should take place and a record should be kept. Problem areas may need continuous monitoring; other areas may be monitored on a less frequent basis. The JCAH has emphasized that all quality assurance activities have a direct impact on patient care. It is not surprising that malpractice insurers and third party health insurance companies are also recommending quality assurance activities.

Quality assurance can be broadly divided into two general areas: those activities aimed at maintaining aspects of health care delivery that are acceptable, and those aimed at correcting deficiencies and improving care. Those responsible for quality assurance must monitor the ongoing care and act on any identified problems.

Some monitoring activities are required by JCAH, some are dictated by the nature of emergency medicine, and some are determined according to the emergency department's needs. Examples of those required by JCAH include daily record review, certain required protocols, inclusion of emergency services in blood and drug utilization review, and review of radiographs, laboratory reports, and electrocardiograms. Monitors indicated by the nature of emergency medicine reflect areas of greatest risk. These include review of all deaths or critically ill patients treated in the emergency department, return visits, parent or patient complaints, and patients leaving against medical advice. Certain monitors are reflective of an individual emergency department and are often instituted by a particular event. This is usually a bad outcome or "near-miss" situation that, when reviewed, demonstrated an area that could be improved and thus prevent a future recurrence. The medical director should be the monitor of the functioning of emergency medical staff by ensuring continuing medical education, and by reviewing complaints and the results of other monitors.

Quality assurance can take a great deal of time, but without it the emergency department is at greater risk of legal action. The results of these activities must be discussed with all appropriate members of the staff, otherwise such activities are wasted. When the staff is involved in setting standards and monitoring, compliance is enhanced.[16]

Risk management and quality assurance should be mutually supportive. The ongoing monitoring of care should alert the hospital risk manager to cases that may result in litigation. This could take the form of a patient complaint, or an unexpected death in the emergency department. The sooner a particular case is investigated, the more accurate is the information regarding the particular case. The defense of a suit filed a year after a patient is examined and treated may depend completely on the often scanty information on the emergency department record. Although it is impossible to predict all the possible lawsuits, a good quality assurance program should identify most. Likewise, a staff member who is constantly identified by quality assurance monitors may require remedial action.

One of the major aspects of risk management is a good defense. Since many suits are brought because of a poor outcome, which in many cases was unavoidable, the documentation of the care becomes critical. An essential part of risk management and quality assurance is knowing which situations, at what times, and which diseases result in a higher incidence of lawsuits. By monitoring these problems, an emergency department can help avoid litigation or have a successful defense.

In emergency medicine, certain diseases produce a high incidence of legal action. In pediatrics, the cause of the largest monetary loss is failure to diagnose meningitis. Thus, the care of the febrile child requires close scrutiny. The most frequent causes of lawsuits, although not resulting in the biggest monetary losses, are missed fractures and retained foreign bodies. This obviously necessitates frequent radiologic evaluation of the injured child, and preventive treatment in unsure cases. Other high-risk concerns in children are failure to diagnose appendicitis, testicular torsion, and ectopic pregnancy. Appropriate and unrestricted use of consultants helps prevent lawsuits.

The emergency department employee works in shifts, and the volume of patients is high and variable. Therefore, certain times demonstrate a higher risk of potential suits, such as during change of shifts when a patient's care is transferred from one physician to another. Thorough documentation on the emergency department record and good staff communication are essential. It is also advisable not to have the entire staff change in a brief period. The end of long shifts and times when patient volume exceeds adequate staffing are other periods of high risk. Most disputed cases occur during the evening and night, and on weekends and holidays; these are times when staffing may be minimal or part-time staff are used.

In teaching hospitals, there is the added liability of physicians who are less well trained evaluating patients. The attending physician on duty has legal responsibility for the care of all the patients in the department managed by residents and students. There is a possibility of the emergency physician sharing responsibility even for those patients managed by private attending physicians in the emergency department.

Most suits involve patients discharged from an emergency department. In retrospect, many of these cases involved conditions that may have warranted admission to the hospital. Emergency physicians should insist on the admission of any child whose condition could worsen before the next evaluation. A physician consulted by phone should not be relied on to make this decision.

EMERGENCY DEPARTMENT MEDICAL RECORD

Thorough documentation on the medical record is often key in the defense of malpractice litigation. In the fast pace of an emergency department, documentation often becomes a secondary priority. It is often difficult to remember the details of a patient seen a month previously; it becomes virtually impossible to remember details of one seen a year or two earlier. The other source of memory in a lawsuit is that of the patient or parent, for whom the details may be clear although somewhat altered by time and intervening events.

The medical record may be viewed as a jigsaw puzzle where every piece should fit and no pieces should be left out. There are essential parts to a good emergency department record. The first is the chief complaint, which in pediatrics is usually brief (Table 141–4); hidden agendas must always be documented as they are discovered. The chief complaint should be in the patient's or parent's own words and should be the main reason that care was sought. This is usually followed by a nursing triage note, which is an abbreviated history and physical examination. The function of this note is to assign a triage category and not propose a diagnosis. Any discrepancies between this note and the physician's note should be addressed. Vital signs are part of the triage note, and any abnormalities should be explained in the remainder of the medical record. If abnormal vital signs are considered to be a result of a child being frightened or crying, it is advisable to repeat these tests at a more opportune time. Axillary temperatures are also unreliable and should not be relied on when evaluating children with potentially febrile illnesses. The remainder of the triage note should include a listing of present medications, allergies, any chronic medical conditions, tetanus immunization status, and the name of the patient's private physician.[17]

The physician's history taking should address the chief complaint and any related disorders. In the emergency department an extensive medical history is not usually indicated nor is time available. Fortunately, for most pediatric patients the entire medical history is brief. It is always advisable to clarify any unclear points in the triage note and again seek any contributing medical history, such as chronic conditions. The physical examination must be directed by the history but should be more complete when the history

TABLE 141–4
ESSENTIAL DOCUMENTATION

Chief complaint
Nursing observations (triage note)
Timed vital signs (including an accurate temperature and weight)
Medications
Immunization status
Allergies
Name of private physician
Chronic medical conditions
Brief history
Pertinent physical examination
Diagnostic evaluation including test results
Therapeutic intervention and results of therapy (Record times)
Discussion with consultant or private physician (Record times)
Physician's final assessment (consider avoiding the term "diagnosis")
Discharge instructions (Be specific regarding follow-up plans, especially concerning the timing of evaluation and criteria for return to the emergency department)

is unclear or confusing. As the history given by children is often inadequate, a complete physical examination is often required in younger children. The diagnostic evaluation is directed by the history and physical examination. The episodic nature of emergency care and the lack of an established patient-doctor relationship often lead to a more extensive workup than would be done in a private doctor's office. While the emergency physician is often criticized for a "shotgun" approach to evaluation, risk management usually justifies the more extensive evaluation. It is best to call the physician's summary of all the above an "assessment" rather than a "diagnosis," as it is often impossible to determine a firm diagnosis. The assessment should address all aspects of the history and physical examination in the order of medical priority. The therapeutic plan should be recorded, and if therapy is performed in the emergency department, the results should be documented. If the patient is discharged, clear discharge instructions should be given, including when and why further medical evaluation should be sought. Therapies given in the emergency department should be timed, and the patient's condition reassessed and documented. Consultations should be obtained as needed either in the emergency department, by phone, or in follow-up consultation. It is always advisable to ask for additional expertise in a difficult or confusing case. Follow-up should be assured in cases requiring medical evaluation within a brief period. This can be accomplished by consultation with the private physician or by directing the patient to return to the emergency department. All telephone calls should be documented on the record.[17]

All records that accompany the patient (EMS records, records from a transferring hospital) should be carefully reviewed and the review documented on the emergency department record. Discrepancies or changes in the clinical condition should be documented. The results of all laboratory and radiology tests should likewise be recorded.

Minutes in the emergency department seem like hours to hospitalized patients. Times should be recorded on time of arrival, triage notes, all orders, repeat examinations, consultation requests, and discharge documents. The emergency department record is a legal document.[18]

It is important that the emergency department record not contain any derogatory remarks regarding the patient, the parent, or other medical personnel. Any corrections on an emergency department record should be made with a single line through the incorrect information, and initialed. This allows anyone to review what was written and by whom and why it was corrected. Nothing makes a jury more suspicious than an altered record. Likewise, all subsequent notes should be dated and timed, especially belated laboratory information.

The medical record can be a physician's best friend or worst enemy. Since handwritten charts are briefer and illegible, dictated and typed charts are preferred. The attending emergency physician is responsible for what is written by other personnel, so notes by consultants, residents, and students should be carefully reviewed.

References

1. MacDonald M, Meyer K, Essig B. Healthcare Law. Albany, NY, Matthew Bender, 1988.
2. Henry GL. Legal rounds: problem: Preventing malpractice lawsuits. Emerg Med 1986; July:53.
3. Pegalis SE, Wachsman HF. Emergency room negligence. Trial 1980; 16:50–53.
4. Ladd RE.: Patients without choices: The ethics of decision-making in emergency medicine. J Emerg Med 1985;3:149.
5. Riley B. Reducing Risks in the Emergency Department. Medical Reports Group, American Health Group, American Health Consultants, 1989.
6. Korin J, Selbst S, Torrey S. Medicolegal issues in pediatric emergency medicine. Pediatric Emerg Care 1985;1:48.
7. George JE (ed). Keeping the lid on malpractice in the E.D. Emergency Physician Legal Bull 1981;7:2.
8. Britton R, Magen B. Preventative measures to limit legal liability in pediatric emergencies: An analysis through cases concerning failure to diagnose meningitis. Pediatr Emerg Care 1986;2:109.
9. Kolber JL. Malpractice law and emergency department medicine. Emerg Med Clin North Am 1985;3:625.
10. Taraska J. Legal Guide for Physicians. Albany, NY, Matthew Bender, 1988.
11. Peters B, Rosenbloom A. The physician's deposition: Preparation and testimony of the medical malpractice defendant. Pediatr Emerg Care 1987;3:194.
12. Selbst S.: Treating minors without their parents. Pediatr Emerg Care 1985;1:168.
13. Dobbs D. Legal responsibilities and liabilities when treating child abuse. Pediatr Emerg Care 1986;2:40.
14. George JE. Consent to Treatment. Law and Emergency Care. St. Louis, CV Mosby, 1980; pp 35–50.
15. George JE (ed). Consent and the emergency physician. Emergency Physician Legal Bull 1979;5:2.
16. Walkerwitz S, Unfer S. Quality assurance in emergency pediatrics. Pediatr Emerg Care 1987;3:121.
17. Fossarelli, P, Baker D. What You don't record can hurt you: Documentation in the emergency department. Pediatr Emerg Care 1985;1:223.
18. George JE, Quattrone MS, Espinosa JA (eds). The emergency department record. Emerg Physician Legal Bull 1992;18:2.

CHAPTER 142

Pediatric Bioethics

Kenneth V. Iserson

INTRODUCTION
Defining Bioethics

Applying values and moral rules to human activities is *ethics*. *Bioethics*, a subset of ethics, uses ethical principles and decision making to solve real or anticipated problems in medicine and biology. It tries to find reasoned and defensible solutions to moral problems.

Since antiquity, ethics has been recognized as having applications to medical practice. Part of the Hippocratic Oath, particularly paragraphs 3 to 7, is devoted to what is now called bioethics (Table 142–1). Subsequent oaths and codes for those practicing medicine also have incorporated ethical issues. The American Medical Association's (AMA) current Principles of Medical Ethics (Table 142–2) is one such code; this code also has been adopted by the American College of Emergency Physicians.

Bioethics and Professional Etiquette

There has always been confusion over what constitutes bioethics and what constitutes professional etiquette. Paragraph 2 of the Hippocratic Oath describes how the practitioner is supposed to behave toward teachers, pupils, and other practitioners (i.e., professional etiquette). The initial

Parts of this chapter were modified by permission from Iserson KV. Bioethics. In Rosen P, Baker FJ, Barkin RM, et al (eds). Emergency Medicine: Concepts and Clinical Practice. 3rd ed. St Louis, CV Mosby, 1992.

Code of Medical Ethics of the AMA, published in 1847, only wished to enhance the then low standing of physicians by establishing their relations with one another and promoting their superiority over lay practitioners. The AMA's current code concentrates on bioethics, with an emphasis on the professional's duty to provide competent care and respect patients' rights (see Table 142–2).

For many years, medical societies did not clarify this confusion: in their bylaws, they mixed bioethics with complaints about strained professional interactions. This, however, was not unusual, because these societies often were formed to deal specifically with professional interactions within specialties.

Bioethics and professional etiquette are two distinct values and standards. Bioethics concerns itself with relationships between practitioners and patients, practitioners and society, and society and patients. Professional etiquette specifically deals with standards that govern relationships and interactions between practitioners. There is some overlap in the two areas on occasion, but they both rely on different values, different standards, and different methods of problem solving.

Problem areas that are specifically within the realm of professional etiquette include billing, advertising, competition, conflicts of interest, referrals, professional courtesy, employment and supervision of auxiliary personnel, use of secret remedies and exclusive methods, and location and appearance of an office, emergency department, or urgent care center. These differ from basic moral values and patient-centered issues that are the concern of bioethics.

TABLE 142–1

HIPPOCRATIC OATH

I swear by Apollo Physician and Asclepius and Hygeia and Panaceia and all the gods and goddesses, making them my witness, that I will fulfill according to my ability and judgement this oath and this covenant:

To hold him who has taught me this art as equal to my parents and to live my life in partnership with him, and if he is in need of money to give him a share of mine, and to regard his offspring as equal to my brothers in male lineage and to teach them this art—if they desire to learn it—without fee and covenant; to give a share of precepts and oral instruction and all the other learning to my sons and to the sons of him who has instructed me and to pupils who have signed the covenant and have taken an oath according to the medical law, but to no one else.

I will apply dietetic measures for the benefit of the sick according to my ability and judgement; I will keep them from harm and injustice.

I will neither give a deadly drug to anybody if asked for it, nor will I make a suggestion to this effect. Similarly I will not give to a woman an abortive remedy. In purity and holiness I will guard my life and my art.

I will not use the knife, not even on sufferers from stone, but will withdraw in favor of such men as are engaged in this work.

Whatever houses I may visit, I will come for the benefit of the sick, remaining free of all intentional injustice, of all mischief and in particular of sexual relations with both female and male persons, be they free or slaves.

What I may see or hear in the course of treatment or even outside of the treatment in regard to the life of men, which on no account one must spread abroad, I will keep to myself holding such things shameful to be spoken about.

If I fulfill this oath and do not violate it, may it be granted to me to enjoy life and art, being honored with fame among all men for all time to come; if I transgress it and swear falsely, may the opposite of all this be my lot.

TABLE 142–2

AMERICAN MEDICAL ASSOCIATION PRINCIPLES OF MEDICAL ETHICS*

Preamble: The medical profession has long subscribed to a body of ethical statements developed primarily for the benefit of the patient. As a member of this profession, a physician must recognize responsibility not only to patients, but also to society, to other health professionals, and to self. The following principles adopted by the American Medical Association are not laws, but standards of conduct which define the essentials of honorable behavior for the physician.

  I. A physician shall be dedicated to providing competent medical service with compassion and respect for human dignity.
 II. A physician shall deal honestly with patients and colleagues and strive to expose those physicians deficient in character or competence or who engage in fraud or deception.
III. A physician shall respect the law and also recognize a responsibility to seek changes in those requirements which are contrary to the best interests of the patient.
 IV. A physician shall respect the rights of patients, of colleagues, and of other health professionals and shall safeguard patient confidences within the constraints of the law.
  V. A physician shall continue to study, apply, and advance scientific knowledge; make relevant information available to patients, colleagues, and the public; obtain consultation; and use the talents of other health professionals when indicated.
 VI. A physician shall, in the provision of appropriate patient care, except in emergencies, be free to choose whom to serve, with whom to associate, and the environment in which to provide medical services.
VII. A physician shall recognize a responsibility to participate in activities contributing to an improved community.

*Also adopted by the American College of Emergency Physicians.
Reprinted from American Medical Association Principles of Modern Ethics, as published by the American Medical Association in Current Opinions: The Council on Ethical and Judificial Affairs of the American Medical Association, Copyright 1989.

THE LAW AND ETHICS

Good ethics makes good law, it has been stated, but good law does not necessarily make good ethics. The values of a society are incorporated both within the law and within ethical principles and decisions. However, laws often vary from locale to locale, whereas bioethical principles do not change because of geography (at least not within one general culture). One reason for an increased interest in bioethics is the time lag between medicine's and society's need for answers to questions raised by new technologies, procedures, treatments, and limitations on resources, and the law's development (accompanied by resulting discrepancies within the law). The need for relatively fast answers and political wariness on the part of legislators are primary reasons why more health laws are being made in the courts than in the legislatures.

There is significant overlap between the law and ethical decision making. Often the two concur on basic issues. Sometimes, clarity within the law can lead to clearer thinking in bioethics, and vice versa. Such is the case concerning the term *rights,* such as in "patients' rights" and "the right to die." Often the term *rights* is used within the context of advancing an ethical argument about medical care, yet it is frequently misunderstood or erroneously applied. A legal "right" is a demand that one person can make on another person (*in personam* rights) or a claim that can be made against the state to recognize and enforce this demand (*in rem* rights). In bioethical discussions, most rights are in rem rights. These are, in general, *negative rights* (i.e., it is someone else's duty to refrain from doing something). Less often involved are *positive rights* (i.e., a right to another person's positive actions), such as the right of an accident victim to be assisted by anyone who is in a position to help.

A common source of ethical conflict is between *active rights*—the right to act or not act as one chooses—and *passive rights*—the right to not be acted on by others in certain ways. In society, the issue often arises because of conflicts between the rights of liberty and safety. One conflict in both law and ethics is the presence of *absolute rights*—complete, exceptionless, and unconditional rights, such as those present in the U.S. Constitution's Bill of Rights. The issue has been debated in both the U.S. Supreme Court and the ethical literature.[1] Specific rights for children have been advocated, in part because of the lack of rights for minors in the legal system. Some of these specific children's rights include the right to be regarded as a person; to receive parental love and affection; to be supported, maintained, and educated; to receive fair treatment; to earn and keep one's own earnings; to be free of legal disabilities; to seek and obtain medical care and treatment and counseling; and to receive special care, consideration, and protection.[2]

It is said that the rights of an individual cannot exist in the absence of the duties of an individual, and vice versa. In general, a *duty* is an action understood to be required, whether by the rights of others, by law, by higher authority, or by conscience.[1] The obligation to perform an action can be based on an individual's personal values, professional position, or other commitment.[3] More specifically for the physician, this has been described as "role responsibility," such that "whenever a person occupies a distinctive place or office in a social organization, to which specific duties are attached to provide for the welfare of others or to advance in some specific way the aims or purposes of the organization, he is properly said to be responsible for the performance of these duties, or for doing what is necessary to fulfill them."[4] In this situation, performance is not predicated on a guarantee of compensation, but rather on concern for another person's welfare.[5] The emergency physician has just such a duty.

Bioethics began emerging as a force in U.S. medicine in the 1970s because the law often did not address, was inconsistent, or was morally wrong on matters important to the biomedical community. The increase in biotechnology, the failure of the legal system and legislatures to deal with or resolve new and pressing issues, and the increasing liability crisis have driven the medical community to seek answers to the difficult questions practitioners confront daily. In some cases, practitioners believe that laws governing their practice are wrong because they do not take into account relevant moral principles. Several generally accepted values have emerged that have guided ethical thinking and have been instrumental in helping to form health care policies.

VALUES

Values are standards by which human behavior is judged. Values are learned from indoctrination into the culture into which one is born. These values are taught, usually at an early age, through secular (including professional) and religious education and from observing the behavior of others. Society's institutions incorporate and promulgate values, often attempting to strictly fix old values, even in a changing society. In a pluralistic society, however, clinicians must be sensitive to the beliefs and traditions of patients whose value systems may be different. Certain values have become generally accepted by the medical community, courts, legislatures, and society at large. Autonomy and individual dignity are two such fundamental values. Although there is some disagreement regarding each of the generally accepted values (Table 142–3), this dissension has not affected the application of these values to medical care.

Societal and Professional Values

The basic tenet, "First, do no harm," is derived from the historical knowledge that patient encounters with physicians can be harmful as well as helpful. Yet even with the physician's fallibility acknowledged, the recognition of patient autonomy is, and has been since the 1970s, the preeminent professional and societal bioethical value. *Autonomy* is the recognition of a competent individual's right to determine the course of his or her medical care, even to the extent of refusing all care. It is the counterbalance to the long-entrenched paternalism of the medical profession, wherein what was "good" for the patient was determined only by the physician.

Beneficence, the act of doing good, and *confidentiality*, the holding of information in confidence, are long-standing tenets in the medical profession. Similarly, *personal integrity*, the adherence to one's own moral and professional standards, is basic to ethical thinking and actions.

On a more global basis, the concept of comparative or distributive justice essentially says that comparable individuals and groups in society should share comparably in the benefits and burdens of the society. Many society-wide decisions that affect the allocation of limited health care resources are based on this principle. However, it is fallacious to extrapolate from this valid principle that simply because there may be a need to limit health care expenditures, individual clinicians can arbitrarily limit or terminate care on a case-by-case basis at the bedside of individual patients.

Fidelity has been espoused by those who believe that the patient, no matter what the circumstances, has the right to know "the truth." Others believe that honesty must be tempered with compassion. Many who espouse truth telling as an important value justifiably complain that it is often done poorly. Requiring that the truth be told with a measure of sensitivity does not lessen the requirement that the truth be told. Nevertheless, truth telling is not universally accepted within the medical profession.

TABLE 142–3

COMMONLY ACCEPTED SOCIETAL AND BIOETHICAL VALUES

Autonomy: Self-determination; a person's ability to make his or her own decisions, including those affecting his or her medical care. Autonomy is opposed by paternalism.

Beneficence: Doing good. A duty to confer benefits or the production of benefit.

Confidentiality: The presumption that what the patient tells the physician will not be revealed to any other person or institution without the patient's permission.

Distributive Justice: Fairness in the allocation of resources and obligations. This value is the basis of and is incorporated into society-wide health care policies.

Nonmaleficence: Not doing harm; the prevention of harm and the removal of harmful conditions.

Personal Integrity: Adhering to one's own reasoned and defensible set of values and moral standards.

Religious Values

Organized religions are recognized as one of society's keepers of values (Table 142–4). Most religions have as a basic tenet, "Do unto others as you would have them do unto you."

Problems arise in applying religious teachings to bioethical situations when more specific religious injunctions are used. Although "thou shalt not kill" is generally accepted, activities that constitute killing can and do vary within the interpretations of the world's religions and can include active or passive euthanasia or merely reasonable medical care.[6]

Some practitioners have a conflict with specific values on a religious, philosophic, or practical basis. When such a conflict arises, it is, within certain constraints, morally and legally acceptable for the practitioner to follow a course of action based on his or her own value system. It is always important to recognize the patient's identity, dignity, and autonomy in order to avoid the blind imposition of one's own values on others. Even when there is agreement with societally accepted values, a different course of action may be taken depending on the circumstances of the case and the hierarchic importance of the values involved. In each specific case, the ethical analysis must recognize all possible courses of action and the benefits and detriments of each. At the same time, the patient's values must be respected.

The following is a modern set of definitions that may help the physician solve ethical problems. *Good* is what no rational person will avoid without a reason. Examples include freedom, pleasure, health, wealth, ability, and knowledge. *Evil* is what all rational persons desire to avoid for themselves and for others about whom they care. Examples include death, pain, disability, and the loss of freedom or pleasure.[7]

BIOETHICAL DILEMMAS

The most straightforward example of an ethical quandary is the *dilemma*. A dilemma occurs when there are two or more courses of action, each representing a conflicting value to which one adheres. An example is the 16-year-old Jehovah's Witness patient, dying from an acute intra-abdominal hemorrhage, who demands that no blood products be given. The patient's autonomy is a major value to which the practitioner may subscribe, and he or she may be willing under that value to forego the lifesaving blood transfusions. However, the practitioner may also believe strongly in, and

have based his or her career in emergency medicine on, the value of beneficence—helping those in need and saving lives when possible. This value suggests that blood products be given. An additional problem in this case is that the patient is a minor. This raises the question of whether the patient has the right or ability to be autonomous. The physician may also be uncertain as to whether the patient will definitely die without blood products. Thus, as can be seen from this example, bioethics deals with problems that are not black or white—only gray.

Resuscitation efforts frequently pose ethical dilemmas, especially when patient or family wishes are unknown or differ from accepted medical practice. The conflict between the societal utility of teaching the next generation of practitioners and the physician beneficence inherent in the individual physician-patient relationship is a constant reality at teaching institutions. Dilemmas also arise in the emergency medical service (EMS) system when administrative rules and good patient care conflict. Also, the increasing number of patients presenting to emergency departments after being denied access to health care elsewhere puts practitioners and institutions into the financial conflict between compassionate service and financial failure. These problems may be recognized as bioethical problems because they require a choice between two or more values intrinsic to good medical care.

BIOETHICS IN PEDIATRIC EMERGENCY MEDICINE

Bioethics and ethical decision making have been recognized as important elements of all pediatric practice.[8] The American Board of Pediatrics (ABP) recommends that every pediatrician should demonstrate a respect for the patient's and family's values, confidentiality, truth telling, a caring attitude, interest in the patient's welfare, a sensitivity to the patient's and family's needs and the resources they have available, and open-mindedness. The ABP also expects the pediatric practitioner to make "a commitment to the patient's/family's best interest without regard to their social background or financial status," and the practitioner "is encouraged to accept whatever self-sacrifice is required to provide comprehensive care for the patient."[8] In addition, the pediatric physician is encouraged to make patient care decisions based on the patient's best interest and in such a manner that decisions can be applied to other similar situations.

The physician in an emergency pediatric practice has a markedly different relationship with patients than other physicians involved principally in primary care pediatrics (Table 142–5).[9, 10] The emergency physician often has the uncomfortable task of caring for unfamiliar patients and for those for whom no institutional medical records exist. Primary care physicians often have an easier time making difficult ethical decisions regarding patients than do emergency physicians because of their greater knowledge about their patients' values. Pediatricians normally operate under less uncertainty than do physicians seeing a patient only for acute care. Emergency physicians, however, still must make ethical decisions (Table 142–6).

BIOETHICAL DECISION MAKING

In bioethics, although there may be disagreements regarding the optimal course of action using a specific set of values, there is often general agreement as to what constitutes ethically wrong actions. One method of ethical case analysis is designed to provide the emergency practitioner prompt assistance in selecting an ethically correct, although not

---

TABLE 142–4

COMMONLY ACCEPTED MORAL RULES

Moral rules govern actions that are immoral to do without an adequate moral reason—and can justifiably be enforced and their violation punished. None of these rules is absolute, but they do require one not to cause evil. Somewhat paradoxically, however, they may not require preventing evil or doing good.

1. Do not kill.
2. Do not cause pain.
3. Do not disable.
4. Do not deprive of freedom.
5. Do not deprive of pleasure.
6. Do not deceive.
7. Keep your promise.
8. Do not cheat.
9. Obey the law.
10. Do your duty.

Adapted from Gert B. Morality: A New Justification of the Moral Rules. New York, Oxford University Press, 1988.

TABLE 142–5

DIFFERENCES BETWEEN EMERGENCY PEDIATRICS AND PRIMARY CARE PEDIATRICS

Emergency Pediatrics	Primary Care Pediatrics
Patient unexpectedly enters medical care system.	Parent or patient chooses to enter medical care system.
Patient often brought by ambulance, police, etc.	Patient often brought by parent.
Parent or patient does not choose physician.	Parent or patient chooses physician.
Physician must gain patient's and parents' trust.	Physician already enjoys parents' and patient's trust.
Physician may evaluate and treat child without parental or guardian permission.	Physician rarely evaluates or treats child without parental or guardian permission.
Physician does not know patient, family, or their values.	Physician knows patient, family, and their values.
Physician specifically evaluates a patient's acute change in health.	Physician evaluates patient's global health care needs and goals.
Anxiety, pain, alcohol, or acutely altered mental status are frequent.	Altered mental status is unusual.
Decisions are made quickly.	Decisions are made after reflection and deliberation.
Physician represents institution and medical staff.	Physician represents self or medical group.
Work environment open and less controlled.	Work environment private and controlled.

Adapted from Sanders AB. Unique aspects of ethics in emergency medicine. *In* Iserson KV, Sanders AB, Mathieu DR, Buchanan AE (eds). Ethics in Emergency Medicine. Baltimore, Williams & Wilkins, 1986, p 9. © 1986, Williams & Wilkins Co.

necessarily the theoretically "best," course of action (see Table 142–6).

Using this algorithm, the simplest solution to an ethical dilemma is to use a known precedent. However, this requires planning, reading, and thinking about ethical problems in advance. Many physicians are unprepared to do this. Emergency physicians should be prepared with a course of action for the ethical dilemmas most likely to occur in the emergency department.

Guidelines for Decision Making

If there is no precedent to rely on, the practitioner must select a possible course of action and test it for ethical viability. The three tests used—the Impartiality Test, the Universalizability Test, and the Interpersonal Justifiability Test—are drawn from three different philosophic theories. The Impartiality Test has the practitioner ask whether he or she would prefer this action if in the patient's place. In essence, this is a form of the Golden Rule ("Do unto others as you would have them do unto you"). The Universalizability Test asks if the practitioner would feel comfortable having all practitioners perform this action in all relevantly similar circumstances. This generalizes the action, asking whether developing a universal rule for the contemplated behavior is reasonable. The Interpersonal Justifiability Test asks if the practitioner can supply good reasons to others for the action. This test uses the basic theory of consensus values as a final screen for a proposed action.[11] If all three tests can be answered in the affirmative, then the practitioner has a reasonable probability that the proposed action falls within the scope of morally acceptable actions.

Decisions in Pediatric Emergency Medicine

In pediatric emergency medicine, there are three types of relationships between the clinician and the patients or parents: (1) physician–parent of an incompetent child (generally younger than 14 years); (2) physician–parent–older child with some decision-making capacity; and (3) physician–child. Unlike in adult emergency medicine, most pediatric patients are not the ones consenting to their emergency treatment.

There are several types of decision makers and decision making involving children. These include parental or guardian surrogacy based on a best-interest or substituted judgment standard. There are also instances (e.g., mature or emancipated minors) or specific illnesses (e.g., venereal disease) in which children can make their own treatment decisions. Finally, there are the frequent scenarios when evaluation and treatment must proceed without the usually necessary parental consent.

Two ethical dilemmas that can arise include patient confidentiality, usually when treating adolescents, and conflicts between the patient's best interests and parental demands.

One goal of society is preserving the family unit. This involves giving parents information about their child's illness and injuries and involving them when possible in the medical decision-making process. In some cases, as in venereal disease and pregnancy, many states have specifically waived parental notification requirements by physicians. However, much information can pass between the child patient and the physician that would be considered confidential and privileged between an adult and a physician. Is it the physician's duty to relate this information to a parent? Confidentiality is a right of minor patients. This right grows stronger in proportion to the minor's willingness and ability

TABLE 142–6

A RAPID APPROACH TO EMERGENCY ETHICAL PROBLEMS

Question: Is this a type of ethical problem for which you have already worked out a rule or is it at least similar enough so that the rule could reasonably be extended to cover it?

YES   **NO**

Follow the rule.   Is there an option that will buy you time for deliberation without excessive risk to the patient?

YES   **NO**

Take that option.   1. Apply Impartiality Test
2. Apply Universalizability Test
3. Apply the Interpersonal Justifiability Test

Adapted from Iserson KV. An approach to ethical problems in emergency medicine. *In* Iserson KV, Sanders AB, Mathieu DR, Buchanan AE (eds). Ethics in Emergency Medicine. Baltimore, Williams & Wilkins, 1986, p 35. © 1986, Williams & Wilkins Co.

to take responsibility for his or her own health care decisions. Physicians, therefore, have a more complex duty to relate to parents or guardians only the normally confidential information that is essential for the child's well-being. There is often tacit agreement on this when parents, at the child's request, leave the child and physician alone to discuss a medical problem.

Conflicts between parents' requests and a minor's best interests can take several forms. Most commonly seen are parental refusals for what clinicians see as essential, often life-preserving diagnostic procedures or therapy (e.g., lumbar punctures or transfusion of blood products). Physician beneficence, although it usually extends to the family, must be primarily directed toward the patient. The child patient should receive the diagnostic and therapeutic maneuvers that standards of care suggest are necessary to reduce morbidity and mortality. No child should suffer from parental decisions that would cause harm. When questions exist as to proper or necessary procedures, however, communication with parents and, frequently, deferral to parental wishes are appropriate.

More infrequently seen in the emergency department is disagreement between the two parents or between the parent and the older child regarding treatment. When the situation demands immediate action, the physician should act in such a way as to lessen the chance for morbidity.

RESUSCITATION ISSUES

Teaching Versus Resuscitation

The emergency department is a major teaching environment for developing physicians and paramedical personnel. Because the sickest and most diverse set of patients enters the hospital through the emergency department, the balance of training and treatment raises some difficult bioethical issues.

The most time dependent of all activities, and arguably the best training periods in the emergency department, occur during resuscitations. Patients needing this care have implicitly been promised that all appropriate medical knowledge and skill will be brought to bear in an attempt to save their life. This leads to the dilemma. If the most proficient individuals always lead the resuscitations and perform procedures, then patients receive the presumed beneficence, as well as nonmaleficence, they thought they would receive. However, by not allowing less proficient individuals to lead the resuscitation effort, future patients are deprived of trained clinicians who could, in turn, bestow beneficence on them.

The appropriate balance seems to be that training in emergency departments, as it does in other areas of medicine, can ethically proceed if safeguards in the form of on-site supervision by highly experienced clinicians are available to ensure that patients get appropriate care. It has also been suggested that medical students and residents be certified in cognitive and procedural skills in a manner similar to that used for other hospital physicians. This would enable faculty to better evaluate and ensure competence in these skills.[12]

Postmortem Teaching

A less well known part of emergency medical teaching is the use of recently deceased patients for the teaching and practice of emergency medical techniques such as intubations and central line placement. Even more controversial is proceeding with resuscitation procedures when the patient is obviously dead in order to give staff members experience in protocol and procedures. Although there is controversy as to whether these practices are ethical,[13] societal utility suggests that the skills learned in these situations can be successfully applied to future patients who may benefit from the clinician's skills. If a patient has died despite reasonable efforts at resuscitation, then the emergency physician's responsibility is to the next patient who may need resuscitative services—that is, the subsequent patient who needs the expertise in resuscitative techniques learned through postmortem practice.

Rawls proposed that decisions on societal rules ideally could be made by individuals who are ignorant of their own societal position, future desires, and immediate needs. From this perspective, social justice demands that medical practitioners be well trained and proficient in lifesaving techniques. Furthermore, the training should, as much as possible, cause minimal harm to people.

This is not to condone the desecration of a body. Instead, this view suggests that experienced clinicians learned on previous patients or cadavers the techniques used during this now-dead patient's resuscitation. This nonresuscitated individual now owes the next patient the same courtesy. Further, the principle of nonmaleficence specifically suggests using dead patients for instruction and practice, rather than the living, who could be harmed.

Implicit in this idea is the fact that the consent of relatives would not be obtained prior to instruction or practice. If such consent were obtained, little in the way of an ethical problem would arise. In at least one pediatric emergency department, it has been decided that postmortem procedures cannot ethically be performed without specific consent. As a result, such consent is not being requested, and the procedures are not being taught or practiced in this fashion. Other emergency departments report that procedures are done after it is clear that the patient will not survive resuscitation attempts, but before death is actually pronounced. The physicians involved claim that this behavior is more morally correct. However, it is necessary to consider that any added financial costs of this admitted charade must be borne by the payors, and any cost in loss of integrity of the profession must be borne by those involved in the practice.

An argument can be made for postmortem teaching practice both as part of a condition of emergency treatment and as part of a broader social contract covering an individual's interaction with and need for physicians skilled in emergency medical techniques. Religious values and the emotional impact of a child's unexpected death on emergency department personnel, however, may make practicing or teaching these procedures problematic.

Resuscitation Research

In a new and advancing specialty such as emergency medicine, there is an obligation to advance the knowledge base. This can only be done through research, a component of which must necessarily be clinically based. Research is defined as "a systematic investigation designed to develop or contribute to generalizable knowledge."[14] This should be differentiated both from validated practice (i.e., procedures and medications that have been scientifically shown to be effective), and from nonvalidated practice (i.e., using medications and techniques with a "lack of suitable validity of the safety or ethics of the practice").[15]

Applications for research involving human subjects are studied by a federally mandated Institutional Review Board (IRB).[14] This includes research that takes place in emergency departments. One major effort of IRBs is to guarantee that an adequate informed consent document is available and prospectively signed by patients or their legal representative. It has been suggested that even when the patient is conscious, it is unclear whether truly free and informed consent can be given in the midst of a medical emergency.[16] In trauma and cardiac resuscitation research, getting informed consent is impossible. Retrospective parental approval, if obtainable, does not solve the problem. Such approval would merely ratify, rather than be a consent for, research.

All patients benefit from prior medical research. Preservation of patient and parental autonomy in this situation when wishes cannot be ascertained mandates following their probable wishes. In assessing the interests of an unknown next patient, a "reasonable person" standard should be used. Given this assumption, most "reasonable" patients would acquiesce to the research, given the basic values of "good" and "evil." (see Table 142–4).[17, 18] In fact, if there is a chance that they could benefit from the research, most people would demand that it be done.

Another function of an IRB is to determine whether an appropriate risk-to-benefit ratio exists in human research. The only caveat here is that IRB approval is insufficient. The individual researcher must ascertain that the proposed study is ethical, especially in those children whose parents, because of the type of research, cannot prospectively sign consent.[19] Furthermore, with the specific concern most bioethicists have with nontherapeutic or non–"customary practice" research on children, special care must be taken in limiting or restricting protocols to nonharmful activities.[20–23]

TREATING INDIGENT CHILDREN

As a result of the increasing burden of health care costs, efforts are being made to reduce expenditures associated with health care. The impact of this is felt most by the nation's 39 million medically indigent patients, a significant proportion of whom are children. In the United States, the poorest children also have the worst health.[24] Governments and private industry are referring many cases to case-management health care organizations that purport to deliver "better" care at lower costs.[25] This is done by utilizing case managers (ideally, the patient's primary care physician). In reality, a nurse or physician who knows nothing about the patient often decides whether a specific element of medical care will be reimbursed. An expressed goal of this system is to decrease the number of relatively expensive visits to emergency departments. A common policy is to approve payment for emergency department treatment only in "life-threatening emergencies."[26] It has been suggested that by increasing access to other health care sites and providers, the use of emergency departments would decrease.[25]

Several studies suggest that the medical resource of last resort, or the "safety net," for indigent patients may be the emergency department. When this source of health care is closed to the parents of pediatric patients, they may not seek alternative care, even when it is available.[27, 28] In addition, it may not be possible to determine how sick a child is without a medical evaluation. The principle of beneficence therefore suggests that, at a minimum, an evaluation by a medically qualified individual should be performed on every child who presents to the emergency department.[25, 27] Additionally, the principle of nonmaleficence dictates that a child be treated whenever possible to avoid unnecessary second examinations (or go without care, if the parent elects not to seek another source of treatment) just to get appropriate therapy for a medical condition.

The question of adequate funding to pay for medical care is a difficult issue for all levels of the government. The societal utility of treating children is balanced against other needs of more vocal and organized segments of the population. It is a difficult issue for politicians to face; however, the physician caring for the child in medical need must press the issue. This issue of cost versus access and the role of the physician in this debate is perhaps the major bioethical dilemma of this generation.[29]

ACTING BEYOND THE LEVEL OF COMPETENCE

Physicians are susceptible to erring in patient care. Ethical issues arise when a physician consciously puts himself or herself in a position to increase the likelihood of making mistakes, thus violating the value of nonmaleficence. An example is depriving oneself of sleep or increasing one's stress level by working too many hours in order to provide more consecutive free days. Although free time is important, and each individual has differing levels of performance under stress conditions, exceeding personal limits potentially puts patients in danger.[30]

ROLE OF CONSULTANTS

One alternative to ethical decision making in emergency care is to "buy time." That time can be used to good effect by requesting assistance from the hospital's bioethics committee or consultant. If a concurrent consultation is impossible, either the bioethics committee or the bioethics consultant can perform a retrospective review of the ethical decision made, to give advice on an appropriate course of action for the future.

BIOETHICS COMMITTEES

Bioethics committees, or institutional ethics committees (IEC), have a relatively short history. With the 1971 Medico-Moral Guide of the Canadian bishops, the 1973 Massachusetts General Hospital Critical Care Committee, and the 1977 Montefiore Medical Center (New York) bioethics committee, the movement was begun to establish a basis for hospital ethical decision making.

There have been some governmental attempts to legislate the functions of hospital ethics committees. In some states, the ethics committee must be consulted in all cases involving life-threatening conditions. The remainder of the legislative charges to these committees is broad and includes "medical decision-making; decisions to withhold medical treatment," including specifically the education of hospital personnel, patients, and families; and the review and recommendation of institutional policies and guidelines concerning the withholding of medical treatment.

Most IECs are located in hospitals. They may serve the entire hospital or a special unit, such as a neonatal intensive care nursery or a cardiac intensive care unit. They usually have four main functions. First, they coordinate education on issues concerning the ethical dimensions of clinical care. The educational programs can be for the committee members, hospital physicians and staff, patients, families, or the local hospital community. Second, these committees assist in the development of institutional policies or guidelines dealing with bioethical issues. These directives generally are for health care professionals and concern decision-making processes in problematic cases and for resource allocation issues. Third, IECs consult prospectively and retrospectively on clinical cases and offer advice and conclusions to those involved. This often involves the treatment or nontreatment of patients who lack decision-making capacities. The committees do not act as the primary decision makers but instead serve in a consultative, informative, and advisory capacity, supporting the primary decision-making role of the patient-family-physician triad. This is especially true for urgent decisions about withholding, withdrawing, or continuing life-sustaining medical care. Finally, the committees counsel hospital staff, patients, and families on ethical issues. This is often done by providing forums for discussion among hospital and medical professionals and for resolving disagreements among staff, patients, and families about clinical decisions. The committee must also act as a source of support when these difficult decisions are made. In essence, the function of the ethics committee is to consider and assist in resolving complicated ethical problems.

The experience of many committees suggests that ethics per se is not the issue in many discussions. Because conflict is an essential element in issues brought before ethics committees, clarifying facts and fostering communication comprise a large part of their work.

Current IEC functions, therefore, closely parallel those of a model bill proposed by the President's Commission in 1983 to establish hospital ethics committees. The suggested scope of authority of such committees would be to review treatment decisions made on behalf of terminally ill competent patients who request committee review, review medical decisions having ethical implications, provide counseling, establish guidelines, and educate.

Pediatric IECs differ from adult IECs in that nearly all patients have identified and interested relatives (parents), and most patients have never expressed independent interests or desires. Most pediatric bioethics committees accept a "best interest" of the child position but must be careful not to appear to have superior morals or values to the patient's family.[32,33] Additionally, most IECs take the position that all members of the committee are advocates for the child, rather than assigning one or more persons to that role, as suggested by the initial "Baby Doe" regulations.[34] In some cases, subcommittees act as smaller consultation teams, with final decisions reviewed by the committee as a whole.[35]

References

1. Feinberg J. Social Philosophy. Englewood Cliffs, NJ, Prentice-Hall, 1973.
2. Foster HH. A Bill of Rights for Children. Springfield, IL, Charles C Thomas, 1974.
3. Black HC. Black's Law Dictionary. 5th ed. St Paul, MN, West Publ Co, 1979.
4. Hart HLA. Punishment and Responsibility. Oxford, England, Oxford University Press, 1976, p 242.
5. Ladd J. Legalism and medical ethics. J Med Philosophy 1979;4:70.
6. McCormick RA. Theology and bioethics. Hastings Center Rep 1989;19:5.
7. Gert B. Morality: A New Justification of the Moral Rules. Oxford, England, Oxford University Press, 1988.
8. Daeschner CW, Anyan WR, Feldt RH, et al. Teaching and evaluation of interpersonal skills and ethical decision making in pediatrics. Pediatrics 1987;79:829.
9. Iserson KV. The problem patient. In Hamilton GC, Sanders AB, Strange GR, Trott AT (eds). Emergency Medicine: An Approach to Clinical Problem-Solving. Philadelphia, WB Saunders, 1991, pp 1133–1139.
10. Iserson KV. The Ethics of Emergency Medicine. J Emerg Med 1985;3:161.
11. Gauthier DP. Morals by Agreement. Oxford, England, Clarendon Press, 1986.
12. Iserson KV. The supervision of physicians in training: An educational and ethical dilemma. Med Teacher 1988;10:195.
13. Iserson KV. Using a cadaver to practice and teach. Hastings Center Rep 1986;16:28.
14. Department of Health and Human Services of the United States. Regulations of the DHHS on the Protection of Human Subjects. Code 45, CFR 46.102. Washington, DC, DHHS, 1978. Revised 8 March 1983.
15. Levine RJ. Clarifying the concepts of research ethics. Hastings Center Rep 1979;9:22.
16. Grimm PS, Singer PA, Gramelspacher GP, et al. Informed consent in emergency research. JAMA 1989;262:252.
17. Iserson KV. Human subjects in trauma research. In Iserson KV, Sanders AB, Mathieu DR, Buchanan AE. Ethics in Emergency Medicine. Baltimore, Williams & Wilkins, 1986, p 82.
18. Fost NC. Human subjects in cardiopulmonary resuscitation research. In Iserson KV, Sanders AB, Mathieu DR, Buchanan AE. Ethics in Emergency Medicine. Baltimore, Williams & Wilkins, 1986, p 77.
19. Iserson KV. Physician ethics in human research: The role of medical publications. Ann Emerg Med 1990;19:828.
20. Redmon RB. How children can be respected as 'ends' yet still be used as subjects in non-therapeutic research. J Med Ethics 1986;12:77.
21. Laor N. Toward liberal guidelines for clinical research with children. Med Law 1987;6:127.
22. Holder AR. Legal Issues in Pediatrics and Adolescent Medicine. 2nd ed. New Haven, CT, Yale University Press, 1985.
23. Koren G, Litwack J, Biggar DW. The use of infants in drug research when there is no direct benefit to them: A survey of Canadian health care professionals serving on ethics committees. Can Med Assoc J 1988;138:899.
24. Miller G (ed). Giving Children a Chance: The Case for More Effective National Policies. Washington, DC, Center for National Policy Press, 1989.
25. Muller HA. Emergency medicine and the health care needs of the indigent child. Ann Emerg Med 1990;19:98.
26. Kerr HD. Access to emergency departments: A survey of HMO policies. Ann Emerg Med 1989;18:274.
27. Shaw KN, Selbst SM, Gill FM. Indigent children who are denied care in the emergency department. Ann Emerg Med 1990;19:59.
28. Dershewitz RA. Patients who leave a pediatric emergency department without treatment. Ann Emerg Med 1986;15:717.
29. President's Commission for the Study of Ethical Problems in Medicine and Biomedical Research. Securing Access to Health Care. Vol 1. The Ethical Implications of Differences in the Availability of Health Services. Washington, DC, US Government Printing Office, 1983.
30. Bock BF. Physician's quality of life versus quality of patient care. In Iserson KV, Sanders AB, Mathieu DR, Buchanan AE. Ethics in Emergency Medicine. Baltimore, Williams & Wilkins, 1986, p 200.
31. Iserson KV, Goffin FB, Markham JJ. The future functions of HECs. Hospital Ethics Committee Forum 1989;1:63.
32. Cross AW, Churchill LR. Pediatric ethics committees: Learning from our experience. J Pediatr 1986;108:242.
33. Leikin S. Children's hospital ethics committees: A first estimate. Am J Dis Child 1987;141:954.
34. Office of the Secretary, Department of Health and Human Services. Child abuse and neglect prevention and treatment program, and services and treatment for disabled infants: Model guidelines for health care providers to establish infant care review committees. Federal Register 1985;50:1478.
35. Michaels RH, Oliver TK. Human rights consultation: A 12-year experience of a pediatric bioethics committee. Pediatrics 1986;78:566.

CHAPTER 143

Brain Death and Organ Donation

Mark G. Goetting
Elizabeth Contreras
Bassam M. Gebara

INTRODUCTION

Organ donation and the concept of brain death developed concurrently in modern medicine. Breakthroughs in the fields of immunology, surgery, organ preservation, and tissue matching propelled organ transplantation into a clinical reality. Patients who "survive" extreme neurologic insults can now be maintained on life support without hope of brain recovery. Despite some ethical controversy, these individuals have become the major source of whole organs for transplantation, thus benefiting the recipient and perhaps society in general.

Early identification and appropriate medical management of the potential donor are key aspects for successful transplantation. The emergency physician is often faced with the decision whether to withhold or terminate life support in the patient with a near-certain fatal neurologic insult. In this situation the patient must be considered a possible organ donor. The emergency physician may then begin the process that leads to the diagnosis of brain death, and may support the patient appropriately to allow retrieval of viable organs.

PATHOPHYSIOLOGY OF BRAIN DEATH

Direct brain injury, such as head trauma and stroke, and indirect injury, such as hypoxia and hypoglycemia, can cause brain death. In both instances, potentially viable tissue can progress to necrosis through a similar process. Damaged tissue loses its normal high-energy state, causing accumulation of sodium and water in the intracellular compartment. This edema creates or exacerbates intracranial hypertension, which diminishes blood flow to the entire brain. The resultant ischemia creates a low-energy state in otherwise healthy tissue, leading to infarction and edema, thus creating a self-perpetuating cycle that ends in brain death. In addition, direct brain injury may produce intra-axial and extra-axial masses that aggravate intracranial hypertension. In virtually all cases there is no significant cerebral blood flow in brain death.

In the agonal stage of intracranial hypertension, there is usually a marked increase in sympathetic output. Systemic hypertension and tachycardia are typical, although bradycardia may occur. Brain stem reflexes are lost, most commonly in a rostrocaudal order. Spontaneous hyperventilation or gasping is often seen. Status myoclonicus is frequently present, especially after hypoxic injury. As the caudal portion of the brain stem dies, blood pressure and heart rate decrease, which may produce hypotension. Ventilatory and myoclonic movements also cease.

DETERMINATION OF BRAIN DEATH

Brain death determination is a complex process that provides the setting for a dignified death and paves the way for the honorable contribution of life through organ donation. Brain death is not a prerequisite for the withdrawal of life-sustaining treatment in patients with a dismal neurologic outcome. However, brain death is required for the retrieval of organs from a potential donor.

In the United States the diagnosis of brain death requires the irreversible cessation of "all functions of the entire brain, including the brain stem," although it is impossible to test the entire brain for function and it is likely that some brain activities continue in many who are determined to be brain dead. Nonetheless, the clinical condition that is recognized as brain death is an accurate predictor of the fact that cardiovascular collapse will inevitably, usually imminently, occur without return of any level of consciousness, brain stem reflexes, or spontaneous ventilation. This diagnosis is based on clinical criteria. Laboratory tests such as electroencephalography (EEG) and radionuclide cerebral angiography (RCA) are confirmatory only and helpful in certain situations, but their routine use is unnecessary. A period of continuous observation for return of neurologic function is required. The determination is made by at least two physicians not on the transplant team (usually the attending physician and a consultant neurologist or neurosurgeon), and is based on community standards of medical practice and regulated by the hospital's medical board policies in accordance with state law.

The Task Force for the Determination of Brain Death in Children published its guidelines in 1987. Previous reports did not address criteria for brain death determination in children under the age of 5 years because of the unique medical issues related to the difficulties of clinical assessment, determination of the proximate cause of coma, and uncertainty concerning the confirmatory laboratory tests in infants and young children. In addition, despite the lack of convincing clinical documentation, it was believed that the brains of infants and young children were more resistant to damage leading to brain death.

Clinical Criteria

History. It is imperative to determine the cause of coma, that this cause produces complete and irreversible brain failure, and that it is consistent with the clinical appearance and course of the patient. Misdiagnosis of brain death is usually attributable to omitting this step. Potentially reversible conditions such as hypothermia, hypotension, shock, drug intoxication, and the use of paralytic and sedative-hypnotic drugs must be excluded. It is often advisable to obtain toxicology and ethanol screening to exclude drug intoxication.

The most accepted confirmatory tests are EEG, RCA, and conventional four-vessel cerebral angiography. Of these three, only conventional angiography assesses the brain stem. Therefore, if the cause of coma is uncertain, irreversibility of brain failure should be demonstrated by lack of perfusion with conventional angiography.

Physical Examination. Formal bedside examination for the determination of brain death is performed at least three times: at the beginning and end of the observation period by the attending physician and once independently by the consultant. The neurologic examination should be performed when the child is hemodynamically stable, normothermic (rectal temperature greater than 35°C), in reasonable metabolic balance, and not receiving any sedating or neuromuscular blocking agents. Residual neuromuscular blockade can be diagnosed by using a peripheral nerve stimulator. The examination should reveal the following:

1. *Absence of cerebral function.* The patient has no purposeful, decorticate, or decerebrate response to noxious stimuli. Spinal reflexes may be preserved. Noxious stimulation should be applied by deep sternal rub and by bilateral supraorbital pressure. Absence of response to auditory stimulation is tested by shouting into each ear.

2. *Absence of brain stem functions.* Pupils are unresponsive to light. Atropine in the recommended dosage for resuscitation does not cause fixed and dilated pupils. The oculocephalic (doll's eye) and oculovestibular (cold caloric) reflexes are absent. The latter reflex is tested with a minimum of 20 ml of of iced water injected into each external auditory canal after ascertaining that the tympanic membrane is intact. There should be no tonic eye deviation or nystagmus. The corneal reflex is absent. There is no response to pharyngeal stimulation with a tongue blade and tracheal stimulation with suctioning.

3. *Absence of spontaneous ventilatory movements.* The patient is continuously observed for spontaneous ventilatory effort. Formal apnea testing is usually postponed to the last step in the final neurologic assessment because it creates hypercarbia, which may be injurious to a patient who is still salvageable. In preparation for apnea testing, the $PaCO_2$ should be normalized by discontinuing hyperventilation. The patient is then ventilated with 100% oxygen for 5 minutes. Mechanical ventilation is discontinued and oxygen is passively insufflated at 6 L/min through a suction catheter in the trachea to avoid hypoxemia. The patient is observed for any ventilatory activity until the $PaCO_2$ reaches 60 mm Hg. The rate of rise of $PaCO_2$ in brain-dead children varies but is approx-

imately 3 to 4 mm Hg/min. The patient should be monitored with a pulse oximeter. The test is discontinued if spontaneous respirations resume, oxygen desaturation below 80% occurs, or cardiovascular instability develops. A $Paco_2$ of 60 mm Hg or greater is documented by arterial blood gas analysis.

Observation Period. A period of observation is required to demonstrate that the cessation of brain function is irreversible. The duration of this period varies with the age of the patient and the cause of coma. It is more difficult to demonstrate irreversibility with some causes of coma (hypoxic-ischemic or metabolic injury) than with others (catastrophic head trauma). This led to the recommendation of longer periods of observation for hypoxic-ischemic coma than for traumatic coma. Demonstration of irreversibility of coma in the very young infant may be more difficult, although this is controversial. Hypoxic-ischemic encephalopathy secondary to perinatal asphyxia accounts for more than 90% of cases of clinical brain death in the newborn. The primary injury has usually occurred in utero under poorly defined circumstances and when the severity and duration of the insult are undetermined. Available brain-imaging techniques do not unequivocally define the severity of hypoxic-ischemic brain injury in the first week of postnatal life. In addition, the clinical, EEG, and perfusion studies used in the determination of brain death are inconclusive and subject to errors, primarily because of maturation-dependent factors in the newborn. With this background in mind, the recommendations for the observation period and laboratory tests are presented according to age:

1. *Full-term neonates under the age of 7 days.* There are no accepted criteria for the determination of brain death in this age group.

2. *Full-term infants between 7 days and 2 months of age.* The observation period is between two EEGs at least 48 hours apart.

3. *Patients between 2 months and 1 year of age.* The observation period is between two EEGs at least 24 hours apart. An EEG is unnecessary if RCA or conventional angiography demonstrates no evidence of cerebral perfusion.

4. *Patients over the age of 1 year.* For direct brain injury the observation period is at least 12 hours; for indirect brain injury, at least 24 hours. This period may be reduced by employment of confirmatory testing.

It is possible to make the diagnosis of brain death in the emergency department, although this is unusual. For example, a child with massive head trauma can be stabilized and neurologically assessed in the resuscitation room. If there is no sign of brain function, conventional angiography can be used to demonstrate absence of blood flow to the cerebrum and brain stem. Provided that the consultant agrees, the patient can then be declared brain dead.

ORGAN DONATION

Statistics from the United Network for Organ Sharing show that during 1990 there were 9560 kidney, 2085 heart, 2656 liver, 549 pancreas, 50 heart-lung, and 262 lung transplants, of which 370 kidney, 78 heart, 405 liver, 6 heart-lung, and 3 lung transplants were performed in children. As of May, 1991 there were 23,069 registered candidates awaiting organ transplantation. This pool of candidates needed 2019 heart, 174 heart-lung, 18,392 kidney, 1447 liver, 443 lung, and 594 pancreas transplants. Long-term survival rates for heart transplant patients exceed 50% and for liver transplant patients 60%.

In 1985, 75% of Americans approved of organ transplantation, but only 17% had signed donor cards. Of the estimated 2 million people who die each year, about 20,000 are considered potential organ donors, yet only 15% to 20% participate as donors. Between one third and one half of all patients awaiting transplantation die before a donor is found. Nationally, 30% to 50% of children under 2 years of age die while waiting.

History of Organ Donation

Systemized organ procurement evolved over several decades. The passage of the Uniform Anatomical Gift Act in 1968, with subsequent adoption in 1973, legalized organ donation in the United States. Established in 1978, the United Network of Organ Sharing initially computerized and matched renal transplant candidates with donor centers, and expanded in 1986 to include other tissues and organs through the joint efforts of the North American Transplant Coordinators to guarantee equitable sharing of organs. The passage of the National Organ Transplant Act in 1984 provided the framework necessary for a national registry and organ procurement-transplantation network, and established a task force to interpret and advise on the laws governing organ donation and address miscellaneous matters of concern, such as reimbursement for immunosuppressive therapy. The request laws adopted by 43 states in 1988 required physicians to offer families the opportunity to participate in organ donation.

ELIGIBILITY OF ORGAN DONORS

The search for potential organ donors requires direction and organization to ensure an expedient and successful retrieval. Delay in recognizing the potential donor dramatically reduces the donor pool secondary to unexpected cardiac arrest, hemodynamic instability, or infection. Patients who are considered donor candidates are those who have suffered severe head injuires, cerebrovascular accidents, cardiopulmonary arrest, primary brain tumors, or drug overdose.

All individuals falling into these categories should first receive intensive resuscitation and supportive measures without regard for the status of the potentially transplantable organs, and establishment of brain death criteria should remain secondary. Usual contraindications to procurement include infection, disseminated malignancy, autoimmune and hematologic disorders, current intravenous drug abuse, and human immunodeficiency virus (HIV) infection.

The criteria for specific organs is limited by factors of age, laboratory parameters, organ size, ischemic time, and certain contraindications particular to that system. Ischemic times are subject to extension by the transplanting surgeon. Acceptable age ranges vary according to the transplantable organ. Kidneys from donors aged 1 to 65 years are acceptable. Hearts and lungs are generally recruited from males under 40 and females under 45 years of age. Livers are accepted from patients as young as 6 months to those aged 55. The range for a transplantable pancreas is 2 to 50 years of age. Ischemic times likewise vary: kidney, 24 hours; heart, 4 hours; lung, 2 to 3 hours; pancreas, 6 to 8 hours; and liver, 7 to 12 hours.

APPROACHING THE FAMILY

Approaching the subject of organ donation is often so difficult for physicians that it is sometimes avoided altogether. Physicians shift their role from primary caregiver to advocate for the potential organ recipient, and addressing this matter with the family that is experiencing shock, disbelief, denial, and grief may be extremely stressful.

Armed with the knowledge that organ donation often eases the grief of surviving family members, physicians should proceed with optimism.

Timing the request is essential to successful procurement. The family should be approached in a sensitive and informative manner only after brain-death determination has been established. They should be assured that all exhaustive measures have been undertaken to ensure the patient's optimal outcome. Accompanying the physician should be a designated requestor who has been trained and is qualified to answer questions regarding policy, procedure, effects on burial arrangements, and cultural and religious orientations as well as to deal with the family's reaction to grief. It is preferable that this individual make the actual request and not the physician who has cared for the deceased.

The matter of organ donation should be addressed once the family has had the opportunity to deal with the reality of death. They should be approached in a dignified and sensitive manner and be allowed to have support persons present for the discussion. Furthermore, a quiet room that allows for open and uninterrupted discussion should be made available so that their decision may be made in privacy.

Religious and cultural beliefs strongly influence the probability of successful organ procurement. Christians are generally receptive to the idea of organ donation. Jehovah's Witnesses do not encourage donation but are unopposed to donation or transplantation, as long as all blood has been drained. Orthodox Jews do not accept brain-death criteria as determination of death, and oppose organ retrieval before the heart has stopped beating. Native Americans, Chinese, and some Southeast Asians consider the body to be sacred and on loan to the individual; to disturb the body is unacceptable. Gypsies generally oppose donation since the soul is believed to retrace its steps over the next year. Christian Scientists rarely participate in the process. Individuals of the Islamic faith will participate in donation if the organs are transplanted immediately, and consider the priority of saving a human life as justification for organ donation.

The opportunity to participate in organ donation should be offered to every family of a potential organ donor, respecting their religious and cultural beliefs. A sensitive, informative, and well-directed approach provides the greatest opportunity for acceptance. Moreover, families' ability to offer the gift of life may lessen their grief.

MANAGEMENT OF THE POTENTIAL ORGAN DONOR

Hemodynamic Instability

Proper management of the potential organ donor is immensely important. Hemodynamic instability may be due to hypovolemia from blood loss, third-spacing, excessive urinary output, or inadequate fluid administration; loss of vasomotor tone from decreased sympathetic output; or primary cardiac failure from damaged myocardium (contraction band necrosis, hypoxia-ischemia, contusion) or dysrhythmias. Usually there is a combination of these factors. Maintenance of an appropriate blood pressure is essential to adequate perfusion of viable organs. It is generally agreed that adult donors should maintain a minimal mean arterial pressure of 65 mm Hg; child donors should have a mean arterial pressure of 50 mm Hg, although lower pressures may suffice. Hypovolemia may be corrected by administration of 0.9 normal saline, Ringer's lactate, or colloid solutions. After the first 20 to 40 ml/kg, colloid administration may hold an advantage over crystalloid because it may minimize interstitial edema and consequent hypoxemia. Hematocrit levels should be maintained between 25% and 35%.

If pharmacologic support is necessary to maintain blood pressure and if the urinary output is less than 0.5 ml/kg/hr, dopamine is the drug of choice, ideally no more than 10 μg/kg/min. Pure vasoconstrictors should be avoided, since they compromise renal and hepatic blood flow.

Impaired Renal Function

Renal insufficiency may be due to previous or current hypotension or to toxic renal injury, e.g., from medications or rhabdomyolysis. A brisk urinary output, probably the equivalent of at least 2 ml/kg/hr in infants and children, is associated with a higher likelihood of successful kidney transplantation in adults. After obstruction is discounted as a cause of oliguria, a fluid challenge is indicated. If there is no urinary output despite normal blood pressure, furosemide (1 mg/kg) may be administered 30 minutes after fluid challenge. Low doses of dopamine (0.5 to 2 μg/kg/min) may be helpful in improving the glomerular filtration rate.

Central Diabetes Insipidus

This candidate is characterized by the excretion of large amounts of free water after hypothalamic injury and resultant inadequate amounts of antidiuretic hormone. This excessive water loss produces hypovolemia, hypernatremia, hypokalemia, hypomagnesemia, and hypophosphatemia. Polyuria with a low urinary sodium concentration and progressive hypernatremia is indicative of diabetes insipidus. Preexisting hypovolemia should be treated with isotonic fluid. The water deficit can rapidly be repaired with a 1.5% to 5.0% glucose in water solution, depending on serum glucose clearance. Ongoing water loss can be replaced with a solution containing glucose (usually about 2%) and potassium in a concentration similar to that measured in the urine. One reasonable approach is to replace all urinary output above 2 ml/kg/hr with this solution, while providing a maintenance infusion of a standard hypotonic saline solution. Intravenous administration of vasopressin is necessary once the diagnosis has been made. A continuous infusion beginning at 50 to 70 μU/kg/min is increased by 10 μU/kg/min every 15 to 30 minutes until a urinary output of about 2 to 3 ml/kg/hr has been achieved.

Pulmonary Dysfunction

Pulmonary dysfunction may result from inadequate ventilation, atelectasis, and pulmonary edema of various causes. The goal is to maintain normal arterial blood gases and acid-base status. The oxygen saturation should be at least 95% with the least possible FIO_2 to avoid oxygen toxicity. A positive end-expiratory pressure of 5 cm H_2O or less is recommended to minimize its adverse effects on cardiac output and renal and hepatic perfusion.

Temperature Instability

Loss of hypothalamic function causes the body temperature to equilibrate with the environment (poikilothermia). Hypothermia may produce a decrease in glomerular filtration rate and "cold diuresis," metabolic acidosis, decreased cardiac output, impaired coagulation, cardiac dysrhythmias, and even cardiac arrest. Temperature monitoring is imperative. Hypothermia usually requires only surface and inspired gas warming.

FUTURE CONSIDERATIONS

The emotional ambiguity of brain death and its legal implications make some health care professionals uncomfortable with the declaration process and subsequent management of the patient. This can diminish the willingness to address the issue of organ donation with surviving family members. Moreover, widespread education of the general public may dispel those beliefs that are cited for failing to sign donor cards. These include reluctance to address the issue of one's own mortality and death in general, and distrust of the moral integrity and motives of the "system." The family's concerns include whether optimal treatment to prevent brain death is delivered, the removal of organs before brain death occurs, and the hastening of the brain-death declaration process to achieve the same purpose. Those most likely to donate are between the ages of 25 and 29 years, Caucasian, and female; they have a higher educational level and belong to a higher socioeconomic status.

Currently, organ donation functions under a voluntary system that relies on individuals who fill out donor cards, write living wills, or sign for organ donation on their driver's licenses. The Uniform Anatomical Gift Act identifies those individuals 18 years or older who in the presence of two witnesses have expressed a desire to participate in organ donation. Although legally binding, the desires of the deceased have been waived when familial objections have been expressed. Only a small percentage of individuals who express interest in organ donation actually leave written expression of their intent. The implementation of two additional means of consent could further expand the donor pool: presumed consent and mandatory consent. Presumed consent laws would authorize the removal of organs unless there is expressed dissent by the donor or surviving family members. Concern regarding "silence" on the part of the presumed donor or family member may be regarded or interpreted as failure to register dissent or understanding. Alternatively, mandatory consent would require all individuals of legal age to register their written consent or dissent to organ donation. The formation of a national registry could be facilitated with information obtained by several means, for example, driver's license issuance and renewal with provisions allowing for easy access for any changes in the donor's status. However, the often distrusting public may interpret this solution as "compulsory," and massive withdrawal from the program as a form of protest would likely occur.

Selected References

Ashwal S, Schneider S. Brain death in children: Part II. Pediatr Neurol 1987;3:69.

Ashwal S, Schneider S. Brain death in the newborn. Pediatrics 1989;84:429.

Broznick BA. Organ procurement: Fulfilling a need. Transplant Proc 1988;20(Suppl):1010.

Childress JF. Ethical criteria for procuring and distributing organs for transplantation. J Health Polit Policy Law 1989;14:87.

Darby JM, Stein K, Grenvik A, Stuart SA. Approach to management of the heartbeating "brain dead" organ donor. JAMA 1989;261:2222.

Evans RW, Manninen DL, Garrison LP, Maier AM. Donor availability as the primary determinant of the future of heart transplantation. JAMA 1986;255:1892.

Fackler JC, Rogers MC. Is brain death really cessation of all intracranial function? J Pediatr 1987;110:84.

Goetting MG, Contreras E. Systemic atropine administration does not cause fixed and dilated pupils after CPR. Ann Emerg Med 1991;20:55.

Jeddoleh NP, Chetterjee SN. Legal problems in organ donation. Surg Clin North Am 1979;58:245.

MacDonald JC. The national organ procurement and transplantation network. N Engl J Med 1988;725.

Malatak JJ, Schaid DJ, Urback JM, et al. Choosing a pediatric patient for orthotopic liver transplantation. J Pediatr 1987;111:479.

Miller M. A proposed solution to the present organ donation crisis based on a hard look at the past. Circulation 1987;75:20.

National Organ Transplant Act. PL 98-507, Section 372, 1985.

President's Commission for the Study of Ethical Problems in Medicine and Biomedical and Behavioral Research: Guidelines for the determination of death. JAMA 1981;246:2184.

Prichard JG, Bale RM, Abou-Samra M, et al. Severe cerebral injury and brain death: Management of the patient's family. J Fam Pract 1985;21:341.

Reitz BH, Wallwork JL, Hunt SA, et al. Heart lung transplantation: Successful therapy for patients with pulmonary vascular disease. N Engl J Med 1982;306:557.

Rivers EP, Buse SM, Bivens BA, Horst HM. Organ and tissue procurement in the acute care setting; principles and practice—Parts 1 and 2. Ann Emerg Med 1990;19:78, 193.

Rowland TW, Donnelly JH, Jackson AH. Apnea documentation for the determination of brain death in children. Pediatrics 1984;74:505.

Starnes VA, Stinson EB, Dyer PE, et al. Cardiac transplantation in children and adolescents. Circulation 1987;76(Suppl):V43.

Task Force for the Determination of Brain Death in Children. Guidelines for the determination of brain death in children. Arch Neurol 1987;44:587.

Tolle SW, Bennett WM, Hichman DH, Benson JA. Responsibilities of primary physicians in organ donation. Ann Intern Med 1987;106:740.

Volpe JJ. Brain death determination in the newborn. Pediatrics 1987;80:293.

Weiss DQ. Organ transplantation, medical ethics and Jewish law. Transplant Proc 1988;20(Suppl 1):1071.

Younger SJ, Landefeld CS, Coulton CJ, et al. Brain death and organ retrieval: A cross-sectional survey of knowledge and concepts among health professionals. JAMA 1989;261:2205.

Zitelli BJ, Malatak JJ, Gartner JC, et al. Evaluation of the pediatric patient for liver transplant. Pediatrics 1986;78:559.

INDEX

Note: Numbers in *italics* refer to illustrations; numbers followed by (t) indicate tables.

1105

ISBN 0-7216-3281-5

Dosing and Dosage Forms of Oral Antibiotics

ORAL ANTIBIOTICS

Drug	Dose	Comments
Amoxicillin (Amoxil)	40 mg/kg/day divided q8 hr; adult dose 250–500 mg q8 hr	Drops 50 mg/ml; suspension 125 mg/5 ml, 250 mg/ 5 ml (50, 100, 150, 200 ml); caps 250, 500 mg; chewable tabs 125, 250 mg
Amoxicillin and clavulanic acid (Augmentin)	40 mg/kg/day divided q8 hr; adult dose 250–500 mg q8 hr	Suspension 125 mg/5 ml, 250 mg/5 ml (75, 150 ml); tabs 125, 250 mg; chewable tabs 125, 250 mg; dose based on amoxicillin component
Ampicillin (Omnipen, Polycillin)	50 mg/kg/day divided q6 hr; adult dose 250–500 mg q6 hr	Drops 100 mg/ml (20 ml); suspension 125 mg/5 ml, 250 mg/5 ml (80, 100, 150, 200 ml), 500 mg/5 ml (100 ml); caps 250, 500 mg
Cefaclor (Ceclor)	40 mg/kg/day divided q8 hr; adult dose 250–500 mg q8 hr	Suspension 125 mg/5 ml, 250 mg/5 ml (75, 150 ml); caps 250, 500 mg
Cefadroxil (Duricef)	30 mg/kg/day divided q12 hr; adult dose 500– 1000 mg q12 hr	Suspension 125 mg/5 ml, 250 mg/5 ml, 500 mg/5 ml (50, 100 ml); caps 500 mg; tabs 1 g
Cephalexin (Keflex)	40 mg/kg/day divided q6 hr; adult dose 250–500 mg q8 hr	Drops 100 mg/ml (10 ml); suspension 125 mg/5 mg, 250 mg/5 ml (100, 200 ml); caps 250, 500 mg; tabs 1 g
Cloxacillin (Tegopen, cloxapen)	50–100 mg/kg/day divided q6 hr; adult dose 250–1000 mg q6 hr	Solution 125 mg/ml (100, 200 ml); caps 250, 500 mg
Dicloxacillin (Dynapen)	40 mg/kg/day divided q6 hr; adult dose 150–500 mg q6 hr	Suspension 62.5 mg/5 ml (80, 100, 200 ml); caps 125, 250, 500 mg
Erythromycin (Pediamycin, E-mycin, Ery-Ped)	40 mg/kg/day divided q6 hr; adult dose 250–500 mg q6 hr	*Erythromycin:* Caps 125, 250 mg; tabs 250, 333, 500 mg *EES:* Drops 100 mg/2.5 ml (50 ml); suspension 200 mg/ 5 ml, 400 mg/5 ml (60, 100, 200 ml); tabs 200, 400 mg
Erythromycin ethylsuccinate (EES) and sulfisoxazole (SXZ) (Pediazole)	EES 40 mg/kg/day; SXZ 120 mg divided q6 hr; maximum dose 6 g SXZ/day	Suspension 200 mg EES and 600 mg SXZ/5 ml (100, 150, 200 ml); *rapid dose formula:* child's weight in kg is total daily dose in ml (e.g., 20-kg child receives 5 ml q6 hr)
Penicillin V potassium (Pen·Vee K)	40 mg (65,000 units) kg/day divided q6 hr; adult dose 250–500 mg q6 hr	Solution 125 mg (200,000 units) 5 ml, 250 mg (400,000 units) 5 ml; tabs 125 mg (200,000 units), 250 mg (400,000 units), 500 mg (800,000 units)
Sulfisoxazole (Gantrisin)	120 mg/kg/day divided q6 hr; adult dose 500 mg q6 hr	Suspension 500 mg/5 ml (120 mg); syrup 500 mg/ 5 ml (472 ml); tabs 500 mg; *otitis media prophylaxis:* 50–75 mg/day divided bid
Trimethoprim (TMP) and sulfamethoxazole (SMZ) (Bactrim, Septra)	10 mg TMP/50 mg SMX/kg/day divided q12 hr; adult dose 80–160 mg TMP/400–500 SMX q12 hr	Suspension 40 mg TMP/200 mg SMX/5 ml; tabs 80 mg TMP/400 mg SMX, 160 mg TMP/800 mg SMX; *rapid dosing formula:* child's weight in kg equals total daily dose in ml (e.g., a 20-kg child receives 10 ml q12 hr); do not use in infants <2 mo old